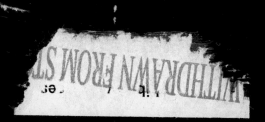
WITHDRAWN FROM STOCK

D1587695

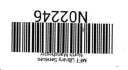
N02246

MFT Library Services
North Manchester

Sleisenger & Fordtran's
GASTROINTESTINAL AND LIVER DISEASE

WI 140
FEL
2006

JACK TAYLOR LIBRARY
ROCHDALE EDUCATION CENTRE
ROCHDALE INFIRMARY
ROCHDALE OL12 0NB

Sleisenger & Fordtran's
GASTROINTESTINAL AND LIVER DISEASE

PATHOPHYSIOLOGY / DIAGNOSIS / MANAGEMENT

8th EDITION   **VOLUME 2**

Edited by

Mark Feldman MD
William O. Tschumy Jr., MD, Chair of Internal Medicine
Presbyterian Hospital of Dallas
Clinical Professor of Internal Medicine
University of Texas Southwestern Medical School
Dallas, Texas

Lawrence S. Friedman MD
Professor of Medicine
Harvard Medical School
Chair, Department of Medicine
Newton-Wellesley Hospital
Assistant Chief of Medicine
Massachusetts General Hospital
Newton, Massachusetts

Lawrence J. Brandt MD
Professor of Medicine and Surgery
Albert Einstein College of Medicine
Chief, Division of Gastroenterology
Montefiore Medical Center
Bronx, New York

Consulting Editor
Marvin H. Sleisenger MD
Professor of Medicine, Emeritus
University of California, San Francisco, School of
  Medicine
Distinguished Physician
Department of Veterans Affairs Medical Center
San Francisco, California

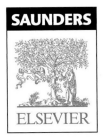

SAUNDERS

ELSEVIER

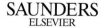

SAUNDERS
ELSEVIER

1600 John F. Kennedy Blvd.
Ste 1800
Philadelphia, PA 19103-2899

SLEISENGER & FORDTRAN'S GASTROINTESTINAL AND LIVER DISEASE
Two-volume set ISBN-10: 1-4160-0245-6
Two-volume set ISBN-13: 978-1-4160-0245-1

Volume 1 ISBN: 9996002551
Volume 2 ISBN: 9996002616

E-dition ISBN-10: 1-4160-3245-2
E-dition ISBN-13: 978-1-4160-3245-8

Copyright © 2006, 2002, 1998, 1993, 1989, 1983, 1978, 1973, by Saunders, an imprint of Elsevier Inc.

All rights reserved. No part of this publication may be reproduced or transmitted in any form or by any means, electronic or mechanical, including photocopying, recording, or any information storage and retrieval system, without permission in writing from the publisher. Permissions may be sought directly from Elsevier's Health Sciences Rights Department in Philadelphia, PA, USA: phone: (+1) 215 239 3804, fax: (+1) 215 239 3805, e-mail: healthpermissions@elsevier.com. You may also complete your request on-line via the Elsevier homepage (http://www.elsevier.com), by selecting 'Customer Support' and then 'Obtaining Permissions'.

Notice

Knowledge and best practice in this field are constantly changing. As new research and experience broaden our knowledge, changes in practice, treatment, and drug therapy may become necessary or appropriate. Readers are advised to check the most current information provided (i) on procedures featured or (ii) by the manufacturer of each product to be administered, to verify the recommended dose or formula, the method and duration of administration, and contraindications. It is the responsibility of the practitioner, relying on their own experience and knowledge of the patient, to make diagnoses, to determine dosages and the best treatment for each individual patient, and to take all appropriate safety precautions. To the fullest extent of the law, neither the Publisher nor the Editors assume any liability for any injury and/or damage to persons or property arising out of or related to any use of the material contained in this book.

The Publisher

Library of Congress Cataloging-in-Publication Data

Sleisenger & Fordtran's gastrointestinal and liver disease : pathophysiology, diagnosis, management / [edited by] Mark Feldman, Lawrence S. Friedman, Lawrence J. Brandt.—8th ed.
    p. ; cm.
  Includes bibliographical references and index.
  ISBN 1-4160-0245-6
  1. Gastrointestinal system—Diseases. 2. Liver—Diseases. I. Title: Sleisenger and Fordtran's gastrointestinal and liver disease. II. Title: Gastrointestinal and liver disease. III. Sleisenger, Marvin H. IV. Feldman, Mark. V. Friedman, Lawrence S. (Lawrence Samuel). VI. Brandt, Lawrence J.
  [DNLM: 1. Gastrointestinal Diseases. 2. Liver Diseases. WI 140 S632 2006]
RC801.G384 2006
616.3'3—dc22   2005049767

Acquisitions Editor: Karen Bowler
Developmental Editor: Melissa Dudlick
Publishing Services Manager: Frank Polizzano
Project Manager: Jeff Gunning
Design Direction: Steven Stave

Printed in Canada
Last digit is the print number: 9 8 7 6 5 4 3 2 1

Working together to grow
libraries in developing countries

www.elsevier.com | www.bookaid.org | www.sabre.org

ELSEVIER   BOOK AID International   Sabre Foundation

The editors dedicate the eighth edition of this book to Marvin H. Sleisenger, MD. Dr. Sleisenger's contributions to gastroenterology and to this textbook are numerous and legendary. Marv Sleisenger, along with John Fordtran (to whom the sixth edition was dedicated), launched this venerable textbook more than 30 years ago. Their emphasis on pathophysiology and on science-based diagnosis and management of gastrointestinal disease established almost immediately the preeminence of this book in the field of gastroenterology. Two of the current editors had the honor and privilege of co-editing previous editions of this book with Dr. Sleisenger, and all of us have the highest regard for his leadership and his devotion to excellence, comprehensiveness, and precision in editing. We hope that this eighth edition, the first for which Dr. Sleisenger has not served as a principal editor, will meet the high standards that he and Dr. Fordtran established for this textbook over the past 3 decades. We also thank Dr. Sleisenger from the bottom of our hearts for the opportunity to continue his work and for his serving as a consulting editor on this, the eighth edition of *Sleisenger & Fordtran*.

Contributors

Rakesh Aggarwal MD, DM
Adjunct Professor, Department of Gastroenterology,
Sanjay Gandhi Postgraduate Institute of Medical
Sciences, Lucknow, India
Hepatitis E

Aijaz Ahmed MD
Assistant Professor of Medicine, Stanford University
School of Medicine, Stanford, California
Liver Chemistry and Function Tests

Jane M. Andrews MBBS, PhD, FRACP
Clinical Senior Lecturer in Medicine, Adelaide
University Faculty of Medicine; Senior Consultant
Gastroenterologist, Repatriation General Hospital,
Adelaide, South Australia, Australia
*Small Intestinal Motor and Sensory Function and
Dysfunction*

Paul Angulo MD
Associate Professor of Medicine, Mayo Clinic College of
Medicine; Senior Associate Consultant, Division of
Gastroenterology and Hepatology, Mayo Clinic and
Foundation, Rochester, Minnesota
Primary Biliary Cirrhosis

Thomas Anthony MD
Chief, Surgical Services, Veterans Affairs North Texas
Health Care System, Dallas, Texas
*Gastrointestinal Carcinoid Tumors and the Carcinoid
Syndrome*

John E. Antoine MD
University of South Florida College of Medicine; Chief,
Radiation Oncology Service, James A. Haley Veterans
Administration Medical Center, Tampa, Florida
Radiation Injury to the Gastrointestinal Tract

Bruce R. Bacon MD
James F. King, MD, Endowed Chair in Gastroenterology
and Professor of Internal Medicine, Saint Louis
University School of Medicine; Director, Division of
Gastroenterology and Hepatology, Saint Louis
University Hospital, St. Louis, Missouri
Hemochromatosis

William F. Balistreri MD
Dorothy M.M. Kersten Professor of Pediatrics,
University of Cincinnati College of Medicine; Medical
Director, Liver Care Center, Cincinnati Children's
Hospital Medical Center, Cincinnati, Ohio
Other Inherited Metabolic Disorders of the Liver

Anne E. Becker MD, PhD, ScM
Associate Professor of Medical Anthropology and
Assistant Professor of Psychiatry, Harvard Medical
School; Director, Eating Disorders Clinical and Research
Program, Massachusetts General Hospital, Boston,
Massachusetts
Eating Disorders

Marina Berenguer MD
Adjunct Professor, Digestive Medicine Service, La Fe
University Hospital, Valencia, Spain
Hepatitis C

L. Ashley Blackshaw PhD
Associate Professor, Nerve Gut Research Laboratory,
Hanson Institute, Adelaide, South Australia, Australia
*Small Intestinal Motor and Sensory Function and
Dysfunction*

Lawrence J. Brandt MD
Professor of Medicine and Surgery, Albert Einstein
College of Medicine; Chief of Gastroenterology,
Montefiore Medical Center, Bronx, New York
*Vascular Lesions of the Gastrointestinal Tract; Intestinal
Ischemia; Complementary and Alternative Medicine
Therapies in Gastrointestinal and Hepatic Disease*

Robert S. Bresalier MD, FACP
Professor of Medicine and Birdie J. and Lydia J. Resoft
Distinguished Professor in Gastrointestinal Oncology;
Chairman, Department of Gastrointestinal Medicine
and Nutrition, The University of Texas M.D. Anderson
Cancer Center, Houston, Texas
Malignant Neoplasms of the Large Intestine

Robert S. Britton PhD
Associate Research Professor, Department of Internal
Medicine, Division of Gastroenterology and Hepatology,
Saint Louis University School of Medicine; Saint Louis
University Hospital, St. Louis, Missouri
Hemochromatosis

Simon J. Brookes PhD
Professor of Human Physiology, Flinders University
School of Medicine, Adelaide, South Australia, Australia
Colonic Motor and Sensory Function and Dysfunction

Jeffrey D. Browning MD
Assistant Professor, Department of Internal Medicine
and Advanced Imaging and Research Center,
University of Texas Southwestern Medical School,
Dallas, Texas
Gallstone Disease

Alan L. Buchman MD, MSPH
Associate Professor of Medicine, Division of
Gastroenterology, Northwestern University Feinberg
School of Medicine; Staff Physician, Northwestern
Memorial Hospital, Chicago, Illinois
Short Bowel Syndrome

J. Steven Burdick MD
Associate Professor of Medicine, University of Texas
Southwestern Medical School; Staff Physician and
Director of Endoscopy, Parkland Health and Hospital
System, and Staff Physician, Zale Lipshy University
Hospital and St. Paul University Hospital, Dallas, Texas
*Anatomy, Histology, Embryology, and Developmental
Anomalies of the Pancreas*

Michael Camilleri MD
Professor of Medicine and Physiology, Mayo Clinic
College of Medicine; Consultant in Gastroenterology,
Mayo Clinic, Rochester, Minnesota
Acute and Chronic Pseudo-obstruction

Robert L. Carithers MD
Professor of Medicine and Head, Section of Hepatology,
Division of Gastroenterology, Department of Medicine,
University of Washington School of Medicine; Director,
Liver Care Line, and Medical Director of the Liver
Transplantation Program, University of Washington
Medical Center, Seattle, Washington
Alcoholic Liver Disease

Julie G. Champine MD
Associate Professor of Radiology, The University of
Texas Southwestern Medical School; Medical Director of
Radiology, Parkland Memorial Hospital, Dallas, Texas
Abdominal Abscesses and Gastrointestinal Fistulas

Francis K.L. Chan MD
Associate Professor, Department of Medicine and
Therapeutics, Prince of Wales Hospital, The Chinese
University of Hong Kong, Shatin, New Territories,
Hong Kong
Treatment of Peptic Ulcer Disease

Eugene B. Chang MD
Professor of Medicine, University of Chicago Pritzker
School of Medicine, Chicago, Illinois
Intestinal Water and Electrolyte Transport

L. Chinsoo Cho MD, MS
Associate Professor of Therapeutic Radiology, University
of Minnesota Medical School, Minneapolis, Minnesota
Radiation Injury to the Gastrointestinal Tract

Daniel C. Chung MD
Assistant Professor of Medicine, Harvard Medical
School; Director, GI Cancer Genetics Service,
Gastrointestinal Unit and Cancer Center, Massachusetts
General Hospital, Boston, Massachusetts
Cellular Growth and Neoplasia

Raymond T. Chung MD
Assistant Professor of Medicine, Harvard Medical
School; Director of Hepatology and Medical Director,
Liver Transplant Program, Massachusetts General
Hospital, Boston, Massachusetts
*Bacterial, Parasitic, and Fungal Infections of the Liver,
Including Liver Abscess*

Robert R. Cima MD
Assistant Professor of Surgery, Mayo Clinic College of
Medicine; Senior Associate Consultant, Division of
Colon and Rectal Surgery, Mayo Clinic, Rochester,
Minnesota
Ileostomy, Colostomy, and Pouches

Ray E. Clouse MD
Professor of Medicine and Psychiatry, Washington
University School of Medicine; Physician,
Barnes-Jewish Hospital, St. Louis, Missouri
*Esophageal Motor and Sensory Function and Motor
Disorders of the Esophagus*

Philip Cole MD
Clinical Professor of Surgery, Department of Surgery,
Louisiana State University Health Sciences Center
School of Medicine Shreveport, Shreveport, Louisiana
Intestinal Obstruction and Ileus

Robert H. Collins, Jr. MD, FACP
Professor, Department of Hematology/Oncology–
Hematopoietic Cell Transplantation, University of Texas
Southwestern Medical School, Dallas, Texas
Gastrointestinal Lymphomas

Ian J. Cook MBBS, MD(Syd), FRACP
Professor of Medicine, University of New South Wales
Faculty of Medicine; Head, Department of
Gastroenterology, St. George Hospital, Sydney, New
South Wales, Australia
Colonic Motor and Sensory Function and Dysfunction

Diane W. Cox PhD, CCMG, FRSC
Professor of Medical Genetics, University of Alberta
Faculty of Medicine, Edmonton, Alberta, Canada
Wilson Disease

Byron Cryer MD
Professor of Medicine, The University of Texas
Southwestern Medical School; Staff Physician,
Gastroenterology Section, Dallas Veterans
Administration Medical Center, Dallas, Texas
Peptic Ulcer Disease

Albert J. Czaja MD
Professor of Medicine, Mayo Clinic College of Medicine;
Consultant, Gastroenterology and Hepatology, Mayo
Clinic, Rochester, Minnesota
Autoimmune Hepatitis

Fredric Daum MD
Professor of Pediatrics, Yale University School of Medicine; Attending Pediatric Gastroenterologist, Yale–New Haven Children's Hospital, New Haven, Connecticut
Anatomy, Histology, Embryology, and Developmental Anomalies of the Small and Large Intestine

Paul A. Dawson PhD
Associate Professor, Department of Internal Medicine, Division of Gastroenterology, Wake Forest University School of Medicine, Winston-Salem, North Carolina
Bile Secretion and the Enterohepatic Circulation

Mark H. DeLegge MD, FACG
Professor of Medicine, Medical University of South Carolina College of Medicine, Charleston, South Carolina
Nutrition in Gastrointestinal Diseases

George D. Demetri MD
Associate Professor of Medicine, Harvard Medical School; Director, Center for Sarcoma and Bone Oncology, Department of Medical Oncology, Dana-Farber Cancer Institute and Brigham and Women's Hospital, Boston Massachusetts
Gastrointestinal Stromal Tumors (GISTs)

Kenneth R. DeVault MD
Professor of Medicine, Mayo Clinic College of Medicine–Jacksonville; Chair, Division of Gastroenterology and Hepatology, Mayo Clinic–Jacksonville, Jacksonville, Florida
Symptoms of Esophageal Disease

Nicholas E. Diamant MD, FRCPC
Professor of Medicine and Physiology (Emeritus), University of Toronto Faculty of Medicine; Staff Physician, Division of Gastroenterology, Department of Medicine, Toronto Western Hospital–University Health Network, Toronto, Ontario, Canada
Esophageal Motor and Sensory Function and Motor Disorders of the Esophagus

David E. Elliott MD, PhD
Associate Professor, Division of Gastroenterology, Department of Internal Medicine, University of Iowa Roy J. and Lucille A. Carver College of Medicine, Iowa City, Iowa
Intestinal Worms

Grace H. Elta MD
Professor of Medicine, University of Michigan Medical School, Ann Arbor, Michigan
Biliary Tract Motor Function and Dysfunction

Geoffrey C. Farrell MD, FRACP
Professor of Hepatic Medicine, Australian National University Medical School; Director of Gastroenterology and Hepatology, The Canberra Hospital, Canberra, Australian Capital Territory, Australia
Liver Disease Caused by Drugs

James J. Farrell MD
Assistant Professor of Medicine, Division of Digestive Diseases, David Geffen School of Medicine at UCLA; Director of Pancreaticobiliary Endoscopy, Division of Digestive Diseases/Gastroenterology, UCLA Healthcare, Los Angeles, California
Digestion and Absorption of Nutrients and Vitamins

Richard J. Farrell MD
Assistant Professor of Medicine, Harvard Medical School; Associate Physician, Gastroenterology Division, Beth Israel Deaconess Medical Center, Boston, Massachusetts
Celiac Sprue and Refractory Sprue

Michael J. G. Farthing DSc(Med), MD, FRCP, FMedSci
Principal and Professor of Medicine, St. George's University of London, London, United Kingdom
Tropical Malabsorption and Tropical Diarrhea

Jordan J. Feld MD, FRCPC
Hepatology Research Fellow, Liver Diseases Section, National Institute of Diabetes and Digestive and Kidney Diseases, National Institutes of Health, Bethesda, Maryland
Hepatitis Caused by Other Viruses

Mark Feldman MD
William O. Tschumy Jr., MD, Chair of Internal Medicine, Presbyterian Hospital of Dallas; Clinical Professor of Internal Medicine, University of Texas Southwestern Medical School, Dallas, Texas
Gastric Secretion; Gastritis and Gastropathies

Carlos Fernández-del Castillo MD
Associate Professor of Surgery, Harvard Medical School; Visiting Surgeon, Massachusetts General Hospital, Boston, Massachusetts
Pancreatic Cancer, Cystic Pancreatic Neoplasms, and Other Nonendocrine Pancreatic Tumors

David R. Fischer MD
Assistant Professor of Surgery and Associate Program Director of Residency Education, University of Cincinnati College of Medicine, Cincinnati, Ohio
Surgical Peritonitis and Other Diseases of the Peritoneum, Mesentery, Omentum, and Diaphragm

J. Gregory Fitz MD
Professor and Chairman, Department of Internal Medicine, University of Texas Southwestern Medical School, Dallas, Texas
Hepatic Encephalopathy, Hepatopulmonary Syndromes, Hepatorenal Syndrome, and Other Complications of Liver Disease

David E. Fleischer MD
Professor of Medicine, Mayo Clinic College of Medicine, Rochester, Minnesota; Chairman, Division of Gastroenterology and Hepatology, Mayo Clinic, Scottsdale, Arizona
Tumors of the Esophagus

Robert J. Fontana MD
Associate Professor of Medicine, University of Michigan Medical School, Ann Arbor, Michigan
Acute Liver Failure

Chris E. Forsmark MD
Professor of Medicine and Chief, Division of Gastroenterology, Hepatology, and Nutrition, University of Florida College of Medicine, Gainesville, Florida
Chronic Pancreatitis

Jeffrey M. Fox MD, MPH
Assistant Clinical Professor of Medicine, University of California, San Francisco, School of Medicine, San Francisco; Staff Physician, Division of Gastroenterology, Kaiser Permanente, San Rafael, California
Diverticular Disease of the Colon

Lawrence S. Friedman MD
Professor of Medicine, Harvard Medical School; Chair, Department of Medicine, Newton-Wellesley Hospital; Assistant Chief of Medicine, Massachusetts General Hospital, Newton, Massachusetts
Bacterial, Parasitic, and Fungal Infections of the Liver, Including Liver Abscess

Ralph A. Giannella MD
Mark Brown Professor of Medicine, Division of Digestive Diseases, University of Cincinnati College of Medicine; Staff Physician, University Hospital, Cincinnati, Ohio
Infectious Enteritis and Proctocolitis and Bacterial Food Poisoning

Gregory G. Ginsberg MD
Professor of Medicine, University of Pennsylvania School of Medicine; Executive Director of Endoscopic Services, University of Pennsylvania Health System, Hospital of the University of Pennsylvania, Philadelphia, Pennsylvania
Foreign Bodies and Bezoars; Tumors of the Esophagus

Robert E. Glasgow MD
Assistant Professor of Surgery, University of Utah School of Medicine; Director, Minimally Invasive Surgery, University of Utah Hospital and Clinics, Salt Lake City, Utah
Acute Abdominal Pain; Treatment of Gallstone Disease

David Y. Graham MD
Professor of Medicine and Molecular Virology and Microbiology, Baylor College of Medicine; Chief of Gastroenterology, Michael E. DeBakey Veterans Affairs Medical Center, Houston, Texas
Helicobacter pylori

David A. Greenwald MD
Associate Professor of Medicine, Albert Einstein College of Medicine; Associate Division Director and Gastroenterology Fellowship Training Program Director, Montefiore Medical Center, Bronx, New York
Protein-Losing Gastroenteropathy

Heinz F. Hammer MD
Associate Professor of Internal Medicine, Medical University of Graz, Graz, Austria
Maldigestion and Malabsorption

William Harford MD
Professor of Internal Medicine, University of Texas Southwestern Medical School; Director, GI Endoscopy Laboratory, Dallas Veterans Affairs Medical Center, Dallas, Texas
Diverticula of the Pharynx, Esophagus, Stomach, and Small Intestine; Abdominal Hernias and Gastric Volvulus

Laura E. Harrel MD
Instructor of Medicine, Section of Gastroenterology, Department of Medicine, University of Chicago Pritzker School of Medicine, Chicago, Illinois
Intestinal Water and Electrolyte Transport

David J. Hass MD
Fellow, Division of Gastroenterology, Albert Einstein College of Medicine and Montefiore Medical Center, Bronx, New York
Complementary and Alternative Medicine Therapies in Gastrointestinal and Hepatic Disease

E. Jenny Heathcote MD, FRCP, FRCPC
Professor of Medicine, University of Toronto Faculty of Medicine; Staff Physician, Toronto Western Hospital, Toronto, Ontario, Canada
Hepatitis Caused by Other Viruses

Maureen Heldmann MD
Associate Professor of Radiology, Louisiana State University Health Sciences Center School of Medicine Shreveport; Director, Body CT and MRI, Louisiana State University Health Sciences Center, Shreveport, Louisiana
Intestinal Obstruction and Ileus

Axel von Herbay MD
Professor and Consultant in Gastrointestinal Pathology, Academic Department of Pathology, St. Mark's Hospital, London, United Kingdom
Whipple's Disease

Christoph Högenauer MD
Associate Professor of Internal Medicine, Medical University of Graz, Graz, Austria
Maldigestion and Malabsorption

JeanMarie Houghton MD, PhD
Associate Professor of Medicine, University of Massachusetts Medical School; UMass Memorial Medical Center, Worcester, Massachusetts
Tumors of the Stomach

Tracy L. Hull MD
Staff Colorectal Surgeon, The Cleveland Clinic Foundation, Cleveland, Ohio
Diseases of the Anorectum

Christopher D. Huston MD
Assistant Professor, Department of Medicine and Microbiology and Molecular Genetics, University of Vermont College of Medicine; Attending Physician, Division of Infectious Diseases, Fletcher Allen Health Care, Burlington, Vermont
Intestinal Protozoa

Steven H. Itzkowitz MD
Dr. Burrill B. Crohn Professor of Medicine, Mount Sinai School of Medicine; Attending Physician and Associate Director, Gastrointestinal Division, The Mount Sinai Hospital, New York, New York
Colonic Polyps and Polyposis Syndromes

Rajeev Jain MD
Clinical Assistant Professor of Medicine, University of Texas Southwestern Medical School; Chief of Gastroenterology, Presbyterian Hospital of Dallas, Dallas, Texas
Gastrointestinal and Hepatic Manifestations of Systemic Diseases

Robert T. Jensen MD
Chief, Cell Biology Section, Digestive Diseases Branch, National Institute of Diabetes and Digestive and Kidney Diseases, National Institutes of Health, Bethesda, Maryland
Endocrine Tumors of the Pancreas and Gastrointestinal Tract

Rohan Jeyarajah MD, FACS
Director of Surgical Oncology, Methodist Dallas Medical Center, Dallas, Texas
Diverticula of the Pharynx, Esophagus, Stomach, and Small Intestine; Abdominal Hernias and Gastric Volvulus

Ramon E. Jimenez MD
Assistant Professor of Surgery, University of Connecticut School of Medicine, Farmington; Attending Surgeon, Hartford Hospital, Hartford, Connecticut
Pancreatic Cancer, Cystic Pancreatic Neoplasms, and Other Nonendocrine Pancreatic Tumors

Ellen Kahn MD
Professor of Pathology and Pediatrics, New York University School of Medicine, New York; Attending Pathologist and Associate Attending Pediatrician, North Shore University Hospital, Manhasset, New York
Anatomy, Histology, Embryology, and Developmental Anomalies of the Small and Large Intestine

Patrick S. Kamath MD
Professor of Medicine, Mayo Clinic College of Medicine; Consultant, Gastroenterology, Hepatology, and Liver Transplantation, St. Mary's Hospital and Rochester Methodist Hospital, Rochester, Minnesota
Portal Hypertension and Gastrointestinal Bleeding

David A. Katzka MD
Associate Professor of Medicine, Gastrointestinal Division, University of Pennsylvania School of Medicine, Philadelphia, Pennsylvania
Esophageal Disorders Caused by Medications, Trauma, and Infection

Emmet B. Keeffe MD
Professor of Medicine, Division of Gastroenterology and Hepatology, Stanford University School of Medicine; Chief of Hepatology and Co-Director, Liver Transplantation Program, Stanford University Medical Center, Stanford, California
Liver Chemistry and Function Tests

Ciarán P. Kelly MD
Associate Professor of Medicine, Harvard Medical School; Director, Gastroenterology Training Program, Beth Israel Deaconess Medical Center, Boston, Massachusetts
Celiac Sprue and Refractory Sprue; Antibiotic-Associated Diarrhea, Pseudomembranous Enterocolitis, and Clostridium difficile-Associated Diarrhea and Colitis

Michael C. Kew MD
Department of Medicine, University of the Witwatersrand Medical School; Staff Physician, Johannesburg Academic and Baragwanath Hospitals, Johannesburg, South Africa
Hepatic Tumors and Cysts

Seema Khan MB, BS
Pediatric Gastroenterologist, Alfred I. duPont Hospital for Children, Wilmington, Delaware
Eosinophilic Disorders of the Gastrointestinal Tract

Lawrence Kim MD
Chief, Surgical Services, Central Arkansas Veterans Healthcare System, Little Rock, Arkansas
Gastrointestinal Carcinoid Tumors and the Carcinoid Syndrome

Michael B. Kimmey MD
Professor of Medicine, Division of Gastroenterology, University of Washington School of Medicine, Seattle, Washington
Complications of Gastrointestinal Endoscopy

Samuel Klein MD
William H. Danforth Professor of Medicine and Nutritional Science, Washington University in St. Louis School of Medicine, St. Louis, Missouri
Obesity

Kris V. Kowdley MD
Professor of Medicine, Division of Gastroeuterology, University of Washington School of Medicine, Seattle, Washington
Sclerosing Cholangitis and Recurrent Pyogenic Cholangitis

Krzysztof Krawczynski MD, PhD
Distinguished Consultant, Division of Viral Hepatitis, Centers for Disease Control and Prevention, Atlanta, Georgia
Hepatitis E

Braden Kuo MD, MSc
Instructor in Medicine, Harvard Medical School; Assistant Physician, Gastrointestinal Unit, Massachusetts General Hospital, Boston, Massachusetts
Chronic Abdominal Pain

Jeanne M. LaBerge MD
Professor of Radiology, University of California, San Francisco, School of Medicine, San Francisco, California
Endoscopic and Radiologic Treatment of Biliary Disease

J. Thomas Lamont MD
Professor of Medicine, Harvard Medical School; Chief of Gastroenterology Division, Beth Israel Deaconess Medical Center, Boston, Massachusetts
Antibiotic-Associated Diarrhea, Pseudomembranous Enterocolitis, and Clostridium difficile-Associated Diarrhea and Colitis

Anne M. Larson MD
Associate Professor of Medicine, University of Washington School of Medicine, Seattle, Washington
Gastrointestinal and Hepatic Complications of Solid Organ and Hematopoietic Cell Transplantation

James Y.W. Lau MD
Endoscopy Centre, Prince of Wales Hospital, The Chinese University of Hong Kong, Shatin, New Territories, Hong Kong
Treatment of Peptic Ulcer Disease

Edward L. Lee MD
Professor and Chairman, Department of Pathology,
Howard University School of Medicine, Washington, DC
Gastritis and Gastropathies

Anthony L. Lembo MD
Assistant Professor of Medicine, Harvard Medical
School; Director, Gastrointestinal Motility Center, Beth
Israel Deaconess Medical Center, Boston, Massachusetts
Constipation

Mike A. Leonis MD, PhD
Research Instructor, Department of Pediatrics,
University of Cincinnati College of Medicine; Staff
Physician, Cincinnati Children's Hospital Medical
Center, Cincinnati, Ottio
Other Inherited Metabolic Disorders of the Liver

Michael D. Levitt MD
Professor of Medicine, University of Minnesota Medical
School; ACOS for Research, VA Medical Center,
Minneapolis, Minnesota
Intestinal Gas

James H. Lewis MD, FACP, FACG
Professor of Medicine, Georgetown University School of
Medicine; Director of Hepatology, Georgetown
University Medical Center, Washington, DC
*Liver Disease Caused by Anesthetics, Toxins, and Herbal
Preparations*

Gary R. Lichtenstein MD
Professor of Medicine, University of Pennsylvania
School of Medicine; Director, Center for Inflammatory
Bowel Diseases, Hospital of the University of
Pennsylvania, Gastroenterology Division, Department
of Medicine, Philadelphia, Pennsylvania
Ulcerative Colitis

Rodger A. Liddle MD
Professor of Medicine, Duke University School of
Medicine; Chief, Division of Gastroenterology, Duke
University Medical Center, Durham, North Carolina
Gastrointestinal Hormones and Neurotransmitters

Steven D. Lidofsky MD, PhD
Associate Professor of Medicine and Pharmacology and
Director of Hepatology, University of Vermont College
of Medicine; Attending Physician, Fletcher Allen Health
Care, Burlington, Vermont
Jaundice

Keith D. Lillemoe MD
Jay L. Grosfeld Professor and Chairman, Department of
Surgery, Indiana University School of Medicine;
Surgeon-in-Chief, Indiana University Hospital,
Indianapolis, Indiana
Tumors of the Gallbladder, Bile Ducts, and Ampulla

Keith D. Lindor MD
Professor of Medicine, Mayo Clinic College of Medicine;
Consultant, Division of Gastroenterology and
Hepatology, Mayo Clinic, Rochester, Minnesota
Primary Biliary Cirrhosis

G. Richard Locke III MD
Professor of Medicine, Mayo Clinic College of Medicine;
Consultant in Gastroenterology and Hepatology, Mayo
Clinic, Rochester, Minnesota
*A Biopsychosocial Understanding of Gastrointestinal Illness
and Disease*

Peter M. Loeb MD
Clinical Professor of Medicine, Department of Internal
Medicine, University of Texas Southwestern Medical
School; Director, Gastroenterology Laboratory,
Presbyterian Hospital of Dallas, Dallas, Texas
Caustic Injury to the Upper Gastrointestinal Tract

John D. Long MD
Associate Professor of Medicine, Department of
Gastroenterology, Wake Forest University School of
Medicine, Winston-Salem, North Carolina
*Anatomy, Histology, Embryology, and Developmental
Anomalies of the Esophagus*

Adair Look MD
Attending Psychiatrist, California Pacific Medical
Center, Department of Psychiatry, San Francisco,
California
Eating Disorders

Matthias Maiwald MD, PhD, FRCPA, D(ABMM)
Associate Professor of Medical Microbiology,
Department of Microbiology and Infectious Diseases,
Flinders University School of Medicine; Consultant in
Medical Microbiology, Flinders Medical Centre,
Adelaide, South Australia, Australia
Whipple's Disease

Carolina Malagelada MD
Fellow in Gastroenterology, Digestive Diseases
Department, Vall d'Hebron University Hospital and
Autonomous University of Barcelona, Barcelona, Spain
Nausea and Vomiting

Juan-R. Malagelada MD
Professor and Chairman, Digestive Diseases
Department, Vall d'Hebron University Hospital and
Autonomous University of Barcelona, Barcelona, Spain
Nausea and Vomiting

Lawrence A. Mark MD, PhD
Dermatology Resident, Indiana University School of
Medicine, Indianapolis, Indiana
*Oral Disease and Oral-Cutaneous Manifestations of
Gastrointestinal and Liver Disease*

Lisa Marr MD
Assistant Professor, Department of Medicine, Division
of Neoplastic Diseases and Related Disorders, Medical
College of Wisconsin; Palliative Medicine Physician,
Medical College of Wisconsin, Milwaukee, Wisconsin
*Palliative Medicine in Patients with Advanced
Gastrointestinal and Hepatic Disease*

Paul Martin MD
Professor of Medicine and Associate Director, Division
of Liver Diseases, Mount Sinai School of Medicine, New
York, New York
Liver Transplantation

Joel B. Mason MD
Associate Professor of Medicine and Nutrition, Tufts University School of Medicine; Physician, Divisions of Clinical Nutrition and Gastroenterology, Tufts–New England Medical Center, Boston, Massachusetts
Nutritional Assessment and Management of the Malnourished Patient

Jeffrey B. Matthews MD
Christian R. Holmes Professor and Chairman, Department of Surgery, University of Cincinnati College of Medicine, Cincinnati, Ohio
Surgical Peritonitis and Other Diseases of the Peritoneum, Mesentery, Omentum, and Diaphragm

Craig McClain MD
Professor of Medicine, Division of Gastroenterology/Hepatology, University of Louisville School of Medicine, Louisville, Kentucky
Alcoholic Liver Disease

George B. McDonald MD
Professor of Medicine, University of Washington School of Medicine; Head, Gastroenterology/Hepatology Section, Fred Hutchinson Cancer Research Center, Seattle, Washington
Gastrointestinal and Hepatic Complications of Solid Organ and Hematopoietic Cell Transplantation

Kenneth R. McQuaid MD
Professor of Clinical Medicine, University of California, San Francisco, School of Medicine; Director of Gastrointestinal Endoscopy, San Francisco Veterans Affairs Medical Center, San Francisco, California
Assistant Editor for Imaging
Dyspepsia

Joseph P. Minei MD
Professor of Surgery, Division of Burn, Trauma, and Critical Care, The University of Texas Southwestern Medical School; Chief, Section of Trauma, University of Texas Southwestern Medical Center; Surgeon-in-Chief and Medical Director of Trauma Services, Parkland Memorial Hospital, Dallas, Texas
Abdominal Abscesses and Gastrointestinal Fistulas

Ginat W. Mirowski DMD, MD
Adjunct Associate Professor, Indiana University School of Dentistry, Indianapolis, Indiana
Oral Disease and Oral-Cutaneous Manifestations of Gastrointestinal and Liver Disease

Sean J. Mulvihill MD
Professor and Chairman, Department of Surgery, University of Utah School of Medicine; Senior Director for Clinical Affairs, Huntsman Cancer Institute, University of Utah Hospital and Clinics, Salt Lake City, Utah
Acute Abdominal Pain; Treatment of Gallstone Disease

Anil B. Nagar MD
Assistant Professor, Department of Internal Medicine, Section of Digestive Diseases, Yale University School of Medicine, New Haven; Endoscopy Director, West Haven VA Hospital, West Haven, Connecticut
Ulcers of the Small and Large Intestine

Satheesh Nair MD
Medical Director, Liver Transplantation, Ochsner Clinic Foundation, New Orleans, Louisiana
Hepatitis B and D

Jeffrey A. Norton MD
Professor of Surgery, Stanford University School of Medicine; Chief, Surgical Oncology, Stanford University Medical Center, Stanford, California
Endocrine Tumors of the Pancreas and Gastrointestinal Tract

Michael J. Nunez MD
Department of Internal Medicine, Division of Gastroenterology, Presbyterian Hospital of Dallas, Dallas, Texas
Caustic Injury to the Upper Gastrointestinal Tract

Hiroki Ohge MD
Assistant Professor of Surgery, Hiroshima University School of Medicine, Hiroshima, Japan
Intestinal Gas

Seamus O'Mahony MD, FRCP
Lecturer, University College Cork; Consultant Gastroenterologist, Cork University Hospital, Cork, Ireland
Enteric Bacterial Flora and Bacterial Overgrowth

Susan R. Orenstein MD
Professor of Pediatrics, University of Pittsburgh School of Medicine, Pittsburgh, Pennsylvania
Eosinophilic Disorders of the Gastrointestinal Tract

Roy C. Orlando MD
Professor of Medicine and Adjunct Professor of Physiology, Tulane University School of Medicine; Chief, Gastroenterology and Hepatology, Tulane University Health Sciences Center, New Orleans, Louisiana
Anatomy, Histology, Embryology, and Developmental Anomalies of the Esophagus

James W. Ostroff MD
Professor of Clinical Medicine and Pediatrics, University of California, San Francisco, School of Medicine; Director, Endoscopy Unit and Gastrointestinal Consultation Service, Moffitt-Long Hospital and Mount Zion Hospital and Cancer Center, San Francisco, California
Endoscopic and Radiologic Treatment of Biliary Disease

Stephen J. Pandol MD
Professor of Medicine, University of California, Los Angeles, School of Medicine; Staff Physician, Veterans Affairs Greater Los Angeles Healthcare System—West Los Angeles, Los Angeles, California
Pancreatic Secretion

Sonal M. Patel MD
Fellow, Division of Gastroenterology, Harvard Medical School and Beth Israel Deaconess Medical Center, Boston, Massachusetts
Constipation

John H. Pemberton MD
Professor of Surgery, Mayo Clinic College of Medicine;
Consultant, Colon and Rectal Surgery, Mayo Clinic,
Rochester, Minnesota
Ileostomy, Colostomy, and Pouches

Robert Perrillo MD
Director, Academic Affairs, Section of Gastroenterology
and Hepatology, Ochsner Clinic Foundation, New
Orleans, Louisiana
Hepatitis B and D

Kimberly M. Persley MD
Assistant Clinical Professor of Medicine, University of
Texas Southwestern Medical School; Staff Physician,
Presbyterian Hospital of Dallas, Dallas, Texas
*Acalculous Cholecystitis, Cholesterolosis, Adenomyomatosis,
and Polyps of the Gallbladder*

Patrick R. Pfau MD
Assistant Professor of Medicine and Director of
Gastrointestinal Endoscopy, Section of Gastroenterology
and Hepatology, University of Wisconsin School of
Medicine and Public Health, Madison, Wisconsin
Foreign Bodies and Bezoars

Daniel K. Podolsky MD
Mallinckrodt Professor of Medicine and Faculty Dean
for Academic Programs at the Partners Healthcare
System, Harvard Medical School; Chief, Gastrointestinal
Unit, Massachusetts General Hospital, Boston,
Massachusetts
Cellular Growth and Neoplasia

Deborah D. Proctor MD
Associate Professor of Medicine and Director,
Gastroenterology Fellowship Training Program,
Department of Internal Medicine, Section of Digestive
Diseases, Yale University School of Medicine; Attending
Physician, Department of Internal Medicine, Section of
Digestive Diseases, Yale–New Haven Hospital, New
Haven, Connecticut
Ulcers of the Small and Large Intestine

Eamonn M.M. Quigley MD, FRCP, FACP, FACG, FRCPI
Professor of Medicine and Human Physiology and Head
of the Medical School, National University of Ireland;
Consultant Gastroenterologist, Cork University
Hospital, Cork, Ireland
*Gastric Motor and Sensory Function and Motor Disorders of
the Stomach*

Carol A. Redel MD
Assistant Professor of Pediatrics, Department of
Pediatrics, Division of Gastroenterology, Hepatology,
and Nutrition, Baylor College of Medicine; Attending
Gastroenterologist, Texas Children's Hospital, Houston,
Texas
*Anatomy, Histology, Embryology, and Developmental
Anomalies of the Stomach and Duodenum*

Andrea E. Reid MD, MPH
Assistant Professor of Medicine, Harvard Medical
School; Assistant Physician and Program Director,
Gastroenterology Training Program, Gastrointestinal Unit,
Massachusetts General Hospital, Boston, Massachusetts
Nonalcoholic Fatty Liver Disease

John F. Reinus MD
Associate Professor of Medicine, Albert Einstein College
of Medicine; Director of Hepatology, Montefiore
Medical Center, Bronx, New York
*Gastrointestinal and Hepatic Disorders in the Pregnant
Patient*

David A. Relman MD
Associate Professor of Medicine and Microbiology and
Immunology, Stanford University School of Medicine,
Stanford; Chief, Infectious Diseases, Veterans Affairs
Palo Alto Health Care System, Palo Alto, California
Whipple's Disease

Joel E. Richter MD
Professor of Medicine and Richard L. Evans Chair,
Department of Medicine, Temple University School of
Medicine, Philadelphia, Pennsylvania
Gastroesophageal Reflux Disease and Its Complications

Caroline A. Riely MD
Professor of Medicine and Pediatrics, University of
Tennessee School of Medicine, Memphis, Tennessee
*Gastrointestinal and Hepatic Disorders in the Pregnant
Patient*

Eve A. Roberts MD, FRCPC
Professor of Paediatrics, Medicine and Pharmacology,
University of Toronto Faculty of Medicine; Staff
Physician and Senior Scientist, Research Institute,
Division of Gastroenterology, Hepatology and
Nutrition, The Hospital for Sick Children, Toronto,
Ontario, Canada
Wilson Disease

Jeremy Rochester MD
GI Fellow, Mount Sinai School of Medicine and The
Mount Sinai Hospital, New York, New York
Colonic Polyps and Polyposis Syndromes

Don C. Rockey MD
Professor of Medicine and Chief, Gastroenterology,
University of Texas Southwestern Medical School,
Dallas, Texas
Gastrointestinal Bleeding

Hugo R. Rosen MD
Waterman Professor of Medicine and Immunology,
University of Colorado School of Medicine, Denver,
Colorado
Liver Transplantation

Jayanta Roy-Chowdhury MD
Professor, Department of Medicine (Liver) and
Department of Molecular Genetics, Albert Einstein
College of Medicine; Scientific Director, Gene
Therapy Facility, Montefiore Medical Center, Bronx,
New York
Liver Physiology and Energy Metabolism

Namita Roy-Chowdhury PhD
Professor, Department of Medicine (Liver) and
Department of Molecular Genetics, Albert Einstein
College of Medicine, Bronx, New York
Liver Physiology and Energy Metabolism

Bruce A. Runyon MD
Professor of Medicine, Loma Linda University School of
Medicine; Chief, Liver Service, and Medical Director,
Liver Transplantation, Loma Linda University Medical
Center, Loma Linda, California
Ascites and Spontaneous Bacterial Peritonitis

Michael A. Russo MD
Assistant Professor of Pediatrics, The University of Texas
Southwestern Medical School; Attending Physician,
Pediatric Gastroenterology, Children's Medical Center of
Dallas, Dallas, Texas
*Anatomy, Histology, Embryology, and Developmental
Anomalies of the Stomach and Duodenum*

Anil K. Rustgi MD
T. Grier Miller Professor of Medicine and Genetics,
University of Pennsylvania School of Medicine; Chief of
Gastroenterology, The Hospital of the University of
Pennsylvania, Philadelphia, Pennsylvania
Small Intestinal Neoplasms

Hugh A. Sampson MD
Professor of Pediatrics and Immunobiology, Mount
Sinai School of Medicine; Staff Physician and Director,
General Clinical Research Center, The Mount Sinai
Hospital, New York, New York
Food Allergies

Bruce E. Sands MD, MS
Assistant Professor of Medicine, Harvard Medical
School; Associate Physician, Massachusetts General
Hospital, Boston, Massachusetts
Crohn's Disease

R. Balfour Sartor MD
Distinguished Professor of Medicine, Microbiology, and
Immunology, University of North Carolina at Chapel
Hill School of Medicine; Director, Multidisciplinary IBD
Center, UNC Hospitals, Chapel Hill, North Carolina
*Mucosal Immunology and Mechanisms of Gastrointestinal
Inflammation*

George A. Sarosi, Jr. MD
Assistant Professor of Surgery, The University of Texas
Southwestern Medical School; Staff Physician, Dallas
Veterans Affairs Medical Center, Surgery Service, Dallas,
Texas
Appendicitis

Lawrence R. Schiller MD
Clinical Professor of Internal Medicine, University
of Texas Southwestern Medical School; Attending
Physician, Baylor University Medical Center, Dallas,
Texas
Diarrhea; Fecal Incontinence

Joseph H. Sellin MD
Professor of Internal Medicine, University of Texas
Medical Branch, Galveston, Texas
Diarrhea

Vijay H. Shah MD
Associate Professor of Medicine, Physiology, and Cell
Biology, Mayo Clinic College of Medicine, Rochester,
Minnesota
Portal Hypertension and Gastrointestinal Bleeding

Fergus Shanahan MD
Professor and Chair, Department of Medicine,
University College Cork, National University of
Ireland; Cork University Hospital, Cork, Ireland
Enteric Bacterial Flora and Bacterial Overgrowth

Maria H. Sjogren MD
Associate Professor of Preventive Medicine, Uniformed
Services University of the Health Sciences F. Edward
Hébert School of Medicine, Bethesda, Maryland;
Associate Professor of Medicine, Georgetown University
School of Medicine, Washington, DC; Chief,
Department of Clinical Investigation, Walter Reed
Army Medical Center, Washington, DC
Hepatitis A

Stuart Jon Spechler MD
Professor of Medicine and Berta M. and Cecil O. Patterson
Chair in Gastroenterology, University of Texas
Southwestern Medical Center; Chief, Division of
Gastroenterology, Dallas Veterans Administration
Medical Center, Dallas, Texas
Peptic Ulcer Disease

Jayaprakash Sreenarasimhaiah MD
Assistant Professor of Internal Medicine, The University
of Texas Southwestern Medical School, Dallas, Texas
Gallstone Disease

William M. Steinberg MD
Clinical Professor of Medicine, George Washington
University School of Medicine and Health Sciences,
Washington, DC
Acute Pancreatitis

William E. Stevens MD
Clinical Faculty, Department of Internal Medicine,
Division of Gastroenterology, Presbyterian Hospital of
Dallas, Dallas, Texas
Vascular Diseases of the Liver

Neil H. Stollman MD
Associate Clinical Professor of Medicine, University of
California, San Francisco, School of Medicine, San
Francisco, California
Diverticular Disease of the Colon

Chinyu Su MD
Assistant Professor of Medicine, University of
Pennsylvania School of Medicine; Attending Physician,
Division of Gastroenterology, Hospital of the University
of Pennsylvania and Penn Presbyterian Medical Center,
Philadelphia, Pennsylvania
Ulcerative Colitis

Frederick J. Suchy MD
Herbert H. Lehman Professor and Chair, Department of
Pediatrics, Mount Sinai School of Medicine;
Pediatrician-in-Chief, The Mount Sinai Hospital, New
York, New York
*Anatomy, Histology, Embryology, Developmental Anomalies,
and Pediatric Disorders of the Biliary Tract*

Joseph J.Y. Sung MD, PhD
Professor of Medicine, The Chinese University of Hong
Kong; Director, Institute of Digestive Disease, Prince of
Wales Hospital, Shatin, New Territories, Hong Kong
Helicobacter pylori

Nicholas J. Talley MD, PhD
Professor of Medicine, Mayo Clinic College of Medicine;
Consultant, Mayo Clinic, Rochester, Minnesota
Irritable Bowel Syndrome

Narci C. Teoh MBBS, PhD, FRACP
Senior Lecturer in Medicine, Australian National
University Medical School; Consultant
Gastroenterologist, The Canberra Hospital, Canberra,
Australian Capital Territory, Australia
Liver Disease Caused by Drugs

Dwain L. Thiele MD
Professor of Medicine, University of Texas Southwestern
Medical School; Vice-Chief, Division of Digestive and
Liver Diseases, and Chief of Hepatology, University of
Texas Southwestern Medical Center; Chief of Liver
Diseases Service, Parkland Health and Hospital System;
Attending Physician, Zale Lipshy University Hospital,
Dallas, Texas
*Gastrointestinal and Hepatic Manifestations of Systemic
Diseases*

Matthew L. Tompson MD
The Methodist Hospital, Houston, Texas
*Anatomy, Histology, Embryology, and Developmental
Anomalies of the Pancreas*

Bruce Y. Tung MD
Assistant Professor of Medicine, Division of
Gastroenterology, University of Washington School of
Medicine, Seattle, Washington
Sclerosing Cholangitis and Recurrent Pyogenic Cholangitis

Richard H. Turnage MD
Professor and Chairman, Department of Surgery,
Louisiana State University Health Sciences Center
School of Medicine Shreveport; Surgeon-in-Chief,
Louisiana State University Health Sciences Center,
Shreveport, Louisiana
Appendicitis; Intestinal Obstruction and Ileus

Arnold Wald MD
Professor of Medicine, University of Wisconsin School
of Medicine and Public Health, Madison, Wisconsin
Other Diseases of the Colon and Rectum

Timothy C. Wang MD
Dorothy L. and Daniel B. Silberberg Professor of
Medicine, Columbia University College of Physicians
and Surgeons; Chief of Gastroenterology, New
York–Presbyterian Hospital—Columbia Campus;
Director, Division of Digestive and Liver Diseases,
Department of Medicine, Columbia University Medical
Center, New York, New York
Tumors of the Stomach

Ian R. Wanless MD, CM, FRCPC
Professor, Department of Pathology, Dalhousie
University Faculty of Medicine; Pathologist, Queen
Elizabeth II Health Sciences Centre, Halifax, Nova
Scotia, Canada
*Anatomy, Histology, Embryology, and Developmental
Anomalies of the Liver*

David E. Weissman MD
Professor of Internal Medicine, Medical College of
Wisconsin; Director, Palliative Care Center, Froedtert
Hospital, Milwaukee, Wisconsin
*Palliative Medicine in Patients with Advanced
Gastrointestinal and Hepatic Disease*

David C. Whitcomb MD, PhD
Giant Eagle Foundation Professor of Cancer Genetics
and Professor of Medicine, Cell Biology and Physiology,
and Human Genetics, University of Pittsburgh School
of Medicine; Chief, Division of Gastroenterology,
Hepatology, and Nutrition, University of Pittsburgh
Medical Center, Pittsburgh, Pennsylvania
*Hereditary, Familial, and Genetic Disorders of the Pancreas
and Pancreatic Disorders in Childhood*

C. Mel Wilcox MD
Professor of Medicine and Director, Division of
Gastroenterology and Hepatology, University of
Alabama at Birmingham School of Medicine,
Birmingham, Alabama
*Gastrointestinal Consequences of Infection with Human
Immunodeficiency Virus*

Teresa L. Wright MD
Professor of Medicine, University of California, San
Francisco, School of Medicine; Chief, Gastroenterology
Section, San Francisco Veterans Affairs Medical Center,
San Francisco, California
Hepatitis C

Foreword

It is now over 35 years since Marvin Sleisenger and John Fordtran decided in their wisdom that something was needed beyond that found in the then-extant clinical textbooks dealing with gastrointestinal diseases. Among other considerations, they felt that it was imperative to incorporate both the physiology and the pathophysiology of diseases. What emerged from their efforts was the first edition of *Gastrointestinal Disease: Pathophysiology/Diagnosis/Management*. Their book soon became what many considered to be the "Bible" of gastroenterology for students, clinical scholars, and practitioners as the primary resource for both the general and the detailed aspects of the specialty.

Marvin Sleisenger and John Fordtran continued their active editorial oversight of the textbook for the next four editions. Subsequently, three new and outstanding editors have come on board—Mark Feldman in the fifth edition (along with Bruce Scharschmidt, assistant editor of the fifth edition), Lawrence S. Friedman in the seventh edition, and now Lawrence J. Brandt. Thus, the eighth edition is the first for which neither of its distinguished founders has served as editor. In my view, the book continues its tradition as the definitive clinical resource in the field of gastroenterology and liver disease. The eighth edition retains its tradition for many reasons, not the least of which is the innovative approaches of its current editors. Their goals and objectives are very much in evidence—namely, to provide the reader with a state-of-the-art resource that is both informative and detailed and yet still very readable.

What in fact is required to achieve and then maintain the overall excellence of a textbook such as this? From my own editorial experience and observations, the answer is straightforward: a focus on excellence at every level. This requires the exercise of rigorous oversight of the editorial content. The planning of a subsequent edition entails the dispassionate analysis of existing chapters by outside reviewers, with the request that they examine the accuracy, content, and quality of presentation. It also demands "in-house" review by the editors and a process that does not avoid self-criticism. The update of an existing chapter by its authors is fairly straightforward, but there is always the risk that the original authors may make only cosmetic rather than substantive changes and that the chapter will in fact become "stale." Therefore, in the long term, an enlightened approach often is achieved by regular and planned rotation of authors. It is evident that the current editors have kept all of these issues very much in mind.

The critical oversight of this textbook by the editors is all the more essential in view of the rapid advances in modern biology and medicine. From my observations, readers of this edition can rest assured that these advances have been thoughtfully included in the subject matter and, when appropriate, incorporated into the latest clinical recommendations. These molecular biological advances apply especially to the development of newer pharmacologic agents that are altering the manner in which we are treating disorders such as inflammatory bowel disease, irritable bowel syndrome, and chronic liver diseases, to mention just a few. In a multi-authored textbook such as this, the editors need to scrutinize the text to make certain that the clinical and therapeutic recommendations are internally consistent, without undue overlap or redundancy. This again obviously requires thorough editorial oversight, which I know has been an important consideration in the development of the eighth edition of *Sleisenger & Fordtran*. Finally, the editors have ensured that the visual material—endoscopic pictures, radiographic images, and histologic representations, all so important to the practice of gastroenterology—are of the highest quality.

I am pleased that the current distinguished editors—Mark Feldman, Lawrence S. Friedman, and Lawrence J. Brandt—have focused on excellence at every level of this textbook. Indeed, with the 8th edition they have succeeded in continuing the high standards of Marvin Sleisenger and John Fordtran and have made this edition the best it can be.

Kurt J. Isselbacher, MD, ScD(Hon)
Director Emeritus, Gastrointestinal Unit, and
*   Director Emeritus, Cancer Center*
Massachusetts General Hospital
Distinguished Mallinckrodt Professor of Medicine
Harvard Medical School
Boston, Massachusetts

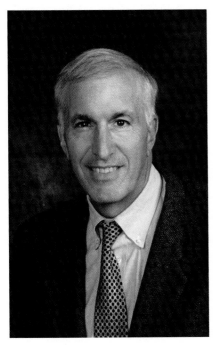

Mark Feldman MD
Editions 5-8

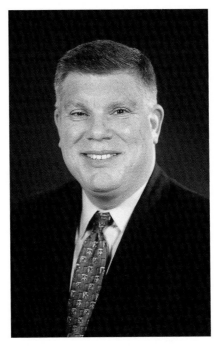

Lawrence S. Friedman MD
Editions 7, 8

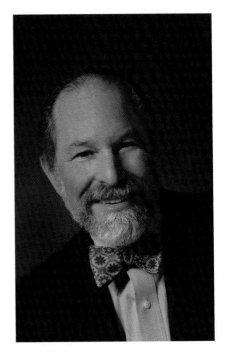

Lawrence J. Brandt MD
Edition 8

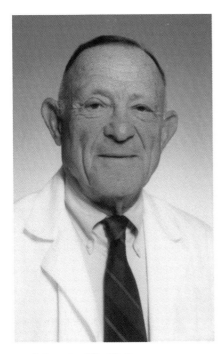

Marvin H. Sleisenger MD
Editions 1-7

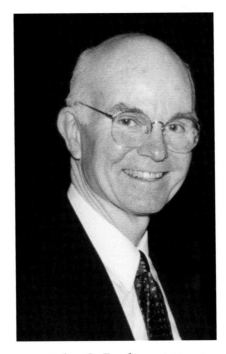

John S. Fordtran MD
Editions 1-5

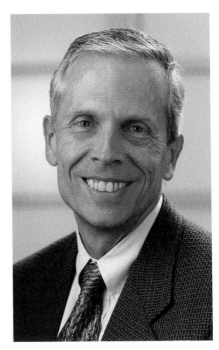

Bruce F. Scharschmidt MD
Editions 5, 6

Preface

The eighth edition of *Sleisenger & Fordtran's Gastrointestinal and Liver Disease* is the first edition for which neither of the founding editors is serving as a principal editor— Dr. Fordtran stepped down as editor after publication of the fifth edition, and for this edition, Dr. Sleisenger is serving as consulting editor. In Dr. Sleisenger's place, one of us, Dr. Lawrence J. Brandt, has become a principal editor. Given the explosion of information in gastroenterology over the past 2 decades and the incorporation of liver disease into the textbook since the sixth edition, we believe that the book is best served by three editors, rather than two. That the book continues to serve as a state-of-the-art, user-friendly source for the spectrum of gastroenterologic and hepatic disorders is a tribute to the vision and efforts of its founding editors, John Fordtran and Marvin Sleisenger. The sixth edition was dedicated to Dr. Fordtran, and this edition is dedicated with equal admiration, appreciation, and affection to Dr. Sleisenger.

As with previous editions, the editors have relied on the gracious advice of reviewers, colleagues, and trainees and have incorporated many improvements and refinements into this edition. Every effort has been made to minimize redundancies, correct deficiencies, and improve the book's flow and organization. Completing an enhancement that was begun in the seventh edition, virtually all endoscopic and histologic figures are now in full color. The color figures are fully integrated with the text in each chapter, not segregated into a separate atlas section as in many other textbooks. To be certain that all figures are of the highest quality and clarity, we were assisted by an imaging editor, Dr. Kenneth R. McQuaid, whose contribution we gratefully acknowledge. Two gastrointestinal pathologists, Drs. Pamela Jensen and Edward L. Lee, helped individual authors and editors find selected classic histologic examples of various diseases. In addition, for the eighth edition, nearly all of the diagrams and algorithms have been redrawn in a uniform and visually appealing style that complements and enhances the text.

The overall organization of the book remains similar to that of previous editions, although several chapters on new topics have been added and the placement of individual chapters has been refined. Moreover, fully one third of the contributing authors are new to this edition, thereby ensuring that the information is fresh, updated, and critically assessed; each contributor was chosen because of his or her expertise in the area covered and

reputation for clarity and effectiveness as a writer. Since publication of the seventh edition in 2002, there has been a remarkable amount of new information in the field of gastroenterology; for example, at least 20 new drugs, including tegaserod for constipation-predominant irritable bowel syndrome, adefovir and entecavir for hepatitis B, and oxaliplatin, bevacizumab, and cetuximab for metastatic colon cancer, have been approved by the U.S. Food and Drug Administration. Every effort has been made to ensure that the content of the book is as current as possible.

Section I contains three chapters that deal with the Biology of the Gastrointestinal Tract and Liver and provides a cogent introduction to basic science relevant to gastroenterology. Basic pathophysiology also is incorporated into the chapters on specific diseases. Section II, as in the previous two editions, presents an Approach to Patients with Symptoms and Signs and includes chapters written by new authors, including Dr. DeVault (Symptoms of Esophageal Disease), the two Drs. Malagelada (Nausea and Vomiting), and Drs. Patel and Lembo (Constipation), as well as the stalwarts from previous editions. New authors for Section III on Nutrition in Gastroenterology—Drs. Mason, DeLegge, Becker, and Look—have joined veteran Dr. Klein to produce a veritable book-within-a-book that now includes separate chapters on Eating Disorders and on Obesity; the chapter on Food Allergies by Dr. Sampson also has been moved to this section. Section IV, Topics Involving Multiple Organs, has been expanded and reorganized. A new chapter has been added on Gastrointestinal Stromal Tumors (GISTs), by Dr. Demetri, and some chapters previously covered elsewhere in the book have been placed more appropriately in this section, including chapters on Eosinophilic Disorders of the Gastrointestinal Tract by Drs. Khan and Orenstein; Gastrointestinal Carcinoid Tumors and the Carcinoid Syndrome by Drs. Anthony and Kim; Vascular Lesions of the Gastrointestinal Tract by Dr. Brandt; Surgical Peritonitis and Other Diseases of the Peritoneum, Mesentery, Omentum, and Diaphragm by Drs. Fischer and Matthews; and Radiation Injury to the Gastrointestinal Tract by Drs. Cho and Antoine. Single chapters by Drs. Jain and Thiele and by Drs. Reinus and Riely now cover Gastrointestinal and Hepatic Manifestations of Systemic Diseases and Gastrointestinal and Hepatic Disorders in the Pregnant Patient, respectively, and an expanded chapter by Drs. Jensen and

Norton covers Endocrine Tumors of the Pancreas and Gastrointestinal Tract. Dr. Kimmey concludes the section with a thoughtful review of Complications of Gastrointestinal Endoscopy.

The next several sections constitute what we like to refer to as the "organ recital" of gastrointestinal and liver diseases: Sections V through X cover the Esophagus, Stomach and Duodenum, Pancreas, Biliary Tract, Liver, and Small and Large Intestine, respectively. Each section begins with a consideration of anatomy, histology, embryology, and developmental abnormalities, as well as basic function of the organ (for example, motility and sensory function of the hollow organs and biochemical function of the solid organs). The highlights and new contributors are many. Among the changes since the seventh edition are incorporation of the discussion of nonsteroidal anti-inflammatory drug–induced gastric ulceration into the chapter on Peptic Ulcer Disease by Drs. Cryer and Spechler (in addition to the chapter on *Helicobacter pylori* by Drs. Graham and Sung); creation of an expanded chapter on Treatment of Peptic Ulcer Disease by Drs. Chan and Lau; revision of the chapter on Acute Pancreatitis by Dr. Steinberg; updating of the chapter on Gallstone Disease by Drs. Browning and Sreenarasimhaiah and of the chapter on Acalculous Cholecystitis, Cholesterolosis, Adenomyomatosis, and Polyps of the Gallbladder by Dr. Persley (both chapters ably written in previous editions by our friend and colleague the late Dr. Lyman Bilhartz); and revision of the chapter on Sclerosing Cholangitis and Recurrent Pyogenic Cholangitis by Drs. Tung and Kowdley. New authors in the section on the Liver include the two Drs. Roy-Chowdhury (Liver Physiology and Energy Metabolism); Drs. Ahmed and Keeffe (Liver Chemistry and Function Tests); Dr. Stevens (Vascular Diseases of the Liver); Drs. Carithers and McClain (Alcoholic Liver Disease); Dr. Reid (Nonalcoholic Fatty Liver Disease); Drs. Shah and Kamath (Portal Hypertension and Gastrointestinal Bleeding); and Dr. Fontana (Acute Liver Failure). The single comprehensive chapter on Viral Hepatitis in the seventh edition has been divided into five separate chapters, which take advantage of the expertise of Drs. Sjogren, Perrillo, Nair, Berenguer, Wright, Krawczynski, Aggarwal, Heathcote, and Feld. In addition, a separate chapter on Liver Disease Caused by Anesthetics, Toxins, and Herbal Preparations, by Dr. Lewis, has been split off from the chapter on Liver Diseases Caused by Drugs by Drs. Teoh and G. Farrell.

New authors in the section on Small and Large Intestine include Drs. Kahn and Daum (Anatomy, Histology, Embryology, and Developmental Anomalies of the Small and Large Intestine); Drs. Harrell and Chang (Intestinal Water and Electrolyte Transport); Drs. O'Mahony and Shanahan (Enteric Bacterial Flora and Bacterial Overgrowth); Dr. Buchman (Short Bowel Syndrome); Dr. Giannella (Infectious Enteritis and Proctocolitis and Bacterial Food Poisoning); Drs. Kelly and Lamont (Antibiotic-Associated Diarrhea, Pseudomembranous Enterocolitis, and *Clostridium difficile*-Associated Diarrhea and Colitis); Drs. Su and Lichtenstein (Ulcerative Colitis); Drs. Fox and Stollman (Diverticular Disease of the Colon); Dr. Talley (Irritable Bowel Syndrome); and Dr. Camilleri (Acute and Chronic Pseudo-obstruction).

Finally, the last section of the book, on Psychosocial Factors in Gastrointestinal Disease, includes a new author, Dr. Locke (A Biopsychosocial Understanding of Gastrointestinal Illness and Disease), and new chapters on Palliative Medicine in Patients with Advanced Gastrointestinal and Hepatic Disease by Drs. Marr and Weissman and on Complementary and Alternative Medicine Therapies in Gastrointestinal and Hepatic Disease by Drs. Hass and Brandt.

As in previous editions, a mini-outline with page citations is included at the start of each chapter, and each major section contains a listing of the chapters with page citations in that section. The high-quality glossy paper for which the book is known has been retained, as have extensive cross-referencing and a comprehensive index.

The eighth edition of this classic textbook is a living tribute to its founding editors, Drs. John Fordtran and Marvin Sleisenger. True to their vision, the eighth edition presents a critical overview of the state of gastrointestinal practice and its scientific basis by eminent authorities in their respective fields. International in scope, with authors from eleven countries, the book remains the definitive resource for all who provide care for patients with gastrointestinal and liver disorders.

Mark Feldman MD
Lawrence S. Friedman MD
Lawrence J. Brandt MD

Acknowledgments

As the editors of the eighth edition of *Sleisenger & Fordtran's Gastrointestinal and Liver Disease*, we are most grateful to the more than 150 contributing authors from eleven countries in North America, Europe, Asia, Africa, and Australia whose knowledge and experience fill its pages. We also appreciate the talented staff at Saunders/Elsevier who made publishing this book possible, particularly Sue Hodgson, Melissa Dudlick, Rolla Couchman, Fiona Foley, Karen Bowler, and Jeff Gunning.

We also acknowledge the valuable assistance of Dr. Kenneth R. McQuaid of the University of California, San Francisco, the editor for imaging, and Drs. Pamela Jensen of Dallas and Edward Lee of Washington, DC, for their help with many pathology photographs.

Tracy Thornburg, Alison Sholock, and Sheila Frenchman provided outstanding administrative support. We are especially grateful to our wives for their constant encouragement and understanding: Barbara Feldman, Mary Jo Cappuccilli, and Lois Brandt.

We also thank Dr. Kurt J. Isselbacher of Harvard Medical School and Massachusetts General Hospital, Boston, for writing the Foreword. Finally, we acknowledge the past efforts and leadership of previous editors, John Fordtran, Bruce Scharschmidt, and of course Marv Sleisenger, to whom this book is dedicated.

Contents

Volume 1

Volume 2

SECTION
IX

Liver

CHAPTER

68 Anatomy, Histology, Embryology, and Developmental Anomalies of the Liver

Ian R. Wanless

Knowledge of normal morphology is basic to an understanding of pathologic processes and the secure practice of hepatobiliary surgery. This chapter is a brief introduction to anatomy of the human liver and its variations. More detailed expositions can be found elsewhere.[1-4] Embryology of the biliary tract and liver is reviewed in Chapter 59.

SURFACE ANATOMY

The normal liver occupies the right upper quadrant and extends from the fifth intercostal space in the midclavicular line to the right costal margin. The lower margin of the liver descends below the costal margin during inspiration. The median liver weight is 1800 g in men and 1400 g in women.[5,6]

Transcutaneous liver biopsy specimens are commonly obtained in the midaxillary line through the third interspace below the upper limit of liver dullness during full expiration; this site is usually in the ninth intercostal space.

The superior, anterior, and right lateral surfaces of the liver are smooth and convex, fitting against the diaphragm. The posterior surface has indentations from the colon, right kidney, and duodenum on the right lobe and the stomach on the left lobe (Fig. 68–1).

The fibrous capsule on the posterior aspect of the liver reflects onto the diaphragm and posterior abdominal wall and leaves a "bare area" where the liver is in continuity with the retroperitoneum. The liver is supported by the peritoneal reflections that form the coronary ligaments, the right and left triangular ligaments, and the falciform ligament (see Fig. 68–1). The lower free edge of the falciform ligament contains the round ligament, which is composed largely of the obliterated umbilical vein. The falciform ligament joins the anterior surface of the liver to the diaphragm. Superiorly, the falciform ligament joins the peritoneal reflections to the left of the vena cava.

The hepatoduodenal ligament connects the liver to the superior part of the duodenum. The free margin of this ligament contains the hepatic artery, portal vein, bile duct, nerves, and lymphatic vessels. These structures connect with the liver in the transverse portal fissure. The caudate lobe of the liver is posterior, and the quadrate lobe anterior, to this fissure. The quadrate lobe is further demarcated on the right by the gallbladder and on the left by the umbilical fissure.

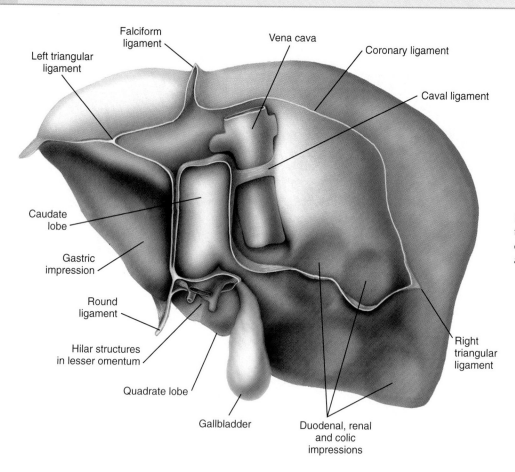

Left triangular
ligament

Falciform
ligament

Vena cava

Coronary ligament

Caval ligament

Caudate
lobe

Gastric
impression

Round
ligament

Hilar structures
in lesser omentum

Quadrate lobe

Gallbladder

Duodenal, renal
and colic
impressions

Right
triangular
ligament

Figure 68–1 Posterior view of the liver. The shape of the liver is determined by molding against adjacent organs.

SEGMENTAL ANATOMY

The liver classically has been divided into left and right lobes by the location of the falciform ligament. Because this location does not correspond to the internal subdivisions of the liver, a more functional nomenclature was developed by Hjortso and Couinaud on the basis of the distribution of vessels and ducts within the liver.[7,8] In this nomenclature, the line extending between the vena cava and the gallbladder (Cantlie's line) demarcates the right and left livers (or hemilivers), each with independent vascular and duct supplies. This line marks a relatively bloodless plane that is of use to the surgeon. The liver can be divided further into eight segments, each containing a pedicle of portal vessels and ducts and drained by hepatic veins situated in the planes (called *scissura*) between the segments (Fig. 68–2).[7] Because branching of the left portal vein is irregular, Strasberg[8] has recommended that the segments be defined by the divisions of the arteries or ducts.

The segments usually have no surface fissures to allow their accurate identification. The left hemiliver is composed of the classic left lobe plus the caudate lobe and the quadrate lobe and its superior extension. There is considerable individual variation in the location of the segments, especially in the right hemiliver.[9,10]

The common resections, using the Strasberg nomenclature, are as follows[7,8]:

- Right hemihepatectomy (segments 5 to 8, or right hepatectomy, right hepatic lobectomy)
- Right trisectionectomy (segments 4 to 8, or right lobectomy, trisegmentectomy of Starzl)
- Left hemihepatectomy (segments 1 to 4, or left hepatectomy, left hepatic lobectomy)
- Left lateral sectionectomy (segments 1 to 3, or left lobectomy, left lateral segmentectomy).

VARIATIONS IN ANATOMY

An elongation of the right lobe (Riedel's lobe) can be mistaken for hepatomegaly. This anomaly and minor variations in the shape of the liver explain why clinical estimation of liver size correlates poorly with more objective measures.

Deep fissures may demarcate supernumerary lobes. Rarely, the left lobe is attached to the right lobe by a narrow pedicle. Accessory livers may be found in the ligaments or mesentery or on the surface of the gallbladder, spleen, or adrenals.

Atrophy of the left lobe is usually an acquired abnormality resulting from thrombosis of the portal or hepatic veins.[11] Coarse lobulations (hepar lobatum) are a result of obliterative lesions in large and medium-sized vessels, typically after invasion by a neoplasm[12] or in syphilis (see Chapter 79).

Right posterior section   Right anterior section   Left medial section   Left lateral section

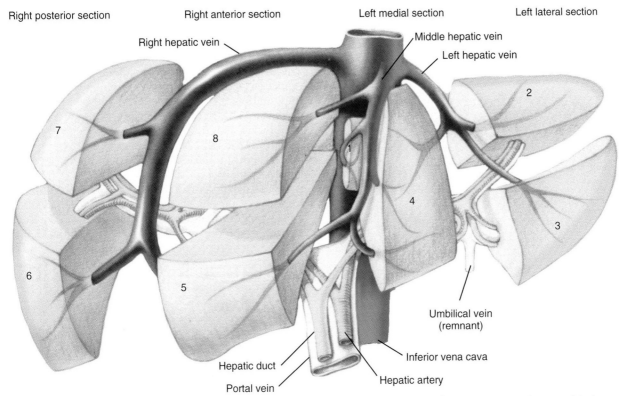

Figure 68–2   Diagram of the functional segments using the nomenclature of Couinaud. For explanation, see text. Segment 1 is the caudate lobe (see Figure 68–1).

LARGE VESSELS OF THE LIVER

PORTAL VEINS

The portal vein normally supplies 70% of the blood flow to the hepatic parenchyma. The portal vein receives almost all of the blood flow from the digestive tract between the proximal stomach and upper rectum as well as from the spleen, pancreas, and gallbladder (Fig. 68–3). The splenic and superior mesenteric veins join behind the pancreas to form the portal vein. The splenic vein sits in a groove of the pancreas and receives the short gastric veins, pancreatic veins, left gastroepiploic vein, and inferior mesenteric vein. The portal vein receives the superior pancreaticoduodenal vein and the left gastric (coronary) vein. The superior mesenteric vein receives the inferior pancreaticoduodenal vein and the right gastroepiploic vein. There is some variation in the veins that drain into the portal system.

The portal trunk bifurcates in the portal fissure. The left branch has a transverse segment that turns caudally to form the umbilical portion, which terminates in the obliterated umbilical vein. The left portal vein supplies the quadrate, caudate, and left lobes of the liver. The right portal vein usually receives the cystic vein.

The periductal venous plexus is a collection of variable veins that arise from the pancreas, duodenum, and stomach. The plexus runs along the common bile duct and drains into the perihilar segments of liver or into large branches of the portal vein.[13] This periduct plexus may explain some examples of focal fatty change and focal fatty sparing because of the variable concentration of insulin delivered to the perihilar parenchyma.[14]

Anomalies of the Portal Venous System

Anomalies of the portal venous system are uncommon. A portion of the right liver may be supplied by a branch of the left portal vein.[15] The ductus venosus usually closes shortly after birth. Persistent ductus venosus prevents the normal development of the portal vein, thereby leading to hypoplasia of the intrahepatic branches, nodular hyperplasia of the liver, and hyperammonemia; atrial septal defect has also been associated with this finding.[16]

Atresia or agenesis of the portal vein may be congenital (and often associated with anomalies of the systemic vasculature)[17,18] or a result of neonatal omphalitis or portal vein thrombosis. Portal vein thrombosis may lead to remodeling of the liver, recognized as nodular hyperplasia or atrophy of the left lobe (see Chapter 80).[19] Aneurysm of the portal trunk or intrahepatic branches can occur.[20]

HEPATIC VEINS

There are three main hepatic veins. In 80% of persons the middle and left hepatic veins join before entering the vena cava. The major veins divide at acute angles into branches of equal diameter to form an axial tree that receives smaller tributaries at right angles. Anastomoses are commonly found between branches of the hepatic veins.

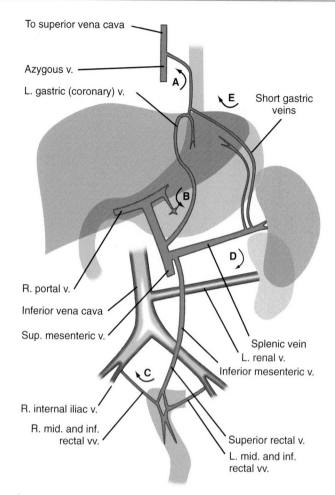

To superior vena cava

Azygous v.

L. gastric (coronary) v.

A

E Short gastric veins

B

R. portal v.

Inferior vena cava

Sup. mesenteric v.

D

Splenic vein

L. renal v.

Inferior mesenteric v.

C

R. internal iliac v.

R. mid. and inf. rectal vv.

Superior rectal v.

L. mid. and inf. rectal vv.

Figure 68–3 Diagram of the portal circulation. The most important sites for the potential development of portosystemic collaterals are shown. A, Esophageal submucosal veins, which are supplied by the left gastric vein and drain into the superior vena cava via the azygous vein. B, Paraumbilical veins, which are supplied by the umbilical portion of the left portal vein and drain into abdominal wall veins near the umbilicus. These veins may form a caput medusae at the umbilicus. C, Rectal submucosal veins, which are supplied by the inferior mesenteric vein through the superior rectal vein and drain into the internal iliac veins through the middle (mid.) and inferior (inf.) rectal veins. D, Splenorenal shunts, which are created spontaneously or surgically. E, Short gastric veins, which are supplied by the esophageal submucosal veins and drain into the splenic vein.

Several additional veins, including those from the caudate lobe, drain directly into the vena cava. The caudate veins usually remain patent when thrombosis affects the main hepatic veins in Budd-Chiari syndrome, thereby allowing the caudate lobe to undergo compensatory hyperplasia.[21] Webs commonly develop in the hepatic veins and vena cava after thrombosis.[22] Rarely, venous webs are congenital malformations (see Chapter 80).

HEPATIC ARTERIES

The common hepatic artery arises from the celiac artery, ascends in front of the portal vein, usually to the left and behind the bile duct, and gives off the left and right

hepatic arteries. The gallbladder is supplied by one or two cystic arteries that arise from the right hepatic artery.

Although the left and right hepatic arteries are end-arteries, they often anastomose within the hilar tissues.[15] There are also abundant collateral channels between branches of the celiac axis and branches of the superior mesenteric artery.[23] Anomalies in these large arteries are common. The right hepatic artery may arise from the superior mesenteric artery, and the left hepatic artery may arise from the left gastric artery.[23,24]

Although arterial ligation is usually well tolerated in persons with normal liver function,[25] the cirrhotic liver is highly dependent on arterial flow because of marked loss of portal vein perfusion. Loss of arterial perfusion after liver transplantation is often followed by ischemic stricturing of the bile duct near the hilum,[26] possibly because of ligation of potential collaterals during extirpation of the donor liver (see Chapter 92).

HEPATIC COLLATERAL CIRCULATION

When portal vein blood flow is impeded by cirrhosis or thrombosis of portal or hepatic veins, dilated collateral veins are found at many sites (see Fig. 68–3). These collaterals are prone to rupture, especially in the submucosa of the esophagus and stomach and less often in the colon and at colostomy sites. The surgeon encounters collateral veins at additional sites, especially in various hepatic ligaments, retroperitoneal attachments of other abdominal organs, and both sides of the diaphragm and the lesser omentum as well as near the bladder and rectum. These veins drain into the systemic circuit mainly via the azygous, renal, adrenal, and inferior hemorrhoidal veins. Dilated paraumbilical veins arise from the umbilical portion of the left portal vein, extend to the umbilicus via the round ligament, and connect with epigastric and internal mammary veins to produce umbilical and abdominal wall varices. Within the cirrhotic liver, there is significant collateral flow in small veins that connect branches of the portal and hepatic veins.[27]

LYMPH VESSELS

Hepatic lymph forms in the connective tissue spaces beneath the sinusoidal endothelial cells (space of Disse), in portal tracts, and around hepatic veins.[28] Recognizable lymphatic vessels are found in small portal tracts and the walls of small hepatic veins. These vessels drain to lymph nodes of the hilum and vena cava, respectively. Additional lymphatics in the liver capsule drain to various ligaments, across the diaphragm to esophageal and xiphisternal nodes, and along the bile duct. The frequent occurrence of pleural effusion in patients with massive ascites may be explained by lymph flow in transdiaphragmatic lymphatics.

NERVE SUPPLY

The liver has a rich sympathetic and parasympathetic innervation.[29,30] Fibers derive from lower thoracic ganglia, the celiac plexus, the vagi, and the right phrenic nerve to form the plexuses about the hepatic artery, portal vein, and bile duct. The arteries are innervated mainly by sympathetic fibers. The bile ducts are innervated by both sympathetic and parasympathetic fibers. Unmyelinated sympathetic fibers send branches to individual hepatocytes.

The denervated state of the transplanted liver persists for years[31] but does not affect liver function significantly.[32]

BILIARY SYSTEM

The common bile duct is usually located anterior to the portal vein and anterior to and to the right of the hepatic artery. There is considerable variation in the position of the duct relative to the vessels and in the branching pattern at the hilum, but intrahepatic bile ducts closely follow the course of intrahepatic portal veins and arteries within the portal tracts.[33]

The common hepatic duct and common bile duct normally have a luminal diameter of 4 to 6 mm. Lobar ducts measure 2 to 4 mm. Segmental bile ducts measure between 0.4 and 0.8 mm in diameter. All of these large ducts have columnar epithelium supported by a well-defined sheath of collagen.[34] Medium-sized (septal) ducts measure 0.1 to 0.4 mm and also have columnar epithelium. Small (interlobular) ducts measure less than 0.1 mm and have cuboidal epithelium. Terminal bile ducts are the smallest biliary radicles to be accompanied by arteries. Bile ductules connect the terminal ducts to the canals of Hering. The canals of Hering connect ductules to hepatocellular canaliculi.[35]

The canals of Hering are composed of both hepatocytes and cholangiocytes and can be identified by cytokeratin 19 staining in the proximal third of the acinus or the choleohepaton (see later).[36] There has been renewed interest in the duct of Hering, which has been identified as the site of hepatic stem cells.[4,35,37,38] Bone marrow–derived stem cells are believed to home to this site. Stem cells are believed to be capable of differentiating into either hepatocytes or duct cells, depending on the nature of local stimuli.

The large intrahepatic ducts and all extrahepatic ducts are accompanied by periductal glands and rarely by ectopic pancreatic acinar tissue.[39]

ANATOMIC VARIATIONS OF THE BILIARY SYSTEM

There is considerable variation in the extrahepatic and primary intrahepatic branches of the biliary tree, which can provide surprises for the surgeon (see Chapter 59).[33,40] Large ducts from one side of the liver may drain into the opposite lobar duct. The cystic duct may drain into the right hepatic duct. The common bile duct may be short or absent, with the right and left ducts joining just before their entry into the duodenum. Medium-sized ducts often anastomose between lobes, sometimes providing spontaneous relief of obstruction after ligation. The ducts of Luschka are ducts in the gallbladder bed that, if tran-

sected during cholecystectomy, may leak bile into the peritoneal cavity.[41]

A choledochal cyst is a focal dilatation of the biliary tree; Caroli's disease is a subtype of choledochal cyst characterized by diffuse intrahepatic dilatation. These conditions may manifest as cholangitis, abscesses, jaundice, or cirrhosis. Common bile duct dilatation is commonly seen after cholecystectomy and is sometimes a feature of polycystic liver disease.[42]

Atresia of the large bile ducts is one of the most common causes of cirrhosis in children (see Chapter 59). Hypoplasia and atresia are often associated with other anomalies and may thus be a congenital malformation. It is possible that acquired infections may also cause atresia.

Periductal glands are prone to inflammation and the formation of retention cysts,[39] which are usually incidental findings but rarely obstruct the bile ducts at the bifurcation.[43]

MICROANATOMY

Hepatocytes are polyhedral with a central spherical nucleus. They are arranged in plates that are one cell thick and have blood-filled sinusoids on each side. The cytoplasmic membrane has specialized domains that provide a canalicular region on the lateral walls and numerous microvilli on the sinusoidal (basolateral) surfaces. The canalicular domains of adjacent hepatocytes are bound together by tight junctions to form bile canaliculi that coalesce and ultimately drain into ducts within portal tracts. The sinusoidal surface is covered with a layer of endothelial cells to enclose the extravascular space of Disse. Within this space are liver-associated lymphocytes and stellate (fat-storing, formerly Ito) cells. The stellate cells normally contain numerous droplets of vitamin A ester. When activated by various cytokines, stellate cells lose their fat droplets and function as the principal hepatic fibroblasts. Kupffer cells are the hepatic macrophages that reside in the sinusoids and have pseudopodia anchored to subendothelial structures.

Hepatic sinusoids differ from systemic capillaries in that the endothelial cells are fenestrated and subendothelial stromal material is scanty, thereby permitting passage of large macromolecules, including lipoproteins. The sinusoidal walls are supported by a delicate network of collagen fibers that stains with the reticulin stain.

Normal and abnormal ultrastructure is discussed in detail in other reviews.[1,35,44]

SINUSOIDAL PATHOLOGY

During the development of cirrhosis the sinusoids acquire some features of systemic capillaries; the space of Disse becomes widened with collagen, basement membrane material is deposited, endothelial fenestrations become smaller and less numerous, and hepatocellular microvilli are effaced. These changes likely reduce transport across the sinusoidal walls.

Weakening of reticulin fibers may predispose to the rupture of sinusoidal walls and the formation of blood-filled cysts, a condition known as *peliosis hepatis* (see Chapter 80).[19]

ORGANIZATION OF HEPATIC PARENCHYMA: THE ACINUS AND THE LOBULE

The organization of the hepatic parenchyma has been conceptualized in two contrasting models, the acinus and the lobule (Fig. 68–4).[45] Terminal portal veins interdigitate with the terminal hepatic venules, with sinusoids bridging the gaps between these vessels. The terminal hepatic venules can be considered as being the center of a lobule or the periphery of several acini. The conceptual advantage of the acinus model is that the blood supply of a small portion of parenchyma and the bile duct draining that parenchyma reside in the same portal triad. Thus, "structural, circulatory, and functional unity is established in this small clump of parenchyma."[3] In contrast, the classic lobule is supplied by several separate portal vein branches, each of which also supplies adjacent lobules.

Portal vein blood is actually distributed by numerous small inlet venules, thereby giving a portal supply that is more diffuse and less granular than pictured by the original description of the acinus.[46] Therefore, acini appear to be subsumed as components of a hedge rather than as individual grapes on a vine.

A smaller conical subunit has been described, the hepatic microcirculatory subunit (HMS).[47] Each HMS is defined by its portal supply from a single inlet venule. Each venule usually is paired with a single ductule. The HMS is a structural unit that includes two functional compartments, the choleon and the hepaton, that reside in a common space. The choleon is composed of hepatocytes from which the bile produced drains into a canal of Hering. The hepaton is composed of the hepatocytes supplied by a single inlet venule. Although the notion of a choleohepaton is conceptually attractive, collateral blood flow between subunits may relegate functional unity to larger units that are the size of acini or primary lobules.

In normal human liver there are no sharp demarcations between adjacent subdivisions, so acini are difficult to visualize. However, acini become evident in pathologic conditions such as nodular regenerative hyperplasia, in which there is a pruning of the portal venous supply. As with a hedge, when individual portal units are pruned, the remaining units undergo hyperplasia to form an array of spherical units, revealing the underlying acinar structure.

Regardless of how one visualizes the vascular arrangements, hepatocytes close to the portal supply (acinar zone 1) are adapted to an environment that is rich in oxygen and nutrients. Cells more distant from the portal supply (acinar zones 2 and 3) have a different enzymatic phenotype and respond differently to hypoxia and toxin exposure.[3,29,48,49]

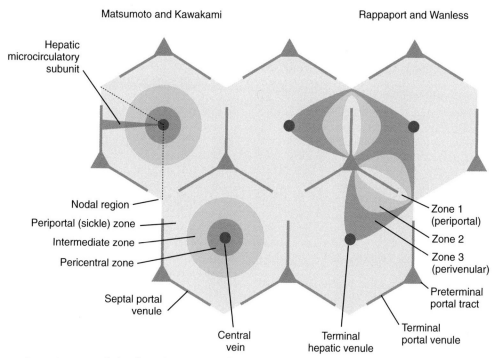

Figure 68–4   The acinar structure of the hepatic microcirculation, as conceived by Rappaport and Wanless[45] and modified by Matsumoto and Kawakami.[46] In both models, the margins of the shaded zones represent planes of equal blood pressure (isobars), oxygen content, or other characteristics. Periportal tissue (zone 1) receives blood that is higher in oxygen content than is the perivenular (zone 3) tissue. The models differ in the shape of the isobars surrounding terminal portal venules. The acinus is bulb shaped, and the classic lobule is composed of several wedge-shaped portions (called primary lobules, indicated by *dotted lines, upper left*), which have cylindrical (*sickle-shaped*) isobars. The hepatic microcirculatory subunit is the smallest functional unit in which there is the potential for countercurrent flow (shown as a *red wedge, left*).

HEPATIC MICROCIRCULATION

The terminal portal twigs supply sinusoids directly and give a constant but sluggish blood flow.[3] The arteries form a peribiliary plexus that surrounds and nourishes small bile ducts. The efferent flow from this plexus drains into terminal portal venules and proximal (zone 1) sinusoids. Some arterioles drain directly into zone 1 sinusoids. The artery gives a pulsatile but small-volume flow that appears to enhance sinusoidal flow, especially in periods of reactive arterial flow, such as the postprandial state. Arterial flow varies inversely with portal vein flow.[50] Local control of the microcirculation may depend on arteriolar sphincters and, at the sinusoidal level, on the state of contraction of endothelial cells and stellate cells.[30]

MICROCIRCULATION IN CHRONIC LIVER DISEASE

After hepatocellular necrosis, the sinusoidal stroma is normally repopulated with hepatocytes. If regeneration is delayed, usually because vessels are obstructed, the stroma becomes fibrotic and cannot support hepatocellular regeneration. The affected acini become extinct and are replaced by a focal scar. When numerous acini become extinct, the fibrotic and regenerative changes are recognized as cirrhosis.[19] In cirrhosis, small portal and hepatic veins are markedly reduced in number,[51] thereby leading to increased intrahepatic resistance and portal hypertension. The cirrhotic liver is predisposed to secondary thrombotic events, unrelated to the original etiology, that lead to the progression of tissue extinction and greater clinical morbidity.[52]

REFERENCES

1. MacSween RNM, Desmet VJ, Roskams T, Scothorne RJ: Developmental anatomy and normal structure. In MacSween RNM, Burt AD, Portmann BC, et al (eds): Pathology of the Liver, 4th ed. Edinburgh, Churchill Livingstone, 2002, p 1.
2. Ishak KG, Sharp HL: Developmental abnormalities and liver disease in childhood. In MacSween RNM, Burt AD, Portmann BC, et al (eds): Pathology of the Liver, 4th ed. Edinburgh, Churchill Livingstone, 2002, p 107.
3. Wanless IR: Physioanatomic considerations. In Schiff L, Schiff ER (eds): Schiff's Diseases of the Liver, 8th ed. Philadelphia, JB Lippincott, 1999, p 3.
4. Saxena R, Theise ND, Crawford JM: Microanatomy of the human liver: Exploring the hidden interfaces. Hepatology 30:1339, 1999.
5. Furbank RA: Conversion data, normal values, nomograms, and other standards. In Simpson K (ed): Modern Trends in Forensic Medicine. New York, Appleton-Century-Crofts, 1967, p 344.
6. Ludwig J: Current Methods of Autopsy Practice. Philadelphia, WB Saunders, 1972.
7. Bismuth H, Chiche L: Surgical anatomy and anatomical surgery of the liver. In Blumgart LH (eds): Surgery of the Liver and Biliary Tract, 2nd ed. Edinburgh, Churchill Livingstone, 1994, p 3.
8. Strasberg SM: Terminology of liver anatomy and liver resections: Coming to grips with hepatic Babel. J Am Coll Surg 184:413, 1997.
9. van Leeuwen MS, Noordzij J, Fernandez MA, et al: Portal venous and segmental anatomy of the right hemiliver: Observations based on three-dimensional spiral CT renderings. AJR Am J Roentgenol 163:1395, 1994.
10. Fasel JHD, Selle D, Everetsz CJG, et al: Segmental anatomy of the liver: Poor correlation with CT. Radiology 206:151, 1998.
11. Benz EJ, Baggenstoss AH, Wollaeger EE: Atrophy of the left lobe of the liver. Arch Pathol 53:315, 1952.
12. Qizilbash A, Kontozoglou T, Sianos J, Scully K: Hepar lobatum associated with chemotherapy and metastatic breast cancer. Arch Pathol Lab Med 111:58, 1987.
13. Couinaud C: The parabiliary venous system. Surg Radiol Anat 10:311, 1988.
14. Battaglia DM, Wanless IR, Brady AP, Mackenzie RL: Intrahepatic sequestered segment of liver presenting as focal fatty change. Am J Gastroenterol 90:238, 1995.
15. Madding GF, Kennedy PA: Trauma of the liver. In Calne RY (ed): Liver Surgery with Operative Color Illustrations. Philadelphia, WB Saunders, 1982, p 5.
16. Wanless IR, Lentz JS, Roberts EA: Partial nodular transformation of liver in an adult with persistent ductus venosus. Arch Pathol Lab Med 109:427, 1985.
17. Odievre M, Pige G, Alagille D: Congenital abnormalities associated with extrahepatic portal hypertension. Arch Dis Child 52:383, 1977.
18. Komatsu S, Nagino M, Hayakawa N, et al: Congenital absence of portal venous system associated with a large inferior mesenteric-caval shunt: A case report. Hepatogastroenterology 42:286, 1995.
19. Wanless IR: Vascular disorders. In MacSween RNM, Burt AD, Portmann BC, et al (eds): Pathology of the Liver, 4th ed. Edinburgh, Churchill Livingstone, 2002, p 539.
20. Itoh Y, Kawasaki T, Nishikawa H, et al: A case of extrahepatic portal vein aneurysm accompanying lupoid hepatitis. J Clin Ultrasound 23:374, 1995.
21. Tavill AS, Wood EJ, Creel L, et al: The Budd-Chiari syndrome: Correlation between hepatic scintigraphy and the clinical, radiological, and pathological findings in 19 cases of hepatic venous outflow obstruction. Gastroenterology 68:509, 1975.
22. Kage M, Arakawa M, Kojiro M, Okuda K: Histopathology of membranous obstruction of the inferior vena cava in the Budd-Chiari syndrome. Gastroenterology 102:2081, 1992.
23. Michels NA: Newer anatomy of liver: Variant blood supply and collateral circulation. JAMA 172:125, 1960.
24. Bengmark S, Rosengren K: Angiographic study of the collateral circulation to the liver after ligation of the hepatic artery in man. Am J Surg 119:620, 1970.
25. Brittain RS, Marchioro TL, Hermann G, et al: Accidental hepatic artery ligation in humans. Am J Surg 107:822, 1964.
26. Hesselink EJ, Slooff MJ, Schuur KH, et al: Consequences of hepatic artery pathology after orthotopic liver transplantation. Transplant Proc 19:2476, 1987.
27. Popper H, Elias H, Petty DE: Vascular pattern of the cirrhotic liver. Am J Clin Pathol 22:717, 1952.
28. Trutmann M, Sasse D: The lymphatics of the liver. Anat Embryol 190:201, 1994.
29. Sasse D, Spornitz UM, Maly IP: Liver architecture. Enzyme 46:8, 1992.
30. McCuskey RS, Reilly FD: Hepatic microvasculature: Dynamic structure and its regulation. Semin Liver Dis 13:1, 1993.
31. Kjaer M, Jurlander J, Keiding S, et al: No reinnervation of hepatic sympathetic nerves after liver transplantation in human subjects. J Hepatol 20:97, 1994.
32. Lindfeldt J, Balkan B, Vandijk G, et al: Influence of periarterial hepatic denervation on the glycemic response to exercise in rats. J Autonom Nerv Syst 44:45, 1993.
33. Smadja C, Blumgart LH: The biliary tract and the anatomy of biliary exposure. In Blumgart LH (ed): Surgery of the Liver and Biliary Tract. Edinburgh, Churchill Livingstone, 1988, p 11.

34. Nakanuma Y, Hoso M, Sanzen T, Sasaki M: Microstructure and development of the normal and pathologic biliary tract in humans, including blood supply. Microsc Res Tech 38:552, 1997.

35. Roskams TA, Theise ND, Balabaud C, et al: Nomenclature of the finer branches of the biliary tree: Canals, ductules, and ductular reactions in human livers. Hepatology 39:1739, 2004.

36. Theise ND, Saxena R, Portmann BC, et al: The canals of Hering and hepatic stem cells in humans. Hepatology 30:1425, 1999.

37. Theise ND, Nimmakayalu M, Gardner R, et al: Liver from bone marrow in humans. Hepatology 32:11, 2000.

38. Roskams T, Libbrecht T, Desmet V: Progenitor cells in diseased human liver. Semin Liver Dis 23:385, 2003.

39. Terada T, Nakanuma Y, Kakita A: Pathologic observations of intrahepatic peribiliary glands in 1000 consecutive autopsy livers: Heterotopic pancreas in the liver. Gastroenterology 98:1333, 1990.

40. Prinz RA, Howell HS, Pickleman JR: Surgical significance of extrahepatic biliary tree anomalies. Am J Surg 131:755, 1976.

41. Braghetto I, Bastias J, Csendes A, Debandi A: Intraperitoneal bile collections after laparoscopic cholecystectomy: Causes, clinical presentation, diagnosis, and treatment. Surg Endosc 14:1037, 2000.

42. Terada T, Nakanuma Y: Congenital biliary dilatation in autosomal dominant adult polycystic disease of the liver and kidneys. Arch Pathol Lab Med 112:1113, 1988.

43. Wanless IR, Zahradnik J, Heathcote EJ: Hepatic cysts of periductal gland origin presenting as obstructive jaundice. Gastroenterology 93:894, 1987.

44. Phillips MJ, Poucell S, Patterson J, Valencia P: The Liver: An Atlas and Text of Ultrastructural Pathology. New York, Raven Press, 1987.

45. Rappaport AM, Wanless IR: Physioanatomic considerations. In Schiff L, Schiff ER (eds): Diseases of the Liver, 7th ed. Philadelphia, JB Lippincott, 1993, p 1.

46. Matsumoto T, Kawakami M: The unit-concept of hepatic parenchyma: A reexamination based on angioarchitectural studies. Acta Pathol Jpn 32(Suppl 2):285, 1982.

47. Ekataksin W, Wake K: New concepts in biliary and vascular anatomy of the liver. In Boyer J, Ockner RK (eds): Progress in Liver Diseases. Philadelphia, WB Saunders, 1997, p 1.

48. Lamers WH, Hilberts A, Furt E, et al: Hepatic enzymic zonation: A reevaluation of the concept of the liver acinus. Hepatology 10:72, 1989.

49. Jungermann K, Kietzmann T: Oxygen: Modulator of metabolic zonation and disease of the liver. Hepatology 31:255, 2000.

50. Lautt WW: Relationship between hepatic blood flow and overall metabolism: The hepatic arterial buffer response. Fed Proc 42:1662, 1983.

51. Popper H: Pathologic aspects of cirrhosis. Am J Pathol 87:228, 1977.

52. Wanless IR, Wong F, Blendis LM, et al: Hepatic and portal vein thrombosis in cirrhosis: Possible role in development of parenchymal extinction and portal hypertension. Hepatology 21:1238, 1995.

CHAPTER

69 Liver Physiology and Energy Metabolism

Namita Roy-Chowdhury and Jayanta Roy-Chowdhury

LIVER CELL TYPES AND ORGANIZATION

Liver cells can be classified into the following three groups: (1) parenchymal cells, which comprise hepatocytes and bile duct epithelia, (2) sinusoidal cells, which comprise hepatic sinusoidal endothelial and Kupffer cells (hepatic macrophages), and (3) perisinusoidal cells, which consist of hepatic stellate cells and pit cells. Hepatocytes account for 60% of the adult liver cell population and represent ≈78% of the tissue volume (see Chapter 68).[1]

PARENCHYMAL CELLS

Hepatocytes

Hepatocytes are large polyhedral cells approximately 20 to 30 μm in diameter.[2] Consistent with their high synthetic and metabolic activity, hepatocytes are enriched in organelles. About 30% of human hepatocytes are binucleate. Hepatocytes are polarized epithelial cells. Their plasma membranes have three distinct domains—(1) the sinusoidal surface (≈37% of the cell surface) that comes in direct contact with plasma through the fenestrae of the specialized hepatic sinusoidal endothelial cells, (2) the canalicular surface (≈13% of the cell surface) that encloses the bile canaliculus, and (3) contiguous surfaces. By analogy with glandular epithelia, the sinusoidal, canalicular, and contiguous plasma membrane domains are also called the basolateral, apical, and lateral surfaces, respec-

tively.[3] The sinusoidal and canalicular surfaces contain microvilli, which greatly extend the surface area of these domains.

The space between the endothelia and the sinusoidal villi is termed the space of Disse. There is a bidirectional exchange of liquids and solutes between the plasma and hepatocytes at the sinusoidal surface. In many cases, the molecular transfer is augmented by proteins that promote facilitated diffusion or energy-consuming active transport. The canalicular domains of two adjacent hepatocytes are sealed at the periphery by tight junctions (desmosomes), thereby delimiting the bile canaliculus, which is the beginning of the biliary drainage system (see Chapter 59). In contrast to the bidirectional flow at the sinusoidal surface, flow from hepatocytes into the bile canaliculi is predominantly unidirectional.

Plasma Membranes

The plasma membranes of hepatocytes consist of lipid bilayers composed of glycerophospholipids, cholesterol, and sphingolipids and provide a barrier to water and most polar substances.[3,4] The inner and outer leaflets of the plasma membrane differ in lipid, protein, and carbohydrate composition, reflecting functional differences. Protein molecules within the leaflets mediate transport of specific molecules and serve as a link with cytoskeletal structures and the extracellular matrix. Hepatocyte plasma membranes are 36% lipid, 54% protein, and 10% carbohydrate by dry weight. The outer leaflets of hepatocyte plasma membranes are enriched in carbohydrates.

Lipid rafts are microdomains (≈50 nm diameter) of the outer leaflets of the plasma membrane that are highly enriched in cholesterol and sphingolipids.[5] These lipid rafts are coupled to cholesterol-rich microdomains in the inner leaflet by an unknown mechanism. Raft lipids and associated proteins diffuse together laterally on the membrane surface. Some surface receptors become associated with the rafts on binding to a ligand or can lead to "clustering" of smaller rafts into larger ones. Lipid rafts are important in signal transduction, apoptosis, cell adhesion and migration, cytoskeletal organization, and protein sorting during both exocytosis and endocytosis (see later). Certain viruses enter cells via the lipid rafts.

Membrane proteins perform receptor, enzyme, and transport functions.[6] Integral membrane proteins traverse the lipid bilayer once or multiple times or are buried in the lipid. Additional "extrinsic" protein molecules are associated with plasma membrane. Membrane proteins can rotate or diffuse laterally but usually do not "flip-flop" from one leaflet to another. The concentration of specific membrane proteins is maintained by a balance between their synthesis and degradation through shedding of membrane vesicles, proteolytic digestion within the membrane, or internalization into the cell. Receptor proteins internalized into the cell may be degraded or recycled to the cell surface.

Cell Junctions. Hepatocytes are organized into sheets (seen as chords in two-dimensional sections) by occluding (tight), communicating (gap), and anchoring junctions (Fig. 69–1). Tight junctions, or desmosomes, form gasket-like seals around the bile canaliculi, thereby permitting a concentration difference of solutes between the cytoplasm and bile canaliculus. Tight junctions are specialized membrane structures that anchor intermediate filaments to the plasma membrane and link cells together. Gap junctions are subdomains of contiguous membranes of hepatocytes that constitute ≈3% of the total surface membrane. They consist of hexagonal particles with hollow cores, termed connexons, each of which is made up of six connexin molecules.[7] Connexons of one cell are joined to those of an adjacent cell to form a radially symmetrical cylinder that can open or close the central channel. Gap junctions are involved in nutrient exchange, synchronization of cellular activities, and conduction of electrical impulses.

The Cytoskeleton

The hepatocyte cytoskeleton supports the organization of subcellular organelles, cell polarity, intracellular movement of vesicles, and molecular transport.[8,9] It consists of microfilaments, microtubules, and intermediate filaments as well as the cytoskeleton-associated proteins.[10] Intermediate filaments are polymers of fibrous polypeptides (cytokeratins and lamins) that provide structural support to the cells. In addition, vimentin is expressed by hepatocytes in tissue culture, and neurofilaments appear in injured hepatocytes and form Mallory bodies. Hepatocytes express two cytokeratins, CK8 and CK18. Bile duct epithelial cells express these proteins and CK19. Plectin is a giant protein that cross-links intermediate filaments to each other and to the plasma membrane, microtubules, and actin filaments.

Microtubules are hollow tubular structures (with a 24-nm outer diameter), consisting of polymerized dimers of α and β tubulin, that are involved in intracellular transport and cellular organization.[11,12] Microtubules serve as tracks for the movement of cytoplasmic vesicles, mediated by adenosine triphosphatase (ATPase)–powered motor proteins, kinesin, dynein, and dynamin. Depolymerization of the microtubules, for example by treatment with colchicine, inhibits plasma protein secretion without affecting protein synthesis. Microtubules participate in cellular organization by interacting with the Golgi apparatus, intermediate filaments, and F-actin.[13] They also maintain the integrity of the surface membrane during canalicular contraction.[14]

Microfilaments are composed of double-helical F-actin strands, which are polymers of G-actin. A large number of actin-associated proteins control the polymerization, depolymerization, and splicing of F-actin. Together with myosins, actins maintain the integrity of the cell matrix, facilitate bile canalicular contraction, and control tight junction permeability. Microfilaments are also important in receptor-mediated endocytosis and various transport processes. Collapse of the cellular structure of hepatocytes during apoptosis and formation of apoptotic bodies may be related to remodeling of the actin cytoskeleton of hepatocytes.[15]

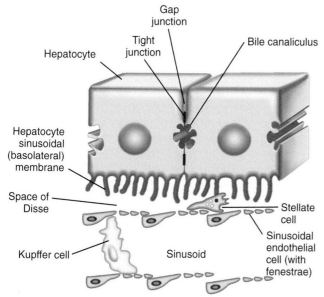

Figure 69–1   The spatial relationship among the different cell types of the liver. Sinusoidal plasma comes in direct contact with hepatocytes in the space of Disse. The endothelial cells are fenestrated and lack a basement membrane. Kupffer cells are located in the lumen of the sinusoid, where they are in direct contact with the sinusoidal endothelial cells and portal blood. Stellate cells are situated between the endothelial cells and hepatocytes and come in direct contact with both cell types. The hepatocytes are joined with each other by tight junctions and the gap junctions. The canalicular domain of the plasma membrane of two adjacent hepatocytes encloses the bile canaliculus.

The Nucleus

Nuclei of hepatocytes are relatively large and have prominent nucleoli. The two concentric nuclear membranes are stabilized by networks of intermediate filaments, one inside the inner membrane and one outside the outer membrane.[16] The outer nuclear membrane is in direct continuity with the endoplasmic reticulum (ER) membranes. The perinuclear space between the two nuclear membranes surrounds the nucleus and is continuous with the ER lumen. The nuclear membrane contains pores, through which molecules are selectively transported to and from the cytoplasm. The ribonuclear protein (RNP) network and the perinucleolar chromatin radiate from the nucleolus.

The nuclear chromatin contains the chromosomes and associated proteins. The chromosomes comprise a series of genes, interspersed with intragenic DNA. The DNA is transcribed into RNA, which undergoes multiple processing steps, giving rise to messenger RNA (mRNA) molecules that are translocated across the nuclear pores into the cytoplasm, where they become associated with ribosomes. Nuclear DNA also encodes additional RNA types that have accessory roles in protein synthesis and other functions. Ribosomal RNAs (rRNAs) are encoded by DNA within the nucleolus. Transfer RNA (tRNA) binds to amino acids and provides a necessary link between the nucleic acid code and sequential amino acid incorporation in the growing protein chain during translation. Other RNAs are involved in the processing of mRNA, rRNA, and tRNA molecules. Just before cell division, both the DNA and protein components of chromatin are duplicated. The two copies of each duplicated chromosome are separated and precisely distributed so that each of the two daughter cells receives a complete set of genes.

Transport Between the Nucleus and the Cytoplasm. Pores of the nuclear envelope are associated with a large number of proteins that are organized in an octagonal symmetry.[17] The nuclear pore complex (NPC) is a large macromolecular assembly that protrudes into both the cytoplasm and the nucleoplasm. Bidirectional nucleocytoplasmic transport occurs through the central aqueous channel in NPCs.[18] Histones, DNA- and RNA-polymerases, transcription factors, and RNA-processing proteins are transported selectively into the nucleus from the cytoplasm where they are synthesized, whereas tRNAs and mRNAs are synthesized in the nucleus and exported to the cytoplasm through the NPCs.

Often, the export and import processes are interrelated. For example, ribosomal proteins are imported into the nucleus from the cytoplasm and, after assembly with ribosomal RNA, are exported to the cytoplasm as a ribosomal subunit. Proteins that contain nuclear localization motifs consisting of specific cationic amino acid sequences are recognized by pore complex receptors, termed importins or karyopherins, and are transported rapidly into the nucleus via an energy-consuming process powered by specific ATPase and guanosine triphosphatase (GTPase) enzymes. In other cases, large molecules diffuse slowly through the nuclear pores and are retained in the nucleus by binding to specific intranuclear sites. Molecules that are smaller than 5 kd diffuse freely across the nuclear pores.

The Endoplasmic Reticulum

The ER, the largest intracellular membrane compartment, comprises membranous tubules or flattened sacs (cisternae) that enclose a continuous lumen or space and extend throughout the cytoplasm.[19] The domain of ER where active protein synthesis occurs has attached ribosomes and is termed the rough ER. The other domain, termed smooth ER, is devoid of ribosomes and is the site of lipid biosynthesis, detoxification, and calcium regulation. The nuclear envelope is a specialized domain of the ER.[20]

The Golgi Complex

The Golgi complex consists of a stack of cisternae that are dilated at the margins.[21] Many proteins synthesized in the rough ER are transported to the Golgi apparatus in protein-filled transition vesicles. The aspect of the Golgi complex facing the ER is the *cis* face; the opposite side is the *trans* face. Glycoproteins are thought to be transported between the Golgi sacs via shuttle vesicles. The highly mannosylated glycosyl moiety of proteins that are N-glycosylated in the ER are processed in the Golgi sacs into mature forms. Some other proteins are O-glycosylated in the Golgi complex. These proteins are then sorted for transport to appropriate cellular organelles (see later discussion of exocytosis and endocytosis).[22]

Lysosomes

Lysosomes consist of a system of membrane-bound sacs and tubules containing hydrolytic enzymes that are active at pH 4.5 to 5.[23,24] The ATPase-powered proton pump maintains the acid pH by importing hydrogen ions into the lysosomal lumen.[23] Lysosomal enzymes are glycoproteins with N-linked oligosaccharides. After synthesis in the ER, the carbohydrate moieties are modified in the Golgi apparatus, where their mannose residues are phosphorylated. Recognition of these mannose-6-phosphate (M6P) groups by the M6P receptor in *trans*-Golgi stacks[25] results in their segregation and translocation into late endosomes, which transform into lysosomes.[26,27]

Mitochondria

Mitochondria constitute about 20% of the cytoplasmic volume of hepatocytes and are responsible for cellular respiration.[28-30] They contain the enzymes of the tricarboxylic acid cycle, fatty acid oxidation, and oxidative phosphorylation.[30,31] Mitochondria conserve the energy generated by oxidation of substrates as high-energy phosphate bonds of ATP. In addition, parts of the urea cycle, gluconeogenesis, fatty acid synthesis, regulation of intracellular calcium concentration, and heme synthesis take place in the mitochondria. Mitochondria play a key role in programmed cell death, or apoptosis (see later).[32]

The outer smooth surface membrane of the mitochondrion is functionally different from the inner membrane, which is highly folded to form cristae. Mitochondria are positioned at major sites of ATP utilization by translocation along microtubules. In addition to soluble enzymes, the mitochondrial matrix includes large intramitochondrial granules that store calcium and other ions and smaller granules that contain mitochondrial ribosomes. Mitochondrial DNA, embedded within the matrix, encodes a number of mitochondrial proteins. The remaining mitochondrial proteins are encoded by nuclear genes.

Glycolysis and fatty acid oxidation in the mitochondria generate chemical intermediates that feed into the citric acid cycle of energy-yielding reactions.[33,34] The citric acid cycle breaks down acetyl coenzyme A (acetyl CoA) into three molecules of reduced nicotinamide adenine dinucleotide (NADH), one molecule of reduced flavin adenine dinucleotide ($FADH_2$), and two molecules of carbon dioxide. Electrons derived from NADH and $FADH_2$ drive an electron transport pathway in the inner mitochondrial membrane, leading to ATP production. Passage of electrons across the inner mitochondrial membrane to the space between the inner and outer membranes generates a proton gradient that drives ATP synthesis.[35]

Peroxisomes

Peroxisomes are spherical-looking structures that enclose a matrix containing a lattice or crystalline core.[36] Peroxisomes are abundant in hepatocytes and are thought to be essential for life. Several oxidative catabolic reactions, as well as anabolic reactions, take place in peroxisomes, which provide important links in the metabolism of carbohydrates, lipids, proteins, fats, and nucleic acids.

Exocytosis and Endocytosis

Exocytosis and endocytosis are pathways involved in exporting, importing, and intracellular trafficking of molecules. The addition of new proteins and lipids to the plasma membrane by exocytosis and removal of membrane components into cytoplasmic compartments by endocytosis keep the cell surface in a state of dynamic polarization. During exocytosis, secreted proteins that are synthesized in the ER pass sequentially through the *cis-*, *medial-*, and *trans-*Golgi stacks and the *trans-*Golgi network (TGN) and finally appear at the cell surface.[37,38] This vectorial transport through the Golgi stacks occurs via vesicles that are coated by proteins termed coatamers or COPs (COPI and COPII), which are distinct from clathrin (see later).[39,40] Guanosine triphosphate–guanosine diphosphate (GTP-GDP) exchange factors and GTP-activating proteins that are specific for each vesicle type stimulate membrane binding and catalytic activation of small GTPases.

Once bound to the membrane, GTPases induce recruitment of COP proteins. In the ER, the first coat protein to be recruited is COPII, and vesicular/tubular clusters are formed. These clusters are thought to coalesce, forming a complex tubular network termed the ER/Golgi intermediate compartment. Acquisition of COPI proteins by the membranes of this tubular network results in the formation of vesicles that carry out bidirectional protein transport to and from the Golgi stacks. Some vesicles emerging from the exit side of the Golgi apparatus, or the TGN, can transport multiple protein molecules simultaneously and release them together into the extracellular medium. However, other types of vesicles that carry membrane proteins and enzymes destined for specific intracellular organelles also pass through this secretory pathway. These vesicles are sorted at the TGN, and vesicles carrying specific cargo are delivered to appropriate target organelles.[41]

Endocytosis is the import of extracellular macromolecules by processes that include pinocytosis, phagocytosis, receptor-mediated endocytosis (RME), and caveolar internalization.[42] Pinocytosis is the nonselective bulk-phase uptake of extracellular fluid via engulfment by plasma membrane invaginations. Phagocytosis is the ingestion of particles as well as regions of the cell surface. In contrast to these nonspecific modes of uptake, RME is a mechanism of uptake of specific molecules (ligands). After the ligands bind to their specific cell surface receptors, the ligand-receptor complexes concentrate in "pits" that are coated on the cytoplasmic surface by three-pronged structures (triskelions) composed of three heavy chains and three light chains of clathrin. The assembled coats consist of a geometric array of 12 pentagons and a variable number of hexagons, depending on the size of the coat. The coated pits pinch off into the underlying cytoplasm as coated vesicles.[43]

In the next step, the vesicles lose their clathrin coat, at which point they are called endosomes. Endosomal vesicles travel along microtubules and can take three distinct pathways. Some endosomes return to the cell surface, and the contained ligand-receptor complexes are secreted out of the cells by a process called diacytosis. Transferrin is a prototype ligand for diacytosis. Some other ligands, such as immunoglobulin A (IgA) oligomers, may traverse the cells to be secreted into bile along with the receptor; this process is called transcytosis.[44]

The best-studied type of RME is the classic endocytotic pathway, in which the interior of the endosome is acidified by the action of a proton pump, thereby leading to ligand-receptor uncoupling.[45] By mechanisms that have not been elucidated fully, the dissociated ligands and receptors are sorted into different vesicles. The ligand-containing vesicles proceed to lysosomes, where the ligand is degraded by lysosomal hydrolases. A majority of the ligand-free receptors translocate to the cell surface and replenish the receptor pool. Some receptors, such as the insulin receptor, do not undergo recycling and are degraded rapidly in lysosomes. In addition to the recruitment of clathrin, initiation of the formation of endocytotic vesicles requires adaptor proteins, particularly AP-2, which localizes between the lipid bilayer and clathrin. Non-scaffold proteins, such as the GTPases and dynamin, are also important in the conversion of a coated pit to a coated vesicle. This function of dynamin requires association with a protein called amphiphysin. Genetic, cell biologic, and biochemical studies are identifying additional proteins that are required for clathrin coat and vesicle formation (reviewed by Stockert[45]). In addition to physiologic ligands, many viruses utilize receptor-mediated endocytosis for entering a cell.

Internalization via caveolae is another pathway by which macromolecules can enter cells. Binding of caveolin to the cytoplasmic aspect of cholesterol-rich lipid rafts on the plasma membrane generates 50- to 60-nm, flask-shaped invaginations of the plasma membrane. These invaginations bud off into the cytoplasm to form vesicles called caveolae or plasmalemmal vesicles. Caveolae provide various functions, including signal transduction, calcium regulation, non–clathrin-dependent internalization, and transcytosis. Glucosyl phosphatidylinositol (GPI)–anchored proteins, the β-adrenergic receptor, and tyrosine kinase are concentrated in caveolae.[46]

Bile Duct Epithelial Cells

Bile duct epithelial cells (BECs), or cholangiocytes, comprise large and small subpopulations of cells, the cell volumes of which correlate roughly with the diameter of the intrahepatic bile ducts (see Chapter 59). The large cholangiocytes have a relatively more developed ER and a lower nucleus-to-cytoplasm ratio than do the small cholangiocytes.[47] The paucity of expression of cytochrome P450–dependent monooxygenase activity imparts a survival advantage to the small cholangiocytes against injury by chemicals. For example, cytochrome P4502E1–mediated formation of toxic intermediates of carbon tetrachloride leads to the loss of large cholangiocyte function after administration of this protoxin, whereas the small cholangiocytes are resistant to the toxic injury.

Bile ducts are not mere passive conduits for biliary drainage; they play an active role in the secretion and absorption of biliary components and regulation of the extracellular matrix composition. Cholangiocytes are highly polarized. A sodium-dependent bile salt transporter (ABAT), located at the apical (luminal) surface of cholangiocytes, mediates the uptake of conjugated bile acids by cholangiocytes, whereas an alternatively spliced truncated form of the protein (ASBT), located at the basolateral surface, mediates the efflux of the bile acids in a sodium-independent manner. The sodium-dependent glucose transporter (SGLT1), located at the apical domain, and GLUT1, a facilitative glucose transporter on the basolateral domain, are responsible for glucose reabsorption from bile. Aquaporin-1 at the apical and basolateral surfaces constitutes water channels that may mediate hormone-regulated transport of water into bile by cholangiocytes. The purinergic receptor (P_{2u}) stimulates chloride ion efflux. Activation of apical P_{2u} by ATP, which is secreted into the bile by hepatocytes, mobilizes Ca^{2+} stores, thereby stimulating Cl^- efflux from cholangiocytes. The large, but not the small, cholangiocytes express secretin and somatostatin receptors, chloride/bicarbonate exchanger, and cystic fibrosis transmembrane regulator, which may enable this population of cholangiocytes to modulate water and electrolyte secretion in response to secretin and somatostatin (see also Chapter 61).[48]

SINUSOIDAL NONPARENCHYMAL CELLS

Hepatic Sinusoidal Endothelial Cells

Hepatic sinusoidal endothelial cells (HSECs) account for 20% of total liver cells. These cells are distinguished by the fenestrae (pores) in their flat, thin extensions that form sieve plates. Unlike capillary endothelial cells, HSECs do not form intracellular junctions and simply overlap one another (see Fig. 69–1). The presence of fenestrae and the absence of a basement membrane permit plasma to enter the space of Disse and come in direct contact with the sinusoidal surfaces of hepatocytes (see Chapter 68).[49] Diameters of the fenestrae are controlled actively by the actin-containing components of the cytoskeleton in response to changes in the chemical milieu.[50] Therefore, the specialized endothelial lining of hepatic sinusoids serves as a selective barrier between the blood and the hepatocytes. HSECs can secrete prostaglandins and a wide variety of proteins, including

interleukin-1 (IL-1) and IL-6, interferon, tumor necrosis factor-α (TNF-α), and endothelin.

Kupffer Cells

Kupffer cells are specialized tissue macrophages that account for 80% to 90% of the total population of fixed macrophages in the body. These cells are derived from bone marrow stem cells or monocytes and are highly active in removing particulate matters and toxic or foreign substances that appear in the portal blood from the intestines.[51] Kupffer cells are located in the sinusoidal lumen and are in direct contact with endothelial cells (see Fig. 69–1). They possess bristle-coated micropinocytic vesicles, fuzzy-coated vacuoles, and worm-like structures that are special features of cells active in pinocytosis and phagocytosis. An abundance of lysosomes reflects the prominent role of Kupffer cells in degrading substances taken up from the blood stream. Kupffer cells secrete a variety of vasoactive toxic mediators that may be involved in host defense mechanisms and in pathophysiologic processes in some liver diseases. Kupffer cells increase in number and activity in response to chemical, infectious, or immunologic injury to the liver.[52]

PERISINUSOIDAL NONPARENCHYMAL CELLS

Hepatic Stellate Cells

Hepatic stellate cells (HSCs)—also known as Ito cells, vitamin A–storing cells, fat-storing cells, and lipocytes—are a part of the stellate cell system, which includes similar cells in the pancreas, lung, kidney, and intestine. HSCs are located between the endothelial lining and hepatocytes (see Fig. 69–1). These mesenchymal cells, which represent 5% to 8% of all liver cells, are important sources of paracrine, autocrine, juxtacrine, and chemoattractant factors that maintain homeostasis in the microenvironment of the hepatic sinusoid. The flat cytoplasmic extensions of quiescent HSCs spread out parallel to the endothelial lining and contact several cells.[53] Their cytoplasmic extensions are enriched in microfilaments and microtubules, and contain characteristic vitamin A–rich lipid droplets. HSCs express receptors for retinol-binding protein (RBP), which mediates the endocytosis of RBP-retinol complexes.[54]

After chronic liver injury, HSCs become activated, as evidenced by the loss of retinoids and up-regulation of the synthesis of extracellular matrix components such as collagen, proteoglycan, and adhesive glycoproteins. HSC activation is the central event in hepatic fibrosis.[55] The activated HSCs metamorphose from the slender star-shaped structure of the quiescent cells to elongated myofibroblasts. Activation of HSCs is initiated by paracrine stimulation by neighboring HSECs, Kupffer cells, and hepatocytes as well as platelets and leukocytes. Endothelial cells participate in activation by producing cellular fibronectin and by converting the latent form of transforming growth factor-β (TGF-β) to its active, profibrogenic form. The three-dimensional structure of the extracellular matrix modulates the shape, proliferation, and function of HSCs, probably by signal transduction via binding to cell surface integrins followed by changes in cytoskeleton assembly.

Activation of HSCs is perpetuated by the continued effect of these stimuli, leading to several discrete changes in cell behavior, such as proliferation, contractility, overexpression of extracellular matrix proteins (e.g., collagens I, III, IV, V, and VI, laminin, tenascin, undulin, hyaluronic acid, and proteoglycans), matrix degradation by release of metalloproteinases, and release of leukocyte chemoattractants and cytokines. The overall number of HSCs rises during fibrosis, because of a change in the balance between proliferation and apoptosis, which is influenced by soluble growth factors and the matrix.

Pit Cells

Pit cells, natural killer (NK) cells of the liver, are located mainly within the sinusoidal lumen, close to Kupffer cells. They have the appearance of large lymphocytes and are adherent to the sinusoidal wall, often anchored with villous extensions (pseudopods).[56] In the human liver, pit cells have pronounced polarity, abundant cytoplasm that contains dense granules, a conspicuous cytocenter (the site in the cells where microtubules converge), and a locomotory shape characterized by hyaloplasmic pseudopods and a uropod (a tail-like structure that forms on the trailing end of a moving cell). The cytoplasmic granules look like pits on microscopy; hence the name pit cells. Pit cells are short-lived and are replenished from extrahepatic sources.

In common with circulating NK cells, the pit cells express OX-8 antigen, and some express asialo-GMr1. However, pit cells do not express the pan-T-cell marker, OX-19, which is expressed by circulating NK cells. Although the source of pit cells continues to be debated, they are antigenically related to NK cells of other viscera. Pit cells have tumor cell–killing activity in the liver and are also thought to remove virus-infected liver cells. Their per-cell cytolytic activity is greater than that of circulating NK cells. Pit cells may also have a role in controlling the growth and differentiation of liver cells and possibly in liver graft rejection.[57]

INTEGRATION OF THE FUNCTIONS OF THE DIFFERENT CELL TYPES

Functional integration of the various groups of liver cells occurs through direct cell-to-cell communication (e.g., via gap junctions), paracrine secretion that affects neighboring cells, cell signaling, interaction with the extracellular matrix, and a generalized response to endocrine and metabolic fluxes.[58] Hepatocytes and HSECs lack a continuous basement membrane, and the spatial relationship of the cells is maintained through interaction with the extracellular matrix. Anchoring to the extracellular matrix is important for the survival of hepatocytes. Anchoring also provides traction for movement and permits liver cells to receive signals from matrix components and matrix-bound growth factors. Hepatic extracellular matrix components are produced during development along the migration path of the hepatocytes and exhibit unique patterns of distribution and organization. HSCs, hepatocytes, and, to some extent,

HSECs are major producers of the extracellular matrix in the liver. Excess deposition of connective tissue causes changes in hemodynamic properties and eventually impairs liver function.[55]

CELL-MATRIX INTERACTIONS

Cell-matrix interactions in the liver are important for maintaining hepatocyte morphology and proliferation. For example, when plated on a flat layer of collagen, hepatocytes synthesize DNA at a level that is four times higher than when they are grown on gels composed of basement membrane proteins. The type of matrix determines the level of expression of albumin and other hepatocyte-specific gene products in cultured hepatocytes.[58,59] On the other hand, cell-cell and cell-matrix interactions determine the level of synthesis and deposition of hepatic extracellular matrix proteins by the various types of liver cells. Such interactions also modulate the production of specific enzymes, and their inhibitors, that mediate remodeling of the extracellular matrix.

Integrin and non-integrin receptors mediate the interaction of liver cells with extracellular matrix. Integrins bind to extracellular matrix proteins at specialized cell attachment sites that often contain the arginine-glycine-aspartate (Arg-Gly-Asp) motif, thereby resulting in attachment of the extracellular matrix to the intracellular cytoskeleton network. This attachment results in changes in cell shape, spreading, and migration. Integrins also influence cell proliferation, differentiation, survival, apoptosis, and gene expression via signal transduction.[60,61] Non-integrin surface receptors mediate cell attachment by different mechanisms.

COMPONENTS OF THE EXTRACELLULAR MATRIX

Components of the extracellular matrix include collagens, noncollagenous glycoproteins, and proteoglycans. The liver contains five types of collagen (I, III, IV, V, and VI) and seven classes of noncollagenous glycoproteins (fibronectin, laminin, entactin/nidogen, tenascin, thrombospondin, SPARC [secreted protein, acidic, and rich in cysteine], and undulin). Hepatic extracellular matrix also contains a large number of proteoglycans and glycosaminoglycans, such as membrane-associated syndecan, thrombomodulin, and betaglycan, and extracellular matrix-associated versican, biglycan, decorin, fibromodulin, and perlecan.[58,62]

REGENERATION AND APOPTOSIS OF LIVER CELLS

LIVER REGENERATION

Normal adult hepatocytes divide infrequently, with fewer than 1 in 10,000 hepatocytes undergoing mitosis at any given time. Yet the liver possesses a unique capacity to replace tissue mass after injury or loss of liver mass. The capacity of the liver to regulate its own growth is evident in liver transplantation, after which the size of the transplanted organ increases or decreases as appropriate to the size of the recipient. Such finely regulated hyperplasia of the liver is also seen after successful single-lobe liver transplantation in children.[63]

Hepatic regeneration has been studied extensively in rodents. After resection of two thirds of the liver in rats, the residual liver cells proliferate and restore the liver mass within days to weeks. Although generally termed "regeneration," this process is in fact restorative hyperplasia, because the total liver mass, rather than the lobulated anatomic configuration, is reconstituted. In the rat, DNA synthesis peaks at 24 hours after partial hepatectomy, when approximately 35% of hepatocytes are in cell cycle. Cell division occurs 6 to 8 hours after DNA synthesis. The time frame of DNA synthesis varies from species to species. For example, in mice, maximum DNA synthesis occurs 36 to 40 hours after hepatic resection. Because 80% to 95% of hepatocytes undergo mitosis, liver mass is restored after one or two cell divisions. All classes of hepatocytes, including diploid, tetraploid, and octaploid cells, participate in this quasi-synchronized proliferation, either by mitosis of mononucleated cells or by cytokinesis of binucleated or tetranucleated hepatocytes, after DNA synthesis in all nuclei. Interestingly, adult hepatocytes, rather than liver progenitor cells, contribute to liver regeneration after partial hepatectomy. Only when the proliferation of adult hepatocytes is inhibited because of certain toxic or physical injuries do progenitor cells, often called oval cells, proliferate. The oval cells are thought to give rise to both hepatocytes and bile duct epithelial cells.[64]

After liver injury, early signals for hepatocyte replication come from nonparenchymal cells (Fig. 69–2B).[65,66] Lipopolysaccharides (LPSs) and gut-derived cytokines stimulate Kupffer cells and hepatic sinusoidal endothelial cells to produce TNF-α and IL-6. Growth factors, such as hepatic growth factor (HGF), are released from stores in hepatic matrix and are secreted by HSCs, whereas epidermal growth factor is secreted by epithelial cells of the proximal small intestine into portal blood and by salivary glands.[65] Hormones and neurotransmitters, such as triiodothyronine (T_3), insulin, and norepinephrine, are important cooperative factors in liver regeneration.[67] Replication of nonparenchymal cells lags behind that of hepatocytes by 24 to 72 hours. Initially, the newly proliferated hepatocytes form clusters, first in zone 1 and later in other zones of the liver (see Chapter 68). Regenerating endothelial cells invade these clusters and restore the single-cell-thick liver plates.

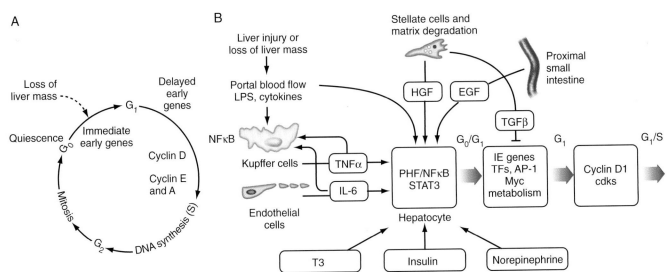

Figure 69–2 *A,* The cell cycle of hepatocytes in response to liver injury or loss of liver mass. Quiescent hepatocytes (G_0) rapidly enter G_1 after loss of liver mass (e.g., partial hepatectomy), along with expression of immediate early genes. This phase is followed sequentially by the expression of delayed early genes and cyclins. DNA synthesis (S phase) reaches a peak in 24 hours in rats and 36–40 hours in mice. Shortly after this, the cell enters G_2 and undergoes mitosis (M). *B,* The sequence of signals that leads to liver regeneration after partial hepatectomy. Gut-derived lipopolysaccharides (LPS) and cytokines activate Kupffer cells and endothelial cells, which release tumor necrosis factor-α (TNFα) and interleukin-6 (IL-6). These signals lead to the activation of nuclear activating factor kappa B (NFκB), also known as posthepatectomy factor (PHF), and STAT3 (signal transducer and activator of transcription-3), without the need for new protein synthesis. Hepatic growth factor (HGF) is released by hepatic stellate cells and also may be derived from storage sites following matrix degradation. Epidermal growth factor (EGF), secreted by the proximal small intestinal and salivary gland epithelial cells, and insulin, triiodothyronine (T3), and norepinephrine serve as cooperative factors for transition of hepatocytes through G_1 to the S phase. Immediate early (IE) genes and transcription factors (TFs) are expressed as the hepatocyte enters the initial phase of G_1. Delayed early genes and cyclins are expressed later in G_1. Transforming growth factor-β (TGFβ), which inhibits hepatocyte DNA synthesis, is blocked during the proliferative phase. Removal of the block at the end of the cell cycle may be one of the factors that permit the hepatocyte to return to the quiescent state. Ap-1, activator protein-1; cdks, cyclin-dependent kinases. (Data from Taub R: Liver regeneration: From myth to mechanism. Nature Reviews 5:836, 2004.)

There are early as well as late changes in the expression of extracellular matrix components and the enzymes that modulate them. The mitotic phase is mostly complete in 3 days, and the liver mass is restituted in about 7 days. Liver cells return to their quiescent state once the liver mass is restored to the original size, give or take ≈10%. A balance between mitosis and apoptosis fine-tunes the restoration of hepatic mass. The strictly self-limited nature of hepatocyte replication suggests the presence of strong regulatory pressures that favor replicative repression. The ability of the liver to regulate its size depends on signals generated outside the liver, such as hormonal or metabolic signals, as well as internal signals generated within the liver.[64] However, signals for cessation of growth of the regenerating liver are understood less well than those governing hepatocellular replication.

Gene Expression during Hepatic Regeneration

The regenerative process is a cascade of events that move cells from their resting G_0 phase through G_1, DNA synthesis (S phase), and G_2 to mitotic cell division (M phase) (Fig. 69–2A). Expression of a large number of genes is induced or down-regulated after partial hepatectomy at transcriptional or post-transcriptional levels.[65,67] The sequence of activation of various genes during liver regeneration has been elucidated by studies using partial hepatectomy and gene knockout mice that lack specific cytokines. These genes include cell cycle genes, metabolic genes, genes that code for extracellular matrix proteins, growth factors, cytokines, and transcription factors. Chronologically, these genes can be grouped into immediate early genes, delayed early genes, and cell cycle–associated genes. Expression of these genes is modulated by signal transduction pathways that receive and transduce stimuli for cell replication and tissue remodeling (see Chapter 3).

Immediate Early Genes

Immediate early genes are activated almost immediately after partial hepatectomy without the need for protein synthesis. More than 70 immediate early genes have been identified, and more are expected to be discovered through microarray analysis of gene expression after partial hepatectomy (see Chapter 3). Many of these immediate early genes are involved in metabolic processes that are not linked directly to DNA synthesis. In addition to the proto-oncogenes c-fos, c-jun, c-myc, and c-ets, the immediate early genes include transcription factors, such as nuclear transactivating factor kappaB (NFκB), STAT3 (signal transducer and activator of transcription), activator protein-1 (AP-1), C/EBPβ (CCAAT enhancer binding protein β), insulin-like growth factor-binding protein-1, phosphatases, cyclic adenosine monophosphate (AMP) responsive promoter element modulator gene (CREM), and X-box-binding protein 1 (XBP-1), as well as metabolic genes such as phospho-enolpyruvate carboxykinase (PEPCK) and glucose-6-phosphatase.

In the quiescent liver, NFκB remains in the cytosol, where it is inactivated by binding to its inhibitor (IκB). Binding of TNF to its cell surface receptor initiates a signaling cascade that culminates in phosphorylation of

IκB, thereby causing the release of NFκB and its translocation to the nucleus, in turn resulting in transcriptional activation of more than a dozen genes likely to be involved in the immediate early response. IL-6 is one of the target genes of NFκB. IL-6 is a strong inducer of STAT3 activation and is thought to play an important role in hepatic regeneration. C/EBPα expression is down-regulated during liver regeneration, whereas C/EBP-β expression is induced. C/EBP-α may repress hepatocyte replication by inhibiting the proteolytic degradation of the cell cycle inhibitor p21 and by reducing E2F complexes containing the retinoblastoma protein p107. On the other hand, C/EBPβ activates the expression of mitogen-activated protein kinase protein phosphatase (MKP-1) and Egr-1 transcription factor as well as the cell cycle proteins cyclin B and E. CREM and XBP-1 participate in the regulation of liver regeneration through their effect on cAMP-responsive genes.

Delayed Early Genes

Delayed early genes are transcribed after the immediate early gene response but before the cell cycle genes reach their maximum level of expression. Expression of these genes occurs during the $G_0 \rightarrow G_1$ phase transition and depends on protein synthesis. This group of genes includes HRS/SRp40 (a splicing factor and modulator of alternative splicing of RNA transcripts) and the anti-apoptotic gene bcl-x. In contrast, the proapoptotic genes BAK, BAD, and BAX are down-regulated initially after partial hepatectomy and are induced at a later point.

Cell Cycle Genes

Cyclins and cyclin-dependent kinases (cdks) are expressed during cell cycle progression from G_1 through the S phase to the M phase. During the G_1 phase, cdks catalyze the phosphorylation of the retinoblastoma gene protein (pRB) and cause its dissociation from the E2F family of proteins. This dissociation eliminates the repression of gene expression by pRB. In regenerating mouse liver, cyclin D1 mRNA is expressed before DNA synthesis, whereas the expression of cyclin E mRNA coincides with DNA synthesis. Cyclin D1 forms a complex with cdk4, which causes phosphorylation of pRB and results in E2F activation. Cyclin D1 also may sequester the cell cycle inhibitor p27.

Integration of Cytokines and Growth Factors in Liver Regeneration

The very early reversible phase in liver regeneration, during which hepatocytes can enter the cell cycle by moving from the quiescent G_0 state to early G_1 phase, is called priming.[65] This phase is initiated by the effect of cytokines, the best studied of which are TNF-α and IL-6. Generation of reactive oxygen species, as a consequence of the acute metabolic changes, and release of lipopolysaccharides, in response to the loss of hepatic functional mass, may have a role in triggering the initial cytokine response. During priming, NFκB and STAT3 are activated, and AP-1 and C/EBP are expressed. Together, these factors lead to the immediate early gene expression response after partial hepatectomy (see earlier). The priming events sensitize hepatocytes to growth factors. In the absence of growth factors, the cells cannot move past a certain "restriction point" in G1.

The second phase of liver regeneration, called progression, requires HGF and TGF-α as well as cyclins D1 and E. During the progression phase, the cells move past the restriction point in G1 to S and beyond.

Once the peak level of cyclin D1 expression is reached, cells progress autonomously through the cell cycle, without further need for growth factors. Expression of HGF, TGF-α, and, probably, epidermal growth factor (EGF) increases after partial hepatectomy. These factors are the direct mitogens for liver regeneration. EGF binds to both the EGF receptor and the TGF-α receptor; c-met is the receptor for HGF. Growth hormone, thyroid hormones, and parathyroid hormone are permissive for liver regeneration, whereas insulin and norepinephrine are considered adjuvant factors.[65]

HGF and c-met

Major sources of HGF in the liver are Kupffer cells and HSCs. HGF is produced as a single 87- to 90-kd protein by nonparenchymal cells and is cleaved into ≈64-kd and ≈32-kd peptides that form heterodimers.[64,65] HGF mRNA levels rise 12 to 24 hours after partial hepatectomy in rats. Elevations of HGF have been observed in the serum of patients with fulminant hepatic failure, thereby suggesting an important role for HGF in regeneration of human liver. The HGF receptor, c-met, is a heterodimer that consists of a 145-kd β-chain and a 45-kd α-chain linked by disulfide bonds. The two polypeptide chains of c-met are also derived from proteolytic cleavage of a single precursor protein. The β-chain contains the transmembrane region and the intracellular tyrosine kinase domain. HGF binding to the extracellular domain of c-met activates tyrosine kinase and thus initiates a signal transduction pathway.

PROGRAMMED CELL DEATH

Programmed cell death, or *apoptosis*, is an integral part of hepatic regeneration. Apoptosis is involved in the fine-tuning and remodeling process that results in reconstruction of the hepatic architecture. Apoptosis results in the removal of damaged, senescent, or supernumerary cells without altering the cellular microenviroment. Loss of function of proapoptotic proteins, overexpression of antiapoptotic proteins, or loss of apoptotic signaling in cells can allow the survival of DNA-damaged cells, thereby giving rise to several forms of cancer (see Chapter 3).[68]

Apoptotic signals can originate within cells through mechanisms that sense DNA damage and inappropriate proliferative signals. In other cases, the apoptotic signals come from other cells in one of at least three ways.[69] First, cells recognized as foreign or as pathogens may receive apoptotic signals from immune mediator cells. Second, the nurturing signals of neighboring cells or extracellular matrix may be lost, thereby resulting in apoptosis of anchor-dependent cells. Third, some cells undergo apoptosis in response to certain growth factors, such as TGF-β1.

In contrast to necrosis, apoptosis is an active process that culminates in cell death. During the latent phase of apoptosis, the cell undergoes molecular and biochemical changes but remains morphologically intact. In the "execution" phase, a series of dramatic structural changes culminates in the fragmentation and condensation of the cell into membrane-enclosed apoptotic bodies. Initially, a variety of stimuli—including DNA damage, growth factor withdrawal, toxins, and radiation—triggers the apoptotic pathway. The signal is transduced by a series of defined protein-protein interactions. Finally, cell death is carried out by the activation of specific proteases, called caspases, that cleave multiple substrates, thereby leading to DNA fragmentation, chromatin condensation, cell shrinkage, and membrane blebbing. The apoptotic cell may be phagocytosed or may simply lose contact with neighboring cells. Apoptosis does not cause an acute inflammatory reaction. All of these morphologic features of apoptosis contrast with those of necrosis, in which the cell swells and releases proinflammatory material into the neighboring space.[68]

The two major apoptotic pathways are activation of cell surface death receptors[69] and mitochondrial permeability transition.[70] At least six different cell surface molecules can function as death receptors. One of the best-characterized death receptors is Fas (also known as Apo1 or CD95). Fas belongs to the family of TNF receptors. Binding of Fas to Fas ligand leads to an interaction between the cytoplasmic domain of the Fas receptor and the death domain of the adaptor protein, FADD, which in turn recruits and activates procaspase-8. Once activated, caspase-8 activates downstream caspases such as caspase-3. The second major pathway involves mitochondria and is triggered by various toxic insults. Either Bax or Bak opens channels, thereby releasing the electron transport protein cytochrome c and other proteins from the intermembranous space into the cytoplasm. Cytochrome c binds the scaffolding protein Apaf-1. The C-terminal portion of Apaf-1 is a negative regulator of apoptosis. The N-terminal region contains a caspase recruitment domain and an ATPase domain. Binding of cytochrome c and deoxyadenosine triphosphate (dATP) removes the negative regulatory influence of the C-terminus of Apaf-1, thereby permitting binding and autoactivation of caspase-9. Activated caspase-9, in turn, activates caspase-3 and caspase-7, thereby initiating cell death. In addition, permeabilization of the mitochondrial outer membrane results in the loss of function of the electron transport chain, which is essential for most mitochondrial function, including ATP generation.

Expression of Genes Involved in Apoptosis during Liver Regeneration

Liver regeneration is a complex process involving a balance of cell replication, apoptosis, and remodeling, orchestrated by a number of molecular mediators. The genes involved in apoptosis are actively expressed in the regenerating liver. They include the inducing genes c-*fos*, c-*jun*, c-*myc*, *p53*, *Bax*, *Bad*, *Bak*, and *TGF-β*; the apoptosis inhibitory genes *Bcl-2*, *Bcl-X_L*, and *TRPM-2/clusterin*; and the *Rb* gene. Some of these genes also are involved in cell proliferation through regulation of the cell cycle (see Chapter 3).

PROTEIN SYNTHESIS AND DEGRADATION IN THE LIVER

HEPATIC GENE EXPRESSION

Compared with most organs, the liver expresses a large number of genes. More than 90% of plasma proteins and about 15% of the total protein mass of the body are produced in the liver.[71] As in all mammalian cells, gene expression is initiated by transcription of the gene into an RNA transcript, a process that is mediated by RNA polymerase II. The nascent RNA is modified by capping of the 5'-terminus with 7-methylguanosine, excision of the noncoding intervening sequences (introns), splicing together of the coding sequences (exons), and, in most cases, addition of polyadenylate at the 3' end. The processed mRNA is transported actively out of the nucleus. In the cytoplasm, association of the mRNA with the 40s ribosomal subunit and methionine tRNA requires several initiation factors, a cap-binding protein, and ATP hydrolysis.

Once this initiation complex is formed, the 60s ribosomal subunit is recruited, and polypeptide chain elongation proceeds as specific tRNAs recognize corresponding codons and attach appropriate amino acids sequentially. Chain elongation requires elongation factors and energy provided by GTP hydrolysis. Cessation of translation at the stop codons requires recognition by a termination factor. In most cases, the nascent protein is processed by cleavage of an amino-terminal signal peptide. Many proteins undergo further proteolytic cleavage, cotranslational glycosylation, and modification of the carbohydrate moieties in the Golgi apparatus before being secreted or transported to other intracellular organelles (see earlier).

Gene expression is regulated at multiple levels. Gene transcription is regulated by the state of the chromatin, which determines the accessibility of specific genes to the transcription machinery, and binding of specific transcription factors that promote or repress gene transcription. Post-transcriptional regulation can involve differential splicing, modulation of mRNA stability and efficiency of translation, protein folding, association with self or other proteins, and phosphorylation or other forms of protein modification. Modulation of protein degradation is another important mechanism that regulates net protein content (see later). All these modes of regulation are active in liver cells and are areas of intensive investigation.

Some genes expressed in hepatocytes, loosely termed "housekeeping genes," are expressed in other organs as well, but the expression of many other genes occurs preferentially or uniquely in the liver. Expression of these liver-specific genes permits the liver to perform essential functions of the body, including secretion of plasma proteins, gluconeogenesis, glycogen storage, glucose metabolism, cholesterol homeostasis, bile salt production, and detoxification of endogenous metabolites and exogenous substances. A series of cis-acting elements in specific genes mediates their hepatocyte-preferred expression.[72] These cis-acting DNA elements bind different families of hepatocyte nuclear factors (HNFs). Although none of these factors is entirely liver-specific, high levels of liver-preferred gene expression occur only in the presence of combinatorial interaction of these transcription factors. Maintenance of hepatocyte-enriched expression of specific transcription factors involves cross-regulation by other unrelated liver-enriched transcription factors. Some of the transcription factors involved in hepatocyte specificity are also important in hepatic tissue specification during embryogenesis. Many of the transcription factors are normally located in the cytoplasm. Binding of hormones or cytokines to their respective cell surface receptors causes conformational changes in the cytoplasmic domain of these receptors, often through phosphorylation. Such conformational changes result in a series of events that eventually lead to the translocation of specific transcription factors to the nucleus and their binding to the respective cis-acting elements in the regulatory regions of genes. Therefore, extracellular signals are transduced to a series of intracellular events, thereby culminating in the induction or repression of gene expression.

Regulation of gene transcription is the most important, but not the only, mechanism for modulating gene expression. The stability of the RNA, translational regulation, and post-translational modifications all can affect the steady-state concentration, intracellular or extracellular location, and activity of a given gene product.

Nuclear Receptors

Modulation of metabolic pathways and detoxicating mechanisms according to the needs of the body often requires coordinated up-regulation or repression of expression of a set of genes. In many cases, such coordination is mediated by nuclear receptors, such as retinoid X-receptor (RXR), liver X-receptor (LXR), farnesoid X-receptor (FXR), constitutive androstane receptor (CAR), peroxisome proliferator activator receptor (PPAR), and thyroid hormone receptor (TR).[73] For example, expression of the proteins that mediate bilirubin uptake by hepatocytes, intracellular storage of bilirubin, bilirubin glucuronidation, and bile canalicular excretion of bilirubin glucuronides may each be regulated by CAR. Nuclear receptors mediate induction or repression of genes by small nonprotein molecules. For example, phenobarbital binds to CAR in the cytoplasm, thereby leading to the translocation of CAR to the nucleus and resulting, in turn, in the simultaneous induction of multiple genes that have CAR-binding elements in their cis-regulatory regions. Similarly, bile acids bind to FXR, fibrates bind to PPAR, and thyroid hormones bind to TR. In most cases, nuclear receptors function by forming heterodimers with RXR, although some nuclear receptors can function as homodimers.

PROTEIN FOLDING

Proteins that are destined for export to intracellular membranes or secretion into the plasma are translocated into the ER, where folding takes place prior to secretion through the Golgi apparatus.[74] The ER contains a number of molecular chaperones and folding catalysts that promote efficient folding. All chaperones enable and promote protein folding and assembly, but their specific functions differ. Many chaperones work in tandem with another chaperone. Some molecular chaperones bind to nascent chains as they emerge from the ribosome and protect aggregation-prone hydrophobic regions. Other chaperones are involved in later stages of folding, particularly for complex proteins, including oligomeric species and multimolecular assemblies.

In addition to promoting proper folding, chaperones play an important role in the "quality control" of proteins by involving a complex series of glycosylation and deglycosylation processes and preventing misfolded proteins from being secreted from the cell.[75] The unfolded or misfolded proteins are targeted for degradation through the ubiquitin-proteosome pathway (see later).[76] Up to half of all polypeptide chains fail to satisfy the quality control mechanism in the ER, and for some proteins, such as the cystic fibrosis conductance regulator (CFTR), the success rate is even lower. The proportion of molecules that misfold is increased greatly in mutant proteins with amino acid substitutions. Some molecular chaperones are able to rescue misfolded proteins to enable them to have a second chance to fold correctly. Under some circumstances, chaperones can solubilize proteins that have aggregated because of misfolding. In some cases, energy for such active intervention may be derived from ATP hydrolysis. Many molecular chaperones, such as the heat shock protein, are up-regulated in stressful situations, in which protein misfolding is more prone to occur.

In addition to molecular chaperones, several classes of folding catalysts accelerate steps in the folding process. For example, peptidylprolyl isomerases increase the rate of *cis/trans* isomerization of peptide bonds involving proline residues, and protein disulfide isomerases enhance formation and reorganization of disulfide bonds within proteins.

PROTEIN CATABOLISM

Like protein synthesis, proteolysis is a major process that contributes to the turnover of protein in the body. The autophagic-lysosomal pathway and the ubiquitin-proteosome pathway are the two major mechanisms of protein degradation. The autophagic-lysosomal mechanism is responsible for bulk degradation of endogenous proteins as well as degradation of other cellular components, such as RNA, carbohydrates, and lipids. This pathway may be seen as a cell restructuring mechanism. The autophagy system is regulated physiologically by plasma levels of the amino acids leucine, glutamine, tyrosine, phenylalanine, proline, methionine, tryptophan, and histidine, probably through binding to cell surface receptors and subsequent intracellular signaling. Protein kinase cascades such as mTOR, Erk, and eIF2a may be involved in the regulation of autophagy. Amino acids may exert their effects through these pathways in combination with insulin.[77]

The ubiquitin-proteosome pathway is the principal mechanism for turnover of normally short-lived proteins in mammalian cells.[78] Ubiquitin is a small protein that can covalently link to itself or to other proteins, either as monomers or as chains of polyubiquitin. Ubiquitin is added to a target protein by ubiquitin-activating, ubiquitin-conjugating, and ubiquitin-ligating enzymes. The first function attributed to ubiquitin was the covalent binding to misfolded proteins, thereby directing proteosome-dependent proteolysis. Now ubiquitin and ubiquitin-related proteins are also known to direct specific proteins through the endocytotic pathway by modifying the cargo proteins as well as by regulating components of the cytoplasmic protein trafficking machinery. By regulating the turnover of mitotic cyclins, ubiquitination plays an important role in cell cycle regulation.[79,80]

Although the ubiquitin-proteosome pathway is generally considered to be separate from the lysosomal proteolysis mechanism, ubiquitination is sometimes required for lysosomal proteolysis. A subset of endocytosed proteins must be conjugated to ubiquitin as a trigger for internalization from the plasma membrane.[81,82] Therefore, ubiquitin conjugation appears to be important in several protein trafficking steps, including endocytosis.

The major plasma proteins synthesized and secreted by the liver are shown in Table 69–1.

HEPATIC NUTRIENT METABOLISM

The liver is at the hub of numerous metabolic pathways. The liver provides energy continuously to the entire body through its ability to store and modulate the availability of systemic nutrients.[83] In turn, the metabolic function of the liver is regulated by hormones secreted by the pancreas, adrenal gland, and thyroid as well as by neuronal inputs. During nutrient absorption (fed state), the liver regulates nutrient flux as the absorbed nutrients are metabolized, modified for storage in the liver and fatty tissue, or made available to other organs as energy source. During nonabsorptive periods (fasting state), the energy supply is maintained from the stored fuel and by synthesis. Detailed reviews of hepatic nutrient metabolism are available elsewhere.[84]

CARBOHYDRATE METABOLISM

Glucose is the primary energy source for the brain, erythrocytes, muscle, and renal cortex. Maintaining adequate circulating levels of glucose is essential for the central nervous system, which normally uses glucose as its major metabolic fuel. After a person fasts for 24 to 48 hours, the brain can utilize ketones as a metabolic fuel, thereby reducing its glucose requirement by 50% to 70%.[84] The liver is the principal organ that maintains total carbohydrate stores by synthesizing glycogen and generating glucose from precursors.[85] Glucose is synthesized from nonoxidative metabolic products of glucose (pyruvate and lactate) that are generated predominantly by red blood cells (RBCs) and from amino acid precursors that are derived predominantly from muscle during prolonged starvation or exercise.

Regulation of Glucose Uptake and Efflux from the Hepatocyte

Glucose is a critical molecule in the metabolic pathway because it can be converted to amino acids, fatty acids,

Table 69–1 Serum Proteins Produced by the Liver

Protein	Molecular Weight (daltons)	Function	Association with Liver Disease	Acute-Phase Response
Albumin	66,500	Binding protein, osmotic regulator	Decreased in chronic liver disease	Decreased
Alpha-fetoprotein	66,300	Binding protein	Increased in hepatocellular carcinoma	Decreased
α_1-antitrypsin (α_1-AT)	54,000	Inhibitor of elastin	Missense mutations associated with liver disease	Increased
Ceruloplasmin	132,000	Ferroxidase	Decreased in Wilson disease	Increased
Fibrinogen	340,000	Precursor to fibrin in hemostasis, wound healing	Decreased in chronic liver disease	Increased
Transferrin	79,500	Iron-binding protein	Increased in iron deficiency	Decreased
Complement C3	185,000	Complement pathway	—	Increased
Complement C4	200,000	Complement pathway	—	Increased
α_1-Acid glycoprotein (orosomucoid)	40,000	Inhibits proliferating response of peripheral lymphocytes to mitogens	—	Increased
α_1-Antichymotrypsin	68,000	Inhibits chymotrypsin-like serine proteinase	—	Increased
Haptoglobin	≈100,000	Binds hemoglobin released by hemolysis	—	Increased
C-reactive protein	118,000	Binds pathogens and damaged cells to initiate their elimination	—	Increased
Serum amyloid A	9,000	Unknown	—	Increased
Ferritin	450,000	Intracellular iron storage	Increased in hemochromatosis	Increased

Data from Katz N, Jungermam K: Metabolic heterogeneity of the liver. In Tavoloni N, Berk PD (eds): Hepatic Transport and Bile Secretion: Physiology and Pathophysiology. New York, Raven Press, 1993, p 55; and Putnan FW: Progress in plasma proteins. In: The Plasma Proteins: Structure, Function, and Genetic Control. Orlando, FL, Academic Press, 1984, p 45.

or glycogen, the major storage form of glucose. Glucose enters hepatocytes via the glucose transporter-2, which facilitates the diffusion of glucose across the sinusoidal membrane.[86] Glucose transporter-2 differs from other members of the glucose transporter family in that it is independent of metabolic conditions and insulin levels. Because of the low-affinity, high-capacity characteristics of glucose transporter-2, intrahepatic glucose concentration is determined by the plasma glucose level, which in turn is regulated by glucokinase (GK) activity (see "Formation of Glucose-6-Phosphate").[87] Glucose transporter-1, which is present in the brain, erythrocytes, and hepatocytes, particularly in zone 3 of the liver lobule, is a high-affinity, low-capacity glucose transporter that permits glucose uptake by hepatocytes when the circulating glucose concentration is low. Increased expression of glucose transporter-1 during fasting enhances glucose uptake by hepatocytes. Hepatocellular glucose homeostasis is maintained by interlinking pathways that are regulated by multiple signals, which prevent competing pathways from operating at the same time.[88] Figure 69–3 illustrates these pathways and the modulating influences that control the metabolic flux of glucose and other sugars, such as fructose.

Formation of Glucose-6-Phosphate

Rapid conversion of glucose to glucose-6-phosphate (glucose-6-P) modulates the glucose concentration within the hepatocyte, thereby regulating influx or efflux of glucose from the hepatocyte.[85] Glucose-6-P is a nodal branch point compound that can enter three independent metabolic pathways: (1) synthesis of glycogen, which can be mobilized rapidly during fasting, (2) anaerobic glycolysis via the Embden-Meyerhof pathway, which generates pyruvate or lactate as a substrate for the tricarboxylic acid (Krebs) cycle in mitochondria, and (3) the pentose-phosphate shunt, which generates reducing equivalents necessary for anaerobic glycolysis and fatty acid synthesis. The pentose-phosphate shunt is regulated by the activity of mitochondrial glucose-6-P dehydrogenase.[86] Conversion of glucose to glucose-6-P is catalyzed by hexokinase, which accepts several different hexose substrates, and GK (also termed hexokinase type 4 or D), which is expressed predominantly in the liver and pancreas and is specific for glucose.[89]

A low-affinity, high-capacity system, GK is not inhibited by the reaction product glucose-6-P. Therefore, the level of GK activity regulates intrahepatocellular glucose concentration, which determines the net uptake of glucose by hepatocytes from hepatic sinusoidal plasma. GK is activated by insulin and inhibited by glucagon.[84] Mutations in the GK gene are associated with some rare cases of maturity-onset diabetes of young adults (MODY).[89] Fructose-1-phosphate modulates GK activity by regulating the inhibitory activity of a GK regulatory protein.[90] The regulation of GK by fructose is thought to prevent futile cycling between glucose and glucose-6-P that consumes ATP. Starvation decreases GK activity, thereby promoting glucose efflux from the hepatocyte.

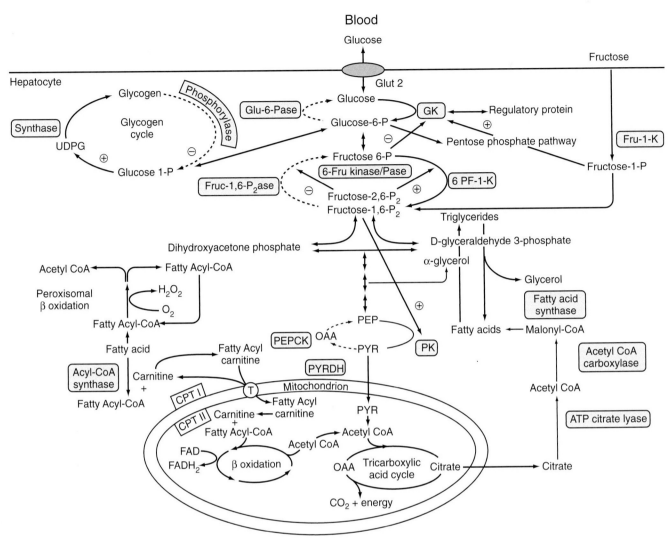

Figure 69–3 Hepatic carbohydrate and lipid metabolism. Gluconeogenic pathways are identified by *dashed lines*. 6-Fru kinase/Pase, 6-phosphofructo-2-kinase/fructose-2,6-biphosphatase; 6 PF-1-K, 6-phosphofructo-1-kinase; ATP, adenosine triphosphate; CoA, coenzyme A; CPT, carnitine palmitoyltransferase; FAD, flavin adenine dinucleotide; $FADH_2$, reduced flavin adenine dinucleotide; Fru-1-K, hepatic fructokinase; Fruc-1,6-P_2ase, fructose-1,6-biphosphatase; Fructose-1-P, fructose-1-phosphate; Fructose-1,6-P_2, fructose-1,6-biphosphate; Fructose-2,6-P_2, fructose-2,6-biphosphate; Fructose 6-P, fructose-6-phosphate; GK, glucokinase; Glu-6-P, glucose-6-phosphate; Glu-6-Pase, glucose-6-phosphatase; Glut 2, glucose transporter 2; OAA, oxaloacetate; PEP, phosphoenol pyruvate; PEPCK, phosphoenol pyruvate carboxykinase; PK, pyruvate kinase; PYR, pyruvate; PYRDH, pyruvate dehydrogenase; T, carnitine:acylcarnitine transferase; UDPG, uridine diphosphate glucose. (Data from Pilkis SJ, Granner DK: Molecular physiology of the regulation of hepatic gluconeogenesis and glycolysis. Annu Rev Physiol 54:885, 1992.)

Conversion of Glucose-6-Phosphate to Glucose

Conversion of glucose-6-P to glucose is catalyzed by glucose-6-phosphatase (glu-6-Pase), a multi-subunit enzyme whose active site is located within the ER lumen.[91] Therefore, glucose-6-P needs to traverse the ER membrane to be dephosphorylated. Inherited deficiency of glu-6-Pase causes glycogen storage disease type Ia (see Chapter 73).[91] Glucose-6-P transport is mediated by a microsomal transport protein, which when defective causes glycogen storage disease type Ib. As expected, glu-6-Pase activity is increased by starvation, which results in an increase in hepatocellular glucose concentration and consequent efflux of glucose into the sinusoidal space by the bidirectional glucose transporter-2.

Glucose-6-P can enter the pentose monophosphate shunt that generates the reduced form of nicotinamide dinucleotide phosphate (NADPH). The other possible metabolic fate of glucose-6-P is conversion to fructose-6-P, which can enter the fructose 6-P-fructose 1,6-diphosphate (fructose-1,6-P_2) pathway. Fructose-1,6-P_2 modulates the activity of pyruvate kinase (PK), which can affect substrate cycling in the subsequent pyruvate (PYR)–phosphoenol pyruvate (PEP) pathway. These opposing enzyme reactions regulate both the formation of gluconeogenesis precursors and glycolysis.

The relative production of fructose-6-P and fructose-1,6-P_2 is regulated by the opposing action of 6-phosphofructo-1-phosphokinase (6-PK-1-K) and fructose-1,6-bisphosphatase (fruc-1,6$_2$Pase).[85] Within this cycle is a unique enzyme: 6-phosphofructo-2-kinase/fructose-2,6-biphosphatase (6-fru kinase/Pase). This enzyme, which combines the properties of both a 6-phosphofructo-2-kinase and its corresponding phosphorylase enzyme activity, produces the regulatory product fructose-2,6-P_2. Fructose-2,6-P_2 is a potent activator of 6-PF-1-K and inhibitor of fruc-1,6$_2$Pase. Moreover, it favors the formation of the fructose-1,6-P_2 product. This enzyme, which is regulated by both hormonal and nutrient factors, serves as another modulator of glucose metabolism. During starvation, when fructose-2,6-P_2 levels are low, gluconeogenesis is enhanced. On the other hand, high levels of fructose-2,6-P_2 found during refeeding and insulin administration promote glycolysis and fatty acid synthesis. The phosphorylation status of the 6-fru kinase/Pase is regulated by both the cAMP-dependent kinase site and phosphatase 2A activity.

From fructose-1,6-P_2, a sequence of four biochemical reactions leads to the formation of PEP with generation of eight molecules of ATP.[83] PEP can then be metabolized into PYR as part of the third regulatory cycle in glucose metabolism. PK, which transforms PEP to PYR, generates two ATP molecules. PYR is another nodal branch point in the metabolic pathway, from which it can undergo further metabolism in mitochondria to form acetyl CoA. Thereafter, it can undergo aerobic metabolism by the tricarboxylic acid cycle. In this pathway, PYR may be metabolized ultimately to water and carbon dioxide, with the production of 15 molecules of ATP per molecule of PYR. Other products of the tricarboxylic acid cycle are also precursors for fatty acid (citrate) or amino acids by means of oxaloacetate formation. Fructose-1,6-P_2 is also an inducer of PK.[92] In the reverse reaction, PYR is metabolized to oxaloacetate, which is a precursor for the amino acid L-aspartate. Oxaloacetate is converted by the energy-dependent activity of phosphoenolpyruvate carboxykinase (PEPCK), an important regulator of gluconeogenesis. PEPCK expression is inhibited by insulin at a transcriptional level[84,92] and is up-regulated during fasting and in diabetes mellitus.

Hepatic Metabolism of Galactose and Fructose

Lactose, a major disaccharide present in human milk and cow's milk, is split into glucose and galactose. Galactose can be converted to glucose-6-P, after which it can be utilized for glycogen synthesis; or it can be oxidized further to form PYR or acetyl-CoA for additional energy generation or fatty acid synthesis.[83] Galactose is initially phosphorylated by galactokinase to form galactose-1-P. In the presence of uridine diphosphoglucose (UDP-glucose), it can then undergo metabolism by uridyltransferase to form glucose-1-phosphate (glucose-1-P) and UDP-galactose. UDP-galactose can be epimerized by UDP-glucose-4-epimerase to form UDP-glucose, which is a precursor for glucose-1-P. Glucose-1-P can be converted to glucose-6-P. Thus, like glucose, galactose can participate in the glycolytic pathway.

Fructose, an abundant sugar in the diet, is absorbed by the intestinal epithelium by a sodium-independent carrier distinct from the intestinal glucose transporter. It is converted to fructose-1-phosphate (fructose-1-P) by hepatic fructokinase (fru-1-K) using either ATP or GTP as a cofactor. Fructose-1-P activates GK activity by removing the inhibitory regulatory protein. Fructose-1-P does not enter the glucogenic pathway but is metabolized by fructose-1-phosphate aldolase to form two trioses, dihydroxylacetone phosphate and glyceraldehyde-3-phosphate. Dihydroxylacetone phosphate may be isomerized to glyceraldehyde phosphate and enter the glycolytic pathway or may be reduced to glyceraldehyde-3-phosphate and provide the glycerol backbone for triacylglycerol and phospholipids. Glyceraldehyde-3-phosphate may be combined with dihydroxylacetone phosphate by aldolase B ultimately to form fructose-1,6-P_2. Depending on the metabolic requirements of the liver, fructose-1,6-P_2 can be used for gluconeogenesis and glycogen synthesis or may be subjected to glycolysis, ultimately resulting in the formation of lactate. Because fructose enters the carbohydrate cycle at the second regulatory step, fructose is a better substrate than glucose for lipogenesis in the liver. Aldolase B deficiency results in hereditary fructose intolerance as a result of excess fructose-1-P build-up. Treatment consists of avoidance of sucrose and fructose in the diet.

Glycogen Formation

Glycogen stored in the liver is the main source of rapidly available glucose for the glucose-dependent tissues such as erythrocytes, retina, renal medulla, and brain.[93] The liver glycogen stores contain up to a 2-day supply of glucose, after which gluconeogenesis occurs mainly from lactate, a three-carbon end-product of anaerobic glucose metabolism.[83,94] Hepatic gluconeogenesis produces up to 240 mg of glucose a day, which is approximately twice the metabolic need of the retina, RBCs, and brain. The three-carbon precursors generated by anaerobic metabolism from muscle, intestine, liver, or RBCs may account for up to 50% of the glycogen pool formed during non-absorptive states. Alanine, another major glucose precursor, is generated by the catabolism of muscle proteins, which is a major cause of muscle wasting during prolonged fasting. Glycogen stored in muscle is utilized locally and cannot be exported out of the cell because muscles lack glu-6-Pase. The relative contribution of each of the precursors to glycogen synthesis depends on the nutritional status, amount and route of glucose administration (oral vs. intravenous), and hormonal regulation.

Rapid switching between glycogen synthesis and breakdown is mediated by a cascade of enzymes that are regulated by local nutrients and hormones.[83] Glycogen phosphorylase, which is activated by phosphorylation, catalyzes the breakdown of glycogen subunits, and glycogen synthase, which is activated by dephosphorylation, catalyzes the addition of UDP-glucose to the expanding glycogen chain. In addition glucose and glucose-6-P are allosteric activators of glycogen synthase, whereas glucose binding inactivates glycogen phosphorylase.

Glycogen exists as two distinct populations that consist of proglycogen, with a molecular weight of approximately 4×10^5, and macroglycogen, with a molecular weight of 1×10^7, the concentrations of which depend on the relative activities of enzymes favoring proglycogen formation (phosphorylase and debranching enzymes) and those favoring glycogenin formation (branching enzymes). The ability of glycogenin to initiate the formation of glycogen is important in hepatic carbohydrate metabolism. The existence of these two distinct pools of glycogen permits subtle control of glucose levels, and their relative contributions could have a physiologic role in disease states such as diabetes mellitus.

Regulation of Glycolytic-Gluconeogenic Pathways

The glycolytic-gluconeogenic pathways are regulated by hormonal signals and the relative availability of nutrients. Insulin up-regulates the expression of genes that encode the glycolytic enzymes and represses the expression of metabolic enzymes responsible for gluconeogenesis. Glucagon, catecholamines, corticosteroids, and growth hormone raise cellular cAMP levels, thereby augmenting the gluconeogenic pathway. In many cases, post-transcriptional mRNA stabilization or degradation, post-translational phosphorylation or end-product inhibition, or allosteric modulation contributes to the relative abundance or activity of specific enzymes.[85,92] Glucose and fructose affect the enzyme activities by directly inhibiting or allosterically modulating the enzymes. In the fed state, high activity of GK, 6-PF-1-K, and PK induced by insulin favors formation of PYR; the activity of PEPCK and other gluconeogenic enzymes is low. During fasting, a drop in plasma insulin levels removes inhibition of the gluconeogenic enzymes PEPCK and fructose-1,6-P_2ase. Simultaneously, an increase in levels of glucagon and β-adrenergic agonists increases intracellular cAMP levels, which inhibit 6-PK-2 kinase activity and stimulate 6-phosphofructo-2-kinase, thereby reducing the fructose-2,6-P_2 concentration and leading to activation of fruc-1,6₂Pase and a net increase in gluconeogenesis. After a prolonged fast, gluconeogenesis is stimulated further by an increase in the supply of substrate and alterations in the concentration of various enzymes.

Carbohydrate Metabolism in Cirrhosis

Patients with cirrhosis have an increased frequency of hyperglycemia and relative hyperinsulinemia.[95] The hyperglycemia may be explained by decreased glucose uptake by muscle and reduced glycogen storage in liver and muscle. These changes lead to insulin resistance, which causes a rise in plasma insulin levels. Other causes of relative insulin resistance include an increase in serum fatty acid levels that can inhibit glucose uptake by muscle; altered second messenger activity after insulin binds to its receptor; and a rise in serum concentrations of cytokines that results from elevated serum levels of lipopolysaccharides. Increased levels of glucagon and catecholamines may be contributing factors. The net result is impaired nonoxidative utilization of glucose with decreased storage of glycogen and impaired uptake of glucose by muscle, thereby causing a relative insulin-resistant state similar to that found in patients with diabetes and obesity.

LIPID METABOLISM

Fatty acids are an important energy source for the liver and serve as an efficient fuel store within and outside the liver, because oxidation of fatty acids yields the highest ATP production of any metabolic fuel.[83] In addition, most organs are capable of utilizing fatty acids as a fuel.[96] The liver plays a central role in regulating the body's total fatty acid needs. Excess glucose can be converted to fatty acid for future use and stored in adipose tissue or delivered by lipoproteins to other organs (see later). Beta oxidation of fatty acids in mitochondria and peroxisomes has different physiologic consequences.[97] Furthermore, fatty acids are structural components of cell membranes and are important in cellular function and cell anchoring. The regulation of fatty acid synthesis and transport of fatty acids to other organs in association with lipoproteins constitute another critical role of the liver in managing the metabolic needs of the entire body.

Fatty Acid Synthesis

Fatty acid synthesis occurs in the cytosol of the hepatocyte and is regulated closely by the availability of acetyl-CoA, which forms the basic subunit of the developing fatty acid carbon chain.[83] Acetyl-CoA is synthesized predominantly in mitochondria and is derived mainly from carbohydrate metabolism, with a small fraction coming from amino acids.[4,12,13] Acetyl-CoA is combined with oxaloacetate to form citrate, which is exported from the mitochondria and is then cleaved by the cytosolic ATP citrate lyase to provide oxaloacetate and acetyl-CoA. Conversion of acetyl-CoA to malonyl-CoA by the action of acetyl-CoA carboxylase is the first step in fatty acid synthesis. Acetyl-CoA carboxylase is the key enzyme in regulating fatty acid synthesis, because it provides the necessary building blocks for elongation of the fatty acid carbon chain.[98]

Malonyl-CoA is utilized by a set of enzymatic activities contained within a single peptide chain that make up the remarkable fatty acid synthase system.[83] Malonyl-CoA binds to acyl carrier protein (ACP). Catalytic activity is contained within two distinct domains that catalyze sequential condensation, reduction, dehydrogenation, and reduction, which constitute the fatty acid synthetic cycle. Two NADPH molecules are required for each two-carbon unit that is added to the growing fatty acid chain. After completion of the first cycle, the 4-carbon butyl group is transferred from ACP to a peripheral thiol, thus allowing it to accept the next malonyl-CoA group to restart the entire cycle. The cycle continues for an additional six or seven rounds until a carbon-16 (palmitate) or carbon-18 (stearate) fatty acid is synthesized. Fatty acid–CoA is then released and used for other metabolic pathways.

Further elongation of the fatty acid chain can occur either in the mitochondrion or within the microsomal membrane.[83] In the mitochondrion, the first step is mediated by enoyl-CoA reductase. Microsomal elongation utilizes malonyl-CoA to increase the size of fatty acyl-CoA in a process that involves four separate enzymatic reactions. The elongation ability of microsomes is tissue dependent and serves the needs of specific organs. The fatty acid chain elongates until an appropriate length has been achieved, and the fatty acid is then esterified with glycerol to form triglycerides. These newly formed triglycerides can be transported by lipoproteins to distal sites for storage and use. In situations of excess carbohydrates, PYR can be converted to acetyl-CoA by the mitochondrial pyruvate dehydrogenase complex to serve as fatty acid precursors, although lipogenesis from carbohydrates consumes about 25% of the energy contained in the carbohydrates.

Beta Oxidation of Fatty Acids

Fatty acid beta oxidation is an important source of energy for many organs, including the liver. Beta oxidation occurs in mitochondria and peroxisomes, and the process requires transport of substrates across the membranes that delimit these organelles.

Mitochondrial Beta Oxidation

Fatty acids are translocated across the mitochondrial membranes by first undergoing fatty acyl-CoA formation by the activity of distinct fatty acyl-CoA synthetases that are specific for short-, medium-, or long-chain fatty acids in the mitochondrial outer membrane.[83,99] In the inner mitochondrial membrane, conjugation of fatty acyl-CoA with carnitine is catalyzed by carnitine palmitoyltransferase I, with formation of fatty acylcarnitine, which is translocated into the mitochondrion in exchange for free carnitine by an integral inner membrane protein, fatty acylcarnitine:carnitine translocase.[100] Inside the mitochondrion, a reverse reaction mediated by carnitine palmitoyltransferase II releases fatty acyl-CoA, which is now a substrate for beta oxidation. The first step that is unique to beta oxidation is formation of *trans*-enoyl fatty acid, which is generated by acyl-CoA dehydrogenase. Acyl-CoA dehydrogenase transfers two electrons to flavin adenine dinucleotide (FAD), which then transfers them to the electron transport chain in the mitochondrion. 3-Keto fatty acyl-CoA then undergoes a series of sequential reactions to acetyl CoA and fatty acyl-CoA, which undergo another round of beta oxidation. Acetyl CoA can enter the tricarboxylic acid cycle, thus generating 12 ATP, or it can enter the 3-hydroxyl methyl glutaryl-CoA cycle to form ketone bodies. Only mitochondria in the liver are capable of forming ketone bodies. Regulation of mitochondrial beta oxidation lies with fatty acylcarnitine formation, which is catalyzed by carnitine palmitoyltransferase I.[100] Malonyl-CoA, the basic subunit of fatty acid synthesis, is a potent inhibitor of carnitine palmitoyltransferase I, thereby preventing beta oxidation and fatty acid synthesis from occurring concurrently.

Peroxisomal Beta Oxidation of Fatty Acids

Peroxisomes have lesser capacity than mitochondria for beta oxidation of fatty acid. The relative contribution of peroxisomes to beta oxidation depends on the length of fatty acid chains and administration of peroxisome proliferators. In contrast to fatty acid oxidation in the mitochondria, initial fatty acyl-CoA formation within the peroxisome does not require fatty acyl carnitine formation for entry into the peroxisomes. During the next metabolic step, in which *trans*-enoyl fatty acyl-CoA is formed, another significant difference between peroxisomes and mitochondria is evident. Two electrons produced by this step are transferred to FAD to form $FADH_2$, which is then transferred directly to oxygen to form hydrogen peroxide. Hydrogen peroxide is detoxified by catalase to form water and oxygen. In the mitochon-

drion, electrons are delivered to the mitochondrial electron transport system that ultimately generates water and ATP. The significance of this difference lies in both loss of ATP production and generation of hydrogen peroxide in the peroxisomes, which in the presence of transitional metals can yield toxic hydroxyl radicals and thus can promote lipid peroxidation and oxidant injury.

NADH generated in subsequent reactions needs to be removed from the peroxisomes, whereas in mitochondria, NADH can enter the electron transport cycle and generate additional ATP molecules. Peroxisomal enzymes can metabolize only long-chain fatty acids with a minimal chain length of 10 carbons and a maximal length of 24 carbons. As in mitochondria, beta oxidation in peroxisomes proceeds similarly by 2-carbon acetyl-CoA cleavage until octanoyl-CoA is formed. Octanoyl is then combined with carnitine to form fatty acyl carnitine, which can be transported by the mitochondrial inner membrane transporter and undergo completion of beta oxidation. Acyl-CoA formed in peroxisomes by beta oxidation of fatty acids can diffuse out of the peroxisomes after formation of acetyl carnitine.[100]

The regulation of peroxisomal metabolism of fatty acids appears to be solely at the level of substrate availability, which may be regulated by a family of soluble fatty acid–binding proteins present in the cytosol of all cells. The peroxisomal pathway provides a supply of acetyl-CoA that does not require citrate formation and that can be used in fatty acid synthesis. However, because the initial electron transfer is not coupled to the mitochondrial electron transport system, peroxisomal fatty acid beta oxidation is less efficient than mitochondrial beta oxidation and may provide a means of eliminating fatty acids with energy loss. Peroxisomes proliferate upon administration of a large number of hypolipidemic agents, such as clofibrate, which can result in a five- to ten-fold increase in the relative contribution of peroxisomal fatty acid beta oxidation. Because peroxisomal beta oxidation produces less ATP than mitochondrial beta oxidation, a relative increase in peroxisomal fatty acid beta oxidation can lead to a reduction in lipid mass and weight loss. This pathway also provides a means of generating hydrogen peroxide, which can be used by catalase for the oxidation of substrates such as ethanol.

Greater triglyceride synthesis, reduced synthesis of lipid transport proteins (see later), and decreased beta oxidation can result in the accumulation of fat within hepatocytes (steatosis). A classic example of this process is alcoholic steatosis, which occurs when a large percentage of the total caloric intake is derived from ethanol. Alteration in the redox potential with excess NADH produced by ethanol metabolism results in an increased NADH/NAD ratio, which favors the formation of α-glycerol phosphate and thereby promotes triglyceride formation. In addition, higher NAD content in the mitochondria may reduce fatty acid beta oxidation, thereby contributing to fatty acid accumulation.[101]

Lipoproteins

Apolipoproteins (apos), which are synthesized by the liver, in combination with triglycerides, phospholipids, cholesterol, and cholesterol esters, constitute circulating lipoproteins, which mediate the transport of lipids from the liver into the plasma and from the plasma into the liver and other tissues. The liver also expresses cell surface receptors for circulating lipoproteins and modulates plasma levels of these important macromolecules. Lipoprotein trafficking has been reviewed elsewhere[102] and is summarized in the following section.

Types of Lipoproteins

Lipoproteins were originally classified according to their relative density, which is inversely related to their particle size. Listed in increasing order of density, they are: chylomicrons, very-low-density lipoproteins (VLDLs), intermediate-density lipoproteins (IDLs), low-density lipoproteins (LDLs), and high-density lipoproteins (HDLs). Density differences in these particles reflect the type and amount of specific lipids and the proportion of protein present within these lipoprotein fractions.[102] Specific apolipoproteins bind lipids to form lipoproteins, which are modified by enzymes in plasma or endothelial cells and act as ligands for specific lipoprotein receptors that mediate their uptake by target tissues.

The lipid components of lipoproteins are in constant dynamic flux because of delivery of lipids and cholesterol to cells, transfer to other lipoproteins (mediated by lipid transfer proteins), and catalysis by lipolytic enzymes. Triglycerides are the major lipids contained in chylomicrons generated in the intestinal epithelial cells and VLDL produced in the liver. They are the energy source for peripheral tissues as well as components of cellular membrane structures. Cholesterol is the major lipid in LDL and HDL. Cholesterol, unlike triglycerides, is used not as a fuel source but as a structural component of membranes and as a precursor for steroid hormones. Trafficking of cholesterol is usually in the form of cholesteryl ester, which is generated in the plasma by the activity of lecithin-cholesterol acyltransferase (LCAT) (see later).

Tangier's disease is a rare autosomal recessive disorder characterized by the accumulation of cholesteryl esters in reticuloendothelial cells, including the tonsils, thymus, and lymph nodes as well as the liver, spleen, and gallbladder, in combination with the near absence of serum HDL cholesterol. It is now recognized to be caused by mutations in the ATP-binding cassette transporter-A1 (ABCA1), a member of the ABC supergene family.[103] Affected patients classically present with enlarged, orange-colored tonsils and have a four- to six-fold higher risk of atherosclerotic heart disease. Although the function of the transporter is not completely known, its location at the plasma membrane suggests that it mediates the active transport ("flipping") of cholesterol ester from the inner to the outer leaflet of the plasma membrane, from which it can be transferred to apolipoproteins and secreted.[103]

Apolipoproteins

The major apolipoproteins associated with triglyceride transport are apoB-100, which is synthesized in the liver, and apoB-48, which is synthesized in the intestine.[104] Both proteins are translated from the same mRNA. In human intestinal epithelium, the apoB mRNA undergoes post-transcriptional RNA editing, which generates a stop codon by cytidine deamination and results in the trans-

lation of a form of apoB that is approximately 48% of the size of the full-length apoB-100 generated in the liver. The carboxy-terminal domain that is absent in apoB-48 is essential for binding to the LDL receptor. Unlike VLDL, which contains apoB-100, chylomicron remnants contain apoB-48, are cleared rapidly from plasma, and do not give rise to LDL.[104]

ApoC is synthesized predominantly in the liver with minor expression in the intestine and other organs. It comprises three different gene products that may inhibit the uptake of chylomicron remnants by the liver. ApoC-1 is a minor component of VLDL, HDL, and IDL, and its function is unknown. ApoC-II, present in VLDL, IDL, HDL, and chylomicrons, is an essential activator of lipoprotein lipase (LPL) (see later). Inherited deficiency of apoC-II causes hypertriglyceridemia. ApoC-III is present in IDL, HDL, and chylomicrons and may be an inhibitor of LPL activity.[105]

ApoE is synthesized in the liver and is found on all lipoproteins. ApoE is important for removal of lipoprotein remnants in the serum, can bind to the LDL receptor and other membrane proteins, and is important in targeting lipoproteins to specific receptors on peripheral cells. Three major alleles of the apoE gene exist (ε2, ε3, and ε4), with the ε3 allele being the most abundant and the ε2/ε3 genotype being the most common. Each allele possesses a different ability to bind to the LDL receptor. Absence of apoE leads to reduced clearance of chylomicron and VLDL remnants and results in elevated plasma values of these lipoproteins and a consequent increase in the risk of atherosclerosis.[106] ApoE is also important in lipid transport in the central nervous system, especially after neuronal injury. Inheritance of a single apoε4 allele is associated with the onset of Alzheimer's disease 6 to 8 years earlier than the onset associated with the ε3/ε3 genotype.[107]

ApoA-I and apoA-II are synthesized in the liver and intestine. ApoA-I is the major component of HDL lipoproteins. In a lipid-poor state, apoA-I accepts cholesterol from cell membranes. ApoA-I is a key activator of LCAT, which enhances cholesterol esterification in the plasma, and the absence of a specific, conserved region in apoA-I causes loss of its LCAT-activating property. ApoA-II is another component of HDL. ApoA-IV is a minor constituent synthesized in the intestine.[108]

Lipolytic Enzymes

Lipoprotein lipase (LPL) is synthesized in fat and muscle cells and is localized to the luminal surfaces of the capillary beds of adipose, lung, and muscle tissues.[109] LPL catalyzes lipolysis of triglycerides present in VLDL, chylomicrons, or HDL. LPL is stimulated by fasting, fatty acids, hormones, and catecholamines. Patients who are homozygous for LPL deficiency present with severe hypertriglyceridemia in childhood and pancreatitis.

Hepatic triglyceride lipase (HTGL) is another member of the lipase gene family. It is synthesized in the liver and binds to the luminal surfaces of hepatic endothelial cells. It is involved in lipolysis of VLDL or IDL and thus plays a major role in LDL formation. HDL may be another substrate for its activity.

Inherited deficiency of LPL leads to accumulation of large particles containing both apoB-100 and apoB-48, with almost complete absence of smaller apoB-containing lipoprotein. In animal studies, inhibition of HTGL results in accumulation of VLDL and IDL, with the enrichment of HDL in triglycerides.

Lipid Transport Proteins

In plasma, lipid exchange between particles is facilitated by the activity of LCAT and cholesteryl ester transfer protein (CETP).[109] LCAT is synthesized in the liver, and apoA-I is a cofactor for LCAT activity. CETP is synthesized predominantly in the liver and circulates in association with HDL. CETP mediates the exchange of cholesteryl esters from HDL with triglycerides from chylomicrons or VLDL. The activity of LCAT in combination with the lipid transfer proteins CETP and phospholipid transfer protein (PLTP) is essential for the transfer of cholesterol from nonhepatic tissue to the liver.[109]

Intestinal and Hepatic Lipid Transport

The liver functions as the hub for receiving fatty acids and cholesterol from the diet and peripheral tissues, packaging them into lipoprotein complexes, and releasing the complexes into the circulation (Fig. 69–4). After absorption by intestinal epithelial cells, fatty acids are formed

into triglycerides, and cholesterol is esterified. Both lipids are packaged into nascent chylomicrons composed predominantly of triglycerides (85% to 92%), phospholipids (6% to 12%), cholesteryl ester (1% to 3%), fat-soluble vitamins, and the apolipoproteins (1% to 3%) apoB-48, apoA-I, apoA-II, and apoA-IV.[110] Nascent chylomicrons enter the interstitial space and are carried into the systemic venous circulation via the thoracic duct. In the interstitial space, chylomicrons acquire apoC-II, which activates LPL, thereby promoting triglyceride release. Triglyceride release may be reduced by acquisition of apoC-III, which may inhibit LPL activity. Addition of apoE is critical for targeting of the chylomicron remnant, which can then be taken up by hepatocytes through the chylomicron remnant receptor.

Release of triglycerides by LPL and extraction by peripheral tissues raises the relative concentration of cholesteryl ester in chylomicron remnants, which are taken up by hepatocytes via a hepatocyte membrane transporter that recognizes a binding domain on apoE. The endocytosed chylomicron remnants are targeted to lysosomes, where they are degraded. Inherited mutations of the binding domain of apoE reduces the clearance of chylomicron remnants. When chylomicron excretion is delayed, as occurs with mutations of the binding domain

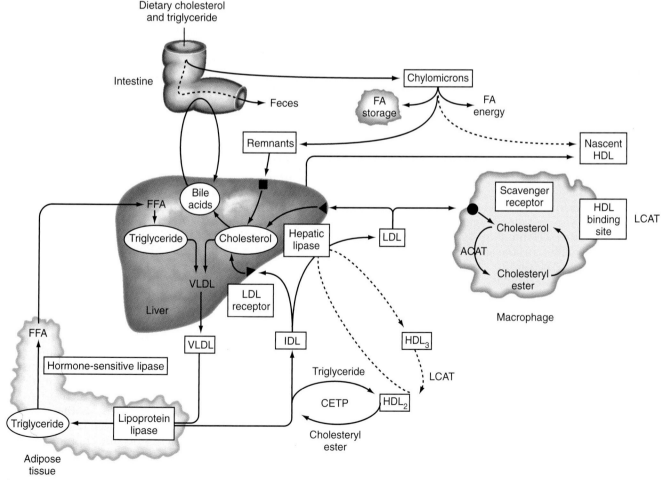

Figure 69–4 Lipoprotein metabolism. ACAT, acylcholesterol acyltransferase; CETP, cholesteryl ester transfer protein; FA, fatty acids; LDL, low-density lipoproteins; FFA, free fatty acids; HDL, high-density lipoproteins; LCAT, lecithin-cholesterol acyltransferase; VLDL, very-low-density lipoproteins. (Modified from Shepherd J: Lipoprotein metabolism: An overview. Drugs 47[Suppl 2]:2, 1994.)

of apoE or with reduced LPL activity or apoC-II levels, chylomicron remnants that accumulate in the serum may be taken up by endothelial cells or macrophages, which transform into foamy cells. The foamy cells are precursors of fatty streaks and atheromas. Increased VLDL secretion resulting from excess fatty acid absorption can also compete with the chylomicron remnant uptake system.

Fatty acids released from adipocytes by the action of intracellular hormone-sensitive lipase are bound to serum albumin and transported to other tissues, including the liver, where they are used for synthesis of phospholipids and triglycerides.[111] The liver synthesizes cholesterol from low-molecular-weight precursors. Hepatic cholesterol synthesis is regulated by the rate-limiting enzyme 3-hydroxy-3-methylglutaryl coenzyme A reductase (HMG-CoA reductase). Lipids are exported from the liver as VLDL particles, which are the major carriers of plasma triglycerides during nonabsorptive states.[83] Lipids may be stored temporarily in the liver as fat droplets and cholesteryl esters, excreted directly into bile, or metabolized into bile acids. The liver is the major site of sterol excretion from the body and is the site of bile acid synthesis (see Chapter 61).

The coordinated input, synthesis, and excretion of sterols require complex regulation of multiple enzymatic pathways. Bile acids returning to the liver via the enterohepatic circulation modulate these enzyme activities. Bile acids recycle 20 to 30 times per day via the enterohepatic circulation; specific transmembrane transporters at apical and basolateral domains of hepatocyte plasma membrane, as well as intracellular binding proteins, are involved in this process.[112] In the terminal ileum, a great majority of the bile acid molecules are reabsorbed via a sodium-dependent bile acid transporter. Bile acids are also important in the micellization of fats for intestinal absorption and as a coactivator of bile acid–dependent lipase activity. FXR, a member of the sterol nuclear receptor family, binds to and is activated by bile salts. Heterodimers of activated FXR and RXR modulate the coordinated regulation of multiple genes expressing key bile salt transporters, such as sodium-dependent taurocholate pump (NTCP) at the sinusoidal domain of hepatocytes, bile salt export pump (BSEP) at the canalicular domain, the intestinal bile acid transporter (IBAT) in the terminal ileum, and cholesterol-7α-hydroxylase in hepatocytes (see Chapter 61).[113]

Transport of ApoB-Containing Lipoproteins
In the fasting state, VLDLs, which are synthesized in the liver, replace chylomicrons as the major transporters of triglycerides and cholesterol. In addition to the full-length apoB-100, VLDL contains triglycerides (taken up from plasma or synthesized in the liver), cholesteryl esters (exogenous or endogenous), and phospholipids.[114] During fasting, fatty acids in VLDL are derived predominantly from the activity of hormone-sensitive lipase in adipocytes, whereas after a meal, dietary fatty acids are the major source. Fatty acids may be taken up by hepatocytes through passive diffusion or via fatty acid transport proteins in the sinusoidal domain of the cell membrane. In hepatocyte cytosol, fatty acids are stored bound to the abundant 12-kd fatty acid–binding protein (FABP) family, which may direct fatty acids to specific subcellular targets, such as the smooth ER for VLDL synthesis or peroxisomes for beta oxidation. FABPs are regulated transcriptionally by peroxisome-proliferating agents (e.g., fibrates), thereby suggesting that they have a physiologic role in global lipid metabolism.

ApoB-100 is the predominant transport carrier in VLDL; apoC-I, apoC-II, apoC-III, and apoE arise from other lipoproteins within the serum. ApoB-100 synthesis and VLDL secretion are regulated by the availability of cotransported lipids and sterols in the smooth ER. ApoB-100 synthesis may change dramatically without an alteration in apoB-100 mRNA levels.[115] After synthesis in the smooth ER, apoB-100 interacts with newly synthesized triglycerides and cholesteryl esters that enter the ER via specific membrane transporters. The apoB-lipid complex is translocated into the lumen, transported through the Golgi apparatus, and secreted into the sinusoidal space as VLDL. When the lipid components are not available, apoB-100 undergoes degradation in the ER. During periods of low triglyceride levels, the liver secretes smaller IDL-like particles or even LDL-type particles.

In the plasma, the activity of LPL and HTGL removes triglycerides from VLDL, thereby generating progressively smaller and denser IDL and LDL particles. Conversion of IDL to LDL requires the activity of apoE. LDL particles become enriched in cholesteryl esters, through both removal of triglycerides and acquisition of cholesteryl ester from other lipoproteins, predominantly HDL, with release of apoC to HDL. LDL subsequently is removed from the circulation by LDL receptors in the liver and peripheral tissues. Subpopulations of VLDL that begin as large VLDL undergo lipolysis to be converted to IDL, which is taken up via the LDL receptor.

Transport of ApoA-Containing High-Density Lipoprotein
HDL, another major class of lipoproteins secreted by the liver, appears to have a protective role against atherosclerosis. HDL is a heterogeneous population of lipoproteins that can be separated by sophisticated analytic centrifugation techniques. Nascent HDL is formed in the liver and intestine by lipolysis from VLDL and chylomicrons, respectively, with modification by peripheral tissue. The major protein constituents of HDL are apoA-I and apoA-II, with minor amounts of apoA-IV, apoC, apoE, and others.[116] In humans, apoA-I is synthesized in the liver and intestine. Nascent apoA-containing lipoprotein complexes that appear as discoid particles can be transformed into HDL particles in the serum by the action of LCAT and the lipid transfer proteins CETP and PLTP.

The HDL_3 subclass is particularly important because the cholesterol-poor particles are able to deliver cholesterol extracted from peripheral membranes and provide a substrate for plasma LCAT activity. Cholesteryl esters formed by LCAT are extremely hydrophobic and move into the core of the lipoprotein complex, thereby providing space on the surface of the lipoprotein for extraction of additional cholesterol from cell membranes. This complex enlarges with increasing amounts of cholesteryl esters, which are able to accommodate apoC-II and apoC-III, thereby resulting in HDL_2 formation. CETP removes esterified cholesterol out of HDL in exchange for triglycerides, which eventually are hydrolyzed by HTGL, thereby regenerating small HDL. Acquisition of apoC-II also promotes LPL activity, thereby increasing lipolysis.[109]

The movement of apolipoproteins between HDL and chylomicrons allows the recycling of lipids and proteins between these two pools. Cholesterol and phospholipids also are transferred to the chylomicrons, as triglycerides are released by LPL activity to local tissues. As the remnant is processed further, apoC-II and apoC-III, phospholipids, and cholesterol are transferred back to HDL. Triglycerides that are transferred from VLDL and chylomicrons to HDL are more accessible to lipolysis by endothelium-based lipases because of their smaller size. With the removal of triglycerides, these particles revert to HDL$_3$ and apoC-II, after which apoC-II and apoE recycle to chylomicrons and VLDL.

Lipoprotein Receptors

The major lipoprotein receptors for LDL, chylomicron remnants, and HDL and the LDL scavenger receptor are members of the larger LDL receptor supergene family.[117] These receptors share the following four major structural features: (1) cysteine-rich complement-type repeats, (2) EGF precursor-like repeats, (3) a transmembrane domain, and (4) a cytoplasmic domain.[118]

LDL Receptor

The LDL receptor exists as an oligomeric surface glycoprotein that plays a pivotal role in LDL clearance and cholesterol homeostasis. It binds ligands at the cell surface, after which the ligand-receptor complex is internalized via the classic endocytotic pathway. The ligand dissociates from the receptor in acidic endosomal vesicles. After this, the ligand is delivered to lysosomes for degradation, and the receptor returns to the surface. The LDL receptor is present on all cell types; however, the liver contains approximately 70% of the total body pool of LDL receptors. The LDL receptor recognizes apoE and apoB-100 but not apoB-48. ApoE-containing chylomicron remnants, VLDL, LDL, IDL, and HDL can all be taken up via the LDL receptor. Approximately two thirds of LDL is cleared by this receptor. Homozygous deficiency of functional LDL receptor occurs in approximately 1 in 1 million persons and is associated with accelerated atherosclerosis, presenting in childhood (familial hypercholesterolemia). LDL receptors are highly conserved among species.[117]

Very-Low-Density Lipoprotein Receptor

The VLDL receptor has a high sequence homology with the LDL receptor but is expressed predominantly in extrahepatic tissues such as heart, muscle, and fat. Unlike the LDL receptor, the VLDL receptor does not bind to apoB, and it may serve to take up specifically triglyceride-rich apoE-containing lipoproteins, such as VLDL and IDL.[117,118]

Chylomicron Remnant Receptor

The chylomicron remnant receptor accepts apoE as a ligand. Chylomicron remnants are removed from the circulation exclusively by the liver, probably because these large complexes can penetrate the unique sinusoidal vascular space. The chylomicron remnant receptor is the multifunctional α_2-macroglobulin/LDL receptor-related protein (LRP).[119] LRP is present in liver, brain, and muscle. In cultured cells, LRP is able to mediate the endocytosis of apoE-containing chylomicron remnants. Mice that lack LRP in the liver do not have hepatic chylomicron remnant uptake, thereby confirming that LRP is the major chylomicron remnant receptor. Unlike the LDL receptor, LRP is able to bind a number of unrelated ligands, such as lipoprotein, proteinase-inhibitor complex, and protein-lipid complex.

Low-Density Lipoprotein Scavenger Receptors

Ligands for the scavenger receptor A (SR-A) include lipopolysaccharides, polyanionic lipids, and LDL in which some of the free lysine residues have been chemically modified.[120] These receptors exist in two forms as trimeric integral membrane glycoproteins in endothelial cells, macrophages, and Kupffer cells. Oxidized LDL is internalized via the scavenger receptors but is metabolized poorly in macrophages, leading to the accumulation of cholesteryl esters within the cell. Monocytes, which migrate into lipid-enriched atherosclerotic lesions, can also be induced to express the scavenger receptor.

High-Density Lipoprotein Receptor

A high-affinity HDL-binding protein has been identified in the plasma membrane of hepatocytes, macrophages, adrenal cells, and adipocytes.[120] These receptors appear to recognize apoA present in HDL particles specifically. The HDL receptor does not mediate endocytosis but allows only selective delivery of lipids to and from the HDL lipoproteins. By mediating the transfer of cholesterol from the plasma membrane to the HDL lipoprotein, the HDL receptor facilitates reverse cholesterol transport. The HDL receptor is a class B scavenger receptor, referred to as SR-B1.[116] This receptor is most abundant in the liver, ovary, and adrenal glands—organs shown previously to be the principal sites of cholesterol uptake from HDL in vivo. HDL is a major source of cholesterol secreted in bile. Overexpression of SR-B1 in mouse liver increases biliary cholesterol secretion and reduces plasma HDL levels.[121] Conversely, deficiency of this receptor results in diminished biliary cholesterol secretion.[122]

Derangement of Lipid Metabolism in Liver Disease

The most common lipid abnormality in chronic liver disease is hypertriglyceridemia (250 to 500 mg/dL), which is found in both alcoholic and viral liver diseases and tends to resolve when the liver disease improves. Excess ethanol ingestion causes predominantly hypertriglyceridemia, as a result of increased fatty acid synthesis and decreased beta oxidation of fatty acids, owing to greater NADH production by alcohol metabolism. Moderate alcohol ingestion is associated with increased HDL$_3$ levels, which may reduce the risk of atherosclerosis. LDL, HDL, and total serum cholesterol levels decrease progressively as cirrhosis advances from Child-Turcotte-Pugh class A to class C (see Chapters 70 and 87). The serum cholesterol level may be a useful prognostic marker in noncholestatic liver diseases.[123]

Cholestatic disorders manifest as a distinct pattern of dyslipoproteinemia because of the retention of cholesterol, phospholipids, and bile salts that are normally secreted in bile.[124] A prolonged increase in total serum cholesterol and lipid levels, as seen in primary biliary cirrhosis, can be associated with xanthoma formation. Within the LDL fraction of the serum of cholestatic patients, three distinct lipoproteins can be identified, namely, β_2-lipoprotein (triglyceride rich), also known as lipoprotein Y (LP-Y), lipoprotein X (LP-X), and normal LDL. LP-Y appears to be a remnant of a triglyceride-rich lipoprotein that is distinct from IDL. Cholestatic patients with elevated serum triglyceride values often have clear serum because most of the triglycerides are contained in LP-Y and LDL. LP-X is a complex composed of equimolar amounts of excess phospholipid and cholesterol in combination with albumin and certain members of the apoC family. The phospholipid flippase activity of multidrug resistance protein-3 (MDR3), also termed ATP-binding cassette protein B4 (ABCB4) (see Chapter 61) is essential for LP-X formation. Mice that lack mdr2 (the murine homolog of MDR3) are unable to form LP-X during cholestasis due to complete bile duct obstruction.[125]

In patients with chronic parenchymal liver disease, plasma cholesteryl ester levels are often reduced, a finding that suggests that LCAT activity is diminished because of impaired hepatic synthesis. Alternatively, decreased LCAT activity may result from reduced apoC-II levels or release of cholesteryl ester hydrolase from damaged hepatocytes, with conversion of cholesteryl esters to cholesterol. Chronic dyslipoproteinemia in affected patients also can lead to alterations in cellular membrane lipids that result in formation of abnormal RBCs, such as echinocytes, and alterations in membrane function with potential pathophysiologic consequences.

REFERENCES

1. Desmet VJ: Organizational principles. In Arias IM, Boyer JL, Chisari FV, et al (eds): The Liver: Biology and Pathobiology, 4th ed. Philadelphia, Lippincott Williams & Wilkins, 2001, p 3.
2. Saxena R, Zucker SD, Crawford JM: Anatomy and physiology of the liver. In Zakim D, Boyer TD (eds): Hepatology: A Textbook of Liver Diseases, 4th ed. Philadelphia, WB Saunders, 2003, p 3.
3. Zegers MMP, Hoekstra D: Mechanisms and functional features of polarized membrane traffic in epithelial and hepatic cells. Biochem J 336:257, 1998.
4. Singer SJ: The molecular organization of membranes. Annu Rev Biochem 43:805, 1974.
5. Simons K, Toomre D: Lipid rafts and signal transduction. Nat Rev Mol Cell Biol 1:31, 2000.
6. Schachter D: The hepatocyte plasma membrane: Organization, differentiation, biogenesis and turnover. In Arias IM, Boyer JL, Chisari FV, et al (eds): The Liver: Biology and Pathobiology, 4th ed. Philadelphia, Lippincott Williams & Wilkins, 2001, p 77.
7. Kumar NM, Gilula NB: The gap junction communication channel. Cell 84:381, 1996.
8. Novikoff PM, Cammer M, Tao L, et al: Three-dimensional organization of rat hepatocyte cytoskeleton: Relation to the asialoglycoprotein endocytosis pathway. J Cell Sci 109:21, 1996.
9. Roma MG, Milkiewicz P, Elias E, Coleman R: Control by signaling modulators of the sorting of canalicular transporters in rat hepatocyte couplets: Role of the cytoskeleton. Hepatology 32:1342, 2000.
10. Moll R, Franke WW, Schiller DL, et al: The catalog of human cytokeratins: Patterns of expression in normal epithelia, tumors and cultured cells. Cell 31:11, 1982.
11. Brinkley BR: Microtubule-organizing centers. Annu Rev Cell Biol 1:145, 1985.
12. Sobel HJ, Marquet E: Zipper-like structure and centrioles in hepatocytes. Ultrastruct Pathol 4:115, 1983.
13. Satir P: Motor molecules. In Arias IM, Boyer JL, Chisari FV, et al (eds): The Liver: Biology and Pathobiology, 4th ed. Philadelphia, Lippincott Williams & Wilkins, 2001, p 47.
14. Tzanakakis ES, Hansen LK, Hu WS: The role of actin filaments and microtubules in hepatocyte spheroid self-assembly. Cell Motil Cytoskeleton 48:175, 2001.
15. Blom WM, de Bont HJ, Meijerman I, et al: Remodeling of the actin cytoskeleton of target hepatocytes and NK cells during induction of apoptosis. Cell Motil Cytoskeleton 49:78, 2001.
16. Newport J, Forbes DJ: The nucleus: Structure, function and dynamics. Annu Rev Biochem 56:535, 1987.
17. Miller M, Park MK, Hanover JA: Nuclear pore complex: Structure, function, and regulation. Physiol Rev 71:909, 1991.
18. Nakielny S, Dreyfuss G: Transport of proteins and RNAs in and out of the nucleus. Cell 99:677, 1999.
19. DePierre JW, Dallner G: Structural aspects of the membrane of the endoplasmic reticulum. Biochim Biophys Acta 415:411, 1975.
20. Sitia R, Meldolesi J: Endoplasmic reticulum: A dynamic patchwork of specialized subregions. Mol Biol Cell 3:1067, 1993.
21. Hauri H-P, Schweizer A: Relationship of the ER-Golgi intermediate compartment to endoplasmic reticulum and Golgi apparatus. Curr Opin Cell Biol 4:600, 1992.
22. Altan-Bonnet N, Sougrat R, Lippincott-Schwartz J: Molecular basis for Golgi maintenance and biogenesis. Curr Opin Cell Biol 16:364, 2004.
23. deDuve C, Wattiaux R: Functions of lysosomes. Ann Rev Physiol 28:435, 1966.
24. Swanson J, Bushnell A, Silverstein SC: Tubular lysosome morphology and distribution within macrophages is dependent on the integrity of cytoplasmic microtubules. Proc Natl Acad Sci U S A 84:1921, 1987.
25. Stein M, Zijderhand-Bleekemolen JE, Geuze H, et al: Mr 46,000 mannose 6-phosphate specific receptor: Its role in targeting of lysosomal enzymes. EMBO J 6:2677, 1987.
26. Mayor S, Presley JF, Maxfield FR: Sorting of membrane components from endosomes and subsequent recycling to the cell surface occurs by a bulk flow process. J Cell Biol 121:1257, 1993.
27. Dunn KW, Maxfield FR: Delivery of ligands from sorting endosomes to late endosomes occurs by maturation of sorting endosomes. J Cell Biol 117:301, 1992.
28. Srere PA: The structure of the mitochondrial inner membrane-matrix compartment. Trends Biochem Sci 7:375, 1982.
29. Ernster L, Kuylenstierna B: Outer membrane of mitochondria. In Racker E (ed): Membranes of Mitochondria and Chloroplasts. New York, Van Nostrand Reinhold, 1970, p 172.
30. Ontko JA, Dashti N: Enzymes of mitochondria. In Altman PI, Katz DD (eds): Cell Biology. Bethesda, MD, Federation of American Societies for Experimental Biology, 1976, p 161.
31. Hinkle PC, Kumar MA, Resetar A, Harris DL: Mechanistic stoichiometry of mitochondrial oxidative phosphorylation. Biochemistry 30:3576, 1991.

32. Newmeyer DD, Ferguson-Miller S: Mitochondria: Releasing power for life and unleashing the machineries of death. Cell 112:481, 2003.

33. Racker E, Hortsman LL: Partial resolution of the enzymes catalyzing oxidative phosphorylation. XIII: Structure and function of submitochondrial particles completely resolved with respect to coupling factor. J Biol Chem 242:2547, 1967.

34. Walker JE: The NADH: Ubiquinone oxidoreductase (complex I) of respiratory chains. Q Rev Biophys 25:253, 1992.

35. Trumpower BL: The protonmotive Q cycle: Energy transduction by coupling of proton translocation to electron transfer by the cytochrome bc1 complex. J Biol Chem 265:11409, 1990.

36. Gould SJ, Raymond GV, Valle D: The peroxisome biogenesis disorders. In Scriver CR, Beaudet AL, Sly WS, Valle D (eds): The Metabolic and Molecular Bases of Inherited Disease, 8th ed. New York, McGraw Hill, 2001, p 3181.

37. Bannykh SI, Rowe T, Balch WE: The organization of endoplasmic reticulum export complexes. J Cell Biol 135:19, 1996.

38. Rothman JE: Mechanisms of intracellular protein transport. Nature 372:55, 1994.

39. Harter C: COP-coated vesicles in intracellular protein transport. FEBS Lett 369:89, 1995.

40. Zhao L, Helms JB, Brugger B, et al: Direct and GTP-dependent interaction of ADP ribosylation factor 1 with coatomer subunit beta. Proc Natl Acad Sci U S A 94:4418, 1997.

41. Saucan L, Palade GE: Membrane and secretory proteins are transported from the Golgi complex to the sinusoidal plasmalemma of hepatocytes by distinct vesicular carriers. J Cell Biol 125:733, 1994.

42. Conner SD, Schmid SL: Regulated portals of entry into the cell. Nature 422:37, 2003.

43. Crowther RA, Pearse BM: Assembly and packing of clathrin into coats. J Cell Biol 91:790, 1981.

44. Hemery I, Durand-Schneider AM, Feldmann G, et al: The transcytotic pathway of an apical plasma membrane protein (B10) in hepatocytes is similar to that of IgA and occurs via a tubular pericentriolar compartment. J Cell Sci 109:1215, 1996.

45. Stockert RJ: Receptor-mediated endocytosis. In Arias IM, Boyer JL, Chisari FV, et al (eds): The Liver: Biology and Pathobiology, 4th ed. Philadelphia, Lippincott Williams & Wilkins, 2001, p 161.

46. Cohen AW, Hnasko R, Schubert W, Lisanti MP: Role of caveolae and caveolins in health and disease. Physiol Rev 84:1341, 2004.

47. Alpini G, McGill JM, Larusso NF: The pathobiology of biliary epithelia. Hepatology 35:1256, 2002.

48. Benedetti A, Bassotti C, Rapino K, et al: A morphometric study of the epithelium lining the rat intrahepatic biliary tree. J Hepatol 24:335, 1996.

49. Ramadori G, Reider H, Knittel T: Biology and pathobiology of sinusoidal liver cells. In Tavoloni N, Berk PD (eds): Hepatic Transport and Bile Secretion: Physiology and Pathophysiology. New York, Raven Press, 1993, p 83.

50. Arias IM: The biology of hepatic endothelial fenestrae. Prog Liver Dis 9:11, 1990.

51. Wake K, Decker K, Kirn A, et al: Cell biology and kinetics of Kupffer cells in the liver. Int Rev Cytol 118:173, 1989.

52. Rogoff TM, Lipsky PE: Role of Kupffer cells in local and systemic immune responses. Gastroenterology 80:854, 1981.

53. Sato M, Suzuki S, Senoo H: Hepatic stellate cells: Unique characteristics in cell biology and phenotype. Cell Struct Funct 28:105, 2003.

54. Senoo H: Structure and function of hepatic stellate cells. Med Electron Microsc 37:3, 2004.

55. Hui AY, Friedman SL: Molecular basis of hepatic fibrosis. Expert Rev Mol Med 14:1, 2003.

56. Doherty DG, O'Farrelly C: Innate and adaptive lymphoid cells in the human liver. Immunol Rev 174:5, 2000.

57. Wisse E, Luo D, Vermijlen D, et al: On the function of pit cells, the liver-specific natural killer cells. Semin Liver Dis 17:265, 1997.

58. Bedossa P, Paradis V: Liver extracellular matrix in health and disease. J Pathol 200:504, 2003.

59. Hynes RO: Integrins: Bidirectional, allosteric signaling machines. Cell 110:673, 2002.

60. Jaeschke H: Cellular adhesion molecules: Regulation and functional significance in the pathogenesis of liver diseases. Am J Physiol 273:G602, 1997.

61. Mitaka T: Reconstruction of hepatic organoid by hepatic stem cells. J Hepatobil Pancreat Surg 9:697, 2002.

62. Greenwal P, Rojkind M: The extracellular matrix of the liver. In Arias IM, Boyer JL, Chisari FV, et al (eds): The Liver: Biology and Pathobiology, 4th ed. Philadelphia, Lippincott Williams & Wilkins, 2001, p 469.

63. Steer CJ: Liver regeneration. FASEB J 9:1396, 1995.

64. Fausto N: Liver regeneration and repair: Hepatocytes, progenitor cells, and stem cells. Hepatology 39:1477, 2004.

65. Taub R: Liver regeneration: From myth to mechanism. Nature Rev 5:836, 2004.

66. Malik R, Selden C, Hodgson H: The role of non-parenchymal cells in liver growth. Semin Cell Dev Biol 13:425, 2002.

67. Michalopoulos GK, DeFrances MC: Liver regeneration. Science 276:60, 1997.

68. Wyllie AH: Apoptosis and carcinogenesis. Eur J Cell Biol 73:189, 1997.

69. Yin XM, Ding WX: Death receptor activation-induced hepatocyte apoptosis and liver injury. Curr Mol Med 3:491, 2003.

70. Kim JS, He L, Qian T, Lemasters JJ: Role of the mitochondrial permeability transition in apoptotic and necrotic death after ischemia/reperfusion injury to hepatocytes. Curr Mol Med 3:527, 2003.

71. Burt AP, Day CP: Pathophysiology of the liver. In MacSween RNM, Burt AD, et al. (eds): Pathology of the Liver, 4th ed. London, Churchill Livingstone, p 67.

72. Cereghini S: Liver-enriched transcription factors and hepatocyte differentiation. FASEB J 10:267, 1996.

73. Karpen SJ: Nuclear receptor regulation of hepatic function. J Hepatol 36:832, 2002.

74. Gething M-J, Sambrook J: Protein folding in the cell. Nature 355:33, 1992.

75. Hammond C, Helenius A: Quality control in the secretory pathway. Curr Opin Cell Biol 7:525, 1995.

76. Bonaficio JS, Lippincott-Schwartz J: Degradation of proteins within the endoplasmic reticulum. Curr Opin Cell Biol 3:592, 1991.

77. Klionsky DJ, Emr SD: Autophagy as a regulated pathway of cellular degradation. Science 290:1717, 2000.

78. Lecker SH, Solomon V, Mitch WE, Goldberg AL: Muscle protein breakdown and the critical role of the ubiquitin-proteosome pathway in normal and disease states. J Nutr 129:227S, 1999.

79. Glotzer M, Murray AW, Kirschner MW: Cyclin is degraded by the ubiquitin pathway. Nature 349:132, 1991.

80. Hershko A: The ubiquitin pathway of protein degradation and proteolysis of ubiquitin-protein conjugates. Biochem Soc Trans 19:726, 1991.

81. Riezman H, Munn A, Geli MI, Hicke L: Actin-, myosin- and ubiquitin-dependent endocytosis. Experientia 52:1033, 1996.

82. Kolling R, Hollenberg CP: The ABC-transporter Ste6 accumulates in the plasma membrane in a ubiquitinated form in endocytosis mutants. EMBO J 13:3261, 1994.

83. Seifter S, Englard S: Energy metabolism. In Arias IM (ed): The Liver: Biology and Pathobiology, 3rd ed. New York, Raven Press, 1994, p 323.

84. Felber JP, Golay A: Regulation of nutrient metabolism and energy expenditure. Metabolism 44:4, 1995.

85. Pilkis SJ, Granner DK: Molecular physiology of the regulation of hepatic gluconeogenesis and glycolysis. Annu Rev Physiol 54:885, 1992.

86. Pessin JE, Bell GI: Mammalian facilitative glucose transporter family: Structure and molecular regulation. Annu Rev Physiol 54:911, 1992.

87. Nordlie RC, Foster JD, Lange AJ: Regulation of glucose production by the liver. Annu Rev Nutr 19:379, 1999.

88. Van Schaftingen E: Glycolysis revisited. Diabetologia 36:581, 1993.

89. Matschinsky FM: Glucokinase as glucose sensor and metabolic signal generator in pancreatic beta-cells and hepatocytes. Diabetes 39:647, 1990.

90. Van Schaftingen E, Detheux M, Veiga da Cunha M: Short-term control of glucokinase activity: Role of a regulatory protein. FASEB J 8:414, 1994.

91. Burchell A: Hepatic microsomal glucose transport. Biochem Soc Trans 22:658, 1994.

92. Vaulont S, Kahn A: Transcriptional control of metabolic regulation genes by carbohydrates. FASEB J 8:28, 1994.

93. McGarry JD, Kuwajima M, Newgard CB, et al: From dietary glucose to liver glycogen: The full circle round. Annu Rev Nutr 7:51, 1987.

94. Foster DW: Banting Lecture 1984: From glycogen to ketones and back. Diabetes 33:1188, 1984.

95. Nolte W, Hartmann H, Ramadori G: Glucose metabolism and liver cirrhosis. Exp Clin Endocrinol Diabetes 103:63, 1995.

96. Coppack SW, Jensen MD, Miles JM: In vivo regulation of lipolysis in humans. J Lipid Res 35:177, 1994.

97. Osmundsen H, Bremer J, Pedersen JI: Metabolic aspects of peroxisomal beta-oxidation. Biochim Biophys Acta 1085:141, 1991.

98. Kim KH, Tae HJ: Pattern and regulation of acetyl-CoA carboxylase gene expression. J Nutr 124:1273S, 1994.

99. Kerner J, Hoppel D: Fatty acid import into mitochondria. Biochim Biophys Acta 1486:1, 2001.

100. Bremer J: The role of carnitine in intracellular metabolism. J Clin Chem Clin Biochem 28:297, 1990.

101. Lieber CS: Biochemical factors in alcoholic liver disease. Semin Liver Dis 13:136, 1993.

102. Miller JP: Liver disease, alcohol and lipoprotein metabolism. In Zakim D, Boyer TD (eds): Hepatology: A Textbook of Liver Diseases, 4th ed. Philadelphia, WB Saunders, 2003, p 127.

103. Oram JF: Tangier disease and ABCA1. Biochim Biophys Acta 1529:321, 2000.

104. Teng B, Burant CF, Davidson NO: Molecular cloning of an apolipoprotein B messenger RNA editing protein. Science 260:1816, 1993.

105. Jong MC, Hofker MH, Havekes LM: Role of ApoCs in lipoprotein metabolism: Functional differences between ApoC1, ApoC2, and ApoC3. Arterioscler Thromb Vasc Biol 19:472, 1999.

106. Mahley RW, Ji ZS: Remnant lipoprotein metabolism: Key pathways involving cell-surface heparan sulfate proteoglycans and apolipoprotein E. J Lipid Res 40:1, 1999.

107. Saunders AM, Trowers MK, Shimkets RA, et al: The role of apolipoprotein E in Alzheimer's disease: Pharmacogenomic target selection. Biochim Biophys Acta 1502:85, 2000.

108. Tall AR: Plasma high-density lipoproteins: Metabolism and relationship to atherogenesis. J Clin Invest 86:379, 1990.

109. Bruce C, Chouinard RA, Tall AR: Plasma lipid transfer proteins, high-density lipoproteins, and reverse cholesterol transport. Annu Rev Nutr 18:297, 1998.

110. Hussain MM: A proposed model for the assembly of chylomicrons. Atherosclerosis 148:1, 2000.

111. Yeaman SJ: Hormone-sensitive lipase: A multipurpose enzyme in lipid metabolism. Biochim Biophys Acta 1052:128, 1990.

112. Meier PJ: Molecular mechanisms of hepatic bile salt transport from sinusoidal blood into bile. Am J Physiol 269:G801, 1995.

113. Sinal CJ, Tohkin M, Miyata M, et al: Targeted disruption of the nuclear receptor FXR/BAR impairs bile acid and lipid homeostasis. Cell 102:731, 2000.

114. Yao Z, McLeod RS: Synthesis and secretion of hepatic apolipoprotein B-containing lipoproteins. Biochim Biophys Acta 1212:152, 1994.

115. Davis RA: Cell and molecular biology of the assembly and secretion of apolipoprotein B-containing lipoproteins by the liver. Biochim Biophys Acta 1440:1, 1999.

116. Krieger M: Charting the fate of the "good cholesterol": Identification and characterization of the high-density lipoprotein receptor SR-BI. Annu Rev Biochem 68:523, 1999.

117. Hussain MM, Strickland DK, Bakillah A: The mammalian low-density lipoprotein receptor family. Annu Rev Nutr 19:141, 1999.

118. Willnow TE: The low-density lipoprotein receptor gene family: Multiple roles in lipid metabolism. J Mol Med 77:306, 1999.

119. Rohlmann A, Gotthardt M, Hammer RE, et al: Inducible inactivation of hepatic LRP gene by cre-mediated recombination confirms role of LRP in clearance of chylomicron remnants. J Clin Invest 101:689, 1998.

120. Fielding CJ, Fielding PE: Molecular physiology of reverse cholesterol transport. J Lipid Res 36:211, 1995.

121. Kozarsky KF, Donahee MH, Rigotti A, et al: Overexpression of the HDL receptor SR-B1 alters plasma HDL and bile cholesterol levels. Nature 387:414, 1997.

122. Rigotti A, Trigatti BL, Penman M, et al: A targeted mutation in the murine gene encoding the high density lipoprotein (HDL) metabolism. Proc Natl Acad Sci U S A 94:12610, 1997.

123. Cicognani C, Malavolti M, Morselli-Labate AM, et al: Serum lipid and lipoprotein patterns in patients with liver cirrhosis and chronic active hepatitis. Arch Intern Med 157:792, 1997.

124. Miller JP: Dyslipoproteinaemia of liver disease. Baillieres Clin Endocrinol Metab 4:807, 1990.

125. Oude Elferink RP, Ottenhoff R, van Marle J, et al: Class III P-glycoproteins mediate the formation of lipoprotein X in the mouse. J Clin Invest 102:1749, 1998.

CHAPTER
70 Liver Chemistry and Function Tests

Aijaz Ahmed and Emmet B. Keeffe

The term "liver function tests" is a misnomer and can be misleading. Biochemical assessment of the liver is provided by true tests of hepatic synthetic function, which consist of the serum albumin level and prothrombin time, liver enzyme values, and the serum bilirubin level, a test of hepatic excretory function. The serum albumin level and prothrombin time can be influenced by nonhepatic factors in the setting of a normally functioning liver. Levels of liver enzymes (serum aminotransferases and alkaline phosphatase) and the serum bilirubin are markers of hepatobiliary disease and also provide useful diagnostic clues to the type of underlying liver disease. The constellation of laboratory tests that involve hepatic synthetic function (serum albumin and prothrombin time), liver enzymes, and the serum bilirubin level is referred to as *liver biochemical tests* or *liver function tests* (LFTs). Clinical evaluation of patients in whom liver disease is suspected involves accurate interpretation of abnormalities in liver biochemical test results in the context of a carefully obtained history and thorough physical examination.[1-5] The severity and pattern of abnormalities in biochemical liver test results can be distinctive or nonspecific. Recognition of characteristic fluctuations in liver biochemical parameters may facilitate a pragmatic clinical evaluation that includes biochemical testing for disease-specific markers, radiologic imaging, and liver biopsy.

BIOCHEMICAL MARKERS OF HEPATIC INJURY

The clinical significance of commonly used liver biochemical tests is summarized in Table 70–1.[3] The pattern of liver biochemical test result abnormalities may suggest predominantly hepatocellular necrosis or cholestatic injury. A substantial number of patients may present with abnormalities that characterize a mixed pattern of hepatic damage. In addition, assessment of hepatic synthetic function provides important information in patients with underlying cirrhosis.

HEPATOCELLULAR NECROSIS

Aminotransferases

Aspartate aminotransferase (AST, or serum glutamic oxaloacetic transaminase [SGOT]) and alanine aminotransferase (ALT, or serum glutamic pyruvic transaminase [SGPT]) are categorized as the aminotransferases. The aminotransferases catalyze the transfer of amino groups from aspartic acid or alanine to ketoglutaric acid to form oxaloacetic acid and pyruvic acid, respectively, during gluconeogenesis. ALT is localized primarily in the liver and is confined to the cytoplasm, whereas AST can be isolated from the liver and a wide variety of extrahepatic sites, including myocardium, skeletal muscle, kidney, brain, pancreas, and blood cells, in both cytoplasm and mitochondria. Normal serum ALT and AST levels correlate with body mass index.

Elevated serum aminotransferase levels indicate hepatocyte injury or hepatocellular necrosis. The leakage of aminotransferases from hepatocytes as a result of hepatocellular injury can be triggered by various types of liver diseases, including viral hepatitis, ischemic injury, and toxin- or drug-induced hepatotoxicity. It is important to confirm the hepatic origin of an isolated serum

Table 70–1   Clinical Significance of Liver Biochemical Tests

Test (Normal Range*)	Basis of Abnormality	Associated Liver Diseases	Extrahepatic Origin
Aminotransferases ALT (10–55 U/L) AST (10–40 U/L)	Leakage from damaged tissue	Mild to moderate elevations: many types of liver disease Marked elevations: hepatitis (viral, toxic, autoimmune, and ischemic) AST/ALT > 2 suggests alcoholic liver disease or cirrhosis of any etiology	ALT, more specific than AST for hepatic injury AST, nonspecific: can originate from skeletal muscle, red blood cell, kidney, pancreas, brain, and myocardium
AP (45–115 U/L)	Overproduction and leakage into serum	Moderate elevations: many types of liver disease Marked elevations: extrahepatic and intrahepatic cholestasis, diffuse infiltrating disease (e.g., tumor, MAC), rarely alcoholic hepatitis	Bone growth or disease (e.g., tumor, fracture, Paget's disease), placenta, intestine, and tumors
GGTP (0–30 U/L)	?Overproduction and leakage into serum	Same as for AP; induced by ethanol and drugs GGTP/AP >2.5 suggests alcoholic liver disease	Kidney, spleen, pancreas, heart, lung, and brain
5'-Nucleotidase (0–11 U/L)	?Overproduction and leakage into serum	Same as for AP	Found in many tissues, but serum elevation is relatively specific for liver disease
Bilirubin (0.0–1.0 mg/dL)	Decreased hepatic clearance	Moderate elevations: many types of liver disease Marked elevations: extrahepatic and intrahepatic bile duct obstruction, viral, alcoholic or drug-induced hepatitis, inherited hyperbilirubinemia	Increased breakdown of hemoglobin (resulting from hemolysis, disordered erythropoiesis, resorption of hematoma) or myoglobin (resulting from muscle injury)
Prothrombin time (PT) (10.9–12.5 seconds) (International Normalized Ratio [INR]: 0.9–1.2)	Decreased synthetic capacity	Acute or chronic liver failure (prolonged PT unresponsive to vitamin K) Biliary obstruction (prolonged PT usually responsive to vitamin K administration)	Vitamin K deficiency (secondary to malabsorption, malnutrition, antibiotics), consumptive coagulopathy
Albumin (3.5–5.0 g/dL)	Decreased synthesis; ?Increased catabolism	Chronic liver failure	Decreased in nephrotic syndrome, protein-losing enteropathy, vascular leak, malnutrition, malignancy, infections, and inflammatory states

ALT, alanine aminotransferase; AP, alkaline phosphatase; AST, aspartate aminotransferase; GGTP, gamma glutamyl transpeptidase; MAC, *Mycobacterium avium* complex.
*The normal values tabulated are for adult men and will vary with the methodology used in testing.

AST elevation by checking the serum ALT level. In patients with isolated or disproportionate elevation of serum AST, an extrahepatic origin of AST, such as myocardial or skeletal muscle injury, may have to be excluded. The serum AST level can be raised several-fold by vigorous physical activity, including hiking, marathon running, weight lifting, and wrestling. Muscle-related diseases, such as rhabdomyolysis, muscular dystrophy, and polymyositis, can be associated with isolated elevation of the serum AST level.[6-8] Rarely, patients with severe rhabdomyolysis can present with elevations of both serum AST and ALT.

Aspartate Aminotransferase and Alanine Aminotransferase Levels

The extent of serum aminotransferase elevations correlates poorly with the severity of hepatocellular necrosis and is a poor predictor of outcome in patients with underlying liver disease. Serum aminotransferase levels can be within the normal range in patients with advanced fibrosis or cirrhosis. Patients with azotemia may have a falsely lowered serum AST level. Rarely, AST may form a macroenzyme complex with albumin that results in persistent elevation of the serum AST level.[9]

The degree of serum aminotransferase elevations can provide important diagnostic clues. Although there is no universal consensus as to how the degree of aminotransferase elevations should be categorized, a working definition has been proposed that categorizes the abnormalities as mild, moderate, and marked (Table 70–2).[10] In general, the majority of liver diseases are characterized by mild to moderate elevations in serum aminotransferase levels (<500 U/L). In the Western world, nonalcoholic fatty liver disease (NAFLD) is the most common cause of mildly elevated serum aminotransferase values (see Chapter 82). Typically, serum aminotransferase levels are less than 300 U/L in patients with alcoholic hepatitis (see Chapter 81) or biliary obstruction, although marked aminotransferase elevations can be transiently noted immediately after acute biliary ductal obstruction (see Chapter 62).[11] The most common cause of marked aminotransferase elevations is acute viral hepatitis (see Chapters 74 to 78),

Table 70–2   Definitions of Mild, Moderate, and Marked Elevations of Liver Enzymes*

Enzyme Measured	Mild Elevation	Moderate Elevation	Marked Elevation
Aspartate or alanine aminotransferase	<2-3×	2-3 to 20×	>20×
Alkaline phosphatase	<1.5-2×	1.5-2 to 5×	>5×
Gamma glutamyl transpeptidase	<2-3×	2-3 to 10×	>10×

*Numbers indicate times (×) upper limit of normal for the individual enzyme.
Adapted from Flora KD, Keeffe EB: Significance of mildly elevated liver tests on screening biochemistry profiles. J Insur Med 22:206, 1990.

followed in frequency by acetaminophen-induced hepatotoxicity (see Chapter 83); both disorders can result in aminotransferase levels higher than 1000 U/L. However, the characteristic serum AST-to-ALT (AST/ALT) ratio of less than 1 remains unchanged. In patients with hepatitis, sudden decline in aminotransferase levels followed by continued worsening of the serum bilirubin level and prolongation of the prothrombin time indicates a poor prognosis and the development of acute liver failure (see Chapter 90).

AST/ALT Ratio

The serum AST/ALT ratio may provide a clue to the diagnosis in patients who present with hepatocellular necrosis. The AST/ALT ratio is less than or equal to 1 in the majority of cases of acute hepatocellular injury, with the notable exception of alcoholic hepatitis (see Chapter 81). Most patients with a history of heavy alcohol consumption but without severe liver disease (alcoholic hepatitis or cirrhosis) do not demonstrate a serum AST/ALT ratio greater than 1,[12] but an AST/ALT ratio greater than 1 is suggestive of alcoholic liver disease (especially alcoholic hepatitis or cirrhosis). In patients with alcoholic hepatitis, the AST/ALT ratio is typically higher than 2. The elevated AST/ALT ratio in patients with alcoholic liver disease is associated with pyridoxine deficiency and a poor nutritional status. Both aminotransferases require pyridoxal 5′-phosphate as a coenzyme, and AST has a significantly greater affinity for pyridoxal 5′-phosphate than ALT. Supplementation with pyroxidine in patients with alcoholic liver disease results in a rise in serum ALT levels and a decrease in the AST/ALT ratio. Other unknown factors or mechanisms may also play a role in the predominant elevation of AST and the AST/ALT ratio greater than 2 seen in alcoholic hepatitis.

Patients with cirrhosis secondary to chronic liver disease of any etiology also may present with an AST/ALT ratio greater than 1,[13] and an AST/ALT ratio greater than 1 in a patient who does not have alcoholic hepatitis may indicate underlying cirrhosis (see Chapter 87).[14]

Acute Wilson disease is a rare situation in which the AST value is elevated disproportionately to the ALT value. In fact, patients with fulminant Wilson disease may present with an AST/ALT ratio greater than 4 (see Chapter 72).[15,16] Patients with nonalcoholic steatohepatitis (NASH) typically present with an AST/ALT ratio less than or equal to 1 in the absence of cirrhosis (see Chapter 82).[17,18]

It is important to emphasize that abnormalities in the AST/ALT ratio must be interpreted in the context of other clinical information. Additional clinical and biochemical clues may confirm or exclude the diagnosis in question.

Lactate Dehydrogenase

Lactate dehydrogenase (LDH) can be isolated from a wide variety of tissues, including liver, skeletal muscle, myocardium, red blood cells, brain, and kidneys. Because of its widespread distribution and lack of specificity, measurement of LDH is rarely used as a first-line test to assess liver function. LDH may be fractionated into its isoenzymes to determine the source of an elevated serum LDH value, but this is rarely done in practice. In some circumstances, serum LDH levels may provide useful diagnostic clues. For example, transient, marked elevations of serum LDH are typically seen in patients with ischemic hepatitis (in whom aminotransferase levels are also markedly elevated), and persistent elevation of serum LDH and alkaline phosphatase levels is characteristic of malignant infiltration of the liver.

CHOLESTASIS

Alkaline Phosphatase

Alkaline phosphatase (AP), an enzyme with widespread tissue distribution, provides catalytic activity in liver and extrahepatic sites, including leukocytes, bone, intestine, kidney, and placenta; the precise action of AP is unknown. Liver and bone are the major source of serum AP activity. In addition, AP can be isolated from several neoplasms. The enzymatic activity of AP is stimulated in tissues during active metabolism. For example, during adolescence, AP activity increases threefold during the developmental phase of rapid bone growth; and during the late stages of pregnancy, AP activity increases as a result of placental growth and higher metabolic activity.[19] Neonates without underlying liver disease have serum alkaline phosphatase levels above the normal adult range. In some persons, there may be a genetic predisposition to abnormal elevation of serum AP of unclear significance.

The serum AP level should be determined in a fasting state because the level can rise after a fatty meal. Chronic renal failure can result in an abnormal elevation of the intestinal AP isoenzyme. The hepatic AP isoenzyme can be isolated from the canalicular side of the hepatocyte plasma membrane and the luminal surface of bile duct epithelium. In patients with biliary obstruction, the elevation of serum AP is triggered by increased synthesis and release of the enzyme into serum rather than by impaired biliary secretion.[20] During cholestasis, bile acids accumulate in hepatocytes and solubilize the plasma membrane, thereby resulting in release of AP. The rise in serum AP after biliary obstruction is delayed by a few days, because it requires synthesis of new enzyme. The half-life of serum AP is 5 to 7 days; therefore serum AP remains elevated for several days after the resolution of biliary ductal obstruction.

A two- to three-fold elevation in serum AP values is nonspecific and can result from a wide variety of pathologic processes involving the liver. Typically, abnormal elevations of serum AP of hepatic origin can be observed in patients with biliary obstruction that is intrahepatic (primary biliary cirrhosis [see Chapter 86], primary sclerosing cholangitis [see Chapter 65]) or extrahepatic (choledocholithiasis, stricture [see Chapter 62]). In addition, infiltrative hepatic disorders (granulomatous disease [see Chapter 34] and primary or metastatic tumor [see Chapter 91]) can be associated with an elevation of the serum AP, most likely as a result of compression, malignant invasion, or both, of small, intrahepatic bile ducts. Patients with focal intrahepatic ductal obstruction from a tumor may present with an isolated rise in the serum AP level without a rise in the bilirubin level. In contrast, serum AP levels may remain within the normal range in the setting of extensive hepatic metastasis or extrahepatic bile duct obstruction.[21] Therefore, the level of serum AP is not a reliable indicator of the severity of underlying liver disease. In rare instances, an elevated serum AP—"Regan isoenzyme"—value may be noted in a patient with underlying malignancy but without identifiable liver or bone involvement. The Regan AP isoenzyme is biochemically distinct from hepatic AP isoenzyme and has been associated with several nonhepatic cancers, such as lung neoplasms. The serum hepatic AP isoenzyme value can be elevated as a result of nonspecific hepatitis ("bystander phenomenon") in patients with Hodgkin's disease and renal cell carcinoma in whom direct liver involvement is not demonstrable.

Gamma Glutamyl Transpeptidase

Hepatic gamma glutamyl transpeptidase (GGTP) can be isolated from hepatocytes and biliary epithelia. GGTP is a microsomal enzyme that can be induced by stimulants such as alcohol and drugs, including anticonvulsants and warfarin.[22] GGTP is also present in various extrahepatic tissues, including kidney, spleen, pancreas, heart, lung, and brain. In Japanese men, elevated serum GGTP levels have been reported to correlate with a higher risk of metabolic syndrome and type 2 diabetes mellitus.[23] The lack of GGTP in bone can be helpful in distinguishing a liver source from a bone source of an elevated serum AP value.

A GGTP/AP ratio greater than 2.5 may be noted in the setting of alcohol use, although more than one third of subjects who consume alcohol in amounts greater than 80 g/day have normal serum GGTP levels. Typically, a rise in GGTP levels is not associated with an alcohol binge, thereby limiting the utility of GGTP testing for assessment of surreptitious alcohol use.[24]

The upper limit of normal for serum GGTP levels is significantly higher in infants than in adults. Some cholestatic liver diseases encountered during infancy, such as benign recurrent intrahepatic cholestasis (BRIC) and progressive familial intrahepatic cholestasis (PFIC; e.g., Byler's disease), are characterized by elevated serum AP values and normal GGTP levels. In these instances, the serum GGTP level is as a diagnostic clue and should thus be checked routinely in pediatric patients with cholestatic liver disease (see Chapter 73).

5'-Nucleotidase

5'-Nucleotidase (5'NT) is found in several tissues, including liver, myocardium, pancreas, brain, and blood vessels. Hepatic 5'NT can be isolated from sinusoidal and canalicular plasma membranes. An elevated serum 5'NT value is commonly associated with liver disease and rarely with an extrahepatic disorder. The sensitivity of the serum 5'NT level is comparable to that of the serum AP level for cholestatic liver disease. However, the rise in serum 5'NT levels is noticeable several days after obstruction of the biliary ductal system and may lag behind elevations in serum AP and GGTP.[25]

Bilirubin

Bilirubin, a pigment, is a breakdown product of hemoglobin catabolism. The normal serum bilirubin level is less than 1 mg/dL (18 mmol/L). Serum bilirubin can be fractionated into two types, direct and indirect. Direct bilirubin is a water-soluble, conjugated form of bilirubin, and indirect bilirubin is a lipid-soluble, unconjugated form. In healthy adults, more than 90% of serum bilirubin is unconjugated; the level of unconjugated bilirubin in serum reflects an equilibrium state between the rates of production and hepatobiliary excretion. Serum conjugated bilirubin values can be elevated as a result of parenchymal liver disease or biliary tract obstruction. Because conjugated bilirubin can be filtered through the glomerulus and excreted in the urine, hepatobiliary disease with jaundice is associated with the presence of bilirubin in urine. The unconjugated form of bilirubin is attached to albumin, resulting in a larger molecule that cannot be filtered through the glomerulus (see Chapter 14).

Unconjugated Hyperbilirubinemia

The pathogenetic mechanisms that may lead to abnormal elevation of serum unconjugated bilirubin levels include increased bilirubin production and defects (inherited or acquired) in hepatic uptake or conjugation. The serum unconjugated bilirubin level can rise as a result of increased production of bilirubin by processes such as hemolysis, ineffective erythropoiesis, resolution of a hematoma, and muscle injury. Careful history taking may provide important diagnostic clues to the presence of hemolysis, such as a history of anemia, previous blood transfusions, and use of certain medications. Tests that may suggest a diagnosis of hemolysis include a complete blood count, peripheral blood smear, reticulocyte count, and measurements of serum LDH and haptoglobin levels. The specific cause of hemolysis can be ascertained by confirmatory tests, including a Coombs test, glucose-6-phosphate dehydrogenase (G6PD) assay, and hemoglobin electrophoresis. Chronic hemolysis typically causes mild persistent hyperbilirubinemia (<5 mg/dL) in the setting of normal hepatic function.[2,4]

Conjugated Hyperbilirubinemia

Values of conjugated bilirubin can be abnormally elevated as a result of hepatobiliary diseases, in which the serum conjugated bilirubin level constitutes more than 50% of the total bilirubin level. The rate-limiting step in bilirubin metabolism is the excretion of bilirubin by the hepatocyte. Inherited or acquired defects that lead to a block in the hepatic excretion of bilirubin into the biliary system result in accumulation of bilirubin in hepatocytes and secretion of conjugated bilirubin from hepatocytes into the serum. As noted earlier, conjugated bilirubin is water soluble and can be excreted by the kidneys. Serum bilirubin levels may be higher than 30 mg/dL in patients with hepatobiliary disease in the setting of hemolysis or renal failure.

The level of serum conjugated bilirubin cannot distinguish biliary obstruction from parenchymal liver disease. However, the serum bilirubin level is an indicator of prognosis (the higher the level, the worse the prognosis) in patients with alcoholic hepatitis, primary biliary cirrhosis, and acute liver failure. Patients with end-stage liver disease who are awaiting liver transplantation obtain a higher listing status on the basis of a formula, the Model for End-stage Liver Disease (MELD), that incorporates the serum bilirubin level (see later).[26,27]

In patients with long-standing cholestasis, a fraction of serum conjugated bilirubin can bind tightly to albumin, thereby preventing the excretion of bilirubin in urine. The albumin-bound conjugated bilirubin ("delta fraction") continues to react directly with the diazo reagent that measures conjugated bilirubin levels.[28] This phenomenon explains several unusual findings that can be noted in patients with long-standing cholestasis in the setting of parenchymal liver disease, including conjugated hyperbilirubinemia without bilirubinuria; resolution of bilirubinuria before the hyperbilirubinemia resolves; and delayed resolution of hyperbilirubinemia.

Bile Acids

Bile acids are synthesized from cholesterol within hepatocytes. Serum bile acid levels have been studied as a test of liver function, but there is no evidence to support the use of serum bile acid levels as a more reliable marker of hepatobiliary disease than standard liver biochemical test results.[29] Therefore, serum bile acid levels are not routinely included in the diagnostic evaluation of patients with hepatobiliary disease (see Chapter 61).

HEPATIC SYNTHETIC FUNCTION

Prothrombin Time

All clotting factors except factor VIII are synthesized by hepatocytes; factor VIII is produced by vascular endothelium and reticuloendothelial cells. The prothrombin time measures the rate of production of thrombin from prothrombin. The prothrombin time provides an estimate of hepatic synthetic function because it depends on the activity of several clotting factors involved in the extrinsic coagulation pathway—factors II, V, VII, and X, which are all synthesized by the liver.

The differential diagnosis of an abnormally prolonged prothrombin time also includes vitamin K deficiency, therapeutic anticoagulation, and a consumptive coagulopathy. Vitamin K is needed for gamma-carboxylation and normal functioning of clotting factors II, VII, IX, and X. Vitamin K deficiency can be associated with malnutrition, malabsorption, or antibiotic use and may lead to prolongation of the prothrombin time. The use of warfarin interferes with the vitamin K–induced gamma-carboxylation. The prothrombin time can be prolonged as a result of disseminated intravascular coagulation (DIC) and congenital deficiency of clotting factors. When prolongation of the prothrombin time is caused by liver disease, levels of factor VIII are normal or increased, whereas in DIC, factor VIII levels are decreased.[30] Measurement of the serum factor V level and administration of vitamin K can be used to differentiate hepatic dysfunction and vitamin K deficiency as a cause of a prolonged prothrombin time. Factor V levels are decreased in liver disease but remain unaffected by vitamin K deficiency. Administration of vitamin K, 10 mg subcutaneously, results in correction of the prothrombin time by at least 30% within 24 hours in patients with vitamin K deficiency, but not in those with liver disease.

Hepatic synthetic function can be assessed in patients with acute liver failure through measurement of the prothrombin time. The level of factor VII, which has the shortest half-life (6 hours) of all the clotting factors, can be monitored in patients with acute liver failure to assess hepatic synthetic function (see Chapter 90).[31] The international normalized ratio (INR), which is a reproducible method used to standardize the monitoring of anticoagulation therapy, is not superior as a prognostic indicator to the prothrombin time in patients with acute liver failure but has been incorporated into several prognostic scoring systems for assessing the severity of liver disease (see later).[32,33]

Albumin

Hepatocytes produce and secrete 10 g of albumin per day. In patients with hepatic decompensation, albumin synthetic capacity decreases, resulting in hypoalbuminemia. However, the serum albumin level also can be lowered by extrahepatic conditions, such as malnutrition, enteropathy, renal disease, and hormonal disturbances. Therefore, hypoalbuminemia is not a specific indicator of hepatic dysfunction. Because the serum half-life of albumin is 20 days, the serum albumin level is not a reliable marker of hepatic synthetic function in patients with acute liver disease. However, the serum albumin level can be used as a prognostic indicator in patients with chronic liver disease.

Prealbumin, like albumin, is synthesized by the liver but has a shorter half-life. Serum prealbumin levels can be influenced by several extrahepatic factors and therefore are not used widely as a marker of liver dysfunction.

PATTERNS AND SEVERITY OF HEPATIC INJURY

The pattern and severity of abnormalities of liver biochemical test results can provide important clues in the differential diagnosis of liver disease. However, patterns of liver biochemical test results are not always distinctive, and "mixed" biochemical pictures can occur. Therefore, a detailed history and careful physical examination must be integrated into the interpretation of abnormal liver biochemical test results (Table 70–3).

HEPATOCELLULAR NECROSIS

Hepatocellular necrosis results predominantly in abnormal elevation of the serum aminotransferase levels. The assessment and interpretation of serum aminotransferase elevations should take into account the rate of rise in the aminotransferase levels, the severity (peak levels), the AST/ALT ratio, coexisting abnormalities in laboratory test results, and the patient's clinical presentation. Data are conflicting on whether serum AST or ALT elevations correlate with the severity of histologic damage to the liver.[34-36]

Mild to Moderate Persistent Aminotransferase Elevations

A mild elevation of serum aminotransferase levels (<250 U/L) is nonspecific and can result from almost any type of liver disease.[37,38] The causes of an asymptomatic, mild elevation in serum aminotransferase values vary with geography and the patient population. In the United States, NAFLD is the most common cause of asymptomatic, mild aminotransferase elevations.[18,39] Other common causes are chronic viral hepatitis, alcoholic liver disease, metabolic liver diseases, and drug-induced liver injury.[40,41] Chronic hepatitis B is more prevalent in the Far East, schistosomiasis in Egypt, and malaria in Africa.

The diagnostic specificity of moderate aminotransferase elevations (250 to 1000 U/L) is also poor, because almost any type of liver disease may present with such abnormalities. The most common causes of moderate aminotransferase elevations are viral and drug-induced

liver injury. Both hepatotropic viruses (hepatitis viruses A to E) and the herpesviruses (Epstein-Barr virus, cytomegalovirus, and herpes simplex virus) may be associated with moderate aminotransferase elevations (see Chapters 74 to 78). Over-the-counter drugs, such as nonsteroidal anti-inflammatory agents, may result in hepatotoxicity characterized by mild to moderate elevations in aminotransferase levels (see Chapter 83). Cocaine and methamphetamines can cause transient, moderate aminotransferase elevations (see Chapter 84). Aminotransferases can be elevated as a result of celiac sprue or adrenocortical insufficiency (Addison's disease) and should be considered in the differential diagnosis when more common causes have been excluded (see Chapter 34).[42,43]

Asymptomatic patients with mild to moderate elevations in serum aminotransferase levels are seen commonly in clinical practice. The elevations are often detected by accident, for example, during blood donor screening or an insurance examination.[37,44] The prevalence of liver disease is low in volunteer blood donors, and the majority of the abnormalities detected are clinically unimportant. In this era of cost containment, a conservative diagnostic approach may be appropriate in a patient population with a low prevalence of liver disease.

The diagnostic approach to asymptomatic patients with elevated serum aminotransferase levels should be individualized according to findings from the patient's history, physical examination, and laboratory test results (Fig. 70–1). First and foremost, any abnormalities should be confirmed. Up to one third of blood donors with asymptomatic aminotransferase elevations demonstrate only a single elevation of the serum ALT on longitudinal follow-up.[44] Typically, the higher the elevation, the less likely that the result is falsely positive.[37] Careful history taking is important in establishing the basis of clinical suspicion for a specific disease. During the physical examination, the patient should be checked for stigmata of advanced liver disease, including a firm liver edge, splenomegaly, ascites, cutaneous stigmata of chronic liver

Table 70–3 General Patterns of Liver Biochemical Values According to Type of Liver Disease*

	Hepatocellular Necrosis			Biliary Obstruction		Hepatic Infiltration
Etiology Examples	Toxin, ischemia Acetaminophen or ischemic hepatitis	Viral hepatitis Hepatitis A or B	Alcohol Alcoholic hepatitis	Complete Pancreatic carcinoma	Partial Hilar tumor, primary sclerosing cholangitis	Infitrative disease Primary or metastatic carcinoma, tuberculosis, sarcoidosis, amyloidosis
Measurements						
Aminotransferases	50–100×	5–50×	2–5×	1–5×†	1–5×†	1–3×
Alkaline phosphatase	1–3×	1–3×	1–10×	2–20×	2–10×	1–20×
Bilirubin	1–5×	1–30×	1–30×	1–30×	1–5×	1–5× (often normal)
Prothrombin time	Prolonged and unresponsive to vitamin K in severe disease			Often prolonged and responsive to parenteral vitamin K		Usually normal
Albumin	Decreased in subacute and chronic diseases			Usually normal; decreased in cirrhosis		Usually normal

*Numbers indicate times (×) upper limit of normal.
†Rapid onset of complete biliary obstruction (e.g., secondary to choledocholithiasis) rarely may result in massive (20–50× normal) but transient elevation of the aminotransferases.

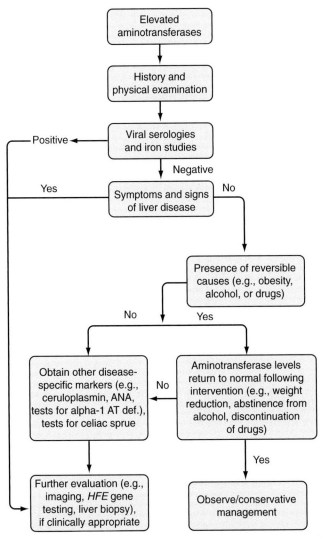

Figure 70–1 Algorithm for the evaluation of mild but sustained aminotransferase elevations. Clinical history taking should focus on risk factors for viral hepatitis, medication, alcohol and illicit drug use, recent weight gain, and a family history of liver disease. The physical examination should focus on the detection of stigmata of liver disease (e.g., splenomegaly, cutaneous spiders), Kayser-Fleischer rings (especially in young patients), and extrahepatic disease that could contribute to elevations of aminotransferases (e.g., signs of right-sided heart failure). ANA, antinuclear antibodies; alpha-1 AT def., alpha-1 antitrypsin deficiency.

disease (spider angiomata, palmar erythema), asterixis, muscle wasting, and bruising. An extrahepatic disorder can be considered in an asymptomatic patient with serum aminotransferase elevations and no evidence of chronic liver disease from the history or physical examination. Patients with an isolated AST elevation and normal ALT value should be evaluated for muscle disease.[37]

During the diagnostic evaluation of patients with elevated aminotransferase levels, known causes of liver disease should be excluded. Every effort should be made to pursue potentially treatable conditions. Therefore, serologic studies for hepatitis B and C should be

obtained, particularly in patients with risk factors for viral hepatitis; iron studies and possibly genetic testing for hemochromatosis should be ordered, particularly in patients with a family history of iron overload or hemochromatosis; quantification of urinary copper and a serum ceruloplasmin measurement are warranted in younger patients (<40 years) with any suspicion of Wilson disease; and markers of autoimmune liver disease should be checked, particularly in young female patients with possible autoimmune hepatitis.

Patients with persistent aminotransferase elevations of unclear etiology should discontinue any potentially hepatotoxic medications, including herbs and supplements, and should abstain from consuming alcohol. For patients with alcoholic liver disease, several weeks of abstinence are needed to lower the serum AST level to the normal range. Discontinuation of hepatotoxic drugs may lead to improvement in aminotransferase levels, with some exceptions.[45] In patients with NAFLD, weight loss is recommended and may lead to stabilization and possibly regression of hepatic fibrosis, if present. Improvement in biochemical abnormalities as a result of weight loss may prevent the risk, inconvenience, and cost of further evaluation, including liver biopsy.[46-48] However, a liver biopsy can be pursued if conservative interventions have been ineffective and aminotransferase values remain persistently elevated (more than 1.5 times the upper limit of normal) for 6 to 12 months.

Marked Aminotransferase Elevations

The differential diagnosis of marked elevation in aminotransferase levels (>2000 U/L) includes acute viral hepatitis, drug hepatotoxicity, toxin-induced hepatic injury, and ischemic liver injury (shock liver). Rarely, choledocholithiasis with acute biliary ductal obstruction can manifest as a marked rise in aminotransferase levels to more than 2000 U/L accompanied by a mild coexisting cholestatic pattern of liver test results, right upper quadrant pain, nausea, and vomiting. Typically, the aminotransferase elevations improve dramatically within 24 to 48 hours and are followed by rises in serum AP and bilirubin levels. Autoimmune hepatitis and giant cell hepatitis can result in striking elevations in serum aminotransferases. Marked aminotransferase elevations in the setting of autoimmune hepatitis indicate aggressive liver disease and a poor prognosis if therapy is delayed.[49]

The most common cause of marked aminotransferase elevations is acute viral hepatitis; the peak elevations are lower, but the duration of abnormalities is longer, than for other causes of marked aminotransferase elevations, such as ischemic hepatitis or hepatitis due to a drug or toxin. Careful history taking generally facilitates prompt diagnosis of acute viral hepatitis. Questioning the patient about potential modes of transmission may provide important diagnostic clues. For example, a history of raw shellfish ingestion is a risk factor for hepatitis A; injection drug use is a risk factor for hepatitis B, C, or D; and travel to Southeast Asia is a risk factor for hepatitis E (see Chapters 74 to 77).

Hepatic injury associated with ischemia results in a marked elevation in serum aminotransferase levels that is abrupt and brief (a few days), compared with elevations seen in viral or drug-induced hepatic dysfunction, which generally are gradual and prolonged (a few weeks). Detailed history taking plays an important role in making the correct diagnosis. Ischemic hepatitis (shock liver) usually occurs in patients who experience a precipitous drop in blood pressure or effective circulating volume, as may occur during or after major surgery or because of heart failure, myocardial infarction, arrhythmias, sepsis, extensive burns, severe trauma, heat stroke, or multiorgan shock.[50] The episode of hypotension may be recognized only in retrospect, after the marked rise in liver enzyme levels. Patients with ischemic hepatitis demonstrate an abrupt, massive elevation in aminotransferase values, usually to more than 2000 U/L, with rapid normalization over 5 to 7 days (unless the patient dies of the underlying cause), followed by mild but transient abnormalities in the prothrombin time and serum AP and bilirubin levels. Elevation of the serum LDH level to more than 5000 U/L and transient renal insufficiency are characteristically associated with ischemic hepatic injury.[51] In contrast, LDH levels are usually unaffected in viral hepatitis. The prognosis of ischemic hepatic injury is associated with the underlying circulatory disorder rather than the severity of enzyme abnormalities (see Chapter 80).

A diagnosis of drug- or toxin-induced liver injury is based on a constellation of findings that prompt a high index of suspicion,[52] including clues in the patient's history, findings on physical examination, and the pattern of liver enzyme abnormalities. The severity and duration of aminotransferase elevations vary with the underlying etiology, but the elevations are usually more prolonged than in ischemic hepatitis. The most common cause of drug-induced liver injury in the Western world is acetaminophen.[53] The dose of acetaminophen needed to cause severe hepatic dysfunction in healthy adults is more than 10 to 12 grams. However, lower doses can cause severe hepatic injury in patients who have been fasting for a prolonged period or who have alcoholic liver disease or possibly cirrhosis. For some drugs, findings on physical examination may provide clues to a diagnosis of drug-induced liver injury; these findings may include fever and rash, as occurs in some cases of halothane hepatitis, often in association with eosinophilia. Other agents associated with severe hepatocellular necrosis and marked aminotransferase elevations are other inhalation anesthetics and solvents such as carbon tetrachloride (see Chapters 83 and 84).

CHOLESTASIS

Cholestasis refers to impairment of bile flow and is characterized biochemically by a predominant elevation in the serum AP, conjugated bilirubin, or both, often in association with pruritus and jaundice. Serum AP and bilirubin elevations are not specific for biliary ductal obstruction but can be associated with a wide variety of liver diseases, including alcoholic hepatitis, hepatitis A, end-stage liver disease, and certain drugs.[54] It is important to differentiate intrahepatic cholestasis from extrahepatic biliary obstruction in patients with cholestasis. The clinical history, physical findings, and laboratory test results provide important diagnostic clues. Diagnostic

imaging of the biliary tree and, in some cases, a liver biopsy may be needed to confirm the diagnosis and assess the severity of the underlying liver disease (see Chapter 14).

Isolated or Predominant Alkaline Phosphatase Elevations

Patients with partial biliary ductal obstruction or hepatic infiltrative disease can present with an isolated elevation of serum AP without a significant rise in serum bilirubin. The underlying pathologic processes typically associated with partial biliary obstruction include biliary strictures of the small intrahepatic ducts and choledocholithiasis. Biliary strictures involving the small bile ducts can result from primary sclerosing cholangitis, primary biliary cirrhosis, recurrent pyogenic cholangitis, and malignant obstruction of either the left or right ductal system at the level of ductal bifurcation (Klatskin tumor) (see Chapters 65, 66, and 86). The bilirubin level remains within normal limits as a result of compensatory secretion of bilirubin by hepatocytes in the distribution of the nonobstructed ductal system. Hepatic infiltrative diseases, such as primary hepatic tumor, metastatic cancer, amyloidosis, mycobacterial infection, and granulomatous disorders, can also be associated with isolated elevation of the serum AP level and a normal bilirubin level (see Chapters 34, 79, and 91). Drug-induced liver injury with a predominantly cholestatic pattern can result from anabolic steroids, estrogens, and antipsychotic medications (see Chapter 83). Isolated elevation of serum AP in the setting of a normal serum GGTP (or 5'NT) level can be associated with rapid bone growth in children, Paget's disease, and pregnancy. Additional rare hepatic disorders associated with an isolated AP elevation are PFIC, BRIC, and hereditary defects of bile acid synthesis. Byler's disease, a form of PFIC, is a lethal autosomal recessive cholestatic disease of unclear pathogenesis for which liver transplantation is the only therapeutic option.[55] BRIC is an idiopathic familial syndrome that manifests as abdominal pain and other nonspecific constitutional symptoms and is characterized by recurrent, benign episodes of intrahepatic cholestasis, which may span several months. Typically, a patient with BRIC presents with elevated serum AP and bilirubin levels accompanied by near-normal aminotransferase and GGTP levels. Both Byler's disease and BRIC type I are caused by a gene defect on chromosome 18q.[56] Other gene defects account for other forms of PFIC. These cholestatic disorders are associated with defects in bile acid synthesis and failure of hepatocytes to secrete bile acids into the canaliculus (see Chapter 73).[55]

A systematic diagnostic evaluation is indicated for patients with a predominant elevation of serum AP (Fig. 70–2). Initially, the hepatic source of the AP elevation can be confirmed by documenting coexisting elevation of the serum GGTP or 5'NT. In patients with an AP elevation of hepatic origin, abdominal ultrasonography or computed tomography (CT) should be ordered to assess the intrahepatic ducts for dilatation and to look for hepatic lesions. Further diagnostic evaluation of patients with biliary ductal dilatation can be performed with magnetic resonance cholangiopancreatography (MRCP), endoscopic retrograde cholangiopancreatography, or percuta-

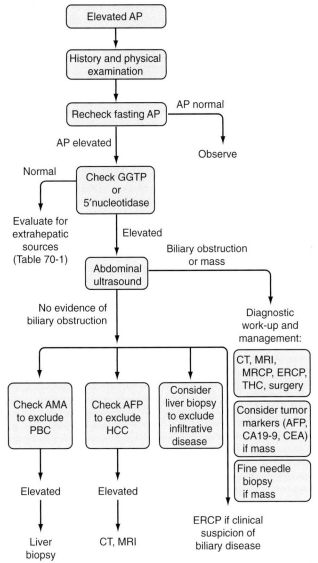

Figure 70–2 Evaluation of an isolated alkaline phosphatase (AP) elevation. Clinical history taking should focus on possible extrahepatic sources of AP (e.g., symptoms of bone disease, pregnancy), medication use, biliary pain, and cholestasis (e.g., pruritus). The physical examination should focus on detection of stigmata of chronic liver disease (e.g., splenomegaly) as well as signs of chronic cholestasis (e.g., excoriations). AFP, alpha fetoprotein; AMA, antimitochondrial antibodies; CEA, carcinoembryonic antigen; CT, computed tomography; ERCP, endoscopic retrograde cholangiopancreatography; GGTP, gamma glutamyl transpeptidase; HCC, hepatocellular carcinoma; MRCP, magnetic resonance cholangiopancreatography; MRI, magnetic resonance imaging; PBC, primary biliary cirrhosis; THC, transhepatic cholangiography.

neous transhepatic cholangiography. Unless a therapeutic intervention is anticipated, MRCP is increasingly preferred as the initial diagnostic modality (see Chapter 67). Patients with a focal hepatic lesion can be evaluated by ultrasound- or CT-guided aspiration biopsy.

In the absence of biliary ductal obstruction or a focal hepatic lesion, a test for antimitochondrial antibodies should be obtained to look for primary biliary cirrhosis. Medications must be reviewed for the possibility of drug-induced cholestasis. Any suspected drugs should be

discontinued, and the serum AP level subsequently monitored periodically until the level normalizes. A liver biopsy may be needed to confirm a diagnosis of an infiltrative disease. In some patients with an isolated elevation of hepatic AP, evaluation is negative, yielding no clear etiology to account for the elevation. Liver biochemical test levels should be monitored in these patients, and selected diagnostic tests should be repeated if the levels rise further.

Isolated or Predominant Bilirubin Elevations

In patients with predominant hyperbilirubinemia, the bilirubin should first be fractionated into its conjugated and unconjugated portions. Patients with predominantly conjugated hyperbilirubinemia may have one of the common causes of liver disease (alcohol, viral, or drugs) or a rare inherited disorder, such as Dubin-Johnson or Rotor's syndrome. Severe extrahepatic bacterial infection may be associated with elevated serum conjugated bilirubin, and less often, a predominant elevation of the serum AP level may be noted.[57]

Patients with predominantly unconjugated hyperbilirubinemia may have an inherited or acquired abnormality in the hepatic uptake or conjugation of bilirubin, including Gilbert's syndrome. In addition, hemolysis as an isolated event or as a manifestation of liver disease, as in acute Wilson disease, can result in predominantly unconjugated hyperbilirubinemia. Gilbert's syndrome is a benign condition that results from a defect in the conjugation of bilirubin, specifically reduced activity of uridine diphosphate glucuronyl transferase. The disorder manifests as mild, intermittent, unconjugated hyperbilirubinemia (from 2 to 5 mg/dL); a rise in the bilirubin level typically occurs in association with a stressful event, such as fasting, trauma, surgery, or infection (see Chapter 14). In fulminant Wilson disease, the predominantly unconjugated hyperbilirubinemia is associated with hemolysis and inhibition of serum AP activity. Hemolysis associated with Wilson disease results from an abrupt rise in serum copper levels and may occur after interruption of chelation therapy (see Chapter 72).[58,59]

Isolated GGTP Elevations

GGTP activity can be induced by alcohol and drugs, such as anticonvulsants and warfarin.[22] Isolated elevation of GGTP with normal levels of AP and other liver biochemical values should raise the clinical suspicion of alcoholic liver disease. Abstinence from alcohol is recommended, and the GGTP level should be monitored periodically. Certain drugs also can result in an isolated GGTP elevation. Conservative management is generally appropriate as long as hepatic synthetic function remains intact.

PREDICTORS OF HEPATIC INJURY

Liver biochemical tests can be used to monitor patients for drug-induced liver injury, assess a patient's risk for surgery, identify candidates for liver transplantation, and prioritize candidates with end-stage liver disease for liver transplantation.[60-64]

DRUG-INDUCED LIVER INJURY

Several commonly prescribed drugs can result in hepatotoxicity and liver dysfunction. Drug-induced liver injury can be idiosyncratic and therefore difficult to predict. However, certain drugs, such as acetaminophen, methotrexate, and isoniazid, are associated with a more predictable hepatotoxicity. Patients who are prescribed potentially hepatotoxic drugs should be monitored, but the efficacy of screening for drug-induced liver injury is controversial, because of the poor ability of liver biochemical tests to predict hepatotoxicity. For example, modest elevations in the serum aminotransferase levels develop in at least 10% of patients taking isoniazid, but the levels generally return to normal with continued use of the drug; serious toxicity is less common. In patients undergoing isoniazid therapy, liver biochemical testing may not be needed routinely unless symptoms of hepatitis develop. On the other hand, patients may have progressive fibrosis and cirrhosis with long-term methotrexate use despite persistently normal liver enzyme levels. In some cases, hepatotoxicity may develop suddenly and with rapid decompensation, making periodic screening for drug-induced liver injury ineffective. Still, the guidelines for screening patients undergoing methotrexate therapy are considered the standard of care and should be followed (see Chapter 83). Other drugs for which screening is recommended and useful are lovastatin and other lipid-lowering drugs, valproate, pyrazinamide, ketoconazole, dantrolene, tacrine, and synthetic retinoids (e.g., isotretinoin). Patients with a baseline elevation in serum aminotransferases are not thought to be at greater risk for hepatotoxicity from hydroxymethyl-coenzyme A reductase inhibitors (statins).[60]

SURGICAL CANDIDACY

Operative risk in a patient with chronic liver disease depends on several factors, and assessment of the risk should be individualized and based on the severity of the underlying liver disease.[61] Factors important in preserving hepatic function during and after surgery include improving the nutritional status in the preoperative period, maintaining hemodynamic stability in the perioperative period, and minimizing the use of hepatotoxic medications (e.g., halothane). In the absence of prospective data, making firm predictions about the risk of surgery in patients with liver disease is difficult. However, rates of postoperative complications and mortality are higher in patients with active or decompensated liver disease. The operative risk is higher with certain types of surgery, such as hepatic resection, biliary surgery, gastric surgery, colectomy, and cardiac surgery. Elective surgical procedures are contraindicated in patients with acute hepatitis, severe chronic hepatitis, and decompensated cirrhosis. Furthermore, elective surgery should be postponed in patients in whom abnormal liver test results are noted incidentally during the preoperative evaluation. Elective surgery can be rescheduled or cancelled once the etiology and severity of underlying liver disease have been established.

In patients with cirrhosis, the Child-Turcotte-Pugh (CTP) scoring classification is used to predict prognosis after surgery. The CTP scoring system was originally formulated to predict the prognosis of patients with liver disease who were undergoing portosystemic shunt surgery (see Table 87–6). In a subsequent retrospective analysis of 92 patients with cirrhosis who underwent abdominal surgery of various types, the mortality rate was 10%, 30%, and 82% for patients with Child's class A, class B, and class C disease, respectively.[62,63] In addition, the CTP scoring system can be used to establish the frequency of postoperative complications, such as renal failure, hepatic encephalopathy, bleeding, infection, intractable ascites, and deterioration in liver failure. Preliminary experience suggests that the MELD score, which is generally used to prioritize candidates for liver transplantation, also may correlate with surgical risk (see Chapter 87).

In patients with well-compensated or Child's class A cirrhosis, the operative risk appears to be increased only modestly, whereas in those with Child's class B and C cirrhosis or decompensated liver disease, the risks associated with surgery are substantial.[61,63] Ideally, elective surgery should be postponed until the complications are treated. In some cases, it may be preferable to proceed with liver transplantation first. In fact, elective surgery is contraindicated in patients with Child's class C cirrhosis; these patients should be considered for surgery only in life-threatening situations, such as an incarcerated hernia, gangrenous cholecystitis, or bowel infarction. When surgery is unavoidable in such patients, meticulous perioperative management is required, including maintenance of hemodynamic stability, improvement in overall nutritional status, coverage with broad-spectrum antibiotic therapy, correction of coagulopathy, avoidance of nephrotoxins and sedatives that may precipitate hepatic encephalopathy, and extended intensive care unit management if needed.

PROGNOSIS

The markers of hepatic synthetic function and the serum bilirubin level are useful for predicting prognosis in certain circumstances. Prolongation of the prothrombin time and an elevation in the serum bilirubin level predict a poor prognosis in non–acetaminophen-related acute hepatic failure (see Chapter 90).[31] The same two parameters—prolonged prothrombin time and hyperbilirubinemia—are associated with greater mortality in patients with alcoholic hepatitis and are useful in identifying candidates for glucocorticoid therapy (see Chapter 81).[65] In patients with primary biliary cirrhosis, prognosis correlates directly with the serum bilirubin level, and a composite score derived from the patient's age, serum bilirubin level, prothrombin time, serum albumin level, and severity of fluid retention is useful for assessing prognosis (see Chapter 86).[66] The role of liver biochemical tests in predicting the prognosis of patients with liver diseases is variable and disease specific. In general, the test results become abnormal only in the late stages of liver disease.

Allocation of allografts for liver transplantation is determined primarily by the patient's MELD score, which is based on the INR, serum bilirubin level, and serum creatinine level (Table 70–4).[64,67] The MELD scoring system has been used successfully to predict early mortality after a transjugular intrahepatic portosystemic shunt (TIPS) and has several advantages over the CTP score. The variables in the CTP scoring system are limited by a lack of consistency and reproducibility and are "operator dependent"; for example, ascites and hepatic encephalopathy are graded subjectively. Furthermore, the CTP scoring system classifies patients into three categories only—low, intermediate, and high risk—without quantifying expected survival. Also, the CTP scoring system is unable to stratify patients with severely decompensated liver disease.

For example, of two patients with Child's class C cirrhosis, one may have a serum bilirubin level of 4 mg/dL and the other a serum bilirubin level of 25 mg/dL; both are classified as having Child's class C disease, but they do not have the same prognosis. The MELD model is able to differentiate levels of severity in advanced liver disease and to provide a more reliable assessment of prognosis (see Chapters 87 and 92).

ADDITIONAL TESTS

Supplemental tests are available to assess hepatic synthetic function and to estimate the extent of hepatic injury. Some of these methods are still undergoing testing to confirm their validity and therefore should be used with caution.

FIBROTEST-ACTITEST

The necessity and timing of a liver biopsy to assess the severity of underlying liver disease is undergoing reassessment, and noninvasive tests of hepatic inflammation and fibrosis are being studied. In 2001, FibroTest-ActiTest (FT-AT) was introduced as a panel of biochemical markers with high diagnostic value for fibrosis (FT range, 0.00 to 1.00) and necroinflammatory histologic activity (AT range, 0.00 to 1.00). On the basis of encouraging preliminary data, the use of the biochemical markers of liver

---

Table 70–4   Model for End-stage Liver Disease (MELD) Scoring Equation*

MELD score for TIPS = $0.957 \times \log_e$(creatinine [mg/dL]) + $0.378 \times \log_e$(bilirubin [mg/dL]) + $1.120 \times \log_e$(INR) + .643 (cause of liver disease)[†]

MELD score for liver transplantation[‡] = $0.957 \times \log_e$(creatinine [mg/dL]) + $0.378 \times \log_e$(bilirubin [mg/dL]) + $1.120 \times \log_e$(INR) + .643

INR, international normalized ratio; TIPS, transjugular intrahepatic portosystemic shunt.
*Laboratory values less than 1.0 are set at 1.0. The maximum serum creatinine level considered in the MELD score equation is 4.0 mg/dL.
[†]0 if cholestatic or alcoholic liver disease, and 1 if other liver disease.
[‡]Multiply by 10 and round to the nearest whole number.

Table 70–5   Quantitative Liver Function Tests

Test	Description*	Comments[†]
Indocyanine green clearance	Concentration of dye, which is taken up almost exclusively by hepatocytes and excreted unchanged into the bile, is measured photometrically in blood samples taken at regular intervals after a bolus intravenous injection (0.5 mg/kg) Clearance of the dye decreases with loss of hepatocyte mass	May help predict death in patients with primary biliary cirrhosis and outcome after liver transplantation Not useful for measuring hepatic blood flow in patients with liver disease Anaphylaxis is rarely reported
Galactose elimination capacity	Metabolism of intravenously administered galactose (0.5 g/kg) is measured with serial blood samples collected 20-50 minutes after intravenous injection	May predict death in primary biliary cirrhosis and outcome in chronic hepatitis Safe, although a large volume of fluid is required
Aminopyrine breath test	Radioactivity ($^{14}CO_2$) is measured in breath at 15-min intervals for 2 hr after oral or intravenous administration of ^{14}C-labeled methyl aminopyrine	May predict death and histology in chronic hepatitis Safety not established Radioactivity exposure
Antipyrine clearance	Metabolite of antipyrine is measured in saliva 24 hr after oral antipyrine administration (15 mg/kg)	Time-consuming to perform Safety not established Drug interactions may influence results
Monoethylglycinexylidide (MEGX)	Lidocaine metabolite is measured in blood sample 15 min after intravenous administration of lidocaine (1 mg/kg)	May predict death and complications before and after liver transplantation May predict donor liver function
Caffeine clearance	Caffeine metabolites are measured in saliva samples over 24 hr after oral administration of caffeine (280 mg)	Safe Drug interactions Relatively easy to perform

*As typically performed; variations may exist.
[†]Usefulness not clearly established for any of the tests listed.

fibrosis (FT) and necrosis (AT) was recommended as an alternative to liver biopsy for the assessment of histologic damage in patients with chronic hepatitis C.[68] Currently, FT-AT remains an experimental tool that should be used with caution until the preliminary data are confirmed in large trials. Other technologies, such as "clinical glycomics" (the generation of profiles of serum *N*-glycans), have also demonstrated that a highly specific set of biomarkers can be used to diagnose cirrhosis.[69]

QUANTITATIVE TESTS OF LIVER FUNCTION

The limitations of liver biochemical tests to precisely predict the severity of liver disease warrants a cautious approach in interpreting the results of these tests. Ideally, diagnostic tests that are more sensitive and quantitative without a subjective bias may predict liver function more accurately in individual patients.[70] Data are insufficient to establish whether such quantitative tests are superior to conventional biochemical tests in predicting the presence, severity, and prognosis of liver disease. The quantitative tests have their own limitations, including expense, availability, invasiveness, and lack of validity (Table 70–5).[71,72] Further controlled, prospective studies are needed to compare quantitative liver function tests with conventional liver biochemical tests, so quantitative liver function tests currently have limited use in clinical practice.

REFERENCES

1. Prati D, Taioli E, Zanella A, et al: Updated definitions of healthy ranges for serum alanine aminotransferase levels. Ann Intern Med 137:1, 2002.
2. Pratt DS, Kaplan MM: Laboratory tests. In Schiff ER, Sorrell MF, Maddrey WC (eds): Schiff's Diseases of the Liver, Vol 1. Philadelphia, Lippincott-Raven, 1999, p 205.
3. Kratz A, Lewandrowski KB: Case records of the Massachusetts General Hospital: Weekly clinicopathological exercises: Normal reference laboratory values. N Engl J Med 339:1063, 1998.
4. Friedman LS, Martin P, Munoz SJ: Liver function tests and the objective evaluation of the patient with liver disease. In Zakim D, Boyer TD (eds): Hepatology: A Textbook of Liver Disease, Vol 1. Philadelphia, WB Saunders, 1996, p 791.
5. Sackett DLHR, Guyatt GH, Tugwell P: Clinical Epidemiology: A Basic Science for Clinical Medicine. Boston, Little, Brown, 1991.
6. Begum T, Oliver MR, Kornberg AJ, Dennett X: Elevated aminotransferase as a presenting finding in a patient with occult muscle disease. J Paediatr Child Health 36:189, 2000.
7. Zamora S, Adams C, Butzner JD, et al: Elevated aminotransferase activity as an indication of muscular dystrophy: Case reports and review of the literature. Can J Gastroenterol 10:389, 1996.
8. Helfgott SM, Karlson E, Beckman E: Misinterpretation of serum transaminase elevation in "occult" myositis. Am J Med 95:447, 1993.
9. Litin SC, O'Brien JF, Pruett S, et al: Macroenzyme as a cause of unexplained elevation of aspartate aminotransferase. Mayo Clin Proc 62:681, 1987.
10. Flora KD, Keeffe EB: Significance of mildly elevated liver tests on screening biochemistry profiles. J Insur Med 22:206, 1990.
11. Fortson WC, Tedesco FJ, Starnes ED, et al: Marked elevation of serum transaminase activity associated with extrahepatic biliary tract disease. J Clin Gastroenterol 7:502, 1985.
12. Nyblom H, Berggren U, Balldin J, et al: High AST/ALT ratio may indicate advanced alcoholic liver disease rather than heavy drinking. Alcohol Alcohol 39:336, 2004.
13. Williams AL, Hoofnagle JH: Ratio of serum aspartate to alanine aminotransferase in chronic hepatitis: Relationship to cirrhosis. Gastroenterology 95:734, 1988.
14. Park SY, Kang KH, Park JH, et al: Clinical efficacy of AST/ALT ratio and platelet counts as predictors of degree of fibrosis in HBV infected patients without clinically evident liver cirrhosis. Korean J Gastroenterol 43:246, 2004.
15. Berman DHLR, Gavaler JS, Cadoff EM, et al: Clinical differentiation of fulminant Wilsonian hepatitis from other causes of hepatic failure. Gastroenterology 100:1129, 1991.
16. Sallie R, Katsiyiannakis L, Baldwin D, et al: Failure of simple biochemical indexes to reliably differentiate fulminant Wilson's disease from other causes of fulminant liver failure. Hepatology 16:1206, 1992.
17. Sorbi D, Boynton J, Lindor KD: The ratio of aspartate aminotransferase to alanine aminotransferase: Potential value in differentiating nonalcoholic steatohepatitis from alcoholic liver disease. Am J Gastroenterol 94:1018, 1999.
18. Clark JM, Brancati FL, Diehl AM: The prevalence and etiology of elevated aminotransferase levels in the United States. Am J Gastroenterol 98:960, 2003.
19. Bacq Y, Zarka O, Brechot JF, et al: Liver function tests in normal pregnancy: A prospective study of 103 pregnant women and 103 matched controls. Hepatology 23:1030, 1996.
20. Seetharam S, Sussman NL, Komoda T, et al: The mechanism of elevated alkaline phosphatase activity after bile duct ligation in the rat. Hepatology 6:374, 1986.
21. McGarrity TJ, Samuels T, Wilson FA: An analysis of imaging studies and liver function tests to detect hepatic neoplasia. Dig Dis Sci 32:1113, 1987.
22. Keeffe EB, Sunderland MC, Gabourel JD: Serum gamma-glutamyl transpeptidase activity in patients receiving chronic phenytoin therapy. Dig Dis Sci 31:1056, 1986.
23. Nakanishi N, Suzuki K, Tatara K: Serum gamma-glutamyl-transferase and risk of metabolic syndrome and type 2 diabetes in middle-aged Japanese men. Diabetes Care 27:1427, 2004.
24. Penn R, Worthington DJ: Is serum gamma-glutamyltransferase a misleading test? Br Med J 286:531, 1983.
25. Reichling JJ, Kaplan MM: Clinical use of serum enzymes in liver disease. Dig Dis Sci 33:1601, 1988.
26. Kamath PS, Wiesner RH, Malinchoc M, et al: A model to predict survival in patients with end-stage liver disease. Hepatology 33:464, 2001.
27. Wiesner R, Edwards E, Freeman R, et al: The United Network for Organ Sharing Liver Disease Severity Score Committee. Model for end-stage liver disease (MELD) and allocation of donor livers. Gastroenterology 124:91, 2003.
28. Weiss JS, Gautam A, Lauff JJ, et al: The clinical importance of a protein-bound fraction of serum bilirubin in patients with hyperbilirubinemia. N Engl J Med 309:147, 1983.
29. Ferraris R, Colombatti G, Fiorentini MT, et al: Diagnostic value of serum bile acids and routine liver function tests in hepatobiliary diseases: Sensitivity, specificity, and predictive value. Dig Dis Sci 28:129, 1983.
30. Mammen EF: Coagulation defects in liver disease. Med Clin North Am 78:545, 1994.
31. O'Grady JG, Alexander GJ, Hayllar KM, et al: Early indicators of prognosis in fulminant hepatic failure. Gastroenterology 97:439, 1989.
32. Kovacs MJ, Wong A, MacKinnon K, et al: Assessment of the validity of the INR system for patients with liver impairment. Thromb Haemost 71:727, 1994.

33. Denson KW, Reed SV, Haddon ME: Validity of the INR system for patients with liver impairment. Thromb Haemost 73:162, 1995.

34. Zechini B, Pasquazzi C, Aceti A: Correlation of serum amino-transferases with HCV RNA levels and histological findings in patients with chronic hepatitis C: The role of serum aspartate transaminase in the evaluation of disease progression. Eur J Gastroenterol Hepatol 16:891, 2004.

35. Toyoda H, Kumada T, Kiriyama S, et al: Influence of age, sex, and degree of liver fibrosis on the association between serum alanine aminotransferase levels and liver inflammation in patients with chronic hepatitis C. Dig Dis Sci 49:295, 2004.

36. Mofrad P, Contos MJ, Haque M, et al: Clinical and histologic spectrum of nonalcoholic fatty liver disease associated with normal ALT values. Hepatology 37:1286, 2003.

37. Pratt DS, Kaplan MM: Evaluation of abnormal liver-enzyme results in asymptomatic patients. N Engl J Med 342:1266, 2000.

38. Daniel S, Ben-Menachem T, Vasudevan G, et al: Prospective evaluation of unexplained chronic liver transaminase abnor-malities in asymptomatic and symptomatic patients. Am J Gastroenterol 94:3010, 1999.

39. Patt CH, Yoo HY, Dibadj K, et al: Prevalence of transaminase abnormalities in asymptomatic, healthy subjects participating in an executive health-screening program. Dig Dis Sci 48:797, 2003.

40. Hultcrantz R, Glaumann H, Lindberg G, et al: Liver investiga-tion in 149 asymptomatic patients with moderately elevated activities of serum aminotransferases. Scand J Gastroenterol 21:109, 1986.

41. Van Ness MM, Diehl AM: Is liver biopsy useful in the evalua-tion of patients with chronically elevated liver enzymes? Ann Intern Med 111:473, 1989.

42. Boulton R, Hamilton MI, Dhillon AP, et al: Subclinical Addison's disease: A cause of persistent abnormalities in transaminase values. Gastroenterology 109:1324, 1995.

43. Bardella MT, Vecchi M, Conte D, et al: Chronic unexplained hypertransaminasemia may be caused by occult celiac disease. Hepatology 29:654, 1999.

44. Friedman LS, Dienstag JL, Watkins E, et al: Evaluation of blood donors with elevated serum alanine aminotransferase levels. Ann Intern Med 107:137, 1987.

45. Murphy EJ, Davern TJ, Shakil AO, et al: Troglitazone-induced fulminant hepatic failure. Acute Liver Failure Study Group. Dig Dis Sci 45:549, 2000.

46. Palmer M, Schaffner F: Effect of weight reduction on hepatic abnormalities in overweight patients. Gastroenterology 99:1408, 1990.

47. de Ledinghen V, Combes M, Trouette H: Should a liver biopsy be done in patients with subclinical chronically elevated transaminases? Eur J Gastroenterol Hepatol 16:879, 2004.

48. Sorbi D, McGill DB, Thistle JL: An assessment of the role of liver biopsies in asymptomatic patients with chronic liver test abnormalities. Am J Gastroenterol 95:3206, 2000.

49. Davis GL, Czaja AJ, Baggenstoss AH, et al: Prognostic and therapeutic implications of extreme serum aminotransferase elevation in chronic active hepatitis. Mayo Clin Proc 57:303, 1982.

50. Henrion J, Schapira M, Luwaert R, et al: Hypoxic hepatitis: Clinical and hemodynamic study in 142 consecutive cases. Medicine 82:392, 2003

51. Gitlin N, Serio KM: Ischemic hepatitis: Widening horizons. Am J Gastroenterol 87:831, 1992.

52. Lucena MI, Camargo R, Andrade RJ, et al: Comparison of two clinical scales for causality assessment in hepatotoxicity. Hepa-tology 33:123, 2001.

53. Ostapowicz G, Fontana RJ, Schiødt FV, et al: Results of a prospective study of acute liver failure at 17 tertiary centers in the United States. Ann Intern Med 137:947, 2002.

54. Gordon SC, Reddy KR, Schiff L, et al: Prolonged intrahepatic cholestasis secondary to acute hepatitis A. Ann Intern Med 101:635, 1984.

55. Jacquemin E, Dumont M, Bernard O, et al: Evidence for defec-tive primary bile acid secretion in children with progressive familial intrahepatic cholestasis (Byler disease). Eur J Pediatr 153:424, 1994.

56. Carlton VE, Knisely AS, Freimer NB: Mapping of a locus for progressive familial intrahepatic cholestasis (Byler disease) to 18q21-q22, the benign recurrent intrahepatic cholestasis region. Hum Mol Genet 4:1049, 1995.

57. Fang MH, Ginsberg AL, Dobbins WOD: Marked elevation in serum alkaline phosphatase activity as a manifestation of sys-temic infection. Gastroenterology 78:592, 1980.

58. Shaver WA, Bhatt H, Combes B: Low serum alkaline phos-phatase activity in Wilson's disease. Hepatology 6:859, 1986.

59. Willson RA, Clayson KJ, Leon S: Unmeasurable serum alkaline phosphatase activity in Wilson's disease associated with ful-minant hepatic failure and hemolysis. Hepatology 7:613, 1987.

60. Chalasani N, Aljadhey H, Kesterson J, et al: Patients with ele-vated liver enzymes are not at higher risk for statin hepato-toxicity. Gastroenterology 126:1287, 2004.

61. Friedman LS: The risk of surgery in patients with liver disease. Hepatology 29:1617, 1999.

62. Mansour A, Watson W, Shayani V, et al: Abdominal operations in patients with cirrhosis: Still a major surgical challenge. Surgery 122:730, 1997.

63. Suman A, Barnes DS, Zein NN, et al: Predicting outcome after cardiac surgery in patients with cirrhosis: A comparison of Child-Pugh and MELD scores. Clin Gastroenterol Hepatol 2:719, 2004.

64. Freeman RB Jr: MELD and liver allocation: Continuous quality improvement. Hepatology 40:787, 2004.

65. Ramond MJ, Poynard T, Rueff B, et al: A randomized trial of prednisolone in patients with severe alcoholic hepatitis. N Engl J Med 326:507, 1992.

66. Dickson ER, Grambsch PM, Fleming TR, et al: Prognosis in primary biliary cirrhosis: Model for decision making. Hepa-tology 10:1, 1989.

67. Malinchoc M, Kamath PS, Gordon FD, et al: A model to predict poor survival in patients undergoing transjugular intrahepatic portosystemic shunts. Hepatology 31:864, 2000.

68. Imbert-Bismut F, Messous D, Thibaut V, et al: Intra-laboratory analytical variability of biochemical markers of fibrosis (Fibrotest) and activity (Actitest) and reference ranges in healthy blood donors. Clin Chem Lab Med 42:323, 2004.

69. Callewaert N, Van Vlieberghe H, Van Hecke A, et al: Nonin-vasive diagnosis of liver cirrhosis using DNA sequencer-based total serum protein glycomics. Nat Med 10:429, 2004.

70. Jalan R, Hayes PC: Review article: Quantitative tests of liver function. Aliment Pharmacol Ther 9:263, 1995.

71. Albers I, Hartmann H, Bircher J, et al: Superiority of the Child-Pugh classification to quantitative liver function tests for assessing prognosis of liver cirrhosis. Scand J Gastroenterol 24:269, 1989.

72. Burra P, Masier A: Dynamic tests to study liver function. Eur Rev Med Pharmacol Sci 8:19, 2004.

CHAPTER
71 Hemochromatosis

Bruce R. Bacon and Robert S. Britton

Trousseau was the first to describe a case of hemochromatosis in the French pathology literature in 1865.[1] Almost 25 years later, in 1889, von Recklinghausen, thinking that the disease was a blood disorder that caused increased skin pigmentation, coined the term *hemochromatosis*.[1] In 1935, Sheldon published a description of all 311 cases of the disease that had been reported in the world's literature to that point, including several from his own records. His conclusions have been borne out over the subsequent years. Sheldon realized that hemochromatosis was an inborn error of iron metabolism and that all the pathologic manifestations of the disease were caused by increased iron deposition in the affected organs.[1] In 1976, Simon and coworkers[2] demonstrated that the gene for hereditary hemochromatosis (HH) was linked to the *HLA* region on the short arm of chromosome 6. The benefit of early diagnosis on survival was shown clearly in a classic paper by Niederau and colleagues,[3] who demonstrated that if HH was identified before the development of cirrhosis or diabetes, survival of affected patients was equivalent to that of an age- and gender-matched population.

In 1996, the *HFE* gene was identified on chromosome 6, thereby permitting genetic testing for the two major mutations (C282Y, H63D) that are responsible for *HFE*-related HH.[4] Several prospective population surveys have shown that the frequency of the C282Y homozygous state is approximately 1 in 250 in white populations of northern European descent.[5] Subsequently, several additional genes and proteins involved in the regulation of iron homeostasis have been identified, contributing to a better understanding of cellular iron uptake and release. Also, numerous clinical and pathophysiologic studies have been performed and have led to improved diagnosis, better family screening, and new insights into normal and abnormal iron homeostasis. *HFE*-related HH is a common autosomal recessive disorder of iron metabolism; if it is diagnosed early and treated appropriately,

every patient with the disorder can have a normal lifespan.

CAUSES OF IRON OVERLOAD

Hereditary hemochromatosis comprises several inherited disorders of iron homeostasis characterized by increased intestinal iron absorption resulting in tissue iron deposition (Table 71–1). The older terms primary hemochromatosis and idiopathic hemochromatosis should no longer be used. The liver is always the principal recipient of most of the absorbed iron and is always involved in symptomatic HH. The most common form of HH by far is *HFE*-related HH.[6-8] It is an autosomal recessive disorder usually identified in adults of northern European ancestry. Most patients who present with HH are homozygous for the C282Y mutation of *HFE*, although some persons who are compound heterozygotes (C282Y/H63D) also have iron overload.

Other inherited forms of iron overload, classified as non-*HFE*-related HH, are juvenile hemochromatosis, African iron overload, and iron overload resulting from mutations in hepcidin,[9] transferrin receptor 2 (*TfR2*),[10] or ferroportin 1.[11] *Juvenile HH* is characterized by rapid iron accumulation. Mutations in two different genes have been shown to cause forms of juvenile HH. The more common mutation occurs in the *HJV* gene on chromosome 1q; this gene encodes a protein called hemojuvelin, the function of which is currently unknown.[12] Mutations in the hepcidin gene (*HAMP*) also produce a form of juvenile HH[9]; hepcidin is a hepatic peptide that acts to downregulate iron absorption. Mutations of the gene *TfR2* produce an autosomal recessive form of HH that is clinically similar to *HFE*-related HH.[10] How these *TfR2* mutations result in iron overload is not yet known, but it is possible that they cause abnormal iron sensing by hepatocytes, the predominant site of TfR2 expression.[13] A rare

Table 71–1   Iron Overload Conditions

Hereditary hemochromatosis	*HFE*-related hereditary hemochromatosis: 　　C282Y homozygosity 　　C282Y/H63D compound heterozygosity 　　Other *HFE* mutations Non–*HFE*-related hereditary 　　hemochromatosis: 　　Hemojuvelin (*HJV*) mutations 　　Hepcidin (*HAMP*) mutations 　　Transferrin receptor 2 (*TfR2*) mutations 　　Ferroportin 1 (*SLC40A1*) mutations 　　African iron overload
Secondary iron overload	Acquired iron overload: 　Iron-loading anemias 　　Thalassemia major 　　Sideroblastic anemia 　　Chronic hemolytic anemia 　　Aplastic anemia 　　Pyruvate kinase deficiency 　　Pyridoxine-responsive anemia 　Parenteral iron overload 　　Red blood cell transfusions 　　Iron-dextran injections 　　Long-term hemodialysis 　Chronic liver disease 　　Hepatitis C 　　Hepatitis B 　　Alcoholic liver disease 　　Nonalcoholic steatohepatitis 　　Porphyria cutanea tarda 　　Portacaval shunt 　Dietary iron overload 　Dysmetabolic iron overload syndrome
Miscellaneous	Neonatal iron overload Aceruloplasminemia Congenital atransferrinemia

autosomal dominant form of HH results from missense mutations in the ferroportin 1 gene.[11] In this disorder, iron loading of periportal hepatocytes as well as reticuloendothelial cells is observed. The mechanism of iron overload caused by mutated ferroportin 1 is not clear.

African iron overload occurs primarily in sub-Saharan Africa and is now considered to be the result of a non–*HFE*-related genetic trait that can be exacerbated by dietary iron loading.[14] Some people who manifest African iron overload consume an iron-rich fermented maize beverage, but iron overload also can occur in people who do not drink this beverage. In most cases, iron-loaded Kupffer cells are prominent in African iron overload; in contrast, Kupffer cells are relatively spared in *HFE*-related HH. It has been suggested that a similar form of iron overload may occur in African-Americans,[15] but further investigations are needed to determine the genetic basis, prevalence, and clinical consequences of this condition. Approximately 20% of a cohort of Africans and African-Americans with iron overload have a novel mutation in the ferroportin 1 gene, suggesting that this mutation may contribute to iron loading.[16]

Persons who absorb excessive amounts of iron as a result of an underlying cause other than any of the previously mentioned inherited defects have *secondary iron overload* (see Table 71–1).[17] Examples are people with dis-

orders of ineffective erythropoiesis, liver disease (in some cases), increased oral intake of iron, or the rare condition congenital atransferrinemia. Both HH and secondary iron overload should be distinguished from *parenteral iron overload*, which is always iatrogenic and which leads to iron deposition that is initially found in the reticuloendothelial system. In patients with ineffective erythropoiesis who require red blood cell transfusions, parenchymal and reticuloendothelial iron overload coexists, because these people have a stimulus to increased iron absorption and receive iron in the form of red blood cell transfusions. A syndrome of *neonatal iron overload* has been described that appears to be distinct from any of the causes mentioned previously.[18]

PATHOPHYSIOLOGY

The pathophysiologic mechanisms of HH fall into the following three main categories: (1) altered function of HFE protein, (2) increased intestinal absorption of dietary iron, and (3) iron-induced tissue injury and fibrogenesis.

HFE PROTEIN

Studies of HFE protein structure and function were a direct consequence of the cloning of the *HFE* gene. The *HFE* gene encodes a 343–amino acid protein consisting of a 22–amino acid signal peptide, large extracellular domain, single transmembrane domain, and short cytoplasmic tail (Fig. 71–1).[4] The extracellular domain of HFE protein consists of three loops (α_1, α_2, and α_3), with intramolecular disulfide bonds within the second and third loops. The structure of the HFE protein is similar to that of other major histocompatibility complex (MHC) class I proteins, but evidence indicates that HFE protein does not participate in antigen presentation.[19] However, like MHC class I molecules, HFE protein is physically associated with β_2-microglobulin (β_2m) (see Fig. 71–1). The major mutation responsible for HH results in the substitution of tyrosine for cysteine at amino acid 282 in the α_3 loop (C282Y) and abolishes the disulfide bond in this domain.[4] Loss of this disulfide bond interferes with the interaction of HFE protein with β_2m, and the C282Y mutant protein demonstrates decreased presentation at the cell surface, increased retention in the endoplasmic reticulum, and accelerated degradation.[20]

The HH-like phenotype of β_2m-knockout mice provides independent evidence of the importance of the HFE protein–β_2m association for normal HFE protein function.[21] A second mutation associated with HH results in the change of a histidine to an aspartate at position 63 in the $\alpha1$ chain (H63D), but this mutation has less biologic impact than the C282Y mutation. Like HH patients, *Hfe*-knockout mice manifest higher hepatic iron levels, elevated transferrin saturation (TS), increased intestinal iron absorption, and relative sparing of iron loading in reticuloendothelial cells.[13]

The first mechanistic link between HFE protein and cellular iron metabolism resulted from the observation that HFE protein forms a complex with the transferrin receptor (TfR1). The physical association of HFE protein with

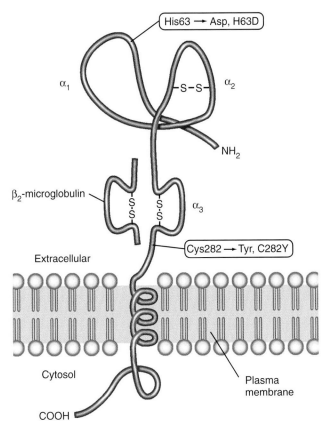

Figure 71–1 Schematic model of HFE protein in association with β_2-microglobulin at the cell surface. The three extracellular domains of HFE protein are designated α_1, α_2, and α_3. β_2-Microglobulin is physically associated with the α_3 domain. HFE protein also contains a transmembrane domain and a short intracellular domain. Positions of the two common HFE mutations, C282Y and H63D, are shown.

TfR1 has been observed in cultured cells and in duodenal crypt enterocytes, the site of regulation of dietary iron absorption. The observation that HFE protein and TfR1 are physically associated has led to a number of investigations on the effect of HFE protein on TfR1-mediated iron uptake and cellular iron status.[13] These studies have yielded conflicting results concerning the effects of HFE protein on cellular iron metabolism, and more research is required to resolve this issue, especially in the duodenum, liver, and reticuloendothelial system.

DUODENAL IRON ABSORPTION

An increase in intestinal iron absorption is a pathogenic characteristic of *HFE*-related HH. Understanding the pathogenesis of HH, therefore, requires a review of the determinants of duodenal iron absorption. Because there are no important physiologic mechanisms to regulate iron loss, iron homeostasis depends on a tight linkage between body iron requirements and intestinal iron absorption. Nearly all absorption of dietary iron occurs in the duodenum, where iron may be taken up as either ionic iron or heme.[13,22] The absorption of both forms of iron is increased in patients with *HFE*-related HH.

Uptake of heme occurs by an as yet unidentified transporter. Absorption of ionic iron across the enterocyte occurs in two stages, uptake across the apical membrane and transfer across the basolateral membrane (Fig. 71–2A). Before uptake, ionic iron must be reduced from the ferric to the ferrous state; this is accomplished by the ferric reductase (duodenal cytochrome b; Dcytb), which is expressed on the luminal surface of duodenal enterocytes. The ferrous iron crosses the apical membrane via

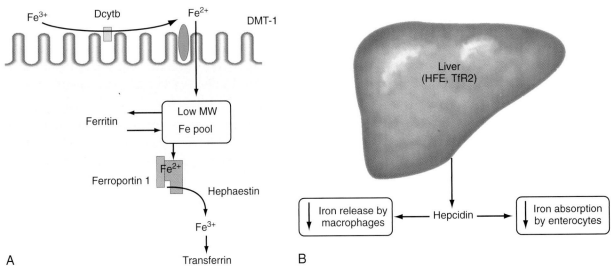

Figure 71–2 Iron absorption pathway in duodenal enterocytes and the role of hepcidin. *A,* Duodenal enterocytes are the major site of iron absorption. Prior to uptake, dietary ionic iron requires reduction from the ferric (Fe^{3+}) to the ferrous (Fe^{2+}) state. This is accomplished by the ferric reductase (Dcytb) that is expressed on the luminal surfaces of enterocytes. Ferrous iron is taken up by the apical transporter, DMT-1. Iron may be stored within the cell as ferritin, and lost with the sloughed senescent enterocyte, or transferred across the basolateral membrane to the plasma. This latter process occurs via the transporter ferroportin 1 and requires oxidation of iron to the ferric state by the molecule hephaestin. MW, molecular weight. *B,* Hepcidin is produced by the liver and secreted into the blood. Both HFE protein and transferrin receptor 2 (TfR2) may participate in the hepatic iron-sensing mechanism that regulates hepcidin expression. Hepcidin acts on macrophages to reduce iron release (and thereby increase macrophage iron stores) and on duodenal enterocytes to reduce the amount of dietary iron absorbed into the circulation. In *HFE*-related hereditary hemochromatosis, loss of functional HFE protein leads to aberrant hepatocellular sensing of plasma iron, inappropriately low levels of hepcidin, diminished macrophage iron stores, and greater duodenal iron absorption.

divalent metal transporter 1 (DMT-1). Iron taken up by the enterocyte may be stored as ferritin (and excreted in the feces when the senescent enterocyte is sloughed) or transferred across the basolateral membrane to the plasma. This latter process occurs via the transporter ferroportin 1. The basolateral transfer of iron requires oxidation of iron to the ferric state by the molecule hephaestin.

In addition to increased uptake of iron from the diet, patients with *HFE*-related HH demonstrate increased basolateral transfer of iron from the enterocytes to the plasma. Some data suggest that the greater basolateral transfer of iron may be the driving force behind the increased intestinal iron absorption observed in *HFE*-related HH. Some studies of patients with *HFE*-related HH and *Hfe*-knockout mice have demonstrated higher duodenal expression of Dcytb, DMT-1, and ferroportin 1.[13]

Duodenal iron absorption is tied to iron requirements by at least two functionally defined regulators.[23] One is the erythropoietic regulator, which adjusts intestinal iron absorption in response to the demands of erythropoiesis independent of body iron stores. The other is the stores regulator, which modulates iron absorption in response to the level of body iron stores. The stores regulator prevents iron overload after ensuring that iron needs are met. In patients with *HFE*-related HH, the stores regulator appears to function, but at a higher set point (i.e., the rate of intestinal iron absorption is excessive relative to the level of liver iron stores). The molecular components of the stores regulator have begun to be identified. One is the small peptide hepcidin, which is produced by the liver and secreted into the plasma.[24,25] Hepcidin acts as a negative regulator of dietary iron absorption, and its expression in the liver is inversely related to liver iron stores.[24]

Two different (but not mutually exclusive) hypotheses have been proposed to explain the effect of mutant *HFE* on intestinal iron absorption: (1) the hepcidin hypothesis and (2) the duodenal crypt cell programming hypothesis. These hypotheses differ as to the proposed cell type in which loss of functional HFE protein leads to downstream changes in body iron homeostasis. In the hepcidin hypothesis, the affected cell is the hepatocyte, whereas in the crypt cell programming hypothesis, the affected cell is the duodenal crypt enterocyte.

As outlined earlier, patients with *HFE*-related HH have excessive dietary iron absorption relative to body iron stores. This observation suggests that normal function of at least one of the components of the iron stores regulator is regulated abnormally in HH. Several lines of evidence point to hepcidin as a candidate for this abnormally regulated component. A phenotype similar to that of *Hfe*-knockout mice develops in mice in which the hepcidin gene is knocked out; features include hepatic iron loading, elevated TS, and reticuloendothelial iron sparing.[24] Furthermore, hepcidin is an acute-phase reactant and plays a central role in the hypoferremia of inflammation (i.e., anemia of chronic disease).[25] Intriguingly, the changes in iron homeostasis observed during inflammation (reduced intestinal iron absorption and larger reticuloendothelial iron stores) are the converse of those observed in *HFE*-related HH.[25] Indeed, patients with *HFE*-related HH have decreased hepatic expression of

hepcidin, as do *Hfe*-knockout mice, despite excess hepatic iron stores.[26,27] Furthermore, patients who carry mutations in the hepcidin gene have a severe form of juvenile HH.[9] Why hepcidin is inappropriately under-expressed, with loss of functional HFE protein, is uncertain. One possibility is that HFE protein is a participant in the process by which hepatocytes sense iron status.[13] The preponderance of current data indicates that abnormally low levels of hepcidin play an important role in the pathogenesis of *HFE*-related HH (see Fig. 71–2*B*).

The duodenal crypt cell programming hypothesis offers an alternative explanation for the increase in iron absorption seen in *HFE*-related HH. Duodenal crypt cells have long been proposed to play a role in sensing of body iron status and thereby influence the level of dietary iron absorption when these cells differentiate into absorptive enterocytes.[28] Expression of HFE protein in association with TfR1 has been demonstrated in duodenal crypt cells.[29] These observations have led to the proposal that HFE protein influences the sensing of circulating iron by the duodenal crypt cells. This model postulates that normal HFE protein in duodenal crypt cells facilitates the uptake of plasma iron by the TfR1-mediated pathway and that mutant HFE protein lacks this facilitating effect.[8,13] Functional loss of HFE protein may thus diminish the regulatory iron pool in crypt cells, thereby resulting in a relatively iron-deficient state in these cells. This sequence could lead to the greater expression of iron transport genes in daughter villus enterocytes and increased dietary iron absorption.

The precise role of HFE in regulating iron homeostasis remains an area of intensive investigation. Ultimately, testing the two hypotheses will require an examination of the consequences of mutant HFE protein in hepatocytes and in duodenal crypt enterocytes.

IRON-INDUCED TISSUE INJURY AND FIBROSIS

The final major pathophysiologic mechanism to consider in HH relates to the liver damage resulting from iron overload. In patients with advanced HH, hepatic fibrosis and cirrhosis are the principal pathologic findings. A number of studies of experimental hepatic iron overload have identified iron-dependent lipid peroxidation, and membrane-dependent functions of mitochondria, microsomes, and lysosomes are abnormal at hepatic iron concentrations at which lipid peroxidation occurs.[30] A relationship between iron-induced lipid peroxidation and fibrosis has been shown in several studies.[31,32] One hypothesis is that iron-induced lipid peroxidation occurs in hepatocytes and causes hepatocellular injury or death. Kupffer cells may become activated by products released from injured iron-loaded hepatocytes and produce profibrogenic cytokines, which can, in turn, stimulate hepatic stellate cells to synthesize larger amounts of collagen, thereby leading to pathologic fibrosis.[31,32]

Studies of iron-induced tissue damage in organs other than the liver, such as the heart, pancreas, and endocrine glands, have been limited. Studies in myocardial cells have shown functional abnormalities resulting from iron-induced peroxidation.[33]

CLINICAL FEATURES

Currently, many patients with *HFE*-related HH come to medical attention without any symptoms or physical findings. They are identified as homozygous relatives of probands during family screening studies or by the results of serum iron studies in routine screening blood chemistry panels (Table 71–2).[34,35] Nonetheless, the clinician should know the typical clinical manifestations in patients who do present with symptomatic disease. Most patients with symptomatic *HFE*-related *HH* are 40 to 50 years of age at the time of detection. Although the defective gene is distributed equally between men and women, most clinical series have identified more men than women, with ratios ranging from 2:1 to 8:1. Therefore, the frequency of *HFE*-related HH in women is often underestimated when the diagnosis is based solely on phenotypic expression, most likely because of iron loss from normal menses and childbirth in women.

When patients present with symptoms, the most common are weakness and lethargy, arthralgias, abdominal pain, and loss of libido or potency in men.[3,36] Hepatomegaly is found on physical examination in a majority of patients; splenomegaly and other complications of chronic liver disease, including ascites, edema, and jaundice, may be present. Diabetes has decreased in frequency with earlier diagnosis of hemochromatosis and is typically not seen in the absence of cirrhosis. Detection of the often subtle bronzed or slate gray skin pigmentation of *HFE*-related HH requires astuteness on the part of the clinician. Organ damage and symptoms are usually related to the extent of iron loading. When patients are identified prospectively by either family or population screening, the frequency of patients who are asymptomatic increases dramatically.

All patients with *HFE*-related HH who have elevated serum ferritin values should also have increased hepatic iron stores, but the extent of hepatic iron loading is often not high enough to cause liver damage. In the late 1960s, cirrhosis was found in more than 50% of the patients identified with HH[3]; in studies from the 1970s through the 1990s, cirrhosis was found in only 5% to 10% of patients.[34,35] Later population screening studies have reported an even lower frequency of liver injury in C282Y homozygotes.[37-39] Serum aminotransferase elevations are usually mild. With regular phlebotomy and depletion of excess iron stores, elevated liver enzyme values typically revert to normal. When *HFE*-related HH is diagnosed and treated before the development of hepatic fibrosis or cirrhosis, long-term hepatic abnormalities do not develop. However, when *HFE*-related HH is detected after cirrhosis has developed, hepatocellular carcinoma can occur even after successful phlebotomy,[40] thus emphasizing the importance of early diagnosis and treatment. Finally, patients with *HFE*-related HH may have nonspecific right upper quadrant abdominal pain that is most likely caused by hepatic capsular distention.

Other clinical manifestations that can occur relate to the level of iron loading in nonhepatic organs. In older series, diabetes was a common complication of pancreatic iron loading,[3] but in later series in which the diagnosis of *HFE*-related HH was made earlier in its course, diabetes has rarely been present.[34,35] Other endocrinologic abnormalities are loss of libido and impotence in men, owing to both primary testicular failure and gonadotropin insufficiency resulting from the effects of iron on

Table 71–2 Clinical Features of Hereditary Hemochromatosis

Variable	Reference		
	3	**34**	**35**
Case selection method	Symptomatic index cases, family screening	Family screening by HLA-typing	Screening chemistry panels, family screening
Dates of study	1959-1983	Before 1990	1990-1995
Number of patients:	163	37	40
Men	145	19	26
Women	18	18	14
Mean age (yrs):	46	Men: 49 Women: 53	Men: 46 Women: 47
Age range (yrs)	18-77	11-79	23-73
Symptoms (%)			
None	9	46	73
Weakness or lethargy	83	19	25
Abdominal pain	58	3	3
Arthralgias	43	40	13
Loss of libido, impotence (% of men)	38	32	12
Findings (%)			
Cirrhosis	69	3	13*
Hepatomegaly	83	3	13
Skin pigmentation	75	9	5
Diabetes mellitus	55	11	5
Elevated liver enzymes	62	27	33

*Five of 40 patients had cirrhosis, but 1 had concomitant chronic hepatitis C and 1 had alcoholic liver disease.

pituitary function,[41] and occasionally hypothyroidism; adrenal function is typically normal. Other endocrinologic effects can occur as a result of complications of cirrhosis (see Chapter 89).

Cardiac manifestations occur rarely because patients are now diagnosed earlier in the course of *HFE*-related HH. Cardiomyopathy, atrial and ventricular dysrhythmias, and congestive heart failure can occur.[42] Characteristic of the arthropathy of *HFE*-related HH are changes in the second and third metacarpophalangeal joints. Joint space narrowing, chondrocalcinosis, subchondral cyst formation, osteopenia, and swelling of the joints may be seen.[3,36,43] Unfortunately, the arthritic symptoms of *HFE*-related HH typically do not improve with phlebotomy. The skin pigmentation of *HFE*-related HH, which can be subtle, is characterized by either a bronze discoloration due to predominant melanin pigmentation or a gray pigmentation resulting from iron deposition in the basal layers of the epidermis.[36] The frequency of certain infections, including those caused by *Vibrio vulnificus*, *Listeria monocytogenes*, *Yersinia enterocolitica*, and *Yersinia pseudotuberculosis*, is more common in iron-loaded patients, although still rare.

DIAGNOSIS

The requirements for diagnosis of HH have changed since the availability of *HFE* mutation analysis. As in the past, the disorder must be considered in any patient with elevated liver enzymes and abnormal screening iron test results. If the results raise suspicions, then the appropriate serum iron tests along with *HFE* mutation analysis should be obtained. With the advent of genetic testing, the need for liver biopsy has diminished. In symptomatic patients, the most common symptoms are fatigue, malaise, right upper quadrant abdominal pain, and arthralgias. Less commonly, symptoms of chronic liver disease, diabetes, and congestive heart failure are identified. Because many of these symptoms are nonspecific or are related to other common diseases, HH is commonly not considered in symptomatic patients at first encounter with the clinician.

In the early 1990s, patients with HH commonly presented after the discovery of abnormal results of screening blood chemistry tests obtained as part of routine health maintenance or for another reason.[35] Many commercial laboratories added iron and total iron-binding capacity (TIBC), with TS calculated as iron ÷ TIBC × 100%, to their panel of screening serum chemistry tests, and in many patients, a TS was obtained inadvertently even though the test had not been specifically ordered. In one series, 62% of patients newly identified between 1990 and 1995 came to medical attention in this way.[35] Another 14% of cases were identified through screening of family members of a known proband. Therefore, as many as 75% of patients came to medical attention by way of screening laboratory tests; the majority of these patients were asymptomatic and had no physical findings for HH, and the frequency of end-stage complications of *HFE*-related HH, such as cirrhosis and diabetes, was much lower than that reported in earlier series of patients who presented with symptoms of the disease.[35] In 1998, the Health Care Finance Administration (HCFA; now Center for Medicare and Medicaid Services [CMS]) stopped providing reimbursement for screening tests of any kind, and since then, fewer American patients with HH have been identified through routine screening.

Once *HFE*-related HH has been considered, the diagnosis is relatively straightforward. Measurements of serum iron and TIBC or transferrin, with calculation of TS, and serum ferritin should be obtained in the fasting state (Table 71–3). Because more than 50% of normal persons have transiently elevated serum iron values after

Table 71–3 Representative Iron Measurements and HFE Mutation Analysis Findings in Patients with HFE-Related Hereditary Hemochromatosis

	Normal Values/Findings	Values/Findings In HFE-Related Hemochromatosis
Serum:		
Iron:		
(µg/dL)	60-180	180-300
(µmol/L)	11-32	32-54
Transferrin saturation (%)	20-45	45-100
Ferritin:		
Men (ng/mL; µg/L)	20-200	300-3000
Women (ng/mL; µg/L)	15-150	250-3000
Liver:		
Iron staining	0, 1+	3+, 4+
Iron concentration		
(µg/g dry weight)	300-1500	3000-30,000
(µmol/g dry weight)	5-27	53-536
Iron index (µmol/g dry weight ÷ age in years)	<1.1	>1.9
HFE mutation analysis	wt/wt	C282Y/C282Y
	C282Y/wt	C282Y/H63D
	H63D/wt	

wt, wild-type.

eating, the blood sample must be drawn with the patient in the fasting state; otherwise, the TS can be elevated in the absence of increased iron stores. In addition, there is a diurnal variation in serum iron concentration, and to establish a diagnosis of HH, blood should be drawn for serum iron studies from fasting patients in the morning.

A TS value greater than 45% is the earliest phenotypic manifestation of *HFE*-related HH. As a result, TS is a more sensitive and specific test for HFE-related HH than serum ferritin, which can be normal in young persons with *HFE*-related HH or elevated in unaffected persons for a variety of reasons, including various types of necroinflammatory liver disease (e.g., chronic viral hepatitis, alcoholic liver disease, nonalcoholic steatohepatitis), certain malignancies, and other inflammatory conditions. An elevated serum ferritin level with a normal TS value in a person who has an inflammatory disorder generally suggests that the person does not have *HFE*-related HH. On the other hand, an elevated TS value with a normal ferritin value in a young person does not exclude *HFE*-related HH. A large population screening study in San Diego demonstrated that 1 in 237 persons was homozygous for the C282Y mutation, but only 64% of these homozygotes had a TS value higher than 45%.[37] This finding indicates

that a much higher proportion of C282Y homozygotes do not express iron overload than had previously been thought. The proportion of the non-expressing cohort that will subsequently show evidence of iron loading is uncertain. In a longitudinal follow-up study of patients identified by genetic screening, progressive iron loading, as indicated by rising serum ferritin levels, developed in 40% of C282Y homozygotes.[44]

Once serum iron parameters have been determined to be abnormal in the appropriate setting, *HFE* mutation analysis should be performed. If the patient is a C282Y homozygote or a compound heterozygote (C282Y/H63D) and has a serum ferritin level lower than 1000 ng/mL, normal liver enzyme values, and no evidence of hepatomegaly, there is no need for a liver biopsy.[45-47] If, however, the serum ferritin value is higher than 1000 ng/mL, liver enzymes are elevated, or hepatomegaly is present, liver biopsy is indicated. When liver biopsy is performed, sufficient tissue for histopathologic evaluation and biochemical measurement of the hepatic iron concentration (HIC) should be obtained. With the advent of genetic testing, liver biopsy is performed solely to assess the damage (if any) to the liver. A proposed algorithm for evaluating people for possible *HFE*-related HH is shown in Figure 71–3.

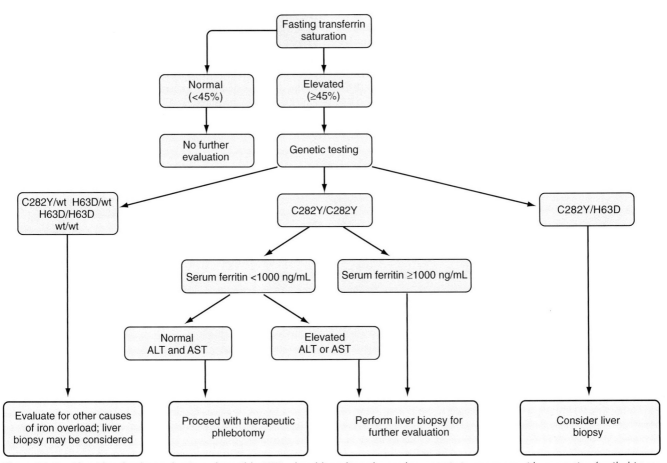

Figure 71–3 Algorithm for the evaluation of possible HFE-related hereditary hemochromatosis in a person with a negative family history. ALT, alanine aminotransferase; AST, aspartate aminotransferase; wt, wild-type.

When liver biopsy is performed, the Perls' Prussian blue stain is used for the determination and localization of storage iron. Iron stores in *HFE*-related HH are typically found in periportal hepatocytes, with little or no iron found in Kupffer cells (Fig. 71–4).[48] In patients with a higher HIC, iron distribution becomes panlobular, and storage iron can be seen in Kupffer cells and bile duct cells. Grade 1 or 2 Perls' Prussian blue staining can be seen in specimens from normal livers or specimens from patients with very early HH, which is confirmed by *HFE* mutation analysis. Grade 3 stainable iron can occasionally be seen in specimens from patients with alcoholic cirrhosis or in end-stage liver disease (ESLD), in which iron staining correlates poorly with HIC. In the absence of other disorders, grade 3 to 4 stainable iron in an *HFE* pattern is consistent with *HFE*-related HH.

In addition to histochemical staining, biochemical iron measurement in the liver is important (see Table 71–3). Typically, patients with *HFE*-related HH who present with symptoms have an HIC greater than 10,000 μg/g (dry weight) (normal < 1500 μg/g); HIC values may be more than 30,000 μg/g. Fibrosis and cirrhosis are usually not seen until the HIC exceeds 20,000 μg/g.[49] In patients with both *HFE*-related HH and other forms of chronic liver disease, such as alcoholic liver disease or chronic viral hepatitis, increased fibrosis or cirrhosis can occur at a much lower HIC and at a younger age.[50-52] In asymptomatic or younger patients with early *HFE*-related HH, HIC is increased to a lesser degree, often being much less than 10,000 μg/g.

A common diagnostic dilemma occurs when it is not clear whether a patient has liver disease with abnormal iron parameters or *HFE*-related HH with elevations in liver enzymes. In this setting, *HFE* mutation analysis is extremely useful. If the patient is a C282Y homozygote or a compound heterozygote (C282Y/H63D), the iron loading is most likely caused predominantly by the genetic abnormality. On the other hand, if the patient has underlying liver disease, is a C282Y heterozygote, or is an H63D heterozygote or H63D homozygote, or has neither mutation, it is likely that the iron loading is caused by the underlying liver disease, perhaps with a minor contribution from the *HFE* genotype. In the past, the hepatic iron index (HIC in μmoles/g ÷ the patient's age in years) was useful for distinguishing HH from secondary iron overload.[49] With *HFE* mutation analysis, the value of the hepatic iron index has diminished.

Computed tomography (CT), magnetic resonance imaging (MRI), and magnetic susceptibility testing have all been proposed as techniques to quantify HIC without the need for a liver biopsy (Fig. 71–5). Magnetic susceptibility testing is available in only a few centers in the United States and Europe as a research tool. In early studies, CT and MRI were generally not reliable for detecting mild iron overload, but a newer MRI technique has shown improved sensitivity.[53]

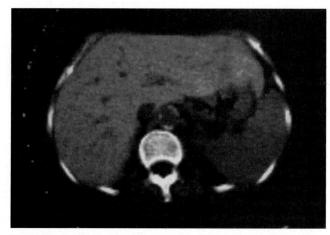

Figure 71–5 Computed tomography (CT) in hemochromatosis. Hepatic density measured by CT scanning is increased in heavily iron-loaded people. The iron-containing liver is much brighter than the spleen.

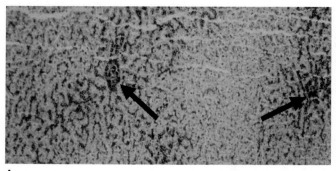
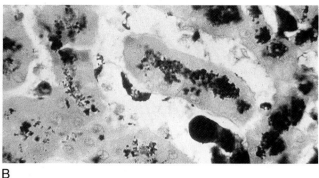

A   B

Figure 71–4 Histology of HFE-related hereditary hemochromatosis. *A,* This liver biopsy specimen was obtained from a 47-year-old C282Y homozygous woman who presented with a transferrin saturation of 63% and a serum ferritin level of 590 ng/mL. The hepatic iron concentration was 9840 μg/g with a calculated hepatic iron index of 3.7. At low power, iron deposition is seen to be much greater in the periportal zone (acinar zone 1) (*arrows*) than in the centrilobular zone (acinar zone 3). (Perls' Prussian blue stain; ×100.) (Courtesy of Elizabeth M. Brunt, MD, St. Louis, Mo.) *B,* At a higher magnification of a specimen from another patient with *HFE*-related hereditary hemochromatosis, iron deposition is seen to be in hepatocytes arranged in cords and not in reticuloendothelial (Kupffer) cells that line the intervening sinusoids. In patients with higher hepatic iron concentrations, iron deposition becomes panlobular, and storage iron can be seen in Kupffer cells and bile duct cells. (Perls' Prussian blue stain.) (Courtesy of Edward Lee, MD, Washington, D.C.)

Table 71–4 Treatment of HFE-Related Hereditary Hemochromatosis

Perform phlebotomy of 500 mL (1 unit) of whole blood weekly until hematocrit value drops below 37%.

Check transferrin saturation and ferritin levels at 2- to 3-month intervals to monitor response (optional).

Once iron stores are depleted (ferritin <50 ng/mL; transferrin saturation <50%), proceed to maintenance phlebotomy of 1 unit of whole blood every 2 to 3 months. Aim to keep transferrin saturation <50%; if successful, ferritin should remain <50 ng/mL.

TREATMENT AND PROGNOSIS

The treatment of HFE-related HH is relatively straightforward; most patients can be treated with routine therapeutic phlebotomy (Table 71–4). Ideally, diagnosis and initiation of treatment should begin before the development of hepatic fibrosis or cirrhosis; if they are, patients will have normal lifespans. Each unit of whole blood (500 mL) contains approximately 200 to 250 mg of iron, depending on the hemoglobin concentration; therefore, C282Y homozygotes who have 10 to 20 g of excess storage iron require extended phlebotomy regimens (40 to 80 units of blood removed). Most patients can tolerate weekly phlebotomy of 1 unit of whole blood, and occasional younger patients can tolerate the removal of 2 or 3 units per week. Some older patients and occasional patients with a coexistent underlying hematologic disorder resulting in anemia can tolerate phlebotomy of only 0.5 unit per week or every other week. The iron-chelating drug deferoxamine is used in patients with HFE-related HH and cardiac manifestations or in patients who cannot tolerate phlebotomy.

Although not absolutely necessary, it is useful to obtain a TS value and serum ferritin level every 2 to 3 months to predict the eventual return of iron stores to normal. Typically, the serum ferritin level falls progressively as hepatic iron stores decrease, whereas TS usually remains elevated until just before iron stores return to normal. In uncomplicated cases, the ferritin level drops about 30 ng/mL with each unit of blood removed. Once the iron stores have reached a level in the low-normal range, the serum ferritin level should be less than 50 ng/mL and the TS less than 50%. At this point, maintenance phlebotomies every 2 to 3 months are required in most patients. The rate of reaccumulation of iron varies in individuals, and patients may require regular maintenance phlebotomy at more or less frequent intervals. Occasional patients do not reaccumulate iron, for reasons that are unknown.

The prognosis for patients with HFE-related HH is improved significantly by therapeutic phlebotomy.[3,54,55] Life expectancy is reduced in patients who present with cirrhosis or diabetes, and the risk of death from hepatocellular carcinoma is higher in patients with HFE-related HH. Hepatocellular cancer is usually seen only in patients who already have cirrhosis. Established cirrhosis typically does not reverse with phlebotomy, but as many as 30% of patients have some reduction of fibrosis with aggressive treatment. Unfortunately, neither arthritis nor hypogonadism improves; however, management of diabetes may become easier after iron removal.

The value of screening for hepatocellular carcinoma in cirrhotic patients with HH is controversial, because the cost-effectiveness of the screening approaches has not been validated. Most authorities suggest ultrasonography or CT scanning and a serum α-fetoprotein measurement every 6 months in cirrhotic patients with HFE-related HH. With improved methods of detection and treatment of small, early hepatocellular carcinomas (e.g., radiofrequency ablation, chemoembolization, resection, and liver transplantation), screening seems to be reasonable (see Chapter 91).

When diagnosis and treatment are delayed and complications of ESLD develop, liver transplantation (LT) may be undertaken (see also Chapter 92). Although experience with LT for HFE-related HH is limited, existing data indicate that LT for this purpose carries a higher mortality than transplantation for other causes of ESLD.[56,57] The higher mortality rate relates to iron overload, whether caused by HFE-related HH or secondary iron overload in conjunction with another liver disease such as chronic hepatitis C or alcoholic liver disease. In fact, only about 10% of patients with iron overload and ESLD are C282Y homozygotes.[58] If iron overload from any cause is diagnosed early, it should be treated in order to reduce the chance of post-transplant death. Post-transplant deaths in patients with iron overload are usually related to infectious or cardiac complications.[58,59]

Unfortunately, HFE-related HH or secondary iron overload is often not diagnosed before LT, and one series has shown a high frequency of primary liver cancer diagnosed incidentally in affected patients only at the time of transplantation.[56] A factor that may account for the increased postoperative mortality in patients with undiagnosed or untreated HFE-related HH is the extent of iron deposition in extrahepatic sites. A high index of suspicion for iron overload in patients with ESLD should lead to improved diagnosis and prompt institution of phlebotomy or iron-chelation therapy before LT. These changes in management should reduce the frequency of postoperative complications and improve long-term post-transplant survival.

FAMILY SCREENING

Once a proband with HFE-related HH has been identified and his or her therapy initiated, there is still a responsibility to the patient's family.[60] For asymptomatic C282Y homozygotes and compound heterozygotes (C282Y/H63D) identified by HFE mutation analysis within a sibship, there is no need for liver biopsy. In family members in whom serum ferritin levels are increased, proceeding to therapeutic phlebotomy is reasonable, with liver biopsy reserved for those patients for whom there is a question of another underlying liver disease. Persons who are C282Y heterozygotes (C282Y/wt) are not at risk for progressive iron overload. If the spouse of a C282Y homozygote is a C282Y heterozygote, there is a 50% chance that their offspring will be homozygous for C282Y. HFE mutation analysis in the children can eliminate the need for subsequent serum iron testing if a genotype of C282Y/C282Y or C282Y/H63D is not found, although the issues of genetic discrimination and stigmatization must be acknowledged and considered. In children who are C282Y homozygotes or compound heterozygotes, serum ferritin measurements should be obtained yearly, and phlebotomy instituted when ferritin values become elevated.

REFERENCES

1. Bacon BR: Joseph H. Sheldon and hereditary hemochromatosis: Historical highlights. J Lab Clin Med 113:761, 1989.
2. Simon M, Bourel M, Fauchet R, et al: Association of HLA-A3 and HLA-B14 antigens with idiopathic hemochromatosis. Gut 17:332, 1976.
3. Niederau C, Fischer R, Sonnenberg A, et al: Survival and causes of death in cirrhotic and noncirrhotic patients with primary hemochromatosis. N Engl J Med 313:1265, 1985.
4. Feder JN, Gnirke A, Thomas W, et al: A novel MHC class 1-like gene is mutated in patients with hereditary haemochromatosis. Nat Genet 13:339, 1996.
5. Bacon BR, Powell LW, Adams PC, et al: Molecular medicine and hemochromatosis: At the crossroads. Gastroenterology 116:193, 1999.
6. Powell LW: Hereditary hemochromatosis. Pathology 32:24, 2000.
7. Harrison SA, Bacon BR: Hereditary hemochromatosis: Update for 2003. J Hepatol 38(Suppl 1):S14, 2003.
8. Pietrangelo A: Hereditary hemochromatosis: A new look at an old disease. N Engl J Med 350:2383, 2004.
9. Roetto A, Papanikolaou G, Politou M, et al: Mutant antimicrobial peptide hepcidin is associated with severe juvenile hemochromatosis. Nat Genet 33:21, 2003.
10. Camaschella C, Roetto A, Cali A, et al: The gene TFR2 is mutated in a new type of haemochromatosis mapping to 7q22. Nat Genet 25:14, 2000.
11. Pietrangelo A: Non-HFE hemochromatosis. Hepatology 39:21, 2004.
12. Papanikolaou G, Samuels ME, Ludwig EH, et al: Mutations in HFE2 cause iron overload in chromosome 1q-linked juvenile hemochromatosis. Nat Genet 36:77, 2004.
13. Fleming RE, Britton RS, Waheed A, et al: Pathogenesis of hereditary hemochromatosis. Clin Liver Dis 8:755. 2004.
14. Gordeuk VR: African iron overload. Semin Hematol 39:263, 2002.
15. Barton JC, Acton RT, Rivers CA, et al: Genotypic and phenotypic heterogeneity of African Americans with primary iron overload. Blood Cells Mol Dis 31:310, 2003.
16. Gordeuk VR, Caleffi A, Corradini E, et al: Iron overload in Africans and African-Americans and a common mutation in the SCL40A1 (ferroportin 1) gene. Blood Cells Mol Dis 31:299, 2003.
17. Bottomley SS: Secondary iron overload disorders. Semin Hematol 35:77, 1998.
18. Knisely AS, Mieli-Vergani G, Whitington PF: Neonatal hemochromatosis. Gastroenterol Clin North Am 32:877, 2003.
19. Lebron JA, Bennett MJ, Vaughn DE, et al: Crystal structure of the hemochromatosis protein HFE and characterization of its interaction with transferrin receptor. Cell 93:111, 1998.
20. Waheed A, Parkkila S, Zhou XY, et al: Hereditary hemochromatosis: Effects of C282Y and H63D mutations on association with β2-microglobulin, intracellular processing, and cell surface expression of the HFE protein in COS-7 cells. Proc Natl Acad Sci U S A 94:12384, 1997.
21. de Sousa M, Reimao R, Lacerda R, et al: Iron overload in β2-microglobulin-deficient mice. Immunol Lett 39:105, 1994.
22. Andrews NC: Disorders of iron metabolism. N Engl J Med 341:1986, 1999.
23. Finch C: Regulators of iron balance in humans. Blood 84:1697, 1994.
24. Nicolas G, Viatte L, Bennoun M, et al: Hepcidin, a new iron regulatory peptide. Blood Cells Mol Dis 29:327, 2002.
25. Ganz T: Hepcidin, a key regulator of iron metabolism and mediator of anemia of inflammation. Blood 102:783, 2003.
26. Bridle KR, Frazer DM, Wilkins SJ, et al: Disrupted hepcidin regulation in HFE-associated haemochromatosis and the liver as a regulator of body iron homoeostasis. Lancet 361:669, 2003.
27. Ahmad KA, Ahmann JR, Migas MC, et al: Decreased liver hepcidin expression in the Hfe knockout mouse. Blood Cells Mol Dis 29:361, 2002.
28. Anderson GJ: Control of iron absorption. J Gastroenterol Hepatol 11:1030, 1996.
29. Waheed A, Parkkila S, Saarnio J, et al: Association of HFE protein with transferrin receptor in crypt enterocytes of human duodenum. Proc Natl Acad Sci U S A 96:1579, 1999.
30. Bacon BR, Britton RS: The pathology of hepatic iron overload: A free radical-mediated process? Hepatology 11:127, 1990.
31. Britton RS, Bacon BR: Role of free radicals in liver diseases and hepatic fibrosis. Hepato-Gastroenterol 41:343, 1994.
32. Pietrangelo A: Iron, oxidative stress and liver fibrogenesis. J Hepatol 28(Suppl 1):8, 1998.
33. Hershko C, Link G, Cabantchik I: Pathophysiology of iron overload. Ann N Y Acad Sci 850:191, 1998.
34. Adams PC, Kertesz AE, Valberg LS: Clinical presentation of hemochromatosis: A changing scene. Am J Med 90:445, 1991.
35. Bacon BR, Sadiq SA: Hereditary hemochromatosis: Presentation and diagnosis in the 1990s. Am J Gastroenterol 92:784, 1997.
36. Edwards CQ, Cartwright GE, Skolnick MH, et al: Homozygosity for hemochromatosis: Clinical manifestations. Ann Intern Med 93:511, 1980.
37. Beutler E, Felitti V, Gelbart T, Ho N: The effect of HFE genotypes on measurements of iron overload in patients attending a health appraisal clinic. Ann Intern Med 133:329, 2000.
38. Beutler E, Felitti VJ, Koziol JA, et al: Penetrance of 845G→A (C282Y) HFE hereditary haemochromatosis mutation in the USA. Lancet 359:211, 2002.
39. Asberg A, Hveem K, Thorstensen K, et al: Screening for hemochromatosis: High prevalence and low morbidity in an unselected population of 65,238 persons. Scand J Gastroenterol 36:1108, 2001.
40. Deugnier YM, Guyader D, Crantook L, et al: Primary liver cancer in genetic hemochromatosis: A clinical, pathological, and pathogenetic study of 54 cases. Gastroenterology 104:228, 1992.
41. Lufkin EG, Baldus WP, Bergstralh EJ, et al: Influence of phlebotomy treatment on abnormal hypothalamic-pituitary function in genetic hemochromatosis. Mayo Clin Proc 62:473, 1987.
42. Olson LJ, Edwards WD, Holmes DR, et al: Endomyocardial biopsy in hemochromatosis: Clinicopathologic correlates in six cases. J Am Coll Cardiol 13:116, 1989.
43. Shumacher HR: Articular cartilage in the degenerative arthropathy of hemochromatosis. Arthritis Rheum 25:1460, 1982.
44. Olynyk JK, Hagan SE, Cullen DJ, et al: Evolution of untreated hereditary hemochromatosis in the Busselton population: A 17-year study. Mayo Clin Proc 79:309, 2004.
45. Guyader D, Jacquelinet C, Moirand R, et al: Noninvasive prediction of fibrosis in C282Y homozygous hemochromatosis. Gastroenterology 115:929, 1998.
46. Bacon BR, Olynyk JK, Brunt EM, et al: HFE genotype in patients with hemochromatosis and other liver diseases. Ann Intern Med 130:953, 1999.

47. Morrison ED, Brandhagen DJ, Phatak PD, et al: Serum ferritin level predicts advanced hepatic fibrosis among U.S. patients with phenotypic hemochromatosis. Ann Intern Med 138:627, 2003.

48. Brunt EM, Olynyk JK, Britton RS, et al: Histological evaluation of iron in liver biopsies: Relationship to *HFE* mutations. Am J Gastroenterol 95:1788, 2000.

49. Bassett ML, Halliday JW, Powell LW: Value of hepatic iron measurements in early hemochromatosis and determination of the critical iron level associated with fibrosis. Hepatology 6:24, 1986.

50. Bonkovsky HL, Banner BF, Rothman AL: Iron and chronic viral hepatitis. Hepatology 25:759, 1997.

51. Diwarkaran HH, Befeler AS, Britton RS, et al: Accelerated hepatic fibrosis in patients with combined hereditary hemochromatosis and chronic hepatitis C infection. J Hepatol 36:687, 2002.

52. Fletcher LM, Dixon JL, Purdie DM, et al: Excess alcohol greatly increases the prevalence of cirrhosis in hereditary hemochromatosis. Gastroenterology 122:281, 2002.

53. St Pierre TG, Clark PR, Chua-Anusorn W, et al: Noninvasive measurement and imaging of liver iron concentrations using proton magnetic resonance. Blood 105:855, 2005.

54. Adams PC, Speechley M, Kertesz AE: Long-term survival analysis in hereditary hemochromatosis. Gastroenterology 101:368, 1991.

55. Niederau C, Fischer R, Pürschel A, et al: Long-term survival in patients with hereditary hemochromatosis. Gastroenterology 110:1107, 1996.

56. Kowdley KV, Hassanein T, Kaur S, et al: Primary liver cancer and survival in patients undergoing liver transplantation for hemochromatosis. Liver Transpl Surg 1:237, 1995.

57. Poulos JE, Bacon BR: Transplantation for hemochromatosis. Dig Dis 14:316, 1996.

58. Brandhagen DJ, Alvarez W, Therneau TM, et al: Iron overload in cirrhosis: *HFE* genotypes and outcome after liver transplantation. Hepatology 31:456, 2000.

59. Tung BY, Farrell FJ, McCashland TM, et al: Long-term follow-up after liver transplantation in patients with hepatic iron overload. Liver Transpl Surg 5:369, 1999.

60. Galhenage SP, Viiala CH, Olynyk JK: Screening for haemochromatosis: Patients with liver disease, families, and populations. Curr Gastroenterol Rep 6:44, 2004.

CHAPTER
72 Wilson Disease

Diane W. Cox and Eve A. Roberts

Copper, a component of several essential enzymes, is toxic to tissues when present in excess. Dietary intake of copper generally exceeds the trace amount required, and mechanisms to control influx and efflux of copper from cells must maintain an appropriate balance. Two disorders of copper transport are known: *Menkes disease*, an X-linked defect in transport of copper from the intestine, and *Wilson disease*, an autosomal recessive disorder of copper overload. Wilson disease was first described, in 1912 by Kinnear Wilson,[1] as a familial disease characterized by progressive, lethal neurologic dysfunction associated with chronic liver disease and a corneal abnormality, the Kayser-Fleischer ring. Wilson also observed that some younger siblings of patients with typical Wilson disease died of severe liver disease without experiencing neurologic abnormalities. In this disease, inadequate hepatic copper excretion leads to accumulation of copper in the liver, brain, kidney, and cornea. The incidence in most populations is on the order of 1 in 30,000.

THE COPPER PATHWAY

Dietary copper is absorbed in the upper intestine and binds to albumin in serum. Albumin and copper-histidine transport copper to a variety of tissues; most copper is transported to the liver. Trace amounts of copper are required for essential enzymes that affect connective tissue and elastin cross-linking (lysyl oxidase), free radical scavenging (superoxide dismutase), electron transfer (cytochrome oxidase), pigment production (tyrosinase), and neurotransmission (dopamine β-monooxygenase). Copper in hepatocytes and other cells is bound to metallochaperones, low-molecular-weight proteins that each deliver copper to a specific target molecule.

In the liver, copper is incorporated into the protein apoceruloplasmin to produce ceruloplasmin (also called holoceruloplasmin). More than 90% of the copper in plasma is an integral part of ceruloplasmin, an α₂-glycoprotein that contains six molecules of copper and has a molecular weight of 132 kd. The normal serum concentration of ceruloplasmin in adults, as measured by immunochemical or enzymatic techniques, is 200 to 400 mg/L, rising from a very low level at birth to 300 to 500 mg/L in the first years of life. Ceruloplasmin is an acute-phase reactant that is elevated by inflammatory hepatic disease, pregnancy, and the use of exogenous estrogen. The majority of ingested copper is excreted via the bile; a small fraction is excreted in urine. When tissues such as the intestine and liver are overloaded with copper, a class of low-molecular-weight cysteine-rich proteins, the metallothioneins, are induced and sequester copper in a nontoxic form. The normal pathways of copper transport in the body and in the hepatocyte are shown in Figures 72–1 and 72–2.

THE BASIC MOLECULAR DEFECT

Our understanding of the basic defect in Wilson disease has increased dramatically with the cloning of the genes, first for X-linked Menkes disease and then for Wilson disease.[2,3] The gene for Menkes disease (*ATP7A*), which was cloned by using a chromosomal breakpoint in an affected female patient, was found to be related to bacterial copper resistance genes. Cloning of the Wilson disease gene (*ATP7B*) was accomplished by a combination of conventional linkage analysis,[4] physical mapping of the relevant region of chromosome 13q14, and recognition of its high homology with the Menkes disease

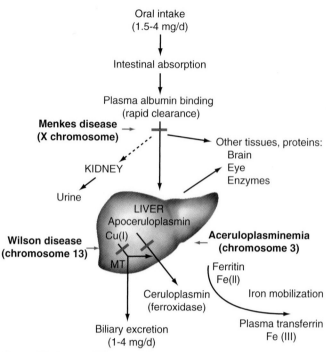

Oral intake
(1.5-4 mg/d)

Intestinal absorption

Plasma albumin binding
(rapid clearance)

**Menkes disease
(X chromosome)**

Other tissues, proteins:
Brain
Eye
Enzymes

KIDNEY

Urine

LIVER
Apoceruloplasmin

**Wilson disease
(chromosome 13)**

Cu(I)

**Aceruloplasminemia
(chromosome 3)**

MT

Ferritin
Fe(II)

Iron mobilization

Ceruloplasmin
(ferroxidase)

Plasma transferrin
Fe (III)

Biliary excretion
(1-4 mg/d)

Figure 72–1 Simplified overview of the pathways for copper ion transport and steps affected in genetic disorders of copper metabolism. MT, metallothioneins. (Modified from Cox DW: Genes of the copper pathway. Am J Hum Genet 56:828, 1995.)

gene.[2,3] The coding region of the Wilson disease gene is 4.1 kilobases in length, with messenger RNA (mRNA) of about 8 kilobases. The product is a membrane P-type adenosine triphosphatase (ATPase) that consists of 1443 amino acid residues and has a molecular mass of 160 kd. There are predicted to be six copper binding domains, a phosphorylation domain, an ATP-binding region, and eight transmembrane domains (Fig. 72–3).[2] All functionally important regions of the gene are conserved between bacteria and yeast. Mutations in the *ATP7B* gene result in retention of copper in the liver as well as impaired incorporation of copper into ceruloplasmin. The LEC (Long-Evans cinnamon) rat and the toxic milk (tx) mouse have mutations in their homologous *Atp7b* genes and are thus suitable models for the study of Wilson disease mechanisms and therapy.[5,6]

Although the gene for Menkes disease is expressed in many tissues, including muscle, kidney, heart, and intestine, the gene for Wilson disease is expressed predominantly in the liver and kidney, with minor expression in brain, lungs, and placenta. Studies in cultured cells show localization of the protein in the trans-Golgi network, with trafficking from the trans-Golgi network to cytoplasmic vesicles in the presence of increased copper.[7] The protein is found at the apical membrane in hepatocytes,

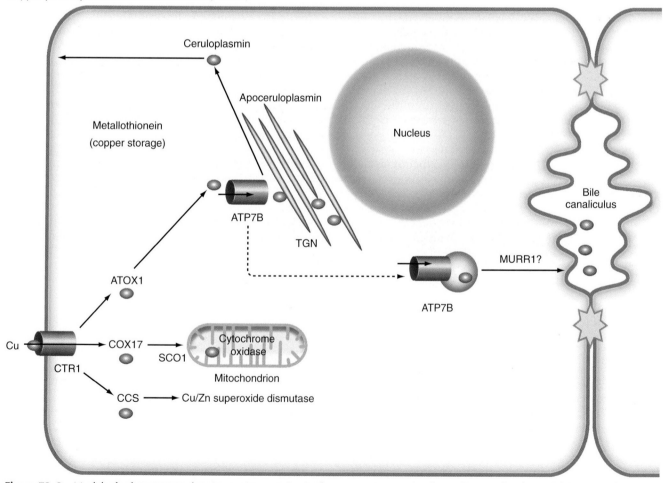

Figure 72–2 Model of a hepatocyte showing major proteins in the copper transport pathway. Low-molecular-weight-copper chaperones (ATOX1, COX17, and CCS) deliver copper to specific target proteins (ATP7B, cytochrome oxidase, and superoxide dismutase, respectively). SCO1 transports copper across the mitochondrial membrane. ATP7B (shown as a channel) traffics from the trans-Golgi network (TGN) to cytoplasmic vesicles that deliver copper to the bile canaliculus. MURR1 may be involved in excretion of copper into bile.

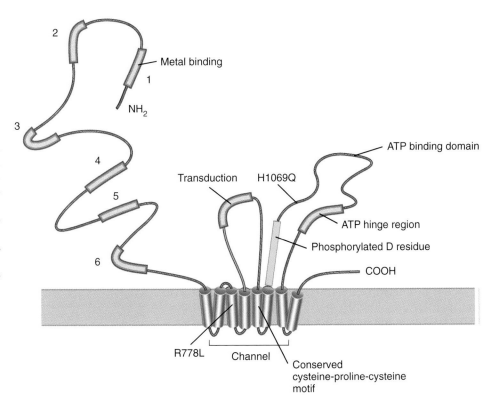

Figure 72–3 A model of the predicted product of the Wilson disease gene, *ATP7B*. Functional domains conserved in the Menkes disease gene are indicated as *blocks*. Numerous mutations occur in functionally important regions. Positions of common missense mutations, H1069Q and R778L, are shown. ATP, adenosine triphosphate. (Model modified from Bull PC, Cox DW: Wilson disease and Menkes disease: New handles on heavy-metal transport. Trends Genet 10:246, 1994.)

consistent with its proposed function of facilitating excretion of copper via bile.[8]

Additional proteins are involved in the intracellular transport of copper. Copper is not free in the cell but is transported to specific proteins by copper chaperones.[9] The chaperone ATOX1 transports copper to ATP7B. The study of inherited copper toxicosis in Bedlington terriers has identified a possible new component of the copper transport system. Affected dogs show clinical variability that ranges from death from hepatic disease at 2 to 3 years of age to less severe chronic disease to a very high level of hepatic copper without clinical consequences. The proposed defective canine gene was identified by positional cloning through the use of markers to identify a region containing the *MURR1* gene.[10] This deletion of one exon of the *MURR1* gene is found in most, but not all, affected dogs.[11] Although MURR1 has been shown to interact with ATP7B and to have a moderate effect on copper transport, the discrepant results in dogs leave the role of MURR1 in the copper transport pathway unconfirmed.

CLINICAL FEATURES

The clinical presentation of Wilson disease is extremely variable. The age at onset of symptoms generally ranges from 6 to about 40 years. Wilson disease with hepatic involvement has been identified in patients younger than 5 years and patients older than 60 years. Patients may present with chronic or fulminant liver disease, a progressive neurologic disorder without clinically prominent hepatic dysfunction, isolated acute hemolysis, or psychiatric illness. The clinical variability often makes confirmation of the diagnosis difficult.

HEPATIC PRESENTATION

A hepatic presentation of Wilson disease is more common in children than in adults. Wilson disease should be considered as a possible diagnosis in any child, symptomatic or not, who has hepatomegaly, persistently elevated serum aminotransferase levels, or evidence of fatty liver. Symptoms may be vague and nonspecific, such as fatigue, anorexia, and abdominal pain. Occasionally patients present with a self-limited clinical illness that resembles *acute hepatitis*, with malaise, anorexia, nausea, jaundice, elevated serum aminotransferases, and abnormal coagulation test results. Some patients have a history of self-limited jaundice, apparently caused by unexplained hemolysis. Patients may present with severe, established *chronic liver disease*—hepatosplenomegaly, ascites, congestive splenomegaly, a low serum albumin level, and persistently abnormal coagulation test results. Some patients have isolated splenomegaly without hepatomegaly. Many of these findings relate more to *portal hypertension* as a consequence of Wilson disease than to the metabolic disorder itself.

Wilson disease may manifest in children and young adults as clinical liver disease indistinguishable from *autoimmune hepatitis*.[12] As in autoimmune hepatitis, the onset may be acute. Fatigue, malaise, arthropathy, and rashes may occur; laboratory findings include elevated serum aminotransferase levels, a greatly increased serum immunoglobulin (Ig) G concentration, and detectable nonspecific autoantibodies such as antinuclear and anti–smooth muscle (anti-actin) antibodies. Wilson disease must be specifically ruled out because the treatment of the two diseases is entirely different. With appropriate treatment, the long-term outlook for patients with Wilson disease that manifests as autoimmune hepatitis appears to be favorable, even if cirrhosis is present.

Wilson disease may also manifest as *fulminant hepatic failure*, with severe coagulopathy and encephalopathy.[13] Acute intravascular hemolysis is usually present, and renal failure may develop. Because the patient typically has not been suspected to have underlying liver disease, fulminant viral hepatitis is usually the working diagnosis. Unlike fulminant viral hepatitis, fulminant Wilson disease is usually characterized by disproportionately low serum aminotransferase levels (usually much less than 1500 U/L) at the onset of clinically apparent disease. The serum alkaline phosphatase level is in the normal range or even low for age, and the serum bilirubin level is often disproportionately high as a result of hemolysis.[14] However, the biochemical profile is nonspecific.[15] Slit-lamp examination of the eyes may demonstrate Kayser-Fleischer rings (see later). Urinary copper excretion is greatly elevated. Affected patients do not show a good response to chelation treatment and require urgent liver transplantation; albumin dialysis and related techniques may serve as temporary procedures until liver transplantation can be performed.[16] This presentation of Wilson disease is more common than initially supposed, and patients with it account for a significant proportion of liver transplant recipients (see Chapters 90 and 92).

Recurrent bouts of hemolysis may predispose to the development of *gallstones*. Cirrhosis, if present, may be a further predisposing factor. Children with unexplained cholelithiasis, particularly with small bilirubinate stones, should be tested for Wilson disease. Unlike other types of chronic liver disease, Wilson disease is rarely complicated by hepatocellular carcinoma.

In patients who have predominantly hepatic disease, evidence of subtle neurologic involvement often can be found. Mood disturbance (mainly depression, but sometimes impulsive or neurotic behavior), deterioration in school performance or handwriting, and clumsiness may be identified through careful questioning of the patient or his or her parents. A soft whispery voice (hypophonia) is another early feature of neurologic involvement.

NEUROLOGIC PRESENTATION

The neurologic presentation of Wilson disease tends to occur in the second and third decades or later but has been reported in children as young as 6 to 10 years. Most patients with a neurologic presentation have hepatic involvement, albeit often asymptomatic. Neurologic involvement follows two main patterns, *movement disorder* and *rigid dystonia*.[17] Movement disorders tend to occur earlier and consist of tremors, poor coordination, and loss of fine motor control. Spastic dystonic disorders generally develop later, with mask-like facies, rigidity, gait disturbance, and pseudobulbar involvement such as dysarthria, drooling, and swallowing difficulty. Intellect is not impaired.

PSYCHIATRIC PRESENTATION

As many as 20% of patients may present with purely psychiatric symptoms.[18] These symptoms are highly variable, although depression is common. Phobias and compulsive behaviors have been reported; aggressive and antisocial behaviors may also be seen.

OCULAR SIGNS

The classic *Kayser-Fleischer ring* is caused by copper deposition in Descemet's membrane of the cornea. Copper is actually distributed throughout the cornea, but fluid streaming favors accumulation near the limbus, especially at the superior and inferior poles and, eventually, circumferentially around the iris. Kayser-Fleischer rings are visible on direct inspection only when iris pigmentation is light and copper deposition heavy. A careful slit-lamp examination is mandatory.

Copper deposition in the lens (*sunflower cataract*), which does not interfere with vision, may be seen on slit-lamp examination and, like Kayser-Fleischer rings, disappears with chelation therapy. Kayser-Fleischer rings may be absent in 15% to 50% of patients with exclusively hepatic involvement and in presymptomatic patients, whereas most patients with a neurologic or psychiatric presentation of Wilson disease have Kayser-Fleischer rings; only 5% do not. Kayser-Fleischer rings are not specific for Wilson disease. They may be found in patients with other types of chronic liver disease, usually with a prominent cholestatic component, such as primary biliary cirrhosis, primary sclerosing cholangitis, autoimmune hepatitis, and familial cholestatic syndromes. Kayser-Fleischer rings have also been reported in patients with nonhepatic diseases.

INVOLVEMENT OF OTHER ORGANS

Wilson disease can be accompanied by various extrahepatic disorders apart from neurologic disease. Episodes of *hemolytic anemia* can result from sudden release of copper into the blood. *Renal disease*, mainly *Fanconi's syndrome*, may be prominent. Findings include microscopic hematuria, aminoaciduria, phosphaturia, and defective acidification of the urine. *Nephrolithiasis* also has been reported. *Arthritis*, affecting mainly the large joints, may occur as a result of synovial copper accumulation. Other musculoskeletal problems are *osteoporosis* and *osteochondritis dissecans*. Vitamin D–resistant *rickets* may develop as a result of the renal damage. Copper deposition in the heart can lead to *cardiomyopathy* or *cardiac arrhythmias*. Sudden death in Wilson disease has been attributed to cardiac involvement but is rare. Copper deposition in skeletal muscle can cause *rhabdomyolysis*. Endocrine disorders can occur. *Hypoparathyroidism* has been attributed to copper deposition. *Amenorrhea* and *testicular problems* appear to result from Wilson disease itself, not from cirrhosis. *Infertility* or *repeated spontaneous abortion* may be a sign of Wilson disease. *Pancreatitis*, possibly resulting from copper deposition in the pancreas, may also occur.

PATHOLOGY

In the earliest stages before cirrhosis develops, histologic findings in the liver consist of steatosis, focal necrosis, glycogenated nuclei in hepatocytes, and sometimes apoptotic bodies. As parenchymal damage progresses, possibly through repeated episodes of lobular necrosis, periportal fibrosis develops. Cirrhosis is usually macronodular but may be micronodular.

Early in the course of Wilson disease, hepatocellular copper is bound mainly to metallothionein and distributed diffusely in the cytoplasm of hepatocytes; therefore, results of histochemical stains for copper are negative. As the disease progresses, copper exceeds the capacity of metallothionein and is deposited in lysosomes. These lysosomal aggregates of copper can be detected by special staining techniques for copper or copper-binding protein (such as rubeanic acid or orcein). Copper is usually distributed throughout the hepatic lobule or nodule, but in the cirrhotic liver, some areas may have no stainable copper at all. If the clinical presentation mimics that of autoimmune hepatitis, liver biopsy specimens reveal classic histologic features of chronic hepatitis, such as interface hepatitis. Inflammation may be severe. Results of Mallory staining for hyalin may be positive, and hepatocellular copper accumulation may be detected. In patients who present with fulminant hepatic failure, liver biopsy confirms preexisting liver disease; cirrhosis may be present; and parenchymal copper is located mainly in Kupffer cells rather than hepatocytes.

Changes in hepatocellular mitochondria, identified with electron microscopy, are an important feature in Wilson disease.[19] The mitochondria vary in size; the numbers of dense bodies in mitochondria may be increased. The most striking change is dilatation of the tips of the mitochondrial cristae as a result of separation of the inner and outer membranes of the cristae, so that the intercristal space is widened to an irregular cystic shape. The crista resembles a tennis racquet if only the tip is dilated. This finding, although not absolutely specific for Wilson disease, can be helpful diagnostically, even in quite young and minimally affected patients. Involvement of hepatocytes may not be uniform, so abnormalities may be found in some hepatocytes in some lobules and not in others. The mitochondrial changes are probably a consequence of oxidative damage from excessive liver copper.

DIAGNOSIS

The patient with the classic combination of chronic liver disease, tremor or dystonia, and Kayser-Fleischer rings is readily diagnosed on clinical grounds, but such patients are uncommon. A diagnostic scoring system has been proposed but has not yet been tested rigorously.[20] Suggestive clinical symptoms are often the main prerequisite for diagnosing Wilson disease, and laboratory investigations may provide confirmation. Kayser-Fleischer rings should be sought through a careful slit-lamp examination, repeated if necessary. Lack of Kayser-Fleischer rings does not exclude the diagnosis of Wilson disease. Routine liver biochemical testing usually yields abnormal results, with mild to moderate elevations of serum aminotransferase values. Serum levels of alanine aminotransferase (ALT) may be much lower than those of aspartate aminotransferase (AST), possibly reflecting damage to hepatocellular mitochondria.

Two major disturbances of copper disposition in Wilson disease are a reduction in the rate of incorporation of copper into ceruloplasmin and a decrease in biliary excretion of copper. A summary of biochemical features of Wilson disease in comparison with those in normal persons is shown in Table 72–1. Traditionally, more than 95% of patients with Wilson disease have been considered to have a low serum ceruloplasmin concentration; however, ceruloplasmin concentrations are within the normal range in many patients with liver manifestations.[21] In these patients, hepatic inflammation may be sufficient to elevate serum ceruloplasmin concentrations. Also, the normal range for serum ceruloplasmin is increased in very young children. Part of the explanation for a normal ceruloplasmin concentration in a patient with Wilson disease may also lie in the method of measurement used. Immunologic methods, commonly used in routine laboratories, measure both apoceruloplasmin and holoceruloplasmin and typically overestimate the true amount of ceruloplasmin in plasma. The oxidase assay, although technically less convenient in automated laboratories, provides a more reliable measure of ceruloplasmin for diagnosis, because it measures enzymatically active, copper-containing ceruloplasmin. This method permits an accurate estimate of non–ceruloplasmin-bound copper[22] and can also indicate possible early copper deficiency.[23]

Serum ceruloplasmin measurement by itself is not a sufficient diagnostic test for Wilson disease. A low serum ceruloplasmin level is not unique to Wilson disease; synthesis of ceruloplasmin may be reduced in other types of chronic liver disease or as a result of intestinal malabsorption, nephrosis, and malnutrition. Furthermore, a low ceruloplasmin concentration is found in at least 10% of heterozygotes for Wilson disease. Nearly complete absence of ceruloplasmin is also seen in hereditary *aceruloplasminemia*, a rare recessive condition that is associated with neurologic, retinal, and pancreatic degeneration due to iron accumulation in the brain, retina, and pancreas, respectively.[24,25] Anemia and a rise in plasma ferritin levels are observed, but the excessive iron storage should not be mistaken for hereditary hemochromatosis. Aceruloplasminemia has confirmed the important function of ceruloplasmin as a ferroxidase that oxidizes iron for transport from ferritin to transferrin, a function proposed

Table 72–1   Biochemical Parameters in Patients with Wilson Disease and in Normal Adults

	Wilson Disease*	Normal Adults
Serum ceruloplasmin (mg/L)	0-200	200-350
Serum copper (µg/L)	190-640	700-1520
(µmol/L)	3-10	11-24
Urinary copper (µg/d)	100-1000	<40
(µmol/d)	>1.6	<0.6
Liver copper (µg/g dry weight)	>200	20-50

*In all assays, there is overlap with heterozygotes in some cases.

in the late 1960s. Targeted disruption of the ceruloplasmin gene in a mouse model has confirmed the critical role of ceruloplasmin in transporting iron out of cells.[26] Theoretically, patients who undergo rigorous, prolonged chelation therapy for Wilson disease could show the same effects if ceruloplasmin oxidase activity is reduced to undetectable levels, but this theory remains to be confirmed.

The serum copper concentration is low, in parallel with the low serum ceruloplasmin level, in most patients with Wilson disease. The non–ceruloplasmin-bound copper concentration is elevated; this concentration can be estimated by subtraction of the amount of copper associated with ceruloplasmin from the total serum copper level. One can estimate the amount of ceruloplasmin-bound copper (in μg/L) by multiplying the serum ceruloplasmin level (in μg/L) by 3.15 (the amount of copper, in mg, per mg of ceruloplasmin). If the total serum copper is reported in μmol/L, one converts this value to μg/L by multiplying it by 63.5, the molecular weight of copper. In normal persons, the non–ceruloplasmin-bound copper concentration is approximately 50 to 100 μg/L. In Wilson disease, the concentration is more than 200 μg/L, or even ten times higher in the presence of fulminant liver failure and intravascular hemolysis. The usefulness of this calculation depends highly on the accuracy of serum copper and ceruloplasmin measurements, and it has not yet been validated as a diagnostic criterion.

Serum uric acid and phosphate concentrations may be low, reflecting renal tubular dysfunction in patients with untreated Wilson disease. Urinalysis may show microscopic hematuria; if possible, aminoaciduria, phosphaturia, and proteinuria should be quantified.

Studies of urinary copper excretion, preferably with three separate 24-hour urine collections, have proven useful for diagnosis. It is critical to ensure that the collection is complete and that precautions are taken to avoid contamination with copper in the collection process. The basal 24-hour urinary copper excretion is elevated to at least two to three times normal in the vast majority of patients. Presymptomatic patients may not necessarily have increased daily urinary copper excretion; however, even borderline elevations (between 0.6 and 1.2 μmol/day) merit further investigation. Heterozygotes usually have a normal 24-hour urinary copper excretion rate, although the level may be borderline abnormal in some. A provocative test of urinary copper excretion in which penicillamine (500 mg orally every 12 hours) is given to the patient while a 24-hour urine collection is obtained sometimes provides useful information.[27] Although a normal person may excrete as much as 20 times the baseline level of copper after administration of penicillamine, a patient with Wilson disease excretes considerably more; urinary copper excretion of 25 μmoles or more of copper per 24 hours is diagnostic of Wilson disease. This provocative test has been suggested to be more reliable than measurement of the hepatic tissue content of copper.[27] In fact, when one biochemical assay result is borderline, others tend to be borderline as well.

Hepatic tissue copper concentration, usually measured by neutron activation analysis or atomic absorption spectrometry, may provide important diagnostic information. Hepatic copper content greater than 250 μg per gram dry weight is considered diagnostic of Wilson disease. A hepatic parenchymal concentration lower than 40 μg per gram dry weight is regarded as strong evidence against the diagnosis of Wilson disease. Liver biopsy samples must be collected without extraneous copper contamination; in general, ordinary disposable liver biopsy needles can be used. In early stages of Wilson disease, when copper is distributed diffusely in the liver cell cytoplasm, this measurement may clearly indicate hepatic copper overload. In later stages of hepatic Wilson disease, the measurement of hepatic copper is less reliable, because copper is distributed unequally in the liver.[28] However, liver biopsy may not be safe in such patients because of coagulopathy or ascites, and therefore this diagnostic parameter may not be available. In some patients with Wilson disease, the hepatic tissue copper concentration is intermediate between normal and definitely elevated (between 100 and 250 μg per gram dry weight). Some heterozygotes have a similarly moderate elevation of the liver tissue copper concentration. An elevated hepatic copper concentration is not specific for Wilson disease; patients with chronic cholestasis or diseases such as Indian childhood cirrhosis may have elevated hepatic copper concentrations.

The impaired incorporation of copper into ceruloplasmin can be measured using radioactive (^{64}Cu, ^{67}Cu) or stable (^{65}Cu) copper isotopes. Patients with Wilson disease show little or no incorporation of labeled copper into plasma or into the ceruloplasmin component after oral or intravenous administration of copper isotope. However, presymptomatic heterozygotes cannot always be differentiated from homozygous patients. This test is rarely used diagnostically at present.

In view of the availability of numerous diagnostic tests, some prioritization is required. Minimum diagnostic criteria for Wilson disease applicable to all patients are difficult to establish. The classic patient, whether displaying hepatic or neurologic findings, may be considered to be someone between 6 and 40 years of age with a serum ceruloplasmin level less than 5 mg/dL (<50 mg/L) and definite Kayser-Fleischer rings. Otherwise, in the presence of chronic liver disease (indicated by hepatomegaly or biochemical abnormalities) or typical neurologic symptomatology, the combination of a subnormal serum ceruloplasmin concentration and an elevated basal 24-hour urinary copper excretion value is highly suggestive of Wilson disease. The measurement of 24-hour urinary copper excretion after administration of penicillamine may be so definitive that the diagnosis of Wilson disease is no longer in doubt.

Typical ocular findings complete the clinical diagnosis but are frequently lacking. A percutaneous liver biopsy has merit for assessing the severity of liver damage and measuring the parenchymal copper concentration, which is regarded by some as the *sine qua non* for the diagnosis of Wilson disease. However, liver biopsy may be hazardous and may have to be delayed in patients with liver dysfunction. Other clinical entities in the differential diagnosis must be appropriately excluded. In the patient who does not have classic manifestations, extensive studies must be pursued meticulously, but ultimately, a gene mutation analysis may be the only convincing diagnostic procedure.

MUTATION ANALYSIS

More than 260 reported mutations in the *ATP7B* gene have been detected in many different populations by single-strand conformation polymorphism analysis or by sequencing of each of the 21 exons.[3,29,30] These mutations are recorded in the Wilson Disease Mutation Database.[31] High-throughput methods are making mutation analysis more feasible for this disease, as for many others. Mutation analysis can be carried out with approaches such as denaturing high-performance liquid chromatography[32] or by high-throughput sequencing of either selected or all exons of the gene. Mutation identification is technically feasible, but care must be taken that the change detected is disease-causing and not a rare normal variant, particularly for missense mutations, in which a single amino acid is substituted. Yeast and cell systems have been developed for functional assessment of variants; such methods are possible because of the similarity between yeast and mammalian copper transport systems.[33,34] The identification of one mutation may be adequate to confirm the diagnosis of Wilson disease, if (1) characteristic clinical symptoms and at least some biochemical features are present and (2) the one mutation detected is clearly established as a disease-causing mutation.

The majority of mutations identified to date in *ATP7B* are missense mutations (57%). Small deletions and insertion (28%), nonsense (7%), and splice site (8%) mutations occur throughout the gene.[31] Large gene deletions, which are found in about 20% of patients with Menkes disease, have not been reported, and the mutation spectrum for the Menkes gene, *ATP7A*, is different from that for *ATP7B*.[35] Various ethnic groups have different specific mutations. The common histidine1069glutamine (His1069Gln) mutation[3] is present at least in the heterozygous state in 35% to 75% of Europeans with Wilson disease; the higher rate is relevant only for Eastern Europe.[36] Exon 8 of the gene is particularly rich in mutations in European populations; depending on the age of onset, at least one mutation can be identified in exon 8 in about 50% to 60% of patients.[37] The mutation arginine778leucine is common in Chinese populations.[29] Because no mutation is present in high frequency in Japanese and Mediterranean populations, mutation detection is more challenging in such populations. In some populations that have ethnic homogeneity or in which the spectrum of mutations is established, testing strategies can identify the mutations in more than 90% of patients, as in Sardinians, among whom Wilson disease occurs with a frequency of 1 in 7000 live births.[38] If the patient is clinically normal, has only slight signs of the disease, or has a late age of onset, that patient could actually be a heterozygote. However, up to now, heterozygotes have not been known to become clinically affected or to require treatment.

Gene deletions, duplications, nonsense mutations, and splice site mutations would be predicted to prevent the formation of the gene product almost completely and, thus, to produce a severe defect. This prediction is true to some extent,[29,39] and the onset of liver disease at age 3 years has been reported in a patient with a severe gene defect that was predicted to abolish the gene product.[40]

The common His1069Gln mutation tends to be associated with neurologic disease and later onset[41]; however, this mutation has been reported in homozygotes as young as 9 years with hepatic disease. The positions of this and other missense mutations (amino acid substitution) are shown in Figure 72–3. Most patients are compound heterozygotes, carrying two different mutations for the gene. Because homozygotes for a single mutation are relatively infrequent, correlating clinical features with specific mutations is difficult.

With the opportunity to confirm a diagnosis of Wilson disease by direct identification of mutations, it is becoming clear that the spectrum of manifestations of Wilson disease is even wider than had been recognized previously. No individual biochemical test is reliable for the identification of patients. In some cases, even all combinations of tests prove inadequate for a diagnosis. For example, Kayser-Fleischer rings, thought to occur inevitably in the presence of neurologic symptoms, are not necessarily present even in conjunction with well-established neurologic symptoms. The serum ceruloplasmin concentration, thought to be reduced in a great majority of patients, may be normal in a major proportion of patients with hepatic manifestations of Wilson disease. The use of molecular tests in patients with any clinical symptoms of the disease may become routine in the near future and is already feasible in some populations.

PRESYMPTOMATIC DIAGNOSIS OF SIBS

Because of the difficulty in distinguishing asymptomatic patients from heterozygotes, mutation analysis is highly recommended. If a mutation has been identified in a patient, analysis is easily carried out in siblings with direct testing for the relevant mutations. If mutations have not been identified, accurate diagnosis can be carried out with the use of markers flanking the gene. The most commonly used type of genetic markers are stretches of dinucleotides or trinucleotides that show such variability in the normal population that most parents within any one family carry different alleles of the markers. This variability allows the tracking of the disease gene as it segregates within families, as shown in the example in Figure 72–4. It is important that informative markers flank the gene, because an erroneous diagnosis could rarely result if markers on only one side of the gene are informative and a recombinant event has occurred close to the gene.

The combination of markers, or haplotype, reliably indicates the genetic status within the family. On the basis of marker studies, an occasional person considered, as a result of biochemical testing, to have a high probability of being a presymptomatic patient has been shown to be a heterozygote.[42] No known heterozygotes have demonstrated overt disease symptoms. Therefore, confirmation of genotype is highly recommended before treatment is initiated. If heterozygotes are found to accumulate copper stores later in life, they may need to be monitored for clinical signs of copper overload.

In the absence of marker analysis, screening should involve physical examination, liver biochemical tests, serum copper and ceruloplasmin measurements, a 24-hour urinary copper measurement, and a careful slit-lamp examination. Children 6 years old or younger who appear to be unaffected should be rechecked at yearly intervals over the next 5 to 10 years. However, genetic screening, with the use of flanking markers or by direct mutation analysis, is the most reliable way to identify affected siblings when the patient's DNA is available. For deceased patients, tissue from autopsy or biopsy material can be used.

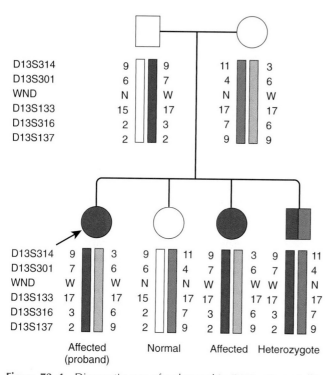

Figure 72–4 Diagnostic use of polymorphic DNA microsatellite markers for siblings of a confirmed patient with Wilson disease in a pedigree. DNA markers are listed in centromeric to telomeric order. Three markers are usually sufficient for an unambiguous result: D13S314, D13S301, and D13S316. Numbers represent alleles of each marker listed. The proband (*arrow*) and presymptomatic sibling confirmed as affected are shown as *filled circles*.

TREATMENT

The following three treatments for Wilson disease are generally recognized: penicillamine, trientine, and zinc (Table 72–2).[43] Chelation with tetrathiomolybdate is a relatively new and still experimental option. With effective chelation treatment, most patients live normal, healthy lives. Early treatment is critical, and the outcome is best for patients in whom the disease is diagnosed and treatment begun when the patient is presymptomatic. However, whether routine institution of chelation therapy in infancy (<2 years) is advantageous or deleterious remains unknown. Likewise, the potential role of gene transfer therapy remains uncertain. Most patients should eliminate copper-rich foods from the diet—organ meats, shellfish, nuts, chocolate, and mushrooms. Vegetarians require specific dietary counseling. If there is reason to believe that the concentration of copper in drinking water is high, the water should be analyzed, and a copper-removing device installed in the plumbing system.

Penicillamine, introduced in 1956 by J. M. Walshe, is effective in most patients with Wilson disease. Penicillamine, which is the sulfhydryl-containing amino acid cysteine substituted with two methyl groups, greatly increases urinary excretion of copper. Studies in the LEC rat model indicate that penicillamine inhibits the accumulation of copper in hepatocyte lysosomes and solubilizes copper for mobilization from these particles, but not from cytoplasmic metallothioneins.[44] In addition to its chelating action, penicillamine inhibits collagen cross-linking and has some immunosuppressant properties.

Table 72–2 Approach to Treatment in Wilson Disease

Drug	Dose*	Tests for Monitoring Efficacy	Tests for Monitoring Side Effects
Penicillamine (+ pyridoxine, 25 mg daily)	Initial: 1-1.5 g/day (adults) or 20 mg/kg/day (children) divided into two or three doses Maintenance: 0.75-1 g/day as needed to maintain cupruresis	24-hour urinary copper: 200-500 μg (3-8 μmol) per day as target; estimated non–ceruloplasmin-bound copper <200 μg/L	Complete blood count; urinalysis; skin examination
Trientine†	Initial: 1-1.2 g/day divided into two or three doses‡ Maintenance: Same	Same as for penicillamine	Complete blood count; iron studies
Zinc	Initial: 50 mg elemental zinc three times daily (adults)§ Maintenance: Titrate dose against efficacy monitoring data¶	24-hour urinary copper: <75 μg (1.2 μmol) per day as target; estimated non–ceruloplasmin-bound copper <100 μg/L	Serum zinc level

*All medications should be taken before or after mealtime if possible, but the timing of the dose may need to be adjusted to enhance compliance.
†Requires refrigeration.
‡The dose of trientine in children is not established (approximately 20 mg/kg/day).
§The dose of zinc in children is not established.
¶The 24-hour urinary copper excretion reflects total body copper load and thus can be used to monitor zinc treatment even though zinc does not cause cupruresis; some groups prefer to use the estimated non–ceruloplasmin-bound copper determination as a guide.

The neurologic status of patients with mainly neurologic symptoms may worsen initially after treatment with penicillamine is started; most, but not all, recover with continued use of penicillamine. Some patients experience a febrile reaction with rash and proteinuria within 7 to 10 days of beginning treatment. Although penicillamine can be restarted slowly, along with glucocorticoids, changing to an alternative chelator may be safer for such patients.

Penicillamine, although effective, can have serious adverse side effects. Adverse reactions involving the skin include various types of rashes, pemphigus, and elastosis perforans serpiginosa. Other side effects vary from minor (loss of taste, gastrointestinal upset, and arthralgias) to severe (proteinuria, leukopenia, and thrombocytopenia). Aplastic anemia occurs rarely and does not always reverse when penicillamine is stopped. Nephrotic syndrome, Goodpasture's syndrome, a myasthenia syndrome, and a systemic disease resembling lupus erythematosus have all been reported. These severe side effects require immediate discontinuation of penicillamine and use of a different chelator. A severe side effect of penicillamine that necessitates a change of treatment develops in up to 30% of patients with Wilson disease.[45] It is not yet apparent whether life-long treatment with penicillamine is free of adverse consequences. Patients who have taken penicillamine for 30 to 40 years may have chronic skin changes with loss of elastic tissue. Whether the antifibrotic effect weakens other connective tissues is not known. Chronic depletion of other trace metals may occur and may not be entirely harmless.

Trientine, or triethylene tetramine dihydrochloride (2,2,2-tetramine), the official short name of which is "trien," is the usual second-line treatment for patients intolerant of penicillamine; it also was introduced by J. M. Walshe.[46,47] Trientine differs chemically from penicillamine in lacking sulfhydryl groups. Copper is chelated by forming a stable complex with the four constituent nitrogens in a planar ring. Trientine increases urinary copper excretion and may interfere with intestinal absorption of copper. Trientine is a less potent chelator than penicillamine, but the difference is not clinically important. Trientine produces little toxicity in patients with Wilson disease, apart from causing occasional gastritis and inducing iron deficiency, apparently by chelating dietary iron. Bone marrow suppression is extremely rare. Adverse effects of penicillamine resolve and do not recur during treatment with trientine.[48] Neurologic worsening after treatment with trientine is begun has been reported rarely.

Oral zinc, used in Europe since the 1970s, has been investigated extensively as a treatment modality in North America.[49] The mechanism of action is entirely different from that of the chelators. Zinc, in pharmacologic doses, interferes with absorption of copper from the gastrointestinal tract and increases copper excretion in the stool. The postulated mechanism of action is through the induction of metallothionein in enterocytes. The metallothionein has a greater affinity for copper than for zinc and preferentially binds copper derived from the intestinal contents. Once bound, the copper is not absorbed but is lost in the feces as enterocytes are shed in normal turnover.[50]

Problems with zinc therapy include gastritis, a common side effect, and uncertainty about dosing. Using salts other than zinc sulfate may minimize gastritis, but any zinc salt is equally acceptable for the treatment of Wilson disease. Food interferes with the effectiveness of zinc, and some investigators recommend that no food be taken for 1 hour before or after a dose of zinc is taken. This dosing regimen tends to increase the severity of gastritis and may be sufficiently inconvenient to compromise adherence, for example, in adolescents. An alternative approach is to be less rigorous about avoiding zinc at mealtimes and to titrate the dose against the serum non–ceruloplasmin-bound copper concentration. Zinc treatment appears to have few adverse side effects.[51] Rare patients experience a deterioration in hepatic Wilson disease when started on zinc. Zinc may have immunosuppressant effects and may reduce leukocyte chemotaxis. Studies in rats suggest a possible interference with bone formation. The long-term effectiveness and adverse side effects of zinc require further investigation, but current data indicate that zinc is effective as maintenance therapy and has low toxicity.

Combining zinc with a more conventional chelator (penicillamine or trientine) has become a relatively popular treatment strategy despite a lack of clinical or laboratory validation. It is important to recognize that the two types of treatments must be temporally separated throughout the day, with at least 4 to 5 hours between the administrations of the two drugs, or else they may neutralize each other. This intensive treatment may be best suited to patients with severe hepatic or neurologic disease, in whom it mainly has been used.[52] Further data are required before this strategy can be recommended firmly.

Ammonium tetrathiomolybdate may be especially suitable for treatment of severe neurologic Wilson disease, because, unlike penicillamine, it is not associated with early neurologic deterioration.[53] Tetrathiomolybdate interferes with copper absorption from the intestine and binds to plasma copper with high affinity. Unlike penicillamine, tetrathiomolybdate has been found to remove copper from metallothionein at low doses in LEC rats; at higher doses, an insoluble copper complex is deposited in the liver.[54] Although tetrathiomolybdate is regarded as nontoxic, bone marrow suppression is a noteworthy adverse side effect. Little is known about where mobilized copper, and molybdate, may be deposited. The optimal dose and length of treatment, as well as long-term side effects, require careful study. Such a potent copper-binding drug could produce copper deficiency.

Antioxidants may be a useful adjunct for preventing tissue damage. Studies in copper-loaded animals and in patients with Wilson disease indicate that copper enhances free radical production in tissues and that this effect may be an important cause of liver damage.[55] Oxidative damage also may be enhanced by low plasma α-tocopherol and ascorbate levels, which have been reported in patients with untreated Wilson disease.[56,57] Oxyradical damage may be reflected in an increase in the frequency of mutations in the p53 tumor suppressor gene and greater activity of nitric oxide synthase reported in the livers of patients with Wilson disease.[58] Antioxidants such as α-tocopherol may help prevent and reverse liver damage, particularly in patients with severe hepatic decompensation. Clinical data relating to this strategy, however, are not available.

For pregnant patients with Wilson disease, treatment must be continued throughout pregnancy. There is a risk of postpartum hepatic decompensation if treatment is stopped altogether during pregnancy. Although many successful pregnancies have occurred during treatment with penicillamine, treatment with zinc may provide less opportunity for adverse effects on developing collagen in the fetus. Occasional reports of severe collagen defects in the offspring of a patient could be caused in part by copper deficiency from prolonged aggressive treatment as well as by teratogenic effects of penicillamine.[59] The absence of enzymatically active ceruloplasmin may be a possible early sign of copper depletion. Judicious reduction of the dose of penicillamine or trientine by approximately 25% of the pre-pregnancy dose is advisable, especially if delivery by cesarean section is anticipated.

Family screening is an important preventive measure. Because the best outcome is associated with treatment begun in the presymptomatic period, screening of the patient's siblings is mandatory when Wilson disease is diagnosed. The approach has been described earlier. The best time to begin treatment in an asymptomatic child has not been established. Treatment of infants and very young children requires careful study to determine the risks of copper depletion during a critical period of growth.

PROGNOSIS

Patients with Wilson disease generally are regarded as having a good prognosis if the disease is diagnosed promptly and treated consistently. An asymptomatic sibling who is diagnosed on biochemical or genetic grounds before any sign of clinical impairment has the best long-term outlook. Patients with early hepatic disease have a generally favorable prognosis as long as treatment is consistent and well-tolerated.[45,60] Severe neurologic disease may not resolve entirely on treatment.

The role of liver transplantation in Wilson disease is limited (see Chapters 90 and 92). Fulminant hepatic failure in a patient with Wilson disease necessitates liver transplantation. Some patients with severe liver disease that is unresponsive to drug therapy also may require early transplantation, although the potential for rescue by antioxidants has not been well explored. Liver transplantation may improve severe neurologic disease, but experience is limited and on balance this approach cannot be recommended.[61,62] Liver transplantation should be reserved for patients who present with severe, decompensated liver disease unresponsive to therapy and for those with fulminant liver failure.[62-64] Live donor transplantation, in which the graft may be from a family member who is a heterozygote, has been found to yield adequately functioning grafts.[65]

Patients who stop taking chelating treatment have a poor prognosis. New neurologic abnormalities, such as dysarthria, may develop. Rapidly progressive hepatic decompensation has been observed and occurs on average within 3 years, although it has been reported as early as 8 months after treatment is stopped. The liver damage is usually refractory to reinstitution of chelation therapy. Affected patients require liver transplantation.

Quality of life in patients with Wilson disease may be compromised by drug toxicity. Anecdotal observations suggest that damage to collagen may accrue over decades in patients maintained indefinitely on penicillamine, but the risk has not been adequately assessed. Deficiencies in trace metals may develop with the use of any chelator, although it is not yet clear whether these deficiencies are clinically important. Abnormal iron metabolism, leading to hepatic iron overload and anemia, can be predicted if ceruloplasmin oxidase activity is reduced to zero.

REFERENCES

1. Wilson SAK: Progressive lenticular degeneration: A familial nervous disease associated with cirrhosis of the liver. Brain 34:295, 1912.
2. Bull PC, Thomas GR, Rommens JM, et al: The Wilson disease gene is a putative copper transporting P-type ATPase similar to the Menkes gene. Nat Genet 5:327, 1993.
3. Tanzi RE, Petrukhin KE, Chernov I, et al: The Wilson disease gene is a copper transporting ATPase with homology to the Menkes disease gene. Nat Genet 5:344, 1993.
4. Frydman M, Bonne-Tamir B, Farrer LA, et al: Assignment of the gene for Wilson disease to chromosome 13: Linkage to the esterase D locus. Proc Natl Acad Sci U S A 82:1819, 1985.
5. Wu J, Forbes JR, Chen HS, et al: The LEC rat has a deletion in the copper transporting ATPase gene homologous to the Wilson disease gene. Nat Genet 7:541, 1994.
6. Theophilos MB, Cox DW, Mercer JF: The toxic milk mouse is a murine model of Wilson disease. Hum Mol Genet 5:1619, 1996.
7. Hung IH, Suzuki M, Yamaguchi Y, et al: Biochemical characterization of the Wilson disease protein and functional expression in the yeast Saccharomyces cerevisiae. J Biol Chem 272:21461, 1997.
8. Schaefer M, Roelofsen H, Wolters H, et al: Localization of the Wilson's disease protein in human liver. Gastroenterology 117:1380, 1999.
9. Field LS, Luk E, Culotta VC: Copper chaperones: Personal escorts for metal ions. J Bioenerg Biomembr 34:373, 2002.
10. van de Sluis B, Rothuizen J, Pearson PL, et al: Identification of a new copper metabolism gene by positional cloning in a purebred dog population. Hum Mol Genet 11:165, 2002.
11. Coronado VA, Damaraju D, Kohijoki R, et al: New haplotypes in the Bedlington terrier indicate complexity in copper toxicosis. Mamm Genome 14:483, 2003.
12. Schilsky ML, Scheinberg IH, Sternlieb I: Prognosis of Wilsonian chronic active hepatitis. Gastroenterology 100:762, 1991.
13. McCullough AJ, Fleming CR, Thistle JL: Diagnosis of Wilson's disease presenting as fulminant hepatic failure. Gastroenterology 84:161, 1983.
14. Hoshino T, Kumasaka K, Kawano K: Low serum alkaline phosphatase activity associated with severe Wilson's disease: Is the breakdown of alkaline phosphatase molecules caused by reactive oxygen species? Clin Chim Acta 238:91, 1995.
15. Sallie R, Katsiyiannakis L, Baldwin D: Failure of simple biochemical indexes to reliably differentiate fulminant Wilson's disease from other causes of fulminant liver failure. Hepatol 16:1206, 1992.
16. Kreymann B, Seige M, Schweigart U, et al: Albumin dialysis: Effective removal of copper in a patient with fulminant Wilson disease and successful bridging to liver transplanta-

tion: A new possibility for the elimination of protein-bound toxins. J Hepatol 31:1080, 1999.

17. Oder W, Prayer L, Grimm G: Wilson's disease: Evidence of subgroups derived from clinical findings and brain lesions. Neurology 43:120, 1993.

18. Dening TR, Berrios GE: Wilson's disease: Psychiatric symptoms in 195 cases. Arch Gen Psychiatry 46:1126, 1989.

19. Sternlieb I: Mitochondrial and fatty changes in hepatocytes of patients with Wilson's disease. Gastroenterology 5:354, 1968.

20. Ferenci P, Caca K, Loudianos G, et al: Diagnosis and phenotypic classification of Wilson disease. Liver Int 23:139, 2003.

21. Steindl P, Ferenci P, Dienes HP, et al: Wilson's disease in patients with liver disease: A diagnostic challenge. Gastroenterology 113:212, 1998.

22. Walshe JM: Wilson's disease: The importance of measuring serum caeruloplasmin non-immunologically. Ann Clin Biochem 40:115, 2003.

23. Macintyre G, Gutfreund KS, Martin WR, et al: Value of an enzymatic assay for the determination of serum ceruloplasmin. J Lab Clin Med 144:294, 2004.

24. Yoshida K, Furihata K, Takeda S, et al: A mutation in the ceruloplasmin gene is associated with systemic hemosiderosis in humans. Nat Genet 9:267, 1995.

25. Harris ZL, Takahashi Y, Miyajima H, et al: Aceruloplasminemia: Molecular characterization of this disorder of iron metabolism. Proc Natl Acad Sci U S A 92:2539, 1995.

26. Harris ZL, Durley AP, Man TK, et al: Targeted gene disruption reveals an essential role for ceruloplasmin in cellular iron efflux. Proc Natl Acad Sci U S A 96:10812, 1999.

27. Martins da Costa C, Baldwin D, Portmann B, et al: Value of urinary copper excretion after penicillamine challenge in the diagnosis of Wilson's disease. Hepatology 15:609, 1992.

28. Faa G, Nurchi V, Demelia L, et al: Uneven hepatic copper distribution in Wilson's disease. J Hepatol 22:303, 1995.

29. Thomas GR, Forbes JR, Roberts EA, et al: The Wilson disease gene: Spectrum of mutations and their consequences. Nat Genet 9:210, 1995.

30. Loudianos G, Dessi V, Lovicu M, et al: Mutation analysis in patients of Mediterranean descent with Wilson disease: Identification of 19 novel mutations. J Med Genet 36:833, 1999.

31. Cox DW: Wilson Disease Mutation Database. Department of Medical Genetics, University of Alberta, Canada. Available online at: *http://www.medicalgenetics.meds.ualberta.ca/wilson/index.php/*

32. Weirich G, Cabras AD, Serra S, et al: Rapid identification of Wilson's disease carriers by denaturing high-performance liquid chromatography. Prev Med 35:278, 2002.

33. Forbes JR, Cox DW: Functional characterization of missense mutations in ATP7B: Wilson disease mutation or normal variant? Am J Hum Genet 63:1663, 1998.

34. Forbes JR, Cox DW: Copper-dependent trafficking of Wilson disease mutant ATP7B proteins. Hum Mol Genet 9:1927, 2000.

35. Hsi G, Cox DW: A comparison of the mutation spectra of Menkes disease and Wilson disease. Hum Genet 114:165, 2004.

36. Caca K, Ferenci P, Kuhn HJ, et al: High prevalence of the H1069Q mutation in East German patients with Wilson disease: Rapid detection of mutations by limited sequencing and phenotype-genotype analysis. J Hepatol 35:575, 2001.

37. Curtis D, Durkie M, Balac (Morris) P, et al: A study of Wilson disease mutations in Britain. Hum Mutat 14:304, 1999.

38. Lovicu M, Dessi V, Zappu A, et al: Efficient strategy for molecular diagnosis of Wilson disease in the sardinian population. Clin Chem 49:496, 2003.

39. Panagiotakaki E, Tzetis M, Manolaki N, et al: Genotype-phenotype correlations for a wide spectrum of mutations in the Wilson disease gene (ATP7B). Am J Med Genet 131A:168, 2004.

40. Wilson DC, Phillips MJ, Cox DW, et al: Severe hepatic Wilson's disease in preschool-aged children. J Pediatr 137:719, 2000.

41. Stapelbroek JM, Bollen CW, van Amstel JK, et al: The H1069Q mutation in ATP7B is associated with late and neurologic presentation in Wilson disease: results of a meta-analysis. J Hepatol 41:758, 2004.

42. Lyon TD, Fell GS, Gaffney D, et al: Use of a stable copper isotope (65Cu) in the differential diagnosis of Wilson's disease. Clin Sci 88:727, 1995.

43. Farinati F, Cardin R, D'Inca R, et al: Zinc treatment prevents lipid peroxidation and increases glutathione availability in Wilson's disease. J Lab Clin Med 141:372, 2003.

44. Klein D, Lichtmannegger J, Heinzmann U, et al: Dissolution of copper-rich granules in hepatic lysosomes by D-penicillamine prevents the development of fulminant hepatitis in Long-Evans cinnamon rats. J Hepatol 32:193, 2000.

45. Walshe JM: Wilson's disease presenting with features of hepatic dysfunction: A clinical analysis of eighty-seven patients. Q J Med 70:253, 1989.

46. Walshe JM: Treatment of Wilson's disease with trientine (triethylenetetramine) dihydrochloride. Lancet 1(8273):643, 1982.

47. Dubois RS, Rodgerson DG, Hambridge KM: Treatment of Wilson's disease with triethylene tetramine hydrochloride (trientine). J Pediatr Gastroenterol Nutrit 10:77, 1990.

48. Scheinberg IH, Jaffe ME, Sternlieb I: The use of trientine in preventing the effects of interrupting penicillamine therapy in Wilson's disease. N Engl J Med 317:209, 1987.

49. Hoogenraad TU, Van Haltum J, Van der Hamer CJA: Management of Wilson's disease with zinc sulphate. J Neurol Sci 77:137, 1987.

50. Yuzbasiyan-Gurkan V, Grider A, Nostrant T, et al: Treatment of Wilson's disease with zinc. X: Intestinal metallothionein induction. J Lab Clin Med 120:380, 1992.

51. Brewer GJ, Dick RD, Johnson VD, et al: Treatment of Wilson's disease with zinc. XV: Long-term follow-up studies. J Lab Clin Med 132:264, 1998.

52. Askari FK, Greenson J, Dick RD, et al: Treatment of Wilson's disease with zinc. XVIII: Initial treatment of the hepatic decompensation presentation with trientine and zinc. J Lab Clin Med 142:385, 2003.

53. Brewer GJ, Dick RD, Johnson V, et al: Treatment of Wilson's disease with ammonium tetrathiomolybdate. I: Initial therapy in 17 neurologically affected patients. Arch Neurol 51:545, 1994.

54. Ogra Y, Suzuki KT: Targeting of tetrathiomolybdate on the copper accumulating in the liver of LEC rats. J Inorg Biochem 70:49, 1998.

55. Sokol RJ, Twedt D, McKim JM, et al: Oxidant injury to hepatic mitochondria in patients with Wilson's disease and Bedlington terriers with copper toxicosis. Gastroenterology 107:1788, 1994.

56. von Herbay A, de Groot H, Hegi U, et al: Low vitamin E content in plasma of patients with alcoholic liver disease, hemochromatosis and Wilson's disease. J Hepatol 20:41, 1994.

57. Shiono Y, Wakusawa S, Hayashi H, et al: Iron accumulation in the liver of male patients with Wilson's disease. Am J Gastroenterol 96:3147, 2001.

58. Hussain SP, Raja K, Amstad PA, et al: Increased p53 mutation load in nontumorous human liver of Wilson disease and hemochromatosis: Oxyradical overload diseases. Proc Natl Acad Sci U S A 97:12770, 2000.

59. Pinter R, Hogge WA, McPherson E: Infant with severe penicillamine embryopathy born to a woman with Wilson disease. Am J Med Genet 128A:294, 2004.

60. Stremmel W, Meyerrose KW, Niederau C, et al: Wilson disease: Clinical presentation, treatment and survival. Ann Intern Med 115:720, 1991.

61. Mason AL, Marsh W, Alpers DH: Intractable neurological Wilson's disease treated with orthotopic liver transplantation. Dig Dis Sci 23:373, 1993.

62. Bellary S, Hassanein T, Van Thiel DH: Liver transplantation for Wilson's disease. J Hepatol 23:373, 1995.

63. Rela M, Heaton ND, Vougas V, et al: Orthotopic liver transplantation for hepatic complications of Wilson's disease. Br J Surg 80:909, 1993.

64. Schilsky ML, Scheinberg IH, Sternlieb I: Liver transplantation for Wilson's disease: Indications and outcome. Hepatology 19:583, 1994.

65. Asonuma K, Inomata Y, Kasahara M, et al: Living related liver transplantation from heterozygote genetic carriers to children with Wilson's disease. Pediatr Transplant 3:201, 1999.

CHAPTER

73 Other Inherited Metabolic Disorders of the Liver

Mike A. Leonis and William F. Balistreri

Inborn errors of metabolism encompass a vast variety of disorders with myriad presentations and complex pathophysiology. Metabolic liver diseases may manifest as acute, life-threatening illnesses in the neonatal period or as chronic liver disease in adolescence or adulthood, with progression to liver failure, cirrhosis, or hepatocellular carcinoma. In one review of 37 transplant centers in the United States, 5.3% of all liver transplants were performed because of complications resulting from metabolic liver disease.[1] When the pediatric population alone is analyzed, this percentage is substantially higher. Nationwide, more than 20% of the liver transplants performed over the 5-year period from 1995 to 2000 were for the complications of metabolic liver disease.[2] Liver transplantation has become a life-saving measure for many patients with metabolic liver diseases. However, new nontransplant treatment options have become available that may, in certain cases, obviate liver transplantation and thereby help alleviate the shortage of donor organs.[3,4]

CLINICAL FEATURES OF METABOLIC LIVER DISEASE

The diverse presenting symptoms of metabolic liver disease are listed in Table 73–1. Such diseases in young

patients may mimic other illnesses, such as acute infections and intoxications. In contrast, the older patient with metabolic liver disease may present with symptoms of chronic disease. Because metabolic diseases can resemble multiple other disorders, a high index of suspicion is required for correct diagnosis.

An infant presenting with cholestasis should undergo an evaluation for metabolic liver disease. (The approach to the patient with jaundice is discussed in detail in Chapter 14.) Any patient with progressive neuromuscular disease, developmental delays, or regression of developmental milestones also requires evaluation. Metabolic liver disease should be an immediate consideration in patients with elevations of serum aminotransferase levels, hepatomegaly, acidosis, hypoglycemia, ascites, bleeding diathesis, hyperammonemia, coma, recurrent vomiting, or failure to thrive.

A detailed history can often raise the possibility of metabolic liver disease and help direct the investigation. A family history of consanguinity, multiple miscarriages, or early infant deaths may suggest a metabolic derangement. Close relatives with undiagnosed liver disease, progressive neurologic or muscle disease, or undiagnosed developmental delays should also raise suspicion. A carefully obtained dietary history is also important in dissecting the nature of the illness; introduction of certain foods may correlate with the onset of symptoms, as in

Table 73–1 Presenting Features of Metabolic Liver Disease

Symptoms	Hyperammonemic symptoms
	Hypoglycemic symptoms
	Recurrent vomiting
	Growth failure
	Neurologic or motor skill deterioration
	Coma
	Seizures
	Developmental delay
Signs	Short stature
	Dysmorphic features
	Unusual odors
	Cataracts
	Hepatomegaly
	Splenomegaly
	Cardiac dysfunction
	Ascites
	Abdominal distention
	Hypotonia
	Jaundice
Other Findings	Acidosis
	Coagulopathy
	Ketosis
	Fulminant hepatic failure
	Cholestasis
	Rickets

Table 73–2 Screening Laboratory Studies for Metabolic Liver Disease*

Serum	Electrolytes
	Anion gap
	Glucose
	Ammonia
	Amino acids
	Aminotransferases
	Albumin
	Fractionated bilirubin
	Alkaline phosphatase
	Gamma glutamyl transpeptidase
	Coagulation profile
	Ferritin
	Peripheral blood smear
	Lactate[†]
	Pyruvate[†]
	Uric acid[†]
Urine	Organic acids
	Orotic acid
	Reducing substances

*Save specimens of serum and urine obtained during acute episodes for later studies.
[†]Obtain if patient is acidotic or has neurologic symptoms.

patients with urea cycle defects, galactosemia, or fructosemia. A history of specific dietary aversions may also be revealing.[5]

Recommended initial screening tests, which should direct further diagnostic evaluation, are listed in Table 73–2. Because patients with metabolic liver disease often present with acute and recurrent symptoms, it is of utmost importance that the physician obtain the diagnostic studies as soon as possible. The laboratory values for many of these illnesses may normalize between acute episodes. In enigmatic cases, serum and urine samples should be obtained during the acute illness and saved (frozen) for definitive studies, if available. A liver biopsy can also be a valuable diagnostic tool. If a metabolic liver disease is suspected, in addition to obtaining specimens for standard histology, a frozen specimen should be saved for an electron microscopic study to look at the subcellular organelles, which may exhibit characteristic changes in some disorders.

α_1-ANTITRYPSIN DEFICIENCY

Deficiency of α_1-antitrypsin (α_1-AT) is transmitted in an autosomal-recessive fashion and leads to an increased risk of lung and liver disease. This deficiency is one of the most common genetic diseases in the world and the most common metabolic disease affecting the liver.[6-8] The following discussion focuses on the effects of α_1-AT deficiency on the liver.

Pathophysiology

The prototypical member of the serpin family of protease inhibitors, α_1-antitrypsin binds with and promotes the degradation of serine proteases in the serum and tissues. The most important of these serine proteases is neutrophil elastase, which is inhibited by α_1-AT through formation of a tight $1:1$ α_1-AT: elastase complex. Loss of serum α_1-AT activity, as occurs in the most common form of α_1-AT deficiency, leads to uninhibited neutrophil elastase activity and is the primary mechanism for the premature development of pulmonary emphysema in affected patients.[9]

Allelic α_1-AT mutant variants produce protease inhibitor (Pi) gene products that can be distinguished from normal by electrophoretic methods; the normal allelic representation is designated PiM. The PiZ variant produces a mutant α_1-ATZ protein. Homozygosity at the PiZ allele is the most common and classic pathologic form of α_1-AT deficiency and is capable of leading to both liver and lung disease. The α_1-ATZ molecule represents a single–amino acid replacement of glutamine with a lysine residue at position 342.[8,10] More than 70 naturally occurring variants of α_1-AT have been described; however, most of these variants are either of no clinical significance or extremely rare.[4,11]

α_1-AT is produced almost exclusively in the rough endoplasmic reticulum (ER) of hepatocytes and is subsequently targeted to the secretory pathway via the Golgi apparatus. Structural misfolding and polymerization of the mutant α_1-ATZ protein causes its aberrant retention in the ER, failure of progression through the secretory pathway, and diminished intracellular degradation. In persons with the phenotype PiZZ, serum α_1-AT activity levels are reduced to less than 15% of normal; this loss of function accounts for the development of pulmonary disease, as mentioned earlier. Studies suggest that the rate of intracellular degradation may itself be genetically determined and may influence the expression of disease; α_1-ATZ appears to be degraded more slowly in the ER of PiZZ patients who are susceptible to liver disease than in PiZZ patients who are not susceptible to liver disease.[12] Conjugation to ubiquitin is a major mechanism of targeting proteins for intracellular degradation, and both ubiquitin-dependent and ubiquitin-independent mechanisms are involved in the degradation of α_1-ATZ.[13,14]

The exact mechanism for α_1-ATZ–induced liver injury is not known, although studies of mice that are transgenic for the human ATZ gene suggest a gain-of-function mechanism by which retention in the ER and accumulation in hepatocytes of mutant α_1-ATZ is responsible for hepatotoxicity.[15] Two distinct signaling pathways are activated by the retention of malformed proteins in the ER, the *unfolded protein response* and the *endoplasmic reticulum overload response*. Both responses influence the transcriptional regulation of genes that could further drive pathologic processes within the hepatocyte.[14,16] An additional downstream alteration in α_1-ATZ deficiency is an increase in the constitutive activation of autophagy, an intracellular degradative pathway that targets proteins and organelles for destruction during development as well as at times of stress or nutrient deprivation. Experimental evidence suggests that the liver in persons with α_1-ATZ deficiency is intolerant of the fasting state because of increased mitochondrial autophagy; this intolerance may be amenable to treatment with cyclosporine, an inhibitor of the mitochondrial permeability transition and mitochondrial autophagy. Mitochondrial permeability transition is a measure of the nonspecific increase in the permeability of the inner mitochondrial membrane. The greater permeability leads to mitochondrial swelling, uncoupling of the electron-transfer chain from the adenosine triphosphate (ATP)–producing translocating ATPase, and release of proapoptotic factors such as cytochrome c and apoptosis-inducing factor.[17,18]

Clinical Features

Although the prevalence of the classic α_1-AT deficiency allele, PiZ, is highest in populations derived from northern European ancestry, many racial subgroups are affected worldwide, and millions of persons have combinations of deficiency alleles (i.e., PiSS, PiSZ, or PiZZ).[6] In the United States, the overall prevalence of deficiency allele combinations is approximately 1 in 490 (i.e., 1 in 1058 for PiSS, 1 in 1124 for PiSZ, and 1 in 4775 for PiZZ).[19] Mounting evidence suggests that numerous heterozygous α_1-AT deficiency states can contribute to the development of cirrhosis and chronic liver failure in adults through mechanisms similar to those encountered with the PiZZ phenotype, although this association needs to be investigated further.[20,21]

In the most unbiased study to date on the epidemiology of liver disease in patients with α_1-AT deficiency, 200,000 Swedish infants were screened for α_1-AT deficiency in a study reported by Sveger[22]; 184 infants were found to have abnormal allelic forms of α_1-AT (127 PiZZ, 2 PiZnull, 54 PiSZ, and 1 PiSnull), and 6 died in early childhood (5 PiZZ and 1 PiSZ), although only 2 from cirrhosis.[22] Although about 10% of newborns with α_1-AT deficiency (PiZZ) present with cholestasis and up to 50%

have elevated serum aminotransferase levels at age 3 months, most are clinically asymptomatic.[11,22-24] Liver disease does not develop in patients with null α_1-AT phenotypes, whereas early-onset emphysema develops in all of them.[25] Therefore, the prognosis for patients with liver disease manifesting in infancy as a result of α_1-AT deficiency (PiZZ) is highly variable. Even those children in whom cirrhosis develops can have a highly variable progression to end-stage liver disease (ESLD), which infrequently leads to liver transplantation (LT).[26]

In the study by Sveger,[22] of 150 patients with α_1-AT deficiency who underwent evaluation at age 16 and 18 years, none had clinical signs of liver disease. Elevated serum aminotransferase or gamma glutamyl transpeptidase (GGTP) levels were found in less than 20% of patients with a PiZZ phenotype and in less than 15% of those with a PiSZ phenotype. Only 2 patients (one PiSZ and the other PiZnull) had abnormal liver biochemical test levels at both visits.[23]

Even though liver disease is often (but not always) mild during infancy and childhood, patients with α_1-AT deficiency have an eight-fold higher risk for development of cirrhosis during adulthood; 37% of all PiZZ patients have histologic evidence of cirrhosis at autopsy.[27,28] Moreover, homozygous α_1-AT deficiency raises the risk for development of hepatocellular carcinoma, especially in men older than 50 years.[29,30] The diagnosis of α_1-AT deficiency should be considered in any patient presenting with noninfectious chronic hepatitis, hepatosplenomegaly, cirrhosis, portal hypertension, or hepatocellular carcinoma.

Histology

Histopathologic features of α_1-AT deficiency change as the affected patient ages. In infancy liver biopsy specimens may show bile duct paucity, intracellular cholestasis with or without giant cell transformation, mild inflammatory changes, or steatosis, with few of the characteristic periodic acid–Schiff (PAS)–positive, diastase-resistant globules. These inclusions are most prominent in periportal hepatocytes but may also be seen in Kupffer cells. Immunohistochemistry with monoclonal antibody to α_1-ATZ can also be performed to verify the diagnosis.[30] As the patient ages, these changes may resolve completely or progress to chronic hepatitis or cirrhosis.[31]

Diagnosis

α_1-AT is considered a hepatic acute-phase reactant, and its release may be stimulated by stress, injury, pregnancy, or neoplasia. Because these factors can influence α_1-AT production, even in patients with PiZZ, the diagnosis of α_1-AT deficiency should be based on phenotype analysis and not solely on the serum α_1-AT level. A liver biopsy, although not universally recommended, should confirm the diagnosis.

Treatment

The initial treatment of α_1-AT deficiency is with symptomatic care. It has been suggested that breast-feeding until the end of the first year of life may decrease the manifestations of cholestatic liver disease, as may the use of ursodeoxycholic acid.[32] The importance of providing fat-soluble vitamins when indicated, adequate nutrition, and counseling about the avoidance of smoking and second-hand smoke cannot be overemphasized. The role of neonatal screening for α_1-AT deficiency is still not settled, although there appears to be a positive effect on smoking practices in patients diagnosed at an early age.[33] If effective therapy for liver disease due to α_1-AT deficiency becomes available, neonatal screening might be even more useful for preventing the need for liver transplantation.

Although progression to ESLD is uncommon, α_1-AT deficiency is the most common metabolic liver disease for which liver transplantation is performed.[7] Besides replacing the injured organ, transplantation corrects the metabolic defect, thereby preventing further progression of systemic disease.

Replacement therapy with purified α_1-AT is the only treatment option approved by the U.S. Food and Drug Administration (FDA) for lung disease associated with α_1-AT deficiency. Patients who receive replacement therapy have a slower rate of decline in lung function than those who do not, although clinical efficacy has not been conclusively demonstrated by a randomized placebo-controlled trial.[34,35] This therapy would not be expected to benefit α_1-AT deficiency–associated liver disease.

Other mechanistically based treatment options aimed at influencing the stability or secretion rates of α_1-ATZ within the hepatocyte ER are being investigated. Chemical chaperones such as phenylbutyric acid (PBA, an agent approved for use in patients with urea cycle defects; see later) and glucosidase and mannosidase inhibitors markedly increase secretion of α_1-ATZ in experimental in vitro and in vivo models of α_1-AT deficiency.[36,37] A small pilot study investigated the potential benefits of PBA in the treatment of children with α_1-AT–deficient liver disease. Unfortunately, no statistically significant increase in serum α_1-AT levels occurred in PBA-treated patients, and the high frequency of side effects they experienced are likely to discourage a trial with higher doses of the drug.[38] Still, this general approach has the potential to be efficacious in humans, given that mutant α_1-ATZ retains approximately 80% of normal antielastase activity and that relatively small increases in plasma α_1-ATZ levels are needed to inhibit destructive proteolysis due to α_1-AT deficiency.[36,39]

α_1-AT deficiency is one of many diseases for which reconstitution of the normal genotype through gene therapy is being studied. Long-term expression of human α_1-AT in murine liver, at therapeutic levels, has been achieved after hydrodynamics-based intravenous injection of nonviral DNA constructs.[40] These results are promising first steps toward the goal of achieving successful gene replacement therapy for this disease; however, alternative strategies are required to repair the endogenous mutant PiZ allele in order to rescue hepatocytes from the burden of α_1-ATZ protein aggregates. Two such methodologies are in early stages of investigation; one employs ribozyme constructs that target the destruction of mutant α_1-ATZ RNA and lead to the expression of a modified, but otherwise normally functioning, α_1-AT protein, and the other involves RNA/DNA oligonucleotide–directed repair of the defective α_1-AT gene.[41,42]

GLYCOGEN STORAGE DISEASES

More than 10 distinct inborn disorders of glycogen metabolism have been described in the literature, but only three are associated with liver disease—glycogen storage disease (GSD) types I, III and IV.[5,43] Other GSDs may cause hepatomegaly or microscopic changes seen on liver histology but generally do not cause clinically important liver disease. The overall incidence of GSD types I, III, and IV is estimated to be between 1 in 50,000 and 1 in 100,000 population.

Glycogen metabolism occurs in many tissues, but the areas of clinical importance are the muscle and liver. The body utilizes glycogen as a storage system for glucose and as a ready reserve for times when systemic glucose is required (see Chapter 69). Glycogen is composed of long-chain glucose molecules arranged in a linear 1,4 linkage. From 8% to 10% of the glucose molecules are attached in a 1,6 linkage to form branching chains, which permit efficient storage of glucose while minimizing the impact on intracellular osmolality. The substrates for glycogen synthesis, glucose-6-phosphate (G6P) and glucose-1-phosphate (G1P), are derived from several pathways, including fructose and galactose metabolic cycles as well as gluconeogenesis and glycogenolysis (Fig. 73–1).

Through the action of uridine diphosphate glucose (UDPG) pyrophosphorylase and glycogen synthase, G1P is metabolized to UDPG and glycogen, sequentially. The 1,4 linkages can be converted to 1,6 linkages by the actions of branching enzymes. Amylo-1,6-glucosidase is a debranching enzyme that can release 8% to 10% of the glucose stored in glycogen. The remaining glucose is released as G1P through the action of phosphorylase *a* and is converted to G6P by phosphoglucomutase. Phosphorylase exists in an active *(a)* and an inactive form *(b)*; protein kinase is responsible for the conversion of phosphorylase *b* to *a*. Protein kinase is stimulated by epinephrine, glucagon, and fasting, thereby increasing

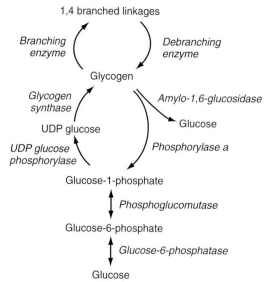

Figure 73–1 The pathway of glycogen synthesis and glycogenolysis. UDP, uridine diphosphate.

glycogenolysis. High levels of glucose influence the conversion of phosphorylase *a* back to phosphorylase *b*, thereby decreasing glycogenolysis. Glycogen synthase also exists in active (*a*) and inactive (*b*) forms. Phosphorylase *a* inhibits the conversion to glycogen synthase *a*, thereby reducing glycogen synthesis. High levels of glycogen favor the formation of glycogen synthase *b*.[44]

TYPE I

GSD type I, the most common inborn error of glycogen metabolism, results from deficiency of a two-component enzyme system involved in the transport of G6P from the cytosol into the ER by G6P translocase and subsequent cleavage of G6P by glucose-6-phosphatase (G6Pase), located on the luminal side of the ER. Clinical and molecular genetic observations have disclosed two subtypes of GSD type I, Ia and Ib, that account for virtually all cases.[45,46] The clinical phenotype with respect to liver disease is similar in the two forms; however, patients with GSD type Ib often have intermittent severe neutropenia and neutrophil dysfunction, making them prone to recurrent episodes of severe bacterial infections and Crohn's-like intestinal disease.[47,48]

Disruption of the function of G6Pase (type Ia) or G6P translocase (type Ib) inhibits the utilization of glucose by gluconeogenesis, glycogenolysis, and the metabolism of fructose or galactose. This inability to release stored glucose leads to hypoglycemia within 90 to 180 minutes of the last ingested glucose. Lactate and fatty acid metabolism and glycolytic pathways are then utilized as sources of energy.

Clinical Features

Most patients with GSD type I present in infancy with symptoms of metabolic derangement, such as lethargy, seizures, or coma due to profound hypoglycemia or metabolic acidosis, a protruding abdomen caused by hepatomegaly, muscular hypotonia, and delayed psychomotor development.[46]

Physical signs invariably include hepatomegaly, usually with a normal-sized spleen. Patients in whom the disease is poorly controlled for a long time exhibit short stature and growth failure and may be prone to adiposity. Delayed bone age and reduced postpubertal bone mineral density are common.[49] Xanthomas can appear after puberty and localize to the elbows, knees, buttocks, or nasal septum, the last leading to epistaxis. Patients with GSD type I are susceptible to a wide spectrum of brain damage that may result in epilepsy, hearing loss, and abnormal neuroradiologic findings, most likely as a result of recurrent episodes of hypoglycemia.[50]

Other metabolic derangements can be seen. Lactic acid levels can reach four to eight times normal; the accompanying metabolic acidosis may manifest as muscle weakness, hyperventilation, malaise, headache, or recurrent fever. Serum ATP and phosphorus levels are low, secondary to an increase in purine synthesis and the inability to release phosphorus from G6P. Hyperuricemia is common and may lead to gout, arthritis, or progressive nephropathy. Nephromegaly secondary to increased glycogen deposition is common, and with advancing age, progressive renal disease, hypertension, and renal failure requiring dialysis and transplantation may develop.[46] Because of hypoglycemia, patients have chronically high serum levels of glucagon with depressed levels of insulin. Hypertriglyceridemia and hypercholesterolemia are present in both GSD Ia and GSD Ib (but more prominently in GSD Ia) and may account for the greater frequency of xanthoma formation.[51]

In addition to the features already noted, patients with GSD type 1b often have severe intermittent neutropenia and neutrophil dysfunction as well as high platelet counts. Crohn's-like inflammatory bowel disease often occurs in patients with GSD type 1b at the time of severe neutropenia, and patients are prone to development of severe bacterial infections, with abscess formation at numerous locations throughout the body.[47]

Hepatic Involvement

Hepatomegaly in GSD type I results from increased glycogen storage in the liver as well as a large degree of fatty infiltration; the latter likely develops because of a wide array of perturbations in lipid metabolism, including increased free fatty acid flux into the liver.[51] Patients demonstrate mild elevations in serum aminotransferase levels but generally do not develop cirrhosis or liver failure.

Hepatic adenomas develop in 22% to 75% of patients, as early as 3 years of age but most commonly in the second decade of life, and tend to increase in both size and number as the patient ages (see Chapter 91).[52] Rarely, adenomas can transform to hepatocellular carcinoma; unfortunately, serum α-fetoprotein levels and features of the lesions on hepatic imaging are not predictive of malignant transformation.[52,53] The pathogenesis of adenoma formation in GSD type I is unknown. Leading theories include chronic exposure of hepatocytes to an imbalance in serum glucagon and insulin levels and increased oxidative stress due to altered fatty acid metabolism.[52,54] In some patients, hepatic adenomas have been demonstrated to regress and disappear after adequate nutritional therapy, but in general, the course is unpredictable.[52-54]

Diagnosis

The hepatic glycogen content is elevated in patients with GSD type I, and the most accurate diagnostic measure is direct analysis of enzyme activity performed on fresh, rather than frozen, liver tissue. Analysis of fresh liver tissue is important to avoid disrupting microsomal G6Pase activity.[55] Fasting serum glucose and lactate levels, a glucagon response test result, and the response to fructose or galactose administration (patients with GSD type I do not show the expected rise in serum glucose concentration after administration of the substance) often provide supportive evidence but may not yield a definitive diagnosis.[44] Intermittent severe neutropenia is noted in most patients with GSD type Ib.[56] DNA analysis–based approaches to diagnosis that integrate biochemical features and the presence or absence of persistent neutropenia have been proposed and may provide a diagnostic alternative to liver biopsy.[57]

Treatment

Patients with undiagnosed or undertreated GSD type I are at increased risk of death, usually from hypoglycemic comas, seizures, metabolic acidosis, or, in those with GSD type Ib, sepsis from neutropenia.[46] Rarely, hepatocellular carcinoma is a cause of death. Management centers on preventing the acute metabolic derangements and potential long-term complications and enabling the patient to attain normal psychologic development and a good quality of life.[55,58]

An early attempt at intervention in patients with GSD type I was surgical portocaval shunting. After the portal blood supply is routed to the systemic circulation, ingested glucose is delivered to the tissues before undergoing hepatic processing. Although this treatment restores normal glucose control to many patients, others still need nutritional supplementation to maintain metabolic control. Because of surgical complications and shunt occlusion, especially in younger patients, this procedure has largely been abandoned.[44]

Consensus guidelines for the management of GSD type I have been proposed.[55,58] Biomedical targets for good metabolic control include a preprandial blood glucose level higher than 3.5–4.3 mmol/L, urine lactate/creatine level lower than 0.06 mmol/L, high-normal serum uric acid level, venous blood base excess higher than –5 mmol/L, bicarbonate level higher than 20 mmol/L, serum triglyceride level lower than 6 mmol/L, and body-mass index (BMI) between 0 and 2 standard deviations from normal. In addition, for GSD type Ib, demonstrating a normal fecal α_1-AT level is desirable.[55,59] Because optimal glycemic control is not always possible and the risk of severe hypoglycemia, if delivery of glucose is interrupted inadvertently, is high, serum lactate levels should be kept at the high end of normal because lactate is an alternative fuel for the brain.

Nutritional supplementation has become the mainstay of therapy for GSD type I. Frequent, high-carbohydrate, daytime feedings, such as uncooked cornstarch, or continuous nighttime drip feedings, or both, allow the steady release of glucose and lead to improved metabolic control and normalized growth and development.[51,59,60] A biochemical target is to maintain the serum glucose level above 70 mg/dL (3.9 mmol/L). Uncooked cornstarch in a dose of 2 g/kg every 6 hours (6 to 8 mg/kg/min) has been suggested; however, alternative regimens have been successfully implemented.

For infants, once the diagnosis of GSD type 1 is confirmed, a formula that does not contain fructose or galactose should be prescribed. Frequent daytime feedings and continuous nocturnal administration are required. The rate of delivery needed to maintain euglycemia has been shown to be ≈8 mg/kg/minute.[61] Morning feedings should be given quickly after discontinuation of the nighttime drip to avoid hypoglycemia. As solids are introduced, high-carbohydrate foods should be emphasized. These patients require special attention during acute illnesses that may affect oral intake or metabolism because they can become hypoglycemic quickly.

Prophylaxis with antibiotics (e.g., cotrimoxazole) is recommended for patients with GSD type 1b and severe neutropenia or recurrent bacterial infections.[58]

Granulocyte-macrophage colony-stimulating factor (GCSF) has been used with success in patients with GSD type 1b to improve hematologic parameters and neutrophil function and reduce the morbidity associated with severe bacterial infections.[62,63] Splenomegaly may worsen with GCSF therapy, and bone marrow aspiration before and during GCSF therapy may be prudent, given rare occurrences of acute myelogenous leukemia (AML) in patients with GSD type 1b.[58] Both GCSF and inflammatory bowel disease raise the risk of osteopenia, and monitoring of bone density is advised.

Liver transplantation has corrected the metabolic error in patients with GSD type I and permitted catch-up growth, even in patients in the third decade of life.[64,65] Moreover, isolated reports have documented improvement in neutrophil counts and function in patients with GSD type 1b after liver transplantation.[66,67] Adenoviral mediated gene replacement therapy of recombinant G6Pase in murine and canine models of GSD type Ia deficiency have led to encouraging results and may be an option for human disease in the future.[68,69]

TYPE III

GSD type III results from deficiency of glycogen-debranching enzyme (GDE) and leads to the accumulation of limit dextrin units, which restrict subsequent glucose release by phosphorylase. Because deficiency of GDE does not interfere with metabolism of G6P, patients with GSD type III still have effective mechanisms for gluconeogenesis. Therefore, affected patients have a milder clinical course than those with GSD type I and are able to fast for longer periods. In infancy, however, GSD type III may be indistinguishable from GSD type I.

GDE is encoded by a single gene and possesses two independent catalytic activities, an amylo-1,6-glucosidase and oligo-1,4→1,4 glucan transferase. Both of these activities are deficient in the two main clinical subtypes of GSD type III, types IIIa and IIIb. Differential expression of four major GDE mRNA isoforms in liver and muscle tissue distinguishes the two types: Type IIIa affects both liver and muscle and accounts for 80% of patients, and type IIIb affects the liver only (15% of patients). The molecular basis for this differential tissue-specific expression of GDE is unknown, although subtype-specific mutations in the GDE gene are being increasingly identified.[70] Rare isolated loss of one of the two GDE activities has been observed (i.e., glucosidase activity in type IIIc and transferase activity in type IIId).

Clinical Features

Persons with GSD type III typically exhibit hypoglycemia, hepatomegaly, and growth failure. Liver enlargement results from increased glycogen deposition and not fatty infiltration. The liver may show fibrotic septa that rarely lead to frank cirrhosis and liver failure. Serum lactate and uric acid levels are normal, and aminotransferase levels are increased only moderately until advanced liver disease occurs. Hyperlipidemia may be present but is not as pronounced as in GSD type I. Patients have normal responses to fructose and galactose loading.

Patients with GSD type III may also display progressive muscle weakness, which worsens with activity, and muscle wasting. Nephromegaly is not seen, but cardiomegaly may be present. The diagnosis can be made by direct enzyme analysis of muscle or liver tissue or peripheral leukocytes[71]; mutation analysis of the GDE gene will be increasingly important for diagnosis in the future.[44,72] Hepatic adenomas develop in approximately 25% of patients, and isolated reports of cirrhosis leading to hepatocellular carcinoma have been reported.[53,73]

Treatment

A high-protein, low-carbohydrate diet has been suggested to normalize metabolic activity, ensure normal growth, normalize muscle function, and minimize hepatomegaly.[74] This diet provides adequate substrates for gluconeogenesis while reducing the need for glycogen storage. Patients with refractory hypoglycemia or persistent hepatomegaly may require a nighttime continuous infusion or cornstarch therapy, as utilized for GSD type I.[74]

TYPE IV

Deficiency of the branching enzyme is seen in GSD type IV, a rare syndrome also known as amylopectinosis. Glycogen and amylopectin accumulate in hepatocytes, leading to hepatomegaly, abdominal distention, and failure to thrive, most commonly during infancy. Signs of liver disease, when present, predominate later in the course of the disease. Several variable forms of GSD type IV have been observed—a severe congenital form that manifests as fetal hydrops, neonatal hypotonia, or fetal death[75]; a childhood subtype that manifests as cardiomyopathy and abnormal neuromuscular development; and other milder, nonprogressive hepatic disease presentations that do not lead to cirrhosis and are not associated with skeletal muscle or neurologic involvement.[76] Genotype:phenotype analyses of the branching enzyme gene have revealed a high degree of molecular heterogeneity without clear clinical associations.[76]

Hypoglycemia is relatively uncommon, and responses to fructose and galactose challenges are normal. Serum lactate and pyruvate levels are normal, and aminotransferase levels are only moderately elevated until more severe liver involvement becomes apparent. Progressive macronodular cirrhosis is present with an abundance of PAS-positive deposits (amylopectin) in hepatocytes. Cirrhosis may progress to liver failure, and adenomas and hepatocellular carcinoma may develop rarely.[77]

The diagnosis of GSD type IV can be made by direct enzyme analysis of liver tissue or fibroblasts. Most patients die within the first 3 years of life if the disease is untreated. Diets high in protein and low in carbohydrate have been associated with improved growth but have had little effect on liver involvement. Liver transplantation has been used successfully and results in correction of the metabolic error and normal growth; however, persistence of amylopectin deposits in the heart (with progressive cardiomyopathy) and leukocytes of affected patients has been described.[64,78]

CONGENITAL DISORDERS OF GLYCOSYLATION

Congenital disorders of glycosylation (CDGs) comprise a group of inherited defects in either the enzymes that synthesize the glycan moiety of glycoproteins or the macromolecules that affect intracellular trafficking and functioning of glycoproteins.[79,80] More than 20 CDGs involving both asparagine (*N*)- and serine/threonine (*O*)-linked protein glycosylation have been reported to date, and many of these disorders lead to dysfunction of the liver, intestine, or both.[79-81] Protein glycosylation is complex and involves multiple enzymatic steps and subcellular compartments.[81] Secretory glycoproteins with altered carbohydrate moieties in CDG include coagulation factors, albumin and other binding proteins, growth hormone, apolipoproteins, insulin, and thyroxine-binding globulin.[82] Because protein glycosylation occurs in all cells, it is not surprising that patients with CDG exhibit multisystemic abnormalities, often dominated by central nervous system manifestations.

Two main groups of protein *N*-glycosylation disorders, groups I and II, have been delineated on the basis of characteristic isoelectric focusing patterns of serum transferrin, a marker protein for this group of disorders.[79] Group I disorders (of which there are 11 types) involve aberrant processing of lipid-linked oligosaccharides before transfer to protein targeted for glycosylation and include the three most common and best-characterized types of CDG, types Ia, Ib, and Ic. Clinical features in common among these three disorders are protein-losing enteropathy, coagulopathy (both procoagulant and anticoagulant states), feeding difficulties, and hepatomegaly.[81,83,84]

CDG type Ia is caused by defects in phosphomannomutase (PMM), an enzyme that converts mannose-6-phosphate to mannose-1-phosphate (Fig. 73–2). Almost

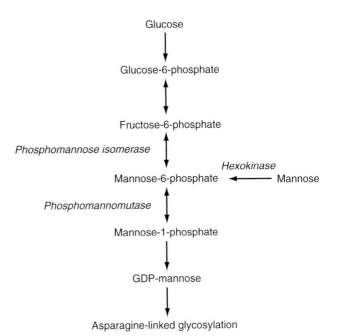

Figure 73–2 Pathway of mannose metabolism. Enzymes are shown in *italics*. GDP, guanosine diphosphate.

60 mutations have been found in the encoding *PMM2* gene, and most patients are compound heterozygotes for mutations that likely preserve some residual PMM enzymatic activity; this observation suggests that complete loss of PMM activity is incompatible with life.[85] Slightly more than 25% of patients with CDG type Ia have the *R141H/F119L* genotype, which carries a mortality rate in childhood of 18% and likely represents the most severe form of the disease.[86,87] Patients typically have severe neurologic abnormalities (ataxia, psychomotor delay, and progressive peripheral neuropathy), dysmorphisms (inverted nipples, abnormal fat distribution, and esotropia) and congenital hepatic fibrosis and steatosis in addition to the features described earlier.[81,83,87] No treatment for CDG type Ia is currently available, although the feasibility of using membrane-permeant derivatives of mannose-1-phosphate, which would represent a potential cure for the disorder, is under investigation.[88]

Patients with *CDG type Ib* have a defect in phosphomannose isomerase (PMI), which converts fructose-6-phosphate to mannose-6-phosphate. In addition to intractable diarrhea, protein-losing enteropathy and congenital hepatic fibrosis, patients with *CDG type Ib* can have recurrent episodes of hyperinsulinemic hypoglycemia and cyclic vomiting. Neurologic symptoms are usually absent, and dysmorphisms are less common than in CDG type Ia.[81,83,84,89,90] Many patients with CDG type Ib have been treated effectively with dietary mannose, making CDG type Ib the only treatable form of CDG to date.[81]

Transient hepatomegaly, without congenital hepatic fibrosis, has been noted in a patient with *CDG type Ic*; otherwise, the clinical features of CDG type Ic are similar to but milder than those of CDG type Ia.[81,83]

Group II CDGs (5 types) involve defects that affect the processing of *N*-linked glycoproteins.[79-81] Most types result from defects in enzymes involved in the trimming of protein-bound oligosaccharides and the subsequent addition of terminal sugars. Patients have marked dysmorphic features and severe developmental retardation. Two infants with hepatosplenomegaly, progressive jaundice, severe epilepsy, recurrent infections, and cardiac insufficiency have been shown to have mutations in a subunit of the conserved oligomeric Golgi complex (COG) that result in disruption of glycosylated protein intracellular trafficking.[80] Therefore, the defects in COG represent a novel mechanism for CDG involving proteins that affect the intracellular trafficking of glycosylated proteins, not just the processing of the glycan moiety. The biochemical and clinical features of the remaining types of CDG are less well characterized.

Isoelectrofocusing of apolipoprotein C-III, which carries a single *O*-linked glycan moiety, has been proposed as a screening method for the *O*-glycan biosynthesis defects (4 types) encountered thus far.[91] Hepatic dysfunction is usually mild in CDG and usually does not lead to symptoms. Mild steatosis and fibrosis typically are seen on light microscopy; on electron microscopy, lysosomal vacuoles with concentric electron-dense membranes and variable electron-lucent and electron-dense material are noted. Patients uncommonly can progress to liver failure, with micronodular cirrhosis noted at autopsy.

Any patient with unexplained congenital hepatic fibrosis, protein-losing enteropathy, or a procoagulant tendency should be evaluated for the possibility of CDG (especially type Ib).[83] An initial screening of serum transferrin with isoelectric focusing should be performed, followed by confirmatory enzymatic analysis in fibroblasts, leukocytes, or liver tissue. If the diagnosis is confirmed, oral mannose therapy should be initiated.[81,90,92]

PORPHYRIAS

A diverse group of metabolic diseases, porphyrias result from deficiencies in enzymes involved in the heme synthetic pathway. In this section, this synthetic pathway and those porphyrias for which the primary site of expression is the liver or direct hepatotoxicity occurs are reviewed.

Pathophysiology

The metabolic pathways for heme synthesis are essentially the same in the two tissues in which heme synthesis primarily occurs, the liver (15% to 20%) and the bone marrow (75% to 80%), although synthetic control may be different in the two tissues. The rate-limiting step in hepatic heme synthesis begins with the conversion of glycine and succinyl CoA to 5-aminolevulinic acid (ALA) by the action of ALA synthase (Fig. 73–3). ALA synthase

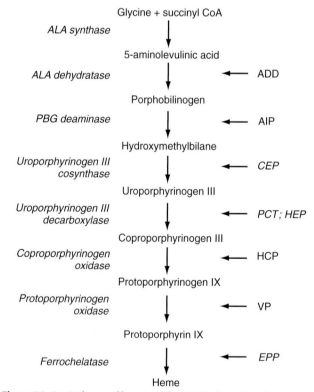

Figure 73–3 Pathway of heme synthesis. The location of enzymatic deficiency in the various porphyrias is noted. On the left, enzymes are shown in *italics*. On the right, abbreviations for cutaneous porphyrias are shown in *italics*, and those for acute porphyrias in normal typeface. ADD, 5-aminolevulinic acid (ALA) dehydratase deficiency; AIP, acute intermittent porphyria; CEP, congenital erythropoietic porphyria; EPP, erythropoietic protoporphyria; HCP, hereditary coproporphyria; HEP, Hepatoerythropoietic porphyria; PCT, porphyria cutanea tarda; PBG, porphobilinogen; VP, variegate porphyria.

Table 73–3   The Porphyrias

	Enzymatic Defect	Mode of Inheritance	Clinical Findings	Site of Expression	Major Biochemical Findings
Acute Porphyrias					
ALA dehydratase deficiency	ALA dehydratase	Autosomal recessive	Neurologic	Liver	Urine: ALA
Acute intermittent porphyria	PBG deaminase	Autosomal dominant	Neurologic	Liver	Urine: ALA < PBG
Hereditary coproporphyria	Coproporphyrinogen oxidase	Autosomal dominant	Neurologic, cutaneous	Liver	Urine: ALA > PBG, coproporphyrin Stool: Coproporphyrin
Variegate porphyria	Protoporphyrinogen oxidase	Autosomal dominant	Neurologic, cutaneous	Liver	Urine: ALA > PBG, coproporphyrin Stool: Coproporphyrin, protoporphyrinogen
Cutaneous Porphyrias					
Porphyria cutanea tarda	Uroporphyrinogen III decarboxylase	Autosomal dominant or acquired	Cutaneous	Liver	Urine: Uroporphyrin, 7-carboxylate porphyrin Stool: Isocoproporphyrin
Hepatoerythropoietic porphyria	Uroporphyrinogen III decarboxylase	Autosomal recessive	Cutaneous	Liver, bone marrow	Urine: Uroporphyrin, 7-carboxylate porphyrin Stool: Isocoproporphyrin
Erythropoietic protoporphyria	Ferrochelatase	Autosomal dominant	Cutaneous, rarely neurologic	Liver, bone marrow	Urine: None Stool: Protoporphyrin, coproporphyrin
Congenital erythropoietic porphyria	Uroporphyrinogen III cosynthase	Autosomal recessive	Cutaneous	Bone marrow	Urine and stool: Coproporphyrin I

ALA, 5-aminolevulinic acid; PBG, porphobilinogen.

activity is decreased by the end-product of the pathway, heme, and is increased by substances that induce the hepatic cytochrome P450 pathway. Six additional enzymatic steps convert ALA to protoporphyrin IX (see Fig. 73-3). In the final step of the pathway, protoporphyrin IX is coupled to ferrous iron by ferrochelatase to create heme. Enzyme deficiencies arising from any of these eight steps of the heme synthetic pathway lead to the clinically apparent diseases known as the porphyrias.

Porphyrias are commonly classified according to clinical features into two main groups, *acute porphyrias*, which are characterized by dramatic and potentially life-threatening neurologic symptoms, and *cutaneous porphyrias*, which typically cause few or no neurologic symptoms but instead give rise to a variety of severe skin lesions (Table 73–3). In five of the porphyrias, the liver is the major site of expression; in two others, both the liver and bone marrow are involved; and in one, only the bone marrow contributes.

Acute Porphyrias

The symptoms and signs of the acute neurovisceral attacks that occur in the four acute porphyrias vary considerably. Abdominal pain is present in more than 90% of patients, followed in frequency by tachycardia and dark urine in about 80% of patients.[93] Neuropsychiatric features include hysteria, depression, psychosis, confusion, hallucinations, seizures, and coma, although there is little evidence that chronic psychiatric illness occurs.[94] Other features are constipation, extremity pain, paresthesias, nausea, vomiting, urinary retention, hypertension, peripheral sensory deficits (often in a "bathing trunk" distribution), and weakness leading to ascending

paralysis or quadriplegia. These neurologic attacks appear to be related to the overproduction of ALA and porphobilinogen (PBG), which leads to higher serum and tissue levels of these products. ALA and PBG have been shown experimentally to elicit neurotoxic reactions, most likely because of their structural similarity to γ-aminobutyric acid (GABA), a major inhibitory neurotransmitter in the central nervous system.[93]

Acute episodes are about five times as common in women as in men and may be precipitated by many factors, most commonly drugs, alcohol ingestion, and smoking.[95] Steroids, sex hormones, and medications that stimulate the hepatic cytochrome P450 system, perhaps by increasing the requirements for heme production, are often identified as precipitants. Other inciting factors are fasting, infections, and pregnancy; some women report greater problems during the luteal phase of their menstrual cycles.[96] The disease is clinically latent in 65% to 80% of patients.

ALA dehydratase deficiency is a rare syndrome with autosomal recessive transmission in which the enzyme activity is less than 3%. The enzyme activity is 50% of normal in carriers, who are asymptomatic. Affected patients have severe, recurrent neurologic attacks that may be life-threatening. They excrete large amounts of ALA in their urine. Liver transplantation was reported to result in complete resolution of symptoms in one patient with ALA dehydratase deficiency.[97]

The three remaining acute porphyrias—*acute intermittent porphyria* (AIP), *hereditary coproporphyria* (HCP), and *variegate coproporphyria* (VP)—result from partial deficiency of the enzymes PBG deaminase, coproporphyrinogen oxidase, and protoporphyrinogen oxidase, respectively. All three disorders are inherited in an autosomal dominant fashion with variable expression. AIP is the most common of the three conditions, occurring in 5 to 10 per 100,000 people, and manifests primarily as derangements in the autonomic nervous system or as a psychiatric disorder.[94] VP is more common in South Africa than elsewhere. Although HCP and VP give rise to neurologic symptoms similar to those of AIP, cutaneous lesions also occur in HCP and VP and predominate in VP.[95]

Cutaneous Porphyrias

The cutaneous porphyrias differ from the acute porphyrias in that affected patients exhibit little or no neurologic symptoms. In these illnesses, excess porphyrins or porphyrinogens are deposited in the upper dermal capillary walls, where these photoreactive compounds cause tissue damage that manifests as cutaneous vesicles and bullae in areas exposed to light or excessive mechanical manipulation. Scarring, infection, pigment changes, and hypertrichosis can follow and even lead to severe mutilation.[98]

Porphyria cutanea tarda (PCT), the most common of the porphyrias, typically involves a 50% reduction in activity of the enzyme uroporphyrinogen decarboxylase. Patients usually present after 20 years of age. Two types of PCT are recognized. Type I PCT affects 80% of patients and is a sporadic (acquired) form with enzyme deficiency restricted to the liver. Type II, which affects the other 20% of patients, is familial, being inherited in an autosomal dominant fashion with incomplete penetrance, and involves enzyme deficiency in all tissues.[99] Symptoms develop in less than 10% of patients with type II PCT. Type I PCT is associated strongly with high alcohol intake, estrogen therapy, and systemic illnesses, including systemic lupus erythematosus, diabetes mellitus, chronic renal failure, and the acquired immunodeficiency syndrome. For unclear reasons, concomitant hepatitis C infection is strongly associated with expression of PCT.[100,101] The frequency of mutations of the *HFE* gene, which causes hereditary hemochromatosis, is increased in patients with PCT types I and II, and these mutations are thus susceptibility factors for clinical expression of the PCT phenotype.[100,102,103] This association is consistent with pathologic findings in liver biopsy specimens from patients with PCT, of whom 80% have siderosis, 15% have cirrhosis, and most have evidence of iron overload.[104] Patients usually do not show signs of overt clinical liver disease, apart from elevated serum aminotransferase levels.

Hepatoerythropoietic porphyria (HEP) is a rare form of porphyria with a pathogenesis similar to that of PCT. HEP results from homozygous uroporphyrinogen decarboxylase deficiency, yielding less than 10% of normal enzyme activity. The cutaneous lesions, which resemble those of PCT, are typically severe and mutilating. The disease usually manifests in the first year of life, and as the patient ages, the dermatologic manifestations may subside, but liver disease, a nonspecific hepatitis, worsens. Mutation analysis of the uroporphyrinogen decarboxylase gene has revealed numerous mutations that are usually unique to an individual family; no clear genotype:phenotype correlations have been observed.[99]

Congenital erythropoietic porphyria (CEP) is a rare form of porphyria with autosomal recessive transmission that is caused by deficiency of uroporphyrinogen III cosynthase, which mainly affects erythropoietic tissue. Affected patients typically present in the first year of life with blisters and disfiguring skin lesions in exposed areas. Infants may present with pink urine and photosensitivity. As patients age, erythrodontia, a pathognomonic red or brownish discoloration of the teeth, is commonly seen. CEP can be distinguished clinically from HEP by the presence in some cases of a Coombs'-negative hemolytic anemia, which can be quite severe. Splenomegaly is common.

Erythropoietic protoporphyria (EPP) is caused by partial deficiency of the enzyme ferrochelatase (FECH), the final step in the heme synthetic pathway. The second most common type of porphyria, EPP is inherited in an autosomal dominant manner with variable penetrance. Patients with EPP and asymptomatic carriers exhibit an FECH enzyme activity of 30% to 40% and 50%, respectively, even though both groups inherit a defective FECH allele. The mechanism for the variable clinical expression is explained by co-inheritance of a "low-expressing" normal FECH allele in symptomatic patients with EPP and a normal FECH allele in asymptomatic patients.[105,106]

Although the bone marrow is the predominant source of excess protoporphyrin, with a variable contribution from the liver and other tissues, the skin is the primary site of deposition of this phototoxic compound. Therefore, the principal clinical manifestation is exquisite photosensitivity, which may present during infancy and can lead to a wide spectrum of symptoms (e.g., itching, burning, or pain) and to scars and lichenification of the skin. Vesicles are rare. Patients with EPP may show a mild hypochromic, microcytic anemia.

Clinical liver disease, which develops in 5% to 10% of patients with EPP, results from progressive hepatic accumulation of protoporphyrin.[107] Liver disease typically occurs after age 30 but has been described in children. The liver appears black and nodular. Of 57 patients with EPP followed up for more than 20 years in one study, 50% had normal serum aminotransferase levels and liver histologic findings. Of the remaining patients, cirrhosis occurred in 7 and liver failure developed in 2.[108] Liver disease is not believed to be secondary to alcohol consumption, viral infections, or external toxins, although these insults can worsen liver function.[109] Genetic heterogeneity in the FECH gene has been noted in multiple studies, including among patients who need liver transplantation.[110]

Diagnosis

The approach to the diagnosis of the porphyrias is shown in Table 73–3.

Clinical features alone are usually not specific enough to confirm a diagnosis or distinguish among the various forms of porphyrias, and biochemical test results must be interpreted correctly for accurate diagnosis and management. The diagnosis of porphyria should be considered in patients with recurrent bouts of severe abdominal pain, dark urine, constipation, and neuropsychiatric disturbances or in patients with typical dermatologic findings. To differentiate among the different porphyrias, urine and stool samples should be obtained for porphyrin studies and a urine specimen collected for quantitative ALA and PBG determinations.

In AIP, excretion of PGB and ALA (PGB more than ALA) in dark urine is common during porphyric attacks, but the levels may be normal during asymptomatic periods and in prepubertal patients.[111] Patients with HCP and VP excrete high levels of ALA and PBG in the urine; in contrast to those with AIP, these patients excrete more ALA than PGB. Fecal coproporphyrins are increased in both HCP and VP, whereas only in VP is the amount of fecal protoporphyrin also increased.

Important advances have been made in the identification of a large number of gene mutations in several of the acute porphyrias, including AIP, VP, and HCP. However, given the high degree of genetic heterogeneity, the lack of clear genotype:phenotype correlations, and the failure to find mutations in 5% to 10% of families with current techniques, genetic testing is not recommended as a general screening tool. If a mutation that causes porphyria has been identified in a particular subject, however, screening of presymptomatic family members has sensitivity and specificity rates of nearly 100% for that family and may be helpful, together with appropriate genetic counseling.

Hepatic Involvement

Hepatic involvement in porphyria is variable; in general, patients with acute porphyria may have elevations of serum aminotransferase and bile acid levels, with further increases during acute episodes. Liver biopsy specimens may show steatosis and iron deposition. Although these changes are minor, patients with acute porphyria are at increased risk for development of hepatocellular carcinoma.[112]

PCT and HEP are more commonly associated with hepatic complications, including liver enlargement with fatty infiltration, inflammation, and granulomatous changes. Siderosis and fibrosis may lead to cirrhosis and liver failure. The risk of hepatocellular carcinoma is increased only slightly in patients with these disorders. The patterns of liver injury in CEP are similar to those in PCT and HEP.[93]

Treatment

The overall survival of patients with acute porphyria is good.[96] Treatment is based on avoidance of drugs and other precipitating factors. Generous fluid and glucose administration is recommended during acute attacks and can elicit the "glucose effect" that diminishes ALA synthase activity. Intravenous administration of hematin, a congener of heme, has been shown to decrease the drive for heme synthesis and its excessive by-products. Hematin can also have a dramatic effect on neurologic symptoms, especially if given early in an attack.[113] Women in whom symptoms are affected by the phases of their menstrual cycle can show improvement while taking oral contraceptives. Liver transplantation has been attempted for several of the porphyrias, with mixed results.[97,114]

Because of the wavelengths of light absorbed by the porphyrins, patients affected by porphyria are at risk from exposure to sunlight as well as to household and fluorescent lights. Patients must use special sunscreen lotions that block rays in the 400- to 410-nm range. Skin trauma should be minimized as much as possible; early treatment of skin infections can decrease scarring. Special screens may be especially useful for protection against indoor lighting. Some patients have incurred severe or lethal internal burns during surgery, an especially noteworthy observation for patients who undergo liver transplantation, and appropriate precautions must be taken.[98]

Treatment of PCT initially consists of removal of any offending agent. Historically, treatment has included phlebotomy to decrease iron overload and hepatic siderosis. This approach may provide relief of cutaneous symptoms in 4 to 6 months. Chloroquine complexes with uroporphyrin and facilitates its excretion, but caution must be used during chloroquine therapy because the drug is potentially hepatotoxic.[98] Chloroquine therapy is ineffective in patients with PCT who are homozygous for mutations in the hemochromatosis *HFE* gene; for them, phlebotomy should be first-line therapy.[115] Treatment strategies for HEP are similar to, but have not been as successful as, those for PCT.

Blood transfusions and administration of hematin, charcoal, and cholestyramine have all led to clinical improvement in patients with EPP, but long-term resolution has not been demonstrated. Liver transplantation has been accomplished in patients with ESLD, with mixed results; the erythropoietic defect persists.[116,117] Therefore, liver transplantation must be considered symptomatic therapy, except in patients with fulminant hepatic failure, given the high risk of recurrent disease in the graft and the added risk of intraoperative photodynamic injury to internal organs.[116,118] Combined bone marrow and liver transplantation may be an option in the future.

Splenectomy, which lengthens the lifespan of circulating red blood cells and decreases the erythropoietic drive, has been shown to be effective in many patients with CEP. Frequent blood transfusions or hematin infusions inhibit the stimulus for heme production, thereby diminishing or eliminating the cutaneous manifestations of the disease.[119] Bone marrow transplantation in severely affected patients has proved curative.[114,119]

TYROSINEMIA

Four known human diseases are caused by enzymatic deficiencies in the catabolic pathway for the amino acid tyrosine: alkaptonuria and hereditary tyrosinemia types I, II, and III. Although all of the enzymes involved in this pathway are found in the liver, only hereditary tyrosinemia type I (HT1) leads to progressive liver dysfunction. Formerly known as *hepatorenal tyrosinemia*, HT1 also affects other organ systems, in particular the kidneys and peripheral nerves. Advances in our understanding of the pathophysiology of the disease process and new treatment options, such as an inhibitor of an early step in the degradation pathway, have improved the clinical course dramatically for affected persons.

A disease with autosomal recessive transmission, HT1 has a worldwide incidence rate of about 1 in 100,000. The incidence rate is much greater in northern Europe (1 per

8000) and the Saguenay-Lac-St. Jean region of Quebec, Canada (1 per 1846), where a founder effect has been documented.[120]

Pathophysiology

The pathway for tyrosine metabolism is shown in Figure 73–4. The enzymatic defect in patients with tyrosinemia has been identified in fumarylacetate hydrolase (FAH), the final step in the degradation process; the gene for FAH has been located on chromosome 15. FAH deficiency leads to accumulation of the upstream metabolites fumarylacetoacetate (FAA) and maleylacetoacetate, which are then converted to the toxic intermediates succinylaceteoacetone (SAA) and succinylacetone (SA). FAA has been shown to deplete blood and liver of glutathione,[121] the consequence of which may be augmentation of the mutagenic potential of FAA.[122] SA inhibits the degradation of ALA to PBG, probably via direct modification of amino acids in enzyme active sites, and also inhibits DNA ligase activity in fibroblasts isolated from patients with HT1.[123] Over time, the combined effects of high levels of FAA and SA on the integrity of DNA and cellular repair mechanisms may account for increased chromosomal breakage in fibroblasts isolated from patients with HT1,[124] as well as a higher risk of hepatocellular carcinoma.

Clinical Features and Pathology

Patients with HTI present either acutely with liver failure or with chronic liver disease, with or without hepatocellular carcinoma. In the *acute* form of HTI, patients present with liver disease in the first 6 months of life; symptoms include those associated with hepatic synthetic dysfunction, such as hypoglycemia, ascites, jaundice, and bleeding diathesis, as well as anorexia, vomiting, and irritability.[125] Laboratory studies show elevations of serum aminotransferase, gamma glutamyl transpeptidase, and bilirubin levels, and decreased levels of coagulation factors. Serum tyrosine, methionine, and α-fetoprotein levels are elevated substantially. Analysis of the urine reveals phosphaturia, glucosuria, hyperaminoaciduria, renal acidosis, and elevated excretion of ALA and phenolic acids. The acute form is usually fatal within the first 2 years of life. In a multicenter study, van Spronsen and associates[125] showed that 77% of patients with tyrosinemia presented before the age of 6 months. The 1- and 2-year survival rates were 38% and 29%, respectively, if patients presented between 0 and 2 months, and 74% and 74%, respectively, if they presented between 2 and 6 months. Survival for both time intervals rose to 96% if the first symptoms appeared after age 6 months. The cause of death was usually recurrent bleeding and liver failure (35 of 47 deaths); however, hepatocellular carcinoma (7 of 47) and neurologic crisis (3 of 47) accounted for some deaths.

Patients with the *chronic* form of HTI classically have symptoms that are similar to but milder than those of the acute presentation. These patients usually present after 1 year of age with hepatomegaly, rickets, nephromegaly, hypertension, and growth retardation. They also are likely to have neurologic problems and hepatocellular carcinoma.

The histologic changes differ in the acute and chronic forms of the disease. In the acute form, the liver may appear enlarged with a pale nodular pattern or may be shrunken, firm, and brown. There may be micronodular cirrhosis, fibrotic septa, bile duct proliferation and plugging, steatosis, pseudoacinar and nodular formations, and giant cell transformation. Varying amounts of FAH enzyme activity have been found in liver tissue from patients with HTI as a result of spontaneous reversion of FAH gene mutations. Patients with the chronic form of the disease have a higher level of reversion and a lower frequency of liver dysplasia.[126] In an analysis of mutations in the FAH gene in members of 13 unrelated families with HT1, no mutation type predominated in the affected families, and no correlation between genotype and phenotype was observed.[127]

In the chronic form of tyrosinemia, the liver appears enlarged, coarse, and nodular. In liver biopsy specimens, micronodular and macronodular cirrhosis may be present, as may steatosis, fibrotic septa, and a mild lymphoplasmacytic infiltrate. Cholestasis is less pronounced than in the acute form of HT1. Large- or small-cell dysplasia may be present, reflecting premalignant changes. Because of the nodular changes, identification of progression to hepatocellular carcinoma can be difficult. Because the serum α-fetoprotein value is elevated before hepatocellular carcinoma develops, measurement of α-fetoprotein is not helpful in the diagnosis of hepatocellular carcinoma in this setting. It has been proposed that visualization of both low- and high-attenuation hepatic nodules on computed tomography (CT) is highly suggestive of hepatocellular carcinoma.[128]

Renal involvement is nearly universal in patients with tyrosinemia. Findings include a decreased glomerular filtration rate, proximal renal tubular dysfunction, nephromegaly, phosphaturia (which is responsible for the development of rickets), glucosuria, and aminoaciduria. The toxic metabolites, SA and SAA, are

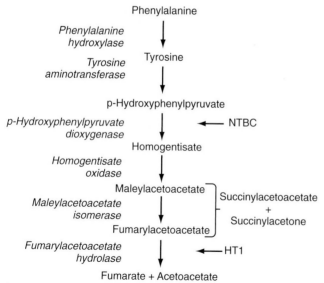

Figure 73–4 Pathway of tyrosine metabolism. The location of the enzymatic defect in hereditary tyrosinemia type 1 (HT1) and the site of action of 2-(2-nitro-4-trifluoro-methylbenzoyl)-1, 3-cyclohexanedione (NTBC) are shown. Enzymes are shown in *italics*.

thought to have a direct effect on kidney function. Some patients progress to renal failure and need renal transplantation.[129,130]

The neurologic manifestations may be the most concerning feature in older patients with tyrosinemia. More than 40% of patients experience porphyria-like symptoms.[131] In a study of 20 children with HTI and 104 neurologic crises, the most common symptoms were pain (96%), hypertonia (76%), vomiting and ileus (69%), weakness (29%), and diarrhea (12%). Eight of the 104 patients required mechanical ventilation. The neurologic crises have been considered to be frequent causes of death,[125] but the onset of a neurologic crisis may not be associated with worsening liver disease. Blockage of the degradation of ALA by SA is thought to be responsible for the neurotoxicity.

Diagnosis

The diagnosis of tyrosinemia should be suspected in any child with neonatal liver disease or a bleeding diathesis or in any child older than 1 year with undiagnosed liver disease or rickets. The diagnosis is suggested by increased tyrosine, methionine, phenylalanine, and α-fetoprotein levels. Elevations of serum and urine SA and urine ALA are regarded as pathognomonic for tyrosinemia. The diagnosis can be confirmed with an assay for FAH in lymphocytes, erythrocytes, or liver tissue.

Treatment

Historically, the treatment of tyrosinemia has been dietary management, with restriction of tyrosine and phenylalanine. Dietary restriction has been shown to reverse renal damage and improve metabolic bone disease; although the liver disease progresses, an adequate intake of these amino acids is needed to ensure normal growth and development. Few studies of the long-term outcome in tyrosinemia treated with strict dietary management alone are available.

Liver transplantation has become a mainstay of therapy for patients with tyrosinemia. The transplant corrects the phenotype and normalizes FAH activity and liver function. Additionally, the biochemical profiles normalize and kidney disease abates, with rapid improvement in glomerular filtration rate, tubular acidosis, and hypercalcemia in most patients. Abnormal renal size and architecture persist after liver transplantation,[132] and many patients continue to excrete SA despite normal serum values.[130]

In 1992, Lindstedt and associates[133] published data on the treatment of tyrosinemia with the herbicide 2-(2-nitro-4-trifluoro-methylbenzoyl)-1,3-cyclohexanedione (NTBC). Later, Holme and Lindstedt[134] published the results of a large long-term study of 220 patients with HT1 who were treated with this agent for up to 7 years. NTBC is a potent inhibitor of 4-hydroxyphenylpyruvate dioxygenase, one of the initial steps in tyrosine metabolism. Blocking the degradation of tyrosine to its downstream toxic metabolites (i.e., FAA, SA, and SAA) was postulated to lead to improved hepatic function. Preliminary results were encouraging, and treated patients exhibited increased liver synthetic function, as reflected by a shortening of the prothrombin time, decreased serum aminotransferase levels, and a reduction in liver parenchymal heterogeneity and nodules on CT. In addition, α-fetoprotein and ALA levels diminished and renal tubular dysfunction reversed.[133] Long-term results showed continued improvement in all parameters noted in the earlier report as well as a lower risk for the development of hepatocellular carcinoma in patients who started therapy and were free of hepatocellular carcinoma before the age of 2 years.[134] No patient withdrew from the study because of adverse side effects of the drug. However, transient thrombocytopenia and neutropenia as well as ocular symptoms suggestive of corneal irritation have been noted rarely.

In another study from Quebec, only 4 of 35 patients treated with NTBC underwent liver transplantation; 1 patient received a transplant because of concern about the heterogeneous texture of the liver shown by ultrasonography (suggestive of cirrhosis) coupled with a persistent moderate elevation in the serum α-fetoprotein value. At resection, this child was found to have a small nodule with hepatocellular dysplasia. The 31 remaining patients were monitored while receiving NTBC therapy for up to 3 years, and none experienced neurologic crises or deterioration of liver disease.[135]

Therefore, therapy with NTBC significantly improves the clinical course of patients treated at an early age. For those in whom therapy is initiated at a later age, NTBC offers a palliative benefit, although the risk of hepatocellular carcinoma is still high in this group of patients. Because the strategy of treating patients with HT1 with NTBC is relatively new, greater experience is required to enable assessment of the relative costs and long-term outcome and recognition of any possible adverse effects of long-term NTBC therapy. Early diagnosis, achieved by inclusion of HT1 in neonatal screening programs, may allow the prompt initiation of effective therapy with NTBC and avoidance of liver transplantation.

UREA CYCLE DEFECTS

Although the syndromes related to the urea cycle defects are not associated with serious liver injury, the basic genetic defect is located within the liver, and the manifestations can mimic those of other metabolic liver diseases. The urea cycle consists of five enzymes that, through several steps, process ammonia derived from amino acid metabolism to urea. Genetic defects in each of these enzymes have been reported, and their overall incidence has been estimated to be 1 in 20,000 to 1 in 30,000.[136]

Pathophysiology

The steps of the urea cycle are illustrated in Figure 73–5. Carbamyl phosphate synthetase (CPS) I forms carbamyl phosphate from ammonium and bicarbonate. This step requires N-acetyl glutamate as a cofactor, which is synthesized from N-acetyl CoA and glutamic acid by N-acetyl glutamate synthetase. Ornithine transcarbamylase (OTC) combines carbamyl phosphate with ornithine to form citrulline. A second nitrogen enters the cycle as aspartate,

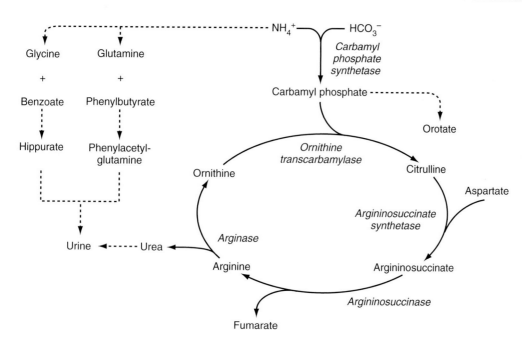

Figure 73–5 The urea cycle. Alternative pathways that are used therapeutically for waste nitrogen disposal are also illustrated. Enzymes are shown in *italics*.

which combines with citrulline by the action of argininosuccinate synthetase (AS) to form argininosuccinate. Argininosuccinate is converted to arginine and fumarate by argininosuccinase, or argininosuccinate lyase (AL). Arginase then catalyzes the breakdown of arginine to urea and ornithine in the final step of the pathway. Several amino acid transporters are involved in shuttling metabolites into the urea cycle, such as citrin, an aspartate/glutamate carrier protein that supplies aspartate to the urea cycle.[137]

CPS II, through the pyrimidine synthetic pathway, leads to the formation of orotic acid. Excess carbamyl phosphate can be used by this pathway if there is a block distal to OTC in the metabolic pathway. Excess nitrogen in the form of amino acids can be shunted to alternative pathways of waste-nitrogen excretion by the medicinal use of sodium benzoate and sodium phenylacetate, leading to the generation of hippurate and phenylacetylglutamine, respectively.

Enzymatic defects have been identified in all five steps involved in the urea cycle. Deficiency of four of these enzymes is transmitted through autosomal recessive inheritance, whereas OTC deficiency is transmitted as an X-linked trait. More than 140 different mutations in the OTC gene give rise to OTC deficiency, the most common urea cycle defect.[138] Numerous defects in the other enzymes or amino acid transporters of the cycle (e.g., *N*-acetylglutamate synthetase or citrin) have been characterized as well.[139,140]

A urea cycle defect has two main biochemical consequences: Arginine becomes an essential amino acid (except in arginase deficiency), and nitrogen accumulates in a variety of molecules, some of which can have deleterious toxic effects.[136]

Clinical Features

The spectra of clinical presentations in patients with any of the urea cycle defects are virtually identical; these dis-

orders usually manifest as acute life-threatening events in the neonatal period. Late-onset adult presentations also have been described. Affected infants appear normal for the first 24 to 72 hours, until they are exposed to their first feeding, which provides the initial protein load that fosters ammonia production. Symptoms include irritability, poor feeding, vomiting, lethargy, hypotonia, seizures, coma, and hyperventilation, all secondary to hyperammonemia.[136] Initially, neonates are often mistakenly thought to have sepsis, despite the absence of perinatal risk factors, and diagnostic laboratory testing is delayed.[141] Plasma ammonia levels should be obtained whenever an evaluation for sepsis is initiated in a neonate; levels may exceed 2000 mmol/L (3400 mg/dL), normal levels being 50 mmol/L (85 mg/dL) or less. Blood gas analysis shows respiratory alkalosis secondary to the hyperventilation caused by the effects of ammonia on the central nervous system. Blood urea nitrogen levels are typically low but can be elevated during times of dehydration or hypoperfusion. Serum levels of liver enzymes are usually normal or minimally elevated. Severe hepatomegaly can occur in early-onset forms of AL deficiency.[136]

As stated earlier, more than 60% of patients with urea cycle defects present in the neonatal period; the rest are diagnosed at variable times from infancy to adulthood. Male patients with OTC deficiency and a varied phenotypic presentation have been diagnosed as late as 40 years of age.[142] As many as 10% of female carriers of OTC deficiency can have symptoms, which may be severe and fatal, although most female carriers have no symptoms or report only nausea after high-protein meals.[143] Late-onset CPS deficiency has also been described,[144] and the adult form of AS deficiency is relatively common in Japan.[145]

Symptoms and signs of late-onset urea cycle defects, especially OTC and CPS deficiencies, include episodic irritability, lethargy, or vomiting; self-induced avoidance of protein such as milk, eggs, and meats; and short stature or growth delays. Neurologic symptoms, which can also be episodic, include ataxia, developmental delays, behavioral abnormalities, combativeness, biting, confusion, hallucinations, headaches, dizziness, visual impairment, diplopia, anorexia, and seizures. Acute hyperammonemic episodes can resemble Reye's syndrome (see Chapter 83).[136] Such episodes can be precipitated by high-protein meals, viral or bacterial infections, medications, trauma, or surgery. Infants may present after being weaned from breast milk to infant formulas, which have higher protein content. Patients with OTC and CPS deficiencies have been reported to present in the postpartum period with acute decompensation and death.[146,147]

Citrin deficiency is associated with both *adult-onset type 2 citrullinemia* and *neonatal intrahepatic cholestasis resulting from citrin deficiency* (NICCD), a syndrome that primarily affects East Asian newborns.[140,148] NICCD is associated with hyperaminoacidemia (e.g., elevated citrulline, methionine, tyrosine levels) and cholestasis.[140,149] Hypergalactosemia also may be observed. In most patients with NICCD all biochemical abnormalities resolve spontaneously or with minimal dietary restrictions (e.g., the use of lactose-free formulas); however, several affected infants have required liver transplantation before age 1 year.[148] Therefore, jaundiced infants with multiple abnormal newborn metabolic screen results (e.g., elevation of blood phenylalanine, methionine, or galactose levels) must be observed closely because of the risk for development of ESLD due to NICCD.[148-150]

Diagnosis

For prompt diagnosis of errors of the urea cycle, a high index of suspicion is required. Symptoms can mimic those of other acute neonatal problems, such as infections and pulmonary or cardiac disease. Later presentations can mimic other behavioral, psychiatric, or developmental disorders. The first clue may be an elevated serum ammonia value with normal serum aminotransferase levels and without metabolic acidosis. Therefore, if a urea cycle defect is considered, the following laboratory measurements should be obtained: serum ammonia, arterial blood gases, urine organic acids, serum amino acids, and urinary orotic acid; Table 73–4 reviews the expected laboratory results.

Urinary organic acid profiles are typically normal in defects of the urea cycle. The plasma amino acid profiles are distinctive, with abnormal levels of arginine, ornithine, and citrulline. Citrulline levels are barely detectable in OTC or CPS deficiencies but markedly raised in AS and AL deficiencies. AS deficiencies can be distin-

guished from AL deficiencies by the finding of argininosuccinic acid in the plasma and urine of patients with AL deficiency. OTC deficiency is differentiated from CPS deficiency by the excessive urinary excretion of orotic acid in OTC deficiency.[136] Direct enzyme analysis can be performed and can be useful in patients who have a partial deficiency or who present in adulthood. Prenatal enzyme and genetic linkage analysis can be carried out in families of known carriers.[149] Early neonatal diagnosis leads to improved survival.[149] An allopurinol loading test, which leads to excretion of orotic acid in amounts that are 10- to 20-fold greater than normal in heterozygote female carriers of OTC deficiency, is nonspecific, and its results must be interpreted with caution; the result can be positive in some patients with mitochondrial disease or defects in pyrimidine metabolism.[151] Liver histology typically shows minimal fatty infiltration.

Treatment

All external protein intake should be discontinued in infants with urea cycle defects presenting acutely. Serum ammonia levels should be restored to normal. The use of oral lactulose to lower the nitrogen load has not been studied in this patient population. Given the extremely high ammonia levels often encountered, continuous arteriovenous hemodialysis or hemofiltration is often required, but exchange transfusions and peritoneal dialysis are ineffective. Alternative pathways for waste nitrogen disposal should be employed, specifically intravenous administration of sodium benzoate and sodium phenylacetate; however, sodium benzoate should be used with caution in patients with cirrhotic liver disease, because a paradoxical rise in blood ammonia levels has been observed.[152] Arginine, carnitine, and long-chain fatty acids are usually at low levels in these patients and should be supplemented.[153] Once the patient stabilizes, low levels of dietary protein, 0.5 to 1.0 gm/kg, may be introduced, with progressive increases as tolerated to provide sufficient protein for growth and tissue repair while minimizing urea production. Long-term therapy and protein restriction are then tailored to the patient; patients with a severe disorder may need essential amino acids to supplement their protein intake. Oral phenylbutyrate can be substituted for phenylacetate to improve palatability.

The outcome for patients who present with hyperammonemic coma and delayed diagnosis is poor. The level of ammonia at the time of the first hyperammonemic episode is a rough guide to the eventual neurodevelopmental outcome.[154] The sooner the hyperammonemia is treated and the correct diagnosis is made, the better the

Table 73–4   Laboratory Values in Urea Cycle Defects

Enzyme Deficiency	Plasma Ammonia	Citrulline (serum)	Argininosuccinate (urine or serum)	Orotic acid (urine)	Arginine/ornithine (serum)
Carbamyl phosphate synthase	↑-↑↑↑	↓	↓	↓	↓
Ornithine transcarbamylase	↑-↑↑↑	↓	↓	↑↑	↓
Argininosuccinate synthase	↑-↑↑↑	↑↑↑	↓	Normal–↑	↓
Argininosuccinase	↑-↑↑↑	↑↑↑	↑↑↑	Normal–↑	↓
Arginase	↑	↑↑	↑↑	Normal–↑	↑↑

long-term survival, although for patients who survive the neonatal period, the median survival without liver transplantation is less than 4 years and is associated with severe developmental delay and neurologic morbidity.[141] With optimal dietary and medical management, patients may still have repeated hyperammonemic crises, often during intercurrent viral infections. Symptomatic OTC heterozygote females also benefit from therapy, which leads to fewer hyperammonemic episodes and a reduced risk of further cognitive decline.[155]

Patients with a urea cycle defect and a deterioration or lack of improvement despite therapy have undergone liver transplantation successfully, with normalization of enzyme activity and ammonia levels and the ability to tolerate a normal diet.[155,156] Liver transplantation, if considered, should be done before neurologic damage is permanent. In a retrospective study of 16 pediatric patients who received liver transplants for urea cycle defects, the neurologic status failed to improve after transplantation. The metabolic condition of the patients normalized completely, however, and in no patient did neurologic status worsen after transplantation. For patients without severe neurologic compromise before transplantation, this therapeutic approach is obviously worthwhile. In addition, the annual cost of care for this group of patients is likely to be reduced dramatically after liver transplantation.[156]

The importance of identifying the deleterious mutation in patients with a urea cycle defect will likely become increasingly important not only as a means of allowing carrier testing and prenatal diagnosis, but also as an aid in treatment decisions. For example, patients with the most severe mutations of OTC deficiency (e.g., abolished enzyme activity) may benefit preferentially from immediate liver transplantation to prevent severe mental retardation or death, whereas those with milder mutations may be better managed medically with dietary restrictions and ammonia scavengers to facilitate growth before possible liver transplantation.[138]

Murine models of urea cycle defects have been developed, and an adenovirally mediated correction of a murine model of OTC deficiency has been achieved.[138] However, successful protocols have not yet been developed for humans. Indeed, gene therapy initiatives are on hold because of concerns that toxicity was unexpectedly excessive in one of the initial trials of the adenovirally mediated correction of partial OTC deficiency in humans.[138]

ARGINASE DEFICIENCY

At least two forms of arginase activity occur in humans: Arginase I (AI) predominates in the liver and red blood cells, and arginase II (AII) is found predominantly in kidney and prostate. Arginase deficiency involving AI is the least common of the urea cycle defects. Hyperammonemia is atypical in affected persons, but hyperammonemic coma and death have been reported.[157] The clinical disorder is distinct from the other urea cycle defects. It is characterized by indolent deterioration of the cerebral cortex and pyramidal tracts, leading to progressive dementia and psychomotor retardation, spastic diplegia progressing to quadriplegia, seizures, and growth failure. The syndrome is often confused with cerebral palsy.

Laboratory studies may reveal elevated arginine values, mild hyperammonemia, and a mild increase in urine orotic acid excretion. Varying amounts of urea are still produced in these patients secondary to the compensatory elevated expression of AII in the kidneys, thereby ameliorating the clinical disorder.[158] The diagnosis is confirmed by enzymatic analysis, which can be performed prenatally on cord blood samples. Treatment consists of protein restriction and, when needed, medical therapy with sodium phenylbutyrate.[136]

BILE ACID SYNTHESIS AND TRANSPORT DEFECTS

The pathways for bile acid synthesis and transport within the hepatobiliary system are complex, involving several enzymes and transport processes located in multiple subcellular fractions of the hepatocyte (see Chapter 61). With technologic advances in molecular biology and mass spectrometry, several different inborn errors in bile acid synthesis and transport have been identified as causes of clinical disease. The definition and classification of these disorders have improved, particularly in the clinically heterogeneous subset of cases comprising *progressive familial intrahepatic cholestasis* (PFIC) syndromes. For some of these disorders, this progress has led to dramatic advances in often life-saving therapy.[159]

The diagnosis of PFIC is imprecise; the accepted criteria are (1) the presence of chronic, unremitting intrahepatic cholestasis, (2) exclusion of identifiable metabolic or anatomic disorders, and (3) characteristic clinical, biochemical, and histologic features.[160,161] Other symptoms and signs are severe pruritus, hepatomegaly, wheezing and cough, short stature, delayed sexual development, fat-soluble vitamin deficiency, and cholelithiasis.[161] Affected patients exhibit severe and progressive intrahepatic cholestasis, usually manifesting within the first few months of life and often proceeding to cirrhosis and ESLD by the second decade of life. Patients with PFIC syndromes have been found to have defects in bile acid synthetic and transport processes.

Some patients believed previously to have idiopathic neonatal hepatitis or an undiagnosed familial hepatitis syndrome may now be diagnosed accurately as having a form of PFIC.[159] It has been estimated that 1% to 2.5% of patients with idiopathic cholestasis may have defects in bile acid metabolism and transport.[162] Table 73–5 lists the known errors of primary and secondary bile acid synthesis and transport.

BILE ACID SYNTHESIS DEFECTS

Bile acid synthetic pathways are discussed in detail in Chapter 61. Only the most common enzyme deficiencies are described here; all can be diagnosed through mass spectrometry of the urine or serum. General principles of therapy rely on the hypothesis that inborn errors of bile acid biosynthesis lead to underproduction of normal

Table 73–5   Inborn Errors of Bile Acid Synthesis and Transport*

Defective bile acid synthesis	
Primary defects	Cerebrotendinous xanthomatosis (C_{27}-steroid-27-hydroxylase deficiency)
	3β-hydroxy-ΔC_{27}-steroid dehydrogenase/isomerase (*HSD3B7*) deficiency
	Δ^4-3-oxosteroid 5β-reductase (*AKR1D1*) deficiency
	C_{24}-steroid-7α-hydroxylase (*CYP7B1*) deficiency
Secondary defects (due to organelle damage)	Peroxisomal biogenesis disorders (PBDs):
	Zellweger's syndrome
	Neonatal adrenoleukodystrophy
	Infantile Refsum's disease
	Zellweger-like syndrome
	Rhizomelic chondrodysplasia punctata
	Other
	Hyperpipecolic acidemia
	Leber's congenital amaurosis
	Disorders with loss of single peroxisomal function:
	X-linked adrenoleukodystrophy
	Thiolase deficiency (pseudo–Zellweger's syndrome)
	Bifunctional protein deficiency
	Acyl-CoA oxidase deficiency
	Hyperoxaluria type I
	Acatalasemia
	Adult Refsum's disease
	Generalized hepatic synthetic dysfunction:
	Fulminant hepatic failure (multiple causes)
	Tyrosinemia
	Neonatal iron storage disease
Defective bile acid or phospholipid transport	FIC1 (*FIC1*) deficiency: progressive familial intrahepatic cholestasis (PFIC) type 1:
	Byler's disease
	Benign recurrent intrahepatic cholestasis (BRIC) syndrome
	Greenland familial cholestasis
	BSEP (*ABCB11*) deficiency: PFIC type 2
	MDR3 (*ABCB4*) deficiency: PFIC type 3
Other	North American Indian childhood cirrhosis (*Cirhin*)
	Cholestasis-lymphedema syndrome (Aagenaes syndrome)
	Alagille's (*Jagged*) syndrome

*Corresponding genes are shown in *italics*.

Modified from Balistreri WF: Inborn errors of bile acid biosynthesis: Clinical and therapeutic aspects. In Hofmann AF, et al (eds): Bile Acids in Gastroenterology. London, Kluwer Academic Publishers, 1995, p 333; and Jonas MM, Perez-Atayde AR: Liver disease in infancy and childhood. In Schiff ER, Sorrell MF, Maddrey WC, et al (eds): Schiff's Diseases of the Liver, 9th ed. Philadelphia, Lippincott Williams & Wilkins, 2003, p 1459.

trophic and choleretic primary bile acids and overproduction of hepatotoxic primitive bile acid metabolites.[159] Bile acids found in patients with inborn errors also act as cholestatic agents by *inhibiting* canalicular ATP-dependent bile acid transport (the rate-limiting step in the overall process of bile acid transport across the canalicular membrane).[163]

Cerebrotendinous xanthomatosis (CTX), C_{27}-steroid-27-hydroxylase deficiency, is characterized by bilateral juvenile cataracts and chronic diarrhea, followed by progressive neurologic dysfunction, hypercholesterolemia, atherosclerosis, and deposition of cholesterol and cholestanol in tissues.[159,162] CTX should be treated with chenodeoxycholic acid. A series of five children with CTX showed dramatic improvement in biochemical and electroencephalographic abnormalities and resolution of diarrhea with this therapy. In addition, no further delay in motor development was noted, and three patients showed an improved intelligence quotient.[164]

Patients with *3β-hydroxy-C_{27}-steroid dehydrogenase/ isomerase* (3β-HSD) deficiency may present with pruritus,

jaundice, hepatomegaly, steatorrhea and fat-soluble vitamin deficiencies. Deficiency of Δ^4-3-oxosteroid 5β-reductase also leads to neonatal cholestasis but rapidly progresses to synthetic dysfunction and liver failure. Both conditions have been treated with a primary bile acid (i.e., cholic acid) and ursodeoxycholic acid supplementation.[159,165] Cholic acid bypasses the enzymatic block and provides negative feedback to earlier steps in the synthetic pathways, and ursodeoxycholic acid displaces toxic bile acid metabolites and serves as a hepatobiliary cytoprotectant. Other known disorders result from 25-hydroxylase, C_{24}-steroid-7α-hydroxylase, and amidation deficiencies.[159]

Many peroxisomopathies have been described; these disorders are associated with multiple abnormalities and up to 50 wide-ranging biochemical abnormalities.[166] They are diagnosed through a combination of specialized tests, such as that for very-long-chain fatty acids (VLCFAs) and ultrastructural analysis of tissue biopsy specimens. Peroxisomes are responsible for beta-oxidation in the final steps of bile acid synthesis to yield the primary bile acids cholic acid and chenodeoxycholic acid. These disorders can be divided into two groups: disorders of peroxisome assembly, which cause multiple abnormalities, and disorders of single proteins, which result in limited dysfunction (see Table 73–5).[166-168] The first group includes *peroxisome biogenesis disorders* (PBDs), which are grouped because they share similar clinical and biochemical features, and *rhizomelic chondrodysplasia punctata* (RCDP), which is characterized by severe rhizomelic shortening of the limbs, severe skeletal abnormalities, cataracts, and facial abnormalities. PBD includes disorders such as *Zellweger's syndrome* (ZS), with the most severe clinical abnormalities, *neonatal adrenoleukodystrophy,* and *infantile Refsum's disease*, with the mildest features.[167]

ZS is a primary disorder of peroxisome biogenesis. The multiple features of ZS include distinctive dysmorphic features (hypertelorism, large anterior fontanelle, deformed earlobes), neonatal hypotonia, impaired hearing, retinopathy, cataracts, seizures, and skeletal changes. Hepatomegaly is common, and the progressive liver disease that develops in patients with ZS is similar to that identified in other errors of bile acid synthesis.[169]

Peroxisome biogenesis involves more than 13 genes and requires the targeting and importation of cytosolic proteins, aided by peroxins (encoded by *PEX* genes), into the peroxisomal membrane and matrix.[166,170] Importation of proteins fated for the peroxisomal matrix requires guidance from one of two peroxisome-targeting signals, PTS1 and PTS2.[166] Patients with PBDs and RCDP display defects in the importation of proteins that use PTS1 and PTS2, respectively. In infantile Refsum's disease, there is a temperature-sensitive block in peroxisome biogenesis, which for four of six patients with the disorder in one series was caused by a temperature-sensitive defect in a protein, PEX1p, that is required for receptor-mediated importation of PTS1-containing proteins.[168] Genotype:phenotype correlations have yet to be established for the transport of peroxisomal membrane proteins, which involves a process separate from that described earlier for matrix proteins.[166]

The most common disorder of peroxisomes, X-linked adrenoleukodystrophy (X-ALD), is included in the second grouping of peroxisomopathies and results from a defect in the peroxisomal adrenoleukodystrophy protein (ALDP), which is a member of the ATP-binding cassette (ABC) superfamily of membrane transporters. Phenylbutyrate induces expression of a protein related to ALDP, thereby leading to correction of VLCFA beta-oxidation and an increase in the number of peroxisomes in fibroblasts isolated from patients with X-ALD and in vivo in the X-ALD transgenic knockout mouse. These findings suggest that phenylbutyrate may play a future role in the therapy of patients with X-ALD.[171]

Historically, the treatment of ZS has been supportive, with most patients not surviving the first year of life. The goals of medical therapy have been to improve nutrition and growth, control central nervous system symptoms, and limit progression of liver disease. Treatment with primary bile acids has been shown to improve biochemical studies and histology, increase growth, and improve neurologic symptoms.[172] In an uncontrolled study, the use of docosahexaenoic acid (DHA) led to improved myelination in patients with peroxisomal disorders; cur-

rently, however, the use of DHA should be limited to controlled clinical trials.[167,170]

BILE ACID TRANSPORT DEFECTS

Intrahepatic cholestasis syndromes caused by defects in canalicular bile acid transport are of great theoretic interest; detailed study of these disorders has enhanced our understanding of hepatic excretory function and bile acid metabolism. The pathogenesis of these diseases has been defined, and the techniques of molecular genetics have been applied to these disorders. Precise terminology of the intrahepatic cholestatic disorders, based on the documented genetic defect, is now possible. These advances will provide clues to the pathophysiology and help establish registries, promote development of new treatments, and allow the institution of valid clinical therapeutic trials.

Byler's disease (or PFIC type 1) was first described in 1965, in an Amish kindred descended from Jacob Byler. Children who have similar clinical features but are unrelated to the Byler family are said to have Byler's syndrome (e.g., PFIC type 2 or type 3), and are genotypically distinct from those with the original Byler's disease. Byler's disease is caused by mutations in a single gene (*FIC1*) located on chromosome 18q21. *FIC1* encodes a P-type adenosine triphosphatase involved in ATP-dependent aminophospholipid transport and is expressed in many organs in addition to the liver and intestine. Defects in *FIC1* also have been found in patients with benign recurrent intrahepatic cholestasis (BRIC type I), which as the name implies gives rise to recurrent episodes of intrahepatic cholestasis beginning in childhood or adulthood that can last days to months and then resolve spontaneously without causing detectable lasting liver damage.[173] Patients with Greenland familial cholestasis have also been reported to have defects in the *FIC1* gene.[174] In all three conditions, serum GGTP and cholesterol levels are normal or mildly elevated, and those of bile acids are elevated in the serum and low in the bile. Serum aminotransferase and bilirubin levels are elevated as well. Impaired bile acid transport in the intestine may account for the striking malabsorption and diarrhea manifested by some patients with PFIC type 1; these intestinal clinical features do not resolve after liver transplantation in such patients.[173] That sweat electrolyte concentrations are frequently abnormal in patients with PFIC type 1 and the *FIC1* gene is expressed widely in epithelium suggest that the FIC1 protein acts globally at sites of secretion and absorption.[173] On electron microscopic evaluation of liver tissue from patients with PFIC type 1, characteristic coarse, granular bile deposits are seen in the canaliculus ("Byler's bile").

A second subset of patients with intrahepatic cholestasis (PFIC type 2) also has high serum bile acid levels but low or low-normal serum GGTP levels. On routine histology of the liver early in the disease, a nonspecific giant cell hepatitis is found, and on electron microscopy, amorphous bile deposits are seen in the canaliculi. The disease-causing gene for PFIC type 2 maps to chromosome 2q24 and encodes an ABC protein that serves as the canalicular bile salt export pump (BSEP).[175] In addition, a genetically distinct form of BRIC (type II) is associated with mutations in *ABCB11* (which encodes BSEP).[176]

Yet another subset, patients with PFIC type 3, have high serum levels of GGTP and bile acids as well as bile ductular proliferation on routine microscopy. The defect in PFIC type 3 has been localized to chromosome 7q21 and is caused by mutations in the *MDR3* gene, also known as the *ABCB4* gene, which encodes a phosphatidylserine translocase located on the canalicular membrane.[177,178] MDR3 deficiency is thought to lead to decreased excretion of cytoprotective biliary phospholipids, leaving an increased pool of cytotoxic biliary bile salts that gives rise to subsequent bile duct damage and proliferation and release of GGTP into the serum. Heterozygous carriers of a mutation in *MDR3* have been found in a group of female patients with familial intrahepatic cholestasis of pregnancy; the mutation likely leads to a genetic predisposition that requires the coexistence of other nongenetic factors for full expression of this disease.[179,180]

Investigations at the molecular genetic level of other chronic intrahepatic cholestatic diseases, such as North American Indian childhood cirrhosis and cholestasis-lymphedema syndrome (Aagenaes syndrome), are at early stages; the disease-causing loci for both conditions are genetically distinct from *FIC1*, BSEP, or *MDR3* mutations.[181,182] A single-point mutation in the *cirhin* gene, which encodes a protein of unknown function, has been identified in patients with North American Indian childhood cirrhosis.[183] Additional series of patients with "PFIC-like" syndromes have been reported but have not been characterized beyond clinical descriptions.[184,185]

Medical treatment of patients with PFIC as a group with phenobarbital, cholestyramine, opioid antagonists, rifampin, and phototherapy has been largely ineffective. Therapy with ursodeoxycholic acid may be effective in reducing pruritus and improving liver biochemical parameters in up to 50% of patients with PFIC, regardless of serum GGTP levels.[186] Surgical approaches such as ileal exclusion and partial external biliary diversion have provided satisfactory symptomatic relief to some patients by decreasing the bile acid pool and pruritus. Long-term marked improvement in pruritus and growth has been reported for 6 pediatric patients treated with biliary diversion.[187] If all else fails, liver transplantation has been shown to normalize bile acid synthesis and growth in selected patients.[188]

CYSTIC FIBROSIS

Cystic fibrosis (CF) is discussed in detail in Chapter 55; here, a brief discussion of the *hepatic complications* seen in this multisystemic disorder is presented. Liver disease can be the presenting symptom of CF in the newborn, and CF-associated liver disease has been seen with meconium ileus syndrome. Although CF has been identified in less than 2% of patients with neonatal cholestasis, the diagnosis should be considered in any infant presenting with neonatal cholestasis.[189]

CF-associated liver disease may become more common as the mean age of survival for patients with CF rises; however, liver involvement is not universal and seems to peak during the adolescent years.[190] Up to 30% of patients may have clinical or symptomatic liver disease after the neonatal period.[191]

Hepatobiliary diseases noted in patients with CF can be grouped into three categories (Table 73–6). The patho-

---

Table 73–6   Spectrum of Hepatobiliary Disease in Patients with Cystic Fibrosis

Lesions specific to cystic fibrosis	Hepatic
	    Focal biliary cirrhosis with inspissation
	    Multilobular biliary cirrhosis with inspissation
	Biliary
	    Microgallbladder
	    Mucous hyperplasia of the gallbladder
	    Mucocele

Lesions secondary to extrahepatic disease	Hepatic lesions associated with cardiopulmonary disease
	    Centrilobular necrosis
	    Cirrhosis
	Pancreatic lesions
	    Pancreatic duct sludge (obstruction)
	    Fibrosis (leading to bile duct compression/stricture)

Lesions that occur with a higher frequency in patients with cystic fibrosis	Hepatic
	    Fatty liver
	    Neonatal cholestasis
	    Drug hepatotoxicity
	    Viral hepatitis
	Biliary
	    Sclerosing cholangitis
	    Biliary sludge
	    Cholelithiasis
	    Cholangiocarcinoma

Modified from Balistreri WF: Liver disease in infancy and childhood. In Schiff ER, Sorrell MF, Maddrey WC (eds): Schiff's Diseases of the Liver, 9th ed. Philadelphia, Lippincott-Raven, 1999, p. 1379.

gnomonic lesion of CF, *focal biliary cirrhosis* (FCC), presumably results from defective function of the cystic fibrosis gene product, which is expressed in bile duct cells. Obstruction of small bile ducts leads to chronic inflammatory changes, bile duct proliferation, and portal fibrosis. At autopsy, FCC has been identified in 25% to 30% of patients more than 1 year of age.[163] Progression to *multilobular biliary cirrhosis* occurs in approximately 10% of patients with CF and leads to symptoms associated with portal hypertension, such as splenomegaly and variceal bleeding.[191] Hepatic steatosis also develops in roughly one half of patients but does not appear to correlate with outcome. Biliary abnormalities range from microgallbladder, which is largely asymptomatic and is found in up to 20% of patients, to cholelithiasis and cholangiocarcinoma.[5]

The variable occurrence and clinical course of liver disease in patients with CF may be related to other genetic factors. For example, elevated concentrations of endogenous ursodeoxycholic acid have been documented in patients with CF without liver disease; this finding suggests that ursodeoxycholic acid may protect against liver injury in these patients.[192]

The diagnosis of liver disease in patients with CF can be difficult because the presenting signs are subtle. Hepatomegaly, which is present in approximately 30% of patients, has been shown to correlate well with the presence of cirrhosis and is often the first finding of liver disease. Liver biochemical test levels may remain relatively normal despite histologic evidence of cirrhosis. Needle biopsy of the liver can be helpful; however, because of the focal distribution of histologic abnormalities, sampling error may occur. Ultrasonography can detect the presence of biliary stones and bile duct or hepatic vein dilatation as well as heterogeneous or nodular liver parenchyma.[191] The latter findings can serve as an early marker of liver disease and a predictor of progressive liver disease.[193]

Treatment of patients with CF with ursodeoxycholic acid improves the biochemical indices of liver injury; however, conclusive evidence that the drug halts the progression to cirrhosis is not yet available.[191,194] Portosystemic shunts can be effective treatment for patients with portal hypertension (see Chapter 87). Liver transplantation is rarely needed for ESLD in patients with CF but has been performed successfully in patients who have portal hypertension and stable pulmonary function.[195]

MITOCHONDRIAL LIVER DISEASES

A growing number of liver diseases has been attributed to defects in mitochondrial function. In addition to defects of mitochondrial enzymes involved in the urea cycle or energy metabolism, several mitochondrial hepatopathies involve respiratory chain/oxidative phosphorylation/electron transport defects or alterations in mitochondrial DNA (mtDNA). The mitochondrial genome is especially vulnerable to oxidative injury, not only because of its spatial relationship to the respiratory chain, but also because of its lack of protective histones and an adequate excision and recombination repair system. Mitochondrial DNA is inherited almost entirely from the maternal

ovum; therefore, primary mitochondrial deficiencies are usually inherited in a dominant fashion. Normal mtDNA and mutant mtDNA are present in varying amounts in a given cell, because of the large number of mitochondria and multiple copies of mtDNA in a mitochondrion. This *heteroplasmy* for mitochondrial DNA mutations often can lead to mixed involvement of organs throughout the body.[196] Heterogeneity of clinical features can lead to a delay or missed diagnosis and can confound therapeutic decision-making, for example, with respect to the merits of liver transplantation.

Neonatal liver failure has been reported in association with *cytochrome c oxidase deficiency*. The key features of this disorder are lactic acidemia and an elevated ratio of lactate to pyruvate. Infants with *Alpers' disease* (progressive neuronal degeneration in childhood with liver disease ascribed to mitochondrial dysfunction) experience vomiting, hypotonia, seizures, and liver failure, often beginning by age 6 months. Frequently, the liver disease is unsuspected clinically and evident late in the course of the disease. Alternatively, in *mtDNA depletion syndrome*, hypoglycemia, acidosis, and liver failure develop early in infancy, and neurologic abnormalities are less prominent. Other multisystemic mitochondrial diseases with liver involvement are *Pearson's marrow-pancreas syndrome* and *chronic diarrhea and intestinal pseudo-obstruction with liver involvement*; these syndromes are still in the early phases of characterization.[196]

The diagnosis of a mitochondrial respiratory chain defect should be considered in a patient with liver disease who has unexplained neuromuscular symptoms, including a seizure disorder, involvement of seemingly unrelated organ systems, and a rapidly progressive course.[196] In about 80% of patients, symptoms appear early in life, before age 2 years.[197]

Liver biopsy specimens typically show macrovesicular and microvesicular steatosis, with increased density and occasional swelling of mitochondria on electron microscopy. Immunohistochemical techniques are being utilized more frequently (e.g., to diagnose cytochrome c oxidase deficiency). Direct measurement of the enzymatic activity of the respiratory chain electron transport protein complexes can be performed on frozen tissue from the organ that expresses the clinical disease, although skin fibroblasts and lymphocytes may also be used. Few academic centers around the world can perform the assays for mitochondrial respiration (polarographic studies) or mtDNA analysis at this time.

There is no effective therapy for respiratory chain disorders that alters the course of disease. Several strategies have been proposed to delay the progression of such disorders, including the use of antioxidants such as vitamin E or ascorbic acid as well as carnitine or succinate supplementation, but the use of these agents is clearly experimental at this time.[196]

REFERENCES

1. Kilpe VE, Krakauer H, Wren RE: An analysis of liver transplant experience from 37 transplant centers as reported to Medicare. Transplantation 56:554, 1993.

2. Arya G, Balistreri WF: Pediatric liver disease in the United States: Epidemiology and impact. J Gastroenterol Hepatol 17:521, 2002.

3. Balistreri WF: Nontransplant options for the treatment of metabolic liver disease: Saving livers while saving lives. Hepatology 19:782, 1994.

4. Teckman J, Perlmutter DH: Conceptual advances in the pathogenesis and treatment of childhood metabolic liver disease. Gastroenterology 108:1263, 1995.

5. Balistreri WF: Liver disease in infancy and childhood. In Schiff ER (ed): Schiff's Diseases of the Liver, 8th ed. Philadelphia, Lippincott-Raven, 1999, p 1357.

6. de Serres FJ: Worldwide racial and ethnic distribution of alpha1-antitrypsin deficiency: Summary of an analysis of published genetic epidemiologic surveys. Chest 122:1818, 2002.

7. Balistreri WF: Transplantation for childhood liver disease: An overview. Liver Transpl Surg 4:S18, 1998.

8. Perlmutter DH: Liver injury in alpha1-antitrypsin deficiency: An aggregated protein induces mitochondrial injury. J Clin Invest 110:1579, 2002.

9. Needham M, Stockley RA: Alpha 1-antitrypsin deficiency. 3: Clinical manifestations and natural history. Thorax 59:441, 2004.

10. Massi G, Chiarelli C: Alpha-1 antitrypsin: Molecular structure and the Pi system. Acta Paediatr Suppl 393:1, 1994.

11. Perlmutter DH: Alpha-1-antitrypsin deficiency. In Schiff ER, Sorrell MF, Maddrey WC (eds): Schiff's Diseases of the Liver, 9th ed. Philadelphia, Lippincott Williams & Wilkins, 2003, p 1207.

12. Wu Y, Whitman I, Molmenti E, et al: A lag in intracellular degradation of mutant alpha 1-antitrypsin correlates with the liver disease phenotype in homozygous PiZZ alpha 1-antitrypsin deficiency. Proc Natl Acad Sci U S A 91:9014, 1994.

13. Teckman JH, Gilmore R, Perlmutter DH: Role of ubiquitin in proteasomal degradation of mutant alpha(1)-antitrypsin Z in the endoplasmic reticulum. Am J Physiol Gastrointest Liver Physiol 278:G39, 2000.

14. Perlmutter DH: The cellular response to aggregated proteins associated with human disease. J Clin Invest 110:1219, 2002.

15. Dycaico MJ, Grant SG, Felts K, et al: Neonatal hepatitis induced by alpha-1 antitrypsin: A transgenic mouse model. Science 242:1409, 1988.

16. Lawless MW, Greene CM, Mulgrew A, et al: Activation of endoplasmic reticulum-specific stress responses associated with the conformational disease Z alpha 1-antitrypsin deficiency. J Immunol 172:5722, 2004.

17. Teckman JH, An JK, Blomenkamp K, et al: Mitochondrial autophagy and injury in the liver in alpha 1-antitrypsin deficiency. Am J Physiol Gastrointest Liver Physiol 286:G851, 2004.

18. Teckman JH, An JK, Loethen S, et al: Fasting in alpha1-antitrypsin deficient liver: Constitutive [correction of consultative] activation of autophagy. Am J Physiol Gastrointest Liver Physiol 283:G1156, 2002.

19. de Serres FJ, Blanco I, Fernandez-Bustillo E: Genetic epidemiology of alpha-1 antitrypsin deficiency in North America and Australia/New Zealand: Australia, Canada, New Zealand and the United States of America. Clin Genet 64:382, 2003.

20. Mahadeva R, Chang WS, Dafforn TR, et al: Heteropolymerization of S, I, and Z alpha-1 antitrypsin and liver cirrhosis. J Clin Invest 103:999, 1999.

21. Graziadei IW, Joseph JJ, Wiesner RH, et al: Increased risk of chronic liver failure in adults with heterozygous alpha1-antitrypsin deficiency. Hepatology 28:1058, 1998.

22. Sveger T: Liver disease in alpha-1 antitrypsin deficiency detected by screening of 200,000 infants. N Engl J Med 294:1316, 1976.

23. Sveger T, Eriksson S: The liver in adolescents with alpha-1 antitrypsin deficiency. Hepatology 22:514, 1995.

24. Mowat AP: Alpha 1-antitrypsin deficiency (PiZZ): Features of liver involvement in childhood. Acta Paediatr Suppl 393:13, 1994.

25. Lee JH, Brantly M: Molecular mechanisms of alpha1-antitrypsin null alleles. Respir Med 94(Suppl C):S7, 2000.

26. Volpert D, Molleston JP, Perlmutter DH: Alpha-1 antitrypsin deficiency-associated liver disease progresses slowly in some children. J Pediatr Gastroenterol Nutr 31:258, 2000.

27. Eriksson S: Alpha-1 antitrypsin deficiency and liver cirrhosis in adults: An analysis of 35 Swedish autopsied cases. Acta Med Scand 221:461, 1987.

28. Elzouki AN, Eriksson S: Risk of hepatobiliary disease in adults with severe alpha-1 antitrypsin deficiency (PiZZ): Is chronic viral hepatitis B or C an additional risk factor for cirrhosis and hepatocellular carcinoma? Eur J Gastroenterol Hepatol 8:989, 1996.

29. Eriksson S, Carlson J, Velez R: Risk of cirrhosis and primary liver cancer in alpha-1 antitrypsin deficiency. N Engl J Med 314:736, 1986.

30. Zhou H, Fischer HP: Liver carcinoma in PiZ alpha-1 antitrypsin deficiency. Am J Surg Pathol 22:742, 1998.

31. Poley JR: Malignant liver disease in alpha-1 antitrypsin deficiency. Acta Paediatr Suppl 393:27, 1994.

32. Deutsch J, Becker H, Aubock L: Histopathological features of liver disease in alpha-1 antitrypsin deficiency. Acta Paediatr Suppl 393:8, 1994.

33. Thelin T, Sveger T, McNeil TF: Primary prevention in a high-risk group: Smoking habits in adolescents with homozygous alpha-1 antitrypsin deficiency (ATD). Acta Paediatr 85:1207, 1996.

34. Juvelekian GS, Stoller JK: Augmentation therapy for alpha(1)-antitrypsin deficiency. Drugs 64:1743, 2004.

35. Wewers MD, Casolaro MA, Sellers SE, et al: Replacement therapy for alpha-1 antitrypsin deficiency associated with emphysema. N Engl J Med 316:1055, 1987.

36. Burrows JA, Willis LK, Perlmutter DH: Chemical chaperones mediate increased secretion of mutant alpha-1 antitrypsin (alpha 1-AT) Z: A potential pharmacological strategy for prevention of liver injury and emphysema in alpha-1 AT deficiency. Proc Natl Acad Sci U S A 97:1796, 2000.

37. Marcus NY, Perlmutter DH: Glucosidase and mannosidase inhibitors mediate increased secretion of mutant alpha-1 antitrypsin Z. J Biol Chem 275:1987, 2000.

38. Teckman JH: Lack of effect of oral 4-phenylbutyrate on serum alpha-1 antitrypsin in patients with alpha-1 antitrypsin deficiency: A preliminary study. J Pediatr Gastroenterol Nutr 39:34, 2004.

39. Campbell EJ, Campbell MA, Boukedes SS, et al: Quantum proteolysis by neutrophils: Implications for pulmonary emphysema in alpha-1 antitrypsin deficiency. J Clin Invest 104:337, 1999.

40. Alino SF, Crespo A, Dasi F: Long-term therapeutic levels of human alpha-1 antitrypsin in plasma after hydrodynamic injection of nonviral DNA. Gene Ther 10:1672, 2003.

41. Ozaki I, Zern MA, Liu S, et al: Ribozyme-mediated specific gene replacement of the alpha-1 antitrypsin gene in human hepatoma cells. J Hepatol 31:53, 1999.

42. Metz R, DiCola M, Kurihara T, et al: Mode of action of RNA/DNA oligonucleotides: Progress in the development of gene repair as a therapy for alpha(1)-antitrypsin deficiency. Chest 121:91S, 2002.

43. Wolfsdorf JI, Holm IA, Weinstein DA: Glycogen storage diseases: Phenotypic, genetic, and biochemical characteristics, and therapy. Endocrinol Metab Clin North Am 28:801, 1999.

44. Ghishan FK, Ballew MP: Inborn errors of carbohydrate metabolism. In Suchy FJ, Sokol RJ, Balistreri WF (eds): Liver

Disease in Children, 2nd ed. Philadelphia, Lippincott Williams & Wilkins, 2001, p 565.

45. Matern D, Seydewitz HH, Bali D, et al: Glycogen storage disease type I: Diagnosis and phenotype/genotype correlation. Eur J Pediatr 161(Suppl 1):S10, 2002.

46. Rake JP, Visser G, Labrune P, et al: Glycogen storage disease type I: Diagnosis, management, clinical course and outcome. Results of the European Study on Glycogen Storage Disease Type I (ESGSD I). Eur J Pediatr 161(Suppl 1):S20, 2002.

47. Visser G, Rake JP, Fernandes J, et al: Neutropenia, neutrophil dysfunction, and inflammatory bowel disease in glycogen storage disease type Ib: Results of the European Study on Glycogen Storage Disease type I. J Pediatr 137:187, 2000.

48. Melis D, Parenti G, Della Casa R, et al: Crohn's-like ileo-colitis in patients affected by glycogen storage disease Ib: Two years' follow-up of patients with a wide spectrum of gastrointestinal signs. Acta Paediatr 92:1415, 2003.

49. Rake JP, Visser G, Huismans D, et al: Bone mineral density in children, adolescents and adults with glycogen storage disease type Ia: A cross-sectional and longitudinal study. J Inherit Metab Dis 26:371, 2003.

50. Melis D, Parenti G, Della Casa R, et al: Brain damage in glycogen storage disease type I. J Pediatr 144:637, 2004.

51. Bandsma RH, Smit GP, Kuipers F: Disturbed lipid metabolism in glycogen storage disease type 1. Eur J Pediatr 161(Suppl 1):S65, 2002.

52. Lee PJ: Glycogen storage disease type I: Pathophysiology of liver adenomas. Eur J Pediatr 161(Suppl 1):S46, 2002.

53. Labrune P, Trioche P, Duvaltier I, et al: Hepatocellular adenomas in glycogen storage disease type I and III: A series of 43 patients and review of the literature. J Pediatr Gastroenterol Nutr 24:276, 1997.

54. Moses SW: Historical highlights and unsolved problems in glycogen storage disease type 1. Eur J Pediatr 161(Suppl 1):S2, 2002.

55. Rake JP, Visser G, Labrune P, et al: Guidelines for management of glycogen storage disease type I. European Study on Glycogen Storage Disease type I (ESGSD I). Eur J Pediatr 161(Suppl 1):S112, 2002.

56. Visser G, Rake JP, Kokke FT, et al: Intestinal function in glycogen storage disease type I. J Inherit Metab Dis 25:261, 2002.

57. Rake JP, ten Berge AM, Visser G, et al: Glycogen storage disease type Ia: Recent experience with mutation analysis, a summary of mutations reported in the literature and a newly developed diagnostic flow chart. Eur J Pediatr 159:322, 2000.

58. Visser G, Rake JP, Labrune P, et al: Consensus guidelines for management of glycogen storage disease type 1b. European Study on Glycogen Storage Disease type 1. Eur J Pediatr 161 Suppl 1:S120-123, 2002.

59. Daublin G, Schwahn B, Wendel U: Type I glycogen storage disease: Favourable outcome on a strict management regimen avoiding increased lactate production during childhood and adolescence. Eur J Pediatr 161(Suppl 1):S40, 2002.

60. Wolfsdorf JI, Crigler JF Jr: Effect of continuous glucose therapy begun in infancy on the long-term clinical course of patients with type I glycogen storage disease. J Pediatr Gastroenterol Nutr 29:136, 1999.

61. Schwenk WF, Haymond MW: Optimal rate of enteral glucose administration in children with glycogen storage disease type I. N Engl J Med 314:682, 1986.

62. Calderwood S, Kilpatrick L, Douglas SD, et al: Recombinant human granulocyte colony-stimulating factor therapy for patients with neutropenia and/or neutrophil dysfunction secondary to glycogen storage disease type 1b. Blood 97:376, 2001.

63. Visser G, Rake JP, Labrune P, et al: Granulocyte colony-stimulating factor in glycogen storage disease type 1b. Results of the European Study on Glycogen Storage Disease Type 1. Eur J Pediatr 161(Suppl 1):S83, 2002.

64. Selby R, Starzl TE, Yunis E, et al: Liver transplantation for type I and type IV glycogen storage disease. Eur J Pediatr 152(Suppl 1):S71, 1993.

65. Matern D, Starzl TE, Arnaout W, et al: Liver transplantation for glycogen storage disease types I, III, and IV. Eur J Pediatr 158(Suppl 2):S43, 1999.

66. Adachi M, Shinkai M, Ohhama Y, et al: Improved neutrophil function in a glycogen storage disease type 1b patient after liver transplantation. Eur J Pediatr 163:202, 2004.

67. Martinez-Olmos MA, Lopez-Sanroman A, Martin-Vaquero P, et al: Liver transplantation for type Ib glycogenosis with reversal of cyclic neutropenia. Clin Nutr 20:375, 2001.

68. Zingone A, Hiraiwa H, Pan CJ, et al: Correction of glycogen storage disease type 1a in a mouse model by gene therapy. J Biol Chem 275:828, 2000.

69. Beaty RM, Jackson M, Peterson D, et al: Delivery of glucose-6-phosphatase in a canine model for glycogen storage disease, type Ia, with adeno-associated virus (AAV) vectors. Gene Ther 9:1015, 2002.

70. Wolfsdorf JI, Weinstein DA: Glycogen storage diseases. Rev Endocr Metab Disord 4:95, 2003.

71. Horinishi A, Okubo M, Tang NL, et al: Mutational and haplotype analysis of AGL in patients with glycogen storage disease type III. J Hum Genet 47:55, 2002.

72. Moses SW: Pathophysiology and dietary treatment of the glycogen storage diseases. J Pediatr Gastroenterol Nutr 11:155, 1990.

73. Siciliano M, De Candia E, Ballarin S, et al: Hepatocellular carcinoma complicating liver cirrhosis in type IIIa glycogen storage disease. J Clin Gastroenterol 31:80, 2000.

74. Goldberg T, Slonim AE: Nutrition therapy for hepatic glycogen storage diseases. J Am Diet Assoc 93:1423, 1993.

75. Maruyama K, Suzuki T, Koizumi T, et al: Congenital form of glycogen storage disease type IV: A case report and a review of the literature. Pediatr Int 46:474, 2004.

76. Moses SW, Parvari R: The variable presentations of glycogen storage disease type IV: A review of clinical, enzymatic and molecular studies. Curr Mol Med 2:177, 2002.

77. de Moor RA, Schweizer JJ, van Hoek B, et al: Hepatocellular carcinoma in glycogen storage disease type IV. Arch Dis Child 82:479, 2000.

78. Rosenthal P, Podesta L, Grier R, et al: Failure of liver transplantation to diminish cardiac deposits of amylopectin and leukocyte inclusions in type IV glycogen storage disease. Liver Transpl Surg 1:373, 1995.

79. Jaeken J, Carchon H: Congenital disorders of glycosylation: A booming chapter of pediatrics. Curr Opin Pediatr 16:434, 2004.

80. Wu X, Steet RA, Bohorov O, et al: Mutation of the COG complex subunit gene COG7 causes a lethal congenital disorder. Nat Med 10:518, 2004.

81. Freeze HH: Congenital disorders of glycosylation and the pediatric liver. Semin Liver Dis 21:501, 2001.

82. Miller BS, Freeze HH: New disorders in carbohydrate metabolism: Congenital disorders of glycosylation and their impact on the endocrine system. Rev Endocr Metab Disord 4:103, 2003.

83. Damen G, de Klerk H, Huijmans J, et al: Gastrointestinal and other clinical manifestations in 17 children with congenital disorders of glycosylation type Ia, Ib, and Ic. J Pediatr Gastroenterol Nutr 38:282, 2004.

84. Babovic-Vuksanovic D, Patterson MC, Schwenk WF, et al: Severe hypoglycemia as a presenting symptom of carbohydrate-deficient glycoprotein syndrome. J Pediatr 135:775, 1999.

85. Kjaergaard S, Skovby F, Schwartz M: Absence of homozygosity for predominant mutations in PMM2 in Danish patients with carbohydrate-deficient glycoprotein syndrome type 1. Eur J Hum Genet 6:331, 1998.

86. Matthijs G, Schollen E, Bjursell C, et al: Mutations in PMM2 that cause congenital disorders of glycosylation, type Ia (CDG-Ia). Hum Mutat 16:386, 2000.

87. Kjaergaard S, Schwartz M, Skovby F: Congenital disorder of glycosylation type Ia (CDG-Ia): Phenotypic spectrum of the R141H/F119L genotype. Arch Dis Child 85:236, 2001.

88. Rutschow S, Thiem J, Kranz C, et al: Membrane-permeant derivatives of mannose-1-phosphate. Bioorg Med Chem 10:4043, 2002.

89. Jaeken J, Matthijs G, Saudubray JM, et al: Phosphomannose isomerase deficiency: A carbohydrate-deficient glycoprotein syndrome with hepatic-intestinal presentation. Am J Hum Genet 62:1535, 1998.

90. Vuillaumier-Barrot S, Le Bizec C, de Lonlay P, et al: Protein losing enteropathy-hepatic fibrosis syndrome in Saguenay-Lac St-Jean, Quebec is a congenital disorder of glycosylation type Ib. J Med Genet 39:849, 2002.

91. Wopereis S, Grunewald S, Morava E, et al: Apolipoprotein C-III isofocusing in the diagnosis of genetic defects in O-glycan biosynthesis. Clin Chem 49:1839, 2003.

92. Westphal V, Kjaergaard S, Davis JA, et al: Genetic and metabolic analysis of the first adult with congenital disorder of glycosylation type Ib: Long-term outcome and effects of mannose supplementation. Mol Genet Metab 73:77, 2001.

93. Bloomer JR, Brenner DA: The porphyrias. In Schiff ER, Sorrell MF, Maddrey WC (eds): Schiff's Diseases of the Liver, 9th ed, Vol 2. Philadelphia, Lippincott Williams & Wilkins, 2003, p 1231.

94. Crimlisk HL: The little imitator—porphyria: A neuropsychiatric disorder. J Neurol Neurosurg Psychiatry 62:319, 1997.

95. Elder GH, Hift RJ, Meissner PN: The acute porphyrias. Lancet 349:1613, 1997.

96. Kauppinen R, Mustajoki P: Prognosis of acute porphyria: Occurrence of acute attacks, precipitating factors, and associated diseases. Medicine (Baltimore) 71:1, 1992.

97. Thunell S, Henrichson A, Floderus Y, et al: Liver transplantation in a boy with acute porphyria due to aminolaevulinate dehydratase deficiency. Eur J Clin Chem Clin Biochem 30:599, 1992.

98. Murphy GM: The cutaneous porphyrias: A review. The British Photodermatology Group. Br J Dermatol 140:573, 1999.

99. Poblete-Gutierrez P, Mendez M, Wiederholt T, et al: The molecular basis of porphyria cutanea tarda in Chile: Identification and functional characterization of mutations in the uroporphyrinogen decarboxylase gene. Exp Dermatol 13:372, 2004.

100. Nagy Z, Koszo F, Par A, et al: Hemochromatosis (HFE) gene mutations and hepatitis C virus infection as risk factors for porphyria cutanea tarda in Hungarian patients. Liver Int 24:16, 2004.

101. Gisbert JP, Garcia-Buey L, Pajares JM, et al: Prevalence of hepatitis C virus infection in porphyria cutanea tarda: Systematic review and meta-analysis. J Hepatol 39:620, 2003.

102. Brady JJ, Jackson HA, Roberts AG, et al: Co-inheritance of mutations in the uroporphyrinogen decarboxylase and hemochromatosis genes accelerates the onset of porphyria cutanea tarda. J Invest Dermatol 115:868, 2000.

103. Harper P, Floderus Y, Holmstrom P, et al: Enrichment of HFE mutations in Swedish patients with familial and sporadic form of porphyria cutanea tarda. J Intern Med 255:684, 2004.

104. Elder GH: Porphyria cutanea tarda. Semin Liver Dis 18:67, 1998.

105. Schneider-Yin X, Gouya L, Meier-Weinand A, et al: New insights into the pathogenesis of erythropoietic protoporphyria and their impact on patient care. Eur J Pediatr 159:719, 2000.

106. Gouya L, Puy H, Robreau AM, et al: The penetrance of dominant erythropoietic protoporphyria is modulated by expression of wildtype FECH. Nat Genet 30:27, 2002.

107. Sarkany RP, Cox TM: Autosomal recessive erythropoietic protoporphyria: A syndrome of severe photosensitivity and liver failure. QJM 88:541, 1995.

108. Doss MO, Frank M: Hepatobiliary implications and complications in protoporphyria, a 20-year study. Clin Biochem 22:223, 1989.

109. Jensen JD, Resnick SD: Porphyria in childhood. Semin Dermatol 14:33, 1995.

110. Bloomer J, Bruzzone C, Zhu L, et al: Molecular defects in ferrochelatase in patients with protoporphyria requiring liver transplantation. J Clin Invest 102:107, 1998.

111. Young JW, Conte ET: Porphyrias and porphyrins. Int J Dermatol 30:399, 1991.

112. Andant C, Puy H, Faivre J, et al: Acute hepatic porphyrias and primary liver cancer. N Engl J Med 338:1853, 1998.

113. Mustajoki P, Nordmann Y: Early administration of heme arginate for acute porphyric attacks. Arch Intern Med 153:2004, 1993.

114. Thomas C, Ged C, Nordmann Y, et al: Correction of congenital erythropoietic porphyria by bone marrow transplantation. J Pediatr 129:453, 1996.

115. Stolzel U, Kostler E, Schuppan D, et al: Hemochromatosis (HFE) gene mutations and response to chloroquine in porphyria cutanea tarda. Arch Dermatol 139:309, 2003.

116. Meerman L, Haagsma EB, Gouw AS, et al: Long-term follow-up after liver transplantation for erythropoietic protoporphyria. Eur J Gastroenterol Hepatol 11:431, 1999.

117. Cox TM, Alexander GJ, Sarkany RP: Protoporphyria. Semin Liver Dis 18:85, 1998.

118. Meerman L, Verwer R, Slooff MJ, et al: Perioperative measures during liver transplantation for erythropoietic protoporphyria. Transplantation 57:155, 1994.

119. Fritsch C, Lang K, Bolsen K, et al: Congenital erythropoietic porphyria. Skin Pharmacol Appl Skin Physiol 11:347, 1998.

120. De Braekeleer M, Larochelle J: Genetic epidemiology of hereditary tyrosinemia in Quebec and in Saguenay-Lac-St-Jean. Am J Hum Genet 47:302, 1990.

121. Stoner E, Starkman H, Wellner D, et al: Biochemical studies of a patient with hereditary hepatorenal tyrosinemia: Evidence of glutathione deficiency. Pediatr Res 18:1332, 1984.

122. Jorquera R, Tanguay RM: The mutagenicity of the tyrosine metabolite, fumarylacetoacetate, is enhanced by glutathione depletion. Biochem Biophys Res Commun 232:42, 1997.

123. Prieto-Alamo MJ, Laval F: Deficient DNA-ligase activity in the metabolic disease tyrosinemia type I. Proc Natl Acad Sci U S A 95:12614, 1998.

124. Gilbert-Barness E, Barness LA, Meisner LF: Chromosomal instability in hereditary tyrosinemia type I. Pediatr Pathol 10:243, 1990.

125. van Spronsen FJ, Thomasse Y, Smit GP, et al: Hereditary tyrosinemia type I: A new clinical classification with difference in prognosis on dietary treatment. Hepatology 20:1187, 1994.

126. Demers SI, Russo P, Lettre F, et al: Frequent mutation reversion inversely correlates with clinical severity in a genetic liver disease, hereditary tyrosinemia. Hum Pathol 34:1313, 2003.

127. Ploos van Amstel JK, Bergman AJ, van Beurden EA, et al: Hereditary tyrosinemia type 1: Novel missense, nonsense and splice consensus mutations in the human fumarylacetoacetate hydrolase gene; variability of the genotype-phenotype relationship. Hum Genet 97:51, 1996.

128. Macvicar D, Dicks-Mireaux C, Leonard JV, et al: Hepatic imaging with computed tomography of chronic tyrosinaemia type 1. Br J Radiol 63:605, 1990.

129. Kvittingen EA, Talseth T, Halvorsen S, et al: Renal failure in adult patients with hereditary tyrosinaemia type I. J Inherit Metab Dis 14:53, 1991.

130. Paradis K, Weber A, Seidman EG, et al: Liver transplantation for hereditary tyrosinemia: The Quebec experience. Am J Hum Genet 47:338, 1990.

131. Mitchell G, Larochelle J, Lambert M, et al: Neurologic crises in hereditary tyrosinemia. N Engl J Med 322:432, 1990.

132. Forget S, Patriquin HB, Dubois J, et al: The kidney in children with tyrosinemia: Sonographic, CT and biochemical findings. Pediatr Radiol 29:104, 1999.

133. Lindstedt S, Holme E, Lock EA, et al: Treatment of hereditary tyrosinaemia type I by inhibition of 4-hydroxyphenylpyruvate dioxygenase. Lancet 340:813, 1992.

134. Holme E, Lindstedt S: Tyrosinaemia type I and NTBC (2-(2-nitro-4-trifluoromethylbenzoyl)-1,3-cyclohexanedione). J Inherit Metab Dis 21:507, 1998.

135. Mitchell GA, Grompe M, Lambert M: Hypertyrosinemia. In Scriver CR, Sly WS, Childs B (eds): The Metabolic and Molecular Bases of Inherited Disease, 8th ed: New York, McGraw-Hill, 2000, p 1777.

136. Brusilow SW, Horwich AL: Urea cycle enzymes. In Scriver CR, Beaudet AL, Sly WS, Valle D (eds): Metabolic and Molecular Basis of Inherited Disease, 8th ed, Vol 2. New York, McGraw-Hill, 2001, p 1909.

137. Palmieri L, Pardo B, Lasorsa FM, et al: Citrin and aralar1 are Ca(2+)-stimulated aspartate/glutamate transporters in mitochondria. EMBO J 20:5060, 2001.

138. Tuchman M, Morizono H, Rajagopal BS, et al: The biochemical and molecular spectrum of ornithine transcarbamylase deficiency. J Inherit Metab Dis 21(Suppl 1):40, 1998.

139. Haberle J, Schmidt E, Pauli S, et al: Mutation analysis in patients with N-acetylglutamate synthase deficiency. Hum Mutat 21:593, 2003.

140. Saheki T, Kobayashi K, Iijima M, et al: Adult-onset type II citrullinemia and idiopathic neonatal hepatitis caused by citrin deficiency: Involvement of the aspartate glutamate carrier for urea synthesis and maintenance of the urea cycle. Mol Genet Metab 81(Suppl 1):S20, 2004.

141. Maestri NE, Clissold D, Brusilow SW: Neonatal onset ornithine transcarbamylase deficiency: A retrospective analysis. J Pediatr 134:268, 1999.

142. Finkelstein JE, Hauser ER, Leonard CO, et al: Late-onset ornithine transcarbamylase deficiency in male patients. J Pediatr 117:897, 1990.

143. Maestri NE, Lord C, Glynn M, et al: The phenotype of ostensibly healthy women who are carriers for ornithine transcarbamylase deficiency. Medicine (Baltimore) 77:389, 1998.

144. Lo WD, Sloan HR, Sotos JF, et al: Late clinical presentation of partial carbamyl phosphate synthetase I deficiency. Am J Dis Child 147:267, 1993.

145. Kobayashi K, Shaheen N, Kumashiro R, et al: A search for the primary abnormality in adult-onset type II citrullinemia. Am J Hum Genet 53:1024, 1993.

146. Wong LJ, Craigen WJ, O'Brien WE: Postpartum coma and death due to carbamoyl-phosphate synthetase I deficiency. Ann Intern Med 120:216, 1994.

147. Arn PH, Hauser ER, Thomas GH, et al: Hyperammonemia in women with a mutation at the ornithine carbamoyltransferase locus: A cause of postpartum coma. N Engl J Med 322:1652, 1990.

148. Tamamori A, Okano Y, Ozaki H, et al: Neonatal intrahepatic cholestasis caused by citrin deficiency: Severe hepatic dysfunction in an infant requiring liver transplantation. Eur J Pediatr 161:609, 2002.

149. Ohura T, Kobayashi K, Abukawa D, et al: A novel inborn error of metabolism detected by elevated methionine and/or galactose in newborn screening: Neonatal intrahepatic cholestasis caused by citrin deficiency. Eur J Pediatr 162:317, 2003.

150. Saheki T, Kobayashi K: Mitochondrial aspartate glutamate carrier (citrin) deficiency as the cause of adult-onset type II citrullinemia (CTLN2) and idiopathic neonatal hepatitis (NICCD). J Hum Genet 47:333, 2002.

151. Bonham JR, Guthrie P, Downing M, et al: The allopurinol load test lacks specificity for primary urea cycle defects but may indicate unrecognized mitochondrial disease. J Inherit Metab Dis 22:174, 1999.

152. Efrati C, Masini A, Merli M, et al: Effect of sodium benzoate on blood ammonia response to oral glutamine challenge in cirrhotic patients: a note of caution. Am J Gastroenterol 95:3574, 2000.

153. Sanjurjo P, Ruiz JI, Montejo M: Inborn errors of metabolism with a protein-restricted diet: effect on polyunsaturated fatty acids. J Inherit Metab Dis 20:783, 1997.

154. Uchino T, Endo F, Matsuda I: Neurodevelopmental outcome of long-term therapy of urea cycle disorders in Japan. J Inherit Metab Dis 21(Suppl 1):151, 1998.

155. Maestri NE, Brusilow SW, Clissold DB, et al: Long-term treatment of girls with ornithine transcarbamylase deficiency. N Engl J Med 335:855, 1996.

156. Todo S, Starzl TE, Tzakis A, et al: Orthotopic liver transplantation for urea cycle enzyme deficiency. Hepatology 15:419, 1992.

157. Picker JD, Puga AC, Levy HL, et al: Arginase deficiency with lethal neonatal expression: Evidence for the glutamine hypothesis of cerebral edema. J Pediatr 142:349, 2003.

158. Iyer R, Jenkinson CP, Vockley JG, et al: The human arginases and arginase deficiency. J Inherit Metab Dis 21(Suppl 1):86, 1998.

159. Balistreri WF: Inborn errors of bile acid biosynthesis and transport: Novel forms of metabolic liver disease. Gastroenterol Clin North Am 28:145, 1999.

160. Bezerra JA, Balistreri WF: Intrahepatic cholestasis: Order out of chaos. Gastroenterology 117:1496, 1999.

161. Whitington PF, Freese DK, Alonso EM, et al: Clinical and biochemical findings in progressive familial intrahepatic cholestasis. J Pediatr Gastroenterol Nutr 18:134, 1994.

162. Setchell KD, O'Connell NC: Disorders of bile acid synthesis and metabolism: A metabolic basis for liver disease. In Suchy FJ, ed. Liver Disease in Children, 2nd ed. Philadelphia, Lippincott Williams & Wilkins, 2001, p 701.

163. Stieger B, Zhang J, O'Neill B, et al: Differential interaction of bile acids from patients with inborn errors of bile acid synthesis with hepatocellular bile acid transporters. Eur J Biochem 244:39, 1997.

164. van Heijst AF, Verrips A, Wevers RA, et al: Treatment and follow-up of children with cerebrotendinous xanthomatosis. Eur J Pediatr 157:313, 1998.

165. Witzleben CL, Piccoli DA, Setchell K: A new category of causes of intrahepatic cholestasis. Pediatr Pathol 12:269, 1992.

166. Raymond GV: Peroxisomal disorders. Curr Opin Pediatr 11:572, 1999.

167. Noetzel MJ: Fish oil and myelin: Cautious optimism for treatment of children with disorders of peroxisome biogenesis. Neurology 51:5, 1998.

168. Imamura A, Tamura S, Shimozawa N, et al: Temperature-sensitive mutation in PEX1 moderates the phenotypes of peroxisome deficiency disorders. Hum Mol Genet 7:2089, 1998.

169. Brown FR 3rd, Voigt R, Singh AK, et al: Peroxisomal disorders: Neurodevelopmental and biochemical aspects. Am J Dis Child 147:617, 1993.

170. Martinez M, Vazquez E: MRI evidence that docosahexaenoic acid ethyl ester improves myelination in generalized peroxisomal disorders. Neurology 51:26, 1998.

171. Kemp S, Wei HM, Lu JF, et al: Gene redundancy and pharmacological gene therapy: Implications for X-linked adrenoleukodystrophy. Nat Med 4:1261, 1998.

172. Setchell KD, Bragetti P, Zimmer-Nechemias L, et al: Oral bile acid treatment and the patient with Zellweger syndrome. Hepatology 15:198, 1992.

173. Bull LN, van Eijk MJ, Pawlikowska L, et al: A gene encoding a P-type ATPase mutated in two forms of hereditary cholestasis. Nat Genet 18:219, 1998.

174. Klomp LW, Bull LN, Knisely AS, et al: A missense mutation in FIC1 is associated with Greenland familial cholestasis. Hepatology 32:1337, 2000.

175. Strautnieks SS, Bull LN, Knisely AS, et al: A gene encoding a liver-specific ABC transporter is mutated in progressive familial intrahepatic cholestasis. Nat Genet 20:233, 1998.

176. van Mil SW, van der Woerd WL, van der Brugge G, et al: Benign recurrent intrahepatic cholestasis type 2 is caused by mutations in ABCB11. Gastroenterology 127:379, 2004.

177. de Vree JM, Jacquemin E, Sturm E, et al: Mutations in the MDR3 gene cause progressive familial intrahepatic cholestasis. Proc Natl Acad Sci U S A 95:282, 1998.

178. Balistreri WF, Bezerra JA, Jansen P, et al: Intrahepatic cholestasis: Summary of an American Association for the Study of Liver Diseases single-topic conference. Hepatology 42:222, 2005.

179. Jacquemin E, Cresteil D, Manouvrier S, et al: Heterozygous non-sense mutation of the MDR3 gene in familial intrahepatic cholestasis of pregnancy. Lancet 353:210, 1999.

180. Dixon PH, Weerasekera N, Linton KJ, et al: Heterozygous MDR3 missense mutation associated with intrahepatic cholestasis of pregnancy: Evidence for a defect in protein trafficking. Hum Mol Genet 9:1209, 2000.

181. Bull LN, Roche E, Song EJ, et al: Mapping of the locus for cholestasis-lymphedema syndrome (Aagenaes syndrome) to a 6.6-cM interval on chromosome 15q. Am J Hum Genet 67:994, 2000.

182. Betard C, Rasquin-Weber A, Brewer C, et al: Localization of a recessive gene for North American Indian childhood cirrhosis to chromosome region 16q22 and identification of a shared haplotype. Am J Hum Genet 67:222, 2000.

183. Chagnon P, Michaud J, Mitchell G, et al: A missense mutation (R565W) in cirhin (FLJ14728) in North American Indian childhood cirrhosis. Am J Hum Genet 71:1443, 2002.

184. Kocak N, Gurakan F, Yuce A, et al: Nonsyndromic paucity of interlobular bile ducts: Clinical and laboratory findings of 10 cases. J Pediatr Gastroenterol Nutr 24:44, 1997.

185. Naveh Y, Bassan L, Rosenthal E, et al: Progressive familial intrahepatic cholestasis among the Arab population in Israel. J Pediatr Gastroenterol Nutr 24:548, 1997.

186. Jacquemin E, Hermans D, Myara A, et al: Ursodeoxycholic acid therapy in pediatric patients with progressive familial intrahepatic cholestasis. Hepatology 25:519, 1997.

187. Ng VL, Ryckman FC, Porta G, et al: Long-term outcome after partial external biliary diversion for intractable pruritus in patients with intrahepatic cholestasis. J Pediatr Gastroenterol Nutr 30:152, 2000.

188. Soubrane O, Gauthier F, DeVictor D, et al: Orthotopic liver transplantation for Byler disease. Transplantation 50:804, 1990.

189. Lykavieris P, Bernard O, Hadchouel M: Neonatal cholestasis as the presenting feature in cystic fibrosis. Arch Dis Child 75:67, 1996.

190. Lindblad A, Glaumann H, Strandvik B: Natural history of liver disease in cystic fibrosis. Hepatology 30:1151, 1999.

191. Sokol RJ, Durie PR: Recommendations for management of liver and biliary tract disease in cystic fibrosis. Cystic Fibrosis Foundation Hepatobiliary Disease Consensus Group. J Pediatr Gastroenterol Nutr 28(Suppl 1):S1, 1999.

192. Smith JL, Lewindon PJ, Hoskins AC, et al: Endogenous ursodeoxycholic acid and cholic acid in liver disease due to cystic fibrosis. Hepatology 39:1673, 2004.

193. Lenaerts C, Lapierre C, Patriquin H, et al: Surveillance for cystic fibrosis-associated hepatobiliary disease: Early ultrasound changes and predisposing factors. J Pediatr 143:343, 2003.

194. Narkewicz MR, Smith D, Gregory C, et al: Effect of ursodeoxycholic acid therapy on hepatic function in children with intrahepatic cholestatic liver disease. J Pediatr Gastroenterol Nutr 26:49, 1998.

195. Noble-Jamieson G, Valente J, Barnes ND, et al: Liver transplantation for hepatic cirrhosis in cystic fibrosis. Arch Dis Child 71:349, 1994.

196. Sokol RJ, Treem WR: Mitochondria and childhood liver diseases. J Pediatr Gastroenterol Nutr 28:4, 1999.

197. Munnich A, Rotig A, Chretien D, et al: Clinical presentation of mitochondrial disorders in childhood. J Inherit Metab Dis 19:521, 1996.

CHAPTER
74 Hepatitis A

Maria H. Sjogren

The development of liver biopsy techniques in the 1930s allowed the recognition of hepatic necroinflammation that characterizes all forms of viral hepatitis. Subsequent experimental work in humans led to the clinical recognition that viruses are etiologic agents of hepatitis A ("infectious hepatitis") and hepatitis B ("serum hepatitis").[1,2] Later, the existence of two hepatitis viruses was demonstrated—hepatitis A virus (HAV) and hepatitis B virus (HBV) (see Chapter 75).[3] Additional viral causes of acute and chronic hepatitis were identified subsequently (see Chapters 76-78). HAV was first characterized in 1973, when scientists detected the virus in stools from human volunteers who were infected with HAV.[4] The ensuing development of sensitive and specific serologic assays for the diagnosis of HAV infection and the isolation of HAV in cell culture[5] were important advances that permitted understanding of the epidemiology of HAV infection and, ultimately, control of the disease.

VIROLOGY

In 1982, HAV was classified as an enterovirus type 72 belonging to the Picornaviridae family. Subsequent determination of the sequence of HAV nucleotides and amino acids led to questioning of this classification, and a new genus, Hepatovirus, was created for HAV.[6]

HAV has an icosahedral shape and lacks an envelope. It measures 27 to 28 nm in diameter, has a buoyant density of 1.33 to 1.34 g/cm^3 in cesium chloride, and has a sedimentation coefficient of 156 to 160S on ultracentrifugation. HAV survives exposure to ether and an acid environment at pH 3. It also survives heat exposure at 60°C for 60 minutes but is inactivated at 85°C for 1 minute. HAV is capable of surviving in sea water (4% survival rate), in dried feces at room temperature for 4 weeks (17% survival), and in live oysters for 5 days (12% survival).[7]

Only one serotype of HAV is known, and there is no antigenic cross-reactivity with the hepatitis B, C, D, E, or G agents. The HAV genome consists of a positive-sense RNA that is 7.48 kb long, single-stranded, and linear (Fig. 74-1). HAV RNA has a sedimentation coefficient of 32 to 33S and a molecular weight of $2.8 \times 10.^4$ The HAV RNA has a long open reading frame, consisting of 6681 nucleotides, and is covalently linked to a 5′ terminal protein and a 3′ terminal polyadenosine tract.

The onset of HAV replication in cell culture systems takes from weeks to months. Primate cells, including African green monkey kidney cells, primary human fibroblasts, human diploid cells (MRC-5), and fetal rhesus kidney cells, are favored for cultivation of HAV in vitro. The virus is not cytopathic, and persistent infection in the cell cultures is the rule. Two conditions control the outcome of HAV replication in cell culture.[8] First, the genetic makeup of the virus is important; HAV strains mutate in distinct regions of the viral genome as they become adapted to cell culture. The second condition is the metabolic activity of the host cell at the time of infection. Cells in culture, although infected simultaneously, initiate HAV replication in an asynchronous manner. This asynchronicity may be caused by differences in the metabolic activity of individual cells, but there is no definitive evidence of cell-cycle dependence of HAV replication.[9]

An initial step in the life cycle of a virus is its attachment to a cell surface receptor. The location and function of these receptors determine tissue tropism. Little is known about the mechanism of entry of HAV into cells. Some work has suggested that HAV could infect cells by a surrogate-receptor binding mechanism (by a nonspecified serum protein). HAV infectivity in tissue culture has been shown to require calcium and to be inhibited by the treatment of the cells with trypsin, phospholipases, and β-galactosidase.[10] A surface glycoprotein, named HAVcr-1, on African green monkey kidney cells has been identified as a receptor for HAV. Blocking of HAVcr-1 with

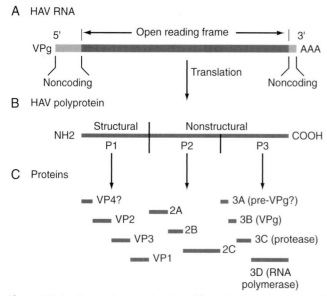

A HAV RNA

Open reading frame

Figure 74–1 Genomic organization of hepatitis A virus. VP, viral protein; VPg, 5′ terminal protein. (From Levine JE, Bull FG, Millward-Sadler GH, et al: Acute viral hepatitis. In Millward-Sadler GH, Wright R, Arther MJP [eds]: Wright's Liver and Biliary Disease, 3rd ed. London, WB Saunders, 1992, p 679.)

specific monoclonal antibodies prevents infection of otherwise susceptible cells. Experimental data suggest that HAVcr-1 not only serves as an attachment receptor but also may facilitate uncoating of HAV and its entry into hepatocytes.[11]

Whatever the entry mechanism, once HAV enters a cell, the viral RNA is uncoated, cell host ribosomes bind to viral RNA, and polysomes are formed. HAV is translated into a large polyprotein of 2227 amino acids. This polyprotein is organized into three regions: P1, P2, and P3. The P1 region encodes structural proteins VP1, VP2, VP3, and a putative VP4. The P2 and P3 regions encode nonstructural proteins associated with viral replication (see Fig. 74–1).

The HAV RNA polymerase copies the plus RNA strand. The RNA transcript in turn is used for translation into proteins, which are used for assembly into mature virions. It appears that down-regulation of HAV RNA synthesis occurs as defective HAV particles appear.[12] In addition, a group of specific RNA-binding proteins has been observed during persistent infection.[13] The origin and nature of these proteins is unknown, but they exert activity on the RNA template and are believed to play a regulatory role in the replication of HAV.[14]

Numerous strains of HAV exist, with considerable nucleotide sequence variability (15% to 25% difference within the P1 region of the genome). Human HAV strains can be grouped in four different genotypes (I, II, III, and VII), whereas simian strains of HAV belong to genotypes IV, V, and VI.[15] Despite the nucleotide sequence heterogeneity, the antigenic structure of human HAV is highly conserved among strains.

The HAV VP1/2A and 2C genes are thought to be responsible for viral virulence, on the basis of experiments in which recombinant HAV caused acute hepatitis in animals after construction of 14 chimeric virus genomes from two infectious cDNA clones that encoded a virulent HAV isolate and an attenuated HAV isolate (HM175 strain) and the genotype and phenotype of each virus were compared.[16]

Among the many strains of HAV, the HM175 and CR326 human HAV strains are important because they were used for production of commercially available vaccines. Strain HM175 was isolated in 1978, from human feces from Australian patients in a small outbreak of hepatitis A. CR326 was isolated from Costa Rican patients infected with HAV. The nucleotide and amino acid sequences showed 95% identity between the two strains. Vaccines prepared from these strains are thought to provide protection against all relevant human strains of HAV.

Variations in the HAV genome are thought to play a role in the development of fulminant hepatic failure (FHF) during acute HAV infection. The 5′ untranslated region of the HAV genome was sequenced in serum samples from 84 patients with HAV infection, including 12 with FHF.[17] The investigators observed fewer nucleotide substitutions in the HAV genome of patients with FHF than in those without FHF ($P < .001$). The differences were most prominent between nucleotides 200 and 500, suggesting that nucleotide variations in the central portion of the 5′ untranslated region influence the clinical severity of HAV infection.

EPIDEMIOLOGY

Acute hepatitis A is a reportable infectious disease in the United States, with a rate of infection of 4 per 100,000.[18] In 2001, 10,616 cases of HAV infection were reported in the United States. With the underreporting of cases and the occurrence of asymptomatic infections taken into consideration, the true number of annual HAV infections has been calculated to be 93,000.[18] The highest rate of reported disease is among children ages 5 to 14 years; 25% of reported cases are among persons 20 years or younger,[19] but HAV infection can occur in any age group.

The epidemiologic risk factors for HAV infection reported for the U.S. population in 2002 were as follows: unknown, 57%; sexual or household contact with a patient who has hepatitis A, 12%; international travel, 9%; male homosexual activity, 8%; injection drug use, 5%; child or employee in a daycare center, 1%; food or waterborne outbreak, 1%; contact with a daycare child or employee, 3%; and other contact with a patient who has hepatitis, 4%.[20]

HAV infection generally follows one of three epidemiologic patterns.[21] In countries where sanitary conditions are poor, most children are infected at an early age. Although earlier seroepidemiologic studies routinely showed that 100% of preschool children in these countries had detectable antibody to HAV (anti-HAV) in serum, presumably reflecting previous subclinical infection, subsequent studies have shown that the average age of infection has risen rapidly to 5 years and older, when symptomatic infection is more likely. For example, 82% of 1393 Bolivian school children were shown to have detectable anti-HAV, but when they were stratified into two groups according to family income, a significant difference was found between the groups: 95% of children from low-income families, but only 56% of children from high-income families, had detectable anti-HAV.[22]

The second epidemiologic pattern is seen in industrialized countries, where the prevalence of HAV infection is low among children and young adults. In the United States, the prevalence of anti-HAV is approximately 10% in children but 37% in adults.[23]

The third epidemiologic pattern is observed in closed or semiclosed communities, such as some isolated communities in the South Pacific, in which HAV is capable (through epidemics) of infecting the entire population, which then becomes immune. Thereafter, newborns remain susceptible until the virus is reintroduced into the community.

Whatever the epidemiologic pattern, the primary route of transmission of HAV is the fecal-oral route, by either person-to-person contact or ingestion of contaminated food or water. Although rare, transmission of HAV by a parenteral route has been documented after transfusion of blood[24,25] or blood products.[26] Cyclic outbreaks among users of injection and noninjection illicit drugs and among men who have sex with men (up to 10% may become infected in outbreak years) have been reported.[27] Table 74–1 provides information about the detection of HAV and its infectivity in human body fluids.[28-35]

Approximately 11% to 22% of patients with acute hepatitis A require hospitalization,[27] with an average cost of $6914 per patient.[36] In one outbreak involving 43 persons, the total cost was approximately $800,000.[27] On average, 27 workdays are lost per adult case of hepatitis A, with a total loss of 829,000 workdays per year in the United States.[27,36] Combined direct and indirect costs associated with HAV infection in the United States totaled more than $200 million in 1989 and approximately $488.8 million in 1997.[27,36]

PATHOGENESIS

Once HAV is ingested and survives gastric acid, it traverses the small intestinal mucosa and reaches the liver via the portal vein. The precise mechanism of hepatic uptake in humans is unknown (see earlier). In an experimental model on African green monkey kidney cells,[11] the puta-tive cellular receptor for HAV has been identified as a surface glycoprotein. Once the virus reaches the hepatocyte, it starts replicating in the cytoplasm, where it is seen on electron microscopy as a fine granular pattern, but it is not present in the nucleus. HAV is distributed throughout the liver. Although HAV antigen has been detected in other organs (lymph nodes, spleen, kidney), the virus appears to replicate exclusively in hepatocytes. Once the virus is mature, it reaches the systemic circulation via the hepatic sinusoids and is released into the biliary tree through bile canaliculi, passed into the small intestine, and eventually excreted in the feces.

The pathogenesis of HAV-associated hepatocyte injury is not completely defined. The lack of injury to cells in cell culture systems suggests that HAV is not cytopathic. Immunologically mediated cell damage is more likely. The emergence of anti-HAV could result in hepatic necrosis during immunologically mediated elimination of HAV.

CLINICAL FEATURES

Infection with HAV does not result in chronic infection, only in an acute self-limited episode of hepatitis. Rarely, acute hepatitis A can have a prolonged or a relapsing course, and occasionally profound cholestasis can occur.[37] The incubation period is commonly 2 to 4 weeks, rarely up to 6 weeks. The mortality rate is low in previously healthy persons. Morbidity can be significant in adults and older children.

The clinical characteristics of cases of hepatitis A reported in 2002 were similar to those in previous years, with a preponderance of cases in men in all age groups. Overall, 72% of patients manifested jaundice, 25% required hospitalization, and 0.5 % died.[20] The need for hospitalization rose with age, from 5% among children younger than 5 years to 34% among persons 60 years or older.[20]

HAV infection usually presents in one of the following five different clinical patterns: (1) asymptomatic without jaundice, (2) symptomatic with jaundice and self-limited to approximately 8 weeks, (3) cholestatic, with jaundice lasting 10 weeks or more,[37] (4) relapsing, with two or more bouts of acute HAV infection occurring over a 6- to 10-week period, and (5) FHF.

Table 74–1 Detection of Hepatitis A Virus (HAV) and Infectivity of Human Secretions or Excretions

Secretion/Excretion	Comment	Reference
Stool	Main source of infection. HAV is detectable during incubation period and for several weeks after the onset of disease. After the onset of symptoms, HAV is detectable in 45% and 11% of fecal specimens collected during the first and second weeks of illness, respectively, whereas HAV RNA (by polymerase chain reaction assay) is detectable for 4 to 5 months.	28,29
Blood	Viremia is present during the incubation period. Blood collected 3 and 11 days before the onset of symptoms has caused post-transfusion infection in recipients. Chronic viremia does not occur.	30,31
Bile	HAV has been detected in the bile of chimpanzees infected with HAV.	32
Urine	HAV is detected in low titer during the viremic phase. A urine sample was reported to be infectious after oral inoculation. Urine contaminated with blood was also infectious.	33,34
Nasopharyngeal secretions	Unknown in humans. HAV has been identified in the oropharynx of experimentally infected chimpanzees.	35
Semen, vaginal fluid	Uncertain. HAV may be detectable during the viremic phase.	—

Children younger than 2 years are usually asymptomatic; jaundice develops in only 20%, whereas symptoms develop in most children (80%) 5 years or older. The rate of symptoms is high in adolescents and adults. HAV infection with prolonged cholestasis is a rare variant but occasionally leads to invasive diagnostic procedures (inappropriately), because the diagnosis of acute hepatitis may not be readily accepted in patients who have jaundice for several months, even in the presence of detectable anti-HAV of the immunoglobulin M (IgM) class (see later).[37] A relapsing course is observed in approximately 10% of patients with acute hepatitis A. Shedding of HAV in stool has been documented during the relapse phase.[38] This variant is benign, and the infection ultimately resolves.[38] Neither the cholestatic variant nor relapsing hepatitis A is associated with greater mortality. In all cases, treatment is symptomatic. Acute hepatitis A, unlike hepatitis E, is not associated with a higher mortality rate in pregnant women.

Prodromal symptoms in patients with acute hepatitis A include fatigue, weakness, anorexia, nausea, vomiting, and abdominal pain. Less common symptoms are fever, headache, arthralgias, myalgias, and diarrhea. Dark urine precedes other symptoms in approximately 90% of infected persons; this symptom occurs within 1 to 2 weeks of the onset of prodromal symptoms. Symptoms of hepatitis may last from a few days to 2 weeks and usually decrease with the onset of clinical jaundice. Right upper quadrant tenderness and mild liver enlargement are found on physical examination in 85% of patients; splenomegaly and cervical lymphadenopathy are each present in 15%. Complete clinical recovery is achieved in 60% of affected persons within 2 months and in almost everyone by 6 months. The overall prognosis of acute hepatitis A in otherwise healthy adults is excellent. Potentially fatal complications (e.g., FHF) develop in a few patients (see later).[39]

Acute HAV infection must be differentiated by appropriate serologic testing from other causes of acute viral hepatitis, autoimmune hepatitis, and other causes of acute hepatitis (see Chapters 14 and 70). However, in some cases the diagnosis may be difficult to make because the patient may harbor another viral infection, such as chronic hepatitis B or chronic hepatitis C, with superimposed acute HAV infection.

FULMINANT HEPATITIS A

FHF due to HAV is rarely seen in children, adolescents, or young adults. However, the case-fatality rate in people older than 49 years with acute hepatitis A is reported to be 1.8%, compared with an overall rate of 0.3% in persons of all ages.[20] Hepatic failure caused by hepatitis A becomes manifest in the first week of illness in about 55% of affected patients and during the first 4 weeks in 90%; FHF is rarely seen after 4 weeks.[39]

The contribution of HAV to acute liver failure has been reported to be greater in populations classified as hyperendemic for HAV. In a report from India, where 276 patients with FHF were seen between 1994 and 1997, 10.6% of the cases among adults were caused by HAV. HAV had been responsible for only 3.5% of cases among

206 patients with FHF seen in the same community from 1978 to 1981.[40]

Certain populations have increased morbidity and a high risk of acute liver failure from HAV infection. Among these groups are the elderly[41] and persons with chronic liver disease. A 1998 report describes the clinical outcome of 256 persons hospitalized for acute hepatitis A in Tennessee from January 1994 through December 1995.[42] On admission, 89% of the patients had experienced prolonged nausea or vomiting, and 26% had a prolonged prothrombin time (>3 seconds); 39 had serious complications (19 hepatobiliary in nature, 20 extrahepatic complications), and 5 (2%) died. Morbidity and mortality correlated with age. Twenty-five percent of patients 40 years and older had at least one complication, compared with 11% of patients younger than 40 years ($P = .014$).

Although two reports since the late 1990s have described a decline in the number of cases of acute viral hepatitis among patients with FHF in the United States,[43,44] this decline is attributable principally to the control of hepatitis B. The contribution of HAV infection to FHF has remained unchanged since the 1970s despite the availability of highly efficacious vaccines.

EXTRAHEPATIC MANIFESTATIONS

Extrahepatic manifestations are less frequent in acute HAV infection than in acute HBV infection and consist most commonly of an evanescent rash (14%) and arthralgias (11%) and less commonly of leukocytoclastic vasculitis, glomerulonephritis, and arthritis, in which immune-complex disease is believed to play an etiologic role. Cutaneous vasculitis is typically seen on the legs and buttocks; skin biopsies reveal the presence of IgM anti-HAV and complement in the blood vessel walls. The arthritis also appears to have a predilection for the lower extremities. Both vasculitis and arthritis have been associated with cryoglobulinemia, although cryoglobulinemia, in general, is more frequently associated with HCV infection. The cryoglobulin has been shown to contain IgM anti-HAV. Other rare extrahepatic manifestations that may be immune-complex related include toxic epidermal necrolysis, fatal myocarditis, renal failure in the absence of liver failure, optic neuritis, transverse myelitis, polyneuritis, and cholecystitis. Hematologic complications include thrombocytopenia, aplastic anemia, and red-cell aplasia. Patients with more protracted illness appear to have a higher frequency of extrahepatic manifestations.

AUTOIMMUNE HEPATITIS AFTER ACUTE HEPATITIS A

Several viruses have been reported to trigger the onset of autoimmune hepatitis (AIH). In rare cases, hepatitis A has been followed by the development of type 1 AIH. Genetic predisposition is thought to play a role (see Chapter 85).[45,46]

DIAGNOSIS

Acute hepatitis A is clinically indistinguishable from other forms of viral hepatitis. The diagnosis of infection is based on the detection of specific antibodies against HAV (anti-HAV) in serum (Fig. 74–2). A diagnosis of acute hepatitis A requires demonstration of IgM anti-HAV in serum. The test result is positive from the onset of symptoms[47] and usually remains positive for approximately 4 months.[48] Some patients may have low levels of detectable IgM anti-HAV for more than a year after the initial infection.[48] IgG anti-HAV is also detectable at the onset of the disease, remains present usually for life, and, after clinical recovery, is interpreted as a marker of previous HAV infection.

Testing for HAV RNA is limited to research laboratories. HAV RNA has been detected in serum, stool, and liver tissue. Viral RNA can be amplified by polymerase chain reaction (PCR) methodology.[49] With a PCR assay, HAV RNA has been documented in human sera for up to 21 days after the onset of illness.[50] The use of HCV RNA testing has been described in a report of 76 French patients with acute HAV infection seen between January 1987 and April 2000; 19 had FHF,[51] 10 of whom required liver transplantation and 1 of whom died while awaiting liver transplantation. The HAV RNA status was determined in 39 of the 50 patients in whom sera and clinical data were available, including the 19 with FHF. HAV RNA was detected in 36 of these 50 patients (72%). The likelihood that HAV RNA was undetectable was greater in patients with FHF than in those with nonfulminant hepatitis ($P < .02$). Of those in whom HAV RNA was detectable, titers were lower in patients with encephalopathy than in patients with nonfulminant hepatitis (3.6 log vs 4.4 log; $P = .02$). These data suggest that detection of IgM anti-HAV coupled with nondetection or finding of low-titer HAV RNA in patients with severe acute hepatitis may signal an ominous prognosis and the need for early referral for liver transplantation. As in other studies, HAV genotype did not seem to play a role in the severity of clinical manifestations.[52]

PREVENTION AND TREATMENT

Recommendations concerning immunoprophylaxis against HAV were published in December 1999 by the Advisory Committee on Immunization Practices.[27] The overall strategy is to protect persons from disease and to lower the incidence of HAV infection in the United States. The available vaccines are not licensed for use in children younger than 2 years. At present, high-risk populations are targeted for immunization; Table 74–2 lists these populations. Because children who reside in high-risk areas are targeted for vaccination, the overall rate of HAV infection has declined steadily; in 2002, it was 3.1 per 100,000, the lowest rate yet recorded. The decline in rates has been greater in children than in adults and in states where routine childhood vaccination is recommended, suggesting that childhood vaccination has had a positive effect.

There are no specific medications to treat acute hepatitis A; symptomatic treatment is the rule. Attention to sanitation and administration of serum immune globulin (IG) are the mainstays of preventing HAV infection. The availability of excellent HAV vaccines has rendered use of IG for preexposure prophylaxis unnecessary. When IG is used for postexposure prophylaxis, it should be given within 2 weeks of exposure. In these cases, the recommended dose is 0.02 mL/kg, given by intramuscular injection. Although considered safe, IG can cause fever, myalgias, and pain at the injection site. Postexposure prophylaxis with IG can be accompanied safely at the same time as initiation of active immunization with the vaccine.[53]

The HAV vaccine was first licensed in the United States in 1995; two inactivated HAV vaccines are commercially

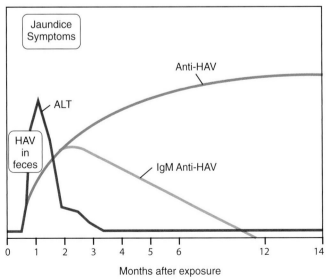

Figure 74–2 Typical course of a case of acute hepatitis A. ALT, alanine aminotransferase; anti-HAV, antibody to hepatitis A virus; HAV, hepatitis A virus; IgM, immunoglobulin M. (From Hoofnagle JH, DiBisceglie AM: Serologic diagnosis of acute and chronic viral hepatitis. Semin Liver Dis 11:73, 1991.)

Table 74–2 Groups at High Risk of Hepatitis A Virus (HAV) Infection

Healthy persons who travel to endemic areas, work in occupations for which the likelihood of exposure is high, are family members of infected patients, or adopt infants or children from endemic areas

Persons with chronic liver disease

Persons who have tested positive for human immunodeficiency virus

Men who have sex with men

Users of injection and noninjection illicit drugs

Persons with clotting factor disorders

Persons who live in communities with high or intermediate rates of HAV infection

Children who live in areas where the rate of HAV infection is at least twice the national average (≥20 cases per 100,000 population)

Table 74–3   Recommended Regimens for Hepatitis A Vaccination*

Vaccine	Age (yr)	Dose	Volume (mL)	Dosing Schedule
HAVRIX	2-18	720 ELU	0.5	0, 6-12 months
	>18	1440 ELU	1.0	0, 6-12 months
VAQTA	2-18	25 U	0.5	0, 6-18 months
	>18	50 U	1.0	0, 6-18 months
TWINRIX	≥18	720 ELU HAV, 20 μg HBV	1.0	0, 1, 6 months

ELU, Enzyme-linked immunoassay (ELISA) units; HBV, hepatitis B virus; U, units.
*Vaccines are injected intramuscularly in the deltoid area.

available. Extensive use of the vaccines in clinical trials and postmarketing surveillance support the safety and efficacy of these products. HAVRIX is manufactured by SmithKline Biologicals, Rixensart, Belgium, and VAQTA by Merck Sharp & Dohme, West Point, Pennsylvania. Both vaccines are derived from HAV grown in cell culture. The final products are purified and formalin-inactivated; they contain alum as an adjuvant. The basic difference between the two commercially available vaccines is the HAV strain used for preparation. HAVRIX was prepared with the HM175 strain, whereas VAQTA was prepared with the CR326 strain.[54,55] The difference is of little practical importance, because both vaccines are safe and immunogenic. The doses and schedule of immunization are shown in Table 74–3. After vaccination with HAVRIX, anti-HAV is estimated to remain detectable in serum for approximately 20 years; immunity may last longer.[56]

From the time the HAV vaccine was licensed in the United States through 1998, more than 6.5 million doses were administered, including 2.3 million pediatric doses. Worldwide, more than 65 million doses of HAV vaccine were administered through 1999. Among adults, the most common local side effects are soreness at the injection site (56%), headache (14%), and malaise (7%). In children, the most common side effects are soreness at the injection site (15%), feeding problems (8%), headache (4%), and injection site induration (4%).

In the United States, through 1998, the national Vaccine Adverse Event Reporting System received 247 reports of unexplained adverse events within 6 weeks of immunization. Approximately one third of these reports occurred with concurrent vaccinations and could not be attributed to the HAV vaccine. Thirteen events in children (0.6 per 100,000 doses distributed) and 85 events in adults (1.4 per 100,000 doses distributed) were considered serious. These events included neurologic, hematologic, and autoimmune syndromes. However, no reported serious event could be attributed definitively to the HAV vaccine, and the reported rates did not exceed the expected background rates. For example, the incidence of Guillain-Barré syndrome ranges from 0.5 to 2.4 cases per 100,000 person-years, and the 5 cases of Guillain-Barré syndrome among adult HAV vaccine recipients represented an incidence of 0.2 cases per 100,000 person-years.[27] Postmarketing reports have not shown a higher incidence rate in vaccine recipients.

A combined formulation of hepatitis A and B vaccines (TWINRIX) is available and has an excellent record of

efficacy and safety.[57] The dosing schedule is shown in Table 74–3.

IMMUNIZATION AGAINST HEPATITIS A VIRUS IN PATIENTS WITH CHRONIC LIVER DISEASE

Persons with chronic liver disease are at increased risk of HAV-related morbidity and mortality if they acquire the infection. Therefore, preexposure prophylaxis with the HAV vaccine has been recommended for patients with chronic liver disease who are susceptible to HAV.[58] This recommendation should be extended to patients awaiting liver transplantation as well as those who have already undergone liver transplantation, although the immunogenicity of the HAV vaccine is reduced in such persons.[59]

An episode of acute hepatitis in a patient with underlying chronic liver disease poses the risk of considerable morbidity and mortality. Although the current guidelines recommend immunization against HAV for all patients with chronic liver disease,[27] the results of several cost-effectiveness analyses have been conflicting. A report published in 2000 found that saving the life of one patient with hepatitis C virus infection through HAV vaccination would cost 23 million Canadian dollars.[60] However, some of the assumptions in this report have been challenged.[61] Two other studies of patients with chronic hepatitis C showed a decided benefit for immunization against HAV.[62,63] The methods used in these studies were dissimilar, and some analyses may have been insensitive to the incidence of HAV or may have underestimated the economic and societal costs of a case of FHF. Universal immunization against HAV during childhood, before the possible occurrence of chronic liver disease, offers the promise of preventing HAV infection.[64]

REFERENCES

1. MacCallum FO, McFarlan AM, Miles JAR, et al (eds): Infective Hepatitis: Studies in East Anglia during the period 1943-1947. Medical Research Council, Special Report No. 273. London, HMSO, 1951, p 1.
2. Havens WP, Ward R, Drill VA, et al: Experimental production of hepatitis by feeding icterogenic materials. Proc Soc Exp Biol Med 57:206, 1944.

3. Krugman S, Ward R, Giles JP, et al: Infectious hepatitis: Detection of virus during the incubation period and in clinically inapparent infections. N Engl J Med 261:729, 1959.

4. Feinstone SM, Kapikian AZ, Purcell RH: Hepatitis A: Detection by immune electron microscopy of a viruslike antigen associated with acute illness. Science 182:1026, 1973.

5. Provost PJ, Hilleman MR: An inactivated hepatitis A virus vaccine prepared from infected marmoset liver. Proc Soc Exp Biol Med 159:210, 1978.

6. Minor PD: Picornaviridae: Classification and nomenclature of viruses: Fifth Report of the International Committee on Taxonomy of Viruses. Arch Virol Suppl 2:320, 1991.

7. Sobsey MD, Shields PA, Hauchman FS, et al: Survival and persistence of hepatitis A virus in environmental samples. In Zuckerman AJ (ed): Viral Hepatitis and Liver Disease. New York, Alan R. Liss, 1988, p 121.

8. Siegl G: Replication of hepatitis A virus and processing of proteins. Vaccine 10:S32, 1992.

9. Harmon SA, Summers DF, Ehrenfeld E: Detection of hepatitis A virus RNA and capsid antigen in individual cells. Virus Res 12:361, 1989.

10. Seganti L, Superti F, Orsi N, et al: Study of the chemical nature of Frp/3 cell recognition units for hepatitis A virus. Med Microbiol Immunol 176:21, 1987.

11. Kaplan G, Totsuka A, Thompson P, et al: Identification of a surface glycoprotein on African green monkey kidney cells as a receptor for hepatitis A virus. EMBO J 15:4282, 1996.

12. Siegl G, Nüesch JPF, de Chastonay J: DI-particles of hepatitis A virus in cell culture and clinical specimens. In Brinton MA, Heinz FX (eds): New Aspects of Positive Strand RNA Viruses. Washington, DC, American Society for Microbiology, 1990, p 102.

13. Nüesch JPF, Weitz M, Siegl G: Proteins specifically binding to the 3′ untranslated region of hepatitis A virus RNA in persistently infected cells. Arch Virol 128:65, 1993.

14. Robertson BH, Jansen RW, Khanna B, et al: Genetic relatedness of hepatitis A virus strains recovered from different geographic regions. J Gen Virol 73:1365, 1992.

15. Mathiesen LR, Feinstone SM, Purcell RH, Wagner JA: Detection of hepatitis A antigen by immunofluorescence. Infect Immun 18:524, 1977.

16. Emerson SU, Huang YK, Nguyen H, et al: Identification of VP1/2A and 2C as a virulence genes of hepatitis A virus and demonstration of genetic instability of 2C. J Virol 76:8551, 2002.

17. Fujiwara K, Yokosuka, Ehata T, et al: Association between severity of type A hepatitis and nucleotide variations in the 5′ non-translated region of hepatitis A virus RNA: Strains from fulminant hepatitis have fewer nucleotide substitutions. Gut 51:82, 2002.

18. Summary of Notifiable Diseases, United States—2001. MMWR Morb Mortal Wkly Rep 50:1, 2001.

19. Centers for Diseases Control and Prevention: Guidelines for Viral Hepatitis Surveillance and Case Management. Atlanta, CDC, 2004.

20. Centers for Disease Control and Prevention. Hepatitis Surveillance Report No. 59. Atlanta, CDC, 2004.

21. Gust ID: Epidemiological patterns of hepatitis A in different parts of the world. Vaccine 10:S56, 1992.

22. Gandolfo GM, Ferri GM, Conti L, et al: Prevalence of infections by hepatitis A, B, C and E viruses in two different socioeconomic groups of children from Santa Cruz, Bolivia. Med Clin (Barc) 120:725, 2003.

23. Prevention of hepatitis A through active or passive immunization: Recommendations of the Advisory Committee on Immunization Practices (ACIP). MMWR Morb Mortal Wkly Rep 45(RR-15):1, 1996.

24. Skidmore SJ, Boxall EH, Ala F: A case report of post-transfusion hepatitis A. J Med Virol 10:223, 1982.

25. Hollinger FB, Khan NC, Oefinger PE, et al: Posttransfusion hepatitis type A. JAMA 250:2313, 1983.

26. Mannucci PM, Gdovin S, Gringeri A, et al: Transmission of hepatitis A to patients with hemophilia by factor VIII concentrates treated with organic solvent and detergent to inactivate viruses. Ann Intern Med 120:1, 1994.

27. Prevention of hepatitis A through active or passive immunization: Recommendations of the Advisory Committee on Immunization Practices (ACIP). MMWR Morb Mortal Wkly Rep 48(RR-12):1, 1999.

28. Coulepis AG, Locarnini SA, Lehmann NI, Gust ID: Detection of HAV in feces. J Infect Dis 141:151, 1980.

29. Rosenblum LS, Villarino ME, Nainan OV, et al: Hepatitis A outbreak in a neonatal intensive care unit: Risk factors for transmission and evidence of prolonged viral excretion among preterm infants. J Infect Dis 164:476, 1991.

30. Francis T Jr, Frisch AW, Quilligan JJ: Demonstration of infectious hepatitis virus in presymptomatic period after transfer by transfusion. Proc Soc Exp Biol Med 61:276, 1946.

31. Harden AG, Barondess JA, Parker B: Transmission of infectious hepatitis by transfusion of whole blood. N Engl J Med 253:923, 1955.

32. Schulman AN, Dienstag JL, Jackson DR, et al: Hepatitis A antigen particles in liver, bile and stool of chimpanzees. J Infect Dis 134:80, 1976.

33. Giles JP, Liebhaber H, Krugman S, Lattimer C: Early viremia and viruria in infectious hepatitis. Virology 24:107, 1964.

34. Findlay GM: Infective hepatitis in West Africa: 1. Mon Bull Ministry Health 7:2, 1948.

35. Cohen JI, Feinstone S, Purcell RH: Hepatitis A virus infection in a chimpanzee: Duration of viremia and detection of virus in saliva and throat swabs. J Infect Dis 160:887, 1989.

36. Berge JJ, Drennan D, Jacobs J, et al: The cost of hepatitis A infections in American adolescents and adults in 1997. Hepatology 31:469, 2000.

37. Gordon SC, Reddy KR, Schiff ER: Prolonged intrahepatic cholestasis secondary to acute hepatitis A. Ann Intern Med 101:635, 1984.

38. Sjogren MH, Tanno H, Fay O, et al: Hepatitis A virus in stool during clinical relapse. Ann Intern Med 106:221, 1987.

39. William R: Classification, etiology and considerations of outcome in acute liver failure. Semin Liver Dis 16:343, 1996.

40. Chadha MS, Walimbe AM, Chobe LP, Arankalle VA: Comparison of etiology of sporadic acute and fulminant viral hepatitis in hospitalized patients in Pune, India during 1978-81 and 1994-97. Indian J Gastroenterol 22:11, 2003.

41. Brown GR, Persley K: Hepatitis A epidemic in the elderly. South Med J 95:826, 2002.

42. Willner IR, Mark DU, Howard SC, et al: Serious hepatitis A: An analysis of patients hospitalized during an urban epidemic in the United States. Ann Intern Med 128:111, 1998.

43. Ostapowicz G, Fontana R, Schiedt FV, et al: Results of a prospective study of acute liver failure at 17 tertiary care centers in the United States. Ann Intern Med 137:947, 2002.

44. Schiodt FV, Atillasoy E, Shakill AO, et al: Etiology and outcome for 295 patients with acute liver failure in the United States. Liver Transpl Surg. 5:29, 1999.

45. Vento S, Cainelli F: Is there a role for viruses triggering autoimmune hepatitis? Autoimmun Rev 3:61, 2004.

46. Tagle Arrospide M, Leon Barua R: Viral hepatitis A as a triggering agent of autoimmune hepatitis report of a case and review of literature. Rev Gastroenterol Peru 23:134, 2003.

47. Liaw YF, Yang CY, Chu CM, Huang MJ: Appearance and persistence of hepatitis A IgM antibody in acute clinical hepatitis A observed in an outbreak. Infection 14:156, 1986.

48. Kao HW, Ashcavai M, Redeker AG: The persistence of hepatitis A IgM antibody after acute clinical hepatitis A. Hepatology 4:933, 1984.

49. Yotsuyanagi H, Iino S, Koike K, et al: Duration of viremia in human hepatitis A viral infection as determined by polymerase chain reaction. J Med Virol 40:35, 1993.

50. Mannucci PM, Gdovin S, Gringeri A, et al: Transmission of hepatitis A to patients with hemophilia by factor VIII concentrates treated with organic solvent and detergent to inactivate viruses. Ann Intern Med 120:1, 1994.

51. Rezende G, Roque-Alsonso M, Samuel D et al: Viral and clinical factors associated with fulminant course of hepatitis A infection. Hepatology 38:613, 2003.

52. Fujiwara K, Yokosuka O, Imazeki F, et al: Analysis of the genotype-determining region of hepatitis A viral RNA in relation to disease severities. Hepatol Res 25:124, 2003.

53. Leentvaar-Kuijpers A, Coutinho RA, Brulein V, Safary A: Simultaneous passive and active immunization against hepatitis A. Vaccine 10:S138, 1992.

54. Andre FE, D'Hondt E, Delem A, Safary A: Clinical assessment of the safety and efficacy of an inactivated hepatitis A vaccine. Vaccine 10 (Suppl 1):S160, 1992.

55. Provost PJ, Hughes JN, Miller WJ, et al: An inactivated hepatitis A viral vaccine of cell culture origin. J Med Virol 19:23, 1986.

56. Van Damme P, Thoelen S, Cramm K, et al: Inactivated hepatitis A vaccine: Reactogenicity, immunogenicity, and long-term antibody persistence. J Med Virol 44:446, 1994.

57. FDA approval for a combined hepatitis A and B vaccine. MMWR Morbid Mortal Wkly Rep September 21, 50:806, 2001.

58. Reiss G, Keeffe EB: Review article: Hepatitis vaccination in patients with chronic liver disease. Aliment Pharmacol Ther 19:715, 2004.

59. Aeslan M, Wiesner RH, Poterucha JJ, Zein NN: Safety and efficacy of hepatitis A vaccination in liver transplantation recipients. Transplantation 72:272, 2001.

60. Myers RP, Gregor JC, Marotta P: The cost-effectiveness of hepatitis A vaccination in patients with chronic hepatitis C. Hepatology 31:834, 2000.

61. Jacobs RJ, Koff, RS: Cost-effectiveness of hepatitis A vaccination in patients with chronic hepatitis C. Hepatology 32:873, 2000.

62. Jacobs RJ, Koff RS, Meyerhoff AS: The cost-effectiveness of vaccinating chronic hepatitis C patients against hepatitis A. Am J Gastroenterol 97:427, 2002.

63. Arguedas MR, Heudebert GR, Fallon MB, Stinnett AA: The cost-effectiveness of hepatitis A vaccination in patients with chronic hepatitis C viral infection in the United States. Am J Gastroenterol 97:721, 2002.

64. Rosenthal P: Cost-effectiveness of hepatitis A vaccination in children, adolescents and adults. Hepatology 37:44, 2003.

CHAPTER
75 Hepatitis B and D

Robert Perrillo and Satheesh Nair

HEPATITIS B

An estimated 400 million persons are carriers of hepatitis B virus (HBV) in the world today, of which 75% reside in Asia and the Western Pacific. Effective vaccines against HBV have been available for more than 20 years, but perinatal and early life exposures continue to be major sources of infection in high–prevalence areas. High-risk behaviors such as promiscuous heterosexual contact and injection drug use account for many new cases in young adults. Fulminant acute hepatitis B accounts for several hundred deaths per year in the United States, and chronic HBV infection accounts for 1 million deaths worldwide each year from complications of end-stage liver disease, including hepatocellular carcinoma (HCC). Hepatitis B is the chief cause of cirrhosis and HCC in the world today, and nationwide vaccination has been shown to greatly diminish the number of new cases of infection and HCC in Taiwanese children.[1] Universal hepatitis B vaccination is likely to have the greatest impact on liver disease–related mortality in future generations.

EPIDEMIOLOGY

Geographic Distribution and Sources of Exposure

The prevalence of hepatitis B varies markedly around the world. In highly endemic regions, such as Southeast Asia (excluding Japan), China, and much of Africa, 8% or more of the population are chronic HBV carriers, and the lifetime risk of infection varies from 60% to 80%.[2,3] In these areas, perinatal transmission and horizontal spread among children are the major sources of infection. Nearly one half of the HBV carriers in the world reside in these highly endemic areas.[4] Areas of intermediate risk include parts of Southern and Eastern Europe, the Middle East, Japan, the Indian subcontinent, much of the former Soviet Union, and Northern Africa. In intermediate-risk areas, the lifetime risk of infection is between 20% and 60%. Persons of all age groups are infected, but as in high-risk areas, most infections occur during infancy or early childhood. Regions of low prevalence are North America, Western Europe, certain parts of South America, and Australia. In these areas, the lifetime risk of HBV infection is less than 20%, and transmission is primarily horizontal (i.e., between young adults). Sexual transmission is the main mode of transmission in Europe and North America, and injection drug use is a major contributor to new cases as well.[5]

Transmission of infection from an HBV carrier mother to her neonate accounts for the majority of new infections in the world today. Sixty percent to 90% of hepatitis B surface antigen (HBsAg)–positive mothers who are hepatitis B e antigen (HBeAg)–positive transmit the disease to their offspring, whereas mothers who are positive for antibody to HBeAg (anti-HBe) do so less frequently (15% to 20%).[6] Other less common sources of infection are household contact with an HBV carrier,[7] hemodialysis,[8] exposure to infected health care workers,[9] tattooing, body piercing,[10] artificial insemination,[11] and receipt of blood products or organs.[12] Since routine screening of the blood supply was implemented in the early 1970s, transfusion-associated hepatitis B has become rare in the United States. Hepatitis B can be transmitted by blood that tests negative for HBsAg but positive for antibody to hepatitis B core antigen (anti-HBc) because of low levels of circulating HBV DNA in such blood.[13] HBsAg-negative blood that is positive for anti-HBc is excluded from the donor pool in the United States and many countries around the world. In 0% to 30% of persons who are seropositive for anti-HBc alone, HBV DNA is detectable in serum by polymerase chain reaction (PCR) testing.[14]

HBV is transmitted efficiently by percutaneous and mucous membrane exposure to infectious body fluids. The virus is 100 times as infectious as human immunodeficiency virus (HIV) and 10 times as infectious as hepatitis C virus (HCV). HBeAg seropositivity indicates a higher risk of transmission from mother to child, after needlestick exposure, and in the setting of household contact.[6,7,15] HBV DNA has been detected by sensitive techniques such as PCR testing in most body fluids, except for stool that has not been contaminated with blood. Although HBV replicates primarily in hepatocytes, the presence of replicative intermediates and virally encoded proteins in other sites, such as the adrenal gland, testis, colon, nerve ganglia, and skin, suggests that there is a vast extrahepatic reservoir for infectious virus.[16] Small amounts of HBV DNA have been demonstrated in peripheral mononuclear cells and liver tissue years after apparent resolution of chronic infection.[17,18] Extrahepatic localization of low levels of replicating virus explains the relatively high rate of transmission of infection from anti-HBc–positive organ donors.[19]

Rates of Infection in the United States

The incidence of hepatitis B has been declining in the United States over the past decade because of vaccination programs, changes in sexual lifestyle, refinements in blood screening procedures, and the availability of virus-inactivated blood components (Fig. 75–1).[20] Most striking has been the decrease among children and health care workers, groups with the highest rates of vaccination. Nonetheless, an estimated 78,000 new HBV infections occurred in 2001, with the highest incidence rates among sexually active young adults (20 to 29 years old) and higher rates occurring among black and Hispanic persons than in white persons.[21] Since 1995, approximately 40% of cases of acute hepatitis B reported to the Centers for Disease Control and Prevention (CDC) were caused by intimate contact among heterosexuals, 15% to 20% were related to intravenous drug use, and 12% occurred in men who have sex with men. No identifiable source of exposure was demonstrated in approximately 15% of cases. Nearly one third of prison inmates have been infected with hepatitis B, and 2% are chronically infected.

According to the third National Health and Nutrition Examination Survey (1988-1994), one or more serologic markers of HBV infection were demonstrated in 4.9% of the U.S. population, and the prevalence of chronic infection was 0.2%.[22] Traditional estimates based on the results of blood donation screening in the late 1970s also indicated a prevalence rate for chronic infection of 0.2% to 0.4% in the United States. Although traditional estimates are that the number of HBV carriers in the United States is between 1.25 and 1.5 million, this figure is likely to be a serious underestimate because of changing immigration patterns and underrepresentation of certain minority groups in field surveys. For example, there are 11 million Asians in the United States and even a conservative estimate that the prevalence in this group is 5% would raise the overall number of HBV carriers in the United States by more than 500,000.

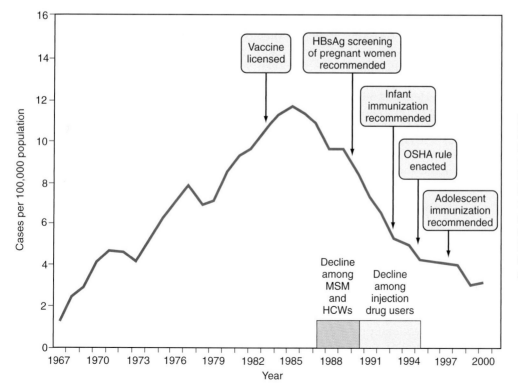

Figure 75–1 Incidence of acute hepatitis B infection in the United States, 1967–2000. Incidence rates for HBV infection have been declining, most notably in health care workers and in neonates. HBsAg, hepatitis B surface antigen; HCWs, health care workers; MSM, men who have sex with men; OSHA, Occupational Safety and Health Administration.

CLINICAL OUTCOMES

Definitions

In common usage, the term *HBV carrier* has often been used to refer to persons persistently infected with HBV who have normal serum aminotransferase levels. (They are sometimes inappropriately referred to as "healthy" HBV carriers.) Because the nomenclature is potentially confusing, the proposal has been made that the carrier state be categorized as inactive or active. *Inactive carriers* are patients who have evidence of HBV replication on a PCR-based assay only (but not with a less sensitive non–PCR-based assay) and normal or only mildly elevated serum aminotransferase values (see later).[23] Long-term follow-up of inactive carriers suggests that the majority of these patients do not have progressive liver disease and do not experience complications. However, some of these patients ultimately have one or more episodes of reactivated hepatitis in which the levels of viremia and serum aminotransferase activity increase. Also, some patients with the inactive carrier state may demonstrate HCC. *Active carriers*, on the other hand, have evidence of HBV replication on non–PCR-based assays for HBV DNA, intermittently or persistently elevated serum aminotransferase levels, and evidence of chronic hepatitis in a liver biopsy specimen.

Clinical Sequelae of Acute Hepatitis B Virus Infection

The age at which a person becomes infected with HBV is a principal determinant of the clinical outcome. HBV infection in adults with intact immune systems is likely to cause clinically apparent acute hepatitis B; only 1% to 5% of these persons become chronically infected.[5] By contrast, as many as 95% of infected neonates become chronic HBV carriers because of immunologic tolerance to the virus.

In adults, fulminant liver failure due to acute hepatitis B occurs in less than 1% of cases, but this group still accounts for 5% of all cases of acute liver failure and approximately 400 deaths annually in the United States.[24] Rapid viral elimination may result in clearance of HBsAg from serum by the time of initial presentation. In these cases, the accurate diagnosis of fulminant hepatitis B may require testing with IgM anti-HBc—immunoglobulin (Ig) M antibody to hepatitis B core antigen (HBcAg) (see section on serologic markers of infection).[25] The rate of spontaneous survival in acute liver failure due to hepatitis B is only approximately 20%.[26] Liver transplantation has resulted in survival rates of 50% to 60%. Recurrent disease in the allograft is now uncommon because of administration of hepatitis B immune globulin (HBIG) and antiviral therapy (see later).

Clinical Sequelae of Chronic Hepatitis B Virus Infection

Chronic hepatitis B develops in 2% to 5% of persons who acquire HBV infection in adulthood. Progressive liver disease (including cirrhosis and HCC) can be expected to develop in one quarter to one third of people chronically infected with HBV. An estimated 15% to 25% of patients older than 40 years with chronic HBV infection die of liver-related causes.

The presence of active viral replication and long-standing necroinflammatory liver disease due to HBV strongly influences the rate of progression to cirrhosis. The major determinant of survival is the extent of the liver disease when the patient first comes to medical attention.[27] Cirrhosis is associated with decreased survival and a higher frequency of HCC. Five- and 20-year survival rates of 55% and 25%, respectively, have been reported in patients with cirrhosis at presentation, whereas rates of 97% and 63%, respectively, have been reported for those with mild disease.[28,29] Survival rates differ most dramatically between patients with compensated and decompensated cirrhosis. In one study, an 84% 5-year survival rate was reported for patients with compensated HBV-related cirrhosis, compared with 14% for patients with ascites, jaundice, encephalopathy, or a history of variceal bleeding.[30] Multivariate analyses in several large cohort studies have identified age, ascites, hyperbilirubinemia, and other features of advanced liver disease as correlating independently with survival in patients with cirrhosis. Interferon-induced clearance of HBeAg (see later) has been associated with prolongation of survival without complications or the need for liver transplantation.[31]

MOLECULAR BIOLOGY OF THE HEPATITIS B VIRUS

HBV is a small DNA virus that belongs to the Hepadnaviridae family. Other members of this virus family are human HBV–like agents that infect the woodchuck, ground and tree squirrels, woolly monkey, crane, heron, Ross goose, and duck. HBV is a small (3.2-kilobase [kb]) virus with a DNA genome that has a relaxed, circular, partially double-stranded configuration (Fig. 75–2). The genome is composed of four open reading frames (ORFs) and has a compact design in which several genes overlap and use the same DNA to encode different viral proteins.[32] The four viral genes are the core, surface, X, and polymerase genes. The core gene encodes the core nucleocapsid protein, which is important in viral packaging and production of HBeAg. The surface gene encodes the pre-S1, pre-S2, and S proteins (large [L], middle [M], and small [S] surface proteins, respectively). The X gene encodes the X protein, which has transactivating properties and may be important in hepatic carcinogenesis. The polymerase gene has a large ORF (approximately 800 amino acids) and overlaps the entire length of the surface ORF. It encodes a large protein with functions that are critical for packaging and DNA replication (including priming, RNA- and DNA-dependent DNA polymerase, and RNase H activities).

Although HBV is a DNA virus, replication occurs through an RNA intermediate and requires an active viral reverse transcriptase/polymerase enzyme. Because the reverse transcriptase lacks a proofreading function, the mutation rate is higher for HBV than for other DNA viruses (an estimated 10^{10}-10^{11} point mutations per day).[33] Complete HBV genomic sequencing has identified a large number of mutations within the HBV genome,

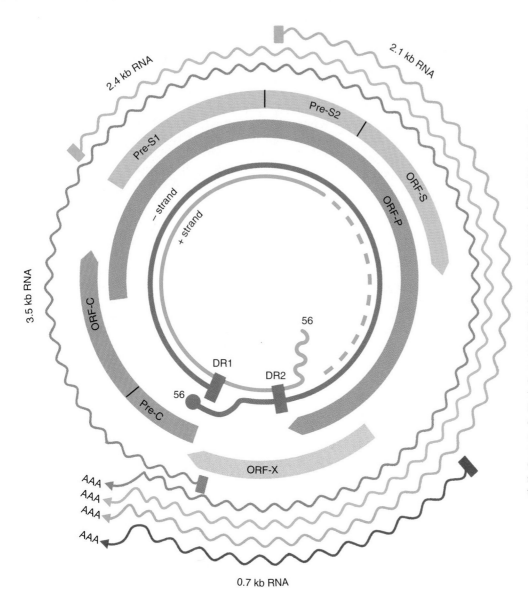

Figure 75–2 Overlapping open reading frames (ORFs) of the hepatitis B virus (HBV) genome and major transcripts. The genome is partially double stranded with four overlapping open reading frames, or genes. The S gene encodes the viral surface envelope proteins (HBsAg) and is composed of the pre-S1, pre-S2, and S regions. The core gene consists of the precore and core regions, which give rise to the hepatitis B e antigen (HBeAg) and core protein, respectively. The polymerase gene overlaps the entire S gene, and mutations in this region may in theory give rise to changes in the HBsAg protein that affect neutralization by antibody to HBsAg. The fourth gene codes for an incompletely understood protein, HBX. Two 11–base-pair direct repeats (DR1 and DR2) are required for strand-specific HBV DNA synthesis during viral replication.

many of which are silent or do not alter the amino acid sequence of encoded proteins. Because of genomic overlap, however, some of the silent mutations in one ORF (for example, the polymerase gene) may result in an amino acid substitution in an overlapping ORF (surface gene), although with currently uncertain clinical implications.

Figure 75–3 illustrates the life cycle of HBV. The initial phase of hepadnaviral infection involves the attachment of mature virions to host cell membranes. The human receptor for HBV remains unknown. Entry of the virus results from fusion of the viral and host membranes as the nucleocapsid is released into the cytoplasm. Mechanisms of intracellular transport of viral genome into the nucleus are poorly understood, but the first step in genomic replication involves conversion of the relaxed circular form of HBV DNA into a double-stranded, covalently closed circular form (cccDNA).[34] The cccDNA, which serves as the template for viral transcription, is the major form of viral DNA in the nucleus of infected hepatocytes. Subgenomic (0.7-2.4 kb) and pregenomic (3.5 kb)

RNA molecules are transcribed from this template. The L protein is translated from the 2.4-kb RNA, the M and S proteins from the 2.1-kb RNA, and the X protein from the 0.7-kb transcript. The pregenomic RNA serves as the template for reverse transcription as well as the messenger RNA (mRNA) for translation of the core and polymerase proteins; the precore RNA codes for the precore gene product.

HBV replication begins with encapsidation of the pregenomic RNA through complex interactions between host and viral proteins. HBV DNA polymerase reverse-transcribes the pregenomic RNA into a negative-strand HBV DNA, which in turn serves as the template for positive-strand synthesis to form a partially double-stranded genome. Concurrent with HBV DNA synthesis, the nucleocapsid undergoes maturation and, through a yet incompletely understood mechanism, interacts with the S protein to initiate viral assembly in the endoplasmic reticulum.

S protein is synthesized in the endoplasmic reticulum, where monomer aggregates that exclude host membrane

Figure 75–3 Life cycle of the hepatitis B virus. The receptor for viral entry has not been identified. Once inside the hepatocyte, the virus undergoes uncoating, and nuclear entry of the HBV genome occurs, followed by repair of the single-stranded DNA strand and formation of the covalently closed circular (ccc) DNA template. Viral transcripts are formed for the hepatitis B surface antigen (HBsAg), DNA polymerase, X protein, and RNA pregenome; the pregenome and polymerase are incorporated into the maturing nucleocapsid. The surface protein enveloping process occurs in the endoplasmic reticulum. Some of the nonenveloped nucleocapsid recirculates back to the nucleus, and the cycle begins again. Excess tubular and spherical forms of HBsAg are secreted in great abundance.

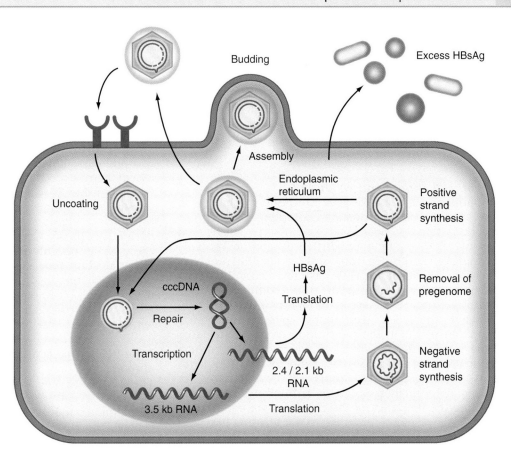

proteins subsequently bud into the lumen as subviral particles. Once formed, HBsAg undergoes glycosylation in the endoplasmic reticulum and the Golgi apparatus. Noninfectious subviral particles (spherical and filamentous forms of HBsAg) are secreted in great abundance when compared with mature virions.

Hepatitis B Virus Genotypes

A genetic classification based on comparisons of complete genomes has demonstrated eight genotypes of HBV, designated A through H (Table 75–1).[35] Several methods have been used for HBV genotyping, including a commercially available line probe assay. Genotypic differences are based on an intergroup divergence of 8% or more in the complete nucleotide sequence. Genotype A is the predominant genotype in northern Europe and the United States. Genotypes B and C are confined to populations in eastern Asia and the Far East, but changes in immigration patterns have resulted in an influx of Asian HBsAg carriers with these genotypes into the United States.[36] Genotype D is found worldwide but is especially prevalent in the Mediterranean area, Middle East, and south Asia. Genotype E is indigenous to western sub-Saharan areas, and genotype F prevails in Central America. Cases of genotype G have been reported in the United States and France. A newly defined genotype, H, has been described in Mexico.

Clinical associations appear to exist with the various genotypes (see Table 75–1). Currently, the strongest clinical associations appear to be that (1) HBeAg seroconversion occurs earlier in patients with genotype B than in those with genotype C, and (2) response to therapy with

Table 75–1 Hepatitis B Genotypes and Their Possible Clinical Associations

Eight Well-Characterized Genotypes (A to H)
Different geographic distributions:
  A: Northwestern Europe, North America, Central Africa
  B: Southeast Asia, including China, Japan and Taiwan (prevalence is increasing in North America)
  C: Southeast Asia (prevalence is increasing in North America)
  D: Southern Europe, Middle East, India
  E: West Africa
  F: Central and South America, American natives, Polynesia
  G: USA, France
  H: Central and South America
Proposed Clinical Associations
Time to HBeAg seroconversion and probability of HBsAg loss: B < C
Response to treatment with interferon alfa: A > B ≥ C > D
Precore/core promoter mutant frequency: precore mutation not selected with A and F
Liver disease activity and risk of progression: B < C
Evolution to chronic liver disease: A < D
Hepatocellular carcinoma risk: B > C in younger age group in Taiwan but B < C in older age group in Japan

HBeAg, hepatitis B e antigen; HBsAg, hepatitis B surface antigen; HBV, hepatitis B virus.

interferon is more common in patients with genotype A than in patients with genotype D.[37] Genotyping also has implications for the prevalence of precore and core mutations (see later) and may have an effect on the frequency of HCC.

Mutations of the Hepatitis B Virus Genome

The inherent mutability of HBV and high production rate of the virus (10^{12}-10^{13} virions per day) could in theory account for all possible single-base mutations in the viral genome made daily. The vast majority of mutations identified by comparing nucleotide sequences with those of wild-type HBV are silent or do not alter the amino acid sequence in a particular ORF. Some mutations have potentially important disease associations.

Hepatitis B Surface Antigen Mutants

Mutations in the surface gene can result in changes in the antibody-binding domain. Accordingly, both virus neutralization by polyclonal antibody to HBsAg and testing for HBsAg by methods that depend on antibody binding can be affected. Large-scale vaccination programs in regions endemic for HBV have revealed a 2% to 3% frequency of vaccine escape mutants resulting from alterations in the "a" determinant of the HBsAg protein, which is the major neutralizable epitope. The typical mutation results in the substitution of glycine for arginine at amino acid position 145, which prevents binding of neutralizing antibodies (i.e., antibody to HBsAg [anti-HBs]). The clinical significance of these mutants for neonatal vaccination programs is highly controversial, because the frequency of these variants among mothers whose infants show response to vaccination has been found to be similar to that of mothers whose infants show no response.[38] The "a" determinant mutants also are proposed to have clinical relevance after liver transplantation for hepatitis B. As many as 50% of patients in whom recurrent HBV infection develops despite the use of HBIG have been shown to have these escape mutants, and the rate at which the mutations are detected appears to correlate with the length of time over which HBIG is repeatedly administered.[39]

Mutations in the Precore, Basal Core Promoter, and Core Genes

Mutations in the precore and basal core promoter regions of the HBV genome can influence the production of HBeAg. A precore mutation results in a stop codon at nucleotide 1896 that abolishes the synthesis of HBeAg,[40] whereas mutations in the basal core promoter at nucleotides 1762 and 1764 decrease HBeAg synthesis by approximately 70% while maintaining pregenomic RNA levels.[41] Both types of mutations have been associated with severe or fulminant hepatitis, which has been attributed to the loss of the immune-tolerizing effects of HBeAg antigen (see later). These two types of HBV mutants have been described in the same patients and are particularly common in Asian and European patients with chronic hepatitis B.[42] A large serosurvey of HBV carriers residing in the United States has found that precore and core promoter mutations are common (frequency 27% and 44%, respectively), depending on the ethnicity and places of birth of the patients. Both mutant forms of HBV were observed to occur far more commonly in HBeAg-negative patients (precore mutation in 38% of HBeAg-negative versus 9% of HBeAg-positive patients; core promoter in 51% versus 36%).[43] In addition to these mutations, upstream mutations in the core gene can influence immunologic responses to HBV. Core gene mutations have been shown to block recognition of HBV by cytotoxic T lymphocytes (CTLs), a key mode of viral clearance. Therefore, the mutations contribute to HBV immune escape and possibly influence the response to interferon.[44,45] Core gene mutations within the immunodominant epitopes of the HBV nucleocapsid also can affect CD4+ T-cell reactivity.[46]

In patients with perinatally acquired chronic hepatitis B, a prolonged immune tolerant phase with minimal to absent hepatic necroinflammatory activity is typically seen for the first 20 to 30 years of HBV infection. Sequencing studies have shown stable core gene sequences during this phase.[47] Precore mutations are also uncommon during this phase. Core gene mutations become more common as patients pass from the immune tolerant phase, at which time a growing number of mutations are observed in the region of the core gene that includes many B and T cell epitopes. Both precore stop codon mutants and core gene mutants have been associated with a poor response to interferon therapy.

Hepatitis B Virus DNA Polymerase Mutants

The polymerase gene product is needed for encapsidation of viral RNA into core particles and conversion of the pregenomic viral RNA into genomic viral DNA. In general, the HBV reverse transcriptase function of the polymerase gene is highly conserved, because major mutations that impair the efficiency of viral replication lead to selection pressure against such variant forms. After prolonged exposure to lamivudine, a nucleoside analog that inhibits HBV DNA polymerase (see later), nucleotide substitutions have been observed in region B (the template-binding site of the polymerase) and region C (the catalytic site of the polymerase). These mutants are referred to collectively as YMDD mutants; the letters stand for the amino acid residues (Y = tyrosine, M = methionine, D = aspartate) in the catalytic domain. The major site of mutation is the methionine residue in the YMDD amino acid motif. Two types of mutations occur at nucleotide position 204 (formerly codon 552) of region C that result in substitution of the amino acid methionine for either isoleucine or valine (designated M204I or M204V, respectively). The M204V mutation tends to occur in conjunction with a mutation in domain B that results in substitution of leucine with methionine (L180M). The M204I mutation or the combined M204V-L180M mutations result in marked resistance to the effect of lamivudine (>10,000-fold reduction in susceptibility).

The inherent mutability of HBV suggests that single and double polymerase mutations of this type preexist in patients and are selected during treatment with lamivudine. Mutations at these sites become more common as the duration of treatment increases; they are found in approximately 15% to 20% of patients after 1 year of treatment, in 30% to 40% after 2 years, in 50% after 3 years, and in more than 65% after 4 years.[48] These mutant viruses appear to be less replication fit, and although patients with these mutants have a lower chance of HBeAg seroconversion than patients infected with wild-type HBV, they may continue to exhibit clinical improvement for a variable period. Persistent infection with the mutant virus, however, is ultimately associated with progression of the disease in many patients and blunting of the histologic response to antiviral therapy.[49] Severe flares of hepatitis have been reported after the emergence of lamivudine-resistant HBV,[50] and acquisition of these mutants may lead to rapidly progressive liver disease after liver transplantation.[51]

PATHOGENESIS

HBV is generally not a cytopathic virus, and the severity of the liver disease is considered to be related to the intensity of host immunologic response to the virus. Whereas both humoral and cellular immune responses are needed for effective viral clearance, the cellular immune response appears to be the arm involved principally in disease pathogenesis. Immunologic response to HBV encompasses both an innate, or nonspecific, response (for example, natural killer cells and interferons) and an adaptive immune response, including antibodies to viral antigens, human leukocyte antigen (HLA) class II–restricted CD4+ T cells, and HLA class I–restricted CD8+ CTLs.[52] Induction of the antigen-specific T cell response is thought to occur in lymphoid organs, where the host T cells encounter viral peptide antigens (or epitopes) that are presented by antigen-presenting cells such as dendritic cells, B cells, and macrophages. This process results in the maturation and expansion of T cells specific for these viral epitopes and is followed by their migration to the liver, where they perform their effector function.

During acute HBV infection, most HBV DNA molecules are cleared rapidly from the liver via noncytopathic mechanisms mediated by cytokines that are released initially by cells of the innate immune system[53] and later by liver-infiltrating HBV-specific CD8+ cells. Cell-mediated immune responses are efficient in self-limited infection, because the responses are vigorous, multispecific, and helper T cell type 1 (T_H1) oriented. Persons with chronic HBV infection, in contrast, exhibit infrequent, narrowly focused, and weak HBV-specific T-cell responses.[54] In chronic hepatitis B, the majority of mononuclear cells in liver infiltrates of patients with chronic hepatitis B at any given time are non–antigen-specific.[55]

CD8+ CTLs are thought to contribute to the disease process in the liver and result in apoptosis of infected hepatocytes. To be recognized by the CD8+ CTLs, targeted hepatocytes must present viral epitopes as short peptides that have been endogenously processed and fit within the peptide-binding groove of the class I major histocompatibility complex (MHC) molecules.[56] The binding of the CTL T-cell receptor (TCR) to the peptide-MHC complex on the hepatocyte surface can then result in the direct killing of the infected cell and release of potent antiviral cytokines by the activated CTL.[57] Recognition by MHC class II–restricted CD4+ T_H cells requires the appropriate presentation of viral peptides in the context of class II MHC molecules. The CD4+ cells produce antiviral cytokines and provide help in neutralizing antibody production. Antibody neutralization limits spread during primary infection and serves an important role in preventing reinfection.

NATURAL HISTORY

Four phases of hepatitis B infection have been described: immune tolerance, immune clearance, low-level replication or nonreplication phase (also referred to as the inactive carrier stage), and reactivation phase (Fig. 75–4). Patients who acquire the infection in the perinatal period often have high serum levels of HBV DNA without biochemical evidence of active hepatitis and are considered to be immunotolerant to HBV. When followed longitudinally, many of these patients ultimately exhibit elevated serum aminotransferase levels in association with histologic evidence of chronic hepatitis. The trigger mechanisms for this apparent change in tolerance are poorly understood but likely reflect changes in the immune reactivity of the host.

Experiments in transgenic mice suggest that HBeAg induces a state of immunologic tolerance to HBV in neonates.[58] Perinatal transmission of HBeAg has been considered to be a potential mechanism for the immunologically tolerant state. As patients enter the immune clearance phase, HBV DNA concentrations diminish, serum alanine aminotransferase (ALT) levels rise, and histologic activity, reflecting immune-mediated lysis of infected hepatocytes, increases. The duration of this second phase varies, often lasting many years.

The third phase (low-level or no replication) occurs after seroconversion from HBeAg to anti-HBe and is usually preceded by a marked reduction in serum HBV DNA to levels that are detectable only by PCR, followed by normalization of serum ALT levels and resolution of liver necroinflammation. Also called the inactive carrier stage, this phase may last a lifetime, but a proportion of patients ultimately undergo spontaneous or immunosuppression-mediated reactivation of HBV replication with reappearance of high levels of HBV DNA in serum, with or without HBeAg seroreversion and a rise in serum ALT levels. For unclear reasons, precore or core promoter mutants that prevent or down-regulate HBeAg production may be selected during or after HBeAg seroconversion.[59]

A key event in the natural history of HBeAg-positive chronic hepatitis is seroconversion of HBeAg to anti-HBe, which is associated with marked reduction in HBV replication and biochemical and histologic remission in the majority of patients. Regression of fibrosis occurs gradually months to year after HBeAg seroconversion.[60] Most studies have found that the mean annual rate of spontaneous HBeAg seroconversion ranges from 8% to 15% in children or adults with serum ALT elevations.

Longitudinal studies of untreated patients with predominantly HBeAg-positive chronic hepatitis B have shown that the frequency of development of cirrhosis ranges from 2 to 5 per 100 person-years, and the 5-year cumulative frequency of progression to cirrhosis from 8% to 20%.[61] The rate of cirrhosis has been suggested to be higher in HBeAg-negative patients than in HBeAg-positive patients. Risk factors for the development of cirrhosis have been identified; of these, older age, the stage of fibrosis at presentation, and ongoing HBV replication with persistent or intermittent detection of HBV DNA by a non-PCR-based assay are perhaps the most important clinically. Combined infection with hepatitis

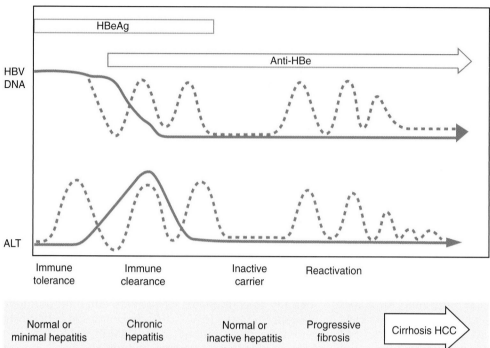

Figure 75–4   Natural evolution and stages of chronic hepatitis B virus (HBV) infection. In some patients, hepatitis B e antigen (HBeAg) seroconversion (to antibody to HBeAg, anti-HBe) is followed by the selection of precore and/or core promoter mutant HBV and continuing chronic hepatitis. Hepatocellular carcinoma (HCC) may complicate cirrhosis or the inactive carrier state. ALT, alanine aminotransferase.

D virus (HDV), hepatitis C virus (HCV), or human immunodeficiency virus (HIV) and concomitant alcohol abuse have also been linked to a higher rate of development of cirrhosis.

Once cirrhosis develops, two major complications may occur: hepatic decompensation and HCC. In a large European cohort with HBV-related compensated cirrhosis, the 5-year cumulative frequency of hepatic decompensation was 16%, and the incidence per 100 person-years was 3.3.[62] Similar rates have been reported in Asians. The cumulative 5-year frequency of HCC varies from 9% to 14%.[62] Factors associated with an increased risk of HCC include male gender, age more than 45 years, having a first-degree relative with HCC, the presence of cirrhosis, HBeAg positivity, and reversion from anti-HBe to HBeAg positivity.[63] HBsAg-positive persons with none of the identified risk factors can still have HCC, but less frequently. In addition, HCC has been described in persons who lose HBsAg. Recommendations about ultrasonography and alpha-fetoprotein screening for HCC are controversial, but screening is generally recommended in patients with cirrhosis and in all HBsAg carriers older than 40 years in whom the likely route of transmission has been perinatal or early childhood exposure; some authorities recommend screening after age 30 years when perinatal acquisition is suspected (see Chapter 91).

CLINICAL FEATURES

Acute Hepatitis B

The incubation period of acute hepatitis B varies from a few weeks to 6 months (average, 60 to 90 days), depending on the amount of replicating virus in the inoculum.

The disease may be more severe in patients coinfected with other hepatitis viruses and in those with established underlying liver disease.[64] Abstention from alcohol is usually recommended, but the chance of an uneventful recovery does not appear to be affected by the consumption of moderate amounts of alcohol (20 to 30 g daily) during the convalescent phase.[65] Acute infections are heralded by a serum sickness–like prodrome of fever, arthralgias/arthritis, and rash, which is most commonly maculopapular or urticarial, in 10% to 20% of patients. This prodrome results from circulating HBsAg–anti-HBs complexes that activate complement and are deposited in the synovium and walls of cutaneous blood vessels.[66] These features generally abate before the manifestations of liver disease and peak serum aminotransferase elevations are observed. Jaundice develops in only about 30% of patients.

Clinical symptoms and jaundice generally disappear after 1 to 3 months, but some patients have prolonged fatigue even after serum ALT levels return to normal. In general, elevated serum ALT levels and serum HBsAg titers decline and disappear together, and in approximately 80% of cases, HBsAg disappears by 12 weeks after the onset of illness.[67] In 5% to 10% of cases, HBsAg is cleared early and is no longer detectable by the time the patient first presents to a healthcare provider. Persistence of HBsAg after six months implies development of a carrier state, with only a small likelihood of recovery during the next 6 to 12 months. Delayed clearance of HBsAg has been reported to be preceded by a decline in HBsAg titers.[68]

Serum aminotransferase levels of 1000 to 2000 U/L are typical, with ALT being higher than aspartate aminotransferase (AST) levels. In patients with icteric hepatitis, the rise in serum bilirubin levels often lags behind that in ALT levels. The peak ALT level does not correlate with prognosis, and the prothrombin time is the best indicator of prognosis.

After clinical recovery from acute hepatitis B and HBsAg seroconversion, HBV DNA often remains detectable in serum as determined by a PCR assay (see later discussion of serologic diagnosis). After resolution of acute hepatitis, the numbers of HBV-specific CD4+ and CD8+ cells in blood and liver decrease rapidly. Nonetheless, T-cell responsiveness remains high on reencounter with HBV antigens, indicating that traces of virus can maintain the CTL response indefinitely after clinical recovery, thereby exerting control over the virus and preventing reactivated infection.[52,69]

Fulminant hepatitis occurs in less than 1% of cases (see Chapter 90). Fulminant hepatitis B generally occurs within 4 weeks of the onset of symptoms and is associated with encephalopathy, multiorgan failure, and a high mortality rate (>80%) if not treated by liver transplantation. Patients older than 40 years appear to be more susceptible than younger persons to "late-onset liver failure," in which encephalopathy, renal dysfunction, and other extrahepatic complications of severe liver insufficiency become manifest over the course of several months.[70] The pathogenic mechanisms of fulminant hepatitis are poorly understood but are presumed to involve massive immune-mediated lysis of infected hepatocytes. This proposed mechanism may explain why many patients with fulminant hepatitis B have no evidence of HBV replication in serum at presentation.

Chronic Hepatitis B

A history of acute or symptomatic hepatitis is often lacking in patients with chronic HBV infection. When symptoms are present, fatigue tends to predominate over other constitutional symptoms, such as poor appetite and malaise. Right upper quadrant pain also may occur but is generally low grade. Patients may remain asymptomatic even during periods of reactivated hepatitis. In other instances, particularly when superimposed on cirrhosis, reactivation of HBV infection may be associated with frank jaundice and signs of liver failure (see later section on acute flares in chronic hepatitis B).

Physical findings may be normal or hepatosplenomegaly may be found. In decompensated cirrhosis, spider angiomata, jaundice, ascites, and peripheral edema are common. Liver biochemical test results are usually completely normal during the inactive HBV carrier state. In contrast with patients in the immune tolerant phase of HBV infection, most patients in the immune clearance phase of chronic HBV infection have mild to moderate elevations in serum AST and ALT levels. During exacerbations of disease, serum ALT levels may be as high as 1000 U/L or more, and the clinical and laboratory picture is indistinguishable from that of acute hepatitis B, including the presence in serum of IgM anti-HBc.[71] Progression to cirrhosis should be suspected whenever hypersplenism, hypoalbuminemia (in the absence of nephropathy), or prolongation of the prothrombin time is found. The serum AST level is typically higher than the serum ALT level in patients with advanced cirrhosis (see Chapter 78).[72]

Extrahepatic Manifestations

Extrahepatic syndromes seen in association with acute or chronic hepatitis B are important to recognize because they may occur without clinically apparent liver disease and can be mistaken for independent disease processes in other organ systems. The pathogenesis of these extrahepatic disorders has not been fully elucidated but likely involves an aberrant immunologic response to extrahepatic viral proteins.[73] Many of the extrahepatic manifestations (e.g., arthritis, dermatitis, glomerulonephritis, polyarteritis nodosa, mixed cryoglobulinemia, papular acrodermatitis, and polymyalgia rheumatica) are observed in association with circulating immune complexes that activate serum complement. Antiviral therapy may be indicated for persistent symptoms.

Arthritis-Dermatitis. The constellation of fever, arthralgias, rash, angioneurotic edema, and, less commonly, hematuria and proteinuria is seen as a prodromal manifestation of acute hepatitis B and rarely in patients with chronic hepatitis B.[74] The proximal interphalangeal joints, knees, ankles, shoulders, and wrists are the joints most commonly affected. During the period of acute joint symptoms, HBsAg titers in the blood are high and complement levels are low. Correspondingly, HBsAg has been detected in synovial membranes, and complement levels in synovial fluid are low. There is evidence for activation of the complement system by HBsAg–anti-HBs complexes. After the joint symptoms subside, complement levels return to normal, and HBsAg titers in serum begin to decline. This syndrome must be distinguished from inflammatory forms of arthritis, because glucocorticoids mistakenly given to patients with such HBV manifestations enhance HBV proliferation, and abrupt withdrawal of these agents may be associated with a flare in disease activity.[75]

Polyarteritis Nodosa. One of the most serious extrahepatic syndromes associated with chronic HBV infection is systemic necrotizing vasculitis, or polyarteritis nodosa. As many as 30% of patients with polyarteritis nodosa are infected with HBV, but the disorder develops in less than 1% of patients with HBV infection,[76] either after acute or recent hepatitis B or, more commonly, in association with chronic HBV infection. Symptoms include arthralgias, mononeuritis, fever, abdominal pain, renal disease, hypertension, central nervous system abnormalities, and rash. Medium to small arteries and arterioles are involved by fibrinoid necrosis and perivascular infiltration. The disease is thought to result from deposition of circulating immune complexes that contain HBsAg; for this reason, therapy with plasmapheresis may be indicated. Good therapeutic responses also have been observed with antiviral agents, given alone or in combination with plasmapheresis.[77] There is no apparent relationship between the severity of the vasculitis and the severity of the hepatic disease, and the hepatic disease often is relatively mild despite high levels of viral replication. The course of polyarteritis nodosa is variable, but the prognosis is gravest for patients with substantial proteinuria (>1 g/day), renal insufficiency (serum creatinine >1.6 mg/dL), gastrointestinal involvement, cardiomyopathy, and involvement of the central nervous system.[78]

Glomerulonephritis. Several types of glomerular lesions have been described in patients with chronic

HBV infection; membranous glomerulonephritis and membranoproliferative glomerulonephritis are the most common.[79] Renal biopsies have demonstrated immune complex deposition and cytoplasmic inclusions in the glomerular basement membrane. The immune complexes activate complement and production of cytokines with a subsequent inflammatory response. Nephrotic syndrome is the most common presentation of HBV-associated glomerulonephritis. In affected children, renal failure at presentation is almost always mild, and a prior history of clinical liver disease is uncommon. Nevertheless, liver biopsy specimens almost always demonstrate varying degrees of chronic hepatitis. The diagnosis of HBV-associated glomerulonephropathy is usually established by serologic evidence of HBV antigens or antibodies, the presence of immune-complex glomerulonephritis in a renal biopsy specimen, and the demonstration of glomerular deposits of one or more HBV antigens, such as HBsAg, HBcAg, or HBeAg, by immunohistochemistry. Most patients have detectable HBeAg in serum and, in addition, demonstrate low serum C3 and occasionally low C4 levels. The renal disease typically resolves in months to several years, especially in children. Often, resolution occurs in conjunction with HBeAg seroconversion. Rarely, however, renal failure may ensue. The natural history of HBV-related glomerulonephritis in adults has not been well defined, but several reports suggest that glomerular disease is often slowly and relentlessly progressive.[80] Successful treatment has been accomplished with interferon alfa and has been linked to long-term control of HBV replication.[81] Therapy with nucleoside analogs has resulted in improved renal function and diminished proteinuria.

Essential Mixed Cryoglobulinemia. Type II cryoglobulins consist of a polyclonal IgG and monoclonal IgM, whereas type III cryoglobulins contain polyclonal IgG and rheumatoid factor. Type II and type III cryoglobulinemia

have been associated with hepatitis B, but the association is uncommon. In a large patient cohort, the frequency of cryoglobulinemia was significantly higher in patients with chronic HCV infection (54%) than in patients with chronic HBV infection (15%) (see Chapter 76).[82] Cryoglobulinemia may be associated with systemic vasculitis (purpura, arthralgias, peripheral neuropathy, and glomerulonephritis) but is often paucisymptomatic or asymptomatic.[83] Interferon has been used successfully to treat symptomatic cryoglobulinemia in association with chronic hepatitis B.[84] Experience with nucleoside analog therapy has not been reported.

Histopathologic Features

Chronic HBV infection is characterized by mononuclear cell infiltration in the portal triads. Periportal inflammation often leads to the disruption of the limiting plate of hepatocytes (interface hepatitis), and inflammatory cells often can be seen at the interface between collagenous extensions from the portal tract and liver parenchyma (referred to as active septa). During reactivated hepatitis B, lobular inflammation is more intense and reminiscent of that seen in acute viral hepatitis. Steatosis is not a feature of chronic hepatitis B, as it is in chromic hepatitis C.

The only histologic feature noted on routine light microscopy that is specific for chronic hepatitis B is the presence of ground-glass hepatocytes (Fig. 75–5). This morphologic finding results from accumulation of HBsAg particles (20–30 nm in diameter) in the dilated endoplasmic reticulum.[85] Because of high levels of cysteine in HBsAg, ground-glass cells have a high affinity for certain dyes, such as orcein, Victoria blue, and aldehyde fuchsin. Ground-glass hepatocytes also may be seen in HBsAg carriers, in whom they may be detected in up to 5% of cells. When present in abundance, ground-glass hepatocytes often indicate active viral replication.[86] Immunofluores-

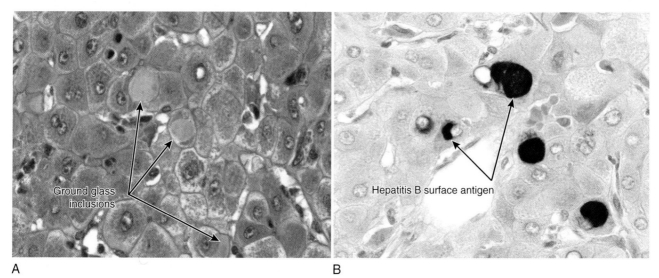

A   B

Figure 75–5 *A,* Liver biopsy specimen showing ground-glass inclusions in hepatocytes. These inclusions represent large amounts of hepatitis B surface antigen (HBsAg) in the endoplasmic reticulum of infected hepatocytes (hematoxylin-eosin, ×630). *B,* Immunohistochemical stain for HBsAg. Note that the brownish inclusions correspond to the ground glass inclusions seen in *A* (×630). (Courtesy of Dr. Gist Farr, New Orleans, La.)

cence and electron microscopic studies have shown HBcAg inside the hepatocyte nuclei of affected cells.[87] During periods of intense hepatitis activity, cytoplasmic core antigen staining is generally observed easily. After successful treatment of HBV infection with nucleoside analogs, the cytoplasmic core antigen staining often disappears, but nuclear core antigen staining may remain, indicating persistence of the HBV cccDNA template.

Acute Flares in Chronic Hepatitis B

Chronic hepatitis B is often punctuated by sudden flares of disease activity that are reflected by a rise in serum aminotransferase levels. Although a uniform definition is lacking, a flare has frequently been described as a rise in serum ALT levels to at least two times the baseline value. Spontaneous flares are an important part of the natural history of hepatitis B, because when they occur repeatedly, they lead to histologic progression. Acute flares in chronic hepatitis B occur in association with a number of circumstances and clinical situations (Table 75–2). Most flares result from a change in the balance between immunologic responses to HBV and the level of viral proliferation. Acute flares in chronic hepatitis B that are not explainable by infection with other hepatotropic viruses often occur as a secondary response to increased levels of replicating wild-type or mutant HBV or as a result of therapeutic intervention with immunologic modifiers such as interferon, glucocorticoids, and cancer chemotherapy. In some instances, the event that initiates an acute exacerbation of chronic hepatitis B may not be readily identifiable, and the flare is considered spontaneous.

Spontaneous Flares

Spontaneous exacerbations of chronic hepatitis B often result from reactivated infection, and an increase in serum HBV DNA levels often precedes an increase in serum aminotransferase levels. Histologic evidence of acute lobular hepatitis superimposed on the changes of chronic viral hepatitis is frequently observed during these flares.[88] IgM anti-HBc, a marker that is often diagnostic of acute viral hepatitis, may also appear in serum at this time.[89]

The reasons for reactivated infection are unknown but likely relate to subtle changes in the immunologic control of viral replication. Reactivation seems to occur more commonly in persons who are infected with HIV.[90] In persons who acquire HBV infection early in life, flares become more common during adulthood presumably due to a breakdown in immune tolerance to HBV.[91]

Fatigue may be reported during flares of chronic hepatitis B, but in many instances, patients remain asymptomatic. Occasionally symptoms and signs of frank liver failure become apparent, particularly when the flare is superimposed on advanced chronic hepatitis B.

Most clinically recognizable flares occur in patients who are in the nonreplicative phase of HBV infection (i.e., initially testing anti-HBe positive and serum HBV DNA negative on a molecular hybridization assay). During such flares, serum HBV DNA levels increase, and HBeAg often reappears in serum (seroreversion). HBV DNA and HBeAg are often detectable in serum when the patient is first seen, but if the flare has been ongoing for several weeks or longer, the accompanying enhancement of the immune response may make it difficult to detect a rise in serum HBV DNA levels. Frequently, these flares of hepatitis are followed by loss of serum HBV DNA and HBeAg.

Flares also can occur in patients who are in the replicative phase of infection (i.e., already positive in serum for HBV DNA and HBeAg). In these instances HBV replication intensifies, serum HBV DNA levels rise, and liver biochemical deterioration occurs, often without the subsequent loss of HBeAg. Multiple episodes of reactivation and remission have been shown to accelerate the progression of chronic hepatitis B and are particularly likely to occur in patients infected with the precore mutant form of chronic hepatitis B.[59]

Table 75–2   Hepatitis Flares in Chronic Hepatitis B

Cause of Flares	Comment
Spontaneous	Factors that precipitate antecedent viral replication are unclear
Immunosuppressive therapy	Flares are often observed during withdrawal; requires preemptive antiviral therapy
Antiviral therapy	
Interferon	Flares are often observed during the second to third month; may herald virologic response
Lamivudine	
During treatment	Flares are no more common than with placebo
YMDD mutant	Can have severe consequences in patients with advanced liver disease
On withdrawal*	Flares are caused by rapid reemergence of wild-type HBV; can have severe consequences in patients with advanced liver disease
HIV treatment	As for lamivudine; flares also can occur with immune reconstitution or secondary to antiretroviral drug hepatotoxicity
Genotypic variation	
Precore and core promoter mutants	Fluctuations in serum ALT levels are common with precore mutant
Superinfection with other hepatitis viruses	May be associated with suppression of HBV replication

ALT, alanine aminotransferase; HIV, human immunodeficiency virus; HBV, hepatitis B virus; YMDD, tyrosine-methionine-aspartate-aspartate.
*Has also been reported with adefovir and entecavir.

Immunosuppressive Therapy–Induced Flares

Reactivation of HBV replication is a well-recognized complication in patients with chronic HBV infection who receive cytotoxic or immunosuppressive therapy.[92] Suppression of the normal immunologic responses to HBV leads to enhanced viral replication and is thought to result in widespread infection of hepatocytes. On discontinuation of immunosuppressive medications, such as cancer chemotherapy, antirejection drugs, and glucocorticoids, immune competence is restored and infected hepatocytes are rapidly destroyed. The more potent the immunosuppression, the higher the level of viral replication and, thus, the greater the potential for serious clinical consequences of sudden withdrawal of the therapy and restoration of immunologic competence. Postmortem studies of liver tissue from patients with severe liver injury have documented sparse staining of viral antigens, suggesting that the patients were in an active state of immune clearance.[93]

The vast majority of patients who experience immunosuppressive therapy–induced flares have been HBsAg positive before treatment, but some studies have described the reappearance of HBsAg in patients who were initially positive for anti-HBs, anti-HBc, or both.[94] Reactivated hepatitis in patients who are HBsAg negative and either anti-HBc or anti-HBs positive is explainable by the possible latency of HBV in liver and mononuclear cells and the large extrahepatic reservoir of HBV. Chemotherapy given to patients with cancer who are chronic HBV carriers is associated with an increased risk of liver-related morbidity and mortality.[95]

Reactivated hepatitis B also occurs in patients who are given immunosuppressive medications to prevent organ transplant rejection. The frequency of reactivated hepatitis appears to be particularly high in patients who undergo bone marrow transplantation, because of extensive immunologic conditioning before transplantation and treatment of graft-versus-host reactions.[96] Rarely, *fibrosing cholestatic hepatitis*, a rapidly progressive form of liver injury associated with inordinately high levels of HBsAg and HBcAg in liver tissue, may develop in such patients.[97]

Acute flares of hepatitis B resulting from cancer chemotherapy and other immunosuppressive drugs are often detected after substantial increases in serum aminotransferase levels have been noted. Initiation of antiviral treatment after detection of such biochemical abnormalities has little effect on reducing liver injury because much of the immunologic response to HBV and viral elimination has already occurred. Instead, the key to management lies in anticipating the occurrence of a flare, initiating antiviral treatment preemptively (e.g., 4 to 6 weeks before the start of chemotherapy), and continuing the treatment until several months after completion of chemotherapy.[98]

Antiviral Therapy–Induced Flares

Antiviral treatment of chronic hepatitis B can be associated with flares of hepatitis in several circumstances. Flares may occur during interferon therapy, after withdrawal of nucleoside analogs or glucocorticoids, and in association with lamivudine-resistant mutants.

Interferon. Interferon-induced flares of chronic hepatitis B occur in approximately one third of treated patients and result from the immunostimulatory properties of the drug. Flares generally occur during the second or third month of treatment with conventional preparations of interferon. Whether or not flares occur as commonly with the newer long-acting (pegylated) forms of interferon is unknown. Serum ALT flares have been shown to be a predictor of sustained virologic response, particularly in patients with high levels of viremia.[99] Flares tend to be particularly common in patients who have decompensated liver disease, with rates as high as 50% reported in one series.[100] Such flares are frequently associated with clinical deterioration in the patient.

Nucleoside Analogs. Serum ALT flares occur in approximately 20% to 25% of patients after withdrawal of nucleoside analogs such as lamivudine and adefovir. These flares probably are caused by rapid resurgence of wild-type virus, and although generally well tolerated, they have been associated with serious clinical exacerbations in patients with advanced liver disease.[101] Reinstitution of therapy is often associated with a decline in serum HBV DNA and aminotransferase levels. Flares have been seen to follow the emergence of YMDD mutant HBV during therapy with lamivudine.[102] Initial reports emphasized the temporal occurrence of these flares at the time of or shortly after detection of lamivudine resistance. However, further follow-up of patients with lamivudine-resistant HBV mutants has indicated that the frequency of moderate or severe serum ALT flares (defined as >5 or >10 times the upper limit of normal, respectively) increases with time after detection of lamivudine resistance. In one long-term study, the cumulative frequencies of such ALT flares were as follows: 24% at less than 1 year, 29% at 1 to 2 years, 30% at 2 to 3 years, 37% at 3 to 4 years, and 61% at more than 4 years after detection of lamivudine resistance.[103]

Glucocorticoid Withdrawal. Serum ALT levels increase, often with inverse declines in HBsAg concentration and HBV DNA levels, after withdrawal of glucocorticoids.[104] In clinical trials, a short course of glucocorticoids used prior to conventional antiviral therapy was reported to enhance virologic response rates.[105,106] The immune rebound following withdrawal of glucocorticoids after a 4- to 8-week course may result from increased activation of lymphocytes that promote T_H1 cytokine responses at a time when viral antigen expression is increased. Serious hepatic decompensation has been reported in patients with advanced disease, and this therapeutic approach is no longer used.

Antiretroviral Therapy. Serum ALT flares occur in patients coinfected with HIV and HBV receiving highly active antiretroviral therapy (HAART).[107] A number of potential causes have been identified. Lamivudine resistance and withdrawal may be associated with ALT flares. HBV infection raises the risk of toxicity from antiretroviral therapy, usually within the first 6 months of treatment initiation. Immune reconstitution resulting from HAART may also be associated with ALT flares. Affected patients may also be particularly susceptible to flares because of infection with other hepatitis viruses.

Hepatitis B Virus Genotypic Variation

Chronic infection with precore mutant HBV (sometimes referred to as HBeAg-negative HBV) often is associated with multiple flares of liver cell necrosis interspersed with periods of normal serum ALT and low serum HBV DNA levels.[59] Approximately 45% of patients have episodic serum ALT flares with normal levels between episodes, and 20% have flares superimposed on persistent ALT elevations.[108] These flares have been attributed to rises in the concentration of precore mutants and changes in the ratio of concentrations of precore to wild-type HBV.[109]

Mutations at the basal core promoter (BCP) region of the HBV genome are associated with greater HBeAg synthesis, histologic evidence of liver inflammation, and increased viral replication.[110] Multiple exacerbations of hepatitis resulting from reactivated HBV infection have been described in patients with BCP mutations, either alone or in association with precore mutations.[111] HBeAg-negative patients who have both precore and core promoter mutants may be particularly predisposed to episodes of severe reactivation after chemotherapy for malignancies.[112]

Infection with Other Viruses

Patients with chronic HBV infection may exhibit severe flares in serum aminotransferase levels and even frank liver failure when superinfected with other hepatotropic viruses, such as hepatitis A virus (HAV), HCV, and HDV. Increased mortality has been reported when HDV superinfection is superimposed on chronic hepatitis B, and chronic HDV infection is often associated with multiple fluctuations in serum aminotransferase levels (see later discussion of HDV).[113] Acute hepatitis C superimposed on chronic hepatitis B has been reported to be as severe as HDV superinfection and has been associated with a high rate of liver failure (34%) and death (10%).[114] A cumulative frequency of cirrhosis and HCC that is higher than that attributable to chronic HDV infection or chronic HBV infection alone has been demonstrated. Acute hepatitis C often leads to chronic HCV infection, and the subsequent course also may be characterized by frequent fluctuations in serum aminotransferase levels.

Patients with chronic hepatitis B who become infected with other hepatotropic viruses (HAV, HCV, HDV, or both HCV and HDV) may test negative for both HBeAg and HBV DNA on non–PCR-based assays because of viral interference.

DIAGNOSIS

HBsAg appears in serum 2 to 10 weeks after exposure to HBV and before the onset of symptoms or elevation of serum aminotransferases. In self-limited acute hepatitis, HBsAg usually becomes undetectable after 4 to 6 months. Persistence of HBsAg for more than 6 months implies progression to chronic HBV infection.

The disappearance of HBsAg is followed several weeks later by the appearance of anti-HBs. In most patients, anti-HBs persists for life and provides long-term immunity. In some patients, anti-HBs may not become detectable after disappearance of HBsAg, but these patients do not appear to be susceptible to recurrent infection.[115] Anti-HBs may not be detectable during a window period of several weeks to months after the disappearance of HBsAg. During this period, the diagnosis of acute HBV infection is made by the detection of IgM anti-HBc in serum.[116]

Coexistence of HBsAg and anti-HBs in serum has been reported in approximately 25% of HBsAg-positive persons and occurs more commonly in individuals with chronic hepatitis B than in those with acute hepatitis B.[117] In most instances, the anti-HBs is present in a low level, non-neutralizing, and heterotypic—that is, directed against a subtype of HBsAg different from the subtype present in the infected patient. The mechanisms behind this finding are not clear but relate to antibody formed against minor variants of the HBsAg protein. The presence of these heterotypic antibodies is not associated with specific risk factors or changes in clinical course and may occur in patients with or without active liver disease and viral replication.[118]

Anti-HBc is detectable in acute and chronic HBV infection. During acute infection, anti-HBc is predominantly of the IgM class and is usually detectable for 4 to 6 months after an acute episode of hepatitis and rarely for up to 2 years. As noted earlier, IgM anti-HBc may become detectable during exacerbations of chronic hepatitis B.[119] Anti-HBc persists in persons who recover from acute hepatitis B and also in association with HBsAg in those who progress to chronic infection.

In areas where HBV is not endemic, isolated anti-HBc in serum has been detected in 1% to 4% of the general population. Isolated reactivity for anti-HBc may occur in the following situations: during the window period of acute hepatitis B, when anti-HBc is predominantly of the IgM class; many years after recovery from acute hepatitis B, when anti-HBs has fallen to undetectable levels; as a false-positive serologic test result; after many years of chronic infection, when the HBsAg titer has fallen below the level of detection; in persons who are coinfected with HCV; and, rarely, as a result of varying sensitivity of HBsAg assays.[120] Evidence for coinfection with HCV has been demonstrated in up to 60% of persons in whom anti-HBc is the only marker of HBV.[121]

Results of PCR testing of sera have shown that 0% to 30% of patients with isolated anti-HBc have HBV DNA in serum. Usually, the HBV DNA is detectable at a low level and not by standard hybridization assays, which are less sensitive than PCR assays.[122] The presence of low-level viremia in these HBsAg-negative subjects has clinical implications with regard to potential infectivity. For example, anti-HBc testing of blood donors prevents some cases of post-transfusion hepatitis B.[123] Also, the risk of transmission of HBV infection from a liver donor with isolated anti-HBc has been found to be as high as 50% to 70% in some series; lower rates of transmission have been observed in other forms of solid organ transplantation.[124,125]

Low-level viral replication also has implications with regard to the possibility of underlying liver disease. HBV DNA in serum and liver tissue has been confirmed by PCR methodology in some HBsAg-negative patients with cirrhosis and HCC and in some patients with fulminant non-A, non-B, non-C hepatitis as defined by conventional serologic testing.[126,127]

HBeAg is a soluble viral protein that is found in serum early during acute HBV infection. HBeAg reactivity usually disappears at or soon after the peak in serum aminotransferase levels, and persistence of HBeAg 3 or more months after the onset of illness indicates a high likelihood of transition to chronic HBV infection. The finding of HBeAg in the serum of an HBsAg carrier indicates greater infectivity, a high level of viral replication, and the need for antiviral therapy. With a commercially available PCR assay, nearly 90% of patients with HBeAg-positive chronic hepatitis B were found to have serum HBV DNA levels persistently above 10^5 copies/mL, with a mean value of 8.37 $\log_{10}$ copies/mL.[128] In contrast, anti-HBe–positive patients had much lower serum HBV DNA levels, higher values being found in those with persistently or intermittently elevated serum ALT levels (mean of 5.1 $\log_{10}$ copies/mL) than in patients with persistently normal ALT levels (3.10 $\log_{10}$ copies/mL).

Most HBeAg-positive patients have active liver disease; the exceptions are HBeAg-positive children and young adults with perinatally acquired HBV infection, who usually have normal serum ALT levels and minimal inflammation of the liver.[23] In general, seroconversion from HBeAg to anti-HBe is associated with a reduction in serum HBV DNA levels of 3 $\log_{10}$ copies/mL or greater and remission of liver disease. Some patients, however, continue to have active liver disease and detectable HBV DNA in serum because of low levels of wild-type virus or the selection of precore or core promoter mutations that impair HBeAg secretion.

HBV DNA can be measured in serum with qualitative or quantitative assays. The clinical utility of testing for serum HBV DNA has been hampered by the absence of a licensed test in the United States as well as an accepted international reference standard. A number of non–PCR-based assays are available with levels of sensitivity ranging from 10^3 to 10^5 genomic copies/mL of serum. Although these assays are less sensitive than those that are PCR-based, their results correlate with clinical response to antiviral therapy, and several of the currently available antiviral therapies were licensed on the basis of clinical trials in which these assays were used (see later). The use of these less sensitive non–PCR-based assays has several shortcomings, however, so most clinical laboratories use one of several commercially available PCR assays with enhanced sensitivity (10^2 genomic copies/mL or less).

The measurement of serum HBV DNA is commonly employed to evaluate a patient's candidacy for antiviral therapy and to monitor response during treatment. Patients with high serum HBV DNA levels at baseline less commonly respond to therapy with conventional interferon than patients with low levels.[129] With the use of solution hybridization testing, a baseline HBV DNA level of 200 pg/mL (roughly equivalent to 56 million copies/mL on a PCR assay) or greater has been found to be associated with a very low rate of response to standard interferon. In contrast, baseline serum HBV DNA levels have not been shown to correlate with response to nucleoside analog therapy, because of the more potent inhibi-

tion of viral replication by these agents. Monitoring of HBV DNA levels at key intervals during therapy allows one to predict the likelihood of HBeAg clearance. Several studies have found that the level of serum HBV DNA at 12 weeks of nucleoside analog treatment may help predict the likelihood of HBeAg seroconversion.[130,131] Other studies have suggested that measuring the HBV DNA level at baseline or during treatment can be used to evaluate the likelihood of both relapse after treatment is discontinued and development of resistance to lamivudine.[132,133] Reappearance of HBV DNA in serum during treatment suggests that drug resistance has occurred,[134] and high pretreatment levels of serum HBV DNA have been shown to correlate with a higher rate of recurrent HBV infection in liver transplant recipients who are treated with lamivudine.[135]

Qualitative PCR is an even more sensitive method of detecting HBV DNA than quantitative PCR. Use of qualitative PCR has altered traditional concepts about the clearance of HBV DNA in acute and chronic HBV infection. Small amounts of HBV DNA can be detected in serum and peripheral mononuclear cells years after recovery from acute hepatitis B.[69] Even after disappearance of HBsAg and apparent loss of HBV DNA from serum in patients with chronic hepatitis B, small amounts of HBV DNA persist in liver tissue and peripheral mononuclear cells years later.[18] Detection of HBV DNA in serum by a qualitative PCR assay before liver transplantation may identify patients who are at increased risk of apparent de novo hepatitis after transplantation and may pinpoint HBV as the cause of liver disease in HBsAg-negative patients.[136,137] Finally, detection of minute amounts of HBV DNA may be particularly important in diagnosing patients with fulminant hepatitis B, who frequently have cleared HBsAg by the time they seek medical attention.[138]

TREATMENT

Virologic End Points and Definitions of Response

The primary goal of treatment for chronic hepatitis B is durable suppression of serum HBV DNA to levels below those associated with liver disease. This goal can be accomplished with either interferon alfa or nucleoside analogs. The level at which serum HBV DNA is suppressed adequately is generally considered to be less than 10^5 copies/mL for patients with HBeAg-positive chronic hepatitis B and often lower for those with HBeAg-negative hepatitis.[23] Definitions of response vary, but the most important clinically is a lasting or durable suppression of serum HBV DNA response when the patient is no longer receiving treatment (Table 75–3). HBeAg seroconversion is an additional end point that can be used to determine the appropriate length of treatment with nucleoside analogs.

Although most experts would agree that achieving HBsAg seroconversion is more desirable than HBV suppression, the former occurs so infrequently with current antiviral therapies that it is considered an impractical end point. Even so, a systematic review of clinical trials with interferon alfa indicates that early HBsAg serocon-

Table 75–3   Treatment of Chronic Hepatitis B: Definitions of Response to Antiviral Therapy

Virologic response	Decrease in serum HBV DNA level to <100,000 copies/mL or <20,000 IU/mL in HBeAg-positive cases and <10,000 copies/mL or <2,000 IU/mL in HBeAg-negative cases
	Loss of HBeAg with or without seroconversion to anti-HBe*
Biochemical response	Normalization of serum ALT levels
On-treatment response	Initial response (suppression of HBV DNA levels to <$10^{4\text{-}5}$ copies/mL with or without loss of HBeAg, in addition to normalization of serum ALT levels)
	Maintained response (requiring continuation of therapy)
Off-treatment response	
Sustained response	Virologic and biochemical response observed for 6-12 months after treatment is discontinued
Durable response	Indefinite virologic and biochemical response after treatment is discontinued

ALT, alanine aminotransferase; HBeAg, hepatitis B e antigen; HBV, hepatitis B virus.
*Pertains to HBeAg-positive patients only.

Table 75–4   Advantages and Disadvantages of Currently Available Antiviral Agents

Agent(s)	Advantages	Disadvantages
Interferon	Finite duration of treatment Durable off-treatment response Loss of HBsAg (5%-8%)	Given by injection Frequent side effects Expensive Low response rate with a high level of viremia
Nucleoside analogs	Negligible side effects Potent inhibition of virus replication Less expensive than interferon	Oral delivery Drug resistance Long or indefinite treatment duration Low rate of HBsAg disappearance Moderately expensive when given long term*

HBsAg, hepatitis B surface antigen.
*Average retail price is approximately $200-$700 (USD) per month, depending on drug.

version occurs significantly more frequently in treated than in nontreated patients. In a meta-analysis of 16 randomized, controlled trials, loss of HBsAg from serum occurred six times as frequently in interferon-treated patients as in nontreated patients.[139] Long-term follow-up (mean, 6.2 years; range, 1–11 years) of HBeAg-positive patients treated with standard interferon alfa demonstrated that 71% of sustained responders became HBsAg negative.[140] By contrast, a 1-year course of lamivudine or adefovir does not result in a higher rate of HBsAg seroconversion than placebo, and the frequency of HBsAg seroconversion with prolonged therapy has yet to be evaluated extensively. The observation that early HBsAg seroconversion occurs often with interferon but not with nucleoside analogs emphasizes that the mechanisms of action of the two treatments differ fundamentally and provides a rationale for the use of combination therapy using both types of drugs (see sections on the individual agents and combination therapy).

Factors Involved in the Choice of Agents

In deciding on the appropriate type of therapy for patients with chronic hepatitis B, the physician should consider the serum ALT level, serum HBV DNA level, and liver histology at baseline as well as the expense of treatment, potential for and ability of the patient to withstand adverse effects, age and other comorbid conditions of the patient, and realistic expectations about the need for monitoring. Interferon and nucleoside analogs each have advantages and disadvantages, and no one therapy is suitable for all patients (Table 75–4). One major advantage of therapy with interferon is that it tends to be time limited, in that durable responses do not require maintenance therapy. In contrast, prolonged treatment with nucleoside analogs is often necessary to maintain viral suppression.

Guidelines for the Management of Hepatitis B

Consensus guidelines for the treatment of hepatitis B have been published by the American Association for the Study of Liver Diseases, Asian-Pacific Association for the Study of the Liver, and European Association for the Study of the Liver.[141-143] In general, the three sets of guidelines are quite similar. As innovations in medical therapy are made, the guidelines are updated, and differences among the guidelines represent, in part, differences in the availability of the various therapeutic agents around the world as well as unavoidable delays in publication that prevent the incorporation of new data. For example, all three guidelines emphasize that interferon may be used as an alternative treatment to nucleoside analogs, but only one of them currently incorporates guidelines on the use of the newer pegylated form of interferon.[142] Also, there are no recommendations about combination therapy with more than one nucleoside analog or interferon and a nucleoside analog. The guidelines do not address the use of antiviral therapy in acute hepatitis B, although many experts recommend use of nucleoside analogs when HBeAg remains detectable in serum for more than 10 to 12 weeks because of the likelihood of evolution to the chronic HBsAg carrier state without treatment. The three guidelines are anticipated to change as new information becomes available.

The recommendations made in the three sets of published guidelines have many similarities. In general, the published guidelines recommend treatment of persons who have serum HBV DNA levels in excess of 20,000 IU/mL or roughly 100,000 copies/mL.[144] Nucleoside analog therapy is recommended specifically in patients with decompensated cirrhosis. Emphasis also is given to the treatment of patients with serum ALT levels that are at least double the upper limit of normal (Table 75–5). (Some experts disagree with these arbitrary serum ALT and HBV DNA thresholds.[144]) The recommendation is based on the observation that rates of sustained virologic response in patients with minimal pretreatment serum ALT elevations are low with either interferon or nucleoside analogs.[129,145] All the guidelines indicate that treatment decisions ideally should be made in the context of liver histologic findings and that treatment should be directed preferentially to patients with histologically moderate to severe hepatitis. Currently, treatment decisions are not based on specific grading or staging of liver histology.

Currently Available Antiviral Agents

Interferon Alfa

Interferon alfa was licensed for the treatment of chronic hepatitis B in 1992. Interferon is effective after a relatively short course of treatment (6 months to 1 year) and, unlike the nucleoside analogs, has not been associated with drug resistance. Also, unlike nucleoside analogs, interferon has direct immunomodulatory properties. Interferon enhances HLA class I antigen expression on the surface of infected hepatocytes and augments CD8+ CTL activity. These effects could be important mechanistically in reducing the amount of the HBV cccDNA (the genomic template for viral transcription) and may thereby explain the loss of HBsAg that occurs in approximately 5% to 8% of interferon-treated patients. The major disadvantages of interferon relate to its poorer acceptance because of side effects (see Chapter 76), lower level of HBV DNA suppression, and greater cost in comparison with nucleoside analogs.

Flares of serum ALT have been described during therapy with interferon alfa, and although these flares are potentially important in achieving a virologic response, they occur unpredictably and are inconsistently associated

Table 75–5 Recommendations for Treatment of Chronic Hepatitis B*

HBeAg Status	Serum HBV DNA Level	Serum ALT Level	Treatment Strategy
+	+[†]	≤2 × ULN	Low efficacy of currently available treatments Observe; consider treatment if serum ALT becomes elevated

+	+	>2 × ULN	Interferon alfa, lamivudine, adefovir, or entecavir may be used as initial therapy
			Duration of therapy:
			    Interferon alfa: 16 weeks
			    Lamivudine: minimum of 1 year; continue for 3-6 months after HBeAg seroconversion
			    Adefovir: minimum of 1 year
			    Entecavir: minimum of 1 year
			For interferon alfa nonresponders or patients with contraindications to interferon alfa, use lamivudine, adefovir, or entecavir
			For lamivudine resistance, use adefovir or entecavir

−	+	>2 × ULN	Interferon alfa, lamivudine, adefovir, or entecavir may be used as initial therapy, but adefovir or entecavir is preferred because of need for long-term therapy
			Endpoints of treatment: Sustained normalization of serum ALT level and undetectable HBV DNA on PCR assay
			Duration of therapy:
			    Interferon alfa: 1 year
			    Lamivudine: >1 year
			    Adefovir: >1 year
			    Entecavir: >1 year
			For interferon alfa nonresponders/contraindications to interferon alfa, use lamivudine, adefovir, or entecavir
			For lamivudine resistance, use adefovir, or entecavir

−	−	≤2 × ULN	No treatment required
+ or −	+	Cirrhosis	Compensated: Lamivudine, adefovir, or entecavir Decompensated: Lamivudine, adefovir, or entecavir; refer for liver transplantation; interferon alfa is contraindicated
+ or −	−	Cirrhosis	Compensated: Observe[‡] Decompensated: Refer for liver transplantation

ALT, alanine aminotransferase; HBeAg, hepatitis B e antigen; PCR, polymerase chain reaction; ULN, upper limit of normal.

*Treatment recommendations for noncirrhotic hepatitis B are intended for patients with moderate to severe hepatitis.

[†]Serum HBV DNA level >10^5 copies/mL.

[‡]Many authorities recommend therapy with a nucleoside analog if the serum HBV DNA level is <10^5 copies/mL.

Adapted from Lok ASF, McMahon BJ; Practice Guidelines Committee, American Association for the Study of Liver Diseases (AASLD): Chronic hepatitis B: Update of recommendations. Hepatology 39:857, 2004.

with antiviral efficacy. The magnitude of an ALT flare has been shown to predict the likelihood of a sustained virologic response in patients with high levels of viremia, suggesting that vigorous cell-mediated immune responses often are required to overcome high levels of viral replication.[99]

Pegylated interferon has been found to be more effective than conventional interferon in the treatment of HBV infection.[146] Doses of 1.0 µg per kg of body weight of pegylated interferon alfa-2b and 180 µg of pegylated interferon alfa-2a given once weekly have been studied in clinical trials.[147,148] No data are yet available for judging whether the increased effectiveness of pegylated interferon is primarily a function of a more pronounced effect on viral replication or of greater immunomodulatory action.

Impact of Genotype on Response. Viral genotype appears to affect the response to interferon. In a report from Taiwan, patients with genotype-B, HBeAg-positive, chronic hepatitis B were found to show response to conventional interferon more frequently than patients with genotype-C chronic hepatitis B.[149] A relationship between virologic response and genotype was recently reaffirmed in a large multicenter study of pegylated interferon alfa-2b. In this study, HBeAg-positive patients with genotype A responded more frequently than those with genotypes B, C, and D (47% versus 44%, 28%, and 25%, respectively).[147] These results confirm and extend those of earlier studies in HBeAg-positive and HBeAg-negative patients suggesting that patients with genotype A respond more frequently than those with genotype D. The effect that genotype exerts on the response to interferon could be particularly relevant to the treatment of North American patients with chronic HBV infection, in light of the influx of Asian HBsAg carriers with genotypes B and C beginning in the last decades of the 20th century.[36]

Nucleoside Analogs

Nucleoside analogs have excellent oral bioavailability, a good safety record, and antiviral efficacy comparable to that observed with interferon alfa-2b. They also are considerably less expensive than interferon when given for 48 weeks, as recommended in the prescribing information. These drugs have proved to be particularly useful in the management of patients with decompensated cirrhosis, in whom even small doses of interferon can lead to worsening liver failure and severe infections. Table 75–6 lists the relative antiviral potencies of the available nucleoside analogs and those under late-stage development.

Nucleoside analogs replace natural nucleosides during the synthesis of the first or second strand (or both) of HBV DNA. They thus serve as competitive inhibitors of the viral reverse transcriptase and DNA polymerase. Because nucleoside analogs partially and reversibly suppress viral replication, they have to be given for more than 1 year in most cases to achieve maximal efficacy. Unfortunately, drug resistance occurs with prolonged monotherapy. Nucleoside analogs have several other limitations as well. With these agents, demonstrating the clearance of HBV cccDNA has been difficult, and in contrast to treatment with interferon, HBsAg clearance rarely

Table 75–6 Relative Antiviral Potencies of Currently Available Drugs for Hepatitis B Virus (HBV) and Drugs under Development*

Drug (Dose)	Level of HBV DNA Suppression (copies/mL)	
	Week 24	**Weeks 48-52**
Lamivudine (100 mg)[†]	≈ –4.4 log	≈ –4.2 log
	≈ –5.2 log	–4.8 log
	NA	–4.7 log
Emtricitabine (200 mg)	– 3.0 log	–2.9 log
Adefovir (10 mg)[†]	≈ –3.0 log	–3.5 log
	≈ –3.6 log	–3.9 log
Tenofovir (300 mg)[†]	–6.6 log[‡]	NA
	–4.3 log[§]	NA
	NA	–4.5 log[‡]
Pegylated interferon[¶] (180 µg)	–3.5 log	NA
	≈ –3.5 log	≈ –4.0 log
Entecavir (0.5 mg, 1 mg)[‡]	≈ –4.6 log	NA
	NA	–4.5, –5.1 log
Telbivudine (600 mg)	NA	–6.1 log

*Studies used a variety of HBV DNA assay methods, and comparisons between studies are thus difficult.
[†]Each line represents the finding of a single study.
[‡]Based on studies in lamivudine-resistant patients.
[§]In human immunodeficiency–coinfected persons.
[¶]Data on pegylated interferon alfa-2a.
NA, not available.

occurs after 1 year of treatment with nucleoside analogs. These problems may result, in part, from the fact that these agents, unlike interferon, do not have a direct, enhancing effect on the immunologic response to HBV.[94] Also, as indicated earlier, post-withdrawal serum ALT flares have been seen in approximately 25% of cases after discontinuation of nucleoside analog therapy.

Lamivudine. The approval of lamivudine in 1998 was a major breakthrough in the treatment of hepatitis B. The drug has been shown to be a relatively potent inhibitor of viral replication, convenient to administer, and free of severe adverse effects. Clinical trials demonstrated that a 1-year course of lamivudine resulted in suppression of viral replication and improvement in histologic findings in the liver.[150] In one study, HBeAg seroconversion and HBeAg loss occurred in 17% and 32% of patients, respectively.[151] A 2-year course of lamivudine proved to be more effective, resulting in an increase in the rate of HBeAg seroconversion from 17% at 1 year to 27% at 2 years.[152] Prolongation of treatment beyond 1 year, however, has been associated with incremental changes in viral resistance (38% at 2 years), and the longer treatment is continued, the more frequently resistance is seen (65% at year 5).[103] Resistance is even more commonly encountered (90% at 4 years) in patients coinfected with HIV, because of the early use of lamivudine in HAART regimens.[107] Lamivudine resistance for more than 2 years has been associated with a blunted histologic response, and patients in whom lamivudine resistance has developed experience more hepatitis flares.[49,103] Fortunately, a number of alternative nucleoside analogs in various phases of development have considerably lower resistance profiles.

Adefovir Dipivoxil. Adefovir dipivoxil is the acyclic phosphonate nucleotide analog of adenosine monophosphate. The drug was approved in 2002 for the treatment of HBeAg-positive and HBeAg-negative chronic hepatitis B on the basis of the findings of randomized, controlled trials in the United States, Europe, and Asia.[153,154] In these pivotal studies, treatment with adefovir for 48 weeks resulted in median serum HBV DNA reductions of 3.52 $\log_{10}$ and 3.91 $\log_{10}$ copies/mL in HBeAg-positive and HBeAg-negative patients, respectively. The rates of HBeAg seroconversion and HBeAg loss were slightly lower than those achieved with lamivudine for 52 weeks (12% and 24%, respectively). A rise in the frequency of HBeAg seroconversion and nondetectability of HBV DNA by PCR methodology has been observed during the second year of adefovir treatment.[155] The level of HBV DNA suppression has been the same irrespective of genotype.[156]

Although the extent of viral suppression is only slightly less with adefovir than with lamivudine, the two drugs differ greatly in their resistance profiles. Point mutations (A181V, N236T) in the B and D domains, respectively, of the HBV polymerase gene affect HBV susceptibility to adefovir but occur in only 3% of patients at 2 years and 6% at 3 years of treatment in initial studies[157,158] and in 18% of patients at 4 years and 29% at 5 years in a subsequent study.[159] In comparison, lamivudine resistance is approximately 15 to 20 times as common at the same time intervals. HBV isolates with the N236T mutation have remained susceptible to lamivudine and appear to be sensitive to entecavir and telbivudine in vitro (see later).[160] The low rate of resistance with prolonged adefovir therapy makes this drug particularly suitable as first-line therapy in patients with HBeAg-negative chronic hepatitis B because of the frequent need for continued viral suppression in this group of patients.

Adefovir is clinically and virologically effective in patients with lamivudine-resistant HBV, whether they have clinically stable disease, decompensated cirrhosis, or recurrent hepatitis B after liver transplantation.[161-163] This agent has been shown to be effective when used alone or in combination with lamivudine maintenance. In one study, 37% of patients infected with lamivudine-resistant HBV experienced serious ALT flares when switched to adefovir monotherapy.[162] These data have led some experts to advise patients with serious underlying liver disease to continue maintenance lamivudine when starting adefovir therapy. Adefovir has the disadvantage of being potentially nephrotoxic, and dose reductions may be necessary in patients likely to experience compromised renal function.[163]

Emtricitabine. Emtricitabine is a fluorinated cytosine analog that inhibits HBV DNA polymerase and HIV reverse transcriptase. This drug is currently licensed in the United States and other countries for the treatment of HIV type 1 (HIV-1) infection. Preliminary results from a placebo-controlled, phase 3 study in previously untreated patients with chronic HBV infection have demonstrated that emtricitabine, 200 mg daily for 48 weeks, reduces serum HBV DNA by a median of 3 $\log_{10}$ copies/mL and improves liver histology significantly.[164] Emtricitabine

treatment of patients coinfected with HBV and HIV has led to levels of suppression of HBV DNA similar to those in treated patients infected with HBV alone.[165] However, the drug is structurally related to lamivudine and has similar mutational sites and rates of resistance. The frequency of YMDD mutations in patients receiving emtricitabine, 200 mg daily, has been shown to be between 9% and 13% at week 48 and 19% at week 96.[166] On the basis of these findings, it is unlikely that this agent will play an important role in the management of chronic hepatitis B except for patients with HBV-HIV coinfection.

Tenofovir Disoproxil Fumarate. Tenofovir, an acyclic nucleotide inhibitor of HBV polymerase and HIV reverse transcriptase, is similar chemically to adefovir dipivoxil. Tenofovir has been licensed for the treatment of HIV infection, and its antiviral activity against HBV has been reported to be greater than that of the 10-mg dose of adefovir in lamivudine-resistant patients.[167] Reports of therapeutic efficacy have come largely from small clinical trials in patients with lamivudine-resistant HBV infection in whom reductions in HBV DNA of 3 $\log_{10}$ to 4 $\log_{10}$ copies/mL have been observed after 1 year of treatment.[167-170] HBV harboring the N236T mutation that confers resistance to adefovir is not sensitive to tenofovir. Despite the possible greater antiviral potency of tenofovir compared with adefovir, large-scale studies of tenofovir in chronic hepatitis B are unlikely to be performed. The U.S. Food and Drug Administration (FDA) has approved a combination formulation of tenofovir and emtricitabine for use in HIV infection. This drug could, in theory, be useful in HBV infection, because HBV that is resistant to emtricitabine remains susceptible to tenofovir, and tenofovir-resistant HBV remains susceptible to emtricitabine.

Entecavir. Entecavir is a deoxyguanine nucleoside analog that inhibits HBV replication selectively. The drug was approved by the FDA in 2005. The drug blocks HBV replication by inhibiting the priming of HBV DNA polymerase and the synthesis of the first and second strands of HBV DNA. It is effective against both wild-type and lamivudine-resistant HBV. An entecavir dose of 0.5 mg given daily for 24 weeks reduced serum HBV DNA levels by an additional 1.28 $\log_{10}$ copies/mL compared with lamivudine in previously untreated HBeAg-positive patients.[171] In phase 3 clinical trials, an entecavir dose of 0.5 mg was used to treat HBeAg-positive and HBeAg-negative patients previously untreated with a nucleoside analog, whereas 1 mg was found to be the more effective dose in patients whose disease was resistant to lamivudine.[172] Entecavir resistance is rare and thus far has been reported only in patients with lamivudine vesistance.[173]

Nucleoside Analogs Under Development

β-ʟ-*Nucleosides*

The ʟ-nucleoside analogs ʟ-deoxythymidine (LdT; telbivudine) and valyl-ʟ-deoxycytidine (val-LdC; valtorcitabine) are promising compounds that are potent and selective inhibitors of HBV replication.[174] Treatment of Hepadnavirus-infected woodchucks with these agents resulted in a reduction in serum viral DNA levels greater than 8 $\log_{10}$ copies/mL, whereas a reduction of only 3 $\log_{10}$ copies/mL was observed in response to lamivudine.[175] Synergism was observed when the animals were treated with both L-nucleosides. Telbivudine has been shown to preferentially inhibit second-strand HBV DNA synthesis in vitro, whereas valtorcitabine inhibits first- and second-strand synthesis, making the drugs potentially complementary.

Data from a phase 2b study of telbivudine has shown that either a 400-mg or 600-mg dose given daily for 52 weeks resulted in an approximate 6 $\log_{10}$ copies/mL reduction in serum HBV DNA levels.[176]

HBeAg loss occurred in 33% of patients treated with telbivudine, compared with 28% receiving lamivudine monotherapy. HBV DNA became undetectable by a PCR assay in 61% of patients treated with telbivudine alone, compared with 32% of those treated with lamivudine. Resistance to telbivudine has been reported to occur in 4% of patients after 1 year of treatment.

Clevudine

Clevudine, a pyrimidine analog, is a potent inhibitor of HBV replication both in vitro and in vivo. This drug has been studied in woodchucks and to a limited extent in humans. In one study, therapy with clevudine given daily for 12 weeks resulted in a greater than 4 $\log_{10}$ copies/mL reduction in serum HBV DNA levels.[177] Rebound to pretreatment HBV DNA levels occurred slowly in this and other studies.[178] The reason for the sustained antiviral activity after discontinuation of the drug is unexplained but may result from the long intracellular half-life of the phosphorylated compound and active metabolites. It may be possible to give this drug less frequently than once daily. Little is known about safety and drug accumulation with long-term use of clevudine.

Innovative Therapeutic Approaches with Available Agents

Lamivudine Maintenance in Patients with Advanced Fibrosis

Nucleoside analog therapy has been associated with improvements in liver histologic findings, including bridging fibrosis and cirrhosis, when treatment is extended beyond 52 weeks.[49] A large, double-blind study of long-term treatment of HBV with lamivudine versus placebo in patients with advanced fibrosis (including cirrhosis) has shown that long-term lamivudine therapy can prevent disease progression.[179] In this study, investigators had intended to treat patients for 5 years, but the study was terminated early (median of 32 months of active treatment) because clinical indicators of disease progression and HCC had become more common in patients in the placebo arm. Among lamivudine recipients, those with YMDD mutant HBV had an intermediate response and reached fewer end points than did untreated controls. If these results are confirmed, long-term nucleoside analog therapy will likely be recommended routinely in patients with advanced disease.

Combination Nucleoside Analog Treatment

It has been proposed that the combination of two or more nucleoside analogs may be more effective therapy

against HBV than a single agent. In vitro data and studies in the woodchuck model of hepatitis B support a role for combination therapy of hepatitis B. It is hoped that combination treatment will prevent or delay the emergence of drug resistance and lead to more rapid clinical stabilization. This outcome could be particularly important for patients with decompensated cirrhosis or those in urgent need of liver transplantation. Disadvantages of combination therapy are the added cost and the potential for greater toxicity. In addition, certain combinations could theoretically lead to multidrug resistance.

Somewhat surprisingly, the results of early clinical trials of combination therapy in previously untreated patients with HBeAg-positive chronic hepatitis B have shown that the combination of 2 nucleoside analogs (telbivudine and lamivudine) or the combination of a nucleoside analog and a nucleotide analog (lamivudine and adefovir) does not lead to greater viral inhibition during the first year of treatment than that seen with monotherapy.[176,180] The reasons for the lack of apparent additive effect in these studies remain unexplained. It is possible that nucleoside analogs like telbivudine and lamivudine compete sterically for binding to the HBV DNA polymerase or compete for phosphorylation enzymes (kinases) required for drug activation. Another possible explanation is that a measurable increase in viral suppression may be difficult to demonstrate whenever a drug with substantially less antiviral activity is added to a more potent drug (for example, when lamivudine is added to telbivudine or when adefovir is added to lamivudine).

Combination Interferon and Nucleoside Analog Treatment

From a conceptual standpoint, treatment with the combination of interferon and a nucleoside analog might prove to be more effective than either drug alone, because these agents have different mechanisms of action, and might also allow for a shorter course of nucleoside analog therapy, thereby reducing the risk of viral resistance. A number of studies in the woodchuck and several clinical trials in humans have provided support for additive or synergistic effects when interferon is used in conjunction with a nucleoside analog. Two large multicenter studies evaluated these effects in patients given a combination of pegylated interferon and lamivudine. In one study, HBeAg-positive patients received pegylated interferon alfa-2b with either lamivudine or placebo for 1 year.[147] At the end of treatment, 44% of the patients who received combination therapy had lost HBeAg, whereas only 29% who received interferon alone had done so; however, response rates in the two groups were no longer significantly different 26 weeks after the end of treatment (35% and 36%, respectively). It is possible that the low dose of pegylated interferon used in this study (100 µg weekly for 8 months followed by 50 µg weekly until the end of treatment) may have contributed to the relatively high relapse rate after remission.

In the second study, patients with HBeAg-negative chronic hepatitis B were treated with pegylated interferon alfa-2a, 180 µg given weekly for 1 year, in combination with either lamivudine or placebo, and these two treatment groups were compared with a group receiving lamivudine monotherapy.[148] Both virologic response and serum ALT normalization were significantly more common at completion of follow-up in patients treated with the interferon-containing regimens, but patients who received the combination therapy did not demonstrate a higher rate of sustained virologic response than those who received pegylated interferon alone. There was, however, a more rapid decline in serum HBV DNA levels and an approximately 1 $\log_{10}$ copies/mL greater reduction in serum HBV DNA levels at the end of treatment in patients who received combination therapy than in the other treatment groups. This study provided proof of the concept that pegylated interferon and lamivudine have additive antiviral effects.

Other Novel Therapies

T_H1 Cytokines

Chronic hepatitis B is an immunologically based liver disorder, and treatments that are directed toward augmenting immune responses could be helpful in viral clearance.[52] The interleukins IL-12 and IL-18 are cytokines secreted by activated macrophages and dendritic cells. These cytokines promote T_H1 cellular responses, which are thought to be important for HBV clearance. The therapeutic administration of these cytokines has shown some efficacy in transgenic mice, but human studies are either lacking or inconclusive.[181,182] IL-28 and IL-29 are cytokines distantly related to interferon-α and IL-10 that have been shown to inhibit HBV replication in a HepG2 cell line These agents induce 2′5′-oligoadenylate synthetase, double-stranded RNA–activated protein kinase, and MxA gene expression in primary hepatocytes.[183] No human studies have been reported.

Thymosin alpha-1 is a thymic-derived peptide that enhances T-cell maturation and augments a number of T-cell functions. This drug is available as therapy for hepatitis B in China, India, Mexico, the Philippines, and several South American countries, on the basis of studies showing that it can improve serum ALT levels and other indicators of viral replication. Published studies of this drug have yielded widely variable results, however, with some suggesting no benefit.[184] A study in patients with HBeAg-negative chronic hepatitis B found significantly higher rates of sustained virologic and biochemical responses in patients treated with a combination of thymosin and interferon alfa-2b followed by interferon alfa-2b alone than in those treated with interferon alone or a combination of interferon and lamivudine.[185] It is possible that thymosin will have a role in combination regimens; side effects have been minimal.

Therapeutic Vaccines

A number of T_H1-promoting vaccine therapeutic strategies are under development, but few have been tested in chronic HBV carriers. On the basis of preclinical data, genetic (DNA) vaccines may one day prove to be highly effective if technical hurdles can be overcome. In contrast, protein-based vaccines with newly developed T_H1 adjuvants are ready to be tested in humans, either alone or in combination with each other.

Small Interfering RNA Molecules

The use of small interfering RNA molecules (siRNAs) is an innovative molecular approach to silencing or suppressing HBV gene expression. The siRNAs are small duplex or hairpin RNA molecules with sequences that match those of target HBV DNA. The activity of these molecules depends on their delivery to the nucleus of HBV-infected cells. The hairpin sequences are exported to the cytoplasm, where they are incorporated into the cytoplasmic RNA–induced silencing complex (RISC) and into HBV mRNA targets, thereby resulting in degradation of the HBV mRNA and inhibition of viral replication.

The feasibility of this approach has been confirmed in vitro and in the mouse model of HBV infection, in which reductions in serum levels of both HBcAg and HBsAg have been observed.[186,187] Further studies are necessary to establish the ideal target sequences to inhibit HBV protein expression and to determine whether these sequences can be incorporated efficiently into human hepatocytes.

Viral Packaging Inhibitors

Several compounds have been developed that have a mechanism of action against HBV that does not involve inhibition of the viral polymerase. Phenylpropenamide derivatives have been shown to reduce the production of encapsidated RNA in both wild-type and lamivudine-resistant HBV without affecting the production of HBV RNA, core protein, or nucleocapsids.[188] However, the safety of these compounds has not been tested, and they may be limited by poor water solubility and extremely low bioavailability.[189] A series of nonnucleoside inhibitors of HBV capsid formation that belong to a unique class of agents referred to as heteroaryldihydropyrimidines (HAPs) have also been developed. These agents interfere directly with viral nucleocapsid formation and have thus far been studied in transgenic mice and the duck model of hepatitis B.

Future Issues in Antiviral Therapy

Despite the many advances in the treatment of chronic hepatitis B, unresolved issues remain. Time-limited treatments that induce a durable virologic response while remaining both safe and easily affordable have not been developed. The treatment of patients with normal or near-normal serum ALT levels, those who are immunosuppressed or are coinfected with HIV, and those with HBeAg-negative chronic hepatitis B pose the greatest clinical challenges. The advent and increasing potency of nucleoside analog therapy since the late 1990s have overshadowed focus on the host immune response for achieving therapeutic end points and has relegated interferon to being considered second-line therapy by many authorities. Data demonstrating the enhanced potency of pegylated interferon now provide reason to reevaluate this issue. The development of better immunologic modifiers and drugs that block viral proliferation independent of viral DNA polymerase would be a great step forward.

PREVENTION

Immunoprophylaxis against HBV is of two types: passive immunization using HBIG and active immunization using inactive HBsAg. Active immunization gives long-term immunity, whereas passive immunization confers only immediate and short-lived protection.

Hepatitis B Immunoglobulin

HBIG is prepared from plasma that is known to contain high titers of anti-HBs. Numerous clinical trials have established the efficacy of HBIG in preventing HBV infection in high-risk persons, such as hemodialysis patients, sexual partners of patients with hepatitis B, and newborn infants of HBsAg-positive mothers.[190-193]

HBIG licensed in the United States has an anti-HBs titer of 1:100,000. In Europe, several preparations of HBIG with different concentrations and pharmacokinetic properties are available. HBIG is safe, although rare anaphylactic reactions can occur. Myalgias, rash, and arthralgias have also been reported and are believed to result from formation of antigen-antibody complexes.

Hepatitis B Vaccine

Currently marketed HBV vaccines make use of DNA recombinant technology by introducing the gene for HBsAg (S gene) into the genome of the yeast *Saccharomyces cerevisiae*. The two vaccines available in the United States are Recombivax HB (Merck, licensed in 1986) and Engerix-B (SmithKline Beecham, licensed in 1989). Aluminum hydroxide is used as an adjuvant in both vaccines. Because thimerosal, a preservative used in the vaccines, contains mercury, thimerosal-free vaccines have become available, especially for use in infants. The HBV vaccine is administered intramuscularly in the deltoid muscle of adults and the anterolateral thigh of infants and neonates. The vaccines induce HBsAg-specific helper T cells and T cell–dependent B cells to produce neutralizing antibody against the "a" epitope (amino acid sequence 124–148) of HBsAg as early as 2 weeks after the first injection.[196,197] HBV vaccines are highly efficacious in preventing HBV infection.[198-200] Because the vaccines contain HBsAg only, anti-HBs is the sole antibody produced. Consequently, a vaccinee who tests positive for anti-HBc after vaccination should be considered to have had a subclinical HBV infection.

The vaccines typically achieve an anti-HBs titer greater than 100 mIU/mL. Antibody titers greater than 100 mIU/mL confer 100% protection against HBV infection, and a lower antibody titer (up to 10 mIU/mL) is seroprotective in most instances. Peak antibody titers and persistence of antibody levels vary among different persons. The titers steadily drop over the first 2 years after vaccination, sometimes to levels less than 10 mIU/mL. Two studies in different populations have demonstrated that anti-HBs titers decrease to nonprotective levels in at least 25% to 50% of recipients over a period of 5 to 10 years.[201,202]

Although protective anti-HBs response rates after HBV vaccination typically exceed 90%, a number of factors can impede an adequate antibody response. Smoking, obesity, injection into the buttock, chronic liver disease, presence of HLA-DR3, DR7, and DQ2 alleles, absence of the HLA-A2 allele, and extremes of age may be associated with reduced immunogenicity. Such "hyporesponders" may benefit from a higher dose of vaccine. Response rates also are lower in immunocompromised patients, such as

transplant recipients, patients receiving chemotherapy, and those with end-stage liver disease. Only 50% to 60% of hemodialysis patients respond adequately to vaccination. Therefore, patients with chronic kidney disease should be vaccinated early in the course of their disease, before renal disease progresses, to ensure optimal response to vaccination.[203]

Five percent to 8% of HBV vaccine recipients do not achieve detectable anti-HBs levels ("nonresponders"). Studies conducted mostly in animals indicate that intradermal injection of the vaccine may produce a stronger humoral and cellular immune response than conventional intramuscular administration.[205-209] Intradermal injection, by recruiting "professional" dendritic cells, stimulates primary MHC class I– and class II–restricted T-cell responses.[204-208] In one study, intradermal vaccination resulted in protective anti-HBs responses in nonresponders to intramuscular administration.[208] Repeated dosing with intradermal vaccination (5 μg every 2 weeks to provide an anti-HBs titer of 1,000 mIU/mL or greater or a total of 52 doses) has resulted in a protective antibody response rate of nearly 100% in patients undergoing long-term hemodialysis.[209] At present there are no recommendations for using intradermal vaccination, in part because of concerns about standardization of the technique for intradermal delivery.

Because HBV vaccination results in strong immunologic memory capable of preventing infection even in patients with low or undetectable antibody titers, there is no role for a booster vaccine dose in immunocompetent adults and children.[210] Current recommendations include booster doses only for patients undergoing hemodialysis, in whom anti-HBs titers should be tested annually and a booster dose given if the titer is lower than 10 mIU/mL.[211]

No serious side effects of the HBV vaccine have been reported. The frequency of neurologic diseases such as aseptic meningitis and Guillain-Barré syndrome is not increased in vaccine recipients.

Targeted High-Risk Groups

Table 75–7 lists the high-risk groups for whom HBV vaccination is recommended. Targeted vaccination has not achieved its objective in certain high-risk groups, such as injection drug users, but has achieved great success among health care workers and newborns.

Vaccination Schedule

The doses of currently available HBV vaccines and recommendations for the schedules of administration are shown in Table 75–8. The typical vaccination schedule is 0, 1, and 6 months. The first two doses have no effect on the final anti-HBs titer. The third dose acts as a booster to achieve a high anti-HBs titer. In immunocompromised patients and patients undergoing hemodialysis, four vaccine doses are recommended, with the fourth dose given to ensure the highest possible anti-HBs titer. If vaccination is interrupted, the second dose should be administered as soon as possible after the first.[211] If the third dose is not given on schedule, it should be given at least 2 months after the second dose.

The HBV vaccine is currently administered to all children and infants as a part of the universal immunization program. Combination HBV vaccines with diphtheria-pertussis-tetanus (DPT) and *Haemophilus influenzae* type B (Hib) (DTPw-HB/Hib), the vaccines in current use for immunization of infants do not reduce the immunogenicity of any of the components of HBV infection.[212] Adolescents who have not been vaccinated in infancy or childhood should also be vaccinated.

Table 75–7 High-Risk Groups for Whom Hepatitis B Virus (HBV) Vaccination Should Be Considered

Heath care workers
Public safety workers with likelihood of exposure to blood
Staff and clients of institutions for developmentally disabled
Hemodialysis patients
Patients who are likely to require multiple transfusions with blood or blood products
Household contacts and sexual partners of HBV carriers or patients with acute hepatitis B
International travelers to areas endemic for HBV who may have intimate contact with the local population or take part in medical activities
Injection drug users
Sexually active men who have sex with men
Sexually active heterosexual men and women, if they have more than one partner
Inmates of correctional facilities
Patients with chronic liver disease
Potential organ transplant recipients

Table 75–8 Recommended Dosing for the Currently Available Hepatitis B Vaccines*

	Recombivax HB (10 µg/mL)	Engerix-B (20 µg/mL)
Infants† and children age <11 yrs	2.5 µg	10 µg
Children age 11-19 yrs	5 µg	20 µg
Adults (≥20 yrs)	10 µg	20 µg
Hemodialysis patients	40 µg (1.0 mL)‡	40 µg (2.0 mL)§
Immunocompromised patients	40 µg (1.0 mL)‡	40 µg (2.0 mL)§

*The standard schedule is 0, 1, and 6 months.
†Infants born to hepatitis B surface antigen–negative mothers.
‡Special formulation.
§Two 1.0-mL doses administered at one site in four-dose schedule (0, 1, 2, 6 months).

Postexposure and Perinatal Prophylaxis

Table 75–9 summarizes recommendations for prevention of perinatal transmission of HBV. Table 75–10 lists recommendations for prophylaxis after exposure to a known HBsAg-positive source. Postexposure vaccination should be considered for any percutaneous, ocular, or mucous membrane exposure. The type of immunoprophylaxis is determined by the HBsAg status of the source and the vaccination-response status of the exposed person.

New Developments

A combined HAV and HBV vaccine has been licensed commercially (Twinrix, Glaxo SmithKline, Research Triangle Park, NC) and has been shown to be highly immunogenic and protective against both infections. This vaccine offers ease of administration for persons at increased risk of both HAV and HBV infection (e.g., world travelers or men who have sex with men) and in patients with underlying chronic liver disease.[213]

Immunogenicity of HBV vaccines may be enhanced by use of more potent adjuvants. HBsAg/AS04 vaccine (which contains 3′-deacylated monophosphoryl lipid A) and MF59-adjuvanted HBV vaccine (which contains surface and pre-S2 antigens) elicit a better immune response than standard HBV vaccines.[214-216] Concomitant administration of granulocyte-macrophage colony–stimulating factor also may enhance the anti-HBs response to vaccination.[217] Immunization using HBV

Table 75–10 Postexposure Prophylaxis of Hepatitis B if the Source Is HBsAg Positive

Vaccination Status of Exposed Person	Immune Prophylaxis
Unvaccinated	HBIG (0.06 mL/kg) and initiate hepatitis B vaccine series
Previously vaccinated:	
Known responder*	No treatment
Known nonresponder	HBIG × 2 doses (one month apart) OR HBIG × 1 dose and initiate revaccination
Antibody response unknown	Test for anti-HBs If adequate*: No treatment If inadequate†: HBIG × 1 dose and give vaccine booster dose

Anti-HBs, antibody to hepatitis B surface antigen; HBIG, hepatitis B immune globulin; HBsAg, hepatitis B surface antigen.
*Anti-HBs titer >10 mIU/mL.
†Anti-HBs titer <10 mIU/mL.

Table 75–9 Hepatitis B Prophylaxis of Infants Born to Hepatitis B Surface Antigen–Positive Mothers

Age of the Infant	HBIG	Vaccination	Vaccine: Give One of the Following:	
			Recombivax HB	Engerix-B
Within 12 hours of birth	0.5 mL IM*	First dose	5 µg (0.5 mL)	10 µg (0.5 mL)
1 month	None	Second dose	5 µg (0.5 mL)	10 µg (0.5 mL)
6 months†	None	Third dose	5 µg (0.5 mL)	10 µg (0.5 mL)

HBIG, hepatitis B immune globulin.
*HBIG should be administered at a site different from that used for the vaccine.
†If four doses of vaccine are administered, the third dose is given at 2 months, and the fourth dose is given at 12-18 months.

DNA encoding for HBsAg and nucleoprotein has generated considerable interest as both a prophylactic and a therapeutic tool.[218] These DNA-based vaccines elicit both humoral and cellular immune responses.

Novel delivery of vaccine to immunize a fetus in utero was accomplished successfully in fetal lambs. HBV DNA vaccine was introduced into the amniotic fluid, thereby resulting in high serum anti-HBs levels and a cell-mediated immune response combined with local immunity in the oral cavity.[219] An edible HBV vaccine is another area of development.

HBV Escape Mutants and Implications for Immunization

As described earlier, mutations in the HBV genome encoding HBsAg can result in mutant HBV virus strains that can escape neutralization by anti-HBs. The mutation involves the "a" determinant and has shown decreased binding to monoclonal anti-a antibodies. Such mutants have been reported worldwide and are particularly common in areas endemic for HBV. These mutant viruses account for some instances in which the HBV vaccine has failed to prevent perinatal transmission. The frequency of this mutation is currently low, but in the future this HBV mutant could emerge as an important threat, in which case HBV vaccines may have to incorporate the mutant antigen in order to remain effective.

HEPATITIS D (DELTA)

Hepatitis D (delta) virus was discovered by Rizzetto and associates in 1977 as a unique nuclear antigen in the hepatocytes of patients infected with HBV.[220] The antigen was identified subsequently as a novel pathogen and was linked to severe chronic hepatitis B and fulminant HBV infection.

EPIDEMIOLOGY

HDV is distributed worldwide with wide variations in prevalence. At least 5% of HBV carriers worldwide are estimated to be infected with HDV, and therefore, the overall burden of HDV infection is between 15 and 20 million cases. The highest prevalence is seen in South America and the Mediterranean basin. The prevalence is low in Northern Europe and North America, where HDV infection is confined to injection drug users. The rate of infection among HBsAg-positive blood donors in the United States has been found to be 3.8%.[221] The incidence of transfusion-associated HDV infection has been declining steadily because of HBV vaccination and screening of donor sera for HBsAg. In fact, many epidemiologists believe that the epidemic of HDV, which started in the 1970s, is coming to an end. For example, epidemiologic data from Italy show that the current prevalence of HDV infection in HBsAg carriers is 8.3%, compared with 25% in the early 1970s.[222-224] However, HDV infection remains an important problem among injection drug users.[225,226]

Among the three genotypes of HDV (I to III), genotype I is the most prevalent and is the most common geno-type in Mediterranean countries, Africa, Europe, and North America.[227,228] Different subtypes within this genotype may exist in certain parts of Africa. Genotype II is reported mostly in Japan and Taiwan and is associated with milder liver disease than that seen with genotype I.[229] Genotype III has been isolated from epidemics in South America.[230] Different genotypes of HDV may interact variably with different HBV genotypes. Whether the interaction between HDV and HBV genotypes specifically increases the severity of HDV infection is unclear, although infection with HDV genotype III and HBV genotype F is reported to cause severe hepatitis. The mode of HDV transmission is linked closely to that of HBV transmission, with the parenteral route being the most efficient. Sexual transmission of HDV has been reported, and familial clustering of cases has been seen in endemic areas.

VIROLOGY

HDV is a unique agent that bears no similarity to other transmissible agents that infect animals. In fact, the 1.7-kb single-strand HDV RNA genome shares several features with plant viroids, such as intramolecular base pairing and autocatalytic RNA segments.[231] However, unlike plant viroids, HDV RNA encodes a protein, hepatitis delta antigen (HDAg). The virion consists of the HDV genome complexed with approximately 70 copies of HDAg in an envelope protein composed of lipids and HBsAg. The protein envelope that is contributed by HBV protects the HDV RNA–HDAg complex. The protein envelope is not required for replication of HDV and is the only helper function provided by HBV. Once HDV with its HBV envelope protein enters the host, the HDV RNA–HDAg complex migrates to the nucleus. Viral replication then proceeds in the nucleus according to a double-rolling model, aided possibly by host DNA–dependent RNA polymerase.[232,233]

During translation, two forms of HDAg (encoded by the same regions of RNA) are produced, a short form (HDAg-S) and long form (HDAg-L). HDAg-L has 19 to 20 more amino acids than HDAg-S. The additional amino acids in HDAg-L are incorporated by a process of RNA editing, another unique aspect of the HDV genome.[234,235] Interestingly, HDAg-S and HDAg-L have opposite effects on viral replication; HDAg-S acts as a facilitator, and HDAg-L as an inhibitor.[236,237] The extent of RNA editing determines the amount of HDAg-L formed and, consequently, influences the rate of replication. In states of high replication, only HDAg-S is produced. Ultimately, the intracellular ratio of HDAg-S to HDAg-L determines the rate of replication, assembly, and transport from infected hepatocytes.

Because it has a unique genome, HDV is classified in a separate genus of the Deltaviridae family. No other virus has been identified in this genus. The current consensus is that HDV is a satellite virus.[238,239] Satellite viruses are subviral particles that carry a distinct nucleic acid, usually RNA, that requires a helper virus for transmission and multiplication. In addition, the nucleic acid of satellite viruses is distinct from the nucleic acid of helper viruses. No other animal virus has been identified as a satellite virus. HDV is not a viroid, as previously believed, because HDV RNA codes for a structural protein, HDAg.[240]

PATHOGENESIS

The pathogenic mechanisms of HDV hepatitis remain poorly understood. Because HBV is not known to be directly cytotoxic, the severity of combined infection with HBV and HDV may be attributed either to a direct cytotoxic effect of HDV or an enhanced immune response against the two viruses. Direct cytotoxicity of HDV has been questioned on the basis of studies in transgenic mice. Mice expressing either HDAg-L or HDAg-S show no evidence of hepatocyte injury.[241] The lack of a direct cytotoxic effect also is supported by the observation that liver transplant recipients who express HDAg in their allografts do not manifest evidence of cellular damage.[242,243] Instead, the pathogenic mechanism of HDV-induced liver damage is most likely related to the immunologic response to HDV. The occurrence of classic necroinflammatory changes in the liver and several autoantibodies, such as antibodies to liver-kidney microsome (anti-LKM), thymocytes, and nuclear lamin C also suggest a role for immune-mediated liver injury. One fact is certain: The ability of HDV to cause hepatic necrosis is determined by expression of HBV, as illustrated after liver transplantation, when HDV infection becomes pathogenic only if HBV infection also recurs.[242,243]

DIAGNOSIS

The most useful markers of HDV infection include HDAg, antibody to HDAg (anti-HDV), HDV RNA, and immunohistochemical staining of HDAg in liver tissue. Detection of HDV RNA by reverse transcriptase PCR amplification (RT-PCR), with a detection limit of 50 to 100 copies/mL, is the most reliable diagnostic technique, with nearly 100% sensitivity.[244,245] HDV RNA is the earliest marker to appear during the course of HDV infection and may be seen in the absence of other markers.[246] Higher levels of HDV RNA in serum may be associated with more severe disease.[247] The level of HDV RNA in serum is a reliable marker for monitoring the efficacy of treatment and documenting viral eradication. HDV RNA also can be detected in liver cells by hybridization techniques, which are generally less sensitive than RT-PCR.

The HDV genomic product, HDAg, is another marker of HDV infection. HDAg can be demonstrated in hepatocytes by immunohistochemical staining, but the reliability of this method decreases as the disease becomes chronic. Measurement of HDAg in serum is also problematic because of the presence of high titers of neutralizing antibodies, which interfere with detection of HDAg.

The most readily available marker of HDV infection has been anti-HDV. Anti-HDV does not confer protection against HDV. Either IgM anti-HDV or total anti-HDV, which is composed of both IgM and IgG anti-HDV, can be detected. IgM anti-HDV appears in serum at the time of acute infection, and IgG anti-HDV develops later in the course.[248-250] IgM anti-HDV often persists as the disease progresses to chronicity and is detectable in high titers in patients with chronic HDV infection. It is frequently regarded as a marker of serious liver damage.[251] As the infection evolves from the acute to the chronic phase, the type of IgM antibody also changes from a monomeric (S) form to a multimeric (19S) form.[252] IgG anti-HDV persists for a long time in immunocompetent persons and may indicate chronic or previous HDV infection. Some patients with IgG anti-HDV may not have active infection and test negative for HDV RNA.[253]

NATURAL HISTORY

Because of the obligate relationship of HDV to HBV infection, the natural history of HDV infection depends on the clinical course of HBV. Two distinct types of HDV infections are possible: One is a coprimary infection, in which there is simultaneous infection of HBV and HDV, and the other is superinfection, in which HDV infection is superimposed on established chronic HBV infection.

Early epidemiologic studies suggested that HDV infection aggravates the severity of HBV infection, but subsequent reports have disputed this claim.[254-256] In a European multicenter study on prognostic factors in 366 patients with chronic hepatitis B and compensated cirrhosis, HDV infection did not influence the prognosis.[257] In a long-term follow-up study of 302 patients with chronic hepatitis B (76 with HDV infection), HDV infection was not an independent predictor of mortality.[258] Therefore, HDV infection appears to have a varying influence on the course of hepatitis B and is not necessarily associated with severe hepatitis. The severity of HDV infection may vary with the frequency of HDV in a population, with the level of HBV viremia, and with interactions between specific HBV and HDV genotypes.

Coprimary infection is seen most often in injection drug abusers (Fig. 75–6). Because HBV infection resolves in a majority of patients, HDV also disappears in most patients, and the risk of chronicity after coprimary infection is less than 5%. However, some data suggest that coinfection with HDV enhances the risk of fulminant hepatitis B.[259-261]

Superinfection of HDV in an HBV carrier can lead to severe hepatitis and acute decompensation of preexisting liver disease. Affected patients often express a high level of HDV viremia, because high serum levels of HBsAg readily protect the replicating HDV genome. Superinfection may also coincide with a decline in serum HBV DNA levels, because HDV replication inhibits HBV replication.[262] In a study involving 185 patients with HDV superinfection, HDV RNA was detectable in 63 of 64 patients with acute HDV infection, but HBV DNA was detectable in only 40% of patients.[262] Rarely, HDV superinfection may lead to disappearance of HBsAg and appearance of anti-HBs.[262] In contrast to coinfection, chronic HDV infection develops frequently after HDV superinfection. HDV superinfection evolves to chronic HDV infection in 70% of patients and is characterized by persistent HDV viremia and detectable HDV RNA in serum. Although the clinical course of chronic HDV infection varies, persistent replication of HDV and HBV often leads to progressive hepatitis and cirrhosis within a few years. More rapid clinical progression leading to end-

Figure 75–6 Serologic results, clinical features, and prognosis of hepatitis D superinfection and coprimary infection. ALT, alanine aminotransferase; Anti-HBc, antibody to hepatitis B core antigen; Anti-HDV, antibody to hepatitis D virus; HBsAg, hepatitis B surface antigen; HBV, hepatitis B virus; HDV, hepatitis D virus.

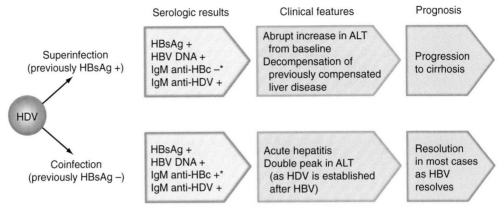

Serologic results	Clinical features	Prognosis

Superinfection (previously HBsAg +)

HBsAg +
HBV DNA +
IgM anti-HBc −*
IgM anti-HDV +

Abrupt increase in ALT from baseline
Decompensation of previously compensated liver disease

Progression to cirrhosis

Coinfection (previously HBsAg −)

HBsAg +
HBV DNA +
IgM anti-HBc +*
IgM anti-HDV +

Acute hepatitis
Double peak in ALT (as HDV is established after HBV)

Resolution in most cases as HBV resolves

* Distinguishing feature between superinfection and coinfection.

stage liver disease within 2 years may be seen in some injection drug users.[263,264]

The clinical course of a triple infection with HBV, HDV, and HCV is usually dominated by the HCV infection. Affected patients often have a severe episode of acute hepatitis at the time of HDV or HCV superinfection, but the chronic stage is slowly progressive and does not differ much from that of chronic HDV and HBV infection.

CLINICAL FEATURES

HDV and HBV coinfection typically manifests as self-limited acute hepatitis. Some patients may demonstrate a double peak in serum aminotransferase levels because of a delay in HDV replication after HBV replication. Markers detectable in serum at the time of acute hepatitis include IgM anti-HBc, IgM anti-HDV, HDV RNA, HBV DNA, and HBsAg. Acute hepatitis usually resolves in a few weeks, with a gradual return of liver biochemical test levels to normal. As the infection resolves, HDV RNA and HBV DNA titers steadily decrease, and anti-HBs appears after the disappearance of HBsAg. Occasionally, IgM anti-HDV may persist after anti-HB appears and serum aminotransferase levels return to normal.

HDV superinfection manifests clinically as acute hepatitis in an otherwise stable chronic HBV carrier. Clinically, HDV superinfection can mimic a spontaneous flare of chronic HBV infection. These two diagnostic possibilities can be differentiated easily, because patients with HDV superinfection have markers of HDV infection, such as HDV RNA and IgM anti-HDV, in serum. IgM anti-HDV is seen in both coinfection and superinfection and is not useful for differentiating the two. Determining whether an HDV infection is a superinfection or coinfection depends on whether the HBV infection is chronic or acute, and the distinguishing serologic feature of coinfection is the presence of IgM anti-HBc in serum.[265]

TREATMENT

Despite developments in the treatment of HBV infection, results of therapy for HDV infection have been disappointing. Interferon has been the only agent to show some promise. Nucleoside analogs, currently the mainstay of treatment for HBV infection, are not effective for HDV infection, probably because nucleoside analogs seldom lead to disappearance of HBsAg, the only HBV protein required by HDV. The superiority of interferon over nucleoside analogs in causing loss of HBsAg makes interferon the preferred treatment for HDV infection.

Several clinical trials have evaluated the efficacy of interferon in the treatment of chronic HDV infection.[266-271] Two major studies conducted in Italy showed that interferon improved serum aminotransferase levels and liver histologic findings but failed to lead to a sustained virologic response.[266,267] In one study, a high dose of interferon alfa (9 million units 3 times weekly for 48 weeks) achieved a 50% end-of-treatment virologic response (absence of HDV RNA in serum as measured by dot blot hybridization assay), but the rate of virologic relapse during follow-up was substantial.[266] In this study, high-dose interferon treatment was associated with a higher response rate than low-dose treatment (3 million units 3 times weekly) or no treatment.[266] In a second clinical trial, lower doses of interferon alfa-2b (5 million units three times weekly followed by 3 million units three times weekly) were compared with no treatment, and sustained virologic responses were not obtained[267]; similar observations have been made in other studies.[268-271]

Long-term follow-up of the original cohort of patients in the Italian studies who were treated with either 9 million units or 3 million units of interferon 3 times weekly for 48 weeks has shown that the patients who were treated with the higher dose of interferon had significantly better survival than the patients who received the lower dose or no treatment.[272] In addition, the high-dose interferon group had a sustained decrease in HDV replication, leading to clearance of HDV RNA and even HBV DNA in some patients.[272] More importantly, hepatic histology improved significantly in the high-dose group, with disappearance of cirrhosis in four of six patients whose initial biopsy specimens showed cirrhosis. The impact of prolonged treatment, which seems logical on the basis of these data, deserves further study.

Controlled studies of pegylated interferons for HDV infection have not been reported. Nucleoside analogs such as lamivudine have not been shown to influence HDV replication and are not recommended for HDV infection.[273-275] Studies in children have demonstrated a disappointing response rate to treatment with interferon. Similarly, patients coinfected with HIV or HCV have had poor rates of response to antiviral therapy.[276,277] Whether antiviral treatment of HDV infection leads to improved liver histology in coinfected patients requires further study.

On the basis of studies to date, HDV infection should be treated with interferon alfa, 9 million units 3 times weekly for at least 1 year. Treatment for a longer duration may be more beneficial and should be considered on the basis of histologic severity, HDV RNA response, and patient tolerability. Whether or not pegylated interferons improve the response rate is not known. However, because pegylated interferon appears to be more effective than conventional interferon for HBV infection, further studies in patients with chronic hepatitis D are certainly warranted.

Advances in molecular biology may help to identify specific inhibitors of HDV replication.[278] Prenylation (addition of prenyl lipids such as farnesyl) of HDAg-L is a critical determinant of HDV particle assembly. In vitro studies have shown that inhibition of prenylation can abolish particle production effectively in a dose-dependent manner.[279]

PREVENTION

Because the ability of HDV to infect a host depends on the preexistence of HBsAg, vaccination against HBV confers protection against HDV. Groups who exhibit a high rate of HDV infection, such as injection drug abusers, should be targeted for vaccination.

REFERENCES

1. Chang MH, Chen CJ, Lai MS, et al: Universal hepatitis B vaccination in Taiwan and the incidence of hepatocellular carcinoma in children. Taiwan Childhood Hepatoma Study Group. N Engl J Med 336:1855, 1997.
2. Maynard JE: Hepatitis B: Global importance and need for control. Vaccine 8(Suppl):S18, 1990.
3. Gust ID: Epidemiology of hepatitis B infection in the Western Pacific and South East Asia. Gut 38(Suppl 2):S18, 1996.
4. Alter MJ: Epidemiology of hepatitis B in Europe and worldwide. J Hepatol 39(Suppl 1):S64, 2003.
5. Lee WM: Hepatitis B virus infection. N Engl J Med 337:1733, 1997.
6. Xu ZY, Liu CB, Francis DP, et al: Prevention of perinatal acquisition of hepatitis B virus carriage using vaccine: Preliminary report of a randomized double-blind placebo-controlled and comparative trial. Pediatrics 76:713, 1985.
7. Perrillo RP, Gelb L, Campbell C, et al: Hepatitis B e antigen, DNA polymerase activity, and infection of household contacts with hepatitis B virus. Gastroenterology 76:1319, 1979.
8. Alter MJ, Ahtone J, Maynard JE: Hepatitis B virus transmission associated with a multiple-dose vial in a hemodialysis unit. Ann Intern Med 99:330, 1983.
9. Harpaz R, Von Seidlein L, Averhoff FM, et al: Transmission of hepatitis B virus to multiple patients from a surgeon without evidence of inadequate infection control. N Engl J Med 334:549, 1996.
10. Limentani AE, Elliott LM, Noah ND, et al: An outbreak of hepatitis B from tattooing. Lancet 2(8133):86, 1979.
11. Berry WR, Gottesfeld RL, Alter HJ, et al: Transmission of hepatitis B virus by artificial insemination. JAMA 257:1079, 1987.
12. Hoofnagle JH: Posttransfusion hepatitis B. Transfusion 30:384, 1990.
13. Dickson RC, Everhart JE, Lake JR, et al: Transmission of hepatitis B by transplantation of livers from donors positive for antibody to hepatitis B core antigen. The National Institute of Diabetes and Digestive and Kidney Diseases Liver Transplantation Database. Gastroenterology 113:1668, 1997.
14. Grob P, Jilg W, Bornhak H, et al: Serological pattern "anti-HBc alone": Report of a workshop. J Med Virol 62:450, 2000.
15. Alter HJ, Seeff LB, Kaplan PM, et al: Type B hepatitis: The infectivity of blood positive for e antigen and HBV DNA polymerase after accidental needlestick exposure. N Engl J Med 295:909, 1976.
16. Mason A, Wick M, White H, et al: Hepatitis B virus replication in diverse cell types during chronic hepatitis B virus infection. Hepatology 18:781, 1993.
17. Mason A, Yoffe B, Noonan C, et al: Hepatitis B virus DNA in peripheral-blood mononuclear cells in chronic hepatitis B after HBsAg clearance. Hepatology 16:36, 1992.
18. Kuhns M, McNamara A, Mason A, et al: Serum and liver hepatitis B virus DNA in chronic hepatitis B after sustained loss of surface antigen. Gastroenterology 103:1649, 1992.
19. Fong TL, Bunnapradist S, Jordan SC, et al: Impact of hepatitis B core antibody status on outcomes of cadaveric renal transplantation: Analysis of United Network of Organ Sharing database between 1994 and 1999. Transplantation 73:85, 2002.
20. Hollinger FB: Comprehensive control (or elimination) of hepatitis B virus transmission in the United States. Gut 38 (Suppl 2):S24, 1996.
21. Alter MJ: Epidemiology and prevention of hepatitis B. Semin Liver Dis 23:39, 2003.
22. McQuillan GM, Coleman PJ, Kruszon-Moran D, et al: Prevalence of hepatitis B virus infection in the United States: The National Health and Nutrition Examination Surveys, 1976 through 1994. Am J Public Health 89:14, 1999.
23. AS Lok, Heathcote EJ, Hoofnagle JH: Management of hepatitis B: 2000—summary of workshop. Gastroenterology 120:1828-1853, 2001.
24. Lee WM. Acute liver failure. N Engl J Med 329:1862, 1993.
25. Schiodt FV, Atillasoy E, Shakil AO, et al: Etiology and outcome for 295 patients with acute liver failure in the United States. Liver Transpl Surg 5:29, 1999.
26. Macagno SG, Rosina F, Rizzetto M: Serologic markers with fulminant hepatitis in persons positive for hepatitis B surface antigen: A worldwide epidemiologic and clinical survey. Ann Intern Med 108:380, 1988.
27. Fattovich G: Natural history of hepatitis B. J Hepatol 39(Suppl 1):S50, 2003.
28. Weissberg JI, Andres LL, Smith CI, et al: Survival in chronic hepatitis B: An analysis of 379 patients. Ann Intern Med 101:613, 1984.
29. Cardenas CL, Soetikno R, Robinson WS, et al: Long-term follow-up of patients with chronic hepatitis B: A 25 year prospective study [abstract]. Hepatology 30:300A, 1999.
30. de Jongh FE, Janssen HLA, de Man RA, et al: Survival and prognostic indicators in hepatitis B surface antigen-positive cirrhosis of the liver. Gastroenterology 103:1630, 1992.
31. Niederau C, Heintgen T, Lange S, et al: Long-term follow-up of HBeAg-positive patients treated with interferon alfa for chronic hepatitis B. N Engl J Med 334:1422, 1996.
32. Tiollais P, Pourcel C, Dejean A: The hepatitis B virus. Nature 317:489, 1985.
33. Nowak MA, Bonhoeffer S, Hill AM, et al: Viral dynamics in hepatitis B virus infection. Proc Natl Acad Sci U S A 93:4398, 1996.

34. Tuttleman JS, Pourcel C, Summers JW: Formation of the pool of covalently closed circular viral DNA in hepadnavirus-infected cells. Cell 47:451, 1986.

35. Bartholomeusz A, Schaefer S: Hepatitis B virus genotypes: Comparison of genotyping methods. Rev Med Virol 14:3, 2004.

36. Chu CJ, Keeffe EB, Han SH, et al: Hepatitis B virus genotypes in the United States: Results of a nationwide study. Gastroenterology 125:444, 2003.

37. Chu CJ, Lok AS: Clinical significance of hepatitis B virus genotypes. Hepatology 35:1274, 2002.

38. Nainan OV, Khristova ML, Byun K-S, et al: Frequency and significance of hepatitis B virus antibody resistant mutants [abstract]. Antiviral Ther 5(Suppl):29, 2000.

39. Ghany MG, Ayola B, Villamil FG, et al: Hepatitis B virus S mutants in liver transplant recipients who were reinfected despite hepatitis B immune globulin prophylaxis. Hepatology 27:213, 1998.

40. Locarnini S, McMillan J, Bartholomeusz A: The hepatitis B virus and common mutants. Semin Liver Dis 23:5, 2003.

41. Li J, Buckwold VE, Hon MW, Ou JH: Mechanism of suppression of hepatitis B virus precore RNA transcription by a frequent double mutation. J Virol 73:1239, 1999.

42. Lindh M, Andersson AS, Gusdal A: Genotypes, nt 1858 variants, and geographic origin of hepatitis B virus: Large scale analysis using a new genotyping method. J Infect Dis 175:1285, 1997.

43. Chu CJ, Keeffe EB, Han SH, et al: Prevalence of HBV precore/core promoter variants in the United States. Hepatology 38:619, 2003.

44. Bertoletti A, Sette A, Chisari FV, et al: Natural variants of cytotoxic epitopes are T-cell receptor antagonist for antiviral cytotoxic T cells. Nature 369:407, 1994.

45. Naoumov NV, Thomas MG, Mason AL, et al: Genomic variations in the hepatitis B core gene: A possible factor influencing response to interferon alfa treatment. Gastroenterology 108:505, 1995.

46. Torre F, Cramp M, Owsianka A, et al: Direct evidence that naturally occurring mutations within hepatitis B core epitope alter CD-4+ T-cell reactivity. J Med Virol 72:370, 2004.

47. Bozkaya H, Akarca US, Ayola B, et al: High degree of conservation in the hepatitis B virus core gene during the immune tolerant phase in perinatally acquired chronic hepatitis B infection. J Hepatol 26:508, 1997.

48. Lai C-L, Dienstag J, Schiff E, et al: Prevalence and clinical correlates of YMDD variants during lamivudine therapy for patients with chronic hepatitis B. Clin Infect Dis 36:687, 2003.

49. Dienstag JL, Goldin RD, Heathcote EJ, et al: Histological outcome during long-term lamivudine therapy. Gastroenterology 124:105, 2003.

50. Liaw YF: Impact of YMDD mutations during lamivudine therapy in patients with chronic hepatitis B. Antivir Chem Chemother 12(Suppl 1):67, 2001.

51. Mutimer D, Pillay D, Shields P, et al: Outcome of lamivudine resistant hepatitis B virus infection in the liver transplant recipient. Gut 46:107, 2000.

52. Rehermann B: Immune responses in hepatitis B virus infection. Semin Liver Dis 23:21, 2003

53. Guidotti LG, Chisari FV: Noncytolytic control of viral infections by the innate and adaptive immune response. Annu Rev Immunol 19:65, 2001.

54. Ferrari C, Missale G, Boni C, Urbani S: Immunopathogenesis of hepatitis Br J Hepatol 39(Suppl 1):S36, 2003.

55. Curry MP, Koziel M: The dynamics of the immune response in acute hepatitis B: New lessons using new techniques. Hepatology 32:117, 2000.

56. Bertoletti A, Ferrari C, Fiaccadori F, et al: HLA class I–restricted human cytotoxic T cells recognize endogenously synthesized hepatitis B virus nucleocapsid antigen. Proc Natl Acad Sci U S A 88:10445, 1991.

57. Koziel M: The immunopathogenesis of HBV infection. Antivir Ther 3(Suppl3):13, 1998.

58. Milich DR, Chen MK, Hughers JL, et al: The secreted hepatitis B precore antigen can modulate the immune response to the nucleocapsid: a mechanism for persistence. J Immunol 160:2013, 1998.

59. Hadziyannis SJ, Vassilopoulos D: Hepatitis B e antigen–negative chronic hepatitis B. Hepatology 34:617, 2001.

60. Perrillo RP, Brunt EM: Hepatic histologic and immunohistochemical changes in chronic hepatitis B after prolonged clearance of hepatitis B surface antigen. Ann Intern Med 115:113, 1991.

61. Fattovich G: Natural history and prognosis of hepatitis B. Semin Liver Dis 23:47, 2003.

62. Fattovich G, Pantalena M, Zagni I, et al: Effect of hepatitis B and C virus infection on the natural history of compensated cirrhosis: A cohort study of 297 patients. Am J Gastroenterol 97:2886, 2002.

63. McMahon BJ: The natural history of chronic hepatitis B virus infection. Semin Liver Dis 24(Suppl 1):17, 2004.

64. Koff RS: Risks associated with hepatitis A and B in patients with hepatitis C. J Clin Gastroenterol 33:20, 2001.

65. Tozun N, Forbes A, Anderson MG, et al: Safety of alcohol after viral hepatitis. Lancet 337:1079, 1991.

66. Gocke DJ: Extrahepatic manifestations of viral hepatitis. Am J Med Sci 270:49, 1975.

67. Krugman S, Overby LR, Mushahwar IK, et al: Viral hepatitis type B: Studies on natural history and prevention-reexamined. N Engl J Med 300:101, 1979.

68. Lindsay KL, Redeker AG, Ashcavai M: Delayed HBsAg clearance in chronic hepatitis B viral infection. Hepatology 1:586, 1981.

69. Rehermann B, Ferrari C, Pasquinelli C, Chisari FV: The hepatitis B virus persists for decades after patients' recovery from acute viral hepatitis despite active maintenance of a cytotoxic T-lymphocyte response. Nat Med 2:1104, 1996.

70. Gimson AE, O'Grady J, Ede RJ, et al: Late onset hepatic failure: Clinical, serologic and histologic features. Hepatology 6:288, 1986.

71. Tassopoulos NC, Sjogren MH, Purcell RH: 19S and 7-8S forms of IgM antibody to hepatitis B core antigen in acute icteric hepatitis superimposed on hepatitis B surface antigen carriage. Infection 18:376, 1990.

72. Williams AL, Hoofnagle JH: Ratio of serum aspartate to alanine aminotransferase in chronic hepatitis: Relationship to cirrhosis. Gastroenterology 95:734, 1988.

73. Prysopoulos NT, Reddy KR: Extrahepatic manifestations of chronic viral hepatitis. Curr Gastroenterol Rep 3:71, 2001.

74. Duffy J, Lidsky MD, Sharp JT, et al: Polyarthritis, polyarteritis and hepatitis B. Medicine (Baltimore) 55:19, 1976.

75. Hoofnagle JH, Davis GL, Pappas SC, et al: A short course of prednisolone in chronic type B hepatitis: Report of a randomized, double-blind, placebo-controlled trial. Ann Intern Med 104:12, 1986.

76. Guillevin L, Lhote F, Jarrousse B, et al: Polyarteritis nodosa related to hepatitis B virus: A prospective study of 66 patients. Ann Med Interne (Paris) 143:63, 1992.

77. Trepo C, Guillevin L: Polyarteritis nodosa and extrahepatic manifestations of HBV infection: The case against immune intervention in pathogenesis. J Autoimmun 16:269, 2001.

78. Guillevin L, Lhote F, Gayraud M, et al: Prognostic factors in polyarteritis nodosa and Churg-Strauss syndrome: A prospective study in 342 patients. Medicine 75:17, 1996.

79. Johnson RJ, Couser WG: Hepatitis B infection and renal disease: Clinical, immunopathogenetic and therapeutic considerations. Kidney Int 37:663, 1990.

80. Lai KN, Li PK, Lui SF, et al: Membranous nephropathy related to hepatitis B virus in adults. N Engl J Med 324:1457, 1991.

81. Conjeevaram HS, Hoofnagle JH, Austin HA, et al: Long-term outcome of hepatitis B virus–related glomerulonephritis after therapy with interferon alfa. Gastroenterology 109:540, 1995.

82. Popp JW, Dienstag JL, Wands JR, et al: Essential mixed cryoglobulinemia without evidence for hepatitis B virus infection. Ann Intern Med 92:379, 1980.

83. Monti G, Galli M, Invernizzi F, et al: Cryoglobulinaemias: A multicenter study of the early clinical and laboratory manifestations of primary and secondary disease. GISC. Italian Group for the Study of Cryoglobulinaemias. Q J Med 88:115, 1995.

84. Lohr H, Goergen B, Welser W, et al: Mixed cryoglobulinemia type II in chronic hepatitis B associated with HBe-minus HBV mutant: Cellular immune reactions and response to interferon treatment. J Med Virol 44:330, 1995.

85. Gerber MA, Hadziyannis S, Vissoulis C, et al: Electron microscopy and immunoelectronmicroscopy of cytoplasmic hepatitis B antigen in hepatocytes. Am J Pathol 75:489, 1974.

86. Shikata T, Uzawa T, Yoshiwara N, et al: Staining methods of Australia antigen in paraffin section detection of cytoplasmic inclusion bodies. Jpn J Exp Med. 44:25, 1974.

87. Gerber MA, Hadziyannis S, Vernace S, et al: Incidence and nature of cytoplasmic hepatitis B antigen in hepatocytes Lab Invest 32:251, 1975.

88. Perrillo RP, Campbell CR, Sanders GE, et al: Spontaneous clearance and reactivation of chronic hepatitis B virus infection among male homosexuals with chronic type B hepatitis. Ann Intern Med 100:43, 1984.

89. Mels GC, Bellati G, Leandro G, et al: Fluctuations in viremia, aminotransferases and IgM antibody to hepatitis B core antigen in chronic hepatitis B patients with disease exacerbations. Liver 14:175, 1994.

90. Di Martino V, Thevenot T, Colin JF, et al: Influence of HIV infection on the response to interferon therapy and the long-term outcome of chronic hepatitis B. Gastroenterology 123:1812, 2002.

91. Liaw YF, Tsai SL: Pathogenesis and clinical significance of spontaneous exacerbations and remissions in chronic hepatitis B virus infection. Viral Hepatitis 3:143, 1997.

92. Xunrong L, Yan AW, Liang R, et al: Hepatitis B virus (HBV) reactivation after cytotoxic or immunosuppressive therapy: Pathogenesis and management. Rev Med Virol 11:287, 2001.

93. Lau JYN, Lai CL, Lin HJ, et al: Fatal reactivation of chronic hepatitis B virus infection following withdrawal of chemotherapy in lymphoma patients. Q J Med 73:911, 1989.

94. Perrillo RP: Acute flares in chronic hepatitis B: The natural and unnatural history of an immunologically mediated liver disease. Gastroenterology 120:1009, 2001.

95. Liang R, Lau GKK, Kwong YL: Chemotherapy and bone marrow transplantation for cancer patients who are also chronic hepatitis B carriers: A review of the problem. J Clin Oncol 17:394, 1999.

96. Lau GKK, Liang R, Chiu EKW, et al: Hepatic events after bone marrow transplantation in patients with hepatitis B infection: A case controlled study. Bone Marrow Transplant 19:795, 1997.

97. Davies SE, Portmann BC, O'Grady JG, et al: Hepatic histological findings after transplantation for chronic hepatitis B virus infection, including a unique pattern of fibrosing cholestatic hepatitis. Hepatology 13:150, 1991.

98. Perrillo RP: Hepatitis B and renal transplantation: Securing the sword of Damocles. Hepatology 36:1041, 2002.

99. Nair S, Perrillo R: Serum alanine aminotransferase flares during interferon treatment of chronic hepatitis B: Is sustained clearance of HBV DNA dependent on levels of pretreatment viremia? Hepatology 34:1021, 2001.

100. Hoofnagle JH, Di Bisceglie AM, Waggoner JG, et al: Interferon alfa for patients with clinically apparent cirrhosis due to chronic hepatitis B. Gastroenterology 104:1116, 1993.

101. Honkoop P, de Man RA, Niesters HG, et al: Acute exacerbation of chronic hepatitis B virus infection after withdrawal of lamivudine therapy. Hepatology 32:635, 2000.

102. Liaw YF, Chien RN, Yeh CT, et al: Acute exacerbation and hepatitis B virus clearance after emergence of YMDD motif mutation during lamivudine therapy. Hepatology 30:567, 1999.

103. Lok ASF, Lai C-L, Leung N, et al: Long-term safety of lamivudine treatment in patients with chronic hepatitis B. Gastroenterology 125:1714, 2003.

104. Perrillo RP, Regenstein FG, Peters MG, et al: Prednisone withdrawal followed by recombinant alpha interferon in the treatment of chronic type B hepatitis: A randomized, controlled trial. Ann Intern Med 109:95, 1988.

105. Krogsgaard K, Marcellin P, Trepo C, et al: Prednisolone withdrawal therapy enhances the effect of human lymphoblastoid interferon in chronic hepatitis B. INTREPED Trial Group. J Hepatol 25:803, 1996.

106. Liaw YF, Tsai SL, Chien RN, et al: Prednisolone priming enhances Th1 response and efficacy of subsequent lamivudine therapy in patients with chronic hepatitis B. Hepatology 32:604, 2000.

107. Thio CL: Hepatitis B in the human immunodeficiency virus-infected patient: Epidemiology, natural history, and treatment. Semin Liver Dis 23:125, 2003.

108. Bonino F, Brunetto MR: Chronic hepatitis B e antigen (HBeAg) negative, anti-HBe positive hepatitis B: An overview. J Hepatol 39(Suppl 1):S160, 2003.

109. Oketani M, Oketani K, Xiaohong C, et al: Low level wild-type and pre-core mutant hepatitis B viruses and HBeAg negative reactivation of chronic hepatitis B. J Med Virol 58:332, 1999.

110. Lindh M, Gustavson C, Mardberg K, et al: Mutation of nucleoside 1,762 in the core promoter region during hepatitis B e seroconversion and its relation to liver damage in hepatitis B e antigen carriers. J Med Virol 55:185, 1998.

111. Gerner P, Lausch E, Friedt M, et al: Hepatitis B virus core promoter mutations in children with multiple anti-HBe/HBeAg reactivations result in enhanced promoter activity. J Med Virol 59:415, 1999.

112. Steinberg JL, Yeo W, Zhong S, et al: Hepatitis B virus reactivation in patients undergoing cytotoxic chemotherapy for solid tumours: Precore/core mutations may play an important role. J Med Virol 60:249, 2000.

113. Hadziyannis SJ: Hepatitis delta: An overview. In Rizzetto M, Purcell RH, Gerin JL, Verme G (eds): Viral Hepatitis and Liver Disease: Proceedings of IX Triennial International Symposium on Viral Hepatitis and Liver Disease. Turin, Edizioni Minerva Medica, 1997, p 283.

114. Liaw YF, Tsai SL, Chang JJ, et al: Displacement of hepatitis B virus by hepatitis C virus as the cause of continuing chronic hepatitis. Gastroenterology 106:1048, 1994.

115. Hoofnagle JH, Schafer DF: Serologic markers of hepatitis B virus infection. Semin Liver Dis 1:6, 1986.

116. Perrillo RP, Chau KH, Overby LR, et al: Anti-hepatitis B core immunoglobulin M in the serologic evaluation of hepatitis B virus infection and simultaneous infection with type B, delta agent, and non-A, non-B viruses. Gastroenterology 85:163, 1983.

117. Shiels MT, Taswell HF, Czaja AJ, et al: Frequency and significance of concurrent hepatitis B surface antigen and antibody in acute and chronic hepatitis B. Gastroenterology 93:675, 1987.

118. Tsang TK, Blei AT, O'Reilly DJ, et al: Clinical significance of concurrent hepatitis B surface antigen and antibody positivity. Dig Dis Sci 31:620, 1986.

119. Bonino F, Colloredo Mels G, Bellati G, et al: Problems in diagnosing viral hepatitis. Gut 34(Suppl 2):S36, 1993.

120. Grob P, Jilg W, Bornhak H, et al: Serological pattern "anti-HBc": Report on a workshop. J Med Virol 62:450, 2000.

121. Weber B, Melchior W, Gehrke R, et al: Hepatitis B virus markers in anti-HBc only positive individuals. J Med Virol 64:312, 2001.

122. Jilg W, Sieger E, Zachoval R, et al: Individuals with antibodies against hepatitis B core antigen as the only serological marker for hepatitis B infection: High percentage of carriers of hepatitis B and C virus. J Hepatol 23:14, 1995.

123. Mosley JW, Stevens CE, Aach RD, et al: Donor screening for antibody to hepatitis B core antigen and hepatitis B virus infection in transfusion recipients. Transfusion 35:5, 1995.

124. Wachs ME, Amend WJ, Ascher NL, et al: The risk of transmission of hepatitis B from HBsAg(–), HBcAb(+), HBIgM(–) organ donors. Transplantation 59:230, 1995.

125. Dodson SF, Issa S, Araya V, et al: Infectivity of hepatic allografts with antibodies to hepatitis B virus. Transplantation 64:1582, 1997.

126. Paterlini P, Gerken G, Nakajima E, et al: Polymerase chain reaction to detect hepatitis B virus DNA and RNA sequences in primary liver cancers from patients negative for hepatitis B surface antigen. N Engl J Med 323:80, 1990.

127. Fukai K, Yokosuka O, Fujiwara K, et al: Etiologic considerations of fulminant non-A, non-B viral hepatitis in Japan: Analyses by nucleic acid amplification method. J Infect Dis 178:325, 1998.

128. Chu C-J, Hussain M, Lok ASF: Quantitative serum HBV DNA levels during different stages of chronic hepatitis B infection. Hepatology 36:1408, 2002.

129. Perrillo RP, Schiff ER, Davis GL, et al: A randomized, controlled trial of interferon alfa-2b alone and after prednisone withdrawal for the treatment of chronic hepatitis B. The Hepatitis Interventional Therapy Group. N Engl J Med 323:295, 1990.

130. Gauthier J, Bourne EJ, Lutz MW, et al: Quantitation of hepatitis B viremia and emergence of YMDD variants in patients with chronic hepatitis B treated with lamivudine. J Infect Dis 180:1757, 1999.

131. Werle B, Cinquin K, Marcellin P, et al: Evolution of hepatitis B viral load and viral genome sequence during adefovir dipivoxil therapy. J Viral Hepat 11:74, 2004.

132. van Nunen AB, Hansen BE, Suh DJ, et al: Durability of HBeAg seroconversion following antiviral therapy for chronic hepatitis B: Relation to type of therapy and pretreatment serum hepatitis B virus DNA and alanine aminotransferase. Gut 52:420, 2003.

133. Lai CL, Dienstag J, Schiff E, et al: Prevalence and clinical correlates of YMDD variants during lamivudine therapy for patients with chronic hepatitis B. Clin Infect Dis 36:687, 2003.

134. Hunt CM, McGill JM, Allen MI, et al: Clinical relevance of hepatitis B viral mutations. Hepatology 31:1037, 2000.

135. Mutimer D, Pillay D, Dragon E, et al: High pre-treatment serum hepatitis B virus titre predicts failure of lamivudine prophylaxis and graft re-infection after liver transplantation. J Hepatol 30:715, 1999.

136. Roche B, Samuel D, Gigou M, et al: De novo and apparent de novo hepatitis B virus infection after liver transplantation. J Hepatol 26:517, 1997.

137. Brechot C, Degos F, Lugassy C, et al: Hepatitis B virus DNA in patients with chronic liver disease and negative tests for hepatitis B surface antigen. N Engl J Med 312:270, 1985.

138. Wright TL, Mamish D, Combs C, et al: Hepatitis B virus and apparent fulminant non-A, non hepatitis. Lancet 339:952, 1992.

139. Wong DKH, Cheung AM, O'Rourke K, et al: Effect of alpha interferon treatment in patients with hepatitis B e antigen–positive chronic hepatitis B: A meta-analysis. Ann Intern Med 119:312, 1993.

140. Lau DT, Everhart J, Keiner DE, et al: Long-term follow up of patients with chronic hepatitis B treated with interferon alfa. Gastroenterology. 113:1660, 1997.

141. Lok ASF, McMahon BJ: Practice Guidelines Committee, American Association for the Study of Liver Diseases (AASLD): Chronic Hepatitis B: Update of recommendations. Hepatology 39:857, 2004.

142. Liaw YF, Leung N, Guan R, et al: Asian-Pacific consensus statement on the management of chronic hepatitis B: A 2005 update. Liver International 25:472, 2005.

143. de Franchis R, Hadengue A, Lau G, et al: EASL Jury: EASL International Consensus Conference on Hepatitis B. 13–14 September 2002, Geneva, Switzerland. Consensus statement (long version). J Hepatol 39:S3, 2003.

144. Keeffe EB, Dieterich DT, Han S-HB, et al: A treatment algorithm for the management of chronic hepatitis B virus infection in the United States. Clin Gastroenterol Hepatol 2:87, 2004.

145. Perrillo RP, Lai CL, Liaw YF, et al: Predictors of HBeAg loss after lamivudine treatment for chronic hepatitis B. Hepatology 36:186, 2002.

146. Cooksley WG: Treatment with interferons in patients with hepatitis B. Semin Liver Dis 24(Suppl 1):45, 2004.

147. Janssen HLA, van Zonneveld M, Senturk H, et al: Pegylated interferon alfa-2b, alone or in combination with lamivudine for HBeAg-positive chronic hepatitis B: A randomized trial. Lancet 365:123, 2005.

148. Marcellin P, Lau GKK, Bonino F, et al: Peginterferon alfa-2a alone, lamivudine alone, and the two in combination in patients with HBeAg-negative chronic hepatitis B. N Engl J Med 351:1206, 2004.

149. Kao JH, Wu NH, Chen PJ, et al: Hepatitis B genotypes and the response to interferon therapy. J Hepatol 33:998, 2000.

150. Lai CL, Chien RN, Leung NW, et al: A one-year trial of lamivudine for chronic hepatitis Engl J Med 339:61, 1998.

151. Dienstag JL, Schiff ER, Wright TL, et al: Lamivudine as initial treatment for chronic hepatitis B in the United States. N Engl J Med 341:1256, 1999.

152. Liaw YF, Leung NWY, Chang TT, et al: Effects of extended lamivudine therapy in Asian patients with chronic hepatitis B. Gastroenterology 119:172, 2000.

153. Marcellin P, Chang TT, Lim SG, et al: Adefovir dipivoxil for the treatment of hepatitis antigen-positive chronic hepatitis B. N Engl J Med 348:808, 2003.

154. Hadziyannis SJ, Tassopoulos NC, Heathcote EJ, et al: Adefovir dipivoxil for the treatment of hepatitis B e antigen-negative chronic hepatitis B. N Engl J Med 348:800, 2003.

155. Marcellin P, Chang T, Lim S, et al: Adefovir dipivoxil (ADV) 10 mg for the treatment of patients with HBeAg+ chronic hepatitis B: Continued efficacy beyond 48 weeks [Abstract 840]. In: Programs and Abstracts from the 53rd Annual Meeting of the American Association for the Study of Liver, November 1–5, 2002, Boston.

156. Westland C, Delaney W 4th, Yang H, et al: Hepatitis B virus genotypes and virologic response in 694 patients in phase III studies of adefovir dipivoxil. Gastroenterology 125:107, 2003.

157. Angus P, Vaughan R, Xiong S, et al: Resistance to adefovir dipivoxil therapy associated with the selection of a novel mutation in the HBV polymerase. Gastroenterology 125:292, 2003.

158. Hadziyannis S, Tassopoulos N, Heathcote EJ, et al: Long-term therapy with adefovir dipivoxil for HBeAg-negative chronic hepatitis B. N Engl J Med 352:2673, 2005.

159. Locarnini S, Qi X, Arterburn S, et al: Incidence and predictors of emergence of adefovir resistant HBV during 4 years of

adefovir dipivoxil (ADV) therapy for patients with chronic hepatitis B [abstract]. J Hepatol 42:17, 2005.

160. Yang H, Westland CE, Das K, et al: In vitro characterization and molecular modeling analysis of adefovir resistance mutation rtN236T in the HBV polymerase [Abstract 054]. In: Programs and Abstracts from the Hep Dart Meeting, December 14–18, 2003, Kauai, Hawaii.

161. Perrillo R, Hann H-W, Mutimer D, et al: Adefovir dipivoxil added to ongoing lamivudine in chronic hepatitis B with YMDD mutant hepatitis B virus. Gastroenterology 126:81, 2004.

162. Peters MG, Hann HW, Martin P, et al: Adefovir dipivoxil alone or in combination with lamivudine in patients with lamivudine-resistant chronic hepatitis B. Gastroenterology 126:91, 2004.

163. Schiff ER, Lai C-L, Hadziyannis S, et al: Adefovir dipivoxil therapy for lamivudine-resistant hepatitis B in pre- and post-liver transplantation patients. Hepatology 38:1419, 2003.

164. Emtriva® Data on file, Gilead Sciences, Inc.

165. Raffi F, Snow A, Borroto-Esoda K, et al: Anti-HBV activity of emtricitabine (FTC) in patients co-infected with HIV and hepatitis B virus [Abstract 215]. In: Programs and Abstracts of the 2nd IAS Conference on Pathogenesis and Treatment, July 13–16, 2003, Paris.

166. Gish R, Leung N, Wang C, et al: Antiviral activity, safety, and incidence of resistance in chronically infected hepatitis B patients (CHB) given once daily emtricitabine for 2 years [abstract]. Hepatology 36:372A, 2003.

167. Van Bommel F, Wunsche T, Mauss S, et al: Comparison of adefovir and tenofovir in the treatment of lamivudine-resistant hepatitis B virus infection. Hepatology 40:1421, 2004.

168. Ristig MB, Crippin J, Aberg JA, et al: Tenofovir disoproxil fumarate therapy for chronic hepatitis B in human immunodeficiency virus/hepatitis B virus-coinfected individuals for whom interferon-alpha and lamivudine therapy have failed. J Infect Dis 186:1844, 2002.

169. Nelson M, Portsmouth S, Stebbing J, et al: An open-label study of tenofovir in HIV-1 and hepatitis B virus co-infected individuals. AIDS 17:F7, 2003.

170. Kuo A, Dienstag JL, Chung RT: Tenofovir disoproxil fumarate for the treatment of lamivudine-resistant hepatitis B. Clin Gastroenterol Hepatol 2:266, 2004.

171. Lai C-L, Rosmawati M, Lao J, et al: Entecavir is superior to lamivudine in reducing hepatitis B virus DNA in patients with chronic hepatitis B infection. Gastroenterology 123:1831, 2002.

172. Chang T-T, Hadziyannis S, Cianciara J, et al: Sustained viral load and ALT reduction following 48 weeks of entecavir treatment in subjects with chronic hepatitis B who have failed lamivudine [abstract]. Hepatology 36:300A, 2002.

173. Colonno RJ, Rose R, Levine S, et al: Infrequent emergence of entecavir resistant variants: Requirement of prior lamivudine resistance [Abstract 049]. In: Programs and Abstracts from the Hep Dart Meeting, December 14–18, 2003, Kauai, Hawaii.

174. Standring DN, Bridges EG, Placidi L, et al: Antiviral β-L-nucleosides specific for hepatis B virus infection. Antivir Chem Chemother 12(Suppl 1):119, 2001.

175. Tennant B, Menne S, Baldwin B, et al: Antiviral activities of β-L-thymidine (LdT), Val-β-L-2′-deoxycytidine (val-LdC), and lamivudine alone and in combination in a 12 week, oral dose study using the woodchuck model of chronic hepatitis B virus infection [Abstract 027]. In: Programs and Abstracts from the Hep Dart Meeting, December 16–20, 2001, Maui, Hawaii.

176. Lai C-L, Leung N, Teo EK, et al: A 1-year trial of telbivudine, lamivudine, and the combination in patients with hepatitis B e antigen-positive chronic hepatitis B. Gastroenterology 129:528, 2005.

177. Lee H-S, Chung YH, Lee KS, et al: A 12-week randomized placebo controlled double blind trial of clevudine in patients with chronic hepatitis B with post-treatment follow up for 24 weeks [Abstract 052]. In: Programs and Abstracts from the Hep Dart Meeting, December 14–18, 2003, Kauai, Hawaii.

178. Marcellin P, Mommeja-Marin H, Sacks SL, et al: A phase II dose-escalating trial of clevudine in patients with chronic hepatitis B. Hepatology 40:140, 2004.

179. Liaw YF, Sung JJY, Chow WC, et al: Lamivudine for patients with chronic hepatitis B and advanced liver disease. N Engl J Med 351:1521, 2004.

180. Sung JJY, Lai JY, Zeuzem S, et al: A randomized double-blind phase II study of lamivudine compared to lamivudine plus adefovir dipivoxil for treatment naive patients with chronic hepatitis B: Week 52 analysis [abstract]. J Hepatol 38(Suppl 2):25, 2003.

181. Cavanaugh VJ, Guidotti LG, Chisari FV: Interleukin-12 inhibits hepatitis B virus replication in the livers of transgenic mice. J Virol 71:3236, 1997.

182. Kimura K, Kakimi K, Wieland S, et al: Interleukin-18 inhibits hepatitis B virus replication in the livers of transgenic mice. J Virol 76:10702, 2002.

183. Klucher K, Kindsvogel V, Henderson K, et al: Interleukin-28 and interleukin-29 have antiviral activity against hepatitis viruses [Abstract 044]. In: Programs and Abstracts from the Hep Dart Meeting, December 14–18, 2003, Kauai, Hawaii.

184. Mutchnick M, Lindsay KL, Schiff ER, et al: Thymosin alpha 1 treatment of chronic hep B: Results of a phase III multi-centre, randomized, double-blind and placebo controlled study. J Viral Hepat 6:397, 1999.

185. Saruc M, Ozden N, Turkel N, et al: Long-term outcomes of thymosin-alpha 1 and interferon alpha-2b combination therapy in patients with hepatitis B e antigen (HBeAg) negative chronic hepatitis B. J Pharm Sci 92:1386, 2003.

186. McCaffrey AP, Nakai H, Pandey K, et al: Inhibition of hepatitis B virus in mice by RNA interference. Nat Biotechnol 21:639, 2003.

187. Klein C, Bock CT, Wedemeyer H, et al: Inhibition of hepatitis B virus replication in vivo by nucleoside analogues and siRNA. Gastroenterology 125:9, 2003.

188. Delaney WE IV, Edwards R, Colledge D, et al: Phenylpropenamide derivatives AT-61 and AT-130 inhibit replication of both wild-type and lamivudine resistant strains of hepatitis B virus in vitro. Antimicrob Agents Chemother 46:3057, 2002.

189. Feld J, Locarnini S: New targets and possible new therapeutic approaches in the chemotherapy of chronic hepatitis B. Hepatology 38:545, 2003.

190. Desmyter J, Bradburne AF, Vermylen C, et al: Hepatitis-B immunoglobulin in prevention of HBs antigenemia in haemodialysis patients. Lancet 2(7931):376, 1975.

191. Redeker AG, Mosley JW, Gocke DJ, et al: Hepatitis immune globulin as a prophylactic measure for spouses exposed to acute type B hepatitis. N Engl J Med 293:1055, 1975.

192. Wong VC, IP HM, Reesink HW, et al: Prevention of the HBsAg carrier state in newborn infants of mothers who are chronic carriers of HBsAg and HBeAg by administration of hepatitis-B vaccine and hepatitis-B immunoglobulin: Double-blind randomised placebo-controlled study. Lancet 1(8383):921, 1984.

193. Kohler PF, Dubois RS, Merrill DA, et al: Prevention of chronic neonatal hepatitis B virus infection with antibody to the hepatitis B surface antigen. N Engl J Med 291:1378, 1974.

194. Dosik H, Jhaveri R: Prevention of neonatal hepatitis infection by high dose hepatitis B immune globulin. N Engl J Med 298:602, 1978.

195. Reesink HW, Reerink-Brongers F, Lafeber-Schut BJ, et al: Prevention of chronic HBsAg carrier state in infants of HBsAg-positive mothers by hepatitis B immunoglobulin. Lancet 2(8140):436, 1979.

196. Bocher WO, Herzog-Hauff S, Herr W, et al: Regulation of the neutralizing anti-hepatitis B surface (HBs) antibody response in vitro in HBs vaccine recipients and patients with acute chronic hepatitis B virus (HBV) infection. Clin Exp Immunol 105:52, 1996.

197. Bocher WO, Herzog-Hauff S, Schlaak J, et al: Kinetics of hepatitis B surface antigen-specific immune responses in acute and chronic hepatitis B or after HBs vaccination: Stimulation of the in vitro antibody response by interferon gamma. Hepatology 29:238, 1999.

198. Szmuness W, Stevens CE, Harley EJ, et al: Hepatitis B vaccine: Demonstration of efficacy in a controlled clinical trial in a high-risk population in the United States. N Engl J Med 303:833, 1980.

199. Francis DP, Hadler SC, Thompson SE, et al: The prevention of hepatitis B with vaccine: Report of the centers for disease control multi-center efficacy trial among homosexual men. Ann Intern Med 97:362, 1982.

200. Szmuness W, Stevens CE, Harley EJ, et al: Hepatitis B vaccine in medical staff of hemodialysis units: Efficacy and subtype cross-protection. N Engl J Med 307:1481, 1982.

201. Hadler SC, Francis DP, Maynard JE, et al: Long-term immunogenicity and efficacy of hepatitis B vaccine in homosexual men. N Engl J Med 315:209, 1986.

202. Wainwright RB, Bulkow LR, Parkinson AJ, et al: Protection provided by hepatitis B vaccine in a Yupik Eskimo population: Results of 10-year study. J Infect Dis 175:674, 1997.

203. Seaworth B, Drucker J, Starling J, et al: Hepatitis B vaccines in patients with chronic renal failure before dialysis. J Infect Dis 157:332, 1988.

204. Bohm W, Schirmbeck R, Elbe A, et al: Exogenous hepatitis B surface antigen particles processed by dendritic cells or macrophages prime murine MHC class I–restricted cytotoxic T lymphocytes in vivo. J Immunol 155:3313, 1995.

205. Schirmbeck R, Melber K, Mertens T, et al: Antibody and cytotoxic T-cell responses to soluble hepatitis B virus (HBV) S antigen in mice: Implication for the pathogenesis of HBV-induced hepatitis. J Virol 68:1418, 1994.

206. Wilson CC, Olson WC, Tuting T, et al: HIV-1 specific CTL responses primed in vitro by blood derived dendritic cells and Th1-biasing cytokines. J Immunol 162:3070, 1999.

207. Bachmann MF, Lutz MB, Layton GT, et al: Dendritic cells process exogenous viral proteins and virus-like particles for class I presentation to CD8+ cytotoxic T lymphocytes. Eur J Immunol 26:2595, 1996.

208. Rahman F, Dahmen A, Herzog-Hauff S, et al: Cellular and humoral immune responses induced by intradermal or intramuscular vaccination with the major hepatitis B surface antigen. Hepatology 31:521, 2000.

209. Charest AF, McDougall J, Goldstein MB: A randomized comparison of intradermal and intramuscular vaccination against hepatitis B virus in incident chronic hemodialysis patients. Am J Kidney Dis 36:976, 2000.

210. Banatvala JE, Van Damme P: Hepatitis B vaccine—do we need boosters? J Viral Hepat 10:1, 2003.

211. Hepatitis B virus: A comprehensive strategy for eliminating transmission in the United States through universal childhood vaccination. Recommendations of the Immunization Practices Advisory Committee (ACIP). MMWR Morb Mortal Wkly Rep 40(RR-13):1, 1991.

212. Lopez P, Rubiano L, del Pilar Rubio M, et al: Immunogenicity and reactogenicity of DTPw-HB/Hib vaccine administered to Colombian infants after a birth dose of hepatitis B vaccine. Expert Rev Vaccines 1:277, 2002.

213. Murdoch DL, Goa K, Figgitt DP: Combined hepatitis A and B vaccines: A review of their immunogenicity and tolerability. Drugs 63:2625, 2003.

214. Jacques P, Moens G, Desombere I, et al: The immunogenicity and reactogenicity profile of a candidate hepatitis B vaccine in an adult vaccine non-responder population. Vaccine 20:3644, 2002.

215. Levie K, Gjorup I, Skinhoj P, et al: A 2-dose regimen of a recombinant hepatitis B vaccine with the immune stimulant AS04 compared with the standard 3-dose regimen of Engerix-B in healthy young adults. Scand J Infect Dis 34:610, 2002.

216. Lewis DJ, Eiden JE, Goilav C, et al: Rapid and frequent induction of protective immunity exceeding UK recommendations for healthcare settings by MF59-adjuvated hepatitis B vaccine. Commun Dis Public Health 6:320, 2003.

217. Kim MJ, Nafziger AN, Harro CD, et al: Revaccination of healthy nonresponders with hepatitis B vaccine and prediction of seroprotection response. Vaccine 21:1174, 2003.

218. Thermet A, Rollier C, Zoulim F, et al: Progress in DNA vaccine for prophylaxis and therapy of hepatitis B. Vaccine 21:659, 2003.

219. Gerdts V, Babiuk LA, van Drunen Littel-van den Hurk S, et al: Fetal immunization by a DNA vaccine delivered into the oral cavity. Nat Med 6:929, 2000.

220. Rizzetto M, Canese MG, Arico S, et al: Immunofluorescence detection of a new antigen-antibody system (delta/anti–delta) associated to hepatitis B virus in liver and in serum of HBsAg carriers. Gut 18:997, 1977.

221. Nath N, Mushawar IK, Fang CT, et al: Antibodies to delta antigen in asymptomatic hepatitis B surface antigen-reactive blood donors in the United States and their association with other markers of hepatitis B virus. Am J Epidemiol 122:218, 1985.

222. Gaeta GB, Stroffolini T, Chiaramonte M, et al: Chronic hepatitis D: A vanishing disease? An Italian multicenter study. Hepatology 32:824, 2000.

223. Sagnelli E, Stroffolini T, Ascione A, et al: Decrease in HDV endemicity in Italy. J Hepatol 26:20, 1997.

224. Navascues CA, Rodriguez M, Sotorrio NG, et al: Epidemiology of hepatitis D virus infection: Changes in the last 14 years. Am J Gastroenterol 90:1981, 1995.

225. Coppola RC, Manconi PE, Piro R, et al: HCV, HIV HBV, and HDV infection in drug addicts. Eur J Epidemiol 10:279, 1994.

226. Tennant F, Moll D: Seroprevalence of hepatitis A, B, C, and D markers and liver function abnormalities in intravenous heroin addicts. J Addict Dis 14:35, 1995.

227. Shakil AO, Hadziyannis S, Hoofnagle JH, et al: Geographic distribution and genetic variability of hepatitis delta virus genotype I. Virology 234:160, 1997.

228. Zhang Y-Y, Tsega E, Hansson BG: Phylogenetic analysis of hepatitis D viruses indicating a new genotype I subgroup among African isolates. J Clin Microbiol 34:3023, 1996.

229. Lee CM, Changchien CS, Chung JC, et al: Characterization of a new genotype II hepatitis delta virus from Taiwan. J Med Virol 49:145, 1996.

230. Casey JL, Niro GA, Engle RE, et al: Hepatitis B virus (HBV)/hepatitis D virus (HDV) coinfection in outbreaks of acute hepatitis in the Peruvian Amazon Basin: The roles of HDV genotype III and HBV genotype F. J Infect Dis 174:920, 1996.

231. Wang KS, Choo QL, Weiner AJ, et al: Structure, sequence and expression of hepatitis delta (delta) viral genome. Nature 323:508, 1986.

232. Taylor JM: The structure and replication of hepatitis delta virus. Annu Rev Microbiol 46:253, 1992.

233. Taylor JM: Hepatitis delta virus: Cis and trans functions needed for replication. Cell 61:371, 1990.

234. Luo GX, Chao M, Hsieh SY, et al: A specific base transition occurs on replicating hepatitis delta virus RNA. J Virol 64:1021, 1989.

235. Casey JL, Bergmann KF, Brown TL, et al: Structural requirements for RNA editing in hepatitis delta virus: Evidence for a uridine-to-cytidine editing mechanism. Proc Natl Acad Sci U S A 89:7149, 1992.

236. Kuo MY, Chao M, Taylor J: Initiation of replication of the human hepatitis delta virus genome from cloned DNA: Role of delta antigen. J Virol 63:1945, 1989.

237. Chao M, Hsieh SY, Taylor J: Role of two forms of hepatitis delta virus antigen: Evidence for a mechanism of self-limiting genome replication. J Virol 64:5066, 1990.

238. Linnen J, Wages J, Zhang-Keck ZY, et al: Molecular cloning and disease association of hepatitis G virus: A transfusion-transmissible agent. Science 271:505, 1996.

239. Diener TO: Hepatitis delta virus-like agents: An overview. Prog Clin Biol Res 382:109, 1993.

240. Mayo MA: Current ideas about the taxonomy of sub-viral virus-like agents. Prog Clin Biol Res 382:117, 1993.

241. Guilhot S, Huang SN, Xia YP, et al: Expression of the hepatitis delta virus large and small antigens in transgenic mice. J Virol 68:1052, 1994.

242. Ottobrelli A, Marzano A, Smedile A, et al: Patterns of hepatitis delta virus reinfection and disease in liver transplantation. Gastroenterology l01:1649, 1991.

243. Samuel D, Zignego AL, Reynes M, et al: Long-term clinical and virological outcome after liver transplantation for cirrhosis caused by chronic delta hepatitis. Hepatology 21:333, 1995.

244. Zignego AL, Deny P, Feray C, et al: Amplification of hepatitis delta virus RNA sequences by polymerase chain reaction: A tool for viral detection and cloning. Mol Cell Probes 4:43, 1990.

245. Madejon A, Castillo I, Bartolome I, et al: Detection of HDV-RNA by PCR in serum of patients with chronic HDV infection. J Hepatol 11:381, 1991.

246. Tang JR, Cova L, Lamelin JP, et al: Clinical relevance of the detection of hepatitis delta virus RNA in serum by RNA hybridization and polymerase chain reaction. J Hepatol 21:953, 1994.

247. Yamashiro T, Nagayama K, Enomoto N, et al: Quantitation of the level of hepatitis delta virus RNA in serum, by real-time polymerase chain reaction—and its possible correlation with the clinical stage of liver disease. J Infect Dis 189:1151, 2004.

248. Smedile AI, Lavarini C, Crivelli O, et al: Radioimmunoassay detection of 1gM antibodies to the HBV-associated delta antigen: Clinical significance in delta infection. J Med Virol 9:131, 1982.

249. Aragona M, Macagno S, Caredda F, et al: Serological response to the hepatitis delta virus in hepatitis D. Lancet 1(8531):478, 1987.

250. Farci P, Gerin JL, Aragona M, et al: Diagnostic and prognostic significance of the 1gM antibody to the hepatitis delta virus. JAMA 255:1443, 1986.

251. Borghesio B, Rosina F, Smedile A, et al: Serum immunoglobulin M antibody to hepatitis D as a surrogate marker of hepatitis D in interferon-treated patients and in patients who underwent liver transplantation. Hepatology 27:873, 1998.

252. Macagno S, Smedile A, Caredda F, et al: Monomeric (7S) immunoglobulin M antibodies to hepatitis delta virus in hepatitis type D. Gastroenterology 98:1582, 1990.

253. Huang YH, Wu JC, Sheng WY, et al: Diagnostic value of anti-hepatitis D virus (HDV) antibodies revisited: A study of total and IgM anti-HDV compared with detection of HDV-RNA by polymerase chain reaction. J Gastroenterol Hepatol 13:57, 1998.

254. Hadziyannis SJ, Hattzakis A, Papaioannou C, et al: Endemic hepatitis delta virus infection in a Greek community. Prog Clin Biol Res 234:181, 1987.

255. Rizzetto M, Ponzetto A, Forzani I: Epidemiology of hepatitis delta virus: Overview. Prog Clin Biol Res 364:1, 1991.

256. Arakawa Y, Moriyama M, Taira M, et al: Molecular analysis of hepatitis D virus in Miyako Island, a small Japanese island. J Viral Hepat 7:375, 2000.

257. Realdi G, Fattovich G, Hadziyannis S, et al: Survival and prognostic factors in 366 patients with compensated cirrhosis type B: A multicenter study. The investigators of the European Concerted Action on Viral Hepatitis (EUROHEP). J Hepatol 21:656, 1994.

258. DiMarco V, Lo Iacono O, Camma C, et al: The long-term course of chronic hepatitis B. Hepatology 30:257, 1999.

259. Krogsgaard K, Mathiesen LR, Aldershvile J, et al: Delta infection and hepatitis B virus replication in Danish patients with fulminant hepatitis B. Scand J Infect Dis 20:127, 1988.

260. Tassopoulos NC, Koutelou MG, Macagno S, et al: Diagnostic significance of IgM antibody to hepatitis delta virus in fulminant hepatitis B. J Med Virol 30:174, 1990.

261. Buti M, Esteban R, Jardi R, et al: Clinical and serological outcome of acute delta infection. J Hepatol 5:59, 1987.

262. Wu J-C, Chen T-Z, Huang Y-S, et al: Natural history of hepatitis D viral superinfection: Significance of viremia detected by polymerase chain reaction. Gastroenterology 108:796, 1995.

263. Shakil AO, Hadziyannis S, Hoofnagle JH, et al: Geographic distribution and genetic variability of hepatitis delta virus genotype I. Virology 234:160, 1997.

264. Tan WI, Zhan MY: Molecular cloning and sequencing of HDAg-coding fragments of six Chinese hepatitis delta virus isolates [Abstract]. Presented at Fifth International Symposium on Hepatitis Delta Virus and Liver Disease, Gold Coast, Australia, 1995, p D10.

265. Farci P, Smedile A, Lavarini C, et al: Delta hepatitis in inapparent carriers of hepatitis B surface antigen: A disease simulating acute hepatitis B progressive to chronicity. Gastroenterology 85:669, 1983.

266. Farci P, Mandas A, Coiana A, et al: Treatment of chronic hepatitis D with interferon alfa-2a. N Engl J Med 330:88, 1994.

267. Rosina F, Pintus C, Meschievitz C, et al: A randomized controlled trial of a 12 mo course of recombinant human interferon-alpha in chronic delta (type D) hepatitis: A multicenter Italian study. Hepatology 13:1052, 1991.

268. Lau JY, King R, Tibbs CJ, et al: Loss of HBsAg with interferon-alpha therapy in chronic hepatitis D virus infection. J Med Virol 39:292, 1993.

269. Gaudin JL, Faure P, Godinot H, et al: The French experience of treatment of chronic type D hepatitis with a 12 month course of interferon alpha-2b: Results of a randomized controlled study. Liver 15:45, 1995.

270. Madejon A, Cotonat T, Bartolome J, et al: Treatment of chronic hepatitis D virus infection with low and high doses of interferon-alpha 2a: Utility of polymerase chain reaction in monitoring antiviral response. Hepatology 19:1331, 1994.

271. DiBisceglie AM, Martin P, Lisker-Melman M, et al: Therapy of chronic delta hepatitis with interferon alfa-2b. J Hepatol 11(Suppl 1):151, 1990.

272. Farci P, Roskams T, Chessa L, et al: Long-term benefit of interferon alpha therapy of chronic hepatitis D: Regression of advanced hepatic fibrosis. Gastroenterology 126:1740, 2004.

273. Lau DT, Doo E, Park Y, et al: Lamivudine for chronic delta hepatitis. Hepatology 30:546, 1999.

274. Wolters LM, van Nunen AB, Honkoop P, et al: Lamivudine-high dose interferon combination therapy for chronic hepatitis B patients coinfected with hepatitis D virus. J Viral Hepat 7:428, 2000.

275. Niro GA, Ciancio A, Tillman HL, et al: Lamivudine therapy in chronic delta hepatitis: A multicentre randomized controlled pilot study. Aliment Pharmacol Ther 22:227, 2005.

276. Puoti M, Rossi S, Forleo MA, et al: Treatment of chronic hepatitis D with interferon alpha-2b in patients with

human immunodeficiency virus infection. J Hepatol 29:45, 1998.

277. Weltman MD, Brotodihardjo A, Crewe EB, et al: Coinfection with hepatitis B and C or B, C and delta viruses results in severe chronic liver disease and responds poorly to interferon-alpha treatment. J Viral Hepat 2:39, 1995.

278. Madejon A, Bartlome J, Carreno V: In vitro inhibition of the hepatitis delta virus replication mediated by interferon and trans-ribozyme or antisense probes. J Hepatol 29:385, 1998.

279. Glenn JS, Marsters JC Jr, Greenberg HB: Use of prenylation inhibitor as a novel antiviral agent. J Virol 72:9303, 1998.

CHAPTER
76 Hepatitis C

Marina Berenguer and Teresa L. Wright

Hepatitis C virus (HCV) is an important human pathogen, not only because of its high prevalence and worldwide burden, but also because of the potentially serious complications of persistent HCV infection. These complications include cirrhosis, hepatocellular carcinoma, and end-stage liver disease necessitating liver transplantation. The incidence rates for all of these complications are expected to rise in the near future.[1,2] Recognition of the importance of HCV infection has led to consensus conferences in both the United States and Europe to establish standards of care for HCV-infected patients and to set research priorities.[3,4] Despite substantial progress, a precise understanding of the mechanisms of HCV replication and persistence, and of the pathogenesis of liver disease caused by HCV, remains elusive. The limited progress in these important areas stems in large part from the lack of an efficient cell culture system, as well as the narrow host range of the virus, with few animal models available for study.

The most striking feature of HCV is its ability to induce persistent infection in at least 85% of affected persons despite vigorous host humoral and cellular immune responses. The natural history of hepatitis C varies greatly; reasons for this heterogeneity are poorly understood but are likely to be related to both viral and host (genetic) variables, as well as environmental factors such as alcohol abuse. Treatment of chronic HCV infection has improved considerably since the early 1990s, particularly with the addition of ribavirin to interferon-based regimens. As a consequence, patient management has been improved substantially, particularly in subpopulations such as those with HCV genotype 2 or 3 infection, in which high rates of sustained viral eradication can be expected (see later). "Difficult-to-treat" patients, such as those who are immunosuppressed or of African-American descent, are clearly in need of improved therapies. Novel therapeutic approaches, including specific inhibitors of HCV replication, ribavirin-like molecules, new interferon molecules, and immune therapies, are in development.

VIROLOGY

Knowledge of the structure and mechanism of replication of HCV is incomplete, largely because of the lack of a productive cell culture system for expression and propagation of HCV and lack of suitable small animal models of HCV infection. Most relevant information has been obtained from the analysis of the HCV genome, expression of its proteins in heterologous expression systems, in vitro and in vivo models, and structural analysis.[5]

STRUCTURE

HCV is an enveloped virus approximately 55 to 65 nm in diameter. It circulates in various forms in the serum of an infected host, including (1) virions bound to very-low-density and low-density lipoproteins to form *lipo-viro-particles*, which appear to represent the infectious fraction; (2) virions bound to immunoglobulins; and (3) free virions. In addition, viral particles that exhibit physicochemical, morphologic, and antigenic properties of nonenveloped HCV nucleocapsids have been detected in plasma.[6] HCV virions have not yet been visualized conclusively by means of electron microscopy; therefore, information on their three-dimensional structure is lacking. By analogy with closely related viruses, HCV is believed to adopt the form of a classic icosahedral scaffold in which its two enveloped proteins are anchored to the host cell–derived double-layer lipid envelope. Underneath the membrane is the nucleocapsid, which is believed to be composed of multiple copies of the core protein and to form an internal icosahedral viral coat that encapsidates the genomic ribonucleic acid RNA.

GENOMIC ORGANIZATION

HCV is a single-stranded positive-sense RNA virus that belongs to the Flaviviridae family and has been classified as the sole member of the genus *Hepacivirus*.[7] The genome of HCV contains approximately 9600 nucleotides with a single open reading frame (ORF) capable of encoding a large viral polypeptide precursor of 3010 to 3033 amino acids (the length of which varies slightly among HCV isolates), with regions at the 5' and 3' ends that are not translated—untranslated regions (UTRs) (Fig. 76–1).[8] The cleavage of this viral polypeptide by cellular and viral proteases results in a series of structural (nucleocapsid [C], or p21; envelope 1 [E1], or gp31; and envelope 2 [E2], or gp70) and nonstructural (NS2, NS3, NS4a, NS4b, NS5a, and NS5b) proteins.[8,9] The structural proteins are separated from the nonstructural proteins by the short membrane peptide p7, which is believed to be a *viroporin*, a protein that plays a role in viral particle release and maturation.[10]

Many of these viral proteins have enzymatic activities that are essential for HCV replication and polyprotein processing.[5,8,9] The NS5b protein functions as an RNA-dependent RNA polymerase. The core proteins and NS5a have been implicated in the pathogenesis of liver damage,[5,8,9,11,12] hepatic steatosis,[11,13-15] and liver cancer[4,7,8,11,12] and in resistance to interferon therapy.[5,8,9,16] In addition to these proteins, ribosomal frameshifts in the core-coding region have been reported to yield alternative forms of the core protein.[5,16,17] The exact role of these proteins is still under debate; they may play a major role in viral morphogenesis, as well as in the regulation of cellular functions critical to the viral life cycle.

The functions of some proteins, such as the integral membrane protein NS4B or the polyphosphorylated NS5A, are unknown. The untranslated noncoding 5'

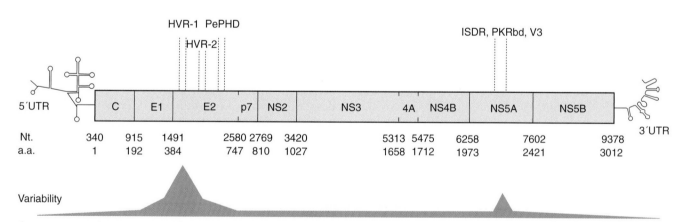

Figure 76–1 Schematic view of the hepatitis C virus (HCV) genome and polyprotein. The genome is flanked by two untranslated regions, the 5' untranslated region (5' UTR) and the 3' UTR, which play important roles in transcription of HCV genomic RNA in ribosomes and in viral replication, respectively. The translated polyprotein is cleaved by host and viral peptidases into the different viral proteins. Structural proteins Core (C), E1, and E2 represent less than one third of the coding region, and nonstructural proteins (viral enzymes such as the NS3 protease, NS3 helicase, and NS5B RNA polymerase) represent the remainder. The genetic variability of the HCV genome is highest in the E2 region, which includes the hypervariable regions (HVRs) and the PKR-eIF2 phosphorylation domain (PePHD). PePHD is similar to the cellular eIF2 phosphorylation domain, the target of the double-stranded RNA-activated protein kinase (PKR), a major mediator of the interferon-induced biological response. Relevant variability also is observed in the NS5A region, which induces the putative interferon sensitivity–determining region (ISDR), the PKR binding domain (PKRbd), and the highly variable V3 region. a.a., amino acid position; Nt., nucleotide position.

terminal region (the 5′ UTR) and portions of the 3′ non-coding region (the 3′ UTR) are the most conserved parts of the HCV genome and contain signals for replication and translation. The 5′ UTR consists of 341 base pairs and has a highly complex secondary RNA structure with four stem loops. It contains an internal ribosomal entry site (IRES) that binds the 40S ribosomal subunit and initiates polyprotein translation in a cap-independent manner (i.e., without the addition of an extra ribonucleotide to the 5′ end of the viral messenger RNA).[5,8,9,18] IRES binding induces a significant conformational change in the 40S ribosomal subunit that leads to a dynamic manipulation of the host translational machinery.[18] The 3′ UTR consists of a varying segment of 40 nucleotides, a poly-(U)-polypyrimidine tract (i.e., a terminal segment of polyuracil), followed by a 98-nucleotide sequence that is highly conserved among HCV genotypes and contains stable stem loop structures. Like the 5′ UTR, this region appears to be essential for RNA synthesis and for translation.[8,9,16]

VIRAL REPLICATION AND LIFE CYCLE

Although hepatocytes, peripheral blood mononuclear cells, and dendritic cells have been reported to support

HCV replication, the liver appears to be the major site of viral replication.[19] Knowledge of the mechanisms of replication comes in part from studies in chimpanzees[20,21] and in part from extrapolation of the mechanisms used by other flaviviruses. The field has advanced with the development of cell culture models for HCV (see later).[22]

Early events in viral binding to the hepatocyte surface are still poorly understood (Fig. 76–2). HCV entry is believed to involve the envelope proteins E1 and E2, which bind to multiple cell surface molecules. Different cell surface molecules appear to mediate binding to specific cells. Two different putative cellular receptors for HCV have been proposed: low-density lipoproteins and CD81. CD81 is a cell surface protein, called tetraspanin, that has four loops (two extracellular and two intracellular) and is expressed on most human cells, except red blood cells and platelets. CD81 serves to attach HCV to the surface of hepatocytes, thereby facilitating subsequent interaction with a specific receptor necessary for viral entry.[16,22] Additional potential receptors include human scavenger receptor and glycosaminoglycans.

After incorporation into the cytoplasm of hepatocytes, the nucleocapsid of HCV is uncoated, probably in acidic endosomes, to release viral RNA. The HCV RNA is translated, and the polyprotein is processed proteolytically into the 10 viral proteins described earlier. The viral

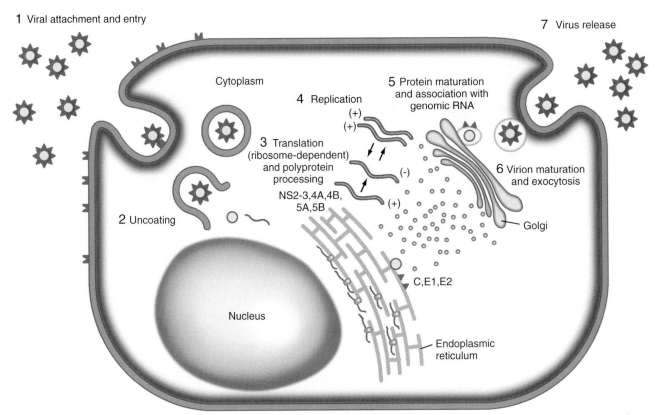

Figure 76–2   Hypothetical life cycle of hepatitis C virus (HCV). Proposed events are as follows: (1) HCV binds to a receptor(s) and enters human hepatocytes. (2) The internalized virus is then uncoated. (3) The viral RNA genome is then translated by the host ribosomes in the endoplasmic reticulum to produce the HCV polyprotein. This HCV polyprotein is processed by both host peptidases and HCV NS2 and NS3 proteases into the structural (C [Core], E1, and E2) and the nonstructural (NS2 to NS5B) viral proteins, which form the replication complex (4) in the so-called membranous web. (5) Structural proteins mature and associate with genomic, positive-strand HCV RNA. (6) and (7) HCV virions eventually are released by exocytosis.

polyprotein is cleaved by a host signal peptidase and two viral proteases, NS2-NS3 zinc-dependent proteinase and NS3 serine proteinase, which cleave the polypeptide at the NS2-3 and NS3-4A regions.[5,8,9,22] After co- and post-translational polyprotein processing, viral proteins remain tightly associated with intracellular membranes to form a complex structure in which the positive-strand RNA genome is used as a template for synthesis of the negative-strand RNA. The negative-strand RNA in turn serves as a template for the synthesis of positive-strand RNA, which combines with core proteins to form the viral nucleocapsid.

Mechanisms of viral packaging and release from the hepatocyte also are poorly understood and probably involve a host secretory mechanism. By analogy with pestiviruses, HCV packaging and release are likely to be inefficient, because much of the virus remains in the cell. Following release, viral particles may either infect adjacent hepatocytes or enter the circulation, where they are available for infection of a new host.

GENOTYPES AND QUASISPECIES

HCV has an inherently high mutational rate that results in considerable heterogeneity throughout the genome.[23] This high mutational rate is in part a consequence of the RNA-dependent RNA polymerase of HCV, which lacks 3'-to-5'-exonuclease proofreading ability that ordinarily would remove mismatched nucleotides incorporated during replication. An average of one error occurs for every 10^4 to 10^5 nucleotides copied. This phenomenon is favored by a high viral turnover rate; the rate of production of HCV virions is on the order of 10^{10} to 10^{12} virions per day.[24] A substantial proportion of newly synthesized viral genomes are defective because of highly deleterious genetic lesions, whereas other genetic alterations confer advantages that lead to the continuous selection of these fittest variants under new environmental conditions. The genetic variability is distributed irregularly along the genome, possibly because of differences in the functional role of the corresponding encoded proteins or the selection of target epitopes by host immune responses or by interactions with cellular proteins. Alignment and sequence comparisons of large collections of HCV sequences are available in both generic databanks (Genbank/EMBL/DDBJ) and specialized databases dedicated to HCV (http://s2as02.genes.nig.ac.jp/ and http://hepatitis.ibcp.fr/). These databases are useful for assessing the degree of conservation of protein sequences among HCV isolates and identifying conserved structural and functional motifs that are essential for survival of HCV.

The first division used to describe the genetic heterogeneity of HCV is the viral *genotype*, which refers to genetically distinct groups of HCV isolates that have arisen during the evolution of the virus. Nucleotide sequencing has shown up to 34% variation between genotypes.[23] The most conserved region (5'UTR) has a maximum nucleotide sequence divergence of 9% between genotypes, whereas the highly variable regions that encode the putative envelope proteins (E1 and E2) exhibit a nucleotide sequence divergence of 35% to 44% between

genotypes. The sequences cluster into 6 major genotypes (designated by Arabic numbers), with sequence similarities of 60% to 70%, and more than 50 subtypes (designated by a lower case letter) within these major genotypes, with sequence similarities of 77% to 80%.[23] In this scheme, the first variant, which was cloned by Choo and colleagues, is designated type 1a. The HCV genotype is an intrinsic characteristic of the infecting HCV strain and does not change over time; therefore, the genotype needs to be tested for only once. Mixed-genotype infections may be seen on occasion and reflect either coinfection with more than one HCV virus or methodologic problems in genotype testing. Global geographic differences exist in the distribution of HCV genotypes, as well as in the mode of acquisition and response to antiviral therapy. For example, genotype 4 is found mainly in Egypt, the Middle East, and several countries in Central Africa.[25] In the United States, 1a is the most prevalent genotype, accounting for approximately 57% of HCV infections, followed by genotype 1b in 17%, genotype 2 in 14%, genotype 3 in 7%; and genotype 4, 5, or 6, or mixed genotypes, in less than 5%.[26] In Europe, the most prevalent genotype is 1b (47%), followed by 1a (17%), 3 (16%), and 2 (13%). The distribution of the genotypes is changing, as are the modes of transmission, however, and since 1995, genotypes 1a and 3a, which are common in injection drug users, have increased in frequency compared with genotype 1b, which is associated most commonly with transmission by blood transfusion.[27]

Another important clinical correlation with HCV genotype is response to treatment (see later). For example, response to therapy with interferon and ribavirin is 1.5 to 2 times more likely in patients with HCV genotype 2 or 3 infection than in those with genotype 1 infection.[28] The reasons for the differences in treatment susceptibility are not fully understood but may be attributable in part to genotype-specific differences in the interaction between certain HCV proteins, such as NS5A and E2, and intracellular pathways that mediate the effects of interferon.[8,9,16] HCV genotype does not influence the severity of liver disease, as defined by the stage of fibrosis, or the likelihood of progression of acute to chronic HCV infection. The more severe outcome associated with genotype 1 observed in early studies probably was confounded by the longer duration of infection in these patients than in those with genotype non-1 infection. A consistent association has been found between HCV genotype 3 infection and liver steatosis, suggesting that HCV genotype 3 may interrupt intracellular metabolism of lipids.[11,13,15]

The second component of genetic heterogeneity is known as *quasispecies*.[23] Quasispecies are closely related, yet heterogeneous sequences of HCV within a single infected person and result from mutations that occur during viral replication. The rate of nucleotide changes varies significantly among the different regions of the viral genome. The highest proportion of mutations has been found in the E1 and E2 regions, particularly in the hypervariable region (HVR) at the amino-terminal end of E2 (E2HVR1). Even though this region represents only a minor part of the E2/NS1 region, it accounts for approximately 50% of the nucleotide changes and 60% of the amino acid substitutions within the envelope region. The quasispecies nature of HCV may be one mechanism by which the virus escapes the host's immune response and establishes persistent infection.[29] It also is implicated in treatment response; patients with fewer changes in viral quasispecies and thus less viral genomic capability after therapy are more likely to achieve viral clearance than are those with significant viral genetic divergence and greater genomic complexity.[23] No intrinsically interferon (IFN)-α–resistant variants of HCV have been defined, however. Genotype 1b infections also have been implicated in a progressive course of post-liver transplantation hepatitis C.[30]

ANIMAL MODELS AND TISSUE CULTURE

The only animal that can readily be infected with HCV is the chimpanzee.[20,21] Unfortunately, major impediments to the use of chimpanzees in medical research have been identified, including cost, availability, and ethical issues.[20] In experimental HCV infection of chimpanzees, HCV RNA is detectable within 3 days and persists in serum during the peak serum alanine aminotransferase (ALT) elevation. Infection is associated with the appearance of viral antigens in hepatocytes, and viral levels in serum peak at 10^5 to 10^7 genome equivalents/mL. As in humans, a substantial proportion of exposed animals fail to clear the virus and become chronically infected despite the presence of both a humoral and a cellular immune response. Although the clinical parameters observed in animals correlate closely with those in humans, liver damage in chimpanzees is not as severe as in humans. Studies in chimpanzees have shown that (1) cell-mediated immunity is essential for viral clearance; (2) viral clearance is not associated with increased reactivity to recombinant E1 and E2 proteins; (3) following viral exposure, significant changes occur in the expression of a large number of genes, particularly interferon-sensitive genes, indicating that the innate immune response plays a major role in HCV clearance; (4) infection with HCV does not provide complete protective immunity to reinfection with homologous or heterologous viruses; and (5) E2HVR1 is not critical for the viability of HCV, because the outcome of an HCV infection in chimpanzees is determined by factors other than the evolution of HVR1 or the immune response to E2. In addition, the rate of viral persistence appears to be similar in chimpanzees infected experimentally with a single strain of HCV to that observed with natural infection,[22] suggesting that viral quasispecies play a minor role if any in viral persistence. The early virologic events are quantitatively (but not qualitatively) different in chimpanzees with acute resolving HCV infection and those with persistent HCV infection. In both groups, the viral titer increases rapidly during the first 2 weeks and is followed by a slower increase during subsequent weeks. Peak viral titers are lower and occur earlier in animals with infection that resolves than in those with persistent infection.[22]

Primary cultures of normal (noninfected) human hepatocytes can be infected in vitro with serum samples from HCV-infected patients in a tissue culture system that is closest to the physiologically infected cell. This system has been used to show that interferon inhibits HCV replication in a dose-dependent manner.[22] In vitro systems that are not limited by low replication levels were reported in 2005 and represent an important breakthrough.

Small animal models and tissue culture models have been developed to study HCV replication and gene expression and to test new antiviral drugs[28]; these approaches include replicons[22] and chimeric viruses.[34] *Replicons* are subgenomic or full-length segments of HCV RNA that are capable of RNA amplification and synthesis of all viral proteins but that do not produce mature viruses.[22] Because replicons carry all known viral enzymes, they can be used to screen compounds directed against these potential targets. *Chimeric viruses* consist of HCV viral sequences under the control of another viral promoter such as poliovirus. Use of such viral sequences allows detailed analysis of the mechanisms of viral replication.

EPIDEMIOLOGY

INCIDENCE AND PREVALENCE

The worldwide seroprevalence of HCV infection, based on detection of antibody to HCV (anti-HCV), is estimated to be 3%, with more than 170 million people infected chronically. Marked geographic variation exists, with seroprevalence rates of 0.4% to 1.1% in North America to 9.6% to 20% in North Africa.[27] Currently, 4 million persons are infected with HCV in the United States, with an estimated prevalence rate of 1.8% in the general population and 0.6% in volunteer blood donors. The prevalence rate is higher in persons ages 30 to 49 years than in older or younger persons and is higher in males than in females (2.5% versus 1.2%) and among certain ethnic groups, such as African Americans and Mexican Americans, than in whites.

Worldwide, three different epidemiologic patterns of HCV infection have emerged.[27] In the United States, Australia, and other developed countries, peak prevalence in persons ages 30 to 49 years and analysis of risk factors suggest that most HCV transmission occurred between the mid-1980s and the mid-1990s, through intravenous drug use. In Japan, southern Europe, and similar areas, the prevalence of HCV infection is highest in older persons, suggesting that the risk of HCV transmission was greatest in the distant past (more than 30 years ago). In these countries, health care–related procedures—particularly unsafe injection practices with reuse of contaminated glass syringes—and folk medicine practices may have played major roles in viral spread. In Egypt and other developing countries, high rates of infection are observed in all age groups, suggesting that an ongoing high risk of acquiring HCV exists.

In the United States, the incidence of acute hepatitis C is falling. The incidence rate was estimated to be 180,000 cases per year in the mid-1980s (peak incidence) but declined to approximately 30,000 new cases per year in 1995.[35] Persons most likely to have HCV infection are those born between 1940 and 1965. Major factors contributing to the falling incidence of acute hepatitis C include widespread blood donor screening programs implemented in the early 1990s, the availability of human immunodeficiency virus (HIV) prevention programs, as well as syringe exchange programs, and the introduction of universal precautions in medical practice aimed at preventing transmission of viral infections. Currently, new HCV infections occur primarily as a result of injection drug use and, to a lesser extent, sex with infected partners.

TRANSMISSION

Modes of transmission of HCV can be divided into *percutaneous* (blood transfusion and needlestick inoculation) and *nonpercutaneous* (sexual contact, perinatal exposure).[36] The nonpercutaneous transmission may represent occult percutaneous exposure. Overall, blood transfusion from unscreened donors and injection drug use are the two risk factors that are documented most clearly. In early studies, HCV was shown to be the etiologic agent in more than 85% of cases of post-transfusion non-A, non-B hepatitis, most of which subsequently was shown to be caused by HCV. Following the introduction of anti-HCV screening of blood donors in 1991, the number of transfusion-related cases of HCV infection declined sharply, and transfusion-related HCV infection is now a rare event (less than 1 case per 200,000 transfusions). Therefore, non–transfusion-related cases of HCV infection have become increasingly important, and injection drug use is now the identified risk factor in more than 60% of cases.[36,37]

Percutaneous Transmission

As a result of the introduction of blood donor screening by first- and second-generation anti-HCV testing, *transfusion*-related hepatitis C now accounts for only 4% of all acute HCV infections.[37]

The frequency of HCV infection in *injection drug users* is 48% to 90%. Although risk factors for hepatitis B virus (HBV) and HIV infection overlap with those for HCV, the prevalence of HCV infection is higher. Fortunately, the number of new cases of HCV infection transmitted through injection drug use is decreasing. A majority of injection drug users become positive for markers of HCV infection within 6 months of initiating injection drug use. Persons infected with HCV who engage in injection drug use should be encouraged to refrain from sharing drug paraphernalia and to practice "safe sex" when possible.

Chronic *hemodialysis* is associated with cases and, occasionally, sporadic outbreaks of HCV infection. The frequency of anti-HCV in patients on hemodialysis ranges from 10% to 20%.[36] Serologic assays for anti-HCV may underestimate the frequency of HCV infection in this relatively immunocompromised population, and virologic assays may be necessary for accurate diagnosis. A correlation has been found between increasing years on dialysis and anti-HCV positivity, suggesting that HCV is transmitted in dialysis units by inadequate infection control procedures.[37]

Anti-HCV seroconversion rates have been 0% to 4% in longitudinal studies of health care workers who have sustained *needlestick exposures* from anti-HCV positive sources. If polymerase chain reaction (PCR) methodology is used to detect HCV RNA in serum, the risk of HCV acquisition after percutaneous exposure is as high as 10%.[36] Regardless of the potential for exposure to HCV, health care professionals, including those with a high likelihood of percutaneous exposure to blood, have seroprevalence rates for anti-HCV that are similar to those in the general population.

Transmission of HCV also may occur from health care worker to patient. Because acute HCV infection often is subclinical, *nosocomial transmission* may occur with greater frequency than has previously been recognized. Strict adherence to universal precautions to protect the health care worker and the patient is critically important.

Nonpercutaneous Transmission

Nonpercutaneous modes of HCV transmission include transmission between sexual partners and perinatal transmission. Available evidence indicates that, in contrast to percutaneous modes of transmission, transmission by nonpercutaneous routes is inefficient. Although 10% of patients with sporadic acute HCV have a history of *sexual exposure* to a partner with HCV infection, most seroepidemiologic studies have demonstrated anti-HCV in only a small number of sexual contacts of infected persons. Anti-HCV is detected in no more than 3% of female sexual partners of male hemophiliacs, the overwhelming majority of whom are infected with HCV. If the index sexual partner also is infected with HIV, the transmissibility of HCV may be increased, probably because of the high serum levels of HCV RNA in co-infected persons. Sexual partners of homosexual men and of heterosexual persons with HCV infection who have multiple partners have an increased frequency of HCV infection. Overall, sexual partners of index patients with anti-HCV have rates of HCV infection ranging from 0% to 27%. Sexual partners of low-risk anti-HCV-positive persons without liver disease and without high-risk behavior (injection drug use or sexual activity with multiple partners) have a frequency of anti-HCV ranging from 0% to 7%. By contrast, sexual partners of persons with liver disease or with high-risk behaviors (or both)—and whose partners may themselves participate in high-risk behavior—have anti-HCV frequency rates of 11% to 27%.[38]

More data are needed to determine the risk for, and factors related to, transmission of HCV. Needed studies include evaluation of long-term steady partners as well as testing of persons with high-risk sexual practices, including those with sexually transmitted diseases that might promote transmission of HCV through increased levels of viremia or breakdown of mucosal barriers. Although the efficiency of sexual transmission of HCV remains controversial, HCV-infected persons commonly are counseled to notify current partners of their HCV status. Although patients typically are told that the risk of sexual transmission is low and that many authorities do not advise use of barrier precautions in stable relationships, "safe sex" practices should be encouraged and barrier precautions recommended in non-monogamous relationships.

Compared with the high efficiency of perinatal transmission of HBV from mothers to infants, the efficiency of *perinatal transmission* of HCV infection is low, with a risk estimated at between 0% and 10%. The frequency of anti-HCV positivity in pregnant women ranges from 0.7% to 4.4%,[36,39] with a rate of HCV RNA detectability in these anti-HCV–positive women of 65% to 72%. Because anti-HCV can be acquired passively by the infant, detection of anti-HCV in the infant does not necessarily imply infection, and virologic tests are required for diagnosis. Therefore, the infant should not undergo testing for anti-HCV before the age of 18 months, because maternal antibodies may persist in the infant's serum. Perinatal transmission occurs exclusively from mothers who are positive for HCV RNA in serum at the time of delivery. As with sexual transmission, high titers of circulating HCV RNA in the mother probably place the infant at increased risk of acquiring HCV infection; the absolute levels of HCV RNA that increase the risk to the infant differ among studies.[36,39] Although the rate of vertical transmission is increased when the mother is coinfected with HIV, studies suggest that for women in whom HIV disease is controlled with use of highly active antiretroviral therapy (HAART), the risk of HCV transmission to the infant is comparable with that for HIV-negative women. Data regarding the risk associated with vaginal delivery as opposed to cesarean delivery are controversial, and routine cesarean section cannot be recommended in HCV-infected women. The risk posed to the infant from breast-feeding is believed to be negligible.[36,37,39] Further studies are needed to delineate the time of perinatal infection (in utero or at the time of delivery), the importance of breast-feeding in neonatal transmission, and the natural history of HCV infection in children.

Sporadic HCV Infection

The source of transmission is considered to be unknown in 10% to 30% of cases of HCV infection. Such "sporadic" HCV infection probably results from "occult" or unidentified percutaneous routes. Intranasal cocaine use has been reported to be associated with acquisition of HCV, although this association is controversial.[36,37] HCV infection probably can be acquired from tattooing and body piercing; transmission by these practices was more common in the past, when less attention was paid to sterile techniques.[36,37] Iatrogenic transmission of HCV is well documented in a variety of circumstances, including delivery of schistosomal treatments with reusable syringes in Egypt.[40] Mini- or single-donor-unit blood transfusions to multiple infant recipients, used in many countries in the past, have been implicated in the transmission of HCV.[41] Often recipients are unaware of the history of transfusions when, decades later, they are asked about HCV exposure. It also is likely that until the implementation of universal precautions in medical practice, HCV was transmitted by inadequately sterilized multi-use instruments and multi-dose vials of vaccines and topical anesthetics. The frequent lack of symptoms in patients with acute HCV infection confounded the identification of these occult parenteral modes of acquiring HCV infection.

PATHOGENESIS

The mechanisms of viral persistence and of hepatocellular injury in patients with chronic HCV infection are poorly understood.

Determinants of *viral persistence* include (1) the quasispecies nature of the virus[23,29]; (2) an inadequate innate immune response; (3) insufficient induction or maintenence of an adaptive immune response; (4) viral evasion from efficient immune responses by several mechanisms, such as infection of immunologically privileged sites, viral interference with antigen processing or other immune responses, and reduction in the effectiveness of antiviral cytokines by the virus; and (5) induction of immunologic tolerance. The net result of the host-virus interplay is the inability to clear the virus despite the development of antibodies against several viral proteins. In addition, immune responses are highly strain-specific, and animals that recover from HCV are susceptible to reinfection.[20] Data from animal studies and from prospective follow-up evaluations of injection drug users to assess the incidence of new HCV infections suggest that *protective* immunity (which controls the infection) exists despite the lack of *sterilizing* immunity (which completely prevents infection).[42] When chimpanzees that have recovered from HCV infection are challenged with homologous and heterologous strains of HCV, reinfection occurs but is clinically milder and shorter in duration, with fast and efficient control of the rechallenge virus.[20] Protection correlates with rapid memory responses of HCV-specific T cells and vigorous proliferation of IFN-γ–producing circulating CD4[+] T cells.

The *pathogenesis of liver damage* in HCV-infected patients is largely immune mediated. Although the immune response clearly is important in preventing viral persistence after acute HCV infection, the immune response also mediates hepatic cell destruction and fibrosis and is not sufficient for eradicating the virus from immunologically privileged sites.

VIRAL MECHANISMS

Viral factors may be important in the pathogenesis of disease caused by HCV, either directly, through cell injury associated with accumulation of the intact virus or viral proteins, or indirectly, through a differential immune response associated with one viral strain but not with another. Severe liver dysfunction has been reported in immunocompromised transplant recipients who demonstrate only moderate inflammation in liver biopsy specimens yet very high levels of HCV RNA in serum, suggesting a *direct cytopathic effect* of HCV.[43] In addition, some histopathologic features, such as steatosis, are compatible with a direct cytopathic effect of the virus. Steatosis is present in 31% to 72% of patients with chronic hepatitis C—a proportion significantly greater than that in patients with chronic hepatitis B (27% to 51%) or autoimmune hepatitis (16% to 19%).[15] Steatosis in these patients may result from the concurrence of different conditions known to induce fatty liver, such as obesity, diabetes, dyslipidemias, and alcohol abuse,[15,44,45] and from virus-induced fatty deposition.[46] A direct role for HCV in the pathogenesis of steatosis is suggested by several findings including: (1) the association of steatosis with HCV genotype 3, suggesting that some specific viral sequences are involved directly in the intracellular accumulation of lipids[46-48]; (2) the association between the severity of steatosis, particularly in patients infected with HCV genotype 3, and the level of HCV replication, both in serum and in the liver[15,46-48]; and (3) the response to antiviral therapy, especially in genotype 3–infected patients, which results in disappearance of steatosis, with reappearance of steatosis following relapse of HCV infection.[48-51]

The mechanisms responsible for the accumulation of HCV-induced fat in hepatocytes are still unknown but may involve the core protein and NS5A.[13-15] Cumulative evidence suggests that steatosis contributes to the progression of fibrosis in HCV-related disease in a pattern similar to that observed in nonalcoholic fatty liver disease (see Chapter 82).[46-48,50,52] Potential mechanisms by which steatosis leads to progression of fibrosis include the increased sensitivity of steatotic livers to oxidative stress and cytokine-mediated injury[11-15] and hyperinsulinemia resulting from steatosis-related hepatic insulin resistance.[53,54]

IMMUNE-MEDIATED MECHANISMS

HCV infection elicits a specific antibody response, as well as circulating and liver-infiltrating virus-specific CD8+ (cytoxic suppressor) and CD4+ T cell and natural killer (NK) cell activity. Although the cellular immune response may play a pivotal role in the pathogenesis of HCV infection, the importance of the antibody response in generating liver damage is less clear.

The HCV-specific CD8+ T cell response is polyclonal and directed against different epitopes of both structural and nonstructural regions of the HCV polyprotein in the context of different major histocompatibility complex (MHC) alleles.[55] Studies have estimated the percentage of HCV-specific CD8+ T cells to range from 0.01% to 1.2% of total CD8+ T cells.[55,56] In persons in whom hepatitis C resolves, the CD8+ T cell response, particularly that of IFN-γ–producing CD8+ T cells, occurs early after resolution of the infection and is durable.[55,57-61] Helper/inducer T cells (CD4+ cells) also may modify hepatocellular damage in chronic HCV infection. The ultimate expression of HCV depends on the balance between type 1 T-helper (T$_H$1) and type 2 T-helper (T$_H$2) CD4+ responses. The T$_H$1 cells secrete interleukin-2 (IL-2) and interferon-γ, which are important stimuli for the host antiviral immune response, including generation of cytotoxic T lymphocytes (CTLs) and activation of NK cells. The T$_H$2 cells produce IL-4 and IL-10, which enhance antibody production and down-regulate the T$_H$1 response. The CD4+ T cell response against HCV also is multispecific (i.e., directed against several viral proteins) and frequently is found in patients with chronic hepatitis C.[55] In persons with chronic hepatitis, however, this CD4+ T cell response is impaired, and the proportion of chronic HCV carriers who are able to mount an effective CD4+ T cell response to HCV is small.[62] In patients in whom acute infection resolves, an early and multispecific CD4+ T cell

proliferative response occurs, with predominance of T$_H$1 CD4+ T cells in the peripheral blood,[55] most of which produce IFN-γ. This "protective" response is still detected 18 to 20 years after infection in a majority of asymptomatic recovered patients, but in only a minority of patients in whom chronic HCV infection develops.[61,62] The reasons for these different early immune responses in acute HCV infection are unknown.

HCV-specific T cells are enriched at the site of viral replication (in the liver) as compared with the peripheral blood.[55,56] CD8+ lymphocytes predominate, suggesting that CTLs are the main perpetrators of hepatocellular injury. Most of the intrahepatic HCV-specific CD8+ T cells express the activation molecule CD69,[56] probably indicating that these cells become activated in the liver after contact with specific HCV antigens. The T cell immune response in the liver may result in direct cytolysis of the infected cells and in the inhibition of viral replication by secreted antiviral cytokines.[55]

The humoral response against HCV is targeted against epitopes within all viral proteins. The role of circulating anti-HCV antibodies in the pathogenesis of hepatocyte injury is unknown. In contrast with the cellular immune response, the antibody response to HCV antigens remains evident in patients with chronic hepatitis C but is lost in most of those who recover, suggesting that T cells and not antibodies effect the resolution of acute hepatitis C.[61]

Other immunologic factors such as human leukologic antigen (HLA) class I and class II alleles probably contribute to HCV-related disease severity and viral persistence.[63,64] Of interest, viral clearance in a homogeneous cohort of women infected with a single-source HCV genotype 1b was associated with the specific class I allele HLA-A*03, -DRB1*0101, or -*0401.[65]

In summary, liver injury probably results from a combination of direct cytopathic effects of viral proteins and immune-mediated mechanisms, including cytolytic and noncytolytic reactions mediated by CTLs and inflammatory cytokines.[66]

CLINICAL FEATURES

ACUTE AND CHRONIC HEPATITIS C

HCV accounts for approximately 20% of cases of acute hepatitis (see Chapters 74, 75, 77, and 78). Acute hepatitis C is rarely seen in clinical practice, because the vast majority of patients are asymptomatic.[67,68] Jaundice occurs in 10% to 20% of patients with acute HCV infection, whereas 20% to 30% present with nonspecific symptoms such as fatigue, nausea, and vomiting. HCV RNA is detectable within 2 to 3 weeks of exposure, and anti-HCV seroconversion occurs between day 15 and month 3. Serum aminotransferase levels peak at about the first month after exposure (Fig. 76–3), exceed 1000 IU/L in 20% of cases, and generally follow a fluctuating pattern for the first few months. In patients in whom jaundice develops, peak serum bilirubin levels usually are less than 12 mg/dL, and jaundice typically resolves within 1 month. Severe impairment of liver function and liver failure are rare. A more severe course of acute hepatitis C may develop in patients who drink large amounts of

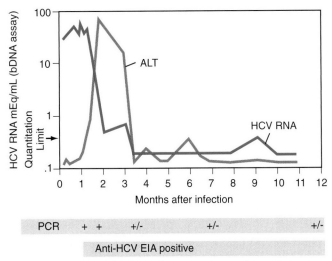

Figure 76–3   Typical course of a case of acute hepatitis C virus (HCV) infection. The changes in HCV RNA and serum ALT levels were manifestations of post-transfusion hepatitis C. Note that viral RNA is detectable for several weeks before anti-HCV conversion. (Courtesy of Chiron Corporation, Emeryville, California.) ALT, alanine aminotransferase; bDNA, branched-chain DNA; EIA, enzyme immunoassay; PCR, polymerase chain reaction (assay).

alcohol or have coinfection with HBV or HIV. HCV infection is self-limited in 10% to 50% of patients, in whom HCV RNA clears and serum ALT levels normalize. In a person suspected of having an acute HCV infection and in whom results of tests for HCV RNA in serum initially are negative, testing should be repeated periodically for up to 12 months.[69] In patients with community-acquired hepatitis C in whom the infection resolves spontaneously, loss of HCV RNA from serum usually occurs within 3 to 4 months of the onset of clinical disease.[70]

The rate of viral persistence varies, ranging from a low of 40% to 50% to a high of 90% to 100%, depending on factors such as the patient's age and gender (younger and female patients have lower rates of chronicity); source of infection and size of inoculum (the rates of chronicity are lower in injection drug users than in those who acquire HCV infection by blood transfusion); immune status of the host (chronicity rates are higher in persons with immunodeficiency states such as agammaglobulinemia and HIV infection); and the patient's race (rates of viral persistence are higher in African Americans than in whites and Hispanic Americans in the United States). Finally, the rate of spontaneous clearance is higher in symptomatic patients in whom jaundice develops during acute infection than in those who remain asymptomatic.[68-72]

A majority of patients with chronic hepatitis C have elevated or fluctuating serum ALT levels, although in one third, serum ALT values are persistently normal, despite continued liver injury and HCV RNA in serum (see later).

Patients with chronic hepatitis C infection are most likely to complain of fatigue, although many patients are asymptomatic. Other frequent manifestations include arthralgias, paraesthesias, myalgias, pruritus, and sicca syndrome. Nonspecific symptoms include depression, nausea, anorexia, abdominal discomfort, and difficulty

with concentration. The severity of these symptoms is not necessarily related to the severity of the underlying liver disease.[73] Many chronically infected patients report a consistent and significant reduction in multiple domains of their health-related quality of life, which may improve with successful antiviral therapy.[73] Once cirrhosis develops, patients with chronic hepatitis C are at risk for complications of portal hypertension (e.g., ascites, gastrointestinal bleeding, encephalopathy) (see Chapters 87 to 89 and 91). Jaundice is rarely seen in patients with chronic hepatitis C until hepatic decompensation has occurred. Referral for liver transplantation should be considered in patients with complications of portal hypertension or evidence of hepatic synthetic failure (e.g., reduction in serum albumin levels, rise in serum bilirubin levels, prolongation of the prothrombin time) (see Chapter 92).

EXTRAHEPATIC MANIFESTATIONS

HCV is increasingly recognized as a cause of extrahepatic diseases, including membranoproliferative glomerulonephritis, essential mixed cryoglobulinemia, porphyria cutanea tarda, leukocytoclastic vasculitis, focal lymphocytic sialadenitis, Mooren's corneal ulcers, lichen planus, rheumatoid arthritis, thyroid disease, non-Hodgkin's lymphoma, and diabetes mellitus.[55,74,75] The strength of these associations with HCV varies. Rheumatologic and skin manifestations are most common. Many HCV-infected patients are seropositive for non–organ-specific autoantibodies (e.g., antinuclear antibodies with a titer greater than 1:40 in 21%, antismooth muscle antibodies with a titer greater than 1:40 in 21%, anti-liver/kidney microsomal antibodies in 5%), cryoglobulins (present in serum in as many as 40% to 50% of patients), and low thyroxine concentrations (10%).[74-76] Disease associated with these abnormalities, however, is much less common.

Anti-HCV is present in serum in 50% to 90% of patients with essential mixed cryoglobulinemia; however, clinical manifestations are reported in only 25% to 30% of these patients. Symptoms and signs include fatigue, arthralgias, arthritis, purpura, Raynaud's phenomenon, vasculitis, peripheral neuropathy, and glomerulonephritis. Treatment with immunosuppressive agents is ineffective. Therapy with IFN-γ has resulted in transient improvement in symptoms and reduction in serum HCV RNA levels (see later). Glomerular disease generally manifests as nephrotic syndrome, non–nephrotic-range proteinuria, or renal insufficiency. Hypocomplementemia is frequent, and in most patients, rheumatoid factor is detected in serum. Therapy in patients with membranoproliferative glomerulonephritis with IFN-γ has been associated with a reduction in proteinuria (65%) but typically no significant improvement in renal function. In about 10% of patients, the disorder progresses to end-stage renal failure requiring dialysis. Use of pulse methylprednisolone therapy may provide some benefit to patients with severe, progressive disease.[74]

HCV infection also has been linked to B cell non-Hodgkin's lymphoma,[75] as suggested by a significantly higher frequency of HCV infection in patients with B cell non-Hodgkin's lymphoma (approximately 15%) than in the general population or in patients with other hematologic malignancies. The mechanisms by which HCV might exert an oncogenic potential are still under investigation. HCV RNA does not integrate into the host genome and cannot be considered a typical oncogenic virus. Rather, HCV shows lymphotropism and may facilitate the development and selection of abnormal B cell clones by chronic stimulation of the immune system. The striking geographic differences in the association between HCV and non-Hodgkin's lymphoma suggest that although HCV infection may be the first step in causing a clonal expansion of infected B cells, additional genetic, environmental, and other viral factors probably are involved in the pathogenesis of non-Hodgkin's lymphoma.

DIAGNOSIS

Several immunologic and molecular assays are used to detect and monitor HCV infection (Table 76–1).[77] The presence of anti-HCV in serum indicates exposure to the virus but does not differentiate among acute, chronic, and resolved infections. Anti-HCV may persist for life in patients with spontaneously resolved infection, although titers decrease and even disappear over time.[61] In patients with chronic hepatitis C, anti-HCV persists in serum for life. Molecular or virologic assays detect specific viral nucleic acid sequences of HCV RNA, which indicate the presence of virus. In patients with persistent HCV infection, serum HCV RNA levels may fluctuate five-fold even in the absence of therapy. Serologic assays typically are used for screening and first-line diagnosis, whereas virologic assays are required for confirming infection and for monitoring response to treatment.[77,78]

INDIRECT ASSAYS

Enzyme immunoassays (EIAs) detect antibodies against different HCV antigens from the core and nonstructural proteins. The time course of the development of symptoms, detection of anti-HCV, and appearance of HCV RNA after acute infection is shown in Figure 76–3. Three generations of EIAs have been developed, with successive assays leading to increasing sensitivity and a progressive decrease in the "window" period between acute exposure to HCV and seroconversion to anti-HCV. The latest, third-generation EIAs detect antibodies against HCV core, NS3, NS4, and NS5 antigens as early as 7 to 8 weeks after infection, with specificity and sensitivity rates of 99%. Despite ongoing viral replication, serologic test results may be negative in patients on hemodialysis or with immune deficiency, as in HIV infection. Because the performance characteristics of third-generation EIAs are so good, confirmation with a recombinant immunoblot assay (RIBA) for antibodies to HCV proteins is rarely used clinically. Use of a RIBA occasionally may establish that a positive anti-HCV EIA result in a person without viremia is attributable to resolved infection, rather than a false-positive EIA result.

DIRECT ASSAYS

HCV RNA can be measured by highly sensitive qualitative and quantitative assays.[77,78]

Qualitative Assays

Detection of HCV RNA may be accomplished by qualitative target amplification methods, such *PCR amplification* or *transcription-mediated amplification* (TMA). Qualitative PCR testing for HCV RNA may detect an HCV RNA level as low as 50 international units (IU)/mL. The manual TMA test has a detection limit of 10 IU/mL (see following discussion). The specificity rate is 99% for both tests. Qualitative testing should be used in the following settings: (1) evaluation of a patient with acute or chronic hepatitis of unknown cause who is seronegative for anti-HCV, particularly if the patient is immunosuppressed; (2) evaluation of a patient with chronic liver disease who is seropositive for anti-HCV but lacks detectable HCV RNA by a quantitative assay for HCV RNA; (3) diagnosis of HCV infection in babies born to HCV-infected mothers; and (4) confirmation of the clearance of HCV RNA from serum after apparently successful antiviral therapy.

Quantitative Assays

Quantitative HCV RNA tests are useful for monitoring antiviral therapy. Testing with a quantitative HCV RNA assay 12 weeks after antiviral treatment is begun can be used to determine whether an early virologic response (EVR) has been achieved (see later).[24,28,77-79] Methods to quantify HCV RNA levels in serum include *signal amplification* and *target amplification*. Signal amplification techniques are represented by the third-generation branched-chain DNA (bDNA) assay. The bDNA assay uses capture and target probes from the conserved 5′ UTR and core regions to detect viral RNA; the bound probe is amplified through a series of synthetic bDNA oligonucleotides (signal amplification) and quantitated. With target amplification techniques, HCV RNA is reverse-transcribed and amplified using primers to the conserved 5′ region of the HCV genome, and the amount of viral RNA present in the amplified sample is estimated from a standardized dilutional series. In the past, the use of quantitative assays was limited by expense and lack of standardization. Universal standardization of HCV RNA quantitation units has been achieved[80] and allows recommendations and guidelines derived from clinical trials to be applied uniformly in clinical practice. Conversion factors for the units previously used in commercial quantitative assays have been calculated, so that 1 IU/mL corresponds to 0.9 copy/mL in the Amplicor HCV Monitor v2.0 Assay, 2.7 copies/mL in the Cobas Amplicor HCV Monitor v2.0 Assay, 3.4 copies/mL in the SuperQuant Assay, 3.8 copies/mL in the LCx HCV RNA Quantitative Assay, and 5.2 copies/mL in the Versant HCV RNA 3.0 Quantitative Assay, respectively (see Table 76–1).

The lower limit of detection of HCV RNA with current assays ranges from 30 to 615 IU/mL. The upper limit of quantification ranges from less than 500,000 to 20,000,000 IU/mL. The accuracy of quantitation dimin-

Table 76–1   Diagnostic Testing for Hepatitis C Virus (HCV) Infection

HCV Marker	Test	Commercial Product(s)*	Limits of Detection†	Use(s)	Comment(s)
Anti-HCV	Third-generation EIA	Various	—	Marker of past or present infection Screening Diagnosis of HCV infection	Seroconversion occurs 7 to 8 weeks after exposure
HCV RNA	Target amplification by PCR or TMA	*PCR:* Amplicor HCV v2.0 and Cobas Amplicor HCV v2.0[a] *TMA:* Versant HCV RNA Qualitative Assay[b]	*Lower limit:* 50 IU of HCV RNA/mL *Lower limit:* 10 IU of HCV RNA/mL	Diagnosis: marker of HCV replication Treatment decision-making Treatment monitoring: assessment of end-of-treatment virologic response and SVR	Detectable 1 to 2 weeks after exposure
Levels of HCV RNA	Target amplification by PCR or TMA Signal amplification by bDNA	Amplicor HCV Monitor v2.0 and Cobas Amplicor HCV Monitor v2.0[a] SuperQuant[c] LCx HCV RNA Assay[d] Cobas TaqMan 48 HCV[a] Versant HCV RNA 3.0 Assay[e]	600-5,000,000 IU/mL 30-1,470,000 IU/mL 25-2,630,000 IU/mL 20-10,000,000 IU/mL 615-7,700,000 IU/mL	Treatment decision-making Choosing optimal treatment regimen Treatment monitoring ("12th week rule" [see text])	Stable levels during chronic infection
HCV core antigen	EIA	EIA[f]	1-2 pg/mL	As for HCV RNA (needs further validation)	1 pg/mL of core antigen is equivalent to 8000 IU/mL of HCV RNA
HCV genotype	Serotyping: competitive EIA testing for type-specific antibodies	Murex HCV serotyping 1-6 assay[g]	Can be determined in 90% of immunocompetent patients	Treatment decision-making	Does not identify subtypes
	Molecular genotyping methods (direct sequencing and phylogenetic analysis, PCR assay with genotype-specific primers, restriction fragment length polymorphism, line-probe or reverse dot-blot hybridization assays)	Trugene HCV 5'NC genotype kit[b] and Inno-Lipa HCV II line probe-test[h]	Subtyping errors in 10%-25% of cases		

*Manufacturers: a, Roche Molecular Systems, Pleasanton, California; b, Bayer Corp., Tarrytown, New York; c, NGI, Los Angeles, California; d, Abbott Diagnostics, Chicago, Illinois; e, Bayer Diagnostics, Tarrytown, New York; f, Ortho-Clinical Diagnostics, Raritan, New Jersey; g, Murex Diagnostics, Dartford, United Kingdom; h, Innogenetics, Ghent, Belgium.
†Dynamic range.
Anti-HCV, antibody to hepatitis C virus; bDNA, branched-chain DNA; EIA, enzyme immunoassay; IU, international unit; PCR, polymerase chain reaction; SVR, sustained virologic response; TMA, transcription-mediated amplification.

ishes substantially when results fall outside the dynamic range of quantification of an assay. Samples that exceed the upper limit should be retested after dilution of serum by 1:10 or 1:100. In the vast majority of serum samples from immunocompetent patients, HCV RNA levels fall between 5×10^4 and 5×10^6 IU/mL. Higher HCV RNA levels are typical of immunosuppressed patients. Variations of less than 0.5 log probably are not clinically significant and reflect patient and test variation. On the basis of dynamic ranges of the different quantitative assays currently available, "real time" PCR technology appears to be the best method for accurate measurement of HCV RNA titers. In addition, because the reaction and measurements with this technique take place in a closed tube, carryover contamination of subsequent samples is minimal.

HCV Core Antigen Assay

HCV core antigen can be detected and quantified with an EIA. The serum HCV core antigen titer correlates closely with the serum HCV RNA level in a ratio of approximately 1 pg/mL to 8000 IU/mL. The lower limit of detection in the HCV core antigen assay is not as sensitive as that for HCV RNA by PCR assay, thus restricting its clinical use.[81]

HCV Genotyping

Differentiation of genotypes is accomplished by several methods that have an overall concordance rate of 90%. Two commercial kits are based on PCR amplification of the 5' UTR region. With these kits, the six genotypes can be identified. Subtype errors occur in 10% to 25% of cases because of variations in the target 5' UTR region.[77,78]

SELECTION OF SEROLOGIC AND VIROLOGIC TESTS

A proposed algorithm for the evaluation of an anti-HCV seropositive person is shown in Figure 76–4. For low-risk patients, a negative result on EIA is sufficient to exclude HCV infection. By contrast, for high-risk patients, including those recently exposed to HCV and immuno-

compromised persons, further testing for HCV RNA is required.

Screening in Blood Banks

The risk of acquiring HCV infection from blood products has declined substantially since blood donors have been screened routinely with serologic tests for HCV and is estimated to be as low as 0.01% to 0.001% per unit transfused.[36,37] With the most recent third-generation EIAs, the number of false or indeterminate test results is extremely low. One major limitation of these assays, however, is the existence of a window period during which the patient may transmit the virus before anti-HCV becomes detectable. For this reason, many blood banks now routinely screen blood with nucleic acid tests, thereby reducing the risk of transfusion-associated HCV infection to as low as 1 per 2 million units transfused.[82]

Diagnosis Following Known Exposure

The diagnosis of HCV infection following an occupational exposure or in the context of mother-to-infant transmission is based on a sensitive HCV RNA detection method. HCV RNA becomes detectable in serum 1 to 2 weeks following exposure. Because spontaneous clearance of HCV RNA from serum is significantly higher in babies than in adults, it is recommended that babies be

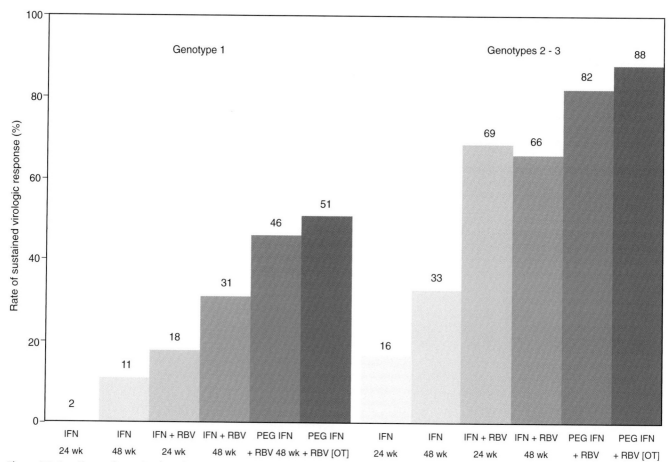

Figure 76–4 Rates of sustained virologic response (SVR) with different therapies for hepatitis C virus (HCV) infection based on the infecting genotype. SVR is defined as HCV RNA–negative by polymerase chain reaction assay 6 months after the discontinuation of therapy. IFN, interferon; OT, optimal treatment; PEG IFN, pegylated interferon; RBV, ribavirin.

tested 6 to 12 months after birth when the mother is infected with HCV.[39]

HISTOPATHOLOGIC FINDINGS AND ROLE OF LIVER BIOPSY

The range of hepatic histologic findings in patients with chronic HCV infection is broad, from minimal periportal lymphocytic inflammation to active hepatitis with bridging fibrosis, hepatocyte necrosis, and cirrhosis.[83] Steatosis, lymphoid aggregates, and bile duct damage are frequent findings. Histologic changes generally are scored for two components—the grade of necroinflammatory changes and the stage of structural alterations—both to assess and compare the efficacy of antiviral and antifibrotic drugs in therapeutic trials and to improve descriptions in routine clinical practice.[83] Available scoring systems have different intraobserver and interobserver variabilities. A frequently used scoring system is the modification, by Ishak and associates, of the Histology Activity Index (HAI) developed by Knodell and colleagues. The Ishak system stages fibrosis from 0 to 6 (1 or 2, portal fibrotic expansion; 3 or 4, bridging fibrosis; 5 or 6, cirrhosis). The necroinflammatory components in this system include periportal inflammation and necrosis (graded as 0 to 10), lobular inflammation and necrosis (0 to 4), and portal inflammation. The other frequently used system is the METAVIR scoring system developed in France, in a simplified version of which inflammation is graded from 0 to 4 (none, mild, moderate, and severe) and fibrosis is staged from 0 to 4 (none, portal fibrosis, portal fibrosis with few septa, bridging fibrosis, and cirrhosis). Agreement is lacking regarding the best scoring system. Although the prognostic implications of specific histologic findings are not clear, mild inflammation and negligible fibrosis are associated with a low risk of progression to cirrhosis, whereas severe necroinflammatory activity and advanced fibrosis are likely to evolve to cirrhosis with time.

The role of liver biopsy in the management of HCV-infected patients is not settled.[84] Although liver biopsy is still considered the gold standard for establishing the severity of liver disease, it has several limitations, including (1) associated morbidity (post-biopsy pain occurs in at least 20% of patients, and major complications such as hemorrhage occur in 0.5%) and mortality, the rate of which may reach 0.1%; (2) substantial cost; (3) poor patient acceptance; (4) intraobserver and interobserver variability, which is higher for grading necroinflammation than for staging fibrosis (with current scoring systems, intraobserver and interobserver variability for staging fibrosis ranges from 60% to 90% and 70% to 90%, respectively); (5) imperfect accuracy, particularly for the diagnosis of cirrhosis, with a mean rate of false-negative results of 24% (10% to 32%); and (6) sampling error of 10% to 40%, especially when small biopsy specimens comprising less than 11 portal triads are analyzed, because of the heterogeneous distribution of the liver lesions.

Because of the limitations of liver biopsy, noninvasive tests for markers of disease severity are under study.[85] An ideal test should be simple, readily available, inexpensive,

and accurate, and the disease marker should be sensitive to the effects of therapy. Individual serum markers of fibrogenesis have limited accuracy in predicting hepatic fibrosis. Composite indices based on a panel of simple serum markers correlate better with histologic fibrosis, but their reliability requires validation by independent investigators. Routine laboratory tests typically used in current indices of hepatic fibrosis include platelet count, serum aspartate aminotransferase (AST)-to-serum ALT ratio, serum bilirubin level, serum cholesterol level, and prothrombin time. These indices can identify patients at both extremes of disease severity (mild inflammatory with mild fibrosis at one end of the spectrum and cirrhosis at the other end) but are, in general, imperfect and lack accuracy and reliability in a substantial proportion of patients in the intermediate zone of histologic severity (Table 76–2).

The following recommendations can be made regarding the role of liver biopsy in the management of patients with chronic hepatitis C (Table 76–3). Regardless of the degree of serum aminotransferase elevations, a baseline liver biopsy is recommended but not mandatory for initial assessment of patients with chronic hepatitis C, especially in those older than 40 years of age and those who wish to defer antiviral therapy. Although the rate of progression of fibrosis appears to be low in patients with normal serum aminotransferase levels, only 20% have a histologically normal liver, and a small percentage (less than 15%) have substantial liver damage.[86,87] A post-treatment liver biopsy is not necessary, because most treatment trials have demonstrated that a sustained virologic response to therapy generally is associated with stable or improved histologic findings. Finally, in patients in whom the diagnosis of cirrhosis is suggested by clinical or ultrasound findings (e.g., ascites, splenomegaly, spider angioma, low platelet count, prolonged prothrombin time, reduction in portal flow, nodularity of the liver), histologic confirmation is not required. A follow-up liver biopsy is recommended to reassess disease severity if re-treatment of a nonresponder to previous therapy is being considered, in view of the low likelihood of achieving a sustained virologic response in these patients. Follow-up biopsies also may be helpful when long-term maintenance therapy to prevent progression of fibrosis is considered (see later). On the basis of the rate of progression of fibrosis in several studies, an interval of at least 5 years between biopsies is required to assess histologic change in patients with initially mild liver disease.[88-94]

NATURAL HISTORY

Progression of chronic hepatitis C is largely silent. Patients often are identified on routine biochemical screening or at blood donation. Several strategies have been used to assess the natural history of chronic HCV infection: (1) cross-sectional studies in which patients with end-stage liver disease are evaluated and assessed for markers of HCV infection; (2) retrospective-prospective studies in which patients with established liver disease are identified and assessed by estimating the time of the initial HCV infection and then determining the natural

Table 76–2 Noninvasive Markers Used for Predicting Liver Fibrosis in Patients with Chronic Hepatitis C

Reference	Predictive Variable(s)	Model	Cutoff Value(s)	S	Sp	PPV	NPV
159	HA, PIIINP	NA	Significant fibrosis predicted by:				
			PIIINP >0.8 kU/L	0.7	0.63	NA	NA
			HA ≥85 µg/L	0.64	0.91	NA	NA
160	HA, PT	NA	Significant fibrosis predicted by:				
			HA ≥60 or	0.97	0.73	0.61	0.98
			PT <85% of control	0.80	0.88	0.74	0.91
161	Age, platelet count (age-platelet index)	Requires table	Significant fibrosis predicted by:				
			Score ≥6	0.29	0.9	0.93	0.32
162	Platelet count, PT, ALT/AST	NA	Significant fibrosis predicted by:				
			Score ≥8	0.46	0.98	NA	NA
163	AST/ALT	AST/ALT	Cirrhosis predicted by:				
			AST/ALT ratio >1	0.53	1	1	NA
164	HA	NA	Significant fibrosis predicted by:			NA	NA
			HA ≥350 g/L	0.85	0.88		
165	TIMP-1, TIMP-2	NA	Significant fibrosis predicted by:			NA	NA
			TIMP-1 ≥500 ng/mL	0.94	0.57		
			TIMP-2 ≥102 ng/mL	0.85	0.47		
166	HA	NA	Lack of significant fibrosis predicted by:				
			HA <60 µg/L	0.88	0.59	0.47	0.93
167	Platelet count	NA	Significant fibrosis predicted by:	NA	NA	0.93	0.99
			Moderate thrombocytopenia (platelet count <20% of normal)				
168	Serum type IV collagen Platelet count	NA	Significant fibrosis predicted by:	0.47	0.89	0.56	0.85
			Type IV collagen >130 ng/mL				
			Platelet count <140,000/mm³				
169	Fibronectin, PT, pseudocholinesterase, ALT, manganese-SOD, N-acetyl-β-glucosaminidase	Complicated	Cirrhosis predicted by:	NA	NA	NA	NA
			Score ≤0.22				
170	Platelet count, AST/ALT	NA	Significant fibrosis predicted by:	0.41	0.99	0.93	0.85
			AST/ALT ratio ≥1				
			Platelet count <150,000/mm³				
171	α₂-Macroglobulin, haptoglobin, gamma globulin, apolipoprotein A₁, GGTP, BR	FibroTest	Score <0.1: lack of fibrosis	1	0.22	0.5	1
			Score >0.6: presence of fibrosis (stage F2–F4, see text)	0.7	0.95	0.91	0.76
172	TIMP-1, HA, α₂-macroglobulin	NA	NA	0.68	0.94	0.81	0.89
173	Platelet count, spider angiomata, AST, gender	Complicated	NA				
174	Age, GGTP, cholesterol, platelet count	Complicated (AGCP)	Lack of significant fibrosis predicted by:				
			AGCP <4.2	0.94	0.51	0.4	0.96
175	Platelet count, AST	APRI (AST-to-platelet ratio index)	APRI <0.5 predicts nonsignificant fibrosis	0.91	0.47	0.61	0.86
			APRI >1.5 predicts significant fibrosis	0.41	0.95	0.88	0.64
176	Age, AST, cholesterol, insulin resistance, past alcohol intake	FPI score	FPI <0.2 predicts nonsignificant fibrosis	0.96	0.44	0.61	0.93
			FPI >0.8 predicts significant fibrosis	0.43	0.94	0.87	0.64
177	PIIINP, MMP-1	PIIINP/MMP-1	Score <0.2 predicts nonsignificant fibrosis	0.91	0.35	—	0.88
			Score >0.4 predicts significant fibrosis	0.35	0.96	0.91	—

AGCP, age–GGTP–cholesterol–platelet count index; ALT, alanine aminotransferase; APRI, AST-to-platelet ratio index; AST, aspartate aminotransferase; BR, bilirubin; FPI, fibrosis probability index; GGTP, gamma glutamyl transpeptidase; HA, hyaluronic acid; MMP-1, matrix metalloproteinase-1; NA, not available/not applicable; NPV, negative predictive value; PIIINP, procollagen type III N-terminal peptide; PPV, positive predictive value; PT, prothrombin time; S, sensitivity; SOD, superoxide dismutase; Sp, specificity; TIMP, tissue inhibitor of metalloproteinase.

history of infection from that time forward; (3) prospective studies in which patients are evaluated at the onset of disease and are followed longitudinally for a defined period; and (4) long-term cohort studies in which the HCV status of persons at the time of a defined parenteral exposure to HCV and outcome were assessed after follow-up periods longer than 15 years. Each approach has its limitations.

As would be predicted, the most severe outcomes have been described in cross-sectional and retrospective studies (Table 76–4). In early cross-sectional studies, anti-HCV was detectable in 50% (range, 8% to 69%) of patients with cryptogenic cirrhosis and in 6% to 76% of those with hepatocellular carcinoma, underscoring the importance of HCV in these diseases. Retrospective-prospective studies subsequently showed that chronic hepatitis, cirrhosis, and hepatocellular carcinoma develop 13 ± 11 years, 21 ± 10 years, and 29 ± 13 years, respectively, after transmission of HCV by blood transfusion.[95] Prospective studies, typically of less than 30 years' duration, have provided unequivocal evidence of the progressive nature of chronic HCV infection. In these studies, death from end-stage liver disease has been uncommon, but clearly liver failure and hepatocellular carcinoma occur. Cohort studies with prolonged follow-up after a defined parenteral exposure allow assessments of not only persons in whom persistent infection and

significant liver disease develop, but also those with mild disease and those who clear infection. In the study by Seeff and colleagues, 568 patients with non-A, non-B post-transfusional hepatitis were compared with 984 matched controls who received transfusions but in whom hepatitis did not develop.[95] After an average of 20 years of follow-up, all-cause mortality rates were no different between cases and controls (51% and 54%, respectively), but the death rate attributable to liver disease was higher in the former than in the latter group (3.3% and 1.5%, respectively). Of the anti-HCV–positive group, 90% had evidence of chronic hepatitis or cirrhosis. The major concepts related to the natural history of post-transfusion HCV infection were derived from this large multicenter study and include the following: (1) approximately one fourth of patients experience spontaneous recovery from HCV infection, with loss of HCV RNA in serum (and in 10% of these patients, concomitant loss of serologic markers of prior HCV infection occurs); and (2) of the 75% of patients with persistent HCV infection, severe progressive liver disease occurs in only 15% to 20%, whereas in the remaining, a benign course is observed.

Iatrogenic outbreaks of HCV infection also have provided insight into the natural history of HCV infection. In 1977, young Irish women were accidentally infected with HCV genotype 1b when a contaminated lot of anti-D immunoglobulin was administered to them. After prolonged follow-up for longer than 18 years, cirrhosis developed in only 2%, and complications of liver disease developed in none.[96] A similar study from Germany involved 152 women infected through contaminated Rh immune globulin.[97] At 15 years after exposure, none of these women had evidence of chronic hepatitis or cirrhosis. These two studies of the natural history of HCV infection in people infected at a young age have important implications for persons infected through injection drug use, a majority of whom are infected in their teens and twenties. Compared with other studies, these two studies document a more slowly progressive course of HCV infection, perhaps because of the gender of the study subjects (disease progression is slower in women than in men), infection at a young age (which also is a predictor of slow disease progression), and the specific route of infection (the inoculum of virus is smaller with injections than with blood transfusions).

A 45-year HCV natural history study of 8568 military recruits, 0.2% of whom tested positive for anti-HCV,

Table 76–3 Value of Liver Biopsy in Patients with Chronic Hepatitis C

Assessment of severity, including grade of hepatic necroinflammation and stage of fibrosis

Exclusion of coexisting diseases, such as hemochromatosis, alcoholic liver disease, and nonalcoholic steatohepatitis

Determination of rate of disease progression in patients with a known date of infection or a previous liver biopsy

Guidance in treatment decision-making:

The presence of mild liver disease may allow treatment to be deferred, particularly in patients in whom treatment efficacy would be limited by a poor host or virologic response profile.

The presence of advanced liver disease may favor treatment, even in patients with a low likelihood of response.

The need for and potential efficacy of maintenance antiviral or antifibrogenic therapy can be established.

Table 76–4 Natural History of Hepatitis C Virus Infection: Summary of Clinical Studies

Type of Study	Duration of Follow-up*	% of Affected Patients		
		Progressing to Cirrhosis	*Developing HCC*	*Dying of Liver-Related Causes*
Retrospective	10-30 years	17-55	1-23	4-15
Retrospective-prospective[†]	9-45 years	0.3-15	0-1.9	0-2.8
Prospective	8-16 years	7-16	0.7-1.3	1.3-3.7

*Years since infection.

[†]In a retrospective-prospective study, patients with established liver disease are assessed by estimating the time of the initial hepatitis C virus infection and then determining the natural history from that point.

HCC, hepatocellular carcinoma.

has the longest follow-up reported to date. In this study, the mortality rate from liver disease in the HCV-positive group was low and only slightly different from that of the control group.[98] These data suggest that HCV is a less progressive disease than was previously believed, and that in only 15% to 20% of HCV-infected persons will the infection eventually progress to potentially serious end-stage liver disease; the remainder will die of causes other than liver disease.

Studies performed in children infected at early ages also point to an overall benign clinical course for HCV infection. In a study performed in Germany, 458 children infected through cardiac surgery before the implementation of blood donor screening were followed for a mean of 17 years; almost one half of the infected children cleared the infection spontaneously, and of the remaining children, only 1 had persistently elevated serum ALT levels. Of the 17 patients who underwent a liver biopsy, only 2 were found to have portal fibrosis, and both of these patients had chronic congestive heart failure, which could have accounted for the more aggressive histologic picture. In another long-term (35 years) follow-up study of 31 adults infected at birth through mini-transfusions from a single infected donor, HCV infection acquired early in life was found to be a slowly progressive disease and associated with a favorable outcome. Most patients had normal or slightly fluctuating ALT levels; none had cirrhosis.[41]

FACTORS ASSOCIATED WITH PROGRESSION OF CHRONIC HEPATITIS C

Many factors contribute to the histologic progression of chronic hepatitis and the development of hepatocellular carcinoma (Table 76–5). Identification of these factors is important so that therapy can be instituted in patients at greatest risk of progressive liver disease, and so that strategies can be aimed at removing the negative predictive factors. Although virus-related factors have little influence on the course of chronic hepatitis C, host and environmental factors play major roles.[67,95,100] *Age at infection* appears to be one of the strongest predictors of outcome. Modeling of the natural history of hepatitis C indicates that progression of fibrosis is not linear over time; rather, the progression is slower at younger ages and increases with each 10- to 15-year period, with the greatest acceleration after the age of 45 to 50 years.[100] The role of aging in progression of fibrosis may be related to a higher vulnerability of older persons to environmental factors (especially oxidative stress), reduction in hepatic blood flow, mitochondrial toxicity, or diminished immune function. *Male gender* is associated with a worse outcome of chronic hepatitis C.[67,95,100] *Race* also has been implicated in disease progression in a few studies, with a lower risk of progression to cirrhosis in African American patients than in whites (2.2% to 22% versus 7.2% to 30%).[101] Polymorphisms in genes implicated in the immune response, such as the genes encoding transforming growth factor (TGF)-β and angiotensin II, play a role in the progression to severe hepatitis.[64]

Alcohol abuse has been shown to increase disease severity, reduce response to therapy with interferon, and enhance development of hepatocellular carcinoma in patients who are chronically infected with HCV. Whether mild to moderate alcohol intake leads to more rapid progression of chronic hepatitis C needs to be defined in further studies. Alcohol enhances HCV replication, possibly through the activation of the nuclear factor κB promoter.[102] In addition, chronic alcohol consumption

Table 76–5   Factors Possibly Associated with Progression of Hepatitis C

Factor	Strength of Association	Potential Intervention
Age at infection	Established: >40 years	
Gender	Established: Male	
Race	Preliminary: White	
Genetic background	Controversial	
Immune status	Established:	
	Immunosuppression (HIV coinfection, agammaglobulinemia, organ transplantation)	
Genotype	Established:* No association	
Level of viremia	Established: No association	
Quasispecies	Controversial	
HBV coinfection	Possibly associated	HBV vaccination
Hemochromatosis heterozygote	Controversial	
NASH/obesity/diabetes	Possibly associated: Hepatic steatosis	Weight loss, control of hyperglycemia, dietary interventions
Schistosomiasis	Possibly associated	
Smoking	Possibly associated	
Alcohol	Established: Intake of >50 g/day	
Iron overload	Possibly associated	Phlebotomy
Serum ALT levels	Possibly associated: Elevated ALT levels	Follow-up schedule based on initial ALT profile and hepatic histologic findings
Histologic degree of necroinflammation	Possibly associated: Moderate to marked necroinflammation	

*Genotype 3 is associated with virus-induced hepatic steatosis, which in turn may lead to progression of fibrosis.
ALT, alanine aminotransferase; HBV, hepatitis B virus; HIV, human immunodeficiency virus; NASH, nonalcoholic steatohepatitis.

increases lipid peroxidation and synergistically increases hepatic tumor necrosis factor (TNF)-α and TGF-β expression, pathways involved in fibrogenesis and development of hepatocellular carcinoma.[103]

Immunosuppression leads to a more aggressive course of chronic hepatitis C. Studies in patients with humoral (hypogammaglobulinemic patients)[104] or cellular immune (liver or kidney transplant recipients,[105] HIV-infected patients with low CD4+ counts)[106] impairment have shown rates of progression of chronic hepatitis C to cirrhosis that are significantly higher than those observed in immunocompetent patients (see later).

Other prognostic factors that have been documented to affect disease progression less consistently include the *mode of transmission* (higher rate of disease progression when infection is acquired through blood transfusion than through injection drug use) and *coinfection with HBV or HIV.* Several *metabolic abnormalities* and comorbid conditions, including type 2 diabetes, obesity, increased hepatic iron stores, and liver steatosis, have been associated in several, but not all, studies with accelerated progression of fibrosis,[45-51,53,54] possibly by enhancement of lipid accumulation in hepatocytes. Of importance, these metabolic conditions tend to increase in frequency with age. The *serum ALT level* also is predictive of outcome; progression of fibrosis occurs mainly in patients with serum ALT levels greater than five times the upper limit of normal.[89,90] Conversely, progression appears to be minimal, at least over a period of 4 to 5 years, in patients with no or mild *degrees of necroinflammation* on initial liver biopsy specimens and accelerated in those with moderate or marked necroinflammation.[89-94] These data support the recommendation that patients with mild disease activity and scant hepatic fibrosis can delay therapy if they wish, until therapeutic regimens that are better tolerated and more effective are available (see later).

Collectively, the data suggest that the course of HCV infection is severe during the first 2 decades of infection in only a small percentage of the entire population of HCV-infected persons. Discrepancies among natural history studies reflect the great heterogeneity of hepatitis C in terms of severity, outcome, and cofactors known to influence the course and progression, particularly age at infection, gender, size of inoculum, and source of infection. The risk of cirrhosis is significantly higher in adult patients, mainly male, who are infected after the age of 45 through blood transfusions (15% to 27%) than in patients with community-acquired hepatitis C (4%), young drug addicts (1%), young women infected by anti-D immunoglobulin preparations (0.4% to 2%), children with hepatitis C (0.3%),[107] and infants with hepatitis C (0%).

CLINICALLY COMPENSATED HEPATITIS C VIRUS–RELATED CIRRHOSIS

Complications may occur once cirrhosis has developed in a patient with chronic hepatitis C (Table 76–6). In the absence of clinical decompensation, actuarial survival rates are as high as 83% to 91% after 5 years and 79% after 10 years. The survival rates drop to 50% at 5 years among patients in whom clinical decompensation occurs. The cumulative probability of development of an episode of decompensation is only 4% to 5% at 1 year but increases to 30% at 10 years from the diagnosis of cirrhosis.[108-111] The risk of hepatocellular carcinoma is 1% to 4% per year once cirrhosis is established. In some, but not all, studies, therapy with interferon has been shown to reduce the risk of hepatic decompensation and hepatocellular carcinoma.[112-115]

DISEASE IN PATIENTS WITH PERSISTENTLY NORMAL AMINOTRANSFERASE LEVELS OR MILD CHRONIC HEPATITIS C

Approximately one third of anti-HCV–positive patients have normal serum ALT levels. Most of these patients have some degree of histologically proved chronic liver damage, ranging from mild chronic hepatitis to significant fibrosis (approximately 22%) and even cirrhosis (1% to 6%).[86,87,90,93,116,117] The wide range of reported disease severity may be related to the lack of consistent characterization of these patients in many studies. Indeed, patients described in various studies have differed with regard to how long the ALT level was normal, whether ALT levels or both aspartate aminotransferase (AST) and ALT levels were normal, and whether or not viremia was detectable. Strictly speaking, patients considered to be HCV carriers are those with persistently normal serum ALT levels over a period of at least 12 months (with measurement of ALT levels on several occasions at least 1 month apart) and with detectable HCV RNA in serum.[86,116] Disease progression appears to be slower in these patients than in those with elevated ALT levels, and progression to cirrhosis is considered a rare event in the

Table 76–6   Natural History of Compensated HCV-Related Cirrhosis: Summary of Clinical Studies

Reference	Duration of Follow-up (years, with range)	% of Affected Patients (annual rate)		
		Developing Hepatic Decompensation	*Developing HCC*	*Dying of Liver-Related Causes*
108 (N = 112)	4.5 (2-7.7)	21.1 (4.4)	8 (2)	12.5 (3.4)
109 (N = 384)	5.1 (0.5-12.8)	18 (3.9)	8 (1.4)	9 (1.9)
110 (N = 103)	3.3 (0.5-6)	14.6 (5)	10.7 (3.3)	14.6 (5.5)
111 (N = 416)	5.7 (0.3-16.6)	—	14.4 (2.7)	15.4 (3.1)

HCC, hepatocellular carcinoma.

absence of alcohol abuse.[86,87,90,93,116,117] Activation of biochemical activity may occur in 15% to 25% of patients during 3 months to 10 years of follow-up.[94] Therefore, these patients require physical examinations and routine laboratory tests every 6 to 12 months.

The management of patients with *mild chronic hepatitis* is controversial. First, a uniform definition of mild chronis hepatitis is lacking, with some studies including only patients with persistently normal serum aminotransferase levels, regardless of histologic findings, and others including only patients with minor histologic changes. We recommend that the term mild chronic hepatitis be applied to HCV infection in persons who show minimal to mild liver histologic abnormalities independent of the serum ALT levels. The natural history in these cases is still an unresolved issue; liver disease in these patients generally is considered to be benign and nonprogressive, but studies based on sequential liver biopsies have demonstrated that progression to more advanced fibrosis occurs in a substantial proportion of patients, particularly in those with elevated serum aminotransferase levels and in those with some degree of fibrosis at baseline (Table 76–7).[96-101] In fact, the cumulative probability of progression to bridging fibrosis or cirrhosis may reach 50% at 10 years in persons with portal fibrosis and an elevated serum ALT level, compared with 2% in those with no fibrosis and a normal serum ALT level at baseline.

DISEASE IN IMMUNOCOMPROMISED PATIENTS

Patients maintained on dialysis and renal transplant recipients have a higher prevalence of HCV infection than that in the general population, in part because of a higher frequency of risk factors in these patients (prior blood transfusion) and in part because of nosocomial spread within dialysis units. As determined by anti-HCV tests, the frequency of HCV infection is 6% to 22%, and the annual incidence is 4.9%.[118] De novo acquisition of HCV from an infected organ or blood products has been well documented. A study of 3078 cadaveric organ donors from eight organ procurement agencies in the United States found a frequency of anti-HCV (by EIA-2) and of HCV RNA (by PCR assay) of 4.2% and 2.4%, respectively.[119] Among recipients of organs from seropositive donors with detectable viremia, the development of

viremia and of liver disease after transplantation was more likely than among recipients of donors lacking these markers. This finding strongly suggests that the presence of HCV RNA in the donor is associated with transmission of HCV. Following renal transplantation, elevated serum aminotransferase levels are more common in anti-HCV–positive than in anti-HCV–negative patients (median rates of 48% and 14%, respectively). In the long term, patient and graft survival rates are lower in anti-HCV–positive than in anti-HCV–negative renal transplant recipients; the increased mortality is related to liver dysfunction.[118,119]

Transmission of HCV to *heart transplant recipients* has been described, particularly in patients who underwent transplantation before 1992. The outcome of de novo hepatitis C in these patients appears to be more favorable than in liver transplant recipients. Although histologic and biochemical signs of chronic hepatitis develop in a majority of patients, long-term survival is similar to that in uninfected controls. In some patients, however, severe cholestatic hepatitis is associated with a poor outcome.[119]

Bone marrow transplant recipients have multiple risk factors for chronic liver disease, including hepatitis virus infections. The cumulative frequency of cirrhosis has been estimated to be 0.6% after 10 years and 3.8% after 20 years. HCV is a major cause of cirrhosis and of liver-related mortality in this population (see Chapter 33).[119]

Chronic HCV infection is the most common indication for *liver transplantation* and is present either alone or in association with alcoholic liver disease in about 40% of patients who undergo liver transplantation in the United States.[120] Recurrence of HCV infection is nearly universal. Typically, levels of viremia increase significantly following transplantation. Histologic evidence of liver injury develops in most patients, but severe graft dysfunction is infrequent in the short term. Two patterns of disease recurrence have been described. The more common response to persistent HCV infection is the evolution of chronic hepatitis and cirrhosis as in the immunocompetent patient but with a level of viremia at least 1 log higher. Compared with that in immunocompetent patients, disease progression in liver transplant recipients is significantly faster, and the time to cirrhosis is shorter.[105,120] In approximately one third of patients with an initial lack of progression, however, a delayed acceleration of fibrosis may occur. The serum ALT level, together with the degree of histologic necroinflammation

Table 76–7 Natural History of Mild Chronic Hepatitis C*: Summary of Clinical Studies

Reference	Mean Interval Between Liver Biopsies (years)	% of Patients with Progression to Fibrosis	
		Overall	*Subset with Advanced Disease[†]*
89 (*N* = 45)	3.8	42	4
90 (*N* = 61)	6.3	33	10
91 (*N* = 110)	3.2	32	2
92 (*N* = 131)	3.6	41	10
93 (*N* = 105)	8.3	60	27
94 (*N* = 214)	2.5	33	6

*Fibrosis stage 0 or 1 at baseline.
[†]Bridging fibrosis or cirrhosis.

at baseline, may predict this sudden change in the course of recurrent hepatitis C, with the highest risk in patients with persistently elevated serum aminotransferase levels and moderate to marked necroinflammation and minimal risk in those with persistently normal aminotransferase levels and no or mild necroinflammation. After 5 to 10 years of follow-up, cirrhosis develops in the graft of 8% to 30% of HCV-infected liver transplant recipients.

The second pattern of recurrent HCV infection, *fibrosing cholestatic hepatitis*, is less common (5%) but severe, leading to graft failure within months of onset. The accelerated course of recurrent hepatitis C also is evident once cirrhosis is established, with a 1-year risk of decompensation of approximately 40%. Both the pattern of recurrence and its severity depend on the interaction among several host, viral, and external factors. High serum HCV RNA levels before or early after liver transplantation, older age of the donor, severe and early acute hepatitis after transplantation, and strong immunosuppression are considered the factors most consistently associated with a poor outcome.[120] Short-term survival is not affected by HCV recurrence in these patients. With continued follow-up, survival rates in patients who undergo liver transplantation for HCV infection are lower than those in patients who undergo liver transplantation for nonviral indications.

Because of shared routes of transmission, *coinfection with HCV and HIV* is common. The efficiency of the transmission of hepatitis viruses and HIV by parenteral or sexual routes appears to differ, however, explaining the wide variation in HCV seropositivity among HIV-infected persons. Indeed, rates of HCV infection ranging from 4% to 100% have been reported in HIV-infected persons, depending on the route of transmission, with higher rates among injection drug users and recipients of blood transfusions than among men who have sex with men and heterosexual contacts of HIV-infected persons.[121] Increasing evidence from the molecular to the clinical level suggests that the effects of HCV infection can be modified by coinfection with HIV. Critical to this interplay has been the change in the natural history of HIV infection, and decline in mortality due to the increased availability of effective antiretroviral therapy, as well as the use of prophylactic therapy to prevent opportunistic infections. As a consequence, chronic hepatitis C is a growing cause of morbidity and mortality in HIV-infected persons (see Chapter 32). Several studies have shown that HIV-HCV–coinfected patients have a higher risk of fibrosis progression,[106] more severe liver injury, and worse prognosis than patients with HCV infection alone.[121] The risk of progression is highest in patients with CD4+ counts less than 200/mm^3 and in persons who abuse alcohol. Additional features of HCV infection that have been proposed to occur more frequently in coinfected patients than in patients infected with HCV alone include (1) reduced sensitivity of serologic assays for diagnosing HCV infection; (2) enhancement of HCV replication, with more than 58% of samples tested with a commercial PCR-based assay exceeding the cut-off level currently used to determine the likelihood of a response to antiviral treatment of HCV (800,000 IU/mL); (3) HCV genotype 1, the least susceptible genotype to viral eradication with current therapies; (4) higher levels of quasispecies

complexity and diversity; and (5) a higher risk of heterosexual and perinatal transmission of HCV infection. Clinical studies that have examined whether HCV influences the progression of HIV infection have shown conflicting results, although considerable evidence suggests that HCV co-infection adversely affects the management of HIV infection by increasing the risk of antiretroviral-associated liver toxicity, in some instances necessitating discontinuation of antiretroviral drug treatment.

Progression of HCV-related disease also is enhanced in patients with *common variable immunodeficiency*. An "iatrogenic accident" provided an opportunity to examine the natural history of infection in patients with impaired humoral immunity. When immune globulin that was contaminated with HCV was infused into patients with various types of hypogammaglobulinemia,[95,104] the rate of transmission of HCV was high (occurring in 85% of recipients of the contaminated immune globulin), and the course was aggressive. During a follow-up period of approximately 10 years, two patients died of liver failure, and one required liver transplantation. Histologic features were abnormal in all 15 patients who underwent liver biopsy, with cirrhosis in 6. In addition, anecdotal evidence suggests that patients with common variable immunodeficiency who undergo liver transplantation for HCV infection have unusually severe post-transplantation recurrence of HCV infection, presumably because of the combined effects of humoral and cellular immunodeficiency.

PREVENTION

GENERAL MEASURES

Because no effective vaccine and no effective postexposure prophylaxis against HCV infection are available, a major effort should be placed on counseling both HCV-infected patients and those at risk for HCV infection.[28,37] In addition, adequate sterilization of medical and surgical equipment is mandatory. Efforts also should be made to modify injection practices among persons involved in folk medicine, rituals, and cosmetic procedures.

Recommendations for HCV screening vary slightly among major entities such as the National Institutes of Health (NIH) Consensus Panel (http://consensus.nih.gov/cons/116/091202116cdc_statement.htm), the Centers for Disease Control and Prevention (ftp://ftp.cdc.gov/pub/Publications/mmwr/rr/rr4719.pdf), and the United States Preventive Services Task Force.[122] Screening for groups at high risk is strongly recommended. Persons at high risk include recipients of blood and blood products before 1990, injection drug users, sexual partners of persons infected with HCV, patients on hemodialysis, infants of infected mothers, people with occupational exposure to HCV-positive blood, and patients with persistently elevated serum ALT levels. Whether household contacts of HCV-infected patients, persons with a history of sexually transmitted diseases, persons with a history of tattooing or body piercing, and persons who share instruments for intranasal cocaine and other noninjection illegal drugs should undergo HCV screening is uncertain.

HCV-infected patients should be instructed to avoid sharing razors and toothbrushes and to cover any open wounds. In addition, "safe sex" practices, such as the use of latex condoms, should be encouraged in persons with multiple sexual partners. By contrast, no recommendation has been issued regarding sexual practices among persons involved in long-term monogamous relationships. Information regarding the risk associated with sexual transmission should be provided to these patients. In view of the low rate of vertical transmission, pregnancy is not contraindicated in HCV-infected women. No recommendations have been issued regarding the mode of delivery. Breast-feeding is not contraindicated. Finally, it is recommended that HCV-infected patients be vaccinated against hepatitis A and B, because of the high risk of severe liver disease if superinfection with either of these viruses occurs.

PASSIVE IMMUNOPROPHYLAXIS

Several lines of evidence suggest that passive immunoprophylaxis with immune globulin is unlikely to be effective. Studies of immune globulin for prophylaxis against post-transfusion non-A, non-B hepatitis in the 1970s failed to demonstrate a clear benefit. In addition, the neutralizing immune response to HCV infection is weak, and it is unlikely that immune globulin would contain sufficient neutralizing antibody to be effective.[20] Finally, HCV has an inherently high mutational rate that facilitates rapid escape from immune recognition and consequent establishment of persistent infection.[23,29] Development of hyperimmune serum containing polyclonal immunoglobulin may be possible through the immunization of healthy adults with HCV proteins. Whether such sera will be protective following exposure to virus remains to be determined.

ACTIVE IMMUNOPROPHYLAXIS

Development of a vaccine against HCV is encountering the same difficulties experienced in the development of a vaccine against HIV. Vaccination of chimpanzees with composite proteins from the envelope regions of HCV (E1/E2 fusion protein) has been demonstrated to be protective against challenge with homologous but not heterologous sequences E1/E2.[123] Neutralizing antibodies to HCV, elicited during natural infection, have been demonstrated to be effective in preventing viral transmission to experimental animals. Active investigation continues in the development of HCV vaccines that may be used prophylactically and therapeutically by potentiating cellular immune response in chronically infected patients.

TREATMENT

Since the early 1990s, substantial progress has been made in the management of patients with chronic hepatitis C. Viral eradication rates have increased from 10% with use of interferon alone for 24 weeks to 56% with use of combination therapy with peginterferon and ribavirin.[124]

GOALS

The primary goal of therapy of HCV infection is to reduce the mortality by preventing liver-related deaths associated with the development of hepatocellular carcinoma and decompensated cirrhosis. These end points, however, are difficult to achieve because of the long course of hepatitis C. Intermediate end points that have been used to assess the success of therapy include normalization of serum aminotransferase levels, loss of HCV RNA from serum, and improvement in hepatic histologic findings. In practice, sustained virologic response (SVR) is used as an indirect measure of these goals. It is likely that the achievement of an SVR will translate into long-term benefit from therapy, as measured by a reduction in the rates of disease progression, need for liver transplantation, and development of hepatocellular carcinoma and by improvement in the rate of survival. In fact, SVR, defined as the clearance of virus (HCV RNA) from serum 6 months after discontinuation of therapy, is an excellent surrogate marker of the resolution of hepatitis. Several studies have clearly demonstrated that the response is durable in the vast majority of patients and is associated with clinical improvement or stabilization of disease progression.[125,126] In addition, retrospective-prospective studies, including a meta-analysis of 3 randomized and 11 nonrandomized studies, have concluded that therapy with interferon reduces the frequency of hepatocellular carcinoma and increases survival by reducing the rate of liver-related mortality; the effect is significant among patients who achieve an SVR.[122-126] Whether interferon therapy is beneficial in nonresponders is still controversial. Additional goals of therapy include a reduction in extrahepatic manifestations and, to a lesser extent, in the secondary spread of HCV infection.

END POINTS

Normalization of serum ALT levels was the end point of therapy in early clinical trials. Following the discovery of HCV, the combination of the loss of HCV RNA from serum and normalization of serum ALT levels has been used as the end point of treatment. These responses usually are evaluated at the end of treatment (end-of-treatment response) and at 6 months after discontinuation of treatment (sustained response). Sustained biochemical and virologic responses, which often are accompanied by histologic improvement, are the current standard therapeutic end points.[124] In addition, response to therapy is associated with improvements in health-related quality of life.

AVAILABLE DRUGS

The treatment of chronic hepatitis C has changed substantially since the mid-1990s. Although interferon-based regimens continue to be the cornerstone of current antiviral therapies, pharmacologic advances, including the addition of ribavirin as adjunctive therapy and the development of pegylated interferons, have made treatment significantly more effective. *Interferons* are naturally occurring proteins that exert a wide array of antiviral, antiproliferative, and immunomodulatory effects. For years, interferon monotherapy was the standard treatment in patients with chronic hepatitis C, with disappointing results.[124] Subsequently, newer formulations of interferon, *peginterferons*, were developed.[127] These pegylated interferons consist of interferon bound to a molecule of polyethylene glycol (PEG) of varying length, which increases the half-life of the interferon and reduces its volume of distribution, allowing once-weekly dosage. With pegylated interferons, more uniform plasma levels can be sustained, as opposed to the fluctuations in viral load observed with every-other-day dosing of standard interferon. As a consequence, pegylated interferons are associated with enhanced viral suppression. Compared with standard interferon, pegylated interferons have a longer half-life, reduced immunogenicity, better pharmacokinetics, enhanced biological activity, and possibly better adherence rates, with a comparable toxicity profile.

Two pegylated interferons are licensed for use in the United States and elsewhere. The first is the 12-kD peginterferon alfa-2b, which is dosed according to weight (1.5 µg/kg, once weekly). The second is the 40-kD peginterferon alfa-2a, which is used at a fixed dose of 180 µg per week. The pharmacokinetic properties of these two pegylated interferons are compared in Table 76–8.

Ribavirin is an antiviral agent with activity against DNA and RNA viruses. It is given orally, making it an attractive alternative to interferon, which must be given by injection. In immunocompetent patients with chronic HCV infection, ribavirin was shown to improve serum ALT levels, but the effect was transient, and no direct antiviral activity was observed. Ribavarin appears to be a pleiotropic agent—that is, it has many intrinsic mechanisms that can influence its overall antiviral properties. Potential mechanisms proposed to explain the synergistic effect of ribavirin when administered in combination with interferon include[128] (1) enhancement of host T cell–mediated immunity against viral infections, (2) inhibition of the host enzyme inosine monophosphate dehydrogenase (IMPDH), (3) direct inhibition of HCV replication, and (4) a role as an RNA mutagen that drives a rapidly mutating RNA virus over the threshold to "error catastrophe."

Ribavirin generally is well tolerated, although clinically important hemolysis occurs with its use. Because of its capability to cause a sudden fall in hemoglobin levels, ribavirin should be used with caution in patients with a history of coronary artery disease or cardiac arrhythmias.

In addition, ribavirin is teratogenic; patients and their partners are required to avoid pregnancy during therapy and for 6 months after cessation of treatment with this agent. Ribavirin has a long cumulative half-life and is excreted by the kidneys, so that severe side effects, particularly hemolysis, can occur in patients with renal failure. Furthermore, ribavirin cannot be removed by hemodialysis. Therefore, ribavirin should be administered with caution to patients with a serum creatinine level greater than 1.5 mg/dL.

Overall, in 10% to 15% of patients receiving ribavirin, the dose must be reduced or discontinued. The rate of dose reduction or drug discontinuation increases significantly when the ribavirin is combined with interferon and taken for 12 months.[129]

EFFICACY

The overall SVR rate has increased successively from 6% to 11% with a 24-week course of interferon alone, to 13% to 16% with a 48-week course, to 25% to 39% with pegylated interferon,[130-132] to 41% with the combination of standard interferon and ribavirin,[133,134] and finally, to 54% to 61% with the combination of pegylated interferon and ribavirin (Tables 76–9 and 76–10).[135-138] Despite differences in the formulation of pegylated interferon used, dose of ribavirin, study design, and patient population, success rates are similar for the two pegylated interferon products in various trials. Overall, the rate of SVR in treatment-naive patients is 54% to 56% and is largely dependent on the genotype of HCV: 42% to 46% in genotype 1–infected patients and 76% to 82% in genotypes 2– and 3–infected patients. When peginterferon alfa-2b plus ribavirin dosed according to body weight (800 to 1400 mg) is used, slight differences in response rates between genotypes 2 and 3 are observed, with SVR rates of 92% to 93% in patients infected with HCV genotype 2 and a rate of 79% in those infected with genotype 3. In patients infected with genotype 3, rates of viral eradication are strongly related to the level of viremia (86% for those with a level less than 600,000 IU/mL and 70% for those with a level of 600,000 IU/mL or greater).[138] These findings suggest that in genotype 3–infected patients, the level of viremia should be taken into account to optimize therapy.

Whereas the dose of peginterferon alfa-2b is based on body weight (1.5 µg/kg per week when administered in combination with ribavirin; 1.0 µg/kg per week if admin-

Table 76–8   Pegylated Interferons: Comparative Pharmacokinetics

Pharmacokinetic Parameter	Interferon-α	Peginterferon alfa-2b (12 kD)	Peginterferon alfa-2a (40 kD)
Absorption after injection	Rapid	Rapid	Sustained
Distribution	Wide	Wide	Blood, organs
Clearance	—	10-fold decrease* (renal and hepatic)	100-fold decrease* (hepatic)
Elimination half-life	3-5 hours	30-50 hours	50-80 hours
Weight-based dosing	No	Yes	No
Increased serum levels with multiple dosing	No	Yes	Yes
Protected from degradation	No	Probably	Yes

*Relative to clearance observed for interferon-α.

Table 76–9 Results of Treatment Trials of Pegylated Interferon Monotherapy for Hepatitis C

Reference	Regimens	Number of Patients	SVR (%) (95% CI)	Variables Associated with Increased SVR*
131 (N = 531)	Interferon alfa-2a, 6 MU 3×/wk for 12 wk, then 3 MU 3×/wk for 36 wk	264	19 (14-24)	Non-1 genotypes,[a] age <40 years, absence of significant fibrosis, lower body mass index, HCV RNA <2 million copies/mL
	Peginterferon alfa-2a, 180 μg/wk for 48 wk	267	39 (33-45)	
132 (N = 271)[‡]	Interferon alfa-2a, 3 MU 3×/wk for 48 wk	88	8 (4-16)	Non-1 genotypes,[b] lower viral levels
	Peginterferon alfa-2a, 90 μg/wk for 48 wk	96	15 (9-23)	
	Peginterferon alfa-2a, 180 μg/wk for 48 wk	87	30 (21-40)	
130 (N = 1219)	Interferon alfa-2b, 3 MU 3×/wk for 48 wk	303	12 (9-16)	Non-1 genotypes[c]
	Peginterferon alfa-2b, 0.5 μg/kg/wk for 48 wk	315	18 (14-23)	
	Peginterferon alfa-2b, 1.0 μg/kg/wk for 48 wk	297	25 (20-30)	
	Peginterferon alfa-2b, 1.5 μg/kg/wk for 48 wk	304	23 (19-28)	

*SVR in genotype 1 patients: a, 28% in the peginterferon treatment group; b, 14% (peginterferon 180 μg) versus 2% (interferon); c, 14% (peginterferon) versus 2% (interferon).
‡Only patients with advanced fibrosis (22%) or cirrhosis (78%) were included. Histologic improvement of at least 2 points in the HAI was significantly greater in the peginterferon arm than in the standard interferon arm (54% versus 31%). The improvement rate was significantly higher among those achieving an SVR than in those without an SVR (90% versus 31%).
CI, confidence interval; HAI, hepatic activity index; HCV, hepatitis C virus; MU, million units; SVR, sustained virologic response.

Table 76–10 Results of Treatment Trials of Pegylated Interferon Plus Ribavirin for Hepatitis C

Reference	Regimens	Number of Patients	SVR (%) (95% CI)	SVR for Genotype 1 versus Non-1 Genotypes (%)	
129 (N = 1121)				Genotype 1	Genotypes 2, 3
	Interferon alfa-2b, 3 MU 3×/wk, + ribavirin, 1000-1200 mg/day, for 48 wk	444	44 (40-49)	36	61
	Peginterferon alfa-2a, 180 μg/wk, + placebo, for 48 wk	224	29 (24-36)	21	45
	Peginterferon alfa-2a, 180 μg/wk, + ribavirin, 1000-1200 mg/day, for 48 wk	453	56 (52-61)	46	76
133 (N = 1530)				Genotype 1	Genotypes 2, 3
	Interferon alfa-2b, 3 MU 3×/wk, + ribavirin, 1000-1200 mg/day, for 48 wk	505	47 (42-51)	33	79
	Peginterferon alfa-2b, 1.5 μg/kg/wk for 4 wk, then 0.5 μg/kg/wk for 44 wk, + ribavirin, 1000-1200 mg/day for 48 wk	514	47 (43-52)	34	80
	Peginterferon alfa-2b, 1.5 μg/kg/wk, + ribavirin, 800 mg/day, for 48 wk	511	54 (49-58)	42	82
137 (N = 1284)				Genotype 1	Non-1 Genotypes
	Peginterferon alfa-2a, 180 μg/wk, + ribavirin, 800 mg/day, for 24 wk	207	NR	29 (21-38)	78 (70-85)
	Peginterferon alfa-2a, 180 μg/wk, + ribavirin, 800 mg/day, for 48 wk	361	NR	40 (34-46)	73 (64-80)
	Peginterferon alfa-2a, 180 μg/wk, + ribavirin, 1000-1200 mg/day, for 24 wk	280	NR	41 (32-50)	78 (71-84)
	Peginterferon alfa-2a, 180 μg/wk, + ribavirin, 1000-1200 mg/day, for 48 wk	436	63 (59-68)	51 (45-57)	77 (70-83)

CI, confidence interval; NR, not reported; SVR, sustained virologic response.

istered as monotherapy), peginterferon alfa-2a is administered in a fixed dose (180 µg per week). The dose of ribavirin and the duration of therapy are based on the HCV genotype. Patients infected with HCV genotypes 2 and 3 require only 24 weeks of therapy with 800 mg daily of ribavirin, whereas patients infected with genotype 1, and possibly those infected with genotype 4, require 48 weeks of treatment and full doses of ribavirin (1000 to 1200 mg daily, depending on body weight, with the lower dose for patients who weigh less than 75 kg and the higher dose for those who weigh 75 kg or greater) (Fig. 76–5).[124,137]

Selection of therapy for patients in whom a first course of antiviral therapy fails to cure the infection should be based on the type of, duration of, and response to the first treatment. Potential candidates for re-treatment comprise four categories: (1) patients who have relapsed after a first course of interferon monotherapy, (2) nonresponders to a first course of interferon monotherapy, (3) those who have relapsed after a first course of interferon in combination with ribavirin, and (4) nonresponders to a prior course of interferon in combination with ribavirin. Response rates using standard or pegylated interferon in combination with ribavirin are acceptable for patients belonging to category 1 (almost the same as for treatment-naive patients) and those in category 3 (with overall SVR rates of approximately 40%).[139] The rate of response for patients who fall into category 2—that is, nonresponders to interferon monotherapy—may reach 12% to 25% with re-treatment with standard interferon plus ribavirin, and up to 25% to 40% with re-treatment with pegylated interferon plus ribavirin, for 48 weeks.[140] Response rates are significantly higher in patients who are infected with genotypes 2 and 3, have lower baseline levels of serum HCV RNA, and have lesser degrees of fibrosis. Viral eradication is less frequently achieved, however, in patients in category 4—that is, nonresponders to prior therapy with interferon plus ribavirin (18%),[140] particularly those infected with genotype 1 or possibly 4. No clear recommendations exist for the treatment of patients in whom pegylated interferon plus ribavirin fails to effect a cure.

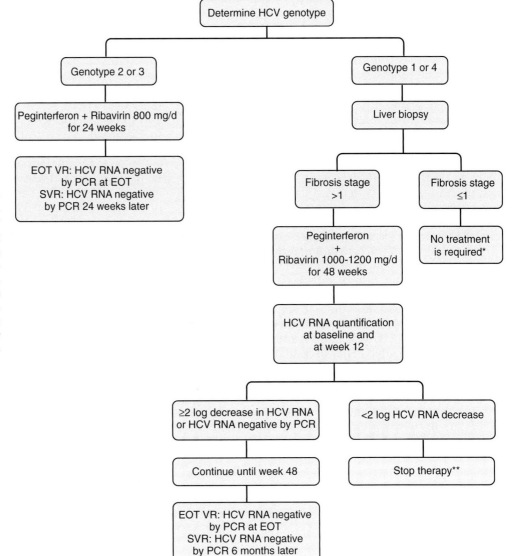

Figure 76–5 Proposed algorithm for the treatment of hepatitis C virus (HCV) infection. EOT VR, end of treatment virologic response; PCR, polymerase chain reaction (assay); SVR, sustained virologic response. *Unless the patient prefers to undergo antiviral therapy. **Continued treatment with interferon may slow progression of liver disease; trials to assess this strategy are in progress.

FACTORS PREDICTIVE OF A SUSTAINED RESPONSE

Factors associated with response to treatment include low serum HCV RNA levels, non–genotype 1, absence of cirrhosis, age younger than 40 years, lack of steatosis or obesity, and white race.[28,124] Although the likelihood of a response to treatment is lower in patients with these negative predictive factors, treatment should not be withheld because of the presence of any or all of these variables. Rather, presence of the predictive factors can be used to counsel patients about treatment options and the likelihood of response, and to tailor the regimens appropriately. Of known predictive variables, the most powerful predictor of response to treatment is the viral genotype, and determination of the viral genotype before therapy is initiated is a critical step in selecting the best treatment regimen.

Additional factors predictive of an antiviral treatment response have been identified. A *body mass index* higher than 30 has been associated with poor response to therapy. Weight reduction, in turn, leads to improved outcomes.[141] *African Americans* have been shown to respond poorly to interferon-based regimens, including pegylated interferon plus ribavirin (with SVR rates ranging from 19% to 26%),[142,143] in part, because of the higher proportion of genotype 1 among African Americans than among whites. In addition, viral kinetic studies have shown that the effectiveness of interferon in inhibiting viral production (first-phase log drop following therapy with interferon) differs between races, with an effectiveness rate of less than 90% in most African Americans and greater than 90% in most whites.[79]

Advanced liver fibrosis has been reported to be a negative predictive factor in studies of the response to interferon-based therapy. Patients with advanced fibrosis, however, are the ones most in need of antiviral therapy. Nevertheless, pegylated interferon has shown promise in such patients. In a multicenter international trial of 271 patients with cirrhosis or bridging necrosis who were randomized to receive peginterferon α-2a, 90 μg or 180 μg weekly for 48 weeks, or conventional IFN-α, the rate of SVR was significantly higher in the patients who received the pegylated formulation of interferon (15% and 30% versus 8%).[132] Of interest, the tolerability of the three regimens was similar, as were the rates of discontinuation (11%, 14%, and 10%) and dose reduction (27%, 28%, and 20%); thrombocytopenia and neutropenia were the most frequent side effects that necessitated discontinuation of the drug or a dose reduction. Data extrapolated from other trials have shown SVR rates ranging from 44% to 52%, (63% to 73% for genotypes 2 and 3 and 29% to 41% for genotype 1) in patients with advanced fibrosis; the best results were obtained in patients given ribavirin in higher doses and for longer durations. Although the results are not as good as those obtained in patients without advanced fibrosis, they are promising. Therefore, clinically compensated cirrhosis should not preclude patients from antiviral therapy.[144]

Finally, strict *adherence to therapy* improves the likelihood of a sustained response, and compliance must be stressed at each visit. Adherence to therapy appears to be particularly relevant in the first months of therapy; the impact of dose reductions is less if they occur after a 3-month virologic response.[145]

INDICATIONS AND CONTRAINDICATIONS

Theoretically, all patients with chronic hepatitis C and persistently elevated serum aminotransferase levels are potential candidates for antiviral therapy.[3,28,124] Because therapy is still imperfect in terms of efficacy and associated with serious side effects, however, and because the clinical course of hepatitis C is benign in a majority of cases, patients and their physicians need to evaluate potential benefits, costs, and risks carefully before therapy is intitiated. Ironically, patients with the lowest likelihood of progression of fibrosis are precisely the ones who are most likely to respond to antiviral therapy. By contrast, those with the least likelihood of responding or with the least tolerance to side effects of treatment often are the ones with the greatest need for antiviral therapy. In patients with a low chance of disease progression (immunocompetent setting, age younger than 40, female gender, no alcohol consumption, and minimal histologic inflammation and fibrosis), arguments for starting treatment and those for waiting for safer and more effective therapies to become available are equally valid. By contrast, all patients infected with genotypes 2 and 3 (particularly genotype 2) should be offered therapy because the SVR rates associated with these genotypes are 93% and 79%, respectively. Therapy in these patients is better tolerated and accepted because of the shorter duration (24 weeks, versus 48 for genotypes other than 2 and 3) and lower daily dose of ribavirin (800 mg, versus 1000 to 1200 mg). A pre-treatment liver biopsy may not be required in patients infected with HCV genotype 2 or 3.

For certain situations, no guidelines regarding treatment have been established. In particular, the management of patients with persistently normal liver enzymes or those with histologically mild chronic hepatitis remains controversial. Although the efficacy of therapy has improved greatly, the tolerability is not yet optimal, and the costs are substantial. Moreover, the natural history of HCV infection is neither homogeneous nor predictable in an individual case. Arguments on either side can be made for these controversial indications. For example, in patients with normal serum aminotransferase levels, liver disease generally is mild, and progression does not occur or is very slow,[116,117] yet antiviral therapy is as effective and safe in these patients as in those with elevated liver enzymes.[146] In addition, biochemical reactivation may occur in as many as 21% of these patients during follow-up; the occurrence of such flares is unpredictable.[87] In patients with mild chronic hepatitis, the course also is relatively benign, at least in the short and intermediate term,[89-94] and therapy can be deferred. The need for continuous monitoring for progression of liver disease may be difficult for the patient to accept, however, particularly if periodic liver biopsies are recommended. Moreover, a proportion of patients with mild chronic hepatitis, particularly those with portal fibrosis and an elevated serum ALT level, are at risk for disease progression. The decision to provide antiviral treatment for these patients should be based on liver histologic features, the patient's age and motivation, the viral genotype and level of viremia, and the presence of comorbid conditions and contraindications. In such cases, some experts recommend immediate antiviral therapy in young, highly motivated patients without contraindications and in those infected with HCV genotypes 2 and 3.

Obese patients with chronic hepatitis C have lower rates of SVR than those achieved in nonobese patients, confirming prior studies suggesting that a high body mass index is an independent negative predictive factor in treatment response.[141] Mechanisms underlying the reduced response to antiviral agents in obese patients include (1) impaired pharmacokinetics of interferon, possibly as a consequence of decreased bioavailability (lower serum concentrations resulting from abnormal lymphatic drainage after subcutaneous administration or from more extensive distribution of the drug because of a larger body size); (2) diminished hepatic response to interferon due to liver steatosis, which is a frequent finding in these patients; and (3) altered immune function mediated in part by resistance to leptin (see Chapter 18). Weight loss may improve the efficacy of antiviral therapy.

Patients with HCV-HIV coinfection should receive the same regimens used for HCV-monoinfected patients. Results are inferior to those obtained in monoinfected patients, however, probably because of a confluence of poor prognostic factors, including high levels of HCV viremia, high frequency of genotype 1 infections, increased genetic complexity and diversity of HCV, high rate of alcohol use, the need for frequent dose reductions because of synergistic or additive drug toxicities, over-representation of racial groups known to have a lower rate of sustained response to antiviral therapy, and low serum $CD4^+$ levels.[147,148] Several studies have shown a decreased rate of sustained eradication of HCV when the $CD4^+$ count is less than $500/mm^3$; response is highly unlikely in patients with $CD4^+$ levels lower than $350 \, mm^3$. Tolerance to therapy is lower, possibly as a consequence of additive drug toxicities. With the pegylated interferons in combination with ribavirin, response rates are lower than those in immunocompetent patients but better than those achieved with standard interferon. SVR rates of 62% to 73% in genotypes 2– and 3–infected patients, and 14% to 29% in genotypes 1– and 4–infected patients, have been reported.[147,148] Results may improve substantially if the patient strictly adheres to therapy. A multidisciplinary approach including experts in addiction medicine, psychologists, psychiatrics, hepatologists, and infectious disease specialists is desirable. Although response rates and tolerance are lower in HCV/HIV–coinfected patients, the benefit-to-risk ratio is higher, in view of their high risk of liver disease progression and high risk of liver toxicity after beginning antiretroviral therapy.

Ideally, HCV antiviral therapy should be started before HAART is initiated, if the stage of HIV infection permits treatment of the HCV infection. A low $CD4^+$ count is associated with a lower rate of sustained response, however, so antiviral therapy of HCV infection should be prescribed only when the $CD4^+$ count is above $350/mm^3$—a threshold easily achievable with current antiretroviral therapies. In patients with $CD4^+$ counts between 200 and $350/mm^3$, additional factors should be taken into consideration before therapy for HCV is initiated, particularly the severity of liver disease and the age of the patient. Finally, therapy of HCV infection should be deferred in patients with a $CD4^+$ count less than $200/mm^3$. Contraindications to antiviral therapy of HCV infection in coinfected patients do not differ from those in monoinfected patients. Although heavy alcohol intake or illegal drug addiction practices should delay therapy, patients on methadone maintenance are acceptable candidates for therapy of HCV infection.[149] In approximately one third of such patients, the dose of methadone will need to be adjusted during antiviral therapy (either upward or downward, depending on the side effects of antiviral therapy).

Interferon has produced short-term remission of the symptoms and signs of cryoglobulinemia when a virologic response is achieved, although recurrence of viremia and cryoglobulinemia is the rule when treatment is discontinued.[74] Interferon also has been used successfully to treat HCV-associated membranoproliferative glomerulonephritis. Although lymphoproliferative disorders typically are treated with immunosuppressive and cytotoxic agents, successful treatment with interferon has been reported in HCV-infected patients.

A strong theoretical rationale for treating patients with acute HCV infection exists: In a substantial proportion of these patients, persistent infection and chronic liver disease will develop, and rates of sustained response to antiviral therapy with high doses of interferon may be as high as 98%. When data from the few studies addressing this issue have been pooled, the rates of disease remission have been higher in patients who received interferon early in the course of infection (median 62%, range 37% to 100%) than in control patients who received no treatment (12%, range 0% to 20%).[150-152] The highest efficacy rates were observed when daily doses of 5 to 10 million units (MU) of IFN-α were used for 8 to 12 weeks, followed by 5 MU given three times weekly for a total of 24 to 52 weeks. SVR rates are similar when pegylated interferon is used with or without ribavirin (85% and 80%, respectively).[151,152]

When to treat patients with acute hepatitis C, and with what regimen, remains to be addressed. The most important question is whether all patients with acute hepatitis C need therapy. Although the rate of chronicity was reported to be as high as 85% in early studies of post-transfusion hepatitis, subsequent studies that focused on different populations reported significantly lower rates of viral persistence, ranging from 50% to 60%. Factors associated with spontaneous resolution of acute hepatitis C have been identified and include young age at infection, female gender, absence of parenteral transmission, and presence of symptoms and jaundice.[68-72] In addition, at least three studies have indicated that delaying therapy until 2 to 4 months after the onset of acute hepatitis C does not compromise efficacy in achieving sustained viral eradication. On the basis of these observations, the most rational approach may be to forego treatment for 3 to 4 months after the onset of acute hepatitis C, to avoid unnecessary, difficult, and costly therapy for many patients who would have recovered on their own without treatment. Therapy then can be started in patients who remain seropositive for HCV RNA. The decision should be made by the patient, who in some instances, particularly after accidental exposure to HCV, may wish to intitate therapy immediately.

In view of the high rate of viral eradication with interferon monotherapy of acute hepatitis C, ribavirin is not required, at least initially, and may be reserved for patients who fail to respond to a 3-month course of interferon alone. The best results have been achieved with high doses of IFN-α (5 to 10 MU daily), particularly during the first 4 weeks, and with pegylated interferon administered weekly. In practice, even if early treatment of acute hepatitis C is effective, identification of patients with acute hepatitis C in the non-transfusion setting is difficult, and early treatment will be limited to a small number of patients.

Response rates in children appear to be similar to those in adults, but data are limited.[107]

MONITORING TREATMENT

Before antiviral therapy is started, blood tests should be obtained to establish the patient's baseline status. Recommended tests include liver biochemical tests, a complete blood count (CBC), and determination of thyroid-stimulating hormone (TSH) level (see Fig. 76–5). A pregnancy test is required in women before ribavirin is started. Determination of the genotype and serum HCV RNA level will help in selecting the best treatment strategy.

During the first month of therapy, a CBC should be done weekly, because most side effects of ribavirin, particularly hemolytic anemia, occur within this period of time. Approximately 10% of patients will have a fall in hemoglobin levels to less than 10 g/dL, with a mean decrease of approximately 3 g/dL. After the first month, serum ALT level determination and a CBC should be performed monthly, and a TSH level should be obtained every 3 months. Drug doses should be adjusted according to the severity of side effects.[28,124]

Assessment of viral kinetics has been shown to help predict the likelihood of an SVR.[24,79] Following interferon or peginterferon therapy with or without ribavirin, the decline in serum HCV RNA levels follows a biphasic curve. The first phase of viral decline, caused by inhibition of viral production and clearance of free virions, is rapid, dose-dependent, and exponential, ending 24 to 48 hours after the initiation of treatment. The second phase of viral decline then ensues; this phase is substantially slower, varies greatly among patients, and is caused mainly by the continued partial inhibition of viral production by interferon, with subsequent loss of virus-producing cells. The change in the level of viremia over a period of time varies, ranging from 1 day to 3 months in different studies, and can predict response to treatment. At 3 months of treatment, for instance, a quantitative HCV RNA test is useful in genotype 1–infected patients for determining whether treatment should be continued. An early virologic response (EVR), defined as a decrease in serum HCV RNA levels at least 2 log-folds, or loss of HCV RNA in patients whose baseline HCV RNA was less than 100 times the detection limit, is useful

for identifying patients who are unlikely to achieve an SVR.[153,154] Patients with an EVR, which occurs at a rate of 69% to 76%, have a high probability of achieving an SVR (67% to 80%) and should continue treatment. By contrast, treatment should be discontinued in patients who do not achieve an EVR, because they have almost no likelihood of achieving an SVR. This strategy is worthwhile for several reasons: (1) it motivates the patient to adhere to therapy during the first critical months of treatment and provides a milepost for assessing the need for continued therapy; (2) it is cost-saving (resulting in a 20% reduction in the cost of therapy); and (3) it permits patients with no chance of viral clearance to avoid the morbidity of extended therapy. In patients infected with HCV genotypes 2 and 3, testing for HCV RNA serum at 12 weeks is not needed, because the SVR rate is higher than 75%.

At the end of treatment and at 6 months after discontinuation of treatment, testing for HCV RNA with a sensitive PCR technique should be repeated to assess response. If a sustained response is achieved, HCV RNA testing should be performed annually for at least 2 years after completion of therapy. A repeat liver biopsy is rarely necessary following treatment. In nonresponders or relapsers in whom no additional treatment is considered, the follow-up regimen should be similar to that in patients who receive no treatment, with at least yearly check-ups and laboratory testing and a repeat liver biopsy every 4 to 5 years to assess disease progression, particularly if re-treatment or maintenance therapy is being considered.

MAINTENANCE THERAPY

The main goal of maintenance therapy is to reduce progression of hepatic fibrosis in patients who do not achieve an SVR on antiviral therapy. The patients who may benefit the most from this theoretical approach are those who have advanced fibrosis and are thus at highest risk of hepatic decompensation and hepatocellular carcinoma and those with rapid rates of fibrosis progression. The rationale behind this approach comes from several retrospective studies of interferon monotherapy in which reduced inflammation and slowing of progression of fibrosis in patients after treatment, including nonresponders, were observed. These findings have been questioned in a meta-analysis of 1013 patients from three randomized trials showing that the reduction in fibrosis after treatment with pegylated interferon and to a lesser extent with standard interferon was limited to sustained responders.[155] By contrast, several studies have demonstrated a reduction in the rates of hepatocellular carcinoma and mortality in patients who received interferon therapy, even in those not achieving a sustained response.[112-115] Ongoing multicenter, prospective randomized studies are assessing the role of maintenance therapy with pegylated interferon in patients with advanced fibrosis.

SAFETY

In clinical trials, withdrawal rates increase with the duration of treatment and the use of combination (pegylated interferon plus ribavirin) therapy.[129-140] For example, therapy was stopped in 13% to 14% of patients receiving interferon monotherapy for 48 weeks and in 19% to 21% of those receiving combination therapy for the same duration. With pegylated interferons, the tolerability and frequency of side effects are similar to those seen with standard interferon, with some exceptions: flu-like symptoms and depression occur less frequently with the pegylated forms, but neutropenia is more frequent. Discontinuation of drugs consequent to an adverse event or laboratory test abnormality occurs in approximately 16% and 5% of patients receiving the combination of pegylated interferon and ribavirin for 48 and 24 weeks, respectively. A reduction in drug dose is required in 26% to 36% of patients for peginterferon and in 19% to 38% for ribavirin, depending on the duration and dose. Neutropenia, anemia, and thrombocytopenia are the most frequent reasons for reductions in dose. To ensure maximal response rates, dose reductions should be avoided, and patient adherence should be promoted.

The most frequent side effects with interferon include flu-like symptoms (in greater than 90% of patients) and alopecia (in 10% to 30%). Minor flu-like side effects are common during the first month of therapy but usually do not necessitate dose adjustments. A mild degree of myelosuppression also is common, particularly when interferon is combined with ribavirin. The most severe adverse events include depression, suicidal ideation, suicide, and sustained hypothyroidism. Because adherence to therapy appears to be an important factor in optimizing efficacy, the various drug-related toxicities—in particular, psychiatric and psychological symptoms and thyroid dysfunction—should be managed proactively.

With ribavirin, anemia and, less frequently, cough and pharyngitis, insomnia, dyspnea, pruritus, rash, nausea, and anorexia are the most common side effects. The most serious side effects are anemia and the teratogenic effect. Hemolytic anemia is reversible and generally occurs within the first month of therapy. Administration of erythropoietin (and granulocyte colony-stimulating factor for interferon-induced severe neutropenia) to the patient makes it possible to continue a full dose of ribavirin without compromising response rates by early dose reductions.[129] Newer ribavirin analogs that result in less severe anemia are under development.

COST-EFFECTIVENESS

Multiple pharmacoeconomic studies have suggested that treatment of HCV infection with pegylated interferon plus ribavirin is cost-effective; the cost of therapy is nearly completely offset by the prevention of future liver-related complications. Applying the 12-week stopping rule (see earlier) further lowers costs and improves the cost-effectiveness of therapy.[156] Certain assumptions in these cost-effectiveness analyses remain to be tested, however. Limitations include an inadequate understanding of the natural history of hepatitis C and a limited understanding of determinants of disease severity that may influence the course. Moreover, in a population of HCV-infected patients that is aging, competing medical conditions, not yet well characterized, may determine life expectancy and, in turn, obviate the need for treatment of the HCV infection.

CONSIDERATIONS IN LIVER TRANSPLANT RECIPIENTS

Special considerations apply to antiviral treatment in liver transplant recipients (see Chapter 92).[157] Preemptive treatment with interferon with ribavirin within the first few weeks after liver transplantation for HCV-related cirrhosis does not appear to modify disease progression, is associated with substantial toxicity, and is not recommended. Pre-transplantation therapy with interferon in patients with advanced cirrhosis is poorly tolerated and may precipitate worsening of hepatic function. In addition, patients with advanced cirrhosis are at increased risk of bone marrow suppression with combination therapy and can experience severe, even life-threatening infections during treatment. Using low doses of the antiviral agents and increasing the doses as tolerated may improve tolerability. The applicability of this approach is limited, however, because few patients meet entry criteria for trials, particularly because of thrombocytopenia and leukopenia, and almost one third of patients need to discontinue therapy because of side effects. If the regimen is tolerated, sustained responses are achievable, leading to a reduced risk of allograft infection with HCV in patients who undergo liver transplantation. Pretransplantation treatment may be most beneficial in select patients with cirrhosis, such as those with Child-Turcotte-Pugh class A or B (see Chapter 87), those who are infected with HCV genotype 2 or 3, or those with genotype 1 and a low level of viremia.

Treatment of recurrent hepatitis attributed to HCV with interferon or ribavirin as a single agent is disappointing. The efficacy is improved when both drugs are administered in combination for 6 to 12 months, with overall sustained response rates of 9% to 33%. The broad range of response rates probably relates to differences in the distribution of genotype (better responses with non-1 genotypes), timing of treatment, and severity of the underlying hepatitis C. With the combination of pegylated interferon and ribavirin, the rate of sustained viral eradication has increased to 26% to 45%. Response generally is associated with resolution of liver histologic changes, particularly necroinflammation and, to a lesser extent, fibrosis. The main predictors of response include the viral genotype and completion of the treatment course. Tolerance remains a limiting factor; up to 90% of patients require dose reductions, and 24% to 49% must discontinue the drugs. Pegylated interferon may carry a higher risk of inducing acute cellular rejection than that observed with standard interferon, particularly if administered as monotherapy. Maintenance therapy with ribavirin is prescribed in some liver transplantation centers, but the efficacy of this approach is unknown. It has been hypothesized that ribavirin, through its immunomodulatory effects, may protect against interferon-induced graft rejection.

FUTURE THERAPIES

Improvements in treatment outcomes in patients who are difficult to treat, including nonresponders to previous therapy, persons coinfected with HIV, African American patients, and organ transplant recipients, will require novel therapeutic approaches.[158] Advances such as the replicon system (see earlier) and structural analysis of HCV components have been essential for the design and evaluation of new antiviral drugs. With the availability of a three-dimensional structure of the three major HCV enzymes—the NS3 serine proteinase, NS3 helicase, and NS5B RNA-dependent RNA polymerase—efforts are being directed to the development of selective inhibitors of HCV replication. The variation in the amino acid sequences of these enzymes suggests that the virus will become resistant to these antiviral agents if they are used as monotherapy. Therefore, combination therapy, similar to that used to treat HIV infection, for which several key molecules essential for viral replication are targeted, will be required to treat chronic HCV infection. Interest also has focused on the 5′ and 3′ UTRs, which contain well-conserved regions, for the development of antisense oligonucleotides and ribozymes. Additional classes of therapeutic interventions include new interferon molecules with enhanced activity and improved pharmacokinetics, ribavirin-like molecules with a better tolerance profile, and immune therapies such as new immunomodulators and therapeutic vaccines. These drugs will be important in managing HCV disease, not just in the Western world but, of greater importance, in developing countries, where HCV is an emerging infection.

REFERENCES

1. El-Serag HB, Mason AC: Rising incidence of hepatocellular carcinoma in the United States. N Engl J Med 340:745, 1999.
2. Davis GL, Albright JE, Cook SF, Rosenberg DM: Projecting future complications of chronic hepatitis C in the United States. Liver Transpl 9:331, 2003.
3. National Institutes of Health Consensus Development Conference statement: Management of hepatitis C 2002 (June 10-12, 2002). Hepatology 36(suppl 1):S3, 2002.
4. Proceedings of the Consensus Conference on Hepatitis C. April 21-22, 2004. Edinburgh, United Kingdom. J Viral Hepat 11(Suppl 1):1, 2004.
5. Penin F, Dubuisson J, Rey FA, et al: Structural biology of hepatitis C virus. Hepatology 39:59, 2004.
6. Maillard P, Krawczynski K, Nitkiewicz J, et al: Nonenveloped nucleocapsids of hepatitis C virus in the serum of infected patients. J Virol 75:8240, 2001.
7. Robertson B, Myers G, Howard C, et al: Classification, nomenclature, and database development for hepatitis C virus (HCV) and related viruses: Proposals for standardization. International Committee on Virus Taxonomy. Arch Virol 143:2493, 1998.
8. Shi ST, Lai MM: Hepatitis C viral RNA: Challenges and promises. Cell Mol Life Sci 58:1276, 2001.
9. Reed KE, Rice CM: Overview of hepatitis C virus genome structure, polyprotein processing and protein properties. Curr Top Microbiol Immunol 242:55, 2000.
10. Sakai A, Claire MS, Faulk K, et al: The p7 polypeptide of hepatitis C virus is critical for infectivity and contains functionally important genotype-specific sequences. Proc Natl Acad Sci U S A 100:11646, 2003.
11. Lerat H, Honda M, Beard MR et al: Steatosis and liver cancer in transgenic mice expressing the structural and nonstructural proteins of hepatitis C virus. Gastroenterology 122:352, 2002.
12. Okuda M, Li K, Beard MR, et al. Mitochondrial injury, oxidative stress and antioxidant gene expression are induced by hepatitis C virus core protein. Gastroenterology 122:366, 2002.
13. Walsh MJ, Vanags DM, Clouston AD, et al: Steatosis and liver cell apopotosis in chronic hepatitis C: A mechanism for increased liver injury. Hepatology 39:1230, 2004.
14. Shi ST, Polyak SJ, Tu H, et al: Hepatitis C virus NS5A colocalizes with the core protein on lipid droplets and interacts with apolipoproteins. Virology 292:198, 2002.
15. Lonardo A, Adinolfi LE, Loria P, et al: Steatosis and hepatitis C virus: Mechanisms and significance for hepatic and extrahepatic disease. Gastroenterology 126:586, 2004.
16. Polyak SJ: Hepatitis C virus-cell interactions and their role in pathogenesis. Clin Liver Dis 7:67, 2003.
17. Choi J, Xu Z, Ou JH: Triple decoding of hepatitis C virus RNA by programmed translational frameshifting. Mol Cell Biol 23:1489, 2003.
18. Spahn CM, Kieft JS, Grassucci RA, et al: Hepatitis C virus IRES RNA-induced changes in the conformation of the 40S ribosomal unit. Science 291:1959, 2001.
19. Lerat H, Hollinger FB: Hepatitis C virus (HCV) occult infection or occult HCV RNA detection? J Infect Dis 189:3, 2004.
20. Bukh J: A critical role for the chimpanzee model in the study of hepatitis C. Hepatology 39:1469, 2004.
21. Major ME, Dahari H, Mihalik K, et al: Hepatitis C virus kinetics and host responses associated with disease and outcome of infection in chimpanzees. Hepatology 39:1708, 2004.
22. Pietschmann T, Bartenschlager R: Tissue culture and animal models for hepatitis C virus. Clin Liver Dis 7:23, 2003.
23. Pawlotsky JM: Hepatitis C virus genetic variability: Pathogenic and clinical implications. Clin Liver Dis 7:45, 2003.
24. Neuman AU, Lam NP, Dahari H, et al: Hepatitis C viral dynamics in vivo and the antiviral efficacy of interferon-alpha therapy. Science 282:103, 1998.
25. Diago M, Hassanein T, Rodes J, et al: Optimized virologic response in hepatitis C virus genotype 4 with peginterferon-alpha2a and ribavirin. Ann Intern Med 140:72, 2004.
26. Blatt LM, Mutchnick MG, Tong MJ, et al: Assessment of hepatitis C virus RNA and genotype from 6807 patients with chronic hepatitis C in the United States. J Viral Hepat 7:196, 2000.
27. Wasley A, Alter MJ: Epidemiology of hepatitis C: Geographic differences and temporal trends. Semin Liver Dis 20:1, 2000.
28. Strader DB, Wright TL, Thomas DL, Seeff LB: Diagnosis, management and treatment of hepatitis C. AASLD practice guideline. Hepatology 39:1147, 2004.
29. Farci P, Shimoda A, Coiana A, et al: The outcome of acute hepatitis C is predicted by the evolution of the viral quasispecies. Science 288:339, 2000.
30. Lopez-Labrador FX, Berenguer M, Sempere A, et al : Genetic variability of hepatitis C virus NS3 protein in human leukocyte antigen-A2 liver transplant recipients with recurrent hepatitis C. Liver Transpl 10:217, 2004.
31. Lindenbach BD, Evans MJ, Syder AJ, et al: Complete replication of hepatitis C virus in cell culture. Science 309:623, 2005.
32. Wakita T, Pietschmann T, Kato T, et al: Production of infectious hepatitis C virus in tissue culture from a cloned viral genome. Nat Med 11:791, 2005.
33. Zhong J, Gastaminza P, Cheng G, et al: Robust hepatitis C virus infection in vitro. Proc Natl Acad Sci U S A 102:9294, 2005.
34. Mercer DF, Schiller DE, Elliott JF, et al: Hepatitis C virus replication in mice with chimeric human livers. Nat Med 7:927, 2001.

35. Armstrong GL, Alter MJ, McQuillan GM, Margolis HS: The past incidence of hepatitis C virus infection: Implications for the future burden of chronic liver disease in the United States. Hepatology 31:777, 2000.
36. Murphy EL, Bryzman SM, Glynn SA, et al: Risk factors for hepatitis C virus infection in United States blood donors. NHLBI Retrovirus Epidemiology Donor Study (REDS). Hepatology 31:756, 2000.
37. Alter MJ: Prevention of spread of hepatitis C. Hepatology 36(suppl 1):S93-S98, 2002.
38. Terrault NA: Sexual activity as a risk factor for hepatitis C. Hepatology 36(suppl 1):S99, 2002.
39. Conte D, Fraquella M, Prati D, et al: Prevalence and clinical course of chronic hepatitis C virus (HCV) infection and rate of HCV vertical transmission in a cohort of 15,250 pregnant women. Hepatology 31:751, 2000.
40. Frank C, Mohamed MK, Strickland GT, et al: The role of parenteral antischistosomal therapy in the spread of hepatitis C in Egypt. Lancet 355:887, 2000.
41. Casiraghi MA, De Paschale M, Romanò L, et al: Long-term outcome (35 years) of hepatitis C after acquisition of infection through mini transfusions of blood given at birth. Hepatology 39:90, 2004.
42. Mehta SH, Cox A, Hoover DR, et al: Protection against persistence of hepatitis C. Lancet 359:1478, 2002.
43. McCaughan GW, Zekry A: Mechanisms of HCV reinfection and allograft damage after liver transplantation. J Hepatol 40:368, 2004.
44. Monto A, Alonzo J, Watson JJ, et al: Steatosis in chronic hepatitis C: Relative contributions of obesity, diabetes mellitus, and alcohol. Hepatology 36:729, 2002.
45. Hu KQ, Kyulo NL, Esrailian E, et al: Overweight and obesity, hepatic steatosis, and progression of chronic hepatitis C: A retrospective study on a large cohort of patients in the United States. J Hepatol 40:147, 2004.
46. Rubbia-Brandt L, Quadri R, Abid K, et al: Hepatocyte steatosis is a cytopathic effect of hepatitis C virus genotype 3. J Hepatol 33:106, 2000.
47. Adinolfi LE, Gambardella M, Andreana A, et al: Steatosis accelerates the progression of liver damage of chronic hepatitis C patients and correlates with specific HCV genotype and visceral obesity. Hepatology 33:1358, 2001.
48. Kumar D, Farrell GC, Fung C, George J: Hepatitis C virus genotype 3 is cytopathic to hepatocytes: Reversal of hepatic steatosis after sustained therapeutic response. Hepatology 36:1266, 2002.
49. Patton HM, Patel K, Behling C, et al: The impact of steatosis on disease progression and early and sustained treatment response in chronic hepatitis C patients. J Hepatol 40:484, 2004.
50. Castera L, Hezode C, Roudot-Thoraval F, et al: Effect of antiviral treatment on evolution of liver steatosis in patients with chronic hepatitis C: Indirect evidence of a role of hepatitis C virus genotype 3 in steatosis. Gut 53:420, 2004.
51. Poynard T, Ratziu V, McHutchison J, et al: Effect of treatment with peginterferon or interferon alfa-2b and ribavirin on steatosis in patients infected with hepatitis C. J Hepatol 38:75, 2003.
52. Castera L, Hezode C, Roudot-Thoraval F, et al: Worsening of steatosis is an independent factor of fibrosis progression in untreated patients with chronic hepatitis C and paired liver biopsies. Gut 52:288, 2003.
53. Hui JM, Sud A, Farrell G, et al: Insulin resistance is associated with chronic hepatitis C virus infection and fibrosis progression. Gastroenterology 125:1695, 2003.
54. Shintani Y, Fujie H, Miyoshi H, et al: Hepatitis C virus infection and diabetes: Direct involvement of the virus in the development of insulin resistance. Gastroenterology 126:840, 2004.
55. Racanelli V. Rehermann B: Hepatitis C virus infection: When silence is deception. Trends Immunol 24:456, 2003.
56. He XS, Rehermann B, López-Labrador FX, et al: Quantitative analysis of hepatitis C virus–specific CD8(+) T cells in peripheral blood and liver using peptide-MHC tetramers. Proc Natl Acad Sci U S A 96:5692, 1999.
57. Cooper S, Erickson AL, Adams EJ, et al: Analysis of a successful immune response against hepatitis C virus. Immunity 10:439, 1999.
58. Lechner F, Wong DK, Dunbar PR. et al: Analysis of successful immune responses in persons infected with hepatitis C virus. J Exp Med 191:1499, 2000
59. Gruner NH, Gerlach TJ, Jung MC, et al: Association of hepatitis C virus–specific CD8+ T cells with viral clearance in acute hepatitis C. J Infect Dis 181:1528, 2000.
60. Cramp ME, Carucci P, Rossol S, et al: Hepatitis C virus (HCV) specific immune responses in anti-HCV positive patients without hepatitis C viraemia. Gut 44:424, 1999.
61. Takaki A, Wiese M, Maertens G, et al: Cellular immune responses persist and humoral responses decrease two decades after recovery from a single-source outbreak of hepatitis C. Nat Med 6:578, 2000.
62. Gerlach JT, Diepolder HM, Jung MC, et al: Recurrence of hepatitis C virus after loss of virus-specific CD4(+) T-cell response in acute hepatitis C. Gastroenterology 117:933, 1999.
63. Asti M, Martinetti M, Zavaglia C, et al: Human leukocyte antigen class II and III alleles and severity of hepatitis C virus–related chronic liver disease. Hepatology 29:1271, 1999.
64. Powell EE, Edwards-Smith CJ, Hay JL, et al: Host genetic factors influence disease progression in chronic hepatitis C. Hepatology 31:828, 2000.
65. McKiernan SM, Hagan R, Curry M, et al: Distinct MHC class I and II alleles are associated with hepatitis C viral clearance, originating from a single source. Hepatology 40:108, 2004.
66. Chang KM: Immunopathogenesis of hepatitis C virus infection. Clin Liver Dis 7:89, 2003.
67. Hoofnagle JH: Course and outcome of hepatitis C. Hepatology 36(suppl 1):S21, 2002.
68. Orland JR, Wright TL, Cooper S: Acute hepatitis C. Hepatology 32:321, 2001.
69. Villano SA, Vlahov D, Nelson KE, et al: Persistence of viremia and the importance of long-term follow-up after acute hepatitis C infection. Hepatology 29:908, 1999.
70. Thimme R, Oldach D, Chang KM, et al: Determinants of viral clearance and persistence during acute hepatitis C virus infection. J Exp Med 194:1395, 2001.
71. Gerlach JT, Diepolder HM, Zachoval R, et al: Acute hepatitis C: High rate of both spontaneous and treatment induced viral clearance. Gastroenterology 125:80, 2003.
72. Lehmann M, Meyer M, Monazahian M, et al: High rate of spontaneous clearance of acute hepatitis C genotype 3 infection. J Med Virol 73:387, 2004.
73. Fontana RJ, Kronfol Z: The patient's perspective in hepatitis C. Hepatology 39:903, 2004.
74. Medina J, Garcia-Buey L, Moreno-Otero R: Hepatitis C virus–related extra-hepatic disease: Aetiopathogenesis and management Aliment Pharmacol Ther 20:129, 2004.
75. Gisbert JP, Garcia-Buey L, Pajares JM, Moreno-Otero R: Prevalence of hepatitis C virus infection in B-cell non-Hodgkin's lymphoma: Systematic review and meta-analysis. Gastroenterology 125:1723, 2003.
76. El-Serag HB, Hampel H, Yeh C, Rabeneck L: Extrahepatic manifestations of hepatitis C among United States male veterans. Hepatology 36:476, 2002.
77. Pawlotsky JM: Use and interpretation of virological tests for hepatitis C. Hepatology 36:S65, 2002.
78. Pawlotsky JM: Molecular diagnosis of viral hepatitis. Gastroenterology 122:1554, 2003.

79. Layden TJ, Layden JE, Ribeiro RM, Perelson AS: Mathematical modelling of viral kinetics: A tool to understand and optimise therapy. Clin Liver Dis 7:163, 2003.

80. Saldanha J, Lelie N, Heath A: Establishment of the first international standard for nucleic acid amplification technology (NAT) assays for HCV RNA. Vox Sang 76:149, 1999.

81. Bouvier-Alias M, Patel K, Dahari H, et al: Clinical utility of total HCV core antigen quantification: A new indirect marker of HCV replication. Hepatology 36:211, 2002.

82. Stramer SL, Glynn SA, Kleinman SH, et al: Detection of HIV-1 and HCV infections among antibody-negative blood donors by nucleic acid-amplification testing. N Engl J Med 351:760, 2004.

83. Scheuer PJ, Standish RA, Dhillon AP: Scoring of chronic hepatitis. Clin Liver Dis 6:335, 2002.

84. Dienstag JL: The role of liver biopsy in chronic hepatitis C. Hepatology 36(5 suppl 1):S152, 2002.

85. Fontana RJ, Lok AS: Noninvasive monitoring of patients with chronic hepatitis C. Hepatology 36(suppl 1):S57, 2002.

86. Prati D, Taioli E, Zanella A, et al: Updated definitions of healthy ranges for serum alanine aminotransferase levels. Ann Intern Med 137:1, 2002.

87. Puoti C, Castellaci R, Montagnese E, et al: Histological and virological features and follow-up of hepatitis C virus carriers with normal aminotransferase levels: The Italian Prospective Study of Asymptomatic C Carriers (ISACC). J Hepatol 37:117, 2002.

88. Poynard T, Bedossa P, Opolon P, for the OBSVIRC, METAVIR, CLINIVIR and DOSVIRC groups: Natural history of liver fibrosis progression in patients with chronic hepatitis C. Lancet 349:825, 1997.

89. Ghany MG, Kleiner DE, Alter HJ, et al : Progression of fibrosis in chronic hepatitis C. Gastroenterology 124:97, 2003.

90. Hui CK, Belaye T, Montegrande K, Wright TL: A comparison in the progression of liver fibrosis in chronic hepatitis C between persistently normal and elevated transaminase. J Hepatol 38:511, 2003.

91. Marcellin P, Asselah T, Boyer N: Fibrosis and disease progression in hepatitis C. Hepatology 36(5 suppl 1):S47, 2002.

92. Zarski JP, McHutchison JM, Bronowicki JP, et al: Rate of natural disease progression in patients with chronic hepatitis C. J Hepatol 38:307, 2003.

93. Alberti A, Noventa F, Benvegnu L, et al: Prevalence of liver disease in a population of asymptomatic persons with hepatitis C virus infection. Ann Intern Med 17:137:961, 2002.

94. Ryder SD, Irving WL, Jones DA, et al, for the Trent Hepatitis C Study Group: Progression of hepatic fibrosis in patients with hepatitis C: A prospective repeat liver biopsy study. Gut 53:451, 2004.

95. Seeff LB: Natural history of chronic hepatitis C. Hepatology 36(suppl 1):S35, 2002.

96. Kenny-Walsh E, for the Irish Hepatology Research Group: Clinical outcomes after hepatitis infection from contaminated antiglobulin. N Engl J Med 340:1228, 1999.

97. Wiese M, Berr F, Lafrenz M, et al: Low frequency of cirrhosis in a hepatitis C (genotype 1b) single-source outbreak in Germany: A 20-year multicenter study. Hepatology 32:91, 2000.

98. Seef LB, Miller RN, Rabkin CS, et al: 45-year follow-up of hepatitis C virus infection in healthy young adults. Ann Intern Med 132:105, 2000.

99. Vogt M, Lang T, Frosner G, et al : Prevalence and clinical outcomes of hepatitis C infection in children who underwent cardiac surgery before the implementation of blood-donor screening. N Engl J Med 341:866, 1999.

100. Poynard T, Ratziu V, Charlotte F, et al: Rates and risk factors of liver fibrosis progression in patients with chronic hepatitis C. J Hepatol 34:730, 2001.

101. Wiley TE, Brown J, Chan J: Hepatitis C virus infection in African Americans: Its natural history and histological progression. Am J Gastroenterol 97:700, 2002.

102. Zhang T, Li Y, Lai P, et al : Alcohol potentiates hepatitis C virus replicon expression. Hepatology 38:57, 2003.

103. Perlemuter G, Letteron P, Carnot F, et al: Alcohol and hepatitis C virus core protein additively increase lipid peroxidation and synergistically trigger hepatic cytokine expression in a transgenic mouse model. J Hepatol 39:1020, 2003.

104. Bjoro K, Froland SS, Yun Z, et al: Hepatitis C infection in patients with primary hypogammaglobulinemia after treatment with contaminated immune globulin. N Engl J Med 331:1607, 1994.

105. Berenguer M, Ferrell L, Watson J, et al: HCV-related fibrosis progression following liver transplantation: Increase in recent years. J Hepatol 32:673, 2000.

106. Benhamou Y, Bochet M, Di Martino V, et al: Liver fibrosis progression in human immunodeficiency virus and hepatitis C virus coinfected patients. The Multivirc Group. Hepatology 30:1054, 1999.

107. Jonas MM: Children with hepatitis C. Hepatology 36(5 suppl 1):S173, 2002.

108. Hu K-Q, Tong MJ: The long-term outcomes of patients with compensated hepatitis C virus related cirrhosis and history of parenteral exposure in the United States. Hepatology 29:1311, 1999.

109. Fattovitch G, Giustina G, Degos F, et al: Morbidity and mortality in compensated cirrhosis type C: A retrospective follow-up study of 384 patients. Gastroenterology 112:463, 1997.

110. Serfarty L, Aumaître H, Chazouillères O, et al: Determinants of outcome of compensated hepatitis C virus–related cirrhosis. Hepatology 27:1435, 1998.

111. Degos F, Christidis C, Ganne-Carrie N, et al : Hepatitis C virus related cirrhosis: Time to occurrence of hepatocellular carcinoma and death. Gut 47:131, 2000.

112. Cammà C, Giunta M, Andreone P, Craxi A: Interferon and prevention of hepatocellular carcinoma in viral cirrhosis: An evidence-based approach. J Hepatol 34:593, 2001.

113. Esteban R: Can interferon prolong life? Hepatology 38:292, 2003.

114. Imazeki F, Yokosuka O, Fukai K, Saisho S: Favorable prognosis of chronic hepatitis C after interferon therapy by long-term cohort study. Hepatology 38:493, 2003.

115. Yoshida H, Arakawa Y, Sata M, et al: Interferon therapy prolonged life expectancy among chronic hepatitis C patients. Gastroenterology 123:483, 2002.

116. Pradat P, Alberti A, Poynard T, et al: Predictive value of ALT levels for histological findings in chronic hepatitis C: A European collaborative study. Hepatology 36:973, 2002.

117. Persico M, Persico E, Suozzo R, et al: Natural history of hepatitis C virus carriers with persistently normal aminotransferase levels. Gastroenterology 118:760, 2000.

118. Meyers CM, Seeff LB, Stehman-Breen O, Hoofnagle JH: Hepatitis C and renal disease: An update. Am J Kidney Dis 42:631, 2003.

119. Keeley S, Lake J: Hepatitis C in the setting of kidney, heart, lung and bone marrow transplants. Curr Hep Rep 2:159, 2003.

120. Berenguer M, Lopez-Labrador FX, Wright TL: Hepatitis C and liver transplantation. J Hepatol 35:666, 2001.

121. Sulkowski MS, Thomas DL: Hepatitis C in the HIV-infected person. Ann Intern Med 138:197, 2003.

122. U.S. Preventive Services Task Force: Screening for hepatitis C virus infection in adults: Recommendation statement. Ann Intern Med 140:462, 2004.

123. Forns X, Bukh J, Purcell RH: The challenge of developing a vaccine against hepatitis C virus. J Hepatol 37:684, 2002.

124. Alberti A, Bevegnu L: Management of hepatitis C. J Hepatol 38:S104, 2003.

125. Marcellin P, Boyer N, Gervais A, et al: Long-term histologic improvement and loss of detectable intrahepatic HCV RNA in patients with chronic hepatitis C and sustained response to interferon-alfa therapy. Ann Intern Med 127: 875, 1997.

126. Poynard T, McHutchison J, Manns M, et al: Impact of pegylated interferon alfa 2b and ribavirin on liver fibrosis in patients with chronic hepatitis C. Gastroenterology 122: 1303, 2002.

127. Zeuzem S, Welsch C, Herrmann E: Pharmacokinetics of peginterferons. Semin Liver Dis 23(suppl)1:23, 2003.

128. Lau JYN, Tam RC, Lian J, Hong Z: Mechanism of action of ribavirin in the combination treatment of chronic HCV infection. Hepatology 35:1002, 2002.

129. Fried MW: Side effects of therapy of hepatitis C and their management. Hepatology 36(5 suppl 1):S237, 2002.

130. Lindsay K, Trepo C, Heintges T, et al: A randomized, double blind trial comparing pegylated interferon alfa-2b to interferon alfa-2b as initial treatment for chronic hepatitis C. Hepatology 34:395, 2001.

131. Zeuzem S, Feinman V, Rasenack J, et al: Peginterferon alfa-2a in patients with chronic hepatitis C. N Engl J Med 343:1666, 2000.

132. Heathcote J, Shiffman M, Cooksley G, et al: Peginterferon alfa-2a in patients with chronic hepatitis C and cirrhosis. N Engl J Med 343:1673, 2000.

133. McHutchinson JG, Gordon SC, Schiff ER, et al. Interferon alfa-2b alone or in combination with ribavirin as initial treatment for chronic hepatitis C. N Engl J Med 339:1485, 1998.

134. Poynard T, Marcellin P, Lee SS, et al: Randomized trial of interferon alfa-2b plus ribavirin for 48 weeks or for 24 weeks versus interferon alfa-2b plus placebo for 48 weeks for treatment of chronic infection with hepatitis C virus. Lancet 352:1426, 1998.

135. Manns MP, McHutchison JG, Gordon SC, et al: Peginterferon alfa-2b plus ribavirin compared with interferon alfa-2b plus ribavirin for initial treatment of chronic hepatitis C: A randomized trial. Lancet 358:958, 2001.

136. Fried MW, Shiffman M, Reddy KR, et al: Peginterferon alpha-2a plus ribavirin for chronic hepatitis C virus infection. N Engl J Med 347:975, 2002.

137. Hadziyannis SJ, Sette H Jr, Morgan TR, for the PEGASYS International Study Group: Peginterferon-alpha2a and ribavirin combination therapy in chronic hepatitis C: A randomized study of treatment duration and ribavirin dose. Ann Intern Med 140:346, 2004.

138. Zeuzem S, Hultcrantz R, Bourliere M, et al: Peginterferon alfa-2b plus ribavirin for treatment of chronic hepatitis C in previously untreated patients infected with HCV genotypes 2 or 3. J Hepatol 40:993, 2004.

139. Davis GL, Esteban-Mur R, Rustgi V, et al: Interferon alfa-2b alone or in combination with ribavirin for the treatment of relapse of chronic hepatitis C. N Engl J Med 339:1493, 1998.

140. Shiffman ML, Di Bisceglie AM, Lindsay KL, for the Hepatitis C Antiviral Long-Term Treatment Against Cirrhosis Trial Group: Peginterferon alfa-2a and ribavirin in patients with chronic hepatitis C who have failed prior treatment. Gastroenterology 126:1015, 2004.

141. McCullough AJ: Obesity and its nurturing effect on hepatitis C. Hepatology 38:557, 2003.

142. Jeffers LJ, Cassidy W, Howell CD, et al: Peginterferon alfa-2a (40 kD) and ribavirin for black American patients with chronic HCV genotype 1. Hepatology 39:1702, 2004.

143. Muir AJ, Bornstein JD, Killenberg PG, for the Atlantic Coast Hepatitis Treatment Group: Peginterferon alfa-2b and ribavirin for the treatment of chronic hepatitis C in blacks and non-Hispanic whites. N Engl J Med 350:2265, 2004.

144. Wright TL: Treatment of patients with hepatitis C and cirrhosis. Hepatology 36(5 suppl 1):S185, 2002.

145. Kleinman L, Barker CM, Revicki DA, et al: Relationship of health-related quality of life to treatment adherence and sustained response in chronic hepatitis C patients. Gastroenterology 35:704, 2002.

146. Zeuzem S, Diago M, Gane E, et al: International, multicenter, randomized, controlled study for the treatment of patients with chronic hepatitis C and persistently normal ALT levels with peginterferon alfa-2a (40 kD) (Pegasys) and ribavirin (Copegus) [abstract #106]. Hepatology 38(suppl):208A, 2003.

147. Chung RT, Andersen J, Volberding P, et al: Peginterferon alfa-2a plus ribavirin versus interferon alfa-2a plus ribavirin for chronic hepatitis C in HIV-coinfected persons. N Engl J Med 351:451, 2004.

148. Torriani FJ, Rodriguez-Torres M, Rockstroh JK, et al: Peginterferon alfa-2a plus ribavirin for chronic hepatitis C virus infection in HIV-infected patients. N Engl J Med 351:438, 2004.

149. Mauss S, Berger F, Goelz J, et al: A prospective controlled study of interferon-based therapy of chronic hepatitis C in patients on methadone maintenance. Hepatology 40:120, 2004.

150. Jaeckel E, Cornberg M, Wedemeyer H, et al: Treatment of acute hepatitis C with interferon alfa-2b. N Engl J Med 345:1452, 2001.

151. Wedemeyer H, Jackel E, Wiegand J, et al: Whom? When? How? Another piece of evidence for early treatment of acute hepatitis C. Hepatology 39:1201, 2004.

152. Kamal SM, Ismail A, Graham CS, et al: Pegylated interferon alfa therapy in acute hepatitis C: Relation to hepatitis C virus-specific T cell response kinetics. Hepatology 39:1721, 2004.

153. Davis GL, Wong JB, McHutchison JG, et al: Early virologic response to treatment with peginterferon alfa-2b plus ribavirin in patients with chronic hepatitis C. Hepatology 38:645, 2003.

154. Davis GL: Monitoring of viral levels during therapy of hepatitis C. Hepatology 36:S145, 2002.

155. Camma C, Di Bona D, Craxi A: The impact of antiviral treatments on the course of chronic hepatitis C: An evidence-based approach. Curr Pharm Des 10:2123, 2004.

156. Sullivan SD, Craxi A, Alberti A, et al: Cost effectiveness of peginterferon alpha-2a plus ribavirin versus interferon alpha-2b plus ribavirin as initial therapy for treatment-naive chronic hepatitis C. Pharmacoeconomics 22:257, 2004.

157. Berenguer M, Wright LT: Treatment strategies for Hepatitis C: Intervention prior to liver transplant, pre-emptively or after established disease. Clin Liver Dis 7:631, 2003.

158. Pawlotsky JM, McHutchison JG: Hepatitis C. Development of new drugs and clinical trials: Promises and pitfalls. Summary of an AASLD hepatitis single topic conference, Chicago, Ill, February 27–March 1, 2003. Hepatology 39:554, 2004.

159. Guechot J, Laudat A, Loria A, et al: Diagnostic accuracy of hyaluronan and type III procollagen amino-terminal peptide serum assays as markers of liver fibrosis in chronic viral hepatitis C evaluated by ROC curve analysis. Clin Chem 42:558, 1996.

160. Oberti F, Valsesia E, Pilette C, et al: Noninvasive diagnosis of hepatic fibrosis or cirrhosis. Gastroenterology 113:1609, 1997.

161. Poynard T, Bedossa P: Age and platelet count: a simple index for predicting the presence of histological lesions in patients with antibodies to hepatitis C virus. METAVIR and CLINVIR Cooperative Study Groups. J Viral Hepat 4:199, 1997.

162. Bonacini M, Hadi G, Govindarajan S, Lindsay KL: Utility of a discriminant score for diagnosing advanced fibrosis or cir-

rhosis in patients with chronic hepatitis C virus infection. Am J Gastroenterol 92:1302, 1997.

163. Sheth SG, Flamm SL, Gordon FD, Chopra S: AST/ALT ratio predicts cirrhosis in patients with chronic hepatitis C virus infection. Am J Gastroenterol 93:44, 1998.

164. Wong VS, Hughes V, Trull A, et al: Serum hyaluronic acid is a useful marker of liver fibrosis in chronic hepatitis C virus infection. J Viral Hepat 5:187, 1998.

165. Walsh KM, Timms P, Campbell S, et al: Plasma levels of matrix metalloproteinase-2 (MMP-2) and tissue inhibitors of metalloproteinases-1 and -2 (TIMP-1 and TIMP-2) as noninvasive markers of liver disease in chronic hepatitis C: comparison using ROC analysis. Dig Dis Sci 44:624, 1999.

166. McHutchison JG, Blatt LM, de Medina M, et al: Measurement of serum hyaluronic acid in patients with chronic hepatitis C and its relationship to liver histology. Consensus Interferon Study Group. J Gastroenterol Hepatol 15:945, 2000.

167. Renou C, Muller P, Jouve E, et al: Relevance of moderate isolated thrombopenia as a strong predictive marker of cirrhosis in patients with chronic hepatitis C virus. Am J Gastroenterol 96:1657, 2001.

168. Murawaki Y, Koda M, Okamoto K, et al: Diagnostic value of serum type IV collagen test in comparison with platelet count for predicting the fibrotic stage in patients with chronic hepatitis C. J Gastroenterol Hepatol 16:777, 2001.

169. Fortunato G, Castaldo G, Oriani G, et al: Multivariate discriminant function based on six biochemical markers in blood can predict the cirrhotic evolution of chronic hepatitis. Clin Chem 47:1696, 2001.

170. Pohl A, Behling C, Oliver D, et al: Serum aminotransferase levels and platelet counts as predictors of degree of fibrosis in chronic hepatitis C virus infection. Am J Gastroenterol 96:3142, 2001.

171. Imbert-Bismut F, Ratziu V, Pieroni L, et al: MULTIVIRC Group: Biochemical markers of liver fibrosis in patients with hepatitis C virus infection: a prospective study. Lancet 357:1069, 2001.

172. Patel K, Gordon SC, Jacobson I, et al: Evaluation of a panel of non-invasive serum markers to differentiate mild from moderate-to-advanced liver fibrosis in chronic hepatitis C patients. J Hepatol 41:935, 2004.

173. Kaul V, Friedenberg FK, Braitman LE, et al: Development and validation of a model to diagnose cirrhosis in patients with hepatitis C. Am J Gastroenterol 97:2623, 2002.

174. Forns X, Ampurdanes S, Llovet JM, et al: Identification of chronic hepatitis C patients without hepatic fibrosis by a simple predictive model. Hepatology 36:986, 2002.

175. Wai CT, Greenson JK, Fontana RJ, et al: A simple noninvasive index can predict both significant fibrosis and cirrhosis in patients with chronic hepatitis C. Hepatology 38:518, 2003.

176. Sud A, Hui JM, Farrell GC, et al: Improved prediction of fibrosis in chronic hepatitis C using measures of insulin resistance in a probability index. Hepatology 39:1239, 2004.

177. Leroy V, Monier F, Bottari S, et al: Circulating matrix metalloproteinases 1, 2, 9 and their inhibitors TIMP-1 and TIMP-2 as serum markers of liver fibrosis in patients with chronic hepatitis C. Am J Gastroenterol 99:271, 2004.

CHAPTER
77 Hepatitis E

Krzysztof Krawczynski and Rakesh Aggarwal

Hepatitis E is a form of acute, icteric, self-limited viral hepatitis caused by the hepatitis E virus (HEV). The disease was first recognized in the 1980s, when sera collected during the first recorded epidemic in Delhi, India, in 1955[1] and during another epidemic in Kashmir, India, in 1978[2] were found to lack serologic markers of hepatitis A and B.[3] The virus was identified in 1983 using immune electron microscopy[4]; its genome was cloned in 1990 and fully sequenced shortly thereafter.[5,6] In retrospect, several epidemics of enterically transmitted hepatitis with epidemiologic features resembling those of hepatitis E outbreaks occurred in Europe in the 18th and 19th centuries.

VIROLOGY

HEV is a small RNA virus, 32 to 34 nm in diameter, nonenveloped, and icosahedral. HEV RNA is approximately 7.2 kilobases in length, single- and positive-stranded, 5′-capped, and polyadenylated. It contains three open reading frames (ORFs) (Fig. 77–1).[6] ORF1 encodes nonstructural proteins, ORF2 encodes the viral capsid protein, and ORF3 encodes a protein of unknown function. Details of attachment and entry of HEV into hepatocytes and its replication and release from infected cells remain unknown. The virus currently is classified in a separate genus named *Hepatitis E–like Viruses* and seems to be related phylogenetically to the Togaviridae.[7] Various geographically distinct isolates of HEV have been classified phylogenetically into at least four distinct genotypes (Table 77–1).[8] The various isolates included in genotype 1 ("Asian strain") have a nucleotide sequence homology of 92% to 99% (amino acid sequence homology 95% to 99%), but a nucleotide homology of 75% (amino acid homology 86%) with the single isolate included in genotype 2 ("Mexico strain"). Isolates from the United States, classified as genotype 3, are 92% identical to each other but only 73.5% to 74.5% identical to genotypes 1 and 2.[9] Genotype 4 comprises isolates from some parts of China and Taiwan. Separate genotypes have

been proposed for single isolates from other non-endemic regions.[8] All genotypes share at least one major serologically cross-reactive epitope.

Swine HEV, an HEV-like virus, was identified in pigs in the midwestern United States[10] and later in other countries. It naturally infects pigs and induces transient viremia and antibodies that react with the capsid protein of human HEV strains. A comparison of swine HEV with the Burmese and Mexican isolates of human HEV has shown approximately 90.2% to 91.7% and 78.9% to 82.9% identity at the amino acid level in the ORF2 and ORF3 regions, respectively. Swine HEV identified in India is genetically different from the HEV in patients from the same geographic region,[11] but swine HEV strains in Taiwan and Spain are more similar genetically to human HEV strains from these regions than to swine and human HEV isolates from other parts of the world. An HEV-like virus has been recovered from chickens and its genome partially sequenced.[12]

EPIDEMIOLOGY

Several epidemics of hepatitis E have occurred on the Indian subcontinent and in southeast and central Asia, where this infection is endemic.[13] Outbreaks of hepatitis E also have been reported from the northern and western parts of Africa and the Middle East. Two small outbreaks were reported in Mexico in 1986 and 1987 (Fig. 77–2). Epidemic hepatitis E occurs as large outbreaks that affect several hundred to several thousand persons.[1,2,14,15] Overall attack rates range from 1% to 15% and are higher for adults (3% to 30%) than for children (0.2% to 10%). The male-to-female ratio among cases has ranged from 1:1 to 4:1. The outbreaks have been characterized by a particularly high attack rate and mortality rate among pregnant women. The epidemics vary in nature, ranging from single-peaked, short-lived outbreaks to prolonged, multipeaked epidemics lasting for more than a year (Table 77–2).

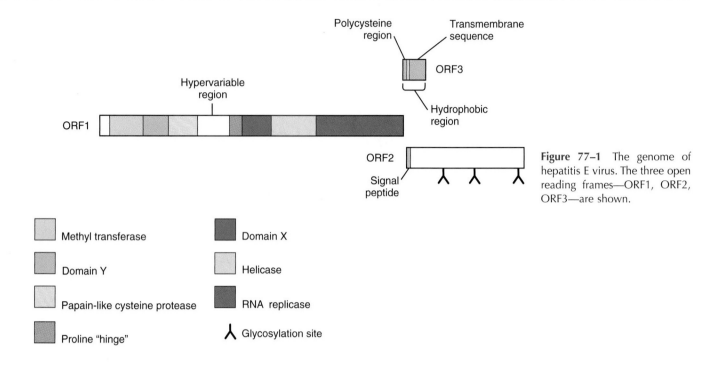

Figure 77–1 The genome of hepatitis E virus. The three open reading frames—ORF1, ORF2, ORF3—are shown.

Table 77–1 Proposed Classification System for Hepatitis E Virus Genotypes*

Genotype	Geographic Origin of Isolates
1	Asia
1A	India, Myanmar (formerly Burma), Nepal
1B	China, Pakistan, countries of the former Soviet Union
1C	Africa
1D	An isolate from a patient with fulminant hepatic failure and a few Indian isolates
2	Mexico; some African strains
3	United States
4	China/Taiwan
5	Italy
6	Greece
7	Greece
8	Argentina (2 isolates)

*Based on phylogenetic analysis of nucleotide sequences.
Adapted from Schlauder GG, Frider B, Sookoian S, et al: Identification of 2 novel isolates of hepatitis E virus in Argentina. J Infect Dis 182:294, 2000.

HEV infection is transmitted predominantly through the fecal–oral route. Most reported outbreaks have been related to consumption of fecally contaminated drinking water. The outbreaks frequently follow heavy rains and floods, but some epidemics occur during the hot summer months, when decreased flow in rivers may increase the risk of water contamination. Recurrent epidemics in endemic regions probably are related to continuous fecal contamination of water, because person-to-person transmission is distinctly uncommon during epidemics,[16] and secondary attack rates among household contacts of persons with hepatitis E are only 0.7% to 2.2%. Continuous contamination of water supplies in endemic regions is suggested by demonstration of HEV RNA in waste water, sewage, and drinking water in endemic regions,[17] and of viable HEV (infectious to primates) in occasional sewage specimens in nonendemic regions.[18]

Mechanisms postulated to contribute to contamination of water sources by HEV and to maintain the virus in endemic areas include the occurrence of continuous subclinical HEV infection, animal reservoirs that harbor HEV-like viral agents, and prolonged fecal shedding of the virus. Subclinical HEV infection has not yet been demonstrated in humans in endemic regions, but viral excretion has been demonstrated in an experimental macaque model of subclinical HEV infection.[19] The existence of other reservoirs of HEV responsible for recurrent outbreaks of hepatitis E is not well established. Zoonotic transmission of HEV infection is not compatible with the rarity of human HEV infection in nonendemic areas despite the high prevalence of antibody to HEV (anti-HEV) among animals, failure of epidemic strains of HEV to induce experimental infection in pigs, and genetic differences between human and animal HEV isolates in endemic regions such as India. The duration of fecal shedding of the virus following acute hepatitis E in humans is much shorter than was previously suggested.[20]

Sporadic hepatitis E, which is demographically and clinically similar to epidemic hepatitis E, accounts for a substantial proportion (as many as 50% to 70%) of cases of acute hepatitis in endemic areas. In nonendemic regions, hepatitis E accounts for less than 1% of sporadic cases of acute viral hepatitis and is related mostly to travel to HEV-endemic regions. Infrequent indigenous cases have been reported; in occasional cases, the source of infection has been identified as undercooked meat.[21] One study showed evidence of transmission of HEV by blood transfusion,[22] but further data are needed to determine the frequency of transmission by this mode.

Prevalence rates of anti-HEV, which is detectable in all geographic areas, are higher among populations in

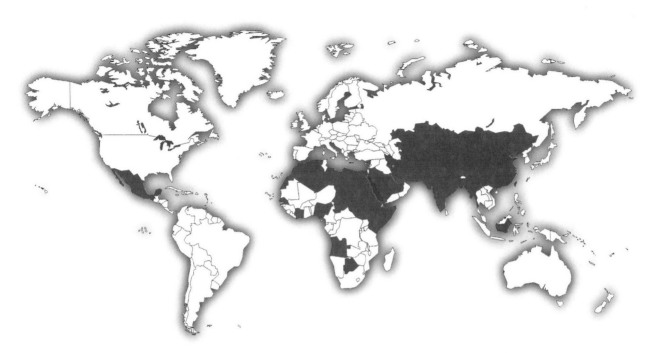

Figure 77–2   Geographic distribution of areas endemic for hepatitis E virus *(red areas)*.

Table 77–2   Epidemiologic Features of Hepatitis E

Large outbreaks involving several thousand persons in developing countries
Sporadic cases:
   Frequent in endemic areas
   Uncommon in nonendemic areas (occur mainly among travelers to endemic areas)
Fecal–oral transmission, usually through contaminated water
Highest attack rates among young adults age 15 to 40 years, with relative sparing of children
Infrequent person-to-person transmission
No evidence of parenteral or sexual transmission
High attack rate in pregnant women, particularly in second and third trimesters
Mother-to-newborn (transplacental) transmission is likely
High mortality rates (15%-25%) in pregnant women, especially in the third trimester

endemic areas (10% to 40%) than among those in nonendemic areas (1% to 5%). Whether anti-HEV seroreactivity in nonendemic areas reflects subclinical HEV infection, serologic cross-reactivity with other agents, false-positive serologic results, or contact with animal reservoirs of HEV-like viruses is unclear.

PATHOGENESIS

Understanding of the pathogenesis of HEV infection, summarized in Figure 77–3, is based on data from both human patients and experimentally infected primates (cynomolgus macaques, rhesus monkeys, and chimpanzees). The virus enters the host primarily through the oral route, although the mechanism(s) by which the virus reaches the liver is unknown. In human volunteers, the incubation period after oral exposure is 4 to 5 weeks.

HEV can be detected in the stool approximately 1 week before the onset of illness and for up to 2 weeks thereafter. HEV RNA can be detected in serum for 2 weeks after the onset of illness in virtually all patients. In experimentally infected primates, HEV RNA has been found in serum, bile, and feces a few days before elevation of the serum alanine aminotransferase (ALT) levels. HEV antigen (HEVAg) is expressed in hepatocytes as early as 7 days after infection[23] and may be identified in more than 50% of the cells, but the number of HEVAg-positive cells decreases sharply when serum ALT levels increase markedly. The onset of ALT elevations in the serum and histopathologic changes in the liver generally corresponds with the appearance of anti-HEV in serum. These findings suggest that liver injury may be largely immune-mediated, especially because the lymphocytes that infiltrate the liver have a cytotoxic/suppression immunophenotype. Preliminary results documenting activation of HEV-specific cellular immunity in patients with hepatitis E have been reported.[24]

Histopathologic features of hepatitis E are similar to those of other forms of acute hepatitis and include ballooned hepatocytes, acidophilic bodies, focal parenchymal necrosis, and inflammatory infiltrates in the lobules and enlarged portal tracts. Nearly one half of patients with hepatitis E have cholestatic hepatitis, characterized by canalicular bile stasis and gland-like transformation of parenchymal cells, with less marked hepatocytic degeneration and necrosis.[25] In patients with severe liver injury, submassive or massive necrosis and collapse of liver parenchyma are seen.

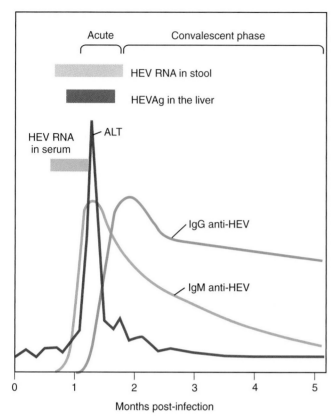

Figure 77–3 The time course of events during hepatitis E virus (HEV) infection (based on studies in human subjects and in experimentally infected primates). ALT, alanine aminotransferase; anti-HEV, antibody to HEV; HEVAg, HEV antigen; IgG, immunoglobulin G; IgM, immunoglobulin M.

Table 77–3 Clinical Features of Hepatitis E

Incubation period of 2 to 10 weeks
Varying clinical manifestations:
   Icteric hepatitis
   Severe hepatitis leading to fulminant hepatic failure
   Anicteric hepatitis
   Inapparent, asymptomatic infection
Clinical illness is similar to that with other types of viral hepatitis
   (except among pregnant women)
Milder illness in children
Low mortality rate (0.07%-0.6%) (except in pregnant
   women, see Table 77–2)
No relation with chronic hepatitis, cirrhosis, or hepatocellular
   carcinoma

CLINICAL FEATURES

The most common recognizable form of HEV infection is acute icteric hepatitis. The clinical manifestations, summarized in Table 77–3, are similar to those observed in patients with acute hepatitis A or B.[26] The illness usually is insidious in onset. An initial prodromal phase lasts 1 to 4 days and is characterized by a varying combination of flu-like symptoms, fever, mild chills, abdominal pain,

anorexia, nausea, aversion to smoking, vomiting, clay-colored stools, dark urine, diarrhea, arthralgias, asthenia, and a transient macular skin rash. Most prodromal symptoms tend to diminish with the onset of jaundice (icteric phase), but dark urine, light stool color, and itching persist for a varying amount of time. Physical examination reveals jaundice and a mildly enlarged, soft, and slightly tender liver. Some patients have splenomegaly. Laboratory test abnormalities include bilirubinuria, conjugated hyperbilirubinemia, and marked elevations in serum aminotransferase and gamma glutamyl transpeptidase levels. Elevation of the serum ALT level may precede symptoms, and the magnitude of the elevation does not correlate with the severity of liver injury. Mild leukopenia and relative lymphocytosis may occur. As the illness subsides, serum aminotransferase levels return to normal, followed by a decline in the serum bilirubin, which usually returns to normal levels by 6 weeks. Ultrasonography may demonstrate normal findings or show a mildly enlarged liver, increase in parenchymal echogenicity, gallbladder wall edema, prominence of portal venules, and a slightly enlarged spleen. The main use of ultrasonography is to exclude biliary obstruction as the cause of jaundice.

Acute hepatitis E usually is self-limited. A few patients have a prolonged course with marked cholestasis (cholestatic hepatitis), including persistent jaundice lasting 2 to 6 months, prominent itching, and marked elevation of the serum alkaline phosphatase level, ultimately with spontaneous resolution. Chronic hepatitis or cirrhosis does not occur as a complication of acute HEV infection. Reported case-fatality rates have ranged from 0.5% to 4%; however, these rates seem to be overestimated because they are based on data from hospitals. Population surveys during outbreaks have reported lower mortality rates of 0.07% to 0.6%.[13]

Some HEV-infected persons may exhibit only nonspecific symptoms resembling those of an acute viral febrile illness with serum aminotransferase elevations but without jaundice (anicteric hepatitis), and some may remain entirely asymptomatic. Asymptomatic and anicteric infections may occur more frequently than icteric disease, because a large proportion of HEV-seropositive persons in endemic areas do not recall ever having had jaundice. The lower attack rates among children than among adults during HEV outbreaks may represent a higher frequency of anicteric or subclinical HEV infections in the younger age group. In a small proportion of patients, the disease is severe and associated with subacute or fulminant hepatic failure. In endemic regions, HEV infection constitutes an important cause of fulminant hepatic failure.

Pregnant women, particularly those in the second or third trimester, are more frequently affected during hepatitis E outbreaks than are others in the population and have a worse outcome, with mortality rates of 5% to 25%. In an epidemic in Kashmir, India,[27] clinical hepatitis E developed in 17.3% of pregnant women, compared with 2.1% of nonpregnant women and 2.8% of men, all ages 15 to 45 years. Among the pregnant women, attack rates during the first, second, and third trimesters were 8.8%, 19.4%, and 18.6%, respectively. Fulminant hepatic failure developed in 22.2% of the affected pregnant women but in only 2.8% and 0% of affected men and nonpregnant women, respectively. The frequency of abortions, still-births, and neonatal deaths also is increased. The pathogenic reason for particularly severe liver damage during pregnancy remains unknown.

DIAGNOSIS

The diagnosis of human HEV infection is based on detection of either HEV RNA in stool and serum specimens using a reverse transcription–polymerase chain reaction assay or the virus-specific host immune response (humoral and cellular). Tests to detect HEV RNA are available only in research laboratories. Enzyme immunoassays (EIAs) for the detection of immunoglobulin M (IgM) and IgG antibodies to HEV have been developed using recombinant HEV antigens expressed in *Escherichia coli* or insect cells, synthetic peptides corresponding to immunogenic epitopes of HEV, and protein expressed from a synthetic gene encoding multiple linear antigenic epitopes from the ORF2 and ORF3 regions.[28-30] The presence in serum of IgM anti-HEV indicates acute infection, whereas detection of IgG anti-HEV may indicate the convalescent phase or past infection. IgM anti-HEV appears in the early phase of clinical illness, lasts 4 to 5 months, and can be detected in 80% to 100% of cases during outbreaks of acute hepatitis E. In one study, 100%, 50%, and 40% of sera collected 1 to 40 days, 3 to 4 months, and 6 to 12 months after the onset of jaundice, respectively, from patients during hepatitis E outbreaks tested positive for IgM anti-HEV. IgG anti-HEV appears in serum a few days after IgM anti-HEV, and the titer of IgG anti-HEV increases during the convalescent phase and remains high for at least 1 to 4.5 years; the exact duration of persistence of IgG anti-HEV in serum is not known. Although several commercial kits for the detection of IgM and IgG anti-HEV are available in various countries, none is currently licensed for clinical use in the United States. Use of different target antigens from different HEV strains and of different expression systems to produce recombinant proteins makes comparison of different tests problematic; the sensitivity of various assays has ranged from 17% to 100% when such assays are applied to specimens from nonendemic areas.[31]

TREATMENT AND PREVENTION

Acute hepatitis E usually is self-limited and requires only supportive care and no specific intervention. Patients with fulminant hepatitis need measures to control cerebral edema and consideration of liver transplantation (see Chapter 90). In pregnant women, no proved benefit to terminating the pregnancy has been confirmed; postpartum hemorrhage resulting from deranged coagulation requires treatment with fresh frozen plasma.

Prevention of hepatitis E in endemic areas depends primarily on the supply of clean drinking water and strict attention to sewage disposal. Measures that improve water quality lead to rapid abatement of an epidemic. Boiling of water appears to reduce the risk of transmission. Isolation of infected persons is not indicated, because person-to-person transmission is uncommon. In the few studies that have evaluated the role of immune globulin manufactured in endemic areas for pre- or post-exposure prophylaxis, no significant reduction in disease rates with use of this agent was found. The occurrence of large epidemics of hepatitis E among adults in endemic areas suggests either that anti-HEV is not fully protective or that antibody levels in serum decline with time and gradually reach a nonprotective level.

Cloning of the HEV genome and subsequent availability of recombinant proteins have encouraged trials of candidate vaccines in HEV-susceptible primates. These studies have shown protection against hepatitis and absence of viremia after immunization with recombinant HEV capsid protein, although viral excretion is not prevented.[32] An experimental HEV DNA vaccine also was tested in cynomolgus macaques and shown to induce serum levels of anti-HEV protective against heterologous HEV strain challenge.[33] Further studies of HEV vaccines are needed, because even short-term protection may be useful for travelers and pregnant women.

REFERENCES

1. Vishwanathan R: Infectious hepatitis in Delhi (1955-56): A critical study: Epidemiology. Indian J Med Res 45(suppl 1):1, 1957.
2. Khuroo MS: Study of an epidemic of non-A, non-B hepatitis: Possibility of another human hepatitis virus distinct from post-transfusion non- A, non-B type. Am J Med 68:818, 1980.
3. Wong DC, Purcell RH, Sreenivasan MA, et al: Epidemic and endemic hepatitis in India: Evidence for a non-A, non-B hepatitis etiology. Lancet 2:876, 1980.
4. Balayan MS, Andjaparidze AG, Savinskaya SS, et al: Evidence for a virus in non-A, non-B hepatitis transmitted via the fecal-oral route. Intervirology 20:23, 1983.
5. Reyes GR, Purdy MA, Kim JP, et al: Isolation of a cDNA from the virus responsible for enterically transmitted non-A, non-B hepatitis. Science 247:1335, 1990.
6. Tsarev SA, Emerson SU, Reyes GR, et al: Characterization of a prototype strain of hepatitis E virus. Proc Natl Acad Sci U S A 89:559, 1992.
7. Berke T, Matson DO: Reclassification of Caliciviridae into distinct genera and exclusion of hepatitis E virus from the family on the basis of comparative phylogenetic analysis. Arch Virol 145:1421, 2000.
8. Schlauder GG, Frider B, Sookoian S, et al: Identification of 2 novel isolates of hepatitis E virus in Argentina. J Infect Dis 182:294, 2000.
9. Erker JC, Desai SM, Schlauder GG, et al: A hepatitis E virus variant from the United States: Molecular characterization and transmission in cynomolgus macaques. J Gen Virol 80:681, 1999.
10. Meng XJ, Purcell RH, Halbur PG, et al: A novel virus in swine is closely related to the human hepatitis E virus. Proc Natl Acad Sci U S A 94:9860, 1997.
11. Arankalle VA, Chobe LP, Joshi MV, et al: Human and swine hepatitis E viruses from western India belong to different genotypes. J Hepatol 36:417, 2002.
12. Haqshenas G, Shivaprasad HL, Woolcock PR, et al: Genetic identification and characterization of a novel virus related to human hepatitis E virus from chickens with hepatitis-splenomegaly syndrome in the United States. J Gen Virol 82:2449, 2001.

13. Aggarwal R, Krawczynski K: Hepatitis E: An overview and recent advances in clinical and laboratory research. J Gastroenterol Hepatol 15:9, 2000.

14. Naik SR, Aggarwal R, Salunke PN, Mehrotra NN: A large waterborne viral hepatitis E epidemic in Kanpur, India. Bull World Health Organization 70:597, 1002.

15. Zhuang H: Hepatitis E and strategies for its control. In Wen YM, Xu ZY, Melnick JL (eds): Viral Hepatitis in China: Problems and Control Strategies. Frankfurt, Karger, 1991, p 126.

16. Aggarwal R, Naik SR: Hepatitis E: Intrafamilial transmission versus waterborne spread. J Hepatol 21:718, 1994.

17. Jothikumar N, Aparna K, Kamtchiammal S, et al: Detection of hepatitis E virus in raw and treated wastewater with the polymerase chain reaction. Appl Environ Microbiol 59:2558, 1993.

18. Pina S, Jofre J, Emerson SU, et al: Characterization of a strain of infectious hepatitis E virus isolated from sewage in an area where hepatitis E is not endemic. Appl Environ Microbiol 64:4485, 1998.

19. Aggarwal R, Kamili S, Spelbring J, Krawczynski K: Experimental studies on subclinical hepatitis E virus infection in cynomolgus macaques. J Infect Dis 184:1380, 2001.

20. Aggarwal R, Kini D, Sofat S, et al: Duration of viraemia and faecal viral excretion in acute hepatitis E. Lancet 356:1081, 2000.

21. Tei S, Kitajima N, Takahashi K, Mishiro S: Zoonotic transmission of hepatitis E virus from deer to human beings. Lancet 362:371, 2003.

22. Khuroo MS, Kamili S, Yattoo GN: Hepatitis E virus infection may be transmitted through blood transfusions in an endemic area. J Gastroenterol Hepatol 19:778, 2004.

23. Krawczynski K, Bradley DW: Enterically transmitted non-A, non-B hepatitis: Identification of virus-associated antigen in experimentally infected cynomolgus macaques. J Infect Dis 159:1042, 1989.

24. Naik S, Aggarwal R, Naik SR, et al: Evidence for activation of cellular immune responses in patients with acute hepatitis E. Indian J Gastroenterol 21:149, 2002.

25. Gupta DN, Smetana HF: The histopathology of viral hepatitis as seen in the Delhi epidemic (1955-56). Indian J Med Res 45(suppl):101, 1957.

26. Vishwanathan R, Sidhu AS: Infectious hepatitis: Clinical findings. Indian J Med Res 45(suppl):49, 1957.

27. Khuroo MS, Teli MR, Skidmore S, et al: Incidence and severity of viral hepatitis in pregnancy. Am J Med 70:252, 1981.

28. Tsarev SA, Tsareva TS, Emerson SU, et al: ELISA for antibody to hepatitis E virus (HEV) based on complete open-reading frame-2 protein expressed in insect cells: Identification of HEV infection in primates. J Infect Dis 168:369, 1993.

29. Dawson GJ, Chau KH, Cabal CM, et al: Solid-phase enzyme-linked immunosorbent assay for hepatitis E virus IgG and IgM antibodies utilizing recombinant antigens and synthetic peptides. J Virol Methods 38:175, 1992.

30. Favorov MO, Khudyakov YE, Mast EE, et al: IgM and IgG antibodies to hepatitis E virus (HEV) detected by an enzyme immunoassay based on an HEV-specific artificial recombinant mosaic protein. J Med Virol 50:50, 1996.

31. Mast EE, Alter MJ, Holland PV, Purcell RH: Evaluation of assays for antibody to hepatitis E virus by a serum panel. Hepatitis E Virus Antibody Serum Panel Evaluation Group. Hepatology 27:857, 1998.

32. Purcell RH, Nguyen H, Shapiro M, et al: Pre-clinical immunogenicity and efficacy trial of a recombinant hepatitis E vaccine. Vaccine 21:2607, 2003.

33. Kamili S, Spelbring J, Carson D, Krawczynski K: Protective efficacy of hepatitis E virus DNA vaccine administered by gene gun in the cynomolgus macaque model of infection. J Infect Dis 189:258, 2004.

CHAPTER

78 Hepatitis Caused by Other Viruses

E. Jenny Heathcote and Jordan J. Feld

A number of recently identified viruses may be hepatotropic in that viremia is occasionally associated with elevations in serum aminotransferase levels and viral replication may occur in hepatocytes, but little, if any, liver disease ensues. Such viruses include hepatitis G virus (HGV) and the GB agents, TT virus (TTV), Sanban virus, Yonban virus, TTV-like mini-virus, and the SEN virus.

Other viral diseases may sometimes involve the liver as part of a systemic infection. The agents of such infections include human immunodeficiency virus (HIV) (see Chapter 32), Epstein-Barr virus (EBV), cytomegalovirus (CMV), herpes simplex virus (HSV), and varicella-zoster virus (VZV). Infection with any of these viruses may rarely lead to severe, sometimes fatal liver disease.

HEPATITIS G AND GB AGENT INFECTION

During the long search for the cause of transfusion-associated non-A, non-B hepatitis (see Chapter 76), the GB agent (GBV) and HGV were discovered and later shown to be two isolates of the same virus. The designation GBV is derived from the initials (GB) of the index patient in whose serum the infectious agent was first identified—a 35-year-old surgeon with acute icteric hepatitis. When his serum was inoculated serially into healthy marmosets, they too developed hepatitis.[1] Analysis of the marmosets infected with derivations of the GB serum led to the identification of two distinct viruses, labeled GBV type A (GBV-A) and GBV type B (GBV-B).[2,3]

A third virus closely related to the GB agents subsequently was identified by the same investigators from a human sample and classified as GBV-C.[4] At approximately the same time, another group of investigators independently identified a virus from the serum of a patient with cryptogenic non–A-to-E hepatitis, which they named HGV.[5] Subsequent studies revealed 96% homology between the genomes of HGV and GBV-C, indicating that they were actually two strains of the same virus.[6] Because large epidemiologic studies have not demonstrated an association between infection with GBV-C/HGV and acute or chronic hepatitis, the use of the term "hepatitis G virus" has been questioned. In fact, even the index patient ("GB") was subsequently shown to be infected not with GBV-C/HGV but rather with hepatitis C virus (HCV). For clarity, GBV-C/HGV is hereafter referred to as GBV-C.

VIROLOGY

GBV-C is a positive-strand RNA virus that has a genome of 9400 nucleotides encoding approximately 2900 amino acids and is classified as a member of the Flaviviridae family. GBV-C shares 44% and 28% nucleotide homology with GBV-A and GBV-B, respectively. Although GBV-C is similar in many respects to HCV, the two viruses share only 27% nucleotide homology and are clearly distinct.

The GBV-C genome is organized like that of HCV. One long open reading frame encodes a single large polyprotein, with structural proteins encoded at the 5' amino terminus and nonstructural proteins encoded at the 3′ carboxyl terminus. A nontranslated region at the 5′ end serves as an internal ribosomal entry site (IRES), allowing translation of the uncapped messenger RNA.[7]

The structural proteins differ between HCV and GBV-C. Two glycoproteins—E1 and E2—predicted to compose the GBV-C viral envelope are cleaved from the polyprotein, probably by a host cell signal peptidase.[5,6] Although HCV E1 and E2 have 5 and 11 N-linked glycosylation sites, respectively, GBV-C E1 and E2 have only 1 and 3 such sites, respectively.[6,8] Perhaps of greater importance, amino acid polymorphisms do not cluster in the hypervariable region of GBC-C E2 as they do in HCV E2.[8] The hypervariable region of HCV E2 is believed to account in part for the ability of HCV to evade immune attack and cause persistent infection. This difference in E2 polymorphisms may account for the 60% to 75% rate of chronic HCV infection, compared with a rate of chronic viremia of only 25% in GBV-C infection.

The GBV-C genome does not encode a core protein, but biophysical and electron microscopic evaluations suggest that the virus does have a nucleocapsid structure, presumably with a core protein.[9] Some GBV-C–infected patients have antibodies in serum that react with a synthetic peptide corresponding to the region immediately proximal to the E1 coding region, suggesting that GBV-C may have a truncated core protein at the amino terminus of the genome.[9]

In contrast with the structural proteins of the two viruses, with their well-recognized differences, the GBV-C nonstructural proteins—designated NS1, NS2, and so on—are similar to those of HCV, including a zinc-dependent thiol protease that cleaves NS2 from NS3,[6] a serine protease at the amino terminus of NS3 that probably cleaves all downstream proteolytic sites, and an RNA helicase (as in all positive-strand RNA viruses) that also is found in NS3 downstream from the protease region. NS4A probably serves as a cofactor for the NS3 protease.[6] The NS5A protein is believed to be involved with double-strand RNA protein kinase, and NS5B serves as the RNA-dependent RNA polymerase.[10] The ability of GBV-C to replicate in cell culture should provide new insights into both GBV-C and HCV replication.

Another important difference between GBV-C and HCV may be tissue tropism. Negative-strand RNA (indicating the presence of active viral replication) has been demonstrated in liver tissue for HCV, implying hepatotropism, but this has not been clearly shown for GBV-C. Negative-strand RNA, however, has been demonstrated in peripheral blood mononuclear cells (PBMCs), bone marrow, and spleens of patients with GBV-C infection, suggesting that GBV-C, like HCV, is a lymphotropic virus.[11] The demonstration of replication of a GBV-C clone in CD4+ T cells confirms that GBV-C is able to replicate in lymphocytes and may help explain the interaction between GBV-C and HIV infection (see later).[12]

GBV-C can be grown in cell culture and has been proposed as a model for studying HCV. Persistent GBV-C infection has been achieved in marmosets, providing a small animal model of HCV infection in which a new serine protease inhibitor targeted to HCV has produced a marked reduction in GBV-C viremia.[13] GBV-B causes acute and rarely chronic hepatitis in tamarins and marmosets,[14] which may be even better small animal models of human HCV infection.

EPIDEMIOLOGY

GBV-C is found worldwide. At least five genotypes have been identified, each with a specific geographic distribution: genotype 1 predominates in West Africa, genotype 2 in Europe and the United States, genotype 3 in parts of Asia, genotype 4 in Southeast Asia, and genotype 5 in South Africa.[15]

The development in serum of antibodies to GBV-C E2 correlates with loss of GBV-C viremia and suggests past exposure and clearance of GBV-C infection.[16] Evidence of current and past GBV-C infection is found frequently in persons with parenteral risk factors and also is common among volunteer blood donors. Between 14% and 38% of persons with frequent exposures to blood are viremic with GBV-C, and 50% to 70% of such persons are seropositive for E2 antibodies.[17,18] Up to 16% of healthy blood donors test positive for antibodies to E2, but their rate of active viremia is much lower.[19] Past or current GBV-C viremia is found as often in blood donors with normal serum alanine aminotransferase (ALT) levels as in donors rejected because of elevated serum ALT levels.[20] Consequently, transmission of GBV-C by transfusion is not prevented by exclusion of donors with elevated serum ALT levels. GBV-C also has been shown to be transmitted sexually and vertically much more frequently than HCV[21,22]; however, the infected babies have no evidence of hepatitis or other clinical sequelae.[23] Because both GBV-C and HCV are transmitted parenterally, it is not surprising that GBV-C–HCV coinfection is common. GBV-C viremia is present in about 20% of HCV-infected persons, and 80% of the remaining subjects are seropositive for antibodies to E2.[10] These findings suggest that the rate of natural clearance of GBV-C is higher (75%) than that for HCV (25% to 50%).

CLINICAL FEATURES

Although GBV-C is detected in many patients with non–A-to-E acute and chronic hepatitis and may persist for years, it does not appear to cause liver (or any other) disease, even in immunocompromised patients.[24-26] In addition, it does not appear to modulate the course or response to treatment of chronic HCV or hepatitis B virus (HBV) infection.[27,28] GBV-C infection also does not interfere with liver transplantation. Although liver transplant recipients have high rates of GBV-C viremia and exposure, probably because of their high transfusion requirements, the outcome of transplantation is unaffected by current or past GBV-C infection.[29]

The duration of GBV-C infection may depend on the immune status and age of the host. As with HBV infection, childhood acquisition of GBV-C is likely to lead to chronic infection, whereas sexual transmission in immunocompetent adults typically leads to rapid clearance of viremia.[30] Chronic GBV-C is more likely to develop in HIV-infected than in noninfected patients.[31] In contrast with HCV infection, the development of antibodies to GBV-C E2 seems to protect against reinfection in most persons.[32] No clear association between GBV-C infection and hepatocellular carcinoma,[33] non-Hodgkin's lymphoma,[34] aplastic anemia,[35] porphyria cutanea tarda,[36] or lichen planus has been documented.[37]

DIAGNOSIS

Because GBV-C rarely causes human disease, diagnostic tests are not widely available and generally are reserved for research purposes. GBV-C RNA can be detected by using polymerase chain reaction (PCR) methodology with commercially available primers. A test for GBV-C antibody, to document past infection, is also available.

GB VIRUS TYPE C AND HUMAN IMMUNODEFICIENCY VIRUS

Once GBV-C was shown not to cause liver disease, interest in this virus diminished. In 1998, however, two independent groups of investigators observed that among a small number of HIV-infected patients, lower HIV viral loads as well as slower progression to acquired immunodeficiency syndrome (AIDS) and death correlated with the presence of GBV-C viremia (Fig. 78–1).[38,39] Subsequent larger studies have confirmed that HIV–GBV-C–coinfected patients have a better prognosis than that observed for HIV–monoinfected patients.[40-42] In addition, coinfected patients respond better to antiretroviral therapy, with a more rapid increase in CD4+ counts and suppression of the HIV viral load.[43] The explanation for the improved response to treatment of coinfected persons remains unknown, although various explanations have been proposed.

HIV replication is diminished in PBMCs infected with both HIV and GBV-C.[44] In addition, a higher inoculum of HIV is required to infect cells already infected with GBV-C.[45] Although virologic inhibition may explain this interaction, immune mechanisms also may be involved. In an Italian study, patients with HIV–GBV-C coinfection maintained a strong T-helper type 1 (T$_H$1) immune profile, whereas HIV-infected patients without GBV-C infection demonstrated a slow waning of T$_H$1 response over time.[46] Vaccination against GBV-C in populations at risk for HIV may be a reasonable experiment to consider.

TREATMENT

Because GBV-C infection is not associated with clinical liver disease, no treatments have targeted GBV-C specifically. In a small series of patients who were coinfected with GBV-C and HCV and received treatment with interferon and ribavirin, GBV-C RNA disappeared from serum during therapy but reappeared in all patients following discontinuation of therapy.[47]

TT VIRUS INFECTION

TTV was first identified in 1977 by using representational difference analysis in a patient (with the initials TT) in Japan who had acute post-transfusion non–A-to-G hepatitis.[48]

VIROLOGY

TTV is a nonenveloped, single-stranded, negative-polarity, circular DNA virus. It is closely related to a family of animal viruses known as Circoviridae, which have not been associated with human disease. TTV is the first human single-stranded circular DNA virus to be identified and does not fit precisely into any known virus family; it may in fact represent a novel virus group.

The TTV genome is 3965 nucleotides long and contains at least 3 overlapping open reading frames. Three messenger RNAs (mRNAs) are expressed by TTV. The protein product of the largest mRNA (3.0 kilobases long) functions as the capsid protein and also serves as a replicase enzyme; the products of the other two mRNAs have not yet been identified. Significant genomic sequence diversity exists among isolates, and at least 16 genotypes have been identified, with greater than 30% sequence divergence. Some genotypes differ in sequence by greater than 50%, and genotype prevalence rates vary geographically.[49]

TTV is believed to be hepatotropic on the basis of the observation that higher viral levels have been found in liver than in the serum of infected patients. TTV also has been identified within hepatocytes, where it has been shown by in situ hybridization and PCR methodology to replicate; however, no or only minor morphologic changes have been seen in cells with positive hybridization signals.[50] TTV also has been shown to replicate in stimulated PBMCs and bone marrow cells.[51]

EPIDEMIOLOGY

TTV is found worldwide, and TTV infection is common. Initial studies documented infection in 1% to 40% of healthy blood donors.[52,53] As more inclusive primers have been used to detect differing genotypes, reported prevalence rates among blood donors have increased dramatically, reaching close to 100% in some studies.[54] TTV also is found in a variety of nonhuman primate species.[55]

TTV is transmitted effectively by all parenteral routes, and high prevalence rates have been documented in hemophiliacs, intravenous drug users, hemodialysis patients, and organ transplant recipients.[56,57] TTV also has been shown to be transmitted enterically, and high TTV DNA titers are present in the feces of viremic patients. Fecal–oral spread may account for the extremely high prevalence rates among low-risk healthy blood donors.[58]

CLINICAL FEATURES

Although TTV was associated with acute hepatitis in the patient in whom it was first identified, other studies have not supported a causal association between TTV and liver disease.[59] In the original study, viremia was detected 6 weeks after exposure and 2 weeks before the rise in serum ALT levels. The viral DNA was cleared from serum, as doc-

A

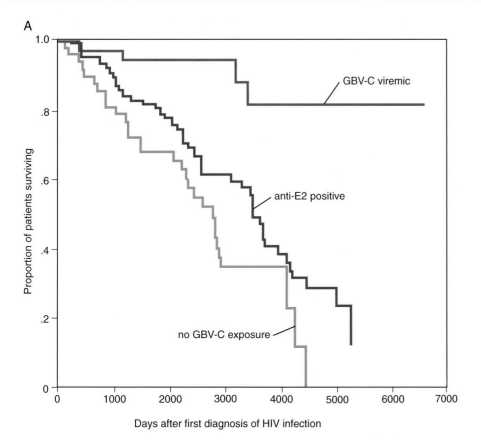

Days after first diagnosis of HIV infection

B

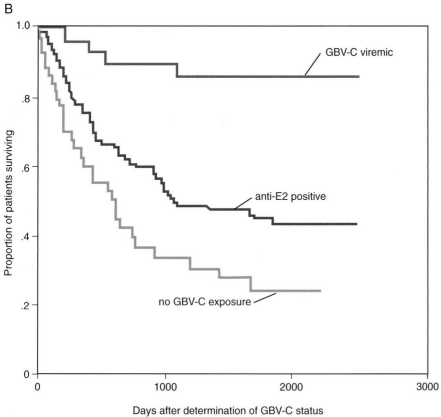

Days after determination of GBV-C status

Figure 78–1 Survival according to GBV-C status in patients with human immunodeficiency virus (HIV) infection. Survival from the time of diagnosis of HIV infection (*A*) and survival from the time the blood sample was drawn to determine the GBV-C status (*B*) are shown in relation to the GBV-C status. For both measures, the patients who were seropositive for GBV-C RNA had significantly better survival. (From Tillmann HL, Heiken H, Knapik-Botor A, et al: Infection with GB virus C and reduced mortality among HIV-infected patients. N Engl J Med 345:715, 2001.)

umented by PCR assay, and serum ALT levels subsequently returned to normal. Viremia may persist for years in both immunocompetent and immunosuppressed persons. Most infected persons have no biochemical or histologic evidence of liver disease.[60,61] Like GBV-C, TTV does not appear to alter the natural history or response to treatment of chronic HCV or HBV infection.[54,62,63] A report that TTV infection may increase the risk of hepatocellular carcinoma in patients with chronic HCV infection remains to be confirmed.[64]

TREATMENT

Formal studies of treatment of TTV infection have not been performed. A small study of HCV-TTV–coinfected patients showed that TTV infection had no affect on the rate of a sustained virologic response to pegylated interferon and ribavirin therapy in HCV infection. Although 6 of 10 patients cleared TTV viremia by the end of therapy, 4 of 6 relapsed within 6 months.[65]

SANBAN, YONBAN, AND SEN VIRUSES AND TTV-LIKE MINI-VIRUS INFECTIONS

Since the discovery of TTV in 1997, several similar viruses with small DNA genomes have been isolated in Japan and named Sanban virus, Yonban virus, and TTV-like mini-virus (TLMV).[66] These viruses have been divided into 29 genotypes with sequence divergence of greater than 30%.[67] Like TTV, they are readily transmitted parenterally and also can be passed by the fecal–oral route. None has been clearly associated with human liver disease to date.

In 1999, a novel virus was identified in an HIV-positive patient (with the initials SEN) who had post-transfusion hepatitis of unknown etiology. This virus was found with the use of degenerative primers from the prototype TTV. The SEN virus is a small, nonenveloped, single-strand DNA virus, but unlike that of TTV, the SEN viral genome is linear. Nucleotide sequencing has shown 50% homology with the prototype TTV, but only 30% of amino acids are homologous. Sequencing of multiple isolates has demonstrated sequence divergence of 15% to 50%.[68]

Like TTV, SEN virus is transmitted both parenterally and by the fecal–oral route. Vertical transmission occurs but in most cases does not lead to chronic infection. Natural clearance of both perinatally and parenterally acquired SEN virus does not appear to protect against reinfection.[69,70] Prevalence rates vary markedly and are highest among patients with parenteral risk factors, particularly those coinfected with HCV.[71,72] The prevalence rate among healthy blood donors is approximately 2% in the United States and 10% in Japan.[73]

The clinical significance of SEN virus infection remains controversial. One study of patients with post-transfusion non–A-to-E hepatitis suggested that SEN virus was the cause in a majority (11 of 12) of patients. SEN viremia persisted for greater than 1 year in 45% of those infected. Clinical hepatitis did not develop in a majority (86%) of transfused patients who acquired SEN virus infection, however, and none of the patients with hepatitis exhib-

ited a fulminant course, nor did chronic liver disease or cirrhosis develop in any of the patients during the study follow-up.[74] Other case reports and case series have identified SEN virus or TTV viremia in patients with both fulminant and chronic hepatitis, but causation has been difficult to establish.[54,75] Most studies have shown no association between SEN or any of the other viruses in this group and human disease[76,77] nor any effect on the course or response to treatment of chronic viral hepatitis.[78-80]

SYSTEMIC VIRAL INFECTIONS THAT MAY INVOLVE THE LIVER

EPSTEIN-BARR VIRUS INFECTION

EBV infection is common and covers a wide spectrum of clinical manifestations. Most affected infants and children either are asymptomatic or have mild, nonspecific complaints, whereas adolescents and adults typically present with the triad of pharyngitis, fever, and lymphadenopathy. Although usually subclinical, liver involvement is nearly universal in patients with EBV mononucleosis and ranges from mild self-limited serum aminotransferase elevations to rare cases of fulminant and even fatal hepatitis.[81]

Up to 90% of patients with acute mononucleosis have serum aminotransferase and lactate dehydrogenase elevations two to three times the upper limit of normal. The enzyme levels typically rise over a 1- to 2-week period, and peak levels are much lower than those normally seen in acute hepatitis A, B, D, or E.[82] Mild elevations of the serum alkaline phosphatase level are common, and mild hyperbilirubinemia is observed in up to 45% of cases. In most patients, liver test results normalize within 1 month, often with complete resolution of clinical symptoms. As with infectious mononucleosis, EBV hepatitis tends to be more severe in adults older than 30 years of age than in younger patients and children. Elderly patients occasionally present with jaundice, fever, and right upper quadrant pain, leading to a clinical diagnosis of extrahepatic biliary obstruction.[83] Although jaundice may be caused by virus-induced cholestasis, autoimmune hemolytic anemia should be excluded in all hyperbilirubinemic patients.[84] Cholestatic jaundice with pruritus may be observed in young women with EBV infection who continue to take oral contraceptive pills.

Rarely, EBV may cause persistent chronic infection with involvement of the liver, lungs, and other organs. In the largest series of fatal mononucleosis, hepatic involvement was universal and was the cause of death in 13 of 30 patients.[85] Granulomatous hepatitis also has been attributed to chronic EBV infection on occasion. Fatal, fulminant hepatitis has been described in both immunocompetent and immunocompromised patients.[86]

The diagnosis of EBV hepatitis is based on clinical features of mononucleosis and laboratory data suggestive of acute EBV infection. Most patients (70%) have a leukocytosis with a predominance of lymphocytes and monocytes, and up to 50% have mild thrombocytopenia. The Monospot test is sensitive for the detection of heterophile antibodies but not very specific for confirmation of EBV infection.[87] Levels of EBV-specific immunoglobulin M (IgM) antibodies peak early in serum and may persist for many months, at which point IgG antibodies develop. Findings on ultrasound examination usually are nonspecific, but features may include hepatosplenomegaly, lymphadenopathy, and possibly gallbladder thickening, which has been reported to portend more severe liver disease. Liver biopsy is rarely necessary for diagnosis but, if done, shows portal and sinusoidal mononuclear cell infiltration with no disruption of hepatic architecture; multinucleated giant cells are not a feature. In more severe cases, focal necrosis may be evident.[88] In situ hybridization or a PCR assay in a biopsy sample may be used to confirm the diagnosis.

No specific treatment for EBV hepatitis exists. Acyclovir inhibits replication of EBV and reduces viral shedding from the nasopharynx but has no effect on clinical symptoms or outcome.[89] Liver transplantation has been performed for fulminant EBV hepatitis.[90] EBV rarely causes hepatitis after liver transplantion but has been associated with post-transplantation lymphoproliferative disease (see Chapter 92).[91]

CYTOMEGALOVIRUS INFECTION

CMV is the largest member of the Herpesviridae family and, like other herpesviruses, persists life-long in a latent, nonreplicative state after resolution of primary infection. Consequently, clinical disease caused by CMV may be the result of a primary infection or, more commonly, reactivation of latent infection.[92]

In immunocompetent children and adults, primary CMV infection usually is subclinical but may cause a mononucleosis-like illness. Liver involvement is common and is characterized by slight to moderate elevations of serum aminotransferase (in 88% of cases) and alkaline phosphatase (in 64%) levels, with or without hepatosplenomegaly.[93] Although the clinical course is benign in most patients, rare instances of granulomatous, cholestatic CMV hepatitis, with or without jaundice, and even massive, fatal hepatic necrosis have been described.[94] In addition to the congenital CMV syndrome (jaundice, hepatosplenomegaly, thrombocytopenic purpura, severe neurologic impairment), CMV is a common cause of neonatal hepatitis.[95]

Disseminated, life-threatening CMV infection with multiorgan involvement may develop in patitents with impaired cell-mediated immunity (see Chapters 32 and 33). Hepatobiliary involvement by CMV is common in patients with AIDS and may manifest acutely as hepatitis, pancreatitis, or acalculous gangrenous cholecystitis.[96] CMV also may cause AIDS-associated cholangiopathy, which manifests with chronic cholestasis and mimics primary sclerosing cholangitis clinically and radiographically.[97] Patients may have papillary stenosis alone or in combination with intra- or extrahepatic (or both) biliary strictures and dilatations (Fig. 78–2; see also Fig. 32–7). Antiviral therapy has no effect on this syndrome, but papillotomy with or without biliary stent placement may lead to symptomatic improvement.[96] Organ transplant recipients also are at risk for aggressive CMV hepatitis, but for unclear reasons, cholangiopathy does not

develop in these patients. CMV hepatitis can be difficult to distinguish from graft rejection in liver transplant recipients.[98]

Diagnosis of CMV infection is based on results of either serologic studies or liver biopsy, or both. In acute primary infection, IgM antibodies to CMV are present. For patients with reactivation of latent CMV, "shell vial" assays, in which monoclonal antibodies are used to detect CMV antigens, or direct CMV antigenemia testing is necessary. Because CMV viremia precedes organ involvement, testing for CMV antigenemia is useful for screening in immunocompromised patients.[99] Multinucleated giant cells with mononuclear portal, parenchymal inflammatory infiltrates, and cholestasis are seen commonly in liver biopsy specimens. Large nuclear inclusions, sometimes referred to as "owl's eye inclusions," may be seen in hepatocytes or biliary epithelial cells (Fig. 78–3).[100]

With mild CMV disease in immunocompetent adults, treatment is unnecessary. In immunocompromised patients, antiviral therapy is indicated. Ganciclovir, a guanosine nucleoside analog with a much longer intracellular half-life than that of acyclovir, has proved to be the most effective agent. The major toxic effect is bone marrow suppression, particularly granulocytopenia. Because viremia correlates with disease outcome, ganciclovir should be continued until CMV antigenemia is undetectable.[101] For patients resistant to or intolerant of ganciclovir, alternative agents include foscarnet and cidofovir.

HERPES SIMPLEX VIRUS INFECTION

HSV typically causes mucocutaneous vesicular oral or genital lesions; visceral involvement may be seen in certain clinical settings. HSV hepatitis occurs in neonates, pregnant women, and immunocompromised persons and can be aggressive and potentially life-threatening.[102] Severe hepatitis with multiorgan involvement and, often, adrenal insufficiency may develop in neonates exposed to infected genital secretions at the time of delivery.[103] In pregnant women, HSV hepatitis usually has a fulminant course. It is most common in late gestation, typically (in 65% of patients) occurring in the third trimester. Mucocutaneous lesions are present in only one half of cases, and a high index of clinical suspicion is important for timely diagnosis.[104] Maternal and perinatal mortality rates approach 40%, and in the largest series, 25% of the cases were diagnosed only at autopsy.[105] Early diagnosis and initiation of antiviral therapy are critical.

Mild, asymptomatic liver enzyme elevations may be seen in 14% of immunocompetent patients with acute genital HSV infection. By contrast, immunocompromised patients may present with fulminant hepatitis.[106] Hepatitis is more common with acute infection than with reactivation and manifests with fever, leukopenia, and markedly elevated serum aminotransferase levels. Coagulopathy, including disseminated intravascular coagulation, and jaundice also may be seen.

Liver biopsy is essential for diagnosis, particularly in pregnancy. The transjugular route may be required because liver failure, precluding a precutaneous biopsy,

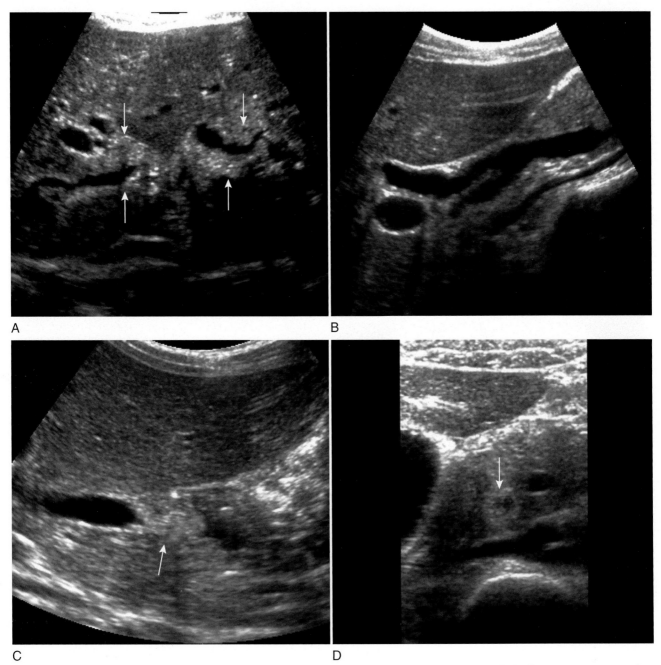

Figure 78–2 Ultrasound findings in AIDS cholangiopathy and cytomegalovirus infection. *A*, A thick rind of echogenic tissue *(arrows)* surrounds the central portal triads and causes irregular narrowing of the intrahepatic bile ducts. *B*, The common bile duct (CBD) is dilated and its wall is minimally irregular. *C*, The dilated CBD tapers abruptly at an echogenic, inflamed ampulla *(arrow)*, indicative of papillary stenosis. *D*, The ampulla *(arrow)* is enlarged and echogenic, as viewed transversely in the caudal aspect of the pancreatic head.

develops rapidly. Focal or extensive hemorrhagic or coagulative necrosis, with few inflammatory infiltrates, is seen. Intranuclear (Cowdry A type) inclusions may be identified in hepatocytes at the margins of the necrosis. In addition, some multinucleated periportal hepatocytes show a ground-glass appearance suggestive of viral inclusions (Fig. 78–4).[107] Electron microscopy, immunohistochemical staining, and PCR techniques can be used to confirm the diagnosis.[108]

HSV hepatitis constitutes an emergency, and empirical treatment should be instituted pending diagnostic confirmation. High-dose intravenous acyclovir (at least 10 mg/kg every 8 hours) is effective and appears to be safe in pregnancy.[109] Successful liver transplantation also has been reported.[110]

VARICELLA-ZOSTER VIRUS INFECTION

Like HSV infection, VZV infection occasionally can be complicated by hepatitis. Liver enzymes may be elevated in up to 3.4% of children with chickenpox; however,

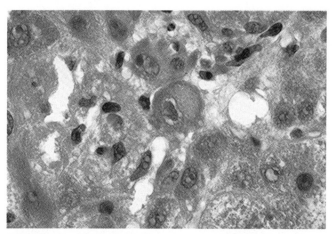

Figure 78–3 Pathologic findings in cytomegalovirus hepatitis. In the *center* is a large hepatocyte with a large nucleus that contains an inclusion. Hematoxylin-eosin. (Courtesy of Maha Guindi, MD, Toronto.)

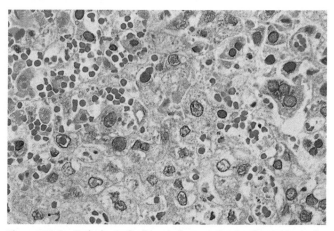

Figure 78–4 Pathologic findings in herpes simplex hepatitis. At the edge of a necrotic zone, some hepatocytes are multinucleated, and many nuclei contain eosinophilic viral (Cowdry type A) inclusions. Hematoxylin-eosin. (From Lucas SB: Other vrial and infectious diseases and HIV-related liver disease. In MacSween RNM, Burt AD, Portmann BC, et al [eds]: Pathology of the Liver, 4th ed. London, Churchill Livingstone, 2001, p 366.)

clinically significant hepatitis has been reported only rarely.[111] Although VZV reactivation in adults usually is limited to the skin, dissemination with liver, lung, and pancreatic involvement may occur.[112] Rarely, visceral involvement has been reported to develop before cutaneous manifestations in bone marrow or solid organ transplant recipients.[113] If visceral involvement is suspected, treatment with high-dose intravenous acyclovir should be instituted.

SEVERE ACUTE RESPIRATORY SYNDROME

During the 2003 outbreak of severe acute respiratory syndrome (SARS), a rapidly progressive respiratory illness, it was not unusual to observe elevated serum aminotransferase levels during the acute illness. Subsequently, cases of SARS hepatitis were reported in which the coronavirus that causes SARS was demonstrated in the liver by reverse transcriptase–PCR techniques in three patients; no viral particles were seen on electron microscopy. All three cases fulfilled the World Health Organization criteria for SARS. Examination of liver tissue revealed marked apoptosis, ballooning of hepatocytes, and moderate lobular lymphocytic infiltration.[114]

REFERENCES

1. Deinhardt F, Holmes AW, Capps RB, Popper H: Studies on the transmission of human viral hepatitis to marmoset monkeys. I. Transmission of disease, serial passages and description of liver lesions. J Exp Med 125:673, 1967.
2. Simons JN, Pilot-Matias TJ, Lery TP, et al: Identification of two flavivirus-like genomes in the GB hepatitis agent. Proc Natl Acad Sci U S A 92:3401, 1995.
3. Muerhoff AS, Leary TP, Simons JN, et al: Genomic organization of GB viruses A and B: Two new members of the Flaviviridae associated with GB agent hepatitis. J Virol 69: 5621, 1995.
4. Simons JN, Leary TP, Dawson GJ, et al: Isolation of novel virus-like sequences associated with human hepatitis. Nat Med 1:564, 1995.
5. Linnen J, Wages J, Zhang-Keck Z-Y, et al: Molecular cloning and disease association of hepatitis G virus A transfusion-transmissible agent. Science 271:505, 1996.
6. Leary TP, Muerhoff AS, Simons JN, et al: Sequence and genomic organization of GBV-C: A novel member of the Flaviviridae associated with human non–A-E hepatitis. J Med Virol 48:60, 1996.
7. Simons JN, Desai SM, Schultz DE, et al: Translation initiation in GB viruses A and C: Evidence for internal ribosome entry and implications for genomic organization. J Virol 70:6126, 1996.
8. Simons JN, Desai SM, Mushahwar IK: The GB viruses. Curr Top Microbiol Immunol 242:341, 2000.
9. Xiang J, Daniels KJ, Soll DR, et al: Visualization and characterization of the GB virus C (hepatitis G virus) particles: Evidence for a a nucleocapsid. J Virol 6:S16, 1999.
10. Stapleton JT: GB virus type C/hepatitis G virus. Semin Liver Dis 23:137, 2003.
11. Tucker TJ, Smuts HE, Eedes C, et al: Evidence that the GBV-C/hepatitis G virus is primarily a lymphotropic virus. J Med Virol 61:52, 2000.
12. George SL, Xiang J, Stapleton JT: Clinical isolates of GB virus type C vary in their ability to persist and replicate in peripheral blood mononuclear cell cultures. Virology 316:191, 2003.
13. Bright H, Carroll AR, Watts PA, Fenton RJ: Development of a GB virus B marmoset model and its validation with a novel series of hepatitis C virus NS3 protease inhibitors. J Virol 78:2062, 2004.
14. Martin A, Bodola F, Sangar DV, et al: Chronic hepatitis associated with GB virus B persistence in a tamarin after intrahepatic inoculation of synthetic viral RNA. Proc Natl Acad Sci U S A 100:9962, 2003.
15. Hattori J, Ibe S, Nagai H, et al: Prevalence of infection and genotypes of GBV-C/HGV among homosexual men. Microbiol Immunol 47:759, 2003.
16. Schaluder GG, Dawson GJ, Simons JN, et al: Molecular and serologic analysis in the transmission of the GB hepatitis agents. J Med Virol 46:81, 1995.
17. Feucht HH, Zollner B, Polywka S, et al: Distribution of hepatitis G viremia and antibody response to recombinant proteins with special regard to risk factors in 709 patients. Hepatology 26:491, 1997.

18. Jarvis LM, Davidson F, Hanley JP, et al: Infection with hepatitis G virus among recipients of plasma products. Lancet 348:1352, 1996.

19. Tacke M, Schmolke S, Schlueter V, et al: Humoral immune response to the E2 protein of hepatitis G virus is associated with long-term recovery from infection and reveals a high frequency of hepatitis G virus exposure among healthy blood donors. Hepatology 26:1626, 1997.

20. Alter HJ, Nakatsuji Y, Melpolder J, et al: The incidence of transfusion-associated hepatitis G virus infection and its relationship to liver disease. N Engl J Med 336:747, 1997.

21. Frey SE, Homan SM, Sokol-Anderson M, et al: Evidence for probable sexual transmission of the hepatitis G virus. Clin Infect Dis 34:1033, 2002.

22. Sathar MA, York DF, Gouws E, et al: GB virus type C coinfection in HIV-infected African mothers and their infants, KwaZulu Natal, South Africa. Clin Infect Dis 38:405, 2004.

23. Wejstal R, Manson AS, Widell A, Norkrans G: Perinatal transmission of hepatitis G virus (GB virus type C) and hepatitis C virus infections: A comparison. Clin Infect Dis 28:816, 1999.

24. Di SR, Ferraro D, Bonura C, et al: Are hepatitis G virus and TT virus involved in cryptogenic chronic liver disease? Dig Liver Dis 34:53, 2002.

25. De Filippi F, Lampertico P, Soffredini R, et al: High prevalence, low pathogenicity of hepatitis G virus in kidney transplant recipients. Dig Liver Dis 33:477, 2001.

26. Alter HJ, Gallagher M, Morris TT, et al: Acute non–A-E hepatitis in the United States and the role of hepatitis G virus infection. N Engl J Med 336:741, 1997.

27. Yuen MF, Chan TM, Yip TP, et al: Prevalence and significance of hepatitis GB virus-C/hepatitis G virus viremia in a large cohort of patients with chronic hepatitis B infection, with chronic hepatitis C infection, and on renal replacement therapy in Hong Kong. Dig Dis Sci 47:432, 2002.

28. Campo N, Brizzolara R, Sinelli N, et al: Hepatitis G virus infection in intravenous drug users with or without human immunodeficiency virus infection. Hepatogastroenterology 47:1385, 2000.

29. Fried MW, Kyudyakov YE, Smallwood GA, et al: Hepatitis G virus co-infection in liver transplant recipients with chronic hepatitis C and non-viral chronic liver disease. Hepatology 25:1271, 1997.

30. Christensen PB, Fisker N, Mygind LH, et al: GB virus C epidemiology in Denmark: Different routes of transmission in children and low- and high-risk adults. J Med Virol 70:156, 2003.

31. Clevenberg P, Durant J, Halfon P, et al: High prevalence of GB virus C/hepatitis G virus infection in different risk groups of HIV-infected patients. Clin Microbiol Infect 4:644, 1998.

32. Tillman HL, Herinlak S, Trauwein C, et al: Antibodies against the GB virus C envelope 2 protein before liver transplantation protect against GB virus C de novo infection. Hepatology 28:379, 1998.

33. Kanda T, Yokosuka O, Imazeki F, et al: GB virus-C RNA in Japanese patients with hepatocellular carcinoma and cirrhosis. J Hepatol 27:464, 1997.

34. Collier J, Zanke B, Moore M, et al: No association between hepatitis C and hepatitis G and B-cell lymphoma in North America. Hepatology 29:1259, 1999.

35. Moriyama K, Okamujra T, Nakano S: Hepatitis GB virus C genome in the serum of aplastic anaemia patients receiving frequent blood transfusions. Br J Haematol 96:864, 1997.

36. Fargion S, Sampietro M, Fracanzani AL, et al: Hepatitis G virus in patients with porphyria cutanea tarda (PCT). J Hepatol 26(suppl):207, 1997.

37. Nagao Y, Sata M, Noguchi S, et al: GB virus infection in patients with oral cancer and oral lichen planus. J Oral Pathol Med 26:138, 1997.

38. Heringlake S, Ockenga J, Tillmann HL, et al: GB virus C/hepatitis G virus infection: A favorable prognostic factor in human immunodeficiency virus–infected patients? J Infect Dis 177:1723, 1998.

39. Toyoda H, Fukuda Y, Hayakawa T, et al: Effect of GB virus C/hepatitis G virus co-infection on the course of HIV infection in hemophilia patients in Japan. J Acquir Immune Defic Syndr 17:209, 1998.

40. Lefrere JJ, Roudot-Thorval F, Morand-Joubert L, et al: Carriage of GB virus C/hepatitis G virus RNA is associated with a slower immunologic, virologic and clinical progression of human immunodeficiency virus disease in co-infected persons. J Infect Dis 179:783, 1999.

41. Yeo AE, Matsumoto A, Hisada M, et al: Effect of hepatitis G virus infection on progression of HIV infection in patients with hemophilia. Multicenter Hemophilia Cohort Study. Ann Intern Med 132:959, 2000.

42. Tillmann HL, Heiken H, Knapik-Botor, et al: Infection with GB virus C and reduced mortality among HIV-infected patients. N Engl J Med 345:715, 2001.

43. Rodriguez B, Woolley I, Lederman MM, et al: Effect of GB virus C coinfection on response to antiretroviral treatment in human immunodeficiency virus–infected patients. J Infect Dis 187:504, 2003.

44. Xiang J, Wunschmann S, Diekama DJ, et al: Effect of co-infection with GB virus C (hepatitis G virus) on survival among patients with HIV infection. N Engl J Med 345:707, 2001.

45. Xiang J, George SL, Wunschmann S, et al: GBV-C infection inhibits CCR5 and CXCR4 HIV strains and alters chemokine and cytokine gene expression in PBMC cultures. Presented at the Conference on Retroviruses and Opportunistic Infections, February 12, 2003, Boston.

46. Nunnari G, Nigro L, Palermo F, et al: Slower progression of HIV-1 infection in persons with GB virus C co-infection correlates with an intact T-helper 1 cytokine profile. Ann Intern Med 139:26, 2003.

47. Cheng PN, Jen CM, Young KC, et al: High-dose interferon-alpha 2b plus ribavirin combination therapy for GB virus-C/hepatitis G virus infection: A study in patients with chronic hepatitis C. Hepatogastroenterology 50:449, 2003.

48. Nishizawa T, Okamato H, Konishi K, et al: A novel DNA virus (TTV) associated with elevated transaminase levels in post-transfusion hepatitis of unknown etiology. Biochem Biophys Res Comm 241:92, 1997.

49. Khudyakov YE, Cong ME, Nichols B, et al: Sequence heterogeneity of TT virus and loosely related viruses. J Virol 74:2990, 2000.

50. Comar M, Ansaldi F, Morandi L, et al: In situ polymerase chain reaction detection of transfusion-transmitted virus in liver biopsy. J Viral Hepat 9:123, 2002.

51. Zhong S, Yeo W, Tang M, et al: Frequent detection of the replicative form of TT virus DNA in peripheral blood mononuclear cells and bone marrow cells in cancer patients. J Med Virol 66:428, 2002.

52. Berg T, Schreier E, Heuft HG, et al : Occurrence of novel DNA virus (TTV) in patients with liver disease and its frequency in blood donors. J Med Virol 59:117,1999.

53. Ali S, Fevery J, Peerlinck K, et al: TTV infection and its relation to serum transaminases in apparently healthy blood donors and in patients with clotting disorders who have been investigated previously for hepatitis C virus and GBV-C/HGV infection in Belgium. J Med Virol 66:561, 2002.

54. Hsu HY, Ni YH, Chen HL, et al: TT virus infection in healthy children, children after blood transfusion, and children with non–A to E hepatitis or other liver diseases in Taiwan. J Med Virol 69:66, 2003.

55. Thom K, Morrison C, Lewis JC, Simmonds P: Distribution of TT virus (TTV), TTV-like minivirus, and related viruses

in humans and nonhuman primates. Virology 306:324, 2003.

56. Boysen T, Christensen JK, Madsen CD, et al: Presence and significance of TT virus in Danish patients on maintenance hemodialysis. Scand J Urol Nephrol 37:259, 2003.

57. Desai SM, Muerhoff AS, Leary TP, et al: Prevalence of TT virus infection in U.S. blood donors and populations at risk for acquiring parenterally transmitted viruses. J Infect Dis 179:1242, 1999.

58. Kato T, Mizokami M, Orito E, et al : High prevalence of TT virus infection in Japanese patients with liver diseases and in blood donors. J Hepatol 31:221, 1999.

59. Naoumov NV, Petrova EP, Thomas MG, Williams R: Presence of a newly described human DNA virus (TTV) in patients with liver disease. Lancet 352:195, 1998.

60. Gimenez-Baracons M, Forns X, Ampurdanes S, et al: Infection with a novel human DNA virus (TTV) has no pathogenic significance in patients with liver diseases. J Hepatol 30:1028, 1999.

61. Charlton M, Adjei P, Poterucha J, et al: TT virus infection in North American blood donors, patients with fulminant hepatic failure and cryptogenic cirrhosis. Hepatology 28:839, 1998.

62. Dai CY, Yu ML, Lin ZY, et al: Clinical significance of TT virus (TTV) infection in chronic hepatitis C patients with high dose interferon-alpha therapy in Taiwan: Re-evaluated by using new set of TTV primers. Hepatol Res 27:95, 2003.

63. Kawanaka M, Niiyama G, Mahmood S, et al: Effect of TT virus co-infection on interferon response in chronic hepatitis C patients. Liver 22:351, 2002.

64. Tokita H, Murai S, Kamitsukasa H, et al: High TT virus load as an independent factor associated with the occurrence of hepatocellular carcinoma among patients with hepatitis C virus–related chronic liver disease. J Med Virol 67:501, 2002.

65. Moreno J, Moraleda G, Barcena R, et al: Response of TT virus to IFN plus ribavirin treatment in patients with chronic hepatitis C. World J Gastroenterol 10:143, 2004.

66. Takahashi K, Hijikata M, Samokhvalov EI, Mishiro S: Full or near full length nucleotide sequences of TT virus variants (types SANBAN and YONBAN) and the TT virus-like mini virus. Intervirology 43:119, 2000.

67. Hijikata M, Takahasahi K, Mishiro S: Complete circular DNA genome of a TT virus variant (isolate name SANBAN) and 44 partial ORF2 sequences implicating a great degree of diversity beyond genotypes. Virology 260:17, 1999.

68. Tanakaa Y, Primi D, Wang RYH, et al: Genomic and molecular evolutionary analysis of a newly identified infectious agent (SEN virus) and its relationship to the TT virus family. J Infect Dis 183:359, 2001.

69. Pirovano S, Bellinzoni M, Ballerini C, et al: Transmission of SEN virus from mothers to their babies. J Med Virol 66:421, 2002.

70. Wilson LE, Umemura T, Astemborski J, et al: Dynamics of SEN virus infection among injection drug users. J Infect Dis 184:1315, 2001.

71. Pfeiffer RM, Tanaka Y, Yeo AE, et al: Prevalence of SEN viruses among injection drug users in the San Francisco Bay area. J Infect Dis 188:13, 2003.

72. Schroter M, Laufs R, Zollner B, et al: A novel DNA virus (SEN) among patients on maintenance hemodialysis: Prevalence and clinical importance. J Clin Virol 27:69, 2003.

73. Shibata M, Wang RY, Yoshiba M, et al: The presence of a newly identified infectious agent (SEN virus) in patients with liver diseases and in blood donors in Japan. J Infect Dis 184:400, 2001.

74. Umemura T, Yeo AE, Sottini A, et al: SEN virus infection and its relationship to transfusion-associated hepatitis. Hepatology 33:1303, 2001.

75. Yusufu Y, Mochida S, Matsui A, et al: TT virus infection in cases of fulminant hepatic failure: Evaluation by clonality based on amino acid sequence of hypervariable regions. Hepatol Res 21:85, 2001.

76. Yoshida H, Kato N, Shiratori Y, et al: Weak association between SEN virus viremia and liver disease. J Clin Microbiol 40:3140, 2002.

77. Umemura T, Tanaka E, Ostapowicz G, et al: Investigation of SEN virus infection in patients with cryptogenic acute liver failure, hepatitis-associated aplastic anemia, or acute and chronic non–A-E hepatitis. J Infect Dis 188:1545, 2003.

78. Lin JG, Goto T, Nakane K, et al: Clinical significance of SEN-virus on interferon response in chronic hepatitis C patients. J Gastroenterol Hepatol 18:1144, 2003.

79. Umemura T, Alter HJ, Tanaka E, et al: SEN virus: Response to interferon alfa and influence on the severity and treatment response of coexistent hepatitis C. Hepatology 35:953, 2002.

80. Rigas B, Hasan I, Rehman R, et al: Effect on treatment outcome of coinfection with SEN viruses in patients with hepatitis C. Lancet 358:1961, 2001.

81. Grotto I, Mimouni D, Huerta M, et al: Clinical and laboratory presentation of EBV positive infectious mononucleosis in young adults. Epidemiol Infect 131:683, 2003.

82. Rosalki S, Jones T, Verney A: Transaminases and liver function studies in infectious mononucleosis. BMJ 1:929, 1960.

83. Edoute Y, Baruch Y, Lachter J, et al: Severe cholestatic jaundice induced by Epstein-Barr virus infection in the elderly. J Gastroenterol Hepatol 13:821, 1998.

84. Hinedi TB, Koff RS: Cholestatic hepatitis induced by Epstein-Barr virus infection in an adult. Dig Dis Sci 48:539, 2003.

85. Markin RS: Manifestations of Epstein-Barr virus-associated disorders in liver. Liver 14:1, 1994.

86. Palanduz A, Yildirmak Y, Telhan L, et al: Fulminant hepatic failure and autoimmune hemolytic anemia associated with Epstein-Barr virus infection. J Infect 45:96, 2002.

87. Schooley A: Epstein-Barr virus. In Mandell G, Bennett J, Dolin R (eds): Principles and Practice of Infectious Diseases, vol 2. Philadelphia, Churchill Livingstone. 2000, p 1599.

88. White NJ, Juel-Jensen BE: Infectious mononucleosis hepatitis. Semin Liver Dis 4:301, 1984.

89. van der Horst C, Joncas J, Ahronheim G, et al: Lack of effect of peroral acyclovir for the treatment of acute infectious mononucleosis. J Infect Dis 164:788, 1991.

90. Feranchak AP, Tyson RW, Narkewicz MR, et al: Fulminant Epstein-Barr viral hepatitis: Orthotopic liver transplantation and review of the literature. Liver Transpl Surg 4:469, 1998.

91. Sokal EM, Antunes H, Beguin C, et al: Early signs and risk factors for the increased incidence of Epstein-Barr virus–related posttransplant lymphoproliferative diseases in pediatric liver transplant recipients treated with tacrolimus. Transplantation 64:1438, 1997.

92. Goodgame R: Gastrointestinal cytomegalovirus disease. Ann Intern Med 119:924, 1993.

93. Wreghitt TG, Teare EL, Sule O, et al: Cytomegalovirus infection in immunocompetent patients. Clin Infect Dis 37:1603, 2003.

94. Eddleston M, Peacock S, Juniper M, Warrell DA: Severe cytomegalovirus infection in immunocompetent patients. Clin Infect Dis 24:52, 1997.

95. Domiati-Saad R, Dawson DB, Margraf LR, et al: Cytomegalovirus and human herpesvirus 6, but not human papillomavirus, are present in neonatal giant cell hepatitis and extrahepatic biliary atresia. Pediatr Dev Pathol 3:367, 2000.

96. Benhamou Y, Caumes E, Gerosa Y, et al: AIDS-related cholangiopathy: Critical analysis of a prospective series of 26 patients. Dig Dis Sci 38:1113, 1993.

97. Mahajani RV, Uzer MF: Cholangiopathy in HIV-infected patients. Clin Liver Dis 3:669, 1999.

98. Sampathkumar P, Paya CV: Management of cytomegalovirus infection after liver transplantation. Liver Transpl 6:144, 2000.

99. St George K, Rinaldo CR Jr: Comparison of cytomegalovirus antigenemia and culture assays in patients on and off antiviral therapy. J Med Virol 59:91, 1999.

100. Espy MJ, Paya CV, Holley KE, et al: Diagnosis of cytomegalovirus hepatitis by histopathology and in situ hybridization in liver transplantation. Diagn Microbiol Infect Dis 14:293, 1991.

101. Nigro G, Krzysztofiak A, Bartmann U, et al: Ganciclovir therapy for cytomegalovirus-associated liver disease in immunocompetent or immunocompromised children. Arch Virol 142:573, 1997.

102. Corey L, Spear PF: Infections with herpes simples viruses. N Engl J Med 314:749, 1986.

103. Overall JC Jr: Herpes simplex virus infection of the fetus and newborn. Pediatr Ann 23:131, 1994.

104. Yaziji H, Hill T, Pitman TC, et al: Gestational herpes simplex virus hepatitis. South Med J 90:347, 1997.

105. Wertheim RA, Brooks BJ Jr, Rodriguez FH Jr, et al: Fatal herpetic hepatitis in pregnancy. Obstet Gynecol 62:38, 1983.

106. Bissig KD, Zimmermann A, Bernasch D, et al: Herpes simplex virus hepatitis 4 years after liver transplantation. J Gastroenterol 38:1005, 2003.

107. Fink CG, Read SJ, Hopkin J, et al: Acute herpes hepatitis in pregnancy. J Clin Pathol 46:968, 1993.

108. Pellise M, Miquel R: Liver failure due to herpes simplex virus. J Hepatol 32:170, 2000.

109. Greenspoon JS, Wilcox JG, McHutchison LB, Rosen DJ: Acyclovir for disseminated herpes simplex virus in pregnancy: A case report. J Reprod Med 39:311, 1994.

110. Twagira M, Hadzic N, Smith M, et al: Disseminated neonatal herpes simplex virus (HSV) type 2 infection diagnosed by HSV DNA detection in blood and successfully managed by liver transplantation. Eur J Pediatr 163:166, 2004.

111. Feldman S, Crout J, Andrew ME: Incidence and natural history of chemically defined varicella-zoster virus hepatitis in children and adolescents. Scand J Infect Dis 29:33, 1997.

112. Fehr T, Bossart W, Wahl C, Binswanger U: Disseminated varicella infection in adult renal allograft recipients: Four cases and a review of the literature. Transplantation 73:608, 2002.

113. Schiller GJ, Nimer SD, Gajerwski JL, Golde DW: Abdominal presentation of varicella-zoster infection in recipients of allogenic bone marrow transplantation. Bone Marrow Transplant 7:489, 1991.

114. Chau TN, Lee KC, Yao H, et al: SARS associated with hepatitis caused by a novel coronavirus: Report of three cases. Hepatology 39:302, 2004.

CHAPTER

79 Bacterial, Parasitic, and Fungal Infections of the Liver, Including Liver Abscess

Raymond T. Chung and Lawrence S. Friedman

The liver serves as the initial site of filtration of absorbed intestinal luminal contents and is particularly susceptible to contact with microbial antigens of all varieties. In addition to infection by viruses (see Chapters 74 to 78), the liver can be affected by (1) spread of bacterial or parasitic infection from outside the liver; (2) primary infection by spirochetal, protozoal, helminthic, or fungal organisms; or (3) systemic effects of bacterial or granulomatous infections.

BACTERIAL INFECTIONS INVOLVING OR AFFECTING THE LIVER

GRAM-POSITIVE AND GRAM-NEGATIVE BACTERIAL INFECTIONS

A number of extrahepatic infections can lead to derangements of hepatic function, ranging from mild abnormalities of liver biochemical tests to frank jaundice and, rarely, hepatic failure.

Staphylococcus aureus Infection: Toxic Shock Syndrome

Toxic shock syndrome is a multisystem disease caused by the staphylococcal toxic shock syndrome toxin. Originally described in association with tampon use, this syndrome is now more frequently a complication of *Staphylococcus aureus* infections in surgical wounds. Typical findings include a scarlatiniform rash, mucosal hyperemia, hypotension, vomiting, and diarrhea. Hepatic involvement is almost always present, can be extensive, and is marked by deep jaundice and high serum aminotransferase levels.[1] Histologic findings in the liver include microabscesses and granulomas. The diagnosis is confirmed by culture of toxigenic *S. aureus* from the wound, blood, or other body sites. Antibiotics effective against *S. aureus* include nafcillin for methicillin-sensitive isolates and vancomycin or linezolid for methicillin-resistant isolates.

Clostridial Infection

Clostridial myonecrosis involving *Clostridium perfringens* usually is a mixed anaerobic infection that results in the rapid development of local wound pain, abdominal pain, and diarrhea. The skin lesions become discolored and even bullous, and gas gangrene spreads rapidly, leading to a high mortality rate. Jaundice may develop in up to 20% of patients with gas gangrene and is predominantly a consequence of massive intravascular hemolysis caused by the exotoxin elaborated by the bacterium.[2] Evidence of liver involvement may include abscess formation and gas in the portal vein. Hepatic involvement does not appear to affect mortality. Presence of clostridial bacteria portends a poor prognosis in persons with cirrhosis.[3] Surgical débridement with wide excision is essential; penicillin and clindamycin are effective antibiotics.

Actinomycosis

Actinomycosis is caused most commonly by *Actinomyces israelii*, a gram-positive anaerobic bacterium. Although cervicofacial infection is the most frequent manifestation of actinomycotic infection, gastrointestinal involvement occurs in 13% to 60% of cases.[4,5] Hepatic involvement is present in 15% of cases of abdominal actinomycosis and is believed to result from metastatic spread from other abdominal sites. Common presenting manifestations of actinomycotic liver abscess include fever, abdominal pain, and anorexia with weight loss.[6,7] The course is more indolent than that seen with the usual causes of pyogenic hepatic abscess. Anemia, leukocytosis, an elevated erythrocyte sedimentation rate, and an elevated serum alkaline phosphatase level are nearly universal.[6] Radiographic findings are nonspecific; multiple abscesses may be seen in both lobes of the liver.

The diagnosis is based on aspiration of an abscess cavity and either visualization of characteristic sulfur granules or positive results on an anaerobic culture. Most abscesses resolve with prolonged courses of intravenous penicillin or oral tetracycline. Large abscesses can be drained percutaneously.[6]

Listeriosis

Hepatic invasion in adult human *Listeria monocytogenes* infection is uncommon. One report described three cases of disseminated listeriosis associated with hepatitis.[8] In almost all cases with overt hepatic involvement, underlying liver disease was present, including cirrhosis, hemochromatosis, or chronic hepatitis. Hepatic histologic features include multiple abscesses and granulomas. The diagnosis of disseminated listerial infection is based on a positive result of blood cultures.[9] Treatment is with ampicillin or penicillin, often with gentamicin for synergy.

Shigellosis and Salmonellosis

Several case reports have described cholestatic hepatitis attributable to enteric infection with *Shigella*.[10,11] Histologic findings in the liver have included portal and periportal infiltration with polymorphonuclear neutrophils, hepatocyte necrosis, and cholestasis.

Typhoid fever, caused by *Salmonella typhi*, is a systemic infection that frequently involves the liver. Some patients may present with an acute hepatitis–like picture, characterized by fever and tender hepatomegaly. Slight elevation of the serum bilirubin level (in up to 16% of cases)

and aminotransferase levels (in 50%) is common.[12] Cholecystitis and liver abscess may complicate hepatic involvement with *S. typhi* infection.[13]

Hepatic damage by *S. typhi* appears to be mediated by bacterial endotoxin, although organisms can be visualized within the liver tissue. Endotoxin may produce focal necrosis, a periportal mononuclear infiltrate, and Kupffer cell hyperplasia in the liver. These changes resemble those seen in gram-negative sepsis. Characteristic typhoid nodules scattered throughout the liver are the result of profound hypertrophy and proliferation of Kupffer cells. The clinical course can be severe, with a mortality rate approaching 20%, particularly with delayed treatment or in patients with other complications of *Salmonella* infection.[12] It has been suggested that severe typhoid fever with jaundice and encephalopathy can be differentiated from acute liver failure by the presence of an elevated serum alkaline phosphatase level, mild hypoprothrombinemia, thrombocytopenia, hepatomegaly, and an aspartate aminotransferase (AST) level greater than the alanine aminotransferase (ALT) level.[14] Ciprofloxacin and ceftriaxone are first-line agents for the treatment of typhoid fever.

S. paratyphi A and B (*Salmonella enterica* serotypes paratyphi A and B) are the predominant causes of paratyphoid fever. As in typhoid fever, abnormalities in liver biochemical tests, with or without hepatomegaly, are common. Serum aminotransferase elevations are frequent (82%); less commonly, elevations in alkaline phosphatase (39%) and bilirubin (19%) levels are seen.[12] Liver abscess is a rare complication.[15] Treatment is with a third-generation cephalosporin or a fluoroquinolone.

Yersiniosis

Infection with *Yersinia enterocolitica* manifests as ileocolitis in children and as terminal ileitis or mesenteric adenitis in adults. Arthritis, cellulitis, erythema nodosum, and septicemia may complicate *Yersinia* infection. Most patients with complicated disease have an underlying comorbid condition, such as diabetes mellitus, cirrhosis, or hemochromatosis. Excess tissue iron, in particular, may be a predisposing factor, because growth of the *Yersinia* bacterium is enhanced by iron.

The subacute septicemic form of the disease resembles typhoid fever or malaria. Multiple abscesses are distributed diffusely in the liver and spleen.[16] In some cases, the occurrence of *Y. enterocolitica* liver abscesses may lead to the detection of underlying hemochromatosis.[17,18] The mortality rate is approximately 50%. Fluoroquinolones are the preferred antibiotics.

Gonococcal Infection

In approximately 50% of patients with disseminated gonococcal infection, serum alkaline phosphatase levels are elevated, and in 30% to 40% of patients, aspartate aminotransferase levels are elevated.[19] Jaundice is uncommon.

The most common hepatic complication of gonococcal infection is the Fitz-Hugh–Curtis syndrome, a perihepatitis that is believed to result from direct spread of the infection from the pelvis.[19] Clinically, patients describe a sudden, sharp pain in the right upper quadrant. The pain may be confused with that of acute chole-cystitis or pleurisy. Most patients have a history of pelvic inflammatory disease. The syndrome is distinguished from gonococcal bacteremia by a characteristic friction rub over the liver and negative blood culture results. The diagnosis is made by vaginal culture for gonococci. The overall prognosis of gonococcal infection appears to be unaffected by the presence of perihepatitis.[20] Ceftriaxone is the antibiotic of choice.

Legionellosis

Legionella pneumophila, a fastidious gram-negative bac-terium, is the cause of legionnaires' disease. Although pneumonia is the predominant clinical manifestation, abnormal liver biochemical test results are frequent, with elevations in serum aminotransferase levels in 50%, alkaline phosphatase levels in 45%, and bilirubin levels in 20% of cases (but usually without jaundice). Involve-ment of the liver does not influence clinical outcome. Liver histologic changes include microvesicular steatosis and focal necrosis; organisms can be seen occasionally. The diagnosis is confirmed by direct fluorescence of antibody in the serum or sputum or of antigen in the urine.[21] The antibiotic of choice is azithromycin or a fluoroquinolone.

Burkholderia pseudomallei Infection (Melioidosis)

Burkholderia pseudomallei is a soil-borne and water-borne gram-negative bacterium that is found predominantly in Southeast Asia. The clinical spectrum of melioidosis ranges from asymptomatic infection to fulminant sep-ticemia with involvement of the lungs, gastrointestinal tract, and liver.[22] Histologic changes in the liver include inflammatory infiltrates, multiple microabscesses, and focal necrosis. Organisms can be visualized with a Giemsa stain of a liver biopsy specimen.[23] With chronic disease, granulomas may be seen. Abscesses may need to be drained or débrided, and ceftazidine or meropenem is the drug of choice.

Brucellosis

Brucellosis may be acquired from infected pigs, cattle, goats, and sheep (*Brucella suis*, *Brucella abortus*, *Brucella melitensis*, and *Brucella ovis*, respectively) and typically manifests as an acute febrile illness. Hepatic abnormali-ties are seen in a majority of infected persons, and jaun-dice may be present in severe cases. Typically, multiple noncaseating hepatic granulomas are found in liver biopsy specimens; less often, focal mononuclear infiltra-tion of the portal tracts or lobules is seen.[24] Rarely, bru-cellosis also may produce hepatosplenic abscesses.[25,26] The diagnosis can be made by isolation of the organism from a culture specimen of liver tissue and is confirmed by serologic testing with use of counterimmunoelec-trophoresis in combination with a history of exposure to animals. Surgical drainage may be required for man-agement of *Brucella* abscesses. The combination of streptomycin and doxycycline is the most effective antimicrobial therapy.

Coxiella burnetii Infection (Q Fever)

Infection by *Coxiella burnetii*, typically acquired by inhalation of animal dusts, causes the clinical syndrome of Q fever, which is characterized by relapsing fevers, headache, myalgias, malaise, pneumonitis, and culture-negative endocarditis. Liver involvement is common.[27] The predominant abnormality is an elevated serum alka-line phosphatase level, with minimal elevations of AST or bilirubin level. The histologic hallmark in the liver is the presence of characteristic fibrin ring granulomas. The diagnosis is confirmed by serologic testing for complement-fixing antibodies.[28] Treatment with doxycy-cline usually is effective.

Bartonellosis

Endemic to Colombia, Ecuador, and Peru, *Bartonella bacil-liformis* is a gram-negative coccobacillus that causes an acute febrile illness accompanied by jaundice, hemolysis, hepatosplenomegaly, and lymphadenopathy.[29] Centri-lobular necrosis of the liver and splenic infarction may occur. As many as 40% of patients die of sepsis or hemol-ysis. Prompt treatment with chloramphenicol or tetra-cycline prevents fatal complications.

Bacillary Angiomatosis and the Acquired Immunodeficiency Syndrome

Bacillary angiomatosis is an infectious disorder that primarily affects persons with the acquired immuno-deficiency syndrome (AIDS) or other immunodeficiency states. The causative agents have been identified as the gram-negative bacilli *Bartonella henselae* and, in some cases, *Bartonella quintana*.[30] Infection frequently is associ-ated with exposure to cats.

Bacillary angiomatosis is characterized most commonly by multiple blood-red papular skin lesions, but dissemi-nated infection with or without skin involvement also has been described.[31] The causative bacilli can infect liver, lymph nodes, pleura, bronchi, bones, brain, bone marrow, and spleen. Additional manifestations include persistent fever, bacteremia, and sepsis. Hepatic infection should be suspected when serum aminotransferase levels are elevated in the absence of other explanations.

Hepatic infection in persons with bacillary angiomato-sis may manifest as peliosis hepatis, or blood-filled cysts (see Chapter 80). Histologically, peliosis in patients with AIDS is characterized by an inflammatory myxoid stroma containing clumps of bacilli surrounding the blood-filled peliotic cysts. Increasingly, diagnosis of *Bartonella* in-fection is by polymerase chain reaction (PCR)-based methods.[32]

Bacillary angiomatosis responds uniformly to therapy with erythromycin. For visceral infection, at least 6 weeks of treatment with erythromycin or doxycycline should be administered.

Bacterial Sepsis and Jaundice

Jaundice may complicate systemic sepsis caused by gram-negative or gram-positive organisms. Exotoxins and endotoxin liberated in overwhelming infection can directly or indirectly, through cytokines such as tumor necrosis factor-α (TNF-α), inhibit the transport of bile acids and other organic anions across the hepatic sinu-soidal and bile canalicular membranes, thereby leading to intrahepatic cholestasis (see Chapter 14).[33,34] Serum bilirubin levels can reach 15 mg/dL or higher. The magnitude of the jaundice does not correlate with mortality. Results of cultures of liver biopsy specimens usually are negative.

RICKETTSIAL INFECTIONS

Rocky Mountain Spotted Fever

Mortality from Rocky Mountain spotted fever, a systemic tick-borne rickettsial illness, has decreased considerably as a result of prompt recognition of the classic maculopapular rash in association with fever and an exposure history. A small subset of patients, however, present with multiorgan manifestations and have a high mortality rate.[35] A characteristic severe vasculitis develops in these patients and is believed to be the result of a microbe-induced coagulopathy. Hepatic involvement is frequent in multiorgan disease. In one postmortem study, rickettsiae were identified in the portal triads of eight of nine fatal cases. Portal tract inflammation, portal vasculitis, and sinusoidal erythrophagocytosis were consistent findings, but hepatic necrosis was negligible. The predominant clinical manifestation was jaundice; elevations of serum aminotransferase and alkaline phosphatase levels varied. Jaundice probably results from a combination of inflammatory bile ductular obstruction and hemolysis and is associated with increased mortality.[27,36]

Ehrlichiosis

Ehrlichiae are rickettsiae that parasitize leukocytes. In the United States, human monocytic ehrlichiosis is caused principally by *Ehrlichia chaffeensis* and, less often, *Ehrlichia canis*. Human granulocytic anaplasmosis (formerly known as human granulocytic ehrlichiosis) is caused by *Anaplasma phagocytophilum*.[27,37] In contrast with Rocky Mountain spotted fever, a rash is often absent. Hepatic involvement is seen in greater than 80% of cases, usually in the form of mild, transient serum aminotransferase elevations. More marked aminotransferase elevations may occur occasionally, in association with cholestasis, hepatosplenomegaly, and liver failure. Liver injury is attributable to proliferation of organisms within hepatocytes and provocation of immune responses. Focal necrosis, fibrin ring granulomas, and cholestatic hepatitis can be observed. A mixed portal tract infiltrate and lymphoid sinusoidal infiltrate usually are seen. The disease generally resolves with appropriate antibiotic therapy (with doxycycline).

SPIROCHETAL INFECTIONS

Leptospirosis

Leptospirosis is one of the most common zoonoses in the world and has a wide range of domestic and wild animal reservoirs. Humans acquire the spirochete by contact with infected urine or contaminated soil or water. In humans, disease can occur as anicteric leptospirosis or as Weil's syndrome (described subsequently).

Anicteric leptospirosis accounts for more than 90% of cases and is characterized by a biphasic illness. The first phase begins, often abruptly, with viral illness–like symptoms associated with fever, leptospiremia, and conjunctival suffusion, which serves as an important diagnostic clue. Following a brief period of improvement, the second phase in 95% of cases is characterized by myalgias, nausea, vomiting, abdominal tenderness, and, in some cases, aseptic meningitis.[38] During this phase, a few patients have elevated serum aminotransferase and bilirubin levels with hepatomegaly.

Weil's syndrome is a severe icteric form of leptospirosis and constitutes 5% to 10% of all cases. The first phase of this illness often is marked by jaundice, which may last for weeks. During the second phase, fever may be high, and hepatic and renal manifestations predominate. Jaundice may be marked, with serum bilirubin levels approaching 30 mg/dL (predominantly conjugated). Serum aminotransferase levels usually do not exceed five times the upper limit of normal.[39] Acute tubular necrosis often develops and can lead to renal failure, which may be fatal. Hemorrhagic complications are frequent and are the result of capillary injury caused by immune complexes.[38] Spirochetes are seen in renal tubules in a majority of autopsy specimens but rarely are found in the liver. Hepatic histologic findings generally are nonspecific and do not include necrosis. Altered mitochondria and disrupted membranes in hepatocytes on electron microscopy suggest the possibility of a toxin-mediated injury.

The diagnosis of leptospirosis is made on clinical grounds in conjunction with a positive result of a blood or urine culture specimen in the first or second phase, respectively. Serologic testing confirms the diagnosis when culture results are unrevealing. Doxycycline is effective if given within the first several days of illness. Most patients recover without residual organ impairment.

Syphilis

Secondary Syphilis

Liver involvement is characteristic of secondary syphilis.[40] The frequency of hepatitis in secondary syphilis ranges from 1% to 50%.[29,40,41] Symptoms and signs usually are nonspecific, including anorexia, weight loss, fever, malaise, and sore throat. A characteristic pruritic maculopapular rash involves the palms and soles.[29] Jaundice, hepatomegaly, and tenderness in the right upper quadrant are less common. Almost all patients exhibit generalized lymphadenopathy.[29] Biochemical testing generally reveals low-grade elevations of serum aminotransferase and bilirubin levels, with a disproportionate elevation of the serum alkaline phosphatase level; isolated elevation of the alkaline phosphatase is common. Proteinuria may be present.

Histologic examination of the liver in syphilitic hepatitis generally discloses focal necrosis in the periportal and centrilobular regions. The inflammatory infiltrate typically includes polymorphonuclear neutrophils, plasma cells, lymphocytes, eosinophils, and mast cells.[29,40,41] Kupffer cell hyperplasia may be seen, but bile ductule injury is rare. Granulomas may be seen. Spirochetes may be demonstrated by silver staining in up to one half of patients. Resolution of these findings without sequelae follows treatment with penicillin.

Tertiary (Late) Syphilis

Tertiary syphilis is now rare. Although hepatic lesions are common in late syphilis, most patients are asymptomatic. Some patients describe anorexia, weight loss, fatigue, fever, or abdominal pain.[29]

The characteristic hepatic lesion in tertiary syphilis is the gumma, which can be single or multiple. It is necrotic centrally, with surrounding granulation tissue consisting of a lymphoplasmacytic infiltrate and endarteritis; exuberant deposition of scar tissue may occur, giving the liver a lobulated appearance (hepar lobatum). If hepatic involvement is unrecognized, hepatocellular dysfunction and portal hypertension with jaundice, ascites, and gastroesophageal varices can ensue.[42] Hepatic gummas may resolve after therapy with penicillin.

Lyme Disease

Lyme disease is a multisystem disease caused by the tick-borne spirochete *Borrelia burgdorferi*. Predominant manifestations are dermatologic, cardiac, neurologic, and musculoskeletal. Hepatic involvement has been described. Among 314 patients, abnormal liver biochemical test results with generally increased serum aminotransferase and lactate dehydrogenase levels were seen in 19%.[43] Clinical findings included anorexia, nausea and vomiting, weight loss, right upper quadrant pain, and hepatomegaly, usually within days to weeks of the onset of illness and often accompanied by the sentinel rash, erythema migrans.[43]

In early stages of the illness, the spirochetes are believed to disseminate hematogenously from the skin to other organs, including the liver.[44] One report has suggested that the Lyme spirochete also can cause acute hepatitis as a manifestation of reactivation,[45] although the possibility of reinfection cannot be fully excluded. Histologic examination of the liver in Lyme hepatitis reveals hepatocyte ballooning, marked mitotic activity, microvesicular fat, Kupffer cell hyperplasia, a mixed sinusoidal infiltrate, and intraparenchymal and sinusoidal spirochetes.[44]

The diagnosis of Lyme disease is confirmed with serologic studies in patients with a typical clinical history. Hepatic involvement tends to be more frequent in disseminated disease but does not appear to affect overall outcome, which is excellent in primary disease after institution of treatment with oral doxycycline, amoxicillin, clarithromycin, or azithromycin.[46] Ceftriaxone is the drug of choice for late disease.[44]

TUBERCULOSIS AND OTHER MYCOBACTERIAL INFECTIONS

Granulomas are found in liver biopsy specimens in approximately 25% of persons with pulmonary tuberculosis and 80% of those with extrapulmonary tuberculosis. Tuberculous granulomas can be distinguished from sarcoid granulomas by central caseation, acid-fast bacilli, and the presence of fewer granulomas, with a tendency to coalesce.[47] Multiple granulomas in the liver also may be seen following vaccination with bacille Calmette-Guérin, especially in persons with an impaired immune response. Patients with multiple granulomas caused by tuberculosis rarely have clinically significant liver disease. Occasionally, tender hepatomegaly is found. Jaundice with elevated serum alkaline phosphatase levels may occur in miliary infection. The treatment of tuberculous granulomatous disease of the liver is the same as that for active pulmonary tuberculosis—namely, four-drug therapy.[47] Hepatic involvement in *Mycobacterium avium* complex infection is discussed in Chapter 32.

PARASITIC INFECTIONS
(Tables 79-1 and 79-2)

PROTOZOAL INFECTIONS (see also Chapter 106)

Malaria

An estimated 300 to 500 million persons in more than 100 countries are infected with malaria each year. The liver is affected during two stages of the malarial life cycle: first in the pre-erythrocytic phase, and then in the erythrocytic phase, which coincides with clinical illness. The life cycle of the prototypical malarial parasite is illustrated in Figure 79–1.

Pathobiology of the Plasmodium Life Cycle

Malarial sporozoites injected by an infected mosquito circulate to the liver and enter hepatocytes. Maturation to schizonts ensues. When the schizont ruptures, merozoites are released into the bloodstream, where they enter erythrocytes. The four major species of *Plasmodium* responsible for malaria differ with respect to the number of merozoites released and the maturation times. Infec-

Table 79–1 Parasitic Infections of the Liver and Biliary Tree: Classification by Pathologic Process

Pathologic Process	Diseases
Hepatocellular Disease	
Granulomatous hepatitis	Schistosomiasis
	Fascioliasis
	Toxocariasis
	Capillariasis
	Strongyloidiasis
Portal fibrosis	Schistosomiasis
Hepatic abscess or necrosis	Amebic abscess
	Toxoplasmosis
Cystic liver disease	Echinococcosis
Peliosis hepatis	Bacillary angiomatosis
Reticuloendothelial Disease	
Kupffer cell infection or hyperplasia	Visceral leishmaniasis
	Malaria
	Babesiosis
	Toxoplasmosis
Biliary Disease	
Cholangitis	Fascioliasis
	Clonorchiasis/opisthorchiasis
Biliary hyperplasia	Ascariasis
	Cryptosporidiosis (see Chapter 106)
	Fascioliasis
	Clonorchiasis
Cholangiocarcinoma	Clonorchiasis/opisthorchiasis

Table 79–2 Parasitic Diseases of the Liver and Biliary Tract

Disease (Cause)	Endemic Areas	Predisposition	Pathophysiology	Manifestations	Diagnosis	Treatment*
Protozoans						
Amebiasis (*Entamoeba histolytica*)	Worldwide, especially Africa, Asia, Mexico, South America	Poor sanitation, sexual transmission	Hematogenous spread and tissue invasion, abscess formation	Fever, RUQ pain, peritonitis, elevated right hemidiaphragm	Cysts in the stool, serology (e.g., ELISA, CIE, IHA), hepatic imaging	Metronidazole 750 mg po or IV tid × 5 d or tinidazole 2 g po × 3 d, followed by diloxanide furoate 500 mg po tid × 10 d or iodoquinol 650 mg po tid × 20 d or paromomycin 25-35 mg/kg/d po in 3 divided doses × 7 d
Malaria (*Plasmodium falciparum, P. malariae, P. vivax, P. ovale*)	Africa, Asia, South America	Blood transfusion, intravenous drug use	Sporozoite clearance by hepatocytes; exoerythrocytic replication in the liver	Tender hepatomegaly: splenomegaly; rarely hepatic failure (*P. falciparum*)	Identification of the parasite on a blood smear	*P. falciparum*: Chloroquine (chloroquine-sensitive); mefloquine; or quinine and either doxycycline or clindamycin; or pyrimethamine-sulfadoxine (Fansidar); or atavaquone/proguanil (chloroquine-resistant) *P. malariae*: Chloroquine *P. vivax, P. ovale*: Chloroquine and primaquine (chloroquine-sensitive) or mefloquine and primaquine (chloroquine-resistant) (eliminate exoerythrocytic forms)
Visceral leishmaniasis (*Leishmania donovani*)	Eurasia, Central America, South America	Immunosuppression (AIDS, organ transplant)	Infection of RE cells	Fever, weight loss, hepatosplenomegaly, secondary bacterial infection, skin hyperpigmentation (kala-azar)	Amastigotes seen in the spleen, liver, or bone marrow	Pentavalent antimonial (Pentostam); or Liposomal amphotericin B IV and aminosidine; or Paromomycin; or Pentamidine; or Gamma-interferon and allopurinol (refractory cases); or Miltefosine po × 4wk (investigational)
Toxoplasmosis (*Toxoplasma gondii*)	Worldwide	Congenital infection, Immunosuppression (AIDS, organ transplant)	Replication in the liver leading to inflammation, necrosis	Fever, lymphadenopathy, occasionally hepatosplenomegaly, atypical lymphocytosis	Serology (IF, ELISA), isolation of the organism in the tissue	Pyrimethamine × 4wk and Sulfadiazine × 4-6wk and Leucovorin
Nematodes						
Ascariasis (*Ascaris lumbricoides*)	Tropical climates	Ingestion of raw vegetables	Migration of larvae to the liver; invasion of the bile ducts by adult worms	Abdominal pain, fever, jaundice, biliary obstruction, perioval granulomas	Ova or adult in stool or contrast study	Albendazole 400 mg × 1 dose; or Mebendazole 100 mg bid × 3d; or Pyrantel pamoate 11 mg/kg up to 1 g
Toxocariasis (*Toxocara canis, T. cati*)	Worldwide	Exposure to dogs or cats, especially in children younger than five years of age	Migration of larvae to the liver (visceral larva migrans)	Granuloma formation with eosinophilia	Larvae in tissue, serology (ELISA)	Diethylcarbamazine 3 mg/kg tid × 21 d; or Thiabendazole 50 mg/kg/d × 5 d; or Albendazole 5-10 mg/kg/d × 5 d

Organism	Geographic distribution	Exposure	Pathogenesis	Clinical manifestations	Diagnosis	Treatment
Hepatic capillariasis (*Capillaria hepatica*)	Worldwide	Exposure to rodents	Migration of larvae to the liver; inflammatory reaction to eggs	Acute, subacute hepatitis, tender hepatomegaly, occasionally splenomegaly, eosinophilia	Adult worms or eggs in a liver biopsy specimen	Supportive; possibly dithiazine iodide, sodium stibogluconate, albendazole, thiabendazole
Strongyloidiasis (*Strongyloides stercoralis*)	Asia, Africa, South America, Southern Europe, United States	Immunosuppression (AIDS, chemotherapy, organ transplant)	Larval penetration from the intestine to the liver	Hepatomegaly, occasionally jaundice, larvae in the portal tract or lobule	Larvae in the stool or duodenal aspirate	Ivermectin 200 µg/kg/d × 2 d; or Albendazole 400 mg/d × 3 d
Trichinosis (*Trichinella spiralis*)	Temperate climates	Ingestion of under-cooked meat	Hematogenous dissemination to the liver	Occasionally jaundice, biliary obstruction, larvae in hepatic sinusoids	History, eosinophilia, fever, muscle biopsy	Glucocorticoids for allergic symptoms Albendazole 400 mg/d × 3 d or mebendazole 200 mg/d × 5 d
Trematodes						
Schistosomiasis (*Schistosoma mansoni, S. japonicum*)	Asia, Africa, South America, Caribbean	Travelers exposed to fresh water	Fibrogenic host immune response to eggs in the portal vein	*Acute*: eosinophilic infiltrate; *chronic*: hepatosplenomegaly, presinusoidal portal hypertension, perioval granuloma formation	Ova in the stool, rectal or liver biopsy	Praziquantel 60 mg/kg in three divided doses × 1 d; or Oxamniquine 15–60 mg/kg/d × 1–2 d. Acute toxemic schistosomiasis: Praziquantel 75 mg/kg in three divided doses × 1 d
Fascioliasis (*Fasciola hepatica*)	Worldwide	Cattle or sheep raising; ingestion of contaminated watercress	Migration of larvae through the liver; penetration of the bile ducts or surgery	*Acute*: fever, abdominal pain, jaundice, hemobilia; *chronic*: hepatomegaly	Ova in the stool, flukes in the bile ducts at ERCP	Triclabendazole 10 mg/kg once
Clonorchiasis/opisthorchiasis (*Clonorchis sinensis, Opisthorchis viverrini, O. felineus*)	Southeast Asia, China, Japan, Korea, Eastern Europe	Ingestion of raw fresh-water fish	Migration through the ampulla; egg deposition in the bile ducts	Biliary hyperplasia, obstruction, sclerosing cholangitis, stone formation, cholangiocarcinoma	Ova in the stool, flukes in the bile ducts at ERCP or surgery	Praziquantel 75 mg/kg in three divided doses × 1 d
Cestodes						
Echinococcosis (*Echinococcus granulosus, E. multilocularis*)	Worldwide	Cattle and sheep raising (*E. granulosus*)	Migration of larvae to the liver; encystment (hydatid cyst)	Tender hepatomegaly, fever, eosinophilia, cyst rupture, biliary obstruction	Serology (ELISA, IHA), hepatic imaging	Surgical resection or percutaneous drainage Perioperative albendazole 400 mg bid × 8 wk

AIDS, acquired immunodeficiency syndrome; CDC, Centers for Disease Control and Prevention; CIE, counter-immunoelectrophoresis; ELISA, enzyme-linked immunosorbent assay; ERCP, endoscopic retrograde cholangiopancreatography; IF, immunofluorescence; IHA, indirect hemagglutination assay; RE, reticuloendothelial; RUQ, right upper quadrant.
*All drugs are given orally unless otherwise specified.

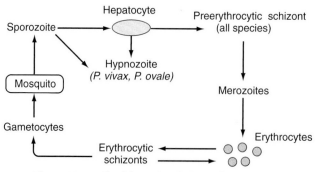

Figure 79–1 The life cycle of *Plasmodium* species.

tion by *Plasmodium falciparum* and *Plasmodium malariae* is not associated with a residual liver stage after the release of merozoites, whereas infection by *Plasmodium vivax* and *Plasmodium ovale* is associated with a persistent exoerythrocytic stage, the hypnozoite, which persists in the liver and, when activated, can divide and mature into schizont forms.

The extent of hepatic injury varies with the malarial species (most severe with *P. falciparum*) and the severity of infection. Unconjugated hyperbilirubinemia most commonly is seen as a result of hemolysis, but hepatocellular dysfunction also is possible, leading to conjugated hyperbilirubinemia. Moderate elevations of serum aminotransferase and 5'-nucleotidase levels may be observed.[48,49] Synthetic dysfunction (e.g., prolongation of the prothrombin time, hypoalbuminemia) may be seen as well. In severe falciparum malaria, hypoglycemia and lactic acidosis are late and life-threatening complications.[50] Reversible reductions in portal venous blood flow have been described during the acute phase of falciparum malaria, presumably as a consequence of micro-occlusion of portal venous branches by parasitized erythrocytes.[50]

Histopathologic Features

In acute falciparum malaria in a previously unexposed person, hepatic macrophages hypertrophy, and large quantities of malarial pigment (the result of hemoglobin degradation by the parasite) accumulate in Kupffer cells, which phagocytose parasitized and unparasitized erythrocytes.[51] Histopathologic features include Kupffer cell hyperplasia with pigment deposition and a mononuclear infiltrate. Hepatocyte swelling and centrizonal necrosis may be seen. All abnormalities are reversible with treatment.

Clinical Features

Only the erythrocytic stage of malaria is associated with clinical illness. Symptoms and signs of acute infection typically develop 30 to 60 days following exposure and include fever, which often is hectic, malaise, anorexia, nausea, vomiting, diarrhea, and myalgias. Jaundice caused by hemolysis is common in adults, especially in heavy infection with *P. falciparum*. In general, hepatic failure is seen only in association with concomitant viral hepatitis or with severe *P. falciparum* infection.[52] One series identified evidence of hepatic encephalopathy in 15 of 86 patients with falciparum malaria and jaundice; four cases were fatal.[52] Tender hepatomegaly with

splenomegaly is common.[51] Cytopenias are common in acute infection. The differential diagnosis includes viral hepatitis, gastroenteritis, amebic liver abscess, yellow fever, typhoid, tuberculosis, and brucellosis.

Diagnosis

The diagnosis of acute malaria rests on the clinical history, physical examination, and identification of parasites on peripheral thin and thick blood smears. Because the number of parasites in the blood may be small, repeated smear examinations should be performed by an experienced examiner when the index of suspicion is high. Serologic assays are more useful for chronic than for acute infection.[48,53]

Treatment

The treatment of acute malaria depends on the species of parasite, and, for falciparum infection, the pattern of chloroquine resistance. Chloroquine generally is effective for *P. malariae*, *P. vivax*, *P. ovale*, and *P. falciparum* in areas endemic for chloroquine-sensitive species. Resistant falciparum infections can be treated with mefloquine alone; quinine and either doxycycline or clindamycin; pyrimethamine-sulfadoxine (Fansidar); or a combination of atovaquone and proguanil. For *P. vivax* and *P. ovale* infections, the addition of primaquine (in persons without glucose-6-phosphate dehydrogenase deficiency) to chloroquine or mefloquine is indicated to eliminate the exoerythrocytic hypnozoites in the liver.[54]

Hyperreactive Malarial Splenomegaly (Tropical Splenomegaly Syndrome)

In endemic areas, repeated exposure to malaria may lead to an aberrant immunologic response characterized by overproduction of B lymphocytes, circulating malarial antibody, and increased levels of circulating immune complexes, resulting in dense hepatic sinusoidal lymphocytosis and stimulation of the reticuloendothelial cell system. The clinical picture includes massive splenomegaly, markedly elevated antimalarial antibody levels, and high serum immunoglobulin M (IgM) levels. Severe debilitating anemia caused by hypersplenism, especially in women of childbearing age, can result. Variceal bleeding may result from portal hypertension consequent to markedly increased splenic and portal venous blood flow but is uncommon.[55] Treatment consists of lifelong antimalarial therapy and blood transfusions.

Babesiosis

Babesiosis, caused by *Babesia* species, is a malaria-like illness transmitted by the tick *Ixodes dammini*. The disease is endemic to coastal areas of the Northeast and areas of the Midwest in the United States. Clinical features include fever, anemia, mild hepatosplenomegaly, abnormalities on liver biochemical tests, hemoglobinuria, and hemophagocytosis on bone marrow biopsy specimen. The disease is especially severe in asplenic and immunocompromised patients. In rare cases, marked pancytopenia occurs. Hepatic involvement reflects the severity of the systemic illness but generally is not severe. Uncomplicated cases are treated with oral clindamycin, 600 mg three times daily, and quinine, 650 mg three times daily for 7 days. In severe cases, the clindamycin may be given intravenously.

Leishmaniasis

Visceral leishmaniasis is caused by *Leishmania donovani* and is endemic in the Mediterranean, central Asia, the former Soviet Union, the Middle East, China, India, Pakistan, Bangladesh, Africa, Central America, and South America.[56] Amastigotes are ingested by the sand fly (*Lutzomyia* in the New World, *Phlebotomus* in the Old World) and become flagellated promastigotes. Following injection into the human host, the promastigotes are phagocytosed by macrophages in the reticuloendothelial system, where they multiply.

Histopathologic Features

In visceral leishmaniasis, organisms usually can be found in mononuclear phagocytes of the liver, spleen, bone marrow, and lymph nodes. Proliferation of Kupffer cells often is seen, and amastigotes can be detected within these cells.[57] Occasionally, parasite-bearing cells aggregate within noncaseating granulomas.[58] Hepatocyte necrosis can range in degree from mild to severe. Healing is accompanied by fibrous deposition, and occasionally the liver takes on a cirrhotic appearance. Nevertheless, complications of chronic liver disease are rare.

Clinical Features

Visceral infection caused by *L. donovani* begins with a papular or ulcerative skin lesion at the site of the sand fly bite. Following an incubation period of 2 to 6 months (sometimes years), intermittent fevers, weight loss, diarrhea (of bacillary, amebic, or leishmanial origin), and progressive painful hepatosplenomegaly develop, often accompanied by pancytopenia and a polyclonal hypergammaglobulinemia. Secondary bacterial infections resulting from suppression of reticuloendothelial cell function are important causes of mortality and include pneumonia, pneumococcal infection, and tuberculosis.

Physical findings include hepatomegaly, massive splenomegaly, jaundice or ascites in severe disease, generalized lymphadenopathy, and muscle wasting. Cutaneous gray hyperpigmentation, which prompted the name *kala-azar* (black fever), is characteristically seen in patients in India. Oral and nasopharyngeal nodules resulting from granuloma formation also may be seen.

Diagnosis

The diagnosis is based on the history, physical examination, and microscopic demonstration of amastigotes by a Wright or Giemsa stain of affected tissue samples. The highest yield (90%) comes from aspiration of the spleen. Liver biopsy is less risky and associated with a yield nearly as great as that of splenic aspiration. The yield of bone marrow aspirates is 80%, and that of lymph node aspirates is 60%.[54] Serologic testing (enzyme-linked immunosorbent assay [ELISA], immunofluorescence, direct agglutination) can be used to support a presumptive diagnosis of visceral leishmaniasis. The leishmanin skin test (Montenegro test) is not helpful in acute visceral disease.

Treatment

Pentavalent antimonial compounds are the drugs of choice for all forms of leishmaniasis. Parenteral sodium stibogluconate (Pentostam) is available through the Centers for Disease Control and Prevention for treatment of infections in the United States. Treatment with antimonials should be administered for at least 4 weeks. Gamma-interferon and allopurinol have been used in combination with antimonials in cases refractory to antimonials alone. Alternative parenteral agents include liposomal amphotericin B and aminosidine.[54] Patients with AIDS and leishmaniasis often fail to respond to or relapse following treatment with conventional regimens.[51] Miltefosine, a phosphocholine analog administered orally, has shown promise in visceral leishmaniasis, with a reported cure rate of 97% in phase II trials.[59]

Toxoplasmosis

Toxoplasmosis, caused by *Toxoplasma gondii*, is found worldwide. In the United States, serologic surveys suggest that 20% to 40% of the population has been exposed to *T. gondii*.[60] The infection may be transmitted congenitally or occur as an opportunistic infection that causes cerebral mass lesions in patients with AIDS. Oocysts of *T. gondii* in soil, water, or contaminated meat are ingested and mature in the intestinal tract of humans to become sporozoites, which penetrate the intestinal mucosa, become tachyzoites, and circulate systemically, invading a wide array of cell types.[61] Hepatic involvement has been observed in severe, disseminated infection.

Clinical Features

Acquired toxoplasmosis can manifest as a mononucleosis-like illness with fever, chills, headache, and regional lymphadenopathy. Hepatomegaly, splenomegaly, and minimal elevations of serum aminotransferase levels are uncommon findings.[62] Infections of immunocompromised hosts can result in pneumonia, myocarditis, encephalitis, and, rarely, hepatitis.[63] Toxoplasmosis can produce atypical lymphocytosis, an otherwise unusual feature of parasitic disease.

Diagnosis

The diagnosis is best made by detecting specific IgM or IgG antibody using highly specific indirect immunofluorescence or an enzyme immunoassay.[64,65] Specialized histologic staining techniques and tissue culture systems can provide adjunctive diagnostic support. PCR analysis of serum and liver also can be helpful in ambiguous cases.[66]

Treatment

Antibiotic therapy should be administered to all persons with severe symptomatic infection and to immunocompromised or pregnant patients with acute uncomplicated infection. Treatment consists of a combination of pyrimethamine for 4 weeks and sulfadiazine for 4 to 6 weeks, plus leucovorin to minimize hematologic toxicity.[64]

HELMINTHIC INFECTIONS (see also Chapter 107)

Nematodes (Roundworms)

Nematodes are nonsegmented roundworms that have a thick cuticle covering the body. Toxocariasis and capillariasis manifest with major hepatobiliary manifestations, whereas ascariasis, strongyloidiasis, and trichinosis affect the liver less frequently or less severely.

Ascariasis

Ascaris lumbricoides infects at least 1 billion persons, particularly in areas of lower socioeconomic standing.[67] Humans are infected by ingesting embryonated eggs, usually adherent to raw vegetables. The eggs hatch in the small intestine, and the larvae penetrate the mucosa, enter the portal circulation, and reach the liver, pulmonary artery, and lungs, where they grow in the alveolar spaces, are regurgitated and swallowed, and become mature adults in the intestine 2 to 3 months after ingestion, whereupon the cycle repeats itself.

Clinical Features. Symptoms generally occur in persons with a large worm burden; most infected persons are asymptomatic. Cough, fever, dyspnea, wheezing, substernal chest discomfort, and hepatomegaly may occur in the first 2 weeks. Chronic infection more frequently is characterized by episodic epigastric or periumbilical pain. If the worm burden is particularly heavy, small bowel complications such as obstruction, intussusception, volvulus, perforation, or appendicitis may occur.[68] Fragments of disintegrating worms within the biliary tree can serve as nidi for the development of biliary calculi.[69] Preexisting disease of the biliary tree or pancreatic duct can predispose the patient to migration of the worm into the bile ducts, with development of obstructive jaundice, cholangitis, or intrahepatic abscesses.[70,71] Chest radiography may show an infiltrate, and eosinophilia may be present.

Diagnosis. A history of regurgitating a worm or passing a large worm (15 to 40 cm long) in the stool suggests ascariasis. In the absence of such a history, the diagnosis is made by identification of characteristic eggs in stool specimens. Larvae also may be identified in sputum and gastric washings and in liver and lung biopsy specimens. In patients with biliary or pancreatic symptoms, ultrasonography, magnetic resonance cholangiopancreatography, or endoscopic retrograde cholangiopancreatography (ERCP) is performed. ERCP also allows extraction of the worm.[72]

Treatment. One of the following regimens may be used: (1) a single dose of albendazole, 400 mg; (2) mebendazole, 100 mg twice daily for 3 days; or (3) pyrantel pamoate, 11 mg/kg to a maximum of 1 g.[72,73] Intestinal or biliary obstruction may require endoscopic or surgical intervention.

Toxocariasis

Toxocara canis and *Toxocara cati* infect dogs and cats, respectively. Infection occurs worldwide, especially in children, and is acquired when embryonated eggs are ingested in soil or contaminated food. The eggs hatch in the small intestine and release larvae that penetrate the intestinal wall, enter the portal vein circulation, and reach the liver and systemic circulation. Blocked by narrowing vascular channels, the immature worms bore through vessel walls and migrate through the tissues, where they cause hemorrhagic, necrotic, and secondary inflammatory responses. When larvae become trapped in tissue, they provoke granuloma formation with a predominance of eosinophils. Tissue larvae may remain in inflammatory capsules or granulomas for months to years.[64] The liver, brain, and eye are affected most frequently.

Clinical Features. Most infected persons are asymptomatic. Two clinical syndromes are recognized: (1) visceral larva migrans and (2) "occult" infections associated with nonspecific symptoms, including abdominal pain, anorexia, fever, and wheezing.[74]

Visceral larva migrans is seen most commonly in children with a history of pica. Findings include fever, hepatomegaly, urticaria, leukocytosis with persistent eosinophilia, hypergammaglobulinemia, and elevated blood group isohemagglutinins.[75] Toxocariasis has been implicated in the development of chronic cholestatic hepatitis,[76] as well as pyogenic liver abscess.[77] Pulmonary manifestations include asthma and pneumonitis. Neurologic involvement can result in focal or generalized seizures, encephalopathy, and abnormal behavior.[75] Ocular larva migrans often is associated with visual loss and strabismus and can manifest as a unilateral raised retinal lesion that resembles an ocular tumor.

Diagnosis. The possibility of toxocariasis should be considered in persons with a history of pica, exposure to dogs or cats, and persistent eosinophilia. Stool studies are not useful for toxocariasis, because these organisms do not produce eggs in humans, nor do they remain in the gastrointestinal tract. A definitive diagnosis is made by identification of the larvae in affected tissues, although blind biopsies are not routinely recommended.[78] The finding of an eosinophilic granuloma may be specific for visceral larva migrans.[79] A liver biopsy may be necessary to differentiate visceral larva migrans from hepatic capillariasis (see later section). A strongly positive result on an ELISA using larval antigens provides support for the diagnosis.

Treatment. Treatment is primarily supportive. Diethylcarbamazine, 3 mg/kg three times daily for 21 days, or thiabendazole, 50 mg/kg/day for 5 days, can be given to kill larvae and prevent migration. Alternatively, albendazole, 5 to 10 mg/kg/day for 5 days, is better tolerated.[80,81] Severe pulmonary, cardiac, ophthalmologic, or neurologic manifestations may warrant use of systemic glucocorticoids.[80]

Hepatic Capillariasis

Human infection with *Capillaria hepatica* is rare. Infection with *C. hepatica* is acquired by ingesting soil, food, or water contaminated with embryonated eggs. Larvae released in the cecum penetrate the intestinal mucosa, enter the portal venous circulation, and lodge in the liver. Four weeks after infection, adult worms disintegrate, releasing eggs into the hepatic parenchyma and producing an intense inflammatory reaction with macrophages, eosinophils, and giant cells. Resolution is accompanied by marked peri-egg fibrosis.

Clinical Features. Hepatic capillariasis typically manifests as acute or subacute hepatitis. Findings include fever, nausea, vomiting, diarrhea or constipation, anorexia, myalgias, arthralgias, tender hepatomegaly, and occasionally splenomegaly. Laboratory investigation may reveal leukocytosis with eosinophilia; mild elevations of serum AST, alkaline phosphatase, and bilirubin levels; anemia; and an increased erythrocyte sedimentation rate. A chest radiograph may show pneumonitis.[82]

Diagnosis. The diagnosis is established by detection of adult worms or eggs in the liver (Fig. 79–2). Histologic findings in the liver include necrosis, fibrosis, and granulomas.[82] A finding of *C. hepatica* eggs in stools is not indicative of acute infection and probably reflects passage of undercooked liver from an infected animal.

Treatment. Treatment of hepatic capillariasis has, in general, been unsuccessful. Anecdotal benefit has been reported in cases identified at end stage with therapy with dithiazanine iodide, sodium stibogluconate, albendazole, and thiabendazole.[83,84]

Strongyloidiasis

Strongyloides stercoralis is prevalent in the tropics and subtropics, southern and eastern Europe, and the United States. Infection usually is asymptomatic. Humans are infected by the filariform larvae, which penetrate intact skin, are carried to the lungs, migrate through the alveoli, and are swallowed to reach the intestine, where maturation ensues. Autoinfection can occur if the rhabditiform larvae transform into infective filariform larvae in the intestine; reinfection occurs by penetration of the bowel wall or perianal skin. Symptomatic infection results from a heavy infectious burden or infection in an immunocompromised patient. In the latter case, a hyperinfection syndrome may result from dissemination of filariform larvae into tissues that usually are not infected.[85]

Clinical Features. Acute infection can lead to a pruritic eruption, followed by fever, cough, wheezing, abdominal pain, diarrhea, and eosinophilia. In immunocompromised patients, the hyperinfection syndrome may be characterized by invasion of any organ, including the liver, lung, and brain. When the liver is affected, features will include jaundice and cholestatic liver biochemical test abnormalities. A liver biopsy specimen may show

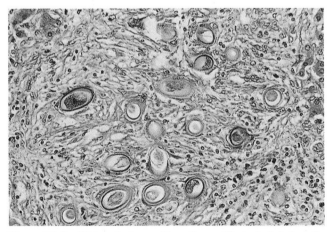

Figure 79–2   Histopathology of hepatic capillariasis. Intrahepatic granulomas surrounding numerous eggs are seen. From MacSween et al: Pathology of the Liver, 4th edition. Churchill Livingstone, 2002, p 386.

periportal inflammation, eosinophilic granulomatous hepatitis, or both. Larvae may be observed in intrahepatic bile canaliculi, lymphatic vessels, and small branches of the portal vein.[85]

Diagnosis. Serologic tests include counterimmunoelectrophoresis and ELISA, but the diagnosis rests on the identification of larvae in the stool or intestinal biopsy specimens. An obstructive hepatobiliary picture in a person with known strongyloidiasis should alert the clinician to the possibility of dissemination.

Treatment. For treatment of acute infection, the drug of choice is ivermectin, 200 mg/kg/day for 2 days. Clearance rates are high. An alternative agent is albendazole, 400 mg/day for 3 days for adults and children older than 2 years of age, but re-treatment may be necessary and this drug is less effective for disseminated disease. The hyperinfection syndrome requires longer courses of treatment than those used for the primary acute infection.[85]

Trichinosis

Humans may be infected with *Trichinella spiralis* by eating raw or undercooked pork bearing larvae, which are released in the small intestine, penetrate the mucosa, and disseminate through the systemic circulation. Larvae can be found in the myocardium, cerebrospinal fluid, brain, and, less commonly, liver and gallbladder. The larvae then re-enter the circulation and reach striated muscle, where they become encapsulated.

Clinical Features. Clinical manifestations occur when the worm burden is high and include diarrhea, fever, myalgias, periorbital edema, and leukocytosis with marked eosinophilia. Rarely, larvae can be seen invading hepatic sinusoids on examination of a liver biopsy specimen. Jaundice may result from biliary obstruction.

Diagnosis. The diagnosis is suggested by a characteristic history in a patient with fever and eosinophilia. Serologic assays for antibody to *Trichinella* may not be helpful in the acute phase of infection but can be useful after 2 weeks.[86] Muscle biopsy may help to confirm the diagnosis. DNA-based tests are investigational.

Treatment. Treatment consists of glucocorticoids to relieve allergic symptoms, followed by antihelminthic treatment with albendazole, 400 mg/day for 3 days, or mebendazole, 200 mg/day for 5 days.[86]

Trematodes (Flukes)

Schistosomiasis (Bilharziasis)

About 200 million persons are infected with trematodes of the genus *Schistosoma* worldwide. *S. mansoni* is found in the western hemisphere, Africa, and the Middle East; *S. haematobium* is found in Africa and the Middle East; *S. japonicum* and *S. mekongi* are found in the Far East; and *S. intercalatum* is found in parts of central Africa. The last two species are much less common than the other three and cause liver disease and colonic disease, respectively.[54]

The infectious cycle is initiated by penetration of the skin by free cercariae in fresh water (Fig. 79–3). The cercariae reach the pulmonary vessels within 24 hours, pass through the lungs, and reach the liver, where they lodge, develop into adults, and mate. Adult worms then migrate to their ultimate destinations in the inferior mesenteric venules (*S. mansoni*), superior mesenteric venules (*S.*

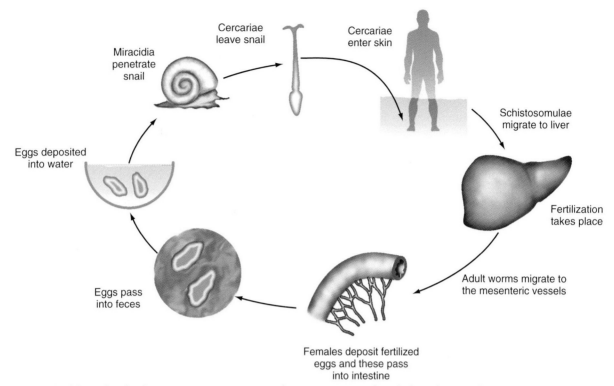

Cercariae
leave snail

Miracidia
penetrate
snail

Cercariae
enter skin

Schistosomulae
migrate to liver

Eggs deposited
into water

Fertilization
takes place

Eggs pass
into feces

Adult worms migrate to
the mesenteric vessels

Females deposit fertilized
eggs and these pass
into intestine

Figure 79–3 The life cycle of *Schistosoma* species. (From Gitlin N, Strauss R: Atlas of Clinical Hepatology. Philadelphia, WB Saunders, 1995, p 72.)

japonicum), or veins around the bladder (*S. haematobium*). These locations correlate with the clinical complications associated with each species. Each female fluke can lay 300 to 3000 eggs daily. The eggs are deposited in the terminal venules and eventually migrate into the lumen of the involved organ, after which they are expelled in the stool or urine. Eggs remaining in the organ provoke a robust granulomatous response. Excreted eggs hatch immediately in fresh water and liberate early intermediate miracidia, which infect their snail hosts. The miracidia transform into cercariae within the snails and then are released into the water, from which they may again infect humans.[87]

Clinical Features. Acute toxemic schistosomiasis (Katayama's syndrome), presumably a consequence of the host immunologic response to mature worms and eggs, occurs approximately 4 to 6 weeks after exposure. Manifestations include headache, fever, chills, cough, diarrhea, myalgias, arthralgias, tender hepatomegaly, and eosinophilia.

Untreated acute schistosomiasis invariably progresses to chronic disease. Mesenteric infection leads to hepatic complications, including periportal fibrosis, presinusoidal occlusion, and, ultimately, portal hypertension, as a result of the inflammatory reaction to eggs deposited in the liver. The development of periportal fibrosis appears to be related to production of TNF-α.[88] The lungs and central nervous system may be affected when eggs or adult worms pass through the liver into the systemic circulation, especially in *S. japonicum* infection; pulmonary hypertension and cor pulmonale may result.[51] With severe schistosomal infection, portal hypertension becomes progressive, leading to gastroesophageal varices, splenomegaly, and rarely ascites.

Chronic schistosomal infection may be complicated by increased susceptibility to *Salmonella* infections.[51] Hepatitis B viral coinfection also is common in persons living in endemic areas and may accelerate the progression of liver disease and development of hepatocellular carcinoma.[51] In African intestinal schistosomiasis, pseudopolyps of the colon may develop, leading in some cases to protein-losing enteropathy and formation of an inflammatory mass in the descending colon.

Laboratory findings in chronic schistosomiasis include anemia from recurrent luminal gastrointestinal bleeding or hypersplenism, leukocytosis with eosinophilia, an elevated erythrocyte sedimentation rate, and increased serum IgE levels. Results of liver biochemical tests generally are normal until the disease is at an advanced stage.

Diagnosis. The possibility of acute schistosomiasis should be considered in a patient with a history of exposure, abdominal pain, diarrhea, and fever. Multiple stool examinations for ova may be required to confirm the diagnosis, because results frequently are negative in the early phase of disease. Serologic testing using counterimmunoelectrophoresis or ELISA has proved useful for early diagnosis.[89] Sigmoidoscopy or colonoscopy may reveal rectosigmoid or transverse colon involvement and may be useful in chronic disease, when few eggs pass in the feces. Ultrasonography and liver biopsy are useful for demonstrating periportal ("pipestem") fibrosis (Fig. 79–4) but not for diagnosing acute infection, because of their insensitivity for detecting schistosomal eggs.

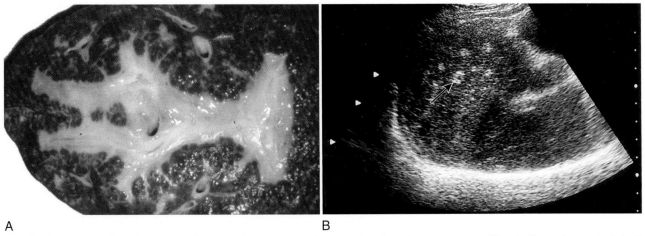

Figure 79–4 Pipestem fibrosis. *A,* Gross liver resection specimen demonstrates characteristic pipestem fibrosis due to long-term infection with *Schistosoma mansoni.* (Courtesy of Dr. Fiona Graeme-Cook, Boston, MA.) *B,* Ultrasound image of liver from a patient with schistosomiasis demonstrates the pipestem fibrosis, seen as echodense circles surrounding vessels *(arrow).* (Courtesy of Dr. Mark Feldman, Dallas, Tex.)

Treatment. Praziquantel, 60 mg/kg given in 1 day in three divided doses 4 hours apart, is the therapeutic agent of choice. Oxamniquine, 15 to 60 mg/kg for 1 to 2 days, is an effective alternative agent in patients who cannot tolerate praziquantel. Treatment of acute toxemic schistosomiasis requires praziquantel, 75 mg/kg in 1 day in three divided doses, in some cases with prednisone for the previous 2 to 3 days to suppress immune-mediated helminthicidal or drug reactions.[54]

Band ligation and injection sclerotherapy of varices are effective in controlling variceal bleeding. Management of advanced chronic schistosomal liver disease may require placement of a distal splenorenal shunt, with or without splenopancreatic disconnection, or esophagogastric devascularization with splenectomy. Fortunately, since the advent of praziquantel, complicated schistosomal liver disease has become uncommon.

Fascioliasis

Fascioliasis is endemic in parts of Europe and Latin America, North Africa, Asia, the Western Pacific, and some parts of the United States. Fascioliasis is caused by the sheep liver fluke *Fasciola hepatica.* Eggs passed in the feces of infected mammals into fresh water give rise to miracidia that penetrate snails and eventually emerge as mobile cercariae, which attach to aquatic plants such as watercress. Hosts become infected when they consume plants containing encysted metacercariae, which then bore into the intestinal wall, enter the abdominal cavity, penetrate the hepatic capsule, and eventually settle in the bile ducts, where they attain maturity. Mature flukes release eggs that are passed in the host's feces to complete the life cycle.[90]

Clinical Features. Three syndromes are recognized: acute or invasive, chronic latent, and chronic obstructive.[51,91] The acute phase corresponds to the migration of young flukes through the liver and is marked by fever, pain in the right upper quadrant, and eosinophilia. Urticaria with dermatographia and nonspecific gastrointestinal symptoms are common. A physical examination often reveals fever and a tender, enlarged liver. Splenomegaly

is seen in up to 25% of cases, but jaundice is rare and liver biochemical test abnormalities are mild. Eosinophilia can be profound, with eosinophils sometimes exceeding 80% of the differential leukocyte count.[90]

The latent phase corresponds with the settling of the flukes into the bile ducts and can last for months to years. Affected patients may experience vague gastrointestinal symptoms. Eosinophilia persists, and fever can occur.

The chronic obstructive phase is a consequence of intrahepatic and extrahepatic bile ductal inflammation and hyperplasia evoked by adult flukes. Recurrent biliary colic, cholangitis, cholelithiasis, and biliary obstruction may result. Blood loss from epithelial injury occurs, but overt hemobilia is rare. Liver biochemical testing commonly demonstrates a pattern suggestive of biliary obstruction.[90] Long-term infection may lead to biliary cirrhosis and secondary sclerosing cholangitis, but no convincing association with biliary tract or hepatic malignancy has been demonstrated.[92,93]

Diagnosis. The diagnosis should be considered in patients with prolonged fever, abdominal pain, diarrhea, tender hepatomegaly, and eosinophilia. Because eggs are not passed during the acute phase, diagnosis depends on the detection of antibody by counterimmunoelectrophoresis or ELISA. In the latent and chronic phases, a definitive diagnosis is based on the detection of eggs in stool, duodenal aspirate specimens, or bile. On occasion, ultrasonography or ERCP will demonstrate flukes in the gallbladder and common bile duct.[93-95]

Hepatic histologic findings include necrosis and granulomas with eosinophilic infiltrates and Charcot-Leyden crystals. Eosinophilic abscesses, epithelial hyperplasia of the bile ducts, and periportal fibrosis may be seen.[90]

Treatment. The drug of choice is now triclabendazole 10 mg/kg given once orally.[96] Praziquantel is not effective for fascioliasis.

Clonorchiasis and Opisthorchiasis

Clonorchis sinensis, Opisthorchis viverrini, and *Opisthorchis felineus* are trematodes of the family Opisthorchioideae.

Infection by *C. sinensis* and *O. viverrini* is widespread in East and Southeast Asia and is linked to lower socioeconomic status. *O. felineus* infects humans and domestic animals in eastern Europe. All three have similar life-cycles and result in similar clinical manifestations. Eggs are passed in the feces into fresh water, consumed by snails, and hatch as free-swimming cercariae, which seek and penetrate fish or crayfish and encyst in skin or muscle as metacercariae. The mammalian host is infected when it consumes raw or undercooked fish. The metacercariae excyst in the small bowel and migrate into the ampulla of Vater and bile ducts, where they mature into adult flukes. Infection can be maintained for 2 decades or longer.[97]

Clinical Features. In general, acute infection is clinically silent. Occasional symptoms include fever, abdominal pain, and diarrhea. Chronic manifestations correlate with the fluke burden and are dominated by hepatobiliary features: fever, pain in the right upper quadrant, tender hepatomegaly, and eosinophilia. If the worm burden in the bile ducts is heavy, chronic or intermittent biliary obstruction can ensue, with frequent cholelithiasis, cholecystitis, jaundice, and, ultimately, recurrent pyogenic cholangitis (see Chapter 65). Liver biochemical test results, especially serum alkaline phosphatase and bilirubin levels, are elevated. Long-standing infection leads to exuberant inflammation, resulting in periportal fibrosis, marked biliary epithelial hyperplasia and dysplasia, and, ultimately, a substantially increased risk of cholangiocarcinoma.[93] Cholangiocarcinoma resulting from clonorchiasis or opisthorchiasis tends to be multicentric and arises in the secondary biliary radicles of the hilum of the liver.[93] Cholangiocarcinoma should be suspected in infected persons with weight loss, jaundice, epigastric pain, or an abdominal mass.

Diagnosis. The diagnosis of clonorchiasis or opisthorchiasis is made by detection of characteristic fluke eggs in the stool, except late in the disease when biliary obstruction has supervened. In these cases, the diagnosis is made by identifying flukes in the bile ducts or gallbladder at surgery or in bile obtained by postoperative drainage or percutaneous aspiration (Fig. 79–5). Endoscopic or intraoperative cholangiography reveals slender, uniform filling defects within intrahepatic ducts that are alternately dilated and strictured, mimicking sclerosing cholangitis. Serologic methods of diagnosis generally are not helpful.[92,98-100]

Treatment. All patients with clonorchiasis or opisthorchiasis should receive praziquantel, which is uniformly effective in a dose of 75 mg/kg in three divided doses over 1 day. Side effects are uncommon and include headache, dizziness, and nausea. After treatment, dead flukes may be seen in the stool or biliary drainage. When the burden of infecting organisms is high, the dead flukes and surrounding debris or stones may cause biliary obstruction, necessitating endoscopic or surgical drainage.[92]

Cestodes (Tapeworms)

Echinococcosis*

Infections with *Echinococcus granulosus* can be found worldwide in areas where dogs are used to help raise live-

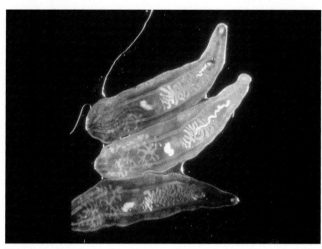

Figure 79–5 *Clonorchis sinensis.* (Courtesy of Dr. Fiona Graeme-Cook, Boston, MA.)

stock. *Echinococcus multilocularis* is distributed in northern North America and Eurasia, whereas *Echinococcus vogeli* is found in scattered areas of Central and Latin America. Infection occurs when humans eat vegetables contaminated by dog feces containing embryonated eggs. The eggs hatch in the small intestine and liberate oncospheres that penetrate the mucosa and migrate via vessels or lymphatics to distant sites. The liver is the most common destination (70%), followed by the lungs (20%), kidney, spleen, brain, and bone. In these organs, a hydatid cyst develops by vesiculation and produces thousands of protoscolices. The cyst wall contains three layers: an outer adventitial layer, which is host-derived and can calcify, and an intermediate acellular layer and inner germinal layer, which are worm-derived. A protoscolex is produced asexually within small secondary cysts that develop from the inner layer. Rupture of the hydatid cyst releases the viable protoscolices, which set up daughter cysts in secondary sites. The adult *Echinococcus* tapeworm consists of a scolex, which contains a rostellum with 20 to 50 hooklets and 4 suckers, a neck, and an immature, mature, and gravid proglottid. Dogs acquire the infection by consuming organs of sheep, cattle, or other livestock bearing the hydatid cyst.

Clinical Features. Most patients with a hydatid cyst in the liver have no symptoms. As the cysts of *E. granulosus* grow within the liver (Fig. 79–6), they begin to cause low-grade fever, pain, tender hepatomegaly (usually affecting the right hepatic lobe), and eosinophilia. If the cysts grow large enough, they may rupture spontaneously or after trauma into the lungs, leading to dyspnea and hemoptysis. More extensive rupture into the peritoneum or lungs may lead to a life-threatening anaphylactic reaction to the cyst contents. Rupture into the biliary tract can cause cholangitis and obstruction; marked eosinophilia may be present. Superinfection of the hepatic cysts can lead to pyogenic liver abscesses in up to 20% of patients with hepatic disease. In fact, echinococcal disease is the most common cause of pyogenic hepatic abscess in Greece and Spain.[101,102] Rare complications of hydatid cysts or cyst rupture include pancreatitis, portal hypertension, and rupture into the pericardial sac.

**Michael C. Kew, M.D. contributed to this section.

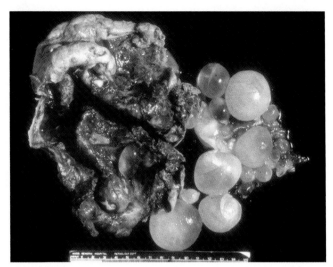

Figure 79–6 Liver resection specimen of a hydatid cyst due to *Echinococcus granulosus*. Multiple daughter cysts can be readily appreciated. (Courtesy of Dr. Fiona Graeme-Cook, Boston, MA.)

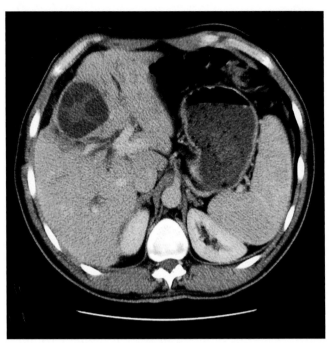

Figure 79–7 Computed tomographic scan showing the typical appearance of a hydatid cyst in the liver. (Courtesy of Dr. Mukesh Harisinghani, Boston, MA.)

E. multilocularis is highly invasive; infection leads to formation of solid masses in the liver that are easily confused with cirrhosis or carcinoma. *Alveolar hydatid disease* is the term applied to hepatic nodules that appear on microscopy as alveoli-like microvesicles.[103] Daughter cysts bud from the germinal membrane in an uncontrolled manner, with "invasion" of the surrounding liver parenchyma by the scolices. Infection of bile ducts and vessels and necrosis of parenchyma may result in cholangitis, liver abscess, sepsis, portal hypertension, hepatic vein occlusion, and biliary cirrhosis. Unfortunately, infection generally is not diagnosed until the lesions are inoperable because of extensive invasion or distant metastatic disease,[103] and mortality rates are high, approaching 90%.[103]

Infection with *E. vogeli* has clinical features intermediate between those of infections caused by the other two species and is characterized by multiple fluid-filled cysts containing daughter cysts and protoscolices. Although not as aggressive as *E. multilocularis* infection, *E. vogeli* infection can spread to contiguous sites.

Diagnosis. A history of exposure in a patient with hepatomegaly and an abdominal mass is highly suggestive of hepatic echinococcosis, but the most important diagnostic tools are radiology and serology. Ring-like calcifications in up to one fourth of hepatic cysts are visible on plain abdominal radiographs in patients infected with *E. granulosus*. The sensitivity and specificity of both ultrasonography and CT in confirming the diagnosis are high (Fig. 79–7).[102,104] Both modalities can demonstrate intracystic septations and daughter cyst formation in about one half of the cysts.[105,106] Contrast-enhanced CT may display avascular cysts with ring enhancement. Percutaneous aspiration of the cyst has traditionally been discouraged because of concern about anaphylactic reactions. Encouraging reports, however, suggest that under carefully controlled conditions, with use of thin needles and concomitant antihelminthic therapy, percutaneous aspiration for diagnosis and therapy may be safe.

The detection of protoscolices or acid-fast hooklets in the cyst fluid confirms the diagnosis.[107] An ELISA or indirect hemagglutination assay also may be used for diagnosis, with sensitivity rates of 90%.[51] Assays for detecting circulating antigen are likely to provide additional diagnostic benefit in the future. The Casoni skin test, used in the past, is nonspecific and no longer recommended.

E. multilocularis infection can be diagnosed with a combination of ELISA and CT, which often shows scattered areas of calcified necrotic tissue. In *E. vogeli* infection, CT demonstrates polycystic lesions in the liver or peritoneal space.

Treatment. In the past, accessible cysts in younger persons were always treated surgically, and surgery is still considered the preferred treatment in many cases. The goal has been removal of the cestode without disruption of cyst contents. Care must be taken to isolate the cyst and to inject cidal agents before the cyst is aspirated. Successful approaches have included cystectomy, endocystectomy, omentoplasty, and marsupialization. A laparoscopic approach is feasible in some cases. In complicated cases, hepatic lobectomy or hemihepatectomy may be necessary. Calcified cysts need not be removed.

Promising data indicate that careful percutaneous drainage is a safe and effective alternative to surgery for the treatment of complicated cysts.[108] In addition to surgery or drainage, administration of an antihelminthic, such as albendazole, 10 mg/kg/day for 8 weeks, is recommended.[108,109] A report from Europe demonstrated that *p*uncture, *a*spiration, *i*njection (of a scolicidal agent), and *r*e-aspiration (PAIR) could be performed safely with long-term control of echinococcal cysts.[110] Injection of hydatid liver cysts with albendazole has also been described.[111] Therefore, nonsurgical approaches are now available for management of hydatid cysts.[112] Cysts that cannot be treated surgically or percutaneously should be treated with albendazole, preferably, or mebendazole. Large doses and prolonged treatment are required (e.g., albendazole 10 mg/kg daily in two divided doses for 28 days, repeated three or four times, with 2-week breaks between courses).

Surgical resection is curative in up to one third of cases of *E. multilocularis* infection. In most cases the disease is advanced when the diagnosis is made. In such cases, palliative drainage procedures or long-term treatment with albendazole or other benzimidazole carbamates may prolong survival.[103,113] Surgery appears to be the most effective approach for management of *E. vogeli* infection.

FUNGAL INFECTIONS

CANDIDIASIS

Candida species may cause invasive systemic infection with hepatic involvement in severely immunocompromised persons (see Chapters 32 and 33). The liver can become infected by *C. albicans* in the setting of disseminated, multiorgan disease. Most disseminated infections occur in leukemic patients undergoing high-dose chemotherapy and become clinically evident during the period of recovery from severe neutropenia. In several series, hepatic candidiasis was present in 51% to 91% of predominantly leukemic patients with disseminated candidiasis.[114,115] Disease often is overwhelming, with high mortality rates.[115]

Other, less frequent presentations in the compromised host include isolated or focal hepatic or hepatosplenic candidiasis.[116] Focal candidiasis is believed to result from colonization of the gastrointestinal tract by *Candida*, which disseminates locally following the onset of neutropenia and mucosal injury caused by high-dose chemotherapy.[116] Resulting fungemia of the portal vein seeds the liver, leading to formation of hepatic microabscesses and macroabscesses.

In either focal or disseminated candidiasis involving the liver, clinical features include fever, abdominal pain and distention, nausea, vomiting, diarrhea, and tender hepatomegaly. The serum alkaline phosphatase level is almost invariably elevated, with varying elevations in serum aminotransferase and bilirubin levels. CT of the abdomen is the most sensitive test to detect hepatic or splenic abscesses, which often are multicentric (Fig. 79–8).[115] In cases diagnosed ante mortem, liver biopsy or laparoscopy reveals macroscopic nodules, necrosis with microabscesses, and characteristic yeast or hyphal forms of *Candida*.[117,118] The results of cultures of biopsy material are negative in most cases. PCR methodology has been used to diagnose hepatic candidiasis.[119]

Response rates to therapy with intravenous amphotericin B, 0.8 to 1.0 mg/kg per day intravenously, are better (almost 60%) for focal hepatic candidiasis than for disseminated disease. The success of treatment is currently far from optimal, however. Alternatives to amphotericin B are fluconazole, 800 mg per day intravenously; liposomal amphotericin, 5 mg/kg per day intravenously;

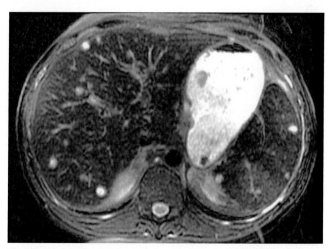

Figure 79–8 T2-weighted magnetic resonance image showing characteristic small high-intensity foci of hepatosplenic candidiasis. (Courtesy of Dr. Mukesh Harisinghani, Boston, MA.)

and, for refractory cases, intravenous caspofungin, 70 mg followed by 50 mg per day.[120]

HISTOPLASMOSIS

Infection with *Histoplasma capsulatum* is acquired through the respiratory tract and in most cases is confined to the lungs. Severely immunocompromised persons (e.g., those with AIDS), however, are predisposed to disseminated histoplasmosis (see Chapter 32). The liver can be invaded in both acute and chronic progressive disseminated histoplasmosis. Fever, oropharyngeal ulcers, hepatomegaly, and splenomegaly may be present in patients with chronic disease.[121] In children with acute hepatic disease, which appears to be an extension of primary pulmonary infection, marked hepatosplenomegaly is universal and is associated with high fever and lymphadenopathy. Serum ALT and alkaline phosphatase levels often are elevated. Hepatosplenomegaly is present in approximately 30% of adults with acute disease (often the AIDS-defining illness).

Yeast forms can be identified in liver biopsy specimens with standard hematoxylin and eosin staining. The silver methenamine method is superior for detecting yeast forms in areas of caseating necrosis or in granulomas. The organism is difficult to culture and almost never grows from biopsy specimens. Serologic testing for complement-fixing antibodies is therefore helpful in confirming the diagnosis. In immunocompromised persons who may not be capable of mounting an antibody response, detection of *H. capsulatum* antigens in urine and serum can be useful.[121] Treatment options include therapy with amphotericin B, fluconazole, or itraconazole.

LIVER ABSCESS

PYOGENIC LIVER ABSCESS

In the past, most cases of pyogenic liver abscess were a consequence of appendicitis complicated by pylephlebitis (portal vein inflammation) in a young patient. This presentation is less common today as a result of earlier diagnosis and effective antibiotic therapy. Most cases now are cryptogenic or occur in older men with underlying biliary tract disease.[122] Predisposing conditions include malignancy, immunosuppression, diabetes, and previous biliary surgery or interventional endoscopy.

Pathogenesis

Infections of the biliary tract (e.g., cholangitis, cholecystitis) are the most common identifiable source of liver abscess. Infection may spread to the liver from the bile duct, along a penetrating vessel, or from an adjacent septic focus (including pylephlebitis). Pyogenic liver abscess may arise as a late complication of endoscopic sphincterotomy for bile duct stones or within 3 to 6 weeks of a surgical biliary–intestinal anastomosis.[122] Pyogenic liver abscesses may complicate recurrent pyogenic cholangitis, which is found predominantly in East and Southeast Asia and is characterized by recurring episodes of cholangitis, intrahepatic stone formation, and, in many cases, biliary parasitic infections (see Chapter 65). Less commonly, liver abscess is a complication of bacteremia arising from underlying abdominal disease, such as diverticulitis, perforated or penetrating peptic ulcer, gastrointestinal malignancy, inflammatory bowel disease, or peritonitis, or rarely from bacterial endocarditis or penetration of a foreign body through the wall of the colon. The risk of liver abscess and associated mortality rate may be increased in patients with cirrhosis.[123] Occasionally, a pyogenic liver abscess may be the presentation of a hepatocellular or gallbladder carcinoma or a complication of chemoembolization or percutaneous ablation of a hepatic neoplasm.[124]

In approximately 40% of cases of pyogenic liver abscess, no obvious source of infection can be identified. Oral flora have been proposed to be a potential source in such cases, particularly in patients (often alcoholics) with severe periodontal disease.

Microbiology

Most pyogenic liver abscesses are polymicrobial.[125] The bacterial organisms that have been cultured from liver abscesses are listed in Table 79–3. The most frequently isolated organisms are *Escherichia coli* and *Klebsiella*, *Proteus*, *Pseudomonas*, and *Streptococcus* species, particularly *Streptococcus milleri*. With improved cultivation methods and earlier diagnosis, the number of cases caused by anaerobic organisms has increased. The most commonly identified anaerobic species are *Bacteroides fragilis* and *Fusobacterium necrophorum*; anaerobic streptococci also have been identified. Pyogenic abscess associated with recurrent pyogenic cholangitis may be caused by *Salmonella typhi*. *Clostridium* and *Actinomyces* species are uncommon causes of liver abscess, and rare cases are caused by *Yersinia enterocolitica*, *Pasteurella multocida*, *Haemophilus parainfluenzae*, and *Listeria* species. Septic melioidosis also has been described. Liver abscesses caused by *Staphylococcus aureus* infection are most common in children and patients with septicemia or other conditions associated with impaired host resistance, including chronic granulomatous disease.[126] Fungal abscesses of the liver may occur in immunocompromised hosts, particularly those with a hematologic malignancy.[114]

Clinical Features and Diagnosis

In the preantibiotic era, patients with a pyogenic liver abscess typically presented with acutely spiking fevers, pain in the right upper quadrant, and, in many cases, shock. After the introduction of antibiotics, the presentation of pyogenic liver abscess became less acute. Today's presentation often is insidious, particularly in elderly patients, and is characterized by malaise, low-grade fever, weight loss, and dull abdominal pain that may increase with movement. Symptoms may be present for 1 month or more before a diagnosis is made. Multiple abscesses are typical when biliary disease is the source and are associated with a more acute systemic presentation, often with sepsis and shock, than is the case with solitary abscesses. When an abscess is situated near the dome of the liver, pain may be referred to the right shoulder, or a cough resulting from diaphragmatic irritation or atelectasis may be present.

A physical examination usually discloses fever, hepatomegaly, and liver tenderness, which is accentuated

Table 79–3   Organisms That May Be Isolated from the Abscess and the Blood in Patients with a Pyogenic Liver Abscess

Gram-Negative Aerobes	Gram-Positive Aerobes	Anaerobes	Others
Escherichia coli	Enterococci	*Bacteroides*	*Candida albicans*
Klebsiella pneumoniae	*Streptococcus pyogenes*	*Fusobacterium*	*Mycobacterium tuberculosis*
Enterobacter	*Staphylococcus aureus*	Streptococci	
Pseudomonas	*Streptococcus milleri*	*Peptostreptococcus*	
Citrobacter	*Listeria monocytogenes**	*Peptococcus*	
Morganella	*Bacillus cereus**	*Prevotella**	
Proteus		*Clostridium**	
Salmonella		*Actinomyces**	
*Serratia marcescens**			
*Yersinia**			
*Burkholderia pseudomallei**			
*Capnocytophaga canimorsus**			
*Pasteurella multocida**			
*Achromobacter xylosoxidans**			

*Rare cause.

by movement or percussion. Splenomegaly is unusual, except with a chronic abscess. Ascites is rare, and in the absence of cholangitis, jaundice is present only late in the course of the illness. Portal hypertension may follow recovery if the portal vein has been thrombosed.

Laboratory findings include anemia, leukocytosis, an elevated erythrocyte sedimentation rate, and abnormal liver biochemical test results, especially an elevated serum alkaline phosphatase level. Blood culture specimens will identify the causative organism in at least 50% of cases. Chest x-rays may show elevation of the right hemidiaphragm and atelectasis.

Ultrasonography and CT are the initial imaging modalities of choice.[127] Abscesses as small as 1 cm in diameter can be detected. Ultrasonography is inexpensive and accurate and can guide needle aspiration of the abscess. Culture specimens of aspirated material yield positive results in 90% of cases (although the yield probably is lower if the patient has been receiving antibiotics). CT also is accurate, with a sensitivity rate approaching 100%, but is more expensive than ultrasonography. Hepatic abscesses are usually hypodense on a CT scan and may display a rim of contrast enhancement in less than 20% of cases (Fig. 79–9). CT permits precise localization of an abscess, assessment of its relationship to adjacent structures, and detection of gas in the abscess, which is associated with increased mortality. An abscess must be distinguished from other mass lesions in the liver, including cystic lesions, benign and malignant neoplasms, soft tissue tumors (neurofibroma, leiomyoma, and malignant fibrous histiocytoma), focal nodular hyperplasia, and hemangiomas (see Chapter 91), as well as inflammatory pseudotumors. Magnetic resonance imaging is more sensitive than CT for detecting small abscesses, which have low signal intensity on T1-weighted images and high signal intensity on T2-weighted images and enhance with gadolinium. ERCP is indicated in patients with imaging evidence of biliary stones or prominent cholesta-

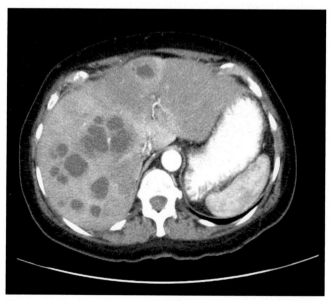

Figure 79–9   Computed tomographic scan showing multiple pyogenic abscesses in the liver. (Courtesy of Dr. Mukesh Harisinghani, Boston, MA.)

sis.[128] Rarely, arteriography may be of value in distinguishing an abscess from a tumor.

Inflammatory pseudotumor of the liver (also called plasma cell granuloma) is a rare, benign lesion characterized by proliferating fibrous tissue infiltrated by inflammatory cells. The cause is unknown. Affected persons (typically young men) often have a history of recent infection, but a causative infectious agent is rarely isolated from the lesion. Additional associated disorders include chronic inflammatory and autoimmune disorders, particularly ascending cholangitis and primary sclerosing cholangitis, as well as diabetes, Sjögren's syndrome, gout, ulcerative colitis, Crohn's disease, HIV infection, Epstein-Barr virus infection, and acute myeloblastic leukemia. Patients typically present with intermittent fever, abdominal discomfort, vomiting, diarrhea, weight loss, and malaise and have hepatomegaly, right upper quadrant tenderness, and jaundice on physical examination. Portal hypertension may develop. Laboratory findings also are similar to those associated with liver abscess, including polyclonal hyperglobulinemia in 50% of cases, and imaging studies generally are interpreted as showing a tumor or an abscess. Treatment generally has been by surgical resection of the lesion, although some patients may recover spontaneously or after treatment with antibiotics or glucocorticoids, once the diagnosis is made on the basis of needle biopsy findings.[129,130]

Prevention and Treatment

Pyogenic liver abscesses are best prevented by prompt treatment of acute biliary and abdominal infections and by adequate drainage of infected intra-abdominal collections under appropriate antibiotic coverage. Treatment of a hepatic abscess requires antibiotic therapy directed at the causative organism(s) and, in most cases, drainage of the abscess, usually percutaneously with radiologic guidance. An indwelling drainage catheter may be placed in the abscess until the cavity has resolved, although intermittent needle aspiration may be as effective as continuous catheter drainage.[131] With multiple abscesses, only the largest abscess may need to be aspirated; smaller lesions often resolve with antibiotic treatment alone, but rarely, each lesion may need drainage. For a small abscess, antibiotic therapy without drainage may suffice. Biliary decompression is essential when a hepatic abscess is associated with biliary tract obstruction or communication and may be accomplished through the endoscopic or transhepatic route (see Chapter 67). Surgical drainage of a hepatic abscess may be necessary in patients with incomplete percutaneous drainage, unresolved jaundice, renal impairment, a multiloculated abscess, or a ruptured abscess.[132] A laparoscopic approach may be feasible in select cases.

Initial antibiotic coverage, pending culture results, should be broad spectrum and include ampicillin and an aminoglycoside (when a biliary source is suspected) or a third-generation cephalosporin (when a colonic source is suspected), plus, in either case, metronidazole, to cover anaerobic organisms. If amebiasis is suspected, metronidazole should be started before aspiration is performed. After culture results and sensitivity profiles have been obtained, antibiotic therapy directed at the specific organism(s) should be administered intravenously for at least 2 weeks and then orally for up to 6 weeks.[133] For streptococcal infections, the use of high-dose oral antibiotics for 6 months may be preferable.

The mortality rate for patients with hepatic abscesses treated with antibiotics and percutaneous drainage has improved over the past 3 decades but remains at least 6%.[132] A worse prognosis is associated with a delay in diagnosis, multiple abscesses, multiple organisms cultured from blood, a fungal cause, shock, jaundice, hypoalbuminemia, a pleural effusion, an underlying biliary malignancy, multiorgan dysfunction, or other associated medical diseases.[122,132,134,135] Complications of pyogenic liver abscess include empyema, pleural or pericardial effusion, portal or splenic vein thrombosis, rupture into the pericardium, thoracic and abdominal fistula formation, and sepsis. Metastatic septic endophthalmitis occurs in up to 10% of diabetic patients with a liver abscess caused by *Klebsiella pneumoniae*.[136]

AMEBIC LIVER ABSCESS

Pathogenesis

Amebiasis occurs in 10% of the world's population and is most common in tropical and subtropical regions (see also Chapter 106).[137,138] In the United States, it is a disease of young, often Hispanic adults. Endemic areas include Africa, Southeast Asia, Mexico, Venezuela, and Colombia. Amebic liver abscess is the most common extraintestinal manifestation of amebiasis. Compared with affected persons who reside in an endemic area, persons in whom an amebic liver abscess develops after travel to an endemic area are older and more likely to be male, have

marked hepatomegaly, and have a large abscess or multiple abscesses. The occurrence of an amebic liver abscess in a person who has not traveled to or resided in an endemic area should raise the suspicion of underlying immunosuppression, particularly AIDS.[139] Other persons at increased risk include inpatients in residential institutions and men who have sex with men. Host factors that contribute to the severity of disease include younger age, pregnancy, malnutrition, alcoholism, glucocorticoid use, and malignancy.

During its life cycle, *Entamoeba histolytica* exists as trophozoite or cyst forms (Fig. 79–10). After infection, amebic cysts pass through the gastrointestinal tract and become trophozoites in the colon, where they invade the mucosa and produce typical "flask-shaped" ulcers. The organism is carried by the portal vein circulation to the liver, where an abscess may develop. Occasionally, organisms travel beyond the liver and can establish abscesses in the lung or brain. Rupture of an amebic liver abscess into the pleural, pericardial, and peritoneal spaces can also occur.

Clinical Features

Amebic liver abscess is 10 times as common in men as in women and is rare in children.[137] An amebic liver abscess is more likely than a pyogenic liver abscess to be associated with an acute presentation. Symptoms are present on average for 2 weeks by the time a diagnosis is made. A latency period between intestinal and subsequent liver infection of up to many years is possible, and less than 10% of patients report an antecedent history of bloody diarrhea with amebic dysentery.

Abdominal pain is typically well localized to the right upper quadrant. Fever is nearly universal but may be intermittent. Malaise, myalgias, and arthralgias are

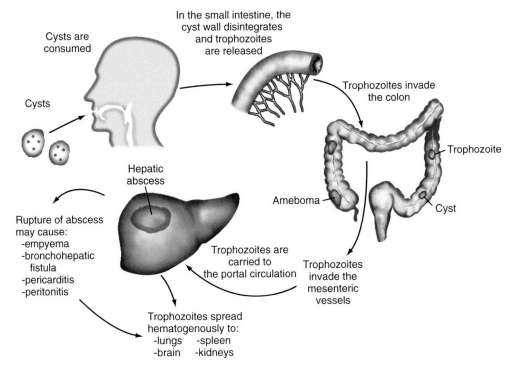

Figure 79–10 The life cycle of *Entamoeba histolytica* in amebiasis. (From Gitlin N, Strauss R: Atlas of Clinical Hepatology. Philadelphia, WB Saunders, 1995, p 64.)

Table 79–4   Pyogenic and Amebic Liver Abscess: Clinical Distinctions

Parameter	Pyogenic Liver Abscess	Amebic Liver Abscess
Number	Often multiple	Usually single
Location	Either lobe of liver	Usually right hepatic lobe, near the diaphragm
Presentation	Subacute	Acute
Jaundice	Mild, if present	Moderate, if present
Diagnosis	US or CT ± aspiration	US or CT and serology
Treatment	IV antibiotics ± drainage	Metronidazole, 750 mg tid for 5 d orally *or* IV, *or* tinidazole, 2 g orally for 3 d, *followed by* iodoquinol, 650 mg orally tid for 20 d; diloxanide furoate, 500 mg orally tid for 10 d; or paromomycin 25-35 mg/kg/d orally in three divided doses for 7 d

CT, computed tomography; IV, intravenous; US, ultrasonography.

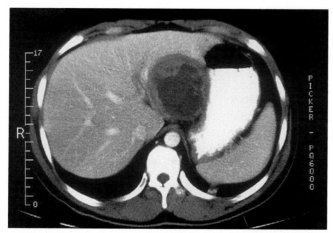

Figure 79–11 Computed tomographic scan showing a large amebic abscess in the left lobe of the liver. (Courtesy of Dr. Mark Feldman, Presbyterian Hospital, Dallas, Tex.)

common. Jaundice is uncommon and signifies a poor prognosis. Pulmonary symptoms and signs may be present, but a pericardial rub and peritonitis are rare. Occasionally a friction rub is heard over the liver. Laboratory features resemble those found in pyogenic abscess.

Diagnosis

The diagnosis of amebic liver abscess is based on clinical suspicion, hepatic imaging, and serologic testing. The organism is isolated from the stool in only 50% of cases. Hepatic imaging studies cannot distinguish a pyogenic from an amebic liver abscess (Fig. 79–11). An amebic abscess is commonly localized to the right hepatic lobe, close to the diaphragm, and usually is single (Table 79–4). Available serologic tests include an ELISA and indirect hemagglutination, cellulose acetate precipitin, counter-immunoelectrophoresis, immunofluorescent antibody, and rapid latex agglutination tests. Serologic test results must be interpreted in the clinical context, because serum antibody levels may remain elevated for years after recovery or cure. The sensitivity of these tests is approximately 95%, and the specificity is over 95%. False-negative results may occur within the first 10 days of infection.[138] PCR-based tests to detect amebic DNA and an ELISA to detect amebic antigens in serum are available in the research setting.[137,138,140]

Aspiration of an amebic abscess should be performed if the diagnosis remains uncertain. The presence of a reddish-brown pasty aspirate ("anchovy paste" or "chocolate sauce") is typical; trophozoites rarely are identified. Aspiration also may be considered in rare cases when no response to antibiotic therapy has occurred after 5 to 7 days or when an abscess in the left lobe of the liver is close to the pericardium.[137]

Treatment

Standard therapy consists of metronidazole, 750 mg three times daily by mouth or, if necessary, intravenously for 5 to 10 days. Tinidazole or chloroquine may be substituted for metronidazole. The response to treatment usually occurs within 96 hours. Following a course of metronidazole, most authorities recommend the addition of an oral luminal amebicide—such as iodoquinol, 650 mg three times daily for 20 days; diloxanide furoate, 500 mg three times daily for 10 days; or paromomycin 25 to 35 mg/kg daily in three divided doses for 7 days—to eradicate residual amebae in the gut. Pyogenic coinfection of an amebic liver abscess is uncommon. Rare complications of amebic abscesses can include intraperitoneal, intrathoracic, and pericardial rupture and multiorgan failure. The development of a vaccine against *E. histolytica* has been hampered in part because natural infection does not result in long-term immunity.

REFERENCES

1. Stevens DL: The toxic shock syndromes. Infect Dis Clin North Am 10:727, 1996.
2. Meer RR, Songer JG, Park DL: Human disease associated with *Clostridium perfringens* enterotoxin. Rev Environ Contam Toxicol 150:75, 1997.
3. Chen YM, Lee HC, Chang CM, et al: *Clostridium* bacteremia: Emphasis on the poor prognosis in cirrhotic patients. J Microbiol Immunol Infect 34:113, 2001.
4. Jonas RB, Brasitus TA, Chowdhury L: Actinomycotic liver abscess: Case report and literature review. Dig Dis Sci 32:1435, 1987.
5. Weese WC, Smith IM: A study of 57 cases of actinomycosis over a 36-year period: A diagnostic "failure" with good prognosis after treatment. Arch Intern Med 135:1562, 1975.
6. Miyamoto MI, Fang FC: Pyogenic liver abscess involving *Actinomyces*: Case report and review. Clin Infect Dis 16:303, 1993.

7. Sharma M, Briski LE, Khatib R: Hepatic actinomycosis: An overview of salient features and outcome of therapy. Scand J Infect Dis 34:386, 2002.

8. Yu VL, Miller WP, Wing EJ, et al: Disseminated listeriosis presenting as acute hepatitis: Case reports and review of hepatic involvement in listeriosis. Am J Med 73:773, 1982.

9. Hof H, Nichterlein T, Kretschmar M: Management of listeriosis. Clin Microbiol Rev 10:345, 1997.

10. Stern MS, Gitnick GL: *Shigella* hepatitis. JAMA 235:2628, 1976.

11. Nasrallah SM, Nassar VH: Enteric fever: A clinicopathologic study of 104 cases. Am J Gastroenterol 69:63, 1978.

12. Pramoolsinsap C, Viranuvatti V: *Salmonella* hepatitis. J Gastroenterol Hepatol 13:745, 1998.

13. Chaudhry R, Mahajan RK, Diwan A, et al: Unusual presentation of enteric fever: Three cases of splenic and liver abscesses due to *Salmonella typhi* and *Salmonella paratyphi* A. Trop Gastroenterol 24:198, 2003.

14. Kamath PS, Jalihal A, Chakraborty A: Differentiation of typhoid fever from fulminant hepatic failure in patients presenting with jaundice and encephalopathy. Mayo Clin Proc 75:462, 2000.

15. Rajagopal A, Ramasamy R, Mahendran G, Thomas M: Hepatic abscess complicating paratyphoid infection. Trop Gastroenterol 23:181, 2002.

16. Strungs I, Farrell DJ, Matar LD, et al: Multiple hepatic abscesses due to *Yersinia enterocolitica*. Pathology 27:374, 1995.

17. Bergmann TK, Vinding K, Hey H: Multiple hepatic abscesses due to *Yersinia enterocolitica* infection secondary to primary haemochromatosis. Scand J Gastroenterol 36:891, 2001.

18. Hopfner M, Nitsche R, Rohr A, et al: *Yersinia enterocolitica* infection with multiple liver abscesses uncovering a primary hemochromatosis. Scand J Gastroenterol 36:220, 2001.

19. Holmes KK, Counts GW, Beaty HN: Disseminated gonococcal infection. Ann Intern Med 74:979, 1071.

20. Ross JD: Systemic gonococcal infection. Genitourin Med 72:404, 1996.

21. Cunha BA: Clinical features of Legionnaires' disease. Semin Respir Infect 13:116, 1998.

22. White NJ: Melioidosis. Lancet 361:1715, 2003.

23. Leelarasamee A: Melioidosis in Southeast Asia. Acta Trop 74:129, 2000.

24. Ablin J, Mevorach D, Eliakim R: Brucellosis and the gastrointestinal tract: The odd couple. J Clin Gastroenterol 24:25, 1997.

25. Colmenero J de D, Queipo-Ortuno MI, Maria Reguera J, et al: Chronic hepatosplenic abscesses in brucellosis: Clinicotherapeutic features and molecular diagnostic approach. Diagn Microbiol Infect Dis 42:159, 2002.

26. Ariza J, Pigrau C, Canas C, et al: Current understanding and management of chronic hepatosplenic suppurative brucellosis. Clin Infect Dis 32:1024, 2001.

27. Zaidi SA, Singer C: Gastrointestinal and hepatic manifestations of tickborne diseases in the United States. Clin Infect Dis 34:1206, 2002.

28. Rice PS, Kudesia G, McKendrick MW, Cullen DR: *Coxiella burnetii* serology in granulomatous hepatitis. J Infect 27:63, 1993.

29. Albrecht H: Bacterial and miscellaneous infections of the liver. In Zakim DS, Boyer TD (eds): Hepatology: A Textbook of Liver Disease, 4th ed. Philadelphia, WB Saunders, 2003, p 1109.

30. Tompkins DC, Steigbigel RT: *Rochalimaea's* role in cat scratch disease and bacillary angiomatosis. Ann Intern Med 118:388, 1993.

31. Cotell SL, Noskin GA: Bacillary angiomatosis: Clinical and histologic features, diagnosis, and treatment. Arch Intern Med 154:524, 1994.

32. Gasquet S, Maurin M, Brouqui P, et al: Bacillary angiomatosis in immunocompromised patients. AIDS 12:1793, 1998.

33. Roelofsen H, Schoemaker B, Bakker C, et al: Impaired hepatocanalicular organic anion transport in endotoxemic rats. Am J Physiol 269(3 pt 1):G427, 1995.

34. Moseley RH: Sepsis-associated jaundice. Hepatology 24:969, 1996.

35. Lee SM: Viscerotropic Rocky Mountain spotted fever in southeastern Texas: Report of a survivor with atypical manifestations and multiple organ failure. South Med J 82:640, 1989.

36. Adams JS, Walker DH: The liver in Rocky Mountain spotted fever. Am J Clin Pathol 75:156, 1981.

37. Katz B, Waites K: Emerging intracellular bacterial infections. Clin Lab Med 24:627, 2004.

38. Sperber SJ, Schleupner CJ: Leptospirosis: A forgotten cause of aseptic meningitis and multisystem febrile illness. South Med J 82:1285, 1989.

39. Feigin RD, Anderson DC: Human leptospirosis. CRC Crit Rev Clin Lab Sci 5:413, 1975.

40. Baker AL, Kaplan MM, Wolfe HJ, McGowan JA: Liver disease associated with early syphilis. N Engl J Med 284:1422, 1971.

41. Feher J, Somogyi T, Timmer M, Jozsa L: Early syphilitic hepatitis. Lancet 2:896, 1975.

42. Klatskin G: Hepatitis associated with systemic infections. In Schiff L (ed): Diseases of the Liver. Philadelphia, JB Lippincott, 1975, p 711.

43. Steere AC, Bartenhagen NH, Craft JE, et al: The early clinical manifestations of Lyme disease. Ann Intern Med 99:76, 1983.

44. Nadelman RB, Wormser GP: Lyme borreliosis. Lancet 352:557, 1998.

45. Goellner MH, Agger WA, Burgess JH, Duray PH: Hepatitis due to recurrent Lyme disease. Ann Intern Med 108:707, 1988.

46. Horowitz HW, Dworkin B, Forseter G, et al: Liver function in early Lyme disease. Hepatology 23:1412, 1996.

47. Alvarez SZ: Hepatobiliary tuberculosis. J Gastroenterol Hepatol 13:833, 1998.

48. World Health Organization: WHO expert committee on malaria: 18th report. Tech Rep Ser 735, WHO, Geneva, 1986.

49. Ghoda MK: Falciparum hepatopathy: A reversible and transient involvement of liver in falciparum malaria. Trop Gastroenterol 23:70, 2002.

50. Molyneux ME, Looareesuwan S, Menzies IS, et al: Reduced hepatic blood flow and intestinal malabsorption in severe falciparum malaria. Am J Trop Med Hyg 40:470, 1989.

51. Dunn M: Parasitic diseases. In Schiff ER, Sorrell MF, Maddrey WC (eds.): Diseases of the Liver, 9th ed. Philadelphia, Lippincott Williams & Wilkins, 2003, p 1509.

52. Kochar DK, Agarwal P, Kochar SK, et al. Hepatocyte dysfunction and hepatic encephalopathy in *Plasmodium falciparum* malaria. Q J Med 96:505, 2003.

53. Strickland G: Malaria. In Strickland GT (ed): Hunter's Tropical Medicine, 7th ed. Philadelphia, WB Saunders, 1991, p 586.

54. Murray H, Pepin J, Nutman T, et al: Tropical medicine. BMJ 320:490, 2000.

55. Bates I: Hyperreactive tropical splenomegaly in preganancy. Trop Doct 21:101, 1991.

56. Smith D: Visceral leishmaniasis: Human aspects. In Gilles HM (ed): Recent Advances in Tropical Medicine. Edinburgh, Churchill Livingstone, 1984, p 797.

57. Sen PG: The liver in kala-azar. Ann Trop Med Parasitol 50:252, 1956.

58. Moreno A, Marazuela M, Yebra M, et al: Hepatic fibrin-ring granulomas in visceral leishmaniasis. Gastroenterology 95:1123, 1988.

59. Jha TK, Sundar S, Thakur CP, et al: Miltefosine, an oral agent, for the treatment of Indian visceral leishmaniasis. N Engl J Med 341:1795, 1999.

60. Sever JL, Ellenberg JH, Ley AC, et al: Toxoplasmosis: Maternal and pediatric findings in 23,000 pregnancies. Pediatrics 82:181, 1988.

61. Frenkel J: Pathophysiology of toxoplasmosis. Parasitol Today 4:273, 1988.

62. Benenson MW, Takafuji ET, Lemon SM, et al: Oocyst-transmitted toxoplasmosis associated with ingestion of contaminated water. N Engl J Med 307:666, 1982.

63. Ruskin J, Remington JS: Toxoplasmosis in the compromised host. Ann Intern Med 84:193, 1976.

64. Bryan R, Michelson M: Parasitic infections of the liver and biliary tree. In Surawicz C, Owen RL (eds): Gastrointestinal and Hepatic Infections. Philadelphia, WB Saunders, 1995, p 405.

65. Vischer TL, Bernheim C, Engelbrecht E: Two cases of hepatitis due to *Toxoplasma gondii*. Lancet 2:919, 1967.

66. Botterel F, Ichai P, Feray C, et al: Disseminated toxoplasmosis, resulting from infection of allograft, after orthotopic liver transplantation: Usefulness of quantitative PCR. J Clin Microbiol 40:1648, 2002.

67. World Health Organization: Prevention and control of intestinal parasitic infections: Report of a WHO expert committee. Tech Rep Ser 749, WHO, Geneva, 1987.

68. Thein H: A profile of ascariasis morbidity in Rangoon Children's Hospital, Burma. J Trop Med Hyg 90:165, 1987.

69. Schulman A: Non-western patterns of biliary stones and the role of ascariasis. Radiology 162:425, 1987.

70. Uflacker R, Duarte D, Silva P: Association of congenital cystic dilatation of the common bile duct and congenital diverticulum of the hepatic duct with concomitant ascariasis. Gastrointest Radiol 3:407, 1978.

71. Javid G, Wani NA, Gulzar GM, et al: Ascaris-induced liver abscess. World J Surg 23:1191, 1999.

72. Khuroo MS: Ascariasis. Gastroenterol Clin North Am 25:553, 1996.

73. Cline BL: Current drug regimens for the treatment of intestinal helminth infections. Med Clin North Am 66:721, 1982.

74. Taylor M, Keane C, O'Connor P, et al: The expanded spectrum of toxocaral disease. Lancet 1:692, 1988.

75. Huntley CC, Costas MC, Lyerly A: Visceral larva migrans syndrome: Clinical characteristics and immunologic studies in 51 patients. Pediatrics 36:523, 1965.

76. Hartleb M, Januszewski K: Severe hepatic involvement in visceral larva migrans. Eur J Gastroenterol Hepatol 13:1245, 2001.

77. Rayes AA, Teixeira D, Serufo JC, et al: Human toxocariasis and pyogenic liver abscess: A possible association. Am J Gastroenterol 96:563, 2001.

78. Nichols RL: The etiology of visceral larva migrans. I. Diagnostic morphology of infective second-stage *Toxocara* larvae. J Parasitol 42(4 section 1):349, 1956.

79. Kaplan KJ, Goodman ZD, Ishak KG: Eosinophilic granuloma of the liver: A characteristic lesion with relationship to visceral larva migrans. Am J Surg Pathol 25:1316, 2001.

80. World Health Organization: WHO model-prescribing information: Drugs used in parasitic diseases, 2nd ed. Geneva: World Health Organization, 1995.

81. Overgaauw PA: Aspects of *Toxocara* epidemiology: Human toxocarosis. Crit Rev Microbiol 23:215, 1997.

82. Grencis RK, Cooper ES: *Enterobius, Trichuris, Capillaria*, and hookworm including *Ancylostoma caninum*. Gastroenterol Clin North Am 25:579, 1996.

83. Berger T, Degremont A, Gebbers JO, Tonz O: Hepatic capillariasis in a 1-year-old child. Eur J Pediatr 149:333, 1990.

84. Sawamura R, Fernandes MI, Peres LC, et al: Hepatic capillariasis in children: Report of 3 cases in Brazil. Am J Trop Med Hyg 61:642, 1999.

85. Mahmoud AA: Strongyloidiasis. Clin Infect Dis 23:949, 1996.

86. Capo V, Despommier DD: Clinical aspects of infection with *Trichinella* spp. Clin Microbiol Rev 9:47, 1996.

87. World Health Organization: The control of schistosomiasis. Tech Rep Ser 728, WHO, Geneva, 1985.

88. Henri S, Chevillard C, Mergani A, et al: Cytokine regulation of periportal fibrosis in humans infected with *Schistosoma mansoni*: IFN-gamma is associated with protection against fibrosis and TNF-alpha with aggravation of disease. J Immunol 169:929, 2002.

89. Hancock K, Tsang V: Development and optimization of the FAST-ELISA for detecting antibodies to *Schistosoma mansoni*. J Immunol 92:167, 1986.

90. Bunnag D, Thanongsak B, Goldsmith R: Fascioliasis. In Strickland GT (ed): Hunter's Tropical Medicine, 7th ed. Philadelphia, WB Saunders, 1991, p 823.

91. Sezgin O, Altintas E, Disibeyaz S, et al. Hepatobiliary fascioliasis: Clinical and radiologic features and endoscopic management. J Clin Gastroenterol 38:285, 2004.

92. Chan CW, Lam SK: Diseases caused by liver flukes and cholangiocarcinoma. Baillieres Clin Gastroenterol 1:297, 1987.

93. Osman M, Lausten SB, El-Sefi T, et al: Biliary parasites. Dig Surg 15:287, 1998.

94. Takeyama N, Okumura N, Sakai Y, et al: Computed tomography findings of hepatic lesions in human fascioliasis: Report of two cases. Am J Gastroenterol 81:1078, 1986.

95. Van Beers B, Pringot J, Geubel A, et al: Hepatobiliary fascioliasis: Noninvasive imaging findings. Radiology 174(3 pt 1):809, 1990.

96. Loutan L, Bouvier M, Rojanawisut B, et al: Single treatment of invasive fascioliasis with triclabendazole. Lancet 2:383, 1989.

97. Bunnag D, Thanongsak B, Goldsmith R: Clonorchiasis. In Strickland GT (ed): Hunter's Tropical Medicine, 7th ed. Philadelphia, WB Saunders, 1991, p 822.

98. Dennis MJ, Dennison AR, Morris DL: Parasitic causes of obstructive jaundice. Ann Trop Med Parasitol 83:159, 1989.

99. Wang KX, Zhang RB, Cui YB, et al: Clinical and epidemiological features of patients with clonorchiasis. World J Gastroenterol 10:446, 2004.

100. Mairiang E, Mairiang P: Clinical manifestation of opisthorchiasis and treatment. Acta Trop 88:221, 2003.

101. Schantz P, Okelo G: Echinococcosis (hydatidosis). In Warren KS, Mahmoud AAF (eds): Tropical and Geographical Medicine. New York, McGraw-Hill, 1990, p 505.

102. Schaefer JW, Khan MY: Echinococcosis (hydatid disease): Lessons from experience with 59 patients. Rev Infect Dis 13:243, 1991.

103. Akinoglu A, Demiryurek H, Guzel C: Alveolar hydatid disease of the liver: A report on thirty-nine surgical cases in eastern Anatolia, Turkey. Am J Trop Med Hyg 45:182, 1991.

104. Kalovidouris A, Pissiotis C, Pontifex G, et al: CT characterization of multivesicular hydatid cysts. J Comput Assist Tomogr 10:428, 1986.

105. Filice C, Di Perri G, Strosselli M, et al: Parasitologic findings in percutaneous drainage of human hydatid liver cysts. J Infect Dis 161:1290, 1990.

106. Mathisen GE, Sokolov RT Jr, Meyer RD: Fever, abdominal pain, and headache in an Iranian woman. Rev Infect Dis 12:529, 1990.

107. Hira PR, Shweiki H, Lindberg LG, et al: Diagnosis of cystic hydatid disease: Role of aspiration cytology. Lancet 2:655, 1988.

108. Khuroo MS, Wani NA, Javid G, et al: Percutaneous drainage compared with surgery for hepatic hydatid cysts. N Engl J Med 337:881, 1997.

109. Horton RJ: Chemotherapy of *Echinococcus* infection in man with albendazole. Trans R Soc Trop Med Hyg 83:97, 1989.

110. Crippa FG, Bruno R, Brunetti E, Filice C: Echinococcal liver cysts: Treatment with echo-guided percutaneous puncture

PAIR for echinococcal liver cysts. Ital J Gastroenterol Hepatol 31:884, 1999.

111. Paksoy Y, Ödev K, Sahin M, et al: Percutaneous treatment of liver hydatid cysts: Comparison of direct injection of albendazole and hypertonic saline solution. AJR 185:727, 2005.

112. Menezes da Silva A: Hydatid cyst of the liver: Criteria for the selection of appropriate treatment. Acta Trop 85:237, 2003.

113. Craig P: *Echinococcus multilocularis.* Curr Opin Infect Dis 16:437, 2003.

114. Lipsett PA, Huang CJ, Lillemoe KD, et al: Fungal hepatic abscesses: Characterization and management. J Gastrointest Surg 1:78, 1997.

115. Myerowitz RL, Pazin GJ, Allen CM: Disseminated candidiasis: Changes in incidence, underlying diseases, and pathology. Am J Clin Pathol 68:29, 1977.

116. Tashjian LS, Abramson JS, Peacock JE Jr: Focal hepatic candidiasis: A distinct clinical variant of candidiasis in immunocompromised patients. Rev Infect Dis 6:689, 1984.

117. Semelka RC, Shoenut JP, Greenberg HM, Bow EJ: Detection of acute and treated lesions of hepatosplenic candidiasis: Comparison of dynamic contrast-enhanced CT and MR imaging. J Magn Reson Imaging 2:341, 1992.

118. Phillips EH, Carroll BJ, Chandra M, et al: Laparoscopic-guided biopsy for diagnosis of hepatic candidiasis. J Laparoendosc Surg 2:33, 1992.

119. Kirby A, Chapman C, Hassan C, Burnie J: The diagnosis of hepatosplenic candidiasis by DNA analysis of tissue biopsy and serum. J Clin Pathol 57:764, 2004.

120. Sora F CP, Piccirillo N, et al: Successful treatment with caspofungin of hepatosplenic candidiasis resistant to liposomal amphotericin B. Clin Infect Dis 35:1135, 2002.

121. Bullock W: *Histoplasma capsulatum.* In Mandell GL, Bennett JE, Dolin R (eds): Principles and Practice of Infectious Diseases, 5th ed. New York, Churchill Livingstone, 1995, p 2340.

122. Rockey D: Hepatobiliary infections. Curr Opin Gastroenterol 17:257, 2001.

123. Molle I, Thulstrup AM, Vilstrup H, Sorensen HT: Increased risk and case fatality rate of pyogenic liver abscess in patients with liver cirrhosis: A nationwide study in Denmark. Gut 48:260, 2001.

124. Shibata T, Yamamoto Y, Yamamoto N, et al: Cholangitis and liver abscess after percutaneous ablation therapy for liver tumors: Incidence and risk factors. J Vasc Interv Radiol 14:1535, 2003.

125. Brook I, Frazier EH: Microbiology of liver and spleen abscesses. J Med Microbiol 47:1075, 1998.

126. Lublin M, Bartlett DL, Danforth DN, et al: Hepatic abscess in patients with chronic granulomatous disease. Ann Surg 235:383, 2002.

127. Ralls PW: Inflammatory disease of the liver. Clin Liver Dis 6:203, 2002.

128. Lam YH, Wong SK, Lee DW, et al: ERCP and pyogenic liver abscess. Gastrointest Endosc 50:340, 1999.

129. Koea JB, Broadhurst GW, Rodgers MS, McCall JL: Inflammatory pseudotumor of the liver: Demographics, diagnosis, and the case for nonoperative management. J Am Coll Surg 196:226, 2003.

130. Papachristou GI, Wu T, Marsh W, Plevy SE: Inflammatory pseudotumor of the liver associated with Crohn's disease. J Clin Gastroenterol 38:818, 2004.

131. Yu SC, Ho SS, Lau WY, et al: Treatment of pyogenic liver abscess: Prospective randomized comparison of catheter drainage and needle aspiration. Hepatology 39:932, 2004.

132. Lee KT, Wong SR, Sheen PC: Pyogenic liver abscess: An audit of 10 years' experience and analysis of risk factors. Dig Surg 18:459, 2001.

133. Ng FH, Wong WM, Wong BC, et al: Sequential intravenous/oral antibiotic vs. continuous intravenous antibiotic in the treatment of pyogenic liver abscess. Aliment Pharmacol Ther 16:1083, 2002.

134. Alvarez JA, Gonzalez JJ, Baldonedo RF, et al: Single and multiple pyogenic liver abscesses: Etiology, clinical course, and outcome. Dig Surg 18:283, 2001.

135. Alvarez Perez JA, Gonzalez JJ, Baldonedo RF, et al: Clinical course, treatment, and multivariate analysis of risk factors for pyogenic liver abscess. Am J Surg 181:177, 2001.

136. Fung CP, Chang FY, Lee SC, et al: A global emerging disease of *Klebsiella pneumoniae* liver abscess: Is serotype K1 an important factor for complicated endophthalmitis? Gut 50:420, 2002.

137. Haque R, Huston CD, Hughes M, et al: Amebiasis. N Engl J Med 348:1565, 2003.

138. Stanley SL Jr: Amoebiasis. Lancet 361:1025, 2003.

139. Hung CC, Chen PJ, Hsieh SM, et al: Invasive amoebiasis: An emerging parasitic disease in patients infected with HIV in an area endemic for amoebic infection. AIDS 13:2421, 1999.

140. Tachibana H, Cheng XJ, Masuda G, et al: Evaluation of recombinant fragments of *Entamoeba histolytica* Gal/GalNAc lectin intermediate subunit for serodiagnosis of amebiasis. J Clin Microbiol 42:1069, 2004.

CHAPTER

80 Vascular Diseases of the Liver

William E. Stevens

Vascular disorders of the liver are relatively uncommon but frequently result in significant liver disease and portal hypertension. The continuously high metabolic activity of the liver makes it particularly susceptible to vascular compromise; however, its complex dual blood supply offers unique protection against ischemic injury. Hypercoagulable states play an important role in the pathogenesis of many of these disorders, and knowledge of them is essential for understanding and treating the associated hepatic vascular conditions. This chapter reviews a heterogeneous group of disorders resulting from hepatic vascular and cardiovascular diseases. Vasculitis involving the liver is discussed in Chapter 34.

BUDD-CHIARI SYNDROME

Hepatic venous outflow obstruction is the hallmark of the Budd-Chiari syndrome. Reductions in hepatic venous outflow can occur anywhere from the right atrium to the small hepatic venules and result in dramatic anatomic and physiologic changes. Classic Budd-Chiari syndrome results from thrombosis of one or more hepatic veins at their opening into the inferior vena cava. The deleterious physiologic changes of hepatic venous obstruction are transmitted directly to the hepatic sinusoids, resulting in sinusoidal congestion, portal vein hypertension, and reduced portal vein blood flow. The result is hepatomegaly,

pain, ascites, and impaired hepatic function. The ascitic fluid typically has a high serum-ascites albumin gradient and a high protein content, as a result of increased filtration of serum proteins through the highly permeable sinusoidal spaces (see Chapter 88). The progression of the disease is rarely fulminant; in most patients, the clinical course is subacute and less than 6 months in duration.[1] In older series, the mortality rate in untreated cases was as high as 90% at 3.5 years.[2] With advances in diagnostic imaging and improved medical, surgical, and radiologic treatments for Budd-Chiari syndrome, however, survival has improved significantly since 1980.

The literature on Budd-Chiari syndrome is extensive. Two major reviews of the world literature collected data on cases reported before 1980.[3,4] Reviews of greater than 100 cases have appeared from Japan, India, China, and South Africa.[5-8] The review from India is especially helpful in demonstrating the geographic diversity of this syndrome.[6]

ETIOLOGY

Anatomically, Budd-Chiari syndrome results from hepatic vein obstruction, inferior vena cava obstruction (above or at the level of the hepatic veins), or both. The main causes of the syndrome are listed in Table 80–1. In Western countries, thrombosis of the hepatic veins is the most common presentation, whereas in Asia and Africa,

Table 80–1 Causes of Budd-Chiari Syndrome

Hypercoagulable States
Antiphospholipid syndrome
Antithrombin deficiency
Essential thrombocytosis
Factor V Leiden mutation
Lupus anticoagulant
Methylenetetrahydrofolate reductase mutation TT677
Myeloproliferative disorder
Oral contraceptives
Paroxysmal nocturnal hemoglobinuria
Polycythemia rubra vera
Postpartum thrombocytopenic purpura
Pregnancy
Protein C deficiency
Protein S deficiency
Prothrombin mutation G20210A
Sickle cell disease
Infections
Amebic or pyogenic liver abscess
Aspergillosis
Filariasis
Hydatid cysts

Pelvic cellulitis
Schistosomiasis
Syphilis
Tuberculosis
Malignancy
Adrenal carcinoma
Bronchogenic carcinoma
Hepatocellular carcinoma
Leiomyosarcoma
Leukemia
Renal carcinoma
Rhabdomyosarcoma
Miscellaneous
Behçet's syndrome
Celiac sprue
Dacarbazine therapy
Inflammatory bowel disease
Laparoscopic cholecystectomy
Membranous obstruction of the vena cava
Polycystic liver disease
Sarcoidosis
Trauma

membranous obstruction of the inferior vena cava (MOVC) accounts for more than 40% of cases.[9] Thrombogenic states can be identified in at least 75% of cases not caused by MOVC. Increasingly sophisticated testing for hypercoagulable states has reduced the frequency of idiopathic cases to less than 10%.[1,10] Hematologic disorders are the most common cause for Budd-Chiari syndrome. Primary myeloproliferative diseases, particularly polycythemia rubra vera, may account for 50% of cases.[1] In addition, latent myeloproliferative disorders may be detectable with use of cell culture techniques.[11] Tumors, infections, and pregnancy each account for about 10% of cases. Other hypercoagulable states associated with Budd-Chiari syndrome include paroxysmal nocturnal hemoglobinuria, antiphospholipid syndrome,[12] and deficiencies of antithrombin, protein C, and protein S.[13] More recently recognized causes include factor V Leiden mutation[14] and mutations of the prothrombin gene and the methylenetetrahydrofolate reductase gene.[15] Oral contraceptive use increases the risk of Budd-Chiari syndrome by greater than two-fold. Greater than one fourth of the patients are found to have a combination of thrombogenic risk factors.[15]

The pathophysiologic characteristics of MOVC are poorly understood. The disorder is much more common in developing countries, especially Asia and Africa, than in Western countries. The clinical presentation usually is subacute or chronic. The membranous webs may be thick or thin and typically occur in the intrahepatic inferior vena cava, often with occlusion of the ostia of the hepatic veins (Fig. 80–1). A congenital origin for the lesion has been proposed, on the basis of the complex embryologic development of the inferior vena cava and reported presentations in childhood. An acquired origin, however, is supported by the peak occurrence in the fourth decade of life and histologic studies suggesting that the membrane

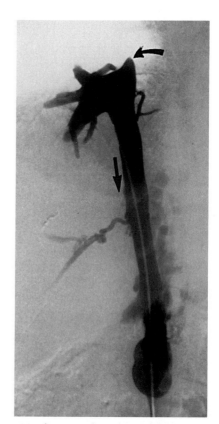

Figure 80–1 Membranous obstruction of the vena cava. Injection of contrast medium into the inferior vena cava demonstrates retrograde flow toward the legs (*downward arrow*), rather than antegrade flow toward the right atrium. The membranous obstruction is nearly complete; only a tiny opening is visible as a small protrusion (*curved arrow*). (Courtesy of Drs. Jeanne LaBerge, Roy Gordon, Robert Kerlin, and Ernest Ring, San Francisco, Calif.)

develops from an organizing thrombus. Hypercoagulability is relatively less common in MOVC than in hepatic vein thrombosis. Therefore, other explanations for thrombosis in MOVC have been proposed, such as chronic infection, endothelial trauma caused by movement of the diaphragm with respiration and coughing, and venous turbulence resulting from the right-angle flow of blood from the hepatic veins into the inferior vena cava. Another feature of MOVC is a propensity for the development of hepatocellular carcinoma, which is extremely rare in classic Budd-Chiari syndrome.[16,17] The distinctive features of MOVC have led some investigators to consider MOVC to be a separate clinical entity termed *obliterative hepatocavopathy*.[18]

CLINICAL FEATURES

The epidemiologic characteristics of Budd-Chiari syndrome (except those cases associated with MOVC) parallel those of its underlying conditions. The syndrome is rare in infants and young children; the largest pediatric series describes South African children with MOVC. More than one half of the cases of classic Budd-Chiari syndrome occur between the ages of 20 and 39 years.[4] Budd-Chiari syndrome occasionally may be identified in asymptomatic persons undergoing evaluation for mildly elevated liver biochemical test levels.[19] In these patients, the lack of symptoms probably is the result of thrombosis of only one hepatic vein or the development of large venous collaterals.

Fulminant Budd-Chiari syndrome is uncommon and occurs most often in women with a hypercoagulable state due to pregnancy, usually in the setting of an additional predisposing factor (e.g., factor V Leiden mutation). Patients present with abrupt and severe abdominal pain and vomiting, marked hepatomegaly, jaundice, ascites, high serum aminotransferase levels (greater than 1000 U/L), and rapid deterioration of hepatic function, with resulting encephalopathy and renal failure. Few of these patients survive without prompt intervention, usually including liver transplantation.

Acute Budd-Chiari syndrome is more common, accounting for 20% to 30% of cases. The clinical findings depend on the location of the thrombus, stage and rapidity of evolution, and percentage of liver tissue deprived of venous drainage. Symptoms and signs develop over 1 to 2 months and include abdominal pain, tender hepatomegaly, and ascites but not hepatic encephalopathy. Typically the serum bilirubin level is less than 5 mg/dL, and the serum aminotransferase levels are elevated two- to three-fold. Some patients may have a remitting course.

Most patients with Budd-Chiari syndrome present with subacute or chronic symptoms and signs evolving over 3 to 6 months. Many of these patients already have cirrhosis and exhibit complications of chronic decompensation. Hepatosplenomegaly and ascites usually are present. If the inferior vena cava also is occluded, then signs of collateral circulation, such as dilated venous collaterals over the flanks and back, will be present, and most patients will have lower extremity edema. Liver biochemical test levels may be nonspecifically, mildly elevated. Some patients will experience variceal bleeding requiring endoscopic therapy.

Because Budd-Chiari syndrome is uncommon and symptoms and signs are nonspecific, misdiagnosis or delays in diagnosis are frequent. The manifestations of Budd-Chiari syndrome are similar to those of other causes of fulminant hepatitis, but massive hepatomegaly and rapid development of ascites are suggestive features. Acute alcoholic hepatitis with prominent hepatomegaly, ascites, and mildly abnormal liver biochemical test levels may be confused with Budd-Chiari syndrome. Right-sided congestive heart failure, severe tricuspid regurgitation, and constrictive pericarditis all are associated with impaired venous return from the liver and may mimic subacute or chronic Budd-Chiari syndrome (see later). These cardiac conditions are suggested by the presence of distended jugular veins and hepatojugular reflux; careful cardiovascular examination and echocardiography will assist in the diagnosis. Patients with Budd-Chiari syndrome presenting with right upper quadrant pain and gallbladder wall thickening on ultrasound examination may be misdiagnosed as having acute cholecystitis. Budd-Chiari syndrome should be considered in patients presenting with decompensated cirrhosis or refractory ascites out of proportion in severity to the magnitude of liver biochemical test abnormalities. In addition, anyone with a hypercoagulable disorder who presents with hepatomegaly and ascites should be evaluated for Budd-Chiari syndrome.

Although the course of Budd-Chiari syndrome may be indolent, few cases ever regress. Some form of intervention is needed in most patients to prevent ongoing hepatic ischemic necrosis and to control ascites and other complications.

PATHOLOGY

Acutely, the hepatic histologic features of centrilobular congestion, hemorrhage, sinusoidal dilatation, and noninflammatory cell necrosis predominate (Fig. 80–2).

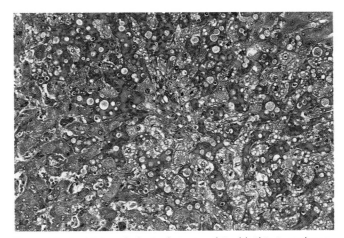

Figure 80–2 Histopathologic features of Budd-Chiari syndrome. This low-power photomicrograph shows the centrizonal congestion, hemorrhage, and hepatocyte necrosis typical of the acute type of Budd-Chiari syndrome. (Courtesy of Edward Lee, MD, Washington, DC.)

Within weeks, fibrosis develops in the centrilobular areas, more so than in periportal areas. Chronically, these lesions evolve into cirrhosis. Large regenerative nodules are common, especially in areas of decreased portal venous perfusion.[20] Indeed, portal vein thrombosis can be seen in 10% of cases and in 50% of hepatic explants at the time of liver transplantation for Budd-Chiari syndrome.[21] Because hepatic vein occlusion is asymmetrical, the pathologic effects may vary in different regions of the lever. Massive caudate lobe hypertrophy is a common feature, probably because of preservation of venous drainage directly into the inferior vena cava, and may contribute to compression of the inferior vena cava. Pathologic changes (except for cirrhosis) can be reversed with adequate decompression of the hepatic sinusoids (see later).

DIAGNOSIS

Liver biochemical test levels may be normal or demonstrate only mild elevations or nonspecific changes. Occasionally, serum aminotransferase levels may be more than five times the upper limit of normal in fulminant and acute cases. Often, the severity of the hepatic illness seems out of proportion to the mild degree of abnormality on liver biochemical tests.

Doppler ultrasonography, with sensitivity and specificity rates greater than 80%, is the diagnostic procedure of first choice.[22,23] It is relatively inexpensive, safe, and available in most hospitals. Typical Doppler ultrasonographic features of Budd-Chiari syndrome include lack of visualization of normal hepatic venous connections to the inferior vena cava, comma-shaped intrahepatic or subcapsular collateral vessels, and absence of flow signal in the hepatic veins. The diagnostic accuracy of ultrasonography is decreased by a large body habitus and also is operator dependent.

Magnetic resonance imaging (MRI) and computed tomography (CT) also may demonstrate characteristic features of Budd-Chiari syndrome but do not add much to the findings on adequate ultrasonographic examination.[24] MRI may be a better second-line test than CT because of the ability to provide accurate angiographic detail of the hepatic vein and inferior vena cava anatomy. The combination of Doppler ultrasonography and MRI or CT imaging should be able to diagnose most cases of Budd-Chiari syndrome.

For years, venography was the gold standard for diagnosis of Budd-Chiari syndrome, but nowadays venography often is unnecessary for diagnostic purposes alone. Venography should be performed in cases of suspected Budd-Chiari syndrome when first- and second-line imaging tests are nondiagnostic and when surgery and other therapeutic interventions are planned. Measurement of the hepatic venous pressure gradient is required when vena cava stenosis is present, to plan for shunt surgery (see Chapter 87). Venography also allows access for transjugular liver biopsy of both the right and left lobes, which can confirm the diagnosis of Budd-Chiari syndrome and guide therapy. Liver biopsy is not essential for making the diagnosis of Budd-Chiari syndrome, however, and clinical staging of hepatic synthetic function (Child-Turcotte-Pugh score) may be better for planning treatment (see later).[25]

TREATMENT

The therapy of Budd-Chiari syndrome depends on the cause, anatomic characteristics, and pace of the disease (Fig. 80–3). The precipitating causes of Budd-Chiari syndrome must be evaluated and treated. Most patients need some form of intervention, and collaboration among a hepatologist, an interventional radiologist, and a hepatobiliary surgeon is desirable. Treatment options consist primarily of combinations of medical therapy with diuretics and anticoagulants, interventional therapy to decompress the hepatic sinusoids and prevent further

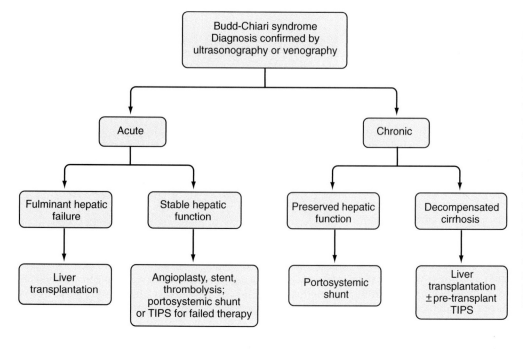

Figure 80–3 Approach to the management of patients with Budd-Chiari syndrome. Although each case must be individualized, this algorithm shows typical treatment options for the various forms of Budd-Chiari syndrome. Patients with fulminant disease or decompensated cirrhosis should be considered for liver transplantation. Patients with clinically stable, acute disease have the most options available to them. Special effort should be made to determine local (nonsystemic) or transient causes of the syndrome that might benefit from less invasive therapies. TIPS, transjugular intrahepatic portosystemic shunt.

hepatic necrosis, and liver transplantation for hepatic failure.

Medical management alone may be appropriate for patients with mild forms of Budd-Chiari syndrome. Treatment typically consists of diuretic therapy with spironolactone and furosemide and dietary sodium restriction to achieve a negative sodium balance (see Chapter 88). Large-volume paracentesis may be needed to relieve tense ascites. Anticoagulation is recommended and consists of intravenous heparin followed by warfarin to achieve an international normalized ratio (INR) for prothrombin of 2.0 to 2.5. Medical therapy is considered successful if ascites is controlled, liver biochemical test results improve or normalize, and symptoms resolve. Most patients with Budd-Chiari syndrome do not respond adequately to medical therapy alone, however, and need some form of intervention to decompress the hepatic sinusoids.

Many case reports and small series have described the use of thrombolytic therapy for acute Budd-Chiari syndrome. Thrombolytics are most effective if given within 3 weeks of the onset of symptoms, if flow is demonstrated in the thrombosed vein, and if the infusion is given directly into the occluded hepatic vein. Systemic and hepatic arterial infusions are less effective.[26] Angioplasty often is performed with thrombolysis to improve vein patency and to reopen an acutely thrombosed stent or transjugular intrahepatic portosystemic shunt (TIPS) (see later).

The role of interventional radiology in the treatment of Budd-Chiari syndrome has expanded greatly. Angioplasty, with or without stenting of short and localized stenoses of the hepatic veins or the inferior vena cava, can relieve symptoms in greater than 80% of patients with MOVC and is the primary treatment for this disorder in many parts of the world.[27-30] The rate of restenosis is high, and regular follow-up with Doppler ultrasonography is required.[31] Angioplasty also can be combined successfully with surgical creation of a portacaval shunt in patients with both inferior vena cava and hepatic vein obstruction (see later).[32]

Use of TIPS has gained popularity as a treatment for refractory complications of portal hypertension (see Chapter 87). Procedural mortality is low, and shunt placement usually is successful,[33] even in complete hepatic vein occlusion, in which a shunt can be placed between the intrahepatic vena cava and portal vein.[34] TIPS also is useful for treating combined hepatic vein and inferior vena cava obstruction. TIPS can be effective in patients with fulminant Budd-Chiari syndrome waiting for a liver transplant; however, short-term mortality rates in this setting may be as high as 50%.[35] TIPS also has been used successfully in patients with acute Budd-Chiari syndrome in whom thrombolytic therapy and angioplasty have failed. Finally, TIPS is an effective "bridge" to liver transplantation in patients with chronic Budd-Chiari syndrome who have liver failure and refractory ascites or variceal bleeding. Unfortunately, TIPS dysfunction requiring revision occurs in up to 70% of patients[36] and seems to be more common in patients with Budd-Chiari syndrome than in those with other indications for TIPS placement. In addition, liver transplantation is made more complicated by previous placement of a TIPS that

extends too far into the portal vein or into the suprahepatic vena cava.

In Western countries, surgical therapy for Budd-Chiari syndrome consists mainly of portosystemic shunting and liver transplantation. Surgical therapy of MOVC that is unsuitable for or refractory to angioplasty and stenting may entail resection or transatrial "finger fracture" of vena cava webs[37] or dorsocranial liver resection with hepaticoatrial anastomosis (the Senning procedure).[38] For classic Budd-Chiari syndrome, portosystemic shunting relieves portal hypertension effectively, thereby alleviating hepatic ischemic necrosis, refractory ascites, and variceal bleeding. When shunt surgery is successful, the portal vein becomes the hepatic outflow tract, hepatomegaly resolves, hepatic histologic findings improve and even normalize, and survival is prolonged in greater than 90% of cases.[39]

The choice of a shunt depends on the degree of hepatomegaly and caudate lobe hypertrophy, presence or absence of inferior vena cava stenosis, and expertise of the surgeon. Portacaval and mesocaval shunts are associated with the best results. With mesocaval shunts, the rate of shunt thrombosis is higher—33% at 5 years[40]—but placement is technically simpler when portal dissection is impeded because of caudate lobe hypertrophy. Thrombosis of portacaval shunts is uncommon, with a rate of only 3% over 13 years,[39] but portacaval shunts increase the technical difficulty of subsequent liver transplantation more than do mesocaval shunts. Placement of a portacaval or mesocaval shunt is contraindicated if inferior vena cava stenosis is present and the vena cava pressure is greater than 20 mm Hg or if the portacaval pressure gradient is less than 10 mm Hg. Surgical options in these patients include placement of a mesoatrial shunt,[41,42] a combined portacaval and cavoatrial shunt,[39] and combinations of surgical shunt creation with vena cava angioplasty and stenting.[32] Because of high rates of shunt thrombosis, however, TIPS may be the best option in these patients.

Liver transplantation is appropriate in patients with liver failure resulting from fulminant or chronic Budd-Chiari syndrome and in patients with a failed surgical shunt (see Chapter 92).[43] In patients with protein C, protein S, or antithrombin deficiency, liver transplantation also cures the underlying hypercoagulable state, although most patients will require lifelong anticoagulation. Underlying myeloproliferative disorders can be managed effectively with hydroxyurea and aspirin after liver transplantation.[44] Recurrent Budd-Chiari syndrome after liver transplantation occurs in 4% to 10% of patients, and the risk of thrombosis of the hepatic artery and portal vein is increased as well.[45,46] In addition, bleeding complications are more common because of anticoagulant therapy. Despite these drawbacks, 5-year survival rates for patients with Budd-Chiari syndrome who undergo liver transplantation are greater than 85%.[46]

The choices of therapy in patients with Budd-Chiari syndrome are complicated, in great part because of the lack of large, controlled studies comparing various treatments and the lack of standardization in classifying Budd-Chiari syndrome into acute, subacute, and chronic forms.[47] One multivariate analysis failed to show a survival advantage in surgically shunted patients compared with those receiving medical treatment alone.[48] No controlled or long-term studies of TIPS as definitive therapy in Budd-Chiari syndrome have been performed. Surgical shunting seems to be most efficacious in patients with acute or chronic Budd-Chiari syndrome with refractory symptoms and preserved hepatic synthetic function (Child-Turcotte-Pugh classes A and B).[49] Patients with fulminant or chronic Budd-Chiari syndrome with impaired hepatic synthetic function (Child-Turcotte-Pugh classes B and C) should be considered for liver transplantation, with or without prior TIPS placement. In patients with acute Budd-Chiari syndrome, attempts should be made to decompress the hepatic sinusoids with combinations of angioplasty, stenting, and thrombolytic therapy, followed by TIPS placement or creation of a surgical shunt in those in whom these treatment approaches fail.

SINUSOIDAL OBSTRUCTION SYNDROME (VENO-OCCLUSIVE DISEASE)

Occlusion of the terminal hepatic venules and hepatic sinusoids resembles the Budd-Chiari syndrome clinically; however, the causes, epidemiologic and pathophysiologic characteristics, and prognosis of this entity are sufficiently distinct to justify a separate designation. In the past, the entity was known as *veno-occlusive disease*. Because the occlusion consistently involves the hepatic sinusoids, the term *sinusoidal obstruction syndrome* has been proposed as a more appropriate name for this disorder.[50]

ETIOLOGY

Liver disease caused by *Senecio* poisoning originally was reported from South Africa in 1920 (see Chapter 84),[51] but the term *veno-occlusive disease* was not used until 1954, when it was related to the ingestion of pyrrolizidine alkaloids contained in plants of the genera *Senecio*, *Crotalaria*, and *Heliotropium* in Jamaica.[52] Ingestion of alkaloids in inadequately winnowed wheat or in "bush tea," especially in malnourished persons, is the main cause of veno-occlusive disease (sinusoidal obstruction syndrome) worldwide. Epidemics have been reported in India, Afghanistan, South Africa, the Middle East, and the United States. More recently, the herbal remedy comfrey (genus *Symphytum*) has been associated with sinusoidal obstruction syndrome. Rare familial clusters have been reported in association with immunodeficiency states.[53]

Since the advent of cancer chemotherapy in the 1950s, sinusoidal obstruction syndrome in Western countries occurs most commonly after bone marrow transplantation.[54] A variety of antineoplastic drugs have been implicated as causes for sinusoidal obstruction syndrome, including gemtuzumab ozogamicin, actinomycin D, dacarbazine, cytosine arabinoside, mithramycin, and 6-thioguanine. Hepatic irradiation and therapy with busulfan plus cyclophosphamide also are established risk factors. In addition, long-term immunosuppression with azathioprine and 6-thioguanine used in patients with inflammatory bowel disease and in kidney and liver transplant recipients has been reported to cause sinusoidal obstruction syndrome.[54] The frequency of this disorder after bone marrow transplantation varies, ranging from 0% to 70%, depending on patient and treatment-related variables.

CLINICAL FEATURES AND COURSE

In the early stages of the disorder, features of portal hypertension predominate. Classically, sinusoidal obstruction syndrome manifests with mild hyperbilirubinemia (bilirubin levels greater than 2 mg/dL), painful hepatomegaly, weight gain of greater than 2%, and development of ascites. Weight gain and painful hepatomegaly usually precede the onset of jaundice, which can be followed by the development of ascites, encephalopathy, and multiorgan failure. Sinusoidal obstruction syndrome occurs most commonly within 10 to 20 days after bone marrow transplantation (see Chapter 33). Serum bilirubin levels typically peak at day 17 after transplantation. Predisposing factors include advanced age, elevated serum aminotransferase levels before transplantation, presence of hepatic metastases, recent systemic bacterial or viral infections, previous bone marrow transplantation, and allogeneic (as opposed to autologous) bone marrow transplantation.[54]

The diagnosis of sinusoidal obstruction syndrome is often based on characteristic clinical features and exclusion of other conditions. Distinguishing this disease from the many other disorders that may complicate bone marrow transplantation is challenging. The most frequent conditions that can mimic sinusoidal obstruction syndrome include graft-versus-host disease, hepatic dysfunction caused by sepsis and drug toxicity, and cholestasis resulting from hemolysis and congestive heart failure. Graft-versus-host disease is rare before day 15 after transplantation, and sepsis and drug toxicity rarely cause painful hepatomegaly and ascites. Routine liver biochemical test results are not specific for sinusoidal obstruction syndrome. Serum alkaline phosphatase and aminotransferase elevations can accompany the hyperbilirubinemia and probably indicate coexistent hepatic ischemic necrosis. Thrombocytopenia is common and may be aggravated by portal hypertension and splenic sequestration. Findings on ultrasound examination, CT, and MRI are nonspecific in early sinusoidal obstruction syndrome but are helpful in excluding biliary obstruction, infiltrative liver lesions, and hepatic vein occlusion. Common findings in sinusoidal obstruction syndrome include gallbladder wall thickening, hepatosplenomegaly, ascites, portal vein enlargement with sluggish or reversed flow, and umbilical vein recanalization. Ultrasound and Doppler findings can predict disease severity noninvasively.[55] Increased uptake of technetium-99m sulfur colloid by the lungs during hepatic scintigraphy may suggest a diagnosis of sinusoidal obstruction syndrome and provides an estimate of its severity.[56] Hepatic scintigraphy is done infrequently in the United States nowadays, however. If the diagnosis is still uncertain, a transjugular liver biopsy and measurement of the hepatic venous pressure gradient can be performed (see Chapter 87). In this setting, a gradient of greater than 10 mm Hg is highly suggestive of sinusoidal obstruction syndrome and predictive of increased disease severity.[57]

Serum levels of a variety of mediators of coagulation, inflammation, and fibrosis have been found to be predictive of sinusoidal obstruction syndrome before it becomes clinically apparent. Levels of protein C, factor VII, and antithrombin are decreased in plasma before onset of sinusoidal obstruction syndrome, whereas levels of plasminogen activator inhibitor type 1, tumor necrosis factor-α, and procollagen type III are increased.[58] In patients who undergo hematopoietic stem cell transplantation, an elevated procollagen type III level even before chemotherapy is a risk factor for the later development of the disorder.[59] It is unclear if these abnormalities cause the occlusion or result from the occlusion or hepatic injury.

In most patients with sinusoidal obstruction syndrome, the disorder gradually resolves over 2 to 3 weeks. The overall mortality rate is 20% to 50%, and more deaths are caused by multiorgan failure than by hepatic failure.[54] Severe sinusoidal obstruction syndrome, which carries a mortality rate of almost 100%, can be predicted by more rapid increases in the serum bilirubin level and weight. Other predictors of severe disease include the presence of ascites, a hepatic venous pressure gradient greater than 20 mm Hg, and the onset of multiorgan failure.[60]

PATHOLOGY

The principal histologic features of sinusoidal obstruction syndrome result from toxic injury to the centrilobular (zone 3) endothelial cells in the hepatic sinusoids and terminal hepatic venules (see Fig. 33–5A and B).[61] The resultant cellular debris, exfoliated hepatocytes, activated coagulation factors, and extravasated red blood cells produce progressive occlusion of the sinusoids and venules, causing sinusoidal dilatation and severe hepatic congestion. Inflammation is notably absent. Progressive venular sclerosis ensues, with deposition of collagen in the sinusoids and venules eventually leading to venular obliteration, hepatocellular ischemic necrosis, and widespread fibrosis. The cause of the endothelial injury is unclear; possibilities include direct endothelial toxicity from causative compounds, toxicity from cytochrome P450–derived metabolic by-products, and glutathione depletion.[62]

TREATMENT

The lack of effective and safe treatment for sinusoidal obstruction syndrome has increased interest in preventive strategies. Recognizing risk factors for the development of the disorder and altering chemotherapeutic regimens and doses can decrease associated morbidity and mortality. Studies of ursodeoxycholic acid, heparin, and low-molecular-weight heparin (LMWH) for the prevention of sinusoidal obstruction syndrome yielded inconclusive results. Ursodeoxycholic acid has minimal toxicity and in two studies reduced the frequency of the disease by greater than 50%, compared with placebo or no treatment, but had no effect on overall survival.[63,64] One large study failed to show any preventive benefit of

ursodeoxycholic acid. Similarly, heparin reduced the frequency of sinusoidal obstruction syndrome in a large prospective randomized trial from 13.7% in control subjects who received no treatment to 2.5% in patients in the group treated with heparin,[65] but two other studies showed no preventive benefit from heparin and a 7% risk of hemorrhagic complications.[64,66] The combination of ursodeoxycholic acid and heparin offers no advantage over heparin alone.[67] Use of LMWH is associated with a lower rate of bleeding complications than those observed with heparin and may be more effective. In a retrospective study in which LMWH was compared with heparin and no treatment, the frequency of sinusoidal obstruction syndrome with LMWH was 4%, compared with 11% with heparin and 22% with no treatment in the control group.[68] Studies of prostaglandin E₁ to prevent sinusoidal obstruction syndrome also have had inconclusive results, and use of this agent is limited by significant toxicity.

Treatment of sinusoidal obstruction syndrome entails primarily supportive care including diuresis, analgesia for pain, paracentesis for tense ascites, and avoidance of nephrotoxins and other hepatotoxins. Survival once multiorgan failure has occurred is dismal. Treatment with tissue plasminogen activator, as described in many case reports and small series, has shown response rates of 30% and a rate of life-threatening hemorrhage of 20% to 30%.[64] Treatment is ineffective in patients in whom multiorgan failure has developed. Other treatments reported in small studies or in trials with inconclusive results include use of high-dose glucocorticoids, N-acetylcysteine, and antithrombin.[64] Defibrotide is a novel oligonucleotide with anti-ischemic, antithrombotic, and thrombolytic activity but no systemic anticoagulant effect. Several studies have shown efficacy of defibrotide in the treatment of sinusoidal obstruction syndrome, with no serious toxicity. A large multi-institutional study of defibrotide for severe sinusoidal obstruction syndrome showed a 36% rate of response (improvement in serum bilirubin levels and multiorgan failure) in a group of patients with an otherwise dismal prognosis.[69]

TIPS has been performed successfully in patients with sinusoidal obstruction syndrome, but with generally poor results. Clinical improvement after TIPS may be seen in one half of the patients, but only 10% survive long term.[70] Until more studies are available, TIPS should be reserved for patients with severe sinusoidal obstruction syndrome who have refractory ascites or who are candidates for liver transplantation. Liver transplantation has been performed successfully for liver failure caused by sinusoidal obstruction syndrome. Most patients with sinusoidal obstruction syndrome, however, are unsuitable for liver transplantation because of underlying malignancy and the severity of the associated multiorgan failure. Because a majority of patients with mild to moderate sinusoidal obstruction syndrome do well with conservative therapy, the focus on future investigation should be directed at prevention and treatment of severe sinusoidal obstruction syndrome. As the ability to predict severe sinusoidal obstruction syndrome improves and as newer agents, such as defibrotide, become available, morbidity and mortality from sinusoidal obstruction syndrome will likely decrease.

PORTAL VEIN THROMBOSIS

Portal vein obstruction results from thrombosis, constriction, or invasion of the portal vein. The resulting portal hypertension leads to splenomegaly and formation of portosystemic collaterals and esophageal, gastric, duodenal, and jejunal varices. Varices proliferate in the porta hepatis and involve the gallbladder and bile duct. As portal vein thrombosis evolves, fibroblasts transform the clot into a firm, collagenous plug in which tortuous venous channels develop. This *cavernous transformation* begins within days after acute thrombosis and continues to evolve over weeks to months. Upstream from the obstruction, the small intestine and colon become congested, and the stomach exhibits changes of portal hypertensive gastropathy. Mesenteric ischemia can occur if the thrombus extends into the mesenteric veins. Downstream from the clot, the liver usually maintains normal function and appears unaffected. Ascites may develop during the initial stages but usually recedes subsequently. As more venous collaterals form, a state of equilibrium is reached in which some portal perfusion is maintained and some portal hypertension persists. Clinically, portal vein thrombosis usually is asymptomatic until variceal bleeding occurs.

ETIOLOGY

Most cases of portal vein thrombosis have an identifiable cause related to hypercoagulability or to local factors such as inflammation, trauma, or malignancy (Table 80–2).

Less than 20% of cases are considered idiopathic. Better understanding of the multiple causes of hypercoagulability has led to the recognition that multiple coexisting risk factors are present in as many as 40% of affected patients.[71] Infection, most often umbilical vein sepsis, is the main cause of portal vein thrombosis in children. Portal vein thrombosis is well documented after neonatal umbilical vein catheterization but resolves in greater than 50% of cases.[72] In adults, cirrhosis or abdominal malignancies are responsible for more than one half of the cases of portal vein thrombosis.[73] The disorder occurs in at least 10% of patients with cirrhosis, presumably as a result of sluggish portal vein blood flow, but acquired and inherited hypercoagulable states can be identified in many patients with cirrhosis and portal vein thrombosis.[74] Hepatocellular and pancreatic carcinomas are the most common malignant causes for portal vein thrombosis,[73] usually because of a combination of hypercoaguability and invasion or constriction of the portal vein. Local inflammatory reactions resulting from acute or chronic pancreatitis are a common cause of portal vein thrombosis. Pylephlebitis, or septic portal vein thrombosis, can complicate intra-abdominal infections such as appendicitis, diverticulitis, and cholangitis. In addition, splenic vein trauma during splenectomy results in portal vein thrombosis in 8% of cases; the risk increases to 40% if a myeloproliferative disorder is present.[75]

CLINICAL FEATURES AND COURSE

Portal vein thrombosis is found with equal frequency in adults (mean age, 40 years) and children (mean age, 6

Table 80–2   Causes of Portal Vein Thrombosis

Hypercoagulable States	**Complications of Therapeutic Interventions**
Antiphospholipid syndrome	Alcohol injection
Antithrombin deficiency	Colectomy
Factor V Leiden mutation	Endoscopic sclerotherapy
Methylenetetrahydrofolate reductase mutation TT677	Fundoplication
Myeloproliferative disorder	Gastric banding
Nephrotic syndrome	Hepatic chemoembolization
Oral contraceptives	Hepatobiliary surgery
Paroxysmal nocturnal hemoglobinuria	Islet cell injection
Polycythemia rubra vera	Liver transplantation
Pregnancy	Peritoneal dialysis
Prothrombin mutation G20210A	Radiofrequency ablation of hepatic tumor(s)
Protein C deficiency	Splenectomy
Protein S deficiency	TIPS procedure
Sickle cell disease	Umbilical vein catheterization
Inflammatory Diseases	**Impaired Portal Vein Flow**
Behçet's syndrome	Budd-Chiari syndrome
Inflammatory bowel disease	Cirrhosis
Pancreatitis	Cholangiocarcinoma
Infections	Hepatocellular carcinoma
Appendicitis	Nodular regenerative hyperplasia
Cholangitis	Pancreatic carcinoma
Cholecystitis	Sinusoidal obstruction syndrome
Diverticulitis	**Miscellaneous**
Liver abscess	Bladder cancer
Schistosomiasis	Choledochal cyst
Umbilical vein infection	Living at high altitude

TIPS, transjugular intrahepatic portosystemic shunt.

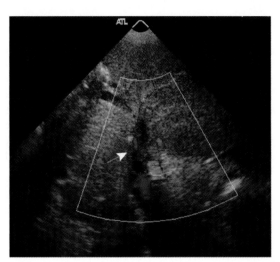

Figure 80–4 Doppler ultrasound image of portal vein thrombosis. The *arrow* points to the portal vein thrombus. The *red coloring* indicates disordered blood flow around the thrombus toward the liver.

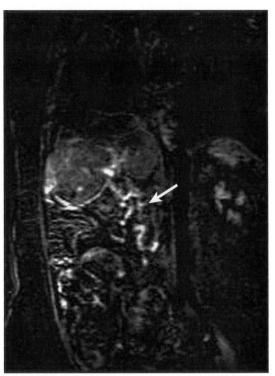

Figure 80–5 Magnetic resonance angiography of cavernous transformation of the portal vein. The *arrow* points to numerous small tortuous collateral vessels replacing the normal portal vein anatomy.

years). The presenting manifestation is almost always hematemesis from variceal bleeding. Abdominal pain is unusual unless the thrombosis involves the mesenteric veins and causes intestinal ischemia. Splenomegaly usually is present, but ascites is uncommon, except in acute portal vein thrombosis or when the thrombosis complicates cirrhosis. Liver biochemical test results usually are normal. Occasionally, common bile duct varices can cause biliary obstruction[76] and even mimic cholangiocarcinoma on endoscopic retrograde cholangiopancreatography.[77] Other unusual locations for ectopic varices in portal vein thrombosis include the gallbladder, duodenum, and rectum. Doppler ultrasonography is highly sensitive for detection of this disorder and reveals an echogenic thrombus in the portal vein (Fig. 80–4), extensive collateral vessels in the porta hepatis, an enlarged spleen, and occasionally nonvisualization of the portal vein. When the diagnosis of portal vein thrombosis is still uncertain, magnetic resonance angiography is better than CT in demonstrating the typical changes of portal vein thrombosis (Fig. 80–5). Portal venography usually is unnecessary unless a surgical shunt is being considered. Evaluation of the patient for precipitating hypercoagulable risk factors may require a consultation with a hematologist.

The natural history of portal vein thrombosis is related primarily to the underlying disorder. In the absence of cirrhosis, cancer, and mesenteric vein thrombosis, the 10-year survival rate for patients with portal vein thrombosis is greater than 80%; only 2% experience fatal variceal hemorrhage.[73] Variceal bleeding caused by portal vein thrombosis has a much better outcome than that observed with variceal bleeding caused by cirrhosis, because of preserved hepatic function and lack of coagulopathy in patients with thrombosis alone. In addition, development of spontaneous portosystemic collaterals can lead to a reduced frequency of recurrent variceal bleeding in patients with portal vein thrombosis.

TREATMENT

Endoscopic band ligation or sclerotherapy is first-line therapy for variceal bleeding in patients with portal vein thrombosis. Sessions should be repeated until the varices are obliterated. Therapy with beta blockers is beneficial in preventing initial[78] and, in combination with endoscopic therapy, recurrent variceal bleeding. Recurrent or refractory variceal bleeding or bleeding from varices distal to the esophagus is an indication for placement of a portosystemic shunt. TIPS is an option if the technical challenge of gaining access to the portal vein can be overcome, but few studies have been performed on use of TIPS for portal vein thrombosis. Focal malignant portal vein obstruction can be stented percutaneously, with successful control of refractory variceal bleeding and ascites.[79] Elective mesocaval and splenorenal shunts[80] and the extended Sugiura procedure (esophagogastric devascularization and transection)[81] also have been performed successfully in patients with portal vein thrombosis, with low mortality and long survival.

Anticoagulation is recommended in patients with acute portal vein thrombosis, to prevent cavernous transformation and complications of portal hypertension. Spontaneous recanalization with acute thrombosis is rare, but therapeutic recanalization can be achieved in greater than 80% of the cases with anticoagulants (intravenous heparin or subcutaneous LMWH, followed by warfarin to achieve an INR of 2.0 to 2.5 for at least 6 months).[82] Prompt use of broad-spectrum antibiotics in cases of septic pylephlebitis also leads to resolution of the thrombosis. Systemic and selective venous infusions of thrombolytic agents have been used successfully in acute portal vein thrombosis[83] and are beneficial when the thrombosis is associated with mesenteric vein thrombosis and intestinal ischemia. Chronic anticoagulation should be considered in patients with portal vein thrombosis and a recognized hypercoagulable state, surgical shunt, or concomitant mesenteric vein thrombosis. The safety of chronic anticoagulation in patients with portal vein thrombosis and varices has been a major concern, but one study has shown that chronic anticoagulation does not increase the risk or severity of variceal bleeding, while preventing further portal and mesenteric venous thrombotic complications.[84] Currently, however, anticoagulants are not recommended for chronic portal vein thrombosis, especially when associated with cavernous transformation. In the past, portal vein thrombosis was an absolute contraindication to liver transplantation, but with improved surgical techniques, liver transplantation for liver failure complicated by portal vein thrombosis is now possible.

ISCHEMIC HEPATITIS

Because *hepatitis* refers to inflammation of the liver, the term *ischemic hepatitis* is somewhat of a misnomer, because inflammation typically is not present. A more physiologic term would be *hypoxic hepatitis*, because the primary cause of this syndrome is tissue hypoxia, which may be the result of hypoperfusion from cardiac failure, systemic hypoxemia from respiratory failure, or increased oxygen requirements from sepsis.[85] The name ischemic hepatitis is used, however, because of clinical similarities to other forms of acute hepatitis and the characteristic pathologic feature of acute centrilobular necrosis. Ischemic hepatitis probably is the most commonly encountered form of vascular liver disease.

ETIOLOGY

Of all cases of extreme serum aspartate aminotransferase (AST) elevation (to greater than 3000 U/L), ischemic hepatitis accounts for about one half.[86] The most common cause of ischemic hepatitis is cardiovascular disease, which accounts for more than 70% of cases, followed in frequency by respiratory failure and sepsis, each of which accounts for less than 15% of cases.[85] Hypotension is documented as a precipitating factor in greater than one half of the patients with ischemic hepatitis but does not need to be evident for ischemic hepatitis to occur. Hypotension often is clinically apparent as a result of acute myocardial infarction, severe congestive heart failure, or sepsis but may be less obvious following a transient arrhythmia or silent coronary ischemic event. The presence of congestive heart failure significantly increases the likelihood that a drop in the cardiac output from any cause will result in ischemic hepatitis. Indeed, greater than 80% of cases of ischemic hepatitis occur in the setting of congestive heart failure.[87] Acute trauma, hemorrhage, burns, and heat stroke also can cause ischemic hepatitis, but the likelihood is substantially less in the absence of underlying heart disease.

DIAGNOSIS

Ischemic hepatitis often is first considered when extreme serum aminotransferase elevations are detected in a patient hospitalized for problems not primarily associated with the liver. Findings on physical examination usually are dominated by the underlying precipitating medical condition. The patient's mental status often is altered becaue of diminished cerebral perfusion. Laboratory studies show extreme elevations of the aminotransferase levels (greater than 3000 U/L). The serum lactate dehydrogenase (LDH) level is profoundly elevated, more so than the alanine aminotransferase (ALT), and an ALT-to-LDH ratio of less than 1.5 is more typical of ischemic hepatitis than of viral hepatitis.[88] The prothrombin time may be prolonged by 2 or 3 seconds, and the serum bilirubin level often is mildly increased, with peak levels seen after the aminotransferase levels peak. The serum creatinine and blood urea nitrogen levels often are elevated because of acute tubular necrosis. Characteristically, serum aminotransferase levels usually peak 1 to 3 days after the hemodynamic insult and return to normal within 7 to 10 days.

The differential diagnosis for this type of severe acute injury includes acute hepatitis caused by viral infections, autoimmunity, toxins, and medications (see also Chapter 70). Liver biopsy specimens—although biopsy usually is unnecessary—reveal bland, centrilobular necrosis with preservation of the hepatic architecture (Fig. 80–6). Occasionally a definitive diagnosis of ischemic hepatitis can be difficult to make, but the typical prompt rise in serum aminotransferase and LDH levels followed by a rapid fall within a few days is more characteristic of ischemic hepatitis than of other causes of severe acute liver injury[88] (Fig. 80–7).

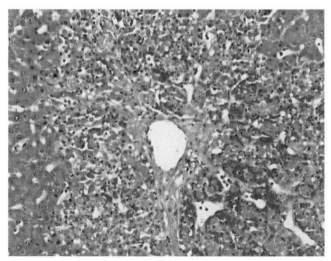

Figure 80–6 Histopathologic features of ischemic hepatitis. This high-power photomicrograph demonstrates centrilobular necrosis, loss of hepatocytes, and sinusoidal congestion with red blood cells, but only scant inflammatory infiltrate. Perivenular fibrosis is evident. Hematoxylin-eosin stain. (Courtesy of Dr. Pamela Jensen, Dallas, Tex.)

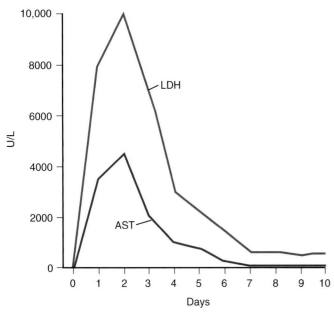

Figure 80–7   The typical course of serum aspartate aminotransferase (AST) and lactate dehydrogenase (LDH) levels in ischemic hepatitis. (Adapted from Gitlin NG, Serio KM: Ischemic hepatitis: Widening horizons. Am J Gastroenterol 7:831, 1992.)

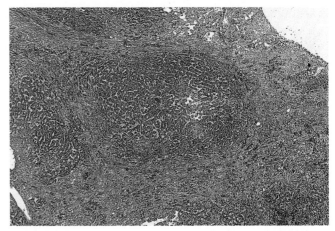

Figure 80–8   Histopathologic features of cardiac cirrhosis. This low-power view shows a portal tract in the center of a regenerative nodule and fibrotic bands bridging central veins. The size of the scar and the presence of the nodule attest to the long-term course of the fibrotic process. Even at low power, the bland nature of the cirrhosis is apparent. No inflammatory cells are evident. The sinusoids are dilated and congested. (Courtesy of Edward Lee, MD, Washington, DC.)

CLINICAL COURSE AND TREATMENT

Most cases of ischemic hepatitis are transient and self-limited. In the most severely affected patients, ischemic hepatitis is just one manifestation of multiorgan failure and carries a poor prognosis. Fulminant hepatic failure resulting from ischemic hepatitis is uncommon but is more likely to occur when chronic congestive heart failure or cirrhosis also is present. The overall prognosis depends primarily on the severity of the underlying predisposing condition, not the severity of the liver disease. No specific therapy exists for ischemic hepatitis, and treatment is directed at improving cardiac output and systemic oxygenation.

CONGESTIVE HEPATOPATHY

The effects of congestive heart failure on the liver predictably include decreased hepatic blood flow, increased hepatic vein pressure, and decreased arterial oxygen saturation.[90] Right-sided heart failure results in transmission of increased central venous pressure from the heart directly to the hepatic sinusoids. The result is centrilobular congestion and sinusoidal edema that further decrease oxygen delivery. The injurious effects of superimposed ischemic hepatitis are common in these patients. The acute and chronic damage results in progressive centrilobular fibrosis. Sinusoidal hypertension and congestion can lead to the development of ascites, with a characteristically high serum–ascites albumin gradient and a high protein concentration (see Chapter 88).

Clinically, the symptoms and signs of congestive heart failure are the predominant features. Dull right upper quadrant pain in association with hepatomegaly is common. The liver may be pulsatile, and hepatojugular reflux often is apparent on compression over the liver. Spider angiomata and varices usually are not present, and variceal bleeding caused by congestive hepatopathy alone does not occur. Mild elevation of the serum bilirubin level (to less than 3 mg/dL) is common, but jaundice is seen in less than 10% of patients, usually those with severe or acute congestive heart failure.[91] The prothrombin time is prolonged in greater than three fourths of cases and usually is resistant to therapy with vitamin K. Other liver biochemical test levels often are normal or only mildly elevated. Liver test results improve slowly or normalize with effective therapy of the underlying congestive heart failure.

The histologic features of congestive hepatopathy include atrophy of hepatocytes, sinusoidal distention, and centrilobular fibrosis (Fig. 80–8). Centrilobular necrosis, consistent with ischemic hepatitis, is frequent in liver biopsy specimens that show congestive hepatopathy and usually correlates with recent hypotension.[92] Bridging fibrosis typically extends between central veins (rather than between portal tracts) to produce a pattern of "reverse lobulation" characteristic of *cardiac cirrhosis*. The distribution of fibrosis throughout the liver is highly variable and correlates with focal sinusoidal thrombosis, with obliteration of central and portal veins that leads in turn to localized ischemia, parenchymal extinction, and fibrosis.[93]

The presence of congestive hepatopathy does not affect the prognosis in patients with heart failure; the mortality rate is determined primarily by the severity of the underlying cardiac disease. Occasionally, paracentesis may be needed to alleviate tense ascites, but therapy generally is directed at the cardiac failure.

PELIOSIS HEPATIS

Peliosis hepatis is characterized by the presence of multiple blood-filled cavities distributed randomly throughout the liver. The cavities range in size from a few millimeters to 3 cm across and usually are seen in association with dilated hepatic sinusoids (Fig. 80–9). Two histologic types of peliosis hepatis occur. In the *parenchymal* type, blood-filled cavities are lined by hepatocytes, and hemorrhagic parenchymal necrosis and congestion usually are present. In the *phlebectatic* type, the cavities are lined by endothelial cells associated with aneurysmal dilatation of the central vein.[94] Fibrosis, cirrhosis, regenerative nodules, and tumors also may be seen with peliosis. In the past, peliosis hepatis was largely a histologic curiosity, but its association with renal transplantation and the acquired immunodeficiency syndrome (AIDS) have increased clinical awareness of this syndrome.

Although jaundice, painful hepatomegaly, liver failure, and fatal hemorrhage may be manifestations of peliosis, more often the disorder is detected during evaluation of abnormal liver biochemical test results in an asymptomatic patient. If the hemorrhagic cavities are large enough, they can be detected by ultrasonography, computed tomography, and magnetic resonance imaging.[95]

The pathogenesis of peliosis hepatis is unknown, but the leading theories include damage to sinusoidal endothelial cells, outflow obstruction of blood flow at the sinusoidal level, and hepatocellular necrosis. Before the 1970s, peliosis was most often identified in patients dying of wasting diseases, particularly tuberculosis and carcinomatosis.[94] Since then, peliosis has been associated with the use of anabolic steroids, oral contraceptives, tamoxifen, danazol, vitamin A, glucocorticoids, 6-thioguanine, and azathioprine and exposure to urethane, vinyl chloride, and thorium dioxide (see Chapter 84). The syndrome can regress with discontinuation of the causative agent. Myeloproliferative diseases such as agnogenic myeloid metaplasia[96] and malignant histiocytosis[97] and infections such as *E. coli* pyelonephritis[98] also have been associated with peliosis.

Bacillary peliosis is caused by the bacterium responsible for cat-scratch disease, in the genus *Bartonella*. Traumatic exposure to cats is a recognized risk factor. The syndrome has been reported in immunocompetent persons but is associated primarily with AIDS (see Chapters 32 and 79).[99] In affected patients, vascular proliferative lesions are found commonly in the skin (where they are termed *bacillary angiomatosis*), or in the liver and spleen (where they are termed *bacillary peliosis*, and where bacilli can be identified histologically adjacent to the peliotic lesions). Symptoms and signs include anorexia, abdominal pain, fever, lymphadenopathy, hepatosplenomegaly, and cutaneous vascular lesions or nodules.[100] Anemia, an elevated serum alkaline phosphatase level, and a $CD4^+$ lymphocyte count of less than 200/mm^3 are typical laboratory findings. Bacillary peliosis responds to antibiotic therapy (e.g., erythromycin, doxycycline) (see Chapter 79).

Peliosis hepatis occurs in 20% of patients after kidney transplantation and is associated mainly with the prolonged use of azathioprine and possibly cyclosporine.[101] The lesions often are asymptomatic or associated with abnormal liver biochemical test levels, but progressive fibrosis, cirrhosis, and portal hypertension may be additional findings. Hepatic lesions may regress on withdrawal of azathioprine, but the overall course is not clearly modified and the risk of transplant rejection is increased substantially.[102]

HEPATIC ARTERY ANEURYSM

Hepatic artery aneurysms (HAAs) are uncommon, but they are the second leading category of visceral artery aneurysms and account for over 20% of cases (after splenic artery aneurysms). A majority of true HAAs are isolated, sacular, extrahepatic lesions involving the full arterial wall. In the past, HAAs were mainly mycotic (infectious) in etiology, but today they typically result from atherosclerosis, mediointimal degeneration, trauma, and less commonly, infection. Other rare causes of true HAA are vasculitides, such as polyarteritis nodosa, systemic lupus erythematosus, Takayasu's arteritis, and Kawasaki disease, and connective tissue disorders, such as Marfan's syndrome, Ehlers-Danlos syndrome, and Osler-Weber-Rendu disease.[103] Approximately one half of HAAs are pseudoaneurysms (aneurysms resulting from injury). Procedures commonly associated with hepatic artery pseudoaneurysms include liver biopsy, transhepatic biliary drainage, cholecystectomy, hepatectomy, and liver transplantation.[104]

Symptoms of HAA include epigastric or right subchondral pain, but most affected persons are asymptomatic until the aneurysm ruptures. Rarely, a pulsatile right upper quadrant mass or thrill may be detected. Patients may present with rupture into the biliary tree, with hemobilia, epigastric pain and icterus; rupture into the portal vein, with portal hypertension and variceal bleeding; or rupture into the peritoneal cavity, with abdominal pain and shock. The mortality rate from rupture of HAA is greater than 30%. Nonatherosclerotic aneurysms

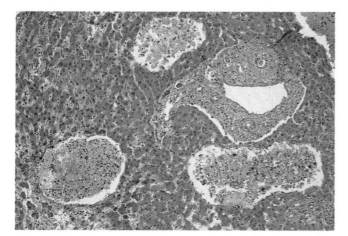

Figure 80–9 Histopathologic features of peliosis hepatis. Note the presence of three blood-filled cysts without lining cells and an adjacent portal tract. Sinusoidal dilatation is also present. (Courtesy of Edward Lee, MD, Washington, DC.)

and multiple HAAs carry an increased risk of rupture and should be treated. Although the risk of rupture of an aneurysm is independent of its size, atherosclerotic aneurysms greater than 2 cm in diameter also should be treated.[103]

Doppler ultrasound studies and computed tomography readily demonstrate HAAs, but angiography is especially useful for defining these lesions, accessing the collateral circulation, and planning treatment. Hepatic artery pseudoaneurysms are treated effectively by angiographic embolization.[104] True extrahepatic aneurysms may be treated with embolization, provided that presence of collateral circulation, distance from the gastroduodenal artery, absence of cirrhosis, and patency of the portal vein can be confirmed, but surgical resection of the aneurysm may be preferable, to minimize the risk of hepatic infarction.[105]

ATHEROSCLEROSIS

Despite its frequency in the general population, atherosclerosis is rarely a cause of liver disease. Intimal thickening and atherosclerosis in hepatic arteries are less common and occur later in life than is typical for the coronary arteries.[106] Hepatic infarction resulting from atherosclerosis alone is rare. The dual blood supply to the liver undoubtedly confers protection from ischemia. Nevertheless, atherosclerosis is the primary cause of approximately one third of hepatic artery aneurysms.[105] In addition, because the common bile duct receives all of its blood from the hepatic artery, atherosclerosis can result in ischemic cholangiopathy with biliary strictures and obstruction.[107] The presence of atherosclerosis also limits the use of livers from older donors for transplantation. Atherosclerosis makes arterial anastomoses technically more difficult to secure and may predispose the liver to ischemic injury during transport and reperfusion.

REFERENCES

1. Valla DC: Hepatic vein thrombosis (Budd-Chiari syndrome). Semin Liver Dis 22:5, 2002.
2. Tavill AS, Wood EJ, Kreel L, et al: The Budd-Chiari syndrome: Correlation between hepatic scintigraphy and the clinical, radiological, and pathological findings in nineteen cases of hepatic venous outflow obstruction. Gastroenterology 68:509, 1975.
3. Mitchell MC, Boitnott JK, Kaufman S, et al: Budd-Chiari syndrome: Etiology, diagnosis and management. Medicine 61:199, 1982.
4. Parker RGF: Occlusion of the hepatic veins in man. Medicine 38:369, 1959.
5. Okuda H, Yamagata H, Obata H, et al: Epidemiological and clinical features of Budd-Chiari syndrome in Japan. J Hepatol 22:1, 1995.
6. Dilawari JB, Bambery P, Chawla Y, et al: Hepatic outflow obstruction (Budd-Chiari syndrome). Medicine 73:21, 1994.
7. Wang Z: Recognition and management of Budd-Chiari syndrome: Experience with 143 patients. Chinese Med J 102:338, 1989.
8. Simson IW: Membranous obstruction of the inferior vena cava and hepatocellular carcinoma in South Africa. Gastroenterology 88:576, 1985.
9. Okuda K, Kage M, Shrestha SM: Proposal of a new nomenclature for Budd-Chiari syndrome: Hepatic vein thrombosis versus thrombosis of the inferior vena cava at its hepatic portion. Hepatology 28:1191, 1998.
10. Menon KV, Shah V, Kamath PS: The Budd-Chiari syndrome. N Engl J Med 350:578, 2004.
11. Valla D, Casadevall N, Lacombe C, et al: Primary myeloproliferative disorder and hepatic vein thrombosis. Ann Intern Med 103:329, 1985.
12. Espinosa G, Font J, Garcia-Pagan JC, et al: Budd-Chiari syndrome secondary to antiphospholipid syndrome. Medicine 80:345, 2001.
13. Mohanty D, Shetty S, Ghosh K, et al: Hereditary thrombophilia as a cause of Budd-Chiari syndrome: A study from Western India. Hepatology 34:666, 2001.
14. Deltenre P, Denninger MH, Hillaire S, et al: Factor V Leiden related Budd-Chiari syndrome. Gut 48:264, 2001.
15. Denninger MH, Chait Y, Casadevall N, et al: Cause of portal or hepatic venous thrombosis in adults: The role of multiple concurrent factors. Hepatology 31:587, 2000.
16. Matsui S, Ichida T, Watanabe M, et al: Clinical features and etiology of hepatocellular carcinoma arising in patients with membranous obstruction of the inferior vena cava: In reference to hepatitis viral infection. J Gastroenterol Hepatol 15:1205, 2000.
17. Havlioglu N, Brunt E, Bacon B: Budd-Chiari syndrome and hepatocellular carcinoma: A case report and review of the literature. Am J Gastroenterol 98:201, 2003.
18. Okuda K: Inferior vena cava thrombosis at its hepatic portion (obliterative hepatocavopathy). Semin Liver Dis 22:15, 2002.
19. Hadengue A, Poliquin M, Vilgrain V, et al: The changing scene of hepatic vein thrombosis: Recognition of asymptomatic cases. Gastroenterology 106:1042, 1994.
20. Ibarrola C, Castellano VM, Colina F: Focal hyperplastic hepatocellular nodules in hepatic venous outflow obstruction: A clinicopathological study of four patients and 24 nodules. Histopathology 44:172, 2004.
21. Cazals-Hatem D, Vilgrain V, Genin P, et al: Arterial and portal circulation and parenchymal changes in Budd-Chiari syndrome: A study in 17 explanted livers. Hepatology 37:510, 2003.
22. Bolondi L, Gaiani S, Li Bassi S, et al: Diagnosis of Budd-Chiari syndrome by pulsed Doppler ultrasound. Gastroenterology 100:1324, 1991.
23. Singh V, Sinha SK, Nain CK, et al: Budd-Chiari syndrome: Our experience in 71 patients. J Gastroenterol Hepatol 15:550, 2000.
24. Kane R, Eustace S: Diagnosis of Budd-Chiari syndrome: Comparison between sonography and MR angiography. Radiology 195:117, 1995.
25. Tang TJ, Batts KP, de Groen PC, et al: The prognostic value of histology in the assessment of patients with Budd-Chiari syndrome. J Hepatol 35:338, 2001.
26. Sharma S, Texeira A, Texeira P, et al: Pharmacological thrombolysis in Budd Chiari syndrome: A single centre experience and review of the literature. J Hepatol 40:172, 2004.
27. Xu K, Feng B, Zhong H, et al: Clinical application of interventional techniques in the treatment of Budd-Chiari syndrome. Chin Med J 116:609, 2003.
28. Zhang, CQ, Fu LN, Xu L, et al: Long term effect of stent placement in 115 patients with Budd-Chiari syndrome. World J Gastroenterol 9:2587, 2003.
29. De BK, Biswas PK, Sen S, et al: Management of the Budd-Chiari syndrome by balloon cavoplasty. Indian J Gastroenterol 20:151, 2001.
30. Wu T, Wang L, Xiao Q, et al: Percutaneous balloon angioplasty of inferior vena cava in Budd-Chiari syndrome-R1. Int J Cardiol 83:175, 2002.

31. Pelage JP, Denys A, Valla D, et al: Budd-Chiari syndrome due to prothrombotic disorder: Mid-term patency and efficacy of endovascular stents. Eur Radiol 13:286, 2003.

32. Mourad FH, Khalifeh M, Al-Kutoubi A, et al: Inferior vena cava obstruction in Budd-Chiari syndrome: Successful treatment by radiological stenting followed by a portosystemic shunt. Eur J Gastroenterol Hepatol 13:275, 2001.

33. Rossle M, Olschewski M, Siegerstetter V, et al: The Budd-Chiari syndrome: Outcome after treatment with the transjugular intrahepatic portosystemic shunt. Surgery 135:394, 2004.

34. Gasparini D, Del Forno M, Sponza M, et al: Transjugular intrahepatic portosystemic shunt by direct transcaval approach in patients with acute and hyperacute Budd-Chiari syndrome. Eur J Gastroenterol Hepatol 14:567, 2002.

35. Mancuso A, Fung K, Mela M, et al: TIPS for acute and chronic Budd-Chiari syndrome: A single-centre experience. J Hepatol 38:751, 2003.

36. Perello A, Garcia-Pagan JC, Gilabert R, et al: TIPS is a useful long-term derivative therapy for patients with Budd-Chiari syndrome uncontrolled by medical therapy. Hepatology 35:132, 2002.

37. Xu PQ, Dang XW: Treatment of membranous Budd-Chiari syndrome: Analysis of 480 cases. Hepatobiliary Pacreat Dis Int 3:73, 2004.

38. Pasic M, Senning A, von Segesser L, et al: Transcaval liver resection with hepatoatrial anastamosis for treatment of patients with the Budd-Chiari syndrome. J Thorac Cardiovasc Surg 106:275, 1993.

39. Orloff MJ, Daily PO, Orloff SL, et al: A 27 year experience with surgical treatment of Budd-Chiari syndrome. Ann Surg 232:340, 2000.

40. Terpstra OT, Ausema B, Bruining HA, et al: Late results of mesocaval interposition shunting for bleeding oesophageal varices. Br J Surg 74:787, 1987.

41. Behera A, Menakuru SR, Thingnam S, et al: Treatment of Budd-Chiari syndrome with inferior vena caval occlusion by mesoatrial shunt. Eur J Surg 168:355, 2002.

42. Slakey DP, Klein AS, Venbrux AC, et al: Budd-Chiari syndrome: Current management options. Ann Surg 233:522, 2001.

43. Ringe B, Lang H, Oldhafer KJ, et al: Which is the best surgery for Budd-Chiari syndrome: Venous decompression or liver transplantation? A single-center experience with 50 patients. Hepatology 21:1337, 1995.

44. Melear JM, Goldstein RM, Levy MF, et al: Hematologic aspects of liver transplantation for Budd-Chiari syndrome with special reference to myeloproliferative disorders. Transplantation 74:1090, 2002.

45. Bahr MJ, Schubert J, Bleck JS, et al: Recurrence of Budd-Chiari syndrome after liver transplantation in paroxysmal nocturnal hemoglobinuria. Transpl Int 16:890, 2003.

46. Parthi S, Mohamed R, Andreas P, et al: Liver transplantation for Budd-Chiari syndrome. Transplantation 73:973, 2002.

47. Janssen HLA, Garcia-Pagan JC, Elias E, et al: Budd-Chiari syndrome: A review by an expert panel. J Hepatol 38:364, 2003.

48. Langlet P, Escolano S, Valla D, et al: Clinicopathological forms and prognostic index in Budd-Chiari syndrome. J Hepatol 39:496, 2003.

49. Murad SD, Valla DC, de Groen PC, et al: Determinants of survival and the effect of portosystemic shunting in patients with Budd-Chiari syndrome. Hepatology 39:500, 2004.

50. DeLeve LD, Shulman HM, McDonald GB: Toxic injury to hepatic sinusoids: Sinusoidal obstruction syndrome (veno-occlusive disease). Semin Liver Dis 22:27, 2002.

51. Willmot FC, Robertson GW: Senecio disease, or cirrhosis of the liver due to *Senecio* poisoning. Lancet 2:848, 1920.

52. Bras G, Jelliffe DB, Stuart KL: Veno-occlusive disease of liver with nonportal type of cirrhosis, occurring in Jamaica. Arch Pathol 57:285, 1954.

53. Mellis C, Bale PM: Familial hepatic venoocclusive disease with probable immune deficiency. J Pediatr 88:236, 1976.

54. Kumar A, DeLeve LD, Kamath PS, et al: Hepatic veno-occlusive disease (sinusoidal obstruction syndrome) after hematopoietic stem cell transplantation. Mayo Clin Proc 78:589, 2003.

55. Lassau N, Auperin A, Leclere J, et al: Prognostic value of Doppler-ultrasonography in hepatic veno-occlusive disease. Transplantation 74:60, 2002.

56. Jacobson AF, Teefey SA, Higano CA, et al: Increased lung uptake of ^{99m}Tc-sulphur colloid as an early indicator of the development of hepatic veno-occlusive disease in bone marrow transplant patients. Nucl Med Commun 14:706, 1993.

57. Shulman HM, Gooley T, Dudley MD, et al: Utility of transvenous liver biopsies and wedged hepatic venous pressure measurements in sixty marrow transplant recipients. Transplantation 59:1015, 1995.

58. Yoshimoto K, Ono N, Okamura T, et al: Recent progress in the diagnosis and therapy for veno-occlusive disease of the liver. Leukemia Lymphoma 44:229, 2003.

59. Tanikawa S, Mori S, Ohhashi K, et al: Predictive markers for hepatic veno-occlusive disease after hematopoietic stem cell transplantation in adults: A prospective single center study. Bone Marrow Transplant 26:881, 2000.

60. Richardson P, Guinan E: Hepatic veno-occlusive disease following hematopoietic stem cell transplantation. Acta Haematol 106:57, 2001.

61. Shulman HM, Fisher LB, Schoch HG, et al: Venoocclusive disease of the liver after marrow transplantation: Histological correlates of clinical signs and symptoms. Hepatology 19:1171, 1994.

62. Wadleigh M, Ho V, Momtaz P, et al: Hepatic veno-occlusive disease: Pathogenesis, diagnosis and treatment. Curr Opin Hematol 10:451, 2003.

63. Essell JH, Schroeder MT, Harman GS, et al: Ursodiol prophylaxis against hepatic complications of allogeneic bone marrow transplantation: A randomized, double-blind, placebo-controlled trial. Ann Intern Med 128:975, 1998.

64. Bearman SI: Avoiding hepatic veno-occlusive disease: What do we know and where are we going? Bone Marrow Transplant 27:1113, 2001.

65. Attal M, Huguet F, Rubie H, et al: Prevention of hepatic veno-occlusive disease after bone marrow transplantation by continuous infusion of low-dose heparin: A prospective, randomized trial. Blood 79:2834, 1992.

66. Reiss U, Cowan M, McMillan A, et al: Hepatic venoocclusive disease in blood and bone marrow transplantation in children and young adults: Incidence, risk factors, and outcome in a cohort of 241 patients. J Pediatr Hematol Oncol 24:746, 2002.

67. Park SH, Lee MH, Lee H, et al: A randomized trial of heparin plus ursodiol vs heparin alone to prevent hepatic veno-occlusive disease after hematopoietic stem cell transplantation. Bone Marrow Transplant 29:137, 2002.

68. Simon M, Hahn T, Ford LA, et al: Retrospective multivariate analysis of hepatic veno-occlusive disease after blood or marrow transplantation: Possible beneficial use of low molecular weight heparin. Bone Marrow Transplant 27:627, 2001.

69. Richardson PG, Murakami C, Jin Z, et al: Multi-institutional use of defibrotide in 88 patients after stem cell transplantation with severe veno-occlusive disease and multisystem organ failure: Response without significant toxicity in a high-risk population and factors predictive of outcome. Blood 100:4337, 2002.

70. Azoulay D, Castaing D, Lemoine A, et al: Transjugular intrahepatic portosystemic shunt (TIPS) for severe veno-occlusive disease of the liver following bone marrow transplantation. Bone Marrow Transplant 25:987, 2000.

71. Janssen HL: Changing perspectives in portal vein thrombosis. Scand J Gastroenterol 232:69, 2000.

72. Kim, JH, Lee YS, Kim SH, et al: Does umbilical vein catheterization lead to portal venous thrombosis? Prospective US evaluation in 100 neonates. Radiology 219:645, 2001.

73. Janssen, HL, Wijnhoud A, Haagsma EB, et al: Extrahepatic portal vein thrombosis: Aetiology and determinants of survival. Gut 49:720, 2001.

74. Amitrano L, Guardascione MA, Brancaccio V, et al: Risk factors and clinical presentation of portal vein thrombosis in patients with liver cirrhosis. J Hepatol 40:736, 2004.

75. Winslow ER, Brunt LM, Drebin JA, et al: Portal vein thrombosis after splenectomy. Am J Surg 184:631, 2002.

76. Lohr JM, Kuchenreuter S, Grebmeier H, et al: Compression of the common bile duct due to portal-vein thrombosis in polycythemia vera. Hepatology 17:586, 1993.

77. Bayraktar Y, Balkanci F, Kayhan B, et al: Bile duct varices or "pseudo-cholangiocarcinoma sign" in portal hypertension due to cavernous transformation of the portal vein. Am J Gastroenterol 87:1801, 1992.

78. Gurakan, F, Eren M, Kocak N, et al: Extrahepatic portal vein thrombosis in children: Etiology and long-term follow-up. J Clin Gastroenterol 38:368, 2004.

79. Yamakado K, Nakatsuka A, Tanaka N, et al: Portal venous stent placement in patients with pancreatic and biliary neoplasms invading portal veins and causing portal hypertension: initial experience. Radiology 220:150, 2001.

80. Boles ET, Wise WE, Birken G: Extrahepatic portal hypertension in children: Long-term evaluation. Am J Surg 151:734, 1986.

81. Dagenais M, Langer B, Taylor BR, et al: Experience with radical esophagogastric devascularization procedures (Sugiura) for variceal bleeding outside Japan. World J Surg 18:222, 1994.

82. Valla DC, Condat B, Lebrec D: Spectrum of portal vein thrombosis in the West. J Gastroenterol Hepatol 17:s224, 2002.

83. Malkowski P, Pawlak J, Michalowicz B, et al: Thrombolytic treatment of portal thrombosis. Hepatogastroenterology 50:2098, 2003.

84. Condat B, Pessione F, Hillaire S, et al: Current outcome of portal vein thrombosis in adults: Risk and benefit of anticoagulant therapy. Gastroenterology 120:490, 2001.

85. Henrion J, Schapira M, Luwaert R, et al: Hypoxic hepatitis: Clinical and hemodynamic study in 142 consecutive cases. Medicine 82:392, 2003.

86. Johnson RD, O'Connor ML, Kerr RM: Extreme serum elevations of aspartate aminotransferase. Am J Gastroenterol 90:1244, 1995.

87. Seeto RK, Fenn B, Rockey DC: Ischemic hepatitis: Clinical presentation and pathogenesis. Am J Med 109:109, 2000.

88. Cassidy WM, Reynolds TB: Serum lactate dehydrogenase in the differential diagnosis of acute hepatocellular injury. J Clin Gastroenterol 19:118, 1994.

89. Gitlin N, Serio KM: Ischemic hepatitis: Widening horizons. Am J Gastroenterol 87:831, 1992.

90. Giallourakis CC, Rosenberg PM, Friedman LS: The liver in heart failure. Clin Liver Disease 6:4, 2002.

91. Richman SM, Delman AJ, Grob D: Alterations in indices of liver function in congestive heart failure with particular reference to serum enzymes. Am J Med 30:211, 1961.

92. Arcidi JM, Moore GW, Hutchins GM: Hepatic morphology in cardiac dysfunction: A clincopathologic study of 1000 subjects at autopsy. Am J Pathol 104:159, 1981.

93. Wanless IR, Liu JJ, Butany J: Role of thrombosis in the pathogenesis of congestive hepatic fibrosis (cardiac cirrhosis). Hepatology 21:1232, 1995.

94. Yanoff M, Rawson AJ: Peliosis hepatis: An anatomical study with demonstration of two varieties. Arch Pathol Lab Med 77:159, 1964.

95. Ferrozzi F, Tognini G, Zuccoli G, et al: Peliosis hepatis with pseudotumoral and hemorrhagic evolution: CT and MR findings. Abdom Imaging 26:197, 2001.

96. Makdisi WJ, Cherian R, Vanveldhuizen PJ, et al: Fatal peliosis of the liver and spleen in a patient with agnogenic myeloid metaplasia treated with danazol. Am J Med 90:317, 1994.

97. Fine KD, Solano M, Polter DE, et al: Malignant histiocytosis in a patient presenting with hepatic dysfunction and peliosis hepatis. Am J Gastroenterol 90:485, 1995.

98. Jacquemin E, Pariente D, Fabre M, et al: Peliosis hepatis with initial presentation as acute hepatic failure and intraperitoneal hemorrhage in children. J Hepatol 30:1146, 1999.

99. Tappero JW, Mohle-Boetani J, Koehler JE, et al: The epidemiology of bacillary angiomatosis and bacillary peliosis. JAMA 269:770, 1993.

100. Mohle-Boetani JC, Koehler JE, Berger TG, et al: Bacillary angiomatosis and bacillary peliosis in patients infected with human immunodeficiency virus: Clinical characteristics in a case-control study. Clin Infect Dis 22:794, 1996.

101. Izumi S, Nishiuchi M, Kameda Y, et al: Laparoscopic study of peliosis hepatis and nodular transformation of the liver before and after renal transplantation: Natural history and aetiology in follow-up cases. J Hepatol 20:129, 1994.

102. Cavalcanti R, Pol S, Carnot F, et al: Impact and evolution of peliosis hepatis in renal transplant recipients. Transplantation 58:315, 1994.

103. Abbas MA, Fowl RJ, Stone WM, et al: Hepatic artery aneurysm: Factors that predict complications. J Vasc Surg 38:41, 2003.

104. Tessier DJ, Fowl RJ, Stone WM, et al: Iatrogenic hepatic artery pseudoaneurysms: An uncommon complication after hepatic, biliary, and pancreatic procedures. Ann Vasc Surg 17:663, 2003.

105. Baggio E, Migliara B, Lipari G, et al: Treatment of six hepatic artery aneurysms. Ann Vasc Surg 18:93, 2004.

106. Krus S, Turjman MW, Fiejka E: Comparative morphology of the hepatic and coronary artery walls. Part 1. Differences in the distribution and intensity of atherosclerotic intimal thickening and atherosclerosis. Med Sci Monit 6:19, 2000.

107. Saiura A, Umekita N, Inoue S, et al: Benign biliary stricture associated with atherosclerosis. Hepatogastroenterology 48:81, 2001.

CHAPTER
81 Alcoholic Liver Disease

Robert L. Carithers and Craig McClain

Alcoholic liver disease remains a challenging enigma for both basic scientists and clinicians. Despite more than 5 decades of research, many important facets of this disease have yet to be resolved. Paramount among these important questions are the following: (1) Why does cirrhosis develop in only a small fraction of heavy alcohol abusers? (2) What is the pathogenesis of severe alcoholic liver disease? (3) What are the most effective treatments for patients with advanced disease?

EPIDEMIOLOGY

Although two thirds of American adults drink alcohol, only a minority are problem drinkers. Nevertheless, the number of alcoholics in the United States is estimated to be 14 million.[1] The total costs of alcohol abuse amount to $185 billion annually, most of which are related to lost productivity and motor vehicle accidents. Alcoholic liver disease also is a major health care problem, accounting for 40% of deaths from cirrhosis and more than 30% of cases of hepatocellular carcinoma in the United States.[1,2] Comparable statistics have been reported from Europe.[3]

Numerous studies have shown that alcoholic liver disease develops in women after a shorter duration of drinking and with a lower daily alcohol intake than in men.[4,5] Population-based surveys have documented that men usually must drink 40 to 80 g of alcohol daily and women 20 to 40 g daily for 10 to 12 years to achieve a significant risk of liver disease.[4-6] Table 81–1 illustrates the alcohol content of various beverages, their typical serving sizes, and the daily alcohol intake, for at least 10 years, that puts both men and women at risk for the development of alcoholic liver disease.

SPECTRUM OF DISEASE

Chronic alcohol abuse can result in a spectrum of liver injury ranging from mild fatty infiltration to cirrhosis and hepatocellar carcinoma[7,8] (Fig. 81–1). Fat accumulation in liver cells, which is the earliest and most predictable response to alcohol ingestion, is seen in 90% of heavy drinkers. Although fatty liver generally is a benign condition and usually quickly reversible with abstinence, perivenular fibrosis, which can progress to cirrhosis, may develop in some affected persons. Fibrosis is particularly likely to develop if the steatosis is severe and present in a mixed micro- or macrovesicular pattern. Much more important is the development of necroinflammation with or without fat infiltration and fibrosis (alcoholic hepatitis), which occurs in approximately 10% to 35% of heavy drinkers. Alcoholic hepatitis is an important clinical entity for two reasons: (1) patients with severe alco-

Table 81–1   Alcohol Content of Various Beverages

Beverage	Alcohol Content	Serving Size	Amount of Alcohol	Daily Intake Needed to Exceed Threshold for Alcoholic Liver Disease*	
				Men	Women
Beer	5%	12 oz	13.85 g	3-6 cans	1.5-3 cans
Wine	12%	4 oz	10.7 g	4-8 glasses	2-4 glasses
Fortified wine	20%	4 oz	17.8 g	2-4 glasses	1-2 glasses
Hard liquor	40%	1.5 oz	13.4 g	3-6 drinks	1.5-3 drinks

*Alcohol intake of 10-40 g/day for women and 40-80 g/day for men for 10 years.

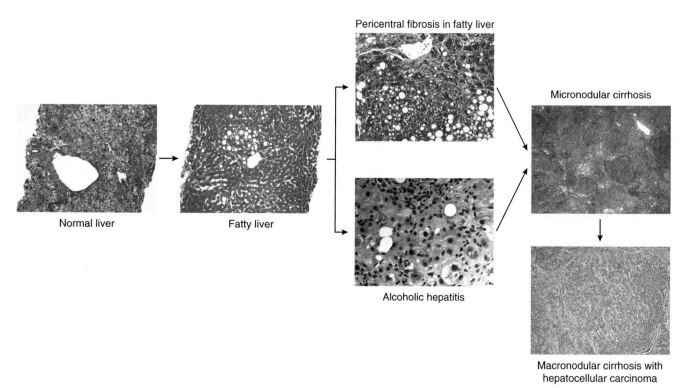

Pericentral fibrosis in fatty liver

Micronodular cirrhosis

Normal liver

Fatty liver

Alcoholic hepatitis

Macronodular cirrhosis with hepatocellular carcinoma

Figure 81–1   Histologic spectrum of alcoholic liver disease.

holic hepatitis have extremely high short-term mortality rates, and (2) alcohol hepatitis is a well-documented precursor of cirrhosis, with a long-term frequency of cirrhosis nine times higher than that for patients with fatty liver alone.[9] With continued alcohol abuse, a fine mesh-like pattern of cirrhosis with prominent involvement of the central vein (micronodular or Laennec's cirrhosis) develops in 8% to 20% of heavy drinkers. Over time, this lesion can evolve to include broad bands of fibrosis that separate large nodules of liver tissue (macronodular cirrhosis). Hepatocellular carcinoma may develop in this setting.

DIAGNOSIS OF ALCOHOL ABUSE

The diagnosis of alcohol abuse is based on a history of heavy alcohol intake and the presence of other organ system damage or an unusual frequency of falls, lacera-

tions, and fractures. Physicians typically identify only 50% of patients with drinking problems, because of both inadequate questioning by the physician and denial by the patient.[10] The uniform application of screening tools such as the AUDIT (*A*lcohol *U*se *D*isorders *I*dentification *T*est) 10-item instrument and the 4-item CAGE (need to *c*ut down, *a*nnoyed by criticism, *g*uilty about drinking, need for an *e*ye-opener in the morning) questionnaire dramatically improves the recognition of patients with problem drinking in primary care clinics.[11]

A number of laboratory studies have been used to identify patients with problem drinking. In most studies, carbohydrate-deficient transferrin (CDT) appears to be the most specific marker for alcohol abuse, although levels can be strongly influenced by body iron stores.[12-14] CDT appears in the serum after regular daily intake of 50 to 80 g of ethanol for at least 1 week and gradually declines during abstinence, with a half-life of approximately 15 days; however, the sensitivity of the test in

Table 81–2   Symptoms and Signs in Hospitalized Patients with Alcoholic Liver Disease*

Symptom or Sign	Patients Affected (%)			
	Mild Disease (n = 89)	*Moderate Disease (n = 58)*	*Severe Disease (n = 37)*	*Overall*
Hepatomegaly	84.3	94.7	79.4	86.7
Jaundice	17.4	100	100	60.1
Ascites	30.3	79.3	86.5	57.1
Hepatic encephalopathy	27.3	55.2	70.3	44.6
Splenomegaly	18.0	30.9	39.4	26.0
Fever	18.0	31.0	21.6	22.8

*Moderate disease was defined by a bilirubin level >5 mg/dL; severe disease, by a bilirubin level >5 mg/dL and a prolonged prothrombin time (>4 seconds).
Data from Mendenhall CL: Alcoholic hepatitis. Clin Gastroenterol 10:420, 1981.

patients who have abstained for longer than 4 days is low.[12] False-positive results are seen most commonly in patients with autoimmune liver diseases and iron deficiency.[12,14] Mean corpuscular erythrocyte volume (MCV), serum gamma glutamyl transpeptidase (GGTP) levels, and the ratio of mitochondrial aspartate aminotransferase (AST) to total AST (mitochondrial AST/total AST) in serum also have been touted as markers of alcohol abuse. No single test or combination of tests, however, has adequate sensitivity and specificity for reliable screening for excessive alcohol use.[15]

DIAGNOSIS OF ALCOHOLIC LIVER DISEASE

HISTORY

Most patients with fatty liver are asymptomatic.[16] Although patients with alcoholic hepatitis and cirrhosis may be asymptomatic, many present with a variety of complaints including anorexia, nausea and vomiting, weakness, jaundice, weight loss, abdominal pain, fever, and diarrhea.[17]

PHYSICAL EXAMINATION

The most extensive demographic information on alcoholic liver disease in the United States is from studies of hospitalized patients who were assigned the diagnosis on the basis of clinical and histologic parameters.[17,18] Although these studies included few asymptomatic patients, they provide a useful guide to diagnosis. The most common physical finding in patients with fatty liver and alcoholic hepatitis is hepatomegaly, which is detectable in more than 75% of patients, regardless of disease severity. Patients with alcoholic hepatitis and cirrhosis also may have hepatic tenderness, an audible bruit over the liver, spider angiomata, splenomegaly, and peripheral edema. Jaundice and ascites, which are found in approximately 60% of patients, are more frequent in patients with severe disease (Table 81–2). Various degrees of hepatic encephalopathy can be seen, usually in the most severely ill patients. Some patients with alcoholic hepatitis have fever with temperatures as high as 104°F, which can persist for weeks.

Table 81–3   Laboratory Values in Hospitalized Patients with Alcoholic Liver Disease*

Laboratory Test	Mean Value		
	Mild Disease (n = 89)	*Moderate Disease (n = 58)*	*Severe Disease (n = 37)*
Hematocrit (%)	38	36	33
MCV (μm³)	100	102	105
WBC count (per mm³)	8,000	11,000	12,000
Serum AST level (U/L)	84	124	99
Serum ALT level (U/L)	56	56	57
Serum alkaline phosphatase level (U/L)	166	276	225
Serum bilirubin level (mg/dL)	1.6	13.5	8.7
Prolongation of prothrombin time (seconds)	0.9	2.4	6.4
Serum albumin level	3.7	2.7	2.4

*Moderate disease was defined by a bilirubin level >5 mg/dL, and severe disease by a bilirubin level >5 mg/dL and a prolonged prothrombin time >4 seconds.
ALT, alanine aminotransferase; AST, aspartate aminotransferase; MCV, mean corpuscular volume; WBC, white blood cell.
Data from Mendenhall CL: Alcoholic hepatitis. Clin Gastroenterol 10:422, 1981.

In patients with well-compensated cirrhosis, findings on the physical examination can be normal; however, most patients have obvious hepatomegaly and splenomegaly. As the disease progresses, the liver decreases in size and has a hard and nodular consistency. Patients with decompensated cirrhosis typically have muscle wasting, ascites, spider angiomata, palmar erythema, and Dupuytren's contractures. Enlarged parotid and lacrimal glands often are seen, and severely ill patients may have Muercke's or white nails. Patients with hepatopulmonary syndrome often have digital clubbing.

LABORATORY FEATURES

Only one third of hospitalized patients with fatty liver have laboratory abnormalities, which usually consist of mild increases in serum AST and alanine aminotransferase (ALT) levels.[16] As illustrated in Table 81–3, surprisingly modest elevations of serum aminotransferase levels are seen in patients with alcoholic hepatitis and cirrhosis, even when the disease is severe.[17,18] Serum AST levels are almost always less than 300 to 500 U/L and typically are associated with trivial elevation of serum ALT levels, resulting in an AST/ALT ratio greater than 2, which is characteristic of alcoholic liver disease. Serum alkaline phosphatase levels can range from normal to values greater than 1000 U/L. Serum bilirubin levels range from normal to 20 to 40 mg/dL, and serum albumin levels may be normal or depressed to a value as low as 1.0 to 1.5 g/dL. Most patients with alcoholic liver disease are anemic and have some degree of thrombocytopenia. By contrast, the white blood cell count usually is normal or elevated, occasionally to levels consistent with a leukemoid state. Severely ill patients usually have marked prolongation of the prothrombin time—often expressed as the international normalized ratio (INR)—and often have elevated serum creatinine values.[17-20]

HISTOPATHOLOGY

The clinical diagnosis of alcoholic liver disease is quite sensitive and specific; therefore, liver biopsy is rarely needed to establish the diagnosis.[21,22] A liver biopsy is essential for determining precisely the severity of hepatic injury, however, and for clarifying the diagnosis in atypical cases. Centrilobular and perivenular fatty infiltration in the liver is seen in most persons who drink more than 60 g of alcohol daily. Classic histologic features of alcoholic hepatitis include ballooning degeneration of hepatocytes, alcoholic hyaline (Mallory bodies) within damaged hepatocytes, and a surrounding infiltrate composed of polymorphonuclear leukocytes. Most patients have moderate to severe fatty infiltration. Varying degrees of fibrosis may be present, and many patients exhibit an unusual perisinusoidal distribution of fibrosis, at times with partial or complete obliteration of the terminal hepatic venules (*sclerosing hyaline necrosis*). Cirrhosis can be identified by the presence of nodules of hepatic tissue that are completely surrounded by fibrous tissue.[7,8]

Alcoholic cirrhosis typically is micronodular or mixed micro- and macronodular. In patients with coexisting alcoholic hepatitis, Mallory bodies are almost universal, and sclerosing hyaline necrosis and moderate to severe fatty infiltration are common.[7,8] In patients with alcoholic cirrhosis who abstain from alcohol for long periods, a frequent finding is a gradual transformation to macronodular cirrhosis, which is indistinguishable from cirrhosis caused by other forms of liver disease.

CLINICAL CHALLENGES

Although the clinical diagnosis of alcoholic liver disease usually is quite straightforward, the similarity of clinical and histologic features of other disorders to those of alcoholic liver disease sometimes causes diagnostic confusion. In addition, occasionally, determining why a patient with stable, well-compensated alcoholic liver disease has suddenly and inexplicably deteriorated may be difficult.

CLINICAL CONDITIONS THAT MAY RESEMBLE ALCOHOLIC LIVER DISEASE

The most commonly encountered conditions that have clinical or histologic features in common with alcoholic liver disease are nonalcoholic fatty liver disease (NAFLD), hereditary hemochromatosis, amiodarone hepatotoxicity, and the Budd-Chiari syndrome.

Nonalcoholic Fatty Liver Disease

The condition that is most challenging to differentiate from alcoholic liver disease is NAFLD. The two conditions are histologically indistinguishable. As a consequence, the differentiation between alcoholic liver disease and NAFLD has to be made on clinical grounds. The strongest evidence in support of a diagnosis of NAFLD rather than alcoholic liver disease is a history of daily alcohol intake less than 20 g. When a patient's alcohol intake is questionable, differentiating the two conditions can be difficult, if not impossible. Patients with NAFLD are more likely than patients with alcoholic liver disease to be asymptomatic women who have peripheral insulin resistance, obesity, hypertension, and dyslipidemias.[23,24] They also are more likely to have relatively normal liver biochemical test results and a serum AST/ALT ratio of less than 1, compared with a ratio of greater than 2 in most patients with alcoholic liver disease. Patients with NAFLD and cirrhosis, however, often have a serum AST/ALT ratio greater than 1. The serum CDT level can be useful for distinguishing heavy drinkers from abstinent patients with NAFLD; however, the accuracy of this test for detecting moderate but clinically significant levels of alcohol intake is less clear (see earlier and Chapter 82).[13,24]

Hereditary Hemochromatosis

On occasion, it can be difficult to distinguish patients with alcoholic liver disease and secondary iron overload from patients with liver disease caused by hereditary hemochromatosis, particularly those with decompensated cirrhosis. Patients with end-stage liver disease from alcoholic cirrhosis may have elevated serum iron and ferritin levels and increased hepatic iron levels suggestive of hereditary hemochromatosis.[25] In fact, more than 20% of patients with end-stage alcoholic cirrhosis have clinically important hepatic siderosis.[26] To complicate matters further, 15% to 40% of patients with hereditary hemochromatosis consume more than 80 g of alcohol daily.[27]

The overlapping clinical features of hereditary hemochromatosis and alcoholic liver disease include hepatomegaly, testicular atrophy, cardiomyopathy, and glucose intolerance. Testing for mutations in the hereditary hemochromatosis gene, *HFE*, is the best method for differentiating the two conditions among Caucasians. Few patients with alcoholic cirrhosis and iron overload are homozygous for *C282Y* or heterozygous for the *C282Y* and *H63D HFE* genes, whereas some have hepatic iron index values greater than 1.9, suggestive of hereditary hemochromatosis[25,28] (see Chapter 71).

Amiodarone Hepatoxicity

Much less common and less difficult than NAFLD to distinguish from alcoholic liver disease is amiodarone hepatotoxicity. Although the hepatic histologic features of this condition may be indistinguishable from those of alcoholic hepatitis with or without cirrhosis, the clinical setting usually distinguishes amiodarone hepatotoxicity from alcoholic liver disease[8,29] (see Chapter 83).

Budd-Chiari Syndrome

Occasional patients with severe alcoholic liver disease can be misdiagnosed as having acute Budd-Chiari syndrome on the basis of rapid clinical deterioration, marked hepatomegaly, caudate lobe hypertrophy, and failure to visualize the hepatic veins by Doppler ultrasonography.[30] Careful evaluation of these patients usually reveals typical clinical and biochemical features of severe alcoholic hepatitis. Patent hepatic veins usually can be demonstrated by venography. Liver biopsy is particularly useful in distinguishing the typical histologic features of alcoholic liver disease from those of Budd-Chiari syndrome. Failure to recognize alcoholic hepatitis as the underlying cause of the liver disease before anticoagulation or portacaval shunt surgery can result in high mortality rates (see Chapter 80).[30]

DIFFERENTIAL DIAGNOSIS OF CLINICAL DETERIORATION

Acetaminophen Hepatotoxicity

The most common cause of severe drug-induced liver injury encountered in the United States is acetaminophen hepatotoxicity (see Chapter 83). Two clinical patterns of liver injury have been identified: (1) suicidal or accidental ingestion of large quantities of acetaminophen sufficient to cause hepatic injury and (2) ingestion of lesser quantities of acetaminophen by patients predisposed to injury because of up-regulation of the hepatic enzymes that convert acetaminophen to a hepatoxic metabolite. The latter type of toxicity is seen most commonly in chronic alcoholics who take excessive acetaminophen over a period of days to weeks for relief of a headache, toothache, or other minor pain.[31] The clinical features in these patients are indistinguishable from those of alcoholic liver disease, with one obvious exception: AST values are typically more than 1000 U/L, much higher than those in patients with alcoholic liver disease. Because liver injury typically has occurred by the time of hospitalization, acetaminophen levels are not helpful for diagnosis or management. Recognition of the cause of the unusually elevated serum aminotransferase levels comes from careful questioning of the patient and family about acetaminophen ingestion in the days to weeks before hospitalization. The morbidity and mortality associated with this condition are considerable.[31] Because many of these patients have a history of recent heavy alcohol use, few are candidates for liver transplantation.

Acute Viral Illness

Patients with alcoholic cirrhosis are vulnerable to decompensation from a variety of viral illnesses. Acute viral hepatitis can result in the sudden onset of liver failure, with extremely high mortality rates[32,33] (see Chapters 74 to 78). Sudden decompensation and liver failure also have been reported during infection with influenza A virus, but the mechanism is unknown.[34] These dramatic cases illustrate the importance of routine immunization against hepatitis A and B and influenza in patients with alcoholic cirrhosis.

Hepatocellular Carcinoma

Occasional patients with alcoholic cirrhosis who have been abstinent for many years decompensate suddenly, with the abrupt onset of hepatic encephalopathy, variceal bleeding, or ascites. Not infrequently, the underlying cause is hepatocellular carcinoma. Unfortunately, the sudden onset of symptoms frequently results from tumor invasion of the portal or hepatic veins; as a result, the prognosis for these patients is dismal.[3] The risk of hepatocellular carcinoma in patients with alcoholic cirrhosis underscores the need for surveillance for this neoplasm in these patients, especially those who abstain from alcohol and in whom the long-term prognosis is otherwise good (see Chapter 91).

COFACTORS THAT MAY INFLUENCE PROGRESSION OF ALCOHOLIC LIVER DISEASE

A number of factors have been reported to have an adverse effect on the progression of liver disease in chronic alcoholics. The most important of these factors are chronic hepatitis C virus (HCV) infection, obesity, and smoking.

CHRONIC HEPATITIS C

The co-factor that influences progression of alcoholic liver disease most profoundly is HCV infection. Between one fourth and one third of patients with alcoholic liver disease have serologic or virologic evidence (or both) of HCV infection.[35] The prevalence of HCV infection is highest in patients who have used injection drugs; however, the risk is high even among those who deny drug use. Histologic features of focal lymphoid aggregates, portal inflammation, and periportal or bridging fibrosis are common in liver biopsy specimens from alcoholics with HCV infection.[36] Of greater importance, liver disease is more severe, advanced disease develops at a younger age, and survival is shorter in patients with both alcoholic liver disease and HCV infection than in patients with alcoholic liver disease and no evidence of HCV infection.[35,37] In one of the more striking examples of the interaction between alcohol abuse and hepatitis C, Corrao and colleagues found that the relative risk of cirrhosis was 10-fold higher among heavy drinkers with chronic hepatitis C than among those who had no evidence of HCV infection[38] (Fig. 81–2). In addition, the risk of hepatocellular carcinoma is two to four times higher in patients with alcoholic cirrhosis and HCV infection than in those with alcoholic cirrhosis alone.[39,40]

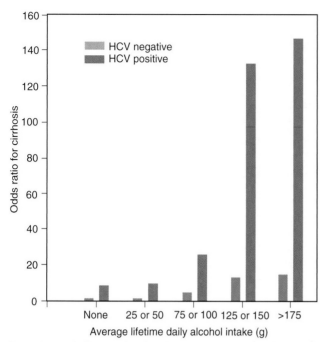

Figure 81–2 Relative risks of cirrhosis in patients who chronically drink varying amounts of alcohol based on the presence or absence of hepatitis C virus (HCV) infection. (Data from Corrao G, Lepore AR, Torchio P, et al: The effect of drinking coffee and smoking cigarettes on the risk of cirrhosis associated with alcohol consumption. A case-control study. Provincial Group for the Study of Chronic Liver Disease. Eur J Epidemiol 10:657, 1994.)

OBESITY AND SMOKING

The risk of liver disease is two to three times higher in drinkers who are obese than that in drinkers who have a normal body mass.[41] Although an increased risk of fatty liver is not surprising in obese persons, obesity also appears to be an independent risk factor for both alcoholic hepatitis and cirrhosis.[41,42] Cigarette smoking also has been shown to accelerate the progression of fibrosis in patients with alcoholic liver disease,[43,44] and smoking appears to accelerate disease progression in patients with HCV infection who drink heavily.[45]

PATHOGENESIS

ETHANOL METABOLISM AND TOXIC METABOLITES

The liver is the main organ responsible for ethanol metabolism; other organs such as the stomach contribute to much lesser degrees. Ethanol is metabolized by three major systems in the liver: alcohol dehydrogenases (ADHs), cytochrome P450 2E1 (CYP2E1), and, of least importance, catalase.[46] The ADHs are cytoplasmic enzymes with multiple isoforms. ADH is the primary enzyme system responsible for ethanol metabolism at low concentrations, whereas CYP2E1 contributes at higher concentrations (greater than 10 mM) and is induced by ethanol exposure. Both ADH and CYP2E1 convert ethanol to acetaldehyde, which is then converted

to acetate by aldehyde dehydrogenase (ALDH). Acetaldehyde is a highly reactive and potentially toxic compound that is responsible for many of the systemic toxic effects of alcohol, such as nausea, headaches, and flushing. The "Oriental flush syndrome" results from impaired metabolism of acetaldehyde caused by inheritance of the ALDH22 allele, which encodes an inactive form of ALDH2. Persons from East Asia who are homozygous for this mutation rarely drink ethanol, because they invariably experience severe toxic systemic effects, such as flushing and tachycardia, when they do drink.

Acetaldehyde also is postulated to play an etiologic role in alcoholic liver disease. Acetaldehyde can form adducts with reactive residues on proteins or small molecules (e.g., cysteines). These chemical modifications can alter or interfere with normal biologic processes and be directly toxic to the cell. Modified molecules also may stimulate the host's immune response and cause autoimmune-like diseases. Antibodies against such oxidatively modified proteins have been reported in both human and animal models of alcoholic liver disease.[47] An example is the hybrid adduct of malondialdehyde and acetaldehyde (MAA), unique to alcohol exposure, which induces an immune reaction both in human alcoholics and in animal models of alcoholic liver disease.[47] Acetaldehyde also has been shown to impair mitochondrial glutathione transport and to sensitize hepatocytes to tumor necrosis factor (TNF)-mediated killing.[48]

In addition to forming cytotoxic metabolites such as acetaldehyde, ethanol metabolism can alter the cellular oxidation-reduction (redox) state, thereby modulating liver injury. Specifically, the oxidation of ethanol utilizes nicotinamide-adenine dinucleotide (NAD^+) as an electron acceptor and thereby causes a shift in the reduced NAD (NADH)/NAD^+ ratio to a more reduced state.[46] This change in the redox state can impair normal carbohydrate and lipid metabolism; multiple effects ensue, including a decrease in the supply of adenosine triphosphate (ATP) to the cell and an increase in hepatic steatosis.

METABOLIC MECHANISMS

Oxidative Stress

Oxidative stress is an imbalance between pro-oxidants and antioxidants. Reactive oxygen species (ROS) and reactive nitrogen species (RNS) are products of normal metabolism and can be beneficial to the host (e.g., by contributing to bacterial killing).[49] Overproduction of ROS and RNS or inadequate antioxidant defenses (e.g., low levels of vitamins, selenium, mitochondrial glutathione), or both, can lead to liver injury. Oxidative stress is well documented in alcoholic liver disease.[50] Studies in normal volunteers have shown that acute alcohol consumption causes a dose-related increase in urinary isoprostane levels (a marker of lipid peroxidation, which is an indirect marker of oxidative stress), and patients with alcoholic hepatitis exhibit high isoprostane levels.[51] Major ROS and RNS include superoxide anion, hydrogen peroxide, and hydroxyl radical (ROS) and nitric oxide, peroxynitrite (RNS), and hypohalous acid.

Oxidative stress usually is documented by detection of one of several indirect markers: (1) protein oxidation (e.g., protein thiol or carbonyl products); (2) lipid oxidation (e.g., isoprostanes, malondialdehyde); (3) DNA oxidation (e.g., oxodeoxyguanosine); or (4) depletion or induction of antioxidant defenses (e.g., vitamin E, glutathione, thioredoxin).

The stimulus for oxidative stress in the liver comes from multiple sources. In hepatocytes, CYP2E1 activity increases after alcohol consumption, in part because of stabilization of messenger RNA (mRNA). The CYP2E1 system leaks electrons to initiate oxidative stress.[49] CYP2E1 is localized in the hepatic lobule in areas of alcohol-induced liver injury. Moreover, overexpression of CYP2E1 in mice and in HepG2 cells (a hepatocyte cell line) in vitro leads to enhanced alcohol hepatotoxicity.[52,53] On the other hand, alcohol-induced liver injury still develops in CYP2E1-knockout mice. These findings suggest that increased CYP2E1 probably plays a role in alcoholic liver injury but is not the sole or dominant factor. In the CYP2E1-knockout mice, other compensatory mechanisms may be operational, such as induction of other microsomal enzymes. Nonparenchymal cells and infiltrating inflammatory cells (e.g., polymorphonuclear neutrophils) are another major source of pro-oxidants that are used for normal cellular processes, such as killing invading organisms. Major enzyme systems for pro-oxidant production in Kupffer cells include nicotinamide-adenine dinucleotide phosphate (NADPH) oxidase and inducible nitric oxide synthase (iNOS). Mice deficient in NADPH oxidase or mice treated with the drug diphenyleneiodonium sulfate, which blocks NADPH oxidase, are resistant to ethanol-induced liver injury.[54,55] Infiltrating neutrophils use enzyme systems such as myeloperoxidase to generate hypochlorus acid ($HOCl^-$, a halide species that causes oxidative stress) and RNS.

Oxidative stress can mediate liver injury through at least two major pathways: direct injury and cell signaling. Direct cell injury is indicated by markers such as lipid peroxidation and DNA damage. An even greater role is played by signaling pathways—for example, activation of transcription factors such as nuclear factor kappa B (NFκB), which plays a critical role in the production of cytokines such as TNF.

The critical role of oxidative stress in the development of alcoholic liver disease has been validated in multiple studies in rats and mice fed alcohol and treated with various antioxidants ranging from ebselen to green tea polyphenols that overexpress both superoxide dismutase I and II. Various antioxidants have been shown to block or attenuate the development of alcoholic liver disease in rodents.[49]

Mitochondrial Dysfunction

Mitochondria are the major consumers of molecular oxygen and major generators of ROS in the liver. Mitochondrial dysfunction is well documented in alcoholic liver disease and contributes to oxidative stress.[56,57]

Mitochondrial abnormalities in alcoholic liver disease include megamitochondria observed on light and electron microscopy and functional mitochondrial abnormalities as documented by an abnormal ^{14}C ketoacid breath test result (ketoacids are metabolized by mitochondria).[58] Short-term alcohol administration causes increased hepatic superoxide generation in liver mitochondria, with an increased flow of electrons along the respiratory electron transport chain. The increased $NADH/NAD^+$ ratio caused by ethanol intake favors superoxide generation.[49] Because hepatic mitochondria lack catalase, glutathione plays a critical role in protecting mitochondria against oxidative stress. Mitochondria do not make glutathione but instead import it from the cytosol. In alcoholic liver disease, the transport of glutathione into mitochondria is impaired, and selective mitochondrial glutathione depletion is observed.[59] Glutathione depletion also sensitizes the liver to the toxic effects of TNF, and TNF also impairs mitochondrial function. Finally, an increase in mitochondrial membrane depolarization and permeability leads to hepatocyte death, especially apoptotic (programmed), rather than necrotic, death.

Hypoxia

The centrilobular area of the hepatic lobule (the functional unit of the liver) has the lowest oxygen tension and greatest susceptibility to hypoxia. Chronic alcohol intake increases oxygen uptake by the liver and increases the lobular oxygen gradient. A chronic intragastric feeding model in rats has been used to define the mechanisms underlying hepatic hypoxia and the association of these mechanisms with cycling of urinary alcohol levels (UALs).[60] At high UALs, hepatic hypoxia is observed, along with reduced ATP levels; the $NADH/NAD^+$ ratio is shifted to the reduced state; and the hypoxia-inducible factor (HIF) 1 and 2 genes are up-regulated. When UALs fall, reperfusion injury occurs, with free radical formation and peak liver enzyme release from hepatocytes. Stimuli for this cycle of events include catecholamines (levels of which coincide with peak UALs) and modulators of vascular tone (e.g., nitric oxide, endothelin-1); modulation of these stimuli offers future therapeutic possibilities.

Impaired Proteasome Function

The 26S ubiquitin-proteasome pathway is the primary proteolytic pathway of eukaryotic cells (see Chapter 69). It controls the levels of numerous proteins involved in gene regulation, cell division, and surface receptor expression, as well as stress response and inflammation. The proteasome system is now considered a cellular defense mechanism, because it also removes irregular and damaged proteins generated by mutations, translational errors, or oxidative stress.[61] This pathway involves two major steps: (1) covalent attachment of multiple ubiquitin molecules to the protein substrate and (2) degradation of the targeted protein by the 26S proteasome complex. The 26S ubiquitin-proteasome pathway may play a pathogenic role in the development of alcoholic liver disease.[62]

Early clinical studies showed that hepatomegaly caused by chronic alcohol consumption resulted in part from accumulation of protein in the liver.[63] Animal studies have demonstrated that chronic ethanol feeding results in a significant decrease in proteolytic activity of the proteasome; this decreased activity can lead to abnormal protein accumulation, including accumulation of oxidized proteins.[64,65] The decrease in proteasome function correlates significantly with the level of hepatic oxidative stress. Patients with alcoholic cirrhosis have increased serum ubiquitin levels, suggesting damaged proteasome function.[66] Also, hepatocytes from alcoholics contain large amounts of ubiquitin in the form of cellular inclusions, or Mallory bodies, which accumulate because they are not degraded efficiently by the proteasome.[67] The formation of Mallory bodies, which occurs when the ubiquitin-proteasome system is inhibited or overwhelmed, is a pathway of liver injury caused by diverse toxins, including alcohol.[67] As hepatocytes die as a result of proteasome inhibition, they inappropriately release cytokines such as interleukin (IL)-8 and IL-18. IL-8 recruits neutrophils and probably plays a role in neutrophil infiltration in alcoholic hepatitis, and IL-18 sustains inflammation in the liver.[68]

Abnormal Metabolism of Methionine, S-adenosylmethionine, and Folate

In mammals, the liver plays a central role in methionine metabolism; nearly one half of the daily intake of methionine is metabolized in the liver (Fig. 81–3). The first step in methionine metabolism is the formation of S-adenosylmethionine (SAM) in a reaction catalyzed by methionine adenosyltransferase (MAT). Activity of this enzyme is depressed in alcoholic liver disease.[69] SAM is the principal biologic methyl donor through the transmethylation pathway; the precursor of aminopropyl groups utilized in polyamine biosynthesis; and a precursor of glutathione through its conversion to cysteine along the transsulfuration pathway. Under normal conditions, most of the SAM generated daily is used in trans-

methylation reactions, in which methyl groups are added to a large number of molecules by means of specific methyltransferases.[70] These compounds include DNA, RNA, biogenic amines, phospholipids, histones, and other proteins; methylation of these compounds may modulate cellular functions and integrity. In this process, SAM is converted to S-adenosylhomocysteine (SAH), which is a potent competitive inhibitor of most methyltransferases. Both an increase in SAH and a decrease in the SAM/SAH ratio are known to inhibit transmethylation reactions.[70-72]

SAM deficiency in alcoholic liver disease was first noted in the early 1980s, when it was observed that alcoholic subjects had delayed clearance of an oral bolus of methionine (presumably because of blocked conversion of methionine to SAM).[73] Functional MAT activity was subsequently shown to be subnormal in liver biopsy specimens from alcoholic subjects.[74] Subnormal hepatic SAM levels also are noted in various experimental models of liver injury. Exogenous administration of SAM corrects the deficiency and attenuates the severity of these experimental forms of liver injury.[69,75]

Because SAM is a precursor of glutathione, SAM deficiency results in glutathione deficiency, which is observed in many forms of liver disease.[76] In animal studies, exogenous SAM corrects hepatic deficiencies of both SAM and glutathione.[77] Because glutathione is required for optimal expression of MAT activity in liver, hepatic deficiency of MAT may be caused in part by glutathione deficiency. Also, hepatic MAT is sensitive to oxidative stress, and the subnormal hepatic MAT activity in patients with alcoholic liver disease could result from oxidation of MAT.[78]

In models of alcohol-induced hepatotoxicity, SAM has been shown to maintain mitochondrial glutathione levels. Depletion of mitochondrial glutathione is thought to be one pathogenic factor in the development of alcoholic liver disease, and SAM, but not other glutathione prodrugs, prevents mitochondrial glutathione depletion in experimental alcoholic liver disease (possibly by protecting mitochondrial glutathione transport systems).[79] SAM also decreases lipopolysaccharide (LPS)-stimulated TNF release and increases IL-10 release in a monocyte cell line.[69] Similarly, in rats fed a diet to induce SAM deficiency, serum TNF levels increase, and sensitivity to endotoxin-induced hepatotoxicity, which can be blocked by SAM injection, increases markedly.[80] These data support the concept that SAM may have direct hepatoprotective functions and may modify LPS-stimulated cytokine production.

Although serum SAM levels are decreased in patients with alcoholic liver disease, levels of the downstream products SAH and homocysteine are elevated. Homocysteine has been postulated to play a role in the pathogenesis of fatty liver seen with alcoholic liver disease, and reduction of homocysteine levels with betaine administration (to convert homocysteine to methionine) in experimental animals attenuates the severity of alcoholic liver disease.[81] Elevated SAH levels recently have been shown to sensitize hepatocytes to TNF-mediated destruction, and SAH may be a critical physiologic sensitizer of TNF-mediated killing in liver injury.[72] Homocysteine and SAH can be removed by giving the drug betaine, which

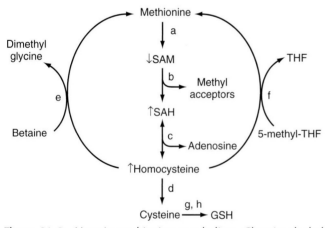

Figure 81–3 Hepatic methionine metabolism. Chronic alcohol consumption causes S-adenosylmethionine (SAM) deficiency and an increase in homocysteine and S-adenosylhomocysteine (SAH) levels. a, methionine adenosyltransferase; b, enzymes involved in transmethylation reactions, including phosphatidylethanolamine N-methyltransferase; c, SAH hydrolase; d, cystathionine B-synthase; e, betaine-homocysteine methyltransferase; f, methionine synthetase; g, glutamate-cysteine synthetase; h, glutathione (GSH) synthetase. ↑↓, effects of alcohol; THF, tetrahydrofolate.

facilitates regeneration of methionine from homocysteine. Folic acid also can play a critical role in the regeneration of homocysteine to methionine by means of 5-methyltetrahydrofolate (5-MTHF).[82] Fatty liver develops in mice lacking the MTHF reductase (MTHFR) gene, and steatohepatitis develops in MAT1A-knockout mice; these findings further support a role for this critical pathway in the development of steatosis and steatohepatitis. Halsted and colleagues have shown that folic acid deficiency enhances the development of alcohol-induced liver injury in micropigs and that alcohol feeding interferes with normal folic acid metabolism in multiple different pathways, from impaired intestinal uptake to increased renal excretion.[82] Collectively, the data support a role for altered methionine-transmethylation-transsulfuration metabolism in alcoholic liver disease and link these pathways to TNF hepatotoxicity.

IMMUNE AND INFLAMMATORY MECHANISMS

Kupffer Cell Activation and Dysregulated Cytokine Production

Cytokines are low molecular weight mediators of cellular communication (see Chapter 2).[83] Multiple cell types in the liver are potential sources of the increased release of pro-inflammatory cytokines observed in alcoholic liver disease.[83] Kupffer cells are prominent producers of pro-inflammatory cytokines such TNF-α, as well as certain anti-inflammatory cytokines such as IL-10. Sinusoidal endothelial cells express adhesion molecules, which modulate white blood cell adhesion and transmigration. Activated stellate cells produce collagen in response to signals such as the profibrotic cytokine transforming growth factor-β (TGF-β). Hepatocytes are a relatively newly recognized source of cytokine production, including IL-8, a major neutrophil chemotactic peptide and angiogenesis factor.

Major stimuli for the observed increase in pro-inflammatory cytokine production in alcoholic liver disease are believed to be ROS and gut-derived LPS.[83] In alcoholic liver disease, intestinal permeability is increased and the frequency of endotoxemia is high.[83] LPS activates the redox-sensitive transcription factor NFκB in Kupffer cells, thereby resulting in the production of certain cytokines such as TNF[83] (Fig. 81–4). TNF can increase gut permeability, induce oxidative stress, and perpetuate this cycle. Generation of ROS through the metabolism of alcohol also can activate NFκB and stimulate proinflammatory cytokine production.[84] Although necrosis has traditionally been thought to be the major mechanism of hepatocyte cell death in alcoholic liver disease, increased apoptosis also has been documented. As hepatocytes die of apoptosis, they can be taken up by Kupffer cells and stimulate TNF production.[85] Moreover, when alcohol-fed rodents are treated with caspase inhibitors to block apoptosis, liver inflammation and injury are markedly attenuated.[86] When hepatocytes die of proteasome inhibition–mediated apoptosis, the dying hepatocytes release IL-8 and IL-18, which cause sustained inflammation.[68] Therefore, in alcoholic liver disease, hepatocyte apoptosis may sustain pro-inflammatory cytokine production and cell injury or death.

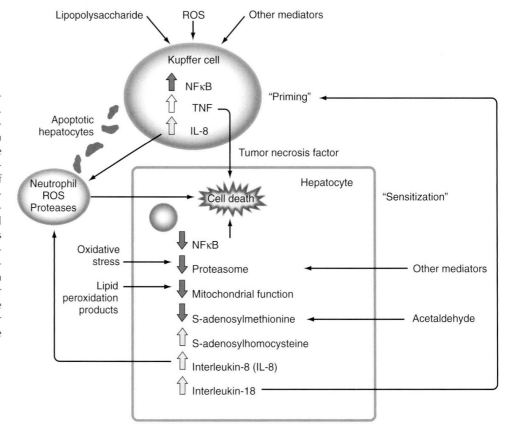

Figure 81–4 Cytokine production in alcoholic liver disease. Kupffer cells are *primed* to overproduce cytotoxic cytokines in response to a lipopolysaccharide stimulus, and hepatocytes are *sensitized* to the hepatotoxic effects of these cytokines through mechanisms such as decreased production of antiapoptotic survival proteins. Hepatocyte death causes increased production of interleukin-8 (neutrophil chemoattractant) and interleukin-18 (which primes tumor necrosis factor release and a T_H1 response) (see text for details). NFκB, nuclear factor kappa B; ROS, reactive oxygen species.

TNF metabolism in alcoholic hepatitis is dysregulated, as suggested by the observation that cultured monocytes (which produce substantial amounts of TNF) from patients with alcoholic hepatitis produce significantly increased amounts of TNF in response to LPS stimulation.[87] Increased serum TNF concentrations in patients with alcoholic hepatitis show a strong correlation with disease severity and risk of mortality.[83] Serum concentrations of TNF-inducible cytokines and chemokines, such as IL-6, IL-8, IL-18, monocyte chemoattractant protein 1 (MCP-1), and others, are elevated in patients with alcoholic hepatitis or cirrhosis, and the levels often correlate with markers of the acute-phase response, reduced liver function, and poor clinical outcomes.[83]

This enhanced cytokine response to a physiologic stimulus such as LPS is termed *priming*. Increased serum or urinary levels of neopterin and other markers indicate that monocytes and Kupffer cells are primed in alcoholic liver disease. This priming for LPS-stimulated TNF production has been reproduced in vitro by culturing monocyte cell lines with relevant concentrations of alcohol. This response appears to be mediated, at least in part, by CYP2E1 induction and oxidative stress.[88]

Studies in rats, mice, and tissue culture have validated a pathogenic role for cytokines (especially TNF) in the development of alcoholic liver disease.[83] Rats chronically fed alcohol are more sensitive to the hepatotoxic effects of injected LPS and have much higher LPS-stimulated plasma levels of TNF in comparison with control rats. Liver injury can be attenuated by giving a prostaglandin analog to down-regulate TNF production.[89] Because rats have a natural aversion to alcohol, an intragastric route often is used to deliver high amounts of alcohol. Studies using the intragastric alcohol-feeding model have demonstrated that the development of liver injury coincides with an increase in TNF mRNA expression in the liver and in isolated Kupffer cells.[90,91] Rats fed ethanol intragastrically also have high blood LPS levels and increased expression of CYP2E1, as well as markers of oxidative stress and lipid peroxidation.

Not only are levels of pro-inflammatory cytotoxic cytokines increased in alcoholic liver disease, but also monocyte and Kupffer cell production of protective anti-inflammatory cytokines such as IL-10 is decreased.[92] The importance of this observation for humans has been confirmed using IL-10–knockout mice, in which more severe ethanol-induced hepatotoxicity develops and increased levels of pro-inflammatory cytokines such as TNF are seen.[93]

Several strategies have been devised to decrease cytokine production or activity in an attempt to block or attenuate liver injury. Examples include antibiotics to modulate gut flora and LPS, gadolinium chloride to destroy Kupffer cells, and antioxidants such as glutathione prodrugs to inhibit cytokine production. Each of these strategies has been successful in attenuating alcohol-induced liver injury in rats.[83] Prebiotics such as oat bran also have been shown to decrease endotoxemia in experimentally induced alcoholic liver injury. Perhaps the most compelling data relating TNF to alcohol-induced liver injury are studies using anti-TNF antibody to prevent liver injury in alcohol-fed rats.[94] Similarly,

alcoholic liver injury does not develop in mice lacking the TNF type I receptor.[95]

Hepatocytes normally are resistant to TNF killing. Hepatocytes from rats fed alcohol or hepatocytes incubated in alcohol are sensitized to TNF killing, however.[52,96] Some potentially relevant mechanisms for this sensitization include mitochondrial glutathione depletion, SAH accumulation, and proteasome inhibition, among others. Therefore, in alcoholic liver disease, monocytes and Kupffer cells are primed to increase TNF production and to sensitize hepatocytes to TNF killing. These processes are closely intertwined with previously described mechanisms such as oxidative stress, mitochondrial dysfunction, abnormal methionine metabolism, and proteasome dysfunction.

Immune Responses to Altered Hepatocellular Proteins

Alcoholic hepatitis may persist histologically for many months after ethanol exposure has ceased, suggesting an ongoing immune or autoimmune response. Autoimmune reactions are now well documented in alcoholic liver disease, with autoantibodies directed against phospholipids, alcohol dehydrogenase, heat shock protein, and other potential antigens.[97] Patients with alcoholic liver disease are at increased risk for the development of immune responses directed at neoantigens generated from the interactions of alcohol metabolites (e.g., acetaldehyde or hydroxyethyl radicals) with liver proteins.[98] Studies have linked genetics and autoimmunity in alcoholic liver disease. Some humans have a genetic mutation in the cytotoxic T lymphocyte–associated antigen 4G (CTLA-4G) allele, which leads to inappropriately activated T cell function. One of the breakdown products of alcohol metabolism, the hydroxyethyl radical, can modify CYP2E1 and, in the presence of the CTLA-4G mutation, increase the risk that anti-CYP2E1 autoantibodies will develop.[99] This is one pathway whereby alcohol abuse may break "self-tolerance" in the liver.

GENDER AND GENETIC FACTORS

Because the development of liver injury varies among people who drink the same amount of alcohol, great interest exists in possible gender and genetic predisposition to alcoholic liver disease.

Female gender is now a well-accepted risk factor for the development and rapid progression of alcoholic liver disease.[4,5] Although rates of metabolism and elimination of alcohol have been reported to be more rapid in women than in men, when adjusted for liver volume, elimination rates are similar between genders.[100] Studies in rats or mice fed alcohol chronically have demonstrated that females are more susceptible than males to liver injury. Risk factors for the development of liver disease in females appear to include increased endotoxemia, lipid peroxidation, activation of the critical transcription factor NFκB, and chemokine (e.g., monocyte chemotactic protein-1) mRNA levels.[101] These risk factors are critical for determining "safe" levels of alcohol consumption in women. Many authorities consider any amount of alcohol above 20 g a day to be a risk factor for the development of liver disease in women; differences between men and women in levels of alcohol dehydrogenase in gastric mucosa are not thought to play a major role in the greater susceptibility of women to alcoholic liver injury.

Genetic polymorphisms in alcohol-metabolizing systems such as CYP2E1 and ADHs have been postulated to play a role in the development of alcoholic liver disease.[102] None of these polymorphisms, however, adequately explains the diverse pathologic responses seen among patients with alcoholic liver disease. Polymorphisms in the promoter regions of cytokines TNF and IL-10 also have been reported to predispose affected persons to the development of alcoholic liver disease and are under active study.[103,104]

EMERGING MECHANISMS

Ethanol metabolism, and the consequent shift in the redox state of the liver (altered NADH/NAD$^+$ redox potential), and inhibition of fatty acid oxidation have long been implicated in the pathogenesis of alcohol-induced hepatic steatosis. Crabb and colleagues have shown that ethanol also can impair fatty acid oxidation by affecting critical enzymes, as well as by inducing lipogenic enzymes and augmenting lipogenesis. Specifically, data obtained from cultured cells and experimental models of alcoholic liver disease strongly suggest that alcoholic fatty liver may be caused by ethanol-induced down-regulation of peroxisome proliferator–activated receptor α (PPARα) and adenosine monophosphate (AMP)–dependent protein kinase (AMPK), as well as up-regulation of sterol regulatory element–binding protein 1 (SREBP-1).[105-107] Ethanol could act directly on these receptors and enzymes or indirectly by affecting adiponectin (an anti-inflammatory cytokine produced in adipocytes) or TNF expression.

MECHANISMS OF FIBROSIS

The development of hepatic fibrosis, leading to cirrhosis, indicates major progression of alcoholic liver disease and represents a maladaptive wound healing response. The development of fibrosis is a dynamic state, with constant remodeling of scar tissue; fibrosis may regress with discontinuation of exposure to alcohol. The stellate cell is the major source of collagen production in the liver. It normally exists in a quiescent state and serves as a major storehouse for vitamin A. Following activation, the stellate cell assumes a myofibroblast-like contractile phenotype and produces collagen. The cytokine TGF-β is a major stimulus for stellate cell activation and collagen production. Other cytokines implicated in activation of stellate cells include platelet-derived growth factor and connective tissue growth factor. Oxidative stress plays a major role in stellate cell activation, and a variety of antioxidants can block both stellate cell activation and collagen production in vitro. Serum levels of 4-hydroxy-nonenal, a specific product of lipid peroxidation, are elevated in patients with alcoholic liver disease, serving to up-regulate both procollagen type I and tissue inhibitor of metalloproteinase-1 (TIMP-1) gene expression. Matrix metalloproteinase-1 plays a major role in degrading type I collagen. TIMP-1 levels also are elevated in alcoholic liver disease. The result appears to be an increase in stellate cell activation and collagen production on the one hand and a decrease in matrix degradation on the other hand.[108-110]

PROGNOSIS

The prognosis for individual patients with alcoholic liver disease depends on the degree of pathologic injury, the patient's nutritional status, presence of complications of advanced liver disease, presence of other comorbid conditions such as HCV infection, and the patient's ability to discontinue destructive patterns of drinking. In studies that have examined the natural history of alcoholic liver disease on the basis of histologic characteristics at diagnosis, patients with fatty liver have had the best outcome (70% to 80% survival rate at 4 to 5 years); those with alcoholic hepatitis or cirrhosis have had an intermediate outcome (50% to 75% survival rate at 4 to 5 years); and those with cirrhosis combined with alcoholic hepatitis have had the worst outcome (30% to 50% survival rate at 4 to 5 years)[111] (Fig. 81–5). Among all patients with alcoholic liver disease, the average 1-year and 5-year survival rates are approximately 80% and 50%, respectively.[18] Alcoholic cirrhosis also appears to be an independent risk factor (albeit a weaker one than viral hepatitis) for hepatocellular carcinoma.[2,3,39,40] Among alcoholics, men older than 50 years of age appear to be most vulnerable to the development of hepatocellular carcinoma.[112]

Estimating the prognosis of patients with alcoholic liver disease is particularly important for (1) determining the need for specific therapy in patients with severe alcoholic hepatitis and (2) determining the need for liver transplantation in patients with alcoholic cirrhosis.

ALCOHOLIC HEPATITIS

The prognosis among patients with alcoholic hepatitis can vary dramatically. In patients with severe disease, the mortality rate is extremely high, approaching that for patients with fulminant hepatic failure. Clinical features associated with severe disease include hepatic encephalopathy, marked prolongation of the prothrombin time, elevation of serum bilirubin levels greater than 25 mg/dL, depressed serum albumin levels, elevated serum creatinine levels, and older age. Maddrey and Boitnott discovered a simple formula they called the *discriminant function* (DF), calculated as

$$[4.6 \times \text{prothrombin time} - \text{control value (seconds)}] + \text{serum bilirubin (mg/dL)}.$$

The DF has proved useful for identifying patients with poor short-term survival rates.[113] Three prospective

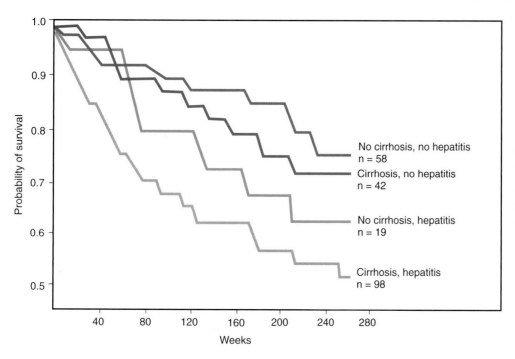

Figure 81–5 Five-year survival of patients with alcoholic liver disease stratified by histologic severity of disease. (From Orrego H, Black JE, Blendis LM, et al: Prognosis of alcoholic cirrhosis in the presence or absence of alcoholic hepatitis. Gastroenterology 92:208, 1987.)

studies have demonstrated that patients with a DF value greater than 32 have a poor prognosis, with 1-month mortality rates of 35% to 45%.[20,114,115] By contrast, patients with DF values less than 32 have short-term survival rates of 90% to 100%.[113,116] Other important prognostic variables in patients with severe alcoholic hepatitis are the presence of spontaneous hepatic encephalopathy and of hepatorenal syndrome.[17,19,20] The 1-month mortality rate in patients with spontaneous hepatic encephalopathy is approximately 50%, and the rate in those with hepatorenal syndrome is 75%[17,19,20,114,115] (Fig. 81–6).

ALCOHOLIC CIRRHOSIS

The clinical tool used most widely to determine prognosis in patients with alcoholic cirrhosis is the Child-Turcotte-Pugh (CTP) classification (see also Chapter 87). This simple classification system, which was designed specifically to assess the risk of requirement for portacaval shunt surgery in cirrhotic patients with variceal bleeding, has gained favor as a rapid method for determining the prognosis of patients with various chronic liver diseases. The CTP classification is as effective as quantitative liver function tests and disease-specific prognostic models for determining short-term prognosis in groups of patients awaiting liver transplantation (see Chapter 92).[117] Despite its limitations, the CTP classification has been adopted widely for risk-stratifying patients with cirrhosis because of its simplicity and ease of use. Five-year survival rates for patients with alcoholic cirrhosis decrease dramatically as the CTP class becomes higher at the time of clinical presentation[117] (Fig. 81–7).

The development of ascites, variceal bleeding, hepatic encephalopathy, spontaneous bacterial peritonitis, or hepatorenal syndrome also has a significant impact on

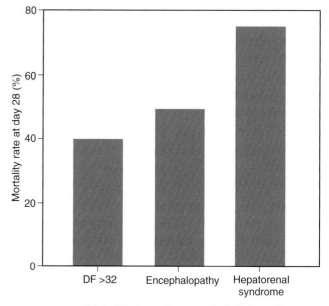

Clinical features of severe alcoholic hepatitis

Figure 81–6 Mortality rate at day 28 in patients with severe alcoholic hepatitis who received no treatment and who had a discriminant function (DF) score greater than 32, spontaneous hepatic encephalopathy, or hepatorenal syndrome. See text for calculation of DF. (Data from references 19, 49, and 50.)

the prognosis of patients with alcoholic cirrhosis. The 5-year survival rate for persons in whom any of these complications develop is only 20% to 50% of that for patients with compensated cirrhosis.[118] The most ominous complications are spontaneous bacterial peritonitis and rapid-onset hepatorenal syndrome (see Chapters 88 and 89). Less than one half of the patients in whom spontaneous bacterial peritonitis develops can be expected to survive

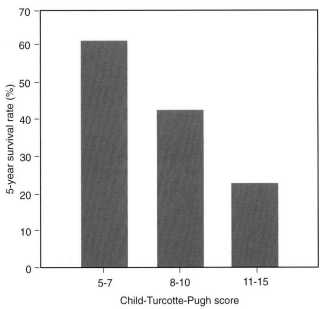

Figure 81–7 Five-year survival rates in patients with alcoholic cirrhosis according to their Child-Turcotte-Pugh scores. (Data from Poynard T, Naveau S, Doffoel M, et al: Evaluation of efficacy of liver transplantation in alcoholic cirrhosis using matched and simulated controls: 5-year survival. Multi-centre group. J Hepatol 30:1130, 1999.)

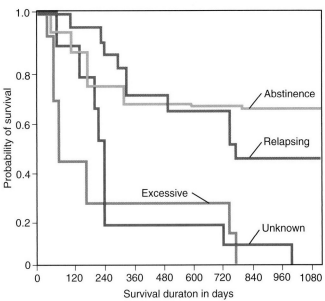

Figure 81–8 Survival curves during the 3 years following hospital discharge according to alcohol consumption: *abstinence*: patients who were abstinent; *relapsing*: patients with one or more periods of abstinence alternating with one or more periods of excessive consumption; *excessive*: patients with excessive consumption of alcohol at the first follow-up point. Survival differed significantly between abstinent and excessively drinking patients (*P* < .001). (Modified with permission of Veldt BJ, Laine F, Guillygomarc'h A, et al: Indication of liver transplantation in severe alcoholic liver cirrhosis: Qualitative evaluation and optimal timing. J Hepatol 36:93, 2002.)

1 year; the median survival of patients with hepatorenal syndrome is less than 2 weeks.[119,120]

Other models that have been used to predict prognosis in patients with alcoholic cirrhosis are the proportional hazards model developed by Poynard and colleagues—the Beclere model—and the prognostic model for end-stage liver disease (MELD) developed by investigators at the Mayo Clinic.[117,121] The Beclere model, which was developed from a database of 818 patients with alcoholic cirrhosis who were followed prospectively for 4 years, includes the serum bilirubin level, serum albumin level, patient's age, and presence or absence of hepatic encephalopathy.[117] The MELD model, which originally was developed to assess short-term prognosis in patients undergoing transjugular intrahepatic portosystemic shunt placement, includes the serum creatinine level, INR, and serum bilirubin level. This model has been shown to be useful for predicting short-term survival in groups of patients with various liver diseases (see Chapter 87).[121]

Abstinence from continued excessive drinking is the most important predictor of survival in patients who survive an initial hospitalization for alcoholic cirrhosis.[122] The rate of survival over the ensuing 2 years is 70% to 80% among patients who abstain or dramatically reduce their excessive drinking, compared with only 20% to 30% in those who continue to drink heavily (Fig. 81–8).[122]

TREATMENT

ABSTINENCE AND LIFESTYLE MODIFICATION

Virtually every study of abstinence in alcoholic liver disease shows beneficial effects on patient survival, even

in patients with decompensated cirrhosis (see Fig. 81–8). Reducing but not completely stopping alcohol consumption also has been shown to improve projected survival in patients with alcoholic liver disease.[57,123,124] So-called brief interventions are a simple form of psychological therapy for alcohol abuse that have been shown to result in a reduction in alcohol consumption from approximately 16 drinks a day to 2.5 drinks per day over a period of 6 years.[124] Abstinence causes resolution of hepatic steatosis; an additional goal of abstinence is to prevent ongoing injury, fibrosis, and the possible development of hepatocellular carcinoma, but few studies have addressed the effects of abstinence on disease progression. Newer drugs to improve abstinence, such as naltrexone and acamprosate (recently approved by the U.S. Food and Drug Administration), have reduced or eliminated alcohol intake in some chronic alcoholics; however, these drugs have not been tested extensively in patients with underlying alcoholic liver disease.

Malnutrition is a regular feature of end-stage alcoholic liver disease.[125] Obesity also is associated with the development of fatty liver, steatohepatitis, and cirrhosis,[41,42] however, and may be a major risk factor for progression of alcoholic liver disease. Patients who drink often smoke cigarettes as well, and smoking is a risk factor for more severe alcoholic liver disease. Therefore, lifestyle modifications including reduction or cessation of alcohol consumption, reduced cigarette smoking, and weight control are important initial approaches to the treatment of alcoholic liver disease.

NUTRITIONAL SUPPORT

A high frequency of malnutrition was documented conclusively in hospitalized patients with alcoholic hepatitis who participated in two large Veterans Administration (now Veterans Affairs [VA]) Cooperative Studies.[126,127] The first of these studies, which included more than 280 patients who underwent complete nutritional assessments, demonstrated that every patient with alcoholic hepatitis had some degree of malnutrition and that patients derived almost 50% of their total energy intake from the consumption of alcohol.[126] Evaluating malnutrition in patients with liver disease can be difficult, because the tests most commonly used to assess nutritional status (e.g., serum albumin concentration, anthropometry, immune status) often are affected by the liver disease. In this study[126] and a follow-up study,[127] the creatinine-height index[126] was found to be an important indicator of loss of muscle mass and was used to demonstrate that patients with more severe liver disease generally had more severe malnutrition (the index was less than 70% of normal in patients with moderate to severe alcoholic hepatitis). In both of these studies,[126,127] patients were encouraged to consume a balanced 2500-kcal diet, but despite careful monitoring by a dietitian, approximately two thirds of patients did not achieve this objective. Of importance, an inverse relationship was noted between energy intake and mortality rate.[126]

Additional interest in the role of nutritional support as therapy for alcoholic liver disease stemmed from early studies by Patek and colleagues demonstrating that a "nutritious diet" improved 5-year outcome in patients with alcoholic cirrhosis, compared with historical controls.[128] Subsequent studies have supported a role for nutritional support in patients hospitalized for alcoholic liver disease. In one trial, liver function, as assessed by serum bilirubin levels and antipyrine clearance, improved significantly in patients who received enteral nutritional supplementation through a feeding tube, compared with that in patients who ate a hospital diet.[129] Patients who received nutritional supplementation also had significantly greater protein and caloric intake. In a pivotal multicenter study by Cabre and co-workers, patients were randomized to receive prednisone, 40 mg daily (see later) or a liver-specific formula containing 2000 calories per day, through a feeding tube.[130] The 1-month mortality rates were similar in both groups, but the 1-year mortality rate was significantly lower in the patients who received the enteral nutrition, in great part because of reduced infectious complications, in comparison with patients who received glucocorticoids (Fig. 81–9). This study clearly demonstrates the important role of enteral nutrition in hospitalized patients with severe alcoholic liver disease.

Tube feeding in patients with alcoholic liver disease probably is underutilized in most hospitals because of concerns about precipitating hepatic encephalopathy or stimulating bleeding from esophageal varices, neither of which has been documented. Most patients probably can tolerate standard enteral products, and only selected patients with overt hepatic encephalopathy require liver-specific products rich in branched-chain amino acids.

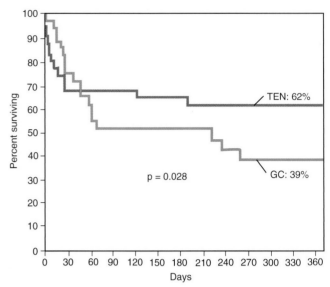

Figure 81–9 Probability of survival for 1 year after randomization of 72 patients to total enteral nutrition (TEN) versus glucocorticoid therapy (GC). (Used with permission of Cabre E, Rodriguez-Iglesias P, Caballeria J, et al: Short- and long-term outcome of severe alcohol induced hepatitis treated with steroids or enteral nutrition: A multicenter randomized trial. Hepatology 32:36, 2000.)

Studies of nutritional support in outpatients are limited, but Hirsch and colleagues demonstrated that patients from an outpatient liver clinic who took an enteral nutrition support product containing 1000 kcal and 34 g of protein had significantly improved protein intake and fewer hospitalizations in comparison with those not receiving the supplement.[131] This group of investigators subsequently showed that an enteral supplement improved nutritional status and immune function in outpatients with alcoholic cirrhosis.[132]

Therefore, nutritional support can improve nutritional status and, in some patients, may enhance liver function and decrease the risk of death. Assessment of nutritional status and nutritional supplementation should be pursued aggressively in both inpatients and outpatients with alcoholic liver disease, especially those with more severe alcoholic hepatitis and cirrhosis.

ANTI-INFLAMMATORY AND ANTICYTOKINE DRUGS

Glucocorticoids

Glucocorticoid therapy has been the most extensively studied and the most controversial treatment for patients with alcoholic hepatitis. A total of 10 small, single-center, placebo-controlled randomized trials of glucocorticoid therapy were published from 1971 to 1984, and only two showed a benefit.[114] Fallon and colleagues demonstrated improved survival only in patients who had hepatic encephalopathy within the first 10 days after hospital admission.[17] Maddrey and colleagues confirmed the prognostic importance of encephalopathy and found that a DF value greater than 32 (see earlier) was as effective as encephalopathy in selecting patients at high risk for early mortality, who appeared to benefit from glucocorticoid therapy.[113] These two prognostic tools—hepatic encephalopathy and an elevated DF—were used to select patients for entry into a subsequent multicenter study that demonstrated a dramatic impact of glucocorticoid therapy on short-term survival.[114] The cumulative 28-day mortality rate for this severely ill group of patients was 35% in the placebo recipients, compared with only 6% in patients who received methylprednisolone. Using the same selection criteria for study entry, Ramond and colleagues confirmed the improvement in short-term survival and also demonstrated a continued survival benefit for up to 6 months after treatment with glucocorticoids[115] (Fig. 81–10). Additional follow-up of these patients revealed that the survival benefit of glucocorticoid therapy persisted for 1 but not 2 years after treatment.[133] No major complications were associated with glucocorticoid therapy in these studies.[114,115] These two clinical trials included only patients with severe disease; patients with gastrointestinal bleeding requiring transfusions and active infection were excluded. Furthermore, none of the patients had evidence of hepatorenal syndrome before entry into the studies.

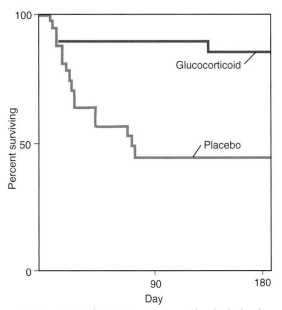

Figure 81–10 Survival in 61 patients with alcoholic hepatitis randomly assigned to receive glucocorticoid therapy or placebo. Survival rates at 6 months were 84% ± 6% in the glucocorticoid treatment group and 45% ± 9% in the placebo group (P = .002). (Used with permission of Raymond MJ, Poynard T, Rueff B, et al: A randomized trial of prednisone in patients with severe alcoholic hepatitis. N Engl J Med 326:507, 1992.)

Since the publication of these two pivotal studies, several meta-analyses of the trials of glucocorticoid therapy in alcoholic hepatitis have been published.[116,134] With one notable exception,[135] the general consensus among these analyses of the published data has been that glucocorticoids improve survival in patients with severe alcoholic hepatitis, particularly in patients with hepatic encephalopathy.

The available evidence suggests that (1) glucocorticoids should not be used in patients with mild alcoholic hepatitis; (2) they also should not be used in patients with gastrointestinal bleeding requiring blood transfusions or with evidence of active infection; (3) a short course of glucocorticoids (e.g., prednisone, 40 mg daily for 28 days, followed by 20 mg daily for 7 days and 10 mg daily for 7 days) may be beneficial in patients with spontaneous hepatic encephalopathy or a DF value greater than 32; and (4) glucocorticoids probably are not effective in patients with hepatorenal syndrome.[19]

Pentoxifylline

Pentoxifylline is a nonselective phosphodiesterase inhibitor that increases intracellular concentrations of adenosine 3′,5′-cyclic monophosphate (cAMP) and guanosine 3′,5′-cyclic monophosphate (cGMP) and may therefore inhibit TNF production. Pentoxifylline also has been shown to decrease gene transcription and to affect multiple steps in the cytokine/chemokine inflammatory pathway, either directly or indirectly by inhibiting TNF.[136] Selected effects of pentoxifylline include inhibition of cytokine/chemokine synthesis (e.g., MCP-1, IL-8, macrophage inflammatory protein [MIP]-1α and MIP-1β), decreased expression of adhesion molecules on endothelial cells, decreased activation of neutrophils, decreased proliferation of lymphocytes and monocytes, and decreased binding and transmigration of leukocytes. Pentoxifylline also reduces fibroblast proliferation and secretion of collagen and other interstitial matrix proteins.

Akriviadis and colleagues performed a prospective, randomized, double-blind clinical trial of pentoxifylline in patients with severe alcoholic hepatitis (DF greater than 32).[20] Forty-nine patients received pentoxifylline, 400 mg orally three times daily, and 52 received placebo (vitamin B_{12}) for 4 weeks. Only 12 patients (24.5%) who received pentoxifylline died, compared with 24 (46%) who received placebo (Fig. 81–11). Pentoxifylline therapy was associated with a significant decrease in the frequency of hepatorenal syndrome as a cause of death and was well tolerated with no major side effects. On the basis of this single trial, pentoxifylline appears to be a viable alternative to glucocorticoids, particularly in patients with clinically important renal dysfunction.

Specific Anti–Tumor Necrosis Factor Therapy

Dysregulated cytokine metabolism was described in alcoholic hepatitis long before it was recognized in inflammatory bowel disease and rheumatoid arthritis. An initial concern in alcoholic liver disease arose from early observations that low ("basal") amounts of TNF were important for liver regeneration.[137] Therefore, many investigators suggested that down-regulating, without

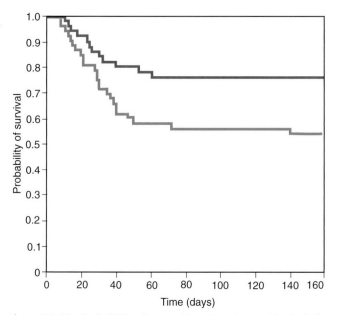

Figure 81–11 Probability of survival in 101 patients with alcoholic hepatitis treated with pentoxifylline *(red line)* or placebo *(blue line).* (Used with permission of Akrividas E, Botla R, Briggs W, et al: Pentoxifylline improves short-term survival in severe acute alcoholic hepatitis: A double blind, placebo-controlled trial. Gastroenterology 119:1637, 2000.)

totally blocking, TNF activity would be a preferred therapeutic intervention. Indeed, many therapies used in alcoholic liver disease (e.g., glucocorticoids, pentoxifylline, *S*-adenosylmethionine) decrease but do not abolish TNF activity.

Because anti-TNF antibody has been shown to block development of alcohol-induced liver injury in rats, it has been studied in small clinical trials in patients with alcoholic hepatitis. In a study from Europe, 12 patients with moderate to severe alcoholic hepatitis were given infliximab (anti-TNF antibody) in a dose of 5 mg/kg as a single 2-hour infusion; 10 of the 12 patients were alive after a median of 15 months.[138] Pilot data from a small U.S. open-label trial of etanercept, a TNF receptor antagonist, also showed safety in patients with less severe alcoholic hepatitis, and a multicenter trial of this agent is being funded by the National Institutes of Health.[139] On the other hand, a large, double-blind, randomized controlled trial from France in which patients with acute alcoholic hepatitis received either prednisolone treatment or prednisolone plus high-dose infliximab was terminated because of an increased rate of infectious complications in the combined therapy group.[140] Etanercept may be more attractive than infliximab in alcoholic liver disease because of its shorter duration of action. Theoretical concerns remain, however, with regard to blocking TNF activity completely for a long duration and a consequent increase in the risk of infections and impairment in liver regeneration. Until more data are available, specific anti-TNF therapy should be used only in the context of a clinical trial.

ANTIOXIDANTS

S-adenosylmethionine

Abnormal methionine metabolism is well documented in alcoholic liver disease, which is characterized by elevated plasma methionine concentrations and decreased clearance of intravenously or orally administered methionine. MAT activity is decreased in alcoholic liver disease, and plasma SAM levels also are decreased.[141] SAM has been reported to protect against experimental liver injury caused by alcohol, acetaminophen, carbon tetrachloride, and galactosamine.[69,75] Theoretical benefits of SAM in alcoholic liver disease include roles as an antioxidant and a critical methyl donor and in maintaining mitochondrial function, decreasing TNF levels, and producing glutathionine. A multicenter clinical study reported that SAM in a dose of 1200 mg significantly reduced the mortality rate and decreased the need for liver transplantation in patients with alcoholic liver disease.[142] SAM has been used in Europe for the treatment of other liver diseases and appears to have a good safety profile.

Silymarin

Silymarin, the active ingredient extracted from *Silybum marianum* (also known as milk thistle), has been shown in experimental animals to protect against various hepatotoxins, including carbon tetrachloride, acetaminophen, iron (in iron overload), and poisonous mushrooms.[143] It has antioxidant properties, protects against lipid peroxidation, and exerts anti-inflammatory and antifibrotic effects. Large controlled trials of silymarin have been performed in Europe, with varying results. Ferenci and co-workers evaluated silymarin, 140 mg three times daily, in 170 patients with cirrhosis for a mean duration of 41 months; they observed a beneficial effect, especially in patients with alcoholic cirrhosis.[144] On the other hand, Pares and colleagues found no beneficial effects of silymarin, 150 mg three times daily, in 200 patients with alcoholic cirrhosis, some of whom also had hepatitis C.[145] Despite these inconsistent results, silymarin has become the most popular form of complementary and alternative medicine therapy for patients with liver disease because of its good safety profile.

Vitamin E

Vitamin E deficiency has been well documented in alcoholic liver disease.[146] Vitamin E has hepatoprotective effects in experimental liver injury induced by carbon tetrachloride or ischemia. Its potential beneficial effects include membrane stabilization, reduced NFκB activation and TNF production, and inhibition of hepatic stellate cell activation and collagen production.[146-148] Unfortunately, the largest randomized study of vitamin E supplementation in patients with alcoholic liver disease did not show a significant benefit, possibly because a relatively low dose was used.[149]

Glutathione Prodrugs

Glutathione is a tripeptide that is synthesized from glutamate, cysteine, and glycine. Glutathione prodrugs have produced beneficial effects in virtually every known experimental model of hepatotoxicity.[150] The glutathione prodrug N-acetylcysteine (given as Mucomyst) is the standard agent to treat acetaminophen toxicity in humans (see Chapter 83). Maintaining adequate hepatocyte glutathione levels has been documented to prevent acetaminophen liver injury, and maintaining mitochondrial glutathione levels is important in preventing experimental alcoholic liver disease. Glutathione prodrugs also can inhibit TNF and IL-8 in alcoholic cirrhosis.[151] Large randomized studies of glutathione prodrugs with death as an outcome have not been performed in patients with alcoholic liver disease, however.

Other Antioxidants

A variety of other antioxidants have been used with success in experimental animal models of alcoholic liver disease. The agents range from zinc to ebselen to gene therapy with superoxide dismutase.[46,49] Clinical trials in humans have yet to be performed, however.

DRUGS WITH UNLIKELY BENEFITS

Colchicine

Colchicine has many potential therapeutic mechanisms of action in alcoholic liver disease, including inhibition of collagen production, enhancement of collagenase activity, and anti-inflammatory activity. Initial positive studies[152] led to a large VA Cooperative Study of colchicine therapy in patients with alcoholic cirrhosis that showed no beneficial effects on overall or liver-related mortality.[153] A smaller study from Europe also showed no beneficial effects of colchicine therapy in patients with alcoholic liver disease.[154]

Propylthiouracil

Chronic alcohol feeding in animal models can induce a hypermetabolic state with increased oxygen consumption similar to the hypermetabolic state associated with hyperthyroidism. This hypermetabolic state may lead to relative hypoxia in the centrilobular area of the liver. Propylthiouracil has been postulated to attenuate the hypermetabolic state, function as an antioxidant, and improve portal blood flow. A Cochrane review of six randomized trials involving more than 700 patients found no beneficial effect of propylthiouracil therapy in patients with alcoholic liver disease, however.[155]

Anabolic Steroids

Anabolic steroids have been shown to decrease fatty infiltration in the liver and are hepatoprotective. As noted earlier, patients with end-stage liver disease frequently are malnourished and often have low circulating levels of the anabolic hormone insulin-like growth factor-1. These observations provide a rationale for using anabolic steroids to treat alcoholic liver disease.[126] Nevertheless, a Cochrane review was not able to demonstrate efficacy for anabolic steroids (specifically oxandrolone) in patients with alcoholic liver disease, although such therapy did appear to be safe.[156]

Polyenylphosphatidylcholine

Polyenylphosphatidylcholine, or lecithin, a lipid extract obtained from soybeans, has been shown to prevent septal fibrosis and cirrhosis in alcohol-fed baboons and to stimulate the release of collagenase activity by cultured hepatic stellate cells. It also has antioxidant effects and decreases TNF production.[157] Multiple positive studies of polyenylphosphatidylcholine in animal models of liver disease led to a VA Cooperative Study that evaluated the effects of this drug in humans with early alcoholic liver disease.[158] Results of this study were negative; however, patients decreased their alcohol use markedly during the trial, thus decreasing the likelihood that a beneficial effect of polyenylphosphatidylcholine could be demonstrated.

LIVER TRANSPLANTATION

The outcome following liver transplantation for alcoholic liver disease is comparable to that in patients who receive transplants for most other conditions, with 7-year survival rates of 60% (see also Chapter 92).[159] Rejection, graft failure, and the need for retransplantation all are less common in patients with alcoholic liver disease than in patients undergoing transplantation for other conditions.[160] Although recidivism rates vary considerably from transplant center to transplant center, graft loss as a consequence of destructive drinking after liver transplantation is uncommon.[40,161] Profound confusion in the early postoperative period is more likely to develop in patients with alcoholic cirrhosis, however, than in those undergoing transplantation for other liver diseases.[162] The result can be a prolonged hospitalization and an increase in the cost of transplantation. In addition, patients with alcoholic liver disease have an increased risk of pharyngeal, esophageal, and gastric malignancies after transplantation.[163]

Many patients with apparently advanced alcoholic liver disease can recover to the degree that transplantation is not required if they reduce their alcohol intake significantly or abstain completely[122] (Fig. 81-12). Because the benefits of abstinence can be so dramatic, requiring a period of abstinence before proceeding with transplantation is reasonable for patients with alcoholic liver disease. Patients who have a CTP score of 11 or greater despite at least 6 months of abstinence have improved survival with liver transplantation, compared with predicted survival based on the Beclere model[117] (Fig. 81-13). Similar, although less impressive, results have been shown using other prognostic models.[164] The optimal length of pretransplant abstinence remains controversial.[40] Some experts have argued that patients with severe alcoholic hepatitis should be abstinent for 1 year before being considered for transplantation, whereas others have argued that patients should be considered for transplantation if they continue to have CTP scores of 11 or greater after only 3 months of abstinence.[122,133]

Evidence of a survival benefit following transplantation is less clear for patients with milder alcoholic liver disease, unless they have hepatocellular carcinoma. Patients with CTP scores of 5 to 7 do not benefit from

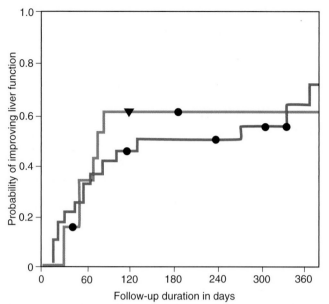

Figure 81–12 Probability that liver function will improve with time in patients with cirrhosis due to alcoholic liver disease who reduce alcohol intake or abstain from alcohol. Improvement was defined as a change from Child-Turcotte-Pugh class C to class B or A. *Red line,* patients who reduced intake; *blue line,* abstinent patients; *circles,* deaths; *triangles,* patients undergoing transplantation. (Used with permission of Veldt BJ, Laine F, Guillygomarc'h A, et al: Indication of liver transplantation in severe alcoholic liver cirrhosis: Qualitative evaluation and optimal timing. J Hepatol 36:93, 2002.)

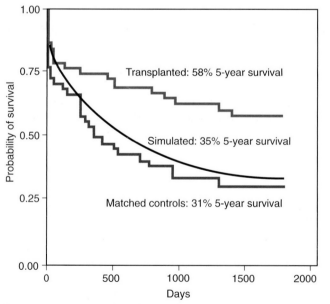

Figure 81–13 Probability of survival over 5 years in patients with Child-Turcotte-Pugh scores of 11 to 15 after 6 months of abstinence from alcohol who underwent liver transplantation *(top line),* compared with matched control subjects (*P* = .008) and simulated control subjects (*P* = .001). (Modified with permission of Poynard T, Naveau S, Doffoel M, et al: Evaluation of efficacy of liver transplantation in alcoholic cirrhosis using matched and simulated controls: 5 year survival. Multi-centre group. J Hepatol 30:1130, 1999.)

liver transplantation.[117] The survival benefit from transplantation for patients with CTP scores of 8 to 10 after 6 months of abstinence is minimal compared with predicted survival using the Beclere and MELD models.[117,164] Furthermore, a trial in which patients with a CTP score of 8 to 10 were randomized to receive immediate transplantation or to be observed expectantly showed a lower 2-year survival rate among the patients randomized to undergo immediate transplantation (73% versus 80%), primarily because of a high risk of postoperative malignancy.[165] Efforts to refine risk scores in patients with severe alcoholic liver disease and incorporate them into standard transplantation selection are ongoing.

OPTIMAL MANAGEMENT OF PATIENTS WITH ALCOHOLIC LIVER DISEASE

The optimal management of patients with alcoholic liver disease begins with a dramatic reduction in or elimination of alcohol intake, which often can be successfully accomplished using "brief interventions" by a nurse, primary care physician, or gastroenterologist. Abstinence can have a profound impact on survival even in patients with decompensated cirrhosis. The next important step is to eliminate other factors, such as cigarette smoking and obesity, that can enhance disease progression. Treatment of concomitant HCV infection may be an important aspect of management in some patients.

Patients with severe alcoholic hepatitis should receive enteral feedings to ensure adequate calorie and protein intake. In patients with spontaneous hepatic encephalopathy who do not have a systemic infection or gastrointestinal bleeding, a short course of glucocorticoid therapy should be considered. An alternative strategy is the use of pentoxifylline, especially in patients with marginal renal function or hepatorenal syndrome.

For patients with alcoholic cirrhosis, no drugs available in the United States have documented efficacy. Many patients already are taking agents such as milk thistle or SAM that may be of benefit and appear to be safe. These agents are not covered by insurance, however, and access to such agents often depends on the socioeconomic status of the patient. Because of the risk of decompensation with superimposed infections, all patients with alcoholic cirrhosis should receive vaccinations for hepatitis A and B and annual vaccinations for influenza. In addition, they should undergo regular screening for hepatocellular carcinoma (see Chapter 91). Screening is particularly important in older patients with cirrhosis who have been abstinent for sustained periods. Finally, liver transplantation has been shown to be effective in carefully selected patients who have discontinued drinking.

REFERENCES

1. Kim WR, Brown RS Jr, Terrault NA, El Serag H: Burden of liver disease in the United States: Summary of a workshop. Hepatology 36:227, 2002.
2. Hassan MM, Hwang LY, Hatten CJ, et al: Risk factors for hepatocellular carcinoma: Synergism of alcohol with viral hepatitis and diabetes mellitus. Hepatology 36:1206, 2002.

3. Schoniger-Hekele M, Muller C, Kutilek M, et al: Hepatocellular carcinoma in Austria: Aetiological and clinical characteristics at presentation. Eur J Gastroenterol Hepatol 12:941, 2000.

4. Fuchs CS, Stampfer MJ, Colditz GA, et al: Alcohol consumption and mortality among women. N Engl J Med 332:1245, 1995.

5. Becker U, Deis A, Sorensen TI, et al: Prediction of risk of liver disease by alcohol intake, sex, and age: A prospective population study. Hepatology 23:1025, 1996.

6. Thun MJ, Peto R, Lopez AD, et al: Alcohol consumption and mortality among middle-aged and elderly U.S. adults. N Engl J Med 337:1705, 1997.

7. MacSween RN, Burt AD: Histologic spectrum of alcoholic liver disease. Semin Liver Dis 6:221, 1986.

8. Ishak KG, Zimmerman H, Ray MB: Alcoholic liver disease: Pathologic, pathogenetic and clinical apects. Alcohol Clin Exp Res 15:45, 1991.

9. Lieber CS: Alcoholic liver injury: Pathogenesis and therapy in 2001. Pathol Biol (Paris) 49:738, 2001.

10. Saitz R, Mulvey KP, Plough A, Samet JH: Physician unawareness of serious substance abuse. Am J Drug Alcohol Abuse 23:343, 1997.

11. Fiellin DA, Reid MC, O'Connor PG: Screening for alcohol problems in primary care: A systematic review. Arch Intern Med 160:1977, 2000.

12. Arndt T: Carbohydrate-deficient transferrin as a marker of chronic alcohol abuse: A critical review of preanalysis, analysis, and interpretation. Clin Chem 47:13, 2001.

13. Fletcher LM, Kwoh-Gain I, Powell EE, et al: Markers of chronic alcohol ingestion in patients with nonalcoholic steatohepatitis: An aid to diagnosis. Hepatology 13:455, 1991.

14. De Feo TM, Fargion S, Duca L, et al: Carbohydrate-deficient transferrin, a sensitive marker of chronic alcohol abuse, is highly influenced by body iron. Hepatology 29:658, 1999.

15. Conigrave KM, Saunders JB, Whitfield JB: Diagnostic tests for alcohol consumption. Alcohol Alcohol 30:13, 1995.

16. Bruguera M, Bordas JM, Rodes J: Asymptomatic liver disease in alcoholics. Arch Pathol Lab Med 101:644, 1977.

17. Helman RA, Temko MH, Nye SW, Fallon HJ: Alcoholic hepatitis: Natural history and evaluation of prednisolone therapy. Ann Intern Med 74:311, 1971.

18. Mendenhall CL: Alcoholic hepatitis. Clin Gastroenterol 10:417, 1981.

19. Depew W, Boyer T, Omata M, et al: Double-blind controlled trial of prednisolone therapy in patients with severe acute alcoholic hepatitis and spontaneous encephalopathy. Gastroenterology 78:524, 1980.

20. Akriviadis E, Botla R, Briggs W, et al: Pentoxifylline improves short-term survival in severe acute alcoholic hepatitis: A double-blind, placebo-controlled trial. Gastroenterology 119:1637, 2000.

21. Van Ness MM, Diehl AM: Is liver biopsy useful in the evaluation of patients with chronically elevated liver enzymes? Ann Intern Med 111:473, 1989.

22. Talley NJ, Roth A, Woods J, Hench V: Diagnostic value of liver biopsy in alcoholic liver disease. J Clin Gastroenterol 10:647, 1988.

23. Marchesini G, Bugianesi E, Forlani G, et al: Nonalcoholic fatty liver, steatohepatitis, and the metabolic syndrome. Hepatology 37:917, 2003.

24. Falck-Ytter Y, Younossi ZM, Marchesini G, McCullough AJ: Clinical features and natural history of nonalcoholic steatosis syndromes. Semin Liver Dis 21:17, 2001.

25. Cotler SJ, Bronner MP, Press RD, et al: End-stage liver disease without hemochromatosis associated with elevated hepatic iron index. J Hepatol 29:257, 1998.

26. Deugnier Y, Turlin B, le Quilleuc D, et al: A reappraisal of hepatic siderosis in patients with end-stage cirrhosis: Practical implications for the diagnosis of hemochromatosis. Am J Surg Pathol 21:669, 1997.

27. Fletcher LM, Powell LW: Hemochromatosis and alcoholic liver disease. Alcohol 30:131, 2003.

28. Press RD, Flora K, Gross C, et al: Hepatic iron overload: Direct HFE (HLA-H) mutation analysis vs quantitative iron assays for the diagnosis of hereditary hemochromatosis. Am J Clin Pathol 109:577, 1998.

29. Simon JB, Manley PN, Brien JF, Armstrong PW: Amiodarone hepatotoxicity simulating alcoholic liver disease. N Engl J Med 311:167, 1984.

30. Janssen HL, Tan AC, Tilanus HW, et al: Pseudo–Budd-Chiari syndrome: Decompensated alcoholic liver disease mimicking hepatic venous outflow obstruction. Hepatogastroenterology 49:810, 2002.

31. Seeff LB, Cuccherine BA, Zimmerman HJ, et al: Acetaminophen hepatotoxicity in alcoholics: A therapeutic misadventure. Ann Intern Med 105:399, 1986.

32. Akriviadis EA, Redeker AG: Fulminant hepatitis A in intravenous drug users with chronic liver disease. Ann Intern Med 110:838, 1989.

33. Feller A, Uchida T, Rakela J: Acute viral hepatitis superimposed on alcoholic liver cirrhosis: Clinical and histopathologic features. Liver 5:239, 1985.

34. Duchini A, Hendry RM, Redfield DC, Pockros PJ: Influenza infection in patients before and after liver transplantation. Liver Transpl 6:531, 2000.

35. Koff RS, Dienstag JL: Extrahepatic manifestations of hepatitis C and the association with alcoholic liver disease. Semin Liver Dis 15:101, 1995.

36. Fong T-L, Kanel GC, Conrad A, et al: Clinical significance of concomitant hepatitis C infection in patients with alcoholic liver disease. Hepatology 19:554, 1994.

37. Mendenhall CL, Seeff L, Diehl AM, et al: Antibodies to hepatitis B virus and hepatitis C virus in alcoholic hepatitis and cirrhosis: Their prevalence and clinical relevance. The VA Cooperative Study Group (No. 119). Hepatology 14:581, 1991.

38. Corrao G, Arico S: Independent and combined action of hepatitis C virus infection and alcohol consumption on the risk of symptomatic liver cirrhosis. Hepatology 27:914, 1998.

39. Yamauchi M, Nakahara M, Maezawa Y, et al: Prevalence of hepatocellular carcinoma in patients with alcoholic cirrhosis and prior exposure to hepatitis C. Am J Gastroenterol 88:39, 1993.

40. Neuberger J, Schulz KH, Day C, et al: Transplantation for alcoholic liver disease. J Hepatol 36:130, 2002.

41. Naveau S, Giraud V, Borotto E, et al: Excess weight risk factor for alcoholic liver disease. Hepatology 25:108, 1997.

42. Raynard B, Balian A, Fallik D, et al: Risk factors of fibrosis in alcohol-induced liver disease. Hepatology 35:635, 2002.

43. Klatsky AL, Armstrong MA: Alcohol, smoking, coffee, and cirrhosis. Am J Epidemiol 136:1248, 1992.

44. Corrao G, Lepore AR, Torchio P, et al: The effect of drinking coffee and smoking cigarettes on the risk of cirrhosis associated with alcohol consumption. A case-control study. Provincial Group for the Study of Chronic Liver Disease. Eur J Epidemiol 10:657, 1994.

45. Pessione F, Ramond MJ, Njapoum C, et al: Cigarette smoking and hepatic lesions in patients with chronic hepatitis C. Hepatology 34:121, 2001.

46. Arteel G, Marsano L, Mendez C, et al: Advances in alcoholic liver disease. Best Pract Res Clin Gastroenterol 17:625, 2003.

47. Thiele GM, Worrall S, Tuma DJ, et al: The chemistry and biological effects of malondialdehyde-acetaldehyde adducts. Alcohol Clin Exp Res 25:218S, 2001.

48. Lluis JM, Colell A, Garcia-Ruiz C, et al: Acetaldehyde impairs mitochondrial glutathione transport in HepG2 cells through

endoplasmic reticulum stress. Gastroenterology 124:708, 2003.

49. Arteel GE: Oxidants and antioxidants in alcohol-induced liver disease. Gastroenterology 124:778, 2003.

50. Reinke LA, Lai EK, DuBose CM, McCay PB: Reactive free radical generation in vivo in heart and liver of ethanol-fed rats: Correlation with radical formation in vitro. Proc Natl Acad Sci U S A 84:9223, 1987.

51. Meagher EA, Barry OP, Burke A, et al: Alcohol-induced generation of lipid peroxidation products in humans. J Clin Invest 104:805, 1999.

52. Wu D, Cederbaum AI: Ethanol cytotoxicity to a transfected HepG2 cell line expressing human cytochrome P4502E1. J Biol Chem 271:23914, 1996.

53. Morgan K, French SW, Morgan TR: Production of a cytochrome P450 2E1 transgenic mouse and initial evaluation of alcoholic liver damage. Hepatology 36:122, 2002.

54. Kono H, Rusyn I, Uesugi T, et al: Diphenyleneiodonium sulfate, an NADPH oxidase inhibitor, prevents early alcohol-induced liver injury in the rat. Am J Physiol Gastrointest Liver Physiol 280:G1005, 2001.

55. Kono H, Rusyn I, Yin M, et al: NADPH oxidase–derived free radicals are key oxidants in alcohol-induced liver disease. J Clin Invest 106:867, 2000.

56. Hoek JB, Cahill A, Pastorino JG: Alcohol and mitochondria: A dysfunctional relationship. Gastroenterology 122:2049, 2002.

57. Adachi M, Ishii H: Role of mitochondria in alcoholic liver injury. Free Radic Biol Med 32:487, 2002.

58. Witschi A, Mossi S, Meyer B, et al: Mitochondrial function reflected by the decarboxylation of [^{13}C]ketoisocaproate is impaired in alcoholics. Alcohol Clin Exp Res 18:951, 1994.

59. Coll O, Colell A, Garcia-Ruiz C, et al: Sensitivity of the 2-oxoglutarate carrier to alcohol intake contributes to mitochondrial glutathione depletion. Hepatology 38:692, 2003.

60. French SW: The role of hypoxia in the pathogenesis of alcoholic liver disease. Hepatol Res 29:69, 2004.

61. Yang Y, Yu X: Regulation of apoptosis: The ubiquitous way. FASEB J 17:790, 2003.

62. Donohue TM Jr: The ubiquitin-proteasome system and its role in ethanol-induced disorders. Addict Biol 7:15, 2002.

63. Baraona E, Leo MA, Borowsky SA, Lieber CS: Pathogenesis of alcohol-induced accumulation of protein in the liver. J Clin Invest 60:546, 1977.

64. Fataccioli V, Andraud E, Gentil M, et al: Effects of chronic ethanol administration on rat liver proteasome activities: Relationship with oxidative stress. Hepatology 29:14, 1999.

65. Donohue TM Jr, Zetterman RK, Zhang-Gouillon ZQ, French SW: Peptidase activities of the multicatalytic protease in rat liver after voluntary and intragastric ethanol administration. Hepatology 28:486, 1998.

66. Takagi M, Yamauchi M, Toda G, et al: Serum ubiquitin levels in patients with alcoholic liver disease. Alcohol Clin Exp Res 23:76S, 1999.

67. Bardag-Gorce F, van Leeuwen FW, Nguyen V, et al: The role of the ubiquitin-proteasome pathway in the formation of Mallory bodies. Exp Mol Pathol 73:75, 2002.

68. Joshi-Barve S, Barve SS, Butt W, et al: Inhibition of proteasome function leads to NF-kappaB–independent IL-8 expression in human hepatocytes. Hepatology 38:1178, 2003.

69. McClain CJ, Hill DB, Song Z, et al: S-adenosylmethionine, cytokines, and alcoholic liver disease. Alcohol 27:185, 2002.

70. Mato JM, Alvarez L, Ortiz P, Pajares MA: S-adenosylmethionine synthesis: Molecular mechanisms and clinical implications. Pharmacol Ther 73:265, 1997.

71. Hoffman DR, Marion DW, Cornatzer WE, Duerre JA: S-adenosylmethionine and S-adenosylhomocystein metabolism in isolated rat liver. Effects of L-methionine, L-homocystein, and adenosine. J Biol Chem 255:10822, 1980.

72. Song Z, Zhou Z, Uriarte S, et al: S-adenosylhomocysteine sensitizes to TNF hepatotoxicity: A possible etiologic factor in alcoholic liver disease. Hepatology 40:989, 2004.

73. Horowitz JH, Rypins EB, Henderson JM, et al: Evidence for impairment of transsulfuration pathway in cirrhosis. Gastroenterology 81:668, 1981.

74. Cabrero C, Duce AM, Ortiz P, et al: Specific loss of the high-molecular-weight form of S-adenosyl-L-methionine synthetase in human liver cirrhosis. Hepatology 8:1530, 1988.

75. Song Z, McClain CJ, Chen T: S-adenosylmethionine protects against acetaminophen-induced hepatotoxicity in mice. Pharmacology 71:199, 2004.

76. Chawla RK, Lewis FW, Kutner MH, et al: Plasma cysteine, cystine, and glutathione in cirrhosis. Gastroenterology 87:770, 1984.

77. Lieber CS, Casini A, DeCarli LM, et al: S-adenosyl-L-methionine attenuates alcohol-induced liver injury in the baboon. Hepatology 11:165, 1990.

78. Sanchez-Gongora E, Ruiz F, Mingorance J, et al: Interaction of liver methionine adenosyltransferase with hydroxyl radical. FASEB J 11:1013, 1997.

79. Colell A, Garcia-Ruiz C, Miranda M, et al: Selective glutathione depletion of mitochondria by ethanol sensitizes hepatocytes to tumor necrosis factor. Gastroenterology 115:1541, 1998.

80. Chawla RK, Watson WH, Eastin CE, et al: S-adenosylmethionine deficiency and TNF-alpha in lipopolysaccharide-induced hepatic injury. Am J Physiol 275:G125, 1998.

81. Ji C, Kaplowitz N: Hyperhomocysteinemia, endoplasmic reticulum stress, and alcoholic liver injury. World J Gastroenterol 10:1699, 2004.

82. Halsted CH, Villanueva JA, Devlin AM, Chandler CJ: Metabolic interactions of alcohol and folate. J Nutr 132:2367S, 2002.

83. McClain CJ, Barve S, Deaciuc I, et al: Cytokines in alcoholic liver disease. Semin Liver Dis 19:205, 1999.

84. Sen CK, Packer L: Antioxidant and redox regulation of gene transcription. FASEB J 10:709, 1996.

85. Canbay A, Feldstein AE, Higuchi H, et al: Kupffer cell engulfment of apoptotic bodies stimulates death ligand and cytokine expression. Hepatology 38:1188, 2003.

86. Deaciuc IV, D'Souza NB, de Villiers WJ, et al: Inhibition of caspases in vivo protects the rat liver against alcohol-induced sensitization to bacterial lipopolysaccharide. Alcohol Clin Exp Res 25:935, 2001.

87. McClain CJ, Cohen DA: Increased tumor necrosis factor production by monocytes in alcoholic hepatitis. Hepatology 9:349, 1989.

88. Zhang Z, Bagby GJ, Stoltz D, et al: Prolonged ethanol treatment enhances lipopolysaccharide/phorbol myristate acetate–induced tumor necrosis factor-alpha production in human monocytic cells. Alcohol Clin Exp Res 25:444, 2001.

89. Honchel R, Ray MB, Marsano L, et al: Tumor necrosis factor in alcohol enhanced endotoxin liver injury. Alcohol Clin Exp Res 16:665, 1992.

90. Kamimura S, Tsukamoto H: Cytokine gene expression by Kupffer cells in experimental alcoholic liver disease. Hepatology 22:1304, 1995.

91. Nanji AA, Zhao S, Sadrzadeh SM, Waxman DJ: Use of reverse transcription–polymerase chain reaction to evaluate in vivo cytokine gene expression in rats fed ethanol for long periods. Hepatology 19:1483, 1994.

92. Le Moine O, Marchant A, De Groote D, et al: Role of defective monocyte interleukin-10 release in tumor necrosis factor-alpha overproduction in alcoholics cirrhosis. Hepatology 22:1436, 1995.

93. Hill DB, D'Souza NB, Lee EY, et al: A role for interleukin-10 in alcohol-induced liver sensitization to bacterial lipopolysaccharide. Alcohol Clin Exp Res 26:74, 2002.

94. Iimuro Y, Gallucci RM, Luster MI, et al: Antibodies to tumor necrosis factor alpha attenuate hepatic necrosis and inflammation caused by chronic exposure to ethanol in the rat. Hepatology 26:1530, 1997.

95. Yin M, Wheeler MD, Kono H, et al: Essential role of tumor necrosis factor alpha in alcohol-induced liver injury in mice. Gastroenterology 117:942, 1999.

96. Pastorino JG, Hoek JB: Ethanol potentiates tumor necrosis factor-alpha cytotoxicity in hepatoma cells and primary rat hepatocytes by promoting induction of the mitochondrial permeability transition. Hepatology 31:1141, 2000.

97. Chedid A, Chadalawada KR, Morgan TR, et al: Phospholipid antibodies in alcoholic liver disease. Hepatology 20:1465, 1994.

98. Clot P, Bellomo G, Tabone M, et al: Detection of antibodies against proteins modified by hydroxyethyl free radicals in patients with alcoholic cirrhosis. Gastroenterology 108:201, 1995.

99. Vidali M, Stewart SF, Rolla R, et al: Genetic and epigenetic factors in autoimmune reactions toward cytochrome P4502E1 in alcoholic liver disease. Hepatology 37:410, 2003.

100. Kwo PY, Ramchandani VA, O'Connor S, et al: Gender differences in alcohol metabolism: Relationship to liver volume and effect of adjusting for body mass. Gastroenterology 115:1552, 1998.

101. Nanji AA, Jokelainen K, Fotouhinia M, et al: Increased severity of alcoholic liver injury in female rats: Role of oxidative stress, endotoxin, and chemokines. Am J Physiol Gastrointest Liver Physiol 281:G1348, 2001.

102. Crabb DW, Matsumoto M, Chang D, You M: Overview of the role of alcohol dehydrogenase and aldehyde dehydrogenase and their variants in the genesis of alcohol-related pathology. Proc Nutr Soc 63:49, 2004.

103. Grove J, Daly AK, Bassendine MF, Day CP: Association of a tumor necrosis factor promoter polymorphism with susceptibility to alcoholic steatohepatitis. Hepatology 26:143, 1997.

104. Grove J, Daly AK, Bassendine MF, et al: Interleukin 10 promoter region polymorphisms and susceptibility to advanced alcoholic liver disease. Gut 46:540, 2000.

105. Fischer M, You M, Matsumoto M, Crabb DW: Peroxisome proliferator–activated receptor alpha (PPARalpha) agonist treatment reverses PPARalpha dysfunction and abnormalities in hepatic lipid metabolism in ethanol-fed mice. J Biol Chem 278:27997, 2003.

106. You M, Fischer M, Deeg MA, Crabb DW: Ethanol induces fatty acid synthesis pathways by activation of sterol regulatory element-binding protein (SREBP). J Biol Chem 277:29342, 2002.

107. Donohue TM Jr, Clemens DL, Galli A, et al: Use of cultured cells in assessing ethanol toxicity and ethanol-related metabolism. Alcohol Clin Exp Res 25:87S, 22001.

108. Friedman SL: Liver fibrosis—from bench to bedside. J Hepatol 38(suppl 1):S38, 2003.

109. Zamara E, Novo E, Marra F, et al: 4-Hydroxynonenal as a selective pro-fibrogenic stimulus for activated human hepatic stellate cells. J Hepatol 40:60, 2004.

110. Reeves HL, Friedman SL: Activation of hepatic stellate cells—a key issue in liver fibrosis. Front Biosci 7:d808, 2002.

111. Orrego H, Blake JE, Blendis LM, Medline A: Prognosis of alcoholic cirrhosis in the presence and absence of alcoholic hepatitis. Gastroenterology 92:208, 1987.

112. Poynard T, Aubert A, Lazizi Y, et al: Independent risk factors for hepatocellular carcinoma in French drinkers. Hepatology 13:896, 1991.

113. Maddrey WC, Boitnott JK, Bedine MS, et al: Glucocorticoid therapy of alcoholic hepatitis. Gastroenterology 75:193, 1978.

114. Carithers RL Jr, Herlong HF, Diehl AM, et al: Methylprednisolone therapy in patients with severe alcoholic hepatitis: A randomized multicenter trial. Ann Intern Med 110:685, 1989.

115. Ramond M-J, Poynard T, Rueff B, et al: A randomized trial of prednisolone in patients with severe alcoholic hepatitis. N Engl J Med 326:507, 1992.

116. Mathurin P, Mendenhall CL, Carithers RL, et al: Glucocorticoids improve short-term survival in patients with severe alcoholic hepatitis (AH): Individual data analysis of the last three randomized placebo controlled double blind trials of glucocorticoids in severe AH. J Hepatol 36:480, 2002.

117. Poynard T, Naveau S, Doffoel M, et al: Evaluation of efficacy of liver transplantation in alcoholic cirrhosis using matched and simulated controls: 5-year survival. Multi-centre group. J Hepatol 30:1130, 1999.

118. Gines P, Quintero E, Arroyo V, et al: Compensated cirrhosis: Natural history and prognosis factors. Hepatology 7:122, 1987.

119. Andreu M, Sola R, Sitges SA, et al: Risk factors for spontaneous bacterial peritonitis in cirrhotic patients with ascites. Gastroenterology 104:1133, 1993.

120. Gines A, Escorsell A, Gines P, et al: Incidence, predictive factors, and prognosis of the hepatorenal syndrome in cirrhosis with ascites. Gastroenterology 105:229, 1993.

121. Kamath PS, Wiesner RH, Malinchoc M, et al: A model to predict survival in patients with end-stage liver disease. Hepatology 33:464, 2001.

122. Veldt BJ, Laine F, Guillygomarc'h A, et al: Indication of liver transplantation in severe alcoholic liver cirrhosis: Quantitative evaluation and optimal timing. J Hepatol 36:93, 2002.

123. Powell WJ, Klatskin G: Duration and survival in patients with Laennec's cirrhosis. Am J Med 44:406, 1968.

124. Lieber CS, Weiss DG, Groszmann R, et al: I. Veterans Affairs Cooperative Study of polyenlyphosphatidylcholine in alcoholic liver disease: Effects on drinking behavior by nurse/physician teams. Alcohol Clin Exp Res 27:1757, 2003.

125. Mendenhall CL, Anderson S, Weesner RE, et al: Protein-calorie malnutrition associated with alcoholic hepatitis. Am J Med 76:211, 1984.

126. Mendenhall CL, Moritz TE, Roselle GA, et al: A study of oral nutritional support with oxandrolone in malnourished patients with alcoholic hepatitis: Results of a Department of Veterans Affairs cooperative study. Hepatology 17:564, 1993.

127. Mendenhall C, Roselle GA, Gartside P, Moritz T: Relationship of protein calorie malnutrition to alcoholic liver disease: A reexamination of data from two Veterans Administration Cooperative Studies. Alcohol Clin Exp Res 19:635, 1995.

128. Patek AJ, Post J, Ralnoff OD: Dietary treatment of cirrhosis of the liver. JAMA 139:543, 1948.

129. Kearns PJ, Young H, Garcia G: Accelerated improvement of alcoholic liver disease with enteral nutrition. Gastroenterology 102:200, 1992.

130. Cabre E, Rodriguez-Iglesias P, Caballeria J, et al: Short- and long-term outcome of severe alcohol-induced hepatitis treated with steroids or enteral nutrition: A multicenter randomized trial. Hepatology 32:36, 2000.

131. Hirsch S, Bunout D, de la Maza P, et al: Controlled trial on nutrition supplementation in outpatients with symptomatic alcoholic cirrhosis. JPEN J Parenter Enteral Nutr 17:119, 1993.

132. Hirsch S, de la Maza MP, Gattas V, et al: Nutritional support in alcoholic cirrhotic patients improves host defenses. J Am Coll Nutr 18:434, 1999.

133. Mathurin P, Duchatelle V, Ramond MJ, et al: Survival and prognostic factors in patients with severe alcoholic hepatitis treated with prednisone. Gastroenterology 110:1847, 1996.

134. Imperiale TF, McCullough AJ: Do glucocorticoids reduce mortality from alcoholic hepatitis? A meta-analysis of the randomized trials. Ann Intern Med 113:299, 1990.

135. Christensen E, Gluud C: Glucocorticoids are ineffective in alcoholic hepatitis: A meta-analysis adjusting for confounding variables. Gut 37:113, 1995.

136. Strieter RM, Remick DG, Ward PA, et al: Cellular and molecular regulation of tumor necrosis factor-alpha production by pentoxifylline. Biochem Biophys Res Commun 155:1230, 1988.

137. Akerman PA, Cote PM, Yang SQ, et al: Long-term ethanol consumption alters the hepatic response to the regenerative effects of tumor necrosis factor-alpha. Hepatology 17:1066, 1993.

138. Tilg H, Jalan R, Kaser A, et al: Anti-tumor necrosis factor-alpha monoclonal antibody therapy in severe alcoholic hepatitis. J Hepatol 38:419, 2003.

139. Menon KV, Stadheim L, Kamath PS, et al: A pilot study of the safety and tolerability of etanercept in patients with alcoholic hepatitis. Am J Gastroenterol 99:255, 2004.

140. Naveau S, Chollet-Martin S, Dharancy S, et al: A double-blind randomized controlled trial of infliximab associated with prednisolone in acute alcoholic hepatitis. Hepatology 39:1390, 2004.

141. Lee TD, Sadda MR, Mendler MH, et al: Abnormal hepatic methionine and glutathione metabolism in patients with alcoholic hepatitis. Alcohol Clin Exp Res 28:173, 2004.

142. Mato JM, Camara J, Fernandez DP, et al: S-adenosylmethionine in alcoholic liver cirrhosis: A randomized, placebo-controlled, double-blind, multicenter clinical trial. J Hepatol 30:1081, 1999.

143. Luper S: A review of plants used in the treatment of liver disease: Part 1. Altern Med Rev 3:410, 1998.

144. Ferenci P, Dragosics B, Dittrich H, et al: Randomized controlled trial of silymarin treatment in patients with cirrhosis of the liver. J Hepatol 9:105, 1989.

145. Pares A, Planas R, Torres M, et al: Effects of silymarin in alcoholic patients with cirrhosis of the liver: Results of a controlled, double-blind, randomized and multicenter trial. J Hepatol 28:615, 1998.

146. McClain C, Hill D, Kugelmas M, Marsano L: Nutrition and liver disease. In Bowman BA, Russell RM, Russell R (eds): Present Knowledge in Nutrition, 8th ed. Washington, DC, International Life Sciences Institute, 2001, p 483.

147. Hill DB, Devalaraja R, Joshi-Barve S, et al: Antioxidants attenuate nuclear factor-kappa B activation and tumor necrosis factor-alpha production in alcoholic hepatitis patient monocytes and rat Kupffer cells, in vitro. Clin Biochem 32:563, 1999.

148. Lee KS, Buck M, Houglum K, Chojkier M: Activation of hepatic stellate cells by TGF alpha and collagen type I is mediated by oxidative stress through c-Myb expression. J Clin Invest 96:2461, 1995.

149. de la Maza MP, Petermann M, Bunout D, Hirsch S: Effects of long-term vitamin E supplementation in alcoholic cirrhotics. J Am Coll Nutr 14:192, 1995.

150. Meister A: Glutathione metabolism and its selective modification. J Biol Chem 263:17205, 1988.

151. Pena LR, Hill DB, McClain CJ. Treatment with glutathione precursor decreases cytokine activity. JPEN J Parenter Enteral Nutr 23:1, 1999.

152. Kershenobich D, Vargas F, Garcia-Tsao G, et al: Colchicine in the treatment of cirrhosis of the liver. N Engl J Med 318:1709, 1988.

153. Morgan TR, Weiss DG, Nemchausky N, et al: Colchicine treatment of alcoholic cirrhosis: A randomized, placebo-controlled clinical trial of patient survival. Gastroenterology 128:882, 2005.

154. Cortez-Pinto H, Alexandrino P, Camilo ME, et al: Lack of effect of colchicine in alcoholic cirrhosis: Final results of a double blind randomized trial. Eur J Gastroenterol Hepatol 14:377, 2002.

155. Rambaldi A, Gluud C: Colchicine for alcoholic and non-alcoholic liver fibrosis and cirrhosis. Cochrane Database Syst Rev CD002148, 2001.

156. Rambaldi A, Iaquinto G, Gluud C: Anabolic-androgenic steroids for alcoholic liver disease: A Cochrane review. Am J Gastroenterol 97:1674, 2002.

157. Cao Q, Mak KM, Lieber CS: Dilinoleoylphosphatidylcholine decreases acetaldehyde-induced TNF-alpha generation in Kupffer cells of ethanol-fed rats. Biochem Biophys Res Commun 299:459, 2002.

158. Lieber CS, Weiss DG, Groszmann R, et al: II. Veterans Affairs Cooperative Study of polyenylphosphatidylcholine in alcoholic liver disease. Alcohol Clin Exp Res 27:1765, 2003.

159. Roberts MS, Angus DC, Bryce CL, et al: Survival after liver transplantation in the United States: A disease-specific analysis of the UNOS database. Liver Transpl 10:886, 2004.

160. Farges O, Saliba F, Farhamant H, et al: Incidence of rejection and infection after liver transplantation as a function of the primary disease: Possible influence of alcohol and polyclonal immunoglobulin. Hepatology 23:240, 1996.

161. Pageaux GP, Bismuth M, Perney P, et al: Alcohol relapse after liver transplantation for alcoholic liver disease: Does it matter? J Hepatol 38:629, 2003.

162. Buis CI, Wiesner RH, Krom RA, et al: Acute confusional state following liver transplantation for alcoholic liver disease. Neurology 59:601, 2002.

163. Bellamy CO, DiMartini AM, Ruppert K, et al: Liver transplantation for alcoholic cirrhosis: Long term follow-up and impact of disease recurrence. Transplantation 72:619, 2001.

164. Young TA, Neuberger J, Longworth L, et al: Survival gain after liver transplantation for patients with alcoholic liver disease: A comparison across models and centers. Transplantation 76:1479, 2003.

165. Miguet JP, Vanlemmens C, Milan C, et al: Impact of liver transplantation on survival in Pugh B alcoholic cirrhotic patients: A multicenter randomized trial. 38(suppl 1):90A, 2003.

CHAPTER

82 Nonalcoholic Fatty Liver Disease

Andrea E. Reid

NONALCOHOLIC FATTY LIVER AND STEATOHEPATITIS

In 1980, Ludwig and colleagues from the Mayo Clinic coined the term *nonalcoholic steatohepatitis* (NASH) to describe a form of liver disease observed in 20 middle-aged patients with abnormal liver biochemical test results and histologic evidence of alcoholic hepatitis but no history of alcohol abuse.[1] No other cause of liver disease was identified. Sixty percent of these patients were women, 90% were obese, 25% had hyperlipidemia, and 25% had adult-onset diabetes mellitus. On examination of liver biopsy specimens, the hallmark feature was moderate to severe macrovesicular steatosis with lobular inflammation; fibrosis was present in 70% and cirrhosis in 15% of specimens.

Much has been learned about NASH since this initial description. It is now clear that NASH is part of the spectrum of *nonalcoholic fatty liver disease* (NAFLD), which encompasses simple fatty liver, NASH, and NAFLD-associated cirrhosis. Many reviews have been written about NAFLD,[2-6] and the entity has emerged as an exciting area of basic and clinical investigation in the field of hepatology.

EPIDEMIOLOGY

Although large epidemiologic studies of NAFLD are lacking and the prevalence of NAFLD in the general population is undefined, NAFLD probably is the most common liver disorder in the world, affecting 2.8% to 24% of the general population,[3,7-9] including overweight children and adolescents.[10] Most cases of NAFLD occur in the fourth to sixth decades of life. In early clinical studies, a majority of patients with NAFLD were female; however, more contemporary data suggest that males and females may be affected equally. The prevalence of NAFLD among different racial groups is not known. Studies suggest that African Americans and Mexican Americans have higher frequencies of unexplained serum aminotransferase elevations than those reported in whites,[8,9,11,12] although they may be given a diagnosis of NAFLD less frequently than expected.[13] Familial clustering of NAFLD may occur,[14] although no genetic markers for NAFLD have been identified definitively. Familial clustering probably reflects both genetic and environmental predisposition to the metabolic conditions associated with NAFLD.

ETIOLOGY

Many different agents and conditions have been associated with NAFLD. The causes may be divided into two broad categories: (1) drugs and toxins and (2) metabolic abnormalities, either acquired or congenital. Potential causes of NAFLD are listed in Table 82–1. Obesity is the condition most often reported in association with NAFLD. The frequency of NAFLD may be as high as 80% in obese persons, with advanced disease (i.e., NASH) seen in 9% to 30%.[15,16] A correlation among body mass index (BMI), degree of steatosis, and severity of liver injury has been demonstrated in several studies; however, the distribution of body fat may be more important than the total adipose mass for the development of hepatic steatosis. Studies have shown a significant correlation between the degree of hepatic steatosis and the waist-to-hip ratio,

Table 82–1 Causes of Nonalcoholic Fatty Liver Disease

Acquired Metabolic Disorders	**Metals**
Diabetes mellitus	Antimony
Obesity	Barium salts
Hyperlipidemia	Chromates
Kwashiorkor and marasmus	Phosphorus
Starvation	Rare earths of low atomic number
Cytotoxic/Cytostatic	Thallium compounds
Drugs	Uranium compounds
L-Asparaginase	**Inborn Errors of Metabolism**
Azacitidine	Abetalipoproteinemia
Methotrexate	Familial hepatosteatosis
Azaserine	Galactosemia
Bleomycin	Glycogen storage disease
Puromycin	Hereditary fructose intolerance
Tetracycline*	Homocystinuria
Other Drugs/Toxins	Systemic carnitine deficiency
Amiodarone	Tyrosinemia
4,4'-diethylaminoethoxyhexestrol	Weber-Christian syndrome
Dichlorethylene	Wilson disease
Ethionine	**Surgical Procedures**
Ethyl bromide	Biliopancreatic diversion
Estrogens	Extensive small bowel resection
Glucocorticoids	Gastric bypass
Highly active antiretroviral	Jejunoileal bypass
therapy	**Miscellaneous Conditions**
Hydrazine	Industrial exposure to petrochemicals
Hypoglycin	Inflammatory bowel disease
Orotate	Partial lipodystrophy
Perhexilene maleate	Jejunal diverticulosis with bacterial overgrowth
Safrole	Severe anemia
Tamoxifen	Total parenteral nutrition

*Tetracycline is cytotoxic by virtue of inhibiting mitochondrial β-oxidation.

highlighting the importance of intra-abdominal or visceral fat as a predictor of fatty liver.[17]

NAFLD also is associated with type 2 diabetes mellitus and glucose intolerance, with or without superimposed obesity. Type 2 diabetes mellitus, hyperglycemia, or glucose intolerance has been described in 20% to 75% of adult patients with NASH and may increase the risk of NASH more than two-fold compared with nondiabetics. The association between type 2 diabetes mellitus and NAFLD appears strongest in morbidly obese patients.[16] NAFLD has been associated with insulin resistance and hyperinsulinemia, even in lean subjects with normal glucose tolerance.[18] Diabetes mellitus may be an independent predictor of advanced NAFLD, including cirrhosis and hepatocellular carcinoma.[19-21]

Hyperlipidemia is found in a substantial proportion of patients with NAFLD. Most patients with NAFLD have multiple risk factors, including obesity, type 2 diabetes mellitus, and hyperlipidemia, although some lack all recognized risk factors. NAFLD has been associated with many drugs and toxins and metabolic, surgical, and genetic conditions (see Table 82–1) that have abnormal fat metabolism and mitochondrial injury or dysfunction in common. NAFLD is now recognized as the hepatic component of the *metabolic syndrome*, which includes hyperlipidemia, glucose intolerance, obesity, and systemic hypertension. The risk and severity of NAFLD increase with the number of components of the metabolic syndrome.[18]

CLINICAL AND LABORATORY FEATURES

The clinical and laboratory features of NAFLD are summarized in Table 82–2. NAFLD usually is discovered incidentally because of elevated liver biochemical test levels or hepatomegaly noted during an evaluation for an unrelated medical condition. Most patients with NAFLD are asymptomatic, but some may describe vague right upper quadrant pain, fatigue, and malaise. Hepatomegaly has been described in up to 75% of patients with NAFLD but often is difficult to appreciate on physical examination because of obesity. Stigmata of chronic liver disease, such as splenomegaly, spider angiomata, and ascites, are rare, except in patients with NAFLD-associated cirrhosis.

Elevated liver biochemical test levels may be found in up to 50% of patients with simple steatosis and are present in approximately 80% of patients with advanced NAFLD. A slight (1.5- to 4-fold) elevation of serum aspartate aminotransferase (AST) or alanine aminotransferase (ALT) level, or both, is usual, and levels seldom exceed 10 times the upper limit of normal. The serum ALT level usually is greater than the AST level, in contrast with the pattern of alcoholic hepatitis, in which the AST is at least two-fold higher than the ALT (see Chapter 81). The alkaline phosphatase and gamma glutamyl transpeptidase (GGTP) levels may be elevated, but the serum bilirubin level, prothrombin time, and serum albumin level typically are normal, except in patients with NAFLD-associated cirrhosis. Up to one

Table 82–2 Clinical and Laboratory Features of Nonalcoholic Fatty Liver Disease

Clinical Features		
Symptoms	*Signs*	**Laboratory Features**
Common		
None (48-100% of patients)	Hepatomegaly	2- to 4-fold elevation of serum ALT and AST levels
		AST/ALT ratio less than 1 in most patients
		Serum alkaline phosphatase level is slightly elevated in one third of patients
		Normal serum bilirubin and serum albumin levels and prothrombin time
		Elevated serum ferritin level
Uncommon		
Vague right upper quadrant pain	Splenomegaly	Low-titer (less than 1:320) ANA
Fatigue	Spider angiomata	Elevated transferrin saturation
Malaise	Palmar erythema	*HFE* gene mutation (C282Y)
	Ascites	

ANA, antinuclear antibodies; ALT, alanine aminotransferase; AST, aspartate aminotransferase.

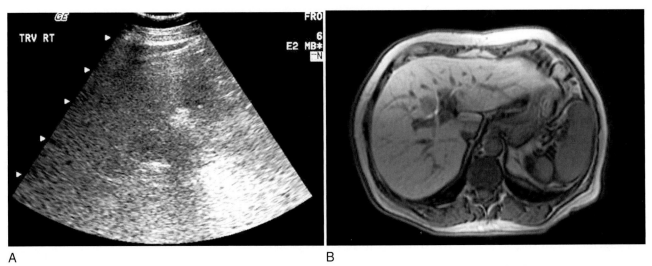

Figure 82–1 Imaging studies of fatty liver. *A*, Ultrasound demonstrating increased echogenicity. *B*, T1-weighted magnetic resonance image demonstrating a bright liver. (Courtesy of Mukesh Harisinghani, MD, Boston, MA.)

fourth of patients with NAFLD may have antinuclear antibodies (ANA) in low titers (less than 1:320).[22] Antimitochondrial antibodies (AMA) and antibody to hepatitis B surface antigen are not detected. Antibody to hepatitis C virus (anti-HCV) must be absent to implicate NAFLD as the sole cause of abnormal liver biochemical test levels; however, steatosis, often in association with visceral obesity, frequently accompanies HCV infection and may be associated with a more aggressive course.[23] Serum ceruloplasmin and α_1-antitrypsin levels are within normal limits. Serum and hepatic iron levels may be elevated in patients with NAFLD. In particular, the serum ferritin level may be elevated in 20% to 50% of patients with NAFLD and may be a marker of more advanced disease.[19,24] Nevertheless, the frequency of genetic hemochromatosis among patients with NAFLD is similar to that in the general population. Clinical and laboratory findings do not correlate with the histologic severity of NAFLD. The entire histologic spectrum of NAFLD, including cirrhosis, can be seen in patients with normal or near-normal serum aminotransferase levels.[21]

Imaging studies often are obtained during the evaluation of unexplained liver biochemical abnormalities or suspected NAFLD. Hepatic ultrasonography, the imaging modality employed most commonly, may reveal a "bright" liver of increased echogenicity, consistent with hepatic steatosis (Fig. 82–1). Fatty liver also can be documented by abdominal computed tomography (CT) scan (a fatty liver is lower in density than the spleen), and by magnetic resonance imaging (MRI), with which fat appears bright on T1-weighted imaging. A study that assessed the sensitivities of MRI, abdominal CT, and ultrasonography for distinguishing advanced NASH from simple steatosis showed that ultrasonography and CT had sensitivity rates of 100% and 93% for detecting hepatic fat involving greater than 33% of the liver, with positive predictive values of 62% and 76%, respectively.[25] No radiologic modality, however, was able to distinguish simple steatosis from more advanced forms of NAFLD. Imaging studies such as ultrasonography may support the diagnosis of NAFLD but cannot predict the severity of disease and cannot replace liver biopsy for establishing the diagnosis with certainty.

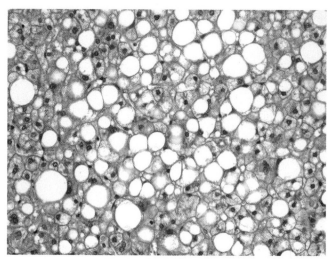

Figure 82–2 Histologic features of simple steatosis (fatty liver). The characteristic feature is diffuse macrovesicular steatosis. Mild lymphocytic, neutrophilic, or mixed inflammatory infiltrates also may be observed, and glycogenated nuclei are common. Hematoxylin-eosin stain. (Courtesy of Gregory Y. Lauwers, MD, Boston, MA.)

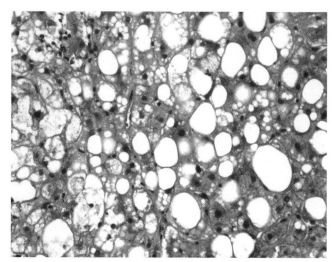

Figure 82–3 Histologic features of nonalcoholic steatohepatitis. Diffuse or perivenular macrovesicular steatosis is present in all cases. Lobular inflammation may consist of lymphocytes, other mononuclear cells, and neutrophils. Hepatocyte ballooning and necrosis of varying degrees are hallmark features. Glycogenated nuclei may be present. Mallory bodies, which may be small, sparse, and inconspicuous, are seen frequently. Pericellular, perisinusoidal, and periportal fibrosis may be present. Hematoxylin-eosin stain. (Courtesy of Gregory Y. Lauwers, MD, Boston, MA.)

HISTOPATHOLOGIC FEATURES

The major histologic features of NAFLD resemble those of alcohol-induced liver disease and include steatosis (fatty liver), steatohepatitis (fatty liver plus parenchymal inflammation with or without accompanying focal necrosis), and varying degrees of fibrosis, including cirrhosis (see Chapter 81). Steatosis is predominantly macrovesicular and usually is distributed diffusely throughout the liver lobule, although prominent microvesicular steatosis and zone 3 (perivenular) steatosis have been reported occasionally (Fig. 82–2). Mild lymphocytic, neutrophilic, or mixed inflammatory infiltrates also may be observed, and glycogenated nuclei are common.

NASH, which is an advanced form of NAFLD, is indistinguishable histologically from alcoholic hepatitis (Fig. 82–3 and Table 82–3). Strict histologic criteria for NASH have not yet been defined. Steatosis is present in all cases and can affect the hepatic lobules either diffusely or primarily in the central zones. The degree of steatosis may correlate with the patient's BMI and generally is more severe in NASH than in alcoholic hepatitis.[26] Lobular inflammation is a hallmark feature of NASH and is characterized by infiltration of lymphocytes, other mononuclear cells, and polymorphonuclear neutrophils. The intensity of the inflammation varies with the severity of steatohepatitis and may be milder in NASH than in alcoholic hepatitis.[6] Glycogenated nuclei may be present. Hepatocyte ballooning and hepatocyte necrosis of varying degrees often are present and may portend a worse prognosis.[27,28] Mallory bodies, which may be small, sparse, and inconspicuous, are seen frequently. Mild stainable iron may be present in up to one half of the patients. Pericellular, perisinusoidal, and periportal fibrosis has been described in 37% to 84% of patients with NASH. The extent of fibrosis varies considerably, ranging

Table 82–3	Histologic Features of Nonalcoholic Steatohepatitis

Features Present in All or Most Cases
Macrovesicular steatosis
  Diffuse or centrilobular steatosis; degree may correlate with BMI
Parenchymal inflammation
  Lymphocytes, polymorphonuclear neutrophils, other mononuclear cells
Hepatocyte necrosis
Ballooning hepatocyte degeneration
Features Observed with Varying Frequencies
Perivenular, perisinusoidal, or periportal fibrosis (37%-84%), moderate to severe in 15%-50%; most prevalent in zone 3 (perivenular)
Cirrhosis (7%-16% on index biopsy specimen)
Mallory bodies
Glycogenated nuclei
Lipogranulomas
Stainable hepatic iron

BMI, body mass index.

from delicate strands surrounding small veins or groups of cells to densely fibrotic septa with distortion of the hepatic architecture. Perisinusoidal fibrosis is most common, especially in adults, is initially mild, and predominates in zone 3 around the terminal hepatic veins.[6] Cirrhosis is found on initial biopsy in 7% to 16% of patients with NAFLD and abnormal liver biochemical test levels.[16,19] The risk of cirrhosis in the setting of NAFLD may be greatest in morbidly obese patients. In NAFLD-associated cirrhosis, the typical histologic features of NAFLD may be minimal or absent, potentially leading to the misdiagnosis of cryptogenic cirrhosis.

PATHOGENESIS

The pathogenesis of NAFLD is poorly understood, in part because of a lack of suitable animal models that mimic human NAFLD. In light of the variety of conditions that have been associated with NAFLD, it is not surprising that no common pathogenic mechanism has been identified. The prevailing theory is the "two-hit hypothesis," first proposed by Day and James in 1998.[29] This hypothesis states that dysregulation of fatty acid metabolism leads to steatosis, which is the first hepatic insult in NAFLD. Steatosis is associated with several cellular adaptations and altered signaling pathways, which render hepatocytes vulnerable to a "second hit." The second insult may be one or more environmental or genetic perturbations, which cause hepatocyte necrosis and inflammation and activate the fibrogenic cascade, thereby leading to fibrosis and cirrhosis in a minority of patients with NAFLD.

Hepatic steatosis is the hallmark histologic feature of NAFLD. Normally, free fatty acids (FFAs) are supplied to the liver through gut absorption (in the form of chylomicron remnants) or from lipolysis of adipose tissue, where FFAs are stored as triglycerides. In the liver, FFAs are oxidized by mitochondria, esterified into triglycerides, synthesized into phospholipids and cholesteryl esters, and secreted from the liver as very-low-density lipoproteins (VLDLs). Under normal circumstances, fatty acid metabolism is under tight regulatory control by catecholamines, glucagon, growth hormone, and insulin (see Chapter 69). Hepatic triglyceride accumulation occurs when fatty acid metabolism shifts to favor net lipogenesis, rather than lipolysis. This shift occurs when the amount of FFA supplied to the liver from the intestine or adipose tissue exceeds the amount needed for mitochondrial oxidation, phospholipid synthesis, and synthesis of cholesteryl esters. Triglycerides also accumulate in the liver when synthesis of lipoprotein decreases or export of lipids from the liver is impeded.

Current evidence points to insulin resistance and hyperinsulinemia as the primary pathogenic factors in steatosis in most patients with NAFLD. Strong laboratory and clinical evidence supports the association of insulin resistance and hyperinsulinemia with NAFLD, even in lean patients without obvious glucose intolerance.[30-32] Diabetes and obesity are associated with increased amounts of FFA in plasma, due in part to abnormal release of FFA by insulin-resistant adipocytes. Excess FFAs contribute to insulin resistance by down-regulating insulin receptor substrate-1 (IRS-1) signaling.[33] Insulin resistance and hyperinsulinemia cause steatosis by means of a number of aberrant mechanisms of FFA disposal. In the liver, insulin stimulates fatty acid synthesis, down-regulates mitochondrial β-oxidation of FFA in the liver, blocks the secretion of triglycerides from hepatocytes by increasing intracellular degradation of VLDL and apolipoprotein B-100 (apoB-100), and blocks exocytosis of VLDL-containing vesicles.[34-36] Also, patients with NASH have impaired hepatic synthesis of apoB-100, which also may contribute to hepatic triglyceride accumulation.[37]

Insulin resistance in NAFLD may be potentiated by aberrant levels or function of several important peptide mediators secreted by adipocytes, including tumor necrosis factor-α (TNF-α), leptin, and adiponectin. In noninflammatory states, TNF-α is derived from adipose tissue, and plasma levels of TNF-α correlate with body fat mass.[3] TNF-α interferes with insulin signaling by down-regulating IRS-1 signaling by means of serine phosphorylation, thereby contributing to the development of insulin resistance in obesity. Elevated TNF-α levels have been demonstrated in several studies of NAFLD,[38,39] although the relative contribution of TNF-α to insulin resistance in NAFLD is not clear.

Adiponectin is secreted by adipocytes in inverse proportion to BMI and is a potent inhibitor of TNF-α. Serum adiponectin levels are reduced in obesity, insulin resistance, diabetes mellitus, and the metabolic syndrome.[40] Delivery of recombinant adiponectin to mice fed a high-fat, alcohol-containing diet and to genetically obese (ob/ob) mice dramatically alleviates hepatomegaly, steatosis, inflammation, and elevated liver biochemical test levels in both murine populations.[41] These therapeutic effects result in part from the ability of adiponectin to enhance hepatic fatty acid oxidation while decreasing fatty acid synthesis. Furthermore, adiponectin treatment suppresses hepatic and plasma concentrations of TNF-α. One study reported an inverse relationship between serum adiponectin levels and the degree of steatosis and hepatocyte injury in humans with NAFLD, independent of insulin resistance.[38] Further studies are needed to determine whether low adiponectin levels in NAFLD are a result of elevated TNF-α levels or have a primary pathogenic role in the development of steatosis and progression of steatohepatitis.

Leptin is a satiety hormone, derived from adipocytes, that controls food intake and energy regulation. Leptin is intimately involved with insulin signaling and regulation of glucose metabolism in peripheral tissues and may play an important role in regulating the partitioning of fat between mitochondrial β-oxidation and triglyceride synthesis in the liver.[42] Severe steatosis and steatohepatitis develop in leptin-deficient (ob/ob) mice. Obesity in humans is associated with relative leptin resistance and high leptin levels, which may contribute to the genesis of steatosis by a negative impact on insulin signaling or may be a consequence of the chronic hyperinsulinemia associated with obesity. Several studies have examined the relationship between serum leptin levels and NAFLD, with conflicting results.[43-45] One study has suggested that serum leptin levels in patients with NASH correlate with the severity of hepatic steatosis independent of BMI but not with the degree of hepatic inflammation or fibrosis.[43] At present, the contribution of leptin to the pathogenesis of NAFLD is unclear.

Although it is clear that insulin resistance and hyperinsulinemia are pivotal to the development of steatosis, consensus is lacking on the subsequent insults that cause steatosis to progress to steatohepatitis and fibrosis in some patients. Similarities in the histologic features and natural history of alcoholic liver disease and NAFLD suggest that common mechanisms may be involved in the pathogenesis of these disorders. Chronic oxidative stress is believed to be central to the pathogenesis of alcohol-related liver damage. Processes that increase the production of oxidants in the liver during chronic alcohol exposure include the metabolism of ethanol to its reactive intermediate acetaldehyde; induction of microsomal ethanol-oxidizing enzymes, such as cytochrome P450 IIE1 (CYP2E1), which generates reactive oxygen species (ROS) that can peroxidize cellular membranes, thereby causing cellular injury[46]; inhibition of mitochondrial electron transport chain activity; and depletion of mitochondrial glutathione[47] (see Chapter 81). Activation of microsomal enzymes, including CYP2E1, in patients with NAFLD[48,49] and mitochondrial production of ROS in murine models of NAFLD[50,51] suggest that chronic oxidative stress and lipid peroxidation also may be central to the pathogenesis of NAFLD.

Increased levels of FFAs can be directly toxic to hepatocytes through a number of mechanisms. An increased FFA concentration leads to lysosomal destabilization and stimulation of TNF-α.[52] FFAs also up-regulate cytochrome P450 isoenzymes, leading to enhanced generation of ROS and lipid peroxidation.[53] An increased intracellular FFA concentration can lead to sustained up-regulation of peroxisomal proliferator–activated receptor-α (PPAR-α), which promotes fatty acid oxidation and disposal but also may increase oxidative stress through the production of dicarboxylic acid derivatives; PPAR-α also may predispose affected persons to carcinogenesis.[54] FFAs can be directly toxic to cellular membranes, lead to the formation of toxic fatty acid ethyl ethers, and cause overall disruption of mitochondrial function, thereby overwhelming the overlapping protective mechanisms designed to combat FFA hepatotoxicity.[3]

Endotoxin and endotoxin-mediated cytokine release are suspected in the pathogenesis of alcoholic steatohepatitis, in which increased serum levels of bacterial endotoxin and lipopolysaccharide (LPS) stimulate hepatic production of TNF-α, interleukin (IL)-6, and IL-8 and activate an inflammatory response that leads to hepatic necrosis.[47] Bacterial endotoxin also may contribute to the development of NAFLD in some circumstances. Portal endotoxemia was believed to contribute to NASH and hepatic failure associated with surgical jejunoileal bypass (performed in the past to treat obesity), the risk of which was reduced with antibiotics. Yang and colleagues have demonstrated that ob/ob mice with steatosis are highly vulnerable to endotoxin-induced hepatocyte damage, and NASH rapidly develops in these animals after exposure to low doses of bacterial LPS.[55] In addition, Zucker diabetic (fa/fa) rats and ob/ob mice demonstrate decreased Kupffer cell function, which may increase the vulnerability of steatotic hepatocytes to TNF-α–mediated liver damage.[56] The roles of bacterial endotoxins and Kupffer cell function in human NAFLD have not been established, however.

A growing body of evidence suggests that mitochondrial changes and altered hepatic energy homeostasis may play roles in the pathogenesis of NAFLD. Studies have shown a decrease in the activity of mitochondrial respiratory chain complexes in steatotic livers, with a concomitant increase in mitochondrial ROS formation; these changes correlate with serum TNF-α levels, insulin resistance, and BMI.[57,58] Ob/ob mice have increased levels of uncoupling protein, UCP-2, an inner mitochondrial membrane protein that mediates proton leak, uncouples adenosine triphosphate (ATP) synthesis, regulates ROS production, and may render fatty hepatocytes vulnerable

to metabolic stressors[50]; however, the role of UCP-2 in NAFLD in humans is unknown. Studies have shown that mice and humans with NAFLD have diminished capacity for replenishing ATP stores after ATP depletion.[59,60] Mitochondrial structural defects may be one cause of reduced ATP stores. Megamitochondria and crystalline mitochondrial inclusions have been identified in patients with NAFLD and may represent an adaptive process to oxidative stress or secondary injury.[61] Limited data in patients with NASH suggest differential expression of several genes important for proper mitochondrial functioning, including genes involved in ROS scavenging, glucose metabolism, and fatty acid metabolism.[62] In addition, mitochondrial DNA damage similar to that found in alcoholic liver disease and Wilson disease also may contribute to the development of NASH.[63] Further animal and human studies are needed to determine whether mitochondrial dysfunction and ATP depletion are causes or consequences of NAFLD.

Fibrosis is a frequent histologic finding in advanced NAFLD but has not been well studied in this disease. Hepatic fibrosis results from activation and proliferation of hepatic stellate cells in the subendothelial space of Disse, with subsequent secretion of extracellular matrix components, including collagen types I and III. Factors proposed to initiate and perpetuate the fibrogenic process in stellate cells include inflammatory cytokines, angiotensin, alterations in the extracellular matrix, growth factors, and oxidative stress. In NAFLD, lipid peroxidation products may enhance hepatic production of transforming growth factor-β (TGF-β), which activates stellate cells.[64] Endothelial cells, leukocytes, and Kupffer cells may stimulate the stellate cells to proliferate, possibly through the release of platelet-derived growth factor (PDGF), TGF-β, and other cytokines.[65] In addition, hyperinsulinemia and hyperglycemia associated with NAFLD may stimulate release of connective tissue growth factor (CTGF), an intermediate molecule involved in fibrogenesis.[66] Finally, animal data suggest that leptin may perpetuate fibrogenesis in NAFLD by stimulating Kupffer cells and sinusoidal endothelial cells to produce TGF-β.[67]

Research into the pathogenesis of NAFLD is proliferating at a rapid pace, but the picture is far from clear (Fig. 82–4). It is unlikely that one of the putative mechanisms discussed here explains the pathogenesis of NAFLD in all affected patients. More likely, NAFLD develops as a consequence of a "multi-hit" process. The first "hit" is steatosis induced primarily by insulin resistance and hyperinsulinemia. After steatosis develops, a number of factors, including lipid peroxidation, oxidative stress, cytokine alterations, mitochondrial dysfunction, and Kupffer cell activation, may incite an inflammatory response and fibrosis in some patients with genetic or environmental susceptibilities. The exact interplay between these and other factors remains to be elucidated, but understanding of the pathogenesis should be enhanced by the development and refinement of appropriate animal models, including the genetically obese, leptin-deficient ob/ob mouse and Zucker diabetic rats, in which steatosis develops; S-adenosylmethionine (SAM)-deficient mice, in which severe steatohepatitis develops[68]; and a high-fat-fed rat model in which insulin resistance,

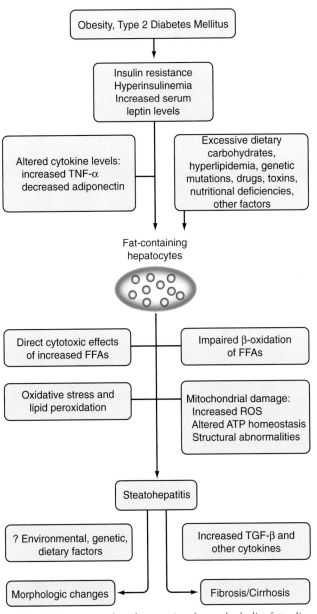

Figure 82–4 Proposed pathogenesis of nonalcoholic fatty liver disease (NAFLD). NAFLD is believed to occur as a result of a multi-hit process. Insulin resistance and hyperinsulinemia are present in many patients with NAFLD and, possibly in association with other metabolic or genetic abnormalities and altered cytokine levels, may lead to hepatic steatosis. Hepatocellular injury occurs in a minority of patients with fatty liver, probably as a result of multiple overlapping insults. Free fatty acids (FFAs), uncompensated oxidative stress, lipid peroxidation, cytokine dysregulation, mitochondrial dysfunction, and other environmental and genetic factors may contribute to the development of hepatocellular injury and fibrosis in susceptible persons. ATP, adenosine triphosphate; ROS, reactive oxygen species; TNF-α, tumor necrosis factor-α; TGF-β, transforming growth factor-β.

elevated serum TNF-α levels, increased oxidative stress, mitochondrial lesions, and early fibrosis develop.[69]

NATURAL HISTORY

The natural history of NAFLD is largely unknown, because no prospective, longitudinal studies with histo-

logic follow-up have been conducted in patients with NAFLD. The available data from retrospective studies suggest that NAFLD is a benign disease in most patients. It is clear that the prognosis for steatosis in the absence of hepatocyte necrosis and fibrosis is favorable, with little potential for histologic or clinical progression. In some patients, however, NAFLD can lead to cirrhosis, liver failure, or hepatocellular carcinoma. Through 2005, five retrospective studies have been published and have included a total of 74 patients with NAFLD and paired liver biopsy specimens, with follow-up periods ranging from 1 to 15 years.[28,70-73] Histologic progression of liver disease was documented in 32% to 50% of the patients, with development of cirrhosis in up to 20%. Histologic progression did not signal clinical deterioration in most cases, and no clinical or laboratory data predicted the course of liver disease. These limited data suggest that NAFLD is an indolent condition, with few clinical sequelae in most patients, but can progress to irreversible, clinically important liver disease over a relatively short period of time.

This conclusion is supported by data from a study of 132 patients with NAFLD evaluated over an 18-year period. The study compared outcomes based on the degree of injury on an index liver biopsy specimen.[74] Each biopsy specimen was assigned to a histologic subgroup, types 1 to 4, which represented progressive severity in steatosis, inflammation, hepatocyte necrosis, and fibrosis. Cirrhosis and liver-related deaths were more common (25% and 11%, respectively) in patients with NAFLD types 3 and 4 (steatosis, inflammation, and necrosis, with or without fibrosis) than in patients with NAFLD types 1 and 2 (steatosis without necrosis), although the mortality difference failed to reach statistical significance. In addition, the liver-related mortality rate of 11% among patients with NAFLD types 3 and 4 was higher than the age-adjusted death rate from chronic liver disease/cirrhosis in the general U.S. population (9.5 per 100,000 per year). These data suggest that the risk of liver-related complications in NAFLD correlates, at least to some extent, with the degree of hepatocellular injury and fibrosis found on an index liver biopsy specimen.

NAFLD and alcoholic hepatitis are identical histologically but differ substantially in clinical outcomes. The 5-year survival rate of patients with alcoholic hepatitis is 50% to 75%, because of the large proportion of patients (greater than 50%) in whom cirrhosis and its complications develop. A study has shown that the long-term survival of patients with NASH is significantly better than the long-term survival of patients with alcoholic hepatitis.[26] In the minority of patients in whom NAFLD-associated cirrhosis develops, however, the outcome may be similar to that for other causes of cirrhosis. NAFLD probably is the cause of most cases of cryptogenic cirrhosis[75] and may be associated with the development of hepatocellular carcinoma.[20,76] One study showed that the 5- to 10-year outcome of NAFLD-associated cirrhosis was similar to that for HCV-associated cirrhosis, although hepatocellular carcinoma was less common in the patients with NAFLD.[77]

Large prospective studies are needed to define the natural history of NAFLD, but emerging evidence con-

Table 82–4 Features of Advanced Nonalcoholic Fatty Liver Disease

Clinical Features
Older age (>50 years)
Obesity
Diabetes mellitus/insulin resistance
Hypertension
Laboratory Features
AST/ALT ratio >1
Serum ALT level > twice the upper limit of normal
Serum triglyceride levels >1.7 mmol/L
Histologic Features
Severe steatosis
Necroinflammatory activity (hepatocyte ballooning, necrosis)
Stainable iron

ALT, alanine aminotransferase; AST, aspartate aminotransferase.

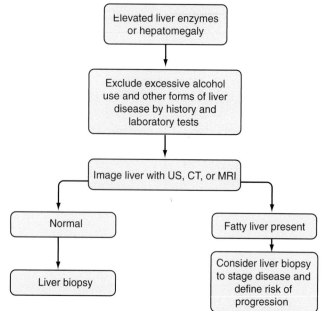

Figure 82–5 Diagnostic approach to patients with suspected non-alcoholic fatty liver disease (NAFLD). The diagnosis of NAFLD is based on clinical and histologic criteria. Most patients are evaluated because of elevated serum aminotransferase levels or hepatomegaly. The diagnosis of NAFLD should be considered when excessive alcohol use is absent and laboratory test results exclude other causes of liver disease. Radiologic studies may demonstrate fatty liver. Liver biopsy is the standard means of diagnosis and the only test that can reliably differentiate simple steatosis from advanced NAFLD (nonalcoholic steatohepatitis). CT, computed tomography; MRI, magnetic resonance imaging; US, ultrasonography.

firms that NAFLD can be progressive and associated with significant morbidity and mortality in some patients. The risks of liver-related morbidity and mortality are greatest in those with evidence of advanced NAFLD (steatohepatitis with necrosis and fibrosis) on the initial liver biopsy specimen.[74] If clinical and biochemical risk factors for progressive disease can be established, a subset of patients can be identified in whom a liver biopsy will have the greatest prognostic and therapeutic value. Several potential risk factors have been identified in different populations (Table 82–4). Women are overrepresented in studies of NAFLD, but it is unclear if gender is an independent risk factor for advanced disease. Older age, obesity, diabetes mellitus, and an AST/ALT ratio greater than 1 were demonstrated in one study to be significant predictors of severe fibrosis (bridging/cirrhosis) in patients with NAFLD.[19] In another study of overweight patients with abnormalities on liver biochemical tests, liver fibrosis was independently associated with hepatic necroinflammatory activity, BMI greater than 28 kg/m², age older than 50 years, serum triglyceride level higher than 1.7 mmol/L, and serum ALT more than twice normal.[28] In another study of morbidly obese patients referred for bariatric surgery, systemic hypertension, an elevated serum ALT level, and a high insulin resistance index were highly predictive of advanced NAFLD.[16] As noted previously, however, the full spectrum of liver damage, including cirrhosis, has been documented in nonobese patients with near-normal liver biochemical test results.

DIAGNOSIS

Establishing a definitive diagnosis of NAFLD requires both clinical and histologic data (Fig. 82–5). Most patients with NAFLD are evaluated because of chronically elevated liver biochemical test levels, with or without hepatomegaly. The combination of the patient's history, physical examination, blood test results, and radiologic findings is useful for excluding other causes of liver disease. Laboratory testing should include liver biochemical tests (see Chapter 70), complete blood count, prothrombin time, anti-HCV, hepatitis B surface antigen, iron indices, ceruloplasmin in persons younger than 40

years of age, α_1-antitrypsin, and AMA. Imaging studies may support the diagnosis (see earlier), but the absence of characteristic findings does not preclude a diagnosis of NAFLD. To establish a diagnosis of NAFLD, alcoholic liver disease must be excluded. Clinical and histologic data unreliably differentiate NAFLD from alcoholic liver disease in ambulatory patients.[26] Therefore, the diagnosis of NAFLD should be entertained only in the absence of significant alcohol use (that is, consumption of less than 20 to 40 g of alcohol per day in most clinical studies).

The Role of Liver Biopsy

The role of liver biopsy in establishing the diagnosis of NAFLD has been debated. Many practitioners consider NAFLD a diagnosis of exclusion, when clinical and laboratory examinations fail to reveal another cause of chronic liver disease. The diagnosis of NAFLD is also suggested when an imaging study provides evidence of fatty liver. Most patients with NAFLD do not undergo a liver biopsy, largely because the results usually will not affect management (therapeutic options are limited). The argument for liver biopsy in all patients with presumed NAFLD is centered on several lines of evidence: The correlation among clinical, laboratory, and histologic findings in NAFLD is poor; liver biopsy is the only diagnostic test that can reliably quantify hepatic steatosis, necrosis, and fibrosis; and the histologic stage of NAFLD is the best prognostic indicator. In addition, understanding of the natural history and treatment of NAFLD has been hampered by the lack of histologic data in most clinical studies. The most prudent approach may be to select patients for whom liver biopsy might influence management. Patients with obesity, long-standing or persistent liver biochemical test abnormalities (even with good glycemic control and after weight loss), older age, multiple components of the metabolic syndrome, an AST/ALT ratio greater than 1, markedly elevated liver biochemical test levels, symptoms and signs of portal hypertension, or evidence of fibrosis on an imaging study are more likely to have advanced disease. The results of a liver biopsy in these patients might lead to a more aggressive treatment strategy, participation in clinical trials, or screening for hepatocellular carcinoma in the setting of cirrhosis.

TREATMENT

The optimal therapy for NAFLD has not been established. To date, no large, randomized treatment trials demonstrating resolution of steatosis, inflammation, and fibrosis have been conducted in patients with NAFLD. Small numbers, varying inclusion criteria, and varying end points have limited the clinical impact of published studies.

Historically, the treatment of NAFLD has consisted of weight loss, removal of offending drugs and toxins, and control of associated metabolic disorders, including diabetes mellitus and hyperlipidemia. Several case reports and small studies of diet and exercise have shown improvements in biochemical, ultrasonographic, and in some cases, histologic abnormalities in children and adults with NASH.[78-80] One case report showed improvements in liver biochemical test levels and remission of fibrosis in a few patients who achieved weight loss with orlistat, a reversible inhibitor of gastric and pancreatic lipases.[81]

Unfortunately, the therapeutic benefit of weight loss achieved with diet, medicinal aids, exercise, or surgery has not been examined in randomized, prospective studies with firm histologic end points. Until such studies are performed, it is reasonable to recommend moderate weight loss to overweight patients with NAFLD, although weight loss is seldom achieved. Rapid weight loss can exacerbate steatohepatitis in morbidly obese patients, especially after bariatric surgery[82]; therefore, the rate of weight loss and serial liver biochemical test results should be monitored carefully in patients on a weight reduction regimen. New therapeutic methods should capitalize on today's improved understanding of the pathogenesis of NAFLD (Table 82–5).

Antioxidants

Medications that minimize oxidative stress may prove useful. Vitamin E, an inexpensive yet potent antioxidant, has been examined as an agent for treatment of NAFLD in several small pediatric and adult studies, with varying results.[80,83-85] In all studies, vitamin E was well tolerated, and most studies showed modest improvements in serum

Table 82–5   Potential Therapies for Nonalcoholic Fatty Liver Disease

Avoidance of toxins
  Discontinue potentially offending medications/toxins
  Minimize alcohol intake
Exercise and diet
  Moderate, sustained exercise and weight loss in overweight patients
  Effects of specific diets are not known
Bariatric surgery for morbid obesity
Antidiabetic/insulin-sensitizing agents
  Metformin
  Thiazolidinediones
Antihyperlipidemic agents
  Gemfibrizol
  Statins
Antioxidants
  Vitamin E
  Betaine
  Superoxide dismutase
  N-acetylcysteine
Iron reduction by phlebotomy
Inflammatory mediators
  Agents that raise adiponectin levels
  Agents that modulate TNF-α activity
  Agents that modulate leptin activity
Agents that increase mitochondrial ATP stores and/or activity

ATP, adenosine triphosphate; TNF-α, tumor necrosis factor-α.

aminotransferase levels, ultrasonographic appearance of the liver, and infrequently, histologic findings. Randomized controlled studies with histologic inclusion criteria and end points are needed, however, to determine if vitamin E leads to histologic improvement in NAFLD.

Betaine, a metabolite of choline that raises SAM levels and decreases cellular oxidative damage, has shown promise in a small pilot study as a therapeutic agent for NASH.[86] N-acetylcysteine, superoxide dismutase (SOD), and PPAR-α agonists such as ragaglitazar also may hold therapeutic promise,[51,87,88] although clinical studies in humans are lacking.

Insulin-Sensitizing Agents

The association between hyperinsulinemic insulin resistance and NAFLD provides a logical target for treatment. Metformin, a biguanide that reduces hyperinsulinemia and improves hepatic insulin sensitivity, reduces hepatomegaly and hepatic steatosis in ob/ob mice,[89] but results in human studies have been less impressive.[90,91] Thiazolidinediones (TZDs), potent PPAR-γ agonists, also are being investigated as possible agents for the treatment of NAFLD. PPAR-γ is a nuclear receptor expressed in adipose tissue, muscle, and liver. In adipocytes, PPAR-γ promotes cell differentiation and decreases lipolysis and FFA release. TZDs improve insulin sensitivity and hyperinsulinemia by increasing glucose disposal in muscle and decreasing hepatic glucose output. Treatment with troglitazone, a first-generation TZD, was associated with biochemical and histologic improvements in patients with NASH,[92] but troglitazone subsequently was withdrawn from the market because of rare but serious hepatotoxicity. Rosiglitazone and pioglitazone, TZDs with low rates of hepatotoxicity, have been investigated in separate 48-week, single-arm treatment trials in patients with histologically proved NASH.[93,94] In both studies, treatment was well tolerated and was associated with improved insulin sensitivity, normalization of values on liver biochemical testing, and histologic improvement in most patients. A drawback of both TZDs, however, was substantial weight gain (4.0% to 7.3%) and increased total body adiposity. In addition, the durability of biochemical and histologic improvements after completion of therapy was not examined in either study. TZDs must be assessed in large, placebo-controlled trials before they can be recommended for routine use in patients with NAFLD.

Iron Reduction

High serum iron and ferritin levels have been identified in some patients with NAFLD, most of whom do not have genetic hemochromatosis or hepatic iron overload. Most investigators believe that increased serum iron indices are a by-product of hepatic inflammation, rather than a contributor to the pathogenesis of NAFLD, but one study has suggested that iron depletion may have a therapeutic role in NAFLD by decreasing plasma insulin, glucose, and serum amintransferase levels.[95] The relationship between iron and insulin is complex, but the insulin-sparing effect of iron depletion may be the result of enhanced skeletal muscle glucose transport and metabolism and increased hepatic extraction and metabolism of insulin.[96] The primary limitation of this study was the lack of histologic inclusion criteria and end points, but the results are intriguing and merit further investigation.

Antihyperlipidemic and Cytoprotective Agents

The usefulness of lipid-lowering and cytoprotective drugs for treatment of NAFLD has been assessed in a few small trials, with varying results. Treatment with gemfibrozil was associated with biochemical improvement in 74% of patients in the treatment group, compared with 30% of control subjects (no treatment), but histologic features were not assessed.[97] Treatment of NASH with atorvastatin, a 3-hydroxy-3-methylglutaryl–coenzyme A (HMG-CoA) reductase inhibitor, showed promise in a small pilot study,[98] but statins have not been assessed in a large clinical trial. Ursodeoxycholic acid, a cytoprotective agent, showed promise in a pilot study of NASH but was not effective in a randomized placebo-controlled trial.[99] Future therapies for NAFLD might include agents that increase adiponectin levels, neutralize TNF-α, improve mitochondrial ATP homeostasis, or alter leptin levels. Assuredly, new therapeutic agents will be developed as the pathogenesis of NAFLD is elucidated further.

Liver Transplantation

Patients with NAFLD in whom end-stage liver disease develops should be evaluated for liver transplantation (see Chapter 92). The outcome of liver transplantation in these patients is good, although NAFLD can recur after liver transplantation.[100] The risk factors for recurrent or de novo NAFLD after liver transplantation probably are multifactorial and include hypertriglyceridemia, obesity, diabetes mellitus, and glucocorticoid therapy.

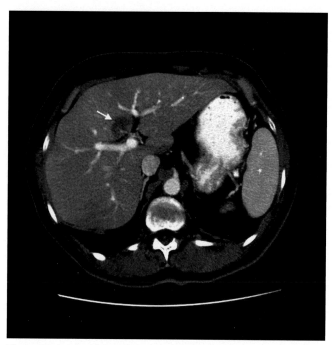

Figure 82–6 Focal fatty liver. Focal fatty liver *(arrow)* on computed tomography (CT) scan. The characteristic features are the nonspherical shape, absence of a mass effect, and CT attenuation values consistent with those of soft tissue. Ultrasound studies and magnetic resonance imaging also may confirm the diagnosis of focal fatty liver. (Courtesy of Mukesh Harisinghani, MD, Boston, MA.)

FOCAL FATTY LIVER

In contrast with NAFLD, which is a diffuse parenchymal process, focal fatty liver is a localized or patchy process that simulates a space-occupying lesion in the liver on imaging studies. This condition is recognized increasingly in adults and children as a result of the improved sensitivity of abdominal imaging. Focal fatty liver has characteristic patterns on CT: usually a nonspherical shape, absence of mass effect, and CT attenuation values consistent with those of soft tissue.[101] The density of focal fatty liver is close to that of water, unlike that of liver metastases, which have a density that is closer to that of hepatocytes. Ultrasonography and MRI can help confirm a diagnosis of focal fatty liver (Fig. 82–6). A presumptive diagnosis of focal fatty liver should not be made when a mass effect, areas of mixed hypo- and hyperechogenicity, an irregular shape, or a history of prior malignancy is present. In such cases, ultrasonographically guided fine-needle biopsy is recommended. No evidence exists to suggest that the pathogenesis of focal fatty liver is similar to that of NAFLD. In fact, the pathogenesis of focal fatty liver is uncertain and may involve altered venous blood flow to the liver, tissue hypoxia, and malabsorption of lipoproteins. Furthermore, in the absence of accompanying or background liver disease, the lesion often regresses. Therefore, no specific treatment is justified.

REFERENCES

1. Ludwig J, Viggiano T, McGill D, Ott B: Nonalcoholic steatohepatitis: Mayo Clinic experiences with a hitherto unnamed disease. Mayo Clin Proc 55:434, 1980.
2. Reid A: Nonalcoholic steatohepatitis. Gastroenterology 121: 710, 2001.
3. Neuschwander-Tetri B, Caldwell S: Nonalcoholic steatohepatitis: Summary of an AASLD single topic conference. Hepatology 37:1202, 2003.
4. Angulo P: Nonalcoholic fatty liver disease. N Engl J Med 346:1221, 2002.
5. Harrison S, Kadakia S, Lang K, Schenker S: Nonalcoholic steatohepatitis: What we know in the new millennium. Am J Gastroenterol 97:2714, 2002.
6. Zafrani E: Nonalcoholic fatty liver disease: An emerging pathological spectrum. Virchows Arch 444:3, 2004.
7. Bellentani S, Saccoccio G, Masutti F, et al. Prevalence of and risk factors for hepatic steatosis in Northern Italy. Ann Intern Med 132:112, 2000.
8. Ruhl C, Everhart J: Determinants of the association of overweight with elevated serum alanine aminotransferase activity in the United States. Gastroenterology 124:71, 2003.
9. Clark J, Brancati F, Diehl A: The prevalence and etiology of elevated aminotransferase levels in the United States. Am J Gastroenterol 98:960, 2003.
10. Roberts E: Nonalcoholic steatohepatitis in children. Curr Gastroenterol Rep 5:253, 2004.
11. Kemmer N, McKinney K, Vuaim S-Y, et al: High prevalence of NASH among Mexican American females with type II diabetes mellitus [abstract]. Gastroenterology 120:A117, 2001.
12. Schwimmer J, Deutsch R, Rauch JB, et al: Obesity, insulin resistance, and other clinicopathological correlates of pediatric nonalcoholic fatty liver disease. J Pediatr 143:500, 2003.
13. Caldwell S, Harris D, Patrie J, Hespenheide E: Is NASH underdiagnosed among African Americans? Am J Gastroenterol 97:1496, 2002.
14. Willner I, Waters B, Patil S, et al: Ninety patients with nonalcoholic steatohepatitis: Insulin resistance, familial tendency, and severity of disease. Am J Gastroenterol 96:2957, 2001.
15. Hsiao T, Chen J, Wang J: Insulin resistance and ferritin as major determinants of alcoholic fatty liver disease in apparently healthy obese patients. Int J Obes Relat Metab Disord 28:167, 2004.
16. Dixon J, Bhathal P, O'Brien P: Nonalcoholic fatty liver disease: Predictors of nonalcoholic steatohepatitis and liver fibrosis in the severely obese. Gastroenterology 121:91, 2001.
17. Stranges S, Dorn J, Muti P, et al: Body fat distribution, relative weight, and liver enzyme levels: A population-based study. Hepatology 39:754, 2004.
18. Marchesini G, Bugianesi E, Forlani G, et al: Nonalcoholic fatty liver, steatohepatitis, and the metabolic syndrome. Hepatology 37:917, 2003.
19. Angulo P, Keach J, Batts K, Lindor K: Independent predictors of liver fibrosis in patients with nonalcoholic steatohepatitis. Hepatology 30:1356, 1999.
20. El-Serag H, Tran T, Everhart J: Diabetes increases the risk of chronic liver disease and hepatocellular carcinoma. Gastroenterology 126:460, 2004.
21. Mofrad P, Contos M, Haque M, et al: Clinical and histologic spectrum of nonalcoholic fatty liver disease associated with normal ALT values. Hepatology 37:1286, 2003.
22. Adams L, Lindor K, Angulo P: The prevalence of autoantibodies and autoimmune hepatitis in patients with nonalcoholic fatty liver disease. Am J Gastroenterol 99:1316, 2004.
23. Lonardo A, Adinolfi L, Loria P, et al: Steatosis and hepatitis C virus: Mechanisms and significance for hepatic and extrahepatic disease. Gastroenterology 126:586, 2004.
24. Bugianesi E, Manzini P, D'Antico S, et al: Relative contribution of iron burden, HFE mutations, and insulin resistance to fibrosis in nonalcoholic fatty liver. Hepatology 39:179, 2004.
25. Saadeh S, Younossi Z, Remer E, et al: The utility of radiological imaging in nonalcoholic fatty liver disease. Gastroenterology 123:745, 2002.
26. Cortez-Pinto H, Baptista A, Camilo M, De Moura M: Nonalcoholic steatohepatitis—a long-term follow-up study: Comparison with alcoholic hepatitis in ambulatory and hospitalized patients. Dig Dis Sci 48:1909, 2003.
27. Gramlich T, Kleiner D, McCullough A, et al: Pathologic features associated with fibrosis in nonalcoholic fatty liver disease. Hum Pathol 35:196, 2004.
28. Ratziu V, Giral P, Charlotte F, et al: Liver fibrosis in overweight patients. Gastroenterology 118:1117, 2000.
29. Day C, James O: Steatohepatitis: A tale of two "hits"? [editorial]. Gastroenterology 114:842, 1998.
30. Chitturi S, Abeygunasekera S, Farrell G, et al: NASH and insulin resistance: Insulin hypersecretion and specific association with the insulin resistance syndrome. Hepatology 35:373, 2002.
31. Pagano G, Pacini G, Musso G, et al: Nonalcoholic steatohepatitis, insulin resistance, and metabolic syndrome: Further evidence of an etiologic association. Hepatology 35:367, 2002.
32. Sanyal A, Campbell-Sargent C, Mirshahi F, et al: Non-alcoholic steatohepatitis: Association of insulin resistance and mitochondrial abnormalities. Gastroenterology 120:1183, 2001.
33. Schmitz-Peiffer C: Signalling aspects of insulin resistance in skeletal muscle: Mechanisms induced by lipid oversupply. Cell Signal 12:583, 2000.
34. Boden G: Interaction between free fatty acids and glucose metabolism. Curr Opin Clin Nutr Metab Care 5:545, 2002.
35. Neuschwander-Tetri B: A resistance movement in NASH. Am J Gastroenterol 96:2813, 2001.
36. Angulo P, Lindor K: Insulin resistance and mitochondrial abnormalities in NASH: A cool look into a burning issue. Gastroenterology 120:1281, 2001.
37. Charlton M, Sreekumar R, Rasmussen D, et al: Apolipoprotein synthesis in nonalcoholic steatohepatitis. Hepatology 35:898, 2002.
38. Hui J, Hodge A, Farrell G, et al: Beyond insulin resistance in NASH: TNF-α or adiponectin? Hepatology 40:46, 2004.
39. Crespo J, Cayon A, Fernandez-Gil P, et al: Gene expression of tumor necrosis factor alpha and TNF-receptors, p55 and p75, in nonalcoholic steatohepatitis patients. Hepatology 34:1158, 2001.
40. Czaja M: Liver injury in the setting of steatosis: Crosstalk between adipokine and cytokine. Hepatology 40:19, 2004.
41. Xu A, Wang Y, Keshaw H, et al: The fat-derived hormone adiponectin alleviates alcoholic and nonalcoholic fatty liver diseases in mice. J Clin Invest 112:91, 2003.
42. Harrison S, Di Bisceglie A: Advances in the understanding and treatment of nonalcoholic fatty liver disease. Drugs 63:2379, 2003.
43. Chitturi S, Farrell G, Frost L, et al: Serum leptin in NASH correlates with hepatic steatosis but not fibrosis: A manifestation of lipotoxicity? Hepatology 36:403, 2002.
44. Uygun A, Kadayifci A, Yesilova Z, et al: Serum leptin levels in patients with nonalcoholic steatohepatitis. Am J Gastroenterol 95:3584, 2000.
45. Chalasani N, Crabb D, Cummings O, et al: Does leptin play a role in the pathogenesis of human nonalcoholic steatohepatitis? Am J Gastroenterol 98:2771, 2003.
46. Kessova I, Cederbaum AI: CYP2E1: Biochemistry, toxicology, regulation and function in ethanol-induced liver injury. Curr Mol Med 3:509, 2003.
47. Hoek J, Pastorino J: Ethanol, oxidative stress, and cytokine-induced liver injury. Alcohol 27:63, 2002.

48. Weltman M, Farrell G, Hall P, et al: Hepatic cytochrome P450 2E1 is increased in patients with nonalcoholic steatohepatitis. Hepatology 27:128, 1998.

49. Chalasani N, Gorski C, Asghar M, et al: Hepatic cytochrome P450 2E1 activity in nondiabetic patients with nonalcoholic steatohepatitis. Hepatology 37:544, 2003.

50. Yang S, Zhu H, Li Y, et al: Mitochondrial adaptations to obesity-related oxidant stress. Arch Biochem Biophys 378:259, 2000.

51. Laurent A, Nicco C, Van Nhieu J, et al: Pivotal role of superoxide anion and beneficial effect of antioxidant molecules in murine steatohepatitis. Hepatology 39:1277, 2004.

52. Feldstein A, Werneburg NW, Canbay A, et al: Free fatty acids promote hepatic lipotoxicity by stimulating TNF-α expression via a lysosomal pathway. Hepatology 40:185, 2004.

53. Leclercq I, Farrell G, Field J, et al: CYP2E1 and CYP4A as microsomal catalysts of lipid peroxides in murine nonalcoholic steatohepatitis. J Clin Invest 105:1067, 2000.

54. Yu S, Rao S, Reddy JK: Peroxisome proliferator-activated receptors, fatty acid oxidation, steatohepatitis and hepatocarcinogenesis. Curr Mol Med 3:561, 2003.

55. Yang S, Lin H, Diehl AM: Fatty liver vulnerability to endotoxin-induced damage despite NF-κB induction and inhibited caspase 3 activation. Am J Physiol Gastrointest Liver Physiol 281:G382, 2001.

56. Diehl A: Nonalcoholic fatty liver disease abnormalities in macrophage function and cytokines. Am J Physiol Gastrointest Liver Physiol 282:G1, 2002.

57. Pérez-Carreras M, Hoyo P, Martín M, et al: Defective hepatic mitochondrial respiratory chain in patients with nonalcoholic steatohepatitis. Hepatology 38:999, 2003.

58. Fromenty B, Robin M, Igoudjil A, et al: The ins and outs of mitochondrial dysfunction in NASH. Diabetes Metab 30:121, 2004.

59. Chavin K, Yang S, Lin H, et al: Obesity induces expression of uncoupling protein-2 in hepatocytes and promotes liver ATP depletion. J Biol Chem 274:5692, 1999.

60. Cortez-Pinto H, Chatham J, Chacko V, et al: Alterations in liver ATP homeostasis in human nonalcoholic steatohepatitis—a pilot study. JAMA 282:1659, 1999.

61. Le T, Caldwell S, Redick J, et al: The zonal distribution of megamitochondria with crystalline inclusions in nonalcoholic steatohepatitis. Hepatology 39:1423, 2004.

62. Sreekumar R, Rosado B, Rasmussen D, Charlton M: Hepatic gene expression in histologically progressive nonalcoholic steatohepatitis. Hepatology 38:244, 2003.

63. Jaeschke H, Gores G, Cederbaum A, et al: Mechanisms of hepatotoxicity. Toxicol Sci 65:166, 2002.

64. Pessayre D, Mansouri A, Fromenty B: Nonalcoholic steatosis and steatohepatitis V. Mitochondrial dysfunction in steatohepatitis. Am J Physiol Gastrointest Liver Physiol 282:G193, 2002.

65. Pinzani M, Rombouts K: Liver fibrosis: From the bench to clinical targets. Dig Liver Dis 36:231, 2004.

66. Paradis V, Perlemuter G, Bonvoust F, et al: High glucose and hyperinsulinemia stimulate connective tissue growth factor expression: A potential mechanism involved in progression to fibrosis in nonalcoholic steatohepatitis. Hepatology 34:738, 2001.

67. Saxena N, Ikeda K, Rockey DC, et al: Leptin in hepatic fibrosis: Evidence for increased collagen production in stellate cells and lean littermates of ob/ob mice. Hepatology 35:762, 2002.

68. Lu SC, Alvarez L, Huang Z-Z, et al: Methionine adenosyltransferase 1A knockout mice are predisposed to liver injury and exhibit increased expression of genes involved in proliferation. Proc Natl Acad Sci U S A 98:5560, 2001.

69. Lieber C, Leo M, Mak K, et al: Model of nonalcoholic steatohepatitis. Am J Clin Nutr 79:502, 2004.

70. Lee R: Nonalcoholic steatohepatitis: A study of 49 patients. Hum Pathol 20:594, 1989.

71. Bacon B, Farahvash M, Janney C, Neuschwander-Tetri B: Nonalcoholic steatohepatitis: An expanded clinical entity. Gastroenterology 107:1103, 1994.

72. Powell E, Cooksley W, Hanson R, et al: The natural history of nonalcoholic steatohepatitis: A follow-up study of forty-two patients for up to 21 years. Hepatology 11:74, 1990.

73. Harrison S, Torgerson S, Hayashi P: The natural history of nonalcoholic fatty liver disease: A clinical histopathological study. Am J Gastroenterol 98:2042, 2003.

74. Matteoni C, Younossi Z, Gramlich T, et al : Nonalcoholic fatty liver disease: A spectrum of clinical and pathological severity. Gastroenterology 116:1413, 1999.

75. Poonawala A, Nair S, Thuluvath P: Prevalence of obesity and diabetes in patients with cryptogenic cirrhosis: A case-control study. Hepatology 32:689, 2002.

76. Marrero J, Fontana R, Su G, et al: NAFLD may be a common underlying liver disease in patients with hepatocellular carcinoma in the United States. Hepatology 36:1349, 2002.

77. Hui J, Kench J, Chitturi S, et al: Long-term outcomes of cirrhosis in nonalcoholic steatohepatitis compared with hepatitis C. Hepatology 38:420, 2003.

78. Hickman I, Jonsson J, Prins J, et al: Modest weight loss and physical activity in overweight patients with chronic liver disease results in sustained improvements in alanine aminotransferase, fasting insulin, and quality of life. Gut 53:413, 2004.

79. Knobler H, Schattner A, Zhornicki T, et al: Fatty liver—an additional and treatable feature of the insulin resistance syndrome. Q J Med 92:87, 1999.

80. Kugelmas M, Hill D, Vivian B, et al: Cytokines and NASH: A pilot study of the effects of lifestyle modification and vitamin E. Hepatology 38:413, 2003.

81. Harrison SA, Ramrakhiani S, Brunt EM, et al: Orlistat in the treatment of NASH: A case series. Am J Gastroenterol 98:926, 2003.

82. Luyckx F, Lefebvre P, Scheen A: Nonalcoholic steatohepatitis: Association with obesity and insulin resistance, and influence of weight loss. Diabetes Metab 26:98, 2000.

83. Hasegawa T, Yoneda M, Nakamura K, et al: Plasma transforming growth factor-β1 and efficacy of alpha-tocopherol in patients with nonalcoholic steatohepatitis: A pilot study. Aliment Pharmacol Ther 15:1667, 2001.

84. Harrison S, Torgerson S, Hayashi P, et al: Vitamin E and vitamin C treatment improves fibrosis in patients with nonalcoholic steatohepatitis. Am J Gastroenterol 98:2485, 2003.

85. Lavine J: Vitamin E treatment of nonalcoholic steatohepatitis in children: A pilot study. J Pediatr 136:734, 2000.

86. Abdelmalek M, Angulo P, Jorgensen R, et al: Betaine, a promising new agent for patients with nonalcoholic steatohepatitis: Results of a pilot study. Am J Gastroenterol 96:2711, 2001.

87. Gulbahar O, Karasu Z, Ersoz G, et al: Treatment of nonalcoholic steatohepatitis with N-acetylcysteine [abstract]. Gastroenterology 118:A1444, 2000.

88. Ip E, Farrell G, Hall P, et al: Administration of the potent PPAR alpha agonist, Wy-14,643, reverses nutritional fibrosis and steatohepatitis in mice. Hepatology 39:1286, 2004.

89. Lin H, Yang S, Chuckaree C, et al: Metformin reverses fatty liver disease in obese, leptin-deficient mice. Nature Med 6:998, 2000.

90. Marchesini G, Brizi M, Bianchi G, et al: Metformin in nonalcoholic steatohepatitis. Lancet 358:893, 2001.

91. Nair S, Diehl AM, Wiseman M, et al: Metformin in the treatment of nonalcoholic steatohepatitis: A pilot open label trial. Aliment Pharmacol Ther 20:23, 2004.

92. Caldwell S, Hespenheide EE, Redick J, et al: A pilot study of a thiazolidinedione, troglitazone, in nonalcoholic steato-hepatitis. Am J Gastroenterol 96:519, 2001.

93. Neuschwander-Tetri B, Brunt E, Wehmeier K, et al: Improved nonalcoholic steatohepatitis after 48 weeks of treatment with the PPAR-γ ligand rosiglitazone. Hepatology 38:1008, 2003.

94. Promrat K, Lutchman G, Uwaifo G, et al: A pilot study of pioglitazone treatment for nonalcoholic steatohepatitis. Hepatology 39:188, 2004.

95. Facchini F, Hua N, Stoohs R: Effect of iron depletion in carbohydrate-intolerant patients with clinical evidence of nonalcoholic fatty liver disease. Gastroenterology 122:931, 2002.

96. Fernandez-Real J, Lopez-Bermejo A, Ricart W: Cross-talk be-tween iron metabolism and diabetes. Diabetes 51:2348, 2002.

97. Basaranoglu M, Acbay O, Sonsuz A: A controlled trial of gemfibrozil in the treatment of patients with nonalcoholic steatohepatitis [letter]. J Hepatol 31:384, 1999.

98. Kiyici M, Gulten M, Gurel S, et al: Ursodeoxycholic acid and atorvastatin in the treatment of nonalcoholic steatohepati-tis. Can J Gastroenterol 17:713, 2003.

99. Lindor K, Kowdley K, Heathcote E, et al:. Ursodeoxycholic acid for treatment of nonalcoholic steatohepatitis: Results of a randomized trial. Hepatology 39:770, 2004.

100. Contos M, Cales W, Sterling RK, et al: Development of non-alcoholic fatty liver disease after orthotopic liver transplan-tation for cryptogenic cirrhosis. Liver Transpl 7:363, 2001.

101. Siegelman E, Rosen MA: Imaging of hepatic steatosis. Semin Liver Dis 21:71, 2001.

CHAPTER

83 Liver Disease Caused by Drugs

Narci C. Teoh and Geoffrey C. Farrell

DEFINITIONS AND IMPORTANCE

Drugs are a relatively common cause of liver injury, which usually is defined by abnormalities on liver biochemical tests, particularly an increase in serum alanine aminotransferase (ALT), alkaline phosphatase, or bilirubin levels to more than twice the upper limit of normal. Drug-induced liver injury can be difficult to define in clinical practice because values of the biochemical tests used to detect liver injury also may be elevated as part of an *adaptive response* to drugs. Furthermore, the severity of drug-induced liver injury varies, ranging from minor nonspecific changes in hepatic structure and function to acute liver failure, cirrhosis, and liver cancer.

Use of the term *drug-induced liver disease* should be confined to cases in which the nature of liver injury has been characterized histologically. With the exception of aceta-

minophen, anticancer drugs, and some botanical or industrial hepatotoxins (see Chapter 84), most cases of drug-induced liver disease represent *adverse drug reactions* or *hepatic drug reactions*. These reactions are noxious, unintentional effects that occur at doses recommended for prophylaxis or therapy. With such reactions, the latent period is longer (typically 1 week to 3 to 6 months) than with toxicity caused by direct hepatotoxins (hours to a few days), and extrahepatic manifestations of drug hypersensitivity may be associated features.

Although drug-induced liver disease is a relatively uncommon cause of jaundice or acute hepatitis in the community, it is an important cause of more severe types of acute liver disease, particularly among older people (see "Epidemiology"). Among patients admitted to the hospital for drug-induced liver diseases, the overall mortality rate is approximately 10%.[1] The reported frequencies of individual hepatic drug reactions often may be underestimated because of the inadequacy of spontaneous (physician and pharmacist) reporting.[2,3] As determined using more reliable prospective and epidemiologic techniques, the frequency of most types of drug-induced liver disease is between 1 per 10,000 and 1 per 100,000 persons exposed.[4] Because these events clearly are rare and unpredictable responses to drug exposure, they often are termed *idiosyncratic drug reactions*. Their rarity blunts diagnostic acumen because most health care practitioners will see few if any cases and therefore will not have an appropriate level of clinical suspicion; this concern applies especially to remedies and herbal products used in complementary and alternative medicine (CAM), as discussed in Chapters 84 and 125. Another challenge is that hepatic drug reactions produce an array of clinical syndromes and pathologic conditions affecting the liver that mimic known hepatobiliary diseases. Furthermore, although individual agents (and some drug classes) typically produce a characteristic "signature syndrome," they also can be associated with other and sometimes multiple clinicopathologic syndromes.

Drug-induced liver injury is the most common reason for withdrawal of an approved drug from the market. The subject therefore has medicoeconomic, legal, and regulatory ramifications. Because of the low frequency of most types of idiosyncratic drug reactions involving the liver, serious hepatotoxicity usually is not detected until postmarketing surveillance is conducted. Historically, drugs that have developed a reputation for potential hepatotoxicity usually have been replaced by more acceptable alternatives. Recent examples include troglitazone, the prototypic thiazolidinedione, and bromfenac, a nonsteroidal anti-inflammatory drug (NSAID); both agents were withdrawn from the market because of several cases of fatal acute liver failure.

The burgeoning number of available conventional medicines and CAM preparations now includes hundreds of substances that can be cited as rare causes of drug-induced liver disease. This increasing number of potentially causative agents poses several challenges to clinicians,[5-7] including concern about what constitutes an adequate level of patient information at the time the drug is prescribed and the reliability of evidence linking an individual agent to a particular type of liver injury.[5-8] Another development is the appreciation that drug toxicity, in the context of complex medical situations, can interact with other causes of liver injury. Noteworthy examples of such situations are bone marrow transplantation; cancer chemotherapy; highly active antiretroviral therapy (HAART) for human immunodeficiency virus (HIV) infections and acquired immunodeficiency syndrome (AIDS); use of antituberculosis drugs in patients with chronic viral hepatitis; and nonalcoholic steatohepatitis (NASH) precipitated by tamoxifen and possibly other drugs in persons with the metabolic syndrome.

EPIDEMIOLOGY

Frequency or *risk*—the number of adverse reactions for a given number of persons exposed—is the best term for expressing how common a drug reaction is. Time-dependent terms such as *incidence* and *prevalence* are not appropriate for drug reactions, because the frequency is not related linearly to the duration of exposure. For most drug reactions, the onset occurs within a relatively short exposure time, or *latent period*, although some rarer types of chronic liver disease occur after many months or years of exposure to a drug. The frequency of drug-induced liver disease usually is based on the reported rate of drug reactions; such reports usually are a voluntary part of postmarketing surveillance and are submitted to pharmaceutical companies or adverse drug reaction monitoring bodies. In the United States, following Food and Drug Administration (FDA) approval, pharmaceutical companies are required to report serious adverse events (any incident resulting in death, a threat to life, hospitalization, or permanent disability). Surveillance becomes a more passive process once a drug is approved for marketing, and physicians and pharmacists are encouraged to file voluntary written reports through the MediWatch program. Similar systems operate in most industrialized countries. Nevertheless, it has been estimated that Medi-Watch receives reports for fewer than 10% of adverse drug reactions[2]; in France, less than 6% of hepatic adverse drug reactions are reported.[3] The situation may be somewhat better in Sweden, but the annual reported incidence of 2.2 per 100,000 in the population older than 15 years of age is still much lower than the predicted incidence of 14 per 100,000.[3] In a prospective surveillance study in Spain, the annual incidence of drug-related acute serious liver disease was 7.4 per 1 million inhabitants.[4]

CASE DEFINITION: WHICH AGENT?

At least 300 agents have been implicated in drug-induced liver injury.[9] The evidence for most drugs is confined to individual or a few case reports, especially in letters to scientific journals or regulatory authorities, or to small observational series. For most agents, the evidence that they could cause liver injury is circumstantial and incomplete. Reports often lack pathologic definition, full exclusion of other disorders (especially in older reports), and logistic imputation of causality, especially with respect to temporal associations (see "A Practical Approach to Diagnosis"). In all, probably fewer than 50 agents have been implicated reliably to cause drug-induced liver disease.

FREQUENCIES OF HEPATIC DRUG REACTIONS

Because of incomplete reporting, the frequency of a hepatic drug reaction often may be underestimated. Case recognition and reporting depend on the skill and motivation of observers. Moreover, the case definition of a drug reaction may be inaccurate (see "A Practical Approach to Diagnosis").[5,8] Increased interest in a drug by prescribers once initial cases of drug-induced liver disease have been described, together with inappropriate prescribing, can give rise to the perception of an epidemic of drug-induced liver disease. More appropriate epidemiologic methods applied to hepatotoxicity have included prescription event monitoring (adverse drug reactions are linked to hospitalizations, death, and prescriptions), record linkage (information about drug exposures is linked to prescribing data), and case-control studies.[10,11]

Epidemiologic studies confirm the rarity of drug-induced liver disease with currently used agents. For NSAIDs, the risk of liver injury lies between 1 and 10 per 100,000 persons exposed[10,11]; amoxicillin–clavulanic acid combinations have been associated with cholestatic hepatitis in 1 to 2 per 100,000 exposed persons[12,13]; and low-dose tetracyclines cause hepatotoxicity in less than 1 case per 1 million persons exposed.[14] The frequency of hepatotoxicity may be higher for agents that cause a metabolic type of hepatotoxicity (see discussion of metabolic idiosyncrasy later). For instance, isoniazid causes liver injury in up to 2% of exposed persons; the risk depends on age, gender, concomitant exposure to other agents, and the presence of chronic hepatitis B virus (HBV) and possibly chronic hepatitis C virus (HCV) infections.[15,16] With some drugs associated with liver injury in which other host factors play a pathogenic role, case-control studies have been used to define attributable risk. Examples include the role of aspirin in Reye's syndrome[17] and the role of oral contraceptive steroids (OCS) in liver tumors[18-20] and hepatic vein thrombosis (Budd-Chiari syndrome).[18]

A relationship between the frequency and degree of serum ALT elevations caused by a drug and the risk of severe hepatotoxicity has been postulated. This relationship was proposed in the 1970s by the late Hyman Zimmerman.[6] According to "Hy's rule," the propensity of a drug to cause acute liver failure is related to the frequency with which it is associated with an elevation of the serum ALT level to eight times the upper limit of normal or higher, or with hyperbilirubinemia. The actual rate of liver failure is approximately 10%. Thus, if 2 cases of jaundice associated with drug-induced liver injury are observed in 2500 patients in phase III clinical trials, 1 case of acute liver failure would be expected for approximately every 12,500 persons who take the drug during the marketing phase.

IMPORTANCE OF DRUGS AS A CAUSE OF LIVER DISEASE

Hepatotoxicity accounts for less than 5% of cases of jaundice or acute hepatitis in the community and for even fewer cases of chronic liver disease.[5,6] Drugs are an important cause of severe liver disease and of liver disease in older people. Drugs account for 10% of cases of severe hepatitis requiring hospitalization in France[6] and for 43% of cases of hepatitis among patients 50 years of age or older.[7] Drugs may account for more than one half of the cases of acute liver failure among patients referred to specialized units in the United States[7] and between 20% and 75% of cases of acute liver failure in other industrialized countries.[4,7]

In most instances of drug-related liver injury, drugs are the sole cause of hepatic damage. In other instances, drugs increase the *relative risk* for types of liver disease that may occur in the absence of drug exposure. Examples of drugs in the latter category are salicylates in Reye's syndrome,[17] OCS in hepatic venous thrombosis,[18]

methotrexate in hepatic fibrosis associated with alcoholic or diabetes-related fatty liver disease, and tamoxifen in NASH. The predisposition of patients with preexisting liver disease to drug-induced injury is minimal, but some potential interactions between chronic HCV infection and several groups of drugs and between chronic HBV infection and antituberculosis chemotherapy are now reasonably established, as discussed later.

INDIVIDUAL RISK FACTORS

For dose-dependent hepatotoxins such as acetaminophen and methotrexate and for some idiosyncratic reactions that are partly dependent on the dose of the drug (bromfenac, tetracyclines, dantrolene, tacrine, oxypenicillins), factors that influence the risk of drug-induced liver disease include the dose, blood level, and duration of intake of the drug. For most idiosyncratic reactions, host determinants are central to liver injury. The most critical host factors are likely to be genetic, but other "constitutional" and environmental factors can influence the risk of liver injury, as summarized in Table 83–1. The most important of these factors are age,[4] gender, exposure to other substances, a history of previous drug reactions, other risk factors for liver disease, and concomitant medical disorders.

Genetic Factors

Genetic determinants predispose affected persons to drug-induced liver disease,[21] as they do in other types of drug reactions, such as penicillin allergy. Although atopic patients have been claimed to have an increased risk of some types of drug hepatitis, this relationship has not been proved. Genetic factors determine the activity of drug-activating and antioxidant pathways, encode pathways of canalicular bile secretion, and modulate the immune response, cell stress response, and cell death pathways. Documented examples of a familial predisposition to adverse hepatic drug reactions are few and include valproic acid and phenytoin hepatitis. Inherited mitochondrial diseases are another risk factor for valproic acid–induced hepatotoxicity.[22] Some forms of drug-induced liver disease, particularly drug-induced hepatitis and granulomatous reactions, can be associated with the *reactive metabolite syndrome* (RMS), which is described in more detail later in the chapter.

Weak associations have been reported between human leukocyte antigen (HLA) haplotype and some types of drug-induced liver disease.[23] Andrade and colleagues[24] found positive associations between class II HLA haplotype and cholestatic or mixed liver damage caused by some drugs. They suggested that no specific HLA allele predisposed affected persons to the overall risk of drug-induced liver disease but that the pattern of liver injury could be influenced by these genetic determinants. Other investigators have found stronger associations between HLA haplotype and cholestatic reactions to amoxicillin–clavulanic acid[25] and tiopronin.[26]

Age

Most hepatic drug reactions are more common in adults than in children. Exceptions include valproic acid hepa-

Table 83–1 Factors Influencing the Risk of Liver Diseases Caused by Drugs

Factor	Examples of Drugs Affected	Influence
Age	Isoniazid, nitrofurantoin, halothane, troglitazone	Age >60 years: increased frequency, increased severity
	Valproic acid, salicylates	More common in children
Gender	Halothane, minocycline, nitrofurantoin	More common in women, especially with chronic hepatitis
	Amoxicillin–clavulanic acid, azathioprine	More common in men
Dose	Acetaminophen, aspirin; some herbal medicines	Blood levels directly related to risk of hepatotoxicity
	Tetracycline, tacrine, oxypenicillins	Idiosyncratic reactions, but partial relationship to dose
	Methotrexate, vitamin A	Total dose, dosing frequency, and duration of exposure related to risk of hepatic fibrosis
Genetic factors	Halothane, phenytoin, sulfonamides	Multiple cases in families
	Amoxicillin–clavulanic acid	Strong HLA association
	Valproic acid	Familial cases, association with mitochondrial enzyme deficiencies
History of other drug reactions	Isoflurane, halothane, enflurane	Instances of cross-sensitivity have been reported among members of each drug class but are rare
	Erythromycins	
	Diclofenac, ibuprofen, tiaprofenic acid	
	Sulfonamides, COX-2 inhibitors	
Other drugs	Acetaminophen	Isoniazid, zidovudine, and phenytoin lower dose threshold and increase severity of hepatotoxicity
	Valproic acid	Other antiepileptics increase risk of hepatotoxicity
	Anticancer drugs	Interactive vascular toxicity
Excessive alcohol use	Acetaminophen hepatotoxicity	Lowered dose threshold, poorer outcome
	Isoniazid, methotrexate	Increased risk of liver injury, hepatic fibrosis
Nutritional status		
Obesity	Halothane, troglitazone, tamoxifen, methotrexate	Increased risk of liver injury; hepatic fibrosis
Fasting	Acetaminophen	Increased risk of hepatotoxicity
Preexisting liver disease	Hycanthone, pemoline	Increased risk of liver injury
	Antituberculosis drugs, ibuprofen	Increased risk of liver injury with chronic hepatitis B and C
Other diseases/conditions		
Diabetes mellitus	Methotrexate	Increased risk of hepatic fibrosis
HIV infection/AIDS	Sulfonamides	Increased risk of hypersensitivity
Renal failure	Tetracycline, methotrexate	Increased risk of liver injury, hepatic fibrosis
Organ transplantation	Azathioprine, thioguanine, busulfan	Increased risk of vascular toxicity

AIDS, acquired immunodeficiency syndrome; COX-2, cyclooxygenase-2; HIV, human immunodeficiency virus; HLA, human leukocyte antigen.

totoxicity, which is most common in children younger than 3 years of age and is rare in adults,[27] and Reye's syndrome, in which salicylates play a key role.[17,28] As discussed later, both may be examples of mitochondrial toxicity.[29] Among adults, the risk of isoniazid-associated hepatotoxicity is greater in persons older than 40 years of age. Similar observations have been made for nitrofurantoin, halothane, etretinate, diclofenac, and troglitazone.[27] The increased frequency of adverse drug reactions in older persons, however, is largely the result of increased exposure, use of multiple agents, and altered drug disposition. In addition, the clinical severity of hepatotoxicity increases strikingly with age, as exemplified by fatalities following reactions to isoniazid and halothane.

Gender

Women are particularly predisposed to drug-induced hepatitis, but not simply because of greater exposure than that among men. Examples of drugs that cause heptotoxicity more often in women than in men include halothane, nitrofurantoin, sulfonamides, flucloxacillin, minocycline, and troglitazone.[5,6] Drug-induced chronic hepatitis caused by nitrofurantoin, diclofenac, or minocycline has a pronounced female preponderance.[6] Conversely, equal gender frequency or even male preponderance is common for some drug reactions characterized by cholestasis, such as amoxicillin–clavulanic acid toxicity, which is more common in men than in women.[12,13] Male renal transplant recipients also are more susceptible than female recipients to azathioprine-induced liver disease.

Concomitant Exposure to Other Agents

Patients taking multiple drugs are more likely to experience an adverse reaction than are those taking a single agent.[5,30,31] One mechanism of increased toxicity is enhanced cytochrome P450 (CYP)-mediated metabolism of the drug to a toxic intermediate (discussed later). Examples of such agents (discussed later) include acetaminophen, isoniazid, valproic acid, other anticonvulsants, and anticancer drugs. Alternatively, drugs may alter the disposition of another drug by reducing bile flow or competing with canalicular pathways for biliary excretion (phase III drug elimination) (see later). This mechanism may account for apparent interactions between OCS and other drugs to produce cholestasis. Drugs or their metabolites also might interact to cause cellular toxicity and cell death by mechanisms that involve mitochondrial injury, effects on intracellular signaling pathways, activation of transcription factors, and regulation of hepatic genes involved in controlling the response to stress and injury.[32,33]

Previous Drug Reactions

A history of an adverse drug reaction generally increases the risk of adverse reactions to the same drug and also to other agents (see later). Nevertheless, instances of cross-sensitivity to related agents in cases of drug-induced liver disease are surprisingly uncommon. Examples include haloalkane anesthetics (see Chapter 84), erythromycins, phenothiazines and tricyclic antidepressants, isoniazid and pyrazinamide, sulfonamides and other sulfur-containing compounds (e.g., some cyclooxygenase-2 [COX-2] inhibitors), and some NSAIDs. A crucial point is that a previous reaction to the same drug is an important predisposing factor to drug-induced liver injury of increased severity.[27]

Alcohol

Chronic excessive alcohol ingestion decreases the dose threshold and enhances the severity of acetaminophen-induced hepatotoxicity and increases the risk and severity of isoniazid hepatitis, niacin (nicotinamide) hepatotoxicity, and methotrexate-induced hepatic fibrosis.

Nutritional Status

Obesity is strongly associated with the risk of halothane hepatitis (see Chapter 84) and appears to be an independent risk factor for the development of NASH and hepatic fibrosis in patients taking methotrexate or tamoxifen. Fasting also predisposes patients to acetaminophen hepatotoxicity,[34] and a role for undernutrition has been proposed in isoniazid hepatotoxicity.[35]

Preexisting Liver Disease

In general, liver diseases such as alcoholic cirrhosis and cholestasis do not predispose affected patients to adverse hepatic reactions to specific drugs. Exceptions include some anticancer drugs, niacin (nicotinamide),[36] pemoline,[37] and hycanthone.[38] Preexisting liver disease also is a critical determinant of methotrexate-induced hepatic fibrosis (discussed later). Patients with chronic HBV infection,[15] and possibly those with chronic HCV infection or HIV infection/AIDS, appear to be at heightened risk for liver injury during antituberculosis or HAART chemotherapy,[39] after exposure to ibuprofen and possibly other NSAIDs,[40] after myeloablative therapy in preparation for bone marrow transplantation (resulting in hepatic veno-occlusive disease, also known as sinusoidal obstruction syndrome),[41] and possibly after taking antiandrogens such as flutamide and cyproterone

acetate.[42] HCV infection (present in 33% of patients with HIV infection/AIDS) is strongly associated with a risk of liver injury during HAART; the risk may be increased 2- to 10-fold.[43-46]

Other Diseases

Rheumatoid arthritis appears to increase the risk of salicylate hepatotoxicity. Diabetes, obesity, and renal failure predispose affected patients to methotrexate-induced hepatic fibrosis, and HIV/AIDS confers a heightened risk of sulfonamide hypersensitivity.[47] A retrospective cohort study of patients with diabetes mellitus in five health maintenance organizations found age- and sex–standardized incidence rates for drug-induced acute liver failure of 0.08 to 0.15 per 1000 person-years irrespective of the agent used to treat diabetes, including insulin (the number of persons using troglitazone was small). The incidence rate was higher (approximately 0.3 per 1000) during the first 6 months of exposure to all agents.[48] Renal transplantation is a risk factor for azathioprine-associated vascular injury[5]; renal failure predisposes affected patients to tetracycline-induced fatty liver.[6] A curious, unexplained observation is that hepatitis associated with sulfasalazine appears to be more common among patients with rheumatoid arthritis than among those with inflammatory bowel disease.[49] Finally, sinusoidal obstruction syndrome induced by anticancer drugs is more common after bone marrow transplantation, as well as in patients with chronic HCV infection.[41]

PATHOPHYSIOLOGY

ROLE OF THE LIVER IN DRUG ELIMINATION

By virtue of the portal circulation, the liver is highly exposed to drugs and other toxins absorbed from the gastrointestinal tract. Most drugs tend to be lipophilic compounds that are taken up readily by the liver but that cannot be excreted easily unchanged in bile or urine. The liver is well equipped to handle these agents by an adaptable (inducible) series of metabolic pathways. These pathways include (1) those that alter the parent molecule (*phase 1*); (2) those that synthesize conjugates of the drug or its metabolite with a more water-soluble moiety, such as a sugar, amino acid, or sulfate molecule (*phase 2*); and (3) energy-dependent pathways to excrete either the parent molecule or its conjugates into bile (*phase 3*). For any given compound, one, two, or all three of these steps may participate in elimination of the drug.

PATHWAYS OF DRUG METABOLISM

Phase 1 pathways of drug metabolism include oxidation, reduction, and hydrolytic reactions. The products can be readily conjugated or excreted without further modification.

Cytochrome P450

Most phase 1 reactions are catalyzed by microsomal drug oxidases, the key component of which is a hemoprotein of the *CYP* gene superfamily. The apparent capability of drug oxidases to metabolize a wide range of drugs, environmental toxins, steroid hormones, lipids, and bile acids results from the existence of multiple, closely related CYP proteins; more than 20 CYP enzymes in the human liver are recognized.

The phase 1 reaction cycle involves binding of molecular oxygen to iron in the heme prosthetic group of CYP, with subsequent reduction of oxygen by acceptance of an electron from the nicotinamide-adenine dinucleotide phosphate (NADPH) cytochrome P450 reductase, a flavoprotein reductase. The resultant "activated oxygen" is incorporated into the drug or other lipophilic compound. Reduction of oxygen and insertion into a drug substrate ("mixed function oxidation") can result in formation of chemically reactive intermediates, including free radicals, electrophilic "oxy-intermediates" (e.g., unstable epoxides, quinone imines), and reduced (and therefore reactive) oxygen species (ROS). A typical example is the CYP2E1-catalyzed metabolite of acetaminophen, *N*-acetyl-*p*-quinone imine (NAPQI), an oxidizing and arylating metabolite that is responsible for liver injury associated with acetaminophen hepatotoxicity. Other quinone compounds are potential reactive metabolites of troglitazone,[50] quinine, and methyldopa. Epoxide metabolites of diterpenoids may be hepatotoxic products of the hepatic metabolism of some plant toxins.[51,52] ROS have broad significance in the production of tissue injury, particularly by contributing to oxidative stress and triggering cell stress responses and cell death pathways, as discussed later.

The hepatic content of CYP proteins is higher in zone 3 of the hepatic acinus than in zones 1 and 2. Localization of CYP2E1 usually is confined to a narrow rim of hepatocytes 1 to 2 cells thick around the terminal hepatic venule. This localization explains in part the zonality of hepatic lesions produced by drugs and toxins, such as acetaminophen and carbon tetrachloride, that are converted to reactive metabolites.

Genetic and Environmental Determinants of Cytochrome P450 Enzymes

Pharmacogenetics and Polymorphisms of Cytochrome P450 Expression

The hepatic expression of each CYP enzyme is genetically determined. This observation largely explains the fourfold or greater difference in rates of drug metabolism among healthy persons. Some CYPs, particularly minor forms, also are subject to polymorphic inheritance; occasional persons completely lack the encoded protein (see later). One example is CYP2D6, the enzyme responsible for metabolism of debrisoquine and perhexiline metabolism. Poor metabolizers lack CYP2D6 and accumulate perhexiline when given usual doses; lack of CYP2D6 is the critical determinant in serious adverse effects of perhexiline, including chronic hepatitis and cirrhosis.[53] Other examples include the CYPs 2C9 and 2C19, which affect metabolism of *S*-warfarin, tolbutamide, phenytoin, and *S*-mephenytoin, respectively; 3% of white populations and 15% of Asians are poor metabolizers of *S*-mephenytoin.

Developmental Regulation and Constitutive Expression

Expression of several CYPs is developmentally regulated. During adult life, the activity of some CYPs may decline slightly (up to 10%) with advancing age,[54] but this change is minor compared with the magnitude of genetic variation, environmental influences, and the effects of liver disease.[55,56] Gender differences in expression of the CYPs 3A4 and 2E1 may explain the slightly enhanced metabolism of certain drugs (erythromycin, chlordiazepoxide, midazolam) in women,[55] but whether this difference contributes to the increased risk of hepatic drug reactions in women is unclear.

Nutrition- and Disease-Related Changes

Nutritional status influences the expression of certain CYPs, in both health and liver disease.[56] CYP2E1 activity is increased by obesity, high fat intake, and fasting. Diseases that alter expression of hepatic CYPs include diabetes mellitus (increased CYP2E1), hypothyroidism (decreased CYP1A), and hypopituitarism (decreased CYP3A4). Severe liver disease (cirrhosis) is associated with both decreased levels of total CYP and reduced hepatic perfusion; the result is a decrease in the clearance of drugs that are rapidly metabolized by the liver. The effects of cirrhosis vary among individual CYP families (e.g., CYP1A levels are unvariably lowered, whereas CYP2C and CYP2D6 levels often are preserved) and with the type of cirrhosis (e.g., CYP3A4 levels are preserved with cholestatic liver disease but lowered with hepatocellular liver disease).[57,58]

Adaptive Response and Enzyme Induction

Exposure to lipophilic substances results in an adaptive response that usually involves synthesis of new CYP protein, a process termed *enzyme induction*. The molecular basis for genetic regulation of constitutive and inducible expression of the principal human hepatic cytochrome P450, CYP3A4, has been determined.[59] Agents such as rifampin interact with the pregnane X receptor (PXR), a member of the orphan nuclear receptor family of transcriptional regulators. Activated PXR and the analogous constitutive androstane receptor (CAR), in turn, bind to cognate nucleotide sequences upstream to the CYP3A4 structural gene within a "xenobiotic-regulatory enhancer module" (XREM).[59] This interaction regulates the CYP3A4 promoter downstream and ultimately the transcription of CYP3A4 protein. Similar control mechanisms apply to several other CYP pathways,[60] particularly those involved with bile acid synthesis, in which the implicated nuclear receptors include PXR and the farnesyl X receptor (FXR) (see Chapter 61).[59]

Common examples of the induction of microsomal enzymes by environmental compounds are the effect of smoking cigarettes and cannabis on CYP1A2[60] and of alcohol on CYP2E1 and possibly CYP3A4. Several drugs are potent inducers of CYP enzymes. Isoniazid induces CYP2E1, whereas phenobarbital and phenytoin increase the expression of multiple CYPs. Rifampin is a potent inducer of CYP3A4, as is hypericum,[61] the active ingredient of St. John's wort, a commonly used herbal medicine, allowing for drug-drug interactions between conventional medicines and CAM preparations. The implications for drug-induced liver disease are two-fold. First, enzyme induction often involves more than the CYP system, possibly because of activation of the nuclear orphan receptor transcriptional regulators; such activation could account for increases in serum alkaline phosphate and gamma glutamyl transpeptidase (GGTP) levels, which are part of the "hepatic adaptation" to chronic drug ingestion. Second, the influence of one drug on expression and activity of drug metabolizing enzymes and drug elimination pathways (phase 3) can alter the metabolism or disposition of other agents. Such drug-drug interactions are important pharmacologically and may be relevant to mechanisms of drug-induced liver injury.

Inhibition of Drug Metabolism

Some chemicals inhibit drug metabolism. In persons taking more than one medication, for example, competition for phase 2 pathways such as glucuronidation and sulfation could facilitate the presentation of unconjugated drug to the CYP system. This mechanism appears to explain in part why agents like zidovudine and phenytoin lower the dose threshold for acetaminophen-induced hepatotoxicity.

Other Pathways of Drug Oxidation

In addition to CYP enzymes, electron transport systems of mitochondria may lead to the generation of tissue-damaging reactive intermediates during metabolism of some drugs. Examples of such reactive intermediates are nitroradicals derived from nitrofurans such as nitrofurantoin and cocaine.[32] Subsequent electron transfer by flavoprotein reductases to molecular oxygen generates superoxide and other ROS. The imidazole antimicrobial agents and some anticancer drugs such as doxorubicin (Adriamycin) can participate in other oxidation-reduction (redox) cycling reactions that generate ROS.

Phase 2 (Conjugation) Reactions

Phase 2 reactions involve formation of ester links to the parent compound or a drug metabolite. The responsible enzymes include glucuronosyl transferases, sulfotransferases, glutathione S-transferases, and acetyl and amino acid N-transferases.[62] The resulting conjugates are highly water soluble and can be excreted readily in bile or urine. The rate of conjugation reactions can be retarded by depletion of rate-limiting cofactors (glucuronic acid, inorganic sulfate), and the relatively low capacity of these enzyme systems can restrict the rate of drug elimination when substrate concentrations exceed enzyme saturation. In general, drug conjugates are nontoxic, and phase 2 reactions are considered to be detoxification reactions, with some exceptions. For example, some glutathione conjugates can undergo cysteine S-conjugate β-lyase–mediated activation to highly reactive intermediates. Little is known about the regulation of such enzymes and their potential significance for drug-induced liver disease or hepatocarcinogenesis.

Phase 3 Pathways of Drug Elimination from the Liver

The general importance of energy-dependent pathways by which drugs, drug metabolites, or their conjugates are excreted from the liver, often referred to as phase 3 of hepatic drug elimination, is now better appreciated. These pathways involve ATP-binding cassette (ABC) transport proteins, which derive the energy for their transport functions from the hydrolysis of adenosine triphosphate (ATP). ABC transport proteins are distributed widely in nature and include the cystic fibrosis transmembrane conductance regulator (CFTR) and the canalicular and intestinal copper transporters (see Chapters 61, 69, and 72).[63-65]

Multidrug resistance protein (MDR), or Mdr-1 in humans (formerly termed p-glycoprotein), is highly expressed on the apical (canalicular) plasma membrane of hepatocytes, where it transports cationic drugs, particularly anticancer agents, into bile. Another family of ABC transporters, the multidrug resistance–associated proteins (MRPs), also are expressed in the liver. At least two members of this family serve to excrete drug (and other) conjugates from hepatocytes; MRP-1 (and probably MRP-3) on the basolateral surface facilitates passage of drug conjugate into the sinusoidal circulation, whereas MRP-2 (formerly known as the canalicular multipurpose organic anion transporter [cMOAT]) is expressed on the canalicular membrane. MRP-2 pumps endogenous conjugates (e.g., bilirubin diglucuronide, leukotriene-glutathionyl conjugates) and drug conjugates into bile. The bile salt export pump (BSEP) and MDR3 (in humans)/Mdr2 (in mice) are two other important canalicular transport proteins, which facilitate energy-dependent bile acid secretion and phospholipid secretion, respectively, into bile. Genetic polymorphisms of these genes are associated with human cholestatic liver disease (see Chapter 61). BSEP interacts with several drugs.[65]

Regulation of the membrane expression and activity of these drug elimination pathways is complex. The possibility that their altered expression or impaired activity (by competition between agents, changes in membrane lipid composition, or damage from reactive metabolites or covalent binding) could lead to drug accumulation, impairment of bile flow, or cholestatic liver injury has been demonstrated for estrogens,[66] troglitazone,[67] terbinafine,[68] and flucloxacillin[69] and may have wider mechanistic importance for drug-induced cholestasis and other forms of liver injury.[65]

TOXIC MECHANISMS OF LIVER INJURY

Direct Hepatotoxins and Reactive Metabolites

Highly hepatotoxic chemicals cause direct, irreversible damage to key subcellular structures of cells in the liver, particularly mitochondria and the plasma membrane. The injury arrests energy generation, dissipates ionic gradients, and disrupts the physical integrity of the cell. This type of overwhelming cellular injury does not apply to currently relevant hepatotoxic drugs, most of which require *metabolic activation* to mediate damage to hepatocytes. The resultant *reactive metabolites* can interact with critical cellular target molecules, particularly those with nucleophilic substituents such as thiol-rich proteins and nucleic acids. Together with ROS, they act as oxidizing species within the hepatocyte to establish *oxidative stress,* a state of imbalance between pro-oxidants and antioxidants. ROS also are key signaling molecules that mediate biologic responses to stress, as discussed later. Alternatively, reactive metabolites bind irreversibly to macromolecules, particularly proteins and lipids. Such *covalent binding* may produce injury by inactivating key enzymes or by forming protein-drug adducts that could be targets for immunodestructive processes that cause liver injury.

Oxidative Stress and the Glutathione System

The liver is exposed to oxidative stress because of the propensity of hepatocytes to reduce oxygen, particularly in mitochondria but also in microsomal electron transport systems (such as CYP2E1), and because of NADPH oxidase–catalyzed formation of ROS and nitroradicals in Kupffer cells, endothelial cells, and stimulated polymorphonuclear neutrophils and macrophages. To combat oxidative stress, the liver is well endowed with antioxidant mechanisms, including micronutrients such as vitamins E and C, thiol-rich proteins (e.g., metallothionein), metal-sequestering proteins (e.g., ferritin), and enzymes that metabolize reactive metabolites (e.g., epoxide hydrolases), ROS (e.g., catalase, superoxide dismutase), and lipid peroxides (e.g., glutathione peroxidases). Glutathione [*N*-(*N*-L-gamma-glutamyl-L-cysteinyl)glycine] is the most important antioxidant in the mammalian liver.[32,70]

Hepatocytes are the exclusive site of glutathione synthesis. Hepatic levels of glutathione are high (5 to 10 mmol/L), and its synthesis can be increased by enhancing the supply of cysteine; this mechanism is the cornerstone of thiol antidote therapy for acetaminophen poisoning (see later). Hepatocyte glutathione synthesis increases in response to pro-oxidants, as occurs when CYP2E1 is overexpressed.[71,72] Glutathione is a critical cofactor for several antioxidant pathways, including thiol-disulfide exchange reactions and *glutathione peroxidase.* Glutathione peroxidase has a higher affinity for hydrogen peroxide than that of catalase and disposes of lipid peroxides, free radicals, and electrophilic drug metabolites. Reduced glutathione is a cofactor for conjugation reactions catalyzed by the *glutathione S-transferases.* Other reactions occur nonenzymatically; the products include glutathione-protein mixed disulfides and oxidized glutathione. The latter can be converted back to reduced glutathione by proton donation catalyzed by *glutathione reductase.*

Normally, most glutathione within the hepatocyte is in the reduced state, indicating the importance of this pathway for maintenance of the redox capacity of the cell. The reduced form of NADPH is an essential cofactor for glutathione reductase; NADPH formation requires ATP, thereby illustrating a critical link between the energy-generating capacity of the liver and its ability to withstand oxidative stress.[70] Glutathione also is compartmentalized within the hepatocyte, with the highest concentrations found in the cytosol. Adequate levels of glutathione are essential within mitochondria, where ROS are constantly being formed as a minor by-product of oxidative respiration and in response to some drugs or metabolites that interfere with the mitochondrial respiratory chain. Levels of mitochondrial glutathione are maintained by active uptake of glutathione from the cytosol, a transport system that is altered by chronic ethanol exposure and is therefore another potential target of drug toxicity.[32]

Biochemical Mechanisms of Cellular Injury

Mechanisms once thought to be central to hepatotoxicity, such as covalent binding to cellular enzymes and peroxidation of membrane lipids, are no longer regarded as exclusive pathways of cellular damage. Rather, oxidation of proteins, phospholipid fatty acyl side chains (lipid peroxidation), and nucleosides appear to be components of the biochemical stress that characterizes toxic liver injury. Secondary reactions also may play a role; these reactions include post-translational modification of proteins through mono-adenosine diphosphate (ADP) ribosylation or protease activation, cleavage of DNA by activation of endogenous endonucleases, and disruption of lipid membranes by activated phospholipases.[33] Some of these catabolic reactions could be initiated by a rise in cytosolic ionic calcium concentration, $[Ca^{2+}]_i$, resulting from increased Ca^{2+} entry into the cell or release from internal stores such as the endoplasmic reticulum and mitochondria.[5]

The concept that hepatotoxic chemicals cause hepatocyte cell death by a *biochemical final common pathway* (e.g., activation of catalytic enzymes by a rise in $[Ca^{2+}]_i$) has proved inadequate to explain the diverse processes that can result in lethal hepatocellular injury. Rather, a variety of processes can damage key organelles, thereby causing intracellular stress that activates signaling pathways and transcription factors. In turn, the balance between these factors can either trigger the onset of cell death or facilitate protection of the cell, as discussed in the following sections.

Cellular Processes Pertinent to Drug- and Toxin-induced Liver Injury: Types of Cell Death

Apoptosis

Apoptosis is an energy-dependent, genetically programmed form of cell death that typically results in controlled deletion of individual cells. In addition to its major roles in developmental biology, tissue regulation, and carcinogenesis, apoptosis is important in toxic, viral, and immune-mediated liver injury.[73] The ultrastructural features of apoptosis are cell and nuclear shrinkage, condensation and margination of nuclear chromatin, plasma membrane blebbing, and ultimately fragmentation of the cell into membrane-bound bodies that contain intact mitochondria and other organelles. Engulfment of these *apoptotic bodies* by surrounding epithelial and mesenchymal cells conserves cell fragments that contain nucleic acid and intact mitochondria. The fragments are then digested by lysosomes and recycled without release of bioactive substances. As a consequence, apoptosis in its purest form (usually found only in vitro) does not incite an inflammatory tissue reaction. The cellular processes that occur in apoptosis are mediated by caspases, a family of proteolytic enzymes that contain a cysteine at their active site and that cleave polypeptides at aspartate residues.

It is now clear that apoptosis is rarely, if ever, the sole form of cell death in common forms of liver injury, such as ischemia-reperfusion, cholestatic, and toxic liver injury, all of which typically are associated with a hepatic inflammatory response. Whether or not activation of pro-death signals causes cell death depends on several factors, including the operation of pro-survival signals, rapidity of the process, availability of glutathione and ATP, and role of other cell types. Some of these issues are discussed briefly here and have been reviewed in more detail elsewhere.[33,73]

Hepatocytes undergo apoptosis when pro-apoptotic intracellular signaling pathways are activated, either because of toxic biochemical processes within the cell (intrinsic pathway) or because cell surface receptors are activated to transduce cell death signals (external pathway) (Fig. 83–1). Pro-apoptotic receptors are members of the tumor necrosis factor-α (TNF-α) receptor superfamily; these receptors possess a so-called death domain. The receptors include the Fas receptor (for which the cognate ligand is Fas ligand [Fas-L]), TNF-R1 receptor (cognate ligand TNF), and *T*NF-*r*elated *a*poptosis-inducing *l*igand (TRAIL) receptor (cognate ligand TRAIL). Some drugs (e.g., acetaminophen, plant diterpenoids) have been shown to be converted into pro-oxidant reactive metabolites, thereby setting in motion the following sequence: CYP-mediated metabolism to form a reactive metabolite→glutathione depletion→mitochondrial injury with release of cytochrome *c* and operation of the mitochondrial membrane permeability transition (MPT)→caspase activation→apoptosis.[51,52,74]

Mitochondria play a pivotal role in pathways that either provoke or oppose apoptosis.[33,73] In the external pathway, activation of the death domain of pro-apoptotic receptors recruits adapter molecules—Fas-associated death domain (FADD), TNF receptor–associated death domain (TRADD)—that bind and activate procaspase-8 to form the *d*eath-*i*nducing *s*ignaling *c*omplex (DISC). In turn, caspase-8 cleaves Bid, a pro-apoptotic member of the B cell lymphoma/leukemia-2 (Bcl-2) family, to tBid. tBid causes translocation of Bax to the mitochondria, where Bax aggregates with Bak to promote permeability of the mitochondria.[75] Release of cytochrome *c* and other pro-death molecules, including Smac (which binds caspase inhibitor proteins, such as inhibitor of apoptosis proteins [IAPs]) and apoptosis-inducing factor (AIF, also known as Apaf),[76] allows formation of the "aptosome," which activates caspase-9 and eventually caspase-3 to execute cell death. Intracellular stresses in various sites release other mitochondrial permeabilizing proteins (e.g., Bmf from the cytoskeleton) that promote mitochondrial permeability, whereas members of the Bcl-2 family, Bcl-2

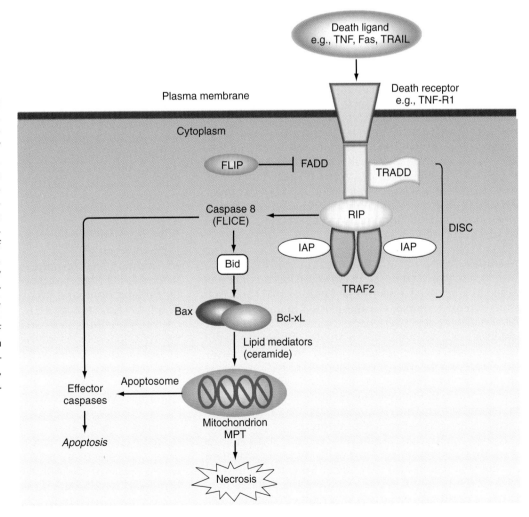

Figure 83–1 Apoptosis and necrosis pathways in mammalian cells. See text for details. Bcl, B cell lymphoma/leukemia family (Bax, Bid, and Bcl-xL are members); DISC, death-inducing signaling complex; FADD, Fas-associated death domain; FLIP, FLICE-inhibitory proteins; IAP, inhibitor of apoptosis proteins; MPT, mitochondrial permeability transition; RIP, receptor-interacting protein; TNF, tumor necrosis factor; TNF-R1 TNF receptor-1; TRADD, TNF receptor–associated death domain; TRAF2, TNF receptor–associated factor-2; TRAIL, TNF-related apoptosis ligand.

and Bcl-X_L, antagonize apoptosis and serve as survival factors by regulating the integrity of mitochondria; the protective mechanism is poorly understood. Stress-ctivated protein kinases, particularly c-jun N-terminal kinase (JNK), also may be pro-apoptotic,[77] by phosphorylating and inactivating the mitochondrial protective protein Bcl-X_L.

Execution of cell death by apoptosis usually occurs through activation of caspase-3, but more than one caspase-independent pathway of programmed cell death has been described. Stresses to the endoplasmic reticulum can bypass mitochondrial events by activation of caspase-12, which in turn activates caspase-9 independently of the apoptosome. The final steps of programmed cell death are energy dependent, and ATP depletion abrogates the controlled attempt at "cell suicide," resulting instead in necrosis or an overlapping pattern of apoptosis and necrosis (necrapoptosis).[73] Furthermore, when apoptosis is massive, the capacity for rapid phagocytosis can be exceeded, and "secondary" necrosis can occur.[78]

Intracellular processes and activation of proapoptotic death receptors are not mutually exclusive pathways of cell death in toxic liver injury.[32] In fact, drug toxicity could predispose the injured hepatocyte to apoptosis mediated by TNF-R–operated or FAS-operated pathways by several mechanisms, including blockade of nuclear factor-kappa B (NFκB), which usually is a hepatoprotective transcription factor in hepatocytes, and inhibition of purine and protein synthesis. Furthermore, activation of Kupffer cells (e.g., by endotoxin) and recruitment of activated inflammatory cells (see later) can increase TNF production, whereas drug-induced oxidative stress can increase synthesis and surface aggregation of Fas (Wu, Farrell, Jones, unpublished data).[73,74]

Inhibition of caspases is an important protective mechanism against cell death. Such anti-apoptotic pathways include chemical blockade of the cysteine thiol group by nitric oxide (NO)[79] or ROS or secondary to cellular depletion of glutathione.[33] Protein inhibitors include IAP family members, heat shock proteins (HSPs), and FLICE (caspase-8)-inhibitory proteins (FLIP).[75-77] FLIP inhibit caspase-8 activation as a decoy for FADD binding. Bcl-2 and Bcl-X_L inhibit mitochondrial permeability, whereas phosphatidylinositol 3-kinase/Akt phosphorylates caspase-9 and activates NFκB.

Necrosis

In contrast with apoptosis, necrosis has been conceptualized as a relatively uncontrolled process that can result from extensive damage to the plasma membrane, with disturbance of ion transport, dissolution of membrane potential, cell swelling, and eventually rupture of the cell (see Fig. 83-1). Drug-induced injury to the mitochondrion can impair energy generation, and MPT can release stored Ca^{2+} into the cytosol and perturb other ionic gradients. Mitochondrial enzymes appear to be a particular target of NAPQI, the reactive metabolite of acetaminophen. Reye's syndrome–like disorders (e.g., toxicity caused by valproic acid; some nucleoside analogs, such as fialuridine, didanosine, zidovudine, and zalcitabine; and possibly "ecstasy") also may result from mitochondrial injury.[80] Mitochondrial injury can result in cell death by either apoptosis or necrosis[81]; determination of the type

of cell death pathway may depend primarily on the energy state of the cell, as well as the rapidity and severity of the injury process. In the presence of ATP, cell death can proceed by apoptosis, but when mitochondria are de-energized, the mechanism of cell death is necrosis. This apparent dichotomy between cell death processes probably is artificial, and apoptosis and necrosis more likely represent the morphologic and mechanistic ends of a spectrum of overlapping cell death processes.[32,82]

One important way in which necrosis differs from apoptosis is that uncontrolled dissolution of the cell liberates macromolecular breakdown products, including lipid peroxides, aldehydes, and eicosanoids. These products act as *chemoattractants for circulating leukocytes*, which enjoin an inflammatory response in the hepatic parenchyma. Even before cell death occurs, oxidative stress produced during drug toxicity can up-regulate *adhesion molecules and chemokines* that are expressed or secreted by endothelial cells.[74] These processes contribute to recruitment of the hepatic inflammatory response, which is prominent in some types of drug-induced liver disease. Lymphocytes, polymorphonuclear leukocytes (neutrophils and eosinophils), and macrophages also may be attracted to the liver as part of a cell-mediated immune reaction.

Roles of Oxidative Stress

Although severe oxidative stress in hepatocytes, particularly that focused on mitochondria, is likely to induce necrosis, lesser (or more gradual) exposure can trigger apoptosis, because ROS and oxidative stress can activate Fas signaling, JNK and other kinases, p53, microtubular assembly, and damage to the endoplasmic reticulum. Oxidative stress also may amplify cell death processes by uncoupling the mitochondrial respiratory chain, cytochrome c release, and export of glutathione, which is required for Fas signaling. Conversely, oxidative stress may protect against apoptosis in some circumstances through inhibition of caspase or activation of NF-κB. As a result of these opposing effects, predicting the consequences of hepatic oxidative stress in terms of liver injury is not easy.

Role of Hepatic Nonparenchymal Cells and the Innate Immune Response

In addition to migratory cells, activation of nonparenchymal liver cell types is likely to play an important role in drug- and toxin-induced liver injury.[83]

Kupffer cells function as resident macrophages and antigen-presenting cells. Some of the toxic effects of activated Kupffer cells, as well as of recruited leukocytes, may be mediated by *release of cytokines*, such as TNF and Fas-L, which under some circumstances present during toxic liver injury can induce cell death of hepatocytes by apoptosis or necrosis.[82] Carbon tetrachloride–induced liver injury in mice requires TNF.[84] Ablation of macrophages modifies the acute hepatotoxicity of acetaminophen, but absence of TNF does not, suggesting a role for other Kupffer cell–derived molecules. Activated Kupffer cells release ROS, nitroradicals, leukotrienes, and proteases.[85,86]

Endothelial cells of the hepatic sinusoids or terminal hepatic veins are vulnerable to injury by some hepatotoxins because of their low glutathione content. Such hepatotoxins include alkaloids, which are an important cause of the sinusoidal obstruction syndrome[87,88] (see Chapters 80 and 84).

Hepatic *stellate cells* (formerly fat-storing or Ito cells) are the principal liver cell type involved in matrix deposition in hepatic fibrosis. Stellate cells are activated in methotrexate-induced hepatic fibrosis. The possibility that vitamin A, ROS, or drug metabolites can transform stellate cells into collagen-synthesizing myofibroblasts is of considerable interest.

IMMUNOLOGIC MECHANISMS

In addition to activation of innate inflammatory processes in the liver by toxic mechanisms, (extrinsic) immunologic mechanisms could account for certain aspects of idiosyncratic drug-induced liver disease. Immune attack involves liganding of death receptors, as discussed earlier, or introduction of the enzyme granzyme into target cells by the pemeabilizing protein porin.[32] The most convincing evidence for drug allergy is a clinical picture that includes (1) delayed onset after initial exposure and accelerated onset after rechallenge; (2) hepatic inflammatory infiltrates with polymorphonuclear neutrophils and eosinophils; and (3) fever, rash, lymphadenopathy, eosinophilia, and involvement of other organs. In some types of drug hepatitis, the liver is clearly implicated as part of a systemic hypersensitivity reaction, as described later for RMS; sulfonamides, phenytoin, nitrofurantoin, minocycline, nevirapine, and some Chinese herbal medicines are examples of causative agents. Why the liver is the predominant site of injury in some persons, whereas different organs are involved in others, is unclear; genetic factors relevant to tissue-specific gene expression could be involved.

One possible immunopathogenic mechanism of drug-induced liver disease is the *altered antigen concept*, in which an initial interaction between drug metabolites and cellular proteins results in the formation of *neoantigens* (haptens) or *drug-protein adducts*. An example is the formation of trifluoroacetylated (TFA) adducts after exposure to halothane or other haloalkane anesthetics (see Chapter 84). For these adducts to initiate tissue-damaging immune responses, (1) they must be presented in an immunogenic form (e.g., by Kupffer cells, in association with major histocompatibility [MHC] molecules); (2) appropriately responsive CD4$^+$ T cells must be present to help induce an immune response; and (3) the drug-derived antigen, together with a class II MHC molecule, must be expressed on the target cells in order to attract CD8$^+$ (cytotoxic) T cells. That bile duct epithelial cells are more likely to express class II MHC antigens may explain why they are possible targets in drug-induced cholestatic hepatitis.

Although antibodies directed against TFA protein adducts circulate in a majority of patients following recovery from halothane-induced liver injury,[89] the specificity and pathogenicity of these antibodies remain in doubt (see Chapter 84). Another way in which circulating drug-induced antibodies could result in immune-mediated lysis of hepatocytes is through molecular mimicry of host enzymes. Experimental evidence suggests that for diclofenac, antibody-dependent cell-mediated immunity could operate as a mechanism for drug-induced liver disease.[90]

A second type of immunopathogenic mechanism that could account for some instances of drug-induced liver disease is dysregulation of the immune system, termed *drug-induced autoimmunity*. This mechanism can lead to formation of drug-induced autoantibodies (e.g., anti-liver-kidney microsome [anti-LKM] antibodies) directed against microsomal enzymes. For tienilic acid, CYP2C9 is the target of anti-LKM antibodies, whereas antibodies that circulate after halothane hepatitis are directed against CYP2E1. Non–tissue-specific autoantibodies, such as antinuclear and anti–smooth muscle antibodies, may be detected in patients with nitrofurantoin, methyldopa, or minocycline hepatitis. Like spontaneous autoimmunity, drug-induced autoimmunity may involve genetic predisposition through anomalies of immune tolerance.[91]

CLINICOPATHOLOGIC FEATURES OF DRUG-INDUCED LIVER DISEASE

CLASSIFICATION

Hepatic drug reactions mimic all known liver diseases, but classification often is difficult because of overlap among categories. Although a classic ("signature") syndrome is associated with many individual agents, a given drug may be associated with more than one clinicopathologic syndrome. Furthermore, the clinical and laboratory features of liver disease and the hepatic histologic findings may be discordant. Therefore, although recognition of specific patterns or syndromes is a vital clinical clue to the diagnosis of drug-induced liver disease, the chronologic relationship between drug administration and liver injury is a more important clue.

Drugs often are divided into dose-dependent, or predictable, hepatotoxins and dose-independent, or unpredictable (idiosyncratic), hepatotoxins. *Dose-dependent hepatotoxins* generally require metabolic activation to a toxic metabolite and interfere with subcellular organelles and biochemical processes at key sites, such as mitochondria or canalicular bile secretion.[64,66] Liver injury produced by dose-dependent hepatotoxins usually occurs after a short latent period (hours), is characterized by zonal necrosis or microvesicular steatosis, and can be reproduced in other species. By contrast, *idiosyncratic hepatotoxins* cause a wide range of histologic changes and do not reliably cause injury in other species; in addition, the latent period before the onset of injury is variable in duration. The distinction between dose-dependent and idiosyncratic hepatotoxins is blurred with agents such as dantrolene, tacrine, perhexiline, flucloxacillin, cyclophosphamide, nucleoside analogs, bromfenac, anticancer drugs, and cyclosporine. Liver injury caused by each of these drugs is partly dose dependent, but reactions occur in only a small proportion of exposed persons.

Two general types of mechanisms have been proposed to account for idiosyncratic hepatotoxicity: metabolic idiosyncrasy and immunoallergy. *Metabolic idiosyncrasy* refers to the susceptibility of rare persons to hepatotoxicity from a drug that, in conventional doses, usually is safe. Such susceptibility may result from genetic or acquired differences in drug metabolism or canalicular secretion, mitochondrial defects, or cell death receptor signaling. *Immunoallergy* indicates that operation of the immune system is involved in mediating the response to a drug. The two mechanisms may be interrelated (see later). Another potential pathogenic mechanism is indirect mediation of liver injury, as occurs when vascular (and possibly hyperthermic) changes are produced by cocaine, "ecstasy," intra-arterial fluroxuridine (to bile ducts), and possibly anesthetics (see Chapter 84).

The most practical classification of drug hepatotoxicity is that based on clinical, laboratory, and hepatic histologic features, as summarized in Table 83–2. This classification provides a framework for discussing drug-induced hepatic disease in comparison with other hepatobiliary disorders but is imperfect because the clinical and pathologic features are not always congruent. Moreover, much overlap between categories exists, particularly in the spectrum from severe necrosis (which may result from dose-dependent or idiosyncratic hepatotoxicity) to focal necrosis with lobular inflammation—*hepatitis*—to cholestasis. Many drugs produce a spectrum of syndromes from hepatitis to cholestasis; some authorities, therefore, include a further category of *mixed cholestatic/hepatocellular reactions*. Granulomatous hepatitis is associated with liver biochemical test abnormalities that usually are indistinguishable from those typical of hepatitis, cholestasis, or mixed reactions.

Drugs can alter liver biochemical test results without causing important liver injury. Such *adaptive responses* include hyperbilirubinemia associated with rifampin and flavaspidic acid (male fern extract) and raised serum GGTP and alkaline phosphatase levels associated with drugs such as phenytoin and warfarin.[5,6] The latter effect probably is attributable to microsomal enzyme induction.

Table 83–2   Clinicopathologic Classification of Drug-Induced Liver Disease

Category	Description	Implicated Drugs: Examples
Hepatic adaptation	No symptoms; raised serum GGTP and AP levels (occasionally raised ALT)	Phenytoin, warfarin
	Hyperbilirubinemia	Rifampin, flavaspidic acid
Dose-dependent hepatotoxicity	Symptoms of hepatitis; zonal, bridging, and massive necrosis; serum ALT level >5-fold increased, often >2000 U/L	Acetaminophen, nicotinic acid, amodiaquine, hycanthone
Other cytopathic toxicity, acute steatosis	Microvesicular steatosis, diffuse or zonal; partially dose dependent, severe liver injury, features of mitochondrial toxicity (lactic acidosis)	Valproic acid, didanosine, HAART agents, fialuridine, L-asparaginase, some herbal medicines
Acute hepatitis	Symptoms of hepatitis; focal, bridging, and massive necrosis; serum ALT level >5-fold increased; extrahepatic features of drug allergy in some cases	Isoniazid, dantrolene, nitrofurantoin, halothane, sulfonamides, phenytoin, disulfiram, acebutolol, etretinate, ketoconazole, terbinafine, troglitazone
Chronic hepatitis	Duration >3 months; interface hepatitis, bridging necrosis, fibrosis, cirrhosis; clinical and laboratory features of chronic liver disease; autoantibodies with some types of reaction (see Table 83–6)	Nitrofurantoin, etretinate, diclofenac, minocycline, nefazodone (see also Table 83–6)
Granulomatous hepatitis	Hepatic granulomas with varying hepatitis and cholestasis; raised serum ALT, AP, GGTP levels	Allopurinol, carbamazepine, hydralazine, quinidine, quinine (see also Table 83–5)
Cholestasis without hepatitis	Cholestasis, no inflammation; serum AP levels >twice-normal	Oral contraceptives, androgens
Cholestatic hepatitis	Cholestasis with inflammation; symptoms of hepatitis; raised serum ALT and AP levels	Chlorpromazine, tricyclic antidepressants, erythromycins, amoxicillin–clavulanic acid
Cholestasis with bile duct injury	Bile duct lesions and cholestatic hepatitis; clinical features of cholangitis	Chlorpromazine, flucloxacillin, dextropropoxyphene
Chronic cholestasis	Cholestasis present >3 months	
Vanishing bile duct syndrome	Paucity of small bile ducts; resembles primary biliary cirrhosis, but AMA negative	Chlorpromazine, flucloxacillin, trimethoprim-sulfamethoxazole
Sclerosing cholangitis	Strictures of large bile ducts	Intra-arterial floxuridine, intralesional scolicidals
Steatohepatitis	Steatosis, focal necrosis, Mallory's hyaline, pericellular fibrosis, cirrhosis; chronic liver disease, portal hypertension	Perhexiline, amiodarone
Vascular disorders	Sinusoidal obstruction syndrome, nodular regenerative hyperplasia, others	Many (see Table 83–8)
Tumors	Hepatocellular carcinoma, adenoma, angiosarcoma, others	Many (see Chapter 91)

ALT, alanine aminotrasferase; AMA, antimitochondrial antibodies; AP, alkaline phosphatase; AST, aspartate aminotransferase; GGTP, gamma glutamyl transpeptidase; HAART, highly active antiretroviral therapy.

With agents such as isoniazid, the distinction between minor injury and adaptation is blurred; adaptation in such cases may in fact occur in response to oxidative injury. Conversely, liver tumors or hepatic fibrosis may develop insidiously without significant liver test abnormalities—the former in association with sex steroids or vinyl chloride monomer and the latter with methotrexate, arsenic, or excessive vitamin A.

The duration of the disorder is another dimension that must be considered in classifying drug-induced liver diseases. In general, chronic liver disease is much less commonly attributable to drugs and toxins than are acute reactions, but not to consider drugs as a possible etiology can lead to a missed diagnosis, with serious clinical consequences.[8,29] In contrast with most other types of hepatic pathobiology, drugs and toxins constitute the most important cause of vascular disorders of the liver (see later). Drugs also have been associated with chronic cholestasis, chronic hepatitis, steatohepatitis, hepatic fibrosis, cirrhosis, and benign and malignant liver tumors.

HISTOPATHOLOGIC FEATURES

Although no pathognomonic hallmarks of drug-induced liver disease exist, certain histologic patterns suggest a drug etiology. These patterns include zonal necrosis or microvesicular steatosis (which accompanies mitochondrial injury) and mixed features of hepatocellular necrosis and cholestasis. Necrotic lesions that are disproportionately severe in comparison with the clinical picture also indicate a possible drug cause. Destructive bile duct lesions and prominent neutrophils and eosinophils (at least 25%) suggest drug-induced cholestatic hepatitis. Hepatic granuloma formation is another common feature of some hepatic drug reactions. In cases of steatohepatitis, hepatic fibrosis, or liver tumors, no specific clues to a drug cause can be identified, although sex steroids increase the vascularity of hepatic tumors and frequently are associated with sinusoidal dilatation or peliosis hepatis. Drug-induced steatohepatitis caused by amiodarone and perhexilene tends to be associated with severe lesions that more closely resemble those of alcoholic hepatitis than of NASH.[92] With other drugs (e.g., tamoxifen, methotrexate), the lesions are identical to those found in NASH attributable to the insulin resistance syndrome.[6,93]

CLINICAL FEATURES

The history and physical examination can provide important clues to the diagnosis of a hepatic drug reaction. The most important feature is the *temporal pattern of disease evolution* in relation to exposure to a drug or toxin. The identification of *specific risk factors for hepatotoxicity* (e.g., chronic excessive alcohol intake in a person taking acetaminophen) and the presence of *systemic features of drug hypersensitivity* may indicate the correct diagnosis. Systemic features may include fever, rash, mucositis, eosinophilia, lymphadenopathy, a mononucleosis-like syndrome, bone marrow suppression, vasculitis, renal failure, pneumonitis, and pancreatitis. These features

may be part of a characteristic syndrome thought to be inherited and mediated by formation of drug metabolites that act as haptens to initiate an immunodestructive tissue reaction; this is the reactive metabolite syndrome (RMS) described earlier.[94]

Reactive Metabolite Syndrome

Several drugs have been implicated as a cause of RMS, including sulfonamides, aminopenicillins, fluoroquinolones, clozapine, anticonvulsants (phenytoin, lamotrigine, phenobarbital, carbamazepine), minocycline, protease inhibitors (nevirapine, abacavir), some NSAIDs, and Chinese herbal medicines.[94] The factors associated with an increased risk of RMS include history of the syndrome in a first-degree relative (increases the risk to 1 in 4); use of other drugs, such as glucocorticoids or valproic acid, at the time the new agent is started (increases the risk 4- to 10-fold); and the presence of a disorder associated with immune dysregulation (e.g., systemic lupus erythematosus increases the risk 10-fold; HIV infection/AIDS increases the risk 100-fold).

The pattern of illness is characteristic. The onset occurs between 1 and 12 weeks (typically 2 to 4 weeks) after the drug is started; "sentinel symptoms" may include fever, pharyngitis, malaise, periorbital edema, headache or otalgia, rhinorrhea, and mouth ulcers. A severe drug rash is an essential feature. Erythematous reactions are usual and may evolve to toxic epidermal necrolysis or erythema multiforme, often with mucositis (Stevens-Johnson syndrome). Early hematologic abnormalities include neutrophilia and mobilization of acute-phase reactants; atypical lymphocytosis and eosinophilia may be noted later.

Hepatic reactions occur in approximately 13% of cases of RMS. Patterns include cholestasis, acute hepatitis, and granuloma formation. Manifestations of involvement of other organs include lymphadenopathy (16%), nephritis (6%), pneumonitis (6%), and more severe hematologic abnormalities (5%).

Latent Period to Onset

For idiosyncratic drug reactions, a *latent period* occurs from the commencement of drug intake to the onset of clinical and laboratory abnormalities. The duration of the latent period is commonly 2 to 8 weeks for immunoallergic types of drug hepatitis (such as RMS) and 6 to 20 weeks or longer for agents such as isoniazid, dantrolene, and troglitazone. Occasionally, liver injury may become evident after discontinuation of the causative agent; for oxypenicillins and amoxicillin-clavulanic acid, the onset of hepatotoxicity may occur as late as 2 weeks after therapy is stopped. In other cases, hepatotoxicity is rare after the first exposure to a drug but increasingly frequent and more severe after subsequent courses. Typical examples are halothane, nitrofurantoin, and dacarbazine. Therefore, history of a reaction to the drug in question (*inadvertent rechallenge*) may be a key to diagnosis of drug-induced liver disease.

Dechallenge and Rechallenge

Another aspect of the temporal relationship between drug ingestion and hepatotoxicity is the response to discontinuation of the drug, or *dechallenge*. Dechallenge should be accompanied by discernible and progressive clinical and biochemical improvement within days or weeks of stopping the incriminated agent. Exceptions to this rule include ketoconazole, troglitazone, coumarol, etretinate, and amiodarone; with these agents, reactions may be severe, and clinical recovery may be delayed for months. Although some types of drug-induced cholestasis also can be prolonged, failure of jaundice to resolve in suspected drug reactions most often indicates an alternative diagnosis. Rarely, *deliberate rechallenge* may be used to confirm the diagnosis of drug-induced liver disease or to prove the involvement of one particular agent when the patient has been exposed to several drugs. This approach is potentially hazardous, however, and should be undertaken only with a fully informed and consenting (in writing) patient, and preferably with the approval of an institutional ethics committee.

A PRACTICAL APPROACH TO DIAGNOSIS

In the absence of specific diagnostic tests, the diagnosis of drug-induced liver disease requires clinical suspicion, exclusion of other disorders, a carefully taken drug history, and consideration of the temporal relationships between ingestion of the drug and the onset of liver disease. The objective weighing of evidence for and against individual agents, *causality assessment*, is a probabilistic form of diagnosis.[95,96] Several clinical scales that incorporate and give weight to various features have been described.[97,98] Although the performance of these scales is modest, the scales serve as a framework for aspects to be addressed in cases of suspected hepatic adverse drug reactions, thereby improving the consistency of diagnosis.[8,99] In some cases, a liver biopsy may be indicated to exclude other diseases and provide further clues to a drug etiology. In the future, in vitro tests may provide confirmatory evidence for particular drugs,[89,98] but rechallenge currently is the gold standard for diagnosis of drug-induced liver disease.

PHYSICIAN AWARENESS

Physician awareness is crucial to the diagnosis of drug-induced liver disease. The sources of potential hepatotoxins include prescribed medications, over-the-counter drugs (e.g., ibuprofen), preparations used in CAM (see Chapter 125), substances taken for recreational use (e.g., cocaine, "ecstasy") or self-poisoning, and environmental contaminants in food and water supplies and in the home, workplace, and community (see Chapter 84). Unfortunately, patients and physicians do not always heed early nonspecific symptoms associated with reactions to hepatotoxic drugs. Isoniazid is a classic example; preventable deaths from liver failure still occur more than 30 years after the recognition that isoniziad can cause drug hepatitis. Continuing education and availability of information about potentially hepatotoxic drugs are important isssues, and physicians have a professional and legal obligation to inform patients about possible adverse drug reactions.

Drug toxicity should be considered in cases of obscure or poorly explained liver disease, including cases characterized by mixed or atypical patterns of cholestasis and hepatitis, unexplained cholestasis (after common causes have been excluded), particularly in the elderly, and histologic features that suggest a drug etiology. It is then mandatory to *address the drug history as a special investigation*, with attention paid to separate sources of information (household members, primary care providers), examination of household drug cupboard contents, use of nonprescribed medications, and exposure to environmental toxins (see Chapter 84).

EXCLUSION OF OTHER DISORDERS

Exclusion of other disorders is essential before hepatobiliary disease can be ascribed to a drug. For acute and chronic hepatocellular reactions, viral and autoimmune causes of hepatitis and vascular and metabolic disorders must be considered.[5] In a study published in 1993,[100] 60% of cases reported as drug-related syndromes were later found to be associated with hepatitis C. On the other hand, some types of drug-induced chronic hepatitis are associated with autoantibodies, thus superficially resembling autoimmune hepatitis, as occurs with nitrofurantoin. Drug-induced cholestasis should be considered only after dilatation of the common bile duct has been excluded by imaging. In older patients, and particularly when the patient has not been taking agents known to cause cholestasis, cholangiography (e.g., magnetic resonance cholangiography or endoscopic retrograde cholangiography [ERCP]) is obligatory, as is liver biopsy. The potential interaction between drugs and metabolic factors is particularly complex in patients with steatohepatitis (see later).

EXTRAHEPATIC FEATURES

Extrahepatic features such as skin rash, eosinophilia, and involvement of other organs are relatively specific for adverse drug reactions (see earlier). The *absence* of these features is not helpful, however, because they are present in only a minority of cases of drug-induced liver disease; in particular, drugs that cause idiosyncratic liver injury by nonimmunologic mechanisms are not usually associated with extrahepatic features. *Specific diagnostic tests* for individual drug-induced liver diseases have been described[89,101] but are not yet widely available or generally accepted. In the case of dose-dependent hepatotoxins, measurement of *blood levels* of the drug or a metabolite may be helpful but is associated with pitfalls, as discussed later.

CHRONOLOGIC RELATIONSHIPS

For most drugs, the chronologic relationship among drug ingestion, onset of liver injury, and resolution of liver disease remains the most important consideration in establishing the diagnosis.[8,97,102,103] The criteria for *temporal eligibility* include relation to onset, course of the reaction after discontinuation of the drug, and response to readministration of the drug.[102] Deliberate rechallenge is rarely indicated, for logistic and ethical reasons, because it can be hazardous, but *inadvertent rechallenge* may have occurred. Results of rechallenge are regarded as positive if the serum ALT or alkaline phosphatase level increases at least two-fold.[102] Deliberate rechallenge may be considered when it is essential to ascertain that a drug that is important for an individual patient is responsible for hepatotoxicity (e.g., amiodarone for refractory ventricular tachycardia). In other cases, it may be desirable to document the propensity of a newer agent, hitherto unrecognized as a hepatotoxin, to cause liver injury. As mentioned earlier, written informed consent is required for a deliberate rechallenge.

WHICH DRUG?

Use of new and nonproprietary compounds by a patient should arouse particular suspicion in investigating the cause of liver injury. For patients taking multiple drugs, the agent most likely responsible for drug hepatotoxicity is the one started most recently before the onset of liver injury. If that agent is unlikely to be the culprit and another well-known hepatotoxin is being taken by the patient, the latter is the more likely culprit. When possible, the most likely hepatotoxin or all therapeutic agents should be discontinued. If the patient improves, the drugs that are unlikely to be responsible can be carefully reintroduced.

INDICATIONS FOR LIVER BIOPSY

Liver biopsy may be helpful in difficult cases, especially when the temporal relationship between the onset of liver injury and ingestion of a known hepatotoxic agent is unclear. In practice, the onset of jaundice within 2 to 6 weeks of initiation of an agent such as amoxicillin–clavulanic acid and the occurrence of acute hepatitis in the presence of other features of RMS in a person taking nevirapine as part of HAART would be contexts in which the suspicion of a drug etiology is so strong that a liver biopsy is unnecessary. Conversely, a substantial rise in liver biochemistry test levels (greater than five-fold elevation of the serum ALT) and detection of one or more autoantibodies suggestive of autoimmune hepatitis in a person who has been taking a statin or cardiovascular drug for 3 to 6 months may constitute a clinical challenge; in such cases, the diagnosis of drug hepatotoxicity may be readily confirmed by liver biopsy.

CONSIDERATIONS IN PATIENTS WITH VIRAL HEPATITIS

Patients with chronic hepatitis B or C may be at increased risk of liver injury from antituberculosis drugs, ibuprofen and possibly other NSAIDs, anticancer drugs, and HAART agents, compared with persons without viral hepatitis.[43-46] A more common clinical problem is the finding of a serum ALT level greater than 300 U/L at a routine clinic visit in a patient with previous levels less than 150 U/L. In patients with hepatitis C, the rise in serum ALT level is more likely to be the result of drug toxicity than to represent a spontaneous change in the activity of the hepatitis C, particularly when the serum ALT level is greater than 1000 U/L. The most commonly implicated agents are acetaminophen taken in moderate dosage under conditions of increased risk (fasting, alcohol excess, other medication; see later) and CAM preparations, typically Chinese herbal medicines. Clinical suspicion is essential for recognizing a drug cause of liver injury so that appropriate management advice can be given. Determination of blood levels of acetaminophen may be useful in difficult cases, but the levels may be undetectable and thus potentially misleading in the context of regular ingestion, as opposed to a single episode of self-poisoning (see later).

PREVENTION AND MANAGEMENT

With the exception of acetaminophen hepatotoxicity (discussed later), little effective treatment for drug-induced liver disease is available. Special emphasis, therefore, must be placed on prevention and early detection of liver injury, as well as on prompt withdrawal of the offending agent. Safe use of self-medication with agents such as acetaminophen and CAM preparations is important. Clear and open communication between physician and patient and appropriate recommendations about dose limitations could prevent most instances of liver injury from these agents.

A majority of drugs associated with drug-induced liver disease are idiosyncratic hepatotoxins; therefore, liver injury is rare. The overall frequency of adverse hepatic reactions can be minimized by avoiding overuse of these drugs; antibiotics such as amoxicillin–clavulanic acid and flucloxacillin are pertinent examples. Similarly, polypharmacy should be avoided when possible. The rarity of adverse drug reactions also means that the hepatotoxic potential of new agents may not be recognized until after their introduction.[104] All physicians share the responsibility of reporting suspected adverse effects to monitoring agencies during postmarketing surveillance of new drugs.

For dose-dependent hepatotoxins, prevention depends on *adherence to dosage guidelines* or *measurement of blood levels*. This approach has virtually eliminated some forms of drug-induced liver injury, such as tetracycline-induced fatty liver, aspirin hepatitis, and methotrexate-induced hepatic fibrosis. When a drug is associated with specific risk factors, strategies to prevent toxicity are essential (e.g., avoid use of valproic acid with other drugs in the very young; do not prescribe methotrexate for persons who consume alcohol to excess). Likewise, moderate acetaminophen dosing is contraindicated in heavy drinkers and after fasting,[34] and administration of halothane should not be repeated within 28 days or in persons suspected of having previous sensitivity to haloalkane anesthetics.

Early detection of drug-induced liver disease is critical. Patients should be warned to report any untoward symptoms, particularly unexplained nausea, malaise, right upper quadrant abdominal pain, lethargy, or fever. These nonspecific features may represent the prodrome of drug-induced hepatitis and constitute an indication for liver biochemical testing and, if the results suggest liver injury, for cessation of treatment.

A more difficult issue is whether regular screening with liver biochemical tests should be performed when a drug is prescribed.[104-106] Although such screening often is recommended by authors and drug manufacturers, the efficiency and cost-effectiveness of this approach are unknown. The onset of liver injury often is rapid, rendering once-a-month or every-second-week screening futile. Furthermore, 7.5% of persons who receive placebo in clinical trials have persistently raised serum ALT levels.[106] If liver biochemical test values are monitored, the level of abnormality at which drugs should be discontinued is uncertain.[104] The challenges to monitoring are illustrated by isoniazid, which causes some liver biochemical test abnormality in 30% of exposed persons. Generally, it is recommended that the drug be stopped if the serum ALT level exceeds 250 U/L or is more than five times the upper limit of normal, but abnormalities in serum bilirubin or albumin levels or of the prothrombin time provide a clearer indication to stop therapy. Conversely, a rise in serum GGTP or a minor elevation of serum alkaline phosphatase does not usually indicate liver injury. Although we do not routinely recommend protocol screening, it could be useful for agents such as valproic acid, isoniazid, pyrazinamide, ketoconazole, dantrolene, tacrine, thiazolidinediones, and synthetic retinoids, either because the onset of liver injury may be delayed and gradual in some cases or because such screening can serve to emphasize the hepatotoxic potential of a particular drug to patients and physicians. Liver biopsy has a role in the assessment for hepatic fibrosis in patients taking methotrexate (see later).

Occupational exposure to hepatotoxic chemicals raises special issues with regard to prevention, including the avoidance of highly toxic solvents, most of which have been abandoned; adequate ventilation; and use of masks and protective clothing. In some cases, liver biochemical tests are performed routinely in persons exposed to certain agents, but abnormalities are more likely to reflect diseases such as chronic hepatitis C, alcoholism, and NASH than toxic liver injury. In the case of vinyl chloride exposure, periodic physical examination (for hepatomegaly) and hepatic imaging with ultrasonography may be useful (see Chapter 84).

Active management of drug-induced liver injury may include removal of the drug and the administration of antidotes and anti-inflammatory and cytoprotective agents. In practice, treatment usually is confined to *discontinuation of the hepatotoxic drug*. Failure to discontinue a drug that is the cause of liver injury is the single most important factor leading to a poor outcome, such as acute liver failure and chronic liver disease.[29] For ingested toxins like metals, poisonous mushrooms, and acetaminophen, *removal of unabsorbed drug* through the aspiration of stomach contents may be appropriate. Methods to remove absorbed hepatotoxins, such as hemodialysis through charcoal columns and forced diuresis, are not effective for hepatotoxins. For chlordecone, an organochlorine insecticide that is lipid-soluble and

excreted in bile, oral administration of cholestyramine enhances removal from the body by interrupting the enterohepatic cycle.[107] Thiol replacement therapy, usually *N*-acetylcysteine (NAC), is the indicated antidote for acetaminophen poisoning. Whether NAC or other antioxidants have a role in other types of acute hepatotoxicity is unclear, but the flavonoid silybin is traditionally used for *Amanita phalloides* toxicity,[108] and tocopherol analogs show promise in experimental hepatotoxicity.

Beyond discontinuing the offending agent, the management of drug hepatitis and cholestasis is symptomatic and supportive. In cases of acute liver failure, liver transplantation should be considered.[7] Ursodeoxycholic acid has some benefit in the management of chronic cholestasis and pruritus, as discussed later. Glucocorticoids have little role in management of drug-induced cholestasis or hepatitis and are ineffective in chlorpromazine-, methyldopa-, and isoniazid-induced hepatitis and in drug-induced fulminant hepatic failure. Case reports attest to the occasional effectiveness of glucocorticoids in protracted cases of hepatitis caused by etretinate, allopurinol, diclofenac, and ketoconazole.[5] Glucocorticoids should be reserved for atypical and refractory cases, particularly those associated with vasculitis. Clinical evidence of the effectiveness of putative hepatoprotective agents, such as prostaglandin analogs, is lacking.

DOSE-DEPENDENT HEPATOTOXICITY

Few dose-dependent hepatotoxins are clinically important today. Examples are acetaminophen, some herbal medicines (CAM preparations), plant and fungal toxins, amodiaquine, hycanthone, vitamin A, methotrexate, cyclophosphamide, anticancer drugs, carbon tetrachloride, phosphorus, and metals (especially iron, copper, and mercury). Acetaminophen is by far the most important of these; hepatotoxicity of CAM preparations and other toxins is discussed in Chapter 84.

Acetaminophen

General Nature, Frequency, and Predisposing Factors

Acetaminophen (paracetamol) is a widely used analgesic available without prescription. It is safe when taken in the recommended therapeutic dose of 1 to 4 g daily, but hepatotoxicity produced by *self-poisoning with acetaminophen* has been recognized since the 1960s. Despite the effectiveness of thiol-based antidotes, acetaminophen remains *the most common cause of drug-induced liver injury in most countries* and an important cause of acute liver failure.[7,109] Suicide or suicide gesture is the usual reason for an overdose.[109,110] Although the concept is controversial,[111,112] hepatologists and pediatricians see cases of acetaminophen poisoning that have arisen through what Zimmerman and Maddrey have termed a *therapeutic misadventure*.[113] This occurrence is especially common in persons who habitually drink alcohol to excess[113] and also has been recognized after daily ingestion of moderate therapeutic doses (10 to 20 g over 3 days) of acetaminophen in adults and children who are fasting or malnourished[34] or who are taking drugs that interact with the metabolism of acetaminophen.[113,114]

Single doses of acetaminophen exceeding 7 to 10 g (140 mg/kg of body weight in children) may cause liver injury, but not inevitably. Severe (as indicated by serum ALT levels greater than 1000 U/L) or fatal liver injury usually involves acetaminophen doses of at least 15 to 25 g, but because of interindividual variability, survival is possible even after ingestion of a single massive dose of acetaminophen (greater than 50 g).[115] Among persons with an untreated acetaminophen overdose, severe liver injury occurred in only 20%, and among those with severe liver injury, the mortality rate was 20%.[115] Conversely, among heavy drinkers, daily doses of 2 to 6 g have been associated with fatal hepatotoxicity.[113]

Risk factors for acetaminophen-induced hepatotoxicity are summarized in Table 83–3. Children are relatively resistant to acetaminophen-induced hepatotoxicity, possibly because of their tendency to ingest smaller doses, greater likelihood of vomiting, or biologic resistance. Therapeutic misadventure involving administration of multiple doses, especially during fasting and when weight-based recommendations have been exceeded, carries a high mortality rate, however.[116] By contrast, the presence of underlying liver disease does not predispose the patient to acetaminophen hepatotoxicity.

Self-poisoning with acetaminophen is most common in young women, but fatalities are more frequent in men, possibly because of alcoholism and late presentation.[109-112] The time of presentation is critical, because thiol therapy given within 12 hours of acetaminophen poisoning virtually abolishes significant liver injury.[109-111] Therapeutic misadventure also is associated with a worse outcome than that observed with self-poisoning.[112] Concomitant use of agents such as phenobarbital, phenytoin, isoniazid,[114,117] and zidovudine is another risk factor for acetaminophen hepatotoxicity. These drugs may promote the oxidative metabolism of acetaminophen to NAPQI by inducing CYP2E1 (for isoniazid) or CYP3A4 (for phenytoin) or by competing with glucuronidation pathways (for zidovudine). Alcohol and fasting have dual effects by enhancing expression of CYP2E1 and by depleting hepatic glutathione. Fasting also may impair conjugation by acetaminophen-depleting cofactors for the glucuronidation and sulfation pathways.[34]

Acetaminophen hepatotoxicity produces zone 3 necrosis, with submassive (bridging) or panacinar (massive) necrosis in severe cases.[93] Inflammation is minimal, and recovery is associated with complete resolution without fibrosis. The zonal pattern of acetaminophen-induced necrosis is related to the localization of CYP2E1, which is expressed in zone 3 of the hepatic acinus, and of glutathione, levels of which are lower in zone 3 than in zones 1 and 2.

Clinical Course, Outcomes, and Prognostic Indicators

In the first 2 days after acetaminophen self-poisoning, features of liver injury are not present. Nausea, vomiting, and drowsiness often are caused by concomitant ingestion of alcohol and other drugs. After 48 to 72 hours, serum ALT levels may be elevated, and symptoms such as anorexia, nausea and vomiting, fatigue, and malaise may occur. Hepatic pain may be pronounced. In severe cases, the course is characterized by repeated vomiting, jaundice, hypoglycemia, and other features of acute liver failure, particularly coagulopathy and hepatic encephalopathy. The liver may shrink as a result of severe necrosis. Levels of ALT are often between 2000 and 10,000 U/L. These high levels, together with those of other intracellular proteins (ferritin, glutathione S-transferases), may provide a clue to the diagnosis in complex settings, including suggestive symptoms in alcoholic persons and those with viral hepatitis.[113]

Indicators of a poor outcome include grade IV hepatic coma, acidosis, severe and sustained impairment of coagulation factor synthesis, renal failure, and a pattern of falling serum ALT levels in conjunction with a worsening prothrombin time[109-112] (see also Chapter 90). Renal failure reflects acute tubular necrosis or the hepatorenal syndrome. Myocardial injury has also been attributable to acetaminophen toxicity.[115] Death occurs between 4 and 18 days after the overdose and generally results from cerebral edema and sepsis complicating hepatic and multiorgan failure. A majority of the patients recover completely. Rare cases of apparent chronic hepatotoxicity have been attributed to continued ingestion of acetaminophen (2 to 6 g per day), usually in a susceptible host such as a heavy drinker or a person with preexisting, unrecognized liver disease.[5,6] Very rare cases of acetaminophen hypersensitivity, typically involving skin or lung, have been reported in association with liver injury.[118-120]

Management

In patients who present within 4 hours of ingesting an excess amount of acetaminophen, the stomach should be

---

Table 83–3   Risk Factors for Acetaminophen-Induced Hepatotoxicity

Factor	Relevance
Age	Children may be more resistant than adults
Dose	Minimal hepatotoxic dose: 7.5 g (≈100 mg/kg) in adults, >150 mg/kg in children
	Severe toxicity possible with dose >15 g
Blood level	Influenced by dose, time after ingestion, gastric emptying
	Best indicator of risk of hepatotoxicity (see text and Fig. 83–2)
Chronic excessive alcohol ingestion	Toxic dose threshold lowered; worsens prognosis (also related to late presentation); nephrotoxicity common
Fasting	Toxic dose threshold lowered—therapeutic misadventure (see text)
Concomitant medication	Toxic dose threshold lowered—therapeutic misadventure; worsens prognosis (e.g., isoniazid, phenytoin, zidovudine)
Time of presentation	Late presentation or delayed treatment (>16 hr) predicts worse outcome

emptied with a wide-bore gastric tube. Osmotic cathartics or binding agents have little if any role in management. Charcoal hemoperfusion has no established role. The focus of management is on identifying patients who should receive thiol-based antidote therapy and, in patients with severe liver injury, assessment of candidacy for liver transplantation.

Blood levels of acetaminophen should be measured at the time of presentation. Because of delayed gastric emptying, however, blood levels within 4 hours of ingestion may underestimate the extent of exposure. After 4 hours, *acetaminophen blood levels give a reliable indicator of the risk of liver injury* in acute overdose (but not with a therapeutic misadventure). The risk of liver injury is then estimated by reference to the Prescott nomogram[115] (Fig. 83–2). Indications for antidote therapy include a reliable history of major poisoning (more than 10 g), blood acetaminophen level in the moderate- or high-risk bands, or both.[110,115] At-risk patients should be hospitalized for monitoring.

Hepatic necrosis occurs only when glutathione concentrations fall below a critical level, thereby allowing NAPQI to produce liver injury. Administration of cysteine donors stimulates hepatic synthesis of glutathione. Many cysteine precursors or thiol donors could be used, but NAC has become the agent of choice. Oral administra-

tion is preferred in the United States,[109,115] with a loading dose of 140 mg/kg, followed by administration of 70 mg/kg every 4 hours, for up to 72 hours. This regimen is highly effective,[121] despite the theoretical disadvantage that delayed gastric emptying and vomiting may reduce absorption of NAC. In Europe and Australia, NAC is administered by slow bolus intravenous injection followed by infusion (150 mg/kg over 15 minutes in 200 mL of 5% dextrose, with a second dose of 50 mg/kg 4 hours later, when the blood acetaminophen levels indicate a high risk of hepatotoxicity, and a total dose over 24 hours of 300 mg/kg).[115] The intravenous route may be associated with a higher rate of hypersensitivity reactions because much higher blood levels are achieved.[5] Adverse reactions to NAC may be severe and include rash, angioedema, and shock, which occasionally is fatal.[5] Therefore, NAC must be administered under close supervision and only for appropriate indications. For patients known to be sensitized to NAC, methionine is probably just as effective but is not available in a commercial preparation; it must be made up fresh, and it often causes vomiting.[115]

Cases of acetaminophen-induced severe liver injury are virtually abolished if NAC is administered within 12 hours and possibly within 16 hours of acetaminophen ingestion.[109,110,115] After 16 hours, thiol donation is unlikely to affect the development of liver injury, because oxidation of acetaminophen to NAPQI, with consequent oxidation of thiol groups, is complete, and mitochondrial injury and activation of cell death pathways are likely to be established. Nevertheless, NAC has been reported to decrease the mortality associated with acetaminophen-induced hepatotoxicity when administered 16 to 36 hours after self-poisoning,[109,110,115] possibly because NAC stabilizes vascular reactivity in liver failure. Therefore, administration of NAC is recommended even for patients with a late presentation after acetaminophen overdose. Other strategies to protect the liver against acetaminophen poisoning that are efficacious in rats, such as inhibition of CYP-dependent metabolism through the use of cimetidine or administration of prostaglandin analogs, have not been established as clinically useful in humans. The constitutive androstane receptor (CAR) has been identified as a regulator of acetaminophen metabolism and hepatotoxicity in mice,[122] and inhibition of CAR activity by administration of androstanol 1 hour after acetaminophen dosing has been shown to block liver injury.

Liver transplantation has been advocated as a therapeutic option for select patients in whom liver failure develops after acetaminophen poisoning.[109,110] The selection of cases is based on the aforementioned prognostic indicators and is strongly influenced by the prospects for successful psychological rehabilitation (see Chapter 92). In several series, approximately 60% of listed patients have received transplants, and survival rates have exceeded 70%.

Prevention

Safe use of acetaminophen involves adherence to the recommended daily maximum dose for healthy adults and children, and education about the risk factors that lower the toxic dose threshold. Acetaminophen doses of more

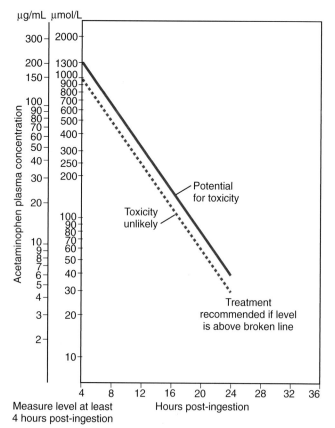

Measure level at least 4 hours post-ingestion

Figure 83–2 Acetaminophen toxicity nomogram. The risk of hepatotoxicity correlates with the plasma acetaminophen level and the time after ingestion. (From Smilkstein MJ, Knapp GL, Kulig KW, et al: Efficacy of oral *N*-acetylcysteine in the treatment of acetaminophen overdose. Analysis of the National Multicenter Study [1976-1985]. N Engl J Med 319:1557, 1988.)

than 2 g each day are contraindicated in heavy drinkers, in persons who take other medications (particularly phenytoin, zidovudine, and isoniazid), and during fasting. Prolonged use of acetaminophen requires caution in patients with severe cardiorespiratory disease or advanced cirrhosis. Use of acetaminophen for self-poisoning continues despite attempts at public education about the risks involved. The chance of harm from suicidal gestures may be reduced by the sale of acetaminophen in smaller packages and in blister packs, which hamper ready access to the tablets or capsules.[124,125]

OTHER TYPES OF CYTOPATHIC LIVER INJURY

Some hepatotoxins are not as clearly dose dependent as acetaminophen but cause cytopathic or cytotoxic changes, such as extensive hydropic change, diffuse or zonal microvesicular steatosis, zonal necrosis, or combinations of these lesions.[5,6] Injury probably represents *metabolic idiosyncrasy* in which the drug or one of its metabolites accumulates and interferes with protein synthesis, intermediary metabolism, or both. The mitochondrion often appears to be the main subcellular target, and other metabolically active tissues also can be injured. For example, pancreatitis and renal tubular injury may accompany severe liver injury caused by valproic acid, tetracycline, and drugs used in highly active antiretroviral therapy (HAART), and metabolic acidosis with a shock-like state is common with toxicity caused by these agents. The first agent recognized to cause this clinicopathologic syndrome was tetracycline administered in high doses (greater than 2 g per day for more than 4 days, usually intravenously) to pregnant women, to men receiving estrogens, or to patients with renal failure.[6] With appropriate dose limitations, this reaction is entirely preventable.

Niacin (Nicotinic Acid)

Hepatotoxicity associated with use of niacin, or nicotinic acid (3-pyridinecarboxylic acid), has been noted since the 1960s. When used to treat hypercholesterolemia, niacin has been an important cause of liver injury.[120,126] It is a dose-dependent hepatotoxin; liver injury usually occurs at doses that exceed 2 g per day, but in rare instances, low-dose (500 mg per day), sustained-release niacin has been implicated in fulminant hepatic failure.[127] Patients taking sulfonylurea drugs and those with preexisting liver disease, particularly alcoholic hepatitis, are at increased risk.[127] No association with age, diet, or insulin-managed diabetes has been recognized. The symptoms of niacin hepatotoxicity begin as early as 1 week to as long as 4 years after the drug is started. The clinicopathologic spectrum encompasses mild and transient increases in serum aminotransferase levels, jaundice, acute hepatitis, and cholestasis. Liver injury resolves completely when the drug is stopped. Liver biopsy specimens show hepatic necrosis and centrilobular cholestasis.[128] Well-documented cases of fulminant hepatitis also have been attributed to niacin, in some cases necessitating liver transplantation.[129] Product substitution without dose adjustment should be avoided; switching from an imme-

diate-release to a sustained-release preparation requires a 50% to 70% reduction in the dose of niacin.

Valproic Acid (Sodium Valproate)

Vaproic acid–associated hepatic injury occurs almost exclusively in children, particularly those younger than 3 years of age.[130] Also at risk are persons with a family history of mitochondrial enzyme deficiencies (particularly involving the urea cycle or long-chain fatty acid metabolism), Friedreich's ataxia, Reye's syndrome, or a history of valproic acid hepatotoxicity in a sibling. Another risk factor is multiple drug therapy. Cases in adults have been described very rarely.[131] The overall risk of liver injury among persons taking valproic acid varies, ranging from 1 per 500 exposed persons among high-risk groups (children younger than 3 years of age, polypharmacy, genetic defects of mitochondrial enzymes) to less than 1 in 37,000 in low-risk groups.[132]

No relationship exists between valproic acid toxicity and dose, but blood levels of valproic acid tend to be high in one half of affected persons. The metabolite, 4-en-valproic acid, produced by CYP-catalyzed metabolism of valproic acid, is a dose-dependent hepatotoxin in animal models and in vitro. The concept has emerged that valproic acid is an occult dose-dependent toxin in which accumulation of a hepatotoxic metabolite (favored by coexposure to CYP-inducing antiepileptic agents) produces mitochondrial injury in a susceptible host (e.g., young children, especially those with partial deficiencies of mitochondrial enzymes).[5,29,133]

Symptoms begin 4 to 12 weeks after valproic acid therapy is started and often are nonspecific, including lethargy, malaise, poor feeding, somnolence, worsening seizures, muscle weakness, and facial swelling. In typical cases, features of hepatotoxicity follow, including anorexia, nausea, vomiting, abdominal discomfort over the region of the liver, and weight loss.[5,29] After jaundice appears, hypoglycemia, ascites, coagulation disorders, and encephalopathy indicate liver failure with imminent coma and death. In some cases, a neurologic syndrome characterized by ataxia, mental confusion, and coma predominates, with little evidence of hepatic involvement.[133] In other cases, fever and tender hepatomegaly suggestive of Reye's syndrome may be present (see later); patients with this latter syndrome tend to have a better prognosis. Additional extrahepatic features may include alopecia, hypofibrinogenemia, thrombocytopenia, and pancreatitis. The terminal phase often is marked by renal failure, hypoglycemia, metabolic acidosis, and severe bacterial infection.

Laboratory features include modest elevations of serum bilirubin and ALT levels; the aspartate aminotransferase (AST) level usually is higher than the ALT level. Profound depression of clotting factor levels, hypoalbuminemia, and raised serum ammonia levels are common. A small liver with increased echogenicity on hepatic imaging is suggestive of steatosis or extensive necrosis. Histologic examination of the liver shows submassive or massive hepatic necrosis in two thirds of cases, with either zonal or generalized microvesicular steatosis. Ultrastructural studies indicate conspicuous abnormalities of the mitochondria.

Treatment is supportive. At least 60 fatalities have been reported, and the mortality rate remains high. Prevention depends on careful adherence to prescribing guidelines, including the avoidance of valproic acid in combination with other drugs in the first 3 years of life and in children who may have mitochondrial enzyme abnormalities. Elevations of liver biochemical test levels develop in at least 40% of patients who take valproic acid and therefore constitute an unreliable predictor of severe hepatotoxicity. It is important to warn patients and parents about the need to report any adverse symptoms during the first 6 months of valproic acid therapy.

Fialuridine

Fialuridine (FIAU) (1-[2′-deoxy-2′-fluoro-β-D-arabinofuranosyl]-5-iodouracil), a nucleoside analog that acts as a chain terminator for DNA synthesis, is a potent inhibitor of HBV replication that showed early promise in short-term trials. A study to examine efficacy and safety of a 6-month course was stopped as soon as toxicity was recognized.[134] The onset of toxicity was delayed. Hepatic and renal dysfunction developed in 14 of 15 patients, often in association with peripheral and autonomic neuropathy, myopathy, and pancreatitis. Severe complications developed in 7 of the 10 patients who received the drug for more than 8 weeks, and 5 died.[134]

The constellation of metabolic acidosis, hepatic failure, and renal failure is best explained as a form of mitochondrial toxicity, as supported by ultrastructural changes.[135] Further work is required to explain completely the delayed onset of hepatic toxicity; phosphorylation of FIAU and inhibition of mitochondrial DNA synthesis are likely to be involved.[136,137]

Antiretroviral Agents

Abnormal liver biochemical test levels and clinical evidence of liver disease are common in patients with HIV infection/AIDS. Underlying reasons include HBV or HCV infection, other hepatobiliary infections, lymphoma and other tumors, and possibly effects of HIV infection itself. Of note, however, the frequency of hepatic injury associated with HAART, which often includes three to four agents, is at least 10%.[39,44,138] The agents used can be broadly categorized as nucleoside (or nucleotide) reverse transcriptase inhibitors, non-nucleoside reverse transcriptase inhibitors, and protease inhibitors. Because co-infection with HBV or HCV increases the risk of toxicity, all patients should be screened for viral hepatitis before starting HAART.

Nucleoside (or Nucleotide) Reverse Transcriptase Inhibitors

Nucleosides and nucleotides that block HIV reverse transcriptase also are weak inhibitors of mitochondrial DNA polymerase gamma in vitro; the order of potency is *zalcitabine > didanosine > stavudine > lamivudine > zidovudine > abacavir*.[139] These drugs may cause deletion of mitochondrial DNA. The mechanism of hepatotoxicity also may involve oxidative stress, resulting in further deletion of mitochondrial DNA and other consequences, including impaired oxidative phosphorylation, fatty acyl β-oxidation, and insulin resistance.

In clinical studies, zidovudine, didanosine, and stavudine are the agents most often implicated in liver injury.[140-146] Risk factors for mitochondrial drug toxicity among persons with HIV infection include obesity, female gender, and absence of an AIDS-defining illness.[147] Hallmarks of mitochondrial hepatotoxicity include extensive microvesicular or macrovesicular steatosis, or both, lactic acidosis, and liver biochemical test abnormalities progressing to acute liver failure. Asymptomatic hyperlactatemia is common (especially with stavudine) among persons receiving HAART,[147] but life-threatening lactic acidosis with hepatic steatosis is rare; the estimated risk is 1.3 per 1000 person-years of antiretroviral drug use. The onset is at a median of 6 months (with a range of 3 to 17 months) after initiation of treatment. The presenting manifestations are nonspecific and include nausea, vomiting, diarrhea, dyspnea, lethargy, and abdominal pain. Extrahepatic manifestations, such as myopathy or peripheral neuropathy and, in severe cases, pancreatitis and renal failure, may follow the onset of lactic acidosis and liver injury. Discontinuation of drugs is mandatory but may not prevent fatalities. Nevertheless, the overall mortality rate is low.[46] One suggested approach to prevention is to monitor therapy with nucleoside reverse transcriptase inhibitors by coupling serum ALT and AST testing with serial measurements of HIV loads and CD4+ counts. Any new serum ALT elevation should be monitored closely in conjunction with measurement of serum lactate and muscle and pancreatic enzyme levels.[145]

Non-Nucleoside Reverse Transcriptase Inhibitors

Non-nucleoside reverse transcriptase inhibitors occasionally may cause hepatitis as part of a hypersensitivity reaction within the first 6 weeks of use.[138,148] Reactions usually are accompanied by peripheral and tissue eosinophilia, skin rash, and lymphadenopathy. Resolution occurs within 4 weeks of discontinuing the drug.[148] *Nevirapine* also has been implicated in several instances of severe hepatotoxicity,[149,150] including cases among health care workers in whom nevirapine was used for postexposure prophylaxis against HIV infection.[150] The FDA received 12 reports of such hepatotoxic reactions from 1997 through 2000: Liver failure developed in one person, who subsequently required hepatic transplantation; seven had clinical features of hepatitis (jaundice, fever, nausea, vomiting, abdominal pain, and/or hepatomegaly); and four had elevated serum ALT levels without symptomatic illness. The recommended 2-week dose escalation regimen was not adhered to in some of the cases.[151] Sequential toxicity with nevirapine followed by *efavirenz* has been reported in an HIV-HCV–co-infected person.[152]

Protease Inhibitors

Elevation of liver enzymes occurs commonly with protease inhibitors, but clinical hepatitis is infrequent. The agents implicated most often in liver injury are *ritonavir* and *indinavir*. The latter also may be associated with unconjugated hyperbilirubinemia in 7% of persons receiving the drug, a finding that is of no clinical consequence but may be striking in patients with Gilbert's syndrome (see Chapter 14).[148] Severe acute hepatitis may occur rarely. The association of hepatotoxicity with peripheral or tissue eosinophilia (in liver biopsy specimens) in some cases suggests an immunoallergic basis for liver injury.[153,154] Acute hepatitis also has been reported in 2.9% to 30% of persons prescribed ritonavir.[155] The course of the illness generally is mild, and the liver injury responds favorably to drug withdrawal. Rarely, acute liver failure may develop; in these cases, liver histologic examination has shown severe microvesicular steatosis, cholestasis, and extensive fibrosis.[156]

Several studies have addressed the potential influence of underlying chronic viral hepatitis on the toxicity of protease inhibitors. Although hepatotoxicity appeared to be more common in patients with chronic viral hepatitis, liver injury was rapidly reversible in most cases, suggesting that toxicity of protease inhibitors is not detrimental in co-infected persons.[157] Many protease inhibitors induce or inhibit CYP3A4, thereby causing important drug-drug interactions.[158] Furthermore, the immune reconstitution that can follow successful HAART may cause a flare-up of previously quiescent chronic hepatitis B (see Chapter 32).[159]

Aspirin

Aspirin occasionally has been associated with major increases in serum ALT levels suggestive of drug hepatitis, but hepatotoxicity occurs only when blood salicylate concentrations exceed 25 mg/dL.[5,160] In addition, individual susceptibility factors include hypoalbuminemia and a diagnosis of active juvenile rheumatoid arthritis or systemic lupus erythematosus. Most cases of aspirin-induced hepatotoxicity have been identified by liver biochemical testing, rather than clinical features. If present, symptoms usually begin within the first few days or weeks of high-dose aspirin therapy. Acute liver failure has rarely been observed, and only one fatality has been reported. Resolution occurs rapidly after drug withdrawal, and salicylates can be reintroduced at a lower dose. All salicylates appear to carry hepatotoxic potential, so there is no advantage to replacing aspirin with another salicylate. Liver biopsy specimens reveal a nonspecific focal hepatitis with hepatocellular degeneration and hydropic changes. Steatosis is not usually present, and the absence of steatosis distinguishes aspirin hepatotoxicity from Reye's syndrome.

Patients with juvenile rheumatoid arthritis (Still's disease) or systemic lupus erythematosus appear to be at peculiar risk for aspirin hepatotoxicity. Clinical or laboratory features of chronic liver disease do not develop in these patients, nor do features of drug allergy. Management centers on suspicion of the correct diagnosis and reduction in the dose (or discontinuation) of aspirin. Recovery is usually rapid. Aspirin can be used again in a lower dose, but other NSAIDs have displaced high-dose aspirin for most conditions.

Reye's syndrome has been linked with aspirin use in febrile children. Although Reye's syndrome is not simply a form of drug-induced liver disease, aspirin plays an important role in its multifactorial pathogenesis. Reye's syndrome usually occurs between 3 and 4 days after an apparently minor viral infection. The syndrome is characterized by acute encephalopathy and hepatic injury that is documented by a three-fold or greater rise in serum aminotransferase or ammonia levels and by characteristic histologic findings. Because of effective public health campaigns warning against the use of aspirin in young febrile children, the incidence of Reye's syndrome has declined markedly.[161]

Other Drugs

L-Asparaginase is an antileukemic drug that often causes hepatotoxicity, which usually is reversible but can result in liver failure associated with diffuse microvesicular steatosis.[162]

Amodiaquine, a 4-aminoquinolone antimalarial agent, has been associated with fatal hepatotoxicity, as well as with agranulocytosis.[163] Toxicity may be related to the total dose of drug. Amodiaquine should be reserved for active treatment of chloroquine-resistant falciparum malaria, and dose recommendations should be strictly observed.

Hycanthone is an antischistosomal agent for which dose is the most important risk factor for hepatotoxicity. Other risk factors for hepatotoxicity include concomitant administration of phenothiazines or estrogens, preexisting liver injury, and bacterial infection.[164]

The hepatotoxic effects of environmental toxins, illicit drug abuse substances, and metals are discussed in Chapter 84.

DRUG-INDUCED ACUTE HEPATITIS

The term *acute hepatitis* is used for lesions characterized by the presence of hepatic inflammation with conspicuous hepatocyte cell death or degeneration. More severe lesions include zonal and bridging necrosis or massive (panlobular) hepatic necrosis; these lesions may be associated with *fulminant* or *subfulminant hepatic failure*.[5,6] Acute hepatitis accounts for nearly one half of reported adverse drug reactions involving the liver,[1-4] and potential causative agents are numerous.[5,6,164]

Two broad types of drug hepatitis are those with clinical and laboratory features consistent with drug allergy (immunoallergic reactions) and those without such features. The latter may be the result of metabolic idiosyncrasy; partial dose dependence, relationship to metabolism of the drug, and histologic or ultrastructural features consistent with chemical toxicity often are found. The clinical and laboratory features that suggest one or the other type of drug hepatitis are summarized in Table 83–4. Nitrofurantoin is discussed next as an example of immunoallergy, whereas isoniazid is used to illustrate metabolic idiosyncrasy. Other relatively frequent examples of drug hepatitis also are described briefly.

IMMUNOALLERGIC REACTIONS

Nitrofurantoin

Nitrofurantoin, a synthetic furan-based compound, is a urinary antiseptic with a range of uncommon adverse effects. The frequency of nitrofurantoin hepatic injury is between 0.3 and 3 cases per 100,000 exposed persons.[165]

Table 83–4 Types of Drug-Induced Acute Hepatitis: Immunoallergic Reactions versus Metabolic Idiosyncrasy

Characteristic	Immunoallergic Type	Metabolic Idiosyncrasy
Frequency	<1 case per 10,000 persons exposed	1 to 50 cases per 10,000 persons exposed
Gender predilection	Women, often ≥2 : 1	Variable, slightly more common in women
Latent period to onset	Fairly constant, 2 to 10 weeks	More variable, 2 to 24 weeks, occasionally longer than 1 year
Relationship to dose	None	Usually none (occasional exceptions)
Interactions with other agents	None	Alcohol; occasionally other drugs (e.g., isoniazid with rifampin)
Course after stopping drug	Prompt improvement (rare exceptions, e.g., minocycline)	Variable; occasionally slow improvement or deterioration (e.g., troglitazone)
Positive rechallenge	Always; often fever within 3 days	Usual (in two thirds of cases), abnormal liver biochemical test levels in 2 to 21 days
Fever	Usual; often initial symptom, part of prodrome	Infrequent, less prominent
Extrahepatic features (rash, lymphadenopathy)	Common	Rare
Eosinophilia:		
Blood	33% to 67% of cases	<10% of cases
Tissue	Usual, pronounced	Common but mild
Autoantibodies	Often present	Rarely present
Examples	Nitrofurantoin, phenytoin, methyldopa, sulfonamides, etretinate, minocycline	Isoniazid, pyrazinamide, ketoconazole, dantrolene, troglitazone

The risk increases with age, particularly after the age of 64 years. Two thirds of acute cases occur in women, and the female-to-male ratio is 8 : 1 for chronic hepatitis.[165,166] The range of liver diseases associated with nitrofurantoin includes acute hepatitis, sometimes with features of cholestasis, hepatic granulomas, chronic hepatitis with autoimmune phenomena, acute liver failure, and cirrhosis.[165,166] Causality has been proved by rechallenge, and no relationship to dose has been observed; cases even have been described after ingestion of milk from a nitrofurantoin-treated cow.[167]

The relative frequencies of hepatocellular versus cholestatic or mixed reactions[165,166] and acute versus chronic hepatitis caused by nitrofurantoin have been a subject of debate.[5] Reactions cover a spectrum of biochemical and histologic features, but these features have no apparent relevance to clinical outcome. Chronicity depends mostly on the duration of drug ingestion, which has been less than 6 weeks in acute cases but more than 6 months in 90% of chronic cases.[165,166] Patients with chronic hepatitis often have continued taking nitrofurantoin despite symptoms attributable to adverse drug effects, or they have been exposed to a second course after previous toxicity. The mortality rate for chronic nitrofurantoin hepatitis is 20%, compared with 5% to 10% for acute hepatitis.[165]

The latent period between initial exposure to the drug and the onset of liver disease lasts from a few days to 6 weeks. Early symptoms and signs may be nonspecific (e.g., fever, myalgias, arthralgias, fatigue, malaise, anorexia, weight loss) and are followed by more specific features of hepatitis, such as nausea and vomiting, hepatic pain or discomfort, dark urine, jaundice, and, occasionally, pruritus. Rash occurs in 20% of affected persons, and lymphadenopathy may be present. Pneumonitis complicated by pulmonary fibrosis can develop concurrently with hepatitis in 20% of cases and is suggested by cough and dyspnea. Rarely, liver failure develops, with ascites, coag-

ulopathy, and encephalopathy. In patients with chronic hepatitis, clinical findings may suggest chronic liver disease, such as spider angiomata, hepatosplenomegaly, muscle wasting, and ascites.

Liver biochemical testing may show pronounced elevation of serum ALT levels, but more often the pattern is mixed, with some increase in the serum alkaline phosphate level as well. In other cases, the pattern suggests cholestasis. Serum bilirubin levels tend to be increased in proportion to the severity of the reaction. In contrast with most types of acute drug hepatitis, serum albumin concentrations often are low. Hyperglobulinemia is more likely in patients with chronic hepatitis than in those with acute hepatitis.[165] Eosinophilia occurs in 33% of cases. Autoantibodies (antinuclear antibodies and anti–smooth muscle antibodies) are present in some patients with acute hepatitis and in 80% of those with chronic disease. In contrast with idiopathic autoimmune hepatitis, the frequency of the human leukocyte antigens HLA-B8 and -DRw3 is not increased.[165,166]

No specific treatment exists. Glucocorticoids have no role, even in chronic hepatitis with autoimmune features. Recovery is rapid after discontinuation of nitrofurantoin. Monitoring liver biochemical test levels in users of nitrofurantoin is unlikely to be useful or cost-effective.

Other Drugs

Methyldopa was one of the first drugs reported to cause immunoallergic drug hepatitis. Cases are now rare, because better antihypertensive agents are available. The spectrum of hepatic reactions to methyldopa includes abnormal liver biochemical test levels, severe acute hepatitis, granuloma formation, cholestasis, chronic hepatitis with bridging necrosis, and cirrhosis. The female predilection, clinical and laboratory changes, course, and extrahepatic features of drug allergy are similar to those for nitrofurantoin.[5,6]

Phenytoin causes severe acute hepatitis in less than 1 per 10,000 persons exposed.[5] Incidence rates are equal in men and women, and cases can occur in childhood. Blacks may be affected more often than whites. Rash, fever, eosinophilia, lymphadenopathy, a pseudomononucleosis syndrome, and other allergic features are common, suggesting immunoallergy as part of RMS. A familial enzymatic defect in the disposal of phenytoin arene oxide has been detected among patients with phenytoin reactions, thereby implicating a possible metabolic factor in predisposition to phenytoin reactions.

The mortality rate is 10% to 40%. Some deaths result from liver failure, whereas others result from severe systemic hypersensitivity, bone marrow suppression, exfoliative dermatitis, or vasculitis involving the skin and kidney. Rarer hepatic associations with phenytoin reactions include cholestatic hepatitis and bile duct injury.[5] The most common association with phenytoin therapy is an adaptive response of the liver with induction of microsomal enzymes; at least two thirds of patients have raised serum GGTP levels, and one third exhibit raised serum alkaline phosphatase levels. On histopathologic examination, ground-glass cytoplasm, which represents hypertrophied smooth endoplasmic reticulum, is usually present in hepatocytes.

Barbiturates, including *phenobarbital*, rarely are associated with acute hepatitis. Described cases have been similar to phenytoin reactions; fever and rash are usual, and the rate of mortality resulting from liver failure is high.[168] Among newer antiepileptic drugs, felbamate[169] and topiramate[170] have been associated with acute liver failure.

Sulfonamides are a cause of drug hepatitis that is relatively common with combination drugs such as co-trimoxazole (sulfamethoxazole plus trimethoprim).[1,171] Trimethoprim alone has been infrequently associated with cholestatic hepatitis; the estimated risk is 1.4 cases per 100,000 exposed persons.[171] Reactions to co-trimoxazole resemble those for trimethoprim more closely than for sulfonamides; cholestasis is more common. Patients with HIV infection/AIDS are predisposed to sulfonamide hypersensitivity.[172]

Some drugs have a sulfa moiety that differs from that of sulfonamides but may increase the risk of cross-sensitivity reactions. For example, the COX-2 inhibitor celecoxib has been observed to cause severe hepatitis in two women with a past history of sulfonamide sensitivity.[172] Likewise, sulfonylureas, such as *gliclazide*, rarely have been associated with drug hepatitis with features of immunoallergy.[173]

The latent period between exposure to the drug and the onset of sulfonamide hepatitis is 5 to 14 days. Clinical features often include fever, rash, and mucositis (Stevens-Johnson syndrome), as well as lymphadenopathy and vasculitis (that is, features of RMS).[5,6] Reactions may be severe, and deaths have occurred. The serum ALT level usually is increased to a greater degree than the serum alkaline phosphatase level, but mixed and cholestatic reactions occur. A few cases of hepatic granulomas and chronic hepatitis have also been associated with sulfonamides.

Sulfasalazine (salicylazosulfapyrine, salazopyrine) also has been associated with rare cases of often severe acute hepatitis.[1,174] Although the sulfonamide moiety has been assumed to be responsible, this assumption has been challenged by the report of one patient in whom hepatitis recurred after exposure to *mesalamine* (mesalazine, 5-aminosalicylate).[175] This implicates the salicylate moiety as the cause, and like salicylate hepatitis (discussed earlier), sulfasalazine hepatotoxicity appears to be more common in patients with rheumatoid arthritis than in those with inflammatory bowel disease.[1-4] A case of mesalamine-induced chronic hepatitis with autoimmune features was diagnosed after 21 months of treatment with the drug.[176]

Minocycline and other tetracyclines used in conventional low doses are rare but important causes of drug hepatitis,[14,177] including cases that have resulted in acute liver failure requiring liver transplantation.[178] Minocycline is one of the few agents in current use that can lead to drug-induced autoimmune hepatitis, as discussed later.

Disulfiram (Antabuse) rarely has been associated with acute hepatitis, occasionally leading to liver failure.[179,180] Disulfiram hepatitis is usually easy to distinguish from alcoholic hepatitis by the ten-fold or greater elevation of serum ALT activity.

β-Adrenergic blocking agents rarely have been incriminated in hepatotoxicity. *Acebutolol*,[181] *labetalol*,[182] and *metoprolol*[183] each have been associated with cases of acute hepatitis; some cases were proved by rechallenge. Reactions were hepatocellular and severe. Data are insufficient to indicate whether or not immunoallergy is likely.

The *calcium channel blockers nifedipine*,[184] *verapamil*,[185] and *diltiazem*[186] have a good safety record, but rare cases of acute hepatitis with a short incubation period (5 days to 6 weeks) and other features of immunoallergy have been reported with their use.

Irbesartan is an angiotensin II receptor blocker used primarily to treat hypertension and heart failure. Two cases of cholestasis with irbesartan have been reported.[187,188] In both patients, jaundice developed within 1 month of starting therapy. Liver biochemical test abnormalities were predominantly cholestatic, and findings on ultrasonographic examination of the liver were normal. Histologic examination revealed marked cholestasis in both patients, with an inflammatory infiltrate and eosinophils in one patient. Clinical resolution occurred once the medication was stopped, but biochemical abnormalities persisted for more than 1 year in one of the patients.

Angiotensin-converting enzyme (ACE) inhibitor–induced liver disease is a rare but important complication of this widely prescribed class of drugs. The incidence has been estimated to be 9 per 100,000 patients treated.[189] Reactions to captopril (the oldest and possibly most hepatotoxic representative) and enalapril usually manifest as cholestatic hepatitis, but hepatocellular or mixed hepatocellular reactions can occur.[128,190-192] Features of hypersensitivity such as fever, skin rashes, and eosinophilia have been observed in patients with captopril hepatotoxicity.[190] Histologic examination reveals marked centrilobular cholestasis with eosinophilic portal tract infiltrates.[193] Liver biochemical abnormalities usually resolve after withdrawal of therapy, but resolution may take up to 6 months in some cases. Fulminant hepatic failure has been attributed to lisinopril,[194] and fosinopril has been associated with bland cholestasis.[195]

Hydroxymethylglutaryl-coenzyme A reductase inhibitors ("statins"), as a class of drugs, are not associated strongly with important hepatic injury, although reports in the literature and data contributed to drug safety surveillance authorities appear to be discordant. The use of these drugs has increased greatly, because new guidelines have lowered the target level for low-density lipoprotein (LDL) cholesterol, thereby resulting in the use of higher doses of statins to achieve the desired LDL level. A dose-related rise in serum aminotransferase levels occurs in 1% to 3% of persons who take statins.[196] A minor rise in serum ALT (to less than twice normal) and AST (also to less than twice normal) levels without symptoms is the most common manifestation of liver injury caused by these compounds. These changes are usually rapidly reversible with discontinuation of the drug, but levels also often normalize if therapy is not interrupted.[197] *Lovastatin*,[198] *pravastatin*,[199] *atorvastatin*,[200] and *simvastatin*[201] have been implicated in a few reports of cholestatic hepatitis. Use of some members of this group of lipid-lowering agents in combination with *gemfibrozil* is associated with a higher rate of myositis than that observed with use of a statin alone, but apparently not with a higher rate of drug-induced liver injury. Prescribing guidelines for statins invariably warn about the risk of liver injury when these agents are prescribed to persons with preexisting liver abnormalities. Nevertheless, evidence that fatty liver (or steatohepatitis), hepatitis C, and other common liver disorders predispose to statin-induced liver disease is lacking.[202,203] Monitoring serum aminotransferase levels often is recommended, but this approach is unlikely to predict toxicity[197,204,205] or to be cost-effective. In the Air Force Texas Coronary Atherosclerosis Prevention Study (AFCAPS/TEXCAPS), increases of more than three times the upper limit of normal were observed in only 18 of 100,000 aminotransferase determinations in users of lovastatin; in none of these instances did hepatitis develop.[204]

Etretinate, a synthetic retinoid, is useful for treating several skin diseases. Unlike vitamin A (see Chapter 84), synthetic retinoids are not predictable hepatotoxins, but etretinate has been associated with abnormal liver biochemical test results in 10% to 25% of patients receiving the drug.[5,206] Levels may normalize with a reduction in drug dose, thereby suggesting partial dose dependency. Approximately 10 cases of severe hepatitis have been attributed to etretinate; some have been proved by rechallenge.[5,206] Most patients were women older than 50 years of age; two cases were associated with chronicity, and one patient appeared to respond to glucocorticoids.

Because etretinate has a half-life of 100 days, it is recommended that serum ALT levels be monitored in users of the drug. Progressive increases in serum ALT levels above twice the upper limit of normal constitute an indication to stop the drug or to perform a liver biopsy.[206] *Acitretin*, another synthetic retinoid, has been associated with a single case of severe acute hepatitis.

Gastric acid suppression drugs have an excellent safety record, although rare adverse hepatic reactions have been reported.[5-7,164] The histamine H_2 receptor antagonist *oxmetidine* was removed from clinical trials because

of hepatotoxicity, and subsequently *ebrotidine* was withdrawn because of many cases of liver injury.[207] *Cimetidine*,[208] *ranitidine*,[209] and *famotidine*[210] have been associated with acute hepatitis, mostly mild and often with cholestatic features. Some cases have been proved by rechallenge. Features of immunoallergy were present in some of the cimetidine reactions. Cases of hepatotoxicity attributed to the proton pump inhibitor *omeprazole* are few, and causality has not been proved.[211,212]

Zafirlukast, a leukotriene receptor antagonist effective against asthma, has been reported to cause severe liver injury, with acute liver failure observed in two of three reported cases.[213]

Ticlopidine and *clopidogrel* are antiplatelet agents that have been incriminated in at least one case of microvesicular steatosis and in another of cholestatic hepatitis.[214]

METABOLIC IDIOSYNCRASY

Isoniazid

Isoniazid-induced liver injury has been characterized since the 1970s, but deaths still occur.[215-217] Hepatitis develops in approximately 21 of 1000 persons exposed to isoniazid; 5% to 10% of cases are fatal. The risk and severity of isoniazid hepatitis increase with age; the risk is 0.3% in the third decade of life and increases to 2% or higher after age 50.[215,216] Overall frequency rates are the same in men and in women, but 70% of fatal cases are in women; black and Hispanic women may be at particular risk.[215,216] The risk of toxicity is not related to the dose or blood level of isoniazid. The role of genetic factors has been controversial. Slow acetylators of isoniazid may be at increased risk of toxicity, but the data are conflicting.[5] Chronic excessive alcohol intake increases the frequency and severity of isoniazid hepatotoxicity,[215,216] as may rifampin and pyrazinamide.[216] Concomitant use of pyrazinamide and acetaminophen has been associated with several cases that were fatal or led to hepatic transplantation.[217] Some studies have found that the risk of liver injury from isoniazid and other antituberculosis drugs is increased among persons with chronic HBV infection,[15] but reports are conflicting.[21] Malnutrition may play a role in some countries.[35] Likewise, in patients with HCV or HIV infection (or both), the risk of significant serum ALT elevations during antituberculosis treatment has been reported to be increased several-fold[15]; successful antiviral treatment of hepatitis C allowed the safe reintroduction of antituberculosis drugs in four patients.

Serum ALT levels increase in 10% to 36% of persons taking isoniazid during the first 10 weeks. Abnormalities typically are minor and resolve spontaneously. In persons in whom hepatitis develops, the latent period from exposure to disease ranges from 1 week to more than 6 months; the median is approximately 8 weeks, and 12 weeks for severe cases.[215,216] Re-exposure may be associated with an accelerated onset, although the experience in India is that gradual reintroduction of isoniazid and rifampin therapy can be achieved in a majority of cases after drug hepatitis has resolved.[35] Prodromal symptoms occur in one third of patients and include malaise, fatigue, and early symptoms of hepatitis such as anorexia, nausea, and vomiting. Jaundice appears several days later and is the only feature in approximately 10% of cases. Fever, rash, arthralgias, and eosinophilia are uncommon.

Liver biochemical testing indicates hepatocellular injury; serum AST levels exceed ALT levels in one half of patients. Serum bilirubin levels usually are elevated; values that are increased more than 10-fold indicate a poor prognosis. In one study,[215] one third of patients had a prolonged prothrombin time, and 60% of these cases were fatal. Liver biopsy samples generally show hepatocellular injury, which is focal in approximately one half of cases, often with marked hydropic change in residual hepatocytes. Liver biopsy specimens in the remaining cases show zonal, submassive, or massive necrosis with inflammation confined to the portal tracts. Cholestasis and lobular regeneration suggestive of early cirrhosis are rare features.

Cases with a fatal outcome have been associated with a longer duration of therapy or continued ingestion of isoniazid after the onset of symptoms.[215,216] Therefore, most deaths from isoniazid hepatitis could be prevented if patients report symptoms early and isoniazid is discontinued.[218,219] In 1993, isoniazid hepatitis was reported to be the most common hepatic drug reaction requiring liver transplantation in New York[219]; acetaminophen has since greatly surpassed isoniazid as the most common drug indication for liver transplantation.

Recovery is rapid if isoniazid is discontinued before severe liver injury is established. Management of liver failure is supportive; transplantation is indicated in the most severe cases. Prevention is the most appropriate way to deal with this problem, and it is critical to determine whether the risks of isoniazid preventive therapy outweigh those of latent tuberculosis.[219] The optimal approach to monitoring patients for isoniazid toxicity is uncertain; monitoring of serum ALT levels once or twice per month will not always be adequate to prevent the rapid onset of severe hepatotoxicity. Effective prevention depends on recognition of early symptoms, no matter how nonspecific, that could indicate drug toxicity.

Other Drugs

Other Antituberculosis Drugs
Most cases in which *rifampin* has been implicated with liver injury have occurred in patients taking isoniazid,[220] but a few cases have been observed when rifampin was given alone to patients with underlying liver disease.[221]

Pyrazinamide (as well as the related *ethionamide*) was known as a dose-dependent hepatotoxin in earlier years.[5,6] It is still used in lower doses (1.5 to 2 g per day), because of the emergence of resistant strains of mycobacteria. Hepatotoxicity may be particularly severe in patients taking combinations that include isoniazid and pyrazinamide.[215] Monitoring serum ALT levels during therapy is recommended. Cross-sensitivity among isoniazid, pyrazinamide, and ethionamide is possible.[5,6]

Antifungal Agents
Ketoconazole is associated with raised liver enzyme levels in 5% to 17% of patients taking this drug.[5,222,223] Symptomatic hepatitis occurs in 7 to 20 per 100,000 exposed persons. Women (female-to-male ratio 2:1) and persons older than 40 years of age are particularly susceptible to ketoconazole-induced liver injury.[220] Reactions usually are mild but can be severe, including rare cases of acute liver failure; the mortality rate is 3% to 7%.[222] The onset is at 6 to 12 weeks after ketoconazole therapy is started, and rarely after the drug is stopped. No relation to dose has been observed. Continued ingestion of the drug after the onset of symptoms leads to an adverse outcome. Jaundice occurs in 50% of persons in whom acute hepatitis develops, but up to one third of affected persons may present with nonspecific symptoms such as nausea, anorexia, and vomiting. Fever, rash, eosinophilia, and other immunoallergic characteristics are rare. The pattern of liver biochemical test results is mostly hepatocellular or mixed, but cholestatic hepatitis or bland cholestasis may occur.[222] Resolution of jaundice is usual within 12 weeks but may take months.[222] The role of glucocorticoids in cases that are slow to resolve is unclear. Fulminant hepatic failure requiring liver transplantation has been reported.[224] Fatal liver failure also has followed the use of ketoconazole to reduce hypercortisolism in patients with Cushing's syndrome.[225]

Terbinafine is an allylamine antifungal agent effective against onychomycosis. Several cases of cholestatic hepatitis have been reported.[226-228] The frequency of hepatotoxicity has been estimated to be 2 to 3 cases per 100,000 persons exposed.[227] The onset is usually within 4 to 6 weeks of beginning treatment. Liver biopsy specimens show hepatocyte degeneration and canalicular cholestasis with variable portal tract inflammation.[228] Recovery is usual with discontinuation of the drug, although prolonged cholestasis with ductopenia has been reported. Fulminant hepatic failure also has been described,[229] and a case of sinusoidal obstruction syndrome (veno-occlusive disease) has been associated with use of terbinafine in a liver transplant recipient.[230] The FDA has received at least 16 reports of fulminant liver failure possibly linked to terbinafine,[231] with an estimated frequency of 1 case per 1 million persons exposed.

Fluconazole and *itraconazole* appear to be less hepatotoxic than ketoconazole and terbinafine; elevations of liver biochemical test levels occur in fewer than 5% of patients, and liver injury has been documented in only a few reports.[232-238] Rare cases of severe hepatic necrosis have been ascribed to fluconazole, but other causes were not excluded. Among more than 69,000 patients who received an oral antifungal agent, ketoconazole and itraconazole were most often associated with liver injury; the relative risks were 228 and 17.7, respectively, in comparison with nonusers.[239]

Antidiabetic Drugs
Thiazolidinediones. *Troglitazone* was the first peroxisome proliferator–activated receptor-γ (PPARγ) agonist used in type 2 diabetes for improving glycemic control and lowering serum lipid levels by reducing insulin resistance. Elevations of serum aminotransferase levels were noted in 0.5% to 1.9% of recipients in early trials, which failed to reveal serious hepatotoxicity.[240,241] Reports of acute liver failure emerged in the postmarketing phase,[240-247] in which troglitazone was associated with more than 75 instances of fatal hepatotoxicity or liver failure requiring hepatic transplantation.[248] In one retrospective epi-

demiologic study, troglitazone was not associated with a higher frequency of acute liver injury than that observed with other hypoglycemic agents,[48] but this study included a small number of troglitazone-treated cases.

Reported cases of troglitazone hepatotoxicity generally were in older women and obese persons—the common phenotype for persons with type 2 diabetes. Detailed epidemiologic studies have not been performed to define the risk factors clearly.[249] Evidence that preexisting liver disease or concomitant use of other drugs predisposed these patients to troglitazone hepatotoxicity is lacking, although a progressive course in one patient was attributed to concurrent use of simvastatin and troglitazone.[250]

The onset of troglitazone hepatotoxicity was often as late as 9 to 12 months after treatment was started[251,252]; rare cases had a much earlier onset (8 days).[253] Presenting symptoms and signs included nausea, fatigue, jaundice, vomiting, and manifestations of liver failure. Progression to acute liver failure often was rapid, and in some cases deterioration continued despite discontinuation of troglitazone.[243] Histologic examination of liver biopsy specimens, explants, or autopsies showed submassive or massive hepatic necrosis with post-collapse scarring, bile duct proliferation, and some eosinophils.[241] Severe cholestasis also was reported.[254]

Serious liver injury appears to be rare with the second-generation thiazolidinediones *rosiglitazone* and *pioglitazone*. In clinical trials, a raised serum ALT level (to greater than three times the upper limit of normal) was reported in 0.25% of patients who received rosiglitazone and in 0.26% of those who received pioglitazone.[248] Hepatotoxicity associated with rosiglitazone has been reported.[255-258] In each case, the onset was earlier (e.g., 8 days, 21 days) than for most cases of troglitazone hepatotoxicity, and the patients survived. An alternative diagnosis of ischemic hepatitis (or ischemia-reperfusion injury) was proposed for one of the cases in which exceptionally high serum levels of ALT (11,000 U/L) and rapid resolution (within 9 days) were described. Pioglitazone has been implicated in one report of acute hepatocellular injury in a person also taking another medication. The liver injury resolved 1 week after pioglitazone was discontinued.[259] An isolated reversible increase in the serum alkaline phosphatase level has been described with pioglitazone.[260]

Before treatment with drugs of this class is begun, the FDA recommends that liver biochemical tests be performed; the pretreatment serum ALT levels should be less than 2.5 times the upper limit of normal. Monitoring the ALT level every 2 months during the first year of therapy and periodically thereafter is advised. If serum ALT levels remain persistently elevated (greater than three times the upper limit of normal), the thiazolidinedione should be discontinued. Symptoms suggestive of hepatitis should be assessed immediately. Persons in whom jaundice developed with troglitazone should not take other thiazolidinediones.[261]

Oral Hypoglycemic Drugs. Hepatocellular liver injury was common with older sulfonylureas, such as *carbutamide, metahexamide,* and *chlorpropamide.*[5,262] *Tolbutamide, tolazamide,* and *glibenclamide,* which are the currrently used sulfonylureas, rarely have been associated with cholestasis or cholestatic hepatitis.[263-266] Hypersensitivity phenomena (fever, skin rash, eosinophilia) were present in

some cases, as would be expected in view of the structural relationship of sulfonylureas to sulfonamides.[267] Most cases resolved after withdrawal of the drug, but chronic cholestasis progressing to vanishing bile duct syndrome has been described with tolbutamide and tolazamide.[265,266] Fatality from liver failure has been reported in at least two patients, one of whom had underlying cirrhosis.[267] *Gliclazide* and *glibenclamide* also have been associated with hepatocellular liver injury, with hepatic granulomas reported as well with the latter.[268,269]

Metformin, acarbose, and *human insulin* rarely have been associated with liver injury.[270-276]

Drugs Used in Neurologic Disorders

Several neuroleptic agents have been associated with drug hepatitis, either an immunoallergic type or an apparent metabolic idiosyncrasy, depending on the structure of the drug. Reactions have been reported to commonly used antidepressants including *fluoxetine,*[277,278] *paroxetine,*[279] *venlafaxine,*[280,281] *trazodone,*[282] *tolcapone,*[283] and *nefazodone*[284-286]; the last two drugs have been implicated in several cases of acute liver failure.

Antidepressants. The *monoamine oxidase inhibitor* (MAOI) iproniazid was one of the first drugs known to be associated with acute hepatitis.[6] Reactions occurred in 1% of recipients and often were severe, including instances of fatal fulminant liver failure. The hydrazine substituent (which iproniazid shares in part with isoniazid, ethionamide, pyrazinamide, and nicotinamide) was deemed to be the hepatotoxic moiety.[287] Hydrazine sulfate can cause severe hepatorenal toxicity.[288] *Phenelzine*[289] and *isocarboxazid* also have been associated with occasional instances of hepatocellular injury, but MAOIs are now rarely prescribed.

Tricyclic antidepressants bear structural resemblance to the phenothiazines and are an occasional cause of cholestatic or, less commonly, hepatocellular injury. Recovery following discontinuation of the drug is usual, but prolonged cholestasis has been observed with amitriptyline[290] and imipramine.[291]

Selective serotinin reuptake inhibitors (SSRIs) and other modern antidepressants have a better overall safety profile than that of tricyclic antidepressants. Liver enzyme elevations in the absence of symptoms have been described with *fluoxetine* and *paroxetine.*[292] A few reports of acute and chronic hepatitis have been attributed to the use of SSRIs.[292-295] *Nefazodone* has been associated with subacute liver failure.[296,297] Recovery is possible with withdrawal of the drug, but two patients have required liver transplantation.[298] Centrilobular hepatic necrosis was observed on liver histologic examination. *Trazodone* has been implicated in cases of acute and chronic hepatocellular injury.[299] The onset can be delayed as long as 18 months after therapy is begun.[300] Occasional reports have noted the occurrence of severe hepatotoxicity with combinations of antidepressants,[301-303] or of antidepressants and other neuroleptics.[282]

Other Neurologic Drugs. Tolcapone, a catechol-O-methyltransferase (COMT) inhibitor used in the treatment of parkinsonism, has been associated with at least four cases of acute liver failure.[304,305] All reported cases occurred in women older than 70 years of age, who presented with jaundice and high serum ALT levels.

Centrilobular necrosis was observed on liver histologic examination at autopsy in one case.[304,305] Serious liver injury has not been reported in users of the drug who have been monitored correctly.[306] Tolcapone has been withdrawn in Europe but not in the United States, where stringent monitoring guidelines are recommended. These guidelines consist of serum ALT testing every 2 weeks during the first year of use, because most cases of liver injury from tolcapone occur within the first 6 months.[305]

Alpidem,[307] *zolpidem*,[308] and *bentazepam*[309] are sedative-hypnotics that have been implicated in hepatotoxicity. In three reported cases of bentazepam hepatotoxicity, the clinicopathologic pattern resembled that in chronic hepatitis but without autoantibodies or other immunologic features.[309]

Tacrine is a reversible choline esterase inhibitor that improves cognition in patients with Alzheimer's disease. In a survey of tacrine-related adverse effects in 2446 patients with Alzheimer's disease, serum ALT elevations more than three times the upper limit of normal occurred in 25% and more often in women than men; levels were elevated more than 20-fold in 2% of users.[310] No dose effect was observed. Serum ALT elevations occurred abruptly, not after a gradual rise, and discontinuation of tacrine led to resolution of the elevations. Symptoms were rare; only nausea and vomiting correlated with major serum ALT elevations. In liver biopsy specimens from three patients, steatosis and mild lobular hepatitis were observed. According to this study, minor degrees of hepatocellular injury occur in one half of users of tacrine, but tolerance to this minor form of liver injury eventually develops. Isolated reports of jaundice indicate a rare potential for tacrine to cause more serious hepatotoxicity.[5,7] Weekly monitoring of serum ALT levels during the first 3 months of tacrine use, with discontinuation if values reach three times the upper limit of normal, should prevent important hepatotoxicity.[310] Although the mechanism of tacrine-induced hepatotoxicity is unclear, metabolic idiosyncrasy is likely. Mitochondrial injury has been implicated in an animal model.[311]

Dantrolene, a skeletal muscle relaxant that is valuable against spasticity, causes hepatitis in approximately 1% of exposed persons, but the case-fatality rate has been approximately 28%.[312] Most afflicted patients have been older than 30 years of age. One third of affected persons are asymptomatic, whereas the remainder present with jaundice and symptoms of hepatitis. Hepatocellular necrosis, often submassive or massive, has been noted on liver biopsy specimens.[5,312] When therapy with dantrolene is initiated, liver biochemical test values should be monitored every 2 weeks. Liver enzyme elevations constitute an indication to stop dantrolene.

Other neurotropic drugs and muscle relaxants implicated as idiosyncratic hepatotoxins include *tizanidine* (a centrally acting muscle relaxant),[313] *alverine* (a smooth muscle relaxant),[314] and *riluzole*.[315,316] *Riluzole* is a glutamate antagonist approved for the treatment of amyotrophic lateral sclerosis. During clinical trials of this drug, increased serum ALT levels were reported in 1.3% to 10% of recipients. Two cases of acute hepatitis with microvesicular steatosis have since been reported, with onset at 4 and 8 weeks, respectively, after the start of treatment.[315,316] Rarely, hepatocellular injury may be delayed for as long as 6 months. Liver biochemical test abnormalities resolve rapidly after riluzole is discontinued.

Nonsteroidal Anti-inflammatory Drugs

NSAIDs rarely cause drug-induced liver disease, with or without immunoallergic features and with varying degrees of hepatocellular injury and cholestasis.[5,164]

Bromfenac is a phenylacetic acid derivative. The drug was withdrawn from the U.S. market in 1998 because of several cases of severe hepatotoxic reactions that resulted in acute liver failure leading to liver transplantation or death.[317-319] Most patients had received therapeutic doses of bromfenac for more than 90 days before experiencing malaise and fatigue, followed by symptoms of severe hepatitis and progressive liver failure over 5 to 37 days; use of the drug had been recommended for only up to 7 days. No features suggestive of immunoallergy were present. Histologic examination showed zonal or confluent necrosis with a predominantly lymphocytic infiltrate.

COX-2 inhibitors appear to be relatively free of hepatic drug reactions, although a small number of cases of hepatotoxicity have been reported in association with nimesulide and celecoxib.[172,320-324] *Celecoxib* has a low potential for liver injury. In a review of 14 controlled trials, the frequency of hepatic dysfunction (0.8%) was not significantly different from that in patients who received placebo (0.9%) and appeared to be lower than that observed with other NSAIDs.[323] Elevations in serum aminotransferase levels often occurred in persons taking diclofenac concurrently.[323] When serious hepatocellular injury was attributed to celecoxib, female gender was a predisposing factor. The onset of symptoms was between 4 days and 4 weeks after the drug was started. Liver biochemical abnormalities were consistent with a pattern of hepatocellular or mixed liver injury. Eosinophilia and skin rash suggestive of RMS occurred in some patients. All patients recovered within 1 to 4 months of discontinuing the drug.[323] The manufacturer currently recommends that celecoxib not be administered to persons with a documented sulfonamide allergy because of published reports of cross-reactivity and toxicity.

Nimesulide, an NSAID that has preferential COX-2 selectivity, has been linked to several cases of acute hepatitis and fatal hepatic failure, especially in women; however, the risk of liver injury is small.[320,325] Time to onset of symptoms has ranged from 1 to 15 weeks, although a delay of up to 8 months is possible.[326,327] Hypersensitivity features with peripheral eosinophilia may be present. Centrilobular or bridging necrosis and occasionally bland cholestasis have been described on liver histologic examination. Resolution usually occurs 2 to 17 months after cessation of nimesulide.[327]

DRUG-INDUCED GRANULOMATOUS HEPATITIS

Granulomatous reactions are a common type of drug-induced liver disease,[328] and drugs account for 2% to 29% of cases of *granulomatous hepatitis* (see also Chapter 34). The number of drugs and foreign compounds associated

Table 83–5 Drug-Induced Granulomatous Hepatitis: Major Causative Agents, Frequency, Clinicopathologic Characteristics, and Outcomes

Causative Agent*	Key Reference	Frequency, Risk Factors	Clinicopathologic Characteristics, Outcome
Allopurinol	329	Rare (<40 cases) Older men, black race, renal failure, use of thiazides	Acute hepatitis, cholestatic hepatitis, bile duct injury also frequent; rash (exfoliative dermatitis), nephritis, vasculitis usual; mortality rate 15%, especially with vasculitis
Carbamazepine	330	16:100,000 treatment years Age >40 yr, no gender predilection	Two thirds of cases show granulomatous hepatitis; remainder show acute hepatitis, cholangitis; no features of drug allergy; no reported fatality, rapid recovery
Phenylbutazone	331	1:5000 exposed No age or gender predilection	Severe acute hepatitis, cholestasis and bile duct injury also reported; features of drug allergy common; occasionally vasculitis; mortality rate 25%, particularly in cases with hepatocellular necrosis
Hydralazine	332	Rare; older patients, possibly slow acetylators	Other types of reaction also common: acute hepatitis, cholestatic hepatitis, cholangitis; features of drug allergy uncommon; vasculitis not described; reactions severe but no mortality reported
Quinine	333	Rare; no recognized risk factors	Acute hepatitis in two thirds of cases; rash, interstitial pneumonitis, positive Coombs' test, thrombocytopenia; vasculitis not described; good prognosis

*Other drugs that have been reliably reported to cause granulomatous hepatitis include quinidine,[334] phenytoin (usually with vasculitis),[335] sulfonamides[32] (usually with vasculitis), nitrofurantoin, aspirin, papaverine, procainamide, sulfasalazine, mesalamine,[336] and glyburide.[337] Single case reports have implicated many other agents, as referred to briefly in the text and detailed in reviews.[4-6,9]

with hepatic granulomas exceeds 40; some are summarized in Table 83–5.[329-337] Not all are associated with systemic inflammation or with persuasive evidence of causality. Many are more commonly associated with other patterns of liver injury (e.g., halothane, methyldopa, nitrofurantoin, troglitazone, amiodarone, amoxicillin–clavulanic acid). Some of these associations may be fortuitous.

The clinical picture is heralded by fever and systemic symptoms (e.g., malaise, headache, myalgia), from 10 days to 4 months after the start of treatment. Hepatomegaly and hepatic tenderness are common; splenomegaly is present in 25% of patients. Extrahepatic features of drug hypersensitivity are common, as is eosinophilia (30%). Liver biochemical test results are typically mixed because of the infiltrative nature of hepatic granulomas and the frequent presence of some hepatocellular necrosis or cholestasis. For several drugs that cause granulomatous hepatitis, continued exposure leads to more severe types of liver disease, such as cholestatic hepatitis, with or without bile duct injury, or hepatic necrosis (see Table 83–5). Small-vessel vasculitis is another potential complication (see Table 83–5) and may involve the kidneys, bone marrow, skin, and lungs; the mortality rate is high.[5]

DRUG-INDUCED CHRONIC HEPATITIS

Chronic hepatitis is defined as hepatitis continuing for more than 6 months. For drug reactions, the definition often has been based inappropriately on hepatic histologic features alone.[338-339] The histologic features include periportal inflammation (piecemeal necrosis), bridging necrosis, and fibrosis. Because these features may be present as early as 6 weeks after the onset of a severe drug reaction, they do not confirm chronicity. The diagnosis of chronic hepatitis is more convincing when clinical or

biochemical evidence of hepatitis has been present for more than 3 months and when clinical and laboratory features of chronic liver disease or histologic evidence of established hepatic fibrosis are present.

Drugs are an uncommon cause of chronic hepatitis (Table 83–6). Implicated agents such as *oxyphenisatin*[5,338,339] and *methyldopa* are now used rarely, and with the increasing importance of chronic viral hepatitis (see Chapters 75 and 76), only a small proportion of cases of chronic hepatitis (2% to 6%, depending on geographic reporting region) are caused by drugs.[5,27] In fact, several cases reported in the past as drug-induced disease subsequently were found to be chronic hepatitis C.[129] Nevertheless, recognition of a drug cause remains important, because a poor outcome usually is attributable to continued ingestion of the drug after clinical onset of the disorder.[27]

Drug-induced chronic hepatitis is approximately four times more likely to develop in women than in men.[338,339] Older patients appear to be at greater risk (as is the case for nitrofurantoin), and the reaction is virtually unknown in children. Drugs associated with chronic hepatitis more commonly cause acute hepatitis, and the latent period to recognition tends to be longer in cases of chronic hepatitis; therefore, the duration of drug ingestion may be a risk factor for chronic hepatitis.

Two syndromes of chronic hepatitis occur. In the first, cases appear to be identical to acute hepatitis but more severe, more prolonged, or later in onset, perhaps as a result of failure of recognition. These cases may be appropriately termed *chronic toxicity*. Clinical and laboratory features of chronic liver disease are rare, and hallmarks of autoimmunity are absent. Management consists of withdrawal of the drug and treatment of liver failure (see Table 83–6).

The second syndrome more closely resembles autoimmune hepatitis by the presence of spider angiomata, firm liver edge, splenomegaly, and potential for liver

Table 83–6 Drug-Induced Chronic Hepatitis: Causative Agents, Risk Factors, Clinicopathologic Characteristics, and Outcomes

Causative Agent*	Risk Factors	Clinicopathologic Characteristics, Outcome
Nitrofurantoin	Age >40 yr; 90% of cases in women; continued ingestion after onset	Clinical features of chronic hepatitis, liver failure; some cases with features of cholestasis; 20% with pneumonitis; hyperglobulinemia usual, ANA, SMA; mortality rate 10%
Methyldopa	Age >50 yr; 80% of cases in women; repeated courses, continued ingestion in sensitized patient	Jaundice, systemic features, diarrhea, liver failure; hyperglobulinemia, ANA, SMA positive; protracted course, high mortality rate
Diclofenac	Age >65 yr; most cases in women	Clinical features of chronic hepatitis, liver failure; ANA, SMA, hyperglobulinemia; response to glucocorticoids in a few cases
Minocycline	Young women; prolonged use of drug	Often part of drug-induced systemic lupus erythematosus syndrome (arthritis, rash, rarely nephritis); ANA, hyperglobulinemia; cases may be severe, with fatal outcome or need for liver transplantation; glucocorticoid treatment may be indicated
Isoniazid	Age >50 yr; continued drug ingestion after onset; duration of therapy	Severe and fatal cases with cirrhosis; no immune phenomena; high mortality rate or need for liver transplantation
Dantrolene	Age >30 yr; dose, duration of therapy	Jaundice, liver failure; no immune phenomena; high mortality rate
Etretinate	Age >50 yr; two thirds in women	Jaundice, weight loss, liver failure; deterioration after stopping drug; response to glucocorticoids in two cases
Acetaminophen	Regular intake at moderate doses (2 to 6 g/day); alcohol, fasting, other drugs	No features of chronic liver disease, no autoimmune phenomena; there are cases of chronic toxicity; rapid normalization of liver biochemical test levels after drug is stopped

*Other drugs include oxyphenisatin and tienilic acid, which are now of historical interest,[5,6] and clometacin, for which many affected patients have now been shown to have had hepatitis C.[100] Several other agents, including sulfonamides, aspirin, halothane, cimetidine, methotrexate, trazadone, fluoxetine, fenfibrate, and germander, have been mentioned as associated with chronic hepatitis, but details are not always convincing.[5]

ANA, antinuclear antibodies; SMA, anti-smooth muscle antibodies.

failure. Ascites, bruising, bleeding esophageal varices, and hepatic encephalopathy are common. In addition to raised serum ALT and bilirubin levels, hypoalbuminemia and hyperglobulinemia are usual. The prothrombin time is prolonged in severe cases. Autoantibodies, particularly antinuclear and anti–smooth muscle antibodies, are frequent. In contrast with idiopathic autoimmune hepatitis, other hallmarks of autoimmunity, such as a history of other autoimmune diseases and genetic predisposition indicated by the HLA-B8 and -DRw3 alleles, are not found. Treatment with immunosuppressants usually is not indicated; the clinical condition improves spontaneously after withdrawal of the causative drug; however, in individual cases (see later), glucocorticoids occasionally appear to hasten recovery.

Diclofenac

Diclofenac is one of the world's most prescribed NSAIDs and appears to be at least as safe as comparable agents.[340] Serious hepatotoxicity occurs in approximately 1 to 5 per 100,000 persons exposed, or 0.4 per 1 million defined daily doses; the latter figure is minimally greater than that for phenylbutazone (0.2 per 1 million) and piroxicam (0.3 per 1 million) but less than that for benoxaprofen (12.6 per 1 million)[10] and bromfenac,[317-319] which was withdrawn from the market (see earlier). At least 30 cases

of diclofenac hepatitis have been reported,[2,340,341] including several confirmed by indavertent rechallenge. Only four cases have been fatalities, and five cases can reasonably be regarded as chronic hepatitis.

The risk of diclofenac hepatotoxicity is increased in women and with aging. A prodromal illness characterized by anorexia, nausea, vomiting and malaise heralds the onset of liver injury, which usually occurs within 3 months (range, 1 to 11 months) of the start of the drug. Fever and rash occur in 25% of patients.[340,341] Liver biochemical test results reflect acute hepatitis with or without cholestasis. Reactions tend to be severe, with jaundice in 50% of cases. Liver biopsy specimens reveal acute lobular hepatitis, but in severe cases, bridging or confluent necrosis, interface hepatitis, and fibrous expansion of the portal tracts have been noted.[342] The prognosis is usually good, with resolution occurring after discontinuation of the drug. Cases of drug-induced chronic hepatitis have been described in which the clinical and laboratory features (ascites, hypoalbuminemia, hyperglobulinemia, and jaundice) suggested autoimmune hepatitis, although the frequency of autoantibodies is unclear. These cases usually have improved spontaneously after discontinuation of the drug, but glucocorticoids have been used successfully in a few protracted cases.[340] Cross-sensitivity between NSAIDs seems to be rare, but one patient with diclofenac hepatitis also experienced an adverse reaction to ibuprofen, and another had an adverse reaction to tiaprofenic acid.[5,340] The rarity of severe diclofenac-induced hepatotoxicity makes liver biochemical monitoring unrealistic. Patients need to be advised to report adverse effects, and clinicians must be aware that diclofenac can cause both acute and chronic hepatitis.

Minocycline

Minocycline has been associated with rare cases of drug-induced systemic lupus erythematosus (rash, polyarthritis, hyperglobulinemia, and antinuclear antibodies), chronic hepatitis with autoimmune features, or both syndromes in the same patient.[177,343,344] The onset often occurs after treatment with minocycline for longer than 6 months, and young women appear to be particularly affected. The reactions are severe; some patients have died or required liver transplantation, and the course may be prolonged after the drug is discontinued. Several patients have been managed with glucocorticoids.[344]

DRUG-INDUCED ACUTE CHOLESTASIS

IMPORTANCE, TYPES OF REACTIONS, AND DIAGNOSIS

Drugs are an important cause of acute cholestasis, with or without hepatitis.[345,346] The full spectrum of drug-related cholestatic disorders includes *cholestatic hepatitis with cholangitis* and *chronic cholestasis* with either a *vanishing bile duct syndrome* resembling primary biliary cirrhosis or with *biliary strictures* reminiscent of sclerosing cholangitis.[5,345] The clinical and biochemical features of drug-induced cholestasis resemble those of several other hepatobiliary disorders, and clinicians must take a thorough drug history from all patients with cholestasis. The prompt discontinuation of the causative agent prevents an adverse outcome and avoids unnecessary invasive investigations or surgery.

The clinical syndrome of cholestasis is indicated by pruritus, dark urine, pale stools, and, often, jaundice. Liver biochemical test results show a predominant elevation of serum alkaline phosphatase level with a lesser increase in serum ALT level, elevation of GGTP and 5'-nucleotidase levels, raised serum bile acid levels, and conjugated hyperbilirubinemia. The serum ALT level may be elevated up to eight-fold, as a result of either the toxic effects of acute bile retention on hepatocellular integrity or concomitant "hepatitis." In such cases, the ratio of the relative increases in serum ALT and serum alkaline phosphatase levels (based on multiples of the upper limit of normal) typically is less than 2:1 in cholestasis.[103] Cases of *mixed cholestasis and hepatitis* are highly suggestive of a drug reaction.

Hepatobiliary imaging is essential to exclude dilatation of the bile ducts produced by biliary obstruction and to exclude a hepatic or pancreatic mass lesion. In the absence of these findings, drug-induced cholestasis is more likely, and a liver biopsy is often advisable. Certain histologic features suggest a hepatic drug reaction, whereas others (e.g., edema of the portal tracts) suggest

biliary obstruction. When the temporal relationship to drug ingestion indicates a high probability of a drug reaction, particularly when the agent is known to be potentially hepatotoxic, the incriminated drug should be discontinued and the patient observed for improvement.

Management is focused on relief of symptoms, with particular attention given to pruritus.[5,345,346] Glucocorticoids have no role. Pruritus often is ameliorated with oral cholestyramine. Phenobarbital and antihistamines usually are ineffective or cause oversedation of the patient. In intractable cases, treatment with oral ursodeoxycholic acid has shown promise.[346,347] Rifampin can be tried; phototherapy, plasmapheresis, and morphine receptor antagonists (e.g., naloxone, naltrexone, nalmefene) have been used as third-line therapies.[346]

CHOLESTASIS WITHOUT HEPATITIS

Cholestatic reactions without hepatitis are characterized by the retention of bile in canaliculi, Kupffer cells, and hepatocytes, with minimal inflammation or hepatocellular necrosis. Synonyms are *pure*, *canalicular*, and *bland cholestasis*. Cholestasis without hepatitis reflects a primary disturbance in bile flow. Sex steroids are the typical causative agents. Some drugs more often associated with cholestatic hepatitis occasionally produce bland cholestasis (e.g., amoxicillin–clavulanic acid, sulfonamides, griseofulvin, ketoconazole, tamoxifen, warfarin, ibuprofen).[5,345] *Cyclosporine* is associated with liver biochemical test abnormalities; the features resemble those of cholestasis, but hyperbilirubinemia usually is predominant.[5] The reaction is mild and is reversed rapidly with a reduction in dose.

Steroid-Induced Cholestasis

Oral Contraceptive Steroids. The frequency of cholestasis with OCS is 2.5 per 10,000 women exposed. The occurrence of cholestasis with OCS is partly dose dependent and less likely with low-dose than with high-dose estrogen preparations.[348] Genetic factors influence the frequency of this complication, with a particularly high rate observed among women in Chile and Scandinavia.[5,6] Persons with a previous history of cholestasis of pregnancy are also at risk (50%).[5] The estrogenic component is most likely responsible. Symptoms develop 2 to 3 months, rarely as late as 9 months, after commencement of OCS. A mild transient prodrome of nausea and malaise may occur and is followed by pruritus and jaundice. The serum alkaline phosphatase level is moderately elevated, and aminotransferases are increased transiently, occasionally to levels exceeding 10 times the upper limit of normal. The GGTP level is often normal. Recovery is usually prompt, within days to weeks, after cessation of the drug. Chronic cholestasis is rare.[345]

Hormonal replacement therapy is safe in patients with liver disease. Jaundiced patients, however, may experience an increase in serum bilirubin levels, and liver biochemical test levels should be monitored in users with liver disease.[345]

Anabolic Steroids. At high doses, anabolic steroids often produce reversible bland cholestasis, usually within 1 to

6 months of beginning treatment. Prolonged jaundice with ductopenia is a rare complication.[349]

Both OCS and the 17-alkylated anabolic steroids also are associated with vascular lesions and hepatic neoplasms (see Chapter 91). The strength of these associations with individual lesions varies. Benign hepatic neoplasms clearly are associated with OCS, whereas their association with hepatocellular carcinoma is controversial. By contrast, hepatocellular carcinoma is well documented in users of anabolic steroids. Likewise, hepatic and portal vein thrombosis is an established adverse effect of OCS, but not of anabolic steroids. Other vascular lesions, such as peliosis hepatis, are observed more often with anabolic steroids than with OCS.

CHOLESTASIS WITH HEPATITIS

Cholestasis with hepatitis is a common type of hepatic drug reaction and is characterized histologically by conspicuous cholestasis and hepatocellular necrosis. Histologic lesions in the liver include lobular and portal tract inflammation, often with neutrophils and eosinophils, as well as mononuclear cells. This type of reaction overlaps with drug-induced acute hepatitis (occasionally resulting in acute liver failure), cholestasis without hepatitis, and cholestasis with bile duct injury. Causative agents include chlorpromazine, antidepressants and other psychotropic agents, erythromycins and other macrolide antibiotics, sulfonamides,[5,6] oxypenicillins,[5,345,350,351] ketoconazole (discussed earlier),[222] sulfonylureas,[5] sulindac,[352] ibuprofen,[352,353] phenylbutazone,[6] piroxicam,[353] captopril,[354] flutamide,[355,356] enalapril,[5] pravastatin,[357] atorvastatin,[358] ticlopidine,[359] ciprofloxacin,[360] norfloxacin,[361] and metformin.[362]

Chlorpromazine

Chlorpromazine hepatitis, the prototypical drug-induced cholestatic hepatitis,[5,363] has been recognized since the 1950s, but cases still occur.[347] The full spectrum of hepatic reactions to chlorpromazine includes asymptomatic liver biochemical test abnormalities in 20% to 50% of those exposed and rare cases of fulminant hepatic necrosis. The reported frequency of cholestatic hepatitis depends on the type of study, ranging from 0.2% to 2.0%; the lower value probably is representative of the risk in the general population.[5] No relationship to dose or underlying liver disease has been recognized. Female predominance is evident. Reactions do not appear to be more common with increasing age but are rare in children.

The onset of cholestatic hepatitis is generally at 1 to 6 weeks after the start of chlorpromazine and occasionally 5 to 14 days after its discontinuation. Accelerated onset occurs with rechallenge. A prodromal illness of fever and nonspecific symptoms is usual and is followed by the development of gastrointestinal symptoms and jaundice. Pruritus is common and occurs later with chlorpromazine hepatitis than with drug-induced cholestasis without hepatitis. In a small proportion of affected patients, right upper quadrant abdominal pain is severe. Rash is infrequent. Liver biochemical test results include an elevation of both serum ALT and alkaline phosphatase levels and

hyperbilirubinemia. Eosinophilia is present in 10% to 40% of patients. Most patients with chlorpromazine hepatitis recover completely—one third within 4 weeks, another third between 4 and 8 weeks, and the remainder after 8 weeks.[363] In approximately 7% of cases, full recovery has not occurred by 6 months (see later).

Amoxicillin–Clavulanic Acid

At least 150 cases of cholestatic hepatitis have been attributed to the use of amoxicillin–clavulanic acid (Augmentin), a commonly prescribed antibiotic. The overall frequency is 1 to 2 cases per 100,000 persons exposed; male gender, increasing age (older than 55 years), and possibly use of the antibiotic for a prolonged period are risk factors.[12,364] The clavulanic acid component has been implicated as the cause, because similar lesions have been noted with ticarcillin–clavulanic acid,[365,366] whereas amoxicillin rarely causes liver disease.

The onset of symptoms is within 6 weeks (mean 18 days) of the start of drug therapy, although rarely the onset of symptoms may be delayed until 6 weeks after discontinuation of treatment. Hypersensitivity features such as fever, skin rash, and eosinophilia are seen in 30% to 60% of patients.[367] Liver biopsy specimens show cholestasis with mild portal inflammation.[368] Bile duct injury, usually mild, and perivenular bilirubinostasis with lipofuscin deposition are often present. Other histologic features include hepatic granulomas and biliary ductopenia.[369-372] Most patients recover completely in 4 to 16 weeks; fatal outcomes are rare.[372] A strong association with the HLRADRB1*1501-DRB5*0101-DQB1*062 haplotype supports the view that an immunologic idiosyncrasy mediated through HLA class II antigens could play a pathogenic role in this form of drug-induced cholestatic hepatitis.[13,25] Nevertheless, the presence of this haplotype has no influence on the clinical characteristics, severity, and outcome of the disease.

CHOLESTATIC HEPATITIS WITH BILE DUCT INJURY

Bile duct (cholangiolytic) injury is observed with several drugs that cause cholestatic hepatitis, such as chlorpromazine[363] and flucloxacillin.[358] The severity of bile duct injury may be a determinant of the development of vanishing bile duct syndrome (see later).[373] The clinical features may resemble those of bacterial cholangitis and include upper abdominal pain, fever, rigors, tender hepatomegaly, jaundice, and cholestasis. Liver biochemical test abnormalities are typical of cholestasis. Compounds associated with this syndrome include arsphenamine,[6] carbamazepine,[374] dextropropoxyphene,[375] and methylenediamine, an industrial toxin responsible for *Epping jaundice*, an outbreak associated with the ingestion of bread made from contaminated flour (see Chapter 84).[376]

Dextropropoxyphene

Dextropropoxyphene, an opioid analgesic used alone or in compound analgesics, has caused cholestasis with bile duct injury in at least 25 reported cases,[375] some proved by inadvertent rechallenge. A female predominance has been recognized. The onset of symptoms is usually within 2 weeks of the start of dextropropoxyphene. Illness often is heralded by abdominal pain, which may be severe and simulate that due to other causes of cholangitis. Jaundice is usual. ERCP shows normal bile ducts. Liver biopsy specimens demonstrate cholestasis with expansion of the portal tracts by inflammation and mild fibrosis; portal tract edema also may be present. Other features include irregularity and necrosis of the biliary epithelium, together with an infiltrate of neutrophils and eosinophils on the outer surface of bile ducts. Bile ductule proliferation is universal. Recovery has occurred in all reported cases.[375] Liver biochemical test results normalize between 1 and 3 months after discontinuation of the drug. This type of hepatic drug reaction must be distinguished from bile duct obstruction and bacterial cholangitis.

DRUG-INDUCED CHRONIC CHOLESTASIS

Drug-induced liver disease is considered to be chronic when typical liver biochemical changes last longer than 3 months[102,103]; earlier definitions required the presence of jaundice for more than 6 months or anicteric cholestasis (raised serum alkaline phosphatase and GGTP levels) for more than 12 months after the implicated agent was stopped. Drug-induced chronic cholestasis is uncommon but has been ascribed to more than 45 compounds,[345,346,363,364,377,378] Chronicity complicates approximately 7% of cases of chlorpromazine hepatitis[347,363] and is a feature in 10% to 30% of cases of flucloxacillin hepatitis.[5,345,358] Chronicity has been reported in less than 5% of cases of erythromycin hepatitis[346,363,377] and in only isolated instances for other agents such as tetracycline,[378] amoxicillin–clavulanic acid,[368] ibuprofen,[379,380] trimethoprim-sulfamethoxazole,[381] and ciprofloxacin.[382]

Chronic cholestasis always is preceded by an episode of acute cholestatic hepatitis. The episode of acute cholestatic hepatitis tends to be severe and occasionally is associated with the Stevens-Johnson syndrome.[380] One study indicated that the severity of bile duct lesions at the time of the initial hepatic reaction is a critical determinant of a chronic course.[371] Other possible mechanisms of chronicity include continuing toxic or immunologic destruction of the biliary epithelium.[372] The histologic lesion is characterized by a paucity of smaller (septal, interlobular) bile ducts and ductules, often with residual cholestasis, and portal tract inflammation directed against injured bile ducts. This process may lead to an irreversible loss of biliary patency and to the vanishing bile duct syndrome.

The clinical features are those of chronic cholestasis. Pruritus is the dominant symptom and is often severe. Continuing jaundice, dark urine, and pale stools are other possible findings, but these features are not invariable and may resolve despite persistence of the biochemical abnormalities. In severe cases, intestinal malabsorption, weight loss, and bruising caused by vitamin K deficiency may occur; xanthelasma, tuberous xanthomas, and other complications of severe hypercholesterolemia also have been noted. Firm hepato-

megaly may be found on physical examination, but splenomegaly is unusual unless portal hypertension develops. Antimitochondrial antibodies are not a feature of drug-induced chronic cholestasis. The outcome usually is favorable, with resolution of jaundice in most instances. Progression to biliary cirrhosis is rare[345] and is associated with a severe reduction in the number of bile ducts.[93]

Flucloxacillin

Flucloxacillin is one of the most important causes of drug-induced hepatitis in Europe, Scandinavia, and Australia.[5,345,350] Flucloxacillin-induced hepatitis is usually severe, and several fatalities have resulted. The course is prolonged, and a high proportion of cases result in chronic cholestasis and vanishing bile duct syndrome.[350] Other oxypenicillins appear to be less prone to cause this complication, but cholestatic hepatitis has been reported with dicloxacillin and cloxacillin.[351]

Drug-Induced Cholestasis with Fibrotic Bile Duct Strictures

Cholestasis caused by some drugs may lead to development of *fibrotic strictures of the larger bile ducts*. This complication has been associated with *intralesional therapy of hepatic hydatid cysts* with formalin[383] and *intra-arterial infusion of floxuridine* for metastatic colorectal carcinoma.[373,384] After several months of floxuridine infusion, the frequency of toxic hepatitis or bile duct injury, or both, is 25% to 55%. Acalculous cholecystitis is another complication.[5] ERCP shows strictures, typically in the common hepatic duct and the left and right hepatic ducts. In contrast with primary sclerosing cholangitis, the common bile duct and the smaller intrahepatic bile ducts are spared. Ischemia has been suspected as a pathogenic factor,[5,384] but toxicity to biliary epithelial cells is another possibility. Recovery may occur after infusion therapy with floxuridine is discontinued. Other patients require dilation or stenting of biliary strictures.

DRUG-INDUCED STEATOHEPATITIS, HEPATIC FIBROSIS, AND CIRRHOSIS

Drug-induced liver disease can produce cirrhosis by a variety of processes; chronic hepatitis and chronic cholestasis with the vanishing bile duct syndrome have already been discussed. *Steatohepatitis* is a form of chronic liver disease in which fatty change is associated with focal liver cell injury, ballooning degeneration, Mallory's hyaline, focal inflammation of mixed cellularity, including polymorphonuclear neutrophils, and progressive hepatic fibrosis in a pericentral (zone 3) and pericellular distribution[385] (see Chapters 81 and 82). Alcohol consumption is a common etiologic factor. NASH is associated with insulin resistance, diabetes, obesity, and several drugs (e.g., perhexiline maleate,[53] amiodarone; see later).[386] In addition to causing steatohepatitis or chronic injury to liver cells or bile ducts, some exogenous compounds appear to promote hepatic fibrogenesis directly, most likely through effects on hepatic nonparenchymal cells; stellate cells are central to this process (see Chapter

68). Compounds that stimulate hepatic fibrosis include arsenic, vitamin A, and methotrexate (see later).

Amiodarone-Induced Liver Disease

Amiodarone is an iodinated benzofuran derivative used for therapy-resistant ventricular tachyarrhythmias. Adverse effects lead to discontinuation of the drug in 25% of patients. These adverse effects include pulmonary infiltrates, worsening cardiac failure, hypothyroidism, peripheral neuropathy, nephrotoxicity, and corneal deposits, but liver disease is one of the most serious. The spectrum of abnormalities includes liver biochemical test abnormalities in 15% to 80% of patients and clinically significant liver disease, including rare cases of acute liver failure, in 0.6%.[387-391] The most typical lesion is steatohepatitis; cirrhosis is present in 15% to 50% of patients with heptotoxicity.[387,388]

A notable feature of amiodarone-induced liver disease is that the disease may progress despite discontinuation of amiodarone.[5,388-392] Amiodarone is highly concentrated in the liver, and after a few weeks of treatment the drug accounts for as much as 1% of the wet weight of the organ. The drug's iodine component absorbs radiation, so that the liver appears opaque on computed tomography.[391] Although odd, this appearance is not clinically significant.

Hepatic storage of amiodarone also produces *phospholipidosis*, a storage disorder characterized by enlarged lysosomes stuffed with whorled membranous material (*myeloid bodies*).[93] In animals fed amiodarone, the development of phospholipidosis is time and dose dependent.[389] Phospholipidosis may result from direct inhibition of phospholipase or formation of nondegradable drug-phospholipid complexes but appears to have no relationship to the development of NASH and hepatocyte injury. Other occasional hepatic abnormalities in patients taking amiodarone include granuloma formation and acute liver failure, apparently caused by severe acute hepatitis or a Reye's syndrome–like illness.[5,393]

Amiodarone is concentrated in mitochondria by virtue of its physicochemical properties and may interrupt mitochondrial electron transport.[394] In rats and mice, treatment with amiodarone produced microvesicular steatosis, augmented mitochondrial production of ROS, and caused lipid peroxidation.[395,396]

Chronic liver disease only is detected 1 year or later (median, 21 months) after amiodarone is started. A relationship between the development of chronic liver disease and the duration of amiodarone therapy, and possibly the total dose[393,397] but not the incremental dose, has been confirmed. The frequency of other toxic effects of amiodarone (most of which are thought to be dose dependent) is increased in patients with liver disease.[397] Patients' complaints include fatigue, nausea and vomiting, malaise, weight loss, and abdominal swelling as a result of the development of ascites. Hepatomegaly, jaundice, bruising, and other features of chronic liver disease may be present. Liver biochemical test abnormalities include increased serum aminotransferase levels, most often to at least five times the upper limit of normal, and minor increases in serum alkaline phosphatase levels. The ratio of serum AST to ALT is close to unity and thus differs from the ratio seen in alcoholic hepatitis. In severe cases of amiodarone-induced liver disease, hyperbilirubinemia, low serum albumin levels, and prolongation of the prothrombin time are evident. Diagnosing the cause of abnormal liver biochemical test results and hepatomegaly often is difficult in patients taking amiodarone, and a liver biopsy may be indicated. The histologic changes in the liver include phospholipidosis, steatosis, focal necrosis with Mallory's hyaline, infiltration with polymorphonuclear neutrophils, and pericellular fibrosis.[93,388] Cirrhosis is often present.

Prevention and management of amiodarone-induced liver disease are problematic because liver biochemical test abnormalities are common in patients taking amiodarone, particularly those with cardiac failure. In asymptomatic or mild cases, abnormalities resolve in 2 weeks to 4 months after amiodarone is discontinued. In cases of severe liver disease, the mortality rate is high.[388,397] Cessation of amiodarone therapy does not always result in clinical improvement, presumably because of prolonged hepatic storage of amiodarone; in one study, the outcome was worse (usually from fatal arrhythmias) in patients who discontinued amiodarone than in those who did not.[388] Although serial liver biochemical tests are recommended in patients taking amiodarone,[397] whether such testing is adequate to prevent serious hepatotoxicity is unknown.

Tamoxifen and Other Causes of Drug-Induced Steatohepatitis

With the various agents reported to be associated with steatohepatitis during the 1990s, causality has been difficult to prove,[386] particularly because NASH is a common disorder among patients with insulin resistance or the metabolic syndrome (see Chapter 82). Calcium channel blockers used to treat arterial hypertension or cardiac arrhythmias rarely have been associated with steatohepatitis,[398,399] and methyldopa has been reported to be associated with cirrhosis in obese middle-aged women[400]; these associations may have been fortuitous. Other drugs, including estrogens[401] and glucocorticoids,[402] may precipitate NASH in predisposed persons because of the effects of these drugs on the risk factors for NASH—insulin resistance, type 2 diabetes, obesity, and hypertriglyceridemia. The association between NASH and *tamoxifen* appears to be much stronger.

Tamoxifen is an estrogen receptor ligand with both agonist and antagonist actions. It is widely used for the prevention and treatment of breast cancer. Several forms of liver injury have been attributed to tamoxifen[403]: cholestasis,[404] hepatocellular carcinoma,[405] peliosis hepatis,[406] acute hepatitis, massive hepatic necrosis,[403] steatosis, and steatohepatitis, occasionally with cirrhosis.[386,407-413] In one series of 66 women with breast cancer who had received tamoxifen for 3 to 5 years, 24 showed radiologic evidence of hepatic steatosis.[410] Seven others were diagnosed with NASH (proven by liver biopsy) after taking tamoxifen for 7 to 33 months.[408,409,411]

The metabolic profile of women with radiologic evidence of hepatic steatosis (or histologic proof of steatohepatitis) during tamoxifen therapy appears to be similar to that of most patients with NASH; one half have been obese, and increase in body mass index (BMI) has correlated with hepatic steatosis among women taking tamoxifen.[414] Tamoxifen also can induce hypertriglyceridemia, another risk factor for NASH. In two women undergoing treatment with bezafibrate, a PPARα stimulator, steatosis, as assessed radiologically, decreased markedly.[414] It therefore seems possible that tamoxifen may play a synergistic role with other factors such as insulin resistance, hyperlipidemia, and obesity to cause steatohepatitis.

Physicians need to be aware of the high frequency (approximately 30%) of hepatic steatosis, as determined by hepatic imaging, or steatohepatitis in women who receive tamoxifen. Monitoring patients for this adverse effect should include physical examination to detect hepatomegaly and liver biochemical tests; some authors also advocate annual hepatic imaging by ultrasonography or computed tomography.[415] Liver biopsy may be indicated to establish the severity of the disorder, particularly if liver biochemical test abnormalities do not resolve after tamoxifen is discontinued, or to exclude metastatic breast cancer. Many cases appear to improve after tamoxifen is discontinued, but whether treatment should always be withdrawn permanently is not clear, particularly because the effect of taximofen on survival from breast cancer is impressive.

Toremifene, an analog of tamoxifen, also has been reported to cause steatosis or steatohepatitis, but with a lower frequency (less than 10%) than that reported for tamoxifen.[415]

Perhexiline maleate and *coralgil* (4,4'-diethyl-aminoethoxyhexestrol) are recognized toxic causes of steatohepatitis but have been withdrawn from the market.[5,6,386]

Methotrexate-Induced Hepatic Fibrosis

Methotrexate is a dose-dependent toxin. In high doses, methotrexate can result in bone marrow suppression, mucocutaneous reactions, pneumonitis, and hepatotoxicity. In the 1950s, it became apparent that previous methotrexate treatment of acute childhood leukemia was complicated by severe hepatic fibrosis and cirrhosis[5,6]; in a few cases, hepatocellular carcinoma developed.[416] In the 1960s, the use of methotrexate for treatment of psoriasis was associated with development of hepatic fibrosis and cirrhosis in as many as 25% of cases.[417] Since then, a clearer picture of methotrexate as a dose-dependent promoter of hepatic fibrosis has emerged, particularly in persons who drink alcohol excessively or have preexisting liver disease. Guidelines have been instituted for scheduled pretreatment and interval liver biopsies to monitor the safety of methotrexate therapy.

Methotrexate is now used most often in a low-dose weekly regimen for the management of rheumatoid arthritis, psoriasis, and other immunologic conditions, including inflammatory bowel disease. The problem of hepatotoxicity has largely been overcome by the avoidance of daily dosing with methotrexate and a reduction in the weekly treatment regimen to a dose of 5 to 15 mg.[418-420]

Risk Factors

Risk factors for methotrexate-induced hepatic fibrosis are listed in Table 83–7; dose, alcohol intake, and preexisting liver disease are the most important.[419,420] Total dose, incremental dose, dosing interval, and duration of methotrexate therapy each influence the risk of

Table 83–7 Risk Factors for Methotrexate-Induced Hepatic Fibrosis

Risk Factor	Importance	Implications for Prevention
Age	Increased risk >60 yr; possibly related to renal clearance and/or biological effect on fibrogenesis	Greater care in use of methotrexate in older people
Dose	Incremental dose	5-15 mg/wk safe
	Dose frequency	Weekly bolus (pulse) safer than daily schedules
	Duration of therapy	Consider liver biopsy every 2 years
	Cumulative (total) dose	Consider liver biopsy after each 2 g methotrexate
Alcohol consumption	Increased risk with daily levels >15 g (1 to 2 drinks)	Avoid methotrexate use if intake not curbed
		Consider pretreatment liver biopsy with relevant history
Obesity	Increased risk	Consider pretreatment and interval liver biopsies
Diabetes mellitus	Increased risk in obese persons (type 2 diabetes mellitus)	Consider pretreatment and interval liver biopsies
Preexisting liver disease	Greatly increased risk	Pretreatment liver biopsy mandatory
	Particularly related to alcohol, obesity, and diabetes (NASH)	Avoid methotrexate, or schedule interval biopsies according to severity of hepatic fibrosis, total dose, and duration of methotrexate therapy
		Monitor liver biochemical tests during therapy
Systemic disease	Possibly risk greater with psoriasis than rheumatoid arthritis (may depend on preexisting liver disease, alcohol intake)	None
Impaired renal function	Increased risk because of reduced clearance of methotrexate	Reduce dose; greater caution with use
Other drugs	Possibly NSAIDs increase risk; vitamin A, arsenic may increase risk	Greater caution with use; monitor liver biochemical tests

NASH, nonalcoholic steatohepatitis; NSAIDs, nonsteroidal anti-inflammatory drugs.

hepatic fibrosis. After the cumulative ingestion of 3 g of methotrexate, the chance of histologic progression is 20%, but only 3% of patients are found to have advanced hepatic fibrosis.[420] Obesity and diabetes mellitus may be important risk factors for fibrosis because they predispose to NASH and are associated with induction of CYP2E1; the strong association between NASH and methotrexate in causing liver injury during long-term low-dose methotrexate treatment has been highlighted,[92] as has the possibility that methotrexate itself can cause a pattern of injury resembling steatohepatitis. Increasing age, impaired renal function, and concomitant use of certain drugs decrease the elimination of methotrexate or facilitate tissue uptake by displacing methotrexate from plasma protein-binding sites.

Psoriasis and rheumatoid arthritis are associated with various hepatic abnormalities that range from liver biochemical test abnormalities (in 25% to 50% of cases) and minor histologic changes (50% to 70%) to fibrosis (11% of patients with psoriasis) and cirrhosis (1% in patients with psoriasis) (see Chapter 34). In patients with psoriasis, alcoholism often is a complicating factor. In a meta-analysis,[420] alcohol consumption was the most important determinant of advanced hepatic fibrosis in patients undergoing methotrexate treatment; the risk of progressive hepatic fibrosis was 73% in persons who drank more than 15 g of alcohol daily, compared with 26% in those who did not.

The possibility that low-dose (5 to 15 mg) methotrexate given as a single weekly dose can cause hepatic fibrosis has been debated.[6,418-420] The available data are limited by a lack of controlled studies in which pretreatment liver histologic appearance was evaluated; the lack of pretreatment liver histologic findings is a particularly serious deficiency in view of the high frequency of liver abnormalities among patients with rheumatoid arthritis and psoriasis. It appears that regimens in current use can promote hepatic fibrosis, at least at the ultrastructural level, but that cases of clinically significant liver disease are now virtually unknown. Indeed, repeat liver biopsies have shown a reduction in hepatic fibrosis despite continuation of methotrexate in lower doses.[421] Therefore, although methotrexate remains a potential cause of liver disease, advanced hepatic fibrosis is in large part preventable.[92]

Clinicopathologic Features

Liver biochemical test abnormalities are common among patients taking methotrexate, but advanced hepatic fibrosis occasionally can develop in the absence of such abnormalities. Likewise, nausea, fatigue, and abdominal pain are common adverse effects of methotrexate, but patients with hepatic fibrosis typically are asymptomatic unless complications of liver failure or portal hypertension, such as bleeding esophageal varices, develop.[5,6] A firm liver edge, hepatomegaly, splenomegaly, or ascites may be noted on physical examination. Liver biochemical test results are either normal or nonspecific and may include minor elevations of the serum ALT and GGTP levels.[5,6] In more advanced cases, hypoalbuminemia is present, but elevations of the serum bilirubin level and coagulation disturbances are rare. Thrombocytopenia may be present in patients with cirrhosis.[6]

Liver histologic findings often are graded according to the system of Roenigk, which has been useful in analyzing the published literature.[93,420] In this system, grades 1 and 2 indicate varying amounts of steatosis, nuclear pleomorphism, and necroinflammatory activity but no fibrosis. Higher grades reflect increasing degrees of fibrosis, as follows: grade 3a, few septa; grade 3b, bridging fibrosis; and grade 4, cirrhosis. The pattern of hepatic fibrosis includes pericellular fibrosis, a feature of both alcoholic steatohepatitis and NASH; the possibility that methotrexate itself causes steatohepatitis or accentuates fibrogenesis among persons with underlying "primary NASH" has been suggested.[92] Cases of hepatic fibrosis in livers with a relative paucity (or complete absence) of portal and lobular inflammation have been reported, however.

Outcome and Prevention

Serious clinical sequelae (portal hypertension, liver failure, hepatocellular carcinoma) resulting from methotrexate-induced liver disease are now rarely seen. In a study of 32 patients with inflammatory bowel disease receiving long-term methotrexate (mean dose of 2.6 g; follow-up period of 131 weeks), minor histologic changes in the liver were common, but advanced hepatic fibrosis was rare.[422] Cases that have come to liver transplantation generally have been associated with suboptimal supervision of methotrexate therapy.[423] Cases of severe hepatic fibrosis (Roenigk grades 3b and 4) often are associated with lack of progression and even improvement after discontinuation of methotrexate or a reduction in the dose.[421] In less severe cases, a balanced judgment must be made about the appropriateness of continuing or discontinuing methotrexate. An interval liver biopsy after an additional 2 years or 2 g of methotrexate may be judicious in a patient who is found to have minor fibrosis on the initial liver biopsy specimen.

Recommendations for preventing methotrexate-induced hepatic fibrosis have been made (see Chapter 34).[419,424] If at all possible, methotrexate should be avoided when the risk of liver injury is high. Patients should abstain from alcohol use during treatment, and those drinking more than 100 g of ethanol per week should not be given methotrexate.[419,420,424] A pretreatment liver biopsy is indicated only if the liver biochemical test results are abnormal or if the history (e.g., alcoholism, risk factors for NASH) and clinical features (e.g., hepatomegaly) indicate possible underlying liver disease.[5,6,92]

The use of liver biochemical testing to monitor progress is recommended but is problematic because of the lack of specificity and sensitivity of the tests; four to six sets of liver biochemical test values often are obtained each year in people undergoing methotrexate treatment. Persistent or recurrent elevation in serum AST or ALT levels, any decrease in the serum albumin level, or the development of hepatomegaly warrants investigation by liver biopsy. Scheduled liver biopsies are recommended after a cumulative methotrexate dose of 4 g or therapy duration of 2 years,[420] but whether a liver biopsy is necessary in patients with normal liver biochemistry test results and without major risk factors for hepatic fibrosis remains unclear.[421,424] Noninvasive serum biochemical tests that indicate progressive hepatic fibrosis, such as the procollagen type III peptide assay, have not proved sufficiently accurate for monitoring patients taking methotrexate.[5]

DRUG-INDUCED VASCULAR TOXICITY

Vascular injury gives rise to several unusual types of liver disease, including hepatic venous outflow obstruction, dilatation and destruction of hepatic sinusoids (peliosis hepatis), noncirrhotic portal hypertension, and nodular regenerative hyperplasia (see Chapter 80). Drugs and chemical toxins are the most common cause of hepatic vascular injury.[18,403] The mechanism is primarily dose-dependent toxicity to sinusoidal and other vascular endothelial cells; additional risk factors include interactions between drugs used in combination and with radiotherapy. Activation of inflammatory cells also may be important. Individual drugs (e.g., azathioprine) have been associated with more than one vascular syndrome, and the individual disorders overlap and may evolve from one type to another. Vascular injury may give rise to a continuum of disorders, each resulting from damage to different components of the hepatic vasculature. The essential features of these disorders are summarized in Table 83–8. Hepatic imaging and measurement of portal pressure play a role in the diagnosis of these conditions, some of which, particularly nodular regenerative hyperplasia, are difficult to confirm in needle biopsy specimens of the liver.

SINUSOIDAL OBSTRUCTION SYNDROME (VENO-OCCLUSIVE DISEASE)

Veno-occlusive disease, now renamed *sinusoidal obstruction syndrome*,[87,88] is the most common type of drug-induced vascular injury and is often fatal (Chapter 80). More than 20 drugs and toxic alkaloids have been identified as causative agents. All contain a strong alkylating agent that can destroy the vascular endothelium of sinu-soids and terminal hepatic venules, as well as surrounding hepatocytes. Hepatotoxicity is at least partly dose dependent. Sinusoidal obstruction syndrome occurs in at least 1% of patients using anticancer drugs, and rates as high as 54% have been reported after bone marrow transplantation, depending on the regimen used.[162] Pyrrolizidine alkaloids are another important cause (see Chapter 84).[87,88]

The onset of sinusoidal obstruction syndrome generally is at 2 to 10 weeks after initiation of therapy. The clinical features are described in Chapter 80. No specific treatment exists. The prognosis generally has been regarded as poor, with death occurring within a few weeks in most patients with liver failure. Recovery is possible, however, particularly in less severe cases.

NODULAR REGENERATIVE HYPERPLASIA

Nodular regenerative hyperplasia of the liver is characterized by the presence of regenerative nodules in the absence of hepatic fibrosis. The critical lesion is obliterative portal venopathy (i.e., obstruction of the terminal radicles of hepatic arterioles and portal venules, possibly secondary to endothelial cell damage). The resulting hepatic ischemia may be responsible for induction of the nodular regenerative change. Nodular regenerative hyperplasia is associated with myeloproliferative and immunologic disorders (see Chapter 33), but cases attributed to the use of anticancer drugs and azathioprine are well documented (see Table 83–8).[287]

The clinical features are described in Chapters 33 and 80. The prognosis is generally good; complete reversal of the abnormalities may occur in some drug-induced cases.

NONCIRRHOTIC PORTAL HYPERTENSION

Noncirrhotic portal hypertension induced by drugs usually results from obstruction of the portal vein or its terminal branches, or of hepatic veins, or from compres-

Table 83–8 Types of Drug-Induced Hepatic Vascular Disorders: Clinicopathologic Features and Major Etiologic Agents

Disorder	Clinicopathologic Features and Outcome	Implicated Etiologic Agents
Sinusoidal obstruction syndrome (veno-occlusive disease)	Abdominal pain, tender hepatomegaly, ascites, liver failure; occasionally chronic liver disease, other signs of portal hypertension; high mortality rate; some cases may evolve into nodular regenerative hyperplasia	Especially in bone marrow transplantation: 6-thioguanine, busulfan; dactinomycin, azathioprine, mitomycin; pyrrolizidine alkaloids (e.g., in comfrey)
Nodular regenerative hyperplasia	Portal hypertension, encephalopathy—especially after variceal bleeding; diagnosed by histology; relatively good prognosis	Anticancer drugs: busulfan, dactinomycin; azathioprine
Noncirrhotic portal hypertension	Splenomegaly, hypersplenism, varices; ascites if associated hepatocellular disease; prognosis depends on cause and associated liver injury	Vitamin A, methotrexate, azathioprine, arsenic, vinyl chloride, anticancer drugs
Peliosis hepatis	Incidental finding, hepatomegaly, hepatic rupture, liver failure; diagnosed from appearances at surgery, vascular imaging; prognosis depends on cause and complications	Anabolic steroids, azathioprine, 6-thioguanine
Sinusoidal dilatation	Hepatomegaly, abdominal pain; may regress after stopping oral contraceptives	Oral contraceptive steroids

sion, damage, and distortion of the hepatic sinusoids. Such distortion may result from processes other than cirrhosis, including compression from swollen hepatocytes and perisinusoidal cells. A variable extent of perisinusoidal fibrosis is usual. Cases with more extensive hepatic fibrosis apparently arising from the portal tracts (*hepatoportal sclerosis*) may be a variant of this type of injury. Agents associated with noncirrhotic portal hypertension include vitamin A, azathioprine,[403] methotrexate, cytotoxic agents,[162] arsenic,[425] and vinyl chloride monomer (see Chapter 84).[426] The clinical features are described in Chapter 80.

PELIOSIS HEPATIS

Peliosis hepatis refers to the presence of blood-filled cavities that do not have an endothelial lining.[18,93] At laparoscopy, bluish-black cystic lesions are seen on the surface of the liver, ranging in diameter from 1 mm to several centimeters. The lesions correspond to dilatation and disruption of the sinusoidal architecture occurring as a result of disintegration of the reticulin framework. Surrounding hepatocytes atrophy. Peliosis hepatis may occur in association with androgens,[5] azathioprine,[403] estrogens, tamoxifen,[427] 6-thioguanine,[428] and possibly vitamin A.[429] It also is a common finding in association with sex steroid–induced liver tumors (see Chapter 91). The clinical features are described in Chapter 80. In some cases, regression of peliosis has been recorded after discontinuation of a causative drug.[428] The diagnosis is rarely suspected before surgery or liver biopsy, but the latter is contraindicated if peliosis is suspected. The clue is unexplained hepatomegaly in a patient taking a drug known to cause this lesion.

AZATHIOPRINE-RELATED VASCULAR INJURY

Hepatic complications of azathioprine, although rare, may be severe, diverse, and often late in onset. The overall frequency is less than 0.1%, but many cases occur in complex medical situations, particularly organ transplantation, in which activation of the immune system, viral infections, and other agents may increase the risk of hepatotoxicity. The central role of azathioprine has been confirmed in some cases that resolved after discontinuation of the drug and others in which a positive rechallenge was documented.[430] Disorders associated with azathioprine include bland cholestasis, cholestatic hepatitis with bile duct injury,[431,432] zonal necrosis, and vascular toxicity,[433,434] which gives rise to the diverse syndromes of sinusoidal obstruction syndrome, peliosis hepatis, nodular regenerative hyperplasia, and noncirrhotic portal hypertension.[434,435] Hepatocellular carcinoma with focal glycogenosis also has been reported in a long-term recipient.[430]

Azathioprine is associated with an extraordinary range of hepatic disorders, including liver biochemical test abnormalities in asymptomatic patients, bland cholestasis, cholestatic hepatitis, bile duct injury, and vascular injury. Cholestatic hepatitis probably is the most common presentation; several cases have been associated with zone 3 necrosis and congestion, suggesting acute vascular injury, and azathioprine shares the vascular toxicity of other thiopurines (see Table 83–8). All of the hepatic syndromes resulting from vascular injury have been associated with use of azathioprine after organ transplantation. Cases of azathioprine-induced nodular regenerative hyperplasia and sinusoidal obstruction syndrome also have been reported with other medical conditions, including inflammatory bowel disease.[437]

No relation to dose or duration of azathioprine therapy has been observed, but men are affected almost exclusively in cases of hepatic vascular injury following renal transplantation.[5,18,403] The onset of cholestatic reactions is 2 weeks to 22 months after the start of azathioprine, but vascular toxicity is recognized later, typically 3 months to 3 years, and occasionally more than 9 years, after transplantation.[438] The presentation and the clinical features depend on the type of reaction. Cases of later onset are the result of delayed recognition and tend to be associated with complications of portal hypertension, ascites, and liver failure. Patients may recover,[438] but the overall mortality rate is high.

In contrast with azathioprine, *6-mercaptopurine* may cause dose-dependent hepatocellular necrosis, which has been fatal in a few cases, and, even more rarely, cholestasis.[5]

REFERENCES

1. Gluud C: Acute, serious drug-induced liver injury. J Hepatol 97:657, 2002.
2. Lasser KE, Allen PD, Woolhandler SJ, et al: Timing of new black box warnings and withdrawals for prescription medications. JAMA 287:2215, 2002.
3. Sgro C, Clinard F, Ouazir K, et al: Incidence of drug-induced hepatic injuries: A French population-based study. Hepatology 36:451, 2000.
4. Ibanez L, Perez E, Vidal X, et al: Prospective surveillance of acute serious liver disease unrelated to infectious, obstructive, or metabolic diseases: Epidemiological and clinical features, and exposure to drugs. J Hepatol 37:592, 2002.
5. Farrell GC: Drug-Induced Liver Disease. Edinburgh, Churchill Livingstone, 1994.
6. Zimmerman HJ: Hepatotoxicity. The Adverse Effects of Drugs and Other Chemicals on the Liver, 2nd ed. Philadelphia, Lippincott Williams & Wilkins, 1999.
7. Ostapowicz G, Fontana RJ, Schiødt FV, et al: Results of a prospective study of acute liver failure at 17 tertiary care centers in the United States. Ann Intern Med 137:947, 2002.
8. Kaplowitz N: Causality assessment versus guilt-by-association in drug hepatotoxicity. Hepatology 33:308, 2001.
9. Biour M, Poupon R, Grange JD, et al: Drug-induced hepatotoxicity. The 13th updated edition of the bibliographic database of drug-related liver injuries and responsible drugs. Gastroenterol Clin Biol 24:1052, 2000.
10. Kromann-Andersen H, Pedersen A: Reported adverse reactions to and consumption of nonsteroidal anti-inflammatory drugs in Denmark over a 17-year period. Dan Med Bull 35:187, 1988.
11. García Rodríguez LA, Gutthann SP, Walker AM, et al: The role of nonsteroidal anti-inflammatory drugs in acute liver injury. BMJ 305:865, 1992.
12. Larrey D, Vital T, Babany G, et al: Hepatitis associated with amoxicillin–clavulanic acid combination. Report of 15 cases. Gut 33:368, 1992.

13. O'Donohue J, Oien KA, Donaldson P, et al: Co-amoxiclav jaundice: Clinical and histological features and HLA class II association. Gut 47:717, 2000.

14. Bjornsson E, Lindberg J, Olsson R: Liver reactions to oral low-dose tetracyclines. Scand J Gastroenterol 32:390, 1997.

15. Wong WM, Wu PC, Yuen MF, et al: Antituberculosis drug–related liver dysfunction in chronic hepatitis B infection. Hepatology 31:201, 2000.

16. Ungo JR, Jones D, Ashkin D, et al: Antituberculosis drug–induced hepatotoxicity. The role of hepatitis C virus and the human immunodeficiency virus. Am J Respir Crit Care Med 157:1871, 1998.

17. Hurwitz ES, Barrett MJ, Bregman D, et al: Public Health Service study of Reye's syndrome and medications. JAMA 257:1905, 1987.

18. Dourakis SP, Tolis G: Sex hormonal preparations and the liver. Eur J Contracept Reprod Health Care 3:7, 1998.

19. Rooks JB, Ory HW, Ishak KG, et al: Epidemiology of hepatocellar adenoma. The role of oral contraceptive use. JAMA 242:644, 1979.

20. Prentice RL: Epidemiologic data on exogenous hormones and hepatocellular carcinoma and selected other cancers. Prev Med 20:38, 1991.

21. Larrey D, Pageaux GP: Genetic predisposition to drug-induced hepatotoxicity. J Hepatol 26(suppl 2):12, 1997.

22. Bryant AE, Dreifuss FE: Valproic acid hepatic fatalities. III. U.S. experience since 1986. Neurology 46:465, 1996.

23. Berson A, Freneaux E, Larrey D, et al: Possible role of HLA in hepatotoxicity. An exploratory study in 71 patients with drug-induced idiosyncratic hepatitis. J Hepatol 20:336, 1994.

24. Andrade RJ, Lucena MI, Alonso A, et al: HLA class II genotype influences the type of liver injury in drug-induced idiosyncratic liver disease. Hepatology 39:1603, 2004.

25. Hautekeete ML, Horsmans Y, Van Waeyenberge C, et al: HLA association of amoxicillin-clavulanate–induced hepatitis. Gastroenterology 117:1181, 1999.

26. Kurosaki M, Takagi H, Mori M: HLA-A33/B44/DR6 is highly related to intrahepatic cholestasis induced by tiopronin. Dig Dis Sci 45:1103, 2000.

27. Aithal PG, Day C: The natural history of histologically proved drug induced liver disease. Gut 44:731, 1999.

28. Belay ED, Bresee JS, Holman RC, et al: Reye's syndrome in the United States from 1981 through 1997. N Engl J Med 340:1377, 1999.

29. Krähenbühl S, Bandner S, Kleinle S, et al: Mitochondrial diseases represent a risk factor for valproate-induced fulminant hepatic failure. Liver 20:346, 2000.

30. Smith DW, Cullity GJ, Silberstein EP: Fatal hepatic necrosis associated with multiple anticonvulsant therapy. Aust N Z J Med 18:575, 1988.

31. Perez Gutthann S, Garcia Rodriguez LA: The increased risk of hospitalizations for acute liver injury in a population with exposure to multiple drugs. Epidemiology 4:496, 1993.

32. Kaplowitz N: Mechanisms of liver cell injury. J Hepatol 32(suppl 1):39, 2000.

33. Kaplowitz N: Biochemical and cellular mechanisms of toxic liver injury. Semin Liver Dis 22:137, 2002.

34. Whitcomb DC, Block GD: Association of acetaminophen hepatotoxicity with fasting and ethanol use. JAMA 272:1845, 1994.

35. Singh J, Garg PK, Tandon RK: Hepatotoxicity due to antituberculosis therapy. Clinical profile and reintroduction of therapy. J Clin Gastroenterol 22:211, 1996.

36. Gray DR, Morgan T, Chretien SD, et al: Efficacy and safety of controlled-release niacin in dyslipoproteinemic veterans. Ann Intern Med 121:252, 1994.

37. Marotta PJ, Roberts EA: Pemoline hepatotoxicity in children. J Pediatr 132:894, 1998.

38. Dennis EW: Fatal hepatic necrosis in association with the use of hycanthone. S Afr Med J 54:137, 1978.

39. Sulkowski MS, Thomas DL, Chaisson RE, Moore RD: Hepatotoxicity associated with antiretroviral therapy in adults infected with human immunodeficiency virus and the role of hepatitis C or B virus. JAMA 283:74, 2000.

40. Riley TR 3rd, Smith JP: Ibuprofen-induced hepatotoxicity in patients with chronic hepatitis C: A case series. Am J Gastroenterol 93:1563, 1998.

41. Strasser SI, Myerson D, Spurgeon CL, et al: Hepatitis C virus infection and bone marrow transplantation: A cohort study with 10-year follow-up. Hepatology 29:1893, 1999.

42. Pu YS, Liu CM, Kao JH, et al: Antiandrogen hepatotoxicity in patients with chronic viral hepatitis. Eur Urol 36:293, 1999.

43. Bonacini M: Liver injury during highly active antiretroviral therapy: The effect of hepatitis C infection. Clin Infect Dis 38(suppl 2):S104, 2004.

44. Sulkowski MS: Drug-induced liver injury associated with antiretroviral therapy that includes HIV-1 protease inhibitors. Clin Infect Dis 38(suppl 2):S90, 2004.

45. Dieterich DT, Robinson PA, Love J, Stern JO: Drug-induced liver injury associated with the use of nonnucleoside reverse transcriptase inhibitors. Clin Infect Dis 38(suppl 2):S80, 2004.

46. Qurishi N, Kreuzberg C, Lüchters G, et al: HAART and the HCV-infected liver: Friend or foe? Lancet 362:1708, 2003.

47. Gordin FM, Simon GL, Wofsy CB, et al: Adverse reactions to trimethoprim-sulfamethoxazole in patients with acquired immunodeficiency syndrome. Ann Intern Med 100:495, 1984.

48. Chan KA, Truman A, Gurwitz JH, et al: A cohort study of the incidence of serious acute liver injury in diabetic patients treated with hypoglycaemic agents. Arch Intern Med 163:728, 2003.

49. Ransford RA, Langman MJ: Sulphasalazine and melsalazine: Serious adverse events reevaluated on the basis of suspected adverse reaction reports to the Committee on Safety of Medicines. Gut 51:536, 2002.

50. Yamazaki H, Shibata A, Suzuki M, et al: Oxidation of troglitazone to a quinone-type metabolite catalyzed by cytochrome P-450 2C8 and P-450 3A4 in human liver microsomes. Drug Metab Dispos 27:1260, 1999.

51. Fau D, Lekehal M, Farrell G, et al: Diterpenoids from germander, an herbal medicine, induce apoptosis in isolated rat hepatocytes. Gastroenterology 113:1334, 1997.

52. Haouzi D, Lekehal M, Moreau A, et al: Cytochrome P450–generated reactive metabolites cause mitochondrial permeability transition, caspase activation, and apoptosis in rat hepatocytes. Hepatology 32:303, 2000.

53. Morgan MY, Reshef R, Shah RR, et al: Impaired oxidation of debrisoquine in patients with perhexiline liver injury. Gut 25:1057, 1984.

54. George J, Byth K, Farrell GC: Age but not gender selectively affects expression of individual cytochrome P450 proteins in human liver. Biochem Pharmacol 50:727, 1996.

55. Hunt CM, Westerkam WR, Stave GM: Effect of age and gender on the activity of human hepatic CYP3A. Biochem Pharmacol 44:275, 1992.

56. George J, Byth K, Farrell GC: Influence of clinicopathological variables on CYP protein expression in human liver. J Gastroenterol Hepatol 11:33, 1996.

57. George J, Murray M, Byth K, Farrell GC: Differential alterations of cytochrome P450 proteins in livers from patients with severe chronic liver disease. Hepatology 21:120, 1995.

58. George J, Liddle C, Murray M, et al: Pre-translational regulation of cytochrome P450 genes is responsible for disease-specific changes of individual P450 enzymes among patients with cirrhosis. Biochem Pharmacol 49:873, 1995.

59. Goodwin B, Hodgson E, Liddle C: Orphan human pregnane X receptor mediates the transcriptional activation of *CYP3A4* by rifampicin through a distal enhancer module. Mol Pharmacol 56:1329, 1999.

60. Liddle C, Goodwin B. Regulation of hepatic drug metabolism: The role of the nuclear receptors PXR and CAR. Semin Liver Dis 22:115, 2002.

61. Moore LB, Goodwin B, Jones SA, et al: St. John's wort induces hepatic drug metabolism through activation of the pregnane X receptor. Proc Natl Acad Sci U S A 97:7500, 2000.

62. Meech R, Mackenzie PI: Structure and function of uridine diphosphate glucuronosyltransferases. Clin Exp Pharmacol Physiol 24:907, 1997.

63. Lee J, Boyer JL: Molecular alterations in hepatocyte transport mechanisms in acquired cholestatic liver disorders. Semin Liver Dis 20:373, 2000.

64. Trauner M, Meier PJ, Boyer JL: Molecular pathogenesis of cholestasis. N Engl J Med 339:1217, 1998.

65. Bohan A, Boyer JL: Mechanisms of hepatic transport of drugs: Implications for cholestatic drug reactions. Semin Liver Dis 22:123, 2002.

66. Huang L, Smit JW, Meijer DK, Vore M: Mrp2 is essential for estradiol-17beta(beta-D-glucuronide)-induced cholestasis in rats. Hepatology 32:66, 2000.

67. Funk C, Ponelle C, Scheuermann G, Pantze M: Cholestatic potential of troglitazone-induced hepatotoxicity: In vivo and in vitro interaction at the canalicular bile salt export pump (BSEP) in the rat. Mol Pharmacol 59:627, 2001.

68. Iverson SL, Uetrecht JP: Identification of a reactive metabolite of terbinafine: Insights into terbinafine-induced hepatotoxicity. Chem Res Toxicol 14:175, 2001.

69. Lakehal F, Dansette PM, Becquemont L, et al: Indirect cytotoxicity of flucloxacillin toward human biliary epithelium via metabolite formation in hepatocytes. Chem Res Toxicol 14:694, 2001.

70. Kaplowitz N, Tsukamoto H: Oxidative stress and liver disease. Prog Liver Dis 14:131, 1996.

71. Jones BE, Liu H, Lo CR, et al: Cytochrome P450 2E1 expression induces hepatocyte resistance to cell death from oxidative stress. Antioxid Redox Signal 4:701, 2002.

72. Nieto N, Mari M, Cederbaum AI: Cytochrome P450 2E1 responsiveness in the promoter of glutamate-cysteine ligase catalytic subunit. Hepatology 37:96, 2003.

73. Patel T, Steer CJ, Gores GJ: Apoptosis and the liver: A mechanism of disease, growth regulation, and carcinogenesis. Hepatology 30:811, 1999.

74. Kaplowitz N: Hepatotoxicity of herbal remedies: Insights into the intricacies of plant-animal warfare and cell death. Gastroenterology 113:1408, 1997.

75. Wei MC, Zong W-X, Cheng EH-Y, et al: Proapoptotic BAX and BAK: A requisite gateway to mitochondrial dysfunction and death. Science 292:727, 2001.

76. Joza N, Susin SA, Daugas E, et al: Essential role of the mitochondrial apoptosis-inducing factor in programmed cell death. Nature 410:549, 2001.

77. Lei K, Davis RJ: JNK phosphorylation of Bim-related members of the Bcl2 family induces Bax-dependent apoptosis. Proc Natl Acad Sci U S A 100:2432, 2003.

78. Maher JJ, Gores GJ: Apoptosis: Silent killer or neutron bomb? Hepatology 28:865, 1998.

79. Dimmeler S, Haendeler J, Sause A, Zeiher AM: Nitric oxide inhibits APO-1/Fas-mediated cell death. Cell Growth Differ 9:415, 1998.

80. Lewis W, Dalakas MC: Mitochondrial toxicity of antiviral drugs. Nat Med 1:417, 1995.

81. Tapner MJ, Jones BE, Wu W, Farrell GC: Toxicity of low-dose azathioprine and 6-mercaptopurine in rat hepatocytes. Roles of xanthine oxidase and mitochondrial injury. J Hepatol 40:454, 2004.

82. Lemasters J: Mechanisms of hepatic toxicity V. Necrapoptosis and the mitochondrial permeability transition: Shared pathways to necrosis and apoptosis. Am J Physiol 276:G1, 1999.

83. Laskin DL: Nonparenchymal cells and hepatotoxicity. Sem Liver Dis 10:293, 1990.

84. Czaja M, Xu J, Alte E: Prevention of carbon tetrachloride–induced rat liver injury by soluble tumor necrosis receptor. Gastroenterology 108:1849, 1995.

85. Laskin DL, Gardner CR, Price VF, Jollow DJ: Modulation of macrophage functioning abrogates the acute hepatotoxicity of acetaminophen. Hepatology 21:1045, 1995.

86. Boess F, Bopst M, Althaus R, et al: Acetaminophen hepatotoxicity in tumor necrosis factor/lymphcytotoxin-α gene knockout mice. Hepatology 27:1021, 1998.

87. DeLeve LD, McCuskey RS, Wang X, et al: Characterization of a reproducible rat model of hepatic veno-occlusive disease. Hepatology 29:1779, 1999.

88. DeLeve LD, Wang X, Kand GC, et al: Decreased hepatocyte NO production contributes to the development of rat sinusoidal obstructive syndrome. Hepatology 38:900, 2003.

89. Smith GCM, Kenna JG, Harrison DJ, et al: Autoantibodies to hepatic microsomal carboxylesterase in halothane hepatitis. Lancet 342:963, 1993.

90. Kretz-Rommel A, Boelsterli UA: Cytotoxic activity of T cells and non-T cells from diclofenac-immunized mice against cultured syngeneic hepatocytes exposed to diclofenac. Hepatology 22:213, 1995.

91. Mackay IR: The immunological mediation of drug reactions affecting the liver. In Farrell GC (ed): Drug-Induced Liver Disease. Edinburgh, Churchill Livingstone, 1994, p 61.

92. Langman G, Hall PM, Todd G: Role of non-alcoholic steatohepatitis in methotrexate-induced liver injury. J Gastroenterol Hepatol 16:1395, 2001.

93. Hall P de la M: Histopathology of drug-induced liver disease. In Farrell GC (ed): Drug-Induced Liver Disease. Edinburgh, Churchill Livingstone, 1994, pp 115.

94. Knowles SR, Uetrecht J, Shear NH: Idiosyncratic drug reactions: The reactive metabolite syndromes. Lancet 356:1587, 2000.

95. Andrade RJ, Camargo R, Lucena MI, Gonzalez-Grande R: Causality assessment in drug-induced hepatotoxicity. Expert Opin Drug Saf 3:329, 2004.

96. Lewis LD, Nierenberg DW: Adverse drug reactions, Medwatch reporting and medical student education. Pharmacoepidemiol Drug Saf 12:93, 2003.

97. Danan G, Benichou C: Causality assessment of adverse reactions to drugs. I. A novel method based on the conclusions of international consensus meetings: Application to drug-induced liver injuries. J Clin Epidemiol 46:1323, 1993.

98. Maria VA, Victorino RM: Development and validation of a clinical scale for the diagnosis of drug induced hepatitis. Hepatology 26:664, 1997.

99. Lucena MI, Camargo R, Andrade RJ, et al: Comparison of two clinical scales for causality assessment in hepatotoxicity. Hepatology 33:123, 2001.

100. Laurent-Puig P, Dussaix E, de Paillette L, et al: Prevalence of hepatitis C RNA in suspected drug-induced liver diseases [letter]. J Hepatol 19:487, 1993.

101. Maria VA, Victorino RM: Diagnostic value of specific T cell reactivity to drugs in 95 cases of drug induced liver injury. Gut 41:534, 1997.

102. Benichou C: Criteria for drug-induced liver disorders. Report of an International Consensus Meeting. J Hepatol 11:272, 1990.

103. Benichou C, Danan G, Flahault A: Causality assessment of adverse reactions to drugs. II. An original model for validation of drug causality assessment methods: Case reports with positive rechallenge. J Clin Epidemiol 46:1331, 1993.

104. Kaplowitz N: Avoiding hepatic injury from drugs. Gastroenterology 117:759, 1999.

105. Amacher DE: Serum transaminase elevations as indicators of hepatic injury following the administration of drugs. Regul Toxicol Pharmacol 27:119, 1998.

106. Rosenzweig P, Miget N, Brohier S: Transaminase elevation on placebo during phase I trials. Br J Clin Pharmacol 48:19, 1999.

107. Cohn WJ, Boylan JJ, Blanke RV, et al: Treatment of chlordecone (Kepone) toxicity with cholestyramine. Results of a controlled clinical trial. N Engl J Med 298:243, 1978.

108. Pond SM, Olson KR, Woo OF, et al: Amatoxin poisoning in Northern California, 1982-1983. West J Med 145:204, 1986.

109. Kaplowitz N: Acetaminophen hepatotoxicity: What do we know, what don't we know, and what do we do next? Hepatol 40:10, 2004.

110. Lee WM: Acetaminophen and the U.S. Acute Liver Failure Study Group: Lowering the risks of hepatic failure. Hepatology 40:6, 2004.

111. Dart RC, Kuffner EK, Rumack BH: Treatment of pain or fever with paracetamol (acetaminophen) in the alcoholic patient: A systematic review. Am J Therapeut 7:123, 2000.

112. Prescott LF: Therapeutic misadventure with paracetamol: Fact or fiction? Am J Therapeut 7:99, 2000.

113. Zimmerman HJ, Maddrey WC: Acetaminophen (paracetamol) hepatotoxicity with regular intake of alcohol: Analysis of instance of therapeutic misadventure. Hepatology 22:767, 1995.

114. Crippin JS: Acetaminophen hepatotoxicity: potentiation by isoniazid. Am J Gastroenterol 88:590, 1993.

115. Prescott LF, Critchley JAJH: The treatment of acetaminophen poisoning. Annu Rev Pharmacol Toxicol 23:87, 1983.

116. Heubi JE, Barbacci MB, Zimmerman HJ: Therapeutic misadventures with acetaminophen: Hepatotoxicity after multiple doses in children. J Pediatr 132:22, 1998.

117. Nolan CM, Sandblom RE, Thummel KE, et al: Hepatotoxicity associated with acetaminophen usage in patients receiving multiple drug therapy for tuberculosis. Chest 105:408, 1994.

118. Vitols S: Paracetamol hepatotoxicity at therapeutic doses. J Intern Med 253:95, 2003.

119. Kurtovic J, Riordan SM: Paracetamol-induced hepatotoxicity at recommended dosage. J Intern Med 253:240, 2003.

120. Stricker BHCH, Meyboom RHB, Linqvist TM: Acute hypersensitivity reactions to paracetamol. BMJ 291:938, 1985.

121. Buckley NA, Whyte IM, O'Connell DL, Dawson AH: Oral or intravenous N-acetylcysteine: Which is the treatment of choice for acetaminophen (paracetamol) poisoning? J Toxicol Clin Toxicol 37:759, 1999.

122. Zhang J, Huang W, Chua SS, et al: Modulation of acetaminophen-induced hepatotoxicity by the xenobiotic receptor CAR. Science 298:422, 2002.

123. Manautou JE: CAR inhibitors: New line of treatment for APAP poisoning? J Hepatol 39:297, 2003.

124. Robinson D, Smith AM, Johnston GS: Severity of overdose after restriction of paracetamol availability: Retrospective study. BMJ 321:926, 2000.

125. Turvill JL, Burroughs AK, Moore KP: Change in occurrence of paracetamol overdose in U.K. after introduction of blister packs. Lancet 355:2048, 2000.

126. McKenny JM, Proctor JD, Harris S, et al: A comparison of the efficacy and toxic effects of sustained- vs immediate-release niacin in hypercholesterolemic patients. JAMA 271:672, 1994.

127. Gray DR, Morgan T, Chretien SD, Kashyap ML: Efficacy and safety of controlled-release niacin in dyslipoproteinemic veterans. Ann Intern Med 121:252, 1994.

128. Lahoti S, Lee WM: Hepatotoxicity of anticholesterol, cardiovascular, endocrine drugs and hormonal agents. Gastroenterol Clin North Am 24:907, 1995.

129. Mullin GE, Greenson JK, Mitchel MC: Fulminant hepatic failure after ingestion of sustained-release nicotinic acid. Ann Intern Med 111:253, 1989.

130. Dreifuss FE, Santilli N, Langer DH, et al: Valproic acid hepatic fatalities: A retrospective review. Neurology 37:379, 1987.

131. Konig SA, Schenk M, Sick C, et al: Fatal liver failure associated with valproate therapy in a patient with Friedreich's disease: Review of valproate hepatotoxicity in adults. Epilepsia 40:1036, 1999.

132. Bryant AE III, Dreifuss FE: Valproic acid hepatic fatalities. III. U.S. experience since 1986. Neurology 46:465, 1996.

133. Appleton RE, Farrell K, Applegarth DA, et al: The high incidence of valproate hepatotoxicity in infants may relate to familial metabolic defects. Canad J Neurol Sci 17:145, 1990.

134. McKenzie R, Fried MW, Sallie R, et al: Hepatic failure and lactic acidosis due to fialuridine (FIAU), an investigational nucleoside analogue for chronic hepatitis B. N Engl J Med 333:1099, 1995.

135. Kleiner DE, Gaffey MJ, Sallie R, et al: Histopathologic changes associated with fialuridine hepatotoxicity. Mod Pathol 10:192, 1997.

136. Klecker RW, Katki AG, Collins JM: Toxicity, metabolism, DNA incorporation with lack of repair, and lactate production for 1-(2'-fluoro-2'-deoxy-β-D-arabinofuranoxyl)-5-iodouracil in U-937 and MOLT-4 cells. Mol Pharmacol 46:1204, 1994.

137. Horn DM, Neeb LA, Colacino JM, Richardson FC: Fialuridine is phosphorylated and inhibits DNA synthesis in isolated rat hepatic mitochondria. Antiviral Res 34:71, 1997.

138. Kontorinis N, Dieterich DT: Toxicity of non-nucleotide analogue reverse transcriptase inhibitors. Semin Liver Dis 23:173, 2003.

139. Kakuda TN: Pharmacology of nucleoside and nucleotide reverse transcriptase inhibitor–induced mitochondrial toxicity. Clin Ther 22:685, 2000.

140. Freiman JP, Helfert KE, Hamrell MR, et al: Hepatomegaly with severe steatosis in HIV-seropositive patients. AIDS 7:379, 1993.

141. Chariot P, Drogou I, de Lacroix-Szmania I, et al: Zidovudine-induced mitochondrial disorder with massive liver steatosis, myopathy, lactic acidosis, and mitochondrial DNA depletion. J Hepatol 30:156, 1999.

142. Lai KK, Gang DL, Zawacki JK, et al: Fulminant hepatic failure associated with 2',3'-dideoxyinosine (ddI). Ann Intern Med 115:283, 1991.

143. Bissuel F, Bruneel F, Habersetzer F, et al: Fulminant hepatitis with severe lactic acidosis in HIV-infected patients on didanosine therapy. J Intern Med 235:367, 1994.

144. Roy PM, Gouello JP, Pennison-Besnier I, Chennebault JM: Severe lactic acidosis induced by nucleoside analogues in an HIV-infected man. Ann Emerg Med 34:282, 1999.

145. Miller KD, Cameron M, Wood LV, et al: Lactic acidosis and hepatic steatosis associated with use of stavudine: Report of four cases. Ann Intern Med 133:192, 2000.

146. Bleeker-Rovers CP, Kadir SW, van Leusen R, et al: Hepatic steatosis and lactic acidosis caused by stavudine in an HIV-infected patient. Neth J Med 57:190, 2000.

147. John M, Moore CB, James IR, et al: Chronic hyperlactemia in HIV-infected patients taking antiretroviral therapy. AIDS 15:717, 2001.

148. Carr A, Cooper DA: Adverse effects of antiretroviral therapy. Lancet 356:1423, 2000.

149. Cattelan AM, Erne E, Slatino A, et al: Severe hepatic failure related to nevirapine treatment. Clin Infect Dis 29:455, 1999.

150. Johnson S, Baraboutis JG, Sha BE, et al: Adverse effects associated with use of nevirapine in HIV postexposure for 2 health care workers [letter]. JAMA 284:2722, 2000.

151. Serious adverse events attributed to nevirapine regimens for postexposure prophylaxis after HIV exposures—worldwide, 1997-2000. JAMA 285:402, 2001.

152. Piroth L, Grappin M, Sgro C, et al: Recurrent NNRTI-induced hepatotoxicity in an HIV-HCV–coinfected patient. Ann Pharmacother 34:534, 2000.

153. Bräu N, Leaf HL, Wieczorek RL, et al: Severe hepatitis in three AIDS patients treated with indinavir [letter]. Lancet 349:924, 1997.

154. Matsuda J, Gohchi K, Yamanaka M: Severe hepatitis in patients with AIDS and haemophilia B treated with indinavir [letter]. Lancet 350:364, 1997.

155. Arribas JR, Ibanez C, Ruiz-Antoran B, et al: Acute hepatitis in HIV-infected patients during ritonavir treatment. AIDS 12:1722, 1998.

156. Picard O, Rosmorduc O, Cabane J: Hepatotoxicity associated with ritonavir [letter]. Ann Intern Med 129:670, 1998.

157. den Brinker M, Wit FW, Wertheim-van Dillen PM, et al: Hepatitis B and C virus co-infection and the risk for hepatotoxicity of highly active antiretroviral therapy in HIV-1 infection. AIDS 14:2895, 2000.

158. Piscitelli SC, Gallicano KD: Interactions among drugs for HIV and opportunistic infections. N Engl J Med 344:984, 2001.

159. Carr A, Cooper DA: Restoration of immunity to chronic hepatitis B infection in HIV-infected patient on protease inhibitor. Lancet 349:995, 1997.

160. O'Gorman T, Koff RS: Salicylate hepatitis. Gastroenterology 72:726, 1977.

161. Orlowski JP: Whatever happened to Reye's syndrome? Did it ever exist? Crit Care Med 27:1582, 1999.

162. Zimmerman HJ: Hepatotoxic effects of oncotherapeutic agents. In Popper H, Schaffner F (eds): Progress in Liver Disease, vol 8. New York, Grune & Stratton, 1986, p 621.

163. Bernuau J, Larrey D, Campillo B, et al: Amodiaquine-induced fulminant hepatitis. J Hepatol 6:109, 1988.

164. Zimmerman HJ: Update of hepatotoxicity due to classes of drugs in common clinical use: Non-steroidal, anti-inflammatory drugs, antibiotics, antihypertensives, and cardiac and psychotropic agents. Semin Liver Dis 10:322, 1990.

165. Stricker BCCH, Blok APR, Claas FHJ, et al: Hepatic injury associated with the use of nitrofurans: A clinicopathological study of 52 reported cases. Hepatology 8:599, 1988.

166. Sharp JR, Ishak KG, Zimmerman HJ: Chronic active hepatitis and severe hepatic necrosis associated with nitrofurantoin. Ann Intern Med 92:14, 1980.

167. Berry WR, Warren GH, Reichen J: Nitrofurantoin-induced cholestatic hepatitis from cow's milk in a teenaged boy. West J Med 140:278, 1984.

168. Mockli G, Crowley M, Stern R, et al: Massive hepatic necrosis in a child after administration of phenobarbital. Am J Gastroenterol 84:820, 1989.

169. Pellock JM, Brodie MJ: Felbamate: 1997 update. Epilepsia 38:1261, 1997.

170. Bjøro K, Gjerstad L, Bentdal Ø, et al: Topiramate and fulminant liver failure. Lancet 352:1119, 1998.

171. Lindgren A, Olsson R: Liver reactions from trimethoprim. J Intern Med 236:281, 1994.

172. Jones B: [Untitled letter]. Med J Aust 174:,368, 2001.

173. Dourakis SP, Tzemanakis E, Sinani C, et al: Gliclazide-induced acute hepatitis. Eur J Gastroenterol Hepatol 12:119, 2000.

174. Besnard M, Debray D, Durand P, et al: Fulminant hepatitis in two children treated with sulfasalazine for Crohn's disease. Arch Pediatr 6:643, 1999.

175. Hautekeete ML, Bougeois N, Potvin P, et al: Hypersensitivity with hepatotoxicity to mesalazine after hypersensitivity to sulfasalazine. Gastroenterology 103:1925, 1992.

176. Deltenre P, Berson A, Marcellin P, et al: Mesalazine (5-aminosalicylic acid) induced chronic hepatitis. Gut 44:886, 1999.

177. Goldstein PE, Deviere J, Cremer M: Acute hepatitis and drug-related lupus induced by minocycline treatment. Am J Gastroenterol 92:143, 1997.

178. Pohle T, Menzel J, Domschke W: Minocycline and fulminant hepatic failure necessitating liver transplantation. Am J Gastroenterol 95:560, 2000.

179. Bartle WR, Fisher MM, Kerenyi N: Disulfiram-induced hepatitis. Report of two cases and review of the literature. Dig Dis Sci 30:834, 1985.

180. Rabkin JM, Corless CL, Orloff SL, et al: Liver transplantation for disulfiram-induced hepatic failure. Am J Gastroenterol 93:830, 1998.

181. Tanner LA, Bosco LA, Zimmerman HJ: Hepatic toxicity after acetabutolol therapy. Ann Intern Med 111:533, 1989.

182. Clark JA, Zimmerman HJ, Tanner LA: Labetalol hepatotoxicity. Ann Intern Med 113:210, 1990.

183. Larrey D, Henrion J, Heller F, et al: Metoprolol-induced hepatitis: Rechallenge and drug oxidation phenotyping. Ann Intern Med 108:67, 1988.

184. Shaw DR, Misan GMH, Johnson RD: Nifedipine hepatitis. Aust N Z J Med 17:447, 1987.

185. Hare DL, Horowitz JD: Verapamil hepatotoxicity: A hypersensitivity reaction. Am Heart J 11:610, 1986.

186. Shallcross H, Padley SPG, Glynn MJ, et al: Fatal renal and hepatic toxicity after treatment with diltiazem. BMJ 295:1236, 1987.

187. Andrade RJ, Lucena MI, Fernandez MC, et al: Cholestatic hepatitis related to use of irbesartan: A case report and a literature review of angiotensin II antagonist–associated hepatotoxicity. Eur J Gastroenterol Hepatol 14:887, 2002.

188. Hariraj R, Stoner E, Jader S, Preston DM: Drug points: Prolonged cholestasis associated with irbesartan. BMJ 321:547, 2000.

189. Bellary SV, Isaacs PET: Captopril and the liver. Lancet 2:514, 1989.

190. Rahmat J, Gelfand RL, Gelfand M, et al: Captopril-associated cholestatic jaundice. Ann Intern Med 102:56, 1985.

191. Rosellini SR, Costa PL, Gaudio M, et al: Hepatic injury related to enalapril. Gastroenterology 97:810, 1989.

192. Todd P, Levison D, Farthing MJG. Enalapril-related cholestatic jaundice. J R Soc Med 83:271, 1990.

193. Rahmat J, Gelfand RL, Gelfand MC, et al: Captopril-associated cholestatic jaundice. Ann Intern Med 102:56, 1985.

194. Larrey D, Babany G, Bernuau J, et al: Fulminant hepatitis after lisinopril administration. Gastroenterology 99:1832, 1990.

195. Nunes AC, Amaro P, Macas F, et al: Fosinopril-induced prolonged cholestatic jaundice and pruritus: First case report. Eur J Gastroenterol Hepatol 13:279, 2001.

196. Farmer JA, Torre-Amione G: Comparative tolerability of the HMG-CoA reductase inhibitors. Drug Saf 23:197, 2000.

197. Tolman KG: Defining patient risks from expanded preventive therapies. Am J Cardiol 85:15E, 2000.

198. Grimbert S, Pessayre D, Degott C, Benhamou JP: Acute hepatitis induced by HMG-CoA reductase inhibitor, lovastatin. Dig Dis Sci 39:2032, 1994.

199. Hartleb M, Rymarczyk G, Januszewski K: Acute cholestatic hepatitis associated with pravastatin. Am J Gastroenterol 94:1388, 1999.

200. Jimenez-Alonso J, Osorio JM, Gutierrez-Cabello F, et al: Atorvastatin-induced cholestatic hepatitis in a young woman with systemic lupus erythematosus. Grupo Lupus Virgen de las Nieves. Arch Intern Med 159:1811, 1999.

201. Ballare M, Campanini M, Catania E, et al: Acute cholestatic hepatitis during simvastatin administration. Recent Prog Med 82:233, 1991.

202. Farrell GC: Hepatitis C, Other Liver Disorders, and Liver Health. Sydney, MacClennan and Petty, 2002, p 1.

203. Chalasani N, Aljadhey H, Kesterson J, et al: Patients with elevated liver enzymes are not at a higher risk for statin hepatotoxicity. Gastroenterology 126:1287, 2004.

204. Downs JR, Clearfield M, Tyroler HA, et al: Air Force/Texas Coronary Atherosclerosis Prevention Study (AFCAPS/TEXCAPS): Additional perspectives on tolerability of long-term treatment with lovastatin. Am J Cardiol 87:1074, 2001.

205. Smith CC, Bernstein LI, Davis RB, et al: Screening for statin-related toxicity: The yield of transaminase and creatine kinase measurements in a primary care setting. Arch Intern Med 163:688, 2003.

206. Roenigk HH Jr: Liver toxicity of retinoid therapy. J Am Acad Dermatol 19:199, 1988.

207. Andrade RJ, Lucena MI, Martin-Vivaldi R, et al: Acute liver injury associated with the use of ebrotidine, a new H_2-receptor antagonist. J Hepatol 31:641, 1999.

208. Kimura H, Akamatsu K, Sakaue H, et al: Fulminant hepatitis induced by cimetidine. J Gastroenterol Hepatol 3:223, 1988.

209. Black M, Scott WE Jr, Kanter R: Possible ranitidine hepatotoxicity. Ann Intern Med 101:208, 1984.

210. Hashimoto F, Davis RL, Egli D: Hepatitis following treatments with famotidine and then cimetidine. Ann Pharmacother 28:37, 1994.

211. Jochem V, Kirkpatrick R, Greenson J, et al: Fulminant hepatic failure related to omeprazole. Am J Gastroenterol 87:523, 1992.

212. Koury SI, Stone CK, La Charite DD: Omeprazole and the development of acute hepatitis. Eur J Emerg Med 5:467, 1998.

213. Reinus JF, Persky S, Burkiewicz JS, et al: Severe liver injury after treatment with the leukotriene receptor antagonist zafirlukast. Ann Intern Med 133:964, 2000.

214. Remy AJ, Heran B, Galindo G, et al: A new drug responsible for microvesicular steatosis: Ticlopidine. Gastroenterol Clin Biol 23:151, 1999.

215. Mitchell JR, Zimmerman HJ, Ishak KG, et al: Isoniazid liver injury: Clinical spectrum, pathology and probable pathogenesis. Ann Intern Med 84:181, 1976.

216. Maddrey WC: Isoniazid-induced liver disease. Semin Liver Dis 1:129, 1981.

217. Durand F, Bernuau J, Pessayre D, et al: Deleterious influence of pyrazinamide on the outcome of patients with fulminant or subfulminant liver failure during antituberculous treatment including isoniazid. Hepatology 21:929, 1995.

218. Hwang SJ, Wu JC, Lee CN, et al: A prospective clinical study of isoniazid-rifampicin-pyrazinamide–induced liver injury in an area endemic for hepatitis B. J Gastroenterol Hepatol 12:87, 1997.

219. Halpern M, Meyers B, Miller C, et al: Severe isoniazid-associated hepatitis—New York, 1991-1993. JAMA 270:809, 1993.

220. Pessayre D, Bentata M, Deggott C, et al: Isoniazid rifampicin fulminant hepatitis: A possible consequence of enhancement of isoniazid hepatotoxicity by enzyme induction. Gastroenterology 72:284, 1977.

221. Bachs L, Parés A, Elena M, et al: Effects of long-term rifampicin administration in primary biliary cirrhosis. Gastroenterology 102:2077, 1992.

222. Lewis JH, Zimmerman HJ, Benson GD, et al: Hepatic injury associated with ketoconazole therapy. Analysis of 33 cases. Gastroenterology 86:503, 1984.

223. Chien RN, Yang LJ, Lin PY, et al: Hepatic injury during ketoconazole therapy in patients with onychomycosis: A controlled cohort study. Hepatology 25:103, 1997.

224. Knight TE, Shikuma CY, Knight J: Ketoconazole-induced fulminant hepatitis necessitating liver transplantation. J Am Acad Dermatol 25:398, 1991.

225. Zollner E, Delport S, Bonnici F: Fatal liver failure due to ketoconazole treatment of a girl with Cushing's syndrome. J Pediatr Endocrinol Metab 14:335, 2001.

226. van't Wout JW, Herrmann WA, de Vries RA, et al: Terbinafine-associated hepatic injury. J Hepatol 21:115, 1994.

227. Gupta AK, del Rosso JQ, Lynde CW, et al: Hepatitis associated with terbinafine therapy: Three case reports and a review of the literature. Clin Exp Dermatol 23:64, 1998.

228. Fernandes NF, Geller SA, Fong TL: Terbinafine hepatotoxicity: Case report and review of the literature. Am J Gastroenterol 93:459, 1998.

229. Agarwal K, Manas DM, Hudson M: Terbinafine and fulminant hepatic failure. N Engl J Med 340:1292, 1999.

230. Walter RB, Lukaschek J, Renner EL, et al: Fatal hepatic veno-occlusive disease associated with terbinafine in a liver transplant recipient. J Hepatol 38:373, 2003.

231. Itraconazole, terbinafine possibly linked to liver failure. Am J Health Syst Pharm 58:1076, 2001.

232. Talwalkar JA, Soetikno RE, Carr-Locke DL, et al: Severe cholestasis related to itraconazole for the treatment of onychomycosis. Am J Gastroenterol 94:3632, 1999.

233. Hann SK, Kim JB, Im S, et al: Itraconazole-induced acute hepatitis. Br J Dermatol 129:500, 1993.

234. Gallardo-Quesada S, Luelmo-Aguilar J, Guanyabens-Calvet C: Hepatotoxicity associated with itraconazole. Int J Dermatol 34:589, 1995.

235. Jacobson MA, Hanks DK, Ferrel LD: Fatal acute hepatic necrosis due to fluconazole. Am J Med 96:188, 1994.

236. Guillaume MP, De Prez C, Cogan E: Subacute mitochondrial liver disease in a patient with AIDS: Possible relationship to prolonged fluconazole administration. Am J Gastroenterol 91:165, 1996.

237. Crerar-Gilbert A, Boots R, Fraenkel D, et al: Survival following fulminant hepatic failure from fluconazole induced hepatitis. Anaesth Intensive Care 27:650, 1999.

238. Munoz P, Moreno S, Berenguer J, et al: Fluconazole-related hepatotoxicity in patients with acquired immunodeficiency syndrome. Arch Intern Med 151:1020, 1991.

239. Garcia Rodriguez LA, Duque A, Castellsague J, et al: A cohort study on the risk of acute liver injury among users of ketoconazole and other antifungal drugs. Br J Clin Pharmacol 48:847, 1999.

240. Watkins PB, Whitcomb RW: Hepatic dysfunction associated with troglitazone [letter]. N Engl J Med 338:916, 1998.

241. Shibuya A, Watanabe M, Yoshikuni F, et al: An autopsy case of troglitazone-induced fulminant hepatitis. Diabetes Care 21:2140, 1998.

242. Gitlin N, Julie NL, Spurr CL, et al: Two cases of severe clinical and histologic hepatotoxicity associated with troglitazone. Ann Intern Med 129:36, 1998.

243. Neuschwander-Tetri BA, Isley WL, Oki JC, et al: Troglitazone-induced hepatic failure leading to liver transplantation. Ann Intern Med 129:38, 1998.

244. Vella A, de Groen PC, Dinneen SF: Fatal hepatotoxicity associated with troglitazone [letter]. Ann Intern Med 129:1080, 1998.

245. Murphy EJ, Davern TJ, Shakil O, et al: Troglitazone-induced fulminant hepatic failure. Dig Dis Sci 45:549, 2000.

246. Kohlroser J, Mathai J, Reichheld J, et al: Hepatotoxicity due to troglitazone: Report of two cases and review of adverse events reported to the United States Food and Drug Administration. Am J Gastroenterol 95:272, 2000.

247. Schiano T, Dolehide K, Hart J, et al: Severe but reversible hepatitis induced by troglitazone. Dig Dis Sci 45:1039, 2000.

248. Bloomgarden ZT: American Diabetes Association 60th Scientific Sessions, 2000: Thiazolidinediones, obesity, and related topics. Diabetes Care 24:162, 2001.

249. Malik AH, Prasad P, Saboorian MH, et al: Hepatic injury due to troglitazone. Dig Dis Sci 45:210, 2000.

250. Caldwell SH, Hespenheide EE, von Borstel RW: Myositis, microvesicular hepatitis, and progression to cirrhosis from troglitazone added to simvastatin. Dig Dis Sci 46:376, 2001.

251. Bell DSH, Ovalle F: Late-onset troglitazone-induced hepatic dysfunction [letter]. Diabetes Care 23:128, 2000.

252. Iwase M, Yamaguchi M, Yoshinari M, et al: A Japanese case of liver dysfunction after 19 months of troglitazone treatment. Diabetes Care 22:1382, 1999.

253. Jagannath S, Rai R: Rapid-onset subfulminant liver failure associated with troglitazone [letter]. Ann Intern Med 132:677, 2000.

254. Menon KVN, Angulo P, Lindor KD: Severe cholestatic hepatitis from troglitazone in a patient with nonalcoholic steatohepatitis and diabetes mellitus. Am J Gastroenterol 96:1631, 2001.

255. Forman LM, Simmons DA, Diamond RH: Hepatic failure in a patient taking rosiglitazone. Ann Intern Med 132:118, 2000.

256. Al-Salman J, Arjomand H, Kemp DG, et al: Hepatocellular injury in a patient receiving rosiglitazone. A case report. Ann Intern Med 132:121, 2000.

257. Bonkovsky HL, Azar R, Bird S, et al: Severe cholestatic hepatitis caused by thiazolidinediones: Risks associated with substituting rosiglitazone for troglitazone. Dig Dis Sci 47:1632, 2002.

258. May LD, Lefkowitch JH, Kram MT, et al: Mixed hepatocellular-cholestatic liver injury after pioglitazone therapy. Ann Intern Med 136:449, 2002.

259. Maeda K: Hepatocellular injury in a patient receiving pioglitazone. Ann Intern Med 135:306, 2001.

260. Hachey DM, O'Neil MP, Force RW: Isolated elevation of alkaline phosphatase level associated with rosiglitazone. Ann Intern Med 133:752, 2000.

261. Lenhard MJ, Funk WB: Failure to develop hepatic injury from rosiglitazone in a patient with a history of troglitazone-induced hepatitis. Diabetes Care 24:168, 2001.

262. Jick SS, Stender M, Myers MW: Frequency of liver disease in type 2 diabetic patients treated with oral antidiabetic agents. Diabetes Care 22:2067, 2000.

263. Saw D, Pitman E, Maung M, et al: Granulomatous hepatitis associated with glyburide. Dig Dis Sci 41:322, 1996.

264. Van Thiel DH, de Belle R, Mellow M, et al: Tolazamide hepatotoxicity. Gastroenterology 67:506 1974.

265. Gregory DH, Zaki GF, Sarosi GA, et al: Chronic cholestasis following prolonged tolbutamide administration. Arch Pathol 84:194, 1967.

266. Nakao NL, Gelb AM, Stenger R, et al: A case of chronic liver disease due to tolazamide. Gastroenterology 89:192, 1985.

267. Clarke BF, Campbell JW, Ewing DJ, et al: Generalized hypersensitivity reaction and visceral arteritis with fatal outcome during glibenclamide therapy. Diabetes 23:739, 1974.

268. Dourakis SP, Tzemanakis E, Sinani C, et al: Gliclazide-induced acute hepatitis. Eur J Gastroenterol Hepatol 12:119, 2000.

269. Chitturi S, Le V, Kench J, et al: Gliclazide-induced acute hepatitis with hypersensitivity features. Dig Dis Sci 47:1107, 2002.

270. Babich MM, Pike I, Shiffman ML: Metformin-induced acute hepatitis. Am J Med 104:490, 1998.

271. Desilets DJ, Shorr AF, Moran KA, et al: Cholestatic jaundice associated with the use of metformin. Am J Gastroenterol 96:2257, 2001.

272. Andrade RJ, Lucenga MI, Rodriguez-Mendizabel M: Hepatic injury caused by acarbose [letter]. Ann Intern Med 124:931, 1996.

273. Carrescasa M, Pascual F, Aresti S: Acarbose-induced acute severe hepatotoxicity [letter]. Lancet 349:698, 1997.

274. Diaz-Gutierrez FL, Ladero JM, Diaz-Rubio M: Acarbose-induced acute hepatitis [letter]. Am J Gastroenterol 93:481, 1998.

275. Andrade RJ, Lucena M, Vega JL, et al: Acarbose-associated hepatotoxicity [letter]. Diabetes Care 21:2029, 1998.

276. Tawata M, Ikeda M, Kodama Y, et al: A type 2 diabetic patient with liver dysfunction due to human insulin. Diabetes Res Clin Pract 49:17, 2000.

277. Cai Q, Benson MA, Talbot TJ, et al: Acute hepatitis due to fluoxetine therapy. Mayo Clin Proc 74:692, 1999.

278. Johnston DE, Wheeler DE: Chronic hepatitis related to use of fluoxetine. Am J Gastroenterol 92:1225, 1997.

279. Benbow SJ, Gill G: Paroxetine and hepatotoxicity [letter]. BMJ 314:1387, 1997.

280. Cardona X, Avila A, Castellanos P: Venlafaxine-associated hepatitis [letter]. Ann Intern Med 132:417, 2000.

281. Horsmans Y, De Clercq M, Sempoux C: Venlaxafine-associated hepatitis [letter]. Ann Intern Med 130:944, 1999.

282. Fernandes NF, Martin RR, Schenker S: Trazodone-induced hepatotoxicity: A case report with comments on drug-induced hepatotoxicity. Am J Gastroenterol 95:532, 2000.

283. Spahr L, Rubbia-Brandt L, Burkhard PR, et al: Tolcapone-related fulminant hepatitis. Electron microscopy shows mitochrondrial alterations. Dig Dis Sci 45:1881, 2000.

284. Aranda-Michel J, Koehler A, Bejarano PA, et al: Nefazodone-induced liver failure: Report of three cases. Ann Intern Med 130:285, 1999.

285. Lucena MI, Andrade RJ, Gomez-Outes A, et al: Acute liver failure after treatment with nefazodone. Dig Dis Sci 44:2577, 1999.

286. Schrader GD, Roberts-Thompson IC: Adverse effect of nefazodone: Hepatitis. Med J Aust 170:452, 1999.

287. Black M, Hussain H: Hydrazine, cancer, the Internet, isoniazid, and the liver. Ann Intern Med 133:911, 2000.

288. Hainer MI, Tsai N, Komura ST, et al: Fatal hepatorenal failure associated with hydrazine sulfate. Ann Intern Med 133:877, 2000.

289. Bonkovsky HL, Blanchette PL, Schned AR: Severe liver injury due to phenelzine with unique hepatic deposition of extracellular material. Am J Med 80:689, 1986.

290. Anderson BN, Henrikson IR: Jaundice and eosinophilia associated with amitriptyline. J Clin Psychiatry 39:730, 1978.

291. Horst DA, Grace ND, LeCompte PM: Prolonged cholestasis and progressive hepatic fibrosis following imipramine therapy. Gastroenterology 79:550, 1980.

292. Cai Q, Benson MA, Talbot TJ, et al: Acute hepatitis due to fluoxetine therapy. Mayo Clin Proc 74:692, 1999.

293. Johnston DE, Wheeler DE: Chronic hepatitis related to use of fluoxetine. Am J Gastroenterol 92:1225, 1997.

294. Helmchen C, Boerner RJ, Meyendorf R, et al: Reversible hepatotoxicity of paroxetine in a patient with major depression. Pharmacopsychiatry 29:223, 1996.

295. Benbow SJ, Gill G: Paroxetine and hepatotoxicity [letter]. BMJ 314:1387, 1997.

296. Lucena MI, Andrade RJ, Gomez-Outes A, et al: Acute liver failure after treatment with nefazodone. Dig Dis Sci 44:2577, 1999.

297. Aranda-Michel J, Koehler A, Bejarano PA, et al: Nefazodone-induced liver failure: Report of three cases. Ann Intern Med 130:285, 1999.

298. Eloubeidi MA, Gaede JT, Swaim MW: Reversible nefazodone-induced liver failure. Dig Dis Sci 45:1036, 2000.

299. Beck PL, Bridges RJ, Demetrick DJ, et al: Chronic active hepatitis with trazodone therapy. Ann Intern Med 118:791, 1993.

300. Fernandes NF, Martin RR, Schenker S: Trazodone-induced hepatotoxicity: A case report with comments on drug-induced hepatotoxicity. Am J Gastroenterol 95:532, 2000.

301. Kim KY, Hwang W, Narendran R: Acute liver damage possibly related to sertraline and venlafaxine ingestion. Ann Pharmacother 33:381, 1999.

302. Cardona X, Avila A, Castellanos P: Venlafaxine-associated hepatitis [letter]. Ann Intern Med 132:417, 2000.

303. Selim K, Kaplowitz N: Hepatotoxicity of psychotropic drugs. Hepatology 29:1347, 1999.

304. Assal F, Spahr L, Hadengue A, et al: Tolcapone and fulminant hepatitis. Lancet 352:958, 1998.

305. Olanow CW: Tolcapone and hepatotoxic effects. Tasmar advisory panel. Arch Neurol 57:263, 2000.

306. Watkins P: COMT inhibitors and liver toxicity. Neurology 55(11 suppl 4):S51, 2000.

307. Ausset P, Malavialle P, Vallet A, et al: Subfulminant hepatitis due to alpiderm, treated by hepatic transplantation. Gastroenterol Clin Biol 19:222, 1995.

308. Karsenti D, Blanc P, Bacq Y, et al: Hepatotoxicity associated with zolpidem treatment. BMJ 318:1179, 1999.

309. Andrade RJ, Lucena MI, Aguilar J, et al: Chronic liver injury related to use of bentazepam. An unusual instance of benzodiazepine hepatotoxicity. Dig Dis Sci 45:1400, 2000.

310. Watkins PB, Zimmerman HJ, Knapp MJ, et al: Hepatotoxic effects of tacrine administration in patients with Alzheimer's disease. JAMA 271:992, 1994.

311. Fromenty B, Robin MA, Igoudjil A, et al: The ins and outs of mitochondrial dysfunction in NASH. Diabetes Metab 30:121, 2003.

312. Wilkinson SP, Portmann B, Williams R. Hepatitis from dantrolene sodium. Gut 20:33, 1979.

313. de Graaf EM, Oosterveld M, Tjabbes T, Stricker BH: A case of tizanidine-induced hepatic injury. J Hepatol 25:772, 1996.

314. Malka D, Pham BN, Courvalin JC, et al: Acute hepatitis caused by alverine associated with anti-lamin A and C autoantibodies. J Hepatol 27:399, 1997.

315. Remy AJ, Camu W, Ramos J, et al: Acute hepatitis after riluzole administration. J Hepatol 30:527, 1999.

316. Castells LI, Gámex J, Cervera C, Guardia J: Icteric toxic hepatitis associated with riluzole [letter]. Lancet 351:648, 1998.

317. Fontana RJ, McCashland TM, Benner KG, et al: Acute liver failure associated with prolonged use of bromfenac leading to liver transplantation. The Acute Liver Failure Study Group. Liver Transpl Surg 5:480, 1999.

318. Moses PL, Schroeder B, Alkhatib O, et al: Severe hepatotoxicity associated with bromfenac sodium. Am J Gastroenterol 94:1393, 1999.

319. Rabkin JM, Smith MJ, Orloff SL, et al: Fatal fulminant hepatitis associated with bromfenac use. Ann Pharmacother 33:945, 1999.

320. Romero-Gomez M, Nevado Santos M, Fobelo MJ, et al: Nimesulide acute hepatitis: Description of 3 cases. Med Clin (Barc) 113:357, 1999.

321. McCormick PA, Kennedy F, Curry M, Traynor O: COX 2 inhibitor and fulminant failure [letter]. Lancet 353:40, 1999.

322. Boersterli UA: Diclofenac-induced liver injury: A paradigm of idiosyncratic drug toxicity. Toxicol Appl Pharmacol 192:307, 2003.

323. Maddrey WC, Maurath CJ, Verburg KM, Geis GS: The hepatic safety and tolerability of the novel cyclooxygenase-2 inhibitor celecoxib. Am J Ther 7:153, 2000.

324. Rostom A, Goldkind L, Laine L: Nonsteroidal anti-inflammatory drugs and hepatic toxicity: A systematic review of randomized controlled trials in arthritis patients. Clin Gastroenterol Hepatol 3:489, 2005.

325. Traversa G, Bianchi C, Da Cas R, et al: Cohort study of hepatotoxicity associated with nimesulide and other non-steroidal anti-inflammatory drugs. BMJ 327:18, 2003.

326. Schattner A, Sokolovskaya N, Cohen J: Fatal hepatitis and renal failure during treatment with nimesulide. J Intern Med 247:153, 2000.

327. Van Steenbergen W, Peeters P, De Bondt J, et al: Nimesulide-induced acute hepatitis: Evidence from six cases. J Hepatol 29:135, 1998.

328. McMaster KR, Hennigar GR: Drug-induced granulomatous hepatitis. Lab Invest 44:61, 1981.

329. Al-Kawas FH, Seeff LB, Berendson RA, et al: Allopurinol hepatotoxicity. Report of two cases and review of the literature. Ann Intern Med 95:588, 1981.

330. Williams SJ, Ruppin DC, Grierson JM, et al: Carbamazepine hepatitis: The clinicopathological spectrum. J Gastroenterol Hepatol 1:159, 1986.

331. Benjamin SE, Ishak KG, Zimmerman HJ, et al: Phenylbutazone liver injury: A clinico-pathological survey of 23 cases and review of the literature. Hepatology 1:255, 1981.

332. Myers JL, Augur NA: Hydralazine-induced cholangitis. Gastroenterology 87:1185, 1984.

333. Mathur S, Dooley J, Scheuer PJ: Quinine induced granulomatous hepatitis and vasculitis [letter]. BMJ 300:613, 1990.

334. Knobler H, Levij IS, Gavish D, et al: Quinidine-induced hepatitis. A common and reversible hypersensitivity reaction. Arch Intern Med 146:526, 1986.

335. Mullick FG, Ishak KG: Hepatic injury associated with diphenylhydantoin therapy. A clinicopathological study of 20 cases. Am J Clin Pathol 74:442, 1980.

336. Braun M, Fraser GM, Kunin M, et al: Mesalamine-induced granulomatous hepatitis. Am J Gastroenterol 94:1973, 1999.

337. Saw D, Pitman E, Maung M, et al: Granulomatous hepatitis associated with glyburide. Dig Dis Sci 41:322, 1996.

338. Maddrey WC, Boitnott JK: Drug-induced chronic liver disease. Gastroenterology 72:1348, 1977.

339. Seeff LB: Drug-induced chronic liver disease; with emphasis on chronic active hepatitis. Semin Liver Dis 1:104, 1981.

340. Scully LJ, Clarke D, Bar J: Diclofenac induced hepatitis: 3 cases with features of autoimmune chronic active hepatitis. Dig Dis Sci 38:744, 1993.

341. Banks AT, Zimmerman HJ, Ishak KG, et al: Diclofenac-associated hepatotoxicity: Analysis of 180 cases reported to the Food and Drug Administration as adverse reactions. Hepatology 22:820, 1995.

342. O'Connor N, Dargan PI, Jones AL: Hepatocellular damage from non-steroidal anti-inflammatory drugs. Q J Med 96:787, 2003.

343. Gough A, Chapman S, Wagstaff K, et al: Minocycline induced autoimmune hepatitis and systemic lupus erythematosus-like syndrome. BMJ 312:169, 1996.

344. Teitelbaum JE, Perez-Atayde Ar, Cohen M, et al: Minocycline-related autoimmune hepatitis: case series and literature review. Arch Pediatr Adolesc Med 152:1132, 1998.

345. Chitturi S, Farrell GC: Drug-induced cholestasis. Semin Gastrointest Dis 12:113, 2001.

346. Chitturi S, Farrell GC: Drug-induced liver disease. Curr Treat Options Gastroenterol 3:457, 2000.

347. Moradpour D, Altorfer J, Flury R, et al: Chlorpromazine-induced vanishing bile duct syndrome leading to cirrhosis. Hepatology 20:1437, 1994.

348. Kreek MJ: Female sex steroids and cholestasis. Semin Liver Dis 7:8, 1987.

349. Glober GA, Wilkerson JA: Biliary cirrhosis following the administration of methyltestosterone. JAMA 204:170, 1968.

350. Koek GH, Sticker BHCH, Blok APR, et al: Flucloxacillin-associated hepatic injury. Liver 14:225, 1994.

351. Gosbell IB, Turnidge JD, Tapsall JW, et al: Toxicities of flucloxacillin and dicloxacillin— is there really a diference? Med J Aust 173:500, 2000.

352. Tarazi EM, Harter JG, Zimmerman HJ, et al: Sulindac-associated hepatic injury: Analysis of 91 cases reported to the Food and Drug Administration. Gastroenterology 104:569, 1993.

353. Hepps KS, Maliha GH, Estrada R, Goodgame RW: Severe cholestatic jaundice associated with piroxicam. Gastroenterology 101:1737, 1991.

354. Crantock L, Prentice R, Powell L: Cholestatic jaundice associated with captopril therapy. J Gastroenterol Hepatol 6:528, 1991.

355. Cetin M, Demirci D, Unal A, et al: Frequency of flutamide induced hepatotoxicity in patients with prostate carcinoma. Hum Exp Toxicol 18:137, 1999.

356. Andrade RJ, Lucena MI, Fernandez MC, et al: Fulminant liver failure associated with flutamide therapy for hirsutism [letter]. Lancet 33:983, 1999.

357. Hartleb M, Rymarczyk G, Januszewski K: Acute cholestatic hepatitis associated with pravastatin. Am J Gastroenterol 94:1388, 1999.

358. Jimenez-Alonso J, Osorio JM, Gutierrez-Cabello F, et al: Atorvastatin-induced cholestatic hepatitis in a young woman with systemic lupus erythematosus. Grupo Lupus Virgen de las Nieves. Arch Intern Med 159:1811, 1999.

359. Iqbal M, Goenka P, Young MF, et al: Ticlopidine-induced cholestatic hepatitis: Report of three cases and review of the literature. Dig Dis Sci 43:2223, 1998.

360. Labowitz JK, Silverman WB: Cholestatic jaundice induced by ciprofloxacin. Dig Dis Sci 42:192, 1997.

361. Lucena MI, Andrade RJ, Sanchez-Martinez H, et al: Norfloxacin-induced cholestatic jaundice. Am J Gastroenterol 93:2309, 1998.

362. Babich MM, Pike I, Shiffman ML: Metformin-induced acute hepatitis. Am J Med 104:490, 1998.

363. Ishak KG, Irey NS: Hepatic injury associated with the phenothiazines. Clinicopathologic and follow-up study of 36 patients. Arch Pathol 93:283, 1972.

364. Thompson JA, Fairley CK, Ugoni AM, et al: Risk factors for the development of amoxycillin–clavulanic acid associated jaundice. Med J Aust 162:638, 1995.

365. Ryan J, Dudley F: Cholestasis with ticarcillin–potassium clavulanate (Timentin). Med J Aust 156:291, 1992.

366. Sweet JM, Jones MP: Intrahepatic cholestasis due to ticarcillin–clavulanic acid [letter]. Am J Gastroenterol 90:675, 1995.

367. Larrey D, Vial T, Micaleff A, et al: Hepatitis associated with amoxycillin-clavulanic acid combination report of 15 cases. Gut 33:368, 1992.

368. Richardet J-P, Mallat A, Zafrani ES, et al: Prolonged cholestasis with ductopenia after administration of amoxicillin/clavulanic acid. Dig Dis Sci 44:1997, 1999.

369. Hautekeete ML, Brenard R, Horsmans Y, et al: Liver injury related to amoxycillin-clavulanic acid: Interlobular bile-duct lesions and extrahepatic manifestations. J Hepatol 22:71, 1995.

370. Chawla A, Kahn E, Yunis EJ, Daum F: Rapidly progressive cholestasis: An unusual reaction to amoxicillin/clavulanic acid therapy in a child. J Pediatr 136:121, 2000.

371. Degott C, Feldmann G, Larrey D, et al: Drug-induced prolonged cholestasis in adults: A histological semiquantitative study demonstrating progressive ductopenia. Hepatology 15:244, 1992.

372. Hebbard GS, Smith KG, Gibson PR, et al: Augmentin-induced jaundice with a fatal outcome. Med J Aust 156:285, 1992.

373. Geubel AP, Sempoux SL: Drug- and toxin-induced bile duct disorders. J Gastroenterol Hepatol 15:1232, 2000.

374. Forbes GM, Jeffrey GP, Shilkin KB, et al: Carbamazepine hepatotoxicity: Another cause of the vanishing bile duct syndrome. Gastroenterology 102:1385, 1992.

375. Rosenberg WMC, Ryley NG, Trowell JM, et al: Dextropropoxyphene induced hepatotoxicity: A report of nine cases. J Hepatol 19:470, 1993.

376. Kopelman H, Scheuer PJ, Williams R: The liver lesion of the Epping jaundice. Q J Med 35:553, 1966.

377. Lazarczyk DA, Duffy M: Erythromycin-induced primary biliary cirrhosis. Dig Dis Sci 45:1115, 2000.

378. Hunt CM, Washington K: Tetracycline-induced bile duct paucity and prolonged cholestasis. Gastroenterology 107:1844, 1994.

379. Alam I, Ferrell LD, Bass NM: Vanishing bile duct syndrome temporally associated with ibuprofen use. Am J Gastroenterol 91:1626, 1996.

380. Srivastava M, Perez-Atayde A, Jonas MM: Drug-associated acute-onset vanishing bile duct and Stevens-Johnson syndromes in a child. Gastroenterology 115:743, 1998.

381. Yao F, Behling CA, Saab S, et al: Trimethoprim-sulfamethoxazone–induced vanishing bile duct syndrome. Am J Gastroenterol 92:167, 1997.

382. Bataille L, Rahier J, Geubel A: Delayed and prolonged cholestatic hepatitis with ductopenia after long-term ciprofloxacin therapy for Crohn's disease. J Hepatol 37:696, 2002.

383. Belghiti J, Benhamou J-P, Houry H, et al: Caustic sclerosing cholangitis. A complication of the surgical treatment of hydatid disease of the liver. Arch Surg 121:1162, 1986.

384. Anderson SD, Holley HC, Berland LL, et al: Causes of jaundice during hepatic artery infusion chemotherapy. Radiology 161:439, 1986.

385. Brunt EM, Janney CG, Di Bisceglie AM, et al: Nonalcoholic steatohepatitis: A proposal for grading and staging the histological lesions. Am J Gastroenterol 94:2467, 1999.

386. Farrell GC: Is bacterial ash the flash that ignites NASH? Gut 48:148, 2001.

387. Rigas B: The evolving spectrum of amiodarone hepatotoxicity. Hepatology 10:116, 1989.

388. Lewis JH, Ranard RC, Caruso A, et al: Amiodarone hepatotoxicity: Prevalence and clinicopathologic correlations among 104 patients. Hepatology 9:679, 1989.

389. Pirovino M, Müller O, Zysset T, et al: Amiodarone-induced hepatic phospholipidosis: Correlation of morphological and biochemical findings in an animal model. Hepatology 8:591, 1988.

390. Breuer HW, Bossek W, Haferland C, et al: Amiodarone-induced severe hepatitis mediated by immunological mechanisms. Int J Clin Pharmacol Ther 36:350, 1998.

391. Beuers U, Heuck A: Images in hepatology. Iodine accumulation in the liver during long-term treatment with amiodarone. J Hepatol 26:439, 1997.

392. Chang CC, Petrelli M, Tomashefski JF, McCullough AJ: Severe intrahepatic cholestasis caused by amiodarone toxicity after withdrawal of the drug: A case report and review of the literature. Arch Pathol Lab Med 123:251, 1999.

393. Richer M, Roberts S: Fatal hepatotoxicity following oral administration of amiodarone. Ann Pharmacother 29:582, 1995.

394. Fromenty B, Fisch C, Labbe G, et al: Amiodarone inhibits the mitochondrial β-oxidation of fatty acids and produces microvesicular steatosis of the liver in mice. J Pharmacol Exp Ther 255:1371, 1990.

395. Letteron P, Fromenty B, Terris B, et al: Acute and chronic hepatic steatosis lead to in vivo lipid peroxidation in mice. J Hepatol 24:200, 1996.

396. Berson A, De Beco V, Letteron P, et al: Steatohepatitis-inducing drugs cause mitochondrial dysfunction and lipid peroxidation in rat hepatocytes. Gastroenterology 114:764, 1998.

397. Hilleman D, Miller MA, Parker R, et al: Optimal management of amiodarone therapy: Efficacy and side effects. Pharmacotherapy 18:138S, 1998.

398. Babany G, Uzzan F, Larrey D, et al: Alcoholic-like liver lesions induced by nifedipine. J Hepatol 9:252, 1989.

399. Beaugrand M, Denis J, Callard P: Tous les inhibiteurs calciques peuvent-ils entrainer des lesions d'hepatite alcoolique? Gastroenterol Clin Biol 1:76, 1987.

400. Sotaniemi EA, Hokkanen OT, Ohakas JT, et al: Hepatic injury and drug metabolism in patients with alpha-methyldopa–induced liver damage. Eur J Clin Pharmacol 12:429, 1977.

401. Seki K, Minami Y, Nishikawa M, et al: Nonalcoholic steatohepatitis induced by massive doses of synthetic estrogen. Gastroenterol Jpn 18:197, 1983.

402. Itoh S, Igarashi M, Tsukada Y, Ichinoe A: Nonalcoholic fatty liver with alcoholic hyaline after long-term glucocorticoid therapy. Acta Hepatogastroenterol (Stuttg) 24:415, 1977.

403. Lee AU, Farrell GC: Drug-induced liver disease. Current Opin Gastroenterol 13:199, 1997.

404. Agrawal BL, Zelkowitz L: Bone "flare" hypercalcemia and jaundice after tamoxifen therapy [letter]. Arch Intern Med 141:2140, 1981.

405. Moffat DF, Oien KA, Dickson J, et al: Hepatocellular carcinoma after long-term tamoxifen therapy. Ann Oncol 11:1195, 2000.

406. Blackburn WR, Amiel SA, Millis RR, Rubens RD: Tamoxifen and liver damage. BMJ 289:288, 1984.

407. Cai Q, Bensen M, Greene R, Kirchner J: Tamoxifen-induced transient multifocal hepatic fatty infiltration. Am J Gastroenterol 95:277, 2000.

408. Pratt DS, Knox TA, Erban J: Tamoxifen-induced steatohepatitis [letter]. Ann Intern Med 123:236, 1995.

409. Cortez-Pinto H, Baptista A, Camilo ME, et al: Tamoxifen-associated steatohepatitis—report of three cases. J Hepatol 23:95, 1995.

410. Ogawa Y, Murata Y, Nishioka A, et al: Tamoxifen-induced fatty liver in patients with breast cancer [letter]. Lancet 351:725, 1998.

411. Van Hoof M, Rahier J, Horsmans Y: Tamoxifen-induced steatohepatitis [letter]. Ann Intern Med 124: 855, 1996.

412. Oien KA, Moffat D, Curry GW, et al: Cirrhosis with steatohepatitis after adjuvant tamoxifen [letter]. Lancet 353:36, 1999.

413. Dray X, Tainturier MH, De La Lande P, et al: Cirrhosis with nonalcoholic steatohepatitis: Role of tamoxifen. Gastroenterol Clin Biol 24:1122, 2000.

414. Saibara T, Ogawa Y, Takahashi M, et al: Tamoxifen-induced nonalcoholic steatohepatitis and benzafibrate [abstract]. J Gastroenterol Hepatol 15(suppl):F96, 2000.

415. Hamada N, Ogawa Y, Saibara T, et al: Toremifene-induced fatty liver and NASH in breast cancer patients with breast-conservation treatment. Int J Oncol 17:1119, 2000.

416. Ruymann FB, Mosijczuk AD, Sayers RJ: Hepatoma in a child with methotrexate-induced hepatic fibrosis. JAMA 238:2631, 1977.

417. Zachariae H, Kragbelle K, Søgaard H: Methotrexate-induced liver cirrhosis: Studies including serial liver biopsies during continued treatment. Br J Dermatol 102:407, 1980.

418. Shergy WJ, Polisson RP, Caldwell DS, et al: Methotrexate-associated hepatotoxicity; retrospective analysis of 210 patients with rheumatoid arthritis. Am J Med 85:771, 1988.

419. Lewis JH, Schiff ER: Methotrexate-induced chronic liver injury: Guidelines for detection and prevention. Am J Gastroenterol 88:1337, 1988.

420. Whiting-O'Keefe QE, Fyfe KH, Sack KD: Methotrexate and histologic hepatic abnormalities: A meta-analysis. Am J Med 90:711, 1991.

421. Zachariae H, Søgaard H: Methotrexate-induced liver cirrhosis: A follow up. Dermatologica 175:178, 1987.

422. Te HS, Schiano TD, Kuan SF, et al: Hepatic effects of long-term methotrexate use in the treatment of inflammatory bowel disease. Am J Gastroenterol 95:3150, 2000.

423. Gilbert SC, Klintmalm G, Menter A, et al: Methotrexate-induced cirrhosis requiring liver transplantation in three patients with psoriasis. Arch Intern Med 150:889, 1990.

424. Kremer JM, Alarcon GS, Lightfoot RW Jr, et al: Methotrexate for rheumatoid arthritis. Suggested guidelines for monitoring liver toxicity. Arthritis Rheum 37:316, 1994.

425. Nevens F, Fevery J, Van Steegbergen W, et al: Arsenic and non-cirrhotic portal hypertension. A report of eight cases. J Hepatol 11:80, 1990.

426. Thomas LB, Popper H, Berk PD, et al: Vinyl-chloride-induced liver disease. From idiopathic portal hypertension (Banti's syndrome) to angiosarcomas. N Engl J Med 292:17, 1975.

427. Loomus GN, Aneja P, Bota RA: A case of peliosis hepatis in association with tamoxifen therapy. Am J Clin Pathol 80:881, 1983.

428. Larrey D, Fréneaux E, Berson A, et al: Peliosis hepatis induced by 6-thioguanine administration. Gut 29:1265, 1988.

429. Zafrani ES, Bernuau D, Feldmann G: Peliosis-like ultrastructural changes of the hepatic sinusoids in human chronic hypervitaminosis A: Report of three cases. Hum Pathol 15:1166, 1984.

430. Sterneck M, Weisner R, Ascher N, et al: Azathioprine hepatotoxicity after liver transplantation. Hepatology 14:806, 1991.

431. Horsmans Y, Rahier J, Geubel AP: Reversible cholestasis with bile duct injury following azathioprine therapy. A case report. Liver 11:89, 1991.

432. Sobesky R, Dusoleil A, Condat B, et al: Azathioprine-induced destructive cholangitis. Am J Gastroenterol 96:616, 2001.

433. Sterneck M, Weisner R, Ascher N, et al: Azathioprine hepatotoxicity after liver transplantation. Hepatology 14:806, 1991.

434. Mion F, Napoleon B, Berger F, et al: Azathioprine induced liver disease: Nodular regenerative hyperplasia of the liver and perivenous fibrosis in a patient treated for multiple sclerosis. Gut 32:715, 1991.

435. Russmann S, Zimmermann A, Krahenbuhl S, et al: Veno-occlusive disease, nodular regenerative hyperplasia and hepatocellular carcinoma after azathioprine treatment in a patient with ulcerative colitis. Eur J Gastroenterol Hepatol 13:287, 2001.

436. Cattan S, Wendum D, Chazouilleres O, et al: Hepatocellular carcinoma and focal hepatic glycogenosis after prolonged azathioprine therapy. Hum Pathol 31:874, 2000.

437. Duvoux C, Kracht M, Lang P, et al: Nodular regenerative hyperplasia of the liver associated with azathioprine therapy. Gastroenterol Clin Biol 15:968, 1991.

438. Gane E, Portmann B, Saxena R, et al: Nodular regenerative hyperplasia of the liver graft after liver transplantation. Hepatology 20:88, 1994.

CHAPTER

84 Liver Disease Caused by Anesthetics, Toxins, and Herbal Preparations

James H. Lewis

Although halothane hepatitis is now largely of historical interest in the United States, it holds an important place in the annals of causality assessment in drug-induced liver disease.[1] In contrast with the largely unpredictable hepatotoxicity seen with anesthetics and most other medicinal agents (as discussed in Chapter 83), liver damage caused by occupationally and environmentally encountered chemical compounds and other toxins often is more predictable, dose related, and predominantly cytotoxic in nature.[1-5] Industrial exposure to hepatotoxic chemicals is a less frequent occupational hazard today than in the past, but reports of toxicity from chemical agents, as well as metals, adulterated cooking oils, and botanical toxins, have not disappeared.[3,4] Additionally, the use of complementary and alternative medicine (CAM) preparations continues to increase, and reports of liver injury from potentially hepatotoxic herbal products continue to appear[6,7] (see Chapter 125).

the original haloalkane anesthetic, has long been abandoned but remains an important experimental hepatotoxin, as does carbon tetrachloride (another chlorinated aliphatic hydrocarbon), which found use as an early vermifuge and is still employed as a household reagent in some parts of the world.[1,8] Halothane, introduced in the 1950s as a safer, nonexplosive alternative to ether, is a haloalkane compound that produced a well-described but rare syndrome of acute hepatotoxicity, usually after repeat exposure.[9] The anesthetics that followed—methoxyflurane, enflurane, isoflurane—all have been implicated as a cause of similar injury, albeit, for enflurane and isoflurane, less commonly than for halothane; even fewer instances have been reported for the newest agents, sevoflurane and desflurane,[10,11] because of their proportionally lower degree of metabolism.[12] Halothane is rarely used today in the United States but continues to be employed in other countries[13] and is a case study in the elucidation of immunologic-mediated liver injury.[14]

ANESTHETIC AGENTS

The volatile inhalational anesthetics in current use are derivatives of some of the most potent chemical hepatotoxins developed for medicinal purposes. Chloroform,

HALOTHANE

The retrospective National Halothane Study, cited in the past as the basis for exonerating halothane as a cause of hepatotoxicity,[15] is now considered flawed.[1] Nearly 1000 cases of halothane hepatoxicity were reported worldwide during the 1960s and 1970s.[1,9,16] A fairly uniform clinical picture of postoperative fever, eosinophilia, jaundice, and hepatic necrosis occurred a few days or weeks after anesthesia, usually after repeat exposure to halothane, and the case-fatality rate was high (Table 84–1). Rare cases of halothane-induced liver injury have occurred after workplace exposure among anesthesiologists, surgeons, nurses, and laboratory staff, and after halothane sniffing for "recreational" use; in affected persons, antibodies to trifluoroacetylated (TFA) proteins can be demonstrated, indicating previous exposure.[17]

Two types of postoperative liver injury have been associated with halothane. A *minor form* is seen in 10% to 30% of patients, in whom mild asymptomatic elevations in serum alanine aminotransferase (ALT) levels develop between the first and tenth postoperative days; the risk of hepatotoxicity is higher after two or more exposures to halothane than with subsequent use of alternative agents such as enflurane, isoflurane, and desflurane. Evidence of immune activation is lacking in these patients,[18] in whom the ALT elevations generally are rapidly reversible. The *major form* of halothane-induced hepatotoxicity is a rare, dose-independent, severe hepatic drug reaction with elements of immunoallergy and metabolic idiosyncrasy (see Table 84–1). After an initial exposure to halothane, the frequency of this form of toxicity is only approximately 1 per 10,000,[19] but the rate increases to approximately 1 per 1000 after two or more exposures, especially when the anesthetic agent is readministered within a few weeks.[1] Typically, zone 3 (centrilobular) hepatic necrosis is seen histologically.[20] The case-fatality rate ranged from 14% to 71% in the pre–liver transplantation era.[1]

Risk Factors for Halothane Hepatitis

Host-related risk factors for halothane hepatitis are listed in Table 84–2. The reaction is rare in childhood[11]; patients younger than 10 years of age represent only about 3% of the total, and cases in persons younger than 30 years account for less than 10%.[11,16] The disease tends to be more severe in persons older than 40 years of age. Two thirds of cases have been in women, and repeat exposure to halothane (especially within a few weeks or months) is documented in as many as 90% of cases.[1] The time between exposures can be as long as 28 years.[21] After repeat exposure, hepatitis is earlier in onset and more severe. Obesity is another risk factor, possibly because of storage of halothane in body fat. The induction of cytochrome P450 (CYP) enzymes (especially CYP2E1) that metabolize halothane to its toxic intermediate has been produced experimentally with phenobarbital, alcohol, and isoniazid; valproate inhibits and phenytoin has no specific effect on halothane hepatotoxicity.[1] Inhibition of CYP2E1 by administration of a single dose of disulfiram has been suggested as a means of preventing halothane hepatitis, through inhibition of the production of the metabolite responsible for neoantigen formation.[22]

Familial predisposition to halothane-induced liver injury has been reported in closely related family members.[23] Serum antibodies to volatile anesthetics have been found in pediatric anesthesiologists,[17] who, like patients with halothane hepatitis, had higher levels of serum autoantibodies to CYP2E1 and to endoplasmic reticulum protein (ERp58) than those found in general anesthesiologists and control subjects who had never been exposed to inhalational anesthetics. The autoantibodies are not thought to have a role in pathogenesis. As yet, no serologic test for halothane hepatitis is readily available.[1]

Table 84–1 Halothane Hepatitis. Clinicopathologic Features

Estimated incidence:
  After first exposure: 0.3 to 1.5 per 10,000
  After multiple exposures: 10 to 15 per 10,000
Female-to-male ratio 2:1
Latent period to first symptom:
  After first exposure: 6 days (11 days to jaundice)
  After multiple exposures: 3 days (6 days to jaundice)
Jaundice as presenting symptom in 25% (range of serum
  bilirubin: 3-50 mg/dL)
Fever in 75% (precedes jaundice in 75%); chills in 30%
Rash in 10%
Myalgias in 20%
Ascites, renal failure, gastrointestinal hemorrhage in 20%-30%
Eosinophilia in 20%-60%
Serum ALT and AST levels: 25-250× ULN
Alkaline phosphatase level: 1-3× ULN
Histologic features
  Zone 3 massive hepatic necrosis in 30%; submassive
    necrosis in 70% (autopsy series)
  Inflammation usually less marked than in viral hepatitis
  Eosinophilic infiltrate in 20%
  Granulomatous hepatitis
Course and outcome
  Mortality rate (pretransplantation era): 10%-80%
  Symptoms can resolve within 5-14 days
  Full recovery can take 12 weeks or longer
  Chronic hepatitis not well documented
Adverse prognostic findings
  Age >40 years
  Obesity
  Short duration to jaundice
  Bilirubin >20 mg/dL
  Coagulopathy

ALT, alanine aminotransferase; AST, aspartate aminotransferase; ULN, upper limit of normal.

Table 84–2 Risk Factors for Halothane Hepatitis

Older age (>40 years)
Female gender
Two or more exposures (documented in 80%-90% of cases)
Obesity
Familial predisposition
Induction of CYP2E1 by phenobarbital, alcohol, or isoniazid

CYP2E1, cytochrome P4502E1.

Pathology

In a study of 77 cases of halothane hepatitis reviewed by the Armed Forces Institute of Pathology,[20] various degrees of liver injury were seen, depending on the severity of the reaction. Massive or submassive necrosis involving zone 3 was present in all autopsy specimens, whereas biopsy material revealed a broader range of injury, from spotty necrosis in about one third of cases to zone 3 necrosis in two thirds. The zone 3 injury is sharply demarcated, and the inflammatory response is less severe than in acute viral hepatitis.

Pathogenesis

Halothane injury occurs by one or more of three potential mechanisms: hypersensitivity, production of hepatotoxic metabolites, and hypoxia, in decreasing order of importance.[1] Evidence for the role of hypersensitivity is found in the increased susceptibility and shortened latency after repeat exposure, the hallmark symptoms and signs of drug allergy (fever, rash, eosinophilia, and granuloma formation), and the detection of neoantigens and antibodies. Halothane oxidation yields trifluoroacetylchloride, which acts on hepatocyte proteins to produce neoantigens that are responsible for the major form of injury. By contrast, reductive pathways produce free radicals that can act as reactive metabolites that may have a role in causing minor injury. A unifying hypothesis set forth by Zimmerman[1] suggests that halothane injury most likely is the result of immunologic enhancement of zone 3 necrosis produced by the reductive metabolite(s). Accordingly, the hepatotoxic potential of halothane depends on the susceptibility of the patient and on factors that promote production of hepatotoxic or immunogenic metabolites.[1]

Course and Outcome

Mortality rates for halothane hepatitis were high in early series; since then, successful treatment has been achieved with liver transplantation in many patients.[13] When spontaneous recovery occurs, symptoms usually resolve within 5 to 14 days, and recovery is complete within several weeks.[1] Immunosuppressive agents have only rarely been reported to improve the outcome.[11] It is doubtful that halothane causes chronic hepatitis.[1]

Adverse prognostic factors include age older than 40 years, obesity, severe coagulopathy, serum bilirubin level greater than 20 mg/dL, and a shorter interval to onset of jaundice.[1,16,19] Halothane hepatitis often can be prevented by attention to the patient's anesthetic history and adherence to safety guidelines.[24]

OTHER ANESTHETIC AGENTS

The likelihood that individual haloalkane anesthetics will cause liver injury appears to be related to the extent to which they are metabolized by hepatic CYP enzymes: 20% to 30% for halothane, greater than 30% for methoxyflurane, 2% for enflurane, 1% for sevoflurane, and 0.2% or less for isoflurane and desflurane.[12] Accordingly, the estimated frequency of hepatitis from the newer agents is much less than that for halothane (Table 84–3).

Methoxyflurane caused hepatotoxicity and a high frequency of nephrotoxicity that led to its withdrawal.[25] *Enflurane* caused a clinical syndrome similar to that for halothane, with the onset of fever within 3 days and jaundice in 3 to 19 days after anesthesia[26,27]; the estimated incidence of enflurane-induced liver injury was about 1 in 800,000 exposed patients.[10]

Despite its low rate of metabolism,[12] numerous instances of *isoflurane*-associated liver injury have been reported.[28,29,30] In one case, cross-sensitivity was suspected 22 years after an initial exposure to enflurane.[29] TFA liver proteins have been detected in patients with suspected isoflurane liver toxicity.[30]

The newest haloalkane anesthetics, *desflurane* and *sevoflurane*, appear to be nearly free of adverse hepatic effects. Desflurane undergoes minimal biotransformation and was not associated with the development of TFA antibodies in exposed rats.[12] Only isolated reports of liver injury in patients receiving desflurane anesthesia have been published.[31] The biotransformation of sevoflurane also is minimal, and only rare reports have implicated this agent in postoperative hepatic dysfunction.[32] Ether, nitrous oxide, and cyclopropane apparently are devoid of significant hepatotoxic potential, owing to their lack of halogen moieties.[1]

JAUNDICE IN THE POSTOPERATIVE PERIOD

From 25% to 75% of patients undergoing surgery experience postoperative hepatic dysfunction, ranging from mild elevations in liver biochemical tests to hepatic failure; jaundice has been reported in nearly 50% of patients with underlying cirrhosis in the postoperative period (see Chapter 70).[33] Patients undergoing upper abdominal surgical procedures are at highest risk of postoperative liver dysfunction, as well as pancreatitis, cholecystitis, and bile duct injury, because of impaired blood flow to the liver.[33] Table 84–4 lists many causes of postoperative jaundice and hepatic dysfunction, broadly

Table 84–3 Hepatotoxic Anesthetics Other than Halothane

Agent	Percent Metabolized	Incidence of Adverse Events	Cross-Reactivity with Other Haloalkanes	Other Features
Methoxyflurane	>30%	Low	Yes	Nephrotoxicity
Enflurane	2%	1 in 800,000	Yes	Similar to halothane
Isoflurane	0.2%	Rare	Yes	Similar to halothane
Desflurane	<0.2%	Isolated reports	Yes	Cardiac toxicity, malignant hyperthermia
Sevoflurane	Minimal	Rare reports	Uncertain	Unknown

divided into hepatocellular injury, cholestasis, and indirect hyperbilirubinemia. Drugs that may cause hepatoxicity in this setting include antibiotics (e.g., erythromycin, telethromycin, amoxicillin-clavulanate, trimethoprim-sulfamethoxazole) and the halogenated anesthetics discussed earlier; most produce injury by hypersensitivity mechanisms within 1 to 2 weeks of administration.[1,2] Table 84–5 contrasts the features of halogenated anesthetic–induced hepatitis, ischemic hepatitis (shock liver), and cholestatic injury in the early postoperative period.

Table 84–4 Causes of Postoperative Hepatic Dysfunction

Hepatocellular Injury (predominant serum ALT elevation, with or without hyperbilirubinemia)
Inhalational anesthetics—halothane, others
Ischemic hepatitis (shock liver)
Other drugs—antihypertensives (e.g., labetalol), heparin
Acute post-transfusion hepatitis
Unrecognized chronic liver disease—NASH, hepatitis C, other disorders
Hepatic allograft rejection
Hepatic artery thrombosis
Cholestatic Jaundice (elevated serum alkaline phosphatase ± ALT; direct hyperbilirubinemia)
Benign postoperative cholestasis
Cardiac bypass of prolonged duration
Sepsis
Acalculous cholecystitis
Common bile duct obstruction—gallstones, pancreatitis
Cholangitis
Bile duct injury—post-cholecystectomy, post–liver transplantation
Microlithiasis (biliary sludge)
Prolonged total parenteral nutrition
Hemobilia
Drugs—amoxicillin-clavulanate, chlorpromazine, erythromycin, telethromycin, trimethoprim-sulfamethoxazole, warfarin, others
Indirect Hyperbilirubinemia (serum alkaline phosphatase and ALT often normal)
Multiple transfusions
Resorbing hematoma
Hemolytic anemia
G6PD deficiency
Gilbert's syndrome

ALT, alanine aminotransferase; G6PD, glucose-6-phosphate dehydrogenase; NASH, nonalcoholic steatohepatitis.

CHEMICALS

COMMERCIAL AND INDUSTRIAL CHEMICALS

Among tens of thousands of chemical compounds in commercial and industrial use, several hundred are listed as causing liver injury by the National Institute for Occupational Safety and Health (NIOSH), as published in their most recent *Pocket Guide to Chemical Hazards*.[34] The National Library of Medicine also maintains a database of chemical toxins in its Toxicology and Environmental Health Information Program (TEHIP).[35]

Toxic exposure to chemical agents occurs most often from inhalation or absorption by the skin and less often from absorption by the gastrointestinal tract after oral ingestion or through a parenteral route. Because most chemical toxins are lipid soluble, once absorbed they can easily cross biologic membranes to reach their target organ(s), including the liver.[3,4] Hepatotoxic chemical exposure (as with carbon tetrachloride and phosphorus) usually results in an acute cytotoxic injury that typically consists of three distinct phases, similar to those observed after an acetaminophen overdose or ingestion of toxic mushrooms[1,3] (Table 84–6). Less commonly, acute cholestatic injury may occur.[36] Many chemicals (e.g., vinyl chloride) also are carcinogenic, and hepatic malignancies have been part of the clinicopathologic spectrum of chemical injury[37] (Table 84–7). Although liver injury is the dominant toxicity for some agents, hepatic damage may be only one facet of more generalized toxicity for other agents.[3]

Table 84–5 Types of Acute Postoperative Liver Injury

Feature	Haloalkane Anesthetic Toxicity	Ischemic Hepatitis	Postoperative Cholestasis
Incidence	Rare	Not uncommon	Common
Latency	2-15 days	Within 24 hours	Few days
Fever, rash, eosinophilia	Present	Absent	Absent
Serum ALT (× ULN)	25-200	Can exceed 200	Minimal or normal
Jaundice	Common	Rare	Common (indirect hyperbilirubinemia)
Histology	Zone 3 necrosis	Coagulative necrosis, sinusoidal congestion	Bile plugs, cholestasis
Mortality	High	Varies with diagnosis	Not from liver disease
Recovery time	Up to 12 weeks	10-12 days with supportive care	Variable, may be prolonged
Risk factors			
Age	Adults, age >40 years	Any	Any
Gender	F > M 2:1	F = M	F = M
Body weight	Obese	Any	Any
Hypotension	May or may not be present	Documented in 50%	Absent

ALT, alanine aminotransferase; F, female; M, male; ULN, upper limit of normal.

Table 84–6   Phases of Acute Hepatic Injury from Chemical Toxins

Feature	Toxin			
	Acetaminophen	*Phosphorus*	*Amanita phalloides*	*Carbon Tetrachloride*
Phase I (1-24 hours)				
Onset	Immediate	Immediate	Delayed 6-20 hr	Immediate
A,N,V,D	+	++++	++++	+
Shock	–	+	±	–
Neurologic symptoms	–	+	±	–
Phase II (24-72 hours)				
Asymptomatic latent period	+	±	+	+
Phase III (>72 hours)				
Jaundice	+	+	+	+
Hepatic failure	+	+	+	+
Renal failure	+	+	+	+
Maximum AST and ALT (× ULN)	1000	<10-100	500	500
Zonal necrosis	3	1	3	3
Steatosis	–	++++	+	+
Case-fatality rate	5-15%	25-50%	20-25%	20-25%

ALT, alanine aminotransferase; AST, aspartate aminotransferase; A,N,V,D, anorexia, nausea, vomiting, diarrhea; ULN, upper limit of normal.
Adapted from Zimmerman HJ: Hepatotoxicity. The Adverse Effects of Drugs and Other Chemicals on the Liver, 2nd ed. Philadelphia, Lippincott Williams & Wilkins, 1999.

Carbon Tetrachloride and Other Chlorinated Aliphatic Hydrocarbons

Carbon tetrachloride (CCl$_4$) is a classic example of a zone 3 hepatotoxin that causes necrosis leading to hepatic failure (see Table 84–6). Injury is mediated by its metabolism to a toxic trichloromethyl radical catalyzed by CYP2E1.[8] Alcohol potentiates the injury through induction of this cytochrome.[1] Most cases have been the result of industrial or domestic accidents, such as inhalation of CCl$_4$-containing dry cleaning fluids that are used as household reagents or ingestion of these compounds by alcoholics who mistake them for potable beverages.[1] At the cellular level, direct damage to cellular membranes results in leakage of intracellular enzymes and electrolytes, leading in turn to calcium shifts and lipid peroxidation.[8] Hepatic steatosis develops as a result of triglyceride accumulation caused by haloalkylation-dependent inhibition of lipoprotein micelle transport out of the hepatocyte.[38] CCl$_4$ is more toxic than other haloalkanes and haloalkenes, because toxicity correlates inversely with the level of bond dissociation energy, number of halogen atoms, and chain length[1,38] (Table 84–8). In older series, complete clinical and histologic recovery from CCl$_4$-induced liver damage was the rule with modest exposures, but supervening acute tubular necrosis and gastrointestinal hemorrhage were associated with a case-fatality rate of 10% to 25%.[1,3]

Chloroform remains an important experimental hepatotoxin, although its use as an anesthetic has long been abandoned[3,38] (see later). Hepatic injury, including chronic hepatitis, has been reported with *1,1,1-trichloroethane*.[39]

Hydrochlorofluorocarbons (HCFCs) have been associated with liver injury in several industrial workers exposed to dichlorotrifluoroethane (HCFC 123) and 1-chlorotetrafluoroethane (HCFC 124), both of which are metabolized to reactive trifluoroacetyl halide intermediates similar to those implicated in halothane toxicity.[40] Zone 3 necrosis is present on liver biopsy specimens, and autoantibodies against CYP2E1 or P58 are detected in the serum of many affected persons. As with halothane, liver toxicity may be potentiated by ethanol.[41]

Vinyl Chloride and Other Chlorinated Ethylenes

In the past, exposure to *vinyl chloride monomer* (VCM), or monochloroethylene, occurred in polymerization plants where vinyl chloride was heated to form polyvinyl chloride (PVC) in the manufacture of plastics; the toxic gas containing VCM was inhaled in this process.[1] Vinyl chloride is ubiquitous in the environment and has been estimated by the Environmental Protection Agency to exist in at least 10% of toxic waste sites.[4] Although PVCs appear to be nontoxic, long-term exposure to VCM has led to chronic liver injury, including nodular subcapsular fibrosis, sinusoidal dilatation, peliosis hepatis, and periportal fibrosis associated with portal hypertension.[3,5] Milder, reversible forms of liver injury also have been described, especially in workers with hepatitis B or C virus infection.[42]

Vinyl chloride is carcinogenic. Angiosarcoma develops after a mean latency of 25 years after exposure; the risk is related to the duration and extent of contact.[43] Alcohol appears to enhance the hepatocarcinogenicity of vinyl chloride in rodents and possibly in humans, by inducing CYP2E1, which converts vinyl chloride to a toxic or carcinogenic metabolite (e.g., 2-chloroethylene oxide).[1] A history of vinyl chloride exposure was found in 15% to 25% of all cases of hepatic angiosarcoma reported in the late 1970s,[3] and strict hygienic measures instituted in 1974 have resulted in a marked decrease in the frequency of angiosarcoma since then[5]; however, persons with the highest exposure still have a fourfold increased risk of developing periportal hepatic fibrosis, which may be a precursor of angiosarcoma.[44] Persons previously exposed to vinyl chloride should undergo regular clinical examination for early detection of liver tumors,[5] and those with known chronic liver disease or high levels of exposure should undergo regular hepatic imaging. Persons who work in PVC plants should undergo regular monitoring

Table 84–7 Clinicopathologic Spectrum of Chemical Hepatotoxins

Acute Injury
Necrosis
Carbon tetrachloride and other haloalkanes
Haloaromatics, nitroaromatics, nitroaliphatics
Hydrochlorofluorocarbons
Phosphorus, iron, copper salts, inorganic arsenic
Cocaine, "ecstasy," phencyclidine
Microvesicular steatosis
Dimethylformamide
Hypoglycin
Hydrazine
Toluene, xylene
Chlordecone
Cocaine
Boric acid
Thallium
Cholestasis
Methylene dianiline
Paraquat
Aniline—rapeseed oil
Dinitrophenol
Alpha-naphthylisocyanate
Subacute Injury
Necrosis
Trinitrotoluene
Sinusoidal obstruction syndrome
Pyrrolizidine alkaloids, arsenic, thorium dioxide
Toxic cirrhosis
Tetrachlorethane
Hexachlorobenzene, polychlorinated biphenyls
Peliosis hepatis
Dioxin
Chronic Injury
Cirrhosis
Chloroaliphatics, trinitrotoluene, arsenic, pyrrolizidine
    alkaloids
Hepatoportal sclerosis
Arsenic, vinyl chloride
Neoplasia
Hepatocellular carcinoma
Arsenic, aflatoxins, thorium dioxide
Angiosarcoma
Vinyl chloride, thorium dioxide, arsenic
Hemangioendothelioma
Arsenic

Data from references 1, 3, 4, 5, 36, 37.

Table 84–8 Relative Hepatotoxicity of Haloalkane Compounds

Compound	Relative Toxicity
Carbon tetrachloride	++++
Tetrachlorethane	++++
Chloroform	++
Trichloroethylene	+ to ++
1,1,2-Trichloroethane	+ to ++
Tetrachloroethylene	+
1,1,1-Trichloroethane	+
Dichloromethane	±
Dibromomethane	±
Methylchloride	–

Scale from ++++, maximal injury to –, trivial or no injury.
Data from references 1, 3, 38.

of liver biochemical test levels, and those with persistent abnormalities should be removed from workplace exposure.[44]

Nonhalogenated Organic Compounds

Benzene has been associated with minor hepatic injury in animals. *Toluene* led to steatosis and necrosis in a "glue sniffer"[45] and has been associated with acute fatty liver during pregnancy; it caused elevations in serum gamma-glutamyl transpeptidase levels after industrial exposure. *Xylene* can cause mild hepatic steatosis, and *styrene* (vinyl benzene) has led to elevated serum aminotransferase levels after prolonged exposure.

Trinitrotoluene and Other Nitroaromatic Compounds

Trinitrotoluene (TNT), or nitroglycerin, was first observed to be hepatotoxic during World War I, when severe acute and subacute hepatic necrosis developed in munitions workers in England, Germany, and the United States; the case-fatality rate was more than 25%.[1,3] The frequency of hepatotoxicity during World War II was lower, with approximately 1 in 500 workers affected, but the estimated frequencies of methemoglobinemia and aplastic anemia were 50 times higher.[3] Subacute hepatic necrosis followed 2 to 4 months of regular exposure to TNT. Percutaneous absorption was the major source of exposure. In some patients, rapidly progressive liver failure and death occurred within days to months, with massive hepatic necrosis at autopsy. In others, the subacute injury progressed over several months to micronodular cirrhosis and portal hypertension. The relatively low incidence of injury suggests that formation of a toxic metabolite was involved.[1]

Nitrobenzene and *dinitrobenzene* also were observed to be hepatotoxic during World War I. As with TNT, excessive exposure led to methemoglobinemia.

Nitroaliphatic Compounds

Nitromethane, *nitroethane*, and *nitropropane* cause variable degrees of hepatic injury. 2-Nitropropane (2-NP) has caused fatal massive hepatic necrosis after occupational exposure as a solvent, fuel additive, varnish remover, and rocket propellant. Toxic hepatitis associated with the chronic inhalation of propane and butane also has been reported.[46]

Polychlorinated Biphenyls and Other Halogenated Aromatic Compounds

Polychlorinated biphenyls (PCBs) are mixtures of trichloro-, tetrachloro-, pentachloro-, and hexachloro- derivatives of biphenyls, naphthalenes, and triphenyls that are used in the manufacture of electrical transformers, condensers, capacitors, insulating materials for electrical cables, and industrial fluids. Acute and chronic hepatotoxicity from PCB exposure seen during World War II resembled that caused by TNT.[3,4] Inhalation of toxic fumes released by the melting of PCBs and *chloronaphthalene* mixtures during soldering of electrical materials was the most common means of exposure.[1] The severity of liver injury correlated with the number of chlorine molecules.[3] Liver damage appeared as early as 7 weeks after ongoing exposure and was accompanied by anorexia, nausea, and edema of the face and hands. Acne-like skin lesions (chloracne) usually preceded hepatic injury. Once jaundice appeared, death occurred within 2 weeks in fulminant cases, which were characterized by massive necrosis (so-called *acute yellow atrophy*), or after 1 to 3 months in the subacute form. Cirrhosis developed in some persons who survived the acute injury.[1]

Polybrominated biphenyls (PBBs) appear to be even more toxic than PCBs. Consumption of milk and meat from livestock given feed mistakenly contaminated by a PBB has led to hepatomegaly and minor elevations in liver enzyme levels in exposed persons.[3]

Miscellaneous Chemical Compounds

Dimethylformamide is a solvent used in the synthetic resin and leather industries that causes dose-related massive hepatic necrosis in animals[47] and is capable of producing focal hepatic necrosis and microvesicular steatosis in humans.[3] Most persons exposed for more than 1 year have symptomatic disease that slowly resolves when they are removed from the workplace. Disulfiram-like symptoms can occur.[48] Alcohol use, hepatitis B virus infection, and a high body mass index are risk factors.[49]

Hydrazine and its derivatives are experimental hepatotoxins and carcinogens and have been reported to cause hepatic steatosis and focal necrosis in humans.[1] *Bromoalkanes* and *iodoalkanes*, used in insecticides and aircraft fuels, have rarely caused hepatic injury.[3] *Ethylene dibromide* (dibromoethane) led to zone 3 hepatic necrosis after ingestion in an attempted suicide. Occupational exposure has been linked to fatal toxicity, which may be potentiated by the concomitant use of disulfiram.[1]

PESTICIDES

Although exposure to insecticides, herbicides, and other pesticides is common, acute liver injury resulting from these compounds, many of which are chlorinated hydrocarbons, is rare.[50] Evidence that *dichlorodiphenyltrichloroethane* (DDT) and other organochlorines (aldrin, amitrole, chlordane, dieldrin, lindane, mirex) lead to liver damage or carcinogenicity is extremely limited.[1] *Agent Orange* (2.4-dichlorophenoxyacetic acid), the defoliant widely used in Vietnam, has been reported to cause acute hepatitis after chronic exposure, however.[51] Contaminating dioxins have been suggested to be responsible for the toxic effects attributed to Agent Orange.[52,53] Nevertheless, chronic liver injury among Vietnam veterans is more likely to have been related to viral infections or alcohol than to Agent Orange,[54] and hepatocarcinogenesis is more likely to have been related to chronic hepatitis B infection.[55]

Ingestion of or dermal exposure to *dichloridedimethyldipyridylium* (*Paraquat*) has been implicated in several instances of hepatotoxicity as a result of attempted suicide and homicide.[56] Patients may present with severe vomiting and profuse diarrhea leading to hypokalemia and often have evidence of oral, pharyngeal, and esophageal caustic injury after ingestion. Death results from a combination of renal, respiratory, cardiac, and hepatic failure; mortality rates are as high as 70%, and death often occurs within the first 48 hours. Treatment

with charcoal hemoperfusion in conjunction with cyclophosphamide, dexamethasone, furosemide, and vitamins B and C—the so-called "Caribbean scheme"—has been attempted, but persons who ingest more than 45 mL are likely to die with or without this treatment.[56] Histopathologic changes include zone 3 necrosis followed by injury to small and medium-sized interlobular bile ducts.[57]

Chlordecone (Kepone) has been shown to impair biliary excretion and lipid transport and storage,[58] but neurologic toxicity appears to dominate the clinical injury. Occupational exposure has led to hepatic steatosis and elevated serum aminotransferase levels. Trivial hepatic enzymes abnormalities have been seen in persons heavily exposed to *chloretone*.[3] *Hexachlorobenzene* in contaminated grain has been associated with an epidemic of porphyria cutanea tarda and liver injury.[3]

Inorganic arsenic has long been used as a homicidal or suicidal agent, and toxic exposure in the past also followed ingestion of Fowler's solution (arsenic trioxide) used as a treatment for psoriasis and asthma.[1,3] Other sources of exposure are contaminated ground and well water and homemade alcohol. Doses greater than 3 g can cause death in 1 to 3 days; hepatic injury generally is overshadowed by gastrointestinal, neurologic, and vascular effects,[1] leading ultimately to central nervous system depression and vascular collapse. A lesion resembling hepatic veno-occlusive disease can develop,[3] and noncirrhotic portal hypertension developed in more than 90% of 248 patients who consumed contaminated drinking water for up to 15 years.[59]

Occupational exposure to arsenic is still observed among vineyard workers, farmers, and gold miners,[60] although its use as an insecticide has been curtailed since the 1940s. Lumber treated with chromated copper arsenate as a preservative may be an additional source of exposure.[61] The clinical syndrome associated with arsenicosis includes skin lesions (blackfoot disease), anemia, diabetes mellitus, hearing loss, neurobehavioral disorders, and cardiovascular diseases, in addition to benign and malignant liver disease.[62] Chronic hepatic injury, including cirrhosis and noncirrhotic portal hypertension, may be precursors to hepatic neoplasms, such as angiosarcomas, hemangioendotheliomas, and hepatocellular carcinomas, after exposure of greater than 10 years.[63] Treatment with thiol chelators has had variable success in cases of prolonged exposure, and coadministration of antioxidants, such as vitamins C and E, may be of added benefit.[64]

METALS

IRON

Most of the 5000 cases of accidental iron poisoning in the United States each year occur in young children who mistake iron supplements for candy.[1] The severity of injury correlates with the dose ingested[3]; ingestion of less than 20 mg/kg of elemental iron is unlikely to produce serious toxicity, whereas doses of more than 200 mg/kg can be fatal.[1] Iron, per se, is not hepatotoxic, but ferric and ferrous ions can act through free radicals and lipid peroxidation to cause membrane disruption and necrosis.[65] Clinically evident liver injury is uncommon, but zone 1 necrosis occurs in the most severe cases.[1] Clinical illness is characterized by sequential phases of gastrointestinal injury, subsidence of symptoms, and overt hepatotoxicity accompanied by renal failure.

PHOSPHORUS

Poisoning by white phosphorus has been rare since its use in firecrackers and matches was outlawed more than 60 years ago.[3] Cases reported since then usually have been the result of ingestion of rat or roach poison.[1] Shortly after ingestion, vomiting, gastrointestinal bleeding, convulsions, shock, and death occur within 24 hours. Phosphorescence of the vomitus and stools and a typical garlic-like odor on the breath are characteristic, when present. The predominant hepatic lesion is steatosis and necrosis, most prominent in the periportal region. Serum aminotransferase levels generally are no higher than 10 times the upper limit of normal.[1]

COPPER SALTS

Acute poisoning by copper leads to a syndrome resembling iron toxicity. Ingestion of toxic amounts (1 to 10 mg) usually is seen with suicidal intent, especially on the Indian subcontinent.[3,65] Vomiting, diarrhea, and abdominal pain accompanied by a metallic taste are seen during the first few hours after ingestion. Gastrointestinal tract erosions, renal tubular necrosis, and rhabdomyolysis often accompany zone 3 hepatic necrosis by the second or third day. Jaundice results from both hepatic injury and acute hemolysis caused by high blood copper levels.[3] The mortality rate is 15%, with early deaths resulting from shock and circulatory collapse and late deaths resulting from hepatic and renal failure.[1]

THORIUM DIOXIDE

Thorium dioxide (Thorotrast) was used as an intravenous contrast medium for radiographic procedures in the first half of the twentieth century; more than 50,000 persons may have been exposed.[1] Thorotrast was subsequently found to cause hepatic angiosarcomas after latency periods of 20 to 40 years. As with arsenic, reports of hepatic veno-occlusive disease and a Budd-Chiari–like syndrome of portal hypertension also have appeared. Given the extraordinarily long half-life (hundreds of years) of the compound, which is a radioactive alpha emitter, exposed persons remain at risk for the development of leukemia, in addition to hepatocellular cancers.[66] Histologically, thorium dioxide is found in Kupffer cells and macrophages as dark brown refractile granules, the identity of which can be confirmed by spectrographic analysis.[37]

OTHER METALS

Although *cadmium* produces hepatic necrosis and cirrhosis in laboratory animals,[1,65] evidence is lacking that exposure to cadmium causes important human injury.[1] *Beryllium* has led to midzonal liver necrosis as a result of phagocytosis of insoluble beryllium phosphate by Kupffer cells.[1] Chronic industrial exposure (usually by inhalation of high concentrations of oxide or phosphorus mixtures) is associated with the formation of hepatic (and pulmonary) granulomas.[3] Therapy with chelating agents and antioxidants has been used in animal models of beryllium toxicity.[67]

ADULTERATED COOKING OILS AND CONTAMINATED FOODS

A number of contaminated foodstuffs and cooking oils have been associated with epidemics of hepatotoxicity, now largely of historical interest only.

The *Spanish toxic oil syndrome* occurred in 1981, after exposure of up to 100,000 Spaniards to rapeseed cooking oil that was contaminated by anilines and acetanilides. Nearly 20,000 persons became ill, many with hepatic injury and jaundice. Approximately 2500 died.[68] Among 332 patients followed for up to 8 years, hepatic injury developed in 43%, usually at the onset of a multisystem disease. A mixed cholestatic-hepatocellular injury pattern was seen, with jaundice or hepatomegaly in less than 20%. After an 8-year follow-up, liver disease persisted in only 4 patients.[69]

Epping jaundice refers to an epidemic of toxic liver injury that occurred in Epping, England, in 1965.[3,36] The outbreak involved 84 persons who had eaten bread contaminated with methylenedianiline that had spilled onto the floor of a van carrying flour. The clinical syndrome consisted of abdominal pain, fever, and chills, followed by cholestatic jaundice resembling that seen with biliary obstruction; eosinophilia was seen in about one half of patients. Liver biopsy specimens revealed Kupffer cell hyperplasia with portal inflammation but little or no necrosis.[3] Most persons recovered in 4 to 6 weeks, with jaundice lasting up to 4 months in a few. The mechanism of injury was thought to be a chemically induced cholangitis, possibly as a result of a hypersensitivity reaction. Cholangiocarcinoma later developed in one patient.[70]

Yusho oil disease in western Japan, and a related epidemic referred to as *yu-cheng* in Taiwan, involved nearly 2000 persons who had eaten rice prepared in oil contaminated by PCBs, dioxins, and polychlorinated dibenzofurans in 1968. The disease was characterized by chloracne, skin hyperpigmentation, eyelid edema, and neuropathy, with jaundice reported in approximately 10% of patients.[71] Exposed persons still harbor high levels of these agents nearly 3 decades after the outbreak.[71]

Hexachlorobenzene contamination of wheat in the 1950s led to an epidemic of toxic porphyria cutanea tarda and severe liver disease involving more than 3000 Turkish Kurds, with a mortality rate that exceeded 10%. This fungicide had been added to seed grain that was used for food during a famine.[3,36]

DRUGS OF ABUSE

Cocaine is a dose-dependent hepatotoxin.[3] Acute cocaine intoxication affects the liver in 60% of patients,[72] and many affected persons have markedly elevated serum ALT levels (greater than 1000 U/L). Associated features include rhabdomyolysis, hypotension, hyperpyrexia, disseminated intravascular coagulation, and renal failure. Hepatic injury probably is the result of toxic metabolites (e.g., norcocaine nitroxide) formed by the CYP system, specifically CYP2E1 and CYP2A,[73] and enhanced hepatotoxicity is seen in persons who regularly consume alcohol.[3] In animals, pretreatment with N-acetylcysteine decreases the risk of cocaine hepatotoxicity,[74] although the usefulness of N-acetylcysteine for treating human cocaine-induced hepatic injury has not been reported.

"Ecstasy" (3,4-methylenedioxymethamphetamine) is a euphorigenic and psychedelic amphetamine derivative that can lead to hepatic necrosis as part of a heat stroke–like syndrome resulting from exhaustive dancing in hot nightclubs ("raves").[75] The injury can be fatal and has necessitated liver transplantation in some instances.[76,77] The role of CYP enzymes in the toxicity of this and other so-called designer drugs may relate to specific genetic polymorphisms of CYP2D6 or other cytochromes.[78]

Phencyclidine ("angel dust") is another stimulant that can lead to hepatic injury as part of a syndrome of malignant hyperthermia that produces zone 3 hepatic necrosis, congestion, and collapse, with high serum AST and ALT levels reminiscent of ischemic hepatitis.[79]

BOTANICAL AND ENVIRONMENTAL HEPATOTOXINS

Examples of hepatotoxic mushrooms, fruits, and other foodstuffs, including grains and nuts contaminated by fungal mycotoxins or other potentially injurious compounds, are listed in Table 84–9.

MUSHROOMS

Poisonous varieties of mushrooms number approximately 100 among the more than 5000 species, and more than 8000 mushroom poisonings were reported in the United States in 2001.[80] Greater than 90% of cases of fatal poisoning are caused by *Amanita phylloides* (death cap) or *Amanita verna* (destroying angel), found in the Pacific Northwest and eastern United States.[81] A fatal outcome can follow ingestion of a single 50-g (2-oz) mushroom; the toxin is one of the most potent and lethal in nature.[82] Alpha-amatoxin is thermostable, can resist drying for years, and is not inactivated by cooking. Rapidly

absorbed through the gastrointestinal tract, the amatoxin reaches hepatocytes through the enterohepatic circulation and inhibits production of messenger RNA and protein synthesis, leading in turn to cell necrosis. A second toxin, phalloidin, is responsible for the severe gastroenteritis that precedes hepatic and central nervous system injury.[83] Phalloidin disrupts cell membranes by interfering with polymerization of actin. A latent period of 6 to 20 hours after ingestion of a mushroom precedes the first symptoms of intense abdominal pain, vomiting, and diarrhea. Hepatocellular jaundice and renal failure occur over the next 24 to 48 hours and are followed by confusion, delirium, convulsions, and eventually coma by 72 hours.[1,83] The characteristic hepatic lesion is steatosis and zone 3 hepatic necrosis, with nucleolar inclusions seen on electron microscopy.[3]

In a case series of eight patients,[83] the mean serum AST level was 5488 U/L (range, 1486 to 12,340), ALT 7618 (range, 3065 to 15,210), and bilirubin 10.5 mg/dL (range, 1.8 to 52), with peak levels on days 4 and 5. Acute renal failure requiring dialysis developed in one patient, and three exhibited encephalopathy. Mortality rates traditionally have been high, especially when the serum ALT level exceeds 1000 U/L, and emergency liver transplantation often is required[84]; however, some patients survive with conservative management, which includes nasogastric lavage with activated charcoal, intravenous penicillin G, N-acetylcysteine (using a standard acetaminophen [N-acetyl-p-aminophenol, or APAP] protocol of a loading dose of 140 mg/kg orally followed by 15 additional doses of 70 mg/kg), and milk thistle (*Silybum marianum*).[83] The use of these therapeutic modalities is not always effective, and in a large review of 2108 cases over a 20-year period in the United States and Europe,[85] penicillin G, either alone or in combination with other therapy, demonstrated limited benefit. Similarly, no role for glucocorticoids was found. The utility of plasmapheresis or hemoperfusion is unproved.

OTHER FOODSTUFFS

The unripe fruit of the *ackee tree* (*Blighia surpida*), native to Jamaica, contains a cholestatic hepatotoxin, hypoglycin A, that produces a clinical syndrome of gastrointestinal distress and microvesicular steatosis known as Jamaican vomiting sickness, which resembles Reye's syndrome (see Chapter 83).[3,36,86] Cholestatic jaundice has been described after chronic ingestion.[87]

Cycasin is a potent hepatotoxin and hepatocarcinogen found in the fruit of the cycad tree (*Cycas circinalis*, *Cycas*

Table 84–9   Botanical and Environmental Hepatotoxins

Agent	Toxic Component	Type of Injury	Comment
Toxic mushrooms	Amatoxin	FHF	Resembles APAP injury
Ackee fruit	Hypoglycin	Microvesicular steatosis	Jamaican vomiting sickness
Cycasin	Methylazoxymethanol	Acute hepatitis	—
Aspergillus flavus	Aflatoxin B1	Acute hepatitis, portal hypertension	Hepatocarcinogenic
Aspergillus tamari	Cyclopiazonic acid	Acute hepatitis	—

APAP, N-acetyl-p-aminophenol (acetaminophen); FHF, fulminant hepatic failure.

revoluta). A small epidemic of acute hepatic injury attributable to the ingestion of cycad nuts was reported from Japan. The purported toxin is methylazoxymethanol, which normally is eliminated or rendered inactive in preparing the nuts before ingestion.[3]

Aflatoxins are a family of mycotoxins found in *Aspergillus flavus* and related fungi that are ubiquitous in tropical and subtropical regions. They contaminate peanuts, cashews, soybeans, and grains stored under warm, moist conditions and are well-known hepatotoxins and hepatocarcinogens.[3,5] Aflatoxin B1, a potent inhibitor of RNA synthesis, is the most hepatotoxic member of the family. Reactive metabolites are formed by the CYP system, and malnutrition is a possible potentiating factor (perhaps because of the depletion of glutathione). When consumed in large quantities, aflatoxin B1 is responsible for a clinical syndrome characterized by fever, malaise, anorexia, and vomiting followed by jaundice. Portal hypertension with splenomegaly and ascites may develop over the next few weeks. In large epidemics, mortality rates have approached 25% and correlate with the dose ingested.[3] Zone 3 hepatic necrosis without inflammation is the characteristic lesion. Other histologic findings include cholestasis, microvesicular steatosis, and bile duct proliferation.[3]

The risk of hepatocellular carcinoma (HCC) is directly related to the amount of aflatoxin consumed, especially in sub-Saharan Africa and eastern China, where wheat often exceeds rice as a staple in the diet[3] (see Chapter 91). Alcohol and possibly exposure to DDT may play an enhancing role in hepatocarcinogenesis.[88] An even more important cofactor may be the hepatitis B virus.[89] The frequency of a mutation in the p53 tumor suppressor gene has been directly correlated with the development of HCC in these regions, but this mutation is rare in HCC from Western countries[89] (see Chapter 91).

VITAMINS AND HERBAL PREPARATIONS

The use of vitamins, dietary supplements, and herbal and nonproprietary remedies is an important aspect of CAM. This field continues to grow in the United States and around the world[90,91] (see Chapter 125). In the United States, alternative medicines were used by 34% of the population in 1990 and 42% in 1997; nearly 20% of the population took complementary medicines at the same time as conventional prescriptions.[92] The use of herbal products is even more popular among patients with chronic liver disease,[93,94] despite the absence of controlled clinical trials to assess safety and efficacy in this setting.[95] Many so-called health foods, dietary and weight loss supplements, and herbal products are potent hepatotoxins that have led to acute liver failure and the need for emergency liver transplantation.[6,7,96,97]

HYPERVITAMINOSIS A

Vitamin A (retinol) is a dose- and duration-dependent hepatotoxin capable of causing injury ranging from asymptomatic elevations in serum liver enzyme levels with minor hepatic histologic changes to perisinusoidal fibrosis leading to noncirrhotic portal hypertension and, in some cases, cirrhosis.[98] Approximately one third of the U.S. population is estimated to take vitamin supplements containing vitamin A, with as many as 3% of products providing a daily dose of at least 25,000 IU. Hypervitaminosis A usually is the result of self-ingestion, rather than intentional overdose, and all age groups are represented.[99] The average daily dose of vitamin A in reported cases of liver disease has been nearly 100,000 IU over an average duration of 7.2 years, for a mean cumulative dose of 229 million IU, but liver injury has been described with daily doses of 10,000 to 45,000 IU,[100] and cirrhosis has occurred after a daily intake of 25,000 IU for at least 6 years.[98,100] Long-term use of low-dose vitamin A supplements (250 to 5000 retinol equivalents per day) does not appear to be toxic.[101]

Because of the long half-life of vitamin A in the liver (50 days to 1 year),[100,102] the fibrotic process may continue due to the slow release of hepatic vitamin A stores despite discontinuation of oral intake of the vitamin. Genetic factors may play a role, and apparent familial hypervitaminosis A occurred in four siblings who ingested large doses as treatment for congenital ichthyosis.[103] Vitamin A toxicity has been reported in native Alaskans who ingest large amounts of fresh polar bear liver.[5] Water-soluble, emulsified, and solid formulations of vitamin A are up to 10 times as toxic as oil-based preparations.[104]

Hepatotoxicity from vitamin A has been attributed to activation of hepatic stellate cells, the body's principal storage site of the vitamin. Resulting hyperplasia and hypertrophy produce sinusoidal obstruction and increased collagen synthesis, leading in turn to portal hypertension.[105] Rare cases of peliosis hepatis also have been attributed to hypervitaminosis A. Beta carotene, a precursor of vitamin A, is involved in the neoplastic transformation of squamous cell lung and tracheal tissues, especially in smokers who consume alcohol.[106]

Liver biopsy specimens show increased storage of vitamin A, seen as characteristic greenish autofluorescence on irradiation with ultraviolet light.[98] The excess vitamin A is stored initially in stellate cells that lie in the space of Disse and become hyperplastic and hypertrophic. The enlarged clear stellate cells compress the hepatic sinusoids, giving rise to a "Swiss cheese," or honeycombed, appearance.[98] Hepatocellular injury usually is minor, with microvesicular steatosis and focal degeneration and without significant necrosis or inflammation. Hepatic fibrosis in a perisinusoidal distribution can arise from activated stellate cells that transform into myofibroblasts.[5] In one series,[98] cirrhosis was present in 59%, chronic hepatitis in 34%, microvesicular steatosis in 21%, perisinusoidal fibrosis in 14%, and peliosis in 3% of cases.

Hypervitaminosis A also can involve the skin and central nervous system.[1] Hepatomegaly is common, and in severe cases, splenomegaly, ascites, and esophageal variceal bleeding may be features.[1,5] Liver biochemical test abnormalities, present in two thirds of cases, are nonspecific, with only modest elevations in serum aminotransferase and alkaline phosphatase levels.

The diagnosis of vitamin A toxicity rests on a dietary and medication history and clinical suspicion. Plasma vitamin A levels may be normal, and the diagnosis is supported by the demonstration of increased hepatic stores of vitamin A and characteristic histologic findings.[107] The diagnosis may be delayed for several years if hepatotoxicity is not recognized or is misdiagnosed.[98,100]

Symptoms resolve and liver enzymes normalize gradually after discontinuation of vitamin A ingestion in less severe cases, but deterioration may continue in cases of severe intoxication, particularly when cirrhosis is already present.[100] Features of liver failure and cirrhosis at the time of diagnosis indicate a poor prognosis, and liver transplantation may be required.[1] Alcohol can potentiate hepatotoxicity and should be avoided. Vitamin A supplements generally should be avoided in other types of liver disease because of possible accentuation of hepatic injury and fibrosis.[106]

HERBAL REMEDIES AND RELATED PRODUCTS

Paralleling the rise in herbal therapy have been reports of hepatotoxicity from many components of these agents.[6,7,108,109] Warnings have been issued for several agents, and in a few instances, the U.S. Food and Drug Administration (FDA) and other health authorities have requested their removal from the marketplace (e.g., kava kava in the United States, germander in France). Any patient with liver disease should be questioned about the ingestion of herbal remedies. Estes and colleagues[96] documented the use of several commonly promoted herbal agents (including Lipokinetix, skullcap, ma huang, chaparral, and kava kava) in 50% of their patients with acute liver failure over a 2-year period. The agents were used by an equal number of men and women, for several months to 15 years. Six of 10 patients underwent emergency liver transplantation (with 2 deaths), 3 died before transplantation, and only 1 patient recovered spontaneously. Table 84–10 lists various herbal remedies according to their toxic constituent and the nature of the associated liver disease.

Pyrrolizidine Alkaloids

Pyrrolizidine alkaloids are found in approximately 3% of all flowering plant species throughout the world, and ingestion of such plants, often as medicinal teas or in other formulations, can produce acute and chronic liver disease, including sinusoidal obstruction syndrome (SOS) (known in the past as veno-occlusive disease), in humans and livestock.[110] SOS was first reported in the 1950s as a disease of Jamaican children, manifesting with acute abdominal distention, marked hepatomegaly, and ascites, a triad that resembled Budd-Chiari syndrome[3] (see Chapter 80). The disease was linked to consumption of "bush tea," made largely from plants of *Senecio*, *Heliotropium*, and *Crotalaria* species and taken as a folk remedy for acute childhood illnesses, and characterized histologically by centrilobular hepatic congestion with occlusion of the hepatic venules leading to congestive cirrhosis. *Comfrey* (*Symphytum officinale*) remains commercially available even though it is a dose-dependent

hepatotoxin.[6,110] In Afghanistan, ingestion of pyrrolizidine alkaloid–contaminated grains and bread led to a large epidemic of SOS, affecting 8000 persons and innumerable sheep.[3]

Hepatotoxic pyrrolizidine alkaloids are cyclic diesters, and some forms (e.g., fulvine, monocrotaline) cause both liver and lung injury.[110] The mechanism of injury is postulated to be impairment of nucleic acid synthesis by reactive metabolites of pyrrolizidine alkaloids generated by hepatic microsomes, leading in turn to progressive loss of sinusoid cells and sinusoidal hemorrhage, as well as injury to the endothelium of the terminal hepatic venule, with deposition of fibrin.[110,111]

SOS causes acute, subacute, and chronic injury. The *acute* form is characterized by zone 3 necrosis and sinusoidal dilatation, leading to a Budd-Chiari–like syndrome with abdominal pain and the rapid onset of ascites within 3 to 6 weeks of ingestion. In Jamaica, the course was rapidly fatal in 15% to 20% of affected persons. Approximately one half of the patients with the acute form recovered spontaneously; transition to a more chronic form of injury occurred in the remainder.[1,3] In the *subacute* and *chronic* forms, central fibrosis and bridging between central veins led to a form of cirrhosis similar to that seen with chronic passive hepatic congestion (so-called cardiac cirrhosis). At one time, this form of injury accounted for one third of the cases of cirrhosis seen in Jamaica, with death often resulting from complications of portal hypertension in as few as 1 to 3 years.[3] Certain pyrrolizidine alkaloids, such as comfrey extracts, are hepatocarcinogenic and, like aflatoxins, induce mutations of the p53 gene.[110]

Germander

The blossoms of plants from the Labiatae family (*Teucrium chamaedrys*) were used for years in herbal teas and in the mid-1980s as capsules for weight reduction in France, until several dozen cases of liver injury, including fatal hepatic failure,[112,113] forced its withdrawal from the French marketplace in 1992.[113] Most patients were middle-aged women who had ingested germander for 3 to 18 weeks, with consequent development of acute hepatocellular injury, often with jaundice.[113] The injury usually resolved within 1.5 to 6 months after the germander was discontinued, with prompt recurrence after rechallenge in many persons. The cause of germander hepatotoxicity is an interplay between toxic metabolites and immunoallergic mechanisms. Germander is composed of several compounds, including glycosides, flavonoids, and furan-containing diterpenoids, all of which are converted by the CYP system (especially CYP3A) to reactive metabolites. Covalent binding to cellular proteins, depletion of hepatic glutathione, apoptosis, and cytoskeleton membrane injury (bleb formation) cause cell disruption in animal models.[6,7] Epoxide hydrolase on plasma membranes is a target of germander antibodies, which have been found in the sera of patients who have consumed germander teas over long periods of time.[114]

Reports of liver injury also have appeared with other species of *Teucrium*, including *Teucrium capitatum*[115] and *Teucrium polium*.[116]

Table 84–10 Hepatotoxic Herbal Remedies

Remedy	Use	Source	Hepatotoxic Component	Type of Liver Injury
Barakol	Anxiolytic	*Cassia siamea*	Uncertain	Reversible hepatitis or cholestasis
Black cohosh	Menopausal symptoms	*Cimicifuga racemosa*	Uncertain	FHF
"Bush tea"	Fever	*Senecio, Heliotropium, Crotalaria* spp.	Pyrrolizidine alkaloids	SOS
Cascara sagrada	Laxative	—	Anthracene glycoside	Cholestatic hepatitis
Chaso/onshido	Weight loss	—	*N*-nitro-fenfluramine	Acute hepatitis, FHF
Chaparral leaf (greasewood, creosote bush)	"Liver tonic," burn salve, weight loss	*Larrea tridenta*	Nordihydroguaiarectic acid	Acute and chronic hepatitis, FHF
Chinese medicines				
Ma-huang	Weight loss	*Ephedra* spp.	Ephedrine	Severe hepatitis, FHF
Jin bu huan	Sleep aid, analgesic	*Lycopodium serratum*	?Levo-tetrahydropalmitine	Acute or chronic hepatitis or cholestasis, steatosis
Syo-saiko-to	Multiple uses	*Scutellaria* root	Diterpenoids	Hepatocellular necrosis, cholestasis, steatosis, granulomas
Shou-wu-pian	Traditional medicine	*Polygonum multiflorum*	Uncertain	Acute hepatitis or cholestasis
Comfrey	Herbal tea	*Symphytum* spp.	Pyrrolizidine alkaloid	Acute SOS, cirrhosis
Germander	Weight loss, fever	*Teucrium chamaedry, T. capitatum, T. polium*	Diterpenoids, epoxides	Acute and chronic hepatitis, ?autoimmune injury, FHF
Greater celandine	Gallstones, IBS	*Chelidonium majus*	Uncertain	Cholestatic hepatitis, fibrosis
Impila	Multiple uses	*Callilepsis laureola*	Potassium atractylate	Hepatic necrosis
Kava kava	Anxiolytic	*Piper methysticum*	Kava lactone, pyrone	Acute hepatitis, cholestasis, FHF
Kombucha	Weight loss	Lichen alkaloid	Usnic acid	Acute hepatitis
Lipokinetix	Weight loss	Lichen alkaloid	Usnic acid	Acute hepatitis, jaundice, FHF
Mistletoe	Asthma, infertility	*Viscus album*	Uncertain	Hepatitis (in combination with skullcap)
Oil of cloves	Dental pain	Various foods, oils	Eugenol	Zonal necrosis
Pennyroyal (squawmint oil)	Abortifacient	*Hedeoma pulegoides Mentha pulegium*	Pulegone, monoterpenes	Severe hepatocellular necrosis
Prostata	Prostatism	Multiple sources	Uncertain	Chronic cholestasis
Sassafras	Herbal tea	*Sassafras albidum*	Safrole	HCC (in animals)
Senna	Laxative	*Cassia angustifolia*	Sennoside alkaloids; anthrone	Acute hepatitis
Skullcap	Anxiolytic	*Scutellaria*	Diterpenoids	Hepatitis
Valerian	Sedative	*Valeriana officinalis*	Uncertain	Elevated liver enzymes

FHF, fulminant hepatic failure; HCC, hepatocellular carcinoma; IBS, irritable bowel syndrome; SOS, sinusoidal obstruction syndrome.

Individual references can be found in Schiano TD: Hepatotoxicity and complementary and alternative medicines. Clin Liver Dis 7:453, 2003; and Stedman C: Herbal hepatotoxicity. Semin Liver Dis 22:195, 2002.

Chaparral

The dried leaf of the desert shrub chaparral (*Larrea tridentata*), also known as greasewood or creosote bush, is ground into a tea or used in capsules or tablets for various ailments. Multiple reports of hepatitis have appeared; most cases have occurred within 1 to 12 months of use and resolved within a few weeks to months of discontinuation.[117] Among 13 cases reported to the FDA,[117] acute hepatocellular or cholestatic injury was observed, with 2 cases of fulminant hepatitis requiring liver transplantation and 4 cases of progression to cirrhosis. Renal toxicity and skin rash can accompany liver injury. The active ingredient, nordihydroguaiaretic acid, an inhibitor of cyclooxygenase and lipoxygenase pathways, is the likely cause of hepatic injury, although the mechanism also may involve phytoestrogen-induced effects on the liver.[96] A case of recurrence on rechallenge suggests a possible role for immunoallergy.[6]

Pennyroyal

The leaves of pennyroyal (the common name for two related plant species, *Hedeoma pulegoides* and *Mentha pulegium*) are used to make oils (squawmint oil), tablets, and home-brewed mint teas. The plant contains pulegone and smaller amounts of other monoterpene ketones. Oxidative metabolites of pulegone (e.g., menthofuran) bind to cellular proteins and deplete hepatic glutathione, thereby leading to liver injury.[118] Cases of hepatocellular injury, including fatal necrosis, were associated with gastrointestinal and central nervous system toxicity within a few hours of ingestion. In animals, inhibition of pulegone metabolism by the CYP system with disulfiram and cimetidine has limited pennyroyal hepatotoxicity.[119] The use of N-acetylcysteine may protect against pennyroyal toxicity in human cases.[118]

Chinese Herbal Medications

Jin bu huan (*Lycopodium serratum*) is a traditional herbal remedy that has been used as a sedative and analgesic for more than 1000 years.[6,7] Numerous cases of hepatic injury have appeared[120,121] with a mean latency of 20 weeks (range, 7 to 52 weeks) after the start of jin bu huan in recommended doses. Associated symptoms and signs included fever, fatigue, nausea, pruritus, abdominal pain, hepatomegaly, and jaundice. Liver biopsy specimens from a small number of patients showed a range of histopathologic changes, including lobular hepatitis with prominent eosinophils, mild hepatitis with microvesicular steatosis, and fibrotic expansion of the portal tracts. The injury resolved within a mean of 8 weeks (range, 2 to 30 weeks) but could recur on rechallenge.[120] The only predisposing factor was female predominance. Serum ALT levels were increased 20- to 50-fold, with minor increases in the alkaline phosphatase levels, except in one patient with cholestasis. Hyperbilirubinemia was prominent in the more severe cases. A case of chronic hepatitis has been described.[6] The mechanism of injury may involve levo-tetrahydropalmatine, a neuroactive metabolite with structural similarity to pyrrolizidine alkaloids. At present, the FDA has banned the importation of jin bu huan anodyne tablets into the United States.[6]

Syo-saiko-to (*xiao-chai-hu-tang*, *dai-saiko-to*) contains *Scutellaria* root (skullcap), which is a postulated hepatotoxin.[122] The spectrum of liver injury has included hepatocellular necrosis, microvesicular steatosis, cholestasis, granuloma formation, and a flare of autoimmune hepatitis.[123] Reversible acute hepatitis or cholestasis has followed the consumption of *shou-wu-pian*, a product derived from *Polygonum multiflorum*.[124]

Ma-huang, derived from plants of *Ephedra* species, has been reported to cause acute, sometimes severe, hepatitis, including acute liver failure.[96,125,126] The active constituent, ephedrine, also has been linked to severe adverse cardiovascular and central nervous system effects, including fatalities, when used as a stimulant and weight loss aid.[127] The FDA has issued a ruling that ephedra-containing products present an unreasonable risk and should be avoided.[128]

Chaso and *onshido* are Chinese herbal dietary weight loss supplements that were reported to cause severe liver injury, with a mean serum ALT level of 1978 U/L (range, 283 to 4074), in 12 patients.[129] Fulminant hepatic failure developed in 2 persons, 1 of whom died and the other of whom survived after receiving a liver transplant. The suspected hepatotoxic ingredient was *N*-nitroso-fenfluramine, a derivative of the appetite suppressant fenfluramine, which was withdrawn from the U.S. market a few years ago.[130]

A related dietary supplement used for weight loss, *Lipokinetix*, which is composed of norephedrine, sodium usniate (usnic acid), diiodothyronine, yohimbine, and caffeine, has been associated with acute hepatitis, including fulminant hepatic failure requiring liver transplantation.[96,131] In a case series of seven previously healthy patients (four women, three men; mean age, 27 years), acute hepatitis developed after a latent period of less than 4 weeks in five patients and 8 to 12 weeks in the other two. Mean serum ALT levels were 4501 U/L (range, 438 to 14,150), and mean serum bilirubin levels were 6.5 mg/dL (range, 2.2 to 14.6). No evidence of immuno-allergy was evident. All of the patients recovered spontaneously, with normalization of serum ALT and bilirubin levels within 4 months.

Fulminant hepatic failure necessitating emergency liver transplantion was reported in a previously healthy 28-year-old nonobese woman who had taken an over-the-counter preparation of usnic acid for weight loss,[132] suggesting that this agent may be the hepatotoxic component of Lipokinetix. Usnic acid also is a component of Kombucha tea, which has been associated with hepatic injury.[6]

In 2003, the Center for Natural Product Research of the FDA hosted a workshop to review the possible mechanisms of injury and predict the frequency of liver injury from these various botanical products.[133]

Kava Kava

Kava kava is a natural sedative and antianxiety agent derived from the root of the pepper plant (*Piper methysticum*). This herbal product has been the subject of an FDA consumer alert[6] after it was banned in the European Union and Canada[134] because of severe hepatotoxicity, including fatal liver failure.[96,135,136] A review of 78 cases of hepatic injury reported to the FDA included 11 cases of liver failure requiring liver transplantation and 4 deaths.[136] Although kavalactone has been shown to inhibit CYP450, deplete hepatic glutathione, and possibly inhibit cyclooxygenase,[136] the hepatotoxic component may be the major kava alkaloid pipermethystine.[137]

REFERENCES

1. Zimmerman HJ: Hepatotoxicity. The Adverse Effects of Drugs and Other Chemicals on the Liver, 2nd ed. Philadelphia, Lippincott Williams & Wilkins, 1999.
2. Lewis JH: Drug-induced liver disease. Med Clin North Am 84:1275, 2000.
3. Zimmerman HJ, Lewis JL: Chemical- and toxin-induced hepatotoxicity. Gastroenterol Clin North Am 24:1027, 1995.
4. Tolman KG, Sirrine RW: Occupational hepatotoxicity. Clin Liver Dis 2:563, 1998.
5. Farrell GC: Drug-Induced Liver Disease. Edinburgh, Churchill Livingstone, 1994.
6. Schiano TD: Hepatotoxicity and complementary and alternative medicines. Clin Liver Dis 7:453, 2003.
7. Stedman C: Herbal hepatotoxicity. Semin Liver Dis 22:195, 2002.
8. Weber LW, Boll M, Stampfl A: Hepatotoxicity and mechanism of action of haloalkanes: Carbon tetrachloride as a toxicological model. Crit Rev Toxicol 33:105, 2003.
9. Inman WH, Mushin WW: Jaundice after repeated exposure to halothane: A further analysis of reports to the Committee on Safety of Medicines. BMJ 2:1455, 1978.
10. Holt C, Csete M, Martin P: Hepatotoxicity of anesthetics and other central nervous system drugs. Gastroenterol Clin North Am 24:853, 1995.
11. Kenna JG: Mechanism, pathology, and clinical presentation of hepatotoxicity of anesthetic agents. In Kaplowitz N,

DeLeve L (eds): Drug-Induced Liver Disease. New York, Marcel Dekker, 2004, p 405.

12. Njoku D, Laster MJ, Gong DH, et al: Biotransformation of halothane, enflurane, isoflurane, and desflurane to trifluoroacetylated liver proteins: Association between protein acylation and hepatic injury. Anesth Analg 84:173, 1997.

13. Lo SK, Wendon J, Mieli-Vergani G, et al: Halothane-induced acute liver failure: Continuing occurrence and use of liver transplantation. Eur J Gastroenterol Hepatol 10:635, 1998.

14. Vergani D, Mieli-Vergani G, Alberti A, et al: Antibodies to the surface of halothane-altered rabbit hepatocytes in patients with severe halothane-associated hepatitis. N Engl J Med 303:66, 1980.

15. Summary of the National Halothane Study. Possible association between halothane anesthesia and postoperative hepatic necrosis. JAMA 197:775, 1966.

16. Neuberger J: Halothane and hepatitis. Incidence, predisposing factors and exposure guidelines. Drug Saf 5:28, 1990.

17. Njoku DB, Greenberg RS, Bourdi M, et al: Autoantibodies associated with volatile anesthetic hepatitis found in the sera of a large cohort of pediatric anesthesiologists. Anesth Analg 94:243, 2002.

18. Sakaguchi Y, Inaba S, Irita K, et al: Absence of antitrifluoroacetate antibody after halothane anaesthesia in patients exhibiting no or mild liver damage. Can J Anaesth 41:398-403, 1994.

19. Cousins MJ, Plummer JL, Hall PD: Risk factors for halothane hepatitis. Aust N Z J Surg 59:5, 1989.

20. Benjamin SB, Goodman ZD, Ishak KG, et al: The morphologic spectrum of halothane-induced hepatic injury: Analysis of 77 cases. Hepatology 5:1163, 1985.

21. Martin JL, Dubbink DA, Plevak DJ, et al: Halothane hepatitis 28 years after primary exposure. Anesth Analg 74:605, 1992.

22. Spracklin DK, Emery ME, Thummel KE, et al: Concordance between trifluoroacetic acid and hepatic protein trifluoroacetylation after disulfiram inhibition of halothane metabolism in rats. Acta Anaesthesiol Scand 47:765, 2003.

23. Farrell GC, Prendergast D, Murray M: Halothane hepatitis. Detection of a constitutional susceptibility factor. N Engl J Med 313:1310, 1985.

24. Neuberger J: Halothane hepatitis. Eur J Gastroenterol Hepatol 10:631, 1998.

25. Joshi PH, Conn HO: The syndrome of methoxyflurane-associated hepatitis. Ann Intern Med 80:395, 1974.

26. Lewis JH, Zimmerman HJ, Ishak KG, et al: Enflurane hepatotoxicity. A clinicopathologic study of 24 cases. Ann Intern Med 98:984, 1983.

27. Eger EI II, Smuckler EA, Ferrell LD, et al: Is enflurane hepatotoxic? Anesth Analg 65:21, 1986.

28. Turner GB, O'Rourke D, Scott GO, et al: Fatal hepatotoxicity after re-exposure to isoflurane: A case report and review of the literature. Eur J Gastroenterol Hepatol 12:955, 2000.

29. Martin JL, Keegan MT, Vasdev GMS, et al: Fatal hepatitis associated with isoflurane exposure and CYP2A6 autoantibodies. Anesthesiology 95:551, 2001.

30. Njoku DB, Shrestha S, Soloway R, et al: Subcellular localization of trifluoroacetylated liver proteins in association with hepatitis following isoflurane. Anesthesiology 96:757, 2002.

31. Berghaus TM, Baron A, Geier A, et al: Hepatotoxicity following desflurane anesthesia. Hepatology 29:613, 1999.

32. Shichinohe Y, Masuda Y, Takahashi H, et al: A case of postoperative hepatic injury after sevoflurane anesthesia. Jpn J Anesth 41:1802, 1992.

33. Faust TW, Reddy KR: Postoperative jaundice. Clin Liver Dis 8:151, 2004.

34. National Institute for Occupational Safety and Health (NIOSH) Pocket Guide to Chemical Hazards January 2003. Publication No. 97-140. Government Printing Office, P.O. Box 371954, Pittsburgh, PA 15250-7954. (www.cdc.gov/niosh/npg/npg.html)

35. Wexler P: The U.S. National Library of Medicine's Toxicology and Environmental Health Information Program. Toxicology 198:161, 2004.

36. Lewis JH, Zimmerman HJ: Drug- and chemical-induced cholestasis. Clin Liver Dis 3:433, 1999.

37. Ishak KG, Zimmerman HJ: Morphologic spectrum of drug-induced hepatic disease. Gastroenterol Clin North Am 24:759, 1995.

38. Recknagel RO, Glende EA Jr, Dolak JH, et al: Mechanisms of carbon tetrachloride toxicity. Pharmacol Ther 43:139, 1989.

39. Croquet V, Fort J, Oberti F, et al: 1,1,1-trichloroethane-induced chronic active hepatitis. Gastroenterol Clin Biol 27:120, 2003.

40. Boucher R, Hanna C, Rusch GM, et al: Hepatotoxicity associated with overexposure to 1,1-dichloro-2,2,2-trifluoroethane (HCFC-123). AIHA J (Fairfax, Va) 64:68, 2003.

41. Hoet P, Buchet JP, Sempoux C, et al: Potentiation of 2,2-dichloro-1,1,1-trifluoroethane (HCFC-123)-induced liver toxicity by ethanol in guinea pigs. Arch Toxicol 76:707, 2002.

42. Hsieh HI, Wang JD, Chen PC, et al: Synergistic effect of hepatitis virus infection and occupational exposures to vinyl chloride monomer and ethylene dichloride on serum aminotransferase activity. Occup Environ Med 60:774, 2003.

43. Du CL, Wang JD: Increased morbidity odds ratio of primary liver cancer and cirrhosis of the liver among vinyl chloride monomer workers. Occup Environ Med 55:528, 1998.

44. Maroni M, Mocci F, Visentin S, et al: Periportal fibrosis and the liver ultrasonography findings in vinyl chloride workers. Occup Environ Med 60:60, 2003.

45. Meadows R, Verghese A: Medical complications of glue sniffing. South Med J 89:455, 1996.

46. Aydin Y, Ozcakar L: Occupational hepatitis due to chronic inhalation of propane and butane gases. Int J Clin Pract 57:546, 2003.

47. Senoh H, Katagiri T, Arito H, et al: Toxicity due to 2- and 13-wk inhalation exposures of rats and mice to N,N-dimethylformamide. J Occup Health 45:365, 2003.

48. Fiorito A, Larese F, Molinari S, et al: Liver function alterations in synthetic leather workers exposed to dimethylformamide. Am J Ind Med 32:255, 1997.

49. Luo JC, Kuo HW, Cheng TJ, et al: Abnormal liver function associated with occupational exposure to dimethylformamide and hepatitis B virus. J Occup Environ Med 43:474, 2001.

50. Guzelian P: Hepatic injury due to environmental agents. Clin Lab Med 4:483, 1984.

51. Leonard C, Burke CM, O'Keane C, et al: "Golf ball liver": Agent Orange hepatitis. Gut 40:687, 1997.

52. Niittynen M, Tuomisto JT, Auriola S, et al: 2,3,7,8-Tetrachlorodibenzo-p-dioxin (TCDD)-induced accumulation of biliverdin and hepatic peliosis in rats. Toxicol Sci 71:112, 2003.

53. Michalek JE, Ketchum NS, Longnecker MP: Serum dioxin and hepatic abnormalities in veterans of Operation Ranch Hand. Ann Epidemiol 11:304, 2001.

54. Tamburro CH: Chronic liver injury in phenoxy herbicide–exposed Vietnam veterans. Environ Res 59:175, 1992.

55. Cordier S, Le TB, Verger P, et al: Viral infections and chemical exposures as risk factors for hepatocellular carcinoma in Vietnam. Int J Cancer 55:196, 1993.

56. Botella de Maglia J, Belenguer Tarin JE: Paraquat poisoning. A study of 29 cases and evaluation of the effectiveness of the "Caribbean scheme." Med Clin (Barc) 115:530, 2000.

57. Mullick FG, Ishak KG, Mahabir R, et al: Hepatic injury associated with paraquat toxicity in humans. Liver 1:209, 1981.

58. Carpenter HM, Hedstrom OR, Siddens LK, et al: Ultrastructural, protein, and lipid changes in liver associated with chlordecone treatment of mice. Fundam Appl Toxicol 34:157, 1996.

59. Santra A, Das Gupta J, De BK, et al: Hepatic manifestations in chronic arsenic toxicity. Indian J Gastroenterol 18:152, 1999.

60. Eisler R: Arsenic hazards to humans, plants, and animals from gold mining. Rev Environ Contam Toxicol 180:133, 2004.

61. Rice KC, Conko KM, Hornberger GM: Anthropogenic sources of arsenic and copper to sediments in a suburban lake, Northern Virginia. Environ Sci Technol 36:4962, 2002.

62. Guha Mazumder DN: Chronic arsenic toxicity: Clinical features, epidemiology, and treatment: experience in West Bengal. J Environ Sci Health A Tox Hazard Subst Environ Eng 38:141, 2003.

63. Chen Y, Ahsan H: Cancer burden from arsenic in drinking water in Bangladesh. Am J Public Health 94:741, 2004.

64. Kannan GM, Flora SJ: Chronic arsenic poisoning in the rat: Treatment with combined administration of succimers and an antioxidant. Ecotoxicol Environ Saf 58:37; 2004.

65. Britton RS: Metal-induced hepatotoxicity. Semin Liver Dis 16:3, 1996.

66. Ito Y, Kojiro N, Nakashima T, et al: Pathomorphologic characteristics of 102 cases of Thorotrast-related hepatocellular carcinoma, cholangiocarcinoma and hepatic angiosarcoma. Cancer 62:1153, 1988.

67. Johri S, Shukla S, Sharma P: Role of chelating agents and antioxidants in beryllium induced toxicity. Indian J Exp Biol 40:575, 2002.

68. Sanchez-Porro Valades P, Posada de la Paz M, de Andres Copa P, et al: Toxic oil syndrome: Survival in the whole cohort between 1981 and 1995. J Clin Epidemiol 56:701, 2003.

69. Solis-Herruzo JA, Vidal JV, Colina F, et al: Nodular regenerative hyperplasia of the liver associated with the toxic oil syndrome. Hepatology 6:687, 1986.

70. Hall AJ, Harrington JM, Waterhouse JA: The Epping jaundice outbreak: A 24 year follow up. J Epidemiol Community Health 46:327, 1992.

71. Yoshimura T: Yusho in Japan. Ind Health 41:139, 2003.

72. Silva MO, Roth D, Reddy KR, et al: Hepatic dysfunction accompanying acute cocaine intoxication. J Hepatol 12:312, 1991.

73. Aoki K, Takimoto M, Ota H, et al: Participation of CYP2A in cocaine-induced hepatotoxicity in female mice. Pharmacol Toxicol 87:26, 2000.

74. Labib R, Abdel-Rahman MS, Turkall R: N-acetylcysteine pretreatment decreases cocaine- and endotoxin-induced hepatotoxicity. J Toxicol Environ Health A 66:223, 2003.

75. Henry JA, Jeffreys KJ, Dawling S: Toxicity and deaths from 3,4-methylenedioxymethamphetamine ("ecstasy"). Lancet 340:384, 1992.

76. Garbino J, Henry JA, Mentha G, et al: Ecstasy ingestion and fulminant hepatic failure: Liver transplantation to be considered as a last therapeutic option. Vet Human Toxicol 43:99, 2001.

77. Lange-Brock N, Berg T, Muller AR, et al: Acute liver failure following the use of ecstasy (MDMA). Z Gastroenterol 40:581, 2002.

78. Maurer HH, Kraemer T, Springer D, et al: Chemistry, pharmacology, toxicology, and hepatic metabolism of designer drugs of the amphetamine (ecstasy), piperazine, and pyrrolidinophenone types: A synopsis. Ther Drug Monit 26:127, 2004.

79. Armen R, Kanel G, Reynolds T: Phencyclidine-induced malignant hyperthermia causing submassive liver necrosis. Am J Med 77:167, 1984.

80. Litovitz L, Klein-Schwartz W, Rodgers GC, et al: 2001 annual report of the American Association of Poison Control Centers Toxic Exposure Surveillance System. Am J Emerg Med 20:391, 2002.

81. Nordt SP, Manoguerra A, Clark RF: 5-year analysis of mushroom exposures in California. West J Med 173:314, 2000.

82. Vetter J: Toxins of *Amanita phalloides*. Toxicon 36:13, 1998.

83. Rengstorff DS, Osorio RW, Bonacini M: Recovery from severe hepatitis caused by mushroom poisoning without liver transplantation. Clin Gastroenterol Hepatol 1:392, 2003.

84. Broussard CN, Aggarwal A, Lacey SR, et al: Mushroom poisoning—from diarrhea to liver transplantation. Am J Gastroenterol 96:3195, 2001.

85. Enjalbert F, Rapior S, Nouguier-Soule J, et al: Treatment of amatoxin poisoning: 20-year retrospective analysis. J Toxicol Clin Toxicol 40:715, 2002.

86. Toxic hypoglycemic syndrome—Jamaica, 1989-1991. MMWR Morb Mortal Wkly Rep 41:53, 1992.

87. Mohi-ud-din R, Lewis JH: Drug- and chemical-induced cholestasis. Clin Liver Dis 8:95, 2004.

88. Angsubhakorn S, Pradermwong A, Phanwichien K, et al: Promotion of aflatoxin B1–induced hepatocarcinogenesis by dichlorodiphenyl trichloroethane (DDT). Southeast Asian J Trop Med Public Health 33:613, 2002.

89. Kew MC: Synergistic interaction between aflatoxin B1 and hepatitis B virus in hepatocarcinogenesis. Liver Int 23:405, 2003.

90. Kessler RC, Davis RB, Foster DF, et al: Long-term trends in the use of complementary and alternative medical therapies in the United States. Ann Intern Med 135:262, 2001.

91. Rhee SM, Garg VK, Hershey CO: Use of complementary and alternative medicines by ambulatory patients. Arch Intern Med 164:1004, 2004.

92. Eisenberg DM, Kessler RC, Van Rompay MI: Perceptions about complementary therapies relative to conventional therapies among adults who use both. Results from a national survey. Ann Intern Med 135:344, 2001.

93. Seeff LB, Lindsay KL, Bacon BR, et al: Complementary and alternative medicine in chronic liver disease. Hepatology 34:595, 2001.

94. Fogden E, Neuberger J: Alternative medicines and the liver. Liver Int 23:213, 2003.

95. Angell M, Kassirer JP: Alternative medicine—the risks of untested and unregulated remedies. N Engl J Med 339:839, 1998.

96. Estes JD, Stolpman D, Olyaei A, et al: High prevalence of potentially hepatotoxic herbal supplement use in patients with fulminant hepatic failure. Arch Surg 138:852, 2003.

97. Stickel F, Egerer G, Seitz HK: Hepatotoxicity of botanicals. Public Health Nutr 3:1134, 2000.

98. Geubel AP, De Galocsy C, Alves N, et al: Liver damage caused by therapeutic vitamin A administration: Estimation of dose-related toxicity in 41 cases. Gastroenterology 100:1701, 1991.

99. Leo MA, Lieber CS: Hypervitaminosis A: A liver lover's lament. Hepatology 8:412, 1988.

100. Kowalski TE, Falestiny M, Furth E, et al: Vitamin A hepatotoxicity: A cautionary note regarding 25,000 IU supplements. Am J Med 97:523, 1994.

101. Johnson EJ, Krall EA, Dawson-Hughes B, et al: Lack of an effect of multivitamins containing vitamin A on serum retinyl esters and liver function tests in healthy women. J Am Coll Nutr 11:682, 1992.

102. Jorens PG, Michielsen PP, Pelckmans PA, et al: Vitamin A abuse: Development of cirrhosis despite cessation of vitamin A. A six-year clinical and histopathologic follow-up. Liver 12:381, 1992.

103. Sarles J, Scheiner C, Sarran M, et al: Hepatic hypervitaminosis A: A familial observation. J Pediatr Gastroenterol Nutr 10:71, 1990.

104. Myhre AM, Carlsen MH, Bohn SK, et al: Water-miscible, emulsified, and solid forms of retinol supplements are more toxic than oil-based preparations. Am J Clin Nutr 78:1152, 2003.

105. Hautekeete ML, Geerts A: The hepatic stellate (Ito) cell: Its role in human liver disease. Virchows Arch 430:195, 1997.

106. Leo MA, Lieber CS: Alcohol, vitamin A, and β-carotene: Adverse interactions, including hepatotoxicity and carcinogenicity. Am J Clin Nutr 69:1071, 1999.

107. Ukleja A, Scolapio JS, McConnell JP, et al: Nutritional assessment of serum and hepatic vitamin A levels in patients with cirrhosis. JPEN J Parenter Enteral Nutr 26:184, 2002.

108. Larrey D: Hepatotoxicity of herbal remedies. J Hepatol 26(suppl 1):47, 1997.

109. Dasgupta A: Review of abnormal laboratory test results and toxic effects due to use of herbal medicines. Am J Clin Pathol 129:127, 2003.

110. Chojkier M: Hepatic sinusoidal-obstruction syndrome: Toxicity of pyrrolizidine alkaloids. J Hepatol 39:437, 2003.

111. Copple BL, Ganey PE, Roth RA: Liver inflammation during monocrotaline hepatotoxicity. Toxicology 190:155, 2003.

112. Perez Alvarez J, Saez-Royuela F, Gento Pena E, et al: Acute hepatitis due to ingestion of *Teucrium chamaedrys* infusions. Gastroenterol Hepatol 24:240, 2001.

113. Larrey D, Vial T, Pauwels A, et al: Hepatitis after germander (*Teucrium chamaedrys*) administration: Another instance of herbal medicine hepatotoxicity. Ann Intern Med 117:129, 1992.

114. De Berardinis V, Moulis C, Maurice M, et al: Human microsomal epoxide hydrolase is the target of germander induced autoantibodies on the surface of human hepatocytes. Mol Pharmacol 58:542, 2000.

115. Dourakis S, Papanikolaou IS, Tzemanakis EN, et al: Acute hepatitis associated with herb (*Teucrium capatatum* L.) administration. Eur J Gastroenterol Hepatol 14:693, 2002.

116. Polymeros D, Kamberoglou D, Tzias V: Acute cholestatic hepatitis caused by *Teucrium polium* (golden germander) with transient appearance of antimitochondrial antibody. J Clin Gastroenterol 34:100, 2002.

117. Sheikh NM, Philen RM, Love LA: Chaparral-associated hepatotoxicity. Arch Intern Med 157:913, 1997.

118. Anderson IB, Mullen WH, Meeker JE, et al: Pennyroyal toxicity: Measurement of toxic metabolite levels in two cases and review of the literature. Ann Intern Med 124:726, 1996.

119. Sztajnkrycer MD, Otten EJ, Bond GR, et al: Mitigation of pennyroyal oil hepatotoxicity in the mouse. Acad Emerg Med 10:1024, 2003.

120. Woolf GM, Petrovic LM, Rojter SE, et al: Acute hepatitis associated with the Chinese herbal product Jin Bu Huan. Ann Intern Med 121:729, 1994.

121. Horowitz RS, Feldhaus K, Dart RC, et al: The clinical spectrum of jin bu huan toxicity. Arch Intern Med 156:899, 1996.

122. Itoh S, Marutani K, Nishijima T, et al: Liver injuries induced by herbal medicine, syo-saiko-to (xiao-chai-hu-tang). Dig Dis Sci 40:1845, 1995.

123. Kamiyama T, Nouchi T, Kojima S, et al: Autoimmune hepatitis triggered by administration of an herbal medicine. Am J Gastroenterol 92:703, 1997.

124. Mazzanti G, Battinelli L, Daniele C, et al: New case of acute hepatitis following the consumption of Shou Wu Pian, a Chinese herbal product derived from *Polygonum multiflorum*. Ann Intern Med 140:W30, 2004.

125. Nadir A, Agarwal S, King PD, et al: Acute hepatitis associated with the use of a Chinese herbal product, ma-huang. Am J Gastroenterol 91:1436, 1996.

126. Bajaj J, Know JF, Komorowski R, et al. The irony of herbal hepatitis: Ma-huang–induced hepatotoxicity associated with compound heterozygosity for hereditary hemochromatosis. Dig Dis Sci 48:1925, 2003.

127. Shekelle PG, Hardy ML, Morton SC, et al: Efficacy and safety of ephedra and ephedrine for weight loss and athletic performance: A meta-analysis. JAMA 289:1537, 2003.

128. Rados C: Ephedra ban: No shortage of reasons. FDA Consumer 38:6, 2004.

129. Adachi M, Saito H, Kobayashi H, et al: Hepatic injury in 12 patients taking the herbal weight loss aids Chaso or Onshido. Ann Intern Med 139:488, 2003.

130. Kawaguchi T, Harada M, Arimatsu H, et al: Severe hepatotoxicity associated with a N-nitrosofenfluramine–containing weight-loss supplement: Report of three cases. J Gastroenterol Hepatol 19:349, 2004.

131. Favreau JT, Ryu ML, Braunstein G, et al: Severe hepatotoxicity associated with the dietary supplement LipoKinetix. Ann Intern Med 136:590, 2002.

132. Durazo FA, Lassman C, Han SHB, et al: Fulminant liver failure due to usnic acid for weight loss. Am J Gastroenterol 99:950, 2004.

133. Willett KL, Roth RA, Walker L: Workshop overview: Hepatotoxicity assessment for botanical dietary supplements. Toxicol Sci 79:4, 2004.

134. Schulze J, Raasch W, Siegers CP: Toxicity of kava pyrones, drug safety and precautions—a case study. Phytomedicine 10(suppl 4):68, 2003.

135. Stickel F, Baumuller HM, Seitz K, et al: Hepatitis induced by kava (*Piper methysticum* rhizome). J Hepatol 39:62, 2003.

136. Clouatre DL: Kava kava: Examining new reports of toxicity. Toxicol Lett 150:856, 2004.

137. Nerurkar PV, Dragull K, Tang CS: In vitro toxicity of kava alkaloid, pipermethystine, in HepG2 cells compared to kavalactones. Toxicol Sci 79:106, 2004.

CHAPTER
85 Autoimmune Hepatitis

Albert J. Czaja

Autoimmune hepatitis (AIH) is an unresolving inflammation of the liver of unknown cause. It is characterized by the presence of interface hepatitis on histologic examination (Fig. 85–1), hypergammaglobulinemia, and autoantibodies.[1] Diagnosis requires the exclusion of other chronic liver diseases that have similar features, including Wilson disease, chronic viral hepatitis, α_1-antitrypsin deficiency, hemochromatosis, drug-induced liver disease, nonalcoholic steatohepatitis, and the immune cholangiopathies of primary biliary cirrhosis (PBC), primary sclerosing cholangitis (PSC), and autoimmune cholangitis. Centrilobular (Rappaport zone 3) necrosis has been described in AIH and may indicate an early stage of the disease before the development of interface hepatitis.[2,3]

DIAGNOSTIC CRITERIA

An international panel codified the diagnostic criteria of AIH in 1992, and an expanded panel updated them in 1999.[4] The propensity for an acute, rarely fulminant, presentation has been recognized; the requirement for 6 months of disease activity to establish chronicity has been waived; and lobular hepatitis is now part of the histologic spectrum[4] (Fig. 85–2). Cholestatic histologic changes, including bile duct injury and ductopenia, are incompatible findings, but trivial biliary changes within the background of classic histologic features do not preclude the diagnosis.[5,6]

The serologic tests essential for diagnosis are assays for antinuclear antibodies (ANA), smooth muscle antibodies (SMA), and antibodies to liver-kidney microsome type 1 (anti-LKM1).[1,7,8] These assays are based on the indirect immunofluorescence of rodent tissues or Hep-2 cell lines or on enzyme immunoassays using microtiter plates with adsorbed recombinant or highly purified antigens. Perinuclear anti-neutrophil cytoplasmic antibodies (pANCAs) are common in type 1 AIH, and assays for pANCAs are routinely available in most clinical laboratories. These antibodies have been useful in evaluating patients who lack the conventional autoantibodies.[7-9] Celiac sprue can be associated with liver disease that resembles AIH and should be excluded in patients with cryptogenic chronic hepatitis by screening for immunoglobulin A (IgA) antibodies to endomysium.[8] Endomysial antibodies are more predictive of celiac sprue in AIH than are IgA antibodies to tissue transglutaminase, which can be stimulated by hepatic inflammation and fibrogenesis.[10]

New autoantibodies continue to be characterized in the hope of improving diagnostic specificity and prognostic value, but none has been incorporated into conventional diagnostic algorithms.[7,8] Antibodies to soluble liver antigen/liver pancreas (anti-SLA/LP), actin (anti-actin), chromatin (anti-chromatin), asialoglycoprotein receptor (ASGPR), and liver cytosol type 1 (anti-LC1) have been

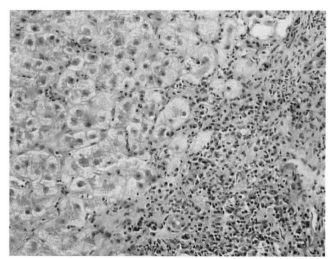

Figure 85–1 Interface hepatitis. The limiting plate of the portal tract is disrupted by a lymphoplasmacytic infiltrate. This histologic pattern is the hallmark of autoimmune hepatitis, but it is not disease specific. Hematoxylin and eosin stain, ×200.

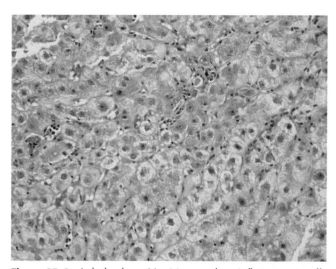

Figure 85–2 Lobular hepatitis. Mononuclear inflammatory cells line the sinusoidal spaces. Typically, lobular hepatitis coexists with interface hepatitis, but it may be pronounced during an acute onset or during a relapse after treatment withdrawal. Hematoxylin and eosin stain, ×200.

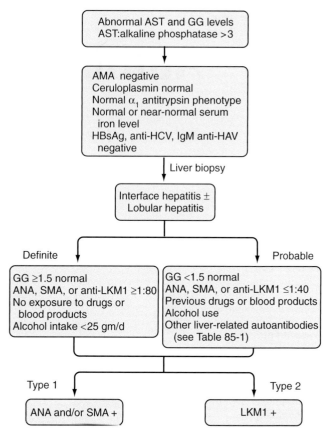

Figure 85–3 Diagnostic algorithm for autoimmune hepatitis. Diagnosis requires predominant elevation of the serum aminotransferase levels, exclusion of other similar disorders (especially Wilson disease, drug-induced hepatitis, and viral hepatitis), interface hepatitis on histologic examination, and manifestations of immunoreactivity, including serum gamma globulin (GG) elevation and seropositivity for antinuclear antibodies (ANA), smooth muscle antibodies (SMA), or antibodies to liver-kidney microsome type 1 (anti-LKM1). The degree of immunoreactivity and the presence of confounding etiologic factors, such as alcohol or drug exposure, distinguish definite from probable autoimmune hepatitis. Classification into one of the descriptive categories of type 1 and type 2 autoimmune hepatitis is based on the nature of the autoantibodies. AMA, antimitochondrial antibodies; AST, aspartate aminotransferase; anti-HAV, antibody to hepatitis A virus; anti-HCV, antibody to hepatitis C virus; HBsAg, hepatitis B surface antigen; IgM, immunoglobulin M.

associated with severe disease, poor treatment response, and relapse after drug withdrawal.[11-17] Their major clinical limitation has been their low individual occurrence in AIH.

CLINICAL CRITERIA

The *definite* diagnosis of AIH requires exclusion of other similar diseases; laboratory findings that indicate substantial immunoreactivity; and histologic features of interface hepatitis (Fig. 85–3).[4] A *probable* diagnosis is justified when findings are compatible with AIH but insufficient for a definite diagnosis (see Fig. 85–3).[4] Patients

who lack conventional autoantibodies but who are seropositive for investigational markers, such as antibodies to ASGPR, SLA/LP, actin, or LC1, are classified as having *probable* disease.

SCORING CRITERIA

A scoring system proposed by the International Autoimmune Hepatitis Group accommodates the diverse manifestations of AIH and renders an aggregate score that reflects the net strength of the diagnosis before and after glucocorticoid treatment (Table 85–1).[4] By weighing each component of the syndrome, discrepant features can be

Table 85–1 Scoring System for the Diagnosis of Autoimmune Hepatitis

Category	Factor	Score
Gender	Female	+2
AP/AST	>3	−2
	<1.5	+2
Gamma globulin or IgG levels above normal	>2.0*	+3
	1.5-2.0*	+2
	1.0-1.5*	+1
	<1.0	0
ANA, SMA, or anti-LKM1 titers	>1:80	+3
	1:80	+2
	1:40	+1
	<1:40	0
AMA	Positive	−4
Viral markers	Positive	−3
	Negative	+3
Illicit drug use	Yes	−4
	No	+1
Alcohol	<25 g/day	+2
	>60 g/day	−2
HLA	DR3 or DR4	+1
Immune disease	Thyroiditis, ulcerative colitis, synovitis, others	+2
Other liver-defined autoantibodies	Anti-SLA/LP, anti-actin, anti-LC1, pANCA	+2
Histologic features	Interface hepatitis	+3
	Plasmacytic infiltrate	+1
	Rosettes	+1
	None of above	−5
	Biliary changes	−3
	Other features	−3
Treatment response	Complete	+2
	Relapse	+3
Pretreatment score		
Definite diagnosis	>15	
Probable diagnosis	10-15	
Posttreatment score		
Definite diagnosis	>17	
Probable diagnosis	12-17	

*Times normal.

AMA, antimitochondrial antibodies; ANA, antinuclear antibodies; anti-LC1, antibodies to liver cytosol type 1; anti-LKM1, antibodies to liver/kidney microsome type 1; anti-SLA/LP, antibodies to soluble liver antigen/liver pancreas; AP/AST (or AP/ALT), ratio of serum alkaline phosphatase level to serum aspartate aminotransferase (or serum alanine aminotransferase) level; HLA, human leukocyte antigen; IgG, serum immunoglobulin G level; pANCA, perinuclear anti-neutrophil cytoplasmic antibodies; SMA, smooth muscle antibodies.

accommodated and biases associated with isolated inconsistencies avoided. The scoring system is rarely used in clinical practice, but it does have investigational value as a means to ensure compatible study populations in clinical trials.[4] The scoring system is not a discriminative diagnostic index, and it should not be used to distinguish AIH from other liver diseases. The components of the scoring system are not unique to AIH, nor has the scoring system been developed on the basis of direct comparisons with other liver diseases.[18]

PATHOGENESIS

The pathogenic mechanisms of AIH are unknown. The most popular hypotheses invoke a constellation of interactive factors that include a triggering agent, genetic predisposition, and various determinants of autoantigen display, immunocyte activation, and effector cell expansion.[19,20] Proposed triggering factors include infectious agents, drugs, and toxins. The lag time between exposure to the trigger and onset of the disease can be long, and the triggering factor may not be needed for perpetuation of the disorder. The CD4+ helper T cell is the principal effector cell, and its activation is the initial step in the pathogenic pathway.

Molecular mimicry of a foreign antigen and a self-antigen is the most common explanation for the loss of self-tolerance, but this mechanism has not been established for any autoimmune disease.[20] Genetic factors influence autoantigen presentation and CD4+ helper T cell recognition. The antigen-binding groove of the class II molecule of the major histocompatibility complex (MHC) is encoded by alleles that determine the groove's configuration and ability to activate immunocytes. The susceptibility alleles of AIH in white North Americans and northern Europeans reside on the *DRB1* gene, and they are *DRB1*0301* and *DRB1*0401*.[21,22]

Different ethnic groups have different susceptibility alleles, a finding that supports a "shared motif hypothesis" of pathogenesis.[22,23] According to this hypothesis, the risk of disease relates to amino acid sequences in the antigen-binding groove of the class II MHC molecule, and multiple alleles encode the same or similar sequence ("shared motif"). The critical shared motif in white North Americans and northern Europeans with AIH is a six-amino-acid sequence represented by the code LLEQKR.[24,25] This sequence is located between positions 67 and 72 of the DRβ polypeptide chain of the class II MHC molecule, and lysine (K) in position 71 is the critical determinant of susceptibility. *DRB1*0301* and *DRB1*0401* encode identical amino acid sequences in the DRβ67-72 region and affect susceptibility similarly.

*DRB1*0404* and *DRB1*0405* are the susceptibility alleles in Mexican, Japanese, and Argentine adults and encode a similar sequence, except for arginine (R) instead of lysine (K) at the DRβ71 position.[22,23,25] Arginine is a positively charged amino acid that is structurally similar to lysine, and its substitution for lysine should not greatly alter the antigen-binding properties of the class II MHC molecule. By contrast, *DRB1*1501* protects against AIH in white North Americans and northern Europeans, and this allele encodes isoleucine (I) instead of leucine (L) at position DRβ67 and alanine (A) instead of lysine (K) at position DRβ71. Alanine is a neutral, nonpolar amino acid that, when substituted for lysine, should greatly affect antigen presentation and immunocyte activation.

Antigenic peptides are selected for display by the nature of the amino acids that interact with residues within the antigen-binding groove.[24-26] The critical six-amino-acid motif in AIH restricts the range of peptides that can be accommodated. Multiple self-antigens or foreign antigens may satisfy the minimal structural requirements and serve as immunogenic peptides. The ideal triggering epitope must have a negatively charged amino acid residue (aspartic acid or glutamic acid) at peptide position P4 to form a salt bridge with the positively charged lysine or arginine at DRβ71.[25] Molecular modeling indicates that a negatively charged P4 residue in the antigenic peptide and the positively charged lysine or arginine at DRβ71 can form a P4-DRβ71 immunoreactive unit that is independent of the other residues within the antigen and antigen-binding groove. This minimal immunoreactive unit can be created by multiple antigenic peptides and class II MHC molecules, and the number of these units may affect susceptibility by a "dose effect."

DRB1*1301 is associated with AIH in Argentine children[27] and Brazilian patients[28,29] and encodes ILEDER at positions DRβ67-72. Glutamic acid (E), aspartic acid (D), and glutamic acid (E) are at positions DRβ69, DRβ70, and DRβ71, respectively, in the class II MHC molecule, and the presence of these critically located but negatively charged amino acid residues argues against the "shared motif" hypothesis of pathogenesis. The findings have generated an alternative "molecular footprint" hypothesis of pathogenesis that holds that susceptibility to AIH in different regions and ethnic groups relates to indigenous factors or agents favored by certain genetic phenotypes.[23] In South America, *DRB1*1301* is associated with protracted hepatitis A virus infection, and persons with this allele may be "selected" from their environment to have prolonged exposure to viral and hepatic antigens that favor the development of AIH.[30] An understanding of the individual susceptibility allele in different geographic regions may allow use of this "footprint" to track the cause of the disease.

The "autoimmune promoter hypothesis" of pathogenesis complements the "shared motif" and "molecular footprint" hypotheses by proposing that genetic promoters inside and outside the MHC can affect disease occurrence, either in synergy with the principal susceptibility factors or in lieu of them.[22,23,25] Polymorphisms of the tumor necrosis factor (TNF)-α gene *(TNFA*2)*[31] and the cytotoxic T lymphocyte antigen 4 gene *(CTLA-4)*[32] have been associated with increased immunoreactivity and disease severity. Constellations of autoimmune promoters, as yet undefined, may affect the occurrence, clinical phenotype, and outcome of AIH.

Liver cell destruction is accomplished by either cell-mediated cytotoxicity or antibody-dependent cell-mediated cytotoxicity, or a combination of both mechanisms.[19] Cell-mediated cytotoxicity depends on the clonal expansion of CD8+ cytotoxic T cells that accomplish liver cell injury through the release of lymphokines. This mechanism is regulated by type 1 cytokines, and the −308 polymorphism of *TNFA*2* may facilitate this pathway.[31] Antibody-dependent cell-mediated cytotoxicity is regulated by type 2 cytokines, and the natural killer cell accomplishes liver cell destruction by binding of its Fc receptor with an antigen-antibody complex on the hepatocyte surface.[19] The predominant mechanism depends on the phenotypical differentiation of the CD4+ helper T cell, which in turn reflects the cytokine milieu. The cytokine milieu may reflect polymorphisms of the cytokine genes that favor excessive production of some modulators, such as TNF-α, or deficient production of others.

CLASSIFICATION

Three types of AIH have been proposed on the basis of serologic markers,[33] but only two types have distinctive serologic profiles. None has been ascribed a unique cause, specific management strategy, or special type of behavior. The International Autoimmune Hepatitis Group has not endorsed this classification of AIH (see Fig. 85–3).

TYPE 1 AUTOIMMUNE HEPATITIS

Type 1 AIH is characterized by SMA and/or ANA in serum (Table 85–2).[33] Antibodies to actin have greater specificity for the diagnosis of AIH than SMA, but less sensitivity.[8,11,15] Perinuclear anti-neutrophil cytoplasmic antibodies, which also occur in PSC and chronic ulcerative colitis, are found in up to 90% of patients with type 1 AIH[9] and typically are absent in type 2 AIH.[34]

Type 1 AIH can occur at any age and in either gender (see Table 85–2).[1,35] Initial studies that suggested a bimodal age distribution probably reflected referral biases to tertiary medical centers.[35] The disease has been described in infants and probably is underdiagnosed in the elderly.[36] Seventy-eight percent of patients are women (female-to-male ratio 3.6:1), and 41% have concurrent extrahepatic immunologic diseases. Autoimmune thyroiditis (occurring in 12% of the cases), Graves' disease (6%), and chronic ulcerative colitis (6%) are the most common associated immune disorders. Rheumatoid arthritis, pernicious anemia, systemic sclerosis, Coombs-positive hemolytic anemia, autoimmune thrombocytopenic purpura, symptomatic cryoglobulinemia, leukocytoclastic vasculitis, nephritis, erythema nodosum, systemic lupus erythematosus, and fibrosing alveolitis also may occur (less than 1% each). Cholangiography is warranted in all patients who have concurrent chronic ulcerative colitis, to exclude PSC.[37]

Type 1 AIH is associated with an abrupt onset of symptoms in 40% of cases and may manifest in a fulminant fashion.[38] Typically, patients who have an acute presentation exhibit clinical (ascites, esophageal varices, or spider angiomata), laboratory (thrombocytopenia, hypoalbuminemia, or hypergammaglobulinemia), and histologic (advanced fibrosis) changes that suggest chronic liver disease. The acute presentation frequently reflects preexisting subclinical disease that is unmasked by progression or represents a spontaneous exacerbation of inflammatory activity. Features of chronicity are lacking in 8% percent of patients, and the presentation of the disorder is indistinguishable from that of acute viral or toxic hepatitis.

The target autoantigen of type 1 AIH is unknown, but the asialoglycoprotein receptor (ASGPR) is a candidate.[39] The ASGPR is expressed on the hepatocyte surface and is associated with high-titer autoantibody (anti-ASGPR) and sensitized liver-infiltrating lymphocytes. Antibodies to ASGPR, especially those directed against human-derived antigen, are specific for AIH. Antibody titers correlate with the laboratory and histologic indices of liver inflammation, and persistence of the antibodies during therapy identifies patients who commonly relapse after withdrawal of medication.[17]

Table 85–2   Classification of Autoimmune Hepatitis Based on Autoantibodies*

Clinical Feature	Type 1	Type 2	Type 3
Signature autoantibodies	Smooth muscle Nuclear	Liver/kidney microsome type 1	Soluble liver antigen/liver-pancreas

Associated autoantibodies	pANCA
	Actin
	Asialoglycoprotein receptor
	Chromatin
	Soluble liver antigen/liver-pancreas
	Liver/kidney microsome type 1
	  (rare)
		*Liver cytosol type 1**
		Recombinant CYP2D6
		  254-271 core motif
			Smooth muscle
			Nuclear
			Actin
			Chromatin

Putative autoantigen	Unknown	CYP2D6	50-kd protein tRNP$^{(Ser)Sec}$
Age (years)	Infants to elderly	Children (2-14)	Adults (30-50)
Women	78%	89%	90%
Concurrent immune diseases (%)	41	34	58
Typical concurrent autoimmune diseases	Autoimmune thyroiditis Graves' disease Ulcerative colitis	Autoimmune thyroiditis Vitiligo Type 1 diabetes APECED	Same as type 1
Organ-specific antibodies	4%	30%	Same as type 1
Gamma globulin elevation	+++	+	++
HLA associations	B8, DR3, DR4	B14, DR3, C4A-Q0, DR7	DR3

Allelic risk factors	*DRB1*0301* and *0401*
	  (white North Americans and
	  northern Europeans)
		*DRB1*07*
		  (Germans and Brazilians)
			*DRB1*0301*

Glucocorticoid responsive	+++	++	+++

*Autoantibodies in *italics* are investigational only and not available for routine clinical use.
APECED, autoimmune polyendocrinopathy–candidiasis–ectodermal dystrophy; CYP2D6, cytochrome P450 2D6; pANCA, perinuclear anti-neutrophil cytoplasmic antibodies; tRNP$^{(Ser)Sec}$, transfer ribonucleoprotein complex involved in serine (Ser) metabolism.

Human leukocyte antigen (HLA)-DR3 *(DRB1*0301)* and HLA-DR4 *(DRB1*0401)* are independent risk factors for type 1 AIH in North Americans and northern Europeans.[21,24] *DRB1*0301* is associated most closely with the disease in white patients of northern European extraction, and *DRB1*0401* has a secondary but independent association with AIH in the same population. More than 80% of white patients in Great Britain and the United States possess either *DRB1*0301* or *DRB1*0401*, compared with 42% of the unaffected white population. These findings indicate that type 1 AIH is a polygenic disorder.

TYPE 2 AUTOIMMUNE HEPATITIS

Type 2 AIH is characterized by the expression of anti-LKM1 (see Table 85–2).[40] Most affected persons are children (ages 2 to 14 years), but in Europe, especially in Germany and France, 20% of patients are adults. In the United States, type 2 AIH is rare, and only 4% of patients older than 18 years of age have anti-LKM1.[41] The regional differences in prevalence may relate to genetic polymorphisms of cytochrome P450 2D6 (CYP2D6), which is the target autoantigen.[26]

Type 2 patients are younger than type 1 patients and may have different clinical and laboratory features[40] (see Table 85–2). An acute or fulminant presentation is possible, and it is essential to screen all patients who experience an acute decompensation for type-specific

autoantibodies.[42] Earlier perceptions that type 2 AIH has a worse outcome than is seen in type 1 disease have not been corroborated, and both types respond well to glucocorticoids.[43] Type 2 AIH is associated with HLA-B14, HLA-DR3, and HLA-C4A-Q0. *DRB1*07* has also been implicated as a susceptibility factor in German and Brazilian patients.[44,45] These findings suggest that type 2 AIH has a distinctive genetic predisposition.

The target antigen of type 2 AIH is CYP2D6.[26] This protein is a 50-kd microsomal drug-metabolizing enzyme, and its expression on the hepatocyte surface can be modulated by interleukins and TNF-α. Antibodies to LKM1 inhibit the activity of CYP2D6 in vitro but not in vivo, and lymphocytes extracted from the liver tissue of patients who have the disease exhibit immunoreactivity specific to the antigen.

Recombinant CYP2D6 has been used to define the epitopes of anti-LKM1, and reactivity is restricted mainly to a short linear 33-amino-acid sequence.[26] Of the sera reactive to this sequence, 50% are reactive to an even shorter eight-amino-acid sequence. Sera from patients with type 2 AIH bind mainly to the peptide sequence 254-271 of recombinant CYP2D6, and this region has been designated as its core motif. Antibodies to LKM1 are present in some patients with chronic hepatitis C, but their reactivities usually are to epitopes outside the core motif.[46]

A distinct form of anti-LKM–positive AIH occurs in association with the syndrome of autoimmune polyendocrinopathy–candidiasis–ectodermal dystrophy (APECED).[47] APECED consists of multiple endocrine organ failure (parathyroids, adrenals, ovaries), mucocutaneous candidiasis, and ectodermal dysplasia in various syndromic combinations that may include autoimmune hepatitis. The syndrome is caused by a single-gene mutation, localized to 21q22.3, that affects the generation of a transcription factor, called the *autoimmune regulator* (AIRE), which is involved in the negative selection of autoreactive immunocytes in the thymus. Unlike other autoimmune diseases, APECED has a mendelian pattern of inheritance, complete penetrance of the gene, no HLA-DR associations, and no female predominance. Patients who have APECED and AIH may have particularly aggressive liver disease that does not respond well to standard immunosuppressive regimens.[48]

TYPE 3 AUTOIMMUNE HEPATITIS

A type 3 AIH was proposed because of the discovery of anti-SLA/LP in some persons[49,50] (see Table 85–2). Subsequent studies indicated that patients with anti-SLA/LP are indistinguishable from patients with type 1 AIH,[51,52] and the designation of a type 3 AIH has not been justified. Anti-SLA/LP, however, may have important diagnostic and prognostic implications that warrant continued investigation.[11-14] The target autoantigen of anti-SLA/LP is a 50-kd protein[53] that may be a transfer ribonucleoprotein complex (tRNP$^{(Ser)Sec}$) involved in the incorporation of selenocysteine into peptide chains.[54] Patients who have anti-SLA/LP have more severe disease than has been observed in seronegative patients[14] and invariably relapse after glucocorticoid wthdrawal.[11,12,55] Furthermore, the expression of anti-SLA/LP is closely associated with HLA-DR3.[12,14,55] This association may explain the low frequency of anti-SLA/LP in Japan, where HLA DR3 is rare,[13] and the refractory nature of the disease in many seropositive patients.[12,14,55] Testing for anti-SLA/LP may be useful in reclassifying patients with cryptogenic chronic hepatitis,[13,52] and a standardized enzyme immunoassay based on recombinant antigen is available as a commercial kit.[11,12,55]

VARIANT FORMS

Patients who have atypical features of AIH currently lack an official designation and confident treatment strategy.[56] They may have manifestations of AIH and another type of chronic liver disease (overlap syndrome) or findings that are incompatible with AIH by current diagnostic criteria (outlier syndrome)[57,58] (Table 85–3).

OVERLAP WITH PRIMARY BILIARY CIRRHOSIS

AIH in patients who also have antimitochondrial antibodies (AMA) and histologic features of cholangitis constitutes an overlap syndrome with PBC (see Table 85–3).[57,58] Typically, affected patients have low titers of AMA and concurrent features of bile duct injury or loss. Antibodies against the PBC-specific M2 mitochondrial antigens may be present[51]; histologic features of cholangitis, including destructive cholangitis, may be seen[5,6,59]; and copper staining of hepatic tissue indicative of cholestasis may be observed.[59] Occurrence rates range from 5% of patients initially diagnosed as having AIH to 19% of patients initially diagnosed as having PBC.[57]

The clinical course of the disease and response to treatment depend mainly on the predominant component of the disease. Patients who have high serum aspartate aminotransferase (AST) levels, serum alkaline phosphatase levels less than twice the upper limit of normal, moderate to severe interface hepatitis on histologic examination, and high diagnostic scores for AIH commonly respond to glucocorticoid therapy.[57,59] By contrast, patients who have serum alkaline phosphatase levels greater than twice normal, serum gamma glutamyl transpeptidase levels at least five times the upper limit of normal, and florid bile duct lesions on histologic examination mainly have PBC and commonly respond to ursodeoxycholic acid in combination with glucocorticoids.[60]

Table 85–3   Variant Forms of Autoimmune Hepatitis

	AIH + PBC	AIH + PSC	Autoimmune Cholangitis	Cryptogenic Chronic Hepatitis
Clinical and laboratory features	AIH features AMA +	AIH features Ulcerative colitis AMA – Abnormal cholangiogram	ANA and/or SMA + AMA – No ulcerative colitis Normal cholangiogram	AIH features No autoantibodies HLA-B8 or DR3
Histology	Cholangitis Cholestasis	Cholestasis Cholangitis	Cholangitis Cholestasis	Interface hepatitis
Treatment	Prednisone if AP ≤2× normal; prednisone and UDCA if AP >2× normal and/or florid duct lesions	Prednisone and UDCA	Prednisone and/or UDCA depending on AP level and histologic features	Conventional regimens for AIH

AIH, autoimmune hepatitis; AMA, antimitochondrial antibodies; ANA, antinuclear antibodies; AP, serum alkaline phosphatase level; HLA, human leukocyte antigen; PBC, primary biliary cirrhosis; PSC, primary sclerosing cholangitis; SMA, smooth muscle antibodies; UDCA, ursodeoxycholic acid.

OVERLAP WITH PRIMARY SCLEROSING CHOLANGITIS

Histologic changes of lymphocytic, pleomorphic, or fibrous cholangitis; cholestatic laboratory findings; concurrent inflammatory bowel disease; or failure to respond to glucocorticoids constitute justification for cholangiography in patients who have AIH.[37,57,58] As many as 41% of these persons have cholangiographic changes of PSC and are classifiable as having an overlap variant (see Table 85–3). Furthermore, 54% of patients who have PSC have aggregate scores that support a probable or definite diagnosis of AIH.[57,61] The absence of characteristic cholangiographic changes does not preclude the diagnosis of PSC, because small-duct disease may be present (see Table 85–3).[37]

Diagnostic difficulty is incurred mainly in children. Autoimmune sclerosing cholangitis is a disorder described in children who have the clinical phenotype of AIH but abnormal findings on cholangiographic studies.[43,62] The concomitant presence of features of AIH and PSC satisfies the criteria for an overlap syndrome. Inflammatory bowel disease, however, frequently is absent, and these children respond as well to glucocorticoid therapy as do their counterparts who have classic AIH. Consequently, they are distinct from the adults who have the overlap syndrome of AIH and PSC and are best categorized separately.

Treatment is empirical and typically ineffective.[57] Glucocorticoids and ursodeoxycholic acid (13 to 15 mg/kg orally daily) alone or in combination can be considered, depending on whether hepatitic or cholestatic features predominate. Preliminary studies have suggested that high-dose ursodeoxycholic acid (20 mg/kg daily) may have some value in typical PSC, and a multicenter treatment trial is under way to evaluate this possibility. Extrapolations from this controlled experience may be applicable to the AIH-PSC variant.

AUTOIMMUNE CHOLANGITIS

Autoimmune cholangitis is a chronic inflammation of the liver that has features of AIH in combination with those of AMA-negative PBC or small-duct PSC[57,58,63] (see Table 85–3). The term is generic and probably encompasses a heterogeneous group of diseases in varying stages of evolution. ANA or SMA (or both) typically are present in conjunction with cholestatic biochemical changes and histologic features of bile duct injury. By definition, findings on the cholangiographic examination are normal (see Table 85–3). Autoimmune cholangitis does not have an established niche in the spectrum of autoimmune liver disease and has been variously categorized as a variant of PBC, PSC, or AIH; a hybrid of each; and a separate disease entity.[63]

Persons who have autoimmune cholangitis are variably responsive to glucocorticoids and ursodeoxycholic acid.[57,63] Preliminary experience suggests that these therapies can help to improve the clinical and laboratory abnormalities but not the histologic changes.

CRYPTOGENIC CHRONIC HEPATITIS

In 13% of adults who have nonviral chronic hepatitis, the findings satisfy international criteria for the diagnosis of AIH, but characteristic autoantibodies are lacking (see Table 85–3). These patients commonly are designated as having cryptogenic chronic hepatitis and may be excluded inappropriately from therapies of potential benefit. Autoantibody-negative patients are similar in age, female predominance, frequency of concurrent immunologic diseases, histologic features, and laboratory findings to patients with classic AIH.[64] Furthermore, they have similar frequencies of HLA-B8, HLA-DR3, and HLA-A1-B8-DR3, and they respond as well to glucocorticoid treatment as do their autoantibody-positive counterparts. These persons probably have a form of AIH that has escaped detection by conventional serologic assays, and they are candidates for a closely monitored treatment trial of glucocorticoids. Assays for pANCA, anti-SLA/LP, and IgA endomysial antibodies occasionally yield positive results in these patients, and successive testing for conventional autoantibodies may demonstrate the late appearance of typical autoimmune markers in some cases (see Table 85–3).[65]

AUTOIMMUNE HEPATITIS AND CHRONIC HEPATITIS C

Eight percent of white North American adults with classic AIH have concurrent infection with hepatitis C virus (HCV), and 52% of patients with chronic hepatitis C have autoantibodies, concurrent immune diseases, or both.[66] Identification of these patients as belonging to one or the other group is important, because interferon therapy can enhance the immune manifestations of persons with AIH and concurrent HCV infection, and immunosuppressive treatment can increase serum viral levels in persons with chronic hepatitis C and background autoimmune features.

The nature and degree of the associated immune manifestations distinguish AIH with background HCV infection from chronic hepatitis C with autoimmune features[66] (Fig. 85–4). Concurrent immune diseases that reflect a cell-mediated response against autoantigens (autoimmune thyroiditis, Graves' disease, inflammatory bowel disease) typify an autoimmune process and occur more commonly in AIH than in chronic hepatitis C. They also are more likely to have clinical consequences if the immune diseases are exacerbated during antiviral therapy. Serum autoantibody titers can increase during antiviral treatment, but this increase is not pathogenic or associated with clinical deterioration. Patients with chronic hepatitis C and background autoimmune features have immune complex diseases (vasculitis, glomerulonephritis, and symptomatic cryoglobulinemia) more frequently than do patients with classic AIH, and these findings support a predominantly viral disease.

Patients with classic AIH typically express multiple antibodies in titers that exceed 1:320.[66] By contrast, patients with chronic hepatitis C typically express one type of autoantibody (ANA or SMA) in titers that are usually less than 1:320. Furthermore, patients with AIH

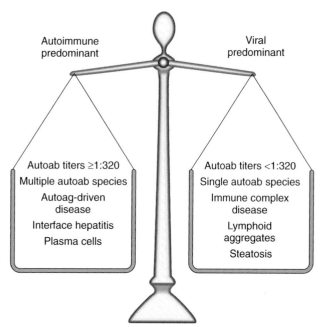

Figure 85–4 Key features for determining the predominant autoimmune or viral nature of autoimmune hepatitis with concurrent hepatitis C infection. Autoimmune-predominant disease is characterized by high-titer (≥1:320) autoantibodies (Autoab), multiple autoantibody species, concurrent autoantigen-driven (Autoag) immune disease (autoimmune thyroiditis, Graves' disease, or ulcerative colitis), and histologic features of interface hepatitis and portal plasma cell infiltration. Virus-predominant disease is characterized by low-titer autoantibodies, single autoantibody expression, concurrent immune complex diseases, and histologic features of portal lymphoid aggregates and hepatic steatosis. Immune complex diseases may include vasculitis, glomerulonephritis, and symptomatic cryoglobulinemia.

have higher serum levels of AST, gamma globulin, and immunoglobulin G (IgG) than those characteristic of patients with chronic hepatitis C. High serum titers (greater than 1:320) of autoantibodies, marked hypergammaglobulinemia, multiple autoantibody types, or the presence of autoantigen-driven concurrent immune diseases indicates an autoimmune-predominant syndrome. Further differentiation requires liver biopsy evaluation.

Patients with classic AIH more commonly have severe interface hepatitis, moderate to severe portal plasma cell infiltration, and panacinar hepatitis in liver biopsy specimens than do patients with typical chronic hepatitis C.[67] By contrast, patients with typical chronic hepatitis C have a higher frequency of portal lymphoid aggregates and steatosis than is seen in patients with classic AIH. The histologic features of moderate to severe interface hepatitis, portal plasma cell infiltration, and panacinar hepatitis constitute an autoimmune pattern that typifies autoimmune hepatitis. The hepatic histologic features of portal lymphoid aggregation and steatosis constitute a viral pattern that typifies chronic hepatitis C. The histologic diagnoses based on these patterns have high specificity (81% and 91%) and predictability (62% and 82%) for AIH and chronic hepatitis C, respectively.[68] Their sensitivity for each clinical diagnosis, however, is

low (40% and 57%, respectively). Treatment for patients with mixed features of AIH and chronic hepatitis C should be appropriate for the predominant disease and must be based on the nature of concurrent immune diseases, number and titers of associated autoantibodies, and histologic pattern. Combined therapies with glucocorticoid and antiviral drugs should be avoided.

EPIDEMIOLOGY

The incidence of AIH among white northern Europeans is 1.9 cases per 100,000 persons per year, and its point prevalence is 16.9 cases per 100,000 persons per year.[69] In the United States, AIH affects 100,000 to 200,000 persons and accounts for 2.6% of the transplantations in the European Liver Transplant Registry and 5.9% in the National Institutes of Health Liver Transplantation Database. The frequency of AIH among patients with chronic liver disease in North America is between 11% and 23%.

The impact of genetic risk factors must be considered in assessing the occurrence of disease in different regions. The prevalence of AIH is greatest among northern European white persons who have a high frequency of HLA-DR3 and HLA-DR4, and AIH is found with similar frequency in the derivative populations of North America and Australia. The Japanese have a low frequency of HLA-DR3, and AIH in Japan is associated with HLA-DR4.[22,23,25] All populations are susceptible to AIH, which has been described in African Americans, Brazilians, Argentinians, Arabs, Japanese, and Indians. The prevalence of AIH among Alaskan natives (43 per 100,000 population) is higher than that reported in a white Norwegian population (16.9 per 100,000).[69,70]

PROGNOSTIC INDICES

The prognosis for AIH relates mainly to the severity of liver inflammation at the initial medical consultation, as reflected in the laboratory indices and the histologic findings. HLA status and ethnicity influence disease occurrence, clinical phenotype, and treatment outcome (Table 85–4).

LABORATORY INDICES

Serum AST and gamma globulin levels reflect the severity of disease and immediate prognosis. Sustained severe derangements indicate a poor outcome unless therapy is started. Less severe laboratory abnormalities are associated with a better prognosis[1] (see Table 85–4).

Spontaneous resolution is possible in 13% to 20% of patients regardless of disease activity. No features predict this outcome, however, and patients should not be managed with this expectation. Of persons who survive the early, most active stage of the disease, inactive cirrhosis develops in 41%. Patients who receive no treatment and who have initially severe disease and survive the first 2 years of illness typically survive long term.

Table 85–4   Prognosis of Autoimmune Hepatitis

	Outcome	
	Cirhosis Rate	**Mortality Rate**
Prognostic Indices before Treatment		
AST ≥10-fold normal OR AST ≥5-fold normal and gamma globulin ≥2-fold	High	50% at 3 years 90% at 10 years
AST <10-fold normal and gamma globulin <2-fold	49% at 15 years	10% at 10 years
Interface hepatitis	17% at 5 years	Normal at 5 years
Bridging necrosis OR Multilobular necrosis	82% at 5 years	45% at 5 years
Cirrhosis	—	58% at 5 years
Prognostic Indices after Treatment	**Characteristics and Outcome**	
HLA-B8, DR3 or *DRB1*0301*	Young age Severe inflammation at presentation Propensity for relapse Treatment failure common Liver transplantation frequent	
HLA-DR4 or *DRB1*0401*	Old age Women Concurrent immunologic diseases Good response to glucocorticoids	
C4A gene deletions	Low serum complement level Early-onset disease Associated with HLA-DR3	
Multilobular necrosis and failure of pretreatment hyperbilirubinemia to improve after 2 weeks	High mortality rate	
Failure to enter remission within 4 years and first sign of decompensation (e.g., ascites)	High mortality rate	

AST, serum aspartate aminotransferase level; HLA, human leukocyte antigen.

HISTOPATHOLOGIC FINDINGS

The histologic findings at presentation also are indices of disease severity, and each pattern of liver cell injury has its own prognostic implication[1] (see Table 85–3). Esophageal varices develop in 54% of patients with cirrhosis, and death from variceal hemorrhage occurs in 20% of those with varices if treatment is not instituted. Hepatocellular carcinoma also can occur in patients with cirrhosis, but the risk is small.[71]

HUMAN LEUKOCYTE ANTIGEN STATUS

White North American and northern European patients who have HLA-B8, which is in tight linkage dysequilibrium with HLA-DR3, typically are younger than patients who have other HLA types and have more active disease[22,23,25] (see Table 85–4). Caucasians with HLA-DR3 respond less well to glucocorticoids than do patients with HLA-DR4, whereas those with HLA-DR4 have different clinical features and better outcomes than those seen in patients with HLA-DR3.[72]

Compared with their counterparts with *DRB1*0301*, white North American and northern European patients who have *DRB1*0401* have less severe disease initially, relapse less frequently after drug withdrawal, frequently have concurrent immune diseases such as autoimmune thyroiditis, and have the disease later in life.[72] Null allotypes at the C4A and C4B loci occur in 90% of patients with early-onset disease, and a 21-hydroxylase A pseudogene in adults has been associated with increased rates of mortality and relapse. By contrast, *DRB1*1501* protects against AIH in white North Americans and northern Europeans.[22-25] At present, the clinical applications of HLA testing in AIH are uncertain, and determinations are not made routinely.

ETHNICITY

Ethnicity may affect disease severity as well as presentation. Cirrhosis is present at accession more commonly in black North American patients with AIH than in white North American patients (85% versus 38%), and hepatic synthetic function, as reflected in the prothrombin time, is decreased more frequently.[73] Both groups respond similarly to glucocorticoids, but black North American patients are younger at presentation than their white counterparts. These findings suggest that black North Americans have more aggressive disease than is seen in white North Americans and that their higher frequency of advanced disease reflects intrinsic disease behavior, rather than delays in diagnosis or difficulties in accessing medical care.

Studies in Alaskan natives,[70] Turks,[74] Japanese,[22,23] South Americans,[27-29] and non-European, non-white patients with AIH[75] also have emphasized clinical and prognostic differences among the racial groups. Alaskan natives have a higher frequency of acute icteric disease, asymptomatic illness, and advanced fibrosis at presentation than is characteristic of their white counterparts.[70] Turkish patients have a clinical phenotype similar to that of their white counterparts with AIH but lack HLA-B8.[74]

The lower frequency of HLA-B8 among Turkish patients with AIH than among the normal Turkish population (0% versus 11%) suggests that HLA-B8, which increases susceptibility for AIH in white North American and northern European populations, may protect against the disease in the Turkish population.

Japanese patients lack the *DRB1*0301* allele, which has been associated with disease occurrence, early age at onset, and poor treatment response in white populations.[22,23,25] The clinical phenotype and treatment requirements in Japanese patients with AIH differ from those in their white counterparts: They typically have mild, late-onset disease that may respond to nonsteroidal medications such as ursodeoxycholic acid.

South American patients in Brazil and Argentina are younger than their North American white counterparts.[27-29] They have more severe laboratory derangements, and *DRB1*1301* is their principal susceptibility allele. African, Asian, and Arab patients also have an earlier age at onset than their white northern European counterparts and a higher frequency of cholestatic laboratory findings, greater occurrence of biliary changes on histologic examination, and poorer initial response to standard therapy than are found for white patients or other ethnic groups.[75]

Indigenous etiologic agents may naturally select patients with genetic predispositions that favor their propagation. The absence of HLA-B8 in Turkish patients and the frequency of *DRB1*1301* in South American patients may be clues to region-specific, triggering factors that are enhanced by these phenotypes. Other autoimmune promoters may be linked to each region-specific susceptibility factor and may further modify the expression and outcome of the disease to a degree that imparts an ethnic or geographic distinction. Interwoven into the natural history of AIH in each ethnic population and geographic region are cultural and socioeconomic factors that may affect the time to diagnosis and access to treatment.

CLINICAL FEATURES

The clinical manifestations of AIH reflect chronic liver inflammation (Table 85–5). Cholestatic features may be present but do not dominate the clinical picture. Similarly, manifestations of liver decompensation, such as ascites, hepatic encephalopathy, and variceal bleeding, are uncommon findings at the initial medical consultation.

Ready fatigability is the most common symptom (seen in 86% of patients) (see Table 85–5). Weight loss is uncommon, and intense pruritus argues against the diagnosis. Hepatomegaly is the most common physical finding (78%), and jaundice is found in 69% of patients. Splenomegaly can be present in patients with and without cirrhosis (56% and 32%, respectively), as can spider angiomata. Thirty-four percent of patients may be asymptomatic at initial consultation; such asymptomatic patients are most commonly men with serum aminotransferase and immunoglobulin levels that are lower than those of symptomatic patients.[76] Histologic features are similar between asymptomatic and symptomatic

Table 85–5 Clinical Features of Autoimmune Hepatitis

	Occurrence (%)
Symptoms	
Fatigue	86
Jaundice	77
Upper abdominal discomfort	48
Pruritus (mild)	36
Anorexia	30
Myalgias	30
Diarrhea	28
Cushingoid features	19
Fever (≤40°C)	18
None (at presentation)	14-34
Physical Findings	
Hepatomegaly	78
Jaundice	69
Splenomegaly	≥32
Spiders	58
Ascites	20
Encephalopathy	14
Concurrent immune disease	≤48
Laboratory Features	
Aspartate aminotransferase elevation	100
Hypergammaglobulinemia	92
Increased immunoglobulin G level	91
Hyperbilirubinemia	83
Alkaline phosphatase ≥2-fold normal	33
Immunoserologic Markers*	
SMA, ANA, or anti-LKM1	100
Perinuclear anti-neutrophil cytoplasmic antibodies	92 (type 1 only)
Anti–asialoglycoprotein receptor	82
Anti-actin	74
Anti-chromatin	42 (ANA+ only)
Anti-liver cytosol 1	32 (type 2 only)
Anti–Saccharomyces cerevisiae	28
Anti–soluble liver antigen/liver-pancreas	11-17

*Autoantibodies in italics are investigational or are not available for routine clinical use.
SMA, smooth muscle antibodies; ANA, antinuclear antibodies; anti-LKM1, antibodies to liver-kidney microsome type 1.

patients, and both groups respond as well to glucocorticoids. Most asymptomatic patients become symptomatic during follow-up, and differences between the asymptomatic and the symptomatic states may reflect variations in disease activity and patient tolerance.

Hyperbilirubinemia is present in 83% of patients, but the serum bilirubin level is greater than three times the upper limit of normal in only 46%.[59] Similarly, the serum alkaline phosphatase level commonly is increased (81%), but elevations of more than two times (33%) or four times (10%) the upper limit of normal are uncommon (see Table 85–5).

The hypergammaglobulinemia of AIH is polyclonal; the IgG fraction predominates. Paraproteins are common, and patients may have diverse, nonspecific serologic findings, including antibodies to bacteria (*Escherichia coli*, *Bacteroides*, and *Salmonella* species) and viruses (measles virus, rubella virus, and cytomegalovirus). Cryoglobulinemia may be present, but symptomatic cryoglobulinemia is rare.

Table 85–6 Treatment Indications in Autoimmune Hepatitis

	Indication		
Findings	**Absolute**	**Relative**	**None**
Clinical	Incapacitating symptoms	Mild or no symptoms	Asymptomatic with mild laboratory changes
	Relentless clinical progression		Previous intolerance of prednisone and/or azathioprine
Laboratory	AST ≥10-fold normal	AST 3- to 9-fold normal	AST <3-fold normal
	AST ≥5-fold normal and gamma globulin ≥2-fold normal	AST ≥5-fold normal and gamma globulin <2-fold normal	Severe cytopenia
Histologic	Bridging necrosis	Interface hepatitis	Inactive cirrhosis
	Multilobular necrosis		Portal hepatitis
			Decompensated cirrhosis with variceal bleeding

AST, serum aspartate aminotransferase level.

Table 85–7 Preferred Treatment Regimens in Autoimmune Hepatitis

Combination Therapy		Single-Drug Therapy
Prednisone (mg/day)	**Azathioprine (mg/day)**	**Prednisone (mg/day)**
30 mg × 1 wk	50 mg until end point	60 mg × 1 wk
20 mg × 1 wk		40 mg × 1 wk
15 mg × 2 wk		30 mg × 2 wk
10 mg until end point		20 mg until end point

Concurrent immunologic diseases are common and involve diverse organ systems, most frequently the thyroid.[1] Smooth muscle antibodies, ANA, and anti-LKM1 are required for the diagnosis, and other autoantibodies may be present, as shown in Table 85–5. These other autoantibodies do not have routine clinical applications.

TREATMENT

INDICATIONS

The indications for treatment are shown in Table 85–6[1,77] and are based on manifestations of inflammation.

TREATMENT REGIMENS

Prednisone, alone or at a lower dose in combination with azathioprine, is effective (Table 85–7).[1,77] No findings at presentation preclude a satisfactory response to therapy. The presence of ascites or hepatic encephalopathy identifies patients with a poor prognosis, but these findings do not preclude a full response to glucocorticoid therapy.[78] Decompensated patients with multilobular necrosis on histologic examination in whom at least one laboratory parameter fails to normalize, or in whom hyperbilirubinemia does not improve, after 2 weeks of treatment have a high immediate mortality rate. These patients should be evaluated for liver transplantation (see

Table 85–4). Patients in whom these parameters improve during the first 2 weeks of therapy have excellent immediate survival rates, and their drug treatment should be continued.[78]

DRUG-RELATED SIDE EFFECTS

Cosmetic changes, such as facial rounding, dorsal hump formation, obesity, acne, and hirsutism, occur in 80% of patients after 2 years of treatment regardless of the regimen used.[1,77] Severe side effects include osteopenia with vertebral compression, diabetes, cataracts, emotional lability, and hypertension. Severe complications are uncommon, but if they develop, they do so after protracted therapy (more than 18 months) and on the schedule with the higher dose of prednisone (20 mg per day). Azathioprine with prednisone is preferred to prednisone alone because the combination produces fewer glucocorticoid-related side effects during comparable periods of treatment (10% versus 44%). Treatment must be discontinued prematurely in 13% of patients, mainly because of intolerable obesity, cosmetic changes, or osteoporosis.

Postmenopausal patients are at risk for vertebral compression and must be selected carefully for therapy before institution of a glucocorticoid regimen.[79] A regular program of exercise and supplementation with calcium and vitamin D may help preserve bone density. Bisphosphonates, such as alendronate (70 mg per week), should be considered for patients with osteopenia. Carefully selected postmenopausal patients respond as well as others to initial therapy, but protracted therapy, especially retreatment after relapse, is associated with an increased risk of complications.

Treatment with azathioprine can be complicated by cholestatic liver disease, nausea, emesis, rash, and cytopenias.[1,77] These side effects occur in less than 10% of patients receiving 50 mg per day and reverse with a reduction in dose or termination of therapy. Teratogenicity and oncogenicity are theoretical complications. A high frequency of birth defects has not been documented in women with AIH who received treatment during pregnancy,[80] and nonhepatic malignancy develops at only a slightly higher frequency than in an age-

and sex-matched normal population.[81] The low but increased risk of malignancy (1.4-fold greater than normal) does not contraindicate azathioprine therapy in AIH but emphasizes the importance of maintaining strict indications for treatment.

Azathioprine is converted in blood to 6-mercaptopurine, which is converted in turn to 6-thioguanines by hypoxanthine guanine phosphoribosyl transferase.[77] The 6-thioguanines are the active metabolites that interfere with purine nucleotide synthesis within the cell cycle and impair proliferation of rapidly dividing T and B lymphocytes. Thiopurine methyltransferase (TPMT) converts 6-mercaptopurine to 6-methylmercaptopurine, which is an inactive end-product of azathioprine metabolism. Blood TPMT levels are significantly lower in patients with AIH and intolerance to azathioprine than in patients with uncomplicated courses of treatment.[82] Similar findings of an association between low blood TPMT levels and drug intolerance have been described in patients with inflammatory bowel disease and rheumatic conditions (see Chapter 108). These observations have suggested that low blood TPMT levels may identify persons with AIH at risk for azathioprine-related complications. The low frequency of nearly absent TPMT activity (0.3%), uncertainty about minimum enzyme requirements for inactivation of low-dose azathioprine, ability of azathioprine therapy to up-regulate TPMT production, and rarity of aplastic anemia in treated patients suggest that routine screening for TPMT deficiency may have limited benefit in AIH.

TREATMENT END POINTS

Glucocorticoid therapy is continued until remission, treatment failure, incomplete response, or drug toxicity occurs[1,77] (Fig. 85–5). *Remission* implies the absence of symptoms, resolution of inflammatory indices (except for a serum AST level no greater than twice the upper limit of normal), and histologic improvement to normal or minimal activity. Histologic resolution lags behind clinical and laboratory resolution by 3 to 8 months, and therapy must be extended to compensate for this lag. Liver biopsy examination before drug withdrawal ensures an optimal end point. Improvement of the liver tissue to normal is associated with a frequency of relapse of only 20% after cessation of treatment.[83] Improvement to portal hepatitis alone is associated with a 50% frequency of relapse. Progression to cirrhosis or persistence of interface hepatitis is associated with a 100% frequency of relapse. The presence of plasma cells within the portal tract may reflect persistent immune reactivity and the propensity for relapse more reliably than other histologic features of inflammation.[84]

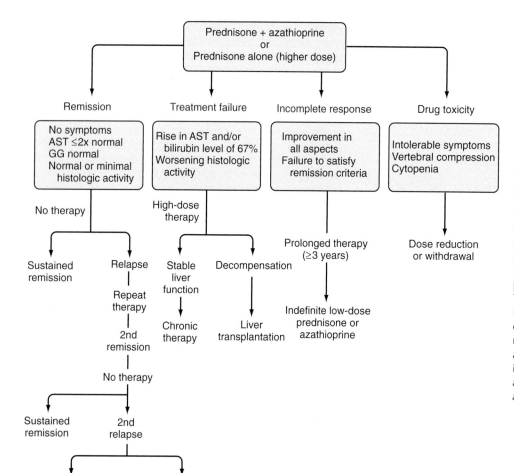

Figure 85–5 Treatment algorithm for autoimmune hepatitis. Patients who satisfy absolute or relative indications for glucocorticoid therapy are given prednisone in combination with azathioprine or a higher dose of prednisone alone (see Table 85–7). Treatment is continued until the criteria for a treatment end point are met. Possible end points are remission, treatment failure, incomplete response, and drug toxicity. Therapy can then be discontinued, increased in dose, or reduced in dose. Responses to the dose adjustments determine the need for other actions. The principal indices of inflammatory activity are serum aspartate aminotransferase (AST) and gamma globulin (GG) levels.

Treatment failure connotes deterioration during therapy.[1,77] It is characterized by worsening of the serum AST or bilirubin levels by at least 67% of previous values, progressive histologic activity, or onset of ascites or encephalopathy. Conventional glucocorticoid therapy should be stopped, and a high-dose regimen should be instituted.

Incomplete response connotes improvement that is insufficient to satisfy remission criteria.[1,77] Failure to achieve remission within 3 years indicates that remission is unlikely and warrants discontinuation of conventional treatment.

Drug toxicity justifies premature withdrawal of medication or a reduction in dose.[1,77] Most side effects are reversible, and some consequences such as cataracts and osteopenia with vertebral compression have effective therapies. Weight gain, acne, edema, and diabetes may be consequences of the disease, rather than of the drugs.

TREATMENT RESULTS

Prednisone alone or in combination with azathioprine induces a clinical, biochemical, and histologic remission in 65% of patients within 3 years.[1,77] The average treatment interval until remission is 22 months. Therapy improves survival: The 10-year life expectancies following treatment for patients with and without cirrhosis at the time of the initial medical consultation are 89% and 90%, respectively. The overall 10-year survival rate is 93% and is comparable to that of an age- and sex-matched cohort from the population at large (94%). Patients who have histologic cirrhosis respond as well as do noncirrhotic patients and should receive similar treatment, with the same expectation of success. Twenty-one percent of patients managed with conventional regimens of prednisone alone or in combination with azathioprine sustain their remission for a median of 76 months after drug withdrawal, and an effort should be made to withdraw all patients from initial therapy after criteria for remission have been satisfied.[85]

Treatment with glucocorticoids also may reduce hepatic fibrosis.[86] Fibrosis scores have improved in 56% of patients followed for 55 ± 9 months, and fibrosis did not progress in 33% of patients followed for 62 ± 14 months. Histologic activity indices decreased concurrently, and patients in whom the histologic activity indices improved had a higher frequency of improvement in the fibrosis scores (80% versus 25%, P = .002). These findings suggest that improvement in hepatic fibrosis occurs in conjunction with reduction in liver inflammation and that glucocorticoids may facilitate the disappearance of fibrosis by suppressing inflammatory activity. Small case studies have also suggested that cirrhosis can disappear during treatment, but this possibility must await confirmation by assays more reliably reflective of cirrhosis than conventional needle biopsy of the liver.

RELAPSE

Patients who enter remission commonly experience an exacerbation after drug withdrawal.[1,77] Relapse occurs in 50% within 6 months, and most patients (70% to 86%) experience exacerbation within 3 years. Reinstitution of the original treatment induces another remission, but relapse commonly recurs after termination of therapy. The major consequence of relapse and retreatment is the development of drug-related complications, which occur in 70% of those who have multiple relapses and retreatments.

Patients who have had at least two relapses should be given either low-dose prednisone or azathioprine as the sole drug (see Fig. 85–5). Eighty-seven percent of patients can be managed long term on prednisone at less than 10 mg per day (median dose, 7.5 mg per day).[87] The dose is titrated to the lowest level needed to prevent symptoms and to maintain serum aminotransferase levels below three times normal. Side effects attributable to previous glucocorticoid therapy resolve in 85% of patients; the immediate survival rate is comparable to that for persons managed with conventional treatment (91% versus 90%), and new complications do not occur.

Continuous azathioprine therapy (2 mg/kg per day) is an alternative strategy that can be used in patients who are not severely cytopenic.[88] Eighty-three percent of persons using this regimen remain in remission for up to 10 years. Symptoms of glucocorticoid withdrawal (arthralgias and myalgias) occur in 56% but are self-limited. Myelosuppression (6%) and nonhepatic malignancies (7%) are infrequent. The low-dose prednisone and azathioprine maintenance regimens have not been compared directly, and no objective basis for preferring one to the other has been recognized.

Treatment after relapse need not be indefinite.[85] Twenty-eight percent of patients who receive another course of treatment after a relapse can enter a sustained long-term remission without medication, and the probability of achieving this outcome after initial or repeated treatments is 47% after 10 years. The frequency of ultimately inducing a sustained remission and the ready ability to diagnose and treat a relapse effectively support the effort to withdraw treatment in all patients with stable inactive disease even after repeated earlier relapses.

TREATMENT FAILURE

Nine percent of patients deteriorate during glucocorticoid therapy (treatment failure)[1,77] (see Fig. 85–5). High doses of prednisone alone (60 mg per day) or prednisone (30 mg per day) in conjunction with azathioprine (150 mg per day) constitute standard treatment in this group. Each schedule induces clinical and biochemical improvement in 70% of patients within 2 years. Histologic resolution, however, occurs in only 20%, and long-term therapy frequently is necessary. These patients are at risk for liver failure and serious drug toxicity. Liver transplantation must be considered at the first sign of hepatic decompensation. The development of ascites typically heralds the need for a transplant evaluation (see Table 85–4).

Alternative management strategies for treatment failure have included the administration of cyclosporine, mycophenolate mofetil, ursodeoxycholic acid, budesonide, 6-mercaptopurine, methotrexate, and cyclophosphamide.[77] In each instance, experience has been limited, and in most reports the preliminary results have been encouraging but uncorroborated. Among the new drugs used in treatment failure, only ursodeoxycholic acid has been evaluated by a randomized controlled clinical trial, and the findings did not support its use.

INCOMPLETE RESPONSE

In 13% of patients, clinical improvement is observed during therapy, but the findings do not satisfy remission criteria[1,77] (see Fig. 85–5). The diminishing benefit-to-risk ratio of protracted therapy justifies an alternative strategy. A low-dose prednisone regimen and the administration of azathioprine (2 mg/kg daily) as the sole drug are reasonable approaches.[87,88] The goal of treatment is to reduce and stabilize disease activity on a drug schedule that is well tolerated.

DRUG TOXICITY

For patients with serious side effects from therapy, treatment usually can be continued with the single tolerated drug (prednisone or azathioprine) in an adjusted dose (see Fig. 85–5). Cyclosporine, 6-mercaptopurine, and cyclophosphamide also have been used successfully after drug toxicity in isolated cases.[1,77]

LIVER TRANSPLANTATION

Liver transplantation is effective in the treatment of decompensated AIH (see Chapter 92).[1,77] Five-year survival rates for patients and grafts range from 83% to 92%, and the actuarial 10-year survival rate after transplantation is 75%. Autoimmune hepatitis recurs in at least 17% of patients, and AIH develops de novo in 3% to 5% of patients undergoing transplantation for nonautoimmune liver disease. Acute rejection, glucocorticoid-resistant rejection, and chronic rejection occur more commonly in patients undergoing transplantation for AIH than for other conditions, and patients with AIH are more difficult to withdraw from glucocorticoids.[89]

Recurrent AIH typically is mild and develops in patients who are inadequately immunosuppressed. Dose adjustments usually are sufficient to suppress the disease, but progression to cirrhosis and graft failure have been reported. De novo AIH is a clinical syndrome that affects mainly children who undergo transplantation for nonautoimmune liver disease. Immunosuppression with cyclosporine is a common feature of the post-transplant regimen, and treatment with prednisone and azathioprine typically is effective. Those patients with de novo AIH in whom glucocorticoid therapy fails experience worsening fibrosis with possible graft loss, and those who do not receive glucocorticoids progress to cirrhosis, require retransplantation, or die of liver failure. De novo AIH in some adults has been associated with severe centrilobular necrosis, and adult patients have been reported to express an atypical anti–liver-kidney cytosolic antibody of uncertain pathogenic significance.[89] Autoimmune hepatitis should be included in the differential diagnosis of allograft dysfunction in all transplant recipients.

FUTURE DIRECTIONS

Future investigations must focus on the clarification of pathogenic mechanisms, characterization of target autoantigens, identification of host susceptibility factors, and assessment of alternative treatment strategies. Future drug trials must include more powerful immunosuppressive agents, novel cytoprotective drugs, and combinations of both.[77] Agents already exist that can interfere selectively with each costimulatory signal of immunocyte activation, and agents that block transendothelial migration of effector T cells into target tissues may become available.[90] Cyclosporine, tacrolimus, sirolimus, and mycophenolate mofetil constitute a core repertoire of new immunosuppressive agents with selective actions that may target critical pathogenic pathways in AIH. The strong rationale for their use justifies their consideration as single agents or as part of combination regimens in clinical trials. A network of collaborating centers must be established to perform these clinical trials in a rapid and statistically powerful fashion.

Site-specific interventions will be possible once the pathogenic mechanisms are clarified.[77] These therapies may include peptides to block autoantigen display within the class II MHC molecules, agents such as cytotoxic T lymphocyte antigen 4 to temper immunocyte response, T cell vaccination, oral tolerance regimens, cytokine manipulations, and gene therapies that can offset the overexpression of dysregulatory cytokines, limit fibrosis, and promote regeneration. Continuing clarification of disease mechanisms and refinement of experimental models will facilitate the emergence of these novel therapies.

REFERENCES

1. Czaja AJ, Freese DK: Diagnosis and treatment of autoimmune hepatitis. Hepatology 36:479, 2002.
2. Pratt DS, Fawaz KA, Rabson A, et al: A novel histological lesion in glucocorticoid-responsive chronic hepatitis. Gastroenterology 113:664, 1997.
3. Okano N, Yamamoto K, Sakaguchi K, et al: Clinicopathological features of acute-onset autoimmune hepatitis. Hepatol Res 25:263, 2003.
4. Alvarez F, Berg P, Bianchi F, et al: International Autoimmune Hepatitis Group report: Review of criteria for diagnosis of autoimmune hepatitis. J Hepatol 31:929, 1999.
5. Czaja AJ, Carpenter HA: Autoimmune hepatitis with incidental histologic features of bile duct injury. Hepatology 34:659, 2001.
6. Czaja AJ, Muratori P, Muratori L, et al: Diagnostic and therapeutic implications of bile duct injury in autoimmune hepatitis. Liver International 24:1, 2004.
7. Czaja A, Homburger H: Antibodies in liver disease. Gastroenterology 120:239, 2001.
8. Czaja AJ, Norman GL: Autoantibodies in the diagnosis and management of liver disease. J Clin Gastroenterol 37:315, 2003.

9. Targan SR, Landers C, Vidrich A, et al: High-titer antineutrophil cytoplasmic antibodies in type 1 autoimmune hepatitis. Gastroenterology 108:1159, 1995.

10. Czaja AJ, Shums Z, Donaldson PT, et al: Frequency and significance of antibodies to *Saccharomyces cerevisiae* in autoimmune hepatitis. Dig Dis Sci 49:611, 2004.

11. Czaja AJ, Shums Z, Norman GL: Nonstandard antibodies as prognostic markers in autoimmune hepatitis. Autoimmunity 37:195, 2004.

12. Czaja AJ, Donaldson PT, Lohse AW: Antibodies to soluble liver antigen/liver pancreas and HLA risk factors in type 1 autoimmune hepatitis. Am J Gastroenterol 97:413, 2002.

13. Baeres M, Herkel J, Czaja AJ, et al: Establishment of standardized SLA/LP immunoassays: Specificity for autoimmune hepatitis, worldwide occurrence, and clinical characteristics. Gut 51:259, 2002.

14. Ma Y, Okamoto M, Thomas MG, et al: Antibodies to conformational epitopes of soluble liver antigen define a severe form of autoimmune liver disease. Hepatology 35:658, 2002.

15. Czaja AJ, Cassani F, Cataleta M, et al: Frequency and significance of antibodies to actin in type 1 autoimmune hepatitis. Hepatology 24:1068, 1996.

16. Czaja AJ, Shums Z, Binder WL, et al: Frequency and significance of antibodies to chromatin in autoimmune hepatitis. Dig Dis Sci 48:1658, 2003.

17. Czaja AJ, Pfeifer KD, Decker RH, et al: Frequency and significance of antibodies to asialoglycoprotein receptor in type 1 autoimmune hepatitis. Dig Dis Sci 41:1733, 1996.

18. Talwalkar JA, Keach JC, Angulo P, et al: Overlap of autoimmune hepatitis and primary biliary cirrhosis: An evaluation of a modified scoring system. Am J Gastroenterol 97:1191, 2002.

19. Czaja AJ: Understanding the pathogenesis of autoimmune hepatitis. Am J Gastroenterol 96:1224, 2001.

20. Vergani D, Choudhuri K, Bogdanos DP, et al: Pathogenesis of autoimmune hepatitis. Clin Liver Dis 6:727, 2002.

21. Strettell M, Donaldson P, Thomson L, et al: Allelic basis for HLA-encoded susceptibility to type 1 autoimmune hepatitis. Gastroenterology 112:2028,1997.

22. Czaja A, Donaldson P: Genetic susceptibilities for immune expression and liver cell injury in autoimmune hepatitis. Immunol Rev 174:250, 2000.

23. Donaldson PT, Czaja AJ: Genetic effects on susceptibility, clinical expression, and treatment outcome of type 1 autoimmune hepatitis. Clin Liver Dis 6:799, 2002.

24. Doherty DG, Donaldson PT, Underhill JA, et al: Allelic sequence variation in the HLA class II genes and proteins in patients with autoimmune hepatitis. Hepatology 19:609, 1994.

25. Czaja AJ, Doherty DG, Donaldson PT: Genetic bases of autoimmune hepatitis. Dig Dis Sci 47:2139, 2002.

26. Manns M, Griffin K, Sullivan K, et al: LKM-1 autoantibodies recognize a short linear sequence in P450IID6, a cytochrome P-450 monooxygenase. J Clin Invest 88:1370, 1991.

27. Pando M, Larriba J, Fernandez GC, et al: Pediatric and adult forms of type 1 autoimmune hepatitis in Argentina: evidence for differential genetic predisposition. Hepatology 30:1374, 1999.

28. Goldberg AC, Bittencourt PL, Mougin B, et al: Analysis of HLA haplotypes in autoimmune hepatitis type 1: Identifying the major susceptibility locus. Hum Immunol 62:165, 2001.

29. Czaja AJ, Souto EO, Bittencourt PL, et al: Clinical distinctions and pathogenic implications of type 1 autoimmune hepatitis in Brazil and the United States. J Hepatol 37:302, 2002.

30. Fainboim L, Velasco VCC, Marcos CY, et al: Protracted, but not acute, hepatitis A virus infection is strongly associated with HLA-DRB1*1301, a marker for pediatric autoimmune hepatitis. Hepatology 33:1512, 2001.

31. Czaja A, Cookson S, Constantini P, et al: Cytokine polymorphisms associated with clinical features and treatment outcome in type 1 autoimmune hepatitis. Gastroenterology 117:645, 1999.

32. Agarwal K, Czaja AJ, Jones DEJ, et al: CTLA-4 gene polymorphism and susceptibility to type 1 autoimmune hepatitis. Hepatology 31:49, 2000.

33. Czaja A, Manns M: The validity and importance of subtypes of autoimmune hepatitis: A point of view. Am J Gastroenterol 90:1206, 1995.

34. Zauli D, Ghetti S, Grassi A, et al: Anti-neutrophil cytoplasmic antibodies in type 1 and type 2 autoimmune hepatitis. Hepatology 25:1105, 1997.

35. McFarlane IG: Autoimmune hepatitis: Clinical manifestations and diagnostic criteria. Can J Gastroenterol 15:107, 2001.

36. Schramm C, Kanzler S, Meyer zum Buschenfelde K-H, et al: Autoimmune hepatitis in the elderly. Am J Gastroenterol 96:1587, 2001.

37. Perdigoto R, Carpenter H, Czaja A: Frequency and significance of chronic ulcerative colitis in severe corticosteroid-treated autoimmune hepatitis. J Hepatol 14:325, 1992.

38. Nikias G, Batts K, Czaja A: The nature and prognostic implications of autoimmune hepatitis with an acute presentation. J Hepatol 21:866, 1994.

39. Poralla T, Treichel U, Lohr H, et al: The asialoglycoprotein receptor as target structure in autoimmune liver diseases. Semin Liver Dis 11:215, 1991.

40. Homberg J, Abuaf N, Bernard O, et al: Chronic active hepatitis associated with anti–liver-kidney microsome antibody type 1: A second type of "autoimmune" hepatitis. Hepatology 7:1333, 1987.

41. Czaja A, Manns M, Homburger H: Frequency and significance of antibodies to liver/kidney microsome type 1 in adults with chronic active hepatitis. Gastroenterology 103:1290, 1992.

42. Porta G, Da Costa Gayotto LC, Alvarez F: Anti–liver-kidney microsome antibody–positive autoimmune hepatitis presenting as fulminant liver failure. J Pediatr Gastroenterol Nutrition 11:138, 1990.

43. Gregorio G, Portmann B, Reid F, et al: Autoimmune hepatitis in childhood: A 20 year survey. Hepatology 25:541, 1997.

44. Czaja A, Kruger M, Santrach P, et al: Genetic distinctions between types 1 and 2 autoimmune hepatitis. Am J Gastroenterol 92:2197, 1997.

45. Bittencourt P, Goldberg A, Cancado E, et al: Genetic heterogeneity in susceptibility to autoimmune hepatitis types 1 and 2. Am J Gastroenterol 94:1906, 1999.

46. Yamamoto A, Cresteil D, Homberg J, et al: Characterization of the anti–liver-kidney microsome antibody (anti-LKM1) from hepatitis C virus–positive and –negative sera. Gastroenterology 104:1762, 1993.

47. The Finnish-German APECED Consortium: An autoimmune disease, APECED, caused by mutations in a novel gene featuring two PHD-type zinc finger domains. Nat Genet 17:399, 1997.

48. Clemente M, Obermayer-Straub P, Meloni A, et al: Cytochrome P450 1A2 is a hepatic autoantigen in autoimmune polyglandular syndrome type 1. J Clin Endocrinol Metab 82:1353, 1997.

49. Manns M, Gerken G, Kyriatsoulis A, et al: Characterization of a new subgroup of autoimmune chronic active hepatitis by autoantibodies against a soluble liver antigen. Lancet 1:292, 1987.

50. Stechemesser E, Klein R, Berg P: Characterization and clinical relevance of liver-pancreas antibodies in autoimmune hepatitis. Hepatology 18:1, 1993.

51. Czaja A, Carpenter H, Manns M: Antibodies to soluble liver antigen, P450IID6, and mitochondrial complexes in chronic hepatitis. Gastroenterology 105:1522, 1993.

52. Kanzler S, Weidemann C, Gerken G, et al: Clinical significance of autoantibodies to soluble liver antigen in autoimmune hepatitis. J Hepatol 31:635, 1999.

53. Wies I, Brunner S, Henninger J, et al: Identification of target antigen for SLA/LP autoantibodies in autoimmune hepatitis. Lancet 355:1510, 2000.

54. Costa M, Rodriques-Sanchez JL, Czaja AJ, et al: Isolation and characterization of cDNA encoding the antigenic protein of the human tRNA(Ser)Sec complex recognized by autoantibodies from patients with type 1 autoimmune hepatitis. Clin Exp Immunol 121:364, 2000.

55. Czaja AJ, Shums Z, Norman GL: Frequency and significance of antibodies to soluble liver antigen/liver pancreas in variant autoimmune hepatitis. Autoimmunity 35:475, 2002.

56. Czaja A: The variant forms of autoimmune hepatitis. Ann Intern Med 125:588, 1996.

57. Czaja A: Frequency and nature of the variant syndromes of autoimmune liver disease. Hepatology 28:360, 1998.

58. Ben-Ari Z, Czaja AJ: Autoimmune hepatitis and its variant syndromes. Gut 49:589, 2001.

59. Kenny RP, Czaja AJ, Ludwig J, et al: Frequency and significance of antimitochondrial antibodies in severe chronic active hepatitis. Dig Dis Sci 31:705, 1986.

60. Chazouilleres O, Wendum D, Serfaty L, et al: Primary biliary cirrhosis–autoimmune hepatitis overlap syndrome: Clinical features and response to therapy. Hepatology 28:296, 1998.

61. Boberg K, Fausa O, Haaland T, et al: Features of autoimmune hepatitis in primary sclerosing cholangitis: An evaluation of 114 primary sclerosing cholangitis patients according to a scoring system for the diagnosis of autoimmune hepatitis. Hepatology 23:1369, 1996.

62. Gregorio GV, Portmann B, Karani J, et al: Autoimmune hepatitis/sclerosing cholangitis overlap syndrome in childhood: A 16-year prospective study. Hepatology 33:544, 2001.

63. Czaja A, Carpenter H, Santrach P, et al: Autoimmune cholangitis within the spectrum of autoimmune liver disease. Hepatology 31:1231, 2000.

64. Czaja A, Carpenter H, Santrach P, et al: The nature and prognosis of severe cryptogenic chronic active hepatitis. Gastroenterology 104:1755, 1993.

65. Czaja A: Behavior and significance of autoantibodies in type 1 autoimmune hepatitis. J Hepatol 30:394, 1999.

66. Czaja AJ: The autoimmune hepatitis/hepatitis C overlap syndrome: Does it exist? In Leuschner U, Broome U, Stiehl A (eds): Cholestatic Liver Diseases: Therapeutic Options and Perspectives. Falk Symposium No. 136. Lancaster, UK, Lancaster Publishing Services, 2004, p 132.

67. Czaja AJ, Carpenter HA: Histological findings in chronic hepatitis C with autoimmune features. Hepatology 26:459, 1997.

68. Czaja AJ, Carpenter HA: Sensitivity, specificity and predictability of biopsy interpretations in chronic hepatitis. Gastroenterology 105:1824, 1993.

69. Boberg K, Aadland E, Jahnsen J, et al: Incidence and prevalence of primary biliary cirrhosis, primary sclerosing cholangitis, and autoimmune hepatitis in a Norwegian population. Scand J Gastroenterol 33:99, 1998.

70. Hurlburt KJ, McMahon BJ, Deubner H, et al: Prevalence of autoimmune hepatitis in Alaska natives. Am J Gastroenterol 97:2402, 2002.

71. Park S, Nagorney D, Czaja A: Hepatocellular carcinoma in autoimmune hepatitis. Dig Dis Sci 45:1944, 2000.

72. Czaja A, Strettell M, Thomson L, et al: Associations between alleles of the major histocompatibility complex and type 1 autoimmune hepatitis. Hepatology 25:317, 1997.

73. Lim KN, Casanova RL, Boyer TD, et al: Autoimmune hepatitis in African Americans: Presenting features and responses to therapy. Am J Gastroenterol 96:3390, 2001.

74. Kosar Y, Kacar S, Sasmaz N, et al: Type 1 autoimmune hepatitis in Turkish patients: Absence of association with HLA B8. J Clin Gastroenterol 35:185, 2002.

75. Zolfino T, Heneghan MA, Norris S, et al: Characteristics of autoimmune hepatitis in patients who are not of European caucasoid ethnic origin. Gut 50:713, 2002.

76. Kogan J, Safadi R, Ashur Y, et al: Prognosis of symptomatic versus asymptomatic autoimmune hepatitis. A study of 68 patients. J Clin Gastroenterol 35:75, 2002.

77. Czaja AJ: Treatment of autoimmune hepatitis. Semin Liver Dis 22:365, 2002.

78. Czaja A, Rakela J, Ludwig J: Features reflective of early prognosis in corticosteroid-treated severe autoimmune chronic active hepatitis. Gastroenterology 95:448, 1988.

79. Wang K, Czaja A: Prognosis of corticosteroid-treated hepatitis B surface antigen–negative chronic active hepatitis in postmenopausal women: A retrospective analysis. Gastroenterology 97:1288, 1989.

80. Heneghan MA, Norris SM, O'Grady JG, et al: Management and outcome of pregnancy in autoimmune hepatitis. Gut 48:97, 2001.

81. Wang K, Czaja A, Beaver S, et al: Extrahepatic malignancy following long-term immunosuppressive therapy of severe hepatitis B surface antigen–negative chronic active hepatitis. Hepatology 10:39, 1989.

82. Langley PG, Underhill J, Tredger JM, et al: Thiopurine methyltransferase phenotype and genotype in relation to azathioprine therapy in autoimmune hepatitis. J Hepatol 37:441, 2002.

83. Czaja AJ, Davis GL, Ludwig J, et al: Complete resolution of inflammatory activity following corticosteroid treatment of HBsAg-negative chronic active hepatitis. Hepatology 4:622, 1984.

84. Czaja AJ, Carpenter HA: Histological features associated with relapse after corticosteroid withdrawal in type 1 autoimmune hepatitis. Liver Int 23:116, 2003.

85. Czaja AJ, Menon KVN, Carpenter HA: Sustained remission after corticosteroid therapy for type 1 autoimmune hepatitis: A retrospective analysis. Hepatology 35:890, 2002.

86. Czaja AJ, Carpenter HA: Decreased fibrosis during corticosteroid therapy of autoimmune hepatitis. J Hepatol 40:644, 2004.

87. Czaja A: Low dose corticosteroid therapy after multiple relapses of severe HBsAg-negative chronic active hepatitis. Hepatology 11:1044, 1990.

88. Johnson P, McFarlane I, Williams R: Azathioprine for long-term maintenance of remission in autoimmune hepatitis. N Engl J Med 333:958, 1995.

89. Czaja AJ: Autoimmune hepatitis after liver transplantation and other lessons of self-intolerance. Liver Transplantation 8:505, 2002.

90. Vierling JM, Flores PA: Evolving new therapies of autoimmune hepatitis. Clin Liver Dis 6:825, 2002.

CHAPTER
86 Primary Biliary Cirrhosis

Paul Angulo and Keith D. Lindor

Primary biliary cirrhosis (PBC) is an autoimmune liver disease that generally affects middle-aged women from a variety of racial groups and represents the most common chronic cholestatic liver disease in adults in the United States. PBC is characterized by ongoing inflammatory destruction of the intralobular bile ducts, which leads to chronic cholestasis and biliary cirrhosis, with consequent complications such as portal hypertension and liver failure. Although the designation *primary biliary cirrhosis* has been used for several decades, the term is potentially misleading, because most patients do not have "cirrhosis" on liver biopsy specimens when the disease is diagnosed. Evidence for an immunologic cause of PBC includes the presence of activated T cells in areas of bile duct destruction, the presence of highly specific autoantibodies that react with antigens localized on biliary epithelial cells, and the association of PBC with other disorders thought to be autoimmune in nature.

Fatigue and pruritus are the most common presenting symptoms of PBC; however, as many as one half of patients are asymptomatic when the disease is diagnosed on the basis of incidentally discovered elevated serum liver enzyme levels in a cholestatic pattern. Rarely, patients present with advanced disease manifested by esophageal variceal hemorrhage, ascites, or hepatic encephalopathy. PBC should be considered in a patient with an elevated serum alkaline phosphatase level, hyper-

cholesterolemia, and an elevated serum immunoglobulin M (IgM) level. The presence of antimitochondrial antibodies in serum is highly characteristic of the disease. Ursodeoxycholic acid (UDCA) is the only medication of proven benefit for patients with PBC, and liver transplantation offers a life-extending alternative for patients with end-stage PBC. Complications of chronic cholestasis such as osteopenic bone disease, fat-soluble vitamin deficiency, hypercholesterolemia, and steatorrhea should be recognized and treated. Survival models are used to help predict the prognosis of patients with the disease and the timing of liver transplantation.

EPIDEMIOLOGY

PBC occurs worldwide and predominantly in women, with a female-to-male ratio of 9:1. The diagnosis of PBC usually is made between the ages of 30 and 60 years, with a range of 21 to 93 years. The disease has been documented in even younger patients—two teenagers 15 and 16 years of age, respectively.[1] Until the early 1970s, PBC was considered a rare condition that manifested with persistent jaundice and almost inevitably progressed to end-stage liver disease. A better understanding of its pathogenesis, along with subsequent clinical and epidemiologic studies, has modified current concepts regarding this condition. PBC seems to be more common than was formerly believed, because of increasing awareness of the disease and because asymptomatic patients are identified through the widespread use of screening tests such as determination of serum cholesterol levels and liver biochemical test levels in otherwise healthy populations.

The reported prevalence of PBC varies among countries, with a range of 19 cases per 1 million population in Israel to 402 cases per 1 million population in Olmsted County, Minnesota.[2] Whether the difference in prevalence is real or a result of different methodologies in detecting the disease among studies is unknown. Inconsistency in case definition and case finding methods, as well as imprecision in defining the study area, the populations evaluated, and the dates of diagnosis, particularly in earlier reports, makes comparisons among studies difficult. Estimates of the annual incidence of PBC range from 0.7 to 49 per 1 million population. The prevalence of PBC seems to have increased over time, without a clear increase in incidence[3]; the increase in prevalence may reflect an increase in survival time in patients with PBC.

In the United States,[4] the age-adjusted reported incidence rate of PBC per 1 million person-years is 45 for women and 7 for men (27 overall). The reported prevalence per 1 million population is 654 for women and 121 for men (402 overall); these figures represent the highest prevalence rates for PBC ever reported.

PATHOGENESIS

Although the cause of PBC remains unknown, several lines of evidence suggest an autoimmune pathogenesis. The evidence includes the intense humoral and cellular response to an intracytoplasmic antigen, presence of highly specific antimitochondrial antibodies (AMA), involvement of T lymphocytes in the destruction of bile ducts, and numerous defects in immunologic regulation. Like other autoimmune diseases, PBC has a clear female predominance and often coexists with other autoimmune diseases. Patients with PBC often have a positive family history of other autoimmune diseases, and the pathogenesis of the condition may involve molecular mimicry and xenobiotics. The disease seems to be triggered by an immune-mediated response to one or more allo- or autoantigens, which leads to progressive destruction of bile ducts, chronic cholestasis, and eventual biliary cirrhosis. Immunohistochemical phenotyping of inflammatory cells surrounding the bile ducts shows a combination of CD4+ and CD8+ T lymphocytes, accompanied by B lymphocytes and natural killer cells.[5,6] Bile duct destruction is induced directly by the cytotoxicity of CD4+ and CD8+ T cells in contact with biliary epithelium. B lymphocytes are relatively uncommon in the inflammatory reaction but sometimes can be seen in clusters. Intracellular adhesion molecules (e.g., intracellular adhesion molecule-1 [ICAM-1]) are strongly expressed on many epithelial cells, particularly in areas of lymphocyte damage[7]; these molecules may facilitate the interaction between destructive lymphocytes and their targets. In the early biliary lesions of PBC, eosinophilic infiltration and granulomas often are seen. Only biliary epithelial cells are affected in patients with PBC, despite the ubiquity of mitochondrial autoantigens. In contrast to other autoimmune diseases, no specific human leukocyte antigen (HLA) associations are recognized, and no spontaneous or induced animal models of PBC have been described.

AUTOANTIBODIES

Much attention has been devoted to the humoral immune system in PBC, in particular, the antigens recognized by AMA have been identified.[8-10] AMA are directed to the E2 component of the pyruvate dehydrogenase complex (PDC-E2), the E2 unit of the branched-chain 2-oxo-acid dehydrogenase complex (BCOADC-E2), and the E2 subunit of the 2-oxo-glutarate dehydrogenase complex (OGDC-E2). Other AMA recognize the E1α subunit of PDC and the dihydrolipoamide dihydrogenase–binding protein (E3BP). These molecules all are located on the inner mitochondrial membranes. At least one of these components usually reacts with AMA in patients with PBC. The most frequent antigen against which AMA are directed is PDC-E2; PDC-E2–reacting antibodies are present in 90% to 95% of PBC sera.

The mechanisms by which AMA are developed against proteins located on the inner surface of mitochondrial membranes are unknown; PDC-E2 or a cross-reactive molecule is overexpressed on biliary cells in PBC, predominantly at the luminal domain, and PDC-E2–specific CD4+ T cells are present in the portal inflammatory infiltrate.[8] Although AMA are predominantly of the IgG1 and IgG3 classes, a characteristic feature of PBC is elevated serum levels of IgM, possibly attributable to faulty switching from IgM to IgG synthesis after exposure to an unknown antigen or to defective suppressor T cell activity. Why the lesions in PBC are confined to the small intrahepatic bile ducts when the antigens on the mitochondrial membrane are found in all tissues of the body is uncertain. Evidence shows that these antigens appear to share a common epitope with antigens in the cytoplasmic region of bile duct epithelial cells in patients with PBC.[11] Similar immunoreactive material also is found on the damaged bile ducts of AMA-negative patients with PBC.[12] The main targets of the immune reactions in PBC are the epithelial cells of interlobular bile ducts. AMA do not appear to be cytotoxic: (1) They persist after liver transplantation without evidence of disease recurrence; (2) disease severity is unrelated to antibody titer; (3) they are not always present in PBC; and (4) they develop in animal models after the injection of recombinant PDC-E2 protein, but bile duct destruction or inflammation does not occur.

AMA are not the only PBC-specific autoantibodies. Antibodies against the nuclear pore protein gp210, a transmembrane glycoprotein, are found in 25% of patients with AMA-positive PBC and in up to 50% of those with AMA-negative PBC. The specificity of antibodies to gp210 (anti-gp210) for PBC when detected by immunoblotting is greater than 99%,[13] and the antibodies seem to have prognostic importance.[14] Antibodies against the nuclear pore protein p62 (anti-p62) are found in approximately 25% of patients with PBC[15] and are highly specific for PBC. Anti-p62 antibodies seem to be mutually exclusive with anti-gp210 antibodies.

GENETIC FACTORS

The occurrence of PBC in relatives of affected persons plus abnormalities of cell-mediated immunity in first-degree relatives of patients suggests a genetic association. Although no link between PBC and a specific HLA class I phenotype has been found, class II HLA molecules may contribute to the development of this condition. An association with HLA-DR8 has been observed most frequently but in only approximately one third of cases.[16] Conversely, the DQA1*0102 haplotype seems to be strongly associated with resistance to the disease.[17] An association with HLA class III genes, which code for complement components C2 and C4 and factor B, has been studied less extensively. An increased frequency of haplotype C4B2 has been reported. Using a genotyping method, an excess frequency of haplotype C4A*Q0 (relative risk, 184) also has been found to be associated with PBC.[18]

MOLECULAR MIMICRY

Molecular mimicry between host autoantigens and unrelated exogenous proteins is one of the hypotheses to explain how autoantibodies to self-proteins arise, break tolerance, and lead to autoimmune disease. Molecular mimicry of an extrinsic protein produced by an infectious agent has long been suggested as a possible initiating event in PBC. Infectious agents incriminated in the immune response in PBC include various bacteria[19] and viruses[20]—most recently *Chlamydia pneumoniae*,[21] *Novospingobium aromaticivorans*,[22] and human betaretrovirus.[23] Microorganisms produce a multitude of foreign antigens that collectively constitute the major determinants recognized by the immune system. These antigens potentially include a variety of carbohydrates, lipids, and proteins that can be recognized by specific receptors on inflammatory cells. In PBC, PDC-E2 appears to be an ideal candidate for foreign antigens to mimic. PDC-E2, particularly its inner lipoyl domain, is highly conserved among bacteria, yeasts, and mammals. Autoimmune phenomena in PBC could result from peptides that mimic T cell epitopes of microbial proteins and that are derived from, and presented by, abnormally expressed HLA class II molecules. Molecular mimicry has been invoked to explain the breaking of tolerance against mitochondrial antigens. Definitive evidence for this theory is still lacking, however.

XENOBIOTICS AND OTHER IMPLICATED AGENTS

Xenobiotics are foreign compounds that may alter self-proteins by inducing a change in the molecular structure of the native protein sufficient to induce an immune response. The immune response may then result in the recognition of both the modified and the native proteins.[24] The continued presence of the self-protein may perpetuate the immune response initiated by the xenobiotic-induced adduct, thereby leading to chronic autoimmunity. Because many xenobiotics are metabolized in the liver, the potential for liver-specific alteration of proteins is substantial. To address the hypothesis that PBC is induced by xenobiotic exposure, Long and colleagues[25] synthesized the inner lipoylated domain of PDC-E2, replaced the lipoic acid moiety with synthetic structures, and quantified the reactivity of these structures with sera from patients with PBC. AMA from all patients reacted more strongly to 3 of the 18 modified organic autoepitopes than to the native domain. Defective sulfoxidation of certain compounds, such as bile acids, estrogen, or drugs, and selenium deficiency have been proposed as underlying mechanisms that may lead to this process. These hypotheses are still far from proved.

CLINICAL FEATURES

ASYMPTOMATIC DISEASE

Widespread use of screening laboratory tests has led to diagnosis of PBC at an asymptomatic stage in up to 60% of patients with this condition. Such patients are found incidentally to have an elevated serum alkaline phosphatase level and AMA during routine health evaluations or during investigation of an unrelated complaint, such as a clinical manifestation of an autoimmune disease known to be associated with PBC. Most asymptomatic persons with AMA and normal results of liver biochemical tests are found to have features on liver biopsy diagnostic of or consistent with PBC; symptoms, signs, and laboratory evidence of chronic cholestasis eventually develop in these persons.[26,27]

SYMPTOMATIC DISEASE

The typical patient with symptomatic disease (Table 86–1) is a middle-aged woman with a complaint of fatigue or pruritus. Other symptoms include right upper quadrant abdominal pain, anorexia, and jaundice. Fatigue, although relatively nonspecific, is considered to be the most disabling symptom by many patients, and it worsens in some patients as the disease progresses. Some reports suggest that fatigue may affect between 70% and 85% of patients with PBC, although this high rate has been questioned.[28,29] Fatigue in patients with PBC does not correlate with several markers of disease severity, or with the patient's age or thyroid status, but does correlate with sleep disturbance and depression.[28]

Pruritus may occur at any point, early or late, in the course of the disease, or intermittently throughout the

Table 86–1   Symptoms and Signs of Primary Biliary Cirrhosis at Presentation

Finding	Frequency (%)
Fatigue	21-85
Pruritus	19-55
Jaundice	3-10
Right upper quadrant pain	8
Hyperpigmentation	25
Hepatomegaly	25
Splenomegaly	15
Xanthelasma	10
None	25-61

course. Pruritus generally is intermittent during the day and is most troublesome in the evening and at night. Pruritus often resolves as the disease progresses, but in some patients, severe, intractable pruritus can develop in earlier stages of the disease and may require liver transplantation for effective management. Most patients with PBC do not have jaundice at the time of diagnosis.

Jaundice occurs later in the course of the disease and usually is persistent and associated with a worse prognosis. Symptoms also may relate to fat-soluble vitamin deficiency, bone pain with or without spontaneous fractures, or an associated autoimmune disease that may occur in patients with PBC (Table 86–2). Symptoms and signs of advanced liver disease, such as ascites, bleeding from gastroesophageal varices, and encephalopathy, usually occur late in the course of PBC.

On physical examination, the most common signs are hyperpigmentation, hepatosplenomegaly, xanthelasma, and, in more advanced disease, jaundice. Symptoms appear to be less frequent in men than in women, and autoimmune manifestations, especially Sjögren's syndrome, also are less frequent in men. Otherwise, PBC is identical clinically in men and in women.

ASSOCIATED DISEASES

Many of the diseases found frequently in patients with PBC (see Table 86–2) are thought to be related to disturbances in immune mechanisms. These associated disorders include Sjögren's syndrome (characterized by dry eyes [keratoconjunctivitis sicca] and dry mouth), scleroderma and its variants, rheumatoid arthritis, some cutaneous disorders, renal tubular acidosis, and thyroiditis.

The frequency of malignancy is increased in patients with PBC. An increased risk of breast cancer in women with PBC was found in earlier studies but was not confirmed by subsequent, larger studies.[30,31] Although hepatocellular carcinoma occurs in only 1% to 2% of patients with PBC, the risk is much higher than that in the general population.[30] Gallstones can be found in up to one third

Table 86–2 Diseases Associated with Primary Biliary Cirrhosis

Disease	Frequency (%)
Keratoconjunctivitis sicca (Sjögren's syndrome)	72-100
Arthritis/arthropathy	4-42
Scleroderma and its variants	15-19
Scleroderma	3-4
CREST or any of its components	7
Raynaud's disease	8
Autoimmune thyroiditis	15-20
Cutaneous disorders—lichen planus,	
discoid lupus, pemphigoid	11
Renal tubular acidosis	50-60
Gallstones	33
Hepatocellular carcinoma	1-2
Pulmonary fibrosis	Rare
Celiac sprue	Rare

CREST, calcinosis–Raynaud's phenomenon–esophageal dysmotility–sclerodactyly–telangiectasia.

of patients with PBC, but inflammatory bowel disease and interstitial pulmonary fibrosis are rare.

DIAGNOSIS

The diagnosis of PBC is established by liver biochemical test results consistent with chronic cholestasis plus the presence in serum of AMA. Liver biopsy helps to confirm the diagnosis of PBC but may not be necessary for establishing the diagnosis in patients with characteristic chronic cholestasis and AMA.[32]

BIOCHEMICAL CHANGES

Liver biochemical test results show a cholestatic picture. Almost all patients have increased serum levels of alkaline phosphatase (three to four times normal) and gamma glutamyl transpeptidase. Serum aminotransferase (aspartate aminotransferase [AST], alanine aminotransferase [ALT]) levels are mildly elevated (usually less than three times normal); marked elevations (more than five times normal) are distinctly unusual and may suggest PBC–autoimmune hepatitis overlap syndrome or coexisting viral hepatitis (see Chapter 85). Serum bilirubin levels usually are normal in early stages and increase slowly over the course of the disease; levels may exceed 20 mg/dL. A high serum bilirubin level, low serum albumin, and prolonged prothrombin time indicate a poor prognosis and advanced disease. Serum immunoglobulin levels, especially IgM, are increased, as are serum levels of bile acids, in particular cholic and chenodeoxycholic acids, and cholesterol.

SEROLOGIC DIAGNOSIS

Indirect immunofluorescence, immunoblotting, and enzyme-linked immunosorbent assay (ELISA) can detect AMA. Indirect immunofluorescence is by far the most commonly used serologic test and detects AMA in 90% to 95% of patients with PBC; however, indirect immunofluorescence testing requires interpretation by a skilled observer, and the result may be erroneously interpreted as negative for AMA in some patients with PBC. Immunoblotting and ELISA have sensitivity and specificity rates higher than 95% for the detection of AMA in PBC and can detect AMA in patients with PBC who are AMA negative by direct immunofluorescence testing. Other autoantibodies found in patients with PBC include rheumatoid factor (70%), anti–smooth muscle antibodies (66%), antithyroid (antimicrosomal, antithyroglobulin) antibodies (41%), and antinuclear antibodies (35%).

HISTOPATHOLOGIC FEATURES

The initial lesion on a liver biopsy specimen in PBC (Figs. 86–1 and 86–2A and B) is damage to epithelial cells of the small bile ducts. The most important and only diagnostic clue in many cases is *ductopenia*, defined as the absence of interlobular bile ducts in greater than 50% of portal tracts. The florid duct lesion, in which the epithe-

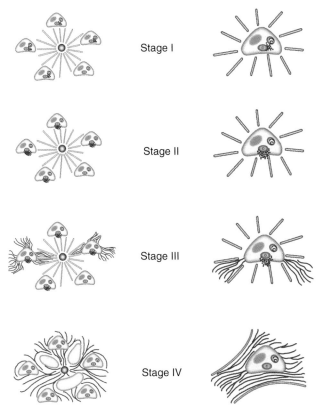

Figure 86–1 Schematic representation of the staging system of primary biliary cirrhosis (Ludwig's classification). The left side of the schematic shows five portal tracts surrounding a central vein at each stage. The right side shows a larger single portal tract at each stage. In stage I the inflammation is confined to the portal space, focused on the bile duct. In stage II the inflammation extends into the hepatic parenchyma (interface hepatitis or piecemeal necrosis). In stage III fibrosis is present, and in stage IV cirrhosis is present.

lium of the interlobular and segmental bile ducts degenerates segmentally, with formation of poorly defined, noncaseating epithelioid granulomas, is nearly diagnostic of PBC but is found in a relatively small number of cases, mainly in early stages. The two most popular histologic staging systems are those proposed by Ludwig and colleagues[33] and Scheuer,[34] which classify the disease in four stages. Both systems describe progressive pathologic changes, beginning initially in the portal areas surrounding the bile ducts and culminating in cirrhosis.

Ludwig stage 1 disease is characterized by inflammatory destruction of the intrahepatic septal and interlobular bile ducts that range up to 100 μm in diameter. These lesions often are focal and described as *florid duct lesions*, characterized by marked inflammation and necrosis around a bile duct. The portal tracts usually are expanded by lymphocytes, with only sparse neutrophils or eosinophils seen. In stage 2 disease (see Fig. 86–2A), the inflammation extends from the portal tract into the hepatic parenchyma, a lesion called *interface hepatitis* or formerly *piecemeal necrosis*. Destruction of bile ducts with proliferation of bile ductules can be seen. Stage 3 disease is characterized by scarring and fibrosis. Lymphocytic involvement of the portal and periportal areas, as well as the hepatic parenchyma, can be seen, but the hallmark of this stage is the presence of fibrosis without regenerative nodules. Stage 4 disease is characterized by cirrhosis with fibrous septa and regenerative nodules (see Fig. 86–2B).

The rate of histologic progression in PBC has been described using the data from 916 liver biopsy specimens obtained from 222 patients with PBC during 779 patient-years of follow-up.[35] In this series, most patients demonstrated progression of the condition; a few patients had a prolonged course of histologic stability, and only rare patients had sustained regression. A time course Markov model was used to describe the rate of histologic progression over time (Table 86–3).

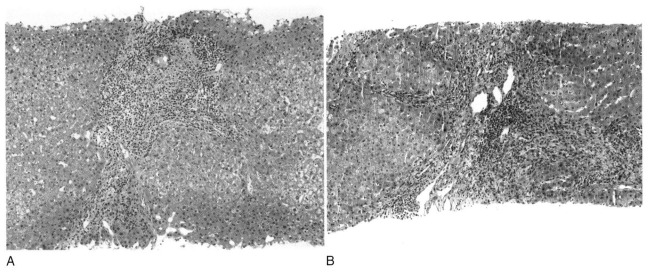

A   B

Figure 86–2 *A,* Photomicrograph of stage II primary biliary cirrhosis (PBC). Mononuclear inflammatory cells expand the portal tracts with some disruption of the limiting plates (interface hepatitis). The bile ducts are surrounded by inflammatory cells, and no fibrosis is evident. (Hematoxylin-eosin, ×100.) *B,* Stage IV PBC. Cirrhosis, with areas of fibrosis surrounding the hepatic parenchyma, is present. A dense mononuclear inflammatory infiltrate is still seen in the portal tract with interface hepatitis. (Hematoxylin-eosin, ×100.)

Table 86–3 Time Course of Histologic Progression to a Higher Stage in Patients with Primary Biliary Cirrhosis

	Initial Histologic Stage		
Rate of Progression	**I**	**II**	**III**
1 year	41%	43%	35%
2 years	62%	62%	50%

*Data from Locke RG III, Therneau TM, Ludwig J, et al: Time course of histological progression in primary biliary cirrhosis. Hepatology 23:52, 1996.

Liver biopsy has been considered necessary for confirming the diagnosis of PBC and excluding other liver diseases. This routine indication for diagnostic purposes has been questioned, however.[32] In a patient with AMA in serum, the combination of a serum alkaline phosphatase level greater than 1.5 times the upper limit of normal plus a serum AST level less than 5 times the upper limit of normal yields a 98.2% positive predictive value for a diagnosis of PBC. Therefore, a liver biopsy is not necessary to confirm the diagnosis in most patients with PBC and should be performed in only the minority of AMA-positive patients with a serum alkaline phosphatase level less than 1.5 times normal or a serum AST level greater than 5 times normal.[32]

IMAGING STUDIES

Cross-sectional imaging with ultrasonography, computed tomography, or, less frequently, magnetic resonance imaging is useful for excluding biliary obstruction. Other than increased liver echogenicity and signs of parenchymal liver disease or portal hypertension, findings on cross-sectional imaging usually are unremarkable. Adenopathy in the portal area is found in approximately 24% of patients with PBC, is not progressive, and is important to recognize so as to avoid confusion about the diagnosis or undue concern about the presence of an underlying malignancy.[36] Large, bulky adenopathy, however, should raise the question of associated malignancy.

NATURAL HISTORY

The natural history of PBC has been described in patients with symptoms attributable to PBC, as well as in asymptomatic patients who have normal or abnormal liver biochemical test levels. Prognostic models useful in predicting survival in an individual patient have been developed.

ASYMPTOMATIC PRIMARY BILIARY CIRRHOSIS

In 1986, Mitchison and colleagues[37] reported on 29 patients with AMA (in a titer of 1 : 40 or greater), normal liver biochemical test levels, and no symptoms of liver disease. Liver histology was compatible with or diagnostic of PBC in 24 patients (83%) and normal in only 2 patients. The entire cohort of patients was followed for a median of 17.8 years (range, 11 to 24 years).[35] Liver biochemical test values became persistently abnormal in 24 patients (83%), and persistent symptoms attributable to PBC, including fatigue, pruritus, and right upper abdominal discomfort, developed in 22 (76%). Five patients died, none because of liver disease, after a median period of 11.7 years (range, 6.4 to 16.8 years) from the first positive AMA titer. The median time from the first positive AMA result to persistent liver biochemical abnormalities was 5.6 years (range, 0.9 to 19 years). Four of 10 patients who underwent a second liver biopsy during a median follow-up of 11.4 years (range, 1.3 to 14.3 years) showed progression of disease stage, but cirrhosis or portal hypertension did not develop in any of the patients during the follow-up period. This study shows clearly that asymptomatic patients who have AMA and normal liver biochemical test levels have early PBC; with time, clinically obvious PBC may develop. These patients may represent a subgroup of patients with PBC whose natural history is different from that in the general PBC patient population.

Several reports have described the natural history of asymptomatic patients who have AMA, abnormal liver biochemical test levels consistent with cholestasis, and liver histologic features diagnostic of or compatible with PBC. Asymptomatic patients have less advanced disease than that typically seen in symptomatic patients.[38] Patients who are asymptomatic at presentation may survive longer, but a majority will eventually have progressive disease. A median survival of approximately 10 years has been reported for this group of patients in several series.[29,37,39,40] Patients who remain asymptomatic for several years may have a significantly longer survival than that in symptomatic patients, but their life expectancy is still less than that of an age- and gender-matched population. Symptoms of PBC will develop in approximately 40% of the initially asymptomatic patients within 5 to 7 years of follow-up, and most asymptomatic patients ultimately will become symptomatic if the follow-up period is long enough (95% after 20 years).[38] Once symptoms develop, life expectancy falls significantly and is the same as that for other symptomatic patients. The mortality rate for liver-related causes is significantly higher in initially symptomatic patients than in initially asymptomatic patients; however, an excess rate of non–liver-related mortality in initially asymptomatic patients has been reported to decrease the median survival in these patients to that in initially symptomatic patients.[38]

SYMPTOMATIC PRIMARY BILIARY CIRRHOSIS

Compared with asymptomatic patients, patients with PBC who have symptoms of chronic cholestasis show a more rapid progression to end-stage liver disease and have a worse prognosis. Several independent predictors of a poor prognosis have been identified in this group of patients[29,40-45] (Table 86–4).

The manifestations of portal hypertension and its complications in patients with PBC are similar to those in other forms of cirrhosis. Most patients with PBC and portal hypertension have cirrhosis; however, portal

Table 86–4 Independent Predictors of Survival in Patients with Primary Biliary Cirrhosis*

Yale[41]	Europe[45]	Mayo Clinic[40]	Oslo[42]	Glasgow[43]	Australia[44]	Newcastle (UK)[29]
Age	Age	Age	Variceal bleeding	Age	Age	Age
Bilirubin	Bilirubin	Bilirubin	Bilirubin	Bilirubin	Bilirubin	Bilirubin
Hepatomegaly	Albumin	Albumin		Ascites	Albumin	Albumin
Fibrosis	Cirrhosis	Prothrombin time		Variceal bleeding		Alkaline phosphatase
Cirrhosis	Cholestasis	Edema		Fibrosis		
				Cholestasis		
				Mallory's hyaline		

*Data summarized from various clinical studies.

Table 86–5 Prognostic Models in Primary Biliary Cirrhosis

Reference	Predictive Variables	Formula (If Used)	Validated by Other Groups
40	Age Total bilirubin Serum albumin Prothrombin time Edema score	$R = 0.871 \log_e$ (bilirubin in mg/dL) $- 2.53 \log_e$ (albumin in g/dL) $+ 0.039$ (age in years) $+ 2.38 \log_e$ (prothrombin time in seconds) $+ 0.859$ edema	Yes
42	Bleeding varices Bilirubin	$\log_e R = 1.68$ (bleeding $- 0.25$) $+ 2.03 \log$ (bilirubin $- 30.3$)	No
45	Bilirubin Ascites Albumin Age Gastrointestinal bleeding Central cholestasis Cirrhosis Immunoglobulin M	Calculated from pocket chart and tables in published article	Yes
29	Age Bilirubin Albumin Alkaline phosphatase	$R = \exp [(0.0742 \times$ age in years) $+ (0.195 \times \log_e$ bilirubin ratio*) $- (2.7878 \times$ albumin ratio*) $+ (0.2610 \times \log_e$ alkaline phosphatase ratio*)]	No

R, risk score.
*Ratio = times lower limit of normal for albumin and times upper limit of normal for bilirubin and alkaline phosphatase.

hypertension can be found in some patients with PBC and moderate to severe inflammation without cirrhosis on a liver biopsy specimen. Development of esophageal varices is an ominous sign that is observed in approximately one third of patients with PBC during extended follow-up. Approximately 40% of these patients will experience one or more episodes of variceal bleeding within 3 years of developing varices and, as a group, have a decreased survival rate.[46]

PREDICTING SURVIVAL

When untreated, PBC may follow a course that extends over a 15- to 20-year period. In patients with a serum bilirubin level greater than 10 mg/dL, however, the average life expectancy is reduced to 2 years. In order to predict survival in patients with PBC, prognostic models, some of which rely on Cox's proportional hazard analysis, have been developed[29,40,42,45] (Table 86–5). Among these models, the Mayo risk score[36,47] has been cross-validated and is widely used in predicting survival and in guiding referral of patients for liver transplantation.

These prognostic models also can be used for monitoring the efficacy of experimental drugs in clinical trials. Although all of the prognostic models are of help in clinical decision-making, they should not replace clinical judgment in determination of the optimal timing of liver transplantation in an individual patient.

TREATMENT

SPECIFIC THERAPY

A large number of published controlled and uncontrolled trials have evaluated various drugs in PBC. These drugs can be separated according to their mechanisms of action as immunosuppressive, anti-inflammatory, cupruretic, antifibrotic, or bile acids.

Glucocorticoids

Only one placebo-controlled trial of glucocorticoids has been conducted.[48] Thirty-six patients who received prednisolone for a period of 1 year showed clinical and biochemical improvement, as well as a decrease in overall inflammation in liver biopsy specimens. The study was continued in a single-blind manner for another 2 years, but the mortality rates were similar in the treatment and the control groups. The main concern about using glucocorticoids in the treatment of PBC is worsening osteopenic bone disease. Therefore, glucocorticoids currently cannot be recommended outside of the context of prospective trials.

Budesonide

Budesonide is a newer steroid structurally related to 16α-hydroxyprednisolone, with extensive first-pass hepatic metabolism and minimal systemic availability. In theory, budesonide is devoid of glucocorticoid-associated systemic effects. Budesonide has been evaluated in combination with UDCA in two studies.[49,50] In previously untreated patients, the combination of budesonide and UDCA led to a greater improvement in serum alkaline phosphatase, AST, and immunoglobulin levels, as well as improvement in the degree of inflammation and fibrosis on liver biopsy specimens, than that seen with UDCA alone.[49] The effect of such combination therapy on important prognostic markers such as serum bilirubin levels and the Mayo risk score was not reported. In the second study,[50] the combination of budesonide and UDCA did not benefit patients who had responded incompletely to UDCA alone for a number of years. In that study,[50] the combination of UDCA and budesonide not only failed to improve serum bilirubin levels or the Mayo risk score but also led to significant worsening of osteoporosis and cosmetic effects, particularly in patients with more advanced liver disease.

D-Penicillamine

Eight controlled trials of D-penicillamine involving more than 700 patients have been reported. D-Penicillamine therapy was associated with a modest and transitory improvement in liver biochemical test values in some studies but was not associated with any effect on survival. Furthermore, serious side effects occurred in approximately one fifth of patients receiving the drug. Accordingly, penicillamine is not used in the treatment of PBC.

Colchicine

Three placebo-controlled trials of colchicine involving a total of 181 patients have been conducted. Colchicine was associated with some improvement in liver biochemical test values, but no effect on symptoms related to cholestasis, histologic progression to cirrhosis, or overall survival was seen.[51] Analysis of these studies suggests that colchicine is not of benefit in patients with PBC.

Azathioprine

Azathioprine was evaluated in a large international study involving 248 patients with PBC. After the first 18 months of follow-up, no significant effects were noted on clinical course, liver biochemical test values, liver histologic findings, or survival. With extended follow-up, and after adjustment for a slight imbalance in mean serum bilirubin levels between the treatment and the control groups, a statistical improvement in survival was shown with this drug.[45] Because of uncertainty about the conclusions of this trial, due to a large number of withdrawals, missing data, and the initially reported negative results, azathioprine is rarely used for treatment of PBC.

Chlorambucil

Chlorambucil was evaluated in a small controlled trial involving 24 patients with a mean follow-up period of 4.1 years.[52] Although improvement in liver biochemical test levels and a decrease in inflammation on liver biopsy specimens were observed, no effect on the stage of disease was seen, and the study was too small to evaluate any benefit in survival. Bone marrow toxicity necessitating discontinuation of the drug occurred in one third of patients, and chlorambucil is an unattractive drug for further evaluation.

Cyclosporine

A large European study involving 349 patients with PBC and a follow-up period of up to 6 years (mean 2.5) with death or liver transplantation as the main end points showed biochemical improvement but no effect on histologic progression or patient survival.[53] A multivariate analysis suggested a reduction in mortality rate among patients who received cyclosporine treatment. The use of this drug, however, is associated with a high frequency of side effects that largely preclude long-term use in PBC.

Methotrexate

Anecdotal reports of patients with PBC who demonstrated clinical, biochemical, and histologic improvement with methotrexate therapy have been published. In a placebo-controlled trial of methotrexate for PBC,[54] methotrexate in a dose of 7.5 mg per week for up to 6 years not only was of no benefit but was also associated with more unfavorable outcomes than were observed with placebo.

URSODEOXYCHOLIC ACID

UDCA, the 7β epimer of chenodeoxycholic acid, occurs naturally in small quantities in human bile (less than 4% of total bile acids). It was first introduced for the dissolution of radiolucent gallstones in the 1970s and is the only medication approved by the U.S. Food and Drug Administration for treatment of PBC. Several mechanisms for the protective actions of UDCA have been proposed, including inhibiting absorption of toxic, hydrophobic, endogenous bile salts; stabilizing hepatocyte membranes against toxic bile salts; replacing endogenous bile acids, some of which may be hepatotoxic, with the nonhepatotoxic UDCA; and reducing expression of major histocompatibility complex (MHC) class I and class II antigens. During UDCA therapy, a variable increase in the concentration of total bile acids in serum is observed. The proportion of UDCA in serum and bile increases to approximately 30% to 60% of total bile acids,[55-58] and the proportion of endogenous bile acids, such as cholic, chenodeoxycholic, deoxycholic, and lithocholic acids, declines consequently. The degree of enrichment of the bile acid pool with UDCA is similar in all histologic stages of PBC and correlates with improvement in liver biochemical test levels and the Mayo risk score.

Because of its safety and patient adherence to treatment with the drug, UDCA has received the most attention of any drug used to treat PBC. Treatment with UDCA leads to rapid improvement in liver biochemical test levels[55-59] and a decrease in the histologic severity of interface hepatitis, inflammation, cholestasis, bile duct paucity, and bile duct proliferation.[56-58,60,61] UDCA significantly decreases the risk of development of gastroesophageal varices[62] and delays progression to cirrhosis.[63,64] The predicted probability that cirrhosis will develop after 5 years of therapy with UDCA for patients with stage 1, 2, or 3 disease at diagnosis is 4%, 12%, and 59% respectively; at 10 years of therapy with UDCA, the probability of cirrhosis is 17%, 27%, and 76% respectively.[64] These figures confirm the beneficial effect of UDCA on delaying progression to cirrhosis, as compared with disease progression in the absence of treatment.[35] Moreover, UDCA reduces proliferation of colonic epithelial cells, and its long-term use in patients with PBC significantly reduces the probability that colorectal adenomas will recur following removal.[65]

The beneficial effect of UDCA on long-term survival in patients with PBC has been questioned recently on the basis of results of two meta-analyses.[66] These meta-analyses had serious methodologic flaws derived primarily from mixing different patient populations, including some in which the duration of treatment—with suboptimal doses of UDCA—was too short to demonstrate an effect.[66] When an effective dose of UDCA has been used (13 to 15 mg/kg per day) and an appropriate number of patients received treatment for an appropriate period of time, UDCA has been shown clearly to improve survival free of liver transplantation[67-69] (Fig. 86–3).

The Mayo risk score, a cross-validated index of survival in PBC, decreases significantly during UDCA therapy.[57-59] With UDCA therapy, the Mayo risk score (recalculated at 6 months of UDCA therapy) retains its validity in predicting survival, just as it does in the absence of effective therapy.[70] The most cost-effective dose of UDCA in patients with PBC is 13 to 15 mg/kg per day,[59] which can be given in one or two divided doses taken with meals. In patients also taking cholestyramine, UDCA should be taken at least 2 hours before or after cholestyramine to ensure intestinal absorption.

COMBINATION THERAPY AND OTHER MEDICATIONS

The use of combination therapy with drugs that have different properties has been evaluated in open and controlled trials. Combinations studied include UDCA and methotrexate, UDCA and colchicine, cyclosporine and prednisone, chlorambucil and prednisolone, UDCA and glucocorticoids, UDCA and budesonide, UDCA and sulindac, and UDCA, prednisone, and azathioprine.

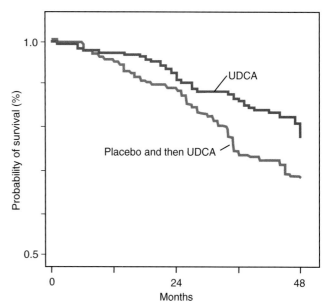

Figure 86–3 Survival in 548 patients with primary biliary cirrhosis. The probability of survival free of liver disease was significantly greater in patients who received treatment with ursodeoxycholic acid (UDCA) for 4 years than in those who first received placebo and then received UDCA (*P* < .001; relative risk, 1.92; 95% confidence interval, 1.30 to 2.82). (Adapted from Poupon R, Lindor KD, Cauch-Dudek K, et al: Combined analysis of French, American and Canadian randomized controlled trials of ursodeoxycholic acid therapy in primary biliary cirrhosis. Gastroenterology 113:884, 1997.)

Although some biochemical benefit in the short term has been reported with some of these combinations, the small numbers of patients enrolled, short follow-up, and risk of drug-related side effects do not allow us to recommend any of these combinations in the treatment of PBC. Furthermore, none of these combinations seems to be more effective than UDCA alone.

A large randomized trial evaluating UDCA (15 mg/kg per day) plus methotrexate (15 mg/m² of body surface area weekly, maximal dose of 20 mg per week) versus UDCA plus placebo has been published.[71] In that study, 265 patients with PBC and a serum bilirubin level below 3 mg/dL were assigned to one of the two treatment groups; the mean period of study was 7.5 years. The hazard ratio for death with or without liver transplantation was no better in the methotrexate-UDCA combination group than in the UDCA-placebo group. Therefore, methotrexate should not be recommended routinely as monotherapy or as an adjuvant to UDCA.

Other medications that have been proposed as potential agents for treatment of PBC include silymarin, malotilate, mycophenolate mofetil, tetracycline, bezafibrate, tacrolimus, and thalidomide. Some of these medications have been tested in patients with PBC but showed no benefit (i.e., silymarin, malotilate, and tetracycline). Mycophenolate mofetil and bezafibrate have shown promising results in small pilot studies and may deserve further evaluation in larger trials.

COMPLICATIONS OF CHRONIC CHOLESTASIS

BONE DISEASE

Osteopenic bone disease with a predisposition to spontaneous fracturing is a common complication of chronic cholestatic liver disease. In North America, most patients with osteopenia from cholestasis have osteoporosis rather than osteomalacia. *Osteoporosis* is defined as defective bone formation, whereas *osteomalacia* is defective bone mineralization resulting from vitamin D deficiency. The cause of osteoporosis associated with PBC is poorly understood, but the pathogenesis seems to be related to cholestasis itself. Women with PBC lose bone mass at a rate approximately twice that seen in age-matched controls,[72] and this accelerated bone loss is the result of decreased formation rather than increased resorption of bone.[73]

The severity and progression of bone disease can be assessed by measurement of bone mineral density in different sites, in particular the lumbar spine and femur. Dual-energy x-ray absorptiometry and dual-photon absorptiometry are noninvasive techniques that quantify bone mass accurately. At the time of referral for or diagnosis of the liver disease, approximately 20% of patients with PBC have osteoporosis, as defined by a T-score below −2.5 in either the lumbar spine or the femoral neck, and approximately 10% have severe bone disease, as defined by a Z-score below −2.[74,75] (The *T-score* is the number of standard deviations below the mean peak value in young gender-matched normal subjects, whereas the *Z-score* is the number of standard deviations below mean normal values corrected for age and gender.) The risk of osteoporosis (T-score below −2.5) is eight times higher in patients with PBC than in a gender-matched population, whereas the risk of severe bone disease (Z-score below −2) is four times higher in patients with PBC than in a healthy gender- and age-matched population.[75]

In patients with PBC, as in the general population, older age, postmenopausal status, and lower body mass index are independent risk factors for the development of osteoporosis. In patients with PBC, however, the severity of osteoporosis increases as liver disease advances; bone mass in patients with stage 1 or 2 PBC is similar to that in a normal age- and gender-matched population, but bone mass is significantly lower in patients with stage 3 or 4 disease.[75] Higher serum bilirubin levels, possibly as an indication of more advanced PBC, correlate significantly with a higher rate of bone loss.[75] One half of patients with PBC who undergo liver transplantation have severe bone disease, and one half of patients with PBC (almost exclusively those with preexisting osteopenia) experience a pathologic fracture during the first months after liver transplantation.[76]

Treatment of the bone disease includes adequate exercise and supplemental calcium (1200 to 1500 mg daily orally) and vitamin D (600 to 800 IU daily orally, or if deficiency is present, 25,000 to 50,000 IU orally once or twice per week). Treatment with estrogens significantly prevents loss of bone mass in postmenopausal patients with PBC[77] and was not associated with worsening cholestasis in a series of 46 patients with PBC who received estrogen treatment for a mean period of almost 5 years.[77] Because of the carcinogenic properties of estrogens, their lack of protective cardiovascular effects, a possible increased risk of dementia, and resumption of menses, however, postmenopausal women are not enthusiastic about taking estrogens.

Raloxifen, a selective estrogen receptor modulator, looks promising as an alternative to estrogen replacement therapy for postmenopausal osteoporosis. Raloxifen is currently under evaluation in patients with PBC. Bisphosphonates also may hold promise in the treatment of osteoporosis in patients with PBC. Although etidronate was no better than placebo in one randomized controlled study,[78] alendronate has been found to improve bone mass significantly after 2 years of treatment when compared with etidronate[79] or placebo.[80] Other bisphosphonates, including residronate and palmidronate, deserve evaluation.

FAT-SOLUBLE VITAMIN DEFICIENCY

Most patients with PBC and fat-soluble vitamin deficiency have advanced liver disease with jaundice. Fat-soluble vitamin deficiency is almost always caused by malabsorption resulting from decreased amounts of bile salts in the intestinal lumen. Vitamin D deficiency should be excluded in patients with PBC by measurement of 25-hydroxyvitamin D, a major metabolite of vitamin D. When vitamin D deficiency is encountered, vitamin D in a dose of 25,000 to 50,000 IU, given once or twice per week, usually is sufficient to achieve a normal serum vitamin D level. Because 25-hydroxylation of vitamin D is normal in patients with PBC, vitamin D, rather than the more expensive 25-hydroxyvitamin D or 1,25-hydroxyvitamin D, can be prescribed.

Vitamin A deficiency, which can cause problems with night vision, can occur in patients with PBC. When blood levels of vitamin A are low and the patient is symptomatic, replacement therapy with oral vitamin A, 100,000 IU daily for 3 days, and then 50,000 IU daily for 14 days, should be instituted. If patients are deficient but asymptomatic, a dose of 25,000 to 50,000 IU two or three times per week is adequate. The adequacy of replacement therapy is assessed by repeating serum vitamin A assays and evaluating the patient for dark adaptation, if indicated.

Vitamin K deficiency occurs with severe cholestasis and is manifested by an increased prothrombin time. A trial of vitamin K, 5 to 10 mg orally, should be given to determine if the prothrombin time improves. If it does, the patient should be maintained on a water-soluble vitamin K, 5 mg per day.

Deficiency of vitamin E has been reported in a few patients with PBC. Typically, vitamin E deficiency causes a neurologic abnormality that primarily affects the posterior columns and is characterized by areflexia, loss of proprioception, and ataxia. In patients with chronic cholestasis and low serum levels of vitamin E, replacement therapy with 100 mg/kg per day may halt progression of neuropathy.

HYPERCHOLESTEROLEMIA AND HYPERLIPIDEMIA

Lipid abnormalities are found in up to 85% of patients with PBC. High-density lipoprotein (HDL)-cholesterol levels usually are most prominently elevated in the early stages of PBC; as the disease progresses, HDL-cholesterol levels decrease and low-density lipoprotein (LDL)-cholesterol levels increase. The risk of atherosclerosis in these patients with hyperlipidemia does not appear to be increased.[81] Xanthelasmas (deposits of cholesterol in the skin) may develop in some patients with hyperlipidemia and can be troublesome. Therapy with UDCA has been shown to lower the LDL-cholesterol levels in patients with PBC and has been useful in some patients with xanthelasmas. Surgical removal of xanthelasmas is seldom successful, and such attempts should be avoided. The use of simvastatin has been evaluated in 6 patients with PBC and hypercholesterolemia.[82] In all patients, serum LDL levels decreased, whereas HDL levels remained largely unchanged after 2 months of therapy; of interest, the serum alkaline phosphatase and gamma glutamyl transpeptidase levels also improved. Further evaluation of simvastatin for PBC is warranted.

PRURITUS

The cause of pruritus in patients with PBC remains an enigma. The bile acid–binding resin cholestyramine was the first medication described to alleviate this symptom. Therapy with cholestyramine is successful in a majority of patients who can tolerate the unpleasant side effects of bad taste, bloating, and occasional constipation. The recommended total dose is 3 to 12 g/day orally, and the drug is most effective when one half of the dose is given 30 minutes before and one half is given 30 minutes after breakfast, to permit maximal bile acid binding as the gallbladder empties. All drugs that can potentially bind to cholestyramine should be taken several hours before or after the cholestyramine.

Not all patients with pruritus are helped by cholestyramine. The antibiotic rifampin also is effective in relieving the pruritus of PBC. A majority of patients respond to rifampin, and benefit occurs within a week of the start of therapy. The starting dose is 150 mg twice daily orally; occasionally, higher doses are needed. Rifampin induces drug-metabolizing enzymes, so caution is needed when concurrent drugs are administered. Rifampin has been associated with liver injury in up to 15% of patients.

Occasionally, treatment with UDCA alleviates pruritus, although on occasion pruritus may worsen with initiation of UDCA.

In warm countries, exposure to ultraviolet light without sun block can alleviate pruritus, and not surprisingly, the pruritus of PBC subsides during the summer months. It has been hypothesized that pruritus may be related to the release of endogenous opioids.[83] Intravenous infusion of the opiate receptor antagonist naloxone has shown a clear benefit in a double-blind trial.[84] Oral opiate receptor antagonists such as nalmefene[85] and naltrexone[86] have led to amelioration of pruritus in patients with PBC, although further trials are needed to evaluate their safety. Because of their sedative effects, antihistamines are helpful for treating the insomnia associated with pruritus; pruritus is always more troublesome at night. Phenobarbital may have the same effect. The pruritus of PBC is almost always cured by liver transplantation, which is a viable option for patients with severe intractable pruritus.

STEATORRHEA

Steatorrhea can occur in patients with advanced PBC. Several causes have been described. The most important cause is decreased bile acid delivery with insufficient micellar concentration of bile acids in the small intestine. Occasionally, exocrine pancreatic insufficiency can be found as part of a widespread glandular dysfunction seen in some patients with PBC. Coexisting celiac sprue has been reported in a small number of patients with PBC, and bacterial overgrowth may be the cause of steatorrhea in some patients with PBC and scleroderma. Because each of these causes has specific and different treatments, determining the exact cause of steatorrhea is important. Patients with decreased intestinal bile acid concentrations usually benefit from substitution of medium-chain triglycerides in their diets for long-chain triglycerides and a decrease in total fat intake. Patients with exocrine pancreatic insufficiency will benefit from pancreatic replacement therapy; patients with celiac sprue require gluten withdrawal from the diet; and patients with bacterial overgrowth should receive intermittent broad-spectrum oral antibiotic therapy.

LIVER TRANSPLANTATION

The best therapeutic alternative for patients with end-stage PBC is liver transplantation. The major manifestations of chronic liver disease that should prompt an evaluation for liver transplantation in patients with other chronic liver diseases also apply for patients with PBC (see Chapter 92). These indications include major complications related to portal hypertension, including bleeding from gastroesophageal varices, diuretic-resistant ascites, hepatorenal syndrome, and hepatic encephalopathy. In patients with PBC, the development of complications associated with chronic cholestasis, such as a poor quality of life secondary to disabling fatigue, intractable pruritus, and severe muscle wasting, as well as persistent increases in the serum bilirubin level in the absence of hepatic malignancy, should prompt clinicians to consider referral for liver transplantation, even in patients without cirrhosis on a liver biopsy specimen.

Liver transplantation clearly improves survival, as well as quality of life. One-year survival rates after liver transplantation are currently higher than 90%, with 5-year survival rates higher than 80% in most transplant centers. The advent of prognostic models has helped identify factors that predict survival (see Table 86–5). The Mayo risk score has been used commonly, but the Model for End-Stage Liver Disease (MELD) scale also is a reliable measure of mortality risk in patients with end-stage liver disease, including PBC, and is used as a disease severity index to determine organ allocation priorities[87] (see Chapter 92).

PBC-specific autoantibodies against mitochondria (AMA) and gp210 protein generally persist after liver transplantation. PBC may recur in the allograft, and the rate of recurrence increases with time, so that by 10 years, histologic recurrence may be found in 30% to 50% of patients. No clear factors identify patients at risk for recurrence, but the pattern and degree of immunosuppression may play a role. Recurrent PBC following liver transplantation seems to follow a benign course, at least in the intermediate term, and cirrhosis has only rarely been reported to develop.[88]

AUTOIMMUNE CHOLANGITIS (AMA-NEGATIVE PRIMARY BILIARY CIRRHOSIS)

Autoimmune cholangitis, or AMA-negative PBC, is the designation for those patients who clinically, biochemically, and histologically appear to have the classic features of PBC but are not found to have AMA in serum by indirect immunofluorescence or immunoblotting techniques. Most of these patients have antinuclear or anti–smooth muscle antibodies (or both) and tend to follow a clinical course, and to demonstrate a therapeutic response to UDCA, similar to those in AMA-positive PBC patients.[89-92] Although these patients may be distinguished by the lack of AMA in serum, the specific AMA antigen PDC-E2 is expressed on the apical region of their biliary epithelium, as occurs in AMA-positive patients—an observation suggesting that the pathogenesis of both conditions may be identical.[12] Of interest, this staining reaction is found before HLA class II expression is detected, and it may be the earliest specific lesion of PBC. Whether a different genetic susceptibility exists for the development of AMA-positive PBC and autoimmune cholangitis is still uncertain. Patients with autoimmune cholangitis should receive UDCA in a dose of 13 to 15 mg/kg per day; however, when histologic features of superimposed autoimmune hepatitis are detected, the combination of glucocorticoids and UDCA should be considered.

REFERENCES

1. Dahlan Y, Smith L, Simmonds D, et al: Pediatric-onset primary biliary cirrhosis. Gastroenterology 125:1476, 2003.
2. Prince M, James OFW: The epidemiology of primary biliary cirrhosis. Clin Liver Dis 7:795, 2003.
3. Metcalf JV, Bhopal RS, Gray J, et al: Incidence and prevalence of primary biliary cirrhosis in the city of Newcastle upon Tyne, England. Int J Epidemiol 26:830, 1997.
4. Kim WR, Lindor KD, Locke GR III, et al: Epidemiology and natural history of primary biliary cirrhosis in a U.S. community. Gastroenterology 119:16, 2000.
5. Bjorkland A, Festin R, Mendel-Hrtvig I, et al: Blood and liver infiltrating lymphocytes in primary biliary cirrhosis: Increased in activated T and natural killer cells and recruitment of primed memory T cells. Hepatology 13:1106, 1991.
6. Nakanuma Y: Distribution of B lymphocytes in nonsuppurative cholangitis in primary biliary cirrhosis. Hepatology 18:570, 1993.
7. Lim AG, Jazrawi RP, Ahmed HA, et al: Soluble intercellular adhesion molecule-1 in primary biliary cirrhosis: Relationship with disease stage, immune activity, and cholestasis. Hepatology 20:882, 1994.
8. Van de Water J, Ansari AA, Surh CD, et al: Evidence for the targeting by 2-oxo-dehydrogenase enzymes in the T cell response of primary biliary cirrhosis. J Immunol 146:89, 1991.
9. Leung PSC, Chuang DT, Wynn RM, et al: Autoantibodies to BCOADC-E2 in patients with primary biliary cirrhosis recognize a conformational epitope. Hepatology 22:505, 1995.
10. Maeda T, Loveland BE, Rowley MJ, et al: Autoantibody against dihydrolipoamide dehydrogenase, the E3 subunit of the 2-oxoacid dehydrogenase complex. Significance for primary biliary cirrhosis. Hepatology 14:994, 1991.
11. Tsuneyuma K, Van De Water J, Leung PSC, et al: Abnormal expression of the E2 component of the pyruvate dehydrogenase complex on the luminal surface of biliary epithelium occurs before major histocompatibility complex class II and BBI-B7 expression. Hepatology 21:1031, 1995.
12. Tsuneyama K, Van De Water J, Van Thiel D, et al: Abnormal expression of PDC-E2 on the apical surface of biliary epithelial cells in patients with antimitochondrial antibody negative primary biliary cirrhosis. Hepatology 22:1440, 1995.
13. Bandin O, Courvalin J, Poupon R, et al: Specificity and sensitivity of gp210 autoantibodies detected using an enzyme-linked immunosorbent assay and a synthetic polypeptide in the diagnosis of primary biliary cirrhosis. Hepatology 23:1020, 1996.
14. Itoh S, Ichida T, Yoshida T, et al: Autoantibodies against a 210 kDa glycoprotein of the nuclear pore complex as a prognostic marker in patients with primary biliary cirrhosis. J Gastroenterol Hepatol 12:257, 1998.
15. Wasleska-Gadek J, Honenauer H, Hitchman E, et al: Autoantibodies against nucleoporin p62 constitute a novel marker of primary biliary cirrhosis. Gastroenterology 110:840, 1996.
16. Underhill J, Donaldson P, Bray G, et al: Susceptibility to primary biliary cirrhosis is associated with HLA-DR8-DQB1*0402 haplotype. Hepatology 16:1404, 1992.
17. Begovich AB, Klitz W, Moosamy PV, et al: Genes within the HLA class II region confer both predisposition and resistance to primary biliary cirrhosis. Tissue Antigens 43:71, 1994
18. Manns MP, Bremm A, Schneider PM, et al: HLA DRw 8 and complement C4 deficiency as risk factor in primary biliary cirrhosis. Gastroenterology 101:1367, 1991.
19. Tanaka A, Prindiville TP, Gish R, et al: Are infectious agents involved in primary biliary cirrhosis? A PCR approach. J Hepatol 31:664, 1999.
20. Mason AL, Xu L, Guo L, et al: Detection of retroviral antibodies in primary biliary cirrhosis and other idiopathic biliary disorders. Lancet 351:1620, 1998.
21. Abdulkarim AS, Petrovic LM, Kim RW, et al: Primary biliary cirrhosis: An infectious disease caused by *Chlamydia pneumoniae*? J Hepatol 40:380, 2004.
22. Selmi C, Balkwill DL, Invernizzi P, et al: Patients with primary biliary cirrhosis react against a ubiquitous xenobiotic-metabolizing bacterium. Hepatology 38:1250, 2003.
23. Xu L, Sakalian M, Shen Z, et al: Cloning the human betaretrovirus proviral genome from patients with primary biliary cirrhosis. Hepatology 39:38, 2004.
24. Medzhitov R, Janeway CA Jr: How does the immune system distinguish self from nonself? Semin Immunol 12:185, 2000.
25. Long SA, Quan C, van de Water J, et al: Immunoreactivity of organic mimeotopes of the E2 component of pyruvate dehydrogenase: Connecting xenobiotics with primary biliary cirrhosis. J Immunol 167:2956, 2001.
26. Mitchison HC, Bassendine MF, Hendrick A, et al: Positive antimitochondrial antibody but normal alkaline phosphatase: Is this primary biliary cirrhosis? Hepatology 6:1279, 1986.

27. Metcalf JV, Mitchison HC, Palmer JM, et al: Natural history of early primary biliary cirrhosis. Lancet 348:1399, 1996.

28. Goldblatt J, Taylor PJS, Lipman T, et al: The true impact of fatigue in primary biliary cirrhosis: A population study. Gastroenterology 122:1235, 2002.

29. Prince M, Chetwynd A, Newman W, et al: Survival and symptom progression in a geographically based cohort of patients with primary biliary cirrhosis: Follow-up for up to 28 years. Gastroenterology 123:1044, 2002.

30. Nijhawan PK, Therneau TM, Dickson ER, et al: Incidence of cancer in primary biliary cirrhosis: The Mayo experience. Hepatology 29:1396, 1999.

31. Loof L, Adami HO, Sparen P, et al: Cancer risk in primary biliary cirrhosis: A population-based study from Sweden. Hepatology 20:101, 1994.

32. Zein CO, Angulo P, Lindor KD: When is liver biopsy needed in the diagnosis of primary biliary cirrhosis? Clin Gastroenterol Hepatol 1:89, 2003.

33. Ludwig J, Dickson ER, McDonald GSA: Staging of chronic non-suppurative destructive cholangitis (syndrome of primary biliary cirrhosis). Virchows Arch 379:103, 1978.

34. Scheuer PJ: Primary biliary cirrhosis: Chronic non-suppurative destructive cholangitis. Am J Pathol 46:387, 1965.

35. Locke RG III, Therneau TM, Ludwig J, et al: Time course of histological progression in primary biliary cirrhosis. Hepatology 23:52, 1996.

36. Lazaridis K, Angulo P, Keach JC, et al: Lymphadenopathy in patients with cholestatic liver disease. Hepatology 32:512A, 2000.

37. Mitchison HC, Lucey MR, Kelly, et al: Symptom development and prognosis in primary biliary cirrhosis: A study of two centers. Gastroenterology 99:778, 1990.

38. Prince M, Chetwynd A, Craig JV, et al: Asymptomatic primary biliary cirrhosis: Clinical features, prognosis, and symptom progression in a large population based cohort. Gut 53:865, 2004.

39. Balasubramaniam K, Grambsch PM, Wiesner RH, et al: Diminished survival in asymptomatic primary biliary cirrhosis. A prospective study. Gastroenterology 98:1567, 1990.

40. Dickson ER, Grambsch PM, Flemming TR, et al: Prognosis in primary biliary cirrhosis: Model for decision making. Hepatology 10:1, 1989.

41. Roll J, Boyer JL, Barry D, et al: The prognostic importance of clinical and histologic features in asymptomatic and symptomatic primary biliary cirrhosis. N Engl J Med 308:1, 1983.

42. Rydning A, Schrumpf E, Abdelnoor M, et al: Factor of prognostic importance in primary biliary cirrhosis. Scand J Gastroenterol 25:119, 1990.

43. Goudie BM, Burt AD, Macfarlane GJ, et al: Risk factors and prognosis in primary biliary cirrhosis. Am J Gastroenterol 84:713, 1989.

44. Jeffrey GP, Reed WD, Shilkin KB: Natural history and prognostic variables in primary biliary cirrhosis (PBC) [abstract]. Hepatology 12:955, 1990.

45. Christensen E, Neuberger J, Crowe J, et al: Beneficial effect of azathioprine and prediction of progression in primary biliary cirrhosis. Final results of an international trial. Gastroenterology 89:1084, 1985.

46. Gores GJ, Wiesner RH, Dickson ER, et al: A prospective evaluation of esophageal varices in primary biliary cirrhosis: Development, natural history and influence on survival. Gastroenterology 96:1552, 1989.

47. Murtaugh PA, Dickson ER, van Dam GM, et al: Primary biliary cirrhosis: Prediction of short-term survival based on repeated patient visit. Hepatology 20:126, 1994.

48. Mitchison HC, Bassendine MF, Malcolm AJ, et al: A pilot double-blind controlled 1-year trial of prednisolone treatment in primary biliary cirrhosis: Hepatic improvement but greater bone loss. Hepatology 10:420, 1989.

49. Leuschner M, Maier KP, Schlichting J, et al: Oral budesonide and ursodeoxycholic acid for treatment of primary biliary cirrhosis: Results of a prospective double-blind trial. Gastroenterology 117:918, 1999.

50. Angulo P, Jorgensen RA, Keach JC, et al: Oral budesonide in the treatment of patients with primary biliary cirrhosis with a suboptimal response to ursodeoxycholic acid. Hepatology 31:318, 2000.

51. Zifroni A, Schaffner F: Long-term follow-up of patients with primary biliary cirrhosis on colchicine therapy. Hepatology 14:990, 1991.

52. Hoofnagle JH, Davis JL, Schafer DF, et al: Randomized trial of chlorambucil for primary biliary cirrhosis. Gastroenterology 91:1327, 1986.

53. Lombard M, Portmann B, Neuberger J, et al: Cyclosporin A treatment in primary biliary cirrhosis: Results of a long-term placebo controlled trial. Gastroenterology 104:519, 1993.

54. Hendrickse MT, Rigney E, Giaffer MH, et al: Low-dose methotrexate is ineffective in primary biliary cirrhosis: Long-term results of a placebo-controlled trial. Gastroenterology 117:400, 1999.

55. Lindor KD, Dickson ER, Baldus WP, et al: Ursodeoxycholic acid in the treatment of primary biliary cirrhosis. Gastroenterology 106:1284, 1994.

56. Heathcote EJ, Cauch-Dudek K, Walker V, et al: The Canadian multicenter double-blind randomized controlled trial of ursodeoxycholic acids in primary biliary cirrhosis. Hepatology 19:1149, 1994.

57. Combes B, Carithers RL, Maddrey WC, et al: A randomized, double-blind, placebo-controlled trial of ursodeoxycholic acid in primary biliary cirrhosis. Hepatology 22:759, 1995.

58. Poupon RE, Balkau B, Eschwege E, et al: A multicenter, controlled trial of ursodiol for the treatment of primary biliary cirrhosis. N Engl J Med 324:1548, 1991.

59. Angulo P, Dickson ER, Therneau TM, et al: Comparison of three doses of ursodeoxycholic acid in the treatment of primary biliary cirrhosis: A randomized trial. J Hepatol 30:830, 1999.

60. Pares A, Caballeria L, Rodes J, et al: Long-term effects of ursodeoxycholic acid in primary biliary cirrhosis: Results of a double-blind controlled multicentric trial. J Hepatol 32:561, 2000.

61. Poupon RE, Lindor KD, Pares A, et al: Combined analysis of the effect of treatment with ursodeoxycholic acid on histologic progression in primary biliary cirrhosis. J Hepatol 39:12, 2003.

62. Lindor KD, Jorgensen RA, Dickson ER, et al: Ursodeoxycholic acid delays the onset of esophageal varices in primary biliary cirrhosis. Mayo Clin Proc 72:1137, 1997.

63. Angulo P, Batts KP, Therneau TM, et al: Long-term ursodeoxycholic acid delays histologic progression in primary biliary cirrhosis. Hepatology 29:644, 1999.

64. Corpechot C, Carrat F, Poupon R, et al: Primary biliary cirrhosis: Incidence and predictive factors of cirrhosis development in ursodiol-treated patients. Gastroenterology 122:652, 2002.

65. Serfaty L, De Leusse A, Rosmorduc O, et al: Ursodeoxycholic acid therapy and the risk of colorectal adenoma in patients with primary biliary cirrhosis: An observational study. Hepatology 38:203, 2003.

66. Lindor KD, Poupon R, Poupon RE, et al: Ursodeoxycholic acid for primary biliary cirrhosis. Lancet 355:657, 2000.

67. Poupon RE, Poupon R, Balkau B, et al: Ursodiol for the long-term treatment of primary biliary cirrhosis. N Engl J Med 330:1342, 1994.

68. Lindor KD, Therneau TM, Jorgensen RA, et al: Effects of ursodeoxycholic acid on survival in patients with primary biliary cirrhosis. Gastroenterology 110:1515, 1996.

69. Poupon R, Lindor KD, Cauch-Dudek K, et al: Combined analysis of French, American and Canadian randomized controlled

trials of ursodeoxycholic acid therapy in primary biliary cirrhosis. Gastroenterology 113:884, 1997.

70. Angulo P, Lindor KD, Therneau TM, et al: Utilization of the Mayo risk score in patients with primary biliary cirrhosis receiving ursodeoxycholic acid. Liver 19:115, 1999.
71. Combes B, Emerson SS, Flye NL, et al: Methotrexate (MTX) plus ursodeoxycholic acid (UDCA) in the treatment of primary biliary cirrhosis. Hepatology 42:1184, 2005.
72. Eastell R, Dickson ER, Hodgson SF, et al: Rate of vertebral bone loss before and after liver transplantation in women with primary biliary cirrhosis. Hepatology 14:296, 1991.
73. Janes CH, Dickson ER, Okazaki R, et al: Role of hyperbilirubinemia in the impairment of osteoblast proliferation associated with cholestatic jaundice. J Clin Invest 95:2581, 1995.
74. Springer JE, Cole DE, Rubin LA, et al: Vitamin D–receptor genotypes as independent genetic predictors of decreased bone mineral density in primary biliary cirrhosis. Gastroenterology 118:145, 2000.
75. Menon N, Angulo P, Weston S, et al: Bone disease in patients with primary biliary cirrhosis: Independent predictors and rate of progression. J Hepatol 35:316, 2001.
76. Porayko M, Wiesner RH, Hay JE, et al: Bone disease in liver transplant recipients: Incidence, timing and risk factors. Transplant Proc 23:1462, 1991.
77. Menon KV, Angulo P, Boe G, et al: Safety and efficacy of estrogen therapy in preventing bone loss in primary biliary cirrhosis. Am J Gastroenterol 98:889, 2003.
78. Lindor KD, Jorgensen RA, Tiegs RD, et al: Etidronate for osteoporosis in primary biliary cirrhosis. A randomized trial. J Hepatol 33:878, 2000.
79. Guanabens N, Pares A, Ros I, et al: Alendronate is more effective than etidronate for increasing bone mass in osteopenic patients with primary biliary cirrhosis. Am J Gastroenterol 98:2268, 2003.
80. Zein OC, Jorgensen RA, Clarke B, et al: Alendronate improves bone mineral density in patients with PBC: Randomized placebo-controlled trial. Gastroenterology 126(suppl 2):A671, 2004.
81. Longo M, Crosignani A, Battezzati PM, et al: Hyperlipidaemic state and cardiovascular risk in primary biliary cirrhosis. Gut 51:265, 2002.
82. Ritzel U, Leonhardt U, Nather M, et al: Simvastatin in primary biliary cirrhosis: Effects on serum lipids and distinct disease markers. J Hepatol 36:454, 2002.
83. Jones EA, Bergasa NV: The pruritus of cholestasis. Hepatology 29:1003, 1999.
84. Bergasa NV, Alling DW, Talbot TL, et al: Effect of naloxone infusion in patients with the pruritus of cholestasis. A double-blind, randomized, controlled trial. Ann Intern Med 123:161, 1995.
85. Bergasa NV, Schmidt JM, Talbot TL, et al: Open-label trial of oral nalmefene therapy for the pruritus of cholestasis. Hepatology 27:679, 1998.
86. Wolfhagen FHJ, Sternieri E, Hop WCJ, et al: Oral naltrexone treatment for cholestatic pruritus: A double-blind, placebo-controlled study. Gastroenterology 113:1264, 1997.
87. Kamath PS, Wiesner RH, Malinchoc M, et al: A model to predict survival in patients with end-stage liver disease. Hepatology 33:464, 2001.
88. Neuberger J: Recurrent primary biliary cirrhosis. Best Pract Res Clin Gastroenterol 14:669, 2000.
89. Mitchieletti P, Wanless IR, Katz A, et al: Antimitochondrial antibody negative primary biliary cirrhosis: A distinct syndrome of autoimmune cholangitis. Gut 35:260, 1994.
90. Lacerda MA, Ludwig J, Dickson ER, et al: Antimitochondrial antibody-negative primary biliary cirrhosis. Am J Gastroenterol 90:247, 1995.
91. Invernizzi P, Crogsinani A, Battezzati PM, et al: Comparison of the clinical features and clinical course of antimitochondrial antibody–positive and negative primary biliary cirrhosis. Hepatology 25:1090, 1997.
92. Kim WR, Poterucha JJ, Jorgensen RA, et al: Does antimitochondrial antibody status affect response to treatment in patients with primary biliary cirrhosis? Outcomes of ursodeoxycholic acid therapy and liver transplantation. Hepatology 26:22, 1997.

CHAPTER

87 Portal Hypertension and Gastrointestinal Bleeding

Vijay H. Shah and Patrick S. Kamath

Variceal hemorrhage, hepatic encephalopathy, and ascites—the major complications of cirrhosis of the liver—result from portal hypertension, defined as an increase in hepatic sinusoidal pressure to 6 mm Hg or greater. Portosystemic collaterals decompress the hypertensive hepatic sinusoids and give rise to varices at the gastroesophageal junction and elsewhere. These portosystemic collaterals also may allow gut-derived ammonia to reach the brain, thereby resulting in hepatic encephalopathy through a pathologic process of several intermediary steps involving the peripheral benzodiazepine-type receptors, neurosteroids, and γ-aminobutyric acid (GABA) receptors (see Chapter 89). Additionally, portal hypertension is associated with renal retention of sodium and water and the formation of ascites (see Chapter 88). Indeed, portal hypertension and its complications remain important clinical problems despite advances in treatment and improved understanding of both the molecular basis and the pathophysiology of portal hypertension.

NORMAL PORTAL CIRCULATION

The portal venous system carries capillary blood from the esophagus, stomach, small and large intestine, pancreas,

gallbladder, and spleen to the liver. The portal vein is formed by the confluence of the splenic vein and the superior mesenteric vein behind the neck of the pancreas.[1] The inferior mesenteric vein usually drains into the splenic vein. The left gastric vein, also called the left coronary vein, usually drains into the portal vein at the confluence of the splenic vein and superior mesenteric vein (Fig. 87–1). The portal vein is approximately 7.5 cm in length and runs dorsal to the hepatic artery and common bile duct into the hilum of the liver. The uppermost 5 cm of the portal vein does not receive any tributaries.[2] In the hilum of the liver, the portal vein divides into the left and right portal vein branches, which supply the left and right sides of the liver, respectively. The umbilical vein drains into the left portal vein. The cystic vein from the gallbladder drains into the right portal vein, whereas the portal venules drain into hepatic sinusoids that, in turn, are drained by the hepatic veins into the inferior vena cava. The left and middle hepatic veins usually join together and drain into the inferior vena cava separately but adjacent to the confluence of the right hepatic vein with the inferior vena cava. The caudate lobe drains separately into the inferior vena cava.

The circulatory system of the normal liver is a high-compliance, low-resistance system that is able to accommodate a large blood volume, as occurs after a meal, without substantially increasing portal pressure. The liver receives a dual blood supply from the portal vein and the hepatic artery that constitutes nearly 30% of total cardiac output. Portal venous blood derived from the mesenteric venous circulation constitutes approximately 75% of total hepatic blood flow, whereas the remainder of blood is derived from the hepatic artery, which provides highly oxygenated blood directly from the celiac trunk of the aorta. Portal vein–derived and hepatic artery–derived blood flow converge in high-compliance, specialized vascular channels termed *hepatic sinusoids*. A dynamic and compensatory interplay occurs between hepatic

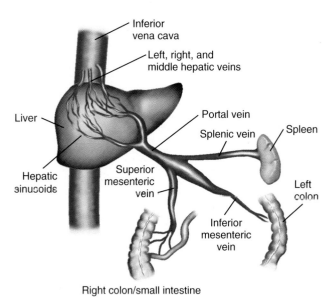

Figure 87–1 Anatomy of the portal circulation. Blood vessels that constitute the portal circulation and hepatic outflow tracts are depicted.

blood flow derived from the portal vein and that from the hepatic artery. Specifically, when portal venous blood flow to the liver is diminished, as occurs in portal vein thrombosis, arterial inflow increases in an attempt to maintain total hepatic blood flow constant. Similarly, after hepatic artery occlusion, portal venous inflow increases in a compensatory manner. This autoregulatory mechanism, aimed at maintaining total hepatic blood flow at a constant level, is termed the *hepatic arterial buffer response*.

The sinusoids are highly permeable and thus facilitate the transport of macromolecules to the parenchymal hepatocytes that reside on the extraluminal side of the endothelial cells. The hepatic sinusoids are highly permeable because they lack a proper basement membrane and because the endothelial cells that line the sinusoids contain fenestrae. Other unique aspects of the hepatic sinusoids are the space of Disse, a virtual space located extraluminal to the endothelial cell and adjacent to the hepatocyte, and its cellular constituents, the hepatic stellate cell (HSC) and the Kupffer cell (Fig. 87–2). These two cell types probably play an important role, in concert with the endothelial cell, in regulating sinusoidal hemodynamics and homeostasis and may contribute to the sinusoidal derangements that occur in portal hypertension. Under basal conditions, HSCs maintain a quiescent phenotype and accumulate vitamin A. On activation, however, as occurs in cirrhosis and portal hypertension, these cells are postulated to develop contractile abilities that permit them to function as sinusoidal pericytes. Kupffer cells contribute to vascular homeostasis by generating cytokines with potent cellular and vasoregulatory actions, including tumor necrosis factor. Endothelial cells and smooth muscle cells in nonsinusoidal hepatic vessels such as the portal venule and the terminal hepatic venule are important in hepatic vasoregulation, particularly in the normal liver, where HSCs are quiescent, unactivated, and presumably less contractile.

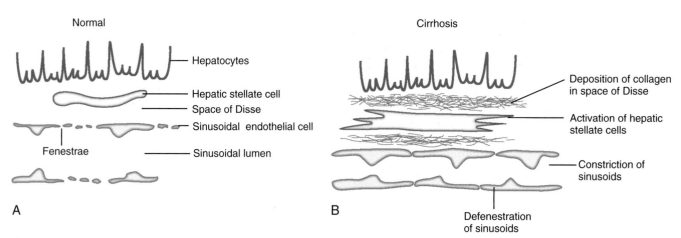

Figure 87–2 Anatomy of the hepatic microvasculature. *A,* Normal sinusoidal microanatomy is depicted. The sinusoidal lumen is lined by fenestrated sinusoidal endothelial cells that allow the transport of macromolecules to the abluminal space of Disse. Quiescent hepatic stellate cells reside within this space, adjacent to both parenchymal cells and endothelial cells. *B,* In cirrhosis, a number of changes occur in the hepatic microcirculation, including loss of fenestrae in endothelial cells (defenestration), constriction of sinusoids, and activation of hepatic stellate cells with ensuing deposition of collagen and increased contractility.

Many studies have established the important role of nitric oxide (NO), derived from endothelial NO synthase (eNOS), in hepatic vasodilatation. Shear stress, caused by the frictional force of blood within the sinusoids, is one of the most potent physiologic stimuli of eNOS-derived NO production in hepatic sinusoids. By contrast, endothelin-1 (ET-1), also released by endothelial cells, promotes hepatic vasoconstriction by binding to ET-A receptors located on HSCs. ET-1 also appears to be generated within HSCs themselves and promotes HSC contraction through an autocrine loop. Of interest, ET-1 may alternatively bind to ET-B receptors on endothelial cells. This signaling pathway paradoxically promotes vasodilatation by activating eNOS. Other vascular mediators implicated in hepatic vasoregulation include carbon monoxide generated by the heme oxygenase system, the sympathetic adrenergic agonist norepinephrine, the renin-dependent vasoconstrictor angiotensin, prostaglandins, thromboxane, and leukotrienes. Of these mediators, angiotensin is of particular interest, because it is a potent constrictor of HSCs and is released in increased amounts in cirrhosis owing to systemic sympathetic hyperactivity. A number of angiotensin receptor blockers are undergoing evaluation for the treatment of portal hypertension.

HEMODYNAMIC PRINCIPLES OF PORTAL HYPERTENSION

In cirrhosis, as well as in most noncirrhotic causes of portal hypertension, portal hypertension results from changes in portal resistance in combination with changes in portal inflow. The influence of flow and resistance on pressure can be represented by the formula for Ohm's law:

$$\Delta P = F \times R$$

in which the pressure gradient in the portal circulation (ΔP) is a function of portal flow (F) and resistance to flow (R). Increases in either portal resistance or portal flow can contribute to increased pressure. Portal hypertension almost always results from increases in both portal resistance and portal flow (Fig. 87–3). One exception is that of an arteriovenous fistula, which in the initial stages causes portal hypertension largely through an increase in portal flow in the absence of an increase in resistance. The mechanism of the increase in portal resistance depends on the site and cause of portal hypertension; in the Western world, the most common cause is liver cirrhosis (see later). Because of the increase in hepatic resistance and decrease in hepatic compliance, small changes in flow that do not increase pressure in the normal liver can have a prominent stimulatory effect on portal pressure in the cirrhotic liver. The increase in portal venous inflow is part of a generalized systemic derangement termed the *hyperdynamic circulatory state*. Collateral vessels that dilate and new vascular sprouts that form connect the high-pressure portal venous system with lower-pressure systemic veins. Unfortunately, this process of angiogenesis

and collateralization is insufficient for normalizing portal pressure and actually causes complications of portal hypertension, such as esophageal varices.[3]

The changes in portal flow and resistance also can be viewed as originating from mechanical and vascular factors. Mechanical factors include the fibrosis and nodularity of the cirrhotic liver with distortion of the vascular architecture and the remodeling that is recognized to occur in the systemic and splanchnic vasculature in response to the chronic increases in flow and shear stress that characterize the hyperdynamic circulatory state. Vascular factors include intrahepatic vasoconstriction, which contributes to increased intrahepatic resistance, and the splanchnic and systemic vasodilatation that accompanies the hyperdynamic circulatory state. The vascular factors that contribute to portal hypertension are particularly important because they are reversible and dynamic and therefore compelling targets for experimental therapies. Conversely, effective therapies for the fixed, mechanical component of portal hypertension caused by scar, regenerative nodules, and vascular remodeling are currently lacking. Indeed, most available therapies for portal hypertension focus on correction of hemodynamic alterations in the portal circulation. Approaches include use of nonselective beta blockers, octreotide, and vasopressin, to reduce the hyperdynamic circulation, portal venous inflow, and splanchnic vasodilatation.[4,5] Alternative agents reduce the increased intrahepatic resistance and include angiotensin receptor blockers and mononitrates.

INCREASED INTRAHEPATIC RESISTANCE

In cirrhosis, increased portal resistance occurs in great part as a result of mechanical factors that reduce vessel diameter. In addition to regenerative nodules and fibrotic bands, these mechanical factors include capillarization of the space of Disse and swelling of cells, including hepatocytes and Kupffer cells. As discussed earlier, however, reduced hepatic vessel diameter resulting in increased portal resistance, even when caused by cirrhosis, is not a purely mechanical phenomenon.[6,7] Hemodynamic changes in the hepatic circulation also contribute to increased intrahepatic resistance.[8,9] These changes are characterized by hepatic vasoconstriction and impaired responses to vasodilatory stimuli. The increase in intrahepatic resistance is determined largely by changes in vessel radius, with small reductions in vessel radius causing prominent increases in resistance. Blood viscosity and vessel length also can influence resistance, albeit to a much smaller extent. The factors that regulate resistance can be viewed in the context of the law of Poiseuille:

$$R = 8\eta L/\pi r^4$$

in which R is resistance, ηL is the product of blood viscosity and vessel length, and r is vessel radius.

Although vasoactive changes were estimated initially to account for 10% to 30% of the increase in portal resistance in cirrhosis, subsequent studies have suggested that these figures actually may underestimate the contribution of hepatic vasoconstriction to the increased resist-

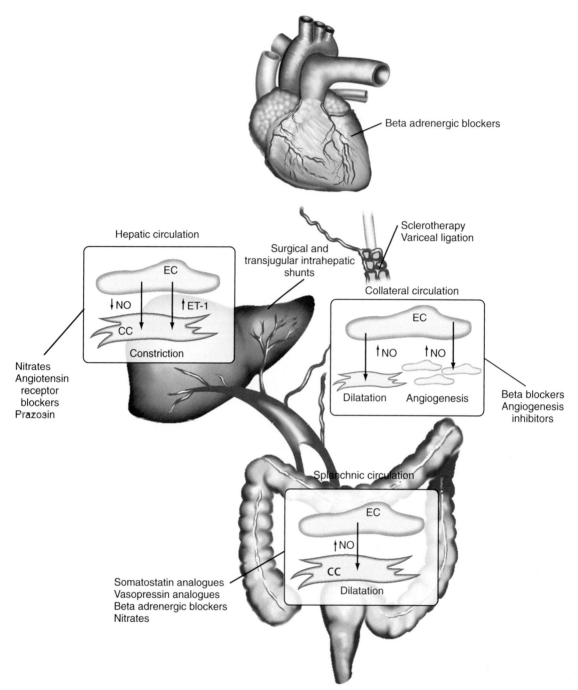

Figure 87–3 Vascular disturbances in portal hypertension and sites of action of portal pressure–reducing therapies. Portal hypertension typically results from increased resistance, usually from within the liver, in combination with increased portal venous flow. The increase in hepatic resistance results from mechanical factors in combination with dynamic vasoconstriction mediated by decreased nitric oxide (NO) production and increased endothelin production. The increase in portal venous flow occurs from vasodilatation in the splanchnic circulation that is mediated by increased NO production. A collateral circulation, including esophageal varices, develops between the hypertensive portal vasculature and systemic venous system; however, these collaterals are inadequate to decompress the hypertensive portal circulation fully. Collateral development is mediated by dilatation of existing collateral vessels, as well as development of new blood vessels and sprouts (angiogenesis). Therapies aimed at the different sites of hemodynamic disturbances are shown. CC, contractile cell; EC, endothelial cell.

ance observed in the cirrhotic liver. In noncirrhotic causes of portal hypertension, the increase in resistance may occur at sites upstream (prehepatic) or downstream (posthepatic) of the liver, as in portal vein thrombosis and hepatic vein thrombosis, respectively (Fig. 87–4). Furthermore, the site of increased intrahepatic resistance

can be further delineated as the sinusoids (sinusoidal), upstream from the sinusoids within the portal venules (presinusoidal), or downstream from the sinusoids in the hepatic venules (postsinusoidal), as in alcoholic cirrhosis, schistosomiasis, and sinusoidal obstruction syndrome, respectively. Pressure is increased only in the portal

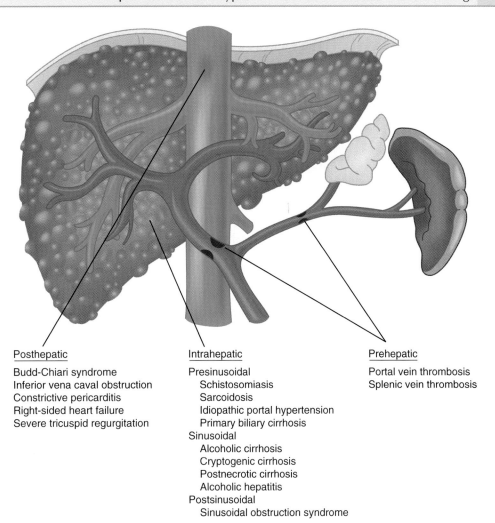

Figure 87–4 Classification of portal hypertension. The different sites of increased resistance to portal flow are shown. Many diseases cause a mixed pattern. Portal hypertension rarely can occur exclusively as a result of increased portal flow, as occurs with arteriovenous shunts *(not shown)*.

Posthepatic

Budd-Chiari syndrome
Inferior vena caval obstruction
Constrictive pericarditis
Right-sided heart failure
Severe tricuspid regurgitation

Intrahepatic

Presinusoidal
  Schistosomiasis
  Sarcoidosis
  Idiopathic portal hypertension
  Primary biliary cirrhosis
Sinusoidal
  Alcoholic cirrhosis
  Cryptogenic cirrhosis
  Postnecrotic cirrhosis
  Alcoholic hepatitis
Postsinusoidal
  Sinusoidal obstruction syndrome

Prehepatic

Portal vein thrombosis
Splenic vein thrombosis

circulation behind the site of increased resistance, and in isolated portal vein thrombosis, hepatic function frequently remains largely preserved despite prominent portal hypertension.

Most evidence suggests that a decrease in the production of the vasodilator NO in combination with an increase in the production of the vasoconstrictor ET-1 jointly contribute to the increase in hepatic vascular resistance. In experimental models of cirrhosis, the bioavailability of hepatic NO is diminished, because of a reduction in the production of NO by endothelial cells.[8,10,11] A similar paradigm is observed in the human cirrhotic liver.[12] Most studies indicate that the reduction in NO production occurs not through a reduction in hepatic eNOS protein levels[10,11] but through defects in the steps necessary to activate existing eNOS protein. For example, increases in the production of the eNOS-inhibiting protein caveolin-1[11] have been observed in experimental models of cirrhosis[11] and in human cirrhosis.[13] Another pathway that contributes to deficient generation of NO by eNOS is a reduction in the level of AKT phosphorylation of eNOS in the cirrhotic liver. Irrespective of the mechanism of deficiency, the lack of availability of NO is thought to allow HSCs, which are activated and highly contractile in liver cirrhosis, to constrict the sinusoids that they envelop, thereby increasing

portal pressure. The role of the HSCs in this process remains controversial, however, because evidence is mixed regarding whether the site of the increase in intrahepatic resistance in cirrhosis is the sinusoids, where stellate cells reside, or the pre- or postsinusoidal venules (or both), which are devoid of stellate cells and in which endothelial cells signal smooth muscle cells.

In clinical practice, NO can be delivered by NO donor agents such as mononitrates. NO donor agents exert their beneficial effects in part by relaxing the actively contractile stellate cells.[14,15] The systemic actions of these agents, however, tend to cause side effects and exacerbate the hyperdynamic circulatory state. In studies utilizing a liver-specific NO donor compound, the increased intrahepatic vascular resistance could be corrected by generation of additional NO and consequent relaxation of HSCs.[16,17] In cirrhosis, however, deficient endothelial cell NO generation may be accompanied by impaired stellate cell relaxation in response to NO,[18] perhaps because of diminished response of the NO second messenger cyclic guanosine monophosphate (cGMP) in activated cells.[14] In this situation, a prominent beneficial effect of NO donors is less predictable.

Excessive ET-1 also contributes to increased intrahepatic vasoconstriction in portal hypertension through vasoconstrictive effects in the liver, presumably by enhancing HSC contractility.[19,20] In experimental models, ET-1 protein and receptor expression are increased most notably in hepatic stellate cells and endothelial cells.[19,21,22] In humans with portal hypertension, plasma and liver ET-1 levels also are increased[23,24] The reason for activation of the ET-1 system in portal hypertension is not known, but this effect may be secondary to transforming growth factor-β (TGF-β), a key fibrogenic growth factor.[22] Clinical trials of ET antagonists in patients with portal hypertension are under way; however, the variable effects of ET modulation in experimental models of portal hypertension, as well as the possible hepatotoxicity of these compounds, have limited enthusiasm for studies in humans.[25] Other therapies for portal hypertension may provide benefit through the ET pathway. For example, somatostatin, which reduces portal pressure by constricting the splanchnic circulation, also may act by inhibiting ET-1–dependent HSC contraction.[26]

Other vasoconstrictive mediators, including cysteinyl leukotrienes, thromboxane, and angiotensin, also have been implicated in the development of increased intrahepatic resistance in cirrhosis.[27,28] Some of these mediators, particularly angiotensin, which causes contraction of HSCs, have been studied in humans. Attempts to reduce portal pressure using pharmacologic agents that inhibit angiotensin activation of HSC contraction have met with mixed results thus far.[29]

HYPERDYNAMIC CIRCULATION

In addition to the increases in portal resistance discussed earlier, a major factor in the development and perpetuation of portal hypertension is an increase in portal venous flow, or the hyperdynamic circulation. The term *portal venous inflow* indicates the total blood that drains into the portal circulation, not the blood flow in the portal vein itself, which may actually be diminished in portal hypertension because of portosystemic collateral shunts. The hyperdynamic circulation is characterized by peripheral and splanchnic vasodilatation, reduced mean arterial pressure, and increased cardiac output. Vasodilatation, particularly in the splanchnic bed, permits an increase in inflow of systemic blood into the portal circulation.[30]

Splanchnic vasodilatation is caused in large part by relaxation of splanchnic arterioles and ensuing splanchnic hyperemia. Studies of experimental portal hypertension have demonstrated that splanchnic vascular endothelial cells are primarily responsible for mediating splanchnic vasodilatation and enhanced portal venous inflow through excess generation of NO.[31-39] This excess generation of NO and ensuing vasodilatation, hyperdynamic circulation, and hyperemia in the splanchnic and systemic circulation contrasts with the hepatic circulation, in which NO deficiency contributes to increased intrahepatic resistance.

The mechanism of excess NO production from the endothelial cells of the systemic and splanchnic arterial circulation is an area of active investigation. Some of the increase in NO production probably occurs from shear stress–dependent and shear stress–independent increases in the expression of eNOS, which can be corrected in part by beta blockers.[37,40-45] Activation of existing eNOS by

cytokines or mechanical factors also seems to contribute to excess systemic and splanchnic NO generation through pathways that include eNOS phosphorylation and protein interactions.[42,46] The physiologic stimuli that mediate this process are not well understood but may include ET-1, which is increased in the serum of patients with portal hypertension, and the cytokine tumor necrosis factor-α (TNF-α), because inhibitors of TNF improve portal pressure and the splanchnic circulatory disturbances in both human and experimental portal hypertension. TNF-α may be derived from intestinal endotoxin, and intestinal decontamination appears to correct the hyperdynamic circulation in humans, suggesting a link with intestinal inflammation.[47] In humans with portal hypertension, therapeutic inhibition of NOS has met with mixed clinical results. In one study, inhibition of NOS corrected altered systemic hemodynamics,[48] but other studies have not demonstrated significant portal pressure–reducing effects of systemic NOS inhibition.[49] Other mediators that may contribute to systemic and splanchnic vasodilatation include anandamide, an endogenous vasodilatory cannabinoid,[50-52] heme oxygenase,[15,53-55] and cyclooxygenase.[56] Compelling evidence also supports a primary defect in smooth muscle cells in portal hypertension, perhaps because of defects in potassium channels.[57-61] In fact, many pharmacologic therapies for portal hypertension target the splanchnic arteriolar smooth muscle cells, rather than endothelial cells, to reduce splanchnic vasodilatation. For example, octreotide, a synthetic analog of somatostatin, causes marked but transient reductions in portal pressure by contracting splanchnic smooth muscle cells, thereby limiting portal venous inflow, especially after meals. Nonselective beta blockers and vasopressin also reduce portal pressure by constricting splanchnic arterioles and thereby reducing portal venous inflow. Because intrahepatic resistance persists, therapies targeted toward the increase in portal venous inflow usually do not normalize portal pressure entirely but often blunt the prominent increases in portal venous inflow that occur in response to a meal. Combination therapy with an agent to reduce increased intrahepatic resistance, such as a nitrate, and an agent to reduce portal venous inflow, such as a beta blocker, are more effective in reducing portal pressure than is either agent alone.

COLLATERAL CIRCULATION AND VARICES

The portal vein–systemic collateral circulation develops and expands in response to elevation of the portal pressure.[62] Blood flow in the low volumes that normally perfuse these collaterals and flow toward the portal circulation is reversed in portal hypertension, because the increased portal pressure exceeds the systemic venous pressure. Therefore, flow is reversed in these collateral vessels, and blood flows out of the portal circulation toward the systemic venous circulation.

The sites of collateral formation are the rectum, where the inferior mesenteric vein connects with the pudendal vein and results in rectal varices; the umbilicus, where the vestigial umbilical vein communicates with the left portal vein and gives rise to prominent collaterals around the umbilicus (caput medusae); the retroperitoneum, where collaterals, especially in women, communicate between the ovarian vessels and iliac veins; and the distal esophagus and proximal stomach, where gastroesophageal varices are the major collaterals formed between the portal venous system and systemic venous system.

Four distinct zones of venous drainage at the gastroesophageal junction are particularly relevant to the formation of esophageal varices.[63] The *gastric* zone, which extends for 2 to 3 cm below the gastroesophageal junction, comprises veins that are longitudinal and located in the submucosa and lamina propria. They come together at the upper end of the cardia of the stomach and drain into short gastric and left gastric veins. The *palisade* zone extends 2 to 3 cm proximal to the gastric zone into the lower esophagus. Veins in this zone run longitudinally and in parallel in four groups corresponding to the esophageal mucosal folds. These veins anastomose with veins in the lamina propria. The perforating veins in the palisade zone do not communicate with extrinsic (periesophageal) veins in the distal esophagus. The palisade zone is the dominant watershed area between the portal and the systemic circulations. More proximal to the palisade zone in the esophagus is the *perforating* zone, where there is a network of veins. These veins are less likely to be longitudinal and are termed "perforating veins" because they connect the veins in the esophageal submucosa and the external veins. The *truncal* zone, the longest zone, is approximately 10 cm in length, located proximally to the perforating zone in the esophagus, and usually characterized by four longitudinal veins in the lamina propria.

Veins in the palisade zone in the esophagus are most prone to bleeding, because no perforating veins at this level connect the veins in the submucosa with the periesophageal veins. Varices in the truncal zone are unlikely to bleed because the perforating vessels communicate with the periesophageal veins, allowing the varices in the truncal zone to decompress. The periesophageal veins drain into the azygous system, and as a result, an increase in azygous blood flow is a hallmark of portal hypertension. The venous drainage of the lower end of the esophagus is through the coronary vein, which also drains the cardia of the stomach, into the portal vein.

The fundus of the stomach drains through short gastric veins into the splenic vein. In the presence of portal hypertension, varices may therefore form in the fundus of the stomach. Splenic vein thrombosis usually results in isolated gastric fundal varices. Because of the proximity of the splenic vein to the renal vein, spontaneous splenorenal shunts may develop and are more common in patients with gastric varices than in those with esophageal varices.[64,65]

The predominant collateral flow pattern in intrahepatic portal hypertension is through the right and left coronary veins, with only a small portion of flow through the short gastric veins. Therefore, most patients with intrahepatic causes of portal hypertension have esophageal varices or gastric varices in continuity with esophageal varices.

Unfortunately, portal hypertension caused by cirrhosis generally persists and progresses despite the development of even an extensive collateral circulation. Progression of portal hypertension results from (1) the prominent obstructive resistance in the liver, (2) resistance within the collaterals themselves, and (3) continued increase in portal vein inflow. The collateral circulatory bed develops through a combination of angiogenesis, the development of new blood vessels, and dilatation and increased flow through preexisting collaterals.[3,66] Experimental evidence suggests that vascular endothelial growth factor (VEGF), a key NO stimulatory growth factor, may contribute to both the angiogenic and the collateral vessel responses.[54,67] Inhibition of either VEGF or NO may attenuate the collateral vessel propagation by inhibiting angiogenic responses in experimental models of portal hypertension and collateralization.[66-71] Some pharmacologic agents used in the management of portal hypertension, such as beta blockers and octreotide, may act in part by constricting collateral vessels.[72-75]

To develop gastroesophageal varices requires a portal pressure gradient of at least 10 mm Hg. Furthermore, a portal pressure gradient of at least 12 mm Hg is thought to be required for varices to bleed; other local factors that increase variceal wall tension also are needed,[76] because all patients with a portal pressure gradient of greater than 12 mm Hg do not necessarily bleed. Factors that influence variceal wall tension can be viewed in the context of the law of Laplace:

$$T = Pr/w$$

where T is variceal wall tension, P is the transmural pressure gradient between the variceal lumen and esophageal lumen, r is the variceal radius, and w is the variceal wall thickness. When the variceal wall thins and the varix increases in diameter and pressure, the tolerated wall tension is exceeded and the varix will rupture. These physiologic observations are manifested clinically by the observation that patients with larger varices (r) in sites of limited soft tissue support (w), with elevated portal pressure (P), tend to be at greatest risk for variceal rupture from variceal wall tension (T) that becomes excessive. One notable site in which soft tissue support is limited is at the gastroesophageal junction. The lack of tissue support and high vessel density may contribute to the greater frequency of bleeding from varices at the gastroesophageal junction. The law of Laplace also has implications for the relevance of pharmacologic therapies aimed at reducing portal pressure. Reductions in portal pressure will reduce the variceal transmural pressure gradient, thereby reducing the risk that variceal wall tension will become excessive and varices will rupture. Clinically, a reduction in the hepatic venous pressure gradient to less than 12 mm Hg almost negates the risk of variceal hemorrhage. The changes in portal pressure and local variceal factors, however, are dynamic and influenced by a number of physiologic (increases in intra-abdominal pressure and meal-induced increases in portal pressure), diurnal (circadian changes in portal pressure), and pathophysiologic (acute alcohol use) factors, and portal pressure and esophageal variceal pressure may vary at different times.

MEASUREMENT OF PORTAL PRESSURE

Portal pressure may be measured indirectly or directly. The most commonly used method of measuring portal pressure is determination of the hepatic vein pressure gradient (HVPG), which is an indirect method. Splenic pulp pressure measurement and direct measurement of the portal vein pressure are invasive, cumbersome, and infrequently used approaches. Variceal pressure also can be measured, although this is not routinely performed in clinical practice.

HEPATIC VEIN PRESSURE GRADIENT

The HVPG is the difference between the wedged hepatic venous pressure (WHVP) and free hepatic vein pressure (FHVP). The HVPG has been used to assess portal hypertension since its first description in 1951[77] and has been validated as the best predictor for the development of complications of portal hypertension.

Measurement of the HVPG requires passage of a catheter into the hepatic vein under radiologic control until the catheter can be passed no further, that is, until the catheter has been "wedged" in the hepatic vein. The catheter can be passed into the hepatic vein either through the femoral vein or using a transjugular venous approach. The purpose of wedging the catheter is to form a column of fluid that is continuous between the hepatic sinusoid and the catheter. Therefore, the measured pressure of fluid within the catheter reflects hepatic sinusoidal pressure. One of the drawbacks of using a catheter that is wedged in the hepatic vein is that the WHVP measured in a more fibrotic area of liver may be higher than the pressure measured in a less fibrotic area, because of regional variation in the degree of fibrosis. Using a balloon-occluding catheter in the right hepatic vein to create a stagnant column of fluid in continuity with the hepatic sinusoids eliminates this variation in measurement of WHVP, because the balloon catheter measures the WHVP averaged over a wide segment of the liver.[78] HVPG is not effective for detecting presinusoidal causes of portal hypertension. For example, in portal hypertension secondary to portal vein thrombosis, the HVPG is normal. Moreover, the HVPG may underestimate sinusoidal pressure in primary biliary cirrhosis and other presinusoidal causes of portal hypertension.[79] Therefore, HVPG is accurate for detecting only sinusoidal and postsinusoidal causes of portal hypertension.

The HVPG represents the gradient between the pressure in the portal vein and the intra-abdominal inferior vena caval pressure. An elevation in intra-abdominal pressure increases both WHVP and FHVP equally, so that the HVPG is unchanged. The advantage of the HVPG is that variations in the "zero" reference point have no impact on the HVPG.[80] The HVPG is measured at least three times to demonstrate that the values are reproducible. Total occlusion of the hepatic vein by the inflated balloon to confirm that the balloon is in a wedged position is demonstrated by injecting contrast into the hepatic vein. A sinusoidal pattern should be seen, with no collateral circulation to other hepatic veins. The contrast washes out promptly with deflation of the balloon. Correct posi-

tioning of the balloon also is demonstrated by a sharp increase in the recorded pressure on inflation of the balloon. The pressure then becomes steady until the balloon is deflated, when the pressure drops sharply. In experienced hands, measurement of the HVPG is highly reproducible, accurate, and safe.

Measurement of the HVPG has been proposed for three indications: (1) to monitor portal pressure in patients on drugs to prevent variceal bleeding; (2) to assess the risk of hepatic resection in patients with cirrhosis; and (3) to delineate the cause of portal hypertension (that is, presinusoidal, sinusoidal, or postsinusoidal), usually in combination with venography, right-sided heart pressure measurements, and transjugular liver biopsy. Although the widest potential indication for HVPG measurement is to monitor the efficacy of therapies to reduce portal pressure, HVPG monitoring is not routinely done in clinical practice, because no controlled trials have yet demonstrated its usefulness.[81]

SPLENIC PULP PRESSURE

Splenic pulp pressure determination is an indirect method of measuring portal pressure and involves puncture of the splenic pulp with a needle catheter. Splenic pulp pressure is elevated in presinusoidal portal hypertension, when the HVPG is normal. Because of the potential risk of complications, especially bleeding, associated with splenic puncture, however, the procedure is rarely used.

PORTAL VEIN PRESSURE

Direct measurement of the pressure in the portal vein is a rarely used method that can be carried out through a percutaneous transhepatic route or a transvenous approach. The transhepatic route requires portal vein puncture performed under ultrasound guidance. A catheter is then threaded over a guidewire into the main portal vein. With increasing use of the transjugular intrahepatic portosystemic shunt (TIPS) (see later), radiologists have gained expertise in puncturing the portal vein and measuring portal vein pressure by a transjugular route. Direct portal pressure measurements are carried out when HVPG cannot be measured, as in patients with occluded hepatic veins caused by the Budd-Chiari syndrome, in whom a surgical portosystemic shunt is being contemplated,[82] or in patients with intrahepatic, presinusoidal causes of portal hypertension, such as idiopathic portal hypertension, in which the HVPG may be normal.

ENDOSCOPIC VARICEAL PRESSURE

Varices rupture and bleed when the expanding force of intravariceal pressure exceeds variceal wall tension. Measurement of the difference between intravariceal pressure and pressure within the esophageal lumen is important, because the derived transmural pressure gradient across the varices is potentially a more important indicator of bleeding risk than measurement of HVPG,[83,84] especially in patients with portal vein thrombosis and other causes of portal hypertension associated with a normal HVPG.

Variceal pressure can be measured by inserting a needle connected to a pressure transducer, through a fluid-filled catheter, into a varix; this approach is currently not justified except when measurement of variceal pressure is followed by variceal injection sclerotherapy. Because variceal sclerotherapy has fallen out of favor (see later), measurement of variceal pressure by variceal puncture is seldom carried out except in research studies.

A miniature pneumatic pressure sensitivity gauge attached to the tip of an endoscope (Varipres Solid Components, Barcelona, Spain) allows noninvasive measurement of variceal pressure. In studies using this device, patients with previous variceal bleeding have been demonstrated to have higher variceal pressures than those in patients without previous bleeding.[85] A variceal pressure greater than18 mm Hg during a bleeding episode is associated with failure to control bleeding and predicts early rebleeding.[86] Moreover, patients on pharmacologic therapy who show a decrease in variceal pressure of greater than 20% from baseline have a low probability of bleeding, as compared with patients who do not demonstrate a greater than 20% decrease in variceal pressure, in whom the risk of variceal bleeding is 46%.[85] Variceal pressure measurements determined with use of Varipres are considered satisfactory when they meet the following criteria: (1) a stable intraesophageal pressure; (2) absence of artifacts caused by esophageal peristalsis; and (3) correct placement of the capsule over the varix, as shown by fine fluctuations in the pressure tracing that correspond to the cardiac cycle and respirations. Therefore, measurement of variceal pressure requires both a skilled endoscopist and a cooperative patient, and, even in expert hands, accurate variceal pressure measurements cannot be obtained in 25% of patients.

Manometry using an endoscopic balloon to measure variceal pressure is subject to observer bias, because it relies on visual appearance to determine whether the varices have collapsed.[87-89] With this technique, a balloon is inserted into the esophagus and inflated until the varices are noted on endoscopy to collapse. The pressure in the balloon required to collapse the varices represents the variceal pressure. In general, techniques of measuring variceal pressure are still considered experimental and not suitable for routine clinical use.

DETECTION OF VARICES

UPPER GASTROINTESTINAL ENDOSCOPY

Upper gastrointestinal endoscopy is the most commonly used method to detect varices. The current consensus is that all patients with cirrhosis of the liver should be screened for esophageal varices by endoscopy. In patients in whom no varices are detected on initial endoscopy, endoscopy to look for varices should be repeated in 2 to 3 years. If small varices are detected on the initial endoscopy, endoscopy should be repeated in 1 to 2 years.[90,91] Various noninvasive methods of determining

which patients benefit most from endoscopic screening have been studied. In patients with primary sclerosing cholangitis, a platelet count less than $150 \times 10^3/dL$ and serum albumin level less than 3.3 g/dL were reported to predict the presence of large varices.[92] Unfortunately, the predictive accuracy of these markers is not high enough to recommend their routine use in clinical practice.[93] The role of noninvasive markers in predicting the risk of large esophageal varices requires study in large multicenter trials. Similarly, the role of capsule endoscopy in screening for esophageal varices is under study (see Chapter 13).

Endoscopic grading of esophageal varices is subjective. Various criteria have been used to try to standardize the reporting of esophageal varices. The best known of these criteria are those compiled by the Japanese Research Society for Portal Hypertension. The descriptors include red color signs, color of the varix, form (size) of the varix, and location of the varix.[94] Red color signs include red "wale" markings, which are longitudinal whip-like marks on the varix; cherry-red spots, which usually are 2 to 3 mm or less in diameter; hematocystic spots, which are blood-filled blisters 4 mm or greater in diameter; and diffuse redness. The color of the varix can be either white or blue. The form of the varix at endoscopy is what is described most commonly. Esophageal varices may be small and straight (grade I); tortuous and occupying less than one third of the esophageal lumen (grade II); or large and occupying more than one third of the esophageal lumen (grade III). Varices can be in the lower third, middle third, or upper third of the esophagus. Of all of the aforementioned descriptors, the size of the varices in the lower third of the esophagus is the most important. The size of the varices in the lower third of the esophagus is determined during withdrawal of the endoscope (Fig. 87–5). As much air as is possible should be aspirated from the stomach while the esophageal lumen is fully inflated. Small varices, that is, those occupying less than one third of the lumen, are less than 5 mm in diameter, whereas large varices are greater than 5 mm in diameter.[94,95] As a point of reference, any varix larger in diameter than an open pinch biopsy forceps is likely to be greater than 5 mm in diameter. Patients with large esophageal varices, Child-Turcotte-Pugh (CTP) class C cirrhosis (see later), and red color signs on varices have the highest risk of variceal bleeding within 1 year.[96] The increase in bleeding risk attributable to the presence of red color signs, however, is not independent of the risk associated with large variceal size. Therefore, prophylactic treatment to prevent variceal bleeding is recommended in all patients with large esophageal varices irrespective of the presence or absence of red color signs.

ULTRASONOGRAPHY

Ultrasound examination of the liver with Doppler study of the vessels has been used widely to assess patients with portal hypertension. Features suggestive of portal hypertension on ultrasonography include splenomegaly, portosystemic collateral vessels, and reversal of the direction of flow in the portal vein (hepatofugal flow). Some studies

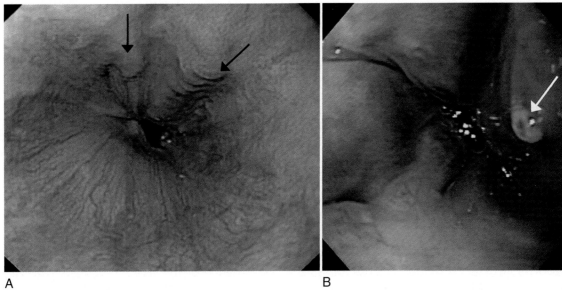

A   B

Figure 87–5 Endoscopic appearances of esophageal varices. *A,* Upper gastrointestinal endoscopy demonstrates dilated and straight veins (small esophageal varices) in the lower esophagus *(arrows). B,* Upper gastrointestinal endoscopy demonstrates large esophageal varices, greater than 5 mm in diameter, with a fibrin plug *(arrow)* representing the site of a recent bleed.

have demonstrated that a portal vein diameter greater than 13 mm and the absence of respiratory variations in the splenic and mesenteric veins are sensitive but nonspecific markers of portal hypertension.[97,98] These criteria are not used routinely in clinical practice in most centers. Ultrasound examination can detect thrombosis of the portal vein, which appears as either nonvisualization or cavernous transformation of the portal vein; the latter finding indicates an extensive collateral network in place of the portal vein.[99] Splenic vein thrombosis also can be demonstrated. Portal blood flow can be measured by Doppler ultrasonography, which is the easiest research method for detecting postprandial increases in splanchnic blood flow.[100] Although Doppler ultrasonography is clinically useful in the initial evaluation of portal hypertension, the technique is not widely used to provide quantitative assessments of the degree of portal hypertension, owing to interobserver variability with the same instrument and intraobserver variability with different instruments.

COMPUTED TOMOGRAPHY

Computed tomography (CT) is useful for demonstrating many features of portal hypertension, including abnormal configuration of the liver, ascites, splenomegaly, and collateral vessels (Fig. 87–6). Detection of varices may be an emerging indication for CT. Diagnosis of fundal varices by multi-detector row CT (MDCT) is at least as accurate as endoscopic ultrasonography (see later). CT is especially helpful in distinguishing submucosal from perigastric fundal varices[101] and is considered a less invasive alternative to conventional angiographic portography in assessing portosystemic collaterals.[102] At present,

however, CT is not a recommended screening method for detecting large esophageal varices.

MAGNETIC RESONANCE IMAGING

Gadolinium-enhanced magnetic resonance imaging (MRI) is becoming recognized as a potentially useful method of detecting esophageal varices.[103] In addition, MRI can be used to measure portal and azygous blood flow, which is increased in patients with portal hypertension.[104] MRI provides excellent detail of the vascular structures of the liver and can detect portal venous thrombosis and portosystemic shunts. The role of MRI in the assessment of portal hypertension requires further study.

ENDOSCOPIC ULTRASONOGRAPHY

Endoscopic ultrasound examination using radial or linear array echo-endoscopes or endoscopic ultrasound miniprobes passed through the working channel of a diagnostic endoscope has been applied as an investigational tool in the evaluation of patients with varices. Endoscopic ultrasonography has been used to study several aspects of esophageal varices, including identification of patients at increased risk of bleeding by assessment of the cross-sectional area of varices[76]; size of and flow in the left gastric vein, azygous vein, and paraesophageal collaterals; changes after endoscopic therapy; and recurrence of esophageal varices following variceal ligation.[105] Endosonography can be combined with endoscopic measurement of transmural variceal pressure to allow estimation of variceal wall tension, which is a predictor of variceal bleeding (see earlier).[106-108]

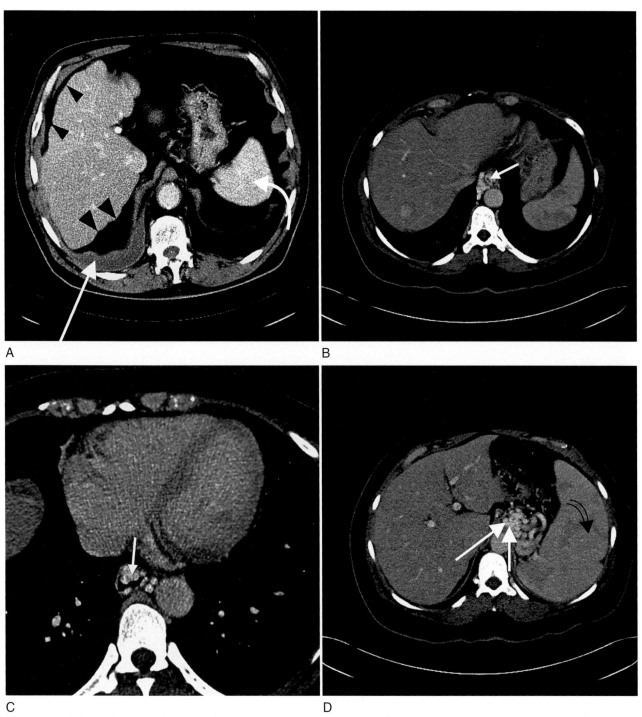

Figure 87–6 Abdominal computed tomography (CT) scans in patients with portal hypertension. *A,* CT scan shows an irregular contour of the liver typical of cirrhosis *(arrowheads).* A small right pleural effusion is evident *(straight arrow).* The liver is hypointense relative to the spleen *(curved arrow),* typical of fatty infiltration of the liver in alcoholic cirrhosis. *B,* CT scan demonstrates contrast-enhanced vessels at the lower end of the esophagus *(arrow)* that suggest esophageal varices and periesophageal collaterals. *C,* Close-up view of the lower end of the esophagus on CT demonstrates a large varix occupying greater than 50% of the esophageal lumen *(arrow). D,* CT scan demonstrates a tuft of gastroesophageal collaterals *(straight arrows).* The enlarged spleen also is seen *(curved arrow).*

CAUSES OF PORTAL HYPERTENSION

The usual classification of causes of portal hypertension is based on the site of increased resistance to portal blood flow—namely, prehepatic, intrahepatic, and posthepatic—and is outlined in Figure 87–4. Intrahepatic sites of increased resistance can be presinusoidal, sinusoidal, or postsinusoidal. Many liver conditions, however, can increase resistance at more than one site. For example, alcoholic cirrhosis may be associated with increased resistance at the presinusoidal, sinusoidal, and postsinu-soidal levels. Therefore, classification based on the site of

Table 87–1   Causes of Portal Hypertension

Common
Cirrhosis
Schistosomiasis
Extrahepatic portal vein thrombosis
Idiopathic portal hypertension
Less Common
Nodular regenerative hyperplasia
Partial nodular transformation of the liver
Congenital hepatic fibrosis
Polycystic liver disease
Sarcoidosis
Splanchnic arteriovenous fistula
Hereditary hemorrhagic telangiectasia
Myeloproliferative disorders
Malignancy

resistance may not be possible for all diseases that cause portal hypertension. A more useful classification is clinically based and considers common and less common causes of portal hypertension (Table 87–1).

COMMON CAUSES

Cirrhosis

Complications related to portal hypertension are the usual clinical manifestations of cirrhosis of the liver. Although all causes of cirrhosis are associated with portal hypertension, some features are disease specific. In alcoholic liver disease, elevation of the portal pressure is accurately reflected by the HVPG; moreover, portal hypertension may occur in the absence of cirrhosis but is more marked when cirrhosis is present. Perivenular lesions implicated in the pathogenesis in noncirrhotic alcoholic liver injury account for a presinusoidal component of portal hypertension in these patients.[109] Autoimmune hepatitis also may be associated with portal hypertension in the absence of cirrhosis[110]; however, the risk of variceal bleeding is low in patients with autoimmune liver disease. In hemochromatosis, portal hypertension may be seen even before cirrhosis; the severity of portal hypertension increases with increasing fibrosis. Patients with hemochromatosis may bleed from varices despite an HVPG less than 12 mm Hg, indicating a presinusoidal component of portal hypertension. Phlebotomy therapy in patients with hemochromatosis may result in a decrease in portal hypertension.[111] In patients with primary biliary cirrhosis, portal hypertension also may occur before cirrhosis has developed. In a prospective evaluation of 265 patients with primary biliary cirrhosis who did not have esophageal varices at entry into this study, esophageal varices developed in one third of the patients during a median follow-up period of 5 to 6 years. Of those in whom varices developed, approximately one half experienced episodes of variceal bleeding. The risk of variceal bleeding was increased with an increase in the histologic stage of the disease; 1-year and 3-year survival rates following a bleed were 83% and 59%, respectively.[112] In earlier stages of primary biliary cirrhosis, portal hypertension is predominantly presinusoidal, but as the disease progresses, a sinusoidal component develops. Therefore,

the HVPG may underestimate portal pressure in patients with primary biliary cirrhosis.[79] Portal hypertension occurs in patients with primary sclerosing cholangitis and in those with biliary strictures. A long duration of biliary obstruction usually is required, although portal hypertension has been known to develop in a few months in patients with chronic bile duct obstruction caused by chronic alcoholic pancreatitis.[113] Portal hypertension in patients with biliary obstruction regresses following relief of the biliary obstruction.

Schistosomiasis

Schistosomiasis may be the most common cause of portal hypertension worldwide (see Chapter 79). Bleeding from esophageal varices is a major cause of death in patients with hepatosplenic schistosomiasis. Portal hypertension results from presinusoidal obstruction caused by deposition of eggs of *Schistosoma mansoni* and *Schistosoma japonicum* in the presinusoidal portal venules. The host reaction results in granulomatous inflammation, which causes presinusoidal and periportal fibrosis.[114] The fibrosis that results is sometimes called "clay pipestem" or simply "pipestem" fibrosis and usually is associated with sustained heavy infection. The periportal collagen deposition leads to progressive obstruction of portal blood flow, portal hypertension, and variceal bleeding, along with splenomegaly and hypersplenism. Lobular architecture usually is preserved. Coinfection with chronic hepatitis B or C in patients with hepatic schistosomiasis can result in hepatic failure and an increased risk of hepatocellular carcinoma.[115,116]

In the initial stages of schistosomiasis, the HVPG is normal owing to the presinusoidal nature of the obstruction. Some patients with schistosomiasis and portal hypertension also may have portal vein thrombosis. Patients with schistosomiasis often undergo surgical portosystemic shunts to treat variceal bleeding, with excellent long-term outcomes.

Extrahepatic Portal Vein Thrombosis

Extrahepatic portal vein thrombosis is a prehepatic, presinusoidal cause of portal hypertension and a common cause of portal hypertension in children (see Chapter 80). The most common causes of portal vein thrombosis include a prothrombotic state, such as antithrombin, protein C, or protein S deficiency; antiphospholipid antibody syndrome; oral contraceptive use; and neoplasm, usually intra-abdominal. Other causes include hematologic disorders, such as polycythemia vera, essential thrombocythemia, and paroxysmal nocturnal hemoglobinuria; inflammatory diseases, such as pancreatitis, inflammatory bowel disease, and diverticulitis; abdominal trauma; and postoperative states, especially postsplenectomy. Cirrhosis of the liver also is a cause of portal vein thrombosis. Older studies suggested that portal vein thrombosis occurs in approximately 6% of patients with cirrhosis and in up to 25% of those with cirrhosis and hepatocellular carcinoma.[117] With improved imaging, portal vein thrombosis is now known to be a more common complication of cirrhosis, and the association with hepatocellular carcinoma is not as strong as previously thought. Isolated splenic vein thrombosis caused by a pancreatic neoplasm or pancreatitis usually is not associated with a thrombophilia. Umbilical vein sepsis may be an etiologic factor in children with portal vein thrombosis, but even in these cases, an associated prothrombotic state may predispose the patient to portal vein thrombosis.

Acute and subacute portal vein thrombosis usually does not manifest with variceal bleeding.[1] Chronic portal vein thrombosis is suggested by nonvisualization of the portal or splenic vein and an extensive collateral circulation. Patients may present with nonspecific symptoms, or with variceal bleeding and hypersplenism. Bleeding usually is from gastroesophageal varices but may be from duodenal varices and, rarely, ectopic sites. Gallbladder varices also have been described in patients with portal vein thrombosis.[118]

The treatment of portal vein thrombosis is symptomatic, with the aim of controlling variceal bleeding or preventing recurrent variceal bleeding. Patients in whom esophageal varices are not large, and a thrombophilia is detected, are best managed with anticoagulation, because in these patients, the benefits of anticoagulation outweigh the risks.[119] Endoscopic therapy is used both to control acute variceal bleeding and to prevent recurrent bleeding. Use of pharmacologic agents to prevent variceal bleeding, such as beta blockers, probably also is effective in patients with portal vein thrombosis, but this approach has not been as well studied. In addition, patients with portal vein thrombosis have lower mortality and morbidity rates from variceal bleeding than those reported in patients with cirrhosis and variceal bleeding, owing to the lack of coagulopathy and synthetic liver dysfunction in patients with portal vein thrombosis. Surgical portosystemic shunt procedures are carried out in patients in whom bleeding cannot be controlled by conservative measures. If a suitable vein is not available for anastomosis, a large venous collateral vein may be anastomosed to a systemic vein.[120] Placement of a TIPS generally is not indicated in patients with chronic portal vein thrombosis.

Idiopathic Portal Hypertension

Idiopathic portal hypertension is uncommon in Western countries but common in parts of Asia such as India and Japan. This disorder is diagnosed when the portal pressure is elevated in the absence of significant histologic changes in the liver or extrahepatic portal vein obstruction.[121] A liver biopsy specimen from affected patients may be entirely normal,[117] although increased concentrations of ET-1 have been noted in the periportal hepatocytes, portal venules, and hepatic sinusoids of patients with idiopathic portal hypertension.[122] Various terms used (rather loosely) to describe idiopathic portal hypertension include hepatoportal sclerosis, noncirrhotic portal fibrosis, and Banti's syndrome.[123,124] Use of the term *idiopathic portal hypertension* probably is best restricted to portal hypertension in patients in whom no hepatic lesion is found on light microscopy. The term *hepatoportal sclerosis* suggests obliterative portal venopathy with subendothelial thickening of the intrahepatic portal veins; thrombosis and recanalization of these veins may follow. Fibrosis of the portal tracts is prominent later in the course.

The cause of idiopathic portal hypertension is unclear in a majority of patients, although chronic arsenic intoxication, exposure to vinyl chloride, and hypervitaminosis A have been implicated (see Chapter 84). These etiologic factors are present in only a minority of patients. The dominant clinical features of the condition are variceal bleeding and hypersplenism related to a markedly enlarged spleen. Liver biochemical test levels are usually normal, although the serum alkaline phosphatase level may be mildly elevated. Ascites is uncommon. The HVPG in this disorder usually is normal, because the site of increased resistance is presinusoidal.[125] Surgical portosystemic shunts are well tolerated in these patients, although hepatic encephalopathy may occur on long-term follow-up evaluation.[117] Liver transplantation is rarely required in these patients.

Idiopathic portal hypertension may be confused with incomplete septal cirrhosis, which probably is an unrelated condition characterized by incomplete septa and liver nodularity.[126] Patients with incomplete septal cirrhosis are clinically similar to patients with cirrhosis and may progress to end-stage liver disease and require liver transplantation.

LESS COMMON CAUSES

Nodular Regenerative Hyperplasia

Nodular regenerative hyperplasia is a histopathologic diagnosis characterized by atrophy of zone 3 hepatocytes and hypertrophy of zone 1 hepatocytes without significant fibrosis (see Chapters 34 and 91).[127] This disorder has been recognized increasingly as a cause of portal hypertension and may even occur after liver transplantation.[128] Similar histologic changes may be seen in well-established Budd-Chiari syndrome.[129] The nodular hyperplasia may not be apparent on histologic examination unless a reticulin stain is carried out to demonstrate the micronodules. These regenerative nodules are believed to result from an imbalance between hyperperfused areas of the liver, with resulting regenerative nodules, and poorly perfused areas, with resulting atrophy. Nodular regenerative hyperplasia is associated with a variety of conditions, predominantly hematologic and rheumatologic. Liver biochemical abnormalities include mild elevation of the serum aminotransferase levels. Portal hypertension manifesting as variceal bleeding is the predominant clinical presentation. Ascites also may develop in these patients, suggesting that an increase in sinusoidal pressure occurs. Hepatocellular carcinoma does not occur, but liver transplantation may be required in some patients.

Partial Nodular Transformation of the Liver

Partial nodular transformation of the liver is an uncommon lesion that is characterized by large nodules in the perihilar region.[130] These nodules may be visible on imaging studies of the liver. The rest of the liver may be normal or may show changes of nodular regenerative hyperplasia. Liver biochemical test levels usually are normal. Like nodular regenerative hyperplasia, partial nodular transformation of the liver is believed to be related to an imbalance in portal perfusion of the liver, but the abnormality is restricted to the hilar branches, whereas in nodular regenerative hyperplasia the abnormality is more diffuse. Variceal bleeding is the predominant presentation in partial nodular transformation of the liver, although patients with large nodules may experience abdominal pain. Treatment with a surgical portosystemic shunt is associated with good long-term results.

Congenital Hepatic Fibrosis

Congenital hepatic fibrosis occurs in association with Caroli's disease of the liver, polycystic disease of the kidney, and medullary sponge kidney (see Chapter 59). The major manifestation of congenital hepatic fibrosis is variceal bleeding.[131] Portosystemic shunts may be placed in these patients to treat refractory variceal bleeding, with a low risk of long-term hepatic encephalopathy.

Polycystic Liver Disease

Patients with polycystic liver disease, whether associated with polycystic kidney disease or not, rarely present with portal hypertension (see Chapter 91).[132] Portal hypertension may decrease after treatment of the cysts.

Sarcoidosis

Portal hypertension is an uncommon manifestation of hepatic sarcoidosis[133] (see Chapter 34). The site of increased intrahepatic resistance in patients with sarcoidosis seems to be postsinusoidal, in view of the elevated HVPG. In early disease, however, the resistance is predominantly at a presinusoidal level. Whether glucocorticoids decrease portal hypertension in patients with hepatic sarcoidosis is unknown.

Myeloproliferative Disorders and Malignancy

Portal hypertension has been associated with myeloproliferative disorders such as leukemias, lymphomas, and systemic mastocytosis[134] (see Chapters 33 and 34). Portal hypertension also may occur in patients with hepatocellular carcinoma independent of the presence of cirrhosis (see Chapter 91). The pathogenesis of portal hypertension in patients with hepatocellular carcinoma is thought to be multifactorial; contributing factors include portal vein thrombosis, pressure by the tumor on the portal vein, and in some cases a hepatic artery–portal vein fistula. Esophageal varices may be seen in patients with hepatic metastases, although variceal bleeding is unusual.[135]

Splanchnic Arteriovenous Fistula

Splanchnic arteriovenous fistula should be suspected when the onset of portal hypertension is acute, with development of ascites and variceal bleeding, especially in the presence of an abdominal bruit. Arteriovenous fistula may occur from the splenic artery to splenic vein or from the hepatic artery to portal vein, as in patients with hereditary hemorrhagic telangiectasia. When a splanchnic artery ruptures into a mesenteric vein, the portal pressure increases acutely, reaching levels of systemic arterial pressure. The result is acute portal hypertension with development of ascites and variceal bleeding. A bruit may be heard in the left upper quadrant of the abdomen with a splenic arteriovenous fistula and in the right upper quadrant with a hepatic artery–portal vein fistula. With a long-standing fistula, secondary hepatic changes of perisinusoidal fibrosis related to an increase in portal venous inflow may be present. In the early stages, embolization or ligation of the fistula will ameliorate the portal hypertension. In late stages, however, portal fibrosis may be advanced, and the portal hypertension may not correct completely with embolization of the fistula.

Hereditary Hemorrhagic Telangiectasia

Hereditary hemorrhagic telangiectasia (HHT), or Osler-Weber-Rendu syndrome, is an unusual cause of portal hypertension (see also Chapter 36). Diagnostic criteria include mucocutaneous telangiectasias, epistaxis, arteriovenous fistulas of the viscera (usually lung or liver), and a family history of the disorder. Manifestations of hereditary hemorrhagic telangiectasia depend on the site of fistula formation. A fistula between the hepatic artery and hepatic vein manifests predominantly as biliary disease, mainly biliary strictures and cholangitis, and high-output cardiac failure. A fistula between the hepatic artery and portal vein results in portal hypertension and biliary strictures, whereas a fistula between the portal vein and hepatic vein, which is rare, results in hepatic encephalopathy.[136,137] Although symptomatic liver disease in hereditary hemorrhagic telangiectasia is rare, involvement of the liver is found in a majority of patients.[138]

CLINICAL ASSESSMENT OF PATIENTS WITH PORTAL HYPERTENSION–RELATED BLEEDING

Gastric or esophageal variceal bleeding manifests as either hematemesis or melena (or both). Chronic blood loss is a more common presentation of portal hypertensive gastropathy or gastrointestinal vascular ectasia. The classic presentation of patients with variceal bleeding is with effortless and recurrent hematemesis; the vomitus is described as dark red in color.

Portal hypertension should be suspected in all patients with gastrointestinal bleeding and peripheral stigmata of liver disease—namely, jaundice, spider telangiectasias, palmar erythema, Dupuytren's contractures, parotid enlargement, testicular atrophy, loss of secondary sexual characters, ascites, and encephalopathy. Splenomegaly is an important clue to the presence of portal hypertension, and the presence of ascites makes the presence of esophageal varices even more likely. Caput medusae, suggestive of an intrahepatic cause of portal hypertension, is present around the umbilicus; the flow of blood is away from the umbilicus. In Budd-Chiari syndrome, by contrast, veins are dilated in the flanks and back, and blood flows in a cephalic direction.[82] A bruit may be heard in either the left or the right upper quadrant in a patient with a splanchnic arteriovenous fistula. A venous hum may be heard in the epigastrium of a patient with portal hypertension and represents collateral flow in the falciform ligament.

Laboratory studies frequently reveal evidence of hepatic synthetic dysfunction, including prolongation of the prothrombin time, hypoalbuminemia, and hyperbilirubinemia, as well as anemia. Thrombocytopenia and leukopenia, reflecting hypersplenism and, in alcoholics, bone marrow suppression, may be noted. Patients with severe bleeding may present with hypovolemic shock, and renal insufficiency. Abdominal imaging studies frequently reveal splenomegaly, collateral vessels, abnormal liver echotexture and contour, and ascites.

TREATMENT OF PORTAL HYPERTENSION–RELATED BLEEDING

The treatment of portal hypertension is aimed either at reducing portal blood flow with pharmacologic agents such as beta blockers or vasopressin and its analogs or at decreasing intrahepatic resistance, either with pharmacologic agents such as nitrates or by radiologic or surgical creation of a portosystemic shunt. Treatment also may be directed at the varices with use of endoscopic methods.

PHARMACOLOGIC THERAPY

The pharmacologic agents used in the treatment of portal hypertension are divided into two groups: those that decrease splanchnic blood flow and those that decrease intrahepatic vascular resistance (Table 87–2). The agents that decrease splanchnic blood flow acutely are vasopressin and its analogs and somatostatin and its analogs. Beta-adrenergic blocking agents also decrease portal blood flow but are used only to prevent variceal bleeding and rebleeding. Agents that target intrahepatic vascular resistance include α-adrenergic blockers, angiotensin receptor blockers, and nitrates, but only nitrates are now considered for clinical use. Diuretics, by decreasing plasma volume, may reduce portal pressure but are not recommended as sole agents for the treatment of portal hypertension. Metoclopramide and cisapride may decrease intravariceal pressure by contracting the lower esophageal sphincter, but these agents have not been evaluated in clinical trials and are not recommended.

Vasopressin and Its Analogs

Vasopressin is an endogenous nonpeptide that causes splanchnic vasoconstriction, reduces portal venous inflow, and reduces portal pressure. This drug is associated with serious systemic side effects, however. By causing constriction of systemic vessels, vasopressin may result in necrosis of the bowel. Additionally, vasopressin has direct negative inotropic and chronotropic effects on the myocardium that lead to reduced cardiac output and bradycardia, respectively. An increase in afterload can result in myocardial infarction, and antidiuresis, resulting from the action of vasopressin on the kidney, can result in hyponatremia.

Terlipressin, or triglycyl-lysine-vasopressin, is a semisynthetic analog of vasopressin that is cleaved by endothelial peptidases to release lysine vasopressin. Compared with vasopressin, terlipressin results in lower circulatory levels of the vasopressin analog and a lower rate of systemic side effects. Both vasopressin and terlipressin have been used in combination with nitrates to decrease the risk of systemic side effects. Terlipressin is preferred over vasopressin because of its superior safety profile. In addition, an increase in survival has been demonstrated in patients with variceal bleeding treated with terlipressin. Terlipressin is not currently available in the United States.

Somatostatin and Its Analogs

Somatostatin is a 14-amino-acid peptide. Five somatostatin receptors—SRTR 1 to SRTR 5—are recognized, but the actual distribution of the receptors in humans is not clear. Following intravenous injection, somatostatin has a half-life in the circulation of 1 to 3 minutes; therefore, longer-acting analogs of somatostatin have been synthesized. The best known of these analogs are octreotide, lanreotide, and vapreotide.[139] Somatostatin decreases portal pressure and collateral blood flow by inhibiting release of glucagon.[140] The optimal dose and duration of use of somatostatin have not been adequately studied. Following a single 250-μg bolus injection of somatostatin, portal and azygous blood flow decrease, but the effect lasts only a few minutes.[141] Use of higher doses is associated with a more impressive decrease in HVPG. Somatostatin also decreases portal hypertension by decreasing postprandial blood flow.[142] Following a variceal bleed, blood in the gastrointestinal tract acts like a meal, leading to an increase in portal flow and elevation in the portal pressure; this elevation in pressure is ameliorated by the use of somatostatin.

Following intravenous administration, octreotide has a half-life in the circulation of 80 to 120 minutes. Its effect on reducing portal pressure is not prolonged, however. Moreover, continuous infusion of octreotide does not decrease portal pressure despite decreasing the postprandial increase in portal pressure.[61,143]

Available evidence is insufficient to prove superiority of somatostatin and its analogs to placebo in the control of acute variceal bleeding.[139] Some randomized controlled trials, however, support the view that somatostatin or octreotide may be equivalent in efficacy to sclerotherapy or terlipressin for controlling of acute variceal bleeding. Also, early administration of vapreotide may be associated with improved control of bleeding but without a significant reduction in mortality rate.[144] In clinical practice, treatment with somatostatin or octreotide is combined with endoscopic management of variceal bleeding.

Table 87–2   Drugs Used in the Treatment of Portal Hypertension

Drugs That Decrease Portal Blood Flow
Nonselective beta-adrenergic blocking agents
Vasopressin
Somatostatin and its analogs
Drugs That Decrease Intrahepatic Resistance
Nitrates
α₁-Adrenergic blocking agents (e.g., prazosin)
Angiotensin receptor blocking agents

β-Adrenergic Blockers

Nonselective β-adrenergic blockers have been used extensively since the landmark study of Lebrec and colleagues demonstrating the efficacy of these agents in preventing variceal rebleeding.[145] Nonselective β-adrenergic blocking agents such as propranolol or nadolol are preferred. Blockade of β_1-adrenergic receptors in the heart decreases cardiac output. Blockade of β_2-adrenergic receptors in the mesenteric circulation, which cause vasodilatation, allows unopposed action of α_1-adrenergic receptors and results in decreased portal flow. The combination of decreased cardiac output and decreased portal flow leads to a decrease in portal pressure. Nadolol has advantages over propranolol in that it is excreted predominantly by the kidney, has low lipid solubility, and is associated with a lower risk of central nervous system side effects such as depression. The effectiveness of beta blockers is assessed most accurately by monitoring the HVPG; this approach is not widely used in clinical practice. The usual method of monitoring the efficacy of beta blockers is to observe a decrease in the heart rate, which is a measure of β_1-adrenergic receptor blockade. Despite adequate β_1-adrenergic receptor blockade, however, some patients might benefit from a further increase in the dose of beta blocker, to increase the degree of β_2-adrenergic blockade. Raising the dose, however, results in more side effects and the likelihood that treatment will need to be withdrawn.[146] The addition of isosorbide mononitrate to beta blockers may result in a further decrease in portal pressure.

Nitrates

Short-acting (nitroglycerin) or long-acting (isosorbide mononitrates) nitrates result in vasodilatation. The vasodilatation results from a decrease in intracellular calcium in vascular smooth muscle cells. Nitrates cause venodilatation, rather than arterial dilatation, and decrease portal pressure predominantly by decreasing portal venous blood flow. The effect on intrahepatic resistance is less impressive than has been generally believed. Nitroglycerin has been used in combination with vasopressin to control acute variceal bleeding. The rate of infusion of nitroglycerin is 50 to 400 μg per minute, provided that the systolic blood pressure is greater than 90 mm Hg. However, the combination of vasopressin and nitroglycerin is seldom used nowadays. Nitrates are no longer recommended, either alone or in combination with a beta blocker, for primary prophylaxis to prevent first variceal bleeds. For secondary prophylaxis (to prevent variceal rebleeding), isosorbide mononitrate may be added to a beta blocker if the beta blocker alone has not resulted in an appropriate decrease in HVPG. In clinical practice, it is unusual for patients to tolerate nitrates for any length of time because of side effects, especially hypotension and headaches.

Drugs that Decrease Intrahepatic Vascular Resistance

The ideal agent for treatment of portal hypertension would be a drug that decreases intrahepatic vascular resistance. Unfortunately, such a drug is not currently available. A desirable drug would be one that selectively decreases intrahepatic vascular resistance without worsening systemic vasodilatation. Agents that may decrease intrahepatic resistance include α_1-adrenergic blockers such as prazosin,[147] but long-term administration of prazosin causes worsening of the systemic hyperdynamic circulation associated with portal hypertension and consequent sodium retention and ascites.[147] The addition of propranolol to prazosin may ameliorate the adverse affects of prazosin on the systemic circulation. Losartan, an angiotensin II receptor type I antagonist, causes a reduction in portal pressure without significant effects on the systemic circulation.[148] In randomized controlled trials of either losartan or another angiotensin II receptor antagonist, irbesartan, portal pressure was not reduced significantly, however. In fact, renal function has worsened in patients given losartan or irbesartan.[149,150] Endothelin receptor blockers and liver-selective NO donors are promising investigational agents for therapies that target intrahepatic vascular resistance.[16]

ENDOSCOPIC THERAPY

Endoscopic therapy is the only treatment modality that is widely accepted for the prevention of variceal bleeding, control of acute variceal bleeding, and prevention of variceal rebleeding. Endoscopic variceal therapy includes variceal sclerotherapy and band ligation.

Sclerotherapy

Endoscopic sclerotherapy has largely been supplanted by endoscopic band ligation, except when poor visualization precludes effective band ligation of bleeding varices. Available evidence does not support emergency sclerotherapy as first-line treatment of variceal bleeding[151] (Table 87–3). The technique involves injection of a sclerosant into (intravariceal) or adjacent to (paravariceal) a varix. Some paravariceal injection usually takes place during attempted intravariceal therapy. The sclerosants used include sodium tetradecyl sulfate, sodium morrhuate, ethanolamine oleate, and absolute alcohol; the choice of a sclerosant is based on availability, rather than on superior efficacy of one agent over another.

Complications of endoscopic sclerotherapy may arise during or after the procedure. During injection, the

Table 87–3   Complications of Endoscopic Variceal Therapy*

During Procedure
Retrosternal chest pain
Aspiration pneumonia
Following Procedure
Local ulcers
Bleeding
Stricture
Dysmotility
Perforation
Mediastinitis
Systemic (Usually with Sclerotherapy)
Sepsis
Pulmonary embolism
Mesenteric venous thrombosis

*Sclerotherapy and band ligation.

patient may experience some degree of retrosternal discomfort, which may persist postoperatively. More serious complications include sclerosant-induced esophageal ulcer-related bleeding, strictures, and perforation. The risk of ulcers caused by sclerotherapy may be reduced by prescribing sucralfate to the patient after sclerotherapy.

Variceal Ligation

Endoscopic variceal ligation is the preferred endoscopic modality for control of acute esophageal variceal bleeding and prevention of rebleeding; however, the utility of band ligation in the treatment of gastric varices is limited. Variceal ligation is simpler to perform than injection sclerotherapy. The procedure involves suctioning of the varix into the channel of an endoscope and deploying a band around the varix. The band strangulates the varix, thereby causing thrombosis. Multi-band devices can be used to apply several bands without requiring withdrawal and reinsertion of the endoscope. Varices at the gastroesophageal junction are banded initially, and then more proximal varices are banded in a spiral manner in intervals of approximately every 2 cm; the endoscope is then withdrawn. Varices in the mid- or proximal esophagus do not need to be banded. Endoscopic variceal ligation is associated with fewer complications than sclerotherapy and requires fewer sessions to achieve variceal obliteration. Moreover, esophageal variceal ligation during an acute bleed is not associated with a sustained elevation in HVPG, as occurs with sclerotherapy.[152]

Endoscopic variceal ligation can cause local complications, including esophageal ulcers (Fig. 87–7), strictures, and dysmotility, albeit less frequently than does sclerotherapy. Banding-induced ulcers can be large and potentially serious if gastric fundal varices are banded. Now that overtubes are no longer used to facilitate repeated insertion of the endoscope during a banding session, the mechanical complications seen in the past (mucosal tears and esophageal perforations) are uncommon.

TRANSJUGULAR INTRAHEPATIC PORTOSYSTEMIC SHUNTS

A *transjugular intrahepatic portosystemic shunt* (TIPS)—also referred to as a *transjugular intrahepatic portosystemic stent shunt* (TIPSS)—reduces elevated portal pressure by creating a communication between the hepatic vein and an intrahepatic branch of the portal vein. A percutaneous transjugular approach is used to insert the shunt. A TIPS functions as a side-to-side portacaval shunt and has been used to treat complications of portal hypertension, mainly variceal bleeding and refractory ascites, as well as Budd-Chiari syndrome, hepatic hydrothorax, and hepatorenal syndrome. A TIPS can be placed by an interventional radiologist, with a mortality rate less than 1% to 2%. TIPS placement usually is carried out with the patient under sedation. A platelet count greater than $60 \times 10^3/\mu L$ and an acceptable prothrombin time as reflected by an international normalized ratio (INR) less than 1.4 usually are recommended but are not essential in an emergency. Broad-spectrum antibiotic coverage is recommended when TIPS placement is carried out in patients with primary sclerosing cholangitis and as an emergency procedure.

For this procedure, the hepatic vein is cannulated through a transjugular approach, and using a Rosch needle, the portal vein is cannulated. A guidewire is then passed to connect the hepatic vein and a branch of the portal vein. Following dilation of the tract, a stent is placed and dilated as required to reduce the portacaval pressure gradient (the pressure difference between the portal vein and the inferior vena cava at the confluence of the hepatic vein) to below 12 mm Hg (Fig. 87–8). Whether a lesser reduction of portacaval pressure gradient, to only 15 mm Hg or so (instead of 12 mm Hg), could be associated with reduced bleeding but a lower frequency of hepatic encephalopathy requires further study.

The stents most commonly used for a TIPS are the Wallstent and the Palmaz stent. A coated stent has become available (Viatorr, from Gore, Flagstaff, Arizona). This stent has an uncoated portion that anchors the stent to the portal vein and a polytetrafluoroethylene-coated portion that lines the tract in the liver parenchyma and the draining hepatic vein. The frequency of shunt stenosis is reduced when coated stents are used instead of uncoated stents.[153]

A TIPS can be placed successfully by an experienced operator in greater than 95% of cases. Complications following the procedure are classified as procedure related, early (occurring before 30 days), or late (after 30 days) (Table 87–4). The prevention and treatment of procedure-

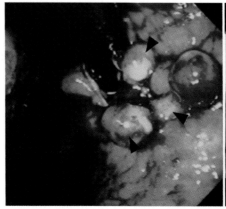
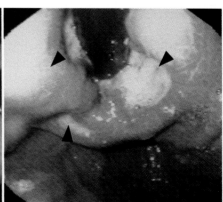

Figure 87–7 Endoscopic view of variceal ligation–related ulcers. *A,* The gastroesophageal junction is seen on a retroflexed view following ligation of multiple gastric varices *(arrowheads),* which resemble polyps. *B,* Upper endoscopy in the same patient 4 weeks later demonstrates multiple ulcers at the sites of prior ligation *(arrowheads).*

A   B

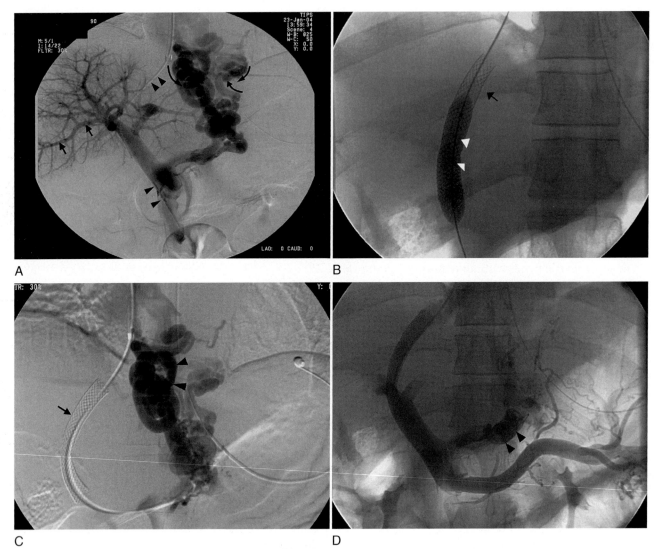

Figure 87–8 Creation of a transjugular intrahepatic portosystemic shunt (TIPS). *A,* Portogram with a catheter in the portal venous system *(arrowheads).* The portal venous system is clearly outlined *(straight arrows).* Gastroesophageal collaterals are also demonstrated *(curved arrows). B,* A stent *(arrow)* has been placed to bridge the hepatic vein and the portal vein. A balloon *(arrowheads)* is being used to dilate the parenchymal tract within the liver. *C,* Following expansion of the stent *(arrow),* injection into the portal vein demonstrates persistence of the gastroesophageal varices *(arrowheads). D,* Following embolization of the varices with steel coils *(arrowheads),* the intrahepatic portal vasculature is no longer demonstrated, indicative of hepatofugal flow of portal blood through the shunt.

related, early, and late post-TIPS complications are outlined in Table 87–5.

Portal Hypertension–Related Bleeding

The most common indication for placement of a TIPS is refractory variceal bleeding. TIPS has been used to control acute variceal bleeding and to prevent variceal rebleeding when pharmacologic and endoscopic therapies have failed, especially in patients with CTP class B or C cirrhosis, in whom bleeding is more likely to be refractory to therapy than that in patients with CTP class A cirrhosis. Refractory ascites and prevention of variceal rebleeding are the only indications for TIPS that have been subjected to controlled trials. When bleeding from varices cannot be controlled after two sessions of endoscopic therapy within a 24-hour period, TIPS placement is the

usual salvage treatment. TIPS also is used to treat bleeding from isolated gastric fundal varices, for both control of bleeding and prevention of rebleeding. A surgical portosystemic shunt may be preferred over a TIPS in patients with preserved synthetic liver function (CTP class A) in centers that have the surgical expertise.

TIPS has been effective in the management of uncontrolled esophageal variceal bleeding in patients with decompensated cirrhosis of the liver.[154] Hemorrhage is controlled in greater than 90% of patients, but the mortality rate in such patients is high—greater than 60% within 60 days. A similar outcome is observed in patients who undergo TIPS placement for refractory gastric variceal bleeding.[155]

Twelve randomized controlled trials have compared TIPS and endoscopic therapy (sclerotherapy or variceal ligation) or pharmacologic therapy (or both) for the pre-

Table 87–4   Complications of Transjugular Intrahepatic Portosystemic Shunt Placement*

Timing of Complication	Complication
Procedure-related (life-threatening)	Intraperitoneal hemorrhage
	Sepsis
	Cardiopulmonary failure
Early post-procedure (1–30 days)	
Major	Shunt thrombosis
	Stent migration
	Hepatic encephalopathy
	Progressive hepatic failure
	Pulmonary artery hypertension
Minor	Hematoma at puncture site
	Pain
	Cardiac arrhythmias
	Fever
	Reactions to contrast media
	Hemolytic anemia
Late post-procedure (>30 days)	Shunt stenosis
	Hepatic encephalopathy
	Portal vein thrombosis
	Progressive hepatic failure

*Modified from Kamath PS, McKusick M: Transjugular portosystemic shunt (TIPS). Bailleres Clin Gastroenterol 11:327, 1997.

vention of recurrent esophageal variceal bleeding. In a meta-analysis of studies that compared TIPS with endoscopic therapy, the rate of rebleeding was reduced by TIPS, but the frequency of encephalopathy was increased, and no effect on survival was observed.[156] Therefore, TIPS cannot be recommended as a first choice of treatment for preventing variceal rebleeding; rather, it is reserved for patients who have failed endoscopic or pharmacologic therapy.

Follow-up Evaluation

The frequency of stenosis of a TIPS is high, ranging from 20% to 78%, depending on the surveillance technique used and definition of stenosis. Neither the optimal interval nor the most cost-effective method of surveillance for TIPS stenosis has been determined. Doppler ultrasound evaluation generally is used to identify TIPS stenosis, but the negative predictive value of this approach is low and the positive predictive value is only acceptable. The best indicator that the shunt has stenosed is recurrence of the problem that necessitated the TIPS. The only certain method of demonstrating shunt patency is by means of a TIPS venogram and measurement of the portacaval pressure gradient. An increase in the gradient to greater than 12 mm Hg warrants dilation of the stent or placement of an additional stent.

Table 87–5   Prevention and Treatment of Transjugular Intrahepatic Portosystemic Shunt–Related Complications*

Complication	Prevention	Treatment
Inadvertent carotid artery puncture during jugular vein access	Perform with ultrasound visualization to guide venous access	Manual compression of carotid puncture site to prevent hematoma
Hepatic capsular laceration during portal vein access	Avoid atrophic lobes and limit needle passes to 3-4 cm of excursion	Usually requires no treatment
		For severe hemorrhage, transfuse with blood products until stable; obtain abdominal CT scan and surgical consultation
Extrahepatic puncture of portal venous system	Delineate bifurcation of portal vein on preprocedure CT scan	Leave catheter in place for portogram; use as a guide for intrahepatic portal vein puncture
		Work quickly to establish a functioning shunt; then remove the errant catheter
Intrahepatic arterial or biliary puncture	Work centrally within the liver	Usually no treatment is required; remove the catheter and continue
		If a fistula develops, embolize the arterial feeder with steel coils
Sepsis after shunt placement	Give prophylactic antibiotics	Broad-spectrum antibiotic coverage
	Adhere to strict sterile technique	
Early shunt thrombosis	Avoid sharp angles when placing the stent	Shunt venogram and clot lysis using tPA delivered by pulse-spray technique
	Ends should not abut against the intima of the vein	Extend the shunt to ensure stent coverage of the intrahepatic tract and to ensure adequate length in both hepatic and portal veins
Uncontrollable encephalopathy after shunt placement	Use narrow shunts in high-risk patients	Reduce the diameter of the shunt with additional concentrically placed stents
		Embolize the shunt with steel coils
Shunt stenosis	Use wider or covered stents	Dilation or atherectomy of the shunt
	Avoid bile duct injury	Placement of an additional stent if necessary
Post-shunt liver failure	Avoid procedure in patients with a MELD score ≥24	Consider early liver transplantation

CT, computed tomography; MELD, Model for End-State Liver Disease; tPA, tissue plasminogen activator.
*Modified from Kamath PS, McKusick M: Transjugular portosystemic shunt (TIPS). Bailleres Clin Gastroenterol 11:327, 1997.

Selection of Patients

Because the presence of a TIPS may worsen liver function by depriving the liver of portal venous blood, thereby increasing the risk of hepatic encephalopathy, with decreased survival in some patients, the procedure should be used selectively. Various studies have reported mortality rates of up to 60% at 3 months in patients who have undergone TIPS placement when endoscopic and pharmacologic treatment have failed to control acute bleeding. Emergency TIPS is clearly associated with high mortality rates.[157,158] In patients in whom TIPS placement has been carried out to prevent variceal rebleeding, 30-day mortality rates are as high as 44%. Factors associated with a poor prognosis include a serum alanine aminotransferase (ALT) level greater than 100 U/L, serum bilirubin level greater than 3 mg/dL, and pre-TIPS hepatic encephalopathy unrelated to bleeding.[158] Patients with a high CTP (Table 87–6) score also have reduced survival. The CTP classification has some limitations, however: For one thing, it does not discriminate survival well among patients within each CTP class. Furthermore, some parameters that make up the CTP score, such as ascites and encephalopathy, are assessed by subjective interpretation. The need for a more accurate method to assess survival in patients undergoing TIPS has led to creation of a new tool to predict survival, the Model for End-Stage Liver Disease (MELD) (see http://www.mayoclinic.org/gi-rst/mayomodel6.html).[157] With data from four centers within the United States, this mathematical model originally was composed of the serum creatinine level, INR as a measure of the prothrombin time, serum bilirubin level, and etiology of liver disease. Subsequently, the MELD formula was modified to include only the first three parameters (creatinine, INR, and bilirubin).[159] The MELD has been widely validated for predicting survival in patients with cirrhosis, including patients who have undergone TIPS placement, and is more accurate for this purpose than the CTP classification.

Patients with a MELD score of 14 or less have an excellent survival rate after TIPS placement; therefore, this procedure may be carried out routinely in such patients when indicated. Patients with a MELD score higher than 24 have reduced survival following TIPS placement, with a mortality rate approaching 30% at 3 months. Because these patients are at high priority for liver transplantation, TIPS should be avoided unless needed to control acute variceal bleeding. In the intermediate group with MELD scores ranging from 15 to 24, TIPS placement can be carried out depending on the patient's preference and the physician's judgment and taking into consideration the likelihood of liver transplantation. This approach has been validated independently.[160]

SURGERY

Surgical treatment of portal hypertension falls into three groups: non-shunt procedures, portosystemic shunt procedures, and liver transplantation. Surgical procedures are used as salvage therapy when standard management with pharmacologic and endoscopic therapy fails in patients with CTP class A cirrhosis. Surgical treatment also may be considered early in the course of portal hypertension in patients who live at a great distance from centers that can manage variceal bleeding adequately or in whom cross-matching blood products (in case of bleeding) is difficult. How failure of standard therapy is defined will depend on the specific circumstances of the patient's presentation, availability of surgical expertise, and, outcome of conservative management.

Liver transplantation should be considered in all patients with variceal bleeding who meet minimal listing criteria for liver transplantation (currently, a CTP score of 7 or greater). Selection and prioritization of patients for liver transplantation are discussed in Chapter 92.

Non-Shunt Procedures

Non-shunt procedures include esophageal transection and gastroesophageal devascularization. They are performed infrequently but may be required in selected cases.

Esophageal Transection

Esophageal transection, in which the esophagus is stapled and transected, is highly effective in controlling variceal bleeding and is associated with a lower risk of encephalopathy than that for portosystemic shunts. Esophageal transection was considered in the past when two sessions of endoscopic therapy had failed to control variceal bleeding within a 24-hour period.[161] Mortality rates are not improved over those observed with endoscopic sclerotherapy, however. With the advent of TIPS, esophageal staple transection is now seldom used. Transection is especially not recommended if the patient is a candidate for liver transplantation, because of the resulting increased risk of operative morbidity at transplantation.

Devascularization Procedures

Devascularization procedures typically have been used to prevent recurrent variceal bleeding in patients with extensive splenic and portal vein thrombosis when a suitable vein is not available for creation of a portosystemic shunt.[162] In the original operation described by Sugiura and Futagawa, both a thoracotomy and a laparotomy were carried out.[163] Subsequently, the operation has been

Table 87–6 Child-Turcotte-Pugh Classification

Parameter	Numerical Score		
	1	*2*	*3*
Ascites	None	Slight	Moderate/severe
Encephalopathy	None	Slight/moderate	Moderate/severe
Bilirubin (mg/dL)	<2.0	2-3	>3.0
Albumin (g/dL)	>3.5	2.8-3.5	<2.8
Prothrombin time (seconds increased)	1-3	4-6	>6.0

Total Numerical Score	Child-Turcotte-Pugh Class
5-6	A
7-9	B
10-15	C

carried out through an abdominal approach and combined with a splenectomy. The procedure consists of total devascularization of the greater curvature of the stomach combined with devascularization of the upper two thirds of the lesser curvature of the stomach and circumferential devascularization of the lower 7.5 cm of the esophagus.

The rate of recurrent bleeding following this procedure is variable but may be as high as 40%, depending on the population being treated and duration of follow-up.

Portosystemic Shunts

With the increasing availability of TIPS, the use of surgical shunts for refractory variceal bleeding has declined markedly. Surgical portosystemic shunts are categorized as *selective shunts* such as distal splenorenal shunts, *partial shunts* such as the side-to-side calibrated portacaval shunt, and *total portosystemic shunts* such as the side-to-side portacaval shunt or end-to-side portacaval shunt.

Selective Shunts

The most widely used selective shunt is the distal splenorenal shunt, originally described by Warren and colleagues.[164] With this shunt, only varices at the gastroesophageal junction and spleen are decompressed, and

portal hypertension is maintained in the superior mesenteric vein and portal vein; therefore, variceal bleeding is controlled, but ascites persists. The shunt procedure involves a portal-azygous disconnection and subsequent anastomosis between the splenic vein and left renal vein in an end-to-side fashion (Fig. 87–9). The entire length of the pancreas must be mobilized, and the left adrenal vein ligated. The distal splenorenal shunt has been associated with control of variceal bleeding in approximately 90% of patients and a lower rate of hepatic encephalopathy than that reported for total shunts.[165]

Partial Portosystemic Shunts

A partial portosystemic shunt is carried out using a synthetic interposition graft between the portal vein and the inferior vena cava. When the shunt diameter is 8 mm, portal pressure is reduced below 12 mm Hg, and antegrade flow to the liver is maintained in most patients.[166] Rates of preventing variceal rebleeding and encephalopathy following the shunt are similar to those seen with a distal splenorenal shunt. As in patients who have had a distal splenorenal shunt, ascites may occur in approximately 20% of patients who have had a partial portosystemic shunt because hepatic sinusoidal pressure is not reduced.[167]

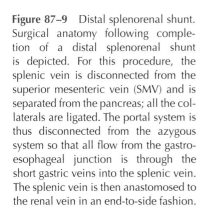

Figure 87–9 Distal splenorenal shunt. Surgical anatomy following completion of a distal splenorenal shunt is depicted. For this procedure, the splenic vein is disconnected from the superior mesenteric vein (SMV) and is separated from the pancreas; all the collaterals are ligated. The portal system is thus disconnected from the azygous system so that all flow from the gastroesophageal junction is through the short gastric veins into the splenic vein. The splenic vein is then anastomosed to the renal vein in an end-to-side fashion.

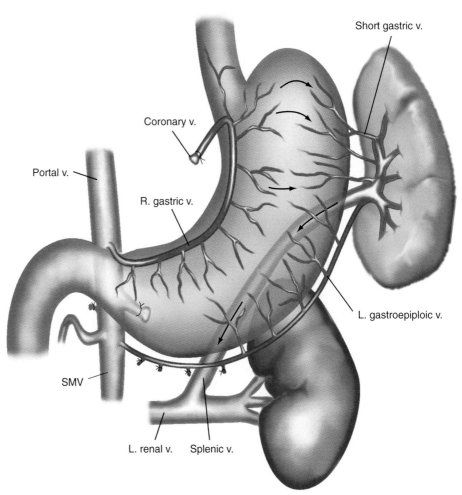

Portacaval Shunts

End-to-side and side-to-side portacaval shunts have been described, but nowadays only the side-to-side portacaval shunt is in common use.[168] Any portacaval shunt that is greater than 12 mm in diameter is likely to result in a total shunt. An interposition graft with a diameter less than 12 mm may be placed, or a direct vein-to-vein anastomosis may be constructed. Variceal bleeding, as well as ascites, is well controlled because the hepatic sinusoids are decompressed. Variceal rebleeding following a total shunt is seen in less than 10% of patients, but hepatic encephalopathy occurs in 30% to 40% of patients.[169] Liver transplantation in patients who have had a portacaval shunt is associated with increased operative morbidity and intraoperative transfusion requirements. The outcome of liver transplantation is not otherwise significantly different, however, from that for patients who have not had a portacaval shunt. Nonetheless, portacaval shunts should be avoided in patients who are potential candidates for liver transplantation.

MANAGEMENT OF SPECIFIC LESIONS

ESOPHAGEAL VARICES

Natural History

Esophageal varices are present in approximately 40% of patients with cirrhosis and in up to 60% of patients with cirrhosis and ascites.[170] In cirrhotic patients who do not have esophageal varices at initial endoscopy, new varices will develop at a rate of approximately 5% per year. In patients with small varices at initial endoscopy, progression to large varices occurs at a rate of 10% to 15% per year and is related predominantly to the degree of liver dysfunction.[171] On the other hand, improvement in liver function in patients with alcoholic liver disease who abstain from alcohol is associated with a decreased risk, and sometimes even disappearance, of varices.[172]

Up to 25% of patients with newly diagnosed varices will bleed at 2 years.[171] The best clinical predictor of bleeding appears to be variceal size: The risk of bleeding in patients with varices less than 5 mm in diameter is 7% at 2 years, and the risk in patients with varices greater than 5 mm in diameter is 30% at 2 years.[171] Even more important, however, is the HVPG, because the risk of bleeding is virtually absent when the HVPG is below 12 mm Hg.[173] Nevertheless, measurement of HVPG is not routinely performed in clinical practice to assess bleeding risk.

The prognosis for variceal bleeding in patients with cirrhosis has improved since the 1980s. Initial treatment is associated with cessation of bleeding in approximately 90% of patients.[171,174] Approximately one half of patients with a variceal bleed stop bleeding spontaneously, because hypovolemia leads to splanchnic vasoconstriction, which results in a decrease in portal pressure. Excessive transfusions may, in fact, increase the chance of rebleeding.[175] Active bleeding at endoscopy, a lower initial hematocrit level, higher serum aminotransferase levels, CPT class, bacterial infection, an HVPG greater than 20 mm Hg, and portal vein thrombosis are associated with failure to control bleeding at 5 days.[174,176-178] Of patients who have stopped bleeding, approximately one third will rebleed within the next 6 weeks. Of all rebleeding episodes, approximately 40% will take place within 5 days of the initial bleed.[179] Predictors of rebleeding include active bleeding at emergency endoscopy, bleeding from gastric varices, hypoalbuminemia, renal insufficiency, and an HVPG greater than 20 mm Hg.[171] The risk of death with acute variceal bleeding is 5% to 8% at 1 week and 20% to 30% at 6 weeks.[171] Patients who rebled early, or those in whom renal failure develops, have the highest risk of death. Alcohol as the cause of cirrhosis, a higher serum bilirubin level, a lower serum albumin level, hepatic encephalopathy, and hepatocellular carcinoma are additional factors associated with an increased 6-week mortality rate.

Treatment of esophageal variceal bleeding is classified as either primary prophylaxis, that is, prevention of variceal hemorrhage in patients who have never bled; control of acute variceal bleeding; or secondary prevention of rebleeding in patients who have survived an initial bleeding episode. Effective treatments to prevent the development of varices and ascites in patients with cirrhosis are not yet available, although beta blockers may slow enlargement of small varices into large varices.

Prevention of Bleeding

Available data suggest that all patients with large varices (diameter greater than 5 mm) should receive prophylactic therapy ("primary prophylaxis") to prevent variceal bleeding. The presence of additional endoscopic signs such as red wales does not influence the decision regarding prophylactic therapy. Twelve trials have addressed the use of nonselective beta blockers for primary prophylaxis of variceal bleeding and have demonstrated a decrease in the risk of variceal bleeding from 25% in patients in the control group to 15% in patients taking beta blockers. The absolute risk reduction is thus approximately 10%, and the number needed to treat to prevent one variceal bleed is approximately 10 patients. The mortality rate is reduced from 28.4% in control patients to 23.9% in patients taking beta blockers; the absolute risk reduction is 4.5%. The number of patients needed to be treated to prevent one death is approximately 22. In patients who do not bleed during therapy and who do not experience side effects, treatment should be continued indefinitely, because withdrawal of beta blockers can result in an increased risk of bleeding.[180]

The side effects of treatment probably are overemphasized, because only approximately 15% of patients need to discontinue treatment.[181] A baseline heart rate and blood pressure recording will help determine whether a patient is a candidate for pharmacologic treatment with beta blockers. A resting heart rate of less than 55 to 60 beats per minute or a systolic blood pressure less than 90 mm Hg indicates that the patient is likely to be intolerant of beta blockers. In other patients, HVPG ideally should be measured at baseline (Fig. 87–10). Either a long-acting preparation of propranolol or nadolol may be started; the usual starting dose of long-acting propranolol is 60 mg once daily and that of nadolol is 20 mg once daily. Because the risk of bleeding is greatest at

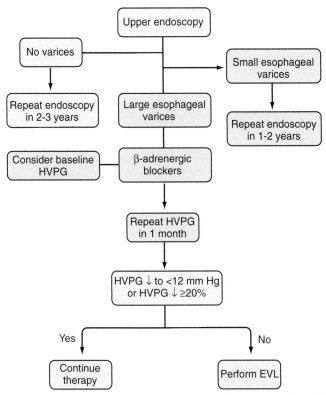

Figure 87–10 Algorithm for primary prophylaxis of esophageal variceal hemorrhage. EVL, endoscopic variceal ligation; HVPG, hepatic venous pressure gradient.

night, the beta blocker should probably be administered in the evening.[104] The dose of propranolol or nadolol can be increased gradually every 3 to 5 days until the target heart rate of 25% below baseline or 55 to 60 beats per minute is reached, provided that the systolic blood pressure remains above 90 mm Hg. The daily dose of long-acting propranolol or nadolol required to reach the target heart rate ranges from 40 to 160 mg. Patients with a decrease in systolic blood pressure below 90 mm Hg are most likely to experience side effects.

In patients on pharmacologic therapy, follow-up endoscopy is unnecessary unless gastrointestinal bleeding occurs. Once the target heart rate is reached, however, a repeat HVPG measurement is recommended within 1 to 3 months, preferably as close to 1 month as possible. In patients in whom the HVPG has decreased to less than 12 mm Hg, the risk of bleeding is virtually eliminated. Patients in whom the HVPG decreases by at least 20% have a risk of variceal bleeding of less than 10%. Unfortunately, only 30% to 40% of patients respond to beta blockers; those with better liver function show the best response.[182] In patients who are intolerant of or have contraindications to beta blockers, isosorbide mononitrate has been tried but is no better than placebo in preventing variceal bleeding.[183] In these patients, endoscopic prophylaxis should be pursued.

Endoscopic Therapy to Prevent a First Variceal Bleed

Prophylactic sclerotherapy for the prevention of variceal bleeding has been studied extensively but cannot be rec-

ommended.[184] The preferred method of endoscopic treatment is variceal band ligation. Variceal band ligation has been compared with no treatment in five trials. A meta-analysis of these studies demonstrates that, as compared with no treatment, endoscopic variceal ligation decreases both the risk of first bleeding and the mortality rate.[185] Patients who do not achieve a decrease in the HVPG to less than 12 mm Hg, or of greater than 20%, on beta blockers may not respond well to endoscopic variceal ligation either.[186] Eight trials have compared endoscopic variceal ligation with beta blockers,[187] and a meta-analysis has shown no difference between endoscopic band ligation and nonselective blocker therapy for either risk of bleeding or mortality rate.[95] A subsequent larger study came to the same conclusion.[188] Therefore, current evidence does not support endoscopic variceal ligation as the preferred method of primary prophylaxis against variceal bleeding. Moreover, beta blockers are cheaper and more convenient to use and may potentially reduce the risk of bleeding from gastric varices and portal hypertensive gastropathy. Band ligation is the only option for patients with high-risk varices who have contraindications to beta blockers or who have not responded to or are intolerant of beta blockers. Combined use of propranolol and endoscopic variceal ligation to prevent primary prophylaxis is under study.

Control of Acute Bleeding

Acute esophageal variceal bleeding constitutes a life-threatening emergency and requires management by a well-trained team of hepatologists, endoscopists, intensive care personnel, radiologists, and surgeons. Treatment is aimed at resuscitating the patient, controlling the bleed, and preventing complications (see Chapter 13). Two large-bore intravenous access lines should be inserted immediately. Red blood cells should be transfused with the goal of maintaining the hematocrit value between 25% and 30%. Intravenous normal saline may be infused until the red blood cells are available for transfusion. In patients with active bleeding, the airway needs to be protected, and endotracheal intubation is advised. Antibiotics should be initiated in all patients to prevent bacteremia and spontaneous bacterial peritonitis. Norfloxacin, 400 mg orally twice daily for 7 days, is the preferred choice.[189] When oral intake is not possible, ciprofloxacin, 400 mg intravenously every 12 hours, or levofloxacin, 500 mg intravenously every 24 hours for 7 days, is recommended.

A combination of endoscopic therapy and pharmacologic therapy of variceal bleeding may be superior to pharmacologic treatment alone. Pharmacologic agents should be started as early as possible; in some centers, they are started while the patient is being transferred by ambulance to the hospital. Somatostatin, octreotide, terlipressin, and vasopressin plus nitroglycerin are the options for pharmacologic therapy. The specific agent chosen depends on availability and physician preference. In the United States, octreotide is the agent most commonly used. Terlipressin is the first choice in many other countries because it is the only drug that has been associated with improved survival.[190] Pharmacologic treatment should be continued for up to 5 days to prevent early rebleeding.

Endoscopic therapy is carried out as soon as the patient is hemodynamically stabilized. At upper endoscopy, bleeding from esophageal varices is diagnosed if active bleeding from the varices is seen; if signs of recent hemorrhage, such as a white fibrin plug or a red blood clot over a varix, are present; if varices with risk signs for bleeding, such as a cherry-red spot, hematocystic spot, or red wale sign, are seen; or if esophageal varices are seen in the absence of any other lesion that could give rise to gastrointestinal bleeding. Endoscopic treatment is recommended at the time of initial endoscopy, and endoscopic variceal ligation is the preferred method.

At upper endoscopy, the actively bleeding varix is ligated (Fig. 87–11). Ligation initially should be at or immediately below the bleeding site. Other large varices also should be banded during the same session. If active bleeding is not seen, ligation should be carried out beginning with varices at the gastroesophageal junction and proceeding proximally at intervals of 2 cm in a spiral fashion. If bleeding obscures the varices, then multiple bands are placed at the gastroesophageal junction cir-

cumferentially until bleeding can be controlled, but the long-term risks of esophageal stricture are increased in such patients. Bleeding can be controlled in up to 90% of patients with a combination of pharmacologic and endoscopic treatment.

Bleeding cannot be controlled in approximately 10% of patients, as defined by any of the following three factors: (1) transfusion of four units of red blood cells or more to maintain the hematocrit value between 25% and 30%; (2) inability to increase the systolic blood pressure by 20 mm Hg or to greater than 70 mm Hg; or (3) persistence of a heart rate greater than 100 beats per minute.[191] *Rebleeding* is defined as recurrence of bleeding after initial control for 24 hours during which the vital signs and hemoglobin level are stable. When two sessions of endoscopic treatment within a 24-hour period have failed to control variceal bleeding, salvage therapies such as TIPS placment should be carried out (Fig. 87–12), although the mortality rate in this group of patients is high. Surgical portosystemic shunts, although extremely effective in controlling variceal bleeding, have largely

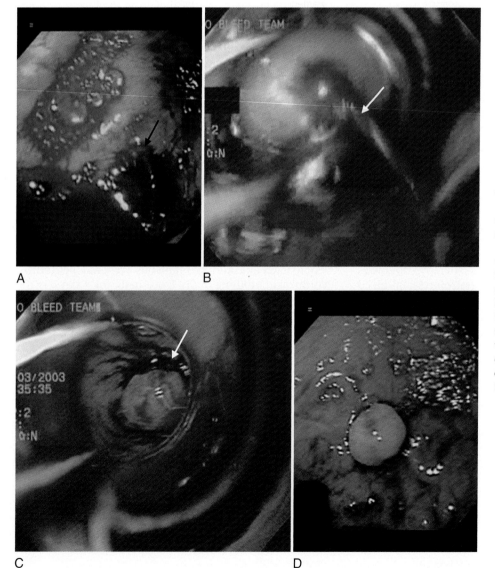

A

B

C

D

Figure 87–11 Band ligation for control of esophageal variceal bleeding. *A,* On upper endoscopy, an actively bleeding varix can be seen at the lower end of the esophagus *(arrow). B,* With the variceal banding device in position, the varix is suctioned into the device at the site of active bleeding *(arrow). C,* After the band is in place *(arrow)* and the varix has been ligated, the bleeding has stopped. *D,* Visualization of the varix with the band in place with complete control of bleeding. (Images courtesy of Dr. Louis M. Wong Kee Song, Rochester, Minn.)

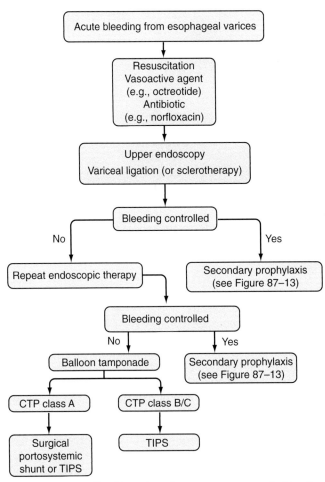

Figure 87–12 Algorithm for the management of bleeding esophageal varices. CTP, Child-Turcotte-Pugh; TIPS, transjugular intrahepatic portosystemic shunt.

been abandoned because of high mortality rates. Balloon tamponade sometimes is used to stabilize the patient until definitive treatment can be carried out.

Prevention of Rebleeding

All patients who have had a variceal bleed should receive prophylactic therapy ("secondary prophylaxis") to reduce the risk of rebleeding, which otherwise occurs in up to 80% of patients at 2 years. Patients with a CTP score of 7 or greater also should be evaluated for liver transplantation. Options for preventing variceal rebleeding are pharmacologic therapy, endoscopic therapy, and portosystemic shunts (either surgical or radiologic), or combinations of these therapies.

Therapy with nonselective beta blockers is the preferred treatment, and either long-acting propranolol or nadolol may be used. Ideally, the hemodynamic response to beta blockers should be monitored with the goal of reducing the HVPG by greater than 20% or to less than 12 mm Hg. If these goals are not achieved, isosorbide mononitrate may be added. The extended-release form of isosorbide mononitrate is preferred, with an initial starting dose of 30 mg per day. Unfortunately, it is unusual for patients in our practice to tolerate nitrates after they have achieved beta blockade. Hypotension and headaches are the usual reasons for discontinuing isosorbide mononitrate.

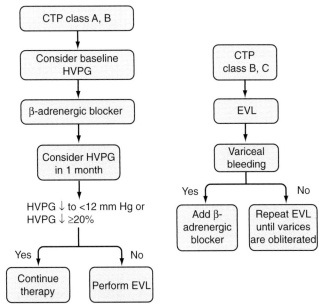

Figure 87–13 Algorithm for the prevention of recurrent variceal bleeding (secondary prophylaxis). CTP, Child-Turcotte-Pugh; EVL, endoscopic variceal ligation; HVPG, hepatic venous pressure gradient.

Endoscopic variceal ligation also may be performed to prevent variceal rebleeding, especially in patients who have poor liver function (Fig. 87–13). In practice, the first endoscopic session is carried out 7 to 14 days after the initial variceal ligation to control bleeding. Endoscopic therapy is then repeated at 3- to 4-week intervals; this approach has been suggested because bands might still be in place if variceal ligation is done earlier. A combination of variceal ligation and pharmacologic treatment is more effective than either variceal ligation or pharmacologic therapy alone. If the HVPG is monitored, however, a reduction in HVPG to less than 12 mm Hg or by greater than 20% should obviate the need for variceal ligation. For patients who bleed during pharmacologic treatment, variceal ligation should be carried out. Conversely, for patients who have undergone variceal ligation and experience recurrent bleeding, beta blockers should be started. Patients who have a variceal rebleed despite receiving optimal pharmacologic and endoscopic treatment require a portosystemic shunt, usually a distal splenorenal shunt in patients with CTP class A cirrhosis and a TIPS in all other patients.

GASTRIC VARICES

The most widely used classification of gastric varices is the Sarin classification.[192] According to this classification, type 1 gastroesophageal varices (GOV1) extend 2 to 5 cm below the gastroesophageal junction and are in continuity with esophageal varices; type 2 gastroesophageal varices (GOV2) are in the fundus of the stomach and in continuity with esophageal varices; varices that occur in the fundus of the stomach in the absence of esophageal varices are called isolated gastric varices type 1 (IGV1), whereas varices that occur in the gastric body, antrum, or pylorus are called isolated gastric varices type 2 (IGV2).

Approximately 25% of patients with portal hypertension have gastric varices, most commonly GOV1, which comprise approximately 70% of all gastric varices. Intrahepatic causes of portal hypertension may be associated with both GOV1 and GOV2. Splenic vein thrombosis usually results in IGV1, but the most common cause of fundal gastric varices may be cirrhosis.

Natural History

Gastric varices typically occur in association with more advanced portal hypertension. Bleeding is thought to be more common in patients with GOV2 and IGV1 than in those with other types of gastric varices; in other words, bleeding is more common from fundal varices than from varices at the gastroesophageal junction. Whereas intraesophageal pressure is negative, intra-abdominal pressure is positive, and the transmural pressure gradient across gastric varices is smaller than that across esophageal varices. Gastric varices, however, tend to be larger in diameter than esophageal varices. Gastric varices are supported by gastric mucosa, whereas esophageal varices tend to be unsupported in the lower third of the esophagus. Therefore, gastric varices are likely to bleed only when they are large, as demonstrated in a study in which larger gastric varices (greater than 5 to 10 mm in diameter) were more likely to bleed than smaller ones.[193] Although gastric varices have been thought to bleed less frequently than esophageal varices, the bleeding rates probably are comparable if patients are matched for the severity of cirrhosis (CTP score).[192] In contrast with esophageal varices, bleeding from gastric varices has been described with an HVPG less than 12 mm Hg.[194,195] Gastric varices in continuity with esophageal varices may regress following treatment of the esophageal varices. When gastric varices persist despite obliteration of esophageal varices, the prognosis is poorer, probably because of the severity of liver disease.

Prevention of Bleeding

Unfortunately, no studies have evaluated pharmacologic or endoscopic treatment for primary prophylaxis of gastric variceal hemorrhage, and recommendations are based primarily on the guidelines for managing esophageal varices. Large gastric varices with red color signs, especially in patients with CTP class C liver disease, are most likely to bleed. Because these gastric varices usually are associated with esophageal varices, pharmacologic treatment with nonselective beta blockers may be initiated to prevent variceal hemorrhage. Neither endoscopic treatment nor TIPS is currently recommended for the primary prevention of gastric variceal bleeding.

Control of Acute Bleeding

The approach to treating esophageal variceal hemorrhage also applies to acute gastric variceal hemorrhage and includes volume resuscitation, avoidance of overtransfusion, and antibiotic prophylaxis with norfloxacin, 400 mg twice daily for 7 days. Upper endoscopy is carried out after patients have been volume resuscitated and stabilized and often following endotracheal intubation to protect the airway. The endoscopic diagnosis of gastric variceal bleeding may be difficult because of pooling

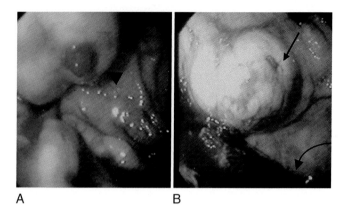

Figure 87–14 Gastric variceal bleeding. *A,* Active bleeding from a gastric varix *(arrowhead)* can be seen. *B,* Bleeding from the varix *(straight arrow)* is controlled following injection of sodium tetradecyl sulfate. Pooling of blood in the stomach is indicated by the *curved arrow.*

of blood in the fundus. A diagnosis of gastric variceal hemorrhage should be considered if bleeding is noted from a gastric varix (Fig. 87–14); blood is found to appear at either the gastroesophageal junction or the gastric fundus; blood is found in the stomach and gastric varices with a "white nipple sign" (indicating a fibrin-platelet plug) are noted in the absence of other causes of bleeding; and gastric varices are noted in the absence of other lesions in the esophagus and stomach.[196]

Because controlled studies evaluating pharmacologic therapy for gastric variceal bleeding are lacking, the agents used are based on extension of the data relating to esophageal varices. Medical management with vasoactive agents should be started as early as possible, preferably at least 30 minutes before endoscopic therapy is carried out. In the United States, octreotide is the vasoactive agent used most frequently in this setting, whereas in many other countries terlipressin is preferred. The preferred endoscopic therapy for gastric variceal bleeding is injection of polymers of cyanoacrylate, usually *N*-butyl-2-cyanoacrylate,[197,198] but these tissue adhesives are not currently available in the United States. Obliteration of the varices occurs when the injected cyanoacrylate adhesive hardens on contact with blood. The mucosa overlying the varix eventually sloughs, and the hardened polymer is extruded. Fortunately, the resulting ulcers occur late, and the risk of bleeding is lower than that associated with sclerotherapy-related ulcers. Cyanoacrylate injection has been found to be superior to both variceal band ligation and sclerotherapy using alcohol.[198] Complications of cyanoacrylate injection include bacteremia and variceal ulceration. Cerebral and pulmonary emboli have been reported on occasion, usually in patients with spontaneous large portosystemic or intrapulmonary shunts. The endoscope may be damaged by the glue, but the risk is minimized if silicone gel is used and suction is avoided for 15 to 20 seconds following injection.[199]

Injection can be carried out using an "end-on" endoscopic view for GOV1. For injection of GOV2 or IGV1, however, a retroflexed endoscopic approach is recommended. Sclerosants such as sodium tetradecyl sulfate, ethanolamine oleate, and sodium morrhuate are not particularly effective for control of gastric variceal bleeding.[200] When sclerotherapy is carried out for gastric varices, the volume of sclerosant required is larger than that used for esophageal varices, and fever and retrosternal pain are more common. It is much easier to obliterate GOV1 than GOV2 or IGV1. IGV1 are the most difficult gastric varices to obliterate and, when present, should prompt early consideration of definitive treatment such as portosystemic shunting.

Although some authors recommend ligation of gastric varices up to 20 mm in diameter,[201] this recommendation is not supported by our experience. Band ligation of varices greater than 10 mm in diameter usually is unsafe. Ligation is safest if the varices are in the cardia of the stomach. Because gastric fundal varices are covered by mucosa, drawing the entire varix into the ligation device is often not possible. Application of bands results in creation of a large ulcer on the varix, sometimes with disastrous results (see Fig. 87–8).

If endoscopic and pharmacologic therapy fail to control gastric variceal bleeding, then a Linton-Nachlas tube, which has a 600-mL balloon, may be passsed as a temporizing measure. The commonly used Minnesota tube and Sengstaken-Blakemore tube, with only 250-mL gastric balloons, are not as effective for controlling bleeding from gastric fundal varices as is the Linton-Nachlas tube.[202,203] Nevertheless, most patients in whom endoscopic and pharmacologic treatment fails to control gastric variceal bleeding will require a TIPS, which can control bleeding in greater than 90% of patients—a rate of efficacy equivalent to that for TIPS in controlling esophageal variceal bleeding[204,205] (Fig. 87–15).

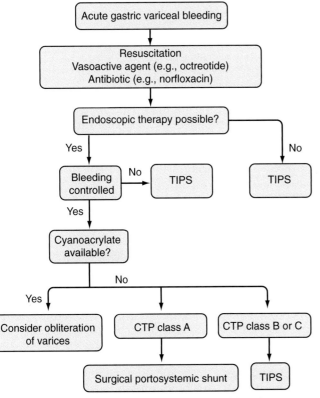

Figure 87–15 Algorithm for the management of bleeding gastric varices. CTP, Child-Turcotte-Pugh; TIPS, transjugular intrahepatic portosystemic shunt.

Prevention of Rebleeding

Endoscopic Therapy

In the absence of large, well-conducted trials, recommendations regarding pharmacologic or endoscopic therapy to prevent gastric variceal rebleeding are derived from retrospective studies. Cyanoacrylate glue has been used to prevent gastric variceal rebleeding, with favorable results.[206] In a small study, the 2-octyl-cyanoacrylate polymer (Dermabond) has been used to prevent gastric variceal rebleeding, with excellent results.[207] Patients require an average of two or three sessions for obturation of gastric varices with cyanoacrylate polymers. The procedure may be carried out under endoscopic ultrasonographic monitoring for greater safety and efficacy.[208]

Detachable snares have been used to ligate gastric varices that may be too large for band ligation.[209]

Transvenous Obliteration of Gastric Varices

Balloon-occluded retrograde transvenous obliteration of gastric fundal varices is carried out in patients with demonstrable splenorenal shunts. Such shunts can be demonstrated on multi-detector CT in a large number of patients with bleeding gastric varices. In these patients, a catheter is passed into the left renal vein, usually through a transfemoral approach, and into the varices, which drain into the renal vein. Following balloon occlusion of the varices, a sclerosant is injected retrograde into the varix under fluoroscopic guidance. An extension of this technique is to occlude the varix through a transfemoral approach while, at the same time, the other end of the varix is approached through a percutaneous transhepatic portal venous route. This technique allows occlusion of the varices at both ends, after which sclerosant can be injected.[210] The use of these techniques, which require considerable radiologic skill, is currently limited to some centers in the Far East.

Portosystemic Shunts

Limited data are available regarding use of surgical portosystemic shunts for the treatment of gastric varices in patients with cirrhosis. Two studies performed in patients with good liver function, most of whom had extrahepatic portal vein thrombosis, demonstrated excellent results, with a low long-term risk of bleeding and encephalopathy, after creation of a surgical shunt.[211,212]

TIPS also is effective in preventing gastric variceal rebleeding. Patients with an HVPG less than 12 mm Hg after TIPS are protected from esophageal variceal bleeding but have been known to bleed from gastric varices. Therefore, if the HVPG is reduced to a level below 12 mm Hg but gastric fundal varices are still prominent when contrast is injected into the portal vein (especially if the patient has bled from gastric fundal varices), the gastric varices should be embolized. Because TIPS for this indication does not always result in a decrease in the size of gastric varices,[213] the target HVPG is uncertain in these patients.[195]

ECTOPIC VARICES

Varices that occur at a site other than the gastroesophageal junction are termed *ectopic varices* and account for less than 5% of all varix-related bleeding episodes. Ectopic varices most commonly manifest with melena or hematemesis. They also may manifest with hemobilia, hematuria, hemoperitoneum, or retroperitoneal bleeding. Ectopic varices may occur with both extrahepatic portal vein obstruction and cirrhosis. The duodenum is a common site of ectopic varices. Duodenal varices typically are associated with portal vein obstruction, but in the West, the usual cause of duodenal varices is cirrhosis. The common occurrence of duodenal varices in patients with portal vein obstruction probably relates to the formation of collateral vessels around the thrombosed portal vein, which connects pancreaticoduodenal veins to retroduodenal veins, which drain into the inferior vena cava.[214] In some of those patients with extrahepatic portal vein obstruction, varices form around the gallbladder and common bile duct.

The other common site of ectopic varices is peristomal, in patients with inflammatory bowel disease and primary sclerosing cholangitis who have undergone a proctocolectomy with creation of an ileostomy.[215] Varices develop at the level of the mucocutaneous border of the stoma and are termed *stomal varices*. They are recognized by a bluish halo surrounding the stoma and by a dusky appearance and friable consistency of the stomal tissue; no obvious variceal lesions are seen.

Anorectal varices are reported in 10% to 40% of cirrhotic patients who undergo colonoscopy. Anorectal varices must be distinguished from hemorrhoids. Rectal varices are dilated superior and middle hemorrhoidal veins, whereas hemorrhoids are dilated vascular channels above the dentate line. Rectal varices collapse with digital pressure, but hemorrhoids do not.

Ectopic variceal bleeding should be considered in all patients with portal hypertension, a fall in the hemoglobin level, and overt gastrointestinal bleeding without an obvious bleeding source on endoscopy; or a drop in the hemoglobin level associated with abdominal pain or worsening ascites. Bleeding from stomal varices is readily apparent on presentation.

Management

In patients suspected of having ectopic variceal bleeding, vasoactive drugs may be administered initially to control the bleeding. If the bleeding ectopic varix is visualized at endoscopy, as typically is the case with duodenal or colonic varices, then endoscopic therapy can be carried out.[216] Endoscopic sclerotherapy or band ligation is the preferred approach for bleeding duodenal varices. Colonic varices tend to be larger in diameter and may require application of hemostatic clips. Patients with bleeding stomal varices can be trained to compress the site locally if bleeding is obvious. Because bleeding from stomal varices is visible and detected early, the mortality rate for bleeding stomal varices is low.[217]

At present, no recommendations support primary prophylaxis to prevent bleeding from ectopic varices. To prevent rebleeding from ectopic varices, pharmacologic treatment with beta blockers usually is tried, although no studies are available to support this approach. If the portal vein is patent, then transhepatic embolization of stomal varices can be carried out (Fig. 87–16). Emboliza-

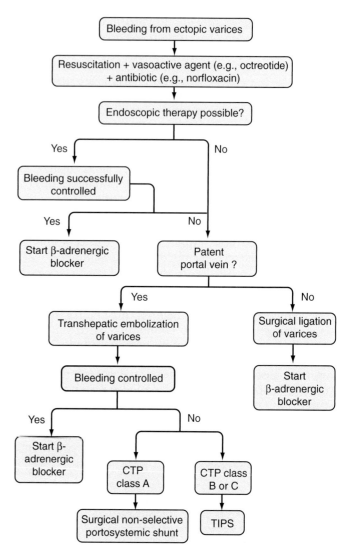

Figure 87–16 Algorithm for the management of bleeding from ectopic varices. CTP, Child-Turcotte-Pugh; TIPS, transjugular intrahepatic portosystemic shunt

tion of varices using a transhepatic approach can control bleeding in most patients with stomal varices. The rate of rebleeding is high, however, because the portal hypertension persists. In patients in whom embolization fails to prevent rebleeding, TIPS placement may be considered. A surgical portosystemic shunt is recommended in patients with CTP class A cirrhosis and in patients with portal hypertension from extrahepatic portal vein thrombosis in whom a vein suitable for a shunt is available. Only placement of a nonselective portosystemic shunt, such as a portacaval shunt, mesocaval shunt, or central splenorenal shunt, should be carried out in patients with stomal varices.

Patients with ectopic varices who present with intraabdominal hemorrhage have a poor outcome, because the diagnosis usually is not considered. The diagnosis often is made at laparotomy. Intra-abdominal bleeding from ectopic varices should be suspected in patients with a sudden increase in ascitic fluid volume associated with abdominal pain, hypotension, and a fall in the hematocrit value. CT of the abdomen demonstrates layering of free fluid in the peritoneal cavity, typical for fresh blood mixed with ascitic fluid. The diagnosis is confirmed by a paracentesis that yields bloody ascitic fluid with clots. The acute bleeding may be controlled by either trans-hepatic obliteration or surgical ligation of the varices. In patients who are critically ill, TIPS placement followed by embolization of the bleeding varix should be carried out.

PORTAL HYPERTENSIVE GASTROPATHY AND GASTRIC VASCULAR ECTASIA

Mucosal changes in the stomach in patients with portal hypertension include portal hypertensive gastropathy (PHG) and gastric vascular ectasia (GVE). In all likelihood, these lesions are distinct, as demonstrated by histologic features and differences in the response to a TIPS. An appearance analogous to PHG in the colon is termed portal hypertensive colopathy (see Chapter 35).

The diagnosis of PHG is based on the presence of a characteristic mosaic-like pattern of the gastric mucosa on endoscopic examination. This pattern is characterized by small polygonal areas with a depressed border. Super-imposed on this mosaic-like pattern may be red point lesions that usually are greater than 2 mm in diameter. PHG is considered mild when only a mosaic-like pattern is present and severe when superimposed discrete red spots also are seen[218] (Fig. 87–17). The etiopathogenesis of PHG is poorly understood. Development of PHG cor-relates with the duration of cirrhosis but not necessarily the degree of liver dysfunction. The frequency of PHG following endoscopic treatment of esophageal varices is increased, possibly a result of longer duration of portal hypertension in these patients.

In GVE, aggregates of ectatic vessels can be seen on endoscopic examination as red spots without a mosaic background.[219] When the aggregates are confined to the antrum of the stomach, the term *gastric antral vascular ectasia* (GAVE) is used (see Chapters 13 and 35). The

aggregates in the antrum can be linear, in which case the term *watermelon stomach* is used to describe the lesion (see Fig. 35–10). When the red spots are distributed diffusely, in both the distal and the proximal stomach, the term *diffuse gastric vascular ectasia* is preferred.[220]

Distinguishing PHG from GVE (or GAVE) is sometimes difficult. A background mosaic pattern and proximal dis-tribution favor PHG (Table 87–7). GVE is less common, occurs in the absence of a background mosaic pattern, and typically is antral in location, although lesions may be present in the proximal stomach. Mucosal biopsies are recommended when the endoscopic diagnosis is uncer-tain. GVE appears histologically as dilated mucosal cap-illaries with focal areas of fibrin thrombi or ectasia in combination with proliferation of spindle cells.[221] Similar ectatic lesions may be seen in the small bowel and may cause acute or chronic gastrointestinal blood loss.

Table 87–7   Comparison of Portal Hypertensive Gastropathy (PHG) and Gastric Vascular Ectasia (GVE)

Feature	PHG	GVE
Distribution	Proximal stomach	Distal stomach*
Mosaic pattern	Present	Absent
Red color signs	Present	Present
Findings on gastric mucosal biopsy		
Thrombi	–	+++
Spindle cell proliferation	+	+ +
Fibrohyalinosis		+ + +
Treatment	β-adrenergic blockers TIPS	?Antrectomy ?Liver transplantation

*Gastric antral vascular ectasia (GAVE).
TIPS, transjugular intrahepatic portosystemic shunt.

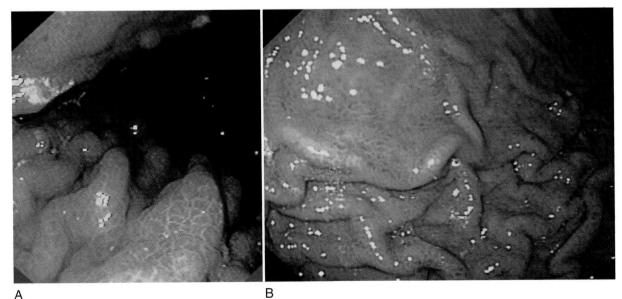

A   B

Figure 87–17   Endoscopic views of portal hypertensive gastropathy. *A,* Mild portal hypertensive gastropathy is characterized by a mosaic appearance without red color signs. *B,* Severe portal hypertensive gastropathy is characterized by a cobblestone appearance with super-imposed red spots.

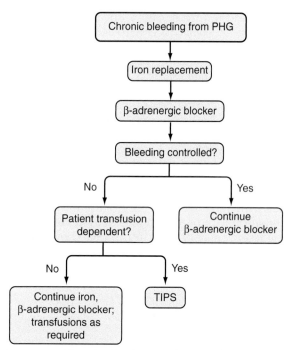

Figure 87–18 Algorithm for the management of chronic bleeding from portal hypertensive gastropathy. TIPS, transjugular intrahepatic portosystemic shunt.

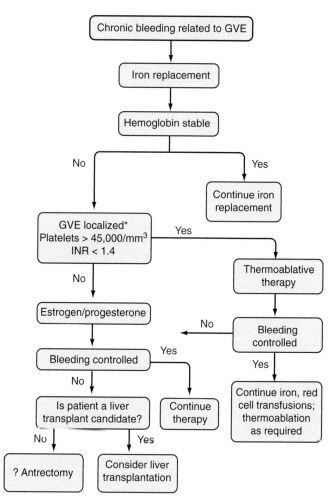

Figure 87–19 Algorithm for the management of chronic bleeding from gastric vascular ectasia (GVE). *Gastric antral vascular ectasia (GAVE). INR, international normalized ratio.

Management

PHG accounts for approximately one fourth of all cases of bleeding (acute and chronic) in patients with portal hypertension, but for less than 10% of all acute bleeding episodes. The more common presentation is one of chronic, slow bleeding and anemia. Pharmacologic therapy to prevent bleeding (primary prophylaxis) in patients with severe portal hypertensive gastropathy is not currently recommended. Small studies have suggested that octreotide may be useful for controlling acute bleeding.[222] Beta blockers are recommended for preventing chronic blood loss in patients who have bled from severe PHG.[223,224] When patients are transfusion-dependent despite beta blockade and iron supplementation, a TIPS may be inserted (Fig. 87–18). A TIPS decreases transfusion requirements and results in reversal of the mucosal lesions on endoscopic examination.[220]

Management of GVE is more problematic. Initial treatment involves repletion of iron and red blood cell transfusions to treat symptomatic anemia. If lesions are localized, the platelet count is greater than approximately 45,000/mm³, and the INR is less than 1.4, thermoablative therapy, as with argon plasma coagulation, may be helpful (Fig. 87–19). The usual settings for argon plasma coagulation are an energy of 60 to 90 watts and a gas flow rate of 1 to 2 L per minute. If the coagulation parameters are suboptimal, thermal coagulation is associated with an increase in mucosal bleeding in many patients. If thermoablation fails, therapy with an oral estrogen-progesterone combination may be useful in reducing transfusion requirements.[225] The usual dose is estradiol, 35 µg, plus norethindrone, 1 mg daily. Because the medication is

taken daily, no risk of breakthrough vaginal bleeding exists. Rarely, painful gynecomastia may limit use of this combination in men. In the patient with preserved hepatic synthetic function who continues to bleed despite thermoablative therapy and estrogen-progesterone combinations, a surgical antral resection may be carried out. TIPS does not reduce the bleeding risk in patients with GVE and is associated with a substantial risk of hepatic encephalopathy.[220] Therefore, TIPS placement is not recommended as therapy for GVE. Nevertheless, GVE is reversed with liver transplantation, even in the presence of portal hypertension, suggesting that GVE is related to liver failure, rather than to portal hypertension.[49,226]

REFERENCES

1. Kumar S, Sarr MG, Kamath PS: Mesenteric venous thrombosis. N Engl J Med 345:1683, 2001.
2. Douglas BE, Baggenstoss AH, Hollingshead WN: The anatomy of the portal vein and its tributaries. Surg Gynecol Obst 91:562, 1950.

3. Sarin S, Groszmann R, Mosca P, et al: Propranolol ameliorates the development of portal-systemic shunting in a chronic murine schistosomiasis model of portal hypertension. J Clin Invest 87:1032, 1991.

4. Angelico M, Carli L, Piat C, et al: Effects of isosorbide-5-mononitrate compared with propranolol on first bleeding and long-term survival in cirrhosis. Gastroenterology 113:1632, 1997.

5. Rodriguez-Perez F, Groszmann R: Pharmacologic treatment of portal hypertension. Gastroenterol Clin North Am 21:15, 1992.

6. Bhathal P, Grossman H: Reduction of the increased portal vascular resistance of the isolated perfused cirrhotic rat liver by vasodilators. J Hepatol 1:325, 1985.

7. Bhathal P, Grossman H: Active contractile and mechanical factors in the pathogenesis of portal hypertension—a study utilizing three experimental models. In Sarin SK, Nayak NC (eds): Animal Models of Portal Hypertension. New Delhi, Kunj Publishing, 1988, p 111.

8. Gupta T, Toruner M, Chung M, Groszmann R: Endothelial dysfunction and decreased production of nitric oxide in the intrahepatic microcirculation of cirrhotic rats. Hepatology 28:926, 1998.

9. Shah V, Garcia-Cardena G, Sessa W, Groszmann R: The hepatic circulation in health and disease: Report of a single-topic symposium. Hepatology 27:279, 1998.

10. Rockey DC, Chung JJ: Reduced nitric oxide production by endothelial cells in cirrhotic rat liver: Endothelial dysfunction in portal hypertension. Gastroenterology 114:344, 1998.

11. Shah V, Toruner M, Haddad F, et al: Impaired endothelial nitric oxide synthase activity associated with enhanced caveolin binding in experimental liver cirrhosis. Gastroenterology 117:1222, 1999.

12. Sarela A, Mihaimeed F, Batten J, et al: Hepatic and splanchnic nitric oxide activity in patients with cirrhosis. Gut 44:749, 1999.

13. Chatila R, Theise N, Shah V, et al: Caveolin-1 in normal and human cirrhotic liver. Gastroenterology 118:A979, 2000.

14. Failli P, DeFranco R, Caligiuri A, et al: Nitrovasodilators inhibit platelet-derived growth factor–induced proliferation and migration of activated human hepatic stellate cells. Gastroenterology 119:479, 2000.

15. Bellis L, Berzigotti A, Abraldes J, et al: Low doses of isosorbide mononitrate attenuate the postprandial increase in portal pressure in patients with cirrhosis. Hepatology 37:378, 2003.

16. Fiorucci S, Antonelli E, Morelli O, et al: NCX-1000, a NO-releasing derivative of ursodeoxycholic acid, selectively delivers NO to the liver and protects against development of portal hypertension. Proc Natl Acad Sci U S A 98:8897, 2001.

17. Loureiro-Silva M, Cadelina G, Iwakiri Y, Groszmann R: A liver-specific nitric oxide donor improves the intra-hepatic vascular response to both portal blood flow increase and methoxamine in cirrhotic rats. J Hepatol 39:940, 2003.

18. Dudenhoefer A, Loureiro-Silva M, Cadelina G, et al: Bioactivation of nitroglycerin and vasomotor response to nitric oxide are impaired in cirrhotic rat livers. Hepatology 36:381, 2002.

19. Rockey DC, Weisiger RA: Endothelin induced contractility of stellate cells from normal and cirrhotic rat liver: Implications for regulation of portal pressure and resistance. Hepatology 24:233, 1996.

20. Pinzani M, Milani S, De Franco R, et al: Endothelin 1 is overexpressed in human cirrhotic liver and exerts multiple effects on activated hepatic stellate cells. Gastroenterology 110:534, 1996.

21. Kamath P, Tyce G, Miller V, et al: Endothelin-1 modulates intrahepatic resistance in a rat model of noncirrhotic portal hypertension. Hepatology 30:401, 1999.

22. Rockey D, Fouassier L, Chung J, et al: Cellular localization of endothelin-1 and increased production in liver injury in the rat: Potential for autocrine and paracrine effects on stellate cells. Hepatology 27:472, 1998.

23. Alam I, Bass NM, Bacchetti P, et al: Hepatic tissue endothelin-1 levels in chronic liver disease correlate with disease severity and ascites. Am J Gastroenterol 95:199, 2000.

24. Salo J, Francitorra A, Follo A, et al: Increased plasma endothelin in cirrhosis. Relationship with systemic endotoxemia and response to changes in effective blood volume. J Hepatol 22:389, 1995.

25. Douggrell S: The therapeutic potential of endothelin-1 receptor antagonists and endothelin-converting enzyme inhibitors on the cardiovascular system. Expert Opin Investig Drugs 11:1537, 2002.

26. Reynaert H, Vaeyens F, Qin H, et al: Somatostatin suppresses endothelin-1 induced rat hepatic stellate cell contraction via somatostatin receptor subtype 1. Gastroenterology 121:915, 2001.

27. Graupera M, Garcia-Pagan J, Titos E, et al: 5-Lipoxygenase inhibition reduces intrahepatic vascular resistance of cirrhotic rat livers: A possible role of cysteinyl-leukotrienes. Gastroenterology 122:387, 2002.

28. Yokoyama M, Xu H, Kresge N, et al: Role of thromboxane A_2 in early BDL-induced portal hypertension. Am J Physiol 284:G453, 2003.

29. Blendis L, Wong F: Does losartan work after all? Am J Gastroenterol 98:1222, 2003.

30. Sikuler E, Groszmann RJ: Hemodynamic studies in long- and short-term portal hypertensive rats: The relation to systemic glucagon levels. Hepatology 6:414, 1986.

31. Atucha N, Shah V, Garcia-Cardena G, et al: Role of endothelium in the abnormal response of mesenteric vessels in rats with portal hypertension and liver cirrhosis. Gastroenterology 111:1627, 1996.

32. Sieber CC, Groszmann RJ: Nitric oxide mediates hyporeactivity to vasopressors in mesenteric vessels of portal hypertensive rats. Gastroenterology 103:235, 1992.

33. Sieber CC, Groszmann RJ: In vitro hyporeactivity to methoxamine in portal hypertensive rats: Reversal by nitric oxide blockade. Am J Physiol 262:G996, 1992.

34. Sieber C, Lopez-Talavera JC, Groszmann RJ: Role of nitric oxide in the in vitro splanchnic vascular hyporeactivity in ascitic cirrhotic rats. Gastroenterology 104:1750, 1993.

35. Niederberger M, Gines P, Martin P, et al: Comparison of vascular nitric oxide production and systemic hemodynamics in cirrhosis versus prehepatic portal hypertension in rats. Hepatology 24:947, 1996.

36. Cahill P, Foster C, Redmond E, et al: Enhanced nitric oxide synthase activity in portal hypertensive rabbits. Hepatology 22:598, 1995.

37. Cahill P, Redmond E, Hodges R, et al: Increased endothelial nitric oxide synthase activity in the hyperemic vessels of portal hypertensive rats. J Hepatol 25:370, 1996.

38. Garcia-Pagan J, Fernandez M, Bernadich C, et al: Effects of continued NO inhibition on portal hypertensive syndrome after portal vein stenosis in rat. Am J Physiol 267:G984, 1994.

39. Sogni P, Sabry S, Moreau R, et al: Hyporeactivity of mesenteric resistance arteries in portal hypertensive rats. J Hepatol 24:487, 1996.

40. Martin P, Xu D, Niederberger M, et al: Upregulation of endothelial constitutive NOS: A major role in the increased NO production in cirrhotic rats. Am J Physiol 270:F494, 1996.

41. Wiest R, Das S, Cadelina G, et al: Bacterial translocation in cirrhotic rats stimulates eNOS-derived NO production and impairs mesenteric vascular contractility. J Clin Invest 104:1223, 1999.

42. Shah V, Wiest R, Garcia-Cardena G, et al: Hsp90 regulation of endothelial nitric oxide synthase contributes to vascular control in portal hypertension. Am J Physiol 277:G463, 1999.

43. Morales-Ruiz M, Jimenez W, Perez-Sala D, et al: Increased nitric oxide synthase expression in arterial vessels of cirrhotic rats with ascites. Hepatology 24:1481, 1996.

44. Tazi K, Barriere E, Moreau R, et al: Role of shear stress in aortic eNOS up-regulation in rats with biliary cirrhosis. Gastroenterology 122:1869, 2002.

45. Pateron D, Tazi K, Sogni P, et al: Role of aortic nitric oxide synthase 3 (eNOS) in the systemic vasodilation of portal hypertension. Gastroenterology 119:196, 2000.

46. Iwakiri Y, Tsai M, McCabe T, et al: Phosphorylation of eNOS initiates excessive NO production in early phases of portal hypertension. Am J Physiol 282:H2084, 2002.

47. Rasaratnam B, Kaye D, Jennings G, et al: The effect of selective intestinal decontamination on the hyperdynamic circulatory state in cirrhosis. A randomized trial. Ann Intern Med 139:186, 2003.

48. La Villa G, Barletta G, Pantaleo P, et al: Hemodynamic, renal, and endocrine effects of acute inhibition of nitric oxide synthase in compensated cirrhosis. Hepatology 34:19, 2001.

49. Spahr L, Villeneuve JP, Dufresne MP, et al: Gastric antral ectasia in cirrhotic patients: Absence of relation with portal hypertension. Gut 44:739, 1999.

50. Ros J, Claria J, To-Figueras J, et al: Endogenous cannabinoids: A new system involved in the homeostasis of arterial pressure in experimental cirrhosis in the rat. Gastroenterology 122:85, 2002.

51. Batkai S, Jarai Z, Wagner J, et al: Endocannabinoids acting at vascular CB1 receptors mediate the vasodilated state in advanced liver cirrhosis. Nat Med 7:827, 2001.

52. Wagner J, Varga K, Ellis E, et al: Activation of peripheral CB$_1$ cannabinoid receptors in haemorrhagic shock. Nature 390:518, 1997.

53. Fernandez M, Lambrecht R, Bonkovsky H: Increased heme oxygenase activity in splanchnic organs from portal hypertensive rats: role in modulating mesenteric vascular reactivity. J Hepatol 34:936, 2001.

54. Fernandez M, Vizzutti F, Garcia-Pagan J, et al: Anti-VEGF receptor-2 monoclonal antibody prevents portal-systemic collateral vessel formation in portal hypertensive mice. Gastroenterology 126:886, 2004.

55. Fallon M, Abrams G, Luo B, et al: The role of eNOS in the pathogenesis of a rat model of hepatopulmonary syndrome. Gastroenterology 113:606, 1997.

56. Hou M, Cahill P, Zhang S, et al: Enhanced cyclooxygenase-1 expression within the superior mesenteric artery of portal hypertensive rats: Role in the hyperdynamic circulation. Hepatology 27:20, 1998.

57. Heinemann A, Stauber RE: Vasodilator responses to nitric oxide are enhanced in mesenteric arteries of portal hypertensive rats. Eur J Clin Invest 26:824, 1996.

58. Heinemann A, Wachter C, Holzer P, et al: Nitric oxide–dependent and –independent vascular hyporeactivity in mesenteric arteries of portal hypertensive rats. Br J Pharmacol 121:1031, 1997.

59. Tazi K, Moreau R, Cailmail S, et al: Altered growth and lack of responsiveness to angiotensin II in aortic vascular smooth muscle cells from cirrhotic rats. Gastroenterology 112:2065, 1997.

60. Tazi K, Moreau R, Heller J, et al: Changes in protein kinase C isoforms in association with vascular hyporeactivity in cirrhotic rat aortas. Gastroenterology 119:201, 2000.

61. Escorsell A, Bandi JC, Andreu V, et al: Desensitization to the effects of intravenous octreotide in cirrhotic patients with portal hypertension. Gastroenterology 120:161, 2001.

62. Gupta T, Chen L, Groszmann R: Pathophysiology of portal hypertension. Baillieres Clin Gastroenterol 11:203, 1997.

63. Vianna A, Hayes PC, Moscoso G: Normal venous circulation of the gastroesophageal junction. A route to understanding varices. Gastroenterology 93:876, 1987.

64. Watanabe K, Kimura K, Matsutani S, et al: Portal hemodynamics in patients with gastric varices. A study in 230 patients with esophageal and/or gastric varices using portal vein catheterization. Gastroenterology 95:434, 1988.

65. Dilawari JB, Chawla YK: Spontaneous (natural) splenoadrenorenal shunts in extrahepatic portal venous obstruction: A series of 20 cases. Gut 28:198, 1987.

66. Sumanovski L, Battegay E, Stumm M, et al: Increased angiogenesis in portal hypertensive rats: Role of nitric oxide. Hepatology 29:1044, 1999.

67. Fernandez-Varo G, Ros J, Morales-Ruiz M, et al: Nitric oxide synthase 3–dependent vascular remodeling and circulatory dysfunction in cirrhosis. Am J Pathol 162:1985, 2003.

68. Sieber C, Sumanovski L, Stumm M, et al: In vivo angiogenesis in normal and portal hypertensive rats: Role of basic fibroblast growth factor and nitric oxide. J Hepatol 34:644, 2001.

69. Lee FY, Colombato LA, Albillos A, Groszmann RJ: Administration of N-omega-nitro-L-arginine ameliorates portal-systemic shunting in portal-hypertensive rats. Gastroenterology 105:1464, 1993.

70. Mosca P, Lee F-Y, Kaumann A, Groszmann R: Pharmacology of portal-systemic collaterals in portal hypertensive rats: Role of endothelium. Am J Physiol 263:G544, 1992.

71. Chan C, Lee F, Wang S, et al: Effects of vasopressin on portal-systemic collaterals in portal hypertensive rats: Role of nitric oxide and prostaglandin. Hepatology 30:630-635, 1999.

72. Huang H, Lee F, Chan C, et al: Effects of somatostatin and octreotide on portal-systemic collaterals in portal hypertensive rats. J Hepatol 36:163, 2002.

73. Huang H, Wang S, Chan C, et al: Chronic inhibition of nitric oxide increases the collateral vascular responsiveness to vasopressin in portal hypertensive rats. J Hepatol 40:234, 2004.

74. Sakurabayashi S, Koh K, Chen L, Groszmann R: Octreotide ameliorates the increase in collateral blood flow during postprandial hyperemia in portal hypertensive rats. J Hepatol 36:507, 2002.

75. Chan C, Wang S, Lee F, et al: Endothelin-1 induces vasoconstriction on portal-systemic collaterals of portal hypertensive rats. Hepatology 33:816, 2001.

76. Escorsell A, Gines A, Llach J, et al: Increased intra-abdominal pressure increases pressure, volume, and wall tension in esophageal varices. Hepatology 36:936, 2002.

77. Myers JD, Taylor WJ: An estimation of portal venous pressure by occlusive catheterization of a hepatic venule. J Clin Invest 30:662, 1951.

78. Groszmann R, Glickman M, Blei AT, et al: Wedged and free hepatic venous pressure measured with a balloon catheter. Gastroenterology 76:253, 1979.

79. Boyer T, Triger D, Horisawa M, et al: Direct transhepatic measurement of portal vein pressure using a thin needle. Comparison with wedged hepatic vein pressure. Gastroenterology 72:584, 1977.

80. Groszmann RJ: Hepatic venous pressure gradient: Anything worth doing should be done right. Hepatology 39:280, 2004.

81. Thalheimer U, Mela M, Patch D, Burroughs AK: Targeting portal pressure measurements: A critical reappraisal. Hepatology 39:286, 2004.

82. Menon KV, Shah VH, Kamath PS: The Budd-Chiari syndrome. N Engl J Med 350:578, 2004.

83. Nevens F, Bustami R, Schley SI, et al: Variceal pressure is a factor predicting the risk of a first variceal bleed. A prospective cohort study in cirrhotic patients. Hepatology 27:15, 1998.

84. Escorsell A, Bordas JM, Castaneda B, et al: Predictive value of the variceal pressure response to continued pharmacological therapy in patients with cirrhosis and portal hypertension. Hepatology 31:1061, 2000.

85. Rigau J, Bosch J, Bordas JM, et al: Endoscopic measurement of variceal pressure in cirrhosis: Correlation of portal pressure and variceal hemorrhage. Gastroenterology 96:873, 1989.

86. Ruiz del Arbul L, Martin de Argila C, Vasquez M: Endoscopic measurement of variceal pressure during hemorrhage from esophageal varices. Hepatology 16:147, 1992.

87. Gertsch P, Fischer G, Kleber G: Manometry as it relates to varices: Comparison of an endoscopic balloon technique with needle puncture. Gastroenterology 105:1159, 1993.

88. Brensing KA, Neubrand M, Textor J: Endoscopic manometry of esophageal varices: Evaluation of balloon technique compared with direct portal pressure measurement. J Hepatol 29:94, 1998.

89. Scheurlen C, Roleff A, Neubrand M, Sauerbruch T: Non-invasive endoscopic determination of intravascular pressure in patients with portal hypertension: Clinical experience with a new balloon technique. Endoscopy 30:326, 1998.

90. Grace ND, Groszmann RJ, Garcia-Tsao G, et al: Portal hypertension and variceal bleeding: An AASLD single topic symposium. Hepatology 28:868, 1998.

91. D'Amico G, Garcia-Tsao G, Cales P, et al: Diagnosis of portal hypertension: How and when? In de Franchis R (ed): Portal Hypertension III. Proceedings of the Third Baveno International Consensus Workshop on Definitions, Methodology and Therapeutic Strategies. Oxford, Blackwell Science, 2001, p 36.

92. Zein CO, Lindor KD, Angula P: Prevalence and predictors of esophageal varices in patients with primary sclerosing cholangitis. Hepatology 39:203, 2004.

93. D'Amico G, Morabito A: Non-invasive markers of esophageal varices: Another round, not the last. Hepatology 39:30, 2004.

94. Beppu K, Inoquachi K, Koyanagi N, et al: Prediction of variceal hemorrhage by esophageal endoscopy. Gastrointest Endosc 27:213, 1981.

95. Bosch J, Abraldes JG, Groszmann R: Current management of portal hypertension. J Hepatol 38:S54, 2003.

96. The North Italian Endoscopic Club for the Study and Treatment of Esophageal Varices (NIEC): Prediction of the first variceal hemorrhage in patients with cirrhosis of the liver and esophageal varices. A prospective multicenter study. N Engl J Med 319:983, 1988.

97. Cottone M, D'Amico G, Maringhini A, et al: Predictive value of ultrasonography in the screening of non-ascitic cirrhotic patients with large varices. J Ultrasound Med 5:189, 1986.

98. Schepis F, Camma C, Niceforo D, et al: Which patients with cirrhosis should undergo endoscopic screening for esophageal varices detection? Hepatology 33:333, 2001.

99. Van Gansbekeb AEF, Delcour C, Engelholm LJS: Sonographic features of portal vein thrombosis. AJR Am J Roentgenol 144:749, 1985.

100. Sabbas S, Ferraioli G, Buanamico P, et al: A randomized study of propranolol on postprandial hyerpemia in cirrhotic patients. Gastroenterology 102:1009, 1992.

101. Willmann JK, Weishaupt D, Bohm T, et al: Detection of submucosal gastric fundal varices with multi-detector row CT angiography. Gut 52:886, 2003.

102. Matsumoto A, Kitamoto M, Imamura M, et al: Three-dimensional portography using multi-slice hellical CT is clinically useful for management of gastric fundal varices. Med J Roentgenol 176:899, 2001.

103. Matsuo M, Kanematsu M, Kim T, et al: Esophageal varices: diagnosis with gadolinium-enhanced MR imaging of the liver for patients with chronic liver damage. AJR Am J Roentgenol 180:461, 2003.

104. Sugano S, Yamamoto K, Sasao K, et al: Daily variation of azygos and portal blood flow and the effect of propranolol administration once an evening in cirrhotics. J Hepatology 34:26, 2001.

105. Konishi Y, Nakamura T, Kida H, et al: Catheter ultrasound probe EUS evaluation of gastric cardia and perigastric vascular structures to predict esophageal variceal recurrence. Gastrointest Endosc 55:1997, 2002.

106. Escorsell A, Bordas JM, Feu F, et al: Endoscopic assessment of variceal volume and wall tension in cirrhotic patients: Effects of pharmacological therapy. Gastroenterology 113:1640, 1997.

107. Leung VK, Sung JJ, Ahuja AT, et al: Large paraesophageal varices on endosonography predict recurrence of esophageal varices and re-bleeding. Gastroenterology 112:1811, 1997.

108. Miller LS, Dai Q, Thomas A, et al: A new ultrasound-guided esophageal variceal pressure–measuring device. Am J Gastroenterol 99:1267, 2004.

109. Pomier-Layrargues GP, Kusielewic ZD, Willems B, et al: Presinusoidal portal hypertension in non-alcoholic cirrhosis. Hepatology 5:415, 1985.

110. Czaja AJ, Wolf AM, Summerskill WH: Development and early prognosis of esophageal varices in severe chronic active liver disease (CALD) treated with prednisone. Gastroenterology 77:629, 1979.

111. Fracanzani AL, Fargion S, Romano R, et al: Portal hypertension and iron depletion in patients with genetic hemochromatosis. Hepatology 22:1127, 1995.

112. Gores GJ, Wiesner RH, Dickson ER, et al: Prospective evaluation of esophageal varices in primary biliary cirrhosis: Development, natural history, and influence on survival. Gastroenterology 96:1552, 1989.

113. Afroudakis A, Kaplowitz N: Liver histopathology in chronic common bile duct stenosis due to chronic alcoholic pancreatitis. Hepatology 1:65, 1981.

114. Ross AJP, Bartley PB, Sleigh AC, et al: Current concepts: Schistosomiasis. N Engl J Med 346:1212, 2002.

115. Badawia F, Michael MS: Risk factors for hepatocellular carcinoma in Egypt: The role of hepatitis B viral infection in schistosomiasis. Anticancer Res 19:4565, 1999.

116. Frank C, Mohammed MK, Strickland GT: The role of parenteral anti-schistosomal therapy in the spread of hepatitis C virus in Egypt. Lancet 355:887, 2000.

117. Okuda K, Kono K, Ohnishi K, et al: Clinical study of 86 cases with idiopathic portal hypertension in comparison with cirrhosis with splenomegaly. Gastroenterology 86:600, 1984.

118. Dilawari JB, Chawla YK: Pseudosclerosing cholangitis in extrahepatic portal venous obstruction. Gut 33:272, 1992.

119. Condat B, Pessione F, Hillar RES: Current outcome of portal vein thrombosis in adults: Risks and benefits of anticoagulant therapy. Gastroenterology 120:4907, 2001.

120. D'Cruz AJ, Kamath PS, Ramachandra C, Jalihal A: Nonconventional portosystemic shunts in children with extrahepatic portal vein obstruction. Acta Paediatr Jpn 37:17, 1995.

121. Ludwig J, Hashimoto E, Obata H, Baldus W: Idiopathic portal hypertension. Hepatology 17:1157, 1993.

122. Kamath PS, Carpenter HA, Lloyd RV, et al: Hepatic localization of endothelin-1 in patients with idiopathic portal hypertension in cirrhosis of the liver. Liver Transpl 6:596, 2000.

123. Sama SK, Bhargava S, Nath NG, et al: Non-cirrhotic portal fibrosis. Am J Med 51:160, 1971.

124. Boyer JL, Sen Gupta KP, Biswas SK, et al: Idiopathic portal hypertension. Comparison with portal hypertension of cirrhosis and extrahepatic vein obstruction. Ann Intern Med 1967, 66:41, 1967.

125. Sarin SK, Selhi KK, Nanda R: Measurement and condition of wedged hepatic, intrahepatic, intrasplenic and intravariceal pressures in patients with cirrhosis of the liver and non-cirrhotic portal fibrosis. Gut 28:260, 1987.

126. Nevens F, Staessen D, Sciot R, et al: Clinical aspects of incomplete septal cirrhosis in comparison with macronodular cirrhosis. Gastroenterology 106:454, 1994.

127. Wanless IR: Micronodular transformation (nodular regenerative hyperplasia) of the liver: A report of 64 cases among 2500 autopsies and a new classification of benign hepatocellular nodules. Hepatology 11:787, 1990.

128. Gane E, Portmann B, Saxena R, et al: Nodular regenerative hyperplasia of the liver graft after liver transplantation. Hepatology 20:88, 1994.

129. Cazals-Hatem D, Vilgrain V, Genin P, et al: Arterial and portal circulation and parenchymal changes in Budd-Chiari syndrome: A study in 17 explanted livers. Hepatology 37:510, 2003.

130. Sherlock S, Feldman CA, Moran B, Scheur PJ: Partial nodular transformation of the liver with portal hypertension. Am J Med 40:195, 1966.

131. Kerrd NS, Okonkwo S, Choa RE: Congenital hepatic fibrosis: The long-term prognosis. Gut 19:514, 1978.

132. Qian Q, Lia R, King BF, et al: Clinical profile of autosomal-dominant polycystic liver disease. Hepatology 37:164, 2003.

133. Johns CJ, Michele TM: The clinical management of sarcoidosis: A 50-year experience at the Johns Hopkins Hospital. Medicine 78:65, 1999.

134. Grundfest A, Cooperman A, Ferguson R: Portal hypertension associated with systemic mastocystosis and splenomegaly. Gastroenterology 78:370, 1980.

135. Hyun B, Singer E, Sharriett R: Esophageal varices and metastatic carcinoma of the liver: A report of three cases and a review of the literature. Arch Pathol 77:292, 1976.

136. Saluja S, White RI: Hereditary hemorrhagic telangiectasia of the liver: Hyperperfusion with relative ischemia—poverty amidst plenty. Radiology 230:25, 2004.

137. Garcia-Tsao G, Korzenik JR, Young L, et al: Liver disease in patients with hereditary hemorrhagic telangiectasia. N Engl J Med 343:931, 2000.

138. Ianora AA, Memo M, Sabba C, et al: Hereditary hemorrhagic telangiectasia: Multi-detector row helical CT assessment of hepatic involvement. Radiology 230:250, 2004.

139. Abraldes JG, Bosch J: Somatostatin and analogs in portal hypertension. Hepatology 35:1305, 2002.

140. Bosch J, Kravetz D, Rodes J: Effects of somatostatin on hepatic and systemic hemodynamics in patients with cirrhosis of the liver: Comparison with vasopressin. Gastroenterology 80:518, 1981.

141. Cirera I, Feu F, Luca A, et al: Effects of bolus injections and continuous infusions of somatostatin and placebo in patients with cirrhosis: A double-blind hemodynamic investigation. Hepatology 22:106, 1995.

142. Villanueve C, Ortiz J, Minna J, et al: Somatostatin treatment and risk stratification by continuous portal pressure monitoring during active variceal bleeding. Gastroenterology 121:110, 2001.

143. Buanamico P, Sabba C, Garcia-Tsao G, et al: Octreotide blunts postprandial splanchnic hyperemia in cirrhotic patients: A double-blind randomized echo Doppler study. Hepatology 21:134, 1995.

144. Cales P, Masliah C, Bernard B, et al: French Club for the Study of Portal Hypertension. Early administration of vapreotide for variceal bleeding in patients with cirrhosis. N Engl J Med 344:23, 2001.

145. Lebrec D, Poynard T, Hillon P, Benhamou JP: Propranolol for prevention of recurrent gastrointestinal bleeding in patients with cirrhosis: A controlled study. N Engl J Med 305:1371, 1981.

146. Lui HF, Stanley AJ, Forrest EH, et al: Primary prophylaxis of variceal hemorrhage: A randomized controlled trial comparing band ligation, propranolol, and isosorbide mononitrate. Gastroenterology 123:735, 2002.

147. Albillos A, Lledo JL, Rossi I, et al: Continuous prazosin administrastion in cirrhotic patients: Effects on portal hemodynamics and on liver and renal function. Gastroenterology 109:1257, 1995.

148. Schneider AW, Friedrich J, Klein CP: Effect of losartan, an angiotensin II receptor antagonist, on portal pressure in cirrhosis. Hepatology 29:334, 1999.

149. Schepke M, Werner E, Biecker E, et al: Hemodynamic effects of the angiotensin II receptor antagonist irbesartan in patients with cirrhosis and portal hypertension. Gastroenterology 121:389, 2001.

150. Gonzalez-Abraldes J, Albillos A, Banares R, et al: Randomized comparison of long-term losartan versus propranolol in lowering portal pressure in cirrhosis. Gastroenterology 121:382, 2001.

151. D'Amico G, Pietrosi G, Tarantino I, Pagliaro L: Emergency sclerotherapy versus vasoactive drugs for variceal bleeding in cirrhosis: A Cochrane meta-analysis. Gastroenterology 124:1277, 2003.

152. Avgerinos A, Armonis A, Stefanidis G, et al: Sustained rise of portal pressure after sclerotherapy, but not band ligation, in acute variceal bleeding in cirrhosis. Hepatology 39:1623, 2004.

153. Bureau C, Garcia-Pagan JC, Otal P, et al: Improved clinical outcome using polytetrafluoroethylene-coated stents for TIPS. Results of a randomized study. Gastroenterology 126:469, 2004.

154. Azoulay D, Castaing D, Majno P, et al: Salvage transjugular intrahepatic portosystemic shunt for uncontrolled variceal bleeding in patients with decompensated cirrhosis. J Hepatology 35:590, 2001.

155. Barange K, Peron JM, Imani K, et al: Transjugular intrahepatic portosystemic shunt in the treatment of refractory bleeding from ruptured gastric varices. Hepatology 30:1139, 1999.

156. Papatheodoridis GV, Goulis J, Leandro G, et al: Transjugular intrahepatic portosystemic shunt compared with endoscopic treatment for prevention of variceal re-bleeding: A meta-analysis. Hepatology 30:612, 1999.

157. Malinchoc M, Kamath PS, Gordon FD, et al: A model to predict poor survival in patients undergoing transjugular intrahepatic portosystemic shunts. Hepatology 31:864, 2000.

158. Chalasani N, Clark WS, Martin LG, et al: Determinants of mortality in patients with advanced cirrhosis after transjugular intrahepatic portosystemic shunting. Gastroenterology 118:138, 2000.

159. Kamath PS, Wiesner RH, Malinchoc M, et al: A model to predict survival in patients with end-stage liver disease. Hepatology 33:464, 2001.

160. Ferral H, Gamboa P, Postoak DW, et al: Survival after elective transjugular intrahepatic portosystemic shunt creation: Prediction with model for end-stage liver disease score. Radiology 231:231, 2004.

161. Burroughs AK, Hamilton G, Phillips A, et al: A comparison of sclerotherapy with staple transection of the esophagus for the emergency control of bleeding from esophageal varices. N Engl J Med 321:857, 1989.

162. Henderson JM: Therapies for refractory variceal hemorrhage. Clin Liver Dis 5:709, 2001.

163. Sugiura M, Futagawa S: Esophageal transection with para-esophagogastric devascularization (Sugiura procedure) in the treatment of esophageal varices. World J Surg 8:673, 1984.

164. Warren WD, Zeppa R, Foman JS: Selective trans-splenic decompression of gastroesophageal varices by distal splenorenal shunts. Ann Surg 166:437, 1967.

165. Rikkers LF, Jin G, Langnas AN: Shunt surgery during the era of liver transplantation. Ann Surg 226:51, 1997.

166. Sarfeh IJ, Rypins E: A systemic appraisal of portacaval H-graft diameters. Clinical and hemodynamic perspectives. Ann Surg 204:356, 1986.

167. Rosemurgy AS, Goode SE, Swiebel BR: A prospective trial of TIPS versus small diameter prosthetic H graft portocaval shunt in the treatment of bleeding varices. Ann Surg 224:378, 1996.

168. Orloff MJ, Orloff MS, Orloff SL: Three decades of experience with emergency portocaval shunt for acute bleeding esophageal varices in 400 unselected patients with cirrhosis of the liver. J Am Coll Surg 180:257, 1995.

169. Stipa S, Balducci G, Ziparo V: Total shunting in elective management of variceal bleeding. World J Surg 18:200, 1994.

170. Bosch J, Abraldes JG, Groszmann R: Current management of portal hypertension. J Hepatol 38:S54, 2003.

171. de Franchis R, Primignani M: Natural history of portal hypertension in patients with cirrhosis. Clin Liver Dis 5:645, 2001.

172. Vorobioff J, Groszmann R, Picabea E, et al: Prognostic value of hepatic venous pressure gradient measurements in alcoholic cirrhosis: A 10-year prospective study. Gastroenterology 111:701, 1996.

173. Escorsell A, Bordas JM, Castaneda B, et al: Predictive value of the variceal pressure response to continued pharmacological therapy in patients with cirrhosis and portal hypertension. Hepatology 31:1061, 2000.

174. D'Amico G, de Franchis R: Upper digestive bleeding in cirrhosis. Post-therapeutic outcome and prognostic indicators. Hepatology 38:599, 2003.

175. Castaneda B, Morales J, Lionette R, et al: Effects of blood volume restitution following a portal hypertensive–related bleeding in anesthetized cirrhotic rats. Hepatology 33:821, 2001.

176. McCormick PA, O'Keefe C: Improving prognosis following a first variceal haemorrhage over four decades. Gut 49:682, 2001.

177. Ben Ari Z, Cardin F, McCormick AP, et al: A predictive model for failure to control bleeding during acute variceal haemorrhage. J Hepatology 31:443, 1999.

178. Goulis J, Armonis A, Patch D, et al: Bacterial infection is independently associated with failure to control bleeding in cirrhotic patients with gastrointestinal hemorrhage. Hepatology 27:1207, 1998.

179. Graham D, Smith J: The course of patients after variceal hemorrhage. Gastroenterology 80:800, 1981.

180. Abraczinskas DR, Ookubo R, Grace ND, et al: Propranolol for the prevention of first esophageal variceal hemorrhage: A lifetime commitment? Hepatology 34:1096, 2001.

181. Garcia-Pagan JC, Villanueve C, Vila MC, et al: Isosorbide mononitrate in the prevention of first variceal bleed in patients who cannot receive beta-blockers. Gastroenterology 121:908, 2001.

182. Escorsell A, Ferayomi L, Bosch J, et al: The portal pressure response to beta-blockade is greater in cirrhotic patients without varices than in those with varices. Gastroenterology 112:2012, 1997.

183. Garcia-Pagan JC, Villanueve C, Vila MC, et al: Isosorbide-5-mononitrate in the prevention of the first variceal bleed in patients who cannot receive beta-blockers. Gastroenterology 121:908, 2001.

184. de Franchis R: Updating consensus in portal hypertension: Report of the Baveno III consensus workshops on definitions, methodology and therapeutic strategies in portal hypertension. J Hepatol 33:846, 2000.

185. Imperiale TF, Chalasani N: A meta-analysis of endoscopic variceal ligation for primary prophylaxis of esophageal variceal bleeding. Hepatology 33:802, 2001.

186. Bureau C, Peron JM, Alric L, et al: "A la carte" treatment of portal hypertension: Adapting medical therapy to hemodynamic response for the prevention of bleeding. Hepatology 36:1361, 2002.

187. de Franchis R: Incidental esophageal varices. Gastroenterology 126:1860, 2004.

188. Schepke M, Kleber G, Willert J, et al: Ligation versus propranolol for the primary prophylaxis of variceal bleeding in cirrhosis. Hepatology 40:65, 2004.

189. Bernard B, Grange JD, Khac EN, et al: Antibiotic prophylaxis for the prevention of bacterial infections in cirrhotic patients with gastrointestinal bleeding: A meta-analysis. Hepatology 29:1655, 1999.

190. Levacher S, Letoumelin P, Pateron D, et al: Early administration of terlipressin plus glyceryl trinitrate to control active upper gastrointestinal bleeding in cirrhotic patients. Lancet 346:865, 1995.

191. de Franchis R: Portal Hypertension II. Proceedings of the Second Baveno International Consensus Workshop on Definitions, Methodology, and Therapeutic Strategies. Oxford, Blackwell Science, 1996.

192. Sarin SK, Lahoti D, Saxena SP, et al: Relevance, classification and natural history of gastric varices: A long-term follow-up study in 568 portal hypertension patients. Hepatology 16:1343, 1992.

193. Kim T, Shijo H, Kokawa H, et al: Risk factors for hemorrhage from gastric fundal varices. Hepatology 25:307, 1997.

194. Tripathi D, Therapondos G, Jackson E, et al: The role of the transjugular intrahepatic portosystemic stent shunt (TIPSS) in the management of bleeding gastric varices: Clinical and haemodynamic correlations. Gut 51:270, 2002.

195. Rinella ME, Shah D, Vogelzang RL, et al: Fundal variceal bleeding after correction of portal hypertension in patients with cirrhosis. Gastrointest Endosc 58:122, 2003.

196. Siringo S, McCormick PA, Mistry P: Prognostic significance of the white nipple sign in variceal bleeding. Gastrointest Endosc 37:51, 1991.

197. Lo G, Lai K, Cheng J, et al: A prospective, randomized trial of butyl cyanoacrylate injection versus band ligation in the management of bleeding gastric varices. Hepatology 33:1060, 2001.

198. Sarin SK, Jain AK, Jain M, Gupta R: A randomized controlled trial of cyanoacrylate versus alcohol injection in patients with isolated fundic varices. Am J Gastroenterol 97:1010, 2002.

199. Binmoeller KF: Glue for gastric varices: Some sticky issues. Gastrointest Endosc 52:298, 2000.

200. Trudeau W, Prindville T: Endoscopic injection sclerosis in bleeding gastric varices. Gastrointest Endosc 32:264, 1986.

201. Ryan BM, Stockbrugger RW, Ryan JM: A pathophysiologic, gastroenterologic, and radiologic approach to the management of gastric varices. Gastroenterology 126:1175, 2004.

202. Panes J, Teres J, Bosch J, Rodes J: Efficacy of balloon tamponade in treatment of bleeding gastric and esophageal varices. Results in 151 consecutive episodes. Dig Dis Sci 33:454, 1988.

203. Teres J, Cecilia A, Bordas JM, et al: Esophageal tamponade for bleeding varices. Controlled trial between the Sengstaken-Blakemore tube and the Linton-Nachlas tube. Gastroenterology 75:566, 1978.

204. Barange K, Peron JM, Imani K, et al: Transjugular intrahepatic portosystemic shunt in the treatment of refractory bleeding from ruptured gastric varices. Hepatology 30:1139, 1999.

205. Chau T, Patch D, Chan YW, et al: "Salvage" transjugular intrahepatic portosystemic shunts: Gastric fundal compared with esophageal variceal bleeding. Gastroenterology 114:981, 1998.

206. Mahadeva S, Bellamy MC, Kessel D, et al: Cost-Effectiveness of N-butyl-2-cyanoacrylate (Histoacryl) glue injections versus transjugular intrahepatic portosystemic shunt in the management of acute gastric variceal bleeding. Am J Gastroenterol 98:2688, 2003.

207. Greenwald B, Caldwell SH, Hespenheide E, et al: N-2-butyl-cyanoacrylate for bleeding gastric varices: A United

States pilot study and cost analysis. Am J Gastroenterol 98:1982, 2003.

208. Lee YT, Chan FK, Ng EK, et al: EUS-guided injection of cyanoacrylate for bleeding gastric varices. Gastrointest Endosc 52:168, 2000.

209. Yoshida T, Harada T, Shigemitsu T, et al: Endoscopic management of gastric varices using a detachable snare and simultaneous endoscopic sclerotherapy and O-ring ligation. J Gastroenterol Hepatol 14:730, 1999.

210. Shiba M, Higuchi K, Nakamura K, et al: Efficacy and safety of balloon-occluded endoscopic injection for sclerotherapy as a prophylactic treatment for high-risk gastric varices: A prospective, randomized, comparative clinical trial. Gastrointest Endosc 56:522, 2002.

211. Orloff MJ, Orloff MS, Girard B, Orloff SL: Bleeding esophagogastric varices from extrahepatic portal hypertension: 40 years' experience with portal-systemic shunt. J Am Coll Surg 194:717, 2002.

212. Thomas PG, D'Cruz AJ: Distal splenorenal shunting for bleeding gastric varices. Br J Surg 81:241, 1994.

213. Sanyal AJ, Freedman AM, Luketic VA, et al: The natural history of portal hypertension after transjugular intrahepatic portosystemic shunts. Gastroenterology 112:889, 1997.

214. Itzchak Y, Glickman MG: Duodenal varices in extrahepatic portal obstruction. Radiology 124:619, 1977.

215. Weisner RH, LaRusso NF, Dozois RR: Peristomal varices after proctocolectomy in patients with primary sclerosing cholangitis. Gastroenterology 90:316, 1986.

216. Norton ID, Andrews J, Kamath PS: Management of ectopic varices. Hepatology 28:1154, 1998.

217. Ackerman NB, Graeber GM, Fey J: Enterostomal varices secondary to portal hypertension: Progression of disease in conservatively managed cases. Arch Surg 115:1454, 1980.

218. Primignani M, Materia M, Preatoni P, et al: Natural history of portal hypertensive gastropathy in patients with liver cirrhosis. Gastroenterology 119:181, 2000.

219. Jabbari M, Cherry R, Lough JO: Gastric antral vascular ectasia: The watermelon stomach. Gastroenterology 87:1165, 1984.

220. Kamath PS, Lacerda M, Ahlquist D, et al: Gastric mucosal responses to intrahepatic portosystemic shunting in patients with cirrhosis. Gastroenterology 118:905, 2000.

221. Payen JL, Cales P, Voigt JJ: Severe portal hypertensive gastropathy and antral vascular ectasia are distinct entities in patients with cirrhosis. Gastroenterology 108:138, 1995.

222. Zhou Y, Qiao WJ, Hu H, Xu C: Control of bleeding in portal hypertensive gastropathy. Comparison of the efficacy of octreotide, vasopressin, and omeprazole in the control of acute bleeding in patients with portal hypertensive gastropathy: A controlled study. J Gastroenterol Hepatol 17:973, 2002.

223. Perez-Ayuso R, Pique J, Bosch J, et al: Propranolol in prevention of recurrent bleeding from severe portal hypertensive gastropathy in cirrhosis. Lancet 337:1431, 1991.

224. Panes J, Bordas JM, Pique J, et al: Effects of propranolol on gastric mucosal perfusion in cirrhotic patients with portal hypertensive gastropathy. Hepatology 17:213, 1993.

225. Tran A, Villeneuve J-P, Blodeau M, et al: Treatment of chronic bleeding from gastric antral vascular ectasia (GAVE) with estrogen-progesterone in cirrhotic patients: An open pilot study. Am J Gastroenterol 94:2909, 1999.

226. Vincent C, Pomier-Layrargues GP, Dagenais M, et al: Cure of gastric antral vascular ectasia by liver transplantation despite persistent portal hypertension: A clue for pathogenesis. Liver Transpl 8:717, 2002.

CHAPTER
88 Ascites and Spontaneous Bacterial Peritonitis

Bruce A. Runyon

Ascites is of Greek derivation ("askos") and refers to a bag or sack. The word is a noun and describes pathologic fluid accumulation within the peritoneal cavity. The adjective *ascitic* is used in conjunction with the word *fluid* to describe the liquid per se.

PATHOGENESIS OF ASCITES

CIRRHOTIC ASCITES

Ascites occurs in the setting of cirrhosis as a result of the sequence of events detailed in Figure 88–1. The most recent theory of ascitic fluid formation, the "peripheral arterial vasodilation hypothesis," proposes that both older hypotheses, the underfill and overflow theories, are correct, but that each is operative at a different stage.[1] The first abnormality that develops appears to be portal hypertension. Portal pressure increases above a critical threshold, and circulating nitric oxide levels increase. Nitric oxide leads to vasodilatation.[2] As the state of vasodilatation worsens, plasma levels of vasoconstrictor, sodium-retentive hormones increase, renal function deteriorates, and ascitic fluid forms—that is, decompensation occurs.

In the setting of volume overload in a patient with cirrhosis and ascites, the explanation for the neurohumoral excitation, which is characteristic of volume depletion, may relate to volume sensors. Animals have sophisticated systems for detecting and preserving vascular perfusion pressures and intravascular osmolality. An organism's ability to detect changes in intravascular volume (especially volume overload) is limited, however, and is linked to pressure receptors. This observation may explain in part the paradox of dramatic volume overload in the face of sympathetic nervous traffic and hormone levels that are indicative of intravascular volume depletion.

NONCIRRHOTIC ASCITES

The mechanism of fluid retention in patients with malignancy-related ascites depends on the location of the tumor. Peritoneal carcinomatosis appears to cause ascites through the production of proteinaceous fluid by tumor cells lining the peritoneum. Extracellular fluid enters the peritoneal cavity to reestablish oncotic balance. Fluid accumulates in patients with massive liver metastases because of portal hypertension caused by stenosis or occlusion of portal veins by tumor nodules or tumor emboli.[3] In patients with hepatocellular carcinoma, ascites arises because of the underlying cirrhosis-related portal hypertension, tumor-induced portal vein thrombosis, or both. Chylous ascites in patients with malignant lymphoma appears to be caused by lymph node obstruction by tumor and rupture of chyle-containing lymphatics.

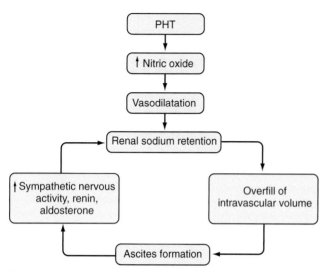

Figure 88–1   Pathogenesis of ascites in the setting of cirrhosis. PHT, portal hypertension.

Table 88–1   Causes of Ascites

Causative Disorder	% of Affected Patients
Cirrhosis (with or without infection)	85
Miscellaneous portal hypertension–related disorder (including 5% with two causes)	8
Cardiac disease	3
Peritoneal carcinomatosis	2
Miscellaneous nonportal hypertension–related disorders	2

Data from Runyon BA, Montano AA, Akriviadis EA, et al: The serum-ascites albumin gradient is superior to the exudate-transudate concept in the differential diagnosis of ascites. Ann Intern Med 117:215, 1992.

Ascites can complicate high-output or low-output heart failure or nephrotic syndrome. As in cirrhosis, effective arterial blood volume appears to be decreased, and the vasopressin, renin-aldosterone, and sympathetic nervous systems are activated.[4] These changes lead to renal vasoconstriction and sodium and water retention. Fluid then "weeps" from the congested hepatic sinusoids as lymph, as in cirrhotic ascites. Tuberculosis, *Chlamydia* infection, and coccidioidomycosis probably cause ascites through the production of proteinaceous fluid, as in peritoneal carcinomatosis. Spontaneous bacterial peritonitis does not appear to cause fluid to accumulate; infection develops only in preexisting ascites.

In patients with pancreatic or biliary ascites, fluid accumulates by leakage of pancreatic juice or bile into the peritoneal cavity or forms secondary to a "chemical burn" of the peritoneum. After abdominal surgery, especially extensive retroperitoneal dissection, lymphatics may be transected and may leak lymph for varying amounts of time.[5] The mechanism of development of ascites in this condition is similar to that for malignant chylous ascites, namely, lymphatic leak.

CLINICAL FEATURES

HISTORY

Most patients (approximately 85%) with ascites in the United States have cirrhosis. The three most common causes of cirrhosis are alcohol, chronic hepatitis C, and nonalcoholic steatohepatitis (NASH) related to obesity. As the obesity epidemic evolves, it is conceivable that NASH could become the most common cause of cirrhosis. Many patients have two of these conditions, and some have all three.[6,7] In approximately 15% of patients with ascites, a nonhepatic cause of fluid retention is identified (Table 88–1).

Ascites frequently develops during a patient's first decompensatory episode of alcoholic liver disease. Ascites can develop early in alcoholic liver disease in the precir-

rhotic, alcoholic hepatitis stage. At this stage, portal hypertension and the resulting predisposition to sodium retention are reversible with abstinence from alcohol.[8] Patients with precirrhotic alcoholic liver disease may lose their predisposition to fluid retention when they reduce or cease consumption of alcohol.

Evidence is accumulating that nonalcoholic cirrhosis also can be reversible with effective therapy.[9] Whether decompensated nonalcoholic cirrhotic livers can revert to a normal liver, however, remains to be seen. Many patients with cirrhosis and ascites will require liver transplantation.

Patients with ascites should be questioned about risk factors for liver disease other than alcohol, such as intravenous drug use, blood transfusions, sex with a same-gender partner, acupuncture, tattoos, ear piercing, and country of origin. Commonly, the cause of ascites in a middle-aged or elderly woman is viral hepatitis–induced cirrhosis resulting from a remote, often forgotten blood transfusion. Another cause of "cryptogenic" cirrhosis and ascites is NASH from long-standing obesity.[10] Many patients who have been obese will spontaneously lose 50 or even 100 pounds after their liver disease decompensates. Unless the physician asks about lifetime maximum body weight and usual adult body weight, the possibility of NASH-related cirrhosis may not be considered. With careful history-taking and appropriate laboratory testing, the percentage of patients with cirrhosis who are now labeled cryptogenic is approaching zero.[10]

Patients with a long history of stable cirrhosis and the sudden development of ascites should be suspected of harboring a hepatocellular carcinoma that has precipitated the decompensation.

Patients with ascites who have a history of cancer should be suspected of having malignancy-related ascites. Cancer in the past, however, does not guarantee a malignant cause of ascites. For example, patients with tobacco-related lung cancer and a history of alcohol abuse may have ascites due to cirrhosis. Breast, lung, colon, and pancreatic cancers are regularly complicated by ascites.[3] Abdominal pain is a helpful distinguishing feature. Malignancy-related ascites frequently is painful, whereas cirrhotic ascites usually is not, unless superimposed bacterial peritonitis or alcoholic hepatitis is present.

A history of heart failure may raise the possibility of cardiac ascites. Alcoholics in whom ascites develops may have alcoholic cardiomyopathy or alcoholic liver disease, but usually not both.

Tuberculous peritonitis usually manifests as fever and abdominal pain. Many affected patients are recent immigrants from an endemic area. In the United States, more than one half of the patients with tuberculous peritonitis have underlying alcoholic cirrhosis, which may contribute to the formation of ascitic fluid.

Ascites may occur in patients with acute hemorrhagic pancreatitis or a ruptured pancreatic duct from chronic pancreatitis or trauma. Often troublesome ascites also may develop in a small percentage of patients on hemodialysis. Fitz-Hugh–Curtis syndrome caused by *Chlamydia* or gonorrhea may cause inflammatory ascites in a sexually active woman.[11] Patients in whom ascites and anasarca develop in the setting of diabetes should be suspected of having nephrotic ascites. Ascites in a patient with symptoms and signs of myxedema should prompt assessment of thyroid function. Serositis in a patient with a connective tissue disease may be complicated by ascites.[12]

PHYSICAL EXAMINATION

On the basis of the history and the appearance of the abdomen, the diagnosis of ascites is readily suspected and usually is confirmed easily on physical examination. The presence of a full, bulging abdomen should lead to percussion of the flanks. If the degree of flank dullness is greater than usual (i.e., if the percussed air-fluid level is higher than that normally found on the lateral aspect of the abdomen with the patient supine), the examiner should check for "shifting." If flank dullness is absent, checking for shifting is unnecessary. Approximately 1500 mL of fluid must be present before dullness is detected.[13] If flank dullness is not present, the chance that the patient has ascites is less than 10%.[13] A fluid wave is not worth testing for.[13]

Gaseous distention of the bowel, a thick panniculus, and an ovarian mass can mimic ascites.[14] Gaseous distention should be readily apparent on percussion. Ovarian masses usually cause tympanic flanks with central dullness. An obese abdomen may be diffusely dull to percussion, and abdominal ultrasonography may be required to determine if fluid is present. Also, the speed of increase in abdominal girth can be helpful; ascites develops in days to weeks, whereas thickening of omentum and panniculus takes months to years. As the percentage of patients with ascites and obesity increases, the use of ultrasound examination to detect the presence or absence of fluid also will increase. Ultrasonographic scans can detect as little as 100 mL of fluid in the abdomen.[15]

The presence of palmar erythema, large pulsatile spider angiomata, large abdominal wall collateral veins, or fetor hepaticus is suggestive of parenchymal liver disease and portal hypertension. The presence of large veins on the patient's back suggests inferior vena cava blockage. An immobile mass in the umbilicus, the Sister Mary Joseph nodule, is suggestive of peritoneal carcinomatosis.

The neck veins of patients with ascites should always be examined. Alcoholic cardiomyopathy with cardiac ascites can mimic cirrhosis with ascites; an elevated jugular venous pressure helps with this aspect of the differential diagnosis. Constrictive pericarditis is one of the few curable causes of ascites. Most patients with cardiac ascites have impressive jugular venous distention. Some have no visible jugular venous distention but such high central venous pressures that their bulging forehead veins rise to the top of their skulls. When present, peripheral edema in patients with liver disease usually is found in the lower extremities and occasionally may involve the abdominal wall. Patients with nephrotic syndrome or cardiac failure may have total body edema (anasarca).

DIAGNOSIS

Although the diagnosis of ascites may be suspected on the basis of the history and physical examination, final confirmation is based on successful abdominal paracentesis or detection of ascites on imaging. Determination of the cause of ascites is based on the results of the history, physical examination, and ascitic fluid analysis. In general, few other tests are required.

ABDOMINAL PARACENTESIS

Indications

Abdominal paracentesis with appropriate ascitic fluid analysis is probably the most rapid and cost-effective method of diagnosing the cause of ascites. Also, because of the possibility of ascitic fluid infection in a cirrhotic patient admitted to the hospital, a surveillance paracentesis performed on admission may detect unexpected infection.[15] Not all patients with ascitic fluid infection are symptomatic; many have subtle symptoms, such as mild confusion noticed only by the family. Detection of infection at an early asymptomatic stage may reduce mortality. Therefore, ascitic fluid should be sampled in all inpatients and outpatients with new-onset ascites and in all patients with ascites who are admitted to the hospital. Paracentesis should be repeated in patients (whether hospitalized or not) in whom symptoms, signs, or laboratory abnormalities suggestive of infection develop (e.g., abdominal pain or tenderness, fever, encephalopathy, hypotension, renal failure, acidosis, peripheral leukocytosis).

Contraindications

Few contraindications to paracentesis have been recognized. Coagulopathy is a potential contraindication; however, most patients with cirrhotic ascites have coagulopathy, and if mild to moderate coagulopathy were viewed as a contraindication to paracentesis, few cirrhotics would undergo this procedure.[16] In my opinion, coagulopathy should preclude paracentesis only when clinically evident fibrinolysis or disseminated intravascular coagulation is present.[16] These conditions occur in fewer than 1 per 1000 taps. No data are available to support a cutoff for coagulation parameters beyond which paracentesis should be avoided. Even after multiple paracenteses, bloody ascites usually does not develop in patients with severe prolongation of the prothrombin time. Cirrhotic patients without clinically obvious coagulopathy simply do not bleed excessively from needlesticks unless a blood vessel is entered.[16]

Studies regarding complications of paracentesis in patients with ascites have documented no deaths or infections caused by paracentesis.[15,16] No episodes of hemoperitoneum or entry of the paracentesis needle into the bowel have been reported in these studies. Complications have included only abdominal wall hematomas in approximately 2% of paracenteses, even though 71% of the patients had an abnormal prothrombin time and 21% had a prothrombin time prolonged by more than 5 seconds.[16] Complication rates may be higher when paracentesis is performed by an inexperienced operator.

Transfusion of blood products (fresh frozen plasma or platelets) routinely before paracentesis in cirrhotic patients with coagulopathy, presumably to prevent hemorrhagic complications, is not supported by data. Because a hematoma that necessitates blood transfusion develops in only approximately 1% of patients who undergo paracentesis without prophylactic transfusion of plasma or platelets, approximately 100 to 200 units of fresh frozen plasma or platelets would have to be given to prevent the transfusion of approximately 2 units of red blood cells.

Patient Position and Choice of Needle Entry Site and Needle

The volume of fluid in the abdomen and the thickness of the abdominal wall determine in part how the patient should be positioned in preparation for the procedure. Patients with a large volume of ascites and thin abdominal walls can be "tapped" successfully in the supine position, with the head of the bed or examining table elevated slightly. Patients with less fluid can be placed in the lateral decubitus position and tapped in the midline or in the right or left lower quadrant while supine (see later). Patients with small amounts of fluid may be tapped successfully only in the face-down position or with ultrasound guidance.[16]

The choice of the site for inserting the needle has changed over the years because of the increasing prevalence of obesity and frequency of therapeutic paracentesis. Paracentesis in obese patients poses special challenges. In obese patients, the abdominal wall usually is substantially thicker in the midline than in the lower quadrants on ultrasound examination.[17] The abdominal wall may be even thicker than the length of a 3.5-inch paracentesis needle. Also, on physical examination, determining whether ascites is present or absent in the obese patient is frequently difficult. Ultrasound examination is helpful in confirming the presence of fluid and in guiding the paracentesis needle to obtain a fluid sample.[18] Preferably, the needle is inserted into the left lower quadrant, rather than the right lower quadrant, because the cecum may be distended with gas from lactulose therapy. Also, the right lower quadrant is more likely to have a surgical scar (e.g., from appendectomy) than the left. When therapeutic paracentesis is performed, more fluid can be obtained using a lower quadrant needle insertion site than a midline site.

The needle must be placed several centimeters from a surgical scar. The bowel may be adherent to the peritoneal surface of the abdomen near a scar, and a needle inserted there may enter the bowel.[15] A long midline scar precludes midline paracentesis. An appendectomy scar precludes a right lower quadrant site, in general.

I usually choose a site in the left lower quadrant two fingerbreadths cephalad and two fingerbreadths medial to the anterior superior iliac spine. In a patient with multiple abdominal scars, ultrasound guidance may be required.

In the patient who is not overweight, I prefer to use a standard metal 1.5-inch, 22-gauge needle. Paracentesis in obese patients requires the use of a longer needle, for example, a 3.5-inch, 22-gauge variety. Steel needles are preferable to plastic-sheathed cannulas because plastic sheaths may shear off into the peritoneal cavity, with the potential to kink and obstruct the flow of fluid after the cannula is removed. Metal needles do not puncture the bowel unless the bowel is adherent to a scar or severe gaseous distention is present.

Technique of Diagnostic Paracentesis

Drapes, gown, hat, and mask are optional, but sterile gloves should be used when paracentesis is performed. The skin is disinfected with an iodine solution. The skin and subcutaneous tissue should be infiltrated with a local anesthetic. The sterile package insert enclosing the gloves can be used as a sterile field on which to place syringes, needles, gauze, and other supplies. When sterile gloves are not used, ascitic fluid cultures frequently grow skin contaminants. A single viable organism will grow to detectable levels in blood culture bottles.

To prevent leakage of fluid after the needle is withdrawn, a special technique is required. The previously used term "Z tract" led to confusion about the precise technique: It does not involve manipulating the needle up and down, as this could lead to tissue injury. This technique of needle insertion is accomplished by displacing (with one gloved hand) the skin approximately 2 cm downward and then slowly inserting the paracentesis needle mounted on the syringe held in the other hand. The hand holding the syringe stabilizes the syringe and retracts its plunger simultaneously. A steady hand and experience are needed. The skin is released only after the needle has penetrated the peritoneum and fluid flows. When the needle is ultimately removed, the skin resumes its original position and seals the needle pathway. (If the needle were inserted straight into the peritoneum from the skin surface, the fluid would leak out easily, because the pathway would be straight.)

The needle should be advanced slowly through the abdominal wall in approximately 5-mm increments. Slow insertion allows the operator to see blood if a vessel is entered, so that the needle can be withdrawn immediately before further damage is done. Slow insertion also allows the bowel to move away from the needle, thereby avoiding bowel puncture. The syringe that is attached to the needle should be aspirated intermittently during insertion. If continuous suction is applied, bowel or omentum may be drawn to the end of the needle as soon as the needle enters the peritoneal cavity, thereby occluding flow and resulting in an apparently unsuccessful tap. Slow insertion also allows time for the elastic peritoneum to "tent" over the end of the needle and be pierced by it. The most common causes of an unsuccessful paracentesis are continuous aspiration during insertion of the needle and rapid insertion and withdrawal of the needle before the peritoneum is pierced. If the operator is certain that the needle tip is inserted far enough but no fluid is apparent, the syringe and needle can be twisted 90 degrees to pierce the peritoneum, thereby permitting flow of fluid.

Approximately 30 mL of fluid is obtained using one or more syringes. I prefer to use a 5- or 10-mL syringe for the initial portion of a diagnostic tap and then twist this syringe off the needle and replace it with a 20- or 30-mL syringe to obtain the remainder of the sample. The initial use of a small syringe allows the operator to have better control and to see fluid more easily as it enters the hub of the syringe. The syringe and attached needle are then pulled out of the abdomen, and the needle is removed and discarded. A sterile needle is then placed on the larger syringe, and an appropriate amount of fluid is inoculated into each of a pair of prepared blood culture bottles (see later). Usually, 5 to 10 mL is inoculated into 50-mL bottles, and 10 to 20 mL into 100-mL bottles. The next aliquot is placed into a "purple-top" ethylenediaminete-tra-acetic acid tube for a cell count, and the final aliquot is placed into a "red-top" tube for chemistries. Inoculating the culture bottles first with a sterile needle minimizes contamination. The fluid must be placed promptly into the anticoagulant-containing tube to avoid clotting; clotted fluid cannot be analyzed for cell count.

Technique of Therapeutic Paracentesis

Therapeutic paracentesis is similar to diagnostic paracentesis except that a larger-bore needle is used and additional equipment is required. In the patient who is not overweight, I prefer to use a standard metal 1.5-inch, 16- to 18-gauge needle. Obese patients may require a longer needle, for example, a 3.5-inch, 18-gauge needle. Recently, 15-gauge five-hole needles have been produced specifically for therapeutic abdominal paracentesis; these needles may replace the spinal needles used currently for paracentesis in obese patients. The new needles have a removable sharp inner component and a blunt outer cannula; they range in length from 3.25 to 5.9 inches.

An old method of using a 60-mL syringe, stopcock, and collection bag is tedious. Use of vacuum bottles (1 or 2 L) connected to the needle with noncollapsible tubing is much faster. Use of a peristaltic pump is even faster than vacuum bottles. Unless the needle is allowed to drift subcutaneously, the needle (or blunt steel cannula) can be left in the abdomen during a therapeutic paracentesis without injury. Larger-bore needles or cannulas permit more rapid removal of fluid but leave larger defects if they enter vessels or the bowel inadvertently.

Once fluid is flowing, the needle should be stabilized to ensure steady flow. It is not unusual for flow to cease intermittently. With respiratory movement, the needle may gradually work its way out of the peritoneal cavity and into the soft tissue, and some serosanguineous fluid may appear in the needle hub or tubing. When this happens, the pump should be turned off or a clamp placed on the tubing connected to the vacuum bottle.

The tubing is removed from the needle, and the needle is twisted a few degrees. If flow does not resume, the needle is twisted a bit more. If flow still does not resume, the needle is inserted in 1- to 2-mm increments until brisk dripping of fluid from the needle hub is seen. The tubing is then reattached, and more fluid is removed. Occasionally, fluid cannot be aspirated but drips from the needle hub. In this situation, fluid is allowed to drip into a sterile container for collection, as in a lumbar puncture.

As the fluid is removed, the bowel and omentum draw closer to the needle and eventually block the flow of ascitic fluid. The patient then must be repositioned so that gravity causes the fluid to pool near the needle. It is useful to reposition the patient a few times during a total paracentesis to maximize the amount of fluid removed. Excessive manipulation of the needle is avoided, to minimize the risk of trauma to the bowel or blood vessels.

After samples of fluid are obtained for testing, 2 to 4 L of fluid is removed to relieve the pressure of tense ascites in patients with new or diuretic-sensitive ascites. A sodium-restricted diet and diuretics are prescribed to further reduce the fluid (see later). If a patient is known to be diuretic-resistant, a "total tap" is performed—that is, all of the fluid that is accessible is removed. If less is removed, the tap will need to be repeated soon (see later section, "Refractory Ascites").

ASCITIC FLUID ANALYSIS

Gross Appearance

Non-neutrocytic (i.e., ascitic fluid neutrophil count less than 250/mm^3 [0.25×10^9/L]) ascitic fluid is transparent and usually slightly yellow (Fig. 88–2). Ascitic fluid with a very low protein concentration may have no pigment and look like water. The opacity of many cloudy ascitic fluid specimens is caused by neutrophils. The presence of neutrophils leads to a shimmering effect when a glass tube containing the fluid is rocked back and forth in front of a light. Fluid with an absolute neutrophil count less than 1000/mm^3 (1.0×10^9/L) may be nearly clear. Fluid with a count greater than 5000/mm^3 (5.0×10^9/L) is quite cloudy, and fluid with a count greater than 50,000/mm^3 (50.0×10^9/L) resembles mayonnaise.

Ascitic fluid specimens frequently are blood-tinged or frankly bloody. A red blood cell count of 10,000/mm^3 (10.0×10^9/L) is the threshold for a pink appearance; smaller concentrations result in clear or turbid fluid. Ascitic fluid with a red blood cell count greater than 20,000/mm^3 (20.0×10^9/L) is distinctly red. Many ascitic fluid specimens are bloody because of a traumatic tap; these specimens are blood-streaked and frequently clot unless the fluid is transferred immediately to the anticoagulant-containing tube (for the cell count). By contrast, nontraumatic or remotely traumatic blood-tinged ascitic fluid is homogeneous and does not clot, because it has already clotted and the clot has lysed. Some patients with portal hypertension have bloody hepatic lymph, resulting in bloody ascitic fluid, perhaps because of rupture of lymphatics that are under high pressure. Samples from patients with hepatocellular carcinoma are regularly bloody, but only about 10% of samples from patients

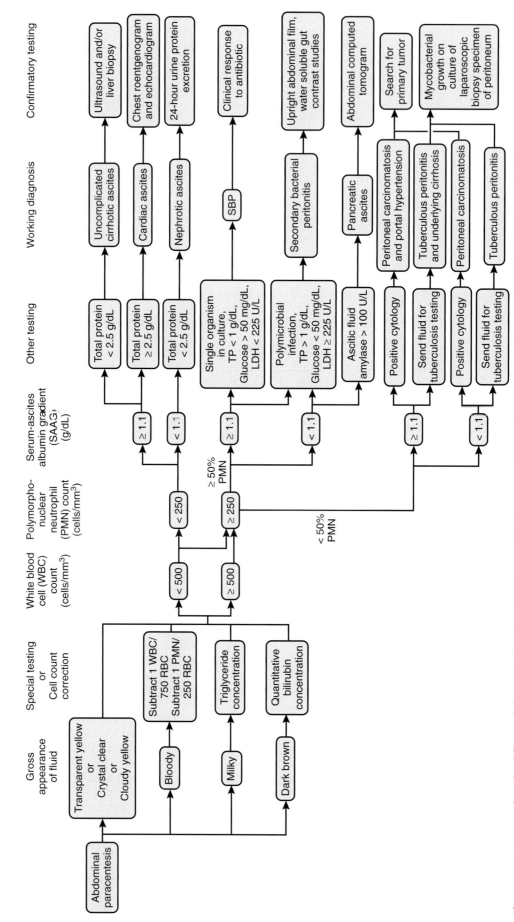

Figure 88–2 Approach to the differential diagnosis of ascites. LDH, lactate dehydrogenase; PMN, polymorphonuclear neutrophil; RBC, red blood cells; SBP, spontaneous bacterial peritonitis; TP, total protein.

with peritoneal carcinomatosis are red.[3] Although many physicians have the impression that tuberculosis results in bloody ascitic fluid, less than 5% of tuberculous samples are hemorrhagic in my experience.

Ascitic fluid frequently is lipid-laden. Lipid opacifies the fluid. The degree of opalescence of ascitic fluid ranges from slightly cloudy to completely opaque and chylous. Most opaque milky fluid samples have a triglyceride concentration greater than 200 mg/dL (2.26 mmol/L), usually greater than 1000 mg/dL (11.30 mmol/L). Fluid that has the appearance of dilute skim milk has a triglyceride concentration between 100 mg/dL (1.13 mmol/L) and 200 mg/dL (2.26 mmol/L). A substantial minority of cirrhotic ascitic fluid samples are neither transparent nor frankly milky. These opalescent samples have slightly elevated triglyceride concentrations ranging from 50 mg/dL (0.56 mmol/L) to 200 mg/dL (2.26 mmol/L).[19] The opacity of these fluids does not have the shimmering characteristics of ascitic fluid with an elevated white blood cell count. The lipid usually layers out when a tube of ascitic fluid is placed in the refrigerator for 48 to 72 hours. In contrast with findings in older published reports, most patients with chylous or opalescent ascites have cirrhosis.[19,20]

Dark-brown fluid with a bilirubin concentration greater than that of serum usually indicates biliary perforation.[21] Deeply jaundiced patients have bile-stained ascitic fluid, but the bilirubin level and the degree of pigmentation are visually less than those of the corresponding serum. Pancreatic ascites may be pigmented because of the effect of pancreatic enzymes on red blood cells. The red blood cells may have to be centrifuged before the discolored supernatant is revealed. The degree of pigmentation ranges from tea-colored to jet black, as in so-called hemorrhagic pancreatitis. Black ascitic fluid also may be found in patients with malignant melanoma.

Ascitic Fluid Tests

The practice of ordering every available body fluid test on every ascitic fluid specimen is expensive and can be more confusing than helpful, especially when unexpectedly abnormal results are encountered. An algorithm for the analysis of ascitic fluid is shown in Figure 88–2. The basic concept is that screening tests are performed on the initial specimen; additional testing is performed only when necessary as indicated by the results of the screening tests. Further testing may require another paracentesis, but because most specimens consist of uncomplicated cirrhotic ascitic fluid, no further testing is needed in a majority of specimens. Also, because laboratories frequently store the fluid for a few days, additional testing often can be ordered on the stored fluid.

On the basis of cost analysis, tests can be classified as routine, optional, unusual, and unhelpful (Table 88–2).[15] The cell count is the single most helpful ascitic fluid test. Only approximately 10 μL of fluid is required for a standard manual hemocytometer count. Therefore, if only one drop of fluid can be obtained, it should be sent for cell count. More fluid is almost always obtainable, however. The fluid should be submitted in an anticoagulant-containing tube (i.e., ethylenediaminetetra-acetic acid) to prevent clotting. Because the decision to begin empirical antibiotic treatment of suspected ascitic fluid infection is based largely on the absolute neutrophil count (which should have a turnaround time of a few minutes), rather than the culture (which takes 12 to 48 hours to demonstrate growth), the cell count is more important than the culture in the early detection and treatment of ascitic fluid infection.

Cell Count

Surprisingly, ascitic fluid cell counts have not been standardized. Some laboratories count mesothelial cells in addition to white blood cells (WBCs) and label the sum as "nucleated cells." The usefulness of mesothelial cell counts is not clear. The WBC count in uncomplicated cirrhotic ascites usually is less than 500 cells/mm³ (0.5 × 10⁹/L)[15,22] (see Fig. 88–2). During diuresis in patients with cirrhotic ascites, the WBC count can concentrate to more than 1000 cells/mm³ (1.0 × 10⁹/L).[22] A diagnosis of diuresis-related elevation of the ascitic fluid WBC count, however, requires that a prediuresis count be available, that normal lymphocytes predominate in the fluid, and that unexplained clinical symptoms or signs (e.g., fever or abdominal pain) be absent.

The upper limit of normal for the absolute polymorphonuclear neutrophil (PMN) count in uncomplicated cirrhotic ascitic fluid usually is stated to be lower than 250/mm³ (0.25 × 10⁹/L).[15,22] The short survival of PMNs results in relative stability of the absolute PMN count during diuresis.[22] Therefore, the 250 cells/mm³ (0.25 × 10⁹/L) "cutoff" remains reliable even after diuresis.

New methods have been developed to estimate or measure the number of ascitic fluid cells.[23] "Dipsticks" can detect an ascitic fluid PMN count greater than 250/mm³ (0.25 × 10⁹/L) in 90 to 120 seconds. Automated cell counters have now been shown to be accurate in this setting. Most of these studies have been performed in Europe. Federal regulations may delay their general use in the United States.

Table 88–2 Ascitic Fluid Laboratory Data

Routine	Optional	Unusual	Unhelpful
Cell count	Culture in blood culture bottles	TB smear and culture	pH
Albumin	Glucose	Cytology	Lactate
Total protein	LDH	Triglyceride	Cholesterol
	Amylase	Bilirubin	Fibronectin
	Gram stain		α₁-Antitrypsin
			Glycosaminoglycans

LDH, lactate dehydrogenase; TB, tuberculosis.

Any inflammatory process can result in an elevated ascitic fluid WBC count. Spontaneous bacterial peritonitis is the most common cause of inflammation of ascitic fluid and the most common cause of an elevated ascitic WBC count (see later). The total WBC count, as well as the absolute PMN count, is elevated in spontaneous bacterial peritonitis, and PMNs usually account for more than 70% of the total WBC count. Also, in tuberculous peritonitis and peritoneal carcinomatosis, the total ascitic WBC count frequently is elevated, but usually with a predominance of lymphocytes.[3]

In most instances, bloody ascitic fluid is the result of a slightly traumatic tap. Leakage of blood into the peritoneal cavity leads to an elevated ascitic fluid WBC count. Because neutrophils predominate in blood, the ascitic fluid differential count may be altered by contamination of ascitic fluid with blood. To correct for this, 1 PMN is subtracted from the absolute ascitic fluid PMN count for every 250 red blood cells[22] (see Fig. 88-2). If the leakage of blood occurred at a remote time, the PMNs will have lysed, and the corrected PMN count will be a negative number. If the corrected PMN count in a bloody specimen is greater than or equal to 250 cells/mm³ (0.25×10^9/L), the patient must be assumed to be infected.

Exudate/Transudate

Before the 1980s, the ascitic fluid total protein concentration was used to classify ascites as either exudative (greater than 2.5 g/dL [25 g/L]) or transudative (less than 2.5 g/dL [25 g/L]). Unfortunately, this classification does not work well in ascitic fluid, and these terms as applied to ascitic fluid were never carefully defined or validated. Attempts at using combinations of lactate dehydrogenase (LDH) and serum–to–ascitic fluid ratios of LDH and protein also have not been shown to classify ascitic fluid accurately into exudates and transudates.[24]

Serum-Ascites Albumin Gradient

The *serum-ascites albumin gradient* (SAAG) has been proved in multiple studies to categorize ascites better than either the total protein concentration or other parameters[25-27] (Table 88-3). The SAAG is based on oncotic-hydrostatic balance.[25] Portal hypertension results

in an abnormally high hydrostatic pressure gradient between the portal bed and ascitic fluid. A similarly large difference must exist between ascitic fluid and intravascular oncotic forces.[25] Albumin exerts greater oncotic force per gram than that exerted by other proteins. Therefore, the difference between the serum and ascitic fluid albumin concentrations correlates directly with portal pressure.[25]

Calculating the SAAG involves measuring the albumin concentration of serum and ascitic fluid specimens and simply *subtracting* the ascitic fluid value from the serum value. Unless a laboratory error has been made, the serum albumin concentration is always the larger value. The gradient is calculated by subtraction and is *not* a ratio. If the SAAG is 1.1 g/dL (11 g/L) or greater, the patient can be considered to have portal hypertension with an accuracy of approximately 97%.[26] Also, if the serum albumin-ascitic fluid *total protein* gradient is 1.1 g/dL (11 g/L) or greater, the patient has portal hypertension, because the ascitic fluid albumin concentration cannot be greater than the ascitic fluid total protein concentration. Conversely, if the SAAG is less than 1.1 g/dL (11 g/L), the patient is unlikely to have portal hypertension. The SAAG does not explain the pathogenesis of ascites formation, nor does it explain where the albumin came from—that is, liver or bowel. It simply gives the physician an indirect but accurate index of portal pressure. The accuracy of the test is excellent, even with ascitic fluid infection, diuresis, therapeutic paracentesis, intravenous infusions of albumin, and various causes of liver disease.[26]

Measurement of the ascitic fluid albumin concentration has been routine in some laboratories for more than 20 years. Nevertheless, before sending ascitic fluid for the first time to a laboratory to measure the albumin concentration, a physician should discuss the test with the laboratory chemist. The accuracy of the albumin assay at low albumin concentrations (e.g., less than 1 g/dL [10 g/L]) should be confirmed, because many patients with ascites have a serum albumin concentration in the range of 2.0 g/dL (20 g/L) and an ascitic fluid albumin concentration in the range of 0 to 1.0 g/dL (0 to 10 g/L). If a patient with cirrhosis has a serum albumin level of less than 1.1 g/dL (11 g/L), as occurs in less than 1% of patients with cirrhotic ascites, the SAAG will be falsely low.

The accuracy of the SAAG also is reduced when specimens of serum and ascites are not obtained nearly simultanously. The specimens should be obtained on the same day, preferably within the same hour. Both serum and ascitic fluid albumin concentrations change over time; however, these values change in parallel, so the difference is stable. Arterial hypotension may result in a decrease in the portal pressure and a narrowing of the SAAG. Lipid interferes with the assay for albumin, and chylous ascites may result in a falsely high SAAG.

Serum hyperglobulinemia (serum globulin level greater than 5 g/dL [50 g/L]) leads to a high ascitic fluid globulin concentration and can narrow the albumin gradient by contributing to the oncotic forces. A narrowed gradient caused by high serum globulin levels occurs in only approximately 1% of ascitic fluid specimens. To correct the SAAG in the setting of a high serum globulin level, the following formula is used[27]:

Table 88–3 Classification of Ascites by Serum-Ascites Albumin Gradient

High Gradient ≥1.1 g/dL (11 g/L)	Low Gradient <1.1 g/dL (11 g/L)
Cirrhosis	Peritoneal carcinomatosis
Alcoholic hepatitis	Tuberculous peritonitis
Cardiac ascites	Pancreatic ascites
"Mixed" ascites	Bowel obstruction or infarction
Massive liver metastases	Biliary ascites
Fulminant hepatic failure	Nephrotic syndrome
Budd-Chiari syndrome	Postoperative lymphatic leak
Portal vein thrombosis	Serositis in connective tissue diseases
Sinusoidal obstruction syndrome	
Myxedema	
Fatty liver of pregnancy	

$$\text{Corrected SAAG} = \text{uncorrected SAAG} \times 0.16 \times$$
$$(\text{serum globulin [in g/dL]} + 2.5)$$

Approximately 5% of patients with ascites have "mixed" ascites (that is, two causes of ascites) (see Table 88–1). Most of these patients have portal hypertension from cirrhosis plus another cause of ascites, such as tuberculosis or peritoneal carcinomatosis.[26] The albumin gradient is high (1.1 g/dL [11 g/L] or greater) in mixed ascites, as a reflection of the underlying portal hypertension.[26]

The presence of a high SAAG does not confirm a diagnosis of cirrhosis; it simply indicates the presence of portal hypertension. Many causes of portal hypertension other than cirrhosis are recognized (see Tables 88–1 and 88–3). A low SAAG does not confirm a diagnosis of peritoneal carcinomatosis. Although peritoneal carcinomatosis is the most common cause of a low SAAG, other causes exist (see Table 88–3). The SAAG needs to be determined only on the first paracentesis specimen in a given patient; it does not need to be repeated on subsequent specimens, if the first value is definitive. If the first result is borderline (e.g., 1.0 or 1.1 g/dL [10 or 11 g/L]), repeating the paracentesis and analysis usually provides a definitive result.

High-albumin-gradient and *low-albumin-gradient* should replace the modifiers "transudative" and "exudative" in the classification of ascites.[25-27]

Culture

In the past, culture methodology for ascitic fluid was based on the notion that most episodes of ascitic fluid infection were polymicrobial with high colony counts, as in surgical peritonitis. The most common bacterial infection of ascitic fluid, spontaneous bacterial peritonitis, is monomicrobial, however, with a low bacterial concentration (median colony count of only 1 organism/mL).[28] The older method of culture consisted of inoculation (in the microbiology laboratory) of each of three agar plates and some broth with a few drops of fluid. This method of culturing ascitic fluid, as if it were urine or stool, is predictably insensitive for detecting monomicrobial infections with low colony counts. Spontaneous bacterial peritonitis is more like bacteremia in terms of numbers of bacteria present; culturing ascitic fluid as if it were blood has a high yield.[15,28,29]

In fact, the sensitivity of culture in detecting bacterial growth in neutrocytic ascites (i.e., ascitic fluid with a PMN count of 250 cells/mm^3 [0.25×10^9/L] or greater) depends on the method of culture used. The older method of culture has been found to detect bacterial growth in approximately 50% of neutrocytic samples, whereas bedside inoculation of blood culture bottles with ascitic fluid detects growth in approximately 80%.[15] Multiple prospective studies have demonstrated the superiority of the blood culture bottle method.[15] Also, bedside inoculation is superior to delayed laboratory inoculation of blood culture bottles in the laboratory.[29] Gene probes are now commercially available for the detection of bacteremia; it is hoped that they also will lead to rapid (30-minute) and accurate detection of organisms in ascitic fluid.[30] Culture will continue to be required, however, for assessment of the susceptibility of the organism to antibiotics.

Total Protein

The antiquated exudate/transudate system of ascitic fluid classification, which is based on ascitic fluid total protein concentration, is problematic. The protein concentration in cirrhotic ascites is determined almost entirely by the serum protein concentration and portal pressure.[25] A patient with cirrhosis and a relatively high serum protein concentration will have a relatively high ascitic fluid protein concentration. Because of this relationship, almost 20% of samples in patients with cirrhosis will have a protein concentration greater than 2.5 g/dL (25 g/L). The ascitic fluid total protein concentration does not increase during spontaneous bacterial peritonitis; it remains stable before, during, and after infection.[31] In fact, patients with the lowest ascitic protein concentrations are the most susceptible to spontaneous peritonitis.[32] During a 10-kg diuresis, the ascitic fluid total protein concentration doubles, and 67% of such patients with cirrhotic ascites have a protein concentration greater than 2.5 g/dL (25 g/L) by the end of diuresis.[22] In almost one third of patients with malignant ascites, the ascites is caused by massive liver metastases or hepatocellular carcinoma, and the ascitic fluid in these patients has a low protein concentration.[3] In cardiac ascites, the ascitic fluid protein concentration is greater than 2.5 g/dL (25 g/L).[33]

Therefore, the exudate/transudate method of classification of ascites places many patients with cirrhosis and ascites and all patients with cardiac ascites in the exudate category, and many patients with malignant ascites and essentially all patients with spontaneously infected ascites in the transudate category. Clearly, this method of classification is not useful. By contrast, the SAAG classifies fluid by the presence or absence of portal hypertension and is much more physiologic and intuitive in nature.[25,26] The albumin gradient classifies cardiac ascites in the high-SAAG category, similar to cirrhotic ascites. The high SAAG of cardiac ascites is presumably the result of high right-sided cardiac pressures. In patients with cardiac ascites, the SAAG may narrow with diuresis; this does not happen in patients with cirrhosis.

The combination of ascitic fluid total protein, glucose, and LDH is of value in distinguishing spontaneous bacterial peritonitis from gut perforation with leakage of gut contents into ascites[34] (Fig. 88–3). Patients who have neutrocytic ascitic fluid, in whom the clinical picture suggests bacterial peritonitis (rather than peritoneal carcinomatosis or tuberculous peritonitis) and who meet two of the following three criteria, are likely to have surgical peritonitis and merit immediate radiologic evaluation to determine if gut perforation with leakage of gut contents into ascites has occurred: total protein greater than 1 g/dL (10 g/L), glucose less than 50 mg/dL (2.8 mmol/L), and LDH greater than the upper limit of normal for serum.[34]

Glucose

The glucose molecule is small enough to diffuse readily into body fluid cavities. Therefore, the concentration of glucose in ascitic fluid is similar to that in serum, unless glucose is being consumed by ascitic fluid WBCs or bacteria.[34] In early spontaneous bacterial peritonitis, the ascitic fluid glucose concentration is similar to that of sterile fluid.[34] By contrast, in spontaneous bacterial peritonitis detected late in its course (as well as in the

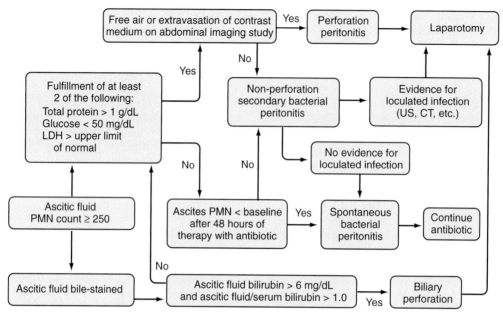

Figure 88–3   Algorithm for differentiating spontaneous from secondary bacterial peritonitis in patients with neutrocytic ascites (i.e., neutrophil count of 250 cells/mm³ [0.25 × 10⁹/L] or greater) in the absence of hemorrhage into ascitic fluid, tuberculosis, peritoneal carcinomatosis, or pancreatitis. CT, computed tomography; LDH, lactate dehydrogenase; PMN, polymorphonuclear neutrophil; US, ultrasound. (Reproduced with permission from Akriviadis EA, Runyon BA: The value of an algorithm in differentiating spontaneous from secondary bacterial peritonitis. Gastroenterology 98:127, 1990. Copyright 1990 by the American Gastroenterological Association.)

setting of gut perforation into ascitic fluid), the ascitic fluid glucose concentration usually drops to 0 mg/dL (0 mmol/L) because of large numbers of stimulated neutrophils and bacteria.[34]

Lactate Dehydrogenase

The LDH molecule is too large to enter ascitic fluid readily from blood,[34] and the ascitic fluid concentration of LDH usually is less than one half of the serum level in uncomplicated cirrhotic ascites. In spontaneous bacterial peritonitis, the ascitic fluid LDH level rises because of the release of LDH from neutrophils, and the ascitic fluid concentration is greater than that of serum. In secondary peritonitis, the LDH level is even higher than that seen in spontaneous bacterial peritonitis and may be several-fold higher than the serum LDH level.[34]

Amylase

In uncomplicated cirrhotic ascites, the ascitic fluid amylase concentration usually is one half that of the serum value, approximately 50 U/L.[35] In patients with acute pancreatitis or gut perforation (with release of luminal amylase into the ascitic fluid), the fluid amylase concentration is elevated markedly, usually greater than 2000 U/L and approximately fivefold greater than simultaneous serum values.[34-36]

Gram Stain

Gram stains of body fluids demonstrate bacteria only when more than 10,000 bacteria/mL are present. The median ascitic concentration of bacteria in spontaneous bacterial peritonitis is only 1 organism/mL, similar to the colony count in bacteremia.[28] Requesting an ascitic fluid Gram stain to detect bacteria in spontaneous bacterial peritonitis is analogous to requesting a Gram stain of blood to detect bacteremia. Bacteria are detected on Gram stain only with overwhelming infection, as in advanced spontaneous bacterial peritonitis or asplenic pneumococcal sepsis. Gram stain of ascitic fluid is most helpful in the diagnosis of free perforation of the gut into ascitic fluid. In this setting, sheets of multiple different bacteria are found. Gram stain of the centrifuged sediment of 50 mL of ascites has a sensitivity rate of only 10% for visualizing bacteria in spontaneous bacterial peritonitis.[28]

Smear and Culture for Tuberculosis

A direct smear of ascitic fluid to detect mycobacteria is almost never positive, because of the rarity of tuberculous peritonitis and the low concentration of mycobacteria in ascitic fluid in tuberculous peritonitis.[37] The older literature suggests that 1 L of fluid should be cultured. The largest centrifuge tube found in most laboratories, however, has a capacity of 50 mL. In general, only one 50-mL aliquot of fluid is centrifuged, and the pellet is cultured. In contrast with a sensitivity rate of approximately 50% for ascitic fluid mycobacterial culture with optimal processing, laparoscopy with histology and culture of peritoneal biopsies has a sensitivity rate approaching 100% for detecting tuberculous peritonitis.[37] Tuberculous peritonitis can easily be confused with spontaneous bacterial peritonitis, because both conditions are associated with abdominal pain and fever, and one half of the patients with tuberculous peritonitis have cirrhosis. A negative bacterial culture and predominance of mononuclear cells in the differential count, however, provide clues to the diagnosis of tuberculous peritonitis. DNA probes are now available to detect mycobacteria and probably will replace older methods of detection.[38]

Nevertheless, cultures still will be required to determine susceptibility to antimicrobial agents.

Cytologic Examination

In the past, malignant ascites was assumed to be caused only by peritoneal carcinomatosis; massive liver metastases and hepatocellular carcinoma superimposed on cirrhosis were not recognized as causes of malignant ascites. These studies did not compare cytologic examination with a "gold standard" diagnostic test, such as autopsy, laparotomy, or laparoscopy, and cytologic study was reported to have a sensitivity rate of only about 60% in detecting malignant ascites.[39] Cytologic studies, however, can be expected to detect malignancy only when tumor cells line the peritoneal cavity and exfoliate into the ascitic fluid—that is, in peritoneal carcinomatosis. Such studies should not be expected to detect tumor when the peritoneum is uninvolved, as in hepatocellular carcinoma or massive liver metastases causing ascites because of portal hypertension or malignant lymphoma causing ascites by lymph node obstruction.[3] In one study in which the location and type of tumor causing ascites were confirmed by a gold standard test, only approximately two thirds of patients with malignancy-related ascites were found to have peritoneal carcinomatosis, but nearly 100% of patients with peritoneal carcinomatosis were reported to have positive findings on cytologic examination of ascitic fluid; the remaining one third of patients with massive liver metastases, chylous ascites caused by lymphoma, or hepatocellular carcinoma had negative cytologic findings.[3] Therefore, the sensitivity rate for cytology is approximately 100% for detecting peritoneal carcinomatosis but much lower for detecting malignancy-related ascites caused by conditions other than peritoneal carcinomatosis. Cytologic studies should not be falsely positive if performed carefully; I have never encountered a false-positive result.

Because hepatocellular carcinoma rarely metastasizes to the peritoneum, a positive ascitic fluid cytology in a patient with hepatocellular carcinoma is unusual enough to be the subject of a case report.[40] Measurement of the serum alpha-fetoprotein concentration (which is always higher in serum than in ascitic fluid) may be of value in detecting hepatocellular carcinoma; serum alpha-fetoprotein is much more sensitive than ascitic cytology for this purpose.[3] In malignancy-related ascites, the fluid may have an elevated PMN count, presumably because dying tumor cells attract neutrophils.[3] The elevated PMN count may cause confusion with spontaneous bacterial peritonitis; however, a predominance of lymphocytes in malignancy-related ascites is usual. Flow cytometry and magnetic enrichment of ascitic fluid as an adjunct to cytology may further increase diagnostic accuracy.[41]

Triglyceride

A triglyceride level should be measured in opalescent or frankly milky ascitic fluid (see Fig. 88–2). By definition, chylous ascites has a triglyceride concentration greater than 200 mg/dL (2.26 mmol/L) and greater than the serum level; usually, the level is greater than 1000 mg/dL (11.30 mmol/L).[42] In sterile cirrhotic ascitic fluid specimens that are slightly cloudy, without an elevated cell count (i.e., opalescent), the triglyceride concentration is elevated—64 ± 40 mg/dL (0.72 ± 0.45 mmol/L), compared with 18 ± 9 mg/dL (0.20 ± 0.10 mmol/L) for clear cirrhotic ascites.[19]

Bilirubin

The bilirubin concentration should be measured in ascitic fluid that is dark brown. An ascitic fluid bilirubin level greater than 6 mg/dL (102 µmol/L) and greater than the serum level of bilirubin suggests biliary or upper gut perforation into ascitic fluid.[21,34]

Tests That Are Seldom Helpful

Tests that have been proposed to be helpful in the analysis of ascitic fluid but shown subsequently to be of no benefit include determination of pH, lactate, fibronectin, and cholesterol. The studies that attempted to validate the value of pH and lactate included small numbers of patients and used suboptimal culture techniques. In the two largest and most recent studies, which did not have some of the deficiencies of the earlier studies, the ascitic fluid pH and lactate were found not to be helpful.[43,44] The pH was found to have no impact on decision-making regarding the use of empirical antibiotic therapy.[43]

Fibronectin and cholesterol have been proposed to be useful in detecting malignant ascites. The basic premise in studies of these markers was that ascitic fluid cytologic examination is insensitive. Unfortunately, the design of the studies was problematic, several subgroups of malignancy-related ascites (e.g., massive liver metastases, hepatocellular carcinoma with cirrhosis) were not considered, and appropriate control groups (e.g., patients with ascites caused by conditions other than cirrhosis or peritoneal carcinomatosis) were not included. Other studies have demonstrated that in patients with massive liver metastases, ascitic fluid fibronectin and cholesterol concentrations are not abnormally elevated.[45,46] Therefore, in patients with malignancy-related ascites and negative cytologic findings, these "humoral tests of malignancy" are usually negative. Additionally, patients with high-protein noncirrhotic ascites nearly always have false-positive ascitic fibronectin and cholesterol elevations.[3,45,46]

Carcinoembryonic antigen (CEA) in ascitic fluid has been proposed as a helpful marker for detecting malignant ascites.[47] However, the study that attempted to validate this proposal was flawed, and more studies, with various subgroups of patients, are required before testing for ascitic fluid CEA can be considered validated.

Measurement of adenosine deaminase has been proposed as a useful test for detecting peritoneal tuberculosis. In the United States, however, where greater than 50% of patients with tuberculous peritonitis have underlying cirrhosis, the adenosine deaminase level has been found to be too insensitive to be helpful.[37]

DIFFERENTIAL DIAGNOSIS

Although cirrhosis is the cause of ascites in most patients evaluated by internists, a cause other than liver disease is found in approximately 15% of patients (see Table 88–1). Approximately 5% of patients have two causes of ascites, that is, "mixed" ascites.[26] Usually, these patients have cirrhosis plus one other cause, such as peritoneal carcinomatosis or peritoneal tuberculosis (see Table 88–1). Because tuberculosis is potentially fatal but curable and frequently occurs in cirrhotic patients with preexisting ascites, the physician must not assume that liver disease is the only cause of ascites in a febrile alcoholic patient if the ascitic fluid analysis is atypical. For example, if the ascitic fluid lymphocyte count is unusually high, peritoneal tuberculosis may be present. Interpretation of the results of ascitic fluid analysis is difficult in patients with mixed ascites but crucial to accurate diagnosis and treatment. Additionally, liver diseases other than cirrhosis (e.g., alcoholic hepatitis or fulminant hepatic failure) may cause ascites (see Table 88–1).

An algorithm for the differential diagnosis of ascites is shown in Figure 88–2. This proposed strategy is applicable to a majority of patients with ascites, including many with the causes listed in Table 88–1. Not every patient (including patients with rare causes of ascites) can be categorized readily with such an algorithm, however. Many patients with enigmatic ascites eventually are found to have two or even three causes of ascites (e.g., heart failure, cirrhosis caused by nonalcoholic steatohepatitis, diabetic nephropathy). In these cases, the sum of predisposing factors leads to sodium and water retention, even though each factor alone may not be severe enough to cause fluid overload.

In most patients with ascites, cirrhosis is the cause. Cirrhotic ascites, especially low-protein cirrhotic ascites, is complicated frequently by spontaneous bacterial peritonitis (see later). Other forms of ascites are complicated by spontaneous peritonitis so rarely that they are the subjects of case reports or small series.[48-50]

The gut can perforate with spillage of contents into the fluid collection in patients with ascites of any cause, cirrhosis or otherwise. The ascitic fluid analysis in gut perforation is dramatically different from that in spontaneous bacterial peritonitis (see Fig. 88–3).[34] Distinguishing spontaneous bacterial peritonitis from surgical peritonitis in a patient with cirrhosis is critical to the patient's survival; spontaneous bacterial peritonitis is treated with antibiotics alone, whereas surgical peritonitis is treated with antibiotics and emergency surgical intervention.

Cancer accounts for less than 10% of cases of ascites (see Table 88–1). Not all cases of malignancy-related ascites are caused by peritoneal carcinomatosis; the characteristics of the ascitic fluid and the treatments vary, depending on the pathophysiology of the ascites—for example, peritoneal carcinomatosis versus massive liver metastases[3] (Table 88–4; see also section "Ascitic Fluid Analysis").

Table 88–4 Classification of Malignancy-Related Ascites

Peritoneal carcinomatosis
Massive liver metastases
Peritoneal carcinomatosis with massive liver metastases
Hepatocellular carcinoma
Malignant lymph node obstruction
Malignant Budd-Chiari syndrome (tumor emboli in hepatic veins)

Heart failure accounts for less than 5% of cases of ascites. Cardiac ascites is characterized by a high albumin gradient, high ascitic fluid protein concentration, and normal blood hematocrit value.[33] Patients with cardiac ascites often have alcoholic cardiomyopathy, with cardiomegaly on a chest x-ray and four-chamber enlargement of the heart on an echocardiogram. Clinically, heart failure may mimic cirrhosis, including the presence of small nonbleeding esophageal varices and hepatic encephalopathy.[51] Cirrhotic ascites is charcterized by a high albumin gradient, as in cardiac ascites, but a low protein concentration, and patients with cirrhosis and ascites have a lower mean blood hematocrit value of 32%.[33]

In the United States, tuberculous peritonitis generally is a disease of Asian and Latin American immigrants to the West Coast, poor African Americans, and the elderly. Tuberculous peritonitis was a rare disease between 1955 and 1985, but it has increased in prevalence because of the acquired immunodeficiency syndrome (AIDS).[52] Fifty percent of patients with tuberculous peritonitis have underlying cirrhosis (i.e., "mixed" ascites). Although most patients with liver disease are not unusually predisposed to the hepatotoxicity of antituberculosis drugs, they tolerate drug toxicity less well than do patients with normal livers.[53] Underdiagnosis can lead to unnecessary deaths from untreated tuberculosis, whereas overdiagnosis and overtreatment of suspected but unproven tuberculous peritonitis may lead to unnecessary deaths from the hepatotoxicity of isoniazid. If the clinical circumstances (e.g., fever in an immigrant from an area endemic for tuberculosis) and results of the initial ascitic fluid analysis (high lymphocyte count) suggest tuberculosis, strong consideration should be given to an urgent laparoscopy with histologic examination and culture of peritoneal biopy specimens. If at laparoscopy the peritoneum demonstrates the typical "millet-seed" and "violin-string" appearance, antituberculosis therapy can be started immediately. Blind peritoneal biopsy may be performed in the patient without cirrhosis; however, in a cirrhotic patient, the predictable presence of peritoneal collateral veins makes blind biopsy potentially hazardous, and laparoscopically guided biopsy is preferable. Suspected tuberculous peritonitis is one of the few principal indications for diagnostic laparoscopy.[54] Peritoneal coccidioidomycosis can mimic tuberculous peritonitis, including its appearance at laparoscopy, and can occur in patients without AIDS.[55]

The high sensitivity rates of cytology for peritoneal carcinomatosis and ultrasound-guided biopsy for focal liver lesions have obviated the need for laparoscopy in detecting tumor, for all practical purposes.[3]

Pancreatic ascites, an uncommon condition, occurs in patients with clinically obvious severe acute pancreatitis or a history of chronic pancreatitis or pancreatic trauma. Ordering an ascitic fluid amylase level on all ascitic fluid samples is unnecessary; the test is indicated only in patients in whom pancreatitis is suspected or the initial ascitic fluid is nondiagnostic (see Table 88–2). Patients with alcohol-related pancreatic ascites also may have underlying alcoholic cirrhosis. Pancreatic ascites frequently is neutrocytic and also may be complicated by bacterial infection. Patients with an ascitic fluid neutrophil count of 250 cells/mm³ (0.25 × 10⁹/L) or greater merit empirical antibiotic coverage, at least until the cause of the elevated neutrophil count is explained.

Nephrogenous ascites is a poorly understood form of ascites that develops in patients undergoing hemodialysis.[56] On careful evaluation, most of these patients are found to have another cause of ascites, usually cirrhosis from alcohol abuse or hepatitis C. The presence of a second cause of fluid overload explains why these patients have ascites whereas a majority of patients on dialysis do not.

Although the nephrotic syndrome used to be a common cause of ascites in children, it is rare in adults.[57] When it occurs in adults, a second cause of ascites usually is present, just as in nephrogenous ascites.[57] The ascitic fluid usually is characterized by a low protein concentration and low albumin gradient and can be complicated by spontaneous bacterial peritonitis.

Chlamydia (or rarely gonococcal) peritonitis should be suspected in sexually active young women with fever and neutrocytic, high-protein, low-gradient ascites and no evidence of liver disease.[11] This infection responds rapidly to oral doxycycline and is one of the few curable causes of ascites.

In some patients, pathologic accumulations of fluid develop in the peritoneal cavity as a result of leakage from a ruptured viscus (e.g., "bile ascites" from a ruptured gallbladder).[21,34] The ascitic fluid analysis is critical to the preoperative diagnosis of this condition (see earlier section, "Ascitic Fluid Analysis," and Fig. 88–3).

Chylous ascites develops when intra-abdominal lymphatics containing chyle rupture. The older literature suggests that this form of ascites is caused by a malignancy in almost 90% of cases.[42] By contrast, cirrhosis is the cause of chylous ascites in more than 90% of the patients that I have encountered (see Table 88–1).[20,26] The high lymphatic flow and pressure are presumed to be the cause of lymphatic rupture in patients with cirrhosis. In addition, retroperitoneal surgery and radical pelvic surgery in patients with cancer can transect lymphatics, leading to chylous ascites.

Additional causes of ascites include ambulatory peritoneal dialysis, Budd-Chiari syndrome, myxedema, connective tissue disease, postoperative ascites, and rare entities. With the iatrogenic form of ascites associated with peritoneal dialysis, the patient usually is not under the care of a gastroenterologist. Although Budd-Chiari syndrome is regularly complicated by ascites, hepatic vein thrombosis is rare and accounts for less than 0.1% of cases of ascites. Ascites in patients with myxedema appears to be related to heart failure[58]; treatment of the hypothyroidism cures the fluid retention. Serositis with development of ascites may complicate systemic lupus erythematosus.[12]

Ascites after abdominal surgery (often after cholecystectomy in the setting of asymptomatic gallstones and abnormal liver tests) is a common mode of presentation of previously undiagnosed cirrhosis.[5] Resection of hepatocellular carcinoma in the setting of cirrhosis regularly leads to hepatic decompensation, which all too often starts a downward spiral ending in death.[59]

Aggressive hormone administration to induce ovulation can lead to ascites from "ovarian hyperstimulation syndrome."[60] Other rare causes of ascites include the POEMS syndrome (polyneuropathy, organomegaly, endocrinopathy, M component, and skin changes) and hemophagocytic syndrome.[61,62] The latter is a rare syndrome that usually occurs in patients with leukemia or lymphoma and can masquerade as decompensated cirrhosis.[62]

Ascites that recurs or does not resolve after liver transplantation appears to be due to relative hepatic venous outflow obstruction or hepatitis C but frequently is enigmatic.[63,64]

COMPLICATIONS

INFECTION

Ascitic fluid infection can be classified into five categories based on ascitic culture results, PMN count, and presence or absence of a surgical source of infection (Table 88–5). An abdominal paracentesis must be performed and ascitic fluid must be analyzed before a confident diagnosis of ascitic fluid infection can be made. A "clinical diagnosis" of infected ascitic fluid without a paracentesis is not adequate.

Classification

Of the three subtypes of spontaneous ascitic fluid infection, the prototype is spontaneous bacterial peritonitis. The diagnosis of *spontaneous bacterial peritonitis* is made when there is a positive ascitic fluid culture and an elevated ascitic fluid absolute PMN count (i.e., at least 250 cells/mm³ [0.25 × 10⁹/L]) without evidence of an intra-abdominal surgically treatable source of infection.[15] When Correia and Conn coined the term "spontaneous bacterial peritonitis" in 1975, their goal was to distinguish this form of infection from surgical peritonitis,[65] an important distinction. Therefore, although many patients with spontaneous bacterial peritonitis have a focus of infection (e.g., urinary tract infection or pneumonia), the diagnosis of spontaneous bacterial peritonitis is still appropriate unless the focus requires surgical intervention (e.g., a ruptured viscus). I have not encountered a convincing case of polymicrobial spontaneous bacterial peritonitis; all of the patients presumed to have spontaneous bacterial peritonitis in whom ascitic fluid cultures initially grew more than one organism eventually were found to have surgical peritonitis or an erroneous culture result (e.g., a pathogen plus a contaminant, or two colony morphologies of one species of bacteria).

The criteria for a diagnosis of *monomicrobial non-neutrocytic bacterascites* (MNB) include (1) a positive ascitic

Table 88–5 Classification of Ascitic Fluid Infection

Spontaneous bacterial peritonitis
Monomicrobial non-neutrocytic bacterascites
Culture-negative neutrocytic ascites
Secondary bacterial peritonitis
Polymicrobial bacterascites (needle perforation of the bowel)

fluid culture for a single organism, (2) an ascitic fluid PMN count lower than 250 cells/mm³ (0.25 × 10⁹/L), and (3) no evidence of an intra-abdominal surgically treatable source of infection.[66] In the older literature, MNB was either grouped with spontaneous bacterial peritonitis or labeled "asymptomatic bacterascites." Because many patients with bacterascites have symptoms, the modifier "asymptomatic" seems inappropriate.

Culture-negative neutrocytic ascites (CNNA) is diagnosed when (1) the ascitic fluid culture grows no bacteria, (2) the ascitic fluid PMN count is 250 cells/mm³ (0.25 × 10⁹/L) or greater, (3) no antibiotics have been given (not even a single dose), and (4) no other explanation for an elevated ascitic PMN count (e.g., hemorrhage into ascites, peritoneal carcinomatosis, tuberculosis, or pancreatitis) can be identified.[67] This variant of ascitic fluid infection seldom is diagnosed when sensitive culture methods are used.[28]

Secondary bacterial peritonitis is diagnosed when (1) the ascitic fluid culture is positive (usually for multiple organisms), (2) the PMN count is 250 cells/mm³ (0.25 × 10⁹/L) or greater, and (3) an intra-abdominal surgically treatable primary source of infection (e.g., perforated gut, perinephric abscess) has been identified.[34] The importance of distinguishing this variant from spontaneous bacterial peritonitis is that secondary peritonitis usually requires emergency surgical intervention (see also Chapter 36).

Polymicrobial bacterascites is diagnosed when (1) multiple organisms are seen on Gram stain or cultured from the ascitic fluid and (2) the PMN count is lower than 250 cells/mm³ (0.25 × 10⁹/L).[68] This diagnosis should be suspected when the paracentesis is traumatic or unusually difficult because of ileus, or when stool or air is aspirated into the paracentesis syringe. Polymicrobial bacterascites is essentially diagnostic of gut perforation by the paracentesis needle.

Clinical Setting

The spontaneous variants of ascitic fluid infection—spontaneous bacterial peritonitis, CNNA, and MNB—occur only in the setting of severe liver disease. The liver disease usually is chronic (cirrhosis), but may be acute (fulminant hepatic failure) or subacute (alcoholic hepatitis). Cirrhosis of all causes can be complicated by spontaneous ascitic fluid infection. Spontaneous infection of noncirrhotic ascites is rare enough to be the subject of case reports.[48-50]

Essentially all patients with spontaneous bacterial peritonitis have an elevated serum bilirubin level and abnormal prothrombin time, and they usually have Child-Turcotte-Pugh class B or C cirrhosis.[15] Ascites appears to be a prerequisite for the development of spontaneous bacterial peritonitis. It is unlikely that the peritonitis precedes the development of ascites. Usually, the infection develops when the volume of ascites is at its maximum.

Secondary bacterial peritonitis and polymicrobial bacterascites can develop with ascites of any type. The only prerequisite, in addition to the presence of ascites, for the development of secondary bacterial peritonitis is an intra-abdominal surgical source of infection.[34] Such an infection can result from penetration of a needle into the bowel during attempted paracentesis.[68]

Pathogenesis

Since the 1990s, the elusive cause of spontaneous bacterial peritonitis has become clearer, and the pathogenesis of spontaneous forms of ascitic fluid infection has been partially elucidated (Fig. 88–4). The body of currently available evidence suggests that the spontaneous forms of ascitic fluid infection are the result of overgrowth of a specific organism in the gut, "translocation" of that microbe from the gut to mesenteric lymph nodes, and resulting spontaneous bacteremia and subsequent colonization of susceptible ascitic fluid[69,70] (see Fig. 88–4).

Once bacteria enter the fluid in the abdomen, by whatever route, a battle ensues between the virulence factors of the organism and the immune defenses of the host.[71] The ascitic fluid protein concentration does not change with development of spontaneous infection.[31] Low-protein ascitic fluid (e.g., protein content less than 1 g/dL [10 g/L]) is particularly susceptible to spontaneous bacterial peritonitis.[32] The endogenous antimicrobial activity (opsonic activity) of human ascitic fluid correlates directly with the protein concentration of the fluid.[71] Patients with deficient ascitic fluid opsonic activity are predisposed to spontaneous bacterial peritonitis.[72] Patients with detectable ascitic fluid opsonic activity appear to be protected from spontaneous bacterial peri-

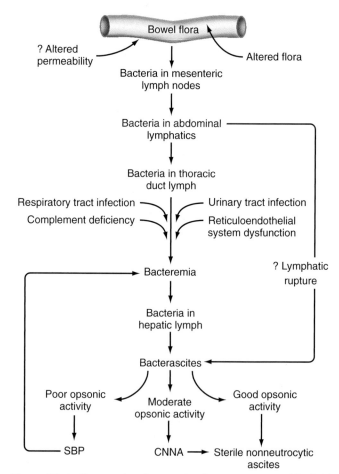

Figure 88–4 Proposed pathogenesis of spontaneous ascitic fluid infection. CNNA, culture-negative neutrocytic ascites; SBP, spontaneous bacterial peritonitis.

tonitis unless they are exposed to a particularly virulent organism (e.g., *Salmonella*).[50,71,72]

Studies in both patients and animals with cirrhosis demonstrate that MNB is common.[66,73] In both humans and rats, most episodes of bacterascites resolve without antibiotic treatment.[66,73] The fluid frequently becomes sterile without a rise in ascitic PMNs. Apparently, the host's defense mechanisms are able to eradicate the invading bacteria on most occasions. Uncontrolled infection probably develops only when the defenses are weak or the organism is virulent (see Fig. 88–4). Bacterascites probably is more common than spontaneous bacterial peritonitis. Conceivably, ascitic fluid in the setting of cirrhosis is regularly colonized by bacteria, and almost just as regularly, the colonization resolves. The entry of PMNs into the fluid probably signals failure of the peritoneal macrophages to control the infection.[74] A majority of episodes of MNB appear to resolve in cirrhotic rats and humans, whereas untreated spontaneous bacterial peritonitis frequently is fatal. In summary, MNB probably represents an early stage of ascitic fluid infection, which can resolve to CNNA or progress to spontaneous bacterial peritonitis.

Most episodes of CNNA are diagnosed by insensitive culture methods for which numbers of bacteria are insufficient to reach the threshold of detectability.[28] Inoculation of ascitic fluid into blood culture bottles can lead to detection of a single organism in the cultured aliquot of fluid, whereas the older method of culture by inoculation of agar plates and broth probably requires at least 100 organisms/mL.[28] Even when optimal culture methods are used, however, a small percentage of specimens of neutrocytic ascitic fluid grow no bacteria. A study of rapid sequential paracenteses (before the initiation of antibiotic treatment) in patients with CNNA demonstrated that in most cases, the PMN count dropped spontaneously and the culture results remained negative in the second specimen.[75] When sensitive culture techniques are used, CNNA probably results from (1) previous antibiotic treatment (even one dose), (2) an inadequate volume of fluid inoculated, or (3) spontaneously resolving spontaneous bacterial peritonitis in which the paracentesis is performed after all bacteria have been killed by host defenses but before the PMN count has normalized.

The pathogenesis of secondary bacterial peritonitis is more straightforward than that of spontaneous bacterial peritonitis. When the gut perforates, billions of bacteria flood into the ascitic fluid. In the absence of a frank perforation, bacteria may cross inflamed tissue planes and enter the fluid. The pathogenesis of polymicrobial bacterascites is also obvious[68]: The paracentesis needle enters the bowel, and the bowel contents are released into the ascites.

Symptoms and Signs

Although 87% of patients with spontaneous bacterial peritonitis are symptomatic at the time the infection is diagnosed, the symptoms and signs of infection are often subtle, such as a slight change in mental status.[66] Without prompt paracentesis, the diagnosis and treatment of infected ascites may be delayed, often resulting in the death of the patient. The symptoms and signs manifested in all five variants of ascitic fluid infection are listed in Table 88–6.

Prevalence

Since the 1980s, routine paracenteses on hospitalization in patients with ascites have provided data regarding the prevalence of ascitic fluid infection. In the 1980s, approximately 10% of patients with ascites were infected at the time of hospital admission; of the subgroup of patients with cirrhosis, about 27% were infected.[15] At present, because of measures to prevent spontaneous bacterial peritonitis, the prevalence has dropped significantly (see later). Of patients with culture-positive ascitic fluid, about two thirds have neutrocytic ascitic fluid (spontaneous bacterial peritonitis), and one third have MNB.[66] The frequency of CNNA depends largely on the culture technique (see earlier). Polymicrobial bacterascites occurs in only 1 in 1000 paracenteses. Secondary bacterial peritonitis is found in only 0% to 2% of patients with ascites at the time of hospital admission.[15,34]

Bacteriology

Escherichia coli, streptococci (mostly pneumococci), and *Klebsiella* cause most episodes of spontaneous bacterial peritonitis and MNB in patients who are not receiving selective intestinal decontamination (Table 88–7; see later); CNNA is by definition culture-negative and polymicrobial bacterascites is by definition polymicrobial. The most apparent difference between the sponta-

Table 88–6   Symptoms and Signs of Ascitic Fluid Infection

Symptom or Sign	Frequency (%)*				
	SBP	*Bacterascites*	*CNNA*	*Secondary Peritonitis*	*Polymicrobial Bacterascites*
Fever	68	57	50	33	10
Abdominal pain	49	32	72	67	10
Abdominal tenderness	39	32	44	50	10
Rebound	10	5	0	17	0
Altered mental status	54	50	61	33	0

*Data presented as % of the total number of patients in that group.
CNNA, culture-negative neutrocytic ascites; SBP, spontaneous bacterial peritonitis.
Data from references 34, 66–68.

Table 88–7 Pathogens in Ascitic Fluid Infection

Organism	Frequency (%)*			
	SBP	**Monomicrobial Non-Neutrocytic Bacterascites**	**Secondary Bacterial Peritonitis**	**SBP with SID**
Monomicrobial				
Escherichia coli	37	27	20	0
Klebsiella pneumoniae	17	11	7	7
Pneumococci	12	9	0	29
Streptococcus viridans	9	2	0	0
Staphylococcus aureus	0	7	13	0
Miscellaneous gram-negative	10	14	7	7
Miscellaneous gram-positive	14	30	0	50
Polymicrobial	1	0	53	7

*Data reported as % of total patients in that group.
SBP, spontaneous bacterial peritonitis; SID, selective intestinal decontamination.
Data from references 28, 66, 76.

neous forms of ascitic fluid infection and the secondary forms (secondary peritonitis and polymicrobial bacterascites) is that the former always are monomicrobial and the latter usually are polymicrobial. Although older papers reported that anaerobic bacteria were present in approximately 6% of cases of spontaneous bacterial peritonitis, the detection of anaerobes probably reflected unrecognized cases of secondary bacterial peritonitis. In more recent series, anaerobes have been found in approximately 1% of cases of spontaneous bacterial peritonitis and MNB.[28,66]

Selective intestinal decontamination causes a change in the bacteria isolated from patients in whom an ascitic infection develops. Gram-positive organisms usually are cultured from the ascitic fluid of these patients (see Table 88–7).[76]

Risk Factors

Patients with cirrhosis are unusually predisposed to bacterial infection because of multiple defects in immune defense. The concept that cirrhosis is a form of acquired immunodeficiency (in the generic sense) is rather new. In a prospective study, a bacterial infection occurred in more than 40% of consecutive cirrhotic patients at the time of admission to the hospital or during the hospitalization.[77] Low ascitic fluid total protein concentrations, as well as the phagocytic (both motile and stationary) dysfunction associated with cirrhosis, are risk factors for bacterial infection.

Paracentesis itself has been proposed as a risk factor for ascitic fluid infection. This theoretical risk has not been substantiated in prospective studies of paracentesis-related complications.[16] Spontaneous bacterial peritonitis is statistically more likely to be diagnosed on the first paracentesis than on subsequent taps.[16] Needle-induced ascitic fluid infections do not occur unless the bowel is penetrated by the paracentesis needle[16,68]; fortunately, this occurs in only one in 1000 taps. One would expect bacteria of the skin flora such as *Staphylococcus aureus* to be isolated more frequently if poor paracentesis technique were the cause of many cases of spontaneous bacterial peritonitis; yet skin flora microorganisms are seldom isolated from ascitic fluid.[28] Iatrogenic peritonitis

Table 88–8 Indications for Empirical Antibiotic Therapy of Suspected Spontaneous Ascitic Fluid Infection

Convincing symptoms or signs of infection
Ascitic fluid neutrophil count ≥250/mm³ (0.25 × 10⁹/L) OR positive "dipstick" test

is most likely to occur when the paracentesis needle enters the bowel during a difficult paracentesis.

Gastrointestinal hemorrhage is an underrecognized risk factor for the development of spontaneous bacteremia and spontaneous bacterial peritonitis. The cumulative probability of infection during a single hospitalization for bleeding is approximately 40%.[78] The risk appears to peak 48 hours after the onset of hemorrhage. The high risk of infection probably is mediated by a shock-induced increase in the translocation of bacteria from the gut to extraintestinal sites. Urinary tract infections also constitute an underrecognized risk factor for spontaneous bacterial peritonitis.[79]

Diagnosis

Timely diagnosis of ascitic fluid infection requires a high index of suspicion and a low threshold for performing a paracentesis. Clinical deterioration, especially fever or abdominal pain, in a patient with ascites should raise the suspicion of infection and prompt a paracentesis. If the ascitic fluid PMN count is elevated, the working diagnosis is ascitic fluid infection until proved otherwise. Although peritoneal carcinomatosis, pancreatitis, hemorrhage into ascites, and tuberculosis can lead to an elevated ascitic fluid PMN count, most cases of neutrocytic ascites are caused by bacterial infection. A predominance of PMNs in the WBC differential count lends further credence to the diagnosis of infection. In patients with peritoneal carcinomatosis, pancreatitis, and tuberculosis, a predominance of PMNs in the ascites would be an unusual finding. An elevated absolute ascitic fluid PMN count with a predominance of neutrophils in a clinical setting compatible with infection should prompt empirical antibiotic therapy (Table 88–8; see also details later in text).

Although spontaneous bacterial peritonitis is approximately six times as common as surgical peritonitis in a patient with ascites, secondary peritonitis should be considered in any patient with neutrocytic ascites (see also Chapter 36). Clinical symptoms and signs do not distinguish patients with secondary peritonitis from those with spontaneous bacterial peritonitis (see Fig. 88–3).[34] Even with free perforation of the colon into ascitic fluid, a classic surgical abdomen does not develop. Peritoneal signs require contact of inflamed visceral and parietal peritoneal surfaces, and such contact does not occur when there is a large volume of fluid separating these surfaces. Gut perforation can be suspected and pursued if a specimen of ascites is neutrocytic and meets two of the following three criteria (see Fig. 88–3): Total protein greater than 1 g/dL (10 g/L), glucose less than 50 mg/dL (2.8 mmol/L), and LDH greater than the upper limit of normal for serum.[34] In the setting of a perforated viscus, cultures of ascitic fluid nearly always disclose multiple organisms, except gallbladder rupture, which is usually monomicrobial.[21] Brown ascitic fluid with a bilirubin concentration that is greater than 6 mg/dL (102 µmol/L) and greater than the serum level is indicative of biliary or upper gut perforation into ascites.[21] An ascitic fluid amylase level that is greater than fivefold that of the serum level also may be indicative of gut rupture (except gallbladder rupture) and the release of luminal amylase.[34,35]

The initial ascitic fluid analysis is helpful in delineating which patients are likely to have a ruptured viscus (see Fig. 88–3). Within minutes of the detection of neutrocytic ascitic fluid, these patients should undergo a radiologic evaluation to confirm and localize the site of rupture. Plain and upright abdominal films and water-soluble contrast studies of the upper and lower gut or abdominal computed tomography should be obtained. If perforation is documented, emergency surgical intervention is the next step. Timing is crucial; after septic shock occurs, death is nearly certain. Antibiotic therapy without surgical intervention in the treatment of a ruptured viscus is predictably unsuccessful.

In contrast with patients with peritonitis resulting from perforation of a viscus, patients with secondary peritoni-

tis unrelated to perforation tend not to have a diagnostic initial ascitic fluid analysis.[34] The need to make the diagnosis of secondary peritonitis in patients without free perforation is less urgent, and there may be time to evaluate the response of the ascitic PMN count and fluid culture to treatment with antibiotics. The best time to repeat the paracentesis to assess the response to treatment is after 48 hours of therapy; by 48 hours, the ascitic PMN count will be lower than the pretreatment value and the ascitic culture will be negative in essentially every patient with spontaneous bacterial peritonitis who has received treatment with an appropriate antibiotic.[34] Before 48 hours of treatment, the ascitic PMN count may rise to a value higher than baseline in either spontaneous bacterial peritonitis or secondary peritonitis.[34] The culture remains positive in secondary peritonitis and becomes rapidly negative in spontaneous bacterial peritonitis (see Fig. 88–3).[34] Whereas antibiotics alone cannot control secondary peritonitis, medical therapy rapidly cures spontaneous bacterial peritonitis.[34]

Treatment

Patients with an ascitic fluid PMN count of 250 cells/mm³ (0.25×10^9/L) or greater and a clinical scenario compatible with ascitic fluid infection should receive empirical antibiotic treatment (Table 88–9; see also Table 88–8).[15,80] Patients with hemorrhage into the ascitic fluid, peritoneal carcinomatosis, pancreatic ascites, or tuberculous peritonitis may have an elevated PMN count that is unrelated to spontaneous bacterial peritonitis and usually do not require empirical antibiotic treatment. If they do receive antibiotics, the ascitic PMN count usually fluctuates randomly, in contrast to the dramatic reduction in PMN count typical of spontaneous bacterial peritonitis. If the clinical picture initially is unclear, the physician should err on the side of antibiotic treatment (with a non-nephrotoxic antibiotic). In patients with uninfected neutrocytic ascitic fluid (except those with hemorrhage), lymphocytes usually predominate in the ascitic fluid differential count, in contrast with spontaneous bacterial peritonitis, in which PMNs predominate. In patients with bloody ascitic fluid, a "corrected" PMN count should be calculated (as discussed earlier). Antibiotic therapy is

Table 88–9   Treatment of Subtypes of Ascitic Fluid Infection

Diagnosis	Treatment
Spontaneous bacterial peritonitis	Five days of intravenous antibiotic to which the organism is highly susceptible (e.g., cefotaxime 2 g q8h empirically followed by more specific therapy after susceptibility results are available)
Monomicrobial non-neutrocytic bacterascites	Five days of intravenous antibiotic to which the organism is highly susceptible, if the patient is symptomatic or persistently culture-positive; not all patients with bacterascites require treatment
Culture-negative neutrocytic ascites	Five days of intravenous third-generation cephalosporin (e.g., cefotaxime 2 g q8h)
Secondary bacterial peritonitis	Surgical intervention plus approximately 2 weeks of intravenous cephalosporin (e.g., cefotaxime 2 g q8h) plus an antianaerobic drug such as metronidazole*
Polymicrobial bacterascites	Intravenous third-generation cephalosporin (e.g., cefotaxime 2 g q8h) plus an antianaerobic drug such as metronidazole* Duration is determined by clinical response and serial ascitic fluid PMN counts and cultures

*Dose of intravenous metronidazole is 15 mg/kg × 1, then 7.5 mg/kg q6h.
PMN, polymorphonuclear neutrophil.

not necessary for patients with bloody fluid unless the corrected ascitic fluid PMN count is 250 cells/mm³ (0.25 × 10⁹/L) or greater.

The decision to begin empirical antibiotic treatment in patients with bacterascites must be individualized. Many episodes resolve without treatment.[66] The hospital mortality rate of 22% to 43% in patients with MNB is attributable at least in part to infection, however.[66,81] Therefore, treatment appears to be warranted in many patients. By definition, the ascitic PMN count is lower than 250 cells/mm³ (0.25 × 10⁹/L) in this variant of ascitic fluid infection, and the PMN count cannot be the only parameter on which to base the decision about empirical therapy. Most patients with MNB in whom the colonization does not resolve progress to spontaneous bacterial peritonitis and have symptoms or signs of infection at the time of the paracentesis that documents bacterascites.[66] Therefore, patients with cirrhotic ascites who have convincing symptoms or signs of infection should receive treatment regardless of the ascitic fluid PMN count. Empirical treatment can be discontinued after only 2 to 3 days if the culture demonstrates no growth. Asymptomatic patients may not need treatment.[66,81] The paracentesis should be repeated for cell count and culture in patients without clinical evidence of infection, once it is known that the initial culture result is positive. If the PMN count has risen to at least 250/mm³ (0.25 × 10⁹/L) or if symptoms or signs of infection have developed, treatment should be started. Culture results usually are negative in patients without a rise in the ascitic fluid PMN count on repeat paracentesis and without clinical evidence of infection, and these persons do not require treatment,[66] because colonization has been eradicated by host immune defenses.

The physician will not know initially that the ascitic fluid culture is destined to be negative in a patient with CNNA; therefore, empirical antibiotic treatment should be started. When the preliminary culture demonstrates no growth, it is helpful to repeat the paracentesis after 48 hours of therapy to assess the response of the PMN count to antibiotics. A dramatic decline in PMN count (always below the baseline pretreatment value and frequently a greater than 80% reduction) confirms a response to treatment. In such cases, a few more days of therapy probably is warranted. A stable ascitic fluid PMN count, especially with a predominance of lymphocytes and monocytes, suggests a nonbacterial (or mycobacterial) cause of ascitic fluid neutrocytosis, and the fluid should be sent for cytologic examination and mycobacterial culture. Because a negative culture result may be due to insensitive culture techniques, the prevalence of CNNA in a hospital that still uses conventional methods of culture can be reduced by convincing the microbiology laboratory to accept and process ascitic fluid submitted in blood culture bottles.[28]

Gram stain of the ascitic fluid is most helpful in detecting secondary peritonitis, in which multiple different bacterial forms are seen. Gram stain is of little value in guiding the choice of empirical antibiotic treatment for spontaneous ascitic infections. I have found that use of the Gram stain did not help narrow the antibiotic coverage in even 1 patient of approximately 500 with spontaneous bacterial peritonitis. Only approximately 10% of Gram stains demonstrate organisms in spontaneous bacterial peritonitis.[28] If a Gram stain indicates secondary peritonitis, coverage of anaerobic flora, in addition to coverage of aerobic and facultative anaerobic flora, is required, as is an emergency search for the source of the infection (see Fig. 88–3 and Table 88–9).[34] Therefore, a positive Gram stain may lead to broader antibiotic coverage, rather than narrower coverage. Choosing narrow coverage (e.g., penicillin alone) based on a misinterpretation of the significance of the results of Gram staining may lead to the patient's death from uncontrolled infection before it becomes apparent that the isolated organism is resistant to the chosen antibiotic.

Until the results of susceptibility testing are available, relatively broad-spectrum antibiotic therapy is warranted in patients with suspected ascitic fluid infection. After sensitivities are known, the spectrum of coverage usually can be narrowed. The antibiotics that have been recommended for empirical treatment have changed over the years. In the late 1970s, the combination of ampicillin and gentamicin was promoted, but this recommendation was not based on susceptibility testing or efficacy data. Subsequently, gentamicin was shown to have an unpredictable volume of distribution in patients with ascites, and the serum creatinine level (and even the creatinine clearance) was found to be a poor index of the glomerular filtration rate in patients with ascites.[82,83] Therefore, determining the appropriate loading and maintenance doses of gentamicin for this patient population is difficult. No evidence-based guidelines are available for the prescribing physician to follow. In my experience, even if high serum levels are avoided, nephrotoxicity still develops in most patients receiving aminoglycosides.[84] One study has documented an adjusted odds ratio of 4.0 for aminoglycosides as a risk factor for renal dysfunction in patients with cirrhosis.[85] Evidence that newer aminoglycosides are less nephrotoxic than gentamicin is lacking.

Several nonaminoglycoside antibiotics are now available for the treatment of ascitic fluid infection. Cefotaxime, a third-generation cephalosporin, has been shown in a controlled trial to be superior to ampicillin plus tobramycin for the treatment of spontaneous bacterial peritonitis.[86] Fully 98% of causative organisms were susceptible to cefotaxime, which did not result in superinfection or nephrotoxicity.[86] Cefotaxime or a similar third-generation cephalosporin appears to be the treatment of choice for suspected spontaneous bacterial peritonitis.[15] Anaerobic coverage is not needed, nor is coverage for *Pseudomonas* or *Staphylococcus*.[28] Cefotaxime, 2 g intravenously every 8 hours, has been shown to result in excellent ascitic fluid levels (20-fold killing power after one dose).[87] In patients with a serum creatinine level greater than 3 mg/dL, the dosing interval may be extended to 12 hours.[87] Neither a loading dose nor an intraperitoneal dose appears to be necessary or appropriate. The clinician should, however, write "first dose STAT" when ordering treatment, to avoid a delay in administration of the life-saving agent.

Other Intravenous Antibiotics

Amoxicillin–clavulanic acid has been shown to be as effective as cefotaxime in a randomized trial but is not available in a parenteral formulation in the United States.[88] Other antibiotics have been recommended as well but have been less well studied than has cefotaxime. Some newer drugs have been used to treat spontaneous bacterial peritonitis (without any data on antibiotic penetration into the ascitic fluid) on the basis of their spectrum of coverage and formulary constraints. Infection with organisms that are resistant to the empirical antibiotic or use of drugs that do not enter the ascitic fluid in high enough concentrations to kill the bacteria may lead to the patient's death.

Intravenous Albumin

Renal impairment occurs in 33% of episodes of spontaneous bacterial peritonitis.[89] Spontaneous bacterial peritonitis leads to increased intraperitoneal nitric oxide production, which in turn further increases systemic vasodilatation and promotes renal failure (see Chapter 89).[90] Intravenous albumin (1.5 g/kg of body weight at the time the infection is detected and 1.0 g/kg on day 3) can increase intravascular volume and, in combination with cefotaxime, has been shown in a large randomized trial to reduce the risk of renal failure and improve survival compared with cefotaxime without albumin.[91] A confirmatory trial is needed. Because of the survival advantage, however, the use of intravenous albumin as an adjunct to antibiotic treatment has been recommended.[92]

Oral Antibiotic Treatment

Oral ofloxacin has been reported in a controlled trial to be as effective as parenteral cefotaxime in the treatment of spontaneous bacterial peritonitis in patients who are not vomiting, in shock, bleeding, or in renal failure.[93] The dose studied was 400 mg twice daily.[93] Another study has demonstrated the efficacy of intravenous ciprofloxacin, 200 mg every 12 hours for 2 days, followed by oral ciprofloxacin, 500 mg every 12 hours for 5 days.[94] Because of the possibility of fluoroquinolone resistance in patients receiving fluoroquinolones to prevent spontaneous bacterial peritonitis (see later), however, the empirical use of a fluoroquinolone to treat suspected spontaneous bacterial peritonitis should be avoided.[95] Fortunately, bacterial isolates from patients with spontaneous bacterial peritonitis who were receiving fluoroquinolones for prophylaxis of this disorder remain susceptible to cefotaxime.[76]

Narrowing the Spectrum of Coverage

After the results of susceptibility testing are available, an antibiotic with a narrower spectrum of activity usually can be substituted for the broad-spectrum drug (e.g., pneumococci usually will be sensitive to penicillin, and most E. coli species usually will be sensitive to ampicillin).

Duration of Treatment

Infectious disease subspecialists generally recommend 10 to 14 days of antibiotic therapy for life-threatening infections. No data are available to support this duration of treatment in spontaneous ascitic fluid infections, however. The ascitic fluid culture becomes sterile after one dose of cefotaxime in 86% of patients.[34] After 48 hours of therapy, the ascitic fluid PMN count is always

less than the pretreatment value in patients with a spontaneous ascitic fluid infection treated with appropriate antibiotics; frequently, an 80% reduction is observed at 48 hours.[34] A randomized, controlled trial involving 100 patients has demonstrated that 5 days of treatment is as efficacious as 10 days in the treatment of spontaneous bacterial peritonitis and CNNA.[96] I have been treating spontaneous bacterial peritonitis and CNNA for 5 days since the early 1990s, with excellent results.

The average duration of oral ofloxacin treatment was 8 days in the only published trial.[93]

Follow-up Paracentesis in Spontaneous Bacterial Peritonitis

On the basis of a large database of repeat paracenteses during and after the treatment of spontaneous bacterial peritonitis,[34,97] a follow-up paracentesis does not appear to be needed if the setting (advanced cirrhosis with symptoms and signs of infection), bacterial isolate (monomicrobial with a typical organism), and response to treatment (dramatic reduction in symptoms and signs of infection) are typical.[97] Paracentesis should be repeated after 48 hours of treatment if the course is atypical.[34,97]

Treatment of Ascitic Fluid Infection Other than Spontaneous Bacterial Peritonitis

Because of the predictable presence of anaerobes, patients with suspected secondary peritonitis require empirical antibiotic coverage that is broader in spectrum than that used for spontaneous bacterial peritonitis. They also require an emergency evaluation to assess the need for surgical intervention (see earlier discussion, and Table 88–8 and Fig. 88–3). Cefotaxime plus metronidazole appears to provide excellent initial empirical therapy of suspected secondary peritonitis.[34]

Polymicrobial bacterascites (from needle perforation of the bowel) is tolerated relatively well. Peritonitis developed in only 1 in 10 patients with a needle perforation of the gut with spillage of gut contents into ascitic fluid in the one relevant study.[68] The single episode of paracentesis-related peritonitis was not fatal. Patients with low-protein ascitic fluid appear to be at most risk for development of a PMN response and clinical peritonitis related to needle perforation of the gut.[68] Most of the patients with a higher ascitic protein concentration (e.g., greater than 1 g/dL [10 g/L]) did not receive antibiotics, yet did well. Many physicians, however, probably would feel uncomfortable withholding antibiotic treatment if needle perforation is suspected. If a decision to treat is made, anaerobic coverage should be included (e.g., cefotaxime and metronidazole; see Table 88–9). Whether or not treatment is begun, a follow-up paracentesis is helpful (if it can be performed safely) to monitor the ascitic fluid PMN count and culture. If a decision is made not to treat and the number of organisms in the ascitic fluid does not decrease or the PMN count rises in the second specimen, antibiotic treatment should be initiated (see Table 88–9).

Prognosis

In the past, 48% to 95% of patients with a spontaneous ascitic fluid infection died during the hospitalization in which the diagnosis was made, despite antibiotic treatment.[15,24] The most recent series report the lowest mortality rates (less than 5% if antibiotics are administered in a timely fashion), probably because of earlier detection and treatment of infection, as well as the avoidance of nephrotoxic antibiotics.[96] The trial in which cefotaxime plus albumin was studied reported the lowest hospitalization mortality rate yet—10%.[91] Even now, however, some patients are cured of their infection but die of liver failure or gastrointestinal bleeding, because of the severity of the underlying liver disease. In fact, spontaneous ascitic fluid infection is a good marker of end-stage liver disease and has been proposed as an indication for liver transplantation in a patient who is otherwise a candidate.

In order to maximize survival, it is important that paracentesis be performed in all patients with ascites at the time of hospitalization, so that infection can be detected and treated promptly. The ascitic fluid cell count should be reviewed as soon as the results are available (approximately 60 minutes), and appropriate treatment should be instituted when indicated. The first dose of antibiotic should be given immediately. Because the "dipstick" test results are available in 90 to 120 seconds, this new tool may speed treatment of spontaneous bacterial peritonitis and improve survival further.[23]

Paracentesis should be repeated during the hospitalization if any manifestation of clinical deterioration develops, including abdominal pain, fever, change in mental status, renal failure, acidosis, peripheral leukocytosis, or gastrointestinal bleeding. If the physician waits to perform a paracentesis until convincing symptoms and signs of infection have developed, the infection is likely to be advanced by the time the diagnosis is made. No survivors of spontaneous bacterial peritonitis have been reported when the diagnosis is made after the serum creatinine level has risen above 4 mg/dL (350 μmol/L) or after shock has developed.

Without surgical intervention, the mortality rate for secondary peritonitis in hospitalized patients with ascites approaches 100%. When secondary peritonitis is diagnosed early and is treated with emergency laparotomy, the mortality rate is approximately 50%.[34]

Prevention

The identification of risk factors for spontaneous bacterial peritonitis (including an ascitic fluid protein concentration less than 1.0 g/dL, variceal hemorrhage, and previous episode of spontaneous bacterial peritonitis) has led to controlled trials of prophylactic antibiotics.[32,98-100] Norfloxacin, 400 mg per day orally, has been reported to reduce the risk of spontaneous bacterial peritonitis in inpatients with low-protein ascites and those with previous spontaneous bacterial peritonitis.[98,99] Norfloxacin, 400 mg orally twice daily for 7 days, helps prevent infection in patients with variceal hemorrhage[100] and is cost-effective in preventing recurrent spontaneous bacterial peritonitis.[101] Oral antibiotics select for resistant organisms in the gut flora, however, thereby potentially causing spontaneous ascitic fluid infection.[76,98-100,102] For the primary prevention of ascitic fluid infection in the setting of low-protein ascites, the use of prophylactic

antibiotics should be restricted to inpatients, with discontinuation of the drug at the time of hospital discharge.[103] According to a randomized trial, this strategy achieves the best compromise in preventing ascitic fluid infection without selecting resistant organisms.[103]

Trimethoprim-sulfamethoxazole also has been shown to prevent spontaneous bacterial peritonitis in an animal model and in patients.[104,105] The recommended dose is one double-strength tablet daily.[105]

Use of parenteral antibiotics to prevent endoscopic sclerotherapy- or banding-related infections does not appear to be warranted, as indicated by a controlled trial.[106] Active bleeding, not the endoscopic treatment, appears to be the risk factor for ascitic fluid infection. On the other hand, bacterial infection is associated with failure to control variceal hemorrhage.[107] This observation provides additional incentive to try to prevent and to detect and treat infection aggressively in this setting to minimize mortality related not only to infection but also to hemorrhage.

CELLULITIS

Cellulitis is a common cause of soft tissue infection in obese patients with edema. One study has documented a 14% cumulative probability of cellulitis during hospitalization of patients with cirrhosis and ascites, compared with only a 4% probability of spontaneous bacterial peritonitis.[108] Risk factors for cellulitis included obesity (which is increasing in frequency in cirrhotic patients), homelessness, and greater degree of edema.[108] A high index of suspicion and low threshold for treating with a first-generation cephalosporin or other antibiotic may help decrease morbidity and mortality from cellulitis.

TENSE ASCITES

Some patients with ascites do not seek medical attention until they can no longer breathe or eat comfortably because of the pressure of the intra-abdominal fluid on the diaphragm. Tense ascites requires urgent therapeutic paracentesis. Contrary to folklore, tense ascites can be drained without untoward hemodynamic effects.[109] "Total paracentesis," even more than 20 L, has been demonstrated to be safe.[109] In the setting of tense ascites, therapeutic paracentesis improves venous return and hemodynamics; the myth of paracentesis-related hemodynamic catastrophes was based on observations in small numbers of patients.

PLEURAL EFFUSIONS

"Sympathetic" pleural effusions are common in patients with cirrhotic ascites. They usually are unilateral and right-sided but occasionally may be bilateral and larger on the right side than on the left. A unilateral left-sided effusion suggests tuberculosis.[110] A large effusion in a patient with cirrhotic ascites is referred to as *hepatic hydrothorax*.[111] Most carefully studied patients with hepatic hydrothorax have been shown to have a small defect in the right hemidiaphragm. Occasionally, the effusion develops acutely, with sudden onset of shortness of breath as the abdomen decompresses. With large diaphragmatic defects, ascites may be undetectable on clinical examination despite a large pleural effusion.

The most common symptom associated with hepatic hydrothorax is shortness of breath. Infection of the fluid can occur, usually as a result of spontaneous bacterial peritonitis and transmission of bacteria across the diaphragm.[112] The analysis of uncomplicated hepatic hydrothorax fluid is similar, but not identical, to that of ascitic fluid, because the pleural fluid is subject to hydrostatic pressures different from those that affect the portal bed. The total protein concentration is higher (by approximately 1.0 g/dL [10 g/L]) in the pleural fluid than in ascitic fluid.[111]

The treatment of hepatic hydrothorax was difficult until the transjugular intrahepatic portosystemic shunt (TIPS) became available (see later).[111] The effusions tend to occur in patients who are the least adherent to treatment regimens or whose hydrothorax is most refractory to therapy. Some authors have recommended chest tube insertion and sclerosing of the pleurae with tetracycline. Chest tubes inserted to treat hepatic hydrothorax usually are difficult to remove, however[113]; shortness of breath may recur when the tube is clamped, and fluid may leak around the insertion site of the tube. Direct surgical repair of the diaphragmatic defect can be considered, but the patients typically are poor operative candidates. A peritoneovenous shunt (see later) can be considered when the patient with hepatic hydrothorax has large-volume ascites, but the shunt usually clots after a short time. Videothoracoscopic suture of the hole in the diaphragm followed by pleurodesis has been reported to be successful in one patient.[114] Sodium restriction plus use of diuretics is the safest and most effective first-line therapy of hepatic hydrothorax. TIPS placement has been reported to be successful and constitutes reasonable second-line treatment.[111] If the patient is a candidate for liver transplantation, proceeding with a transplantation evaluation may be the best approach.

ABDOMINAL WALL HERNIAS

Abdominal wall hernias are common in patients with ascites. They usually are umbilical or incisional but occasionally are inguinal. Little published information on these hernias is available. In one study, almost 20% of cirrhotic patients with ascites were found to have umbilical hernias at the time of hospitalization.[115] Some of these hernias incarcerate or perforate. Because of these potential complications, elective surgical treatment should be considered in all patients with hernias and ascites. The ascitic fluid should be medically removed preoperatively, because the hernia recurs in 73% of patients who have ascites at the time of hernia repair but in only 14% of those who have no ascitic fluid at the time of repair[116]; however, hernia repair is not without hazard. Successful laparoscopic repair of a recurrent strangulated umbilical hernia has been described.[117] TIPS also has been reported to lead to such good control of symptoms that surgical repair was not needed.[118] Many transplant surgeons prefer

to avoid repair of the hernia or postpone it until the time of liver transplantation.

Surgical repair of a hernia should be performed semi-emergently in patients with skin ulceration, crusting, or black discoloration and emergently for refractory incarceration or rupture. Rupture is the most feared complication of umbilical hernias.

TREATMENT OF ASCITES

Appropriate treatment of ascites depends on the cause of fluid retention. Accurate determination of the etiology of ascites is crucial. The SAAG is helpful diagnostically and for therapeutic decision-making. Patients with a low SAAG usually do not have portal hypertension and do not respond to salt restriction and diuretics (except for those with nephrotic syndrome). Conversely, patients with a high SAAG have portal hypertension and usually are responsive to these measures.[15]

LOW-ALBUMIN-GRADIENT ASCITES

Peritoneal carcinomatosis is the most common cause of low-albumin-gradient ascites.[3] Peripheral edema in affected patients can be managed with diuretics. By contrast, patients without peripheral edema who receive diuretics lose only intravascular volume, without loss of ascitic fluid. The mainstay of treatment of nonovarian peritoneal carcinomatosis is outpatient therapeutic paracentesis. Patients with peritoneal carcinomatosis usually live only a few months. Patients with ovarian malignancy are an exception to this rule and may exhibit a good response to surgical debulking and chemotherapy.

Ascites caused by tuberculous peritonitis (without cirrhosis) is cured by antituberculosis therapy. Diuretics do not speed weight loss unless the patient has underlying portal hypertension from cirrhosis. Pancreatic ascites may resolve spontaneously, require endoscopic placement of a stent in the pancreatic duct or operative intervention, or respond to treatment with somatostatin.[119] A postoperative lymphatic leak from a distal splenorenal shunt or radical lymphadenectomy also may resolve spontaneously but on occasion may require surgical intervention or peritoneovenous shunting. *Chlamydia* peritonitis is cured by tetracycline.[11] Ascites caused by lupus serositis may respond to glucocorticoids.[12] Dialysis-related ascites may respond to aggressive dialysis.[56]

HIGH-ALBUMIN-GRADIENT ASCITES

Cirrhosis is the most common cause of liver disease that leads to high-albumin-gradient ascites (see Table 88–1). Many patients with cirrhosis experience multiple insults to the liver, including those from excessive alcohol use, NASH, and chronic hepatitis C.[6,7] One of the most important steps in treating high-albumin-gradient ascites in a patient with alcoholic liver disease is to convince the patient to stop drinking alcohol. In a period of months, abstinence from alcohol can result in healing of the reversible component of alcoholic liver disease,[8] and the ascites may resolve or become more responsive to medical therapy. Similarly, patients with other forms of treatable liver disease (e.g., autoimmune hepatitis, hemochromatosis, Wilson disease) should receive specific therapy for these diseases. Occasionally, nonalcoholic cirrhosis is reversible[9]; however, these diseases are less reversible than alcoholic liver disease, and by the time ascites is present, these patients may be better candidates for liver transplantation than for protracted medical therapy.

Hospitalization

Outpatient treatment of patients with small-volume ascites can be attempted initially. However, patients with large-volume ascites and those who are resistant to outpatient treatment usually require hospitalization for definitive diagnosis and management of the fluid overload and the underlying liver disease.[15,24] Many of these patients also have gastrointestinal hemorrhage, encephalopathy, infection, or hepatocellular carcinoma. An intensive period of inpatient education and treatment may be required to convince the patient that the diet and diuretics actually are effective and worth the effort required to follow the regimen at home.

Precipitating Cause

Determining the precipitating cause of ascites formation (e.g., dietary indiscretion or nonadherence to therapy with diuretics) may be of value. Further education about diet may help prevent future hospitalizations for ascites. Ascites may be precipitated by saline infusions given perioperatively or to treat variceal hemorrhage, in which case the ascites may resolve without the need for long-term treatment.

Diet Education

Fluid loss and weight change are related directly to sodium balance in patients with portal hypertension–related ascites. In the presence of avid renal retention of sodium, dietary sodium restriction is essential. The patient and the food preparer should be educated by a dietitian about a sodium-restricted diet. Severely sodium-restricted diets (e.g., 500 mg, or 22 mmol, of sodium per day) are feasible (but not palatable) in an inpatient setting but unrealistic for outpatients. The dietary sodium restriction that I recommend for both inpatients and outpatients is 2 g (88 mmol) per day. Protein is not restricted unless the patient has refractory hepatic encephalopathy.

Fluid Restriction

Indiscriminate restriction of fluid in treatment of cirrhotic ascites is inappropriate and serves only to alienate patients, nurses, and dietitians; moreover, hypernatremia may result.[120] Sodium restriction, not fluid restriction, results in weight loss; fluid follows sodium passively. The chronic hyponatremia usually seen in patients with cirrhotic ascites is seldom morbid. Attempts to correct hyponatremia rapidly in this setting can lead to more complications than those related to the hyponatremia. Severe hyponatremia (e.g., serum sodium concentration less than 120 mmol/L) does warrant fluid restriction in the patient with cirrhotic ascites.[120,121] Unless the decline in sodium concentration is rapid, symptoms of hyponatremia usually do not develop in cirrhotic patients until the serum sodium concentration is below 110 mmol/L.

No Bed Rest

Although it is traditional to order bed rest, no controlled trials support this practice; bed rest was part of the treatment of heart failure in the past and was extrapolated to the treatment of cirrhosis without data.[122] An upright posture may aggravate the plasma renin elevation found in most cirrhotic patients with ascites and, theoretically, increase renal sodium retention. In all likelihood, however, strict bed rest is unnecessary and may lead to decubitus ulcer formation in these emaciated patients.

Urine Sodium Excretion

The 24-hour urinary sodium excretion is a helpful parameter to follow in patients with portal hypertension–related ascites. The completeness of the urine collection can be assessed by measuring the urinary creatinine excretion. Cirrhotic men should excrete 15 to 20 mg/kg per day of creatinine, and women should excrete 10 to 15 mg/kg per day.[15,123] Excretion of less creatinine indicates an incomplete collection. Only the 10% to 15% of patients who have significant spontaneous natriuresis can be considered for dietary sodium restriction as sole therapy of ascites (i.e., without diuretics).[15,24] When given a choice, however, most patients would prefer to take some diuretics with a more liberal intake of sodium than to take no pills with severe restriction of sodium intake. Contrary to popular belief, most patients, including outpatients, can comply with instructions to collect complete 24-hour specimens.

Because urine is the most important route of excretion of sodium in the absence of diarrhea or hyperthermia, and because dietary intake is the only source of nonparenteral sodium, dietary intake and urinary excretion of sodium should be roughly equivalent, if the patient's weight is stable. Nonurinary sodium losses are less than 10 mmol per day in these patients.[124] A suboptimal decline in body weight may be the result of inadequate natriuresis, failure to restrict sodium intake, or both. Monitoring 24-hour urinary sodium excretion and daily weight will clarify the issue. Patients who are adherent to an 88–mmol-per-day sodium diet and who excrete more than 78 mmol per day of sodium in the urine should lose weight. If the weight is increasing despite urinary losses in excess of 78 mmol per day, one can assume that the patient is consuming more sodium than is prescribed in the diet.

Urine Sodium/Potassium Ratio

Although 24-hour urine specimens constitute the diagnostic gold standard, one study has demonstrated that when a random urine specimen has a sodium concentration greater than the potassium concentration, a 24-hour specimen will reveal sodium excretion greater than 78 mmol per day in approximately 90% of cases.[125] Therefore, a random urine sodium/potassium concentration ratio greater than 1 predicts that the patient should lose weight if a sodium-restricted diet is followed. Patients who do not lose weight despite a random urine sodium/potassium ratio greater than 1 probably are not adherent to the diet.

Avoid Use of Urinary Bladder Catheters

Many physicians promptly insert a bladder catheter in hospitalized patients with cirrhosis to monitor urine output accurately. Unfortunately, these immunocompromised patients regularly have urinary tract infections on hospital admission.[79] Urethral trauma from insertion of the catheter in the setting of cystitis can lead to bacteremia. Prolonged catheterization predictably leads to cystitis and possibly sepsis in these patients. I insert urinary catheters only briefly and only in the intensive care unit setting; these portals of entry for bacteria should be removed as soon as possible. Twenty-four-hour urine specimens almost always can be collected completely without catheters.

Diuretics

Spironolactone is the mainstay of treatment for patients with cirrhosis and ascites but increases natriuresis slowly. Single-agent diuretic therapy with spironolactone requires several days to induce weight loss. Although spironolactone alone has been shown to be superior to furosemide alone in the treatment of cirrhotic ascites,[126] I prefer to start spironolactone and furosemide together on the first hospital day in initial doses of 100 mg and 40 mg, respectively, each taken once in the morning.[15] Amiloride, 10 mg per day, can be substituted for spironolactone; amiloride is less widely available and more expensive than spironolactone but more rapidly effective, and it does not cause gynecomastia. A new potassium-sparing diuretic, eplerenone, has been used in the treatment of heart failure and does not cause gynecomastia, but studies of its use in cirrhosis are lacking.[127] The half-life of spironolactone is approximately 24 hours in normal control subjects but is markedly prolonged in patients with cirrhosis; almost 1 month is required to reach a steady state.[128] In view of its long half-life, dosing the drug multiple times per day is unnecessary. A loading dose may be appropriate but has not been studied. Single daily doses maximize adherence; 25-, 50-, and 100-mg spironolactone tablets are available generically. Furosemide also should be given once a day.[129]

If the combination of spironolactone, 100 mg per day (or amiloride, 10 mg per day) and furosemide, 40 mg per day orally, is ineffective in increasing urinary sodium or decreasing body weight, the doses of both drugs should be increased simultaneously, as needed (e.g., spironolactone, 200 mg plus furosemide, 80 mg, then 300 mg plus 120 mg, and finally 400 mg plus 160 mg). In my experience, starting both drugs at once speeds the onset of diuresis; slowly increasing the daily dose of spironolactone to 400 mg or even higher before adding furosemide delays diuresis and results in hyperkalemia.

The 100:40 ratio of the daily doses of spironolactone and furosemide usually maintains normokalemia. The ratio of doses can be adjusted to correct abnormal serum potassium levels. Occasionally, an alcoholic patient who has had no recent food intake will have hypokalemia at the time of admission and for a variable interval thereafter. Such a patient should receive spironolactone alone until the serum potassium normalizes; furosemide can then be added.

When combined with a sodium-restricted diet in a study of almost 4000 patients, the regimen of spironolactone and furosemide has been demonstrated to achieve successful diuresis in more than 90% of cirrhotic patients.[130]

Intravenous diuretics cause acute decreases in the glomerular filtration rate in patients with cirrhosis and ascites and generally should be avoided.[131] Many patients are given intravenous furosemide when they are hospitalized because of failure of outpatient treatment of ascites in the setting of cirrhosis. The approach of switching from oral to intravenous administration is effective for heart failure, but in patients with cirrhosis, repeated doses of intravenous furosemide regularly lead to crescendo azotemia and then to an erroneous diagnosis of hepatorenal syndrome. (The correct diagnosis is diuretic-induced azotemia that resolves when the diuretics are withheld and fluid is given intravenously.) Repeated intravenous dosing of furosemide appears to be too "harsh" for the patient with cirrhosis; oral diuretics are better tolerated. On the other hand, a single intravenous 80-mg dose of furosemide has been reported to effectively separate patients with diuretic-resistant ascites from those with diuretic-sensitive ascites on the basis of the 8-hour sodium excretion: less than 50 mmol in the former and greater than 50 mmol in the latter.[132]

If rapid weight loss is desired, therapeutic paracentesis should be performed (see later). No limit has been identified for acceptable daily weight loss in patients who have massive edema. Once the edema has resolved, a reasonable maximum weight loss probably is 0.5 kg per day.[133] Encephalopathy, a serum sodium concentration less than 120 mmol/L despite fluid restriction, and a serum creatinine level greater than 2.0 mg/dL (180 mmol/L) are indications to discontinue diuretics and reassess the patient. Abnormalities in potassium levels almost never prohibit diuretic use, because the ratio of the two diuretics can be readjusted. Patients with parenchymal renal disease (e.g., diabetic nephropathy) usually require relatively higher doses of furosemide and lower doses of spironolactone; otherwise, they develop hyperkalemia. Patients in whom complications develop despite a careful attempt at diuretic treatment usually require second-line therapy. Prostaglandin inhibitors (e.g., nonsteroidal anti-inflammatory drugs) should be avoided in patients with cirrhosis and ascites, because they inhibit diuresis, may promote renal failure, and may cause gastrointestinal bleeding.[134]

Reducing the quantity of fluid in the abdomen can improve the patient's comfort and prevent hepatic hydrothorax and hernias. Also, by concentrating the ascitic fluid, diuresis increases the opsonic activity of ascitic fluid 10-fold and theoretically may be of value in preventing spontaneous ascitic fluid infection.[135]

In the past, patients with ascites frequently occupied hospital beds for prolonged durations, because of uncertainty regarding the diagnosis and optimal treatment and because of iatrogenic complications. Although a "dry" abdomen is a reasonable ultimate goal, complete resolution of ascites should not be a prerequisite for discharge from the hospital. Patients who are stable, with ascites as their major problem, can be discharged after they are demonstrated to be responding to the medical regimen and are normokalemic, are not azotemic, and have a normal or slightly to moderately reduced serum sodium level. Following discharge from the hospital, a patient should be seen in the outpatient setting within 7 to 14 days.

No Sodium Bicarbonate

Mild renal tubular acidosis develops in a substantial minority of patients with cirrhosis and ascites. Although oral sodium bicarbonate administration has been recommended in this setting, such treatment increases sodium intake dramatically and cannot be advocated in the absence of evidence to support its use.

Aquaretics

The *aquaretics* are a new class of drugs that have been used in animals and preliminarily in patients with cirrhosis to increase urinary water excretion and to increase the serum sodium concentration. Patients with mild hyponatremia (serum sodium less than 130 mmol/L) can respond with an increase in the serum sodium level, although dose reductions were common in a randomized trial.[136] Whether these drugs will improve severe hyponatremia without causing hypotension awaits further investigation.

Outpatient Management

After discharge from the hospital, the patient's body weight, orthostatic symptoms, and serum electrolyte, urea, and creatinine levels should be monitored. Twenty-four-hour or random urine specimens for sodium/potassium ratios can be collected to assist with treatment decisions. It is my experience that adherent outpatients can collect complete specimens successfully, when adequate written and oral instructions are provided. The subsequent frequency of follow-up evaluations is determined by the response to treatment and stability of the patient. I usually evaluate these patients every 1 to 4 weeks until they clearly are responding to treatment and are not experiencing problems. Intensive outpatient follow-up helps prevent subsequent hospitalizations.

Diuretic doses and dietary sodium intake are adjusted to achieve weight loss and negative sodium balance. Patients who are gaining fluid weight despite diuretic therapy should not be considered to have diuretic-resistant ascites until they are demonstrated to be adherent to the diet. Monitoring the urine sodium concentration provides insight into adherence. Patients who excrete more than 78 mmol per day of sodium in the urine or have a random urine sodium/potassium ratio greater than 1 should be losing weight if they are consuming less than 88 mmol of sodium per day. In my experience, most patients who initially are thought to be diuretic-resistant eventually are found to be nonadherent to the diet; they demonstrate weight gain and urinary sodium excretion as high as 500 mmol per day or more. Diet education is crucial to the successful management of such patients. Patients with truly diuretic-resistant ascites excrete nearly sodium-free urine despite maximal doses of diuretics.

During long-term follow-up, abstinent alcoholic patients may become more sensitive to diuretics, the dose of which may be tapered and even discontinued.

REFRACTORY ASCITES

Refractory ascites is defined as ascites unresponsive to a sodium-restricted diet and high-dose diuretic treatment. Refractoriness may manifest as minimal or no weight loss despite diuretics or the development of complications of diuretics.[137] Several studies have shown that cirrhotic ascites is refractory to standard medical therapy in less than 10% of patients.[126,130]

In the 1960s, portacaval shunts were used to treat refractory ascites, but operative hemorrhagic complications and portosystemic encephalopathy led to abandonment of this approach.[122] In Europe in the 1970s, the Paris pump was used to ultrafilter ascitic fluid and reinfuse it intravenously.[122] Unfortunately, this approach was complicated by disseminated intravascular coagulation and was abandoned.

Viable options for patients refractory to routine medical therapy include liver transplantation, serial therapeutic paracenteses, TIPS, and peritoneovenous shunts (Fig. 88–5).[15]

Liver Transplantation

Liver transplantation should be considered among the treatment options for patients with cirrhosis and ascites—whether the fluid is diuretic-sensitive or diuretic-refractory (see also Chapter 92). In many areas of the United States, patients are not offered transplantation until hepatorenal syndrome has developed (see Chapter 89). The 12-month survival rate for patients with ascites refractory to medical therapy is only 25%.[138] The survival rate for liver transplantation is much higher.

In patients who are candidates for transplantation, procedures that could make transplantation difficult should be avoided. Surgery in the right upper quadrant causes adhesions that become vascularized and difficult to remove during transplant surgery. Even peritoneovenous shunting can lead to the formation of a "cocoon" in the right upper quadrant that can involve the bowel and liver.[139]

Serial Paracenteses

Therapeutic abdominal paracentesis is one of the oldest medical procedures. In the 1980s, after 2000 years of use, scientific data regarding large-volume paracentesis were reported, and patients were documented to tolerate large-volume paracentesis well, just as patients had in the 1940s and earlier.[140-143] In one large randomized, controlled trial, therapeutic paracentesis plus intravenous infusion of colloid led to fewer minor (asymptomatic) changes in serum electrolyte and creatinine levels than those reported with diuretic therapy.[140] No differences in morbidity or mortality rates could be demonstrated, however.[140] Therapeutic paracentesis now appears to be first-line therapy for patients whose ascites is tense and second-line therapy for cirrhotic patients whose ascites is refractory to diuretics (see Fig. 88–5).[15] The world record

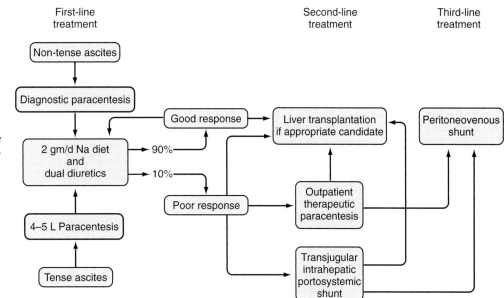

First-line treatment   Second-line treatment   Third-line treatment

Figure 88–5 Algorithm for the treatment of patients with cirrhotic ascites.

for volume of fluid removed at one time appears to be 41 L.[144]

Colloid Replacement

A controversial issue regarding therapeutic paracentesis is that of colloid replacement. In one study, patients with tense ascites were randomized to receive intravenous albumin (10 g/L of fluid removed) or no albumin after therapeutic paracentesis.[143] More statistically significant (asymptomatic) changes in serum electrolyte, plasma renin, and serum creatinine levels developed in the patients who did not receive albumin than in those who received albumin, but no greater frequency of clinical morbidity or mortality was seen. Although another study has documented that the patients who have a postparacentesis rise in plasma renin levels have a decreased life expectancy compared with those who have stable renin levels, no study has demonstrated a decreased survival rate in patients not given a plasma expander compared with patients given albumin after paracentesis.[145] A new phrase, "paracentesis-induced circulatory dysfunction," has been coined to describe the rise in plasma renin levels after paracentesis.[146] Despite the lack of benefit of albumin infusion on survival, the authors of the two studies cited previously recommend routine infusion of albumin after therapeutic paracentesis.[143,145] Albumin infusions markedly increase the degradation of albumin, however, and albumin is expensive.[147,148] In a study performed 40 years ago, 58% of infused albumin was offset by increased degradation, and a 15% increase in the serum albumin level led to a 39% increase in degradation.[147] Increasing the concentration of albumin in cell culture media has been shown to decrease albumin synthesis.[149] In view of the cost ($2 to $25/g or $100 to $1250/tap), it is difficult to justify the expense of routine infusions of albumin based on the available data.

The confusion regarding albumin infusion relates in part to the design of the relevant studies. In the studies

from Barcelona, patients with "tense" ascites could be entered into the trial of albumin versus no albumin, and 31% of these patients were not even receiving diuretics.[143] It seems more appropriate to study the population in which chronic paracenteses are really needed, specifically the diuretic-resistant group, rather than all patients with tense ascites.[150] Another group of investigstors has shown that patients with cirrhosis and diuretic-resistant ascites tolerate a 5-L paracentesis without a change in plasma renin levels.[151] My approach to patients with tense ascites is to take off enough fluid (4 to 5 L) to relieve intra-abdominal pressure and then to rely on diuretics to eliminate the remainder. To remove all of the fluid by paracentesis when most of it can be removed with diuretics seems inappropriate, in part because paracentesis removes opsonins, whereas diuresis concentrates opsonins.[135] Patients with early cirrhosis and diuretic-sensitive ascites should be managed with diuretics, not large-volume paracentesis; these patients may be more sensitive to paracentesis-related volume depletion than are patients with advanced cirrhosis.[152] Chronic therapeutic paracenteses should be reserved for the 10% of patients in whom diuretic treatment fails to relieve the ascites.

Other studies have compared less expensive plasma expanders with albumin. No differences in electrolyte imbalance or clinically relevant complications between the groups have been found.[153] In addition, some authors advocate giving one half of the plasma expander immediately after the paracentesis and the other half 6 hours later.[145,153] This approach converts an otherwise simple outpatient procedure into an all-day clinic visit or even a brief hospitalization and seems unwarranted. A colloid that specifically should be avoided is hetastarch, which can accumulate in Kupffer cells and cause portal hypertension in patients without preexisting liver disease.[154]

Consensus statements and systematic reviews have pointed out some of the hazards of albumin infusion and have recommended against its liberal use.[155,156] Until more convincing data involving appropriate groups of patients are available, it seems reasonable to (1) avoid serial large-volume paracenteses in patients with diuretic-sensitive ascites; (2) withhold albumin after taps of 5 L or less; and (3) consider albumin infusion optional after taps of larger volume in patients with diuretic-resistant ascites.[15]

Transjugular Intrahepatic Portosystemic Shunt

TIPS is a side-to-side portacaval shunt that is placed by an interventional radiologist (or hepatologist), usually with the use of local anesthesia. TIPS placement was first used for the treatment of refractory variceal bleeding, but it also has been advocated for diuretic-resistant ascites[157] (see Chapter 87). TIPS was received with great enthusiasm in the 1990s, similar to the enthusiasm for the peritoneovenous shunt in the 1970s. Just as with peritoneovenous shunting, TIPS was overused until serious complications and suboptimal efficacy were reported. Four large-scale randomized trials in diuretic-resistant patients have demonstrated consistent superiority of TIPS over repeated paracentesis but no survival advantage.[158-161] A meta-analysis has confirmed efficacy but no difference in survival; hepatic encephalopathy was more common in the TIPS group.[162] Although TIPS dysfunction is common and must be managed with repeated manipulation of the stent, maintaining a TIPS is logistically less challenging than large-volume paracenteses performed every 2 weeks. New polytetrafluoroethylene-coated stents have been reported to improve patency and survival when compared with uncoated stents in a nonrandomized study and to improve patency, with no survival advantage, when compared with uncoated stents in a randomized trial.[163,164] Also, the four older TIPS trials preceded development and implementation of the Model for End–stage Liver Disease (MELD) score, which predicts 90-day mortality after TIPS placement; new trials using the covered stent and selecting patients according to their MELD scores may demonstrate a survival advantage for TIPS compared with repeated taps.

TIPS also is useful in the treatment of hepatic hydrothorax and umbilical hernia.[111,118] The direct intrahepatic portosystemic shunt (DIPS) connects the portal vein directly to the inferior vena cava and has applicability in patients with Budd-Chiari syndrome.[165]

Peritoneovenous Shunt

In the mid-1970s, the peritoneovenous shunt was promoted as a new "physiologic" treatment for the management of ascites. Reports of shunt failure, fatal complications following shunt insertion, and randomized trials demonstrating no survival advantage have led to the relegation of this procedure to third-line therapy in patients with cirrhosis and ascites[15,130] (see Fig. 88–5). Patients who are not candidates for liver transplantation and who have a scarred abdomen that is not amenable to repeated paracenteses, who are not candidates for TIPS, or in whom an attempt at TIPS placement has failed make up the small subset of candidates for a peritoneovenous shunt. A randomized trial has shown that even an uncoated TIPS stent has better "assisted patency" than the peritoneovenous shunt.[166]

Novel Treatments

Novel treatment options for patients with refractory ascites include peritoneal-urinary drainage of the fluid using a surgically implanted pump and percutaneous placement of a peritoneovenous shunt by an interventional radiologist.[167,168]

SUMMARY OF THE TREATMENT OF ASCITES IN PATIENTS WITH CIRRHOSIS

The mainstay of the treatment of ascites in patients with cirrhosis is dietary sodium restriction and diuretics (see Fig. 88–5). Standard medical therapy is effective in 90% of patients. Evaluation for liver transplantation should be considered at the time of first hepatic decompensation. Psychosocial issues, however, frequently preclude transplantation. A therapeutic paracentesis should be performed promptly in patients with tense ascites and as second-line treatment in the 10% of patients in whom cirrhotic ascites is refractory to medical therapy. Therapeutic paracenteses can be repeated indefinitely or until a more definitive treatment is provided. TIPS placement is a second-line treatment that should be reserved for (1) diuretic-resistant patients who are not candidates for liver transplantation, as well as those who are awaiting transplantation, and (2) patients with hepatic hydrothorax. Peritoneovenous shunting is a third-line therapy and should be reserved for special and unusual circumstances. For patients with no psychosocial contraindications, evaluation for liver transplantation is even more urgent once ascites has become diuretic-resistant.

PROGNOSIS

Cirrhosis complicated by ascites is associated with significant morbidity and mortality, related in part to the severe underlying liver disease and in part to the ascites per se. In one half of the patients in whom cirrhosis is detected before decompensation (i.e., development of ascites, jaundice, or encephalopathy or gastrointestinal hemorrhage), ascites occurs within 10 years.[169] Once ascites appears, the expected mortality rate is approximately 50% in just 2 years.[170] With liver transplantation, survival is improved dramatically.

REFERENCES

1. Martin P-Y, Gines P, Schrier RW: Nitric oxide as a mediator of hemodynamic abnormalities and sodium and water retention in cirrhosis. N Engl J Med 339:533, 1998.
2. Rockey D: Vascular mediators in the injured liver. Hepatology 37:4, 2003.
3. Runyon BA, Hoefs JC, Morgan TR: Ascitic fluid analysis in malignancy-related ascites. Hepatology 8:1104, 1988.
4. Schrier RW: Pathogenesis of sodium and water retention in high-output and low-output cardiac failure, nephrotic syndrome, cirrhosis, and pregnancy. N Engl J Med 319:1065, 1988.
5. Brown MW, Burk RF: Development of intractable ascites following upper abdominal surgery in patients with cirrhosis. Am J Med 80:879, 1986.

6. Naveau S, Giraud V, Borotto E, et al: Excess weight risk factor for alcoholic liver disease. Hepatology 25:108, 1997.

7. Hourigan LF, MacDonald GA, Purdie D, et al: Fibrosis in chronic hepatitis C correlates significantly with body mass index. Hepatology 29:1215, 1999.

8. Reynolds TB, Geller HM, Kuzma OT, et al. Spontaneous decrease in portal pressure with clinical improvement in cirrhosis. N Engl J Med 263;734, 1960.

9. Malekzadeh R, Mohamadnejad M, Rakhshani N, et al: Reversibility of cirrhosis in chronic hepatitis B. Clin Gastroenterol Hepatol 2:34, 2004.

10. Caldwell SH, Oelsner DH, Iezzoni JC, et al: Cryptogenic cirrhosis: Clinical characterization and risk factors for underlying disease. Hepatology 29:664, 1999.

11. Muller-Schoop JW, Wang SP, Munzinger J, et al: *Chlamydia trachomatis* as possible cause of peritonitis and perihepatitis in young women. BMJ 1:1022, 1978.

12. Weinstein PJ, Noyer CM: Rapid onset of massive ascites as the first presentation of systemic lupus erythematosus. Am J Gastroenterol 95:302, 2000.

13. Cattau El, Benjamin SB, Knuff TE, et al: The accuracy of the physical exam in the diagnosis of suspected ascites. JAMA 247:1164, 1982.

14. Fiedorek SC, Casteel HB, Reddy G, et al: The etiology and clinical significance of pseudoascites. J Gen Intern Med 6:77, 1991.

15. Runyon BA: Management of adult patients with ascites caused by cirrhosis. Hepatology 39:841, 2004.

16. Runyon BA: Paracentesis of ascitic fluid: A safe procedure. Arch Intern Med 146:2259, 1986.

17. Sakai H, Sheer TA, Mendler MH, Runyon BA: Choosing the location for non-image guided abdominal paracentesis. Liver International 25:984, 2005.

18. Bard C, Lafortune M, Breton G: Ascites: ultrasound guidance or blind paracentesis. Can Med Assoc J 135:209, 1986.

19. Runyon BA, Akriviadis EA, Keyser AJ: The opacity of portal hypertension-related ascites correlates with the fluid's triglyceride concentration. Am J Clin Pathol 96:142, 1991.

20. Rector WG: Spontaneous chylous ascites of cirrhosis. J Clin Gastroenterol 6:369, 1984.

21. Runyon BA: Ascitic fluid bilirubin concentration as a key to the diagnosis of choleperitoneum. J Clin Gastroenterol 9:543, 1987.

22. Hoefs JC: Increase in ascites WBC and protein concentrations during diuresis in patients with chronic liver disease. Hepatology 1:249, 1981.

23. Runyon BA: Strips and tubes: Improving the diagnosis of spontaneous bacterial peritonitis. Hepatology 37:745, 2003.

24. Runyon BA: Approach to the patient with ascites. In Yamada T, Alpers D, Kaplowitz N, et al (eds): Textbook of Gastroenterology, 4th ed. Philadelphia, Lippincott Williams & Wilkins, 2003, p 948.

25. Hoefs JC: Serum protein concentration and portal pressure determine the ascitic fluid protein concentration in patients with chronic liver disease. J Lab Clin Med 102:260, 1983.

26. Runyon BA, Montano AA, Akriviadis EA, et al: The serum-ascites albumin gradient is superior to the exudate-transudate concept in the differential diagnosis of ascites. Ann Intern Med 117:215, 1992.

27. Hoefs JC: Globulin correction of the albumin gradient: Correlation with measured serum to ascites colloid osmotic gradient. Hepatology 16:396, 1992.

28. Runyon BA, Canawati HN, Akriviadis EA: Optimization of ascitic fluid culture technique. Gastroenterology 95:1351, 1988.

29. Runyon BA, Antillon MR, Akriviadis EA, et al: Bedside inoculation of blood culture bottles with ascitic fluid is superior to delayed inoculation in the detection of spontaneous bacterial peritonitis. J Clin Microbiol 28:2811, 1990.

30. Davis TE, Fuller DD: Direct identification of bacterial isolates in blood cultures using a DNA probe. J Clin Microbiol 29:2193, 1991.

31. Runyon BA, Hoefs JC: Ascitic fluid analysis before, during, and after spontaneous bacterial peritonitis. Hepatology 5:257, 1985.

32. Runyon BA: Low-protein-concentration ascitic fluid is predisposed to spontaneous bacterial peritonitis. Gastroenterology 91:1343, 1986.

33. Runyon BA: Cardiac ascites: A characterization. J Clin Gastroenterol 10:410, 1988.

34. Akriviadis EA, Runyon BA: The value of an algorithm in differentiating spontaneous from secondary bacterial peritonitis. Gastroenterology 98:127, 1990.

35. Runyon BA: Amylase levels in ascitic fluid. J Clin Gastroenterol 9:172, 1987.

36. Haas LS, Gates LK Jr: The ascites to serum amylase ratio identifies two distinct populations in acute pancreatitis with ascites. Pancreatology 2:100, 2002.

37. Hillebrand DJ, Runyon BA, Yasmineh W, et al: Ascitic fluid adenosine deaminase insensitivity in detecting tuberculous peritonitis. Hepatology 19:731, 1994.

38. Altamirano M, Kelly MT, Wong A, et al: Characterization of a DNA probe for detection of *Mycobacterium tuberculosis* complex in clinical samples by polymerase chain reaction. J Clin Microbiol 30:2173, 1992.

39. Motherby H, Nadjari B, Friegel P, et al: Diagnostic accuracy of effusion cytology. Diagn Cytopath 20:350, 1999.

40. Chetty R, Learmonth GM, Taylor DA: Giant cell hepatocellular carcinoma. Cytopathology 1:233, 1990.

41. Kielhorn E, Schofield K, Rimm DL: Use of magnetic enrichment for detection of carcinoma cells in fluid specimens. Cancer 94:205, 2002.

42. Press OW, Press NO, Kaufman SD: Evaluation and management of chylous ascites. Ann Intern Med 96:358, 1982.

43. Runyon BA, Antillon MR: Ascitic fluid pH and lactate: Insensitive and nonspecific tests in detecting ascitic fluid infection. Hepatology 13:929, 1991.

44. Albillos A, Cuervas-Mons V, Millan I, et al: Ascitic fluid polymorphonuclear cell count and serum to ascites albumin gradient in the diagnosis of bacterial peritonitis. Gastroenterology 98:134, 1990.

45. Runyon BA: Elevated ascitic fluid fibronectin: A non-specific finding. J Hepatol 3:219, 1986.

46. Runyon BA: Editorial: Malignancy-related ascites and ascitic fluid "humoral tests of malignancy." J Clin Gastroenterol 18:94, 1994.

47. Loewenstein MS, Rittgers RA, Feinerman AE, et al: CEA assay of ascites and detection of malignancy. Ann Intern Med 88:635, 1978.

48. Runyon BA: Spontaneous bacterial peritonitis associated with cardiac ascites. Am J Gastroenterol 79:796, 1984.

49. Kurtz RC, Bronzo RL: Does spontaneous bacterial peritonitis occur in malignant ascites? Am J Gastroenterol 77:146, 1982.

50. Wolfe GM, Runyon BA: Spontaneous *Salmonella* infection of high protein non-cirrhotic ascites. J Clin Gastroenterol 12:430, 1990.

51. Arora A, Seth S, Acharya SK, et al: Hepatic coma as a presenting feature of constrictive pericarditis. Am J Gastroenterol 88:430, 1993.

52. Cappell MS, Shetty V: A multicenter, case-controlled study of the clinical presentation and etiology of ascites and of the safety and clinical efficacy of diagnostic abdominal paracentesis in HIV seropositive patients. Am J Gastroenterol 89:2172, 1994.

53. Wong W-M, Wu P-C, Yuen M-F, et al: Antituberculosis drug-related liver dysfunction in chronic hepatitis B infection. Hepatology 31:201, 2000.

54. De Groen PC, Rakela J, Moore C, et al: Diagnostic laparoscopy in gastroenterology: A 14-year experience. Dig Dis Sci 32:677, 1987.

55. Weisman IM, Moreno AJ, Parker AL, et al: Gastrointestinal dissemination of coccidioidomycosis. Am J Gastroenterol 81:589, 1986.

56. Han S-HB, Reynolds TB, Fong T-L: Nephrogenic ascites: Analysis of 16 cases and review of the literature. Medicine 77:233, 1998.

57. Ackerman Z: Ascites in nephrotic syndrome: Incidence, patients' characteristics and complications. J Clin Gastroenterol 22:31, 1996.

58. Mauer K, Manzione NC: Usefulness of the serum-ascites albumin gradient in separating transudative from exudative ascites: Another look. Dig Dis Sci 33:1208, 1988.

59. Ikeda Y, Kanematsu T, Matsumata T, et al: Liver resection and intractable postoperative ascites. Hepatogastroenterology 40:14, 1993.

60. Schenker JG, Weinstein D: Ovarian hyperstimulation syndrome: A current survey. Fertil Steril 30:255, 1978.

61. Case records of the Massachusetts General Hospital. Case 39-1992. A 49-year-old woman with peripheral neuropathy, hepatosplenomegaly, and intermittent abdominal pain. N Engl J Med 327:1014, 1992.

62. de Kerguenec C, Hillaire S, Molinie V, et al: Hepatic manifestations of hemophagocytic syndrome: A study of 30 cases. Am J Gastroenterol 96:852, 2001.

63. Cirera I, Navasa M, Rimola A, et al: Ascites after liver transplantation. Liver Transpl 6:157, 2000.

64. Stewart C, Wertheim J, Olthoff K, et al.: Ascites after liver transplantation—a mystery. Liver Transpl 10:654, 2004.

65. Correia JP, Conn HO: Spontaneous bacterial peritonitis in cirrhosis: Endemic or epidemic? Med Clin North Am 59:963, 1975.

66. Runyon BA: Monomicrobial nonneutrocytic bacterascites: A variant of spontaneous bacterial peritonitis. Hepatology 12:710, 1990.

67. Runyon BA, Hoefs JC: Culture-negative neutrocytic ascites: A variant of spontaneous bacterial peritonitis. Hepatology 4:1209, 1984.

68. Runyon BA, Canawati HN, Hoefs JC: Polymicrobial bacterascites: A unique entity in the spectrum of infected ascitic fluid. Arch Intern Med 146:2173, 1986.

69. Guarner C, Runyon BA, Young S, et al: Intestinal bacterial overgrowth and bacterial translocation in an experimental model of cirrhosis in rats. J Hepatol 26:1372, 1997.

70. Runyon BA, Squier SU, Borzio M: Translocation of gut bacteria in rats with cirrhosis to mesenteric lymph nodes partially explains the pathogenesis of spontaneous bacterial peritonitis. J Hepatol 21:792, 1994.

71. Runyon BA, Morrissey R, Hoefs JC, et al: Opsonic activity of human ascitic fluid: A potentially important protective mechanism against spontaneous bacterial peritonitis. Hepatology 5:634, 1985.

72. Runyon BA: Patients with deficient ascitic fluid opsonic activity are predisposed to spontaneous bacterial peritonitis. Hepatology 8:632, 1988.

73. Runyon BA, Sugano S, Kanel G, et al: A rodent model of cirrhosis and spontaneous bacterial peritonitis. Gastroenterology 100:1737, 1991.

74. Dunn DL, Barke RA, Knight NB, et al: Role of resident macrophages, peripheral neutrophils, and translymphatic absorption in bacterial clearance from the peritoneal cavity. Infect Immun 49:257, 1985.

75. McHutchison JG, Runyon BA: Spontaneous bacterial peritonitis. In Surawicz CM, Owen RL (eds): Gastrointestinal and Hepatic Infections. Philadelphia, WB Saunders, 1994, p 455.

76. Llovet J, Rodriguez-Iglesias P, Moitinho E, et al: Spontaneous bacterial peritonitis in patients with cirrhosis undergoing selective intestinal decontamination. J Hepatol 26:88, 1997.

77. Caly WR, Strauss E: A prospective study of bacterial infections in patients with cirrhosis. J Hepatol 18:353, 1993.

78. Bernard B, Cadranel J-F, Valla D, et al: Prognostic significance of bacterial infection in bleeding cirrhotic patients: A prospective study. Gastroenterology 108:1828, 1995.

79. Cadranel J-P, Denis J, Pauwels A, et al: Prevalence and risk factors of bacteriuria in cirrhotic patients: A prospective case-control multicenter study in 244 patients. J Hepatol 31:464, 1999.

80. Rimola A, Garcia-Tsao G, Navasa M, et al: Diagnosis, treatment and prophylaxis of spontaneous bacterial peritonitis: A consensus document. J Hepatol 32:142, 2000.

81. Pelletier G, Lesur G, Ink O, et al: Asymptomatic bacterascites: Is it spontaneous bacterial peritonitis? Hepatology 14:112, 1991.

82. Gill MA, Kern JW: Altered gentamicin distribution in ascitic patients. Am J Hosp Pharm 36:1704, 1979.

83. Papadakis MA, Arieff AI: Unpredictability of clinical evaluation of renal function in cirrhosis: Prospective study. Am J Med 82:945, 1987.

84. Cabrera J, Arroyo V, Ballesta AM, et al: Aminoglycoside nephrotoxicity in cirrhosis. Gastroenterology 82:97, 1982.

85. Hampel H, Bynum GD, Zamora E, et al: Risk factors for the development of renal dysfunction in hospitalized patients with cirrhosis. Am J Gastroenterol 96:2206, 2001.

86. Felisart J, Rimola A, Arroyo V, et al: Randomized comparative study of efficacy and nephrotoxicity of ampicillin plus tobramycin versus cefotaxime in cirrhotics with severe infections. Hepatology 5:457, 1985.

87. Runyon BA, Akriviadis EA, Sattler FR, et al: Ascitic fluid and serum cefotaxime and desacetylcefotaxime levels in patients treated for bacterial peritonitis. Dig Dis Sci 36:1782, 1991.

88. Ricart E, Soriano G, Novella MT, et al: Amoxicillin–clavulanic acid versus cefotaxime in the therapy of bacterial infections in cirrhotic patients. J Hepatol 32:596, 2000.

89. Follo A, Llovet JM, Navasa M, et al: Renal impairment after spontaneous bacterial peritonitis in cirrhosis: Incidence, clinical course, predictive factors and prognosis. Hepatology 20:1495, 1994.

90. Such J, Hillebrand DJ, Guarner C, et al: Nitric oxide in ascitic fluid is an independent predictor of renal impairment in patients with cirrhosis and spontaneous bacterial peritonitis. Eur J Gastroenterol Hepatol 16:1, 2004.

91. Sort P, Navasa M, Arroyo V, et al: Effect of intravenous albumin on renal impairment and mortality in patients with cirrhosis and spontaneous bacterial peritonitis. N Engl J Med 341:403, 1999.

92. Runyon BA: Albumin infusion for spontaneous bacterial peritonitis. Lancet 354:1838, 1999.

93. Navasa M, Follo A, Llovet JM, et al: Randomized, comparative study of oral ofloxacin versus intravenous cefotaxime in spontaneous bacterial peritonitis. Gastroenterology 111:1011, 1996.

94. Terg R, Cobas S, Fassio E, et al: Oral ciprofloxacin after a short course of intravenous ciprofloxacin in the treatment of spontaneous bacterial peritonitis: Results of a multicenter, randomized study. J Hepatol 33:564, 2000.

95. Aparicio JR, Such J, Pascual S, et al: Development of quinolone-resistant strains of *Escherichia coli* in stools of patients with cirrhosis undergoing norfloxacin prophylaxis: Clinical consequences. J Hepatol 31:277, 1999.

96. Runyon BA, McHutchison JG, Antillon MR, et al: Short-course vs long-course antibiotic treatment of spontaneous bacterial peritonitis: A randomized controlled trial of 100 patients. Gastroenterology 100:1737, 1991.

97. Akriviadis EA, McHutchison JG, Runyon BA: Follow-up paracentesis is usually not necessary in patients with typical

spontaneous bacterial peritonitis. Hepatology 26:288A, 1997.

98. Soriano G, Teixedo M, Guarner C, et al: Selective intestinal decontamination prevents spontaneous bacterial peritonitis. Gastroenterology 100:477, 1991.

99. Gines P, Rimola A, Planas R, et al: Norfloxacin prevents spontaneous bacterial peritonitis recurrence in cirrhosis: Results of a double-blind, placebo-controlled trial. Hepatology 12:716, 1990.

100. Soriano G, Guarner C, Tomas A, et al: Norfloxacin prevents bacterial infection in cirrhotics with gastrointestinal hemorrhage. Gastroenterology 103:1267, 1992.

101. Younossi Z, McHutchison JG, Ganiats TG: An economic analysis of norfloxacin against spontaneous bacterial peritonitis. J Hepatol 27:295, 1997.

102. Runyon BA, Borzio M, Young S, et al: Effect of selective bowel decontamination with norfloxacin on spontaneous bacterial peritonitis, translocation, and survival in an animal model of cirrhosis. Hepatology 21:1719, 1995.

103. Novella M, Sola R, Soriano G, et al: Continuous versus inpatient prophylaxis of the first episode of spontaneous bacterial peritonitis with norfloxacin. Hepatology 25:532, 1997.

104. Guarner C, Runyon BA, Heck M, et al: Effect of long-term trimethoprim-sulfamethoxazole prophylaxis on ascites formation, bacterial translocation, spontaneous bacterial peritonitis and survival in cirrhotic rats. Dig Dis Sci 44:1957, 1999.

105. Singh N, Gayowski T, Yu VL, et al: Trimethoprim-sulfamethoxazole for the prevention of spontaneous bacterial peritonitis in cirrhosis: A randomized trial. Ann Intern Med 122:595, 1995.

106. Rolando N, Gimson A, Philpott-Howard J, et al: Infectious sequelae after endoscopic sclerotherapy of oesophageal varices: Role of antibiotic prophylaxis. J Hepatol 18:290, 1993.

107. Goulis J, Armonis A, Patch D, et al: Bacterial infection is independently associated with failure to control bleeding in cirrhotic patients with gastrointestinal hemorrhage. Hepatology 27:1207, 1998.

108. Rongey CA, Runyon BA: Cellulitis in patients with cirrhosis and edema: An under-recognized complication that may be more common than spontaneous bacterial peritonitis. Hepatology 36:528A, 2002.

109. Tito L, Gines P, Arroyo V, et al: Total paracentesis associated with intravenous albumin management of patients with cirrhosis and ascites. Gastroenterology 98:146, 1990.

110. Mirouze D, Juttner HU, Reynolds TB: Left pleural effusion in patients with chronic liver disease and ascites: Prospective study of 22 cases. Dig Dis Sci 26:984, 1981.

111. Strauss RM, Boyer TD: Hepatic hydrothorax. Semin Liver Dis 17:227, 1997.

112. Xiol X, Castellote J, Baliellas C, et al: Spontaneous bacterial empyema in cirrhotic patients: Analysis of eleven cases. Hepatology 11:365, 1990.

113. Runyon BA, Greenblatt M, Ming RHC: Hepatic hydrothorax is a relative contraindication to chest tube insertion. Am J Gastroenterol 81:566, 1986.

114. Temes RT, Dacis MS, Follis FM, et al: Videothoracscopic treatment of hepatic hydrothorax. Ann Thorac Surg 64:1468, 1997.

115. Belghiti J, Durand F: Abdominal wall hernias in the setting of cirrhosis. Semin Liver Dis 17:219, 1997.

116. Runyon BA, Juler GL: Natural history of umbilical hernias in patients with and without ascites. Am J Gastroenterol 80:38, 1985.

117. Sarit C, Eliezer A, Mizrahi S: Minimally invasive repair of recurrent strangulated umbilical hernia in cirrhotic patient with refractory ascites. Liver Transpl 9:621, 2003.

118. Bajaj JS, Varma RR: TIPSS as therapeutic modality for umbilical hernia in patients with advanced liver disease. Liver Transpl 10:159, 2004.

119. Oktedalen O, Nygaard K, Osnes M: Somatostatin in the treatment of pancreatic ascites. Gastroenterology 99:1520, 1990.

120. Adrogue HJ, Madias NE: Hypernatremia. N Engl J Med 342:1493, 2000.

121. Adrogue HJ, Madias NE: Hyponatremia. N Engl J Med 342:1581, 2000.

122. Runyon BA: Historical aspects of treatment of patients with cirrhosis and ascites. Semin Liver Dis 17:163, 1997.

123. Pirlich M, Selberg O, Boker K, et al: The creatinine approach to estimate muscle mass in patients with cirrhosis. Hepatology 24:1422, 1996.

124. Eisenmenger WJ, Blondheim SH, Bongiovanni AM, et al: Electrolyte studies on patients with cirrhosis of the liver. J Clin Invest 29:1491, 1950.

125. Stiehm AJ, Mendler MH, Runyon BA: Detection of diuretic-resistance or diuretic-sensitivity by the spot urine Na/K ratio in 729 specimens from cirrhotics with ascites: Approximately 90% accuracy as compared to 24-hour urine Na excretion. Hepatology 36:222A, 2002.

126. Perez-Ayuso RM, Arroyo V, Planas R, et al: Randomized comparative study of efficacy of furosemide vs. spironolactone in nonazotemic cirrhosis with ascites. Gastroenterology 84:961, 1983.

127. Pitt B, Remme W, Zannad F, et al: Eplerenone, a selective aldosterone blocker, in patients with left ventricular dysfunction after myocardial infarction. N Engl J Med 348:1309, 2003.

128. Sungaila I, Bartle WR, Walker SE, et al: Spironolactone pharmacokinetics and pharmacodynamics in patients with cirrhotic ascites. Gastroenterology 102:1680, 1992.

129. Cohn JN: The management of chronic heart failure. N Engl J Med 335:490, 1996.

130. Stanley MM, Ochi S, Lee KK, et al: Peritoneovenous shunting as compared with medical treatment in patients with alcoholic cirrhosis and massive ascites. N Engl J Med 321:1632, 1989.

131. Daskalopoulos G, Laffi G, Morgan T, et al: Immediate effects of furosemide on renal hemodynamics in chronic liver disease with ascites. Gastroenterology 92:1859, 1987.

132. Spahr L, Villeneuve J-P, Tran HK, et al: Furosemide-induced natriuresis as a test to identify cirrhotic patients with refractory ascites. Hepatology 33:28, 2001.

133. Pockros PJ, Reynolds TB: Rapid diuresis in patients with ascites from chronic liver disease: The importance of peripheral edema. Gastroenterology 90:1827, 1986.

134. Mirouze D, Zipser RD, Reynolds TB: Effect of inhibitors of prostaglandin synthesis on induced diuresis in cirrhosis. Hepatology 3:50, 1983.

135. Runyon BA, Antillon MR, Montano AA: Effect of diuresis versus therapeutic paracentesis on ascitic fluid opsonic activity and serum complement. Gastroenterology 97:158, 1989.

136. Wong F, Blei AT, Blendis LM, et al: A vasopressin receptor antagonist (VPA-985) improves serum sodium concentration in patients with hyponatremia: A multicenter, randomized, placebo-controlled trial. Hepatology 3:182, 2003.

137. Arroyo V, Gines P, Gerbes AL, et al: Definition and diagnostic criteria of refractory ascites and hepatorenal syndrome in cirrhosis. Heptology 23:164, 1996.

138. Bories P, Garcia-Compean D, Michel H, et al: The treatment of refractory ascites by the LeVeen shunt: A multi-center controlled trial (57 patients). J Hepatol 3:212, 1986.

139. Stanley MM, Reyes CV, Greenlee HB, et al: Peritoneal fibrosis in cirrhotics treated with peritoneovenous shunting for ascites. Dig Dis Sci 41:571, 1996.

140. Gines P, Arroyo V, Quintero E, et al: Comparison of paracentesis and diuretics in the treatment of cirrhotics with

tense ascites: Results of a randomized study. Gastroenterology 93:234, 1987.

141. Kao HW, Rakov NE, Savage E, et al: The effect of large volume paracentesis on plasma volume—a cause of hypovolemia? Hepatology 5:403, 1985.

142. Pinto PC, Amerian J, Reynolds TB: Large-volume paracentesis in nonedematous patients with tense ascites: Its effect on intravascular volume. Hepatology 8:207, 1988.

143. Gines P, Tito L, Arroyo V, et al: Randomized comparative study of therapeutic paracentesis with and without intravenous albumin in cirrhosis. Gastroenterology 94:1493, 1988.

144. Smith GS, Barnard GF: Massive volume paracentesis (up to 41 liters) for the outpatient management of ascites. J Clin Gastroenterol 25:402, 1997.

145. Gines A, Fernandez-Esparrach G, Monescillo A, et al: Randomized trial comparing albumin, dextran 70 and polygeline in cirrhotic patients with ascites treated by paracentesis. Hepatology 111:1002, 1996.

146. Ruiz-del-Arbol L, Monescillo A, Jimenez W, et al: Paracentesis-induced circulatory dysfunction: Mechanism and effect on hepatic hemodynamics in cirrhosis. Gastroenterology 113:579, 1997.

147. Rothschild M, Oratz M, Evans C, et al: Alterations in albumin metabolism after serum and albumin infusions. J Clin Invest 43:1874, 1964.

148. Wilkinson P, Sherlock S: The effect of repeated albumin infusions in patients with cirrhosis. Lancet 2:1125, 1962.

149. Pietrangelo A, Panduro A, Chowdhury JR, et al: Albumin gene expression is down-regulated by albumin or macromolecule infusion in the rat. J Clin Invest 89:1755, 1992.

150. Runyon BA: Patient selection is important in studying the impact of large-volume paracentesis on intravascular volume. Am J Gastroenterol 92:371, 1996.

151. Peltekian KM, Wong F, Liu PP, et al: Cardiovascular, renal, and neurohumoral responses to single large-volume paracentesis in patients with cirrhosis and diuretic-resistant ascites. Am J Gastroenterol 92:394, 1997.

152. Moller S, Bendtsen F, Henriksen JH: Effect of volume expansion on systemic hemodynamics and central and arterial blood volume in cirrhosis. Gastroenterology 109:1917, 1995.

153. Planas R, Gines P, Arroyo V, et al: Dextran-70 versus albumin as plasma expanders in cirrhotic patients with tense ascites treated with total paracentesis. Gastroenterology 99:1736, 1990.

154. Christidis C, Mal F, Ramos J, et al: Worsening of hepatic dysfunction as a consequence of repeated hydroxyethylstarch infusions. J Hepatol 35:726, 2001.

155. Vermeulen LC, Ratko TA, Erstad BL, et al: The University Hospital Consortium guidelines for the use of albumin, nonprotein colloids, and crystalloid solutions. Arch Intern Med 155:373, 1995.

156. The SAFE Study Investigators: A comparison of albumin and saline for fluid resuscitation in the intensive care unit. N Engl J Med 350:2247, 2004.

157. Ochs A, Rossle M, Haag K, et al: The transjugular intrahepatic portosystemic stent-shunt procedure for refractory ascites. N Engl J Med 332:1192, 1995.

158. Rossle M, Ochs A, Gulberg V, et al: A comparison of paracentesis and transjugular intrahepatic portosystemic shunting in patients with ascites. N Engl J Med 342:1701, 2000.

159. Gines P, Uriz J, Calahorra B, et al: Transjugular intrahepatic portosystemic shunting versus paracentesis plus albumin for refractory ascites in cirrhosis. Gastroenterology 123:1839, 2002.

160. Sanyal AJ, Genning C, Reddy KR, et al: The North American Study for the Treatment of Refractory Ascites. Gastroenterology 123:634, 2003.

161. Salerno F, Merli M, Riggio O, et al: Randomized controlled study of TIPS vs paracentesis with albumin in cirrhosis with refractory ascites. Hepatology 40:629, 2004.

162. Saab S, Niets JM, Ly D, et al: TIPS versus paracentesis for patients with refractory ascites may benefit from transjugular intrahepatic portosystemic stent-shunts. Cochrane Database Syst Rev 3:CD004889, 2004.

163. Angermayr B, Cejna M, Koenig F, et al: Survival in patients undergoing transjugular intrahepatic portosystemic shunt: ePTFE-covered stentgrafts versus bare stents. Hepatology 38:1043, 2003.

164. Bureau C, Garcia-Pagan JC, Otal P, et al: Improved clinical outcome using polytetrafluoroethylene-coated stents for TIPS: Results of a randomized study. Gastroenterology 126:469, 2004.

165. Petersen B: Intravascular ultrasound-guided direct intrahepatic portacaval shunt: Description of technique and technical refinements. J Vasc Interv Radiol 14:21, 2003.

166. Rosemurgy AS, Zervos EE, Clark WC, et al: TIPS versus peritoneovenous shunt in the treatment of medically intractable ascites: A prospective randomized trial. Ann Surg 239:883, 2004.

167. Rozenblit GN, Del Guercio LRM, Rundback JH, et al: Peritoneal-urinary drainage for treatment of refractory ascites: A pilot study. J Vasc Interv Radiol 9:998, 1998.

168. Park JS, Won JY, Park SI, et al: Percutaneous peritoneovenous shunt creation for the treatment of benign and malignant refractory ascites. J Vasc Interv Radiol 12:1445, 2001.

169. Gines P, Quintero E, Arroyo V, et al: Compensated cirrhosis: Natural history and prognostic factors. Hepatology 7:12, 1987.

170. D'Amico G, Morabito A, Pagliaro L, Marubini E: Survival and prognostic indicators in compensated and decompensated cirrhosis. Dig Dis Sci 31:468, 1986.

CHAPTER

89 Hepatic Encephalopathy, Hepatopulmonary Syndromes, Hepatorenal Syndrome, and Other Complications of Liver Disease

J. Gregory Fitz

The liver plays a central role in the regulation of other organ systems by virtue of its functions in nutrition, metabolism, and secretion of xenobiotics and endobiotics. Consequently, chronic liver disease can lead to a broad range of systemic manifestations that may dominate the clinical course and represent principal indications for liver transplantation. Some of these complications result from a decrease in the number of functioning hepatocytes and concomitant loss of synthetic and metabolic capacity. Others reflect the increased pressure in the portal circulation, leading to opening of vascular collaterals and shunting of blood away from hepatic lobules. These manifestations of cirrhosis—decreased synthetic reserve and altered perfusion—are functionally interrelated and can change over time in response to varying physiologic

demands. Consequently, effects of cirrhosis on other organ systems also are dynamic, and symptoms frequently develop in the absence of obvious deterioration as manifested in the standard biochemical tests of liver function.

Despite the diverse organ systems affected by cirrhosis, in the early stages the extrahepatic complications share a common mechanistic bond in that they are largely functional in nature, representing a secondary effect of cirrhosis and not a primary abnormality of the target organ(s). Thus, replacing a failing liver by transplantation can lead to full restoration of associated neurologic, renal, or other abnormalities. Specific diagnostic features are not always present, however, and patients with liver disease also are susceptible to other disease processes.

In certain systemic diseases such as cystic fibrosis (pulmonary) or Wilson disease (brain), multiple organ systems are targeted by the same pathophysiologic process that affects the liver. This chapter provides an overview of the pathophysiology of the most common systemic manifestations of chronic liver disease and focuses in particular on their diagnosis and management.

HEPATIC ENCEPHALOPATHY

Hepatic encephalopathy (HE), or portosystemic encephalopathy, represents a reversible decrease in neurologic function caused by liver disease.[1,2] It occurs most notably in patients with portal hypertension and shunting of blood away from the liver. In the setting of chronic liver disease, the onset of encephalopathy often is insidious and is characterized by subtle and sometimes intermittent changes in memory, personality, concentration, and reaction times.[3,4] Typically, early changes are subclinical—in which case the disorder is termed *minimal hepatic encephalopathy* (MHE)—and are recognized only in retrospect, but MHE can be clinically significant. For example, studies of compensated cirrhotic patients without clinical evidence of HE indicate that more than one half perform abnormally on number connection tests or auditory-evoked responses,[5] and more than one half may be unfit to drive an automobile, as assessed by a battery of psychometric tests.[1] Although these results cannot be extended to all patients with cirrhosis,[6] the implications for patients and for society are important in view of the prevalence of cirrhosis.

With progression of encephalopathy, the neurologic abnormalities become more apparent and commonly are graded on a numerical scale that reflects increasing degrees of neurologic dysfunction, as described in Table 89–1.[1] The manifestations of stage 1 encephalopathy reflect involvement of higher cortical functions, with decreases in attention span, changes in personality, irritability, and impaired computational and construction skills. The patient's sleep pattern changes, with wakefulness at night and drowsiness during the day. Findings on the electroencephalogram (EEG) usually are normal, but the EEG tracing may show subtle slowing of the dominant frequency.

Progression to stage 2 encephalopathy is characterized by an exaggeration of these cortical manifestations, with more drowsiness and lethargy, and by the appearance of movement disorders that reflect increasing involvement of the descending reticular system or other neurologic structures. These movement disorders include tremors, incoordination, and asterixis.[7,8] In cooperative patients, asterixis is commonly evaluated by asking the patient to hold the arms extended with the wrists dorsiflexed; an abrupt loss of flexor tone and a characteristic wristdrop occur in a periodic manner every 2 to 3 seconds. Alternatively, the periodic relaxations become apparent when the examiner grips the patient's hand and holds the wrist lightly in a dorsiflexed position. In a patient with mental confusion, drowsiness, and personality changes, the presence of asterixis is highly suggestive of underlying hepatic encephalopathy. An EEG performed in stage 2 usually shows slower rhythms and the appearance of triphasic waves in the frontal regions.

Progression to stage 3, defined as increasing obtundation in a still arousable patient, or to stage 4, in which the patient is comatose, reflects either severe bilateral cortical dysfunction or involvement of the brainstem and reticular activating system. Asterixis may be lost, and hyperreflexia and muscle rigidity become apparent.[1] The EEG shows severe slowing, with frequencies in the theta and delta ranges. Even though the clinical features may be fully reversible with treatment (see later), encephalopathy of this degree generally is a manifestation of advanced liver disease and is associated with a poor long-term prognosis.[9]

These clinical features of HE are nonspecific. Similar manifestations can accompany hypoxia, acidosis, drug toxicity, and other metabolic and toxic insults. These possibilities should be excluded by appropriate drug screens and testing. The neurologic manifestations of HE are generally (but not always) symmetrical, and the appearance of focal neurologic motor or sensory abnormalities, such as cranial nerve dysfunctions or paresis, should always prompt investigation for other causes of structural neurologic disease, such as intracranial hemorrhage.

Histologic examination of the brains of patients with chronic liver disease and recurrent or chronic encephalopathy has identified several abnormalities, the most notable of which are neuronal cell swelling and a change

Table 89–1 Clinical Stages of Hepatic Encephalopathy

| Clinical Stage | Impairment | |
	Intellectual Function	Neuromuscular Function
Subclinical	Normal examination findings, but work or driving may be impaired	Subtle changes on psychometric or number connection tests
Stage 1	Impaired attention, irritability, depression, or personality change	Tremor, incoordination, apraxia
Stage 2	Drowsiness, behavioral changes, poor memory and computation, sleep disorders	Asterixis, slowed or slurred speech, ataxia
Stage 3	Confusion and disorientation, somnolence, amnesia	Hypoactive reflexes, nystagmus, clonus, and muscular rigidity
Stage 4	Stupor and coma	Dilated pupils and decerebrate posturing; oculocephalic ("doll's eye") reflex; absence of response to stimuli in advanced stages

in astrocytes referred to as Alzheimer type II astrocyto-sis.[2,10,11] These histologic changes suggest that HE is a disease that affects neurons or astrocytes or, more likely, both cell types. Whether these changes represent a cause or an effect of encephalopathy is unclear, however. Evidence for and against increased signal intensity in T1-weighted magnetic resonance images of the globus pallidus has been presented.[12] That most cases of early encephalopathy are fully reversible with treatment argues against a structural basis for encephalopathy and for a toxic or neurohumoral cause, particularly in the early stages.

PATHOPHYSIOLOGY

Despite the frequency and characteristic clinical features of HE, the precise pathogenic mechanisms are not fully defined. Decades of experience with animal models, including dogs with a surgically created Eck fistula (end-to-side portocaval shunt),[13] have identified the essential pathophysiologic elements. In the setting of porto-systemic shunting, by which portal blood is diverted away from the liver and into the vena cava, ingestion of a protein meal is associated with the onset of encepha-lopathy and progression to coma and death. Although the precise mechanisms are not established, these find-ings suggest that absorption of nitrogenous by-products of proteins from the colon into the portal circulation plays a key role.

This pathophysiologic model of hepatic encepha-lopathy is simplistic in some ways and does not account for other potentially important parameters, such as changes in central neurotransmitters and the blood-brain barrier,[2,11,14] but the model fits well with clinical experi-ence and makes no assumptions about the precise iden-tity of the toxin(s) involved. For example, even though creation of a portocaval shunt is highly effective for treat-ment of bleeding associated with portal hypertension (see Chapter 87), the clinical consequence is increased shunting and an increase in the frequency and severity of encephalopathy.[15,16] Therefore, recognition of these key features—portosystemic shunting and defective hepatic clearance of nitrogenous metabolites—continues to form the basis of standard treatments for HE.

Is ammonia the toxin responsible for HE? Yes, but not the only one, and the mechanisms whereby ammonia produces neuropsychiatric abnormalities are not fully defined.[17,18] In most relevant clinical series, elevated blood ammonia levels are detected in 60% to 80% of patients with cirrhosis and encephalopathy, and therapy aimed at decreasing the concentration of ammonia results in resolution of encephalopathy.[3,5,8,19,20] It is clear, however, that multiple metabolic abnormalities coexist, including changes in the profile of circulating amino acids, mercaptans, and central nervous system levels of dopamine and other neurotransmitters.[2,14,21,22] These alterations, as summarized in Table 89–2, are present to a variable extent in different clinical scenarios of HE and probably work in a complementary manner to modify neurologic function in cirrhosis.[14,17] Even if ammonia is not the only cause, or even the predominant cause, of

Table 89–2   Pathogenesis of Hepatic Encephalopathy

Mechanism	Hypothesis
Accumulation of toxins (ammonia, mercaptans)	Levels of ammonia and mercaptans produced by the action of intestinal bacteria on urea and protein are elevated in blood and brain as a result of defective hepatic clearance, leading to impaired neural function through cytotoxicity, cell swelling, and depletion of glutamate
Enhanced GABAergic neurotransmission	Defective hepatic clearance of GABA produced by intestinal bacteria, increased neuronal GABA synthesis, and increased production of benzodiazepine receptor agonists lead to neuronal inhibition through stimulation of the GABA receptor complex in postsynaptic membranes
Accumulation of false neurotransmitters	Increase in the ratio of plasma aromatic amino acids to branched-chain amino acids results in an increase in brain levels of aromatic amino acid precursors of false neurotransmitters

GABA, γ-aminobutyric acid.

HE, it is a clinically useful marker of the production of enteric toxins from nitrogenous substrates.

Detailed reviews of the pathogenesis and molecular mechanisms of HE have been published.[1-3,18] In the fol-lowing sections, emphasis is placed on a brief review of the role of ammonia and on the potential role of inhibitory neurotransmission through γ-aminobutyric acid (GABA) receptors in the central nervous system. The focus on these two mechanisms is based on the impor-tance of ammonia as a guide to therapy and the emerg-ing support for the GABA receptor complex as a target for newer therapies. Mechanisms involving changes in central neurotransmitters and circulating amino acids also are relevant, but their therapeutic implications are not as well defined. It is notable, for example, that in an animal model of HE, exploratory studies using micro-array technology to detect messenger RNA (mRNA) levels have demonstrated a two-fold increase in 16 mRNA tran-scripts and a two-fold decrease in 15 transcripts.[23] Some of these transcripts are derived from genes involved in neurotransmitter receptors, transporters, signal transduc-tion, and the cellular response to oxidative stress.[23] Evi-dence for reproducible alterations in soluble guanylate cyclase, nitric oxide (NO), and related pathways also has been published.[2,24] These multiple changes and the lack of unanimity regarding which one is primary underscore the need for continued efforts to improve our under-standing of this important complication of liver failure.

Ammonia Hypothesis

Ammonia is a key intermediate in nitrogen and protein metabolism, and the dynamics of ammonia handling in humans are well defined.[25,26] The gastrointestinal tract is the primary site of ammonia production. Nitrogenous compounds in the colon, which include ingested proteins and secreted urea, are degraded by bacteria with liberation of ammonia, which is then absorbed into the portal circulation, where concentrations are 5- to 10-fold greater than in mixed venous blood.[26] The first-pass extraction of ammonia by the liver is high,[25] resulting in clearance of ammonia from the portal system and prevention of its entry into the systemic circulation. Within hepatocytes, ammonia is converted rapidly by a series of enzymatic reactions to nontoxic glutamine and is synthesized in separate reactions into urea for secretion by the kidneys. Abnormalities in urea cycle enzymes occur in congenital syndromes (see Chapter 73), but enzyme deficiencies are not the major concern in most patients with cirrhosis, in whom ammonia bypasses the liver as a result of portosystemic shunting.

In addition to their role in urea transport, the kidneys are a site of ammonia generation and actively secrete ammonia into the urine.[25] Indeed, a net increase in the concentration of ammonia is observed in the renal veins as compared with the renal arteries, and the concentration of ammonia in the renal veins is increased by hypokalemia and use of diuretics.[26,27] Clinical studies support a role for hypokalemia in precipitating HE through an effect on renal ammoniagenesis.[28]

Following bolus injection of radiolabeled ammonia, the liver, bladder, and brain show appreciable uptake.[25] In encephalopathy, arterial ammonia levels increase and the rate of accumulation of ammonia in the brain also increases from 32 ± 3 μmol/min to 53 ± 7 μmol/min.[25] Because muscle is an important site of ammonia clearance, the muscle atrophy seen in advanced cirrhosis may contribute to the increase in the uptake of ammonia by the brain.[25]

Although the implications of these observations regarding ammonia metabolism, portosystemic shunting, and the pathogenesis of HE are not fully defined, in aggregate the observations indicate a clear relationship between HE and abnormal ammonia handling.

Difficulties in the measurement and interpretation of blood ammonia levels include (1) substantial variations in venous as compared with arterial ammonia levels; (2) exercise-induced release of ammonia from skeletal muscle; (3) a poor correlation between the absolute value of the blood ammonia level and the degree of encephalopathy; and (4) differences in the time course between the rise in blood ammonia levels and the onset of symptoms of encephalopathy.[29] Despite these limitations, measures to lower arterial ammonia levels remain a cornerstone of the management of hepatic coma.[19,30,31]

Patients with cirrhosis are subject to changes in systemic fluid and electrolyte balance by virtue of the sodium and water retention that accompanies cirrhosis and the frequent use of potent diuretics. Because encephalopathy commonly is precipitated by metabolic events,[32] it is instructive to consider how abnormalities in acid-base and electrolyte balance influence ammonia metabolism, with the assumption that increases in blood ammonia levels increase the severity of encephalopathy. The effects of uremia are predictable, because urea diffuses into the colon, where it is metabolized to liberate ammonia after bacterial degradation. The effects of

hypokalemia and alkalosis are more subtle. Hypokalemia frequently develops in cirrhotic patients as a consequence of diuretic-induced urinary losses, diarrhea, vomiting, and nutritional deficiencies. First, hypokalemia increases ammonia production by the kidney.[27,28] Second, hypokalemia and alkalosis favor cellular uptake of ammonia.[29] Because most of the body's K^+ stores are found in the intracellular space, lowering K^+ concentrations in the extracellular fluid stimulates efflux of K^+ out of cells to restore extracellular concentrations. Cells compensate for the loss of K^+ by a net uptake of Na^+ and H^+ ions to maintain electroneutrality, thereby leading to relative alkalinization of the extracellular space and acidification of the intracellular space.[29] Because ammonia (NH_3) and ammonium ion (NH_4^+) exist in equilibrium, the extracellular alkalosis increases the portion of membrane-permeable NH_3, whereas the intracellular acidosis serves to trap NH_4^+ within the cell. Therefore, the net effect of hypokalemia is a shift of ammonia into neurons or other cells, where it exerts its toxic effects. Consequently, normalizing hypokalemia is therapeutic.[33]

Despite the strong evidence that implicates ammonia as an important contributor to HE, the precise cellular mechanisms involved remain elusive.[18] Several potential mechanisms of ammonia-induced neuronal dysfunction have been described. Ammonia has been reported to decrease the concentration of glycogen in cultured astrocytes,[10] impair glial-neuronal communication,[34] and interfere with synaptic transmission.[21] Over longer periods, sustained elevation of ammonia levels induces pathologic changes in perineural astrocytes.[2,21] Because glycogen stores in astrocytes represent an important energy reserve for the brain, disruption of glial-neuronal signaling may play a role on the pathogenesis of HE.[10,35] Observations in animal models of HE and hyperammonemia support these general conclusions,[30] although the multiple effects of ammonia and its metabolites have not been fully resolved. In addition, ammonia modulates cell signaling through effects on glutamate and GABA signaling,[17,18] and alterations in ammonia metabolism and GABA signaling are thus related.

γ-Aminobutyric Acid Hypothesis

Ammonia causes some of the symptoms and signs of HE only after it is metabolized by glutamine synthetase in the brain. In an animal model of HE, portacaval shunting has been shown to lead to increases in plasma and brain ammonia concentrations, as well as increases in brain glutamine and tryptophan levels as a result of the action of glutamine synthetase.[36] Inhibition of glutamine synthetase results in normalization of brain glutamine concentrations and normalization of glucose consumption, supporting a role for glutamine synthesis in the development of cerebral metabolic abnormalities in hyperammonemic states.[36] Therefore, ammonia alone does not explain the central nervous system abnormalities in HE.

Studies in humans and animal models have implicated the GABA receptor complex as a key contributor to neuronal inhibition in HE.[18,22,37] The GABA receptor complex (Fig. 89–1) is localized to postsynaptic membranes and constitutes the principal inhibitory network in the

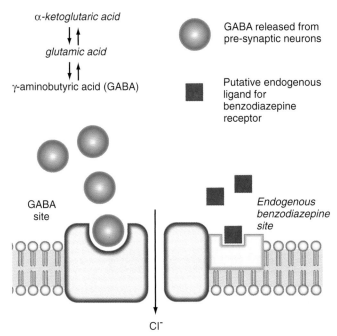

α-ketoglutaric acid

glutamic acid

γ-aminobutyric acid (GABA)

○ GABA released from pre-synaptic neurons

■ Putative endogenous ligand for benzodiazepine receptor

GABA site

Endogenous benzodiazepine site

Cl⁻

Figure 89–1 γ-Aminobutyric acid (GABA) receptor–chloride (Cl⁻) channel complex in the postsynaptic membrane.

central nervous system. The complex consists of (1) a GABA-binding site that faces the extracellular surface; (2) a Cl⁻-selective pore that opens in response to GABA binding to permit influx of Cl⁻ and produce membrane hyperpolarization; and (3) closely associated barbiturate and benzodiazepine receptor sites that potentiate the effects of GABA. The endogenous ligands for the benzodiazepine receptor have not been clearly identified.

Theoretically, increases in GABAergic transmission could result from increased availability of extracellular GABA or benzodiazepine receptor ligands. The liver contains high concentrations of GABA and GABA transaminase.[38] Liver injury disrupts GABA homeostatic mechanisms and may thereby contribute to the pathogenesis of HE. In addition, ammonia combines with α-ketoglutarate in the central nervous system to form glutamate, which, in turn, is amidated to produce GABA. Therefore, increased production of GABA would be expected to correlate with ammonia levels.[1,30]

The evidence for the role of endogenous benzodiazepine receptor ligands in increasing GABAergic transmission, however, is stronger.[22,37,39] In the absence of known ligands, putative benzodiazepine receptor agonists are identified by their competitive inhibition of flumazenil (a benzodiazepine receptor antagonist) binding.[22,40] In both animal[41] and human[40] models, HE is associated with an increase in levels of benzodiazepine receptor ligands. Similarly, benzodiazepine-like activity is increased in cerebrospinal fluid, blood, and urine in humans with HE.[3] Several additional points merit emphasis. First, gut bacteria provide precursors of benzodiazepine receptor ligands, just as they produce ammonia.[42] Impairment of hepatic clearance of such ligands in patients with cirrhosis parallels the reduced clearance of ammonia, and treatment to lower ammonia levels would be expected to have similar effects on levels of benzodi-

azepine receptor ligands. Second, the concentration of these ligands correlates roughly with the stage of HE.[40] Finally, HE is ameliorated in some patients by flumazenil[39] or its structurally related analogs Ro 15-3505 and Ro 15-4513.[37]

The efficacy of flumazenil in the treatment of HE has been studied in several clinical trials. In general, intravenous infusion of flumazenil (0.4 to 1 mg) results in modest but rapid improvement in the EEG and a more delayed improvement in the patient's mental status.[43,44] Some of the responders in these trials had received pharmaceutical benzodiazepines. Other studies, including blinded cross-over trials, have failed to identify a beneficial effect of flumazenil.[45] The reasons for the different results are not clear. In a literature review encompassing 13 trials and 805 patients, short-term improvement was detectable following treatment with flumazenil, but no appreciable change in rates of recovery or mortality was observed.[46] Therefore, most beneficial responses usually are incomplete, without full recovery to normal mental status, and are short-lived, perhaps because flumazenil-like drugs are incomplete benzodiazepine receptor blockers, or, more likely, other factors such as ammonia, mercaptans, and amino acids also contribute to HE.[1]

These studies support a role for benzodiazepine receptor ligands in the pathogenesis of HE and suggest that flumazenil or other benzodiazepine receptor antagonists may be useful in the treatment of HE. Clearly, these agents are of benefit in reversing the effects of exogenous benzodiazepines, may provide useful prognostic information, and may aid in the differential diagnosis of coma.[37] Although the findings in animal models are not necessarily generalizable to all forms of liver injury, the implications are intriguing: Encephalopathy may be caused in part by an increase in inhibitory neurotransmitter tone in the central nervous system. It merits emphasis that ammonia potentiates GABAergic transmission, thereby supporting the concept that the ammonia hypothesis and the GABA hypothesis are functionally related.[18]

DIAGNOSIS

Hepatic encephalopathy manifests as a spectrum of neurologic abnormalities, but each of the individual principal clinical features is nonspecific. Subtle impairments of memory, consciousness, and personality are easily overlooked if the underlying liver disease is not recognized. Alternatively, even if well-defined periods of encephalopathy have been documented, it may be difficult to assess whether recovery has been complete. By contrast, the clinical features of advanced encephalopathy and asterixis in a patient with known cirrhosis and portal hypertension are quite characteristic, and the combination of asterixis, hyperammonemia, and other clinical features permits confident recognition of portosystemic encephalopathy.

The recognition of MHE is of particular importance in view of the prevalence of cirrhosis. In the absence of characteristic features, subtle abnormalities of neuropsychiatric function generally are assessed by more specialized neuropsychiatric tests such as the trail-making test, block

Table 89–3 Common Clinical Factors That May Precipitate Hepatic Encephalopathy in Patients with Cirrhosis

Nitrogenous Encephalopathy	Non-Nitrogenous Encephalopathy
Uremia/azotemia	Sedatives, benzodiazepines
Gastrointestinal bleeding	Barbiturates
Dehydration	Hypoxia
Metabolic alkalosis	Hypoglycemia
Hypokalemia	Hypothyroidism
Constipation	Anemia
Excessive dietary protein	
Infection	

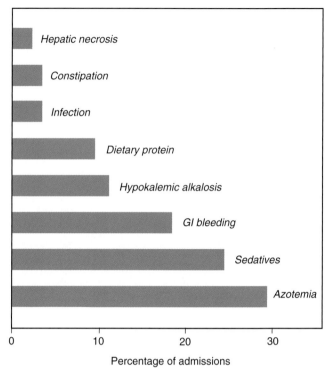

Figure 89–2 Clinical causes of hepatic encephalopathy. GI, gastrointestinal. (From Fessel JM, Conn HO: An analysis of the causes and prevention of hepatic coma. Gastroenterology 62:191, 1972.)

design and digit symbol tests, and visual reaction times[6] (see later). In addition, some evidence supports the use of brainstem auditory-evoked responses and somatosensory-evoked responses for the diagnosis of HE.[5,47] Some of these specialized tests are not readily performed in the clinical setting. Therefore, outside of the research setting, a high index of suspicion in patients at risk of HE, such as those with a recent surgical or transjugular portosystemic shunt,[15,48,49] and a beneficial response to a therapeutic trial are clinically more useful diagnostic approaches.

Special attention has been paid to the cerebral functional defects of latent or subclinical HE with regard to the patient's fitness to drive and quality of life. Driving requires complex response and spatial recognition skills, and in a series of cirrhotic patients without clinical signs of portosystemic encephalopathy, psychometric testing indicated that 60% were unfit to drive and an additional 25% had questionable driving skills.[4] Some, but not all, studies have confirmed a reasonably high frequency of subclinical encephalopathy in patients with cirrhosis, but no consensus has been reached on whether the ability to drive is significantly impaired in the absence of major abnormalities on neuropsychiatric testing.[6,50-53] Therefore, decisions regarding driving should be made on a case-by-case basis, with no clear support to strictly prohibit driving in patients with compensated cirrhosis and no overt evidence of encephalopathy. Administration of lactulose does seem to be beneficial in improving psychometric performance.[50]

Progression to clinically apparent HE is commonly associated with two modes of presentation. Encephalopathy may be acute in onset, with rapid deterioration of mental function and coma in the absence of previous symptomatology, or chronic and relapsing, as usually occurs in patients with more pronounced portal hypertension. In either case, HE typically is reversible, and a precipitating cause for the deterioration usually can be identified and corrected, as summarized in Table 89–3. The relative contributions of different precipitating factors were analyzed by Fessel and Conn in 100 patients requiring hospitalization and are illustrated in Figure 89–2.[32] Many of these precipitating factors are readily understood on the basis of their effects on ammonia. An increase in nitrogenous substances as a result of azotemia and gastrointestinal hemorrhage together accounted for

almost one half of the admissions. Medications also figured prominently, and causative mechanisms for the precipitation of coma were either direct, from increased sensitivity to tranquilizers and sedatives, or indirect, through hypokalemia, dehydration, and alkalosis associated with diuretic use. Identification and correction of these causes constitute the cornerstone of effective therapy, and in very few patients with chronic cirrhosis is encephalopathy the result of an irreversible loss of hepatocyte mass and synthetic capacity.

Blood ammonia levels may be measured when hepatic encephalopathy is suspected, both for diagnostic purposes and as a general guide to treatment. Normal ammonia values do not exclude the diagnosis and should not delay initiation of ammonia-lowering therapy. Measurable differences exist between arterial and venous levels of ammonia. In practice, venous levels are measured most often for convenience and because no evidence is available to suggest that the accuracy of measurement or outcome of the patient depends on the source of the blood sample. Approximately one fourth of patients will have non-nitrogenous precipitants of encephalopathy, such as adverse reactions to sedatives and fluid and electrolyte imbalances. In view of the potential involvement of the GABA receptor complex and the abnormalities in multiple other signaling pathways in HE, it is not surprising that patients with normal ammonia values respond to treatment in a manner similar to those with elevated ammonia levels. Measurement of glutamine levels in the cerebrospinal fluid and an EEG can provide confirmation of the clinical impression of HE but are neither sensitive nor specific.

The clinical stages of HE provide a general index of severity in the acute setting but are not sufficiently quantitative to assess subtle changes in clinical performance. Consequently, the need remains for a reliable, reproducible test that can be easily administered. The trail-making test provides a semiquantitative measure of encephalopathy. In this test, the subject connects 25 consecutively numbered circles, and the number of seconds required to complete the task is recorded.[8] An alternative figure-making test also has been introduced and validated for patients who cannot recognize numbers, and detects subclinical encephalopathy in 48% of subjects.[54] None of these measures alone is entirely satisfactory, and they are best utilized when administered serially to assess changes over time. The overall assessment provided by the Portosystemic Encephalopathy Index introduced by Conn in the 1970s and based on an arbitrary measure of the degree of abnormality of five factors—clinical assessment of mental state, trailmaking time, EEG, asterixis, and arterial ammonia—is still unsurpassed as a clinical research tool.[8] Although complex, the Index emphasizes the need for taking multiple parameters into account in the overall assessment and diagnosis of HE.

In the near future, the diagnosis of HE is likely to include cerebral imaging studies as well. Currently, computed tomography (CT) and magnetic resonance imaging (MRI) are used to exclude structural causes of altered mental status such as intracerebral bleeding. However, MRI and ^{1}H spectroscopy of the brain of patients with cirrhosis detect abnormalities in brain metabolites that correlate with encephalopathy and are completely reversed 3 to 7 months after liver transplantation.[2,55] The overall sensitivity of these and other techniques is not yet established, but they offer promise for real-time imaging of encephalopathy-specific brain metabolic changes in the future.

TREATMENT

The principles involved in management of HE are straightforward: identify and correct the precipitating cause(s), initiate ammonia-lowering therapy, and minimize the potential medical complications of cirrhosis and depressed consciousness (Table 89–4). Among these, careful scrutiny for and correction of the underlying cause of the deterioration, such as bleeding, tranquilizers, electrolyte abnormalities, or azotemia, is the most important. These basic steps are relatively easy and effective, with excellent recovery to basal function in most patients when comorbid factors are absent.

Correction of the precipitating factor for encephalopathy depends on a careful review of potential contributors, many of which, such as gastrointestinal bleeding, dehydration, hypokalemia, and azotemia, are readily apparent from the initial physical examination and basic laboratory studies. Particular attention should be paid to the possibility of gastrointestinal bleeding because of the high risk of bleeding in the setting of portal hypertension and the need for specific therapeutic intervention. Catabolism of blood in the intestine liberates ammonia and presumably benzodiazepine receptor ligands and

Table 89–4   Treatment of Hepatic Encephalopathy

1. Identify and correct the precipitating cause(s).
   a. Assess volume status, vital signs.
   b. Assess for gastrointestinal bleeding.
   c. Eliminate sedatives, tranquilizers, and similar drugs.
   d. Perform screening tests for hypoxia, hypoglycemia, anemia, hypokalemia, and other potential metabolic or endocrine factors, and correct as indicated.
2. Initiate ammonia-lowering therapy.
   a. Nasogastric lavage, cathartics, or enemas can be used to remove the source of ammonia from the colon.
   b. Minimize or eliminate dietary protein.
   c. Initiate treatment with lactulose or lactitol to produce 2 to 4 bowel movements per day.
   d. Consider giving oral nonabsorbable antibiotics to reduce intestinal bacterial counts.
   e. Consider giving flumazenil and other benzodiazepine receptor antagonists (see text).
3. Minimize the potential complications of cirrhosis and depressed consciousness; provide supportive care with attention to airway, hemodynamics, and metabolic status.

other mediators and is a classic cause of nitrogenous encephalopathy.

Action should be taken as soon as potential precipitating factors are identified. If azotemia is the cause, rehydration with concomitant attention to other prerenal factors is indicated. If bleeding is the precipitant, it must be controlled. Medications should be reviewed in detail, with specific attention to tranquilizers and sedatives and to the adverse effects of diuretics. Any potentially contributing medicines should be discontinued. Moreover, general measures to correct and maintain serum glucose levels, oxygenation, and acid-base balance are essential.

The second step in treatment involves measures directed at lowering elevated blood ammonia levels. Therapy involves removing the source of the ammonia from the intestinal tract, trapping ammonia in the colon to prevent systemic absorption, and, in some patients, decreasing the number of ammonia-producing bacteria in the colon. In patients with gastrointestinal bleeding, removing the source of ammonia involves eliminating blood from the gastrointestinal tract. For hemorrhage in the upper gastrointestinal tract, nasogastric lavage to remove blood and initiation of lactulose or other cathartics to speed transit through the colon are appropriate. In patients with more chronic encephalopathy that is not associated with bleeding, excessive ingestion of protein or constipation may elevate blood ammonia to levels high enough to cause encephalopathy.[32] In such cases, dietary protein intake should be decreased to approximately 60 g per day, and lactulose or other laxatives should be prescribed to eliminate protein from the colon (see later). In addition, substitution of vegetable protein for other protein sources appears to be of some advantage, because of a lower rate of ammonia production with such foods.[56] In severe encephalopathy, dietary protein should be eliminated completely until the patient improves sufficiently to allow institution of a stable therapeutic regimen.

The synthetic disaccharides lactulose (1,4-galacto-sidofructose)[8] and lactitol (beta-galactosidosorbitol)[57] have been the mainstays of medical therapy of nitrogenous hepatic encephalopathy for decades. Debate continues as to their efficacy, however.[20] These agents target the production and absorption of ammonia and benzodiazepine receptor ligands in the gut. Lactulose was introduced in the 1970s as an agent for therapy of HE on the basis of the concept that the drug would acidify the contents of the colon, thereby favoring trapping of NH_4^+ in the lumen and prevention of absorption. In the colon, lactulose is metabolized by bacteria to release lactic, acetic, and other organic acids and decreases stool pH to approximately 5.5.[8] In most relevant studies, treatment with lactulose is clinically effective in greater than 80% of patients, in whom serum ammonia levels decrease and the encephalopathic changes abate[8,19,57] (including patients with subclinical encephalopathy revealed by psychometric testing).[50] Treatment with lactulose is well tolerated, and the principal toxic effects are abdominal cramping, diarrhea, and flatulence. When administered orally to normal adults in amounts up to 160 g per day, lactulose decreases fecal ammonia production and increases fecal nitrogen excretion approximately fourfold, as a result of an increase in stool volume.[31] An increase in the number of bowel movements to two to four soft stools per day is an important therapeutic goal. In comparative clinical trials, lactulose and lactitol have been equally effective, but a trend toward better palatability and fewer side effects with lactitol has been observed.[57] Over longer periods in the outpatient setting, evidence suggests that efforts to modulate colonic bacterial flora to increase the proportion on non–urease-producing *Lactobacillus* species can lower blood ammonia levels, with subsquent abatement of encephalopathy.[5]

Several antibiotics, including neomycin, ampicillin, and rifaximin, also are effective in lowering blood ammonia levels.[8,19,58] The effect of these antibiotics on ammonia is the result in large part of a decrease in the number of colonic bacteria and a concomitant decrease in bacterial urease and protease activity, the main enzymes responsible for generation of ammonia.[58] In addition, decreasing colonic bacteria appears to decrease the production of benzodiazepine receptor ligands.[42] In most patients, the response to antibiotics is equivalent to that of lactulose, and in small series, use of antibiotics has been associated with improved patient compliance.[8,19] Nonspecific use of antibiotics in the absence of an established or suspected infection raises concerns, however. For example, neomycin can be absorbed systemically in concentrations sufficient to induce ototoxicity and nephrotoxicity, particularly when the drug is given over long periods. Furthermore, the alterations in gut flora associated with antibiotic use can contribute to diarrhea, malabsorption, and staphylococcal and other bacterial overgrowth syndromes. Therefore, chronic therapy with antibiotics should be reserved for patients who cannot tolerate oral lactulose or lactitol therapy, and neomycin should be avoided.

The relative benefit of nonabsorbable disaccharides as compared with antibiotics for acute HE has been evaluated in a review of 22 randomized clinical trials.[20] Although effective alone, lactulose and lactitol were not as effective as antibiotics, but it was unclear whether the difference was clinically important.

Treatment of HE in the absence of elevated blood ammonia levels follows the same principles as those for nitrogenous HE, including a careful review of the patient's use of sedatives and analgesics. Prolonged recovery from sedatives given for endoscopy or other procedures is characteristic of patients with HE. Therapy to lower blood ammonia levels appears to be effective in these patients, perhaps because of the effects on GABA-ergic transmission.[1,42]

The role of flumazenil and other benzodiazepine receptor antagonists is not yet defined.[37] In clinical trials, evidence for[43,44] and against[45] a clinical benefit with these agents has been presented. Even when the response was favorable, the recovery was rarely complete and was short-lived because of the pharmacokinetic properties of the drug. A review of 13 trials concluded that the short-term beneficial effect was not associated with significant improvement in the rates of recovery and mortality.[46] Much remains to be learned regarding the origin, overall contribution, and therapy of increased GABAergic transmission in HE. At present, as suggested by Jones and others, therapy with flumazenil should be limited to (1) reversing the effects of exogenous benzodiazepines; (2) aiding in the differential diagnosis of encephalopathy; and (3) providing information about prognosis in HE.[1,37,39] These indications are likely to evolve with additional clinical experience and the development of more selective and effective benzodiazepine receptor analogs.

There is a long history of clinical trials involving other more experimental approaches to the treatment of HE. These approaches have included use of levodopa, branched-chain amino acids, charcoal hemoperfusion, and molecular adsorbents[1,3,59] (see Chapter 90). Although anecdotal reports have been encouraging, none of these therapies has been sufficiently beneficial to lead to widespread application.

HEPATOPULMONARY SYNDROMES

Cirrhotic patients are at increased risk for specific abnormalities of pulmonary mechanics, hemodynamics, and ventilation-perfusion matching. These derangements can adversely affect the patient's quality of life and longevity (Table 89–5). In the early stages, subtle symptoms such as exertional dyspnea and tachypnea are commonly attributed to poor conditioning and nonspecific effects of chronic disease. With progression, dyspnea occurs at rest and may be associated with clubbing of the digits, cyanosis, spider angiomata, and pulmonary arteriovenous malformations. The degree of liver dysfunction does not predict the severity of the pulmonary disorder.[60] Hypoxemia and intrapulmonary shunting are common in patients with cirrhosis, however, and affect 20% to 40% of cirrhotic patients tested. Hypoxemia may be severe (PaO_2 less than 60 mm Hg) in selected patients.[60-62] Therefore, the development of hypoxia as a complication of cirrhosis indicates a high-risk patient with a poor long-term prognosis in the absence of definitive therapy.

Three of the most common pulmonary manifestations of cirrhosis are (1) alterations in lung mechanics

Table 89–5 Pulmonary Syndromes Associated with Cirrhosis

Pulmonary Manifestation	Diagnostic Features
Systemic diseases that affect both lung and liver	
Cystic fibrosis	Juvenile onset, obstructive airway disease, positive sweat chloride test
α_1-Antitrypsin deficiency	Emphysematous changes, phenotype (e.g., ZZ)
Sarcoidosis	Black race, hilar adenopathy, granulomatous inflammation
Drug toxicity	Exposure history, restrictive airway disease, chest x-ray
Mechanical effects of ascites	Tense ascites ± pleural effusion(s); decreased lung volumes
	Therapeutic response to large-volume paracentesis
Hepatopulmonary syndrome	Presence of liver disease
	Absence of primary cardiopulmonary disease
	Normal chest x-ray findings except for basilar shadowing
	Pulmonary gas exchange defects including an increased $D(A-a)O_2$ with or without hypoxemia; evidence for intrapulmonary vascular shunting
Pulmonary hypertension	Loud pulmonic component of second heart sound
	Right ventricular heave
	Right ventricular dilatation or hypertrophy on echocardiography
	Elevated pulmonary artery pressure (to greater than 40 mm Hg) by echocardiography

$D(A-a)O_2$, alveolar-arterial oxygen content difference.

caused by *ascites*, (2) intrapulmonary shunting and gas exchange abnormalities that together are referred to as the *hepatopulmonary syndrome*; and (3) *portopulmonary hypertension*. Of course, other important causes of pulmonary dysfunction may be present in patients with cirrhosis. Some reflect involvement of both lung and liver in specific disease processes, such as primary biliary cirrhosis, cystic fibrosis, and sarcoidosis.[26] Others result from adverse effects of therapy, such as sclerotherapy for bleeding esophageal varices, which has been reported to decrease PaO_2 and vital capacity in some patients, possibly secondary to the development of a restrictive lung defect caused by embolization of sclerosant to the lung.[63]

PATHOPHYSIOLOGY

Mechanical Effects of Ascites

Accumulation of ascites can lead to abnormal pulmonary mechanics through effects on intra-abdominal and intrathoracic pressure and accompanying alterations in thoracic volumes. Generally, the clinical findings are not subtle; the onset of respiratory symptoms and hypoxia is associated with worsening of ascites and fluid accumulation. In some patients, the ascitic fluid may cross the diaphragm through dilated lymphatics or holes in the diaphragm and accumulate in the intrapleural space. Thus, pleural fluid can represent an "ascites equivalent" and require treatment aimed at controlling portal hypertension, rather than at a specific pulmonary process.

When the diaphragm is compressed by ascitic fluid, standard pulmonary function tests show a decrease in mean lung volumes, including functional residual capacity and total lung capacity.[64,65] In addition, the diffusion capacity is decreased in many patients.[64,66] Air flow dynamics such as the forced expiratory volume (FEV_1 or FEV_{25-75}) generally are not affected unless coexisting airway disease is present.[64,65] With substantial ascites, dyspnea is attributable in large part to an increase in the work of breathing. Indeed, many patients improve symptomatically after large-volume paracentesis, even without an appreciable change in PaO_2.[65] The progressive loss of lung volumes and functional alveolar surface area, however, can result in overt hypoxemia.

Hepatopulmonary Syndrome

The hepatopulmonary syndrome (HPS) is more complex pathophysiologically than diaphragmatic compression by ascites and frequently is not as obvious clinically.[67] From 15% to 25% of patients with cirrhosis have HPS, which, when present, has a striking effect on survival.[68] In a series of well-characterized cirrhotic patients, careful evaluation by contrast echocardiography (see later) detected HPS in 24% of patients, and its presence was associated with a decrease in median survival from 41 months to 11 months.[69] In individual patients, HPS may coexist with mechanical pulmonary dysfunction from ascites. Pulmonary vascular dilatation that results in intrapulmonary shunting is the main determinant of impaired gas exchange in HPS and can develop in the absence of ascites or other evidence of advanced liver disease.[67] The pulmonary symptoms may be of sufficient severity to warrant liver transplantation even when the other clinical manifestations of cirrhosis are stable and well compensated.[70] Impaired hypoxic vasoconstriction and ventilation-perfusion mismatching also contribute to the hypoxia of the HPS to varying degrees.[62]

The HPS generally is associated with a hyperdynamic circulatory state, with elevation of cardiac output, cardiac index, oxygen delivery, and oxygen consumption. Both pulmonary vascular resistance and systemic vascular resistance are low.[62,71] Clinically, the low-resistance vascular channels in the pulmonary circuit reflect shunt pathways, through which blood from the pulmonary arteries bypasses functional alveoli and returns to the systemic circulation without full oxygenation, leading to desaturation of arterial blood[66] (Fig. 89–3). The effects of intrapulmonary shunting may be severe. In a series of nine cirrhotic patients with an average PaO_2 of 64 mm Hg, the shunt fraction determined during breathing of pure

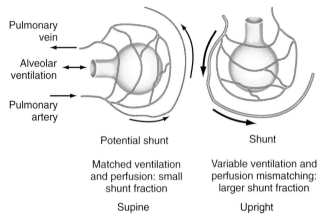

Pulmonary vein

Alveolar ventilation

Pulmonary artery

Potential shunt

Matched ventilation and perfusion: small shunt fraction

Supine

Shunt

Variable ventilation and perfusion mismatching: larger shunt fraction

Upright

Figure 89–3 Intrapulmonary shunting of blood from pulmonary artery to pulmonary vein in the hepatopulmonary syndrome. Changing from a supine to upright position can result in preferential perfusion of basilar regions with increased shunting and hypoxia (orthodeoxia).

oxygen averaged 20%.[62] In other words, 20% or more of the cardiac output bypassed functioning alveoli. The shunt fraction can increase with exercise. Postural changes also reduce oxygen saturation, a condition referred to as *orthodeoxia*.[62,72] When a patient assumes an upright position, blood shifts to the dilated precapillary beds in the bases of the lungs because of the effect of gravity, thereby increasing shunting and exacerbating hypoxemia[72] (see Fig. 89–3). The underlying pathophysiology has not been fully defined experimentally,[73] although the mechanisms involved have been reviewed.[67]

Several theories have been proposed to account for the circulatory changes associated with cirrhosis. In human studies, elevated plasma catecholamine (epinephrine) levels correlate positively with the hyperkinetic circulation, suggesting a causal role.[74] In animal studies, glucagon also has been found to have potent vasodilatory actions.[75] Plasma glucagon levels increase in chronic bile duct–ligated rats, and the degree of elevation correlates positively with the cardiac index and negatively with systemic vascular resistance.[75] These animals also have impaired hypoxic pulmonary vasoconstriction, consistent with a role for glucagon in HPS.[75] More recently, elevated blood endothelin-1 levels have been detected in some models of cirrhosis and associated with vasodilatation.[76] In one of these models, endothelin-1 levels are increased, and the interaction of endothelin-1 with its receptors stimulates an increase in NO production and pulmonary vasodilatation.[77] In the same study, blockade of the endothelin B receptor decreased pulmonary NO production and normalized pulmonary vascular dynamics.[77] These and other findings identify endothelin-1 and NO as important in the pathophysiology of HPS, but studies of other potential mediators, including somatostatin and thromboxane A_2, suggest that more than one factor will ultimately be implicated.[66,68,78]

Portopulmonary Hypertension

The underlying pathophysiology of portopulmonary hypertension is quite distinct from that of HPS. Pulmonary artery pressures are elevated and contrast with the pulmonary vascular dilatation and intrapulmonary shunting in HPS. Little is known about the pathogenesis of portopulmonary hypertension. Primary pulmonary hypertension is quite rare, but the general consensus among transplant centers is that the frequency of pulmonary hypertension is increased in patients with cirrhosis. Unfortunately, few studies have assessed the frequency of pulmonary hypertension in this population. It is attractive to speculate that pulmonary hypertension develops in some patients when vasoactive molecules bypass the cirrhotic liver because of portal hypertension and shunting and then mediate vasoconstriction when they reach the pulmonary circulation. Unfortunately, neither this nor any other theory has withstood critical appraisal in the absence of definitive clinical studies. Although much additional study is needed, it is important to emphasize that portopulmonary hypertension probably is underdiagnosed. Case studies suggest that portopulmonary hypertension can be reversed in some cases by liver transplantation and restoration of normal portal dynamics.

Cardiac Dysfunction

Cirrhosis per se also may be linked to significant impairment of myocardial contractility. The cellular mechanisms are not fully defined. In many animal models, elevated plasma catecholamine levels result in gradual impairment of myocardial function and emergence of heart failure over time, and blockade of adrenergic receptors is associated with improvement of contractility. Elevated blood catecholamine levels are characteristic of patients with cirrhosis, but no direct link between blood catecholamine levels and cardiac dysfunction has been established. The clinical distinction between a primary pulmonary process and myocardial dysfunction rests on the diagnostic approach described later.

DIAGNOSIS

Because of the increased morbidity and mortality rates associated with pulmonary syndromes in patients with cirrhosis, a high index of suspicion for the presence of such syndromes and a systematic approach to their diagnosis and management are essential. In patients with known cirrhosis, the worsening fatigue or dyspnea should not be ascribed to chronic liver disease without further evaluation. Initially, *oxygen saturation* should be measured noninvasively at rest and with exercise to identify patients at risk. *Arterial blood gases* provide a more definitive measure of oxygen delivery and help to categorize the defect in oxygenation as mild (PaO_2 greater than 80 mm Hg), moderate (PaO_2 60 to 80 mm Hg) or severe (PaO_2 less than 60 mm Hg). Exercise-induced oxygen desaturation is common in affected patients, and the severity of pulmonary disease may be underestimated if gas exchange is assessed under basal conditions only. Similarly, *orthodeoxia*, defined as a decrease in PaO_2 of at least 5% when the patient changes from a supine to upright position, is highly suggestive of HPS.[73] *Spirometry* can assess pulmonary volumes and diffusion capacity and helps to exclude other causes of hypoxia, such as restrictive or obstructive airway disease, particularly in disorders such as primary biliary cirrhosis, in which the lungs represent a primary target of injury.[79]

Tense ascites or pleural effusions on physical examination suggest that lung volumes may be decreased and the work of breathing may be increased. After measurement of oxygen saturation and assessment of the possibility of coexisting pleural effusions or pulmonary parenchymal disease, the best diagnostic information often is provided by the therapeutic response to a large-volume paracentesis (see later). Symptoms characteristically resolve within several hours of fluid removal when the diaphragm is compressed by massive ascites.[64]

The presence of digital clubbing, cyanosis, and spider angiomata is suggestive of HPS, rather than ascites alone, as the cause of dyspnea. Four diagnostic criteria that emphasize the functional nature of HPS have been proposed[60] (see Table 89–5): (1) the presence of chronic liver disease; (2) the absence of intrinsic cardiopulmonary disease (normal findings on chest radiograph, absence of nodular shadows in the lung bases attributable to vascular redistribution); (3) pulmonary gas exchange abnormalities, including an increased alveolar-arteriolar oxygen gradient with or without hypoxemia; and (4) evidence of intrapulmonary vascular shunting. Notably, these criteria make no assumptions about the severity of the underlying liver disease. Cardiac echocardiography is the most reliable approach to assessing myocardial function and detecting myocardial disease related to cirrhosis.

HPS is much more common than portopulmonary hypertension. The index of suspicion for pulmonary hypertension should be increased by a loud pulmonic component of the second heart sound and a right ventricular heave on physical examination. Additional evaluation by echocardiography usually is sufficient to confirm the diagnosis in the presence of right ventricular dilatation, right ventricular hypertrophy, and pulmonary artery pressures greater than 40 mm Hg. When pulmonary hypertension is suspected, patients should be referred to a transplantation center for definitive management (see later).

Several options are available for assessing the degree of intrapulmonary shunting in patients with suspected HPS, but contrast echocardiography generally is viewed as the best screening test (see later).[68] Alternatively, inert gas elimination techniques to assess the ventilation-perfusion ratio, arterial blood gas measurements, and measurement of shunt fraction and alveolar-arterial oxygen content difference [D(A-a)O$_2$] are standard techniques that are available through most hospital-based pulmonary function laboratories.[62,66,71] The presence of a large intrapulmonary shunt fraction in the setting of cirrhosis and hypoxemia is highly suggestive of HPS. The effect of postural changes on shunt fraction, oxygenation, and D(A-a)O$_2$ can be used to document the basis of orthodeoxia and provide further support for the presence of intrapulmonary shunts in a basilar distribution.[62,72] Right-sided heart catheterization with measurement of pulmonary artery pressures and hemodynamics is an important adjunctive diagnostic procedure in many patients.[71] In patients with severe hypoxia, a pulmonary

angiogram should be considered to look for large, dominant shunts. Certain centers have developed expertise in embolization or other therapeutic approaches for closing dominant shunts and thereby improving oxygenation.

Noninvasive measures, including whole-body radionuclide scanning with technetium-99m (^{99m}Tc)-labeled macroaggregated albumin and contrast echocardiography, have proved useful for detecting intrapulmonary shunting.[60,80,81] Under normal conditions, ^{99m}Tc-labeled macroaggregated albumin spheres are approximately 20 nm in diameter and are trapped in pulmonary capillaries, thereby providing a reliable measure of lung perfusion. In cirrhosis and other conditions associated with intrapulmonary shunting, opening of low-resistance vascular pathways allows the albumin spheres to bypass the capillary beds and appear in the systemic circulation, where they can be detected by whole-body imaging. Enhanced uptake of isotope by extrapulmonary organs is indicative of the presence of an intrapulmonary shunt.[80]

By an entirely different approach, contrast echocardiography also can detect dilatation of intrapulmonary vascular beds. Because of its availability and convenience, contrast echocardiography is now the screening test of choice for suspected HPS or portopulmonary hypertension.[68] When compared directly to radionuclide scanning, contrast echocardiography has proven to be a more useful screening test because of its greater sensitivity.[61] In one study,[61] 38% of cirrhotic patietns had a positive contrast echocardiography result, and 18% had both positive echocardiography results and gas-exchange abnormalities. No patient had a positive lung scan and negative echocardiography result. Even in normoxemic patients with cirrhosis, contrast echocardiography detects pulmonary vasodilatation in up to 10% of cases.[82]

The tests described above focus primarily on the detection of intrapulmonary shunting; it is important to emphasize that shunting is not the sole cause of hypoxemia in patients with HPS. Ventilation-perfusion mismatching, impaired oxygen diffusion, reduced cardiac output, and altered systemic hemodynamics all can play a role.[60,73] Detection of intrapulmonary shunting is the central focus for establishing the diagnosis of HPS, however.

TREATMENT

Mechanical Effects of Ascites

The clinical management of patients with a mechanical abnormality of ventilatory function focuses on control of ascites and fluid retention. In the short term, oxygen supplementation provides symptomatic relief. A careful clinical assessment is necessary to assure the adequacy of intravascular volume and the absence of pneumonia or other contributing factors. Blood is obviously the best treatment for a low intravascular volume when the hemoglobin level is less than 10 mg per day. In addition, careful investigation for hepatopulmonary shunting is warranted in most patients.

Large-volume paracentesis with removal of 3 L or more of ascitic fluid has proved to be safe and effective in patients with dyspnea associated with tense ascites.[64] Following paracentesis, lung volumes increase significantly, with the greatest increase (10%) in expiratory reserve volume, and significant increases in vital capacity, functional residual capacity, and total lung capacity as well.[64,65] Air flow generally is not affected by paracentesis, and effects on oxygenation are variable.[64,65,83] Nevertheless, the reduced work of breathing and increase in lung volumes lead to marked symptomatic improvement in most patients. The improvement is detectable within hours and sustained as long as the ascites does not reaccumulate.[65] The response to paracentesis is so reliable that the absence of significant improvement should prompt a more rigorous search for other causes of dyspnea.

In patients with pleural effusions resulting from ascites, therapeutic thoracentesis is required only if the effusion is unusually large or if the nature of the effusion is uncertain. A majority of such effusions improve over several days or weeks with control of the ascites. When the pleural effusion seems to be out of proportion to the ascites, free communication between the intrathoracic and intra-abdominal spaces can be documented by injection of a marker such as methylene blue or a radioisotope label into the ascitic fluid. The rapid appearance of the marker in the pleural space indicates the presence of low-resistance pathways between the pleural and peritoneal cavities. Isotopes have the advantage that they can be detected by nuclear imaging without the need for thoracentesis.

Although paracentesis is effective in the short term and can be repeated when needed, long-term management requires control of ascites through sodium restriction, diuretics to promote natriuresis and diuresis, and measures to lower portal pressure (see Chapter 88). Several medical regimens have been demonstrated to be effective.[84] In the absence of renal impairment, dietary sodium restriction and bed rest are successful in only approximately 10% of patients. The addition of spironolactone in doses up to 400 mg per day to antagonize the effects of aldosterone increases the proportion of responding patients to approximately 65%, and addition of furosemide or other loop diuretics allows effective control of ascites in up to 90% of patients.[84,85] The two-drug regimen is preferred (see Chapter 88). The goal of medical therapy is to minimize fluid accumulation and prevent pulmonary symptoms from developing. In ascites refractory to medical management, early consideration of liver transplantation is warranted. In the interim, placement of a transjugular intrahepatic portosystemic shunt (TIPS) to lower portal pressure may improve fluid balance in approximately two thirds of patients and help prevent recurrent pleural and abdominal fluid[86]; several weeks may be required before the ascites improves. Ultimately, the associated risks of worsening encephalopathy and shunt stenosis reduce the desirability of TIPS as a long-term management strategy unless all other conservative measures have failed.[15,16,87]

Hepatopulmonary Syndrome

Because the pathophysiology underlying the HPS is complex, involving intrapulmonary shunting, ventilation-perfusion mismatching, and impaired oxygen diffusion, clinical management can be challenging.[60,67,68] The

Table 89–6 Guide to the Management of Hypoxemia in Cirrhosis

Supplemental oxygen to maintain PaO_2 above 60 mm Hg
Large-volume paracentesis and medical therapy of ascites; consider diagnostic or therapeutic thoracentesis
Spirometry and radiographic evaluation to identify intrinsic pulmonary disease
Quantitation of gas exchange abnormalities, including alveolar-arterial oxygen gradient
Echocardiography to evaluate right ventricular function and to estimate pulmonary artery pressure
Assessment of evidence for intrapulmonary vascular shunting through inert gas elimination, arterial blood gas measurements, and estimation of shunt fraction using contrast echocardiography, pulmonary scanning, or other approaches
Consider right heart catheterization, pulmonary angiography
Liver transplantation

therapeutic approach is largely supportive (Table 89–6). Oxygen supplementation is required to overcome any contribution of ventilation-perfusion mismatching and hypoxic vasoconstriction and to improve tissue oxygen delivery. In addition, control of ascites and optimization of systemic and pulmonary hemodynamics are important adjunctive measures.[60] Small series have reported beneficial responses to pharmacologic agents such as almitrine, methylene blue, and even garlic powder (*Allium sativum*), which increase pulmonary vascular resistance, pulmonary artery pressures, and arterial oxygenation.[71] No standard pharmacologic approach, however, has proved to be effective over prolonged periods.[62,66,72] Occasional patients, particularly those anticipating surgery or other procedures, will benefit from right-sided heart catheterization and measurement of pulmonary pressures, to optimize cardiac filling pressures and oxygen delivery. Some authorities consider a pulmonary angiogram to be part of the evaluation of patients with severe hypoxemia, to permit detection and correction of dominant intrapulmonary shunts.

With supportive therapy, the prognosis of patients with the HPS is poor, with an overall mortality rate of 41% after 2.5 years in a representative series[72] and a median survival of only 11 months in a second study.[69] Liver transplantation can reverse intrapulmonary shunting effectively and correct the associated hypoxia,[60,76,80,88,89] but the risk of transplantation is increased by coexisting hypoxia.[62,80] In selected patients, however, transplantation is the only effective therapeutic option. Consequently, patients with suspected HPS should be referred to a transplantation center early in the clinical course. This recommendation is particularly important in children with biliary atresia, a disorder that appears to increase the risk of pulmonary arteriovenous shunting.[80] In general, patients with a PaO_2 less than 60 mm Hg should undergo transplantation as soon as possible, before the intrapulmonary shunting becomes more severe. Those with advanced disease marked by a PaO_2 less than 60 mm Hg require careful evaluation by the transplant team with respect to their operative candidacy and risk.[67,88] Successful liver transplantation is followed by gradual improvement in the alveolar-arterial oxygen gradient and PaO$_2$ (see Chapter 92).[70]

Portopulmonary Hypertension

Optimal treatment of portopulmonary hypertension has not been defined because of limited clinical experience. Ensuring tissue oxygen delivery by supplemental oxygen represents the mainstay of therapy. Experimental interventions have focused on the use of endothelin receptor antagonists (e.g., bosentan) to counteract the vasoconstrictor effects of endothelin and related peptides. Successful liver transplantation for treatment of portopulmonary hypertension has been described in a few reports. The challenge, however, is to focus efforts at transplantation primarily on those patients with reversible increases in pulmonary pressure, because fixed pulmonary hypertension carries a poor prognosis.

HEPATORENAL SYNDROME

The hyperkinetic changes in the circulatory system that are characteristic of cirrhosis and portal hypertension exist as a spectrum. At the extreme lies the *hepatorenal syndrome* (HRS), which is defined as functional renal failure in the setting of cirrhosis in the absence of intrinsic renal disease.[90,91] The HPS is characterized by intense constriction of the renal arterial vasculature with resulting oliguria and avid sodium retention.[87,92,93] Histologically, the kidneys are normal,[87,94] and function can be restored when the kidneys are removed and transplanted into a noncirrhotic recipient[94,95] or following correction of portal hypertension by liver transplantation.[96]

Unfortunately, the probability that HRS will develop in a patient with cirrhosis and ascites is relatively high. In a series of 234 nonazotemic patients with cirrhosis and ascites, HRS developed in 18% within 1 year and 39% within 5 years.[97] Typically, HRS occurs in the setting of portal hypertension and ascites and is characterized by a rise in the serum creatinine level and oliguria with a urine output of 400 to 800 mL/day. The course generally is progressive, and laboratory studies demonstrate (1) relatively hyperosmolar urine, (2) a high ratio, typically greater than 30, of urinary to plasma creatinine, and (3) a very low urine sodium concentration, usually less than 10 mEq/L, even in the presence of diuretics.[94] Of importance, central filling pressures must be normal. In a retrospective evaluation of nonazotemic patients with cirrhosis and ascites, multivariate analysis revealed only three factors that were independent predictors of HRS: a low serum sodium concentration, high plasma renin activity, and absence of hepatomegaly.[97] Other predictive factors identified on univariate analysis included ascites, nutritional status, and esophageal varices.[97]

Patients with cirrhosis are also at increased risk for development of other causes of renal insufficiency, related in part to involvement of both liver and kidney by the same disease process. Primary biliary cirrhosis, for example, is associated with lymphocytic infiltration of the renal parenchyma and interstitial nephritis, and renal tubular damage in Wilson disease frequently leads to renal tubular acidosis and impaired renal potassium secretion. Renal tubular acidosis and impaired acid secretion are relatively common in patients with cirrhosis of many causes. A greater clinical concern is hypovolemia associated with diuretic use, lactulose, or bleeding. The clinical features of hypovolemia may be difficult to assess with confidence in the setting of low systemic vascular resistance, and the laboratory features of prerenal azotemia are indistinguishable from those of HRS. Consequently, a beneficial response to volume expansion often is diagnostic.

PATHOPHYSIOLOGY

The liver plays an important role in the regulation of renal function under normal conditions.[98] In the absence of cirrhosis, uptake of amino acids by the liver stimulates an increase in renal blood flow, glomerular filtration rate, and urine volumes.[98,99] Mediators that have been proposed to link liver and kidney function include glucagon, intrarenal prostaglandins, NO, and angiotensin II, but their respective roles remain controversial.[99,100] Other factors that are released by the liver and target the kidney, and collectively referred to as *liver-borne diuretic factors* or *glomerulopressin*, have been proposed but have not been isolated and identified.[98] Such factors could account for the effect of protein loading on the glomerular filtration rate, and their absence in liver failure could contribute to impaired renal function.[98]

Functional renal failure in cirrhosis is characterized by sodium retention, water retention, and renal vasoconstriction[90,91]; it is associated with decreases in renal blood flow, glomerular filtration rate, and urinary output that contribute to the azotemia.[90,93] The pathophysiologic mechanisms responsible for these functional changes are not fully defined, however. HRS appears to represent a final stage in the complex hemodynamic derangements associated with portal hypertension and ascites that include systemic vasodilatation, effective hypovolemia, and a hyperkinetic circulation.[91,92]

Three main hypotheses to explain the pathogenesis of ascites formation have been proposed: vascular underfilling, vascular overflow, and peripheral arterial vasodilatation[91,94] (see Chapter 88). These hypotheses are not mutually exclusive, and each probably contributes at some stage in the process.[90] The traditional underfilling hypothesis focuses on intrahepatic blockade of hepatic blood flow, which leads to an increase in hydrostatic pressure within the hepatic and splanchnic circulation. Ascites develops when hepatic lymph production exceeds the capacity for lymphatic return, and contraction of blood volume and underfilling lead to secondary renal dysfunction. The vascular overflow model is based on the observation that renal sodium retention often precedes the onset of ascites and can lead to an increase in blood volume. The increased blood volume, in turn, leads to ascitic fluid formation and reflex vasodilatation to compensate for the increased volume.[90]

The peripheral arterial vasodilatation model, illustrated in Figure 89–4, was proposed because many of the pathophysiologic features of ascites and renal dysfunction could not be fully explained by the underfilling and overflow hypotheses.[90,101,102] Arterial hypotension is nearly

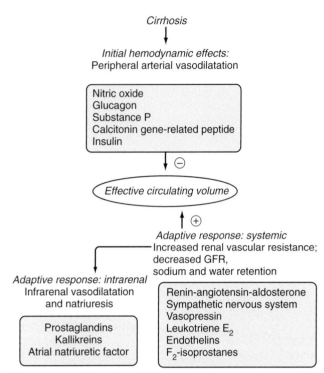

Figure 89–4 Pathogenesis of hepatorenal syndrome. Peripheral arterial vasodilatation appears to be an early event in the pathogenesis of fluid retention and the hepatorenal syndrome. Following initial vasodilatation, maintenance of normal renal perfusion depends on a balance between vasodilatory and vasoconstricting factors. Hepatorenal syndrome represents an imbalance favoring vasoconstrictive over vasodilating factors, the consequences of which are a marked increase in renal vascular resistance, decrease in GFR, and avid sodium and water retention. –, decrease; +, increase; GFR, glomerular filtration rate.

universal in advanced liver disease because of peripheral vasodilatation. According to this model, the initial abnormality is peripheral and splanchnic arterial vasodilatation related to portal hypertension. This vasodilatation initiates adaptive reponses that stimulate renal vasoconstriction and renal sodium and water retention. These adaptive responses include stimulation of the sympathetic nervous system, activation of the renin-angiotensin-aldosterone system, and nonosmotic release of arginine vasopressin as well as intrarenal responses. Ultimately, the balance between these various factors is lost, and striking increases in renal vascular resistance and functional renal failure result (see Fig. 89–4). The vasoconstrictor-mediated increase in proximal renal tubular sodium absorption accounts in part for diminished delivery of sodium to the distal tubule, which is the site of action of aldosterone and atrial natriuretic peptide.[101-103]

The precise factors involved in initiating peripheral arterial vasodilatation remain obscure.[104] A role for chronic increases in NO, a highly reactive diffusible gas,[93,105] has been proposed as a cause of both the hyperdynamic circulatory changes[106] and the renal failure.[94] Similarly, plasma levels of glucagon,[105] substance P,[93] and calcitonin gene–related peptide are elevated. Calcitonin gene-related peptide is a potent vasodilator, and circulat-

ing levels are increased in patients with alcoholic cirrhosis and ascites, but not in healthy controls or cirrhotic patients without ascites.[107]

Regardless of the precise mechanism, peripheral arterial vasodilatation and underfilling of the arterial compartment initiates a sequence of responses aimed at restoring the arterial filling pressure.[92,101] Activation of the sympathetic nervous system,[108,109] and the renin-angiotensin-aldosterone system[97,110] and release of vasopressin,[111,112] and other factors cause increases in renal vascular resistance[92] and renal sodium and water retention.[101,113]

Nonosmotic stimulation of arginine vasopressin release appears to account for the impaired ability to excrete a water load that is characteristic of advanced cirrhosis.[111] In patients with cirrhosis and in animal models of cirrhosis, serum levels of arginine vasopressin are elevated, and the metabolic clearance rate and half-time in serum of vasopressin are reduced.[111,112] In addition, some evidence suggests increased expression of the genes for vasopressin-regulated water channels.[114] The increase in plasma vasopressin levels and increase in the number of water channels would be expected to increase reabsorption of water in the distal nephron, thereby contributing to fluid retention and dilutional hyponatremia.

Levels of the vasoconstrictor endothelin-1 have been found to be elevated in several pathologic conditions characterized by sodium retention.[115,116] In heathy subjects, infusion of low doses of endothelin-1 decreases renal sodium excretion by 36%, and infusion of high doses decreases sodium excretion further and increases renal vascular resistance by 37%.[115] These effects are partially blocked by the calcium channel blocker nifedipine.[115] Arterial and hepatic venous levels of endothelin-1 and endothelin-3 are increased in patients with cirrhosis[116]; values are higher when ascites is present than when ascites is absent.[117] In addition, plasma levels of endothelin-1 and endothelin-3 show a significant correlation with elevations in the serum creatinine level[116-118] and a negative correlation with central and arterial blood volume, diastolic blood pressure, and serum sodium concentrations.[116,118]

F_2-isoprostanes, including 8-epi-prostaglandin $F_{2\alpha}$, also have been implicated in renal vasoconstriction through effects on endothelin release.[119,120] The F_2-isoprostane 8-epi-prostaglandin $F_{2\alpha}$ is an extremely potent renal vasoconstrictor, and plasma levels are markedly elevated in patients with HRS, but not in those with compensated cirrhosis, normal controls, or patients with other forms of renal disease.[120] The F_2-isoprostanes are generated in response to oxidative stress by a free radical–catalyzed lipid peroxidation mechanism that does not require cyclooxygenase.[119] In cultured endothelial cells, the F_2-isoprostanes bind to specific receptors that are closely related to thromboxane receptors and stimulate the release of endothelin-1.[119] The stimulation of F_2-isoprostane production in response to hypoxia suggests a potential role for this mediator in HPS, alcoholic liver injury, and other forms of oxidative stress.

In patients with cirrhotic ascites, both local and systemic factors counterbalance renal vasoconstriction to promote a natriuresis. For example, expansion of intravascular volume causes release of atrial natriuretic factor.[103,109] Initially, the release of atrial natriuretic factor may be sufficient to counteract the antinatriuretic influences at the expense of an expanded intravascular volume. As fluid retention progresses, the elevated levels of atrial natriuretic factor are inadequate to counteract the sodium-retaining effects of aldosterone, because of diminished delivery of sodium to the distal renal tubule.[101] Epstein and colleagues have concluded that the role of atrial natriuretic factor in cirrhosis is primarily beneficial in that it successfully compensates for antinatriuretic forces in patients with compensated cirrhosis. Renal resistance to atrial natriuretic factor develops in later stages,[95,103] however, and abnormalities of atrial natriuretic factor are not likely to represent a primary cause of HRS.

Renal vasoconstriction also leads to intrarenal production of vasodilating prostaglandins and kallikreins.[92] Ultimately, when the balance between renal vasoconstriction and vasodilatation is lost, renal vascular resistance increases dramatically (renal blood flow decreases), and HRS with uremia develops (see Fig. 89–4).

The balance between the different regulatory and counterregulatory signals leads to a spectrum of disorders. The approach to therapy of HRS in patients with advanced cirrhosis can best be understood, however, by remembering the following sequence of events: (1) dilatation of the splanchnic arteries; (2) underfilling of the arterial circulation; and (3) severe constriction of the renal vasculature and presumably of other systemic arterial beds as well.[121-123]

DIAGNOSIS

Diagnostic Criteria for Hepatorenal Syndrome

HRS should be suspected in any patient with acute or chronic liver disease and portal hypertension when the serum creatinine level rises above 1.5 mg/dL. In general, HRS occurs in the setting of relatively advanced liver disease, and the risk of HRS is increased in patients with hyponatremia, high plasma renin activity, and small liver size.[124] Nevertheless, neither the etiology of the liver disease nor the Child-Turcotte-Pugh score (see Chapter 87) has significant predictive value.[124]

Criteria for the diagnosis of HRS have been summarized by the International Ascites Club and are shown in Table 89–7.[90] Major criteria must be present for a diagnosis of HRS, and minor criteria provide support for the diagnosis. The *major criteria* include (1) the presence of chronic or acute liver disease with advanced hepatic failure and portal hypertension; (2) a low glomerular filtration rate, as indicated by a serum creatinine level higher than 1.5 mg/dL or a creatinine clearance less than 40 mL/min; (3) the absence of nephrotoxic drugs, shock, infection, recent fluid losses, or other potential causes of nephrotoxicity; (4) lack of sustained improvement in renal function following withdrawal of diuretics and volume expansion with 1.5 L isotonic saline; and (5) absence of evidence of significant proteinuria, renal obstruction, or parenchymal renal disease.[90]

The *minor criteria* are based largely on functional evidence of low glomerular filtration rate and avid sodium

---

Table 89–7   Criteria for the Diagnosis of Hepatorenal Syndrome

Major Criteria
1. Chronic or acute liver disease with advanced hepatic failure and portal hypertension
2. Low glomerular filtration rate, indicated by a serum creatinine level >1.5 mg/dL or creatinine clearance <40 mL per minute
3. Absence of treatment with nephrotoxic drugs, shock, infection, and substantial recent fluid losses
4. Lack of sustained improvement in renal function following diuretic withdrawal and volume expansion with 1.5 L of isotonic saline
5. Urinary protein level <500 mg/dL and lack of ultrasonographic evidence of parenchymal renal disease and obstruction

Additional Criteria
1. Urine volume <500 mL/day
2. Urine sodium <10 mEq/L
3. Urine osmolality greater than plasma osmolality
4. Urine red blood cells <50 per high-power field
5. Serum sodium concentration <130 mEq/L

From Arroyo V, Gines P, Gerbes AL, et al: Definition and diagnostic criteria of refractory ascites and hepatorenal syndrome in cirrhosis. Hepatology 23:164, 1996.

---

retention and include (1) urine volume less than 500 mL per day, (2) a urinary sodium concentration less than 10 mEq/L, (3) urine osmolality greater than plasma osmolality; (4) absence of significant hematuria, and (5) a serum sodium concentration less than 130 mEq/L. Although not required for the diagnosis of HRS, these associated features are sufficiently common that their absence should raise doubts about the diagnosis and prompt further investigation.

The diagnostic criteria require that patients with suspected HRS be evaluated for other causes of renal insufficiency (including a careful urinalysis) and undergo a thorough physical examination to evaluate their volume status. A renal ultrasound examination should be performed to look for renal parenchymal disease and exclude obstruction, and a post-void residual bladder volume should be measured if any question of bladder outlet obstruction exists.

HRS is classified into two types on the basis of severity and progression. *Type I HRS* is characterized by severe and rapidly progressive renal failure, defined as doubling of the serum creatinine to a level greater than 2.5 mg/dL in less than 2 weeks. Type I HRS usually occurs in patients with severe liver failure (jaundice, encephalopathy, coagulopathy) and often following a precipitating event, such as bleeding or an infection. *Type II HRS* has a more indolent course with a median survival of 6 months. The clinical picture is one of moderate stable renal disease in a patient with refractory ascites. The treatment trials discussed later in the chapter generally have included patients with type I HRS.

Limitations of Creatinine Measurements

Significant limitations exist regarding the use of the serum creatinine level as a marker of renal function in patients with cirrhosis. In general, estimates of glomerular filtration rate based on serum creatinine levels and creatinine clearance tend to overestimate the actual glomerular filtration rate in the presence of cirrhosis.[125] For example, in comparison with inulin clearance, the sensitivity rates of the serum creatinine (18%) and creatinine clearance (74%) for detecting renal insufficiency in 56 cirrhotic patients were marginal; the actual glomerular filtration rate was overestimated by about 50% in patients with a reduced inulin clearance.[125] The overestimation appears to result from increased tubular secretion of creatinine.[125]

The serum creatinine and creatinine clearance may be inadequate markers of renal function, even in patients with well-compensated cirrhosis.[126] In 68 nonazotemic patients with uncomplicated cirrhosis, evidence of renal dysfunction was detected in nearly two thirds,[127] including 21 patients with a creatinine clearance of 50 to 80 mL/min and 25 patients with a creatinine clearance less than 50 mL/min. Detection of renal insufficiency is clinically important, because patient mortality is substantially increased. With a mean follow-up period of 180 days, the mortality rate was 24% in patients with a creatinine clearance of 50 to 80 mL/min and 36% in those with a creatinine clearance less than 50 mL/min, as compared with 9% in those with normal renal function.[127]

Alternative Methods for Early Detection of Hepatorenal Syndrome

Ideally, in cirrhotic patients the glomerular filtration rate should be measured with techniques more sensitive than the creatinine clearance, such as iothalamate clearance, but such testing is not feasible in most settings.[90] Because HRS is characterized by renal vasoconstriction that appears before clinically recognized disease, several studies have evaluated alternative diagnostic approaches. One of the most promising approaches is the use of Doppler ultrasonography to assess the *resistive index*, a measure of resistance to blood flow in the renal vasculature.[124,128] In 180 patients with liver disease in the absence of azotemia, renal vascular waveform analysis indicated an increase in the resistive index in 42%.[124] Renal dysfunction subsequently developed in 55% of these patients, as compared with only 6% of those with a normal resistive index, and HRS occurred in 26% of those with an elevated resistive index, as compared with only 1% of those with a normal index.[124] In cirrhotic patients with renal failure, the resistive index correlates with the glomerular filtration rate, arterial blood pressure, plasma renin activity, and free water clearance[129] and has rates of sensitivity and specificity for the detection of kidney failure of 71% and 80%, respectively.[129] Therefore, measurement of the resistive index is an effective and noninvasive method for detecting hemodynamic changes characteristic of HRS.[128]

Can measurement of the resistive index identify high-risk patients when standard tests of renal function are still normal? The resistive index increases progressively from normal values in control patients (0.53 ± 0.03) to higher values in nonascitic cirrhotic patients without ascites (0.67 ± 0.06) and in those with ascites. Values also are higher in patients with Child-Turcotte-Pugh class B and class C cirrhosis than in those with class A cirrhosis.[130] Although an abnormal resistive index may help identify high-risk patients,[124] operator experience is important, and considerably more information is required before the resistive index can be recommended as a standard approach. Nonetheless, an increased resistive index measured in the presence of normal renal function does appear to identify a subgroup of cirrhotic patients at higher risk for development of HRS.[128]

TREATMENT

In general, HRS occurs in the setting of diuretic treatment of portal hypertension and ascites. Typically, patients are on strict dietary sodium restriction and an intensive diuretic regimen of spironolactone, in doses of up to 400 mg per day, and, usually, furosemide, in doses of up to 160 mg per day.[84,85] As noted earlier, these measures lead to control of ascites in up to 90% of patients but pose the risk of prerenal azotemia, hypokalemia, and encephalopathy.[84,85] Patients who fail to respond with a natriuresis and diuresis after 1 week of intensive therapy can be considered to have refractory ascites, which is a frequent prelude to HRS.[90] In a retrospective review of 46 patients, the factors that precipitated HRS most commonly were infection in 48%, gastrointestinal bleeding in 33%, and a recent paracentesis in 27%.[131]

Management of a rise in the serum creatinine level to greater than 1.5 mg/dL in a cirrhotic patient with ascites on an intensive diuretic regimen is a demanding clinical challenge. Initially, all potential nephrotoxic agents including nonsteroidal anti-inflammatory drugs, aminoglycosides, and, if possible, other antibiotics must be discontinued. Because prerenal azotemia can mimic the clinical and laboratory features of HRS, including oliguria, a low urine sodium concentration, and high urine–to–plasma osmolality ratio, and because cirrhotic patients are at risk of prerenal azotemia from diuretics, bleeding, and other volume losses, an intravascular volume challenge is required in most patients. A volume challenge is one of the major diagnostic criteria for HRS according to the International Ascites Club, which advocates withdrawal of diuretics and a volume challenge of 1.5 L of isotonic saline.[90] Ultimately, the diagnosis of HRS remains one of exclusion of other causes of renal failure. When doubt about the diagnosis persists, central filling pressures should be assessed by right-sided heart catheterization.

The emergence of diuretic resistance[102] represents a major limitation of current treatments of HRS. Moreover, use of diuretics in the setting of an elevated serum creatinine level increases the risk that the glomerular filtration rate will worsen because of further decreases in plasma volume. Consequently, alternative therapies often are considered. Large-volume paracentesis causes a significant increase in cardiac output and a rapid fall in portal pressure, as well as a fall in plasma renin and aldosterone levels, and has been reported to improve serum creatinine and blood urea nitrogen levels in patients with HRS.[132] The creatinine clearance may decrease following a large-volume paracentesis, however, even when the serum creatinine and blood urea nitrogen levels remain unchanged, presumably because the intravascular volume is decreased.[127] Limited evidence has supported the use of extracorporeal albumin dialysis[133] and pharmacologic treatment with low-dose dopamine, combination therapy with norepinephrine and dopamine,[134] terlipressin (a long-acting vasopressin analog) alone,[135] or the vasopressin analog ornipressin alone.[84,92,136] Results of studies of these agents are not sufficiently compelling to warrant widespread application to clinical practice.

The 2000s have seen renewed interest in the use of combination therapy with intravenous albumin for circulatory support and potent vasoconstrictors to reverse the vasodilatation of the splanchnic bed.[123,137] The goal of this approach is to reverse the functional decrease in effective arterial blood volume and to improve renal perfusion. Intravenous infusion of albumin has been used for some time to prevent renal failure associated with large-volume paracentesis. In 21 consecutive cirrhotic patients with HRS, the combination of albumin plus terlipressin reversed the syndrome in 12 patients (57%), whereas terlipressin alone had no effect.[138] Similar results have been obtained with albumin plus intravenous norepinephrine or midodrine, an alpha agonist.[139,140] In view of the poor prognosis for HRS, these reports of reversal are encouraging, but care in using these approaches is warranted because of the lack of apparent benefit in some studies, risk of inducing myocardial ischemia, and need for broader experience.[141]

Several case reports also have proposed a role for TIPS in reversing HRS.[87,142] In a series of patients with refractory ascites, TIPS increased the mean urinary sodium excretion and improved the serum creatinine level and glomerular filtration rate.[114] This response was associated with a decrease in plasma aldosterone levels and renin activities. Clinical improvement with control of ascites was detected in 74% of patients, and the mean use of diuretics was decreased by one half.[114] A majority of patients, however, did not have overt HRS. Consequently, the use of TIPS may be appropriate for some patients with diuretic-resistant ascites, and in selected patients with HRS who have responded to pharmacologic therapy, but the overall role of TIPS in the treatment of HRS remains to be established.[140]

Beginning decades ago, head-out water immersion of patients proved to be a valuable model for studying both the pathogenesis and the treatment of diuretic-resistant ascites.[95,109] In patients with ascites, head-out water immersion increases central blood volume and promotes marked natriuresis and diuresis, leading to an increase in urine volume and urine sodium output by two- to three-fold.[109,143] Plasma levels and urinary excretion of norepinephrine decrease, and plasma levels of immunoreactive atrial natriuretic factor increase promptly.[109] When facilities are available, the hemodynamic response to immersion is favorable, but this approach is used uncommonly.

The onset of renal failure in patients with cirrhosis carries a poor prognosis. The plasma renin activity, plasma concentration of antidiuretic hormone, and serum sodium concentration have some value as predictors of survival,[129] but in the absence of a clearly reversible cause of renal failure, treatment is largely supportive. The traditional view is that dialysis is futile in HRS except as a bridge to liver transplantation.[144] In patients with preexisting liver disease and acute renal failure (including HRS) requiring dialysis, the relative risk of dying has been shown to be increased substantially in those with thrombocytopenia (platelet count less than $100,000/mm^3$), HE, or a prolonged prothrombin time. Even in the absence of these features, the 1-year survival rate was only 38%.[144] The investigators concluded that renal failure alone, in the absence of contraindications, does not preclude dialysis, but the risks of dialysis are significant.[144]

Liver transplantation remains the ultimate treatment for HRS. When transplantation is successful, full recovery from functional renal failure can be expected. Delaying transplantation until the onset of renal failure imposes great risks, however. Liver transplant recipients with HRS have a significantly decreased survival at 5 years as compared with those without HRS.[96] In addition, transplant recipients with HRS require longer stays in the intensive care unit, longer hospitalizations, and more dialysis sessions. Therefore, early transplantation is preferable whenever possible.[96]

ENDOCRINE DYSFUNCTION

Advanced cirrhosis invariably leads to abnormal regulation and function of multiple endocrine systems.[145] The effects of cirrhosis are complex, however, as anticipated from the diverse roles of the liver as a target organ whose function is regulated by circulating hormones and as a site for the uptake and metabolism of hormones and the production of serum hormone-binding globulins.[146-148] The frequency and severity of endocrine dysfunction are increased in diseases that affect both the liver and endocrine organs by a common pathophysiologic process. For example, iron accumulation in the testes, hypothalamus, and pancreatic beta cells leads to hypogonadism and diabetes in patients with hemochromatosis,[149] and autoimmune damage to the thyroid gland frequently accompanies primary biliary cirrhosis (Table 89–8). Cirrhosis per se, however, can alter regulation along the hypothalamic–pituitary–endocrine gland axis,[150] and the clinical manifestations of feminization and hypogonadism, including gynecomastia, spider angiomata, and palmar erythema, are so common that they are considered to be characteristic of advanced liver disease.

In this section, emphasis is placed on the effects of cirrhosis on sex and thyroid hormone functions because of their frequency and clinical impact.[145,148,151,152] These endocrine abnormalities frequently are overlooked, but approximately 60% of cirrhotic patients have a history of diminished libido, loss of well-being, and impotence.[149,153,154] Diabetes also merits mention because of its frequency in patients with cirrhosis. The detection and management of insulin resistance, however, are similar in patients with and those without cirrhosis, except for a higher risk of complications of oral hypoglycemic medications in patients with cirrhosis because of prolonged drug half-lives and secondary hypoglycemia.[155]

Table 89–8   Endocrine and Metabolic Abnormalities Associated with Cirrhosis

Disorder	Manifestations
Systemic diseases affecting both endocrine organ(s) and liver	
Hemochromatosis	Gonadal insufficiency
	Hypothalamic dysfunction
	Diabetes mellitus
Primary biliary cirrhosis	Autoimmune thyroid disease
	Metabolic bone disease
Alcoholic cirrhosis	Gonadal insufficiency
	Hypothalamic dysfunction
Feminization and hypogonadism	Elevated estrone level
	Decreased total and free testosterone levels
	Loss of diurnal variation
	Elevated sex hormone–binding globulin level
	Hypothalamic dysfunction
	Testicular atrophy
Hypothyroidism	Decreased triiodothyronine level
	Normal or increased thyroxine-binding globulin level
Diabetes mellitus	Elevated fasting glucose level
	Insulin resistance

PATHOPHYSIOLOGY

Normal regulation of both thyroid and sex hormone levels depends on an intact hypothalamic-pituitary axis and on peripheral factors, including the level of hormone-binding globulins, which influence the availability and distribution of free (non–protein-bound) hormone.

Feminization and Hypogonadism

Feminization and hypogonadism in men with cirrhosis result from a decrease in serum testosterone levels and a relative increase in circulating estrogen levels. The abnormalities can be striking in patients with advanced cirrhosis, as illustrated in a study in which serum free testosterone levels were lower (0.11 ± 0.02 versus 0.22 ± 0.03 nmol/L) and the estrogen/free testosterone ratio was significantly higher (10.3 ± 2.5 versus 2.6 ± 0.5) in cirrhotic men than in noncirrhotic controls.[156] In a similar study of cirrhotic men, the endocrine status was invariably abnormal, with a decrease in testosterone levels in 90% and in free testosterone levels in 100%.[157] The decrease in testosterone levels results in part from diminished testicular synthesis of testosterone, and the increase in estrone or estradiol levels appears to be related to an increase in the peripheral conversion of weak androgens to estrogens.[158] In addition, a general decrease in sensitivity occurs throughout the hypothalamic-pituitary-gonadal hormone axis. These changes often normalize after liver transplantation.[157]

The clinical features of feminization, which include loss of libido, a decreased sperm count,[150] decreased muscle mass, testicular atrophy, appearance of spider angiomata, and changes in hair distribution, presumably reflect effects of the increased estrogen/free testosterone

ratio on target organs that express androgen and estrogen receptors. An exception may be gynecomastia, for which the frequency among cirrhotic patients of 44% does not appear to differ from that of nonobese controls without cirrhosis.[156] Moreover, estradiol levels are not different in cirrhotic patients with and those without gynecomastia.[156] Therefore, factors other than estrogen excess may contribute to the development of gynecomastia and perhaps other features of feminization as well.

Interpretation of the significance of sex hormone levels depends in large part on simultaneous measurements of levels of sex hormone–binding globulin (SHBG), a glycoprotein with high-affinity binding for 17α-hydroxysteroid hormones, including testosterone and estradiol.[147] SHBG is produced in the liver, and plasma concentrations are regulated by androgen-estrogen balance, thyroid hormones, and insulin.[147] The amount of free (biologically active) hormone is a function of the amount of SHBG present in the circulation. SHBG levels are increased significantly in patients with compensated cirrhosis,[152,159] although not in all studies.[160] Therefore, total estrogen and testosterone levels may be normal or only slightly decreased when free levels of these hormones are low, because of the increase in SHBG levels. With progression of cirrhosis, serum free testosterone levels and the testosterone/SHBG ratio decrease, and serum estradiol, free estradiol levels, and the estradiol/testosterone ratio increase.[152] The net effect is estrogen excess and loss of androgen stimulation.

Several other factors contribute to alterations in the estrogen/testosterone balance in cirrhosis. First, the normal circadian rhythm of testosterone release is lost.[158] Second, hepatic uptake of sex steroids, which accounts for 20% to 50% of their metabolic clearance, is altered, consistent with a significant role of the liver in the bioavailability of these hormones.[146] Finally, and importantly, production of testosterone is decreased as a result of impaired hypothalamic regulation. Typically, plasma luteinizing hormone (LH) and follicle-stimulating hormones (FSH) levels are normal or slightly increased in patients with cirrhosis, but the increase is not to the degree expected on the basis of the low testosterone levels.[153] Stimulation of pituitary gonadotropin release with clomiphene[158] or gonadotropin-releasing hormone (GnRH) increases release of LH and FSH.[153] Therefore, pituitary and gonadal function are relatively preserved in patients with compensated cirrhosis, and defective hypothalamic sensing of low hormone levels or defective release of GnRH appears to contribute importantly to gonadal insufficiency. This interpretation is consistent with the finding of elevated prolactin levels seen in some patients with cirrhosis. Pituitary secretion of prolactin is under tonic inhibitory regulation by the hypothalamus by way of dopamine, a prolactin inhibitory factor. Loss of hypothalamic dopamine regulation leads to release of prolactin.[161]

Similar effects occur in women with cirrhosis, but they have not been as well studied, because feminization is not as great a clinical concern in the early stages in women as in men. In postmenopausal women, in whom the effects of menstrual cycle variations are minimized, both estradiol levels and the estradiol/testosterone ratio are increased over those in control patients.[162] Testosterone,

LH, and FSH levels typically are decreased.[160,162] In younger women, these endocrine abnormalities can lead to amenorrhea.[163] Injection of GnRH stimulates an increase in LH and FSH levels, indicating preservation of pituitary responsiveness.[160,163] Moreover, the findings in women are consistent with those in men, in whom the hypothalamus, rather than the pituitary, represents a primary site of disturbance in gonadotropin secretion.[163]

The complicating effects of alcohol merit mention. Alcohol, even in moderate amounts, can have substantial effects on estradiol, testosterone, and estrogen-responsive pituitary hormone levels in normal postmenopausal women.[164] These effects are exaggerated in the presence of cirrhosis.[164] In addition, SHBG levels are elevated in most patients with cirrhosis, but the increase is greater with alcoholic cirrhosis than with other causes of cirrhosis.[158] These abnormalities of sex hormone regulation are not limited to alcohol-related disease, and the degree of endocrine regulatory dysfunction tends to correlate with the severity of liver disease[162] and portal hypertension,[150,151,164,165] rather than the cause of the liver disease.

Hypothyroidism

Changes in free thyroxine levels parallel those of sex hormones in patients with cirrhosis, in that the levels also are influenced by thyroxine-binding globulin (TBG), which frequently are increased in patients with cirrhosis.[166] Although the changes in TBG levels limit interpretation of standard thyroid tests, hypothyroidism is thought to be relatively common in patients with cirrhosis; however, few studies have examined the frequency and mechanisms involved early in cirrhosis. Uncertainty about the true frequency of hypothyroidism exists in part because the clinical features of advanced liver disease and of hypothyroidism (loss of energy, decreased appetite, and depressed affect) are similar. Moreover, the sick-euthyroid state may develop in patients with advanced cirrhosis.

In nonalcoholic cirrhotic patients with HE, serum triiodothyronine (T_3) and free T_4 levels typically are decreased,[167] and TBG and total thyroxine levels are elevated.[166] Clinical interpretation of these findings requires measurement of thyroid-stimulating hormone (TSH) levels, which usually are normal in patients with compensated cirrhosis and elevated in those with true hypothyroidism.[166] In 73 men with alcoholic cirrhosis, the decrease in serum T_3 concentrations and increase in serum TSH levels correlated with the degree of liver dysfunction and serum testosterone levels, suggesting a possible relationship between testosterone and thyroid function.[168] Available evidence suggests both central and peripheral defects in thyroid secretion in cirrhosis. Alcohol in particular appears to have a direct toxic effect on the thyroid gland.[169] In addition, in patients with cirrhosis and low total T_3 and T_4 levels, the TSH response to injected thyrotropin-releasing hormone (TRH) frequently is subnormal or delayed.[170]

Is hypothyroidism in a patient with cirrhosis good or bad? An intriguing clinical study has suggested that relative hypothyroidism paradoxically may have beneficial effects on the outcome of cirrhosis.[148] In a retrospective analysis, a significant negative correlation was found between blood TSH levels and tests of liver function. Because many of the synthetic and metabolic functions of the liver are regulated by thyroid hormones, subtle hypothyroidism may minimize the rate of progression of liver disease and decrease the frequency of bleeding, ascites, and encephalopathy.[148] These findings are highly theoretical and require considerable additional investigation.

DIAGNOSIS

Feminization and hypogonadism typically are suspected on the basis of clinical findings of estrogen excess, including palmar erythema, spider angiomata, and an altered secondary hair pattern. In affected men, decreased libido and a history of impotence are common, and physical examination shows testicular atrophy and a loss of muscle mass. In women, decreased libido and amenorrhea or menstrual irregularity are frequent.

The laboratory evaluation begins with measurement of total and free testosterone and estrogen levels to assess gonadal release and of LH and FSH levels to evaluate the pituitary response. In the early stages of compensated cirrhosis, the only findings are increases in the mean serum concentrations of estrone and SHBG.[165] With progression, low levels of free and total testosterone may become apparent, and estrone levels increase markedly.[165] Large increases in LH and FSH are uncommon and, when present, suggest primary gonadal failure. By contrast, suppression of LH and FSH in the setting of low testosterone levels implies a central regulatory defect. When the diagnosis of hypogonadism is uncertain, the effects of GnRH on LH, FSH, and testosterone can be assessed, and the hypothalamic-pituitary axis imaged by CT, but these tests are rarely indicated.

The clinical features of hypothyroidism are nonspecific and are easily attributable to the systemic manifestations of cirrhosis. Consequently, every patient with cirrhosis, regardless of etiology, should have screening studies to assess thyroid hormone levels and TSH. An increased risk of hypothyroidism is widely recognized in diseases such as primary biliary cirrhosis. The risk also is increased in many patients with cryoglobulinemia and chronic hepatitis C and in those receiving interferon therapy (see Chapter 76). Low blood levels of free T_3 are suggestive of hypothyroidism, but clinically significant hypothyroidism may be difficult to distinguish from the sick-euthyroid state. Typically, the TSH level is normal or slightly decreased in sick-euthyroid disease and increased in hypothyroidism. When doubt about the presence of hypothyroidism exists, pituitary responsiveness can be assessed with a TRH stimulation test or a clinical trial of thyroid hormone replacement initiated. Clinical improvement and normalization of thyroid hormone and TSH levels would support continuation of therapy.

TREATMENT

The endocrine abnormalities associated with cirrhosis become more frequent and more severe as liver disease and portal hypertension progress.[150] Patients with advanced disease (Child-Turcotte-Pugh class C) are more likely to have severe feminization, hypogonadism, and hypothyroidism. In view of the poor prognosis with advanced liver disease, it is understandable that little definitive information is available regarding the effects of hormone replacement on survival, quality of life, or disease progression. Consequently, treatment decisions must be individualized according to the patient's response and often are based on criteria developed for other diseases.

Treatment of hypothyroidism with synthetic T_4 aims to relieve the fatigue and correct the metabolic abnormalities and other systemic manifestations of decreased thyroid hormone levels. Therapy is initiated in conventional doses of 50 to 100 mg per day, and the dose is adjusted gradually to achieve the desired clinical effect and to maintain thyroid hormone and TSH levels in the normal range. No large controlled clinical series have evaluated the efficacy of prolonged therapy in patients with cirrhosis. Early detection of thyroid disease and initiation of therapy before progression to advanced cirrhosis is likely to improve outcomes in affected patients.

Several clinical trials have evaluated the role of testosterone replacement therapy in cirrhotic men with feminization and hypogonadism. In some studies, testosterone enanthate, 250 mg intramuscularly every 4 weeks, has been shown to be safe and to improve libido, well-being, and sexual potency.[149] In larger series, however, testosterone in different forms has shown no consistent benefit with respect to liver function, hemodynamics, general well-being, sexual function, or survival.[159,171] Oral testosterone therapy, 200 mg three times daily, appears to decrease the frequency of gynecomastia.[171] As with thyroid disease, it is likely that early recognition of hypogonadism, before the development of advanced liver disease, may identify patients who would benefit from replacement therapy. Short-term treatment with clomiphene increases LH and FSH levels and increases testicular androstenedione release,[158] but no long-term trials of the safety or efficacy of clomiphene have been conducted.

The long-term effects of liver transplantation on recovery of endocrine function are not fully defined. In two small series, liver transplantation resulted in clear trends toward normalization of total and free testosterone levels and SHBG levels.[153,157] The beneficial effects appear be greater in patients with alcohol-related liver disease than in those with nonalcoholic liver disease.[172] Endocrinologic recovery is incomplete in some patients, however, suggesting the presence of residual damage to the hypothalamic-pituitary-gonadal axis that persists despite liver replacement.[153,172] Therefore, continued clinical and laboratory monitoring of the patient's endocrine status is required following liver transplantation, until the precise etiology and natural history of these important disorders are better defined.

COAGULATION DISORDERS

The risk of bleeding in patients with cirrhosis is increased greatly with the development of specific disorders of coagulation. The pathogenesis of these disorders is complex and involves abnormalities of platelets, the intrinsic and extrinsic coagulation cascades, and fibrinolysis.[50] When acute bleeding occurs, correction of these coagulation abnormalities constitutes a principal goal of therapy. In the absence of bleeding, coagulation disorders cause no specific symptoms and are detected only by screening laboratory studies. In general, the severity of the hemostatic defects tends to increase as the liver disease advances, and their detection identifies a subset of cirrhotic patients with a high risk of a poor outcome. For example, decreases in factor VII levels, decreases in platelet counts, and increases in fibrinolysis each have been shown to increase the probability of bleeding and to affect survival adversely in different clinical scenarios.[173-175] Consequently, standard measures of hemostasis, including the platelet count, prothrombin time, and partial thromboplastin time, should be monitored in cirrhotic patients and assessed if the patient bleeds and before liver biopsy or other invasive procedure. Moreover, the prothrombin time serves as a key element in most of the grading systems that aim to quantitate disease severity for the purpose of determining liver donor organ allocation priorities[176] (see Chapters 87 and 92).

PATHOPHYSIOLOGY

The parenchymal cells of the liver produce most of the factors involved in coagulation and fibrinolysis, and the reticuloendothelial cells of the liver play an active role in the clearance of endotoxins, fibrin degradation products, and other factors that contribute to the balance between thrombin deposition and removal. A variety of hemostatic disorders have been described in cirrhotic patients. In general, these disorders can be categorized as abnormalities of platelet number or function, increased fibrinolysis, or deficient synthesis of clotting factors (Table 89–9). Because these abnormalities frequently coexist in individual patients, a systematic approach to their evaluation is warranted.

Platelet Abnormalities

Cirrhosis is associated with both quantitative and qualitative platelet abnormalities. Approximately 40% of cirrhotic patients have abnormal prolongation of the

Table 89–9 Coagulation Abnormalities in Cirrhosis

Abnormality	Laboratory Features
Thrombocytopenia and coagulopathy	Platelet count < 80,000/mm³ Bleeding time > 9 min Impaired platelet aggregation
Altered synthesis of vitamin K–dependent coagulation factors	Prolonged prothrombin time Decreased factor VII levels Normal factor VIII levels
Dysfibrinogenemia	Fibrinogen level normal or low Increase in levels of fibrin degradation products, D-dimer Prolonged thrombin time Prolonged reptilase time

bleeding time to greater than 10 minutes and platelet counts of less than 100,000/mm³.[177] The severity of the thrombocytopenia increases with the patient's Child-Turcotte-Pugh score, and platelet counts less than 50,000/mm³ are common.[178] This decrease in the number of circulating platelets is related in part to pooling of platelets in the spleen as a result of portal hypertension and splenomegaly and in part to immunologic destruction of platelets. In a representative study of 31 cirrhotic patients with an average platelet count of 46,000/mm³, splenic uptake of the radiolabeled platelet pool ranged from 43% to 54%, and platelet survival decreased from control values of 9.3 days to 6.5 days.[179] Several studies have confirmed the presence of platelet-associated immunoglobulin G (IgG) in patients with cirrhosis, and serum immunoglobulin levels increase in proportion to the severity of the liver disease.[178-180] This phenomenon is a particular concern in chronic hepatitis C, in which levels of platelet-associated IgG are increased and thrombocytopenia is observed in 41% of patients (versus 19% of patients with chronic hepatitis B).[181] In addition, hepatitis C virus may act directly to reduce the platelet count, because viral RNA can be detected in circulating platelets.[181] The relative contributions of splenic sequestration and immune-mediated destruction of platelets are difficult to assess in individual patients. In addition, the role of thrombopoietin is uncertain, with evidence of both decreased production of and decreased sensitivity to thrombopoietin. Elucidating the precise mechanisms involved in thrombocytopenia is of great interest because thrombopoietin could be used to treat some patients. The key point is that, generally, the lower the platelet count, regardless of the cause, the poorer the clinical outcome.

Cirrhosis also is associated with functional abnormalities in which circulating platelets are not activated in a normal manner, resulting in defective clot formation.[182,183] The decrease in platelet aggregation, as measured by the ristocetin test, may be related to decreases in glycoprotein Ib levels in the platelet membrane[184] or to defective signal transduction within the platelets.[185] Patients with bleeding times longer than 7 minutes or a clinical history of bleeding have the lowest glycoprotein Ib levels.[184] Other mechanisms to account for defective platelet function are likely to be involved as well.[186]

Dysfibrinogenemia

Dysfibrinogenemia represents an activation of fibrinolysis and is detected by increased blood levels of fibrin degradation products, D-dimer, and tissue plasminogen activator in patients with cirrhosis. Fibrinogen levels may be normal, but the thrombin time and reptilase time generally are prolonged. Enhanced fibrinolysis increases the risk of gastrointestinal hemorrhage[175] and presumably other causes of bleeding as well. Increased levels of both tissue plasminogen activator and plasminogen activator inhibitors frequently are detected and appear to contribute to the underlying disorder.[187-190] The mechanisms involved are not clear, however. Proposed mechanisms include an exchange between plasma and ascitic fibrinolytic proteins that regulates plasma fibrinolytic potential[189] and entry of endotoxin derived from intestinal bacteria into blood, with activation of the fibrinolytic

cascade.[191] The relative contributions of these and other factors appear to vary from patient to patient. In more severe cases, dysfibrinogenemia may progress to disseminated intravascular coagulation. The plasma concentration of antithrombin appears to be an important determinant of this progression.[192] Thrombin formation is increased in patients with cirrhosis, but if the antithrombin level is sufficient, the formation of thrombin is controlled. When levels of antithrombin are low (less than 0.3 U/mL), thrombin is not inactivated, potentially leading to sustained interactions with fibrin and an increase in the risk of disseminated intravascular coagulation.[192]

Clotting Factor Deficiencies

With loss of functioning liver parenchymal cells, clotting factor deficiencies develop and may be quite severe.[193] Vitamin K–dependent factors, including factors II, VII, IX, and X, and protein S and C are affected early.[193] Factor VII, with a half-life of only 4 to 7 hours, is particularly important clinically,[83] and recombinant factor VII is now available commercially (see later). After synthesis, vitamin K serves as a cofactor for a hepatic carboxylase that modifies these factors to provide a site for Ca^{2+} binding, an essential step in the function of these factors. As factor VII levels decrease, the prothrombin time increases progressively, reflecting decreased function of the extrinsic coagulation cascade. Prolongation of the prothrombin time occurs with sufficient frequency that the prothrombin time is a standard component of the Child-Turcotte-Pugh score used to assess the severity of cirrhosis (see Chapter 87).

DIAGNOSIS

Acquired hemostatic abnormalities associated with cirrhosis have important clinical implications, but the lack of specific clinical findings necessitates a laboratory-based approach to their evaluation. Generally, the diagnosis is straightforward, and standard laboratory tests are readily available. Consequently, surveillance studies, including the platelet count, prothrombin time, and partial thromboplastin time, should be performed at regular intervals in patients with cirrhosis or whenever hemorrhage is suspected. A low platelet count commonly is associated with physical manifestations of portal hypertension, including ascites and splenomegaly. Generally, platelet counts above 70,000/mm³ are well tolerated and do not cause prolongation of the bleeding time unless qualitative platelet abnormalities are present as well. Other causes of thrombocytopenia, including bone marrow suppression from alcohol or interferon or other medications, must be excluded by history and bone marrow examination if necessary. Splenic sequestration is most often a diagnosis of exclusion, but when uncertainty exists, increased platelet trapping can be visualized directly using indium-111 (^{111}In) tropolone–labeled platelets.[180] Platelet-associated IgG levels (antiplatelet antibodies) should be measured in most patients, especially those with chronic hepatitis C and autoimmune hepatitis, to assess the possible contribution of immune-mediated platelet destruction.[180] Prolongation of the bleeding time also can reflect impaired platelet function in vivo.[177] When necessary, formal studies of platelet aggregation induced by ristocetin can be performed.[184]

Dysfibrinogenemia involves activation of fibrinolysis and is detected by increased blood levels of fibrin degradation products and D-dimer. Fibrinogen levels may be normal, but the thrombin time and reptilase time generally are prolonged. In patients with compensated cirrhosis, levels of thrombin-antithrombin complexes are increased.[192] The presence of overt disseminated intravascular coagulation should prompt a rigorous evaluation for endotoxemia and other reversible causes.

Deficiencies in vitamin K–dependent clotting factors are detected by prolongation of the prothrombin time.[193] Direct measurement of factor VII levels is a more sensitive method of detecting clotting factor deficiency, because factor VII has a comparatively short half-life and levels must decrease to less than 60% of control levels before the prothrombin time becomes abnormal. Decreases in levels of other vitamin K–dependent factors and of protein S and protein C also can contribute to a prolonged prothrombin time. A therapeutic trial of vitamin K is important for evaluating the role of vitamin K deficiency, as opposed to diminished hepatic parenchymal synthetic capacity, in prolonging the prothrombin time.

TREATMENT

Management strategies differ according to the urgency of the clinical situation. In a patient with acute bleeding or in whom an invasive procedure is planned, the goal is to improve hemostasis in the short term. The detection of coagulopathy identifies a high-risk subset of cirrhotic patients who should be evaluated for liver transplantation early in their clinical courses.

In urgent settings, prolonged bleeding times related to thrombocytopenia and thrombopathies generally can be managed by platelet transfusions. In addition, administration of desmopressin may improve the bleeding time,[194] shorten the activated partial thromboplastin time, and increase factor VIII, XI, and XII levels[194] but does not generally affect the prothrombin time.

For thrombocytopenia related to portal hypertension and splenic sequestration, reports of some clinical experience with splenic embolization have described a 40% to 60% reduction in splenic blood flow. The procedure is associated with some short-term morbidity but effectively prolongs platelet survival time and decreases the spleen/liver platelet uptake ratio.[180] In addition, splenic embolization decreases platelet-associated IgG levels, suggesting that the improvement in platelet counts results not only from an effect on splenic pooling but also from immunologic mechanisms.[178,180,195] The clinical experience with splenic embolization has decreased as the availability of liver transplantation has increased.

From a theoretical perspective, TIPS represents an attractive approach to the treatment of splenic platelet sequestration by lowering portal pressures. Clinical studies of TIPS for this indication have been few in number and have included limited numbers of patients,

however, and do not yet allow definitive conclusions. In a retrospective analysis of 21 patients, a significant rise in platelet counts following TIPS placement was observed in patients who had a post-shunt portal pressure gradient less than 12 mm Hg.[196] In a larger prospective series, however, TIPS had no beneficial effect on thrombocytopenia.[197] Therefore, TIPS cannot be advocated as a definitive treatment for thrombocytopenia in the absence of further investigation.

The treatment of dysfibrinogenemia is clinically challenging. Generally, when the underlying cirrhosis is severe enough to cause dysfibrinogenemia, other hematologic abnormalities are present as well. Therefore, the therapy of dysfibrinogenemia is largely supportive, directed at minimizing any effects of endotoxemia, through surveillance cultures and antibiotics, and correcting associated platelet and coagulation factor deficiencies. Enhanced fibrinolysis has a poor prognosis but multiple causes,[174] and results of the clinical studies of antifibrinolytic therapy have not been compelling enough to allow recommendations to use these therapies except in certain situations such as during liver transplantation or for management of perioperative bleeding.[193]

Factor deficiencies related to decreased hepatic synthesis are detected by prolongation of the prothrombin time and quantitation of the levels of individual factors, particularly factor VII. In the urgent setting, factor deficiencies can be corrected by administration of fresh frozen plasma in amounts sufficient to lower the prothrombin time and control bleeding. Fresh frozen plasma generally is preferable to specific replacement of factor VII (or other concentrated factors) because the synthetic defects associated with cirrhosis cause multiple abnormalities in the coagulation cascade, and other important factors, such as protein S and protein C, are not readily quantitated. In addition, vitamin K should be administered to optimize hepatic carboxylation of vitamin K–dependent factors, even when malabsorption or malnutrition is not suspected on clinical grounds.[193]

REFERENCES

1. Basile AS, Jones EA, Skolnick P: The pathogenesis and treatment of hepatic encephalopathy: evidence for the involvement of benzodiazepine receptor ligands. Pharm Rev 43:27, 1991.
2. Butterworth RF: Pathogenesis of hepatic encephalopathy: Update on molecular mechanisms. Indian J Gastroenterol 22(suppl 2):S11, 2003.
3. Rodes J: Clinical manifestations and therapy of hepatic encephalopathy. Adv Exp Med Biol 341:39, 1993.
4. Schomerus H, Hamster W, Blunck H, et al: Latent portasystemic encephalopathy. I. Nature of cerebral functional defects and their effect on fitness to drive. Dig Dis Sci 26:622, 1981.
5. Liu Q, Duan ZP, Ha DK, et al: Synbiotic modulation of gut flora: Effect on minimal hepatic encephalopathy in patients with cirrhosis. Hepatology 39:1441, 2004.
6. Srivastava A, Mehta R, Rothke SP, et al: Fitness to drive in patients with cirrhosis and portal-systemic shunting: A pilot study evaluating driving performance. J Hepatol 21:1023, 1994.

7. Conn HO: Asterixis in non-hepatic disorders. Am J Med 29:647, 1960.
8. Conn HO, Leevy CM, Vlachevic ZR, et al: Comparison of lactulose and neomycin in the treatment of chronic portal-systemic encephalopathy. Gastroenterology 72:573, 1977.
9. Said A, Williams J, Holden J, et al: Model for end stage liver disease score predicts mortality across a broad spectrum of liver disease. J Hepatol 40:897, 2004.
10. Dombro RS, Hutson DG, Norenberg MD: The action of ammonia on astrocyte glycogen and glycogenolysis. Mol Chem Neuropathol 19:259, 1993.
11. Mousseau DD, Perney P, Latrargues GP, Butterworth RF: Selective loss of pallidal dopamine D2 receptor density in hepatic encephalopathy. Neurosci Lett 162:192, 1993.
12. Thuluvath PJ, Edwin D, Yue NC, et al: Increased signals seen in globus pallidus in T1-weighted magnetic resonance imaging in cirrhotics are not suggestive of chronic hepatic encephalopathy. Hepatology 21:440, 1995.
13. Fischer JE, Funovics JM, Aquirre A: The role of plasma amino acids in hepatic encephalopathy. Surgery 78:276, 1975.
14. Zieve L, Doizaki WM, Zieve FJ: Synergism between mercaptans and ammonia or fatty acids in the production of coma: A possible role in the pathogenesis of hepatic coma. J Lab Clin Med 83:16, 1974.
15. Somberg KA, Riegler JL, LaBerge JM, et al: Hepatic encephalopathy after transjugular intrahepatic portosystemic shunts: Incidence and risk factors. Am J Gastroenterol 90:531, 1995.
16. Boyer TD: Transjugular intrahepatic portosystemic shunt: Current status. Gastroenterology 124:1700, 2003.
17. Monfort P, Munoz MD, ElAyadi A, et al: Effects of hyperammonemia and liver failure on glutamatergic neurotransmission. Metab Brain Dis 17:237, 2002.
18. Jones EA: Ammonia, the GABA neurotransmitter system, and hepatic encephalopathy. Metab Brain Dis 17:275, 2002.
19. Bucci L, Palmieri GC: Double blind, double dummy comparison between treatment with rifaximin and lactulose in patients with medium to severe degree hepatic encephalopathy. Curr Med Res Opin 13:109, 1993.
20. Als-Nielsen B, Gluud LL, Gluud C: Non-absorbable disaccharides for hepatic encephalopathy: Systematic review of randomised trials. BMJ 328:1046, 2004.
21. Szerb JC, Butterworth RF: Effect of ammonium ions on synaptic transmission in the mammalian central nervous system. Prog Neurobiol 39:135, 1992.
22. Basile AS, Hughes RD, Harrison PM, et al: Elevated brain concentrations of 1,4-benzodiazepines in fulminant hepatic failure. N Engl J Med 325:473, 1991.
23. Song G, Dhodda VK, Blei AT, et al: GeneChip analysis shows altered mRNA expression of transcripts of neurotransmitter and signal transduction pathways in the cerebral cortex of portacaval shunted rats. J Neurosci Res 68:730, 2002.
24. Rodrigo R, Montoliu C, Chatauret N, et al: Alterations in soluble guanylate cyclase content and modulation by nitric oxide in liver disease. Neurochem Int 45:947, 2004.
25. Lockwood AH, McDonald JM, Reiman RE, et al: The dynamics of ammonia metabolism in man. J Clin Invest 63:449, 1979.
26. McDermott WV: Metabolism and toxicity of ammonia. N Engl J Med 257:1076, 1957.
27. Conn HO: Effects of high-normal and low-normal serum potassium levels on hepatic encephalopathy: Facts, half-facts or artifacts? Hepatology 20:1637, 1994.
28. Gabuzda GJ, Hall PW: Relation of potassium depletion to renal ammonium metabolism and hepatic coma. Medicine 45:481, 1966.
29. Conn HO: Hepatic encephalopathy. In Schiff L, Schiff ER (eds): Diseases of the Liver. Philadelphia, JB Lippincott, 1993, p 1036.
30. Mullen KD, Birgisson S, Gacad RC, Conjeevaram H: Animal models of hepatic encephalopathy and hyperammonemia. Adv Exp Med Biol 368:1, 1994.
31. Mortensen PB: The effect of oral-administered lactulose on colonic nitrogen metabolism and excretion. Hepatology 16:1350, 1992.
32. Fessel JM, Conn HO: An analysis of the causes and prevention of hepatic coma. Gastroenterology 62:191, 1972.
33. Zavagli G, Ricci G, Bader G, et al: The importance of the highest normokalemia in the treatment of early hepatic encephalopathy. Miner Electrolyte Metab 19:362, 1993.
34. Norenberg MD, Neary JT, Bender AS, Dombro RS: Hepatic encephalopathy: A disorder in glial-neuronal communication. Prog Brain Res 94:261-269, 1992.
35. Albrecht J, Faff L: Astrocyte-neuron interactions in hyperammonemia and hepatic coma. Adv Exp Med Biol 368:45, 1994.
36. Hawkins RA, Jessy J, Mans AM, De Joseph MR: Effect of reducing brain glutamine synthesis on metabolic symptoms of hepatic encephalopathy. J Neurochem 60:1000, 1993.
37. Jones EA, Basile AS, Yurdaydin C, Skolnich P: Do benzodiazepine ligands contribute to hepatic encephalopathy? Adv Exp Med Biol 341:57, 1993.
38. Minuk GY: Gama-aminobutyric acid and the liver. Dig Dis 11:45, 1993.
39. Hoffman EJ, Warren EW: Flumazenil: A benzodiazepine antagonist. Clin Pharm 12:641, 1993.
40. Basile AS, Harrison PM, Hughes RD, et al: Relationship between plasma benzodiazepine receptor ligand concentrations and severity of hepatic encephalopathy. Hepatology 19:112, 1994.
41. Yurdaydin C, Gu ZQ, Nowak G, et al: Bezodiazepine receptor ligands are elevated in an animal model of hepatic encephalopathy: Relationship between brain concentration and severity of encephalopathy. J Pharm Exp Ther 265:565, 1993.
42. Yurdaydin C, Walsh TJ, Engler HD, et al: Gut bacteria provide precursors of benzodiazepine receptor ligands in a rat model of hepatic encephalopathy. Brain Res 679:42, 1995.
43. Cadrenal JF, el Younsi M, Pidoux B, et al: Flumazenil therapy for hepatic encephalopathy in cirrhotic patients: A double-blind pragmatic randomized, placebo study. Eur J Gastroenterol Hepatol 7:325, 1995.
44. Pomier-Layrargues G, Giguere JF, Lavoie J, et al: Flumazenil in cirrhotic patients in hepatic coma: A randomized double-blind placebo-controlled crossover trial. Hepatology 19:32, 1994.
45. Van der Rijt CC, Schalm SW, Meulstee J, Stijnen T: Flumazenil therapy for hepatic encephalopathy. A double-blind crossover study. Gastroenterol Clin Biol 19:572, 1995.
46. Als-Nielsen B, Gluud LL, Gluud C: Benzodiazepine receptor antagonists for hepatic encephalopathy. Cochrane Database Syst Rev CD002798, 2004.
47. Kullmann F, Hollerbac S, Holstege A, Scholmerich J: Subclinical hepatic encephalopathy: The diagnostic value of evoked potentials. J Hepatol 22:101, 1995.
48. Chalasani N, Clark WS, Martin LG, et al: Determinants of mortality in patients with advanced cirrhosis after transjugular intrahepatic portosystemic shunting. Gastroenterology 118:138, 2000.
49. Pomier-Layrargues G: TIPS and hepatic encephalopathy. Semin Liver Dis 16:315, 1996.
50. Dhiman RK, Sawhney MS, Chawla YK, et al: Efficacy of lactulose in cirrhotic patients with subclinical hepatic encephalopathy. Dig Dis Sci 45:1549, 2000.
51. Hartmann IJ, Groeneweg M, Quero JC, et al: The prognostic significance of subclinical hepatic encephalopathy. Am J Gastroenterol 95:2029, 2000.

52. Groeneweg M, Moerland W, Quero JC, et al: Screening of subclinical hepatic encephalopathy. J Hepatol 32:748, 2000.

53. Groeneweg M, Quero JC, De B, et al: Subclinical hepatic encephalopathy impairs daily functioning. Hepatology 28:45, 1998.

54. Dhiman RK, Saraswat VA, Verma M, Naik SR: Figure connection test: A universal test for assessment of mental state. J Gastroenterol Hepatol 10:14, 1995.

55. Naegele T, Grodd W, Viebahn R, et al: MR imaging and (1)H spectroscopy of brain metabolites in hepatic encephalopathy: Time-course of renormalization after liver transplantation. Radiology 216:683, 2000.

56. Conn HO: Animal versus vegetable protein diet in hepatic encephalopathy. J Int Ned 233:369, 1993.

57. Camma C, Fiorello F, Tine F, et al: Lactitol in treatment of chronic hepatic encephalopathy. A metaanalysis. Dig Dis Sci 38:916, 1993.

58. Alexander T, Thomas K, Cherian AM, Kanakasabapathy A: Effect of three antibacterial drugs in lowering blood and stool ammonia production in hepatic encephalopathy. Indian J Med Res 96:292, 1992.

59. Schmidt LE, Tofteng F, Strauss GI, Larsen FS: Effect of treatment with the Molecular Adsorbents Recirculating System on arterial amino acid levels and cerebral amino acid metabolism in patients with hepatic encephalopathy. Scand J Gastroenterol 39:974, 2004.

60. Rodriguez-Roisin R, Agusti AG, Roca J: The hepatopulmonary syndrome: New name, old complexities. Thorax 47:897, 1992.

61. Abrams GA, Jafffe CC, Hoffer PB, et al: Diagnostic utility of contrast echocardiography and lung perfusion scan in patients with hepatopulmonary syndrome. Gastroenterology 109:1283, 1995.

62. Andrivet P, Cadranel J, Housset B, et al: Mechanisms of impaired arterial oxygenation in patients with liver cirrhosis and severe respiratory insufficiency. Chest 103:500, 1993.

63. Samuels T, Lovett MC, Campbell IT, et al: Respiratory function after injection sclerotherapy of oesophageal varices. Gut 35:1459, 1994.

64. Berkowitz KA, Butensky MS, Smith RL: Pulmonary function changes after large volume paracentesis. Am J Gastroenterol 88:905, 1993.

65. Angeuira CE, Kadakia SC: Effects of large volume paracentesis on pulmonary function in patients with tense cirrhotic ascites. Hepatology 20:825, 1994.

66. Soderman C, Juhlin-Dannfelt A, Lagerstrand L, Eriksson LS: Ventilation-perfusion relationships and central hemodynamics in patients with cirrhosis. Effects of a somatostatin analogue. J Hepatol 21:52, 1994.

67. Fallon MB, Abrams GA: Hepatopulmonary syndrome. Curr Gastroenterol Rep 2:40, 2000.

68. Gaines DI, Fallon MB: Hepatopulmonary syndrome. Liver Int 24:397, 2004.

69. Schenk P, Schoniger-Hekele M, Fuhrmann V, et al: Prognostic significance of the hepatopulmonary syndrome in patients with cirrhosis. Gastroenterology 125:1042, 2003.

70. Taille C, Cadranel J, Bellocq A, et al: Liver transplantation for hepatopulmonary syndrome: A ten-year experience in Paris, France. Transplantation 75:1482, 2003.

71. Nakos G, Evrenoglou D, Vassilakis N, Lampropoulos S: Haemodynamics and gas exchange in liver cirrhosis: The effect of orally administered almitrine bismesylate. Respir Med 87:93, 1993.

72. Krowka MJ, Dickson ER, Cortese DA: Hepatopulmonary syndrome. Clinical observations and lack of response to somatostatin analogue. Chest 104:515, 1993.

73. Gomez FP, Martinez-Palli G, Barbera JA, et al: Gas exchange mechanism of orthodeoxia in hepatopulmonary syndrome. Hepatology 40:660, 2004.

74. Braillon A, Gaudin C, Poo JL, et al: Plasma catecholamine concentrations are a reliable index of sympathetic vascular tone in patients with cirrhosis. Hepatology 15:58, 1992.

75. Ohara N, Jaspan J, Chang SW: Hyperglucagonemia and hyperdynamic circulation in rats with biliary cirrhosis. J Lab Clin Med 121:142, 1993.

76. Luo B, Abrams GA, Fallon MB: Endothelin-1 in the rat bile duct ligation model of hepatopulmonary syndrome: Correlation with pulmonary dysfunction. J Hepatol 29:571, 1998.

77. Ling Y, Zhang J, Luo B, et al: The role of endothelin-1 and the endothelin B receptor in the pathogenesis of hepatopulmonary syndrome in the rat. Hepatology 39:1593, 2004.

78. Chang SW, Ohara N: Increased pulmonary vascular permeability in rats with biliary cirrhosis: Role of thromboxane A_2. Am J Physiol 264:L245, 1993.

79. Costa C, Sambataro A, Baldi S, et al: Primary biliary cirrhosis: Lung involvement. Liver 15:196, 1995.

80. Barbe T, Losay J, Gromin G, et al: Pulmonary arteriovenous shunting in children with liver disease. J Pediatr 126:571, 1995.

81. Aller R, Moya JL, Moreira V, et al: Diagnosis and grading of intrapulmonary vascular dilatation in cirrhotic patients with contrast transesophageal echocardiography. J Hepatol 31:1044, 1999.

82. Mimidis KP, Karatza C, Spiropoulos KV, et al: Prevalence of intrapulmonary vascular dilatations in normoxaemic patients with early liver cirrhosis. Scand J Gastroenterol 33:988, 1998.

83. Chang SC, Chang HI, Chen FJ, et al: Effects of ascites and body position on gas exchange in patients with cirrhosis. Proc Natl Sci Counc Repub China B 19:143, 1995.

84. Gerbes AL: Medical treatment of ascites. J Hepatol 17:S4, 1993.

85. Arroyo V, Gines P, Planas R: Treatment of ascites in cirrhosis. Diuretics, peritovenous shunt, and large-volume paracentesis. Gastroenterol Clin North Am 21:237, 1992.

86. Somberg KA, Lake JR, Tomlanovich SJ, et al: Transjugular intrahepatic portosystemic shunts for refractory ascites: Assessment of clinical and hormonal response and renal function. Hepatology 21:709, 1995.

87. Spahr L, Fenyves D, N'Guyen VV, et al: Improvement of hepatorenal syndrome by transjugular intrahepatic portosystemic shunt. Am J Gastroenterol 90:1169, 1995.

88. Hobeika J, Houssin D, Bernard O, et al: Orthotopic liver transplantation in children with chronic liver disease and severe hypoxemia. Transplantation 57:224, 1994.

89. Koneru B, Admed S, Weisse AB, et al: Resolution of pulmonary hypertension of cirrhosis after liver transplantation. Transplantation 58:1133, 1994.

90. Arroyo V, Gines P, Gerbes AL, et al: Definition and diagnostic criteria of refractory ascites and hepatorenal syndrome in cirrhosis. Hepatology 23:164, 1996.

91. Gines P: Diagnosis and treatment of hepatorenal syndrome. Baillieres Best Pract Res Clin Gastroenterol 14:945, 2000.

92. Badalamenti S, Graziani G, Salerno F, Ponticelli C: Hepatorenal syndrome. New perspectives in pathogenesis and treatment. Arch Intern Med 153:1957, 1993.

93. Lang F, Gerok W, Haussinger D: New clues to the pathophysiology of hepatorenal failure. Clin Invest 71:93, 1993.

94. Epstein M: Hepatorenal syndrome: Emerging perspectives of pathophysiology and therapy. J Am Soc Nephrol 4:1735, 1994.

95. Epstein M: Renal sodium retention in liver disease. Hosp Prac 30:33-37, 1995.

96. Gonwa TA, Klintmalm GB, Levy M, et al: Impact of pretransplant renal function on survival after liver transplantation. Transplantation 59:361, 1995.

97. Gines A, Escorsell A, Gines P, et al: Incidence, predictive factors, and prognosis of the hepatorenal syndrome. Gastroenterology 105:229, 1993.

98. Lang F, Tschernko E, Haussinger D: Hepatic regulation of renal function. Exp Physiol 77:663, 1992.

99. Lang F, Ottl I, Haussinger D, et al: Renal hemodynamic response to intravenous and oral amino acids in animals. Semin Nephrol 15:415, 1995.

100. DeSanto NG, Cirillo M, Anastasio P, et al: Renal response to an acute oral protein load in healthy humans and in patients with renal disease or liver disease. Semin Nephrol 15:433, 1995.

101. Abraham WT, Schrier RW: Body fluid volume regulation in health and disease. Adv Intern Med 39:23, 1994.

102. Schrier RW: Peripheral arterial vasodilation in cirrhosis and impaired mineralocorticoid escape. Gastroenterology 102:2165, 1992.

103. Warner L, Skorecki K, Blendis LM, Epstein M: Atrial natriuretic factor and liver disease. Hepatology 17:500, 1993.

104. Castro M, Krowka MJ, Schroeder DR, et al: Frequency and clinical implications of increased pulmonary artery pressures in liver transplant patients. Mayo Clin Proc 71:543, 1996.

105. Michielsen PP, Pelckmans PA: Haemodynamic changes in portal hypertension. Acta Gastroenterol Belg 57:194, 1994.

106. Abrams GA, Nathanson MH: Nitric oxide and liver disease. Gastroenterologist 3:220, 1995.

107. Gupta S, Morgan TR, Gordan GS: Calcitonin gene–related peptide in hepatorenal syndrome. A possible mediator of peripheral vasodilation? J Clin Gastroenterol 14:122, 1992.

108. Henriksen JH, Ring-Larsen H: Hepatorenal disorders: Role of the sympathetic nervous system. Sem Liver Dis 14:35, 1994.

109. Grossman E, Goldstein DS, Hoffman A, et al: Effects of water immersion on sympathoadrenal and dopa-dopamine systems in humans. Am J Physiol 262:R993, 1992.

110. Bernardi M, Trevisani F, Gasbarrini A, Gasbarrini G: Hepatorenal disorders: Role of the renin-angiotensin-aldosterone system. Semin Liver Dis 14:23, 1994.

111. Kim JK, Sumner SN, Schrier RW: Vasopressin gene expression in rats with experimental cirrhosis. Hepatology 17:143, 1993.

112. Solis-Herruzo JA, Gonzalez-Gamarra A, Castellano G, Munoz-Yague MT: Metabolic clearance rate of arginine vasopressin in patients with cirrhosis. Hepatology 16:974, 1992.

113. Gines P, Arroyo V, Rodes J: Ascites and hepatorenal syndrome: Pathogenesis and treatment strategies. Adv Intern Med 43:99, 1998.

114. Asahina Y, Izumi N, Enomoto N, et al: Increased gene expression of water channel in cirrhotic rat kidneys. Hepatology 21:169, 1995.

115. Rabelink TJ, Kaasjager KA, Boer P, et al: Effects of endothelin-1 on renal function in humans: Implications for physiology and pathophysiology. Kidney Int 46:376, 1994.

116. Moller S, Gulberg V, Henriksen JH, Gerbes AL: Endothelin-1 and endothelin-3 in cirrhosis: Relations to systemic and splanchnic haemodynamics. J Hepatol 23:135, 1995.

117. Ucihara M, Izumi N, Sato C, Marumo F: Clinical significance of elevated plasma endothelin concentrations in patients with cirrhosis. Hepatology 16:95, 1992.

118. Moller S, Emmeluth C, Henriksen JH: Elevated circulating plasma endothelin-1 concentrations in cirrhosis. J Hepatol 19:285, 1993.

119. Fukunaga M, Yura T, Badr KF: Stimulatory effect of 8-Epi-PGF2 alpha, an F2-isoprostane, on endothelin-1 release. J Cardiovasc Pharmacol 26:S51, 1995.

120. Morrow JD, Moore KP, Awad JA, et al: Marked overproduction of non-cyclooxygenase derived prostanoids (F_2-isoprostanes) in the hepatorenal syndrome. J Lipid Mediat 6:417, 1993.

121. Guevara M, Rodes J: Hepatorenal syndrome. Int J Biochem Cell Biol 37:22, 2005.

122. Cardenas A, Arroyo V: Hepatorenal syndrome. Ann Hepatol 2:23, 2003.

123. Gines P, Torre A, Terra C, Guevara M: Review article: Pharmacological treatment of hepatorenal syndrome. Aliment Pharmacol Ther 20(suppl 3):57, 2004.

124. Platt JF, Elis JH, Rubin JM, et al: Renal duplex Doppler ultrasonography: A noninvasive predictor of kidney dysfunction and hepatorenal failure in liver disease. Hepatology 20:362, 1994.

125. Caregaro L, Menon F, Angeli P, et al: Limitations of serum creatinine level and creatinine clearance as filtration markers in cirrhosis. Arch Intern Med 154:201, 1994.

126. DeSanto NG, Anastasio P, Loguercio C, et al: Creatinine clearance: An inadequate marker of renal filtration in patients with early posthepatic cirrhosis (Child A) without fluid retention and muscle wasting. Nephron 70:421, 1995.

127. Amarapurkar DN, Dhawan P, Kalro RH: Role of routine estimation of creatinine clearance in patients with liver cirrhosis. Indian J Gastroenterol 13:79, 1994.

128. Kastelan S, Liubicic N, Kastelan Z, et al: The role of duplex-Doppler ultrasonography in the diagnosis of renal dysfunction and hepatorenal syndrome in patients with liver cirrhosis. Hepatogastroenterology 51:1408, 2004.

129. Maroto A, Gines A, Salo J, et al: Diagnosis of functional kidney failure or cirrhosis with Doppler sonography: Prognostic value of resistive index. Hepatology 20:839, 1994.

130. Sacerdoti D, Bolognesi M, Merkel C, et al: Renal vasoconstriction in cirrhosis evaluated by duplex Doppler ultrasonography. Hepatology 17:219, 1993.

131. Watt K, Uhanova J, Minuk GY: Hepatorenal syndrome: Diagnostic accuracy, clinical features, and outcome in a tertiary care center. Am J Gastroenterol 97:2046, 2002.

132. Luca A, Feu F, Garcia-Pagan JC, et al: Favorable effects of total paracentesis on splanchnic hemodynamics in cirrhotic patients with tense ascites. Hepatology 20:30, 1994.

133. Mitzner SR, Stange J, Klammt S, et al: Improvement of hepatorenal syndrome with extracorporeal albumin dialysis MARS: Results of a prospective, randomized, controlled clinical trial. Liver Transpl 6:277, 2000.

134. Durkin RJ, Winter SM: Reversal of hepatorenal syndrome with the combination of norepinephrine and dopamine. Crit Care Med 23:202, 1995.

135. Hadengue A, Gadano A, Moreau R, et al: Beneficial effects of the 2-day administration of terlipressin in patients with cirrhosis and hepatorenal syndrome. J Hepatol 29:565, 1998.

136. Guevara M, Gines P, Fernandez-Esparrach G, et al: Reversibility of hepatorenal syndrome by prolonged administration of ornipressin and plasma volume expansion. Hepatology 27:35, 1998.

137. Gines P, Guevara M, De Las HD, Arroyo V: Review article: Albumin for circulatory support in patients with cirrhosis. Aliment Pharmacol Ther 16(suppl 5):24, 2002.

138. Ortega R, Gines P, Uriz J, et al: Terlipressin therapy with and without albumin for patients with hepatorenal syndrome: Results of a prospective, nonrandomized study. Hepatology 36:941, 2002.

139. Duvoux C, Zanditenas D, Hezode C, et al: Effects of noradrenalin and albumin in patients with type I hepatorenal syndrome: A pilot study. Hepatology 36:374, 2002.

140. Wong F, Pantea L, Sniderman K: Midodrine, octreotide, albumin, and TIPS in selected patients with cirrhosis and type 1 hepatorenal syndrome. Hepatology 40:55, 2004.

141. Pomier-Layrargues G, Paquin SC, Hassoun Z, et al: Octreotide in hepatorenal syndrome: A randomized, double-blind, placebo-controlled, crossover study. Hepatology 38:238, 2003.

142. Sturgis TM: Hepatorenal syndrome: Resolution after transjugular intrahepatic portosystemic shunt. J Clin Gastroenterol 20:241, 1995.

143. Yersin B, Burnier M, Magnenat P: Improvement of renal failure with repeated head-out water immersions in patients

with hepatorenal syndrome associated with alcoholic hepatitis. Am J Nephrol 15:260, 1995.

144. Keller F, Heinze H, Jochimsen F, et al: Risk factors and outcome of 107 patients with decompensated liver disease and acute renal failure: The role of hemodialysis. Ren Fail 17:135, 1995.

145. Madersbacher S, Ludvik G, Stulnig T, et al: The impact of liver transplantation on endocrine status in men. Clin Endocrinol 44:461, 1996.

146. Guechot J, Vaubourdolle M, Ballet F, et al: Hepatic uptake of sex steroids in men with alcoholic cirrhosis. Gastroenterology 92:203, 1987.

147. Selby C: Sex hormone binding globulin: Origin, function and clinical significance. Ann Clin Biochem 27:532, 1990.

148. Oren R, Brill S, Dotan I, Halpern Z: Liver function in cirrhotic patients in the euthyroid versus the hypothyroid state. J Clin Gastroenterol 27:339, 1998.

149. Kley HK, Stremmel W, Kley JB, Schlaghecke R: Testosterone treatment of men with idiopathic hemochromatosis. Clin Invest 70:566, 1992.

150. Kaymakoglu S, Okten A, Cakaloglu Y, et al: Hypogonadism is not related to the etiology of liver cirrhosis. J Gastroenterol 30:745, 1995.

151. Wang YJ, Lee SD, Lin HC, et al: Changes in sex hormone levels in patients with hepatitis B virus–related postnecrotic cirrhosis: Relationship to the severity of portal hypertension. J Hepatol 18:101, 1993.

152. Maruyama Y, Adachi Y, Aoki N, et al: Mechanism of feminization in male patients with non-alcoholic liver cirrhosis: Role of sex hormone binding globulin. Gastroenterol Jpn 26:435, 1991.

153. Handelsman DJ, Strasser S, McDonald JA, et al: Hypothalamic-pituitary-testicular function in end-stage non-alcoholic liver disease before and after liver transplantation. Clin Endocrinol 43:331, 1995.

154. Wang YJ, Wu JC, Lee SD, et al: Gonadal dysfunction and changes in sex hormones in postnecrotic cirrhotic men: A matched study with alcoholic cirrhotic men. Hepatogastroenterology 38:531, 1991.

155. Vidal J, Ferrer JP, Esmatjes E, et al: Diabetes mellitus in patients with liver cirrhosis. Diabetes Res Clin Pract 25:19, 1994.

156. Cavanaugh J, Niewoeher CB, Nuttall FQ: Gynecomastia and cirrhosis of the liver. Arch Intern Med 150:563, 1990.

157. Madersbacher S, Ludvik G, Stulnig T, et al: The impact of liver transplantation on endocrine status in men. Clin Endocrinol (Oxf) 44:461, 1996.

158. Martinex-Riera A, Santolaria-Fernandez F, Gonzalez Riemers E, et al: Alcoholic hupogonadism: Response to clomiphene. Alcohol 12:581, 1995.

159. Gluud C: Testosterone and alcoholic cirrhosis. Epidemiologic, pathophysiologic and therapeutic studies in men. Dan Med Bull 35:564, 1988.

160. Bell H, Raknerud N, Falch JA, Haug E: Inappropriately low levels of gonadotrophins in amenorrhoeic women with alcoholic and non-alcoholic cirrhosis. Eur J Endocrinol 132:444, 1995.

161. Molitich ME: Pathologic hyperprolactinemia. Endocrinol Metab Clin North Am 21:877, 1992.

162. Gavaler JS, Van Thiel DH: Hormonal status of postmenopausal women with alcohol-induced cirrhosis: Further findings and review of the literature. Hepatology 16:312, 1992.

163. Bell H, Rakerud N, Falch JA, Haug E: Inappropriately low levels of gonadotrophins in amenorrheic women with alcoholic and non-alcoholic cirrhosis. Eur J Endocrinol 132:444, 1995.

164. Gavaler JS: Alcohol effects on hormone levels in normal postmenopausal women and in postmenopausal women with alcohol-induced cirrhosis. Recent Dev Alcohol 12:199, 1995.

165. De Besi L, Zucchetta P, Zotti S, Mastrogiacomo I: Sex hormones and sex hormone binding globulin in males with compensated and decompensated cirrhosis of the liver. Acta Endocrinol 120:271, 1989.

166. Huang MJ, Liaw YF: Clinical associations between thyroid and liver disease. J Gastroenterol Hepatol 10:344, 1995.

167. Guven K, Kelestimur F, Yucesoy M: Thyroid function tests in non-alcoholic patients with hepatic encephalopathy. Eur J Med 2:83, 1993.

168. Becker U, Gluud C, Bennett P: Thyroid hormones and thyroxine-binding globulin in relation to liver function and serum testosterone in men with alcoholic cirrhosis. Acta Med Scand 224:367, 1988.

169. Hegedus L, Rasmussen N, Ravn V, et al: Independent effects of liver disease and chronic alcoholism on thyroid function and size: The possibility of a toxic effect of alcohol on the thyroid gland. Metabolism 37:229, 1988.

170. Huang TS, Wu HP, Huang LS, et al: A study of thyroidal response to thyrotropin (TSH) in decompensated liver cirrhosis. Thyroidology 1:119, 1989.

171. Testosterone treatment of men with alcoholic cirrhosis: A double-blind study. The Copenhagen Study Group for Liver Diseases. Hepatology 6:807, 1986.

172. Van Thiel DH, Kumar S, Gavaler JS, Tarter RE: Effect of liver transplantation on the hypothalamic-pituitary-gonadal axis of chronic alcoholic men with advanced liver disease. Alcohol Clin Exp Res 14:478, 1990.

173. Plevris JN, Dhariwal A, Elton RA, et al: The platelet count as a predictor of variceal hemorrhage in primary biliary cirrhosis. Am J Gastroenterol 90:959, 1995.

174. Violi F, Ferro D, Basili S, et al: Prognostic value of clotting and fibrinolytic systems in a follow-up of 165 liver cirrhotic patients. CALC Group. Hepatology 22:96, 1995.

175. Violi F, Ferro D, Basili S, et al: Hyperfibrinolysis increases the risk of gastrointestinal hemorrhage in patients with advanced cirrhosis. Hepatology 15:672, 1992.

176. Kamath PS, Wiesner RH, Malinchoc M, et al: A model to predict survival in patients with end-stage liver disease. Hepatology 33:464, 2001.

177. Violi F, Leo R, Vezza E, et al: Bleeding time in patients with cirrhosis: Relation with degree of liver failure and clotting abnormalities. C.A.L.C. Group. J Hepatol 20:531, 1994.

178. Kajiwara E, Akagi K, Azuma K, et al: Evidence for an immunological basis of thrombocytopenia in chronic liver disease. Am J Gastroenterol 90:962, 1995.

179. Aoki Y, Hirai K, Tanikawa K: Mechanism of thrombocytopenia in liver cirrhosis: Kinetics of indium-111 tropolone labelled platelets. Eur J Nucl Med 20:123, 1993.

180. Noguchi H, Hirai K, Aoki Y, et al: Changes in platelet kinetics after a partial splenic arterial embolization in cirrhotic patients with hypersplenism. Hepatology 22:1682, 1995.

181. Nagamine T, Ohtuka T, Takehara K, et al: Thrombocytopenia associated with hepatitis C viral infection. J Hepatol 24:135, 1996.

182. Laffi G, Marra F, Gresele P, et al: Evidence for a storage pool defect in platelets from cirrhotic patients with defective aggregation. Gastroenterology 103:641, 1992.

183. Laffi G, Cinotti S, Filimberti E, et al: Defective aggregation in cirrhosis is independent of in vivo platelet aggregation. J Hepatol 24:436, 1996.

184. Sanchez-Roig MJ, Rivera J, Moraleda JM, Garcia VV: Quantitative defect of glycoprotein Ib in severe cirrhotic patients. Am J Hemat 45:10, 1994.

185. Laffi G, Marra F, Failli P, et al: Defective signal transduction in platelets from cirrhotics is associated with increased cyclic nucleotides. Gastroenterology 105:148, 1993.

186. Beer JH, Clerici N, Baillod P, et al: Quantitative and qualitative analysis of platelet GPIb and von Willebrand factor in liver cirrhosis. Thromb Haemost 73:601, 1995.

187. Leiper K, Croll A, Moore NR, et al: Tissue plasminogen activator, plasminogen activator inhibitors, and activator-inhibitor complex in liver disease. J Clin Pathol 47:214, 1994.

188. Cimminiello C, Soncini M, Gerosa MC, et al: Lipoprotein a and fibrinolytic system in liver cirrhosis. Coagulation Abnormalities in Liver Cirrhosis (CALC) Study Group. Biomed Pharmacother 49:364, 1995.

189. Toschi V, Rocchini GM, Motta A, et al: The hyperfibrinolytic state of liver cirrhosis: Possible pathogenetic role of ascites. Biomed Pharmacother 47:345, 1993.

190. Violi F, Ferro D, Basili S, et al: Hyperfibrinolysis resulting from clotting activation in patients with different degrees of cirrhosis. The CALC Group. Hepatology 17:78, 1993.

191. Violi F, Ferro D, Basili S, et al: Association between low grade disseminated intravascular coagulation and endotoxemia in patients with liver cirrhosis. Gastroenterology 109:531, 1995.

192. Bakker CM, Knot EA, Stibbe J, Wilson JH: Disseminated intravascular coagulation in liver cirrhosis. J Hepatol 15:330, 1992.

193. Mammen EF: Coagulation defects in liver disease. Med Clin North Am 78:545, 1994.

194. Agnelli G, Parise P, Levi M, et al: Effects of desmopressin on hemostasis in patients with liver cirrhosis. Haemostasis 25:241, 1995.

195. Sangro B, Bilbao I, Herrero I, et al: Partial splenic embolization for the treatment of hypersplenism in cirrhosis. Hepatology 18:309, 1993.

196. Lawrence SP, Lezotte DC, Durham JD, et al: Course of thrombocytopenia after transjugular intrahepatic portosystemic shunts (TIPS). A retrospective analysis. Dig Dis Sci 40:1575, 1995.

197. Sanyal AJ, Freedman AM, Purdum PP, et al: The hematological consequences of transjugular intrahepatic portosystemic shunts. Hepatology 23:32, 1996.

CHAPTER
90 Acute Liver Failure

Robert J. Fontana

Acute liver failure is a rare clinical syndrome that results from the sudden loss of hepatic parenchymal and metabolic functions and manifests as coagulopathy and encephalopathy. The etiology of this disorder varies widely throughout the world, with drug, infectious, and immunologic diseases reported most commonly. Acute liver failure constitutes a medical emergency associated with a high mortality rate because of the development of cerebral edema, bleeding, and infectious complications. Despite advances in medical management, mortality rates in patients with acute liver failure remain high in the absence of emergency liver transplantation.

DEFINITION

Acute liver failure is defined as the rapid development of hepatocellular dysfunction—specifically, coagulopathy—and mental status changes (encephalopathy) in a patient without known preexisting liver disease.[1] It is a clinical syndrome that represents the final common pathway of severe liver injury resulting from various infectious, immunologic, metabolic, vascular, and infiltrative disorders. The mechanism of liver injury in this disorder is most often hepatocellular necrosis, as occurs with acetaminophen toxicity or viral hepatitis. Acute liver failure also can result from severe cellular or mitochondrial dysfunction, as seen with some forms of drug toxicity (e.g., antiretroviral agents), Wilson disease, and acute fatty liver of pregnancy.[2]

Acute liver failure (or fulminant hepatic failure) originally was defined by an interval between the onset of illness and appearance of encephalopathy of 8 weeks or less.[3] In an attempt to predict prognosis and outcome better, O'Grady and colleagues divided patients into three groups based on the time interval between the onset of jaundice and encephalopathy: those with hyperacute liver failure (up to 7 days), those with acute liver failure (between 8 and 28 days), and those with subacute liver failure (after 4 to 24 weeks).[4] In general, patients with hyperacute liver failure are more likely to develop cerebral edema and to recover without liver transplantation. By contrast, patients with subacute or late-onset hepatic failure are more likely to present with evidence of portal hypertension such as ascites and to have a low rate of survival without transplantation.[5-7] Although the duration of illness may help predict prognosis, great overlap exists among patients with varying presentations of acute failure, and the duration of symptoms is related largely to the etiologic disorder. The original definition of acute liver failure—encephalopathy and coagulopathy within 8 weeks of the onset of illness—is used in this chapter, because this definition is the most widely used in clinical studies and in criteria for liver transplantation in the United States.[3]

The diagnosis of acute liver failure is made clinically on the basis of the physical examination (altered mental status) and supportive laboratory findings (hyperbilirubinemia, prolonged prothrombin time). Infrequently, the condition may be confused with other clinical entities that manifest as jaundice, coagulopathy, and encephalopathy, such as sepsis, systemic disorders with liver and brain involvement (e.g., systemic lupus erythematosus, thrombotic thrombocytopenic purpura), and an

Table 90–1 Percentages of Various Causes of Acute Liver Failure Worldwide

Country	Hepatitis A	Hepatitis B	Acetaminophen	Drug/Toxin	Other	Indeterminate
United States (N = 308)[8]	4	7	39	13	24	13
United Kingdom (N = 941)[9]	9	9	53	7	5	17
France (N = 330)[10]	4	47	2	15	10	22
Japan (N = 93)[11]	4	44	0	0	11	41
India (N = 458)[12]	2	16	0	5	30	47
OVERALL (N = 2130)	**6**	**18**	**29**	**8**	**14**	**25**

All causes reported as % of total cases.

acute decompensation of chronic liver disease. In particular, sepsis and acute liver failure are associated with similar hemodynamic profiles, and severe sepsis is frequently accompanied by mental status changes; in this situation, jaundice and coagulopathy may result from intrahepatic cholestasis and disseminated intravascular coagulation (DIC), respectively. Measurement of factor VIII levels may help differentiate sepsis (low factor VIII level) from acute liver failure (factor VIII level generally not reduced). Finally, alcoholic hepatitis and flares of chronic viral hepatitis occasionally may be mistaken for acute liver failure. In these instances, a careful review of the patient's medical history, laboratory and imaging studies, and liver biopsy results in selected cases is helpful.

ETIOLOGY

The underlying cause of acute liver failure in an individual case is established by the patient's history, serologic test results, and characteristic radiologic and histologic features. The predominant etiologic form of acute liver failure differs markedly throughout the world. In the United States and the United Kingdom, medications, including acetaminophen and idiosyncratic drug toxicity, are the most commonly identified etiologic agents of acute liver failure[8,9] (Table 90–1). In France, Japan, and India, however, severe acute hepatitis B virus (HBV) infection is a leading cause of acute liver failure.[10-12] In addition to these causes, numerous other, often rare, conditions can lead to acute liver failure (Table 90–2).

ACETAMINOPHEN TOXICITY

Acetaminophen is a known dose-dependent hepatotoxin that can lead to characteristic, life-threatening hepatocellular injury when ingested in excessive doses (see Chapter 83). Because of its widespread availability, intentional acetaminophen overdose (greater than 10 g) is a common mode of attempted suicide, with greater than 100,000 cases of intentional acetaminophen overdose reported each year in the United States.[13] Although most patients with an intentional acetaminophen overdose recover, in a minority of cases progression to acute liver failure is seen, and acetaminophen has become the leading cause of this disorder in both the United States and the United Kingdom (Fig. 90–1).[8,9] An increasing

Table 90–2 Uncommon Causes of Acute Liver Failure

Wilson disease (initial presentation)
Other infections (e.g., Epstein-Barr virus, herpes simplex virus, cytomegalovirus)
Vascular abnormalities (e.g., Budd-Chiari syndrome, sinusoidal obstruction syndrome)
Toxins (e.g., *Amanita phalloides* ingestion, sea anenome sting, carbon tetrachloride)
Acute fatty liver of pregnancy
Autoimmune hepatitis (initial presentation)
Malignant infiltration (e.g., lymphoma, hematologic malignancy, lung cancer)
Ischemia (e.g., hypotension, heat stroke)
Primary graft nonfunction following liver transplantation

frequency of cases of "nonintentional" acetaminophen overdose leading to acute liver failure also has been reported since the mid-1990s.[14-16] In many of these "therapeutic misadventures," patients ingested over-the-counter products containing acetaminophen along with narcotic-acetaminophen congeners prescribed for an acute medical condition. Chronic heavy alcohol consumption may lower the threshold for acetaminophen toxicity in some patients by inducing cytochrome P450 enzyme activity.[17] In addition, preexisting hepatic dysfunction and glutathione depletion may predispose some patients to acetaminophen toxicity.[18] Most evidence suggests, however, that the recommended dose of acetaminophen of less than 4 g in a 24-hour period probably is safe in a majority of patients.[8,9]

In the United Kingdom, restrictions on the quantity of acetaminophen dispensed, as well as blister packaging of products, were introduced in 1998 to reduce the incidence of acetaminophen toxicity. Since that time, the rates of hospitalization, acute liver failure, and liver transplantation for acetaminophen toxicity have declined.[19,20] In the United States, black-box warnings for and package labeling of acetaminophen products have been instituted, but the impact of these measures on the incidence and severity of acute liver failure caused by acetaminophen has not been evaluated.

IDIOSYNCRATIC DRUG TOXICITY

Numerous prescription drugs, including various antibiotics, nonsteroidal anti-inflammatory drugs, and antiseizure medications, have been implicated in acute

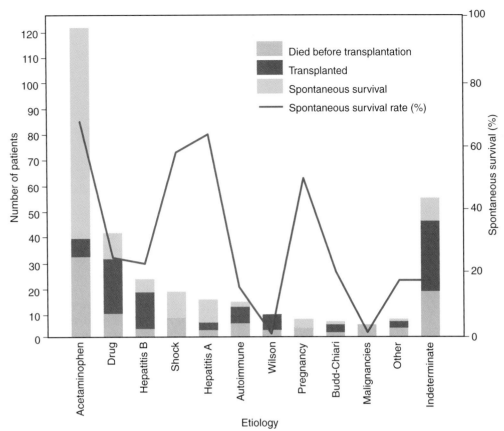

Figure 90–1 Outcomes in acute liver failure in the United States by etiology. The U.S. Acute Liver Failure Study Group identified acetaminophen toxicity (in 39% of the cases) and idiosyncratic drug reactions (in 13%) as the leading causes of this disorder among 308 adults between 1998 and 2001. In patients in whom the etiology was indeterminate and in those with Wilson disease, autoimmune hepatitis, or hepatitis B, the 3-week spontaneous survival rate was less than 25% in the absence of emergency liver transplantation. By contrast, in patients with acetaminophen toxicity-, hepatitis A-, or pregnancy-related acute liver failure, the 3-week survival rate exceeded 50%. Rapid identification of the etiologic disorder is recommended, to facilitate transfer of patients with a poor prognosis to a liver transplantation center. (Data adapted from Ostapowicz G, Fontana RJ, Schiodt FV, et al: Results of a prospective study of acute liver failure at 17 tertiary care centers in the United States. Ann Intern Med 137:947, 2002, with permission from William M. Lee, MD.)

liver failure.[21] In most instances, occurrence of the drug-related disorder is a rare and unpredictable event resulting from metabolic idiosyncrasy that occurs in 1 in 10,000 to 1 in 1 million patient-exposure years. Affected patients frequently are female (70%), and jaundice typically develops within 6 months of starting the suspected agent.[8,21] In a series of 141 U.S. liver transplant recipients with drug-induced acute liver failure, isoniazid (16%), propylthiouracil (9%), phenytoin (7%), and valproate (7%) were the most commonly identified causative medications (see also Chapter 83).[22] Various nonprescription herbal products also have been implicated; these products include kava kava, weight loss supplements, and ephedra, all of which have been withdrawn from the market (see also Chapter 84).[23-25] Establishing a diagnosis of drug-induced acute liver failure usually is difficult because of the lack of specific laboratory markers, inability to rechallenge the patient, and limitations of causality assessment instruments.[26] Nonetheless, the outcome of drug-induced acute liver failure generally is poor unless liver transplantation is performed.

HEPATOTROPIC VIRUSES

Hepatitis A virus (HAV) and HBV are major causes of acute liver failure in many parts of the world, including India and other developing countries (see Table 90-1 and Chapters 74 and 75). Acute infection with HAV rarely leads to acute liver failure (in less than 0.01% of cases), and when it does, the prognosis is relatively good (see Fig. 90-1). Although HBV is the most common viral cause, acute liver failure is an uncommon outcome of acute HBV infection. Infection with hepatitis D virus (HDV) requires co-infection with HBV and accounts for 4% of cases of acute liver failure in areas endemic for HBV infection.[27] Earlier studies suggested that virologic factors including infection with a pre-core or core-promoter variant of HBV may account for the development of acute liver failure in some patients,[28] but subsequent studies have failed to demonstrate unique mutants or variants associated with acute liver failure. Nevertheless, the role of HBV genotypes requires further investigation.[29,30] Acute hepatitis E infection (HEV) is a leading cause of acute liver failure in India and other tropical countries but is rarely seen in

Western countries.[12,31] Pregnant women may be at particular risk for the development of acute liver failure with acute HEV infection.

MISCELLANEOUS CAUSES

Acute liver failure occasionally develops in pregnant women, particularly in the third trimester (see Table 90–2).[32] Acute fatty liver of pregnancy occurs in 0.0008% of all pregnancies and is associated with preeclampsia in greater than 50% of cases[33] (see also Chapter 37). Some affected women with fatty liver of pregnancy have an inherited deficiency in a fatty acid oxidation enzyme that can be identified by genetic testing.[33] Wilson disease, a rare autosomal recessive disorder in which biliary excretion of copper is impaired, can manifest with acute liver failure in up to 25% of cases (see Chapter 72). Most patients so affected present in the second or third decade of life and have prominent hemolysis, low serum alkaline phosphatase levels, elevated urinary copper excretion, and Kayser-Fleischer rings. Prompt recognition and listing for liver transplantation are essential in this otherwise fatal disorder. Other infrequent causes of acute liver failure include mushroom (*Amanita phalloides*) poisoning (see Chapter 84), Budd-Chiari syndrome (see Chapter 80), new-onset autoimmune hepatitis (see Chapter 85), and malignant infiltration of the liver (see Chapter 34). All of these causes combined account for only 5% to 30% of the cases of acute liver failure (see Table 90–1).

INDETERMINATE ACUTE LIVER FAILURE

Acute liver failure of unknown etiology, defined by negative results on serologic testing for hepatitis A, B, C, D, and E and the absence of other known causes, constitutes 15% to 44% of cases of this disorder worldwide (see Table 90–1). Because many of these patients present with a viral prodrome, it has been hoped that new sensitive molecular laboratory methods would identify a viral etiology for acute liver failure of unknown cause. For example, occult HBV infection has been identified in the sera or livers of some patients with acute liver failure of unknown etiology by some[28,34] but not all investigators.[29,30] Although hepatitis C virus (HCV) has been implicated as a cause of acute liver failure in a few patients, HCV appears to be an exceedingly rare cause of the condition in Western countries.[34-37]

Despite the identification of hepatitis G virus (HGV) in patients with the indeterminate form, HGV does not appear to cause acute liver failure.[38] Togavirus-like particles have been identified by electron microscopy in 7 of 18 liver explants from patients who underwent transplantation for indeterminate acute liver failure[39] but are unlikely to be responsible for a substantial proportion of these cryptogenic cases. The transfusion-transmitted virus (TTV) was found in the sera of patients with acute liver failure in early studies, but TTV infection is not thought to be pathogenic.[40,41] Finally, a link between parvovirus B19 or SEN infection and indeterminate acute liver failure has not been demonstrated (see Chapter 78).[42,43]

CLINICAL FEATURES

The clinical features of acute liver failure may result directly from the loss of critical hepatocellular functions (e.g., protein synthesis, intermediary metabolism, detoxification) and from effects on organs other than the liver. The major complications of this disorder, as well as their pathogenesis and medical management, are outlined in Table 90–3. The initial presentation usually includes nonspecific complaints such as nausea, vomiting, and malaise, and jaundice usually develops soon after. Hepatocellular injury leads to impaired elimination of bilirubin; depressed synthesis of coagulation factors I, II, V, VII, IX, and X; and diminished glucose synthesis. In addition, decreased uptake and increased generation of intracellular lactate occur as a result of anaerobic glycolysis. These derangements manifest clinically as jaundice, coagulopathy, hypoglycemia, and metabolic acidosis. Besides portending liver failure, coagulopathy increases the risk of gastrointestinal and intracranial hemorrhage; hypoglycemia can contribute to brain injury; and acidosis can contribute to hypotension.

HEPATIC ENCEPHALOPATHY AND CEREBRAL EDEMA

Hepatic encephalopathy is a defining criterion for acute liver failure. Encephalopathy in acute liver failure is thought to arise primarily from the development of cerebral edema and resulting intracranial hypertension, rather than portosystemic shunting of toxins. In addition to cerebral edema, many of the complications of acute liver failure, including hypoglycemia, sepsis, fever, hypoxemia, and hypotension, may contribute to neurologic abnormalities. The grading of encephalopathy in this disorder is similar to that used for patients with cirrhosis (see Chapter 89). In stage 1, patients have subtle changes in affect, altered sleep patterns, or difficulties with concentration. Stage 2 is characterized by drowsiness, disorientation, and confusion, and stage 3 is marked by somnolence and incoherence. In stage 4, frank coma with minimal (4A) or no (4B) response to noxious stimuli is detected. On physical examination, many patients have asterixis or tremors in stage 1 or 2 and hyperreflexia, clonus, and muscular rigidity in stages 3 and 4. Although worrisome, these upper motor neuron signs do not portend a poor prognosis and can be reversed with recovery or replacement of the failing liver.

Cerebral edema is found in up to 80% of patients who die of acute liver failure and is nearly universal among patients with coma.[44] The pathogenesis of cerebral edema in this disorder is poorly understood. It has been proposed to result in part from the actions of gut-derived neurotoxins that escape hepatic clearance and are released into the systemic circulation.[44,45] The demonstration of swollen endothelial and astroglial cells in the brains of patients with acute liver failure suggests a potential role for cytotoxic edema, possibly resulting from

Table 90–3 Pathogenesis and Management of the Major Complications of Acute Liver Failure

Major Complications	Pathogenesis	Management
Hypoglycemia	Diminished glucose synthesis	Blood glucose monitoring
		Intravenous glucose supplementation
Encephalopathy	Cerebral edema	CT scan (if advanced encephalopathy)
		ICP monitoring (if stage 3 or 4 encephalopathy)
		Head of the bed >30°
		Consider osmotherapy (mannitol) or barbiturates
		Treat other contributing factors (e.g., hypoglycemia, hypoxemia, fever)
		Avoid benzodiazepines and other sedative medications
		? Moderate hypothermia (see text)
Infections	Reduced immune function	Aseptic medical/nursing care
	Invasive procedures	Daily surveillance cultures of blood, urine, and sputum
		High index of suspicion for bacterial and fungal infection
		Preemptive antibiotics
Hemorrhage (e.g., gastrointestinal)	Stress ulceration	Nasogastric tube placement
		Intravenous H_2-receptor antagonists or proton pump inhibitors
Coagulopathy	Reduced clotting factor synthesis	Parenteral vitamin K
	Thrombocytopenia, DIC	Platelet infusions for bleeding and before procedures
	Fibrinolysis	Cryoprecipitate for bleeding with hypofibrinogenemia
		? Recombinant factor VIIa (see text)
Hypotension	Hypovolemia	Hemodynamic monitoring of central pressures
	Decreased vascular resistance	Volume repletion with blood or colloid
		α-Adrenergic agents
Respiratory failure	ARDS	Hemodynamic monitoring of central pressures
		Mechanical ventilation
Pancreatitis	? Hypoxia	Supportive care, including supplemental oxygen if needed
		Abdominal CT scan to exclude necrotizing pancreatitis
Renal failure	Hypovolemia	Hemodynamic monitoring of central pressures
	Hepatorenal syndrome	Volume repletion with blood or colloid
	Acute tubular necrosis	Avoid nephrotoxic agents (e.g., aminoglycosides, NSAIDs, contrast dye)
		Hemofiltration/dialysis

ARDS, acute respiratory distress syndrome; CT, computed tomography; ICP, intracranial pressure; DIC, disseminated intravascular coagulation; NSAIDs, nonsteroidal anti-inflammatory drugs.

increased brain glutamine levels. On the other hand, vacuolization in the basement membranes of capillaries, consistent with disruption of the blood-brain barrier, suggests a vasogenic mechanism of cerebral edema in acute liver failure. In any event, increased production of glutamine in the central nervous system as a result of high circulating levels of ammonia and intracerebral lactate is believed to be critical to the pathogenesis of cerebral edema. In one study, arterial ammonia levels were associated with the risk of uncal herniation and death in patients with acute liver failure.[46]

Progressive cerebral edema associated with the development of intracranial hypertension also can result in cerebral hypoperfusion and consequent cerebral hypoxia that can lead to irreversible neurologic damage, uncal herniation, and brain death. Loss of intracranial vascular tone can lead to surges in intracranial pressure (ICP), with changes in systemic hemodynamics based on the equation

Cerebral perfusion pressure = mean arterial pressure – intracranial pressure.

Because of the complexity of cerebral edema, systemic hemodynamic monitoring and direct intracranial pressure monitoring frequently are recommended in patients with acute liver failure and stage 3 or 4 encephalopathy and in those undergoing liver transplantation.

COAGULOPATHY AND BLEEDING

The liver is the major site of synthesis of coagulation factors and related inhibitory proteins. The reticuloendothelial system of the liver also is involved in the clearance of activated clotting factors and their degradation products. Therefore, it is not surprising that patients with acute liver failure frequently have a multifactorial coagulopathy and a resulting increased risk of bleeding and of clotting. Laboratory features of fibrinolysis, hypofibrinogenemia, dysfibrinogenemia, and DIC frequently are identified in patients with acute liver failure.[47] Thrombocytopenia, which also develops in a majority of these patients, may result from increased destruction of platelets from a consumptive coagulopathy or various combinations of reduced production of thrombopoietin, bone marrow dysfunction, and medication effects.[48] Clinically significant bleeding has been reported to occur in up to 20% of patients with acute liver failure; the upper gastrointestinal tract, nasopharynx, and skin puncture sites are the most common sources of bleeding. Critically ill patients have a particular propensity for gastrointestinal bleeding caused by acute portal hypertension, increased intracranial pressure, and coagulopathy.[49] To monitor the associated coagulopathy, most experts advise obtaining serial assessments of the platelet count, hemoglobin value, international normalized ratio (INR), fibrinogen level, and factor V level. Although measurement of the INR has limitations, the INR can be readily obtained in most hospitals. Because factor V has the shortest serum half-life of the clotting factors synthesized in the liver, serial factor V levels have been proposed as a sensitive measure of recovery of the liver over time.

INFECTION

Bacterial infections may develop in as many as 80% of patients with acute liver failure, and bacteremia is present in up to 25% of patients with a bacterial infection.[45,50] Uncontrolled infection accounts for exclusion of approximately 25% of the patients from liver transplantation and for approximately 40% of post-transplantation deaths.[51] At least three factors place patients with acute liver failure at increased risk for infection. First, gut-derived microorganisms may enter the systemic circulation from portal venous blood as a result of damage to hepatic macrophages (Kupffer cells). Second, impaired polymorphonuclear neutrophil function may result from reduced hepatocellular synthesis of acute-phase reactants, including components of the complement cascade. Third, patients with this disorder often are subjected to invasive procedures (e.g., intravascular and urethral catheterization, endotracheal intubation), and physical barriers to infection, including skin and airway, are thus breached. Indeed, the major sites of infection are the respiratory and urinary tracts.[45] It is not surprising, therefore, that the most common bacteria isolated are staphylococcal and streptococcal species and gram-negative rods.[52]

Fungal infections develop in up to one third of patients with acute liver failure.[53] A majority of these infections are caused by *Candida albicans* and typically develop after the second or third week of hospitalization. Although *Aspergillus* infections have been thought to be uncommon in the setting of acute liver failure, they may be more prevalent than was previously appreciated, and aspergillosis may account for up to one half of fatal infections in the post-transplantation period.[54] Risk factors for fungal infections are renal failure, prolonged antibiotic therapy for bacterial infections, and use of invasive monitoring devices. Characteristically, fungal infection is associated with fever or leukocytosis refractory to broad-spectrum antibiotics.[53] Patients in whom symptoms and signs of the systemic inflammatory response syndrome develop in association with bacterial or fungal infection are more prone to experience worsening encephalopathy and to die; this observation highlights the importance of infections in the outcome of acute liver failure.[55,56]

MULTIPLE ORGAN FAILURE SYNDROME

The multiple organ failure syndrome manifests clinically as peripheral vasodilatation with hypotension, pul-

monary edema, renal failure, and DIC. Liver failure may trigger the microcirculatory derangements that underlie this syndrome by two mechanisms. First, polymerization of actin (released from dying hepatocytes) and platelet activation within the capillary lumen may produce endothelial injury.[57] Second, impaired hepatic clearance may lead to the accumulation of vasoactive substances in the systemic circulation.[58] Multiple organ failure is an important contributor to patient mortality and constitutes a major contraindication to liver transplantation.

Hypotension frequently is observed in patients with acute liver failure and can result from reduced vascular resistance or intravascular volume depletion. Acute pancreatitis also may develop in patients with acute liver failure, particularly those with acetaminophen overdose, because of tissue hypoxia and hypoperfusion. In one series, 44% of patients who died of acute liver failure had pancreatitis.[59] Acute pancreatitis is not a contraindication to liver transplantation unless evidence of extensive pancreatic necrosis is seen on a computed tomography (CT) scan.

Respiratory failure also is commonly associated with acute liver failure. In one series, 37% of patients with acute liver failure had pulmonary edema.[60] In another study, acute respiratory distress syndrome (ARDS) was present in 33% of patients with acetaminophen-associated acute liver failure.[61] Furthermore, ARDS was associated with intracranial hypertension, the requirement for vasopressor agents, and, of most importance, a higher mortality rate.

The cause of renal failure that develops in 30% to 50% of patients with acute liver failure usually is multifactorial.[58] Hepatorenal syndrome often is difficult to distinguish from intravascular volume depletion, because both entities are associated with oliguria, azotemia, and a low fractional excretion of sodium. Acute tubular necrosis is associated with a 50% decrease in survival among patients with acetaminophen-induced acute liver failure,[62] and the mortality rate is more than doubled in patients with multiple organ failure.[63]

PREDICTORS OF OUTCOME

Patients with acute liver failure fall into two broad categories: (1) those in whom intensive medical care enables recovery of hepatic function through regeneration and (2) those who require liver transplantation to survive. Rapid identification of patients with an unfavorable prognosis is critical. The etiology of acute liver failure and clinical presentation are important correlates of prognosis. For example, patients with acute liver failure caused by acetaminophen have a better prognosis than those with the indeterminate form of the disorder[8] (see Fig. 90–1). Similarly, patients who reach stage 3 or 4 encephalopathy tend to do worse than those who remain at only stage 1 or 2.[4] These indicators, however, do not allow accurate prediction of the need for liver transplantation in an individual patient.

Investigators at King's College in London performed a multivariate analysis of clinical and biochemical variables in 588 patients with acute liver failure to determine which variables were the best predictors of mortality.[61] In

Table 90-4   King's College Criteria for Liver Transplantation in Acute Liver Failure

Acetaminophen Cases	Non-Acetaminophen Cases
Arterial pH < 7.3*	INR > 6.5 (PT > 100 seconds)
or	or
Arterial lactate level >3.5 mmol/L at 4 hours	any 3 of the following:
	Age <10 or >40 years
or	Duration of jaundice >7 days
Arterial lactate level >3.0 mmol/L at 12 hours*	Etiology: idiosyncratic drug reaction; non-A, non-B hepatitis; halothane
or	hepatitis; indeterminate
INR > 6.5 (PT > 100 seconds)	Serum bilirubin >17.5 mg/dL
Serum creatinine >3.4 mg/dL	INR > 3.5 (PT > 50 seconds)
Stage 3 or 4 encephalopathy	

*Measured after fluid resuscitation.
Adapted from O'Grady et al[62] and Bernal et al.[64]
INR, International normalized ratio; PT, prothrombin time.

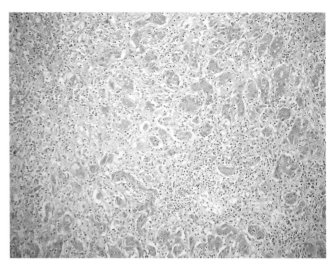

Figure 90-2   Liver histologic features of acute liver failure. The severity and pattern of necrosis are highly variable in liver biopsy specimens from patients with this disorder, compared with explanted whole liver specimens. In addition, the extent of liver injury does not reliably correlate with outcome.[66] Therefore, unless treatable etiologic conditions (e.g., autoimmune hepatitis, herpes simplex hepatitis) can be identified, liver biopsy is not recommended in patients with acute liver failure. The specimen shown is from a 59-year-old man who underwent a transjugular liver biopsy for presumed amoxicillin-clavulanic acid liver toxicity. Findings include severe acute hepatitis with confluent areas of necrosis predominating in the central zones, consistent with but not diagnostic of an idiosyncratic drug reaction. Despite supportive care, multiorgan failure developed, culminating in death. (Hematoxylin-eosin, ×40.)

this analysis, a major distinction was made between patients with acetaminophen toxicity and those with other causes of acute liver failure (Table 90-4). For patients with acetaminophen-induced liver failure, the presence of any single adverse characteristic was associated with a mortality rate of at least 55%, and severe acidosis was associated with a mortality rate of 95%. In a 2002 study, the addition of arterial lactate levels was shown to improve the positive and negative predictive values in patients with acetaminophen-induced acute liver failure.[64] Among patients with non–acetaminophen-related acute liver failure, the presence of any single adverse prognostic factor was associated with a mortality rate of 80%, and the presence of three adverse characteristics was associated with a mortality rate greater than 95%. These mortality rates vastly exceed those associated with liver transplantation. Therefore, the presence of any single indicator of a poor prognosis should prompt early referral to a liver transplantation center. These selection criteria are simple, and acquisition of the necessary data requires only a brief history, routine laboratory studies, and serologic testing for hepatitis A and B. Moreover, the utility of these criteria has been confirmed, albeit with slightly lower predictive accuracy, at another center,[65] although a study from the U.S. Acute Liver Failure Study Group demonstrated lower sensitivity and negative predictive value in 108 patients with acetaminophen-induced acute liver failure.[15]

Liver histologic study in acute liver failure is associated with substantial sampling artifact and potential complications and does not predict outcome reliably.[66] Therefore, transjugular or percutaneous biopsy is not recommended for purposes of prognosis or staging in patients with this disorder[66] (Fig. 90-2). The predictive value of serum Gc-globulin levels is comparable to that of the King's College criteria, but the assay for Gc-globulin is technically difficult and not generally available.[67] Other investigators have examined the prognostic utility of measuring plasma factor V levels[68] and hepatic volumetry,[69] but these parameters do not appear to add significantly to the assessment of outcome. The U.S. Acute Liver Failure Study Group and others have reported on the potential utility of elevated serum phos-

phate levels as a marker of impaired hepatic regeneration in identifying patients with acetaminophen-induced acute liver failure who have a poor prognosis.[70,71] Specifically, the risk of death or need for liver transplantation in patients with a serum phosphate level greater than 3.7 mg/dL on admission was predicted with a sensitivity of 42%, specificity of 84%, and positive predictive value of 53%; these results were similar to those for the King's College criteria in the same cohort of 218 patients.[70]

TREATMENT

A variety of therapies have been proposed and studied in patients with acute liver failure. Therapeutic interventions include glucocorticoid therapy, administration of prostaglandins, and exchange transfusions. Only liver transplantation, however, has led to salvage of patients with irreversible liver failure. Unfortunately, many patients with irreversible acute liver failure do not undergo transplantation, because of late referral, contraindications, or the lack of a donor liver. Therefore, patients with acute liver failure should be evaluated for transplantation as soon as possible and, if no contraindications are identified, placed on a liver transplant waiting list. If and when a donor organ becomes available, patients listed for transplantation should be reassessed for their continued need for transplantation.

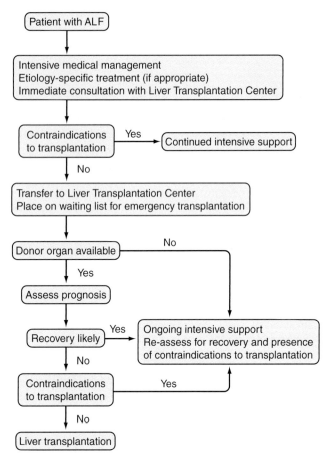

Figure 90–3   Algorithm for the management of acute liver failure. The initial approach to management includes rapid identification and treatment of reversible causes of acute liver failure. Supportive care with careful monitoring for complications of the disorder in an intensive care unit is recommended. Contact with a liver transplantation center should be established promptly, for potential transfer and transplantation evaluation as early as possible. ALF, acute liver failure.

An algorithm depicting the management of acute liver failure is shown in Figure 90–3.

INITIAL EVALUATION AND MANAGEMENT

The initial management of acute liver failure should include rapid identification of the underlying cause, with an emphasis on treatable conditions. For example, acetaminophen toxicity is treated initially with gastric lavage, oral charcoal, and prompt institution of oral *N*-acetylcysteine[72] (see also Chapter 83). For patients with severe nausea and vomiting, the oral formulation of *N*-acetylcysteine can be administered safely as a continuous intravenous infusion in a monitored setting.[73] Similarly, patients with *Amanita* mushroom poisoning should undergo immediate gastric lavage and instillation of charcoal, in an attempt to reduce the toxin loading[74] (see also Chapter 84); in addition, hemodialysis can remove toxins from the serum. The value of intravenous pencillin, cytochrome *c*, and silymarin in lowering the entero-hepatic toxin load further is uncertain.[75] Herpes simplex virus–induced acute liver failure has been reported to respond to intravenous acyclovir[76] (see Chapter 78). Rapid delivery and supportive care constitute the treatment of choice for pregnant women with acute fatty liver of pregnancy, the hemolysis–elevated liver enzymes–low platelets (HELLP) syndrome, and preeclampsia (see Chapter 37).

Patients with acute liver failure should be cared for in an intensive care unit, because they can deteriorate rapidly and require continuous monitoring. Serial laboratory studies to assess the severity and trends in biochemical parameters, such as determination of acid-base status, arterial ammonia levels, and INR, are essential. Urgent transfer to a liver transplantation center is advisable before the development of advanced encephalopathy or other complications of acute liver failure.

ENCEPHALOPATHY AND CEREBRAL EDEMA

The encephalopathy associated with acute liver failure tends to be progressive, unless liver failure is reversed. Sedative-hypnotic drugs, which may exacerbate encephalopathy, should be avoided unless patients require mechanical ventilation. Lactulose is of uncertain benefit and may be associated with bowel ischemia. Reversible conditions that may contribute to altered mental status (e.g., hypoglycemia, hypoxemia) should be treated immediately. Hypoglycemia generally responds to parenteral administration of glucose. Similarly, underlying infection and sepsis should be treated aggressively with fluids and antibiotics, because systemic cytokines may alter brain function (see Table 90–3).

Patients with stage 3 or 4 encephalopathy should undergo elective endotracheal intubation and mechanical ventilation for protection of the airway, particularly before being transported to a liver transplantation center. Many mechanically ventilated patients are also deeply sedated or paralyzed, and evidence of generalized seizure activity that can worsen encephalopathy may be concealed. Therefore, continuous electroencephalographic monitoring of deeply sedated or paralyzed patients with acute liver failure has been proposed. Treatment of subclinical seizures with phenytoin or other antiepileptic medications is appropriate, but the efficacy of prophylactic therapy to prevent seizure activity has not been established.[77]

Intracranial hypertension may be suspected on the basis of noninvasive evaluation or may be detected by direct measurement. Noninvasive approaches such as physical examination and radiologic imaging have important limitations. Impaired pupillary responses, posturing, and seizures, which may suggest the presence of intracranial hypertension, are not sensitive signs, particularly when sedatives or neuromuscular blocking agents have been used in mechanically ventilated patients. CT scanning of the head is valuable for identifying mass lesions, intracranial hemorrhage, and evidence of brainstem herniation; because these diagnoses may affect clinical decision-making, a CT scan of the head should be obtained in all patients with advanced encephalopathy. Nevertheless, the correlation between CT evidence of cerebral edema and measured ICP is imperfect, with a sensitivity rate ranging from 60% to 75%.[78,79]

Monitoring of ICP represents the most accurate way to detect intracranial hypertension but has several potential limitations. First, placement of an ICP transducer requires correction of underlying coagulopathy. Second, the ICP transducer represents a potential portal of entry for infectious organisms. Third, placement of the transducer can precipitate intracranial hemorrhage, which can be fatal. The frequency of major complications ranges from 4% to 20%. Parenchymally placed catheters are associated with a higher rate of complications than that associated with use of subdural or epidural transducers.[80] Nevertheless, ICP transducers can provide invaluable physiologic data that influence management and decisions regarding transplantation. For patients with refractory intracranial hypertension, technetium perfusion brain scans are useful for detecting irreversible brain death that may have developed in a sedated patient.

Elevation of the head of the bed to at least 30 degrees from horizontal (and avoidance of the head-down position) is a simple measure to reduce ICP. If this maneuver fails, specific treatment is required. Osmotherapy and barbiturates are two options for treating intracranial hypertension. Osmotherapy with intravenous mannitol (1 g/kg) requires preserved renal function (or hemofiltration, if necessary) and is effective in controlling intracranial hypertension in approximately 60% of cases.[81] Therapy with intravenous hypertonic saline to maintain serum sodium levels of 145 to 155 mEq/L also may be of value in patients with cerebral edema, but controlled trials are needed.[82] Uncontrolled data support the use of intravenous thiopental, a barbiturate; its efficacy is similar to that of mannitol.[83] Thiopental has two relative advantages: its onset of action is rapid, and its use does not require preserved renal function. Potential drawbacks of thiopental are hypotension and, of greater importance, masking of clinical indicators of neurologic recovery or deterioration. In general, use of mannitol is reasonable as first-line therapy; barbiturates can be reserved for patients with renal insufficiency or refractory intracranial hypertension. Glucocorticoids are of no benefit.[80]

Pilot studies have suggested that moderate hypothermia (e.g., 32° to 33°C) achieved by the use of external cooling blankets may be of benefit in patients with acute liver failure and refractory cerebral edema.[84,85] All patients treated with hypothermia require the placement of an ICP monitor, because paralytic agents must be administered to prevent shivering. The effect of moderate hypothermia on the risk of bleeding and infection requires further study. The potential role of prophylactic hypothermia also requires further study.

COAGULOPATHY AND BLEEDING

Placement of a nasogastric tube to monitor bleeding and gastric pH is recommended in intubated patients with acute liver failure. The risk of upper gastrointestinal hemorrhage can be reduced by intravenous H_2 receptor antagonists,[86] and proton pump inhibitors probably provide similar reasonable benefit. Subcutaneous administration of vitamin K to treat reversible hypoprothrombinemia also is reasonable. Coagulation parameters including INR, plasma factor V levels, platelet counts, and plasma fibrinogen levels should be assessed serially in all patients with acute liver failure.

The decision to administer fresh frozen plasma or clotting factors prophylactically in nonbleeding patients should be tempered by the fact that the infusion will obscure the value of INR as a prognostic factor. Furthermore, infusion of plasma can lead to volume overload and respiratory failure, particularly in patients with renal failure. Moreover, prophylactic administration of plasma has not been shown to improve the clinical outcome of patients with acute liver failure. Therefore, unless the patient is bleeding actively or about to undergo an invasive procedure, prophylactic infusions of plasma are not recommended.

For patients undergoing invasive procedures in whom the INR fails to improve with plasma, recombinant factor VIIa has been shown to be efficacious in improving the coagulopathy; however, factor VIIa should be used cautiously, because the optimal dose has not been established and use of this agent carries a risk of thrombosis.[87] Cryoprecipitate, plasma, and platelets should be given to patients with acute liver failure and hypofibrinogenemia, DIC, and active bleeding.

INFECTION

Clinical recognition of infection may be difficult, because the usual signs such as hypotension, leukocytosis, and acidosis may reflect the underlying liver failure. Accordingly, daily surveillance cultures of blood, urine, and ascitic fluid are recommended in patients with acute liver failure. The advisability of prophylactic antibiotic therapy for these patients is debatable. On one hand, prophylactic antibiotics may prevent or delay the development of infections that limit the applicability of liver transplantation. On the other hand, antibiotics may increase the risk of superinfection with resistant bacteria or fungi. This issue has been addressed in a small randomized trial.[88] Patients who received prophylactic treatment with intravenous cefuroxime demonstrated a significant reduction in the rate of documented infections (from 61% to 32%), compared with those who received conservative treatment, and a modest (but statistically insignificant) increase in the rate of survival (from 45% to 67%). Intestinal decontamination with orally administered antibiotics (in addition to systemic antibiotics) does not appear to alter the clinical outcome in patients with acute liver failure, compared with that observed with systemic antimicrobial agents alone.[89] The utility of systemic prophylactic antibiotics warrants further investigation. At the least, a high level of suspicion for infection and a low threshold for administering antibiotics are required in managing patients with acute liver failure. If infection is suspected, the choice of antibiotics should be based on the spectrum of likely bacterial pathogens (e.g., *Staphylococcus*, gram-negative aerobes) and local hospital patterns of microbial sensitivity. A reasonable empirical regimen in a patient with acute liver failure and a suspected infection consists of intravenous vancomycin and a third-generation cephalosporin or fluoroquinolone.

MULTIPLE ORGAN FAILURE SYNDROME

The fundamental goal of management of multiple organ failure syndrome in patients with acute liver failure is similar to that in patients with other causes of multiple organ failure: to optimize arterial pressure and tissue oxygenation. Ideally, the mean arterial pressure (MAP) should be kept above 60 mm Hg to maintain cerebral perfusion.[44] A central venous or pulmonary arterial catheter may be useful for monitoring the patient's intravascular volume status. Hypotension resulting from intravascular volume depletion should be corrected with blood or colloids. If hypotension is caused by reduced vascular resistance, administration of α-adrenergic agonists may be useful. Although pressors can be used to maintain MAP within a physiologic range, they have the potential to impair tissue oxygenation further; terlipressin may worsen cerebral edema.[90,91] In small, short-term studies, N-acetylcysteine has been shown to improve tissue oxygenation without adverse effects on hemodynamics[92]; however, the impact of this agent on overall patient outcome has not yet been investigated.

Endotracheal intubation and mechanical ventilation frequently are necessary for patients with acute liver failure. Hypoxemia can result from respiratory depression caused by coma, or from impaired gas exchange caused by ARDS or superimposed pneumonia. Vigorous suctioning and Valsalva maneuvers should be avoided, to prevent surges in ICP. Patients with acute liver failure tolerate volume overload poorly, because of their propensity to develop ARDS and cerebral edema. Early measurement of central venous or pulmonary arterial pressure in oliguric patients is preferable to empirical administration of fluid boluses. If oliguria persists in the face of adequate central filling pressures, continuous renal replacement therapy should be initiated. Continuous venovenous hemofiltration has been shown to be superior to intermittent hemodialysis, with less hemodynamic instability and improved tissue oxygen delivery, in oliguric patients.[93] Nephrotoxic drugs such as aminoglycosides and nonsteroidal anti-inflammatory agents should be avoided in all patients with acute liver failure, and precautions should be taken if intravenous contrast dye is required.

LIVER TRANSPLANTATION

Liver transplantation has transformed the management of patients with acute liver failure and is discussed in greater detail in Chapter 92. Before the availability of liver transplantation, less than 30% of patients with this disorder survived with supportive care. By contrast, survival rates for patients with acute liver failure who undergo liver transplantation have been substantially higher, with a short-term survival rate of 80% and a 1-year survival rate of 70% when the results of several major transplantation centers are combined (Table 90–5).[8,94-100] The decision to perform liver transplantation in a patient with acute liver failure must balance the likelihood of spontaneous recovery with the risks of surgery and long-term immunosuppression. Furthermore, contraindications to transplantation, particularly irreversible brain damage, active extrahepatic infection, and multiple organ failure syndrome, must be considered. In countries where cadaveric livers are not readily available, living-related liver transplantation has been performed successfully in selected instances but is not routinely recommended because of concerns about donor coercion and safety.[101,102]

Although changes in the rules governing the allocation of donor livers have shortened waiting times for patients with acute liver failure in the United States, the decision to place a patient on the waiting list for transplantation must still be made promptly.[103] Furthermore, frequent assessments of the patient's clinical status are needed to determine if the patient is likely to recover or if a contraindication to transplantation has developed. In one series, contraindications developed in 22% of liver transplantation candidates, whereas 12% of the patients improved and were removed from the list.[8] The shorter median waiting time among transplant recipients compared with the time that nontransplanted patients were determined not to be transplant candidates because of progression (3 versus 5 days) highlights the critical, ongoing shortage of donor organs.

OUTCOMES

Because of the shortage of donor organs, patients with acute liver failure are more likely to receive an ABO-

Table 90–5 Results of Liver Transplantation for Acute Liver Failure in the United States

Center	Number of Patients	Study Period	Early Patient Survival (%)*	One-Year Patient Survival (%)
Pittsburgh[99]	42	1980-1987	74	59
Chicago[98]	19	1984-1988	74	58
Michigan[97]	19	1985-1990	NR	68
Nebraska[100]	30	1986-1991	75	42
San Francisco[95]	35	1988-1992	94	92
Philadelphia[94]	18	1985-1990	65	65
USA (Multicenter)[96]	121	1994-1996	NR	76
USA (Multicenter)[8]	89	1998-2001	84	NR
OVERALL	**373**	—	**80** (187/233)	**70** (198/284)

*Early patient survival reflects discharge from the hospital following transplantation.
NR = Not reported.

incompatible than an ABO-compatible or ABO-identical graft.[104] In addition, marginal donor grafts, from persons who were older or steatotic, or both, are more frequently utilized in patients undergoing transplantation for acute liver failure than for other causes. These factors may explain in part the higher rate of primary graft nonfunction and rejection among transplant recipients in whom the indication for transplantation was acute liver failure than among those with other indications.[103,105] Post-transplantation seronegative chronic hepatitis also is more common in recipients with acute liver failure than in recipients with cirrhosis (41% versus 14% at 1 year).[106] The long-term functional and cognitive outcomes of recipients with acute liver failure have not been well studied but may be inferior to those of transplant recipients with cirrhosis.[107]

INVESTIGATIONAL APPROACHES

Treatment strategies, such as charcoal hemoperfusion and administration of prostaglandin E_1, that showed early promise have not been shown to be superior to standard care when analyzed in randomized controlled studies.[108,109] Plasmapheresis and hepatectomy have been suggested as possible "bridges" to liver transplantation, but prospective trials have not yet been performed.[110,111] Three additional forms of therapy may provide a bridge to liver transplantation or to regeneration of the native liver with spontaneous recovery: auxiliary liver transplantation, extracorporeal liver support devices, and hepatocyte transplantation.

AUXILIARY LIVER TRANSPLANTATION

Auxiliary liver transplantation, in which the donor graft is implanted either orthotopically beside the surgically reduced native liver or heterotopically inferior to the native liver, has been investigated by a number of centers.[112,113] The advantage of this procedure is that, by providing a temporary auxiliary liver, the severely diseased native liver may be allowed to regenerate. Ideally, immunosuppressive drugs may then be gradually withdrawn, allowing the transplanted liver to undergo involution or surgical removal. The utility of this operation is limited by technical complications, however, as well as by difficulty in predicting which patients with acute liver failure are likely to experience hepatic regeneration. Although early results appeared promising, the benefits of this procedure do not appear to justify the increased risk, and this approach should be undertaken only in centers with specialized expertise.

EXTRACORPOREAL LIVER SUPPORT

Extracorporeal liver support devices fall into two broad categories: hemodiadsorption systems and bioartificial livers.[114] Hemodiadsorption systems employ hemodialysis in combination with perfusion of the patient's plasma or blood through hollow-fiber filters impregnated with charcoal, resins, or albumin. Although these devices may remove circulating toxins, they do not replace other functions of the liver. Albumin dialysis (e.g., the molecular adsorbent recirculating system, or MARS) utilizes hemodialysis of whole blood in series with an albumin dialyzer and charcoal filter. This technology is simpler to use than plasmapheresis and has shown some promise in small trials in cirrhotic patients with hepatic encephalopathy.[115] Information about the safety and efficacy of these systems in patients with acute liver failure is limited, however.[116]

Bioartificial liver devices contain liver cells grown within specialized hollow-fiber cartridges through which the patient's plasma is perfused. The success of such devices depends largely on the mass of cells they contain, the extent to which these cells maintain liver-specific functions, and the duration for which these functions are maintained. Because the devices under clinical investigation contain only hepatocytes, derangements attributable to nonparenchymal cells, such as Kupffer cells and biliary epithelia, are not corrected. In 2004, the results of the HepatAssist bioartificial liver device trial were reported.[117] This device utilizes a dialysis cartridge loaded with approximately 100 g of cryopreserved porcine hepatocytes, or 7 billion cells, and also has a charcoal filter. The 85 patients with acute liver failure in whom this device was used did not experience an improvement in 30-day survival compared with the 86 patients who received standard care (71% versus 62%; $P = 0.26$). Treatment with the device was well tolerated, however, and the rates of thrombocytopenia, hypotension, and other adverse events were not significantly greater in patients in the HepatAssist device treatment group than in control patients. Furthermore, neither inadvertent transmission of porcine retroviruses nor development of xenogenic antibodies was reported for patients in the treatment group.[118] Although this pioneering trial failed to demonstrate a significant benefit in outcome, the proof of the concept that an extracorporeal device with porcine hepatocytes can be utilized and can lead to a trend toward improvement in metabolic, hemodynamic, and clinical parameters was realized. Future devices with a larger hepatocyte mass, simplified circuitry, and differentiated hepatocyte function are eagerly awaited.

HEPATOCYTE TRANSPLANTATION

The potential role of hepatocyte transplantation in patients with acute liver failure is likely to be similar to that of the bioartificial liver devices just described—that is, as a bridge to liver transplantation or regeneration.[119] Human hepatocyte transplantation has demonstrated efficacy in preliminary studies of patients with metabolic disorders and decompensated cirrhosis.[119,120] Stable expression of transplanted hepatocytes has been difficult to achieve, however. In one trial, 3 of 6 patients with acute liver failure survived 14, 20, and 52 days after transplantation of 10^9 to 10^{10} hepatocytes, representing 1% to 10% of normal liver cell mass.[121] Although metabolic parameters improved within 72 hours of transplantation, transient respiratory insufficiency was observed in several patients. This report demonstrates that transplanted human hepatocytes can engraft into a regenerating liver, but further work to enhance graft function, native liver regeneration, and cell delivery is needed. In addition, reliable methods of isolating and storing viable human hepatocytes are needed.

Pluripotent hepatocyte stem cells derived from bone marrow may prove useful for hepatocyte transplantation. In one study, liver biopsy specimens from human recipients of gender-discordant bone marrow or liver transplants were analyzed for marrow-derived hepatocytes and cholangiocytes.[122] The extent of engraftment was associated with the degree of liver injury, thereby suggesting a possible role for bone marrow–derived stem cells in the treatment of severe acute hepatitis, acute liver failure, and metabolic defects. Further studies that identify and isolate pluripotent liver stem cells from human bone marrow and that clarify the factors that govern cellular differentiation and liver regeneration are needed.

REFERENCES

1. Hoofnagle JH, Carithers RL Jr, Shapiro C, et al: Fulminant hepatic failure: Summary of a workshop. Hepatology 21:240, 1995.
2. Riordan SM, Williams R: Mechanisms of hepatocyte injury, multi-organ failure, and prognostic criteria in acute liver failure. Semin Liver Dis 23:203, 2003.
3. Trey C, Davidson C: The management of fulminant hepatic failure. Prog Liver Dis 3:292, 1970.
4. O'Grady JG, Schalm SW, Williams R: Acute liver failure: Redefining the syndromes. Lancet 342:273, 1993.
5. Dhiman RK, Makharia GK, Jain S, et al: Ascites and spontaneous bacterial peritonitis in fulminant hepatic failure. Am J Gastroenterol 95:233, 2000.
6. Gimson AE, O'Grady J, Ede RJ, et al: Late-onset hepatic failure: Clinical, serological and histological features. Hepatology 6:288, 1986.
7. O'Grady JG, Alexander GJ, Thick M, et al: Outcome of orthotopic liver transplantation in the aetiological and clinical variants of acute liver failure. Q J Med 68:817, 1988.
8. Ostapowicz G, Fontana RJ, Schiodt FV, et al: Results of a prospective study of acute liver failure at 17 tertiary care centers in the United States. Ann Intern Med 137:947, 2002.
9. Makin AJ, Wendon J, Williams R: A 7-year experience of severe acetaminophen-induced hepatotoxicity (1987-1993). Gastroenterology 109:1907, 1995.
10. Bernau J, Rueff B, Benhamou JP: Fulminant and subfulminant liver failure: Definitions and causes. Semin Liver Dis 6:97, 1986.
11. Fujiwara K, Mochida S: Indications and criteria for liver transplantation for fulminant hepatic failure. J Gastroenterol 37:74, 2002.
12. Acharya SK, Panda SK, Saxena A et al: Acute hepatic failure in India: A perspective from the east. J Gastroenterol Hepatol 15:473, 2000.
13. Litovitz TL, Klein-Schwartz W, White S, et al: 2000 Annual report of the American Association of Poison Control Centers toxic exposure surveillance system. Am J Emer Med 19:337, 2001.
14. Zimmerman HJ, Maddrey WC: Acetaminophen (paracetamol) hepatotoxicity with regular intake of alcohol: Analysis of instances of therapeutic misadventure. Hepatology 22:767, 1995.
15. Lee WM: Acute liver failure in the United States. Semin Liver Dis 23:217, 2003.
16. Schiodt FV, Rochling FJ, Casey DL, et al: Acetaminophen toxicity in an urban county hospital. N Engl J Med 337:1112, 1997.
17. Schmidt LE, Dalhoff K, Poulsen HE: Acute versus chronic alcohol consumption in acetaminophen-induced hepatotoxicity. Hepatology 35:876, 2002.
18. Whitcomb DC, Block GD: Association of acetaminophen hepatotoxicity with fasting and ethanol use. JAMA 272:1845, 1994.
19. Bernal W: Changing patterns of causation and the use of liver transplantation in the United Kingdom. Semin Liver Dis 23:227, 2003.
20. Hawton K, Townsend E, Deeks J, et al: Effects of legislation restricting pack sizes of paracetamol and salicylate poisoning in the United Kingdom: Before and after study. BMJ 322:1203, 2001.
21. Lee WM: Drug-induced hepatotoxicity. N Engl J Med 349:474, 2003.
22. Russo MW, Shrestha R, Fried MW, et al: Liver transplantation for acute liver failure from drug induced liver injury in the United States. Liver Transpl 10:1018, 2004.
23. Stickel F, Baumuller HM, Seitz K, et al: Hepatitis induced by kava. J Hepatol 39:627, 2003.
24. Favreau JT, Ryu ML, Braunstein G, et al: Severe hepatotoxicity associated with the dietary supplement Lipokinetix. Ann Intern Med 136:590, 2002.
25. Palmer ME, Haller C, McKinney PE, Klein-Schwartz W, et al: Adverse events associated with dietary supplements: An observational study. Lancet 361:101, 2003.
26. Lucena MI, Camargo R, Andrade RJ, et al: Comparison of two clinical scales for causality assessment in hepatotoxicity. Hepatology 33:123, 2001.
27. Feray C, Chitnis DS, Artwani KK, et al: Prevalence of anti-delta antibodies in central India. Trop Gastroenterol 20:29, 1999.
28. Sato S, Suzuki K, Akahane Y, et al: Hepatitis B virus strains with mutations in the core promoter in patients with fulminant hepatitis. Ann Intern Med 122:241, 1995.
29. Teo EK, Ostapowicz G, Hussain M, et al: Hepatitis B Infection in patients with acute liver failure in the United States. Hepatology 33:972, 2001.
30. Wai CT, Fontana RJ: Clinical significance of hepatitis B virus genotypes, variants, and mutants. Clin Liver Dis 8:321, 2004.
31. Lee WM, Brown KE, Young NS, et al: Testing the putative role of parvovirus B19 or hepatitis E virus in acute liver failure in the U.S. [abstract]. Gastroenterology 126(suppl 2):A-706, 2004.
32. Knox TA, Olans LB: Liver disease in pregnancy. N Engl J Med 335:569, 1996.
33. Ibdah JA, Bennett MJ, Rinaldo P, et al: A fetal fatty-acid oxidation disorder as a cause of liver disease in pregnant women. N Engl J Med 340:1723, 1999.
34. Feray C, Gigou M, Samuel D, et al: Hepatitis C virus RNA and hepatitis B virus DNA in serum and liver of patients with fulminant hepatitis. Gastroenterology 104:549, 1993.
35. Kuwada SK, Patel VM, Hollinger FB, et al: Non-A, non-B fulminant hepatitis is also non-E and non-C. Am J Gastroenterol 89:57, 1994.
36. Theilmann L, Solbach C, Toex U, et al: Role of hepatitis C virus infection in German patients with fulminant and subacute hepatic failure. Eur J Clin Invest 22:569, 1992.
37. Farci P, Alter HJ, Shimoda A, et al: Hepatitis C virus–associated fulminant hepatic failure. N Engl J Med 335:631, 1996.
38. Hadziyannis SJ: Fulminant hepatitis and the new G/GBV-C flavivirus. J Viral Hepat 5:15, 1998.
39. Fagan EA, Ellis DS, Tovey GM, et al: Toga virus–like particles in acute liver failure attributed to sporadic non-A, non-B

hepatitis and recurrence after liver transplantation. J Med Virol 38:71, 1992.

40. Charlton M, Adjei P, Poterucha J, et al: TT-virus infection in North American blood donors, patients with fulminant hepatic failure, and cryptogenic cirrhosis. Hepatology 28:839, 1998.

41. Das K, Kar P, Gupta RK, et al: Role of transfusion-transmitted virus in acute viral hepatitis and fulminant hepatic failure of unknown etiology. J Gastroenterol Hepatol 19:406, 2004.

42. Karetnyi YV, Beck PR, Markin RS, et al: Human parvovirus B19 infection in acute fulminant liver failure. Arch Virol 144:1713, 1999.

43. Umemura T, Tanaka E, Ostapowicz G, et al: Investigation of SEN virus infection in patients with cryptogenic acute liver failure, hepatitis-associated aplastic anemia, or acute and chronic nonA-E hepatitis. J Infect Dis 188:1545, 2003.

44. Blei AT, Larsen FS: Pathophysiology of cerebral edema in fulminant hepatic failure. J Hepatol 31:771, 1999.

45. Rolando N, Harvey F, Brahm J, et al: Prospective study of bacterial infection in acute liver failure: An analysis of fifty patients. Hepatology 11:49, 1990.

46. Clemmesen JO, Larsen FS, Kondrup J, et al: Cerebral herniation in patients with acute liver failure is correlated with arterial ammonia concentration. Hepatology 29:648, 1999.

47. Pereira SP, Langley PG, Williams R: The management of abnormalities of hemostasis in acute liver failure. Semin Liver Dis 16:403, 1996.

48. Schiodt FV, Balko J, Schilsky M, et al: Thrombopoietin in acute liver failure. Hepatology 37:558, 2003.

49. Cook DJ, Fuller HD, Guyatt GH, et al: Risk factors for gastrointestinal bleeding in critically ill patients. Canadian Critical Care Trials Group. N Engl J Med 330:377, 1994.

50. Wyke RJ, Canalese JC, Gimson AE, et al: Bacteraemia in patients with fulminant hepatic failure. Liver 2:45, 1982.

51. Lidofsky SD: Fulminant hepatic failure. Crit Care Clin 11:415, 1995.

52. Wade J, Rolando N, Philpott-Howard J, et al: Timing and aetiology of bacterial infections in a liver intensive care unit. J Hosp Infect 53:144, 2003.

53. Rolando N, Harvey F, Brahm J, et al: Fungal infection: A common, unrecognised complication of acute liver failure. J Hepatol 12:1, 1991.

54. Castells A, Salmeron JM, Navasa M, et al: Liver transplantation for acute liver failure: Analysis of applicability. Gastroenterology 105:532, 1993.

55. Rolando N, Wade J, Davalos M, et al: The systemic inflammatory response syndrome in acute liver failure. Hepatology 32:734, 2000.

56. Vaquero J, Polson J, Chung C, et al: Infection and the progression of hepatic encephalopathy in acute liver failure. Gastroenterology 125:755, 2003.

57. Lee WM, Galbraith RM: The extracellular actin-scavenger system and actin toxicity. N Engl J Med 326:1335, 1992.

58. Bihari DJ, Gimson AE, Williams R: Cardiovascular, pulmonary and renal complications of fulminant hepatic failure. Semin Liver Dis 6:119, 1986.

59. Parbhoo SP, Welch J, Sherlock S: Acute pancreatitis in patients with fulminant hepatic failure. Gut 14:428, 1973.

60. Trewby PN, Warren R, Contini S, et al: Incidence and pathophysiology of pulmonary edema in fulminant hepatic failure. Gastroenterology 74:859, 1978.

61. Baudouin SV, Howdle P, O'Grady JG, et al: Acute lung injury in fulminant hepatic failure following paracetamol poisoning. Thorax 50:399, 1995.

62. O'Grady JG, Alexander GJ, Hayllar KM, et al: Early indicators of prognosis in fulminant hepatic failure. Gastroenterology 97:439, 1989.

63. Pitre J, Soubrane O, Dousset B, et al: How valid is emergency liver transplantation for acute liver necrosis in patients with multiple-organ failure? Liver Transpl Surg 2:1, 1996.

64. Bernal W, Donaldson N, Wyncoll D, et al: Blood lactate as an early predictor of outcome in paracetamol-induced acute liver failure: A cohort study. Lancet 359:558, 2002.

65. Anand AC, Nightingale P, Neuberger JM: Early indicators of prognosis in fulminant hepatic failure: An assessment of the King's criteria. J Hepatol 26:62, 1997.

66. Hanau C, Munoz SJ, Rubin R: Histopathological heterogeneity in fulminant hepatic failure. Hepatology 21:345, 1995.

67. Schiodt FV, Bondesen S, Petersen I, et al: Admission levels of serum Gc-globulin: Predictive value in fulminant hepatic failure. Hepatology 23:713, 1996.

68. Pauwels A, Mostefa-Kara N, Florent C, et al: Emergency liver transplantation for acute liver failure. Evaluation of London and Clichy criteria. J Hepatol 17:124, 1993.

69. Sekiyama K, Yoshiba M, Inoue K, et al: Prognostic value of hepatic volumetry in fulminant hepatic failure. Dig Dis Sci 39:240, 1994.

70. Davern TJ, Brown RS, Shakil AO, et al: Serum phosphate as a predictor of clinical outcome in acetaminophen-induced acute liver failure [abstract]. Hepatology 38:212A, 2003.

71. Schmidt LE, Dalhoff K: Serum phosphate is an early predictor of outcome in severe acetaminophen-induced hepatotoxicity. Hepatology 36:659, 2002.

72. Harrison PM, Keays R, Bray GP, et al: Improved outcome of paracetamol-induced fulminant hepatic failure by late administration of acetylcysteine. Lancet 335:1572, 1990.

73. Kao LW, Kirk MA, Furbee RB, et al: What is the rate of adverse events after oral N-acetylcysteine administered by the intravenous route to patients with suspected acetaminophen poisoning? Ann Emerg Med 42:741, 2003.

74. Busi C, Fiume L, Costantino D, et al: Amanita toxins in gastroduodenal fluid of patients poisoned by the mushroom Amanita phalloides. N Engl J Med 300:800, 1979.

75. Bartoloni SO, Giannini A, Botti P, et al: Amanita poisoning: A clinical histopathological study of 64 cases of intoxication. Hepatogastroenterology 32:299, 1985.

76. Klein NA, Mabie WC, Shaver DC, et al: Herpes simplex virus hepatitis in pregnancy. Two patients successfully treated with acyclovir. Gastroenterology 100:239, 1991.

77. Ellis AJ, Wendon JA, Williams R: Subclinical seizure activity and prophylactic phenytoin infusion in acute liver failure: A controlled clinical trial. Hepatology 32:536, 2000.

78. Lidofsky SD, Bass NM, Prager MC, et al: Intracranial pressure monitoring and liver transplantation for fulminant hepatic failure. Hepatology 16:1, 1992.

79. Muñoz SJ, Robinson M, Northrup B, et al: Elevated intracranial pressure and computed tomography of the brain in fulminant hepatocellular failure. Hepatology 13:209, 1991.

80. Blei AT, Olafsson S, Webster S, et al: Complications of intracranial pressure monitoring in fulminant hepatic failure. Lancet 341:157, 1993.

81. Canalese J, Gimson AE, Davis C, et al: Controlled trial of dexamethasone and mannitol for the cerebral oedema of fulminant hepatic failure. Gut 23:625, 1982.

82. Murphy N, Auzinger G, Bernel W, et al: The effect of hypertonic sodium chloride on intracranial pressure in patients with acute liver failure. Hepatology 39:464, 2004.

83. Forbes A, Alexander GJ, O'Grady JG, et al: Thiopental infusion in the treatment of intracranial hypertension complicating fulminant hepatic failure. Hepatology 10:306, 1989.

84. Jalan R, Olde Damink SWM, Deutz NEP, et al: Restoration of cerebral blood flow autoregulation and reactivity to carbon dioxide in acute liver failure by moderate hypothermia. Hepatology 34:50, 2001.

85. Jalan R, Olde Damink SWM, Deutz NEP, et al: Moderate hypothermia prevents cerebral hyperemia and increase in

intracranial pressure in patients undergoing liver transplantation for acute liver failure. Transplantation 75:2034, 2003.

86. Martin LF, Booth FV, Karlstadt RG, et al: Continuous intravenous cimetidine decreases stress-related upper gastrointestinal hemorrhage without promoting pneumonia. Crit Care Med 21:19, 1993.

87. Shami VM, Caldwell SH, Hespenheide EE, et al: Recombinant activated factor VII for coagulopathy in fulminant hepatic failure compared with conventional therapy. Liver Transplant 9:138, 2003.

88. Rolando N, Gimson A, Wade J, et al: Prospective controlled trial of selective parenteral and enteral antimicrobial regimen in fulminant liver failure. Hepatology 17:196, 1993.

89. Rolando N, Wade JJ, Stangou A, et al: Prospective study comparing the efficacy of prophylactic parenteral antimicrobials, with or without enteral decontamination, in patients with acute liver failure. Liver Transpl Surg 2:8, 1996.

90. Wendon JA, Harrison PM, Keays R, et al: Effects of vasopressor agents and epoprostenol on systemic hemodynamics and oxygen transport in fulminant hepatic failure. Hepatology 15:1067, 1992.

91. Shawcross DL, Davies NA, Mookerjee RP, et al: Worsening of cerebral hyperemia by the administration of terlipressin in acute liver failure with severe encephalopathy. Hepatology 39:471, 2004.

92. Harrison PM, Wendon JA, Gimson AE, et al: Improvement by acetylcysteine of hemodynamics and oxygen transport in fulminant hepatic failure. N Engl J Med 324:1852, 1991.

93. Davenport A, Will EJ, Davidson AM: Improved cardiovascular stability during continuous modes of renal replacement therapy in critically ill patients with acute hepatic and renal failure. Crit Care Med 21:328, 1993.

94. Muñoz SJ, Moritz MJ, Martin P, et al: Liver transplantation for fulminant hepatocellular failure. Transplant Proc 25:1773, 1993.

95. Ascher NL, Lake JR, Emond J, et al: Liver transplantation for fulminant hepatic failure. Arch Surg 128:677, 1993.

96. Schiodt FV, Atillasoy E, Shakil AO, et al: Etiology and outcome for 295 patients with acute liver failure in the United States. Liver Transpl Surg 5:29, 1999.

97. Campbell DA, Ham JM, McCurry KR: Liver transplant for fulminant hepatic failure. Am Surg 57:546, 1991.

98. Emond JC, Aran PP, Whitington PF, et al: Liver transplantation in the management of fulminant hepatic failure. Gastroenterology 96:1583, 1989.

99. Iwatsuki S, Steiber AC, Marsh HW, et al: Liver transplantation for fulminant hepatic failure. Transplant Proc 21:2431, 1989.

100. Schafer DF, Shaw BW: Fulminant hepatic failure and orthotopic liver transplantation. Semin Liver Dis 9:189, 1989.

101. Uemoto S, Inomata Y, Sakurai T, et al: Living donor liver transplantation for fulminant hepatic failure. Transplantation 70:152, 2000.

102. Miwa S, Hashikura Y, Mita A, et al: Living-related liver transplantation for patients with fulminant and subfulminant hepatic failure. Hepatology 30:1521, 1999.

103. Higgins PDR, Fontana RJ: Liver transplantation in acute liver failure. Panminerva Med 52:93, 2002.

104. Detre K, Belle S, Beringer K, et al: Liver transplantation for fulminant hepatic failure in the United States: October 1987 through December 1991. Clin Transplant 8:274, 1994.

105. Devlin J, Williams R: Transplantation for fulminant hepatic failure. Transplantation 62:151, 1996.

106. Mohamed R, Hubscher SG, Mirza DF, et al: Posttransplantation chronic hepatitis in fulminant hepatic failure. Hepatology 25:1003, 1997.

107. Jackson EW, Zacks S, Zinn S, et al: Delayed neuropsychologic dysfunction after liver transplantation for acute liver failure: A matched, case-controlled study. Liver Transplant 8:932, 2002.

108. O'Grady JG, Gimson AE, O'Brien CJ, et al: Controlled trials of charcoal hemoperfusion and prognostic factors in fulminant hepatic failure. Gastroenterology 94:1186, 1988.

109. Sterling RK, Luketic VA, Sanyal AJ, et al: Treatment of fulminant hepatic failure with intravenous prostaglandin E_1. Liver Transpl Surg 4:424, 1998.

110. Larsen FS, Hansen BA, Jorgensen LG, et al: High-volume plasmapheresis and acute liver transplantation in fulminant hepatic failure. Transplant Proc 26:1788, 1994.

111. Ejlersen E, Larsen FS, Pott F, et al: Hepatectomy corrects cerebral hyperperfusion in fulminant hepatic failure. Transplant Proc 26:1794, 1994.

112. Sudan DL, Shaw BW Jr, Fox IJ, et al: Long-term follow-up of auxiliary orthotopic liver transplantation for the treatment of fulminant hepatic failure. Surgery 122:771, 1997.

113. van Hoek B, de Boer J, Boudjema K, et al: Auxiliary versus orthotopic liver transplantation for acute liver failure. EURALT Study Group. European Auxiliary Liver Transplant Registry. J Hepatol 30:699, 1999.

114. Allen JW, Hassanein T, Bhatia SN: Advances in bioartificial liver devices. Hepatology 34:447, 2001.

115. Heemann U, Treichel U, Loock J, et al: Albumin dialysis in cirrhosis with superimposed acute liver injury: A prospective, controlled study. Hepatology 36:949, 2003.

116. Schmidt LE, Wang LP, Hansen BA, et al: Systemic hemodynamic effects of treatment with the molecular adsorbents recirculating system in patients with hyperacute liver failure: A prospective, controlled trial. Liver Transplant 9:290, 2003.

117. Demetriou AA, Brown RS, Busuttil RW, et al: Prospective, randomized, multicenter controlled trial of a bioartificial liver in treating acute liver failure. Ann Surg 239:660, 2004.

118. Pitkin Z, Switzer W, Chapman L: An interim analysis of PERV infection in 74 patients treated with a bioartificial liver in a prospective, randomized, multicenter controlled trial [abstract]. Hepatology 34:249A, 2001.

119. Strom SC, Fisher RA, Thompson MT, et al: Hepatocyte transplantation as a bridge to orthotopic liver transplantation in terminal liver failure. Transplantation 63:559, 1997.

120. Fox I, Chowdhury J, Kaufman S, et al: Treatment of the Crigler-Najjar syndrome type I with hepatocyte transplantation. N Engl J Med 338:1422, 1998.

121. Bilir B, Guinette D, Karrer F, et al: Hepatocyte transplantation in acute liver failure. Liver Transpl 6:32, 2000.

122. Petersen BE, Bowen WC, Patrene KD, et al: Bone marrow as a potential source of hepatic oval cells. Science 284:1168, 1999.

CHAPTER

91 Hepatic Tumors and Cysts

Michael C. Kew

Mass lesions of the liver occur sufficiently often that clinicians interested in liver diseases should have a thorough understanding of their presentations, diagnosis, and treatment. Hepatic mass lesions include tumors, tumor-like lesions, abscesses, cysts, hematomas, and confluent granulomas. The frequency with which each is seen varies in different geographic regions and different populations. The more common hepatic tumors and cysts and those important for other reasons are reviewed in this chapter.

HEPATIC TUMORS

Hepatic tumors may either originate in the liver—from hepatocytes, bile duct epithelium, or mesenchymal tissue—or spread to the liver from primary tumors in remote or adjacent organs. In adults in most parts of the world, hepatic metastases are more common than primary malignant tumors of the liver, whereas in children, primary malignant tumors outnumber both metastases and benign tumors of the liver. Except for cavernous hemangiomas, benign hepatic tumors are rare in all geographic regions and in all age groups.

PRIMARY MALIGNANT TUMORS

Hepatocellular Carcinoma

Incidence and Geographic Distribution

Hepatocellular carcinoma is the commonest primary malignant tumor of the liver. It is the fifth most common cancer in men and the eighth most common in women, and it ranks fourth in annual cancer mortality rates.[1,2] Information on incidence is derived from an increasing but still limited number of cancer registries, which makes it possible to classify countries into broad risk categories only. Moreover, in low-income (developing) countries,

especially in sub-Saharan Africa, hepatocellular carcinoma is underdiagnosed and underreported, in some instances by as much as 50%. Despite these sources of inaccuracy, hepatocellular carcinoma clearly has an unusual geographic distribution[1,2] (Fig. 91–1). Moreover, the tumor is not necessarily uniformly common throughout countries with a high incidence, such as China[3] and Mozambique.[4] The incidence of hepatocellular carcinoma has increased considerably in Japan during the past 3 decades,[5] and lesser increases have been recorded in North America, the United Kingdom, a number of European countries, and Australia.[1,2]

Migrants from countries with a low incidence of hepatocellular carcinoma to those with a high incidence usually retain the low risk of their country of origin, even after several generations in the new environment.[2] The consequences for migrants from countries with a high incidence to those with a low incidence differ, depending on the major risk factors for the tumor in their country of origin and whether chronic hepatitis B virus (HBV) infection, if this is the major risk factor, is acquired predominantly by the perinatal or the horizontal route.[2,6,7]

Gender Distribution

Men are generally more susceptible than women to hepatocellular carcinoma. Male predominance is, however, more obvious in populations at high risk for the tumor (mean male-to-female ratio, 3.7:1.0) than in those at low or intermediate risk (2.4:1.0).[1,2] In industrialized (high-income) countries, the numbers of men and of women with hepatocellular carcinoma in the absence of cirrhosis are almost equal.

Age Distribution

The incidence of hepatocellular carcinoma increases progressively with advancing age in all populations, although it tends to level off in the oldest age groups.[1,2]

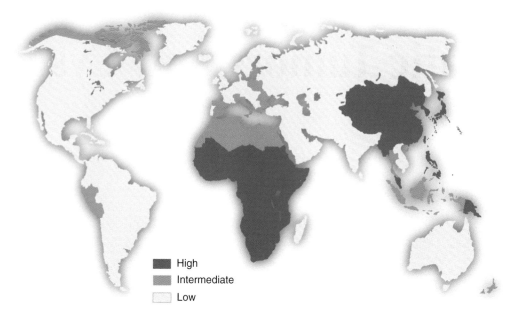

Figure 91–1 Incidence of hepatocellular carcinoma in different parts of the world. High, age-adjusted rate of greater than 15 cases per 100,000 population per year; intermediate, age-adjusted rate of 5 to 15 cases per 100,000 per year; low, age-adjusted rate of fewer than 5 cases per 100,000 per year.

High
Intermediate
Low

In Chinese and particularly in black African populations, however, the mean age of patients with the tumor is appreciably younger than it is in other populations. This phenomenon is most striking in Mozambique, where more than 50% of Shangaan men with hepatocellular carcinoma are younger than 30 years of age, and their mean age is 33 years.[8] Hepatocellular carcinoma is rare in children.[9]

Clinical Features

In far-advanced disease, patients with hepatocellular carcinoma usually present with typical symptoms and signs, and diagnosis is easy. Before this late stage is reached, however, clinical recognition often is difficult. The liver is relatively inaccessible to the examining hand, and its large size dictates that the tumor must reach a substantial size before it can be felt or before it invades adjacent structures. Moreover, because of the functional reserve of the liver, jaundice and other signs of hepatic dysfunction do not appear until a large part of the organ has been replaced by tumor. The ease of recognizing hepatocellular carcinoma clinically also differs among geographic regions. In countries in which hepatocellular carcinoma is common, clinicians are especially mindful of the tumor and its diverse presentations. Consequently, they are likely to recognize hepatocellular carcinoma with greater facility than that typical for clinicians in countries where the tumor is rare. In addition, hepatocellular carcinoma often coexists with cirrhosis,[10] and this association influences detection differently in regions with different incidence rates of the tumor. In regions of low incidence (but also in Japan, a country where the incidence is high), hepatocellular carcinoma commonly develops as a complication of long-standing *symptomatic* cirrhosis, and the patient has few, if any, symptoms attributable specifically to the tumor.[10] If the tumor is small (as it often is in a cirrhotic liver), it may not be obvious in the presence of advanced cirrhosis. One circumstance that should alert the clinician to the possibility that hepatocellular carcinoma has supervened in a cirrhotic liver is a sudden

Table 91–1 Symptoms and Signs of Hepatocellular Carcinoma

Symptom	Frequency (%)	Sign	Frequency (%)
Abdominal pain	59-95	Hepatomegaly	54-98
Weight loss	34-71	Hepatic bruit	6-25
Weakness	22-53	Ascites	35-61
Abdominal swelling	28-43	Splenomegaly	27-42
		Jaundice	4-35
Nonspecific gastrointestinal symptoms	25-28	Wasting	25-41
		Fever	11-54
Jaundice	5-26		

unexplained change in the patient's condition: He or she may complain of abdominal pain or weight loss; ascites may become more severe, the ascitic fluid may become blood-stained, or the condition may become more difficult to treat; the liver may enlarge rapidly or develop an arterial bruit; or hepatic failure may ensue. By contrast, in populations at high risk for hepatocellular carcinoma, the symptoms, if any, of the coexisting cirrhosis are overshadowed by those of the tumor. Hepatocellular carcinomas generally are considerably larger in these populations, and their symptoms and signs are, accordingly, more florid, thereby facilitating diagnosis.[11]

Symptoms. Patients with hepatocellular carcinoma often are unaware of its presence until the tumor has reached an advanced stage. Black Africans, in particular, seek treatment late in the illness.[11,12] The most common, and frequently first, symptom is right hypochondrial or epigastric pain (Table 91–1). Although sometimes severe, the pain usually is a dull continuous ache that becomes more intense in the later stages of the illness. It may be accompanied by weakness and weight loss. Less common complaints are an awareness of a lump or fullness in the upper abdomen, poor appetite, early satiety or discomfort after eating, generalized abdominal swelling, diarrhea, and constipation. Jaundice is an infrequent initial complaint. When jaundice is deep, the cause is likely to be biliary obstruction.[13] When the extent of the tumor burden is appreciated, these symptoms may be of surprisingly short duration, especially in black African and Chinese patients, who often describe symptoms of only 4 to 6 weeks' duration. Rarely, hepatocellular carcinoma manifests as an "acute abdomen" when the tumor ruptures, causing hemoperitoneum. Other rare presentations are with bone pain resulting from skeletal metastases, sudden paraplegia secondary to vertebral destruction, and cough or dyspnea caused by multiple pulmonary metastases or a markedly raised right hemidiaphragm.[14]

The course of hepatocellular carcinoma typically is rapid in black African and Chinese patients but is less so in patients in industrialized countries.

Physical Examination. Physical findings vary with the stage of disease. Early in the course, either evidence of cirrhosis alone may be present, or abnormal findings may be absent (see Table 91–1). More often, the tumor is advanced at the time of the first visit, and the liver is then almost always enlarged, sometimes massively, particularly in black African and Chinese patients. Hepatic tenderness is common and may be profound, especially in the latter stages. The surface of the enlarged liver is smooth, irregular, or frankly nodular. Although the consistency is characteristically stony hard, it may be only firm. An arterial bruit may be heard over the tumor[12,15,16]; the bruit is heard in systole, rough in character, and not affected by changing the position of the patient. Although not pathognomonic, a bruit is a useful clue to the diagnosis of hepatocellular carcinoma. Less often, a friction rub is heard over the tumor, but this sign is more characteristic of hepatic metastases or abscesses.

Ascites may be present when the patient is first seen or may appear with progression of the tumor. In most patients, ascites is the result of long-standing cirrhosis and portal hypertension, but in some cases it is caused by invasion of the peritoneum by the primary tumor or metastases (in which case the ascitic fluid may be bloodstained). In a small proportion of patients, hepatocellular carcinoma invades the hepatic veins, and tense ascites results.[14] Splenomegaly, if present, reflects coexisting cirrhosis and portal hypertension.

The patient may exhibit slight or moderate wasting when first seen. Thereafter, progressive muscle wasting is the rule, and patients typically are emaciated in the final stages of the illness. Jaundice is unusual at first presentation and, when present, is mild; it commonly appears or deepens with progression of the disease. A low to moderate, intermittent or remittent fever may be present, and in rare instances the tumor may masquerade as a fever of unknown origin.

Physical evidence of cirrhosis is common in patients in industrialized countries but unusual in black African and Chinese patients. Severe pitting edema extending up to the groins occurs when hepatocellular carcinoma has invaded the hepatic veins and propagates into and obstructs the inferior vena cava.[14] A Virchow-Trosier node, Sister Mary Joseph's nodule, or enlarged axillary lymph node is rarely present.

Paraneoplastic Manifestations. Some of the deleterious effects of hepatocellular carcinoma are not caused by

Table 91–2 Paraneoplastic Syndromes Associated with Hepatocellular Carcinoma

Hypoglycemia
Polycythemia (erythrocytosis)
Hypercalcemia
Sexual changes: isosexual precocity, gynecomastia, feminization
Systemic arterial hypertension
Watery diarrhea syndrome
Porphyria
Carcinoid syndrome
Osteoporosis
Hypertrophic osteoarthropathy
Thyrotoxicosis
Thrombophlebitis migrans
Polymyositis
Neuropathy

either local effects of the tumor or metastases (Table 91–2). These systemic or remote sequelae result, directly or indirectly, from synthesis and secretion of biologically active substances by the tumor. Most often, clinically recognizable effects are caused by the secretion of hormones or hormone-like substances. Paraneoplastic phenomena may antedate the local effects of the tumor and direct attention to its presence. Moreover, some effects, such as hypoglycemia and hypercalcemia, require treatment in their own right.

Each of the paraneoplastic syndromes in hepatocellular carcinoma is rare or uncommon. One of the more important is type B hypoglycemia, which occurs in less than 5% of patients and manifests as severe hypoglycemia early in the course of the disease.[14] Characteristically, hypoglycemia is the reason for hospitalization. The clinical presentation may include confusion, delirium, acute neuropsychiatric disturbances, convulsions, stupor, or coma; the presence of an underlying tumor is easily overlooked. Type B hypoglycemia is believed to result from the defective processing by malignant hepatocytes of the precursor to insulin-like growth factor II (pro-IGF-II).[17] The resulting *big* IGF-II circulates in 60-kd complexes that are appreciably smaller than the normal complexes. They transfer more readily across capillary membranes and increase access of IGF-II to IGF-I and IGF-II receptors and to insulin receptors. The effect is to greatly increase glucose uptake by tissues. By contrast, type A hypoglycemia is a milder form of glycopenia that occurs in the terminal stages of hepatocellular carcinoma (and other malignant tumors of the liver). It results from the inability of a liver extensively infiltrated by tumor, and often cirrhotic, to satisfy the demands for glucose by both a large, often rapidly growing tumor and the other tissues of the body.

Another important paraneoplastic syndrome is polycythemia (erythrocytosis), which occurs in less than 10% of patients with hepatocellular carcinoma.[18] If polycythemia develops in a patient known to have cirrhosis, hepatocellular carcinoma should be suspected. This syndrome appears to be caused by the synthesis of erythropoietin or an erythropoietin-like substance by malignant hepatocytes.[18]

Patients with hepatocellular carcinoma, especially the sclerosing variety, may present with hypercalcemia in the absence of osteolytic metastases. When hypercalcemia is severe, the patient is drowsy and lethargic and may be stuporous. The probable cause is secretion of parathyroid hormone–related protein (PTHrP) by the tumor.[19]

Cutaneous paraneoplastic manifestations of hepatocellular carcinoma are rare except for *pityriasis rotunda (circumscripta)*, which may be a useful marker of the tumor in black Africans. The rash consists of single or multiple, round or oval, hyperpigmented, scaly lesions on the trunk and thighs that range in diameter from 0.5 to 25 cm.[20]

Diagnosis

Conventional tests of hepatic function do not distinguish hepatocellular carcinoma from other hepatic mass lesions or cirrhosis. Although not specific, an elevated serum cholesterol level occurs in 11% to 38% of patients with hepatocellular carcinoma,[21] and its presence in a patient with noncholestatic liver disease should raise suspicion of hepatocellular carcinoma. Increased de novo cholesterol biosynthesis by malignant hepatocytes results from the absence in these cells of the normal feedback inhibition of the rate-limiting enzyme β-methylglutaryl–coenzyme A reductase.[21]

Serum Tumor Markers. Many of the substances synthesized and secreted by hepatocellular carcinoma are not biologically active. Nevertheless, a few are produced by a sufficiently large proportion of tumors to warrant their use as serum markers for hepatocellular carcinoma (Table 91–3). The most helpful of these is alpha-fetoprotein.

Alpha-Fetoprotein

Alpha-fetoprotein is an α_1-globulin normally present in high concentrations in fetal serum but in only minute amounts thereafter. Reappearance of high serum levels of alpha-fetoprotein strongly suggests the diagnosis of hepatocellular carcinoma (or hepatoblastoma).[22,23] This holds especially true in populations in which hepatocellular carcinoma is most prevalent: The great majority of Chinese and black African patients have a raised serum concentration of alpha-fetoprotein (greater than 10 ng/mL [10 mg/L]), and approximately 75% have a diagnostic level (greater than 500 ng/mL [500 mg/L]). These percentages are lower in populations at low or intermediate

risk for the tumor; consequently, alpha-fetoprotein is a less useful tumor marker in these patients. The mean serum value of alpha-fetoprotein in affected patients in regions with a high incidence of hepatocellular carcinoma is 60,000 to 80,000 ng/mL, compared with approximately 8000 ng/mL in regions with a low or intermediate incidence of the tumor. Raised serum values range over six orders of magnitude, although concentrations of greater than 1 million ng/mL are rare. A value of 500 ng/mL (500 mg/L) is used as a diagnostic level because levels below this value may be found in patients with a variety of acute and chronic benign liver diseases, such as acute and chronic hepatitis and cirrhosis.[22,23] False-positive results also may occur in patients with tumors of endodermal origin and nonseminomatous germ cell tumors[22,23] A progressively rising serum alpha-fetoprotein concentration, even if below the diagnostic level, is highly suggestive of hepatocellular carcinoma.

Not all hepatocellular carcinomas produce alpha-fetoprotein, which is not essential to hepatocarcinogenesis, and evidence indicating that tumors that do not secrete alpha-fetoprotein are biologically different from the tumors that do is lacking. Synthesis of alpha-fetoprotein by a tumor is permanent and age related: The younger the patient, the more likely the serum value is to be raised and the higher the level attained. Provided that patients are age-matched, no gender difference is observed in the production of alpha-fetoprotein. Nor does an obvious correlation exist between the serum concentration of alpha-fetoprotein and any clinical or biochemical feature of the tumor or the survival time after diagnosis. Small presymptomatic tumors, however, are associated with an appreciably lower serum level than that measured with symptomatic tumors.[24] Attempts to correlate the degree of differentiation of hepatocellular carcinoma with production of alpha-fetoprotein have produced conflicting results.

Because both false-positive and false-negative results are obtained when alpha-fetoprotein is used as a serum marker for hepatocellular carcinoma, the search for an ideal marker continues. Alternative markers have not proved to be more useful than alpha-fetoprotein.

Fucosylated Alpha-Fetoprotein

Alpha-fetoprotein is heterogeneous in structure. Its microheterogeneity results from differences in the

Table 91–3 Tumor Markers of Hepatocellular Carcinoma*

Marker	Sensitivity (%)	Specificity (%)	Comments
Alpha-fetoprotein	*High-incidence populations*: 80-90 *Low-incidence populations*: 50-70	90	Relatively quick and easy to measure; most extensively studied Relatively expensive
Des-γ-carboxyprothrombin	58-91	84	Quick and easy to measure Much more expensive than α-fetoprotein
α-L-Fucosidase	75	70-90	Quick and easy to measure; relatively inexpensive

*Note that sensitivity and specificity rates vary both with the population under study and with the absolute level of the marker. Thus, the specificity of a markedly elevated alpha-fetoprotein level in patients with cirrhosis greatly exceeds the sensitivity of mildly elevated levels in persons without cirrhosis.

oligosaccharide side chain and accounts for the differential affinity of the glycoprotein for lectins. Alpha-fetoprotein secreted by malignant hepatocytes contains unusual and complex sugar chains that are not found in alpha-fetoprotein produced by nontransformed hepatocytes. The sugar chains have the same core structure, but the number of the outer chain trisaccharides differ. Several reports have attested to the usefulness of the reactivity of alpha-fetoprotein with *Lens culinaris* agglutinin A in differentiating hepatocellular carcinoma from benign hepatic parenchymal disease and, to a lesser extent, of the reactivity with concanavalin A in distinguishing hepatocellular carcinoma from other tumors that produce alpha-fetoprotein.[25] This refinement is particularly useful in the differential diagnosis for hepatocellular carcinoma when the serum alpha-fetoprotein concentration is less than 500 ng/mL (500 mg/L).[26] In addition, it may improve the diagnostic yield of alpha-fetoprotein testing in surveillance programs for small presymptomatic tumors. Unfortunately, the method used to measure fucosylated alpha-fetoprotein remains complex and costly.

Des-γ-Carboxy Prothrombin

Serum concentrations of des-γ-carboxy prothrombin (also known as prothrombin produced by vitamin K absence or antagonism II [PIVKA II]) are raised in a majority of patients with hepatocellular carcinoma.[27] In populations in which the incidence of hepatocellular carcinoma is low, the abnormal prothrombin might arguably be a better marker than alpha-fetoprotein, and it could be used as a first-line tumor marker. In black Africans, however, des-γ-carboxy prothrombin is less sensitive and less specific than alpha-fetoprotein.[28] Moreover, if the diagnostic cutoff level of des-γ-carboxy prothrombin is increased in an attempt to eliminate false-positive results seen in benign hepatic parenchymal diseases, the sensitivity for detecting hepatocellular carcinoma declines from 91% to 67%.[28]

α-L-Fucosidase and Others

A number of isomers of α-L-fucosidase, including two hepatic forms, have been identified in human tissue. α-L-Fucosidase initially was reported to have a sensitivity of 75% and a specificity of 90% in the diagnosis of hepatocellular carcinoma.[29] In a subsequent study, however, the marker failed to distinguish cirrhosis from hepatocellular carcinoma.[30] Moreover, in black Africans, this marker is less sensitive and less specific and has a lower predictive value than alpha-fetoprotein.[31] When the specificity of each of these markers was increased to 95% by raising the diagnostic cutoff level, the sensitivity of α-L-fucosidase decreased to 21%, whereas that of alpha-fetoprotein remained at 78%.[31]

None of a number of other substances claimed to be serum markers of hepatocellular carcinoma has a sufficiently high sensitivity or specificity to warrant routine use in the diagnosis of this tumor.[23] CA-125, tissue polypeptide antigen, and tumor-associated isoenzymes of 5'-nucleotide phosphodiesterase have high sensitivities but poor specificities. Tumor-associated isoenzymes of gamma-glutamyl transpeptidase and variant alkaline phosphatase have high specificities but low sensitivities, whereas ferritin, carcinoembryonic antigen, CA 19-9, and calcitonin have low sensitivities and specificities. Two tumor markers—abnormal vitamin B_{12}–binding protein and neurotensin—have been linked specifically to the fibrolamellar variant of hepatocellular carcinoma (see later). When present, they provide useful confirmatory evidence of this variant, although the sensitivities of both markers are low.

Hematologic Changes

More than one half of Chinese and black African patients with hepatocellular carcinoma are anemic when they are first seen, although anemia is less common in other populations. Severe anemia is rare, however, and should suggest the possibility of intraperitoneal or variceal bleeding. Slight or moderate leukocytosis may be present. Polycythemia is an infrequent paraneoplastic complication of hepatocellular carcinoma.

Chest Radiograph. Pulmonary metastases may be seen on plain chest radiography, particularly in black African and Chinese patients.[32] They almost always are multiple and may enlarge rapidly. The right hemidiaphragm or, rarely, the left hemidiaphragm may be raised.[32] Skeletal metastases are seen occasionally.

Hepatic Imaging. The imaging modalities used most often for the diagnosis of symptomatic hepatocellular carcinoma are ultrasonography and computed tomography (CT). Magnetic resonance imaging (MRI) also is useful.

Ultrasonography

Ultrasonography detects a majority of hepatocellular carcinomas but does not distinguish this tumor from other solid lesions in the liver. Advantages of ultrasonography include safety, availability, and cost effectiveness, although it has the drawbacks of being nonstandardized and examiner dependent. Approximately two thirds of symptomatic hepatocellular carcinomas are uniformly hyperechoic, whereas the remainder are partly hyperechoic and partly hypoechoic[33,34] (Fig. 91–2). Small tumors are uniformly hypoechoic. The ultrasonographic appearance is influenced by the presence of fat, calcium, and necro-

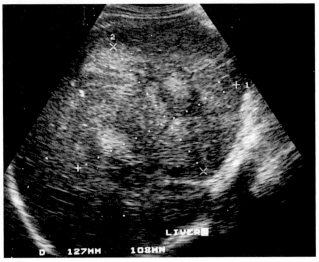

Figure 91–2   Ultrasonogram in a patient with hepatocellular carcinoma showing a nodular hyperechoic pattern with scattered hypoechoic areas. The edges of the tumor are ill-defined.

sis. Tumors located immediately under the right hemidi-aphragm may be difficult to detect. In Japanese patients in particular, hepato-cellular carcinoma may have a well-defined, even thick capsule, which can be seen on ultra-sonography. Ultrasonography with Doppler technology is useful for assessing the patency of the inferior vena cava, portal vein and its larger branches, hepatic veins, and biliary tree.[33,34]

Dynamic contrast-enhanced Doppler ultrasonography with intra-arterial infusion of CO_2 microbubbles and intravenous enhanced color Doppler ultrasonography are refinements that, by characterizing hepatic arterial and portal venous flow in tumorous nodules, facilitate the diagnosis of malignant and benign hepatic nodules.[35]

Computed Tomography

Multiphase helical CT and CT during arterial portogra-phy are the imaging techniques of choice in the diagno-sis of hepatocellular carcinoma.[34-36] The tumor appears hypervascular during the hepatic arterial phase and rela-tively hypodense in the delayed phases. CT is especially helpful in defining the extent of the tumor within and beyond the liver (Fig. 91–3) and in showing the course, caliber, and patency of blood vessels. Because iodized poppy seed oil (Lipiodol) is concentrated and retained in hepatocellular carcinoma tissue, injection of this material at the end of hepatic arteriography can be used in con-junction with CT, performed after a suitable delay, to detect very small tumors.

Magnetic Resonance Imaging

MRI provides another way of distinguishing hepatocellu-lar carcinoma from normal liver tissue. Most tumors have a low signal intensity on T1-weighted images and a high signal intensity on T2-weighted images.[34,35,37] The use of a contrast agent, such as gadopentetate dimeglumine or superparamagnetic iron oxide, increases the accuracy of MRI, especially in detecting small hepatocellular carci-nomas in cirrhotic livers and in distinguishing small hepatocellular carcinomas from hemangiomas discov-ered in surveillance programs.[35] Tissue-specific contrast agents, however, cannot differentiate among well-differentiated hepatocellular carcinomas, regenerative or dysplastic nodules, hepatocellular adenomas, and focal nodular hyperplasia.[34,35,37]

Hepatic Angiography

Since the advent of CT and MRI, the diagnostic role of hepatic angiography has decreased. Digital subtraction angiography is helpful in recognizing small hypervascu-lar hepatocellular carcinomas but may miss early, well-differentiated hypovascular tumors. Hepatocellular carcinomas often are densely vascular, although multi-nodular tumors may be relatively avascular.[38] The arter-ies in the tumor are irregular in caliber and do not taper in the usual way, and the smaller branches may show a bizarre pattern[38] (Fig. 91–4). The hepatic veins fill early, and retrograde filling of the portal veins results from the presence of arteriovenous anastomoses within the tumor. An additional finding is a delay in capillary emptying, which is seen as a blush. The center of some large tumors may be avascular as a result of necrosis or, less often, hem-orrhage. Dynamic contrast-enhanced ultrasonography with intra-arterial infusion of CO_2 microbubbles can be used to detect hypovascular tumors and to differentiate hepatocellular carcinoma from other hepatic nodules.[34] Angiography is essential in delineating the hepatic arte-rial anatomy in planning surgical resection, liver trans-plantation, embolization or chemoembolization of the tumor, or infusion of cytotoxic drugs directly into the hepatic artery or its branches. Angiography also will confirm the patency of the portal vein.

Tumor invasion of the portal vein may be demon-strated during recirculation after celiac axis arteriography or during portal venography.[38] Less often, invasion of the hepatic veins can be demonstrated.

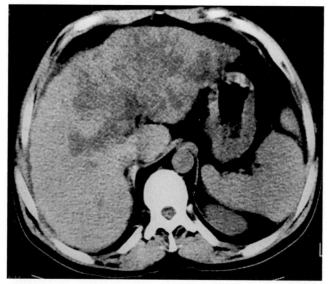

Figure 91–3   Computed tomographic scan of a patient with hepato-cellular carcinoma involving much of the left lobe and the adjacent part of the right lobe of the liver.

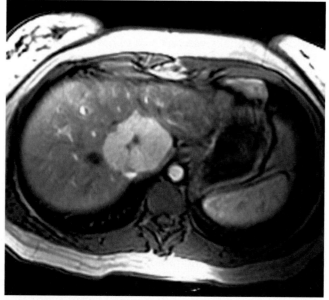

Figure 91–4   Hepatic arteriogram showing the typical features of a highly vascular hepatocellular carcinoma.

Laparoscopy

Laparoscopy can be used to detect peritoneal and other extrahepatic spread, to ascertain whether the nontumorous part of the liver is cirrhotic, and to obtain a biopsy under direct vision.

Pathology. Definitive diagnosis of hepatocellular carcinoma depends on demonstrating the typical histologic features. Suitable samples generally can be obtained by percutaneous biopsy or fine-needle aspiration. The yield and safety of the procedure can be increased by directing the needle under ultrasonographic guidance. Laparoscopically di-rected biopsy is an alternative approach. Because of the risk of local, regional, or systemic dissemination of hepatocellular carcinoma by needle biopsy or fine-needle aspiration of the tumor, many clinicians believe that these procedures should be avoided if the tumor is thought to be operable.

Gross Appearance. Hepatocellular carcinoma may take one of three forms: nodular, massive, or diffuse.[39-41] The nodular variety accounts for about 75% of hepatocellular carcinomas and usually coexists with cirrhosis. It is characterized by numerous round or irregular nodules of various sizes scattered throughout the liver, some of which are confluent. The massive type is characterized by a large circumscribed mass, often with small satellite nodules. This type of tumor is most prone to rupture and is more common in younger patients with a noncirrhotic liver. In the rare diffusely infiltrating variety, a large part of the liver is infiltrated homogeneously by indistinct minute tumor nodules, which may be difficult to distinguish from the regenerating nodules of cirrhosis that are almost invariably present. In the nodular and massive varieties, the tumor tissue usually is soft and bulges above the surrounding cut surface of the liver. Areas of necrosis and hemorrhage are common. Well-differentiated tumors are light brown, whereas anaplastic tumors are yellowish-white or gray. Bile production may cause greenish-brown discoloration of the tumor. The portal vein and its branches are infiltrated by tumor in up to 70% of cases seen at autopsy; the hepatic veins and bile ducts are invaded less often.

Hepatocellular carcinoma rarely, if ever, umbilicates. The tumor may be monoclonal (with intrahepatic metastases) or polyclonal (with multiple primary tumors in the liver).

Microscopic Appearance. Hepatocellular carcinoma is classified histologically into well-differentiated, moderately differentiated, and undifferentiated (pleomorphic) forms.[39-41]

Well-Differentiated Appearance

Despite the aggressive nature and poor prognosis of hepatocellular carcinoma, most tumors are well differentiated. Trabecular and acinar (pseudoglandular) varieties occur, sometimes in a single tumor. In the *trabecular* variety, the malignant hepatocytes grow in irregular anastomosing plates separated by often inconspicuous sinusoids lined by flat cells resembling Kupffer cells. The trabeculae resemble those of normal adult liver but often are thicker and may be composed of several layers of cells. Scanty collagen fibers may be seen adjacent to the sinusoid walls. The malignant hepatocytes are polygonal, with abun-

dant, slightly granular cytoplasm that is less eosinophilic than that of normal hepatocytes. The nuclei are large and hyperchromatic, with prominent nucleoli. Bile production is the hallmark of hepatocellular carcinoma, regardless of the pattern.

Gland-like structures are present in the *acinar* variety. They are composed of layers of malignant hepatocytes surrounding the lumen of a bile canaliculus, which may contain inspissated bile. A tubular or pseudopapillary appearance may be produced by degeneration and loss of cells, or cystic spaces may form in otherwise solid trabeculae. The individual cells may be more elongated and cylindrical than in the trabecular variety.

Moderately Differentiated Appearance

Solid, scirrhous, and clear cell varieties of hepatocellular carcinoma are described. In the solid variety, the cells usually are small, although they vary considerably in shape. Pleomorphic multinucleated giant cells occasionally are present. The tumor grows in solid masses or cell nests. Evidence of bile secretion is rare, and connective tissue is inconspicuous. Central ischemic necrosis is common in larger tumors. In the scirrhous variety, the malignant hepatocytes grow in narrow bundles separated by abundant fibrous stroma. Duct-like structures occasionally are present. In most tumors, the cells resemble hepatocytes. In an occasional tumor, the malignant hepatocytes are predominantly or exclusively clear cells. More often, tumors contain areas of clear cells. The appearance of these cells results from a high glycogen or, in some cases, fat content.

Undifferentiated Appearance

The cells are pleomorphic, varying greatly in size and shape. The nuclei also are extremely variable. Large numbers of bizarre-looking giant cells are present. The cells may be spindle-shaped, resembling those of sarcomas. Globular hyaline structures may be seen in all types of hepatocellular carcinoma. These reflect the presence of alpha-fetoprotein, α_1-antitrypsin, or other proteins. Mallory's hyaline occasionally is present.

Metastases

Extrahepatic metastases are present at autopsy in 40% to 57% of patients with hepatocellular carcinomas.[42] They are more common in patients without coexisting cirrhosis (approximately 70%) than in those with cirrhosis (approximately 30%). The most common sites are the lungs (up to 50% in some populations) and regional lymph nodes (approximately 20%). The adrenal glands are frequently involved.

Fibrolamellar Hepatocellular Carcinoma

The fibrolamellar variant of hepatocellular carcinoma typically occurs in young patients, has an approximately equal gender distribution, does not secrete alpha-fetoprotein, is not caused by chronic hepatitis B or C, and almost always arises in a noncirrhotic liver.[40] Fibrolamellar hepatocellular carcinoma is more often amenable to surgical treatment and therefore generally carries a better prognosis than that for conventional hepatocellular car-

Table 91–4 Risk Factors for Hepatocellular Carcinoma

Major Risk Factors
Chronic hepatitis B virus infection
Chronic hepatitis C virus infection
Cirrhosis
Dietary exposure to aflatoxin B_1
Minor Risk Factors
Oral contraceptive steroids
Cigarette smoking
Dietary iron overload in persons of black African ancestry
Hereditary hemochromatosis
Wilson disease
α_1-Antitrypsin deficiency
Type 1 hereditary tyrosinemia
Type 1 and type 2 glycogen storage disease
Hypercitrullinemia
Ataxia-telangiectasia
Membranous obstruction of the inferior vena cava

cinoma. It does not, however, respond to chemotherapy any better than do other forms of hepatocellular carcinoma. The hepatocytes are characteristically plump, deeply eosinophilic, and encompassed by abundant fibrous stroma composed of thin, parallel fibrous bands that separate the cells into trabeculae or nodules. The cytoplasm is packed with swollen mitochondria and, in approximately one half of the tumors, contains pale or hyaline bodies. Nuclei are prominent, and mitoses are rare.

Etiology and Pathogenesis

Hepatocellular carcinoma is multifactorial in etiology and complex in pathogenesis. Four major and several minor causal associations of the tumor have been identified (Table 91–4). The differing blend of risk factors in different parts of the world may explain in part the diverse biologic characteristics of hepatocellular carcinoma in various populations.[43]

Hepatitis B Virus. Some 387 million carriers of HBV exist in the world today, and hepatocellular carcinoma will develop in as many as 25% of them (see Chapter 75). HBV accounts for up to 80% of hepatocellular carcinomas, which occur with high frequency in Chinese and black African populations.[43,44] Persistent HBV infection antedates the development of hepatocellular carcinoma by several to many years, an interval commensurate with a cause-and-effect relationship between the virus and the tumor. Indeed, in Chinese and black Africans, the carrier state is largely established in early childhood, by either perinatal or horizontal infection.[45,46] Approximately 90% of children infected at this stage of life become chronic carriers of the virus, and these early-onset carriers face a lifetime relative risk for developing hepatocellular carcinoma greater than 100.[47]

An effective vaccine against HBV has been available for about 30 years, and in countries in which this vaccine has been included in the Expanded Program of Immunization for a sufficient length of time, the carrier rate among children has decreased by 10-fold or more. Studies in Taiwan, where universal immunization was started in 1984 and where the rate of HBV carriage among children has decreased by more than 10-fold, have already shown

a 70% reduction in the mortality rate from hepatocellular carcinoma among children in the vaccinated age groups.[48] This finding gives promise for the ultimate eradication of HBV-induced hepatocellular carcinoma and provides further evidence for the causal role of the virus in the development of this tumor.

HBV DNA is integrated into cellular DNA in approximately 90% of HBV-related hepatocellular carcinomas.[43,44] The sites of chromosomal insertion appear to be random, and whether viral integration is essential for hepatocarcinogenesis is still uncertain. The virus appears to be both directly and indirectly carcinogenic.[49] Possible direct carcinogenic effects include *cis*-activation of cellular genes as a result of viral integration, changes in the DNA sequences flanking the integrated viral DNA, transcriptional activation of remote cellular genes by HBV-encoded proteins, particularly the X protein, and effects resulting from viral mutations. The transcriptional activity of the HBV X protein may be mediated by interaction with specific transcription factors, activation of the mitogen-activated protein (MAP) kinase and Janus kinase–signal transducer and activator of transcription (JAK/STAT) pathways, an effect on apoptosis, and modulation of DNA repair.[49] Indirect carcinogenic effects are the result of the chronic necroinflammatory hepatic disease, in particular cirrhosis, induced by the virus. The increased hepatocyte turnover rate resulting from continuous or recurring cycles of cell necrosis and regeneration acts as a potent tumor promoter.[49] In addition, the distorted architecture characteristic of cirrhosis contributes to the loss of control of hepatocyte growth, and hepatic inflammation generates mutagenic reactive oxygen species. The transgenic mouse model of Chisari and coworkers has provided indirect support for the role of prolonged hepatocyte injury in hepatocarcinogenesis.[50]

Hepatitis C Virus. Approximately 170 million people in the world today are chronically infected with hepatitis C virus (HCV) and are at greatly increased risk for the development of hepatocellular carcinoma.[44] In Japan, Italy, and Spain, HCV is the cause of as many as 83% of hepatocellular carcinomas, and in other industrialized countries HCV infection is emerging as a major cause of the tumor, often in combination with alcohol abuse.[44] Patients with HCV-induced hepatocellular carcinoma generally are older than those with HBV-related tumors, and it is likely that the HCV infection is acquired mainly in adult life.

Almost all HCV-induced hepatocellular carcinomas arise in cirrhotic livers, and most of the exceptions are in livers with chronic hepatitis. This observation strongly suggests that chronic hepatic parenchymal disease plays a key role in the genesis of HCV-related tumors.[49] Emerging evidence suggests, however, that this virus also may be directly oncogenic.[49] Because the HCV genome does not integrate into host DNA, the virus would have to exert its direct carcinogenic effect from an extrachromosomal position, and a number of possible mechanisms have been suggested.

Cirrhosis. In all parts of the world, hepatocellular carcinoma frequently coexists with cirrhosis.[10] In Chinese and black African populations, cirrhosis typically is macronodular and is attributed to chronic HBV infection, whereas in other populations, cirrhosis is commonly mixed macronodular-micronodular or solely micronodular and results from chronic HCV infection, alcohol abuse, or both. All etiologic forms of cirrhosis may be complicated by tumor formation.[10] Male gender, age, and duration of cirrhosis are the major risk factors for hepatocellular carcinoma in cirrhotic patients. Cirrhosis contributes to hepatocarcinogenesis mainly by acting as a potent tumor promoter.[49]

Aflatoxin B_1. Dietary exposure to aflatoxin B_1, derived from the fungi *Aspergillus flavus* and *Aspergillus parasiticus*, is an important risk factor for hepatocellular carcinoma in parts of Africa and Asia. These molds are ubiquitous in nature and contaminate a number of staple foodstuffs in tropical and subtropical regions (see Chapter 84). Epidemiologic studies have shown a strong correlation between the dietary intake of aflatoxin B_1 and incidence of hepatocellular carcinoma.[51] Moreover, aflatoxin B_1 and HBV interact synergistically in the pathogenesis of hepatocellular carcinoma. Heavy dietary exposure to aflatoxin B_1 may contribute to hepatocarcinogenesis through an inactivating mutation of the third base of codon 249 of the p53 tumor suppressor gene.[52,53]

Minor Risk Factors. Hepatocellular carcinoma develops in as many as 45% of patients with hemochromatosis (see Chapter 71).[54] Malignant transformation was thought to occur only in the presence of cirrhosis (and is certainly more likely to do so), but this complication also has been reported in patients without cirrhosis,[55] and it is possible that excessive free iron in tissue per se may be carcinogenic, perhaps by generating mutagenic reactive oxygen species.[56] Further support for this theory comes from the observations that black Africans with dietary iron overload are at increased risk of hepatocellular carcinoma[57] and that rats fed a diet high in iron develop iron-free dysplastic foci and hepatocellular carcinoma in the absence of cirrhosis.[58] Hepatocellular carcinoma develops occasionally in patients with Wilson disease, but only in the presence of cirrhosis (see Chapter 72).[59] Malignant transformation has been attributed to the cirrhosis but also may result from oxidant stress secondary to the accumulation of copper in the liver.[60] Hepatocellular carcinoma also may develop in patients with other inherited metabolic disorders that are complicated by cirrhosis, such as α_1-antitrypsin deficiency and type 1 hereditary tyrosinemia, and in patients with certain inherited diseases in the absence of cirrhosis, for example, type 1 glycogen storage disease (see Chapter 73).

A statistically significant correlation between the use of oral contraceptive steroids and the occurrence of hepatocellular carcinoma has been demonstrated in countries in which the incidence of hepatocellular carcinoma is low and no overriding risk factor for devlopment of the tumor is present.[61] Affected patients constitute an extremely small proportion of women who are taking or have taken oral contraceptive steroids and a small proportion of all patients with hepatocellular carcinoma. The risk increases with increasing duration of usage and persists for longer than 10 years after the agents are discontinued.[62] Epidemiologic evidence of a link between cigarette smoking and the occurrence of hepatocellular carcinoma is conflicting, although most of the evidence suggests that smoking is a minor risk factor.[63] Heavy smokers have an approximately 50% higher risk than that in nonsmokers. The cytochrome P450 enzyme system, which is responsible for the metabolic activation of a number of chemical carcinogens, is highly inducible by smoking.

Hepatocellular carcinoma develops in approximately 40% of patients with membranous obstruction of the inferior vena cava, a rare congenital or acquired anomaly. Continuous cycles of hepatocyte necrosis followed by regeneration resulting from the severe and unremitting hepatic venous congestion render the cells susceptible to environmental mutagens, as well as to spontaneous mutations.[64,65]

Natural History and Prognosis

Symptomatic hepatocellular carcinoma carries a grave prognosis; in fact, the annual incidence and mortality rates for the tumor are virtually identical. The main reasons for the poor outcome are the extent of tumor burden when the patient is first seen and the frequent presence of coexisting cirrhosis and hepatic dysfunction. The natural history of hepatocellular carcinoma in its florid form is one of rapid progression with increasing hepatomegaly, abdominal pain, wasting, and deepening jaundice. In black African and Chinese populations, death often ensues within 4 months,[11,12] although in industrialized countries, the tumor generally runs a more indolent course with longer survival times.[16] Rare instances of spontaneous tumor regression have been reported.

Treatment

No form of treatment for symptomatic hepatocellular carcinoma has been shown conclusively or consistently to be better than no treatment, or superior, in terms of survival, to any other form of management.[66] Treatment of hepatocellular carcinoma depends on the extent of the disease, presence or absence of cirrhosis, and degree of hepatic dysfunction. The many patients who show evidence of liver failure seldom are suitable candidates for any specific treatment.

Surgical Resection. Tumor resection or liver transplantation offers the best chance of cure for hepato-cellular carcinoma (Table 91–5). For resection to be considered, the tumor must be confined to one lobe of the liver and be favorably located, and ideally, the nontumorous liver tissue should not be cirrhotic. Resection can be considered, however, if the tumor is limited to the left lobe and hepatic dysfunction from cirrhosis is not severe, or if favorable tumor location in either lobe allows the surgeon to perform a segmentectomy or limited nonanatomic resection. Unfortunately, the proportion of symptomatic patients with resectable tumors is small in countries where hepatocellular carcinoma is most common,[67,68] although the situation is less bleak in industrialized countries.[69] Overall, resection is feasible in only approximately 15% of patients. Resection carries an operative mortality rate of approximately 5% in noncirrhotic and 10% to 15% in cirrhotic livers. One of the most disappointing aspects of resecting hepatocellular carcinomas is the high recurrence rate.[70,71]

Liver Transplantation. Liver transplantation is performed in patients in whom the tumor is not resectable but is confined to the liver or in whom advanced cirrhosis and poor liver function preclude resection.[72] Even

Table 91–5 Treatment Options for Hepatocellular Carcinoma

Modality	Comments
Surgical resection	Offers best chance for cure but is seldom possible when the tumor is symptomatic
	May be technically difficult
	High recurrence rate after resection
Liver transplantation	May be successful in selected patients
	Requires transfer to a transplantation center and, postoperatively, lifelong immunosuppression
	High recurrence rate
	Expensive
Alcohol injection or radiofrequency ablation	Palliative for small (usually multiple) tumors that cannot be resected
	Confirmation that all the malignant cells have been destroyed may be difficult
Chemoembolization	May shrink selected tumors to the point that they may become resectable
	Effect is palliative for localized but unresectable tumors
Chemotherapy	Palliative only; can be used as an adjunct to surgical resection or transplantation
	Drug toxicity is common

patients with well-compensated cirrhosis may be better served by transplantation than by resection.[72] The early experience with transplantation was disappointing, with unacceptably high recurrence rates and short survival times after recurrence.[73] With more careful selection of patients, particular attention to tumor size and vascular invasion, and improved surgical techniques, perhaps with contributions from adjunctive anticancer treatment, better results have been obtained.[72,74,75] Nevertheless, relatively few patients are suitable for transplantation. Moreover, because of undetected spread of the tumor before transplantation, the rate of tumor recurrence remains high, particularly in patients with an unresectable tumor in a noncirrhotic liver.

Ablation and Embolization. Small tumors not amenable to resection because they are multiple or inaccessible or because of severe hepatic dysfunction have been treated with a variety of intralesional ablative techniques.[76] The first of these was ethanol injection, a relatively effective and safe technique that is still used.[77] Establishing that necrosis of tumor tissue is complete may be difficult after ethanol injection. An associated risk is dissemination of tumor by facilitating the passage of malignant cells into the bloodstream. More recently, radiofrequency ablation of the tumor has been shown to ablate these tumors effectively and is now widely used. Its complications and safety, however, have yet to be fully documented.

Arterial embolization and chemoembolization are additional palliative methods in selected patients.[78-81] They also are used to reduce the size of the tumor to make resection possible, or to allow a more conservative resection.

Chemotherapy. A large number of anticancer drugs, including alkylating agents, antitumor antibiotics, antimetabolites, plant alkaloids, platinum derivatives, and procarbazine, have been tried alone and in various combinations and by different routes of administration in the treatment of hepatocellular carcinoma, but response rates have invariably been less than 20%.[82] Because single agents have limited value in treating hepatocellular carcinoma, it is not surprising that combinations of these agents are also disappointing. Multidrug resistance is an important factor in the poor outcomes, and drugs that reverse this resistance are undergoing testing. Biologic response modifiers tested to date have not proved to be of value.

Screening for Small Presymptomatic Hepatocellular Carcinomas

Because symptomatic hepatocellular carcinoma seldom is amenable to surgical cure and responds poorly to conservative treatments, a pressing need exists either to prevent the tumor or to diagnose it at a presymptomatic stage when surgical intervention is still possible. Programs for detecting subclinical hepatocellular carcinomas are of two kinds: (1) screening whole populations with a high incidence of the tumor and (2) case-finding and long-term surveillance of persons at high risk for the development of hepatocellular carcinoma.[24] Mass population screening has rarely been attempted.[83] Case-finding and surveillance of high-risk persons are more feasible,[24] and these approaches have been shown to be cost-effective in countries with a high incidence of the tumor. Programs designed to detect and treat presymptomatic hepatocellular carcinomas should not be undertaken in countries that do not have the financial and human resources to treat the early tumors that are discovered. Case-finding and surveillance involves periodic ultrasonographic examination of the liver and testing of serum for alpha-fetoprotein, but difficulties are encountered. In addition to the limited sensitivity of serum alpha-fetoprotein levels in detecting presymptomatic hepatocellular carcinoma, slightly raised serum levels are difficult to interpret, because benign hepatic diseases that may be complicated by tumor formation also produce slight elevations.[24]

Ultrasonography is used for initial screening because it is noninvasive, carries no radiation hazard, and can be done quickly, cheaply, and repeatedly. With experienced operators and sophisticated equipment, tumors smaller than 1 cm in diameter can be visualized. Hepatocellular carcinomas discovered in this way frequently are hypoechoic, although the pattern changes as the tumor grows.[84] For persons at high risk (Table 91–6), ultrasonography and serum alpha-fetoprotein measurement should be performed at 4- or 6-month intervals, and for those at moderate risk, alpha-fetoprotein levels should be measured every 6 months and ultrasonography should be performed annually. Other imaging modalities (CT, MRI) similar in sensitivity to ultrasonography are used in doubtful cases or special circumstances. One problem encountered in monitoring programs is differentiating

Table 91–6   Factors Influencing Screening for Hepatocellular Carcinomas

Factor	Risk			Screening	
	High	**Moderate**	**Low**	**Yes**	**No**
HBV carriage					
Early onset	+			+	
Later onset		+			
Chronic HCV infection	+			+	
Hemochromatosis	+			+	
Membranous obstruction of the inferior vena cava (in black Africans)	+			+	
Cirrhosis of most other causes			+		+

HBV, hepatitis B virus; HCV, hepatitis C virus.

small hepatocellular carcinomas from benign hepatic lesions, especially regenerating nodules in cirrhotic livers and hemangiomas.[24]

Persons at risk for hepatocellular carcinoma should be counseled about (1) their chances of developing the tumor; (2) the limited treatment options available if a tumor develops; (3) the natural history and prognosis of the tumor; (4) the availability, advantages, and short-comings of surveillance programs; and (5) the results of treating subclinical tumors discovered in surveillance programs. Persons who agree to be monitored should be enrolled in a program. If the tumor detected during mon-itoring is small and accessible to surgery, and if hepatic function is adequate, surgical resection offers the best chance of cure.[24] Five-year survival rates of up to 68% have been achieved, although tumor recurrence, both intrahepatic and extrahepatic, is disturbingly frequent.

Prevention

Although great progress has been achieved in the primary prevention of HBV-induced hepatocellular carcinoma with the incorporation of vaccination against HBV in the Expanded Program of Immunization in many countries in which this virus is endemic and hepatocellular carci-noma is common, the full impact of this vaccination on the occurrence of the tumor will not be realized for many years. In the meantime, the huge numbers of existing HBV carriers worldwide remain at risk for hepatocellular carcinoma, and little progress has been made in prevent-ing malignant transformation in persons with chronic viral hepatitis. Nor has much progress has been made on other fronts. A vaccine against HCV will not be available in the near future, and prevention of aflatoxin-induced tumors is far from a becoming a reality in spite of ongoing trials of chemopreventive agents.

Intrahepatic Cholangiocarcinoma

Cholangiocarcinomas originate from small intrahepatic bile ducts (intrahepatic or peripheral cholangiocarcino-mas), large intrahepatic bile ducts (perihilar cholangio-carcinomas, or Klatskin tumors), or extrahepatic ducts (bile duct carcinomas) (see Chapter 66). Perihilar cholan-giocarcinomas are the most common, and peripheral cholangiocarcinomas are the least common.

Epidemiology and Etiology

The occurrence of intrahepatic cholangiocarcinoma shows geographic variation,[85,86] although not to the same extent as with hepatocellular carcinoma. Frequency rates relative to those for hepatocellular carcinoma range from 5% to 30%. The higher ratios are found in parts of the Far East, most notably northeastern Thailand, Hong Kong, Canton, Laos, and Cambodia, as well as in Eastern Europe and Russia. In all of these regions, chronic infes-tation of the biliary tree with one of the liver flukes (*Clonorchis sinensis* or *Opistorchis viverrini*) is causally related to the tumor.[87]

Although the etiology of intrahepatic cholangiocarci-noma is not known in most global cases, a number of risk factors, in addition to liver flukes, have been identified. Cholangiocarcinoma occasionally occurs years after patients have received the radiographic contrast agent thorium dioxide (Thorotrast) (see Chapter 84).[88] The tumor also may complicate long-standing primary scle-rosing cholangitis,[89] biliary atresia,[90] von Meyenburg complexes,[91] Caroli's disease,[86] choledochal cyst,[86] and intrahepatic cholelithiasis.[92] HBV or HCV infections, alcoholic cirrhosis, and aflatoxin exposure are not risk factors. For unknown reasons, the incidence of cholan-giocarcinoma has been increasing over the past 2 decades in Europe and North America.

At the molecular level, the most frequent changes in cholangiocarcinomas are mutations of the K-ras gene, and allelic loss or mutations of the p53, p16, and p73 genes also have been described.[86] In addition, increased telomerase activity may contribute to malignant trans-formation, as may overexpression of the mucin-1 antigen (MUC-1) gene.[86]

Intrahepatic cholangiocarcinomas are more common in older persons: The average age at presentation is between 50 and 60 years.[85,86] The occurrence rates in males and females are approximately equal.[85,86]

Clinical Features

Peripheral cholangiocarcinoma seldom produces symp-toms until the tumor is advanced. The clinical features are then similar to those of hepatocellular carcinoma, except that jaundice may be more frequent and promi-nent and occurs earlier in the course.[85,86] In addition, the liver tends not to be as enlarged, a bruit is not heard, and ascites, fever, and extrahepatic metastases are less common. The clinical presentation of perihilar cholan-giocarcinoma is one of progressive obstructive jaundice, with or without weight loss.[93]

Diagnosis

In perihilar cholangiocarcinoma, the biochemical picture is that of obstructive jaundice.[93] Elevated serum alkaline phosphatase, gamma glutamyl transpeptidase, and biliru-bin levels are more frequent in peripheral cholangiocarci-noma than in hepatocellular carcinoma, but the results of other liver biochemical tests are similar.[85,86] The tumors occasionally cause hypercalcemia in the absence of oste-olytic metastases, as a result of ectopic production of immunoreactive parathormone by the tumor.[94] Only occasionally is alpha-fetoprotein produced by cholangio-carcinoma.[85,86,93] CA 19-9 levels are raised in about 80% of affected patients, however, and CEA levels in about 50%.[86]

The appearance of peripheral cholangiocarcinoma on ultrasonography and CT is similar to that of hepatocellular carcinoma.[85,95] Gadolinium-enhanced MRI also is useful in defining these tumors.[96] Larger perihilar tumors and the resulting ductal dilatation can be seen with these imaging techniques. Endoscopic retrograde or transhepatic cholangiography localizes the site of perihilar tumors. In peripheral cholangiocarcinomas, a characteristic picture is evident on hepatic arteriography[85,96]; the marked desmoplastic reaction that typifies this tumor causes the branches of the hepatic artery to appear scanty, stretched, and attenuated.

Pathology

Peripheral cholangiocarcinoma usually is a large and solitary tumor, but it may be multinodular.[40,41,97] It is grayish-white, firm, and occasionally umbilicated. The tumor is poorly vascularized and rarely bleeds internally or ruptures. Vascular invasion and tumor necrosis also are less common than with hepatocellular carcinoma. Peripheral cholangiocarcinoma arises in a noncirrhotic liver. Perihilar cholangiocarcinoma may take the form of a firm, intramural tumor encircling the bile duct, a bulky mass centered on the duct or hilar region that radiates into the hepatic tissue, or a spongy friable mass within the lumen of the duct.[40,41,97] Metastatic nodules may be distributed irregularly throughout the liver. The bile ducts peripheral to the tumor may be dilated, and in long-standing cases, biliary cirrhosis may be present.

Microscopically, cholangiocarcinoma exhibits acinar or tubular structures resembling those of other adenocarcinomas.[40,41,97] Most tumors are well differentiated. Secretion of mucus may be demonstrable, but bile production is not seen. The tumor cells provoke a variable desmoplastic reaction, and in many tumors, the collagenized stroma may be the most prominent feature.

Peripheral cholangiocarcinoma often is complicated by intrahepatic metastases and tumor growth along the biliary tracts.[97] Metastases in regional lymph nodes occur in about 50% of cases.[97]

Treatment and Prognosis

Early diagnosis of peripheral cholangiocarcinoma is unusual, and the tumor carries the same poor prognosis as for hepatocellular carcinoma, with an annual mortality rate that is virtually identical to its annual incidence.[85,86] Resection is rarely possible, and the results of radiation therapy and chemotherapy are disappointing. Liver transplantation has been performed successfully in some patients. Recurrence rates are high after both resection and liver transplantation, however. Resection of a perihilar cholangiocarcinoma may be feasible, depending on its position and size, if it has not spread. Inoperable perihilar cholangiocarcinomas tend to progress more slowly than peripheral tumors.[94] For inoperable cases, biliary drainage must be established, usually by an endoscopic or radiologic approach (see Chapter 67). Photodynamic therapy also may be palliative.

Hepatoblastoma

Epidemiology

In children, hepatoblastoma is the third most common malignant tumor and the most common malignant hepatic tumor. It occurs almost exclusively in the first 3 years of life; boys are affected twice as often as girls.[40,41,98,99]

Clinical Features

Most children with hepatoblastoma come to medical attention because of abdominal swelling.[40,41,98,99] Other reasons include failure to thrive, weight loss, poor appetite, abdominal pain, irritability, and intermittent vomiting and diarrhea. The tumorous liver almost always is enlarged and firm and may be tender. Its surface is smooth or nodular. Pallor is common, but the patient seldom has jaundice. Hepatoblastomas rarely rupture. Distant metastases are evident, usually in the lung, in 20% of patients at the initial visit.[99] The tumor occasionally causes isosexual precocity in boys, as a result of the ectopic production of human chorionic gonadotropin.[100]

Diagnosis

Alpha-fetoprotein is present in high concentrations in the serum of 80% to 90% of patients with hepatoblastoma and is a useful clue to diagnosis.[98-101] Anemia is common, as is thrombocytosis, which is attributed to raised serum thrombopoietin levels.[98,99] Pulmonary metastases and, rarely, mottled calcification in the tumor may be seen on plain radiography. Ultrasonography is the most widely used initial imaging technique, although the findings are not specific. CT and MRI are used to define the extent of the tumor and to plan for definitive surgery. The tumor is seen as an avascular mass on hepatic arteriography.[98,99]

Pathology

Hepatoblastomas are the malignant derivatives of incompletely differentiated hepatocyte precursors. Their constituents are diverse, reflecting both the multipotentiality of their mesodermal origin and the progressive stages of embryonic and fetal development. Hepatoblastomas are classified morphologically into an *epithelial type*, composed predominantly of epithelial cells of varying maturity, and a *mixed epithelial and mesenchymal type*, which contains, in addition, tissues of mesenchymal derivation.[40,41,98,99] The tumors usually are solitary, ranging in diameter from 5 to 25 cm, and always well circumscribed (about one half are encapsulated). They vary in color, ranging from tan to grayish-white, and contain foci of hemorrhage, necrosis, and calcification. Vascular channels may be prominent on the capsular surface. Epithelial hepatoblastomas are solid, whereas tumors of the mixed variety often are separated into lobules by white bands of collagen tissue.

Two types of epithelial cells are present in the tumor.[40,41,98,99] Cells of the first type resemble *fetal* hepatocytes and are arranged in irregular plates, usually two cells thick, with bile canaliculi between individual cells and sinusoids between plates. The cytoplasm of the cells is eosinophilic and appears granular or vacuolated. Few mitotic figures are seen. Extramedullary hematopoiesis generally is present. Cells of the second type are *embryonal* and are less differentiated than the fetal type. They are weakly cohesive and usually arranged in sheets or ribbons. Individual cells are small, fusiform, and dark-staining with irregular, ill-defined outlines and scanty and amphophilic cytoplasm. The nuclei contain abundant chromatin and large nucleoli.

Mixed hepatoblastomas contain mesenchymal tissue consisting of areas of a highly cellular primitive type of mesenchyme intimately admixed with epithelial elements. The cells are elongated and spindle-shaped, with delicate processes arising from the tapering ends. The cytoplasm is scanty, and the nuclei are elongated but plump. In some areas of the tumor, the cells are intermediate between primitive mesenchyme and the acellular collagen of fibrous septa. The cells in these areas show parallel orientation, with collagen fibers between the cells. Cartilage and striated muscle may be present. Hepatoblastomas may show foci of squamous cells, with or without keratinization, and with foreign body–type giant cells. Vascular invasion may be evident. Metastases most commonly involve lung, abdominal lymph nodes, and brain.

Etiology and Pathogenesis

Environmental risk factors for hepatoblastoma have not been identified, and the pathogenesis is unclear. Reports of the co-occurrence of hepatoblastoma with familial adenomatous polyposis (FAP) and Beckwith-Wiedman syndrome suggest a possible role for chromosomes 5 and 11 in the genesis of the tumor.[99] The FAP tumor suppressor gene down-regulates β-catenin. Most patients with hepatoblatoma have mutations of the FAP gene, and a similar number have activating mutations of the β-catenin gene, raising the possibility that the wnt signaling pathway plays a role in the development of the tumor.

Treatment and Prognosis

Hepatoblastomas are rapidly progressive.[98,99] The *fetal* variety carries the least favorable prognosis; the *embryonal* and *mixed* types are associated with a slightly better outlook. If the lesion is solitary and sufficiently localized to be resectable, surgery often is curative, with 5-year survival rates as high as 75%.[98,99] The current practice is to pretreat the patient with cisplatin and doxorubicin. When the tumor is judged to be inoperable, neoadjuvant chemotherapy may reduce the size of the tumor sufficiently to permit resection.[99,102] Encouraging results also have been obtained with liver transplantation in patients with bilobar, multifocal tumors without extrahepatic extension.[103] If surgery is not an option, the prognosis generally is poor.

Angiosarcoma

Epidemiology

Although rare, angiosarcoma (also known as malignant hemangioendothelioma, hemangioendothelial sarcoma, or Kupffer cell sarcoma) is the most common malignant mesenchymal tumor of the liver.[40,41,104,105] It occurs almost exclusively in adults and is most prevalent in the sixth and seventh decades of life.[40,41,104,105] Men are affected four times as often as women.[40,41,104,105]

Pathogenesis

Despite its rarity, hepatic angiosarcoma is of special interest because specific risk factors have been identified, although no cause is discerned in the majority of tumors. In early reports, the tumor became evident approximately 20 years after the patient had been exposed to thorium dioxide (see Chapter 84).[106] Angiosarcoma also has occurred in German vintners who used arsenic-containing insecticides and drank wine adulterated with arsenic.[107] A few patients with angiosarcoma had taken potassium arsenite (Fowler's solution) for many years to treat psoriasis.[108] Hepatic angiosarcoma in workers exposed to vinyl chloride monomer (VCM) was first reported in 1974.[104,109,110] The monomer is converted by enzymes of the endoplasmic reticulum to reactive metabolites that form DNA adducts and G-to-A transitions in the *ras* and p53 genes.[110] Angiosarcomas have occurred after exposures of 11 to 37 years (or after shorter periods with a heavy initial exposure).[104,106,109] The mean age of patients at diagnosis is 48 years. In addition to angiosarcoma, persons exposed to VCM may be at increased risk of hepatocellular carcinoma and soft tissue sarcoma.[110]

Clinical Features

The most common presenting symptom is upper abdominal pain. Other frequent complaints are abdominal swelling, rapidly progressing liver failure, malaise, weight loss, poor appetite, and nausea.[104-106,110] Vomiting occurs occasionally. The duration of symptoms generally is between 1 week and 6 months, but a few patients have had symptoms for as long as 2 years before seeking medical attention.

The liver almost always is enlarged and usually is tender. Its surface may be irregular, or a definite mass may be felt.[104-106,110] An arterial bruit occasionally is heard over the enlarged liver. Splenomegaly may be present and is attributed to the hepatic fibrosis and consequent portal hypertension that also may complicate exposure to VCM. Ascites is frequent, and the fluid may be blood-stained. The patient often has jaundice. Fever and dependent edema are less common. Approximately 15% of patients present with acute hemoperitoneum following tumor rupture. Rarely, pulmonary or skeletal metastases are present.

Diagnosis

A rising serum bilirubin level and other evidence of progressive hepatic dysfunction may be present, especially in the later stages of the tumor.[104-106,110] Plain radiography may show pulmonary metastases, a raised right hemidiaphragm, or rarely, skeletal metastases. In patients who received thorium dioxide, radiopaque deposits of the material may be evident in the liver and spleen.[104-106,110] One or more mass lesions may be demonstrated on ultrasonography, CT, or MRI, but diffusely infiltrating tumor may not be visualized. Hepatic arteriography reveals a characteristic appearance[111]: The hepatic arteries are displaced by the tumor, which shows a blush and "puddling" during the middle of the arterial phase that persist for many seconds, except in the central area, which may be hypovascular.[111]

Complications and Prognosis

Hepatic angiosarcomas grow rapidly, and the prognosis is poor; death ensues within 6 months.[104-106,110] Patients may have thrombocytopenia resulting from entrapment of platelets within the tumor (Kasabach-Merritt syndrome),[105] disseminated intravascular coagulation with secondary fibrinolysis,[112] or microangiopathic hemolytic anemia as a result of fragmentation of erythrocytes within the tumor circulation.[113]

Pathology

Angiosarcomas usually are multicentric.[40,41,114] Their hallmark is the presence of blood-filled cysts, although solid growth also is seen. The lesions are fairly well circumscribed but not encapsulated. Larger masses are spongy and bulge beneath Glisson's capsule.

The earliest microscopic change is the presence of hypertrophic sinusoidal lining cells with hyperchromatic nuclei in ill-defined loci throughout the liver.[40,41,114] With progression of the lesion, sinusoidal dilatation and disruption of hepatic plates occur, and the malignant cells become supported by collagen tissue. Enlarging vascular spaces lined by malignant cells cause the tumor to become cavernous. The malignant endothelial cells usually are multilayered and may project into the cavity in intricate fronds and tufts supported by fibrous tissue. The fronds commonly are elongated, with ill-defined borders.[40,41,114] The cytoplasm is clear and faintly eosinophilic. Nuclei are hyperchromatic and vary greatly in size and shape; some cells are multinucleated. Evidence of phagocytosis may be seen. Foci of extramedullary hematopoiesis are common, and invasion of the portal and central veins occurs in most cases. Distant metastases are present in 50% of tumors.

Treatment

Operative treatment usually is precluded by the advanced stage of the tumor.[104,106] Even when surgery is undertaken, the patient commonly survives only 1 to 3 years,[104,106] although long-term survival may be achieved in the few patients with a solitary tumor. The results of irradiation and chemotherapy are poor.

Hepatic Metastases

The liver is the most frequent target for metastatic spread of tumors. Hepatic metastases occur in 40% to 50% of adult patients with extrahepatic primary malignancies.[40,115] Foremost among the reasons for the high frequency of hepatic metastases are the double blood supply of the liver and the presence of fenestrations in the sinusoidal endothelium that facilitate penetration of malignant cells into the hepatic parenchyma.[116] Hepatic metastases commonly originate from primary sites in the distribution of the portal venous system. Outside this distribution, tumors of the lung and the breast are the most common origins of hepatic metastases.[40,115]

Clinical Features

Symptoms resulting from hepatic metastases often are either absent or overshadowed by those of the primary tumor. Occasionally, the symptoms and signs attributable to metastases are the presenting manifestations of an asymptomatic primary tumor. In such cases, the likely symptoms are malaise, weight loss, and upper abdominal pain. Jaundice, when present, is seldom attributable to replacement of hepatic tissue by metastases. Depending on the extent of the metastatic disease, the liver may be enlarged, sometimes markedly. Its surface may be irregular, and umbilicated nodules may be felt by the examiner. A friction rub may be heard over hepatic metastases.

Diagnosis

Ultrasonography generally is used for initial screening, although CT is the most useful imaging technique.[117]

Multiphase helical CT and CT during arterial portography are more sensitive than conventional CT. Dynamic contrast-enhanced Doppler ultrasonography with intra-arterial infusion of CO_2 microbubbles also is useful in the diagnosis of hepatic metastases.[34] T1-weighted MRI also may be helpful, and iron oxide–enhanced MRI is even better. Hepatic arteriography shows most hepatic metastases to have a poor blood supply.

Pathology

Macroscopic Appearance. Hepatic metastases almost always are multiple.[40,115] Their pathologic features vary, depending on their site of origin. Metastases are expansive when they are discrete, or infiltrative. Individual metastases may reach a large size, and with multiple metastases, the liver may be greatly enlarged. Metastases commonly are gray-white and may show scattered hemorrhages or central necrosis. Individual metastases may be surrounded by a zone of venous stasis. Subcapsular lesions often are umbilicated. The dictum that cirrhotic livers are less likely than noncirrhotic livers to harbor metastatic deposits remains to be verified.

Microscopic Appearance. The microscopic features, including the degree of stromal growth, of most hepatic metastases duplicate those of the tumor of origin. Metastatic deposits usually are easily delineated from the surrounding liver tissue. Invasion of portal or hepatic veins may be seen, although less often than with hepatocellular carcinoma.[40,115]

Treatment and Prognosis

The extent of replacement of liver tissue by metastases generally determines the patient's prognosis. The greater the tumor burden, the worse the outlook, with only approximately 50% of patients surviving for 3 months after the onset of symptoms and less than 10% surviving more than 1 year.[118] Improved imaging modalities, advances in surgical techniques for resection and transplantation, and new chemotherapeutic agents and regional therapies have made it possible to achieve long-term survival in individual patients.[118] Long-term survival has been accomplished most often by resection of hepatic metastases in patients with colorectal cancer, a substantial number of whom have been cured or have obtained up to 20 years of disease-free survival.[118-120] If the primary tumor has been removed completely and metastases are confined to the liver, resection of hepatic metastases should be considered. Liver transplantation, with or without chemotherapy, has been performed in a few patients. Radiofrequency ablation is a valid alternative method to surgical resection in colorectal metastases. Other invasive methods of destroying metastases, such as ethanol injection, freezing with cryoprobes, and laser vaporization warrant further study. Radiation therapy and intra-arterial infusion of cytotoxic drugs have limited roles.

BENIGN LIVER TUMORS

Hepatocellular Adenoma

Epidemiology and Pathogenesis

Hepatocellular adenomas were extremely rare before the use of oral contraceptive steroids became widespread.

They are still rare in men, but the number of women in whom this tumor develops while they are taking contraceptive steroids, or thereafter, strongly implies a cause-and-effect relationship.[121-124] Nevertheless, in light of the large number of women who use this form of contraception, the risk of hepatocellular adenoma is small, and its occurrence implies some form of genetic predisposition.[124] The association is particularly strong with prolonged use of oral contraceptive steroids; the estimated risk for women who use oral contraceptive agents continuously for 5 to 7 years is 5 times the normal rate, and this risk increases to 25 times with use for longer than 9 years. Using preparations with a high hormone potency further increases the risk. Contraceptive pill–associated hepatocellular adenomas are more likely to develop in older than younger women.[121-124]

Hepatocellular adenomas have been linked to both types of synthetic estrogen and all forms of progestogen contained in oral contraceptive preparations.[121-124] Current evidence favors estrogens as the culprit, although progestogens may contribute through their enzyme-inducing properties. The growth of hepatocellular adenomas appears to be hormone dependent,[121-124] as evidenced by an increase in size during pregnancy and occasional instances of regression (and even disappearance) of the tumor after cessation of oral contraceptive use. Although hormonal replacement therapy has not proved to be associated with the development of hepatic adenoma, avoidance of this form of therapy in women with a history of oral contraceptive–related hepatic adenoma is prudent, unless compelling reasons to the contrary exist.

Hepatocellular adenomas and adenomatosis also may occur in persons receiving long-term anabolic androgenic steroids[40] and in those with certain inherited metabolic disturbances, especially type 1 glycogen storage disease, in which one or more hepatocellular adenomas occur in approximately 60% of patients.[123] Liver adenomatosis with maturity-onset diabetes of the young is associated with germ-line mutations in hepatocyte nuclear factor 1α.

Clinical Features

Hepatocellular adenomas manifest in a number of ways.[121-124] They may produce no symptoms and be discovered during routine physical examination if large, or during imaging of the upper abdomen for other reasons if small. Approximately one quarter of patients experience pain in the right hypochondrium or epigastrium. The pain usually is mild and ill defined but may be severe as a result of bleeding into or infarction of the tumor. If the liver is enlarged, the surface usually is smooth, and the liver may be slightly tender. The most alarming presentation is with an acute hemoperitoneum following rupture of the adenoma. This complication is not uncommon, especially with tumors linked to oral contraceptive use, and carries an appreciable mortality rate.[121-124] Tumors that rupture generally are large and solitary, although the most important determinant of rupture is a superficial location. Often, the affected woman is menstruating at the time.

Diagnosis

Serum alpha-fetoprotein concentrations are normal. Ultrasonography is used for initial imaging. Tissue harmonic imaging, which is obtained by receiving the second harmonic frequency signals, is capable of increased spatial and contrast resolution, with less acoustic artifact, in comparison with that on standard ultrasound examination, and has facilitated the detection of these (and other) tumors in obese persons.[34] Multiphase helical CT also may be used, although hepatic angiography is the most helpful aid to diagnosis.[124] Approximately 50% of hepatocellular adenomas are avascular, with draping of the hepatic arteries around the lesion; the remainder are hypervascular. The tumor has a clearly defined margin and, often, nearly parallel vessels entering it from the periphery ("spoke-wheel appearance"). Alternatively, the lesion may contain tortuous vessels coursing irregularly through it. When hypervascular, the adenoma may have focal avascular areas as a result of hemorrhage or necrosis. MRI may be a useful alternative to hepatic angiography in the diagnosis of hepatocellular adenomas. Because adenomas mimic normal liver tissue microscopically, needle biopsy and fine-needle aspiration may be of limited value.

Pathology

Hepatocellular adenoma generally occurs as a solitary, relatively soft, light brown to yellow tumor. It is sharply circumscribed but does not have a true capsule, although a pseudocapsule is formed by compression of the surrounding liver tissue[40,41,124,125] (Fig. 91–5A). Hepatocellular adenomas arise in an otherwise normal liver. Occasionally, two or more tumors are present. Adenomas range in diameter from 1 to 30 cm and are commonly 8 to 15 cm in diameter. They are larger on average in women taking contraceptive steroids than in those not taking contraceptive steroids and usually occupy a subcapsular position and project slightly from the surface of the liver. A pedunculated variety is seen occasionally. The cut surface of the tumor may show ill-defined lobulation but is never nodular or fibrotic. Foci of hemorrhage or necrosis are frequent, and bile staining may be evident.

Microscopically, hepatocellular adenoma may mimic normal liver tissue to an astonishing degree[40,41,124,125] (see Fig. 91-5B). The tumor is composed of sheets or cords of normal-looking or slightly atypical hepatocytes that show no features of malignancy. The cells occasionally have an acinar arrangement. The hepatocytes usually are slightly larger and may be paler than normal, with cytoplasm that is finely vacuolated or granular and may be loaded with glycogen. Eosinophilic inclusions containing α_1-antitrypsin often are present. The nuclei show minimal variation in structure or size. Sinusoids are focally dilated, and Kupffer cells are either markedly reduced in number or absent. Few or no portal tracts or central veins are present, and bile ducts are conspicuously absent. Only an infrequent fibrous or vascular septum traverses the lesion. An essentially normal reticulin pattern is demonstrable throughout the adenoma. The walls of arteries and veins are thickened. Some areas with vascular abnormalities are infarcted, and thrombi may be seen. Peliosis hepatis may be found in relation to the tumor.

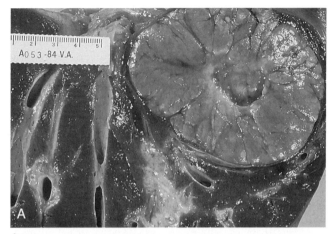

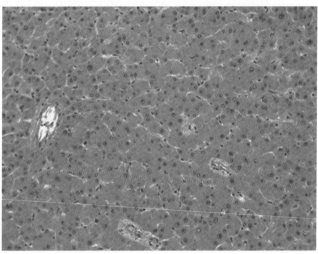

Figure 91–5 *A,* Surgical specimen of a large hepatocellular adenoma. The tumor is yellowish and slightly lobular with a central cavitation and a pseudocapsule. (Courtesy of Edward Lee, MD, Washington, DC.) *B,* Photomicrograph of a hepatocellular adenoma showing the resemblance to normal liver tissue, with cords of normal-looking, although generally slightly larger, hepatocytes as well as Kupffer cells (but fewer in number than normal) lining the sinusoids. Bile ducts and central veins are not seen, but the presence of abnormal vascular structures is evident. (Courtesy of Professor A. C. Paterson, Johannesburg, South Africa.)

Treatment and Prognosis

Because of the danger that a hepatocellular adenoma may rupture, surgical treatment is recommended.[125] Resection usually is feasible in an uncomplicated case. When rupture has occurred, emergency resection should be performed if possible. (It may be necessary to clamp the hepatic artery first to stop the bleeding.) If resection cannot be accomplished, the hepatic artery should be ligated. Whether or not the tumor is removed, the patient must refrain from taking oral contraceptive steroids. If the adenoma is not resected, pregnancy should be avoided.

Hepatocellular carcinoma occurs in a small number of women taking oral contraceptive steroids,[61,126] and it is speculated that hepatocellular adenomas might undergo malignant transformation. Indeed, this sequence has been documented in a few instances.[127] Therefore, managing hepatocellular adenomas merely by discontinuing the use of contraceptive steroids carries the risk that malignant transformation may still occur.

Cavernous Hemangioma

Epidemiology

Cavernous hemangioma is the most common benign tumor of the liver and is found in as many as 7% of autopsies.[40,125] The lesion is thought to be a congenital malformation or hamartoma that increases in size, initially with growth of the liver and thereafter by ectasia. Cavernous hemangiomas affect persons of all ages, although they manifest most often in the third, fourth, and fifth decades of life. Women are predominantly affected (4:1 to 6:1) and often present at a younger age and with larger tumors, in comparison with men.[40,125] Cavernous hemangiomas increase in size with pregnancy or the administration of estrogens and are more common in multiparous than in nulliparous women.[40,125]

Clinical Features

The great majority of cavernous hemangiomas are small and asymptomatic and are discovered incidentally during imaging of the liver for another reason, at autopsy, or at laparotomy.[40,125] Larger or multiple lesions produce symptoms. Those larger than 4 cm in diameter are called *giant cavernous hemangiomas,* which may be as large as 27 cm. Upper abdominal pain is the most common complaint and results from partial infarction of the lesion or pressure on adjacent tissues. Early satiety, nausea, and vomiting also may occur. Cavernous hemangiomas occasionally rupture. The only physical finding may be an enlarged liver. Occasionally, an arterial bruit is heard over the tumor. Arteriovenous shunting has been described with cavernous hemangiomas.

Diagnosis

The ultrasonographic appearance is variable and nonspecific, although the lesion usually is echogenic.[128] Provided that the cavernous hemangioma is larger than 3 cm in diameter, single photon emission computed tomography (SPECT) with colloid ^{99m}Tc-labeled red blood cells shows the tumor to be highly vascular and has a sensitivity and accuracy similar to that of MRI[129] (Fig. 91–6). Almost all cavernous hemangiomas can be diagnosed by bolus-enhanced CT with sequential scans.[128] The center of the lesion remains hypodense, whereas the peripheral zone, which varies in thickness and may have a corrugated inner margin, is enhanced. MRI has a high degree of specificity and a central role in the diagnosis of small hemangiomas (Fig. 91–7).[130] Another useful investigation is hepatic arteriography.[128] The branches of the hepatic artery may be displaced and crowded together or stretched around the lesion; however, they taper normally. Early opacification of irregular areas, or lakes, is seen and the contrast material persists in these lakes long after arterial emptying. With small hemangiomas, the contrast material may assume a ring-shaped or C-shaped configuration, with an avascular center resulting from fibrous obliteration; this appearance is pathognomonic.

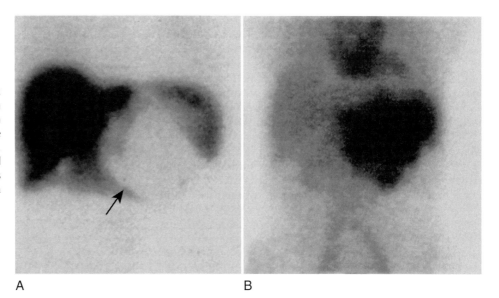

Figure 91–6 *A,* Anterior view of a conventional tin-colloid liver scan showing the presence of a mass lesion *(arrow)* replacing the left lobe of the liver and part of the right lobe. *B,* Anterior view of a ⁹⁹ᵐTc-labeled red blood cell scan performed 48 hours later showing that the mass lesion is a giant cavernous hemangioma.

A   B

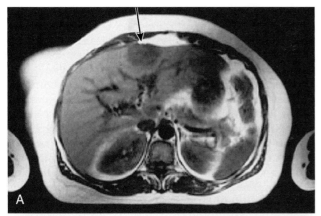

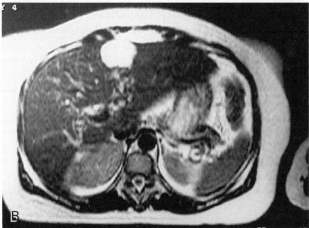

Figure 91–7 Magnetic resonance image of a small cavernous hemangioma in the liver *(arrow)*. *A,* A T1-weighted image shows a rounded mass with a uniform increase in T1 signal intensity (low signal). *B,* A heavily T2-weighted image shows a mass with a uniform increase in signal intensity (bright signal relative to the water signal of cerebrospinal fluid). (Courtesy of Dr. P. Sneider, Johannesburg, South Africa.)

Thrombocytopenia resulting from sequestration and destruction of platelets in large hemangiomas (Kasabach-Merritt syndrome) is seen occasionally in children but rarely in adults.[131] Hypofibrinogenemia, attributed to fibrin deposition in the tumor with secondary fibrinolysis, also is described.[132] Malignant transformation has not been reported.

Because of the risk of severe bleeding, percutaneous needle biopsy should not be performed if a cavernous hemangioma is suspected. Moreover, a needle biopsy is of limited diagnostic value.

Pathology

Cavernous hemangiomas usually are solitary lesions, although multiple tumors occur in 10% of patients.[40,41,125] Reddish-purple or bluish masses are seen under Glisson's capsule or deep in the substance of the liver. The larger lesions may be pedunculated. Cavernous hemangiomas are well circumscribed but seldom encapsulated. They may show central necrosis, and in some instances, the whole tumor is firm in consistency and grayish-white in appearance. Microscopically, hemangiomas are composed of multiple vascular channels of varying sizes lined by a single layer of flat epithelium and supported by fibrous septa.[40,41,125] The vascular spaces may contain thrombi.

Occasionally, cavernous hemangiomas are associated with hemangiomas in other organs. They also may coexist with cysts in the liver or pancreas,[133] von Meyenburg complexes (see later),[134] or focal nodular hyperplasia (see later).[135]

Treatment

The great majority of cavernous hemangiomas can safely be left alone. A cavernous hemangioma that is large but localized, and the cause of incapacitating symptoms, should be resected.[136] If resection is not feasible, reduction in the size of the tumor with relief of symptoms is rarely achieved with irradiation, arterial ligation, arteriographic embolization, or systemic glucocorticoids.[137,138]

Radiofrequency ablation has been used with some success. If a cavernous hemangioma has ruptured, it may be necessary to embolize or clamp the hepatic artery to stop bleeding before proceeding to resection.

Infantile Hemangioendothelioma

Epidemiology and Clinical Features

Although rare, benign infantile hemangioendothelioma (also known as multinodular hepatic hemangiomatosis) is the most common tumor of the liver in infants. Its importance stems from the high incidence of congestive heart failure in infants with this tumor and the resulting 70% mortality rate. The tumor almost invariably manifests in the first 6 months of life and is twice as common in girls as in boys.[40,123,139,140] Hepatic hemangioendothelioma often coexists with hemangiomas in other organs, especially the skin (in approximately 50% of patients). When hemangiomas are present in three or more organs, the condition is referred to as diffuse neonatal hemangiomatosis.

Small hemangioendotheliomas invariably are asymptomatic.[123,139,140] The presence of a large lesion is recognized clinically by the diagnostic triad of an enlarged liver, high-output cardiac failure, and multiple cutaneous hemangiomas.[123,139,140] The liver is larger than expected on the basis of the severity of the cardiac failure, and hepatomegaly persists after the heart failure has been treated successfully. When hemangioendotheliomas occur diffusely throughout the liver, as they usually do, their combined effect is to act as a large peripheral arteriovenous shunt. Shunts of this size are responsible for the cardiac failure.[123,139,140] Approximately one third of patients have jaundice. Patients may be anemic, owing in part to the dilutional effect of the increased circulating plasma volume that develops with large peripheral arteriovenous fistulas. A microangiopathic hemolytic anemia may contribute.[140] In addition, thrombocytopenia may be present (Kasabach-Merritt syndrome).[140] Malignant change is a rare complication.[40]

Diagnosis

Ultrasonography may show one or more echogenic masses in the liver. Hepatic angiography is particularly helpful in diagnosis and shows stretching, but not displacement, of the intrahepatic arteries.[141] Abnormal vessels arise from the hepatic arteries and promptly opacify the liver, thereby giving rise to the characteristic blush of an arteriovenous shunt. The circulation time through the liver is short. Focal avascular areas may be evident when hemorrhage into or necrosis of the tumor has occurred. CT with enhancement and MRI are as specific as hepatic arteriography for the diagnosis of hemangioendotheliomas. Percutaneous biopsy is contraindicated because of the danger of bleeding.

Pathology

Infantile hemangioendotheliomas typically are multifocal and produce a nodular deformity of the entire liver.[40,41,125,139,140] The nodules range in size from a few millimeters to many centimeters and are well demarcated but not encapsulated. At laparotomy, the nodules can be seen to pulsate. They are reddish purple, although large tumors are gray to tan. They may show hemorrhages, fibrosis, or calcification.

Microscopically, infantile hemangioendothelioma is composed of layers of plump endothelial cells.[40,41,125,139,140] A single layer characterizes a *type I pattern*, whereas several layers characterize a *type II pattern*. In some areas of the tumor, solid masses of mesoblastic primordial cells that differentiate early into vascular structures are observed. Fibrous septa may be prominent, and extramedullary hematopoiesis occurs frequently. Thrombosis may be followed by scarring and calcification.

Treatment and Prognosis

The course of infantile hemangioendothelioma is characterized by tumor growth during the early months of life, followed by gradual involution.[140] If the child survives, the tumor involutes completely. Life-threatening aspects of the disorder are intractable congestive heart failure and, to a lesser extent, consumptive coagulopathy or rupture of the tumor. Cardiac failure should be treated by conventional means initially, but if these measures fail, more aggressive forms of treatment, such as embolization, ligation of the hepatic artery, surgical resection, or liver transplantation should be considered.[139,140,142] Use of glucocorticoids has been successful in many (but not all) patients,[143] whereas irradiation has seldom been beneficial. When the tumor is confined to one lobe, surgical resection is curative, even in the presence of cardiac failure.[140,141]

TUMOR-LIKE HEPATIC LESIONS

FOCAL NODULAR HYPERPLASIA

Focal nodular hyperplasia is a circumscribed, usually solitary lesion composed of nodules of benign hyperplastic hepatocytes surrounding a central stellate fibrous scar.[39,40]

Epidemiology and Pathogenesis

Although rare, focal nodular hyperplasia is more common than hepatocellular adenoma. The lesion is seen more often in women than in men, although the gender difference is less striking than that with hepatocellular adenoma.[121-123] Focal nodular hyperplasia occurs at all ages, but most patients present in the third and fourth decades of life[121-123]; the age distribution is similar to that of hepatocellular adenomas. The two lesions may coexist.

The cause of focal nodular hyperplasia is unknown. Abnormalities in arteries in small and medium-sized portal tracts have been described, and an ischemic origin, related to vascular malformation, is probable. A role for oral contraceptive steroids in the development of the lesion was suggested, but no unequivocal evidence is available to support this association.[121-123] Nevertheless, some evidence suggests that focal nodular hyperplasia is hormone dependent.[121-123,144] Contraceptive steroids may accentuate the vascular abnormalities in focal nodular hyperplasia and cause the lesion to enlarge, become more symptomatic, and, rarely, rupture.

Clinical Features

Most of these lesions do not produce symptoms and are discovered during upper abdominal imaging for other reasons or because an enlarged liver is felt on routine examination or found during abdominal surgery or at autopsy.[121-123] Patients may experience mild pain, particularly with bleeding into or necrosis of the lesion. This presentation is more common in patients taking contraceptive steroids than in those not taking these drugs.[121-123] Focal nodular hyperplasia seldom ruptures, even in patients taking oral contraceptive steroids.

Diagnosis

Serum alpha-fetoprotein levels are normal. The mass lesion seen on ultrasonography and CT is not specific for focal nodular hyperplasia,[124] although the central scar may be seen (Fig. 91–8). The picture obtained with dynamic contrast-enhanced Doppler ultrasonography with intra-arterial infusion of CO_2 microbubbles is, however, characteristic.[34] Selective hepatic arteriography shows one or more highly vascular lesions.[124,145] The vessels within the lesion are tortuous. In approximately 50% of the cases, septation of the mass is visible during the capillary phase, which also is characterized by irregular granularity. Distinguishing focal nodular hyperplasia from hepatocellular adenoma on the basis of the arteriographic findings is often impossible, however.

Pathology

Focal nodular hyperplasia manifests as a firm, coarsely nodular light brown or yellowish-gray mass of variable size with a dense, central stellate scar and radiating fibrous septa that divide the lesion into lobules.[40,41,121-123,145] The nodule may be small, resembling a cirrhotic nodule, or extremely large. The lesion of focal nodular hyperplasia usually occupies a subcapsular position and may be pedunculated. It generally is solitary. Larger lesions may show foci of hemorrhage or necrosis, although these features are seen less frequently than in hepatocellular adenomas. The fibrous septa sometimes are poorly developed, and the central scar may be absent. The lesion is sharply demarcated from the surrounding liver tissue, which is normal, but a true capsule is absent. Focal nodular hyperplasia is associated with hepatic hemangiomas in as many as 20% of cases.

Microscopically, focal nodular hyperplasia closely resembles inactive cirrhosis.[40,41,121-123,145] Individual hepatocytes are indistinguishable from those of normal liver but lack the normal cord arrangement in relation to sinusoids, central veins, and portal tracts. The cytoplasm is finely granular but may be vacuolated. Kupffer cells are present. Characteristically, the fibrous septa contain numerous bile ductules and vessels. Other features include heavy infiltrations of lymphocytes and, to a lesser extent, plasma cells and histiocytes. Bile duct proliferation in portal tracts also may be evident. Branches of the hepatic artery and portal vein show various combinations of intimal and smooth muscle hyperplasia, subintimal fibrosis, thickening of the wall, occlusive luminal lesions, and, at times, occluding thrombosis. Whether these vascular changes are primary or secondary is not known. Peliosis hepatis may be an associated lesion. The histologic features almost always make it possible to distinguish focal nodular hyperplasia from hepatocellular adenoma, although the distinction may be extremely difficult in a few instances.

Treatment

Large symptomatic or complicated lesions should be resected, usually by segmental resection or enucleation. Recurrence after resection is rare. Otherwise, focal nodular hyperplasia should be left alone. If the lesion is not resected, discontinuation of contraceptive steroids is recommended and may result in regression of the lesion. Periodic ultrasonography should be performed if a firm diagnosis of focal nodular hyperplasia has not been made, and a lesion seen to increase substantially in size should be resected. The available evidence militates against a concept of focal nodular hyperplasia as a premalignant condition.

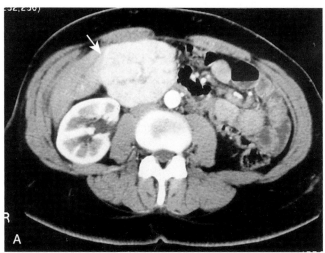

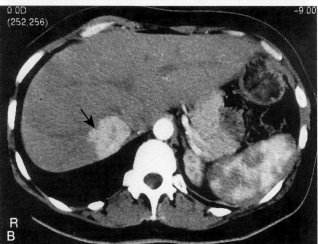

Figure 91–8 Contrast-enhanced computed tomography scans in a 41-year-old woman with two lesions of focal nodular hyperplasia, one (arrow) in the left hepatic lobe (A), the other (arrow) in the right (B). The central stellate scar with radiating bands of fibrosis can be seen in each of the lesions.

OTHER NODULAR DISORDERS

Nodular regenerative hyperplasia is characterized by nodularity of the liver without fibrosis[40] (see Chapter 34). This rare condition may be associated with a number of diseases, such as rheumatoid arthritis and Felty's syndrome. Although generally diffuse, the nodularity occasionally is focal, in which case the lesion may be mistaken for a tumor. Patients with nodular regenerative hyperplasia typically present clinically with portal hypertension. Partial nodular transformation is characterized by nodules that are limited to the perihilar region of the liver. These patients also present with portal hypertension.[40,41]

Macroregenerative nodules may occur in advanced cirrhosis or after massive hepatic necrosis. They are believed to be premalignant conditions and may, in addition, be mistaken for hepatic tumors during hepatic imaging. Inflammatory pseudotumor is a rare entity, resulting from focal infection, that may be mistaken for a hepatic tumor (see Chapter 79).[41] It occurs particularly in young men, who present with intermittent fever, abdominal pain, jaundice, vomiting, and diarrhea. Leukocytosis, an elevated erythrocyte sedimentation rate, and polyclonal hyperglobulinemia are present in approximately 50% of the patients. The lesion may be solitary or multiple and shows a mixture of chronic inflammatory cells, with plasma cells predominating. Focal fatty infiltration, or focal fatty sparing in the presence of diffuse fatty infiltration, may also be mistaken for a hepatic tumor (see Chapter 82).[146]

HEPATIC CYSTS

Hepatic cysts are of three main types: hydatid cysts, a group of conditions collectively known as fibrocystic disease of the liver, and solitary congenital cysts. Hydatid cysts are discussed in Chapter 79.

FIBROCYSTIC DISEASES OF THE LIVER

Fibrocystic diseases of the liver originate from abnormal persistence or defects in the progressive remodeling of the ductal plate. The result is ductal plate malformation, with variations that give rise to a spectrum of congenital diseases of the intrahepatic bile ducts[147,148] (see also Chapter 59). Fibrocystic disorders of the liver described here include polycystic liver disease, solitary congenital cysts, Caroli's disease (type V choledochal cyst), and von Meyenburg complexes. (The other diseases are congenital hepatic fibrosis and type IV choledochal cysts.)

Polycystic Liver Disease

Polycystic liver disease may manifest in childhood as an autosomal recessive disorder that is usually rapidly fatal as a consequence of the associated (autosomal recessive) polycystic kidney disease (ARPKD).[149,150] A proportion of the patients maintain renal function into adulthood, however, and complications of the associated liver disease then predominate. The liver cysts are microscopic, rather than macroscopic, and present a clinical picture indistinguishable from that of congenital hepatic fibrosis. Complications of portal hypertension are the usual hepatic manifestations of the disease.[149,150] The gene responsible for this disease, *PKHD1*, has been

identified at chromosomal locus 6p21-cen, and the ARPKD protein, fibrocystin, is predicted to be an integral receptor-like protein.[151] Many different mutations throughout the gene have been identified in patients with ARPKD.

More commonly, multiple cysts of the liver are diagnosed in adulthood. They present either in association with autosomal dominant polycystic kidney disease (ADPKD)[149,150] or as isolated polycystic liver disease.[152,153] The gene affected in ADPKD1 is located on the short arm of chromosome 16 at locus q13-q23 and expresses a ubiquitous protein, polycystin-1.[154,155] The gene responsible for ADPKD2 is located on chromosome 4 and expresses polycystin-2.[154,155] The two polycystins are believed to work in concert to regulate calcium flux and cell signaling. Isolated polycystic liver disease has been shown in North American and Finnish families to be linked to chromosomal locus 19p13.2-13.1,[155] although other loci undoubtedly exist.

ADPKD carries a better prognosis than that for the recessive variety.[149,150,152,153] Polycystic kidney disease has a more deleterious effect on kidney function than that of polycystic liver disease on hepatic function and largely determines the outcome. Hepatic cysts, which manifest later in life than do the renal cysts, usually are diagnosed in the fourth or fifth decade of life.[149,150,152,153,156] The size and number of cysts correlate with the patient's age, severity of renal disease, and worsening renal function. Women tend to have larger and more numerous cysts, and a correlation with the number of pregnancies has been found. The use of exogenous female sex hormones may accelerate the rate of growth and size of the cysts. In the autosomal dominant variety, cysts also may be present in the pancreas, spleen, and, less often, other organs. In addition, autosomal dominant polycystic liver disease may coexist with the other fibropolycystic liver diseases, such as congenital hepatic fibrosis (in which the patient is likely to present with portal hypertension), Caroli's disease, or von Meyenburg complexes,[149,150,152,153,156] as well as other conditions such as berry aneurysms, mitral valve prolapse, diverticular disease, and inguinal hernias.

The hepatic cysts in polycystic liver disease, whether or not they occur in association with renal cysts, rarely cause morbidity, and many affected patients are asymptomatic.[149,150,152,153,156] The livers of these patients contain only a few cysts or cysts smaller than 2 cm in diameter. With the more widespread use of hepatic imaging, asymptomatic cysts are being discovered more often now than in the past. Symptoms occur in patients with more numerous and larger cysts (10% to 15% of patients, almost always women), usually as abdominal discomfort or pain, postprandial fullness, awareness of an upper abdominal mass, a protuberant abdomen, and shortness of breath. Severe pain may be experienced with rupture or infection of a cyst, bleeding into a cyst, or torsion of a pedunculated cyst. The liver is enlarged in approximately 80% of patients. The associated polycystic kidneys also often are palpable. Jaundice is evident in approximately 5% of patients and is caused by compression of the major intrahepatic or extrahepatic bile ducts. Ascites, if present, is the result of portal hypertension, which generally is caused by the associated congenital hepatic fibro-

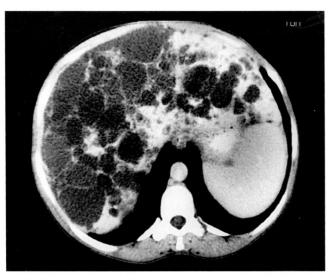

Figure 91–9 Computed tomography scan of the abdomen in a patient with severe autosomal dominant (adult) polycystic liver disease.

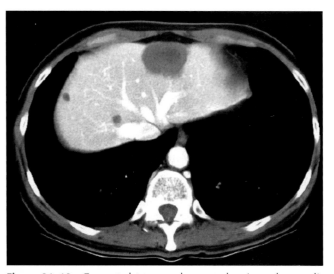

Figure 91–10 Computed tomography scan showing a large solitary congenital cyst in the liver.

sis but occasionally by compression of the hepatic veins by the cysts.

Liver biochemical test results generally are not abnormal, although serum alkaline phosphatase and gamma glutamyl transpeptidase levels may be increased. A raised right hemidiaphragm may be evident on a plain radiograph of the chest in severe polycystic liver disease. The diagnosis of polycystic liver disease is confirmed by ultrasound examination or CT (Fig. 91–9). Hepatic arteriography shows multiple avascular lesions with displacement of the vessels.

The cysts range in diameter from a few millimeters to 10 cm or more. They contain clear, colorless, or straw-colored fluid and are lined by a single layer of cuboidal or columnar epithelium, resembling that of bile ducts.[149,150,152,153,156] Rarely, the cysts may be lined by squamous epithelium, and these cysts may be complicated by the development of squamous cell carcinoma. In addition to the nature of the lining epithelium, evidence for a biliary origin of these cysts is suggested by the composition of the cystic fluid, which has a low glucose content and contains secretory immunoglobulin A and gamma glutamyl transpeptidase. The cysts are thought to arise as a result of ductal plate malformation. This process gives rise to von Meyenburg complexes, which become disconnected from the biliary tree during development and growth and dilate progressively to form cysts.[149,150,152,153,156]

On the rare occasions when a cyst requires treatment, fenestration (unroofing) should be performed.[149,157] Cyst fenestration originally was done at laparotomy but is now performed laparoscopically. A high recurrence rate is observed for cysts treated in this way. Cysts also have been treated by percutaneous injection of sclerosing substances such as alcohol or doxycycline, but most patients have too many cysts of small size to warrant this approach. Patients who fail to respond to cyst fenestration may be considered for partial hepatic resection or liver transplantation (sometimes combined with renal transplantation). Patients with severe symptoms also may be considered for transarterial embolization.

Solitary Non-Parasitic Cysts

Solitary non-parasitic hepatic cysts are congenital in origin and relatively common, occurring in up to 3.6% of the population. They generally are less than 5 cm in diameter (Fig. 91–10) and typically are asymptomatic.[158] The cysts usually are discovered incidentally during upper abdominal imaging. Solitary cysts occur more often in women than in men, and their diagnosed prevalence increases with age. Larger cysts or those complicated by intracystic bleeding or infection may produce discomfort or pain. Complications of intracystic bleeding or infection, rupture, or compression of adjacent organs are rare.

Asymptomatic solitary hepatic cysts should be left alone. If intervention is required, percutaneous aspiration and sclerosis with alcohol or doxycycline will almost always ablate the cyst, but recurrence is frequent.[158] An alternative approach is laparoscopic (or, rarely, open surgical) fenestration, which is seldom followed by recurrence.

Von Meyenburg Complexes

Von Meyenburg complexes (also known as biliary microhamartomas) are common and do not produce symptoms; they are small and usually multiple. Each complex is composed of cystically dilated intra- and interlobular bile ducts embedded in a fibrous stroma.[41,66] The cysts are lined by cuboidal or flat epithelium. They occur in almost all patients with congenital hepatic fibrosis and may coexist with Caroli's disease or ADPKD. Von Meyenburg complexes are found in or adjacent to portal tracts and are believed to arise as a result of malformation of the ductal plate (see Chapter 59). They may be complicated by the development of peripheral cholangiocarcinoma.[92]

Caroli's Disease

Caroli's disease is a rare disorder characterized by congenital nonobstructive gross dilatation of the segmental intrahepatic bile ducts.[40,158-160] It has been included in the classification of choledochal cysts (type V)[149,158] and may occur in association with either medullary sponge kidney (in 60% to 80% of patients) or congenital hepatic fibrosis (see Chapter 59).[40] Caroli's disease is believed to be caused by an intrauterine event that arrests ductal plate remodeling at the level of the larger intrahepatic bile ducts.[148] The resulting bile duct ectasia may be diffuse or localized. Both autosomal recessive and autosomal dominant modes of inheritance have been proposed. Caroli's disease affects men and women equally and usually becomes symptomatic in early adulthood; greater than 80% of patients present with symptoms before the age of 30 years.

Patients typically present with recurrent episodes of fever and abdominal pain caused by cholangitis. The liver often is enlarged. Ductal ectasia predisposes to bile stagnation, which in turn may lead to cholangitis, abscess formation, and septicemia.[159,160] Gallstones form in the ectatic ducts in one third of patients.[159,160] The result of these complications may be cholangiocarcinoma, which develops in less than 10% of patients.

Caroli's disease usually is discovered when the liver is imaged during investigation of suspected cholangitis. Irregular dilatations of the larger intrahepatic bile ducts are seen.

Attacks of cholangitis require treatment with antibiotics. Endoscopic retrograde catheterization of the biliary system may be used to remove sludge or stones from the accessible part of the biliary system, and the cysts may be drained by means of an endoscopic or percutaneous route. Localized forms of the disease may be treated by surgical resection.[161] Liver transplantation has been performed in patients with recurrent bouts of cholangitis unresponsive to endoscopic or radiologic intervention or with complications of associated congenital hepatic fibrosis.

OTHER CYSTIC DISEASES OF THE LIVER

Peliosis Hepatis

Peliosis hepatis is characterized by the presence of blood-filled lakes of various sizes in the hepatic parenchyma that may or may not be lined by epithelium.[41,162] The lesions may be diffuse or focal. They occur in a variety of chronic diseases, such as malnutrition, tuberculosis, acquired immunodeficiency syndrome, and a number of malignant diseases and also are associated with long-term administration of anabolic androgenic steroids and estrogens (see also Chapters 32 and 83).

Mild forms of the disease produce no symptoms or signs, but severe peliosis hepatis manifests with hepatomegaly, hepatic failure, rupture with hemoperitoneum, ascites, and esophageal varices and is associated with a poor prognosis. Treatment is directed to the underlying cause, including drug withdrawal, with partial hepatic resection or liver transplantation occasionally required.

APPROACH TO THE PATIENT WITH A HEPATIC MASS LESION

The approach to the diagnosis of a liver harboring a mass lesion will be influenced by the age and gender of the patient and the presence or absence of symptoms (Fig. 91–11). Making a definite diagnosis of a mass lesion in the liver solely on clinical grounds is seldom possible. Nevertheless, a detailed history will provide important clues to the probable benign or malignant nature of the lesion. Additional clues may be obtained by assessment for various risk factors, such as chronic infection with hepatitis B or C virus, a diet contaminated by aflatoxin or with a high iron content, hemochromatosis, long-term use of oral contraceptive or anabolic androgenic steroids, exposure to VCMs, or residence in a region where amebic liver abscesses are common. Likewise, certain diagnoses can be excluded in the absence of a particular risk factor, as with hydatid cysts in the absence of contact with a definitive host for the causative worm.

Patients known to have chronic hepatic parenchymal disease in whom a solid liver mass develops should be presumed to have hepatocellular carcinoma until proven otherwise. Neoplastic and non-neoplastic masses may mimic each other in their clinical presentations. For example, patients with an amebic (or pyogenic) liver abscess and those with hepatocellular carcinoma may present with a short history of upper abdominal pain, fever, and tender hepatomegaly (see Chapter 79). Although a liver enlarged by a mass lesion may show features that favor a particular pathologic condition, such as umbilication with hepatic metastases, an arterial bruit with hepatocellular carcinoma, or a friction rub with metastases or abscesses, these findings usually are insufficient to support a firm diagnosis. Severe muscle wasting obviously favors a malignant tumor but does not specify its nature. Moreover, some benign hepatic diseases, such as tuberculous hepatitis and chronic amebic abscess, also can cause wasting. Evidence of extrahepatic metastases indicates that the patient has a malignant disease, although the primary tumor may not necessarily be in the liver. The presence of cutaneous hemangiomas in a child with mass lesions in the liver points strongly to a diagnosis of infantile hemangioendothelioma.

The circumstances in which the mass lesion becomes evident also must be considered. With the increasing use of sophisticated imaging modalities, more asymptomatic hepatic lesions are being discovered. Although these lesions may prove to be malignant, the great majority are benign. Subclinical malignant tumors must not be missed, because they are the ones most amenable to cure. Likewise, subclinical benign lesions should be diagnosed, because some may cause life-threatening complications, such as rupture of a hepatocellular adenoma.

Because making a specific diagnosis at the bedside is difficult, available investigations must be used rationally to arrive at the correct diagnosis with the least delay and without undue cost. The approach must take into consideration the likely diagnosis and the expected treatment and prognosis. Plain radiographs of the chest should always be obtained, because they may show a raised right hemidiaphragm (especially with hepatocellular carcinoma and amebic liver abscess), pulmonary metastases, hydatid cysts, or calcification in the liver. Conventional liver biochemical tests are of limited use in the differential diagnosis. Raised serum alkaline phosphatase and gamma glutamyl transpeptidase levels in the presence of normal or slightly elevated serum bilirubin

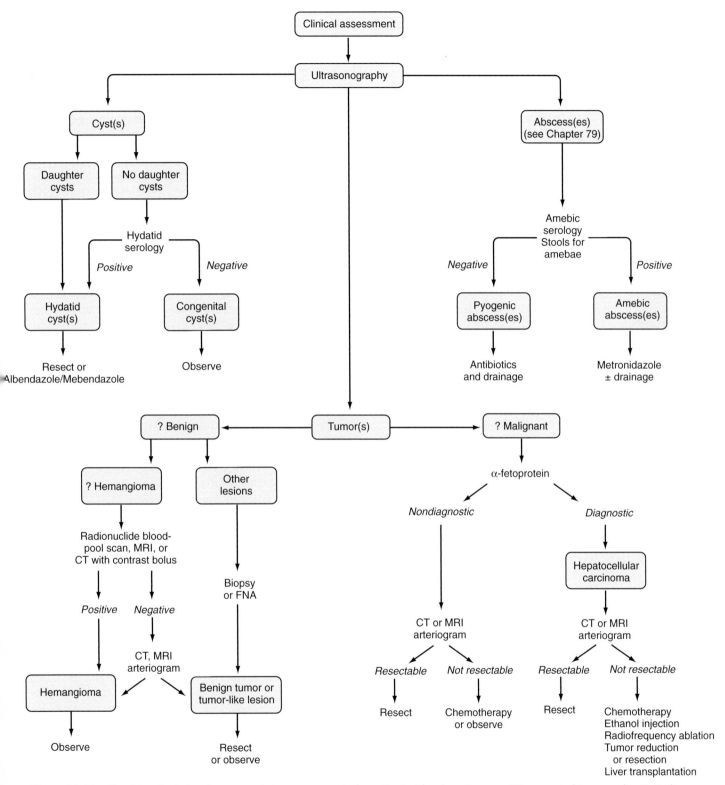

Figure 91–11 Algorithm depicting the approach to management of a patient with a hepatic mass. CT, computed tomography; FNA, fine-needle aspiration; MRI, magnetic resonance imaging.

and aminotransferase levels, however, suggest the presence of a space-occupying or infiltrative lesion in the liver.

Ultrasonography generally is the first imaging study performed and determines if the lesion is cystic or solid and if the intrahepatic bile ducts are dilated. It is the cheapest and most widely available of the several hepatic imaging modalities now in use but is operator dependent. Congenital cysts are completely anechoic and have a clearly defined thin wall; no further investigations are needed to confirm this diagnosis. Ultrasonography also is an effective way to demonstrate the presence of daughter cysts within hydatid cysts. If daughter cysts are not seen, serologic tests may help distinguish hydatid from congenital cysts. Although abscesses are hypoechoic and have a thick irregular wall, an early amebic abscess may be hyperechoic and may be mistaken for a solid hepatic mass. If an abscess is suspected on clinical grounds, treatment should be commenced and the ultrasonography repeated after 3 or 4 days, by which time an abscess will have become hypoechoic. Some tumors such as biliary cystadenoma and cystadenocarcinoma may be partly cystic. In addition, solid tumors may show hypoechoic areas interspersed with the expected hyerechoic picture. The hypoechoic areas result from the histologic characteristics of the tumor or from necrosis or hemorrhage in the lesion. Focal fatty change produces focal hypoechoic areas that also are hypodense on CT. Hemangiomas typically are hyperechoic.

Ultrasonography does not enable a specific diagnosis of hepatic tumors to be made, and additional information needs to be obtained by dynamic contrast-enhanced ultrasonography with intra-arterial infusion of CO_2 microbubbles, CT, or MRI. Each of these techniques has limitations, however, and at present, no ideal method for imaging the liver is available. Cavernous hemangiomas larger than 3 cm in diameter may be recognized on scintigraphy following the injection of radiolabeled red blood cells. Hepatic arteriography may show the typical features of vascular malignant tumors but is not always helpful. If hepatocellular carcinoma or hepatoblastoma is suspected, the serum alpha-fetoprotein concentration should be measured. Laparoscopy may demonstrate unsuspected tumor seeding or the presence of cirrhosis.

Definitive diagnosis of solid hepatic lesions depends on demonstrating the typical histologic features of the tumor. Histologic confirmation usually can be achieved by percutaneous needle biopsy or fine-needle aspiration.

REFERENCES

1. Parkin DM, Muir CS, Whelan SL, et al: Cancer Incidence in Five Continents, vol 5. IARC Publication No. 120. Lyon, International Agency for Research on Cancer, 1997.
2. Bosch FX, Ribes J, Borras J: Epidemiology of primary liver cancer. Semin Liver Dis 13:271, 1999.
3. Terry WD: Primary cancer of the liver. In Kaplan HS, Tsuchtani PJ (eds): Cancer in China. New York, Alan R. Liss, 1978, p 101.
4. Harington JS, McGlashan ND, Bradshaw E, et al: A spatial and temporal analysis of four cancers in African goldminers from southern Africa. Br J Cancer 31:665, 1976.
5. Okuda K, Fugimoto J, Hanai A, et al: Changing incidence of hepatocellular carcinoma in Japan. Cancer Res 7:4976, 1987.
6. Kew MC, Kassianides C, Hodkinson J, et al: Hepatocellular carcinoma in urban-born blacks: Frequency and relation to HBV infection. BMJ 293:1339, 1986.
7. Kew MC, Kassianides C, Berger EL, et al: Prevalence of chronic hepatitis B virus infection in pregnant black women living in Soweto. J Med Virol 22:263, 1987.
8. Prates MD, Torres EO: A cancer survey in Lourenco Marques, Portuguese East Africa. J Natl Cancer Inst 35:729, 1965.
9. Shorter RG, Baggenstoss AH, Logan GB, et al: Primary carcinoma of the liver in infancy and childhood. Pediatrics 25:191, 1960.
10. Kew MC: The role of cirrhosis in hepatocarcinogenesis. In Bannasch P, Keppler D, Weber G (eds): Liver Cell Carcinoma. Dordrecht, Kluwer Academic, 1989, p 37.
11. Bagshawe A, Cameron HM: The clinical problem of liver cell cancer in a high incidence area. In Cameron HM, Linsell DA, Warwick GP (eds): Liver Cell Cancer. Amsterdam, Elsevier, 1976, p 45.
12. Kew MC, Geddes EW: Hepatocellular carcinoma in rural southern African blacks. Medicine (Baltimore) 61:98, 1982.
13. Lau WY, Leung WY, Ho S, et al: Obstructive jaundice secondary to hepatocellular carcinoma. Surg Oncol 4:308, 1995.
14. Kew MC, Paterson AC: Unusual clinical presentations of hepatocellular carcinoma. J Trop Gastroenterol 6:10, 1985.
15. Clain D, Wartnaby K, Sherlock S: Abdominal arterial bruits in liver disease. Lancet 2:516, 1966.
16. Kew MC, Dos Santos HA, Sherlock S: Diagnosis of primary cancer of the liver. BMJ 4:408, 1971.
17. Zapf J, Futo E, Martina P, et al: Can *big* insulin-like growth factor-II in the serum of a tumor patient account for the development of extrapancreatic tumor hypoglycemia? J Clin Invest 90:2574, 1990.
18. Kew MC, Fisher JW: Serum erythropoietin concentrations in patients with hepatocellular carcinoma. Cancer 58:2485, 1986.
19. Yen T-C, Hwang S-J, Lee S-D, et al: Hypercalcemia and parathyroid hormone–related protein in hepatocellular carcinoma. Liver 13:311, 1993.
20. DiBisceglie AM, Hodkinson HJ, Berkowitz I, et al: Pityriasis rotunda—a cutaneous sign of hepatocellular carcinoma in southern African blacks. Arch Dermatol 122:802, 1986.
21. Danilewitz MD, Herrera G, Kew MC, et al: Autonomous cholesterol biosynthesis in murine hepatoma: A receptor defect with normal coated pits. Cancer 54:1562, 1984.
22. Alpert E: Human α_1-fetoprotein. In Okuda K, Peters RL (eds): Hepatocellular Carcinoma. New York, Wiley, 1976, p 353.
23. Kew MC: Tumor markers in hepatocellular carcinoma. J Gastroenterol Hepatol 4:373, 1989.
24. Kew MC: The detection and treatment of small hepatocellular carcinoma. In Hollinger FB, Lemon SM, Margolis H (eds): Viral Hepatitis and Liver Disease. Baltimore, Williams & Wilkins, 1991, p 515.
25. Taketa A, Sekiya C, Namiki M, et al: Lectin-reactive profiles of α-fetoprotein characterizing hepatocellular carcinoma and related conditions. Gastroenterology 99:508, 1990.
26. Du M-Q, Hutchinson WL, Johnson PJ, et al: Differential α-fetoprotein lectin binding in hepatocellular carcinoma: Diagnostic utility at low levels. Cancer 67:476, 1991.
27. Liebman HA, Furie B, Tong MJ, et al: Des-γ-carboxy (abnormal) prothrombin as a serum marker of primary hepatocellular carcinoma. N Engl J Med 310:427, 1984.
28. King MA, Kew MC, Kuyl JM, et al: A comparison between des-γ-carboxy prothrombin and α-fetoprotein as markers of hepatocellular carcinoma in southern African blacks. J Gastroenterol Hepatol 4:17, 1989.
29. Deugnier Y, David V, Brissot P, et al: Serum α-L-fucosidase: A new marker for the diagnosis of primary liver cancer? Hepatology 4:889, 1984.
30. Di Coccio RA, Barlow JJ, Motta KL: Evaluation of α-L-fucosidase as a marker of primary liver cancer. IRCS Med Sci 23:849, 1985.
31. Bukofzer S, Stass PM, Kew MC, et al: α-L-Fucosidase as a serum marker of hepatocellular carcinoma in southern African blacks. Br J Cancer 59:417, 1989.
32. Levy JI, Geddes EW, Kew MC: The chest radiograph in primary liver cancer. S Afr Med J 15:1323, 1976.
33. Kudo M: Ultrasound. In Okuda K, Tabor E (eds): Liver Cancer. New York, Churchill Livingstone, 1997, p 331.
34. Yu SCH, Yeung GDT, So NMC: Imaging features of hepatocellular carcinoma. Clin Radiol 59:145, 2004.

35. Kudo M: Imaging diagnosis of hepatocellular carcinoma and premalignant/borderline lesions. Semin Liver Dis 19:291, 1999.

36. Choi BI: CT diagnosis of liver cancer. In Okuda K, Tabor E (eds): Liver Cancer. New York, Churchill Livingstone, 1997, p 516.

37. Ebara M: MRI diagnosis of hepatocellular carcinoma. In Okuda K, Tabor E (eds): Liver Cancer. New York, Churchill Livingstone, 1997, p 361.

38. Takayasu K: Hepatic angiography. In Okuda K, Tabor E (eds): Liver Cancer. New York, Churchill Livingstone, 1997, p 347.

39. Kojiro M: Pathology of hepatocellular carcinoma. In Okuda K, Tabor E (eds): Liver Cancer. New York, Churchill Livingstone, 1997, p 165.

40. Craig JR, Peters RL, Edmondson HA, et al: Fibrolamellar carcinoma of the liver: A tumor of adolescents and young adults with distinctive clinicopathologic features. Cancer 46:372, 1980.

41. Anthony PP: Tumors and tumor-like lesions of the liver and biliary tract. In MacSween RNM, Anthony PP, Scheuer PJ, et al (eds): Pathology of the Liver. Edinburgh, Churchill Livingstone, 1994, p 635.

42. Yuki K, Hirohashi S, Sakamoto M, et al: Growth and spread of hepatocellular carcinoma. A review of 240 autopsy cases. Cancer 66:2174, 1990.

43. Kew MC: Clinical, pathologic, and etiologic heterogeneity in hepatocellular carcinoma: Evidence from southern Africa. Hepatology 1:366, 1981.

44. Hepatitis viruses. IARC Monographs on the Evaluation of Carcinogenic Risks to Humans, vol 59. Lyon, International Agency for Research on Cancer, 1994, p 202.

45. Stevens CE, Szmuness W: Vertical transmission of hepatitis B and neonatal hepatitis B. In Bianchi LO, Gerock W, Sickinger K, et al (eds): Virus and the Liver. Lancaster, MTP Press, 1980, p 285.

46. Botha JA, Ritchie MJJ, Dusheiko GM, et al: Hepatitis B virus carrier state in black children in Ovamboland: Role of perinatal and horizontal infection. Lancet 2:1209, 1984.

47. Beasley RP, Hwang L-Y: Hepatocellular carcinoma and hepatitis B virus. Semin Liver Dis 4:113, 1984.

48. Chang M-H. Decreasing incidence of hepatocellular carcinoma among children following universal hepatitis B immunization. Liver Int 23:309, 2003.

49. Arbuthnot P, Kew MC: Hepatitis B virus and hepatocellular carcinoma. Int J Exp Pathol 82:77, 2001.

50. Chisari FV, Filippe P, Buras J, et al: Structural and pathological effects of synthesis of hepatitis B virus large envelope polypeptide in transgenic mice. Proc Natl Acad Sci U S A 84:6909, 1987.

51. Wogan GN: Aflatoxin exposure as a risk factor in the etiology of hepatocellular carcinoma. In Okuda K, Tabor E (eds): Liver Cancer. New York, Churchill Livingstone, 1997, p 51.

52. Hsu IC, Metcalf RA, Sun T, et al: Mutational hotspot in the p53 gene in human hepatocellular carcinomas. Nature 350:427, 1991.

53. Bressac B, Kew MC, Wands JR, et al: Selective G to T mutation in the p53 gene in hepatocellular carcinoma from southern Africa. Nature 350:429, 1991.

54. Deugnier YM, Guyader D, Crantock L, et al: Primary liver cancer in genetic hemochromatosis: A clinical, pathological, and pathogenetic study of 54 cases. Gastroenterology 104:228, 1993.

55. Kew MC: Pathogenesis of hepatocellular carcinoma in hereditary hemochromatosis: Occurrence in non-cirrhotic patients. Hepatology 11:806, 1990.

56. Loeb LA, James EA, Waltersdorff AM, et al: Mutagenesis by the auto-oxidation of iron with isolated DNA. Proc Natl Acad Sci U S A 85:3918, 1988.

57. Mandishona E, McPhail AP, Gordeuk VR, et al: Dietary iron overload as a risk factor for hepatocellular carcinoma in black Africans. Hepatology 27:1563, 1998.

58. Asare GA, Paterson AC, Kew MC, et al: Iron-free neoplastic nodules and hepatocellular carcinoma without cirrhosis in Wistar rats fed a diet high in iron. J Pathol 208:82, 2006.

59. Polio J, Enriquez RE, Chow A, et al: Hepatocellular carcinoma in Wilson's disease: Case report and review of the literature. J Clin Gastroenterol 11:220, 1989.

60. Tokol RJ, Twedt T, McKim JM, et al: Oxidant injury to mitochondria in patients with liver disease and Bedlington terriers with copper toxicosis. Gastroenterology 107:1788, 1994.

61. Collaborative MILTS Project Team: Oral contraceptives and liver cancer. Results of a multicenter international liver tumor study (MILTS). Contraception 56:275, 1997.

62. Thomas DB: Exogenous steroid hormones and hepatocellular carcinoma. In Tabor E, DiBisceglie AM, Purcell RH (eds): Etiology, Pathology, and Treatment of Hepatocellular Carcinoma in North America. Houston, Gulf Publishing Co., 1991, p 77.

63. Austin A: The role of tobacco use and alcohol consumption in the etiology of hepatocellular carcinoma. In Tabor E, DiBisceglie AM, Purcell RH (eds): Etiology, Pathology, and Treatment of Hepatocellular Carcinoma in North America. Houston, Gulf Publishing Co., 1991, p 57.

64. Simson IM: Membranous obstruction of the inferior vena cava and hepatocellular carcinoma in South Africa. Gastroenterology 82:171, 1982.

65. Kew MC, McKnight A, Hodkinson HJ, et al: The role of membranous obstruction of the inferior vena cava in the etiology of hepatocellular carcinoma in southern African blacks. Hepatology 9:121, 1989.

66. Johnson PJ: Benign and malignant tumors of the liver. In Bacon BR, DiBisceglie AM (eds): Liver Disease: Diagnosis and Management. New York, Churchill Livingstone, 2000, p 310.

67. Balasegaram M: Management of primary liver cancer. Am J Surg 130:33, 1975.

68. Maraj J, Kew MC, Hyslop RJ: Resectability rate of hepatocellular carcinoma in rural southern African blacks. Br J Surg 75:335, 1988.

69. Foster JA, Berman MM: Solid Liver Tumors. Philadelphia, WB Saunders, 1977.

70. Bathe OF, Scudamore CH, Caron NR, et al: Resection of hepatocellular carcinoma. In Okuda K, Tabor E (eds): Liver Cancer. New York, Churchill Livingstone, 1997, p 511.

71. Tang Z-Y: Surgery of hepatocellular carcinoma—current status and future prospects. J Gastroenterol Hepatol 15(suppl):11, 2000.

72. Bismuth H, Majno PE, Adam R: Liver transplantation for hepatocellular carcinoma. Semin Liver Dis 19:311, 1999.

73. Yokoyama Y, Carr B, Saitsu H, et al: Accelerated growth rates of hepatocellular carcinoma after liver transplantation. Cancer 68:2095, 1991.

74. Ringe BR, Wittekind C, Bechstein WO, et al: The role of liver of recurrent transplantation in hepatobiliary malignancy: A retrospective study of 95 patients with particular regard to tumor stage and recurrences. Am Surg 209:88, 1989.

75. Rolles K: Transplantation for liver cancer. In Okuda K, Tabor E (eds): Liver Cancer. New York, Churchill Livingstone, 1997, p 531.

76. Okada S: Local ablation of hepatocellular carcinoma. Semin Liver Dis 19:323, 1999.

77. Livraghi T: Ethanol injection for the treatment of hepatocellular carcinoma. In Okuda K, Tabor E (eds): Liver Cancer. New York, Churchill Livingstone, 1997, p 497.

78. Wu C-C, Ho Y-Z, Ho WL, et al: Preoperative transcatheter arterial chemoembolization for resectable large hepatocellular carcinoma: A reappraisal. Br J Surg 82:122, 1985.

79. Stephanini GF, Amorati P, Bisseli M, et al: Efficacy of transarterial targeted treatments on survival in patients with hepatocellular carcinoma. Cancer 75:2927, 1995.

80. Nakamura H, Murakami T: Arterial embolization. In Okuda K, Tabor E (eds): Liver Cancer. New York, Churchill Livingstone, 1997, p 449.

81. Bronowicki J-P, Vetter D, Doffoel M: Chemoembolization of hepatocellular carcinoma. In Okuda K, Tabor E (eds): Liver Cancer. New York, Churchill Livingstone, 1997, p 463.

82. Falkson G, Falkson CI: Current approaches in the management of patients with hepatocellular carcinoma. Oncol Res 4:87, 1992.

83. Tang Z-Y: Sub-clinical Hepatocellular Carcinoma. Historical Aspects and General Considerations. Beijing, China Academic Publishers, 1985, p 1.

84. Ebara M, Ohto M, Shinagawa T, et al: Natural history of minute hepatocellular carcinoma smaller than 3 cm complicating cirrhosis. Gastroenterology 90:289, 1986.

85.. Nakanuma Y, Hoso M, Terada T: Clinical and pathologic features of cholangiocarcinoma. In Okuda K, Tabor E (eds): Liver Cancer. New York, Churchill Livingstone, 1997, p 279.

86. Yalcin S: Diagnosis and management of cholangiocarcinonomas: A comprehensive review. Hepatogastroenterology 51:43, 2004.

87. Srivatanakul P, Parkin DM, Yiang Y-Z, et al: The role of infection by *Opistorchis viverrini*, hepatitis B virus, and aflatoxin exposure in liver cancer in Thailand. Cancer 68:2411, 1991.

88. Wogan AM: The induction of liver cancer by chemicals. In Cameron H, Linsell CA, Warwick GP (eds): Liver Cell Cancer. New York, Wiley, 1976, p 6.

89. Stauffer MH, Sauer WG, Dearing WH, et al: The spectrum of cholestatic liver disease. JAMA 191:829, 1965.

90. Kulkarny PB, Beatty EC: Cholangiocarcinoma associated with biliary atresia. Am J Dis Child 31:442, 1977.

91. Dekker A, Ten Kate FJW, Terpstra OT: Cholangiocarcinoma associated with multiple bile duct hamartomas of the liver. Dig Dis Sci 34:592, 1989.

92. Sane S, MacCallum JD: Primary carcinoma of the liver: Cholangiocarcinoma in hepatolithiasis. Am J Pathol 18:675, 1942.

93. Klatskin G: Adenocarcinoma of the hepatic duct at its bifurcation within the porta hepatis. Am J Med 38:241, 1965.

94. Knill-Jones RP, Buckle RM, Parsons V, et al: Hypercalcemia and parathyroid activity in primary hepatoma. N Engl J Med 282:704, 1970.

95. Kaude J, Rian R: Cholangiocarcinoma. Radiology 100:573, 1971.

96. Low RN: Magnetic resonance imaging of the abdomen in the oncology patient. Oncology 14(suppl 6):5, 2000.

97. Sugihara S, Kojiro M: Pathology of cholangiocarcinoma. In Okuda K, Ishak KG (eds): Neoplasms of the Liver. Tokyo, Springer Verlag, 1987, p 143.

98. Stocker JT, Ishak KG: Hepatoblastoma. In Okuda K, Ishak KG (eds): Neoplasms of the Liver. Tokyo, Springer Verlag, 1987, p 127.

99. Exelby PR, Filler RM, Groshield JM: Liver tumors in children with particular reference to hepatoblastoma and hepatocellular carcinoma. J Pediat Surg 10:329, 1975.

100. McArthur JW, Toll GD, Russfield AB, et al: Sexual precocity attributed to ectopic gonadotropin secretion by hepatoblastoma. Am J Med 54:390, 1973.

101. Hasegawa H, Mukojima T, Hattori N, et al: Embryonal carcinoma and α-fetoprotein. Cancer Res 14:129, 1973.

102. Reynolds M, Douglass EC, Finegold M, et al: Chemotherapy can convert unresectable hepatoblastoma. J Pediatr Surg 27:1080, 1992.

103. Koneru B, Flye MW, Busitill RW, et al: Liver transplantation for hepatoblastoma: The American experience. Ann Surg 213:118, 1991.

104. Tamburro CH: Relationship of vinyl chloride to liver cancers: Angiosarcoma and hepatocellular carcinoma. Semin Liver Dis 4:158, 1984.

105. Locker GY, Duroshaw JH, Zwelling IA, et al: The clinical features of hepatic angiosarcoma: A report of four cases and a review of the literature. Medicine (Baltimore) 58:48, 1979.

106. Visfeldt J, Polse H: Of the histopathology of the liver and liver tumors in thorium dioxide patients. Acta Pathol Microbiol Scand 80A:97, 1972.

107. Roth F: Arsen-leber-tumoren hemangioendotheliom. Arch Pathol 60:493, 1955.

108. Regelson W, Kim U, Ospina J, et al: Hemangioendothelial sarcoma of the liver from chronic arsenic intoxication by Fowler's solution. Cancer 21:514, 1968.

109. Creech JL, Johnson MN: Angiosarcoma of the liver in the manufacture of polyvinyl chloride. J Occup Med 16:150, 1974.

110. Kielhorn J, Melber C, Wahnschaffe U, et al. Vinyl chloride: Still a cause for concern. Environ Health Perspect 108:200, 2000.

111. Whelan JG, Creech JL, Tamburro CH: Angiographic and radionuclide characteristics of hepatic angiosarcoma found in vinyl chloride workers. Radiology 118:549, 1976.

112. Truell JE, Peck SD, Reiguam CW: Hemangiosarcoma of the liver complicated by disseminated intravascular coagulation. Gastroenterology 65:936, 1973.

113. Alpert LI, Benisch B: Hemangioepithelioma of the liver associated with microangiopathic hemolytic anemia. Am J Med 48:624, 1970.

114. Ishak KG: Malignant mesenchymal tumors of the liver. In Okuda K, Ishak KG (eds): Neoplasms of the Liver. Tokyo, Springer Verlag, 1987, p 159.

115. Pickren JW, Tsukada Y, Lane WW: Liver metastasis: Analysis of autopsy data. In Weiss L, Gilbert HA (eds): Liver Metastases. Boston, CK Hall, 1982, p 2.

116. Dingemans KP, Roos E: Ultrastructural aspects of the invasion of the liver by cancer cells. In Weiss L, Gilbert HA (eds): Liver Metastases. Boston, CK Hall, 1982, p 51.

117. Ward BA, Miller DL, Frank JA, et al: Prospective evaluation of hepatic imaging studies in the detection of colorectal metastases: Correlation with surgical findings. Surgery 105:180, 1989.

118. Sheiner PA, Brower ST: Treatment of metastatic cancer. Semin Liver Dis 14:169, 1994.

119. Hughes K, Scheele J: Surgery for colorectal cancer metastatic to the liver. Surg Clin North Am 69:339, 1989.

120. Barr LC, Skene AI, Thomas JN: Metastectomy. Br J Surg 79:1268, 1992.

121. Prentice RL, Thomas DB: On the epidemiology of oral contraceptives and disease. Adv Cancer Res 49:285, 1987.

122. Vessey MP, Kay CR, Baldwin JA, et al: Oral contraceptives and benign liver tumors. BMJ 1:164, 1977.

123. Nagorney DM: Benign hepatic tumors, focal nodular hyperplasia, and hepatocellular adenoma. World J Surg 19:13, 1995.

124. Knowles DM, Casarella WJ, Johnson PM, et al: The clinical, radiologic, and pathologic characterization of benign hepatic adenomas. Alleged association with oral contraceptives. Medicine (Baltimore) 57:223, 1978.

125. Goodman ZD: Benign tumors of the liver. In Okuda K, Ishak KG (eds): Neoplasms of the Liver. Toyko, Springer Verlag, 1987, p 105.

126. Tavani A, Negri E, Parazinni F, et al: Female hormone utilization and risk of hepatocellular carcinoma. Br J Cancer 67:635, 1993.

127. Gyoffy E, Bredfeldt JE, Black WC: Transformation of hepatic cell adenoma to hepatocellular carcinoma due to oral contraceptive use. Ann Intern Med 110:489, 1989.

128. Freeny PC, Vimant TR, Barnett TC: Cavernous hemangioma of the liver: Ultrasonography, arteriography, and computed tomography. Radiology 132:143, 1979.
129. Krause T, Hauenstein K, Studier-Fischer B, et al: Improved evaluation of technetium 99m red blood cell SPECT in hemangioma of the liver. J Nucl Med 34:375, 1993.
130. Yamauchi T, Minami M, Yshiro N: Non-invasive diagnosis of small hemangioma of the liver: Advantage of magnetic resonance imaging. Radiology 145:1195, 1985.
131. Cooper WH, Martin JF: Hemangioma of the liver with thrombocytopenia. Am J Radiol 88:751, 1962.
132. Martinez J, Shapiro SS, Halbrun RR, et al: Hypofibrinogenemia associated with hemangioma of the liver. Am J Clin Pathol 29:160, 1958.
133. Feldman M: Hemangioma of the liver. Special reference to its association with cysts of the liver and pancreas. Am J Clin Pathol 29:160, 1958.
134. Chung EB: Multiple bile duct hamartomas. Cancer 26:287, 1970.
135. Banz EJ, Baggenstoss AH: Focal cirrhosis of the liver: Its relation to the so-called hamartoma (adenoma, benign hepatoma). Cancer 6:743, 1953.
136. Hanson SW, Gray HK, Dockerty MB: Benign tumors of the liver. II. Hemangiomas. Surg Gynecol Obstet 103:327, 1956.
137. Park WC, Phillips R: The role of radiation therapy in the management of hemangiomas of the liver. JAMA 21:1496, 1970.
138. Schwartz S, Husser WC: Cavernous hemangioma of the liver. Ann Surg 2905:456, 1987.
139. McLean RH, Moller JH, Warwick J, et al: Multinodular hemangiomatosis of the liver in infancy. Pediatrics 49:563, 1972.
140. Holcomb GW, O'Neill JA, Mahboubi S, et al: Experience with hepatic hemangioendothelioma in infancy and childhood. J Pediat Surg 23:661, 1988.
141. Mortensen W, Petersonn H: Infantile hemangioendothelioma. Angiographic considerations. Acta Radiol (Diagn) (Stockh) 20:161, 1979.
142. Rake MO, Liberman MM, Dawson JL: Ligation of the hepatic artery in the treatment of heart failure due to hepatic hemangiomatosis. Gut 11:512, 1970.
143. Frost NC, Esterley NB: Successful treatment of juvenile hemangiomas with prednisone. J Pediat 72:351, 1968.
144. Ross D, Pinna J, Mirza M, et al: Regression of focal nodular hyperplasia after discontinuation of oral contraceptives. Ann Intern Med 85:203, 1976.
145. Knowles DM, Wolff M, Johnson PM: Focal nodular hyperplasia and liver cell adenoma: Radiologic and pathologic differentiation. Am J, Radiol 131:393, 1978.
146. Wang SS, Chiang J, Tsai Y, et al: Focal hepatic fatty infiltration as a cause of pseudotumors: Ultrasonographic patterns and clinical differentiation. J Clin Ultrasound 18:401, 1990.
147. Jorgensen MJ: The ductal plate malformation. Acta Pathol Microbiol Scand Suppl A 257:1, 1977.
148. Desmet VJ: Congenital diseases of intrahepatic bile ducts; variations on the theme "ductal plate malformation." Hepatology 16:1069, 1992.
149. D'Agata ID, Jonas MM, Perez-Atayde AR, et al: Combined cystic disease of the liver and kidney. Semin Liver Dis 14:215, 1994.
150. Summerfield JA, Nagafuchi Y, Sherlock S, et al: Hepatobiliary fibropolycystic diseases: A clinical and histologic review. J Hepatol 2:141, 1986.
151. Harris PC, Rossetti S: Molecular genetics of autosomal recessive polycystic kidney disease. Mol Genet Metab 81: 75, 2004.
152. Karhunen PJ, Tenhu M: Adult polycystic liver and kidney diseases are separate entities. Clin Genet 30:29, 1985.
153. Pirson Y, Lannoy N, Peters D, et al: Isolated polycystic liver disease as a distinct genetic disease, unlinked to polycystic kidney disease 1 and polycystic kidney disease 2. Hepatology 23:249, 1996.
154. Tahvanainen P, Tahvanainen E, Reijonen H, et al: Polycystic liver disease is genetically heterogenous: Clinical and linkage studies in eight Finnish families. J Hepatol 38:39, 2003.
155. Li A, Davila S, Furu L, et al Mutations in PRKCSH cause isolated autosomal dominant polycystic liver disease. Am J Hum Genet 72: 691, 2003.
156. Everson GT: Hepatic cysts in autosomal dominant polycystic kidney disease. Am J Kidney Dis 22:520, 1993.
157. Que F, Nagorney DM, Gross TB, et al: Liver resection and cyst fenestration in the treatment of severe polycystic liver disease. Gastroenterology 108:407, 1995.
158. Cowles RA, Mulholland MW: Solitary hepatic cysts. J Am Coll Surg 191:311, 2001.
159. Caroli S: Diseases of the intrahepatic biliary tree. Clin Gastroenterol 2:147, 1973.
160. Mathias K, Waldmann D, Daikeler G, et al: Intrahepatic cystic duct dilatations and stone formation: A new case of Caroli's disease. Acta Hepatogastroenterol 25:30, 1978.
161. Ramond JM, Huequet C, Danan G, et al: Partial hepatectomy in the treatment of Caroli's disease. Dig Dis Sci 29:67, 1984.
162. Valla D, Benhamou JP: Disorders of the hepatic venous system, peliosis, and sinusoidal dilatation. In Bacon BR, DiBisceglie AM (eds): Liver Disease: Diagnosis and Management. New York, Churchill Livingstone, 2000, p 331.

CHAPTER
92 Liver Transplantation

Paul Martin and Hugo R. Rosen

Despite continued advances in antiviral therapy and the medical management of chronic liver disease, liver transplantation remains the only prospect for long-term survival in patients with decompensated cirrhosis, unresectable primary hepatic malignancies, and fulminant hepatic failure in which spontaneous recovery is not anticipated. In turn, liver transplantation has continued to evolve in response to the continued shortage of deceased donor organs and the frequency of recurrent disease. The availability of a wider array of immunosuppressive agents has now made graft rejection a lesser concern than disease recurrence.[1] Recurrence of hepatitis C virus (HCV) infection, because of its frequency as an indication for liver transplantation, high rate of graft reinfection and failure, and lack of effective prophylaxis, has become a major problem in the care of transplant recipients.[2] By contrast, effective prophylaxis to prevent hepatitis B virus (HBV) infection has allowed use of liver transplantation in instances of this previously controversial indication, with a low likelihood of graft reinfection.[3] Recurrence of nonviral liver disease also poses a threat to the graft, albeit of an order of magnitude less than that in HCV-infected recipients.[4] Because immunosuppression has a proviral effect, a number of transplantation centers have attempted earlier reduction in dose or withdrawal of glucocorticoids in recipients with chronic HBV or HCV infection. By contrast, more intensive immunosuppression is maintained in disorders of putative autoimmune etiology, including primary biliary cirrhosis (PBC), primary sclerosing cholangitis (PSC), and autoimmune hepatitis, with increased recognition of their recurrence following transplantation.[5]

The unremitting shortage of deceased-donor organs continues to be reflected in deaths on the liver transplantation waiting list. Concerns about lack of an equitable system of allocation of available organs has led to implementation of the Model for End-Stage Liver Disease (MELD), which may have achieved its stated aim of reducing deaths on the waiting list (see Chapters 70 and 87 and later in this chapter).[6] This method of allocation assigns organs to recipients on the basis of an objective, continuous measure of the severity of their liver disease, obviating time spent on the waiting list. Extension of live-donor transplantation to adult recipients has increased the organ pool, despite a tempering of enthusiasm following increased appreciation of potential risks to the donor.[7] Other innovations such as splitting deceased-donor grafts to benefit two recipients and use of so-called marginal grafts, including those from older and non–heart-beating donors, also have modestly expanded the organ supply.[8] Unfortunately, the shortage of deceased-donor organs will continue to be the rate-limiting step in substantially increasing the number of transplant recipients.

The number of persons listed for liver transplantation in the United States and elsewhere has increased exponentially despite the relatively static donor supply before the introduction of MELD. The resulting discrepancy is reflected in the increasing number of patients who succumb to complications of liver disease, as waiting times for liver transplantation become more protracted (Fig. 92–1). Following the introduction of the MELD system, particular priority was given to patients with hepatocellular carcinoma, who as a group may have less decompensated liver disease than that typical for candidates with advanced cirrhosis and without tumor.[9] This strategy may have lessened perioperative mortality rates in the recipient population as a whole, but longer follow-up is needed to determine whether recurrence of tumor will reduce overall survival. Despite ongoing debates about organ allocation and concerns about recurrence of disease, the prospects for long-term survival are very good to excellent for most liver transplant recipients, who otherwise would succumb to their liver disease. For instance, the likely 1-year survival rate for patients with decompensated cirrhosis is less than 10% without liver transplantation but approximately 85% to 90% at 1 year and 75% at 5 years after transplantation for most indications (see later).[10]

A major factor in patient survival following transplantation is the degree of hepatic decompensation and associated debility at the time of transplantation; in some potential recipients, a protracted wait for a liver transplant results in such profound deterioration that surgery is no longer feasible by the time a suitable donor is identified.[11] Although access to transplantation has transformed the management of advanced liver disease, it has resulted in an expanding cohort of increasingly decom-

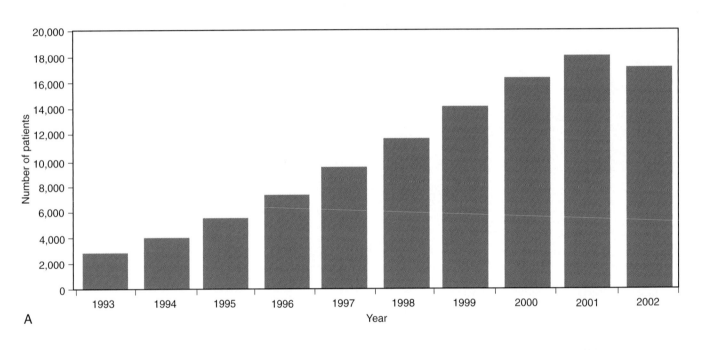

A

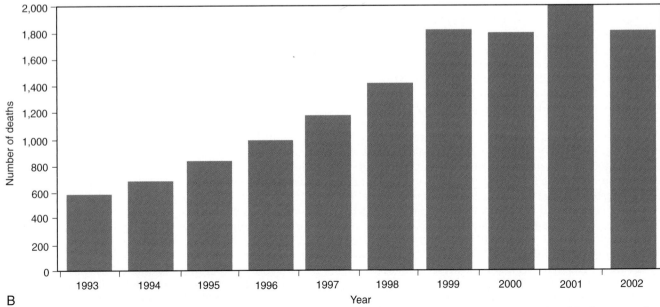

B

Figure 92–1 *A,* Patients listed for liver transplantation in the United States, 1993 to 2002. *B,* Deaths in patients listed for liver transplantation in the United States, 1993 to 2002. (From http://www.UStransplant.org.)

pensated potential recipients who require intensive medical attention. Because the best outcomes following liver transplantation are obtained in patients who have not already experienced multiple complications of liver disease,[12] it is appropriate to refer a patient for transplantation evaluation after an index complication, such as the onset of ascites. For some potential recipients, access to live-donor transplantation may avoid a lengthy waiting period with the risk of further and potentially life-threatening complications of their liver disease.[7]

In parallel with the evolution of liver transplantation, the care of transplantation candidates with advanced disease has become a major clinical challenge. The transplant hepatologist must combine the skills to practice gastroenterology, multidisciplinary internal medicine, and intensive care.[13]

INDICATIONS

The major indications for liver transplantation in adults reflect the most frequent causes of adult liver disease, notably chronic hepatitis C, alcoholic liver disease, and, to a lesser extent, chronic hepatitis B, PBC, PSC, and autoimmune hepatitis (Table 92–1). Other indications include fulminant hepatic failure (FHF) and cirrhosis of other causes, including increasingly nonalcoholic fatty liver disease (NAFLD) and hemochromatosis. The role of transplantation in patients with hepatic malignancy has become better defined in recent years; a clear subset of patients with hepatocellular carcinoma who have a high likelihood of cure with transplantation have been recognized, although the role of adjunctive therapies such as transarterial chemoembolization remains unclear.[14] The other major primary adult hepatic malignancy, cholangiocarcinoma, had been regarded as a contraindication to liver transplantation because of its rapid and almost invariable recurrence subsequently. More recent reports, however, have described improved outcomes in a subset

of patients who receive adjuvant external beam irradiation.[15] The major indication for pediatric liver transplantation is biliary atresia following a failed Kasai procedure (portoenterostomy) or delayed recognition of the diagnosis. Other major pediatric indications include α_1-antitrypsin deficiency and other metabolic disorders.[16]

A key issue in managing a cirrhotic patient is deciding whether liver transplantation will be needed in the future and recognizing the appropriate time to refer the patient for evaluation. An important aspect of the management of a compensated cirrhotic patient is the anticipation of complications such as variceal hemorrhage, which may be prevented by endoscopic surveillance to identify high-risk varices and begin prophylaxis, either pharmacologic or endoscopic, to prevent an initial gastrointestinal bleed (see Chapter 87).[17] Surveillance for hepatocellular carcinoma, although difficult to justify in the absence of controlled clinical trials proving enhanced patient outcomes, is now regarded as the standard of care in a cirrhotic patient (see Chapter 91). Discovery of a hepatic mass suggestive of hepatocellular carcinoma in a cirrhotic patient should prompt an evaluation to determine whether hepatic resection or transplantation is the most appropriate approach to curative surgery. In general, liver transplantation should be a consideration only when the limits of medical therapy have been reached, particularly when live-donor transplantation is an option. The risk of surgery must always be weighed against a realistic assessment of the potential recipient's prognosis without transplantation. For instance, in florid hepatic decompensation caused by alcoholic hepatitis, dramatic recovery is possible with abstinence from alcohol. Similarly, in a patient with decompensated cirrhosis caused by HBV infection, effective suppression of viral replication by one of the newer antiviral agents may result in impressive clinical improvement, thereby delaying the need for liver transplantation.[18] The course of chronic liver disease remains unpredictable, however, and it is sobering to observe that an apparently well-compensated patient can deteriorate dramatically because of an intercurrent complication such as variceal bleeding. Anticipation of complications of cirrhosis may permit prophylactic intervention.

A patient with well-compensated cirrhosis can remain stable for many years, so cirrhosis per se is not an indication for liver transplantation. For example, Fattovich and colleagues[19] observed that in well-compensated cirrhosis caused by hepatitis C virus (HCV) infection, rates of major complications of portal hypertension, such as ascites and variceal hemorrhage, were less than 30% at 10 years, and in the absence of a complication, survival was excellent (Fig. 92–2). Once an index complication has occurred, however, the chance for survival rapidly diminishes. For example, after the development of ascites refractory to diuretics, only 25% of patients survive beyond 1 year.[20]

Predictive models based on the natural history of primary biliary cirrhosis (PBC)[21] (see Chapter 86) and primary sclerosing cholangitis (PSC)[22] (see Chapter 65) have helped in clinical decision-making in patients with these disorders, which tend to progress in a fairly stereotypical fashion. Before the introduction of MELD, analogous models had not been available for the

Table 92–1   Liver Diseases of Adult Transplant Recipients in the United States

Primary Liver Disease	Number	%
Chronic hepatitis C	5155	20.7
Alcoholic liver disease	4258	17.1
Alcoholic liver disease and hepatitis C	1106	4.4
Chronic hepatitis B	1368	5.5
Cryptogenic cirrhosis	2719	10.9
Primary biliary cirrhosis	2317	9.3
Primary sclerosing cholangitis	2178	8.7
Autoimmune hepatitis	1194	4.8
Acute liver failure	1555	6.2
Hepatic malignancy	951	3.8
Metabolic diseases	923	3.7
Other	1050	4.2
Unknown	126	0.5

Note: United Network for Organ Sharing Database 1987-1998; N = 24,900 patients.

Adapted and reprinted with permission from Keeffe EB: Liver transplantation: Current status and novel approaches to liver replacement. Gastroenterology 120:749, 2001.

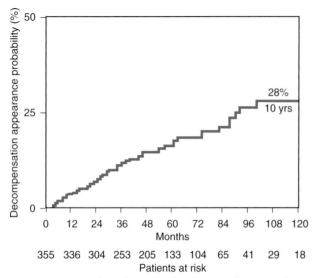

Figure 92–2 Rate of development of major complications (decompensation) in patients with well-compensated cirrhosis due to hepatitis C. (From Fattovich G, Giustina G, Degos F, et al: Morbidity and mortality in compensated cirrhosis type C: A retrospective follow-up study of 384 patients. Gastroenterology 112:463, 1999.)

noncholestatic forms of cirrhosis, and the decision to refer a patient for liver transplantation generally had been based on disease severity as assessed by some objective parameters, such as the serum albumin level, as well as more subjective factors, such as the presence of hepatic encephalopathy.

On clinical grounds, important indications for liver transplantation remain disease severity reflective of hepatocellular failure, such as coagulopathy and jaundice; complications of portal hypertension, such as refractory ascites and recurrent variceal bleeding; or the combination of portosystemic shunting and diminished hepatocellular function, as occurs in hepatic encephalopathy. Predictive models for the natural history of PBC and PSC allow prediction of an individual patient's course on the basis of simple clinical and laboratory parameters, the most ominous of which is a rising serum bilirubin level. Although deterioration in a patient's quality of life may not be reflected adequately in predictive models, including MELD, the presence of potentially disabling symptoms such as pruritus and osteopenia in patients with cholestatic and other forms of cirrhosis, as well as recurrent bacterial cholangitis in those with PSC, are important considerations in deciding when to refer a patient for transplantation. MELD exceptions in which points are added to the MELD score to increase the likelihood that liver transplantation will be performed require approval by a regional review board that includes representatives from local transplantation programs. That points can be added to the MELD score indicates that, although the allocation system based on MELD is a major advance in organ allocation, at least some patients may be disadvantaged by its purely objective parameters and exclusion of factors such as intractable ascites or encephalopathy that were incorporated into older allocation schemes. Ideally, transplantation should occur before a protracted period of disability reduces the likelihood of subsequent post-transplantation rehabilitation to full employment

and social functioning. The potential burden of advanced liver disease for many transplantation candidates includes loss of employment, and referral for transplantation evaluation should be discussed before a patient becomes incapacitated.[23]

LISTING CRITERIA AND POLICIES OF THE UNITED NETWORK FOR ORGAN SHARING

Organ allocation in the United States is administered by the United Network for Organ Sharing (UNOS), which now considers only disease severity in determining a patient's priority for liver transplantation. MELD is a mathematical formula (see www.unos.org) that incorporates the serum bilirubin level, creatinine level, and internationalized normalized ratio (INR) and provides a more objective and accurate way to stratify transplantation candidates for organ allocation and to eliminate time waiting for a donor organ as a determining factor than did clinical and biochemical measures (including the Child-Turcotte-Pugh class) used in the past.[24] The Child-Turcotte-Pugh classification has inherent limitations, including limited discriminatory ability, subjective interpretation of parameters such as presence or absence of ascites on the basis of the physical examination, and the "ceiling effect" of the score (e.g., no greater weight is given to a serum bilirubin level of 35 mg/dL than to a level of 3.5 mg/dL, even though a patient with the higher bilirubin level clearly has more advanced liver disease). Inclusion of the serum creatinine level reflects the major prognostic importance of renal dysfunction in advanced liver disease. Adoption of the MELD system has been a major step in achieving an equitable organ allocation system in the United States, although the MELD will undoubtedly continue to undergo refinement.

ABSOLUTE AND RELATIVE CONTRAINDICATIONS

Contraindications to liver transplantation also have evolved in concert with innovations in surgical technique and postoperative care. For example, effective prophylaxis against recurrent HBV infection now allows excellent graft and patient survival rates in patients with HBV-related cirrhosis.[3] Greater experience has highlighted the futility of liver retransplantation in many debilitated recipients with a failing graft caused by recurrent HCV infection. By contrast, the introduction of highly effective antiretroviral therapy (HAART) now allows consideration of liver transplantation in human immunodeficiency virus (HIV)-infected patients with decompensated liver disease, typically caused by either HCV or HBV infection.[25]

Still, relative and absolute contraindications to liver transplantation remain. An *absolute* contraindication (Table 92–2) is a clinical circumstance in which the likelihood of a successful outcome is so remote that transplantation should not be offered. A *relative* contraindication implies a suboptimal likelihood of a good outcome, although liver transplantation may still be considered in some patients.

Table 92–2   Contraindications to Liver Transplantation

Acquired immunodeficiency syndrome
Extrahepatic malignancy
Cholangiocarcinoma
Hemangiosarcoma
Uncontrolled sepsis
Active alcoholism or substance abuse
Fulminant hepatic failure with sustained ICP >50 mm Hg or
    CPP <40 mm Hg*
Advanced cardiac or pulmonary disease
Child-Turcotte-Pugh score <7
Anatomic abnormality precluding liver transplantation
Persistent noncompliance

*ICP is intracranial pressure; CPP is cerebral perfusion pressure and equals the mean arterial pressure minus ICP.

The role of liver transplantation in the management of hepatocellular carcinoma has become better defined with the recognition that a large tumor burden in patients with hepatocellular carcinoma is associated with a high probability of metastatic spread within a short time after transplantation.[14] The role of adjuvant therapies in transplantation candidates, such as transarterial chemoembolization, has been difficult to establish. Tumor characteristics predictive of a poor outcome, most notably vascular invasion, may be apparent only after the explanted liver has been examined, despite the sophistication of imaging techniques performed preoperatively. For cholangiocarcinoma, which almost inevitably recurs even if discovered as an incidental finding in the explant, a protocol involving external beam irradiation and chemotherapy before transplantation has yielded encouraging results.[15] The results of liver transplantation remain poor for angiosarcoma, and the presence of this tumor remains an absolute contraindication. On the other hand, some patients with epithelioid hemangioendothelioma have undergone transplantation successfully, despite an extensive tumor burden, with documented regression of extrahepatic metastases.

For a transplantation candidate with a previous extrahepatic malignancy, therapy needs to have been curative, with the resection specimen indicating a low likelihood of metastatic spread. A 2-year recurrence-free period before transplantation is adequate for most nonhepatic malignancies, although, for breast cancer, colon cancer, and malignant melanoma, a longer period following resection is desirable. Myeloproliferative disorders are frequent causes of Budd-Chiari syndrome, but fortunately, evolution to acute leukemia is not accelerated following transplantation.[26]

Ongoing alcohol or recreational drug use remains an absolute contraindication to liver transplantation. If the possibility of continued use is a concern, random toxicology screens are appropriate. Although marijuana is used medicinally for palliation, most transplantation programs discourage its use because of concerns about the overall compliance of users, as well as possible pulmonary side effects. A history of prescription narcotic abuse also is a cause for concern, because it may portend difficulties with pain management after transplantation; non-narcotic alternatives should be attempted for chronic pain, although nonsteroidal anti-inflammatory drugs (NSAIDs) also are contraindicated in persons with end-stage liver disease because of potential renal and gastrointestinal complications. Cigarette smoking also is prohibited in transplantation candidates because of the multiple adverse effects of smoking, not the least of which is an increased risk of malignancy following transplantation.[27] With the increasing use of herbal products and other complementary and alternative medicine (CAM) health products, it is appropriate to discuss their unproven efficacies and unknown toxicities with transplantation candidates and to caution them against use of such products in the post-transplantation setting because of the potential for drug interactions (see Chapter 125).[28]

The careful medical workup necessary before liver transplantation frequently uncovers important comorbid conditions, most typically cardiac and pulmonary. The frequency of coronary artery disease in adult patients who present for an evaluation for liver transplantation has been estimated to range from 5% to 10%. In one study of patients with coronary artery disease who underwent transplantation, including a subset of patients who had undergone coronary artery bypass grafting 6 months to 12 years before the procedure, mortality and morbidity rates were found to be 50% and 81%, respectively.[29] Discrete coronary artery stenoses can be managed by angioplasty. Although surgical bypass grafting may be contraindicated because of the significant perioperative risk of excessive bleeding in a patient with decompensated cirrhosis, such surgery, if successful, may render the patient an acceptable candidate for liver transplantation. Pretransplantation cardiac evaluation may overestimate cardiac performance, and impaired cardiac function may become apparent only after the protective effect of the decreased systemic vascular resistance that characterizes cirrhosis is lost after transplantation, when cardiac afterload increases because of the hypertensive effects of the primary immunosuppressive agents and when intravascular volume may be repleted too vigorously. Emerging data suggest that dobutamine stress echocardiography is the screening test of choice, in terms of sensitivity, specificity, and cost, for assessing cardiac function before transplantation.[30] Specific forms of cirrhosis may have extrahepatic manifestations that diminish long-term survival. For example, lethal cardiac arrhythmias may result in poorer survival for patients who undergo liver transplantation for decompensated cirrhosis caused by hemochromatosis than for those who undergo transplantation for other diseases.[31]

A pulmonary evaluation in the liver transplantation candidate also may reveal abnormal arterial oxygenation (see Chapter 89). Although severe chronic obstructive pulmonary disease or pulmonary fibrosis precludes liver transplantation, respiratory restriction caused by ascites or diminished respiratory muscle strength as a result of chronic illness is reversible and should not preclude transplantation. Even patients who undergo liver transplantation for α_1-antitrypsin deficiency may show improvement in pulmonary function test values postoperatively.

The *hepatopulmonary syndrome* is characterized by the triad of chronic liver disease, pulmonary vascular dilations (with right-to-left shunting), and hypoxemia, and was formerly considered an absolute contraindication to liver transplantation.[32] The diagnosis is suggested by the finding of a PaO_2 value less than 70 mm Hg measured on arterial blood gas obtained with the patient in the supine position. Definitive diagnosis is made by the demonstration of intrapulmonary vascular dilatations by contrast-enhanced echocardiography, perfusion lung scanning with technetium 99m–labeled macroaggregated albumin, or pulmonary arteriography.[33] Detection of contrast in the left side of the heart within several beats after its appearance in the right atrium indicates intrapulmonary shunting. Predictors of potential reversibility of the hepatopulmonary syndrome following transplantation include a younger age, lesser degree of preoperative hypoxemia, and adequate correction of hypoxemia with inspiration of 100% oxygen (PaO_2 greater than 200 mm Hg).[32] In a majority of patients with hepatopulmonary syndrome, hypoxemia resolves within several months after transplantation, although a protracted period of ventilatory support may be required in the immediate postoperative period. Because of the potential for improvement with liver transplantation, an increased MELD score may be allocated to a patient with the hepatopulmonary syndrome who otherwise would have a lower priority for transplantation.

It is critical to distinguish the hepatopulmonary syndrome from *portopulmonary hypertension*, which is associated with a high perioperative mortality rate and frequently unchanged pulmonary hemodynamics after liver transplantation. Specifically, a mean pulmonary artery pressure greater than 35 mm Hg, pulmonary vascular resistance greater than 300 dynes/s/cm^{-5}, and cardiac output less than 8 L/minute are indicative of a high perioperative risk, because the patient will be unable to increase cardiac output appropriately in response to altered intraoperative and postoperative hemodynamics.[34]

Hepatic hydrothorax is a not infrequent manifestation of portal hypertension; transudative fluid collects in the pleural cavity, usually on the right side, often with relatively little ascitic fluid remaining in the abdominal cavity (see Chapter 88). Hepatic hydrothorax can be particularly difficult to treat; often, repeated thoracentesis or placement of a transjugular intrahepatic portosystemic shunt (TIPS) is required.[35] The temptation to insert a permanent chest tube needs to be resisted, because presence of the tube can lead to infection in the pleural cavity, with the risk of fistula formation.

Active uncontrolled extrahepatic infection is an absolute contraindication to transplantation, which needs to be deferred if any suspicion of sepsis exists. Liver transplantation may be the only option, however, for a patient with recurrent bacterial cholangitis in the setting of PSC who is allocated a higher MELD score than otherwise reflected by the liver biochemical test levels. Similarly, spontaneous bacterial peritonitis needs to be controlled by antibiotic therapy before transplantation. A particularly ominous finding is fungemia, which typically is impossible to eradicate in a debilitated cirrhotic patient and precludes transplantation.

An important technical consideration in the candidate for liver transplantation is the presence of vascular abnormalities that may increase the difficulty of surgery,

although with increased surgical experience, the importance of these abnormalities, most notably portal vein thrombosis, as obstacles to transplantation has declined. Nevertheless, more extensive vascular thrombosis with involvement of the superior mesenteric vein may still prevent liver transplantation because of lack of a suitable venous anastomosis for the graft. The presence of a previously placed portosystemic shunt, particularly a nonselective (side-to-side or end-to-side) portacaval shunt, increases the technical complexity of liver transplantation but is no longer regarded as a contraindication. With the widespread use of TIPS to control manifestations of portal hypertension, including variceal hemorrhage, intractable ascites, and hydrothorax without disruption of the vascular anatomy, TIPS is now the most frequently encountered shunt in transplant recipients and usually does not present any additional challenges intraoperatively.[36]

Although age restrictions have been relaxed, in evaluating an older transplantation candidate close attention must be paid to comorbid conditions that not only increase the risk of perioperative mortality but also may decrease the likelihood that after transplantation the candidate will be able to return to an active lifestyle, particularly because severe liver disease may cause more debility in older than in younger patients.[37] Because a subset of robust older recipients have good outcomes after liver transplantation, however, candidates in their late 60s who are otherwise in good health should not be precluded a priori from transplantation.

An important consideration in the differential diagnosis of renal insufficiency in patients with advanced liver disease is hepatorenal syndrome, which is potentially reversible (see Chapter 89). Renal failure remains an important predictor of a poor outcome after liver transplantation.[38] Typically, renal dysfunction in a patient with decompensated cirrhosis reflects a variety of insults, including sepsis, hypotension, and nephrotoxic medications. In transplant recipients with decompensated cirrhosis, renal insufficiency severe enough to require dialysis or combined liver-kidney transplantation has been associated consistently with poorer patient and graft outcomes. Assessment of the potential for improvement in renal function following transplantation is key. Inclusion of the serum creatinine level in the MELD score reflects the major prognostic importance of renal insufficiency in advanced liver disease.

A major systemic manifestation of decompensated cirrhosis is malnutrition. Loss of muscle mass increases the likelihood of perioperative morbidity with protracted ventilatory support and poor patient survival. Peripheral edema and ascites make changes in body weight or anthropometric measurements unreliable for assessing nutritional status in patients with advanced cirrhosis. Some specific forms of cirrhosis can be associated with more profound nutritional deficiencies, as in the malnourished alcoholic patient with multiple vitamin and electrolyte deficiencies or the patient with cholestatic liver disease and depletion of fat-soluble vitamins secondary to intestinal malabsorption. Evaluation by a dietitian is an integral part of the evaluation of the transplantation candidate. The nutritional status of these patients may be improved by enteral and parenteral feeding, but the improvement is modest at best. An increasing cause for concern in transplantation candidates is obesity, both as a factor in the pathogenesis of nonalcoholic fatty liver disease (NAFLD) and as a risk factor for postoperative mortality from cardiovascular events.[39]

TRANSPLANTATION EVALUATION AND LISTING

Although the details of a formal multidisciplinary transplantation evaluation differ from transplantation center to transplantation center, the process is designed to provide an opportunity for the patient and his or her family to become acquainted with the procedure and demands of liver transplantation, as well as for the patient to undergo a rigorous medical assessment to confirm that transplantation constitutes the best option for managing the patient's liver disease and that no absolute contraindications exist. The patient typically is seen by a transplant surgeon, hepatologist, psychiatrist, and social worker, with additional consultations as clinically indicated. As increasingly frailer and older candidates are evaluated, it is imperative to identify potential causes of perioperative morbidity, such as carotid artery stenosis. Abdominal imaging is performed both to identify any potential technical problems such as portal vein thrombosis and to detect additional complications such as hepatocellular carcinoma. Disease-specific issues may need to be addressed, such as the likelihood of recidivism in the alcoholic patient or of cure in the patient with hepatocellular carcinoma. The appropriateness of transplantation for each candidate is then discussed formally at a patient selection committee with input from all the members of the transplant team. If the patient is deemed to be an appropriate candidate, the patient is matched by blood type and weight to potential deceased donors and "listed" formally for transplantation.

The patient's priority for liver transplantation is now based on disease severity as reflected by MELD score, rather than on duration of the wait for transplantation, as was done in the past. Although the MELD score is derived from objective variables, the MELD score may differ when different laboratory methodologies, particularly for the INR, are used, and such differences in MELD score may affect the transplant priority of patients.[40] With the critical and seemingly intractable shortage of cadaveric donor organs, a major challenge for UNOS and other organ allocation agencies throughout the world has been to develop an equitable system of allocation in an effort to ensure that hepatic allografts are not used for patients whose prognosis without transplantation remains good. In this regard, patients with a MELD score of less than 15 appear to have a better survival rate without a transplant than with a transplant. As shown in Figure 92–3, the MELD score has been shown to correlate with the 3-month survival rate in patients with cirrhosis.[24]

Once the evaluation process is complete and the patient is accepted for transplantation, financial clearance is sought from the patient's private, state, or federal payor to fund the procedure. The criteria for coverage for

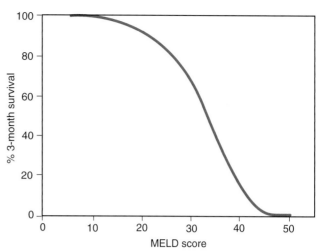

Figure 92–3   Relationship between the 3-month survival rate and MELD score in patients with cirrhosis.

liver transplantation vary among payors, and the transplantation center must have expertise in funding issues.

DISEASE-SPECIFIC INDICATIONS

ALCOHOLIC LIVER DISEASE

Alcoholic liver disease (ALD) is the most frequent cause of decompensated chronic liver disease in the United States (see Chapter 81). Decompensated alcoholic cirrhosis is now firmly established as a legitimate indication for liver transplantation. Major concerns in the past had included recidivism following transplantation, as well as potentially poor adherence of patients to immunosuppressive drug therapy. In addition, it was thought that the large number of patients with ALD would outstrip the donor supply. These fears have not been confirmed, although patients with acute alcoholic hepatitis generally have had a poor outcome following transplantation and a high rate of recidivism. Excellent graft and patient survival rates are the rule following liver transplantation for ALD.

Key factors in determining an alcoholic patient's suitability for liver transplantation include recognition by the patient of the key role alcohol has played in the genesis of the liver disease, participation in some form of alcohol rehabilitation such as attendance at Alcoholics Anonymous, stable social support, and a defined period of abstinence from alcohol, conventionally 6 months. Despite these strategies, a substantial proportion of alcoholic recipients resume drinking after transplantation, although graft loss or death attributable to alcohol abuse has been uncommon.[41] A higher rate of return to alcohol use is elicited by use of anonymous questionnaires or toxicology screening than by direct questioning of patients, and at least 10% to 15% of alcoholic transplant recipients are found to consume alcohol. A particularly difficult dilemma arises in the alcoholic patient with severely decompensated liver disease, recent use of alcohol, and little likelihood of surviving without prompt liver transplantation. Clearly enunciated criteria, including a contractual commitment by the patient to sobriety and active involvement in some form of alcohol rehabilitation, such as the Alcoholics Anonymous program, ensure that the selection process is equitable under these circumstances. Patients who return to pathologic drinking after liver transplantation appear to have a higher rate of medical problems, including pneumonia, cellulitis, and pancreatitis, that require hospitalization and occasionally lead to graft loss and death. In addition, alcoholic transplant recipients are prone to develop de novo oropharyngeal and lung tumors, probably reflecting other aspects of an alcoholic lifestyle, most notably cigarette consumption.

HEPATITIS B

Management of the HBV-infected transplantation candidate has been one of the major triumphs of liver transplantation. During the 1980s, HBV recurrence was frequent and resulted in reduced patient and graft survival rates. Key factors in improving outcomes have included recognition of the key role of active viral replication occurring before liver transplantation, as demonstrated by detection in serum of hepatitis B e antigen or HBV DNA by molecular hybridization, as a predictor of recurrent hepatitis B in the graft, and the protective effect of long-term, high-dose hepatitis B immunoglobulin (HBIG). The transplantation candidate with chronic HBV infection is now readily accepted for liver transplantation, with the requirement for long-term immunoprophylaxis following transplantation, with its attendant inconvenience and expense. In a seminal study, Samuel and colleagues observed that patients with a fulminant presentation of acute HBV infection or hepatitis D (delta) virus co-infection had a lower risk of recurrent hepatitis B after liver transplantation than that observed in patients undergoing liver transplantation for HBV-related cirrhosis in the absence of immunoprophylaxis, because of a lower level of HBV replication.[42] The widespread use of high-dose HBIG, initially administered intravenously, resulted in markedly reduced rates of recurrent hepatitis B following transplantation, and in combination with lamivudine has further decreased HBV recurrence further. Lamivudine initially was used for monotherapy to prevent recurrent HBV infection after transplantation but caused frequent mutations of the HBV polymerase gene, which led to viral resistance to the drug and consequent graft reinfection (see Chapter 75).

The optimal dosing regimen for HBIG has been difficult to establish in the absence of controlled clinical data. Some groups of investigators have titrated HBIG doses to maintain a minimal trough serum level of antibody to hepatitis B surface antigen (anti-HBs). More recently, intramuscular administration of HBIG used in combination with lamivudine has been found to be an efficacious and less expensive alternative to chronic intravenous HBIG plus lamivudine.[43] HBV infection that recurs despite use of HBIG may reflect inadequate dosing or a genomic mutation in the "a" determinant of the hepatitis B surface antigen (HBsAg) that results in less avid binding of the virus to HBIG (see Chapter 75). Lamivudine resistance acquired before transplantation also has

been implicated in HBV recurrence, despite apparently adequate immunoprophylaxis with HBIG after transplantation. The nucleotide analog adefovir dipivoxil, which is efficacious in patients with HBV infection resistant to lamivudine, is another antiviral agent that is being used increasingly in HBV-infected patients before and after transplantation.[44] A large multicenter trial demonstrated that adefovir administered for 48 weeks resulted in significant improvements in virologic, biochemical, and clinical parameters in patients with chronic hepatitis B who were resistant to lamivudine before and after transplantation (see Chapter 75).

Despite the complexities of managing HBV infection in the transplant recipient, excellent graft and patient survival rates are now routine, in contrast with the gloomy picture for HBV-infected liver transplantation candidates before the use of HBIG. An ever-expanding list of oral antiviral agents, including entecavir, promises to improve outcomes further, even in patients in whom resistance develops.

HEPATITIS C

After HCV was identified, early reports suggested that recurrent HCV infection before and after liver transplantation, based on detection of viremia, was frequent but did not have an adverse impact on overall patient or graft survival in the first several years after transplantation. With more extensive clinical experience, it has become clear that in a subset of HCV-infected recipients, severe graft injury and failure may develop as a result of recurrent hepatitis C. Analysis of serial liver biopsy specimens from transplant recipients with recurrent hepatitis C has demonstrated accelerated fibrosis and progression to cirrhosis when compared with the course of HCV infection in immunocompetent patients. In a report from King's College in London, approximately 20% of HCV-infected liver transplant recipients had evidence of allograft cirrhosis on 5-year-protocol biopsy specimens.[45] Although studies with longer follow-up are required to determine the proportion of patients in whom allograft cirrhosis related to recurrent hepatitis C will ultimately develop, it appears that less than 10% of patients with mild hepatitis at 1 year progress to allograft cirrhosis at 5 years. By contrast, two thirds of the patients with at least moderate hepatitis at 1 year progress to cirrhosis by 5 years.[46] Concern has been raised, however, that with more prolonged follow-up, initially benign mild hepatitis may evolve to a late-onset aggressive course in some patients. In a study from Valencia, Spain, the histologic outcome of 57 HCV genotype 1b–infected transplant recipients with initially mild hepatitis, defined as histologic fibrosis stage F0 or F1 (early fibrosis) during the first 3 years following transplantation, was evaluated (see Chapter 76). Progression to fibrosis stage F3 or F4 (late fibrosis) occurred in 35% of these patients. Variables associated with progression to advanced fibrosis on univariate analysis were fibrosis stage and inflammatory activity grade at baseline, recipient female gender, serum alanine aminotransferase (ALT) level at 1 year following transplantation, and serum aspartate aminotransferase (AST) and ALT levels at baseline. By multivariate analysis, the only variable retained in the model was fibrosis stage at baseline (relative risk, 11; 95% confidence interval, 3 to 41; $P = .0007$). Therefore, delayed HCV-related severe liver damage appears to occur in as many as one third of transplant recipients with initially mild recurrent hepatitis C. The presence of some fibrosis at baseline appears to predict this sudden change in the natural history of recurrent hepatitis C.[46] In some cases, an ominous early finding is prominent biochemical and histologic cholestasis, which appears to be a precursor to rapid allograft failure. One report has suggested that antiviral therapy for patients with cholestatic HCV reinfection may need to be administered indefinitely, because discontinuation of antiviral therapy leads to a rapid relapse of the cholestatic syndrome and death (see later).[47]

A number of viral and nonviral predictors of recurrent HCV infection after transplantation have been proposed (Table 92–3). Infection with HCV genotype 1b has been suggested as one such predictor, but this observation has not been universal. Higher serum viral levels before

and immediately after transplantation and possibly more rapid HCV quasispecies evolution have been described in patients with more aggressive recurrent hepatitis C (see Chapter 76). Older deceased donor age also has been implicated. Episodes of acute cellular graft rejection, particularly if multiple, lead to a greater likelihood of severe recurrent hepatitis C. A major challenge is to distinguish recurrent hepatitis C from graft rejection, particularly because many of the histologic hallmarks of acute rejection, including bile duct injury, also are consistent with recurrent hepatitis C (Table 92–4). Serial liver biopsies may help clarify this issue. The use of the antirejection agent OKT3 to treat glucocorticoid-resistant rejection also has been recognized to increase the severity of recurrent hepatitis C (see later discussion).[48] The immunosuppressant tacrolimus does not appear to lead to more severe recurrent hepatitis C when compared with cyclosporine-based immunosuppression.[49]

A study by Berenguer and associates evaluated the natural history of HCV-related graft cirrhosis to define the rates of clinical decompensation and mortality.[50] Thirty-nine patients with clinically compensated allograft cirrhosis were studied; at least one episode of decompensation developed in 18 patients (46%) after a mean follow-up period of approximately 8 months (Fig. 92–4). This rate of decompensation was considerably higher than that reported by Fattovich and colleagues in immunocompetent cirrhotic patients.[19] Moreover, patient survival rates after the development of allograft decompensation were poor: 93%, 61%, and 41% at 1, 6, and 12 months, respectively. Variables associated with decompensation and death included a short interval between transplantation and development of allograft cirrhosis and a high Child-Turcotte-Pugh score (class B or C). The investigators concluded that retransplantation, if considered, should be performed promptly once decompensation develops. Furthermore, an analysis has demonstrated that to achieve maximal utility, retransplantation for HCV-related allograft failure should be performed when the MELD score is 21 to 24, whereas maximal utility for primary liver transplantation occurs at MELD scores greater than 35.[51]

Table 92–3 Factors Associated with More Severe HCV Recurrence Following Liver Transplantation

Viral
High hepatitis C viral RNA levels before transplantation and within 2 wk after transplantation
Viral genotype 1b
Absence of pretransplantation hepatitis B viral coinfection
Cytomegalovirus coinfection
Immunosuppression
Multiple episodes of rejection (indicating a high cumulative prednisone dose)
Use of OKT3 to treat rejection
Other
High tumor necrosis factor-α production in the graft
Impaired HCV-specific CD4[+] T-cell responses
Nonwhite recipients
Ischemic-preservation injury

HCV, hepatitis C virus.

Table 92–4 Histologic Features of Recurrent Hepatitis C Virus Infection versus Acute Cellular Rejection

Feature	HCV Recurrence	Rejection
Time of onset after liver transplantation	Anytime; onset usually within the first yr	Usually within the first 2 months
Portal inflammation	Most cases	Always
Lymphocytes	Bland, uniform	Activated
Lymphoid aggregates	Usually	Occasionally
Lymphoid follicles	50% of cases	Very rarely
Eosinophils	Inconspicuous	Almost always
Steatosis	Often	Never
Acidophilic bodies	Common	Uncommon
Bile ductule damage	About 50% of cases	Very common
Atypical features	Cholestasis, ballooning degeneration without significant inflammation, marked ductular proliferation mimicking obstruction, granulomas	Prominent periportal and lobular necroinflammatory activity without subendothelial venular inflammation

HCV, hepatitis C virus.
From Rosen HR, Martin P: Liver transplantation. In Schiff ER, Sorrell MF, Maddrey WC (eds): Schiff's Diseases of the Liver, 8th ed. Philadelphia, Lippincott-Raven, 1999, p 1589.

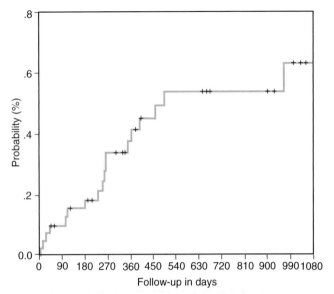

Figure 92–4 High rate of hepatic decompensation in patients with cirrhosis due to recurrent hepatitis C following liver transplantation. (From Berenguer M, Prieto M, Rayon JM, et al: Natural history of clinically compensated hepatitis C virus–related graft cirrhosis after liver transplantation. Hepatology 32:852, 2000.)

In contrast with recurrent HBV infection, universally effective prophylaxis against recurrent HCV infection has not been identified. Interferon-α monotherapy generally has been ineffective in treating established recurrent hepatitis C. When interferon is used with ribavirin, the rate of virologic response is increased, but at the cost of frequent and potentially severe side effects (see Chapter 76). Leukopenia is a particularly vexing problem in patients who undergo such treatment, and adjunctive granulocyte colony-stimulating factor (G-CSF) may be beneficial in permitting continuation of standard doses of interferon. The use of longer-acting, pegylated interferons is the focus of ongoing clinical trials. On the basis of earlier reports of rejection and graft loss in renal transplant recipients who received interferon, as well as preliminary experience in liver transplant recipients, a concern has been that interferon therapy increases the risk of liver graft rejection, although, as noted earlier, the distinction between recurrent HCV infection and rejection is difficult even on histologic grounds.[52] A phase III, randomized open-label study evaluated the efficacy and tolerability of combination therapy with interferon alfa-2b (3 million units three times a week) plus ribavirin (1000 to 1200 mg per day) for 12 months in 52 liver transplant recipients with HCV infection, in comparison with patients in an untreated control group.[53] The end-of-treatment response rate was 32%, and the rate of sustained clearance of serum HCV RNA was 21%. A relationship between viral factors, such as serum levels of HCV RNA and genotype, and response to therapy could not be established because of the small number of patients and the fact that 83% of the patients were infected with HCV genotype 1b. Of interest, all 6 of the patients with a sustained viral response were infected with HCV genotype 1b, and 5 had levels of viremia greater than 2 million copies/mL at the start of therapy; both factors (genotype 1b and a high level of

viremia) usually are considered to be predictors of low virologic response rates. Among the patients with sustained viral response, 2 were still seropositive for HCV RNA at 12 weeks, but all were seronegative for HCV RNA at week 24 following initiation of therapy.

Recurrent hepatitis C is an increasingly frequent cause of graft failure in transplant recipients, and the dilemma arises as to whether repeat liver transplantation is justified in these patients. As discussed later, a subset of patients who undergo retransplantation for graft loss caused by recurrent hepatitis C have a reasonable survival rate if they do not have deep jaundice or renal failure at the time of transplantation.[51]

ACUTE LIVER FAILURE

Acute liver failure, or fulminant hepatic failure, is defined as the onset of hepatic encephalopathy within 8 weeks of the initial symptoms of liver disease of various causes (see Chapter 90). This definition reflects not only the abrupt onset of illness but also the absence of antecedent chronic liver disease and potential reversibility. Acute liver failure is an important but infrequent indication for liver transplantation.[54] In the past, transplantation for acute liver failure resulted in poorer patient survival rates than those for benchmark indications, such as PBC. Subsequent experience, however, has shown that excellent patient survival rates are possible if acute liver failure is recognized promptly and the patient is referred for transplantation before irreversible complications, especially neurologic, have supervened.[54] The absence of papilledema on funduscopy and of typical signs on computed tomography (CT) scanning of the head does not preclude cerebral edema, which may complicate worsening encephalopathy; therefore, direct intracranial pressure monitoring may be required to detect and manage this frequently lethal complication of acute liver failure.

Specific criteria to identify patients with acute liver failure who are unlikely to recover spontaneously without liver transplantation are shown in Table 92–5. A challenge in managing patients with acute liver failure is to avoid unnecessary transplantation in those who will recover spontaneously, while not jeopardizing those whose only option for survival is a new liver by delaying a decision to proceed with transplantation. The role of liver-assist devices in managing acute liver failure, either as definitive therapy or as a "bridge to transplantation," remains an area of active investigation.[55]

CHOLESTATIC LIVER DISEASE

Although encountered less frequently outside referral centers than are other major causes of cirrhosis, PBC and PSC have been relatively common indications for liver transplantation in many transplantation centers and have had a key role in the evolution of disease models for liver disease, with PBC serving as a benchmark for patient and graft survival. Development of the Mayo disease models to predict the course of cholestatic disorders led to improved decision-making regarding timely referral for transplantation (see Chapters 65 and 86).[21,22]

Table 92–5   Criteria for Liver Transplantation in Acute Liver Failure

Criteria of King's College, London
Acetaminophen cases
  Arterial pH <7.3, or
  INR >6.5 and serum creatinine >3.4 mg/dL
Nonacetaminophen cases
  INR >6.5, or
  Any three of the following:
    Age <10 yr or >40 yr
    Duration of jaundice before encephalopathy >7 days
    Etiology: non-A, non-B hepatitis; halothane hepatitis;
      idiosyncratic drug reaction; indeterminate
    Serum bilirubin >17.6 mg/dL
    INR >3.5 (PT >50 seconds)
Criteria of Hôpital Paul-Brousse, Villejuif
Hepatic encephalopathy, and
Factor V level <20% in patients <age 30 yr, or
Factor V level <30% in patients ≥age 30 yr

INR, International Normalized Ratio.
Reprinted with permission from Keeffe EB: Liver transplantation: Current status and novel approaches to liver replacement. Gastroenterology 120:749, 2001.

Patients with PBC and PSC should be referred for transplantation evaluation if their Mayo risk scores predict a 1-year survival rate of less than 95%. The Mayo model for PBC includes serum bilirubin, serum albumin, patient age, prothrombin time, and presence of edema, whereas the model for PSC includes serum bilirubin, patient age, splenomegaly, and edema. These models do not take into account other prominent and frequently disabling complications of cholestatic liver disease, such as pruritus, osteopenia, or, in PSC, recurrent bouts of bacterial cholangitis, and have been superseded by the MELD score for determination of organ allocation.

Despite the generally excellent results of liver transplantation for these disorders, the possibility of recurrence of disease in the graft is an increasing concern.[5,56] Biliary stricturing similar to that in the native diseased liver can be identified in a minority of patients following liver transplantation for PSC and may represent recurrent disease. Differentiation of recurrent disease from other important causes of graft injury such as chronic rejection or ischemia may be difficult. Graft loss caused by recurrent PBC and PSC has been recognized but remains uncommon. Management is limited to excluding other causes of hepatic dysfunction and possibly modifying immunosuppression, to attempt to arrest disease recurrence in at least some recipients. Primary immunosuppression with tacrolimus has been implicated in recurrence of PBC.[57]

HEPATIC MALIGNANCY

Hepatocellular carcinoma is the most common primary hepatic malignancy and usually occurs with cirrhosis as a precursor (see Chapter 91). Tumors discovered incidentally in the explanted liver with diameters of less than 2 cm typically do not have an adverse impact on patient survival. The likelihood of tumor recurrence, however, increases markedly with tumor burden, vascular invasion, and presence of multiple lesions. On the basis of a large European experience reported by Mazzaferro and colleagues, generally accepted criteria for liver transplantation in patients with hepatocellular carcinoma have included a tumor diameter of less than 5 cm if the tumor is solitary or, if multiple, three or fewer lesions, with the largest lesion having a diameter of no greater than 3 cm.[58] Survival rates comparable with those for transplantation for decompensated cirrhosis in the absence of complicating hepatocellular carcinoma (75% at 4 years) have been reported. The preoperative metastatic workup should include a bone scan and chest CT, in addition to abdominal imaging. Portal vein occlusion in a patient with hepatocellular carcinoma is regarded as evidence of metastatic spread and precludes liver transplantation.

Some groups of investigators[59,60] have suggested that disease-free survival may be compatible with a larger tumor burden than that proposed by Mazzaferro and colleagues. On adoption of the MELD scoring system, increased priority was given to patients with hepatocellular carcinoma who met the Mazzaferro criteria, in recognition of the potential for cure of their cancers by liver transplantation and the concern that a protracted wait for a transplant could result in an increase in tumor burden and metastatic spread. This change resulted in proportionally more patients with hepatocellular carcinoma undergoing liver transplantation.[6] In addition, the waiting time for patients with hepatocellular carcinoma to receive a donor organ decreased significantly, and the number of patients who dropped off the waiting list because of advanced hepatocellular carcinoma also decreased.[9] In a more recent modification of the MELD scoring system, less advantage has been conferred to patients with hepatocellular carcinoma because of the relatively good short-term prognosis in patients with small tumors (less than 2 cm in diameter).

Use of a variety of adjuvant interventions has been reported in patients undergoing transplantation for hepatocellular carcinoma.[61] Recurrent tumor occurs frequently in the graft, and the rationale for adjuvant therapy has been to eliminate micrometastatic disease, which typically is disseminated by means of the vascular system. Systemic chemotherapy given perioperatively, as well as for a variable duration before and after transplantation, and usually incorporating doxorubicin, has been reported by a number of transplantation centers, although the benefit of this approach has been difficult to establish in the absence of controlled data. More recently, transarterial chemoembolization has found favor with the aim of reducing tumor burden during the often protracted wait for a transplant. This intervention can be hazardous in patients with decompensated cirrhosis, and its benefit in patients with favorable tumor characteristics remains to be determined. Confounding the management of the transplantation candidate with hepatocellular carcinoma is the frequent observation that the tumor burden in the explant is significantly underestimated by preoperative imaging studies.[58] Despite these caveats, the available data clearly identify a subset of patients with hepatocellular carcinoma who can be cured by liver transplantation and who cannot tolerate surgical resection of the tumor because of associated cirrhosis.

The fibrolamellar variant of hepatocellular carcinoma manifests in younger adults without underlying cirrhosis, often when the tumor burden is already large. Extensive resection can be tolerated because cirrhosis is absent. Liver transplantation still may be performed in patients who have recurrent tumor after resectional surgery. With post-transplantation recurrence, the tumor may be relatively indolent, although recurrences are not as infrequent as was once thought.[62]

Hepatoblastoma is a rare pediatric tumor that also occurs in the absence of underlying parenchymal liver disease. Initial management consists of surgical resection; adjuvant chemotherapy is indicated for metastatic disease. Liver transplantation is an option when the tumor cannot be resected.

Cholangiocarcinoma remains the only major tumor of primarily hepatic origin for which a definitive role for liver transplantation has been difficult to establish (see Chapter 66). The results of liver transplantation for cholangiocarcinoma diagnosed preoperatively have been so poor that its presence has been regarded as a contraindication to transplantation, and even tumors discovered only in the explant have a high recurrence rate. Recurrence is almost invariable and prompt in transplant recipients. Only a subset of patients with a hilar location of the tumor and absence of nodal involvement have been reported to have a good 5-year survival rate. The cholangiocarcinoma frequently is more extensive than suspected on pretransplantation imaging; often local, lymphatic, and perineural spread is found. The addition of en bloc pancreaticoduodenectomy has not resulted in improved survival following liver transplantation. Other approaches to treatment include preoperative irradiation and chemotherapy, with careful intraoperative tumor staging followed by transplantation; preliminary results with this approach are encouraging.[15]

METABOLIC DISORDERS

Patients with congenital hepatic enzyme deficiencies and other inborn errors of metabolism may be cured by implantation of a normal liver[63] (see Chapters 71 to 73). Metabolic disorders considered for hepatic transplantation fall into two broad categories: diseases dominated clinically by obvious hepatocyte injury (e.g., Wilson disease, hemochromatosis) and those without any evidence of clinical or histologic hepatic injury (e.g., primary hyperoxaluria, familial hypercholesterolemia).

Although metabolic disorders are most prominent as indications for liver transplantation in the pediatric population, important adult diseases managed by liver transplantation include Wilson disease and hemochromatosis. Substantial neurologic improvement can occur following transplantation for Wilson disease that manifests with decompensated cirrhosis and neurologic involvement.[64] Wilsonian crisis with severe hemolysis is an indication for urgent liver transplantation; chelating therapy is ineffective in such cases.

Hemochromatosis has been associated with poorer outcomes following transplantation than those observed in other forms of cirrhosis, because of cardiac and infectious complications.[65] Ongoing studies will clarify whether

iron depletion before transplantation will improve post-transplantation survival. Iron reaccumulation in the grafts of patients undergoing transplantation for hemochromatosis is at least a theoretical concern, although continued iron depletion therapy typically is not required.[31]

Liver transplantation also has been performed for a variety of systemic disorders and is a curative procedure in combination with renal transplantation for primary hyperoxaluria, in which end-organ damage is confined to the kidney but the metabolic defect is hepatic. Liver transplantation has been successful in arresting manifestations of familial amyloid polyneuropathy; the explant, which is the source of the abnormal protein, is available for use in a "domino" fashion in an older liver transplant recipient who will not live long enough for consequent neurologic injury to develop.[66] The biliary type of cirrhosis associated with cystic fibrosis also has been managed with transplantation.

NONALCOHOLIC FATTY LIVER DISEASE

NAFLD has been recognized increasingly as a major cause of chronic liver disease, including cirrhosis and hepatocellular carcinoma, and is implicated in many cases of what was formerly termed cryptogenic cirrhosis (see Chapter 82). Many of the key precipitants of NAFLD, including obesity, hyperlipidemia, and diabetes mellitus, are exacerbated by the post-transplantation immunosuppressive regimen.[67] Recurrence of NAFLD has been described, as has de novo NAFLD, following transplantation; this problem will be a major challenge for transplantation programs in the future. In the absence of effective drug therapy, efforts to treat NAFLD after transplantation focus on weight control, optimal diabetic management, and a lipid-lowering regimen.

VASCULAR DISORDERS

Budd-Chiari syndrome is characterized by hepatic venous outflow obstruction of the liver; its presentation often mimics decompensated cirrhosis (see Chapter 80).[68] Important associations are myeloproliferative disorders, hypercoagulable states, and inferior vena cava webs. Medical approaches to management often are disappointing and fail to retard the progression to liver failure and death. Liver biopsy may be helpful in determining whether the therapeutic approach should be decompression with a portosystemic shunt or liver transplantation. Good long-term results have been described in patients who undergo prompt portosystemic shunt surgery, but patients with advanced fibrosis on a liver biopsy specimen generally should undergo liver transplantation. Although many affected patients have an underlying myeloproliferative disorder, accelerated progression to leukemia typically is not observed after transplantation. Long-term anticoagulation is prescribed in patients who undergo transplantation for Budd-Chiari syndrome.

Sinusoidal obstruction syndrome (veno-occlusive disease) is manifested by necrosis of zone 3 hepatocytes and fibrous obliteration of the sinusoids and lumens of central venules in the liver (see Chapters 33 and 80).

Most commonly seen after bone marrow transplantation (BMT), sinusoidal obstruction syndrome may lead to hepatic failure and death in up to 25% of patients, despite an otherwise successful BMT. Although the experience with liver transplantation for hepatic complications of BMT is limited,[69] liver transplantation appears to be the only intervention that consistently alters the course of advanced sinusoidal obstruction syndrome. Similarly, liver transplantation has been shown to be effective in the management of severe post-BMT graft-versus-host disease with predominantly hepatic involvement (see also Chapter 33). Both hypocoagulable (e.g., hemophilia A and B) and hypercoagulable (e.g., protein C and protein S deficiency) hematologic disorders have been cured with liver transplantation.[70]

AUTOIMMUNE HEPATITIS

Failure of immunosuppressive therapy to arrest progression of severe autoimmune hepatitis with the development of hepatic decompensation is an indication to consider liver transplantation (see Chapter 85). Human leukocyte antigen (HLA)-DR3 is associated with a lower likelihood of a therapeutic response to immunosuppression in patients with autoimmune hepatitis than is obtained with other HLA associations. Excellent long-term survival is usual after liver transplantation. The autoimmune diathesis may result in higher rates of acute cellular rejection, however. In addition, recurrent autoimmune hepatitis has been recognized increasingly in recent years and may require higher-than-usual maintenance doses of immunosuppressive agents.[4] Graft survival generally is not diminished by recurrent autoimmune hepatitis. Recurrent autoimmune hepatitis mimics the features of disease in the native liver and is associated with hypergammaglobulinemia and autoantibodies.

OTHER INDICATIONS

A variety of other diagnoses have been reported as indications for liver transplantation. Adult polycystic disease with marked abdominal distention resulting from multiple hepatic cysts that are not amenable to resection has been treated successfully by transplantation (see Chapter 91). If renal failure also is present, combined liver-kidney transplantation is indicated. Cerebral imaging is indicated to exclude intracranial aneurysms, which are a feature of this syndrome. Liver transplantation also is indicated in cases of multiple adenomas associated with glycogen storage disease and not only eliminates the risk of progression to hepatocellular carcinoma but also corrects the underlying metabolic disease (see Chapter 73). Multiorgan diseases for which liver transplantation has been performed include Alagille's syndrome, amyloidosis, and sarcoidosis.

SURGICAL ASPECTS OF LIVER TRANSPLANTATION

Once a potential deceased organ donor is identified, the local organ procurement organization coordinates har-

vesting and supplies pertinent donor medical information to centers with suitable potential recipients listed with UNOS. In contrast with other types of organ transplants, including kidney and bone marrow, absence of HLA incompatibility does not appear to reduce liver graft survival, and donor-recipient matching is based only on ABO blood compatibility and physical characteristics such as recipient weight. In critically ill recipients, an ABO-incompatible organ may be implanted, with the recognition that graft survival may be diminished and hemolytic anemia can develop. In addition to screening serologic studies and routine liver biochemical testing, particular attention is paid to the donor's medical history, including cardiovascular instability and need for pressor support before determination of brain death.[71]

With the critical shortage of deceased organ donors, expansion of the donor pool has included acceptance of donors aged 70 years and older. As noted earlier, however, use of organs from older donors in recipients with HCV infection may lead to more severe recurrence of HCV infection, thereby potentially limiting use of such donor organs in at least some recipients.

The typical donor has had a catastrophic head injury or an intracerebral bleed with brain death but without multiorgan failure. Electrolyte imbalance and hepatic steatosis are particular concerns, because they are predictors of subsequent graft nonfunction. Livers from non–heart-beating donors have been used successfully for transplantation, but long-term graft survival may be diminished in the recipients.

The harvesting team makes a visual and, if necessary, histologic assessment of the donor organ. The organ is preserved in University of Wisconsin (or a similar) solution, which contains free radical scavengers and maintains osmotic stability of the organ, thereby maintaining its viability during transport to the transplant center and for up to 24 hours. Particular note is made during the harvesting procedure of anatomic variants in the hepatic arterial supply that need to be preserved to ensure graft viability. Once the circulation is interrupted, the organ is infused rapidly with cold University of Wisconsin solution to help preserve it before hepatectomy. Donor iliac arteries and veins also are retrieved in case vascular grafting is required. After arrival of the organ at the recipient institution, further vascular dissection, with arterial reconstruction if necessary, is performed before implantation.

Splitting cadaveric donor livers either in situ during harvesting or ex vivo on return to the transplantation center allows two recipients to receive portions of the same liver, if the volume and quality of each portion are sufficient. An adult cadaveric liver is divided into two functioning grafts. The left lateral segments (segments 2 and 3) are used for a pediatric recipient, and the right trisegment (segments 4 to 8) is used for an adult recipient (see Chapter 68). Acceptable graft and patient survival rates can be obtained with split grafts, although high-risk unstable recipients may have poorer outcomes with this technique. Figure 92–5 shows the segmental anatomy of the liver, which forms the basis of dissection for both split and living-donor liver transplantation. Combined data suggest that in vivo split liver transplantation may yield superior survival rates and lower complication rates than those achieved with the ex vivo technique.

Superior view

Inferior view

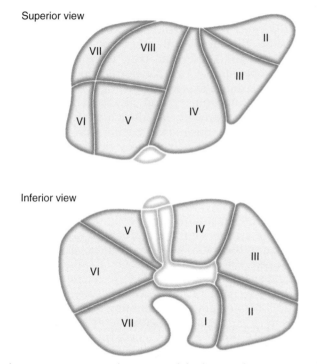

Figure 92–5 Segmental anatomy of the liver in the superior and inferior views. Segment VIII is visible only on the superior view, and segment I (caudate lobe) is visible only on the inferior view. (From Keeffe EB: Liver transplantation: Current status and novel approaches to liver replacement. Gastroenterology 120:749, 2001.)

NATIVE HEPATECTOMY

Removal of the native liver is the most technically challenging part of deceased donor transplantation. Previous abdominal surgery, especially creation of a portosystemic shunt, and severe portal hypertension add to the complexity of hepatectomy. Hepatectomy is technically easier, however, after placement of a TIPS than after surgical creation of a portosystemic shunt, and TIPS is now regarded as a better choice for treatment of intractable variceal bleeding in a patient who ultimately will require transplantation (see Chapter 87).[36] Hilar dissection is performed to permit access to the major hepatic vessels and to devascularize the liver.

Clamping of the portal vein during hepatectomy and liver implantation results in increased bleeding during dissection, mesenteric congestion, and production of lactate, whereas clamping of the inferior vena cava aggravates venous stasis and causes renal hypertension, with diminished venous return to the heart. To circumvent these problems, venovenous bypass is achieved by cannulation of the portal vein and inferior vena cava through the femoral vein and return of blood through the axillary vein to the right side of the heart. This technique commonly is performed in adult and older pediatric transplant recipients. In some recipients, only a suprahepatic anastomosis to the vena cava is performed, and the inferior vena cava is ligated below the graft. This is called the "piggyback" technique, in contrast with the more usual circumstance, in which anastomosis to the vena cava is performed above and below the graft. The piggyback technique may be applicable if uninter-

rupted caval flow during transplantation is particularly beneficial, as in a recipient with cardiac instability, if a previous portosystemic shunt obviates the need for portal bypass, or if the recipient is a pediatric patient in whom venovenous bypass may not be possible.

The portal venous anastomosis is performed after portal bypass is terminated and is followed by the hepatic arterial anastomosis. The bile duct anastomosis is then fashioned directly, duct to duct, with or without a T-tube. Hepaticojejunostomy is the preferred anastomosis if intrinsic bile duct disease is present, as in primary sclerosing cholangitis, or with a major discrepancy in donor and recipient bile duct diameters. Microscopic surgical techniques facilitate the donor-recipient biliary and vascular anastomoses. Vascular anatomic anomalies increase the complexity of surgery further. In the past, direct duct-to-duct anastomosis typically was facilitated by placement of a T-tube in the bile duct to drain bile percutaneously, with the added advantages of easy assessment of bile flow and quality and potential access for cholangiography postoperatively. The risk of a bile leak during subsequent removal of the T-tube, however, has led many transplantation programs to abandon its routine placement.

The use of a live donor involves implantation of a portion of the liver (see later), which is even more technically challenging than use of a whole cadaveric organ (orthotopic liver transplantation). Auxiliary cadaveric liver transplantation is the placement of a graft without removal of the native liver. This technique usually has been performed in critically ill patients, such as those with acute liver failure, who are too unstable to tolerate native hepatectomy.

Irrespective of the type of graft used, after the anastomoses are complete, the newly implanted graft is reperfused, with restoration of normal blood flow. The resulting release of vasoactive agents from pooled blood in the lower half of the body can lead to potentially lethal cardiovascular instability and tachyarrhythmias. Prompt bile production should occur if graft function is adequate. Hyperacute rejection is a rare but devastating complication after liver transplantation and leads to rapid graft necrosis within hours, with the need for urgent retransplantation.

LIVE-DONOR LIVER TRANSPLANTATION

A major surgical advance has been the extension of live-donor liver transplantation (LDLT) from pediatric recipients to adult recipients. The role of LDLT in adult transplant recipients continues to be debated, because of the magnitude of the risk to the donor. The potential donor must be a healthy adult, typically a family member or close friend of the recipient, who volunteers to be evaluated. A series of checks and balances is necessary to ensure that the potential donor undergoes an adequate medical assessment and is not proceeding only as a result of pressure from the patient or family.[72] It is crucial that the potential recipient not be privy to details of the potential donor's evaluation. In most centers, a hepatologist not involved in the care of the recipient performs an assessment of the donor. Often, an independent advocate is also appointed to safeguard the donor's interests. At each stage of the process, the potential donor is given the opportunity to withdraw from consideration. Morbidity and mortality rates in donors undergoing hepatic resection are 10% and 0.5%, respectively, and carefully obtained informed consent is essential. Preoperative evaluation of the donor at a typical transplantation center is performed in four stages over a period of 1 to 3 months; the more invasive testing such as liver biopsy is undertaken later in the evaluation (Table 92–6). After undergoing a complete evaluation, only a relatively small proportion of potential donors are deemed to be satisfactory candidates. One consequence of the evaluation of many potential donors has been the recognition that anatomic abnormalities in the biliary and vascular system and unsuspected abnormalities on liver biopsy specimens are frequent in apparently healthy persons.[73]

Right lobes (segments 5 to 8), extended right grafts (segments 4 to 8), or left hepatic grafts (segments 2 to 4) have been used successfully in adult-to-adult LDLT (see Fig. 92–5). Adult LDLT provides obvious advantages to the recipient, including a reduction in the mortality rate for patients awaiting a donor organ. An expected reduction in the risk of rejection related to use of a graft from a relative has been not realized, and some evidence suggests that recurrence of HCV infection actually may be accelerated.[74] The overriding concern remains the short-term and long-term consequences for the donor, including the risk of immediate perioperative morbidity and mortality. Additional concerns relate to the financial losses resulting from time lost from work, an adverse effect on insurability in the future, and a lack of long-term follow-up data to ensure that hepatic resection and subsequent regeneration do not result in biliary or other abnormalities.

IMMUNOSUPPRESSION

Administration of immunosuppressive agents following liver transplantation is divided into induction (initial) and maintenance (long-term) phases. In addition, episodes of acute cellular and chronic ductopenic rejection require therapy. A wide array of immunosuppressive agents are currently used.[75] In practice, newer immunosuppressive agents are introduced first for renal transplantation before they are used for liver transplantation, reflecting the need for effective antirejection regimens in renal and other nonhepatic solid organ transplant recipients. The primary goal of immunosuppression is to prevent graft rejection and loss; a secondary goal is to avoid the adverse consequences of the antirejection therapy.

A list of the commonly used immununosuppressive agents, routes of administration, methods of monitoring, and common adverse effects is presented in Table 92–7.

Table 92–6 Protocol for Evaluation of Potential Living-Related Donors

Stage 1	Complete history and physical examination
	Laboratory blood tests: liver biochemical tests, blood chemistry, hematology, coagulation profile, urinalysis, alpha-fetoprotein, carcinoembryonic antigen, and serologic tests for hepatitis A, B, and C, cytomegalovirus, Epstein-Barr virus, and human immunodeficiency virus
	Imaging studies: abdominal ultrasound examination, chest x-ray
Stage 2	Complete psychiatric and social evaluation
	Imaging studies: computed tomography scan of the abdomen
	Other studies: pulmonary function tests, echocardiography
Stage 3	Histology: liver biopsy
	Imaging studies: celiac and superior mesenteric angiography with portal phase
Stage 4	Imaging studies: magnetic resonance cholangiogram
	Informed consent

From Ghobrial RM, Amersi F, Busuttil RW: Surgical advances in liver transplantation. Clin Liver Dis 4:553, 2000.

Table 92–7 Major Immunosuppressive Agents

Agent	Mode of Action	Monitoring	Toxic Effects
Cyclosporine	Calcineurin inhibitor: suppresses IL-2–dependent T cell proliferation	Blood level	Renal, neurologic, hyperlipidemia, hypertension, hirsutism
Tacrolimus	Same as cyclosporine	Blood level	Renal, neurologic, diabetes mellitus
Prednisone	Cytokine inhibitor (IL-1, IL-2, IL-6, TNF, and IFN gamma)	None	Hypertension, diabetes mellitus, obesity, osteoporosis, infection, depression, psychosis
Azathioprine	Inhibition of T and B cell proliferation by interfering with purine synthesis	White blood cell count	Bone marrow suppression, hepatotoxicity
Mycophenolate mofetil	Selective inhibition of T and B cell proliferation by interfering with purine synthesis	White blood cell count	Diarrhea, bone marrow suppression
Sirolimus	Inhibition of late T cell functions	Blood level	Neutropenia, thrombocytopenia, hyperlipidemia
OKT3	Blocking of T cell CD3 receptor, preventing stimulation by antigen	CD3+ count	Cytokine release syndrome, pulmonary edema, increased risk of infections
IL-2 receptor blocker	Competitive inhibition of IL-2 receptor on activated lymphocytes	None	Hypersensitivity reactions with basiliximab

IFN, interferon; IL, interleukin; TNF, tumor necrosis factor.
Adapted from Everson GT, Karn I: Immediate postoperative care. In Maddrey WC, Schiff ER, Sorrell MF (eds): Transplantation of the Liver, 3rd ed. Philadelphia, Lippincott Williams & Wilkins, 2001, p 131.

Table 92–8 Clinically Relevant Drug Interactions with Immunosuppressive Drugs

Drugs that increase blood levels of cyclosporine and tacrolimus:
  Antifungals: fluconazole, ketoconazole, itraconazole
  Antibiotics: erythromycin, clarithromycin
  Calcium channel blockers: diltiazem, verapamil
  Others: bromocriptine, metoclopramide, allopurinol
Drugs that decrease levels of cyclosporine and tacrolimus:
  Anticonvulsants: phenytoin, phenobarbitone
  Antibiotics: rifampin, nafcillin
Drugs that increase nephrotoxicity of cyclosporine and tacrolimus:
  Gentamicin, ketoconazole, nonsteroidal anti-inflammatory drugs
Drugs that interact with mycophenolate mofetil:
  Acyclovir, ganciclovir
  Antacids
  Cholestyramine (inhibits absorption)
Drugs that interact with azathioprine:
  Allopurinol, angiotensin-converting enzyme (ACE) inhibitors, warfarin

Common drug-drug interactions are shown in Table 92–8. The calcineurin inhibitors cyclosporine and tacrolimus are the basis for a majority of induction and maintenance immunosuppressive regimens, and both agents have substantial toxicity. Tacrolimus is now used frequently for primary immunosuppression instead of cyclosporine. In addition, the patient's antirejection regimen may be converted from cyclosporine to tacrolimus following glucocorticoid- or OKT3-refractory rejection, late rejection (after 6 months following transplantation), histologically diagnosed chronic rejection, severe cholestasis, intestinal malabsorption of cyclosporine, or cyclosporine toxicity (e.g., hirsutism, gingivitis, severe hypertension). Tacrolimus used for rescue therapy in chronic rejection is less effective in the subgroup of patients with a serum total bilirubin level greater than 10 mg/dL, underscoring that early recognition of chronic rejection is imperative if a favorable outcome is to be achieved. Use of sirolimus, which has been implicated in hepatic artery thrombosis, as well as in delayed wound healing and infections,[76] has been restricted in transplant recipients.

Considerable differences are observed from transplantation center to transplantation center in the rate at which the level of induction immunosuppression is reduced to avoid toxicity and lessen the risk of recurrent disease. Generally, the strategy includes tapering and in some cases discontinuation of maintenance glucocorticoids.[75]

POSTOPERATIVE COURSE

INITIAL PHASE TO DISCHARGE FROM HOSPITAL

Because of the complexity of liver transplantation and the often markedly decompensated state of transplant recipients, invasive monitoring with arterial and pulmonary venous lines is necessary in the first few postoperative days. If a T-tube has been placed, hepatocellular recovery can be monitored at the bedside; dark copious bile output provides reassuring evidence of good graft function. The patient's overall status, including neurologic recovery from anesthesia, urinary output, and cardiovascular stability, also reflects graft function. Routine antimicrobial prophylaxis includes bowel decontamination with oral nonabsorbable antibiotics, and perioperative administration of systemic broad-spectrum antibiotics, antifungal agents, and, to prevent cytomegalovirus infection, ganciclovir. Markedly abnormal liver biochemical test levels are typical during the initial 48 to 72 postoperative hours and reflect a number of insults to the graft, including ischemia following harvesting, preservation, and subsequent reperfusion. The overall trend in serum aminotransferase levels should be downward, with a corresponding improvement in indices of coagulation and a fall in the serum bilirubin level. Thrombocytopenia in the immediate postoperative period reflects a variety of processes including residual splenomegaly, the effect of medications, and, of importance, reduced graft function.

Worrisome clinical features in the post-transplantation period include scanty, pale bile, metabolic acidosis, depressed mentation, and continued need for pressor support with worsening liver biochemical test levels. Hepatic artery thrombosis needs to be excluded promptly by a Doppler ultrasound study and necessitates urgent retransplantation. Hepatic artery thrombosis is more common in pediatric recipients because of the smaller size of the vessels. Primary nonfunction of the graft also is an indication for urgent retransplantation and is suggested by the absence of bile production in the first several hours after transplantation, as well as an unstable overall clinical status. Donor characteristics that are associated with an increased likelihood of primary graft nonfunction include marked hepatic steatosis and profound hyponatremia. If graft function is adequate, pressor support can be tapered and respiratory weaning parameters can be monitored to facilitate extubation, although the recipient who is markedly debilitated from advanced cirrhosis may require several days of ventilatory support. Poor graft function and renal insufficiency also can impede weaning from the ventilator.

Within the first week after transplantation, liver biochemical test levels should steadily improve as ischemia and reperfusion injury resolve. Acute cellular rejection becomes an important and frequent cause of graft dysfunction at 1 week and beyond and is suggested by a rise in serum aminotransferase, alkaline phosphatase, and bilirubin levels. Because the biochemical features are nonspecific, the threshold for performing liver biopsy to evaluate other diagnostic possibilities, which include slowly resolving reperfusion injury, biliary tract obstruction, and cholestasis related to sepsis, should be low. Histologic findings characteristic of acute cellular rejection are bile duct injury, portal tract inflammation with eosinophils, and, with more severe injury, endotheliitis (Fig. 92–6). High doses of glucocorticoids (1000 mg of methylprednisolone or the equivalent) followed by gradually decreasing doses (from 200 to 20 mg per day, extending over several days) constitute first-line therapy. A response is suggested by a return of liver biochemical test levels toward normal values.

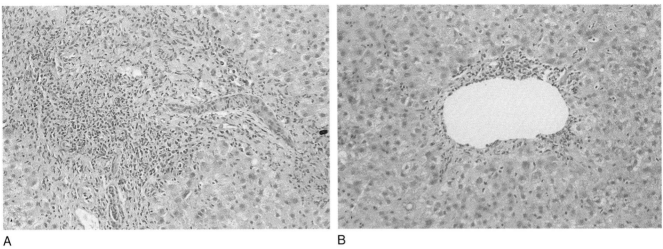

A   B

Figure 92–6   Acute cellular rejection of a liver graft. *A*, The portal tract shows a lymphocytic and plasma cell infiltrate that spills over into the periportal hepatocytes and bile duct. An atypical bile duct also is present. *B*, The central vein shows attachment of lymphocytes to the endothelium (endotheliitis). (From Cotran RS, Kumar V, Collins T [eds]: Robbins' Pathologic Basis of Disease, 6th ed. CD-ROM. Philadelphia, WB Saunders, 1999.)

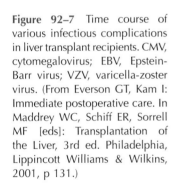

Figure 92–7 Time course of various infectious complications in liver transplant recipients. CMV, cytomegalovirus; EBV, Epstein-Barr virus; VZV, varicella-zoster virus. (From Everson GT, Kam I: Immediate postoperative care. In Maddrey WC, Schiff ER, Sorrell MF [eds]: Transplantation of the Liver, 3rd ed. Philadelphia, Lippincott Williams & Wilkins, 2001, p 131.)

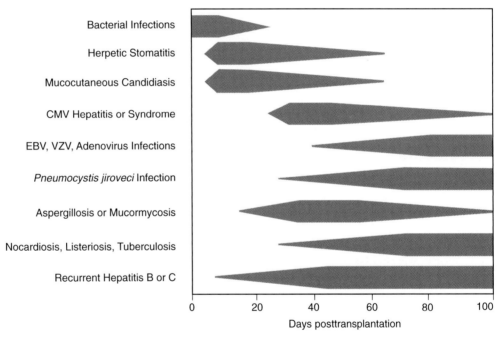

For the occasional patient with presumed acute cellular rejection who fails to have a biochemical response to glucocorticoids, enhancement of immunosuppression may be necessary with the monoclonal antibody OKT3. Liver biopsy should be repeated to confirm a lack of histologic response before more intensive therapy is initiated and to exclude other important causes of graft dysfunction such as ischemia.

The ability of recurrent HCV infection to mimic virtually all of the histologic features of acute cellular rejection has led to a reevaluation of the need to treat apparent acute cellular rejection aggressively in all circumstances. Routine (protocol) liver biopsies also have fallen out of favor, because histologic evidence of acute cellular rejection can be noted in the absence of worsen-

ing graft function and is of no apparent clinical significance. A routine cholangiogram is obtained before the T-tube, if one is present, is clamped; a nonsustained rise in liver biochemical test levels can be anticipated as a result. The timing of various infectious complications following liver transplantation is shown in Figure 92–7. In the first 3 to 4 weeks after transplantation, infections typically are bacterial and related to surgical complications such as intra-abdominal bleeding, bile leak, or wound infection.

A number of other important medical issues are common in the first weeks following transplantation (Table 92–9). Neurologic dysfunction can manifest clinically as an acute confusional state or seizures, and the differential diagnosis may include the lingering effects of hepatic encephalopathy, electrolyte imbalance,

Table 92–9 Medical Complications Occurring in the Immediate Postoperative Period

Infections
  Bacterial
  Viral
    Cytomegalovirus
    Epstein-Barr virus
  Fungal
    Candidiasis, torulopsosis
    Pneumocystis jiroveci pneumonia
    Aspergillosis, mucormycosis
Respiratory complications
  Pneumonia
  Pulmonary edema
  Acute respiratory distress syndrome
  Portopulmonary hypertension
  Hepatopulmonary syndrome
Renal failure
Cardiovascular disease
  Hypertension
  Myocardial ischemia
  Valvular heart disease
  Cardiomyopathy
    Idiopathic hypertrophic subaortic stenosis
    Hemochromatosis
Neurologic complications
  Central pontine myelinolysis
  Seizures
  Central nervous system hemorrhage
  Ischemic events
Coagulopathy
  Thrombocytopenia
  Disseminated intravascular coagulation
Diabetes mellitus

From Everson GT, Karn I: Immediate postoperative care. In Maddrey WC, Schiff ER, Sorrell MF (eds): Transplantation of the Liver, 3rd ed. Philadelphia, Lippincott Williams & Wilkins, 2001.

poor graft function, sepsis, uremia, and side effects of medications. A particular concern is the development of neurologic toxicity caused by the major immunosuppressive agents, the most dramatic presentation of which is central pontine myelinolysis. Overly rapid correction of hyponatremia perioperatively has been implicated in the genesis of central pontine myelinolysis, with evidence of demyelination demonstrable on magnetic resonance imaging of the brain. Management includes correcting the electrolyte imbalance if present and reducing the dose of calcineurin inhibitors, which can be facilitated by the use of mycophenolate mofetil. Diabetes mellitus, which is common in persons with cirrhosis, can occur for the first time in the postoperative period and usually requires insulin for control. HCV infection further increases the risk of post-transplantation diabetes.[77] Renal impairment following transplantation may reflect a number of factors, including pre-transplantation hepatorenal syndrome or renal failure of other causes, intraoperative hypotension resulting in acute tubular necrosis and, of importance, the nephrotoxic effects of cyclosporine and tacrolimus, which cause renal afferent arteriolar vasoconstriction and a corresponding fall in the glomerular filtration rate. Adjunctive therapy with

mycophenolate mofetil allows a reduction in the doses of cyclosporine and tacrolimus while providing adequate immunosuppression. Short-term hemodialysis may be necessary until renal function improves.

FOLLOWING DISCHARGE FROM HOSPITAL

If the initial postoperative course is smooth, planning for discharge is possible by the second week after transplantation. Recovery often is more protracted, however, particularly in debilitated recipients. Once discharged, patients are seen at frequent intervals during the first postoperative month. Liver biochemical test levels should fall to normal within a few weeks following transplantation. Further graft dysfunction is an indication for prompt liver biopsy, because acute cellular rejection remains a concern during this time; in addition, cytomegalovirus (CMV) infection becomes an important consideration three or more weeks after transplantation. Histologic features suggestive of CMV hepatitis include "owl's eye" inclusions in the hepatocytes, as well as neutrophilic abscesses with focal necrosis of the parenchyma[78] (see Chapter 78 and Fig. 78–3). Recipients who have had no prior exposure to CMV are at particularly high risk for CMV infection, particularly if they receive a graft from a CMV-seropositive donor, and are candidates for more intensive antiviral prophylaxis. A distinction is made between CMV viremia and CMV disease with systemic manifestations such as diarrhea, because viremia does not invariably imply the disease. Early recurrence of HCV infection also may become apparent, and as noted earlier, it is crucial to recognize that many of the histologic features of acute cellular rejection, such as bile duct inflammation and endotheliitis, are mimicked by HCV infection (see Table 92–4).

In addition to graft hepatitis, other important manifestations of de novo CMV infection include pneumonitis and diarrhea. Reactivation of CMV in a previously infected recipient tends to be less clinically severe than de novo infection. The diagnosis of CMV infection is confirmed by culture of tissue or blood, but not by isolation from urine.[79] Many transplantation centers now have access to rapid tissue culture techniques with indirect immunofluorescence that allow prompt diagnosis. High-dose intravenous ganciclovir is highly effective in the treatment of CMV infection, but viral resistance has been described. Other useful therapeutic agents include a CMV hyperimmune globulin and foscarnet. Not only is CMV infection an important cause of morbidity and mortality in transplant recipients, but it also has been implicated in other complications, notably chronic graft rejection and recurrent HCV infection.

If a liver biopsy specimen shows features to suggest biliary obstruction or if graft dysfunction is associated with clinical features of cholangitis such as fever and abdominal pain, a cholangiogram is obtained through the T-tube, if present, by endoscopic retrograde cholangiopancreatography (ERCP) if a T-tube is not present and the anastomosis is duct to duct, or by percutaneous transhepatic cholangiography if choledochojejunostomy has been performed. Magnetic resonance cholangiopancreatography is increasingly being used in transplant recipients. A stricture in a choledochocholedochostomy at the site of anastomosis usually is managed initially by balloon dilation at the time of cholangiography, followed by placement of a temporary internal stent. Surgical intervention is reserved for patients who do not respond to this approach, in which case the anastomosis is converted to a Roux-en-Y anastomosis. Anastomotic stricturing also can occur at the site of a choledochojejunostomy and requires access, usually by a percutaneous approach, to dilate the stenotic area.

A critical issue in management is to distinguish anastomotic stricturing from stricturing caused by ischemia. The bile duct in the transplant recipient is prone to ischemia because of its relatively tenuous arterial blood supply, and the development of a biliary stricture (unless it is obviously anastomotic) may reflect hepatic artery thrombosis. Ischemic stricturing generally is diffuse but can be predominantly hilar. Although temporizing measures such as balloon dilation may have some utility, if hepatic artery thrombosis is present or stricturing is widespread, such efforts generally are futile, and retransplantation will be required. Other causes of nonanastomotic stricturing include the use of an ABO-incompatible graft and protracted cold ischemia after harvesting. Biliary stricturing also can be a feature of recurrent PSC.

A T-tube, if present, is removed by the sixth postoperative month, and removal is best performed at the transplantation center, because bile leaks are common. When a bile leak occurs, prompt ERCP with nasobiliary drainage or stenting usually allows the tear in the bile duct to heal uneventfully.

In addition to prophylaxis against CMV infection in the early postoperative months, long-term antibiotics, most frequently trimethoprim-sulfamethoxazole, are prescribed to prevent infection with *Pneumocystis jiroveci*. In patients intolerant of sulfa drugs, alternative options are dapsone tablets and inhaled pentamidine. Because *Pneumocystis* infection occurs most commonly in the first postoperative year, prophylaxis needs to be continued for at least this period of time.

Fungal infections pose a major threat to the transplant recipient, particularly in the setting of marked debilitation, intensive immunosuppression for rejection, or retransplantation. Major sites of infection are mucocutaneous (oral and esophageal), pulmonary, and intracerebral. Despite prolonged therapy with amphotericin or, more recently, itraconazole, a fatal outcome is usual. A diagnosis of a brain abscess in a patient with invasive *Aspergillus* infection implies a dismal prognosis. It is important to distinguish superficial skin infections and simple colonization from invasive fungal infections, because topical antifungal agents such as nystatin or clotrimazole can eradicate the former. Similarly, bladder irrigation with amphotericin can cure candidal cystitis without the need for systemic antifungal therapy.

Opportunistic infections remain a concern in the transplant recipient during long-term follow-up. Patients need prompt assessment of symptoms of infection. Standard antibiotic therapy is appropriate for community-acquired respiratory infections, but a more extensive workup is indicated for unusually severe symptoms or failure of an infection to resolve rapidly with treatment. Enteric bacteremia may be an initial clue to hepatic artery throm-

bosis in an otherwise stable recipient. Reactivation of tuberculosis may manifest in an atypical fashion following transplantation. Bronchoscopy or lumbar puncture with cultures may be necessary, as clinically indicated.

LONG-TERM MANAGEMENT

GENERAL PREVENTIVE MEDICINE

Satisfactory long-term management of the liver transplant recipient requires cooperation and communication between the primary care physician and the transplantation center. Many of the disorders that affect long-term survival after transplantation are common diseases, including systemic hypertension, hyperlipidemia, and diabetes.[80] Regular determination of a complete blood count, electrolytes, liver biochemical test levels and immunosuppressive drug levels should be arranged and the results forwarded to the transplantation center. Generally, the frequency of bloodwork can be reduced after the first postoperative year in recipients with stable graft function.

Systemic hypertension is a frequent complication of liver transplantation and is related to calcineurin inhibitor–induced renal vasoconstriction, as well as to effects of other drugs such as glucocorticoids. Reduction in the level of immunosuppression unfortunately is generally ineffective in ameliorating hypertension. Other contributing factors include mild renal insufficiency, which is frequent following transplantation even when absent preoperatively. Initial antihypertensive therapy usually consists of use of a calcium channel blocker. Because blood cyclosporine and tacrolimus levels are increased by verapamil and diltiazem, nifedipine is the calcium channel blocker of choice. Angiotensin-converting enzyme inhibitors and potassium-sparing diuretics are relatively contraindicated because of their propensity to accentuate hyperkalemia, which is frequent in transplant recipients because of renal tubular acidosis caused by the calcineurin inhibitors. Diuretics also are generally avoided because of concern about exacerbating renal insufficiency in the transplant recipient. Beta blockers are the second-line antihypertensive agents used. Furosemide is the diuretic of choice if fluid overload is present. In the minority of patients in whom hypertension is not controlled, a centrally acting agent such as clonidine is introduced. For the occasional patient with intractable hypertension on cyclosporine-based immunosuppression, substitution of tacrolimus for cyclosporine may aid blood pressure control. Both cyclosporine and tacrolimus are nephrotoxic, however, and will accentuate renal impairment that existed perioperatively. Although acute nephrotoxicity may respond to interruption of or a reduction in the dose of these drugs, chronic renal impairment usually is irreversible, and drastic dose reductions should be avoided for fear of precipitating graft rejection. Cofactors implicated in the progression to chronic dialysis include recurrent HCV infection with associated glomerulonephritis, diabetes, and systemic hypertension. Renal transplantation may be performed successfully in transplant recipients who become dialysis dependent after otherwise successful liver transplantation.[81]

Osteopenia is a frequent cause of morbidity in transplant recipients.[80] Although hepatic osteodystrophy typically is associated with the cholestatic liver diseases, it also is common in patients with other forms of cirrhosis. Factors implicated in the pathogenesis include poor nutritional status, immobility, the calciuric effect of many diuretics, hypogonadism, and glucocorticoid use in patients with autoimmune hepatitis. In the initial several months after transplantation, osteopenia is accelerated further by high-dose glucocorticoid therapy, as well as by use of the other major immunosuppressive agents. Atraumatic fractures may occur in trabecular bone such as vertebrae or ribs. Patients begin to rebuild bone mass, however, after the doses of immunosuppressants are reduced and the patient's mobility increases. Supplemental calcium and vitamin D frequently are prescribed for patients with symptomatic osteopenia, as is a bisphosphonate.

De novo malignancies are increased in frequency following transplantation.[27] Post-transplantation lymphoproliferative disorder (PTLD) ranges in severity from a low-grade indolent process to an aggressive neoplasm. Uncontrolled proliferation of B cells following transplantation, typically in response to primary Epstein-Barr virus infection, can be polyclonal or monoclonal. Pediatric recipients are at particular risk because of absence of prior Epstein-Barr viral infection. Intensive immunosuppression with OKT3 for severe rejection increases the risk of PTLD, which can manifest as a mononucleosis-like syndrome, lymphoproliferation, or malignant lymphoma. Clinical features suggestive of the diagnosis of PTLD include lymphadenopathy, unexplained fever, and systemic symptoms such as weight loss. After the diagnosis is made histologically by biopsy of involved areas (which can include the liver graft and gastrointestinal tract, as well as lymph nodes), therapy includes a reduction in the levels of immunosuppressive and antiviral treatment with ganciclovir directed against Epstein-Barr virus infection. Systemic chemotherapy may be required in patients who present with a malignant lymphoma. The higher frequency of PTLD in pediatric recipients has led to surveillance by polymerase chain reaction methodology for Epstein-Barr viremia and reduction of immunosuppression in patients with a positive result, before clinical features of PTLD occur. Antiviral prophylaxis also is prescribed for high-risk recipients, including those who are seronegative for Epstein-Barr virus and receive a liver from a seropositive donor. Chronic graft rejection is increased in frequency in survivors of PTLD because of the deliberate reduction in the level of immunosuppression, which may be cautiously increased after PTLD is contained (see Chapter 33).

Screening for prostate carcinoma should be performed by yearly digital rectal examination in male transplant recipients older than 40 years of age, in conjunction with serum prostate-specific antigen (PSA) testing. Screening for colorectal cancer also should be performed by colonoscopy every 3 to 5 years after age 50 years in asymptomatic recipients; in patients with a history of PSC and ulcerative colitis, yearly colonoscopy with surveillance mucosal biopsies should be considered.[82] In the setting of chronic immunosuppression, it seems appropriate to screen female transplant recipients older than 40 years of age for breast cancer by yearly mammography, although the cost-effectiveness of this approach is undefined. Other malignancies that are increased in frequency in organ transplant recipients include skin, female genital tract, and perineal cancers; alcoholic patients may be particularly prone to malignancies of the oropharynx. Patients should be encouraged to wear sunscreen and undergo appropriate surveillance for these malignancies.

Hyperlipidemia is observed in up to one half of transplant recipients and reflects a number of factors, including diabetes mellitus, obesity, renal dysfunction, and use of immunosuppressive agents, especially cyclosporine. Pharmacologic therapy is indicated if hypercholesterolemia fails to respond to weight reduction and tight diabetic control. Pravastatin, a 3-hydroxy-3-methylglutaryl–coenzyme A (HMG-CoA) reductase inhibitor, is well tolerated and efficacious in transplant recipients. Diabetes mellitus is common in these patients and occurs postoperatively for the first time in approximately one third of patients. The pathogenesis is multifactorial; immunosuppressive therapy is a major factor because of the hyperglycemic effects of prednisone, cyclosporine, tacrolimus, azathioprine, and mycophenolate mofetil. In most diabetic recipients, therapy with insulin is required. The high frequency of diabetes following liver transplantation has led to the development of glucocorticoid-sparing immunosuppressive regimens.

A related problem is obesity, which is frequent even in transplant recipients who were profoundly malnourished preoperatively. Factors responsible for weight gain following transplantation include glucocorticoid use, increased caloric intake, and decreased physical activity during recuperation from surgery. Immunosuppression with tacrolimus has been reported to result in less weight gain than with cyclosporine; to a large extent, this difference may reflect the lower glucocorticoid doses employed with tacrolimus. Management of obesity in transplant recipients includes a reduction in the dose of glucocorticoids and even complete withdrawal if possible. The advent of mycophenolate mofetil has permitted maintenance immunosuppression without glucocorticoids.

IMMUNIZATIONS AND PROPHYLAXIS OF BACTERIAL INFECTIONS

Immunization against hepatitis A and B, influenza, pneumococcal infection, tetanus, and diphtheria is part of the standard pretransplantation evaluation. A substantial proportion of patients may be unable to mount adequate antibody responses because of the immunosuppression associated with end-stage liver disease. Vaccines based on live or attenuated microorganisms (e.g., measles, mumps, rubella; oral polio; bacille Calmette-Guérin [BCG]; vaccinia) are contraindicated because of the risk of reactivation. It is recommended that patients take prophylactic antibiotics for any dental procedure, even basic cleaning.

WHEN TO CALL THE TRANSPLANTATION CENTER

A number of common symptoms, signs, and laboratory abnormalities warrant a call by the local physician to the transplantation center. These problems include fever, abdominal pain, neurologic symptoms, anticipated surgery, and a possible change in the patient's immunosuppressive regimen. When an unexplained abnormality of liver biochemical tests occurs, a complete workup for possible causes is imperative. Although a liver biopsy can be obtained by the patient's local physician, a local pathologist may be inexperienced in allograft interpretation, and it is critical that the specimen be reviewed at the transplantation center so that appropriate decisions regarding management can be obtained. Additionally, many transplantation programs prefer to perform indicated interventional biliary tract studies, because therapeutic intervention often is required, and immediate access to the transplantation team permits more rapid decision making. Any evidence of graft failure needs to be attended to immediately by referral to the transplantation center.

HEPATIC RETRANSPLANTATION

Although improved immunosuppressive regimens have led to a lower rate of graft loss because of chronic rejection, recurrence of the underlying liver disease has been recognized increasingly as a cause of graft failure, as illustrated most strikingly in HCV-infected recipients. The rates and severity of recurrent disease are highly variable and probably are related to a complex interplay of host factors (including the underlying liver disease), therapeutic decisions (e.g., immunosuppression, antiviral treatment), and possibly genetic variability of the allograft (perhaps through effects on the nature and magnitude of the inflammatory response within the graft).

Understanding the full impact of recurrent disease, especially nonviral disease, on patient and graft survival will require long-term follow-up studies. For example, although the rate of histologic recurrence of viral hepatitis is greatest in the first year after transplantation, recurrent PBC or PSC develops in less than 5% of patients by the first year, whereas more than 20% of patients undergoing transplantation for these disorders demonstrate histologic recurrence 10 years after transplantation. As patients enter their second and third decades after transplantation, it is possible that the number of patients needing retransplantation will deplete the deceased donor pool further. This issue is compounded by the

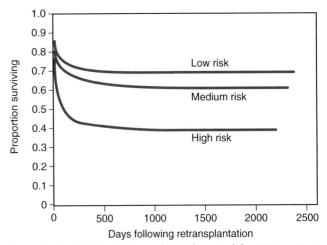

Figure 92–8 Kaplan-Meier analysis of survival for 1356 patients undergoing hepatic retransplantation stratified into low-risk, medium-risk, and high-risk groups using prognostic predictive factors listed in Table 92-10 ($P < .00001$ by Wilcoxon rank sum). (From Rosen HR, Madden JP, Martin P: A model to predict survival following hepatic retransplantation. Hepatology 29:365, 1999.)

Table 92–10 Multivariate Models Developed to Predict Survival Following Liver Retransplantation

Reference	No. of Patients	Prognostic Predictive Factors	Comments
83	1356	Recipient age, bilirubin, creatinine, UNOS status, and cause of graft failure	UNOS database used; HCV positivity, donor age significant predictors by univariate analysis
84	70	Recipient age, UNOS status, inpatient status, creatinine, and bilirubin	Single site: King's College
85	418	Recipient age, mechanical ventilatory status, creatinine, and bilirubin	Single site: University of Pittsburgh
86	150	Recipient age group (pediatric vs. adult), mechanical ventilatory status, organ ischemia time >12 hr, creatinine, bilirubin	Single site: UCLA
87	447	Interval to retransplantation (better prognosis if within 30 days)	Single site: Mayo Clinic; limited to patients with PBC or PSC
88	207	Creatinine; bilirubin	UNOS database used; limited to HCV-positive patients retransplanted for causes other than primary nonfunction

HCV, hepatitis C virus; PBC, primary biliary cirrhosis; PSC, primary sclerosing cholangitis; UNOS, United Network for Organ Sharing.
From Rosen HR: Disease recurrence following liver transplantation. Clin Liver Dis 4:675, 2000.

observation that patients who undergo retransplantation experience an approximately 20% overall reduction in the rate of survival but consume an increased amount of resources when compared with primary transplant recipients. On the basis of these considerations, a number of investigators have developed models to predict survival following retransplantation, especially for HCV infection (Table 92–10 and Fig. 92–8). Preoperative serum bilirubin and creatinine levels consistently provide prognostic information. Although these models estimate only the probability of survival for an individual patient and do not take into account the patient's quality of life, they can be used as adjuncts to clinical judgment. Retransplantation in low-risk patients is associated with survival comparable with that for primary liver transplantation; whether retransplantation is justified in patients with high risk scores will require prospective studies.

REFERENCES

1. Perry I, Neuberger J: Immunosuppression: Towards a logical approach in liver transplantation. Clin Exp Immunol 139:2, 2005.
2. Burton JR Jr, Rosen HR: Retransplantation for hepatitis C: What do we really know? Liver Transpl 10:1504, 2004.
3. Samuel D: Management of hepatitis B in liver transplantation patients. Semin Liver Dis 24(suppl 1):55, 2004.
4. Vogel A, Heinrich E, Bahr MJ, et al: Long-term outcome of liver transplantation for autoimmune hepatitis. Clin Transplant 18:62, 2004.
5. Kugelmas M, Spiegelman P, Osgood MJ, et al: Different immunosuppressive regimens and recurrence of primary sclerosing cholangitis after liver transplantation. Liver Transpl 9:727, 2003.
6. Freeman RB, Wiesner RH, Edwards E, et al: Results of the first year of the new liver allocation plan. Liver Transpl 10:7, 2004.
7. Thuluvath PJ, Yoo HY: Graft and patient survival after adult live donor liver transplantation compared to a matched cohort who received a deceased donor transplantation. Liver Transpl 10:1263, 2004.
8. D'Alessandro AM, Fernandez LA, Chin LT, et al: Donation after cardiac death: The University of Wisconsin experience. Ann Transplant 9:68, 2004.
9. Sharma P, Balan V, Hernandez JL, et al: Liver transplantation for hepatocellular carcinoma: The MELD impact. Liver Transpl 10:36, 2004.
10. Keeffe EB: Liver transplantation: Current status and novel approaches to liver replacement. Gastroenterology 120:749, 2001.
11. Freeman RB Jr, Wiesner RH, Roberts JP, et al: Improving liver allocation: MELD and PELD. Am J Transplant 4(suppl 9):114, 2004.
12. Desai NM, Mange KC, Crawford MD, et al: Predicting outcome after liver transplantation: Utility of the model for end-stage liver disease and a newly derived discrimination function. Transplantation 77:99, 2004.
13. Rosen HR, Fontana RJ, Brown RS, et al: Curricular guidelines for training in transplant hepatology. Liver Transpl 8:85, 2002.
14. Llovet JM, Fuster J, Bruix J: The Barcelona approach: Diagnosis, staging, and treatment of hepatocellular carcinoma. Liver Transpl 10(2 suppl 1):S115, 2004.
15. Heimbach JK, Gores GJ, Haddock MG, et al: Liver transplantation for unresectable perihilar cholangiocarcinoma. Semin Liver Dis 24:201, 2004.
16. Kelly DA: Managing liver failure. Postgrad Med J 78:660, 2002.
17. Menon KV, Kamath PS: Managing the complications of cirrhosis. Mayo Clin Proc 75:501, 2000.
18. Perrillo RP, Wright T, Rakela J, et al: A multicenter United States–Canadian trial to assess lamivudine monotherapy before and after liver transplantation for chronic hepatitis B. Hepatology 33:424, 2001.
19. Fattovich G, Giustina G, Degos F, et al: Morbidity and mortality in compensated cirrhosis type C: A retrospective follow-up study of 384 patients. Gastroenterology 112:463, 1997.
20. Heuman DM, Abou-Assi SG, Habib A, et al: Persistent ascites and low serum sodium identify patients with cirrhosis and low MELD scores who are at high risk for early death. Hepatology 40:802, 2004.
21. Kim WR, Wiesner RH, Poterucha JJ, et al: Adaptation of the Mayo primary biliary cirrhosis natural history model for application in liver transplant candidates. Liver Transpl 6:489, 2000.
22. Kim WR, Poterucha JJ, Wiesner RH, et al: The relative role of the Child-Pugh classification and the Mayo natural history model in the assessment of survival in patients with primary sclerosing cholangitis. Hepatology 29:1643, 1999.
23. Bravata DM, Keeffe EB: Quality of life and employment after liver transplantation. Liver Transpl 7(11 suppl 1):S119, 2001.
24. Kamath PS, Wiesner RH, Malinchoc M, et al: A model to predict survival in patients with end-stage liver disease. Hepatology 33:464, 2001.
25. Neff GW, Sherman KE, Eghtesad B, Fung J: Review article: Current status of liver transplantation in HIV-infected patients. Aliment Pharmacol Ther 20:993, 2004.
26. Menon KV, Shah V, Kamath PS: The Budd-Chiari syndrome. N Engl J Med 350:578, 2004.
27. Herrero JI, Lorenzo M, Quiroga J, et al: De novo neoplasia after liver transplantation: An analysis of risk factors and influence on survival. Liver Transpl 11:89, 2004.
28. Neff GW, O'Brien C, Montalbano M, et al: Consumption of dietary supplements in a liver transplant population. Liver Transpl 10:881, 2004.
29. Plotkin JS, Johnson LB, Rustgi V, Kuo PC: Coronary artery disease and liver transplantation: The state of the art. Liver Transpl 6(4 suppl 1):S53, 2000.
30. Keeffe BG, Valantine H, Keeffe EB: Detection and treatment of coronary artery disease in liver transplant candidates. Liver Transpl 7:755, 2001.
31. Crawford DH, Fletcher LM, Hubscher SG, et al: Patient and graft survival after liver transplantation for hereditary hemochromatosis: Implications for pathogenesis. Hepatology 39:1655, 2004.
32. Krowka MJ, Mandell MS, Ramsay MA, et al: Hepatopulmonary syndrome and portopulmonary hypertension: A report of the multicenter liver transplant database. Liver Transpl 10:174, 2004.
33. Hoeper MM, Krowka MJ, Strassburg CP: Portopulmonary hypertension and hepatopulmonary syndrome. Lancet 363:1461, 2004.
34. Arguedas MR, Abrams GA, Krowka MJ, Fallon MB: Prospective evaluation of outcomes and predictors of mortality in patients with hepatopulmonary syndrome undergoing liver transplantation. Hepatology 37:192, 2003.
35. Garcia N Jr, Mihas AA: Hepatic hydrothorax: Pathophysiology, diagnosis, and management. J Clin Gastroenterol 38:52, 2004.
36. Rosado B, Kamath PS: Transjugular intrahepatic portosystemic shunts: An update. Liver Transpl 9:207, 2003.
37. Keswani RN, Ahmed A, Keeffe EB: Older age and liver transplantation: A review. Liver Transpl 10:957, 2004.
38. Narayanan Menon KV, Nyberg SL, Harmsen WS, et al. MELD and other factors associated with survival after liver transplantation. Am J Transplant 4:819, 2004.

39. Nair S, Verma S, Thuluvath PJ: Obesity and its effect on survival in patients undergoing orthotopic liver transplantation in the United States. Hepatology 35:105, 2002.

40. Trotter JF, Brimhall B, Arjal R, Phillips C: Specific laboratory methodologies achieve higher model for endstage liver disease (MELD) scores for patients listed for liver transplantation. Liver Transpl 10:995, 2004.

41. Jauhar S, Talwalkar JA, Schneekloth T, et al: Analysis of factors that predict alcohol relapse following liver transplantation. Liver Transpl 10:408, 2004.

42. Samuel D, Muller R, Alexander G, et al: Liver transplantation in European patients with the hepatitis B surface antigen. N Engl J Med 329:1842, 1993.

43. Han SH, Martin P, Edelstein M, et al: Conversion from intravenous to intramuscular hepatitis B immune globulin in combination with lamivudine is safe and cost-effective in patients receiving long-term prophylaxis to prevent hepatitis B recurrence after liver transplantation. Liver Transpl 9:182, 2003.

44. Schiff ER, Lai CL, Hadziyannis S, et al: Adefovir dipivoxil therapy for lamivudine-resistant hepatitis B in pre- and post-liver transplantation patients. Hepatology 38:1419, 2003.

45. Gane EJ, Portmann BC, Naoumov NV, et al: Long-term outcome of hepatitis C infection after liver transplantation. N Engl J Med 334:815, 1996.

46. Berenguer M, Aguilera V, Prieto M, et al: Delayed onset of severe hepatitis C–related liver damage following liver transplantation: A matter of concern? Liver Transpl 9:1152, 2003.

47. Gopal DV, Rosen HR: Duration of antiviral therapy for cholestatic HCV recurrence may need to be indefinite. Liver Transpl 9:348, 2003.

48. Rosen HR, Shackleton CR, Higa L, et al: Use of OKT3 is associated with early and severe recurrence of hepatitis C after liver transplantation. Am J Gastroenterol 92:1453, 1997.

49. Martin P, Busuttil RW, Goldstein RM, et al: Impact of tacrolimus versus cyclosporine in hepatitis C virus–infected liver transplant recipients on recurrent hepatitis: A prospective, randomized trial. Liver Transpl 10:1258, 2004.

50. Berenguer M, Prieto M, Rayon JM, et al: Natural history of clinically compensated hepatitis C virus–related graft cirrhosis after liver transplantation. Hepatology 32(4 pt 1):852, 2000.

51. Burton JR Jr, Sonnenberg A, Rosen HR: Retransplantation for recurrent hepatitis C in the MELD era: Maximizing utility. Liver Transpl 10(10 suppl 2):S59, 2004.

52. Stravitz RT, Shiffman ML, Sanyal AJ, et al: Effects of interferon treatment on liver histology and allograft rejection in patients with recurrent hepatitis C following liver transplantation. Liver Transpl 10:850, 2004.

53. Samuel D, Bizollon T, Feray C, et al: Interferon-alpha 2b plus ribavirin in patients with chronic hepatitis C after liver transplantation: A randomized study. Gastroenterology 124:642, 2003.

54. Gow PJ, Jones RM, Dobson JL, Angus PW: Etiology and outcome of fulminant hepatic failure managed at an Australian liver transplant unit. J Gastroenterol Hepatol 19:154, 2004.

55. Demetriou AA, Brown RS Jr, Busuttil RW, et al: Prospective, randomized, multicenter, controlled trial of a bioartificial liver in treating acute liver failure. Ann Surg 239:660, 2004.

56. Sylvestre PB, Batts KP, Burgart LJ, et al: Recurrence of primary biliary cirrhosis after liver transplantation: Histologic estimate of incidence and natural history. Liver Transpl 9:1086, 2003.

57. Neuberger J, Gunson B, Hubscher S, Nightingale P: Immunosuppression affects the rate of recurrent primary biliary cirrhosis after liver transplantation. Liver Transpl 10:488, 2004.

58. Mazzaferro V, Regalia E, Doci R, et al: Liver transplantation for the treatment of small hepatocellular carcinomas in patients with cirrhosis. N Engl J Med 334:693, 1996.

59. Yao FY, Ferrell L, Bass NM, et al: Liver transplantation for hepatocellular carcinoma: Expansion of the tumor size limits does not adversely impact survival. Hepatology 33:1394, 2001.

60. Gondolesi GE, Roayaie S, Munoz L, et al: Adult living donor liver transplantation for patients with hepatocellular carcinoma: Extending UNOS priority criteria. Ann Surg 239:142, 2004.

61. Schwartz M: Liver transplantation for hepatocellular carcinoma. Gastroenterology 127(5 suppl 1):S268, 2004.

62. Pinna AD, Iwatsuki S, Lee RG, et al: Treatment of fibrolamellar hepatoma with subtotal hepatectomy or transplantation. Hepatology 26:877, 1997.

63. Tung BY, Kowdley KV: Liver transplantation for hemochromatosis, Wilson's disease, and other metabolic disorders. Clin Liver Dis 1:341, 1997.

64. Sutcliffe RP, Maguire DD, Muiesan P, et al: Liver transplantation for Wilson's disease: Long-term results and quality-of-life assessment. Transplantation 75:1003, 2003.

65. Tung BY, Farrell FJ, McCashland TM, et al: Long-term follow-up after liver transplantation in patients with hepatic iron overload. Liver Transpl Surg 5:369, 1999.

66. Azoulay D, Samuel D, Castaing D, et al: Domino liver transplants for metabolic disorders: Experience with familial amyloidotic polyneuropathy. J Am Coll Surg 189:584, 1999.

67. Burke A, Lucey MR: Non-alcoholic fatty liver disease, non-alcoholic steatohepatitis and orthotopic liver transplantation. Am J Transplant 4:686, 2004.

68. Srinivasan P, Rela M, Prachalias A, et al: Liver transplantation for Budd-Chiari syndrome. Transplantation 73:973, 2002.

69. Rosen HR, Martin P, Schiller GJ, et al: Orthotopic liver transplantation for bone-marrow transplant-associated veno-occlusive disease and graft-versus-host disease of the liver. Liver Transpl Surg 2:225, 1996.

70. Gordon FH, Mistry PK, Sabin CA, Lee CA: Outcome of orthotopic liver transplantation in patients with haemophilia. Gut 42:744, 1998.

71. Wood KE, Becker BN, McCartney JG, et al: Care of the potential organ donor. N Engl J Med 351:2730, 2004.

72. Brown RS Jr, Russo MW, Lai M, et al: A survey of liver transplantation from living adult donors in the United States. N Engl J Med 348:818, 2003.

73. Trotter JF: Selection of donors for living donor liver transplantation. Liver Transpl 9(10 suppl 2):S2, 2003.

74. Garcia-Retortillo M, Forns X, Llovet JM, et al: Hepatitis C recurrence is more severe after living donor compared to cadaveric liver transplantation. Hepatology 40:699, 2004.

75. Everson GT, Trotter JF, Kugelmas M, Forman L: Immunosuppression in liver transplantation. Minerva Chir 58:725, 2003.

76. Fisher A, Seguel JM, de la Torre AN, et al: Effect of sirolimus on infection incidence in liver transplant recipients. Liver Transpl 10:193, 2004.

77. Zein NN, Abdulkarim AS, Wiesner RH, et al: Prevalence of diabetes mellitus in patients with end-stage liver cirrhosis due to hepatitis C, alcohol, or cholestatic disease. J Hepatol 32:209, 2000.

78. Lefkowitch JH: Diagnostic issues in liver transplantation pathology. Clin Liver Dis 6:555, 2002.

79. Norris S, Kosar Y, Donaldson N, et al: Cytomegalovirus infection after liver transplantation: viral load as a guide to treating clinical infection. Transplantation 74:527, 2002.

80. Muñoz SJ, Rothstein KD, Reich D, Manzarbeitia C: Long-term care of the liver transplant recipient. Clin Liver Dis 4:691, 2000.

81. Coopersmith CM, Brennan DC, Miller B, et al: Renal transplantation following previous heart, liver, and lung transplantation: An 8-year single-center experience. Surgery 130:457, 2001.

82. Vera A, Gunson BK, Ussatoff V, et al: Colorectal cancer in patients with inflammatory bowel disease after liver transplantation for primary sclerosing cholangitis. Transplantation. 75:1983, 2003.

83. Rosen HR, Madden JP, Martin P: A model to predict survival following liver retransplantation. Hepatology 29:365, 1999.

84. Wong T, Devlin J, Rolando N, et al: Clinical characteristics affecting the outcome of liver retransplantation. Transplantation 64:878, 1997.

85. Doyle HR, Morelli F, McMichael J, et al: Hepatic retransplantation: An analysis of risk factors associated with outcome. Transplantation 61:1499, 1996.

86. Markmann JF, Gornbein J, Markowitz JS, et al: A simple model to estimate survival after retransplantation of the liver. Transplantation 67:422, 1999.

87. Kim WR, Wiesner RH, Poterucha JJ, et al: Hepatic retransplantation in cholestatic liver disease: Impact of the interval to retransplantation on survival and resource utilization. Hepatology 30:395, 1999.

88. Rosen HR, Martin P: Hepatitis C infection in patients undergoing liver retransplantation. Transplantation 66:1612, 1998.

CHAPTER

93 Anatomy, Histology, Embryology, and Developmental Anomalies of the Small and Large Intestine

Ellen Kahn and Fredric Daum

ANATOMY

MACROSCOPIC FEATURES

Small Intestine

The small intestine is a specialized tubular structure within the abdominal cavity in continuity with the stomach proximally and the colon distally. The small bowel increases 20 times in length with aging, from 200 cm in the newborn to almost 6 m in the adult, and its length is approximated by three times the length of the infant, or height of the child or adult.[1]

The *duodenum*, the most proximal portion of the small intestine, begins at the duodenal bulb, travels in the retroperitoneal space around the head of the pancreas, and ends on its return to the peritoneal cavity at the ligament of Treitz. The remainder of the small intestine is suspended within the peritoneal cavity by a thin, broad-based mesentery that is attached to the posterior abdominal wall and allows free movement of the small intestine within the abdominal cavity. The proximal 40% of the mobile small intestine is the *jejunum*, and the remaining 60% is the *ileum*. The jejunum occupies the left upper portion of the abdomen, and the ileum is positioned in the right abdomen and upper part of the pelvis. No distinct anatomic demarcation exists between jejunum and ileum.

Visual examination of the luminal surface of the small intestine reveals mucosal folds, the *plicae circulares*. More numerous in the proximal jejunum, the plicae circulares decrease in number in the distal small bowel and are absent in the terminal ileum. Aggregates of lymphoid follicles are scattered throughout the small intestine but are found in highest concentration within the ileum, where they are designated *Peyer's patches*. Peyer's patches normally are more prominent during infancy and childhood than they are in adulthood.

The small bowel is in continuity with the colon at the ileocecal valve, which comprises two semilunar lips that protrude into the cecum. The ileocecal valve provides a barrier to the retrograde flow of colonic contents into the small intestine. This barrier appears to be a function of the angulation between the ileum and cecum that is maintained by the superior and inferior ileocecal ligaments,[2] and a true tonic, sphincter-type pressure does not appear to be present in this region.

Colon and Rectum

The colon is a tubular structure approximately 30 to 40 cm in length at birth in the full-term infant. In the adult, the colon measures 1.5 m, about one quarter of the length of the small bowel. The diameter of the colon is greatest in the cecum (7.5 cm) and narrowest in the sigmoid (2.5 cm). The colon is continuous with the small intestine proximally at the ileocecal valve and ends distally at the anal verge (Fig. 93–1). The external appearance of the colon differs from that of the small bowel, because the longitudinal muscle fibers of the colon coalesce into three discrete bands called *teniae*, located at 120-degree intervals about the colonic circumference: tenia liberis, tenia omentalis, and tenia mesocolica. The teniae start at the base of the appendix and extend continuously to the proximal rectum. Outpouchings of the colon, the *haustra*, are found between the teniae. Semilunar folds characterize the mucosa between the haustra.

Sacs of peritoneum filled with adipose tissue, the *appendices epiploicae*, are found on the surface of the colon.

The first portion of the colon, the *cecum*, lies in the right iliac fossa and projects downward as a blind pouch below the entrance of the ileum. The cecum is a sacculated structure 6 to 8 cm in length and breadth. Because of its large diameter, it is the part of the colon most apt to rupture with distal obstruction, and cecal tumors can grow to be quite large without producing symptoms of obstruction. The mobility of the cecum normally is fixed by a small mesocecum; an anomaly in fixation exists in 10% to 20% of people, predisposing them to cecal volvulus. The *vermiform appendix* is a blind outpouching of the cecum that begins inferior to the ileocecal valve. Appendiceal anatomy is discussed further in Chapter 113.

The *ascending colon* extends from the cecum for 12 to 20 cm along the right side of the peritoneal cavity to the hepatic flexure. The ascending colon is covered with peritoneum anteriorly and on both sides and thus constitutes a retroperitoneal organ.

At the hepatic flexure, the colon turns medially and anteriorly to emerge into the peritoneal cavity as the *transverse colon*. This longest portion of the colon (40 to 50 cm) is the most mobile segment of the colon and

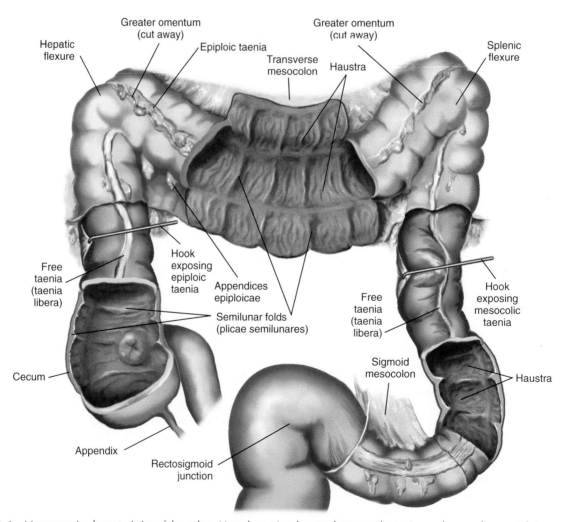

Figure 93–1 Macroscopic characteristics of the colon. Note the teniae, haustra between the teniae and appendices epiploicae on the outer surface, and the semilunar folds on the luminal side. (From Netter FH: The Netter Collection of Medical Illustration, vol 3. Teterboro, NJ, Icon Learning System, 2002.)

drapes itself across the anterior abdomen between the hepatic and splenic flexures. When a person assumes the upright position, the transverse colon may actually dip down into the pelvis. The transverse colon may become fixed in this festooned position by adhesions, most commonly resulting from hysterectomy and potentially leading to a technically difficult colonoscopy.

The *descending colon*, about 30 cm in length, travels posteriorly and then inferiorly in the retroperitoneal compartment to the pelvic brim. There, it emerges into the peritoneal cavity as the *sigmoid colon*. This is an S-shaped redundant segment of variable length, tortuosity, and mobility, which challenges the endoscopist and radiologist and causes it to be susceptible to volvulus. Because the sigmoid is the narrowest part of the colon, tumors and strictures of this region cause symptoms early in the course of disease.

The *rectum*, 10 cm in length in the adult, begins at the peritoneal reflexion and follows the curve of the sacrum ending at the anal canal.

Anal Canal

The *anal canal*, 5 cm in length in the adult, has discrete upper and lower demarcations. The *anorectal ring* is located proximally and is composed of the upper portion of the internal sphincter, the longitudinal muscle of the rectum, the deep portion of the external sphincter, and the puborectalis portion of the levator ani muscle; distally the *anal verge* represents the transition of anal skin to true skin. The mucosa of the distal 3 cm of the rectum and the anal canal contains 6 to 12 redundant longitudinal folds called the *columns of Morgagni*, which terminate in the anal papillae. These columns are joined together by mucosal folds called the *anal valves*, which are situated at the dentate line. The muscularis mucosae disappears in the anorectal canal, and the inner circular coat of muscularis propria thickens to form the internal anal sphincter.[3] The sphincter ani externus muscle constitutes the external anal sphincter and surrounds the anal canal. The fibers of the external sphincter blend with those of the levator ani muscle and are attached posteriorly to the coccyx and anteriorly to the perineal body. The anatomy and function of these muscles are described in more detail in Chapter 122.

Intestinal Vasculature

The superior mesenteric artery delivers oxygenated blood to the distal duodenum, the entire jejunum and ileum, the ascending colon, and the proximal two thirds of the transverse colon. The remainder of the colon is supplied by branches of the inferior mesenteric artery. The anal canal is supplied by the paired middle and inferior rectal (hemorrhoidal) arteries. The rectal arteries are branches of the internal iliac (hypogastric) arteries. Veins follow the arterial distribution. The superior and inferior mesenteric veins join the splenic vein to form the portal vein. (See Chapter 111 for additional discussion of the intestinal blood supply.)

Intestinal Lymphatic Drainage

The lymphatic drainage of both the small bowel and colon follows their respective blood supplies to lymph nodes in the celiac, superior preaortic, and inferior preaortic regions. Lymphatic drainage proceeds to the cisterna chyli and then via the thoracic duct into the left subclavian vein. The perianal region drains to the inguinal lymph nodes.

Intestinal Extrinsic Innervation

The autonomic nervous system—sympathetic, parasympathetic and enteric—innervates the gastrointestinal tract. The sympathetic and parasympathetic nerves constitute the extrinsic nerve supply and connect with the intrinsic nerve supply, which is composed of ganglion cells and nerve fibers within the intestinal wall. Innervation of the small intestine and colon is discussed in detail in Chapters 94 and 95, respecturely.

MICROSCOPIC FEATURES

General Considerations

The small and large intestine share certain histologic characteristics.[3] The wall of the small intestine and colon is composed of four layers: mucosa (or mucous membrane), submucosa, muscularis (or muscularis propria), and adventitia (or serosa) (Fig. 93–2).

Mucosa

The *mucosa* is the innermost layer formed by *glandular epithelium*, *lamina propria*, and *muscularis mucosae* (Fig. 93–3A and B). The *glandular epithelium* forms cylindrical structures, called *crypts*. The *lamina propria*, which supports the epithelium, is a layer of reticular connective tissue with elastin, reticulin, and collagen fibers, lymphocytes, plasma cells, and eosinophilic granulocytes, as well as lymphatics and capillaries. The *muscularis mucosae* consists of a thin layer of smooth muscle at the boundary of the mucosa and submucosa.

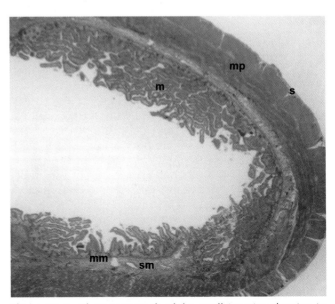

Figure 93–2 Photomicrograph of the small intestine showing its general microscopic architecture. m, mucosa; mm, muscularis mucosae; mp, muscularis propria; s, serosa; sm, submucosa. Hematoxylin-eosin stain, ×25.

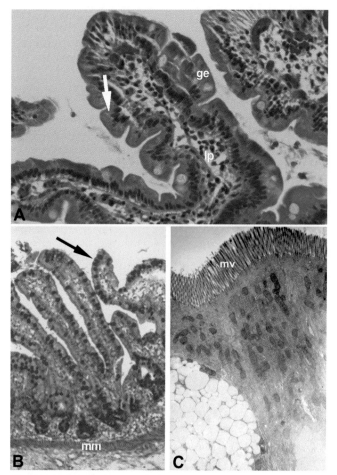

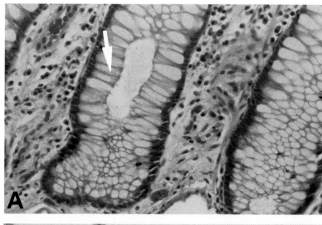

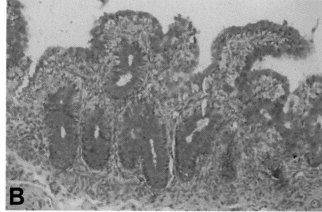

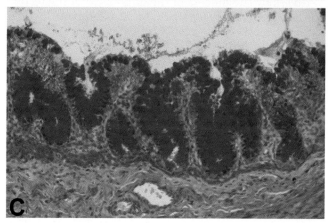

Figure 93–3 Histologic and electron microscopic photographs of the small intestine. *A,* Components of the mucosa: ge, glandular epithelium; lp, lamina propria. Note the absorptive cells which appear as high columnar cells with eosinophilic cytoplasm *(arrow).* Hematoxylin-eosin stain, ×250. *B,* Goblet cells *(arrow)* are stained red. mm, muscularis mucosae. Periodic acid–Schiff stain, ×150. *C,* Microvilli (mv) are seen as delicate finger-like projections on electron microscopic examination. ×9000. (Courtesy of S. Teichberg, PhD.)

Figure 93–4 Photomicrographs of the small intestine demonstrating goblet cells. *A,* Clear, empty-looking cytoplasm and basal nuclei *(arrow)* are seen with use of the hematoxylin-eosin stain. ×250. *B,* Metachromatic staining of the cytoplasm results with use of the alcian blue stain. ×150. *C,* The cells demonstrate red staining with use of the periodic acid–Schiff stain. ×150.

The glandular epithelium is composed of various cell types: stem cells, undifferentiated crypt cells, absorptive cells (also called columnar cells), goblet cells, Paneth cells, enteroendocrine cells, and M cells.

Stem cells are pluripotential cells located at the base of the crypt. *Undifferentiated cells* have fewer intracellular organelles and microvilli than do absorptive cells. The *absorptive cells* (Fig. 93–3A) are high columnar cells with oval, basal nuclei, eosinophilic cytoplasm, and a periodic acid–Schiff (PAS)–positive free surface, the brush border (see Fig. 93–3B). On electron microscopic examination, the brush border is seen to be composed of *microvilli* (see Fig. 93–3C), which are more numerous in the small intestinal than in the colonic epithelium. Small bowel enterocyte microvilli are estimated to increase the luminal surface area of the cell 14- to 40-fold.[5] *Goblet cells* are oval or round, with flattened basal nuclei (Fig. 93–4A); their cytoplasm is basophilic, metachromatic (see Fig. 93–4B), and PAS positive (see Fig. 93–4C). *Paneth cells* are flask-shaped and have an eosinophilic granular cytoplasm and a broad base positioned against the basement membrane (Fig. 93–5). Paneth cells contain zinc, antimicrobial pep-

tides, and growth factors and secrete lysoenzymes.[6] The mucosa also contains specialized cells that because of their specific endocrine function are called *enteroendocrine* or *neuroendocrine cells.*

These neuroendocrine cells historically have been divided into *argentaffin cells* (granules able to reduce silver nitrate) and *argyrophilic cells* (granules that reduce silver nitrate only in the presence of a chemical reducer). Argentaffin cells stain positive with bichromate salts and also are called *enterochromaffin cells.* These cells are oval or triangular (also called "halo cells") and have a basal position in relation to the remaining epithelial cells (Fig. 93–6A) and a pale cytoplasm filled with dark-stained granules.[7] Variation in shapes and cell types has been detected with immunohistochemical staining.[8] The unifying APUD concept[9]—amino acid precursor, uptake, and *decarboxylation*—ascribes common characteristics to these neuroendocrine cells. APUD cells are a group of cells with a common embryonic neural crest origin and with similar cytochemical and electron microscopic features; however, embryologic and morphologic data support an endodermal origin of these cells.[10]

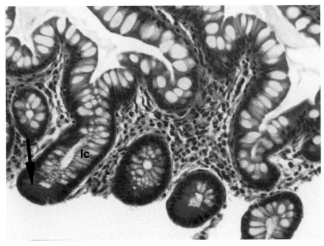

Figure 93–5 Photomicrograph of the small intestinal mucosa demonstrating the crypts of Lieberkühn (lc) and Paneth cells (*arrow*) which are characterized by granular eosinophilic cytoplasm. Hematoxylin-eosin stain, ×250.

Ultrastructurally, enteroendocrine cells contain membrane-bound granules with variably sized electrodense cores (see Fig. 93–6B), averaging 100 to 250 nm in diameter, and comprising large dense-core vesicles and smaller, synaptic-type microvesicles. Neurosecretory granules can be demonstrated with the Grimelius stain by light microscopy as dark granules (see Fig. 93–6C) or more specifically by immunofluorescence, with immunohistochemical stains such as neuron-specific enolase. Chromogranin enables visualization of the large-dense core vesicles, and synaptophysin targets the small synaptic-like microvesicles (see Fig. 93–6D).[11] VMAT1 and VMAT2 are two isoforms of the ATP-dependent vesicular monoamine transporters. These antigens, derived from both the large and small dense-core vesicles, are expressed differentially in small dense-core vesicles. Both are expressed in neuroendocrine cells, but VMAT1 is restricted to serotinin-producing enterochromaffin cells, and VMAT2 is expressed in histamine-producing cells, enterochromaffin-like cells, and pancreatic islet cells.[12] Specific immunohistochemical stains allow for identification of individual protein products of the neuroendocrine cells.

Besides releasing hormones in the blood, neuroendocrine cells also regulate secretion, absorption, motility, mucosal cell proliferation, and possibly immunobarrier control.[11] Electron microscopy and immunohistochemistry have led to the identification of a variety of cell types (Table 93–1). Designation according to the nature of the stored peptide is preferable to characterization of neuroendocrine cells by letters. Serotonin-producing enterochromaffin cells, vasoactive intestinal polypeptide

Figure 93–6 Microscopic characteristics of neuroendocrine cells of the small intestine. *A,* Features include clear cytoplasm and a round nucleus (*arrow*). Hematoxylin-eosin stain, ×250. *B,* Neurosecretory granules are seen as electron-dense, round black bodies (*arrow*) on electron microscopic examination. ×20,000. (Courtesy of S. Teichberg, PhD.) *C,* Black granules can be seen with use of the Grimelius stain (*arrow*). ×150. *D,* Cells stained with synaptophysin have brown cytoplasm (*arrow*). ×250.

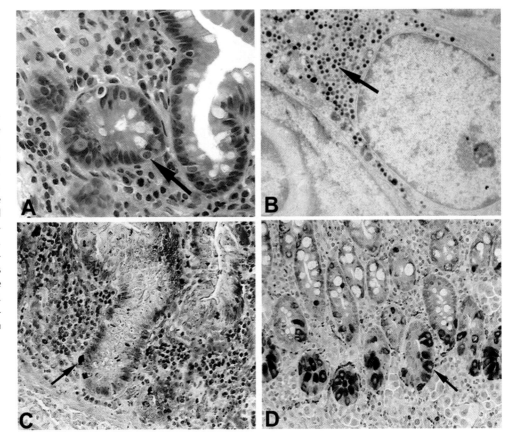

Table 93–1   Enteroendocrine Cells of the Gastrointestinal Tract: Cell Types, Hormones Produced, Vesicle Markers, and Distribution

Cell Type	Hormones		Vesicle Markers		Pancreas	Stomach		Intestine					
								Small			Large		
	Peptide	Amine	LDCV	SLMV		B	An	D	J	I	Ap	C	R
P/D₁	Ghrelin		CgA, VMAT2		e,f	+	f	f	f	f			
EC		5HT	CgA, VMAT1	Syn	f	+	+	+	+	+	+	+	+
D	Som		CgA	Syn	+	+	+	+	+	f	f	f	f
L	GLI/PYY		SgII > CgA	Syn				f	+	+	+	+	+
A (alpha)	Glucagon		CgA > SgII, VMAT2	Syn	+	e							
PP	PP		CgA, SgII, VMAT2	Syn	+			e					
B (beta)	Insulin		CgA, VMAT2, NESP55	Syn	+								
ECL		Histamine	CgA, VMAT2	Syn		+							
G	Gastrin		CgA	Syn			+	+					
CCK	Cholecystokinin							+	+	f			
S	Secretin	5HT	CgA					+	+				
GIP	GIP/Xenin		CgA					+	+	f			
M	Motilin		CgA					+	+	f			
N	Neurotensin		CgA					f	+	+			

An, gastric antrum; Ap, appendix; B, gastric body; C, colon; CgA, chromogranin A; D, duodenum; e, presence of cells in fetus and newborn; EC, enterochromaffin cell, 5HT, 5-hydroxytryptamine (serotonin); ECL, enterochromaffin-like cell; f, presence of few cells; GIP, gastric inhibitory polpypeptide; GLI, glucagon-like immunoreactants (glicentin, glucagon-37, glucagon-29, GLP-1, GLP-2); I, ileum; J, jejunum; LDCV, large dense-core vesicles; NESP55, neuroendocrine secretory protein 55; PP, pancreatic polypeptide; PYY, PP-like peptide with N-terminal tyrosine amide; R, rectum; SgII, secretogranin II (also known as chromogranin C); SLMV, synaptic-like microvesicles; Som, somatostatin; Syn, synaptophysin; VMAT1, VMAT2, vesicular monoamine transporter 1,2; +, presence of cells; >, heavier staining than.

Adapted from Solcia E, Capela C, Fiocca R, et al: Disorders of the endocrine system. In: Pathology of the Gastrointestinal Tract. Ming SC, Goldman H (eds): Philadelphia, Williams & Wilkins, 1998, p 295. Table reflects the current status of knowledge, which, especially for the vesicle markers, is largely incomplete.

(VIP), and somatostatin D cells are distributed throughout the small and large intestine.[12,13]

M cells are specialized epithelial cells overlying lymphoid follicles in the small intestine and colon. M cells selectively bind, process, and deliver pathogens directly to lymphocytes, macrophages, or other components of the mucosal lymphoid system.[14]

Interstitial cells of Cajal are present in both the small intestine and the colon and are mesenchymal cells, located in the myenteric plexus, the muscularis propria and the submucosa.[15] The distribution of the interstitial cells of Cajal is similar in children and in adults (Fig. 93–7) although a difference in their distribution is seen in fetuses of different gestational ages.[16] Recognized as the pacemaker cells of the intestine, they regulate intestinal motility. The interstitial cells of Cajal are spindle-shaped or stellate, with long ramified processes, and have large, oval, light-staining nuclei with sparse perinuclear cytoplasm.[15] The interstitial cells of Cajal express the receptor for tyrosine kinase (c-kit) or CD117. Immunohistochemical stains that utilize antibodies against c-kit allow the interstitial cells of Cajal to be labeled. The distribution and onset of appearance of these cells in the gastrointestinal tract have been described.[16]

Submucosa

The *submucosa*, between the muscularis mucosae and the muscularis propria, is a fibrous connective tissue layer that contains fibroblasts, mast cells, blood and lymphatic vessels, and a nerve fiber plexus—Meissner's plexus—com-

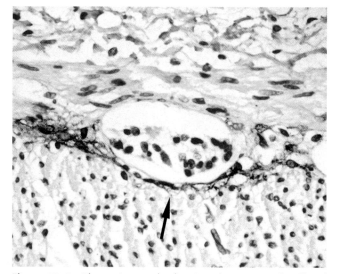

Figure 93–7   Photomicrograph showing the interstitial cells of Cajal in the small intestine. Brown-staining, elongated cells are evident around the myenteric plexus *(arrow)*. CD117 immunostain, ×250.

posed of nonmyelinated, postganglionic sympathetic fibers, and parasympathetic ganglion cells.

Muscularis or Muscularis Propria

The *muscularis propria*, mainly responsible for contractility, consists of two layers of smooth muscle: an inner

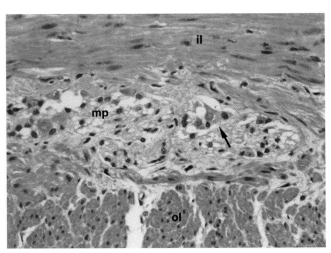

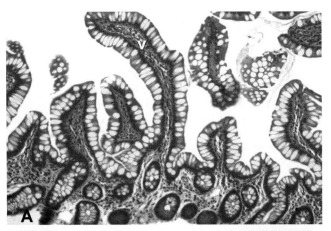

Figure 93–8 Photomicrograph of the muscularis propria of the small intestine. The myenteric plexus (mp) is seen as a pale area between the inner and outer layers (il, ol) of the muscularis propria with ganglion cells *(arrow)*. Hematoxylin-eosin stain, ×250.

circular coat and an outer longitudinal coat arranged in a helicoidal pattern. A prominent nerve fiber plexus called the *myenteric plexus*, or Auerbach's plexus, is found between these two muscle layers (Fig. 93–8). Parasympathetic and postganglionic sympathetic fibers terminate in parasympathetic ganglion cells, and postganglionic parasympathetic fibers terminate in smooth muscle.

Adventitia or Serosa
The *adventitia* is the outermost layer of connective tissue. When covered by a single layer of mesothelial cells, it is called the *serosa*.

Small Intestine
The mucosa of the small intestine is characterized by mucosal folds (plicae circulares, or valves of Kerckring) and villi. The *mucosal folds* are composed of mucosa and submucosa. *Villi* are mucosal folds that decrease in size from the proximal to distal small intestine and are of different shapes in the various segments of the small intestine: they may be broad, short, or leaf-like in the duodenum, tongue-like in the jejunum, and finger-like more distally (Fig. 93–9A). The villous pattern also may vary in different ethnic groups. Thus, for example, biopsy specimens from Africans, Indians, South Vietnamese, and Haitians have shorter and thicker villi, an increased number of leaf-shaped villi, and more mononuclear cells in comparison with specimens from North Americans.

Various methods have been suggested to determine normal villus height. The height of the normal villus is 0.5 to 1.5 mm; villus height should be more than one half of the total thickness of the mucosa,[17] and three to five times the length of the crypts.

Two types of glands are present in the small intestine: *Brunner's glands* and *crypts of Lieberkühn (intestinal crypts)*. The first are submucosal glands (see Fig. 93–9B) found primarily in the first portion of the duodenum and in decreased numbers in the distal duodenum. In children, these glands also may be present in the proximal

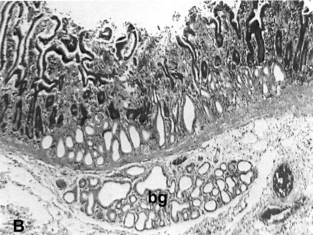

Figure 93–9 Photomicrograph of the duodenal mucosa. *A,* Villi are seen as finger-like projections. Hematoxylin-eosin stain, ×250. *B,* Brunner glands (bg) are found below the mucosa. Hematoxylin-eosin stain, ×150.

jejunum. Brunner's glands open into the intestinal crypts and morphologically resemble pyloric glands. Crypts of Lieberkühn are tubular glands that extend to the muscularis mucosae (see Fig. 93–5).

Absorptive, goblet, Paneth, and enteroendocrine cells are observed in the crypts of Lieberkühn. Paneth and columnar cells predominate in the base of the crypt. Above the base are absorptive cells and oligomucin cells; the latter originate from undifferentiated cells and differentiate into goblet cells. Goblet cells predominate in the upper half of the crypt. Enteroendocrine cells are admixed with goblet cells. A certain number of CD3+ intraepithelial T lymphoctes (30 per 100 epithelial cells) normally are present in the villi. Smooth muscle is found in the lamina propria of the small intestinal villus, extending from the muscularis mucosae vertically. Plasma cells containing primarily IgA, and mast cells also are present. Lymphoid tissue is prominent in the lamina propria as solitary nodules and as confluent masses—Peyer's patches—and also is seen in the submucosa. Peyer's patches are distributed along the antimesenteric border and are most numerous in the terminal ileum; their numbers decrease with age.

Most types of enteroendocrine cells are present in the duodenum.[18] Cells that produce ghrelin, gastrin, cholecystokinin, motilin, neurotensin, gastric inhibitory polypeptide, and secretin are restricted to the small intestine.[11]

The proportions of these cells differ in the villi and crypts, as well as in different segments of the intestine. Ninety percent of the villus epithelial cells are absorptive cells intermingled with goblet and enteroendocrine cells. The proportion of goblet to absorptive cells increases aborad toward the ileum. The interstitial cells of Cajal are more abundant in the myenteric plexus of the small bowel than in the colon.[16]

Large Intestine

The mucosa of the large intestine is characterized by the presence of crypts of Lieberkühn, associated predominantly with goblet cells intermixed with a few absorptive and enteroendocrine cells (see Fig. 93–4). GLI (glucagon-like immunoreactant)/pancreatic polypeptide–like peptide (PYY) with N-terminal tyrosine amide–producing L cells predominate in the large intestine. Enterochromaffin, enterochromaffin-like, and pancreatic polypeptide–producing cells also are found.[13] Paneth cells are scarce and normally are noted only in the proximal colon. The lamina propria of the large intestine contains solitary lymphoid follicles extending into the submucosa. These follicles are more developed in the rectum and decrease in number with age. Confluent lymphoid tissue is present in the appendix. Macrophages (muciphages) predominate in the subepithelial portion of the lamina propria. These cells are weakly PAS positive and are associated with stainable lipids.

Anal Canal

Microscopically, the anal canal[3] is divided into three zones: proximal, intermediate or pectin, and distal or anal skin. The proximal zone is lined by stratified cuboidal epithelium, and the transition with the rectal mucosa, lined by high columnar mucus-producing cells, is called the *anorectal histologic junction* (Fig. 93–10A). The *intermediate* or *pectin zone* is lined by stratified squamous epithelium but without adnexae (e.g., hair, sebaceous glands). Its proximal margin, in contact with the proximal zone, is called the *dentate line*; its distal margin, in contact with the anal skin, constitutes the *pectinate line*, also referred to as the *mucocutaneous junction* (see Fig. 93–10B). The anal skin is lined by squamous stratified epithelium and contains hair and sebaceous glands.

Intestinal Vasculature

Large arterial branches enter the muscularis propria and pass to the submucosa, where they branch to form large plexuses. In the small intestine, two types of branches arise from the submucosal plexuses: some arteries branch on the inner surface of the muscularis mucosae and break into a capillary meshwork that surrounds the crypts of Lieberkühn. Other arteries are destined for villi, each receiving one or two arteries, and set up the anatomic arrangement that allows a countercurrent mechanism during absorption. These vessels enter at the base of the villus and form a dense capillary network immediately underneath the epithelium of the entire villus structure.

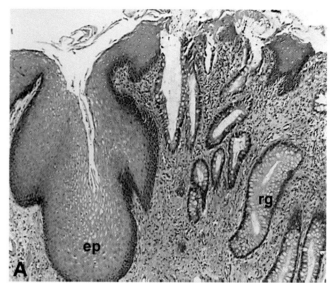

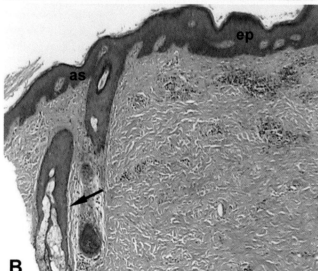

Figure 93–10 Photomicrograph of the anal canal. *A,* Anorectal histologic junction: Transition from rectal glandular mucosa (rg) to proximal anal mucosa lined by stratified squamous epithelium (ep) is evident. Hematoxylin-eosin stain, ×150. *B,* The pectinate line is characterized by anal mucosa with stratified squamous epithelium (ep) and anal skin containing adnexae *(arrow)*. Hematoxylin-eosin stain, ×150.

One or several veins originate at the tip of each villus from the superficial capillary plexus, anastomose with the glandular venous plexus, and then enter the submucosa joining the submucosal venous plexus. In the colon, branches from the submucosal plexus extend to the surface, giving rise to capillaries supplying the submucosa, and there branch to form a capillary meshwork around the crypts of Lieberkühn. From the periglandular capillary meshwork, veins form a venous plexus between the base of the crypts and the muscularis mucosae. From this plexus, branches extend into the submucosa and form a venous plexus, from which large veins follow the distribution of the arteries and pass through the muscularis propria into the serosa.[19]

Lymph Vessels of the Intestine

The lymphatics of the small intestine are called *lacteals* and become filled with milky-white lymph called *chyle* after eating. Each villus contains one central lacteal, except in the duodenum where two or more lacteals per villus may be present. The wall of the lacteal consists of endothelial cells, reticulum fibers, and smooth muscle cells. The central lacteals anastomose at the base of the villus with the lymphatic capillaries between the crypts of Lieberkühn. They also form a plexus on the inner surface of the muscularis mucosae. Branches of this plexus extend through the muscularis mucosae to form a submucosal plexus. Branches from the submucosal plexus penetrate the muscularis propria, where they receive branches from plexuses between the inner and outer layers.[20] Lymphatic vessels are absent in the colonic mucosa, but the distribution of lymphatics in the remaining colonic layers is similar to that in the small intestine.

Nerves of the Intestine[4]

The intrinsic nervous system (enteric nervous system) consists of subserosal, muscular, and submucosal plexuses. The *subserosal plexus* contains a network of thin nerve fibers, without ganglia, that connects the extrinsic nerves with the intrinsic plexus. The *myenteric plexus*, or *Auerbach's plexus*, is situated between the outer and inner layers of the muscularis propria (see Fig. 93–8); it consists of ganglia and bundles of unmyelinated axons that connect with the ganglia forming a meshwork. These axons originate from processes of the ganglion cells and extrinsic vagus and sympathetic ganglia. The *deep muscular plexus* is situated on the mucosal aspect of the circular muscular layer of the muscularis propria. It does not contain ganglia; it innervates the muscularis propria and connects with the myenteric plexus. The *submucosal plexus*, or *Meissner's plexus*, consists of ganglia and nerve bundles. The nerve fibers of this plexus innervate the muscularis mucosae and smooth muscle in the core of the villi. Fibers from this plexus also form a *mucosal plexus* that is situated in the lamina propria and provides branches to the intestinal crypts and villi. The ganglion

cells of the submucosal plexus are distributed in two layers: One is adjacent to the circular muscular layer of the muscularis propria; the other is contiguous to the muscularis mucosae. Ganglion cells are large cells, isolated or grouped in small clusters called *ganglia* (Fig. 93–11). Ganglion cells have an abundant basophilic cytoplasm, a large vesicular round nucleus, and a prominent nucleolus. Ganglion cells are scarce in the physiologic hypoganglionic segment 1 cm above the anal verge.

EMBRYOLOGY

The embryo begins the third week of development as a bilaminar germ disk. During week 3, in a process called *gastrulation*, this disk becomes a trilaminar disk. The surface facing the yolk sac becomes the definitive *endoderm*; the surface facing the amniotic sac becomes the *ectoderm*. The middle layer is called *mesoderm*. The long axis and left-right axis of the embryo also are established at this time. The oral opening is marked by the buccopharyngeal membrane; the future openings of the urogenital and the digestive tracts become identifiable as the cloacal membranes.[5] At 4 weeks of gestation, the alimentary tract is divided into three parts: *foregut, midgut,* and *hindgut.*

The endoderm forms the intestinal tube, which communicates only with the yolk sac. Narrowing of the communication of the yolk sac with the endoderm forms the vitelline duct. With folding of the embryo during the fourth week of development, the mesodermal layer splits. The portion that adheres to endoderm forms the visceral peritoneum, whereas the part that adheres to ectoderm forms the parietal peritoneum. The space between the two layers becomes the peritoneal cavity.[5]

MOLECULAR REGULATION OF INTESTINAL MORPHOGENESIS

Differentiation of the gastrointestinal tract depends on the interaction between the endoderm and mesoderm through the *Hox code.* Signaling from the mesoderm to endoderm is regulated by the *Hox* genes, which encode homeodomain-containing transcription factors. Induction of the *Hox* code in the mesoderm results from expression of Sonic hedgehog (SHH) through the endoderm of the midgut and hindgut. SHH is a signaling molecule that acts as a morphogen or form-producing substance in a variety of organ systems. The mesoderm prompted by this code instructs the endoderm to form the various components of the midgut and hindgut regions, such as the small bowel, cecum, colon, and cloaca.[21] As indicated by animal studies, *Hox* genes contribute to the subdivision of the intestine, with formation of the ileocecal valve that separates the small and the large intestine.[22]

The primitive gut results from incorporation of the endoderm-lined yolk sac cavity into the embryo, following embryonal cephalocaudal and lateral folding. The primitive gut is composed of a blind-ended tube in the cephalic and caudal portions of the embryo, which is the progenitor of the *foregut* and *hindgut*; the *midgut* (Fig.

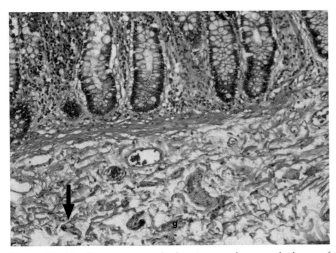

Figure 93–11 Photomicrograph showing a submucosal plexus of the colon. The ganglia (g) are identified by their oval structure and thin nerve trunks *(arrow)*. Hematoxylin-eosin stain, ×150.

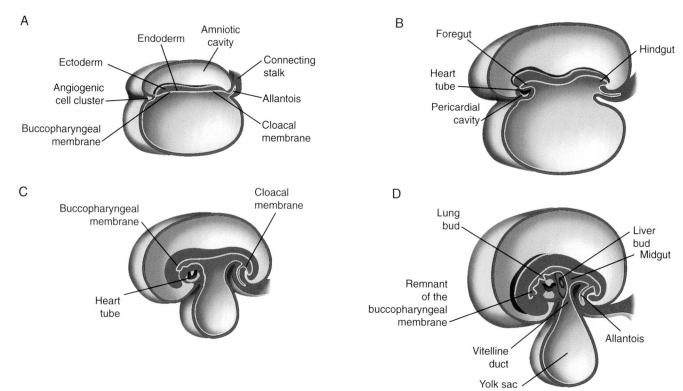

Figure 93–12 Formation of the foregut, midgut, and hindgut (see text for details). (From Sun B [ed]: Langman's Medical Embryology, 9th ed. Philadelphia, Lippincott Williams & Wilkins, 2004.)

93–12) is connected to the yolk sac by the vitelline duct. The endoderm gives rise to the epithelial lining of the gastrointestinal tract; muscle, connective tissue, and peritoneum originate from the splanchnic mesoderm. During week 9 of development, the epithelium begins to differentiate from the endoderm with villus formation and differentiation of epithelial cell types. Organogenesis is complete by 12 weeks of gestation.

Initially, the foregut, midgut, and hindgut are connected to the mesenchyma of the posterior abdominal wall. By week 5 of embryonic development, after narrowing of the connective tissue, the caudal portions of the foregut, the midgut, and most of the hindgut, are suspended from the abdominal wall by the *dorsal mesentery* extending from the duodenum to the cloaca. The dorsal mesentery forms the *mesoduodenum* in the duodenum, the *dorsal mesocolon* in the colon, and the *mesentery proper* in the region of the jejunum and ileum.[21]

SPECIFIC STRUCTURES AND SYSTEMS

Duodenum

The duodenum originates from the terminal portion of the foregut and cephalic part of the midgut. With rotation of the stomach, the duodenum becomes C-shaped and rotates to the right, and the fourth portion becomes fixed in the left upper abdominal cavity. The mesoduo-

denum fuses with the adjacent peritoneum; both layers disappear, and the duodenum becomes fixed in its retroperitoneal location. The lumen of the duodenum is obliterated during the second month of development by proliferation of its cells; this phenomenon is shortly followed by recanalization. Because the foregut is supplied by the celiac artery and the midgut by the superior mesenteric artery, the duodenum is supplied by both arteries.[21]

Midgut

The midgut gives rise to the duodenum distal to the ampulla, to the entire small bowel, and to the cecum, appendix, ascending colon, and the proximal two thirds of the transverse colon. The midgut rapidly elongates with formation of the primary intestinal loop. The cephalic portion of this loop, which communicates with the yolk sac by the narrow vitelline duct, gives rise to the distal portion of the duodenum, the jejunum and a portion of the ileum; the distal ileum, cecum, appendix, ascending colon, and proximal two thirds of the transverse colon originate from the caudal limb. During week 6 of embryonic development, the primary intestinal loop enters the umbilical cord (physiologic umbilical herniation) (Fig. 93–13), and by week 10 it re-enters the abdominal cavity. The proximal portion of the jejunum is the first portion of the intestine to re-enter the abdominal cavity and becomes located on the left side; the subsequent loop that re-enters the abdominal cavity locates to

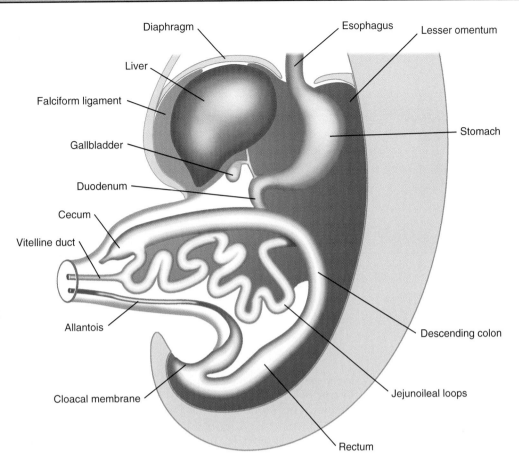

Figure 93–13 Umbilical herniation of the intestinal loop during normal development. Coiling of the small intestinal loops and formation of the cecum occur during the herniation. The first 90 degrees of rotation occur during herniation; the remaining 180 degrees occur during the return of the gut to the abdominal cavity. (From Sun B [ed]: Langman's Medical Embryology, 9th ed. Philadelphia, Lippincott Williams & Wilkins, 2004.)

the right. The cecal bud is the last segment to re-enter the abdominal cavity. It originates as a small dilatation of the caudal limb of the primary intestinal loop by approximately 6 weeks of development. Initially, it lies in the right upper quadrant; then it descends to the right iliac fossa, placing the ascending colon and hepatic flexure in the right side of the abdominal cavity. The appendix originates from the distal end of the cecal bud. Because the appendix develops during descent of the colon, its final position frequently is retrocecal or retrocolonic.

The primary intestinal loop rotates counterclockwise for approximately 270 degrees around an axis formed by the superior mesenteric artery (Fig. 93–14A). This rotation occurs in three stages: first stage between 6 to 8 weeks (90 degrees); second stage at 9 weeks (180 degrees); and third stage (270 degrees) at 12 weeks of gestation (see Fig. 93–14B). Elongation of the bowel continues, and the jejunum and ileum form a number of coiled loops.[21]

Mesentery

When the caudal limb of the primitive intestine moves to the right side of the abdominal cavity, the dorsal mesentery twists around the origin of the superior mesenteric artery. After the ascending and the descending portions of the colon reach their final destinations, their mesenteries fuse with the peritoneum of the poste-

rior abdominal wall, and they become retroperitoneal organs. The appendix, cecum, and descending colon retain their free mesentery. The transverse mesocolon fuses with the posterior wall of the greater omentum. The mesentery of the jejunum and ileum at first is in continuity with the ascending mesocolon; after the ascending colon becomes retroperitoneal, the mesentery only extends from the duodenum to the ileocecal junction.[21]

Hindgut

The distal third of the transverse colon, the descending colon and sigmoid, the rectum, and the upper part of the anal canal originate from the hindgut. Initially, the urinary, genital, and rectal tracts empty into a common channel, the cloaca. They become separated by the caudal descent of the urorectal septum into an anterior urogenital sinus and a posterior intestinal canal. The lateral fold of the cloaca moves to the midline, and the caudal extension of the urorectal septum develops into the perineal body. In the male, the lateral genital ridges coalesce to form the urethra and scrotum; in the female, no fusion occurs, and the labia minora and majora evolve.[23] The cloaca is lined by endoderm and covered anteriorly by ectoderm. The most distal portion of the hindgut enters into the posterior region of the cloaca, the primitive *anorectal canal*. The boundary between the endoderm and

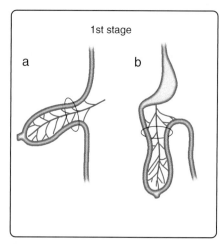
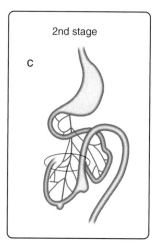
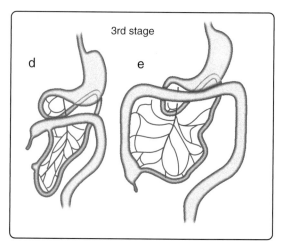

Figure 93–14 The three stages of normal intestinal rotation (see text for details). (From Gosche JR, Touloukian RJ: Congenital anomalies of the midgut. In Wyllie R, Hyams JS [eds]: Pediatric Gastrointestinal Disease. Pathophysiology, Diagnosis, Management, 2nd ed. Philadelphia, WB Saunders, 1999.)

the ectoderm forms the *cloacal membrane*. This membrane ruptures by week 7 of embryonic development, creating the anal opening for the hindgut. This portion is obliterated by the ectoderm but recanalizes by week 9. Thus, the distal portion of the anal canal originates from the ectoderm and is supplied by the inferior rectal artery; the proximal portion of the anal canal originates from the endoderm and is supplied by the superior rectal artery. The pectinate line is situated at the junction of the endoderm and the ectoderm.

Arterial System

Vascular endothelial growth factor (VEGF)-A and its receptors, VEGFR-1 and VEGFR-2, are important for endothelial cell proliferation, migration, and sprouting.[24] Angiopoietins and their receptors, Tie1 and Tie2, play a role in remodeling and maturation of the developing vasculature.[25] Mutation in Tie2 has been reported in vascular dysmorphogenesis.[26] Vascular malformation is briefly discussed in Chapter 35.

Arteries of the dorsal mesentery, originating from fusion of the vitelline arteries, give rise to the celiac, superior mesenteric, and inferior mesenteric arteries. Their branches supply the foregut, midgut, and hindgut, respectively.

Venous System

Vitelline veins give rise to a periduodenal plexus that develops into a single vessel, the portal vein. The superior mesenteric vein originates from the right vitelline vein that receives blood from the primitive intestinal loop.

Lymphatic System

Lymphatics originate from endothelial budding of veins, after which the peripheral lymphatic system spreads by endothelial sprouting into the surrounding tissues and

organs. Flt4 (also known as VEGFR-3), a receptor for VEGF, plays a role in development of both the vascular and the lymphatic systems.[27] Overexpression of VEGF-C, a ligand of Flt4, results in hyperplasia of lymphatic vessels in transgenic mice. The homeobox gene *Prox1* is essential for normal development of the lymphatic system based on animal studies. Homeobox genes contain a conserved sequence of 183 nucleotides. The proteins encoded by homeobox-containing genes act as regulatory molecules that control the expression of other genes. Several families of homeobox-containing genes are known, including the murine *Hox* family that has been implicated in pattern formation during embryogenesis. Disruption of this gene in mice causes chyle-filled intestine. Abnormalities in the development of the lymphatic system can result in lymphangiectasia (see Chapter 27).

Enteric Nervous System

The enteric nervous system originates from *vagal, truncal,* and *sacral* neural crest cells. Most of the enteric nervous system cells derive from the vagal and truncal neural crest, enter the foregut mesenchyma, and colonize the developing intestine in a cephalocaudal direction. The truncal neural crest gives rise to ganglia of the proximal stomach, whereas the vagal neural crest supplies ganglia to the entire intestine including the rectum; this colonization is complete by 13 weeks of embryonic development. A small component of the enteric nervous system originates from sacral neural crest cells. These cells form extraintestinal pelvic ganglia that colonize the hindgut mesenchyma before the arrival of the vagal-derived neural crest cells.[28] The normal development of the enteric nervous system depends on the survival of cells developed from the neural crest, and their proliferation, movement, and differentation into neurons and glial cells. Microenvironmental, genetic, or molecular mechanisms may intervene in these processes (see "Disturbance in the Enteric Nervous System").

CLINICAL IMPLICATIONS

Table 93–2 summarizes the different clinical congenital entities that result from disturbances in embryologic development. Gastrointestinal malformations can be associated with extraintestinal defects when genes such as those that determine left-right asymmetry are involved.[29] The *CFC1* gene plays a role in establishing left-right axis. Mutations of this gene have been reported in extrahepatic biliary atresia, in the polysplenia syndrome (inferior vena cava abnormalities, preduodenal portal vein, intestinal malrotation, and situs inversus), and in right-sided stomach and congenital heart disease.[30,31]

ABNORMALITIES IN NORMAL EMBRYOLOGIC DEVELOPMENT

BODY WALL

Omphalocele

Current theories suggest that a teratogenic event during the first 3 weeks of gestation prevents return of the bowel to the abdomen and failure of lateral embryonic fold development, which results in an omphalocele. Omphalocele occurs with a frequency of 2.5 in 10,000 births. Associated anomalies including sternal defects result from failure of closure of the cephalic folds; failure of caudal fold development results in exstrophy of the bladder and, in extreme cases, exstrophy of the cloaca.

Omphalocele is a congenital hernia that involves the umbilicus and that usually is covered by an avascular sac composed of the fused layers of amnion and peritoneum (Fig. 93–15). The umbilical cord usually is inserted into the apex of the sac, and the blood vessels radiate within the sac wall. Although a central defect is present in the skin and the linea alba, the remainder of the abdominal wall is intact, including the surrounding musculature.[32] Because a small occult omphalocele of the umbilical cord may not be observed at birth, it is recommended that the umbilical cord be tied at least 5 cm from the abdominal wall at the time of delivery.[33] Close inspection of the umbilical cord before clamping will avoid clamping an occult omphalocele.

In the large omphalocele, the liver and spleen frequently are outside of the abdominal cavity. Associated anomalies include incomplete intestinal rotation, intestinal obstruction, exstrophy of the bladder, vesicoenteric fistulae, renal anomalies, and cardiovascular defects.

Table 93–2   Causes of Abnormalities in Normal Embryologic Development

Abnormality	Cause
Mesentery	
Mobile cecum	Persistence of mesocolon
Volvulus	Failure of fusion of mesocolon with posterior abdominal wall
Body wall	
Omphalocele	Failure of the intestine to return to the abdominal cavity after its physiologic herniation
Gastroschisis	Weakening of the abdominal wall by a regressing right umbilical vein
Vitelline duct	
Meckel's diverticulum	Persistence of the vitelline duct
Patent omphalomesenteric duct	Total failure of vitelline duct obliteration
Omphalomesenteric cyst	Focal failure of vitelline duct obliteration
Rotation	
Nonrotation	Failure of stage 2 rotation
Reverse rotation	Rotation of 90 degrees instead of 270 degrees
Malrotation	Failure of rotation of the proximal midgut; distal midgut rotates 90 degrees clockwise
Proliferation	
Duplication	Abnormal proliferation of the intestinal parenchyma
Intestinal atresia and stenosis	
Duodenum	Lack of recanalization
Small and large intestine	Vascular "accident"
"Apple peel" atresia	Coiling of proximal jejunum distal to the atresia around the mesenteric remnant
Anorectum	Disturbance in hindgut development
Enteric nervous system	
Hirschsprung's disease	Failure of migration of ganglion cells; microenvironment changes
Intestinal neuronal dysplasia	Controversial
Pseudo-obstruction	Multifactorial (see Chapter 117)
Miscellaneous	
Microvillus inclusion disease	Not known
Tufting enteropathy	Not known
Other genetic defects	
Glucose/galactose malabsorption	Absence of Na^+/glucose cotransporter
Sucrase/isomaltase deficiency	Abnormal intracellular transport, aberrant processing and defective function of sucrose/isomaltase
Lactase deficiency	Decrease in lactase-phlorizin hydrolase
Chloridorrhea	Abnormal Cl^--HCo_3^- exchanger in the ileum and colon
Cystic fibrosis	Defect in the cystic fibrosis transmembrane regulator

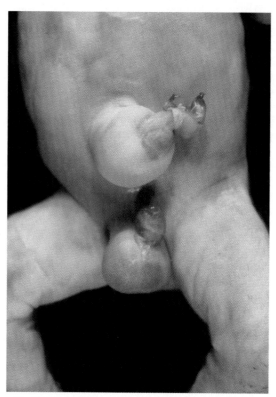

Figure 93–15 A newborn with an omphalocele. Note the translucent sac-like structure with its attached umbilical cord.

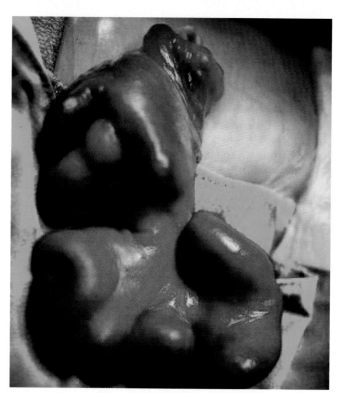

Figure 93–16 Gastroschisis. In this newborn, there are full-thickness disruption of the abdominal wall and protruding viscera without accompanying peritoneum. (From Feldman's online Gastro Alas, Current Medicine.)

Infants with the Beckwith-Wiedemann syndrome (mental retardation, hepatomegaly, large body stature, hypoglycemia in early infancy) may be born with omphalocele. An unusual combination of anomalies including omphalocele, exstrophy of the bladder, imperforate anus, and absence of a major portion of the colon is called *vesicointestinal fissure and omphalocele*.[32] Three of four patients with omphalocele have extraintestinal birth defects, most commonly trisomy 13 or 18 or the Beckwith-Wiedemann syndrome.

Prenatally, increased levels of maternal serum alpha-fetoprotein suggest the presence of possible omphalocele.[34] Ultrasound examination during pregnancy allows the diagnosis of this abdominal wall defect in most infants.

Fetal management including possible termination of pregnancy is determined by the physician in consultation with the family. If pregnancy is continued, mode of delivery and provision for care of a child with possibly coexisting anomalies should be considered before labor and delivery. Operative treatment is required in all patients with omphalocele. The size of the omphalocele determines whether a primary repair or delayed primary closure is selected as the surgical approach. In rare situations in which it is crucial to avoid an operation in the neonatal period, escharification of the intact omphalocele sac has been employed.[35] Reoperation is necessary in up to 25% of cases of omphalocele, either for reclosure of stomas or for subsequent bowel obstruction.[35]

Gastroschisis

Gastroschisis is a small defect most commonly located to the right of an intact umbilical cord (Fig. 93–16). The incidence of gastroschisis is approximately 1 in 10,000 births overall but approaches 7 in 10,000 among mothers younger than 20 years of age. In gastroschisis, a sac is absent, and the extruded bowel is "padded" and thickened along its length from its extended exposure to amniotic fluid. Histologically, the bowel usually is normal, although atresia is a possible finding, thought to be secondary to vascular compromise caused by the small defect itself or by volvulus of the bowel. Almost all patients with gastroschisis exhibit malrotation. Whereas prematurity is more common in children born with gastroschisis than it is in children with omphalocele, extraintestinal anomalies are much more common with omphalocele than they are with gastroschisis.[32] The morbidity and mortality in omphalocele tend to be the result of extraintestinal anomalies, whereas the morbidity and mortality in patients with gastroschisis are largely related to the presence or absence of intestinal atresia. Atresia occurs in 10% to 15% of children with gastroschisis. Gastroschisis also may be complicated by necrotizing enterocolitis, with all of its attendant short-term and long-term complications.[32]

Increased maternal levels of alpha-fetoprotein are suggestive of gastroschisis, as well as omphalocele.[34,36]

Most children with gastroschisis can undergo primary closure safely; however, for the child with significant intestinal atresia as a complication of gastroschisis, bowel exteriorization and secondary closure often constitute the preferred treatment.[37] It is crucial to try to conserve intestinal length in these children. Long-term total parenteral nutrition in children with either gastroschisis or omphalocele may result in chronic liver disease.[37]

VITELLINE DUCT

Persistence of the duct communication between the intestine and the yolk sac beyond the embryonic stage may result in several anomalies of the omphalomesenteric or vitelline duct (Fig. 93–17), including (1) a blind *omphalomesenteric duct*, or *Meckel's diverticulum*; (2) a central cystic dilatation in which the duct is closed at both ends but patent in its center, called an *omphalomesenteric* or *vitelline cyst*; (3) an *umbilical-intestinal fistula* (see Fig. 93–17A), resulting from the duct's remaining patent throughout its length; and (4) complete obliteration of the duct, resulting in a fibrous cord or ligament extending from the ileum to the umbilicus, known as an *omphalomesenteric band*.[32] In approximately 1% to 4% of all infants, a remnant of the embryonic yolk sac is retained, making the omphalomesenteric or vitelline duct the most common site of congenital gastrointestinal anomaly. Between weeks 5 and 7 of gestation, the omphalomesenteric duct, which has connected the embryo to the yolk sac, attenuates, involutes, and separates from the intestine. Before this separation, the epithelium of the yolk sac develops an appearance similar to that of the gastric mucosa.[38] A partial or complete failure of involution of the duct results in a variety of retained structures, as described.

Meckel's Diverticulum

A *Meckel's diverticulum* is an antimesenteric outpouching of the ileum that usually is found approximately 2 feet from the ileocecal junction (see Fig. 93–17B). It occurs in 2% of the population and is more common in males, with a male-to-female ratio of 3:1. Length of the diverticulum varies, ranging from 1 to 10 cm.[32] Ectopic gastrointestinal mucosa or aberrant pancreatic tissue is present in about 50% of all persons. From 80% to 85% of ectopic tissue in the diverticulum is gastric (see Fig. 93–17C), but ectopic tissue may be duodenal, colonic, or bile duct mucosa.[39]

Painless bleeding per rectum is the most common manifestation of a Meckel's diverticulum. Blood in the stool usually is maroon-colored, even in patients with massive bleeding and hypovolemic shock. Bright red blood per rectum, as might be seen with bleeding from the left colon, is almost never encountered, but melena may be seen in patients with intermittent or continuous, less severe bleeding. The cause of bleeding is peptic ulceration secondary to acid production by the ectopic gastric mucosa within the Meckel's diverticulum. A "marginal" ulcer often develops at the junction of the gastric and ileal mucosa.[40] Although *Helicobacter pylori* has been observed in the gastric mucosa within a Meckel's diverticulum, a relationship between bleeding from a Meckel's diverticulum and presence of this organism is unlikely.[41] Despite massive bleeding, death from this cause seldom, if ever, occurs in children with a Meckel's diverticulum. Once hypovolemia occurs from blood loss, the splanchnic blood vessels contract, and bleeding tends to diminish or cease.

Intestinal obstruction is the next most common manifestation of a Meckel's diverticulum. This obstruction is caused either by intussusception with the diverticulum as a lead point or by herniation through or volvulus around a persistent fibrous cord remnant of the vestigial vitelline duct. In children older than 4 years of age, intussusception almost always is secondary to a lead point, and in this age group Meckel's diverticulum is the most common lead point. Diverticulum-related intestinal obstruction may occur at any age, however, and volvulus around a vitelline duct cord may occur in the neonatal period.[32] Bilious vomiting and abdominal distention usually are the initial signs of obstruction. Intestinal obstruction in these patients, as with other causes of obstruction, can lead to ischemia and death.[40]

Diverticulitis of a Meckel's diverticulum occurs as a result of acute inflammation. Most commonly, affected patients are diagnosed as having acute appendicitis, and the diagnosis of Meckel's diverticulitis is made at exploratory laparotomy. Perforation occurs in approximately one third of patients with Meckel's diverticulitis and also may result from peptic ulceration. The mechanism of Meckel's diverticulitis is similar to that of appendicitis.[40] The *chronic* form of Meckel's diverticulitis (Meckel's ileitis) may mimic the presentation of Crohn's disease of the ileum.[42]

The presence of a Meckel's diverticulum always should be considered in an infant or child with significant painless rectal bleeding. Standard abdominal plain films, barium contrast, and sonographic imaging rarely are helpful in making the diagnosis of a Meckel's diverticulum. Because bleeding almost always is from ectopic gastric mucosa within the diverticulum, the Meckel's scan, which can visualize gastric mucosa, should be the initial diagnostic study[40] (see Fig. 93–17D). The uptake of the ^{99m}Tc-pertechnetate is by the mucus-secreting cells of the gastric mucosa, not the parietal cells. Unfortunately, this study has only a 85% sensitivity and 95% specificity.[43] Cimetidine has been used to enhance the diagnostic yield of the Meckel's scan, because it decreases gastric secretion and minimizes enhancement of the second part of the duodenum, which occupies an area similar to that of a Meckel's diverticulum.[44]

When the diagnosis of a bleeding Meckel's diverticulum is entertained and the Meckel's scan results are negative, although superior mesenteric artery angiography[45] and ^{99m}Tc-labeled red blood cell studies may be utilized, diagnosis usually is made at laparotomy. Before laparotomy, it is reasonable to perform esophagogastroduodenoscopy and colonoscopy, to rule out other possible etiologic disorders.

Omphalomesenteric (or Vitelline) Cyst

Omphalomesenteric (or vitelline) cyst is characterized by a mucosa-lined cystic mass in the center of a fibrous cord. Infection of the cyst or intestinal obstruction may result.[40]

Patent Omphalomesenteric (Vitelline) Duct

Patent omphalomesenteric (vitelline) duct represents a persistent connection between the distal ileum and the

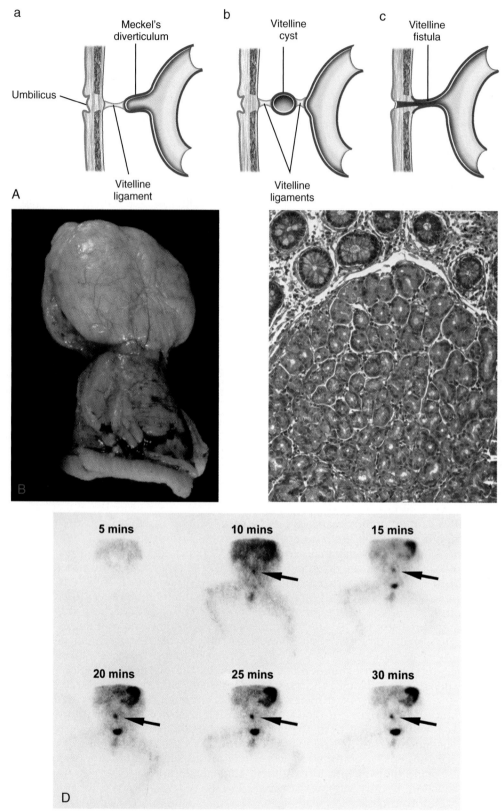

Figure 93–17 Vitelline duct abnormalities. *A,* Schematic representations of a Meckel's diverticulum (a), vitelline cyst (b), and vitelline fistula (c). (From Sun B [ed]: Langman's Medical Embryology, 9th ed. Philadelphia, Lippincott Williams & Wilkins, 2004) (see text for details). *B,* Surgical specimen revealing an outpouching of the ileum (Meckel's diverticulum). *C,* Photomicrograph showing replacement of the small intestinal mucosa by ectopic oxyntic mucosa lining the Meckel's diverticulum. Hematoxylin-eosin stain, ×150. *D,* Meckel's diverticulum scan demonstrating uptake of ^{99m}technetium-pertechnetate *(arrow)* by the diverticulum by 10 minutes. (Courtesy of Dr. I. Zanzi.)

umbilicus. This fistula occurs predominantly in males, with a male-to-female ratio of 5:1, and accounts for 2.5% to 6% of omphalomesenteric duct remnants. The diagnosis usually is made in the first few weeks of life after separation of the umbilical cord from the newborn umbilicus. Drainage from the umbilicus occurs with the characteristics of intestinal fluid. Examination of the umbilicus reveals either an opening or a polypoid mass resulting from limited prolapse of the patent omphalomesenteric duct. Definitive diagnosis can be made by a fistulogram. Complications of this type of fistula include prolapse through the umbilicus of the patent duct, or of the duct and the attached ileum, which may lead to partial intestinal obstruction. Prolapse should not be mistaken for an umbilical polyp, because excision of involved tissue might result in perforation.[40]

Omphalomesenteric Band

In omphalomesenteric band, the solid cord connecting the ileum to the umbilicus remains intact. This cord may result in intestinal obstruction from an internal hernia or volvulus.[40]

Vitelline Blood Vessel Remnants

Failure of involution of vitelline blood vessel remnants results in complications similar to those seen with a retained fibrous cord within the peritoneal cavity. Intestinal obstruction occurs when a portion of the small intestine wraps itself around the band.[40]

Treatment of all vitelline duct abnormalities is surgical.

ROTATION

Rotation defects result from errors in the normal embryonic development of the midgut. The distal duodenum, jejunum, ileum, cecum, and appendix, as well as the ascending colon and proximal two thirds of the transverse colon, all are derived from the midgut. Therefore, aberrations in midgut development may result in a variety of anatomic anomalies, including (1) areas of rotation and fixation, (2) atresias and stenoses, (3) duplications, and (4) persistence of embryonic structures. These congenital anomalies may cause symptoms not only in the newborn or neonatal period but also in later childhood and adulthood. Therefore, considerations in the differential diagnosis of intestinal obstruction and ischemia should include anomalies of the midgut in patients of all ages.

Because anomalies of intestinal rotation may remain asymptomatic throughout life, their true incidence is unknown.[46] Symptoms usually manifest within the first month of life, with bilious emesis and abdominal distention, but presentation may be delayed in mild cases to the fourth decade of life. The patient may have cramping abdominal pain, abdominal tenderness, and blood or even mucosal tissue in the stool from ischemia. If ischemia is allowed to progress, peritonitis and hypovolemic shock may develop, potentially culminating in death.[46] Delay in surgery in patients with ischemia may result in a short bowel, necessitating chronic TPN therapy and eventually small bowel transplantation, with or without liver transplantation.

Classification

Usually anomalies of rotation are characterized by the stage in the rotational process at which normal embryonic development of the midgut has been interrupted. Most anomalies of midgut rotation occur during the second stage of rotation and have been characterized as nonrotation, reverse rotation, and malrotation (Figure 93–18).[47] Of these, *nonrotation* is most common and reflects a complete failure of the second stage of rotation. With this anomaly, the intestinal tract occupies the same position in the abdomen as it does in an 8-week-old embryo; the small intestine is located to the right of the midline, the colon on the left.

Defects in the first and third stages of rotation are uncommon. Abnormalities in the first stage are associated with extroversion of the cloaca; abnormalities of the third stage cause failure of cecal elongation, the cecum remaining in the right upper quadrant.

In adults, *reverse rotation* of the midgut loop is the most commonly diagnosed defect of the midgut.[48] Reverse rotation of the midgut loop is rare, however, and accounts for only 4% of all rotational anomalies. In reverse rotation, the midgut rotates 180 degrees clockwise during the second stage of rotation, resulting in a net 90 degrees of clockwise rotation.[46] This may produce either the retroarterial colon type or the liver and entire colon ipsilateral type of reverse rotation.

Malrotation of the midgut loop, better defined as an anomaly of mixed rotation or of complete rotation, occurs when the proximal midgut fails to rotate around the mesenteric vessels during the second stage of rotation. The distal midgut does rotate 90 degrees in a counterclockwise direction, however, with the result that the jejunum and ileum remain to the right of the superior mesenteric artery and the cecum is situated in the subpyloric region.[46]

Associated Abnormalities

Associated anomalies are seen in 30% to 60% of patients with defects in intestinal rotation. Nonrotation of the midgut is a significant finding in patients with omphalocele, gastroschisis, and diaphragmatic hernia. Rotation defects also are seen in approximately 30% to 50% of infants with duodenal or jejunal atresia and in 10% to 15% of children with intestinal pseudo-obstruction and are associated with a variety of other conditions including Hirschsprung's disease, esophageal atresia, biliary atresia, annular pancreas, meconium ileus, intestinal duplications, mesenteric cysts, Meckel's diverticulum, and imperforate anus.[46]

Anomalies of rotation can cause acute or chronic intermittent obstruction from *volvulus* (see Fig. 93–18C). Venous and lymphatic obstruction, also from volvulus, can lead to malabsorption and abnormalities in intestinal motility. Patients may fail to thrive and present with chylous ascites and other symptoms and signs of lymphangiectasia secondary to chronic lymphatic obstruction.

Duodenal obstruction can occur as the result of midgut volvulus, but also as the result of peritoneal bands between a malpositioned cecum in the subpyloric region and the peritoneum. These bands, called *Ladd's bands*,

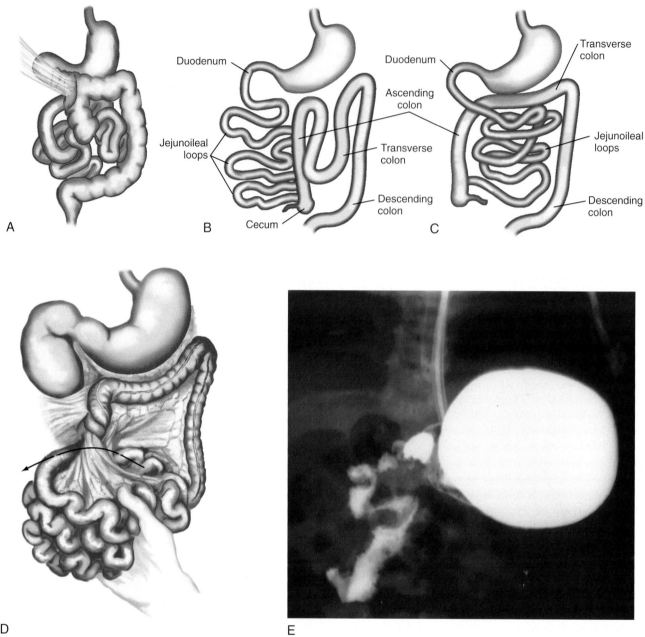

A

B

C

D   E

Figure 93–18 Rotation defects. *A* and *B*, two examples of nonrotation. In *A*, Ladd's bands are seen crossing the duodenum; some authors would refer to this as a "mixed rotation." In nonrotation, the small intestine is located to the right of the midline, the colon is to the left of the midline. (From Gosche JR, Touloukian J: Congenital anomalies of the midgut. In Wyllie R, Hyams JS (eds): Pediatric Gastrointestinal Disease. Pathophysiology, Diagnosis, Management, ed 2. Philadelphia, WB Saunders, 1999.) *C*, Reverse rotation. The transverse colon passes behind the duodenum. (From Sun B [ed]: Langman's Medical Embryology, 9th ed. Philadelphia, Lippincott Williams & Wilkins, 2004.) *D*, Malrotation with volvulus characterized by a clockwise twist of the mesentery and strangulation. (From Netter FH: The Netter Collection of Medical Illustration, vol 3. Teterboro, NJ, Icon Learning System, 2002.) *E*, Radiologic appearance of malrotation depicting the duodenum on the right of the spine, with a volvulus. (Courtesy of Dr. J. Levenbrown.)

cross the second or third portion of the duodenum and cause obstruction by compression or kinking.[46] Ladd's bands are an anomaly of peritoneal embryogenesis and persist throughout life.

Diagnosis

If time allows, diagnosis can be made by upper gastrointestinal contrast examination and delineation of the site of the duodenojejunal junction. Findings on ultrasonog-

raphy may suggest malrotation if the superior mesenteric vein is seen located to the left of the superior mesenteric artery, in contradistinction to the normal anatomy. In the child with acute onset of bilious vomiting and peritoneal signs, no diagnostic studies should be performed if they delay surgical intervention. In the full-term infant with bilious emesis, anomalies of rotation should be considered first and foremost, to avoid the morbidity and mortality associated with these lesions.[46]

PROLIFERATION

Enteric Duplication

Enteric duplications are rare, with an incidence of 2 in 9000 children reported in one autopsy study.[49] Enteric duplications are either spherical or tubular; the former type has no communication with the normal intestinal tract, whereas the latter does communicate. Tubular duplications may join the intestine at one or at both of its ends. Except for duodenal duplications, duplications occur on the mesenteric side of the bowel, and a common blood supply and muscular coat are shared by the duplicated segment and the adjacent bowel. Small bowel duplications often contain gastric mucosa and may be diagnosed by ^{99m}Tc radioisotopic imaging.[46]

The exact etiology of duplications is unclear but may involve a defect in intestinal recanalization. Enteric duplications occur throughout the gastrointestinal tract but are most common in the ileum. Gastric duplications occur least commonly. Depending on the site of the duplication, and whether ectopic gastric mucosa is present (seen in approximately 30% of the cases), complications include intestinal hemorrhage, ulceration, perforation, intestinal obstruction, pancreatitis, jaundice, hematobilia, and cutaneous enteric fistulas.[32]

Duplication of the rectum is the most common of the large bowel duplications and may be associated with constipation or obstipation. Colonic duplications frequently involve the entire colon. Occasionally, large bowel duplications affect variable segments of the colon, leaving "skip areas" of normal colon. Adenocarcinoma and squamous carcinoma have been associated with small bowel and colonic duplications. Carcinoid has been described with duplications of the rectum.

Neuroenteric cysts attach posteriorly to the spinal cord, are associated with asymptomatic hemivertebrae, and may occur at any level of the gastrointestinal tract.[32]

An intra-abdominal mass may be appreciated in a child with intestinal duplication, either by abdominal palpation or on rectal examination. Stool may contain occult blood. Preoperative diagnosis by radiographic evaluation is problematic, but radioisotope studies may prove diagnostic if ectopic mucosa is present in sufficient quantities.

Intestinal duplications may undergo malignant transformation in adults.

INTESTINAL ATRESIA AND STENOSIS

Of all of the congenital anomalies of the midgut, atresias and stenoses occur most frequently. Intestinal atresia refers to a congenital complete obstruction of the intestinal lumen, whereas stenosis indicates a partial or incomplete obstruction. Atresias occur more commonly than do stenoses, and small bowel atresias have a reported incidence rate of 1 in 300 to 1 in 1500 live births. Small bowel atresias are more common in black infants, low birth weight infants, and twins. Jejunoileal atresias are distributed equally throughout the jejunum and ileum, and multiple atresias are found in up to 20% of children. Jejunoileal atresia may occur with maternal use of ergotamine (in Cafergot for headaches) or cocaine taken during pregnancy and also is associated with congenital rubella. Colonic atresia occurs infrequently and accounts for fewer than 10% of all atresias.

In the *duodenum*, atresia results from failure of recanalization of the solid stage of duodenal development, whereas in the remaining small intestine and colon, atresia is the result of intestinal ischemia. Evidence of a vascular "accident" is noted in 30% to 40% of infants with atresia; proposed mechanisms include volvulus, constriction of the mesentery in a tight abdominal wall defect such as gastroschisis, internal hernia, intussusception, and obstruction with perforation.[32] Atresias also may result from low-flow states; in such cases, evidence of a vascular accident will be absent.

Duodenal obstruction is the result of *atresia* (in 40% to 60% of cases), *stenosis* (35% to 40%), or an intestinal *web* (5% to 15%). Eighty percent of these atresias are contiguous to or distal to the ampulla of Vater, and virtually all webs are within a few millimeters of the ampulla. Atresias on occasion may be multiple. The incidence varies, ranging between 1 in 10,000 and 1 in 20,000 live births. About 30% of children with duodenal atresia will have Down syndrome. Stenosis most often is due to extrinsic duodenal obstruction from an annular pancreas, Ladd's bands associated with malrotation, an anterior or preduodenal portal vein, or aberrant intramural pancreatic tissue.

Clinically, the presentation is that of a proximal intestinal obstruction with bilious vomiting on the first day of life, usually without abdominal distention. With gastric dilatation, the epigastrium may appear to be full by inspection and palpation. Excessive retention of gastric aspirate may be a feature, and the fluid typically is bile stained. Duodenal obstruction is diagnosed easily by abdominal films revealing a typical "double bubble" sign with a paucity of small intestinal air (Fig. 93–19).

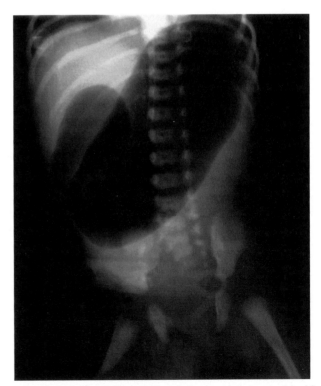

Figure 93–19 Plain film of the abdomen showing a "double bubble," typical of duodenal atresia. The larger bubble is the gastric bubble; the smaller bubble is the duodenal bubble. (Courtesy of Dr. J. Levenbrown.)

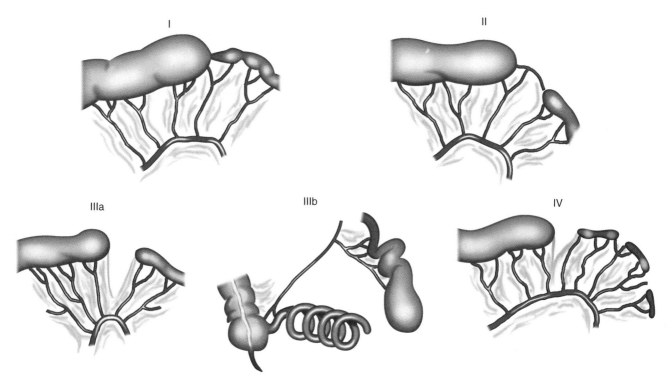

Figure 93–20 Classification of jejunoileal atresias. *Type I*: The mucosa and submucosa form a web or intraluminal diaphragm, resulting in obstruction. A defect in the mesentery is not present, and the intestine is not shortened. *Type II*: The dilated proximal intestine has a bulbous blind end connected by a short fibrous cord to the blind end of the distal bowel. The mesentery, however, is intact and the overall length of the small bowel is not usually shortened. *Type IIIa*: The defect in type IIIa is similar to that in type II in that both types have blind proximal and distal ends. In type IIIa, however, complete disconnection exists. In addition, a V-shaped mesenteric defect is present. The proximal blind end is usually markedly dilated and not peristaltic. The compromised intestine undergoes intrauterine absorption, and as a result, the intestine is shortened. *Type IIIb*: In addition to a large defect of the mesentery, the bowel is significantly shortened. This lesion is also known as Christmas tree deformity because the bowel wraps around a single perfusing vessel, like the tinsel coil wrapped around a Christmas tree; it also has been called an apple peel deformity; The distal ileum receives its blood supply from a single ileocolic or right colic artery because most of the superior mesenteric artery is absent. *Type IV*: Multiple small intestinal atresias are present of any combination of types I to III. This defect often takes on the appearance of a string of sausages because of the multiple lesions. (From Grosfeld JL, Ballantine TVN, Shoemaker R: Operative management of intestinal atresia and stenosis based on pathologic findings. J Pediatr Surg 14:368, 1979.)

Mothers of infants with duodenal obstruction often have polyhydramnios, and uterine ultrasonography may even demonstrate a "double bubble" in the unborn fetus.[32]

Treatment of duodenal webs, atresias, and stenotic lesions is surgical.

The classification system of Grosfeld and colleagues comprises five different types of *jejunoileal* and *colonic* atresias[50] (Fig. 93–20). In the "apple peel" atresia or Christmas tree deformity (type IIIb), proximal atresia with wide separation of the bowel loops is associated with absence of the distal superior mesenteric artery. The distal ileum receives its blood supply by retrograde perfusion through the ileocolic artery.[46] Type IIIb atresias account for fewer than 5% of all atresias.[51] Atresias are far more common than stenoses, with a frequency ratio of 15:1. With the exception of multiple atresias and perhaps the "apple peel" atresia, heredity appears to be of little significance in most cases.[32]

Approximately 50% of patients with duodenal atresia have associated malformations. Of this group, 30% have Down syndrome. Major anomalies occur less frequently with jejunoileal atresias and colonic atresias. Most common of the anomalies are malrotation, meconium ileus, volvulus, and gastroschisis, all of which might have caused intestinal ischemia in utero. Extragastrointestinal anomalies associated with atresias include cardiovascular, pulmonary, and renal malformations and skeletal deformities.[46] Prematurity is common, ranging in incidence from 25% in ileal atresias to 40% in jejunal lesions. Fifty percent of babies with multiple atresias are born prematurely. If the obstruction occurs beyond the ampulla of Vater, bilious and/or feculent vomiting with abdominal distention is seen; at surgery, the presence of meconium in the colon is uncommon, but variable amounts may be noted.[32] In patients with distal obstruction, abdominal films may demonstrate multiple dilated air-filled bowel loops. If perforation has occurred in utero, extraluminal air and intraperitoneal calcifications or calcifications within the scrotal sac may be present, suggesting meconium peritonitis. A "soap bubble" appearance of the ileum may suggest meconium ileus (cystic fibrosis). Air-fluid levels rarely are seen in meconium ileus.

Considerations in the differential diagnosis of distal bowel obstruction include small intestinal and colonic atresias, meconium ileus, Hirschsprung's disease, and meconium plug with or without small left colon syndrome. Contrast studies of the colon are helpful in making a proper diagnosis. An upper gastrointestinal contrast study also may provide additional important information.

Surgery is required to relieve the intestinal obstruction in the atretic or narrowed segment. When the segment proximal to the obstruction is long, with significant dilatation, resection may not be possible. Postoperative complications include fluid and electrolyte disorders, nutritional and feeding problems often requiring long-term use of parenteral nutrition, diarrhea, and failure to thrive. Short bowel syndrome often complicates the postoperative course.

ANORECTUM

The term *anorectal malformation* actually refers to a spectrum of anomalies that vary significantly in their complexity and prognosis.[52] Anorectal malformations occur in 1 in 4000 to 1 in 5000 newborns[53] and are more common among males and in children with Down syndrome.

During normal development, after appearance of the urorectal septum, it is controversial whether a migration of the primitive anus down the posterior wall of the cloaca occurs, whereas others postulate a craniocaudal fusion of the lateral urorectal ridges arising from the walls of the cloaca. The migration of the anus is completed when the urorectal septum reaches the perineum. Ano-malformations during weeks 4 to 12 of gestation are believed to result from failure of migration of the anus and excessive fusion,[54] although their precise cause is unknown; vascular accidents, maternal diabetes, and maternal ingestion of thalidomide, phenytoin, and trimethadione all have been proposed.[5]

Different types of anorectal malformations are illustrated in Figure 93–21. Anorectal malformations are divided into low (infra- or translevator), high (supralevator), and intermediate categories. A functional and practical classification of these malformations, the Wingspread classification, is summarized in Table 93–3A.[55] The classification in Table 92–3B is designed, according to Pena,[52] to increase the physician's awareness of the possibility of the presence of these lesions, as well as to establish therapeutic priorities.

Anocutaneous Fistula

In anocutaneous fistula, the rectum traverses normally through most of the anal sphincter, but its lower portion deviates anteriorly and ends as a perineal, cutaneous fistula anterior to the center of the external anal sphincter (*anocutaneous* or *perineal fistula*). These anomalies are similar in the male and the female. The perineal fistula is the most benign of anorectal defects. Associated urologic defects are uncommon (10%). All patients achieve bowel control after proper surgical treatment. Examination of the perineum may demonstrate features indicative of a perineal fistula, including prominent midline skin ridge ("bucket-handle" malformation) and subepithelial midline raphe fistula having the appearance of a black ribbon because of its meconium content. Surgery consists of a simple anoplasty, usually done without a protective colostomy.

Rectourethral Fistula

In rectourethral fistula, by far the most frequent anorectal malformation in males, the rectum descends through

Table 93–3   Classification of Anorectal Malformations

A. Wingspread Classification[55]

Male	Female
Low*	
Anocutaneous fistula	Anovestibular fistula
Anal stenosis	Anocutaneous fistula
	Anal stenosis
Intermediate†	
Rectobulbar urethral fistula	Rectovestibular fistula
Anal agenesis without fistula	Rectovaginal fistula
	Anal agenesis without fistula
High‡	
Anorectal agenesis	Anorectal agenesis
With rectoprostatic urethral	With rectovaginal fistula
fistula	Without fistula
Without fistula	
Rectal agenesis	Cloaca

B. Classification Based on the Need for Colostomy[52]

Male	Female
Colostomy not required	*Colostomy not required*
Perineal (cutaneous) fistula	Perineal (cutaneous fistula)
Colostomy required	*Colostomy required*
Rectourethral fistula	Vestibular fistula
Bulbar	
Prostatic	
Rectovesical fistula	Persistent cloaca
Imperforate anus without fistula	Imperforate anus without fistula
Rectal atresia	Rectal atresia

*Low, infra-, or translevator.
†Intermediate, between high and low.
‡High, supralevator.

a portion of the pelvic floor musculature but focally deviates anteriorly and communicates with the posterior urethra. This fistula may end in the lower posterior (*bulbar*) or in the upper posterior (*prostatic*) urethra.[52] Children with prostatic urethral fistulas more commonly have sacral and urologic defects (60%) than do children with bulbar prostatic fistula (30%).[56] Eighty-five percent of children with rectourethral bulbar fistula achieve fecal continence after repair, compared with 60% of children with rectoprostatic fistula.[57]

Rectovesical Fistula

In rectovesical fistula, the most proximal anorectal defect seen in males, the rectum opens into the bladder neck. Ninety percent of these malformations are associated with significant urologic defects,[56] and only 15% of children achieve bowel control after surgical repair.[57]

Vestibular Fistula

In vestibular fistula, the most common anorectal defect of females, the rectum opens into the vestibule of the genitalia. The rectum and the vagina share a thin common wall. Thirty percent of affected children have associated urologic defects,[56] and approximately 90% of these children achieve bowel control after surgery.[57] In the *vaginal fistula*, the rectum opens in the lower or, less frequently, the upper half of the vagina.

A

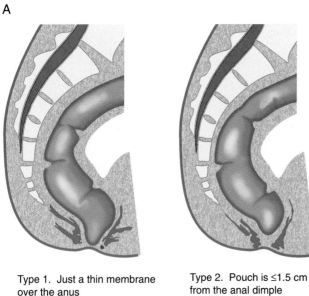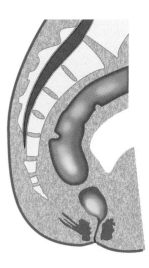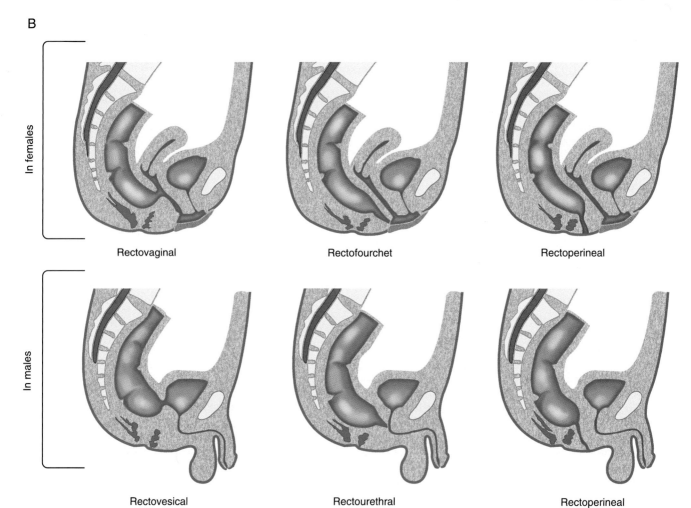

Type 1. Just a thin membrane over the anus

Type 2. Pouch is ≤1.5 cm from the anal dimple

Type 3. A blind pouch >1.5 cm from the anal dimple

Type 4. Atresia of the rectum with a normal anus

B

In females

Rectovaginal

Rectofourchet

Rectoperineal

In males

Rectovesical

Rectourethral

Rectoperineal

Figure 93–21 Anorectal malformations. *A,* Types of imperforate anus. *B,* Types of associated fistulas. (From Netter FH: The Netter Collection of Medical Illustration, vol 3. Teterboro, NJ, Icon Learning System, 2002.)

Anorectal Agenesis (Imperforate Anus) without Fistula

In anorectal agenesis, the rectum ends blindly without a fistula approximately 1 to 2 cm above the perineum. Sphincter function usually is preserved, with 80% of these patients achieving bowel control after surgery.[57] Approximately 50% of children with imperforate anus have Down syndrome. Conversely, 95% of children with Down syndrome who have anorectal malformations will have this specific type.[52]

Rectal Agenesis (Atresia)

Rectal agenesis occurs more frequently in the female than in the male, and it consists of complete (atresia) or partial (stenosis) interruption of the rectal lumen between the anal canal and the rectum. On visual inspection of the perineum, the anus appears normal; however, an obstruction located 1 to 2 cm above the mucocutaneous junction of the anus can be found with apprpriate studies. Sphincter function is normal in these patients, and associated urologic defects are rare. In these children, prognosis is excellent, with 100% achieving full bowel control after anorectoplasty.[57]

Anal Stenosis

Anal stenosis, a fibrous ring located at the anal verge, causes stricture. The patient is constipated, and the stool has a ribbon-like appearance.

Persistent Cloaca

In the complex defect *persistent cloaca*, the rectum, vagina, and urethra are fused into a single common channel that opens into one perineal orifice situated at the site of what should be the opening of the normal urethra. Prognosis depends on the intactness of the sacrum and the length of the common channel. Prognosis is better in those children with a shorter common channel (less than 3 cm).[52] Associated urologic problems are an important consideration with persistent cloaca. For example, urologic emergencies from obstructive uropathy are common, and hydrocolpos may compress the opening of the ureters, resulting in bilateral megaureters and massive vesicoureteral reflux.[58]

Associated Abnormalities

The higher and more complex the anorectal defect, the greater the chance of a dangerous associated defect, especially a urologic anomaly (Table 93–4). Urogenital defects occur in 48% of patients with anorectal malformations and in 72% of children with higher anorectal malformations; sacral abnormalities are more frequent in higher anorectal malformations. Children with a persistent cloaca or rectovesical fistula have a 99% chance of having an associated genitourinary anomaly, whereas fewer than 10% of children with low fistula have these abnormalities.[23]

Anorectal malformation also may manifest in a syndromic form such as in the VACTERL sequence (vertebral, anal, cardiac, tracheal, esophageal, renal and limb abnormalities).

In the first 24 hours of life, decision should be made about whether a child needs a colostomy or simple anoplasty. The presence of an associated defect, either urologic or cardiac, that might be life-threatening requires immediate evaluation.

Table 93–4   Abnormalities Associated with Anorectal Malformations

Sacral and spinal
   Deformed or reduced number of sacral vertebrae
   Hemisacrum
   Higher level of hemivertebrae with scoliosis
   Vertebral agenesis, spina bifida
Skeletal
   Polydactyly
   Clubfoot
   Radial aplasia or hypoplasia
Urogenital
   Renal agenesis
   Vesicoureteral reflux
   Cryptorchidism
   Ureteral duplication
   Hypospadias
   Rotated kidney
   Neurogenic bladder
   Renal dysplasia
   Renal ectopia, hypoplasia, aplasia
   Megaureter
   Hydronephrosis
   Ureterovesical obstruction
Spinal cord
   Tethered cord
   Syrinx
Presacral masses
   Anterior meningocele
   Lipoma
   Dermoid
   Teratoma
Gastrointestinal
   Esophageal atresia and/or fistula
   Small intestinal atresia or stenosis
   Gastroschisis
   Omphalocele
   Meckel's diverticulum
   Malrotation
Cardiac
   Ventricular and atrial septal defects
   Tetralogy of Fallot
Sensory
   Sensorineural deafness
   Ocular malformations

Data from references 5, 23, 54.

ENTERIC NERVOUS SYSTEM

Hirschsprung's Disease

Hirschsprung's disease is due to a congenital absence of ganglion cells in both the submucosal (Meissner's) and myenteric (Auerbach's) plexuses. This absence of ganglia extends continuously for a variable distance proximal to the internal anal sphincter. It may extend up to the splenic flexure or even more proximally, involving the entire colon, as well as portions of the small intestine (long-segment Hirschsprung's disease); it may be restricted to the rectum and sigmoid (short-segment

Hirschsprung's disease); or it may involve only a few centimeters proximal to the dentate line (ultra-short-segment Hirschsprung's disease). With an incidence of 1 in 5000 live births, approximately 700 new cases of Hirschsprung's disease occur each year in the United States. Familial occurrence has been reported in about 7% of cases, particularly in those with long aganglionic segments. Hirschsprung's disease is seen most commonly in full-term infants but, on occasion, does occur in premature births. In the short-segment type, a 4:1 male preponderance is observed, and in the long-segment type, the ratio is reduced to about 2:1. Short-segment Hirschsprung's disease accounts for nearly 90% of cases in childhood, and long-segment Hirschsprung's disease accounts for the remainder. It is rare that ultra-short-segment Hirschsprung's disease manifests in the pediatric population, but it does explain certain cases of chronic constipation that come to attention in adulthood.[59]

Twelve percent of children with Hirschsprung's disease have chromosomal abnormalities, 2% to 8% of which are trisomy 21 (Down syndrome); other associated congenital birth defects and syndromes are noted in Table 93–5.[60]

Pathogenesis

Two pathogenetic mechanisms have been proposed for Hirschsprung's disease: (1) failure of migration and (2) alteration of the colonic microenvironment. Genetic, vascular, and infectious factors are invoked to explain these alterations.

Failure of Migration. The genetics of Hirschsprung's disease have now been characterized.[28] Inheritance of the disease can be either autosomal dominant, autosomal recessive, or polygenic. Three genetic characteristics have

been identified: the penetration of mutations generally is low, a gender difference in the penetrance and expression of mutations has been observed, and the penetrance of the gene mutation depends on the extent of aganglionosis in affected family members. It appears that the mutation, while increasing the child's odds of having Hirschsprung's disease, is not predictive of the specific abnormality. Alterations of several genes have been implicated: *RET* proto-oncogene, *c-kit*, *endothelin*, *SOX10*, and *ErbB2* (Table 93–6).[61] Mutation of the *RET* proto-oncogene, a gene that codes for a receptor tyrosine kinase protein, has been noted in familial Hirschsprung's disease and in sporadic cases. A reduced c-kit level in the colon of patients with Hirschsprung's disease has been observed.[62] Identified gene mutations currently account for only approximately half of all cases of Hirschsprung's disease, but it is recommended that *RET* exon 10 mutation analysis be done in all children with Hirschsprung's disease[28]; germline *RET* mutations also can cause multiple endocrine neoplasia type IIA (MEN II), and although the test results will be negative in the vast majority of cases, the significance of identifying *MENIIA* mutation carrier status for that individual and family may appear to justify such testing.

Microenvironment Changes. A basic defect in the microenvironment necessary for the migration, development, and survival of ganglion cells has been postulated. Levels of various substances such as laminin, NADPH-diaphorase, and neural cell adhesion molecules,[63] as well as other polypeptides, have been shown to be reduced in the aganglionic segment,[59] and some investigators postulate that an alteration in the extracellular matrix with decreased concentrations of laminin and collagen IV constitutes a barrier to neutrophin 3, thereby perhaps impairing the neuroblastic migration and colonization.[64,65] Neutrophin 3 promotes survival of sympathetic and sensory neurons in vitro and supports growth and survival of differing subsets of neurons. Nitric oxide synthase is reduced in the aganglionic segment in Hirschsprung's disease, explaining

---

Table 93–5 Congenital Anomalies and Syndromes Associated with Hirschsprung's Disease

Congenital Anomalies
Genitourinary (5.6%)
Cardiac (4.5%)
Central nervous system (3.9%)
Gastrointestinal (3.9%)
Syndromes
Shah-Waardenburg (regional hyperpigmentation, white forelock, bicolored irides, sensorineural deafness)
Movat-Wilson (characteristic facies, microcephaly, mental retardation)
Smith-Lemli-Opitz (anteverted nostrils, ptosis of eyelids, syndactyly of second and third toes, hypospadias and cryptorchidism in males)
Congenital central hypoventilation
Syndromes with limb abnormalities (metaphyseal dysplasia, McKusick-type—mild bowing of legs, irregular metaphyses, fine sparse hair)
MEN II (medullary thyroid cancer, pheochromocytoma, parathyroid hyperplasia)
Piebaldism (hypopigmentation of skin and hair)

MEN, multiple endocrine neoplasia.
Data from Skinner M: Hirschsprung disease. Curr Probl Surg 32:393, 1996; and Ryan ET, Ecker JL, Christakis NA, et al: Hirschsprung disease: Associated anomalies and demography. J Pediatr Surg 27:76, 1992.

Table 93–6 Genetic Bases of Hirschsprung's Disease

Gene	Associated Syndromes*	Pathogenesis
RET	MEN IIA	Abnormal development of enteric nervous system
c-kit	Piebaldism Waardenburg type 4 (Shah-Waardenburg)	
SOX10	Shah-Waardenburg	Reduced survival of neural cells
ZFHXIB	Movat-Wilson	
ErbB2		Impaired maintenance of enteric nervous system[61]

*See Table 93–5 for details of the named syndromes.
Data from Gariepy E: Developmental disorders of the enteric nervous system: Genetic and molecular bases. J Pediatr Gastroenterol Nutr 39:5, 2004; and Skinner M: Hirschsprung disease. Curr Probl Surg 32:393, 1996.

the failure of relaxation of the affected colonic segment.[66] Isolated case reports have linked the destruction of ganglion cells in segmental Hirschsprung's disease to cytomegalovirus infection[67] and muscular hyperplasia of pericolonic vessels.[68]

Clinical Features

Most children with Hirschsprung's disease should be diagnosed in the newborn nursery. Any full-term infant who does not pass meconium within the first 48 hours of life should be suspected of having the disorder. Frequently, such infants will have abdominal distention and feeding difficulties. They also may have bilious emesis from partial bowel obstruction. Dilation of the empty rectum by the first examiner usually results in the explosive expulsion of retained fecal material and decompression of the proximal normal bowel.[69] Hirschsprung's disease–associated enterocolitis occurs more frequently in the first 3 months of life, in patients with delayed diagnosis, in trisomy 21, and with long-segment involvement; females and patients with a positive familial history also are more frquently affected. Enterocolitis develops secondary to ischemia from colonic distention proximal to the aganglionic segment, with secondary infection from bacteria of the colonic content, but isolated cases also have been reported of Hirschsprung's disease–associated enterocolitis in the aganglionic segment. No specific bacteria have been isolated.[70] Mortality rates of up to 30% have been reported for enterocolitis, which remains the major cause of death in Hirschsprung's disease. Colonic perforation, most frequently involving the cecum and rarely the appendix, may occur even in utero.

Most commonly, infants younger than 6 months of age with Hirschsprung's disease will continue to have variable but significant constipation, punctuated by recurrent obstructive crises or impaction, often with failure to thrive. The abdomen may be distended with fecal masses, and peristaltic waves may be visible. Anemia and hypoalbuminemia are common. Blood-flecked diarrhea should suggest the presence of enterocolitis, and immediate evaluation should be undertaken. As the child with Hirschsprung's disease grows older, these problems continue, and fecal soiling occasionally may occur.[69] An infant with Hirschsprung's disease who is breast-fed may have fewer difficulties with defecation because the high concentration of lactose in breast milk produces watery stools that are passed more easily. Once breast milk is discontinued, symptoms of Hirschsprung's disease may increase.

Diagnosis

The child with symptomatic Hirschsprung's disease usually demonstrates signs and symptoms of bowel obstruction. The diagnosis may be made by one or a combination of the following tests: barium enema, rectal biopsy, and anal manometry. Flexible sigmoidoscopy plays a complementary role in diagnosis.

A *barium enema* performed on the unprepared colon will show the distal narrowed hypertonic segment of bowel (usually seen best in a lateral projection). The transition zone between the narrowed distal and dilated proximal intestine will be seen in the most common form of Hirschsprung's disease—the rectosigmoid form (Fig. 93–22A)—but may not be seen with long- or ultra-short-segment intestinal involvement. In ultra-short-segment

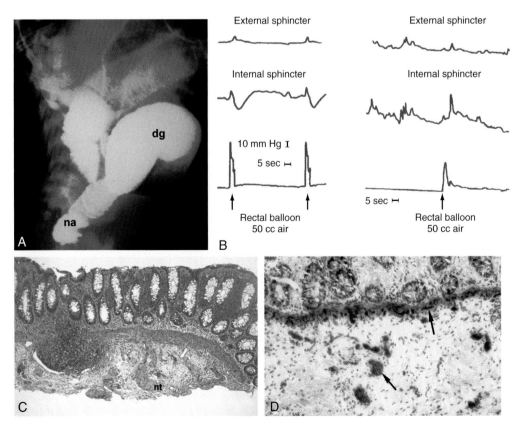

Figure 93–22 Hirschsprung's disease. *A,* Film from a barium enema examination showing the transition zone between the narrowed distal aganglionic segment (na) and the proximal dilated ganglionic segment (dg). *B,* Anal manometry. *Left tracing* illustrates normal function. In the *right tracing* note the lack of relaxation of the internal sphincter in Hirschsprung's disease upon rectal distention. (From Markowitz J: Gastrointestinal motility. In Silverberg M, Daum F [eds]: Textbook of Pediatric Gastroenterology, 2nd ed. Chicago, Year Book Medical Publishers, 1988.) *C,* Photomicrograph of a rectal suction biopsy specimen showing the absence of ganglion cells and thickened nerve trunks (nt) characteristic of Hirschsprung's disease. Hematoxylin-eosin stain, ×125. *D,* Acetylcholinesterase–positive fibers stained brown *(arrows)* in the muscularis mucosae and lamina propria. ×250.

Hirschsprung's disease, a radiologic picture indistinguishable from that in functional constipation with dilated bowel extending to the anus usually is seen. The transition zone may not be evident in rectosigmoid Hirschsprung's disease if the patient has undergone cleansing enemas or colonic irrigation before the study. Although it has been suggested that the transition zone also may not be evident in the first 6 weeks of life, it almost always is noted in the neonate with partial bowel obstruction.[69]

Flexible sigmoidoscopy reveals a normal but empty rectum. The dilated proximal bowel, if within reach of the scope, is traversed easily, except for abundant feces in the lumen; occasionally stercoral ulcers may be seen.

Anal manometry is the most reliable method by which the gastroenterologist can make the diagnosis of ultra-short-segment Hirschsprung's disease. A normal physiologic response to distention of the rectum is relaxation of the smooth muscle internal sphincter pressure. In Hirschsprung's disease, not only does rectal distention fail to induce internal sphincter relaxation, but a paradoxical rise in external sphincter pressure often is seen (see Fig. 93–22B). Sufficient volumes of air must be used to stimulate rectal distention for a reliable study. A false-positive result most commonly is caused by a capacious rectum in constipation or with megacolon, in which case balloon distention may not stimulate the reflex. Up to 20% of normal children have a falsely absent reflex, especially if they are premature or of low birth weight. Nonetheless, a positive response, such as internal sphincter relaxation, is strong evidence against Hirschsprung's disease.

A *suction biopsy* of the rectal mucosa is the most reliable method of diagnosis, except in patients with ultra-short-segment Hirschsprung's disease. The biopsy capsule should be placed at least 2 cm above the mucocutaneous junction in infants and 3 cm above the junction in older children to avoid the physiologic hypoganglionic zone. To be certain of the absence of ganglion cells in the submucosal plexus, an experienced pathologist may need to review many serial sections. Hyperplastic sympathetic nerve fibers and proliferating Schwann cells are associated findings (see Fig. 93–22C), but can be absent in total aganglionosis.

Controversy exists regarding the type of stains necessary to make a diagnosis of Hirschsprung's disease. Because acetylcholinesterase is increased in the muscularis mucosae and lamina propria in the aganglionic segment (see Fig. 93–22D), staining for this enzyme has been used for many years.[71] This technique requires fresh, non–formalin-fixed tissue and technical expertise; at best, this stain is confirmatory. False-positive and false-negative reports have been documented in total colonic aganglionosis.[72] A variety of histochemical staining methods have been proposed for the identification of ganglion cells,[73] but all are expensive, time-consuming, and unnecessary.

In all instances, biopsy of the muscularis propria of the bowel is indicated at the time of surgery to assess for the presence of ganglion cells in the myenteric plexus and to delineate the proximal extension of aganglionosis. A full-thickness biopsy of the anorectal wall performed by a surgeon is diagnostic of ultra-short-segment

Hirschsprung's disease, in contrast with the suction biopsy, which is not as reliable.

In the neonate, considerations in the differential diagnosis in Hirschsprung's disease include other causes of intestinal obstruction, such as meconium ileus, ileal atresia, meconium plug syndrome, and the microcolon seen in infants of diabetic mothers.[69] When symptoms and signs of enterocolitis are present, diagnostic possibilities in the neonate also include primary necrotizing enterocolitis, Hirschsprung's disease–associated enterocolitis, milk protein–induced colitis (see Chapter 19), and sepsis with possible disseminated intravascular coagulation.[69]

In the older child, Hirschsprung's disease must be differentiated from functional constipation (stool withholding, fecal retention). In the latter condition, history indicates that the child did pass meconium in the newborn nursery and that the clinical problems did not arise until the child usually was 18 months of age or older. Fecal impaction almost always is present in fecal retention, and fecal soiling is characteristic. Children with anterior displacement of the anus may be more prone to fecal retention.[69] Idiopathic pseudo-obstruction and intestinal neuronal dysplasia generally can be distinguished from Hirschsprung's disease by rectal biopsy.

Management

Definitive treatment of Hirschsprung's disease is surgical. All full-term babies with meconium plug in the newborn nursery should be evaluated for this disorder before discharge because approximately 15% of children with Hirschsprung's disease have a history of meconium plug. Discharge of any newborn with undiagnosed Hirschsprung's disease with consequent delay in operative intervention may result in a greater frequency of enterocolitis, with resultant morbidity and even mortality.

The specific method of surgery is operator dependent. In general, long-term results are good, but 10% to 20% of children have residual problems, usually with fecal soiling. Long-term prognosis varies and may depend on the length of the aganglionic segment. Even in the most common form of Hirschsprung's disease (short-segment), it is usual to see older children continue to have defecatory issues with fecal retention and encopresis. The exact reasons for these continuing problems remain unclear, but the mechanism may involve an intrinsic abnormality in what is described as normal colon or in the pacemaker system of the colon.

Intestinal Neuronal Dysplasia

Intestinal neuronal dysplasia (IND) is a motility disorder that manifests with intestinal obstruction or severe chronic constipation; characteristic biopsy findings include a two- to five-fold increase in the number of enlarged ganglia and neural hypertrophy (Fig. 93–23A). In addition, acetylcholinesterase activity is increased in the lamina propria and muscularis mucosae.[74] A full-thickness surgical biopsy specimen is necessary to diagnose IND. It has been reported as an isolated lesion affecting especially premature infants, or infants with a history of formula protein intolerance, ileal stenosis, or

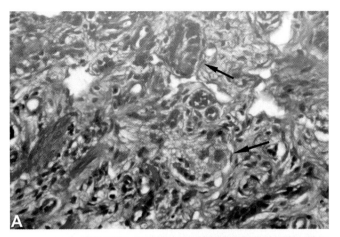

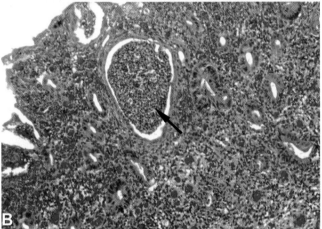

Figure 93–23 Photomicrographs of a rectal biopsy specimen from a patient with intestinal neuronal dysplasia. *A,* Increased number of enlarged ganglia *(arrows).* Hematoxylin-eosin stain, ×250. *B,* Active inflammation of the rectal mucosa with crypt abscess *(arrow).* Hematoxylin-eosin stain, ×250.

small left colon–meconium plug syndrome.[75] IND also can be seen in association with other syndromes such as neurofibromatosis or MEN IIB (or III), or in proximal-segment Hirschsprung's disease.[76]

Three types of IND have been defined. IND type A usually manifests acutely in the neonatal period as severe constipation and enterocolitis. Biopsy features include mucosal inflammation (see Fig. 93–23B), ulceration with hyperplastic neural changes limited to the myenteric plexus, and increased acetylcholinesterase activity in the lamina propria and muscularis mucosae. The submucosal plexus in this type of IND is histologically normal.

IND type B usually is seen in children between 6 months and 6 years of age who have chronic constipation and megacolon. Histopathologic findings include hyperplastic submucosal ganglia with increased acetylcholinesterase-positive fibers in the muscularis mucosae and lamina propria. Ectopic ganglion cells in the muscularis mucosae and lamina propria also have been described. No changes are seen in the myenteric plexus. The histologic features of type B disease must be distinguished from those in MEN III, which carries important implications for medical intervention and screening. Significant interobserver variation has been documented for the pathologic diagnosis of IND type B by rectal suction biopsies. Some reports have speculated that some of the

morphologic features described in type B are normal age-related phenomena. A third, mixed type of IND has an acute presentation and involves both the submucosal and the myenteric plexuses.[76]

The pathogenesis of IND is controversial.[77] In some patients, it constitutes a congenital malformation,[78] whereas in others, it is an acquired phenomenon.[74] Associated conditions include cystic fibrosis, intestinal microvillus atrophy (see later), congenital anomalies, lipoblastomatosis, and inflammatory bowel disease. Therefore, IND may not represent a well-defined entity but rather may constitute a secondary phenomenon related either to age or to obstruction or inflammation.[79] The dysplasia can resolve with maturation.

Chronic Intestinal Pseudo-obstruction

Congenital forms of neuropathic and myopathic pseudo-obstruction are both rare and sporadic, perhaps representing new mutations (see Chapter 117). In these situations, a family history of pseudo-obstruction is lacking, as are any associated syndromes and evidence of other predisposing factors such as toxins, infections, ischemia, or autoimmune disease.[80] Children with chromosomal abnormalities such as Down syndrome, as well as those with MEN III or with Duchenne's muscular dystrophy, may suffer from pseudo-obstruction.[80]

MISCELLANEOUS

Microvillus Inclusion Disease

Congenital microvillus atrophy, also known as microvillus inclusion disease (MID), is an autosomal recessive disorder that may manifest with severe diarrhea shortly after birth and is characterized by atrophy of the intestinal villi and characteristic electron microscopic findings.[81] Although the prevalence of MID is not known, it is reported to be the most common cause of familial intractable diarrhea.[82] A female predominance has been observed, and consanguinity is reported in 20% of cases.[83] The incidence of MID may be higher among Navajo Indians and persons from the Middle East.[84] The pathogenesis is uncertain. Secretory diarrhea is severe, with intolerance to oral feeding and unresponsiveness to most therapeutic modalities.

Three variants of MID are recognized: *congenital,* the most frequent and severe, manifesting within the first week of life; *late-onset,* starting at 6 to 8 weeks; and *atypical,* with either early or late onset.

The wall of the small intestine is paper-thin in MID. The mucosa of the duodenum and small bowel is characterized by villus atrophy, hypoplastic or normal crypts, and normal or decreased cellularity of the lamina propria[85] (Fig. 93–24A). The absence of the brush border membrane is demonstrated by lack of staining with PAS and carcinoembryonic antigen (CEA); intracytoplasmic inclusions also are seen by these stains, because they are surrounded by apical membrane material.

Evaluation by electron microscopy reveals ultrastructural abnormalities of the microvillus membrane including disruption or absence of the brush border membrane, shortening and absence of the microvilli, and microvil-

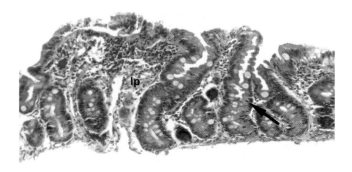

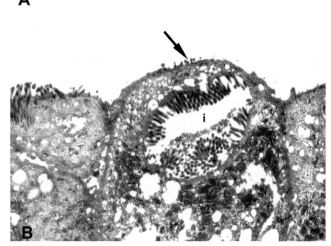

Figure 93–24　Photomicrographs of the duodenum from a patient with microvillus inclusion disease. *A,* Villus atrophy with crypt hyperplasia *(arrow)* and decreased cellularity of the lamina propria (lp). Hematoxylin-eosin stain, ×250. *B,* On electron microscopy, lack of or shortened microvilli *(arrow)* and a cytoplasmic inclusion (i), composed of a vesicle lined by microvilli, can be seen. ×15,000. (Courtesy of S. Teichberg, PhD.)

lus inclusions (see Fig. 93–24*B*). Although these lesions are most commonly noted in biopsy specimens from the small intestine, microvillus inclusions also may be seen in specimens from the colon, rectum, and other extraintestinal sites.[86]

Total parenteral nutrition must be utilized to prolong survival. Small bowel transplantation should be considered. Prognosis is poor, and the disorder usually is fatal.

Tufting Enteropathy

In tufting enteropathy, the surface epithelium is disrupted. Surface epithelial cells are arranged in tufts with a round apex. These epithelial cells have an abnormal expression of E-cadherin and do not contain inclusions on electron microscopic examination.[87] Diarrhea is secretory, and malabsorption is intractable, and unresponsive to medical therapies.[88] This entity may be more common than MID in the Middle East.

OTHER GENETIC

Congenital Glucose/Galactose Malabsorption

Familial glucose/galactose malabsorption, transmitted as an autosomal recessive trait, is characterized by an absence of the active transport carrier protein (Na$^+$/glucose cotransporter) for glucose and galactose. Ingestion of any formula containing glucose or galactose results in severe watery diarrhea in the newborn period. Stools are strongly positive for reducing substances. Neither blood nor white blood cells are present in the stool. Findings on biopsy of the small bowel and colon are normal. Discontinuation of formula containing lactose, glucose, or galactose (lactose is metabolized to glucose and galactose) and institution of a fructose-containing formula with therapeutic benefit usually are sufficient to make a clinical diagnosis of glucose/galactose malabsorption. Diarrhea abruptly ceases and the newborn begins to thrive when fructose-containing formula feedings are instituted.[89] Some reports indicate that the severity of the diarrhea from glucose/galactose diminishes with age because of the increased capacity of the intestinal flora to metabolize glucose.[90]

Congenital Sucrase/Isomaltase Deficiency

Because sucrose is not a common dietary carbohydrate during the first 6 months of life, watery stools generally do not develop in children with this disorder until sucrose is administered in baby food. An exception to this rule would be in the newborn receiving a formula (usually with soy protein) with sucrose as the carbohydrate. Alimentum, a casein hydrolysate formula, also contains small amounts of sucrose. To make the diagnosis in such infants, the stool must be hydrolyzed by boiling it with IN hydrochloric acid for 20 minutes, thereby changing sucrose to glucose and fructose, because sucrose itself is not a reducing substance. Congenital sucrase/isomaltase deficiency, although extremely rare, is the most common congenital disaccharidase deficiency.[89]

Congenital Lactase Deficiency

Congenital absence of lactase is extremely rare. Babies receiving a lactose-containing formula develop severe watery diarrhea, which resolves with the institution of a non–lactose-containing formula. Biopsies of the small intestine reveal diminished or absent lactase.[89]

Congenital Chloridorrhea

Congenital chloridorrhea is a transport defect that may result in chronic diarrhea from birth. The chloride-bicarbonate exchange mechanism in the ileum and colon is reversed, and chloride is actively secreted, resulting in secretory diarrhea. The increased absorption of bicarbonate may result in alkalosis, hyponatremia, and marked hypokalemia. The stool is extremely watery, and no blood, white blood cells, or reducing substances are noted. Findings on biopsies of the small intestine and colon are normal.[89] Treatment is fluid and electrolyte replacement. Acid reduction with proton pump inhibitors has been tried, with variable results.

Cystic Fibrosis

Cystic fibrosis is an autosomal recessive disorder of cyclic adenosine monophosphate chloride transport that results from a defect in the cystic fibrosis transmembrane regulator (CFTR).[91]

Approximately 10% to 15% of newborns with cystic fibrosis present with neonatal meconium ileus or its complications.[92] Meconium plug syndrome also may occur, resulting in colonic obstruction, rather than small bowel obstruction, as is seen with meconium ileus. Antenatally, small bowel ischemia and perforation may occur, resulting in meconium cyst, intestinal atresia, or meconium peritonitis with intra-abdominal or scrotal calcifications.[91]

REFERENCES

1. Montgomery RK, Grand RJ: Development of the human gastrointestinal system. In Timonium MD (ed): The Undergraduate Teaching Project in Gastroenterology and Liver Disease. Timonium, Md., American Gastroenterological Association/Milner-Fenwick, 1999, p 1.
2. Kumar D, Phillips SF: The contribution of external ligamentous attachments to function of the ileocecal junction. Dis Colon Rectum 6:410, 1987.
3. Kahn E: Morphology of the gastrointestinal tract. In Silverberg M, Daum F (eds): Textbook of Pediatric Gastroenterology, 2nd ed. Chicago, Year Book Medical Publishers, 1988, p 1.
4. Fawcett DW: Intestine-nerves of the intestinal tract. In Bloom W, Fawcett DW (eds): Bloom & Fawcett—A Textbook of Histology, 11th ed. Philadelphia, WB Saunders, 1986, p 671.
5. Keljo DJ, Gariepy CE: Anatomy, histology, embryology, and developmental anomalies of the small and large intestine. In Feldman M, Friedman LS, Sleisenger MH (eds): Sleisenger and Fordtran's Gastrointestinal and Liver Disease, 7th ed. Philadelphia, WB Saunders, 2002, p 1643.
6. Ouellette A, Hsieh MM, Nosek MT, et al: Mouse Paneth cell defensins: Primary structures and antibacterial activities of numerous cryptidin isoforms. Infect Immunol 62:5040, 1994.
7. Rubin W: Endocrine cells in the normal human stomach. A fine structural study. Gastroenterology 63:784, 1972.
8. Sjolund K, Sanden G, Hakanson R, Sundler F: Endocrine cells in human intestine: An immunocytochemical study. Gastroenterology 85:1120, 1983.
9. Pearse AG: The APUD cell concept and its implications in pathology. Pathol Annu 9:27, 1974
10. Sidhu GS: The endodermal origin of digestive and respiratory APUD cells. Histopathologic evidence and a review of the literature. Am J Pathol 96:5, 1979.
11. Rindi G, Leiter AB, Kopin AS, et al: The "normal" endocrine cell of the gut. Changing concepts and new evidence. Ann N Y Acad Sci 1014:1, 2004.
12. Jakobsen AM, Andersson P, Saglik G, et al: Differential expression of vesicular monoamine transporter (VMAT) 1 and 2 in gastrointestinal endocrine tumors. J Pathol 195:463, 2001.
13. Lauffer JN, Zhang T, Modlin IM: Review article: Current status of gastrointestinal carcinoids. Aliment Pharmacol Ther 13:271, 1999.
14. Neutra MR, Kraehenbuhl JP: The role of transepithelial transport by M cells in microbial invasion and host defense. J Cell Sci 17(suppl):209, 1993.
15. Faussone-Pellegrine MS, Thuneberg L: Guide to the identification of interstitial cells of Cajal. Micros Res Tech 47:248, 1999.
16. Ahmed A, Yee H, Greco MA, Kahn E: Distribution of c-Kit positive interstitial cells of Cajal in the gastrointestinal tract of fetuses and children. Modern Pathol 14:3P, 2001.
17. Fontaine JL, Navarro J: Small intestinal biopsy in cow's milk protein allergy and infancy. Arch Dis Child 50:357, 1975.
18. Pollak JM, Pearse AGE, Garaud JC, et al: Cellular localization of vasoactive intestinal peptides in the mammalian and avian gastrointestinal tract. Gut 15:720, 1974.
19. Fawcett DW: Intestine-blood vessels of the gastrointestinal tract. In Bloom W, Fawcett DW (eds): Bloom & Fawcett—A Textbook of Histology, 11th ed. Philadelphia, WB Saunders, 1986, p 668.
20. Fawcett DW: Intestine-lymph vessels of the gastrointestinal tract. In Bloom W, Fawcett DW (eds): Bloom & Fawcett—A Textbook of Histology, 11th ed. Philadelphia, WB Saunders, 1986, p 669.
21. Sadler TW: Digestive system. In Sun B (ed): Langman's Medical Embryology, 9th ed. Philadelphia, Lippincott Williams & Wilkins, 2004, p 285.
22. Zakany J, Duboule D: Hox genes and the making of sphincters. Nature 401:761, 1999.
23. Pena A: Pediatric surgical problems. In Corman M (ed): Colon and Rectal Surgery, 4th ed. Philadelphia, Lippincot & Raven, 1998, p 449.
24. Flamme I, Frolich T, Risau W: Molecular mechanisms of vasculogenesis and embryonic angiogenesis. J Cell Physiol 173:206, 1997.
25. Gale NW. Yancopoulos GD: Growth factors acting via endothelial cell–specific receptor tyrosine kinases: VEGFs, angiopoietins, and ephrins in vascular development. Genes Dev 13:1055, 1999.
26. Vikkula M, Boon LM, Carraway KL, et al: Vascular dysmorphogenesis caused by an activating mutation in the receptor tyrosine kinase TIE2. Cell 87:1181, 1996.
27. Kukk E, Lymboussaki A, Taira S, et al: VEGF-C receptor binding and pattern of expression with VEGFR-3 suggests a role in lymphatic vascular development. Development 122:3829, 1996.
28. Gariepy E: Developmental disorders of the enteric nervous system: Genetic and molecular bases. J Pediatr Gastroenterol Nutr 39:5, 2004.
29. Kioussi C, Rosenfeld MG: Body's left side. Cell Mol Biol 45:517, 1999.
30. Jacquemin E, Cresteil D, Raynaud N, Hadchouel M: CFC1 gene mutation and biliary atresia with polysplenia syndrome. J Pediatr Gastroenterol Nutr 34:323, 2002.
31. Bamford RN, Roessler E, Burdine RD, et al: Loss-of-function mutations in the EGF-CFC gene CFC1 are associated with human left-right laterality defects. Nat Genet 26:365, 2000.
32. Schwartz, DL: Congenital malformations and surgical intestinal emergencies of infancy. In Silverberg M, Daum F (eds): Textbook of Pediatric Gastroenterology, 2nd ed. Chicago, Year Book Medical Publishers, 1988, p 194.
33. Vassy LE, Boles TE Jr: Iatrogenic ileal atresia secondary to clamping of an occult omphalocele. J Pediatr Surg 10:797, 1975.
34. Grob M: Lehrbuch der Kinderchirurgie. Stuttgart, George Thieme, 1957, p 311.
35. Tunell WP, Puffinbarger NK, Tuggle DW: Abdominal wall defect in infants: Survival and implications for adult life. Ann Surg 221:525, 1995.
36. Palomaki GE, Hill LE, Knight GJ, et al: Second-trimester maternal serum alpha-fetoprotein levels in pregnancy associated with gastroschisis and omphalocele. Obstet Gynecol 71:906, 1988.
37. Tunell WP: Anterior abdominal wall defects. In Wyllie R, Hyams JS (eds): Pediatric Gastrointestinal Disease. Pathophysiology, Diagnosis, Management, 2nd ed. Philadelphia, WB Saunders, 1999, p 515.
38. Gray SE, Skanddalakis JE: Embryology for Surgeons. Philadelphia, WB Saunders, 1972, p 156.
39. Yammaguchi M, Tacheuchi S, Awazu S: Meckel's diverticulum, investigation of 600 patients in Japanese literature. Am J Surg 136:247, 1978.
40. Schwartz MZ: Meckel's diverticulum and other omphalomesenteric duct remnant. In Wyllie R, Hyams JS (eds): Pediatric Gastrointestinal Disease. Pathophysiology, Diagnosis, Management, 2nd ed. Philadelphia, WB Saunders, 1999, p 483.

41. Bemelman WA, Bosma A, Wiersman PH, et al: Role of *Helicobacter pylori* in the pathogenesis of complications of Meckel's diverticula. Eur J Surg 159:171, 1993.

42. Andreyev HJ, Owen RA, Thompson I, et al: Association between Meckel's diverticulum and Crohn's disease: A retrospective review. Gut 35:788, 1994.

43. Cooney DR, Duszynski DO, Camboa E, et al: The abdominal technetium scan (a decade of experience). J Pediatr Surg 17:611, 1982.

44. Petrokubi RJ, Baum S, Rohrer GV: Cimetidine administration resulting in improved pertechnetate imaging of Meckel's diverticulum. Clin Nucl Med 3:385, 1978.

45. Okazaki M, Higashihara H, Yamasaki S, et al: Arterial embolization to control life-threatening hemorrhage from Meckel's diverticulum. AJR Am J Roentgenol 154:1257, 1990.

46. Gosche JR, Touloukian RJ: Congenital anomalies of the midgut. In Wyllie R, Hyams JS (eds): Pediatric Gastrointestinal Disease. Pathophysiology, Diagnosis, Management, 2nd ed. Philadelphia, WB Saunders, 1999, p 505.

47. Dott NM: Anomalies of intestinal rotation: Their embryology and surgical aspects with report of five cases. Br J Surg 11:251, 1923.

48. Berardi RS: Anomalies of midgut rotation in the adult. Surg Gynecol Obstet 151:113, 1980.

49. Potter EL (ed): Pathology of the Fetus and Infant. Chicago, Year Book, 1961.

50. Grosfeld JL, Ballantine TVN, Shoemaker R: Operative management of intestinal atresia and stenosis based on pathologic findings. J Pediatr Surg 14:368, 1979.

51. Seashore JH, Collins FS, Markowitz RI, et al: Familial apple peel jejunal atresia: Surgical, genetic, and radiologic aspects. Pediatrics 80:540, 1987.

52. Pena A: Imperforate anus. In Wyllie R, Hyams JS (eds): Pediatric Gastrointestinal Disease. Pathophysiology, Diagnosis, Management, 2nd ed. Philadelphia, WB Saunders, 1999, p 499.

53. Trusler GA, Wilkinson RH: Imperforate anus: A review of 147 cases. Can J Surg 5:169, 1962.

54. Nixon H: Congenital deformities of the anorectal region. In Golinger J (ed): Surgery of Anus, Rectum and Colon, 5th ed. Bailliere Tindall, 1984, p 285.

55. Stephens FD, Smith ED: Classification, identification and assessment of surgical treatment of anorectal anomalies. Pediatr Surg Int 1:200, 1986.

56. Rich MA, Brock WA, Pena A: Spectrum of urogenital malformations in patients with imperforate anus. Pediatr Surg Int 3:110, 1988.

57. Pena A: Posterior sagittal anorectoplasty: Results in the management of 322 cases of anorectal malformations. Pediatr Surg Int 3:4, 1988.

58. Pena A: The surgical management of persistent cloaca: Results in 54 patients treated with a posterior sagittal approach. Pediatr Surg Int 24:590, 1989.

59. Skinner M: Hirschsprung disease. Curr Probl Surg 32:393, 1996.

60. Ryan ET, Ecker JL, Christakis NA, et al: Hirschsprung disease: Associated anomalies and demography. J Pediatr Surg 27:76, 1992.

61. Crone SA, Negro A, Trumpp A, et al: Colonic epithelial expression of ErbB2 is required for postnatal maintenance of the enteric nervous system. Neuron 37:29, 2003.

62. Yamataka A, Kato Y, Tibboel D, et al: A lack of intestinal pacemaker (c-Kit) in aganglionic bowel of patients with Hirschsprung disease. J Pediatr Surg 30:441, 1995.

63. Romanska HM, Bishop AE, Brereton RJ, et al: Increased expression of muscular neural cell adhesion molecule in congenital aganglionosis. Gastroenterology 105:1104, 1993.

64. Kapur RP: Contemporary approaches toward understanding the pathogenesis of Hirschsprung disease. Pediatr Pathol 13:83, 1993.

65. Parikh DH, Tam PKH, Velzen DV, Edgar D: Abnormalities in the distribution of laminin and collagen type IV in Hirschsprung disease. Gastroenterology 102:1236, 1992.

66. Vanderwinden JM, De Laet MH, Schiffmann SN, et al: Nitric oxide synthase distribution in the enteric nervous system of Hirschsprung disease. Gastroenterology 105:969, 1993.

67. Dimmick JE, Bove KE: Cytomegalovirus infection of the bowel in infancy: Pathogenetic and diagnostic significance. Pediatr Pathol 2:95, 1984.

68. Taguchi T, Tanaka K, Ikeda K: Fibromuscular dysplasia of arteries in Hischsprung's disease. Gastroenterology 88:1099, 1985.

69. Markowitz J: Gastrointestinal motility. In Silverberg M, Daum F (eds): Textbook of Pediatric Gastroenterology, 2nd ed. Chicago, Year Book Medical Publishers, 1988, p 149.

70. Fraser GC, Berry C: Mortality in neonatal Hirschsprung disease: With special reference to enterocolitis. J Pediatr Surg 2:205, 1967.

71. Wakely PE, McAdams AJ: Acetylcholinesterase histochemistry and the diagnosis of Hirschsprung disease: A 3 1/2-year experience. Pediatr Pathol 2:35, 1984.

72. Sun CCJ, Caniano DA, Hill JL: Intestinal aganglionosis: A histologic and acetylcholinesterase histochemical study. Pediatr Pathol 7:421, 1987.

73. Tam PKH, Owen G: An immunohistochemical study of neuronal microtubule-associated proteins in Hirschsprung disease. Hum Pathol 24:424, 1993.

74. Reifferscheid P, Flach A: A particular form of Hirschsprung disease: neuronal dysplasia of the intestine. In Holschneider A (ed): Hirschsprung's Disease. New York, Thieme Stratton, 1982, p 133.

75. Schofield DE, Yunis EJ: What is intestinal neuronal dysplasia? Pathol Annu 1:249, 1992.

76. Simpser E, Kahn E, Kenigsberg K, et al: Neuronal intestinal dysplasia: Quantitative diagnostic criteria and clinical management. J Pediatr Gastroenterol Nutr 12:61, 1991.

77. Lake BD: Intestinal neuronal dysplasia: Does it exist, or has it been invented? Virchows Arch 426:537, 1995.

78. Meier-Ruge W: Hirschsprung disease: Its etiology, pathogenesis and differential diagnosis. Curr Top Pathol 59:31, 1974.

79. Sacher P, Briner J, Hanimann B: Is neuronal intestinal dysplasia (NID) a primary or secondary phenomenon? Eur J Pediatr Surg 3:228, 1993.

80. Hyman PE: Chronic intestinal pseudoobstruction. In Wyllie R, Hyams JS (eds): Pediatric Gastrointestinal Disease. Pathophysiology, Diagnosis, Management, 2nd ed. Philadelphia, WB Saunders, 1999, p 433.

81. Schofield DE, Agostini RM, Yunis EJ: Gastrointestinal microvillus inclusion disease. Am J Clin Pathol 98:119, 1992.

82. Bell SW, Kerner JA, Sibley RK: Microvillous inclusion disease. The importance of the electron microscopy for diagnosis. Am J Pathol 15:1157, 1991.

83. Cutz R, Rhoads JM, Drumm B, et al: Microvillous inclusion disease: An inherited defect of brush-border assembly and differentiation. N Engl J Med 320:646, 1989.

84. Pohl JF, Shub PD, Trevelline EE, et al: A cluster of microvillous inclusion disease in the Navajo population. J Pediatr 134:103, 1999.

85. Phillips AD, Schmitz J: Familial villous atrophy: A clinicopathological survey of 23 cases. J Pediatr Gastroenterol Nutr 14:380, 1992.

86. Nathavitharana KA, Green NJ, Raafat F, et al: Siblings with microvillous inclusion disease. Arch Dis Child 71:71, 1994.

87. Cutz E, Sherman PM, Davidson GP: Enteropathies associated with protacted diarrhea in infancy. Clinicopathologic features, cellular and molecular mechanisms Pediatr Pathol Lab Med 17:335, 1997.

88. Goulet O, Kedinger M, Brousse N, et al: Intractable diarrhea of infancy with epithelial and basement membrane abnormalities. J Pediatr 127:212, 1995.

89. Vanderhoof JA: Diarrhea. In Wyllie R, Hyams JS (eds): Pediatric Gastrointestinal Disease. Pathophysiology, Diagnosis, Management, 2nd ed. Philadelphia, WB Saunders, 1999, p 32.

90. Wells RG, Mohandas TK, Hediger MA: Localization of the Na^+/glucose transporter gene SGLT2 to human chromosome 16 close to the centromere. Genomics 17:787, 1993.

91. Rothbaum RH: Cystic fibrosis and congenital anomalies of the exocrine pancreas. In Wyllie R, Hyams JS (eds): Pediatric Gastrointestinal Disease. Pathophysiology, Diagnosis, Management, 2nd ed. Philadelphia, WB Saunders, 1999, p 665.

92. Rescorla F, Grosfeld J, West K, Vane D: Changing pattern of treatment and survival in neonates with meconium ileus. Arch Surg 124:837, 1989.

CHAPTER

94 Small Intestinal Motor and Sensory Function and Dysfunction

Jane M. Andrews and L. Ashley Blackshaw

The two most important goals of small intestinal motor and sensory function are the efficient absorption of nutrients and the maintenance of orderly aboral movement of chyme and indigestible residues along the small intestine. Small intestinal motility also is critically important in preventing bacterial overgrowth within the gut. This is achieved by net aboral flow of luminal contents during both the fed and the fasting states, probably with the assistance of the "gatekeeper" function of the ileocecal junction, which prevents backflow of cecal contents and keeps small intestinal bacterial concentrations at their usual relatively low levels.

Net movement of contents along the small intestine is antegrade, but retrograde flow also occurs normally, over short distances. Optimal progression of luminal contents allows optimal mixing of digested food with gut secretions and contact of contents with the epithelium; such contact is important for both the absorption and "sensing" of nutrients within the lumen. Both absorption and mucosal sensing of nutrients exert significant feedback control on gastric and small intestinal motor func-

tion. This interplay is thought to optimize the rate at which additional nutrient is presented to the absorptive epithelium, and to minimize the amount of nutrient lost to the colon. Preceding emesis, and in association with nausea, gross retrograde movement of small intestinal contents occurs over long distances, when a unique pattern of a strong zone of phasic small intestinal contractions travels in an oral direction over a large proportion of the small intestine. These contractions deliver luminal contents back to the stomach for ejection into the esophagus during emesis. This coordinated motor pattern underscores the versatile modulation of small intestinal motility according to physiologic need.

The motor function of the small intestine depends directly on smooth muscle in the gut wall, which contains the basic control mechanisms that initiate contractions and control their frequency. Overlying these basic control mechanisms are the enteric nervous system (ENS) and the autonomic nervous system (ANS). In addition, a number of hormones modulate the frequency and patterning of small intestinal contractions. Each of these factors plays a role in the motility of the small intestine in health, and specific damage of each component in some diseases has helped to define their discrete roles.

This chapter concentrates on the physiology of normal small intestinal motility. Anatomy is considered first, with emphasis on elements that control sensory and motor activity. Neurophysiology, integrative control, and patterning of small intestinal motility are reviewed next, along with some insights into possible mechanisms underlying motor and sensory dysfunction. Measurement techniques and limitations in evaluation of motility then are discussed, followed by descriptions of commonly recognized motor patterns. Finally, more clinically directed commentary on specialized tests used to assess small intestinal motility, disease states in which small intestinal motor and/or sensory function is disturbed, and a general approach to the patient with suspected small intestinal motor dysfunction are presented.

ANATOMY (see also Chapter 93)

The small intestine is approximately 3 to 7 meters long, extending from the duodenal side of the pylorus to the ileocecal valve. It is divided into three regions—duodenum, jejunum, and ileum—based on structural and functional considerations. Although some structural and functional differences exist among these three regions, they exhibit similar motor characteristics. At each end of the small intestine, however, physiologic sphincters—the pylorus and the ileocecal valve—have distinctly different motor patterns that give them the ability to act as controllers of flow between the antrum and duodenum and the ileum and colon, respectively. The motor function of the pylorus is discussed in Chapter 46 and the ileocecal region is discussed in Chapter 95. The duodenum is a fixed, largely retroperitoneal structure located in the upper abdomen, and the distal ileum generally is anchored in the right iliac fossa by its attachment to the cecum. Except for these regions, the small intestine is mobile within the peritoneal cavity.

STRUCTURAL ELEMENTS AND THEIR ROLE IN SMALL INTESTINAL MOTOR AND SENSORY FUNCTION

SMOOTH MUSCLE

The wall of the small intestine comprises the mucosa, consisting of the epithelium and lamina propria; submucosa; muscular layer (muscularis); and serosa (Fig. 94–1). The muscularis is composed of inner circular and outer longitudinal layers of smooth muscle, which are present in continuity along the length of the small intestine. Contractions within these layers are responsible for gross small intestinal motility. A much smaller additional muscular layer, the muscularis mucosae, is present between the mucosa and the submucosa and plays a role in mucosal or villus motility[1] but does not contribute to

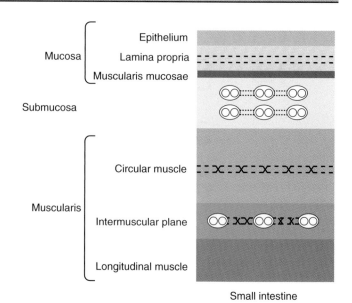

Figure 94–1   Diagram showing the layers and components of the small intestinal wall. (Modified from Christensen J: Intestinal motor physiology. In Feldman M, Scharschmidt BF, Sleisenger MH [eds]: Sleisenger & Fordtran's Gastrointestinal and Liver Disease, 6th ed. Philadelphia, WB Saunders, 1997, p 1438.)

gross motility and is not considered further in this chapter.

The smooth muscle cells within each muscle layer form a *syncytium*. Myocytes communicate electrically with each other through physically specialized areas of cell-to-cell contact, called *gap junctions*, which are visible on electron microscopy. This intimate contact between adjacent myocytes gives low-resistance electrical contact or coupling among them, thereby enabling them to be excited as a unit. Mechanical connections among myocytes in each layer enable them to function as a contractile unit. At a cellular level, the mechanical connections are provided by *intermediate junctions*, and at a tissue level, mechanical connections are provided by the dense extracellular stroma of collagen filaments between bundles of smooth muscle cells.[2] Within each layer, the smooth muscle cell bodies are arranged in parallel, so that the circular muscle layer encircles the lumen, and the longitudinal layer extends axially along the small intestine. Hence, small intestinal muscle contractions can reduce luminal diameter and shorten small intestinal length.[3]

The myocytes themselves are spindle-shaped cells that derive their contractile properties from specialized cytoplasmic filaments and from the attachment of these filaments to cytoskeletal elements (Fig. 94–2). On electron microscopy, condensations of electron-dense, amorphous material are noted around the inner aspect of the cell membrane (dense bands) and throughout the cytoplasm (dense bodies). The contractile filaments—actin and myosin—are arranged in a fashion similar to that in skele-

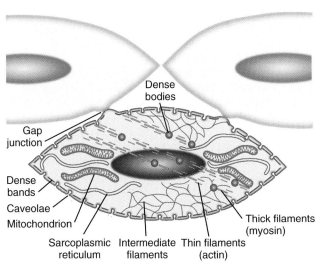

Gap junction

Dense bodies

Dense bands

Caveolae

Mitochondrion

Sarcoplasmic reticulum

Intermediate filaments

Thin filaments (actin)

Thick filaments (myosin)

Figure 94–2 Diagram of a smooth muscle cell showing ultrastructural features discussed in the text. (From Christensen J: Gastrointestinal motility. In West JB [ed]: Best and Taylor's Physiologic Basis for Medical Practice. Baltimore, Williams & Wilkins, 1990, p 614.)

tal muscle and insert onto the dense bands and bodies approximately in parallel with the long axis of the cell. Thus, when the contractile filaments are activated to slide over each other, cell shortening results. Activation of the contractile filaments is triggered by an increase in free intracellular calcium, which results from both release of calcium from intracellular stores and entry of extracellular calcium.

INTERSTITIAL CELLS OF CAJAL

The *interstitial cell of Cajal* (ICC) is another specialized type of cell within the smooth muscle layer that, in recent years, has been recognized as vital for normal small intestinal motor function.[4] They are pleomorphic mesenchymal cells that form an interconnecting network via long, tapering cytoplasmic processes. ICCs lie in close proximity to both nerve axons and myocytes, with which they form electrical gap junctions. ICCs serve two roles in control of small intestinal motility: first, they generate the electrical slow wave that plays an important pacemaker role in determining the basic rhythmicity of small intestinal contractions[4]; second, they transduce both inhibitory and excitatory neural signals to the myocytes[5,6] and thus have the power to vary the myocyte membrane potential and, in turn, contractile activity. This transduction occurs by virtue of the fact that ICCs are interposed functionally between nerve terminals and the smooth muscle that the nerves supply. The small intestinal neuroeffector junctions are not simple contacts between nerve terminals and smooth muscle cells, but between enteric nerve terminals and ICCs, and from there with myocytes by means of electrical gap junctions. Thus, effective neurotransmission results from the activation of specific sets of receptors on ICCs, rather than by direct action on smooth muscle cells.

At least three separate functional groups of ICCs exist. Cells of the ICC_{MY} (myenteric) population form a

dense, electrically coupled network within the intermuscular space at the level of the myenteric plexus between the circular and longitudinal muscle layers. $ICCs_{MY}$ are the pacemaker cells in the small intestine that trigger the generation of slow waves in the smooth muscle. These cells possess a specialized mechanism that uses their oxidative metabolism to generate an inward (pacemaker) current, resulting from the flow of cations through nonselective cation channels in the plasma membrane. A "primary" pacemaker initiates slow waves, and depolarization from the primary event entrains the spontaneous activity of other ICCs within the network. This sequence results in a propagation-like phenomenon where slow waves spread, without decrement, through the ICC network by means of gap junctions. The second population of ICC, ICC_{IM} (intramuscular), is distributed within the muscle layers. $ICCs_{IM}$ are innervated preferentially by intrinsic enteric motor neurons. In the small intestine, a subpopulation of $ICCs_{IM}$ is concentrated at the inner surface of the circular muscle layer at the region of the deep muscular plexus. This third population, ICC_{DMP}, also receives preferential innervation and may be a specialized type of ICC_{IM} in the small intestine. Both inhibitory and excitatory enteric nerve terminals selectively target intramuscular ICCs. Their responses are transduced, in turn, to smooth muscle cells through gap junctions. Inputs from enteric excitatory motor neurons are mediated mainly by muscarinic acetylcholine receptors (M2 and M3) that result in increased inward currents, thereby causing depolarization. When depolarization reaches smooth muscle, it increases the opening of L-type Ca^{2+} channels during slow waves. These conditions result in greater Ca^{2+} entry and more forceful phasic contractions. Inputs from inhibitory enteric motor neurons are mediated by neurotransmitters including nitric oxide and vasoactive intestinal polypeptide which activate both receptor and non-receptor mechanisms in $ICCs_{IM}$. The result of these inputs is increased opening of K^+ channels, and, in turn, a stabilizing effect on membrane potential, reduced Ca^{2+} channel opening, and less forceful contractions. Therefore, the mechanical response of small intestinal muscle to the ongoing slow wave activity depends strongly upon regulation of its excitability by the enteric nervous system via $ICCs_{IM}$. ICCs, in general, play broadly similar roles in the small intestine and colon, and the reader is referred to Chapter 95 for a discussion of their roles in the large bowel (see also Figs. 95–2, 117–2), as well as recent reviews by Sanders and colleagues[7] and Ward and associates.[8] Absence or inactivity of ICCs has been implicated in a number of clinical disorders that manifest as disturbed gut motility.

NEURONS

The small intestine is innervated richly with both extrinsic and intrinsic neurons. Intrinsic neurons have their cell bodies within the wall of the small intestine and constitute the ENS. These instrinsic neurons greatly outnumber the neurons of the extrinsic supply. Extrinsic neurons have their cell bodies outside the gut wall, but have projections that end within the gut wall. Extrinsic neurons can be classified anatomically according to the location of their cell bodies and the route along which their projections travel. Extrinsic motor neurons belong to the ANS and connect the central nervous system (CNS) with the ENS and from there the small intestinal smooth muscle through ICCs. Some extrinsic motor neurons may terminate directly in the muscle layers. Extrinsic sensory neurons from the small intestine do not belong to the ANS and are classified as spinal or vagal, depending on the route they follow to the CNS (Fig. 94–3).

Neurons supplying the gut are designated as either *afferent* or *efferent*, depending on the direction in which they conduct information. By convention, information is conducted centrally by afferent neurons and peripherally by efferent neurons. Thus, the term *afferent* in regard to neural supply is used to describe pathways conducting information that is detected in the gut, although in most texts this is interchangeable with the term *sensory*, despite the fact that most sensory information from the small intestine is not perceived at a conscious level. The terms *efferent* and *motor* in regard to neural supply are used to describe pathways conducting signals toward the effector small intestinal smooth muscle. Although the importance of motor innervation for motility is self-evident, the pivotal role of afferent function in determining motor responses has been less well appreciated. The importance of the extrinsic afferent innervation is emphasized by the observation that at least 80% of vagal fibers are afferent.[9]

Intrinsic Neurons

Small intestinal ENS elements can be subdivided into three major functional groups: primary sensory (afferent) neurons, motor (efferent) neurons, and interneurons. Other categories of neurons, including secretomotor and vasomotor neurons and motor neurons to endocrine cells, are recognized, but these are not considered further

in this chapter. Many distinct groups of enteric neurons are now well characterized both structurally and functionally and are reviewed in detail elsewhere.[10]

The cell bodies of ENS neurons are grouped together in ganglia (clusters of cell bodies) of the two main intramural plexuses. These plexuses lie in the submucosa (submucosal plexus) and between the two muscle layers (myenteric plexus). A deep plexus exists within the circular muscle but does not contain ganglia. The ganglia in the submucosal and myenteric plexuses are connected by interganglionic fascicles. These fascicles are composed predominantly of the axons of motor and interneurons, because sensory nerve processes do not often extend for any distance outside the ganglia. The myenteric plexus consists of ganglia spaced at regular intervals connected by a network of interganglionic fascicles. This major network is known as the *primary plexus*. Within this main structure, smaller branches of nerve bundles arise from the primary plexus and form the *secondary plexus*; and still smaller branches form the *tertiary plexus*. The submucosal plexus has two layers, one close to the mucosa and another nearer to the circular muscle layer. These two layers are connected by interganglionic fascicles. The submucosal plexus does not have a hierarchy of subordinate plexuses.

Intrinsic Afferent Supply

The primary afferent neurons of the ENS are morphologically Dogiel type II neurons (neurons with numerous processes). Intrinsic primary afferent neurons responding to mucosal chemical stimuli have their cell bodies in the myenteric plexus, although the location of their endings has not yet been defined anatomically.[10] The myenteric plexus also contains the cell bodies of intrinsic afferent neurons that fire in response to mechanical stimulation of the muscle layer induced by muscle activity or stretch.[10] Intrinsic afferent neurons that respond to mechanical stimulation of the mucosa also are believed to exist, based on enteric reflexes seen in extrinsically denervated preparations. The cell bodies and processes of these neurons have not yet been identified definitively, although available evidence is consistent with the presence of their cell bodies in the submucosal ganglia.[10] Intrinsic sensory neurons synapse in the intramural plexuses with intrinsic motor and interneurons, where they excite inter- and motor neurons, mainly by means of release of acetylcholine and substance P. A more detailed account of the function and role of intrinsic afferent neurons can be found in a recent review by Furness and coworkers.[11]

Intrinsic Efferent Supply

The axons of the intrinsic motor neurons that supply small intestinal smooth muscle exit the intramural ganglia and enter either the circular or the longitudinal muscle layer, where they pass in close proximity to both the myocytes and the ICCs. No specific neuromuscular junctions are present in small intestinal smooth muscle as in skeletal muscle, although the multiple varicosities along the motor axons probably represent specialized areas of neurotransmission. The motor axons discharge along their length, potentially activating large numbers of myocytes through ICCs, but possibly also directly

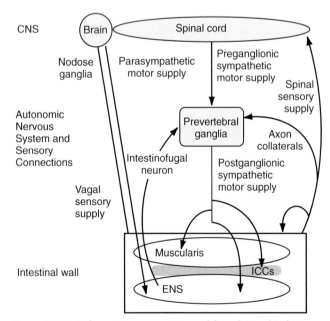

Figure 94–3 Schematic representation of the relationship between the components of the small intestinal motor control system. For further details, see text. CNS, central nervous system; ENS, enteric nervous system; ICCs, interstitial cells of Cajal.

activating them. The lack of exclusive, specific neuro-muscular junctions, the electrical gap junctions among myocytes, and the overlap of innervation of myocytes from more than one motor axon mean that functionally discrete motor units in the gut smooth muscle do not appear to exist, in contrast with skeletal muscle. The ENS motor supply itself is both inhibitory and excitatory, and intrinsic motor neurons generally contain both a fast and a slow neurotransmitter. The predominant excitatory transmitters are acetylcholine (fast) and substance P (slow), and the predominant inhibitory transmitters are nitric oxide (fast), vasoactive intestinal polypeptide (VIP) (slow), and adenosine triphosphate (ATP) (fast).

Intrinsic Interneurons

Interneurons connect ENS neurons of the same class, or of different classes, with one another. They permit local communication within limited lengths of gut wall (measured in millimeters or centimeters) and are implicated in simple local responses by means of release of acetylcholine or nitric oxide, depending on their oral or aboral direction of projection. Some evidence also suggests the presence of connections within the gut wall along greater distances, but these neural pathways are not well defined. These connections may be provided anatomically by the ENS or by connections between the ENS and ANS.

A special type of interneuron, *the intestinofugal neuron,* may be important for local reflex control. Intestinofugal neurons have cell bodies within the myenteric plexus that receive input from several local enteric neurons, and project to the prevertebral ganglia, where they synapse with sympathetic motor neurons (see Fig. 94–3).

Extrinsic Neurons

Extrinsic Afferent Supply

The small intestine is innervated by vagal and spinal extrinsic afferents. The pathway of small intestinal vagal afferent innervation is relatively straightforward. The vagal afferent neurons have endings in the intestinal wall and cell bodies within the nodose and jugular ganglia, which deliver input directly to the brainstem. Spinal afferent fibers travel along perivascular nerves to the prevertebral ganglia, where neurons do not end but may give off an axon collateral that synapses on postganglionic sympathetic motor neurons; these fibers then pass into the thoracic spinal cord along the splanchnic nerves. Spinal afferent neurons have their cell bodies throughout the thoracic dorsal root ganglia and enter the spinal cord through the dorsal roots. They synapse mainly on neurons of the superficial laminae of the spinal gray matter. These neurons, in turn, send projections to numerous areas of the brain involved in sensation and pain control. Spinal afferent neurons also may give off axon collaterals closer to the gut wall, which synapse on components of the ENS, blood vessels, smooth muscle, or secretory elements (see Fig. 94–3). The different stimulus response profiles of vagal and splanchnic mechanoreceptors are generally interpreted as evidence that vagal afferents subserve physiologic regulation while splanchnic afferents mediate pain.[13-15]

The peripheral terminals of vagal and spinal afferents can be localized within the small intestine using neuronal tracing techniques. Functionally, three distinct and characteristic patterns of terminal distribution can be identified within the gut wall. Serosal afferent fibers have responsive endings in the outer, serosal layer and in the mesenteric connections, often in association with mesenteric blood vessels. Muscular afferents form endings either in the muscle layers or in the myenteric plexus.[16] Mucosal afferents form endings in the lamina propria, where they are positioned to detect substances absorbed across the mucosal epithelium or released from epithelial and subepithelial cells, including enterochromaffin and immunocompetent cells.[16]

These three different populations of afferent endings have different sensory modalities, responding to both mechanical and chemical stimulation.[15,17] Serosal afferents are activated by distortion of the mesenteric attachments, suggesting that they do not signal distention or contraction of the bowel wall, unless it is strong enough to cause mesenteric or serosal distortion. Muscular afferents respond to distention and contraction with lower thresholds for activation and reach maximal responses within levels of distention that are encountered normally during digestion. Vagal muscular afferents show maintained responses to distention, whereas splanchnic muscular afferents may be more rapidly adapting; data are currently available only for the colon.[15,18] Small intestinal mucosal afferents have been found in the vagal supply, but their existence in the spinal supply can be inferred only from the fact that they exist in the colon. Mucosal afferents do not respond to distention or contraction but are exquisitely sensitive to mechanical deformation of the mucosa such as might occur with particulate material within the lumen.[13,19]

Nerve terminals in the longitudinal and circular muscle layers have been described as intramuscular arrays (IMAs), consisting of several long (up to a few millimeters) and rather straight axons running parallel to the respective muscle layer and connected by oblique or right-angled short connecting branches.[16,20] IMAs are proposed to be in-series tension receptor endings, possibly responding to both passive stretch and active contraction of the muscle,[21] although direct evidence for this proposal is currently lacking.

Vagal afferent terminals in the myenteric plexus throughout the gastrointestinal tract have been described as intraganglionic laminar endings (IGLEs).[16,20,21] These endings are in intimate contact with the connective tissue capsule and enteric glial cells surrounding the myenteric ganglia and have been hypothesized to detect mechanical shearing forces between the orthogonal muscle layers.[22] Evidence for such a mechanosensory function of IGLEs has been elaborated by mapping the receptive field of vagal afferent endings in the esophagus, stomach, and large intestine, showing morphologically that individual "hot spots" of mechanosensitivity correspond with single IGLEs.[23] IGLEs also may respond to chemical stimuli such as acetylcholine and ATP, raising the possibility that these endings play a key sensory role in detecting release of mediators from within the synaptic neuropil of the myenteric ganglia or surrounding tissues[24]; evidence that such chemosensory mechanisms contribute to mechanotransduction, however, is lacking.

In the rat duodenum and jejunum, vagal afferent fibers penetrate the circular muscle layer and submucosa to form networks of multiply branching axons within the lamina propria of both crypts and villi.[16] Terminal axons are in close contact with but do not seem to penetrate the basal lamina and thus are in an ideal position to detect substances including absorbed nutrients and mediators that are released from both epithelial cells and other structures within the lamina propria. These fibers, also called polymodal receptors, are characterized by low thresholds to mechanical stimuli such as stroking with a fine brush, relatively rapid adaptation to continuous stimulation, and, in most cases, sensitivity to a variety of chemical stimuli.[13-15] Serosal and mesenteric receptors also frequently show evidence of chemosensitivity. This observation hints at potential responsiveness to circulating or locally released factors, especially in view of the localization of these receptors on or near blood vessels.[25]

Extrinsic Efferent Supply

The extrinsic efferent pathways to the small intestine are supplied by the sympathetic and parasympathetic divisions of the ANS. The small intestinal parasympathetic supply is cranial and cholinergic, whereas the sympathetic supply is spinal (thoracic) and adrenergic. These two motor pathways are not entirely separate, however, because postganglionic sympathetic fibers arising from cervical ganglia sometimes are found within the vagus nerve.

The small intestinal parasympathetic motor neurons have cell bodies within the dorsal motor nuclei of the vagi in the CNS. Their axons extend through the vagi to the intestinal intramural plexuses, where they synapse with motor neurons of the ENS. The sympathetic motor supply is more complex: Primary motor neurons within the intermediolateral horn of the thoracic spinal cord synapse with second-order neurons in the prevertebral ganglia, which then synapse with ENS motor neurons within the intestinal intramural plexuses, directly with smooth muscle, or possibly with ICCs.

Both excitatory and inhibitory extrinsic motor outputs to the small intestine are recognized. Excitatory outputs depolarize, and inhibitory outputs hyperpolarize the smooth muscle, thereby facilitating and impeding the development of contractions, respectively. In general, the sympathetic motor supply is inhibitory to the ENS, and this ENS inhibition leads to decreased smooth muscle activity, with the opposite effect seen in sphincter regions. Direct sympathetic inhibitory and excitatory outputs to smooth muscle also exist. The parasympathetic motor output to the ENS is more diffuse, with each primary motor neuron supplying a large area. Excitatory parasympathetic motor output occurs to either inhibitory or excitatory ENS motor neurons, through which parasympathetic efferents may selectively inhibit or excite smooth muscle.

Central Connections of Neural Control Elements

Centrally, the sensory and motor supplies to the small intestine are closely interrelated; the vagal sensory input and the parasympathetic motor output are closely located, as are the spinal sensory input and the sympa-

thetic motor output. Both the vagal/parasympathetic and the spinal/sympathetic supplies have widespread connections to many other areas throughout the CNS that are implicated in feeding, arousal, mood, and other "reflex" behaviors. The proximity of these CNS areas involved in small intestinal regulation, and their interconnections make it likely that the vagal/parasympathetic and the spinal/sympathetic control mechanisms are interconnected and may function less independently than has been previously thought.

The parasympathetic primary motor neurons originate from the ipsilateral dorsal motor nucleus of the vagus in the brainstem. The dorsal motor nucleus of the vagus lies close to, and receives a substantial input from, the nucleus tractus solitarius, which receives the vagal sensory (afferent) fibers through the nodose ganglia and the tractus solitarius. The nucleus tractus solitarius also has extensive connections to other CNS regions, and several of these same regions have input to the dorsal motor nucleus of the vagus, thereby influencing vagal motor output to the gut.

The central connections of the spinal and sympathetic supply to the gut are less well described. The spinal sensory neurons enter the spinal cord, where they synapse ipsilaterally on a second-order sensory neuron and also provide direct feedback to sympathetic primary motor neurons through axon collaterals. The second-order sensory neurons then cross the spinal cord to ascend contralaterally, where they terminate in numerous areas,[14] including the raphe nuclei and periaqueductal gray in the brainstem and the thalamus. The thalamus has extensive ramifications throughout the CNS. The central influence on sympathetic motor output is complex and not well understood, but stress and arousal level play a role. These influences have their output through the brainstem and descending tracts to the sympathetic primary motor neurons in the intermediolateral horn of the spinal cord, which send their axons to the prevertebral ganglia.

INTEGRATIVE CONTROL OF MOTILITY

So far we have considered the structure and function of individual anatomic components of the small intestinal neuromuscular apparatus. When we consider how these components operate together to produce known motility patterns, several gaps are revealed in our knowledge, because the evidence for contribution of specific mechanisms is often circumstantial. Two important examples of motility patterns—peristalsis and the interdigestive motor cycle (IDMC)—are described next. These motor patterns illustrate the involvement of integrated hierarchical levels of control and our current level of understanding of the control systems.

Peristalsis is the fundamental integrated motility pattern of the small intestine and can be coordinated entirely within the ENS and muscular layers. It may be initiated in response to a number of mechanical and chemical stimuli in the lumen and consists of progression of contractile activity usually, but not always, in an aboral direction. Therefore, both sensory and motor aspects to peristalsis are recognized. The populations of intrinsic primary afferent neurons described earlier probably are responsible for detection of luminal stimuli, either directly or following release of mediators from mucosal enteroendocrine cells. Their activation results in transmitter release onto neighboring inter- and motor neurons whose activity is coordinated subsequently as a network to provide synchronous activation of circular and longitudinal muscles on one side of the bolus (usually the oral side) and synchronous inhibition of muscle on the other side. This networked activity normally travels aborally, but the mechanism of propagation is not yet understood. It may be due to patterns of activity in interneurons that may project over distances of several millimeters and thus mediate a general descending excitation. The mechanism by which peristalsis is reversed—for example, in conditions of luminal toxicity—is not known, but the fact that reverse peristalsis does occur in the small intestine illustrates that the pattern is not a totally polarized phenomenon. Debate is ongoing about the precise interactions of transmitters and mediators in the normal function of peristalsis, but it is known to be affected by exogenous activation of several pre- and postsynaptic mechanisms, some of which also may be active endogenously. Of particular interest are serotonergic mechanisms, which have been shown to have involvement in initiation of peristalsis and modulation of transmission between subclasses of enteric neurons.

Whereas other aspects of the IDMC are described later in this chapter, here it serves to demonstrate the extraordinary integrative capacity of the ENS. The *IDMC* is a complex series of periods of variable contractile activity with distinct phases showing different contractile amplitudes, propagation, and regularity. The pattern as a whole sweeps slowly down the small intestine in the fasting state and recurs at regular intervals. Although a number of candidate gut hormones are proposed to be involved in its initiation and recurrence, the switch between quiescent and active phases and their orderly migration along the bowel are functions of the ENS; this ENS function is demonstrated by occurrence of the IDMC in extrinsically denervated or autotransplanted intestine. The ENS is therefore capable of controlling large segments of the small intestine independently of extrinsic input, probably by virtue of its extensive interneuronal connections and constant sensory feedback.

Although the ENS has this regulatory capacity, normal function is modulated by ANS efferent output, which in turn may be influenced by locally or centrally processed information gathered from primary spinal or vagal afferents. Synapses outside the CNS in the spinal sensory and sympathetic motor arms of the extrinsic neural supply to the small intestine are capable of subserving inhibitory intestino-intestinal reflexes that are potentially important in the minute-to-minute regulatory control of motility.[12] Small intestinal neuromuscular function also is influenced by a number of hormones acting in either endocrine or paracrine fashion. Most of this integration of function occurs subconsciously but is perceived sometimes.[13,14]

Little direct information is available on the precise contribution of each extrinsic pathway to small intestinal motor function in humans. Vagal reflexes generally are

thought to make an important contribution in the integration of major homeostatic functions, such as motility, secretion, and the control of food and water intake.[13,14,26] The role of sympathetic reflexes is not so well studied, particularly in control of small intestinal function, because selective nerve recordings and lesioning of the sensory and motor innervation present an extraordinary technical challenge. Previously, spinal pathways were thought to be concerned primarily with responses to noxious stimuli[14] that are evoked by stimulation of afferent endings outside the lumen in the serosal and mesenteric attachments, rather than in normal small intestinal functions; these concepts are now being challenged as investigators examine spinal sensory input from the gut in more detail.

MECHANISMS UNDERLYING ABNORMAL MOTOR AND SENSORY FUNCTION

Much of the evidence for the mechanisms involved in dysfunction of the small intestine is derived from animal models in which mucosal inflammation or infection has been induced, and alterations in physiology, pharmacology, and anatomy of motor and sensory elements then are assessed. These models provide some clues to the underlying mechanisms involved in motor abnormalities seen clinically; however, because many clinical manifestations are of unknown etiology, this approach is limited in the extent to which basic findings can be translated directly.

Infection and inflammation of the gut may result in long-term changes in all elements, including myocytes, ICCs, and intrinsic and extrinsic neurons. Symptoms in functional gastrointestinal diseases such as functional dyspepsia and irritable bowel syndrome (IBS) may be attributable partly to specific sensorimotor abnormalities occurring locally in the gut, but also are attributable to alterations in the extrinsic neural control system of the gut, and possibly to alterations in central perception, processing of afferent information, or both. Abnormalities in pain control systems in the brain and disordered processing of affective components of visceral sensations also have been described in these conditions[27] and may lead to symptom production through the central connections described in the preceding sections. These conditions are dealt with in greater detail elsewhere (see Chapters 7, 8, 10, 46, and 115). Some clinical scenarios in which discrete abnormalities have been identified or hypothesized in small intestinal motility are outlined in Table 94–1.

SMOOTH MUSCLE DYSFUNCTION

It is often difficult to separate pathologic changes in the function of smooth muscle from those in neural control mechanisms; however, a number of changes can be attributed directly to alterations in smooth muscle. Cytokines play an important role in the abnormal smooth muscle function associated with gastrointestinal inflammation and infection. Different insults induce different patterns of cytokines, which in turn determine the type of infiltrating immune or inflammatory cells, which

Table 94–1 Disorders Associated with Abnormal Small Intestinal Motility

Disorders	Smooth Muscle Abnormalities	Neural Abnormalities	Sensory Abnormalities	Potential Outcomes
Irritable bowel syndrome			Increased visceral sensitivity	Alterations in fasting phase III (IDMC), increased clustered contractions
Acute illness	Decreased strength of contractions	Altered neurotransmission		Ileus
Pregnancy	Decreased strength of contractions			Slowed transit
Diabetes		Altered neurotransmission	Enhanced perception of gastrointestinal stimuli	Abnormal patterning of contractions; slow or rapid transit
Metabolic disturbances	Possible decreased strength of contractions	Altered neurotransmission	Nausea, altered sensory perception	Ileus, rapid transit
Drugs	Possible decreased strength of contractions	Altered neurotransmission		Ileus; slow or rapid transit; disordered contractions
Intestinal obstruction	Hypertrophy if chronic			High-amplitude forceful contractions
Pseudo-obstruction syndromes	Hollow visceral myopathy	Multiple neural abnormalities, neuron loss, plexus abnormalities, altered distribution of neurotransmitters		Feeble contractions, absent phase III (IDMC); failure of transit
Scleroderma and other connective tissue diseases	Ischemia and fibrosis	Nerve loss in intestinal wall; extrinsic neural supply also may be lost due to vasculitis		Feeble contractions; thickening of bowel wall; slow transit
Neurologic syndromes		Neural absence or loss	Loss of afferent information for reflex control lost	Disorganized IDMC, failure to convert to "fed" pattern, transit failure
Rare myopathies	Myocyte and mitochondrial abnormalities; inadequate contractile force			Insufficient force for transit and mixing

IDMC, interdigestive motor cycle.

in turn release specific mediators. Thus, the resultant effect on smooth muscle function depends on the origin of disease. For example, nematode infection induces mastocytosis and eosinophilia, which lead to activation of intracellular signaling pathways in smooth muscle by IL-4 and IL-13, ultimately resulting in hypercontractility of smooth muscle.[28] By contrast, chemically induced inflammation is characterized by the presence of neutrophils and macrophages among other cells. Inflammation and infection can lead to changes at sites in the small intestine distant from the affected site, and the functional effects of inflammation in smooth muscle can persist following recovery from the acute insult. Smooth muscle hyperresponsiveness may be characterized by enhanced responses to cholinergic and noncholinergic excitation and are observable in human inflammatory bowel disease.[29]

DYSFUNCTION OF INTRINSIC NEURAL CONTROL

Several abnormalities of small intestinal intrinsic control are attributable to developmental dysfunction and are dealt with separately in Chapter 93. Changes in the

ENS also occur after a bout of intestinal infection or inflammation. Many of these changes are centered on the intrinsic primary afferent neurons. These neurons become more excitable because of changes in the expression of ion channels that initiate action potential generation and those that determine recovery of membrane potential after an action potential. Thus, the long afterhyperpolarization that characterizes intrinsic primary afferent neurons from other classes is shortened, and they are able to fire in longer trains. This ability directly affects the responses of other inter- and motor neurons that receive inputs from these afferent neurons, and which therefore are involved in intrinsic (ENS) reflexes. Changes in excitability may be observed during an acute phase of infection or inflammation,[29] or for several weeks afterward (Mawe, unpublished observations). These longer-term changes are referred to as *plasticity* and may explain partly the occurrence of exaggerated motor responses to a given stimulus both in the acute phase and after recovery of mucosal lesions. Changes may result from alterations in gene expression in enteric neurons persisting beyond the initial insult, persisting increases in locally released mediators following alterations in mucosal cell types, or to both responses.[30]

In animals models of insulin-dependent diabetes mellitus, altered levels of neuropeptides may be seen, which may explain the disordered motility noted clinically in diabetes mellitus. The only reported neuroanatomic human study in a patient with type 1 diabetes mellitus showed that ICCs were decreased markedly throughout the entire thickness of the jejunum. A decrease in neuronal nitric oxide synthase, VIP, pituitary adenyl cyclase–activating peptide (PACAP), and tyrosine hydroxylase–immunopositive nerve fibers was observed in the circular muscle layer, whereas substance P immunoreactivity was increased.[31] Although patients with type 1 diabetes mellitus and sympathetic denervation have abnormally slow gastric emptying (see Chapter 46), their transit of a liquid meal through the distal small intestine is more rapid, which may play a part in the production of diarrhea. Diabetic patients also showed abnormal duodenal motility patterns such as early recurrence of phase III after a meal (see later). No consistent correlation, however, has been found between changes in manometric parameters and the degree of cardiac autonomic neuropathy, nor has any correlation yet been established between changes in enteric neurotransmitters and ICCs and manometric and transit observations.

EXTRINSIC AFFERENT DYSFUNCTION

Mechanisms leading to extrinsic afferent dysfunction after infection or inflammation probably are similar to those involved in intrinsic primary afferent and smooth muscle dysfunction. It is well established that a wide range of chemical mediators may influence mechanosensitivity of extrinsic primary afferents, in addition to evoking direct responses as detailed earlier. These chemical mediators can be released in conditions of inflammation, injury, or ischemia from a variety of cell types including platelets, neutrophils, lymphocytes, macrophages, mast cells, glial cells, fibroblasts, blood vessels, muscles, and neurons. Each of these specific cells may release several modulating agents, some of which may act directly on the sensory nerve terminal, whereas others may act indirectly, causing release of other agents from other cells in a series of cascades. The end result of these actions is that the response properties of extrinsic afferents, like their intrinsic counterparts, are subject to plasticity, usually resulting in an increased sensitivity of the afferent endings; this process is described as *peripheral sensitization*.

Some evidence supports the involvement of algesic mediators, including prostaglandins and purines, in changes leading to peripheral sensitization.[24] Other endogenous chemical mediators, including somatostatin, may down-regulate small intestinal afferent sensitivity such that an imbalance in pro- and anti-sensitizing mechanisms leads to a disordered sensory signal. Such mechanisms are of likely clinical relevance to functional bowel disorders, such as IBS, in which increased perception of both mechanical and chemical stimulation is apparent. Moreover, because these afferents also serve to trigger reflex mechanisms that control and coordinate gut motor function, their sensitization may contribute toward chronic dysmotility, resulting in a cycle of disordered sensory and motor function.

EVALUATION OF SMALL INTESTINAL MOTILITY

SPATIOTEMPORAL MEASUREMENTS

The outcomes of small intestinal motor activity basically depend on the patterning of small intestinal contractions in both space and time; that is, *where and when do the contractions occur with respect to each other?* Measurement methods for assessing small intestinal motor physiology must address substantial technical challenges to gather functionally relevant information on the temporospatial organization of small intestinal motility, especially in humans. These challenges arise from the great length of the small intestine, the spatial and temporal complexity of motor events, and the time frame of several hours over which small intestinal motor activity determines the successful absorption and movement of nutrients.

In the healthy small intestine, the occurrence and patterning of a large number of individual motor events determine the outcomes of absorption and transit, so that "whole-animal" measures of transit and absorption yield a gross, or summary, report of motor function. More detailed descriptions of small intestinal motility report great variability in the patterning of individual contractile events, depending in part on the technique used to assess motility, the time frame over which it is observed, and the temporal and spatial resolution of the measurements themselves.

To understand the relationship between individual motor events and transport in the small intestine, the temporal resolution of the measurement technique must be greater than the duration of each discrete motor event. Based on similar principles, the spatial resolution of measurement techniques also is an important parameter to consider if relationships between motor events and intraluminal flow are to be defined. The importance of spatiotemporal resolution can be appreciated by considering Figure 94–4. Direct evaluation of small intestinal motility requires methods of measurement with a time resolution of at least 2 seconds, because in humans, the intrinsic frequency of small intestinal contractions in the duodenum is up to 12 per minute. Although the optimal spatial resolution for studies of small intestinal motor function has not been determined, the spatial patterning of pressures is known to vary over relatively small distances,[32] with most propagating pressure wave sequences traveling less than 6 cm. Spatial resolution also is complicated by the fact that one ideally seeks high spatial resolution between measurement points combined with a long span over which measurements are made.

EVALUATION OF SINGLE-CELL FUNCTIONS

At a cellular level, a number of techniques can be used to yield insights into small intestinal motor physiology. Intracellular recordings of electrical potential can be

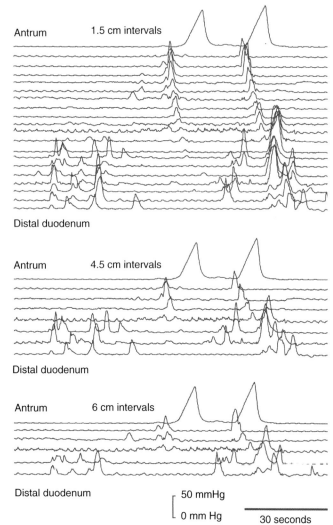

Figure 94–4 Multichannel manometric recordings of the human antrum and duodenum, with recording points placed at various intervals: 1.5 cm *(top panel)*, 4.5 cm *(middle panel)*, and 6 cm *(bottom panel)*. These data demonstrate some of the limitations of varying the interval between recording points: As a phasic contraction travels along a section of intestine, the associated rise in pressure is detected only at each measurement point. If the interval between recording points is too wide, unrelated pressures may be judged to be related to the propagated pressure wave, or a propagated pressure wave sequence may be judged to be a limited phasic event. Spatial detail is lost as the recording interval is widened.

obtained from a number of cell types within the small intestine and its extrinsic neural control system. These recordings give detailed information about the signals received and transmitted by individual cells, with excellent temporal resolution, but generally cannot be applied concurrently over a significant length of gut and therefore have limited real-time spatial resolution with regard to motor events.

An integrated functional and neuroanatomic approach that combines imaging of specific neurons with intra- or extracellular recordings and chemical coding using immunohistochemistry has allowed important correlations to be made between structure and function. In particular, this approach has led to understanding of the function of IGLEs and IMAs (see "Extrinsic Afferent Supply" earlier).

Although electrophysiologic and anatomic methods provide information on structure, neurotransmitters used, and proximity to other elements, they cannot describe precisely how these relate to the actual resulting motility and its temporospatial organization. Although these single-cell techniques generally have been applied to animal tissues, the results probably also are applicable to humans, because a similar structural organization of the control elements is found in human tissue.

RECORDING OF MUSCLE CONTRACTIONS

Direct recording of increased muscle tension generally is done with strain gauges. These can be used in muscle strips, isolated loops of intestine, and whole-organ preparations or even chronically implanted in animals. Strain gauges are capable of excellent temporal resolution of motor events, but the spatial resolution is limited by the size and number of strain gauges that are used concurrently in the selected preparation. Over short lengths of intestine, a spatial resolution of approximately 1 cm is possible. Unfortunately, strain gauges are not suitable for use in human subjects, although they have provided much valuable information on the organization of motor events in animals.[33] Muscle contractions also can be recorded by surrogate measurement techniques that record phenomena associated with contractions. One such approach is the fluorescence measurement of "calcium transients" (rapid increases in free intracellular calcium) in smooth muscle.[34] Over short sections of gut (1 to 2 mm), such measurements provide excellent temporospatial resolution but are likely to be more helpful in elucidating neurophysiologic control than in describing whole-organ function. Other measurement techniques that record phenomena resulting from contractions of the smooth muscle include luminal manometry, fluoroscopy, and transit studies performed by a number of approaches.

Luminal manometry measures the change in intraluminal pressure that results mainly from lumen-occlusive or near–lumen-occlusive contractions. Fortunately, because the small intestine is tubular, with a relatively small diameter, a large proportion of motor events are recognized as pressure rises. Moreover, it has been hypothesized that contractions not resulting in a detectable change in intraluminal pressure are less important in determining the movement of intraluminal contents, and that, therefore, little mechanical information is lost by failure to detect them with manometry. Nevertheless, small changes in intraluminal pressure can be pivotal in producing flows in some regions of the small intestine,[35] and not all manometry systems are appropriately sensitive to these. Manometry can be applied in several settings, ranging from short isolated intestinal segments in the laboratory to clinical use in humans. Appropriately designed manometric assemblies can be placed in any part of the human small intestine and are moderately well tolerated. Modern computer-based recording systems give excellent temporal resolution (10 Hz is routinely achieved), and spatial resolution can be tailored either to give close resolution (1- to 2-cm intervals) over a 20- to 40-cm length or to be wider, to cover an even longer segment of the small intestine. Perfused side-hole manometric assemblies now are capable of routinely recording at up to 22 sites.

WALL MOTION AND TRANSIT STUDIES

Contrast fluoroscopy is the most widely available wall motion study. It yields detailed information on the time and space patterning of motor events in vivo and useful insights into associated movements of luminal contents. When this technique is used in combination with other techniques, such as manometry, intraluminal impedance or strain gauges, useful correlations can be made between contractions or luminal pressures and transit of contents, particularly in animals. These insights are likely to lead to improved understanding of pressure patterns, which may in turn enable us to better interpret less intrusive techniques such as manometry and impedance in humans. Improving the interpretation of these other techniques is important, because radiation exposure severely restricts the usefulness of fluoroscopy in humans, and many other measures of motility are too invasive for use in humans.

Other in vivo imaging methods that can view small intestinal wall motion and associated movement of intraluminal contents include magnetic resonance imaging (MRI), ultrasonography, and intraluminal impedance recording. These approaches are used in research studies, and although suitable for human use and capable of good temporal resolution, they have significant practical limitations when applied to the small intestine, restricting their use outside of research centers as an alternative to contrast fluoroscopy. MRI allows prolonged observation but currently provides inadequate spatial resolution of the small intestine and is prohibitively expensive. Further development may at least partly overcome these limitations, but at present, MRI is restricted to research use for the study of small intestinal motility. Ultrasonography also allows prolonged observation, but only of short segments of the small intestine, and has relatively poor spatial resolution. It is limited in many instances by patient factors such as body habitus and intestinal gas and is operator dependent.

Multichannel intraluminal impedance (MII), described initially by Silny,[36] is a relatively new technique for assessing small intestinal transit. The technique is based on the different conductivities of intraluminal air and liquids as compared with that of opposed sections of wall. Voltage is applied to a recording assembly along which several electrodes are sited. The current recorded between electrode pairs depends on the conductivity and thickness of any air or fluid bolus straddling the electrode pair. In this fashion, MII sequentially measures the transit of a conducting bolus between pairs of electrodes. Thus, the technique measures movement of contents along the bowel, rather than directly measuring motility. The recordings in the small intestine are therefore dependent on the state of filling, and motility in an empty bowel may not be assessed accurately. Esophageal motility has been widely assessed with MII, and in recent times it has

been applied to the proximal small intestine with success.[37] In combination with manometry, MII has the potential to provide real-time pressure-flow relationships.

Other transit and absorption measurements demonstrate whether mass transit occurs but give no information on the mechanical pattern by which the transport of contents is achieved. Methodology for transit studies includes breath tests and scintigraphy. Breath tests are based on the exhalation of gases such as H_2 or with CO_2 labeled with ^{13}C or ^{14}C, both of which are generated when a test meal reaches the colon and undergoes bacterial degradation. Scintigraphic tests visually assess the arrival of a labeled meal into the cecum. These transit techniques yield the lowest temporospatial resolution in assessing small intestinal motility but nonetheless sometimes are clinically useful and are further discussed later in the chapter.

In vitro techniques for detailed assessment of small intestinal wall movements have advanced rapidly over recent years, so that they now reveal subtle motility patterns that cannot be detected with manometry or in vivo wall motion studies. The latest methods are able to measure changes in diameter and length of an immobilized segment of intestine by using digitized video recording.[38] This technique has the unique capacity for changes in the longitudinal and circular muscle layers to be appreciated discretely.

CLINICAL MEASUREMENT OF SMALL INTESTINAL MOTILITY

The broader issues of measurement of small intestinal motor function have been considered earlier, and the discussion that follows is limited to the clinical techniques used to assess small intestinal motor function. Additional techniques, available in specialized centers (such as MRI and MII), are not considered here.

SMALL INTESTINAL TRANSIT STUDIES

Small intestinal transit time can be measured with breath tests or scintigraphic observation of the movement of intraluminal contents. Unless the test substance is delivered past the pylorus by tube, these techniques also include gastric emptying (and thus gastric function) in their measurements. Therefore, they are imprecise about actual small intestinal transit time and are more accurately termed tests of orocecal transit time. Because each technique measures a different aspect of motility, the results obtained from different techniques are not directly comparable.

The lactulose breath test is perhaps the best known and most widely used of these techniques. Lactulose is nonabsorbable and is fermented on reaching the bacteria-laden environment of the colon. The H_2 gas that is formed is rapidly absorbed and exhaled from the lungs. Samples of exhaled gases are taken at baseline and at regular intervals after the ingestion of lactulose. The orocecal transit time is taken as the time at which a sustained rise in exhaled H_2 is seen. An early rise, or a high baseline level, may be evidence of small bowel bacterial overgrowth, but this measure is relatively insensitive for bacterial overgrowth. Similar principles are used in ^{13}C or ^{14}C breath tests, which measure gastric emptying combined with the evaluation of small intestinal absorption of specific nutrients. Acetate, octanoic acid, and triolein have been used in this regard. Acetate appears to be a good liquid marker, octanoic acid is better suited for solids, and triolein is useful in suspected cases of malabsorption. This nutrient-focused assessment of small intestinal function can be combined with the H$_2$ breath test to measure orocecal transit time as well. These methods still are being refined and are confined to laboratories with a special interest in human small intestinal function.

The more familiar visual/anatomic scintigraphic measurement of small intestinal transit also is technically challenging but more widely available. The major difficulty with these studies is the lack of a reliable anatomic landmark for the cecum. The cecum either is defined arbitrarily as the right iliac fossa and a skin marker is used or is considered retrospectively as the area in which radioisotope accumulates. Two approaches are used to report the scintigraphic orocecal transit time. In the simpler approach, the time of first appearance of isotope in the cecum is given; in the other, the initial activity of the radiolabeled meal is quantified in the stomach, and the orocecal transit time is reported as the time taken for 50% of this initial gastric activity to reach the cecum. Values obtained vary depending on which of these methods is used, and each laboratory should set its own normal range.

FLUOROSCOPY

Contrast fluoroscopy is useful for detecting mucosal disease and fixed narrowings of the lumen that may induce secondary changes in motility, transit, and absorption. Fluoroscopy is insensitive for detection of abnormal nutrient absorption and measurement of transit time. Clinical fluoroscopy is limited by short observation times because of radiation exposure; therefore, only gross disturbances of motor activity may be detected. Once a substantial amount of contrast has entered the small intestine, the usefulness of fluoroscopy is reduced further, because overlying loops of bowel hinder the interpretation of the movement of contrast.

MANOMETRY

Small intestinal manometry gives the most direct measurement of the forces that are applied to luminal contents as a result of motor function in humans. Manometry can be performed over hours or even days and over long or short segments and is capable of excellent spatial resolution, although it has major practical limitations. Placement of a manometric assembly along the small intestine is demanding even in healthy persons but is especially challenging in patients who have major abnormalities of motor function. Manometry allows recognition of some abnormal patterns of pressure over time at individual recording points, but no studies have yet performed a critical evaluation of the best spacing of pressure recording points, and of diagnostic criteria

for abnormal pressure patterns to distinguish between health and disease. This lack of specific criteria reflects the current, limited understanding of the relationship between small intestinal intraluminal time-space pressure patterning and the achievement of mixing and propulsion within the small intestine. Because of practical limitations on the number of recording points that can be included on an assembly, the choice must be made between high spatial resolution over a short segment and lower spatial resolution over a longer segment of intestine. Both approaches are likely to be necessary in achieving an accurate understanding of small intestinal motor physiology, perhaps in conjunction with a technique to assess wall motion or intraluminal flow.

NORMAL SMALL INTESTINAL MOTILITY

CONTRACTIONS AT A FIXED POINT

The increased smooth muscle tension arising from contractions can result in increased intraluminal pressure, decreased intraluminal diameter, or small intestinal shortening, or a combination of these effects. Smooth muscle contractions can be tonic or phasic, but common usage has labeled tonic contractions as *tone* and phasic motor events as *contractions*. Human phasic small intestinal contractions generally last from 0.8 to 6.0 seconds.

Small intestinal electrical recordings reveal the presence of a continuous cyclic oscillation in electrical potential, referred to as the *slow wave, basic electrical rhythm,* or *pacesetter potential*. This slow wave is generated by the ICCs (see earlier). In humans, the slow-wave frequency decreases from a peak of 12 per minute in the duodenum to approximately 7 per minute in the distal ileum. A small intestinal contraction arises when an electrical action potential, or spike burst, is superimposed on the slow wave (Fig. 94–5). Spike bursts may be caused by the intrinsic motor output from the ENS to the ICCs and are likely also to be modulated by the extrinsic motor supply. Except during phase III of the IDMC (or migrating motor complex), not every slow wave leads to a phasic contraction. The region-specific frequency of the slow wave thus controls small intestinal rhythmicity by determining the timing and maximal frequency of contractions.

Smooth muscle contraction results from a rapid increase in free intracellular calcium that activates actin and myosin filaments to move over each other and shorten (see Fig. 94–2). These calcium transients can be visualized with fluorescence techniques and appear to spread in a coordinated fashion over an area of smooth muscle and extend over variable distances of the bowel wall. These calcium transients are extinguished by collision with each other or by encountering locally refractory regions.[34]

CONTRACTIONS THAT TRAVEL ALONG THE SMALL INTESTINE

The electrical slow wave migrates along the small intestine in an aboral direction so that each subsequent site

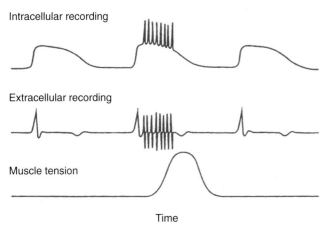

Figure 94–5 Schematic representation of the relationship among slow waves, spike bursts, and muscle contraction. The *top tracing* is from an intracellular electrode in the muscle; the *middle tracing* is from an extracellular electrode; and the *bottom tracing* shows muscle tension. The cyclic fluctuation in membrane potential in the *top tracing* is the slow wave. When spike bursts are superimposed on the peak of the slow wave, the muscle depolarizes and contraction occurs. (From Christensen J: Gastrointestinal motility. In West JB [ed]: Best and Taylor's Physiologic Basis for Medical Practice. Baltimore, Williams & Wilkins, 1990, p 614.)

along the gut is depolarized sequentially. When a slow wave results in contraction, the propagation of the slow wave along the small intestine also will lead to the propagation of the contraction along the small intestine. The propagation velocity of the slow wave thus determines the maximal rate at which contractions can travel along the small intestine. Because not every slow wave leads to a contraction, however, contractions will not always travel at this maximal rate. Additionally, the distance over which muscular excitation or inhibition spreads also appears to be determined by ENS influences mediated through local inhibitory and excitatory circuits.[34]

Contraction sequences may travel aboard (in an antegrade direction) or orad (in a retrograde direction). Little accurate information has been accumulated on the length and direction of travel of small intestinal contractions in humans because of the low spatial resolution of most motility recordings. From animal data and some recent high-spatial-resolution human studies, however, it is known that a large proportion of contractions travel along the small intestine, rather than remaining static, but most contractions are limited to only a few centimeters in extent.[32,33] Further data are needed to determine the contribution that these short contraction sequences make to overall transit compared with the less frequent, longer sequences.

MOTILITY PATTERNS

From experiments on isolated small intestinal segments, ascending excitation and descending inhibition are the simplest well-recognized patterns of motility. *Ascending excitation* refers to the contraction that occurs proximal (oral) to a stimulus, and *descending inhibition* refers to the inhibition of motor activity that occurs distal to a stimulus. These simple reflexes can be demonstrated in the absence of any extrinsic innervation and are thus subserved entirely by the ENS, although extrinsic influences may modulate their occurrence. These two patterns are thought to be responsible for peristalsis and retroperistalsis when they travel in a coordinated fashion along the gut.

Recordings of human small intestinal motility show isolated (stationary) phasic contractions, but frequently spatial patterns are more complex. The limited spatial resolution of many recording techniques may lead to overreporting of the proportion of stationary contractions. Frequently, phasic motor activity consists of a recognizable group of contractions associated along the small intestine in space and time; phase III activity of the IDMC (see later) is a good example of this association. Several other types of grouped small intestinal contractions have been described and include those associated with emesis[39] and discrete clustered contractions, which are said to be common in IBS[40] (see Chapter 115). The most commonly observed motor patterns in the healthy small intestine, however, are described simply as the *postprandial*, or fed, pattern and the *fasting* (interdigestive) pattern, or IDMC (Fig. 94–6).

The pattern at any given time is determined by the presence or absence of a significant amount of nutrient within the small intestine. Despite a large number of studies on fasting motility, very few studies on human postprandial small intestinal motility have been performed; this paucity probably exists because of the difficulty in knowing which aspects of postprandial motility to study, in contrast with fasting motility, which has an easily recognized cyclic pattern and thus easily studied parameters. The fed motor pattern ensures transit of small intestinal contents at a rate consistent with normal digestion and absorption. The fasting motor pattern is less concerned with orderly luminal transport and is thought to serve important roles in clearing the upper gut of solid residues, which otherwise may accumulate and form bezoars; in maintaining relative sterility of the small intestine by keeping it empty; and in preventing net oral migration of colonic bacteria.

Within 10 to 20 minutes of the consumption of a meal, the IDMC in progress at the time of eating is interrupted.[41] The presence of intraluminal nutrients is "sensed" by mucosal nutrient contact, as evidenced by the fact that portal or intravenous nutrients do not have the same effects as those consumed orally.[42] Several neural and humoral signals result from mucosal nutrient contact and are implicated in the induction of the fed motor pattern, including vagal afferent signals, cholecystokinin, and glucagon-like peptide-1 (GLP-1). Moreover, the sensing of intraluminal nutrients is relatively complex, because different types of nutrients, or variable amounts of the same nutrient, generate recognizably different motor responses.[32,33,43,44] In general, the presence of unabsorbed small intestinal nutrients slows small intestine transit by decreasing the frequency and length of travel of phasic contractions, so that the rate at which a substance is absorbed limits its transit rate. In the absence of sufficient proximal small intestinal nutrient stimulation, the fasting motor pattern re-emerges 4 to 6 hours after a meal. In the absence of its interruption by intraluminal nutrients, the IDMC repeats continuously.

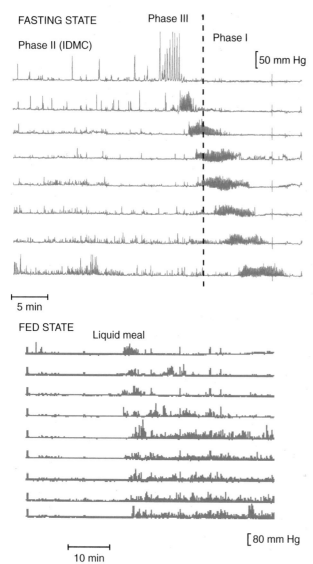

Figure 94–6 Manometric tracings demonstrating small intestinal motility in the fasting (*top*) and fed (*bottom*) state. The three phases of the interdigestive motor cycle (IDMC) (J. M. Andrews, unpublished data) and the conversion to a fed motor pattern by the presence of small intestinal nutrients (data by kind permission of Dr. R. J. Fraser) are shown. In the *top* set of tracings, at a given time point (*dashed vertical line*), all three phases of the IDMC can be encountered at different points along the small intestine. The similarity of phase II and the fed motor pattern can be appreciated by comparing the *top* (fasting) and *bottom* (fed) sets of tracings.

Distention, intraluminal pH changes, and hyperosmolar contents are capable of stimulating small intestinal motor activity. Hyperosmolar contents and pH changes probably are sensed by receptors in the mucosa, whereas distention is signaled by receptors in the muscle. In the normal course of events, these stimuli occur concurrently with the presence of nutrients, and the significance of their isolated effects in healthy subjects is unclear.

The small intestine also exerts negative feedback control on the rate of gastric emptying through neural and humoral means. This negative feedback is achieved by the release of neural signals and gut hormones that suppress phasic gastric motor activity, relax the gastric

fundus, and increase tonic and phasic pyloric pressures subsequent to mucosal sensing of small intestinal nutrients.[45] This process indirectly also prolongs "whole-meal" small intestine transit time by slowing the input of small intestinal chyme. The small intestine, in particular the duodenum, also is thought to offer direct mechanical resistance to gastric emptying by acting as a capacitance resistor[46] and by reaugmenting gastric contents as a result of duodenogastric reflux.[47]

FED MOTOR PATTERN

Radiologic Observations

Early radiologic observations of the small intestine in animals described several different patterns of wall motion and transit of intestinal contents. Cannon[39,48] observed both localized contractions over short segments of intestine in association with to-and-fro movement of contents and intermittent episodes of propulsion of contents over greater distances caused by aborally traveling waves of peristalsis. In the fed state, the most common pattern of wall motion observed in a number of species was termed *rhythmic segmentation*, whereby short columns of chyme were recurrently divided and united into new aliquots by localized circular contractions that caused temporary local occlusion of the lumen over distances of less than 1 to 2 cm.[39,48] These contractions did not travel along the small intestine and did not result in much, if any, net oral movement of contents.[39,48] Peristalsis also was commonly observed, often in combination with segmentation. During small intestinal nutrient loading, peristalsis was noted to have two forms: (1) a slow advance of chyme over short distances in association with segmentation and (2) rapid transit of chyme over longer distances, sometimes several loops, of the small intestine. This "fast peristalsis" frequently was seen in the cat duodenum.[48] Similar observations have been made in other animal species[33,39] and correlate with some of the motor patterns seen during clinical radiologic studies in humans (although these studies usually are performed when the subject is fasting and show the rapid peristaltic pattern more than the segmenting postprandial activity).

Transit Time Observations

The small intestinal transit time for a meal varies greatly according to the amount and nature of what is consumed, because both caloric content and physical form of a meal determine the gastric emptying rate and the rate of transport along the intestine.[49-52] Depending on the test and parameter used, postprandial orocecal transit time usually is less than 6 hours. As assessed by lactulose breath testing, however, orocecal transit time can be as rapid as approximately 70 minutes with low nutrient loads. A systematic evaluation of the optimal conditions for nutrient loading to reveal abnormal small intestinal motor function, using transit studies, is much needed.

Manometric Observations

Postprandial small intestinal motility is characterized by irregular phasic pressure waves without a discernible cyclic pattern. Most small intestinal motility data are quite limited in spatial resolution (interval between sensors and length of small intestine spanned by sensors) because of the length of the small intestine. Nevertheless, most phasic pressures (pressure wave sequences) are thought to travel only a short distance[32,33] and represent the mixing contractions noted in earlier radiologic studies.[39,48] In animal studies, postprandial small intestinal motility is more "segmenting" than is fasting phase II activity, and phasic pressures occur less frequently and travel shorter distances along the bowel, resulting in slower transit of the contents.[33] A similar suppression in the frequency of pressure wave sequences has now been found in the human duodenum.[32] This segmenting motor pattern is thought to assist in mixing food with digestive enzymes and in maximizing the exposure of food to the mucosa to optimize absorption.

FASTING MOTOR PATTERN: INTERDIGESTIVE MOTOR CYCLE

During fasting, small intestinal motor activity adopts a repetitive cyclic motor pattern, the IDMC. The IDMC is absent in a number of disease states, presumably because of a primary neuropathic process. This absence is associated clinically with stasis of small intestinal contents, malabsorption, and small bowel bacterial overgrowth. For detailed reviews, see the articles by Husebye and Sarna.[40,41]

Radiologic Observations

Contrast agents may stimulate small intestinal mucosal receptors sensitive to pH, caloric content, and osmolarity changes. It is possible, therefore, that radiologic studies of "fasting" motility are not truly representative of the fasting state. Nonetheless, in general, contrast agents appear to move more swiftly through the small intestine during fasting than during the postprandial state and to be associated with more episodes of peristalsis over one or more loops and fewer segmenting contractions. When the phase of the IDMC is assessed concurrently (see later), little net movement of small intestinal contents is seen during phase I, but residual luminal contents are swept through the small intestine and into the terminal ileum during late phase II and phase III of the IDMC. This finding is not surprising, because by definition, phase I is the absence of measurable phasic pressure waves, which are likely to be necessary to generate a sufficient intraluminal pressure gradient to cause intraluminal flow.

Transit Time Observations

Studies of small intestine transit time also probably do not represent a true assessment of fasting motor function, because most of the substrates used to measure transit also interact with small intestinal mucosal receptors. The lower the caloric content, the more closely fasting motility will be assessed (see earlier).

Manometric Observations

The IDMC is defined manometrically and comprises three main phases. Phase I is defined as motor quiescence (less than three pressure waves per 10 minutes at any one site); phase II is characterized by random pressure waves at less than the maximal rate; and phase III is characterized by pressure waves at the maximal rate (for the region) for longer than 2 minutes and, ideally, extending over greater than 40 cm. Some authors also include a fourth phase (phase IV) as a transitional period between phases III and I, although this approach is not universal. Phases I and III are quite distinctive and easily recognized, whereas phase II can be recognized reliably only when sandwiched between phases I and III, because it superficially resembles the fed pattern. The phases of the IDMC start proximally and migrate distally over variable distances, few phase IIIs reaching the ileum.[53] Moreover, phase III of each IDMC may start at a variable location; approximately one third of IDMCs have a gastroduodenal component, and most onsets of phase III occur near the proximal jejunum.[53] Because of the length of the small intestine and the velocity of travel of the IDMC, one part of the small intestine can be in phase I while other parts are in phase II or III (see Fig. 94–6). The normal periodicity of the IDMC varies greatly both within and between subjects; however, its median duration is 90 to 120 minutes.

CLINICAL CONSEQUENCES OF DISORDERED SMALL INTESTINAL MOTOR FUNCTION

Most of the time, the overall outcome of small intestinal motility is achieved without conscious awareness; a range of symptoms may arise, however, when an optimal outcome is not attained. Fortunately, like other organs, the small intestine has a substantial reserve capacity and copes with many insults, including infection, resection, inflammation, and denervation, before clinical problems become manifest. In IBS, the most common clinical syndrome in which altered motility is implicated, the sufferer's physical well-being rarely is threatened even when symptoms are considerable. Infrequently, the motor disturbances are severe enough to disrupt a person's ability to maintain oral nutrition.

The most important diseases and clinical settings associated with abnormal small intestinal motility are listed in Table 94–1. Because these disorders are covered elsewhere in this book, they are mentioned here only with regard to the associated small intestinal motor disturbances.

In IBS, a number of abnormalities of visceral sensation have been documented. These sensory abnormalities probably also lead to disordered motility; however, whereas motor abnormalities have been documented in some patients with IBS, such abnormalities are absent in other patients with this syndrome (see Chapter 115). Because it appears likely that IBS is an as-yet undefined generalized enteric neuropathy, failure to define motor abnormalities may result from a poor understanding of normal small intestinal motor physiology and the relatively gross measures by which motility in patients with IBS has been assessed.

Small intestinal motility is severely disrupted in acutely ill persons and is increasingly recognized as an important factor to consider in patients in the intensive care unit. The disturbances are likely to result from several factors, including sepsis and drugs, which disrupt the slow wave rhythm; abdominal trauma and surgery, which stimulate reflex motor responses; and inflammatory mediators, which affect neurotransmission within the CNS, ANS, and ENS. For a more detailed review, see the article by Ritz and colleagues.[54]

Pregnancy is known to alter lower esophageal sphincter function, delay gastric emptying, and disturb the frequency of gastric slow waves. It also is associated frequently with constipation. In view of these widespread complaints and findings related to altered gut motility, it is likely that small intestinal motor function also is altered. In guinea pigs, the strength of the contraction of intestinal circular smooth muscle has been shown to be impaired during pregnancy by down-regulation of Galphaq-11 proteins (which mediate contraction) and up-regulation of $G_s$alpha protein (which mediates relaxation).[55] It is intriguing that G protein associations now are also being reported in IBS sufferers, perhaps hinting at a final common pathway for sensorimotor gut disturbances.[56,57]

Diabetes has widespread effects on the motility of the gastrointestinal tract. Acute effects are the result of changes in blood glucose levels but also may result from the autonomic neuropathy that develops in patients with long-standing disease. As indicated predominantly by studies of the stomach, hyperglycemia may alter the rhythm of the slow wave, modulate sensory signaling, lead to changes in the temporospatial pattern of phasic contractions, and even stimulate inappropriate phase III–like IDMC activity in the small intestine.

Metabolic disturbances of potassium, magnesium, and calcium homeostasis are likely to impair small intestinal motor function because these chemicals are vital for normal neuromuscular function. The effects of abnormal levels of these electrolytes on normal human small intestinal function have not been studied specifically, but in organ bath experiments, their alterations have caused gross disturbances in neural and muscular function. Renal and hepatic failure also are likely to alter small intestinal motility because of the multiple homeostatic inputs of the affected organs; however, altered motility usually is not a prominent clinical feature of these conditions.

Many drugs affect small intestinal motility, especially those that alter ion transport, such as antidepressants, calcium channel blockers, and beta blockers. Sedatives and narcotic analgesics also alter motility but usually do not cause clinically important small intestinal motor dysfunction, except in critically ill patients or those with acute severe pain.

Pseudo-obstruction, scleroderma and other connective tissue diseases, dysautonomia, visceral myopathies, and other rare diseases in which abnormal small intestinal motor function occurs are discussed in detail in other chapters. These diseases may be the most uncommon causes of disordered small intestinal motility, but they have increased our understanding of normal motility, because in some cases, the neural and myopathic processes are impaired separately.

APPROACH TO PATIENTS WITH POSSIBLE SMALL INTESTINAL MOTOR DYSFUNCTION

Taking a thorough history is a vital first step in approaching a patient who may have abnormal small intestinal motility. A review of exposures to drugs and toxins, the family history, and, in the younger patient, milestones of growth and development are especially important to consider. Findings on physical examination in this setting often are unremarkable. First-line investigations generally are suggested by the history, physical examination, and age of the patient and may include a plain abdominal film (to look for dilated small intestinal loops, thickened wall, or air-fluid levels), complete blood count with determination of red blood cell indices (to look for evidence of malabsorption), measurement of serum albumin and electrolyte levels, and random testing of blood glucose or glycosylated hemoglobin level. How much further to proceed with investigation depends on these results and on the severity of the patient's condition.

Special investigations may be indicated to answer particular questions. No standard approach has been recognized, however, and local interest and expertise often determine which investigations are available. Fluoroscopy is widely available and may help exclude medically or surgically treatable problems. Endoscopy with small bowel biopsy or aspiration is useful if celiac sprue, small intestinal bacterial overgrowth, or intestinal infection is considered likely. Analysis of the stool may be necessary to exclude malabsorptive or secretory causes of small intestinal diarrhea. Small intestinal manometry, if available, may help distinguish neuropathic from myopathic forms of disordered motility, although in many settings the abnormalities associated with these two forms overlap (see Table 94–1). Manometry may show features typical of intestinal obstruction, although abdominal imaging by a variety of radiologic techniques is a better tool to identify an obstruction. In selected cases, a full-thickness biopsy of the small intestine will be necessary, but biopsy should be performed only in centers with expertise in immunohistochemistry of gut neurons, because standard histologic approaches often yield little useful information.

REFERENCES

1. Lee JS: Relationship between intestinal motility, tone, water absorption, and lymph flow in the rat. J Physiol (Lond) 345: 489, 1983.
2. Christensen J: Intestinal motor physiology. In Feldman M, Friedman LS, Sleisenger MH (eds): Sleisenger & Fordtran's Gastrointestinal and Liver Disease, 6th ed. Philadelphia, WB Saunders, 1997, p 1437.
3. Sarna SK: Gastrointestinal longitudinal muscle contractions. Am J Physiol 265:G156, 1993.
4. Sanders KM: A case for interstitial cells of Cajal as pacemakers and mediators of neurotransmission in the gastrointestinal tract. Gastroenterology 111:492, 1996.
5. Ward SM, Morris G, Reese L, et al: Interstitial cells of Cajal mediate enteric inhibitory neurotransmission in the lower esophageal and pyloric sphincters. Gastroenterology 115:314, 1998.

6. Ward SM, Beckett EA, Wang X, et al: Interstitial cells of Cajal mediate cholinergic neurotransmission from enteric motor neurons. J Neurosci 20:1393, 2000.

7. Sanders KM, Koh S D, Ördög T, Ward SM: Ionic conductances involved in generation and propagation of electrical slow waves in phasic gastrointestinal muscles. Neurogastroenterol Motil 16(suppl 1):100, 2004.

8. Ward SM, Sanders KM, Hirst GDS: Role of interstitial cells of Cajal in neural control of gastrointestinal smooth muscles. Neurogastroenterol Motil 16(suppl 1):112, 2004.

9. Agostini E, Chinnok JE, Daly MD, Murray JG: Functional and histological studies of the vagus nerve and its branches to the heart, lungs and abdominal viscera. J Physiol (Lond) 135:182, 1957.

10. Furness JB: Types of neurons in the enteric nervous system. J Auton Nerv Syst 81:87, 2000.

11. Furness JB, Jones C, Nurgali K, Clerc N: Intrinsic primary afferent neurons and nerve circuits within the intestine. Prog Neurobiol 72:143, 2004.

12. Furness JB: Intestinofugal neurons and sympathetic reflexes that bypass the central nervous system. J Comp Neurol 455:281, 2003.

13. Grundy D, Scratcherd T: Sensory afferents from the gastrointestinal tract. In Schultz SA (ed): Handbook of Physiology: The Gastrointestinal System. Washington DC, Raven Press, 1989, p 593.

14. Cervero F: Sensory innervation of the viscera: Peripheral basis of visceral pain. Physiol Rev 74:95, 1994.

15. Blackshaw LA, Gebhart GF: The pharmacology of gastrointestinal nociceptive pathways. Curr Opin Pharmacol 2: 642, 2002.

16. Berthoud HR, Blackshaw LA, Brookes SJ, Grundy D: Neuroanatomy of extrinsic afferents supplying the gastrointestinal tract. Neurogastroenterol Motil 16(suppl 1):28, 2004.

17. Grundy D: Neuroanatomy of visceral nociception: Vagal and splanchnic afferent. Gut 51(suppl 1):2, 2002.

18. Brierley SM, Jones RC 3rd, Gebhart GF, Blackshaw LA: Splanchnic and pelvic mechanosensory afferents signal different qualities of colonic stimuli in mice. Gastroenterology 127:166, 2004.

19. Cottrell D, Iggo A: Mucosal enteroceptors with vagal afferent fibres in the proximal duodenum of sheep. J Physiol 354:497, 1984.

20. Berthoud HR, Powley TL: Vagal afferent innervation of the rat fundic stomach: Morphological characterisation of the gastric tension receptor. J Comp Neurol 319:261, 1992.

21. Powley TL, Phillips RJ: Musings on the wanderer: What's new in our understanding of vago-vagal reflexes? I. Morphology and topography of vagal afferents innervating the GI tract. Am J Physiol Gastrointest Liver Physiol 283:G1217, 2002.

22. Neuhuber WL: Sensory vagal innervation of the rat esophagus and cardia: A light and electron microscopic anterograde tracing study. J Auton Nerv Syst 20:243, 1987.

23. Zagorodruk UP, Brookes SJH: Transduction sites of vagal mechanoreceptors in the guinea pig oesophagus. J Neurosci 20:6249, 2000.

24. Kirkup AJ, Brunsden AM, Grundy D: Receptors and transmission in the brain-gut axis: Potential for novel therapies. I. Receptors on visceral afferents. Am J Physiol Gastrointest Liver Physiol 280:G787, 2001.

25. Hicks GA, Coldwell JR, Schindler M, et al: Excitation of rat colonic afferent fibres by 5-HT3 receptors. J Physiol 544:861, 2002.

26. Berthoud HR, Kressel M, Raybould HE, Neuhuber WL: Vagal sensors in the rat duodenal mucosa: Distribution and structure as revealed by in vivo DiI-tracing. Anat Embryol 191:203, 1995.

27. Mayer EA, Naliboff BD, Chang L, Coutinho SV: Stress and the gastrointestinal tract: V. Stress and irritable bowel syndrome. Am J Physiol Gastrointest Liver Physiol. 280:G519, 2001.

28. Zhao A, McDermott J, Urban JF Jr, et al: Dependence of IL-4, IL-13, and nematode-induced alterations in murine small intestinal smooth muscle contractility on Stat 6 and enteric nerves. J Immunol 171:948, 2003.

29. Vermillion DL, Huizinga JD, Riddell RH, Collins SM: Altered small intestinal smooth muscle function in Crohn's disease. Gastroenterology 104:1692, 1993.

30. Coates MD, Mahoney CR, Linden DR, et al: Molecular defects in mucosal serotonin content and decreased serotonin reuptake transporter in ulcerative colitis and irritable bowel syndrome. Gastroenterology 126:1657, 2004.

31. He CL, Soffer EE, Ferris CD, et al: Loss of interstitial cells of Cajal and inhibitory innervation in insulin-dependent diabetes. Gastroenterology 121:427, 2001.

32. Andrews JM, Doran SD, Hebbard GS, et al: Nutrient-induced spatial patterning of human duodenal motor function. Am J Physiol Gastrointest Liver Physiol 280:G501, 2001.

33. Huge A, Weber E, Ehrlein HJ: Effects of enteral feedback inhibition on motility, luminal flow, and absorption of nutrients in proximal gut of minipigs. Dig Dis Sci 40:1024, 1995.

34. Stevens RJ, Publicover NG, Smith TK: Induction and organisation of Ca^{2+} waves by enteric neural reflexes. Nature 399:62, 1999.

35. Hausken T, Mundt M, Samsom M: Low antroduodenal pressure gradients are responsible for gastric emptying of a low caloric liquid meal in humans. Neurogastroenterol Motil 14:97, 2002.

36. Silny J: Intraluminal multiple electric impedance procedure for measurement of gastrointestinal motility. J Gastrointest Motil 3:151, 1991.

37. Silny J, Knigge KP, Fass J, et al: Verification of the intraluminal multiple electrical impedance measurement for the recording of gastrointestinal motility. J Gastrointest Motil 5:107, 1993.

38. Hennig GW, Costa M, Chen BN, Brookes SJH: Quantitative analysis of peristalsis in the guinea-pig small intestine using spatio-temporal maps. J Physiol 517:575, 1999.

39. Cannon WB: The Mechanical Factors of Digestion. London, Edward Arnold, 1911, p 131.

40. Husebye E: The patterns of small bowel motility: Physiology and implications in organic diseases and functional disorders. Neurogastroenterol Motil 11:141, 1999.

41. Sarna SK: Cyclic motor activity: Migrating motor complex. Gastroenterology 89:894, 1985.

42. Gielkins HAJ, van den Biggelaar A, Vetch J, et al: Effect of intravenous amino acids on interdigestive antroduodenal motility and small bowel transit time. Gut 44:240, 1999.

43. Rao SSC, Safadi R, Lu C, Schulze-Delrieu K: Manometric responses of human duodenum during infusion of HCl, hyperosmolar saline, bile, and oleic acid. Neurogastroenterol Motil 8:35, 1996.

44. Rao SSC, Lu C, Schulze-Delrieu K: Duodenum as an immediate brake to gastric outflow: A videofluoroscopic and manometric assessment. Gastroenterology 110:740, 1996.

45. Horowitz M, Dent J: The study of gastric mechanics: A Mad Hatter's Tea Party starting to make sense. Gastroenterology 107:37, 1994.

46. Shirazi S, Schulze-Delrieu K, Brown CK: Duodenal resistance to the emptying of various solutions from the isolated cat stomach. J Lab Clin Med 111:654, 1988.

47. Hausken T, Odegaars S, Matre K, Berstad A: Antroduodenal motility and movements of luminal contents studied by duplex sonography. Gastroenterology 102:1583, 1992.

48. Cannon WB: The movements of the intestines studied by means of the röntgen rays. Am J Physiol 6:251, 1902.

49. Hunt JN, Smith JL, Jiang CL: Effect of meal volume and energy density on the gastric emptying of carbohydrates. Gastroenterology 89:1326, 1985.

50. Benini L, Castellani G, Brighenti F, et al: Gastric emptying of a solid meal is accelerated by the removal of dietary fibre naturally present in food. Gut 36:825, 1995.

51. Lin HC, Doty JE, Reedy TJ, Meyer JH: Inhibition of gastric emptying by sodium oleate depends on length of intestine exposed to nutrient. Am J Physiol 259:G1031, 1990.

52. Lin HC, Zhao XT, Wang L: Jejunal brake: Inhibition of intestinal transit by fat in the proximal small intestine. Dig Dis Sci 41:326, 1996.

53. Kellow J, Borody TJ, Phillips SF, et al: Human interdigestive motility: Variations in patterns from oesophagus to colon. Gastroenterology 91:386, 1986.

54. Ritz MA, Fraser R, Tam W, et al: Impacts and patterns of disturbed gastrointestinal function in critically ill patients. Am J Gastroenterol 95:3044, 2000.

55. Chen Q, Xiao ZL, Biancani P, Behar J: Downregulation of G-alpha q-11 protein expression in guinea pig antral and colonic circular muscle during pregnancy. Am J Physiol 276:G895, 1999.

56. Holtmann G, Grote E, Braun-Lang U, et al: G-Protein B3 subunit 825 CC genotype and the manifestations of functional gastrointestinal disorders. Gastroenterology 126(suppl 2)162:S1094, 2004.

57. Holtmann G, Suffert W, Haag S, et al: G-Protein beta 3 subunit 825 CC genotype is associated with unexplained (functional) dyspepsia. Gastroenterology 126:1193, 2004.

CHAPTER

95 Colonic Motor and Sensory Function and Dysfunction

Ian J. Cook and Simon J. Brookes

Each day, 1200 to 1500 mL of ileal effluent enter the colon, and 200 to 400 mL are finally excreted as stool. The colon mixes its contents to facilitate the transmural exchange of water, electrolytes, and short-chain fatty acids and stores stool for extended periods. The mixing process involves rhythmic to-and-fro motions, together with short stepwise movements of contents, resulting in an overall net aboral flow rate that averages approximately 1 cm per hour. When dehydration threatens survival, such as with water deprivation or severe diarrhea, the ability of the colon to reabsorb fluid is of major physiologic significance; appropriate motility patterns are important in achieving this function. For example, the colon has the capacity to increase its fluid absorption fivefold, when required, but this ability is greatly impaired when transit is accelerated. Under normal circumstances, viscous contents occasionally are propelled aborally at a rapid rate, and if circumstances are appro-

priate, stool is evacuated under voluntary control. Thus, the colon is capable of showing a diverse range of motor patterns that are suited for particular physiologic functions. The generic term *motility* describes the range of motor patterns and the mechanisms that control them.

Common sensorimotor symptoms, such as constipation, diarrhea, bloating, abdominal pain, or rectal urgency, can arise from disturbances of ileocolonic delivery, colonic propulsion, or stool expulsion. Clearly, these symptoms and dysmotility must be linked, although our current understanding of these links is limited, largely because of technical difficulties involved in studying the human colon. Interspecies differences require care in extrapolating data from animal studies to humans. For many years, intraluminal motility recordings in humans were obtained mainly from the rectum and sigmoid. It is now clear that the motor activity of these distal regions is not representative of the colon as a whole. The contents of the colon become increasingly viscous distally, and this alteration complicates the relationship between propulsion and the contractile activity of the smooth muscle. Colonic movements are much less frequent and transit is considerably slower than in other regions of the gastrointestinal tract. The highly propulsive, stereotypical motor patterns that are associated with stool expulsion generally occur only once or twice daily. Hence, in vivo study of the motor patterns in the human cannot be achieved using contrast radiography. Prolonged recording techniques must be used to capture such infrequent motor patterns.

Recording of intraluminal pressure, by means of manometric catheters inserted per rectum, requires prior bowel cleansing, which may modify colonic motility. Furthermore, interpretation of intraluminal pressure measurements is complicated, because many contractions of the colonic wall do not occlude the lumen and therefore are detectable by manometry only if they cause significant pressure changes. Smooth muscle electromyography gives good insight into the patterning of muscle activity but generally requires access to the muscular wall of the colon, which ethically is problematic in humans. Scintigraphy with suitably high frame rates can resolve discrete movements of the contents but is suboptimal for measuring actual wall motion. In vitro study of the cellular basis of motility using isolated specimens of colon faces fewer technical and ethical limitations; however, data obtained at the cellular level, often under highly nonphysiologic conditions, can be difficult to relate to the more complex situation in vivo. Nonetheless, although each of these approaches has intrinsic limitations, in combination they have provided important insights into the relationships among muscle activity, wall motion, intraluminal pressure, and flow.

ANATOMY AND BASIC CONTROL MECHANISMS

MACROSCOPIC STRUCTURE OF THE COLON
(see also Chapter 93)

The human colon is just over 1 meter long and is divided anatomically into the cecum; the ascending, transverse, descending, and sigmoid colon; and the rectum, which lies between the rectosigmoid junction and the anal canal. The outer longitudinal smooth muscle layer forms three thick, cord-like structures called the teniae coli, which are spaced evenly around the circumference of the colon. Between the teniae, the longitudinal smooth muscle is much thinner, allowing the wall to bulge noticeably. In addition, irregularly spaced circumferential constrictions pinch the colon into a series of pockets, called haustra, which give the colon a sacculated appearance for much of its length. Haustra are not fixed structures and appear to be caused by sustained contractions of the circular muscle. Myogenic activity alone, however, does not seem sufficient to explain haustration, and neural input is likely to contribute to their formation; haustra move, disappear, and re-form during the propulsion of colonic contents. The teniae fuse to form a continuous outer longitudinal smooth muscle layer at the

rectosigmoid junction, which then continues down to the distal margin of the anal canal, insinuating itself between the internal and the external anal sphincters. Throughout the length of the colon, the circular smooth muscle layer consists of thick bundles of cells, which are separated by connective tissue septa. The internal anal sphincter consists of a thickening of the circular muscle layer over the last 2 to 4 cm of the anal canal.

STRUCTURE AND ACTIVITY OF COLONIC SMOOTH MUSCLE

Smooth muscle cells in the human colon, as in other muscular organs, are spindle-shaped, nucleolated cells with tapered ends. The surface area of the smooth muscle cell membrane is increased greatly by numerous caveolae, or small pits. Individual smooth muscle cells are connected to neighboring cells by gap junctions, which allow ions and small molecules (with molecular weights of up to approximately 1000 kd) to diffuse between the cells, thereby ensuring that the cells are electrically coupled to one another. Therefore, the smooth muscle cells do not contract as individual cells; rather, they contract together in large, coordinated assemblies, i.e., a syncytium.

Like smooth muscle throughout the gastrointestinal tract, colonic smooth muscle shows spontaneous, oscillatory electrical activity, even when all neural activity is blocked. Two types of rhythmic myoelectrical activity occur.[1] The first type of oscillations have been termed *myenteric potential oscillations* (MPOs) and are small-amplitude, rapid oscillations, with a frequency of 12 to 20 per minute, that originate from the plane of the myenteric plexus. These small oscillations spread, by means of gap junctions, into both the longitudinal and the circular smooth muscle layers and often reach the threshold potential for generating smooth muscle action potentials in both muscle layers. In the circular muscle layer, MPOs, with superimposed action potentials, generate small phasic contractions of the circular muscle layer. When the muscle is strongly excited by neurotransmitters released by enteric excitatory motor neurons, each MPO evokes an action potential, and the phasic contractions summate into powerful contractions, which last several seconds. Although the functions of the colon circular smooth muscle are well understood, the role that the longitudinal muscles play in colonic motility, mixing, and propulsion is a matter of some controversy. The longitudinal muscle probably acts in some ways in an antagonistic role relative to circular muscle (preventing excessive lengthening when the circular muscle contracts—which would be mechanically disadvantageous); it may contribute to propulsion by "pulling" the gut over the contents, so that circular muscle contractions gain more purchase on the contents; and some evidence from modeling suggests that it also may play a role in mixing of liquid contents, at least in the small intestine.

A second pacemaker region is located at the submucosal border of the circular muscle. This region produces larger-amplitude, slower myogenic oscillations in membrane potential called *slow waves*, which also spread through the thickness of the circular smooth muscle by means of gap junctions. Slow waves also often reach the threshold for triggering smooth muscle action potentials and can evoke strong contractions. Slow waves occur throughout the colon at a frequency of approximately 2 to 4 per minute. In the small intestine, a gradient of slow wave intrinsic frequencies causes slow waves to propagate predominantly aboral. This is not the case in the colon: Slow waves propagate over short distances up or down the colon, with complex interactions as waves coming from different initiation sites collide, leading to mixing of contents with little propulsion. The currents produced by pacemaker cells at the myenteric and submucosal borders decay as they spread through the thickness of the circular muscle layer. Thus, operating in the middle of the circular smooth muscle layer is complex spontaneous electrical activity consisting of a mixture of MPOs and slow waves, with superimposed smooth muscle action potentials. Most of the time, slow waves determine the contractile activity of the smooth muscle and cause non-propulsive mixing movements. During times of strong enteric neuronal activity, however, MPO-related contractions summate, giving rise to powerful patterned contractions of much longer duration than those produced by slow waves, and which can propagate for long distances along the colon (propagating sequences). Action potentials in the smooth muscle can be recorded in vivo with electrodes attached to the serosal surface, thereby giving a high-resolution measurement of myoelectric activity or "spike bursts."

ION CHANNELS IN COLONIC SMOOTH MUSCLE

The membrane of colonic smooth muscle cells contains a variety of ion channels, including several types of potassium channels, calcium channels, chloride channels, and nonselective cation channels.[2] Although the exact physiologic roles of many of these ion channels currently are unknown, the high-threshold, voltage-operated calcium channels (L-type calcium channels) play a crucial role in colonic muscle contractility. These channels open when the membrane potential of smooth muscle cells is depolarized beyond a voltage threshold, and they are respon-

sible for the rapid upstroke of smooth muscle action potentials. The influx of calcium through L-type calcium channels during action potentials is a major trigger for activation of the contractile apparatus. It is not surprising that pharmacologic blockade of L-type calcium channels by dihydropyridine drugs such as nifedipine can reduce the contractility of colonic smooth muscle substantially; release of calcium from intracellular stores, which is triggered by excitatory neurotransmitters, also may play a role in muscle contraction.

INTERSTITIAL CELLS OF CAJAL: SMOOTH MUSCLE PACEMAKERS

Since 1991, the interstitial cells of Cajal (ICCs) have been shown to play at least two important roles in the control of gastrointestinal motility: control of myogenic activity and mediating or amplifying the effects of motor neurons on the smooth muscle apparatus. ICCs are non-neuronal in origin and are derived from common progenitors of smooth muscle cells. Mutant mice and rats that are deficient in ICCs have profoundly disturbed intestinal motility, an observation that provides insight into the roles of ICCs in the human gastrointestinal tract. In the human colon, three types of ICCs are recognized, which are named according to their location: ICCs in the plane of the myenteric plexus (ICC$_{MY}$), ICCs near the submucosal plexus (ICC$_{SM}$), and intramuscular ICCs located between the circular and the longitudinal muscle layers (ICC$_{IM}$). ICC$_{MY}$ and ICC$_{SM}$ form extensive networks along the colon and are electrically coupled to one another and to the smooth muscle layers by gap junctions (Figs. 95–1 and 95–2). ICC$_{MY}$ probably are the pacemakers for the small, rapid (12 to 20 per minute) oscillations in membrane potential (MPOs) of longitudinal and circular smooth muscle layers. ICC$_{SM}$ are the pacemakers for the large-amplitude, slow waves (2 to 4 per minute) originating in the plane of the submucosal plexus; these slow waves have a powerful influence on the patterning of circular muscle contraction. The exact ionic basis of rhythmicity in ICC$_{MY}$ and ICC$_{SM}$ that gives rise to MPOs and slow waves is not entirely clear; however, oscillations

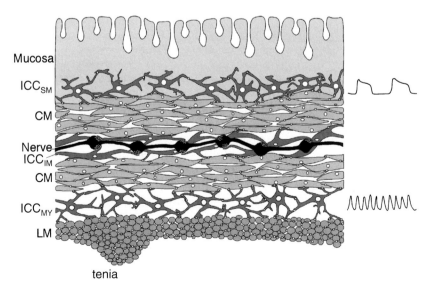

Figure 95–1 Schematic cross section of the muscularis externa of the human colon. The outer longitudinal smooth muscle layer (LM) is thickened at the teniae. In the plane of the myenteric plexus *(not shown)* is a network of interstitial cells of Cajal (ICCs), which generate a rapid myenteric potential oscillation (ICC$_{MY}$; see lower waveform on the *right*). The circular muscle layer (CM) is innervated by axons of enteric motor neurons with transmitter release sites (clusters of clear vesicles) that are associated with specialized intramuscular ICCs (ICC$_{IM}$). At the outer border of the circular muscle is another network of submucosal ICCs, which generate slow waves (ICC$_{SM}$; see upper waveform on the *right*). Also present are axons of motor neurons in the longitudinal muscles and ICC$_{IM}$ (not shown in this cross section). The *tiny white squares* represent gap junctions, which electrically couple cells.

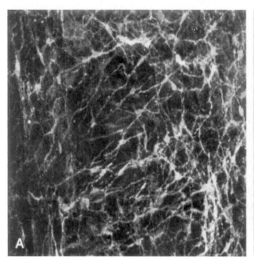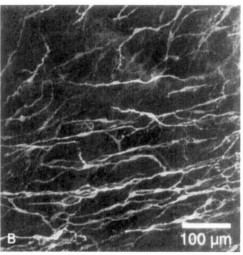

Figure 95–2 Micrographs of interstitial cells of Cajal (ICCs) in the human colon, labeled by c-Kit immunohistochemistry. *A,* ICCs in the plane of the myenteric plexus (ICC$_{MY}$) have an irregular shape, form a dense network of cells, and probably function as pacemakers. *B,* A different plane of focus of the same region shows spindle-shaped intramuscular ICCs (ICC$_{IM}$) in the overlying circular muscle layer. These cells probably are involved in neuromuscular transmission to the smooth muscle. (Courtesy of Liz Murphy and David Wattchow.)

in membrane potential are an intrinsic property of both ICC$_{MY}$ and ICC$_{SM}$. Intramuscular ICCs (ICC$_{IM}$) are a major target of neurotransmitters released from the axons of excitatory and inhibitory enteric motor neurons. Acetylcholine and nitric oxide (and probably several other motor neuron transmitters) evoke changes in the membrane potential of ICC$_{IM}$, which then spread through the smooth muscle by means of gap junctions. ICC$_{IM}$ also may be involved in amplifying the slow waves as they spread through the muscle layers. Thus, these cells appear to be key players in integrating both non-neuronal pacemaker activity and neuronal inputs to the smooth muscle.

The discovery that cellular mechanisms long considered to be the properties of smooth muscle cells actually are mediated by ICCs may have important clinical implications. For example, in the distal bowel, reduced numbers of ICCs, or a reduction in the total volume of ICCs, has been associated with anorectal malformations, colonic manifestations of Chagas' disease, and possibly some cases of slow-transit constipation.[3] Some reports have suggested that the density of ICCs may be affected in the aganglionic segments of colon in Hirschsprung's disease, but this finding has not been consistent.[3]

INNERVATION OF THE COLON

THE ENTERIC NERVOUS SYSTEM

Direct neuronal control of colonic motility is mediated mostly by the enteric nervous system (ENS). Although the ENS is capable of expressing a diverse repertoire of motor patterns, its functions are modulated by sympathetic, parasympathetic, and extrinsic afferent pathways (Fig. 95–3). In terms of numbers of nerve cells, the ENS is by far the largest component of the autonomic nervous system, with considerably more neurons than those of the parasympathetic and sympathetic divisions combined. The nerve cell bodies of the ENS are located in plexuses of myenteric ganglia (Auerbach's plexus), which are located between the longitudinal and the circular muscle layers of the muscularis externa, or in the sub-

mucosal ganglia, which lie between the circular muscle and the mucosa (Fig. 95–4).

The submucosal plexus is divisible into at least two networks: *Meissner's plexus,* which lies closer to the mucosa, and *Schabadasch's plexus,* which lies adjacent to the circular muscle. Internodal strands that contain hundreds of axons run within and between the different plexuses. Finer nerve trunks innervate the various target tissues of the gut wall, including the longitudinal muscle layer, circular muscle, muscularis mucosae, mucosal crypts, and mucosal epithelium. Within the ganglia of each plexus, different functional classes of enteric nerve cell bodies are intermingled, although differences in the proportions of cell types among the plexuses have been observed. It has become clear that an exquisite degree of organization is characteristic of the ENS, with each class of nerve cell making highly specific and precise projections to its particular target.

Enteric Primary Afferent Neurons

Much of the motor and secretory activity of the bowel can be conceptualized as a series of reflexes evoked by mechanical or chemical stimuli. These reflexes involve activation of enteric primary afferent neurons, integration by interneurons, and execution of appropriate responses by motor neurons. The first neurons in these reflex circuits are primary afferent neurons (sometimes called "sensory" neurons, although they do not give rise to conscious sensation). These neurons are located in both myenteric and submucosal plexuses and characteristically have several long axonal processes. Some primary afferents fire action potentials in response to stretch or tension in the bowel wall; others are activated by chemical or mechanical stimuli of the mucosa. These mucosal stimuli probably work, at least in part, by activating specialized enteroendocrine cells in the mucosal epithelium, such as the serotonin-containing enterochromaffin cells. The primary afferent neurons then release synaptic transmitters (acetylcholine or tachykinins or other peptides) to excite other classes of enteric neurons in nearby ganglia. Enteric primary afferent neurons also make excitatory synaptic contacts onto

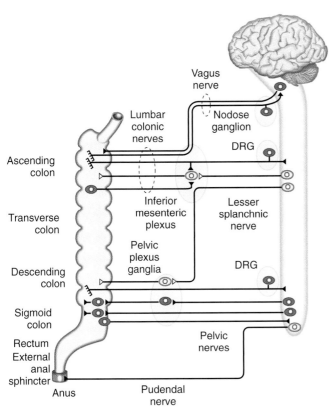

Figure 95–3 The extrinsic innervation of the human colon. Parasympathetic efferent pathways (*filled* cell bodies) arise from the dorsal motor nucleus of the vagus in the brainstem and pass through the vagus nerve and prevertebral sympathetic ganglia, through the lumbar colonic nerves to the proximal colon. Parasympathetic pathways also extend from nuclei in the sacral spinal cord that run through the pelvic nerves and either synapse in the pelvic plexus ganglia or run directly into the gut wall. Sympathetic pathways (*open* cell bodies) consist of preganglionic neurons in the thoracic spinal cord that synapse with sympathetic postganglionic neurons either in the inferior mesenteric plexus or in the pelvic plexus. Enteric nerve cell bodies in the colon receive input from both parasympathetic and sympathetic pathways. Viscerofugal enteric neurons project out of the bowel to the prevertebral ganglia. Afferent pathways consist of vagal afferent neurons from the proximal colon with cell bodies in the nodose ganglion. In addition, spinal afferents with cell bodies in lumbar dorsal root ganglia (DRG) run through both the lesser splanchnic and colonic nerves to the colon and mediate nociception. Another population of spinal afferents, with cell bodies in the sacral DRG, run through the pelvic nerves and pelvic ganglia to the rectum. These include populations of sensory neurons that transmit non-nociceptive information about the distention of the rectum. Finally, the striated muscles of the pelvic floor (including the external anal sphincter) are supplied by motor neurons with cell bodies in the spinal cord and axons that run in the pudendal nerves. *Triangles* represent transmitter release sites; "*combs*" represent sensory transduction sites.

other neurons of their own class, so that they fire in coordinated assemblies.

Enteric Motor Neurons

Enteric motor neurons typically have a smaller cell body than that typical for afferent neurons, with a few short dendrites and a single long axon. Separate populations of motor neurons innervate the circular and longitudinal muscle layers. *Excitatory motor neurons* synthesize acetylcholine, which they release from their varicose endings in the smooth muscle layers. In addition, some of them also release the tachykinin peptides, substance P and neurokinin A, which excite smooth muscle. Typically, the axons of excitatory motor neurons project either directly to the smooth muscle close to their cell bodies or orad for up to 10 mm.[4] Once in the smooth muscle layers, the axons turn and run parallel to the smooth muscle fibers for several millimeters; they branch extensively and form many small varicosities, or transmitter release sites, closely associated with intramuscular ICCs (ICC$_{IM}$).

Inhibitory motor neurons typically are slightly larger than excitatory motor neurons but fewer in number. They also have short dendrites and a single axon, but unlike excitatory motor neurons, they project aborally to the smooth muscle layer for distances of 1 to 15 mm in the human colon.[4] Once the axon reaches the smooth muscle, it branches extensively to form multiple varicose release sites. Inhibitory motor neurons release a "cocktail" of transmitters that inhibit smooth muscle cells, including nitric oxide, adenosine triphosphate (ATP), and peptides, such as vasoactive intestinal polypeptide (VIP) and pituitary adenyl cyclase–activating peptide (PACAP). The varicose transmitter release sites of inhibitory motor neurons also are associated with ICC$_{IM}$, just as are the release sites of excitatory motor neurons. Inhibitory motor neurons can be tonically active, modulating the ongoing contractile activity of the colonic circular smooth muscle. Inhibitory motor neurons are particularly important in relaxing sphincteric muscles in the ileocecal junction and internal anal sphincter.

Enteric Interneurons

When a region of colon is stimulated, as by a bolus that distends it, intrinsic primary afferent neurons (IPANs) are activated. These neurons then activate excitatory and inhibitory motor neurons, which, because of their polarized projections, cause contraction of the muscle orad to the bolus and relaxation aborally. These effects tend to propel the contents aborally. From the new position of the bolus, another set of polarized reflexes is triggered, and peristaltic propulsion results. The *ascending excitatory reflex* and the *descending inhibitory reflex* sometimes are called "the law of the intestine." These reflexes spread farther than is predicted by the projections of the excitatory and inhibitory motor neurons, because interneurons also are involved in these reflex pathways. Ascending cholinergic interneurons in the human colon have axons that project up to 40 mm orad and extend the spread of ascending excitatory reflex pathways. In addition, several classes of descending interneurons are present in the human colon, with axons that project up to 70 mm aborally. Some of these interneurons are involved in spreading descending inhibition along the colon, but others are likely to be involved in the propagation of migratory contractions. Recent evidence suggests that some interneurons may themselves be stretch-sensitive, thereby functioning as primary afferent neurons. In addition to the sensory, inter-, and motor neurons, viscerofugal nerve cells project to the sympathetic prevertebral ganglia,

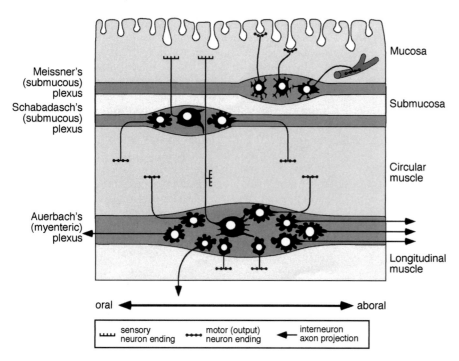

Figure 95–4 Diagram showing the layers and components of the intestinal wall. The lumen is at the *top* and the longitudinal muscle layer is at the *bottom*. Auerbach's myenteric plexus and the submucosal plexuses (Meissner's and Schabadasch's plexuses) are shown, along with some of their major classes of enteric neurons. The networks of interstitial cells are shown separately in Figure 95–1.

vasomotor neurons innervate blood vessels, and secreto-motor neurons stimulate secretion from the colonic epithelium.

SYMPATHETIC INNERVATION

The major sympathetic innervation of the proximal colon arises from the inferior mesenteric ganglion and projects through the lumbar colonic nerves to the ascending and transverse colon (see Fig. 95–3). A small number of sympathetic neurons in the celiac and superior mesenteric ganglia, in the paravertebral chain ganglia, and in the pelvic plexus ganglia also project to the colon (see Fig. 95–3). These neurons receive a powerful cholinergic drive from preganglionic nerve cell bodies in the inter-mediolateral column of the spinal cord (segments L2 to L5). This is a major pathway by which the central nervous system modifies bowel activity, for example, during exercise. Sympathetic efferent neurons also receive input from the enteric viscerofugal neurons and from extrinsic, spinal sensory neurons with cell bodies in the dorsal root ganglia, forming several reflex loops with the distal bowel.

Sympathetic nerve fibers from prevertebral ganglia cause vasoconstriction of the mucosal and submucosal blood vessels. Other cells project to the enteric ganglia, where they cause presynaptic inhibition of synaptic activity in the ENS and thus depress reflex motor activity. Another target for sympathetic axons is the circuitry of the submucosal plexus (largely Meissner's plexus) involved in controlling epithelial secretion. Hence, these pathways inhibit colonic motor activity, reduce blood flow, and inhibit secretion to limit water loss from the body during times of sympathetic activation. In addition, some sympathetic axons innervate the smooth muscle directly, particularly the ileocecal junction and internal anal sphincter, where they cause contraction. These effects also are consistent with closing down enteric motor activity during sympathetic arousal.

PARASYMPATHETIC INNERVATION

The colon receives parasympathetic innervation from both the vagus nerve and pathways in the sacral spinal cord. Branches of the vagus nerve reach the prevertebral ganglia and then run with sympathetic axons to the ceco-ascending and transverse colon. The distal colon is supplied largely by sacral parasympathetic axons via the pelvic nerves. Some of these axons synapse first onto nerve cell bodies in the pelvic plexus, whereas others project directly to the colon. From their point of entry into the colon, many of the axons run in an oral direction and form thick trunks called *shunt fascicles*. Parasympathetic axons project to the enteric ganglia in the colon, where they make excitatory cholinergic synapses onto enteric nerve cell bodies. Sacral parasympathetic pathways play an important role in increasing the propulsive activity of the distal colon before defecation and also may be involved in triggering the propagating complexes that start more proximally before defecation.

EXTRINSIC AFFERENT PATHWAYS

Sensation from the colon is mediated by primary afferent neurons with cell bodies outside the bowel wall. Vagal afferent neurons, with nerve cell bodies located in the nodose and jugular ganglia, project to the proximal colon and run with the vagal efferent parasympathetic pathways. Currently, their exact role in reflex control and sensation is not clear, but they are unlikely to be involved in the transmission of pain sensation from the colon.

The entire colon also is innervated by spinal primary afferent neurons with nerve cell bodies in the lumbar dorsal root ganglia. Lumbar spinal afferents project along the lumbar splanchnic nerves, through the prevertebral inferior mesenteric ganglion and through the lumbar colonic nerves to the colon, where they terminate in sensory endings in the mesentery, serosa, muscular layers, and mucosa throughout the entire colon and rectum. In adition, a population of spinal afferents, with cell bodies in the sacral dorsal root ganglia, project along the pelvic nerves to the colon and traverse the pelvic plexus en route. Evidence indicates that some of these sacral spinal afferents form a functionally different population from the lumbar spinal afferents, encoding different types of information, particularly from the rectum. Sacral afferents include many low-threshold, wide-dynamic-range mechanoreceptors, which probably are responsible for graded sensations of rectal filling and for activating defecatory reflexes.[5] By contrast, lumbar spinal afferents probably are involved in generating pain sensations from all regions of the colon and rectum. They respond to gross distention of the bowel wall, traction on the mesenteric membranes, powerful colonic contractions, or chemical stimulation of the mucosa by bile acids, high osmolarity, and other stimuli. It is well established that the sensitivity of many spinal afferents is increased greatly by inflammation in the gut wall. In addition to their role in sensation, spinal afferents also have axon branches (collaterals) in enteric ganglia and prevertebral sympathetic ganglia and on mucosal blood vessels, where they may play a role in generating peripheral reflex responses to noxious stimuli.

RELATIONSHIPS AMONG CELLULAR EVENTS, PRESSURE, AND FLOW

Smooth muscle activation often is divided into two components. The first component is the tonic, ongoing activation that gives smooth muscle its basal resistance to stretch (i.e., its "tone"). The second component comprises the dynamic, phasic contractions that mix and propel contents. *Compliance* is a term used to describe the extent to which the bowel wall can stretch to accommodate contents. For example, a muscle that is very distensible (e.g., because of powerful inhibitory motor neuron activity) is said to have a high compliance. During phasic contractions, a transient increase occurs in the resistance of the bowel wall to stretch (i.e., a decrease in its compliance). If bowel contents are fluid and no downstream resistance is present to impede flow, the smooth muscle will shorten rapidly. The contents will then be propelled, with a minimal increase in intraluminal pressure. By contrast, if resistance to forward flow of contents, as by a lumen-occluding contraction occurring distally, is encountered, the smooth muscle will not shorten significantly, but its tension will increase. This increase in tension will increase intraluminal pressure but will not cause propulsion. In most situations in vivo, smooth muscle contraction causes a mixture of shortening, increased tension, increased pressure, and propulsion.

In light of the complex, dynamic relationships among smooth muscle length and tension, intraluminal pressure, tone, and compliance, it can be difficult to relate complex motility patterns to the cellular events; a few features, however, appear to be explicable. The frequency of nonpropagating, mixing, or segmenting contractions of the colon in vivo often is 2 to 4 cycles per minute, similar to the frequency of the spontaneous myogenic slow waves generated by ICC_{SM} at the submucosal border of the circular muscle.[1,6] The timing of these nonpropagating contractions probably is affected relatively little by enteric motor neural activity but is very dependent on the degree of wall distention. By contrast, when excitatory motor neurons are active, contractions evoked by MPOs summate, giving rise to powerful, lumen-occlusive contractions that can last longer than slow waves and that may propagate substantial distances along the colon.

The process of propagation is controlled both by pathways intrinsic to the enteric neural circuitry and by triggering sequences of polarized reflexes that cause peristaltic propulsion. The neuropharmacologic basis of propagating colonic contractions seen in the intact human colon is only partially understood, with much of the available evidence being derived from animal studies. In both the mouse colon and the human colon, a tonic nitrergic inhibition of enteric neurons is seen; removal of this inhibition (for example, by administering inhibitors of nitric oxide synthesis) leads to an immediate increase in the frequency of colonic propagating pressure waves.[7,8] Physiologic stimuli capable of triggering these colonic propagating contractions include food, waking from sleep, and stimulants such as laxatives or bile acids that act by means of mucosal receptors.[9]

REGULATION OF COLONIC FILLING, TRANSPORT, AND DEFECATION

THE COLON AS A STORAGE ORGAN

The region of preferential storage of colonic content is not entirely settled. In 1902, Cannon proposed on the basis of radiologic observations that the proximal colon is the site of storage and mixing, whereas the distal colon acts as a conduit for expulsion. Subsequent studies, however, found no difference in the dwell time for radiopaque markers in the middle, proximal, and distal colon (roughly 11 hours in each).[10] Dietary composition influences regional transit and probably accounts for some of the discrepancies among studies. With a liquid diet, the right colon empties rapidly (1 to 2 hours), whereas the transverse colon retains isotope for 20 to 40 hours.[11] A solid diet retards transit through the cecum and ascending colon. With a mixed diet, particulate matter and liquids are stored in both the ascending and the transverse colon, as suggested by Cannon's earlier observations.[12]

REGULATION OF COLONIC FILLING: THE CONTRIBUTION OF THE ILEOCECAL JUNCTION

In humans, the ileocolonic junction regulates colonic filling and prevents coloileal reflux, thereby avoiding contamination of the small bowel by colonic bacteria. In the fasted state, cecal filling is slow and erratic, and ileal chyme is retained in the distal ileum for prolonged periods.[13] The close physical link between the terminal ileum and the cecum by the ileocecal ligaments behaves functionally as a valve and is responsible in part for continence of the ileocolonic junction. A specialized band of muscle forms a low-pressure tonic sphincter.[14] Prominent 6 cycles-per-minute (cpm) phasic contractions contribute to the regulatory function of the ileocolonic junction. Phasic and tonic activity are inhibited concurrently with episodic terminal ileal flow or distention of the ileum, and the tone of the ileocolonic junction increases in response to cecal distention.[14] Phase III of the interdigestive motor cycle (IDMC) (or migrating myoelectric/motor complex [MMC]), a motor pattern that occurs every 90 to 120 minutes in the upper intestine during fasting (see Chapter 94), does not contribute to ileocecal transit, because it rarely reaches the terminal ileum in the human. Most ileal chyme, driven by ileal propagating contractions in synchrony with inhibition of phasic contractions of the ileocolonic junction, enters the cecum in a pulsatile fashion within 90 minutes of a meal. Prolonged studies correlating ileocecal movement of isotope with intraluminal pressures show that 87% of episodes of ileocecal transport are due to monophasic, ileal propagating pressure waves.[15] Furthermore, 85% of such episodes of cecal filling are followed immediately by cecal propagating pressure waves, suggesting that episodic cecal filling is one of the triggers for colonic propagating pressure waves (Fig. 95–5).

REGULATION OF EMPTYING OF THE PROXIMAL COLON

Emptying of the proximal colon occurs more rapidly when wall tone is increased (e.g., by fatty acids) than when the tone is low; the volume and consistency of the contents also affect the rate of emptying.[16] Isotonic fluid infused into the proximal colon stimulates proximal colonic emptying, suggesting that distention per se can activate propulsive motor patterns. Irritant laxatives (which act by stimulating mucosal receptors) in the proximal colon, however, trigger propagating contractions much more reliably than does distention alone.[17] Hence, proximal colonic emptying is influenced by a combination of increased wall tone and the initiation of propagating contractions, probably under the influence of both chemical and mechanical factors.

It has been suggested, from animal studies, that "antiperistaltic" waves of contraction occur in the proximal colon and may contribute to the retention of contents. Retrograde movement of contents was first demonstrated in the feline proximal colon, and subsequently, retrograde-migrating myoelectrical activity was demonstrated. Time-lapse cineradiography suggested that such retrograde movements were infrequent in the human colon; however, combined scintigraphic and manometric studies show that these events, although the colonic contents traversed only short distances, are quite common in the human colon. Retrograde movements probably serve a mixing function and, particularly when the colon is loaded or when defecation is voluntarily suppressed, serve to minimize challenges to continence,

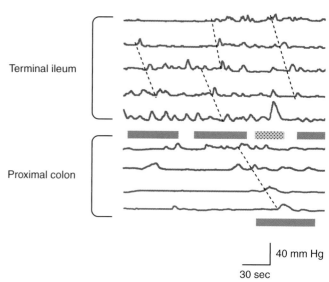

Figure 95–5 Propagating pressure wave sequences identified in the terminal ileum and proximal colon during prolonged combined scintigraphic and manometric recordings. The *filled bars* indicate forward flow of colonic contents across the ileocolonic junction *(center)* or along the proximal colon *(bottom)*. The *stippled bar* represents retrograde flow across the ileocolonic junction. Each burst of cecal filling is preceded by a propagating ileal pressure wave sequence. The second ileal propagating pressure wave sequence triggers a colonic propagating sequence, which arises from the cecum during an episode of cecal filling. (With permission from Dinning PG: Doctoral thesis. Sydney, University of New South Wales, 2004.)

because they are more prevalent in the loaded bowel than in the partially filled colon.[18]

REGIONAL VARIATION IN PRESSURE PATTERNS AND FLOW

Mass movements, recorded using radiologic techniques, are associated with the movement of stool over long distances, and high-amplitude propagating pressure waves are associated with defecation.[19] Mass movements and defecation, however, are relatively infrequent events. By contrast, movements of colonic contents occur in a stepwise fashion over short distances episodically throughout the day.[12,20]

Using a combination of pancolonic manometry and high-frame-rate scintigraphy, it has become possible to record intraluminal pressure and colonic flow with high temporal resolution. This methodology has identified some of the motor patterns that give rise to propulsion and has demonstrated differences in motor patterns among the various regions of the colon in terms of prevalence, amplitude, velocity, distance covered, and ability to propel contents[20] (Fig. 95–6). For example, propagating pressure waves originate nearly four times as frequently in the proximal colon as in the distal colon (see Fig. 95–6). The mean distance covered by antegrade pressure waves starting in the cecum is 50 cm, compared with only 20 cm for sequences originating in the descending and the sigmoid colon. Still, pressure waves arising prox-

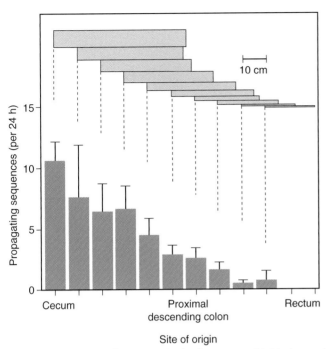

Figure 95–6 Regional variation in the frequency of initiation and extent of propagation of propagating sequences. The histogram at the *bottom* shows the distribution of antegrade propagating sequences grouped according to the site of origin. The *horizontal bars* at the *top* show the mean extent of propagation by sequences originating at the same site. Note that propagating sequences originate significantly more frequently in the proximal than in the distal colon, and that the extent of propagation is much greater for sequences originating in the proximal colon. The vertical thickness of each horizontal bar at the *top* is proportional to the propagating sequence frequency shown at the *bottom* and indicates that the "density" of component pressure waves is highest in the midcolon and lowest in the distal colon. (From Cook IJ, Furukawa Y, Panagopoulos V, et al: Relationships between spatial patterns of colonic pressure and individual movements of content. Am J Physiol 278:G329, 2000.)

imally generally do not propagate beyond the midcolon (see Fig. 95–6). It is now clear that slower propagation rates favor the effective propulsion of contents. The conduction velocity of pressure waves increases as the waves migrate caudally (Fig. 95–7). Indeed, such events frequently accelerate to the point of synchronicity, which arrests the progress of contents. In addition, nonpropagating (segmenting) pressure waves make up a higher proportion of activity in the distal colon than in more proximal regions. Thus, most motor activity in the distal colon functions to retard forward flow, perhaps to minimize challenges to continence.

WHAT DETERMINES WHETHER A PRESSURE WAVE IS PROPULSIVE?

Combined scintigraphic and prolonged manometric studies have shown that propagating pressure wave sequences account for 40% to 50% of discrete movements of isotope-labeled colonic contents within the unprepared colon[20] (see Fig. 95–7). The strength of association is region dependent, being stronger in the transverse than in the cecum and ascending colon; this difference prob-

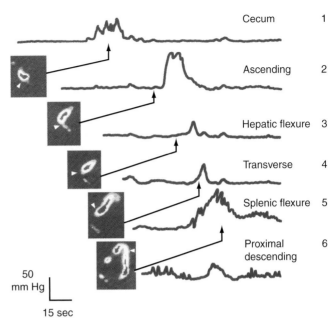

Figure 95–7 Intracolonic pressure measurements and corresponding scintiscans that show a clear correlation between a propagating pressure wave sequence and discrete movement of colonic contents from the cecum to the sigmoid colon. This particular movement of contents was not associated with defecation or sensation. The *vertical arrows* (scintiscan images) correspond to the time (horizontal axis) of acquisition of each 15-second scintigraphic frame. *Small arrowheads* on the scintiscans indicate the location of the manometric side hole from which the corresponding pressure tracing was recorded. In the proximal colon and midcolon (channels 2, 3, and 4 from the top), a close temporal relationship exists between movement of the isotope and the onset of the propagating pressure wave upstroke. When the pressure wave reaches the splenic flexure, however, the proximal descending colon is seen to expand to accommodate the isotope, consistent with loss of lumen occlusion at this region. The pressure waves in channels 5 and 6 do not appear to correspond to lumen-occluding contractions. Note also that propagating pressure wave amplitudes in channels 3 and 4 are only 30 and 39 mm Hg, respectively, yet the motor pattern is clearly propulsive. (From Cook IJ, Furukawa Y, Panagopoulos V, et al: Relationships between spatial patterns of colonic pressure and individual movements of content. Am J Physiol 278:G329, 2000.)

ably is due to the inability of intraluminal manometry to detect all propagating pressure waves in the more capacious cecum. Approximately 25% of episodic movements of colonic contents are related to repetitive, nonpropagating pressure waves that move contents only short distances in either direction; however, roughly a quarter of the remaining episodic movements of content cannot be linked with any measurable changes in intraluminal pressure, a finding that may reflect the occurrence of contractions at points remote from the recording sites. Alternatively, propulsion sometimes may be caused by motor events that do not affect intraluminal pressure significantly, such as longitudinal muscle shortening, non–lumen-occluding circular muscle contractions, or alterations in regional wall tone.

When propagating pressure wave sequences are observed, the likelihood that they will be propulsive of content is greatest in the proximal colon and lowest in the distal colon. Up to 90% of all propagating sequences originating in the cecum and ascending colon are propulsive, whereas only 30% of sequences originating distal to the hepatic flexure propel significant quantities of intraluminal material.[20] This relative, distal propulsive "inefficiency" may be desirable, by limiting challenges to continence and retaining content for appropriate durations to allow optimal fluid and electrolyte absorption. Still to be resolved is why some propagating sequences are propulsive and others are not. It appears that a higher-pressure wave amplitude and slower conduction velocity favor propulsion (see Fig. 95–7). Sequences recorded proximally have these characteristics.

In summary, the distal colon displays a combination of fewer propagating sequences, shorter extent of propagation, higher conduction velocity, and lower probability of content propulsion than are observed in the proximal colon. In addition, proportionally more nonpropagating (segmenting) pressure waves occur in the distal colon than proximally. Considered together, these features would be expected to result in retardation of flow into the distal sigmoid and rectum, thus minimizing challenges to continence while maximizing the mixing of content more proximally.

COLONIC FUNCTION RELATING TO DEFECATION

Variations in propagating motor activity along the colon, as just described, would limit or might even prevent colonic contents from ever reaching the rectum and being expelled. Clearly, additional mechanisms must occur from time to time that lead to defecation. Traditionally, defecation was conceptualized as an exclusively rectoanal function; however, evidence for the integration of colonic motor activity with defecation has come from several sources. Radiopaque markers and scintigraphic recordings confirm that the greater proportion of the entire colonic contents may be evacuated in some cases.[12,21] Furthermore, pancolonic manometric studies have demonstrated that the preparatory phase of defecation not only involves the greater part of the colon but also commences up to 1 hour before stool expulsion.[22] In this predefecatory phase, a characteristic progressive increase occurs in the frequency of propagating pressure wave sequences. These sequences start first in the proximal colon, with each successive sequence originating slightly more distal to the preceding one. These "priming" sequences do not evoke conscious sensation. By contrast, in the 15 minutes leading up to defecation, a dramatic increase occurs in the frequency of these propagating sequences, which leads to a strong defecatory urge. In the last 15 minutes of the predefecatory phase, propagating pressure waves begin to originate in the distal colon; however, in this late phase, each successive propagating sequence originates from a site *proximal* to the preceding one. Each sequence also tends to run for a slightly longer distance and has a higher amplitude in comparison with the preceding propagating sequence (Fig. 95–8). These final sequences provide potent forces to fill and distend the rectum, activating specialized low-threshold sacral spinal afferent mechanoreceptors. These mechanoreceptors then give rise to the defecatory urge,

prompting the expulsive phase in which the anorectum comes into play.

ANORECTAL MOTILITY

ANORECTAL ANATOMY AND INNERVATION
(see also Chapters 93 and 122)

Before considering anorectal function during defecation, it is necessary to understand the gross morphology of the anorectum. Although the rectum is in direct continuity with the colon, the longitudinal muscle layer is not organized into teniae. Rather, it forms a continuous outer longitudinal muscle layer, uniformly encircling the rectum, insinuating distally between the internal and external anal sphincters, and extending to the distal end of the 3- to 4-cm-long anal canal. The narrowed distal rectum, or anorectal junction, is formed by the longitudinal muscle coat of the rectum, which is joined by the sling fibers of the puborectalis muscle, attachments of the levator ani muscles, and proximal margins of the internal and external anal sphincters. The puborectalis and levator ani muscles have important roles in maintaining continence and in defecation. These striated muscles form part of the pelvic floor and are in a state of constant tone that serves to pull the rectum anteriorly and elevate it, thereby reducing the anorectal angle. This mechanical effect tends to prevent entry of stool into the upper anal canal. The *internal anal sphincter* is a thickened band of smooth muscle, with relatively high spontaneous tone, which is in continuity with the circular smooth muscle of the rectum. By contrast, the *external anal sphincter* is a striated muscle and is located distal to, but partly overlying, the internal sphincter. The external sphincter also has a high resting tone, but unlike that of its internal counterpart, its tone can be influenced by voluntary efforts, to help maintain continence.

As expected, the sources of innervation of the internal anal sphincter and of the external anal sphincter are different. The internal sphincter is innervated extrinsically, through the pelvic plexus, by lumbar sympathetic and sacral parasympathetic nerves and receives a powerful inhibitory innervation from enteric inhibitory motor neurons, the cell bodies of which are in the enteric ganglia. The external anal sphincter and other pelvic floor muscles are innervated, through the pudendal nerve (S3-S4), by motor neurons with cell bodies in the spinal cord. The rectum and proximal anal canal are richly supplied with sensory receptors that respond to rectal stretch and the composition of the intraluminal contents. These receptors are important for detecting rectal filling, triggering sensations of urgency, facilitating rectal accommodation, and differentiating the composition (stool or gas) of rectal content.

RECTAL FILLING, CAPACITANCE, AND ACCOMMODATION AND MOTILITY OF THE ANAL SPHINCTERS

If stool or gas enters the rectum, the rectal wall is stretched, thereby simultaneously activating an enteric

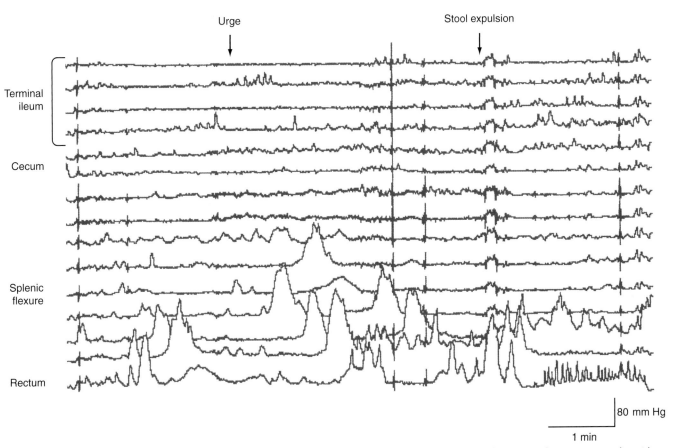

Figure 95–8 Intracolonic pressures leading to spontaneous defecation by the healthy human colon. Recordings were made with a Silastic-perfused catheter passed transnasally so that 15 recording sites at 7.5-cm intervals extended from the terminal ileum *(top)* to the rectum *(bottom)*. Four propagating pressure wave sequences lead up to actual stool expulsion. Each propagating sequence originates from a site more proximal than the preceding sequence. Note also the increase in amplitude and slowing of propagation velocity with successive sequences leading to stool expulsion, which in this example is achieved by a combination of voluntary straining and colonic propulsion. (From Bampton PA, Dinning PG, Kennedy ML, et al: Spatial and temporal organization of pressure patterns throughout the unprepared colon during spontaneous defecation. Am J Gastroenterol 95:1027, 2000.)

descending inhibitory reflex that causes relaxation of the internal anal sphincter and an extrinsic reflex pathway that leads to contraction of the external anal sphincter. The rectoanal inhibitory reflex can be demonstrated and tested by balloon distention of the rectum. Because the reflex is mediated by intramural enteric neural circuits, its presence reflects the integrity of enteric neural pathways. For example, the rectoanal inhibitory reflex is absent in Hirschsprung's disease, which is characterized by loss of enteric ganglia in the rectal myenteric plexus. In health, this reflex permits entry of a small amount of content into the upper anal canal, while continence is maintained by the reflexive contraction of the external anal sphincter. This "sampling" of the content by sensory receptors in the proximal anal canal permits the distinction between solid or liquid stool and gas. "Sampling reflexes" of this kind occur many times each day in response to low-volume rectal distentions, are not registered consciously, and do not cause an urge to defecate. A large-volume rectal distention causes an internal sphincter relaxation of longer duration, which is registered consciously and which necessitates extra voluntary contraction of the external anal sphincter to maintain continence while the person decides how best to deal with the intraluminal content

(stool or gas). Suppression of the defecation urge at this time, together with receptive accommodation of the rectum (see later), results in temporary storage of stool or gas in the rectum or retrograde transport of the stool or gas back to the sigmoid colon.

Although the rectum generally is empty, it has the capacity to temporarily store feces until convenient evacuation can be arranged. More prolonged rectal storage is made possible by the ability of the rectum to accommodate an increasing volume without a corresponding increase in intrarectal pressure, in a manner similar to gastric fundic relaxation.[23] This adaptive increase in rectal compliance, mediated by inhibitory nerves, is important for maintaining continence by permitting prolonged fecal storage without a constant urge to defecate. Such rectal distention also has negative feedback effects on the proximal bowel and inhibits gastric emptying, slows small bowel transit, reduces the frequency of proximal colonic propagating pressure waves, and delays colonic transit. Typically, rectal tone is increased following a meal. A pathologic reduction of rectal compliance, as seen, for example, after pelvic radiotherapy, causes rectal urgency. Conversely, excessive compliance, as in megarectum, attenuates the urge to defecate.

ANORECTAL MOTILITY DURING DEFECATION

If the processes just described give rise to the urge to defecate and the social circumstances are appropriate, the full defecation process is activated. This process involves a combination of pelvic reflexes coordinated in the medulla and pons. Rectal distention by a large volume of stool stimulates reflex relaxation of the internal anal sphincter, and the stool moves into the upper anal canal, heightening the sense of urge. Postural changes and straining facilitate this process in several ways: Sitting or squatting causes descent of the anorectal junction, and straining produces further rectal descent. Both activities serve to increase the anorectal angle, thereby reducing resistance to outflow. At this point, if the person wishes to proceed to expel stool, the external anal sphincter is relaxed voluntarily. At the same time, the puborectalis muscle is relaxed (further increasing the anorectal angle); the levator ani muscles contract; the perineum descends further; and stool is funneled into the anal canal and expelled by increasing strain-induced, intrarectal pressure (Fig. 95–9). Once the expulsion phase has commenced, evacuation of stool can proceed in some cases without further straining, as a consequence of colonic contrac-tions propagating toward the anus[24] (see Fig. 95–8). Expulsion of stool is possible in response to strain alone without rectosigmoid contractions, although a contribution from increased rectal wall tone cannot be excluded.

MODULATORS OF COLONIC MOTILITY

PHYSIOLOGIC MODULATORS: FOOD, SLEEP, AND STRESS

Twenty-four hour recordings of myoelectric activity or intraluminal pressure show that colonic phasic and tonic activity predictably is increased 1 to 2 hours after a meal (the "gastrocolonic response") and is markedly suppressed at night.[9,19,25] The entire colon responds to the meal, with an increase in colonic wall tone, migratory long spike bursts, and propagating and segmenting contractile patterns. It is interesting that a minimum caloric load of approximately 300 kcal is required to generate the colonic response to a meal,[25] and the response also is highly dependent on the fat content of the caloric load. For example, 600 kcal of fat induces the response, whereas equal caloric loads of protein or carbohydrate do

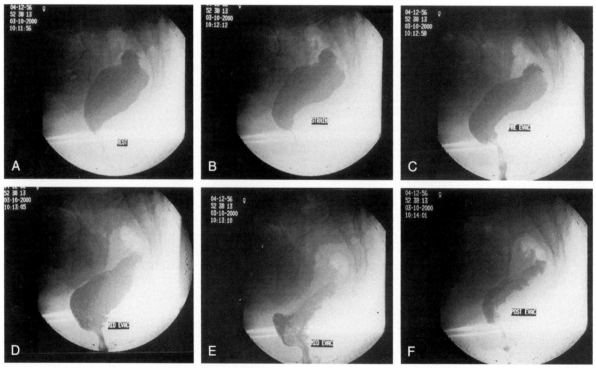

Figure 95–9   Some of the mechanical processes that facilitate stool expulsion, as illustrated by sequential films of a simulated defecation of thickened barium during defecation proctography. *A,* The rectum at rest with a normal resting angle of approximately 90 degrees; the anal canal is closed. *B,* On straining, as the anterior rectal wall begins to flatten, the proximal anal canal begins to funnel as barium contrast is forced into it. *C,* As more pressure is exerted, the anterior rectal wall flattens further, contrast fills the anal canal, and evacuation begins. At this time, the puborectalis muscle and external anal sphincter are relaxing, resulting in the onset of descent of the rectoanal junction. At the same time, the levator ani muscles are activated and help control the descent of the rectoanal junction (e.g., note the posterior indentation resulting from pubococcygeus muscle contraction). *D,* The puborectalis is fully relaxed; this, in combination with vigorous straining, has resulted in nearly complete descent of the rectoanal junction. Note the position of the rectoanal junction, which in this frame is well below the *horizontal pale artifact* (due to the water-filled toilet seat), compared with that in the previous frame, in which the junction is level with this artifact. This descent has now opened up the anorectal angle, thereby reducing further the resistance to outflow through the anal canal. *E,* Rectal emptying continues, and anterior rectal compression is more obvious. *F,* After evacuation, the anorectal junction has ascended to its original position, and the anorectal angle has returned to its more acute resting angle. (Courtesy of Prof. D. Z. Lubowski.)

not. The mechanism of the response to the meal remains unclear, but it is known that neither the stomach nor the spinal cord need to be intact to display the response. Non-nutrient gastric distention, by balloon or water, also can stimulate rectosigmoid motility, yielding a similar response to that with intraduodenal lipid infusion. Both of these responses are markedly attenuated by prior intravenous administration of the 5-hydroxytryptamine-3 (5-HT₃) receptor antagonist granisetron, which suggests that 5-HT₃ receptors on vagal afferents may be involved in the gastrocolic response.[26] Cholecystokinin (CCK), which is released by fats and fatty acids in the duodenum, can reproduce the gastrocolic response but only at doses exceeding those occurring postprandially. The CCK-A antagonist loxiglumide blocks the effects of CCK on the colon but does not abolish the gastrocolic response, thus making CCK an unlikely mediator of the response.

Colonic myoelectric and pressure activities are profoundly suppressed at night.[9,19,25] During stable sleep, propagating pressure waves virtually cease, thereby reducing the challenges to continence at a time when anal sphincter tone and awareness of colorectal sensations are minimal. If the subject moves to a lighter level of sleep, even without actually awakening, an immediate increase occurs in propagating and nonpropagating pressure waves (Fig. 95–10). Forced awakening at night and spontaneous early-morning awakening both stimulate an immediate increase in colonic propagating pressure waves.[9,19] This phenomenon clearly is linked with the readily identifiable habit of defecation soon after awakening in the morning and demonstrates the potential for profound modulation of colonic motor activity by the central nervous system. Stress and emotional factors long have been assumed to influence colonic motility, but evidence for this influence is conflicting, possibly because of reliance on distal colonic recording sites. In light of the profound waking response, it is likely, but unproved, that stress does induce propagating pressure waves.

PHARMACOLOGIC MODULATORS

Laxatives exert their diarrheal actions by increasing mucosal secretion or by stimulating colonic propulsive activity. For example, the irritant laxative bisacodyl and the bile acid chenodeoxycholic acid both stimulate colonic propagating sequences, thereby leading to mass movements. Bisacodyl exerts its motor effect through afferent nerve fibers in the mucosa, because the response can be blocked by topical application of lidocaine to the mucosa. In addition to the local response, these agents, when administered rectally, also can induce an increase in motor activity in the proximal colon, a finding that indicates the existence of long reflex pathways between the rectum and proximal colon.

Serotonin (5-HT) is an important mediator of bowel physiology, and both 5-HT₃ and 5-HT₄ receptors play a role in colonic peristalsis and transit. For example, the 5-HT₃ receptor antagonists granisetron and ondansetron blunt the gastrocolic response and delay colonic transit, respectively.[26] Alosetron, another antagonist of the 5-HT₃ receptor, exerts a significant constipating affect by slowing colonic transit.[27] By contrast, the 5-HT₄ agonists, such as tegaserod, induce colonic propagating contractions and accelerate colonic transit, thereby showing promise in the treatment of constipation.[28,29]

Opiates are well known to have an antidiarrheal effect, but their mechanism of action is less clear. In the human colon in vivo, morphine increases phasic segmenting activity, which is likely to retard flow, and may promote

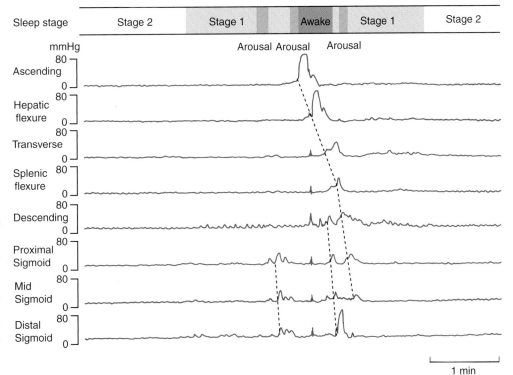

Figure 95–10 Relationship of propagating pressure wave sequences to nocturnal arousals. An arousal represents a lightening of the level of sleep and need not necessarily culminate in waking. This example demonstrates an arousal-induced event propagating from the proximal to the distal sigmoid colon and followed by another arousal-induced event propagating from the ascending colon to the sigmoid. Only the second arousal culminated in a brief period of wakefulness. Repetitive propagating sequences of this type are seen also on early-morning awakening. (From Furukawa Y, Cook IJ, Panagopoulos V, et al: Relationship between sleep patterns and human colonic motor patterns. Gastroenterology 107:1372, 1994.)

mixing and enhance absorption. Barostat studies have shown that morphine also reduces colonic tone and attenuates the bowel's response to a meal.[30] Opiates are known to inhibit both presynaptic and postsynaptic enteric neural circuitry. Therefore, it seems likely that these drugs reduce neurally dependent propagating contractions and favor myogenic mixing movements—both effects contributing to the constipating effect.

DISORDERS OF COLONIC MOTILITY

Disorders attributable to disturbed colonic motor function are discussed elsewhere in this book (see Chapter 117). It is useful, however, to consider how disturbances in the mechanisms of colonic motility described in this chapter may relate to symptoms or pathophysiologic phenomena.

CONSTIPATION (see Chapter 12)

Intuitively, one would expect that constipation and diarrhea should be manifestations of hypomotility and hypermotility, respectively. Sometimes this is true, but in the distal colon, at least, the converse may be true. A paradoxical increase in nonpropagating (segmenting) contractions and myoelectrical short spike bursts has been reported in the rectosigmoid region in constipated patients. Conversely, patients with diarrhea have hypomotility in this region.[31] It is likely that segmenting activity retards forward flow, whereas suppression of such activity permits unrestricted access of stool to the rectum, where a defecatory urge is initiated. Thus, constipation may be a consequence either of infrequent or ineffective propagating pressure waves or of an increase in segmenting distal colonic pressure waves, or perhaps both.

In severe slow-transit constipation, prolonged manometric studies have confirmed a reduction in the overall number of high-amplitude propagating pressure waves. The underlying pathogenesis of severe slow transit constipation is unclear, but changes in the populations of enteric excitatory motor neurons to the smooth muscle in patients with severe slow transit constipation are likely to underpin this disorder.[32] By contrast, in patients with obstructed defecation (outlet delay), normal numbers of propagating pressure waves are demonstrated throughout the colon, and the defecatory urge is preserved, although during the urge, the normal stereotypical increase in frequency and amplitude of these propagating pressure waves is lacking.

DIARRHEA (see also Chapter 9)

Detailed scintigraphic studies in patients with diarrhea have shown the dominant feature to be early and rapid transit through the ascending and transverse colon.[33] Normally, propagating sequences are more frequent in these proximal regions than elsewhere. Manometric data from the entire colon in patients with diarrhea, to help explain these observations, are lacking. A relative lack of distal colonic segmenting activity, perhaps in combination with increased proximal colonic propagating pressure waves, may explain this preferential acceleration of proximal colonic transit, but proof of this hypothesis is awaited.

IRRITABLE BOWEL SYNDROME
(see also Chapter 115)

Although colonic transit generally is slower in constipation-predominant irritable bowel syndrome (IBS) and faster in diarrhea-predominant IBS, no colonic motor pattern is specific for IBS. Exaggerated responses to stimuli such as meals, CCK, and mechanical stimuli have been reported, but a consistent disturbance has not emerged, probably because of the heterogeneity of the disease and the methodologies used for characterization. In addition, remarkably little study of the proximal colon in IBS has been conducted to date. At present, compelling evidence regarding the pathophysiology of IBS suggests a major contribution by afferent hypersensitivity, in addition to a variable alteration in colonic motor function.

COLONIC MOTILITY DISTURBANCES SECONDARY TO NONMOTOR INTESTINAL DISORDERS

Altered motility secondary to underlying inflammation or a hormonal disturbance can contribute to the colonic symptoms of a nonmotor disease. The diarrhea of idiopathic inflammatory bowel disease, for example, results from a combination of enhanced secretion, reduced absorption, and altered colonic motor function. In ulcerative colitis, rectosigmoid-segmenting, nonpropagating pressure waves are diminished, whereas postprandial propagating pressure waves are increased.[12,34] Rectal compliance also is reduced, and together, these effects may exacerbate diarrhea, as suggested by studies demonstrating rapid rectosigmoid transit in ulcerative colitis.[12] The motility of the healthy colon also can be perturbed by ileal diseases. For example, exposure of the healthy proximal colon to supranormal concentrations of bile salts (resulting, for example, from terminal ileal disease or resection) not only stimulates net colonic secretion but also initiates high-amplitude propagating pressure waves, thereby accelerating colonic transit.[12]

REFERENCES

1. Rae MG, Fleming N, McGregor DB, et al: Control of motility patterns in the human colonic circular muscle layer by pacemaker activity. J Physiol 510(pt 1):309, 1998.
2. Farrugia G: Ionic conductances in gastrointestinal smooth muscles and interstitial cells of Cajal. Annu Rev Physiol 61:45, 1999.
3. Sanders KM, Ordog T, Torihashi S, Ward SM: Development and plasticity of interstitial cells of Cajal. Neurogastroenterol Motil 11:311, 1999.
4. Porter AJ, Wattchow DA, Brookes SJ, Costa M: The neurochemical coding and projections of circular muscle motor

neurons in the human colon. Gastroenterology 113:1916, 1997.

5. Lynn PA, Olsson CA, Zagorodnyuk VP, et al: Rectal intraganglionic laminar endings are transduction sites of extrinsic mechanoreceptors in the guinea pig rectum. Gastroenterology 125:786, 2003.

6. Sarna SK: Physiology and pathophysiology of colonic motor activity: Part 1. Dig Dis Sci 36:827, 1991.

7. Spencer NJ, Bywater RAR, Taylor GS: Disinhibition during myoelectric complexes in the mouse colon. J Auton Nerv Syst 71:37, 1998.

8. Dinning PG, Szczesniak M, Cook IJ: Removal of tonic nitrergic inhibition is a potent stimulus for human proximal colonic propagating sequences. Neurogastroenterol Motil 18:37, 2006.

9. Furukawa Y, Cook IJ, Panagopoulos V, et al: Relationship between sleep patterns and human colonic motor patterns. Gastroenterology 107:1372, 1994.

10. Martelli H, Devroede G, Arhan P, et al: Mechanisms of idiopathic constipation: Outlet obstruction. Gastroenterology 75:623, 1978.

11. Metcalf AM, Phillips SF, Zinsmeister AR, et al: Simplified assessment of segmental colonic transit. Gastroenterology 97:40, 1987.

12. O'Brien MD, Phillips SF: Colonic motility in health and disease. Gastroenterol Clin North Am 25:147, 1996.

13. Spiller RC, Brown ML, Phillips SF: Emptying of the terminal ileum in intact humans. Influence of meal residue and ileal motility. Gastroenterology 92:724, 1987.

14. Dinning PG, Bampton PA, Kennedy ML, et al: Basal pressure patterns and reflexive motor responses in the human ileocolonic junction. Am J Physiol 276:G331, 1999.

15. Dinning PG, Bampton PA, Kennedy ML, Cook IJ: Relationship between terminal ileal pressure waves and propagating proximal colonic pressure waves. Am J Physiol 277:G983, 1999.

16. Hammer J, Phillips SF: Fluid loading of the human colon: Effects on segmental transit and stool composition. Gastroenterology 105:988, 1993.

17. Hardcastle JD, Mann CV: Physical factors in the stimulation of colonic peristalsis. Gut 11:41, 1970.

18. Dinning PG, Bampton PA, Kennedy ML, et al: The frequency of retrograde colonic propagating sequences may depend upon colonic loading. [abstract] *Neurogastroenterol Motil* 15:591, A:330, 2003.

19. Bassotti G, Crowell MD, Whitehead WE: Contractile activity of the human colon: Lessons from 24-hour studies. Gut 34:129, 1993.

20. Cook IJ, Furukawa Y, Panagopoulos V, et al: Relationships between spatial patterns of colonic pressure and individual movements of content. Am J Physiol 278:G329, 2000.

21. Lubowski DZ, Meagher AP, Smart RC, Butler SP: Scintigraphic assessment of colonic function during defecation. Int J Colorect Dis 10:91, 1995.

22. Bampton PA, Dinning PG, Kennedy ML, et al: Spatial and temporal organization of pressure patterns throughout the unprepared colon during spontaneous defecation. Am J Gastroenterol 95:1027, 2000.

23. Bell AM, Pemberton JH, Hanson RB, Zinsmeister AR: Variations in muscle tone of the human rectum: Recordings with an electromechanical barostat. Am J Physiol 260:G17, 1991.

24. Bampton PA, Dinning PG, Kennedy ML, et al: Spatial and temporal organization of pressure patterns throughout the unprepared colon during spontaneous defecation. Am J Gastroenterol 95:1027, 2000.

25. Frexinos J, Bueno L, Fioramonti J: Diurnal changes in myoelectric spiking activity of the human colon. Gastroenterology 88:1104, 1985.

26. Bjornsson ES, Chey WD, Ladabaum U, et al: Differential 5-HT$_3$ mediation of human gastrocolonic response and colonic peristaltic reflex. Am J Physiol 275:G498, 1998.

27. Houghton LA, Foster JM, Whorwell PJ: Alosetron, a 5-HT$_3$ receptor antagonist, delays colonic transit in patients with irritable bowel syndrome and healthy volunteers. Aliment Pharmacol Ther 14:775, 2000.

28. Schiller LR: New and emerging treatment options for chronic constipation. Rev Gastroenterol Disord 4:S43, 2004.

29. Johanson J, Wald A, Tougas G, et al: Effect of tegaserod in chronic constipation: A randomized, double-blind, controlled trial. Clin Gastroenterol Hepatol 2:796, 2004.

30. Kamath PS, Phillips SF, O'Connor MK, et al: Colonic capacitance and transit in man: Modulation by luminal contents and drugs. Gut 31:443, 1990.

31. Connell AM: The motility of the pelvic colon. II. Paradoxical motility in diarrhoea and constipation. Gut 3:342, 1962.

32. Porter AJ, Wattchow DA, Hunter A, Costa M: Abnormalities of nerve fibres in the circular muscle of patients with slow transit constipation. Int J Colorect Dis 13:208, 1998.

33. Vassallo MJ, Camilleri M, Phillips SF, et al: Transit through the proximal colon influences stool weight in the irritable bowel syndrome. Gastroenterology 102:102, 1992.

34. Bassotti G, deRoberto G, Chistolini F, et al: Twenty-four hour manometric study of colonic propulsive activity in patients with diarrhea due to inflammatory (ulcerative colitis) and non-inflammatory (irritable bowel syndrome) conditions. Int J Colorectal Dis 19:493, 2004.

CHAPTER
96 Intestinal Water and Electrolyte Transport

Laura E. Harrell and Eugene B. Chang

Little thought is given to the complex and wonderful functions of the digestive tract, particularly in ensuring efficient digestion and absorption of a meal and in meeting the metabolic needs of the body. In view of the substantial variations in the composition and volume of daily oral intake, the capability of the gut to adapt to most physiologic perturbations is remarkable. Digestive functions generally proceed without conscious effort and without problems, a fact often taken for granted until abdominal symptoms or digestive diseases arise. Diarrhea results when the intestinal absorptive capacity is exceeded. Under normal circumstances, this is rare because the intestine is able to tightly control absorptive and secretory processes through an intricate network of regulatory systems. Aberrations in cellular functions or in the homeostatic regulation of intestinal transport functions, however, can result in serious clinical manifestations.

As a system of organs connected in series, the digestive tract has many highly specialized regions that both absorb and secrete water and electrolytes. Secretion is necessary to provide an aqueous phase for food digestion and delivery of important digestive enzymes and antibodies. Absorption, which is carefully regulated, is required to meet the body's metabolic demands and to prevent excessive loss of fluid (diarrhea).

On average, the luminal fluid load of the gut is approximately 9 L per day, composed of oral intake and endogenous secretions. Of this volume, approximately 8.8 L per day or more is absorbed: 7 L per day in the small intestine and 1.8 L per day in the colon. Less than 0.2 L is excreted as a component of the normal stool output (with a typical Western, low-roughage diet). This process represents a highly efficient rate of absorption of greater than 98%, most of which occurs in the small intestine (Fig. 96–1). This efficiency is possible because of the presence of a proximal-to-distal gradient of mucosal permeability to passive flux of water and electrolytes (Fig. 96–2); the small bowel is "leakier," allowing it to accommodate rapid changes in water and electrolyte fluxes that occur after a meal.

In contrast with the small intestine, the colon typically receives about 2 L of fluid per day, most of which must be absorbed against high electrochemical gradients to make solid stool. For this process to be possible, the permeability of the colon and rectum must be less—they must be less "leaky," to prevent back-flux of absorbed water and electrolytes. When rapid changes in dietary intake or endogenous secretions occur, the intestinal mucosa can modulate its overall transport functions to compensate acutely. If the perturbations are large and persistent, however, other adaptive responses that significantly enhance the overall absorptive capacity of the intestines can be called into play to prevent the development of diarrhea or malabsorption. The colon, for example, can increase its maximal absorptive capacity greater than twofold over time.

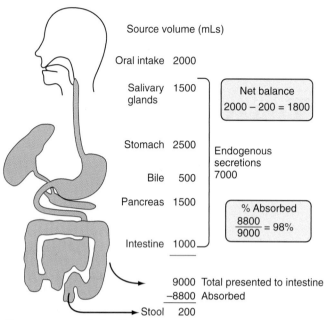

Figure 96–1 Daily fluid load presented to the gastrointestinal tract.

Surface property	Amplification factor	Estimated surface area (cm²)
Cylinder	1	3,300
Plices conniventes	3	10,000
Villi	10	100,000
Microvilli	20	2,000,000

Estimated total surface area—200 m²

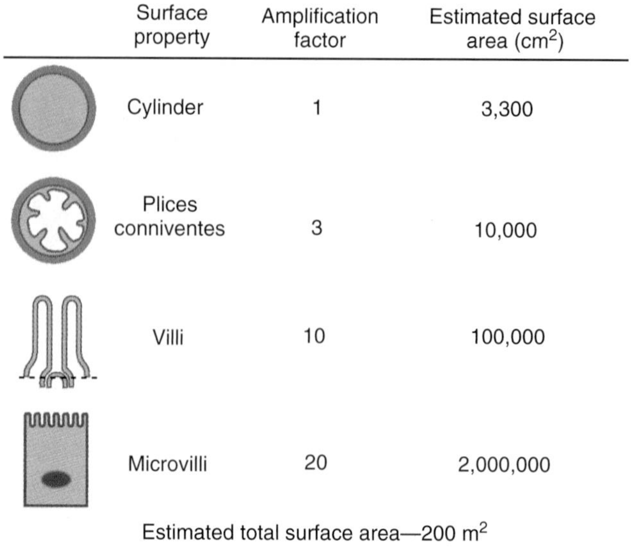

Figure 96–3 Topographic features of the small intestine and the degree to which each factor amplifies the absorptive surface area.

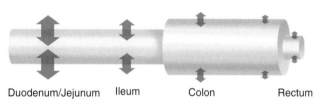

Figure 96–2 Gradient of mucosal permeability to the passive diffusion of water and electrolytes in the small intestine and colon. Passive diffusion of water and electrolytes is greatest in the proximal small intestine and diminishes progressively in the more distal regions of the bowel. This relationship is essential for efficient digestion, secretion, and absorption, and for formation of solid stool.

The tremendous absorptive capacity of the gastrointestinal tract also can be attributed to the large absorptive surface area achieved through the unusual topography of the intestinal mucosa, which is composed of plicae conniventes (folds), villi, and microvilli (Fig. 96–3). Each component contributes an amplification factor that increases the absorptive surface area by almost 600 times that of a simple cylinder. The entire surface area of the small intestine is estimated to be 200 m², or roughly the size of a doubles tennis court (175 m²). Thus, absorption can remain efficient despite changes in transit time, intestinal content, or other physiologic perturbations.

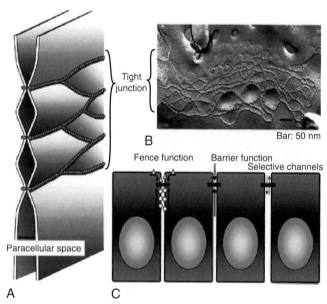

Figure 96–4 Structure and function of the intestinal epithelial tight junction. *A,* The tight junction is formed by points of intercellular contact regulated by several integral membrane proteins. *B,* Freeze-fracture view of the tight junction. *C,* Tight junctions function as molecular fences and selective barriers. See text for details. (Reproduced with permission from Sawada N, Murata M, Kikuchi K, et al: Tight junctions and human diseases. Med Electron Microsc 36:147, 2003.)

FEATURES OF THE INTESTINAL MUCOSA ESSENTIAL FOR WATER AND ELECTROLYTE TRANSPORT

EPITHELIAL BARRIER FUNCTION

An essential feature of the intestinal mucosa is the presence of intercellular tight junctions, which prevent free permeation of substances that otherwise would be harmful to the body or lead to losses of bodily fluids and electrolytes (Fig. 96–4*A* and *B*). Tight junctions are selective and dynamic in function and are regulated by a number of signaling pathways and cellular processes that can determine size selectivity and flow of molecules across this barrier. The tight junction also functions as a molecular fence that restricts plasma membrane proteins of the apical and basolateral membranes to their proper domains, an essential feature for efficient vectoral transport of water, nutrient, and electrolytes and digestive functions (see Fig. 96–4*C*).

The belt-like arrangement of tight junctions is similar to that of a plastic holder for a beverage six-pack. The basic structure of the tight junction complex is shown in Figure 96-4*B*. The intercellular connections are made at points regulated by at least three major intercellular proteins, including occludin, claudin, and junction adhesion molecules (JAMs).[1-3] Occludin and claudin have four membrane-spanning domains, whereas JAMs have only one.[4] Associated with these proteins are several cytoskeletal proteins including isoforms of zonulin, MAGI (membrane-associated guanyl kinase inverted proteins), and PAR (partitioning-defective protein), many having PDZ domains that serve as sites of binding and interaction with other proteins, particularly integral membrane proteins of the tight junction.[4] The coxsackievirus and adenovirus receptor (CAR) is another protein that appears to be associated with the tight junction; however, it appears to be specifically targeted by pathogenic viruses, bacteria, and parasites, allowing these organisms to infect the cell.[5]

For many years, the tight junction was viewed as a static structure. More recent studies, however, have clearly shown that several signaling pathways and effector proteins regulate them, thereby greatly influencing paracellular permeability. One interesting example is the regulation of tight junction permeability by myosin light chain kinase (MLCK), which is activated under a number of physiologic and pathophysiologic circumstances. The absorption of glucose by means of the Na^+-glucose cotransporter results in the activation of MLCK.[6]

EPITHELIAL CELLS

Intestinal epithelial cells line the intestinal surface and represent the largest population of mucosal cells. Intestinal epithelial cells play a major role in barrier, digestive, defensive, absorptive, and secretory functions. Four major types of intestinal epithelial cells are recognized (Fig. 96–5): (1) columnar, polarized epithelial cells capable of vectoral transport of nutrients and electrolytes; (2) mucous or goblet cells; (3) mucosal endocrine cells; and (4) Paneth cells, found at the base of intestinal crypts, which secrete defensins, molecules with antimicrobial properties. Intestinal epithelial cells originate from the proliferative zone near the base of the crypt. With the exception of Paneth cells, these cells differentiate as they migrate up the villus axis and eventually slough off into the intestinal lumen. This process takes 3 to 5 days, during which time crypt cells mature into villus cells.

The columnar cells have polarity—their luminal and basolateral membranes differ in their functional and physical properties. As discussed later, these differences are essential for vectoral transport of water and electrolytes. In addition, columnar cells form a physical barrier between luminal contents and the host and are essential for the protection of the host against pathogens and harmful agents and for efficient transport of water, electrolytes, and nutrients. Villus and crypt cells are different in appearance and also serve different functions (Fig. 96–6). Crypt cells are relatively immature, short, cuboidal cells that have rudimentary microvilli, terminal webs (cytoskeletal structures located at the luminal pole), and tight junction complexes. Villus cells are tall, mature columnar cells that have well-developed microvilli, ter-

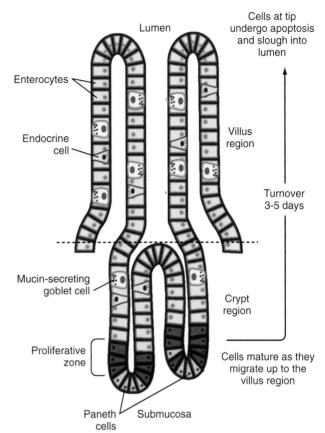

Figure 96–5 Types of epithelial cells of the intestinal mucosa: enterocytes, endocrine cells, goblet cells, and Paneth cells. All of these cell types originate from the proliferative zone near the base of the intestinal crypt. With the exception of Paneth cells, these cells migrate up the villus axis, mature during this process, and eventually undergo apoptosis and slough after 3 to 5 days at the tip of the villus. Paneth cells remain at the base of the crypt and make defensins, which are important in host defense.

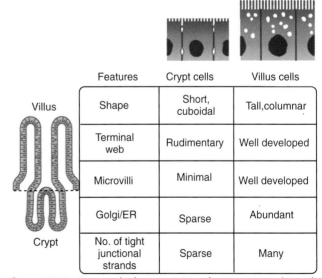

Features	Crypt cells	Villus cells
Shape	Short, cuboidal	Tall, columnar
Terminal web	Rudimentary	Well developed
Microvilli	Minimal	Well developed
Golgi/ER	Sparse	Abundant
No. of tight junctional strands	Sparse	Many

Figure 96–6 Structural characteristics of enterocytes along the crypt-villus axis. Crypt cells exhibit a less differentiated phenotype, with less well-developed microvilli, terminal webs, and tight junctional complexes than villus cells. Villus cells have more differentiated features, being more columnar-shaped and more well-developed microvilli, terminal webs, and tight junctional complexes. ER, endoplasmic reticulum.

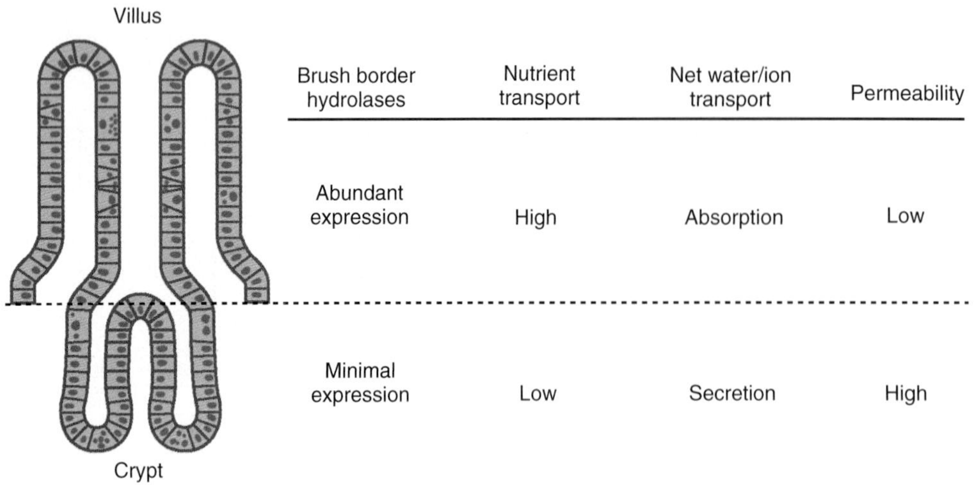

	Brush border hydrolases	Nutrient transport	Net water/ion transport	Permeability
Abundant expression		High	Absorption	Low
Minimal expression		Low	Secretion	High

Figure 96–7 Functional characteristics of enterocytes along the crypt-villus axis. Crypt enterocytes are more secretory, whereas villus cells are more absorptive. (Reproduced with permission from Chang EB, et al [eds]: Gastrointestinal, Hepatobiliary, and Nutritional Physiology. Philadelphia, Lippincott-Raven, 1996.)

minal webs, and tight junctions, features required for efficient absorption of nutrients and electrolytes. The Golgi-endoplasmic reticulum, which is essential for synthesis of membrane and secreted proteins, also is more developed in villus cells.

As shown in Figure 96–7, villus and crypt cells have different functional characteristics. Crypt cells are primarily secretory cells and have little absorptive capacity. The mucosal permeability in this region also is greater, to accommodate the rapid water and electrolyte fluxes that accompany active anion secretion. By contrast, villus cells exhibit a variety of absorptive processes for nutrients and electrolytes. They also express brush border proteins such as hydrolases that are involved in the digestion of micronutrients. Finally, the passive permeability of this region of the mucosa is less than in the crypt region, in order to prevent back-flux of absorbed nutrients, electrolytes, and water.

CAPILLARIES AND LYMPHATICS

Blood capillaries and lymphatics have an important role in intestinal water and electrolyte transport. Flow through these structures is regulated in coordination with other digestive functions such as mucosal transport and motor functions, an effect made possible by the complex enteric neural network and hormonal signals that integrate these functions.[7-12] Thus, during absorption, blood capillaries carry away nutrients, water, and electrolytes in amounts commensurate with the load received from absorbing enterocytes.[13,14] During active secretion, blood flow and capillary filtration increase and villus lymphatic pressure and lymphatic flow decrease.[10,11] These changes are necessary to deliver fluid and electrolytes at a sufficient rate to meet the demands for luminal digestive processes. Just as in the kidney, a countercurrent flow mechanism has been proposed to exist in the villus core between efferent and afferent blood capillaries, resulting in a concentration gradient that further enhances net fluid and electrolyte transport; little substantive evidence is available, however, to support the existence of a countercurrent mechanism.[12]

INTESTINAL MOTILITY

Intestinal motility and water and electrolyte transport are very much interdependent functions of the digestive tract. This interdependence was observed as early as 1912 by Babkin and Ishikawa, who noted that the periodicity of intestinal motor activity paralleled that of intestinal secretion.[15] The integration of these processes is a major function of enteric neural reflexes, which, in the initial phases of digestion, rapidly stimulate intestinal secretion, to liquify luminal contents and activate digestive enzymes. The concomitant stimulation of mixing and propulsive motor functions is important for proper mixing of digestive juices with food, and also increases the exposure of luminal fluid with the absorptive surface area.

It commonly is assumed that increased propulsive motor activity of the gastrointestinal tract is a major cause of diarrhea; however, this is unlikely to be true except in unusual circumstances. Rather, increased propulsive activity can contribute to the severity of diarrhea, which largely arises from decreased net absorption of water and electrolytes. Decreasing propulsive activity can increase contact time between luminal fluid and the absorptive surface area, thereby allowing increased net absorption.[16-18] Such slowing of propulsion is largely the basis for the pharmacologic and antidiarrheal actions of agents such as opiates, loperamide, and α_2-adrenergic agonists.

MUCOSAL COMPONENTS INVOLVED IN THE REGULATION AND MODULATION OF INTESTINAL WATER AND ELECTROLYTE TRANSPORT

Figure 96–8 illustrates the numerous mucosal components and cells that play a role in the physiologic regulation of intestinal water and electrolyte transport; all have specific actions that are integrated to ensure efficient digestive, secretory, motor, and absorptive functions.

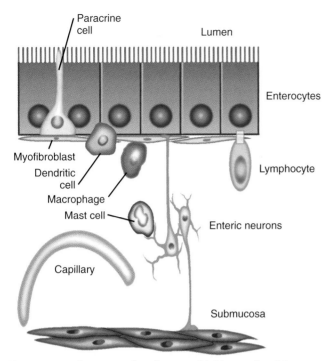

Figure 96–8 Enterocyte functions are highly regulated by many components of the intestinal mucosa. Each component has a specific action and target, but the effects of all the components are integrated to ensure efficient digestive and transport functions of the intestinal mucosa. For example, dendritic and paracrine cells are capable of sensing changes in the luminal compartment, to which they respond by elaborating activating substances that may affect enterocyte functions directly or indirectly by influencing other processes such as blood flow and motility.

MUCOSAL ENDOCRINE CELLS

Endocrine cells are key players in the regulation of intestinal fluid and electrolyte transport and are interspersed between epithelial cells of the gastric and intestinal mucosa. These cells allow the mucosa to sense and quickly respond to changes in luminal contents. Activated cells release hormonal peptides and active amines, which, through paracrine control, alter blood and lymphatic flow, intestinal motility, and ion transport function of nearby cells. Paracrine control is said to occur when a producer cell, such as a mucosal endocrine cell, releases signaling molecules that affect a single cell type in close proximity, such as intestinal epithelial cells. Well-defined microvilli, located on the apical (luminal) surface of the endocrine cells, sense alterations in luminal factors including pH, osmolality, and chemical contents of the luminal milieu.[19,20] In response, secretory granules containing active amines and polypeptide hormones are released at the basal surface of the cell. Although the contents of the secretory granules of these cells are very similar to amines and polypeptides found in the nerve cells of the enteric nervous system, it is likely that the endocrine cells have a unique and independent role in modulating various mucosal functions. Many of the amines and peptides released by endocrine cells have been shown to stimulate net secretion or absorption of intestinal fluids and electrolytes.

Active amines and hormonal polypeptides are distributed regionally throughout the gastrointestinal tract. For instance, cells containing gastrin, cholecystokinin (CCK), and secretin are found in the stomach and proximal small intestine; neurotensin-containing cells are located in the ileum; serotonin-containing enterochromaffin cells are found throughout the gastrointestinal tract, but predominantly in the crypt regions[20-22]; and guanylyl cyclase C (GC-C), a receptor for *Escherichia coli* heat-stable enterotoxin (STa) and the circulating peptides guanylin and uroguanylin,[23,24] is distributed throughout the brush border membrane of the small intestine and the colon, although it is most abundant in the proximal small intestine.[25] STa receptors also have been found on the basolateral membrane of colonocytes, suggesting that circulating guanylin and uroguanylin function through these receptors.[26]

ENTERIC NEURONS

The gastrointestinal tract is richly innervated by the intrinsic and extrinsic nervous systems (see Chapters 94 and 95). Neural regulation of the gastrointestinal tract integrates the processes of intestinal water and electrolyte transport, motility, and blood flow. The intrinsic and enteric nervous systems are composed of afferent neurons, interneurons, and efferent neurons, all of which have cell bodies located within the bowel wall. Numerous neurotransmitters are released by these nerves, including active amines (e.g., serotonin, acetylcholine), neuropeptides (e.g., substance P, neurotensin, CCK, neuropeptide Y, somatostatin, calcitonin gene–related peptide, vasoactive intestinal polypeptide, galanin), and purinergic neurotransmitters (e.g., adenosine, adenosine triphosphate [ATP]). Sensory neurons are capable of sensing mechanical stimuli (e.g., touch, pressure, tension), temperature, noxious stimuli, and changes in luminal contents (including changes in pH, osmolality, and amino acids). Activated afferent neurons stimulate interneurons, nerves that integrate afferent signals and efferent motor neurons. Efferent motor neurons may directly stimulate intestinal epithelial cells, affecting water and electrolyte transport. Sensory signals also are relayed to motor neurons, which affect the motor activity of intestinal smooth muscle, allowing for the mixing of the intestinal contents and digestive juices. The enteric nervous system is capable of functioning independently but also may be modified by the autonomic nervous system.

The extrinsic autonomic nervous system is composed of the parasympathetic and sympathetic nerve pathways. Preganglionic sympathetic fibers synapse in the celiac, mesenteric, and pelvic ganglia with postganglionic fibers, which mostly terminate in the enteric ganglia. A few postganglionic sympathetic fibers also have been reported to synapse with intestinal epithelial cells.[27-29] When norepinephrine is released from these neurons, α_2-adrenergic receptors on the basolateral membranes of the enterocytes are stimulated, resulting in a combination of increased electroneutral absorption of sodium chloride (NaCl) and inhibition of electrogenic anion secretion.[29-31] The role of the parasympathetic system in the regulation of intestinal electrolyte and water transport is less well understood. Some vagal postganglionic fibers modulate the responses of enteric neurons.[32] These postganglionic fibers, probably emanating from myenteric and submucosal neural plexuses, might stimulate net secretion through the secretion of anions, mainly bicarbonate (HCO_3^-) and Cl^-, and the inhibition of electroneutral NaCl absorption, also causing propulsive motor activity and decreasing intestinal transit time.

MESENCHYMAL CELLS OF THE LAMINA PROPRIA

Mesenchymal cells of the lamina propria, including subepithelial fibroblasts, endothelial cells, and innate immune cells such as neutrophils, dendritic cells, resident macrophages, mast cells, eosinophils, and T and B lymphocytes, the latter primarily IgA-bearing,[33] are important in the modulation of intestinal mucosal transport, blood flow, and motor function. The roles of each of these cells in the regulation of intestinal water and electrolyte transport under normal physiologic states, and during pathophysiologic conditions such as infection and inflammatory processes, are not understood precisely.[34]

These cells help regulate intestinal transport of water and electrolytes through a juxtacrine pathway. Juxtacrine control is said to occur when a producer cell, often an innate immune cell within the lamina propria, releases signaling molecules that target multiple cell types such as enteric neuronal cells, endothelial cells, or enterocytes. The mesenchymal cells release a number of mediators, which act on nearby neurons or epithelial cells, influencing the function of these cells.[33] For example, mast cells may release a number of inflammatory mediators such as histamine, adenosine, platelet-activating factor, serotonin, and arachidonic acid metabolites in response to exposure of the mast cell to food antigens or helminth parasites.[33,34] These inflammatory mediators activate nearby enteric neurons, as well as epithelial receptors, with the net result that electroneutral NaCl absorption is decreased and electrogenic anion secretion is increased.[35-40] The secretory response also may be amplified by the release of neurotransmitters from activated enteric neurons.[41]

Macrophages and dendritic cells present in the intestinal mucosa account for 10% to 20% of the cells of the lamina propria.[42] Monocytes continuously travel from the bloodstream to the intestinal mucosa and there mature into macrophages, providing constant turnover of macrophages.[43] The intestinal environment sensitizes the macrophages by continuous exposure to foreign antigens and pathogens present in the colon, after which they are able to react in a rapid manner to various stimuli, allowing them to function as a first line of defense against antigens and pathogens.[44,45] Macrophages initiate the immune and inflammatory response, releasing various mediators, including reactive oxygen, cyclooxygenase, and 5-lipoxygenase metabolites; cytokines such as interleukin-1 (IL-1), IL-6, and granulocyte-macrophage colony-stimulating factor (GM-CSF); and inflammatory mediators such as platelet-activating factor and purinergic agents.[46,47] Many of these mediators are known to modulate water and electrolyte transport and to affect the

motor function of the intestine, capillary blood flow, and permeability.[33,34,41,48-51]

NEUROHUMORAL REGULATION OF INTESTINAL SECRETION AND ABSORPTION

Net intestinal secretion or absorption is the result of interaction of the effects of many different factors, including peptides, active amines, hormones, and neurotransmitters, that circulate in the blood or are released locally from mucosal epithelial cells, lamina propria cells, or enteric neurons. These factors can be classified as secretagogues or pro-absorptive agents, depending on the overall effect of the agent on intestinal cells. Secretagogues cause a net increase in intestinal secretion either by stimulating secretory processes or by inhibiting absorption, whereas pro-absorptive agents promote absorption of fluid and electrolytes. Table 96–1 lists a number of regulators of intestinal water and electrolyte transport and the putative signaling pathways that mediate their actions.

The list is not all-inclusive, and the relative roles of each agent under physiologic or pathophysiologic circumstances are not known. Various sources for these agents have been recognized, including many of the mucosal cells described earlier. In many cases, these cells are strategically placed so that the release of their active agents can stimulate numerous cell targets, thereby integrating their functions. For instance, release of endocrine agents by paracrine cells, in response to certain luminal stimuli, results in stimulation of adjacent epithelial cells, smooth muscle cells, and possibly enteric neurons to produce a coordinated response such as net secretion, motor activity, and blood flow.

Enterocytes have intracellular receptors, as well as receptors on their apical and basolateral membranes. The distribution of the receptors varies throughout the different regions of the gastrointestinal tract. In addition, the existence of multiple isotypes of the different receptors is likely. Differences in receptor isotypes probably allow for different ligand-receptor interactions, resulting in different durations of response. For example, prostaglandins and calcium-dependent secretagogues have a short-lived response, which is in part a result of receptor tachyphylaxis.[52-56] These short-lived responses probably are important reactions to the immediate changes that occur in the gut milieu. Other agents are important in mediating long-term adaptive responses. Changes in physiologic conditions, such as dehydration, may necessitate more lasting alterations in intestinal water and electrolyte transport. Factors released in response to such changes can stimulate and increase recruitment of specific transporters to the enterocyte membrane and the synthesis of transport proteins, thereby modulating the absorptive or secretory capacity of the epithelium. Steroids are an example of factors involved in longer-duration responses.[57,58]

Ion transport is regulated by a number of signal transduction pathways. Secretagogues and pro-absorptive agents activate second messengers, which in turn activate their respective protein kinases, which phosphorylate proteins integral to the process of ion transport. Pro-

Table 96–1 Prosecretory and Proabsorptive Agents Involved in the Regulation of Intestinal Water and Electrolyte Transport*

Agents That Stimulate Net Secretion

Increase cAMP	Increase cGMP	Increase Ca$_i$ and/or Activate Protein Kinase C	Other Pathways (Tyrosine Kinase, MAPK, Gene Regulation)
Vasoactive intestinal polypeptide	Nitric oxide	Acetylcholine	Interferon-γ
Adenosine	Guanylin	Serotonin	TNF-α
Prostaglandins	Uroguanylin	Substance P	Interleukin-1
Histamine		Histamine	Interleukin-6
Bradykinin		Bradykinin	Epidemal growth factor
		ATP	
		Adenosine	
		Neurotensin	

Agents That Stimulate Net Absorption

Inhibit Increases in cAMP	Coupled Transport	Other Pathways
Norepinephrine	Short-chain fatty acids	Aldosterone
Epinephrine	Glucose, amino acids	Glucocorticoids
Dopamine	Dipeptides/tripeptides	Somatostatin
Enkephalins		GLP-2
Neuropeptide Y		
Somatostatin		

*Several agents activate multiple pathways.
ATP, adenosine triphosphate; Ca$_i$, intracellular calcium [concentration]; cAMP, cyclic adenosine monophosphate; cGMP, cyclic guanosine monophosphate; GLP-2, glucagon-like peptide 2; MAPK, mitogen-activated protein kinase; TNF, tumor necrosis factor.

absorptive agents may activate pathways such as the inhibitor G protein (G$_i$) cascade, the inhibitory arm of the adenylate cyclase cascade, or the phosphatidylinositol (PI) cycle. Secretagogues act through signal transduction cascades such as cyclic adenosine monophosphate (cAMP), cyclic guanosine monophosphate (cGMP), Ca^{2+}, or PI. The mechanism by which the second messengers are activated may determine the duration and type of biologic response that ensues.[59] For example, cholera toxin is involved in an irreversible covalent modification of the stimulatory G protein (G$_s$). This stimulation of the G$_s$ protein results in activation of Cl$^-$ secretion, which persists until the enterocyte is sloughed off at the end of its normal life span.[60-64] In vitro, VIP also stimulates secretory processes that are sustained until the hormone is degraded.[65] By contrast, prostaglandins typically result in secretion for only a short duration, because their receptors are susceptible to tachyphylaxis.[54]

Interactions also occur between signaling mechanisms of different signaling pathways. For example, cAMP and Ca^{2+} interact in a synergistic manner, as do cGMP (ST$_a$) and Ca^{2+}.[66,67] The secretion resulting from the synergism of these intracellular mediators results in a greater effect than would result if these mediators acted alone. Phorbol esters, by contrast, have no effect when acting alone but attenuate Cl$^-$ secretion in the presence of cAMP.[68]

Mediators also may alter paracellular permeability, greatly affecting both absorptive and secretory processes. The activation of protein kinase C by different agonists or the *Vibrio cholerae* zonula occludens toxin (ZOT) may result in alterations of the perijunctional actin ring that constitutes the tight junction apparatus.[69] Such changes in tight junctions can significantly affect intracellular transport processes.

MUCOSAL WATER AND ELECTROLYTE TRANSPORT PROCESSES

WATER TRANSPORT

Water transport appears to be largely a passive process that occurs through both paracellular and transcellular routes in the intestine, coupled with solute movement. It is likely, however, that the predominant pathway for water transport is paracellular. The extent and routes of transcellular transport remain controversial. Studies have shown that certain water channel proteins, aquaporins (AQPs), are expressed in the intestinal mucosa, providing water transfer across the cellular membrane. Of the six aquaporin isoforms reported to be expressed in the gastrointestinal tract, AQP3, 4, 5, 8, and 9 have been localized to mucosal cells, although their distribution and expression vary considerably among different cell types and regions of the bowel.[70-72] Other transporters such as the Na$^+$-dependent glucose cotransporter (SGLT1) also have been proposed as important transepithelial routes for water transport. The relative contributions of water channels to overall water flux in the intestine, however, remain unknown.

ELECTROLYTE TRANSPORT

A variety of transport proteins are required for intestinal transport of water and electrolytes. As illustrated in Figure 96–9, ion transporters can be grouped into three major classes: pumps, channels, and carriers. *Pumps* are energy driven and capable of transporting ions against large electrochemical gradients. For instance, the Na$^+$ pump, or

Na$^+$,K$^+$-ATPase, is essential for establishing and maintaining cellular electrochemical gradients required for the other transport processes. *Channels* generally are ion selective and conductive. Examples include the cystic fibrosis transmembrane regulator (CFTR) and electrogenic Na$^+$ channel, both apical or luminal membrane protein transporters found in the intestinal epithelial cells. Because of their ion selectivity, activation of channels involved in vectoral transport often are associated with the development of a mucosal potential difference, which promotes requisite passive diffusion of a counterion. Absorption of Na$^+$ in the rectum through the epithelial Na$^+$ channel, for example, causes a potential difference that promotes passive transport of Na$^+$, resulting in NaCl absorption. *Carrier transport proteins* facilitate ion and nutrient transport across cell membranes. Because this is not an active process, transport rate and direction are determined by the existing electrochemical gradients for the substrate.

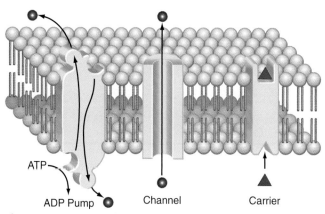

Figure 96–9 Types of membrane transport proteins for carrying nutrients and electrolytes into and out of intestinal cells: pumps, channels, and carriers.

As shown in Figure 96–10, several types of carriers exist: uniporters, symporters, and antiporters (exchangers). *Uniport transporters*, such as the facilitated glucose transporter Glut-2, found in the basolateral membranes of small intestinal villus cells, facilitate the transport of a single ion or nutrient. *Symporters* carry multiple molecules across the cell membrane. In some instances, such as the Na$^+$-dependent glucose cotransporter SGLT1, the 2:1 sodium-glucose stoichiometry exploits the Na$^+$ electrochemical gradient to drive intracellular glucose concentrations above the chemical equilibrium—a requisite for developing a driving force for the exit through Glut2 across the basolateral membrane. Finally, *antiporters*, such as anion and cation exchangers, exchange one molecule for another. Again, the rate of exchange is dependent on existing electrochemical gradients for the substrates.

Expression of the many transporters involved in intestinal water and electrolyte transport is regionally specific. As shown in Figure 96–11, several types of pathways exist for Na$^+$ absorption, Cl$^-$ absorption, and K$^+$ transport, their region-specific expression playing important roles in optimizing conditions for digestion, secretion, absorption, and eventual solidification of feces.

INTESTINAL NA$^+$ ABSORPTION

Na$^+$ absorption is one of the most important functions of the gastrointestinal tract, because Na$^+$ is the predominant ion that determines relative rates of fluid absorption. Na$^+$ is absorbed by several different pathways, each having region-specific expression along the craniocaudal axis, and also along the villus-crypt axis. With regard to the latter, most Na$^+$ absorptive functions are found primarily in mature small intestinal villus cells or the surface absorptive cells of the colon (see Fig. 96–11*A*), although some pathways for Na$^+$ absorption have been reported in crypts.[73]

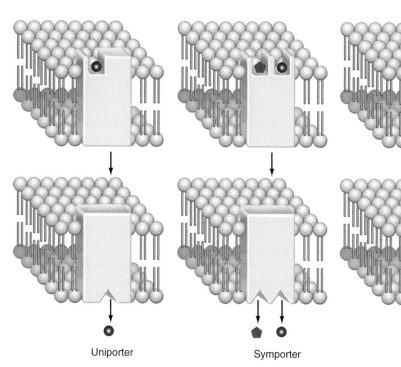

Uniporter   Symporter   Antiporter

Figure 96–10 Examples of ion transport carriers: uniporters, symporters, and antiporters. (Reproduced with permission from Chang EB, et al [eds]: Gastrointestinal, Hepatobiliary, and Nutritional Physiology. Philadelphia, Lippincott-Raven, 1996.)

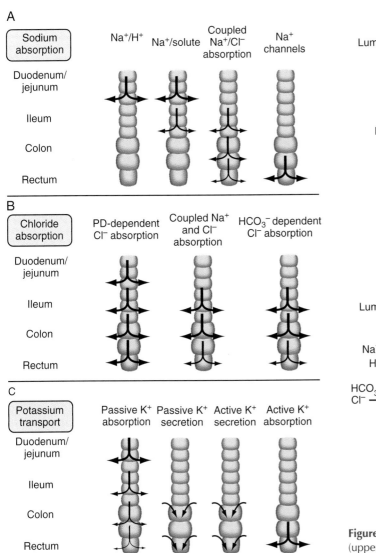

Figure 96–11 Pathways for absorption and transport of electrolytes throughout the gastrointestinal tract: *A*, sodium absorption; *B*, chloride absorption; and *C*, potassium transport. Many transporters are involved and each is expressed in specific regions of the intestine. PD, potential difference. (Reproduced with permission from Chang EB, et al [eds]: Gastrointestinal, Hepatobiliary, and Nutritional Physiology. Philadelphia, Lippincott-Raven, 1996.)

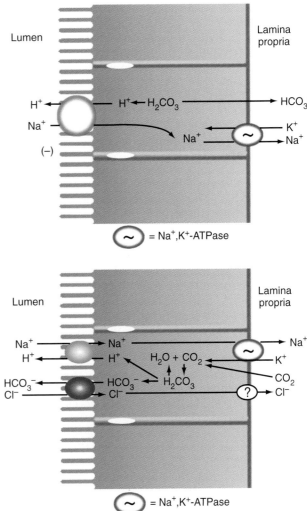

Figure 96–12 Luminal exchangers. In the upper small intestine (upper panel) the Na^+H^+ exchangers is uncoupled, whereas in the lower small intestine and colon (lower panel) Na absorption occurs through two transporters (Na^+-H^+, $Cl^--HCO_3^-$) that are coupled to each other. The one-for-one exchange process is electroneutral, because no net transfer of charge occurs. Na^+ enters the cell from the lumen driven by its electrochemical gradient *(upper panel)* and is extruded from the cell by the Na^+,K^+-ATPase pump *(lower panel)*, which is located on the basolateral membrane.

Non–Nutrient-Coupled Na⁺ Absorption

Non–nutrient-dependent, electroneutral Na^+ absorption is mediated by luminal Na^+-H^+ exchangers (NHEs) and represents a major pathway for intestinal Na^+ absorption.[74] In the small and large intestines, both NHE2 and NHE3 are found in the luminal membranes of surface enterocytes.[75-78] As shown in Figure 96–12, these exchangers mediate one-for-one exchange between Na^+ and H^+, a process that is electroneutral because no net transfer of charge occurs. Na^+ enters the cell driven by its electrochemical gradient and is extruded out of the cell by the Na^+,K^+-ATPase pump that is located in the basolateral membrane. Protons that are exchanged for Na^+ are generated from carbonic acid or from cellular metabolism. In the proximal small intestine, NHE activity appears to function independently of anion absorption, as evidenced by acidification of the lumen in the presence of luminal Na^+.[60] In the ileum and colon, however, these Na^+-H^+ exchangers appear to be functionally coupled with anion exchangers (e.g., $Cl^--HCO_3^-$ exchange), although the specific type of exchanger has not yet been identified.[79-81] Functional coupling is mediated by simultaneous generation of H^+ and HCO_3^- ions by carbonic anhydrase activity. Two anion exchangers, AE1 and DRA (Down-Regulated in Adenoma), have been implicated in functional coupling with apical NHEs,[82,83] the latter being more likely because mutations in the DRA result in congenital chloridorrhea.[84] A third Na^+-H^+ exchanger, NHE1, is expressed by most intestinal epithelial cells but is confined to the basolateral membrane and is not involved in net Na^+ absorption; it functions primarily to regulate intracellular pH and volume.[75] Coordination must exist between NHEs at the apical and the basolateral membranes; it is imperative that these exchangers work in concert and do not cancel out the actions of one another.

Counterproductive activation of apical and basolateral NHEs does not occur, because the respective isoforms respond differently to intracellular signals—for example, increases in cytosolic Ca^{2+} and the activation of protein kinase C inhibit luminal Na^+-H^+ exchangers but activate basolateral NHE1.[75]

To date, it remains unclear why two Na^+-H^+ exchangers are present in the intestinal brush border membrane, because both exchangers have identical functions and substrate specificity. Some insights are provided by the fact that gene-targeted deletion of NHE3, but not NHE2, results in diarrhea.[85] In addition, estimates of the relative contribution of both transporters to overall Na^+ absorptive capacity have shown that NHE3 appears to be the predominant Na^+ transporter.[78] Ileal NHE3 and proximal colon NHE3 also are more sensitive than NHE2 to regulation by aldosterone and glucocorticoids, suggesting that NHE3 may be more important in fine-tuning Na^+ absorptive processes to meet metabolic demands.[57,58,86] To further underscore differences between NHE2 and NHE3, their regulation by various signaling pathways and extracellular stimuli differ substantially. NHE2 activity, for instance, is not affected by activation of protein kinase C or increases in cGMP.[77,87]

The mechanism of NHE3 regulation by cAMP and Ca^{2+} has been elucidated partially and appears to involve two key adapter proteins, the Na^+-H^+ exchanger regulatory factors NHERF-1 and NHERF-2; both possess PDZ-binding domains believed to be important in their physical coupling with NHE3 and with the actin cytoskeleton.[88,89] NHERF-1 appears to be essential for cAMP inhibition of NHE3, whereas NHERF-2 mediates Ca^{2+} regulation of the isoform.[90] In addition, NHERF proteins appear to regulate DRA activity, which possibly is important for the functional coupling between NHE3 and DRA.[91] How these signaling pathways cause NHE3 inhibition is still a matter of debate. Some evidence supports the direct phosphorylation of NHE3, regulating inhibited activity,[89] whereas other reports have implicated stimulated intracellular uptake of apical membrane NHE3 through membrane endocytosis.[92] CFTR also may have a role in regulating apical NHE activity, through an interaction with NHERF PDZ domains.[93] In patients with cystic fibrosis and CFTR-knockout mice, for instance, increases in cAMP appear to stimulate electroneutral Na^+ absorption.[94,95]

Nutrient-Coupled Na^+ Absorption

Amino acids and hexoses stimulate intestinal Na^+ absorption, which in most instances is associated with the development of transepithelial potential differences (i.e., it is an electrogenic process). As shown in Figure 96–13, following ingestion of glucose or starch (the latter is converted to glucose by pancreatic, salivary, and brush border enzymes), D-glucose (and D-galactose) is absorbed with Na^+ through a luminal membrane Na^+-glucose cotransporter (SGLT1) in a stoichiometry of 2 Na:1 glucose (*not shown* in the figure). This process is driven by the electrochemical gradient for Na^+ created by the Na^+ pump and basolateral membrane K^+ channels (they maintain the inside of the cell electronegative with low Na^+). Glucose exits the cell by a facilitative transporter called Glut2, whereas Na^+ exits the cell by means of the Na^+ pump.

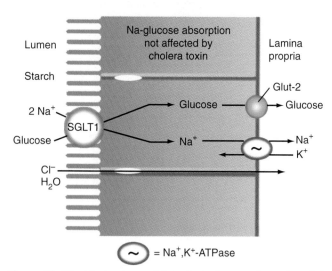

Figure 96–13 Mechanisms of intestinal glucose absorption. Following ingestion of glucose or starch (which is converted to glucose by pancreatic, salivary, and brush border enzymes), D-glucose (and D-galactose) is absorbed with Na^+ by means of a luminal membrane Na^+-glucose cotransporter (SGLT1) in a stoichiometric Na^+-glucose ratio of 2:1. Glut-2, a facilitated glucose transporter; SGLT1, the Na^+-dependent glucose cotransporter.

Of interest, the activation of SGLT1 has several other consequences. One involves the contraction of the perijunctional actin-mysosin ring, which increases tight junctional permeability and facilitates paracellular transport of water and other small molecules. This pathway appears to involve the activation of protein kinase C and MLCK.[6,96,97] Activation of SGLT1 also appears to stimulate NHE3 activity, further enhancing Na^+ absorptive capacity of the gut.[98]

In contrast with other Na^+-absorptive pathways, glucose- and amino acid–stimulated Na^+ absorption are not affected by enterotoxins such as cholera toxin and STa (heat-stable enterotoxin of *E. coli*). This property is the rationale for using sugar- or amino acid–based oral rehydration solutions (ORSs) for the treatment of cholera and traveler's diarrhea.[99] Rice-based electrolyte solutions also have been effective, because rice starch is rapidly converted to glucose by pancreatic amylase and brush border hydrolases. ORS has saved millions of lives and is highly cost-effective. Similarly, this is the basis for sports drinks, which essentially are sugar-based electrolyte solutions.

Electrogenic Na^+ Absorption

A luminal membrane, amiloride-sensitive, electrogenic (capable of developing a transepithelial potential difference), Na^+-selective channel called ENaC mediates Na^+ absorption in the human distal colon and rectum. ENaC is composed of several subunits and is expressed only by surface and upper crypt colonocytes.[100] Luminal Na^+ enters the cell driven by an extremely favorable electrochemical gradient—namely, the presence of a negative cell membrane voltage and low intracellular [Na^+]. ENaC channel activity is both autoregulated and modulated by various signaling pathways. Autoregulation occurs through feedback inhibition initiated by rising intracellular Na^+ concentrations, an effect that appears to be mediated by C-terminal PY motifs in all three ENaC sub-units.[101,102] This process serves as an important mechanism to limit excessive Na+ conductance that might overwhelm volume regulatory mechanisms and other cellular processes. Several signaling pathways also modulate ENaC activity, although the type of response appears to be tissue-specific. In renal cells, for instance, increases in cytosolic calcium and activation of protein kinase C inhibit its activity, whereas increases in cyclic AMP are stimulatory[103]; however, these effects are not observed in ENaC expressed by colonic epithelium. For instance, increases in cAMP appear to have little effect on ENaC conductance.[104,105] In fact, electrogenic Na absorption appears to be unaffected by most gut peptides and neurotransmitters, in contrast with electroneutral Na+-Cl− absorption or electrogenic anion secretion;[106,107] ENaC expression and total activity can be increased significantly by both mineralo- and glucocorticoids, resulting in a chronic and progressive increase in net Na+ absorption and K+ secretion.[57,108-110] These effects appear to be transcriptionally mediated but also involve the up-regulation of the serum and glucocorticoid–regulated kinase SGK, which appears to enhance ENaC activity.[111,112]

Once Na+ enters the cell, it is extruded by the basolateral Na+ pump. Because this is an electrogenic process, Cl− is passively absorbed, followed by water (Fig. 96–14). Some evidence suggests that CFTR may mediate transcellular transport of Cl− in this process, but the relative contribution of this pathway is unknown. The electrogenic ENaC pathway is extremely important in the distal colon and rectum, capable of extracting NaCl against unfavorable luminal-to-serosal gradients. Such a process is required to solidify stool.

Chloride Absorption

Chloride absorption in the jejunum is passive and dependent on transmural potential differences and concentration gradients. In the ileum and proximal colon, Cl− absorption is coupled to Na+ absorption and is electroneutral. This coupled exchange probably occurs through the coordination of two exchangers, the Na+-H+ exchange protein and the Cl−-HCO3− exchange protein.

In the ileum and colon, Cl− also is absorbed by means of a Cl−-HCO3− exchanger independent of Na+. It has been suggested that ClC-2 channels present in the basolateral membrane of the distal colon epithelial cells serve as an exit pathway for Cl−.[113]

CELLULAR ANION SECRETION

Intestinal water and electrolyte secretion primarily involves secretion of Cl− or HCO3− ions. Very little is known about the mechanism of HCO3− secretion in the intestine except that it occurs, and that HCO3− is one of the major ions lost in diarrheal fluid. Several pathways have been proposed for bicarbonate secretion, including electroneutral exchange with luminal Cl− or short-chain fatty acids (SCFAs), CFTR, or coupling of these processes whereby Cl− exchanged for HCO3− is recycled to the lumen through CFTR. Based on observations in both human cystic fibrosis[114] and the CFTR-knockout mouse,[115] intestinal HCO3− transport appears to be highly dependent on the expression of CFTR. Several studies have shown that CFTR is able to transport HCO3−,[116-118] although others have refuted this.[119] CFTR also has been shown to regulate Cl−-HCO3− exchange[120,121] and to enhance DRA expression,[122] representing alternative mechanisms of CFTR-dependent HCO3− secretion.

By contrast, the mechanism of Cl− secretion is much better characterized and appears to involve the integration of several luminal and basolateral membrane transporters (Fig. 96–15). Cl− enters the cell by means of the basolateral membrane Na+-K+-2Cl− cotransporter (NKCC1) and exits by luminal membrane Cl− channels, one of which is CFTR. Na+ exits the cell by means of the Na+,K+-ATPase pump, and K+ exits through K+-selective channels, both processes serving to increase electronegativity of the cell. Na+ secretion that accompanies active Cl− secretion is passive, driven by the transepithelial potential difference resulting from Cl− secretion. The

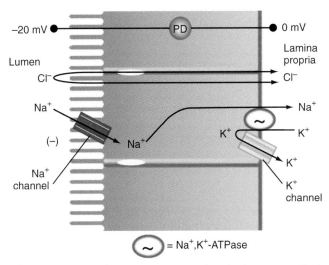

Figure 96–14 In electrogenic intestinal Na+ absorption, Cl− is passively absorbed, followed by water.

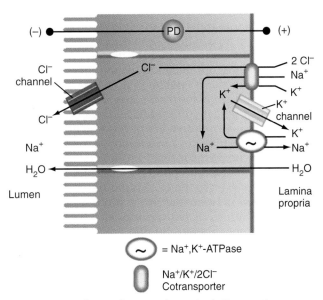

Figure 96–15 The mechanism of intestinal Cl− secretion appears to involve the integration of several luminal and basolateral membrane transporters.

$Na^+ : K^+ : 2Cl^-$ stoichiometry of NKCC1 favors a strong driving force to achieve an intracellular Cl^- activity above its electrochemical equilibrium. By raising Cl^- activity above its electrochemical equilibrium, the cell achieves a sufficient driving force for Cl^- secretion when Cl^- conductance is activated by various signaling pathways, including cyclic nucleotides and calcium.[123] Several apical membrane Cl^- channels have now been reported: CFTR, members of the CLC family of transporters,[124,125] Ca^{2+}-activated Cl^- channels,[126] and intermediate-conductance outwardly rectifying channels[127-129] have been detected in intestinal epithelia. CFTR probably is the major transporter for calcium- and cyclic nucleotide–regulated electrogenic anion secretion in the intestine, based on observations in tissues from patients with cystic fibrosis and CF-knockout animals.[130-132] Genetic differences among individuals may determine the relative role of transporters such as Ca^{2+}-activated Cl^- channels, as evidenced by the fact that a particular inbred strain of CF-knockout mice that lacks CFTR activity expresses Ca^{2+}-activated Cl^- secretion.[126] Of interest, these mice do not manifest intestinal pathology and have normal survival.

The opening of apical membrane Cl^- channels is modulated by numerous neurotransmitters and gut peptides that activate specific signaling pathways. In many cases, these agents stimulate specific membrane receptors that exist on the apical or basolateral membranes of intestinal epithelial cells. The guanylate cyclase receptor for guanylin is an example of the former, which on activation increases cellular levels of cGMP, resulting in a biochemical cascade leading to the opening of apical membrane Cl^- conductance.[133,134] Adenosine A2b receptors also are found in the apical membrane and serve an important role in activating Cl^- secretion in areas of crypt abscesses.[135] Adenosine is formed in the intestinal lumen during active inflammation from neutrophil-derived 5'-AMP. By contrast, agents such as acetylcholine, vasoactive intestinal polypeptide (VIP), and bradykinin stimulate specific receptors on the basolateral membrane of enterocytes. Activation of these receptors results in increases in cyclic nucleotides, calcium, and other pathways (e.g., phosphatidyl inositol, protein kinase C), all of which favor increases in Cl^- and HCO_3^- secretion.[123] In the case of CFTR, part of the activation process involves insertion of transporters into the apical membrane from a subapical endosomal pool—a process that is dependent on adapter proteins such as syntaxin 1A,[136] NHERF1,[137,138] Yes-associated protein 65 (YAP65),[139] and AKAP (PKA-anchoring protein).[140,141] Many of these adapter proteins anchor CFTR in the apical membrane or are involved in associating it with effector molecules or cytoskeletal elements that are essential for membrane trafficking. Some evidence also suggests that CFTR activity may be regulated directly—for example, by protein kinase A through phosphorylation-mediated changes in allosteric confirmation of the channel.[142,143]

POTASSIUM TRANSPORT

Potassium is mostly absorbed passively in the gastrointestinal tract. In the colon, however, active K^+ secretion and absorption are seen in the proximal and distal colon, respectively. Active K^+ absorption is mediated by apical membrane H^+,K^+-ATPases that are members of the gene family of P-type ATPases.[144] The existence of at least two distinct H^+,K^+-ATPases is recognized, which differ in cell-specific expression: one that is the ouabain-sensitive isoform, expressed primarily by crypt cells, and another that is ouabain-insensitive and expressed by surface cells. The latter has been cloned and appears to be composed of an alpha subunit (HKc_{alpha1}) and a beta subunit (HKc_{beta}).[145] Both aldosterone and dietary K^+ depletion stimulate active K^+ absorption, but only the former regulates HKc_{alpha1} at a post-transcriptional level.[144]

Less is known about mechanisms for K^+ secretion in the proximal colon. The prevailing evidence supports a role for luminal K^+ channels, which can be up-regulated by chronic dietary K^+ loading.[146,147] Although little is known about the molecular nature of the apical membrane K^+ channel, it is regulated by changes in intracellular Ca^{2+}, pH, and membrane potential.[146-149] It also appears to differ from the K^+ channels found in the basolateral membrane with regard to cAMP stimulation.[150] Increases in mineralo- or glucocorticoid levels will up-regulate luminal K^+ activity, as well as ENaC.[57]

SHORT-CHAIN FATTY ACID ABSORPTION

SCFAs are monocarboxylic hydrocarbons produced by colonic bacterial digestion of poorly absorbed carbohydrates. SCFAs include acetate, propionate, and butyrate, which are produced along with carbon dioxide and hydrogen in the colon by microbial fermentation of dietary fiber and resistant starches. SCFAs are by far the major anions in colonic fluid and, to a lesser extent, in distal ileum, with an estimated total between 60 and 150 mmol/kg.[151] Despite differences in concentration, however, a nearly constant ratio of 60:25:15 for acetate, propionate, and butyrate, respectively, is maintained.[151] Butyrate, however, is preferentially oxidized compared with propionate and acetate, accounting for 70% to 90% of the energy utilized by the colon[152-155] and 70% of its oxygen consumption.[152-154]

The absorption of SCFAs appears to occur both passively and actively, although the relative contributions of these pathways in overall SCFA transport by the colon and ileum remain controversial.[156,157] It is clear, however, that SCFA absorption promotes short- and long-term electroneutral Na^+ and Cl^- absorption.[158] At least two potential mechanisms mediating the acute effect have been proposed—one involving a specific apical membrane Na-SCFA cotransporter[159] and the other being an SCFA-anion exchange functionally coupled to luminal Na^+-H^+ exchange.[160] In addition, monocarboxylate transporter 1 has been demonstrated to play a role in butyrate transport into the colonocyte.[161] As discussed later, SCFAs also stimulate the overall capacity for NaCl absorption through the induction of apical NHE3 expression and membrane insertion.

CHANGES IN WATER AND ELECTROLYTE TRANSPORT IN DISEASE

Intestinal transport is a dynamic process capable of alteration in response to different pathophysiologic processes.

Ideally, this system aids in the defensive and healing mechanisms and contributes to the body's attempt to meet metabolic demands caused by disease or stress. The following discussion reviews the effects of several disease processes on ion and water transport. Oftentimes the changes in electrolyte and water transport in the face of disease maintain physiologic processes or serve to purge the lumen of noxious stimuli or pathogens. Other times, disease causes aberrations in intestinal transport, which can lead to complications such as malabsorption of water, nutrients, and electrolytes.

DIABETES MELLITUS

Diabetes is an example of a disease process that significantly affects electrolyte and nutrient transport in the intestinal tract. Changes in intestinal transport of nutrients and electrolytes occur in part because of the body's attempt to adapt to the perceived state of starvation and the increased metabolic demands that are characteristic of diabetes. In models of experimentally induced diabetes, the cell number of the crypt-villus columns is increased, resulting in a 1.5- to 2-fold increase in mucosal mass, with a concomitant increase in overall absorptive surface area.[162,163] Cellular turnover is decreased, allowing for greater stromal support of these taller villi. Not only does the increase in surface area result in an increase in absorptive area, but evidently the number of brush border digestive enzymes—including sucrase-isomaltase, lactase, and peptidases—and of ion and nutrient transporters also increases.[164,165] The resulting increase in these enzymatic breakdown products provides substrate for solute-dependent Na^+ absorption in a more rapid manner.

An uncommon but debilitating complication of diabetes is diabetic diarrhea. This condition is a result of several aberrations in intestinal water and electrolyte transport. Autonomic and possibly enteric neuropathy in diabetes probably impairs the neural regulation of salt and water transport. Diabetic rats treated with streptozocin have shown impaired regulation of intestinal ion transport by the enteric nerves.[166] This impairment results in altered Na^+ and Cl^- transport as a result of loss of noradrenergic tone. This in turn causes an imbalance in processes involved in regulation of mucosal water and electrolyte transport, favoring net secretion and development of diarrhea. Capillary blood flow and intestinal motility also are affected by diabetes and contribute to changes in fluid and electrolyte transport. Antidiarrheal medications may be helpful in the treatment of chronic diabetic diarrhea. When antidiarrheal medications are not adequate to control chronic diarrhea in diabetics, use of an α_2-adrenergic receptor agonist such as clonidine or a somatostatin analog such as octreotide may be considered.

INFLAMMATION

Mucosal inflammation of the small and large intestines is an important host response to pathogens and noxious stimuli. When the mucosa is inflamed, the large number of infiltrating inflammatory cells dramatically alters or diminishes the interactions and effects of the factors and cellular components that normally regulate ion transport. These cells secrete large amounts of immune and inflammatory mediators, causing a net increase in intestinal secretion. Whereas the inflammatory response is intended to protect the host and purge the intestines of harmful elements, this response may adversely affect the mucosal integrity and function. Diarrhea may ensue, resulting in dehydration and metabolic disturbances.

Arachidonic acid metabolites, derived from neutrophils, fibroblasts, and activated macrophages, play a major role in stimulating net secretion. These metabolites exert this effect through several different mechanisms. For example, prostaglandin E_2 is believed to activate specific epithelial cell receptors, which in turn stimulate anion secretion and block Na^+ and Cl^- absorption.[37,167,168] Other arachidonic acid metabolites such as prostaglandin D_2, prostacyclin, and the peptidoleukotriene LTC_4 stimulate net secretion through the activation of secretomotor neurons.[168-170] Some variation of response among species has been observed. Some immune and inflammatory mediators also are believed to stimulate intestinal net secretion through the activation of arachidonic acid metabolism in submucosal cells. IL-1 and IL-3 have been shown to stimulate anion secretion, probably through the stimulation of prostaglandin formation.[50] Bradykinin, a potent secretagogue, is a strong inducer of Cl^- secretion. This mediator stimulates secretion through second messengers such as prostaglandins, intracellular Ca^{2+}, and cAMP.[171] Nitric oxide, a regulatory factor produced by activated neutrophils and macrophages, is abundantly produced in inflamed tissue and has been found to increase Cl^- secretion in the human colon. In a manner not entirely understood, nitric oxide stimulates intestinal secretion through the production of cyclooxygenase metabolites, as well as through the stimulation of enteric secretomotor neurons.[172]

Many inflammatory mediators influence secretomotor neurons of the enteric nervous system. It is speculated that the neurocrine response probably represents an attempt to further enhance the secretory response by potentiating the stimulation to target tissues or expanding the area of tissue stimulated. Neurons not only stimulate enterocytes but also influence capillary blood flow, lymphatic flow, and smooth muscle function.

Inflammatory Bowel Disease

Although many inflammatory and immune mediators have been shown to stimulate intestinal secretion, resulting in diarrhea, the mechanisms responsible for inflammatory bowel disease (IBD)-associated diarrhea may be related primarily not to an increase in intestinal secretion but rather to a decrease in intestinal absorption. Clinical observations have suggested that impaired or downregulated nutrient and electrolyte absorption and decreased barrier function may be responsible for IBD-associated diarrhea.[173,174] In one study, rats chronically treated with IFN-γ were observed to have a downregulation of apical membrane exchangers NHE2 and NHE3.[175] The investigators also treated human Caco-

2/bbe cells with IFN-γ and found down-regulated expression of NHE2 and NHE3 that was both dose and time related. The down-regulation of these Na$^+$ transporters suggests that in the presence of IFN-γ, Na$^+$ and thus water absorption is impaired, resulting in a greater luminal fluid volume. In a similar study, T-84 colonic epithelial cells were treated with IFN-γ. After 24 hours of such treatment, decreased expression of several transport- and barrier-related proteins, including the Na$^+$,K$^+$-ATPase α-subunit, Na$^+$/K$^+$/2Cl$^-$, occludin, and Z0-1, was observed; CFTR and the β-subunit of Na$^+$,K$^+$-ATPase were unchanged. The down-regulation of these selective barrier and transport proteins results in an increase in intracellular Na$^+$ and cell volume, ultimately affecting mucosal permeability and epithelial function. These changes may explain the development of diarrhea in patients with IBD, in whom the bowel mucosa is chronically inflamed.[176]

The mechanisms of IBD-associated mucosal T cell activation and diarrhea also have been explored. In mice, T cells were activated with anti-CD3 mAB, resulting in profound diarrhea. T cell activation resulted in increased mucosal permeability and decreased epithelial Na$^+$,K$^+$-ATPase activity that led to decreased intestinal Na$^+$ and water absorption. The findings of this study also suggest that diarrhea in IBD is related to malabsorptive rather than secretory processes.[177]

INFECTIOUS DIARRHEA

The intestinal tract has several mechanisms intended to protect the host from enteric pathogens. Nonetheless, diarrhea commonly results from enteric infection (see Chapters 99, 104, 106, and 107). The pathophysiologic mechanism of the development of diarrhea is complex and may be the result of a number of effects of specific pathogens on the mucosa. Pathogens may cause diarrhea through destruction of mucosa, thereby affecting intestinal absorptive capacity or binding of specific enterocyte receptors, induction of an inflammatory response, or alteration of luminal membrane function. Additionally, malabsorbed or maldigested nutrients may increase luminal fluid loads through osmotic effects. For example, the brush border enzyme lactase is vulnerable to mucosal disruption, and when brush border lactase activity is decreased, levels of lactose in the lumen are increased, creating an osmotic force that draws fluid into the lumen.

Many pathogenic enteric organisms cause diarrhea by increasing secretion of ions such as chloride. Some pathogens have been associated with increased generation of second messengers such as cAMP, cGMP, nitric oxide, and calcium. Various secretagogues produced during inflammatory responses also increase concentrations of these intracellular mediators. These second messengers interact with downstream pathways, which ultimately inhibit NaCl-coupled transport and increase Cl$^-$ secretion.[178] CFTR, a major anion channel, often is targeted by these intracellular mediators.[179-181] Cryptidins secreted from Paneth cells located in the base of the crypts also play a role in intestinal secretion. Cryptidins are antimicrobial cationic proteins that form anion-selective channels in pathogen membranes, increasing the membrane permeability and osmolar stress of the pathogenic organism. These cryptidins also may insert into the luminal membrane of the host intestinal epithelial cells, increasing anion secretion.[182]

A point of interest is that anion secretion does not appear to be increased in bowel mucosa that is inflamed chronically (e.g., for longer than 24 hours). In chronic inflammatory states, the effects of mediators such as IFN-γ and TNF-α predominate and affect the expression of essential transport and barrier-related proteins, ultimately reducing the intestinal absorptive capacity.

Specific Enteric Pathogens

Some pathogens increase intestinal secretion through enterotoxin-mediated increases in intracellular cAMP. For example, *Vibrio cholerae* releases cholera toxin that binds to the G$_{M1}$-ganglioside receptor found on the luminal membrane of the enterocyte, which in turn activates adenosine diphosphate ribosylation of an arginine residue on the guanosine triphosphate (GTP)-binding regulatory protein G$_s$. The binding of the cholera toxin to G$_s$ results in the irreversible activation of G$_s$, thereby causing an increase of cytosolic cAMP, which ultimately results in the inhibition of NaCl-coupled transport and increased Cl$^-$ secretion.[183-185] Cholera toxin also appears to activate enteric secretomotor neurons by stimulating the release of acetylcholine, which results in the opening of basolateral K$^+$ channels. The effects of acetylcholine probably are synergistic with the direct effects of cholera toxin on Cl$^-$ secretion.[186]

STa, the *Escherichia coli* heat-stable enterotoxin, causes diarrhea by increasing intracellular levels of cGMP. STa binds to GC-C on the luminal surface of the enterocyte. The binding of GC-C by STa or its endogenous ligands, guanylin or uroguanylin, results in the production of cGMP. The generated cGMP activates cGMP-sensitive anion channels, cGMP phosphodiesterases, or cGMP-regulated protein kinases.[187,188]

Rotavirus releases the enterotoxin NSP4, a transmembrane endoplasmic reticulum glycoprotein.[189] NSP4 appears to activate a signaling pathway that leads to an increase in intracellular calcium levels, thereby affecting calcium-sensitive anion channels.[190,191] *Salmonella typhimurium* infection of the intestinal epithelial cells leads to an acute inflammatory response, which probably is the result of the increased secretion of IL-8 and other proinflammatory mediators. Invasion by this organism appears to result in tyrosine phosphorylation of the epidermal growth factor receptor, which in turn signals events leading to the production of leukotriene metabolites, which may increase membrane permeability to calcium influx.[192] This rise in intracellular Ca^{2+} might ultimately activate NF-κB and IL-8 secretion.[193]

Although many pathogenic organisms cause diarrhea through the increase of intracellular mediators such as cAMP, cGMP, or calcium, some pathogens or their toxins exhibit their pathogenic effects through the disruption of the cytoskeletal elements. Although by different mechanisms, both *Clostridium difficile* toxins A and B and *E. coli* cytotoxic necrotizing factor 1 modify the Rho family of GTPases that are critical for the cell cytoskeletal architecture. The modified Rho proteins lead to disrupted actin filaments and thereby to disrupted tight junction integrity and decreased transepithelial resistance.[194-196]

ADAPTATION FOLLOWING EXTENSIVE SMALL INTESTINAL RESECTION OR INTESTINAL FAILURE

Intestinal adaptation is a process in which the normal physiologic functions of the bowel are recovered after surgical resection or intestinal failure (see Chapter 100). Following a significant loss of mucosal absorptive surface area, an increase in epithelial cell renewal and migration rate occurs, to increase the absorptive capacity of the intestine. Mucosal hyperplasia is not the only adaptive mechanism noted. A functional adaptation by individual enterocytes evidently also occurs. Studies have reported up-regulation of pumps, transporters, and channels including the Na^+,K^+-ATPase pump, the Na^+-glucose cotransporter, SGLT1, and several aquaporins.[197-199] One study demonstrated that in rats that had undergone massive small bowel resection, expression of apical Na^+-H^+ exchangers was increased in segments of bowel distal to the anastomosis.[200]

SCFAs may be important players in the process of intestinal adaptation. SCFAs are trophic to the small intestine after extensive bowel resection and are known to promote Na^+ absorption in both acute and chronic settings. This property may hold particular value in situations in which the absorptive ability of the intestine is compromised. Although this mechanism is not clearly defined, previous work has demonstrated evidence supporting the presence of an electroneutral Cl^--butyrate exchanger coupled with an Na^+-H^+ exchanger.[201] One group of investigators demonstrated that SCFAs increased apical membrane NHE3 activity in a time-dependent manner in rats and human colonic C2/bbe cells.[202] Other investigators have demonstrated that SCFAs increase glucose transporter expression in the normal small intestines of rats.[203] SCFAs, especially butyrate, also have been shown to affect intestinal cell proliferation. This regulation of cell proliferation probably occurs secondary to the release of growth factors and the direct effects of SCFAs on genes influencing cell proliferation.[204]

Studies still are needed to clarify the role of SCFAs in humans following extensive bowel resection or intestinal failure. The data accrued from in vitro and animal studies stress the importance of SFCAs in the adaptive process.

REFERENCES

1. Furuse M, Fujita K, Hiiragi T, et al: Claudin-1 and -2: Novel integral membrane proteins localizing at tight junctions with no sequence similarity to occludin. J Cell Biol 141:1539, 1998.
2. Furuse M, Hirase T, Itoh M, et al: Occludin: A novel integral membrane protein localizing at tight junctions. J Cell Biol 123(6 pt 2):1777, 1993.
3. Martin-Padura I, Lostaglio S, Schneemann M, et al: Junctional adhesion molecule, a novel member of the immunoglobulin superfamily that distributes at intercellular junctions and modulates monocyte trans-migration. J Cell Biol 142:117, 1998.
4. Schneeberger EE, Lynch RD: The tight junction: A multifunctional complex. Am J Physiol Cell Physiol 286:C1213, 2004.
5. Philipson L, Pettersson RF: The coxsackie-adenovirus receptor—a new receptor in the immunoglobulin family involved in cell adhesion. Curr Top Microbiol Immunol 273:87, 2004.
6. Turner JR, Rill BK, Carlson SL, et al: Physiological regulation of epithelial tight junctions is associated with myosin light-chain phosphorylation. Am J Physiol 273(4 pt 1):C1378, 1997.
7. Granger DN, Perry MA, Kvietys PR, Taylor AE: Permeability of intestinal capillaries: Effects of fat absorption and gastrointestinal hormones. Am J Physiol 242:G194, 1982.
8. Harper SL, Barrowman JA, Kvietys PR, Granger DN: Effect of neurotensin on intestinal capillary permeability and blood flow. Am J Physiol 247(2 pt 1):G161, 1984.
9. Gallavan RH Jr, Chen MH, Joffe SN, Jacobson ED: Vasoactive intestinal polypeptide, cholecystokinin, glucagon, and bile-oleate-induced jejunal hyperemia. Am J Physiol 248(2 pt 1):G208, 1985.
10. Granger DN, Cross R, Barrowman JA: Effects of various secretagogues and human carcinoid serum on lymph flow in the cat ileum. Gastroenterology 83:896, 1982.
11. Cedgard S, Hallback DA, Jodal M, et al: The effects of cholera toxin on intramural blood flow distribution and capillary hydraulic conductivity in the cat small intestine. Acta Physiol Scand 102:148, 1978.
12. Granger DN, Kvietys PR, Korthuis RJ, Premen AJ: Mucosal microcirculation of the intestinal mucosa. In Wood JD (ed): Handbook of Physiology, Section 6. The Gastrointestinal System I, Part 2. Bethesda, Md, American Physiological Society, 1987, p 1045.
13. Granger DN: Intestinal microcirculation and transmucosal fluid transport. Am J Physiol 240:G343, 1981.
14. Granger DN, Perry MA, Kvietys PR, Taylor AE: Interstitium-to-blood movement of macromolecules in the absorbing small intestine. Am J Physiol 241:G31, 1981.
15. Babkin BP, Ishikawa H: Einiges zur frage uberdies periodische arbeit des verdauungskanals. Pflugers Arch 147:335, 1912.
16. Schiller LR, Santa Ana CA, Morawsk SG, Fordtran JS: Mechanism of the antidiarrheal effect of loperamide. Gastroenterology 86:1475, 1984.
17. Schiller LR, Davis GR, Santa Ana CA, et al: Studies of the mechanism of the antidiarrheal effect of codeine. J Clin Invest 70:999, 1982.
18. Schiller LR, Santa Ana CA, Morawski SG, Fordtran JS: Studies of the antidiarrheal action of clonidine. Effects on motility and intestinal absorption. Gastroenterology 89:982, 1985.
19. Eklund S, Fahrenkrug J, Jodal M, et al: Vasoactive intestinal polypeptide, 5-hydroxytryptamine and reflex hyperaemia in the small intestine of the cat. J Physiol 302:549, 1980.
20. Buffa R, Capella C, Fontana P, et al: Types of endocrine cells in the human colon and rectum. Cell Tissue Res 192:227, 1978.
21. Sjolund K, Sanden G, Hakanson R, Sundler F: Endocrine cells in human intestine: An immunocytochemical study. Gastroenterology 85:1120, 1983.
22. Polak JM, DeMay J, Bloom SR: 5-Hydroxytryptamine in mucosal endocrine cells of the gut and lung. In DeClerck F, Vanhoutte PM (eds): 5-Hydroxytryptamine in Peripheral Reactions. New York, Raven Press, 1982, p 22.
23. Currie MG, Fok KF, Kato J, et al: Guanylin: An endogenous activator of intestinal guanylate cyclase. Proc Natl Acad Sci U S A 89:947, 1992.
24. Schulz S, Chrisman TD, Garbers DL: Cloning and expression of guanylin. Its existence in various mammalian tissue. J Biol Chem 267:16019, 1992.

25. Krause WJ, Callingford GL, Freeman RH, et al: Distribution of heat-stable enterotoxin/guanylin receptors in the intestinal tract of man and other mammals. J Anat 184(pt 2):407, 1994.

26. Albano F, Brasitus T, Mann EA, et al: Colonocyte basolateral membranes contain *Escherichia coli* heat-stable enterotoxin receptors. Biochem Biophys Res Commun 284:331, 2001.

27. Newson B, Ahlman H, Dahlstrom A, et al: On the innervation of the ileal mucosa in the rat—a synapse. Acta Physiol Scand 105:387, 1979.

28. Thomas EM, Templeton D: Noradrenergic innervation of the villi of rat jejunum. J Auton Nerv Syst 3:25, 1981.

29. Chang EB, Field M, Miller RJ: Enterocyte alpha 2-adrenergic receptors: Yohimbine and *p*-aminoclonidine binding relative to ion transport. Am J Physiol 244:G76, 1983.

30. Field M, McColl I: Ion transport in rabbit ileal mucosa. 3. Effects of catecholamines. Am J Physiol 225:852, 1973.

31. Chang EB, Field M, Miller RJ: Alpha 2-adrenergic receptor regulation of ion transport in rabbit ileum. Am J Physiol 242:G237, 1982.

32. Cooke HJ: Neurobiology of the intestinal mucosa. Gastroenterology 90:1057, 1986.

33. Ciancio MC, Chang EB: Epithelial secretory response to inflammation. In Stead RP, Perdue M, Cooke HJ, Powell D, Barrett K (eds): Neuro-immuno-physiology of the Gastrointestinal Tract: Implications for Inflammatory Diseases. Ann N Y Acad Sci 664:210–221, 1992.

34. Wilson KT, Musch MU, Chang EB: Diarrhea in inflammatory bowel disease. In MacDermott RP, Stensan WF (eds): Inflammatory Bowel Disease. New York, Elsevier, 1991, p 273.

35. Kimberg DV, Field M, Johnson J, et al: Stimulation of intestinal mucosal adenyl cyclase by cholera enterotoxin and prostaglandins. J Clin Invest 50:1218, 1971.

36. Caldraro VG, DeSimone A, Camussi B, et al: Arachidonic acid metabolites and chloride secretion in rabbit distal colonic mucosa. Am J Physiol 261:G443, 1991.

37. Racusen LC, Binder HJ: Effect of prostaglandin on ion transport across isolated colonic mucosa. Dig Dis Sci 25:900, 1980.

38. Barrett KE, Huott PA, Shah SS, et al: Differing effects of apical and basolateral adenosine on colonic epithelial cell line T84. Am J Physiol 256(1 pt 1):C197, 1989.

39. Hirose R, Chang EB: Effects of serotonin on Na/H exchange and intracellular calcium in isolated chicken enterocytes. Am J Physiol 256:G891, 1988.

40. Cooke HJ, Carey HV: Pharmacological analysis of 5-hydroxytryptamine actions on guinea-pig ileal mucosa. Eur J Pharmacol 111:329, 1985.

41. Hinterleitner TA, Powell DW: Immune system control of intestinal ion transport. Proc Soc Exp Biol Med 197:249, 1991.

42. Pavli P, Woodhams CE, Doe WF, Hume DA: Isolation and characterization of antigen-presenting dendritic cells from the mouse intestinal lamina propria. Immunology 70:40, 1990.

43. Pavli P, Doe WF: Intestinal macrophages. In MacDermott RF, Stenson WF (eds): Inflammatory Bowel Diseases. New York, Elsevier, 1992, p 177.

44. Raz A, Wyche A, Siegel N, Needleman P: Regulation of fibroblast cyclooxygenase synthesis by interleukin-1. J Biol Chem 263:3022, 1988.

45. Doerfler ME, Danner RL, Shelhamer JH, Parrillo JE: Bacterial lipopolysaccharides prime human neutrophils for enhanced production of leukotriene B₄. J Clin Invest 83:970, 1989.

46. Johnston RB Jr: Current concepts: Immunology. Monocytes and macrophages. N Engl J Med 318:747, 1988.

47. Tanner AR, Arthur MJ, Wright R: Macrophage activation, chronic inflammation and gastrointestinal disease. Gut 25:760, 1984.

48. Cooke H: Neuro-modulation of ion secretion by inflammatory mediators. In Stead RP, Perdue M, Cooke HJ, Powell D, Barrett BK (eds): Neuro-immuno-physiology of the Gastrointestinal Mucosa: Implications for Inflammatory Bowel Diseases. Ann N Y Acad Sci 664:346, 1992.

49. Musch MW, Kachur JF, Miller RJ, et al: Bradykinin-stimulated electrolyte secretion in rabbit and guinea pig intestine. Involvement of arachidonic acid metabolites. J Clin Invest 71:1073, 1983.

50. Chang EB, Musch MW, Mayer L: Interleukins 1 and 3 stimulate anion secretion in chicken intestine. Gastroenterology 98:1518, 1990.

51. Tamai H, Gaginella TS, Kachur JF, et al: Ca-mediated stimulation of Cl secretion by reactive oxygen metabolites in human colonic T84 cells. J Clin Invest 89:301, 1992.

52. Chang E, Rao MC: Intracellular mediators of intestinal electrolyte transport. In Field M (ed): Current Topics in Gastroenterology. Diarrheal Diseases. New York, Elsevier, 1991, p. 49-72.

53. Chang EB, Sitrih MD, Blach DD: Gastrointestinal, Hepatobiliary, and Nutritional Physiology. Lippincott-Raven Series in Physiology. In Ganong W (ed): Philadelphia, Lippincott-Raven, 1996, p 91.

54. Musch MW, Field M, Miller RJ, Stoff JS: Homologous desensitization to prostaglandins in rabbit ileum. Am J Physiol 252(1 pt 1):G120, 1987.

55. Roden M, Turnheim K: Sodium pump quantity and turnover in rabbit descending colon at different rates of sodium absorption. Pflugers Arch 413:181, 1988.

56. Clauss W, Arnason SS, Munck BG, Skadhauge E: Aldosterone-induced sodium transport in lower intestine. Effects of varying NaCl intake. Pflugers Arch 401:354, 1984.

57. Binder HJ, McGlone F, Sandle GI: Effects of corticosteroid hormones on the electrophysiology of rat distal colon: Implications for Na⁺ and K⁺ transport. J Physiol 410:425, 1989.

58. Binder HJ: Effect of dexamethasone on electrolyte transport in the large intestine of the rat. Gastroenterology 75:212, 1978.

59. Servin AL, Rouyer-Fessard C, Balasubramaniam A, et al: Peptide-YY and neuropeptide-Y inhibit vasoactive intestinal peptide–stimulated adenosine 3',5'-monophosphate production in rat small intestine: Structural requirements of peptides for interacting with peptide-YY–preferring receptors. Endocrinology 124:692, 1989.

60. Field M, Rao MC, Chang EB: Intestinal electrolyte transport and diarrheal disease (1). N Engl J Med 321:800, 1989.

61. Moss J, Vaughan M: Mechanism of action of choleragen. Evidence for ADP-ribosyltransferase activity with arginine as an acceptor. J Biol Chem 252:2455, 1977.

62. Moss J, Vaughan M: ADP-ribosylation of guanyl nucleotide–binding regulatory proteins by bacterial toxins. Adv Enzymol Relat Areas Mol Biol 61:303, 1988.

63. Cassel D, Pfeuffer T: Mechanism of cholera toxin action: Covalent modification of the guanyl nucleotide–binding protein of the adenylate cyclase system. Proc Natl Acad Sci U S A 75:2669, 1978.

64. Moss J, Vaughan M: Guanine nucleotide–binding proteins (G proteins) in activation of adenylyl cyclase: Lessons learned from cholera and "travelers' diarrhea." J Lab Clin Med 113:258, 1989.

65. Schwartz CJ, Kirnberg DV, Sheerin HE, et al: Vasoactive intestinal peptide stimulation of adenylate cyclase and active electrolyte secretion in intestinal mucosa. J Clin Invest 54:536, 1974.

66. Cartwright CA, McRoberts JA, Mandel KG, Dharmsathaphorn K: Synergistic action of cyclic adenosine monophosphate– and calcium-mediated chloride secretion in a colonic epithelial cell line. J Clin Invest 76:1837, 1985.

67. Levine SA, Donowitz M, Watson AJ, et al: Characterization of the synergistic interaction of *Escherichia coli* heat-stable toxin and carbachol. Am J Physiol 261(4 pt 1):G592, 1991.

68. Warhurst G, Higgs NB, Lees M, et al: Activation of protein kinase C attenuates prostaglandin E_2 responses in a colonic cell line. Am J Physiol 255(1 pt 1):G27, 1988.

69. Fasano A, Baudry B, Pumplin DW, et al: *Vibrio cholerae* produces a second enterotoxin, which affects intestinal tight junctions. Proc Natl Acad Sci U S A 88:5242, 1991.

70. Matsuzaki T, Tajika Y, Ablimit A, et al: Aquaporins in the digestive system. Med Electron Microsc 37:71, 2004.

71. Ma T, Verkman AS: Aquaporin water channels in gastro-intestinal physiology. J Physiol 517(pt 2):317, 1999.

72. Koyama Y, Yamamoto T, Tani T, et al: Expression and localization of aquaporins in rat gastrointestinal tract. Am J Physiol 276(3 pt 1):C621, 1999.

73. Singh SK, Binder HJ, Geibel JP, Boron WF, et al: Fluid absorption in isolated perfused colonic crypts. J Clin Invest 96:2373, 1995.

74. Maher MM, Gontarer JD, Bess RS, et al: The Na^+/H^+ exchange isoform NHE3 regulates basal canine ileal Na^+ absorption in vivo. Gastroenterology 112:174, 1997.

75. Bookstein C, DePaoli AM, Xie Y, et al: Na^+/H^+ exchangers, NHE-1 and NHE-3, of rat intestine. Expression and localization. J Clin Invest 93:106, 1994.

76. Hoogerwerf WA, et al: NHE2 and NHE3 are human and rabbit intestinal brush-border proteins. Am J Physiol 270(1 pt 1): G29, 1996.

77. McSwine RL, Musch MW, Bookstein C, et al: Regulation of apical membrane Na^+/H^+ exchangers NHE2 and NHE3 in intestinal epithelial cell line C2/bbe. Am J Physiol 275(3 pt 1):C693, 1988.

78. Wormmeester L, Sanchez de Medina F, Kokke F, et al: Quantitative contribution of NHE2 and NHE3 to rabbit ileal brush-border Na^+/H^+ exchange. Am J Physiol 274(5 pt 1):C1261, 1998.

79. Knickelbein R, Aronson PS, Schron CM, et al: Sodium and chloride transport across rabbit ileal brush border. I. Evidence for Na-H exchange. Am J Physiol 245:G504, 1983.

80. Field M, Fromm D, McColl I: Ion transport in rabbit ileal mucosa. I. Na and Cl fluxes and short-circuit current. Am J Physiol 220:1388, 1971.

81. Sellin JH, DeSoignie R: Rabbit proximal colon: A distinct transport epithelium. Am J Physiol 246(5 pt 1):G603, 1984.

82. Rajendran VM, Black J, Ardito TA, et al: Regulation of DRA and AE1 in rat colon by dietary Na depletion. Am J Physiol Gastrointest Liver Physiol 279:G931, 2000.

83. Schweinfest CW, Henderson KW, Suster S, et al: Identification of a colon mucosa gene that is down-regulated in colon adenomas and adenocarcinomas. Proc Natl Acad Sci U S A 90:4166, 1993.

84. Hoglund P, Haila S, Socha J, et al: Mutations of the Down-Regulated in Adenoma (*DRA*) gene cause congenital chloride diarrhoea. Nat Genet 14:316, 1996.

85. Shull GE, Miller ML, Schultheis PJ: Lessons from genetically engineered animal models VIII. Absorption and secretion of ions in the gastrointestinal tract. Am J Physiol Gastrointest Liver Physiol 278:G185, 2000.

86. Cho JH, Musch MW, Bookstein CM, et al: Aldosterone stimulates intestinal Na^+ absorption in rats by increasing NHE3 expression of the proximal colon. Am J Physiol 274(3 pt 1):C586, 1998.

87. Bookstein C, Musch MW, Xie Y, et al: Regulation of intestinal epithelial brush border Na^+/H^+ exchanger isoforms, NHE2 and NHE3, in C2bbe cells. J Membr Biol 171:87, 1999.

88. Weinman EJ, Minkoff C, Shenolikar S: Signal complex regulation of renal transport proteins: NHERF and regulation of NHE3 by PKA. Am J Physiol Renal Physiol 279(3):F393, 2000.

89. Weinman EJ, Steplock D, Donowitz M, Shenolikar S: NHERF associations with sodium-hydrogen exchanger isoform 3 (NHE3) and ezrin are essential for cAMP-mediated phosphorylation and inhibition of NHE3. Biochemistry 39:6123, 2000.

90. Lamprecht G, Weinman EJ, Yun CH: The role of NHERF and E3KARP in the cAMP-mediated inhibition of NHE3. J Biol Chem 273:29972, 1998.

91. Lamprecht G, Heil A, Baisch S, et al: The down regulated in adenoma (dra) gene product binds to the second PDZ domain of the NHE3 kinase A regulatory protein (E3KARP), potentially linking intestinal Cl^-/HCO_3^- exchange to Na^+/H^+ exchange. Biochemistry 41:12336, 2002.

92. Cavet ME, Akhter S, Murtazina R, et al: Half-lives of plasma membrane $Na(+)/H(+)$ exchangers NHE1-3: Plasma membrane NHE2 has a rapid rate of degradation. Am J Physiol Cell Physiol 281:C2039, 2001.

93. Ahn W, Kim KH, Lee JA, et al: Regulatory interaction between the cystic fibrosis transmembrane conductance regulator and HCO_3^- salvage mechanisms in model systems and the mouse pancreatic duct. J Biol Chem 276:17236, 2001.

94. O'Loughlin EV, Hunt DM, Gaskin KJ, et al: Abnormal epithelial transport in cystic fibrosis jejunum. Am J Physiol 260(5 pt 1):G758, 1991.

95. Clarke LL, Harline MC: CFTR is required for cAMP inhibition of intestinal Na^+ absorption in a cystic fibrosis mouse model. Am J Physiol 270(2 pt 1):G259, 1996.

96. Nusrat A, Turner JR, Madara JL: Molecular physiology and pathophysiology of tight junctions. IV. Regulation of tight junctions by extracellular stimuli: Nutrients, cytokines, and immune cells. Am J Physiol Gastrointest Liver Physiol 279:G851, 2000.

97. Turner JR, Angle JM, Black ED, et al: PKC-dependent regulation of transepithelial resistance: Roles of MLC and MLC kinase. Am J Physiol 277(3 pt 1):C554, 1999.

98. Turner JR, Black ED, Ward J, et al: Transepithelial resistance can be regulated by the intestinal brush-border $Na(+)/H(+)$ exchanger NHE3. Am J Physiol Cell Physiol 279:C1918, 2000.

99. Rao MC: Oral rehydration therapy: New explanations for an old remedy. Annu Rev Physiol 66:385, 2004.

100. Kunzelmann K, Mall M: Electrolyte transport in the mammalian colon: Mechanisms and implications for disease. Physiol Rev 82:245, 2002.

101. Garty H, Benos DJ: Characteristics and regulatory mechanisms of the amiloride-blockable Na^+ channel. Physiol Rev 68:309, 1988.

102. Turnheim K: Intrinsic regulation of apical sodium entry in epithelia. Physiol Rev 71:429, 1991.

103. Shimkets RA, Lifton R, Canessa CM: In vivo phosphorylation of the epithelial sodium channel. Proc Natl Acad Sci U S A 95:3301, 1998.

104. Bridges RJ, Cragoe EJ, Frizzell RA, Benos DJ: Inhibition of colonic Na^+ transport by amiloride analogues. Am J Physiol 256(1 pt 1):C67, 1989.

105. Briel M, Greger R, Kunzelmann K: Cl^- transport by cystic fibrosis transmembrane conductance regulator (CFTR) contributes to the inhibition of epithelial Na^+ channels (ENaCs) in *Xenopus* oocytes co-expressing CFTR and ENaC. J Physiol 508(pt 3):825, 1988.

106. Brown DR, O'Grady SM: Regulation of ion transport in the porcine intestinal tract by enteric neurotransmitters and hormones. Comp Biochem Physiol A Physiol 118:309, 1997.

107. Hansen MB, Skadhauge E: New aspects of the pathophysiology and treatment of secretory diarrhoea. Physiol Res 44:61, 1995.

108. Binder HS, Sandle GI: Electrolyte transport in the mammalian colon. In Johnson L (ed): Physiology of the Gastrointestinal Tract. New York, Raven, 1994, p 2133.

109. Rossier BC: Lose salt and gain a friend! A tribute to Gerhard Giebisch. Wien Klin Wochenschr 109:504, 1997.

110. Turnamian SG, Binder HJ: Regulation of active sodium and potassium transport in the distal colon of the rat. Role of the aldosterone and glucocorticoid receptors. J Clin Invest 84:1924, 1989.

111. Brennan FE, Fuller PJ: Rapid upregulation of serum and glucocorticoid-regulated kinase (SGK) gene expression by corticosteroids in vivo. Mol Cell Endocrinol 166:129, 2000.

112. Chen SY, Bhargava A, Mastroberardino L, et al: Epithelial sodium channel regulated by aldosterone-induced protein sgk. Proc Natl Acad Sci U S A 96:2514, 1999.

113. Catalan M, Niemeyer MI, Cid LP, Sepulveda FV: Basolateral ClC-2 chloride channels in surface colon epithelium: Regulation by a direct effect of intracellular chloride. Gastroenterology 126:1104, 2004.

114. Pratha VS, Hogan DL, Martensson BA, et al: Identification of transport abnormalities in duodenal mucosa and duodenal enterocytes from patients with cystic fibrosis. Gastroenterology 118:1051, 2000.

115. Cuthbert AW, Hickman ME, MacVinish LJ: Formal analysis of electrogenic sodium, potassium, chloride and bicarbonate transport in mouse colon epithelium. Br J Pharmacol 126: 358, 1999.

116. Poulsen JH, Fischer H, Illek B, Machen TE: Bicarbonate conductance and pH regulatory capability of cystic fibrosis transmembrane conductance regulator. Proc Natl Acad Sci U S A 91:5340, 1994.

117. Illek B, Yankaskas JR, Machen TE: cAMP and genistein stimulate HCO_3^- conductance through CFTR in human airway epithelia. Am J Physiol 272(4 pt 1):L752, 1997.

118. Seidler U, Blumenstein I, Kretz A, et al: A functional CFTR protein is required for mouse intestinal cAMP-, cGMP- and Ca^{2+}-dependent HCO_3^- secretion. J Physiol 505(pt 2):411, 1997.

119. O'Reilly CM, Winpenny JP, Argent BE, Gray MA: Cystic fibrosis transmembrane conductance regulator currents in guinea pig pancreatic duct cells: Inhibition by bicarbonate ions. Gastroenterology 118:1187, 2000.

120. Lee MG, Choi JY, Luo X, et al: Cystic fibrosis transmembrane conductance regulator regulates luminal Cl^-/HCO_3^- exchange in mouse submandibular and pancreatic ducts. J Biol Chem 274:14670, 1999.

121. Lee MG, Wigley WC, Zeng W, et al: Regulation of Cl^-/HCO_3^- exchange by cystic fibrosis transmembrane conductance regulator expressed in NIH 3T3 and HEK 293 cells. J Biol Chem 274:3414, 1999.

122. Wheat VJ, Shumaker H, Burnham C, et al: CFTR induces the expression of DRA along with Cl^-/HCO_3^- exchange activity in tracheal epithelial cells. Am J Physiol Cell Physiol 279: C62, 2000.

123. Field M: Intestinal ion transport and the pathophysiology of diarrhea. J Clin Invest 111:931, 2003.

124. Waldegger S, Jentsch TJ: From tonus to tonicity: Physiology of CLC chloride channels. J Am Soc Nephrol 11:1331, 2000.

125. Jentsch TJ, Friedrich T, Schriever A, Yamada H: The CLC chloride channel family. Pflugers Arch 437:783, 1999.

126. Rozmahel R, Wilschanski M, Matin A, et al: Modulation of disease severity in cystic fibrosis transmembrane conductance regulator deficient mice by a secondary genetic factor. Nat Genet 12:280, 1996.

127. Sakmann B, Neher E: Patch clamp techniques for studying ionic channels in excitable membranes. Annu Rev Physiol 46:455, 1984.

128. Greger RK, Kunzelmann K, Gerlach KL: Mechanisms of chloride transport in secretory epithelia. Ann N Y Acad Sci 574:403, 1990.

129. Hayslett JP, Gogelein H, Kunzelmann K, Greger R: Characteristics of apical chloride channels in human colon cells (HT29). Pflugers Arch 410:487, 1987.

130. Bohme M, Diener M, Rummel W: Calcium- and cyclic-AMP-mediated secretory responses in isolated colonic crypts. Pflugers Arch 419:144, 1991.

131. Mall M, Bleich M, Schurlein M, et al: Cholinergic ion secretion in human colon requires coactivation by cAMP. Am J Physiol 275(6 pt 1):G1274, 1998.

132. Mall M, Wissner A, Seydewitz HH, et al: Defective cholinergic Cl^- secretion and detection of K^+ secretion in rectal biopsies from cystic fibrosis patients. Am J Physiol Gastrointest Liver Physiol 278:G617, 2000.

133. Vaandrager AB, Tilly BC, Smolenski A, et al: cGMP stimulation of cystic fibrosis transmembrane conductance regulator Cl^- channels co-expressed with cGMP-dependent protein kinase type II but not type Ibeta. J Biol Chem 272:4195, 1997.

134. Swenson ES, Mann EA, Jump ML, et al: The guanylin/STa receptor is expressed in crypts and apical epithelium throughout the mouse intestine. Biochem Biophys Res Commun 225:1009, 1996.

135. Sitaraman SV, Merlin D, Si-Tahar M, et al: Neutrophil-epithelial crosstalk at the intestinal luminal surface mediated by reciprocal secretion of adenosine and IL-6. J Clin Invest 107:861, 2001.

136. Ganeshan R, Di A, Nelson DJ, et al: The interaction between syntaxin 1A and cystic fibrosis transmembrane conductance regulator Cl^- channels is mechanistically distinct from syntaxin 1A-SNARE interactions. J Biol Chem 278:2876, 2003.

137. Moyer BD, Duhaime M, Shaw C, et al: The PDZ-interacting domain of cystic fibrosis transmembrane conductance regulator is required for functional expression in the apical plasma membrane. J Biol Chem 275:27069, 2000.

138. Wang S, Raab RW, Sehatz PJ, et al: Peptide binding consensus of the NHE-RF-PDZ1 domain matches the C-terminal sequence of cystic fibrosis transmembrane conductance regulator (CFTR). FEBS Lett 427:103, 1998.

139. Mohler PJ, Kreda SM, Boucher RC, et al: Yes-associated protein 65 localizes p62(c-Yes) to the apical compartment of airway epithelia by association with EBP50. J Cell Biol 147:879, 1999.

140. Sun F, Hug MJ, Bradbury NA, Frizzell RA: Protein kinase A associates with cystic fibrosis transmembrane conductance regulator via an interaction with ezrin. J Biol Chem 275:14360, 2000.

141. Sun F, Hug MJ, Lewarchik CM, et al: E3KARP mediates the association of ezrin and protein kinase A with the cystic fibrosis transmembrane conductance regulator in airway cells. J Biol Chem 275:29539, 2000.

142. Gadsby DC, Nairn AC: Control of CFTR channel gating by phosphorylation and nucleotide hydrolysis. Physiol Rev 79(1 suppl):S77, 1999.

143. Kunzelmann K: The cystic fibrosis transmembrane conductance regulator and its function in epithelial transport. Rev Physiol Biochem Pharmacol 137:1, 1999.

144. Binder HJ, Sangan P, Rajendran VM: Physiological and molecular studies of colonic H^+,K^+-ATPase. Semin Nephrol 19:405, 1999.

145. Abrahamse SI, De Jonge HR, Bindels RJ, Van Os CH: Two distinct K(+)-ATPase activities in rabbit distal colon. Biochem Biophys Res Commun 207:1003, 1975.

146. Butterfield I, Warhurst G, Fones MN, Sandle GI: Characterization of apical potassium channels induced in rat distal colon during potassium adaptation. J Physiol 501(pt 3):537, 1997.

147. Sandle GI, Butterfield I: Potassium secretion in rat distal colon during dietary potassium loading: Role of pH regulated apical potassium channels. Gut 44:40, 1999.

148. Foster ES, Sandle GI, Hayslett JP, Binder HJ: Dietary potassium modulates active potassium absorption and secretion in rat distal colon. Am J Physiol 251(5 pt 1):G619, 1986.

149. Sandle GI, Foster ES, Leur SA, et al: The electrical basis for enhanced potassium secretion in rat distal colon during dietary potassium loading. Pflugers Arch 403:433, 1985.

150. Diener M, Hug F, Strabel D, Scharrer E: Cyclic AMP–dependent regulation of K^+ transport in the rat distal colon. Br J Pharmacol 118:1477, 1996.

151. Cummings JH: Colonic absorption: The importance of short chain fatty acids in man. Scand J Gastroenterol Suppl 93:89, 1984.

152. Roediger WE: Role of anaerobic bacteria in the metabolic welfare of the colonic mucosa in man. Gut 21:793, 1980.

153. Roediger WE: Utilization of nutrients by isolated epithelial cells of the rat colon. Gastroenterology 83:424, 1982.

154. Scheppach W, Bartram P, Rechter A, et al: Effect of short-chain fatty acids on the human colonic mucosa in vitro. JPEN J Parenter Enteral Nutr 16:43, 1992.

155. Marsman KE, McBurney MI: Dietary fiber increases oxidative metabolism in colonocytes but not in distal small intestinal enterocytes isolated from rats. J Nutr 125:273, 1995.

156. Tyagi S, Venugopalakrishnan J, Ramaswamy K, Dudeja PK: Mechanism of *n*-butyrate uptake in the human proximal colonic basolateral membranes. Am J Physiol Gastrointest Liver Physiol 282:G676, 2002.

157. Schmitt MG Jr, Soergel KH, Wood CM, Steff JJ: Absorption of short-chain fatty acids from the human ileum. Am J Dig Dis 22:340, 1977.

158. Charney AN, Micic L, Egnor RW: Nonionic diffusion of short-chain fatty acids across rat colon. Am J Physiol 274(3 pt 1):G518, 1998.

159. Harig JM, Ng EK, Dudeja PK, et al: Transport of *n*-butyrate into human colonic luminal membrane vesicles. Am J Physiol 271(3 pt 1):G415, 1996.

160. Sellin JH, DeSoignie R: Short-chain fatty acid absorption in rabbit colon in vitro. Gastroenterology 99:676, 1990.

161. Hadjiagapiou C, et al: Mechanism(s) of butyrate transport in Caco-2 cells: Role of monocarboxylate transporter 1. Am J Physiol Gastrointest Liver Physiol 279:G775, 2000.

162. Miller DL, Hanson W, Schedl HP, Osborne JW: Proliferation rate and transit time of mucosal cells in small intestine of the diabetic rat. Gastroenterology 73:1326, 1977.

163. Mayhew TM: Striated brush border of intestinal absorptive epithelial cells: Stereological studies on microvillous morphology in different adaptive states. J Electron Microsc Tech 16:45, 1990.

164. Fedorak RN, Chang EB, Madara JL, Field M, et al: Intestinal adaptation to diabetes. Altered Na-dependent nutrient absorption in streptozocin-treated chronically diabetic rats. J Clin Invest 79:1571, 1987.

165. Karasov WH, Diamond JM: Adaptive regulation of sugar and amino acid transport by vertebrate intestine. Am J Physiol 245:G443, 1983.

166. Perdue MH, Davison JS: Altered regulation of intestinal ion transport by enteric nerves in diabetic rats. Am J Physiol 254(3 pt 1):G444, 1988.

167. Field M, Musch MW, Stoff JS: Role of prostaglandins in the regulation of intestinal electrolyte transport. Prostaglandins 21(suppl):73, 1981.

168. Diener M, Bridges RJ, Knobloch SF, Rummel W: Neuronally mediated and direct effects of prostaglandins on ion transport in rat colon descendens. Naunyn Schmiedebergs Arch Pharmacol 337:74, 1988.

169. Bern MJ, Sturbaum CW, Karayalem SS, et al: Immune system control of rat and rabbit colonic electrolyte transport. Role of prostaglandins and enteric nervous system. J Clin Invest 83:1810, 1989.

170. Traynor TR, Brown DR, O'Grady SM: Effects of inflammatory mediators on electrolyte transport across the porcine distal colon epithelium. J Pharmacol Exp Ther 264:61, 1993.

171. Gaginella TS, Kachur JF: Kinins as mediators of intestinal secretion. Am J Physiol 256(1 pt 1):G1, 1989.

172. Stack WA, Filipowicz B, Hawkey CJ: Nitric oxide donating compounds stimulate human colonic ion transport in vitro. Gut 39:93, 1996.

173. Bell CJ, Gall DG, Wallace JL: Disruption of colonic electrolyte transport in experimental colitis. Am J Physiol 268(4 pt 1):G622, 1995.

174. Sandle GI, Higgs N, Crowe P, et al: Cellular basis for defective electrolyte transport in inflamed human colon. Gastroenterology 99:97, 1990.

175. Rocha F, Musch MW, Lishanskiy L, et al: IFN-gamma down-regulates expression of Na^+/H^+ exchangers NHE2 and NHE3 in rat intestine and human Caco-2/bbe cells. Am J Physiol Cell Physiol 280:C1224, 2001.

176. Sugi K, Musch MW, Field M, Chang EB: Inhibition of Na^+,K^+-ATPase by interferon gamma down-regulates intestinal epithelial transport and barrier function. Gastroenterology 120:1393, 2001.

177. Musch MW, Clarke LL, Mamah D, et al: T cell activation causes diarrhea by increasing intestinal permeability and inhibiting epithelial Na^+/K^+-ATPase. J Clin Invest 110:1739, 2002.

178. Chang EB, Brookstein C: Mechanisms of intestinal absorption and secretion: an abbreviated review and update. In Domschke W, Stoll R (eds): Intestinal Mucosa and Its Diseases—Pathophysiology and Clinics. Falk Symposium 110. Dordrecht, The Netherlands, Kluwer Academic Publishers, 1999.

179. Anderson MP, Sheppard DN, Berger HA, Welch MJ: Chloride channels in the apical membrane of normal and cystic fibrosis airway and intestinal epithelia. Am J Physiol 263(1 pt 1):L1, 1992.

180. Anderson MP, Gregery RJ, Thompson S, et al: Demonstration that CFTR is a chloride channel by alteration of its anion selectivity. Science 253:202, 1991.

181. Berger HA, Anderson MP, Gregery RJ, et al: Identification and regulation of the cystic fibrosis transmembrane conductance regulator–generated chloride channel. J Clin Invest 88:1422, 1991.

182. Lencer WI, Cheung G, Strohmeier FR, et al: Induction of epithelial chloride secretion by channel-forming cryptidins 2 and 3. Proc Natl Acad Sci U S A 94:8585, 1997.

183. Dominguez P, Barros F, Lazo PS: The activation of adenylate cyclase from small intestinal epithelium by cholera toxin. Eur J Biochem 146:533, 1985.

184. Lynch CJ, Morbach L, Blackmore PF, Exton JH: Alpha-subunits of Ns are released from the plasma membrane following cholera toxin activation. FEBS Lett 200:333, 1986.

185. Field M, Semrad CE: Toxigenic diarrheas, congenital diarrheas, and cystic fibrosis: Disorders of intestinal ion transport. Annu Rev Physiol 55:631, 1993.

186. Banks MR, Golder M, Farthing MJ, Burleigh DE: Intracellular potentiation between two second messenger systems may contribute to cholera toxin induced intestinal secretion in humans. Gut 53:50, 2004.

187. Vaandrager AB, Bot AG, Ruth P, et al: Differential role of cyclic GMP–dependent protein kinase II in ion transport in murine small intestine and colon. Gastroenterology 118:108, 2000.

188. Schulz S, Green CK, Yaen PS, Garbers DL: Guanylyl cyclase is a heat-stable enterotoxin receptor. Cell 63:941, 1990.

189. Zhang M, Zeng CQ, Morris AP, Estes MK: A functional NSP4 enterotoxin peptide secreted from rotavirus-infected cells. J Virol 74:11663, 2000.

190. Ball JM, Tian P, Zeng CQ, et al: Age-dependent diarrhea induced by a rotaviral nonstructural glycoprotein. Science 272:101, 1996.

191. Tian P, Hu Y, Schilling WP, et al: The nonstructural glycoprotein of rotavirus affects intracellular calcium levels. J Virol 68:251, 1994.

192. Pace J, Hayman MJ, Galan JHE: Signal transduction and invasion of epithelial cells by *S. typhimurium*. Cell 72:505, 1993.

193. Gewirtz AT, Rao AS, Simon PO, et al: *Salmonella typhimurium* induces epithelial IL-8 expression via Ca^{2+}-mediated activation of the NF-kappaB pathway. J Clin Invest 105:79, 2000.

194. Kelly CP, LaMont JT: *Clostridium difficile* infection. Annu Rev Med 49:375, 1998.

195. Nusrat A, van Eichel-Streiber C, Turner JR, et al: *Clostridium difficile* toxins disrupt epithelial barrier function by altering membrane microdomain localization of tight junction proteins. Infect Immun 69:1329, 2001.

196. Hopkins AM, Li D, Mrsny RJ, et al: Modulation of tight junction function by G protein–coupled events. Adv Drug Deliv Rev 41:329, 2000.

197. Tsujikawa T, Itoh A, Fukunaga T, et al: Alteration of aquaporin mRNA expression after small bowel resection in the rat residual ileum and colon. J Gastroenterol Hepatol 18:803, 2003.

198. Hines OJ, Bilchik AJ, Zinner MJ, et al: Adaptation of the Na^+/glucose cotransporter following intestinal resection. J Surg Res 57:22, 1994.

199. Hines OJ, Bilchik AJ, McFadden DW, et al: Up-regulation of Na^+,K^+ adenosine triphosphatase after massive intestinal resection. Surgery 116:401, 1994.

200. Musch MW, Bookstein C, Rocha F, et al: Region-specific adaptation of apical Na/H exchangers after extensive proximal small bowel resection. Am J Physiol Gastrointest Liver Physiol 283:G975, 2002.

201. Rajendran VM, Binder HJ: Apical membrane Cl-butyrate exchange: Mechanism of short chain fatty acid stimulation of active chloride absorption in rat distal colon. J Membr Biol 141:51, 1994.

202. Musch MW, Bookstein C, Xie Y, et al: SCFA increase intestinal Na absorption by induction of NHE3 in rat colon and human intestinal C2/bbe cells. Am J Physiol Gastrointest Liver Physiol 280:G687, 2001.

203. Tappenden KA, Drozdowski LA, Thomson AB, McBurney MI: Short-chain fatty acid-supplemented total parenteral nutrition alters intestinal structure, glucose transporter 2 (Glut2) mRNA and protein, and proglucagon mRNA abundance in normal rats. Am J Clin Nutr 68:118, 1998.

204. Blottiere HM, Buecher B, Galmiche JP, Cherbut C: Molecular analysis of the effect of short-chain fatty acids on intestinal cell proliferation. Proc Nutr Soc 62:101, 2003.

CHAPTER
97 Digestion and Absorption of Nutrients and Vitamins

James J. Farrell

Most nutrients are absorbed with remarkable efficiency: Less than 5% of ingested carbohydrate, fat, and protein usually is excreted in the stool of adults who consume normal diets.[1] Even much of the "indigestible" dietary fiber is absorbed from the colon as short-chain fatty acids that are liberated by bacterial breakdown of the fiber.[2] The intestinal tract of neonates is less efficient: Infants fail to absorb 10% to 15% of their dietary fat, and in prematurity, as much as 25% to 35% may be lost in the stool.[3,4] In old age, nutrient absorption remains highly efficient unless the intestine becomes diseased.

Despite considerable variations in types of food and nutritional intake across national and racial groups, intestinal absorption remains efficient. Good evidence suggests that absorptive mechanisms adapt to the nature and amount of various nutrients presented to the intestinal tract. Such changes occur not only during early development[5] but throughout life and at times of specific need, as during pregnancy.[6] In achieving the overall objective of nutrient absorption, the different parts of the gastrointestinal tract act in a closely integrated and coordinated manner under the control of neural and humoral regulatory mechanisms.

Elucidation of intestinal digestion and absorption at a molecular level has improved our knowledge of the integration and coordination of these functions within the gastrointestinal tract. The pharmacokinetics and pharmacodynamics of several key carbohydrate, fat, peptide, amino acid, vitamin, and nutrient transporters are being increasingly understood. In this chapter, the integration of intestinal function including the dietary intake, digestion, and absorption of major nutrients (fat, carbohydrate and protein) and essential micronutrients (vitamins and trace elements), as well as the genetic and molecular basis of these functions, are discussed. New insights into the effect of bariatric surgery on key absorptive functions also are presented.

DIGESTION AND ABSORPTION OF NUTRIENTS: AN OVERVIEW

The cerebral phase of digestion, whether triggered by the sight, smell, or thought of food, initiates the digestive process. Salivary and gastric secretory responses to these types of stimuli are mediated by the autonomic nervous system, with modest stimulation of pancreaticobiliary secretion by the vagus nerve.[7] Further stimulus by the presence of nutrients in the mouth and upper gastrointestinal tract markedly potentiates secretion by both humoral (Table 97–1) and local neural mechanisms (see Chapter 1).[8]

The speed at which food normally is chewed and swallowed affords little time for significant oral digestion of nutrients; however, good mastication and mixing of foods with saliva initiate digestion of starch by salivary amylase. In infants, digestion of fat is begun by gastric lipase. Gastric acid would switch off these enzymes promptly were it not for the buffering capacity of food that allows some digestion to continue. The optimal pH of gastric lipases is 4.5 to 6.0, and it has been suggested that a considerable proportion of dietary triglyceride may be digested by these lipases.[9,10] Protein digestion begins in the stomach with secretion of gastric pepsinogens and their rapid conversion to pepsins by gastric acid. Pepsins are not catalytically active at pH higher than 4. Therefore, the digestive action of pepsins on proteins is restricted to the stomach. The acidic stomach contents are neutralized by the pancreatic and intestinal secretions when they enter the duodenum, consequently leading to inactivation of pepsins.

During ingestion of food, the stomach distends, but intragastric pressure rises little because of neurally mediated receptive relaxation. The mechanisms by which people perceive satiety and therefore cease eating are complex and are explained only partly by the sensation of fullness. Although a myriad of enzymes and hormones are secreted by the gastrointestinal tract in response to the presence of food in the lumen, only a few are able to influence food intake directly. Satiety signals are relayed to the hindbrain, either indirectly along nerves such as the vagus nerve or directly through the blood. Most factors that influence how much food is eaten during

individual meals act by changing the sensitivity to satiety signals.[11]

Cholecystokinin (CCK), gastrin-releasing peptide, and apolipoprotein A-IV (apo A-IV) all have been implicated as messengers that transmit the satiety signal to the central nervous system (CNS).[12-14] They potentiate each other's actions, and a combination of these agents may participate in the satiety signal. The administration of exogenous CCK or other satiety mediating factors causes consumption of smaller meals, whereas blocking the action of endogenous CCK and other satiety signals allows ingestion of larger meals.[11,15,16] Additional peptides, known as the anorectic peptides, including peptide tyrosine-tyrosine (PYY), pancreatic polypeptide (PP), glucagon-like peptide 1 (GLP-1), and oxyntomodulin, also have been shown to decrease appetite and promote satiety in both animal and human models.[17]

Apo A-IV is a glycoprotein synthesized by the enterocytes of human intestine and the hypothalamus, especially the arcuate nucleus. Intestinal apo A-IV synthesis is markedly stimulated by fat absorption and the signal for the induction of intestinal apo A-IV synthesis is the local formation of chylomicrons; apo A-IV synthesis does not appear to be mediated by the uptake or re-esterification of fatty acids to form triglycerides. Intestinal apo A-IV synthesis also is enhanced by a factor from the ileum (probably PYY), as well as neuropeptide Y (NPY) and PP.[18] Inhibition of food intake by apo A-IV is mediated centrally. The stimulation of intestinal synthesis and secretion of apo A-IV by lipid absorption is rapid, as a result of which apo A-IV plays a role in the short-term regulation of food intake. Evidence also suggests that apo A-IV may be involved in long-term regulation of food intake and body weight, because it is regulated by both leptin and insulin. Leptin can cause a rapid activation of signal transducer and activator of transcription 5 (STAT5) in jejunum, which is associated with a reduction of the apo AIV transcript levels 90 minutes after ingestion of a pure fat load. This observation suggests that leptin might play a physiologic role in lipid handling at this site in vivo. Under physiologic conditions, postprandial rises in plasma leptin could function as a buffer system to reduce the plasma chylomicron triglyceride levels by reducing apo A-IV. It also is possible that leptin may serve as a tonic inhibitory mechanism on the apo A-IV system to reduce the levels of secreted triglycerides. Chronic ingestion of a high-fat diet blunts both the intestinal and the hypothalamic apo A-IV responses to lipid feeding.[19] The hypothalmic apo A-IV level is reduced by food deprivation and restored by lipid feeding.[20,21] At the enterocyte level, the specific mechanism by which leptin mediates reduction in apo A-IV messenger RNA (mRNA) levels needs to be defined.

Leptin, a hormone released from fat cells, is an important peripheral signal from fat stores that modulates food intake. Leptin deficiency and leptin receptor defects produce massive obesity. This peptide signals a variety of central mechanisms by acting on receptors in the arcuate nucleus and hypothalamus.[22] Only one gastrointestinal signal, ghrelin, has been shown to increase appetite.[11]

The major digestive processes are initiated in the duodenum. Delivery of chyme from the stomach is adjusted delicately so that it enters the duodenum at a controlled

Table 97–1	Hormones, Neuropeptides, and Neurotransmitters Involved in the Brain-Gut Axis

Stimulatory	**Inhibitory**
Cholecystokinin (CCK)	Pancreatic polypeptide (PP)
Secretin	Leptin
Gastrin	Peptide YY
Gastrin-releasing peptide (GRP)	Neuropeptide Y
Ghrelin	Calcitonin gene–related
Insulin	peptide
Vasoactive intestinal	Somatostatin
polypeptide (VIP)	Glucagon
Cyclase-activating peptide	Glucagon-like peptides
Substance P and other tachykinins	1 and 2 (GLP-1 and -2)
Adenosine 5′-triphosphate (ATP)	Thyrotropin-releasing
Uridine triphosphate (UTP)	hormone (TRH)
Histamine	Enkephalin (Met- or Leu-)
Pancreatic phospholipase A$_2$	Nitric oxide (NO)
	Dopamine

Adapted with permission from Konturek SJ, Pepera J, Zabielski K, et al: Brain-gut axis in pancreatic secretion and appetite control. J Physiol Pharmacol 54:293, 2003.

rate, thereby allowing efficient mixing with pancreaticobiliary secretions; control of gastric emptying is critical to ensuring optimal digestion (see Chapter 46). The characteristics of gastric contents that determine this rate of emptying include their consistency, pH, osmolality, and lipid and calorie content[23] (Fig. 97–1).

The pylorus is selective in that it allows rapid passage of liquids but retains solid particles with diameters of 2 mm or larger.[24] Thus, large particles are retained and progressively reduced in size by the gastric "mill," a process referred to as *trituration*; trituration ensures that particles will be small enough to allow reasonably close apposition to digestive enzymes once the nutrient is allowed to enter the duodenum. Meals of high viscosity empty more slowly than do those of low viscosity.

Duodenal mucosal receptors for pH and osmolality trigger a delay in gastric emptying when the gastric effluent is acidic or hyper- or hypotonic.[25,26] When duodenal luminal contents are neutralized by pancreaticobiliary bicarbonate and osmolality is adjusted by water fluxes,

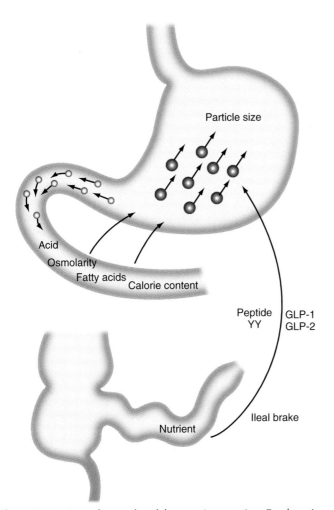

Figure 97–1 Some factors that delay gastric emptying. Food particles larger than 2 mm in diameter are rejected by the antrum. Receptors for pH, osmolarity, fatty acids, and other nutrients in the duodenum signal gastric delay by means of neurohumoral mechanisms. Nutrients in the ileum and colon also influence gastric emptying by the so-called ileal brake mechanism, which may involve peptide tyrosine-tyrosine (PYY) and glucagon-like peptides GLP-1 and GLP-2.

gastric emptying is encouraged once more. This careful titration in the duodenal lumen ensures that nutrients are presented in an optimal fashion to the pancreatic enzymes, which function best at neutral pH.

The total caloric content of meals also controls gastric emptying rates; on average, the human stomach delivers approximately 150 kcal per hour to the duodenum.[27] An increase in the size or energy density of a meal leads to a corresponding increase in the rate of delivery. Duodenal mucosal receptors for fatty acids, amino acids, and carbohydrates are involved in this response, which probably is mediated by both neural and humoral feedback mechanisms.[28]

Gastric emptying also is controlled by a mechanism involving the ileum and colon. If much nutrient escapes digestion and absorption in the jejunum, its presence in the ileum and colon delays gastrointestinal transit, and this again provides more time for digestion and absorption.[29,30] This "ileal brake" probably is mediated by a neurohumoral mechanism; various neurotransmitters and hormones have been implicated, including peptide YY and the glucagon-like peptides GLP-1 and GLP-2.[31,32]

GLP-1 and GLP-2 are synthesized in and cosecreted from enteroendocrine cells in the small and large intestine in response to intraluminal carbohydrate and fat. Both peptides promote efficient nutrient assimilation by decreasing appetite and slowing gastric emptying; GLP-1 also enhances glucose-induced insulin secretion. Circulating levels of GLP-1 and GLP-2 are low in the fasted state and increase rapidly following nutrient ingestion.[33-37]

Simultaneously, in response to the presence of nutrients in the duodenal lumen, CCK and secretin are released into the portal circulation, respectively causing the gallbladder to contract and the pancreas to secrete. Exocrine pancreatic secretion is controlled by the coordination of cephalic (the vagus nerve), gastric (acid and pepsin secretion and gastric emptying), and intestinal (secretin and CCK) mechanisms (see Chapter 54).

CCK and other enterohormones stimulate the pancreas by exciting sensory nerves and triggering of long vagovagal or enteropancreatic reflexes. Numerous neurotransmitters, such as acetylcholine and nitric oxide, and certain neuropeptides, such as gastrin-releasing peptide (GRP), generated by neurons of the enteric nervous system, have been implicated in the regulation of the exocrine pancreas. CCK is distributed widely throughout the gastrointestinal tract and central nervous system and mediates a diverse number of biologic functions. Two receptor subtypes, CCK-A and CCK-B, have been identified; CCK-A receptor is the predominant peripheral CCK receptor subtype, and CCK-B receptor is the predominant central CCK receptor. CCK appears to act through vagal cholinergic pathways to mediate pancreatic enzyme secretion. Human pancreatic acini lack functional CCK-A receptors, explaining why a CCK infusion that produces plasma CCK levels similar to those seen postprandially stimulates pancreatic exocrine secretion by an atropine-sensitive pathway.[38] Under physiologic conditions, cholinergic vagal afferent pathways, rather than pancreatic acinar cells, represent the primary targets on which CCK acts as a major mediator of postprandial pancreatic secretion.[38]

Serotonin, or 5-hydroxytryptamine (5-HT), is released from enterochromaffin cells in the intestinal mucosa and nerve terminals of the enteric nervous system and the intra-pancreatic nerves; through its various receptor subtypes, 5-HT may be involved in both stimulation and inhibition of various digestive processes. 5-HT also mediates the action of secretin and CCK. A synergistic interaction between CCK and 5-HT at the level of the nodose ganglion may explain robust postprandial pancreatic secretion despite a modest postprandial increase in plasma CCK. Peptides affecting appetite behavior that orginate from the intestine (e.g., leptin, ghrelin) or from the pancreas (e.g., PP, neuropeptide Y) appear to modulate the exocrine pancreas through hypothalamic centers.[39,40]

Pancreatic juice provides both positive and negative feedback regulation of pancreatic secretion through mediation of both secretin- and CCK-releasing peptides. Three CCK-releasing peptides have been purified: monitor peptide from pancreatic juice, diazepam-binding inhibitor from porcine intestine, and luminal CCK-releasing factor from rat intestinal secretion. All three have been shown to stimulate CCK release and pancreatic enzyme secretion. Pancreatic phospholipase A_2 (PLA_2) from pancreatic juice and intestinal secretions appears to function as a secretin-releasing peptide.[41]

The simultaneous release of bile salts, pancreatic enzymes, and bicarbonate provides optimal conditions for further nutrient digestion. The simultaneous release of enteropeptidase (enterokinase) from duodenal mucosa is critically important to the activation of pancreatic proteolytic enzymes. Enterokinase releases trypsin from trypsinogen, thus encouraging proteolysis within the duodenal lumen rather than inside the pancreatic duct. That these three factors—bile, pancreatic enzymes, and enteropeptidase—remain separate until they are mixed in the intestinal lumen ensures that they become operational at the site of nutrient delivery.

Adequate lipid digestion is dependent on the presence of bile salts and pancreatic lipase-colipase at nearly neutral luminal pH,[42] whereas digestion of carbohydrate and protein depends on the combined actions of intraluminal secreted enzymes and then brush border and mucosal enzymes. The close physical relationship, at the brush border, between the sites for terminal digestion of protein and carbohydrate and the active absorption of digestive products provide a very efficient mechanism for dealing with these nutrients.

Two other simultaneous phenomena encourage efficient digestion and absorption. Ingestion of a meal stimulates salt and water secretion by the jejunal mucosa, and this maintains luminal contents in a sufficiently fluid state for proper mixing and digestion[43] (see Chapter 96). The other phenomenon is the motor response of the intestine. After feeding, the characteristic repetitive motility pattern that occurs during fasting is disrupted. Instead, an apparently disordered pattern is seen that presumably ensures that nutrient is well mixed and brought into close contact with intestinal mucosa (see Chapter 94). The neurohumoral control mechanisms involving the motor and secretory responses of the intestine are closely integrated.[44] For rapidly absorbed molecules, intestinal blood flow may be the rate-limiting step.[45]

Efficient conservation and recycling mechanisms ensure that gastrointestinal secretions are not entirely lost. Gastric acid secretion is balanced to a large extent by pancreaticobiliary bicarbonate secretion, so that overall acid-base balance is not disturbed. Although intact digestive enzymes are reabsorbed only in trace amounts, the nitrogen they contain is reabsorbed after their digestion. Finally, efficient enterohepatic circulation recycles bile salts several times each day, so that they are utilized approximately twice for each meal.[46] Although bile salts are reabsorbed passively throughout the small intestine, most reach the terminal ileum, where they are reabsorbed through specific active absorptive mechanisms. Thus, bile salts remain in the lumen, where they are needed for lipid digestion, but are largely reabsorbed at the last moment to avoid being lost by the colon (Fig. 97–2) (see Chapter 61).

Once intestinal chyme leaves the ileum and enters the colon, most nutrients have been digested and absorbed, and colonic function serves largely to dehydrate luminal contents by absorbing salt and water and to store the residuum. Dietary fiber may be digested by bacteria, with release of short-chain fatty acids, which are avidly absorbed; however, short-chain fatty acids usually do not have much nutritional significance, other than in areas of the world where the major source of energy is a high-fiber diet. Short-chain fatty acids are an important source of nutrition for the colonocyte.

FAT

DIETARY INTAKE

Approximately 40% of adult energy requirements is supplied by lipids, of which triglycerides account for a major portion.[47] The average daily intake of fat in the United

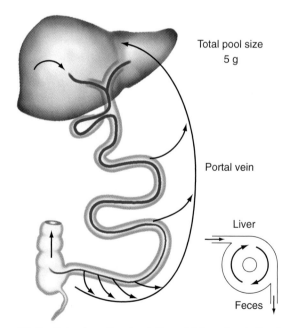

Figure 97–2 Enterohepatic circulation of bile salts. Active transport in the ileum retrieves most bile salts, and the small fraction lost into the colon is compensated for by fresh hepatic synthesis.

States in the 1960s was approximately 150 g per day, two thirds of which was derived from animal fat and one third from vegetable fat.[48] Available evidence suggests that the average fat intake is falling; in the United Kingdom it has now reached 90 g per day, compared with 120 g per day in 1969,[47] and similar trends have been observed in the United States. The proportion of dietary fat contributed by saturated fatty acids also appears to be declining (from 45% in 1980 to 41% in 1990 in the United Kingdom), whereas the proportion of polyunsaturates has increased from 10% to 15%.[47]

Oleic and palmitic acids (C18:1 and C16:0, respectively) account for most of the fatty acids present in dietary triglyceride.[49] In animal triglycerides, most fatty acids are long-chain saturated ones (i.e., longer than C14 chain length) (Fig. 97–3). Polyunsaturated fatty acids such as linoleic and linolenic acids are derived from phospholipid of vegetable origin and, because they cannot be synthesized de novo, they are considered essential fatty acids (Table 97–2).

The average range of phospholipid ingestion lies between 2 and 8 g per day. The most common ingested phospholipid is phosphatidylcholine (lecithin), and the predominant fatty acids in phospholipid are linoleate and arachidonate (see Fig. 97–3). More phospholipid is found in the duodenal lumen (10 to 22 g per day) than is ingested, most of which is derived from endogenous sources, particularly bile.

Cholesterol intake varies widely but averages approximately 200 to 250 mg per day[49]; one unusual patient has been described who for many years consumed 25 eggs per day (almost 5000 mg of cholesterol) without apparent harm.[50]

Hydrogenation of unsaturated bonds in the fatty acids of natural oils raises their melting points, thus allowing commercial production of margarines and spreads of variable consistency. Hydrogenation, in addition to saturation, results in isomerization of *cis* to *trans* double bonds.[51] Although many commercial products contain partially hydrogenated fats, the content of *trans* fatty acids in some margarines exceeds 60%, thus raising concern about their relationship to cancer induction.[52]

DIGESTION AND ABSORPTION

Most dietary lipid is absorbed in the upper two thirds of jejunum. The rate and extent of absorption are

Table 97–2   Common Dietary Fatty Acids*

Saturated	
Butyric	C4:0
Caproic	C6:0
Lauric	C12:0
Myristic	C14:0
Palmitic	C16:0
Stearic	C18:0
Monounsaturated	
Palmitoleic	C16:1
Oleic	C18:1
Polyunsaturated	
Linoleic	C18:2
Linolenic	C18:3
Arachidonic	C20:4

*By convention, the number of carbon atoms in the chain is given by the first figure, and the number of double bonds in the chain by the second figure.

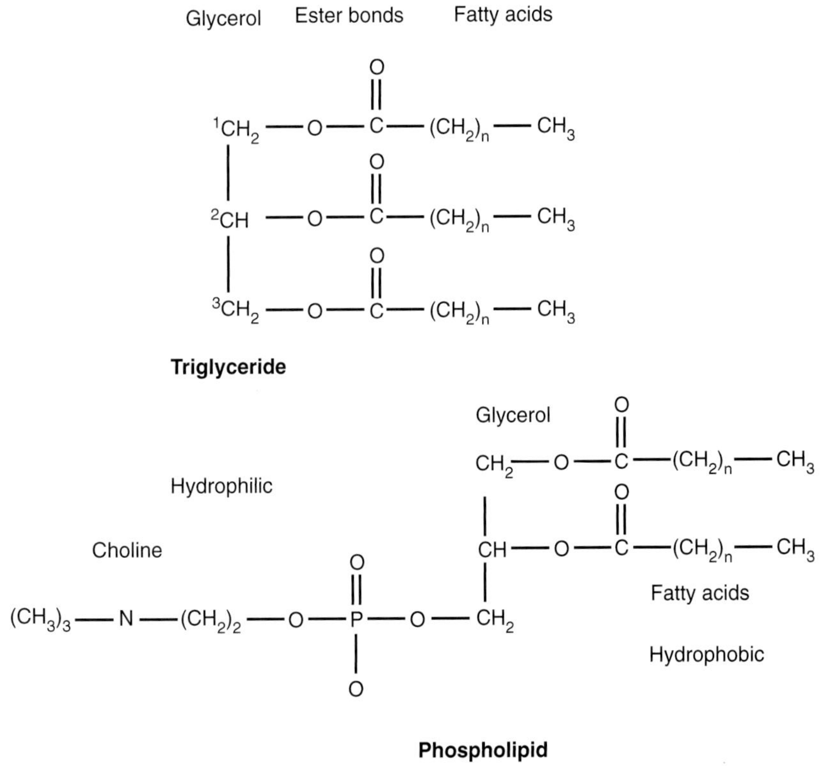

Figure 97–3 General molecular structure of triglycerides and a phospholipid (phosphatidyl choline/lecithin).

influenced by the presence of other foods, particularly dietary fiber, which reduces the rate of absorption.[53] The type of ingested fats also appears to influence the absorptive process, both by modifying the morphologic structure of the intestinal mucosa and by influencing its absorptive function for other nutrients such as carbohydrate.[54]

The problem of the insolubility of fat in water dominates the mechanisms that have been developed to digest and absorb lipid. Within the lumen, ingested fat must be physically released and broken down into emulsion droplets. The products of such digestion are then transported across the bulk (lumen) water phase to the lipid epithelial cell membrane. Transfer across the lipid membrane is followed, within the epithelium, by reconstitution into larger lipid molecules, predominantly triglyceride, which then require specialized processing to permit export from the cell. Thus, after digestion, lipid goes through three phases: water in the lumen, lipid in the epithelial membrane, and water in the lymphatics and bloodstream. Despite these potential barriers to absorption, more than 95% of ingested fat is absorbed in adults.

Triglyceride Digestion

Liberation of fatty acids from the glycerol backbone of triglycerides (lipolysis) is achieved by lipases acting at the surface of emulsified droplets. This occurs initially in the stomach and then in the small intestine. Studies suggest that normal intragastric lipolysis may account for 20% to 30% of total intraluminal lipid digestion[55]; gastric lipase, which is of fundic origin, has been demonstrated in the gastric contents of premature neonates and in mucosal biopsy specimens from adults up to 80 years of age. For either gastric or small intestinal lipolysis to occur, two conditions are critical: first, a stable emulsion of fat droplets of such a size that they present a large surface area to the digestive enzyme, and second, a mechanism for bringing enzyme and triglyceride into close apposition within the emulsion.

Emulsification

A number of factors assist in optimal production of an emulsion. Physical release of fat by mastication and gastric "milling" of food produces a relatively unstable emulsion that is delivered into the duodenum. To permit its stabilization, the droplets in this emulsion have to be coated, and *phospholipid* in the diet provides one such coat. The ratio of ingested phospholipid to triglyceride is approximately 1:30, and more phospholipid is added in the duodenum from bile.[56] In breast milk (Table 97–3), emulsion droplets are smaller and already have proteins as well as phospholipid incorporated into their surface trilayer.[57] Emulsification also is enhanced by the fatty acids liberated by intragastric lipolysis and, within the duodenum, by bile salts (Fig. 97–4). The final emulsification product in the duodenum consists predominantly of triglyceride, together with cholesterol esters and some diglyceride, coated by phospholipid, partially ionized fatty acids, monoglyceride, and bile salts.

Table 97–3   Characteristics of Lipases in Infancy

Milk-Derived Lipase
Stimulated by bile salts
Optimal pH of 7.0 (inactivation by acid is reversible)
Active against ester bonds in positions 1, 2, and 3
Gastric Lipase
Optimal pH of 4.0-6.0
Inhibited by pancreatic proteolysis
Preference for ester bond in position 1
Pancreatic Lipase
Optimal pH of 7.0
Active against ester bonds in positions 1 and 3

Lipase

This stable emulsion then is presented to pancreatic triglyceride lipase. Unlike other soluble enzymes, which can act in a three-dimensional solution, lipase has to act at the two-dimensional surface of the emulsion droplet; this requirement presents particular problems.[58] Certain characteristics of the enzyme itself are important. Thus, the lipolytic "zone" of the molecule is hydrophobic and lies deep within it, shielded from the aqueous phase. It is revealed to the lipid only on close apposition to its surface. The presence of a coat on the lipid droplet thus poses a barrier to the action of lipase, and assistance is required to bring it into close contact with the triglyceride. The presence of colipase, secreted by the pancreas with lipase (molar ratio 1:1), is critical in approximating lipase to triglyceride (see Fig. 97–4). Colipase attaches to the ester bond region of the triglyceride, lipase then binding strongly to colipase by electrostatic interactions.[56] Digestion of the phospholipid on the surface of the lipid emulsion by PLA_2 allows exposure of the triglyceride core to the colipase-lipase complex, further enhancing colipase-dependent anchoring of lipase to the lipid emulsion. PLA_2 digestion requires bile salts and Ca^{2+} for activation, which may assist colipase-lipase–mediated triglyceride lipolysis further by providing a mechanism for removal of lipolytic products. In the absence of colipase, bile salts on the surface of the emulsion droplet inhibit lipase activity.

The colipase gene is located in chromosome 6, and the amino acid sequence of the lipid-binding domain, the lipase-binding domain, and the activation peptide appear to be highly conserved.[59] Colipase is secreted by the pancreas as procolipase,[60] which is activated when trypsin cleaves a pentapeptide from its N terminus after it enters the small intestinal lumen. Of interest, the pentapeptide cleaved from the procolipase by trypsin, called enterostatin, seems to be a specific satiety signal for the ingestion of fat.[61]

Because pancreatic lipase is most active at nearly neutral pH, secretion of bicarbonate by the pancreas and biliary tree is important to neutralize gastric acid; luminal pH falls to approximately 6 in the jejunum, however, and here, it may be significant that bile salts lower the pH optimal for lipase activity from 8 to 6. In the presence of colipase and optimal pH, lipase activity releases fatty acids and monoglyceride extremely rapidly and efficiently (see Fig. 97–4). Pancreatic triglyceride lipase also binds strongly to the mucosal brush border membrane,[62]

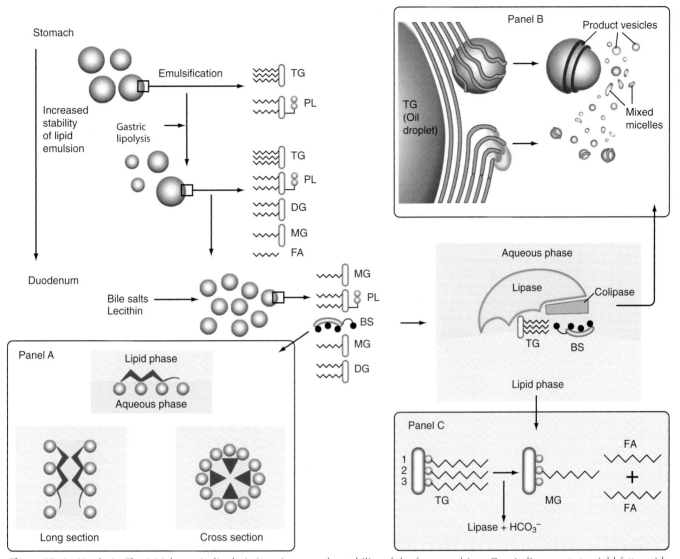

Figure 97–4   Lipolysis. The initial step in lipolysis is to increase the stability of the fatty emulsion. Gastric lipase acts to yield fatty acids (FA) and diglyceride (DG); the latter enhances emulsification. This step is further enhanced in the duodenum by bile salts (BS) and phospholipid (PL), which enable lipase, in the presence of colipase, to act at the surface of the emulsion droplet, bringing it close to the triglyceride molecule and resulting in the release of monoglyceride (MG) and fatty acids. Lipolysis in the duodenum yields two fatty acid molecules and a monoglyceride molecule and occurs in a rapid and efficient manner at nearly neutral pH. *Panel A* is a diagrammatic representation of bile salt molecules *(top)* oriented at an oil-water interface with a hydrophobic sterol backbone in oil phase and its hydrophilic hydroxyl and either taurine or glycine conjugates in aqueous phase. At concentrations above critical micellar concentration (CMC), bile salts aggregate as simple micelles in water with their hydrophilic groups facing into the water. In this diagram, three hydroxyl groups (cholate) are shown as *circles*, and a fourth polar group represents either taurine or glycine. *Panel B* is a diagrammatic representation of the dispersion of the products of lipolysis into lamellae at the surface of the oil phase, each about 4 to 5 nm thick, with water spacings up to 8 nm, and from there into vesicles approximately 20 to 130 nm in diameter. *Panel C* shows fatty acids and monoglyceride within the vesicles pass on into mixed micelles.

where it may participate in lipolysis of cholesteryl esters or triglyceride, releasing fatty acids, monoglyceride, and free cholesterol in proximity to the brush border membrane, where they undergo rapid uptake.

In addition to pancreatic triglyceride lipase and its protein cofactor, colipase, pancreatic acini also synthesize two pancreatic lipase-related proteins, PLRP-1 and PLRP-2, which have strong nucleotide and amino acid sequence homology with pancreatic triglyceride lipase. PLRP-1 has no known activity; PLRP-2 has lipase activity. Similar to pancreatic triglyceride lipase, PLRP-2 cleaves triglycerides, but in comparison with pancreatic triglyceride lipase, it has a broader substrate specificity. PLRP-2 also hydrolyzes phospholipids and galactolipids, two fats that are not substrates for pancreatic triglyceride lipase. It also differs from pancreatic triglyceride lipase with respect to sensitivity to bile salts and its response to colipase. PLRP-2 mRNA appears before birth and persists into adulthood, whereas pancreatic triglyceride lipase mRNA first appears at the suckling-weaning transition, suggesting that PLRP-2 plays a critical role in the digestion of breast milk fats.[63,64]

Micelles and Other Lipid-Containing Particles

The products of lipolysis are distributed among aqueous, oil, and intermediate phases in a number of forms prepared for transfer across the lumen to the mucosal brush border membrane. Shuttling of these products is dependent in part on the formation of micelles with bile salts. The concentration of bile salts in bile is approximately 35 mM, a concentration that is decreased further by dilution to 10 to 20 mM in the duodenum. This concentration lies well above the critical concentration for micelle formation. Mixed micelle production depends on a number of other factors, including pH, presence or absence of lipids, and types of bile salts that are secreted[42] (see Chapter 61).

Bile salts are capable of forming micelles because they are amphipathic (having in their molecules both water-soluble and lipid-soluble parts), and because they have a particular three-dimensional structure (see Fig. 97–4). They orient themselves at an oil-water interface and thus are ideal emulsifying agents. In addition, micelles are formed when bile salt levels are above critical concentrations for micelle formation and therefore are able to aggregate in disk-like particles surrounding the insoluble lipid with their hydrophobic sterol backbones oriented toward each other and their hydrophilic polar groups facing outward into the aqueous phase. Bile salt micelles have the capacity to "dissolve" fatty acids, monoglycerides, and cholesterol, but not triglycerides.[65] Mixed micelles are approximately 50 to 80 nm in diameter and, unlike emulsion droplets, are too small to scatter light. Thus, micellar solutions are clear. The presence of phospholipid in bile enlarges mixed micelles and makes them more efficient in the dissolution of fat.

Other lipid-containing particles participate in the transfer of lipid to the mucosa. As the emulsion droplet shrinks during lipolysis, liquid crystalline structures are formed at its surface.[66,67] These vesicular structures with multilamellar and unilamellar forms can be seen under the electron microscope, budding off the surface of emulsion droplets, and occasionally, close to the brush border membrane of the intestinal mucosa.[68] This physical phase of lipid within the lumen may provide a significant mechanism for transfer of lipid to the mucosa, beyond that provided by bile salt micelles. The presence of these particles could explain the observation that, in the absence of bile salts, some 50% or more of dietary triglyceride still may be absorbed. In the presence of adequate concentrations of bile salts, however, these vesicles undergo rapid spontaneous dissolution and release their lipid into micelles, which are likely to be the major route for lipid trafficking (see Fig. 97–4). Numerically, micelles are much more common than lipid vesicles.

Importance of Intraluminal pH

Lipid digestion and absorption depend on intraluminal pH at several steps in the chain. Pancreatic lipase operates best in the presence of bile salts and at pH 6 or above. It therefore functions well at the pH of the luminal duodenum, where most lipid digestion occurs. Glycine-conjugated bile salts precipitate below pH 5; furthermore, fatty acids are in their protonated form below approximately pH 6 and have limited solubility in bile salt micelles. When intraluminal pH falls, such as in Zollinger-Ellison syndrome or exocrine pancreatic insufficiency, intraluminal precipitation of bile acid crystals or greater passive absorption of bile acids, particularly the glycine conjugates, is seen. The normal glycine-to-taurine ratio is 3:1, and when glycine precipitates, the (optimal) ratio is reduced, thereby decreasing the overall concentration of intraluminal bile acids available for fat digestion and further contributing to the steatorrhea seen with these disorders.

Biologic characteristics of lipases, including effect of pH on activities, are detailed in Table 97–3.

Unstirred Water Layer

An unstirred water layer is present on the surface of the intestinal epithelium that in humans is approximately 40 μm thick.[69] This layer may be rate limiting for uptake of long-chain fatty acids, but not for short- or medium-chain fatty acids, the limiting step for which occurs at the brush border membrane.[56] The provision of a high concentration of fatty acid in the microenvironment adjacent to the epithelium is dependent on the diffusion of micelles into this region. The microclimate here is slightly acidic, owing to activity of a sodium-hydrogen (Na^+-H^+) exchanger at the brush border membrane, and at pH between 5 and 6, the solubility of fatty acids in micelles decreases, thus encouraging liberation of fatty acids close to the mucosa. The high concentration of fatty acids necessary for diffusion across the mucosal membrane is thus achieved, and evidence for this model is increasingly persuasive.[70] The low pH microclimate also encourages the fatty acids to be presented in an undissociated, protonated form. Thus, the pH partition hypothesis would predict that fatty acids could diffuse passively into the cell as protonated species and, at the near-neutral intracellular pH, become trapped in the ionized form.

A surfactant-like material has been discovered close to the brush border membrane, although its role in absorption, if any, is uncertain.[71] It is secreted by enterocytes, contains phosphatidylcholine and alkaline phosphatase, and appears as flat lamellae or vesicles adjacent to the brush border membrane.

Digestion of Other Lipids

Phosphatidylcholine, the major dietary phospholipid, is hydrolyzed by pancreatic phospholipase A_2 (PLA_2) to yield fatty acid from the 2 position and lysophosphatidylcholine. Pancreatic PLA_2 is secreted as an anionic zymogen, which is activated in the small intestine by tryptic cleavage of an N-terminal heptapeptide; it has a molecular weight of approximately 14,000 and requires calcium for activation and bile salts for its activity. Pancreatic PLA_2 has multiple isoforms and apparently requires a 2:1 bile salt–to–phosphatidylcholine molar ratio for optimal activity. Although the bulk of intestinal PLA_2 activity is derived from pancreatic secretions, some contribution comes from the intestinal mucosa, where the enzyme is concentrated in the brush border.[72]

Cholesterol esters, in the presence of bile salts and calcium, are hydrolyzed by carboxyl ester lipase (CEL) (also known as pancreatic cholesterol esterase) to release the free sterol, in which form it is absorbed. Although cell culture and other in vitro studies have defined the potential functions of CEL in the digestion of cholesteryl ester, phospholipids and triglycerides, only its cholesteryl ester hydrolytic activity is unique in the digestive tract.[73] CEL belongs to the α/β-hydrolase family of enzymes, is well conserved, and shares 78% homology in both the rat and human.[74] It is secreted primarily by the pancreatic acinar cells and lactating mammary glands. Using site-directed mutagenesis, the serine at position 194, the histidine at position 435, and the aspartic acid at position 320 are important for its catalytic activity.[73,75-77] The hydrolysis of water-insoluble substrates by CEL requires bile salt–containing 3α- or 7α-hydroxy groups (e.g., cholate or chenodeoxycholate and their conjugates).[78] The arginine 63 and arginine 423 sites play an important role in this bile salt–dependent process, but not in the bile salt–independent lysophospholipid hydrolytic activity of CEL.[79]

Both hydrolytic enzymes (PLA$_2$ and CEL) act on the emulsion phase at the surface of droplets, and the products of digestion are released into multilamellar and unilamellar vesicles and then into mixed micelles. Fatty acids and monoglycerides increase the solubility of cholesterol in micelles, thereby promoting its absorption. The products of phospholipid and cholesterol hydrolysis thus pursue the same route to the brush border membrane as that for the fatty acids and monoglyceride, which originate from dietary triglyceride.

Unabsorbed long-chain fatty acids that enter the colon are not absorbed by this organ, and they undergo a series of bacterial modifications, principally hydroxylation. In healthy persons, no undigested triglyceride is found in the stool, and the standard fecal fat estimate of approximately 7 g per day reflects the cumulative total excretion of saponification products (i.e., fatty acids) that arise principally from membrane phospholipid and bacteria.

Transfer across the Brush Border Membrane

Much of the current understanding of the micellar solubilization and uptake of dietary lipids comes from the work of Hofmann and Borgstroem, who described the uptake of lipid digestion products by enterocytes.[80] Further work by Carey and colleagues revealed the coexistence of unilamellar liposomes with bile salt–lipid mixed micelles in the small intestine.[81] Although the uptake of lipid digestion products by enterocytes has been accepted as a passive process, more recent work has raised the possibility that some lipids may be taken up by enterocytes through carrier-mediated processes that are energy dependent.[82]

Studies with brush border membrane vesicles suggest that linoleic acid uptake occurs by facilitated diffusion.[83] Absorption of oleic and arachidonic acid also appears to occur by a saturable process, suggesting the possibility of active transport. Several membrane proteins have been identified that increase the uptake of long-chain fatty acids when overexpressed in cultured mammalian cells. The most prominent and best-characterized of these are FAT/CD36, long-chain fatty acyl-CoA synthetases (LACS), and fatty acid transport proteins (FATPs/solute carrier family 27).[84-87] The FATPs are transmembrane proteins that enhance the cellular uptake of long-chain and very-long-chain fatty acids. In humans, FATPs comprise a family of six highly homologous proteins, hsFATP1 to hsFATP6, which are found in all fatty acid–utilizing tissues of the body.[84,88,89] Although hsFATP1 is the best characterized of the FATPs, hsFATP4 is the only FATP expressed in the small intestine; it is localized to the apical brush border of the epithelial cells, where it is responsible for absorption of dietary lipids. Studies with FATP4-overexpressing cell lines and with isolated enterocytes demonstrated that FATP4 is both necessary and sufficient for efficient uptake of long-chain and very-long-chain fatty acids.[90] Detailed substrate studies based on ^{14}C-labeled fatty acids have been presented for FATP1 and FATP4[87,90] and showed that uptake of fatty acids shorter than 10 carbon atoms, such as butyric and octanoic acids, was unaffected by FATP expression, whereas uptake of long-chain fatty acids, such as palmitate and oleate, was enhanced.[90]

Nutrients, hormones, and cytokines have been reported to regulate FATP expression. Rats fed a high-fat diet showed increased FATP expression in the heart but not in the liver. Several reports have shown a positive regulation of mouse FATP by ligands that activate either PPAR-γ, PPAR-α, or PPAR-γ/RXR heterodimers in hepatoma cell lines, the liver, and the intestine. Furthermore, a PPAR-binding site was identified in the murine FATP1 promoter. The different PPARs can be considered key messengers responsible for the translation of nutritional, pharmacologic, and metabolic stimuli into changes in genes, specifically those genes involved in lipid metabolism. PPAR-associated induction of FATP may contribute to overall homeostasis by increasing fatty acid transport to compensate for the increase in fatty acid catabolism they also cause. TNF-α is a negative regulator of FATP expression and down-regulates FATP mRNA in liver and FATP1 and FATP4 proteins in adipocytes.[88]

The exact mechanism of FATP-mediated transport of long-chain fatty acids into the intestinal cell is unknown. It has been postulated that extracellular long-chain fatty acids might directly bind to FATP complexes and be transported into cells. Alternatively, long-chain fatty acids could bind first to CD36, which "hands off" the long-chain fatty acids to FATP dimers. Intracellular long-chain fatty acids are coupled to CoA by long-chain acyl-CoA synthetase (LACS), preventing their efflux, whereas fatty acid–binding proteins (FABPs) act as a cytoplasmic buffer for incorporated long-chain fatty acids[88] (Fig. 97–5).

Cholesterol, unlike beta-sitosterol (a plant sterol that is part of the human diet), is well absorbed by the proximal jejunum.[91] The second-order kinetics of cholesterol absorption, its sterol specificity, and its inhibition by drugs such as ezetimibe all suggest that cholesterol is mediated by specific transport proteins at the brush border membrane.[92,93] Thurnhofer and Hauser first described the presence of a possible binding protein in the small intestinal brush border that facilitates the uptake of cholesterol by the small intestine[94]; this 14 kd protein was later identified as sterol carrier protein-2 (SCP-2), which is an intracellular protein.[95] The adenosine triphosphate (ATP)-binding cassette (ABC) A1 transporter and scavenger receptor type B1 (SR-B1) also were postulated to play roles in cholesterol absorption, but targeted inactivation of these genes in mice has had no effect on cholesterol uptake.[96-98]

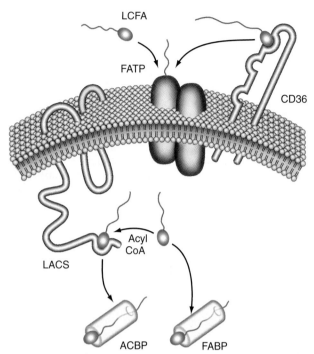

Figure 97–5 Mechanisms of long-chain and very-long-chain fatty acid transport. Extracellular long-chain fatty acid (LCFA) might directly bind to fatty acid transport protein (FATP) complexes and be transported into cells. Alternatively, LCFA could bind first to CD36, which "hands off" the LCFA to FATP dimers. Intracellular LCFAs are coupled to coenzyme A by long-chain fatty acyl-coenzyme A (Acyl CoA) synthetases (LACS), thereby preventing their efflux, whereas fatty acid–binding proteins (FABPs) act as a cytoplasmic buffer for incorporated LCFAs. ACBP, acyl CoA binding proteins. (Adapted with permission from Stahl A: A current review of fatty acid transport proteins [SLC27]. Pflugers Arch 447:722, 2004.)

Evidence favoring a cholesterol membrane transporter also is seen in persons with beta-sitosterolemia, a condition in which the intestine fails to discriminate between cholesterol and beta-sitosterol. Major findings in patients homozygous for sitosterolemia include elevated concentrations of plasma plant sterols, xanthomatosis, and accelerated, often fatal, premature atherosclerosis. The genetic defect of beta-sitosterolemia is linked to chromosomal locus 2p21.[99] Seven different mutations in two adjacent genes have been described that are responsible for encoding new members of the ABC transporter (ABCG5 and ABCG8) in patients with sitosterolemia. The defect in ABCG5 or ABCG8 cotransporter gene locus causes an increased intestinal absorption and a decreased biliary elimination of all sterols (plant sterols and cholesterol), leading to a 50- to 200-fold increase in plasma plant sterol concentrations. Feeding cholesterol to mice up-regulated these genes, thus suggesting that ABCG5 and ABCG8 work together to limit intestinal cholesterol absorption by cholesterol efflux from small intestinal epithelial cells.[100] These two genes are expressed almost exclusively in the liver and intestine and are co-regulated by the nuclear hormone receptor liver X receptor (LXR)[101]; however, these transporters provide the apparatus for efficient shunting of sterols away from the transfer pathway that directs the production of choles-

teryl esters by acyl-CoA cholesterol acyl transferase 2 (ACAT2) and do not appear to be involved in the initial uptake of cholesterol.

Recently, Niemann-Pick C1–like 1 protein (NPC1L1) has been suggested as a key component of intestinal cholesterol transport. Niemann-Pick C1 (NPC1), the defective protein in the cholesterol storage disease Niemann-Pick type C (NP-C), is highly abundant in a variety of tissues and functions in intracellular cholesterol trafficking.[102,103] By contrast, NPC1L1 has 50% amino acid homology with NPC1; has several predicted features of a plasma membrane–expressed transporter; and is expressed in high levels in the small intestine, especially in the brush border membrane of enterocytes. NPC1L1-deficient mice show a substantial reduction in absorbed cholesterol that is unaffected by dietary supplementation of bile acids.[104]

Intracellular Processing

Once within the cell, fatty acids bind to specific fatty acid–binding proteins (FABPs), which are found predominantly in the jejunum and in greater abundance in villus cells than in crypt cells. The small intestine has three distinct proteins belonging to the intracellular lipid-binding protein family: the liver-type FABP (L-FABP), the intestinal FABP (I-FABP), and the ileal lipid-binding protein (ILBP).[105,106] All three proteins have greater affinity for unsaturated fatty acids than for saturated ones and very little affinity, if any, for short-chain or medium-chain fatty acids.[42] On the basis of nuclear magnetic resonance (NMR) binding studies, it is suggested that the binding of I-FABP is involved in the intracellular transport of fatty acids, whereas the L-FABP is involved in the intracellular transport of monoglycerides and lysophosphatidylcholine.[107] They may assist transfer across the cytoplasm to the endoplasmic reticulum for triglyceride resynthesis, modulate intracellular lipid metabolism, and regulate gene expression.

In addition, two sterol carrier proteins, SCP-1 and SCP-2, have been isolated and characterized. SCP-1 is important in the microsomal conversion of squalene to lanosterol,[108] whereas SCP-2 participates in the microsomal conversion of lanosterol to cholesterol, as well as the intracellular transport of cholesterol from cytoplasmic lipid droplets to mitochondria.[109]

In the endoplasmic reticulum, triglyceride is resynthesized by two processes[110] (Fig. 97–6). In the first, monoglyceride is re-esterified with absorbed fatty acid after the latter has been activated to form acyl-coenzyme A (CoA) (the monoglyceride pathway). Microsomal acyl-CoA ligase is necessary to synthesize acyl-CoA from the fatty acid before esterification. Diglyceride and then triglyceride are formed sequentially in reactions that favor long-chain fatty acid absorption from the lumen. This route, involving monoglyceride esterification, accounts for most of the triglyceride synthesized during the absorptive phase, no more than 4% being formed by acylation of absorbed glycerol. It is thought that the synthesis of triglyceride from diglyceride is catalyzed by the enzyme acyl-CoA–diglyceride acyl transferase.[111] The gene for this enzyme has been isolated, and a knockout mouse model for this gene synthesized triglyceride in

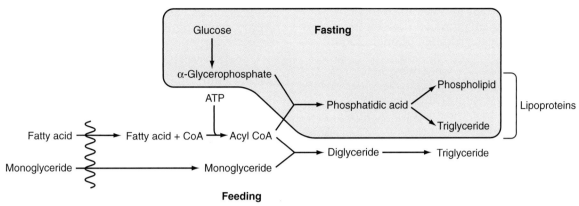

Figure 97–6   Metabolic fate of absorbed fatty acid and monoglyceride in enterocytes. During feeding, triglyceride is resynthesized largely from absorbed fatty acid and monoglyceride. During fasting, triglyceride and phospholipid are synthesized from α-glycerophosphate, derived from glucose entering across the basolateral membrane, and fatty acids. Unsaturated fatty acids tend to form the phospholipid.

the intestinal mucosa, suggesting that another enzyme may be involved in the formation of triglyceride from diglyceride.[112,113]

During fasting, triglyceride (and phospholipid) is synthesized through the second route, which involves acylation of α-glycerophosphate with the formation of phosphatidic acid and, then, triglyceride (or phospholipid) (see Fig. 97–6). The α-glycerophosphate is synthesized largely in the cytoplasm, from glucose. The relative importance of the monoglyceride pathway and the α-glycerophosphate pathway depends on the availability of 2-monoacylglycerol and fatty acid. During normal lipid absorption, when sufficient 2-monoacylglycerol is present, the monoglyceride pathway facilitates the conversion of 2-monoacylglycerol and fatty acid to form triglyceride and aids in inhibiting the α-glycerophosphate pathway. Conversely, when the supply of 2-monoacylglycerol is lacking or insufficient, the α-glycerophosphate pathway becomes the major pathway for formation of triglyceride.

Some absorbed lysophosphatidylcholine is reacylated to form phosphatidylcholine. The remaining absorbed lysophosphatidylcholine is hydrolyzed to form glycero-3-phosphorylcholine. The liberated fatty acids are used for triglyceride synthesis, whereas the glycero-3-phosphorylcholine is transported in the portal blood for use in the liver.

Absorbed dietary cholesterol enters a free cholesterol pool within enterocytes that also contains cholesterol from endogenous sites (non–dietary-absorbed sources [e.g., biliary cholesterol], cholesterol derived from plasma lipoproteins, and cholesterol synthesized de novo). Cholesterol is transported mainly as esterified cholesterol and almost exclusively by the lymphatic system. Cholesterol esterase and acyl-CoA cholesterol acyltransferase (ACAT) are thought to be predominantly responsible for cholesterol esterification. ACAT is stimulated by the feeding of a high-cholesterol diet and appears to play a more important role in mucosal cholesterol esterification than does cholesterol esterase.[114] Two ACAT proteins have been identified: ACAT-1 and ACAT-2.[115,116] The role of ACAT-2 in intestinal cholesterol absorption is supported by resistance to diet-induced hypercholesterolemia due to defec-

tive cholesterol esterification and absorption by the small intestine in the ACAT-2–knockout mouse model.[117]

Once synthesized, triglyceride, cholesterol and its esters, and phospholipids are packaged for export in the form of chylomicrons and very-low-density lipoproteins (VLDLs). During fasting, VLDLs are the major triglyceride-rich lipoproteins that emerge from the epithelium; after feeding, chylomicrons predominate. VLDL triglycerides have a different fatty acid composition from that of triglycerides in chylomicrons, different pathways being involved in their formation. Furthermore, the fatty acids derived from dietary triglyceride go predominantly into the formation of chylomicrons, whereas those derived from phospholipid appear to be utilized in the formation of VLDLs.[56]

The diameter of chylomicrons ranges between 750 and 6000 nm. Their cores consist of triglycerides, whereas cholesterol ester and phospholipid form more than 80% of the surface coat. Forming a smaller proportion of the surface of chylomicrons is the essential component, apolipoprotein. Apo A is an important apoprotein for all lipoproteins, including chylomicrons, VLDLs, and high-density lipoproteins (HDLs). It is synthesized in the small intestine and is found in bile.[118] Apo B probably is synthesized in the Golgi cysterni and is found in the rough endoplasmic reticulum. After feeding, apo B is found in association with the chylomicrons in the smooth endoplasmic reticulum. The absence of apo B prevents synthesis and secretion of chylomicrons; however, data suggest that the supply of apo B is not rate limiting for chylomicron formation. For example, the apo B output in lymph does not change after intraduodenal infusion of lipid, despite the fact that lymphatic triglyceride output increases seven- to eightfold.[119,120]

Abetapolipoproteinemia is a rare genetic disorder resulting in complete failure of the liver and intestine to make triglyceride-rich lipoproteins.[121] Previously it was thought that abetalipoproteinemic patients have a problem synthesizing apo B. Actually, apo B synthesis is reduced, but not abolished, and abetalipoproteinemia results from mutations of the microsomal triglyceride transfer protein gene.[120,122,123] This gene's lipid transfer activity is primarily responsible for the lipidation of the primordial particle (the initial step in chylomicron formation, whereby the addition of phospholipids to the apo B molecule is followed by the addition of small amounts of triglyceride).

Anderson's disease (also known as chylomicron retention disorder) is another small intestinal disorder involving the formation or secretion of chylomicrons. No defect is observed in genes that carry known apoproteins or microsomal triglyceride transfer protein,[124] suggesting that the disease is caused by an unknown factor central to secretion of chylomicrons.

Once chylomicrons have formed in the smooth endoplasmic reticulum, they are transferred to the Golgi apparatus. Golgi-derived chylomicron vesicles are then incorporated into the basolateral membrane and secreted by means of exocytosis into the lymphatic circulation (Fig. 97–7). During absorption, lacteals distend, and endothelial cells, which overlap each other in the fasting state, move apart, opening gaps through which chylomicrons can pass readily.[125]

Medium-chain fatty acids are absorbed by way of the portal vein, but as the chain length of saturated fatty acids increases, they are increasingly absorbed through the lymphatics. Polyunsaturated fatty acids may pass directly across the basolateral membrane and into the portal circulation.

LXR Receptors and Lipid Homeostasis

The liver X receptors—LXR-α and LXR-β—are nuclear receptor transcription factors that are activated by certain derivatives of cholesterol.[126] Hence, LXR activity may be up-regulated by cellular lipid load or dietary cholesterol intake. The identification of a large list of LXR target genes and their response to LXR activation (Table 97–4) indicates that the LXRs play an important role in the response to excess cholesterol, and that their activation may protect against tissue cholesterol overload.[127]

Both LXR-α and LXR-β form obligate heterodimers with the retinoid X receptor (RXR) to result in ligand-activated transcription factors that can be activated by ligands (i.e., lipids) for either RXR or LXR. RXR-LXR heterodimers bind to a specific DNA sequence called the LXR response element (LXRE), which consists of two hexanucleotide sequences separated by four bases[128] (Fig. 97–8). A specific group of LXR agonists have been identified that

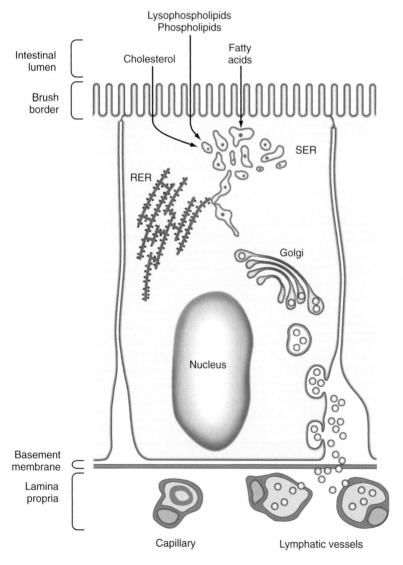

Figure 97–7 Pathway of lipids during passage across the enterocyte. Triglyceride and phospholipid are synthesized in the smooth endoplasmic reticulum (SER) and accumulate there as dense droplets. Apolipoproteins, synthesized in the rough endoplasmic reticulum (RER), assist in the formation of chylomicrons in the tubular endoplasmic reticulum and Golgi apparatus; these lipoproteins finally are released across the basolateral membrane by exocytosis.

Table 97–4   LXR Gene Targets and Functions

Target Gene	Target Sites	Function	Gene Sequence of LXRE
CYP7A1	Liver	Bile acid synthesis	TGGTCActcaAGTTCA
			TGGTCAcccaAGTTCA
			TGGTCAtccaAGTTCA
			TTGTCAaccaAGCTCA*
ABCA1	Macrophage	Cholesterol efflux	AGGTTActatCGGTCA*
	Intestine		GGATCAcctgAGGTCA
			AGATCActtgAGGTCA
			AGGTTActgaAGGCCA
ABCG5/G8	Liver, intestine	Sterol transport	Not known
ABCG1	Macrophage	Cholesterol efflux	TGGTCActcaAGTTCA*
			AGTTTAtaatAGTTCA
APOE	Macrophage	Component of lipoprotein particles	GGGTCActggCGGTCA*
	Adipocyte		GAATCActtaAGGTCA
LPL	Liver	Triglyceride hydrolysis	AGGTCAccacCGGTCA
	Macrophage		AGGTGActgcAGGTCA*
CETP	—	Cholesterol ester transfer	GGGTCAttgtCGGGCA*
SREBP-1c	Liver, fat	Fatty acid synthesis	GGGTTActggCGGTCA
	Intestine		GGGTTActagCGGGCG
LXR	Macrophage	Cholesterol sensor	AGGTTActgcTGGTCA*
YZ2	Liver	?Pyrimidine metabolism	Not known

LXR, liver X receptor; LXRE, LXR response element.
LXRE sequences are from various species. *Denotes a human sequence.

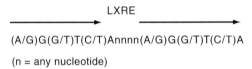

LXRE

(A/G)G(G/T)T(C/T)Annnn(A/G)G(G/T)T(C/T)A

(n = any nucleotide)

Figure 97–8   The consensus DNA sequence that defines the LXR (liver X receptor) response element (LXRE) to which functional LXRs bind to promote transcription. The LXRE consists of a direct repeat of the indicated hexanucleotide sequence, separated by four bases.

are intermediates in cholesterol metabolic pathways. Furthermore, using mouse models lacking LXR-α or LXR-β, or both, LXRs have been generated, thus revealing the key role of LXRs in regulating the expression of genes involved in cholesterol catabolism, absorption, and transport, as well as in fatty acid synthesis (see Table 97–4).

Cholesterol 7α-hydroxylase (CYP7A1) is the rate-limiting enzyme of the classic pathway that converts cholesterol into bile acids.[129,130] The soluble bile acids, produced primarily in the liver, promote the secretion of cholesterol into bile for excretion in feces. In some species (e.g., rodents), but not humans, expression of the CYP7A1 gene is induced in response to dietary cholesterol, thereby accelerating the conversion of cholesterol into bile acids, to promote the net excretion of cholesterol. LXR-α up-regulates the transcription of CYP7A1 by directly binding to an LXRE in the promoter of this gene.[131,132] Furthermore, the liver-specific expression of CYP7A1 requires LRH-1 (liver receptor homolog-1; also called CPF and FTF), a monomeric orphan nuclear receptor. The transcription of CYP7A1 also is regulated by means of feedback inhibition. Specifically, the bile acid receptor FXR (farnesoid X receptor) binds bile acids and induces the expression of SHP (small heterodimer partner), an orphan nuclear receptor that preferentially

dimerizes with LRH-1 and represses a number of enterohepatic genes involved in synthesis and transport of bile acids, including CYP7A1.[133] In this way, LXR and FXR act together to regulate bile acid homeostasis tightly, respectively functioning, with a cholesterol precursor and cholesterol metabolite, to up- and down-regulate CYP7A1.

Dietary and secreted biliary cholesterol enter the intestinal lumen and are absorbed by enterocytes in the proximal bowel. In the mouse, LXR and RXR agonists, which are metabolic indicators of active cholesterol turnover, decrease cholesterol absorption.[134] This net reduction in cholesterol uptake is associated with an RXR/LXR-mediated up-regulation of LXRE-containing genes that encode ATP-binding cassette (ABC) transporters.[135] In the small intestine, at least three ABC transporters are transcriptionally regulated by LXRs and putatively limit cholesterol absorption by pumping cholesterol back into the lumen of the intestine.[134]

ABCA1 is a full transporter protein containing two symmetrical halves, each composed of a six-transmembrane domain and an ABC. Mutations in the ABCA1 gene result in Tangier disease, which is characterized by a low plasma concentration of HDL and the accumulation of cholesterol esters in tonsils, liver, spleen, intestinal mucosa, and macrophage foam cells.[136-138] ABCA1 is up-regulated by LXRs in both intestine and macrophages.

ABCG5 and ABCG8 are half-transporters, each composed of a single transmembrane domain and ABC, and are coexpressed exclusively in the liver and intestine.[100] Mutations in either gene cause a rare autosomal recessive disorder called sitosterolemia, which is characterized by increased absorption of cholesterol and toxic plant sterols and decreased biliary sterol secretion (see earlier discussion). In vivo and in vitro experiments indicate that ABCG5 and ABCG8 are direct targets of LXRs. These findings strongly support the hypothesis that LXRs promote cholesterol loss by increasing biliary cholesterol secretion and limiting cholesterol absorption.[100]

CARBOHYDRATE

DIETARY INTAKE

In Western societies, approximately 45% of total energy requirement is provided by carbohydrate, making it the major source of calories at all stages of life.[139] The volume of carbohydrate ingestion appears to be declining, owing in part to a reduction in the intake of purified sugar.[47,125] Overall, total caloric intake is on the decline because of reductions in dietary fat and carbohydrate by affluent, but diet-conscious, Western societies. The proportion of carbohydrate ingested as fruit and vegetables is rising as the intake of raw fiber is increasing.

In adults who consume a "Western" diet, the amount of glucose produced by digestion is approximately 180 g per day (approximately 1 mol). An ever-increasing amount of fructose is added to our diets (frequently in excess of 50 g per day) through the widespread use of corn syrup as a sweetener. All ingested glucose and galactose is absorbed normally, but the capacity to absorb fructose is limited in both young children and adults. This was evident in healthy young adults (medical students in the United States and the United Kingdom) in whom ingestion of 50 g of fructose produced abdominal pain, bloating, borborygmi, flatus, and positive results on hydrogen breath testing in 70% of the subjects studied[140]; two 12-ounce cans of some popular soft drinks contain approximately 50 g of fructose in the form of corn syrup.

Approximately half of the digestible carbohydrate in an average Western diet is starch derived from cereals and plants, in which it is the major storage form. Starch (as either amylose or amylopectin) is made up of long chains of glucose molecules. Amylose, a linear polymer in which each glucose molecule is coupled to its neighbor by α1-4 linkage, has a molecular weight of 10^6. Amylopectin, by contrast, is a branched-chain polymer in which α1-6 links provide the angulations between adjacent chains of α1-4–linked glucose molecules (Fig. 97–9): It has a molecular weight greater than 10^9. The ratio in starches varies widely; most starches, however, usually contain more amylopectin than amylose. Although starches are relatively easily digested, food preparation can influence

their biologic utilization. Utilization may also be determined by the protein associated with the starch, particularly gluten.[1]

Other major sources of dietary carbohydrate include sugars derived from milk (lactose), contained within the cells of fruit and vegetables (fructose, glucose, sucrose), or purified from cane or beet sources (sucrose). Processed foods form a major source of dietary sugars, particularly fructose and corn syrup; the latter contains not only fructose but oligosaccharides and polysaccharides). The sugar alcohol sorbitol is used widely in the manufacture of "diabetic" sweets and preserves. Sorbitol is formed by hydrogenating the aldehyde group of glucose to an alcohol group, which slows its rate of absorption, thereby diminishing its effect on blood sugar concentrations.[49]

Glycogen is the major storage form of polysaccharide in animals, but the amounts ingested in a normal human diet are small. Its structure is similar to that of amylose and consists of straight chains of α1-4–linked glucose monomers.

Nonstarch polysaccharides form a majority of the "unavailable" carbohydrates. The dietary fiber component of unavailable carbohydrate is found most abundantly in cereals, peas, beans, carrots, and peanuts, and in the United Kingdom, some 10 to 15 g of dietary fiber, consisting predominantly of celluloses and hemicelluloses, is consumed by each person every day.[47] Cellulose is made up of α1-4–linked glucose molecules in straight chains, and hemicelluloses are pentose and hexose polymers with both straight and branched chains. Both forms are resistant to digestion in the small intestine because the α1-4 bond, unlike the α bond in starch, is resistant to amylases. They are, however, broken down to some extent by colonic bacteria to yield short-chain fatty acids, which are absorbed avidly by colonic mucosa.[141] The quantity of cellulose and hemicelluloses in vegetables and fruit varies markedly and depends on their age and "ripeness."

Other unavailable-type carbohydrates include pectins, gums, and alginates, which are metabolized only partially in the colon. Lignins, elaborated by plants in the process of becoming woody, are completely indigestible.[49]

It is well recognized that increased intake of dietary fiber eases constipation by increasing fecal bulk, mainly as a result of the increase in the mass of fecal flora. Dietary fiber has other roles, however, and also affects the absorption of other nutrients. It delays absorption of

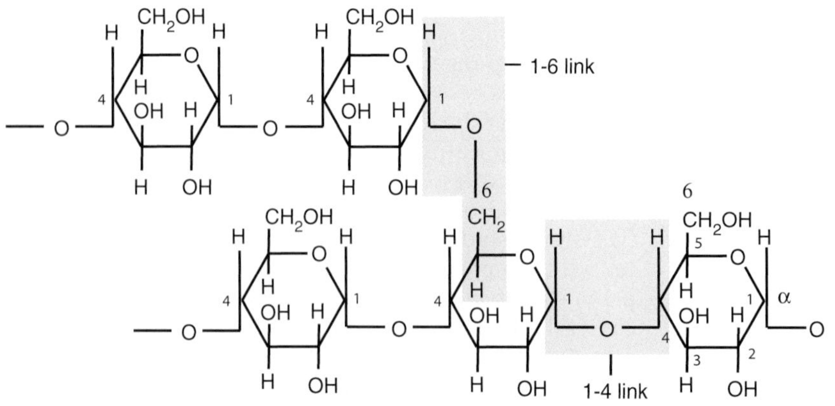

Figure 97–9 Part of an amylopectin molecule indicating the α1-4 and α1-6 linkages between glucose molecules.

sugars and fats and curtails the insulin response to a carbohydrate meal. Some fiber, such as lignins, may lower serum cholesterol by binding bile salts. It may be these other effects that have led to the widespread recommendation of a high-fiber diet for management or prevention of such diseases as diabetes mellitus and atherosclerosis. Satiety is achieved more rapidly from a diet rich in fiber than from a low-fiber diet, and it takes longer to ingest a high-fiber meal; these properties are useful in the management of obesity.

INTRALUMINAL DIGESTION

Salivary and Pancreatic Amylase

Salivary and pancreatic amylases are endoenzymes; that is, they cleave the α1-4 links internal to, or at the second or third bond from, the end of the polysaccharide chain. The products of amylase digestion, therefore, consist of short, linear oligosaccharides with maltotriose and maltose (Fig. 97–10). Because α1-6 links, and the adjacent α1-4 bonds, in the branched chains of amylopectin are not hydrolyzed by amylase, the products of amylopectin digestion include short, branched oligosaccharides, termed α-limit dextrins. Amylase proteins are encoded by a clustered gene family located on human chromosome 1 and mouse chromosome 3.[142] In humans, the *AMY1* gene is expressed in the parotid gland, and the *AMY2* gene is expressed in the pancreas.[143] The sequences of the pancreatic and salivary complementary DNAs (cDNAs) are 94% similar, coding for polypeptides with the same number of amino acids.[144]

The effect of salivary amylase depends on its proximity to the ingested starches and the time they spend within the mouth. Thus, careful, slow chewing affords a good start to digestion, whereas rapid swallowing of poorly chewed foods—often a problem for edentulous persons—may result in suboptimal salivary amylase action.

Salivary amylase is inactivated rapidly by gastric acid, but some activity may persist within the food bolus; short-chain oligosaccharides offer further protection for the enzyme against inactivation at acid pH. Despite these protective factors, it is uncertain what proportion of dietary starch is digested before it reaches the duodenum.

Pancreatic amylase is the major enzyme of starch digestion and, as with salivary amylase, produces short oligosaccharides, maltotriose, maltose, and α-limit dextrins; glucose monomer is not produced. Most of this hydrolysis occurs within the intestinal lumen, but because amylase also attaches itself to the brush border membrane of enterocytes, some digestion may occur at this site as well. Amylase concentration becomes limiting for starch hydrolysis only in severe cases of pancreatic insufficiency, when luminal amylase activity levels are reduced to below 10% of normal.[145] Human milk contains amylase activity, which may be important for carbohydrate digestion in infants.[146]

Brush Border Membrane Hydrolases

The terminal products of luminal starch digestion, together with the major disaccharides in the diet (sucrose and lactose), cannot be absorbed intact and are hydrolyzed by specific brush border membrane hydrolases that are maximally expressed in the villi of the duodenum and jejunum. Several types of carbohydrases have been identified[147] (Table 97–5).

Lactase hydrolyzes lactose to produce one molecule of glucose and one of galactose.

Sucrase-isomaltase, or sucrase–α-dextrinase, possesses two subunits of the same molecule, each with distinct enzyme activity. Sucrase hydrolyzes sucrose to yield one molecule of glucose and one of fructose. Both enzymes remove glucose molecules from the nonreducing end of α-limit dextrins. Isomaltase ("debrancher" enzyme) is critical to hydrolyze the 1-6 glycosidic linkage in α-limit dextrins. The concerted action of sucrase and isomaltase thus yields monomeric glucose molecules from sucrose and α-limit dextrins (Fig. 97–11).

Table 97–5 Characteristics of Brush Border Membrane Carbohydrases

Enzyme	Substrate	Product(s)
Lactase	Lactose	Glucose Galactose
Maltase (glucoamylase)	α-1,4-Linked oligosaccharides; up to 9 residues	Glucose
Sucrase-isomaltase (sucrose α-dextrinase)		
Sucrase	Sucrose	Glucose Fructose
Isomaltase	α-Limit dextrin α-1,6 Link	Glucose
Both enzymes	α-Limit dextrin α-1,4 Link at nonreducing end	Glucose
Trehalase	Trehalose	Glucose

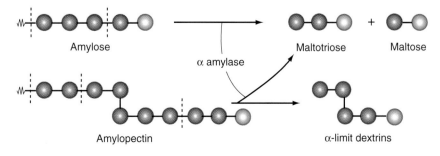

Figure 97–10 Action of pancreatic α-amylase on amylose and amylopectin molecules. Because the α1-6 link in the latter is resistant to amylase, the products include α-limit dextrin. ●, glucose units; ○, reducing glucose units. (From Gray GM: Carbohydrate absorption and malabsorption. In Johnson LR [ed]: Physiology of the Gastrointestinal Tract. New York, Raven Press, 1981, p 1064.)

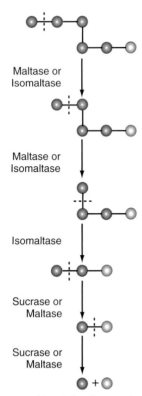

Figure 97–11   Actions of brush border membrane hydrolases. The combined actions of maltase, isomaltase, and sucrase yield glucose molecules from α-limit dextrins. Isomaltase is necessary to split the α1-6 link. ●, glucose units; ○, reducing glucose units.

In addition, two other carbohydrases participate in terminal hydrolysis of starch products. Maltase (glucoamylase) acts on 1-4–linked oligosaccharides containing as many as nine glucose residues, liberating glucose monomers. It has been suggested that although isomaltase hydrolyzes the smallest α-limit dextrin, another enzyme, α-limit dextrinase, is responsible for rapid hydrolysis of penta- and hexa-α-limit dextrins.[148]

The combination of sucrase-isomaltase, maltase, and α-limit dextrinase serves to liberate glucose monomers very rapidly and in proximity to hexose carriers, thus encouraging efficient absorption. Because free hexoses are found in the intestinal lumen, it is likely that the transport process, rather than the actions of the carbohydrases, is the rate-limiting step for uptake of monomers into the epithelium. Trehalose is a disaccharide found predominantly in mushrooms. It is therefore an insignificant element for digestion of the normal diet, but nevertheless, the existence of a specific brush border enzyme, trehalase, for its hydrolysis has been recognized.

Disaccharidase Biosynthesis and Regulation

Much has been learned about the gene regulation, biosynthesis, and processing of the disaccharidases.[149-152] Human sucrase-isomaltase is encoded by a single gene,[153] *SI*, which is located on chromosome 3 at locus 3q25-26.[154] The 5'-flanking region of the *SI* gene has a number of DNA regulatory regions that control initiation of gene transcription[155,156]; all four epithelial cell types in the mouse small intestinal mucosa have the transcriptional machinery to express the *SI* gene.[157] The elements necessary to direct intestinal epithelial cell–specific expression are embodied in a 201-nucleotide, evolutionarily conserved 5'-flanking regions of the gene.[158] At least two types of transcriptional proteins are involved in sucrase-isomaltase promoter transcription: hepatocyte nuclear factor 1 (HNF-1)[159,160] and caudal-related homeodomain proteins (Cdx).[161] The interaction of tissue-specific and tissue-restricted transcription factors facilitates the transcription of genes in a single cell type. It has been suggested that the ratio of HNF-1α to HNF-1β may determine the degree of HNF-1–induced transcription.[159,160]

Congenital sucrase-isomaltase deficiency (CSID) is an intestinal disease of autosomal recessive inheritance that is characterized by absence of the sucrase and most of the maltase digestive activity within the sucrase-isomaltase enzyme complex; the isomaltase activity ranges from absent to normal. Clinically, the disease is manifested as an osmotic-fermentative diarrhea on ingestion of disaccharides and oligosaccharides. Analysis of this disorder at the molecular and subcellular levels has unraveled a number of phenotypes of CSID, which are characterized by perturbations in the intracellular transport, aberrant processing, and defective function of sucrase-isomaltase.[162,163]

Changes in diet have a marked effect on the expression of sucrase-isomaltase. Starvation leads to a decline in brush border sucrase-isomaltase proteins and consequent reduction in sucrase-isomaltase activity; the decline in sucrase-isomaltase expression in the brush border is restored rapidly after refeeding. The type of carbohydrate ingested is important for regulation of sucrase-isomaltase expression: Starch and sucrose both induce sucrase-isomaltase activity, but sucrose is a more potent inducer.[164] Study of the intestinal cell line Caco-2 has shown that a promoter region of the human sucrase gene (nucleotides –370 to + 30) can down-regulate sucrase-isomaltase transcription in the presence of glucose.[165]

The human lactase gene is approximately 55 kilobases (kb) long, with 17 exons, and is located on the long arm of chromosome 2.[166,167] Studies in intestinal cell lines have identified functional DNA elements in the lactase gene promoter that interact with nuclear transcription factors.[168] Cdx proteins and GATA 5, a member of the GATA-type zinc-finger transcription factor family, have been shown to interact with the human lactase gene promoter and to activate transcription.

Lactose intolerance is the most common manifestation of disaccharidase deficiency and results from absent or drastically reduced levels of lactase. In humans, lactase is expressed in fetal small intestine at a time in gestation just after the onset of sucrase-isomaltase expression. Lactase expression is maintained throughout development and during childhood, although sometime during childhood, lactase activity declines to 5% to 10% of early childhood levels in most of the world's populations. This decline occurs at the same time that intestinal sucrase-isomaltase activity is increasing. Ingestion of milk or milk products by persons with diminished lactase activity leads to flatulence, abdominal cramping, and diarrhea. This pattern of reduction in lactase activity has been termed late-onset lactase deficiency, or adult-type hypolactasia. It initially was thought that the regulation of lactase–phlorizin hydrolase (LPH), the gene that produces lactase, was post-translational and associated with altered structural features of the enzyme. More recent studies, however, suggest that the major mechanism of regulation of LPH is transcriptional (see later). Other forms of lactose intolerance include the rare congenital lactase deficiency and secondary forms, such as those caused by mucosal injury, resulting from infectious gastroenteritis, celiac disease, parasitic infection, drug-induced enteritis, and Crohn's disease.

Differential activation of both the lactase and the sucrase-isomaltase promoter is effected by multiple similar transcription factors including GATA factors, HNF-1α, and Cdx-2, alone and in combination. This synergistic activation may be a method whereby higher levels of tissue-specific expression might be possible.[169]

Disaccharidase synthesis occurs within the endoplasmic reticulum, and the proenzymes then follow the path for secretory proteins through the Golgi complex, before being inserted into the brush border membrane. All are glycoproteins, and all undergo extensive intracellular processing with removal of redundant segments of the molecule. Final processing of sucrase-isomaltase occurs on insertion into the brush border membrane after exposure to luminal pancreatic proteases (Fig. 97–12), at which point it is cleaved into its two active subunits. By contrast, lactase already is completely processed before its insertion.

In their final active form, the carbohydrases project into the lumen, forming part of the glycocalyx, and they are attached to the membrane by a hydrophobic anchor that represents approximately 10% of the total mass of the molecule. Evidence suggests that MYO1A (Brush Border Myosin I), a group of monomeric actin-based motors that are known to associate with membranes in intestinal villi, are involved in sucrase-isomaltase retention within the brush border.[170]

Disaccharidases are synthesized by both crypt and villus cells but are expressed only on the latter. The expression of disaccharidase genes in the intestine exhibits a complex spatial pattern along the vertical (crypt-to-villus) and horizontal (proximal-to-distal) axes.[171] Little sucrase-isomaltase activity is present in the crypts and villus tip cells, and maximal activity is in the lower and mid-villus regions.[172] The major mechanism for regulating the expression of sucrase-isomaltase along the crypt-villus axis is the steady-state level of sucrase-isomaltase mRNA, although post-transcriptional and post-translational regulation probably play a role in the expression of the functional sucrase-isomaltase along the intestinal crypt-villus axis.[173]

A functional difference also exists between the jejunum and distal ileum that reflect a difference in the expression of different genes, or gradients of gene expression, along the proximal-distal axis of the intestine. For example, sucrase-isomaltase activity is four- to fivefold greater in the jejunum than in the ileum,[174] although sucrase-isomaltase mRNA appears to be similar in the two areas. Although minor differences are present in the pattern of glycosylation in the Golgi apparatus, the major difference in regulation between the jejunum and ileum appears to be at the level of mRNA translation.[175]

Pancreatic proteolytic enzymes shorten the half-lives of the carbohydrases.[176] Sucrase-isomaltase half-life may

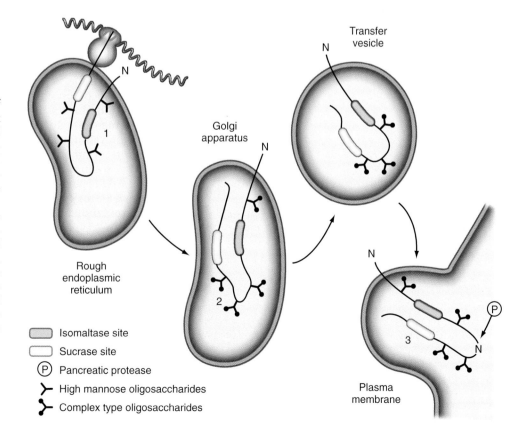

Figure 97–12 Biosynthesis of sucrose isomaltase. The nascent polypeptide is translocated across the endoplasmic reticulum membrane after ribosomal messenger RNA (mRNA) translation (1). Oligosaccharide side chains join the polypeptide, which are transferred to the Golgi apparatus for further processing (2). After transfer to and incorporation in the plasma membrane, luminal proteases cleave the molecule into its active subunits (3). (From Lloyd ML, Olsen WA: Intestinal carbohydrases. Viewpoints Dig Dis 3:13, 1991.)

Transfer vesicle

Golgi apparatus

Rough endoplasmic reticulum

Plasma membrane

⬭ Isomaltase site

▭ Sucrase site

Ⓟ Pancreatic protease

⌁ High mannose oligosaccharides

⌁ Complex type oligosaccharides

drop as low as 4.5 hours after meals, compared with more than 20 hours during fasting. Presumably, proteolysis, as largely determined by meals, is responsible for the diurnal variation in carbohydrase activity.[49]

The levels of sucrase-isomaltase and other saccharidases also may decrease with infection and inflammation. In some cases, a decline in enzyme activity leads to malabsorption of carbohydrates and signs and symptoms of diarrhea, flatulence, and weight loss. In most disease processes, however, the diminished levels of sucrase-isomaltase are associated with global dysfunction of small intestinal mucosa.

Transport across the Mucosa

The three major diet-derived monosaccharides—glucose, galactose, and fructose—are absorbed by saturable carrier-mediated transport systems located in the brush border membrane of enterocytes in the proximal and mid-small intestine.[177] The active transport of glucose and galactose is achieved by the same transport protein that acts as a sodium cotransporter (primarily SGLT1)[178]. Active glucose transport is driven by the sodium gradient across the apical cell membrane (Fig. 97–13). First, a low intracellular sodium concentration is generated by the sodium pump sodium-potassium–adenosine triphosphatase (Na^+,K^+-ATPase) located in the basolateral membrane of the enterocyte, which transports 3 Na^+ out of the cell and

2 K^+ into the cell, resulting in a low intracellular Na^+ concentration. Then 2 Na^+ ions bind to the outer face of the transporter, which produces a conformational change that permits subsequent sugar binding. The 2 Na^+ ions and the glucose molecule then are transferred to the cytoplasmic face of the membrane through another conformational change involving a coordinated rotation or tilt of transmembrane helices.[179] At the cytoplasmic surface, glucose dissociates first, and then the 2 Na^+ ions dissociate into the cytosol to produce a ligand-free transporter. The low affinity of the cytosolic sites for glucose and Na^+, and the low intracellular Na^+ concentration relative to the extracellular concentration (10 versus 140 mEq/L), promote these dissociations. The ligand-free transporter then relaxes to the outward-facing conformation, to complete the cycle. The complete enzymatic turnover of the transporter occurs approximately 1000 times a second at 37°C.

Although some of this glucose fuels cellular metabolism, a sizable fraction passes out of the cell across the basolateral membrane by facilitated diffusion (uniport). The net result is that for every glucose molecule that is transported across the brush border, 2 Na^+ ions (and 2 accompanying anions) also are transported across the epithelium. This, in turn, draws approximately 1100 water molecules across the epithelium to maintain iso-omolarity of the absorbate. How and why water is "dragged" across epithelia is not well understood but may be explained by any of three mechanisms: (1) a localized, intracellular osmotic gradient that drives water across the relatively impermeable membranes; (2) the existence of specialized transmembrane proteins called aquaporins; or (3) because the epithelium is relatively impermeable, that most water movement in the intestine occurs by the paracellular route and is regulated by the tight junctions. Ion and nutrient absorption across the intestine does not increase the osmolarity of the fluid remaining in the gut lumen. The coupling between glucose, salt, and water absorption provides the explanation for the finding that water absorption across the upper and mid-intestine is glucose dependent and constitutes the rationale for oral rehydration therapy (ORT), used to great effect in the management of patients with secretory diarrhea.[180]

The prevailing opinion is that two types of glucose transport occur across brush borders. One is a high-affinity sodium-dependent, phlorizin-sensitive transporter, SGLT1, and the other is a low-affinity transporter that may or may not be sodium dependent and phlorizin sensitive; candidates for the latter role in humans include GLUT2, SGLT4, and SGLT6.[181]

The sodium-glucose cotransporter (SGLT1) has been characterized extensively.[182-184] Activity of this 73-kd cotransporter in the intestinal brush border membrane depends on the presence of four independent, identical subunits arranged in a homotetramer. After cloning and sequencing the sodium-glucose cotransporter and demonstrating that the gene for this resides on chromosome 22, investigators demonstrated that a single missense mutation resulting in a change of amino acid residue 28 from an aspartate to an asparaginase was responsible for the defective sodium-glucose cotransporter in familial glucose/galactose malabsorption. The cloned cDNA codes for transport activity with the same

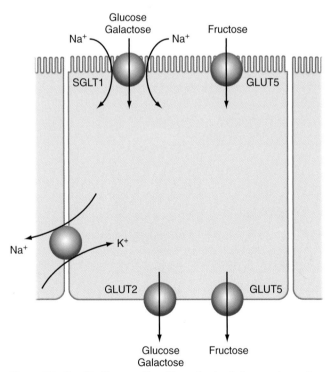

Figure 97–13   "Sodium gradient" hypothesis of glucose absorption. The sodium pump (Na^+,K^+-ATPase) at the basolateral membrane generates a low intracellular sodium concentration. Sodium passes down the concentration gradient thus created and across the apical membrane coupled to glucose (or galactose) on a common carrier. The sodium pump thus generates the energy for this system. Glucose (or galactose) leaves the cell by means of facilitated diffusion across the basolateral membrane. SGLT1, sodium glucose transporter 1; GLUT2, GLUT5, glucose transporter.

relative specificity as for the previously characterized native transport system: D-glucose > α-methyl-D-glucose > D-galactose > 3-O-methyl-D-glucopyranose >>> L-glucose.[185] The cDNA encodes a 662-amino-acid protein with a predicted molecular weight that correlates well with the biochemically defined size. SGLT1 is predicted to have 14 membrane-spanning domains, with one asparagine-linked carbohydrate group on the third extracytoplasmic loop.[186]

The expression and activity of glucose transport in the intestinal brush border are regulated by both short-term and longer-term processes. In the short term, activity of glucose transport is increased by both protein kinase A– and C–dependent processes.[187] The mechanism of this enhanced activity is an increase in the number of membrane transporters, mediated by changes in exocytosis and endocytosis of membrane vesicles that contain the transport protein. Longer-term regulation of glucose transport is mediated by changes in the expression of SGLT, which is controlled by changes in the nutrient environment.[188]

Glucose-galactose malabsorption is characterized by the neonatal onset of severe diarrhea. Multiple distinct mutations in the SGLT1 gene are responsible, including the missense mutation described earlier. Most mutations are responsible for defective passage of the SGLT1 through the biosynthetic machinery from the endoplasmic reticulum, or poor trafficking from the Golgi apparatus to the brush border membrane. Rarely do mutant SGLT1 proteins reach the brush border at a normal rate. In this case, the glucose transport is defective.[181]

Debate has developed over the mechanism of the passive or "diffusive" component of intestinal glucose absorption and, indeed, whether it exists.[189] Pappenheimer and Reiss proposed that paracellular solvent drag contributes a passive component, which, at high concentrations of sugars similar to those in the jejunal lumen immediately after a meal, is several-fold greater than the active component mediated by the sodium-glucose cotransporter SGLT1.[190] Other investigators have argued that the kinetics of glucose absorption can be explained solely in terms of SGLT1 and that a passive or paracellular component plays little, if any, part.[191] More recent data suggest that the passive component of glucose absorption exists but is in fact facilitated, because it is mediated by the rapid, glucose-dependent activation and recruitment of the facilitative glucose transporter GLUT2 to the brush border membrane. This facilitation is regulated through a protein kinase C–dependent pathway activated by glucose transport through SGLT1 and also involves mitogen-activated protein kinase (MAP kinase) signaling pathways.[192]

Fructose absorption occurs by facilitated diffusion; that is, transport occurs not against a concentration gradient, but with a carrier protein to achieve transport rates greater than one would expect from simple diffusion; this process is completely independent of glucose absorption. Studies in humans have demonstrated the existence of a saturable, facilitative transport system for fructose in the intestinal epithelium that has a lower activity than that for transport of glucose and galactose. The protein responsible for most apical membrane fructose transport is a member of the facilitative monosaccharide transporter family called GLUT5. This 501-amino-acid protein in humans has 12 membrane-spanning domains, as do other GLUT molecules, and transports fructose exclusively.[193] Little fructose is metabolized in the enterocytes. Fructose is transported across the basolateral membrane and is taken up and metabolized rapidly by the liver, resulting in low postabsorptive blood levels of fructose. More than one type of fructose transport system may exist. Malabsorption of fructose in humans can be prevented by the simultaneous administration of glucose, suggesting the presence of another, glucose-responsive system in the enterocytes. No inherited disorders of fructose transport (GLUT5) have been reported yet.

Exit from the Epithelium

Most hexoses are exported from the epithelial cell by way of the basolateral membrane, although small amounts are utilized for intracellular metabolism. Exit across the basolateral membrane depends on facilitated diffusion (not requiring energy) mediated by a specific carrier. Two genes that are expressed in the small intestine encode the facilitative sugar transport proteins GLUT2, the basolateral membrane–associated glucose transporter, and GLUT5, an apical membrane fructose transporter.[194] *GLUT2* has molecular structural characteristics similar to those of the other members of this family of genes. The protein has 500 amino acids, with many hydrophobic residues that predict a total of 12 membrane-spanning domains. One long extracellular loop is present between membrane-spanning domains 1 and 2, containing an asparagine that is *N*-glycosylated, and one long cytoplasmic loop is present between membrane-spanning domains 6 and 7. Once the hexoses have entered the interstitial space, they pass onward by diffusion into the portal circulation.

A congenital defect in glucose transport by GLUT2 has been identified and is called the *Fanconi-Bickel syndrome*. Because GLUT2 normally is expressed in the liver, pancreas, and kidney, as well as in the intestine, defects in this transporter are expected to have a widespread effect on glucose homeostasis. Indeed, patients with the Fanconi-Bickel syndrome exhibit tubular nephropathy, fasting hypoglycemia, rickets, stunted growth, and hepatomegaly secondary to glycogen accumulation.[195,196]

The accepted dogma of intestinal glucose absorption at the basolateral membrane by glucose transporters has been challenged by studies of intestinal glucose absorption in GLUT2-null mice and in patients with GLUT2 deficiency. In both cases, no impairment of glucose absorption was observed. Additional work has suggested the presence of two separate pathways for the exit of sugar from enterocytes: one that involves GLUT2 and another that requires glucose phosphorylation, the transfer of glucose-6-phosphate into the endoplasmic reticulum, and the release of free glucose into the blood. The release mechanism is unclear, but it has been proposed to involve vesicle trafficking. This postulate is supported by oral tolerance tests in a patient with congenital deficiency in glucose-6-phosphate translocase 1 in whom glucose absorption was impaired but not eliminated.[196]

Not all potentially digestible carbohydrate is absorbed in the small intestine. As much as 20% of dietary starch may escape into the colon, particularly that derived from cereals and potatoes.[2] Most of this, however, is metabolized by colonic bacteria, and the short-chain fatty acids thus derived are absorbed readily. Hydrogen and methane also are generated, contributing to flatus.

PROTEIN

DIETARY INTAKE

Dietary proteins are the major source of amino acids, and in the average Western diet they provide approximately 10% to 15% of energy intake. Affluent populations ingest more protein than they need to maintain their normal balance. An average adult in a Western country consumes at least 70 g of protein per day, whereas the poor in Asia and Africa consume 50 g or less per day.[49] Recommended dietary requirements vary, ranging from 0.75 to 1 g/kg of body weight per day, but deficiency states are rare even with intakes of 0.5 g/kg per day or less. In the United Kingdom, protein intake has remained fairly steady since the mid-1970s, but with the marked declines in fat and carbohydrate ingestion, the ratio of protein to nonprotein energy intake has risen.[49] Little harm appears to occur in the unusual subgroups of society that consume very large amounts of protein, although renal function can be impaired. The Masai tribes of Africa and the Gaucho of South America, who consume 250 to 300 g (largely of animal origin) per day, suffer no obvious untoward effects.[49]

The variety of types of animal and plant proteins is enormous. Generally, plant proteins are less digestible than those derived from animals, but some fibrous animal proteins, such as keratin and collagen, also are relatively indigestible. High-proline proteins such as the glutenins are less thoroughly digested than are others. The "quality" of proteins depends largely on their amino acid composition; proteins rich in essential amino acids are regarded as being of high quality.

Food processing, by heat, for example, may cause inter- and intramolecular bonding in the proteins to produce polymeric forms that are relatively resistant to hydrolysis.[1] Other constituents of the diet also may interfere with protein digestion, for example, starch and reducing sugars that have the potential to impair digestion.[49] Despite these interferences, digestion and absorption of proteins are remarkably complete, and only approximately 3% to 5% of ingested nitrogen is lost in the stool, probably because of the resistance of some peptide bonds to hydrolysis.[1] A few specific proteins are resistant to proteolysis in the small bowel, including secretory IgA and intrinsic factor. Among the 20 common amino acids that form animal and plant proteins, 8 cannot be synthesized by animals. These 8 "essential" amino acids must be ingested and usually are eaten as plant-derived foods. The essential amino acids are leucine, isoleucine, lysine, methionine, phenylalanine, threonine, tryptophan, and valine. Histidine also is required for growth in infants.

PROTEINS OF ENDOGENOUS ORIGIN

Almost half of all protein that enters the intestine is derived from endogenous sources. Of this endogenous protein, approximately 20 to 30 g per day are derived from secretions of salivary, gastric, biliary, pancreatic, and mucosal origin. Another 30 g per day of protein are provided by epithelial cells desquamated from the villus tips, and 2 g of plasma proteins are delivered into the intestinal lumen each day.

INTRALUMINAL DIGESTION

Pepsins

Digestion of proteins begins in the stomach with the action of pepsins secreted by gastric mucosa. Pepsins are released from their precursor pepsinogens by autoactivation in an acid pH with the loss of a small basic peptide. Pepsinogen release from chief cells is stimulated by gastrin and histamine and also from cholinergic stimulation. Pepsinogen release closely mirrors acid secretion.[197]

The pepsins are a family of proteolytic enzymes that can be distinguished electrophoretically and immunologically. Two immunologically distinct groups are recognized (groups 1 and 2), whereas electrophoresis reveals eight fractions. Both immunologically separated species are secreted by chief cells, but group 2 isoforms also are present in the mucus cells of the oxyntic and pyloric areas of the stomach and in Brunner's glands of the duodenum. Their substrate specificities vary little, but their pH optima differ slightly (between 1.8 and 3.5); all are irreversibly inactivated in alkali.

Pepsins remain active at the acid pH of gastric contents to produce a mixture of peptides with a small proportion of amino acids. The completeness of gastric proteolysis depends in part on the rate of gastric emptying, the pH of intragastric contents, and the types of protein ingested. Persons who are achlorhydric or in whom control of gastric emptying has been lost as a result of pyloroplasty or partial gastrectomy do not appear to have a problem with assimilation of protein, suggesting that gastric proteolysis is not an essential component of digestion.

Pancreatic Proteases

Each of the pancreatic proteases is secreted as a proenzyme and therefore must be activated within the lumen, in contradistinction to amylase and lipase, which are secreted in their active forms. Enterokinase (enteropeptidase) plays a key role in proteolysis. It is liberated from its superficial position in the brush border membrane by the action of bile acids,[198] its action being to convert trypsinogen to trypsin by removing the hexapeptide N terminus of trypsinogen. Trypsin in turn activates the other proteases and continues to split more trypsin from trypsinogen (Fig. 97–14).

The proteases are classified as endo- and exopeptidases, according to the sites of the peptide bonds against which they are most active. Endopeptidases include trypsin, chymotrypsin, and elastase, and exopeptidases include carboxypeptidase A and B (Table 97–6).

Trypsin, chymotrypsin, and elastase have specificity for peptide bonds adjacent to certain specific amino acids and split peptide bonds in the protein molecule; exopeptidases remove a single amino acid from the C-terminal end of the peptide. Trypsin produces short-chain

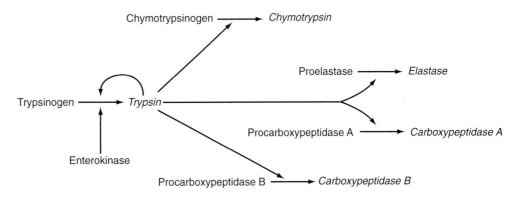

Figure 97–14 Activation of pancreatic proteolytic enzymes. Enterokinase (enteropeptidase) plays a critical role in activating trypsinogen to form trypsin. Trypsin in turn activates not only more trypsinogen, but also the other proteolytic enzyme precursors.

Table 97–6   Pancreatic Proteolytic Enzymes and Some of Their Characteristics

Enzyme	Action	Products
Trypsin	Endopeptidase; cleaves internal bonds at lysine or arginine residues; cleaves other pancreatic proenzymes	Oligopeptides and proteolytic enzymes
Chymotrypsin	Endopeptidase; cleaves bonds at aromatic or neutral amino acid residues	Oligopeptides
Elastase	Endopeptidase; cleaves bonds at aliphatic amino acid residues	Oligopeptides
Carboxypeptidase A	Exopeptidase; cleaves aromatic amino acids from C-terminal end of proteins and peptides	Aromatic amino acids and peptides
Carboxypeptidase B	Exopeptidase; cleaves arginine or lysine from C-terminal end of proteins and peptides	Arginine, lysine, and peptides

oligopeptides, which are hydrolyzed further by the exopeptidases, carboxypeptidase A acting on aromatic and aliphatic C termini, and carboxypeptidase B acting on peptides containing basic C termini. The final products of intraluminal digestion thus are produced by cooperative activity of endo- and exopeptidases and consist of a number of neutral and basic amino acids together with peptides of 2 to 6 amino acids in length. Approximately 30% of luminal amino nitrogen is found in amino acids and approximately 70% is found in oligopeptides.[199]

In addition to nutrient protein hydrolysis, pancreatic proteases have other functions: They split vitamin B_{12} from the R protein to which it is linked, so that it can then bind intrinsic factor; they increase the turnover of brush border membrane hydrolytic enzymes, and as discussed earlier, they initiate the final steps in the processing of the sucrase-isomaltase complex; and finally, they may have a role in the inactivation of some organisms.[1]

Digestion at the Brush Border Membrane and in the Cytoplasm

In contrast with the absorption of carbohydrate, which is restricted largely to uptake of hexose monomers across the brush border membrane, amino acids can be absorbed either as monomers or as di- or tripeptides. Indeed, amino acid absorption is achieved more efficiently in the form of peptides than as single amino acids[200] (Fig. 97–15). The fact that the vast majority of the end-products of protein digestion that reach the portal circulation are amino acids, however, speaks strongly in favor of the presence of peptidases in the epithelium.

In patients with cystinuria and Hartnup's disease, who have specific defects in the absorption of basic and neutral amino acids, respectively, protein deficiency states do not develop, because the absorption of peptides in these patients is normal.[201] The discovery that di- and tripeptides are actively transported by the brush border membrane of enterocytes has been valuable in explaining this observation, and it emphasizes the need for critical evaluation of the supposed nutritional advantage provided by elemental diets that consist only of free amino acids.

A range of peptidases are present in the brush border membrane and in the cytoplasm of villus epithelial cells for the hydrolysis of oligopeptides up to approximately eight amino acid residues in length[202-204] (Table 97–7). The peptidases on the brush border membrane differ in several important respects from those within the cytoplasm (Table 97–8). Approximately 90% of the dipeptidases are found in the cytoplasm and only approximately 10% in the brush border, whereas the distribution of hydrolases for tetrapeptides is the reverse of this. Peptidases for pentapeptides and larger molecules are confined almost entirely to the brush border membrane. Cytoplasmic enzymes are much more heat labile than those in the brush border, and differences in the electrophoretic mobility patterns have been demonstrated for the two sets of enzymes.[75]

Most oligopeptidases appear to be aminopeptidases; that is, they act by removing residues from the N terminus of the peptide. The chain length of the peptides is an important factor that determines not only whether the site at which hydrolysis occurs is at the brush border or within the cell, but also its rate. Thus, rates of brush border membrane hydrolysis for tripeptides are most rapid, and for dipeptides least rapid, whereas tetra- and pentapeptide hydrolysis rates occupy intermediate positions.[200]

Table 97–7   Peptidases Found on the Brush Border Membrane and in the Cytoplasm of Villus Epithelial Cells

Peptidase	Action	Products
Brush Border Membrane Peptidases		
Amino-oligopeptidases (at least two types)	Cleave amino acids from C terminal end of 3 to 8 amino acid peptides	Amino acids and dipeptides
Aminopeptidase A	Cleaves dipeptides with acidic amino acids at N terminal end	Amino acids
Dipeptidase I	Cleaves dipeptides containing methionine	Amino acids
Dipeptidase III	Cleaves glycine-containing dipeptides	Amino acids
Dipeptidyl aminopeptidase IV	Cleaves proline-containing peptides with free α-amino groups	Peptides and amino acids
Carboxypeptidase P	Cleaves proline-containing peptides with free C terminal end	Peptides and amino acids
Gamma glutamyl transpeptidase	Cleaves gamma-glutamyl bonds and transfers glutamine to amino acid or peptide acceptors	Gamma-glutamyl amino acid or peptide
Folate conjugase	Cleaves pteroyl polyglutamates	Monoglutamate
Cytoplasmic Peptidases		
Dipeptidases (several types)	Cleave most dipeptides	Amino acids
Aminotripeptidase	Cleaves tripeptides	Amino acids
Proline dipeptidase	Cleaves proline-containing dipeptides	Proline and amino acids

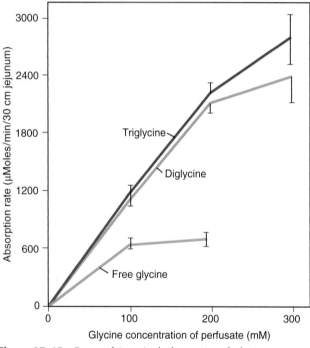

Figure 97–15 Rates of intestinal absorption of glycine (mean ± standard error of mean) from perfusion solutions containing equivalent amounts of glycine in free or peptide form. Results are from studies in the jejunum of four normal humans. (Adibi SA, Morse EL, Masilamani SS, Amin PM: Evidence for two different modes of tripeptide disappearance in human intestine. Uptake by peptide carrier systems and hydrolysis by peptide hydrolases. J Clin Invest 56:1355, 1975.)

At least three other peptidases are distinct from the amino oligopeptidases. Aminopeptidase A has specificity for peptides with acidic amino acids at their N termini. Aminopeptidases 1 and 3 (distinguished on electrophoretic mobility) have specificities for different substrates with different amino acid peptide bonds.[1]

Proline-containing oligopeptides are not hydrolyzed readily by most proteases, despite the fact that many proteins—including collagen, gliadin, and casein—are rich in proline. Two proline-specific carboxypeptidases,

Table 97–8   Relative Distribution of Peptidase Activity Based on Substrate

Substrate	Brush Border Membrane (%)	Cytoplasm (%)
Dipeptides	5-10	80-95
Tripeptides	10-60	30-60
Tetrapeptides	90	1-10
Higher peptides	98	Nil

however, have been demonstrated in the brush border membrane; they have slightly different substrate specificities.[205] Together with a cytoplasmic proline dipeptidase, these are likely to be responsible for hydrolysis of proline-rich peptides.

A number of other brush border membrane peptidases should be mentioned. Gamma-glutamyl transpeptidase hydrolyzes gamma-glutamyl peptide bonds, with the transfer of the gamma-glutamyl group to another amino acid to form a gamma-glutamyl amino acid or peptide derivative.[1] The role of this brush border membrane in the intestine is not yet clear. Folate conjugase, an enzyme concerned with hydrolysis of dietary folate, is considered later on. The recent demonstration of angiotensin 1-converting enzyme (ACE) in intestinal mucosa suggests that it, too, may hydrolyze dietary peptides.[206] Indirect evidence indicates that endopeptidases also may be present on the brush border membrane, because protein digestion occurs even in the complete absence of pancreatic function; these enzymes have yet to be isolated.

As with other proteins, synthesis of each specific peptidase occurs in the rough endoplasmic reticulum, and following transfer to the Golgi apparatus, the proteins are transported to the brush border membrane, where they are inserted by exocytic fusion.[207,208] They are attached to this membrane by short anchoring pieces in a manner analogous to the attachment of disaccharidases[209]; however, unlike with the latter enzymes, little post-translational processing occurs, either within the cytoplasm or by pancreatic enzymes on the brush border.

Of the cytoplasmic dipeptidases, the most abundant appears to be one with broad specificity for neutral amino acid–containing dipeptides. The tripeptidase isolated has broad specificity for N-terminal residues and high specificity toward tripeptides containing proline as the N-terminal residue, a characteristic that distinguishes it from the brush border membrane amino oligopeptidase. Other characteristics of the tripeptide that are required for rapid hydrolysis include a free alpha amino group, an alpha carboxyl group, and an L-configuration for the two amino acid residues.[210]

ABSORPTION

Peptides

Substrate inhibition studies indicate that tri- and dipeptides inhibit uptake of either from the lumen, but that neither is affected by single amino acids. Such evidence suggests that small peptides utilize a separate transporter system from those used by single amino acids. By contrast, tetrapeptide absorption is inhibited by single amino acids but not by di- and tripeptides, suggesting that tetrapeptides are split before absorption.

The advantage of dipeptide absorption over single-amino-acid absorption has been largely demonstrated experimentally with single peptides containing a single amino acid, usually glycine.[200] Several studies, however, have demonstrated the kinetic advantage of peptides over amino acids, even in complex mixtures of partial digests of proteins.[211,212] Absorption was greater from tryptic hydrolysates of proteins than from a mixture of amino acids. Furthermore, the wide variation in absorption rates seen with different individual amino acids was reduced when they were presented as a tryptic hydrolysate.

A number of other factors influence digestion and absorption. The presence of amino acids in the lumen inhibits peptide hydrolysis (product inhibition), whereas luminal glucose and luminal acidification each inhibit amino acid and peptide absorption.[200] Good evidence suggests that di- and tripeptides are taken up by a single type of transporter with some stereospecificity, because the length of the amino acid side chains on the di- or tripeptides is important; the longer the side chain, the more preferred the substrate for the absorption site[213] (Table 97–9). The L-isomers of the amino acids in dipeptides are much preferred to the D-isomers, whereas the presence of acidic and basic amino acid residues in dipeptides reduces affinity for the transport system, compared with neutral amino acid residues. Affinity also is greater for dipeptides than for tripeptides, at least in the example

of peptides containing glycine. The transporter for peptides is not dependent on sodium, but cotransport with protons may occur instead.[214]

The peptide transporter for human small intestine has been cloned[215,216] and is a member of a superfamily of H^+-coupled peptide transporters. The human protein consists of 708 amino acids, with a predicted core molecular size of 79 kd, that contains 12 transmembrane domains. The gene is located on chromosome 13. In humans, it is expressed in the small intestine (duodenum, jejunum, and ileum) but not in the esophagus, stomach, or colon. In the small intestine, it is expressed only in absorptive epithelium. It recognizes a variety of neutral, anionic, and cationic dipeptides as substrates,[217,218] which explains the broad substrate specificity of the intestinal peptide transport system.

The most interesting feature of this transport process is that it uses a transmembrane electrochemical H^+ gradient, rather than a transmembrane electrochemical Na^+ gradient, as its driving force.[219] The acid pH microclimate that characterizes the luminal surface of the intestinal brush border membrane creates a H^+ gradient across the brush border membrane in vivo. This acid pH microclimate is generated and maintained by the combined action of the Na^+-H^+ exchanger in the brush border membrane and Na^+,K^+-ATPase in the basolateral membrane of the enterocyte. The mechanism of the transport process is a simultaneous translocation of H^+ and peptide substrate involving a single H^+-binding site on the protein[220,221] (Fig. 97–16).

A multitude of processes are involved in the absorption of peptides. The well-established processes include (1) an Na^+-H^+ exchanger located in the brush border membrane that maintains an intracellular alkaline pH; (2) an Na^+,K^+-ATPase located in the basolateral membrane that maintains an inside negative membrane potential; and (3) several cytoplasmic peptidases that prevent intracellular accumulation of absorbed peptides. These enzymes convert most of the absorbed oligopeptides to amino acids that either are used by the absorbing cells or are released into the portal circulation via the amino acid transporters located on the basolateral membrane of these cells. The oligopeptides that escape hydrolysis by the cytoplasmic peptidases are transported across the basolateral membrane into the portal circulation by a peptide transporter that appears to differ from Pept-1. Oligopeptide transport could be regulated by alteration in activity or abundance of Pept-1, Na^+-H^+ exchanger, Na^+,K^+-ATPase, cytoplasmic peptidases, and basolateral oligopeptide transporter.[222,223]

Studies of individual substrates and hormones in cell culture have shown that the membrane population of Pept-1 is increased by dipeptides, certain amino acids, insulin, and leptin and decreased by epidermal growth factor and triiodothyronine. In the case of dipeptides, epidermal growth factor (EGF), and thyroid hormone, parallel changes occur in the gene expression brought about by alteration of transcription or stability of Pept-1 mRNA. By contrast, treatment with insulin and leptin does not induce any alteration in Pept-1 gene expression, and the mechanism of increased protein expression appears to be increased trafficking from a pre-formed cytoplasmic pool to the apical membrane.[222,223]

Table 97–9	Relative Specificities of the Intestinal Peptide Transporters for Dipeptides and Tripeptides
Dipeptides	**Tripeptides**
L Form of amino acids in peptide	D Form of amino acids in peptide
Neutral amino acids in peptide	Acidic or basic amino acids in peptide
Long-side-chain amino acids in peptides	Short-side-chain amino acids in peptides

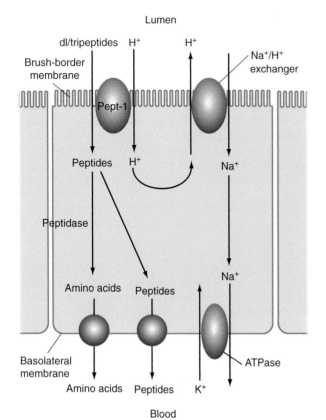

Figure 97–16 Peptide and amino acid transport across the intestinal epithelium. This transport process uses a transmembrane H^+ gradient rather than a transmembrane electrochemical Na^+ gradient as its driving force. The acidic microclimate on the luminal surface of the intestinal brush border membrane is generated and maintained by the combined action of the Na^+-H^+ exchanger in the brush border membrane and Na^+,K^+-ATPase in the basolateral membrane of the enterocyte. The mechanism of the transport process is a simultaneous translocation of H^+ and peptide substrate involving a single H^+-binding site on the protein.

Amino Acids

Although only one type of dipeptide transporter in the brush border membrane for the 400 different possible dipeptides has been recognized, a multiplicity of transport mechanisms are available for the 20 amino acids. In adults, these mechanisms are located on villus enterocytes and involve carrier-mediated active transport or facilitated diffusion processes; a small proportion may be absorbed by simple diffusion. Some difficulty has been encountered in defining the number and types of transporters because they have overlapping specificities; several amino acids utilize a number of different transport systems (Table 97–10). On the basis of kinetic studies, at least four active processes have been identified for transport of *neutral* amino acids across the apical cell membrane. Each is electrogenic and sodium dependent. One has broad specificity for a number of neutral amino acids (NBB system); a second provides another route for phenylalanine and methionine (PHE system); a third provides a mechanism for imino acid absorption (IMINO system); and the fourth transports beta amino acids. Separate sodium-dependent, active transport processes for *basic* and *acidic* amino acids also have been demon-

Table 97–10   Major Amino Acid Transport Systems Detected in Intestinal Epithelial Cells

Transport System	Substrates
Brush Border Membrane	
Neutral amino acids	
NBB (SLC6A19)	Broad specificity for neutral amino acids
PHE	Phenylalanine and methionine
IMINO (SLC36A1)	Imino acids; proline, hydroxyproline
Basic amino acids	Lysine, cysteine, basic amino acids
Acidic amino acids	Glutamate, aspartate
X-GA (SLC1A1)	
Basolateral Membrane	
L	Broad selectivity
A	Broad selectivity
ASC (SLC1A5)	Neutral amino acids, alanine, serine, cysteine
N	Glutamine, histidine, asparagine

strated, and some evidence suggests that facilitated diffusion of these types of amino acids also occurs, although this is likely to be a minor pathway.

Recent genomic advances have allowed most mammalian amino acid transport functions to be attributed to specific gene products; at least 52 amino acid transporter–related gene products are grouped within 12 solute carrier families, with their own new nomenclature.[224] Despite this wealth of information, some intestinal brush border membrane amino acid transport systems (as characterized by functional studies) have yet to be identified at the molecular level. For example, the classic sodium-dependent imino acid transporter has been identified recently as the human PAT1 (human *p*roton-coupled *a*mino acid *t*ransporter 1) or solute carrier SLC36A1. This high-capacity imino acid carrier has been localized at the small intestinal luminal membrane and transports imino and amino acids (glycine, praline, alanine, taurine).[225,226] Human PAT1 mediates 1:1 symport of protons and small neutral amino acids. The acid microclimate of the brush border membrane drives transport of the amino acids into the cytosol. Transport activity is independent of Na^+ and Cl^- (Fig. 97–17).

Hartnup's disease is a disorder of renal and gastrointestinal neutral amino acid transport that is inherited as an autosomal recessive trait. The gene causing Hartnup's disease has been localized to 5p (it had previously been localized to chromosome 19), and a new gene, *SLC6A19*, for a sodium-dependent and chloride-independent neutral amino acid transporter, has been suggested as the defective gene by two separate groups of investigators.[227,228] This transporter has been shown to be expressed in the intestine and has properties of system B0. System B0 refers to a broad range of amino acids with neutral (0) charge. Acidic amino acid transporters that have been identified in the intestinal mucosa include members of the SLC1 family. SLC1A1 is proposed as being an acidic amino acid X-GA transporter of glutamate and aspartate, whereas SLC1A5 is the proposed alanine, serine, cysteine (ASC) carrier for neutral amino acids: alanine, serine, and cysteine.[229] The SLC1A1 carrier cotransports 3 Na^+ and 1 H^+ with countertransport of

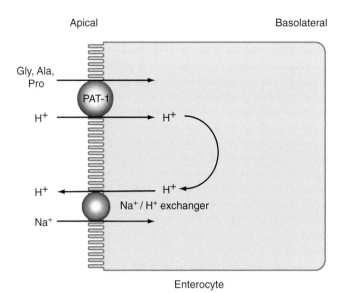

Figure 97–17   Amino acid transport across the intestinal epithelium. The human protein-coupled amino acid transporter (PAT-1) is involved in the absorption of small amino acids across the apical membrane. The acid microenvironment generated by an Na^+-H^+ exchanger provides the electrochemical proton gradient that drives amino acids to the cytosol. (From Boll M, Daniel H, Gasnier B: The SLC36 family: Proton-coupled transporters for the absorption of selected amino acids from extracellular and intracellular proteolysis. Pflugers Arch 447:776, 2004.)

1 K^+; the SLC1A5 transporter mediates sodium-dependent transport. Further clarification of these separate transport systems and their substrate specificity in the gastrointestinal tract is awaited.

Several hormones have been shown to alter the amino acid and peptide transport process in the intestine. Somatostatin and vasoactive intestinal polypeptide decrease these transport processes, whereas EGF, neurotensin, CCK, and secretin enhance them. Human Pept1 appears to be inhibited by protein kinase C[230] and cyclic adenosine monophosphate (cAMP).[231] Expression of the intestinal peptide transporter also is modulated by dietary protein content.[232] Even though the peptide transporter is expressed along the entire small intestine, the diet-induced changes in the expression of the transporter are specific to certain regions. A high-protein diet for example, increases the steady state levels of the transporter specific mRNA in the middle and distal regions of the small intestine. Expression of the brush border peptidases dipeptidylcarboxypeptidase and dipeptidylaminopeptidase IV, which releases dipeptides from oligopeptides, also are enhanced by a high-protein diet.

Exit from the Epithelium

Exit through the basolateral membrane operates through a number of different mechanisms that involve active transport and passive diffusion.[233] Active, sodium-dependent processes exist at this membrane for the uptake of neutral amino acids, which presumably supplies nutrients for crypt cells and for villus enterocytes during fasting when a luminal source is unavailable (see Table 97–10). Villus enterocytes receive the amino acids necessary for production of their own protein from luminal nutrients, whereas crypt cells obtain their supply from the portal circulation. Of all of the amino acids, glutamine appears to be a unique, major source of energy for enterocytes; ammonia is an important metabolic by-product of this process. Active uptake of glutamine at the basolateral membrane, as well as through apical membrane processes, is therefore particularly important.

It has been estimated that approximately 10% of amino acids are utilized in the production of enterocyte protein. Some of these proteins are secreted across the basolateral membrane specifically by villus enterocytes, including the apolipoproteins A1 and A1v, secretion of which increases many-fold after a fatty meal.[49]

The intestinal basolateral membrane possesses a set of amino acid transport systems that differ from those in the brush border membrane. The amino acid transport systems in the basolateral membrane serve to export amino acids from the enterocytes into the portal circulation during feeding. They also participate in importing amino acids into the enterocyte from the portal circulation for cellular metabolism when amino acids are not available from the intestinal lumen, such as between meals. The intestinal basolateral membrane also possesses a peptide transporter system that probably is identical to that in the brush border membrane. This transport system facilitates the exit of hydrolysis-resistant small peptides from the enterocyte into the portal circulation.

Whereas very small amounts of dipeptides have been detected in the portal circulation after a meal, the great majority of absorbed products of protein digestion that reach the circulation are in the form of single amino acids. A somewhat surprising finding is that digestion of protein continues into the ileum, with approximately 40% of ingested protein undergoing transport in this segment of small intestine.[234]

VITAMINS

WATER-SOLUBLE VITAMINS

Although it had been thought that the absorption of water-soluble vitamins was dependent simply on passive diffusion across the intestinal mucosa, recognition of the importance of specific carrier-mediated processes has been increasing (Table 97–11). Furthermore, several of these vitamins are present in the diet as conjugates or coenzymes that require hydrolysis before or during their absorption.

Ascorbic Acid (Vitamin C)

Although most species synthesize all of their vitamin C requirements, primates, guinea pigs, and some birds have lost this capacity and thus are dependent on diet for their needs. Vitamin C is found in a wide range of foods, but the most abundant sources are fresh fruits and fruit juices. Black currants are particularly rich in vitamin C (200 mg/100 g); apples and pears less so (5 mg/100 g). Of animal sources, raw liver contains approximately 20 mg/100 g, and milk, approximately 2 mg/100 g; fresh meat contains only traces of vitamin C. Ingestion of as little ascorbic acid as 10 mg per day prevents scurvy, and

Table 97–11 Water-Soluble Vitamins

Vitamin	Reference Nutrient Intake*	Transport Mechanism
Ascorbic acid	40 mg/day	Active; sodium-dependent process at BBM
Folic acid	200 mg/day	Hydrolysis of dietary polyglutamates by folate conjugase at BBM; sodium-dependent active transport or facilitated diffusion of monoglutamate at BBM
Cobalamin (vitamin B$_{12}$)	1.5 µg/day	Intrinsic factor binding; uptake of intrinsic factor–B$_{12}$ complex at BBM by a specific receptor
Thiamine	1 mg/day	Sodium-dependent active transport; absorption includes hydrolytic and phosphorylation steps
Riboflavin	1.3 mg/day	Absorption includes hydrolytic and phosphorylation steps
Pantothenic acid	3-7 mg/day†	?
Biotin	10-200 µg/day†	?
Pyridoxine	1.5 mg/day	Simple diffusion
Niacin	18 mg/day	?

*Reference nutrient intakes are calculated as 2 SD above the estimated average intake for normal adult men. These amounts provide an adequate intake for nonpregnant adults.
†Nutrient intakes for pantothenic acid and biotin are given as "safe intake" values because insufficient data are available on human needs. These amounts provide a range over which the risk of deficiency or toxicity is absent.
BBM, brush border membrane.

the recommended daily intake is 40 mg.[139] Absorption of ascorbic acid decreases with increased intake and varies from 16% at high (greater than 10 g) to 98% at low (less than 20 mg) intakes. From what is known, 80% to 90% of dietary ascorbic acid is absorbed.

Cooking destroys some of the ascorbic acid contained in food, but destruction can be minimized by shortening cooking times and not keeping foods hot for prolonged periods before they are eaten. Prolonged storage of foods also depletes vitamin C content.

With the loss of the capacity for hepatic synthesis of vitamin C, a specific absorptive mechanism has developed in humans (and guinea pigs). Transport across the apical membrane of small intestinal enterocytes occurs by an active, sodium-dependent process.[235] The active absorption mechanism becomes saturated when the mucosal concentration of vitamin C is greater than 6 mmol/L; this may account for the fact that the proportion of dietary vitamin C absorbed decreases with increasing intake of vitamin C. Electrically neutral, uphill transport of vitamin C probably occurs in the form of sodium ascorbate, through a concentrative, carrier-mediated sodium-dependent mechanism. Two distinct isoforms of these sodium-dependent vitamin C transporters have been described in humans: hSVCT1 and hSVCT2.[236,237] The intestinal ascorbic acid uptake process is regulated by extracellular substrate levels and by an intracellular protein kinase C–mediated pathway.[238] A variable proportion of luminal vitamin C is present in the oxidized form as dehydroascorbic acid, which also is actively absorbed. Within the intestinal cell, dehydroascorbate is rapidly reduced back to ascorbic acid by the reduced glutathione-requiring enzyme dehydroascorbate reductase. It is through this mechanism that the intracellular level of dehydroascorbate is believed to be maintained at low, nontoxic levels.

Folic Acid

Folic (pteroyl monoglutamic) acid consists of the complex pterin molecule conjugated to para-aminobenzoic acid and glutamic acid. Although much dietary folate is in the form of polyglutamates consisting of at least six glutamic acid residues, much is present as formyl- and methylhydrofolate. The folates are distributed widely in the diet, particularly rich sources being spinach (200 mg/100 g), liver (140 mg/100 g), and peanuts and beans (100 mg/100 g). Meat, chicken, potatoes, and fruit (except orange juice) are poor sources of folate (less than 15 mg/100 g). Food preparation, especially prolonged cooking, destroys its value. Recommended dietary intakes are of the order of 200 mg per day in adults and 400 mg per day during pregnancy.[139] The adult body contains only 2 to 3 mg of folate; therefore, in cases of poor intake (or malabsorption of folate) for just a short period, folate depletion occurs relatively rapidly.

Absorption of dietary polyglutamates depends on hydrolysis to monoglutamate at the brush border membrane, followed by transport into the cytoplasm.[239,240] The apical membrane hydrolase (conjugate) in human intestine is expressed predominantly in the proximal jejunum and is a folylpoly-gamma-glutamate carboxypeptidase that cleaves a single glutamic acid residue at a time. This brush border form of folate hydrolase has been cloned and shown to be up-regulated in dietary folate deficiency.[241,242] Also recognized is a cytoplasmic folate hydrolase, an endopeptidase prominent in several species and present in humans; its role in the latter is uncertain.

Uptake is achieved by a specific carrier-mediated, concentrative, sodium-dependent, pH-sensitive process that is active at acid pH.[243] It is inhibited by diphenylhydantoin and sulfasalazine; the latter also depresses hydrolysis. Prolonged exposure to ethanol inhibits hydrolysis (but not uptake), which may be relevant to the folate deficiency sometimes found in alcoholics.

The intestine also is exposed to a second source of folate—the folate that is synthesized by the normal microflora of the large intestine. Significant amounts of folate from this source have been shown to exist in the absorbable monglutamate form. The colon is capable of absorbing some of this folate.[244]

Vitamin B$_{12}$ (Cobalamin)

Cobalamin exists largely as hydroxycobalamin, methyl-cobalamin, and adenosylcobalamin, cobalamin analogs that are found almost entirely in animal sources. Liver, kidney, beef, fish, eggs, and milk provide most of the cobalamin in a normal diet.[49] Vegetables are almost entirely lacking in the vitamin; therefore, the cobalamin intake of strict vegans may be inadequate. Approximately 10 to 20 μg is ingested per day in an average diet, and of this, approximately 1 to 2 μg is required to provide for normal daily needs.[245]

Three types of binding proteins are concerned with the absorption of cobalamin—one in saliva, one in gastric juice, and one in the circulation.[245] The vitamin is released by gastric acid from the various dietary proteins with which it is associated (Fig. 97–18). The first specific binding protein secreted in saliva, the R protein (transcor-rin [TC]), takes up the free cobalamin and binds it with strong affinity in the stomach. At intragastric pH values below 3, intrinsic factor has much weaker affinity for the vitamin than does R protein.[246] It is only in the duodenum, where the R protein is hydrolyzed by pancreatic enzymes, that intrinsic factor is able to bind to the released cobalamin.[247]

In humans, intrinsic factor is secreted from parietal cells in response to the same agonists that stimulate acid secretion—histamine, gastrin, and cholinergic agonists. Unlike R proteins, of which several can bind a wide variety of cobalamin analogs, intrinsic factor is much more selective and specific for cobalamin. It has been suggested that the nonspecificity of binding to the R protein

that exists in plasma may offer an advantage in binding potentially harmful compounds.[248] Intrinsic factor has a very strong affinity for cobalamin and binds it tightly by enclosing the vitamin in its cuplike interior. This complex resists pancreatic proteolysis by undergoing molecular conformational changes and glycosylation, passes down the intestine to the terminal ileum, and there binds to specific receptors (cubilin-amnionless complex) on ileal enterocytes. Distribution of ileal receptors is patchy,[249] and estimates of approximately 300 to 400 receptors per enterocyte, or one per microvillus, located deeply between the microvilli, have been suggested.[250] The number of receptors available determines how much vitamin can be absorbed; absorption doubles during pregnancy by a doubling of the number of available receptors.[251]

After binding to the receptor, the intrinsic factor–cobalamin complex probably enters the cell intact by translocation (see Fig. 97–18). Intracellular events have not been elucidated fully, but B$_{12}$ accumulates in the mitochondria, and the complex is split at some point within the enterocyte. Free cobalamin leaves the base of the cell, where it is immediately bound to an ileal pool of transcobalamin II, which transports it into the portal circulation.

It is clear that this complicated series of events can be interrupted at a number of different points in the pathway. Lack of pancreatic proteolysis would lead to a defect in the release of the vitamin from the R protein for intrinsic factor binding; lack of intrinsic factor would fail to provide the complex necessary for binding and absorption at the ileal mucosa; loss of ileal receptors would

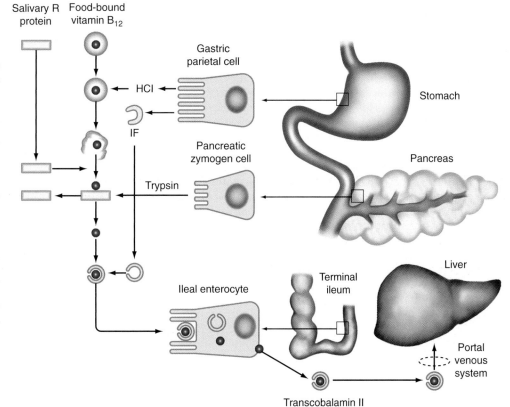

Figure 97–18 Sequence of steps leading to the binding of vitamin B$_{12}$ to intrinsic factor (IF). Food-bound B$_{12}$ is released by gastric acid and pepsin and binds preferentially by salivary R protein in the stomach. Proteolysis of R protein by trypsin releases B$_{12}$ for binding to IF. The subsequent binding and uptake of the IF-B$_{12}$ complex occurs through a specific receptor-mediated process on the brush border membrane of ileal enterocytes. Vitamin B$_{12}$ is released at an intracellular site, transported across the basolateral membrane, and taken up by transcobalamin II for transport to the portal circulation.

Salivary R protein

Food-bound vitamin B$_{12}$

HCl

IF

Gastric parietal cell

Stomach

Pancreatic zymogen cell

Pancreas

Trypsin

Ileal enterocyte

Terminal ileum

Liver

Portal venous system

Transcobalamin II

prevent absorption; and defects within ileal enterocytes may prevent release of the vitamin into the circulation.

Other Water-Soluble Vitamins[49,252]

Thiamine (vitamin B₁) is distributed widely, but the only important dietary sources are seeds of plants. Germs of cereals, nuts, peas, beans, and pulses (legumes) are major sources, whereas green vegetables and fruit are relatively poor ones. White flour or bread and polished (white) rice have virtually no thiamine. Thiamine is water soluble and readily lost in the cooking water. Thiamine occurs almost entirely in phosphorylated form in animal foods but exists in its free form in foods of plant origin and enriched cereal. Dephosphorylation results from the action of phosphatases, present in the intestinal lumen, before absorption. The rate of thiamine absorption approaches a limit as the dosage increases. Absorption can be active or passive, depending upon concentration of the vitamin. Thiamine absorption is greatest in the jejunum and ileum, regardless of whether absorption is active or passive. With low intraluminal concentrations, thiamine is absorbed by a sodium-independent active process, and two human thiamine transporters, SLC19A2 and SLC19A3, have been cloned.[253-256] At high concentrations (greater than 8 mg in a single dose) thiamine is absorbed by passive diffusion.[257] Thiamine is then phosphorylated in the enterocyte after absorption and is transported out of the cell, possibly by the basal membrane Na⁺,K⁺-ATPase. This exit step is inhibited by ethanol.

Niacin (nicotinic acid) and nicotinamide are distributed widely in foods, but their availability in foods varies. About half of the North American and European dietary intake of niacin is supplied in meat and fish. The niacin content of legumes, however, is largely bound and unavailable, although it can be released by treatment with alkali; food preparation methods widely employed in Asia and Africa, such as for maize, do not render the niacin available. Nicotinic acid can be synthesized in humans from tryptophan, 60 mg of the latter being required for the synthesis of 1 mg of niacin. The concept of the "nicotinic acid equivalent" thus has arisen, and foods lacking in niacin may remain valuable in preventing pellagra because of high tryptophan content; such is the case with milk and eggs.

Both nicotinic acid and nicotinamide are absorbed rapidly from the stomach and the small intestine. At low concentrations, absorption occurs through sodium-dependent facilitated diffusion, but at higher concentrations, passive diffusion predominates. Niacin occurs mostly in its coenzyme forms, which are hydrolyzed in the intestinal lumen by pyrophosphatase to nicotinamide; nicotinamide is absorbed as such, without further hydrolysis in the gastrointestinal tract.

Riboflavin (vitamin B₂) is linked with phosphoric acid in most animal and plant tissues to form flavin mononucleotide, and with adenosine monophosphate (AMP) to form flavinadenine dinucleotide. The richest dietary sources of riboflavin are liver, eggs, milk, green vegetables, and beer. It also is synthesized by colonic bacteria, but its availability from the colon is uncertain. Cooking does not destroy much riboflavin, but exposure to sunlight may. Riboflavin is presented to the mucosa in the form of coenzymes, so these must be hydrolyzed at the brush border membrane before active transport into the cell occurs. Studies suggest that riboflavin uptake occurs mainly in the proximal portion of the small intestine and involves a specialized sodium-independent carrier mediated system. This system is regulated by extracellular substrate levels and by a specific intracellular protein kinase–mediated pathway.[258,259] Once within the cell, rephosphorylation occurs.

Biotin is so widely available that spontaneous deficiency states in humans have been described only rarely. Many yeasts and bacteria contain biotin and may provide a sufficient supply in normal foods. Liver, legumes, nuts, and vegetables also are reasonable sources. Little is known about the mechanism of absorption of biotin in humans. Animal studies have indicated that most absorption of the free vitamin occurs in the jejunum and upper ileum by two mechanisms: a saturable facilitated diffusion process that operates at low concentrations and a nonsaturable linear diffusion process operating at higher luminal concentrations of the vitamin.

Further studies have shown that the intestinal biotin transport system also is utilized by two unrelated micronutrients: namely, the water-soluble vitamin pantothenic acid and the metabolically important substrate lipoate. For these reasons, the biotin transport system is now referred to as the sodium-dependent multivitamin transporter (SMVT).[260] It is unclear how cells regulate transport of the individual vitamin by means of this common transport system and how the substrate level of the individual substrate affects SMVT function in these cells.

Pantothenic acid usually is found as its calcium salt and is derived largely from animal tissues, especially liver, kidney, and egg yolk, and from wheat germ and peanuts. It is almost completely lacking in many processed foods but is not lost in normal cooking. The intestine also is exposed to bacterial sources of pantothenic acid. In the diet, pantothenic acid exists mainly in the form of CoA, which is hydrolyzed to free pantothenic acid in the intestinal lumen before absorption. Transport of free pantothenic acid then occurs into the absorptive cells through the SMVT.[260]

Pyridoxine occurs in the diet in one of three forms: pyridoxamine phosphate, pyridoxal phosphate, and pyridoxine phosphate. Its presence is widespread in plant and animal tissues; cereals, peanuts, bananas, and liver are good sources. The phosphorylated form must be dephosphorylated before absorption can occur. The latter is achieved by means of a membrane-bound alkaline phosphatase, found in the intestinal brush border. All three forms of pyridoxine are freely absorbed by passive diffusion in the jejunum and ileum.

FAT-SOLUBLE VITAMINS

Vitamins A, D, E, and K are structurally different from each other, but all can be classified as polar, nonswelling, insoluble lipids. Although their chemical structures are known, the retention of a letter to signify their individuality is valuable, because each consists of a number of closely related compounds with similar properties[49] (Table 97–12).

Vitamin A

Vitamin A (retinol) is found in the diet in milk and milk products, egg yolk, and fish oils. Carotenoids are defined by their chemical structure: the hydrocarbon carotenoids are known as carotenes, and the oxygenated derivatives of these hydrocarbons are referred to as xanthophylls. Beta-carotene, the principal carotenoid in carrots, consists of two conjoined molecules of retinol and is a precursor of the active vitamin (Fig. 97–19).

Many other dietary carotenoids are recognized, but they contain only one retinol molecule. The carotenoids are found predominantly in green vegetables and carrots, and in the United States and Europe, these sources account for approximately half the dietary intake. Retinol and the carotenes are stable with normal cooking. Lycopene is the carotenoid that gives tomatoes and other red fruits and vegetables their color. Although it is similar in structure to carotene, lycopene lacks a beta-ionone ring structure and thus cannot form vitamin A or retinol. Its biologic effects in humans have been attributed to mechanisms other than those for vitamin A.

Both retinol and carotene are absorbed in the small bowel, carotene less readily than retinol.[261,262] Dietary retinal (vitamin A aldehyde) esters first are hydrolyzed to retinol in the intestinal lumen before being absorbed into the intestinal mucosa. Carotenes, by contrast, are converted into retinol, primarily in the enterocytes. Before entering the mucosal layer of the intestine, however, carotenes first are solubilized into micellar solution, along with other fat-soluble compounds. Hence, bile salts and dietary fats are need for the absorption of carotenes in the upper small intestine. The biosynthetic process for converting carotene to retinol in the enterocyte involves two soluble cytosolic enzymes. The first enzyme is responsible for the oxidative split of the beta-carotene molecule to produce the cleavage product of retinal (vitamin A aldehyde), which is then reduced to retinol by a second and reduced nicotinamide-adenine dinucleotide (NADH)-dependent enzyme. Transport across the apical membrane appears to occur by passive diffusion, but facilitated diffusion cannot be excluded. Free retinol (from retinyl ester and carotenes) in the mucosal cells is re-esterified, mainly with palmitic acid, before being incorporated into chylomicrons, which is how vitamin A mostly leaves the mucosa.

Vitamin D

Vitamin D comprises a group of sterols that have antirachitic properties, but the only two nutritionally important members are vitamins D_2 (ergocalciferol) and D_3 (cholecalciferol). Both are produced by ultraviolet irradiation of their precursor sterols, ergosterol and 7-dehydrocholesterol, respectively (see Fig. 97–16). Ergosterol, found in fungi and yeasts, is an unusual constituent of the normal diet, whereas vitamin D_3 is the major dietary form. Vitamin D_3 is found in a restricted range of foods, predominantly the oils of fatty fish, which themselves ingest it in plankton found near the surface of the sea.[49] Human breast milk contains sufficient vitamin D to prevent rickets, but cow's milk is a poor source of this vitamin. Most of a person's requirement for vitamin D, however, is supplied by endogenous synthesis in the skin during exposure to sunlight, and dietary intake becomes critical only when such exposure is inadequate (see Table 97–12).

As with vitamin A, vitamin D absorption occurs by simple passive diffusion in the small intestine.[263] Bile salts are unnecessary, but luminal pH influences absorption. Absorption is reduced at neutral pH and increased in acid.[264] Most absorbed vitamin D passes into the lymphatics unchanged in chylomicrons.

Vitamin E

Vitamin E is still seeking a role in humans. It comprises a group of eight or so tocopherols, the most potent of which in animals is α-tocopherol[106] (see Fig. 97–19). It is distributed widely in the diet; vegetable oils, cereals, eggs, and fruit are good sources. Margarines are particularly rich in vitamin E, and breast milk contains much more vitamin E than that found in cow's milk. Although a variety of diseases can result from deficiency of vitamin E in multiple species of animals, it has proved difficult to ascribe a human disease to E deficiency.

Vitamin E is absorbed passively across the intestinal mucosa.[265] The ester form, in which many vitamin preparations are presented, is hydrolyzed by pancreatic or duodenal esterases, before absorption, but the ester can be absorbed intact.[266] Vitamin E is transported into the lymphatics largely unchanged.

Vitamin K

Vitamin K is found in two forms: K_1, derived largely from plants, is phytomenadione; K_2 comprises a group of bacteria-produced compounds, the multiprenyl menaquinones. K_1, the major dietary form, is found in green vegetables, but beef liver is another good source. K_2 is produced by colonic bacteria, and although some K_2 may

Table 97–12 Fat-Soluble Vitamin Absorptive Mechanisms

Vitamin	Reference Nutrient Intake*	Mechanism of Absorption
Vitamin A (retinol)	700 µg/day	Passive diffusion
Vitamin D (cholecalciferol)	10 µg/day[†]	Passive diffusion
Vitamin E (α-tocopherol)	>4 mg/day[‡]	Passive diffusion
Vitamin K	1 µg/kg/day[‡]	
Phytomenadione (K_1)		Carrier-mediated uptake[267]
Menaquinones (K_2)		Passive diffusion

*Reference nutrient intakes are calculated as 2 SD above the average intake in normal men.
[†]Normal adults with normal exposure to sunlight require no dietary intake of vitamin D.
[‡]Figures for vitamins E and K are "safe intake" values that provide adequate amounts for normal nutrition. Excessive intake of vitamins A and D produces toxic effects, and the listed values are safe in normal men, but not necessarily in infants.

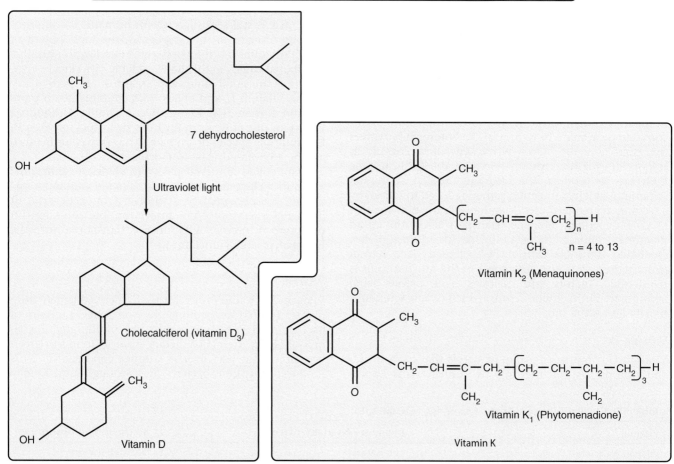

Figure 97–19   Structural formulas of the fat-soluble vitamins A, D, E, and K.

be absorbed from the colon, this absorption alone is an inadequate source if K_1 absorption is impaired. Absorption of K_1 from the small intestine is dependent on luminal bile salts, and uptake is achieved by a carrier-mediated process[267]; K_2 absorption is entirely passive.[268]

MINERALS

Various divalent ions are essential nutrients; some are absorbed in milligram amounts and are major constituents of the body, whereas others are necessary only in trace amounts. Iron, calcium, magnesium, phosphorus, and sulfur are in the former category, and specialized absorptive mechanisms are concerned with their assimilation.

CALCIUM

Milk and cheese are the most valuable sources of calcium, although cereals, legumes, and other vegetables contain significant amounts of calcium. Phytate or oxalate in vegetables binds strongly to calcium, thereby reducing its availability. Dietary fiber also binds calcium and may interfere with its absorption. By contrast, dietary lactose enhances its absorption.[269] Fractional, or true, absorption of calcium accounts for 20% to 30% of total dietary calcium; the remainder is excreted in stool.

Absorption across the intestinal mucosa is achieved by two parallel processes: an active, transcellular transport process and a passive, paracellular diffusive process.[270-272] Under normal dietary conditions, the duodenum is the major site for active transport, whereas passive, paracellular transfer occurs throughout the small intestine. Quantitatively, more calcium may be absorbed in the jejunum and ileum than in the duodenum because of the relative amounts of time luminal contents spend in these regions of the intestine. The human jejunum absorbs calcium faster than the ileum, and absorption rates in both sites are increased by vitamin D treatment.[273]

The paracellular route, through the tight junctions, may be capable of modifying calcium transport, because passive transport increases in response to treatment with vitamin D.[274] Furthermore, evidence suggests that tight junction permeability increases during sugar transport, and this may provide another mechanism for control of paracellular transport.[275]

The transcellular route involves transport across the apical membrane, transfer across the cytoplasm, and exit across the basolateral membrane (Fig. 97-20). Entry probably occurs through specific calcium channels in the apical membrane and down the prevailing electrochemical gradient. Within the cytoplasm, binding to calbindin, a calcium-binding protein, is a key step.[276] Maximal transport rates correlate closely with calbindin concentrations. This protein, present in concentrations of 0.1 to 0.2 mM, must rapidly take up the calcium entering the cell, because intracellular free calcium concentrations are carefully maintained at very low values (approximately 10^{-7} M). Transient rises in intracellular calcium act as key second messenger signals for secretory responses in enterocytes. Absorbed calcium presumably

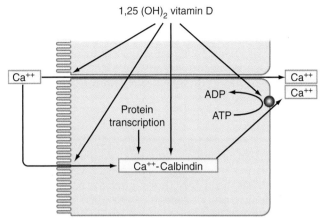

Figure 97-20   Mechanisms of calcium transport across the intestinal epithelium. A paracellular route allows bidirectional flux, although only absorption is shown here. Transport into the epithelial cell occurs through specific channels down an electrochemical gradient. A critical step is the binding to calbindin, which then presents calcium for export by means of a calcium-dependent ATPase on the basolateral membrane. Each of these processes appears to be influenced by 1,25-dihydroxyvitamin D_3, although the greatest effect of vitamin D is on the synthesis of calbindin.

is thereby segregated from the calcium concerned with cell signaling, and calbindin plays a vital role by bringing calcium to the transporter at the basolateral membrane.[277] A calcium-dependent ATPase then is responsible to actively drive calcium uphill against the electrochemical gradient.[276] Calcium arrives at the basolateral pole bound to a site at the cytoplasmic aspect of the calcium-dependent ATPase that spans the basolateral membrane, after which a phosphorylation-induced change occurs in the conformation of the calcium-dependent ATPase, and the calcium ion is extruded through the channel formed by the enzyme transmembrane elements.[278]

The rate-limiting step in the absorption process of calcium is the intracellular calbindin concentration. Calbindin concentrations are regulated by a metabolite of vitamin D, 1,25-dihydroxyvitamin D_3 (1,25[OH]$_2$D$_3$), produced in the kidneys from 25-hydroxyvitamin D (25[OH]D); the latter is converted from absorbed vitamin D by the liver.[271] Vitamin D also has a modest effect on the calcium entry step and enhances activity of the basolateral calcium ATPase. Up-regulation of the calbindin gene in response to vitamin D occurs largely in villus cells.[279]

Some evidence supports colonic absorption of calcium, which also can be enhanced by vitamin D.[280] The presence of the colon has advantages for calcium absorption in patients with short bowel syndrome.[281]

Active duodenal calcium absorption is increased in calcium deficiency states and reduced in calcium repletion states. Increased production of the active 1,25(OH)$_2$D metabolite in response to a small drop in plasma calcium concentration is responsible for increasing calcium absorption, and this change occurs within 1 day of changing from a high-calcium to a low-calcium diet.[282] This same mechanism is likely to be the cause of the enhanced calcium absorption seen during late pregnancy and lactation.

At birth, the active, vitamin D–dependent, absorptive mechanisms are present in the human duodenum. Ingestion of large amounts of calcium, together with lactose, in breast milk ensures adequate intake at this critical stage of life. Calcium absorption declines with age, but this may result in part from a lack of vitamin D.[269]

MAGNESIUM

An average diet provides approximately 300 to 500 mg of magnesium per day in a wide range of vegetables. Its absorption has been less thoroughly investigated than that of calcium, but it seems likely that the mechanisms involved are different. In contrast with calcium absorption, magnesium absorption in the basal state is greater in the human ileum than in the jejunum.[273] Jejunal absorption is increased by vitamin D, whereas ileal absorption is not. Ileal transport involves both a paracellular, diffusive pathway and a transcellular, carrier-mediated, saturable process.[283] Some competition from calcium has been observed for the diffusive pathway but not for the saturable, presumably carrier-mediated process.[283] Quantitatively, magnesium fluxes across ileal mucosa are several-fold greater than those for calcium.

IRON

Meat-eating, affluent societies ingest approximately 20 to 30 mg of iron per day, largely as myoglobin or hemoglobin. Vegetarian societies in less affluent countries ingest much less than this, in wheat and vegetables; moreover, iron in these foods is less readily available for absorption. A careful balance of absorption and loss is maintained in normal adults: Both inputs and losses are approximately 1 mg per day. Developing children and adolescents need to absorb approximately 0.5 mg or more daily, to build up total body iron to adult values. Iron is present in breast milk in the form of lactoferrin, for which a specific brush border membrane receptor has been demonstrated.[284,285] This facilitates absorption of iron in neonates. During reproductive life, females need to compensate for menstrual losses, which are of the order of 5 to 50 mg per month and approximately 500 mg for each pregnancy.

Because dietary intake often markedly exceeds the body's need for iron, it is necessary to absorb only a small portion of that ingested. Overall, a positive and linear relationship has been demonstrated between the *amount* ingested and that absorbed, but the *proportion* absorbed decreases as more is taken in.[286]

Total body iron content is regulated by controlling the level of absorption from the diet. Under normal circumstances, only approximately 10% (1 to 2 mg per day) of dietary iron is absorbed. Most absorption occurs in the proximal small intestine, and the ferrous (Fe^{2+}) form is absorbed better than the ferric (Fe^{3+}) form. The latter is insoluble at pH values above 3, and gastric acid and some sugars and amino acids render it more available for absorption. The presence of some anions, such as oxalate, phosphate, and phytate, precipitate iron out of solution and reduce its absorption. The presence of bile enhances

absorption, but the mechanism of this enhancement is unclear.

Dietary iron is found predominantly in the ferric form, but Fe^{3+} is highly insoluble under physiologic conditions. Therefore, during uptake, ferric iron (Fe^{3+}) is converted to the ferrous (Fe^{2+}) form at the apical membrane before it attaches to an acceptor protein in the membrane. The ability of intestinal mucosa to reduce Fe^{3+} to Fe^{2+} has been documented,[287] and a ferrireductase activity has been characterized for intestinal Caco-2 and HuTu-80 cell lines.[287,288] A functional role for Fe^{3+} reduction in iron transport across the brush border is implicated by the fact that inhibition of ferrireductase activity reduces Caco-2 cell apical iron uptake. Furthermore, increased ferrireductase activity correlates with enhanced iron uptake induced by iron deficiency and hypoxia.[288,289]

Iron uptake into the body occurs at two interfaces of the intestinal epithelium: the apical and the basolateral plasma membranes.[290] The apical plasma membrane of the differentiated enterocyte is specialized for transport of heme and ferrous iron into the cell. Three major pathways of iron transport across the apical membrane have been proposed. The best-characterized pathway is through the divalent metal transporter 1 (DMT1; also known as Nramp2 or DCT1).[291] Two splice variants of DMT1 yield two mRNAs—one containing an iron-responsive element (IRE) termed DMT1 (IRE) mRNA and another without an IRE designated DMT1 (non-IRE) mRNA. DMT1 is a proton symporter that transports ferrous iron and other divalent metals from the intestinal lumen into the enterocyte (Fig. 97–21).

In order of substrate preference, DMT1 can mediate import of Fe^{2+}, Zn^{2+}, Mn^{2+}, Co^{2+}, Cd^{2+}, Cu^{2+}, Ni^{2+}, and Pb^{2+}. The idea that the transporter responsible for dietary iron absorption recognizes other divalent cations agrees well with observations that Zn^{2+}, Mn^{2+}, Cd^{2+} and Cu^{2+} all can inhibit iron absorption. DMT1 mRNA is found in many different tissues, but the protein and its mRNA are most abundant in the proximal duodenum, with decreasing

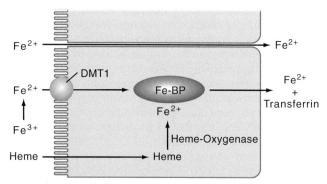

Fe-BP = Iron bonding proteins

Figure 97–21 Mechanisms of iron transport in the intestine. A small amount of inorganic iron may pass through the paracellular route. Inorganic iron is converted into its ferrous form (Fe^{2+}) at the brush border membrane before transport into the cell. Heme iron is transported into the cell by a separate mechanism. Within the cell, one or more iron-binding proteins (Fe-BP) take up iron and transfer it to the basolateral membrane for delivery across the membrane and subsequent binding to transferrin. DMT1, divalent metal transporter 1.

absorption along the distal axis, localizations that are consistent with a function in intestinal iron absorption.[292] Furthermore, iron depletion results in increased DMT1 mRNA levels in the intestine, which suggests that iron-responsive elements (IREs) in its 3' untranslated region bind and stabilize the DMT1 mRNA.[292] Although the major route for dietary iron absorption likely is to be mediated by DMT1, this transporter is found only in the apical surface of enterocytes. Thus, other factors must be involved in the transfer across the intestinal epithelium.

DMT-1 may be involved in the pathogenesis of hereditary hemochromatosis (HH). *HFE* is the gene responsible for HH. HFE protein is found in the crypt cells of the duodenum associated with β_2-microgobulin and transferrin receptor. It is hypothesized that HFE protein may facilitate transferring receptor-dependent iron uptake into crypt cells and that mutant HFE protein may lose this ability, leading to a "relative" iron deficiency in duodenal crypt cells. In turn, this may lead to an increase in the expression of DMT-1, resulting in increased iron absorption in HH. Up-regulation of DMT-1 expression has been confirmed in the HFE-knockout mouse and in humans with HH[293] (see Chapter 71).

Iron also can be absorbed in the form of heme iron (in hemoglobin and myoglobin), which is transported readily across the brush border of the enterocytes as an intact heme moiety. Once within the cell, heme is broken down by heme oxygenase and the iron is released. The molecular mechanisms of heme iron transport have not been established.[294,295]

Another iron-absorptive pathway has been proposed involving intestinal mucins, a 56-kd protein designated mobilferrin, an integrin, and a ferric reductase. This pathway is regulated and dependent on metabolic energy and appears to be encouraged by nonessential fatty acids.[288,296,297] A small proportion of the iron crossing the mucosa utilizes a paracellular route by simple diffusion (see Fig. 97–21).

Iron transport across the basolateral plasma membrane of villus enterocytes involves at least two proteins: a basolateral iron transporter termed ferroportin 1 (or iron-regulated protein 1 or metal transport protein 1) and a ferroxidase called hephaestin. These proteins may work in close conjunction with each other, ferroportin 1 transporting ferrous iron out of the cell and hephaestin oxidizing the ferrous iron to ferric iron, which binds avidly to circulating transferrin.[290]

Intestinal iron absorption is regulated in at least three ways. The long-standing concept of "mucosal block" is based on the observation that after a large oral dose of iron, enterocytes do not absorb additional iron for several days. A second regulatory mechanism of iron absorption is termed the "stores regulator." It acts on a pathway that facilitates a slow accumulation of nonheme dietary iron. The functioning of the stores regulator is of great physiologic importance, because it prevents iron overload after ensuring iron needs are met. The exact molecular mechanism of the stores regulator has not been established. It has been proposed to involve soluble factors such as transferrin-bound iron, serum ferritin, serum transferrin, and hepcidin. The erythropoietic regulator is a third regulatory mechanism that adjusts intestinal iron absorption in response to the demands of erythropoiesis, independent of body iron stores. This regulator must signal directly between the hematopoietic bone marrow and the duodenum. Although the erythropoietic regulator has been proposed to be a soluble component of plasma, it is distinct from the stores regulator, as evidenced by the rate of iron uptake in anemic persons, which is much greater (20 to 40 mg per day) than could be produced by the stores regulator alone.

The stores and erythropoietic regulators are circulating factors that maintain iron homeostasis for the entire organism. Within individual cells, the iron regulatory proteins (IRPs) IRP-1 and IRP-2 act to control iron availability by translational control of the synthesis of proteins such as transferrin and ferritin. IRPs are cytoplasmic RNA-binding proteins that function on mRNAs that contain IREs. Functional IREs are present in the 3'-untranslated region of mRNAs for transferring, in 1 of the 2 isoforms of DMT1 (DMT1 IRE), and in the 5'-untranslated region of mRNAs for ferritin, ferroportin 1, mitochondrial aconitase, and the erythroid-specific form of δ-aminolevulinic acid synthase. IRPs functionally connect intracellular iron availability with cellular iron utilization, and IRP function can also be altered by inflammation and oxidative stress.

Basolateral iron uptake from the plasma by cryptal enterocytes plays an important role in sensing body iron stores. Indeed, considerable evidence indicates that the iron concentration within the cryptal enterocyte is an important determinant of iron absorption. The mechanism by which the intracellular iron concentration may respond to body iron needs is poorly understood. What is clear is that cells in the crypts of Lieberkühn always express transferrin, and the endocytic mechanism imparts information about body iron storage based on plasma transferrin saturation. It also is well recognized that acute changes in body iron status, whether overload or deficiency, are not reflected by changes in iron absorption for a period of 2 to 3 days. This lag response time probably correlates with the migration time for proliferating cells in the crypts to differentiate and migrate into functional, mature enterocytes of villi. Thus, the luminal epithelial cells may be pre-programmed in the crypts in accordance with body iron needs. This pre-programming would, in turn, initiate synthesis of iron transport proteins that are required for dietary iron uptake across the membranes of the villus enterocyte.

TRACE ELEMENTS

The importance of zinc, copper, and iodine in human nutrition has long been recognized, and they have received increasing attention in recent years as their roles in defined enteral and parenteral forms of nutrition have been demonstrated. The value of selenium also has been emphasized, and the need for manganese and chromium is receiving attention. Despite initial observations regarding these interesting trace elements, surprisingly few systematic studies of their absorption have been undertaken.

Zinc is present in the body in approximately half the amount of iron (approximately 2 g), and largely in a wide variety of enzymes. It also plays important roles in maintaining configuration of gene transcription proteins and the integrity of membranes. It is found particularly in meat, shellfish, cereals, and legumes. Daily requirements are approximately 12 to 15 mg per day in adults. Persons who consume a low-energy diet may take in marginal amounts of zinc; requirements are increased during pregnancy and lactation. Absorption is impaired by phytic acid, phytates, and oxalates in the diet, and food processing may render it less available for absorption.[49,298]

Enterohepatic circulation of zinc is recognized, and reabsorption appears to be maximal in the distal small intestine.[299] Studies with vesicles of jejunal brush border membranes of pigs have identified two uptake processes: a saturable, carrier-mediated process and a nonsaturable, diffusive process[300]; the relative importance of each is not known. The recently characterized zinc transporters (ZnTs)[3] have increased our understanding of the interrelationships of cellular zinc uptake and efflux but do not yet account for observations at the whole-body level.[301,302] ZnT-1 is a ubiquitously expressed protein that has been found to be present in the villi of the proximal small bowel. Expression of ZnT-1 in rats was increased in response to zinc supplementation but not to zinc restriction.[303] These and other observations have led to the current consensus that ZnT-1 functions mainly as a zinc exporter and may play a role in zinc homeostasis as a mechanism for zinc acquisition and elimination under conditions of excess zinc.[301]

The role of metallothionein (MT), an intracellular metal-binding protein, in the regulation of zinc absorption, particularly in conjunction with zinc transporters, also remains unclear. This binding protein may be concerned with absorption of zinc, because changing dietary loads of zinc rapidly affect protein synthesis and zinc-binding capacity.[304] Persons on a low-zinc diet respond by decreasing their urinary excretion rate of zinc and by increasing its absorption rate.[299,305] Absorption increases in pregnancy and during lactation.[306]

In experiments with knockout and transgenic mice, the rise in serum zinc after a single dose of zinc was much greater than in the control animals. By contrast, the serum zinc response of the MT-transgenic animals was blunted compared with that of the control animals. The expression of ZnT-1 is directly related to serum zinc levels but is unaffected by MT levels.[307] Thus, MT may function in cellular responses to limit free zinc concentrations within narrow ranges and function as a zinc pool.[301,307] Another transporter potentially involved in zinc and other metal uptake is DMT1, a transmembrane polypeptide that is found in the crypts and lower villi of the duodenal epithelium and may be available for the uptake of several metal ions.[302]

Copper is found in green vegetables and fish, and the average Western diet provides 1 to 3 mg per day, which is adequate for a daily requirement of approximately 1 mg per day. Dietary copper is absorbed from the stomach and small intestine. Although the precise mechanisms involved in copper absorption remain incomplete, within physiologic ranges of intake, absorption probably is by active transport. Competition between copper and zinc for absorption may be demonstrable with large doses of copper but not with normal dietary intakes.[308] Absorption of copper may increase in pregnancy.[309]

In humans, one candidate copper transport protein has been identified and termed hCtr1. A human complementary DNA (cDNA) encoding this putative high-affinity protein copper transport protein was isolated by complementation of yeast cells that are defective in copper transport because of inactivation of both the *CTR1* and *CTR3* genes.[310] Human Ctr1 is a 190-amino-acid protein with three transmembrane domains, and significant homology to yeast Ctr1 and Ctr3, suggesting that mammalian high-affinity copper transporters may have evolved from both Ctr1 and Ctr3. RNA blotting analysis has demonstrated that that hCtr1 is expressed in all organs and tissues examined, with liver, heart, and pancreas exhibiting the highest levels of expression; intermediate levels of expression were found in the intestine, and expression in the brain and muscle was low. Whether hCtr1 plays an important role in copper uptake into intestinal mucosal cells has yet to be firmly established.[311] Two putative low-affinity mammalian copper transporters, hCtr2 and Nramp2, also have been identified. It is unclear what role hCtr2 plays in copper homeostasis, because its mRNA levels are highest in the placenta and very low in liver, intestine, and colon.[310,311] The Nramp2 protein also has been identified as a proton-coupled metal ion transporter that transports a broad range of metal ions.[292]

Acting as a permease or by endocytosis, Ctr1 delivers Cu^{2+} within cells. The mechanism for copper ion reduction before uptake remains unknown. If uncontrolled, this pool of cuprous ions could lead to reactive oxygen species generation, however, very few, if any, free copper ions exist in the cytoplasm. The deliver of copper to target cuproenzymes depends on an elegant metallochaperone system. Several cytoplasmic chaperones have been described: Atox1, CCS (*c*opper *c*haperone for *Cu*²⁺), Zn superoxide dismutase, and Cox 17, as well as membrane-associated copper-transporting ATPases (ATP7A and ATP7B).[312] MNK is a P-type ATPase defective in patients with Menkes disease, in which copper accumulates in intestinal cells.[313]

Once entering the plasma, copper is bound with albumin and histidine in the portal blood and rapidly deposited in the liver, where hCtr1 may play a role in this process. Ceruloplasmin, a major copper-containing protein in plasma, is synthesized in the liver. The incorporation of copper into ceruloplasmin and the excretion of copper into bile are mediated by the Wilson disease gene (*ATP7B*), which is similar to the gene for Menkes disease (*ATP7A*). When the Wilson disease gene is defective, copper accumulates in the liver (see Chapter 72).

Iodine is present in variable amounts in a wide range of foods, depending on the soil content where animals were reared and the vegetation grown. Seafoods are particularly rich in iodine. Iodine is absorbed largely as inorganic iodide, but some iodine also is transported as amino acid complexes.[314]

Selenium is found mainly in association with amino acids, and approximately 60% of dietary selenium is absorbed. Selenium deficiency states have been reported from China (Keshan disease), where very little selenium is present in soil and water,[315] but not in New Zealand, where intake is equally sparse.[316] Absorption of selenium occurs rapidly when it is associated with amino acids, as in selenomethionine, probably by active transport mechanisms operative for the amino acid.[317] Inorganic selenium is absorbed more slowly, possibly by simple diffusion.

The mechanisms underlying the absorption of other trace elements, including manganese and chromium, are largely unknown.[314] Trace element deficiencies are rare in normal persons, even in those with poor protein and calorie intake. Exceptions occur when local geographic availability is suboptimal, as may occur with iodine, and possibly with selenium.

ADAPTATION TO CHANGES IN NEED OR LOAD

One of the most fascinating aspects of intestinal function, observed for more than 30 years, is the phenomenon of adaptation. Two specific forms of intestinal adaptation have been identified in the intestine: (1) mucosal hypertrophy[6] leading to a global increase in absorption of all nutrients and (2) an increase in specific transport mechanisms induced in response to specific dietary needs or availability.[318]

MUCOSAL HYPERTROPHY

Resection of greater than 50% of the human intestine results in increased fecal nitrogen losses, which slowly return toward normal, thus implying that mucosal adaptation has occurred. Normalization is explained largely by hypertrophy of intestinal mucosa, which manifests by increases in the number of villus enterocytes and in villus height without obvious increase in the absorption rate per individual cell.[153] Absorption increases for all nutrients, and absorptive capacity may be enhanced up to five-fold in response to intestinal resection. Jejunal adaptation following ileal resection appears to be less efficient than ileal adaptation in response to jejunal resection.

Although hypertrophy occurring in response to intestinal resection is the best-characterized example of adaptation, other causes also have been discerned, at least in experimental animals. Thus, during lactation and pregnancy,[319] in diabetes,[320] and in the physiologic response to extreme cold,[321] hypertrophy is evident, but this may be a result, at least in part, to the hyperphagia that accompanies these conditions.

The mechanisms by which hypertrophy occurs have been the subject of much study (Fig. 97–22). Signals of adaptation may relate to levels of various hormones, transcription factors, ATP, or changes in the concentration of luminal solutes.[322] The signals and mechanisms of the adaptive process may be different for the jejunum and the ileum, as well as in the crypt and at the villus tip, thus explaining the site-specific alterations and differences between crypt and villus enterocytes.[322,323] Luminal nutrition[6] and pancreaticobiliary secretions[324] are major stimuli to growth. Certain peptide hormones also have been implicated, particularly enteroglucagon and glucagon-like peptides.[325] Gastrin and CCK display trophic effects on the gastrointestinal tract,[326] but more recently, other trophic factors have been identified.[327,328] It is uncertain whether these trophic factors act as local paracrine mediators or as circulating hormones.

Polyamines are other important local mediators of mucosal hypertrophy,[329] because epithelial production of polyamines follows intestinal resection, and inhibiting their synthesis prevents the hypertrophy usually associated with resection. Polyamines also may play a role in the maintenance of normal mucosal structure, because their mucosal level in the intestines of experimental animals decreases rapidly in response to a 24-hour fast and increases within a few hours of refeeding.[330] Although certain prostaglandins have been shown to enhance cell proliferation in the stomach and intestine, their role in adaptation is uncertain at present.[331]

SPECIFIC REVERSIBLE ADAPTATION

Pancreatic Enzyme Secretion

That the digestive capacity of pancreatic juice can be altered by changes in nutritional intake has long been known, but it is now clear that rather specific responses

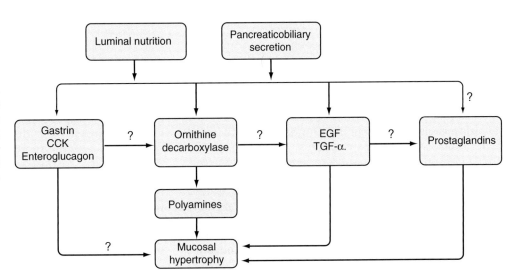

Figure 97–22 Intestinal adaptation. Interrelationships of the major factors concerned with inducing mucosal hypertrophy, as may follow intestinal resection. CCK, cholecystokinin; EGF, epidermal growth factor; TGF-α, transforming growth factor-α.

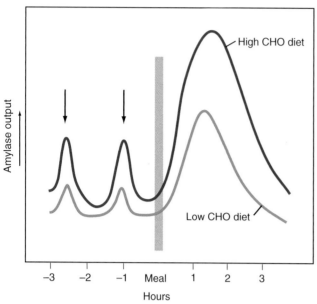

Figure 97–23 Pancreatic enzyme adaptation to dietary manipulation. Diagram of typical pancreatic amylase outputs in normal subjects fed either a high- or a low-carbohydrate (CHO) diet for 2 weeks. Greater amylase secretion rates occur, both during the interdigestive phasic periods (↓) and in response to a standard meal, in subjects given a high-carbohydrate diet.

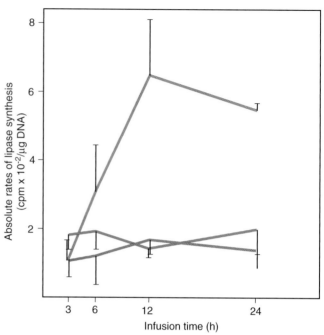

Figure 97–24 Pancreatic enzyme responses to prolonged hormone infusion in rats. The lipase synthesis rate rose in response to secretin (16 units/kg/hour) (*orange line*), but not to cerulein (0.25 µg/kg/hour) (*blue line*) or saline (*purple line*) infused for up to 24 hours. (From Rausch U: Synthesis of lipase in the rat pancreas is regulated by secretin. Pancreas 1:522, 1986.)

occur after different types of dietary manipulation.[332] A high-protein diet enhances proteolytic enzyme production; a high-carbohydrate diet enhances amylase secretion; and a high-fat diet stimulates lipase secretion (Fig. 97–23). In part, these changes appear to depend on specific polypeptide hormone release. Prolonged administration of cerulein (an analog of CCK) stimulates trypsinogen and inhibits amylase secretion,[332] whereas secretin stimulates lipase secretion[333] (Fig. 97–24). Insulin released from pancreatic beta cells, in response to carbohydrate ingestion, appears to be involved indirectly in enhancing amylase secretion.[332] A high-fat diet also induces increased capacity to secrete gastric lipase, but the mechanisms involved are not known.[334]

The underlying molecular biologic events that lead to pancreatic adaptation have been studied, and as might be expected, responses depend on the period over which a dietary stimulus is applied. Responses to short-term stimulation, as after a single meal, appear to depend on enhanced translation of mRNAs for enzymes.[332] Protein synthesis increases within the first 2 hours of hormonal stimulation and appears to be due entirely to translational events; however, more prolonged stimulation—over several days—increases mRNA production by increased transcription, leading to enhanced biochemical commitment to enzyme secretion.[335] A single stimulus after a prolonged period of high protein intake, therefore, results in much greater proteolytic enzyme output than it does in persons whose protein intake is low. The polypeptide hormones secretin, CCK, and possibly insulin, liberated in response to a meal, not only cause immediate release of pancreatic enzymes but also stimulate gene expression over the longer term and thus increase secretory capacity.

Mucosal Responses

Adaptive responses to changes in dietary intake influence mucosal digestive and absorptive processes. Activity of the disaccharidase enzymes sucrase and maltase increases in response to high carbohydrate intake over several days, but not to manipulation of protein intake.[336] Sucrase levels increase first in crypt cells, about 24 hours after refeeding sucrose following a period of starvation. Synthesis of the disaccharidases is stimulated, but their breakdown also is diminished. Conversely, lactase is an enzyme that appears not to respond to manipulation of dietary intake of lactose.[337]

Absorptive function also adapts to dietary manipulation.[192] It has been assumed that there is a considerable reserve of absorptive function under normal circumstances, but Diamond and colleagues argued eloquently that it would be inefficiently costly in biosynthetic energy for the intestine to have a large spare capacity.[192,338] Furthermore, a fairly close match between absorptive capacity for many nutrients and dietary load has been demonstrated. A clear need, therefore, exists for adaptation to occur in response to changes in load, and good evidence suggests that most nutrients regulate their specific mucosal transporter.

Two major mucosal adaptive responses are discernible[192] (Fig. 97–25). In the first type of mucosal response, as exemplified by sugars, peptides, and nonessential amino acids, transport activity rises in response to increased dietary loads. Experimental animals fed diets high or low in glucose increase or decrease their maximum capacity for glucose transport, respectively, over a twofold range, probably by changing the number

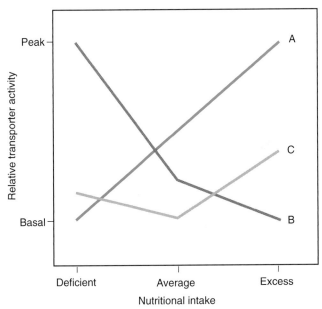

Figure 97–25 Diagram of three types of adaptive responses of intestinal transporters to variation in nutritional intake. Type A response characterizes hexose and nonessential amino acid transport; type B response typifies elements such as iron and calcium and some vitamins; and type C response is a mixed pattern seen with some essential amino acids. (Adapted from Ferraris RP, Diamond JM: Specific regulation of intestinal nutrient transporters by their dietary substrates. Annu Rev Physiol 51:125, 1989, with permission.)

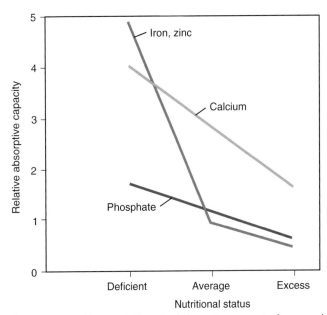

Figure 97–26 Changes in intestinal absorptive capacity for several nutrients in relation to nutritional status. (Adapted from Ferraris RP, Diamond JM: Specific regulation of intestinal nutrient transporters by their dietary substrates. Annu Rev Physiol 51:125, 1989, with permission.)

of transporters. An analogous response to increased dietary load is seen with protein ingestion, in which peptide transporters and some amino acid transporters are increased.

In the second type of mucosal response, as exemplified by a number of vitamins and trace elements, absorptive mechanisms are switched on by low dietary loads and switched off by a large load. Here absorption is enhanced in nutrient deficiency but inhibited with nutrient excess, when potentially toxic effects may result.

A mixed pattern is seen with other types of nutrients, as with essential, predominantly basic, and neutral amino acids, when absorption, presumably in an effort to ensure adequate intake, is enhanced at very low dietary levels. Absorptive mechanisms are at their minimum with average dietary intake but rise as dietary ingestion increases above that range.[192]

The signal for up-regulation of brush border membrane glucose absorption is glucose itself, although an actively transported but unmetabolized sugar also stimulates glucose uptake.[338] Fructose stimulates its own absorption by a separate mechanism from that which stimulates glucose transport.[339] Regulation of mucosal transport of acidic amino acids and imino acids follows the same pattern as that for sugars; that is, an increase in dietary load up-regulates transport. An interesting cross-induction of transport mechanisms by certain types of amino acid with other types has been recognized to occur. Thus, for example, the basic amino acid arginine up-regulates acidic as well as basic amino acid transport, and the acidic amino acid aspartate induces maximal transport of basic amino acids as well as acidic ones.[340]

This cross-stimulation occurs between amino acids and peptides, each of which stimulates the absorption of the other.

Enhanced absorption could result from increased numbers of transporters or from increased activity of each transporter.[192] Evidence in favor of both mechanisms exists, although the former probably predominates. It is uncertain whether an increase in transporter number is caused by increased synthesis, secondary to either transcription or translation, decreased degradation, or an increase in the insertion of preformed transporters into the brush border membrane. Because dietary regulation of glucose and amino acid transporters takes 2 to 3 days, it is likely that regulation occurs at the level of crypt cells.

In diabetes mellitus, the persistent hyperglycemia stimulates both basolateral and apical membrane glucose transport that can be inhibited by protein synthesis inhibitors such as cyclohexamide, suggesting a role for increased synthesis of new glucose transporters.[341]

VITAMINS AND TRACE ELEMENTS

Deficiencies of vitamins and trace elements are associated with up-regulation of their absorptive mechanisms. Upregulation is seen, for example, with biotin, thiamine, and ascorbic acid and with iron, calcium, zinc, and phosphate[192] (Fig. 97–26). Because some of these moieties are potentially toxic, most down-regulate their transport mechanisms when present in higher concentrations. Furthermore, low body stores of iron, zinc, calcium, and phosphate signal enhanced absorptive mechanisms. Zinc deficiency enhances zinc absorption approximately fivefold by increasing transport capacity. Dietary calcium deficiency stimulates calcium uptake in the proximal intestine by a vitamin D–dependent mechanism involving increases in a cytosolic calcium-binding protein and by stimulating transport across the brush border membrane and at the basolateral membrane. These changes occur within a few hours, suggesting that mature enterocytes on the villi are capable of being regulated. By contrast, the effects of dietary regulation of glucose and amino acids take 2 to 3 days to become apparent.

The difference in time scales over which gastrointestinal responses to stimulation by various nutrients occur provides fascinating insights into the molecular and biologic events underlying these phenomena. Immediate responses seen within seconds to a few minutes after exposure are likely to involve release, or activation, of pre-formed proteins. Adaptive responses found within 2 to 3 hours of stimulation probably are due to increased translation; responses that take several hours or days are likely to result from increased transcription and production of more mRNA.[342]

SIGNALING FOR INTESTINAL ADAPTATION AND IMPLICATIONS FOR THERAPY

A variety of signals have been described as possibly playing a role in the process of intestinal adaptation. These include growth hormone (GH), epidermal growth factor (EGF) and EGF receptor, prostanoids, uncoupling proteins, peroxisome proliferator-activated receptor-α (PPAR-α), insulin-like growth factor-1 (IGF-1) receptors and IGF-binding proteins, transforming growth factor-α, SPARC (secreted protein, acidic and rich in cystine), Bcl-2, endothelin-1, erythropoietin, keratinocyte growth factor, the GATA family of zinc finger transcription factors, hepatocyte growth factor, the early-response genes (*ERG*), ornithine decarboxylase (ODC), PC4/TIS7, epimorphin, and AP-1, a transcription factor composed of Fos and JUN family proteins.[322] Several of these signals may lend themselves to be modified in a clinical setting, to enhance the intestinal adaptive response.

For example, evidence from animal intestinal resection models suggests that the enhancing influence of corticosteroids on sugar uptake may be achieved by post-translational processes that involve signaling with *c*-jun, ODC, proglucagon, and other, as-yet unknown signals.[343,344] In a model of extensive intestinal resection (50% enterectomy), prednisone had no effect on the uptake of glucose or fructose in these animals. By contrast, the locally acting steroid budesonide increased by greater than 120% the value of the jejunal maximal transport rate for the uptake of glucose and also increased the ileal uptake of fructose by greater than 150%.[343,345]

GH has been suggested to possess pro-adaptive properties.[346] In animal models, the administration of GH results in an increase in small intestinal length and function per unit length.[347] In hypophysectomized rats, mucosal hypoplasia of the small bowel develops following resection, with a reduced adaptive response that is restored by GH, whereas in transgenic mice expressing elevated levels of GH, hypertrophy of the small intestine develops.[347] IGF-1 expression in the small bowel is regulated by GH and is believed to induce enterotrophic effects following resection. Human and rabbit studies

have indicated that increased nutrient transport activity not associated with morphologic changes may be the method of GH-induced intestinal adaptation.[348] In home parenteral nutrition–dependent patients with short-bowel syndrome, the use of high-dose recombinant human GH (0.4 mg/kg per day) in controlled and uncontrolled studies has led to variable results.[349-351]

GLP-2 increases the adaptive response to massive intestinal resection in rats.[352] The non–placebo-controlled study of Jeppesen and colleagues in eight patients with short bowel syndrome and an end-enterostomy type of anastomosis (six had Crohn's disease, and four were not receiving home parenteral nutrition) showed a significant increase in the absolute and percentage intestinal absorption of net weight, and a significant increase in the percentage but not the absolute, absorption of energy and nitrogen in response to the use of GLP-2.[353]

THE NEONATAL INTESTINE

DEVELOPMENT AND ADAPTATION OF NUTRIENT DIGESTION AND ABSORPTION

Nutrient requirements vary markedly during early postnatal development, and this is mirrored by alterations in digestive and absorptive capacity. Some of these changes are genetically determined and programmed and do not appear to be greatly influenced by changes in dietary load.[5] Thus, for most of the world's population, excluding white persons, the decline in activity of the disaccharidase lactase, which occurs after infancy, cannot be prevented by maintaining a high milk intake.[192]

Some early postnatal responses and most responses in adult life, however, appear to be purposeful and reversible, paralleling changes in dietary intake, for digestive enzyme production and absorptive capacity; such adaptations may occur in response to changes in dietary load or altered body needs.[192,332]

DEVELOPMENTAL CHANGES

Approximately 50% of the total calorie requirement of infants is provided by the fat in milk. Breast milk contains 3.5% to 4% lipid, of which 95% is in the form of triglyceride.[176] The fatty acid composition is a mixture of medium- and long-chain fatty acids. In neonates, pancreatic lipase secretion is low, and the digestion of triglyceride in milk relies on the other lipases present in the milk or secreted by the tongue or gastric mucosa. Pancreatic lipase secretion rises after weaning, because milk-derived lipase no longer is available[342] (Fig. 97–27).

Protein digestion is incomplete in infancy, and many proteins, such as human milk protein (whey), may partially escape digestion.[354] This relative immaturity also may have advantages for the infant because some biologically important peptides and immunoglobulins remain intact. Proteolytic enzymes are derived from a variety of sources, which also are changing during early neonatal life. Thus, several specific proteases, including trypsin and elastase, are present in breast milk.[354] Gastric acid and pepsin are secreted at birth and increase toward

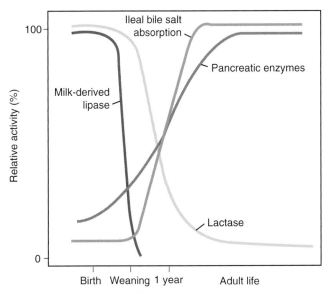

Figure 97–27 Diagram of the major changes in digestive function between the newborn period and adulthood.

adult values over the ensuing 3 to 4 months. Nonetheless, little protein digestion occurs in the stomach during the first few weeks of life, possibly owing to the presence of protease inhibitors in milk. Likewise, luminal proteolytic machinery in the small intestine is not fully developed at birth, although enterokinase and pancreatic proteolytic enzymes are easily detectable. Rates of chymotrypsin and trypsin secretion are slower in infancy than in adult life, and responses to stimulation with CCK are depressed.[355] Low rates of pancreatic enzyme secretion at birth may be attributable in part to the retarded display of polypeptide hormone receptors on the basolateral membrane of acinar cells. Digestive enzymes appear at different times after birth, suggesting that the genes that code for these enzymes may be activated at different times during development.[355]

The human population can be divided into two groups with respect to the ability to digest lactose: lactase-persistent persons, who are able to digest lactose throughout their lifespan, and lactase-nonpersistent (lactose-intolerant, adult-type hypolactasia) persons. Lactase nonpersistence is caused by a decrease in the expression of the small intestine–specific enzyme lactase–phlorizin hydrolase (LPH) at the age of approximately 5 to 10 years. Persons with lactase nonpersistence have a limited ability to digest lactose as adults; however, in both the lactase-nonpersistent and the lactase-persistent phenotypes, high LPH expression after birth is observed. The lactase-persistent phenotype is found most frequently among Northern Europeans, Indians from Punjab, Bedouins, and some nomadic tribes in Africa.[356,357]

The mechanism behind the developmental down-regulation of LPH expression in humans has been shown to be mainly transcriptional, with several transcription factors (Cdx-2, GATA factors, and HNF-1) mutually interacting and activating LPH expression.[358,359] The binding sites for these factors are clustered within 100 base pairs upstream of a TATA box.

The molecular mechanisms behind the developmental down-regulation of LPH expression remain unknown,

although the regulation of LPH expression in both humans and animals has been studied extensively. No differences have been described in the DNA sequence of the *LPH* gene that are correlated with the lactase phenotype; however, recently a T/C polymorphism at position –13910 and an A/G polymorphism at position –22018 from the start codon of the *LPH* gene have been identified. Although these nucleotide variants are located in introns 8 and 13 of the neighboring *MCM6* gene, the –13910C polymorphism associates 100% and the –22018G polymorphism associates approximately 97% with the lactase-nonpersistent phenotype in the Finnish population.[360] Furthermore, it has been shown that the two single-nucleotide polymorphisms are associated with the transcriptional regulation of the *LPH* gene.[361] The –13910 T/C polymorphism is located in a transcriptional enhancer sequence, which strongly activates the LPH promoter activity. Furthermore, the –13910T variant isolated from a lactase-persistent individual has a higher enhancer activity than the corresponding –13910C variant isolated from a lactase-nonpersistent individual. Analyses of the binding of nuclear factors to the –13910 polymorphic sequences show that the –13910T sequence binds nuclear factors with higher affinity compared with the –13910C sequence. The –22018 region polymorphism does not possess enhancer activity and, in fact, results in a very small but significant reduction in reporter gene activity. The reduction of the reporter gene level by the –22018 region is greater in the presence of the enhancer of the –13910 region. It has been suggested that the lactase-persistent phenotype is caused by a mutation in the –13910 position, creating a strong enhancer that is able to keep the *LPH* gene active during adulthood[357] (Fig. 97–28).

Based on these results, a model explaining the mechanisms behind the postweaning down-regulation of LPH expression and adult-type hypolactasia has been proposed. Transcription factors necessary for LPH expression are present in excess during childhood and before weaning in mammals. After the weaning period, the expression of some intestinal transcription factors is changed (e.g., HNF-1α). Also, the availability of some of these factors may be decreased, because genes necessary for digestion of a starch-rich diet (e.g., sucrase-isomaltase) are up-regulated after weaning. Many of these intestinal-specific genes are dependent on the same transcription factors (Cdx-2, HNF-1, and GATA factors) as those for the LPH promoter; competition for these transcriptional activators is higher after weaning. These changes result in a lower LPH expression owing to the weak nature of the LPH promoter, however, the strong enhancer effect of the –13910T variant compensates for these changes and is able to keep the *LPH* gene active throughout adulthood, thereby giving the phenotype of lactase persistence (see Fig. 97–28).

Changes in epithelial membrane transport of nutrients take place when the intestine is suddenly and rapidly expected to assume the role of the placenta in providing nutrients at the moment of birth and immediately thereafter. Brush border membrane glucose and most amino acid transporters are present in the human fetal intestine well before birth,[5] when, in contrast with adult intestine, they are found throughout the crypt-villus axis. Fructose-

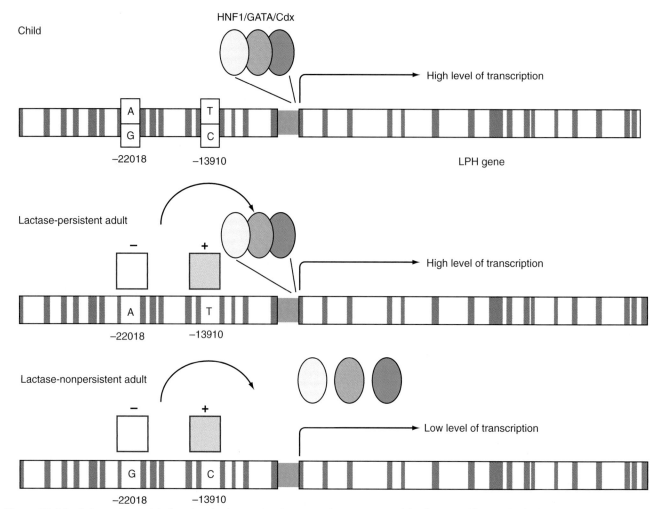

Figure 97–28   Schematic model showing the interaction between the promoter of the lactase-phlorizin hydrolase (LPH) gene and polymorphic −13910 and −22018 regions in the neighboring *MCM6* gene in children and in lactase-persistent and lactase-nonpersistent adults. During childhood and before weaning in other mammals, the level of *LPH* expression is high because the transcription factors (HNF1α, GATA factors, Cdx-2) known to regulate *LPH* expression are available in excess. The expression of *LPH* is therefore not dependent on the −13910 enhancer activity. In adulthood, the accessibility to the transcription factors is reduced. The strong enhancer activity of the −13910T variant ensures an active *LPH* gene throughout life (lactase persistence). The lower activity of the −13910C variant fails to activate/recruit the transcription factors, which results in a low *LPH* gene activity in nonpersistent adults. Although the −22018 region represses LPH transcription, the role of the −22018 region is unclear; the repression does not seem to be related to the A/G polymorphism. (From Troelsen JT: An upstream polymorphism associated with lactase persistence has increased enhancer activity. Gastroenterology 125:1686, 2003.)

absorptive capacity rises rapidly after weaning when this sugar is presented in the diet. Transporters for bile salts are not programmed to appear on ileal enterocytes until weaning.[318]

TRIGLYCERIDE DIGESTION

Some differences have been recognized between how infants digest triglyceride, which they receive in milk, and how adults digest this same fatty substrate. In contradistinction to other dietary sources, the triglyceride in milk is packaged in smaller emulsion droplets, and each is surrounded by a trilaminar membrane that includes both phospholipid and proteins (albumin and beta-lactoglobulin).[342] The newborn infant relies on milk-derived triglyceride for greater than 50% of energy

requirements—but at that point, pancreatic lipase secretion rates are only approximately half those in adults, when expressed in terms of body surface area. Only at weaning does pancreatic lipase secretion begin to rise to adult levels.[362]

Two other lipases are important at this early stage in life (see Table 97–3). The first is secreted by the mammary gland but is inactive in milk and requires the presence of bile salts to activate it. It begins to function, therefore, on entering the duodenum.[342] The second lipase is secreted either from serous glands at the base of the tongue, from gastric mucosa, or from both, depending on the species. In humans, this "preduodenal" lipase is largely, if not entirely, derived from chief cells in the mucosa of the body of the stomach.[363] In the rat, it is derived from the tongue. This lipase has optimal pH of 4 to 6, which is lower than that of pancreatic lipase. It preferentially cleaves the α1 position on triglyceride and releases fatty acid and diacylglycerol, as opposed to the release of monoglyceride by pancreatic lipase. It is not stimulated by bile salts and is released during feeding by autonomic nervous stimulation. Gastric lipase appears to be particularly active at the surface membrane of droplets derived from milk; pancreatic lipase is less so. Although the amount of lipolysis that occurs within the stomach is relatively small, the release of even modest amounts of fatty acids, particularly from the shorter- and medium-chain triglycerides, may be important in the emulsification of fat in the duodenum and in enhancing pancreatic lipase activity. Gastric lipase is rapidly inactivated in the duodenum by proteolytic enzymes. The available evidence is conflicting, however, regarding the importance of intragastric lipolysis. Some investigators have suggested that as much as 30% of fat may be digested here,[57] but the rapid "product" inhibition of gastric lipase activity by released fatty acids makes this unlikely.

Each of the three lipases has a different specificity for the ester bonds in triglyceride. Gastric lipase preferentially cleaves the bond in the 1a position, and pancreatic lipase cleaves the bonds in the 1 and 3α positions; milk-derived, bile salt-stimulated, lipase is nonselective and splits the bonds at the 1, 2, and 3α positions. Thus, luminal contents in a newborn comprise more fatty acids and less monoglyceride and diglyceride than in the adult intestinal lumen; this different makeup probably is advantageous for absorption. Smaller amounts of bile salts are available in newborns than in adults, at least in part because active ileal reabsorption is immature.[342] Under these conditions, fatty acids are likely to be absorbed more readily than is monoglyceride. In addition, the low bile salt availability makes it likely that transfer of fat to the brush border membrane depends more on unilamellar liquid crystalline vesicles.

Gastric lipase persists into adult life, and the amounts found in biopsy specimens of adult gastric mucosa are similar to those found in infant gastric mucosa. Studies suggest gastric lipase may hydrolyze as many as one in four triglyceride acyl chains during digestion of a meal.[10]

CARBOHYDRATE DIGESTION AND ABSORPTION

Lactose is the major carbohydrate in breast milk, and the need for an amylase before weaning is therefore minimal. An α-amylase is present in milk, however, and an amylase also is secreted in saliva at birth.[356] Both of these amylases are inactivated by gastric acid but may resume their activity at nearly neutral pH on reaching the duodenum. It has been estimated that 15% to 40% of amylase activity in the duodenum of infants is of salivary origin.[362] Pancreatic amylase secretion is low, and stimulation with exogenous agonists produces little response, indicating the prematurity of the pancreas at this stage. In any event, the need for any amylase in neonates is small unless starch is introduced into the diet early. Most infant formula feeds do not contain starches, but some contain glucose polymers.

Digestion of any starch ingested during the first 2 or 3 months of life relies on salivary amylase and mucosal α-glucosidases, as well as colonic "salvage" by fermentation of undigested carbohydrate by bacteria.

Mucosal lactase is present at birth in high concentration, as are the other glucosidases.[364] Nevertheless, lactose absorption may be incomplete in neonates, particularly in premature neonates. Estimates of the amount of lactose that reaches the colon vary and have been based on indirect measurements of breath hydrogen concentrations. Probably less than 20% of ingested lactose reaches the colon, but a much smaller proportion is lost in the stool because of bacterial hydrolysis and absorption of the products.

The glucose/galactose transporter in the apical membrane of villus enterocytes is well developed in full-term infants but may be suboptimal in premature infants. This phenomenon is unlikely, however, to pose a significant barrier to nutrition.

PROTEIN DIGESTION AND ABSORPTION

Although acid and pepsinogens are secreted in neonates, little intragastric proteolysis occurs during the first 2 to 6 weeks of life. A renin-like protease is secreted during the first 10 days of life, which causes protein precipitation.[354]

Pancreatic proteolytic enzymes are secreted at birth, although at slower rates than in adults. Trypsinogen secretion is low and, particularly in preterm infants, does not respond to feeding. Furthermore, stimulation with pancreozymin has little effect on pancreatic enzyme secretion for the first 1 to 2 months of life.[177] Enterokinase (enteropeptidase) is present at birth and is capable of activating trypsinogen. Despite the apparent immaturity of the proteolytic machinery, it has been estimated that duodenal proteolysis can cope with as much as 3 or 4 g of protein per kg of body weight of casein, and infants seem not to be prone to defective nitrogen nutrition.

A number of proteases have been found in breast milk, including plasmin, which is most active against casein.[365] The importance of these milk-derived proteases or the protease inhibitors also found in milk[366] in overall nutrition is not known. Transport systems for amino acids and small peptides appear to be well developed in newborns.

The infant intestine has greater capacity than that of the adult intestine to absorb intact macromolecules, including proteins. Transport by pinocytosis or receptor-mediated endocytosis probably accounts for the ability of infants to take in biologically important whole proteins, such as the immunoglobulins, during this phase of life. This mechanism disappears after the first 3 months of life, when "closure" is said to have occurred[367]; however, uptake of intact proteins continues throughout life, albeit in trace amounts, and the role of M cells on Peyer's patches is of major importance in this process. Such uptake is likely to be an important mechanism by which dietary antigens are presented for immune surveillance later in life but is of little nutritional significance.

DIET-GENE INTERACTIONS

Growing evidence points to the interplay among diet, disease, and genetic diversity. Clear evidence is available to support the concept that the diet-disease link is moderated by genetic variation. Important candidate genes studied include those responsible for the synthesis of apo E, 5,10-methylenetetrahydrofolate reductase (MTHFR), and PPAR-γ.[368] Despite the growing knowledge of the various transporters and mediators in lipid, protein, and carbohydrate digestion and absorption, however, little is known about the influence of polymorphic gene changes on these functions and subsequent effects on overall nutritional balance.[368] For example, apolipoprotein A-IV plays a role in lipid absorption and chylomicron assembly. Two genetic polymorphisms of apolipoprotein A-IV, Q360H and T347S, are known to occur at high frequency. The Q360H isoprotein displays high lipid affinity, is associated with increased postprandial hypertriglyceridemia, a reduced low-density lipoprotein response to dietary cholesterol in the settting of a moderate fat intake, an increased high-density lipoprotein response to changes in total dietary fat content, and lower body mass and adiposity. By contrast, T347S displays less lipid affinity and opposite effects compared with the Q360H polymorphism.[369] Of interest, a study of 1144 French subjects showed that an A/G polymorphism in intron 8 of the FATP1 gene (which is not the primary FATP expressed in the intestine) is associated with increased plasma triglyceride levels.[370] Further population studies will be required to evaluate the influence of polymorphic changes in the critical genes involved in digestion and absorption.[371]

BARIATRIC SURGERY: EFFECT ON DIGESTION AND ABSORPTION

During the past several years, the number of bariatric surgical procedures performed has tripled, reaching more than 60,000 in 2002, and it is estimated that this will continue to rise to 100,000 persons per year. At present, the Roux-en-Y gastric bypass (RYGB) is the most widely performed weight loss procedure in the United States. In a 2003 survey, RYGB was preferred by 73% of members of the American Society of Bariatric Surgery, followed by vertical banded gastroplasty (VBG) or laparoscopic gastric banding (15%) and biliopancreatic diversion (BPD) with or without duodenal switch (12%).[372] The exact mechanism of weight loss associated with each treatment modality and how they affect intestinal digestion and absorption are not clearly understood.

Operations for weight loss generally have been classified as either malabsorptive or restrictive, or both, based on the proposed mechanism for the induction of weight loss. The jejunoileal bypass (JIB) and its more recent modifications, the BPD and the distal gastric bypass with duodenal switch (DGB-DS), are classified as malabsorptive procedures; the gastroplasties (horizontal, vertical, and VBG) are restrictive; and RYGB represents a combination of these two mechanisms.

The results of surgical treatment of severe obesity differ considerably and largely can be correlated with the mechanisms of weight loss. Malabsorptive procedures, especially JIB, produce the greatest degree of weight loss but can be associated with serious and potentially life-threatening metabolic and nutritional complications.[373] BPD and DGB-DS produce significant weight loss that

persists and is associated with fewer metabolic complications than those seen with JIB.[372,373] Restrictive procedures produce moderate degrees of weight loss and are associated with the lowest incidence of metabolic and nutritional complications.[372] RYGB has been shown consistently to produce greater and more sustained weight loss than that achieved with VBG, while avoiding the severe metabolic and nutritional consequences of intestinal bypass.

The mechanism of weight loss following VBG appears to be similar to that with other forms of caloric restriction, although the weight loss tends to be more pronounced and to persist for a longer period of time. The role of the regulation of central satiety mechanisms has been studied for both restrictive and malabsorptive surgeries. Ghrelin is a gastric peptide with potent orexigenic effects. Circulating ghrelin concentrations are increased in obese persons and increase further after weight loss. In patients undergoing RYGB, however, a decrease in ghrelin levels has been reported (compared with patients undergoing VBG or BPD) and appears to be dependent on the surgically induced bypass of the ghrelin-producing cell populations of the fundus.[374] Several mechanisms have been suggested to account for the more substantial weight loss after JIB, RYGB and BPD. These mechanisms can be divided into three groups: caloric restriction, changes in energy metabolism, and alterations in gastrointestinal hormones and nutrient absorption

Caloric restriction seems to play a prominent role in JIB and RYGB, with numerous studies documenting significantly decreased caloric intake after each procedure. Animal studies, however, have shown that rats subjected to intestinal bypass maintained lower weights despite caloric intakes comparable with those of sham-operated controls, suggesting an increase in energy expenditure. Human data suggest a relative increase in the mean resting energy expenditure in patients undergoing RYGB.[375,376]

Malabsorption leading to a loss of lean body mass, diarrhea, and vitamin, mineral, and electrolyte deficiencies contributes prominently to weight loss after JIB, and less so after BPD and DGB-DS. After JIB, malabsorption results from the drastically reduced intestinal surface in contact with nutrients (common channel) and from rapid transit time. It has been suggested that the enhanced weight loss after BPD is related to the combination of a short common channel (approximately 50 cm) that limits fat absorption, and a long afferent limb that is not in direct contact with food. Therefore, the effect of the alimentary (Roux) limb, where protein and carbohydrates are absorbed, is limited.

The documented changes in absorption may result from alterations in the hormonal milieu of the gastrointestinal tract. Dumping syndrome, evidenced by lightheadedness, sweating, palpitations, and diarrhea following a test meal containing a high carbohydrate load, results from operations that bypass the normal pyloric functions and has been documented in patients with RYGB.[377,378] These symptoms are temporally associated with changes in levels of intestinal peptides, especially an increase in enteroglucagon, which is secreted by the ileum. Increased enteroglucagon and neurotensin after ileal transposition in rats is associated with weight loss equivalent to that achieved with caloric restriction. These findings suggest that rapid transport of undigested and unabsorbed nutrients into the ileum after these procedures stimulates the secretion of intestinal peptides (e.g., enteroglucagon), which then produce or serve as a marker for full-blown or subclinical "dumping" that in turn contributes to the observed weight loss.[377,379] Peptide YY (PYY) is a hormone secreted by the L-cells lining the terminal small bowel and colon, in response to intestinal nutrients, especially long-chain fatty acids.[21,380] PYY decreases gastric and intestinal emptying and improves intestinal absorption. This mechanism is termed the *ileal brake*.[32] PYY also is a potent anorexigenic hormone and acts by modulating appetite circuits in the hypothalamus, and by stimulating Apo A-IV which plays an important role in upper gastrointestinal function and satiety.[21,381] It has been shown that PYY serum levels are higher in patients who underwent JIB.[382] The role that intestinal adaptation plays after bariatric surgery is not yet understood.

REFERENCES

1. Alpers D: Digestion and obsorption of carbohydrates and proteins. In Johnson L (ed): Physiology of the Gastrointestinal Tract, 2nd ed. New York, Raven Press, 1987, p 1469.
2. McNeil M: Nutritional implications of human and mammalian large intestinal function. World Rev Nutr Diet 56:1, 1988.
3. Fallstrom SP, Nygren CO, Olegard R: Plasma triglyceride increase after oral fat load in malabsorption during early childhood. Acta Paediatr Scand 66:111, 1977.
4. Fomon SJ, Ziegler EE, Thomas LN, et al: Excretion of fat by normal full-term infants fed various milks and formulas. Am J Clin Nutr 23:1299, 1970.
5. Buddington RK, Diamond JM: Ontogenetic development of intestinal nutrient transporters. Annu Rev Physiol 51:601, 1989.
6. Karasov W, Diamond J: Adaptation of intestinal nutrient transport. In Johnson L (ed): Physiology of the Gastrointestinal Tract, 2nd ed. New York, Raven Press, 1987, p 1489.
7. Sarles H, Dani R, Prezelin G, et al: Cephalic phase of pancreatic secretion in man. Gut 9:214, 1968.
8. Brown JC, Harper AA, Scratcherd T: Potentiation of secretin stimulation of the pancreas. J Physiol 190:519, 1967.
9. DiPalma J, Kirk CL, Hamosh M, et al: Lipase and pepsin activity in the gastric mucosa of infants, children, and adults. Gastroenterology 101:116, 1991.
10. Carriere F, Barrowman JA, Verger R, Laugier R: Secretion and contribution to lipolysis of gastric and pancreatic lipases during a test meal in humans. Gastroenterology 105:876, 1993.
11. Woods SC: Gastrointestinal satiety signals I. An overview of gastrointestinal signals that influence food intake. Am J Physiol Gastrointest Liver Physiol 286:G7, 2004.
12. Lieverse RJ, Jansen JB, Masclee AA, Lamers CB: Satiety effects of a physiological dose of cholecystokinin in humans. Gut 36:176, 1995.
13. Gibbs J, Smith GP, Kirkham TO: Gastrin-releasing peptide and satiety. Gastroenterology 106:1374, 1994.
14. Apo A-I: A new satiety signal. Nutr Rev 51:273, 1993.
15. Moran TH, Kinzig KP: Gastrointestinal satiety signals II. Cholecystokinin. Am J Physiol Gastrointest Liver Physiol 286:G183, 2004.
16. Hayes MR, Moore RL, Shah SM, Covasa M: 5-HT$_3$ receptors participate in CCK-induced suppression of food intake by delaying gastric emptying. Am J Physiol Regul Integr Comp Physiol 287:R817, 2004.
17. Stanley S, Wynne K, Bloom S: Gastrointestinal satiety signals III. Glucagon-like peptide 1, oxyntomodulin, peptide YY, and pancreatic polypeptide. Am J Physiol Gastrointest Liver Physiol 286:G693, 2004.
18. Liu M, Doi T, Tso P: Regulation of intestinal and hypothalamic apolipoprotein A-IV. Exp Biol Med (Maywood) 228:1181, 2003.
19. Tso P, Sun W, Liu M: Gastrointestinal satiety signals IV. Apolipoprotein A-IV. Am J Physiol Gastrointest Liver Physiol 286:G885, 2004.
20. Stan S, Delvin E, Lambert M, et al: Apo A-IV: An update on regulation and physiologic functions. Biochim Biophys Acta 1631:177, 2003.
21. Tso P, Liu M: Ingested fat and satiety. Physiol Behav 81:275, 2004.
22. Bray GA: Afferent signals regulating food intake. Proc Nutr Soc 59:373, 2000.
23. Malagelada J-R, Azpiroz F: Determinants of gastric emptying and transit in the small intestine. In Schultz S (ed): Handbook of Physiology. The Gastrointestinal System, vol 1. Bethesda, American Physiological Society, 1989, p 909.
24. Meyer JH, Thomson JB, Cohen MB, et al: Sieving of solid food by the canine stomach and sieving after gastric surgery. Gastroenterology 76:804, 1979.
25. Cooke A: Localisation of receptors inhibiting gastric emptying in the gut. Gastroenterology 72:875, 1977.
26. Meeroff JC, Go VL, Phillips SF: Control of gastric emptying by osmolality of duodenal contents in man. Gastroenterology 68:1144, 1975.
27. Hunt JN, Smith JL, Jiang CL: Effect of meal volume and energy density on the gastric emptying of carbohydrates. Gastroenterology 89:1326, 1985.
28. Mayer E: The physiology of gastric storage and emptying. In Johnson L (ed): Physiology of the Gastrointestinal Tract, 3rd ed. New York, Raven Press, 1994, p 929.
29. Read NW, McFarlane A, Kinsman RI, et al: Effect of infusion of nutrient solutions into the ileum on gastrointestinal transit and plasma levels of neurotensin and enteroglucagon. Gastroenterology 86:274, 1984.
30. Nightingale JM, Kamm MA, van der Sijp JR, et al: Disturbed gastric emptying in the short bowel syndrome. Evidence for a "colonic brake." Gut 34:1171, 1993.
31. Pironi L, Stanghellini V, Miglioli M, et al: Fat-induced ileal brake in humans: A dose-dependent phenomenon correlated to the plasma levels of peptide YY. Gastroenterology 105:733, 1993.
32. Teixeira FV, Pera M, Kelly KA: Enhancing release of peptide YY after near-total proctocolectomy: Jejunal pouch vs. ileal pouch-distal rectal anastomosis. J Gastrointest Surg 5:108, 2001.
33. Drucker DJ: Gut adaptation and the glucagon-like peptides. Gut 50:428, 2002.
34. Brubaker PL, Crivici A, Izzo A, et al: Circulating and tissue forms of the intestinal growth factor, glucagon-like peptide-2. Endocrinology 138:4837, 1997.
35. Xiao Q, Boushey RP, Drucker DJ, Brubaker PL: Secretion of the intestinotropic hormone glucagon-like peptide 2 is differentially regulated by nutrients in humans. Gastroenterology 117:99, 1999.
36. Hartmann B, Johnsen AH, Orskov C, et al: Structure, measurement, and secretion of human glucagon-like peptide-2. Peptides 21:73, 2000.
37. Drucker DJ: Glucagon-like peptides. Diabetes 47:159, 1998.
38. Owyang C, Logsdon CD: New insights into neurohormonal regulation of pancreatic secretion. Gastroenterology 127:957, 2004.

39. Konturek SJ, Zabielski R, Konturek JW, Czarnecki J: Neuroendocrinology of the pancreas; role of brain-gut axis in pancreatic secretion. Eur J Pharmacol 481:1, 2003.

40. Konturek SJ, Pepera J, Zabielski K, et al: Brain-gut axis in pancreatic secretion and appetite control. J Physiol Pharmacol 54:293, 2003.

41. Chey WY, Chang T: Neural hormonal regulation of exocrine pancreatic secretion. Pancreatology 1:320, 2001.

42. Tso P: Intestinal lipid absorption. In Johnson L (ed): Physiology of the Gastrointestinal Tract, Vol 3, 3rd ed. New York, Raven Press, 1994, p 1873.

43. Wright JP, Barbezat GO, Clain JE: Jejunal secretion in response to a duodenal mixed nutrient perfusion. Gastroenterology 76:94, 1979.

44. Greenwood B, Davison JS: The relationship between gastrointestinal motility and secretion. Am J Physiol 252:G1, 1987.

45. Winne D: Influence of blood flow on intestinal absorption of drugs and nutrients. Pharmacol Ther 6:333, 1979.

46. Northfield TC, Hofmann AF: Biliary lipid output during three meals and an overnight fast. I. Relationship to bile acid pool size and cholesterol saturation of bile in gallstone and control subjects. Gut 16:1, 1975.

47. Household Food Consumption and Expenditure. Annual Report of the National Food Survey Committee. London: Ministry of Agriculture, Fisheries and Food, 1989.

48. Rizek R, Risek R, Friend B, Page L: Fat in today's food supply: Level of use and source. J Am Oil Chem Soc 51:244, 1974.

49. Davidson S, Passmore R, Brock J, Truswell A: Human Nutrition and Dietetics. Edinburgh, Churchill Livingstone, 1979.

50. Kern F Jr: Normal plasma cholesterol in an 88-year-old man who eats 25 eggs a day. Mechanisms of adaptation. N Engl J Med 324:896, 1991.

51. Report of the Task Force on Trans Fatty Acids. London, British Nutrition Foundation, 1987.

52. Enig MG, Munn RJ, Keeney M: Dietary fat and cancer trends—a critique. Fed Proc 37:2215, 1978.

53. Borel P, Lairon D, Senft M, et al: Wheat bran and wheat germ: Effect on digestion and intestinal absorption of dietary lipids in the rat. Am J Clin Nutr 49:1192, 1989.

54. Thomson AB, Keelan M, Garg M, Clandinin MT: Dietary effects of omega 3-fatty acids on intestinal transport function. Can J Physiol Pharmacol 66:985, 1988.

55. Abrams CK, Hamosh M, Lee TC, et al: Gastric lipase: Localization in the human stomach. Gastroenterology 95:1460, 1988.

56. Thomson AB, Schoeller C, Keelan M, et al: Lipid absorption: Passing through the unstirred layers, brush-border membrane, and beyond. Can J Physiol Pharmacol 71:531, 1993.

57. Hernell O, Blackberg L, Bernback S: Digestion of human milk fat in early infancy. Acta Paediatr Scand 351:57, 1989.

58. Blow D: Enzymology. Lipases reach the surface. Nature 351:444, 1991.

59. Sims HF, Lowe ME: The human colipase gene: Isolation, chromosomal location, and tissue-specific expression. Biochemistry 31:7120, 1992.

60. Renaud W, Dagorn JC: cDNA sequence and deduced amino acid sequence of human preprocolipase. Pancreas 6:157, 1991.

61. Erlanson-Albertsson C, Larsson A: A possible physiological function of pancreatic pro-colipase activation peptide in appetite regulation. Biochemie 70:1245, 1988.

62. Bosner M, Gulick T, Riley DJ, et al: Heparin-modulated binding of pancreatic lipase and uptake of hydrolyzed triglycerides in the intestine. J Biol Chem 264:2021, 1989.

63. Lowe ME: The triglyceride lipases of the pancreas. J Lipid Res 43:2007, 2002.

64. Lowe ME: Properties and function of pancreatic lipase related protein 2. Biochimie 82:997, 2000.

65. Carey MC, Small DM: The characteristics of mixed micellar solutions with particular reference to bile. Am J Med 49:590, 1970.

66. Holt PR, Fairchild BM, Weiss J: A liquid crystalline phase in human intestinal contents during fat digestion. Lipids 21:444, 1986.

67. Hernell O, Staggers JE, Carey MC: Physical-chemical behavior of dietary and biliary lipids during intestinal digestion and absorption. 2. Phase analysis and aggregation states of luminal lipids during duodenal fat digestion in healthy adult human beings. Biochemistry 29:2041, 1990.

68. Rigler MW, Honkanen RE, Patton JS: Visualization by freeze fracture, in vitro and in vivo, of the products of fat digestion. J Lipid Res 27:836, 1986.

69. Strocchi A, Levitt MD: A reappraisal of the magnitude and implications of the intestinal unstirred layer. Gastroenterology 101:843, 1991.

70. Shiau YF: Mechanism of intestinal fatty acid uptake in the rat: The role of an acidic microclimate. J Physiol 421:463, 1990.

71. DeSchryver-Kecskemeti K, Eliakim R, Carroll S, et al: Intestinal surfactant–like material. A novel secretory product of the rat enterocyte. J Clin Invest 84:1355, 1989.

72. Subbaiah PV, Ganguly J: Studies on the phospholipases of rat intestinal mucosa. Biochem J 118:233, 1970.

73. Hui DY, Howles PN: Carboxyl ester lipase: Structure-function relationship and physiological role in lipoprotein metabolism and atherosclerosis. J Lipid Res 43:2017, 2002.

74. Kumar BV, Aleman-Gomez JA, Colwell N, et al: Structure of the human pancreatic cholesterol esterase gene. Biochemistry 31:6077, 1992.

75. DiPersio LP, Fontaine RN, Hui DY: Identification of the active site serine in pancreatic cholesterol esterase by chemical modification and site-specific mutagenesis. J Biol Chem 265:16801, 1990.

76. DiPersio LP, Fontaine RN, Hui DY: Site-specific mutagenesis of an essential histidine residue in pancreatic cholesterol esterase. J Biol Chem 266:4033, 1991.

77. DiPersio LP, Hui DY: Aspartic acid 320 is required for optimal activity of rat pancreatic cholesterol esterase. J Biol Chem 268:300, 1993.

78. Blackberg L, Duan RD, Sternby B: Purification of carboxyl ester lipase (bile salt-stimulated lipase) from human milk and pancreas. Methods Enzymol 284:185, 1997.

79. Liang Y, Medhekar R, Brockman HL, et al: Importance of arginines 63 and 423 in modulating the bile salt–dependent and bile salt–independent hydrolytic activities of rat carboxyl ester lipase. J Biol Chem 275:24040, 2000.

80. Hofmann AF, Borgstroem B: The intraluminal phase of fat digestion in man: The lipid content of the micellar and oil phases of intestinal content obtained during fat digestion and absorption. J Clin Invest 43:247, 1964.

81. Carey MC, Small DM, Bliss CM: Lipid digestion and absorption. Annu Rev Physiol 45:651, 1983.

82. Phan CT, Tso P: Intestinal lipid absorption and transport. Front Biosci 6:299, 2001.

83. Ling KY, Lee HY, Hollander D: Mechanisms of linoleic acid uptake by rabbit small intestinal brush border membrane vesicles. Lipids 24:51, 1989.

84. Stremmel W: Uptake of fatty acids by jejunal mucosal cells is mediated by a fatty acid binding membrane protein. J Clin Invest 82:2001, 1988.

85. Chiu HC, Kovacs A, Ford DA, et al: A novel mouse model of lipotoxic cardiomyopathy. J Clin Invest 107:813, 2001.

86. Coburn CT, Hajri T, Ibrahimi A, Abumrad NA: Role of CD36 in membrane transport and utilization of long-chain fatty acids by different tissues. J Mol Neurosci 16:117, 2001.

87. Schaffer JE, Lodish HF: Expression cloning and characterization of a novel adipocyte long chain fatty acid transport protein. Cell 79:427, 1994.

88. Stahl A: A current review of fatty acid transport proteins (SLC27). Pflugers Arch 447:722, 2004.

89. Gore J, Hoinard C: Linolenic acid transport in hamster intestinal cells is carrier-mediated. J Nutr 123:66, 1993.

90. Stahl A, Hirsch DJ, Gimeno RE, et al: Identification of the major intestinal fatty acid transport protein. Mol Cell 4:299, 1999.

91. Sylven C: Influence of blood supply on lipid uptake from micellar solutions by the rat small intestine. Biochim Biophys Acta 203:365, 1970.

92. Schulthess G, Compassi S, Boffelli D, et al: A comparative study of sterol absorption in different small-intestinal brush border membrane models. J Lipid Res 37:2405, 1996.

93. Rosenblum SB, Huynh T, Afonso A, et al: Discovery of 1-(4-fluorophenyl)-(3R)-[3-(4-fluorophenyl)-(3S)-hydroxypropyl]-(4S)-(4-hydroxyphenyl)-2-azetidinone (SCH 58235): A designed, potent, orally active inhibitor of cholesterol absorption. J Med Chem 41:973, 1998.

94. Thurnhofer H, Hauser H: Uptake of cholesterol by small intestinal brush border membrane is protein-mediated. Biochemistry 29:2142, 1990.

95. Wouters FS, Markman M, de Graaf P, et al: The immunohistochemical localization of the non-specific lipid transfer protein (sterol carrier protein-2) in rat small intestine enterocytes. Biochim Biophys Acta 1259:192, 1995.

96. McNeish J, Aiello RJ, Guyot D, et al: High density lipoprotein deficiency and foam cell accumulation in mice with targeted disruption of ATP-binding cassette transporter-1. Proc Natl Acad Sci U S A 97:4245, 2000.

97. Drobnik W, Lindenthal B, Lieser B, et al: ATP-binding cassette transporter A1 (ABCA1) affects total body sterol metabolism. Gastroenterology 120:1203, 2001.

98. Hauser H, Dyer JH, Nandy A, et al: Identification of a receptor mediating absorption of dietary cholesterol in the intestine. Biochemistry 37:17843, 1998.

99. Patel SB, Salen G, Hidaka H, et al: Mapping a gene involved in regulating dietary cholesterol absorption. The sitosterolemia locus is found at chromosome 2p21. J Clin Invest 102:1041, 1998.

100. Berge KE, Tian H, Graf GA, et al: Accumulation of dietary cholesterol in sitosterolemia caused by mutations in adjacent ABC transporters. Science 290:1771, 2000.

101. Berge KE: Sitosterolemia: A gateway to new knowledge about cholesterol metabolism. Ann Med 35:502, 2003.

102. Davies JP, Levy B, Ioannou YA: Evidence for a Niemann-Pick C (NPC) gene family: Identification and characterization of NPC1L1. Genomics 65:137, 2000.

103. Carstea ED, Morris JA, Coleman KG, et al: Niemann-Pick C1 disease gene: Homology to mediators of cholesterol homeostasis. Science 277:228, 1997.

104. Altmann SW, Davis HR Jr, Zhu LJ, et al: Niemann-Pick C1 Like 1 protein is critical for intestinal cholesterol absorption. Science 303:1201, 2004.

105. Boord JB, Fazio S, Linton MF: Cytoplasmic fatty acid–binding proteins: Emerging roles in metabolism and atherosclerosis. Curr Opin Lipidol 13:141, 2002.

106. Agellon LB, Toth MJ, Thomson AB: Intracellular lipid binding proteins of the small intestine. Mol Cell Biochem 239:79, 2002.

107. Storch J, Thumser AE: The fatty acid transport function of fatty acid–binding proteins. Biochim Biophys Acta 1486:28, 2000.

108. Noland BJ, Arebalo RE, Hansbury E, Scallen TJ: Purification and properties of sterol carrier protein2. J Biol Chem 255:4282, 1980.

109. Scallen TJ, Noland BJ, Gavey KL, et al: Sterol carrier protein 2 and fatty acid-binding protein. Separate and distinct physiological functions. J Biol Chem 260:4733, 1985.

110. Shiau YF: Mechanisms of intestinal fat absorption. Am J Physiol 240:G1, 1981.

111. Lehner R, Kuksis A: Triacylglycerol synthesis by purified triacylglycerol synthetase of rat intestinal mucosa. Role of acyl-CoA acyltransferase. J Biol Chem 270:13630, 1995.

112. Smith SJ, Cases S, Jensen DR, et al: Obesity resistance and multiple mechanisms of triglyceride synthesis in mice lacking Dgat. Nat Genet 25:87, 2000.

113. Oelkers P, Tinkelenberg A, Erdeniz N, et al: A lecithin cholesterol acyltransferase–like gene mediates diacylglycerol esterification in yeast. J Biol Chem 275:15609, 2000.

114. Field FJ, Cooper AD, Erickson SK: Regulation of rabbit intestinal acyl coenzyme A–cholesterol acyltransferase in vivo and in vitro. Gastroenterology 83:873, 1982.

115. Chang CC, Sakashita N, Ornvold K, et al: Immunological quantitation and localization of ACAT-1 and ACAT-2 in human liver and small intestine. J Biol Chem 275:28083, 2000.

116. Miyazaki A, Sakkashita N, Lee O, et al: Expression of ACAT-1 protein in human arteriosclerotic lesions in cultured human monocyte-macrophages. Arterioscler Thromb Vasc Biol 18:1568, 1998.

117. Buhman KK, Accad M, Novak S, et al: Resistance to diet-induced hypercholesterolemia and gallstone formation in ACAT2-deficient mice. Nat Med 6:1341, 2000.

118. Go MF, Schonfeld G, Pfleger B, et al: Regulation of intestinal and hepatic apoprotein synthesis after chronic fat and cholesterol feeding. J Clin Invest 81:1615, 1988.

119. Davidson NO, Magun AM, Brasitus TA, Glickman RM: Intestinal apolipoprotein A-I and B-48 metabolism: Effects of sustained alterations in dietary triglyceride and mucosal cholesterol flux. J Lipid Res 28:388, 1987.

120. Hayashi H, Fujimoto K, Cardelli JA, et al: Fat feeding increases size, but not number, of chylomicrons produced by small intestine. Am J Physiol 259:G709, 1990.

121. Ohashi K, Ishibashi S, Osuga J, et al: Novel mutations in the microsomal triglyceride transfer protein gene causing abetalipoproteinemia. J Lipid Res 41:1199, 2000.

122. Glickman RM, Glickman JN, Magun A, Brin M: Apolipoprotein synthesis in normal and abetalipoproteinemic intestinal mucosa. Gastroenterology 101:749, 1991.

123. Bouma ME, Beucler I, Aggerbeck LP, et al: Hypobetalipoproteinemia with accumulation of an apoprotein B–like protein in intestinal cells. Immunoenzymatic and biochemical characterization of seven cases of Anderson's disease. J Clin Invest 78:398, 1986.

124. Dannoura AH, Berriot-Varoqueaux N, Amati P, et al: Anderson's disease: Exclusion of apolipoprotein and intracellular lipid transport genes. Arterioscler Thromb Vasc Biol 19:2494, 2000.

125. Sabesin SM, Frase S: Electron microscopic studies of the assembly, intracellular transport, and secretion of chylomicrons by rat intestine. J Lipid Res 18:496, 1977.

126. Mangelsdorf DJ, Thummel C, Beato M, et al: The nuclear receptor superfamily: The second decade. Cell 83:835, 1995.

127. Millatt LJ, Bocher V, Fruchart JC, Staels B: Liver X receptors and the control of cholesterol homeostasis: Potential therapeutic targets for the treatment of atherosclerosis. Biochim Biophys Acta 1631:107, 2003.

128. Repa JJ, Mangelsdorf DJ: Nuclear receptor regulation of cholesterol and bile acid metabolism. Curr Opin Biotechnol 10:557, 1999.

129. Russell DW, Setchell KD: Bile acid biosynthesis. Biochemistry 31:4737, 1992.

130. Vlahcevic ZR, Pandak WM, Stravitz RT: Regulation of bile acid biosynthesis. Gastroenterol Clin North Am 28:1, 1999.

131. Lehmann JM, Kliewer SA, Moore LB, et al: Activation of the nuclear receptor LXR by oxysterols defines a new hormone response pathway. J Biol Chem 272:3137, 1997.

132. Peet DJ, Turley SD, Ma W, et al: Cholesterol and bile acid metabolism are impaired in mice lacking the nuclear oxysterol receptor LXR alpha. Cell 93:693, 1998.

133. Lu TT, Makishima M, Repa JJ, et al: Molecular basis for feedback regulation of bile acid synthesis by nuclear receptors. Mol Cell 6:507, 2000.

134. Repa JJ, Turley SD, Lobaccaro JA, et al: Regulation of absorption and ABC1-mediated efflux of cholesterol by RXR heterodimers. Science 289:1524, 2000.

135. Schwartz K, Lawn RM, Wade DP: *ABC1* gene expression and ApoA-I–mediated cholesterol efflux are regulated by LXR. Biochem Biophys Res Commun 274:794, 2000.

136. Brooks-Wilson A, Marcil M, Clee SM, et al: Mutations in *ABC1* in Tangier disease and familial high-density lipoprotein deficiency. Nat Genet 22:336, 1999.

137. Bodzioch M, Orso E, Klucken J, et al: The gene encoding ATP-binding cassette transporter 1 is mutated in Tangier disease. Nat Genet 22:347, 1999.

138. Rust S, Rosier M, Funke H, et al: Tangier disease is caused by mutations in the gene encoding ATP-binding cassette transporter 1. Nat Genet 22:352, 1999.

139. Dietary Reference Values for Food Energy and Nutrients for the United Kingdom. Report of the Panel on Dietary Reference Values of the Committee on Medical Aspects of Food Policy. London: Department of Health, HMSO, 1991, p 72.

140. Montes RG, Gottal RF, Bayless TM, et al: Breath hydrogen testing as a physiology laboratory exercise for medical students. Am J Physiol 262:S25, 1992.

141. McNeil NI: The contribution of the large intestine to energy supplies in man. Am J Clin Nutr 39:338, 1984.

142. Gumucio DL, Wiebauer K, Dranginis A, et al: Evolution of the amylase multigene family. YBR/Ki mice express a pancreatic amylase gene which is silent in other strains. J Biol Chem 260:13483, 1985.

143. Horii A, Emi M, Tomita N, et al: Primary structure of human pancreatic alpha-amylase gene: its comparison with human salivary alpha-amylase gene. Gene 60:57, 1987.

144. Nishide T, Emi M, Nakamura Y, Matsubara K: Corrected sequences of cDNAs for human salivary and pancreatic alpha-amylases [corrected]. Gene 28:263, 1984.

145. Layer P, Zinsmeister AR, DiMagno EP: Effects of decreasing intraluminal amylase activity on starch digestion and postprandial gastrointestinal function in humans. Gastroenterology 91:41, 1986.

146. Heitlinger LA, Lee PC, Dillon WP, Lebenthal E: Mammary amylase: A possible alternate pathway of carbohydrate digestion in infancy. Pediatr Res 17:15, 1983.

147. Van Beers E, Buller H, Grand R: Intestinal brush border glycohydrolases: Structure, function, and development (review). Crit Rev Biochem Mol Biol 30:197, 1995.

148. Dahlquist A, Semenza G: Disaccharidases of small-intestinal mucosa. J Pediatr Gastroenterol Nutr 4:857, 1985.

149. Sterchi EE, Lentze MJ, Naim HY: Molecular aspects of disaccharidase deficiencies. Baillieres Clin Gastroenterol 4:79, 1990.

150. Naim HY, Sterchi EE, Lentze MJ: Biosynthesis and maturation of lactase–phlorizin hydrolase in the human small intestinal epithelial cells. Biochem J 241:427, 1987.

151. Naim HY, Sterchi EE, Lentze MJ: Structure, biosynthesis, and glycosylation of human small intestinal maltase-glucoamylase. J Biol Chem 263:19709, 1988.

152. Leeper LL, Henning SJ: Development and tissue distribution of sucrase-isomaltase mRNA in rats. Am J Physiol 258:G52, 1990.

153. Wu GD, Wang W, Traber PG: Isolation and characterization of the human sucrase-isomaltase gene and demonstration of intestine-specific transcriptional elements. J Biol Chem 267:7863, 1992.

154. West LF, Davis MB, Green FR, et al: Regional assignment of the gene coding for human sucrase-isomaltase (SI) to chromosome 3q25-26. Ann Hum Genet 52:57, 1988.

155. Traber PG, Silberg DG: Intestine-specific gene transcription. Annu Rev Physiol 58:275, 1996.

156. Traber PG: Epithelial cell growth and differentiation. V. Transcriptional regulation, development, and neoplasia of the intestinal epithelium. Am J Physiol 273:G979, 1997.

157. Markowitz AJ, Wu GD, Bader A, et al: Regulation of lineage-specific transcription of the sucrase-isomaltase gene in transgenic mice and cell lines. Am J Physiol 269:G925, 1995.

158. Tung JM, AJ Silberg DG: Developmental expression of SI in transgenic mice is regulated by an evolutionary conserved promoter. Am J Physiol G83:273, 1997.

159. Wu GD, Chen L, Forslund K, Traber PG: Hepatocyte nuclear factor-1 alpha (HNF-1 alpha) and HNF-1 beta regulate transcription via two elements in an intestine-specific promoter. J Biol Chem 269:17080, 1994.

160. Boudreau F, Zhu Y, Traber PG: Sucrase-isomaltase gene transcription requires the hepatocyte nuclear factor-1 (HNF-1) regulatory element and is regulated by the ratio of HNF-1 alpha to HNF-1 beta. J Biol Chem 276:32122, 2001.

161. Suh E, Chen L, Taylor J, Traber PG: A homeodomain protein related to caudal regulates intestine-specific gene transcription. Mol Cell Biol 14:7340, 1994.

162. Jacob R, Zimmer KP, Schmitz J, Naim HY: Congenital sucrase-isomaltase deficiency arising from cleavage and secretion of a mutant form of the enzyme. J Clin Invest 106:281, 2000.

163. Ritz V, Alfalah M, Zimmer KP, et al: Congenital sucrase-isomaltase deficiency because of an accumulation of the mutant enzyme in the endoplasmic reticulum. Gastroenterology 125:1678, 2003.

164. Cezard JP, Broyart JP, Cuisinier-Gleizes P, Mathieu H: Sucrase-isomaltase regulation by dietary sucrose in the rat. Gastroenterology 84:18, 1983.

165. Rodolosse A, Chantret I, Lacasa M, et al: A limited upstream region of the human sucrase-isomaltase gene confers glucose-regulated expression on a heterologous gene. Biochem J 315:301, 1996.

166. Boll W, Wagner P, Mantei N: Structure of the chromosomal gene and cDNAs coding for lactase–phlorizin hydrolase in humans with adult-type hypolactasia or persistence of lactase. Am J Hum Genet 48:889, 1991.

167. Kruse TA, Bolund L, Grzeschik KH: The human lactase-phlorizin hydrolase gene is located on chromosome 2. FEBS Lett 240:123, 1988.

168. Troelsen JM, C Spodsberg, N: Regulation of lactase-phlorizin hydrolase gene expression by the caudal-related homeodomain protein Cdx-2. Biochem J 322:833, 1997.

169. Krasinski SD, Van Wering HM, Tannemaat MR, Grand RJ: Differential activation of intestinal gene promoters: Functional interactions between GATA-5 and HNF-1 alpha. Am J Physiol Gastrointest Liver Physiol 2001;281:G69-84.

170. Tyska MJ, Mooseker MS: A role for myosin-1A in the localization of a brush border disaccharidase. J Cell Biol 165:395, 2004.

171. Gordon JI: Intestinal epithelial differentiation: New insights from chimeric and transgenic mice. J Cell Biol 108:1187, 1989.

172. Dahlqvist A, Nordstrom C: The distribution of dissacharidases in the villi and crypts of the small intestinal mucosa. Biochim Biophys Acta 113:624, 1966.

173. Traber PG, Yu L, Wu GD, Judge TA: Sucrase-isomaltase gene expression along crypt-villus axis of human small intestine is regulated at level of mRNA abundance. Am J Physiol 262:G123, 1992.

174. Hoffman L, Chang EB: Regional expression and regulation of intestinal sucrase-isomaltase. J Nutr Biochem 4:130, 1992.

175. Hoffman LR, Chang EB: Determinants of regional sucrase-isomaltase expression in adult rat small intestine. J Biol Chem 266:21815, 1991.

176. Das B, Gray C: Intestinal sucrase: In vivo synthesis and degradation. Clin Res 18, 1970.

177. Stevens BR, Kaunitz JD, Wright EM: Intestinal transport of amino acids and sugars: Advances using membrane vesicles. Annu Rev Physiol 46:417, 1984.

178. Desjeux J: Metabolic Basis of Inherited Disease. New York, McGraw-Hill, 1989.

179. Turk E, Martin MG, Wright EM: Structure of the human Na+/glucose cotransporter gene SGLT1. J Biol Chem 269:15204, 1994.

180. Hirschhorn N, Greenough WB 3rd: Progress in oral rehydration therapy. Sci Am 264:50, 1991.

181. Wright EM, Martin MG, Turk E: Intestinal absorption in health and disease—sugars. Best Pract Res Clin Gastroenterol 17:943, 2003.

182. Birnir B, Lee H, Hediger M, Wright E: Expression and characterization of the intestinal Na+/glucose contransporter n COS-7 cells. Biochim Biophys Acta 1048:100, 1990.

183. Umbach JA, Coady MJ, Wright EM: Intestinal Na+/glucose cotransporter expressed in Xenopus oocytes is electrogenic. Biophys J 57:1217, 1990.

184. Stevens BR, Fernandez A, Hirayama B, et al: Intestinal brush border membrane Na+/glucose cotransporter functions in situ as a homotetramer. Proc Natl Acad Sci U S A 87:1456, 1990.

185. Hediger MA, Coady MJ, Ikeda TS, Wright EM: Expression cloning and cDNA sequencing of the Na+/glucose cotransporter. Nature 330:379, 1987.

186. Turk E, Zabel B, Mundlos S, et al: Glucose/galactose malabsorption caused by a defect in the Na+/glucose cotransporter. Nature 350:354, 1991.

187. Wright EM, Hirsch JR, Loo DD, Zampighi GA: Regulation of Na+/glucose cotransporters. J Exp Biol 200:287, 1997.

188. Dyer J, Hosie KB, Shirazi-Beechey SP: Nutrient regulation of human intestinal sugar transporter (SGLT1) expression. Gut 41:56, 1997.

189. Kellet G: The facilitated component of intestinal glucose absorption. J Physiol 531:585, 2001.

190. Pappenheimer JR, Reiss KZ: Contribution of solvent drag through intercellular junctions to absorption of nutrients by the small intestine of the rat. J Membr Biol 100:123, 1987.

191. Ferraris RP, Diamond JM: Specific regulation of intestinal nutrient transporters by their dietary substrates. Annu Rev Physiol 51:125, 1989.

192. Kellett GL: The facilitated component of intestinal glucose absorption. J Physiol 531:585, 2001.

193. Burant CF, Takeda J, Brot-Laroche E, et al: Fructose transporter in human spermatozoa and small intestine is GLUT5. J Biol Chem 267:14523, 1992.

194. Thorens B: Facilitated glucose transporters in epithelial cells. Annu Rev Physiol 55:591, 1993.

195. Santer R, Steinmann B, Schaub J: Fanconi-Bickel syndrome—a congenital defect of facilitative glucose transport. Curr Mol Med 2:213, 2002.

196. Santer R, Hillebrand G, Steinmann B, Schaub J: Intestinal glucose transport: Evidence for a membrane traffic-based pathway in humans. Gastroenterology 124:34, 2003.

197. Samloff IM: Pepsins, peptic activity, and peptic inhibitors. J Clin Gastroenterol 3:91, 1981.

198. Nordstrom C: Release of enteropeptidase and other brush border enzymes from the small intestinal wall in the rat. Biochim Biophys Acta 289:376, 1972.

199. Nixon SE, Mawer GE: The digestion and absorption of protein in man. 2. The form in which digested protein is absorbed. Br J Nutr 24:241, 1970.

200. Adibi S: Glycyl-dipeptides: New substrates for protein nutrition. J Lab Clin Med 113:665, 1989.

201. Adibi S: Peptide absorption and hydrolysis. In Johnson L (ed): Physiology of the Gastrointestinal Tract. New York, Raven Press, 1981, p 1073.

202. Tobey N, Heizer W, Yeh R, et al: Human intestinal brush border peptidases. Gastroenterology 88:913, 1985.

203. Erickson R, Bella A, Brophy E: Purification and molecular characterization of rat intestinal brush border membrane dipeptidyl aminopeptidase IV. Biochim Biophys Acta 756:258, 1983.

204. Ferraci H, Maroux S: Rabbit intestinal amino peptidase N. Purification and molecular properties. Biochim Biophys Acta 448:599, 1980.

205. Erickson RH, Song IS, Yoshioka M, et al: Identification of proline-specific carboxypeptidase localized to brush border membrane of rat small intestine and its possible role in protein digestion. Dig Dis Sci 34:400, 1989.

206. Duggan KA, Mendelsohn FA, Levens NR: Angiotensin receptors and angiotensin I–converting enzyme in rat intestine. Am J Physiol 257:G504, 1989.

207. Ahnen D, Mircheff A, Santiago N: Intestinal surface amino-oligopeptidase. Distinct molecular forms during assembly in intracellular membranes in vivo. J Biol Chem 258:5960, 1983.

208. Danielson E, Cowell G, Noren O, Sjostrom H: Biosynthesis of microvillar proteins. Biochem J 221:1, 1984.

209. Kenny AJ, Maroux S: Topology of microvillar membrane hydrolases of kidney and intestine. Physiol Rev 62:91, 1982.

210. Doumeng C, Maroux S: Aminotripeptidase, a cytosol enzyme from rabbit intestinal mucosa. Biochem J 177:801, 1979.

211. Crampton RF, Gangolli SD, Simson P, Matthews DM: Rates of absorption by rat intestine of pancreatic hydrolysates of proteins and their corresponding amino acid mixtures. Clin Sci 41:409, 1971.

212. Silk D, Marrs T, Addison J: Absorption of amino acids from an amino acid mixture simulating casein and a tryptic hydrolysate of casein in man. Clin Sci Mol Med 45:715, 1973.

213. Asatoor A, Chadra A, Milne M, Prosser D: Intestinal absorption of sterioisomers of dipeptides in the rat. Clin Sci Mol Med 45:199, 1973.

214. Miyamoto Y, Thompson YG, Howard EF, et al: Functional expression of the intestinal peptide-proton co-transporter in Xenopus laevis oocytes. J Biol Chem 266:4742, 1991.

215. Liang R, Fei YJ, Prasad PD, et al: Human intestinal H+/peptide cotransporter. Cloning, functional expression, and chromosomal localization. J Biol Chem 270:6456, 1995.

216. Fei YJ, Kanai Y, Nussberger S, et al: Expression cloning of a mammalian proton-coupled oligopeptide transporter. Nature 368:563, 1994.

217. Amasheh S, Wenzel U, Boll M, et al: Transport of charged dipeptides by the intestinal H+/peptide symporter PepT1 expressed in Xenopus laevis oocytes. J Membr Biol 155:247, 1997.

218. Steel A, Nussberger S, Romero MF, et al: Stoichiometry and pH dependence of the rabbit proton-dependent oligopeptide transporter PepT1. J Physiol 498:563, 1997.

219. Leibach FH, Ganapathy V: Peptide transporters in the intestine and the kidney. Annu Rev Nutr 16:99, 1996.

220. Mackenzie B, Loo DD, Fei Y, et al: Mechanisms of the human intestinal H+-coupled oligopeptide transporter hPEPT1. J Biol Chem 271:5430, 1996.

221. Nussberger S, Steel A, Trotti D, et al: Symmetry of H+ binding to the intra- and extracellular side of the H+-coupled oligopeptide cotransporter PepT1. J Biol Chem 272:7777, 1997.

222. Adibi SA: Regulation of expression of the intestinal oligopeptide transporter (PepT-1) in health and disease. Am J Physiol Gastrointest Liver Physiol 285:G779, 2003.

223. Daniel H: Molecular and integrative physiology of intestinal peptide transport. Annu Rev Physiol 66:361, 2004.

224. Hediger MA, Romero MF, Peng JB, et al: The ABCs of solute carriers: Physiological, pathological and therapeutic implications of human membrane transport proteins. Introduction. Pflugers Arch 447:465, 2004.

225. Anderson CM, Grenade DS, Boll M, et al: H+/amino acid transporter 1 (PAT1) is the imino acid carrier: An intestinal nutrient/drug transporter in human and rat. Gastroenterology 127:1410, 2004.

226. Chen Z, Fei YJ, Anderson CM, et al: Structure, function and immunolocalization of a proton-coupled amino acid transporter (hPAT1) in the human intestinal cell line Caco-2. J Physiol 546:349, 2003.

227. Seow HF, Broer S, Broer A, et al: Hartnup disorder is caused by mutations in the gene encoding the neutral amino acid transporter SLC6A19. Nat Genet 36:1003, 2004.

228. Kleta R, Romeo E, Ristic Z, et al: Mutations in *SLC6A19*, encoding BOAT1, cause Hartnup disorder. Nat Genet 36:999, 2004.

229. Kanai Y, Hediger MA: The glutamate/neutral amino acid transporter family SLC1: Molecular, physiological and pharmacological aspects. Pflugers Arch 447:469, 2004.

230. Brandsch M, Miyamoto Y, Ganapathy V, Leibach FH: Expression and protein kinase C–dependent regulation of peptide/H+ co-transport system in the Caco-2 human colon carcinoma cell line. Biochem J 299:253, 1994.

231. Muller U, Brandsch M, Prasad PD, et al: Inhibition of the H+/peptide cotransporter in the human intestinal cell line Caco-2 by cyclic AMP. Biochem Biophys Res Commun 218:461, 1996.

232. Erickson RH, Gum JR Jr, Lindstrom MM, et al: Regional expression and dietary regulation of rat small intestinal peptide and amino acid transporter mRNAs. Biochem Biophys Res Commun 216:249, 1995.

233. Ganapathy V, Brandsch M, Leibach F: Intestinal transport of amino acids and peptides. In Johnson L (ed): Physiology of the Gastrointestinal Tract. New York, Raven Press, 1994, p 1782.

234. Chung YC, Kim YS, Shadchehr A, et al: Protein digestion and absorption in human small intestine. Gastroenterology 76:1415, 1979.

235. Siliprandi L, Vanni P, Kessler M, Semenza G: Na+-dependent, electroneural L-ascorbate transport across brush border membrane vesicles from guinea pig small intestine. Biochim Biophys Acta 552:129, 1979.

236. Tsukaguchi H, Tokui T, Mackenzie B, et al: A family of mammalian Na+-dependent L-ascorbic acid transporters. Nature 399:70, 1999.

237. Wang Y, Mackenzie B, Tsukaguchi H, et al: Human vitamin C (L-ascorbic acid) transporter SVCT1. Biochem Biophys Res Commun 267:488, 2000.

238. Liang WJ, Johnson D, Ma LS, et al: Regulation of the human vitamin C transporters expressed in COS-1 cells by protein kinase C [corrected]. Am J Physiol Cell Physiol 283:C1696, 2002.

239. Halsted C: The intestinal absorption of dietary folates in health and disease. J Am Coll Nutr 8:651, 1989.

240. Rosenberg IH: 1989 Herman Award lecture. Folate absorption: Clinical questions and metabolic answers. Am J Clin Nutr 51:531, 1990.

241. Devlin AM, Ling EH, Peerson JM, et al: Glutamate carboxypeptidase II: A polymorphism associated with lower levels of serum folate and hyperhomocysteinemia. Hum Mol Genet 9:2837, 2000.

242. Said HM, Chatterjee N, Haq RU, et al: Adaptive regulation of intestinal folate uptake: Effect of dietary folate deficiency. Am J Physiol Cell Physiol 279:C1889, 2000.

243. Schron CM, Washington C Jr, Blitzer BL: The transmembrane pH gradient drives uphill folate transport in rabbit jejunum. Direct evidence for folate/hydroxyl exchange in brush border membrane vesicles. J Clin Invest 76:2030, 1985.

244. Rong N, Selhub J, Goldin BR, Rosenberg IH: Bacterially synthesized folate in rat large intestine is incorporated into host tissue folyl polyglutamates. J Nutr 121:1955, 1991.

245. Seetharam B: Gastrointestinal absorption and transport of coobalamin. In Johnson L (ed): Physiology of the Gastrointestinal Tract, 3rd ed. New York, Raven Press, 1994, p 1997.

246. Marcoullis G, Parmentier Y, Nicolas JP, et al: Cobalamin malabsorption due to nondegradation of R proteins in the human intestine. Inhibited cobalamin absorption in exocrine pancreatic dysfunction. J Clin Invest 66:430, 1980.

247. Allen RH, Seetharam B, Podell E, Alpers DH: Effect of proteolytic enzymes on the binding of cobalamin to R protein and intrinsic factor. In vitro evidence that a failure to partially degrade R protein is responsible for cobalamin malabsorption in pancreatic insufficiency. J Clin Invest 61:47, 1978.

248. Kolhouse JF, Allen RH: Absorption, plasma transport, and cellular retention of cobalamin analogues in the rabbit. Evidence for the existence of multiple mechanisms that prevent the absorption and tissue dissemination of naturally occurring cobalamin analogues. J Clin Invest 60:1381, 1977.

249. Hagedorn C, Alpers D: Distribution of intrinsic factor vitamin B_{12} receptors in human intestine. Gastroenterology 73:1010, 1977.

250. Donaldson R, Small D, Robbins S, Mathan V: Receptors for vitamin B_{12} related to ileal surface area and absorptive capacity. Biochim Biophys Acta 311:477, 1973.

251. Robertson JA, Gallagher ND: Effect of placental lactogen on the number of intrinsic factor receptors in the pregnant mouse. Gastroenterology 77:511, 1979.

252. Rose R: Intestinal absorption of water soluble vitamins. In Johnson L (ed): Physiology of the Gastrointestinal Tract, 2nd ed. New York, Raven Press, 1987, p 1581.

253. Diaz GA, Banikazemi M, Oishi K, et al: Mutations in a new gene encoding a thiamine transporter cause thiamine-responsive megaloblastic anaemia syndrome. Nat Genet 22:309, 1999.

254. Labay V, Raz T, Baron D, et al: Mutations in *SLC19A2* cause thiamine-responsive megaloblastic anaemia associated with diabetes mellitus and deafness. Nat Genet 22:300, 1999.

255. Dutta B, Huang W, Molero M, et al: Cloning of the human thiamine transporter, a member of the folate transporter family. J Biol Chem 274:31925, 1999.

256. Rajgopal A, Edmondson A, Goldman ID, Zhao R: *SLC19A3* encodes a second thiamine transporter ThTr2. Biochim Biophys Acta 1537:175, 2001.

257. Basu TK, Donaldson D: Intestinal absorption in health and disease: Micronutrients. Best Pract Res Clin Gastroenterol 17:957, 2003.

258. Said HM, Ma TY, Grant K: Regulation of riboflavin intestinal uptake by protein kinase A: Studies with Caco-2 cells. Am J Physiol 267:G955, 1994.

259. Said HM, Ma TY: Mechanism of riboflavine uptake by Caco-2 human intestinal epithelial cells. Am J Physiol 266:G15, 1994.

260. Said HM: Cellular uptake of biotin: Mechanisms and regulation. J Nutr 129:490S, 1999.

261. Goodman DS, Blomstrand R, Werner B, et al: The intestinal absorption and metabolism of vitamin A and beta-carotene in man. J Clin Invest 45:1615, 1966.

262. Hollander D: Intestinal absorption of vitamins A, E, D, and K. J Lab Clin Med 97:449, 1981.

263. Hollander D, Rim E, Morgan D: Intestinal absorption of 25-hydroxyvitamin D_3 in unanesthetized rat. Am J Physiol 236:E441, 1979.

264. Hollander D, Muralidhara KS, Zimmerman A: Vitamin D_3 intestinal absorption in vivo: Influence of fatty acids, bile salts, and perfusate pH on absorption. Gut 19:267, 1978.

265. Hollander D, Rim E, Muralidhara KS: Mechanism and site of small intestinal absorption of alpha-tocopherol in the rat. Gastroenterology 68:1492, 1975.

266. Nakamura T, Aoyama Y, Fujita T, Katsui G: Studies on tocopherol derivatives: V. Intestinal absorption of several d,1-3,4-$^3H_2$-alpha-tocopheryl esters in the rat. Lipids 10:627, 1975.

267. Hollander D: Vitamin K_1 absorption by everted intestinal sacs of the rat. Am J Physiol 225:360, 1973.

268. Hollander D, Rim E, Ruble PE Jr: Vitamin K_2 colonic and ileal in vivo absorption: Bile, fatty acids, and pH effects on transport. Am J Physiol 233:E124, 1977.

269. Armbrecht H: Effect of age and the milk sugar lactose on calcium absorption by the small intestine. Adv Exp Med Biol 249:185, 1989.

270. Wasserman RH, Fullmer CS: Vitamin D and intestinal calcium transport: Facts, speculations and hypotheses. J Nutr 125:1971S, 1995.

271. Bronner F: Intestinal calcium transport: The cellular pathway. Miner Electrolyte Metab 16:94, 1990.

272. Calcium phosphate and magnesium absorption. In Johnson L (ed): Physiology of the Gastrointestinal Tract, 3rd ed. New York, Raven Press, 1994, p 2175.

273. Krejs GJ, Nicar MJ, Zerwekh JE, et al: Effect of 1,25-dihydroxyvitamin D_3 on calcium and magnesium absorption in the healthy human jejunum and ileum. Am J Med 75:973, 1983.

274. Karbach U: Segmental heterogeneity of cellular and paracellular calcium transport across the rat duodenum and jejunum. Gastroenterology 100:47, 1991.

275. Madara JL: Loosening tight junctions. Lessons from the intestine. J Clin Invest 83:1089, 1989.

276. Feher JJ: Facilitated calcium diffusion by intestinal calcium-binding protein. Am J Physiol 244:C303, 1983.

277. Carafoli E, James P, Strehler E: Structure-function relationship in the calcium pump of plasma membrane. In Peterlik M, Bronner R (eds): Molecular and Cellular Regulation of Calcium and Phosphate Metabolism. New York, Wiley-Liss 1990, p 181.

278. Bronner F, Pansu D: Nutritional aspects of calcium absorption. J Nutr 129:9, 1999.

279. Walters JR, Weiser MM: Calcium transport by rat duodenal villus and crypt basolateral membranes. Am J Physiol 252:G170, 1987.

280. Favus MJ, Kathpalia SC, Coe FL: Kinetic characteristics of calcium absorption and secretion by rat colon. Am J Physiol 240:G350, 1981.

281. Hylander E, Ladefoged K, Jarnum S: Calcium absorption after intestinal resection. The importance of a preserved colon. Scand J Gastroenterol 25:705, 1990.

282. Freund T, Bronner F: Regulation of intestinal calcium-binding protein calcium intake in the rat. Am J Physiol 228:861, 1975.

283. Karbach U, Rummel W: Cellular and paracellular magnesium transport across the terminal ileum of the rat and its interaction with the calcium transport. Gastroenterology 98:985, 1990.

284. Cox T, Mazurier G, Spik G: Iron binding proteins and influx across the duodenal brush border. Evidence for specific lactotransferrin receptors in human intestine. Biochim Biophys Acta 588:120, 1969.

285. Davidson LA, Lonnerdal B: Fe-saturation and proteolysis of human lactoferrin: Effect on brush-border receptor–mediated uptake of Fe and Mn. Am J Physiol 257:G930, 1989.

286. Conrad M: Iron absorption. In Johnson L (ed): Physiology of the Gastrointestinal Tract, 2nd ed. New York, Raven Press, 1987, p 1437.

287. Riedel HD, Remus AJ, Fitscher BA, Stremmel W: Characterization and partial purification of a ferrireductase from human duodenal microvillus membrane. Biochem J 309:745, 1995.

288. Wessling-Resnick M: Iron transport. Annu Rev Nutr 20:129, 2000.

289. Nunez MT, Alvarez X, Smith M, et al: Role of redox systems on Fe^{3+} uptake by transformed human intestinal epithelial (Caco-2) cells. Am J Physiol 267:C1582, 1997.

290. Parkkila S, Niemela O, Britton RS, et al: Molecular aspects of iron absorption and HFE expression. Gastroenterology 121:1489, 2001.

291. Andrews N: Disorders of iron metabolism. N Engl J Med 341:1986, 1999.

292. Gunshin H, Mackenzie B Berger UV, et al: Cloning and characterization of a mammalian proton-coupled metal-ion transporter. Nature 388:482, 1997.

293. Bacon B: Hemochromatosis: Diagnosis and management. Gastroenterology 120:718, 2001.

294. Parmley R, Barton J, Conrad M: Ultrastructural cytochemistry and radio-autography of hemoglobin iron absorption. Exp Mol Pathol 34:131, 1991.

295. Raffin SB, Woo CH, Roost KT, et al: Intestinal absorption of hemoglobin iron—heme cleavage by mucosal heme oxygenase. J Clin Invest 54:1344, 1974.

296. Simpson R, Raja K, Peters T: Mechanisms of intestinal brush border iron transport. Adv Exp Med Biol 149:27, 1989.

297. Umbreit JN, Conrad ME, Moore EG, Latour LF: Iron aborption and cellular transport: The mobilferrin/paraferritin paradigm. Semin Hematol 35:13, 1998.

298. Sandstrom B: Factors influencing the uptake of trace elements from the digestive tract. Proc Nutr Soc 47:161, 1988.

299. Taylor CM, Bacon JR, Aggett PJ, Bremner I: Homeostatic regulation of zinc absorption and endogenous losses in zinc-deprived men. Am J Clin Nutr 53:755, 1991.

300. Tacnet F, Watkins D, Ripoche P: Studies of zinc transport into brush border membrane vesicles isolated from pig small intestine. Biochim Biophys Acta 1024:323, 1990.

301. Krebs N: Overview of zinc absorption and excretion in the human gastrointestinal tract. J Nutr 130:1374S, 2000.

302. McMahon R, Cousins RJ: Mammalian zinc transporters. J Nutr 128:667, 1998.

303. McMahon R, Cousins RJ: Regulation of the zinc transporter ZnT-1 by dietary zinc. Proc Natl Acad Sci U S A 95:4841, 1998.

304. Menard MP, McCormick CC, Cousins RJ: Regulation of intestinal metallothionein biosynthesis in rats by dietary zinc. J Nutr 111:1353, 1981.

305. Steel L, Cousins RJ: Kinetics of zinc absorption by luminally and vascularly perfused rat intestine. Am J Physiol 248:G46, 1985.

306. Davies NT, Williams RB: The effect of pregnancy and lactation on the absorption of zinc and lysine by the rat duodenum in situ. Br J Nutr 38:417, 1977.

307. Davis SM, McMahon RJ, Cousins RJ: Metallothionein knockout and transgenic mice exhibit altered intestinal processing of zinc with uniform zinc-dependent zinc transporter-1 expression. J Nutr 128:825, 1998.

308. Stuart MA, Johnson PE: Copper absorption and copper balance during consecutive periods for rats fed varying levels of dietary copper. J Nutr 116:1028, 1986.

309. Davies T, Williams R: The effects of pregnancy on uptake and distribution of copper in the rat. Proc Nutr Soc 35:4A, 1976.

310. Zhou B, Gitschier J: hCTR1: A human gene for copper uptake identified by complementation in yeast. Proc Natl Acad Sci U S A 94:7481, 1997.

311. Pena M, Lee J, Thiele DJ: A delicate balance: Homeostatic control of copper uptake and distribution. J Nutr 129:1251, 1999.

312. Prohaska JR, Gybina AA: Intracellular copper transport in mammals. J Nutr 134:1003, 2004.

313. Chelly J, Tumer Z, Tonnesen T: Isolation of a candidate gene for Menkes disease that encodes a potential heavy metal binding protein. Nat Genet 3:14, 1993.

314. Rucker R, Lonnerdal B, Keen C: Intestinal absorption of nutritionally important trace elements. In Johnson L (ed): Physiology of the Gastrointestinal Tract, 3rd ed. New York, Raven Press, 1994, p 2195.

315. Yan G, Ge K, Chen J, Chen X: Selenium-related endemic diseases and the daily requirements of humans. World Rev Nutr Diet 55:98, 1988.

316. Thomson CD, Rea HM, Doesburg VM, Robinson MF: Selenium concentrations and glutathione peroxidase activities in whole blood of New Zealand residents. Br J Nutr 37:457, 1977.

317. Reasbeck PG, Barbezat GO, Weber FL Jr, et al: Selenium absorption by canine jejunum. Dig Dis Sci 30:489, 1985.

318. Heubi JE, Fellows JL: Postnatal development of intestinal bile salt transport. Relationship to membrane physico-chemical changes. J Lipid Res 26:797, 1985.

319. Cripps AW, Williams VJ: The effect of pregnancy and lactation on food intake, gastrointestinal anatomy and the absorptive capacity of the small intestine in the albino rat. Br J Nutr 33:17, 1975.

320. Olsen WA, Rosenberg IH: Intestinal transport of sugars and amino acids in diabetic rats. J Clin Invest 49:96, 1970.

321. Jacobs L, Dowling R: Intestinal adaptation to hypothermic hyperphagia. Clin Sci Mol Med 48:14, 1975.

322. Thiesen A, Drozdowski L, Iordache C, et al: Adaptation following intestinal resection: Mechanisms and signals. Best Pract Res Clin Gastroenterol 17:981, 2003.

323. Ferraris RP, Carey HV: Intestinal transport during fasting and malnutrition. Annu Rev Nutr 20:195, 2000.

324. Weser E, Heller R, Tawil T: Stimulation of mucosal growth in the rat ileum by bile and pancreatic secretions after jejunal resection. Gastroenterology 73:524, 1977.

325. Bloom S, Polak J: The hormonal pattern of intestinal adaptation: A major role for enteroglucagon. Scand J Gastroenterol 115:2176, 1984.

326. Johnson LR: The trophic action of gastrointestinal hormones. Gastroenterology 70:278, 1976.

327. Goodlad RA, Wilson TJ, Lenton W, et al: Intravenous but not intragastric urogastrone-EGF is trophic to the intestine of parenterally fed rats. Gut 28:573, 1987.

328. Lund PK, Ulshen MH, Rountree DB, et al: Molecular biology of gastrointestinal peptides and growth factors: Relevance to intestinal adaptation. Digestion 46:66, 1990.

329. Dowling RH: Polyamines in intestinal adaptation and disease. Digestion 46:331, 1990.

330. Bamba T, Vaja S, Murphy GM, Dowling RH: Effect of fasting and feeding on polyamines and related enzymes along the villus:crypt axis. Digestion 46:424, 1990.

331. Johnson L: Regulation of gastrointestinal growth. In Johnson L (ed): Physiology of the Gastrointestinal Tract, 2nd ed. New York, Raven Press, 1987, p 301.

332. Scheele G: Regulation of gene expression in the exocrine pancreas. In Go V, Brooks F, DiMagno E, et al (eds): The Exocrine Pancreas, Biology, Pathobiology, and Diseases. New York, Raven Press, 1986, p 55.

333. Rausch U, Rudiger K, Vasiloudes P, et al: Lipase synthesis in the rat pancreas is regulated by secretin. Pancreas 1:522, 1986.

334. Borel P, Armand M, Senft M, et al: Gastric lipase: Evidence of an adaptive response to dietary fat in the rabbit. Gastroenterology 100:1582, 1991.

335. Renaud W, Giorgi D, Iovanna J, Dagorn JC: Regulation of concentrations of mRNA for amylase, trypsinogen I and chymotrypsinogen B in rat pancreas by secretagogues. Biochem J 235:305, 1986.

336. Goda T, Koldivsky O: Dietary regulation of small intestinal disaccharidases. World Rev Nutr Diet 57:275, 1988.

337. Flatz G: Genetics of lactose digestion in humans. Adv Human Gen 177:487, 1987.

338. Diamond J: Evolutionary design of intestinal nutrient absorption: Enough but not too much. Persp News Physiolol Sci 6:92, 1991.

339. Solberg DH, Diamond JM: Comparison of different dietary sugars as inducers of intestinal sugar transporters. Am J Physiol 252:G574, 1987.

340. Stein ED, Chang SD, Diamond JM: Comparison of different dietary amino acids as inducers of intestinal amino acid transport. Am J Physiol 252:G626, 1987.

341. Maenz D, Cheeseman C: Effect of hyperglycemia on D-glucose transport across the brush border and basolateral membranes of rat small intestine. Biochim Biophys Acta 860:277, 1986.

342. Hernell O: Specificity of human milk bile salt–stimulated lipase. J Pediatr Gastroenterol Nutr 4:517, 1985.

343. Thiesen A, Wild GE, Tappenden KA, et al: The locally acting glucocorticosteroid budesonide enhances intestinal sugar uptake following intestinal resection in rats. Gut 52:252, 2003.

344. Thiesen AL, Tappenden KA, McBurney MI, et al: Dietary lipids alter the effect of steroids on the transport of glucose after intestinal resection: Part I. Phenotypic changes and expression of transporters. J Pediatr Surg 38:150, 2003.

345. Diamond JM, Karasov WH, Cary C, et al: Effect of dietary carbohydrate on monosaccharide uptake by mouse small intestine in vitro. J Physiol 349:419, 1984.

346. Thompson JS: Can the intestine adapt to a changing environment? Gastroenterology 113:1402, 1997.

347. Ulshen MH, Dowling RH, Fuller CR, et al: Enhanced growth of small bowel in transgenic mice overexpressing bovine growth hormone. Gastroenterology 104:973, 1993.

348. Iannoli P, Miller JH, Ryan CK, et al: Human growth hormone induces system B transport in short bowel syndrome. J Surg Res 69:150, 1997.

349. Szkudlarek J, Jeppesen PB, Mortensen PB: Effect of high dose growth hormone with glutamine and no change in diet on intestinal absorption in short bowel patients: A randomised, double blind, crossover, placebo controlled study. Gut 47:199, 2000.

350. Scolapio JS, Camilleri M, Fleming CR, et al: Effect of growth hormone, glutamine, and diet on adaptation in short-bowel syndrome: A randomized, controlled study. Gastroenterology 113:1074, 1997.

351. Byrne TA, Persinger RL, Young LS, et al: A new treatment for patients with short-bowel syndrome. Growth hormone, glutamine, and a modified diet. Ann Surg 222:243, 1995.

352. Scott RB, Kirk D, MacNaughton WK, Meddings JB: GLP-2 augments the adaptive response to massive intestinal resection in rat. Am J Physiol 275:G911, 1998.

353. Jeppesen PB, Hartmann B, Thulesen J, et al: Glucagon-like peptide 2 improves nutrient absorption and nutritional status in short-bowel patients with no colon. Gastroenterology 120:806, 2001.

354. Britton J, Koldovsky O: Development of luminal protein digestion: Implications for biologically active dietary polypeptides. J Paed Gastroenterol Nutr 9:144, 1989.

355. Scheele G, Kern H: Selective regulation of gene expression in the exocrine pancreas. In Schultz S (ed): Handbook of Physiology: The Gastrointestinal System, Section 6. Vol 1, Part 2. Bethesda, American Physiological Society, 1989, p 499.

356. Kien C, Heitlinger L, Li B, Murray R: Digestion, absorption, and fermentation of carbohydrates. Semin Pernatol 13:78, 1989.

357. Troelsen JT, Olsen J, Moller J, Sjostrom H: An upstream polymorphism associated with lactase persistence has increased enhancer activity. Gastroenterology 125:1686, 2003.

358. Wang Y, Harvey CB, Pratt WS, et al: The lactase persistence/non-persistence polymorphism is controlled by a cis-acting element. Hum Mol Genet 4:657, 1995.

359. Fang R, Santiago NA, Olds LC, Sibley E: The homeodomain protein Cdx2 regulates lactase gene promoter activity during enterocyte differentiation. Gastroenterology 118:115, 2000.

360. Enattah NS, Sahi T, Savilahti E, et al: Identification of a variant associated with adult-type hypolactasia. Nat Genet 30:233, 2002.

361. Kuokkanen M, Enattah NS, Oksanen A, et al: Transcriptional regulation of the lactase–phlorizin hydrolase gene by polymorphisms associated with adult-type hypolactasia. Gut 52:647, 2003.

362. Zoppi G, Andreotti G, Pajno-Ferrara F, et al: Exocrine pancreas function in premature and full term neonates. Pediatr Res 6:880, 1972.

363. Moreau H, Laugier R, Gargouri Y, et al: Human preduodenal lipase is entirely of gastric fundic origin. Gastroenterology 95:1221, 1988.

364. Antonowicz I, Lebenthal E: Developmental pattern of small intestinal enterokinase and disaccharidase activities in the human fetus. Gastroenterology 72:1299, 1977.

365. Korychka-Dahl M, Ribadeau D, Chene N, Martal J: Plasmin activity in milk. J Dairy Sci 66:704, 1983.

366. McGilligan KM, Thomas DW, Eckhert CD: Alpha-1-antitrypsin concentration in human milk. Pediatr Res 22:268, 1987.

367. Udall JN, Walker WA: The physiologic and pathologic basis for the transport of macromolecules across the intestinal tract. J Pediatr Gastroenterol Nutr 1:295, 1982.

368. Gibney MJ, Gibney ER: Diet, genes and disease: implications for nutrition policy. Proc Nutr Soc 63:491, 2004.

369. Weinberg RB: Apolipoprotein A-IV polymorphisms and diet-gene interactions. Curr Opin Lipidol 13:125, 2002.

370. Meirhaeghe A, Martin G, Nemoto M, et al: Intronic polymorphism in the fatty acid transport protein 1 gene is associated with increased plasma triglyceride levels in a French population. Arterioscler Thromb Vasc Biol 20:1330, 2000.

371. Zhang EY, Fu DJ, Pak YA, et al: Genetic polymorphisms in human proton-dependent dipeptide transporter PEPT1: Implications for the functional role of Pro586. J Pharmacol Exp Ther 310:437, 2004.

372. Flancbaum L: Mechanisms of weight loss after bariatric surgery. J Laparoendosc Adv Surg Tech A 13:215, 2003.

373. O'Leary JP: Gastrointestinal malabsorptive procedures. Am J Clin Nutr 55:567S, 1992.

374. Fruhbeck G, Rotellar F, Hernandez-Lizoain JL, Gil MJ, et al: Fasting plasma ghrelin concentrations 6 months after gastric bypass are not determined by weight loss or changes in insulinemia. Obes Surg 14:1208, 2004.

375. Flancbaum L, Choban PS, Bradley LR, Burge JC: Changes in measured resting energy expenditure after Roux-en-Y gastric bypass for clinically severe obesity. Surgery 122:943, 1997.

376. Atkinson RL, Brent EL, Wagner BS, Whipple JH: Energy balance and regulation of body weight after intestinal bypass surgery in rats. Am J Physiol 245:R658, 1983.

377. Sugerman HJ, Londrey GL, Kellum JM, et al: Weight loss with vertical banded gastroplasty and Roux-Y gastric bypass for morbid obesity with selective versus random assignment. Am J Surg 157:93, 1989.

378. Kellum JM, Kuemmerle JF, O'Dorisio TM, et al: Gastrointestinal hormone responses to meals before and after gastric bypass and vertical banded gastroplasty. Ann Surg 211:763, 1990.

379. Brolin RL, Robertson LB, Kenler HA, Cody RP: Weight loss and dietary intake after vertical banded gastroplasty and Roux-en-Y gastric bypass. Ann Surg 220:782, 1994.

380. Teixeira FV: Ghrelin and gastric bypass. Obes Surg 14:1283, 2004.

381. Batterham RL, Cohen MA, Ellis SM, et al: Inhibition of food intake in obese subjects by peptide YY3-36. N Engl J Med 349:941, 2003.

382. Ockander L, Hedenbro JL, Rehfeld JF, Sjolund K: Jejunoileal bypass changes the duodenal cholecystokinin and somatostatin cell density. Obes Surg 13:584, 2003.

CHAPTER

98 Maldigestion and Malabsorption

Christoph Högenauer and Heinz F. Hammer

In the past, it was believed that most malabsorptive diseases manifested clinically with diarrhea and steatorrhea. It is now recognized that many malabsorptive disorders, such as celiac disease, may have subtle clinical presentations. An extraintestinal manifestation of malabsorption, such as anemia, bone loss, or menstrual disturbance, may even be the presenting symptom. In other cases, gastrointestinal symptoms, such as bloating or changes in bowel habits, may be subtle, so that other much more common disorders such as irritable bowel syndrome may be diagnosed erroneously. Awareness also is increasing that subtle malabsorption of single nutrients, such as calcium or vitamin B$_{12}$, may, if unrecognized, lead to complications that may be difficult to reverse or that may not be reversible at all. Therefore, the clinical challenge today is to recognize and treat malabsorption despite its subtle manifestations.

Classically, *maldigestion* is defined as defective hydrolysis of nutrients, and *malabsorption* is defined as defective mucosal absorption. Although this distinction may be useful on pathophysiologic grounds, the clinical presentation and complications of maldigestion and of malabsorption are similar. Moreover, physiologic processes other than digestion and absorption, such as solubilization, intestinal motility, or hormone secretion, contribute to the normal absorption of nutrients, vitamins, and minerals. Therefore, the classic definitions of maldigestion and malabsorption do not cover the pathophysiologic spectrum of the malabsorption syndrome.

In this chapter, the terms *digestion* and *absorption*, or *maldigestion* and *malabsorption*, are used separately only in the discussion of pathophysiology. When the distinction between these terms is not of clinical relevance, only the terms *absorption* and *malabsorption* are used.

Table 98–1 Diseases Causing Nutrient Malabsorption

Gastric Diseases
Autoimmune gastritis (pernicious anemia)
Atrophic gastritis
Gastric resection
Pancreatic Diseases
Pancreatic insufficiency
  Chronic pancreatitis
  Cystic fibrosis
  Johanson-Blizzard syndrome
  Pearson's marrow-pancreas syndrome
  Shwachman's syndrome
Congenital pancreatic enzyme deficiencies
  Colipase deficiency
  Lipase deficiency
  Trypsinogen deficiency
Pancreatic tumors
Liver Diseases
Inborn errors of bile acid biosynthesis and transport
Cirrhosis
Parenchymal liver diseases
Portal hypertension
Obstructive Biliary Diseases
Biliary tumors
Primary and secondary sclerosing cholangitis
Primary biliary cirrhosis
Intestinal Diseases
Amyloidosis
Autoimmune enteropathy
Bacterial overgrowth syndrome
Celiac sprue
Collagenous sprue
Congenital enterocyte defects (see Table 98-14)
Crohn's disease
Enterokinase deficiency
Eosinophilic gastroenteritis
Fistulas
Food allergy
Graft-versus-host disease
Hypolactasia
Ileal bile acid malabsorption
Intestinal infections
  AIDS (HIV infection)
    Cryptosporidiosis
    Mycobacterium-avium-complex
    Viral infections
  Giardiasis

Helminthic infections
Tuberculosis
Whipple's disease
Intestinal ischemia
Intestinal lymphoma
Intestinal resections or bypass
Immune dysregulation–polyendocrinopathy–enteropathy–
  X-linked syndrome (IPEX)
Immunoproliferative small intestinal disease (IPSID)
Mastocytosis
Microvillus inclusion disease
Nongranulomatous chronic idiopathic enterocolitis
Primary immunodeficiency diseases
Postinfectious malabsorption
Radiation enteritis
Refractory sprue
Sarcoidosis
Tropical sprue
Tufting enteropathy
Lymphatic Disease
Intestinal lymphangiectasia
  Primary
  Secondary
    Lymphoma
    Solid tumors
    Trauma, damage, or obstruction to thoracic duct
Neuroendocrine Tumors
  Carcinoid syndrome
  Glucagonoma
  Somatostatinoma syndrome
  Zollinger-Ellison syndrome
Cardiac and Vascular Diseases
Congestive heart failure
Constrictive pericarditis
Endocrine Causes
Addison's disease
Autoimmune polyglandular syndrome type 1
Diabetes mellitus
Hyperthyroidism
Systemic Diseases
Cronkhite-Canada syndrome
Mixed connective tissue disease (MCTD)
Neurofibromatosis type 1
Protein-calorie malnutrition
Scleroderma
Systemic lupus erythematosus

AIDS, acquired immunodeficiency syndrome; HIV, human immunodeficiency virus.

Malabsorption can be caused by many diseases of the small bowel and also by diseases of the pancreas, the liver, the biliary tract, and the stomach (Table 98–1). Whereas in some of these diseases malabsorption may be the presenting feature, in others malabsorption may be only a minor clinical problem or may be detected only as a laboratory abnormality.

This chapter provides an overview of basic pathophysiologic mechanisms leading to symptoms or complications of maldigestion or malabsorption; reviews the clinical manifestations and complications of malabsorption; describes tests that can be used clinically to evaluate digestive and absorptive function and provides a rational diagnostic approach to the individual patient; and discusses malabsorptive diseases and general meas-

ures in the treatment of malabsorption syndrome that are not covered in other chapters of this book.

ETIOLOGY AND PATHOPHYSIOLOGY

From a pathophysiologic point of view, mechanisms causing malabsorption can be divided into premucosal (luminal) factors, mucosal factors, and postmucosal factors (vascular and lymphatic). For clinical purposes, this approach is of limited value, because the various clinical pictures caused by malabsorption syndromes are determined mainly by the nature of the substrates malabsorbed. We therefore discuss the mechanisms causing malabsorption on the basis of the malabsorbed substrate. A separate section is devoted to the role of mechanisms compensating for the consequences of malabsorption.

Normal uptake of nutrients, vitamins, and minerals by the gastrointestinal tract requires several steps, each of which can be compromised in disease. (Normal digestion and absorption are discussed in Chapter 97.) These steps are as follows:

Solubilization is a prerequisite for the absorption of nutrients like fat or calcium. Fat and fat-soluble vitamins are solubilized by the formation of micelles, and calcium is solubilized through acidification of the gastrointestinal lumen. Alternatively, increased solubilization of the components of intestinal chyme may contribute to the manifestations of gastrointestinal diseases (e.g., increased absorption of oxalate, which may result in the development of kidney stones in patients with short bowel syndrome).

Digestion of macromolecular compounds, such as polysaccharides, triglycerides, and proteins, to their molecular components, such as monosaccharides, fatty acids, and amino acids, respectively, is achieved by soluble or membrane-bound digestive enzymes. Absorption of undigested or partially digested macromolecular compounds occurs to a very minor degree in health and may be increased slightly in various intestinal diseases. Although such absorption does not play a nutritive role, it may be important for the normal function of the immune system and for the pathogenesis of diseases such as food allergy (see Chapter 19).

Liberation of substrate, such as vitamin B_{12}, from binding sites in food or, conversely, *binding* to factors such as intrinsic factor allows absorption to take place.

Chemical changes to nutrients may be required for absorption, such as changing the charge of iron.

Mucosal absorption may occur by active or passive carrier-mediated transport or by diffusion.

Postmucosal transport of absorbed substrates also is important.

Intestinal sensory and motor function permits detection of the presence of nutrients, facilitates adequate mixing of nutrients with intestinal secretions and delivery to absorptive sites, and provides adequate time for nutrient absorption (see Chapter 94).

Neural and hormonal functions are required to stimulate and coordinate digestive secretions, mucosal absorption, and intestinal motility.

An overview of pathophysiologic mechanisms of maldigestion and malabsorption is provided in Table 98–2. This table also shows the ingested substrates primarily affected by the individual pathophysiologic mechanisms and lists examples of etiologic disorders for these mechanisms.

FAT MALABSORPTION

Defective Mixing

For sufficient digestion and absorption of lipids, dietary fat must adequately mix with digestive secretions. Gastric resections or gastrointestinal motility disorders that result in rapid gastric emptying or rapid intestinal transit, such as autonomic neuropathy due to diabetes mellitus or amyloidosis, may cause fat malabsorption consequent to impaired gastrointestinal mixing of dietary fat.[1]

Reduced Solubilization of Fat

Fat malabsorption due to decreased micelle formation occurs if the luminal concentrations of conjugated bile acids are lower than the critical concentration required for micelle formation.[2,3] Table 98–3[1,4] shows causes of luminal bile acid deficiency.

Decreased Lipolysis (Lipid Hydrolysis)

If exocrine pancreatic function is severely reduced, impairment of pancreatic lipase and colipase secretion results in decreased luminal hydrolysis of dietary fat.[5] Chronic pancreatitis, cystic fibrosis, pancreatic duct obstruction by pancreatic and ampullary tumors, and pancreatic resections are the most common causes of pancreatic insufficiency.[1] Even when pancreatic enzyme concentrations are normal, reduced pancreatic lipase *activity* due to a low luminal pH,[6] excessive calcium ingestion,[7] or the specific lipase inhibitor orlistat[8] may cause pancreatic steatorrhea. Finally, selective congenital lipase or colipase deficiency is a rare cause of pancreatic fat malabsorption.[9]

Decreased Mucosal Absorption and Chylomicron Formation

Generalized mucosal diseases, such as celiac disease or tropical sprue, often are associated with fat malabsorption. Defective uptake of free fatty acids and monoglycerides is due to a reduction of the mucosal surface area secondary to villus shortening, reduced enterocyte function, and mucosal inflammation.[1] Intestinal fat absorption also is impaired in diseases that result in disturbance of intracellular formation of chylomicrons and accumulation of lipids within the enterocytes, as in abetalipoproteinemia, hypobetalipoproteinemia, and chylomicron retention disease.[10]

Defective Lymphatic Transport of Chylomicrons

Impairment of lymphatic transport of chylomicrons is a cause for postmucosal malabsorption of dietary fat. Decreased lymphatic transport can result from congenital diseases such as primary intestinal lymphangiectasia or from obstruction of lymphatic vessels due to metastatic solid tumors, lymphoma, Whipple's disease, retroperitoneal fibrosis, or trauma[6] (see Chapter 27). Usually, lymphatic vessels in the mucosa become dilated (lymphangiectasia), and chylomicrons are lost into the intestinal lumen postprandially and also in the fasting state[11]; steatorrhea in these situations usually is only mild to moderate.[1]

PROTEIN AND AMINO ACID MALABSORPTION

Defective absorption and/or digestion of dietary proteins has to be differentiated from excessive loss of serum proteins into the gastrointestinal tract, which is termed *protein-losing enteropathy* (see Chapter 27).

Table 98–2 Pathophysiologic Mechanisms of Malabsorption, with Affected Substrates and Representative Etiologic Disorders

Mechanism	Malabsorbed Substrate(s)*	Examples of Etiologic Disorders
Maldigestion		
Conjugated bile acid deficiency	**Fat** **Fat-soluble vitamins** **Calcium** Magnesium	Hepatic parenchymal disease Biliary obstruction Bacterial overgrowth with bile acid deconjugation Ileal bile acid malabsorption CCK deficiency
Pancreatic insufficiency	**Fat** **Protein** **Carbohydrate** Fat-soluble vitamins Vitamin B_{12} (cobalamin)	Congenital defects Chronic pancreatitis Pancreatic tumors Inactivation of pancreatic enzymes (e.g., Zollinger-Ellison syndrome)
Reduced mucosal digestion	**Carbohydrate** Protein	Congenital defects (see Table 98–14) Acquired lactase deficiency Generalized mucosal disease (e.g., celiac sprue, Crohn's disease)
Intraluminal consumption of nutrients	**Vitamin B_{12}** (cobalamin)	Bacterial overgrowth Helminthic infections (e.g., *Diphyllobothrium latum* infection)
Malabsorption		
Reduced mucosal absorption	**Fat** **Protein** **Carbohydrate** **Vitamins** **Minerals**	Congenital transport defects (see Table 98-14) Generalized mucosal diseases (e.g., celiac sprue, Crohn's disease) Previous intestinal resection or bypass Infections Intestinal lymphoma
Decreased transport from the intestine	**Fat** **Protein**	Intestinal lymphangiectasia Primary Secondary (e.g., solid tumors, Whipple's disease, or lymphomas) Venous stasis (e.g., with congestive heart failure)
Other Mechanisms		
Decreased gastric acid and/or intrinsic factor secretion	**Vitamin B_{12}**	Pernicious anemia Atrophic gastritis Previous gastric resection
Decreased gastric mixing and/or rapid gastric emptying	Fat Calcium Protein	Previous gastric resection Autonomic neuropathy
Rapid intestinal transit	Fat	Autonomic neuropathy Hyperthyroidism

*Substrates in **boldface** are those mainly affected.
CCK, cholecystokinin.

Table 98–3 Pathophysiologic Mechanisms Resulting in Deficiency of Luminal Conjugated Bile Acids

Pathophysiologic Mechanism	Disease(s)
Decreased synthesis and/or secretion of conjugated bile acids	Parenchymal liver diseases (e.g., cirrhosis) Biliary obstruction (e.g., primary biliary cirrhosis, tumors) Biliary fistulas Inborn errors of bile acid synthesis CCK deficiency
Intestinal loss of conjugated bile acids	Ileal resection Severe ileal mucosal disease Congenital defects of the ileal sodium–bile acid cotransporter
Luminal deconjugation of bile acids	Bacterial overgrowth
Binding of bile salts or insolubilization of bile salts due to low luminal pH	Cholestyramine (binding) Zollinger-Ellison syndrome (low pH) Exocrine pancreatic insufficiency (low pH)

Data from Wilson FA, Dietschy JM: Differential diagnostic approach to clinical problems of malabsorption. Gastroenterology 61:911, 1971; and Oelkers P, Kirby LC, Heubi JE, et al: Primary bile acid malabsorption caused by mutations in the ileal sodium-dependent bile acid transporter gene (*SLC10A2*). J Clin Invest 99:1880, 1997.
CCK, cholecystokinin.

Defective Intraluminal Proteolysis (Protein Hydrolysis)

Protein digestion may be impaired in patients who have undergone partial or total gastric resection,[12] presumably as a result of poor mixing with digestive secretions, although gastric pepsin deficiency could be contributory. Defective proteolysis also occurs with exocrine pancreatic insufficiency.[1,13,14] In congenital diseases, pancreatic proteolysis can be impaired either by inborn errors in synthesis of proteolytic enzymes (trypsinogen deficiency)[14] or by defective activation of pancreatic proenzymes due to congenital deficiency of intestinal enterokinase (see below).[15]

Defective Mucosal Hydrolysis of Peptides and Decreased Absorption of Oligopeptides and Amino Acids

Generalized mucosal diseases, such as celiac disease and tropical sprue, result in global malabsorption, which includes malabsorption of oligopeptides and amino acids due to lack of mucosal hydrolysis of oligopeptides and defective mucosal absorption.[14] Reduction of intestinal absorptive surface, as in short bowel syndrome or jejunoileal bypass, also results in protein and amino acid malabsorption.[14,16] Congenital defects of amino acid transporters on the enterocytes (e.g., Hartnup's disease, lysinuric protein intolerance) can lead to selective malabsorption of a subgroup of amino acids (see later on).

CARBOHYDRATE MALABSORPTION

Defective Intraluminal Hydrolysis of Carbohydrates

Pancreatic α-amylase normally is secreted in excess into the intestinal lumen. In mild forms of pancreatic insufficiency, carbohydrate digestion usually is at least partially preserved,[17] whereas severe pancreatic insufficiency results in clinically apparent carbohydrate malabsorption and diarrhea due to decreased luminal hydrolysis of ingested starch.[18]

Mucosal Defects of Carbohydrate Digestion and Absorption

The most common cause of carbohydrate malabsorption is late-onset lactose malabsorption due to decreased levels of the intestinal brush border enzyme lactase (adult-type hypolactasia, acquired primary lactase deficiency). Depending on ethnic background, lactase is present in less than 5% to more than 90% of the adult population; its deficiency results in a selective malabsorption of lactose. Acquired malabsorption of carbohydrates occurs commonly after extensive intestinal resections, in diffuse mucosal diseases such as celiac disease or Crohn's disease, or temporarily after gastrointestinal infections (postinfectious carbohydrate malabsorption).[17-19] The pathophysiologic mechanisms of carbohydrate malabsorption are reduction of the intestinal mucosal surface area and a reduced activity or expression of intestinal oligo- and disaccharidases or transport proteins for monosaccharides.[17] Congenital disaccharidase deficiencies (lactase, sucrase-isomaltase, and trehalase)[20] and congenital deficiency or malfunction of transport molecules as in congenital glucose-galactose malabsorption[21] can cause early onset of malabsorption of mono- or disaccharides (see later on). Intolerance of fructose is discussed in a subsequent section.

VITAMIN MALABSORPTION

Fat-Soluble Vitamins (Vitamins A, D, E, and K)

Diseases causing malabsorption of dietary fat commonly cause malabsorption of fat-soluble vitamins, because they require similar absorptive mechanisms. This is especially important in diseases that result in impaired micelle formation due to bile salt deficiency.[22] Fat-soluble vitamins also are malabsorbed in diffuse diseases of the mucosal surface area, in diseases affecting chylomicron formation and transport,[12,23] and in exocrine pancreatic insufficiency[24]; some authors have suggested that absorption of fat-soluble vitamins is less affected by exocrine pancreatic insufficiency than by small intestinal diseases resulting in steatorrhea.[25]

Vitamin B$_{12}$ (Cobalamin)

Decreased release of dietary vitamin B$_{12}$ due to impaired pepsin and acid secretion as in atrophic gastritis[26] or use of acid inhibitory drugs such as proton pump inhibitors[27] usually results in only mild cobalamin malabsorption. By contrast, deficiency of gastric intrinsic factor secretion, as occurs in pernicious anemia or after gastric resections, or secretion of an abnormal intrinsic factor, as in some congenital diseases, results in severe vitamin B$_{12}$ malabsorption with clinical consequences.[26] Autoimmune gastritis of pernicious anemia is the most common cause of vitamin B$_{12}$ malabsorption.[28] Cobalamin malabsorption in pernicious anemia is caused both by decreased intrinsic factor secretion due to parietal cell destruction in the stomach and by blocking autoantibodies that inhibit intrinsic factor binding to vitamin B$_{12}$.[28] Mild cobalamin malabsorption may be found in patients with pancreatic insufficiency, and in patients with Zollinger-Ellison syndrome, owing to decreased proteolytic release of vitamin B$_{12}$ from its complex with R-binding protein[26,29] (see Chapters 31 and 97). In bacterial overgrowth syndrome (see Chapter 99) or helminthic infections such as with *Diphyllobothrium latum* (see Chapter 107), dietary cobalamin is made unavailable to the host or is consumed by the microorganisms or parasites in the intestinal lumen and therefore is not available for intestinal absorption.[26] Diseases and conditions affecting the ileal mucosa, such as Crohn's disease or ileal resection, lead to a reduction of specific absorptive sites for the intrinsic factor–vitamin B$_{12}$ complex.[26] Ileal resections of more than 60 cm usually result in clinically significant vitamin B$_{12}$ malabsorption. Imerslund-Gräsbeck syndrome, a disease of autosomal recessive inheritance due to malfunction of the cubilin-amnionless (AMN) complex, is characterized by selective ileal malabsorption of the intrinsic factor–vitamin B$_{12}$ complex despite normal ileal morphology.[26,30] Finally, congenital diseases affecting transcobalamin II also result in malabsorption of cobalamin.[26,31] In previously healthy persons it usually takes several years of vitamin B$_{12}$ malabsorption before cobalamin deficiency develops, because the body stores contain large amounts of cobalamin and the daily requirement is relatively small.

Folate

Folate malabsorption occurs in mucosal diseases affecting the proximal small intestine, such as celiac disease, Whipple's disease, and tropical sprue.[32,33] Folate deficiency is common in chronic alcoholism, in which it is postulated to be caused by decreased dietary intake as well as decreased intestinal absorption of folate.[34] As discussed later in this chapter, several drugs result in impaired intestinal uptake of folate, and an inherited form of selective folate malabsorption has been described. In contrast with cobalamin, body stores of folate are small relative to the daily requirements; therefore, folate deficiency states develop faster in the setting of malabsorption. Increased serum folate levels resulting from bacterial formation of tetrahydrofolate have been reported in small intestinal bacterial overgrowth states.[35]

Other Water-Soluble Vitamins

Other water-soluble vitamins, such as ascorbic acid and the B complex vitamins, are absorbed in the small intestine either by carrier-mediated transport or by passive diffusion. Generalized malabsorption syndromes of intestinal causes impair the absorption of these vitamins, thereby leading to deficiency states.[36,37] Deficiency of these water-soluble vitamins also occurs in chronic alcoholism, probably owing to decreased oral intake and also reduced intestinal absorption.[34]

MINERAL MALABSORPTION

Calcium

Severe calcium malabsorption may occur in diseases affecting the small intestinal mucosa, such as celiac disease. In these disease states, calcium absorption is impaired directly because of the reduction of the intestinal surface area and indirectly because of formation of insoluble calcium soaps with malabsorbed long-chain fatty acids.[38] Therefore, diseases causing malabsorption of long-chain fatty acids by other mechanisms, such as bile acid deficiency, also may result in calcium malabsorption.[23] In many of these diseases, malabsorption and deficiency of vitamin D also contribute to intestinal calcium malabsorption.[23] Selective intestinal malabsorption of calcium (i.e., without fat malabsorption) may occur in renal disease, hypoparathyroidism, and inborn defects in either 1α,25-dihydroxyvitamin D formation or the intestinal vitamin D receptor.[23] Calcium malabsorption also occurs commonly after gastric resections (see subsequent section, "Malabsorption after Gastric Resection").

Magnesium

In many generalized malabsorptive disorders, magnesium malabsorption may result in magnesium deficiency.[39] Malabsorption is due to the reduction in mucosal absorptive surface area and to luminal binding of magnesium by malabsorbed fatty acids. A congenital form of selective intestinal magnesium malabsorption also has been reported.[40]

Iron

Iron deficiency is common in patients with gastric resection. Reduction in the mucosal surface area of the small intestine due to diffuse mucosal diseases, intestinal resections, or intestinal bypass also may result in impaired iron absorption, potentially leading to iron deficiency.[41] Intestinal loss of iron from chronic gastrointestinal bleeding is, however, the most common gastrointestinal cause of iron deficiency.[42]

Zinc

Zinc, like other minerals, is malabsorbed in generalized mucosal diseases of the small intestine.[43] A congenital selective defect of zinc absorption, acrodermatitis enteropathica, is caused by a defect in the zinc transport protein hZIP4.[44]

Other Minerals

Generalized malabsorption can cause deficiency of copper and selenium.[45,46] In Menkes disease (kinky hair disease), an inherited disorder of cellular copper transport, selective intestinal copper malabsorption results (see later on). It is uncertain whether malabsorptive diseases result in deficiencies of chromium and manganese.[43]

MECHANISMS COMPENSATING FOR MALABSORPTION

Role of the Colon

The colon has the capacity to absorb a limited variety of nutrients and minerals. Although colonic nutrient absorption does not play a major role in health, the nutritive role of the colon in patients with severe malabsorption is increasingly appreciated.[47] Alternatively, colonic preservation of malabsorbed nutrients also may result in symptoms and complications of malabsorption,[48] and colonic hyperabsorption of oxalate contributes to renal stone formation (see later on).

Colonic Salvage of Incompletely Absorbed Carbohydrates

In healthy people, between 2% and 20% of ingested starch escapes absorption in the small intestine[49]; pancreatic insufficiency or severe intestinal disorders further increase this amount.[18] Carbohydrates that reach the colon cannot be absorbed by the colonic mucosa but can be metabolized by the bacterial flora. Anaerobic bacterial metabolism results in the breakdown of oligosaccharides and polysaccharides to mono- and disaccharides, which are metabolized further to lactic acid and short-chain (C2 to C4) fatty acids, such as acetate, propionate, and butyrate, and to odorless gases, including hydrogen, methane, and carbon dioxide.[50]

Studies in normal subjects have suggested that the bacterial metabolism of starch to small carbohydrate moieties is a rapid process in the normal colon. The rate-limiting step in the overall conversion of polysaccharides to short-chain fatty acids appears to be the conversion of monosaccharides to short-chain fatty acids.[18] Colonic absorption of short-chain fatty acids[51] results in a reduction of the osmotic load and, as a result, in mitigation of osmotic diarrhea. In normal subjects, more than 45 g of carbohydrates must reach the colon to cause diarrhea, and up to 80 g of carbohydrates per day can be metabolized by bacteria to short-chain fatty acids; approximately 90% of these short-chain fatty acids are absorbed by colonic mucosa[52] (Fig. 98–1). Chronic carbohydrate malabsorption causes adaptive changes in bacterial metabolic activity that result in an even higher efficiency of the bacterial flora to digest carbohydrates,[53] although at the expense of increased flatus production (see later).

Because short-chain fatty acids have caloric values between 3.4 and 5.95 kcal/g,[54] colonic absorption of these acids may contribute positively to overall calorie balance. In patients with short bowel syndrome, colonic salvage of malabsorbed carbohydrates can contribute up to 700 to 950 kcal per day, provided that a substantial part of the colon remains in continuity with the small bowel.[55] Not all short-chain fatty acids are absorbed by the colon, and those that are not absorbed contribute to osmotic diarrhea.

The beneficial effects of colonic bacterial carbohydrate metabolism may be accompanied by side effects due to gas production (see Chapter 10). Up to 10-fold differences in the volume of gas produced in the colon have been observed in normal persons.[56] The colon also can absorb gas. If intracolonic gas volumes are low, up to 90% of the volume of intracolonic gas can be absorbed; if gas volumes are high, however, this proportion decreases to 20%[56] (Fig. 98–2). Therefore, those persons who have the disadvantage of producing more gas in their colon have an additional disadvantage of absorbing a smaller fraction of the gas. Gas produced from bacterial carbohydrate metabolism is odorless. The odor of flatus is due to volatile sulfur-containing substrates that result from bacterial metabolism of protein.[57]

Impaired colonic salvage of carbohydrates has been suggested to contribute to the diarrhea in Crohn's disease[58] and ulcerative colitis.[59] Bacterial carbohydrate metabolism may be lessened by antibiotic treatment.[60] In some patients, antibiotic-associated diarrhea may be the result of impaired colonic salvage of carbohydrates that normally are not absorbed or dietary fiber, which may accumulate in stool because of decreased bacterial fermentation.[61]

Colon in Fat Malabsorption

Long-chain triglycerides or fatty acids, which constitute most dietary fat, cannot be absorbed by the human colon. Long-chain fatty acids bind calcium in the colon, thereby increasing the amount of sodium oxalate that is absorbed.[62] Fatty acids with chain lengths longer than 12 carbons may cause diarrhea, because they increase mucosal permeability and inhibit colonic absorption of fluid and electrolytes.[63] An increase in colonic perme-

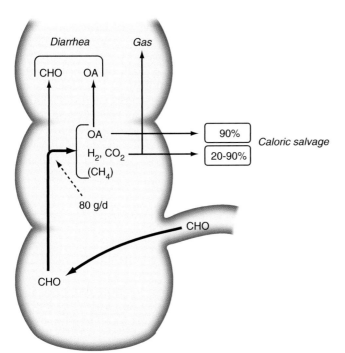

Figure 98–1 Carbohydrate (CHO) metabolism and absorption of metabolic products in the colon. Up to 80 g of CHO that reaches the colon can be metabolized by colonic bacteria to organic acids (OA)—lactic acid and the short-chain fatty acids acetate, butyrate, and propionate—and to hydrogen, carbon dioxide, and methane. Approximately 90% of the OA is absorbed by colonic mucosa, which permits salvage of calories. With accumulation in the stool of OA that escape absorption and CHO that escapes bacterial metabolism, osmotic diarrhea results. Between 20% and 90% of gases produced in the colon is absorbed by the colonic mucosa; the remainder is excreted as flatus.

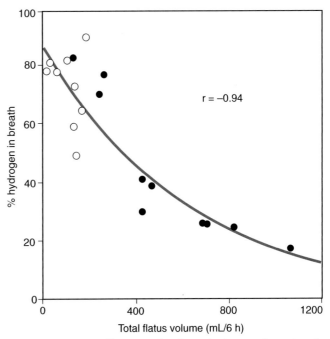

Figure 98–2 The efficiency of colonic hydrogen absorption is inversely related to the amount of gas in the colon: At high flatus volumes, the proportion of hydrogen that is excreted in breath decreases to approximately 20% of total hydrogen excretion. The remaining 80% is excreted in flatus. *Open circles*, fasting state; *closed circles*, after ingestion of 12.5 grams of lactose. (From Hammer HF: Colonic hydrogen absorption: quantification of its effect on hydrogen accumulation caused by bacterial fermentation of carbohydrates. Gut 34:818, 1993.)

ability due to long-chain fatty acids also may be a contributing factor for the increased colonic oxalate absorption seen in patients with steatorrhea and hyperoxaluria.[64]

Patients with short bowel syndrome can gain caloric energy from colonic absorption of medium-chain fatty acids, coming from medium-chain triglyceride supplementation, if they have at least part of the colon in continuity with the remaining small bowel.[65] In the rat colon, absorption of octanoate is not affected by the simultaneous presence of other luminal substrates.[66]

Colonic Salvage of Calcium

Although most unabsorbed calcium is insoluble when it reaches the terminal ileum,[67] preservation of at least half of the colon in patients with extensive small bowel resection improves calcium absorption by about 40%, compared with calcium absorption in patients who have an ileostomy.[68] Absorption of calcium requires solubilization of calcium salts. Bacterial metabolism of dietary fibers or incompletely absorbed carbohydrates may help solubilize calcium by causing a decrease in the pH of luminal contents in the colon. Once calcium is solubilized, it may contact the cecal mucosa, which in the rat has been demonstrated to be the site with the highest calcium absorption rate per surface area in the whole intestine.[69] Calcium solubilization in the colon from bacterial fermentation of malabsorbed lactose also may occur in patients with lactose malabsorption, because in this condition, the bioavailability of calcium from milk is greater than that from mineral water.[70] In addition to their effect on luminal pH, the short-chain fatty acids acetate and propionate, which are products of bacterial metabolism of lactose, have been shown to enhance calcium absorption directly in the human colon.[71]

Role of Intestinal Transit in the Salvage of Malabsorbed Nutrients

The lower parts of the gastrointestinal tract do not normally contact nutrients, and when they do, intestinal transit time is prolonged.[72-75] This delay in transit could contribute to the compensation mechanisms in malabsorptive diseases; however, nutritional salvage by this mechanism has not been quantitated.

CLINICAL FEATURES AND EVALUATION

Diagnosis of malabsorption requires, first, suspecting its presence; second, confirming its existence; and third, demonstrating its cause. Malabsorption usually is suspected on the basis of the patient's history, signs and symptoms, or findings on routine laboratory evaluations. Malabsorption of an ingested nutrient or substrate can be confirmed by measuring its increased stool concentration or its decreased serum concentration or urinary excretion. Finding the cause of malabsorption often requires tests such as endoscopy or small intestinal biopsy, although under certain clinical circumstances, noninvasive tests or radiologic imaging may be helpful in providing a specific diagnosis.

SUSPECTING AND CONFIRMING THE PRESENCE OF MALABSORPTION

History and Physical Examination

Table 98–4 lists symptoms and signs suggestive of malabsorption. Virtually all of the symptoms and signs may have causes other than malabsorption. For example, greasy stools may be indicative of malabsorption, but a greasy appearance also can be due to mucus in stool. Floating of stool in the toilet water can be due to a high stool fat content but also can be caused by high gas content. Nevertheless, these symptoms and signs are helpful in raising the clinician's index of suspicion and in guiding the physician in ordering specific laboratory tests, structural evaluations, or function tests.

Laboratory Findings

Certain blood tests may yield abnormal results in malabsorption, but with rare exceptions they are not specific for malabsorptive diseases. Blood tests also can be used as a screening tool to help the physician decide on how vigorously to evaluate malabsorption. Table 98–5 lists blood tests in which abnormal results should raise the suspicion of malabsorption and stool tests that should be used to confirm the suspicion of malabsorption.

Quantitative fecal fat measurement followed by measurement of fecal chymotrypsin or elastase concentration may be helpful, both in establishing malabsorption and in differentiating between pancreatic and intestinal causes of malabsorption. Low levels of serum β-carotene, cholesterol, triglycerides, and calcium and a prolonged prothrombin time suggest malabsorption of fat and fat-soluble vitamins. Low levels of vitamin B_{12}, folate, iron, and albumin suggest malabsorption of water-soluble substances and therefore indicate intestinal disease rather than pancreatic or biliary disease. Severe deficiency of fat-soluble vitamins may indicate intestinal or biliary disorders. Low levels of plasma citrulline are associated with destructive small intestinal disease, such as celiac disease, or may follow intestinal resection.[76]

DIAGNOSTIC APPROACH TO ESTABLISH THE CAUSE OF MALABSORPTION

Clinical Clues to the Presence of Specific Diseases Causing Malabsorption

Clinical clues (Table 98–6) or results of laboratory tests (Table 98–7)[77] may indicate the presence of a specific underlying disease or may help in the differential diagnosis for malabsorption. In addition, the following evaluations may be helpful.

History and Physical Examination

The following questions should be asked as part of the history before physical examination:

- Has the patient undergone previous surgery, such as gastric or small bowel resection or a gastrointestinal bypass operation?
- Is there a family or childhood history of celiac disease?
- Is there a history of travel to endemic areas of tropical sprue, giardiasis, or other gastrointestinal infections?

Table 98–4   Symptoms and Signs of Malabsorption and Relevant Pathophysiology

Symptom or Sign	Pathophysiologic Explanation
Gastrointestinal	
Diarrhea	Osmotic activity of carbohydrates or short-chain fatty acids
	Secretory effect of bile acids and fatty acids
	Decreased absorptive surface
	Ileal resection
	Severe ileal mucosal disease
	Intestinal loss of conjugated bile acids
	Ileal resection
	Severe ileal mucosal disease
	Congenital defects of the ileal sodium–bile acid cotransporter
Abdominal distention, flatulence	Bacterial gas production from carbohydrates in colon, small intestinal bacterial overgrowth
Foul-smelling flatulence or stool	Malabsorption of proteins or intestinal protein loss
Pain	Gaseous distention of intestine (see above)
Ascites	Protein loss or malabsorption
Musculoskeletal	
Tetany, muscle weakness, paresthesia	Malabsorption of vitamin D, calcium, magnesium, and phosphate
Bone pain, osteomalacia, fractures	Protein, calcium, or vitamin D deficiency; secondary hyperparathyroidism
Skin and Mucous Membranes	
Easy bruisability, ecchymoses, petechiae	Vitamin K and vitamin C (scurvy) deficiency
Glossitis, cheilosis, stomatitis	Deficiency of vitamin B complex, vitamin B_{12}, vitamin C, folate, and iron
Edema	Protein loss or malabsorption
Acrodermatitis, scaly dermatitis	Zinc and essential fatty acid deficiency
Follicular hyperkeratosis	Vitamin A deficiency
Hyperpigmented dermatitis	Niacin deficiency (pellagra)
Thin nails with spoon-shaped deformity	Iron deficiency
Finger clubbing	Severe nutrient malabsorption
Other	
Weight loss, hyperphagia	Nutrient malabsorption
Growth and weight retardation, infantilism	Nutrient malabsorption in childhood and adolescence
Anemia	Iron, folate, or vitamin B_{12} deficiency
Kidney stones	Increased colonic oxalate absorption
Amenorrhea, impotence, infertility	Multifactorial (including protein malabsorption, secondary hypopituitarism, anemia)
Night blindness, xerophthalmia	Vitamin A deficiency
Peripheral neuropathy	Vitamin B_{12} or thiamine deficiency
Fatigue, weakness	Calorie depletion, iron and folate deficiency, anemia
Neurologic symptoms, ataxia	Vitamin E deficiency

- Is there excessive alcohol consumption?
- Does the patient have a history of chronic pancreatitis or symptoms suggestive of a pancreatic tumor?
- Does the patient have clinical features of thyrotoxicosis, Addison's disease, Whipple's disease, biliary or liver disease, or diabetic neuropathy?
- Does the patient eat a diet high in poorly absorbable carbohydrates (sweeteners such as sorbitol or fructose) or fat substitutes or an unbalanced diet that could result in malnutrition?
- Is there an increased likelihood of human immunodeficiency virus infection?
- Is the patient receiving treatment with a drug that may cause malabsorption?
- Does the patient have a history of organ transplantation or abdominal radiation exposure?

A rational approach to establishing the cause of malabsorption may require several diagnostic steps. Depending on the clinician's background, the availability of different tests, and the patient's preferences, different diagnostic approaches may be used. If time constraints are not a consideration, a stepwise approach may be used, starting with noninvasive evaluations that may guide further invasive procedures or even provide a diagnosis.

In other instances, the physician may choose a more invasive test, in hopes of reaching a diagnosis with the fewest possible tests in the shortest possible time. Diagnostic approaches differ depending on the epidemiologic or ethnic background of an individual patient. For example, if parasitic infections are a likely possibility, stool examination may provide a rapid diagnosis by noninvasive testing. In populations with a very low prevalence of lactose intolerance, a secondary cause of lactose malabsorption is more likely, necessitating additional tests, than it is in populations with a high prevalence of acquired primary lactase deficiency.

The sequence of tests, therefore, depends on the affected person's symptoms and history, as well as results of previous testing (Table 98–8). Tests that may detect the most common causes of malabsorption or are noninvasive or inexpensive usually should be performed initially (first-line tests). In some patients, testing for rarer causes of malabsorption and use of more invasive or more expensive tests may be necessary to establish the diagnosis (second-line tests). For unusually difficult cases, additional tests may be required that may be available only in specialized centers (third-line tests).

Table 98–5 Laboratory Tests Useful for Suspected Malabsorption and for Establishing Possible Nutrient Deficiencies and Consequences of Malabsorption

Test	Comment(s)
Blood Cell Count	
Hematocrit, hemoglobin	Decreased in iron, vitamin B_{12}, and folate malabsorption or with blood loss
Mean corpuscular hemoglobin (MCH) or mean corpuscular volume (MCV)	Decreased in iron malabsorption; increased in folate and vitamin B_{12} malabsorption
White blood cells, differential	Decreased in vitamin B_{12} and folate malabsorption; low lymphocyte count in lymphangiectasia
Biochemical Tests (Serum)	
Triglycerides	Decreased in severe fat malabsorption
Cholesterol	Decreased in bile acid malabsorption or severe fat malabsorption
Albumin	Decreased in severe malnutrition, lymphangiectasia, protein-losing enteropathy
Alkaline phosphatase	Increased in calcium and vitamin D malabsorption (severe steatorrhea)
Calcium, phosphorus, magnesium	Decreased in extensive mucosal disease, after extensive intestinal resection, or in vitamin D deficiency
Zinc	Decreased in extensive mucosal disease or intestinal resection
Iron, ferritin	Decreased in celiac sprue, in other extensive mucosal diseases, and with chronic blood loss
Other Serum Tests	
Prothrombin time	Prolonged in vitamin K malabsorption
β-Carotene	Decreased in fat malabsorption due to hepatobiliary or intestinal diseases
Immunoglobulins	Decreased in lymphangiectasia, diffuse lymphoma
Folic acid	Decreased in extensive small intestinal mucosal diseases, with anticonvulsant use, in pregnancy; may be increased in small intestinal bacterial overgrowth
Vitamin B_{12}	Decreased in postgastrectomy, pernicious anemia, terminal ileal disease, and in small intestinal bacterial overgrowth
Methylmalonic acid	Markedly elevated in vitamin B_{12} deficiency
Homocysteine	Markedly elevated in vitamin B_{12} or folate deficiency
Citrulline	Decreased in destructive mucosal small intestinal disease or resection
Stool Tests	
Fat	Qualitative or quantitative parameter for fat malabsorption
Elastase, chymotrypsin	Decreased concentration and output in exocrine pancreatic insufficiency
pH	Less than 5.5 in carbohydrate malabsorption

Table 98–6 Cardinal Clinical Features of Specific Malabsorptive Diseases

Disease	Cardinal Clinical Features
Adrenal insufficiency	Skin darkening, hyponatremia, hyperkalemia
Amyloidosis	Renal disease, nephrotic syndrome, cardiomyopathy, neuropathy, carpal tunnel syndrome, macroglossia, hepatosplenomegaly
Bacterial overgrowth	Previous intestinal surgery, motility disorder (scleroderma, pseudo-obstruction), diverticula, strictures
Bile acid deficiency	Ileal resection or disease, liver disease
Carcinoid	Flushing, cardiac murmur
Celiac sprue	Variable symptoms, from mono- or oligosymptomatic (e.g., mild iron deficiency) to dermatitis herpetiformis, alopecia, aphthous mouth ulcers, arthropathy, neurologic symptoms, and life-threatening malnutrition; abnormal liver chemistry test results
Crohn's disease	Arthritis, aphthous mouth ulcers, episcleritis, erythema nodosum, laboratory signs of inflammation, abdominal mass, fistulas, pyoderma gangrenosum, primary sclerosing cholangitis (PSC)
Cystic fibrosis	Chronic sinopulmonary disease, meconium ileus, distal intestinal obstruction syndrome (DIOS), elevated sweat chloride
Cystinuria, Hartnup's disease	Kidney stones, dermatosis
Diabetes mellitus	Long history of diabetes and diabetic complications
Disaccharidase deficiency	Bloating and cramping, intermittent diarrhea
Fistulas	Previous intestinal surgery or trauma, Crohn's disease
Glucagonoma	Migratory necrolytic erythema
Hyperthyroidism, hypothyroidism	Specific symptoms of thyroid disease
Hypogammaglobulinemia	Recurrent infections
Intestinal ischemia	Other ischemic organ manifestations; abdominal pain with eating
Lymphoma	Mesenteric or retroperitoneal lymph nodes, abdominal mass, abdominal pain, fever
Mastocytosis	Urticaria pigmentosum, peptic ulcer
Mycobacterium-avium complex infection	Acquired immunodeficiency syndrome (AIDS)
Pancreatic insufficiency	History of pancreatitis, abdominal pain or alcoholism, large-volume fatty stools
Parasitic infection	History of travel to endemic areas
Primary biliary cirrhosis	Jaundice, itching
Scleroderma	Dysphagia, Raynaud's phenomenon, skin tightening
Tropical sprue	History of travel to endemic areas
Tuberculosis	Specific history of exposure, endemic areas, immunosuppression, abdominal mass or obstruction, ascites
Whipple's disease	Lymphadenopathy, fever, arthritis, cerebral symptoms, heart murmur
Zollinger-Ellison syndrome	Peptic ulcers

Table 98–7 Laboratory Tests Useful in the Differential Diagnosis of Malabsorption

Test	Comment
Blood Cell Count	
Acanthocytes	Abetalipoproteinemia
Nuclear remnants in erythrocytes (Howell-Jolly bodies)	Splenic atrophy in celiac sprue, inflammatory bowel disease, radiation, amyloidosis
White blood cells, differential	Eosinophilia in eosinophilic gastroenteritis and parasitic disease
	Low lymphocyte count in lymphangiectasia, tuberculosis
	Low CD4$^+$ count in AIDS
Platelets	Increased in inflammatory diseases
Other Tests	
ESR, C-reactive protein	Increased in Crohn's disease, Whipple's disease, lymphoma
Ferritin	Increased in inflammatory diseases
Iron	Decreased in celiac sprue, chronic occult intestinal bleeding, chronic inflammatory diseases
Liver enzymes, bilirubin	Increased in primary biliary cirrhosis and liver diseases, celiac sprue
Immunologic Markers	
Anti-tissue TG/EMA	Celiac sprue
Immunoglobulins	IgA deficiency, immunodeficiency syndromes
Allergen-specific IgE	IgE-mediated hypersensitivity
Autoantibodies (e.g., ANA)	Connective tissue diseases
HLA-DQ2 or -DQ8	Celiac sprue, refractory sprue
Antimitochondrial autoantibodies	Primary biliary cirrhosis
HIV antibodies	AIDS
Neuroendocrine Markers	
ACTH, cortisol	Abnormal values in Addison's disease
Basal TSH	Decreased in hyperthyroidism
Chromogranin A	Elevated in neuroendocrine tumors
5-Hydroxyindoleacetic acid in urine	Elevated in carcinoid syndrome
Gastrin*	Elevated in Zollinger-Ellison syndrome
Glucagon*	Elevated in glucagonoma
Somatostatin*	Elevated in somatostatinoma
Stool Tests	
Occult blood test	Erosive or ulcerative intestinal disease, tumor or celiac sprue
Ova and parasites	Repeated samples may be needed to detect *Giardia lamblia*
Leukocytes	Present in some inflammatory diseases

*To be performed if there is a strong suspicion of an underlying neuroendocrine tumor.[77]
ACTH, adrenocorticotropic hormone; AIDS, acquired immunodeficiency syndrome; ANA, antinuclear antibodies; EMA, endomysial antibodies; ESR, erythrocyte sedimentation rate; HIV, human immunodeficiency virus; HLA, human leukocyte antigen; IgA, IgE, immunoglobulins A and E; TG, transglutaminase; TSH, thyroid-stimulating hormone.

For some disorders, such as bile acid malabsorption, lactose malabsorption, and bacterial overgrowth, it may be difficult to establish a causal link between symptoms and the malabsorbed substrate. In these conditions, observation of the response to therapy may be an important tool to prove or disprove a causal relationship.

ANATOMIC INVESTIGATIONS

Endoscopic examination of the stomach, duodenum, or ileum and histologic examination of mucosal biopsy specimens can establish a diagnosis of the conditions causing malabsorption. The role of radiologic imaging examinations is limited mostly to answering questions about abdominal regions not easily accessible to endoscopy, such as parts of the small intestine, parenchymatous organs, the peritoneal cavity, the mesentery, or the retroperitoneum. Capsule endoscopy and magnetic resonance imaging (MRI) are contributing to making these areas more accessible to diagnostic evaluation. Radiologic studies of the small bowel can show evidence of stasis, blind loops, diverticula, fistulas, rapid transit, and other abnormalities that may assist in diagnosis (see later on).

ENDOSCOPIC EXAMINATION, MUCOSAL BIOPSY, AND ASPIRATION OF INTESTINAL SECRETIONS

Endoscopic inspection of the duodenal mucosa may provide clues to some causes of malabsorption. Aphthae may be suggestive of Crohn's disease, and small, diffuse, white, punctate lesions can be seen in primary or secondary lymphangiectasia. Mosaic, granular, or nodular mucosa, scalloping of duodenal folds (Fig. 98–3), and reduction in number of duodenal folds are highly suggestive of villus atrophy in celiac disease, although these abnormalities may be seen in other diseases.[78] Villus atrophy may be visualized endoscopically using magnification endoscopy and chromoendoscopy with indigo-carmine staining; however, a normal duodenal fold pattern should not deter the endoscopist from taking

Table 98–8   Tests to Establish the Cause of Malabsorption Based on Main Symptoms

Tests in Patients with Weight Loss, Osteomalacia/Osteopenia, Diarrhea, Suspected Steatorrhea, or Deficiency of Fat-Soluble Vitamins

First-line tests
  Laboratory tests (complete blood cell count, white blood cell differential, cholesterol, triglycerides, electrolytes, calcium, magnesium, ALT, AST, AP, bilirubin, prothrombin time, albumin, erythrocyte sedimentation rate/C-reactive protein, TSH)
  Endomysial antibodies/tissue transglutaminase antibodies
  Esophagogastroduodenoscopy with small intestinal biopsies
  Ova, parasites, and leukocytes in stool
  Chymotrypsin and/or elastase concentration in stool
  Abdominal ultrasound
Second-line tests
  Small bowel series
  Capsule endoscopy
  Abdominal computed tomography, MRI
  Special staining of small intestinal biopsies (e.g., Congo red for amyloid, staining for lymphomas, chromogranin A for neuroendocrine tumors)
  Endoscopic examination of the terminal ileum, including ileal biopsies
  Quantitative small intestinal culture or breath tests for bacterial overgrowth
  More extensive laboratory investigation (immunoglobulins, human immunodeficiency virus antibodies, antinuclear antibodies, ferritin, food allergen-specific IgE, adrenocorticotropic hormone, cortisol, chromogranin A, gastrin, urinary 5-HIAA)
  Quantitative fecal fat
  Endoscopic retrograde cholangiopancreatography/MRCP
  Therapeutic trial of pancreatic enzymes, antibiotics (tetracycline, metronidazole), or a gluten-free diet
Tests in unusually difficult cases (third-line tests)
  Glucagon, somatostatin in serum/plasma
  Tube test for exocrine pancreatic secretion (secretin, cholecystokinin, or Lundh test)
  Tests for bile acid malabsorption
  Spiral computed tomography of the pancreas for tumor
  Enteroscopy, including biopsies
  Endoscopic ultrasound
  Somatostatin (octreotide) scan
  Positron emission tomography
  Abdominal angiogram
  Magnetic resonance angiography

Tests in Patients with Bloating, with or without Diarrhea

First-line tests
  Lactose H_2 breath test
  Lactose tolerance test
  Fructose H_2 breath test
  Stool pH (in patients with diarrhea)
Second-line tests
  Esophagogastroduodenoscopy with duodenal biopsies
  Endomysial antibodies/tissue transglutaminase antibodies
  Quantitative small intestinal culture or breath tests for bacterial overgrowth
  Chymotrypsin and/or elastase concentration in stool

Tests in Patients with Anemia and Suspected Malabsorption

Microcytic or hypochromic anemia (low MCV, MCH)
  Iron, ferritin, and transferrin in serum
  Exclude gastrointestinal and nongastrointestinal blood loss
  Endomysial antibodies/tissue transglutaminase antibodies
  Esophagogastroduodenoscopy with duodenal biopsies
  Ova and parasites in stool
  Capsule endoscopy
Macrocytic anemia (high MCV, MCH)
  First-line tests
    Folic acid in serum or red blood cells
    Vitamin B_{12} in serum
  Second-line tests in cases of vitamin B_{12} deficiency
    Schilling test (with and without intrinsic factor)
    Ova and parasites in stool
    Evaluation of ileum
      Endoscopy
      Computed tomography, capsule endoscopy, small bowel series, enteroclysis
    Esophagogastroduodenoscopy with gastric and duodenal biopsies
    Endomysial antibodies/tissue transglutaminase antibodies
    Quantitative small intestinal culture or breath tests for bacterial overgrowth
  Second-line tests in cases of folate deficiency
    Endomysial antibodies/tissue transglutaminase antibodies
    Esophagogastroduodenoscopy with duodenal biopsies

ALT, alanine aminotransferase; AP, alkaline phosphatase; AST, aspartate aminotransferase; 5-HIAA, 5-hydroxyindoleacetic acid; IgE, immunoglobulin E; MCH, mean corpuscular hemoglobin; MCV, mean corpuscular volume; MRCP, magnetic resonance cholangiopancreatography; MRI, magnetic resonance imaging; TSH, thyroid-stimulating hormone.

mucosal biopsy specimens. Endocrine tumors causing malabsorption such as duodenal gastrinomas or somatostatinomas or ampullary tumors obstructing the pancreatic duct also can be detected during endoscopy. If malabsorption is suspected to be caused by ileal disease, visual examination and biopsy of the ileal mucosa may be required to establish a diagnosis.

Examination of endoscopic biopsy specimens from the level of the duodenal ampulla may be diagnostic or highly suggestive (Table 98–9) of a variety of small bowel disorders resulting in malabsorption. A follow-up small intestinal biopsy can be used to assess treatment effects. Duodenal biopsy specimens should be obtained from patients with atypical or nonspecific gastrointestinal symptoms, including abdominal pain, bloating, and weight loss, and should not be limited only to patients with diarrhea.[79,80] Endoscopic biopsy is an adequate substitute for jejunal suction biopsy,[81] and its advantage over capsule biopsy[82] is that focal or patchy lesions can be seen and targeted for sampling.[83] The adequacy of mucosal biopsy specimens is a function of their size and the number obtained.[84] If large specimens can be obtained using "jumbo" biopsy forceps, they can be oriented on a piece of filter paper before they are put into a fixing solution[85]; two or three "jumbo" biopsy specimens usually are sufficient to allow histologic sectioning parallel to the villi and crypts. Specimens also may be obtained with smaller forceps, although the number of specimens obtained must then be increased to four to six. Specimens can be inspected with a low-power dissecting microscope or by magnification endoscopy to obtain an initial impression of the villus architecture.

The diagnostic yield of biopsy is influenced by the distribution of histologic abnormalities, which in some diseases is diffuse but in other diseases is patchy. Tropical diarrhea malabsorption syndrome (tropical sprue; see Chapter 102), abetalipoproteinemia, and immunodeficiency usually result in a diffuse alteration of small intestinal mucosa. Thus, a completely normal appearance of a duodenal biopsy specimen rules out these disorders. Primary lymphangiectasia has a patchy distribution, so that a single mucosal biopsy may not rule out the disorder (see Chapter 27). Patchy distribution also has been described for the histologic changes in some patients with celiac disease, although this disorder usually affects the small intestine diffusely.[86] Other possible sources of error and misdiagnosis include poorly oriented specimens and those obtained too proximally, where peptic injury can be the cause of mucosal alterations. Additional biopsy specimens from the stomach may help the pathol-

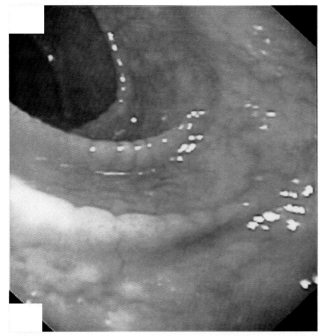

Figure 98–3 Endoscopic image showing scalloping of duodenal folds in a patient with celiac sprue.

Table 98–9 Causes of Malabsorption That Can Be Diagnosed by Small Bowel Biopsy

Cause of Malabsorption	Main Histologic Features
Generalized Histologic Abnormalities	
Abetalipoproteinemia, hypobetalipoproteinemia	Lipid accumulation and vacuolization of enterocytes
Collagenous sprue	Collagenous band below atrophic epithelium
Mycobacterium-avium complex infection	Acid-fast bacilli, foam cells
Whipple's disease (Chapter 103)	Foamy macrophages with PAS-positive inclusion bodies
Patchy Histologic Abnormalities	
Amyloidosis	Congo red–stained deposits with apple-green birefringence in polarized light
Crohn's disease (Chapter 108)	Epithelioid granulomas and characteristic focal inflammation
Eosinophilic gastroenteritis (Chapter 26)	Eosinophilic infiltration
Lymphangiectasia	Ectatic lymph vessels
Lymphoma (Chapter 28)	Clonal expansion of lymphocytes
Mastocytosis (Chapter 34)	Diffuse infiltration with mast cells
Parasites (*Giardia lamblia*, *Strongyloides*, coccidia) (Chapter 106)	Parasites may be seen on histologic examination

PAS, periodic acid–Schiff [stain].
Modified from Riddell RH: Small intestinal biopsy: Who? How? What are the findings? In Barkin JS, Rogers AI (eds): Difficult Decisions in Digestive Diseases. Chicago, Year Book Medical Publishers, 1989, p 326; and Riley SA, Marsh MN: Maldigestion and malabsorption. In Feldman M, Scharschmidt BF, Sleisenger MH (eds): Sleisenger & Fordtran's Gastrointestinal and Liver Disease, 6th ed. Philadelphia, WB Saunders, 1998, p 1501.

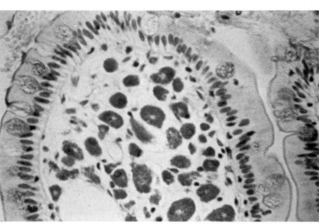

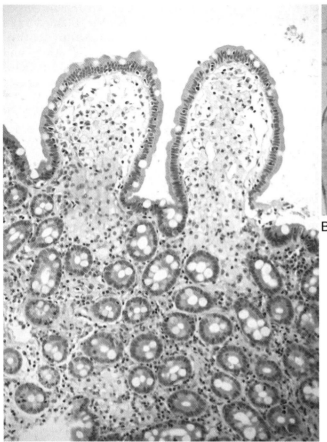

B

A

Figure 98–4 Duodenal biopsy specimen from a patient with Whipple's disease. *A,* Hematoxylin-eosin staining shows villus blunting. The lamina propria is infiltrated with pale-staining foamy macrophages. (Courtesy of Cord Langner, MD.) *B,* High-power view demonstrates purple-red macrophages. Periodic acid–Schiff stain. (Courtesy of Günter J. Krejs, MD, Graz, Austria.)

ogist to establish the extent of peptic injuries in the upper gastrointestinal tract and to interpret inflammatory changes in the duodenum in relation to these lesions. Distortion of villus architecture over Brunner's glands or lymphoid aggregates, common in the duodenum, should be interpreted with caution.

Specific histologic features may be diagnostic for some rare causes of malabsorption (see Table 98–9),[87,88] such as Whipple's disease (Fig. 98–4), abetalipoproteinemia or hypobetalipoproteinemia, intestinal lymphangiectasia, giardiasis (Fig. 98–5), lymphoma, or collagenous sprue. In most patients with small bowel disorders, however, histologic examination is not diagnostic[87,88] (Table 98–10) and reveals a spectrum of mucosal responses ranging from infiltration by lymphocytic cells to a flat mucosa with villus atrophy and crypt hyperplasia (Fig. 98–6). In many parts of the world, celiac disease is by far the most common cause of this type of histologic alteration, but a definite diagnosis of celiac disease cannot be established by mucosal biopsy alone (see Chapter 101).

Some disease states can be identified only with use of special histologic stains, such as a Congo red stain for diagnosis of intestinal amyloidosis, or immunohistochemical techniques for detection of small intestinal lymphomas or enteroendocrine insufficiency (see later on). Polymerase chain reaction analysis of intestinal biopsy specimens for *Tropheryma whippelii* performed in special laboratories may be helpful in the evaluation of patients suspected of having Whipple's disease (see Chapter

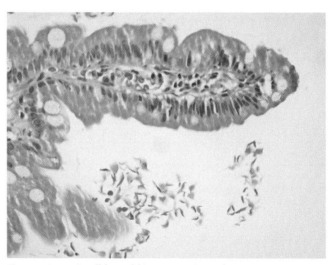

Figure 98–5 Small bowel biopsy specimen from an immunocompetent patient with giardiasis. A normal-appearing villus and adjacent pear-shaped organisms with red-staining nuclei are evident. (Courtesy of Cord Langner, MD.)

103).[89] In cases in which these diseases are a possibility, the clinician has to request these specific tests. Measurement of mucosal enzyme activities in a jejunal biopsy can be used to confirm the diagnosis of disaccharidase deficiency, although this is neither recommended nor available for routine clinical use.

Table 98-10	Malabsorptive Diseases with Abnormal but Not Diagnostic Small Intestinal Histologic Findings

Increased Lymphocyte Infiltration with or without Crypt Hypertrophy
AIDS enteropathy (Chapter 32)
Celiac sprue (Chapter 101)
Infection (due to *Giardia lamblia*, cryptosporidia [Chapter 106]; viral enteritis) (Chapter 104)
Tropical sprue (Chapter 102)

Flat Lesion with or without Mucosal Inflammation
Celiac sprue (Chapter 101)
Drug induced enteropathy (NSAIDs, colchicine, neomycin)
Food protein hypersensitivity (rye, barley, egg, fish, rice, poultry) (Chapter 26)
Immunodeficiency (hypogammaglobulinemia) (Chapter 2)
Immunoproliferative small intestinal disease (IPSID) (Chapters 28, 101, and 112)
Infection (due to *Giardia lamblia*, cryptosporidia) (Chapter 106)
Lymphoma (Chapter 28)
Prolonged folate or cobalamin deficiency
Protein-calorie malnutrition
Transplantation
Traumatic injury
Tropical sprue (Chapter 102)

Atrophic Lesion
Chronic radiation damage (Chapter 38)
Cicatrizing Crohn's disease (Chapter 108)
Diffuse lymphoma (Chapter 28)
Idiopathic diarrhea of infancy (microvillus inclusion disease) (Chapter 93)
Unresponsive gluten sensitivity (lymphoma or ulcerative jejunitis) (Chapter 101)

AIDS, acquired immunodeficiency syndrome; NSAIDs, nonsteroidal anti-inflammatory drugs.
Modified from Riddell RH: Small intestinal biopsy: Who? How? What are the findings? In Barkin JS, Rogers AI (eds): Difficult Decisions in Digestive Diseases. Chicago, Year Book Medical Publishers, 1989, p 326; Riley SA, Marsh MN: Maldigestion and malabsorption. In Feldman M, Scharschmidt BF, Sleisenger MH (eds): Sleisenger & Fordtran's Gastrointestinal and Liver Disease, 6th ed. Philadelphia, WB Saunders, 1998, p 1501.

Fluid aspirated from the descending part of the duodenum may be examined microscopically for *Giardia lamblia* (see Chapter 106) or cultured to detect bacterial overgrowth in patients with diffuse small bowel motility disorders (see Chapter 99).

Capsule Endoscopy

Capsule endoscopy is a new tool for diagnosing diseases of the small bowel. Initially this method was introduced for the evaluation of suspected small bowel bleeding, but studies have suggested a potential benefit of this diagnostic procedure in the diagnosis of small bowel Crohn's disease and other malabsorptive disorders such as complicated celiac disease. In several studies, lesions suggestive of Crohn's disease that were detected by capsule endoscopy had been missed by conventional diagnostic procedures.[90-93] These reports need to be interpreted carefully, because no biopsy specimens were obtained, and long-term evaluations to confirm the diagnosis are lacking. Capsule endoscopy appears to be superior to

conventional or computed tomography (CT) with small bowel enteroclysis in detection of subtle mucosal changes such as aphthous or erosive lesions of the small bowel.[91-93] This test may be used in patients with established malabsorption in whom no diagnosis has been established despite extensive diagnostic workup.

ABDOMINAL IMAGING

Small Bowel Follow-through Studies and Small Bowel Enteroclysis

The principal role of small bowel radiologic series in the evaluation of malabsorption is to identify focal or diffuse abnormalities and alterations that predispose to bacterial overgrowth, such as diverticula, stagnant loops of intestine, or generalized intestinal hypomotility or dilatation; intestinal fistulas; and tumors.[94]

Small bowel enteroclysis is preferred to small bowel follow-through studies, because distention of the lumen results in better visualization of the small bowel contour.[95] Double-contrast enteroclysis, in which intubation of the upper jejunum is used to instill contrast material directly into the upper jejunum, has a higher sensitivity for detecting mucosal changes, although it is less acceptable to the patient and may miss focal changes in the duodenum, such as diverticula.

Alterations associated with diffuse, localized, or distal mucosal changes that might have been missed by proximal mucosal biopsy also may be identified. Normal findings on small bowel series do not rule out intestinal causes of malabsorption and should not dissuade the clinician from performing small bowel biopsy.

Ulcerations and strictures may be seen in various malabsorptive disorders, such as Crohn's disease, radiation enteritis, celiac disease, intestinal lymphoma, and tuberculosis. Aphthous ulcers and cobblestoning of mucosa, either alone or with thickened and distorted folds, are features of Crohn's disease but also can be present in other conditions. Reduced numbers of jejunal folds and an increased number of and thickening of ileal folds may be suggestive of celiac disease.[96] Mass lesions can be found with intestinal lymphoma or, rarely, with hormone-producing tumors.

The disadvantage of conventional enteroclysis is that direct imaging of the bowel wall and surrounding structures is not possible, and overlapping bowel loops potentially may impair complete visualization of the whole small bowel—hence the rationale for combining enteroclysis with CT scanning.[97]

Abdominal Computed Tomography

Abdominal CT for small bowel investigation is performed after administration of oral and/or intravenous contrast agents.[98] Small bowel CT scan is useful for detecting focal intestinal lesions such as thickening of the small bowel wall in Crohn's disease or small intestinal lymphoma, intestinal fistula, and dilated bowel loops; however, mild mucosal changes such as aphthae in Crohn's disease or villus atrophy of various causes are missed by this technique. Diffuse thickening of the small bowel may be seen in Whipple's disease, and graft-versus-

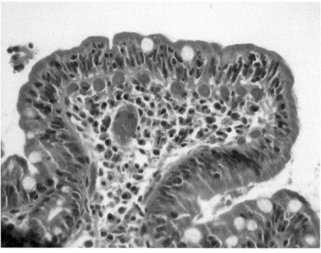

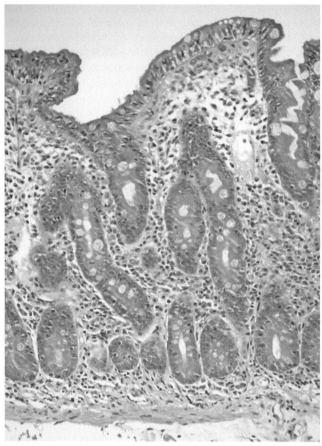

A

Figure 98–6 Duodenal biopsy specimen from a patient with untreated celiac sprue. *A,* Subtotal villus atrophy, crypt elongation, and lymphoplasmacytic infiltration of the lamina propria can be seen. *B,* High-power view demonstrates villus blunting with increased intraepithelial lymphocytes. (Courtesy of Cord Langner, MD.)

host disease.[98] In some cases of celiac disease, reversal of the jejunoileal fold pattern is observed.[99] CT is a sensitive test for detecting enlarged abdominal lymph nodes, which can be present in disorders such as Whipple's disease, small bowel lymphoma, or small intestinal inflammatory diseases such as Crohn's disease. Evidence for pancreatic disease that may be detected on CT includes calcifications of the pancreas, dilatation of the pancreatic duct, and pancreatic atrophy. Tumors obstructing the pancreatic duct or hormone-secreting neuroendocrine tumors also can be located by CT.

Magnetic Resonance Imaging (MRI) of the Small Bowel

A new method for visualizing the small bowel is MRI with use of oral contrast solutions or MRI enteroclysis. Segmental bowel wall thickening with inflammatory involvement of the mesentery, cobblestoning, and ulcerations may be seen in Crohn's disease; this method is very sensitive for demonstrating complications of Crohn's disease, such as intestinal fistula formation. In celiac disease, small bowel MRI with oral contrast may demonstrate dilated small bowel loops, mucosal thickening, and an increased number of folds.[100] A limitation of small bowel MRI with oral contrast and MRI enteroclysis is that subtle mucosal changes in these diseases might be missed, which can be evident on conventional small bowel enteroclysis,[101,102] or capsule endoscopy. Future development will show if MRI or CT imaging of the small bowel will replace "classic" small bowel enteroclysis completely in the radiologic investigation of the small bowel.

Other Radiologic Studies

A plain film of the abdomen may be helpful to detect pancreatic calcifications if exocrine pancreatic insufficiency is suspected. It should be noted, however, that morphologic signs of chronic pancreatitis alone do not prove a pancreatic cause of malabsorption, because the function of the exocrine pancreas must be impaired severely before malabsorption becomes evident. A plain film of the abdomen also may document dilated loops of intestine, predisposing to small bowel bacterial overgrowth or suggesting the presence of an obstruction.

Endoscopic retrograde pancreatography (ERCP) may be helpful in establishing the cause of pancreatic insufficiency (see Chapter 57). It can help distinguish between chronic pancreatitis and pancreatic tumor or document pancreatic duct stones. ERCP is the method of choice for documenting various causes of biliary obstruction. Noninvasive magnetic resonance cholangiography is increasingly being used to replace diagnostic endoscopic retrograde cholangiography. If malabsorption is suspected to be caused by a neuroendocrine tumor (e.g., gastrinoma, somatostatinoma), an indium-111 octreotide scintigraphic scan,[18] fluorodeoxyglucose positron emission tomography (FDG-PET), or an endoscopic ultrasound examination of the pancreas may be helpful in establishing the diagnosis or demonstrating the extent of disease (see Chapters 30 and 31).

Transabdominal ultrasound examinations are very operator dependent. They have the advantage of no radiation exposure and therefore can be used in pregnant patients. Ultrasonography frequently is used to investigate the pancreas, although the sensitivity for the detection of pancreatic tumors is lower than that of ERCP or CT. Nevertheless, obstruction of the biliary tract, pancreatic calcifications, dilatation of the pancreatic duct, or stones within the pancreatic duct may be demonstrated. Ultrasound examination also may be used to document thickening of the bowel wall, abscesses, and fistula in Crohn's disease.

NONINVASIVE EVALUATION OF GASTROINTESTINAL ABSORPTIVE AND DIGESTIVE FUNCTION

Some conditions causing malabsorption can be diagnosed by the use of noninvasive tests, although, as pointed out in Table 98–11, diagnostic accuracy may be limited, and further tests may be necessary to identify underlying diseases or to differentiate between primary and secondary causes. Apart from providing a diagnosis, tests evaluating gastrointestinal absorptive and digestive function may be helpful in the evaluation of complex disease presentations. For most or all of the following tests, the potential benefits with regard to the costs of workup or to patient acceptability have not been established. Because test procedures and analytical methods may vary among laboratories,[103] each should establish its own reference values for these tests.

FAT MALABSORPTION

Quantitative Fecal Fat Analysis

The van de Kamer method is the quantitative titration of fatty acid equivalents in which the results are expressed as fecal output of fat in grams per 24 hours. This method is considered to be the gold standard for fecal fat analysis.[104] Modifications in which the extracted fats are weighed rather than titrated[105,106] have an excellent correlation with the results of the van de Kamer method.[101] Near-infrared reflectance analysis may be a less cumbersome method to quantify fecal fat output in stool collections,[107] because it requires less handling of stool by the laboratory personnel, but it still requires a 48- to 72-hour stool collection to exclude the influence of day-to-day variability and mixing of the stool before a sample is obtained for analysis. In our (unpublished) experience, the accuracy of the near-infrared reflectance analysis technology is influenced by stool consistency—in watery stools, the accuracy of the method decreases.

Fecal fat excretion of less than 7 g per day with a fat intake of 100 g per day usually is considered to be normal. It is, however, important to note that the volume effect of diarrhea by itself increases fecal fat output to levels of up to 14 g per day (secondary fat malabsorption)[108] (Fig. 98–7); this latter normal value could be used in patients with diarrhea.

Quantitative fecal fat analysis is available routinely only in a few centers. Reasons for the limited clinical use of quantitative fecal fat measurements are as follows. First, if the main symptom of malabsorption is chronic diarrhea, measurement of fecal fat may not influence the subsequent workup, because the diagnostic tests performed to establish the etiology of diarrhea are similar to the tests for the workup of steatorrhea. Second, an elevated fecal fat level usually cannot be used to differentiate among biliary, pancreatic, and enteric causes of malabsorption. Third, in many patients with severe steatorrhea, the stools have the characteristic porridge-like appearance, and quantitative studies are not necessary to establish fat malabsorption. Fourth, fat absorption may be normal despite malabsorption of other nutrients, so that a normal fat balance does not imply normal absorptive function of the gastrointestinal tract. Finally, accuracy depends on quantitative stool collections for 48 to

Table 98–11   Malabsorptive Diseases or Conditions in Which Noninvasive Tests Can Establish Malabsorption or Provide a Diagnosis

Disease or Condition	Diagnostic Test(s)*	Comment(s)
Lactose malabsorption	Lactose hydrogen breath test Lactose tolerance	Tests do not differentiate between primary and secondary lactose malabsorption
Fructose malabsorption	Fructose hydrogen breath test	Questionable clinical relevance
Small intestinal bacterial overgrowth (see Chapter 99)	^{14}C-D-xylose breath test Glucose hydrogen breath test Schilling test plus antibiotics	Search for predisposing factor if results of any of the tests are positive
Bile acid malabsorption	SeHCAT test, ^{14}C-TCA test	Does not differentiate between primary and secondary causes
Exocrine pancreatic insufficiency	Quantitative fecal fat	To establish malabsorption in chronic pancreatitis
	Fecal elastase or chymotrypsin, tubeless tests (see Chapters 54 and 57)	Variable sensitivity and specificity, depending on type of test and stage of the disease
Vitamin B$_{12}$ malabsorption	Schilling test	Test is performed without intrinsic factor and depending on result with intrinsic factor, with antibiotics or with pancreatic enzymes (see text). Further tests are needed if small intestinal bacterial overgrowth, terminal ileal disease, or pancreatic disease is suspected

*See text for diagnostic accuracy of the different tests mentioned.
SeHCAT, selenium-75-homotaurocholic acid test; TCA, taurocholic acid.

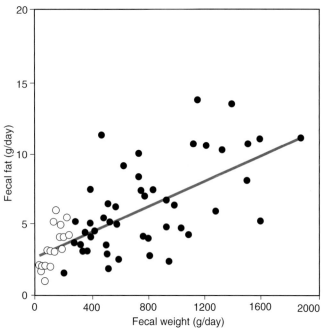

Figure 98–7   Graph showing fecal fat output (average of a 3-day stool collection) plotted as a function of fecal weight from normal subjects (○) and from subjects with induced diarrhea (●). The washout effect of diarrhea increases fecal excretion of fat to levels above the upper limit of normal (7 g/day). In diarrhea, therefore, a fecal fat excretion of 14 g/day should be used as the upper limit of normal. (From Fine KD, Fordtran JS: The effect of diarrhea on fecal fat excretion. Gastroenterology 102:1936, 1992.)

72 hours, adherence to an 80- to 100-g fat diet, and a diet diary to determine fat intake.

Despite the limitations of quantitative fecal fat analysis, it nevertheless is still useful in several clinical circumstances: to establish malabsorption and avoid nutritional deterioration[109] when overt features of intestinal or pancreatic disorders are lacking, such as in some cases of osteoporosis, osteomalacia, anemia, or weight loss; to monitor treatment in patients with established malabsorptive disorders, such as exocrine pancreatic insufficiency or short bowel syndrome; to estimate fecal calorie loss in patients with severe malabsorption syndromes; and to quantitate fecal fat excretion in patients with diarrhea who have undergone ileal resection, to distinguish steatorrhea due to bile acid deficiency from secretory diarrhea caused by bile acid loss, because treatments for these conditions differ.[110] Elevated fecal fat values can be observed in patients consuming a diet rich in the fat substitute Olestra.[105]

Semiquantitative Fat Analysis

For the acid steatocrit test,[111] a sample of stool is diluted 1:3 with distilled water in a test tube. The diluted stool is homogenized, and a 500-µL aliquot is pipetted into a tube. Then 100 mL of 5M HClO₄ is added to allow better fat extraction and separation of the lipid layer. An aliquot of the diluted stool-HClO₄ mixture is put into a nonheparinized microcapillary tube and sealed on one end. After centrifugation of this aliquot at 13,000 rpm for 15 minutes, the fatty layer (FL) and the solid layer (SL) are

measured, and the acid steatocrit (AS) is determined according to the following equation:

$$AS\ (\%) = [FL/(FL + SL)] \times 100$$

An acid steatocrit of less than 31% is normal. In a small study, the acid steatocrit for random spot stool samples had a high sensitivity and specificity for detection of steatorrhea, compared with the van de Kamer method, which is performed on a 72-hour stool collection. A linear correlation also was found between results obtained with the acid steatocrit and those of the van de Kamer method, although results were quite divergent in some patients.[111] Quantitative fecal fat measurements, however, usually are based on 48- to 72-hour stool collections, to minimize the effect of day-to-day variability in fecal fat excretion; therefore, the acid steatocrit cannot be expected to replace quantitative measurement of fat output in borderline cases, or in cases in which exact measurements of fecal fat loss are required.

Qualitative Fecal Fat Analysis

Fat analysis by microscopic examination of random stool samples may provide a clue to the presence of steatorrhea, although it cannot be used to exclude steatorrhea. Its advantage is that it is easy to perform. A sample of stool is placed on a glass slide to which several drops of glacial acetic acid and Sudan III stain are added. Acidification of stool samples improves fat extraction and separation of the lipid layer.[111] The slide is held over a burner and the acidified mixture heated to boiling and examined while still warm for presence of orange fat globules. A count of up to 100 globules with a diameter less than 4 mm per high-power field is normal.[6] Results of qualitative fat analysis by this method and of quantitative fat analysis do not correlate very well.[112] In a small study, Sudan staining of spot stool samples had a sensitivity of 78% and a specificity of 70% for the detection of steatorrhea,[111] but another quantitative microscopic method of counting and measuring fat globules has been shown to correlate with chemically measured fecal fat output.[113]

Breath Tests for Fat Malabsorption

The principle of the ¹⁴C-triolein breath test is to measure $^{14}CO_2$ in breath after ingestion of a triglyceride that has been radiolabeled with ¹⁴C. Fat malabsorption results in decreased pulmonary excretion of $^{14}CO_2$.[114] Because of erroneous results in a variety of metabolic and pulmonary diseases, lack of sensitivity in mild malabsorption, radiation exposure to the patient, cost of the substrate, and the need for expensive equipment, this test has not found widespread acceptance for clinical use; the nonradioactive isotope ¹³C has been used to label triglycerides (see later on).

Serum Tests for Fat Malabsorption

Experience with the measurement of the serum concentration of β-carotene for the qualitative assessment of fat malabsorption is limited. It has been suggested as a useful screening test for steatorrhea, with values below 100 mg/100 mL suggesting the presence of steatorrhea and values less than 47 mg/100 mL strongly indicative of steatorrhea. β-Carotene can be measured photometrically at 456 nm.[115] Concentrations in excess of 100 mg/100 mL do not exclude mild steatorrhea, although they make steatorrhea with fat losses in excess of 16 g per day very unlikely. Normal values also have been established in the pediatric population.[116] β-Carotene can be falsely low in patients with liver disease or in alcoholics who consume a β-carotene–deficient diet. Disorders in lipoproteins or intake of carotene-containing food additives also can influence the results.

CARBOHYDRATE MALABSORPTION

The hydrogen breath test is a noninvasive test that takes advantage of the fact that in most people, bacterial carbohydrate metabolism results in accumulation of hydrogen, which then is absorbed by the colonic mucosa and excreted in the breath. Using different carbohydrates, such as lactose or fructose, the hydrogen breath test can be used to detect malabsorption of these carbohydrates. Measurement of breath hydrogen excretion after ingestion of lactulose has been used to assess orocecal transit time, and glucose has been used as a substrate to detect small bowel bacterial overgrowth, although sensitivity and specificity are poor.[117] Unfortunately, up to 18% of persons are hydrogen nonexcretors,[118] and in these persons, hydrogen breath test results may be falsely negative because hydrogen is metabolized by bacteria to methane.

The diagnosis of lactose malabsorption is established if an increase in breath hydrogen concentration of greater than 20 parts per million over baseline occurs after ingestion of 20-50 g of lactose. An increase within the first 30 minutes after ingestion of lactose has to be disregarded, because it may be due to bacterial degradation of lactose in the oral cavity. Up to 4 hours may be required for the increase in breath hydrogen concentration to occur. Breath hydrogen measurements obtained before and at 30, 60, 90, 180, and 240 minutes after ingestion of 50 g of lactose provide the best diagnostic yield, with the least possible number of measurements.[118]

The lactose hydrogen breath test still is considered to be the gold standard for the clinical evaluation of lactose malabsorption by many researchers, but this test may miss the disorder in hydrogen nonexcretors. In these patients, a lactose tolerance test, that is, measurement of blood glucose before and 30 minutes after ingestion of 50 g of lactose, can be used. An increase in glucose concentration of less than 20 mg/dL over baseline within 30 minutes of ingestion of 50 g of lactose is indicative of lactose malabsorption. The lactose tolerance test has a lower sensitivity to diagnose lactose malabsorption compared with the lactose hydrogen breath test.[118]

Lactase deficiency in acquired primary lactase deficiency (adult-type hypolactasia) is not caused by mutations in the gene coding for intestinal lactase (*LPH* gene). Publications have reported, however, that a single-nucleotide polymorphism (SNP) –13910 T/C upstream of the *LPH* gene is involved in the regulation of intestinal lactase expression.[119] A CC genotype at the SNP –13910 T/C is associated with acquired primary lactase deficiency (adult-type hypolactasia), whereas TC and TT

genotypes are linked with lactase persistence.[120,121] This polymorphism can be used as a diagnostic test for adult-type hypolactasia.[121]

In patients with diarrhea, a stool test to detect a fecal pH lower than 5.5 can serve as a qualitative indicator of carbohydrate malabsorption.[122] In the research setting, fecal carbohydrates can be measured by the anthrone method, which measures carbohydrates on a weight basis.[123] By contrast, the reducing sugar method gives results on a molar basis and therefore provides information about the osmotic activity of malabsorbed carbohydrates.[18] Total short-chain fatty acids and lactic acid, which are the products of bacterial carbohydrate metabolism, can be measured in stool by titration.[124] Individual short-chain fatty acids can be determined by gas chromatography.[125]

PROTEIN MALABSORPTION

The classic test to quantify protein malabsorption, measurement of fecal nitrogen content in a quantitatively collected stool specimen,[13] rarely is used today. For research purposes, a combined ^{14}C-octanoic acid–[13]C-egg white breath test, accompanied by measurement of the urinary output of phenol and *p*-cresol, which are specific metabolites of tyrosine, has been used to assess the effect of gastric acid on protein digestion.[126] In this method, labeling of the ^{13}C-egg protein test meal with ^{14}C-octanoic acid allowed the simultaneous measurement of protein assimilation and gastric emptying rate. Phenol and *p*-cresol result from protein that has escaped digestion and absorption in the small intestine. They are rapidly absorbed, detoxified, and excreted in urine. Recovery of higher amounts of urinary phenols observed after omeprazole treatment in the study of this test indicated an increased availability of protein in the colon.

VITAMIN B₁₂ (COBALAMIN) MALABSORPTION

Schilling Test

The Schilling test is used clinically to distinguish between gastric and ileal causes of vitamin B_{12} deficiency and to evaluate the function of the ileum in patients with diarrhea or malabsorption. The results of the test are not influenced by vitamin B_{12} replacement therapy. The Schilling test does not have an important clinical role for the assessment of pancreatic insufficiency or bacterial overgrowth, because more direct approaches to diagnose these disorders are available. Because both intrinsic factor and hydrochloric acid are produced by parietal cells in humans, alternative approaches to diagnosing pernicious anemia are to document atrophic gastritis by endoscopy and biopsy; to confirm achlorhydria by acid secretion analysis and increased serum gastrin levels; and to look for antibodies directed against parietal cells or intrinsic factor in the serum.[28,33,127] Because the intrinsic factor used in the Schilling test is of bovine origin, the test is not commercially available in some countries.

The Schilling test is performed by administering a small oral dose of radiolabeled vitamin B_{12} and, simultaneously or within 1 or 2 hours, a large intramuscular "flushing dose" of nonradiolabeled vitamin B_{12}. The latter saturates vitamin B_{12} carriers; thus, radioactive vitamin B_{12} absorbed by the intestine is excreted in the urine. If less than 7% to 10% of the administered dose is recovered in urine within 24 hours, vitamin B_{12} malabsorption is confirmed. To specify the site of vitamin B_{12} malabsorption, a second phase of the Schilling test has to be performed subsequently with oral administration of intrinsic factor. In patients with pernicious anemia, the results of the Schilling test normalize after oral administration of intrinsic factor.[26,127]

Patients with pancreatic exocrine insufficiency may have an abnormal result on the Schilling test, with or without added intrinsic factor, but results normalize with the addition of pancreatic enzymes (Chapter 57). In ileal disease or following ileal resection, abnormal results of the Schilling test persist despite use of intrinsic factor. Schilling test results are normal in patients with dietary vitamin B_{12} deficiency, in protein-bound (food-bound) vitamin B_{12} malabsorption,[26,33] and sometimes in congenital transcobalamin II deficiency.[128] In patients with food-bound cobalamin malabsorption, a modified Schilling test using cobalamin bound to eggs, chicken serum, or various meats can be used to detect cobalamin malabsorption.[33]

False-positive results on the Schilling test may be due to renal dysfunction or inadequate urine collection.[127] The value of this test is diminished by the need for accurately timed urine collections. Results in the 5% to 10% excretion range often are difficult to interpret. A variation of the standard Schilling test is the dual-isotope or "single-stage" Schilling test, in which two different cobalamin isotopes are given simultaneously, one of them bound to intrinsic factor. This makes it possible to perform the first two phases of the Schilling test in one day; however, the results of this test are not as accurate as those obtained with the standard protocol.[26,127]

Serum Test for Vitamin B_{12} and Folate Deficiency

Measurements of serum cobalamin and folate concentrations commonly are used to detect deficiency states of these vitamins. The sensitivity and specificity of these tests are unknown, because no gold standard test has been established, and because serum levels do not always correlate with body stores.[26,129] Some authors suggest that the disappearance of symptoms after cobalamin or folate replacement probably is the most sensitive marker for deficiency of these vitamins.[127] Several causes of misleading serum cobalamin levels have been established. Serum vitamin B_{12} levels can be normal despite depleted body stores in small intestinal bacterial overgrowth (as a result of production of inactive cobalamin analogs by the bacteria), liver disease, myeloproliferative disorders, and congenital transcobalamin II deficiency. By contrast, use of oral contraceptives, pregnancy, and folate deficiency can cause low serum cobalamin levels despite normal body stores.[127] Serum folate concentrations decrease within a few days of dietary folate restriction, even if tissue stores are normal. Feeding also influences serum folate levels;

therefore, determination of folate in the fasting state is recommended. Measurement of red blood cell folate concentration has been considered a better estimate of folate tissue stores than serum folate levels by some authors.[33,127]

In cobalamin deficiency, serum concentrations of methylmalonic acid and total homocysteine are elevated.[33,127,129] Folate deficiency results only in an increase in serum homocysteine concentration.[33,127,129] In patients with slightly low or borderline serum cobalamin levels, determination of methylmalonic acid and homocysteine may therefore be helpful in establishing the diagnosis of a deficiency state. Levels of these metabolites tend to normalize within 1 to 2 weeks after institution of replacement therapy, and some authors have suggested that their measurement can be used to distinguish between cobalamin and folate deficiency states.[129] The distinction is important, because in cobalamin-deficient patients, supplemental replacement of folate may correct hematologic changes despite progression of neurologic disease.

BACTERIAL OVERGROWTH

Tests for the diagnosis of bacterial overgrowth are covered in more detail in Chapter 99. Briefly, tests used to diagnose bacterial overgrowth are the quantitative culture of a small intestinal aspirate (which is considered to be the gold standard diagnostic test) and several breath tests, including the ^{14}C-glycocholate breath test, the ^{14}C-D-xylose breath test, the lactulose hydrogen breath test, and the glucose hydrogen breath test. The rationale for the breath tests is the production by intraluminal bacteria of volatile metabolites (i.e., $^{14}CO_2$ or H_2), from the administered substances, which can be measured in the exhaled breath.

EXOCRINE PANCREATIC INSUFFICIENCY

Pancreatic function tests are discussed in detail in Chapters 54 and 57. Invasive pancreatic function tests require duodenal intubation and measurement of pancreatic enzyme, volume, and bicarbonate output after pancreatic stimulation by a liquid test meal (the Lundh test) or by injection of cholecystokinin (CCK) or secretin. Noninvasive tests include measurement of fecal chymotrypsin or elastase concentration, the fluorescein dilaurate test, and the N-benzoyl-L-tyrosyl para-aminobenzoic acid (NBT-PABA) test. In many clinical settings, the measurement of fecal concentration of chymotrypsin or elastase may be sufficient to diagnose or exclude exocrine pancreatic insufficiency. Elastase has a higher sensitivity for the detection of exocrine pancreatic insufficiency compared with chymotrypsin,[130] but the specificity of elastase is low,[131] and fecal elastase levels can be elevated in diseases of the small bowel with villus atrophy.[132]

Measurement of pancreatic enzymes and components of pancreatic fluid in duodenal aspirates obtained during endoscopy and after intravenous stimulation with secretin and CCK may have an excellent correlation with the more classic intubation tests for secretory function.[133,134]

BILE SALT MALABSORPTION

In patients with steatorrhea due to ileal disease or resection, bile salt malabsorption usually is present, but measurement of bile acid malabsorption is of limited clinical value. In patients with diarrhea without steatorrhea, bile salt malabsorption may be present in the absence of overt ileal disease, and in such cases, measurement of bile salt absorption is helpful.

Measurement of Fecal Bile Acid Output

Elevated fecal bile acid concentrations or output can indicate intestinal bile acid malabsorption.[135] Under steady-state conditions, the increased fecal bile acid output reflects increased hepatic synthesis of bile acids.[136] In severe bile acid malabsorption, fecal bile acid output can be reduced, however, if hepatic synthesis of bile acids is impaired. The measurement can be performed by either enzymatic methods or gas chromatography. This test requires a quantitative stool collection, and the analytic techniques are time consuming and require considerable expertise. Enzymatic methods may be unreliable in severe steatorrhea.[137]

^{14}C-Taurocholate Bile Acid Absorption Test

The ^{14}C-taurocholate bile acid absorption test requires a 72-hour stool collection after ingestion of radioactively labeled bile acid. The rate of intestinal bile acid absorption is calculated from the fecal recovery of ^{14}C-labeled taurocholic acid (^{14}C-TCA). Normal values for this test have been established in normal persons with laxative-induced diarrhea, because diarrhea by itself can increase fecal losses of bile acids,[136] presumably because of accelerated intestinal transit.[138] Clinical limitations of this test are that it requires substantial analytical work, access to a gamma camera, and a time-consuming stool collection.

Therapeutic Trial of Bile Acid–Binding Resins (Cholestyramine)

A therapeutic trial of cholestyramine or other bile acid–binding resins can be used to diagnose bile acid malabsorption as a cause of diarrhea. It is, however, controversial to what extent a clinical response to cholestyramine correlates with the presence of bile acid malabsorption, because cholestyramine may have a non-specific constipating effect in patients with diarrhea from other causes. Failure of diarrhea to remit within 3 days of initiation of cholestyramine makes bile acid malabsorption an unlikely cause of diarrhea; however, some patients respond only to large doses of cholestyramine.

In patients with established bile acid malabsorption in whom no improvement is obtained with bile acid–binding resins, it is very unlikely that bile acid malabsorption is the cause of diarrhea. In these patients, bile acid malabsorption is considered a secondary phenomenon due to a "washout effect."[136] In patients with severe bile acid malabsorption resulting in steatorrhea, cholestyramine may even aggravate fat malabsorption and diarrhea.[3] Therefore, without further testing for bile acid malabsorption, neither a positive nor a negative result of a therapeutic trial of cholestyramine constitutes proof of the presence or absence, respectively, of bile acid malabsorption.

Selenium-75–Labeled Homotaurocholic Acid Test

The radioactive taurocholic acid analog used for this test is resistant to bacterial deconjugation. After it has been administered orally, the patient undergoes serial gamma scintigraphy to measure whole-body bile acid retention or, as suggested by some authors, bile acid retention in the gallbladder.[139] A limitation of this test is that normal values for bile acid retention, which are used to compare normal and abnormal bile acid absorption, were obtained only in healthy persons without diarrhea.[140] As mentioned earlier, however, "secondary" bile acid malabsorption can be induced by diarrhea itself and is proportional to the stool weight, as demonstrated with the ^{14}C-TCA test.[136,138] For this test to be clinically useful, normal values need to be established for patients with diarrhea. Finally, this test is very time consuming, because bile acid retention needs to be measured either 4 or 7 days (depending on the protocol) after the bile acid administration.

D-XYLOSE TEST

Absorption of the pentose D-xylose is facilitated by passive diffusion. Approximately 50% of the absorbed D-xylose is metabolized, and the remainder is excreted in urine. After an overnight fast, a 25-g dose of D-xylose is swallowed, and the patient is encouraged to drink sufficient volumes of fluid to maintain good urine output. Urine is collected for the next 5 hours. As an alternative, 1 hour after ingestion of D-xylose, a venous sample may be taken.[141] Less than 4 g (16% excretion) of D-xylose in the urine collection or a serum xylose concentration below 20 mg/dL is indicative of abnormal intestinal absorption. The traditional urine test appears to be more reliable than the 1-hour blood test.

False-positive results occur if the duration of urine collection is too short or if the patient is dehydrated or has renal dysfunction, significant ascites, delayed gastric emptying, or portal hypertension. D-Xylose absorption may be normal in patients with only mild impairment of mucosal function or with predominantly distal small bowel disease. Because D-xylose is susceptible to bacterial metabolism, absorption is diminished in patients with bacterial overgrowth, although the test has a poor sensitivity for detection of this condition.[142] The test is of limited clinical value today and mostly has been replaced by small bowel biopsy.[143]

INTESTINAL PERMEABILITY TESTS

Intestinal permeability tests mostly are used in studies of the pathophysiology of intestinal disorders; they do not provide a specific diagnosis.[144]

Most current permeability tests are based on the differential absorption of mono- and disaccharides. Mucosal damage results in an increased permeability for disaccharides and oligosaccharides, consequent to epithelial injury, and a decreased permeability of monosaccharides, due to reduction of mucosal surface area.[145] Absorption is measured by urinary excretion. Expression of results as the absorption ratio of the mono- and disaccharide minimizes the influences of gastric emptying, intestinal transit, renal and hepatic function, and variations in time of urine collections.[146]

Increased intestinal permeability has been shown to predict the development of Crohn's disease or relapse in patients with this disease.[147,148] In celiac disease, the finding of considerably increased permeability is a sensitive marker for advanced disease; permeability tests also have been used to judge response to a gluten-free diet.[149] Elevated serum aminotransferase levels in patients with celiac disease correlate with increased intestinal permeability.[150] Disturbances of intestinal permeability have been documented in users of nonsteroidal anti-inflammatory drugs,[151] in inflammatory joint disease,[152] and in diabetic diarrhea.[153]

^{13}C BREATH TESTS

The increasing availability of stable isotopes has raised interest in replacing the radioactive ^{14}C by nonradioactive ^{13}C for breath tests.[117,154-156] In diseases with malabsorption, ^{13}C-labeled substrates have been evaluated for the diagnosis of steatorrhea,[157] evaluation of the digestibility of egg protein,[126] and the diagnosis of small bowel bacterial overgrowth and exocrine pancreatic insufficiency.[158] In general, because of concerns about diagnostic accuracy, costs of the substrates, and the equipment and limited availability, these tests have not gained widespread acceptance.

MALABSORPTION IN SPECIFIC DISEASE STATES

LACTOSE MALABSORPTION AND INTOLERANCE

Deficiency of the intestinal brush border enzyme lactase may lead to lactose malabsorption, which may result in lactose intolerance. Several causes for lactase deficiency in infants have been recognized. Unlike other intestinal disaccharidases, which develop early in fetal life, lactase levels remain low until the 34th week of gestation.[159] *Transient lactase deficiency in premature infants* may lead to symptoms of lactose malabsorption, such as diarrhea, until normal intestinal lactase activity develops. In rare cases in which enzyme deficiency is manifest at the time of birth and is permanent, *congenital lactase deficiency* (MIM 223000)* is diagnosed. *Reversible lactase deficiency*

may occur at all ages as a result of transient small bowel injury associated with acute diarrheal illnesses.

Acquired primary lactase deficiency (adult-type hypolactasia, MIM 223100) is the most common form of lactase deficiency worldwide. Most populations lose considerable lactase activity in adulthood.[160] The decline in lactase activity is a multifactorial process that is regulated at the gene transcription level[161] and leads to decreased biosynthesis or retardation of intracellular transport or maturation of the enzyme lactase–phlorizin hydrolase.[162] In white persons, a single-nucleotide polymorphism (SNP) –13910 T/C upstream of the gene coding for the enzyme lactase–phlorizin hydrolase (*LPH* gene) has been found to be involved in the regulation of lactase–phlorizin hydrolase.[119] The CC genotype of the SNP –13910 T/C upstream of the *LPH* gene is associated with adult-type hypolactasia; TC and TT genotypes are linked with lactase persistence.[120] Because it is present in most of the adult human population, this form of lactase deficiency has to be considered normal, rather than abnormal. Lactase deficiency usually produces symptoms only in adulthood, although lactase levels in affected persons start to decline during childhood.[163] Lactase activity persists in most adults of Western European heritage[164] (Table 98–12). Even in this group, the activity of lactase is only approximately half the activity of sucrase and less than 20% of the activity of maltase.[163] Accordingly, in these persons lactase activity is much more susceptible to a reduction in mucosal digestive function with acute or chronic gastrointestinal illnesses.

In lactose malabsorbers, it may be unclear whether lactose malabsorption is from acquired primary lactase deficiency or is the consequence of another small bowel disorder. Therefore, in the individual lactose malabsorber, especially with an ethnic background associated with a low prevalence of acquired primary lactase deficiency, it may be necessary to exclude other malabsorptive small bowel disorders, such as celiac disease. The main symptoms of lactose intolerance are bloating, abdominal cramps, increased flatus, and diarrhea. The development of bloating and abdominal cramps presumably is associ-

---

*The MIM (Mendelian Inheritance in Man) system assigns numbers to specific diseases according to a continuously updated catalog of human genes and genetic disorders, available on line as Online Mendelian Inheritance in Man (OMIM) (http://www.ncbi.nlm.gov/omim). OMIM is based on the book *Mendelian Inheritance in Man* (authored and edited by Dr. Victor A. McKusick and a team of science writers and editors at Johns Hopkins University and elsewhere and published by McKusick-Nathans Institute for Genetic Medicine, Johns Hopkins University, Baltimore, and National Center for Biotechnology Information, National Library of Medicine, Bethesda, 2000), which focuses primarily on inherited, or heritable, genetic diseases.

Table 98–12 Prevalence of Acquired Primary Lactase Deficiency (Adult-Type Hypolactasia)

Lactase Deficiency–Predominant Ethnic Groups (60% to 100% lactase deficient)

Middle East and Mediterranean: Arabs, Israeli Jews, Greek Cypriots, southern Italians

Asia: Thais, Indonesians, Chinese, Koreans

Africa: South Nigerian, Hausa, Bantu

North and South America: Eskimos, Canadian and U.S. Indians, Chami Indians

Lactase Persistence–Predominant Ethnic Groups (2% to 30% lactase deficient)

Northern Europeans

Africa: Hima, Tussi, Nomadic Fulani

India: Indians from Punjab and New Delhi areas

Data from Johnson JD: The regional and ethnic distribution of lactose malabsorption. In Paige DM, Bayless TM (eds): Lactose Digestion. Clinical and Nutritional Implications, 1st ed. Baltimore, Johns Hopkins University Press, 1981, p 11.

ated with increased perception of luminal distention by gas,[165] because no clear relation has been observed between the amount of lactose ingested and the severity of symptoms.[166] Ingestion of as little as 3 g of lactose to as much as 96 g of lactose may be required to induce symptoms in persons with lactose malabsorption.[167] Gastrointestinal symptoms, including diarrhea, have been shown to be more severe in adults with shorter small bowel transit time,[168] but no such relation between intestinal transit and symptoms is observed in children.[169] Also, in pregnant women and in thyrotoxic patients with Graves' disease, changes in intestinal motility play a role in the clinical manifestation of lactose malabsorption.[170,171] In view of the poor correlation between lactose malabsorption and lactose intolerance, it is very important to monitor symptoms during a lactose hydrogen breath test, to confirm that symptoms during the test are truly representative of the patient's symptoms (Fig. 98–8).

Adult-type hypolactasia also may be a risk factor for development of osteoporosis and bone fractures, owing to patients' avoidance of dairy products[172] or interference with calcium absorption.[173]

Patients in whom a clear association between symptoms and lactose malabsorption can be established should be educated about a lactose-reduced or lactose-free diet. Yogurt may be better tolerated by these patients,[174] and these products provide a good source of calcium. Consumption of whole milk or chocolate milk, rather than skim milk, and drinking milk with meals may reduce symptoms of lactose intolerance, presumably as a result of prolongation of gastric emptying. Alternatively, supplementation of dairy products with lactase of microbiologic origin may be suggested.[175] Furthermore, because many carbohydrates other than lactose are incompletely absorbed by the normal small intestine,[49] and because dietary fiber also may be metabolized by colonic bacteria, persistence of some symptoms while the patient is on a lactose-free diet is not uncommon. It also must be kept in mind that symptoms arising after ingestion of dairy products may instead be due to milk protein allergy or to intolerance of fat.

INCOMPLETE ABSORPTION AND INTOLERANCE OF FRUCTOSE

Fructose is found in modern diets either as a constituent of the disaccharide sucrose or as the monosaccharide, used as a sweetener in a variety of food items. Fructose as a constituent of sucrose is absorbed by a well-characterized absorptive system integrating enzymatic hydrolysis of the disaccharide by sucrase and transfer of the resulting two monosaccharides through the apical membrane of the epithelial cell. The absorptive capacity for fructose that is not accompanied by glucose, however, is relatively small.[176]

Ingestion of food that contains fructose in excess of glucose may result in symptoms such as abdominal bloating or diarrhea[177] and also may provoke symptoms in patients with irritable bowel syndrome[178]; it has been suggested that as little as 3 g of fructose may precipitate symptoms in functional bowel disorders.[179] Fructose malabsorption usually is identified by a positive result on a breath hydrogen test after ingestion of 25 or 50 g of fructose. Because fructose content in fruit and in soft drinks usually is below 8 g/100 g of fruit or drink, the amounts of fructose used in the breath hydrogen test are unphysiologic, and no data are available on how many asymptomatic people would have a positive test result. Nevertheless, fructose contents of 30 to 40 g/100 g can be present in chocolate, caramel and pralines.[180]

In a group of patients with isolated fructose malabsorption, no defect of the gene encoding the luminal fructose transporter (*GLUT5*) could be detected.[181] It is therefore unlikely that patients who present with gastrointestinal symptoms really have a defect of intestinal fructose absorption; it is more likely that they belong to a subset of people in whom ingestion of foods rich in fructose provokes symptoms related to other disorders, such as irritable bowel syndrome. Patients in whom symptoms develop after ingestion of fructose-rich food also may represent a subset of persons with unique, but not necessarily abnormal, colonic bacterial activity.[182]

In conclusion, testing for fructose malabsorption by the hydrogen breath test may be useful in identifying a

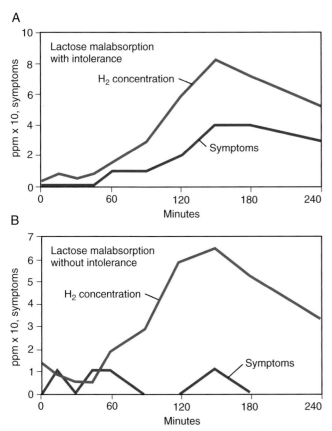

Figure 98–8 The clinical relevance of an abnormal lactose hydrogen breath test should be assessed by monitoring abdominal symptoms (bloating, cramps, pain) during the test. Breath hydrogen concentration in parts per million [ppm] and symptom scores for two different patients are plotted on the graphs. *A,* The patient has symptoms associated with an increase in breath hydrogen concentration and therefore can be considered to have lactose intolerance. *B,* The patient has no increase in symptoms, although the breath hydrogen concentration increases considerably; therefore, the patient has lactose malabsorption without lactose intolerance.

subset of patients in whom dietary restriction of foods with excessive fructose content may be beneficial in the treatment of bloating and diarrhea. Symptoms in these persons probably are the result of ingestion of unphysiologic amounts of fructose and not the consequence of a defect in fructose absorption.

STEATORRHEA DUE TO ILEAL BILE ACID MALABSORPTION

Bile acid malabsorption usually is present in patients who have undergone ileal resection or bypass operations, or who have severe disease of the ileum, where specific bile acid transport proteins normally are located. The clinical consequences of bile acid malabsorption depend on whether bile acid loss can be compensated by increased hepatic synthesis.[183] Ileal resection of greater than 100 cm usually results in severe bile acid malabsorption that cannot be compensated by increased hepatic synthesis; therefore, steatorrhea will result from impaired micelle formation due to decreased luminal concentrations of conjugated bile acids.[3,183] In ileal resections of less than 100 cm, bile acid malabsorption usually can be compensated by increased hepatic synthesis, and malabsorbed bile acids cause secretory diarrhea rather than steatorrhea.[3,183] Secretory diarrhea caused by or associated with bile acid malabsorption is discussed in detail in Chapter 9.

The differing pathophysiology of steatorrhea and of secretory diarrhea due to bile acid malabsorption not only determines the clinical picture but also is important for choosing the appropriate therapy. In patients with compensated bile acid malabsorption, binding of bile salts in the lumen of the intestine by cholestyramine reduces diarrhea. By contrast, in decompensated bile acid malabsorption, cholestyramine further depletes the bile acid pool, thereby worsening steatorrhea. In several cases of decompensated bile acid malabsorption after extensive ileal resections, intestinal fat absorption was improved markedly by the oral administration of conjugated bile acids.[110,184,185] Cholylsarcosine taken in a dose of 2 to 3 g per meal has been reported to enhance fat absorption and nutritional status in patients with short bowel syndrome who have residual colon.[110,186,187] Natural conjugated bile acids lessen severity of steatorrhea in these patients to a smaller extent.[187] Improved fat absorption also was associated with decreased urinary oxalate excretion.[186]

A syndrome of primary bile acid malabsorption with normal ileal morphology has been reported in children. At the time of birth, bile acid malabsorption causes severe diarrhea and steatorrhea, failure to thrive, and reduced plasma cholesterol levels.[188] A study in an index case has shown that this type of bile acid malabsorption is caused by mutations in the ileal sodium–bile acid cotransporter gene (*SLC10A2*).[4] By contrast, adult-onset idiopathic bile acid malabsorption is not caused by *SLC10A2* mutations.[189] The exact pathophysiology of bile acid malabsorption in these patients is unknown, although accelerated intestinal transit may be a causative factor.[190]

AMYLOIDOSIS

Malabsorption has been reported in AL-type amyloidosis, AA-type amyloidosis, and hereditary amyloidosis.[191-193] Fat malabsorption occurs in less than 5% of patients with AL amyloidosis,[191] whereas it was present in 58% of Swedish patients with familial amyloidosis.[192] Fecal fat excretion can reach levels up to 60 g per day.[192] Gastrointestinal absorption of D-xylose and vitamin B[12] can be reduced,[192,194] and protein-losing enteropathy may develop.[195] Amyloid deposits are found in the muscle layers, the stroma of the lamina propria and the submucosa, the wall of mucosal and submucosal blood vessels in the gastrointestinal tract, and enteric and extraenteric nerves.[196,197]

In many patients with amyloidosis who have diarrhea or malabsorption, or both, symptoms suggestive of autonomic neuropathy are present.[138,192] Autonomic neuropathy causes rapid intestinal transit, which in turn leads to severe diarrhea and malabsorption despite normal transport capacity of the intestinal mucosa.[138] Other suggested mechanisms of malabsorption in amyloidosis are decreased absorption due to a physical barrier effect of amyloid deposits[198] and small intestinal bacterial overgrowth, which also might be a consequence of autonomic neuropathy.[194] Bile acid malabsorption is found in many patients with amyloidosis associated with autonomic neuropathy[199] and is caused by rapid intestinal transit, rather than impaired absorptive transport in the terminal ileum.[138] Diarrhea in these patients usually fails to respond to bile acid–binding agents.[138] Findings on gastrointestinal barium studies in patients with amyloidosis usually are normal, but such studies may show thickened folds, nodular lesions, filling defects, dilatation of bowel segments, or altered transit.[193] The endoscopic appearance of the gastrointestinal mucosa can show a fine granular appearance, polypoid protrusions, erosions, ulcerations, atrophic changes, and mucosal friability, but in many affected patients, no macroscopic changes are seen.[193,197] Histologic examination demonstrates amyloid deposits in 72% of esophageal, 75% to 95% of gastric, 83% to 100% of small intestinal, and 75% to 95% of colorectal biopsy specimens.[191,197,200] Subcutaneous fat pad aspiration or biopsy may make the diagnosis more safely without having to resort to endoscopic biopsy and the potential risk of intestinal bleeding. Amyloid deposits may not be seen with routine histologic stains and may be revealed only by a Congo red stain. Therapy of diarrhea in amyloidosis includes attempts to prolong intestinal transit time by means of opioids or octreotide and to avoid further amyloid deposition in the tissue, by treating the underlying disorder in AA amyloidosis, using melphalan and prednisone in AL amyloidosis, and administering colchicine in familial Mediterranean fever.

MALABSORPTION CAUSED BY DRUGS AND FOOD SUPPLEMENTS

Table 98–13[23,26,27,34,108,127,201-219] lists drugs and food supplements reported to induce malabsorption of vitamins, minerals, or nutrients, as well as the suggested pathophysiologic mechanisms by which this occurs.

Table 98–13 Drugs and Dietary Products Causing Malabsorption

Substance	Substrate Malabsorbed	Suggested Mechanism	Reference(s)
Acarbose	Carbohydrates	Inhibition of α-glucosidase	201
Antacids	Phosphate, iron, vitamin A	Luminal binding of substrates	202
Azathioprine	Generalized malabsorption	Villus atrophy	203
Biguanides (metformin, phenformin)	Cobalamin, folate, glucose	Inhibition of intestinal glucose or folate absorption; reduced ileal absorption of IF-cobalamin complex	202, 204, 205
Carbamazepine	Folate	Inhibition of intestinal folate absorption	206
Cholestyramine	Fat, fat-soluble vitamins, bile acids	Binding of conjugated bile salts	202
Colchicine	Fat, xylose, nitrogen, cobalamin, carotene	Mucosal damage and villus atrophy at high doses (impaired processing of IF-cobalamin receptor [the cubilin-AMN complex])	26, 202, 207
Contraceptives, oral*	Folate	Inhibition of pteroylpolyglutamate hydrolase (folate conjugase)	202
Ethanol	Xylose, fat, glucose, nitrogen, thiamine, cobalamin, folate	Mucosal damage; decreased disaccharidase activity; decreased pancreatic exocrine function and bile secretion	34, 202
Fiber, phytates	Iron, calcium, magnesium, zinc	Chelating agents	208
Glucocorticoids	Calcium	Inhibition of calcium absorption	23
Histamine H_2 receptor antagonists*	Cobalamin	Impaired release of food-bound B_{12} due to reduced gastric acid and pepsin secretion (and reduced IF secretion)	209
Irritant laxatives (phenolphthalein, bisacodyl, anthraquinones)	Fat, glucose, xylose	Washout effect; toxic effect on the mucosa	108, 202
Methotrexate	Folate, fat, cobalamin, xylose	Mucosal damage; inhibition of intestinal folate transport	202, 208
Methyldopa†	Generalized malabsorption	Mucosal damage	210
Neomycin	Fat, nitrogen, fat-soluble vitamins, cobalamin, mono- and disaccharides, iron	Mucosal damage; disruption of micelle formation	202, 207, 208
Olestra*	Fat-soluble vitamins	Binding of fat-soluble vitamins	211, 212
Orlistat	Fat, fat-soluble vitamins	Inhibition of pancreatic lipase	201
Para-aminosalicylate	Fat, cobalamin, folate	Unknown	26, 202
Phenytoin	Folate, calcium	Inhibition of folate and calcium absorption due to luminal alkalinization; impaired vitamin D metabolism	23, 208, 213
Proton pump inhibitors*	Cobalamin	Impaired release of food-bound cobalamin due to reduced gastric acid secretion; small intestinal bacterial overgrowth	27
Pyrimethamine	Folate	Competitive inhibition of intestinal folate absorption	214
Somatostatin analogs (e.g., octreotide)	Fat	Inhibition of hepatobiliary bile acid secretion; inhibition of pancreatic enzyme secretion; inhibition of CCK release	215, 216
Sulfonamides, including sulfasalazine	Folate	Inhibition of pteroylpolyglutamate hydrolase and folate transport	127, 208
Tetracycline	Calcium	Precipitation of luminal calcium	323
Thiazides	Calcium	Decreased $1,25(OH)_2D$ synthesis	324
Triamterene*	Folate	Competitive inhibition of intestinal folate absorption	214, 325

*Malabsorption usually does not result in deficiency states.
†Findings in case reports.
AMN, amnionless; CCK, cholecystokinin; IF, intrinsic factor; $1,25(OH)_2D$, 1,25-dihydroxyvitamin D.

MALABSORPTION AFTER GASTRIC RESECTION

Severe steatorrhea after total and partial gastric resections has been a long-observed complication of these operations.[12] Fecal fat excretion rates usually are between 15 and 20 g per day,[1] but values of up to 60 g per day have been reported.[217,218] Suggested mechanisms include defective mixing of nutrients with digestive secretions, lack of gastric acid and gastric lipase secretion, decreased small bowel transit time, small intestinal bacterial overgrowth, and pancreatic insufficiency.[1,219] Studies have shown that pancreatic enzyme supplements[220] and antibiotic treatment[219] do not improve fat absorption or relieve symptoms after gastric resection. Total and partial gastric resections also can result in significant protein malabsorption,[12] whereas absorption of carbohydrates seems not to be significantly impaired. Nutrient malabsorption in these patients can result in gastrointestinal symptoms such as diarrhea and severe weight loss.[221]

Loss of parietal cells after total gastric resection results in diminished intrinsic factor secretion, which in turn leads to malabsorption of vitamin B_{12} and, in approximately 30% of patients, vitamin B_{12} deficiency; lack of release of food-bound cobalamin by diminished gastric acid and pepsin secretion and bacterial overgrowth have been implicated as additional pathogenetic factors. Iron malabsorption resulting in iron deficiency anemia also is commonly present in patients who have undergone gastric resection, although the mechanisms for iron malabsorption are not fully established; lack of acid secretion with resultant decreased solubilization of iron salts has been suggested as a possible cause. Calcium absorption can be severely impaired in patients with gastric resections, resulting in reduced bone density.[222] The mechanisms for calcium malabsorption probably are several, including decreased solubilization of calcium salts due to the loss of gastric acid secretion, rapid intestinal transit, low calcium intake secondary to milk intolerance, and malabsorption of vitamin D. Studies in gastrectomized rats have suggested that diminished calcium absorption after gastric resections is due mainly, if not entirely, to decreased calcium solubilization.[223] By contrast, studies in humans have shown that calcium absorption is normal in patients with atrophic gastritis and in persons in whom acid secretion was inhibited by acid-inhibiting drugs.[224] Treatment for patients who have undergone gastric resection should include the adequate supplementation of malabsorbed vitamins and minerals, to prevent serious long-term complications.[225]

MALABSORPTION IN THE ELDERLY

Malabsorption in elderly persons should not be ascribed to the aging process; it should be evaluated just as malabsorption occurring in younger patients. In healthy elderly persons, small bowel histologic features are normal despite a decline in cell turnover and continual cell renewal.[226,227] Malabsorption of fat has been described in chronic congestive heart failure[228] and in chronic intestinal ischemia (see Chapter 111), but this is not due to aging per se. Elderly persons may be more susceptible to gastrointestinal insult and subsequent decompensation of gastrointestinal function.[229]

Deficiencies of some nutrients, presumably caused by malabsorption, however, may be present in elderly persons with no overt gastrointestinal disease. An increased risk of deficiency of folate and vitamin B_{12}, despite adequate intake of these vitamins, has been reported in the elderly.[230] Malnutrition in the elderly can contribute considerably to morbidity and mortality, although it may be difficult to ascertain whether weight loss is due to altered appetite, increased catabolism, or malabsorption.

Small bowel bacterial overgrowth in elderly persons with gastric hypochlorhydria secondary to atrophic gastritis or treatment with a proton pump inhibitor usually is not associated with clinically significant malabsorption,[231] but an improvement in nutritional status after antibiotic treatment has been described in some elderly patients.[232]

CONNECTIVE TISSUE DISEASES

Scleroderma

The gastrointestinal tract is involved to a variable degree in most patients with systemic sclerosis. Early pathologic changes are characterized by vasculopathy, which results in ischemia and progressive organ dysfunction.[233] The typical histologic findings include atrophy of the muscle layers with increased deposition of elastin and collagen in the submucosa and serosa and between smooth muscle bundles of the muscularis externa.[234] Small bowel biopsy may reveal an increased number of plasma cells within the lamina propria and collagen deposits around and between lobules of Brunner's glands in the submucosa of the duodenum.[235]

Malabsorption in scleroderma usually results from bacterial overgrowth secondary to ineffective motility in the small bowel,[236] but other factors, such as decreased mucosal blood flow,[237] also may contribute. Malabsorption and bacterial overgrowth are not limited to patients with diffuse disease but also may occur in patients with long-standing limited cutaneous systemic sclerosis.[238] Elevated serum concentrations of motilin and CCK have been described in patients with scleroderma and fat malabsorption[239] but are thought to be secondary to myogenic or neurogenic disturbances of intestinal or gallbladder contractions.[240] In addition to antibiotic treatment of bacterial overgrowth, low doses of octreotide (50 μg subcutaneously every evening for 3 weeks) have been shown to induce intestinal migrating motor complexes, reduce bacterial overgrowth, and relieve abdominal symptoms.[236]

Lupus Erythematosus and Other Connective Tissue Diseases

Excessive fecal fat excretion associated with abnormalities on D-xylose breath testing may be found in some patients with lupus erythematosus. These findings may be accompanied by flattened and deformed villi with an inflammatory infiltrate on duodenal biopsy.[241] Malabsorption that resolved after treatment with prednisolone also has been described in association with the hypereosinophilic syndrome in lupus erythematosus.[242] Malabsorption is an uncommon feature of mixed connective tissue disease and polymyositis.[243,244]

CONGENITAL DEFECTS CAUSING MALABSORPTION

Table 98–14[4,10,26,30,40,44,128,245-269] lists congenital intestinal diseases that result in malabsorption of specific substrates or in a generalized malabsorption syndrome. Most of these diseases are very rare, but some occur with an increased frequency in certain ethnic groups.

Amino Acid Transport Defects

Amino acids are absorbed by the enterocyte as oligopeptides, dipeptides, and free amino acids. In several inborn

Table 98–14 Congenital Disorders of the Gastrointestinal Mucosa Resulting in Malabsorption

Disorder	Suggested Mode of Inheritance	Malabsorbed Substrates	Causative Gene	Suggested Mechanism of Malabsorption	Clinical Features	Reference(s)
Malabsorption of Amino Acids						
Hartnup's disorder* (MIM 234500)	AR	Neutral amino acids (tryptophan, leucine, methionine, phenylalanine, tyrosine, valine, ?histidine, ?lysine)	?	Decreased intestinal absorption of free neutral amino acids	Most patients are asymptomatic; some patients may have photosensitive skin rash, intermittent ataxia, psychotic behavior, mental retardation, and diarrhea	245
Cystinuria (types I to III) (MIM 220200)	AR (type I) and incomplete AR (types II, III)	Cystine and/or dibasic amino acids (lysine, ornithine, arginine)	Type I: *SLC3A1* Types II, III: *SLC7A9*	Decreased intestinal absorption of specific free amino acids due to a defective amino acid transporter located at the brush border membrane. *Type I:* no transport of cystine, lysine or arginine; *type II:* no transport of lysine and arginine and reduced transport of cystine; *type III:* reduced or normal cystine transport and reduced lysine and arginine transport	Aminoaciduria, cystine stones in the urinary tract	246
Lysinuric protein intolerance (MIM 222700)	AR	Dibasic amino acids (lysine, ornithine, arginine)	*SLC7A7*	Defect of the basolateral transporter (y+LAT-1) for dibasic amino acids (also malabsorption of di- and oligopeptides)	Sparse hair, hyperammonemia, nausea, vomiting, diarrhea, protein malnutrition, failure to thrive, and aversion to protein-rich food	247, 248
Isolated lysinuria*	?	Lysine	?	Decreased intestinal absorption of lysine	Mental retardation, malnutrition, and failure to thrive	248
Iminoglycinuria (MIM 242600)	AR	L-Proline	?	Impaired intestinal absorption of L-proline in a subgroup of subjects	Aminoaciduria, benign disorder	255
Blue diaper syndrome* (MIM 211000)	AR	Tryptophan	?	Intestinal tryptophan absorption defect	Blue discoloration of diapers, failure to thrive, hypercalcemia, and nephrocalcinosis	249
Methionine malabsorption syndrome* (Oasthouse syndrome) (MIM 250900)	AR	Methionine	?	Intestinal methionine absorption defect	Mental retardation, convulsions, diarrhea, white hair, hyperpnea; urine has characteristic sweet smell of dried celery	250
Oculocerebral syndrome of Lowe (MIM 309000)	XR	Lysine, arginine	*OCRL1*	Impaired intestinal lysine and arginine absorption	Aminoaciduria, mental retardation, cataracts, rickets, choreoathetosis, and renal disease	252

(Continued)

Table 98–14   Congenital Disorders of the Gastrointestinal Mucosa Resulting in Malabsorption—*cont'd*

Disorder	Suggested Mode of Inheritance	Malabsorbed Substrates	Causative Gene	Suggested Mechanism of Malabsorption	Clinical Features	Reference(s)
Malabsorption of Carbohydrates						
Congenital lactase deficiency (MIM 223000)	AR	Lactose	?	Permanent very low lactase activity	Diarrhea, bloating, and dehydration in the first days of life	253
Sucrase-isomaltase deficiency (MIM 222900)	AR	Sucrose, starch	Genetic heterogeneity	Sucrase activity is absent; isomaltase activity is absent or reduced; reduced maltase activity	Osmotic diarrhea after starch or sucrose ingestion; failure to thrive	253
Trehalase deficiency (MIM 275360)	AR	Trehalose	?	Lack of intestinal trehalase activity	Diarrhea and/or vomiting after mushroom ingestion	253
Glucose-galactose malabsorption (MIM 606824)	AR	Glucose, galactose	*SLC5A1*	Defect of the brush border sodium-glucose cotransporter (SGLT1)	Neonatal onset of osmotic diarrhea, dehydration, intermittent or constant glycosuria	254
Malabsorption of Fat						
Abetalipoproteinemia (MIM 200100)	AR	Fat, fat-soluble vitamins	*MTP*	Defective lipoprotein assembly due to a lack of MTP, resulting in triglyceride accumulation in the enterocytes and no chylomicron formation	Steatorrhea, diarrhea, neurologic symptoms, retinitis pigmentosa, failure to thrive, absence of chylomicrons and VLDL in the blood, and acanthocytosis	10
Familial hypobeta-lipoproteinemia (MIM 107730)	Incomplete AD	Fat, fat-soluble vitamins	*APOB*	Triglyceride accumulation in the enterocytes in homozygotes is due to formation of a truncated apolipoprotein B	*Homozygotes:* clinical manifestations as for abetalipoproteinemia *Heterozygotes:* fat absorption probably normal; hypolipidemia, and neurologic manifestations	10
Chylomicron retention disease (MIM 246700), Andersen's disease (MIM 607689)	AR	Fat	*SARA2*	Defective chylomicron formation and accumulation in the enterocytes	Steatorrhea, failure to thrive, absence of chylomicrons and reduced LDL levels in the blood; neurologic symptoms in some patients	10, 256
Wolman's disease, cholesteryl ester storage disease (MIM 278000)	AR	Fat	*LIPA (LAL)*	Deficient activity of hLAL/cholesterol ester hydrolase, causing accumulation of cholesteryl esters and triglycerides in various body tissues; infiltration of intestinal mucosa with foamy cells, intestinal damage	Steatorrhea, hepatosplenomegaly, abdominal distention; failure to thrive, and adrenal calcifications	257, 258
Malabsorption of Vitamins						
Congenital intrinsic factor deficiency (congenital pernicious anemia) (MIM 261000)	AR	Cobalamin (vitamin B$_{12}$)	*GIF*	Defective synthesis of IF or synthesis of an abnormal IF with either reduced affinity for cobalamin or for the ileal IF receptor, or increased susceptibility to proteolysis	Megaloblastic anemia, neurologic symptoms, and delayed development	31, 128, 259

Disease (MIM)	Inheritance	Nutrient	Gene	Defect	Clinical Features	References
Imerslund-Gräsbeck syndrome (ileal B$_{12}$ malabsorption, megaloblastic anemia type I) (MIM 261100)	AR	Cobalamin (vitamin B$_{12}$)	CUBN or AMN	Impaired ileal absorption of IF-cobalamin complex due to defects in the cubilin-AMN complex (IF-cobalamin receptor)	Megaloblastic anemia, neurologic symptoms, and proteinuria	26, 30, 128
Transcobalamin II deficiency (MIM 275350)	AR	Cobalamin (vitamin B$_{12}$)	TCN2	Defective transport of cobalamin out of enterocytes into the portal blood due to absence or malfunction of transcobalamin II	Vomiting, diarrhea, failure to thrive, anemia, immunodeficiency, and neurologic symptoms	31, 128
Malabsorption of Minerals						
Acrodermatitis enteropathica (MIM 201100)	AR	Zinc	SLC39A4	Defective zinc absorption in the small intestine due to a defect in the zinc transport protein (hZIP4)	Diarrhea, scaling erythematous dermatitis, alopecia, and neuropsychatric symptoms; onset after weaning	44
Isolated magnesium malabsorption (hypomagnesemia with secondary hypocalcemia [HOMG1]) (MIM 602014)	AR	Magnesium	TRPM6	Selective defect in intestinal magnesium absorption	Tetany, convulsion, diarrhea, and hypomagnesemia with secondary hypocalcemia	40, 261
Menkes disease (MIM 309400)	XR	Copper	ATP7A	General copper transport disorder; intestinal copper malabsorption with copper accumulation in the intestinal mucosa due to a defective transmembrane copper-transporting ATPase (MNK)	Cerebral degeneration, diarrhea, abnormal hair, hypopigmentation, arterial rupture, thrombosis, hypothermia, and bone changes	262
Occipital horn syndrome (X-linked cutis laxa) (MIM 304150)	XR	Copper	ATP7A	Milder form of same defect as in Menkes disease; low levels of functional MNK	Inguinal hernias, bladder and ureteral diverticula, skin and joint laxity, chronic diarrhea, and bone changes	262, 263
Hereditary selective deficiency of 1α,25(OH)$_2$D (pseudo–vitamin D deficiency rickets) (MIM 264700)	AR	Calcium	CYP27B1	Defective 25(OH)D 1α-hydroxylase, resulting in 1α,25(OH)$_2$D deficiency and reduced intestinal calcium absorption	Bone pain, deformities and fractures, muscle weakness	264

(Continued)

Table 98–14 Congenital Disorders of the Gastrointestinal Mucosa Resulting in Malabsorption—cont'd

Disorder	Suggested Mode of Inheritance	Malabsorbed Substrates	Causative Gene	Suggested Mechanism of Malabsorption	Clinical Features	Reference(s)
Hereditary generalized resistance to 1α,25(OH)$_2$D (vitamin D–resistant rickets) (MIM 277440)	AR	Calcium	VDR	Malfunction of the vitamin D receptor due to defective hormone binding, defective receptor translocation to nucleus, or defective receptor binding to DNA, resulting in malabsorption of calcium	Bone pain, deformities and fractures, muscle weakness, and alopecia	264
Other Defects						
Enterokinase deficiency (MIM 226200)	AR	Protein, fat	PRSS7	Defective activation of pancreatic proenzymes due to lack of intestinal enterokinase	Diarrhea, failure to thrive, hypoproteinemia, edema, and anemia	15, 265, 266
Congenital bile acid malabsorption (MIM 601295)	AR	Bile acids, fat	SLC10A2	Defect of the ileal ASBT	Steatorrhea, diarrhea, and failure to thrive	4
Microvillus inclusion disease (MIM 251850)	AR	Carbohydrates, fat, cobalamin, electrolytes, water	?	Villous atrophy with microvillus inclusions in enterocytes, absent or shortened brush border microvilli	Severe watery diarrhea and steatorrhea requiring total parenteral nutrition	267
Hyperinsulinism, with enteropathy and deafness (MIM 606528)	AR	Generalized malabsorption	USH1C, ABCC8, and KCNJ11	Enteropathy with villus atrophy and inflammation	Hyperinsulinism, profound congenital sensorineural deafness, enteropathy, and renal tubular dysfunction	268

*Reported in only a few case reports.

AD, autosomal dominant; AR, autosomal recessive; ASBT, sodium bile acid cotransporter; hLAL, human lysosomal acid lipase; LDL, low-density lipoprotein; MIM, Mendelian Inheritance in man (see page 2220 for a detailed explanation); MTP, microsomal triglyceride transfer protein; 1α,25(OH)$_2$D, 1α,25-dihydroxyvitamin D; 25(OH)D, 25-hydroxyvitamin D; VLDL, very-low-density lipoprotein; XR, X-linked recessive.

diseases, transport defects for different groups of amino acids have been identified in the intestine and kidney (see Table 98–14). In *iminoglycinuria, Hartnup's disorder,* and *cystinuria,* the intestinal transport defect seems to be of no or only minor clinical significance, because the amino acids affected by the transporter defects still can be absorbed as oligo- and dipeptides, and protein malnutrition can be avoided.[245,246,255] The manifestations in these diseases therefore are due mainly to amino acid transport defects in the kidney. In *lysinuric protein intolerance,* however, the transport defect is located on the basolateral membrane of the enterocytes, leading to malabsorption of cationic amino acids in both their mono- and dipeptide forms.[247] Patients with lysinuric protein intolerance are therefore intolerant to high-protein foods, with consequent development of protein malnutrition. Malabsorption of lysine with resultant deficiency of this essential amino acid is thought to be an important factor in the development of several disease manifestations in these patients[248] (see Table 98–14). Treatment consists of protein restriction and supplementation with oral citrulline. In *Hartnup's disorder,* oral administration of nicotinamide and a high-protein diet have been shown to relieve symptoms to some extent.[245]

Disaccharidase Deficiency and Transport Defects for Monosaccharides

In *sucrase-isomaltase deficiency,* affected infants usually become symptomatic after weaning with the introduction of starch and sucrose to the diet. Symptoms and signs include osmotic diarrhea, failure to thrive, excess flatus, and occasional vomiting. The diagnosis can be established by an oral sucrose absorption test. Treatment includes dietary avoidance of starch and sucrose.[253] Patients with this disease tend to experience spontaneous resolution of their symptoms with age.

Patients with *glucose-galactose malabsorption* suffer from severe diarrhea, leading to dehydration in the first days of life. The diarrhea stops only if glucose and galactose are eliminated from the diet. Older children and adults tolerate the offending carbohydrates better, but the transport defect is lifelong. The diagnosis can be established with an oral glucose tolerance test or by in vitro glucose absorption tests performed on intestinal biopsy specimens. Therapy consists of a fructose-based diet free of glucose and galactose. After the age of 3 months, the addition of foods containing low quantities of glucose or galactose (e.g., vegetables, fruits, cheese) is considered to be safe.[254]

Congenital Disorders of Lipid Absorption

Abetalipoproteinemia is a disorder of autosomal recessive inheritance characterized by triglyceride accumulation in the enterocytes. This disease seems to be caused by mutations in the gene for microsomal triglyceride transfer protein (MTP) resulting in a defective assembly of triglyceride-rich lipoproteins.[10] In the homozygous state, the disorder *familial hypobetalipoproteinemia,* of autosomal dominant inheritance, has clinical manifestations similar to those of abetalipoproteinemia (see Table 98–14). This disease seems to be caused by mutations of the apolipoprotein B gene in most cases.[10]

Chylomicron retention disease and *Anderson's disease* are caused by defective release of chylomicrons by enterocytes due to a defect in the same gene (*SARA2*).[256] General treatment measures in all three diseases include the replacement of triglycerides containing long-chain fatty acids with medium-chain triglycerides and dietary supplementation with tocopherol.[10]

Wolman's disease and the milder, late-onset *cholesteryl ester storage disease* are seemingly caused by mutations in different parts of the *LIPA* gene resulting in infiltration of intestinal mucosa with foam cells and intestinal damage.

Congenital Disorders of Cobalamin Absorption

Several congenital diseases can result in vitamin B_{12} malabsorption. Absence of intrinsic factor synthesis is the most common cause of congenital cobalamin deficiency; abnormal results on Schilling tests normalize with the coadministration of intrinsic factor.[26,128] In some patients, an abnormal (nonfunctional) intrinsic factor is secreted that has a decreased affinity for cobalamin, a decreased affinity for the ileal intrinsic factor cobalamin receptor (cubilin-AMN complex), or an increased susceptibility to proteolysis.[26,128]

Imerslund-Gräsbeck syndrome is a congenital disease characterized by malabsorption of the cobalamin–intrinsic factor complex despite normal ileal morphology. This syndrome can be caused by mutations in two genes that code for the cubilin and AMN proteins, which are colocalized in the ileal mucosa and form the intrinsic factor–cobalamin receptor.[30]

In *transcobalamin II deficiency,* serum levels of cobalamin commonly are normal, although in most patients intestinal cobalamin absorption is abnormal.[128] Diagnosis can be established by demonstrating the absence of transcobalamin II in the plasma.[128] All congenital disorders of cobalamin absorption are treated by the parenteral administration of cobalamin, although high-dose oral cobalamin also may suffice.

Intestinal Enterokinase Deficiency

Enterokinase is an enzyme, secreted by the intestinal mucosa, that initiates the activation of pancreatic proenzymes. Several patients have been reported to have an inborn deficiency of this enzyme, with resultant diarrhea, failure to thrive, and hypoproteinemia due mainly to protein malabsorption. These patients respond well to pancreatic enzyme replacement, and some patients show a tendency to improve with age.[265] Secondary enterokinase deficiency also has been reported in patients with villus atrophy, although patients with celiac disease seem not to be affected.[15]

PRIMARY IMMUNODEFICIENCY DISEASES

Malabsorption commonly occurs in different entities that are characterized by deficiencies in humoral or cellular immunity[270] (see Chapter 2). The immunodeficiency syndromes most commonly associated with malabsorption are *selective IgA deficiency, common variable immunodeficiency (CVID),* and *severe combined immunodeficiency.* The etiology of the malabsorption varies for the different syndromes.

Selective IgA Deficiency

Selective IgA deficiency is the most common primary immunodeficiency disorder and is characterized by a selective near-absence of secretory and serum IgA, leading to susceptibility to respiratory, urogenital, and gastrointestinal infections. Autoimmune and allergic diseases also commonly develop in patients with this disorder. A 10- to 16-fold increased incidence of gluten-sensitive enteropathy in patients with IgA deficiency has been reported[271]; however, at least a subgroup of patients have sprue-like small intestinal lesions, leading to severe diarrhea and malabsorption, that are unresponsive to a gluten-free diet.[272] Improvement with immunosuppressive therapy has been described in one case report.[273] Pernicious anemia, giardiasis, and secondary disaccharidase deficiencies also are seen with increased frequency in persons with selective IgA deficiency.[272,274]

Common Variable Immunodeficiency

Common variable immunodeficiency (CVID), or CVID-acquired hypogammaglobulinemia, comprises a group of immunodeficiency disorders characterized by decreased serum IgG levels; decreased serum levels of other immunoglobulin subclasses and T cell defects commonly are present. Onset of the disease usually is in adulthood, with recurrent respiratory and gastrointestinal infections. Affected patients also are at increased risk for autoimmune and neoplastic diseases. Malabsorption and diarrhea occur in 9% to 40% of patients with CVID[272]; the malabsorption involves dietary fat, carbohydrates, vitamin B_{12}, and folate.[270,275] Small intestinal biopsy specimens show either sprue-like features, including villus shortening with increased numbers of lymphocytes in the epithelium and in the lamina propria, or a pattern similar to that in graft-versus-host disease (see Chapter 33).[272,276] Some specific histologic features, namely, a near-absence of plasma cells, are observed. No response to a gluten-free diet is obtained, and it appears that the sprue-like syndrome in CVID is a distinct entity,[275] sometimes referred to as "hypogammaglobulinemic sprue."[277] In some patients with CVID, foamy macrophages are present, as in Whipple's disease, but in contrast with Whipple's disease, the macrophages do not contain periodic acid–Schiff–positive material.[276] In addition, nodular lymphoid hyperplasia can be detected in the gastrointestinal tract in a high proportion of CVID patients, however, the presence of nodular lymphoid hyperplasia does not correlate with the presence of malabsorption. The incidence of small bowel lymphoma is increased in CVID and this disorder also has to be considered as a potential cause of malabsorption in these patients. *Giardia* organisms often are isolated from patients with CVID, and small bowel bacterial overgrowth frequently is present. Unfortunately, only some of these patients respond to antimicrobial treatment.[276] Some patients with sprue-like intestinal changes have benefited from glucocorticoids[274] or immunoglobulins. Patients with CVID have a higher prevalence of atrophic gastritis with cobalamin malabsorption, although antibodies against parietal cells and intrinsic factor are absent.[272,275]

X-Linked Infantile Agammaglobulinemia (Bruton's Agammaglobulinemia)

X-linked infantile agammaglobulinemia (Bruton's agammaglobulinemia; MIM 300300) is caused by mutations in the gene for Bruton tyrosine kinase.[278] This disease usually manifests after the first 6 months of life and is characterized by recurrent severe bacterial infections. Severe gastrointestinal problems seem to be less common than in CVID.[276] The prevalence of chronic gastroenteritis was 10% in one large series.[279] In affected patients, the possibility of giardiasis and bacterial overgrowth needs to be evaluated.[276,279]

Immune Dysregulation–Polyendocrinopathy–Enteropathy–X-Linked Syndrome (IPEX)

The immune dysregulation–polyendocrinopathy–enteropathy–X-linked syndrome (IPEX) (MIM 304790) is a disorder of early childhood, characterized by protracted diarrhea, dermatitis, insulin-dependent diabetes mellitus, thyroiditis, thrombocytopenia and hemolytic anemia. It is a disorder of X-linked recessive inheritance caused by mutations in the *FOXP3* gene.[280] The diarrhea and malabsorption are secondary to severe villus atrophy with inflammation. Antienterocyte antibodies commonly are present. The enteropathy usually does not respond to a gluten-free diet, but immunosuppressive therapy has been shown to be of some benefit.[280] IPEX usually is lethal in childhood. Successful bone marrow transplantation with amelioration of enteropathy has been reported in some cases.[281]

Other Congenital Immunodeficiency Syndromes

In *severe combined immunodeficiency*, diarrhea and malabsorption are common. Symptoms are associated with stunting of intestinal villi or their complete absence. The pathophysiology of malabsorption is unknown, and the syndrome usually fails to respond to antimicrobial treatment.[272,274] Malabsorption also has been reported in *DiGeorge's syndrome* (thymic hypoplasia, MIM 188400) and *chronic granulomatous disease of childhood* (MIM 306400), but little is known about its etiology.[272]

NEUROFIBROMATOSIS TYPE 1 (VON RECKLINGHAUSEN'S DISEASE)

Malabsorption can be an intestinal complication of neurofibromatosis type 1 (MIM 162200). Mechanisms of malabsorption include periampullary duodenal tumors, which are mainly somatostatin-containing neuroendocrine tumors, and pancreatic carcinomas with resultant pancreatic duct obstruction; tumors may cause exocrine pancreatic insufficiency and biliary obstruction.[282,283] Duodenal somatostatinomas in von Recklinghausen's disease usually do not increase plasma somatostatin levels, although one case of somatostatinoma syndrome has been reported.[284] Infiltrating mesenteric plexiform neurofibromas and vascular damage caused by proliferation of nerves can cause lymphatic and/or vascular obstruction resulting in abdominal pain, protein-losing enteropathy, diarrhea, steatorrhea, and bowel ischemia.[285,286] In patients with von Recklinghausen's disease, an increased incidence of neuroendocrine tumors in other locations has been observed; gastrinomas with Zollinger-Ellison syndrome also have been reported in these patients.[287]

NONGRANULOMATOUS CHRONIC IDIOPATHIC ENTEROCOLITIS

Nongranulomatous chronic idiopathic enterocolitis is an entity that is distinct from refractory celiac disease and inflammatory bowel disease.[288] The etiology of this disease is unknown, and chronic infection and an autoimmune cause have been suggested. Severe diarrhea and malabsorption occur as a result of diffuse villus atrophy, and ulcerations may be present in the small and large bowel. Small bowel villus atrophy and neutrophilic inflammation of the mucosa with crypt abscesses may be seen in biopsy specimens from the small bowel and colon (Fig. 98–9); the number of intraepithelial lymphocytes is not increased.[288,289] Patients respond dramatically to glucocorticoids, and most require long-term low-dose maintenance therapy.[288,289] Improvement with cyclosporine has been reported in one patient and response to long-term antibiotic therapy in another patient.[290] The condition is associated with a high mortality rate.[288,289]

ENDOCRINE AND METABOLIC DISORDERS

Adrenal Insufficiency (Addison's Disease)

Fat malabsorption is observed in some patients with adrenal insufficiency, independent of its etiology; fecal fat excretion of up to 30 g per day has been observed.[291] Fat malabsorption also is observed in rats after adrenalectomy.[292] The pathophysiologic mechanism of malabsorption in this disease is unknown. Fat absorption normalizes after steroid replacement.

Isolated autoimmune Addison's disease has been associated with pernicious anemia[293] and celiac disease.[294] An increased incidence of celiac disease and pernicious anemia also is found in autoimmune polyglandular syndrome (APS) type 2 (Schmidt's syndrome), which is characterized by the association of autoimmune Addison's disease with other autoimmune endocrine disorders, except hypoparathyroidism.[295]

Hypoparathyroidism (Autoimmune Polyglandular Syndrome Type 1)

Autoimmune polyglandular syndrome type 1 (APS 1) (MIM 240300) is characterized by failure of multiple endocrine organs due to autoimmune destruction (especially hypoparathyroidism and adrenal insufficiency), with ectodermal dystrophy and susceptibility to chronic

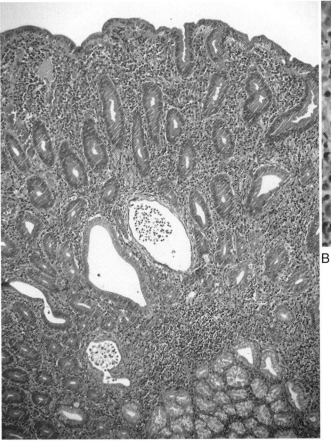

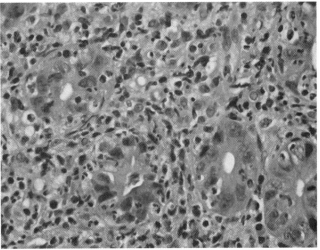

B

Figure 98–9 Duodenal biopsy specimen from a patient with nongranulomatous chronic idiopathic enterocolitis. *A,* Histopathologic features include villus atrophy, diffuse infiltration of the lamina propria with inflammatory cells, and crypt abscesses. *B,* High-power view demonstrates crypt infiltration by neutrophils. (Courtesy of Cord Langner, MD.)

A

Candida infections.[295] APS type 1 is inherited as an autosomal recessive disorder and is caused by mutations in the *AIRE* gene.[296] Severe malabsorption, which tends to be recurrent, develops in approximately 20% of patients with APS type 1. In one patient, the malabsorption was caused by a transient and selective destruction of small intestinal enteroendocrine cells, leading to a transient deficiency of enteroendocrine hormones (especially CCK).[297] These patients have autoantibodies to tryptophan hydroxylase, which are directed against enteroendocrine cells (including CCK-producing cells).[298,299] The long-known association between hypoparathyroidism and steatorrhea may be caused by the same mechanism, because in most reports of this association, the patient fulfills the diagnostic criteria for APS type 1.[300,301] Selective absence of small intestinal enteroendocrine cells can be diagnosed by special immunohistochemical stains for these cells (e.g., immunohistochemical stains for chromogranin A or CCK; Fig. 98–10) or by measurements of postprandial serum levels of the affected hormones. Patients with APS type 1 also have an increased incidence of vitamin B_{12} malabsorption due to autoimmune gastritis.[295]

Hyperthyroidism and Autoimmune Thyroid Disease

Some reports suggest that up to 25% of hyperthyroid patients have at least some degree of fat malabsorption, but data from large series of patients are lacking. Fecal fat values in hyperthyroid patients can reach 35 g per day.[302] The mechanism of steatorrhea in this entity has not been established. Motility studies in hyperthyroid patients (including patients with and without diarrhea) have demonstrated accelerated small bowel and whole-gut transit times[303]; however, fecal fat values were not reported in these patients. It can be hypothesized that more pronounced disturbances of intestinal transit may lead to decreased mixing of food and digestive secretions and reduced intestinal absorption of nutrients. Some of the steatorrhea in hyperthyroid patients might be due to hyperphagia with increased dietary intake of fat.[304] An increased number of lymphocytes and plasma cells and some degree of edema in small intestinal biopsy specimens have been found in patients with steatorrhea and hyperthyroidism; villus architecture, however, is normal.[302] Absorption of glucose and D-xylose is normal in hyperthyroid patients with and without malabsorption.[304] Fat malabsorption tends to normalize when patients attain a euthyroid state.[302,304,305]

In patients with autoimmune thyroid diseases, an increased prevalence of celiac disease[294] and primary biliary cirrhosis,[293] both of which can result in fat malabsorption, has been recognized. The prevalence of celiac disease in patients with autoimmune thyroid disease is approximately 2% to 4%.[294] Cobalamin malabsorption due to autoimmune gastritis is found in a considerable number of patients with thyrotoxicosis and hypothyroidism.[28,293]

Diabetes Mellitus

Chronic diarrhea is common in patients with diabetes mellitus, especially in those with long-standing diabetes mellitus type 1.[306] Mild steatorrhea often is present in patients with diabetic diarrhea and in diabetic patients who do not complain of diarrhea.[307] Although the pathophysiologic mechanism of malabsorption and diarrhea in patients with diabetes mellitus is unknown, poor glycemic control is an important cofactor.[308] Most of these patients have signs of autonomic neuropathy such as orthostatic hypotension, impotence, bladder dysfunction, incontinence, decreased heart rate variability, and abnormal sweating.[310] Therefore, in some patients, the cause of diarrhea and malabsorption has been attributed to rapid gastric emptying and rapid intestinal transit, causing impaired mixing of nutrients with digestive secretions and decreased contact time between nutrients and the intestinal mucosa. The clinician has to be aware that certain treatable diseases, such as celiac disease,[309,311] small intestinal bacterial overgrowth,[310] and pancreatic insufficiency,[313] can be associated with diabetes mellitus. In patients with diabetes mellitus type 1, a high prevalence (3% to 8%) of celiac disease has been reported from screening studies; however, most patients

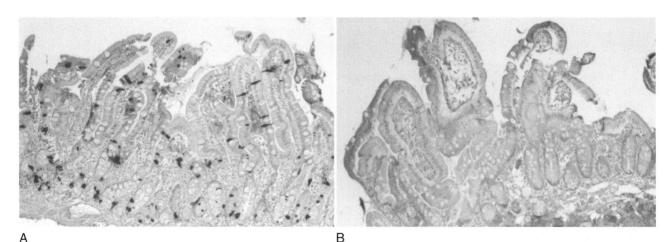

A   B

Figure 98–10   Chromogranin A immunohistochemical staining of enteroendocrine cells in duodenal biopsy specimens obtained from a normal subject *(A)* and from a patient with malabsorption associated with autoimmune polyglandular syndrome type 1 *(B)*. In *B*, enteroendocrine cells are absent. See text for details.

identified were asymptomatic.[312] Markedly reduced pancreatic exocrine function, as determined by fecal elastase measurement, has been reported in 30% of patients with type 1 diabetes and 17% with type 2 diabetes, compared with 5% of control subjects. In 40% of diabetic patients with reduced fecal elastase levels, fat malabsorption with fecal fat output of greater than 10 g per day was detected.[313] Gastrointestinal symptoms and steatorrhea in these patients, however, did not correlate with fecal elastase levels.[313,314] In addition, the unresolved specificity of elastase raises the possibility that not all of these patients truly had pancreatic insufficiency.[131] Cobalamin malabsorption caused by autoimmune atrophic gastritis is more prevalent in patients with diabetes mellitus type 1.[315]

Ingested carbohydrates are malabsorbed in patients receiving acarbose as an antidiabetic treatment, which in turn can lead to symptoms of diarrhea and malabsorption. Dietary foods rich in fructose or sorbitol also may result in bloating and diarrhea.

Metabolic Bone Disease

Special consideration has to be given to osteoporosis and osteomalacia in malabsorptive diseases. Patients with these metabolic bone diseases usually do not present with symptoms or abnormalities on physical examination or on routine laboratory examinations. Reduced bone mineral density is a common finding in patients with gastric resection,[316] celiac disease,[317] or lactose malabsorption.[172] Osteoporosis has been suggested to result from calcium malabsorption or reduced calcium intake, which leads to secondary hyperparathyroidism, which in turn increases bone turnover and cortical bone loss. Vitamin D malabsorption probably is of lesser importance. Although up to one half of patients on a gluten-free diet may have osteoporosis,[318] some studies have shown significant improvement in bone mineral density 1 year after starting a gluten-free diet.[319] In inflammatory bowel diseases such as Crohn's disease, which may be accompanied by malabsorption, other factors such as glucocorticoid use or testosterone deficiency[320] may contribute to the decrease in bone mass. In addition to treating the underlying cause of malabsorption, calcium supplementation is needed, to ensure a daily intake of 1500 mg of calcium, and vitamin D deficiency must be corrected; if osteoporosis is present, bisphosphonate treatment is suggested.[317] Nutritional management is discussed in more detail in Chapters 15 and 16.

GENERAL APPROACH TO THE MANAGEMENT OF MALABSORPTION

Treatment of malabsorptive diseases must be directed against the underlying condition, if possible. In addition, nutritional deficits must be corrected. The reader is referred to the relevant chapters of this book to read about the treatment of specific diseases and their nutrition management.

In severe pancreatic diseases, in disorders of intestinal fat absorption, and in short bowel syndrome, medium-chain triglycerides can be used as a source of dietary calories. In patients with short bowel syndrome and some remaining colon, colonic salvage capacity can be used to regain calories from carbohydrates[321]; these patients, therefore, should consume a diet rich in carbohydrates and medium-chain triglycerides.

In bile acid malabsorption after extensive ileal resections, intestinal fat absorption can be improved markedly by oral administration of natural conjugated bile acids,[184,185] or of synthetic cholylsarcosine at a dose of 2 to 3 g per meal.[110,186,187] Replacement of conjugated bile acids also reduces urinary oxalate excretion and therefore should protect against development of kidney stones.[186]

In patients with malabsorption and an intact colon, fluid depletion must be avoided, to prevent kidney stones associated with hyperoxaluria.[322] In patients with malabsorption syndrome, special care should be given to the replacement of vitamins, iron, calcium, and trace elements, to avoid deficiency syndromes (see Chapters 15 and 16).

In patients with diarrhea, symptomatic treatment with opiates or loperamide may increase the time available for nutrient absorption.

ACKNOWLEDGMENT

We thank Dr. John S. Fordtran for his valuable advice.

REFERENCES

1. Wilson FA, Dietschy JM: Differential diagnostic approach to clinical problems of malabsorption. Gastroenterology 61: 911, 1971.
2. Van Deest BW, Fordtran JS, Morawski SG, et al: Bile salt and micellar fat concentration in proximal small bowel contents of ileectomy patients. J Clin Invest 47:1314, 1968.
3. Hofmann AF, Poley JR: Role of bile acid malabsorption in pathogenesis of diarrhea and steatorrhea in patients with ileal resection. Gastroenterology 62:918, 1972.
4. Oelkers P, Kirby LC, Heubi JE, et al: Primary bile acid malabsorption caused by mutations in the ileal sodium-dependent bile acid transporter gene (SLC10A2). J Clin Invest 99:1880, 1997.
5. Di Magno EP, Go VLW, Summerskill WHJ: Relations between pancreatic enzyme outputs and malabsorption in severe pancreatic insufficiency. N Engl J Med 288:813, 1973.
6. Ryan ME, Olsen WA: A diagnostic approach to malabsorption syndromes: A pathophysiological approach. Clin Gastroenterol 12:533, 1983.
7. Graham DY: Pancreatic enzyme replacement. The effect of antacids or cimetidine. Dig Dis Sci 27:485, 1982.
8. Heck AM, Yanovski JA, Calis KA: Orlistat, a new lipase inhibitor for the management of obesity. Pharmacotherapy 20:270, 2000.
9. Gaskin KJ, Durie PR, Hill RE, et al: Colipase and maximally activated pancreatic lipase in normal subjects and patients with steatorrhea. J Clin Invest 69:427, 1982.
10. Kane JP, Havel RJ: Disorders of the biogenesis and secretion of lipoproteins containing the B apolipoproteins. In Scriver CR, Beaudet AL, Sly WS, et al (eds): The Metabolic and Molecular Bases of Inherited Disease, 8th ed. New York, McGraw-Hill, 2001, p 2717.
11. Mistilis SP, Skyring AP, Stephen DD: Intestinal lymphangiectasia: Mechanism of enteric loss of plasma-protein and fat. Lancet 1:77, 1965.

12. Volwiler W: Gastrointestinal malabsorptive syndromes. Am J Med 23:250, 1957.

13. Comfort MW, Wollaeger EE, Power MH: Total fecal solids, fat and nitrogen. A study of patients with chronic relapsing pancreatitis. Gastroenterology 11:691, 1948.

14. Freeman HJ, Sleisenger MH, Kim YS: Human protein digestion and absorption: Normal mechanisms and protein-energy malnutrition. Clin Gastroenterol 12:357, 1983.

15. Lebenthal E, Antonowicz I, Shwachman H: Enterokinase and trypsin activities in pancreatic insufficiency and diseases of the small intestine. Gastroenterology 70:508, 1976.

16. Ladefoged K, Nicolaidou P, Jarnum S: Calcium, phosphorus, magnesium, zinc, and nitrogen balance in patients with severe short bowel syndrome. Am J Clin Nutr 33:2137, 1980.

17. Ravich WJ, Bayless TM: Carbohydrate absorption and malabsorption. Clin Gastroenterol 12:335, 1983.

18. Hammer HF, Fine KD, Santa Ana CA, et al: Carbohydrate malabsorption. Its measurement and its contribution to diarrhea. J Clin Invest 86:1936, 1990.

19. Ushijima K, Riby JE, Kretchmer N: Carbohydrate malabsorption. Pediatr Clin North Am 42:899, 1995.

20. Gudmand-Hoyer E, Skovbjerg H: Disaccharide digestion and maldigestion. Scand J Gastroenterol 31(suppl 216):111, 1996.

21. Wright EM: I. Glucose galactose malabsorption. Am J Physiol 275:G879, 1998.

22. Sokol RJ: Fat-soluble vitamins and their importance in patients with cholestatic liver diseases. Gastroenterol Clin North Am 23:673, 1994.

23. Bilke DD: Calcium absorption and vitamin D metabolism. Clin Gastroenterol 12:379, 1983.

24. Marotta RB, Floch MH: Dietary therapy of steatorrhea. Gastroenterol Clin North Am 18:485, 1989.

25. Evans WB, Wollaeger EE: Incidence and severity of nutritional deficiency states in chronic exocrine pancreatic insufficiency: Comparison with nontropical sprue. Am J Dig Dis 11:594, 1966.

26. Seetharam B: Gastrointestinal absorption and transport of cobalamin (vitamin B_{12}). In Johnson LR (ed): Physiology of the Gastrointestinal Tract, 3rd ed. New York, Raven Press, 1994, p 1997.

27. Howden CW: Vitamin B_{12} levels during prolonged treatment with proton pump inhibitors. J Clin Gastroenterol 30:29, 2000.

28. Toh BH, van Driel IR, Gleeson PA: Pernicious anemia. N Engl J Med 337:1441, 1997.

29. Glasbrenner B, Malfertheiner P, Büchler M, et al: Vitamin B_{12} and folic acid deficiency in chronic pancreatitis: A relevant disorder? Klin Wochenschr 69:168, 1991.

30. Fyfe JC, Madsen M, Hojrup P, et al: The functional cobalamin (vitamin B_{12})–intrinsic factor receptor is a novel complex of cubilin and amnionless. Blood 103:1573, 2004.

31. Rosenblatt DS, Whitehead VM: Cobalamin and folate deficiency: Acquired and hereditary disorders in children. Semin Hematol 36:19, 1999.

32. Gallagher ND: Importance of vitamin B_{12} and folate metabolism in malabsorption. Clin Gastroenterol 12:437, 1983.

33. Zittoun J, Zittoun R: Modern clinical testing strategies in cobalamin and folate deficiency. Semin Hematol 36:35, 1999.

34. Green PHR: Alcohol, nutrition and malabsorption. Clin Gastroenterol 12:563, 1983.

35. Hoffbrand AV, Tabaqchali S, Mollin DL: High serum-folate levels in intestinal blind loop syndrome. Lancet 1:1339, 1966.

36. Pollack S, Enat R, Haim S, et al: Pellagra as the presenting manifestation of Crohn's disease. Gastroenterology 82:948, 1982.

37. Reinken L, Zieglauer H: Vitamin B-6 absorption in children with acute celiac disease and in control subjects. J Nutr 108:1562, 1978.

38. Pak CYC, Fordtran JS: Disorders of mineral metabolism. In Sleisenger MH, Fordtran JS (eds): Gastrointestinal Disease, 2nd ed. Philadelphia, WB Saunders, 1978, p 251.

39. Booth CC, Babouris N, Hanna S, et al: Incidence of hypomagnesaemia in intestinal malabsorption. BMJ 5350:141, 1963.

40. Milla PJ, Aggett PJ, Wolff OH, et al: Studies in primary hypomagnesaemia: Evidence of defective carrier-mediated small intestinal transport of magnesium. Gut 20:1028, 1979.

41. de-Vizia B, Poggi V, Conenna R, et al: Iron absorption and iron deficiency in infants and children with gastrointestinal diseases. J Pediatr Gastroenterol Nutr 14:21, 1992.

42. Goddard AF, McIntyre AS, Scott BB: Guidelines for the management of iron deficiency anaemia. Gut 46(suppl IV):iv1, 2000.

43. Goldschmid S, Graham M: Trace element deficiencies in inflammatory bowel disease. Gastroenterol Clin North Am 18:579, 1989.

44. Wang K, Zhou B, Kuo YM, et al: A novel member of a zinc transporter family is defective in acrodermatitis enteropathica. Am J Hum Genet 71:66, 2002.

45. Chariot P, Bignani O: Skeletal muscle disorders associated with selenium deficiency in humans. Muscle Nerve 27:662, 2003.

46. Goyens P, Brasseur D, Cadranel S: Copper deficiency in infants with active celiac disease. J Pediatr Gastroenterol Nutr 4:677, 1985.

47. Basilisco G, Phillips SF: Colonic salvage in health and disease. Eur J Gastroenterol Hepatol 5:777, 1993.

48. Nightingale JM, Lennard-Jones JE, Gertner DJ, et al: Colonic preservation reduces need for parenteral therapy, increases incidence of renal stones, but does not change high prevalence of gall stones in patients with short bowel. Gut 33:1493, 1992.

49. Stephen AM, Phillips SF: Passage of carbohydrate into the colon. Direct measurements in humans. Gastroenterology 85:589, 1983.

50. Cummings JH, Macfarlane GT: Role of intestinal bacteria in nutrient metabolism. JPEN J Parenter Enteral Nutr 21:357, 1997.

51. Ruppin H, Bar Meir S, Soergel KH, et al: Absorption of short-chain fatty acids by the colon. Gastroenterology 78:1500, 1980.

52. Hammer HF, Santa Ana CA, Schiller LR, et al: Studies of osmotic diarrhea induced in normal subjects by ingestion of polyethylene glycol and lactulose. J Clin Invest 84:1056, 1989.

53. Florent C, Flourie B, Leblond A, et al: Influence of chronic lactulose ingestion on the colonic metabolism of lactulose in man (an in vivo study). J Clin Invest 75:608, 1985.

54. Yang MG, Manoharan K, Mickelsen O: Nutritional contribution of volatile fatty acids from the cecum of rats. J Nutrition 100:545, 1970.

55. Jeppesen PB, Mortensen PB: Significance of a preserved colon for parenteral energy requirements in patients receiving home parenteral nutrition. Scand J Gastroenterol 33:1175, 1998.

56. Hammer HF: Colonic hydrogen absorption: Quantification of its effect on hydrogen accumulation caused by bacterial fermentation of carbohydrates. Gut 34:818, 1993.

57. Moore JG, Jessop LD, Osborne DN: A gas chromatographic and mass spectrometric analysis of the odor of human feces. Gastroenterology 93:1321, 1987.

58. el-Yamani J, Mizon C, Capon C, et al: Decreased faecal exoglycosidase activities identify a subset of patients with active Crohn's disease. Clin Sci Colch 83:409, 1992.

59. Rao SS, Read NW, Holdsworth CD: Is the diarrhoea in ulcerative colitis related to impaired colonic salvage of carbohydrate? Gut 28:1090, 1987.

60. Högenauer C, Hammer HF, Krejs GJ, et al: Mechanisms and management of antibiotic-associated diarrhea. Clin Infect Dis 27:702, 1998.

61. Kurpad Av, Shetty PS: Effects of antimicrobial therapy on faecal bulking. Gut 27:55, 1986.

62. Hatch M, Freel RW: Alterations in intestinal transport of oxalate in disease states. Scanning Microsc 9:1121, 1995.

63. Ammon HV, Phillips SF: Inhibition of colonic water and electrolyte absorption by fatty acids in man. Gastroenterology 65:744, 1973.

64. Dobbins JW, Binder HJ: Effect of bile salts and fatty acids on the colonic absorption of oxalate. Gastroenterology 1096, 1976.

65. Jeppesen PB, Mortensen PB: The influence of a preserved colon on the absorption of medium chain fat in patients with small bowel resection. Gut 43:478, 1998.

66. Jorgensen JR, Fitch MD, Mortensen PB, et al: Absorption and metabolism of octanoate by the rat colon in vivo: Concentration dependency and influence of alternative fuels. Gut 51:76, 2002.

67. Sheikh MS, Schiller LR, Fordtran JS: In vivo intestinal absorption of calcium in humans. Miner Electrolyte Metab 16:130, 1990.

68. Hylander E, Ladefoged K, Jarnum S: Calcium absorption after intestinal resection. The importance of a preserved colon. Scand J Gastroenterol 25:705, 1990.

69. Karbach U, Feldmeier H: The cecum is the site with the highest calcium absorption in rat intestine. Dig Dis Sci 38:1815, 1993.

70. Halpern GM, Van-de-Water J, Delabroise AM, et al: Comparative uptake of calcium from milk and a calcium-rich mineral water in lactose intolerant adults: Implications for treatment of osteoporosis. Am J Prev Med 7:379, 1991.

71. Trinidad TP, Wolever TM, Thompson LU: Effects of calcium concentration, acetate, and propionate on calcium absorption in the human distal colon. Nutrition 15:529, 1999.

72. Hammer J, Hammer K, Kletter K: Lipids infused into the jejunum accelerate small intestinal transit but delay ileocolonic transit of solids and liquids. Gut 43:111, 1998.

73. Spiller RC, Trotman IF, Higgins BE: The ileal brake—inhibition of jejunal motility after ileal fat perfusion in man. Gut 25:365, 1984.

74. Jain NK, Boivin M, Zinsmeister AR, et al: Effect of perfusing carbohydrates and amylase inhibitor into the ileum on gastrointestinal hormones and gastric emptying of homogenized meal. Gastroenterology 96:377, 1989.

75. Hammer J, Pruckmayer M, Bergmann H, et al: The distal colon provides reserve storage capacity during colonic fluid overload. Gut 41:658, 1997.

76. Crenn P, Vahedi K, Lavergne-Slove A, et al: Plasma citrulline: A marker of enterocyte mass in villous atrophy-associated small bowel disease. Gastroenterology 124:1210, 2003.

77. Schiller LR, Rivera L, Santangelo WC, et al: Diagnostic value of fasting plasma peptide concentrations in patients with chronic diarrhea. Dig Dis Sci 39:2216, 1994.

78. Shah VH, Rotterdam H, Kotler DP, et al: All that scallops is not celiac disease. Gastrointest Endosc 51:717, 2000.

79. Hopper AD, Cross SS, McAlindon ME, et al: Symptomatic giardiasis without diarrhea: Further evidence to support the routine duodenal biopsy? Gastrointest Endosc 58:120, 2003.

80. Green PH, Murray JA: Routine duodenal biopsies to exclude celiac disease? Gastrointest Endosc 58:92, 2003.

81. Mee A, Burke M, Vallon AG, et al: Small bowel biopsy for malabsorption: Comparison of the diagnostic accuracy of endoscopic forceps and capsule biopsy specimens. BMJ 291:769, 1985.

82. Flick AL, Quinton WE, Rubin CE: A peroral hydraulic biopsy tube for multiple sampling at any level of the gastrointestinal tract. Gastroenterology 40:120, 1961.

83. Dickey W, Hughes D: Prevalence of celiac disease and its endoscopic markers among patients having routine upper gastrointestinal endoscopy. Am J Gastroenterol 94:2182, 1999.

84. Dandalides SM, Cavey W, Petras R, et al: Endoscopic small bowel mucosal biopsy: A controlled trial evaluating forceps size and biopsy location in the diagnosis of normal and abnormal mucosal architecture. Gastrointest Endosc 35:197, 1989.

85. Ladas SD, Tsamouri M, Kouvidou C, et al: Effect of forceps size and mode of orientation on endoscopic small bowel biopsy evaluation. Gastrointest Endosc 40:51, 1994.

86. Siegel LM, Stevens PD, Lightdale CJ, et al: Combined magnification endoscopy with chromoendoscopy in the evaluation of patients with suspected malabsorption. Gastrointest Endosc 46:226, 1997.

87. Riddell RH: Small intestinal biopsy: Who? How? What are the findings? In Barkin JS, Rogers AI (eds): Difficult Decisions in Digestive Diseases. Chicago, Year Book Medical Publishers, 1989, p 326.

88. Riley SA, Marsh MN: Maldigestion and malabsorption. In Feldman M, Scharschmidt BF, Sleisenger MH (eds): Sleisenger & Fordtran's Gastrointestinal and Liver Disease, 6th ed. Philadelphia, WB Saunders, 1998, p 1501.

89. Ramzan NN, Loftus E, Burgart LJ, et al: Diagnosis and monitoring of Whipple disease by polymerase chain reaction. Ann Intern Med 126:520, 1997.

90. Ge ZZ, Hu YB, Xiao SD: Capsule endoscopy in diagnosis of small bowel Crohn's disease. World J Gastroenterol 10:1349, 2004.

91. Voderholzer WA, Ortner M, Rogalla P, et al: Diagnostic yield of wireless capsule enteroscopy in comparison with computed tomography enteroclysis. Endoscopy 35:1009, 2003.

92. Eliakim R, Fischer D, Suissa A, et al: Wireless capsule video endoscopy is a superior diagnostic tool in comparison to barium follow-through and computerized tomography in patients with suspected Crohn's disease. Eur J Gastroenterol Hepatol 15:363, 2003.

93. Fireman Z, Mahajna E, Broide E, et al: Diagnosing small bowel Crohn's disease with wireless capsule endoscopy. Gut 52:390, 2003.

94. Herlinger H: Malabsorption. In Gore RM, Levine MS, Laufer I (eds): Textbook of Gastrointestinal Radiology. Philadelphia, WB Saunders, 7994, p 863.

95. Herlinger H: Enteroclysis in malabsorption: Can it influence diagnosis and management? Radiologe 33:335, 1993.

96. Herlinger H: Small bowel malabsorption: Clinical and radiologic perspectives. How we see it. Radiology 184:297, 1992.

97. Umschaden HW, Szolar D, Gasser J, et al: Small-bowel disease: Comparison of MR enteroclysis images with conventional enteroclysis and surgical findings. Radiology 215:717, 2000.

98. Horton KM, Corl FM, Fishman EK: CT of nonneoplastic diseases of the small bowel: spectrum of disease. J Comput Assist Tomogr 23:417, 1999.

99. Tomei E, Marini M, Messineo D, et al: Computed tomography of the small bowel in adult celiac disease: The jejunoileal fold pattern reversal. Eur Radiol 10:119, 2000.

100. Laghi A, Paolantonio P, Catalano C, et al: MR imaging of the small bowel using polyethylene glycol solution as an oral contrast agent in adults and children with celiac disease: Preliminary observations. AJR Am J Roentgenol 180:191, 2003.

101. Albert J, Scheidt T, Basler B, et al: Magnetic resonance imaging in diagnosis and follow-up of Crohn's disease—is conventional enteroclysis still necessary? Z Gastroenterol 40:789, 2002.

102. Prassopoulos P, Papanikolaou N, Grammatikakis J, et al: MR enteroclysis imaging of Crohn disease. Radiographics 21:S161, 2001.

103. Fine KD, Schiller LR: AGA technical review on the evaluation and management of chronic diarrhea. Gastroenterology 116:1464, 1999.

104. Van de Kamer JH, Ten Bokkel Huinink H, Weyers HA: Rapid method for the determination of fat in feces. J Biol Chem 177:347, 1949.

105. Balasekaran R, Porter JL, Santa AC, et al: Positive results on tests for steatorrhea in persons consuming Olestra potato chips. Ann Intern Med 132:279, 2000.

106. Jeejeebhoy KN, Ahmad S, Kozak G: Determination of fecal fats containing both medium and long chain triglycerides and fatty acids. Clin Biochem 3:157, 1970.

107. Picarelli A, Greco M, DiGiovambattista F: Quantitative determination of faecal fat, nitrogen and water by the means of a spectrophotometric technique: Near infrared reflectance analysis (NIRA). Assessment of accuracy and reproducibility compared with chemical methods. Clin Chim Acta 234:147, 1995.

108. Fine KD, Fordtran JS: The effect of diarrhea on fecal fat excretion. Gastroenterology 102:1936, 1992.

109. Dumasy V, Delhaye M, Cotton F, et al: Fat malabsorption screening in chronic pancreatitis. Am J Gastroenterol 99:1350, 2004.

110. Gruy-Kapral C, Little KH, Fordtran JS, et al: Conjugated bile acid replacement therapy for short-bowel syndrome. Gastroenterology 116:15, 1999.

111. Amann ST, Josephson SA, Toskes PP: Acid steatocrit: A simple, rapid gravimetric method to determine steatorrhea. Am J Gastroenterol 92:2280, 1997.

112. Romano TJ, Dobbins JW: Evaluation of the patient with suspected malabsorption. Gastroenterol Clin North Am 18:467, 1989.

113. Fine KD, Ogunji F: A new method of quantitative fecal fat microscopy and its correlation with chemically measured fecal fat output. Am J Clin Pathol 113:528, 2000.

114. Pedersen NT, Halgreen H: Simultaneous assessment of fat maldigestion and fat malabsorption by a double-isotope method using fecal radioactivity. Gastroenterology 88:47, 1985.

115. Lembcke B, Geibel K, Kirchhoff S, et al: Serum beta-carotene: A simple static laboratory parameter for the diagnosis of steatorrhea. Dtsch Med Wochenschr 114:243, 1989.

116. Leung AK, Siu TO, Chiu AS, et al: Serum carotene concentrations in normal infants and children. Clin Pediatr Phila 29:575, 1990.

117. Romagnuolo J, Schiller D, Bailey RJ: Using breath tests wisely in a gastroenterology practice: An evidence-based review of indications and pitfalls in interpretation. Am J Gastroenterol 97:1113, 2002.

118. Hammer HF, Petritsch W, Pristautz H, et al: Assessment of the influence of hydrogen nonexcretion on the usefulness of the hydrogen breath test and lactose tolerance test. Wien Klin Wochenschr 108:137, 1996.

119. Troelsen JT, Olsen J, Moller J, et al: An upstream polymorphism associated with lactase persistence has increased enhancer activity. Gastroenterology 125:1686, 2003.

120. Enattah NS, Sahi T, Savilahti E, et al: Identification of a variant associated with adult-type hypolactasia. Nat Genet 30:233, 2002.

121. Högenauer C, Hammer HF, Mellitzer K, et al: Evaluation of a new DNA test compared with the lactose hydrogen breath test for the diagnosis of lactase non-persistence. Eur J Gastroenterol Hepatol 17:371, 2005.

122. Eherer AJ, Fordtran JS: Fecal osmotic gap and pH in experimental diarrhea of various causes. Gastroenterology 103:545, 1992.

123. Ameen VZ, Powell GK: A simple spectrophotometric method for quantitative fecal carbohydrate measurement. Clin Chim Acta 152:3, 1985.

124. Collin DP, McCormick PG: Determination of short chain fatty acids in stool ultrafiltrate and urine. Clin Chem 20:1173, 1974.

125. Hoverstad T, Fausa O, Bjorneklett A, et al: Short-chain fatty acids in the normal human feces. Scand J Gastroenterol 19:375, 1984.

126. Evenepoel P, Claus D, Geypens B, et al: Evidence for impaired assimilation and increased colonic fermentation of protein, related to gastric acid suppression therapy. Aliment Pharmacol Ther 12:1011, 1998.

127. Snow CF: Laboratory diagnosis of vitamin B_{12} and folate deficiency. Arch Intern Med 159:1289, 1999.

128. Rosenblatt DS, Fenton WA: Inherited disorders of folate and cobalamin transport and metabolism. In Scriver CR, Beaudet AL, Sly WS, et al (eds): The Metabolic and Molecular Bases of Inherited Disease, 8th ed. New York, McGraw-Hill, 2001, p 3897.

129. Allen RH, Stabler SP, Savage DG, et al: Diagnosis of cobalamin deficiency I: Usefulness of serum methylmalonic acid and total homocysteine concentrations. Am J Hematol 34:90, 1990.

130. Loeser C, Moellgaard A, Foelsch UR: Faecal elastase 1: A novel, highly sensitive, and specific tubeless pancreatic function test. Gut 39:580, 1996.

131. Gredal C, Madsen LG, Larsen S: The Lundh test and faecal elastase 1 determination in chronic pancreatitis: A comparative study. Pancreatology 3:389, 2003.

132. Walkowiak J, Herzig KH: Fecal elastase-1 is increased in villous atrophy regardless of the underlying disease. Eur J Clin Invest 31:425, 2001.

133. Conwell DL, Zuccaro G Jr, Vargo JJ, et al: An endoscopic pancreatic function test with synthetic porcine secretin for the evaluation of chronic abdominal pain and suspected chronic pancreatitis. Gastrointest Endosc 57:37, 2003.

134. Conwell DL, Zuccaro G Jr, Vargo JJ, et al: An endoscopic pancreatic function test with cholecystokinin-octapeptide for the diagnosis of chronic pancreatitis. Clin Gastroenterol Hepatol 1:189, 2003.

135. Schiller LR, Bilhartz LE, Santa Ana CA, et al: Comparison of endogenous and radiolabeled bile acid excretion in patients with idiopathic chronic diarrhea. Gastroenterology 98:1036, 1990.

136. Schiller LR, Hogan RB, Morawski SG, et al: Studies of the prevalence and significance of radiolabeled bile acid malabsorption in a group of patients with idiopathic chronic diarrhea. Gastroenterology 92:151, 1987.

137. Porter JL, Fordtran JS, Santa AC, et al: Accurate enzymatic measurement of fecal bile acids in patients with malabsorption. J Lab Clin Med 141:411, 2003.

138. Guirl MJ, Högenauer C, Santa AC, et al: Rapid intestinal transit as a primary cause of severe chronic diarrhea in patients with amyloidosis. Am J Gastroenterol 98:2219, 2003.

139. Hofmann AF, Bolder U: Detection of bile acid malabsorption by the SeHCAT test. Principles, problems, and clinical utility. Gastroenterol Clin Biol 18:847, 1994.

140. Sciarretta G, Vicini G, Fagioli G, et al: Use of 23-selena-25-homocholyltaurine to detect bile acid malabsorption in patients with ileal dysfunction or diarrhea. Gastroenterology 91:1, 1986.

141. Peled Y, Doron O, Laufer H, et al: D-Xylose absorption test. Urine or blood? Dig Dis Sci 36:188, 1991.

142. Riordan SM, McIver CJ, Duncombe VM, et al: Factors influencing the 1-g ^{14}C-D-xylose breath test for bacterial overgrowth. Am J Gastroenterol 90:1455, 1995.

143. Uil JJ, van-Elburg RM, van-Overbeek FM, et al: Clinical implications of the sugar absorption test: Intestinal permeability test to assess mucosal barrier function. Scand J Gastroenterol Suppl 223:70, 1997.

144. Bjarnason I, Macpherson A, Hollander D: Intestinal permeability: An overview. Gastroenterology 108:1566, 1995.

145. Bai JC: Malabsorption syndromes. Digestion 59:530, 1998.

146. Cobden I, Hamilton I, Rothwell J, et al: Cellobiose/mannitol test: Physiological properties of probe molecules and influence of extraneous factors. Clin Chim Acta 148:53, 1985.

147. Wyatt J, Vogelsang H, Hubl W, et al: Intestinal permeability and the prediction of relapse in Crohn's disease. Lancet 341:1437, 1993.

148. Meddings JB: Review article: Intestinal permeability in Crohn's disease. Aliment Pharmacol Ther 11:47, 1997.

149. Smecuol E, Bai JC, Vazquez H, et al: Gastrointestinal permeability in celiac disease. Gastroenterology 112:1129, 1997.

150. Novacek G, Miehsler W, Wrba F, et al: Prevalence and clinical importance of hypertransaminasaemia in coeliac disease. Eur J Gastroenterol Hepatol 11:283, 1999.

151. Sigthorsson G, Tibble J, Hayllar J, et al: Intestinal permeability and inflammation in patients on NSAIDs. Gut 43:506, 1998.

152. Rooney PJ, Jenkins RT, Buchanan WW: A short review of the relationship between intestinal permeability and inflammatory joint disease. Clin Exp Rheumatol 8:75, 1990.

153. Cooper BT, Ukabam SO, O'Brien IA, et al: Intestinal permeability in diabetic diarrhoea. Diabet Med 4:49, 1987.

154. Kato M, Asaka M, Ohara S, et al: Clinical studies of ^{13}C urea breath test in Japan. J Gastroenterol 33:36, 1998.

155. Braden B, Caspary WF, Lembcke B: Nondispersive infrared spectrometry for $^{13}CO_2/^{12}CO_2$ measurements: A clinically feasible analyzer for stable isotope breath tests in gastroenterology. Z Gastroenterol 37:477, 1999.

156. de Meer K, Roef MJ, Kulik W, et al: In vivo research with stable isotopes in biochemistry, nutrition and clinical medicine: An overview. Isotopes Environ Health Stud 35:19, 1999.

157. Loser C, Brauer C, Aygen S, et al: Comparative clinical evaluation of the ^{13}C mixed triglyceride breath test as an indirect pancreatic function test. Scand J Gastroenterol 33:327, 1998.

158. Braden B, Picard H, Caspary WF, et al: Monitoring pancreatin supplementation in cystic fibrosis patients with the ^{13}C-triolein breath test: Evidence for normalized fat assimilation with high dose pancreatin therapy. Z Gastroenterol 35:123, 1997.

159. Antonowicz I, Lebenthal E: Developmental patterns of small intestinal enterokinase and disaccharidase activities in the human fetus. Gastroenterology 72:1299, 1977.

160. Welsh JD, Poley JR, Bhatia M, et al: Intestinal disaccharidase activities in relation to age, race, and mucosal damage. Gastroenterology 75:847, 1978.

161. Sahi T: Genetics and epidemiology of adult-type hypolactasia. Scand J Gastroenterol 29(suppl 202):7, 1994.

162. Escher JC, de Koning ND, van Engen CG, et al: Molecular basis of lactase levels in adult humans. J Clin Invest 89:480, 1992.

163. Sterchi EE, Mills PR, Fransen JA, et al: Biogenesis of intestinal lactase-phlorizin hydrolase in adults with lactose intolerance. J Clin Invest 86:1329, 1990.

164. Johnson JD: The regional and ethnic distribution of lactose malabsorption. In Paige DM, Bayless TM (eds): Lactose Digestion. Clinical and Nutritional Implications, 1st ed. Baltimore, Johns Hopkins University Press, 1981, p 11.

165. Hammer HF, Petritsch W, Pristautz H, et al: Evaluation of the pathogenesis of flatulence and abdominal cramps in patients with lactose malabsorption. Wien Klin Wochenschr 108:175, 1996.

166. Gudmand-Hoyer E, Simony K: Individual sensitivity to lactose in lactose malabsorption. Am J Dig Dis 22:177, 1977.

167. Bedine MS, Bayless TM: Intolerance of small amounts of lactose by individuals with low lactase levels. Gastroenterology 65:735, 1973.

168. Ladas SD, Papanikos J, Arapakis G: Lactose malabsorption in Greek adults: Correlation of small bowel transit time with the severity of lactose intolerance. Gut 23:968, 1982.

169. Roggero P, Offredi ML, Mosca F, et al: Lactose absorption and malabsorption in healthy Italian children: Do the quantitiy of malabsorbed sugar and the small bowel transit time play a role in symptom production? J Pediatr Gastroenterol Nutr 4:82, 1985.

170. Szilagyi A, Salomon R, Martin M, et al: Lactose handling by women with lactose malabsorption is improved during pregnancy. Clin Invest Med 19:416, 1996.

171. Szilagyi A, Lerman S, Barr RG, et al: Reversible lactose malabsorption and intolerance in Graves' disease. Clin Invest Med 14:188, 1991.

172. Obermayer-Pietsch BM, Bonelli CM, Walter DE, et al: Genetic predisposition for adult lactose intolerance and relation to diet, bone density, and bone fractures. J Bone Miner Res 19:42, 2004.

173. Lee MF, Krasinski SD: Human adult-onset lactase decline: An update. Nutr Rev 56:1, 1998.

174. Kolars JC, Levitt MD, Aouji M, et al: Yogurt: An autodigesting source of lactose. N Engl J Med 310:1, 1984.

175. Moskovitz M, Curtis C, Gavaler J: Does oral enzyme replacement therapy reverse intestinal lactose malabsorption? Am J Gastroenterol 82:632, 1987.

176. Riby JE, Fujisawa T, Kretchmer N: Fructose absorption. Am J Clin Nutr 58:748S, 1993.

177. Hoekstra JH, van-Kempen AA, Kneepkens CM: Apple juice malabsorption: Fructose or sorbitol? J Pediatr Gastroenterol Nutr 16:39, 1993.

178. Evans PR, Piesse C, Bak YT, et al: Fructose-sorbitol malabsorption and symptom provocation in irritable bowel syndrome: Relationship to enteric hypersensitivity and dysmotility. Scand J Gastroenterol 33:1158, 1998.

179. Rumessen JJ, Gudmand-Hoyer E: Functional bowel disease: malabsorption and abdominal distress after ingestion of fructose, sorbitol, and fructose-sorbitol mixtures. Gastroenterology 95:694, 1988.

180. Mishkin D, Sablauskas L, Yalovsky M, et al: Fructose and sorbitol malabsorption in ambulatory patients with functional dyspepsia: Comparison with lactose maldigestion/malabsorption. Dig Dis Sci 42:2591, 1997.

181. Wasserman D, Hoekstra JH, Tolia V, et al: Molecular analysis of the fructose transporter gene (GLUT5) in isolated fructose malabsorption. J Clin Invest 98:2398, 1996.

182. Born P, Zech J, Lehn H, et al: Colonic bacterial activity determines the symptoms in people with fructose-malabsorption. Hepatogastroenterology 42:778, 1995.

183. Fromm H, Malavolti M: Bile acid–induced diarrhoea. Clin Gastroenterol 15:567, 1986.

184. Fordtran JS, Bunch F, Davis GR: Ox bile treatment of severe steatorrhea in an ileectomy-ileostomy patient. Gastroenterology 82:564, 1982.

185. Little KH, Schiller LR, Bilhartz LE, et al: Treatment of severe steatorrhea with ox bile in an ileectomy patient with residual colon. Dig Dis Sci 37:929, 1992.

186. Emmett M, Guirl MJ, Santa AC, et al: Conjugated bile acid replacement therapy reduces urinary oxalate excretion in short bowel syndrome. Am J Kidney Dis 41:230, 2003.

187. Kapral C, Wewalka F, Praxmarer V, et al: Conjugated bile acid replacement therapy in short bowel syndrome patients with a residual colon. Z Gastroenterol 42:583, 2004.

188. Heubi JE, Balistreri WF, Partin JC, et al: Refractory infantile diarrhea due to primary bile acid malabsorption. J Pediatr 4:546, 1979.

189. Montagnani M, Love MW, Rossel P, et al: Absence of dysfunctional ileal sodium–bile acid cotransporter gene mutations in patients with adult-onset idiopathic bile acid malabsorption. Scand J Gastroenterol 36:1077, 2001.

190. Sadik R, Abrahamsson H, Ung KA, et al: Accelerated regional bowel transit and overweight shown in idiopathic bile acid malabsorption. Am J Gastroenterol 99:711, 2004.

191. Kyle RA, Gertz MA: Primary systemic amyloidosis: Clinical and laboratory features in 474 cases. Semin Hematol 32:459, 1995.

192. Steen LE, Ek BO: Familial amyloidosis with polyneuropathy. Aspects of the relationship between gastrointestinal symptoms, EMG findings, and malabsorption studies. Scand J Gastroenterol 19:480, 1984.

193. Lovat LB, Pepys MB, Hawkins PN: Amyloid and the gut. Dig Dis 15:155, 1997.

194. Feurle GE: Pathophysiology of diarrhea in patients with familial amyloid neuropathy. Digestion 36:13, 1987.

195. Hunter AM, Campbell IW, Borsey DQ, et al: Protein-losing enteropathy due to gastrointestinal amyloidosis. Postgrad Med J 55:822, 1979.

196. Carrizosa J, Lin KY, Myerson RM: Gastrointestinal neuropathy in familial amyloidosis. Report of a case with severe diarrhea without steatorrhea or malabsorption. Am J Gastroenterol 59:541, 1973.

197. Tada S, Iida M, Iwashita A, et al: Endoscopic and biopsy findings of the upper digestive tract in patients with amyloidosis. Gastrointest Endosc 36:10, 1990.

198. Herskovic T, Bartholomew LG, Green PA: Amyloid and malabsorption syndrome. Arch Intern Med 114:629, 1964.

199. Suhr O, Danielsson A, Steen L: Bile acid malabsorption caused by gastrointestinal motility dysfunction? An investigation of gastrointestinal disturbances in familial amyloidosis with polyneuropathy. Scand J Gastroenterol 27:201, 1992.

200. Steen L, Börje E: Familial amyloidosis with polyneuropathy. A long-term follow-up of 21 patients with special reference to gastrointestinal symptoms. Acta Med Scand 214:387, 1983.

201. Chassany O, Michaux A, Bergmann JF: Drug-induced diarrhoea. Drug Saf 22:53, 2000.

202. Longstreth GF, Newcomer AD: Drug-induced malabsorption. Mayo Clin Proc 50:284, 1975.

203. Ziegler TR, Fernandez-Estivariz C, Gu LH, et al: Severe villus atrophy and chronic malabsorption induced by azathioprine. Gastroenterology 124:1950, 2003.

204. Adams JF, Clark JS, Ireland JT, et al: Malabsorption of vitamin B_{12} and intrinsic factor secretion during biguanide therapy. Diabetologia 24:16, 1983.

205. Bauman WA, Shaw S, Jayatilleke E, et al: Increased intake of calcium reverses vitamin B_{12} malabsorption induced by metformin. Diabetes Care 23:1227, 2000.

206. Hendel J, Dam M, Gram L, et al: The effects of carbamazepine and valproate on folate metabolism in man. Acta Neurol Scand 69:226, 1984.

207. Race TF, Paes IC: Intestinal malabsorption induced by oral colchicine. Am J Med Sci 259:32, 1970.

208. Lembcke B, Caspary WF: Malabsorption syndromes. Baillieres Clin Gastroenterol 2:329, 1988.

209. Force RW, Nahata MC: Effect of histamine H_2-receptor antagonists on vitamin B_{12} absorption. Ann Pharmacother 26:1283, 1992.

210. Shneerson JM, Gazzard BG: Reversible malabsorption caused by methyldopa. BMJ 2:1456, 1977.

211. Peters JC, Lawson KD, Middleton SJ, et al: Assessment of the nutritional effects of Olestra, a nonabsorbed fat replacement: Summary. J Nutr 127:1719S, 1997.

212. Thornquist MD, Kristal AR, Patterson RE, et al: Olestra consumption does not predict serum concentrations of carotenoids and fat-soluble vitamins in free-living humans: Early results from the sentinel site of the Olestra post-marketing surveillance study. J Nutr 130:1711, 2000.

213. Shafer RB, Nuttall FQ: Calcium and folic acid absorption in patients taking anticonvulsant drugs. J Clin Endocrinol Metab 41:1125, 1975.

214. Zimmerman J, Selhub J, Rosenberg IH: Competitive inhibition of folate absorption by dihydrofolate reductase inhibitors, trimethoprim and pyrimethamine. Am J Clin Nutr 46:518, 1987.

215. Nakamura T, Kudoh K, Takebe K, et al: Octreotide decreases biliary and pancreatic exocrine function, and induces steatorrhea in healthy subjects. Intern Med 33:593, 1994.

216. Witt K, Pedersen NT: The long-acting somatostatin analogue SMS 201-995 causes malabsorption. Scand J Gastroenterol 24:1248, 1989.

217. Bragelmann R, Armbrecht U, Rosemeyer D, et al: Nutrient malassimilation following total gastrectomy. Scand J Gastroenterol Suppl 218:26, 1996.

218. Wollaeger EE, Comfort MW, Weir JF, et al: The total solids, fat and nitrogen in the feces: II. A study of persons who had undergone partial gastrectomy with anastomosis of the entire cut end of the stomach and the jejunum (polya anastomosis). Gastroenterology 6:93, 1946.

219. Griffiths A, Taylor RH: Postgastrectomy pancreatic malabsorption: Is there a case for intervention? Eur J Gastroenterol Hepatol 11:219, 1999.

220. Bragelmann R, Armbrecht U, Rosemeyer D, et al: The effect of pancreatic enzyme supplementation in patients with steatorrhoea after total gastrectomy. Eur J Gastroenterol Hepatol 11:231, 1999.

221. Bae JM, Park JW, Yang HK, et al: Nutritional status of gastric cancer patients after total gastrectomy. World J Surg 22:254, 1998.

222. Nilas L, Christiansen C, Christiansen J: Regulation of vitamin D and calcium metabolism after gastrectomy. Gut 26:252, 1985.

223. Hara H, Suzuki T, Kasai T, et al: Ingestion of guar gum hydrolysate, a soluble fiber, increases calcium absorption in totally gastrectomized rats. J Nutr 129:39, 1999.

224. Bo-Linn GW, Davis GR, Buddrus DJ, et al: An evaluation of the importance of gastric acid secretion in the absorption of dietary calcium. J Clin Invest 73:640, 1984.

225. Eagon JC, Miedema BW, Kelly KA: Postgastrectomy syndromes. Surg Clin North Am 72:445, 1992.

226. Lipski PS, Bennett MK, Kelly PJ, et al: Ageing and duodenal morphometry. J Clin Pathol 45:450, 1992.

227. Madjumdar AP, Jaszewski R, Dubick MA: Effect of aging on the gastrointestinal tract and the pancreas. Proc Soc Exp Biol Med 215:134, 1997.

228. King D, Smith ML, Chapman TJ, et al: Fat malabsorption in elderly patients with cardiac cachexia. Age Ageing 25:144, 1996.

229. Lovat LB: Age related changes in gut physiology and nutritional status. Gut 38:306, 1996.

230. Quinn K, Basu TK: Folate and vitamin B_{12} status of the elderly. Eur J Clin Nutr 50:340, 1996.

231. Saltzman JR, Kowdley KV, Pedrosa MC, et al: Bacterial overgrowth without clinical malabsorption in elderly hypochlorhydric subjects. Gastroenterology 106:615, 1994.

232. Haboubi NY, Montgomery RD: Small-bowel bacterial overgrowth in elderly people: Clinical significance and response to treatment. Age Ageing 21:13, 1992.

233. Sjogren RW: Gastrointestinal features of scleroderma. Curr Opin Rheumatol 8:569, 1996.

234. Hoskins LC, Norris HT, Gottlieb LS, et al: Functional and morphologic alterations of the gastrointestinal tract in progressive systemic sclerosis (scleroderma). Am J Med 33:459, 1962.

235. Rosson RS, Yesner R: Peroral duodenal biopsy in progressive systemic sclerosis. N Engl J Med 272:391, 1965.

236. Soudah HC, Hasler WL, Owyang C: Effect of octreotide on intestinal motility and bacterial overgrowth in scleroderma. N Engl J Med 325:1461, 1991.

237. Kaye SA, Seifalian AM, Lim SG, et al: Ischaemia of the small intestine in patients with systemic sclerosis: Raynaud's phenomenon or chronic vasculopathy? Q J Med 87:495, 1994.

238. Kaye SA, Lim SG, Taylor M, et al: Small bowel bacterial overgrowth in systemic sclerosis: Detection using direct and indirect methods and treatment outcome. Br J Rheumatol 34:265, 1995.

239. Akesson A, Ekman R: Gastrointestinal regulatory peptides in systemic sclerosis. Arthritis Rheum 36:698, 1993.

240. Folwaczny C, Rothfuss U, Riepl RL, et al: Gastrointestinal involvement in progressive systemic scleroderma. Z Gastroenterol 33:654, 1995.

241. Mader R, Adawi M, Schonfeld S: Malabsorption in systemic lupus erythematosus. Clin Exp Rheumatol 15:659, 1997.

242. Markusse HM, Schravenhoff R, Beerman H: Hypereosinophilic syndrome presenting with diarrhoea and anaemia in a patient with systemic lupus erythematosus. Neth J Med 52:79, 1998.

243. Marshall JB, Kretschmar JM, Gerhardt DC, et al: Gastrointestinal manifestations of mixed connective tissue disease. Gastroenterology 98:1232, 1990.

244. Narayanaswamy AS, Akhtar M, Kumar N, et al: Polymyositis—a review and follow up study of 24 cases. J Assoc Physicians India 41:354, 1993.

245. Levy HL: Hartnup disorder. In Scriver CR, Beaudet AL, Sly WS, et al (eds): The Metabolic and Molecular Bases of Inherited Disease, 8th ed. New York, McGraw-Hill, 2001, p 4957.

246. Palacin M, Goodyer P, Nunes V, et al: Cystinuria. In Scriver CR, Beaudet AL, Sly WS, et al (eds): The Metabolic and Molecular Bases of Inherited Disease, 8th ed. New York, McGraw-Hill, 2001, p 4909.

247. Torrents D, Mykkanen J, Pineda M, et al: Identification of SLC7A7, encoding y+LAT-1, as the lysinuric protein intolerance gene. Nat Genet 21:293, 1999.

248. Simell O: Lysinuric protein intolerance and other cationic aminoacidurias. In Scriver CR, Beaudet AL, Sly WS, et al (eds): The Metabolic and Molecular Bases of Inherited Disease, 8th ed. New York, McGraw-Hill, 2001, p 4933.

249. Thier SO, Alpers DH: Disorders of intestinal transport of amino acids. Am J Dis Child 117:13, 1969.

250. Hooft C, Timmermans J, Snoeck J, et al: Methionine malabsorption in a mentally defective child. Lancet 2:20, 1964.

251. Desjeux JF: Congenital transport defects. In Walker WA (ed): Pediatric Gastrointestinal Disease, 2nd ed. St. Louis, Mosby, 1996, p 792.

252. Leahey AM, Charnas LR, Nussbaum RL: Nonsense mutations in the OCRL-1 gene in patients with the oculocerebrorenal syndrome of Lowe. Hum Mol Genet 2:461, 1993.

253. Semenza G, Auricchio S, Mantei N: Small-intestinal disaccharidases. In Scriver CR, Beaudet AL, Sly WS, et al (eds): The Metabolic and Molecular Bases of Inherited Disease, 8th ed. New York, McGraw-Hill, 2001, p 1623.

254. Wright EM, Martin MG, Turk E: Familial glucose-galactose malabsorption and hereditary renal glycosuria. In Scriver CR, Beaudet AL, Sly WS, et al (eds): The Metabolic and Molecular Bases of Inherited Disease, 8th ed. New York, McGraw-Hill, 2001, p 4891.

255. Chesney RW: Iminoglycinuria. In Scriver CR, Beaudet AL, Sly WS, et al (eds): The Metabolic and Molecular Bases of Inherited Disease, 8th ed. New York, McGraw-Hill, 2001, p 4971.

256. Jones B, Jones EL, Bonney SA, et al: Mutations in a Sar1 GTPase of COPII vesicles are associated with lipid absorption disorders. Nat Genet 34:29, 2003.

257. Assmann G, Seedorf U: Acid lipase deficiency: Wolman disease and cholesteryl ester storage disease. In Scriver CR, Beaudet AL, Sly WS, et al (eds): The Metabolic and Molecular Bases of Inherited Disease, 7th ed. New York, McGraw-Hill, 1995, p 2563.

258. Anderson RA, Bryson GM, Parks JS: Lysosomal acid lipase mutations that determine phenotype in Wolman and cholesterol ester storage disease. Mol Genet Metab 68:333, 1999.

259. Yassin F, Rothenberg SP, Rao S, et al: Identification of a 4-base deletion in the gene in inherited intrinsic factor deficiency. Blood 103:1515, 2004.

260. van Wouwe JP: Clinical and laboratory diagnosis of acrodermatitis enteropathica. Eur J Pediatr 149:2, 1989.

261. Schlingmann KP, Weber S, Peters M, et al: Hypomagnesemia with secondary hypocalcemia is caused by mutations in TRPM6, a new member of the TRPM gene family. Nat Genet 31:166, 2002.

262. Cizewski Culotta V, Gitlin JD: Disorders of copper transport. In Scriver CR, Beaudet AL, Sly WS, et al (eds): The Metabolic and Molecular Bases of Inherited Disease, 8th ed. New York, McGraw-Hill, 2001, p 3105.

263. Dagenais SL, Adam AN, Innis JW, et al: A novel frameshift mutation in exon 23 of ATP7A (MNK) results in occipital horn syndrome and not in Menkes disease. Am J Hum Genet 69:420, 2001.

264. Liberman UA, Marx SJ: Vitamin D and other calciferols. In Scriver CR, Beaudet AL, Sly WS, et al (eds): The Metabolic and Molecular Bases of Inherited Disease, 8th ed. New York, McGraw-Hill, 2001, p 4223.

265. Ghishan FK, Lee PC, Lebenthal E, et al: Isolated congenital enterokinase deficiency. Recent findings and review of the literature. Gastroenterology 85:727, 1983.

266. Holzinger A, Maier EM, Buck C, et al: Mutations in the proenteropeptidase gene are the molecular cause of congenital enteropeptidase deficiency. Am J Hum Genet 70:20, 2002.

267. Davidson GP: Enteropathies of unknown origin. In Walker WA (ed): Pediatric Gastrointestinal Disease, 2nd ed. St. Louis, Mosby, 1996, p 862.

268. Bitner-Glindzicz M, Lindley KJ, Rutland P, et al: A recessive contiguous gene deletion causing infantile hyperinsulinism, enteropathy and deafness identifies the Usher type 1C gene. Nat Genet 26:56, 2000.

269. Auricchio S: Genetically determined disaccharidase deficiencies. In Walker WA (ed): Pediatric Gastrointestinal Disease, 2nd ed. St. Louis, Mosby, 1996, p 761.

270. Spickett GP, Misbah SA, Chapel HM: Primary antibody deficiency in adults. Lancet 337:281, 1991.

271. Cataldo F, Marino V, Ventura A, et al: Prevalence and clinical features of selective immunoglobulin A deficiency in coeliac disease: An Italian multicentre study. Italian Society of Paediatric Gastroenterology and Hepatology (SIGEP) and "Club del Tenue" Working Groups on Coeliac Disease. Gut 42:362, 1998.

272. Ament ME: Immunodeficiency syndromes and gastrointestinal disease. Pediatr Clin North Am 22:807, 1975.

273. McCarthy DM, Katz SI, Gazze L, et al: Selective IgA deficiency associated with total villous atrophy of the small intestine and an organ-specific anti-epithelial cell antibody. J Immunol 120:932, 1978.

274. Doe WF, Hapel AJ: Intestinal immunity and malabsorption. Clin Gastroenterol 12:415, 1983.

275. Cunningham-Rundles C: Clinical and immunologic analyses of 103 patients with common variable immunodeficiency. J Clin Immunol 9:22, 1989.

276. Washington K, Stenzel TT, Buckley RH, et al: Gastrointestinal pathology in patients with common variable immunodeficiency and X-linked agammaglobulinemia. Am J Surg Pathol 20:1240, 1996.

277. Lewin KJ, Riddell RH, Weinstein WM: Gastrointestinal Pathology and Its Clinical Implications, 1st ed. New York, Igaku-Shoin, 1992.

278. Vetrie D, Vorechovsky I, Sideras P, et al: The gene involved in X-linked agammaglobulinaemia is a member of the src family of protein-tyrosine kinases. Nature 361:226, 1993.

279. Lederman HM, Winkelstein JA: X-linked agammaglobulinemia: An analysis of 96 patients. Medicine (Baltimore) 64:145, 1985.

280. Wildin RS, Smyk-Pearson S, Filipovich AH: Clinical and molecular features of the immunodysregulation, polyendocrinopathy, enteropathy, X linked (IPEX) syndrome. J Med Genet 39:537, 2002.

281. Baud O, Goulet O, Canioni D, et al: Treatment of the immune dysregulation, polyendocrinopathy, enteropathy, X-linked syndrome (IPEX) by allogeneic bone marrow transplantation. N Engl J Med 344:1758, 2001.

282. Wormsley KG, Logan WF, Sorrell VF, et al: Neurofibromatosis with pancreatic duct obstruction and steatorrhoea. Postgrad Med J 43:432, 1967.

283. Dayal Y, Tallberg KA, Nunnemacher G, et al: Duodenal carcinoids in patients with and without neurofibromatosis. A comparative study. Am J Surg Pathol 10:348, 1986.

284. Green BT, Rockey DC: Duodenal somatostatinoma presenting with complete somatostatinoma syndrome. J Clin Gastroenterol 33:415, 2001.

285. Partin JS, Lane BP, Partin JC, et al: Plexiform neurofibromatosis of the liver and mesentery in a child. Hepatology 12:559, 1990.

286. Tatemichi M, Nagata H, Morinaga S, et al: Protein-losing enteropathy caused by mesenteric vascular involvement of neurofibromatosis. Dig Dis Sci 38:1549, 1993.

287. Garcia JC, Carney JA, Stickler GB, et al: Zollinger-Ellison syndrome and neurofibromatosis in a 13-year-old boy. J Pediatr 93:982, 1978.

288. Soergel KH: Nongranulomatous chronic idiopathic enterocolitis: A primary histologically defined disease. Dig Dis Sci 45:2085, 2000.

289. Ruan EA, Komorowski RA, Hogan WJ, et al: Nongranulomatous chronic idiopathic enterocolitis: Clinicopathologic profile and response to corticosteroids. Gastroenterology 111:629, 1996.

290. Sakoulas G, Anastopoulos H: Successful use of cyclosporine in the treatment of glucocorticoid-resistant nongranulomatous chronic idiopathic enterocolitis. Gastroenterology 117:1259, 1999.

291. McBrien DJ, Vaughan Jones R, Creamer B: Steatorrhea in Addison's disease. Lancet 1:26, 1963.

292. Rodgers JB, Riley EM, Drummey GD, et al: Lipid absorption in adrenalectomized rats: The role of altered enzyme activity in the intestinal mucosa. Gastroenterology 53:547, 1967.

293. Su AY, Bilhartz LE: Endocrine-related gut dysfunction. Semin Gastrointest Dis 6:217, 1995.

294. Collin P, Kaukinen K, Valimaki M, et al: Endocrinological disorders and celiac disease. Endocrine Rev 23:464, 2002.

295. Brosnan P, Riley WJ: Autoimmune polyglandular syndrome. In Sperling MA (ed): Pediatric Endocrinology. Philadelphia, WB Saunders, 1996, p 509.

296. The Finnish-German APECED Consortium: An autoimmune disease, APECED, caused by mutations in a novel gene featuring two PHD-type zinc-finger domains. Nat Genet 17:399, 1997.

297. Högenauer C, Meyer RL, Netto GJ, et al: Malabsorption due to cholecystokinin deficiency in a patient with autoimmune polyglandular syndrome type I. N Engl J Med 344:270, 2001.

298. Ekwall O, Hedstrand H, Grimelius L, et al: Identification of tryptophan hydroxylase as an intestinal autoantigen. Lancet 352:279, 1998.

299. Ekwall O, Rorsman F, Kampe O: Malabsorption due to cholecystokinin deficiency in a patient with autoimmune polyglandular syndrome type I. N Engl J Med 345:65, 2001.

300. Jackson WP: Steatorrhea and hypoparathyroidism. Lancet 272:1086, 1957.

301. Sjoberg KH: Moniliasis—an internal disease? Three cases of idiopathic hypoparathyroidism with moniliasis, steatorrhea, primary amenorrhea and pernicious anemia. Acta Med Scand 179:157, 1966.

302. Hellesen C, Friis T, Larsen E, et al: Small intestinal histology, radiology and absorption in hyperthyroidism. Scand J Gastroenterol 4:169, 1969.

303. Wegener M, Wedmann B, Langhoff T, et al: Effect of hyperthyroidism on the transit of a caloric solid-liquid meal through the stomach, the small intestine, and the colon in man. J Clin Endocrinol Metab 75:745, 1992.

304. Thomas FB, Caldwell JH, Greenberger NJ: Steatorrhea in thyrotoxicosis. Relation to hypermotility and excessive dietary fat. Ann Intern Med 78:669, 1973.

305. Goswami R, Tandon RK, Dudha A, et al: Prevalence and significance of steatorrhea in patients with active Graves' disease. Am J Gastroenterol 93:1122, 1998.

306. Hammer J, Howell S, Bytzer P, et al: Symptom clustering in subjects with and without diabetes mellitus: A population-based study of 15,000 Australian adults. Am J Gastroenterol 98:391, 2003.

307. Schiller LR, Santa Ana CA, Schmulen AC, et al: Pathogenesis of fecal incontinence in diabetes mellitus: Evidence for internal-anal-sphincter dysfunction. N Engl J Med 307:1666, 1982.

308. Bytzer P, Talley NJ, Hammer J, et al: GI symptoms in diabetes mellitus are associated with both poor glycemic control and diabetic complications. Am J Gastroenterol 97:604, 2002.

309. Rensch MJ, Merenich JA, Lieberman M, et al: Gluten-sensitive enteropathy in patients with insulin-dependent diabetes mellitus. Ann Intern Med 124:564, 1996.

310. Goldstein F, Wirts CW, Kowlessar D: Diabetic diarrhea and steatorrhea. Microbiologic and clinical observations. Ann Intern Med 72:215, 1970.

311. Blumenthal HT: Interrelationships of diabetes mellitus and pancreatitis. Arch Surg 87:844, 1963.

312. Hanukoglu A, Mizrachi A, Dalal I, et al: Extrapancreatic autoimmune manifestations in type 1 diabetes patients and their first-degree relatives: A multicenter study. Diabetes Care 26:1235, 2003.

313. Hardt PD, Hauenschild A, Jaeger C, et al: High prevalence of steatorrhea in 101 diabetic patients likely to suffer from exocrine pancreatic insufficiency according to low fecal elastase 1 concentrations: A prospective multicenter study. Dig Dis Sci 48:1688, 2003.

314. Hardt PD, Krauss A, Bretz L, et al: Pancreatic exocrine function in patients with type 1 and type 2 diabetes mellitus. Acta Diabetol 37:105, 2000.

315. De-Block CE, De-Leeuw I, Van-Gaal LF: High prevalence of manifestations of gastric autoimmunity in parietal cell antibody–positive type 1 (insulin-dependent) diabetic patients. The Belgian Diabetes Registry. J Clin Endocrinol Metab 84:4062, 1999.

316. Klein KB, Orwoll ES, Lieberman DA, et al: Metabolic bone disease in asymptomatic men after partial gastrectomy with Billroth II anastomosis. Gastroenterology 92:608, 1987.

317. Scott EM, Gaywood I, Scott BB: Guidelines for osteoporosis in coeliac disease and inflammatory bowel disease. British Society of Gastroenterology. Gut 46(suppl 1):i1, 2000.

318. McFarlane XA, Bhalla AK, Reeves DE, et al: Osteoporosis in treated adult coeliac disease. Gut 36:710, 1995.

319. Valdimarsson T, Lofman O, Toss G, et al: Reversal of osteopenia with diet in adult coeliac disease. Gut 38:322, 1996.

320. Farthing MGJ, Dawson AM: Impaired semen quality in Crohn's disease—drugs, ill health or undernutrition? Scand J Gastroenterol 18:57, 1983.

321. Jeppesen PB, Mortensen PB: Colonic digestion and absorption of energy from carbohydrates and medium-chain fat in small bowel failure. JPEN J Parenter Enteral Nutr 23:S101, 1999.

322. Wharton R, D'Agati V, Magun AM, et al: Acute deterioration of renal function associated with enteric hyperoxaluria. Clin Nephrol 34:116, 1990.

323. Oliver MR, Scott RB: Drug-induced bowel injury. In Walker WA (ed): Pediatric Gastrointestinal Disease, 2nd ed. St. Louis, Mosby, 1996, p 882.

324. Zerwekh JE, Pak CY: Selective effects of thiazide therapy on serum 1 alpha,25-dihydroxyvitamin D and intestinal calcium absorption in renal and absorptive hypercalciurias. Metabolism 29:13, 1980.

325. Mason JB, Zimmerman J, Otradovec CL, et al: Chronic diuretic therapy with moderate doses of triamterene is not associated with folate deficiency. J Lab Clin Med 117:365, 1991.

CHAPTER

99 Enteric Bacterial Flora and Bacterial Overgrowth

Seamus O'Mahony and Fergus Shanahan

Increasing recognition of the role of the intestinal flora in the development and function of the gastrointestinal tract has led to a resurgence of scientific and clinical interest in the enteric ecosystem. The contribution of the flora to mucosal homeostasis is so profound that it is no longer acceptable to study intestinal pathophysiology without consideration of the activities of the indigenous bacteria. The lesson of *Helicobacter pylori* in the genesis of peptic ulcer disease and gastric cancer has been a sobering reminder of the potential pathogenic role of luminal bacteria. The contribution of the intestinal flora to health and disease, however, is complex and influenced by a variety of host-related factors, including diet, antibiotic exposure, and immunologic and genetic status. As discussed in this chapter, the enteric bacterial flora are critical to health and host defense, but under conditions such as those favoring bacterial overgrowth, components of the flora may become a liability.

COMPOSITION AND MOLECULAR ANALYSIS OF THE ENTERIC FLORA

Most human enteric bacteria cannot be cultured, because of a lack of truly selective growth media. Nonetheless, molecular profiling has shown that whereas the flora appears distinct in different persons, its composition is relatively stable after infant weaning and throughout adulthood. Evidence from studies of twins suggests that the individuality of human flora may be under genetic control,[1] but environmental variables including diet and sanitation appear to have profound effects on early intestinal colonization with bacteria.[2,3] In adulthood, dietary fluctuations appear to induce changes in bacterial enzymes and metabolic activity, rather than changes in the relative populations of the flora.[2,4,5]

The composition of the flora varies quantitatively and qualitatively over both the long and the cross-sectional axes of the alimentary tract. Beyond the oral cavity, which harbors approximately 200 different bacterial species, the size and diversity of the flora increases distally along the digestive tract (Fig. 99–1). Gastric acid restricts bacterial numbers within the stomach to fewer than 10^3 colony-forming units (CFU)/mL. The gradient in bacterial density is greatest across the ileocecal valve, with approximately 10^8 bacteria per gram of ileal contents and up to 10^{12} per gram of colonic contents, comprising over 400 different bacterial species.[2,4-6] Most (greater than 99%) of the culturable bacteria in the ileum and the colon are obligate anaerobes, but the composition of the flora at the mucosal surface differs from that within the lumen; ratios of anaerobes to aerobes are lower at mucosal surfaces. Furthermore, culture-independent methods, such as the various molecular approaches described below, suggest that mucosa-associated bacteria differ from those recovered from feces, thus supporting the idea that host-related factors have a role in determining the enteric flora[7] and implying that bacterial aspirates from the lumen may be an incomplete reflection of mucosa-associated bacteria.

The flora of the proximal small bowel consists predominantly of gram-positive facultative bacteria,

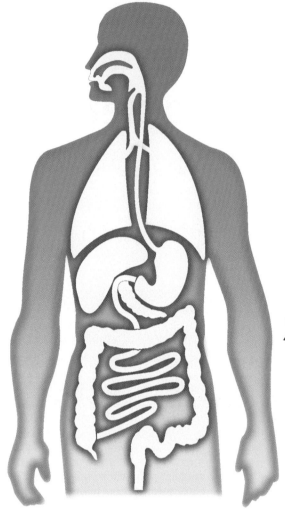

Oral cavity
200 species

Stomach
Helicobacter pylori

Duodenum
and proximal jejunum
$10^2 - 10^3$ bacteria/mL

Ileum
10^8 bacteria/mL

Colon
$10^{10} - 10^{11}$ bacteria/g

400-500 species including

Bacteroides
Eubacterium
Peptostreptococcus
Bifidobacterium
Ruminococcus
Bacillus
Fusobacterium
Clostridium
Lactobacillus
Enterococcus
Enterobacter

Figure 99–1 Composition and distribution of bacterial flora within the human alimentary tract.

although enterobacteria and *Bacteroides* also may be present. Peristalsis is the principal factor restricting bacterial numbers in the small bowel. In the distal small bowel, the composition of the flora resembles that of the colon, with a preponderance of gram-negative anaerobes. The most prominently represented genera in the distal bowel include *Bacteroides, Clostridium, Lactobacillus, Fusobacterium, Bifidobacterium, Eubacterium, Peptococcus,* and *Escherichia*.[2,6]

The impact of diet on the composition of the enteric flora has been studied by several investigators, with varying results. The consensus is that breast-fed babies have a greater proportion of bifidobacteria in their fecal flora than that observed in infants who are formula fed; high-carbohydrate and high-fiber diets are associated with increased bifidobacteria, whereas a high-fat diet is linked with an increase in *Bacteroides*. It is the metabolic activity of the flora, however, rather than its composition, that exhibits the greatest response to dietary changes in a given person.

Detailed analysis of the enteric flora has been confounded by the limitations of traditional culture-dependent microbiology. First, obtaining representative material from different niches within the intestine is problematic; because most of the indigenous flora are obligate anaerobes, major methodologic difficulties with sampling, contamination, transport, and storage are encountered.[8] Second, the lack of truly selective growth media precludes culture of most components of the flora. In this respect, it is noteworthy that culture of *H. pylori* and *C. difficile* was accomplished only within the past 2 to 3 decades. This difficulty has led to a shift in emphasis from conventional bacterial phenotyping toward genotyping and molecular approaches to study the "unculturables."[9,10]

Bacterial nucleic acid extracted from feces or mucosal biopsy samples can provide a profile of the composition of the indigenous flora. The small ribosomal subunit RNA (16S rRNA in bacteria) contains highly conserved regions of base sequences that reflect an absence of evolutionary change. These conserved sequences are interspersed with hypervariable regions, which contain mutational changes reflecting the evolutionary divergence of different species. Sequencing of 16S rRNA, therefore, represents a method for identification and phylogenetic classification of intestinal bacteria. For rapid profiling of the dominant culturable and nonculturable organisms within a complex ecosystem such as that in the intestinal tract, 16S rRNA can be amplified by polymerase chain reaction (PCR) with universal primers spanning conserved and

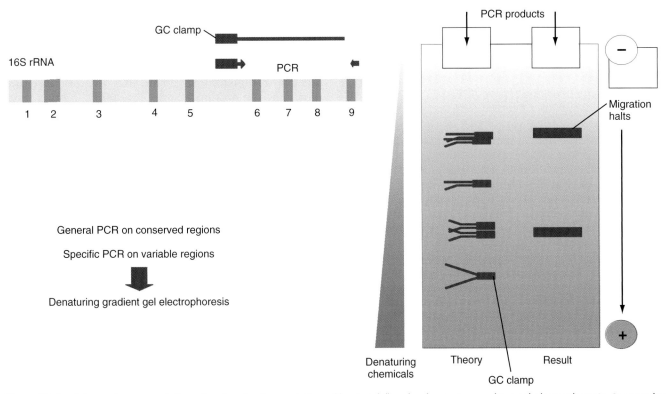

Figure 99–2   Schematic representation of molecular fingerprinting of bacterial flora by denaturing gradient gel electrophoresis. See text for details. GC, guanosine-cytosine; PCR, polymerase chain reaction.

variable regions. The mixture of hypervariable RNA fragments can then be separated by a chemical denaturing gradient or a temperature gradient gel electrophoresis (DGGE and TGGE). Complete denaturation of the RNA fragments is prevented by incorporating a GC-rich 5′ end to one of the primers (a GC clamp)[11] (Fig. 99–2). Variations in migration distance through the denaturing gradients reflect the diversity of 16S "species" in the sample (Fig. 99–3). Theoretically, the technique is semiquantitative, because the more dominant the organism, the more abundant the specific PCR product. The specific PCR product can be cut from the gel and further amplified, cloned, and sequenced to identify individual bacterial strains without requiring a conventional culture step. Further refinements of the technique can be achieved by using PCR primers that are species specific.

In addition to PCR-based approaches, other molecular techniques for analysis of specific bacterial species now are possible because of the increasing availability of genomic sequence data for the major components of the bacterial flora. These techniques include fluorescence in situ hybridization (FISH), flow cytometry (FISH-FLOW), and bacterial DNA microarrays. In disorders such as inflammatory bowel disease, immunologic reactivity against components of the flora has been used to identify microbes that may be etiologic in the pathogenesis of disease. Marker antibodies generated by hybridoma or phage display technology have been used as reagents to identify microbial antigens. For example, anti-neutrophil cytoplasmic antibody (pANCA) associated with ulcerative colitis has been used to identify colonic bacteria expressing a pANCA-related epitope.[12,13] In addition, candidate

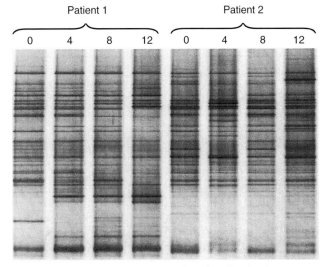

Figure 99–3   Representative examples of molecular fingerprinting profiles. Denaturing gradient gel electrophoresis analysis of the intestinal microbiota in two patients tested over time, at 0, 4, 8, and 12 months. Although the profile for each patient is unique, it also is stable.

microbes can be identified by the presence of unique bacterial nucleic acid sequences associated with a particular lesion or disease location, using subtractive cloning using genomic representational difference analysis. With use of this technique, a sequence representing a bacterial transcription factor from an apparent commensal organism, *Pseudomonas fluorescens*,[14-16] was found in lesions of

Crohn's disease compared with adjacent nonlesional mucosa. Serologic expression cloning also has been used to identify bacterial flagellin as a dominant antigen in Crohn's disease.[17]

HOST-FLORA INTERACTIONS

The flora exerts both positive and negative regulatory effects on the development and function of the intestine. This influence first was shown in comparative studies of germ-free and conventionally colonized animals. A sterile intestine is associated with reductions in mucosal cell turnover, digestive enzyme activity, cytokine production, lymphoid tissue, lamina propria cellularity, vascularity, muscle wall thickness, and motility, but with an increase in enterochromaffin cell area.[18] The molecular events underpinning this regulatory signaling from the lumen currently are being explored using modern techniques such as laser capture microdissection and gene array analysis; such studies promise to reveal new molecular targets to be exploited for the design of novel therapeutics.[19,20] Thus, for example, when applied to animals colonized with only a single bacterial strain, *Bacteroides thetaiotaomicron*, this combined approach has illustrated the impact of bacteria-derived signaling on the expression of host genes controlling mucosal barrier function, nutrient absorption, angiogenesis, and development of the enteric nervous system.

Incoming bacterial signals include secreted chemoattractants, such as the formylated peptide f-Met-Leu-Phe, cellular constituents such as lipopolysaccharide (LPS) and peptidoglycans, flagellin, and bacterial nucleic acids (i.e., CpG DNA). Detection of bacterial stimuli by the host and discrimination of pathogens from commensals are mediated in part by pattern recognition receptors such as Toll-like receptors (TLRs) that are present on epithelial and immune (dendritic) cells. In health, engagement of TLRs by ligands from the commensal flora appears to be required for mucosal homeostasis.[21,22] Thus, not only are bacterial signals required for optimal mucosal and immune development, but they actually are required to maintain and condition the mucosa for responses to injury.[22]

The immune system mediates the sense of microbial danger and responses to injury. Although the primary lymphoid organs are developed at birth, mucosal immune functions require continual education and fine-tuning of cytokine balances and T cell responses; this process is achieved by microbial colonization and sporadic mucosal infections. Without the flora, mucosal lymphoid tissue is rudimentary, and induction of mucosal immune responses and tolerance is suboptimal.[23,24] With a surface area similar to that of a tennis court (approximately 400 m^2) and only one cell layer separating the internal milieu from the lumen, the enteric mucosa is well adapted to immunologic sampling of the intraluminal microbial community. Sampling of the flora across the epithelial "barrier" is mediated by M cells, which deliver particulate and microbial antigens to underlying immune cells, and by mucosal dendritic cells, which appear to extend processes into the lumen between the surface enterocytes without disrupting tight junctions.[25]

It appears that intestinal dendritic cells can ingest and retain intact live commensal bacteria and then undergo transit to the mesenteric lymph node, where immune responses to commensals are induced locally.[26] Thus, the mesenteric lymph node acts as a gatekeeper, preventing access of commensal bacteria to the internal milieu and protecting the host from harmful systemic immune reactivity. The immunosensory function of dendritic cells is facilitated by their plasticity and versatility of responses,[27] depending on whether they are presented with commensals or pathogens; moreover, they appear to exhibit tissue-specific specialization in the intestine.[23,24]

In addition to specific immune responses to enteric bacteria, the surface epithelial cells serve a sensory function to detect microbial danger by production of chemokines that activate the host immune response and recruit it to any breach in the mucosal barrier caused by pathogenic infection.[28]

Transduction of bacterial signals into host immune responses after engagement of TLRs may proceed along more than one molecular pathway. The transcription factor nuclear factor-κB (NF-κB) is the pivotal regulator of epithelial responses to invasive pathogens, but nonpathogenic bacteria can attenuate inflammatory responses by delaying the degradation of IκB, which is counterregulatory to NF-κB.[29] Other signal transduction pathways are likely to emerge to account for the anti-inflammatory effects of probiotics and other commensal organisms such as *Bacteroides thetaiotaomicron*. This anaerobic commensal can antagonize the proinflammatory effects of NF-κB within the epithelial cell by enhancing the nuclear export of its transcriptionally active subunit (RelA), in a peroxisome proliferator–activated receptor-γ (PPAR-γ)-dependent manner.[30]

METABOLIC ACTIVITY OF THE FLORA

The enteric flora is tantamount to a hidden metabolic organ (Table 99–1). Although our understanding of indigenous bacterial metabolites is still superficial, co-evolution with this living inner mass of bacteria has several apparent benefits for the host. In addition to the production of regulatory signals for mucosal homeostasis as discussed earlier, the flora exhibits important metabolic properties not possessed by the host. These include biotransformation of bile acids; degradation of oxalate; breakdown of otherwise indigestible dietary components,

Table 99–1 Examples of Metabolic Activities of Intestinal Microbiota

Biotransformation of bile acids
Breakdown of dietary oxalate
Conversion of prodrugs to active metabolites
Degradation of polysaccharides of plant origin
Production of folate and B vitamins and vitamin K
Production of nutrient short-chain fatty acids
Production of regulatory signals for mucosal and immune homeostasis
Regulation of fat storage

such as plant polysaccharides; and production of short-chain fatty acids, a major energy source for colonic epithelium, from fermentable carbohydrates. Other activities include synthesis of biotin, folate, and vitamin K.[2,20] Clinicians also have exploited enteric bacterial enzymes such as azoreductase to convert prodrugs such as sulfasalazine to active drug metabolites (e.g., aminosalicylate). Other examples of bacterial action on drug bioavailability include the metabolism of L-dopa to dopamine and degradation of digoxin. Not all of the metabolic changes induced by the enteric flora are beneficial to the host, and although bacteria in the flora probably degrade some carcinogens, they also may promote the production of carcinogens from dietary procarcinogens.[31]

A striking example of the importance of bacterial metabolism is exemplified by the regulatory effect that the enteric flora exerts on fat storage.[32] It has long been known that germ-free animals need a significantly greater caloric intake to sustain a body weight similar to that of normal colonized animals. Thus, the normal host-flora relationship has nutritional benefit, in contrast with the negative nutritional effect associated with bacterial overgrowth syndromes. Elegant studies with germ-free mice have shown that on colonization, body weight increases despite a reduced caloric intake. The bacteria in the flora colonizing the intestine promote storage of dietary calories in fat by increasing absorption of monosaccharides and suppressing epithelial-derived fasting-induced adipocyte factor (FIAF).[32] Thus, the composition and activity of the intestinal microbiota should be considered as a variable influenced by Western diets that may influence susceptibility to obesity.

One of the outcomes of bacterial metabolic activity is gas production. Of the five gases—N_2, O_2, CO_2, H_2, CH_4—that comprise 99% of flatus, the latter three are produced by the enteric bacteria, and bacteria are the sole source of hydrogen and methane in the intestine. Hydrogen production by bacterial action on carbohydrates and, to lesser extent, on protein, normally occurs in the colon. In patients with small bowel bacterial overgrowth, however, the small bowel also becomes a site of H_2 production. Bacterial methanogens occur in the colon and produce methane from H_2 and CO_2, with significantly detectable excretion in approximately 30% of humans.[33-37] The principal gases produced are odorless, but bacterial metabolism also is responsible for production of various trace and odiferous gases in flatus such as hydrogen disulfide.[38,39] Qualitative and quantitative variability in gas production with diet illustrates the fluctuations in bacterial metabolic activity despite the apparent stability of the flora in adulthood.

SMALL INTESTINAL BACTERIAL OVERGROWTH

Small intestinal bacterial overgrowth (SIBO) is characterized by malabsorption and overgrowth of bacteria in the small intestine. The syndrome frequently is referred to as *blind loop syndrome*, because the disorder initially was rec-

ognized in patients with predisposing anatomic abnormalities. Other terms that have been used to describe the disorder include stagnant loop syndrome, contaminated small bowel, small intestinal colonization, and small bowel stasis. In 1939, Barker and Hummel[40] reported macrocytic anemia in association with intestinal strictures and anastomoses and postulated that the anemia was secondary to bacterial overgrowth, or "putrefaction." SIBO is not confined to humans and is well recognized in dogs.[41] The syndrome is associated with a variety of anatomic disturbances, such as blind loops,[42] and motility disorders, such as scleroderma,[43] but may occur in the absence of any specific predisposing factor. It is likely that the condition is underdiagnosed, particularly in the elderly.[44]

Patients with SIBO do not necessarily present with a florid malabsorption syndrome. Symptoms may be minor and nonspecific, and considerable debate has concerned the relationship between irritable bowel syndrome (IBS) and SIBO.[45] Bacterial overgrowth has been documented in asymptomatic elderly persons in the community.[46,47] It is debatable whether this phenomenon is of any significance,[48] and in the absence of malabsorption or other symptoms, the overgrowth probably should not be considered to represent true SIBO; such asymptomatic SIBO may be termed "simple colonization" and probably is a result of achlorhydria and abnormal fasting intestinal motility (see later).

The diagnosis of SIBO usually is made by noninvasive breath testing,[49] even though studies on the accuracy of these tests report very variable results. For this reason, culture of small intestinal aspirate must be regarded as the diagnostic gold standard. Unfortunately, much of the published literature on SIBO is based on breath tests, rather than on culture, and the findings must be interpreted with caution.

ETIOLOGY AND PREDISPOSING FACTORS

The upper small intestine is a relatively sterile environment because of the combined effects of normal peristalsis and the antibacterial action of gastric acid. Bacterial counts in aspirates from the normal upper small intestine generally are lower than 1000/mL. A variety of anatomic abnormalities, both iatrogenic and disease-related, lead to stagnation of small intestinal contents, with resulting bacterial overgrowth. The bacterial flora in SIBO is similar to that found in the normal colon, and the following organisms are common: (aerobic) *Streptococcus*, *Escherichia coli*, *Staphylococcus*, *Micrococcus*, *Klebsiella*, and *Proteus*; and (anaerobic) *Lactobacillus*, *Bacteroides*, *Clostridium*, *Veillonella*, *Fusobacterium*, and *Peptostreptococcus*.[50] The classic association of SIBO is with a "blind loop" resulting from abdominal surgery, such as Billroth II partial gastrectomy; other anatomic abnormalities include intestinal strictures and small bowel diverticulosis. Disorders affecting small intestinal peristalsis, such as diabetes mellitus[51] and scleroderma,[43] constitute the next most common cause of SIBO after anatomic abnormalities; other motility disorders affecting small intestinal peristalsis complicated by SIBO include chronic idiopathic intestinal pseudo-obstruction.[52]

The ileocecal valve prevents reflux of colonic bacteria into the small intestine, and resection of the valve or development of fistulas between the colon and upper gastrointestinal tract may lead to reflux of colonic contents into the small intestine, with ensuing bacterial overgrowth.[53,54]

Achlorhydria is known to be a predisposing factor for SIBO, and SIBO has been described in patients after vagotomy,[55] in those with atrophic gastritis, and in those taking acid-suppressant medication.[56-59] SIBO occurs more frequently in patients taking proton pump inhibitors (PPIs) than in those taking histamine H_2 receptor antagonists,[58] but clinical malabsorption does not appear to occur in this situation.[59]

Advancing age seems to be an independent risk factor for SIBO, but it is not clear if overgrowth results from the aging process itself and changes in intestinal motility or is a consequence of achlorhydria. Early studies in this area found that SIBO was a common (and frequently unrecognized) cause of malabsorption in the elderly,[44,60] and that many such patients did not have an obvious predisposing factor, such as a blind loop. More recent studies have reported SIBO in asymptomatic elderly persons residing in the community. These patients, although asymptomatic, had lower weights and body mass indices (BMI) than expected, and treatment with antibiotics increased both weight and BMI.[46,47]

SIBO appears to be common in patients with chronic liver disease.[61,62] SIBO is more common in patients with advanced (Child class C) liver disease[62] and may be an independent risk factor for spontaneous bacterial peritonitis,[63] although this latter association is controversial.[64] No association with any particular cause of chronic liver disease has been found,[65] but SIBO does not occur in cirrhotic patients if portal hypertension is absent.[66] The etiology of SIBO in patients with chronic liver disease is likely to be related to disturbances in motility[66] and possibly to the use of antacids, which might permit proliferation of bacteria, resulting in decreased gastric acidity.[64] Small intestinal dysmotility is more severe in cirrhotic patients with a history of spontaneous bacterial peritonitis,[63] and treatment of SIBO improves motility.[67] Liver transplantation also helps to correct small bowel dysmotility in cirrhotic patients.[68] Both antibiotics and prokinetics (cisapride) are effective in SIBO associated with cirrhosis.[68] SIBO in cirrhosis is associated with systemic endotoxemia.[69] Oral conjugated bile acids reduce bacterial overgrowth and endotoxemia in cirrhotic rats.[70]

SIBO is well recognized in scleroderma; the overgrowth occurs mainly in patients with small bowel involvement[71] and limited cutaneous systemic sclerosis. Diarrhea is the most important symptom. The somatostatin analog octeriotide is effective in the management of SIBO associated with scleroderma.[72]

SIBO has been described in association with several other chronic conditions (Table 99–2):

- SIBO may complicate diabetes mellitus. Although small intestinal dysmotility is thought to be the main predisposing factor, SIBO in diabetics is not especially associated with autonomic neuropathy.[73] Treatment of SIBO in diabetics improves orocecal transit time.[74]
- Many patients with celiac sprue who have persistent symptoms despite their adherence to a gluten-free

Table 99–2 Conditions Associated with Bacterial Overgrowth

Condition(s)	Pathophysiologic Mechanism
Blind loop (Billroth II gastrectomy, end-to-side anastomosis)	Disordered anatomy
Small intestinal diverticulosis	
Small intestinal stricture (Crohn's disease)	
Diabetes	Disordered motility
Idiopathic intestinal pseudo-obstruction	
Scleroderma	
Acid-lowering medications	Reduced gastric acid secretion
Atrophic gastritis	
Vagotomy	
Gastrocolic or enterocolic fistula	Abnormal connection between colon and proximal bowel
Resection of ileocecal valve	
Celiac sprue	Miscellaneous
Chronic pancreatitis	
Chronic renal failure	
Cirrhosis	
Old age	
Rheumatoid arthritis	
Radiation enteritis	

diet have SIBO.[75] It is not clear why this should be so, but a motility disturbance seems the most likely explanation.

- SIBO is common in Crohn's disease, particularly in patients who have had previous intestinal resection, and orocecal transit time has been reported to be prolonged in Crohn's patients with SIBO.[76] Positive results on glucose hydrogen breath tests are particularly associated with the presence of a small bowel stricture.[77]
- SIBO is common in chronic pancreatitis.[78] SIBO in this setting may be caused by small bowel dysmotility, resulting from chronic opioid use, and achlorhydria. Furthermore, pancreatic juice may have an antibacterial effect, so its absence might allow enteric bacteria to proliferate more freely.[79,80]
- More recently, SIBO with rheumatoid arthritis has been described; the syndrome is associated with high disease activity and does not appear to be related to achlorhydria.[81]
- SIBO occurs in late radiation enteritis and appears to be related to intestinal dysmotility.[82]
- SIBO is common in chronic renal failure, which is associated with neuropathic-type abnormalities of small intestinal motility.[83]

Many patients with SIBO may have more than one predisposing factor. For example, SIBO may develop in patients with scleroderma who receive PPI therapy for gastroesophageal reflux.

MECHANISMS OF MALABSORPTION

SIBO classically causes a combination of megaloblastic anemia (due to vitamin B_{12} deficiency) and steatorrhea (due to fat malabsorption). Megaloblastic anemia was described in association with intestinal strictures as long ago as 1897.[84] Vitamin B_{12} deficiency is caused by bacterial consumption of the vitamin within the intestinal lumen before it can be absorbed across the mucosa.[85] Anerobic organisms mainly are responsible for the vitamin B_{12} deficiency, and in animal studies, only antianerobic therapy reversed the deficiency.[86] Unlike aerobic bacteria, anerobes can use vitamin B_{12} both in its free form and as a complex with intrinsic factor.[87] Anerobic bacteria deprive the host of ingested vitamin B_{12} and exacerbate its deficiency by using the B_{12} to produce inactive cobamides, which then may compete with dietary B_{12} for ileal binding sites, thereby decreasing absorption of the vitamin.[88] Deficiencies of thiamine[89] and nicotinamide also have been reported in SIBO.[90] Folate levels tend to be high in SIBO, because the bacteria synthesize folate,[91] which then is absorbed and utilized by the host.[92]

Much of our knowledge on the mechanisms of malabsorption in SIBO is derived from animal models of blind loop.[93,94] Malabsorption of fat and fat-soluble vitamins results mainly from deconjugation of bile acids,[95] and administration of conjugated bile acids has been reported to reverse steatorrhea in human and animal studies.[96] Deficiencies of vitamins A, D,[97] and E[98] have been reported, but vitamin K deficiency is uncommon, because of production of vitamin K by luminal bacteria.

SIBO leads to carbohydrate malabsorption by reducing brush border disaccharidase levels.[99-101] In animal studies, bacterial extracts of cultures from experimentally created blind loops contain proteases that are capable of removing components of the intestinal surface membrane.[102] These proteases appear to have elastase-like substrate specificity and may be etiologic in disaccharidase deficiency. Lactose intolerance is common, and contributes to the diarrhea that typifies SIBO. Bacterial fermentation of carbohydrates contributes to abdominal discomfort and bloating in SIBO and is the basis for the various breath tests used to diagnose the condition.

Protein malabsorption in SIBO is caused by a number of factors: (1) decreased absorption of amino acid and peptides, which has been described in animal models and may result from mucosal damage[103]; (2) low levels of enterokinase, which may impair the activation of pancreatic proteases[104]; and (3) protein-losing enteropathy.[105] Although hypoproteinemia is common in SIBO, manifestations of severe hypoproteinemia, such as edema, are rare.

Small intestinal histologic findings generally are normal in patients with SIBO, and in one study, morphometric findings in small bowel also were described as normal.[106] Abnormalities of the small intestinal mucosa (villus atrophy, cellular infiltration of the lamina propria, intraepithelial lymphocytosis) have been described in some patients with SIBO,[107] however, and these changes revert to normal following antibiotic treatment.[108] Electron microscopy studies of experimental animals with SIBO have described enterocyte abnormalities, such as vacuolization of micovillus membranes and mitochondrial swelling.[109]

CLINICAL FEATURES

SIBO may be difficult to diagnose, because symptoms associated with the predisposing disorder may predominate. The classic clinical presentation of SIBO is that of a malabsorptive state characterized by steatorrhea and vitamin B_{12} deficiency that is not reversible with intrinsic factor. Patients with vitamin B_{12} deficiency may present with neurologic symptoms, central or peripheral neuropathy, and symptoms of anemia, such as fatigue and breathlessness. Patients with steatorrhea may report weight loss, diarrhea, and abdominal bloating and discomfort. Associated fat-soluble vitamin deficiency may occur, leading to night blindness (in vitamin A deficiency), and metabolic bone disease (in vitamin D deficiency). Osteoporosis is a well-recognized complication of SIBO.[110,111]

The clinical presentation of SIBO appears to be changing. Older references to clinical features of SIBO emphasized steatorrhea, megaloblastic anemia, and a history of surgery leading to blind loop syndrome. In a more modern series, Toskes and Kumar reported data for 100 consecutive, albeit highly selected, symptomatic patients referred for ^{14}C-xylose breath testing[112] and found a history of gastrointestinal surgery in only 15%; the three most common associated conditions, which accounted for greater than 90% of the positive results on ^{14}C-xylose breath tests for the patients in their referral center, were gastroparesis, chronic pancreatitis, and irritable bowel syndrome. Diarrhea, bloating, and flatulence were the most common symptoms. Although flawed in terms of patient selection and methods used to diagnose SIBO, more recent studies demonstrate that the clinical presentation in SIBO may be a less dramatic one, with milder symptoms, than the classic description of SIBO. It is likely that the wide use of breath tests is one reason this "newer" type of SIBO patient is being found.

Many patients with SIBO fulfill the Rome Criteria for IBS, and considerable debate on the relationship between IBS and SIBO has ensued since a study in 2000 reported that 78% of Rome Criteria–positive IBS patients in a cohort of patients tested positive for SIBO by lactulose-hydrogen breath testing.[113] Antibiotic therapy led to clinical improvement and normalization of the breath test. This study also has provoked criticism of its selection criteria and study design and raised concerns regarding the accuracy of the lactulose hydrogen breath test,

Considerable interest also has arisen in the putative association between SIBO and nonalcoholic steatohepatitis (NASH). It has been postulated that SIBO might play a role in the pathogenesis of NASH,[114] because NASH is a common complication of jejunoileal bypass surgery for morbid obesity and can be reversed with metronidazole treatment. Furthermore, antibiotic treatment prevents hepatic and bile duct injury in genetically susceptible rats with surgically created blind loops and SIBO.[115,116] The pattern of liver and biliary injury in this experimental situation, however, was histologically and radiologically more compatible with primary sclerosing cholangitis (PSC) than with NASH. Wigg and colleagues[117] postulated that SIBO might lead to NASH by altering small intestinal permeability and thereby increasing absorption of endotoxin. They studied 22 patients with NASH and found SIBO (by lactulose hydrogen breath testing) in 50% of subjects; serum endotoxin levels and small intestinal permeability, measured by the lactulose/rhamnose test, however, were normal in the patients with SIBO.

DIAGNOSIS

The diagnosis of SIBO should be considered in any patient with malabsorption and a predisposing anatomic or functional disturbance. As mentioned earlier, however, most patients today do not have a predisposing surgically induced anatomic disturbance. It is likely that SIBO is overlooked commonly in patients without predisposing factors and in patients who have nonspecific symptoms. Blood tests in patients with SIBO typically reveal a macrocytic anemia: Vitamin B_{12} levels are low, and folate levels may be high. Steatorrhea may be confirmed by 3-day fecal fat collection; this test has understandably fallen from favor with patients and laboratory staff, and microscopic examination of fresh stool for fat globules may suffice.[118,119] If an anatomic defect is suspected as the cause of SIBO, appropriate barium studies may be used to define the anatomy.

The gold standard test for the diagnosis of SIBO is aspiration of small intestinal fluid with culture and bacterial counts of the aspirate; presence of more than 10^5 CFU/mL of duodenal aspirate is considered diagnostic. Unfortunately, such aspiration is invasive and time-consuming. Moreover, although it still is recommended by most experts, some investigators have raised doubts that the test may miss bacterial overgrowth occurring more distally in the small intestine. Corazza and colleagues,[120] however, collected intestinal juice at two different levels of the proximal jejunum and reported a highly significant correlation between the bacterial counts at these sites. Other potential problems with aspiration of small intestinal fluid include contamination of the aspirate with mouth flora and technical difficulties with transport and culture of the aspirate. Contamination with oropharyngeal bacteria may be controlled for by simultaneous culture of saliva and jejunal aspirate.[121] Several techniques for collecting small intestinal contents have been described, including duodenal intubation with fluoroscopic guidance and endoscopic collection of fluid,[122] and brushing of the duodenal mucosa with a cytology brush.[123] Culture of unwashed small intestinal mucosal biopsy specimens is an alternative to culture of small intestinal aspirate, although this method appears to have a lower sensitivity compared with culture of aspirates.[124] Aspirate can be collected easily during routine endoscopy, and this is probably the easiest method in routine clinical practice. Small intestinal aspirate is collected by placing a sterile suction catheter inside a sterile overtube, which is passed through the suction channel of the endoscope. The aspirate then should be placed immediately in an anerobic transport vial, and the aspirate plated for both aerobic and anerobic organisms.

High levels of jejunal fluid volatile fatty acids, such as acetate and propionate, have been reported in SIBO.[125] These acids may be measured by gas-liquid chromatography; although the technique is highly specific, the sensitivity is low,[120] and this test is rarely used. The presence of deconjugated bile salts in small intestinal aspirates is another indicator of SIBO but has given way to breath testing (see later).

A variety of noninvasive tests have been developed for the diagnosis of SIBO. The ^{14}C-glycocholic acid breath test was one of the first breath tests used for this purpose and is based on the ability of bacteria to deconjugate bile salts. ^{14}C-glycine is produced and metabolized, resulting in a peak of $^{14}CO_2$ in the expired air. The test has a low sensitivity, because not all bacteria are capable of deconjugation, and a low specificity, because increased colonic deconjugation of bile salts may occur with ileal disease or following ileal resection.[126] The test therefore cannot distinguish between SIBO and ileal malabsorption and has largely fallen out of favor.

The currently used breath tests are based on the ability of bacteria to produce hydrogen or radiolabeled carbon dioxide after metabolizing a substrate such as glucose, lactulose, or xylose. Breath tests are simple and noninvasive and therefore are more attractive than is duodenal intubation or endoscopy for collection of intestinal aspirates. These tests, however, do have several potential problems[49]: (1) 15% of the population are methane producers (in persons who are colonized with *Methanobrevibacter smithii*, hydrogen reacts with carbon dioxide to form methane, so they produce less hydrogen than is typical for non–methane producers); (2) both slow and rapid small intestinal transit may affect the accuracy of these tests; (3) an acidic environment in the colon, as occurs with ingestion of nonabsorbable carbohydrates (e.g., lactulose), inhibits bacterial carbohydrate metabolism[127]; and (4) several patient-related factors, such as recent diet, smoking, and exercise, may influence baseline levels of breath hydrogen (see later). The literature on breath tests in SIBO is confusing, with wide variations in sensitivity and specificity (Tables 99–3 to 99–5).

The glucose hydrogen breath test probably is the most widely used breath test in clinical practice: The substrate is inexpensive, and the hydrogen meter is economical, portable, and easy to use. The glucose hydrogen breath test first was reported as a diagnostic test for SIBO in 1972 by Bond and Levitt.[128] Normally, glucose is absorbed entirely in the upper small intestine; with bacterial over-

Table 99–3 Sensitivity and Specificity of Glucose Hydrogen Breath Testing in the Diagnosis of Small Intestinal Bacterial Overgrowth: Summary of Clinical Studies

| Reference | Number of Patients | | Sensitivity (%) | Specificity (%) |
	Total	With Overgrowth		
131	45	27	93	78
120	77	44	62	83
132	30	20	75	30
133	40	29	27-52	36-80
134	46	24	58	86

Table 99–4   Sensitivity and Specificity of Lactulose Hydrogen Breath Testing in the Diagnosis of Small Intestinal Bacterial Overgrowth: Summary of Clinical Studies

| Reference | Number of Patients | | Sensitivity (%) | Specificity (%) |
	Total	With Overgrowth		
135	27	9	89	100
120	77	44	68	44
136	28	18	17	70

Table 99–5   Sensitivity and Specificity of [^{14}C]D-Xylose Breath Testing in the Diagnosis of Small Intestinal Bacterial Overgrowth: Summary of Clinical Studies

| Reference | Number of Patients | | Sensitivity (%) | Specificity (%) |
	Total	With Overgrowth		
138	12	12	100	—
139	60	23	65	59
140	30	20	95	100
141	10	6	60	40
142	20	10	60	90
143	47	14	79	85
134	46	24	42	86

growth, however, the glucose is cleaved by bacteria into carbon dioxide and hydrogen. The hydrogen is measured in the exhaled breath (at baseline and then every 30 minutes for 2 hours); a rise of 20 parts per million (ppm) above the baseline is regarded as diagnostic of SIBO. Fasting breath hydrogen levels of more than 20 ppm also are considered positive, but high baseline hydrogen levels are common in untreated celiac disease and normalize after gluten withdrawal for as-yet-unproven reasons.[129] Patient preparation is important for this test[130]: Patients must avoid smoking and ingestion of nonfermentable carbohydrates such as pasta and bread the night before the test, because these factors may raise baseline breath hydrogen values. In addition, exercise may induce hyperventilation, thereby reducing baseline breath hydrogen values, and should be avoided for 2 hours before the test. Some authors recommend an antibacterial mouth rinse before testing to prevent premature hydrogen or carbon dioxide production from the action of the oral flora on the glucose substrate. A number of studies have compared the glucose hydrogen breath test against the gold standard of culture of intestinal aspirate (see Table 99–3). Sensitivity levels from 27% to 52% have been reported, with specificity rates between 30% and 83%[120,131-134]; the largest study, by Corazza and colleagues,[120] reported sensitivity of 62% and specificity of 83%. Very rapid intestinal transit may lead to a false-positive test result, because glucose may reach the colon before it can be absorbed.

The lactulose hydrogen breath test is based on a principle similar to that of the glucose hydrogen breath test: Lactulose is a starch that is not absorbed by the small intestine but is cleaved by bacteria in the proximal colon into hydrogen, producing a late peak in exhaled hydrogen. In the presence of bacterial overgrowth, an early hydrogen peak is observed. Results of this test may be difficult to interpret with either slow or fast intestinal transit, and sensitivity and specificity have been disappointing[120,135,136] (see Table 99–4); Corazza and associates reported sensitivity and specificity rates of 68% and 44%, respectively.[120] Sensitivity of the test may be increased by the addition of scintigraphy, to correct for abnormalities of intestinal transit,[136] but the lactulose hydrogen breath test cannot be recommended for routine clinical use.

The ^{14}C-xylose and ^{13}C-xylose breath tests measure labeled carbon dioxide that is produced by breakdown of labeled substrates by bacteria. The isotope may be radioactive (^{14}C) or stable (^{13}C). The stable isotope has been used in children.[137] D-Xylose 1 g is the most widely used substrate. D-Xylose is absorbed entirely in the small intestine and is metabolized minimally. It is catabolized by gram-negative bacteria and is therefore a good substrate for breath testing for SIBO. The ^{14}C-D-xylose breath test appears to perform better than the glucose or lactulose hydrogen breath test (see Table 99–5), but as with these other breath tests, widely differing levels of accuracy have been reported, with sensitivity rates ranging from 42% to 100%, and specificity rates between 40% and 100%.[134,138-143] The ^{14}C-D-xylose breath test result is considered positive when the "cumulated dose at 4 hours exceeds 4.5% of the administered radioactivity." Disturbances in intestinal transit particularly affect the performance of this test, and accuracy may be improved by the addition of a transit marker (such as barium or diatrizoate meglumine–diatrizoate sodium [Gastrografin]).[143]

Other noninvasive tests described for SIBO include measurement of urinary cholyl-PABA and serum bile acids. Cholyl-PABA is a synthetic substrate made by conjugating cholic acid with para-aminobenzoic acid (PABA), which is hydrolyzed by the bacterial enzyme cholyl hydrolase to release PABA[144]; this PABA-based test, however, does not accurately distinguish between SIBO and other causes of malabsorption.[145] Elevated free serum bile acids have been reported in SIBO, but the test depends on the presence of bacteria that deconjugate bile salts, such as *Bacteroides*.[146]

It is our view that duodenal intubation with collection and culture of small intestinal aspirate remains the gold standard test for the diagnosis of SIBO. Small intestinal juice can be collected easily during standard endoscopy, and we recommend endoscopy with duodenal biopsy and collection of small intestinal juice for culture as a standard diagnostic approach in patients with malabsorption. It is common practice, however, to provide empiric antibiotic treatment for patients with suspected SIBO, without either breath testing or culture of small intestinal aspirate.

TREATMENT

Attention should be given to the patient's nutritional state, and any vitamin deficiency should be corrected (see Chapters 15 and 97). A lactose-free diet may ameliorate the diarrhea. If possible, any predisposing anatomic or functional abnormality should be corrected, but in practice, this is unlikely to be an option. Acid-lowering medication should be discontinued, if possible. A variety of antibiotics have been reported to be effective in SIBO, but little in the way of evidence exists to favor one agent over another. Antibiotics that have been reported to be effective include metronidazole, amoxicillin, amoxicillin-clavulanate, ciprofloxacin, tetracycline, and co-trimoxazole. One randomized cross-over trial reported that norfloxacin and amoxicillin-clavulanate were effective agents in SIBO.[147] In another study, rifaximin and chlortetracycline normalized results on glucose hydrogen breath testing in 70% and 27%, respectively, of patients with SIBO.[148] Both ciprofloxacin and metronidazole were found to be highly effective in SIBO associated with Crohn's disease, and although these antibiotics have been used for primary therapy in Crohn's disease, breath test result normalization occurred in a majority of patients in this study.[149]

Therapy usually is given initially for 2 weeks, and then clinical response is assessed, although it may be useful to repeat breath test or culture. Many patients with an underlying anatomic or motility disorder may require permanent antibiotic treatment; in such patients, it is usual to rotate antibiotic treatment every 2 weeks or, alternatively, to give antibiotics for 2 of every 4 weeks. Continuous treatment with a single agent may lead to antibiotic resistance or to side effects associated with long-term usage, such as peripheral neuropathy in patients given metronidazole.

The somatostatin analog octreotide stimulates intestinal motor activity. Given subcutaneously at low dose (50 µg once daily for 3 weeks), it has been reported to be effective in SIBO associated with scleroderma.[72] At higher doses (200 µg three times daily), octreotide paradoxically may *cause* SIBO by inducing hypomotility.[150] The prokinetic agent cisapride has been reported to be effective in SIBO associated with cirrhosis[151] but the drug is no longer available in the United States, and its use in several countries is strictly controlled because of risk of drug interactions and cardiac arrhythmias.

Probiotic therapy would seem a logical and attractive approach to the management of SIBO, but only a few studies have examined probiotic therapy in SIBO. *Saccharomyces boulardii* does not appear to be effective,[152] and in one double-blind cross-over study, *Lactobacillus fermentum* KLD showed no advantage over placebo.[153] A small, uncontrolled trial showed that *Lactobacillus plantarum* 299V and *Lactobacillus* GG benefited children with SIBO associated with short bowel syndrome.[154]

SIBO probably is second only to celiac disease as the most common cause of malabsorption in developed countries. The condition no longer manifests commonly with the classic features of steatorrhea and megaloblastic anemia, and most patients do not have a blind loop or other predisposing anatomic abnormality. Many patients may have nonspecific symptoms similar to those of IBS. Although the glucose hydrogen and ^{14}C-xylose breath tests are simple and noninvasive, the gold standard test for diagnosis is culture of small intestinal aspirate. The aspirate may be collected easily at endoscopy, which usually is performed to obtain biopsy specimens of the small intestine during evaluation of malabsorption. Treatment with one of several broad-spectrum antibiotics is simple and effective.

REFERENCES

1. Van de Merwe JP, Stegeman JH, Hazenberg MP: The resident faecal flora is determined by genetic characteristics of the host. Implications for Crohn's disease? Antonie van Leeuwenhoek 49:119, 1983.
2. Berg RD: The indigenous gastrointestinal microflora. Trends Microbiol 4:430, 1996.
3. Sonnenburg JL, Angenent LT, Gordon JI: Getting a grip on things: How do communities of bacterial symbionts become established in our intestine? Nat Immunol 5:569, 2004.
4. Bengmark S: Ecological control of the gastrointestinal tract. The role of probiotic flora. Gut 42:2, 1998.
5. Gordon JI, Hooper LV, McNevin SM, et al: Epithelial cell growth and differentiation III. Promoting diversity in the intestine: conversations between the microflora, epithelium, and diffuse GALT. Am J Physiol Gastrointest Liver Physiol 273:G565, 1997.
6. Xu J, Gordon JI: Honor thy symbionts. Proc Natl Acad Sci U S A 100:10452, 2003.
7. Zoetendal EG, Von Wright A, Vilpponen-Salmela T, et al: Mucosa-associated bacteria in the human gastrointestinal tract are uniformly distributed along the colon and differ from the community recovered from the feces. Appl Environ Microbiol 68:3401, 2000.
8. Borriello SP, Hudson M, Hill M: Investigation of the gastrointestinal bacteria flora. In Russell RD (ed): Clinics in Gastroenterology, vol 7. Philadelphia, WB Saunders, 1978, p 329.
9. Vaughan EE, Schut F, Heilig HG, et al: A molecular view of the intestinal ecosystem. Curr Issues Intest Microbiol 1:1, 2000.
10. Akkermans ADL, Zoetendal EG, Favier CF, et al: Temperature and denaturing gradient gel electrophoresis analysis of 16S rRNA from human faecal samples. Bioscience Microflora 19:93, 2000.
11. Collins K, O'Mahony J: The "unculturables". In Hart AL, Stagg AJ, Graffner H, et al (eds): Gut Ecology. London, Martin Dunitz Ltd., 2002, p 25.

12. Dalwadi H, Wei B, Braun J: Defining new pathogens and non-culturable infectious agents. Curr Opin Gastroenterol 16:56, 2000.

13. Cohavy O, Bruckner D, Gordon LK, et al: Colonic bacteria express an ulcerative colitis pANCA-related protein epitope. Infect Immun 68:1542, 2000.

14. Wei B, Dalwadi H, Gordon LK, et al: Molecular cloning of a *Bacteroides caccae* TonB-linked outer membrane protein identified by an inflammatory bowel disease marker antibody. Infect Immun 69:6044, 2001.

15. Dalwadi H, Wei B, Kronenberg M, et al: The Crohn's disease-associated bacterial protein I2 is a novel enteric T cell superantigen. Immunity 15:149, 2001.

16. Sutton CL, Kim J, Yamane A, et al: Identification of a novel bacterial sequence associated with Crohn's disease. Gastroenterology 119:23, 2000.

17. Lodes MJ, Cong Y, Elson CO, et al: Bacterial flagellin is a dominant antigen in Crohn disease. J Clin Invest 113:1296, 2004.

18. Midtvedt T: Microbial functional activities. In Hanson LA, Yolken RH (eds): Intestinal Microflora. Nestle Nutrition Workshop Series No. 42. Philadelphia, Lippincott-Raven, 1999, p 79.

19. Hooper LV, Wong MH, Thelin A, et al: Molecular analysis of commensal host-microbial relationships in the intestine. Science 291:881, 2001.

20. Hooper LV, Midvedt T, Gordon JI: How host-microbial interactions shape the nutrient environment of the mammalian intestine. Annu Rev Nutr 22:283, 2002.

21. Rakoff-Nahoum S, Paglino J, Eslami-Varzaneh F, et al: Recognition of commensal microflora by Toll-like receptors is required for intestinal homeostasis. Cell 118:229, 2004.

22. Madara J: Building an intestine—architectural contributions of commensal bacteria. N Engl J Med 351:1685, 2004.

23. Shanahan F: Nutrient tasting and signaling mechanisms in the gut: V. Mechanisms of immunologic sensation of intestinal contents. Am J Physiol Gastrointest Liver Physiol 278: G191, 2000.

24. Shanahan F: Pathophysiologic basis and prospects for probiotic therapy in inflammatory bowel disease. Am J Physiol Gastrointest Liver Physiol 288:G417, 2005.

25. Rescigno M, Urbano M, Valzasina B, et al: Dendritic cells express tight junction proteins and penetrate gut epithelial monolayers to sample bacteria. Nat Immunol 2:361, 2001.

26. Macpherson AJ, Uhr T: Induction of protective IgA by intestinal dendritic cells carrying commensal bacteria. Science 303:1662, 2004.

27. Huang Q, Liu D, Majewski P, et al: The plasticity of dendritic cell responses to pathogens and their components. Science 294:870, 2001.

28. Kagnoff MF, Eckmann L: Epithelial cells as sensors for microbial infection. J Clin Invest 100:6, 1997.

29. Neish AS, Gewirtz AT, Zeng H, et al: Prokaryotic regulation of epithelial responses by inhibition of IκB-α ubiquitination. Science 289:1560, 2000.

30. Kelly D, Campbell JI, King TP, et al: Commensal anaerobic gut bacteria attenuate inflammation by regulating nuclear-cytoplasmic shuttling of PPAR-gamma and RelA. Nat Immunol 5:104, 2004.

31. Rafter J: Probiotics and colon cancer. Best Pract Res Clin Gastroenterol 17:849, 2003.

32. Backhed F, Ding H, Wang T, et al: The gut microbiota as an environmental factor that regulates fat storage. Proc Natl Acad Sci U S A 101:15718, 2004.

33. Levitt MD: Volume and composition of human intestinal gas determined by means of an intestinal washout technic. N Engl J Med 284:1394, 1971.

34. Levine AS, Bond JH, Prentiss RA, et al: Metabolism of carbon monoxide by the colonic flora of humans. Gastroenterology 83:633, 1982.

35. Levitt, MD, Engel RR: Intestinal gas. Adv Intern Med 20:151, 1975.

36. Levitt MD: Intestinal gas production—recent advances in flatology. N Engl J Med 302:1474, 1980.

37. Levitt MD: Methane production in the gut. N Engl J Med 291:528, 1974.

38. Moore JG, Jessop LD, Osborne DN: Gas-chromatographic and mass-spectrometric analysis of the odor of human feces. Gastroenterology 93:1321, 1987.

39. Suarez FL, Springfield J, Levitt MD: Identification of gases responsible for the odour of human flatus and evaluation of a device purported to reduce this odour. Gut 43:100, 1998.

40. Barker WH, Hummel LE: Macrocytic anemia in association with intestinal strictures and anastomoses. Bull Johns Hopkins Hosp 46:215, 1939.

41. Batt RM, McLean L, Riley JE: Response of the jejunal mucosa of dogs with aerobic and anaerobic overgrowth to antibiotic therapy. Gut 29:473, 1988.

42. Wirts CW, Goldstein F: Studies of the mechanism of postgastrectomy steatorrhea. Ann Intern Med 58:25, 1963.

43. Kahn IJ, Jeffries GH, Sleisenger MH: Malabsorption in intestinal scleroderma: correction by antibiotics. N Engl J Med 274:1339, 1966.

44. Roberts SH, James O, Jarvis EH: Bacterial overgrowth without "blind loop": A cause for malnutrition in the elderly. Lancet 10:1193, 1977.

45. O'Leary C, Quigley EMM: Small bowel bacterial overgrowth, celiac disease and IBS: What are the real associations? Am J Gastroenterol 98:720, 2003.

46. Lewis SJ, Potts LF, Malhotra R, Mountford R: Small bowel bacterial overgrowth in subjects living in residential care homes. Age Ageing 28:181, 1999.

47. Parlesak A, Klein B, Schecher K, et al: Prevalence of small bowel bacterial overgrowth and its association with nutrition intake in nonhospitalised older adults. J Am Geriatr Soc 51:768, 2003.

48. Lipski PS, Kelly PJ, James OFW: Bacterial contamination of the small bowel in elderly people: Is it necessarily pathological? Age Ageing 21:5, 1992.

49. Romagnuolo J, Schiller D, Bailey RJ: Using breath tests wisely in a gastroenterology practice: An evidence-based review of indications and pitfalls in interpretation. Am J Gastroenterol 97:2113, 2002.

50. Bouhnik Y, Alain S, Attar A, et al: Bacterial populations contaminating the upper gut in patients with small intestinal bacterial overgrowth syndrome. Am J Gastroenterol 94:1327, 1999.

51. Goldstein F, Wirts CW, Kowlessar OD: Diabetic diarrhea and steatorrhea: Microbiologic and clinical observations. Ann Intern Med 72:215, 1970.

52. Pearson AJ, Brezechwa-Ajdukiewicz A, McCarthy CF: Intestinal pseudo-obstruction with bacterial overgrowth in the small intestine. Am J Dig Dis 14:200, 1969.

53. Griffin WO Jr, Richardson JD, Medley, E.S: Prevention of small bowel contamination by ileocecal valve. South Med J 64:1056, 1971.

54. Atwater JS, Butt HR, Priestly JT: Gastrojejunocolic fistulae with special reference to associated nutritional deficiencies and certain surgical aspects. Ann Surg 117:414, 1943.

55. Browning GG, Buchan KA, Mackay C: The effect of vagotomy and drainage on the small bowel flora. Gut 15:139, 1974.

56. Ruddell WSJ, Losowsky MS: Severe diarrhoea due to small intestinal colonization during cimetidine treatment. BMJ 281:273, 1980.

57. Fried M, Siegrist H, Frei R, et al: Duodenal bacterial overgrowth during treatment in outpatients with omeprazole. Gut 35:23, 1994.

58. Thorens J, Froehlich F, Schwizer W, et al: Bacterial overgrowth during treatment with omeprazole compared with

cimetidine: A prospective randomised double blind study. Gut 39:54, 1996.

59. Pereira SP, Gainsborough N, Dowling RH: Drug-induced hypochlorhydria causes high duodenal bacterial counts in the elderly. Aliment Pharmacol Ther 12:99, 1998.

60. McEvoy A, Dutton J, James OF: Bacterial contamination of the small intestine is an important cause of occult malabsorption in the elderly. Br Med J (Clin Res Ed) 287:789, 1983.

61. Shindo K, Machida M, Miyakawa K, et al: A syndrome of cirrhosis, achlorhydria, small intestinal bacterial overgrowth, and fat malabsorption. Am J Gastroenterol 88:2084, 1993.

62. Morencos FC, de las Heras Castano G, Martin Ramos L, et al: Small bowel bacterial overgrowth in patients with alcoholic cirrhosis. Dig Dis Sci 40:1252, 1995.

63. Chang CS, Chen GH, Lien HC, et al: Small intestinal dysmotility and bacterial overgrowth in cirrhotic patients with spontaneous bacterial peritonitis. Hepatology 28:1187, 1998.

64. Bauer TM, Steinbruckner B, Brinkmann FE, et al: Small intestinal bacterial overgrowth in patients with cirrhosis: Prevalence and relation with spontaneous bacterial peritonitis. Am J Gastroenterol 96:2962, 2001.

65. Yang CY, Chang CS, Chen GH: Small-intestinal bacterial overgrowth in patients with liver cirrhosis, diagnosed with glucose H_2 and CH_4 breath tests. Scand J Gastroenterol 33:867, 1998.

66. Gunnarsdottir SA, Sadik R, Shev S, et al: Small intestinal motility disturbances and bacterial overgrowth in patients with liver cirrhosis and portal hypertension. Am J Gastroenterol 98:1362, 2003.

67. Madrid AM, Hurtado C, Venegas M, et al: Long-term treatment with cisapride and antibiotics in liver cirrhosis: Effect on small intestinal motility, bacterial overgrowth and liver function. Am J Gastroenterol 96:1251, 2001.

68. Madrid AM, Brahm J, Buckel E, et al: Orthotopic liver transplantation improves small bowel motility disorders in cirrhotic patients. Am J Gastroenterol 92:1044, 1997.

69. Bauer TM, Schawacha H, Steinbruckner B, et al: Small intestinal bacterial overgrowth in human cirrhosis is associated with systemic endotoxemia. Am J Gastroenterol 97:2364, 2002.

70. Lorenzo-Zuniga V, Bartoli R, Planas R: Oral bile acids reduce bacterial overgrowth, bacterial translocation and endotoxemia in cirrhotic rats. Hepatology 37:551, 2003.

71. Kay SA, Lim SG, Taylor M, et al: Small bowel bacterial overgrowth in systemic sclerosis: Detection using direct and indirect methods and treatment outcome. Br J Rheumatol 34:265, 1995.

72. Soudah HC, Hasler WL, Owyang C: Effect of octreotide on intestinal motility and bacterial overgrowth in scleroderma. N Engl J Med 325:1461, 1991.

73. Virally-Monod M, Tielmans D, Kevorkian JP, et al: Chronic diarrhoea and diabetes mellitus: Prevalence of small intestinal bacterial overgrowth. Diabetes Metab 24:530, 1998.

74. Cuoco L, Montalto M, Jorizzo RA, et al: Eradication of small intestinal bacterial overgrowth and oro-cecal transit in diabetics. Hepatogastroenterology 49:1582, 2002.

75. Tursi A, Brandimarte G, Giorgetti G: High prevalence of small intestinal bacterial overgrowth in celiac patients with persistence of gastrointestinal symptoms after gluten withdrawal. Am J Gastroenterol 98:839, 2003.

76. Castiglione F, Del Vecchio Blanco G, Rispo A, et al: Orocaecal transit time and bacterial overgrowth in patients with Crohn's disease. J Clin Gastroenterol 31:63, 2000.

77. Mishkin D, Boston FM, Blank D, et al: The glucose breathtest: A diagnostic test for small bowel strictures in Crohn's disease. Dig Dis Sci 47:489, 2002.

78. Lembeke B, Kraus B, Lankisch PG: Small intestinal function in chronic relapsing pancreatitis. Hepatogastroenterology 32:149, 1985.

79. Rubinstein E, Mark Z, Haspel J, et al: Antibacterial activity of the pancreatic fluid. Gastroenterology 88:927, 1985.

80. Minelli EB, Benini A, Bassi C, et al: Antimicrobial activity of pancreatic juice and its interaction with antibiotics. Antimicrob Agents Chemother 40:2099, 1996.

81. Henriksson AE, Blomquist L, Nord CE, et al: Small intestinal bacterial overgrowth in patients with rheumatoid arthritis. Ann Rheum Dis 52:503, 1993.

82. Husebye E, Skar V, Hoverstad T, et al: Abnormal intestinal motor patterns explain enteric colonization with gram-negative bacilli in late radiation enteropathy. Gastroenterology 109:1078, 1995.

83. Strid H, Simren M, Stotzer PO, et al: Patients with chronic renal failure have abnormal small intestinal motility and a high prevalence of small intestinal bacterial overgrowth. Digestion 67:129, 2003.

84. Faber K: Perniciöse Anämie bei Dunndarmstricturen. Berl Klin Wochenschr 34:643, 1897.

85. King CE, Toskes PP: Small intestinal bacterial overgrowth. Gastroenterology 76:1035, 1979.

86. Giannella RA, Broitman SA, Zamchek N: Competition between bacteria and intrinsic factor for vitamin B_{12}: Implications for vitamin B_{12} malabsorption in intestinal bacterial overgrowth. Gastroenterology 62:255, 1972.

87. Welkos SL, Toskes PP, Baer H: Importance of anaerobic bacteria in the cobalamin malabsorption of the experimental rat blind loop syndrome. Gastroenterology 80:313, 1981.

88. Brandt LJ, Bernstein LH, Wagle A: Production of vitamin B_{12} analogues in patients with small bowel bacterial overgrowth. Ann Intern Med 87:546, 1977.

89. Lervol L, Eugene C, Anciaux ML, et al: Polynévrite compliquant une colonisation bacteriénne chronique du grêle au cours d'une diverticulose jéjunale. Gastroenterol Clin Biol 12:585, 1988.

90. Tabaqchali S, Pallis C: Reversible nicotinamide deficiency encephalopathy in a patient with jejunal diverticulosis. Gut 11:1024, 1970.

91. Hoffbrand AV, Tabaqchali S, Moilin DL: High serum folate levels in intestinal blind loop syndrome. Lancet 1:1339, 1966.

92. Camilo E, Zimmerman J, Mason JB, et al: Folate synthesized by bacteria in the human upper small intestine is assimilated by the host. Gastroenterology 110:991, 1996.

93. Cameron DG, Watson GM, Witts LJ: The experimental production of macrocytic anemia by operations of the intestinal tract. Blood 4:803, 1949.

94. King CE, Toskes PP: The experimental rat blind loop preparation: a model for small-intestine bacterial overgrowth in man. In Pfeiffer CJ (ed): Animal Models for Intestinal Disease. Boca Raton, Fla, CRC Press, 1985, p 217.

95. Tabaqchali S, Hatzioanuou J, Booth CC: Bile salt deconjugation and steatorrhoea in patients with the stagnant loop syndrome. Lancet 2:12, 1968.

96. Kim YS, Spritz N, Blum M, et al: The role of altered bile acid metabolism in the steatorrhea of experimental blind-loop syndrome. J Clin Invest 45:956, 1966.

97. Schonsby H: Osteomalacia in the stagnant loop syndrome. Acta Med Scand Suppl 603:39, 1977.

98. Brin MF, Fetell MR, Green PHA, et al: Blind loop syndrome, vitamin E malabsorption and spinocerebellar degeneration. Neurology 35:338, 1985.

99. Riepe SP, Goldstein J, Alpers DH: Effect of secreted *Bacteroides* proteases on human intestinal brush border hydrolases. J Clin Invest 66:314, 1980.

100. Sherman P, Wesley A, Forstner G: Sequential disaccharidase loss in rat intestinal blind loops: impact of malnutrition. Am J Physiol 248:G626, 1985.

101. Giannella RA, Rout WR, Toskes PP: Jejunal brush border injury and impaired sugar and amino acid uptake in the blind loop syndrome. Gastroenterology 67:95, 1974.

102. Jonas A, Krishnan C, Forstner G: Pathogenesis of mucosal injury in the blind loop syndrome: Release of disaccharidases from brush border membrane extracts of bacteria obtained from intestinal blind loops in rats. Gastroenterology 75:791, 1978.

103. Jones EA, Craigie A, Tavill AS, et al: Protein metabolism in the intestinal stagnant loop syndrome. Gut 9:466, 1968.

104. Rutgeerts L, Mainguet P, Tytgat G, et al: Enterokinase in contaminated small-bowel syndrome. Digestion 10:249, 1974.

105. King CE, Toskes PP: Protein-losing enteropathy in the human and experimental rat blind-loop syndrome. Gastroenterology 80:834, 1981.

106. Riordan SM, McIver CJ, Wakefield D, et al: Small intestinal mucosal immunity and morphometry in luminal growth of indigenous gut flora. Am J Gastroenterol 96:494, 2001.

107. Ament ME, Shimoda SS, Saunders DR, et al: Pathogenesis of steatorrhea in three cases of small intestinal stasis syndrome. Gastroenterology 63:728, 1972.

108. Haboubi NY, Lee GS, Montgomery RD: Duodenal mucosal morphometry of elderly patients with small intestinal bacterial overgrowth: Response to antibiotic treatment. Age Ageing 20:29, 1991.

109. Toskes PP, Giannella RA, Jervis HR, et al: Small intestinal mucosal injury in the experimental blind loop syndrome. Light- and electron-microscopic and histochemical studies. Gastroenterology 68:193, 1975.

110. Di Stefano M, Veneto G, Malservisi S, Corazza GR: Small intestinal bacterial overgrowth and metabolic bone disease. Dig Dis Sci 46:1077, 2001.

111. Stotzer PO, Johansson C, Mellstrom D, et al: Bone mineral density in patients with small intestinal bacterial overgrowth. Hepatogastroenterology 50:1415, 2003.

112. Toskes PP, Kumar A: Enteric bacterial flora and bacterial overgrowth syndrome. In Feldman M, Scharschmidt BF, Sleisenger MH (eds): Sleisenger & Fordtran's Gastrointestinal and Liver Disease, 6th ed. Philadelphia, WB Saunders, 1998, p 1523.

113. Pimentel M, Chow EJ, Lin HC: Eradication of small intestinal bacterial overgrowth reduces symptoms of irritable bowel syndrome. Am J Gastroenterol 95:3503, 2000.

114. Farrell GC: Is bacterial ash the flash that ignites NASH? Gut 48:148, 2001.

115. Lichtman SN, Keku J, Clark RL, et al: Biliary tract disease in rats with experimental small bowel bacterial overgrowth. Hepatology 13:766, 1991.

116. Lichtman SN, Keku J, Schwab JH, et al: Hepatic injury associated with small bowel bacterial overgrowth in rats is prevented by metronidazole and tetracycline. Gastroenterology 100:513, 1991.

117. Wigg AJ, Roberts-Thomson IC, Dymock RB: The role of small intestinal bacterial overgrowth, intestinal permeability, endotoxaemia, and tumour necrosis factor alpha in the pathogenesis of non-alcoholic steatohepatitis. Gut 48:206, 2001.

118. Simco V: Fecal fat microscopy. Acceptable predictive value in screening for steatorrhea. Am J Gastroenterol 75:204, 1981.

119. Fine KD, Ogunji F: A new method of quantitative fecal fat microscopy and its correlation with chemically measured fecal fat output. Am J Clin Pathol 113:528, 2000.

120. Corazza GR, Menozzi MG, Strocchi A, et al: The diagnosis of small bowel bacterial overgrowth. Reliability of jejunal culture and inadequacy of breath hydrogen testing. Gastroenterology 98:302, 1990.

121. Hamilton I, Worsley BW, Cobden I, et al: Simultaneous culture of saliva and jejunal aspirate in the investigation of small bowel bacterial overgrowth. Gut 23:847, 1982.

122. Bardhan PK, Gyr K, Beglinger C, et al: Diagnosis of bacterial overgrowth after culturing proximal small bowel aspirate obtained during routine upper gastrointestinal endoscopy. Scand J Gastroenterol 27:253, 1992.

123. Leon-Barua R, Gilman RH, Rodriguez C, et al: Comparison of three methods to obtain upper small bowel contents for culture. Am J Gastroenterol 88:925, 1993.

124. Riordan SM, McIver CJ, Duncombe VM, et al: Bacteriologic analysis of mucosal biopsy specimens for detecting small-intestinal bacterial overgrowth. Scand J Gastroenterol 30:681, 1995.

125. Chernov AJ, Doe WF, Gompertz D: Intrajejunal volatile fatty acids in the stagnant loop syndrome. Gut 13:103, 1972.

126. Ferguson J, Walker K, Thomson AB: Limitations in the use of ^{14}C-glycocholate breath and stool bile acid determinations in patients with chronic diarrhea. J Clin Gastroenterol 8:258, 1986.

127. Perman JA, Modler S, Olson AC: Role of pH in production of hydrogen from carbohydrates by colonic bacterial flora. J Clin Invest 67:643, 1981.

128. Bond JH, Levitt MD: Use of pulmonary hydrogen [H_2] measurements to quantitate carbohydrate absorption. Study of partially gastrectomized patients. J Clin Invest 51:1219, 1972.

129. Corazza GR, Strocchi A, Gasbarrini G: Fasting breath hydrogen in celiac disease. Gastroenterology 93:53, 1987.

130. Thompson DG, Binfoeld P, DeBelder A, et al: Extraintestnal influences on exhaled breath hydrogen measurements during the investigation of gastrointestinal disease. Gut 26:1349, 1985.

131. Kerlin P, Wong L: Breath hydrogen testing in bacterial overgrowth of the small intestine. Gastroenterology 95:982, 1988.

132. MacMahon M, Gibbons N, Mullins E, et al: Are breath hydrogen tests valid in the elderly? Gerontology 42:40, 1996.

133. Bauer TM, Schwacha H, Steinbruckner B et al: Diagnosis of small intestinal bacterial overgrowth in patients with cirrhosis of the liver: Poor performance of the glucose breath hydrogen test. J Hepatol 33:382, 2000.

134. Stotzer PO, Kilander AF: Comparison of the 1-gram ^{14}C-D-xylose breath test and the 50 gram hydrogen glucose breath test for diagnosis of small intestinal bacterial overgrowth. Digestion 61:165, 2000.

135. Rhodes JM, Middleton P, Jewell DP: The lactulose hydrogen breath test as a diagnostic test for small bowel bacterial overgrowth. Scand J Gastroenterol 14:333, 1979.

136. Riordan SM, McIver CJ, Walker BM, et al: The lactulose breath hydrogen test and small intestinal bacterial overgrowth. Am J Gastroenterol 91:1795, 1996.

137. Dellert SF, Nowicki MJ, Farrell MK, et al: The ^{13}C-xylose breath test for the diagnosis of small bowel bacterial overgrowth in children. J Pediatr Gastroenterol Nutr 25:153, 1997.

138. King CE, Toskes PP, Guilarte TR, et al: Comparison of the one-gram D-^{14}C]xylose breath test to the ^{14}C]bile acid breath test in patients with small-intestine bacterial overgrowth. Dig Dis Sci 25:53, 1980.

139. Rumessen JJ, Gudmand-Hoyer E, Bachmann E, et al: Diagnosis of bacterial overgrowth of the small intestine. Comparison of the ^{14}C-D-xylose breath test and jejunal cultures in 60 patients. Scand J Gastroenterol 20:1267, 1985.

140. King CE, Toskes PP: Comparison of the 1-gram ^{14}C]xylose, 10-gram lactulose-H_2, and 80-gram glucose-H_2 breath tests in patients with small intestinal bacterial overgrowth. Gastroenterology 91:1447, 1986.

141. Valdovinos MA, Camilleri M, Thomforde GM, et al: Reduced accuracy of ^{14}C-D-xylose breath test for detecting bacterial overgrowth in gastrointestinal motility disorders. Scand J Gastroenterol 28:963, 1993.

142. Chang CS, Chen GH, Kao CH, et al: Increased accuracy of the carbon-14 D-xylose breath test in detecting small-

intestinal bacterial overgrowth by correction with the gastric emptying rate. Eur J Nucl Med 22:1118, 1995.

143. Lewis SJ, Young G, Mann M, et al: Improvement in specificity of [^{14}C]D-xylose breath test for bacterial overgrowth. Dig Dis Sci 42:1587, 1997.

144. Bardhan PK, Feger A, Kogon M, et al: Urinary cholyl-PABA excretion in diagnosing small intestinal bacterial overgrowth: Evaluation of a new non-invasive method. Dig Dis Sci 45:474, 2000.

145. Toskes P: Bacterial overgrowth of the gastrointestinal tract. Adv Intern Med 38:387, 1993.

146. Setchell KD, Harrison DL, Gilbert JM, et al: Serum unconjugated bile acids: Qualitative and quantitative profiles in ileal resection and bacterial overgrowth. Clin Chem Acta 152:297, 1985.

147. Attar A, Flourie B, Rambaud JC, et al: Antibiotic efficacy in small intestinal bacterial overgrowth-related chronic diarrhea: A crossover, randomised trial. Gastroenterology 117:794, 1999.

148. Di Stefano M, Malservisi S, Veneto G, et al: Rifaximin versus chlortetracycline in the short-term treatment of small intes-tinal bacterial overgrowth. Aliment Pharmacol Ther 14:551, 2000.

149. Castiglione F, Rispo A, Di Girolamo E, et al: Antibiotic treatment of small bowel bacterial overgrowth in patients with Crohn's disease. Aliment Pharmacol Ther 18:1107, 2003.

150. Witt K, Pedersen NT: The long-acting somatostatin analogue SMS 201-995 causes malabsorption. Scand J Gastroenterol 24:1248, 1989.

151. Pardo A, Bartoli R, Lorenzo-Zuniga V, et al: Effect of cisapride on intestinal bacterial overgrowth and bacterial translocation in cirrhosis. Hepatology 31:858, 2000.

152. Attar A, Flourie B, Rambaud JC, et al: Antibiotic efficacy in small intestinal bacterial overgrowth-related diarrhea: A crossover, randomized trial. Gastroenterology 117:794, 1999.

153. Stotzer PO, Blomberg L, Conway PL, et al: Probiotic treatment of small intestinal bacterial overgrowth by *Lactobacillus fermentum* KLD. Scand J Infect Dis 28:615, 1996.

154. Vanderhoof JA, Young RJ, Murray N, et al: Treatment strategies for small bowel bacterial overgrowth in short bowel syndrome. J Pediatr Gastroenterol Nutr 27:155, 1998.

CHAPTER
100 Short Bowel Syndrome

Alan L. Buchman

Short bowel syndrome (SBS) is defined as a malabsorption due to insufficient intestinal surface area such that the affected person is unable to absorb sufficient fluid, energy, or nutrients to sustain life in the absence of specialized nutritional support. This syndrome, also known as *intestinal failure*, occurs in adults in whom less than 200 cm of intestine is present. The spectrum of SBS, however, ranges from limited ileocolonic resections with moderate nutritional compromise to extensive small intestinal and colonic resections, resulting in duodenostomy, proximal jejunostomy, or jejunocolonic anastomosis, with severe nutritional consequences. SBS also may be a congenital condition or result from a variety of congenital causes.

ETIOLOGY

The major causes of SBS in adults are Crohn's disease for which multiple intestinal resections have been performed; mesenteric infarction from venous or arterial thrombosis, arterial embolism, or midgut volvulus; massive enterectomy performed to manage traumatic injuries or tumor resection, and radiation injury (Table 100–1). The causes of SBS in the pediatric population are congenital abnormalities (see Chapter 93), including gastroschisis, intestinal atresia, malrotation, aganglionosis, and necrotizing enterocolitis. Greater than 90% of infants now survive the extensive intestinal resections required for these conditions and need careful follow-up for their SBS as they mature to adulthood. Intestinal failure also may result from chronic intestinal pseudo-

obstruction syndrome in both adults and children (see Chapter 117), as well as from unclassified sprue (in adults) and congenital villus atrophy (in children).

INCIDENCE AND PREVALENCE

The incidence of SBS is difficult to assess in the United States, because of a lack of both a national registry for affected persons and prospective studies in defined populations of patients who have undergone extensive intestinal resections. The incidence of severe SBS necessitating long-term parenteral nutrition is estimated to be 2 to 4 cases per 1 million persons per year, based on multinational European data.[1] It is estimated that between 10,000 and 20,000 patients in the United States are on a home parenteral nutrition regimen for SBS. Approximately 50% to 70% of patients with SBS who initially require parenteral nutrition can be weaned from this therapy and therefore may not be reflected in the prevalence estimates.[2,3] Such patients often still require aggressive nutritional monitoring. The incidence and prevalence of SBS associated with Crohn's disease are decreasing now that infliximab and strictureplasty have become commonplace.

PATHOPHYSIOLOGY

The major consequence of extensive intestinal resection is loss of absorptive surface area, which results in malab-

Table 100–1   Causes of Short Bowel Syndrome and
              Intestinal Failure

In Adults
Catastrophic vascular accidents
    Superior mesenteric venous thrombosis
    Superior mesenteric arterial embolism
    Superior mesenteric arterial thrombosis
Chronic intestinal pseudo-obstruction*
Intestinal resection for tumor
Midgut volvulus
Multiple intestinal resections for Crohn's disease
Radiation enteritis*
Refractory sprue*
Scleroderma and mixed connective tissue disease*
Trauma
In Children
Congenital villus atrophy*
Extensive aganglionosis*
Gastroschisis
Jejunal or ileal atresia
Necrotizing enterocolitis

*Functional short bowel syndrome also may occur in conditions
associated with severe malabsorption, in which the bowel length
often is intact.

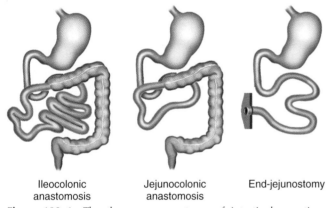

Figure 100–1   The three common types of intestinal resection
and anastomosis observed in patients with short bowel syndrome: ileocolonic anastomosis, jejunocolonic anastomosis, and
end-jejunostomy.

sorption of macronutrients, micronutrients, electrolytes,
and water.[4] The degree of malabsorption is determined by
the length of the remnant intestine; the specific portions
of small and large intestine resected, along with their site-
specific transport processes and endocrine cells; and the
adequacy of adaptive processes in the residual intestine
over time. Three types of intestinal resections typically
are encountered: limited ileal resection for Crohn's
disease, often with cecectomy or right hemicolectomy;
extensive ileal resection with or without partial colectomy and with jejunocolonic anastomosis; and extensive
small intestinal resection and total colectomy resulting in
proximal jejunostomy (Fig. 100–1). Patients in the two
latter groups commonly suffer from Crohn's disease or
had mesenteric infarction.

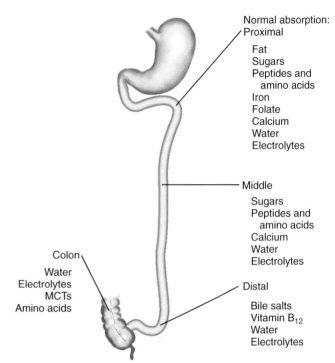

Figure 100–2   Specific areas of absorption of dietary constituents
and secretions in the small intestine and colon. Macronutrients
and micronutrients are absorbed predominantly in the proximal
jejunum. Bile acids and vitamin B_{12} (cobalamin) are absorbed only
in the ileum. Electrolytes and water are absorbed in both the small
and the large intestine. Medium-chain triglycerides (MCTs),
calcium, and some amino acids can be absorbed in the colon.

LOSS OF ABSORPTIVE SURFACE AREA

Nutrient Malabsorption

The length of the small intestine is estimated at 3 to 8
meters, and nutrient absorption is preserved until more
than one half of the small intestine is resected.[5-9] Most
macronutrients (carbohydrates, fat, and nitrogen) are
absorbed in the proximal 100 to 150 cm of intestine.[10]
Specific areas of absorption in the small intestine of nutrients, minerals, vitamins, electrolytes, and trace elements
are discussed in Chapters 96 to 98 and are illustrated
in Figure 100–2. Enterocytes lining the small intestine
appear uniform from the duodenum to the ileocecal
valve, but a distinct proximal-to-distal gradient exists
in both morphology and function.[11] Villi are taller and
crypts are deeper in the jejunum than in the ileum, and
the activity of microvillus enzymes and nutrient absorptive capacity per unit length of intestine are several-fold
higher in the proximal than in the distal small intestine;
loss of part of the jejunum initially will compromise
nutrient absorption more than will loss of an ileal
segment of similar length, because of these morphologic
and functional differences. The ileum, however, eventually is able to compensate for jejunal loss, whereas the
jejunum is unable to compensate for ileal absorption of
bile salts and vitamin B_{12}.

Normal digestion and absorption depend on the
gradual gastric emptying of partially digested nutrients,
mixing of these nutrients with bile and pancreatic

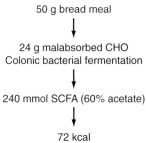

50 g bread meal

↓

24 g malabsorbed CHO
Colonic bacterial fermentation

↓

240 mmol SCFA (60% acetate)

↓

72 kcal

Figure 100–3   Colonic absorption of malabsorbed carbohydrates (CHO) in a hypothetical patient with short bowel syndrome following ingestion of a 50-gram bread meal. Unabsorbed carbohydrates, nonstarch polysaccharides, and soluble fibers are fermented by colonic bacterial flora to hydrogen, methane, carbon dioxide, sulfides, and short-chain fatty acids (SCFAs), including acetate; butyrate, and propionate. By comparison, normal individuals absorb 220-720 mmol SCFA from fermentation of 30-60 g nonstarch polysaccharides.

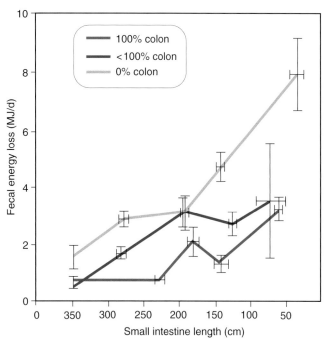

Figure 100–4   The role of the colon as an important digestive organ in patients with short bowel syndrome. Upwards of 1000 kcal (4.2 millijoules [MJ]) per day can be assimilated by means of the metabolism of short-chain fatty acids (SCFAs) synthesized during carbohydrate fermentation; as more of the colon is sacrificed, more energy is lost in the stool.

Table 100–2	Daily Stomal or Fecal Losses of Electrolytes, Minerals, and Trace Elements in Severe Short Bowel Syndrome*	
Sodium	90-100 mEq/L	
Potassium	10-20 mEq/L	
Calcium	772 (591-950) mg/day	
Magnesium	328 (263-419) mg/day	
Iron	11 (7-15) mg/day	
Zinc	12 (10-14) mg/day	
Copper	1.5 (0.5-2.3) mg/day	

*For sodium and potassium, the average concentration per liter of stomal effluent is given. The values for minerals and trace elements are mean 24-hour losses, with the range in parentheses. See text for details.

enzymes in the duodenum, and rapid digestion and absorption of the digestive products in the proximal small intestine. Patients with a proximal jejunostomy have rapid gastric emptying of liquids and rapid intestinal transit, which may compromise the gastric digestive phase, result in inadequate mixing with biliary and pancreatic secretions, insufficient enzymatic digestion, and resultant nutrient maldigestion. Rapid intestinal transit decreases nutrient-enterocyte contact time, and therefore, segmental absorption is decreased. In addition, patients with a high jejunostomy are net secretors of salt and fluid, because jejunal fluid secretion is stimulated by oral intake and subsequent gastric emptying of nutrients—so they excrete more fluid than they ingest.[12] Accordingly, fluid management in these patients may be challenging.

Most patients with a jejunal length of less than 100 cm and no colon will require long-term parenteral nutrition. Preservation of even some colon at surgery is highly beneficial for nutrient absorption. The ileocecal valve acts as a "brake" to slow intestinal transit, thereby increasing nutrient-enterocyte contact time and enhancing absorption. In addition, malabsorbed carbohydrates are fermented by bacterial enzymes in the colon to short-chain fatty acids (SCFAs), which are readily absorbed and utilized by colonocytes (Fig. 100–3). It has been estimated that this intracolonic digestive process can generate up to 1000 kcal (4.2 megajoules [MJ]) per day; in energy supply (Fig. 100–4), 1.0 megajoule (MJ) equals 238.8 kcal[13-15]; small intestine should be anastomosed to colon as soon as the patient is stable.

Water and Electrolyte Malabsorption

Loss of intestinal absorptive surface area may result in significant stomal or fecal losses of electrolytes and water (Table 100–2). The proximal small bowel receives approximately 7 to 9 L daily of water and electrolytes from food and secretions, of which 6 to 8 L is reabsorbed in the small intestine (see Chapter 96). On unrestricted diets, patients with a proximal jejunostomy cannot reabsorb such large volumes; as a consequence, voluminous diarrhea develops, often complicated by hypovolemia, hyponatremia, and hypokalemia. For example, in one study,[12] the diarrheal volume in six jejunostomy patients with a mean jejunal length of 50 cm ranged from 3.2 to 8.3 L/day when they were allowed free access to food and water. All six patients were in negative sodium and water balance, four of the six were in negative potassium balance, and all six required parenteral nutrition with electrolyte replacement and restriction of oral intake of food and water to avoid unacceptable stomal losses. Seven of nine other jejunostomy patients in the same study[12] who had a mean jejunal length of 120 cm were able to maintain positive water and sodium balance under the same conditions. The absorption of water, sodium, and potassium in these 15 jejunostomy patients was correlated with jejunal length. At least 100 cm of intact jejunum is required to maintain positive water and electrolyte balance, similar to the length of jejunum required for nutrient absorption.

In general, patients with a proximal jejunostomy lose 90 to 100 mEq sodium and 10 to 20 mEq potassium/L of stomal effluent[16] (see Table 100–2). Some of these patients will require long-term parenteral electrolyte and water supplements, often administered overnight, whereas others can maintain a positive balance by sipping a glucose-saline oral rehydration solution (ORS) throughout the day. The tight junctions of the jejunum are relatively leaky compared with tight junctions of the ileum and colon; therefore, a high sodium chloride concentration (greater than 90 mmol/L) is required in the glucose-saline solution to achieve net sodium and water absorption.[17,18] Actively absorbed solutes promote intestinal ion transport. Solutes also may be absorbed passively by means of solvent drag once active electrogenic sodium absorption occurs. Water transport into the enterocyte is directly proportional to Na^+ transport. Na^+ also is absorbed by means of an active electrogenic mechanism coupled with Cl^- and H^+ exchange and solvent drag. Absorptive and secretory processes occur simultaneously. Active Na^+ secretion occurs against a concentration gradient from the enterocyte by means of the sodium pump, activated by Na^+,K^+-adenosine triphosphatase in the basolateral membrane (Fig. 100–5). A mixture of 90 to 120 mmol/L sodium chloride and 50 mmol/L glucose is recommended, although such a solution may not be palatable. This mixture takes advantage of the coupled active transport of sodium with glucose and amino acids in the jejunum (see Chapter 96). Electrolyte and water absorption continue in the colon, and in normal humans only 100 to 150 mL of water is lost in the stool each day. The colon has a large reserve absorptive capacity for electrolytes and water, estimated to be 3 to 4 L of isotonic salt solution per day. Preservation of even part of the colon can significantly reduce fecal electrolyte and water losses in patients with SBS. A comparison of two groups of patients with similar jejunal length and jejunum either ending in a jejunostomy or anastomosed to colon showed that patients in the latter group were less likely to require oral or intravenous supplements.[19]

LOSS OF SITE-SPECIFIC TRANSPORT PROCESSES

Nutrient absorption potentially may take place at any level of the small intestine, albeit at different rates, owing to the proximal-to-distal gradient in functional activity of microvillus enzymes and transporters. The absorption of some compounds is restricted to certain areas of the small intestine (see Fig. 100–2); thus, calcium, magnesium, phosphorus, iron, and the water- and fat-soluble vitamins are absorbed predominantly in the duodenum and proximal jejunum (see Chapters 96 and 97). Most patients with SBS have an intact duodenum and a variable length of jejunum, so the development of iron, phosphorus, or water-soluble vitamin deficiency, even in patients with a proximal jejunostomy, is relatively uncommon. Calcium absorption was found to be highly variable in a large study of patients with small intestinal resections.[20] The net absorption of calcium (intake minus fecal loss) ranged from +573 to –268 mg per day, with a median of +65 mg per day; 64% of the patients, however, were in a negative calcium balance (balance = intake – fecal and urinary loss). In a study of 25 patients with a mean jejunal length of 128 cm, large-volume diarrhea (2 to 6 L per day) and steatorrhea,[21] hypocalcemia developed in 13 patients, and hypomagnesemia in 18, during a trial of enteral hyperalimentation despite supplementation with calcium, magnesium, and vitamin D. Malabsorption of calcium and magnesium is a consequence of fat malabsorption, because these minerals are precipitated intraluminally by unabsorbed long-chain fatty acids. Both calcium and magnesium absorption improve on a low-fat diet in patients with small intestinal resections.[22]

The active absorption of vitamin B_{12} and bile acids is restricted to the ileum. The B_{12}–intrinsic factor complexes and bile acids are taken up by specific transport proteins in ileal enterocytes (see Chapters 61 and 97). Most patients with SBS have lost part or all of the ileum, as a result of which vitamin B_{12} and bile acid malabsorption develops. The degree of malabsorption depends on the length of resected ileum. Vitamin B_{12} malabsorption usually is demonstrable when more than 60 cm of ileum has been resected.[4] Resection of less than 100 cm of ileum causes moderate bile acid malabsorption and increased bile acid loss to the colon or in stomal effluents.[23] The increased loss of bile acids to the colon induces electrolyte and water secretion and may exacerbate diarrhea. More extensive ileal resections (of greater than 100 cm) cause severe bile acid malabsorption, which, if bile acid

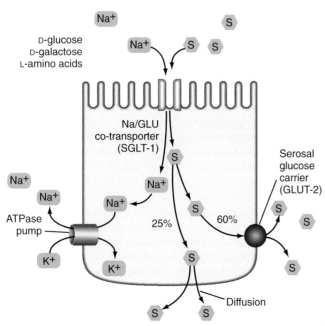

Figure 100–5 Mechanism of solute-coupled Na^+ cotransport. Sodium contained in oral rehydration solutions replaces diarrhea-associated Na^+ losses and promotes water absorption by means of solvent drag. This schematic diagram illustrates the active, Na^+-coupled cotransport of solute into the jejunal enterocyte, where the solute may be glucose (GLU), glucose polymers, galactose, oligopeptides, or L-amino acids. S, solute.

loss exceeds hepatic synthesis, may result in a reduced bile acid pool size, with insufficient micellar solubilization of lipolytic products. Following extensive ileal resection, fat malabsorption develops, as may fat-soluble vitamin deficiency; essential fatty acid (linoleic) deficiency is rare. Loss of unabsorbed long-chain fatty acids to the colon may exacerbate diarrhea if the fatty acids are hydroxylated by colonic bacteria, because hydroxylated fatty acids stimulate colonic electrolyte and water secretion.[24]

LOSS OF SITE-SPECIFIC ENDOCRINE CELLS AND GASTROINTESTINAL HORMONES

The synthesis of gastrointestinal hormones in the intestinal mucosa is distributed in a site-specific manner along the gastrointestinal tract (see Chapter 1). Gastrin, cholecystokinin (CCK), secretin, gastric inhibitory polypeptide, and motilin are produced by endocrine cells in the proximal gastrointestinal tract and regulate secretory processes and motility. The area within which these hormones are synthesized is usually intact in patients with SBS, and hormonal profiles are normal. In approximately 50% of patients with extensive intestinal resections, however, hypergastrinemia and increased gastric acid secretion temporarily develop in the early postoperative phase.[25,26] The cause of this postoperative hypergastrinemia is not known but could be loss of inhibitory signals, because it resolves spontaneously. Glucagon-like peptides 1 and 2 (GLP-1 and GLP-2), neurotensin, and peptide YY (PYY) are produced in the ileum and proximal colon, and these intestinal segments are frequently lost in SBS patients.[27] GLP-1 and GLP-2 and PYY are released by intraluminal fat and carbohydrates, cause a delay in gastric emptying, and slow intestinal transit (the ileal "brake").[28,29] Jejunostomy patients demonstrate impaired release of these hormones in response to a meal, rapid gastric emptying, and rapid intestinal transit of liquids.[30,31] Patients with SBS and preserved colon have increased GLP-1 and GLP-2 concentrations and demonstrate normal gastric emptying[32]; of note, these three hormones also have been shown to inhibit gastric acid secretion and to promote intestinal growth in animal models.

LOSS OF THE ILEOCECAL VALVE

The primary functions of the ileocecal valve are to separate ileal and colonic contents, thereby minimizing bacterial colonization of the small intestine, and to regulate emptying of ileal contents into the colon. The ileocecal valve is removed in most ileal resections, as a consequence of which intestinal transit time decreases, with a risk of bacterial overgrowth if the ileum is anastomosed to the colon. Bacterial overgrowth may worsen nutrient and cobalamin malabsorption (see Chapters 97 and 99), because bacteria compete with the enterocyte for nutrient assimilation. Rapid intestinal transit in these patients, however, may counteract the risk of bacterial colonization. Studies to document the role of bacterial overgrowth in malabsorption in patients with SBS are lacking.

INTESTINAL ADAPTATION TO RESECTION

Adaptive changes in the remaining intestine after intestinal resection have been studied extensively in animal models and to a limited extent in humans[33,34]; adaptive changes are more pronounced in the ileum than in the jejunum. After jejunectomy and duodenoileal anastomosis, the ileum attains the morphologic characteristics of the jejunum, with taller villi and deeper crypts[35]; with time, an increase in ileal diameter and length also occurs. A prospective study of seven patients with jejunoileal bypass operation (20 cm of jejunum anastomosed to 25 cm of ileum) showed an increase in jejunal (80%) and ileal (128%) length and diameter (40% and 50%, respectively, for jejunum and ileum) after 18 months of observation.[36] An increase in absorptive capacity was demonstrated in another study of 41 patients with SBS (mean jejunal length, 119 cm) in whom the mean stool volume decreased from 2.5 to 0.9 L per day over a period of 3 months with continuous oral intake[37]; patients gained weight, and nitrogen balance increased from +3.2 g in the first month to +7.8 g in the second month. The same study also demonstrated a gradual increase in intestinal transit time, which was most pronounced for ileal transit. The result of all of these changes is an increase in absorptive surface area, with an increase in microvillus enzyme activity and absorptive capacity per unit length.[38] An improvement in mineral absorption with time also has been observed in a series of 30 patients with SBS (mean jejunal length, 81 cm) in whom fractional calcium absorption was correlated with time after surgery.[39] In humans, these adaptive changes may take 1 to 2 years to develop fully. The younger the patient, the more profound the adaptive response. Adaptive changes depend on the presence of food and biliary and pancreatic secretions in the intestinal lumen,[40] and adaptive hyperplasia of the ileum failed to develop in jejunectomized animals fed only by parenteral alimentation.[41] To induce these adaptive processes, patients with SBS are encouraged to start oral intake as early as possible in the postoperative phase. Patients with SBS whose colon is in continuity demonstrate qualitative and quantitative changes in colonic flora that result in an increased capacity to metabolize carbohydrate and in an increased fecal bacterial mass.[42]

Adaptive hyperplasia is the result of an increase in crypt cell production rate, presumably mediated by growth factors released by the presence of food and secretions in the intestinal lumen. Vascular endothelial growth factor (VEGF), CCK, gastrin, insulin, neurotensin, GLP-2, and L-glutamine have been shown to stimulate intestinal growth in experimental animals,[43-45] although studies in humans have not indicated any value of supplemental glutamine to enhance intestinal adaptation.[46,47] These extracellular growth factors stimulate polyamine synthesis in crypt cells, which in turn induces increased DNA synthesis and mitotic activity.[48] Inhibition of polyamine synthesis in jejunectomized animals prevents adaptive changes in the ileum.[49] Elucidation of the mediators regulating enterocyte proliferation eventually may lead to development of pharmacologic interventions that can accelerate intestinal adaptation in patients with SBS. The presence of comorbid conditions and the health of the residual bowel and its blood flow are important factors in the prognosis for patients who have undergone massive enterectomy.

MEDICAL MANAGEMENT

The initial management of the patient with SBS involves primarily supportive care designed to enhance the potential for survival. This care includes achievement of hemodynamic stability and appropriate fluid and electrolyte management. In the immediate postoperative phase, most patients with extensive intestinal resections are kept fasting and are supported with TPN, with careful monitoring of weight and volume status and measurement of stomal, fecal, and urinary losses of water, sodium, and potassium, to ensure optimal electrolyte and water balance. Histamine H_2 receptor blockers or proton pump inhibitors are given intravenously to suppress gastric acid hypersecretion from hypergastrinemia and to limit volume losses.[50,51] Patients with jejunostomies have stomal effluents up to several liters per day in this early phase, with obligatory losses of sodium, potassium, and possibly magnesium. Enteral tube feeding, followed by oral feeding, is begun in the late postoperative phase once the patient is hemodynamically stable, adequate intestinal blood flow has been restored, and postoperative ileus has resolved. Patients with extensive resections are kept fasting up to 5 to 10 days to allow for a second-look operation at 24 to 48 hours, and for the healing of enteric anastomoses, and to assess basal losses of water and electrolytes.

LIMITED ILEAL RESECTION

Patients with limited ileal resection (of less than 100 cm), with or without right hemicolectomy, can resume intake of solid food in the late postoperative phase. The response to solid food is determined mainly by the length of ileum removed and whether or not the right colon was resected. These patients may develop diarrhea or steatorrhea with consumption of a regular diet. Secretory diarrhea without steatorrhea is the typical finding in limited ileal resections. Treatment with a bile acid–binding resin, such as cholestyramine or colestipol, in a dose of 2 to 4 g taken with meals, often will ameliorate diarrhea if bile acid malabsorption is the main cause. Colestipol often is better tolerated than is cholestyramine. The diarrhea of some patients with limited ileal resection and right hemicolectomy does not respond to cholestyramine or colestipol despite documented bile acid malabsorption and presumably is due to loss of intestinal absorptive capacity for sodium chloride.[52] Patients with documented fat malabsorption on a regular diet may have less severe steatorrhea while on a low-fat (40 g), high-carbohydrate diet; however, oral energy intake also will be reduced, because fat is calorically dense (9 kcal/g). Patients maintained on such a diet experience a decrease in diarrhea and steatorrhea and improve their net absorption of calcium, magnesium, and zinc.[4] If necessary, medium-chain triglycerides (MCTs), which do not require micellar solubilization, can be added as a fat calorie source.

The possibility of vitamin B_{12} malabsorption should be assessed with a Schilling test, and if this is documented, parenteral B_{12}, usually in a dose of 1 mg intramuscularly monthly, will be required for life.

Malabsorption of fat-soluble vitamins, calcium and magnesium is a risk in patients with fat malabsorption. Fourteen of 27 patients with ileal resections of 50 to 150 cm and an intact colon were in negative calcium balance when studied on a fixed daily calcium intake of 800 mg supplemented with 400 to 800 IU of vitamin D daily.[21] Supplementation with vitamins, calcium, and possibly magnesium should be initiated before overt signs of vitamin deficiency or hypocalcemia and hypomagnesemia develop. Magnesium supplementation by mouth may be unrewarding, because magnesium is a cathartic. Although magnesium gluconate is water soluble and therefore may be the most readily absorbed magnesium salt, some patients still may require periodic parenteral replacement, despite the need for TPN or intravenous fluids. Magnesium deficiency may occur despite a normal serum concentration, because most Mg^{2+} is present in the intracellular space. Therefore, measurement of 24-hour urine Mg^{2+} concentration is prudent in subjects with suspected magnesium deficiency, but normal serum Mg^{2+} concentration. Magnesium deficiency may result in calcium deficiency, because the release of parathyroid hormone is impaired in the presence of hypomagnesemia.[53]

Most patients with SBS already are in a negative calcium balance[54]; therefore, an oral supplement of calcium at a daily dose of 800 to 1500 mg is recommended. The tests to assess vitamin and mineral balance and recommended dosages in malabsorption are discussed in Chapters 96 and 97. Absorption of water-soluble vitamins, carbohydrates, and proteins is, in general, not compromised in patients with limited ileal resections.

EXTENSIVE SMALL INTESTINAL RESECTION AND PARTIAL COLECTOMY

Fluid and Electrolyte Management

Massive enterectomy is associated with gastric hypersecretion for the initial 6 months or so postoperatively. These patients will benefit from the use of intravenous H_2 antagonists or oral or intravenous proton pump inhibitors; absorption of orally ingested medications may be impaired, and more than the usual doses may be required (Table 100–3). Rapid intestinal transit contributes to malabsorption and diarrhea, and use of antidiarrheal drugs is common (see Table 100–3). These medications should be taken 1 hour before meals, and their effect on diarrheal volume should be evaluated before they are recommended for long-term treatment. Use of antimotility agents is important to control fluid losses; such agents include loperamide hydrochloride and diphenoxylate (4 to 16 mg per day), codeine (30 to 180 mg per day), tincture of opium, and the somatostatin analog octreotide (50 to 100 mg three times a day) (see Table 100–3). Most studies have shown these agents to reduce stoma output by up to 50%, but a positive water

Table 100–3 Therapeutic Agents Used to Decrease Intestinal Transit and Diarrheal Volume

Agent	Dosage
Loperamide*	4-6 mg four times daily
Diphenoxylate/atropine*	2.5-5 mg four times daily
Codeine phosphate*	15 mg two-to-four times daily
Ranitidine†	300 mg twice daily
Omeprazole‡	40 mg twice daily
Octreotide	50-100 µg SC twice daily

*The antidiarrheal agents loperamide, diphenoxylate/atropine, and codeine are given 1 hour before meals and at bedtime. Dosages may be increased over those recommended, because of incomplete absorption in patients with short bowel syndrome.
†Cimetidine, famotidine, and nizatidine in appropriate doses are alternatives.
‡Esomeprazole, lansoprazole, rabeprazole, and pantoprazole are alternatives.
SC, subcutaneously.

Table 100–4 Macronutrient Requirements in Patients with a Short Bowel Syndrome

	Colon Present	Colon Absent
Carbohydrate	Complex carbohydrate 30-35 kcal/kg per day Soluble fiber	Variable types 30-35 kcal/kg per day
Fat	MCT/LCT 20%-30% of caloric intake ± Low fat/high fat	LCT 20%-30% of caloric intake ± Low fat/high fat
Protein	Intact protein 1.0-1.5 g/kg per day ± Peptide-based formula	Intact protein 1.0-1.5 g/kg per day ± Peptide-based formula

LCT, long-chain triglycerides; MCT, medium-chain triglycerides.

and electrolyte balance rarely is achieved. Octreotide usually is not necessary except for some patients with a proximal jejunostomy. Octreotide may slow intestinal transit and increase sodium and water absorption,[55-58] but it also decreases splanchnic protein synthesis, thereby inhibiting postresectional intestinal adaptation[57]; the risk of cholelithiasis also is increased with octreotide.[58]

Glucose polymer–based ORSs should be provided to patients to improve hydration and thereby reduce TPN requirements. Glucose and sodium are absorbed through the same active transport mechanism and stimulate absorption of each other. In addition, glucose promotes sodium and water absorption by means of solvent drag[59] (see Fig. 100–5). Therefore, because the jejunum is permeable to both sodium and chloride, passively absorbed solutions that have a high sodium chloride concentration are absorbed to a significant degree; sodium is not as readily absorbed from isotonic or hypotonic solutions. A simple solution developed by the World Health Organization (WHO) can be formulated by dissolving 2.5 g of table salt, 1.5 g of KCl (requires a prescription), 2.5 g of sodium bicarbonate ($NaHCO_3$), and 1.5 g of table sugar (sucrose) in 1 L of water. This solution will provide a sodium concentration of approximately 90 mmol/L. Additional salt may be added to increase the osmolarity as tolerated, to 100 to 120 mmol/L or more, which may be more effective.[60] Sodium losses actually increase when solutions containing less sodium than is in the small bowel effluent (90 mmol/L) are consumed. The use of ORS is not as critical in patients in whom the colon is intact, provided that sufficient dietary sodium is present, because of the colon's ability to absorb sodium and water. For patients who have had significant jejunal resections, the addition of glucose to the ORS is not critical, because glucose does not enhance ileal water absorption.[61] In addition to sodium losses, significant quantities of bicarbonate and magnesium are lost in feces.

Dietary Management

Special Diets

Patients with SBS should be encouraged to eat substantially more than usual (a "hyperphagia" diet) to compensate for malabsorption; they may need to consume two to three times as much energy as that normally ingested before their abdominal catastrophe. This may be the single most important dietary intervention to reduce parenteral nutrition requirements. It has been suggested that patients may counterbalance the discomfort associated with increased fecal volume by the satisfaction of recovering relatively normal eating habits and requiring less parenteral nutrition.[21] Patients also should be encouraged to eat small portions throughout the day, rather than at defined meal times. Separation of liquid and solid portions of meals is impractical and not associated with decreased fecal wet weight loss.

Patients with SBS whose colon is in continuity should be provided a high–complex carbohydrate diet that includes starch, nonstarch polysaccharides, and soluble fiber (Table 100–4). These foodstuffs typically are not absorbed by the human small intestine[62]; however, when they pass undigested into the colon, colonic bacteria will ferment these foodstuffs into SCFAs such as butyrate, acetate, and propionate. Approximately 75 mmol of SCFAs are produced from 10 g of unabsorbed carbohydrate (see Fig. 100–3). Butyrate is the preferred fuel for the colonocyte.[63] A patient with an intact colon may absorb up to 310 to 740 kcal (1.3 to 3.1 megajoules [MJ]) daily when fed a 60% carbohydrate diet.[15] Other studies have indicated that up to 525 to 1170 kcal (2.2 to 4.9 MJ) daily can be absorbed by an intact colon from fermentation of unabsorbed carbohydrate and soluble fiber.[13] The amount of energy absorbed is proportional to the amount of residual colon[15,19] (see Fig. 100–4) and may increase as part of the adaptive response to enterectomy.[43,64] During this adaptive period, colonic bacteria increase and β-galactosidase and other enzymes appear to increase in concentration or activity.[42] Sodium and water absorption are stimulated by SCFAs as well, although decreased fecal fluid and sodium losses have not been documented clinically.[15]

When greater than 100 cm of terminal ileum has been resected, fat maldigestion may develop, because bile salt malabsorption leads to decreased micelle formation, which results in poor fat solubilization. Use of bile salt replacement therapy with ox bile or a synthetic conjugated bile acid (cholylsarcosine) has been reported only in a few patients,[65,66] decreasing fecal fat in most, but leaving fecal volume either unchanged or increased. The bile acid–sequestering agent cholestyramine may be useful in decreasing bile salt–related diarrhea in patients with less than 100 cm of terminal ileum resected but may worsen steatorrhea in those patients who have undergone a more significant resection, because of its binding to dietary lipid[67]; fat-soluble vitamin deficiency also may develop. In addition, cholestyramine binds to many medications, including warfarin, antibiotics, beta blockers, diuretics, oral hypoglycemia agents, and others.

Limited data are available to support the use of low-fat diets in patients with massive enterectomy,[68] although fat restriction often does lead to decreased steatorrhea in patients with limited terminal ileal resections. Because fat is energy concentrated (9 kcal/g), however, dietary fat restriction results in decreased energy intake and may worsen the patient's energy balance; a low-fat diet also may be unpalatable. A high-fat diet, although having greater energy content than that of a high-carbohydrate diet, is associated with increased loss of divalent cations (Ca^{2+}, Mg^{2+}, and Zn^{2+}),[69] will slow gastric emptying, and may induce early satiety, leading to reduced total energy intake. Diets high in fat also may lead to water secretion from the colon.

Because MCTs (C8 to C10, 8.3 kcal/g) are absorbed in the colon, dietary supplementation with MCTs may lead to increased energy absorption.[70] MCT supplementation is of much more limited benefit in patients with an end-jejunostomy. MCTs also do not supply essential fatty acids, and excessive intake is associated with nausea, vomiting, and ketosis.

Experience with long-term parenteral nutrition mainly has been gained in patients with severe SBS (see Chapter 16). Despite the limited adaptive capacity of the jejunum, approximately 50% of patients on a home parenteral nutrition regimen can discontinue TPN and resume oral intake after 1 to 2 years.[71] The diet composition for patients with a jejunostomy on oral intake can be more liberal, because the percentages of energy absorption are similar for a low-fat, high-carbohydrate and a high-fat, low-carbohydrate diet.[72,73] The average daily stomal losses of electrolytes, minerals, and trace elements in severe SBS are listed in Table 100-2.[22,69,72,74,75]

Water-soluble vitamins, except for vitamin B_{12}, are absorbed in the proximal jejunum, as are macronutrients. It is unusual for deficiencies of these vitamins to develop, except in patients with a proximal jejunostomy or duodenostomy; these patients invariably will require TPN with vitamin supplementation. Loss of the ileum results in bile acid and vitamin B_{12} malabsorption, but these patients and those with extensive jejunal resection also are at risk for more pronounced nutrient, mineral, vitamin, and electrolyte and water malabsorption than is seen in patients with limited ileal resection, because of the greater loss of absorptive surface area and rapid intestinal transit. Fat-soluble vitamin (A, D, E, K) deficiency is much more commonly encountered as a result of concurrent fat malabsorption than as a result of loss of absorptive surface area. Most of the human vitamin K requirement is synthesized by colonic bacterial flora,[76] so patients with any residual colon are a lower risk for development of vitamin K deficiency than are those whose colon has been resected; patients who have received broad-spectrum antibiotics also are at risk for vitamin K deficiency. Zinc and selenium are lost in significant concentrations in the feces. The concentration of zinc is 12 mg/L in the small bowel effluent and 16 mg/L in the stool.[77] Oral vitamin, mineral, and trace element supplementation generally is required for patients who do not require TPN (Table 100–5).

Medication malabsorption also occurs in patients with SBS.[78,79] Many medications are absorbed in the jejunum, but medication malabsorption still may occur in patients who have undergone ileal resections alone, because of decreased intestinal transit time.

The loss of the ileocecal valve increases the risk of bacterial overgrowth in the small intestine, which may worsen nutrient absorption and make management more difficult. The ultimate goal is to ensure a stable condition in which all nutritional needs are met, preferably by oral intake alone. In a series of 38 patients with a jejunal length less than 200 cm and in continuity with the colon, all persons with a jejunal length of more than 100 cm could be managed on oral intake alone.[19]

In the late postoperative phase, the liquid diet is replaced by solid food, and the absorptive capacity of the remaining intestine is assessed again by measurement of fecal fat, volume, weight, and electrolytes while the patient is on a known nutrient and liquid intake. Fat absorption is, in general, more compromised than are nitrogen and carbohydrate absorption in these patients. The optimal diet composition for patients with SBS has been debated, but a low-fat, high-carbohydrate diet is of documented advantage in patients whose colon is in continuity with the remaining small intestine.

Nitrogen is the least affected macronutrient in SBS. Because absorption of dietary protein in the form of di- and tripeptides occurs in the very proximal bowel, only patients with short segments of residual jejunum may benefit from the use of hydrolyzed protein or free amino

Table 100–5	Vitamin and Mineral Requirements* in Patients with a Short Bowel Syndrome
Vitamin A	10,000-50,000 units daily*
Vitamin B_{12}	1000 µg SC monthly for patients with terminal ileal resection or disease
Vitamin C	200 mg daily
Vitamin D	1600 units daily as 25 (OH_2)- or 1,25(OH_2)-D_3
Vitamin E	30 IU daily
Vitamin K	10 mg weekly
Calcium	1000-1500 mg daily
Magnesium	See text
Iron	As needed
Selenium	60-150 µg daily
Zinc	220-440 mg daily (sulfate or gluconate form)
Bicarbonate	As needed

Note: The table lists rough guidelines only. Vitamin and mineral supplementation must be monitored routinely and tailored to the individual patient, because relative absorption and requirements may vary. Supplements may be taken orally unless otherwise indicated.
*Use cautiously in patients with cholestatic liver disease, because of the potential for liver toxicity.

acid–based enteral formulas. McIntyre and colleagues compared energy, nitrogen, and fat absorption in a group of seven patients with an end-jejunostomy when they were provided with either a polymeric formula or a peptide-based formula. The length of residual jejunum in these patients ranged between 6 and 150 cm. No differences in nutrient absorption were observed.[72] Similar uncontrolled observations were reported by Levy and coworkers.[80] Contrary to these results, however, were those of Cosnes and associates, who reported modest improvement in patients with end-jejunostomy (mean residual small bowel length 90 to 150 cm) in six patients who received a peptide-based diet, although energy absorption was unaffected.[81] The patient populations in these studies were somewhat heterogeneous, and the peptide chain length and relative concentrations varied between formulas, making it difficult to compare the two studies.

Dietary Restrictions

Lactose malabsorption due to substantial loss of jejunal length may worsen diarrhea, but a study of 14 patients with SBS on either a lactose-free diet or a diet with 20 g of lactose per day showed no significant differences in stool volumes.[82] Patients with SBS whose colon is in continuity should receive an oxalate-restricted diet (see "Calcium Oxalate Kidney Stones" under "Complications") (Table 100–6).

HOME PARENTERAL NUTRITION

For the patient who requires long-term TPN, infusions typically are given on a continuous basis in the hospital until postoperative recovery has progressed and fluid and other metabolic issues have stabilized. Patients should be encouraged to adopt a hyperphagic diet while TPN volume and nutrient support are adjusted, to maintain reasonable weight, fluid status, and nutrient sufficiency. As a patient gains weight or retains additional fluid, TPN fluid volume and nutrient composition can be decreased. It is important not to suppress the hypothalamic hunger center. Even if patients are unable to increase their oral intake significantly, they should still be encouraged to eat, to stimulate normal gallbladder contraction (if the gallbladder is in situ) and to prevent biliary complications (see later on).

To prepare the patient for home TPN, the TPN regimen should be compressed gradually in 2- to 4-hour daily increments so that the total volume can be infused over a 10- to 12-hour period, typically overnight. Occasional patients with hyperglycemia or renal or congestive heart failure may require a more prolonged infusion. The TPN infusion generally is tapered off over a 30- to 60-minute period, to avoid hypoglycemia. Patients with a proximal jejunostomy may require additional fluid before or following completion of home TPN and, in some cases, during the day as well. Because TPN solutions are hypertonic, they must be infused into a central vein, such as the superior or inferior vena cava, through a tunneled catheter, to decrease the risks of infection and thrombosis.[83,84] Percutaneously inserted central catheters (PICCs) should be reserved for short-term use (less than 6

months). For the patient to qualify for Medicare benefits, home TPN must be required for at least 3 months, and failed enteral nutritional support and fat malabsorption must be documented.

The patient should be instructed properly about the indications for TPN, appropriate catheter care and dressing changes, the pump, preparation of TPN solutions, and acute complications of TPN, including air embolism, hypoglycemia, and catheter-related infection. Instruction on self-glucose monitoring also should be included if hyperglycemia has been a problem or if insulin is required. The patient will need to add multivitamins, insulin, and possibly other additives to the TPN solution each night, because these other medications are not sufficiently stable to be added by the home TPN pharmacy. TPN solution typically is delivered in 1- to 2-week batches, so the patient will need a refrigerator dedicated for TPN.

The patient's home environment should be assessed. An appropriate location for setting up the TPN infusion and storing supplies, catheter cleaning, and hookup should be identified. This should not be a "contaminated" area such as a bathroom or kitchen.

Patients often find it helpful to contact a local support group of the Oley Foundation (1-800-776-OLEY or www.oley.org). This independent, nonprofit organization includes patients and their families, as well as health care providers, and provides information, outreach services, emotional support, and conference activities. Physicians caring for patients on a home TPN regimen also should be familiar with TPN- and catheter-related complications and their recognition and treatment. These topics are beyond the scope of this chapter but have been reviewed in Chapter 16 and elsewhere[85,86] (Figs. 100–6 and 100–7).

Patients in whom the frequency of TPN infusions can be reduced to fewer than 5 nights per week should have their micronutrient status monitored two to three times yearly to detect deficiencies. At the clinical visit, particular attention should be paid to the catheter exit site for evidence of erythema, purulent discharge, warmth, or tenderness. A catheter may remain in place indefinitely if properly maintained.[87]

COMPLICATIONS

GALLSTONES

Interruption of the enterohepatic circulation of bile acids by ileal resection results in decreased hepatic bile acid secretion and altered composition of hepatic bile in terms of its organic components: bile acid, cholesterol, and phospholipids (see Chapters 61 and 69). Hepatic bile becomes supersaturated with cholesterol, with subsequent formation of cholesterol crystals and gallstones in gallbladder bile (see Chapter 62). Most gallstones in patients with SBS, however, are composed of calcium bilirubinate; the pathophysiology is unclear. A prevalence of 44% of asymptomatic gallstones was documented in a study of 84 patients with severe SBS who required TPN.[19] Formation of biliary sludge and gallbladder hypomotility probably contribute to the high prevalence, because many of these patients are on long-term parenteral nutri-

Table 100–6   Dietary Recommendations for Patients Requiring an Oxalate-Restricted Diet

Food Group	Foods Classified by Oxalate Content		
	Little or None (<3 mg/serving) Eat as desired	Moderate (2-10 mg/serving) Limit: two 1/2-cup servings/day	High (>10 mg/serving) Avoid completely
Beverages	Apple or pineapple juice	Cranberry juice (4 oz.)	Draft beer
	Bottled beer	Grape juice (4 oz.)	Juices containing berries
	Colas (12 oz. limit/day)	Nescafe powder	Tea
	Distilled alcohol		Cocoa
	Orange juice (4 oz.)		Lemonade or limeade
	Wine, red, rosé		Tomato juice
	Tap water		
	Milk, yogurt		
	Coffee		
Meats, Fish	Lean lamb, beef, pork	Sardines	
	Poultry		
	Seafood		
Fruits/Vegetables	Asparagus	Broccoli	Beans
	Avocado	Cauliflower	Beets
	Brussels sprouts	Cucumber	Carrots
	Cauliflower	Green peas	Celery
	Cabbage	Lettuce	Swiss chard
	Mushrooms	Lima beans	Chives
	Onions	Tomato, 1 small	Collards
	Potatoes	Turnips	Dandelion greens
	Radishes	Eggplant	Endive
	Sweet corn	Apples	Escarole
	Bananas	Apricots	French fries
	Cherries, Bing	Black currants	Kale
	Grapefruit	Cherries, red sour	Leeks
	Grapes, white	Fruit cocktail	Okra
	Mangos	Orange	Berries
	Melons	Peaches	Concord grapes
	Nectarines	Plums, red	Red currants
	Pears	Prunes	Parsnips
	Pineapple	Squash	Sweet potato
	Plums, green/golden	Vegetable soup	Tangerines
Breads, pasta, cereal	Macaroni	Cornflakes	Grits, white corn
	Noodles	Sponge cake	Soybean crackers
	Oatmeal	Spaghetti, canned in tomato	Wheat germ
	Rice	sauce	Bran cereal
	Spaghetti		
	White bread		
Miscellaneous	Eggs	Chicken noodle soup, dehydrated	Peanut butter
	Cheese, cheddar		Soybean curd (tofu)
	Mayonnaise		Nuts
	Salad dressing	Fruitcake	Pretzels
	Vegetable oils		Chocolate
	Jelly or preserves (made with allowed fruits)		Pepper (>1 tsp/day)
	Butter		
	Soups made with allowed ingredients		
	Sugar		

For low-oxalate diet, restrict to 40-50 mg daily.

tion.[88] Postprandial CCK concentration is decreased in some patients with SBS,[89] and injections of CCK have been used experimentally to induce gallbladder contraction; this therapy is not always successful and results in nausea, vomiting, and abdominal pain in some patients.[90,91]

LIVER DISEASE

Liver disease often develops in patients who require long-term TPN. After 5 years of TPN, greater than 50% of these patients will be found to have severe liver disease defined as grade 2 fibrosis, cirrhosis, or one of the following: total serum bilirubin greater than 3.5 mg/dL for longer than 1 month, ascites, portal hypertension, hepatic encephalopathy, or liver failure with a factor V concentration less than 50% of normal.[92] Liver failure will develop in approximately 15% of all TPN-dependent patients.[93] The incidence, prevalence, and severity of liver disease in young children and infants, in particular, are much greater than in adults.[94] The incidence and prevalence of liver disease and liver failure in patients with SBS requiring TPN are unknown. Although these disorders

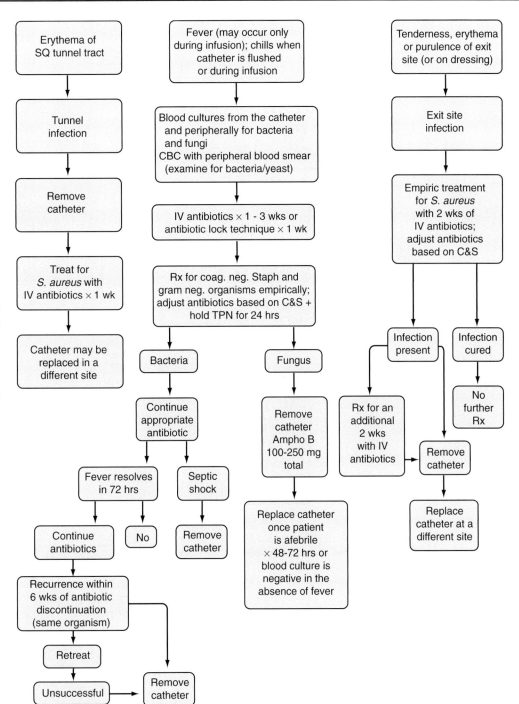

Figure 100–6 Algorithm for the diagnosis and management of catheter-related infection. ampho B, amphotericin B; coag.-neg., coagulase-negative; CBC, complete blood count; C&S, culture and sensitivity testing; Rx, treatment; SC, subcutaneous; TPN, total parenteral nutrition.

often are referred to as "TPN-associated liver disease," in reality, the pathogenesis probably is related to malabsorption of nutrients such as choline[95] and to the route of nutrient assimilation, namely, through the central axis, rather than the portal circulation.[96] Patients with the least amount of residual intestine are at greatest risk for development of liver disease.[97,98]

Diagnosis of liver disease related to intestinal failure in the patient with SBS requires the exclusion of other potential causative disorders. SBS-related liver disease may manifest as cholestasis, steatosis, or steatohepatitis; cholestasis is more common in infants. Studies have suggested benefit from oral lecithin, although it is poorly absorbed, and from intravenous choline (investigational)

and, to a lesser extent, ursodeoxycholic acid.[98-103] Dextrose overfeeding (greater than 40 kcal/kg per day) and excessive fat emulsion infusion (2.5 g/kg per day, possibly only 1.0 g/kg per day) should be avoided.[92] A minimum of 2% to 4% of total calories, however, should be provided as linoleic fatty acid (50% of most lipid emulsions), to prevent essential fatty acid deficiency. Carnitine supplementation is not useful.[104]

CALCIUM OXALATE KIDNEY STONES

Fat malabsorption secondary to bile acid deficiency in patients with extensive ileal resection is associated with

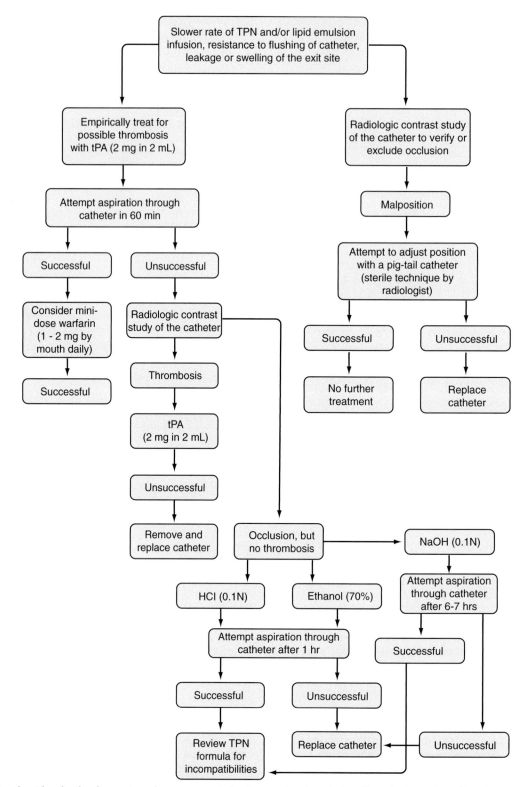

Figure 100–7   Algorithm for the diagnosis and management of catheter-related occlusion (thrombotic and nonthrombotic). HCl, hydrochloric acid; NaOH, sodium hydroxide; tPA, tissue plasminogen activator; TPN, total parenteral nutrition.

an increased risk of oxalate kidney stones if the colon is preserved. Oxalate in food usually precipitates as calcium oxalate in the intestinal lumen and is lost in the stool. Lipolysis in patients with SBS and fat malabsorption is normal, and unabsorbed long-chain fatty acids compete with oxalate for available luminal calcium. Consequently,

a larger amount of free oxalate is lost to the colon, where it is absorbed and ultimately excreted by the kidney (Fig. 100–8), manifesting as just hyperoxaluria or with calcium oxalate stone formation. Patients with SBS who do not have a colon in continuity are not at increased risk. In one study, symptomatic kidney stones developed within

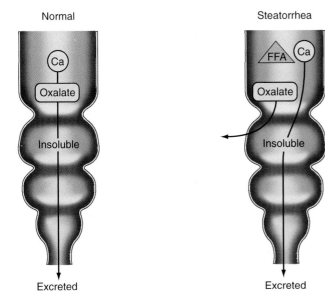

Normal   Steatorrhea

Figure 100–8 Mechanism of oxalate hyperabsorption in patients with steatorrhea. Normally, oxalate in food is precipitated out as calcium oxalate in the intestinal lumen and lost in the stool. Lipolysis in patients with short bowel syndrome with fat malabsorption is normal, and unabsorbed long-chain fatty acids (FFA) compete with oxalate for the available calcium. Consequently, a larger amount of free oxalate is lost to the colon, where it is absorbed and ultimately excreted by the kidney.

2 years of enterectomy in 9 of 38 patients (24%) with SBS and an intact colon.[19] Urinary oxalate excretion should be monitored regularly in these patients. Treatment of hyperoxaluria consists of restriction of oxalate-containing food products (see Table 100–6). If hyperoxaluria persists, then oral administration of calcium citrate should be tried, the extra calcium precipitating dietary oxalate, and the citrate preventing stone growth in the urine. A single case report describes the use of conjugated bile acid supplementation to reduce hyperoxaluria.[105] Hyperoxaluria also may be related to the metabolism of the vitamin C in TPN solution in the presence of light.[106]

D-LACTIC ACIDOSIS

D-Lactic acidosis is a rare complication of SBS and in this setting is observed only in patients with a preserved colon. The episodes of acidosis usually are precipitated by increased oral intake of refined carbohydrates and can be induced in the patient with SBS by carbohydrate overfeeding.[107] Malabsorbed carbohydrate is metabolized by colonic bacteria to SCFAs and lactate, which lower the intracolonic pH. A lower pH inhibits the growth of the predominant *Bacteroides* species and promotes the growth of acid-resistant, gram-positive anaerobes (*Bifidobacterium*, *Lactobacillus*, and *Eubacterium*), which have the capacity to produce D-lactate. D-Lactate is absorbed from the colon and is metabolized to only a limited extent in humans because of the lack of D-lactate dehydrogenase. The main excretory route for D-lactate is the kidney.[108] Absorbed D-lactate results in the development of a metabolic acidosis and characteristic neurologic signs and

symptoms of nystagmus, ophthalmoplegia, ataxia, confusion, and inappropriate behavior. Patients with D-lactate acidosis often are suspected of being inebriated, but their blood alcohol levels are normal. Blood tests will confirm a metabolic acidosis and a normal lactate level; however, the clinical laboratory should be notified that the D-lactic acid rather than the L-lactic acid concentration is requested. The constellation of specific neurologic symptoms and metabolic acidosis in a patient with SBS should raise the suspicion of possible D-lactic acidosis. The diagnosis is confirmed by measurement of wholeblood D-lactate concentration, which will be elevated significantly (to greater than 3 mmol/L, compared with the normal level of less than 0.5 mmol/L).

Treatment consists of correcting the acidosis with sodium bicarbonate and stopping oral intake, which usually results in rapid abatement of the neurologic symptoms. The potential benefit of antibiotic treatment to change the colonic flora is debated. Substitution of refined carbohydrates for starch has prevented recurrent D-lactic acidosis in a few patients.[109] The mediator of the neurologic symptoms still is unknown, and infusion of D-lactic acid in normal subjects to achieve blood levels commonly observed in patients with D-lactic acidosis does not cause any neurologic symptoms. The neurologic symptoms have a striking resemblance to those of Wernicke's encephalopathy, and in one patient with SBS, recurrent D-lactic acidosis was prevented by thiamine supplementation.[110]

OTHER COMPLICATIONS

Renal dysfunction,[111] metabolic bone disease,[112] memory deficits,[113] and neurologic abnormalities[114] all have been described in patients with SBS who require long-term TPN.

SURGICAL MANAGEMENT

INTESTINAL LENGTHENING PROCEDURES

The most important surgical procedure is reanastomosis of the residual small bowel to the residual colon. This procedure carries relatively low mortality and morbidity rates and allows for enhanced energy absorption from SCFAs produced from the bacterial fermentation of unabsorbed carbohydrate. A number of other surgical procedures, such as tapering enteroplasty, construction of intestinal valves, creation of recirculating loops, reversal of a short intestinal segment, or colonic interposition, have been attempted to increase intestinal transit time. These procedures are considered experimental, and the experience with each is limited; outcomes generally are not optimal.[1] Longitudinal intestinal lengthening and tailoring (Bianchi procedure) (Fig. 100–9) may be useful in patients who have segmental dilation and nonfunctional intestine due to dysmotility and bacterial overgrowth. In this procedure, the surgeon divides the dilated bowel and performs an end-to-end anastomosis, thereby doubling the

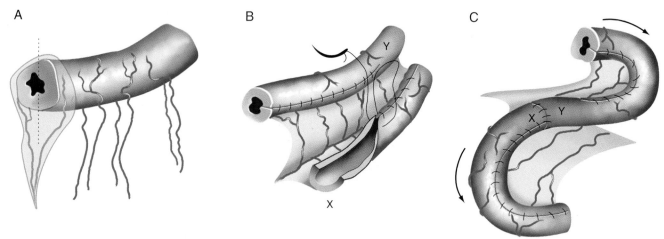

Figure 100–9 The Bianchi procedure for intestinal lengthening depicted in a schematic diagram. *A,* The bowel is split lengthwise; *B,* two hemi-loops are created; *C,* the hemi-loops are anastomosed end to end.

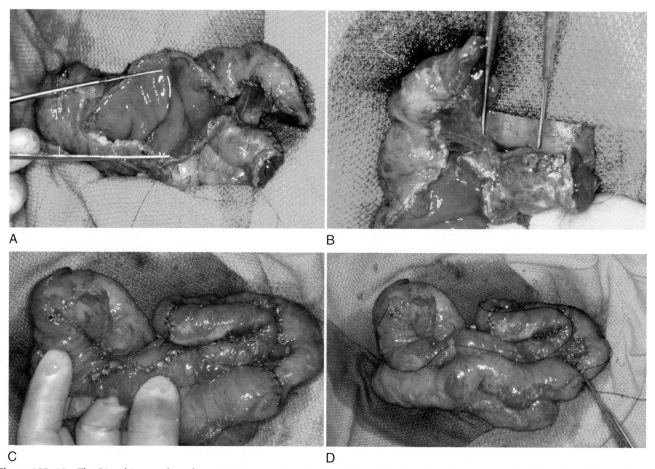

Figure 100–10 The Bianchi procedure shown in intraoperative photographs. *A,* The tips of the forceps are within the dilated loop of intestine, which has been opened; the beginning of each hemi-loop is evident *(right side). B,* A blood vessel can be seen going to the left hemi-loop. *C,* Completed anastomosis. *D,* The suture shows the gain in the length of intestine. The first hemi-loop extends from the tip of the forceps to the first perpendicular suture line. From that point to the end of the thread represents the gain in intestinal length (approximately 26 cm in this infant). (Photographs kindly provided by Kishore R. Iyer, MD, Chicago, IL.)

bowel length[115] (Fig. 100–10). Although the surface area is not truly increased, bowel function may improve, allowing reduction or elimination of TPN. Nearly all of the approximately 100 operations reported have been undertaken in children. This procedure should be attempted only as a last resort before intestinal transplantation, and it should be performed only in centers with significant experience in this area. To date, no studies have been conducted to compare medical and surgical therapies.

INTESTINAL TRANSPLANTATION

Intestinal transplantation is being performed by an increasing number of centers worldwide. The main indication for transplantation in children and adults is TPN-dependent SBS complicated by progressive liver disease. Combined intestine-liver transplantation is the only alternative for patients in whom end-stage liver disease has developed. Isolated intestinal transplantation may be considered for patients with clinically significant liver disease that has not yet progressed to cirrhosis.[116] Patients who have significant fluid losses and who experience frequent episodes of severe dehydration despite appropriate medical management also may be candidates for isolated intestinal transplantation. Medicare has approved other indications, including two-major-vessel thrombosis, a single episode of fungemia, a single episode of bacterial sepsis with shock, and two lifetime episodes of catheter sepsis; the preponderance of evidence, however, does not support these as appropriate indications for transplantation.

Survival has improved considerably since intestinal transplantation was initiated. As of 2001 (most recent data from the International Small Bowel Transplant Registry), 696 transplantation procedures had been performed worldwide in 651 patients, 335 of whom are still alive. This experience included 291 isolated intestine, 310 intestine-liver, and 95 multi-visceral transplants. Patients who have undergone transplantation more recently generally have better survival because of improved technique and optimized immunosuppressive regimens. Mean hospitalization was 59.5 ± 56 days (range, 8 to 431) for isolated intestine, 81.8 ± 79 days (range, 17 to 827) for intestine-liver, and 83.5 ± 56 days (range, 13 to 260) for multi-visceral transplant recipients. Additional information can be found in the International Intestinal Transplant Registry website, http://intestinal-transplant.org, which is updated every 2 years (last time in 2003). Current (2003) patient and graft survival data for the United States are presented in Table 100–7.

The mortality rate for patients waiting for an intestinal-liver transplant is significantly greater than for those waiting for an isolated liver transplant.[1] Therefore, early referral to an intestinal transplantation center at the first sign of liver disease is recommended, even if a transplant does not ultimately become necessary. Intestinal and multiorgan transplantations are expensive and generally cost between $250,000 and $3 million per case. Post-transplantation complications, and the most common causes of death afterward, include acute rejection, chronic rejection, cytomegalovirus infection, sepsis (often complicating rejection), and post-transplantation lymphoproliferative disease (PTLD).[117] Antirejection medications amount to another $10,000 yearly, in addition to repeated hospitalizations for infection and rejection. For those patients who do well, however, nearly all are successfully weaned from TPN, although a few may require some maintenance intravenous fluids. This expense compares with a charge of $100,000 to $150,000 per year for home TPN, in addition to the costs of hospitalization for complications. The actual costs of TPN (including pharmacists' time) however, are closer to $18 to $25 per day. Intestinal transplantation has reached a stage at which it is a feasible, but not yet practical, alternative to conservative treatment of the patient with SBS.

PHARMACOLOGIC ENHANCEMENT OF BOWEL ADAPTATION

The growing knowledge on growth factors has stimulated several clinical studies in patients with SBS. The promising results with the use of growth hormone and dietary L-glutamine in a large uncontrolled study of TPN-dependent patients with SBS[118] raised hopes that intestinal mucosal growth could be enhanced beyond the adaptive period.[6] Two placebo-controlled studies of identical growth hormone and L-glutamine supplementation failed to show any beneficial effect on absorption,[46,47] however, and two other studies showed marginal improvements in fluid and nutrient retention.[119,120]

GLP-2 is intestinotrophic and has been used in a small uncontrolled study of eight patients with SBS, who received GLP-2 400 mg subcutaneously twice a day for 35 days.[121] The treatment resulted in an increase in several absorptive parameters, body weight, and mucosal growth. Use of a synthetic analog of GLP-2 (teduglutide) was associated with increased villus height and increased fluid absorption, with more modest improvements in energy and nitrogen absorption, which regressed once the medication was discontinued.[122] The rapid advance in our knowledge of epithelial growth factors undoubtedly will lead to discovery of still other growth factors that can stimulate intestinal epithelial growth and thus benefit these patients.

A recent double-blinded, randomized, controlled trial of growth hormone (0.1 mg/kg per day for 4 weeks) in 41 TPN-dependent patients showed that TPN requirements in treated patients could be reduced by an additional 2 L per week (or one night weekly) over the reduction with standard therapy described earlier in this chapter.[123] It is unclear whether these effects were related to improved absorption or appetite stimulation. This study led to the FDA approval of growth hormone

| Table 100–7 | Patient and Graft Survival (%) for Isolated Intestine, Combined Intestine/Liver, and Multivisceral Transplants Performed from 1988 to 2004 in the United States |

Transplant Type	1 Year		3 Years		4 Years	
	Patient	Graft	Patient	Graft	Patient	Graft
Isolated intestine n = 351	83.4	78.4	64.7	53.3	58.3	46.2
Intestine/Liver n = 317	60.4	58.2	49.5	47.0	46.4	44.1
Multivisceral n = 253	69.4	65.6	55.7	51.2	54.6	49.4

Based on Organ Procurement and Transplantation Network (http://www.optn.org) data as of November 30, 2005. This work was supported in part by Health Resources and Services Administration contract 231-00-0115.

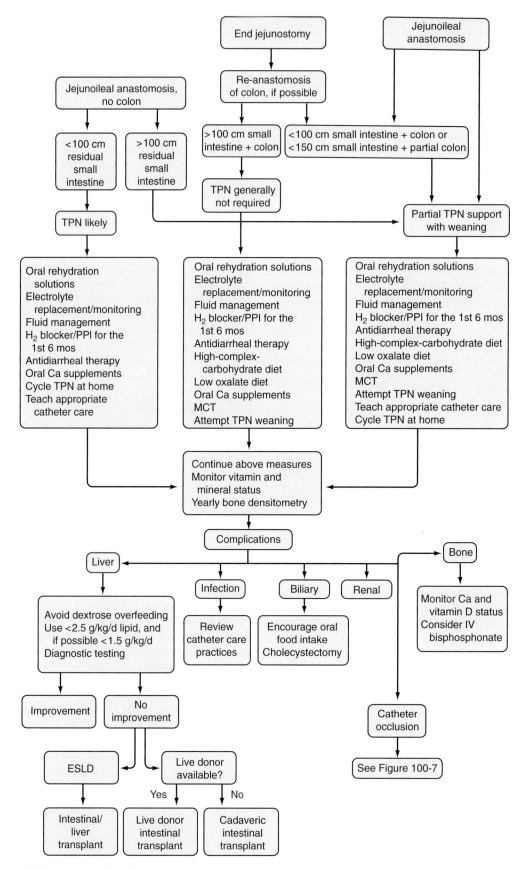

Figure 100–11 Algorithm for management of the patient with short bowel syndrome. Ca, Calcium; ESLD, end-stage liver disease; HCl, hydrochloric acid; MCT, medium-chain triglycerides; NaOH, sodium hydroxide; PPI, proton pump inhibitor; tPA, tissue plasminogen activator; TPN, total parenteral nutrition.

injections for the treatment of TPN-dependent SBS. The benefit from this therapy lasted nearly 4 months following completion of 3 weeks of daily growth hormone injections. It is unclear whether "booster" injections will be required. The benefits of this therapy must be weighed against the potential side effects, which include fluid retention edema, arthralgias, and carpal tunnel syndrome; it also is unknown whether any of the potential growth factor therapies would be more effective if administered during the adaptive phase following enterectomy.

SURVIVAL AND QUALITY OF LIFE

The prognosis for patients with SBS is determined primarily by the type and extent of intestinal resection and by the underlying disease. Patients with limited small intestinal resections, in general, have an excellent prognosis with careful management of their specific malabsorptive defects. Patients with high jejunostomies and severe malabsorption present difficult management problems, and their long-term care poses a challenge for surgeons, gastroenterologists, and dietitians. The rate of survival, prognosis, and quality of life are, however, steadily improving even in this group of patients because of increasing experience with long-term parenteral nutrition and better methods to assess nutritional needs.

The probability of survival and TPN dependence has been assessed in a prospective study of 124 patients with SBS.[71] Most of these patients had intestinal resection for either mesenteric infarction or radiation enteritis. The probability of survival was 86% at 2 years and 75% at 5 years. TPN dependence rates were 49% at 2 years and 45% at year 5, suggesting that most patients requiring long-term TPN can actually be weaned successfully within 2 years using conventional techniques. In a multivariate analysis, survival was related negatively to high jejunostomy, small bowel length less than 50 cm, and mesenteric infarction as a cause for intestinal resection. TPN dependence was related primarily to small bowel length. Remnant bowel length less than 100 cm was highly predictive of permanent intestinal failure and lifelong TPN dependence. Similar results were reported in a study of 225 patients from the Mayo Clinic.[124]

Most patients with SBS have a good quality of life and can work full time. Figure 100–11 depicts an algorithm for management of the patient with SBS.

REFERENCES

1. Buchman AL, Scolapio J, Fryer J: AGA technical review on SBS and intestinal transplantation. Gastroenterology 124:1111, 2003.
2. Messing B, Crenn P, Beau P, et al: Long-term survival and parenteral nutrition dependence in adult patients with SBS. Gastroenterology 117:1043, 1999.
3. Carbonnel F, Cosnes J, Chevret S, et al: The role of anatomic factors in nutritional autonomy after extensive small bowel resection. JPEN J Parenter Enteral Nutr 20:275, 1996.
4. Andersson H, Bosaeus I, Brummer R-J, et al: Nutritional and metabolic consequences of extensive bowel resection. Dig Dis 4:193, 1986.
5. Crenn P, Haniche M, Valleur P, et al: Surgical versus radiological evaluation of remaining small bowel length in SBS. Gastroenterology 110:A321, 1996.
6. Bryant J: Observations upon the growth and length of the human intestine. Am J Med Sci 167:499, 1924.
7. Slater G, Aufses AH Jr: Small-bowel length in Crohn's disease. Am J Gastroenterol 8:1037, 1991.
8. Fanucci A, Cerro P, Fraracci L, Letto F: Small-bowel length measured by radiology. Gastrointestinal Radiol 9:349, 1984.
9. Nightingale JMD, Bartram CI, Lennard-Jones JE: Length of residual small bowel after partial resection: correlation between radiographic and surgical measurements. Gastrointestinal Radiol 16:305, 1991.
10. Borgstrom B, Dahlqvist A, Lundh G, Sjovall J: Studies of intestinal digestion and absorption in the human. JCI 36:1521, 1957.
11. Clarke RM: Mucosal architecture and epithelial cell production rate in the small intestine of the albino rat. J Anat 107:519, 1970.
12. Nightingale JM, Lennard-Jones JE, Walker ER, Farthing MJ: Jejunal efflux in SBS. Lancet 336:765, 1990.
13. Nordgaard I, Hansen BS, Mortensen PB: Importance of colonic support for energy absorption as small-bowel failure proceeds. Am J Clin Nutr 64:222, 1996.
14. Royall D, Wolever TMS, Jeejeebhoy KN: Evidence for colonic conservation of malabsorbed carbohydrate in SBS. Am J Gastroenterol 87:751, 1992.
15. Nordgaard I, Hansen BS, Mortensen PB: Colon as a digestive organ in patients with short bowel. Lancet 343:373, 1994.
16. Ladefoged K, Olgaard K: Fluid and electrolyte absorption and renin-angiotensin-aldosterone axis in patients with severe short-bowel syndrome. Scand J Gastroenterol 14:729, 1979.
17. Spiller RC, Jones BJM, Silk DBA: Jejunal water and electrolyte absorption from two proprietary enteral feeds in man: Importance of sodium content. Gut 28:681, 1987.
18. Lennard-Jones JE: Oral rehydration solutions in SBS. Clin Ther 12:129, 1990.
19. Nightingale JMD, Lennard-Jones JE, Gertner DJ, et al: Colonic preservation reduces need for parenteral therapy, increases incidence of renal stones, but does not change high prevalence of gall stones in patients with a short bowel. Gut 33:1493, 1992.
20. Hylander E, Ladefoged K, Madsen S: Calcium balance and bone mineral content following small-intestinal resection. Scand J Gastroenterol 16:167, 1981.
21. Cosnes J, Gendre J-P, Evard D, et al: Compensatory enteral hyperalimentation for management of patients with severe SBS. Am J Clin Nutr 41:1002, 1985.
22. Hessov I, Andersson H, Isaksson B: Effects of a low-fat diet on mineral absorption in small-bowel disease. Scand J Gastroenterol 18:551, 1983.
23. Andersson H: Effects of a fat-reduced diet on the faecal excretion of radioactivity following administration of ^{14}C-cholic acid and on the duodenal concentration of bile salts in patients with ileal disease. Nutr Metab 20:254, 1976.
24. Bright-Asare P, Binder H: Stimulation of colonic secretion of water and electrolytes by hydroxy fatty acids. Gastroenterology 64:81, 1973.
25. Williams NS, Evans P, King RF: Gastric acid secretion and gastrin production in the SBS. Gut 26:914, 1985.
26. Hyman PE, Everett SL, Harada T: Gastric acid hypersecretion in SBS in infants: Association with extent of resection and enteral feeding. J Pediatr Gastroenterol Nutr 5:191, 1986.
27. Nightingale JMD, Kamm MA, van der Sijp JR: Gastrointestinal hormones in SBS. Peptide YY may be the colonic brake to gastric emptying. Gut 39:267, 1996.
28. Spiller RC, Trotman IF, Higgins BE: The ileal brake—inhibition of jejunal motility after ileal perfusion in man. Gastroenterology 25:365, 1984.

29. Holgate AM, Read NW: Effect of ileal infusion of intralipid on gastrointestinal transit, ileal flow rate and carbohydrate absorption in humans after ingestion of a liquid meal. Gastroenterology 88:1005, 1985.

30. Nightingale JMD, Kamm MA, van der Sijp JR, et al: Disturbed gastric emptying in the SBS: evidence for a "colonic brake." Gut 34:1171, 1993.

31. Jeppesen PB, Hartmann B, Hansen BS, et al: Impaired meal stimulated glucagon-like peptide 2 response in ileal resected short bowel patients with intestinal failure. Gut 45:559, 1999.

32. Jeppesen PB, Hartmann B, Thulesen J, et al: Elevated plasma glucagon-like peptide 1 and 2 concentrations in ileum resected short bowel patients with a preserved colon. Gut 47:370, 2000.

33. Williamson RCN, Chir M: Intestinal adaptation. I. Structural, functional and cytokinetic changes. N Engl J Med 298:1393, 1978.

34. Williamson RCN, Chir M: Intestinal adaptation. II. Mechanisms of control. N Engl J Med 298:1444, 1978.

35. Appleton GVN, Bristol JB, Williamson RCN: Proximal enterectomy provides a stronger systemic stimulus to intestinal adaptation than distal enterectomy. Gut 28:165, 1987.

36. Solhaug JH, Tvete S: Adaptive changes in the small intestine following bypass operation for obesity. Scand J Gastroenterol 13:401, 1978.

37. Levy E, Frileux P, Sandrucci S, et al: Continuous enteral nutrition during the early adaptive stage of the SBS. Br J Surg 75:549, 1988.

38. Chaves M, Smith MW, Williamson RCN: Increased activity of digestive enzymes in ileal enterocytes adapting to proximal small bowel resection. Gut 28:981, 1987.

39. Gouttebel MC, Saint Aubert B, Colette C, et al: Intestinal adaptation in patients with SBS. Dig Dis Sci 34:709, 1989.

40. Dowling RH: Small bowel adaptation and its regulation. Scand J Gastroenterol 17:53, 1982.

41. Johnson LR, Copeland EM, Diedrich SJ: Structural and hormonal alterations in the gastrointestinal tract of parenterally fed rats. Gastroenterology 68:1177, 1975.

42. Briet F, Flourie B, Achour L, et al: Bacterial adaptation in patients with short bowel and colon in continuity. Gastroenterology 109:1446, 1995.

43. Drucker DJ, Ehrlich P, Asa SL, et al: Induction of intestinal epithelial proliferation by glucagon-like peptide 2. Proc Natl Acad Sci U S A 93:7911, 1996.

44. Rhoads JM, Argenzio RA, Chen W, et al: L-Glutamine stimulates intestinal cell proliferation and activates mitogen-activated protein kinases. Am J Physiol 272:G943, 1997.

45. Sham J, Martin G, Meddings JB, Sigalet DL: Epidermal growth factor improves nutritional outcome in a rat model of SBS. J Pediatric Surg 37:765, 2002.

46. Scolapio JS, Camilleri M, Fleming CR, et al: Effect of growth hormone, glutamine, and diet on adaptation in short-bowel syndrome: A randomized, controlled trial. Gastroenterology 113:1074, 1997.

47. Szkudlarek J, Jeppesen PB, Mortensen PB: Effect of high dose growth hormone with glutamine and no change in diet on intestinal absorption in short bowel patients: A randomised, double blind, crossover, placebo controlled study. Gut 47:199, 2000.

48. Luk G, Baylin SB: Polyamines and intestinal growth–increased polyamine biosynthesis after jejunectomy. Am J Physiol 245:G656, 1983.

49. Luk G, Baylin SB: Inhibition of intestinal epithelial DNA synthesis and adaptive hyperplasia after jejunectomy in the rat by suppression of polyamine biosynthesis. J Clin Invest 74:698, 1984.

50. Nightingdale JMD, Walker ER, Farthing MJG, Lennard-Jones JE: Effect of omeprazole on intestinal output in the SBS. Aliment Pharmacol Therap 5:405, 1991

51. Jeppesen PB, Staun M, Tjellesen L, Mortensen PB: Effect of intravenous ranitidine and omeprazole on intestinal absorption of water, sodium, and macronutrients in patients with intestinal resection. Gut 43:763, 1998.

52. Arrambide KA, Santa Ana CA, Schiller LR, et al: Loss of absorptive capacity for sodium chloride as a cause of diarrhea following partial ileal and right colon resection. Dig Dis Sci 34:193, 1989.

53. Anast CS, Winnacker JL, Forte LR, Burns TW: Impaired release of parathyroid hormone in magnesium deficiency. Clin Endocrinol Metab 42:707, 1976.

54. Hylander E, Ladefoged K, Madsen S: Calcium balance and bone mineral content following small-intestinal resection. Scand J Gastroenterol 16:167, 1981.

55. O'Keefe SJD, Peterson ME, Fleming CR: Octreotide as an adjunct to home parenteral nutrition in the management of permanent end-jejunostomy syndrome. J Parenter Enter Nutr 18:26, 1994.

56. Ladefofed K, Christensen KC, Hegnhoj J, Jarnum S: Effect of a long-acting somatostatin analogue SMS 201-995 on jejunostomy effluents in patients with severe SBS. Gut 30:943, 1989.

57. Niv Y, Charash B, Sperber AD, Oren M: Effect of octreotide on gastrostomy, duodenostomy, and cholecystostomy effluents: A physiologic study of fluid and electrolyte balance. Am J Gastroenterol 92:2107, 1997.

58. Catnach SM, Anderson JV, Fairclough PD, et al: Effect of octreotide on gallstone prevalence and gallbladder motility in acromegaly. Gut 34:270, 1993.

59. Fortran JS: Stimulation of active and passive sodium absorption by sugars in the human jejunum. J Clin Invest 55:728, 1975.

60. Pfeiffer A, Schmidt T, Kaess H: The role of osmolality in the absorption of a nutrient solution. Aliment Pharmacol Ther 12:281, 1998.

61. Davis GR, Santa Ana CA, Morawski SG, Fortran JC: Permeability characteristics of human jejunum, ileum, proximal colon, and distal colon: Results of potential difference measurements and unidirectional fluxes. Gastroenterology 83:844, 1982.

62. Englyst HN, Trowell H, Southgate DAT, Cummings JH: Dietary fibre and resistant starch. Ann J Clin Nutr 46:873, 1987.

63. Bond JH, Currier BE, Buchwald H, Levitt MD: Colonic conservation of malabsorbed carbohydrate. Gastroenterology 78:444, 1980.

64. Florent C, Flourie B, Leblond A, et al: Influence of chronic lactulose ingestion on the colonic metabolism of lactulose in man (an in vivo study). J Clin Invest 75:608, 1985.

65. Little KH, Schiller LR, Bilhartz LE, Fortran JS: Treatment of severe steatorrhea with ox bile in an ileectomy patient with residual colon. Dig Dis Sci 37:929, 1992.

66. Fordtran JS, Bunch F, Davis GR: Ox bile treatment of severe steatorrhea in an ileectomy-ileostomy patient. Gastroenterology 82:564, 1982.

67. Hoffman AF, Poley R: Role of bile acid malabsorption in pathogenesis of diarrhea and steatorrhea in patients with ileal resection. Gastroenterology 62:918, 1972.

68. Woolf GM, Miller C, Kurian R, Jeejeebhoy KN: Diet for patients with a short bowel: High fat or high carbohydrate? Gastroenterology 84:823, 1983.

69. Ovesen L, Chu R, Howard L: The influence of dietary fat on jejunostomy output in patients with severe SBS. Am J Clin Nutr 38:270, 1983.

70. Jeppesen PB, Mortensen PB: The influence of a preserved colon on the absorption of medium chain fat in patients with small bowel resection. Gut 43:478, 1998.

71. Messing B, Crenn P, Beau P, et al: Long-term survival and parenteral nutrition dependence in adult patients with the SBS. Gastroenterology 117:1043, 1999.

72. McIntyre PB, Fitchew M, Lennard-Jones JE: Patients with a high jejunostomy do not need a special diet. Gastroenterology 91:25, 1986.

73. Woolf GM, Miller C, Kurian R, et al: Nutritional absorption in SBS. Dig Dis Sci 32:8, 1987.

74. Ladefoged K: Intestinal and renal loss of infused minerals in patients with severe SBS. Am J Clin Nutr 36:59, 1982.

75. Engels LGJ, van den Hamer CJA, van Tongeren JHM: Iron, zinc, and copper balance in short bowel patients on oral nutrition. Am J Clin Nutr 40:1038, 1984.

76. Conly JM, Stein K, Worobetz L, et al: The contribution of vitamin K_2 (menaquinones) produced by the intestinal microflora to human nutritional requirements for vitamin K. Am J Gastroenterol 89:915, 1994.

77. Wolman SL, Anderson GH, Marliss EB, Jeejeebhoy KN: Zinc in total parenteral nutrition: requirements and metabolic effects. Gastroenterology 76:458, 1979.

78. McFadden MA, Delegge MH, Kirby DF: Medication delivery in the SBS. JPEN J Parenter Enteral Nutr 17:180, 1993.

79. Ehrenpreis ED, Guerriero S, Nogueras JJ, Carroll MA: Malabsorption of digoxin tablets, gel tabs, and elixir in a patient with an end jejunostomy. Ann Pharmacother 28:1239, 1994.

80. Levy E, Frileux P, Sandrucci S, et al: Continuous enteral nutrition during the early adaptive stage of the SBS. Br J Surg 75:549, 1988.

81. Cosnes J, Evard D, Beaugerie L, et al: Improvement in protein absorption with a small peptide-base diet in patients with high jejunostomy. Nutrition 8:406, 1992.

82. Marteau P, Messing B, Arrigoni E, et al: Do patients with short-bowel syndrome need a lactose-free diet? Nutrition 13:13, 1997.

83. Buchman AL, Moukarzel A, Goodson B, et al: Catheter-related infections associated with home parenteral nutrition and predictive factors for the need for catheter removal in their treatment. JPEN J Parenter Enteral Nutr 18:297, 1994.

84. Buchman AL, Goodson B, Herzog F, Ament ME: Catheter thrombosis and superior/inferior vena cava syndrome are rare complications of long-term parenteral nutrition. Clin Nutr 13:356, 1994.

85. Buchman AL: Complications of long-term home total parenteral nutrition: Their identification, prevention and treatment. Dig Dis Sci 46:1, 2001.

86. Buchman AL: Practical Nutrition Support Techniques. Thorofare, NJ: Slack, Inc., 2003.

87. Buchman AL, Ament ME: Fifteen-year survival of a Broviac catheter used for home parenteral nutrition. JPEN J Parenter Enteral Nutr 17:489, 1993.

88. Roslyn JJ, Pitt HA, Mann LL, et al: Gallbladder disease in patients on long-term parenteral nutrition. Gastroenterology 84:148, 1983.

89. Ling PR, Sheikh M, Boyce P, et al: Cholecystokinin (CCK) secretion in patients with severe SBS (SSBS). Dig Dis Sci 46:859, 2001.

90. Sitzman JV, Pitt HA, Steinborn PA, et al: Cholecystokinin prevents parenteral nutrition induced biliary sludge in humans. Surg Gynecol Obstet 170:25, 1990.

91. Apelgren KN, Willard DA, Vargish T: TPN alters gallbladder responsivity to cholecystokinin. JPEN J Parenter Enteral Nutr 12:11S, 1988.

92. Cavicchi M, Beau P, Crenn P, et al: Prevalence of liver disease and contributing factors in patients receiving home parenteral nutrition for permanent intestinal failure. Ann Intern Med 132:525, 2000.

93. Chan S, McCowen KC, Bistrian BR, et al: Incidence, prognosis, and etiology of end-stage liver disease in patients receiving home total parenteral nutrition. Surgery 126:28, 1999.

94. Kelly DA: Liver complications of pediatric parenteral nutrition—epidemiology. Nutrition 14:153, 1998.

95. Buchman AL: Total parenteral nutrition–associated liver disease. JPEN J Parenter Enteral Nutr 26:S43, 2002.

96. Stegnick LD, Besten LD: Synthesis of cysteine from methionine in normal adult subjects: Effect of route of alimentation. Science 178:514, 1972.

97. Stanko RT, Nathan G, Mendelow H, Adibi SA: Development of hepatic cholestasis and fibrosis in patients with massive loss of intestine supported by prolonged parenteral nutrition. Gastroenterology 92:197, 1987.

98. Bowyer BA, Fleming CR, Ludwig J, et al: Does long-term parenteral nutrition in adult patients cause chronic liver disease? JPEN J Parenter Enteral Nutr 9:11, 1985.

99. Buchman AL, Dubin M, Jenden D, et al: Lecithin supplementation causes a decrease in hepatic steatosis in patients receiving long term parenteral nutrition. Gastroenterology. 102:1363, 1992.

100. Buchman AL, Dubin MD, Moukarzel AA, et al: Choline deficiency: A cause of hepatic steatosis during parenteral nutrition that can be reversed with intravenous choline supplementation. Hepatology 22:1399, 1995.

101. Buchman AL, Sohel M, Dubin M, et al: Choline deficiency causes reversible hepatic abnormalities in patients during parenteral nutrition: Proof of a human choline requirement; a placebo-controlled trial. JPEN J Parenter Enteral Nutr 25:260, 2001.

102. Spagnuolo MI, Iorio R, Vegnente A, Guarino A: Ursodeoxycholic acid for treatment of cholestasis in children on long-term total parenteral nutrition: A pilot study. Gastroenterology 111:716, 1996.

103. Lindor KD, Burnes J: Ursodeoxycholic acid for the treatment of home parenteral nutrition–associated cholestasis. Gastroenterology 101:250, 1991.

104. Bowyer BA, Miles JM, Haymond MW, Fleming CR: L-Carnitine therapy in home parenteral nutrition patients with abnormal liver tests and low plasma carnitine concentration. Gastroenterology 94:434, 1988.

105. Emmett M, Guirl MJ, Santa Ana CA, et al: Conjugated bile acid replacement therapy reduces urinary oxalate excretion in SBS. Am J Kidney Dis 41:230, 2003.

106. Rockwell GF, Campfield T, Nelson BC, Uden PC: Oxalogenesis in parenteral nutrition solution components. Nutrition 14:836, 1999.

107. Dahlquist NR, Perrault J, Callaway CW, et al: D-Lactic acidosis and encephalopathy after jejunoileostomy: Response to overfeeding and to fasting in humans. Mayo Clin Proc 59:141, 1984.

108. Oh MS, Uribarri J, Alveranga D, et al: Metabolic utilization and renal handling of D-lactate in men. Metabolism 34:621, 1985.

109. Mayne AJ, Handy DJ, Preece MA, et al: Dietary management of D-lactic acidosis in SBS. Arch Dis Child 65:229, 1990.

110. Hudson M, Pocknee R, Mowat AG: D-Lactic acidosis in SBS—an examination of possible mechanisms. Q J Med 74:157, 1990.

111. Buchman AL, Moukarzel A, Ament ME, et al: Serious renal impairment is associated with long-term parenteral nutrition. J Parent Enteral Nutr 17:438, 1993.

112. Buchman AL, Moukarzel A: Metabolic bone disease associated with total parenteral nutrition. Clin Nutr 19:217, 2000.

113. Buchman AL, Sohel M, Brown M, et al: Verbal and visual memory improve after choline supplementation in long-term total parenteral nutrition: A pilot study. JPEN J Parenter Enteral Nutr 25:30, 2001.

114. Idoate MA, Martinez AJ, Bueno J, et al: The neuropathology of intestinal failure and small bowel transplantation. Acta Neuropathol 97:502, 1999.

115. Bianchi A: Intestinal loop lengthening—a technique for increasing small intestinal length. J Pediatr Surg 15:145, 1980.

116. Fishbein TM, Kaufman SS, Florman SS, et al: Isolated intestinal transplantation: Proof of clinical efficacy. Transplantation 76:636, 2003.

117. Grant D: Intestinal transplantation: 1997 report of the international registry. Transplantation 67:1061, 1999.

118. Byrne TA, Persinger RL, Young LS, et al: A new treatment for patients with short-bowel syndrome—growth hormone, glutamine, and a modified diet. Ann Surg 222:243, 1995.

119. Ellegard L, Bosaeus I, Nordgren S, Bengtsson BA: Low-dose recombinant growth hormone increases body weight and lean body mass in patients with SBS. Ann Surg 225:88, 1997.

120. Seguy D, Vahedi K, Kapel N, et al: Low dose growth hormone in adult home parenteral nutrition-dependent SBS patients: A positive study. Gastroenterology 124:293, 2003.

121. Jeppesen PB, Hartmann B, Thulesen J, et al: Treatment of short bowel patients with glucagon-like peptide 2 (GLP-2), a newly discovered intestinotrophic, anti-secretory, and transit modulating peptide. Gastroenterology 118:A178, 2000.

122. Palle B, Jeppesen PB, Consuelo M, et al: ALX-0600, a dipeptidyl peptidase-IV resistant glucagon-like peptide-2 (GLP-2) analog, improves intestinal function in SBS patients. Gastroenterology 122:A191, 2002.

123. Byrne TA, Wilmore DW, Iyer K, et al: Growth hormone, glutamine, and an optimal diet reduces parenteral nutrition in patients with short bowel syndrome: A prospective, randomized, placebo-controlled, double-blind clinical trial. Ann Surg 242:655, 2005.

124. Scolapio JS, Fleming CR, Kelly DG, et al: Survival of home parenteral nutrition–treated patients: 20 years of experience at the Mayo Clinic. Mayo Clin Proc 74:217, 1999.

CHAPTER
101 Celiac Sprue and Refractory Sprue

Richard J. Farrell and Ciarán P. Kelly

DEFINITIONS

Celiac sprue is characterized by (1) small intestinal malabsorption of nutrients following the ingestion of wheat gluten or related proteins from rye and barley; (2) a characteristic, though not specific, villus atrophy of the small intestinal mucosa; (3) prompt clinical and histologic improvement following strict adherence to a gluten-free diet; and (4) clinical and histologic relapse when gluten is reintroduced.[1] The many other names used to identify patients with this condition (*nontropical sprue, celiac syndrome, adult celiac disease, idiopathic steatorrhea, primary malabsorption,* and so on) are testimony to the confusion of the past. The term *celiac sprue* is recognized widely and is used in this chapter—*celiac disease* and *gluten-sensitive enteropathy* are acceptable alternative terms. Celiac sprue exhibits a spectrum of disease (Fig 101–1), with *atypical celiac sprue* (fully expressed gluten-sensitive enteropathy found in association with atypical manifestations including short stature, anemia, and infertility) and *silent celiac sprue* (fully expressed gluten-sensitive enteropathy found after serologic screening in asymptomatic patients) being more common than *classic* or *typical celiac sprue* (fully expressed gluten-sensitive

enteropathy found in association with the classic features of malabsorption). A combination of serologic, genetic, and histologic data also has led to the identification of two other types of celiac sprue. The term *latent celiac sprue* refers to patients who have normal villus architecture on a gluten-containing diet, but who, at another time, have had or will have villus atrophy that recovered or will recover on a gluten-free diet. For example, a patient who had celiac sprue in childhood and recovered completely on a gluten-free diet may have "latent celiac sprue" later in life on resumption of a normal diet. The term *potential celiac sprue* refers to disease in patients who have never had a biopsy consistent with celiac sprue but show immunologic abnormalities characteristic for the disease, such as a positive IgA to endomysium (or tissue transglutaminase [tTG]) or increased intraepithelial lymphocytes (IELs) in the small intestine. These patients often have a genetic predisposition to celiac sprue, especially human leukocyte antigen class II DQ (HLA-DQ2), an affected first-degree relative, or both; the probability of their developing celiac sprue may be as high as 50%.[2] *Refractory sprue*, also known as *unclassified* or *intractable celiac sprue*, is defined as symptomatic, severe small intestinal villus atrophy that mimics celiac sprue but does not

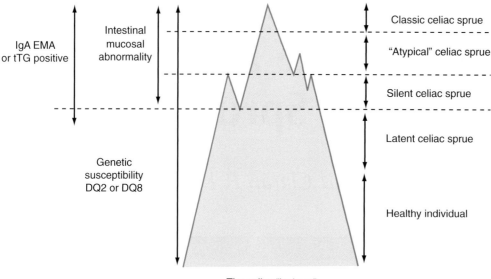

Figure 101–1 The celiac "iceberg" and the spectrum of celiac sprue. EMA, endomysial antibody; tTG, tissue transglutaminase.

respond to at least 6 months of a strict gluten-free diet. This is a diagnosis of exclusion that is not accounted for by inadvertent gluten ingestion, other causes of villus atrophy, or overt intestinal lymphoma.[1,3]

HISTORY

Celiac sprue first was recognized as a clinical entity by Aretaeus the Cappadocian in the 1st century AD.[4] The name *sprue* was coined in the 18th century and is derived from the Dutch word *spruw*, which means aphthous disease, so named because of the high prevalence of aphthous mouth ulcers in these patients. In 1888, Samuel Gee published his paper "On the Coeliac Affection," which describes many of the clinical features of celiac sprue in patients of all age groups and ends by stating that "if the patient can be cured at all it must be by means of the diet."[5] It was not until the middle of this century, however, that the link between certain cereals and celiac sprue was made by Willem Karel Dicke, a Dutch pediatrician. He became convinced that the consumption of bread and wheat flour was directly responsible for the deterioration in patients suffering from this condition.[6] During World War II, cereals used to make bread were particularly scarce in the Netherlands, and during this time, children with celiac sprue improved, only to relapse after the supply of cereal was re-established at the end of the war. It was this serendipitous observation that led to the finding that wheat indeed exacerbated celiac sprue. Subsequent work by van de Kamer and coworkers[7] showed that it was the water-insoluble portion, or gluten moiety, of wheat that produced malabsorption in patients with celiac sprue. In 1954, Paulley[8] provided the first accurate description of the characteristic intestinal lesion in patients with celiac sprue. With the development of effective peroral suction biopsy instruments in the late 1950s, Rubin and coworkers[9] demonstrated that celiac sprue in children and idiopathic or nontropical sprue in adults were identical diseases with the same clinical and pathologic features.

The past 20 years have seen substantial advances in our understanding of the genetic, immune, and molecular mechanisms fundamental to the pathogenesis of celiac sprue and refractory sprue. In 1986, Howell and associates[10] observed that celiac sprue was associated with specific HLA-DQ2 haplotypes. In 1993, Lundin and colleagues[11] demonstrated that the DQ gene products preferentially present gluten-derived gliadin peptides to intestinal mucosal T cells in celiac patients. More recently, the search for the "celiac autoantigen" has focused on the enzyme tTG, leading to more accurate serologic diagnostic tests.[12] In 1998, Molberg and colleagues[13] reported that host tTG modification of gliadin enhances gliadin-specific celiac sprue T cell responses. The identification of specific tTG-modified peptides as dominant α-gliadin T cell epitopes[14] has highlighted the pivotal role played by tTG in the pathogenesis of celiac sprue and may pave the way for antigen-specific immunotherapy. The key role played by IELs in the development of refractory sprue and enteropathy-associated T cell lymphoma (EATL) continues to evolve.[15] Studies also point to the importance of interleukin (IL)-15, a potent proinflammatory cytokine at the interface between innate and adaptive immunity in the pathogenesis of both celiac sprue and refractory sprue.[16]

EPIDEMIOLOGY

The term *celiac iceberg* was coined to describe the wide variations in the nature and intensity of clinical presentation of which overt celiac sprue is only the emerging peak (see Fig 101–1). The discovery of the large immersed part of the celiac iceberg has transformed the status of celiac sprue, long considered a rare disease, particularly in adults, to that of a common health problem. Because we are uncertain of the depth and breadth of the celiac iceberg, the true prevalence of celiac sprue remains unknown. Serologic testing has demonstrated that silent celiac sprue, characterized by positive serology and villus atrophy with no or mild symptoms, is approximately seven times more common than symptomatic celiac sprue.[17] A Finnish study of 3654 schoolchildren ages 7 to 16 years using two serologic screens with antiendomysial and tTG antibodies in 1994 and 2001 demonstrated the heterogeneity of the celiac iceberg.[18] The prevalence of biopsy-proved celiac sprue among schoolchildren was 1:99, whereas the prevalence in schoolchildren of the HLA-DQ2 or HLA-DQ8 haplotype (which is strongly associated with celiac sprue) who also were antibody positive was 1:67. Of note, only 10 of 56 subjects with a positive serology in 1994 developed overt symptoms of celiac sprue before the second screen in 2001; 27 subjects with a positive serology in 1994 continued to have no symptoms in 2001, despite a flat mucosal biopsy; and 10 subjects were symptom free with normal biopsies. Two subjects with positive antibodies in 1994 and 2001 and at risk for celiac sprue because of HLA-DQ2 haplotype had normal mucosa, but both had increased epithelial expression of HLA-DR suggestive of ongoing inflammation, and one had high counts of IELs. These patients might represent cases of latent disease susceptible to evolving into overt celiac sprue after several years. Finally, 5 patients with HLA-DQ2 and positive antibodies in 1994 had negative antibodies in 2001; their intestinal biopsies were normal, but all had increased HLA-DR expression, and 4 of 5 had markedly increased numbers of IELs. This latter finding might indicate a variation in the natural history of celiac sprue, occasionally seen in teenagers, in whom gluten sensitivity fluctuates with time.

Celiac sprue shows a marked geographic variation, with the highest incidence in Western Europe. The condition is significantly more common in Scandinavian and Celtic populations, where the prevalence has been reported to be as high as 1:99[18] and 1:122,[19] respectively. The prevalence is similarly high in Italy[17] and the southeastern region of Austria.[20] The prevalence in Denmark is 40-fold lower than that in Sweden,[21] suggesting considerable variation in prevalence among geographically proximate populations. Factors such as predominant HLA haplotype, timing of introduction of gluten into the diet, significant differences in the gliadin concentration of infant formulas, and interobserver variation in interpreting small intestinal biopsy findings may explain the differences in prevalence.[22]

Celiac sprue also is found in those countries to which Europeans have emigrated, notably North America and Australia. Recent epidemiologic studies in the United States, where the disease only recently has attracted much attention, underscore the varying clinical presentation of celiac sprue and indicate that the prevalence of celiac sprue in the United States is comparable with that in Western Europe. In 1998, a study of 2000 healthy blood donors reported a prevalence of antiendomysial antibodies of 1 in 250 subjects.[23] A large multicenter study by Fasano and coworkers[24] determined the prevalence of antiendomysial antibodies in more than 13,000 at-risk and not-at-risk American subjects and found the prevalence of antiendomysial antibodies to be 1:22 and 1:39 among first-degree and second-degree relatives of subjects with celiac sprue, respectively.[24] A prevalence of 1:56 was documented among patients with gastrointestinal symptoms of celiac sprue or associated disorders. Of most significance, they found a prevalence of antien-

domysial antibodies of 1:133 among 4126 not-at-risk individuals.

Although celiac sprue is rare in the predominantly rice-eating area of southern India, it is prevalent in the Bengal and Punjab provinces of northwest India, where wheat rather than rice has, for many generations, formed part of the staple diet. The condition has been reported in blacks, Arabs, Hispanics, Israeli Jews, Sudanese of mixed Arab-black descent, and Cantonese and is particularly high among the Saharawi population in Northwest Africa.[25] The condition rarely, if ever, affects people of purely African-Caribbean, Chinese, or Japanese descent. Some authors have suggested a female-to-male ratio of 2:1, whereas others have reported ratios as low as 1.3:1.

PATHOLOGY

Celiac sprue affects the mucosa of the small intestine; the submucosa, muscularis propria, and serosa usually are not involved. The mucosal lesion of the small intestine in celiac sprue may vary considerably in both severity and extent.[9] This spectrum of pathologic involvement helps explain the striking variations in the clinical manifestations of the disease. Examination, by hand lens or dissecting microscope, of the mucosal surface of biopsy specimens from untreated celiac sprue patients with severe lesions reveals a flat mucosal surface with complete absence of normal intestinal villi. Histologic examination of tissue sections confirms this loss of normal villus structure (Fig. 101–2A). The intestinal crypts are markedly elongated and open onto a flat absorptive surface. The total thickness of the mucosa is reduced only slightly in most cases, because crypt hyperplasia compensates for the absence or shortening of the villi. These architectural changes decrease the amount of epithelial surface available for digestion and absorption.[9] The remaining absorptive cells, which appear columnar in normal biopsy specimens, are cuboidal or, at times, squamoid in celiac sprue biopsy specimens. Their cytoplasm is more basophilic (RNA rich), the basal polarity of the nuclei is lost, and the brush border is markedly attenuated. When viewed with the electron microscope, the microvilli of the absorptive cells appear shortened and often fused. The number of free ribosomes is increased, reflecting impaired differentiation and resulting in the increase in cytoplasmic basophilia evident on histologic examination. Degenerative changes, including cytoplasmic and mitochondrial vacuolization and the presence of many large lysosomes, are obvious. Structural abnormalities of tight junctions between damaged absorptive cells provide a morphologic explanation for the observed increased permeability of the mucosal barrier in celiac sprue.[26] The endoplasmic reticulum is sparse, reflecting the low level of synthesis of digestive enzymes including disaccharidases and peptidases. Thus, mature absorptive cells are reduced in number and functionally compromised.

Unlike the absorptive cells, the undifferentiated crypt cells are markedly increased in number in patients with severe untreated celiac sprue, and the crypts are therefore lengthened. Moreover, the number of mitoses in crypts is strikingly increased. Cytologic features and histochemistry of the crypt cells are normal by both light and

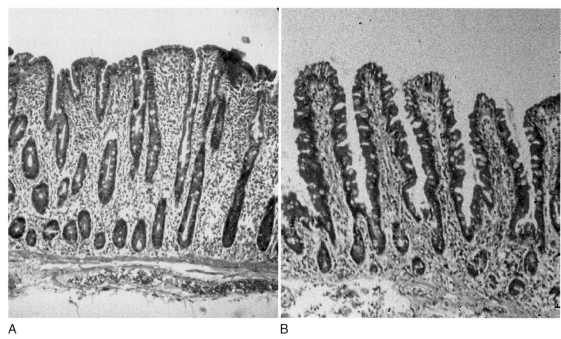

A   B

Figure 101–2 Mucosal pathology in celiac sprue. *A,* Duodenal biopsy specimen of a patient with untreated celiac sprue. The histologic features of severe villus atrophy, crypt hyperplasia, enterocyte disarray, and intense inflammation of the lamina propria and epithelial cell layer are evident. *B,* Repeat duodenal biopsy after 6 months on a strict gluten-free diet. There is marked improvement, with well-formed villi and a return of the mucosal architecture toward normal.

electron microscopy. Studies of epithelial cell kinetics in untreated celiac sprue suggest that "villus atrophy" is a misnomer because there is evidence for an actual increase in "enteropoiesis" in the crypts. Wright and colleagues[27] estimated that intestinal mucosa from patients with celiac sprue produces six times as many cells per hour per crypt as does normal small intestine and that the cell cycle time is halved, reflecting premature shedding. The experimental evidence suggests, therefore, that the central mechanism of villus shortening in celiac sprue is a gliadin-associated toxic effect on maturing enterocytes that results in their premature loss into the intestinal lumen and a compensatory increase in enterocyte replication in the crypts. Such a mechanism would explain many of the histologic abnormalities described earlier.

The cellularity of the lamina propria is increased in the involved small intestine. The cellular infiltrate consists largely of plasma cells and lymphocytes. The number of IgA-, IgM-, and IgG-producing cells is increased twofold to sixfold, but, as in normal mucosa, IgA-producing cells predominate.[28] Polymorphonuclear leukocytes, eosinophils, and mast cells also may contribute substantially to the increased cellularity of the lamina propria. Although the number of IELs per unit length of absorptive epithelium is increased in untreated celiac sprue, the total number of IELs may not be increased, because the absorptive surface is markedly reduced.[9] In the normal small intestinal mucosa, lamina propria T cells are predominantly CD4+ (helper/inducer cells), whereas the IELs are mainly CD8+ (cytotoxic/suppressor) cells. In untreated celiac sprue this distribution of T cells is main-

tained but the density of cells in both compartments is increased.

Marsh[29] pioneered the theory of a sequence of progression of the celiac lesion in the small intestinal mucosa. Starting with a preinfiltrative (stage 0) mucosa, the initial observed event is an increase in IELs, followed by infiltration of the lamina propria with lymphocytes (stage 1). Crypt hyperplasia (stage 2) precedes villus atrophy (stage 3) and is observed only in the presence of lamina propria lymphocytosis, suggesting that IELs are not sufficient to induce intestinal architectural changes in celiac sprue. Finally, total mucosal atrophy (stage 4) develops and is characterized by complete loss of villi, enhanced apoptosis, and crypt hyperplasia.

In untreated patients, the length of small intestinal involvement by the celiac sprue lesion varies among individuals and correlates with the severity of clinical symptoms. Thus, the patient with a severe lesion that involves the full length of the small intestine has more severe malabsorption than the patient with a severe duodenal lesion, a milder jejunal lesion, and a normal ileum. When the intestinal lesion does not involve the entire length of small bowel, the proximal intestine is most severely involved and the lesion decreases in severity distally. Sparing of the proximal intestine with involvement of the distal small intestine does not occur. In some untreated patients with mild celiac sprue, not even the proximal intestine shows the typical severe flat lesion. Rather, some villus structure remains and the absorptive surface, although less than normal, is largely preserved.[9] An increase in IEL count alone is not sufficient to support the histologic diagnosis of celiac sprue, because this finding is nonspecific; some shortening of the villi, crypt hyperplasia, cytologically abnormal surface cells, and increased lamina propria cellularity must be present to establish the diagnosis firmly.

Treatment with a gluten-free diet results in significant improvement in intestinal structure (see Fig. 101–2*B*). The cytologic appearance of the surface absorptive cells improves first, often within a few days. Tall, columnar absorptive cells with basal nuclei and well-developed brush borders replace the abnormal, immature cuboidal surface cells; the ratio of IELs to absorptive cells decreases. Subsequently, villus architecture reverts toward normal, with lengthening of the villi and shortening of the crypts; the lamina propria decreases in cellularity. The mucosa of the distal small intestine improves more rapidly than that of the more severely involved proximal bowel.[30] In some patients, months or even years of gluten withdrawal may be required before the mucosa reverts to normal; indeed, some residual abnormality, which may be striking or subtle, often persists, possibly because of inadvertent gluten indigestion.[31] In the debilitated patient with severe untreated celiac sprue and associated nutritional deficiency states, pathologic changes may be present in many other organ systems besides the digestive tract. Finally, the mucosal lesion of celiac sprue can be identical histologically to the mucosal response to injury typical of a wide range of other enteropathies (see "Differential Diagnosis").

PATHOGENESIS

The interaction of the water-insoluble protein moiety (gluten) of certain cereal grains with the mucosa of the small intestine in susceptible individuals is central to the pathogenesis of celiac sprue. Although the exact molecular mechanism by which gluten damages the mucosa has not been established, our knowledge of the pathogenesis of celiac sprue has accelerated recently. Celiac sprue is now considered to be an immune disorder that is triggered by an environmental agent (gliadin) in genetically predisposed persons. The wide spectrum of clinical manifestations is the result of a complex interplay of varying environmental, genetic, and immune factors.

How these environmental, genetic, and immune factors control expression of celiac sprue and passage from latent to overt disease remains unknown.

ENVIRONMENTAL FACTORS

Celiac sprue is a model for immunologic diseases with a defined environmental trigger. Early work involving physiologic digestion with pepsin and trypsin, followed by separation according to solubility properties, identified several wheat proteins as being responsible for the grain toxicity in celiac sprue Wheat protein exists in a number of storage forms that can be categorized into four general groups based on their solubility characteristics: prolamins (soluble in ethanol), glutenins (partially soluble in dilute acid or alkali solutions), globulins (soluble in 10% NaCl), and minor albumins (soluble in water). The term *gluten* encompasses the prolamins (ethanol-soluble fraction) and the glutenins. Although most toxicity studies have been performed with prolamins, there are data to suggest that glutenins also can damage the celiac intestinal mucosa.[32] The prolamins of wheat are referred to as *gliadins*. Prolamins from other cereals also are considered to be gluten and are named according to their source (*secalins* from rye, *hordeins* from barley, *avenins* from oats, and *zeins* from corn). The taxonomic relationships of the major cereal grain families provide a framework on which their toxicities in celiac sprue can be predicted (Fig. 101–3). Wheat, rye, and barley belong to the tribe known as Triticinae, whereas oats belong to a neighboring tribe known as Aveneae. Avenin is genetically less similar to gliadin than gliadin is to secalin and hordein. Despite their genetic differences, however, prolamins from oats, barley, wheat, and rye still have immunologic cross-reactivity because of their common ancestry.[33] Grains that do not activate disease (rice, corn, sorghum, and millet) are separated still further from wheat, rye, and barley in terms of their derivation from the primitive grasses.

Gliadin can be separated electrophoretically into four major fractions that range in molecular weight from 20 to 75 kd and exist as single polypeptide chains. These have been designated α-, β-, γ-, and ω-gliadins,[34] and all

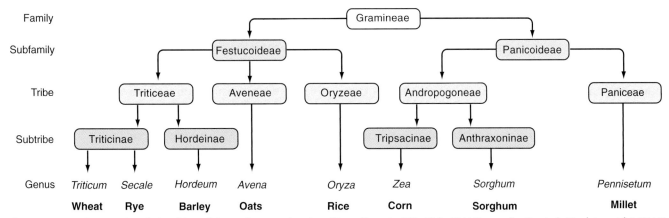

Figure 101–3 Taxonomic relationships of the major cereal grains. (From Kasarda DD, Okita TW, Bernardin JE, et al: Nucleic acid [cDNA] and amino acid sequences of α-type gliadin from wheat [*Triticum aestivum*]. Proc Natl Acad Sci U S A 81:4712, 1984.)

four fractions appear to be toxic to patients with celiac sprue.[35] The complete amino acid sequence of several of the gliadins and related prolamins in grains other than wheat is known.[36] In 2000, Anderson and colleagues[14] identified a partially deamidated peptide, consisting of amino acids 56-75 of α-gliadin as the putative dominant epitope responsible for the T cell response in celiac sprue. Vader and associates,[37] however, demonstrated that the complexity and diversity of the gliadin-specific T cell response is far greater than was previously appreciated and that children and adults with celiac sprue can respond to a diverse repertoire of native gluten peptides and non-deaminated peptides. The authors hypothesized that celiac sprue results from a multistep process of intermolecular and intramolecular epitope spreading. With disease progression, an increased release of intracellular tTG may lead to a progressive deamidation of glutens and an enhancement of a demonstrated gliadin-specific response.

In organ cultures, a synthetic peptide corresponding to amino acids 31-49 of α-gliadin has been shown to be toxic to intestinal mucosa and to induce epithelial lesions via recruitment of IELs. Peptide 31-49 does not activate intestinal CD4+ T cells from patients with celiac sprue in vitro, but a related peptide corresponding to amino acids 31-43 is capable of activating peripheral CD4+ T cells isolated from patients with celiac sprue and of inducing epithelial cell apoptosis and activating macrophages, thereby indicating a likely role for innate immune responses in disease pathogenesis.[38] Gianfrani and colleagues[39] reported that the α-gliadin-derived peptide corresponding to amino acids 123-132 is recognized by CD8+ T lymphocytes from patients with celiac sprue and is associated with cytotoxic activity. By contrast, another peptide corresponding to amino acids 57-68 appears to function in adaptive immunity via stimulation of intestinal T cells in vivo but does not appear to be directly toxic to the intestinal mucosa of patients in vitro.[37]

It also is possible that immunologic similarities between gliadin protein motifs and enteric pathogens may be involved in the pathogenesis of an immunologic response to gluten antigens. This hypothesis was supported by a study in which analysis of α-gliadin demonstrated an amino acid region that was homologous to the 54-kd E1b protein coat of adenovirus 12, suggesting that exposure to the virus in a susceptible person could be involved in celiac sprue pathogenesis.[40] Although patients with celiac sprue have been reported to have a significantly higher prevalence of past adenovirus 12 infection than do control subjects,[41] the role of adenovirus molecular mimicry in the pathogenesis of celiac sprue has not been confirmed. Nieuwenhuizen and coworkers[42] showed some similarities with peptides from *Candida albicans* but have not provided evidence to support the role of this infectious agent in celiac sprue.

The reason why oats may be tolerated by patients with celiac sprue is not obvious because the prolamin fraction of oats contains the same amino acid sequences (QQQPF)* that in wheat gliadin have been shown to be toxic.[43] A possible explanation for this paradox is that oats contain a relatively smaller proportion of this toxic prolamin moiety than do other gluten-containing cereals. Although a feature common to prolamins of wheat, rye, and barley is a high content of glutamine (>30%) and proline (>15%), the prolamins of oats have an intermediate content of these amino acids, and the nontoxic prolamins of rice, corn, and millet have an even lower content of them.[44] This hypothesis is supported by collectively considering the studies on oat challenge in patients with celiac sprue; these studies suggest that tolerance to oats depends at least in part on the total amount consumed.[45] Daily oats consumption of less than 40 to 60 g/day by patients whose celiac sprue is in remission appears to be well tolerated. The data on oats also highlight the important relationship between the amount of gluten consumed and the severity of disease manifestation. A 5- to 10-fold higher incidence of overt celiac sprue in children from Sweden compared with Denmark (two populations with similar genetic backgrounds) has long been cited as evidence of the importance of environmental over genetic factors in celiac sprue pathogenesis. Subsequent studies found as much as a 40-fold difference in the gliadin concentration of Swedish compared with Danish infant formula.[22] This finding suggests that early exposure of the immature immune system to significant amounts of gliadin is a prominent cofactor for the development of overt celiac sprue, possibly by skewing the intestinal immune response to gliadin toward a T helper 1 (Th1) T cell response.

GENETIC FACTORS

Family studies demonstrating frequent intrafamilial occurrence of celiac sprue reflect the importance of genetic factors in its pathogenesis.[44] Concordance for celiac sprue in first-degree relatives ranges between 8% and 18% and reaches 70% in monozygotic twins.[46] Our understanding of the nature of this genetic predisposition began with the significant observation by Howell and coworkers[10] that celiac sprue was associated with specific HLA-DQ2 haplotypes. HLA class II molecules are glycosylated transmembrane heterodimers (α and β chains) that are organized into three related subregions—DQ, DR, and DP—and encoded within the HLA class II region of the major histocompatibility complex on chromosome 6p. The HLA-DQ (α1*501,β1*02) heterodimer, known as *HLA-DQ2*, is found in 95% of patients (compared with 30% of controls) and the related DQ (α1*0301,β1*0302) heterodimer, known as *HLA-DQ8*, is found in most of the remaining patients with celiac sprue. An important link to a genetic predisposition was provided by the isolation of gliadin-specific HLA-DQ2-restricted T cell clones from celiac sprue mucosa.[11] A further advance was the finding that the HLA-DQ2 heterodimer is encoded in either *cis* or *trans*, explaining its association with HLA-DR3 or HLA-DR5/7, respectively.[47] The α and β chains of the DQ2 heterodimer are encoded by two alleles: DQ α1* 0501 and DQ β1* 0201. The two alleles may be inherited in *cis* from one parent on the DQ2-DR3 haplotype or in *trans* from both parents on the DQ2-DR5 and DQ2-DR7 haplotypes. A gene is encoded in *cis* if the alleles that encode the gene

---

*Q, glutamine; P, proline; F, phenylalanine.

are inherited on the same strand of DNA and *trans* if one allele is inherited on one strand of DNA and the other gene is inherited from a complementary strand of DNA. It is now known that after gluten is absorbed, lamina propria antigen-presenting cells (probably dendritic cells) that express HLA-DQ2 or HLA-DQ8 present gliadin peptides on their α/β heterodimer antigen-presenting grooves to sensitized T lymphocytes expressing the α/β T cell receptor (TCR). These lymphocytes then activate B lymphocytes to generate immunoglobulins and other T lymphocytes to secrete cytokines, predominantly interferon (IFN)-γ, and to a lesser degree, IL-4, IL-5, IL-6, IL-10,

tumor necrosis factor (TNF)-α, and transforming growth factor (TGF)-β.[48] These cytokines not only damage enterocytes but also induce expression of aberrant HLA class II cell-surface antigens on the luminal surface of enterocytes, possibly facilitating additional direct antigen presentation by these cells to the sensitized lymphocytes (Fig. 101–4).

Only a few individuals who express DQ2 actually develop celiac sprue. In fact, HLA-DQ2 is common in Europeans and is expressed in 25% to 30% of the normal population. The search for other HLA genes has been complicated by the *strong linkage disequilibrium*, or *non-*

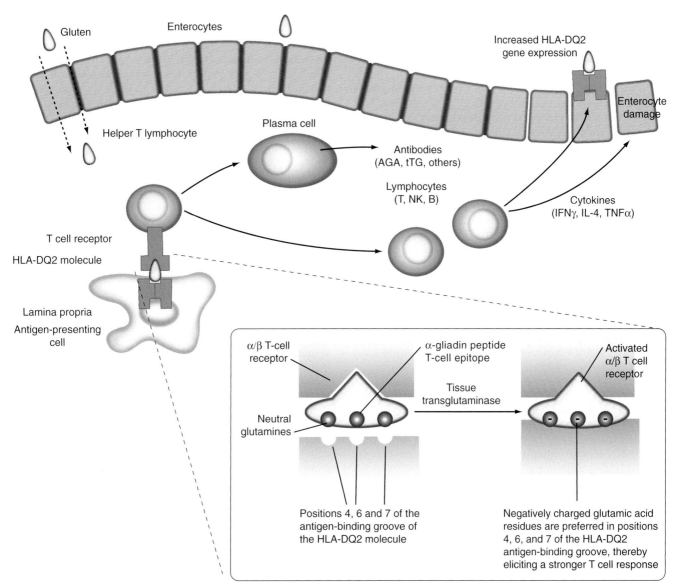

Figure 101–4 Proposed pathogenesis of celiac sprue. Gluten is absorbed into the lamina propria and presented in conjunction with HLA-DQ2 (or DQ8) cell-surface antigens by antigen-presenting cells, probably dendritic cells, to sensitized T lymphocytes expressing the α/β T cell receptor (afferent limb). Tissue transglutaminase deamidates gliadin peptides, generating acidic negatively charged glutamic acid residues from neutral glutamines (*insert*). Because negatively charged residues are preferred in positions 4, 6, and 7 of the antigen-binding groove of HLA-DQ2, deamidated gliadin elicits stronger T-lymphocyte responses. These lymphocytes then activate other lymphocytes to generate immune products (cytokines) that damage the enterocytes, resulting in villus atrophy (efferent limb). Induction of aberrant HLA class II cell-surface antigens on the enterocytes may permit additional gluten antigen presentation by these cells to the sensitized lymphocytes. AGA, antigliadin antibody; HLA, human leukocyte antigen; IFN-γ, interferon gamma; IL-4, interleukin-4; NK, natural killer; TNF-α, tumor necrosis factor alpha; tTG, tissue transglutaminase.

random association, within the HLA region, a term implying the tendency of genes to be inherited as a group. In patients with DR3, an as-yet-unidentified gene in the region telomeric to the HLA-F locus modifies susceptibility to celiac sprue and diabetes type 1.[49] Studies of Irish celiac sprue patients have indicated an additional predisposing role for TNF genes, an association independent of DQ2 that has been demonstrated using a microsatellite polymorphism of the TNF-α gene promoter.[50] Although a Finnish study failed to reproduce the finding of a DQ2-independent association of TNF microsatellites,[51] these discrepant results may relate to population differences.

Sibling studies indicate that the HLA region contributes approximately 35% to 40% to familial aggregation, thus leaving a potential important role for non-HLA-linked genes.[52] Whereas genome searches have failed to identify any new susceptibility locus unambiguously, the collaborative effort of the European Genetics Cluster (a research partnership) clearly has established evidence for a risk factor located in the 5q31-33 region, which encompasses many candidate susceptibility genes.[53] It is reasonable to assume that some of these unidentified genes control the immune response; several studies of candidate genes suggest the role of the gene encoding CTLA-4 (2q33), a negative regulator of the immune response.[54] Other disease associations have been reported with chromosome 15q26, which contains a diabetes type 1 susceptibility locus with chromosome 5q and possibly 11q.[55] Another major site has also been found on chromosome 6p, although the gene has not been identified yet.[55]

IMMUNE FACTORS

The evidence is substantial implicating both humoral- and cell-mediated immune responses to gliadin and related prolamins in the pathogenesis of celiac sprue. There is a twofold to sixfold increase in the numbers of immunoglobulin-producing B cells in the lamina propria of the small intestine in untreated celiac sprue patients.[28] In addition, IgA and IgG serum antibodies to purified gliadin and to all major fractions of gliadin can be detected in the sera of most patients with untreated celiac sprue, in some patients with treated celiac sprue, and in some patients with subclinical disease.[56] Antigliadin antibodies (AGAs), however, do not appear to be essential for the pathogenesis of celiac sprue and may simply reflect a nonspecific response to the passage of incompletely digested antigenic gluten proteins across an abnormally permeable intestinal epithelium. Furthermore, many normal individuals have increased IgA, IgG antigliadin levels or both.[57] Many individuals with celiac sprue have increased levels of serum antibodies against other food proteins such as β-lactoglobulin, casein, and ovalbumin.[58] It is unclear whether this reflects a general aberrant immune responsiveness to food antigens in patients with celiac sprue or enhanced systemic exposure to these proteins because of increased small intestinal permeability. Gluten can be absorbed across normal epithelium, but it is unclear if this results in immune tolerance in individuals who are not genetically predisposed to develop celiac sprue.

The identification of more specific autoantibody responses has altered our understanding of the pathogenesis of celiac sprue. IgA antibodies to endomysium, a connective tissue structure surrounding smooth muscle, are virtually pathognomonic for celiac sprue and are rarely found in the absence of disease.[59] It is now known that the target autoantigen contained within the endomysium is the enzyme tTG.[12] Gliadin is a preferred substrate for this ubiquitous calcium-dependent intracellular enzyme, and it has been shown that tTG deamidates key neutral glutamine residues in gliadin and converts them into negatively charged glutamic acid residues, which are preferred in positions 4, 6, and 7 of the nonapeptide antigen-binding groove of the HLA-DQ2 heterodimer (see Fig 101–4),[13,60] thereby facilitating antigen presentation. Thus, tTG-mediated modification of gliadin plays a pivotal role in eliciting a stronger proliferative response by gliadin specific T cell clones, or, stated differently, tTG makes gliadin "tastier" for the T cells. With gliadin serving as glutamine donor, tTG also can generate additional novel antigenic epitopes by crosslinking molecules of the extracellular matrix with gliadin or with tTG-gliadin complexes.[61] As evidence of the fundamental role of tTG in celiac sprue pathogenesis, one of the dominant epitopes responsible for the T cell response contains a deamidated glutamine residue (Q65E) of α-gliadin.[14] It also has been observed that tTG is necessary for the bioactivation of TGF-β that is required for epithelial differentiation. In a T 84-crypt epithelial cell culture system, autoantibodies to tTG blocked TGF-β-mediated enterocyte differentiation,[62] a finding that suggests release of tTG from cells during inflammation may not only potentiate gliadin presentation by HLA-DQ2 and HLA-DQ8 but that local production of autoantibodies to tTG may contribute to the lack of epithelial differentiation observed in the active celiac lesion.

Given the marked infiltration of lymphocytes into the small intestinal mucosal epithelium and lamina propria in active disease, it is not surprising that cell-mediated immune responses are also important in the pathogenesis of celiac sprue. Recent work supports an interplay between adaptive immunity, characterized by a specific and memory T cell response to gluten peptides, and innate immunity, involving less specific mechanisms. Many of the T cells in the small intestine mucosa are activated in untreated celiac sprue and release potent proinflammatory mediators such as IFN-γ, TNF-α, IL-2, IL-6, and TGF-β.[48] Activated T lymphocytes, most of which are CD4+ cells , are abundant in the lamina propria of the small intestine.[63] In contrast, IELs, which are present in large numbers in untreated celiac sprue, are CD8+ T cells.[64] The increased expression of CD45RO on T cells in the mucosa of untreated patients supports the theory that there is an influx of primed memory cells.[65] In healthy individuals, more than 90% of IELs express the α/β TCR, whereas expression of the γ/δ TCR by IELs in patients with untreated celiac sprue is increased as much as sixfold (to 35%) and is considered a hallmark of the disease.[66] These primitive lymphocytes recognize bacterial nonpeptide antigens and unprocessed stress-related proteins. They appear to act as mucosal guardians and may protect the intestinal mucosa from chronic exposure to dietary gluten in gluten-tolerant individuals by secreting IL-4, which dampens T_H1 in favor of T_H2 reactivity.[67] Their continuous presence in patients on a gluten-free diet may indicate inadvertent gluten ingestion. Patients with refractory sprue also have aberrant IELs with restricted γ/δ TCR gene rearrangements, and the pathogenetic role of these lymphocytes, compared with lamina propria lymphocytes, continues to evolve (see "Refractory Sprue").[68]

Work by the French Coeliac Disease Study Group[15] and by Maiuri and colleagues[69] suggests that IL-15 plays a key role in bridging the innate and adaptive immune responses in celiac sprue pathogenesis. This enterocyte- and macrophage-derived proinflammatory cytokine is increased massively in the mucosa of patients with active celiac sprue and refractory sprue. Although the mechanisms that lead to its overproduction remain unknown, IL-15 regulates IEL homeostasis by promoting migration, preventing apoptosis, and enhancing the capacity of dendritic cells to function as the antigen-presenting cells.[69] In response to gliadin peptides, IL-15 triggers an adaptive $CD4^+$ T cell response in the lamina propria and also is capable of inducing direct epithelial cell injury by inducing IEL secretion of IFN-γ.[16]

CLINICAL FEATURES

Samuel Gee's classic description, with its evocative account, was concerned largely with the gross manifestations of the disorder.[5] This florid presentation, however, is now unusual in the Western world, constituting only the extreme tip of the celiac iceberg. Although some patients still present with severe illness, most have few, subtle, or no symptoms at diagnosis. Such cases may be identified by screening relatives of patients during research studies or from screening patients with associated disorders, such as diabetes mellitus, hypothyroidism, or Down syndrome. Incidental hematologic or biochemical abnormalities may also lead to a diagnosis of celiac sprue.

CHILDHOOD

The classic presentation of celiac sprue in infancy is not easily missed. The typical history is of steatorrhea with or without vomiting and occasional cramping abdominal pain that may occur anytime after weaning when cereals are introduced into the diet, but especially in the first and second years of life. Classically, the child fails to thrive, is apathetic and irritable, and has muscle wasting, hypotonia, and abdominal distention. Watery diarrhea or occasionally constipation may be reported. Diagnosis is more difficult when gastrointestinal features are less prominent, and the possibility of gluten sensitivity should be considered in all children of relevant ethnic backgrounds who present with short stature or failure to thrive, even when there are no other symptoms to suggest an enteropathy. Once a gluten-free diet is commenced, catch-up growth is well documented.[70] Nutritional deficiencies, particularly anemia, are another common mode of presentation, especially in older children. With earlier diagnosis, clinical rickets now is an

uncommon complication but is seen occasionally, especially among Asian children with untreated celiac sprue. Many childhood patients enjoy a temporary, spontaneous remission of symptoms during adolescence, and it is unusual for celiac sprue to present during the teens.

Considerable debate continues as to why celiac sprue tends to be diagnosed later and with milder signs and symptoms than in the past. Early work suggested that breast-feeding could significantly delay the onset of symptoms[71]; however, more recent work found that neither breast-feeding, age at introduction of cow's milk products, or gluten consumption had any significant bearing on the onset of symptoms.[72] The impact of changes in infant feeding practices remains unclear, and the varying effect of gluten on the immature gastrointestinal system also may be important.

ADULTHOOD

In the past, celiac sprue was perceived to be a pediatric disorder, but the diagnosis now is being made increasingly in adult life; currently, the mean age at presentation is approximately 45 years of age. Furthermore, manifesting clinical symptoms also have changed during the past 50 years. Diarrhea is now reported less frequently, and many patients now present with higher body mass indices and even with obesity. The unmasking of asymptomatic disease by surgery that induces rapid gastric emptying (e.g., gastric resection, pyloroplasty) or the finding of the typical lesion in asymptomatic relatives of celiac sprue patients suggests that adults may have silent celiac sprue for some time. A proportion of these adult patients are of short stature or give a history consistent with unrecognized gluten-sensitive enteropathy in childhood. In many, however, there is nothing to suggest previous disease, and it is possible that celiac sprue may develop for the first time in adult life. Celiac sprue is being diagnosed increasingly in later life now, with approximately 25% of cases diagnosed in patients older than 60 years.[73]

GASTROINTESTINAL

The clinical manifestations of celiac sprue vary tremendously from patient to patient. Because most of the symptoms result from intestinal malabsorption, they are not specific for celiac sprue and resemble those seen in other malabsorptive disorders. Many adults present with gastrointestinal symptoms including diarrhea, steatorrhea, flatulence, and weight loss similar to those seen in childhood celiac sprue. Diarrhea often is episodic rather than continuous. Nocturnal or early morning diarrhea is common. Patients with extensive intestinal involvement may have more than 10 stools per day. Because of their high fat content, the stools of patients with celiac sprue may be light tan or grayish and greasy in appearance, with a tendency to float and to be difficult to flush from the toilet bowl; this pallor of the stools is reflected in the ancient Latin term *diarrhea alba*, *alba* meaning white. Steatorrhea often is absent in patients with disease limited to the proximal small intestine.

Several factors contribute to the diarrhea associated with celiac sprue. The stool volume and osmotic load delivered to the colon are increased by the malabsorption of fat,[74] carbohydrate, protein, electrolytes, and other nutrients. In addition, the delivery of excessive dietary fat into the large bowel results in the production by bacteria of hydroxy fatty acids, which are potent cathartics. Electrolytes actually are secreted into, rather than absorbed from, the lumen of the severely damaged upper small intestine in symptomatic patients. This secretion further increases luminal fluid in an intestine with already compromised absorptive capacity. There also is evidence that secretin and cholecystokinin release in response to a meal are impaired in celiac sprue, diminishing delivery of bile and pancreatic secretions into the gut lumen and possibly compromising intraluminal digestion.[75] Alterations in the secretion of other gut peptides have been noted and may contribute to the observed diarrhea. Finally, if the disease extends to and involves the ileum, patients may experience the direct cathartic action of malabsorbed bile salts on the colon.[74]

The amount of weight loss in a patient with celiac sprue depends on the severity and extent of the intestinal lesion and on the ability of the patient to compensate for the malabsorption by increasing dietary intake. Some celiac sprue patients with substantial malabsorption have enormous appetites and lose little or no weight. Rarely, in severe disease, anorexia may develop with associated rapid and severe weight loss. In such debilitated patients, some of the weight loss may be masked by fluid retention caused by hypoproteinemia. Malaise, lassitude, and fatigue also are common even when anemia is absent. Occasionally, severe hypokalemia resulting from the loss of potassium in the stool may cause severe muscle weakness.

Vague abdominal discomfort and especially abdominal bloating are extremely common and may lead to a mistaken diagnosis of irritable bowel syndrome (IBS). Because of the difficulty in distinguishing celiac sprue with mild gastrointestinal manifestations from symptoms of IBS, serologic testing by IgA endomysial antibodies (EMAs) or IgA tTG should be considered in patients with symptoms suggestive of diarrhea-predominant IBS. In a U.K. study, Sanders and colleagues[76] evaluated 300 consecutive new patients who fulfilled Rome II criteria for IBS and 300 healthy age- and sex-matched controls for celiac sprue using IgA AGA, IgG AGA, and EMA; 2 matched controls (0.7%) (both EMA positive) and 14 IBS patients (4.6%) had celiac sprue (11 EMA positive, three EMA negative; $P = 0.004$; odds ratio = 7.0 [95% confidence interval [CI], 1.7-28.0]). Severe abdominal pain may occur but is uncharacteristic in uncomplicated celiac sprue; its occurrence may suggest the presence of intestinal lymphoma. Abdominal distention with excessive amounts of malodorous flatus is a common complaint. Nausea and vomiting are uncommon in uncomplicated celiac sprue. Recurrent severe aphthous stomatitis affects a significant proportion of celiac patients and may be their sole presenting complaint. It is important to exclude celiac sprue in cases of recurrent aphthous stomatitis because a significant proportion of these patients respond to dietary treatment.[77]

EXTRAINTESTINAL

As patients with celiac sprue get older, they tend to present with complaints not directly referable to the gastrointestinal tract. These extraintestinal symptoms and clinical findings often result from nutrient malabsorption and may involve virtually all organ systems (Table 101–1). Extraintestinal features, including anemia, osteopenia, neurologic symptoms, and menstrual abnor-

Table 101–1   Extraintestinal Manifestations of Celiac Sprue

Organ System	Manifestation	Probable Cause(s)
Hematopoietic	Anemia	Iron, folate, vitamin B_{12}, or pyridoxine deficiency
	Hemorrhage	Vitamin K deficiency; rarely, thrombocytopenia due to folate deficiency
	Thrombocytosis, Howell-Jolly bodies	Hyposplenism
Skeletal	Osteopenia	Malabsorption of calcium and vitamin D
	Pathologic fractures	Osteopenia
	Osteoarthropathy	Unknown
Muscular	Atrophy	Malnutrition due to malabsorption
	Tetany	Calcium, vitamin D, and/or magnesium malabsorption
	Weakness	Generalized muscle atrophy, hypokalemia
Hepatic	Elevated liver enzymes	Unknown
Nervous	Peripheral neuropathy	Vitamin deficiencies such as vitamin B_{12} and thiamine
	Ataxia	Cerebellar and posterior column damage
	Demyelinating central nervous system lesions	Unknown
	Seizures	Unknown
Endocrine	Secondary hyperparathyroidism	Calcium/vitamin D malabsorption causing hypocalcemia
	Amenorrhea, infertility, impotence	Malnutrition, hypothalamic-pituitary dysfunction
Integument	Follicular hyperkeratosis and dermatitis	Vitamin A malabsorption, vitamin B complex malabsorption
	Petechiae and ecchymoses	Vitamin K deficiency; rarely, thrombocytopenia
	Edema	Hypoproteinemia
	Dermatitis herpetiformis	Unknown

Modified from Trier JS: Celiac sprue and refractory sprue. In Feldman M, Scharschmidt BF, Sleisenger MH (eds): Gastrointestinal and Liver Disease, 6th ed. Philadelphia, WB Saunders, 1997, p 1557.

malities, often prove more distressing to the patient than do the gastrointestinal symptoms.

Anemia is a common manifestation in both children and adults with celiac sprue and usually is caused by impaired iron or folate absorption from the proximal intestine; in severe disease with ileal involvement, vitamin B_{12} absorption also is impaired. Patients with extensive disease may bleed into the skin or mucous membranes or may develop hematuria, epistaxis, vaginal or gastrointestinal bleeding. Bleeding may aggravate pre-existing anemia and most often is caused by a coagulopathy resulting from impaired intestinal absorption of fat-soluble vitamin K. Evidence of hyposplenism of unknown cause, with thrombocytosis, deformed erythrocytes, and splenic atrophy, occurs in up to 50% of adults with celiac sprue but only rarely in children.[78] In most patients, evidence of hyposplenism disappears with elimination of gluten from the diet.[78]

Osteopenia is the most common complication of celiac sprue, and its prevalence increases with age at diagnosis. More than 70% of patients with untreated celiac sprue have osteopenia,[79] and osteoporosis occurs in more than one quarter of all celiac sprue patients.[80] Osteopenia develops as a result of impaired calcium absorption (secondary to defective calcium transport by the diseased small intestine), vitamin D deficiency (caused by impaired absorption of this fat-soluble vitamin), and binding of intraluminal calcium and magnesium to unabsorbed dietary fatty acids (forming insoluble soaps, which are then excreted in the feces). Patients may present with bone pain, especially of the lower back, rib cage, and pelvis. Calcium and magnesium depletion may cause paresthesias, muscle cramps, and even frank tetany. With prolonged calcium malabsorption, patients may develop secondary hyperparathyroidism resulting in mobilization of calcium from the bones, further exacerbating the osteopenia. Osteopenia is less common in patients with silent celiac sprue, where prevalence rates between 30% and 40% have been reported.[81] Whereas bone disease generally is more severe among patients with symptomatic disease, severe osteopenia has been reported in up to one third of symptom-free adults diagnosed with celiac sprue during childhood who resumed a normal diet during adolescence.[82] A key unanswered question is the functional consequence of osteopenia. An increased risk of fractures was observed in patients with overt celiac sprue in one study[81] but not in another.[83] The fracture risk among patients with silent celiac also remains unclear.

Neurologic symptoms caused by lesions of the central or peripheral nervous system occasionally occur in patients with severe disease and are poorly understood. Ataxia is the commonest neurologic manifestation of celiac sprue, and progressive gait and limb ataxia may be the sole manifestations of disease in some patients. These abnormalities are believed to result from immunologic damage to the cerebellum, posterior columns of the spinal cord, and peripheral nerves, and the term *gluten ataxia* has been proposed to describe this disorder.[84] Muscle weakness and paresthesias with sensory loss also are encountered occasionally, and pathologic evidence of peripheral neuropathy and patchy demyelinization of the spinal cord, cerebellar atrophy, and capillary proliferation suggestive of Wernicke's encephalopathy have been described rarely. Although potential causative roles for specific vitamin deficiencies (including vitamin B_{12}, thiamine, riboflavin, and pyridoxine) have not been established, neurologic symptoms have been reported to improve in some patients receiving multivitamins, including vitamins A, B, and E, or calcium. Night blindness is a clear indication for vitamin A therapy. Peripheral neuropathy and ataxia, however, often appear unrelated to specific vitamin deficiency states and usually do not respond to gluten withdrawal.[85] The associations of celiac sprue and epilepsy, frequently complex partial seizures, and bilateral parieto-occipital cerebral calcification are well recognized.[86] In one series, the epilepsy was reported in approximately 5% of children and young adults with celiac sprue.[87] The cause of the epilepsy remains unclear, and the prognosis appears to depend on how early in the course of the disease a gluten-free diet is started. Although most patients with celiac sprue do not appear psychologically abnormal, many affected subjects report a striking improvement in mood after commencing a gluten-free diet.[88]

Gynecologic and obstetric problems are common in women with untreated celiac sprue.[89] Amenorrhea occurs in one third of women of childbearing age, and there frequently is a delayed menarche (typically by 1 year) in untreated subjects. Women with untreated celiac sprue may present with infertility, and it is common for infertile women with celiac sprue to become pregnant shortly after commencing a gluten-free diet.[90] A high prevalence of silent celiac sprue has been reported in women with recurrent spontaneous abortions, intrauterine fetal growth retardation, and unfavorable outcome of pregnancy, underlining the need to test for celiac sprue in these situations.[91] Infertility secondary to impotence or an abnormally low sperm count often is found in adult men with untreated celiac sprue.[92] Although malnutrition related to malabsorption may contribute to male infertility, abnormalities in hypothalamic-pituitary regulation of gonadal function and gonadal androgen resistance that disappears on gluten withdrawal also have been incriminated.[92]

PHYSICAL EXAMINATION

Physical findings, like symptoms, vary considerably among patients with celiac sprue. Patients with mild disease frequently have a completely normal physical examination. In more severe disease, physical abnormalities usually result from malabsorption and therefore are not specific for celiac sprue. Growth retardation commonly occurs in children, but when they commence a gluten-free diet before puberty, a compensatory growth spurt occurs so the effect on adult height potentially can be minimized. Persons with celiac sprue are, on average, 3 inches shorter than their peers. Tall patients are seen, however, and a height of more than 6 feet does not preclude the diagnosis. In patients with severe celiac sprue, emaciation with evidence of recent weight loss, including loose skin folds and muscle wasting, may be prominent. It is common for adults with celiac sprue to experience a weight gain of more than 6 kg following institution of a gluten-free diet. Clubbing of the fingers occurs occasionally, and koilonychia may be associated with long-standing iron deficiency anemia. There may be pitting edema of the lower extremities secondary to hypoproteinemia. Hypotension may be related to fluid and electrolyte depletion, and the skin may be dry with poor turgor if there is dehydration. Occasionally a low-grade fever associated with anemia is found in untreated celiac sprue, but this finding may indicate a concurrent complication, such as infection or malignancy, particularly lymphoma. Increased skin pigmentation may be obvious in severely ill patients. In addition to dermatitis herpetiformis (DH) (see later), other dermatologic findings may include spontaneous ecchymoses related to hypoprothrombinemia, hyperkeratosis follicularis caused by vitamin A deficiency, and pallor caused by anemia.

Examination of the mouth may show aphthous stomatitis, angular cheilosis, and glossitis with decreased papillation of the tongue. Dental enamel defects are common.[93] The abdomen may be protuberant and tympanic with a characteristic doughy consistency owing to distention of intestinal loops with fluid and gas. Hepatomegaly and abdominal tenderness are uncommon, but ascites may be detected in patients with significant hypoproteinemia. Peripheral lymphadenopathy is unusual in the absence of complicating lymphoma.

The extremities may reveal loss of various sensory modalities, including light touch, vibration, and position, usually resulting from peripheral neuropathy and, rarely, demyelinating spinal cord lesions. If neuropathy is severe, deep tendon reflexes are diminished or even absent. Hyperpathia may be present. A positive Chvostek's or Trousseau's sign may be elicited in patients with severe calcium or magnesium depletion. In such individuals, bone tenderness related to osteopenia may be elicited, especially if collapsed vertebrae or other fractures are present.

DIAGNOSTIC STUDIES

The laboratory findings in celiac sprue, like the symptoms and signs, vary with the extent and severity of the intestinal lesion. Serum IgA EMA or tTG antibody and small bowel biopsy are the most accurate diagnostic tests for celiac sprue. Stool studies, hematologic and biochemical tests, and radiologic studies may be abnormal but seldom provide a specific diagnosis because similar abnormalities are often seen in patients with other diseases that produce intestinal malabsorption (see Chapter 98).

STOOL EXAMINATION

If malabsorption is sufficient to produce significant steatorrhea, a watery or bulky, semi-formed, light tan or grayish, malodorous greasy-appearing stool results. Microscopic evaluation of the fat content of a stool suspension stained with Sudan III or IV after hydrolysis with glacial acetic acid and heat is a helpful test. To document steatorrhea unequivocally, the amount of fat in a 3-day collection of stool may be determined quantitatively, using the reliable van de Kamer chemical method.

HEMATOLOGY AND BIOCHEMISTRY TESTS

A variety of hematologic and biochemical abnormalities may be found in individuals with untreated celiac sprue, including deficiencies of iron, folic acid, and vitamin D. These abnormalities reflect nutritional deficiency states secondary to enteropathy-induced malabsorption. Iron deficiency anemia is common in both children and adults with celiac sprue, and combined iron and folate deficiency is characteristic, especially in children. With the exception of pregnancy, severe anemia is uncommon, usually develops with extensive disease, and should raise the suspicion of a complication such as lymphoma. The peripheral blood film may reveal target cells, siderocytes, Heinz bodies, and crenated red blood cells. Howell-Jolly bodies, which are suggestive of splenic atrophy, frequently are seen.[78] Although relevant to patient evaluation and management, none of these hematologic or biochemical tests is sufficiently sensitive or specific to serve as useful screening or diagnostic tools.[94] Similarly, although an oral D-xylose test and fecal fat evaluation also may be abnormal in untreated celiac sprue, they, too, do not provide a specific diagnosis and no longer have a place as routine investigations in suspected celiac sprue. Furthermore, the absorption and urinary excretion of D-xylose can be normal in up to 20% of patients with untreated celiac sprue, whereas a 3-day fecal fat estimation is a relatively crude test that is subject to errors because of varying dietary fat intake and incomplete stool collection. Chronically elevated serum aminotransferase levels in the range of 1.5 to twice normal values have been reported in 9% to 40% of patients with untreated celiac sprue, and in most patients, the elevated levels resolve on a gluten-free diet.

SEROLOGY

In current clinical practice, there are many serologic studies available to aid in the diagnosis of celiac sprue; however, the most powerful and clinically useful are the IgA EMA and IgA tTG assays. IgA EMA and IgA tTG are based on the target antigen tTG, whereas IgA and IgG AGAs are based on the target antigen gliadin.[1] The approximate sensitivity and specificity of these serum antibody tests are outlined in Table 101–2. A working group of 13 European laboratories has attempted to improve standardization by establishing standard curves on reference sera and protocols for calibration of quality controls. This collaboration has reported that IgA EMA has a sensitivity of 90%, specificity of 99%, and reproducibility of 93% and currently remains the gold standard. IgA antihuman tTG is slightly less reliable (sensitivity 93%, specificity 95%, reproducibility 83%), and the anti-IgG AGA and IgA AGA are the least reliable.[95] In addition to laboratory variation, the reported sensitivity and specificity of these tests depend on the prevalence of the disease in the tested population and the severity of the disease. In one study of 101 patients with biopsy-proved celiac sprue, the sensitivity of IgA EMA among patients with total villus atrophy was 100% compared with only 31% in those with partial villus atrophy. [96]

Table 101–2   Sensitivity, Specificity, and Positive and Negative Predictive Values of Serologic Tests for Untreated Celiac Sprue

Serologic Test	Sensitivity,* %	Specificity,* %	Positive Predictive Value, %	Negative Predictive Value, %
IgA antiendomysial antibody				
Indirect immunofluorescence assay	85-98	97-100	98-100	80-95
ELISA guinea pig tissue transglutaminase†	95-98	94-95	91-95	96-98
ELISA human tissue transglutaminase‡	95-100	97-100	80-95	100
IgA antigliadin antibodies	75-90	82-95	28-100	65-100
IgG antigliadin antibodies	69-85	73-90	20-95	41-88

*Wide variations in test sensitivity and specificity rates are reported among different laboratories.[95]
†The guinea pig tissue transglutaminase antibodies data are based on two large studies.[100,101]
‡The human tissue transglutaminase antibodies data are based on two large studies.[102,103]
ELISA, enzyme-linked immunosorbent assay.

IgA Endomysial Antibody

Serum IgA EMA binds to connective tissue (endomysium), surrounding smooth muscle cells, producing a characteristic staining pattern that is visualized by indirect immunofluorescence.[59] As mentioned earlier, the target antigen has been identified as tTG. Frozen sections of monkey esophagus initially were used for the assay, but currently, most laboratories use sections of human umbilical cord, which are more readily available.[97] The test result is reported simply as positive or negative because even low titers of serum IgA EMA are highly specific for celiac sprue. IgA EMA has a sensitivity of 90% or greater and a specificity approaching 100% in untreated celiac sprue.[59,98] Antibody levels fall on a gluten-free diet, with the test often becoming negative in treated patients.[99] The clinical applications of EMA and other serologic tests are discussed in the following sections.

Anti-Tissue Transglutaminase Antibody

The epitope against which EMA is directed has been identified as tTG.[12] An IgA enzyme-linked immunosorbent assay (ELISA) that uses guinea pig tTG now is widely available, less costly, and easier to perform than the immunofluorescence assay used to detect IgA EMA. IgA guinea pig tTG assays are proving to be highly sensitive and specific for the diagnosis of celiac sprue.[100,101] In one study, anti-tTG was present in 98% of patients with biopsy-proven celiac sprue compared with 5% of controls.[100] In another study that included 136 patients with celiac sprue and 207 controls, the sensitivity and specificity of IgA guinea pig tTG were 95% and 94%, respectively[101]; however, IgA guinea pig tTGs are responsible for many false-positive results, particularly in at-risk individuals with autoimmune diseases or liver disease and in patients with other inflammatory bowel diseases.[95] ELISAs are now available using human recombinant tTG, and in several studies these have proved to be more specific than the ELISA using guinea pig tTG.[102,103] In contrast with the false-positive results of IGA guinea pig tTG, a false-positive EMA is highly unlikely and in the setting of a normal biopsy may indicate a future predisposition to development of clinical celiac sprue (i.e., potential celiac sprue). Although it had been hoped that IgG and IgM tTG assays would prove useful in patients with IgA deficiency, they lack sensitivity and specificity.

Antigliadin Antibody

Purified gliadin, a component of the wheat storage protein gluten, is readily available and is used as the antigen for ELISA assays to detect serum AGAs. Although serum IgA and IgG AGA levels frequently are elevated in untreated celiac sprue, and AGA assays have been used for some years as a diagnostic aid, unfortunately these tests have only moderate sensitivity and specificity.[56,94,104] Thus, testing for AGA is no longer recommended as a primary test for untreated celiac disease—IgA EMA or IgA tTG testing is preferable. The sensitivity and specificity of IgA AGA are marginally superior to those of IgG AGA; however, many clinicians test simultaneously for both IgA and IgG AGA, an approach that gives a small incremental increase in sensitivity but reduces specificity further. IgG AGA testing is particularly useful in the 2% of patients with celiac sprue who have IgA deficiency. The positive predictive value of AGA in a general population is relatively poor. In one series, for example, the positive predictive value for IgG AGA corrected for the expected prevalence in the general population was less than 2%.[105] AGA test results are reported as a titer—a high titer of AGA being somewhat more specific for celiac sprue than a low titer—but as mentioned earlier, some normal individuals have high AGA levels.[57]

Clinical Application of Serologic Tests

Clinical applications of serologic tests include evaluation of patients with suspected celiac sprue, monitoring adherence and response to a gluten-free diet, and potentially, screening asymptomatic individuals for the disease.

An approach to diagnosing celiac sprue is outlined in Figure 101–5. When the index of suspicion is low, (i.e., the pretest probability is < 10%), a negative result for either IgA EMA, IgA tTG, or IgA AGA tests has a high negative predictive value and may obviate the need for small bowel biopsy. In this setting, the IgA EMA has the highest diagnostic accuracy but is more expensive and less widely available than the IgA tTG. Falsely negative IgA EMA and IgA tTG test results are more likely to occur in very young children (<2 years of age), those with mild celiac enteropathy, and, of course, in IgA deficiency. The AGA tests have lower diagnostic accuracy and are no longer recommended for initial diagnosis of celiac sprue.[98] Because the specificities of IgA EMA and IgA tTG tests are

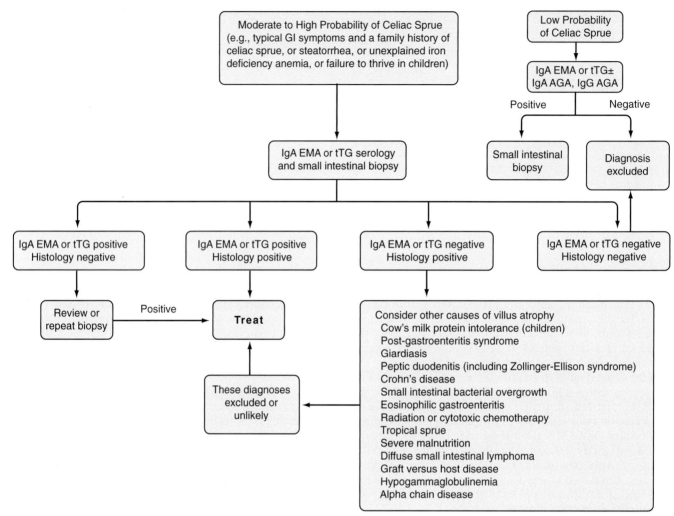

Figure 101–5 Diagnosis of celiac sprue. A false-positive IgA EMA or tTG is rare; a false-negative IgA EMA and tTG can occur in mild enteropathy, in children younger than 2 years of age, and in patients with IgA deficiency. AGA, antigliadin antibody; EMA, endomysial antibody; GI, gastrointestinal; tTG, tissue transglutaminase. (From Farrell RJ, Kelly CP: Diagnosis of celiac sprue. Am J Gastroenterol 96:3237, 2001.)

high, their positive predictive values are high even in low-risk populations.[98,106] In contrast, the specificities of IgA and IgG AGA are lower, and positive results have a low positive predictive value in low-risk populations.[98,106]

When the index of suspicion is moderate to high (i.e., the pretest probability is >10%), the very high specificity of IgA EMA and IgA tTG has led to debate as to whether a positive result in the appropriate clinical setting can be considered diagnostic and eliminate the need for small bowel biopsy. We recommend that both IgA EMA (or anti-tTG) *and* a small bowel biopsy be performed before dietary treatment is recommended. This approach provides the best means of making a definitive diagnosis of celiac sprue at the outset. In contrast, AGA tests are not helpful when there is a moderate or high probability of celiac sprue. A positive or negative result will not alter the need for small bowel biopsy. Because AGA tests have a high false-positive rate, there is no role for a trial of a gluten-free diet for presumed celiac sprue based on the finding of an elevated IgA or IgG AGA level.

Similar to IgA AGA levels,[56] IgA tTG levels decrease in the months following a gluten-free diet and are useful in assessing dietary compliance and excluding inadvertent gluten ingestion.[107] IgA AGA and IgA tTG currently are the most widely used tests for monitoring adherence and response to gluten-free diet among patients whose antibody levels are elevated prior to therapy.[104,107] Hence, a pretreatment antibody level should be determined at the time of diagnosis. Serial samples should be sent to one laboratory for testing to keep interlaboratory assay variation to a minimum. A normal baseline value is typically reached within 3 to 6 months (Fig. 101–6). If the levels do not fall as anticipated, the patient may be continuing to ingest gluten either intentionally or inadvertently; however, minor fluctuations in IgA AGA *and* IgA tTG levels are the norm, and their importance should not be overinterpreted. The decline in IgG AGA after initiating a gluten-free diet is more gradual than the decline of IgA AGA.[56,104]

The advent of highly sensitive and specific serologic tests has changed the epidemiology of celiac sprue radically by revealing the high incidence of silent celiac sprue; this awareness in turn has led to debate on the merits of mass screening. To date, the benefit of screen-

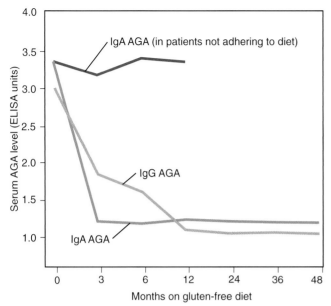

Figure 101–6   Antigliadin antibody (AGA) levels in patients with celiac sprue on a gluten-free diet. Serum AGA levels decrease during treatment with a gluten-free diet and are useful in assessing dietary compliance and excluding inadvertent gluten ingestion. IgA AGA is the most widely used test for monitoring adherence and response to a gluten-free diet among patients with elevated antibody levels before therapy. Hence, a pretreatment level should be determined at the time of diagnosis. A normal baseline value typically is reached within 3 to 6 months. If the levels do not fall as anticipated, the patient may be continuing to ingest gluten either intentionally or inadvertently. The decline in IgG AGA is more gradual than the decline in IgA AGA.[56] ELISA, enzyme-linked immunosorbent assay.

ing for asymptomatic celiac sprue, usually using IgA EMA, has not been demonstrated.[108] The potential advantages of screening for asymptomatic celiac sprue include a reduction in risk for enteropathy-associated T cell lymphoma (EATL), a reversal of unrecognized nutritional deficiency states, resolution of mild or ignored intestinal symptoms, avoidance of other autoimmune disorders, and an improvement in general well-being.[109] All of these hypothetical benefits, however, depend on compliance with a difficult dietary regimen. Asymptomatic individuals may not be motivated sufficiently to adhere to a strict gluten-free diet.[110] There also may be adverse psychological effects when asymptomatic individuals receive a diagnosis of celiac sprue. Furthermore, the natural history of undetected celiac sprue and the consequences of screening and treating silent celiac sprue are unknown. For these reasons, mass screening of asymptomatic individuals generally is not advocated at this time, even in populations in which the prevalence of celiac sprue is high. The current standard of care is a "case-finding" approach, which targets at-risk subjects such as first- and second-degree relatives of patients with celiac sprue; patients with anemia, IBS, diabetes type 1 and autoimmune thyroid, connective tissue, and liver disorders; and subjects with either Down syndrome or selective IgA deficiency, all instances in which the value of serologic testing for celiac disease is accepted widely. Simply by

case finding among at-risk subjects in a primary care setting, Hin and colleagues[111] observed a fourfold increase in the number of celiac sprue diagnoses during a 1-year period. Thus, for now, increased awareness of the typical and atypical presentations of celiac sprue, coupled with a low threshold for serologic testing in at-risk subjects, can uncover a substantial portion of the submerged iceberg.

RADIOLOGY

Barium studies of the small bowel are seldom required in evaluating patients suspected of having untreated celiac sprue. Abnormal roentgen findings include dilation of the small intestine and replacement of the normal delicate feathery mucosal pattern with either marked thickening or complete obliteration of the mucosal folds and straightening of the valvulae conniventes. Even with modern, less viscous barium preparations, flocculation, segmentation, and clumping of contrast occasionally may be seen in severe cases. In patients with mild or moderate disease, the distorted mucosal pattern usually is confined to the proximal small intestine, whereas patients with severe disease have an abnormal mucosal pattern through the entire small intestine. Excessive secretion of fluid into the proximal small intestine, coupled with defective absorption of intraluminal contents, causes dilution of the barium, resulting in decreased contrast in the distal small intestine. Small bowel studies are most useful in suggesting diagnoses other than celiac sprue such as Crohn's disease (terminal ileitis), scleroderma (hypotonicity), bacterial overgrowth (small bowel diverticulosis), or collagenous sprue (bowel wall rigidity). Patients with mild celiac sprue may have a normal small bowel barium study, and these studies are not as sensitive as small intestinal biopsy or serology in providing diagnostic information. Routine small bowel barium studies are unnecessary in most celiac sprue patients and may be considered primarily to exclude complications such as lymphoma, carcinoma, ulcerative jejunoileitis, or stricture. Abdominal computed tomography (CT) or magnetic resonance imaging may provide a diagnostic clue to the presence of celiac sprue or refractory sprue by revealing hyposplenism, ascites, lymphadenopathy, and the presence of cavitating mesenteric lymph nodes. A bone survey may reveal diffuse demineralization with a generalized decrease in bone density. Occasionally, the secondary effects of osteopenic bone disease, including vertebral body compression fractures and pseudofractures (Milkman's lines), are seen.

SMALL INTESTINE BIOPSY

Although the diagnosis of celiac sprue may be suspected on clinical grounds or as a result of abnormal serologic tests, the current recommendation for confirmation of the diagnosis remains biopsy of the small intestine. Since its introduction in the mid-1950s, small intestine biopsy has remained the standard test to establish a diagnosis of celiac sprue. Originally, biopsy specimens were obtained with a suction biopsy tube using a Crosby-Krugler,

Watson, or similar suction biopsy capsule.[9] Capsule biopsy had the advantage of obtaining relatively large distal duodenal or proximal jejunal biopsies, but correct positioning of the capsule was difficult, often time consuming, and required radiologic verification of position and was not always successful. Consequently, the technique has been abandoned in favor of endoscopic biopsy, particularly for older children and adults. Advantages of endoscopic biopsy include the widespread availability and ease of performance of endoscopy and that endoscopic examination of the upper gastrointestinal tract may, in itself be indicated (e.g., in the investigation of iron deficiency anemia).[112] Several biopsies should be obtained from the distal duodenum (second or third parts) to avoid the mucosal architectural distortion produced by Brunner's glands and changes caused by peptic duodenitis, both of which can cause difficulty in histopathologic diagnosis.[9] Although endoscopic biopsies are smaller than capsule biopsies, this problem can be reduced by taking multiple samples. Scalloping or absence of duodenal folds has been noted in some patients with celiac sprue (Fig. 101–7).[113] However, scalloping is not specific for celiac sprue, and other conditions that can cause duodenal scalloping include eosinophilic enteritis, giardiasis, amyloidosis, tropical sprue, and human immunodeficiency virus enteropathy.[114] In addition to scalloping or atrophy of the mucosal folds, the duodenal mucosa in untreated celiac sprue may be marked by multiple fissures. A mosaic appearance also has been described where the fissures circumscribe areas

of mucosal nodularity in a manner similar to the grouting around mosaic tile. These mucosal features (atrophy and scalloping of the folds, fissures, nodularity, or a mosaic appearance) should alert the endoscopist to the need for small intestinal biopsy to evaluate for possible celiac sprue. The mucosa of celiac sprue, however, often appears normal at endoscopy, and absence of the macroscopic features described earlier does not obviate the need for biopsy and histologic examination if celiac sprue is suspected based on clinical grounds or positive serology.

Once the biopsy tissue has been obtained, handling should be minimized to avoid causing artifactual damage. By gently floating the tissue in a small amount of saline, an experienced observer can examine even small endoscopic biopsies using a dissecting microscope or magnifying lens. The villous structure of normal small intestinal mucosa is readily apparent. In severe untreated celiac sprue, a flat, featureless mucosa is recognized easily. The mosaic pattern of less complete forms of villous atrophy also may be recognized, although differentiation from the normal is more difficult and requires some experience.

GLUTEN CHALLENGE

In the past, gluten challenge (discontinuation of treatment with gluten-free diet) followed by repeat biopsy of the small intestine was considered an important confirmatory step in the diagnosis of celiac sprue. In current practice, however, gluten challenge is reserved for the few patients in whom the diagnosis remains in doubt after a period of treatment with a gluten-free diet. Gluten challenge is seldom necessary for patients who present with typical signs or symptoms of celiac sprue and have documented abnormalities consistent with a celiac lesion on small bowel biopsy. A positive IgA EMA or IgA tTG test prior to treatment lends further support to the diagnosis of celiac sprue and makes a gluten challenge superfluous.

A gluten challenge should be considered in patients who began a gluten-free diet empirically without documentation of a characteristic intestinal lesion or the presence of IgA EMA antibody. In such individuals, symptomatic response to a gluten-free diet may indicate the presence of gluten-sensitive enteropathy or simply reflect a change in gastrointestinal function in response to a major dietary change. Individuals with IBS, for example, may experience improvement in symptoms such as abdominal bloating, cramping, or diarrhea after beginning a gluten-free diet. Changes in mild, nonspecific gastrointestinal symptoms are not a reliable method to diagnose celiac sprue and may only reflect the low-residue nature of a gluten-free diet. Gluten challenge also should be considered if a diagnosis of celiac sprue was made during childhood based on small intestinal biopsy abnormalities in the absence of a positive IgA EMA or IgA tTG, because a number of transient childhood enteropathies can mimic the celiac lesion (see later).

Before embarking on a gluten challenge, patients should be evaluated to determine their current response to treatment with a gluten-free diet. This should include a careful nutritional history including their symptomatic responses to previous episodes of inadvertent or pur-

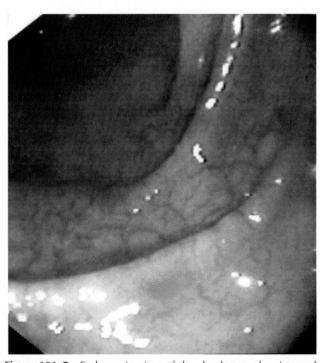

Figure 101–7 Endoscopic view of the duodenum showing scalloping of the folds in a patient with celiac sprue; if present, this finding should alert the endoscopist to the possibility of this diagnosis. Scalloping, however, is not specific for celiac sprue and has been seen in other conditions including eosinophilic gastroenteritis, giardiasis, amyloidosis, tropical sprue, and human immunodeficiency virus enteropathy.

poseful ingestion of gluten-containing foods. Patients who experience substantial symptoms following gluten ingestion are unlikely to tolerate formal gluten challenge and may prefer to remain on a gluten-free diet despite diagnostic uncertainty. Serologic studies should be performed, and a small bowel biopsy should be obtained as a baseline. Gluten challenge must be initiated with caution because occasionally patients are exquisitely sensitive to small amounts of gluten.[115] Other patients may require prolonged challenge before symptoms or significant histologic abnormalities recur. If a small amount of gluten, such as a cracker or one quarter of a slice of bread, is well tolerated, the amount can be doubled every 3 days until the equivalent of at least four slices of bread is ingested daily. The challenge should then be continued for at least 6 weeks or until symptoms redevelop, at which time both serum IgA EMA or IgA tTG and small bowel biopsy should be performed. Ten grams of gluten daily for a period of 6 to 8 weeks are usually sufficient to result in definite histologic deterioration. If serologic tests and small bowel biopsy both are negative, the patient should be monitored for signs and symptoms of celiac sprue on a normal diet for at least 6 months, after which serologic testing should be repeated and rebiopsy considered.

DIFFERENTIAL DIAGNOSIS

The differential diagnosis of celiac sprue includes other causes of malabsorption and gastrointestinal disorders that are associated with changes in proximal small bowel morphology. In both children and adults, the high positive predictive value of a positive IgA EMA or IgA tTG test result means that celiac sprue usually can be diagnosed with a high degree of certainty from the outset, thereby avoiding the need for an in-depth evaluation of alternative diagnoses and for formal gluten challenge. Malabsorption and steatorrhea may result from pancreatic insufficiency, cholestatic liver disease, terminal ileal disease or resection, or small intestinal bacterial overgrowth. In some patients, pancreatic insufficiency or microscopic colitis may be present concurrently with celiac sprue. It is important to exclude this possibility in patients who do not respond to treatment with a gluten-free diet.[116] In adults, celiac sprue is distinguished easily from Whipple's disease, which is a multisystem disease, and from malabsorption secondary to infiltration of the mucosa with *Mycobacterium avium* complex, because the histologic findings on small intestine biopsy are different in these diseases.

Although changes in mucosal morphology also can be seen in parasitic infections other than *Giardia*, such as strongyloidiasis, coccidiosis, and hookworm disease, these changes rarely include villus atrophy. Although villus atrophy is characteristic of untreated celiac sprue, it is by no means pathognomonic and may be seen in varying degrees in a wide variety of other enteric disorders (see Fig. 101-2); villus atrophy on small intestinal biopsy is not sufficient to diagnose celiac sprue. Crypt cell activity, enterocyte characteristics, and the nature of the inflammatory infiltrate also must be examined and in some instances will point toward another diagnosis. For example, patients with hypogammaglobulinemia may have an architectural lesion that resembles celiac sprue, but plasma cells are absent or markedly diminished in the lamina propria, not increased as in celiac sprue. Absence of the other histologic features of celiac sprue often suggests an alternative diagnosis. After an acute viral gastroenteritis, however, the morphologic abnormalities may be indistinguishable from those of celiac sprue. In infants and young children, cow's milk or soy protein intolerance also may result in biopsy findings identical to those of celiac sprue.[117,118] For this reason, morphologic improvement on gluten withdrawal with subsequent deterioration on gluten rechallenge forms the basis for a definitive diagnosis of celiac sprue in children. Soy protein frequently is used as a substitute for milk protein in cow's milk protein intolerance, but some children also develop mucosal abnormalities resembling those of celiac sprue following ingestion of soy protein.[118] In adults, the differential diagnosis is less challenging; consequently, gluten challenge is performed less commonly.

A rare condition that may cause confusion is collagenous sprue (see later discussion of refractory sprue). Patients with collagenous sprue may present initially with symptoms and biopsy findings consistent with celiac sprue; however, their symptoms fail to respond to gluten withdrawal and, with time, extensive deposition of collagen in the lamina propria develops just beneath the absorptive epithelium.[119] The relationship between celiac sprue and both collagenous sprue and the microscopic colitides (lymphocytic and collagenous colitis) is discussed later.

Finally, in some patients with potential celiac sprue, diarrhea develops on gluten ingestion, but the small intestinal mucosa is normal or only mildly edematous, with a minimal inflammatory cell infiltrate. Such gluten-sensitive diarrhea responds to a gluten-free diet, and in many of these patients classic celiac sprue develops subsequently.[120] Other patients have characteristic findings of celiac sprue, but symptoms fail to respond to a gluten-free diet. In most cases, the problem is the inadvertent presence of gluten in the diet or the patient's failure to adhere to a strict gluten-free diet[121]; however, a small number of these patients have refractory sprue or a complication such as lymphoma, ulcerative jejunitis, or collagenous sprue (see later).

DISEASES ASSOCIATED WITH CELIAC SPRUE

A large number of diseases occur more frequently among patients with celiac sprue and are delineated in Table 101-3. In addition to an association with autoimmune disorders, many of the associated diseases have similar HLA haplotype associations.

DERMATITIS HERPETIFORMIS

DH is a skin disease characterized by papulovesicular lesions that occur symmetrically over the extensor surfaces of the extremities and the buttocks, trunk, neck, and scalp. Unlike celiac sprue, DH rarely is diagnosed in childhood and usually presents in early or middle adult life.

Table 101–3   Disorders Associated with Celiac Sprue

Definite Association
Dermatitis herpetiformis
Type 1 diabetes mellitus
Hypothyroidism/hyperthyroidism
IgA deficiency
Epilepsy with cerebral calcification
Inflammatory bowel disease
Microscopic colitis
IgA mesangial nephropathy
Rheumatoid arthritis
Sarcoidosis
Down syndrome
Bird-fancier's lung
Fibrosing alveolitis
Recurrent pericarditis
Idiopathic pulmonary hemosiderosis
Possible Association
Congenital heart disease
Cavitary lung disease
Sjögren's syndrome
Systemic and cutaneous vasculitis
Systemic lupus erythematosus
Polymyositis
Myasthenia gravis
Iridocyclitis or choroiditis
Cystic fibrosis
Macroamylasemia
Addison's disease
Autoimmune thrombocytopenic purpura
Autoimmune hemolytic anemia
Schizophrenia
Autoimmune liver diseases

Modified from Mulder CJ, Tytgat GN: Coeliac disease and related disorders. Neth J Med 31:286, 1987.

DH is slightly more common in males (3:2), although in patients younger than 20 years of age, females predominate (3:2).[122] The rash is intensely pruritic, and scratching off the vesicle relieves the itching; hence, intact vesicles may not be present except for the earliest lesions. The diagnosis of DH requires demonstration by immunofluorescence of granular or speckled IgA deposits in an area of skin close to a lesion but not affected by blistering.[122] Two thirds of patients have a patchy enteropathy indistinguishable from celiac sprue that may require multiple intestinal biopsies to demonstrate; the remaining one third have associated features of gluten sensitivity (increased IELs and γ/δ T cells or the induction of villus atrophy with gluten challenge).[122] DH-associated enteropathy tends to be less severe than celiac sprue, and fewer than 10% of patients have intestinal symptoms.[122] A 10- to 40-fold increased risk of lymphoma has been reported, however, as in celiac sprue,[123] with most lymphomas occurring in patients whose DH was not controlled by a strict gluten-free diet or in those who had been treated with a gluten-free diet for fewer than 5 years.[124]

Approximately 5% to 15% of patients with DH-like skin lesions have linear IgA deposits along the dermoepidermal junction. This condition has been termed *linear IgA disease* and is distinguished from DH on the basis of its unique immunofluorescent finding; the presence of circulating IgA antibasement membrane antibody, which binds to a 97-kd protein found in normal human skin[125]; the absence of circulating IgA EMA[59] or autoantibodies to tTG[126]; different HLA susceptibility genes; and most important, the lack of any associated gluten-sensitive enteropathy.

Sardy and colleagues[127] shed light on the pathogenesis of DH by demonstrating that a related enzyme epidermal (type 3) transglutaminase (eTG) rather than tTG is the dominant autoantigen in DH. This explains why skin symptoms appear in only a portion of patients having celiac sprue. They also showed that the IgA precipitates in the papillary dermis of patients with DH, the defining manifestation of the disease, contain eTG, but not tTG or keratinocyte transglutaminase. Elevated circulating levels of IgA, lowered IgM, and varying changes in IgG occur in DH similar to the pattern observed in celiac sprue. Similarly, the prevalences of HLA-DQ2, HLA-B8, and HLA-DR3 and circulating AGA, antireticulin, and EMA parallel those observed in patients with celiac sprue without DH.[122] Although patients with DH have elevated IgA tTG antibodies, confirming its pathogenic relation with celiac sprue, the prevalence in DH (75%) is lower than that found in celiac sprue (95% to 98%) paralleling the prevalence of EMA in both diseases and also reflecting the milder enteropathy in DH.[128]

Thus, DH and celiac sprue are two very closely related gluten-sensitive disorders but are nonetheless distinct clinical disease entities. Most, if not all, patients with DH also have at least latent celiac sprue, whereas fewer than 10% of patients with celiac sprue have DH. Whereas dapsone treatment at a dose of 1 to 2 mg/kg daily is effective and often diagnostic in its ability to heal the rash of DH and relieve the pruritus rapidly, the enteropathy associated with DH does not improve with dapsone. Six to 12 months of gluten withdrawal, however, usually reverses not only the intestinal but also the skin lesions in most patients with DH, and strict gluten-free diet allows most patients to reduce or discontinue dapsone.[129] Patients with DH, just like those with celiac sprue, can include moderate amounts of oats in their gluten-free diet without deleterious effects to their skin or intestine.[130]

OTHER DISEASE ASSOCIATIONS

Autoimmune disease is associated strongly with celiac sprue and has a prevalence of approximately 20% in adult patients. There is an established association between celiac sprue and insulin-dependent diabetes mellitus (IDDM), reflecting, in part, the increased frequency of the celiac-associated DQ alleles in patients with IDDM. The frequency of celiac sprue in IDDM patients ranges from 3% to 8%[131-133] and the frequency of IDDM in celiac sprue is approximately 5%[134] Most patients with IDDM who have celiac sprue are asymptomatic from the point of view of their celiac sprue, but unexpected episodes of hypoglycemia or diarrhea in patients with IDDM should alert clinicians to the possibility of coexisting celiac sprue. Control of diabetes in patients with celiac sprue can be difficult because of varying nutrient absorption. There is also a high prevalence of autoimmune thyroid disease among patients with celiac sprue, hypothyroidism being more common than hyperthyroidism.[135] Celiac sprue also may be associated with a variety of other autoimmune connective tissue diseases,[136] including systemic lupus erythematosus,[137] Sjögren's syndrome,[138] and polymyositis.[139] Although the relationship between celiac sprue and many autoimmune disorders has been explained by the sharing of a common genetic factor, Ventura and colleagues[140] suggested an increased frequency of autoimmune disease with increased age at diagnosis and lack of diet therapy. The role of a gluten-free diet in preventing the development of autoimmune disease, however, has been challenged by more recent studies.[141]

Although many patients with celiac sprue exhibit lactose and sucrose intolerances at the time of diagnosis, only a small percentage have persistent disaccharidase deficiency following gluten withdrawal. These patients experience abdominal pain and diarrhea with lactose or sucrose intake and can usually be diagnosed by history or by an appropriate sugar tolerance test or hydrogen breath test. Should concomitant disaccharidase deficiency be present, the relevant disaccharide should be excluded from the diet. Selective IgA deficiency occurs 10 times as often in patients with celiac sprue, and as many as 2% of patients with celiac sprue are IgA deficient.[142] Hyposplenism and splenic atrophy have been noted frequently in patients with celiac sprue; the frequency increases with advancing age, duration of exposure to dietary gluten, and disease activity.[78] The underlying mechanism is unknown, but affected patients are at increased risk of developing bacterial infections[143] and should take antibiotics prophylactically for invasive procedures, including dental procedures; they also may benefit from pneumococcal vaccination.

Evidence also supports associations between celiac sprue and inflammatory bowel disease (particularly ulcerative proctitis),[144] chronic hepatitis,[145] sclerosing cholangitis,[145] primary biliary cirrhosis,[145] IgA nephropathy,[146] interstitial lung disease (including chronic fibrosing alveolitis),[147] idiopathic pulmonary hemosiderosis,[148] and Down syndrome.[149]

Finally, there is the curious but well-established relationship between celiac sprue and the microscopic colitides (see Chapter 121).[150] Mild to moderate small intestinal lymphocytosis, and occasionally partial or subtotal villus atrophy, is common in both lymphocytic and collagenous colitis,[151] whereas mild colonic lymphocytosis occurs in patients with untreated celiac sprue.[152] Rectal gluten challenge in patients with celiac sprue has been shown to induce a mild proctitis characterized by lymphocytosis of the rectal lamina propria and epithelium.[153] Furthermore, a gluten-free diet has been reported to be an effective therapy in some patients with refractory collagenous colitis.[154] The demonstration that patients with celiac sprue and microscopic colitis share a set of predisposing HLA-DQ genes[155] underscores the overlap between both diseases. Confusion also can arise in patients with refractory sprue, who have a higher prevalence of colonic lymphocytosis than patients with celiac sprue. Colonic lymphocytosis can be difficult to distinguish from lymphocytic colitis, although most colonic IELs in lymphocytic colitis are CD8[+], whereas those in the colonic lymphocytosis of refractory sprue rarely are CD8[+].[116]

TREATMENT

GLUTEN-FREE DIET

Removal of gluten from the diet is essential for the treatment of patients with celiac sprue (Table 101–4). The importance of gluten withdrawal was established by Dicke's, van de Kamer's, and Weijers' astute studies in the early 1950s when the toxicity of wheat protein in children with celiac sprue was demonstrated.[6,7] In 1962, Rubin and colleagues[30] showed that instillation of wheat, barley, and rye flour into the histologically normal small intestine of persons with treated celiac sprue rapidly induced sprue-like symptoms and that these symptoms were accompanied by the development of the typical celiac sprue lesions in the exposed mucosa.

In reality, complete dietary elimination of all gluten-containing cereal grains is extremely difficult for most patients to achieve and maintain. "Hidden" gluten is present in a wide variety of processed foods because wheat flour is used widely in the food industry as a thickener and inexpensive filler for many commercial products, precooked meals, and convenience foods, including ice cream, pasta, sausages, fish sticks, cheese spreads, salad dressings, soups, sauces, mixed seasonings, mincemeat for mince pies, and some medications[156] and vitamin preparations (Table 101–5). To this end, listings of gluten-free products have been drawn up and a gluten-free symbol (a crossed ear of wheat) has been devised; it is used widely by food manufacturers in Europe but, unfortunately, less so in the United States. Although gluten-free wheat is available for baking, grains that are naturally gluten free can become contaminated with wheat, particularly when mills use the same production lines and equipment to process both gluten-containing and gluten-free products. All beers, lagers, ales, and stout should be avoided, but wines, liqueurs, ciders as well as spirits, including brandy, malt, and scotch whiskey, can

---

Table 101–4 Principles of Initial Dietary Therapy for Patients with Celiac Sprue

Avoid all foods containing wheat, rye, and barley gluten.
Avoid all oats initially.
Use only rice, corn, maize, buckwheat, potato, soybean, tapioca flours, meals, or starches.
Wheat starch from which gluten has been removed can be tried after the diagnosis is established.
Read all labels and study ingredients of processed foods.
Beware of gluten in medications, food additives, emulsifiers, or stabilizers.
Limit milk and milk products initially.
Avoid all beers, lagers, ales, and stouts.
Wine, liqueurs, ciders, and spirits, including whiskey and brandy, are allowed.

Modified from Trier JS: Celiac sprue and refractory sprue. In Feldman M, Scharschmidt BF, Sleisenger MH (eds): Gastrointestinal and Liver Disease, 6th ed. Philadelphia, WB Saunders, 1997, p 1557.

Table 101–5   Potential Sources of Hidden Gluten

Beers, ales, other fermented beverages (distilled beverages are acceptable)
Bouillon/soups
Candy
Communion wafers
Drink mixes/herbal tea
Gravy/sauces
Imitation meat/seafood
Lipstick/lip balms
Medications (pills and capsules)
Nutritional supplements
Play-Doh
Salad dressings/marinades
Self-basting turkeys
Soy sauce

Table 101–6   Key Elements in the Management of Celiac Sprue

Consultation with a skilled dietitian
Education about the disease
Lifelong adherence to a gluten-free diet
Identification and treatment of nutritional deficiencies
Access to an advocacy group
Continuous long-term follow-up by a multidisciplinary team

From the National Institutes of Health Consensus Development Conference Statement on Celiac Disease, June 28-30, 2004 (http://consensus.nih.gov/cons/118/118celiac.htm).

be consumed. Helpful recipes as well as detailed instructions regarding gluten-free diets have been published in excellent, inexpensive books that are of great value to patients with celiac sprue.[157] National celiac societies in many countries publish regularly updated handbooks that list the available gluten-free products. Food lists are applicable for use only in the country in which they were compiled. Similar foods with well-known brand names may be made under franchise using slightly different recipes in different countries and may be gluten free in one country and not in others. Consequently, patient education is crucial, and the institution of an effective gluten-free diet requires extensive and repeated instruction of the patient by the physician and dietitian, as well as a motivated and basically suspicious, label-reading patient. The importance of patient education and support by a multidisciplinary team of health care providers was emphasized in the recently published National Institutes of Health consensus development conference statement (Table 101–6).[158]

There is considerable variation among patients with celiac sprue in their ability to tolerate gluten. Some patients can ingest small amounts of gluten without developing symptoms. Others are exquisitely sensitive to ingestion of even minute amounts of gluten and may develop massive watery diarrhea reminiscent of acute cholera within hours of eating a small piece of bakery bread. Occasionally, the diarrhea may be so severe that it can induce acute dehydration, termed *gliadin shock*.[115]

Patients with untreated celiac sprue may have accompanying brush border lactase deficiency secondary to damage to surface epithelial cells. Therefore, milk and dairy products should be avoided at the initiation of a gluten-free diet. After response to the diet, however, these products can be reintroduced, if they are tolerated. It is now apparent that moderate amounts of oats, at least in the short term, are not toxic in patients with celiac sprue. In a carefully conducted randomized clinical trial, adults with celiac sprue who consumed 50 to 70 g of oats per day for 6 to 12 months did not differ in regard to symptoms, nutritional status, or duodenal mucosal histology compared with patients maintained on an oat-restricted, gluten-free diet.[159] In a smaller follow-on study, the same group has subsequently shown no harm in celiac sprue from 5 years of ingestion of oats.[160] Patients with DH also can include moderate amounts of oats in their gluten-free diet without deleterious effects to the skin or intestine,[130] and an open-labeled study showed that a 6-month trial of commercial oat breakfast cereal also was safe for children with newly diagnosed celiac sprue beginning a gluten-free diet.[161] It should be stressed, however, that oat products obtained from the grocery store shelf may be contaminated with small amounts of other grains, especially wheat. Consequently, oats initially should be avoided in all newly diagnosed patients until remission is achieved on a gluten-free diet. Subsequently, up to 2 ounces of oats per day from a reliable source can be introduced and continued if tolerated.

Because a gluten-free diet represents a lifetime commitment for patients with celiac sprue, is more expensive than a normal diet, and carries a social liability, especially in children and teenagers, it should not be undertaken casually as a therapeutic trial. Rather, the diagnosis should be established first by serologic studies and small intestinal biopsy. Thereafter, institution of a gluten-free diet serves two functions: (1) treatment (followed by clinical improvement) and (2) confirmation of the histologic diagnosis of celiac sprue.

After starting a gluten-free diet, most patients improve within a few weeks. In many, symptomatic improvement is noticed within 48 hours, although it may take weeks or months to achieve full clinical remission. Pink and Creamer[162] reported that 70% of patients with celiac sprue begun on a gluten-free diet returned quickly to normal health and reported improvement in their symptoms within 2 weeks. The speed and eventual degree of histologic improvement are unpredictable but invariably lag behind the clinical response. Although an increase in enterocyte height may be evident within a week of gluten withdrawal, the return of villus architecture toward normal takes considerably longer and may not be evident on rebiopsy for 2 or 3 months. In some patients, histologic improvement may take up to 2 years, the main reason for this slow or partial recovery being inadvertent exposure to gluten.[31] Although a return to normal is common in children, in approximately 50% of adults on a gluten-free diet, biopsies show only partial improvement; the less severely damaged distal intestine recovers more rapidly than the maximally damaged proximal intestine.[163]

If a patient fails to improve on a gluten-free diet, it is much more likely that either the diet is inadequate or the mucosal lesion is caused by another disease causing villus atrophy than the patient has true refractory sprue.[121] It is also important to note that dietary failure is not always the cause of persistent symptoms. Other disorders such as IBS, lactose intolerance, or pancreatic insufficiency may coexist.[121] In the study by Pink and Creamer,[162] the 30% of patients who failed to respond to a gluten-free diet fell into three groups: Patients in the first group experienced progressive deterioration, which was halted in some cases by treatment with glucocorticoids but which progressed to death in others. Patients in the second group had an associated pancreatic disorder. Those in the third group were poorly compliant with a strict gluten-free diet, but even when this problem was addressed, their minor abdominal symptoms, including diarrhea, sometimes persisted.

IMMUNOSUPPRESSANTS

In vitro studies have shown that the addition of glucocorticoids prevented the harmful effects of gluten on biopsies from patients with celiac sprue.[164] In addition to its anti-inflammatory effects, glucocorticoids also may exert a local beneficial effect on the mucosal transport of water and sodium. Although celiac sprue can be treated with glucocorticoids, with rapid improvement in symptoms, the effect rarely persists once treatment is stopped.[165] Therefore, glucocorticoids are not indicated in the routine management of celiac sprue but are reserved for severely ill patients who present with acute celiac crisis manifested by severe diarrhea, dehydration, weight loss, acidosis, hypocalcemia, and hypoproteinemia.[166] These few patients may benefit from a short course of glucocorticoids until the gluten-free diet takes effect. Glucocorticoids also can be used in the rare instances of gliadin shock that occurs occasionally in treated patients who are subject to gluten challenge.[115]

Glucocorticoid treatment also may be necessary in patients with refractory sprue (see later). Azathioprine or 6-mercaptopurine can be used as a glucocorticoid-sparing agent if a dose of 10 mg of prednisolone or more per day is required to keep the condition under control.[167] Although cyclosporine therapy has been reported to be lifesaving in occasional patients with refractory sprue-like disease and may result in reversal of glucocorticoid resistance, its efficacy remains unproved.[168] There has been one published report on the efficacy of infliximab, a chimeric antibody to TNF-α in refractory sprue.[169]

SUPPLEMENTS

In addition to a gluten-free diet, patients with severe disease should receive appropriate supplemental therapy to help correct nutritional deficiencies caused by malabsorption. Anemic patients should receive supplemental iron and folate. Rarely, treatment with vitamin B_{12} may be required. Patients with purpura, bruising, or other evidence of bleeding may have prolongation of their prothrombin time and require supplemental vitamin K. Patients with severe diarrhea and dehydration require vigorous intravenous replacement of fluids and electrolytes. Intravenous calcium gluconate, 1 to 2 g, should

be administered promptly to the patient with tetany. If there is no response, the tetany may be caused by hypomagnesemia and require magnesium replacement.

The risks of osteopenia and osteoporosis should be explained to all patients with celiac sprue and general advice given about exercise (particularly weight bearing), smoking, alcohol excess, and adequate dietary calcium. The importance of adhering strictly to a gluten-free diet should be stressed because there is compelling evidence that this protects against further bone loss and initially is associated with an increase in bone mineral density (BMD).[170] A total daily calcium intake of 1500 mg should be ensured—a pint of skim milk provides 700 mg. If dietary calcium is inadequate, 500 to 1000 mg of supplemental calcium should be given. Vitamin D deficiency should be sought and treated if found, particularly in patients with significant steatorrhea, to prevent mobilization of skeletal calcium until the malabsorption has responded to gluten withdrawal. Whereas 1 year of gluten withdrawal has been shown to reverse osteopenia in most patients, including postmenopausal women and patients with incomplete mucosal recovery,[171] patients who have secondary hyperparathyroidism at the time celiac sprue is diagnosed tend to have more refractory osteopenia, and their BMD may not normalize even after several years of gluten withdrawal.[172] Clinicians often rely on serum calcium, phosphate, and alkaline phosphatase measurements, but osteomalacia still may exist even if these tests are normal. If these tests are normal and osteomalacia still is suspected, serum 25-hydroxy vitamin D usually is measured; this test is expensive, however, and the cheaper parathormone assay should be considered. A low normal calcium and an elevated parathormone level indicates secondary hyperparathyroidism, and treatment with calcium (500 to 1000 mg daily) together with vitamin D (400 to 800 units daily) should be given.[173] The serum calcium level must be monitored and supplementation promptly discontinued if hypercalcemia develops. All patients should have their BMD measured at diagnosis. Recent guidelines suggest that patients with celiac sprue who have osteoporosis should be offered oral biphosphonate therapy and have their BMD checked every 1 to 2 years.[173]

Vitamin A, thiamine, riboflavin, niacin, pyridoxine, vitamin C, and vitamin E, in the form of a multivitamin preparation, probably should be administered to newly diagnosed celiac sprue patients with clinically evident malabsorption; however, there is no need for long-term supplementation of these vitamins once intestinal absorption has normalized. Some patients have reported symptomatic improvement with correction of magnesium, copper, and zinc deficiencies.[174] Finally, it is important to note that drugs, like nutrients, may be absorbed capriciously by patients with severe celiac sprue. Medications considered essential for the patient's well-being may need to be administered parenterally until absorption improves in response to treatment with a gluten-free diet.

COMPLICATIONS

Malignancy, ulcerative jejunoileitis, and collagenous sprue are the major complications of celiac sprue. In the past, patients with celiac sprue or DH had been reported to have a 10-fold increased risk for certain gastrointestinal tract malignancies and a 40- to 70-fold increased risk for non-Hodgkin's lymphoma (NHL).[123,175] Recent studies, however, indicate that the risk of malignancy and particularly lymphoma is much less than initially believed. A large retrospective Swedish study followed up 12,000 hospitalized patients with either celiac sprue or DH between 1964 and 1994, with a mean follow-up of 10 years.[176] The authors reported that the overall cancer and malignant lymphoma risk was increased only modestly (standardized incidence ratio [SIR], 1.3; 95% CI, 1.2-1.5 and SIR, 5.9; 95% CI, 4.3-7.9, respectively). In a prospective Italian study, patients with celiac sprue had a 3.1-fold increased risk of NHL,[177] whereas the prospective BioMed European Working Group on Celiac Disease and Malignancy, which reviewed data from 10 countries, has reported that the prevalence of celiac sprue was increased 2.6-fold in 1446 patients with NHL compared with 9659 control subjects.[178] Furthermore, the European study suggested that the risk of NHL is even less evident in silent celiac sprue.

Small intestinal lymphoma, often multifocal and diffuse, accounts for one half to two thirds of the malignancies complicating celiac sprue and typically occurs after 20 to 40 years of disease (see Chapters 28 and 112).[175,176] Whereas in the general population, most small intestinal lymphomas are of B cell origin, intestinal lymphoma in celiac sprue is typically of T cell origin, and the term *EATL* was coined to describe both the intestinal and extraintestinal lymphomas that complicate celiac sprue. The European multicenter study indicated that intestinal T cell lymphomas and chiefly EATL are highly characteristic of, if not specific for, celiac sprue with an odds ratio of 28. The clinical onset of EATL may be insidious, and its initial presentation and small bowel biopsy appearance may mimic those of untreated celiac sprue. EATL commonly is accompanied by nonspecific mucosal ulceration, similar to that seen in ulcerative jejunoileitis, and these ulcers are sometimes the only endoscopic manifestation of lymphoma (see Chapter 112). Although some patients with EATL may have a partial or temporary response to a strict gluten-free diet, most are unresponsive to gluten withdrawal. In patients previously controlled on a gluten-free diet, the recurrence of gastrointestinal symptoms such as abdominal pain, weight loss, diarrhea, and intestinal bleeding should always raise the clinical suspicion of lymphoma. In some patients with lymphoma, mucosal histology adjacent to and distant from the lymphoma is indistinguishable from that of untreated celiac sprue, yet the patient's symptoms do not respond to gluten withdrawal.[179] There is long-standing controversy as to whether such patients have latent celiac sprue that becomes evident after lymphoma has developed, refractory sprue complicated by lymphoma, or refractory enteropathy induced by primary intestinal T cell lymphoma and indistinguishable by histologic criteria from celiac sprue.[15] Molecular and immunohistochemical studies that have advanced our understanding of the relationships among celiac sprue, refractory sprue, and EATL are discussed in the section on refractory sprue.

Other features suggesting lymphoma include obstruction, intestinal bleeding, fever, hypoalbuminemia, lym-phadenopathy, and erythrophagocytosis. Small bowel radiology, small bowel enteroscopy with biopsy of the mucosa at multiple levels, capsule endoscopy, double-balloon enteroscopy, and CT scanning may be helpful. Mesenteric lymphadenopathy with central cavitation has been described in celiac sprue, both with[180] and without[181] lymphoma. If the index of suspicion is high and studies are not diagnostic, full-thickness biopsy specimens of the small intestine should be obtained at laparoscopy or laparotomy with careful examination of the entire length of the small bowel and examination of mesenteric lymph nodes. Even with such an aggressive approach, EATL can be extremely difficult to diagnose. EATL commonly is fatal: Overall 1-year and 5-year survival rates of 31% and 11%, respectively, were reported in one small series, with long-term survival almost exclusively confined to those treated with chemotherapy.[182]

Carcinoma, particularly of the oropharynx, esophagus, and small intestine, account for one third of the remaining malignancies complicating celiac sprue. The average patient so affected is older than 50 years of age. The Swedish study reported elevated risks for small intestinal (SIR, 10), oropharyngeal (SIR, 2.3), esophageal (SIR, 4.2), as well as primary liver cancers (SIR, 2.7).[176] Patients with DH had a slightly increased overall cancer risk (SIR, 1.2) owing to excesses of lymphoma and leukemia but no increases in gastrointestinal carcinomas.[176] The mechanisms responsible for the increased prevalence of malignancy in celiac sprue are unknown. Increased crypt mitotic activity, increased turnover of lymphoid cells within the mucosa, penetration of the damaged jejunal mucosa by carcinogens, infection with oncogenic viruses, and underlying abnormalities in the mucosal immune system and surface epithelium all are potential factors. In the Swedish study, the excess risk of malignancies, which was confined to adults, disappeared after a 10-year follow-up.[176] This declining risk of malignancies with increased duration of follow-up and thus with the length of gluten-free diet supports the results of a previous study, which indicated that a strict gluten-free diet for 5 years reduced the risk of all malignancies, not just EATL, to that of the general population.[123]

Ulcerative jejunoileitis, also known as *chronic nongranulomatous ulcerative enterocolitis*, or nongranulomatous jejunitis, is a rare but serious complication of celiac sprue characterized by ulceration and strictures of the small intestine (see Chapter 112). Whether ulcerative jejunoileitis truly is a discrete entity has been questioned, because lymphoma ultimately is diagnosed in many of these patients.[183] Indeed, ulcerative jejunoileitis in association with EATL was previously designated *malignant histiocytosis*. It should be suspected in patients with celiac sprue who present with abdominal pain, weight loss, and diarrhea that do not respond to gluten-free diet. Typically, patients experience recurrent episodes of intestinal ulceration and obstruction with gradual weight loss despite surgery and strict adherence to a gluten-free diet. Areas of intestinal ulceration and stricture formation typically cause obstruction and hemorrhage (Fig. 101–8). Perforation with peritonitis also may occur. Diagnosis is made by contrast studies of the small bowel, abdominal CT, or, most frequently, laparotomy. Although some patients may respond to a gluten-free diet, surgical exci-

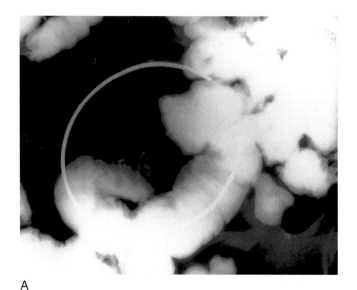

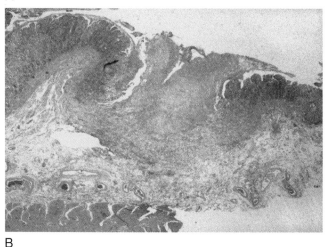

Figure 101–8 A small bowel barium contrast study from a patient with ulcerative jejunoileitis complicating celiac sprue. *A,* a segmental area of fixed narrowing with associated mucosal distortion and ulceration in the distal jejunum/proximal ileum is seen. *B,* Histology of a segment of resected small intestine showing ulcerated mucosa with adjacent diffuse villus atrophy and lymphocytic infiltrate consistent with celiac sprue. Lymphocytes within the epithelium and lamina propria were positive for T cell antigen (CD3); no overt lymphoma was evident, but Southern blot analysis revealed clonal TCR gene rearrangements in both the involved and uninvolved small intestine and an adjacent mesenteric lymph node consistent with cryptic enteropathy-associated T cell lymphoma. TCR, T cell receptor.

sion of the worst affected segments of small bowel has so far proved to be the most effective treatment. There is a high risk for transition to diffuse or multifocal EATL, and there are a few patients with well-documented celiac sprue and localized jejunoileitis in whom no evidence of malignant disease develops and there is a response to either surgical resection or therapy with glucocorticoids and azathioprine.[184] Even in the absence of malignant transformation, however, the 5-year survival rate for patients with ulcerative jejunoileitis is less than 50%.

Collagenous sprue is characterized by the development of a subepithelial collagen band thicker than 10 mm in the small intestine. Although collagenous sprue has been regarded as an entity distinct from celiac sprue,[119] deposition of collagen under the intestinal epithelial cells has been noted in up to 36% of patients with classic celiac sprue.[185] Furthermore, there are several reports of patients with collagenous sprue who have EMA[186] and complications of refractory sprue, specifically ulcerative jejunoileitis[187] and lymphoma.[15] Although collagenous sprue frequently is refractory to therapy, the presence of subepithelial collagen does not, a priori, preclude a successful response to gluten withdrawal.[185,188] Collagenous sprue should be distinguished from collagenous colitis, which rarely may accompany celiac sprue and should be considered in the differential diagnosis of refractory sprue.[154] Compared with both celiac sprue and collagenous colitis, the prognosis in collagenous sprue is grim, with most reported patients dying from the disease.

REFRACTORY SPRUE

Refractory sprue, also known as *unclassified* or *intractable celiac sprue,* is defined as symptomatic severe small intestinal villus atrophy that mimics celiac sprue but does not respond to at least 6 months of a strict gluten-free diet and is not accounted for by other causes of villus atrophy or overt intestinal lymphoma.[1] Refractory sprue is uncommon in adults, extremely rare in children, and largely a diagnosis of exclusion (Fig. 101–9). Symptoms may persist in treated celiac sprue patients for a variety of reasons, the commonest of which is lack of strict compliance with a gluten-free diet, often through inadvertent ingestion of dietary gluten.[189] Other causes of villus atrophy should be excluded, as should coexisting conditions including disaccharidase deficiency, bacterial overgrowth, pancreatic insufficiency, inflammatory bowel disease, and the microscopic colitides. Other exclusion diets also should be considered to uncover other food protein enteropathies such as milk, egg, or soy.[121]

In patients with celiac sprue and no demonstrable cause for lack of response to a gluten-free diet, a variety of treatments (based mostly on small, uncontrolled studies) have been described; these include elimination diets, dietary supplementation with zinc and copper,[174] and immunosuppressive therapy. Evidence supporting the use of immunosuppressive therapy in the treatment of refractory sprue is based mainly on anecdotal reports, and to date no controlled trials have been performed.[190] Some patients with refractory sprue have responded to treatment with glucocorticoids, whereas others had success with immunosuppressive drugs such as azathioprine,[167] cyclosporine,[168] and infliximab.[169] In one open pilot study 13 adult patients with refractory celiac sprue treated for 2 months with oral cyclosporine in doses titrated to achieve serum levels of 100 to 200 ng/mL, small intestinal histology improved in 8 patients (61%), with normalization of villi in 5 (38%).[191] Although a trial of immunosuppressive therapy is worth considering in all patients with refractory sprue, caution must be used, because these patients often are malnourished,

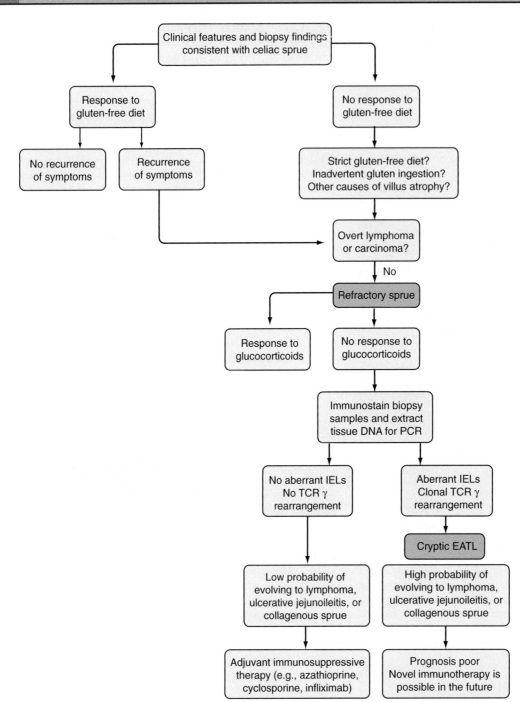

Figure 101–9 Approach to the diagnosis and management of refractory sprue. EATL, enteropathy-associated T cell lymphoma; IEL, intraepithelial lymphocyte; PCR, polymerase chain reaction; TCR, T cell receptor.

have hyposplenism, and hence may be prone to opportunistic infections.[167] Unfortunately, some patients have only partial or no response to immunosuppressive therapy, and the clinical course is characterized by progressive malabsorption necessitating total parenteral nutrition.

It has long been appreciated that patients with refractory sprue are at high risk of developing uncommon but frequently fatal complications such as lymphoma, ulcerative jejunoileitis, and collagenous sprue. Until recently, the precise link between refractory sprue and these complications as well as between refractory sprue and celiac

sprue remained controversial. The spectrum of autoimmune enteropathy was implicated in a handful of adult refractory sprue patients by the presence of antienterocyte antibodies.[192] It is now becoming clear, however, that refractory sprue, EATL, ulcerative jejunoileitis, and possibly collagenous sprue represent a heterogenous but related group of clinical conditions at the extreme end of the celiac sprue spectrum. Moreover, there is now a growing realization that many of these patients have a cryptic intestinal T cell lymphoma, characterized by phenotypically abnormal IELs that have monoclonal rearrangements of the *TCR* γ gene.[15]

Early immunophenotypical studies demonstrated that the normal cell counterpart of EATL was the IEL.[179] It was not until 1995, however, when Murray and colleagues[193] made the remarkable observation that lymphocytes from adjacent nonlymphomatous mucosa in patients with overt EATL contained the identical monoclonal *TCR* gene rearrangement as the overt lymphoma and that the term *cryptic intestinal T cell lymphoma* was coined. Ashton-Key and colleagues[194] later confirmed this finding and showed that both the inflammatory ulcers and the intact (nonlymphomatous) mucosa in cases of ulcerative jejunoileitis harbored a monoclonal T cell population and that the lymphomas that later develop in these patients consisted of the identical T cell clone. Cellier and colleagues[68] showed that the IELs in refractory sprue patients make up a monoclonal population that, in particular, lack expression of CD8, which is consistently found on most normal or celiac sprue IELs. Subsequent work confirmed this finding and showed that the monoclonal IEL in ulcerative jejunoileitis and nonlymphomatous mucosa in EATL shared not only the genotype but also the immunophenotype of the lymphoma.[195] Cellier and colleagues[15] detected aberrant clonal IELs (similar to those in most cases of EATL) in 16 (84%) of 19 patients with refractory sprue, 7 (37%) of whom had collagenous sprue, 6 (32%) of whom had ulcerative jejunoileitis, 6 (32%) of whom had mesenteric lymph nodes cavitation, and 3 (16%) of whom who developed overt EATL that was clonally identical to the IELs of the preexisting refractory sprue. All 3 patients (16%) without aberrant clonal IELs made a complete clinical and histologic recovery with glucocorticoid therapy plus a gluten-free diet. Thus, the cumulative evidence now points to refractory sprue being a manifestation of an aberrant clonal IEL-mediated neoplastic process. These cells have destructive properties, possible related to their cytotoxic phenotype,[196] which leads to mucosal ulceration, and lymph node cavitation and they sometimes, but not always, undergo further molecular and clinical progression to lymphoma. As noted earlier, the proinflammatory cytokine IL-15 is massively increased in the intestine of patients with refractory sprue. IL-15 induces IEL secretion of IFN-γ and increases IEL cytotoxicity against epithelial cells, thereby favoring the severe enteropathy characteristic of refractory sprue.[16] Furthermore, increasing evidence suggests that IL-15, through its key role in modulating IEL homeostasis, ultimately may lead to lymphomatous transformation because IL-15 provides signals mandatory for the survival or expansion of the abnormal clonal IELs. Based on this evidence, patients with suspected refractory sprue should have TCR and monoclonal antibody studies performed on their small bowel biopsy samples. In the future, early recognition of the malignant potential of the intestinal infiltrate may permit curative surgery. Alternatively, novel anti-IL-15 biological agents may prevent the development of refractory sprue and lymphoma.

PROGNOSIS

Celiac sprue has an excellent prognosis if diagnosed early and the patient adheres to a lifelong gluten-free diet. Conversely, if not recognized and properly treated,

patients may develop marked malnutrition and debilitation and even die of complications such as intercurrent infection or hemorrhage. Although earlier studies reported 1.9-fold[197] and 3.4-fold[198] increases in mortality, these studies lacked patients with latent celiac sprue and included patients who were not adhering to a gluten-free diet as well as patients with refractory sprue and intestinal lymphoma. A study of 335 adults with celiac sprue from Finland, at least 83% of the whom adhered strictly to a gluten-free diet, showed that the 5-year survival was comparable with that of the general population.[134] Growth and development in infants and children with celiac disease proceed normally despite continued gluten withdrawal. In adults, absorptive functions usually return, and many of the manifestations of disease disappear after initiation of a gluten-free diet. Complications of the disease, however, such as peripheral neuropathy, ataxia, or pathologic fractures secondary to severe osteopenic bone disease, particularly in the setting of secondary hyperparathyroidism, may not be completely reversible. Studies have questioned the protective effect of gluten-free diet against the development of other autoimmune diseases, and the functional consequences of a gluten-free diet in silent celiac sprue remain unknown, particularly regarding osteopenia and osteoporosis.

Several lines of evidence, gathered during recent years, suggest that celiac sprue is not always a lifelong condition. First, the long-term follow-up of children with proved celiac sprue shows that 10% to 20% develop latent celiac sprue and become "tolerant" (defined on clinical, biological, and histologic grounds) to gluten during adolescence. Second, it has also been shown, in individual cases, that the mucosal lesions typical of the disease may appear de novo during adulthood.[199] The factors leading to the appearance or disappearance of gluten-sensitive enteropathy, however, are still unknown. Although adolescent patients may stray from their gluten-free diet, often without apparent ill effects, their inability to tolerate gluten remains, and many asymptomatic adolescent patients can be shown to have persistent hematologic, biochemical, and morphologic abnormalities.[82] If gluten ingestion continues into adult life, most patients with celiac disease eventually develop recurrent clinical evidence of celiac sprue. Therefore, patients with unequivocal evidence of celiac sprue in childhood should be encouraged to remain on a gluten-free diet indefinitely if recurrent clinical disease is to be avoided during adult life.

FUTURE THERAPIES

Our improved knowledge of celiac sprue pathogenesis allows us to envision several alternatives to the gluten-free diet. The increasingly precise knowledge of the immunostimulatory peptides has suggested several strategies. Genetic modification of wheat to delete toxic peptides is complicated by the large number of T cell epitopes and by the complexity of wheat genetics. An alternative strategy might be to develop peptide analogs capable of interfering with HLA-DQ binding and T cell activation to redirect the immune response toward tolerance. In mice, a vaccine based on the intranasal administration of whole gliadin or of one of its isoforms partially inhibited the systemic T cell response to parenteral challenge by whole gliadin.[200] This approach is not easy to transpose into humans, however, because of the risk of enhancing immunization instead of promoting tolerance. Another strategy, suggested by Maiuri and colleagues,[38] is blockade of signals derived from the cytokine IL-15. This proposal may be premature in uncomplicated celiac sprue in the absence of data concerning the consequence of IL-15 blockade in vivo in humans. Blocking IL-15 and its signals, however, is an attractive possibility in refractory sprue, when patients have become unresponsive to the diet and do not experience a response to conventional anti-inflammatory therapy.

Finally, one interesting suggestion was made by Shan and colleagues,[201] who showed that treating a recombinant α-gliadin with a combination of digestive enzymes in conditions mimicking the in vivo situation released a highly resistant 33-amino acid peptide (33-mer) encompassing a cluster of three immunodominant T cell epitopes. The resistance of this peptide to digestive enzymes was ascribed to its high proline content, because rapid hydrolysis could be obtained in the presence of a bacterial prolyl-endopeptidase.[201] The authors suggested that a bacterial endoprotease could be used therapeutically to cleave gliadin peptides left uncut by gastric acid and digestive and brush border enzymes. Data indicating that the defective intraluminal digestion of gliadin peptides is compensated largely by their efficient epithelial processing in treated patients with celiac sprue do not entirely argue against this possibility.[202] It might be useful to decrease the intraluminal concentration of peptides to reduce further the tiny amounts of gliadin peptides that can escape epithelial processing. Because celiac sprue is, in most cases, a benign disease fully treated by a safe, established diet, any alternative treatment must meet high standards of efficiency and safety. The creation of good animal models for the investigation of celiac sprue would be useful to confirm the new pathogenic hypotheses and to test novel therapeutic approaches.

REFERENCES

1. Farrell RJ, Kelly CP: Celiac sprue. N Engl J Med 346:180, 2002.
2. Arranz E, Ferguson A: Intestinal antibody pattern of celiac disease: Occurrence in patients with normal jejunal biopsy histology. Gastroenterology 104:1263, 1993.
3. Trier JS: Diagnosis of celiac sprue. Gastroenterology 115:211, 1998.
4. Adams F: The extant works of Aretaeus of Cappodocian. London, Sydenham Society, 1856.
5. Gee S: On the coeliac affection. St Barth Hosp Rep 24:17, 1888.
6. Dicke W: Coeliac disease: Investigation of Harmful Effects of Certain Types of Cereal on Patients with Coeliac Disease. University of Utrecht, Netherlands, 1950.
7. van de Kamer JH, Weijers NA, Dicke WK: Coeliac disease: IV. An investigation into the injurious constituents of wheat in connection with their action in patients with coeliac disease. Acta Paediatr 42:223, 1953.
8. Paulley L: Observations on the aetiology of idiopathic steatorrhea. BMJ 2:1318, 1954.
9. Rubin CE, Brandborg LL, Phelps PC, Taylor HC Jr: Studies of celiac disease: I. The apparent identical and specific nature of the duodenal and proximal jejunal lesion in celiac disease and idiopathic sprue. Gastroenterology 38:28, 1960.
10. Howell MD, Austin RK, Kelleher D, et al: An HLA-D region restriction fragment length polymorphism associated with celiac disease. J Exp Med 164:333, 1986.
11. Lundin KE, Scott H, Hansen T, et al: Gliadin-specific, HLA-DQ(alpha 1*0501,beta 1*0201) restricted T cells isolated from the small intestinal mucosa of celiac disease patients. J Exp Med 178:187, 1993.
12. Dieterich W, Ehnis T, Bauer M, et al: Identification of tissue transglutaminase as the autoantigen of celiac disease. Nat Med 3:797, 1997.
13. Molberg O, McAdam SN, Korner R, et al: Tissue transglutaminase selectively modifies gliadin peptides that are recognized by gut-derived T cells in celiac disease. Nat Med 4:713, 1998.
14. Anderson RP, Degano P, Godkin AJ, et al: In vivo antigen challenge in celiac disease identifies a single transglutaminase-modified peptide as the dominant α-gliadin T-cell epitope. Nat Med 6:337, 2000.
15. Cellier C, Delabesse E, Helmer C, et al: Refractory sprue, coeliac disease, and enteropathy-associated T-cell lymphoma. French Coeliac Disease Study Group. Lancet 356:203, 2000.
16. Mention JJ, Ben Ahmed M, Begue B, et al: Interleukin 15: A key to disrupted intraepithelial lymphocyte homeostasis and lymphomagenesis in celiac disease. Gastroenterology 125:730, 2003.
17. Catassi C, Fabiani E, Ratsch IM, et al: The coeliac iceberg in Italy: A multicentre antigliadin antibodies screening for coeliac disease in school-age subjects. Acta Paediatr Suppl 412:29, 1996.
18. Maki M, Mustalahti K, Kokkonen J, et al: Prevalence of celiac disease among children in Finland. N Engl J Med 348:2517, 2003.
19. Johnston SD, Watson RG, McMillan SA, et al: Coeliac disease detected by screening is not silent—simply unrecognized. Q J Med 91:853, 1998.
20. Rossipal E: Incidence of coeliac disease in children in Austria. Z Kinderheilkd 119:143, 1975.
21. Cavell B, Stenhammar L, Ascher H, et al: Increasing incidence of childhood coeliac disease in Sweden: Results of a national study. Acta Paediatr 81:589, 1992.
22. Weile B, Cavell B, Nivenius K, Krasilnikoff PA: Striking differences in the incidence of childhood celiac disease between Denmark and Sweden: A plausible explanation. J Pediatr Gastroenterol Nutr 21:64, 1995.
23. Not T, Horvath K, Hill ID, et al: Celiac disease risk in the USA: High prevalence of antiendomysium antibodies in healthy blood donors. Scand J Gastroenterol 33:494, 1998.
24. Fasano A, Berti I, Gerarduzzi T, et al: Prevalence of celiac disease in at-risk and not-at-risk groups in the United States: A large multicenter study. Arch Intern Med 163:286, 2003.
25. Catassi C, Ratsch IM, Gandolfi L, et al: Why is coeliac disease endemic in the people of the Sahara? Lancet. 354:647, 1999.
26. Madara JL, Trier JS: Structural abnormalities of jejunal epithelial cell membranes in celiac sprue. Lab Invest 43:254, 1980.
27. Wright NA, Watson AJ, Morley AR, et al: Cell production rate in mucosa of untreated coeliac disease. Gut 13:846, 1972.
28. Baklien K, Brandtzaeg P, Fausa O: Immunoglobulins in jejunal mucosa and serum from patients with adult coeliac disease. Scand J Gastroenterol 12:149, 1977.
29. Marsh MN: Gluten, major histocompatibility complex, and the small intestine: A molecular and immunobiologic

approach to the spectrum of gluten sensitivity ("celiac sprue"). Gastroenterology 102:330, 1992.

30. Rubin CE, Brandborg LL, Flick AL, et al: Biopsy studies on the pathogenesis of celiac sprue. In Wolstenholme GEW, Cameron MP (eds): Intestinal Biopsy. Boston, Little, Brown, 1962, p 67.

31. Grefte JM, Bouman JG, Grond J, et al: Slow and incomplete histological and functional recovery in adult gluten-sensitive enteropathy. J Clin Pathol 41:886, 1988.

32. De Vincenzi M, Luchetti R, Peruffo AD, et al: In vitro assessment of acetic acid–soluble proteins (glutenin) toxicity in celiac disease. J Biochem Toxicol 11:205, 1996.

33. Troncone R, Auricchio S, De Vincenzi M, et al: An analysis of cereals that react with serum antibodies in patients with coeliac disease. J Pediatr Gastroenterol Nutr 6:346, 1987.

34. Autran JC, Ellen J, Law L, et al: N-terminal amino acid sequencing of prolamins of wheat and related species. Nature 282:527, 1979.

35. Ciclitira PJ, Ellis HJ: Investigation of cereal toxicity in coeliac disease. Postgrad Med J 63:767, 1987.

36. Kasarda DD, Okita TW, Bernardin JE, et al: Nucleic acid (cDNA) and amino acid sequences of α-type gliadins from wheat (Triticum aestivum). Proc Natl Acad Sci U S A 81:4712, 1984.

37. Vader W, Kooy Y, Van Veelen P, et al: The gluten response in children with celiac disease is directed toward multiple gliadin and glutenin peptides. Gastroenterology 122:1729, 2002.

38. Maiuri L, Ciacci C, Ricciardelli I, et al: Association between innate response to gliadin and activation of pathogenic T cells in celiac disease. Lancet 362:30, 2003.

39. Gianfrani C, Troncone R, Mugione P, et al: Celiac disease association with CD8+ T cell responses: Identification of a novel gliadin-derived HLA-A2-restricted epitope. J Immunol 170:2719, 2003.

40. Kagnoff MF, Paterson YJ, Kumar PJ, et al: Evidence for the role of a human intestinal adenovirus in the pathogenesis of coeliac disease. Gut 28:995, 1987.

41. Arato A, Kosnai I, Szonyi L, Toth M: Frequent past exposure to adenovirus 12 in coeliac disease. Acta Paediatr Scand 80:1101, 1991.

42. Nieuwenhuizen WF, Pieters RH, Knippels LM, et al: Is Candida albicans a trigger in the onset of coeliac disease? Lancet 361:2152, 2003.

43. Shidrawi RG, Day P, Przemioslo R, et al: In vitro toxicity of gluten peptides in coeliac disease assessed by organ culture. Scand J Gastroenterol 30:758, 1995.

44. Schuppan D: Current concepts of celiac disease pathogenesis. Gastroenterology 119:234, 2000.

45. Schmitz J: Lack of oats toxicity in coeliac disease. BMJ 314:159, 1997.

46. Ellis A: Coeliac disease: Previous family studies. In McConnel RB (ed): The Genetics of Coeliac Disease. Lancaster, England, MTP Press, 1981, p 197.

47. Sollid LM, Markussen G, Ek J, et al: Evidence for a primary association of celiac disease to a particular HLA-DQ alpha/beta heterodimer. J Exp Med 169:345, 1989.

48. Nilsen EM, Lundin KE, Krajci P, et al: Gluten-specific, HLA-DQ-restricted T cells from coeliac mucosa produce cytokines with Th$_1$ or Th$_0$ profile dominated by interferon-γ. Gut 37:766, 1995.

49. Lie BA, Sollid LM, Ascher H, et al: A gene telomeric of the HLA class I region is involved in predisposition to both type 1 diabetes and coeliac disease. Tissue Antigens 54:162, 1999.

50. McManus R, Wilson AG, Mansfield J, et al: TNF-2, a polymorphism of the tumour necrosis-α gene promoter, is a component of the celiac disease major histocompatibility complex haplotype. Eur J Immunol 26:2113, 1996.

51. Polvi A, Maki M, Collin P, Partanen J: TNF microsatellite alleles a2 and b3 are not primarily associated with celiac disease in the Finnish population. Tissue Antigens 51:553, 1998.

52. Petronzelli F, Bonamico M, Ferrante P, et al: Genetic contribution of the HLA region to the familial clustering of coeliac disease. Ann Hum Genet 61:307, 1997.

53. Babron MC, Nilsson S, Adamovic S, et al: Genetics cluster on coeliac disease: Meta and pooled analysis of European coeliac disease data. Eur J Hum Genet 11: 828, 2003.

54. Djlali-Saiah I, Schmitz J, Harfouch-Hammoud E, et al: CTLA-4 gene polymorphism is associated with predisposition to celiac disease. Gut 43:187, 1998.

55. Sollid L: Celiac disease: Dissecting a complex inflammatory disorder. Nat Rev Immunol 9:647, 2002.

56. Kelly CP, Feighery CF, Gallagher RB, et al: Mucosal and systemic IgA anti-gliadin antibody in celiac disease: Contrasting patterns of response in serum, saliva, and intestinal secretions. Dig Dis Sci 36:743, 1991.

57. Uibo O, Uibo R, Kleimola V, et al: Serum IgA anti-gliadin antibodies in an adult population sample: High prevalence without celiac disease. Dig Dis Sci 38:2034, 1993.

58. Hvatum M, Scott H, Brandtzaeg P: Serum IgG subclass antibodies to a variety of food antigens in patients with coeliac disease. Gut 33:632, 1992.

59. Chorzelski TP, Beutner EH, Sulej J, et al: IgA anti-endomysium antibody: A new immunological marker of dermatitis herpetiformis and coeliac disease. Br J Dermatol 111:395, 1984.

60. van de Wal Y, Kooy Y, van Veelen P, et al: Selective deamidation by tissue transglutaminase strongly enhances gliadin-specific T cell reactivity. J Immunol 161:1585, 1998.

61. Szabolcs M, Sipka S, Csorba S: In vitro cross-linking of gluten into high-molecular-weight polymers with transglutaminase. Acta Paediatr Hung 28:215, 1987.

62. Halttunen T, Maki M: Serum immunoglobulin A from patients with celiac disease inhibits human T84 intestinal crypt epithelial cell differentiation. Gastroenterology 116:566, 1999.

63. Halstensen TS, Scott H, Fausa O, Brandtzaeg P: Gluten stimulation of coeliac mucosa in vitro induces activation (CD25) of lamina propria CD4+ T cells and macrophages but no crypt-cell hyperplasia. Scand J Immunol 38:581, 1993.

64. Brandtzaeg P, Halstensen TS, Kett K, et al: Immunobiology and immunopathology of human gut mucosa: Humoral immunity and intraepithelial lymphocytes. Gastroenterology 97:1562, 1989.

65. Halstensen TS, Scott H, Brandtzaeg P: Human CD8+ intraepithelial T lymphocytes are mainly CD45RA-RB+ and show increased co-expression of CD45R0 in celiac disease. Eur J Immunol 20:1825, 1990.

66. Halstensen TS, Scott H, Brandtzaeg P: Intraepithelial T cells of the TcR gamma/delta+ CD8- and V delta 1/J delta 1+ phenotypes are increased in coeliac disease. Scand J Immunol 30:665, 1989.

67. Mak TW, Ferrick DA: The gamma/delta T-cell bridge: Linking innate and acquired immunity. Nat Med 4:764, 1998.

68. Cellier C, Patey N, Mauvieux L, et al: Abnormal intestinal intraepithelial lymphocytes in refractory sprue. Gastroenterology 114:471, 1998.

69. Maiuri L, Ciacci C, Ricciardelli I, et al: Association between innate response to gliadin and activation of pathogenic T cells in celiac disease. Lancet 362:30, 2003.

70. Damen GM, Boersma B, Wit JM, Heymans HS: Catch-up growth in 60 children with celiac disease. J Pediatr Gastroenterol Nutr 19:394, 1994.

71. Ansaldi N, Tavassoli K, Dell'Olio D, et al: Clinical data on celiac disease with an early or late onset. Minerva Pediatr 43:377, 1991.

72. Ascher H, Krantz I, Rydberg L, et al: Influence of infant feeding and gluten intake on coeliac disease. Arch Dis Child 76:113, 1997.

73. Beaumont DM, Mian MS: Coeliac disease in old age: "A catch in the rye." Age Ageing 27:535, 1998.

74. Vuoristo M, Miettinen TA: The role of fat and bile acid malabsorption in diarrhoea of coeliac disease. Scand J Gastroenterol 22:289, 1987.

75. Maton PN, Selden AC, Fitzpatrick ML, Chadwick VS: Defective gallbladder emptying and cholecystokinin release in celiac disease: Reversal by gluten-free diet. Gastroenterology 88:391, 1985.

76. Sanders DS, Carter MJ, Hurlstone DP, et al: Association of adult coeliac disease with irritable bowel syndrome: A case-control study in patients fulfilling ROME II criteria referred to secondary care. Lancet. 358:1504, 2001.

77. O'Farrelly C, O'Mahony C, Graeme-Cook F, et al: Gliadin antibodies identify gluten-sensitive oral ulceration in the absence of villous atrophy. J Oral Pathol Med 20:476, 1991.

78. O'Grady JG, Stevens FM, Harding B, et al: Hyposplenism and gluten-sensitive enteropathy: Natural history, incidence, and relationship to diet and small bowel morphology. Gastroenterology 87:1326, 1984.

79. Corazza GR, Di Sario A, Cecchetti L, et al: Bone mass and metabolism in patients with celiac disease. Gastroenterology 109:122, 1995.

80. Kemppainen T, Kroger H, Janatuinen E, et al: Osteoporosis in adult patients with celiac disease. Bone 24:249, 1999.

81. Vasquez H, Mazure R, Gonzalez D, et al: Risk of fractures in celiac disease patients: A cross-sectional, case-control study. Am J Gastroenterol 95:183, 2000.

82. Cellier C, Flobert C, Cormier C, et al: Severe osteopenia in symptom-free adults with a childhood diagnosis of coeliac disease. Lancet 355:806, 2000.

83. Thomason K, West J, Logan RF, et al: Fracture experience of patients with coeliac disease: A population-based survey. Gut 52:518, 2003.

84. Hadjivassiliou M, Grunewald RA, Chattopadhyay AK, et al: Clinical, radiological, neurophysiological, and neuropathological characteristics of gluten ataxia. Lancet 352:1582, 1998.

85. Lewis PD, Pallis CA (eds): Neurological complications of coeliac disease and tropical sprue. In The Neurology of Gastrointestinal Disease. London, WB Saunders, 1974, p 138.

86. Gobbi G, Bouquet F, Greco L, et al: Coeliac disease, epilepsy, and cerebral calcifications. The Italian Working Group on Coeliac Disease and Epilepsy. Lancet 340:439, 1992.

87. Ferroir JP, Fenelon G, Billy C, et al: Epilepsy, cerebral calcifications, and celiac disease. Rev Neurol (Paris) 153:354, 1997.

88. Addolorato G, Capristo E, Ghittoni G, et al: Anxiety but not depression decreases in coeliac patients after one-year gluten-free diet: A longitudinal study. Scand J Gastroenterol 36:502, 2001.

89. Molteni N, Bardella MT, Bianchi PA: Obstetric and gynecological problems in women with untreated celiac sprue. J Clin Gastroenterol 12:37, 1990.

90. Collin P, Vilska S, Heinonen PK, et al: Infertility and coeliac disease. Gut 39:382, 1996.

91. Gasbarrini A, Torre ES, Trivellini C, et al: Recurrent spontaneous abortion and intrauterine fetal growth retardation as symptoms of coeliac disease. Lancet 356:399, 2000.

92. Farthing MJ, Rees LH, Dawson AM: Male gonadal function in coeliac disease: III. Pituitary regulation. Clin Endocrinol (Oxf) 19:661, 1983.

93. Aine L, Maki M, Collin P, Keyrilainen O: Dental enamel defects in celiac disease. J Oral Pathol Med 19:241, 1990.

94. Kelly CP, Feighery CF, Gallagher RB, Weir DG: Diagnosis and treatment of gluten-sensitive enteropathy. Adv Intern Med 35:341, 1990.

95. Stern M: Comparative evaluation of serologic tests for celiac disease: A European initiative toward standardization. J Pediatr Gastroenterol Nutr 31:513, 2000.

96. Rostami K, Kerckhaert J, Tiemessen R, et al: Sensitivity of antiendomysium and antigliadin antibodies in untreated celiac disease: Disappointing in clinical practice. Am J Gastroenterol 94:888, 1999.

97. Volta U, Molinaro N, de Franceschi L, et al: IgA anti-endomysial antibodies on human umbilical cord tissue for celiac disease screening: Save both money and monkeys. Dig Dis Sci 40:1902, 1995.

98. Ferreira M, Davies SL, Butler M, et al: Endomysial antibody: Is it the best screening test for coeliac disease? Gut 33:1633, 1992.

99. Kapuscinska A, Zalewski T, Chorzelski TP, et al: Disease specificity and dynamics of changes in IgA class anti-endomysial antibodies in celiac disease. J Pediatr Gastroenterol Nutr 6:529, 1987.

100. Dieterich W, Laag E, Schopper H, et al: Autoantibodies to tissue transglutaminase as predictors of celiac disease. Gastroenterology 115:1317, 1998.

101. Sulkanen S, Halttunen T, Laurila K, et al: Tissue transglutaminase autoantibody enzyme-linked immunosorbent assay in detecting celiac disease. Gastroenterology 115:1322, 1998.

102. Carroccio A, Vitale G, Di Prima L et al: Comparison of anti-transglutaminase ELISAs and an anti-endomysial antibody assay in the diagnosis of celiac disease: A prospective study. Clin Chem 48:1546, 2002.

103. Gillett HR, Freeman HJ: Comparison of IgA endomysium antibody and IgA tissue transglutaminase antibody in celiac disease. Can J Gastroenterol 14:668, 2000.

104. Kilander AF, Dotevall G, Fallstrom SP, et al: Evaluation of gliadin antibodies for detection of coeliac disease. Scand J Gastroenterol 18:377, 1983.

105. Corrao G, Corazza GR, Andreani ML, et al: Serological screening of coeliac disease: Choosing the optimal procedure according to various prevalence values. Gut 35:771, 1994.

106. Grodzinsky E, Hed J, Skogh T: IgA antiendomysium antibodies have a high positive predictive value for celiac disease in asymptomatic patients. Allergy 49:593, 1994.

107. Tonutti E, Visentini D, Bizzaro N, et al: French-Italian Laboratory Study Group on Coeliac Disease. The role of antitissue transglutaminase assay for the diagnosis and monitoring of coeliac disease: A French-Italian multicentre study. J Clin Pathol 56:389, 2003.

108. Kumar PJ: European and North American populations should not be screened for celiac disease. Gut 52:170, 2002.

109. Fasano A: European and North American populations should be screened for celiac disease. Gut 52:168, 2002.

110. Fabiani E, Taccari LM, Ratsch IM, et al: Compliance with gluten-free diet in adolescents with screening-detected celiac disease: A 5-year follow-up study. J Pediatr 136:841, 2000.

111. Hin H, Bird G, Fisher P, et al: Celiac disease in primary care: Case finding study. BMJ 318:164, 1999.

112. Achkar E, Carey WD, Petras R, et al: Comparison of suction capsule and endoscopic biopsy of small bowel mucosa. Gastrointest Endosc 32:278, 1986.

113. Jabbari M, Wild G, Goresky CA, et al: Scalloped valvulae conniventes: An endoscopic marker of celiac sprue. Gastroenterology 95:1518, 1988.

114. Shah VH, Rotterdam H, Kotler DP, et al: All that scallops is not celiac disease. Gastrointest Endosc 51:717, 2000.

115. von Krainick HG, Debatin F, Gautier F, et al: Additional research on the injurious effect of wheat flour in coeliac disease: Acute gliadin reactions (gliadin shock). Helv Paediatr Acta 13:432, 1958.

116. Fine KD, Lee EL, Meyer RL: Colonic histopathology in untreated celiac sprue or refractory sprue: Is it lymphocytic colitis or colonic lymphocytosis? Hum Pathol 29:1433, 1998.

117. Walker-Smith J, Harrison M, Kilby A, et al: Cows' milk-sensitive enteropathy. Arch Dis Child 53:375, 1978.

118. Ament ME, Rubin CE: Soy protein–another cause of the flat intestinal lesion. Gastroenterology 62:227, 1972.

119. Weinstein WM, Saunders DR, Tytgat GN, Rubin CE: Collagenous sprue—an unrecognized type of malabsorption. N Engl J Med 283:1297, 1970.

120. Cooper BT, Holmes GK, Ferguson R, et al: Gluten-sensitive diarrhea without evidence of celiac disease. Gastroenterology 79:801, 1980.

121. Abdulkarim AS, Burgart LJ, See J, Murray JA: Etiology of non-responsive celiac disease: Results of a systematic approach. Am J Gastroenterol 97:2016, 2002.

122. Fry L: Dermatitis herpetiformis: Problems, progress and prospects. Eur J Dermatol 12:523, 2002.

123. Holmes GK, Prior P, Lane MR, et al: Malignancy in coeliac disease–effect of a gluten-free diet. Gut 30:333, 1989.

124. Lewis HM, Renaula TL, Garioch JJ, et al: Protective effect of gluten-free diet against development of lymphoma in dermatitis herpetiformis. Br J Dermatol 135:363, 1996.

125. Smith EP, Zone JJ: Dermatitis herpetiformis and linear IgA bullous dermatosis. Dermatol Clin 11:511, 1993.

126. Rose C, Dieterich W, Brocker EB, et al: Circulating autoantibodies to tissue transglutaminase differentiate patients with dermatitis herpetiformis from those with linear IgA disease. J Am Acad Dermatol 41:957, 1999.

127. Sardy M, Karpati S, Merkl B, et al: Epidermal transglutaminase (TGase3) is the autoantigen of dermatitis herpetiformis. J Exp Med 195:747, 2002.

128. Porter WM, Unsworth DJ, Lock RJ, et al: Tissue transglutaminase antibodies in dermatitis herpetiformis. Gastroenterology 117:749, 1999.

129. Garioch JJ, Lewis HM, Sargent SA, et al: Twenty-five years' experience of a gluten-free diet in the treatment of dermatitis herpetiformis. Br J Dermatol 131:541, 1994.

130. Hardman CM, Garioch JJ, Leonard JN, et al: Absence of toxicity of oats in patients with dermatitis herpetiformis. N Engl J Med 337:1884, 1997.

131. Sjoberg K, Eriksson KF, Bredberg A, et al: Screening for coeliac disease in adult insulin-dependent diabetes mellitus. J Intern Med 243:133, 1998.

132. Talal AH, Murray JA, Goeken JA, Sivitz WI: Celiac disease in an adult population with insulin-dependent diabetes mellitus: Use of endomysial antibody testing. Am J Gastroenterol 92:1280, 1997.

133. Cronin CC, Feighery A, Ferriss JB, et al: High prevalence of celiac disease among patients with insulin-dependent (type I) diabetes mellitus. Am J Gastroenterol 92:2210, 1997.

134. Collin P, Reunala T, Pukkala E, et al: Coeliac disease-associated disorders and survival. Gut 35:1215, 1994.

135. Counsell CE, Taha A, Ruddell WS: Coeliac disease and autoimmune thyroid disease. Gut 35:844, 1994.

136. Collin P, Maki M: Associated disorders in coeliac disease: Clinical aspects. Scand J Gastroenterol 29:769, 1994.

137. Rustgi AK, Peppercorn MA: Gluten-sensitive enteropathy and systemic lupus erythematosus. Arch Intern Med 148:1583, 1988.

138. Iltanen S, Collin P, Korpela M, et al: Celiac disease and markers of celiac disease latency in patients with primary Sjögren's syndrome. Am J Gastroenterol 94:1042, 1999.

139. Henriksson KG, Hallert C, Norrby K, Walan A: Polymyositis and adult coeliac disease. Acta Neurol Scand 65:301, 1982.

140. Ventura A, Magazzu G, Greco L: Duration of exposure to gluten and risk for autoimmune disorders in patients with celiac disease. Gastroenterology 117:297, 1999.

141. Sategna Guidetti C, Solerio E, Scaglione N, et al: Duration of gluten exposure in adult coeliac disease does not correlate with the risk for autoimmune disorders. Gut 49:502, 2001.

142. Collin P, Maki M, Keyrilainen O, et al: Selective IgA deficiency and coeliac disease. Scand J Gastroenterol 27:367, 1992.

143. O'Donoghue DJ: Fatal pneumococcal septicaemia in coeliac disease. Postgrad Med J 62:229, 1986.

144. Shah A, Mayberry JF, Williams G, et al: Epidemiological survey of coeliac disease and inflammatory bowel disease in first-degree relatives of coeliac patients. Q J Med 74:283, 1990.

145. Freeman HJ: Hepatobiliary tract and pancreatic disorders in celiac disease. Can J Gastroenterol 11:77, 1997.

146. Fornasieri A, Sinico RA, Maldifassi P, et al: IgA-antigliadin antibodies in IgA mesangial nephropathy (Berger's disease). BMJ 295:78, 1987.

147. Smith MJ, Benson MK, Strickland ID: Coeliac disease and diffuse interstitial lung disease. Lancet 1:473, 1971.

148. Reading R, Watson JG, Platt JW, Bird AG: Pulmonary haemosiderosis and gluten. Arch Dis Child 62:513, 1987.

149. Simila S, Kokkonen J: Coexistence of celiac disease and Down syndrome. Am J Ment Retard 95:120, 1990.

150. DuBois RN, Lazenby AJ, Yardley JH, et al: Lymphocytic enterocolitis in patients with "refractory sprue." JAMA 262:935, 1989.

151. Moayyedi P, O'Mahony S, Jackson P, et al: Small intestine in lymphocytic and collagenous colitis: Mucosal morphology, permeability, and secretory immunity to gliadin. J Clin Pathol 50:527, 1997.

152. Wolber R, Owen D, Freeman H: Colonic lymphocytosis in patients with celiac sprue. Hum Pathol 21:1092, 1990.

153. Loft DE, Marsh MN, Crowe PT: Rectal gluten challenge and diagnosis of coeliac disease. Lancet 335:1293, 1990.

154. McCashland TM, Donovan JP, Strobach RS, et al: Collagenous enterocolitis: A manifestation of gluten-sensitive enteropathy. J Clin Gastroenterol 15:45, 1992.

155. Fine KD, Do K, Schulte K, et al: High prevalence of celiac sprue-like HLA-DQ genes and enteropathy in patients with the microscopic colitis syndrome. Am J Gastroenterol 95:1974, 2000.

156. Miletic ID, Miletic VD, Sattely-Miller EA, Schiffman SS: Identification of gliadin presence in pharmaceutical products. J Pediatr Gastroenterol Nutr 19:27, 1994.

157. Dennis M, Case S: Going gluten free: A primer for clinicians. Pract Gastroenterol 28:86, 2004.

158. http://consensus.nih.gov/cons/118/118celiac.htm

159. Janatuinen EK, Pikkarainen PH, Kemppainen TA, et al: A comparison of diets with and without oats in adults with celiac disease. N Engl J Med 333:1033, 1995.

160. Janatuinen EK, Kemppainen TA, Julkunen RJ, et al: No harm from five-year ingestion of oats in coeliac disease. Gut 50:332, 2002.

161. Hoffenberg EJ, Haas J, Drescher A, et al: A trial of oats in children with newly diagnosed celiac disease. J Pediatr 137:361, 2000.

162. Pink IJ, Creamer B: Response to a gluten-free diet of patients with the coeliac syndrome. Lancet 1:300, 1967.

163. MacDonald WC, Brandborg LL, Flick AL, et al: Studies of celiac sprue: IV. The response of the whole length of the small bowel to a gluten-free diet. Gastroenterology 47:573, 1964.

164. Katz AJ, Falchuk ZM, Strober W, Shwachman H: Gluten-sensitive enteropathy: Inhibition by cortisol of the effect of gluten protein in vitro. N Engl J Med 295:131, 1976.

165. Mitchison HC, al Mardini H, Gillespie S, et al: A pilot study of fluticasone propionate in untreated coeliac disease. Gut 32:260, 1991.

166. Lloyd-Still JD, Grand RJ, Khaw KT, Shwachman H: The use of corticosteroids in celiac crisis. J Pediatr 81:1074, 1972.

167. Vaidya A, Bolanos J, Berkelhammer C: Azathioprine in refractory sprue. Am J Gastroenterol 94:1967, 1999.

168. Longstreth GF: Successful treatment of refractory sprue with cyclosporine. Ann Intern Med 119:1014, 1993.

169. Gillett HR, Arnott ID, McIntyre M, et al: Successful infliximab treatment for steroid-refractory celiac disease: A case report. Gastroenterology 122:800, 2002.

170. Valdimarsson T, Lofman O, Toss G, Strom M: Reversal of osteopenia with diet in adult coeliac disease. Gut 38:322, 1996.

171. Sategna-Guidetti C, Grosso SB, Grosso S, et al: The effects of one-year gluten withdrawal on bone mass, bone metabolism, and nutritional status in newly diagnosed adult coeliac disease patients. Aliment Pharmacol Ther 14:35, 2000.

172. Valdimarsson T, Toss G, Lofman O, Strom M: Three years' follow-up of bone density in adult coeliac disease: Significance of secondary hyperparathyroidism. Scand J Gastroenterol 35:274, 2000.

173. Bernstein CN, Leslie WD, Leboff MS: AGA Medical Position Statement: Guidelines on osteoporosis in gastrointestinal diseases. Gastroenterology 124:791, 2003.

174. Jones PE, Peters TJ: Oral zinc supplements in non-responsive coeliac syndrome: Effect on jejunal morphology, enterocyte production, and brush border disaccharidase activities. Gut 22:194, 1981.

175. Corrao G, Corazza GR, Bagnardi V, et al: Mortality in patients with coeliac disease and their relatives: A cohort study. Lancet 358:356, 2001.

176. Askling J, Linet M, Gridley G, et al: Cancer incidence in a population-based cohort of individuals hospitalized with celiac disease or dermatitis herpetiformis. Gastroenterology 123:1428, 2002.

177. Catassi C, Fabiani E, Corrao G, et al: Risk of non-Hodgkin lymphoma in celiac disease. JAMA 287:1413, 2002.

178. Cerf-Bensussan N, Cellier C, Heyman M, et al: Coeliac disease: An update on facts and questions based on the 10th International Symposium on Coeliac Disease. J Pediatr Gastroenterol Nutr 37:412, 2003.

179. Spencer J, Cerf-Bensussan N, Jarry A, et al: Enteropathy-associated T cell lymphoma (malignant histiocytosis of the intestine) is recognized by a monoclonal antibody (HML-1) that defines a membrane molecule on human mucosal lymphocytes. Am J Pathol 132:1, 1988.

180. Freeman HJ, Chiu BK: Small bowel malignant lymphoma complicating celiac sprue and the mesenteric lymph node cavitation syndrome. Gastroenterology 90:2008, 1986.

181. Matuchansky C, Colin R, Hemet J, et al: Cavitation of mesenteric lymph nodes, splenic atrophy, and a flat small intestinal mucosa: Report of six cases. Gastroenterology 87:606, 1984.

182. Egan LJ, Walsh SV, Stevens FM, et al: Celiac-associated lymphoma: A single-institution experience of 30 cases in the combination chemotherapy era. J Clin Gastroenterol 21:123, 1995.

183. Baer AN, Bayless TM, Yardley JH: Intestinal ulceration and malabsorption syndromes. Gastroenterology 79:754, 1980.

184. Enns R, Lay T, Bridges R: Use of azathioprine for nongranulomatous ulcerative jejunoileitis. Can J Gastroenterol 11:503, 1997.

185. Bossart R, Henry K, Booth CC, Doe WF: Subepithelial collagen in intestinal malabsorption. Gut 16:18, 1975.

186. Freeman HJ: Hyposplenism, antiendomysial antibodies, and lymphocytic colitis in collagenous sprue. Can J Gastroenterol 13:347, 1999.

187. Guller R, Anabitarte M, Mayer M: Collagenous sprue and ulcerative jejuno-ileitis in a patient with gluten-induced enteropathy. Schweiz Med Wochenschr 116:1343, 1986.

188. Holtmann M, von Herbay A, Galle PR, Stremmel W: Long-term collagenous sprue: Remission with a gluten-free diet. Z Gastroenterol 37:1163, 1999.

189. Ciacci C, Mazzacca G: Unintentional gluten ingestion in celiac patients. Gastroenterology 115:243, 1998.

190. Ryan BM, Kelleher D: Refractory celiac disease. Gastroenterology 119:243, 2000.

191. Wahab PJ, Crusius JB, Meijer JW, et al: Cyclosporin in the treatment of adults with refractory coeliac disease: An open pilot study. Aliment Pharmacol Ther 14:767, 2000.

192. Corazza GR, Biagi F, Volta U, et al: Autoimmune enteropathy and villous atrophy in adults. Lancet 350:106, 1997.

193. Murray A, Cuevas EC, Jones DB, Wright DH: Study of the immunohistochemistry and T cell clonality of enteropathy-associated T cell lymphoma. Am J Pathol 146:509, 1995.

194. Ashton-Key M, Diss TC, Pan L, et al: Molecular analysis of T-cell clonality in ulcerative jejunitis and enteropathy-associated T-cell lymphoma. Am J Pathol 151:493, 1997.

195. Bagdi E, Diss TC, Munson P, Isaacson PG: Mucosal intra-epithelial lymphocytes in enteropathy-associated T-cell lymphoma, ulcerative jejunitis, and refractory celiac disease constitute a neoplastic population. Blood 94:260, 1999.

196. de Bruin PC, Connolly CE, Oudejans JJ, et al: Enteropathy-associated T-cell lymphomas have a cytotoxic T-cell phenotype. Histopathology 31:313, 1997.

197. Logan RF, Rifkind EA, Turner ID, Ferguson A: Mortality in celiac disease. Gastroenterology 97:265, 1989.

198. Nielsen OH, Jacobsen O, Pedersen ER, et al: Non-tropical sprue: Malignant diseases and mortality rate. Scand J Gastroenterol 20:13, 1985.

199. Schmitz J: Is celiac disease a lifelong disorder? Clin Invest Med 19:352, 1996.

200. Maurano F, Siciliano RA, De Giulio B, et al: Intranasal administration of one α-gliadin can downregulate the immune response to whole gliadin in mice. Scand J Immunol 53:290, 2001.

201. Shan L, Molberg O, Parrot I, et al: Structural basis for gluten intolerance in celiac sprue. Science 297:2218, 2002.

202. Matysiak Budnik T, Candalh C, Dugave C, et al: Alterations of the intestinal transport and processing of gliadin peptides in celiac disease. Gastroenterology 125;696, 2003.

CHAPTER

102 Tropical Malabsorption and Tropical Diarrhea

Michael J. G. Farthing

Malabsorption of dietary nutrients by the small intestine has special relevance for people living in the tropics and subtropics. The causes of intestinal malabsorption differ from those commonly seen in the industrialized world, and the clinical impact often is substantially greater because many persons in the developing world, particularly infants and young children, exist in a state of borderline undernutrition. Tropical malabsorption and diarrhea are not limited to the indigenous population but commonly affect travelers, particularly those from the industrialized world.[1] Acute infectious diarrhea, most commonly caused by enterotoxigenic *Escherichia coli*, is the most common affliction of travelers, although chronic diarrhea and malabsorption also occur as a result of specific infections and tropical sprue.

Tropical malabsorption can be considered to be caused either by *specific* causes, such as known infections and inflammatory and neoplastic disorders, or *nonspecific* conditions, such as tropical enteropathy and tropical sprue, for which the etiology has not been determined (Table 102–1). Acute diarrhea in the tropics without overt intestinal malabsorption is usually caused by acute infection with one or more of a variety of enteropathogens that include bacteria, viruses, protozoa, and helminths (Table 102–2). These organisms are not discussed in detail in this chapter and are dealt with in Chapters 32, 104, 106, and 107.

SPECIFIC CAUSES OF TROPICAL MALABSORPTION

INTESTINAL INFECTION

Most infections that cause intestinal malabsorption in the tropics produce an enteropathy with varying degrees of villus atrophy, crypt hyperplasia, and inflammatory infiltrates in the lamina propria and in some cases in the epithelium.[2] *Giardia lamblia* is the most common human protozoan enteropathogen and is well recognized to cause chronic diarrhea and intestinal malabsorption. Infection with *G. lamblia* is considered a contributory factor in the retardation of growth and development in infants and young children. *Isospora belli* also produces chronic diarrhea and enteropathy but is geographically restricted to the tropics and subtropics, unlike *Giardia*, which is found worldwide. *Cyclospora cayetanensis* is a recently recognized intracellular protozoan that has been identified in a number of tropical and subtropical locations as a cause of chronic diarrhea and enteropathy in both immunocompetent and immunocompromised persons.[3] It was first recognized in travelers in Nepal who presented with diarrhea that persisted for many weeks, often in association with profound weight loss. The more commonly recognized intracellular protozoan, *Cryptosporidium parvum*, is a well-known cause of chronic diarrhea worldwide in immunocompetent persons, in whom the diarrhea is usually is self-limited. *C. parvum* is, however, a major cause of chronic, intractable diarrhea in patients with human immunodeficiency virus (HIV) infection or acquired immunodeficiency syndrome (AIDS). In the developed world, where highly active antiretroviral therapy (HAART) is available, the clinical impact of infection with *C. parvum* has declined dramatically, whereas in the tropics, cryptosporidiosis continues to be a major cause of morbidity and mortality in patients with AIDS. The Microsporida species have emerged as important causes of persistent diarrhea in HIV-infected patients in the tropics. *Enterocytozoon bieneusi* was the first Microsporida to be identified as an important cause of human diarrheal disease, followed by *Encephalitozoon intestinalis*; both species occur in the tropics,

Table 102–1 Tropical Malabsorption

Causes	Specific Organisms
Specific	
Infection	
Protozoa	*Giardia lamblia*
	Isospora belli
	Cryptosporidium parvum
	Enterocytozoon bieneusi
	Encephalitozoon intestinalis
	Cyclospora cayetanensis
Helminths	*Capillaria philippinensis*
	Strongyloides stercoralis
Bacteria	Enteropathogenic *Escherichia coli*
	Mycobacterium tuberculosis
Viruses	Rotavirus
	Enteric adenoviruses (types 40, 41)
	Small, round, structured viruses (e.g., Norovirus)
	Measles virus
	Human immunodeficiency virus
Celiac sprue	
Lymphoma	
Severe undernutrition (kwashiorkor, marasmus)	
Primary hypolactasia	
Nonspecific	
Tropical enteropathy	
Tropical sprue	

Table 102–2 Tropical Diarrhea: Major Enteropathogens

Type of Pathogen	Specific Pathogen
Bacteria	Enterotoxigenic *Escherichia coli* (ETEC)
	Enteropathogenic *E. coli* (EPEC)
	Enteroaggregative *E. coli* (EAggEC)
	Enteroinvasive *E. coli* (EIEC)
	Salmonella
	Shigella
	Campylobacter jejuni
	Mycobacterium tuberculosis (and *Mycobacterium bovis*)
	Aeromonas and *Plesiomonas*
Viruses	Rotavirus
	Enteric adenoviruses (types 40, 41)
	Measles virus
	Human immunodeficiency virus
Protozoa	
Ciliophora	*Balantidium coli*
Mastigophora	*Giardia lamblia*
Coccidia	*Cryptosporidium parvum*
	Isospora belli
Microspora	*Enterocytozoon bieneusi*
	Encephalitozoon intestinalis
Cyclospora	*Cyclospora cayetanensis*
Helminths	*Strongyloides stercoralis*
	Schistosoma

and *E. intestinalis* is notable for its susceptibility to albendazole.[4,5]

Helminths are not a major cause of intestinal malabsorption, although heavy infection with *Strongyloides stercoralis*, including the hyperinfection syndrome, should be included in the differential diagnosis of diarrhea in populations that tend to have multiple coincident infections. *Capillaria philippinensis* is an important cause of intestinal malabsorption in a highly restricted geographic area in Southeast Asia.

Rotavirus, enteric adenoviruses, and the small, round, structured viruses such as Norwalk virus (recently renamed Norovirus) all produce enteropathy, but the illness is usually self-limited, and a chronic malabsorptive state virtually never occurs. The relationship of HIV to enteropathy is controversial, although there is evidence to suggest that the virus itself may be responsible for small intestinal damage, even in the absence of other enteropathogens. The precise mechanisms responsible have not been fully elucidated, although T cell activation does not appear to play a major role, as it does in other forms of enteropathy such as celiac sprue.[6] HIV-related enteropathy appears to be more severe in Africa than in Western Europe, suggesting that background tropical enteropathy may be a risk factor for enteropathy in AIDS (see Chapter 32).

Most bacterial infections of the small intestine produce acute diarrhea and a self-limited illness. Some enteropathogenic *E. coli* strains, however, produce chronic diarrhea and malabsorption in infants and young children; diffuse small intestinal involvement with *Mycobacterium tuberculosis* can produce a similar picture.

CELIAC SPRUE

Celiac sprue (gluten-sensitive enteropathy) is uncommon in the tropics but is described in Africa and India, particularly northern India, where wheat-containing foods form an important part of the diet. Celiac sprue may manifest for the first time in the tropics in European and North American expatriates and thus should be included in the differential diagnosis of such persons who develop persistent diarrhea. Distinguishing celiac sprue from tropical sprue can be difficult in the tropical setting. The morphologic changes in the jejunum usually are more profound in celiac sprue than in tropical sprue and will almost inevitably respond to gluten withdrawal but not to broad-spectrum antibiotics. Testing for antiendomysial or tissue transglutaminase antibodies is now recognized to be a sensitive and specific screen for celiac sprue and should be performed in travelers returning from the tropics with chronic diarrhea with or without overt malabsorption. Clearly, a patient with tropical malabsorption should not be committed to a lifelong gluten-free diet unless the diagnosis of celiac sprue is absolutely secure (see Chapter 101).

LYMPHOMA

Immunoproliferative small intestinal disease (IPSID) and primary upper small intestinal lymphoma (PUSIL) are found predominantly in areas of socioeconomic deprivation (see Chapter 28). Although commonly known as *Mediterranean lymphoma*, the condition has been described in other parts of the world, including the Middle East, South Africa, and South America. Current evidence suggests that these conditions are related; IPSID may progress to PUSIL, and IPSID is, therefore, a premalignant condition. These two disorders usually occur in a younger age group, in contrast to primary intestinal lymphoma, which occurs worldwide, mostly in elderly people.

SEVERE UNDERNUTRITION

Although it is clearly established that luminal nutrients are vital for maintaining mucosal integrity in the gut, the role of undernutrition in the pathogenesis of intestinal malabsorption and small intestinal enteropathy remains controversial. Steatorrhea and villus atrophy have been described in children who have severe kwashiorkor and marasmus, with reversion toward normal following nutritional rehabilitation. Current evidence suggests, however, that less severe degrees of undernutrition do not have a major impact on small intestinal structure and function and are unlikely to explain the abnormalities of villus architecture commonly seen in residents of the tropics.

PRIMARY HYPOLACTASIA

Lactase activity in the small intestine is high in neonates of all ethnic groups. In many such groups, however, particularly those indigenous to the tropics, lactase activity declines rapidly within 3 to 4 months after weaning. Adult hypolactasia is found throughout most countries in Southeast Asia, but it is less common in the Middle East and uncommon in Northern Europe. The practical implication of hypolactasia is small, though, because African and Asian adults avoid milk unless they wish to use it as a purgative; milk-based products cannot be used reliably in these regions as a nutritional supplement. Secondary hypolactasia that occurs after infections that produce enteropathy is usually short-lived and self-limited. Sucrase activity also is reduced in black South Africans living in Johannesburg but not to the same degree to which lactase levels are reduced.[7] If healthy, these persons have normal villus and crypt morphology, and sucrase deficiency cannot be attributed to tropical enteropathy; whether sucrose deficiency is acquired or genetically determined remains to be established.

NONSPECIFIC TROPICAL MALABSORPTION

In addition to the known specific causes of intestinal malabsorption in the tropics, malabsorption also occurs in association with two conditions of unknown etiology: tropical enteropathy and tropical sprue. Although it has been suggested that tropical enteropathy and tropical sprue may represent the two ends of a clinical and pathologic spectrum, the evidence to support this view is far from compelling. Tropical enteropathy, for example, occurs in Africa, where tropical sprue is extremely uncommon. Thus, the widespread nature of tropical enteropathy and the geographic restriction of tropical sprue continue to challenge epidemiologists and clinical investigators. Despite intensive investigation during the

latter half of the 20th century, the cause of both conditions still remains obscure.

TROPICAL ENTEROPATHY

Definition

Enteropathy is characterized by a varying reduction in villus height, usually in association with a hyperplastic response in the crypt.[2] There is, therefore, a decrease in the villus-to-crypt ratio that is accompanied inevitably by a decrease in the surface area of the small intestine. There also may be evidence of damage to the surface epithelial cells with a reduction in their height and therefore a change in shape from columnar to cuboidal. The changes in villus morphology and enterocyte height are associated almost invariably with inflammatory cell infiltrates in the lamina propria and the epithelium.

Epidemiology

Tropical enteropathy has been detected in most tropical regions of Asia, Africa, the Middle East, the Caribbean, and Central and South America (Fig. 102–1). The disorder is acquired; newborn infants in the developing world have villi of heights similar to those of infants in the industrialized world, but by 4 to 6 months of age, the villus architectural abnormalities and inflammatory infiltrates begin to appear. The onset at 4 to 6 months is consistent with the view that the postweaning environment in many countries in the developing world is relatively hostile to the small intestinal epithelium and leads to abnormalities of the villus and crypt architecture. It has been argued, however, that these features are the "normal" state for persons living in these locations. In a longitudinal cohort study of Zambian adults, however, we found substantial fluctuations in villus height with time, possibly influenced by season and certain infectious agents.[8] Tropical enteropathy is not limited to the indigenous population but may be acquired by travelers from the industrialized world and seen in expatriates living and working in the tropics.

Evidence from migrant studies of people traveling from the developed to the industrialized world has suggested that tropical enteropathy is a reversible process. A survey of small bowel morphology in British Indian and British

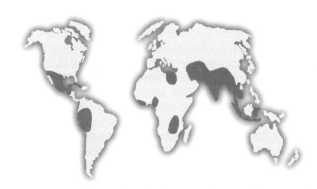

Figure 102–1 Geographic distribution of tropical enteropathy (*orange areas*).

African-Caribbean subjects who have lived in the United Kingdom for more than 30 years, however, has raised the question of genetic predisposition to the development of enteropathy.[9] In both immigrant groups, villus height was reduced compared with that of indigenous British whites, although there was no obvious correlation between the reduction in villus height and the duration of residence in the United Kingdom. In the British Indian subjects, however, there was a relationship between villus height and the time since the last visit to the Indian subcontinent, suggesting that reexposure to the tropical environment was involved in maintaining the enteropathy. Such a relationship was not apparent in the African-Caribbean subjects, further suggesting that the persisting mild abnormality of villus architecture is more likely to be related to genetic factors rather than to reexposure to the tropical environment.

Pathophysiology

Formal investigation of small intestinal absorption in apparently healthy persons in India, Africa, and Central and South America has revealed reduced absorption of D-xylose, glucose, vitamin B$_{12}$, and fat compared with their absorption in healthy Western controls. In addition, intestinal perfusion studies of the transport of glucose, amino acids, and small peptides have confirmed reduced absorption rates, compared with the rates of healthy Europeans.[10,11] For example, 50% of healthy Southern Indian adults had reduced D-xylose absorption, 10% had mild impairment of fat absorption, and 3% had reduced vitamin B$_{12}$ absorption. It should be stressed, however, that these functional abnormalities were mild, were indicative of a subclinical malabsorptive state, and did not correlate with overt manifestations of clinical disease. Such minor abnormalities appear to be more common in persons living in rural or poor periurban locations than in more affluent city dwellers. We have demonstrated a clear difference in intestinal villus height between healthy black residents in a Johannesburg township, in whom mean villus height was indistinguishable from that of healthy Johannesburg whites or British whites, and relatively deprived blacks living in a poor periurban development in Lusaka, Zambia, in whom the mean villus height was substantially lower (Fig. 102–2).[12]

Etiology and Pathogenesis

Current epidemiologic evidence indicates that tropical enteropathy occurs as a result of environmental factors. Climate alone cannot explain these abnormalities, because tropical enteropathy has not been found in locations like Singapore where water quality, sanitation, and nutritional status are similar to those of industrialized countries. The major contributors to enteropathy appear to be intestinal infection or continuing bacterial contamination of the upper small intestine and nutritional insufficiency. In the developing world, it is difficult to separate these factors and to explore in a controlled way their independent and combined effects on intestinal structure and function. Evidence from human and animal studies indicates, however, that the small intestine, in general, is relatively resistant to nutritional insufficiency, except when it is severe; insufficiency

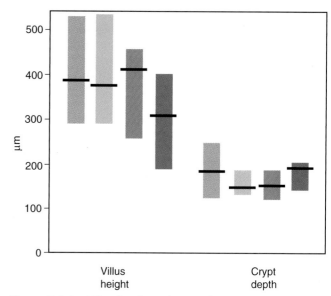

Figure 102–2   Villus height and crypt depth in black Zambians with tropical enteropathy (*red bars*) and black South Africans (*purple bars*) from Johannesburg with normal villus-crypt architecture. *Orange bars,* white British subjects; *blue bars,* white South Africans.

of riboflavin in utero can program villus and crypt architecture in the fetus and result in an irreversible, riboflavin-resistant defect in the neonatal small intestinal epithelium. These relatively subtle influences of micronutrient deficiency on small intestinal structure require further evaluation.

The major emphasis in the study of the pathogenesis of tropical enteropathy has been on the microbiological milieu of the small intestine. Studies in southern Indians have identified a number of "infective factors" that may be important. Apparently healthy, asymptomatic persons have heavy colonization of the small intestine by aerobic and anaerobic organisms and, in addition, they excrete a range of established, classic enteropathogens in their feces.[13] These findings suggest that the persistence of either established enteropathogens or the colonization of the small intestine by excessive numbers of commensal bacteria can result in subclinical small intestinal damage (see Chapter 99). Studies in germ-free animals clearly have shown the importance of the luminal and mucosal bacterial flora in modulating villus architecture and the inflammatory infiltrate, and there is compelling circumstantial evidence to support the view that the increased bacterial load of commensal and pathogenic microorganisms leads to the mucosal abnormalities in many parts of the developing world.

We have tested the hypothesis that the inflammatory response in the epithelium and submucosa, specifically the presence of activated T cells, is important in the pathogenesis of villus atrophy. The T cell activation marker CD69 was increased in black Zambians with tropical enteropathy and was associated with human leukocyte antigen (HLA)-DR expression.[12] These findings suggest that T cell activation in the lamina propria may be involved in the genesis of the villus architectural abnormalities in tropical enteropathy.

The mucosal abnormalities in tropical enteropathy are not limited to the small intestine. There also are subclinical abnormalities of colonocyte structure and function, which can be called *tropical colonopathy*.[14]

The broad geographic distribution of tropical enteropathy indicates that environmental factors are most important in its etiology, and there is little support for a genetic basis for this condition. Still, the recent description of mild, persisting enteropathy in British African-Caribbean subjects who have not returned to their country of origin for many years suggests that there also may be a genetic component.[9]

TROPICAL SPRUE

Although few would dispute the existence of the clinical entity of idiopathic chronic malabsorption in the tropics, commonly referred to as *tropical sprue*, the condition continues to be surrounded by epidemiologic, clinical, and etiopathogenetic controversies.[15] The epidemiology is perplexing because of the restrictive geographic distribution of tropical sprue within the tropics and, unlike most other diarrheal diseases, its relatively low prevalence in children. Its etiology is unknown, but there is no lack of hypotheses; the varied clinical presentation makes it difficult to establish a unifying hypothesis on etiology. One major problem has been the failure to agree on a universally accepted definition of the syndrome.

Definition

The Wellcome Trust collaborative study, "Tropical Sprue and Megaloblastic Anaemia," published in 1971, concluded that "tropical sprue is a syndrome of intestinal malabsorption which occurs among residents in or visitors to certain regions of the tropics."[16] The definition was modified further by Baker and Mathan, working in Vellore, southern India, by including "malabsorption of two or more substances in people in the tropics when other known causes have been excluded."[16] Cook noted that tropical sprue often followed an acute diarrheal illness, and on the basis of this observation and the evidence that the small intestine in sprue was colonized by aerobic and anaerobic bacteria, he recommended that the term *postinfective tropical malabsorption* be used in preference to tropical sprue.[17] Tompkins and Booth opposed this change on the basis that not all episodes of tropical sprue follow an acute diarrheal illness and that the syndrome may remain latent for many years, even after an expatriate has returned to his or her homeland.[18] They proposed the definition "malabsorption in defined areas of the tropics in which no bacterial, viral, or parasitic infection can be detected," which carefully excludes any assumptions about etiopathogenesis. Although the etiology of tropical sprue remains unknown, it would seem wise to resist including speculation on its etiology in the definition.

Historical Aspects

A malabsorptive illness in the tropics was described in an ancient treatise on medicine, *The Charakasamhida*, which was written before 600 BC. William Hillary published the first clear clinical description of the disease in the European literature in 1759, when he described his observations on chronic diarrhea and malabsorption in Barbados in the Caribbean.[19] Reports of similar illness soon followed, largely associated with the colonization of India and Southeast Asia by the European maritime powers. British military physicians referred to the illness as the "white flux," "diarrhea alba," or "chronic diarrhea of the tropics." The disorder was subsequently described among the Dutch in Java, the French in Indochina, and Europeans in China. In 1880, Manson introduced the word *sprue*, which was derived from the Dutch term "sprouw," which describes the oral aphthous ulceration often associated with this form of chronic diarrhea in children.[20] It became apparent that tropical sprue was not confined to Asia when, following the Spanish-American War, it was seen among American expatriates in the Philippines and Puerto Rico. By the beginning of the 20th century, it became evident that tropical sprue was associated with morphologic abnormalities in the small intestine, although all the early observations were made at autopsy, and the significance of the abnormalities remained controversial. Sir Philip Manson-Bahr, in 1924, was convinced that the primary lesion in sprue was in the small intestinal mucosa,[21] and this speculation was confirmed when peroral jejunal biopsy was introduced in the 1950s by Margot Shiner.

Epidemiology

Unlike most infectious diarrheas in the tropics, tropical sprue is markedly geographically restricted. It is predominantly a disease of southern and Southeast Asia, the Caribbean islands, and, to a much lesser extent, Central and South America (Fig. 102–3).[22-24] It almost never occurs in expatriates in Africa, although there have been sporadic reports from South Africa, Zimbabwe, and Nigeria.[25-27] Thus, *endemic* tropical sprue is not found universally in tropical and subtropical regions, a finding that strongly suggests that the etiologic factor or factors similarly are geographically restricted. The prevalence of endemic tropical sprue has not been clearly defined, although in Europeans living in Ceylon, it was estimated to be 0.5%, and in North Americans living in Puerto Rico, the prevalence is 8%.[28] During World War II, tropical sprue was a major cause of morbidity among British

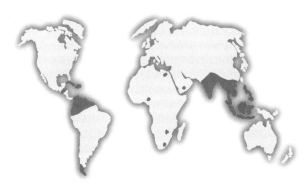

Figure 102–3 Geographic distribution of tropical sprue (*orange areas*).

troops serving in India and Burma[29] but was rare among American forces operating in the islands of the Pacific; it was noted subsequently to be common among British troops serving in Malaya and Hong Kong.[30] Tropical sprue was common among Europeans traveling overland in Asia,[31] although an unexpectedly low prevalence was found in American forces serving in Vietnam[32] and Peace Corps volunteers working in tropical areas. These data and the apparent decline in the incidence of tropical sprue in European overland travelers have been attributed to the widespread early use of antibiotics for acute traveler's diarrhea.

Epidemic tropical sprue has been documented most clearly in villages around Vellore in southern India.[33-35] Such epidemics differ from other causes of acute diarrhea, because the epidemic evolves over many months, with new cases continuing to appear after a year or more. Attack rates are high in adults and relatively low in children; exposure during the first wave of an epidemic appears to offer protection during subsequent waves. Epidemics also have been described in northern India and Burma. During the major epidemics in southern India between 1960 and 1962, an estimated 100,000 people were affected, and tropical sprue was directly related to the deaths of at least 30,000 people.[35] In southern India, epidemics do not exhibit seasonality, although in Puerto Rico, cases commonly manifest during the first 3 months of the year, which is not a time of high rainfall. Clinical impressions worldwide suggest that the incidence of tropical sprue is declining in both the indigenous population and visitors to endemic areas.

Clinical Features

Tropical sprue is a syndrome consisting of chronic diarrhea, often with clinical features of steatorrhea, anorexia, abdominal cramps, bloating, and prominent bowel sounds.[16,18,36-39] In expatriates and during epidemics in the indigenous population, the illness often begins with an acute attack of watery diarrhea associated with fever and malaise. After 1 week, the acute symptoms resolve and are followed by milder chronic diarrhea or overt steatorrhea, usually accompanied by progressive weight loss.[40] This particular form of the illness is found most commonly in persons who travel overland from Europe to India. Lactose intolerance is commonly described as part of this illness and may be associated with deficiencies of vitamin B_{12} and folic acid and occasionally hypocalcemia and hypomagnesemia. Physical findings during the early phase of the illness usually are limited to signs of weight loss and hyperactive bowel sounds.

Chronic atrophic gastritis is a common finding in tropical sprue, particularly in subjects studied in southern India. Affected persons have reduced secretion of gastric acid and intrinsic factor, resulting in vitamin B_{12} malabsorption, which can be corrected by administration of intrinsic factor. The gastritis may persist even after the enteropathy has resolved and clinical symptoms have improved markedly. These observations were made, however, before the discovery of *Helicobacter pylori*, and in view of the extremely high prevalence of *H. pylori* in the developing world, it is possible that the abnormalities observed in the stomach of patients with tropical sprue are not specific to sprue but related to coinfection with *H. pylori*.

In some persons, the acute phase of tropical sprue evolves into a chronic phase with persistent diarrhea and steatorrhea. After months or even years, the clinical picture becomes dominated by nutritional deficiencies that result in anemia (vitamin B_{12}, folate), stomatitis (iron), glossitis (vitamin B_{12}), pigmentation of the skin (vitamin B_{12}), and edema caused by hypoproteinemia. In southern India, 1% of patients with endemic tropical sprue present with nutritional deficiencies in the absence of diarrhea. Occasionally, vitamin B_{12} deficiency produces subacute combined degeneration of the spinal cord. Vitamin A deficiency may manifest as night blindness. In general, the long-term nutritional impact of chronic tropical sprue is more evident in the indigenous population than in visitors, because the natives are more likely already to be borderline undernourished.

A number of case reports have described patients in whom the initial presentation of tropical sprue involved only a mild or subclinical illness and in whom chronic diarrhea and nutritional deficiencies developed months or even years after leaving the tropics.[18,28] This form of the illness has been called *latent sprue*. It has been described in Puerto Ricans living in New York and in Anglo-Indians in London, who typically present with steatorrhea and megaloblastic anemia.

Pathology

The morphologic changes in the gastrointestinal tract in tropical sprue are highly varying but generally correlate with the duration and severity of the clinical presentation.

Enteropathy

Tropical sprue is noted for the broad spectrum of histopathologic abnormalities that can be observed in the jejunal mucosa.[16,41,42] In the early stages, the jejunal mucosa may be normal, but in persons with persistent diarrhea, there usually is a reduction in villus height, increase in crypt depth, and an associated inflammatory cell infiltrate in both the lamina propria and epithelium. The changes are similar to those in celiac sprue (see Figure 101–2) and also in tropical enteropathy but generally are more severe than those in tropical sprue. There is a moderately close relationship between abnormalities of intestinal structure and function, in that the extent of nutrient malabsorption increases with the severity of the villus architectural abnormalities. Ultrastructural studies have suggested that an abnormality in stem cells in the small intestinal crypts may be the primary lesion in tropical sprue.[43,44] Thus, although the rates of crypt cell production and enterocyte migration up the villus are increased in tropical sprue,[45] the cells that are produced are damaged and thus extruded more rapidly than normal from the villus.

Electron microscopy shows distortion and grouping of the microvilli, fragmentation of the terminal web, an increased number of lysosomes, and mitochondrial changes in the enterocytes. In the crypts, cell nuclei show megalocytic changes and argentaffin cells are increased;

Paneth cells are normal in number. The basement membrane usually appears thickened and stains as collagen on light microscopy. Light and electron microscopy demonstrate an accumulation of lipid droplets immediately adjacent to the surface epithelium. The pattern of lipid accumulation in tropical sprue is different from that in normal subjects and patients with celiac sprue but reverts to normal following clinical recovery. The precise significance of this abnormality in tropical sprue is uncertain.

Colonopathy

Colonic epithelial cells show structural abnormalities similar to those described in the small intestine. Sodium and water absorption by the colon are impaired, in part because of increased concentrations of unsaturated free fatty acids in the stool.[46] The free fatty acids have a variety of effects on colonic structure and function, including inhibition of sodium-potassium adenosine triphosphatase, which promotes sodium and water absorption by the colonic epithelium.

Pathophysiology

Although tropical sprue generally is considered to be a disease primarily of the proximal small intestine, pathophysiologic disturbances also occur in the stomach and colon. The mechanisms by which gastric acid secretion and intrinsic factor production are reduced is not clear, and it is uncertain as to whether these changes are primary manifestations of the disease or merely secondary phenomena resulting from severe undernutrition. *H. pylori* is likely to be extremely common in the indigenous populations with endemic tropical sprue and is well recognized to cause acute gastritis, which generally progresses to gastric atrophy and impaired gastric acid secretion. The relationship between *H. pylori* infection and tropical sprue has not been investigated. Similarly, the mechanisms of colonic dysfunction in tropical sprue are not entirely clear and also may be related to the secondary effects of undernutrition and impaired absorption of long-chain fatty acids by the small intestine. The major pathophysiologic disturbances in tropical sprue occur predominantly in the small intestine. Early on, in acute sprue, the jejunum is predominantly affected, whereas in chronic sprue the ileum is progressively involved.

Impaired Small Intestinal Transport

Perfusion studies of the jejunum indicate that some patients with tropical sprue in Puerto Rico have a net secretory state for water that is reversed by treatment with antibiotics.[47] Patients with tropical sprue in southern India, however, were not found to have a secretory state, and they absorb water and electrolytes to the same extent as do local healthy control subjects.[48] Impaired absorption of amino acids and dipeptides has been shown in proximal small intestine.[49,50] D-Xylose absorption is commonly reduced in patients with tropical sprue from all geographic locations as are lactase and disaccharidase activities. One of the most consistent findings in tropical sprue from both Asia and the Caribbean is impaired fat absorption; more than 90% of subjects in southern India have increased fecal fat excretion. These abnormalities of fat and carbohydrate absorption have been shown to impair energy balance significantly in subjects with tropical sprue.[51] Absorption of micronutrients, particularly folic acid, also is impaired, and as the enteropathy progresses to involve the ileum, vitamin B_{12} malabsorption often follows.

Disturbed Intestinal Motility

Small bowel transit time is increased in some patients with tropical sprue,[52] whereas in others it has been found to be normal.[53] In a small group of patients with delayed transit, transit time returned toward normal after treatment with tetracycline and folic acid. It is unclear whether the increase in small intestinal transit is part of the primary pathophysiology of tropical sprue, reflects gastrointestinal peptide hormone abnormalitites (see later), or whether it is secondary to bacterial colonization of the small intestine. Fat malabsorption, which leads to increased concentrations of fat in the distal ileum and colon, is known to increase small intestinal transit time and may be an important factor in modulating small intestinal transit in tropical sprue.

Pancreatic Insufficiency

It is recognized that exocrine pancreatic insufficiency can result from small intestinal disease. Evidence using an indirect test of pancreatic function (pancreolauryl test) indicates that 64.2% of 56 patients from Mexico with tropical sprue had low values[54] and it has been suggested that this dysfunction may be due to impaired pancreatic stimulation from intestinal damage as has been described in celiac sprue. Exocrine pancreatic insufficiency may contribute to energy deficits in tropical sprue.

Gastrointestinal Peptide Hormone Abnormalities

Fasting serum concentrations of motilin and enteroglucagon are increased in patients with acute tropical sprue,[55] and after a standard test meal, there are marked increases in the concentrations of both gut hormones. There also is a relationship between the plasma enteroglucagon concentration and mouth-to-cecum transit time, indicating that enteroglucagon is a candidate hormonal mediator of the increase in small intestinal transit time. Infusion of triglyceride or oleic acid into the distal small intestine increases plasma concentrations of enteroglucagon, neurotensin, and peptide YY (PYY). Serum PYY concentrations have not been measured in patients with tropical sprue, but PYY concentrations correlate closely with changes in small intestinal transit, and PYY is now considered to have a major role in mediating the effects of fat on small intestinal transit, via the so-called ileal brake.

Theories of Etiopathogenesis

The cause of tropical sprue has not been clearly defined, although epidemiologic evidence indicates that, like tropical enteropathy, it relates to factors in the tropical environment.[16,56,57] Nutritional insufficiency and intestinal infection, possibly with the liberation of secretory or cytopathic toxins, have been implicated as causes.

Nutritional deficiencies of folate, vitamin B_{12}, or protein, which can cause small bowel abnormalities under certain circumstances, do not appear to play a primary role in the pathogenesis of the disease, which commonly develops in well-nourished persons as well as in those with varying degrees of undernutrition. Thus, although the disease can have a major effect on macronutrient and micronutrient status, there is little evidence to suggest that undernutrition has a major role in initiating the disease process. Considerable evidence, however, favors the concept that tropical sprue is an infectious disease caused by persistent, chronic intestinal contamination with one or more enteropathogens.

In most instances, either in isolated individual cases or in epidemic outbreaks, tropical sprue follows an episode of acute diarrhea for which no enteric pathogen can be identified. In epidemic outbreaks in southern Indian villages, the acute diarrhea often involves multiple persons within the same household and spreads within families.[34] Chronic diarrhea develops in approximately 50% of such persons but remits spontaneously within 3 months of onset in most persons; diarrhea persists in approximately 10% and develops into overtly recognizable tropical sprue. In similar annual seasonal epidemics of acute diarrhea among American military personnel in the Philippines, the illness resolves spontaneously in some but persists in others, to become tropical sprue with chronic diarrhea and with abnormalities of intestinal structure and function.[58] Studies of epidemics in the Vellore in southern India are entirely consistent with an infectious etiology, and in one outbreak, there was epidemiologic evidence that protection against the condition appeared to emerge during the later phases of the epidemic, consistent with the development of protective immunity.[34]

A variety of bacteria has been isolated from the jejunum of patients with tropical sprue.[59-63] In northern India, Puerto Rico, and Haiti and in Europeans traveling to India, coliforms are present in increased numbers in the jejunum. In the Europeans, *Alcaligenes fecalis, Enterobacter aerogenes,* and *Hafnia* species have been found. In patients from India and the Caribbean, *Klebsiella pneumoniae, E. coli,* and *Enterobacter cloacae* are common. In southern India, however, the prevalence of coliforms in patients with tropical sprue is the same as in healthy controls. Thus, in some geographic areas, there is bacterial colonization of the proximal small intestine with coliforms, but no single species has emerged to explain tropical sprue in all geographic locations. Colonization of the small intestine with coliforms can change villus architecture in animal models, and similar histopathologic lesions have been described in patients with bacterial overgrowth of other causes. *Klebsiella* and other coliform bacteria isolated from patients with tropical sprue in Puerto Rico have been found to produce secretory enterotoxins and to induce structural abnormalities in the small intestine in experimental models.[61,64,65] Although these organisms might be incriminated in the structural and functional disturbances seen in patients in the Caribbean, it seems unlikely that they account for the disease in southern India, where coliform contamination is uncommon.

Viruses have been sought as a cause of tropical sprue, and viral particles resembling orthomyxoviruses and coronaviruses have been found in the feces of patients with tropical sprue[66]; these viruses, however, also were found in similar numbers of asymptomatic control subjects.

It seems possible that the syndrome of tropical sprue may have more than one cause. In the Caribbean, tropical sprue always is associated with vitamin B_{12} malabsorption, is strongly linked to the presence of enterotoxin-producing coliforms, and responds well to broad-spectrum antibiotics. Disease patterns and the bacterial profile in the small intestine differ in patients from southern India and in overland travelers, and the responses of these patients to treatment are less predictable than those of patients with Caribbean tropical sprue.

Possible Model for Etiopathogenesis

Although the etiology of tropical sprue is unknown, it is difficult to develop a clear model of pathogenesis. Cook suggested that the primary event in the pathogenesis of tropical sprue is acute intestinal infection involving the small and possibly large intestine.[16] He has proposed that this infection produces nonspecific mucosal injury, which leads to elevated plasma levels of enteroglucagon,[55] which in turn is responsible for slowing small intestinal transit, thereby resulting in bacterial overgrowth. The transit abnormality amplifies the mucosal injury, which slows further the transit cycle. Although attractive, this hypothesis does not explain all cases of tropical sprue. It is not always possible, for example, to identify an acute diarrheal illness in cases of tropical sprue, although one could postulate that subclinical infection had occurred. In addition, the relationship between the raised plasma enteroglucagon levels and retardation of small intestinal transit is not a universally accepted concept. Finally, the effect of bacterial overgrowth on the small intestine is not clear-cut, and some studies have demonstrated that motility actually may be increased by bacterial overgrowth.

Whatever the initial injury or predisposing factor, an increased number of coliforms in the small intestine does seem to be an observation in many patients studied[59-63]; the response to broad-spectrum antibiotics, at least in some patients, would support the clinical importance of this finding. The importance of fat malabsorption, with respect to the ileal brake, slowing of intestinal transit, and the effect of fatty acids on colonocyte function, is another possible mechanism in the pathogenetic cascade. Possible routes by which these factors may interact to perpetuate the chronic diarrhea–malabsorption cycle are outlined in Figure 102–4.

Diagnosis

Investigation of chronic diarrhea with or without overt clinical malabsorption in persons who have recently returned from the tropics must be targeted at excluding specific causes of malabsorption, namely intestinal infections (Fig. 102–5). Multiple stool specimens obtained on separate days should be examined by light microscopy, using appropriate stains to search for the parasites *G. lamblia, C. parvum,* and *C. cayetanensis;* in an immunocompromised person, special attention should be paid

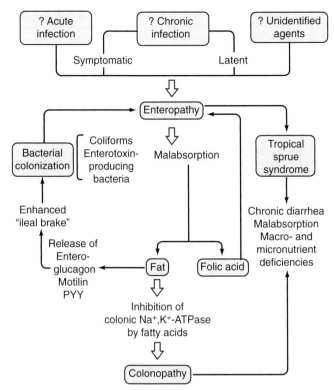

Figure 102–4   A model that relates the many factors that have been proposed to explain the pathogenesis of tropical sprue. PYY, peptide YY.

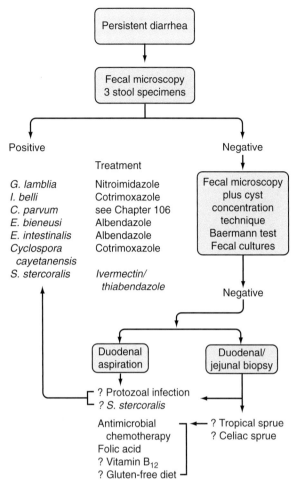

Figure 102–5   Investigation of patients with persistent tropical diarrhea and malabsorption. The Baermann test is a concentration procedure designed to recover *Strongyloides stercoralis* larvae from fecal specimens.

to the identification of *C. parvum*, the microsporidia (*E. bieneusi* and *E. intestinalis*), and *I. belli*. Stool microscopy should include cyst and oocyst concentration techniques if fecal saline wet mounts are negative. Fecal examination is a relatively insensitive method to detect *S. stercoralis*, but detection of larvae can be improved by using the Baermann test or fecal culture. The best test for *S. stercoralis* is enzyme-linked immunosorbent assay (ELISA) for IgG antibodies against the parasite.

If fecal microscopy is negative and any of these infections are strongly suspected, then it is often worthwhile to perform jejunal aspiration and jejunal mucosal biopsy to search for parasites in intestinal fluid or associated with the small intestinal mucosa. *Giardia* often can be identified in fluid or in mucosal smears produced from jejunal biopsies, whereas the intracellular protozoa (*C. parvum*, *I. belli*, and the microsporidia) can be seen in Giemsa-stained specimens of small intestinal mucosa examined by light microscopy. Occasionally, celiac sprue manifests for the first time in persons returning from the tropics, and this disease can now be screened for serologically by testing for the presence of antiendomysial or tissue trans-glutaminase antibodies. Confirmation of the diagnosis by jejunal biopsy is usually required, and if diagnostic uncertainty between celiac sprue and tropical sprue persists, then it may be wise to perform a gluten challenge after recovery of the jejunal mucosa with gluten withdrawal (see Chapter 101).

Small bowel series in tropical sprue usually shows an increase in the caliber of the small intestine and thickening of the folds (Fig. 102–6).[67] These changes are present throughout the small intestine, and the exami-

nation usually is notable for the slow transit of the barium column through the gut.

A barium examination of the small intestine or capsule endoscopy, computed tomographic scanning, and multiple small bowel biopsies by endoscopy or enteroscopy are necessary to exclude small intestinal lymphoma or IPSID.

Once the specific causes of diarrhea and malabsorption have been excluded, fat, vitamin B_{12}, and possibly D-xylose malabsorption are established, and a jejunal biopsy shows partial villus atrophy, the diagnosis of tropical sprue can be assumed.

Treatment

General Measures

Restoration of water and electrolyte balance and replacement of nutritional deficiencies are the priorities in the initial management of persons with tropical sprue. These interventions alone are believed to have been responsible for the marked decrease in mortality in epidemic sprue in southern India. Vitamin B_{12} should be given parenterally, but iron and folic acid are effective when provided orally. These interventions usually result in a prompt hematologic remission of the megaloblastic anemia, disappearance of glossitis, and return of appetite,

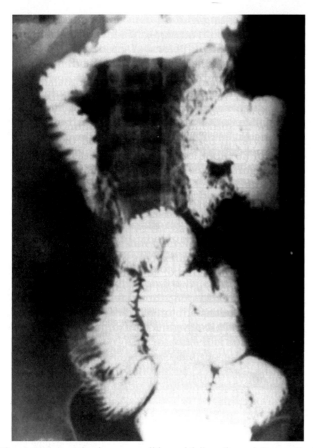

Figure 102–6   Film from a small bowel follow-through in a patient from southern India with chronic tropical sprue showing jejunal dilatation and thickening of the folds.

which results in the onset of weight gain even before improvements in intestinal absorption are apparent.[68-72] Improvements in jejunal structural abnormalities, particularly in the crypts, are evident within 3 to 6 days in those who have marked abnormalities but may be delayed for as long as several weeks in those who have mild abnormalities. The results of treatment with folic acid appear to depend on the chronicity of the intestinal lesions.[29,73] Treatment can be curative in those who have had the disease for only a few months, whereas in those with chronic disease, notably indigenous residents, folic acid alone usually does not correct the intestinal abnormalities.[68]

Antimicrobial Chemotherapy

The role of broad-spectrum antibiotics in the treatment of tropical sprue remains controversial. Overland travelers, such as those from the United Kingdom, and patients in Puerto Rico are reported to improve on tetracycline, 250 mg four times daily, usually given over a period of several months.[28,74,75] In a controlled trial in southern India, the addition of antibiotics to vitamin B[12] and folic acid supplementation did not appear to improve the rate of recovery. Spontaneous recovery does occur, possibly related to a change in environment and the oral bacterial load. Symptomatic treatment with an antidiarrheal preparation such as loperamide often is advised. However, if intestinal stasis and bacterial colonization are

important in the pathogenesis of this syndrome, one might argue that slowing small intestinal transit with an antidiarrheal preparation may delay recovery.

The prognosis in expatriates is good, with most experiencing complete and permanent recovery.[27] Recovery may be more rapid in expatriates who leave the tropics and return to a temperate climate. There is some evidence that tropical sprue can recur in treated patients of the indigenous population in the tropics. Significant malabsorption was detected in 50% of a group of Puerto Ricans examined 5 years after their intestinal abnormalities apparently had been cured by antimicrobial chemotherapy.[76]

Prevention

Other than the usual advice to travelers regarding the avoidance of contaminated food and water, there are no specific preventive measures for tropical sprue. The incidence of this disease appears to be declining in overland travelers and expatriates, perhaps because of the more liberal use of antibiotics for traveler's diarrhea. The epidemics of tropical sprue in southern India also appear to be on the decline, presumably because of improving water quality and sanitary conditions and the widespread availability of antibiotics.

REFERENCES

1. Thielman NM, Guerrant RL: Persistent diarrhea in the returned traveler. Infect Dis Clin North Am 12:489, 1998.
2. Farthing MJG, Kelly MP, Veitch AM: Recently recognised microbial enteropathies in HIV infection. J Antimicro Chemother 37(Suppl B):61, 1996.
3. Hoge CW, Shlim DR, Ghimire M, et al: Placebo-controlled trial of co-trimoxazole for cyclospora infections among travellers and foreign residents in Nepal. Lancet 345:691, 1995.
4. Kelly MP, McPhail J, Ngwenya B, et al: *Septata intestinalis*: A new microsporidian in Africa. Lancet 344:271, 1994.
5. Zulu I, Veitch A, Sianongo S, et al: Albendazole chemotherapy for AIDS-related diarrhoea in Zambia: Clinical, parasitological and mucosal responses. Aliment Pharmacol Ther 16:595, 2002.
6. Veitch AM, Kelly P, Zulu I, et al: Lack of evidence for small intestinal mucosal T-cell activation as a pathogenic mechanism in Africa HIV-associated enteropathy. Dig Dis Sci 46:1133, 2001.
7. Veitch AM, Kelly P, Segal I, et al: Does sucrase deficiency in black South Africans protect against colonic disease [research letter]? Lancet 351:183, 1998.
8. Kelly P, Menzies I, Crane R, et al: Responses of small intestinal architecture and function over time to environmental factors in a tropical population. Am J Trop Med Hyg 70:412, 2004.
9. Wood GM, Gearty JC, Cooper BT: Small bowel morphology in British Indian and Afro-Caribbean subjects: Evidence of tropical enteropathy. Gut 32:256, 1991.
10. Cook GC: Impairment of D-xylose absorption in Zambian patients with systemic intestinal infection. Am J Clin Nutr 25:490, 1972.
11. Cook GC: Tropical Gastroenterology. Oxford, Oxford University Press, 1980, p 271.
12. Veitch AM, Kelly P, Zulu IS, et al: Tropical enteropathy: A T cell-mediated crypt hyperplastic enteropathy. Eur J Gastroenterol Hepatol 13:1175, 2001.
13. Bhat P, Shantakumari S, Rajan D, et al: Bacterial flora of the gastrointestinal tract in Southern Indian control subjects

and patients with tropical sprue. Gastroenterology 62:11, 1972.

14. Ramakrishna BS, Mathan VI: Absorption of water and sodium and activity of adenosine triphosphatases in the rectal mucosa in tropical sprue. Gut 29:665, 1988.

15. Haghighi P, Wolf PL: Tropical sprue and subclinical enteropathy: A vision for the nineties. Crit Rev Clin Lab Sci 34:313, 1997.

16. Baker SJ, Mathan VI: Tropical sprue in Southern India. In Wellcome Trust Collaboration Study 1961-1969. London, Churchill Livingstone, 1971, p 453.

17. Cook GC: Aetiology and pathogenesis of post-infective tropical malabsorption (tropical sprue). Lancet 1:721, 1984.

18. Tomkins A, Booth CC: Tropical sprue. In Disorders of the Small Intestine. Oxford, Blackwell Scientific, 1985, p 311.

19. Booth CC: The first description of tropical sprue. Gut 5:45, 1964.

20. Manson P: Notes on sprue. Med Rep China Imp Marit Customs 19:33, 1880.

21. Manson-Bahr PH: The morbid anatomy and pathology of sprue and their bearing upon aetiology. Lancet 1:1148, 1924.

22. Mathan VI, Baker SJ: The epidemiology of tropical sprue. In Wellcome Trust Collaborative Study 1961-1969. London, Churchill Livingstone 1971, p 15.

23. Klipstein FA, Beauchamp I, Corcino JJ, et al: Nutritional status and intestinal function among rural populations of the West Indies: II. Barrio Nuevo, Puerto Rico. Gastroenterology 63:758, 1971.

24. Klipstein FA, Samloff IM, Smarth G, Schenk EA: Malabsorption in rural Haiti. Am J Clin Nutr 21:1042, 1968.

25. Moshal MG, Hirst W, Kallicburum S, Pillay K: Enteric tropical sprue in Africa. J Trop Med Hyg 78:2, 1975.

26. Thomas G, Clain DJ: Endemic tropical sprue in Rhodesia. Gut 12:877, 1976.

27. Falaiye JM: Tropical sprue in Nigeria. J Trop Med Hyg 73:119, 1970.

28. Klipstein FA, Falaiye JM: Tropical sprue in expatriates from the tropics living in the continental United States. Medicine 48:475, 1969.

29. Keele KD, Bound JP: Sprue in India: Clinical survey of 600 cases. BMJ 1:77, 1946.

30. O'Brien W, England NWJ: Tropical sprue amongst British servicemen and their families in South-East Asia. In Tropical Sprue and Megaloblastic Anaemia. London, Churchill Livingstone, 1971, p 25.

31. Walters AM, James WPT, Cole ACE, Walters JH: Malabsorption in overland travellers to India. BMJ 3:380, 1974.

32. Sheehy TW: Digestive disease as a national problem: VI. Enteric disease among United States troops in Vietnam. Gastroenterology 55:105, 1968.

33. Mathan VI, Baker SJ: An epidemic of tropical sprue in Southern India: I. Clinical features. Ann Trop Med Parasitol 64:439, 1970.

34. Baker SJ, Mathan VI: Epidemic tropical sprue: II. Epidemiology. Ann Trop Med Parasitol 64:453, 1970.

35. Mathan VI, Baker SJ: Epidemic tropical sprue and other epidemics of diarrhea in South Indian villages. Am J Clin Nutr 21:1077, 1968.

36. Baker SJ: Idiopathic small-intestinal disease in the tropics. In Critical Reviews in Tropical Medicine. New York, Plenum, 1982, p 197.

37. Klipstein FA, Falaiye JM: Tropical sprue in expatriates from the tropics living in the continental United States. Medicine 48:475, 1969.

38. Klipstein FA: Tropical sprue in travellers and expatriates living abroad. Gastroenterology 80:590, 1981.

39. Mathan VI: Tropical sprue in Southern India. Trans R Soc Trop Med 82:10, 1988.

40. Klipstein FA, Corcino JJ: Factors responsible for weight loss in tropical sprue. Am J Clin Nutr 30:1703, 1977.

41. Swanson VL, Thomassen RW: Pathology of the jejunal mucosa in tropical sprue. Am J Pathol 46:511, 1963.

42. Wheby MS, Swanson VL, Bayless TM: Comparison of ileal and jejunal biopsies in tropical sprue. Am J Clin Nutr 24:117, 1971.

43. Mathan M, Mathan VI, Baker SJ: An electron microscope study of jejunal mucosal morphology in control subjects and in patients with tropical sprue in Southern India. Gastroenterology 68:17, 1975.

44. Brunser O, Eidelman S, Klipstein FA: Intestinal morphology of rural Haitians: A comparison between overt tropical sprue and asymptomatic subjects. Gastroenterology 58:655, 1970.

45. Mathan MM, Ponniah J, Mathan VI: Epithelial cell renewal and turnover and relationship to morphologic abnormalities in jejunal mucosa in tropical sprue. Dig Dis Sci 31:586, 1986.

46. Ramakrishna BS, Mathan VI: Water and electrolyte absorption by the colon in tropical sprue. Gut 23:843, 1982.

47. Corcino JJ, Maldonado M, Klipstein FA: Intestinal perfusion studies in tropical sprue: I. Transport of water, electrolytes, and D-xylose. Gastroenterology 65:192, 1983.

48. Hellier MD, Bhat P, Albert J, Baker SJ: Intestinal perfusion studies in tropical sprue: II. Movement of water and electrolytes. Gut 18:480, 1977.

49. Hellier MD, Radhakrishnan AN, Ganapathy V, et al: Intestinal perfusion studies in tropical sprue: I. Amino acid and dipeptide absorption. Gut 17:511, 1976.

50. Hellier MD, Ganapathy C, Gammon A, et al: Impaired intestinal absorption of dipeptide in tropical sprue patients in India. Clin Sci 58:431, 1980.

51. Chacko A, Begum A, Mathan VI: Absorption of nutrient energy in southern Indian control subjects and patients with tropical sprue. Am J Clin Nutr 40:771, 1984.

52. Cook GC: Delayed small intestinal transit in tropical malabsorption. BMJ 2:238, 1978.

53. Jayanthi V, Chacko A, Gain IK, Mathan VI: Intestinal transit in healthy southern Indian subjects and in patients with tropical sprue. Gut 30:35, 1989.

54. Morales M, Galvan E, Mery CM, et al: Exocrine pancreatic insufficiency in tropical sprue. Digestion 63:30, 2001.

55. Besterman HS, Cook GC, Sarson DL: Gut hormones in tropical malabsorption. BMJ 2:1252, 1979.

56. Glynn J: Tropical sprue: Its aetiology and pathogenesis. J R Soc Med 79:599, 1986.

57. Tomkins A: Tropical malabsorption: Recent concepts in pathogenesis and nutritional significance. Clin Sci 60:131, 1981.

58. Jones TC, Dean AG, Parker GW: Seasonal gastroenteritis and malabsorption at an American military base in the Philippines: II. Malabsorption following the acute illness. Am J Epidemiol 95:128, 1972.

59. Gorbach SL, Mitra R, Jacobs B, et al: Bacterial contamination of the upper small bowel in tropical sprue. Lancet 1:74, 1969.

60. Gorbach SL, Banwell JG, Jacobs B, et al: Tropical sprue and malnutrition in West Bengal: I. Intestinal microflora and absorptions. Am J Clin Nutr 23:1545, 1970.

61. Klipstein FA, Haldeman LV, Corcino JJ, Moore WEC: Enterotoxigenic intestinal bacteria in tropical sprue. Ann Intern Med 79:632, 1973.

62. Tomkins AM, Drasar BS, James WPT: Bacterial colonisation of jejunal mucosa in acute tropical sprue. Lancet 1:59, 1975.

63. Ghoshal UC, Ghoshal U, Ayyagari A, et al: Tropical sprue is associated with contamination of small bowel with aerobic bacteria and reversible prolongation of orocecal transit time. J Gastroenterol Hepatol 18;540, 2003.

64. Klipstein FA, Engert RF, Short HB: Enterotoxigenicity of colonising coliform bacteria in tropical sprue and blind-loop syndrome. Lancet 2:342, 1978.

65. Klipstein FA, Horowitz IR, Engert RF, Schenk EA: Effect of *Klebsiella pneumoniae* enterotoxin on intestinal transport in the rat. J Clin Invest 56:799, 1975.

66. Baker SJ, Mathan M, Mathan VI, Swaminathan SP: Chronic enterocyte infection with coronavirus: One possible cause of the syndrome of tropical sprue? Dig Dis Sci 11:1039, 1982.

67. McLean AM, Farthing MJG, Kurian G, Mathan VI: The relationship between hypoalbuminaemia and the radiological appearances of the jejunum in tropical sprue. Br J Radiol 55:725, 1982.

68. Sheehy TW, Baggs B, Perez-Santiago E, Floch MH: Prognosis of tropical sprue: A study of the effect of folic acid on the intestinal aspects of acute and chronic sprue. Ann Intern Med 57:892, 1962.

69. Klipstein FA, Schenk EA, Samloff IM: Folate repletion associated with oral tetracycline therapy in tropical sprue. Gastroenterology 51:317, 1966.

70. Tomkins AM, Smith T, Wright SG: Assessment of early and delayed responses in vitamin B_{12} absorption during antibiotic therapy in tropical malabsorption. Clin Sci Mol Med 55:533, 1978.

71. Spies TD, Milanes F, Menandez A, et al: Observations on treatment of tropical sprue with folic acid. J Lab Clin Med 31:223, 1946.

72. Spies TD, Suarez RM: Responses of tropical sprue to vitamin B_{12}. Blood 3:1213, 1948.

73. Sheehy TW, Cohen WH, Wallace DK, Legtens LJ: Tropical sprue in North Americans. JAMA 194:1069, 1965.

74. Guerra R, Whelby MS, Bayless TM: Long-term antibiotic therapy in tropical sprue. Ann Intern Med 63:619, 1965.

75. Sheehy TW, Perez-Santiago E: Antibiotic therapy in tropical sprue. Gastroenterology 41:208, 1961.

76. Rickles FR, Klipstein FA, Tomasini J, et al: Long-term follow-up of antibiotic-treated tropical sprue. Ann Intern Med 76:203, 1972.

CHAPTER
103 Whipple's Disease

*Matthias Maiwald, Axel von Herbay, and
David A. Relman*

Whipple's disease is a chronic systemic infection caused by a gram-positive bacterium, *Tropheryma whipplei*. The small intestine is affected most often, but a variety of other organs also may be involved, including the joints, the central nervous system (CNS), and the heart. The clinical symptoms and findings are protean, and include weight loss, diarrhea, malabsorption, fever, arthralgias, skin hyperpigmentation, and dementia. The disease was considered to be uniformly fatal in the preantibiotic era, but today, treatment with antibiotics usually leads to clinical remission. Many open questions still surround the pathogenesis of this disease; it is presumed that host immunologic factors influence susceptibility to the disease.

HISTORY

In 1907, the pathologist George H. Whipple reported in detail the case of a 36-year-old male physician-missionary who died after a 5-year illness involving arthritis, chronic cough, weight loss, and chronic diarrhea.[1] At autopsy, Whipple found lipid deposits in the intestinal mucosa as well as in mesenteric and retroperitoneal lymph nodes. Microscopic examination further revealed a large number of macrophages with foamy cytoplasm in the lamina propria of the small intestine. Whipple suspected a disorder of fat metabolism and proposed the term *intestinal lipodystrophy* for this disease.

In the following decades, only a few cases were reported and the diagnosis uniformly was made at autopsy. The first antemortem diagnosis was made in 1947, based on findings in a mesenteric lymph node removed at laparotomy[2] and the first diagnosis by peroral intestinal biopsy was made in 1958.[3] In 1949, Black-Schaffer[4] introduced

the periodic acid-Schiff (PAS) stain to the histopathologic diagnosis of Whipple's disease. Inclusions in macrophages stained red using this stain, thus documenting that intracellular material was glycoprotein rather than lipid.

The first report of successful antibiotic treatment (using chloramphenicol) was published in 1952.[5] In 1961, two groups independently visualized bacteria by electron microscopy in affected tissues[6,7]; subsequent reports confirmed these observations. Bacteria associated with Whipple's disease were rod-shaped and of uniform size. Consistent positive therapeutic effects were achieved with antibiotic treatment.[8] These findings and the positive PAS reaction[4] suggested that the disease was unlikely to be a primary disorder of fat metabolism, as previously suspected, and that instead it was a bacterial disease; however, efforts to cultivate this bacterium prior to 2000 failed to yield reproducible or consistent results.

The nature of the bacterium remained obscure until the early 1990s, when its 16S ribosomal DNA (rDNA) sequence was determined and phylogenetic analysis established the relationship of the bacterium to the actinomycetes.[9,10] The name *Tropheryma whippelii* was introduced,[10] and the novel 16S rDNA sequence provided the basis for sensitive diagnostic testing using the polymerase chain reaction (PCR). In situ hybridization experiments showed that the unique bacterial 16S ribosomal RNA (rRNA) sequence colocalized with areas of pathology, thus confirming its relevance.[11] Further advancement came when successful propagation of the Whipple's disease bacterium in co-culture with human fibroblast cells was achieved.[12] At that point, the bacterium formally was described as a new species, and its name was modified to *Tropheryma whipplei*.[13] With the availability of adequate amounts of purified genomic DNA, the complete genome sequences of two different bacterial isolates were determined and published in 2003.[14,15]

EPIDEMIOLOGY

Whipple's disease is a rare disorder. The first comprehensive epidemiologic survey was performed by Dobbins in 1987.[8] In this monograph, he compiled information on 696 patients, comprising 617 published and 79 unpublished cases recorded through 1986. According to this analysis, Whipple's disease is a sporadic disorder with a predilection for middle-aged white men. Data on age and sex were available for 664 patients; 86% were male, and the mean age at diagnosis was 49 years. Most patients were white; only 10 were African, one was a native American, 3 patients were from India, and 1 was Japanese. Most of the patients originated from Europe (373 patients) or from the United States (246 patients). Within Europe, Germany (114 patients) and France (91 patients) were strongly represented. Relatively few cases originated from South America (11 patients) and Australia (13 patients).

A small epidemiologic study from western Switzerland calculated the incidence of Whipple's disease to be approximately 0.4 per million of the population per year.[16] Similarly, the International Whipple's Disease Registry at www.whipplesdisease.net calculates an incidence of 0.4 per million per year for Germany.[17] An epidemiologic analysis of 110 patients in Germany, diagnosed between 1965 and 1995, noted a relatively stable incidence of cases of Whipple's disease over 3 decades and a relatively even geographic distribution of the patients' residences.[18] There are only a few observations of geographically confined case clusters (up to 7 cases).[19-21]

Several studies[18,22,23] indicate a statistically significant[18] increase in recent decades in the age of patients at diagnosis. Presently, patients are diagnosed at a mean age of 56 years, and approximately 80% are men.[24] It has been speculated that the increasing use of antibiotics for unrelated complaints may be a contributing factor in delaying the age of onset of Whipple's disease.

One remarkable epidemiologic feature in Dobbins' analysis[8] was the strong representation of patients with occupations in the farming and building trades involving work outdoors or frequent contact with animals or soil; of 191 patients for whom data were available, 43 (22%) were farmers and 10 (5%) were carpenters. Patients in all farming-related trades accounted for 34% of the total. By comparison, the proportion of farm workers among the total workforce in the analyzed countries was approximately 10%.

MICROBIOLOGY

Many attempts have been undertaken to cultivate the bacterium associated with Whipple's disease, a significant number of which probably have not been reported in the literature.[8] A number of reports of allegedly successful cultivation have not been reproducible or represented isolation of contaminants.[8]

Finally, in 2000, successful propagation of *T. whipplei* from infected heart valve tissue in coculture with human fibroblast cells was reported.[12] Seven culture passages were performed, over a period of 285 days, and the 16S rDNA sequence of *T. whipplei* was detected after each passage. The initial estimate of the doubling time of the bacterium was 18 days, which is extremely slow growth in comparison with other pathogenic bacteria. Since the initial report, at least 8 additional strains of *T. whipplei* have been isolated from infected heart valves, duodenal biopsy specimens, ocular vitreous fluid, and cerebrospinal fluid (CSF).[25-29] Growth and identity of the bacterium were determined using immunofluorescence,[25,28] nucleic acid staining (Fig. 103–1),[29] PCR and sequencing,[25,28,29] quantitative PCR,[27,29] electron microscopy (Fig. 103–2),[29] and in situ hybridization.[29] Subsequent data have indicated shorter doubling times, between 32 hours and 4 days.[27,29] More recently, growth of *T. whipplei* was reported in a cell-free medium, supplemented with amino acids.[30] Despite all these experimental advances, culture of *T. whipplei* at present is feasible only in specialized laboratories and remains unavailable for routine diagnostic purposes.

Phylogenetic analysis of the *T. whipplei* 16S rDNA sequence, initially amplified by broad-range PCR from

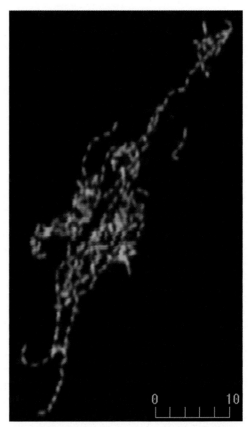

Figure 103–1 Photomicrograph of supernatant from a culture of *Tropheryma whipplei* from cerebrospinal fluid. Bacteria were stained with YO-PRO-1 nucleic acid dye. Note the distinctive appearance of small rods arranged in chains. (Scale bar represents micrometers.) (From Maiwald M, von Herbay A, Fredricks DN, et al: Cultivation of *Tropheryma whipplei* from cerebrospinal fluid. J Infect Dis 188:801, 2003.)

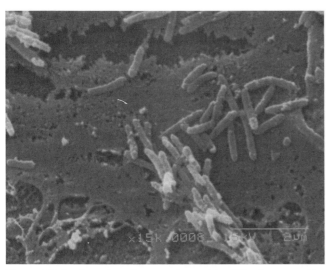

Figure 103–2 Scanning electron micrograph of *Tropheryma whipplei* from cerebrospinal fluid in fibroblast cell culture. Note the small, rod-shaped bacteria outside of cells, arranged in cords. Original magnification ×20,000. (From Maiwald M, von Herbay A, Fredricks DN, et al: Cultivation of *Tropheryma whipplei* from cerebrospinal fluid. J Infect Dis 188:801, 2003.)

infected tissue, established that the bacterium is an actinomycete (i.e., a member of the class *Actinobacteria*).[9,10] A subsequent, more detailed analysis placed the organism in an intermediate phylogenetic position between the genus *Cellulomonas* (with the common group A peptidoglycan) and a rare group of actinomycetes with group B peptidoglycan (i.e., a different linkage of cell wall components).[31] Both groups of organisms consist predominantly of environmental bacteria that are found in soil and water and on plants. Nevertheless, the relationships of *T. whipplei* to any of the other known actinomycetes are quite distant (<92% 16S rRNA sequence similarity).

First steps toward a molecular typing system for different strains of *T. whipplei* were the determination of the 16S-23S rDNA intergenic spacer sequence,[31] followed by the rRNA operon of the bacterium.[32] Seven different 16S-23S rRNA spacer sequence types have been described so far.[32-34] The two most common types, "1" and "2," were found in a similar ratio (≈1:2) in the United States, Germany, and Switzerland. In any given patient, the same spacer type was found in different anatomic compartments (e.g., intestine, blood, CSF),[32] which argues for systemic dissemination of a single bacterial strain in an individual with Whipple's disease. Additional variability between strains was found in a 23S rRNA insertion sequence,[35] in the *groEL* heat-shock protein gene,[36] and at a series of variable number of tandem repeat (VNTR) loci in *T. whipplei*.[37] The question of whether different strains are associated with different clinical features has not been addressed yet.

GENOMICS

The genome of *T. whipplei* is quite small for a bacterium; with approximately 926,000 base pairs, it is the smallest

of all known actinomycete genomes, and its guanine (G) + cytosine (C) content of 46% is unusually low for actinomycetes, which generally are organisms with high genomic G + C content.[14,15] Genome size contraction is believed, in this case, to have resulted from gene loss and is a general feature of bacteria that are highly host adapted. The bacterium has a lack of metabolic capabilities, such as deficiencies in carbohydrate and energy metabolism, and a lack of biosynthesis genes for amino acids, which makes it an organism that is dependent on supplies from other cellular sources. Two more features of the *T. whipplei* genome are quite remarkable. The organism devotes a relatively large amount of its genome to the biosynthesis of cell surface molecules, and it appears to have multiple "built-in" mechanisms for antigenic variation. The latter include VNTR sequences, known from other organisms to be associated with antigenic phase variation, as well as two unusual, large genomic regions of noncoding repetitive DNA that are thought to contribute to genetic variability.[14] In addition, a comparative analysis revealed that the two sequenced strains are distinguished by inversion of a large segment of the genome (≈57%), which is a further indication of genomic plasticity and variability.[15] All these traits suggest that interaction with its host and evasion of a host immune response play major roles in the organism's lifestyle, and all may be factors contributing to its ability to sustain a chronic infection.

PATHOGENESIS AND IMMUNOLOGY

The exact source of infection and the sequence of events leading to bacterial multiplication and pathologic changes are still unclear. Because of the prominence of intestinal manifestations, an oral route of acquisition generally is assumed,[8] but this is unproven. Current concepts hold that once *T. whipplei* has been acquired, it enters the proximal small intestine where the bacteria invade the mucosa. Evidence for this is provided by electron microscopy.[38-40] Fluorescent in situ hybridization further indicates that most viable bacteria are extracellular and located just below the epithelial basement membrane in the lamina propria mucosae (see later).[11] From the intestinal mucosa, bacteria are thought to spread via the lymphatic drainage into the mesenteric lymph nodes[39] and from there into the mediastinal lymph nodes, the thoracic duct, and the blood.

Little is known about the natural habitats of *T. whipplei*. Only humans seem to be affected, with outdoor workers more strongly represented than other professional groups.[8] A PCR-based search in effluent from a German sewage treatment plant revealed positive results for *T. whipplei* DNA in 25 of 38 samples from five different plants; this is the only published evidence of bacterial detection outside of a human host.[41] From within the human host, some investigators have detected *T. whipplei* DNA in saliva, gastric juice, and intestinal biopsies of asymptomatic persons.[42-44] Several large PCR-based studies of intestinal biopsy samples, however, have provided little or no evidence of infection in persons without the histologic features of Whipple's disease (see later).[45-49] There also is no evidence for person-to-person transmission,[8] and there are only a few reports of the disease in relatives of persons with the disease.[50-52] The genome sequence suggests that the organism is highly dependent on nutrients from other sources.[14,15] The proposed extracellular location at the villous tips below the intestinal basement membrane,[11] a site with rich influx of nutrients, would fit these requirements well. Such requirements also would be met, however, if a second environmental lifestyle in association with other cells existed, such as in polymicrobial communities or with free-living protozoa.

Transient (i.e., during active disease) as well as persistent (i.e., after therapy) abnormalities of immune function have been observed in patients with Whipple's disease.[8,53,54] The persistent defects are presumed to serve as predisposing factors for development of disease. Precisely defined immune defects, however, such as the complete absence of specific cell types, mediators, or receptors, have not been identified. Small case series[55,56] have described an over-representation of the HLA-B27 haplotype in patients with Whipple's disease, but others[57,58] have not supported this association. Humoral immunity grossly appears to be normal, although patient antisera have failed to react with areas of pathology in tissue sections of the intestinal mucosa.[8,59]

During active disease, reduced CD4/CD8 T-cell ratios (both in the lamina propria and in peripheral blood), reduced proliferation of peripheral T cells to stimulating agents (e.g., phytohemagglutinin, concanavalin A), and reduced delayed-type hypersensitivity reactions to common antigens in skin tests have been observed.[53,55,60] The extent to which these immune disturbances are a consequence of malnutrition in active Whipple's disease, rather than preexisting factors, remains unclear. The monocytes of one patient exhibited an impaired ability to degrade bacterial antigens after ingestion,[61] which would be consistent with the prolonged persistence of bacterial remnants in intestinal macrophages after therapy, as observed in histologic studies of Whipple's disease.[8,62] Other abnormalities also have been found that persist after therapy: reduced numbers of peripheral blood monocytes that express the alpha chain of complement receptor 3 (CD11b)[53]; a reduced capability of peripheral blood monocytes to produce interleukin-12 on stimulation with bacterial antigens[54]; and a dysregulation of mononuclear cell function, such that the components of a Th1 type immune response are reduced and those of a Th2 immune response increased.[63] All these features and activities play roles in microbial phagocytosis, antigen processing, and the regulation of a cellular immune response.[53,54,63]

Several reports describe opportunistic infections in patients with Whipple's disease, but this is not a generally observed phenomenon. Such secondary or opportunistic agents have included *Giardia lamblia*, *Pneumocystis carinii*, *Cryptosporidium parvum*, *Nocardia* spp., *Mycobacterium tuberculosis*, *Serratia marcescens*, *Candida* spp., dermatophytes, and *Strongyloides stercoralis*.[62,64-66] In addition, *T. whipplei* infection has been detected in a patient with acquired immunodeficiency syndrome (AIDS) on one occasion.[67] A role of the immune system for clearing *T. whipplei* infection was further suggested by the report of one patient without

adequate response to treatment with various antibiotics who eventually benefited from adjuvant interferon-gamma treatment[68]; however, this effect could not be reproduced in several other patients.[17] Taken together, all these observations and laboratory findings suggest that host immunologic factors play a role in determining the occurrence of Whipple's disease.

CLINICAL FEATURES

Whipple's disease is a systemic disorder, and almost any organ or organ system can be affected.[8] Manifestations in the intestinal tract are reported most commonly and are largely responsible for the classic clinical features of Whipple's disease.[20,69] In many patients, arthralgias precede intestinal symptoms by several years (1 to 10 years; up to 30 years reported), and in some cases, low-grade, intermittent fever also occurs for years before the diagnosis is made.[23,70] More recent reports provide a wider spectrum of extraintestinal manifestations, probably reflecting advances in diagnostic procedures. As a result of earlier detection, patients tend to have less advanced disease at the time of diagnosis.[8,23]

INTESTINE AND LYMPHATIC SYSTEM

Bacterial and macrophage-predominant inflammatory cell infiltration of the small intestinal mucosa and obstruction of mesenteric lymph nodes lead to a malabsorption syndrome with weight loss, diarrhea, and abdominal pain as the dominant signs and symptoms.[20,23,69-71] Weight loss in amounts of 5 to 15 kg occurs gradually, usually over a period of at least 1 year, sometimes leading to severe cachexia in the terminal stage of untreated disease.[8,20,70] Diarrhea may consist of voluminous steatorrheic stools or may be watery.[20] Occult gastrointestinal bleeding is not infrequent, and in some cases gross gastrointestinal bleeding occurs.[8,20]

Abdominal (mesenteric and retroperitoneal) as well as peripheral lymphadenopathy are common,[20,23,70,71] and in some instances, enlarged abdominal lymph nodes have raised the suspicion of malignancy.[71] In rare instances, malignant lymphomas have occurred in patients with Whipple's disease.[72-74]

Barium examination of the intestinal tract may reveal nonspecific abnormalities that also are found in other malabsorption syndromes,[8,70] such as prominent and edematous duodenal and jejunal folds and intestinal dilatation (Fig. 103–3). Computed tomography (CT) (Fig. 103–4) or magnetic resonance imaging (MRI) may detect retroperitoneal or para-aortic lymphadenopathy.[70,75] Enlarged abdominal lymph nodes have a hypodense appearance on CT scans and are hyperechoic on ultrasonograms.[65,76]

Laboratory examinations in patients with intestinal Whipple's disease often reveal increased erythrocyte sedimentation rates, decreased serum carotene levels, decreased serum iron concentration, anemia, decreased serum protein levels, proteinuria, and elevated stool fat content.[8,70]

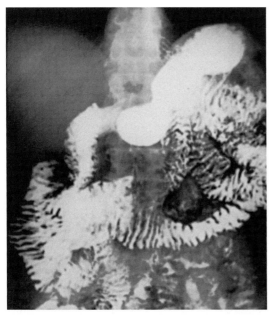

Figure 103–3 Barium contrast study of the small intestine from a patient with Whipple's disease. There is marked thickening of the plicae circulares and a loss of the normal delicate mucosal relief pattern. The small intestine is slightly dilated. (Courtesy of Elihu Schimmel, MD, Boston, MA.)

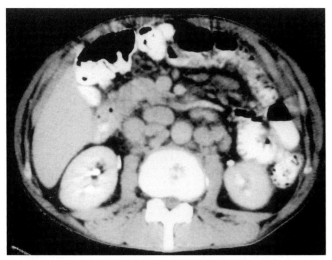

Figure 103–4 CT scan showing extensive retroperitoneal and mesenteric adenopathy caused by Whipple's disease, and simulating lymphoma. (Courtesy of Mark Feldman, MD, Dallas, TX.)

CENTRAL NERVOUS SYSTEM

Symptomatic CNS manifestations have been reported in 10% to 43% of patients with intestinal Whipple's disease.[20,23,70,71] Neurologic disease can occur concurrently with intestinal manifestations at the time of diagnosis, but it is more frequent at the time of clinical relapse, which can occur during or after treatment.[8,77] It is hypothesized that bacteria enter the CNS early in the course of disease and that because most drugs do not penetrate the CNS well, the bacteria persist during drug treatment. The net result is the impression of (intestinal) disease remission initially and the subsequent onset

of (neurologic) disease even while antibiotics continue to be given. Relapses affecting the CNS are ominous, because they can be refractory to renewed antibiotic treatment.[8,78] Although rare, several cases of isolated primary neurologic Whipple's disease have been reported in patients without intestinal manifestations.[79,80]

Two reviews summarized the neurologic findings of 84 and 122 published cases, respectively.[81,82] Common findings are progressive dementia and cognitive changes (28% to 71%), supranuclear ophthalmoplegia (32% to 51%), and altered level of consciousness (27% to 50%). Other less frequent signs are psychiatric symptoms, hypothalamic manifestations (e.g., polydipsia, hyperphagia, insomnia),[83] cranial nerve abnormalities, nystagmus, seizures, and ataxia. Two signs are considered to be characteristic of CNS Whipple's disease—oculomasticatory myorhythmia and oculofacial skeletal myorhythmia—these have not yet been documented in other CNS diseases.[81] Both consist of slow rhythmic and synchronized contractions (≈1/sec) of ocular, facial, or other muscles; both occur in less than 20% of patients with CNS Whipple's disease.[81,82]

Results of neuroimaging (CT or MRI scans) may be normal or may reveal mild to moderate brain atrophy or focal lesions without a predilection for specific sites.[81,82,84] These abnormalities are not specific for Whipple's disease, but focal lesions may be used to guide stereotactic biopsies, which in most cases reveal characteristic histology.[81] MRI appears to be more sensitive than CT scans.[82] Results of standard CSF examinations most often are normal, although sometimes there is mild pleocytosis.[8,81] CSF cytology reveals PAS-positive sickleform particle-containing cells, and PCR often yields positive results for *T. whipplei* DNA, even in a considerable proportion of neurologically asymptomatic patients.[85]

CARDIOVASCULAR SYSTEM

Cardiac manifestations of Whipple's disease include endocarditis, myocarditis, and pericarditis.[23] In one autopsy series from the preantibiotic era,[69] valvular endocarditis with vegetations was noted in 58% of cases. In contrast, in a more recent series,[23] clinically apparent endocarditis was less frequent (3 of 52 patients). All valves may be affected, but the mitral valve is most frequently pathologically altered, and involvement of the aortic valve leads to the most significant symptoms[8]; some patients require valve replacement. PAS-positive macrophages and bacteria have been documented in native[86] and porcine prosthetic[87,88] valve tissue and in the myocardium[89] by histology and electron microscopy, respectively. By PCR testing of excised heart valve tissue, *T. whipplei* is increasingly being recognized as an agent of "blood culture-negative endocarditis," even in patients with only minor or no apparent intestinal Whipple's disease.[88,90-93]

MUSCULOSKELETAL SYSTEM

Oligoarthralgias or polyarthralgias, usually involving the ankles, knees, elbows, or fingers, are a common complaint of patients with Whipple's disease.[8] Rheumatoid factor usually is absent. Destructive joint changes or synovial fluid accumulation are rare, but, if present, are accompanied by PAS-positive macrophages (by histology), bacteria (by electron microscopy), or DNA of *T. whipplei* (by PCR) in synovial tissue or joint fluid.[8,94,95] Sacroiliitis and spondylitis may occur, but ankylosing forms are rare, and there does not seem to be a strong association of these manifestations with HLA-B27.[8] Rare manifestations are infectious spondylodiskitis[96] and prosthetic joint infection.[97]

OTHER MANIFESTATIONS

One common feature of Whipple's disease is skin hyperpigmentation, which has been found in 17% to 66% of patients.[20,23,69-71] This finding tends to occur in light-exposed areas of the skin and is unrelated to adrenal dysfunction or hyperbilirubinemia. Histopathologic changes in the skin, however, are extremely rare,[98] and the nature of the pigment is unknown.

Ocular manifestations of Whipple's disease have been described and are diverse but rare. These include uveitis, vitritis, retinitis, retrobulbar neuritis, and papilledema.[8] They usually are associated with CNS disease, and almost all reported patients also had clinical or histologic evidence of intestinal involvement. PAS-positive macrophages or DNA of *T. whipplei* may be detected in vitrectomy specimens.[99] One case of uveitis has been reported in which the vitreous fluid and one intestinal biopsy specimen yielded positive PCR results, although intestinal histology was normal.[100] Another uveitis case was a source for a positive culture.[26]

Chronic cough was a symptom in Whipple's original patient and was reported relatively frequently in earlier series[69] but infrequently since then.[23] Some patients have pleuritis with effusion or granulomatous pulmonary disease resembling sarcoidosis.[8]

PATHOLOGY

SMALL INTESTINE

The histopathologic features of intestinal Whipple's disease are quite distinctive. On gross inspection, the mucosa of the distal duodenum and jejunum is abnormal in most patients. Whitish to yellow plaque-like patches are observed in approximately three quarters of patients (Fig. 103–5); alternatively, the mucosa may appear pale yellow.[62,101] Abnormal villus structure and mild mucosal flattening become evident using magnifying optics. Viewed with light microscopy, the visible patches reflect lipid deposits or lymphangiectasia, whereas villus distention results from infiltration by macrophages in the lamina propria (Fig. 103–6). The swollen cytoplasm of macrophages appears foamy when stained with hematoxylin-eosin, but numerous granular particles become visible when the PAS stain is used (see Fig. 103–6). These particles correspond to phagolysosomes filled with numerous *T. whipplei*, and the positive reaction with PAS reflects the glycoprotein content of the

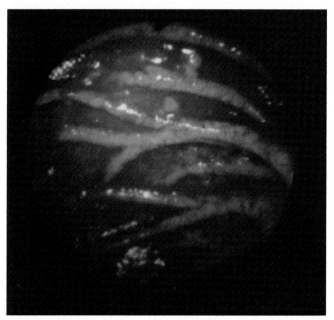

Figure 103–5 Endoscopic view of the distal duodenum in a patient with untreated Whipple's disease. The plicae circulares appear swollen, and the mucosal surface is intact. Numerous whitish patches, reflecting lipid deposits, are present within the mucosa. (Courtesy of Hans Jörg Meier-Willersen, MD, Heidelberg, Germany.)

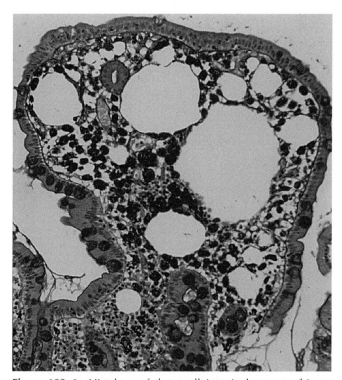

Figure 103–6 Histology of the small intestinal mucosa (biopsy specimen from the same patient as in Fig. 103–5). A villus is distended by an infiltrate of macrophages that contain periodic acid–Schiff-positive granular particles (type 1 cells), and by lipid droplets. The epithelial layer is intact. Original magnification ×84.

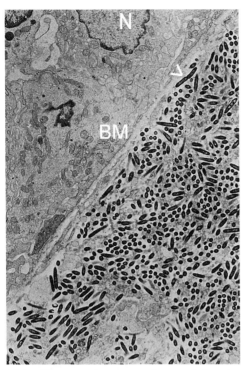

Figure 103–7 Electron microscopy of a small intestinal biopsy specimen in a patient with untreated Whipple's disease. Just beneath the epithelial basement membrane (BM), the lamina propria is densely infiltrated by extracellular rod-shaped bacteria. The bacteria are uniform in size and structure. Some of them are dividing (*arrowhead*). N, nucleus of enterocyte.

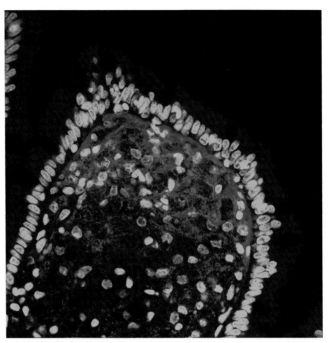

Figure 103–8 Fluorescent in situ hybridization of a small intestinal biopsy specimen in a patient with Whipple's disease. In this confocal micrograph, nuclei of human cells are green, the intracellular cytoskeletal protein vimentin is red, and *Tropheryma whipplei* ribosomal RNA (rRNA) is blue. The *T. whipplei* rRNA signal is most intense in the extracellular spaces of the lamina propria, immediately subjacent to the basal membrane. ×200. (Courtesy of David N. Fredricks, MD, Palo Alto, CA.)

bacterial cell walls. Single extracellular bacteria barely are visible with conventional light microscopy because of their small size, but they become evident in the mucosal stroma with high-resolution light microscopy and electron microscopy (Fig. 103–7). Their number varies greatly among patients.

Electron microscopy shows uniformity in size and shape of the bacteria, with an external diameter of 0.2 to 0.25 μm and a length of up to 2.5 μm.[40,102] There is an electron-dense outer layer that is not found in other bacteria; some authors have speculated that this unusual membrane may be of host origin.[102] Most of the structurally intact bacteria, including dividing forms, are found outside of host cells in the lamina propria (see Fig. 103–7).[8,102] In contrast, the intracellular bacteria in macrophages often are found in various stages of degradation. Findings based on fluorescent in situ hybridization using specific *T. whipplei* 16S rDNA probes support and extend the findings derived from electron microscopy[11]; the 16S rRNA signal from metabolically active bacteria is found in the intestinal lamina propria, just beneath the basement membrane, but is absent from the PAS-positive macrophages (Fig. 103–8). Thus, *T. whipplei* appears to prefer extracellular environments within the host, despite its association with eukaryotic cells.

On immunohistology, the PAS-positive inclusions in tissue react with heterologous antisera against several *Streptococcus* species, *Shigella flexneri,* and a few other species.[59,103,104] More recently, antisera were raised against cultivated *T. whipplei* and used for testing small intestinal,

lymph node, heart, and brain tissue.[12,105,106] Observed staining patterns generally were similar to those of PAS staining, and the *T. whipplei*-specific antisera did not react with a number of control bacteria and tissues affected by other diseases. It remains to be seen, however, whether the specificity of these antibodies is sufficient for routine diagnostic purposes.

Mucosal infiltration with PAS-positive cells usually is diffuse, but in some patients patchy lesions may be present. The inflammatory reaction generally is dominated by macrophages, whereas neutrophils and eosinophils are more scarce, as are lymphocytes and plasma cells.[62,107] This cellular composition is unusual for an invasive bacterial infection, a feature that suggests a disturbance of mobilization and chemotaxis of leukocytes.[62]

Variants of the usual histologic findings occur in some patients. These include rare cases with PAS-positive macrophages that are located exclusively in the submucosa and rare cases with epithelioid granulomas in the affected mucosa.[62] Taken together, the intestinal histopathology of Whipple's disease demonstrates some heterogeneity.

During treatment, the histologic findings in the intestinal mucosa change substantially but slowly, over several months or more.[39,62,108] In addition to a continuous decrease in the number of PAS-positive macrophages, the pattern of cellular infiltration of the mucosa changes with time from diffuse to patchy. This feature demands multiple biopsies during follow-up endoscopic examinations.

Mucosal infiltration shifts from the upper (i.e., villi) to the lower part of the mucosa (i.e., pericryptal lamina propria) and submucosa. More significantly, the cytologic aspects of the PAS-positive macrophages undergo changes.[62] Before treatment, most macrophages have numerous granular particles in the cytoplasm that stain intensely red with PAS (type 1 macrophages; see Fig. 103–6). Within 1 to 6 months of treatment, the percentage of type 1 macrophages gradually decreases, and, in parallel, cells with only some coarse granular inclusions and a background of diffuse or fine granular more faintly PAS-positive cytoplasm (type 2 macrophages) increase in number. After 6 to 15 months, most macrophages that are still present have diffuse and faintly PAS-positive material in their cytoplasm but lack granular inclusions (type 3 macrophages). Type 3 macrophages contain only filamentous remnants of bacteria.[62] Thus, their positive PAS reaction reflects the presence of glycoprotein residue of degraded bacterial cell walls. In adequately treated patients, some type 3 macrophages usually persist, even for more than 10 years; in fact, the finding of type 3 macrophages alone is consistent with intestinal remission. Despite documented clinical remission of intestinal disease, however, some patients still may harbor viable *T. whipplei* and may later develop extraintestinal Whipple's disease. Thus, the prognostic value of intestinal histology during the follow-up of patients is limited.[62]

EXTRAINTESTINAL PATHOLOGY

Autopsy reports of untreated patients with Whipple's disease have revealed involvement of virtually any organ and tissue.[69,109] As with intestinal disease, the histologic hallmark of extraintestinal involvement is the presence of intracellular PAS-positive granular particles; the diagnostic significance of these lesions in extraintestinal tissues is limited, however, and additional evidence is required for the diagnosis of Whipple's disease. Rod-shaped bacteria have been documented by electron microscopy in many extraintestinal organs, including colon, liver, heart, lung, brain, eye, lymph nodes, bone marrow, and spleen.[8]

Two different types of lymph node lesions are common in Whipple's disease. Abdominal nodes generally contain lipid deposits that induce a granulomatous foreign body type of reaction.[1] Peripheral lymph nodes (inguinal, axillary, cervical) generally do not contain lipids but feature a toxoplasmosis-like lymphadenitis with small clusters of epithelioid macrophages, some of which have PAS-positive particles that correspond to inclusions with *T. whipplei*. Rarely, a third type of lymph node reaction may be observed that resembles sarcoidosis; it occurs most commonly in the mediastinum.

Whipple's disease affects diverse regions of the brain. Most commonly, perivascular infiltrates of PAS-positive macrophages are present, as well as tumor-like granulomas of variable size, consisting of glial cells with intensely PAS-positive granular particles.[8] Occasionally, granulomas in the ventricular system cause occlusive hydrocephalus. PAS-positive macrophages frequently can be detected free in the CSF, even in patients without neurologic or psychiatric symptoms (see later).

DIAGNOSIS

Almost all patients with Whipple's disease suffer from involvement of the intestinal tract by this infection, regardless of whether gastrointestinal symptoms are present.[23,70,71] Thus, the primary diagnostic approach to a patient with clinically suspected Whipple's disease is upper endoscopy (see Fig. 103–5) with mucosal biopsy. To avoid sampling errors in patients with patchy lesions, one should obtain approximately five biopsy specimens from regions as far distal as possible within the small intestine.[17] Histologic examination with routine hematoxylin-eosin and PAS stains is usually sufficient to reach a diagnosis (see earlier). In some cases, findings may be corroborated with silver stains[1]; in contrast, the Gram stain is less useful in this infection. Traditionally, electron microscopy has been used as the gold standard for confirming the diagnosis of Whipple's disease.[8] Currently, PCR analysis serves in this capacity.[45,46]

Since the molecular characterization of *T. whipplei*, several PCR-based assays have been developed for diagnostic purposes,[10,35,45-47,96,100,110,111] only some of which have been thoroughly validated. In almost all patients with a histologic diagnosis of Whipple's disease, well-standardized PCR assays detect *T. whipplei* DNA in the intestinal mucosa.[45,46] In contrast, intestinal biopsies with normal histology almost always are negative for DNA of *T. whipplei*.[49] PCR from feces has been proposed for use in a noninvasive screening method,[110] but currently there are no clinical data supporting its usefulness. In practical terms, normal intestinal histology in the absence of extraintestinal disease suggestive of Whipple's disease excludes the diagnosis, provided that multiple biopsy specimens are examined.

Extraintestinal manifestations warrant the examination of specimens from affected sites. Histology and cytology with PAS staining, electron microscopy, and PCR all are useful for this purpose. Since the introduction of PCR for *T. whipplei*,[10] some patients have been reported with a PCR-based diagnosis of *T. whipplei* infection in extraintestinal samples and intestinal histology (when tested) that was negative for PAS-positive macrophages. Examples of such cases include febrile illness with erythrocyte-associated bacteria[112]; uveitis[100]; and valvular heart disease.[92] The number of such reported cases is still small (see earlier). PCR testing of peripheral blood samples has been proposed as a potential noninvasive screening method,[113] but its diagnostic usefulness has been questioned.[114]

Considering the systemic nature of the disorder, it is important to evaluate commonly involved organ systems when a new diagnosis of Whipple's disease has been established. Ultrasound examination may reveal enlarged mesenteric lymph nodes that have unusually high echogenicity due to lipid deposits.[65] Neurologic examination is indicated, including routine sampling of CSF.[85] Based on cytologic or PCR analysis of the spinal fluid, 70% of patients with intestinal Whipple's disease in one study were found to have CNS infection with *T. whipplei*, even though they had no neurologic or psychiatric symptoms.[85] Imaging studies of the brain generally are not helpful in the absence of neurologic symptoms. In selected patients with Whipple's disease and anemia, wireless capsule endoscopy appears to be suitable to detect the site of bleeding in the small intestine.[115]

During treatment, one should repeat diagnostic assessments at regular intervals. Endoscopic lesions usually resolve within months but may last for up to a year.[101] Intestinal histology improves within several months,[62] and PCR assays on intestinal biopsy tissues convert to negative within a time range of about 1 to 12 months after institution of appropriate therapy.[45] Some PAS-positive macrophages may persist for years,[62] even while the patient remains in clinical remission (see earlier). Regression of enlarged abdominal lymph nodes may require more than a year and may result in fibrosis. Follow-up examination of the CSF is performed most effectively with inclusion of PCR analysis.[85] As has been documented in a culture-positive case, *T. whipplei* may persist in a viable state in the CNS despite prolonged administration of antibiotics.[29]

DIFFERENTIAL DIAGNOSIS

Almost all symptoms and findings of Whipple's disease are nonspecific. The broad spectrum of possible clinical presentations generates a wide differential diagnosis, involving several subspecialties of medicine—gastroenterology, infectious diseases, rheumatology, cardiology, hematology, neurology, psychiatry, and ophthalmology.

Disorders that mimic the histology of Whipple's disease are uncommon.[24] PAS-positive cells in intestinal biopsies may include mucosal smooth muscle cells that are rich in glycogen or plasma cells that contain immunoglobulin (Russell bodies) in the setting of chronic duodenitis. Rarely, these PAS-positive cells reflect intestinal infection with *Mycobacterium avium* complex, histoplasmosis, macroglobulinemia, intestinal xanthelasmas, or pseudomelanosis duodeni. Differentiation from Whipple's disease usually is possible by means of histochemical stains (e.g., stains for acid-fast bacteria and use of diastase) and by immunocytochemistry.[24]

Sarcoid-like granulomas are rare in Whipple's disease but may occur in the stomach,[116] small intestine,[62,117] liver,[118] and lymph nodes. A possible relationship between Whipple's disease and sarcoidosis remains unresolved.[119] By means of PCR analysis, thoracic sarcoidosis[120] and intestinal sarcoidosis[121] tissues were both found to be negative for *T. whipplei* DNA.

Most patients with Whipple's disease have enlarged abdominal lymph nodes. This became more apparent with the advent of abdominal ultrasonography and CT scanning.[72] Only rare cases of Whipple's disease associated with metachronous or synchronous malignant lymphomas have been observed.[72-74] The relationship of *T. whipplei* infection and lymphoma, if any, remains unclear.

TREATMENT AND PROGNOSIS

The initial response of Whipple's disease to antibiotic treatment usually is prompt.[122] Diarrhea often resolves within several days; arthralgias within a few weeks; and

significant weight gain occurs within a few months.[20] In the 1970s and early 1980s, long-term tetracycline therapy usually was given,[23,71] however, it became increasingly clear that patients treated in this manner frequently suffered from relapses, many of which affected the CNS.[123,124] CNS relapses have a poor prognosis, because they are often refractory to renewed treatment.[77] It therefore was suggested that the treatment of Whipple's disease include antibiotics that cross the blood-brain barrier. Since the mid-1980s, trimethoprim-sulfamethoxazole has been used commonly.[77,125]

Current recommendations for the treatment of Whipple's disease are based on observations from numerous case reports,[8] several clinical series,[23,70,71] and retrospective analyses of antibiotic regimens.[77,122] Evidence from a randomized prospective study is not available to date. In a retrospective analysis of 88 patients,[77] relapses were most common after monotherapy with tetracyclines. Of 49 patients treated with tetracycline alone, 21 relapsed, including 9 with CNS relapses. Only a small number of relapses (2 of 15 patients treated), none of which involved the CNS, were observed after initial parenteral treatment with penicillin plus streptomycin, followed by long-term oral tetracycline (the "Duke regimen"). Tetracyclines and trimethoprim-sulfamethoxazole were compared in another series of 30 patients.[122] Trimethoprim-sulfamethoxazole was superior to tetracyclines in inducing remission (12 of 13 vs. 13 of 22 treatment courses; includes remissions after relapse). Relapses in the CNS occurred in 2 of 22 patients receiving tetracycline and in 1 of 13 receiving trimethoprim-sulfamethoxazole. Despite its clinical efficacy and ability to cross the blood-brain barrier, several reports indicate that relapses can occur after use of trimethoprim-sulfamethoxazole, including CNS relapses.[126-128] Some patients appear to have benefited from repeated intravenous courses of third-generation cephalosporins.[85]

Based on these clinical observations, the current recommendation for treatment of Whipple's disease is to begin with an induction phase using either penicillin G plus streptomycin or a third-generation cephalosporin, such as ceftriaxone, followed by treatment with at least one drug that efficiently crosses the blood-brain barrier (e.g., trimethoprim-sulfamethoxazole) for at least 1 year. An overview of antibiotic treatment, including suggested doses, is given in Table 103–1.

New data regarding antibiotic susceptibility are becoming available from in vitro experiments with *T. whipplei* in culture as well as from genome analysis. Several *T. whipplei* strains were cultivated with MRC-5 human fibroblasts and their growth kinetics measured by real-time PCR in the presence of antibiotics.[27,129] According to these analyses, *T. whipplei* appears sensitive to doxycycline, penicillins, macrolides, rifampin, teicoplanin, and trimethoprim-sulfamethoxazole; variably sensitive to imipenem; and only moderately sensitive or resistant to vancomycin, cephalosporins, and fluoroquinolones.[129] Analysis of the quinolone resistance-determining regions in *gyrA* and *parC* genes revealed amino acids that are commonly associated with resistance in other bacteria.[27] The *T. whipplei* genome is lacking the gene for dihydrofolate reductase, which is the target for trimethoprim action,[130] so that the susceptibility to trimethoprim-sulfamethoxa-

Table 103–1 Overview of Antibiotics Used to Treat Whipple's Disease

Drugs	Dosage	Comments	References
Penicillin G + streptomycin	6-24 million units IV daily (in divided doses) + 1 g IM once daily	Induction therapy (first 10-14 days)	8, 20, 77
Ceftriaxone	2 g IV once daily	Induction therapy (first 10-14 days) or salvage therapy; less widely used than penicillin G + streptomycin	85, 131, 132
Trimethoprim-sulfamethoxazole	160 mg/800 mg PO twice daily	Long-term therapy; first-line drug; good CNS penetration, but CNS relapses may occur	77, 122, 124, 124
Penicillin VK	500 mg PO four times daily	Alternative for long-term therapy; limited experience	8, 77
Doxycycline (or tetracycline)	100 mg PO twice daily (500 mg PO four times daily)	Used for many years, but clinical relapses, including CNS, are well-described	20, 77, 122
Cefixime	400 mg PO twice daily	Alternative for long-term therapy; limited experience	126
Rifampin	600 mg PO once daily	Second-line drug; good CNS penetration	80, 127, 133
Chloramphenicol	500 mg PO four times daily	Second-line drug; worrisome side effects	5, 8, 80
Erythromycin	500 mg PO four times daily	Second-line drug; limited experience	8, 123, 131, 133
Pefloxacin	400 mg PO twice daily	Second-line drug; limited experience	133

CNS, central nervous system; IM, intramuscular; IV, intravenous; PO, oral.

zole most likely is dependent on its sulfamethoxazole component only.

FUTURE PROSPECTS

Significant new knowledge regarding Whipple's disease and its pathogen has been learned during the last decade, culminating in the first successful culture and the sequencing and analysis of the pathogen's genome. Despite these advances, the perception of enigma still surrounds Whipple's disease and *T. whipplei*. The disease produces a wide spectrum of clinical manifestations; its true prevalence is unknown; but its apparent rarity and its epidemiology suggest that as yet unknown host defects predispose toward disease manifestation. Important questions remaining to be addressed include the basis for pathogenicity of the organism; the organism's natural reservoir; and the interpretation and utilization of the vast information that has become available through the sequenced genomes. Regardless of the magnitude of the burden imposed by this organism on human health, the study of *T. whipplei* and Whipple's disease will continue to reveal important principles in intestinal pathophysiology, actinomycete biology and pathogenicity, and the human immune system.

REFERENCES

1. Whipple GH: A hitherto undescribed disease characterized anatomically by deposits of fat and fatty acids in the intestinal and mesenteric lymphatic tissues. Bull Johns Hopkins Hosp 18:382, 1907.
2. Oliver-Pascual E, Galan J, Oliver-Pascual A, Castillo E: Un caso de lipodistrofia intestinal con lesiones gangliones mesentericas de granulomatosis lipofagica (Enfermedad de Whipple). Rev Esp Enferm Apar Dig 6:213, 1947.
3. Bolt RJ, Pollard HM, Standaert L: Transoral small-bowel biopsy as an aid in the diagnosis of malabsorption states. N Engl J Med 259:32, 1958.
4. Black-Schaffer B: The tinctoral demonstration of a glycoprotein in Whipple's disease. Proc Soc Exp Biol Med 72:225, 1949.
5. Paulley JW: A case of Whipple's disease (intestinal lipodystrophy). Gastroenterology 22:128, 1952.
6. Chears WC, Ashworth CT: Electron microscopic study of the intestinal mucosa in Whipple's disease: Demonstration of encapsulated bacilliform bodies in the lesion. Gastroenterology 41:129, 1961.
7. Yardley JH, Hendrix TR: Combined electron and light microscopy in Whipple's disease. Bull Johns Hopkins Hosp 109:80, 1961.
8. Dobbins WO III: Whipple's Disease. Springfield, IL, Charles C Thomas, 1987.
9. Wilson KH, Blitchington R, Frothingham R, Wilson JAP: Phylogeny of the Whipple's disease-associated bacterium. Lancet 338:474, 1991.
10. Relman DA, Schmidt TM, MacDermott RP, Falkow S: Identification of the uncultured bacillus of Whipple's disease. N Engl J Med 327:293, 1992.
11. Fredricks DN, Relman DA: Localization of *Tropheryma whippelii* rRNA in tissues from patients with Whipple's disease. J Infect Dis 183:1229, 2001.
12. Raoult D, Birg ML, LaScola B, et al: Cultivation of the bacillus of Whipple's disease. N Engl J Med 342:620, 2000.
13. La Scola B, Fenollar F, Fournier PE, et al: Description of *Tropheryma whipplei* gen. nov., sp. nov., the Whipple's disease bacillus. Int J Syst Evol Microbiol 51:1471, 2001.
14. Bentley SD, Maiwald M, Murphy LD, et al: Sequencing and analysis of the genome of the Whipple's disease bacterium *Tropheryma whipplei*. Lancet 361:637, 2003.
15. Raoult D, Ogata H, Audic S, et al: *Tropheryma whipplei* twist: A human pathogenic actinobacteria with a reduced genome. Genome Res 13:1800, 2003.
16. Salomoni I: La maladie de Whipple en Suisse occidentale entre 1960 et 1983. [Whipple's disease in Western Switzerland between 1960 and 1983: Observation of a case, comparison of a series of 11 cases diagnosed in Western Switzerland between 1960 and 1983 with data from the literature]. Rev Med Suisse Romande 104:655, 1984.
17. von Herbay A: Whipple's disease online (2005) URL: http://www.WhipplesDisease.net.

18. von Herbay A, Otto HF, Stolte M, et al: Epidemiology of Whipple disease in Germany: Analysis of 110 patients diagnosed in 1965-95. Scand J Gastroenterol 32:52, 1997.

19. Capron JP, Thevenin A, Delamarre J, et al: Whipple's disease: Study of three cases and epidemiological and radiological remarks. Lille Med 20:842, 1975.

20. Maizel H, Ruffin JM, Dobbins WO III: Whipple's disease: A review of 19 patients from one hospital and a review of the literature since 1950. Medicine (Baltimore) 49:175, 1970.

21. Lopatin RN, Grossman ET, Horine J, et al: Whipple's disease in neighbors. J Clin Gastroenterol 4:223, 1982.

22. Ectors NL, Geboes KJ, Devos RM, et al: Whipple's disease: A histological, immunocytochemical, and electron-microscopic study of the small-intestinal epithelium. J Pathol 172:73, 1994.

23. Vital Durand D, Lecomte C, Cathébras P, et al: Whipple disease: Clinical review of 52 cases. Medicine (Baltimore) 76:170, 1997.

24. von Herbay A: Morbus Whipple: Histologische Diagnostik nach der Entdeckung von *Tropheryma whippelii*. Pathologe 22:82, 2001.

25. Raoult D, La Scola B, Lecocq P, et al: Culture and immunological detection of *Tropheryma whippelii* from the duodenum of a patient with Whipple disease. JAMA 285:1039, 2001.

26. Drancourt M, Raoult D, Lepidi H, et al: Culture of *Tropheryma whippelii* from the vitreous fluid of a patient presenting with unilateral uveitis. Ann Intern Med 139:1046, 2003.

27. Masselot F, Boulos A, Maurin M, et al: Molecular evaluation of antibiotic susceptibility: *Tropheryma whipplei* paradigm. Antimicrob Agents Chemother 47:1658, 2003.

28. Fenollar F, Birg ML, Gauduchon V, Raoult D: Culture of *Tropheryma whipplei* from human samples: A 3-year experience (1999 to 2002). J Clin Microbiol 41:3816, 2003.

29. Maiwald M, von Herbay A, Fredricks DN, et al: Cultivation of *Tropheryma whipplei* from cerebrospinal fluid. J Infect Dis 188:801, 2003.

30. Renesto P, Crapoulet N, Ogata H, et al: Genome-based design of a cell-free culture medium for *Tropheryma whipplei*. Lancet 362:447, 2003.

31. Maiwald M, Ditton HJ, von Herbay A, et al: Reassessment of the phylogenetic position of the bacterium associated with Whipple's disease and determination of the 16S-23S ribosomal intergenic spacer sequence. Int J Syst Bacteriol 46:1078, 1996.

32. Maiwald M, von Herbay A, Lepp PW, Relman DA: Organization, structure, and variability of the rRNA operon of the Whipple's disease bacterium (*Tropheryma whippelii*). J Bacteriol 182:3292, 2000.

33. Hinrikson HP, Dutly F, Nair S, Altwegg M: Detection of three different types of *Tropheryma whippelii* directly from clinical specimens by sequencing, single-strand conformation polymorphism (SSCP) analysis and type-specific PCR of their 16S-23S ribosomal intergenic spacer region. Int J Syst Bacteriol 49:1701, 1999.

34. Geissdörfer W, Wittmann I, Röllinghoff M, et al: Detection of a new 16S-23S rRNA spacer sequence variant (type 7) of *Tropheryma whippelii* in a patient with prosthetic aortic valve endocarditis. Eur J Clin Microbiol Infect Dis 20:762, 2001.

35. Hinrikson HP, Dutly F, Altwegg M: Evaluation of a specific nested PCR targeting domain III of the 23S rRNA gene of "*Tropheryma whippelii*" and proposal of a classification system for its molecular variants. J Clin Microbiol 38:595, 2000.

36. Morgenegg S, Dutly F, Altwegg M: Cloning and sequencing of a part of the heat shock protein 65 gene (*hsp65*) of "*Tropheryma whippelii*" and its use for detection of "*T. whippelii*" in clinical specimens by PCR. J. Clin. Microbiol. 38:2248, 2000.

37. Maiwald M, Lepp PW, Relman DA: Analysis of conserved non-rRNA genes of *Tropheryma whipplei*. Syst Appl Microbiol 26:3, 2003.

38. Kent TH, Layton JM, Clifton JA, Schedl HP: Whipple's disease: Light and electron microscopic studies combined with clinical studies suggesting an infective nature. Lab Invest 12:1163, 1963.

39. Dobbins WO III, Ruffin JM: A light- and electron-microscopic study of bacterial invasion in Whipple's disease. Am J Pathol 51:225, 1967.

40. Dobbins WO III, Kawanishi H: Bacillary characteristics in Whipple's disease: An electron microscopic study. Gastroenterology 80:1468, 1981.

41. Maiwald M, Schuhmacher F, Ditton HJ, von Herbay A: Environmental occurrence of the Whipple's disease bacterium (*Tropheryma whippelii*). Appl Environ Microbiol 64:760, 1998.

42. Street S, Donoghue HD, Neild GH: *Tropheryma whippelii* DNA in saliva of healthy people. Lancet 354:1178, 1999.

43. Ehrbar HU, Bauerfeind P, Dutly F, et al: PCR-positive tests for *Tropheryma whippelii* in patients without Whipple's disease. Lancet 353:2214, 1999.

44. Amsler L, Bauernfeind P, Nigg C, et al: Prevalence of *Tropheryma whippelii* DNA in patients with various gastrointestinal diseases and in healthy controls. Infection 31:81, 2003.

45. von Herbay A, Ditton HJ, Maiwald M: Diagnostic application of a polymerase chain reaction assay for the Whipple's disease bacterium to intestinal biopsies. Gastroenterology 110:1735, 1996.

46. Ramzan NN, Loftus E, Burgart LJ, et al: Diagnosis and monitoring of Whipple disease by polymerase chain reaction. Ann Intern Med 126:520, 1997.

47. Müller C, Petermann D, Stain C, et al: Whipple's disease: Comparison of histology with diagnosis based on polymerase chain reaction in four consecutive cases. Gut 40:425, 1997.

48. Pron B, Poyart C, Abachin E, et al: Diagnosis and follow-up of Whipple's disease by amplification of the 16S rRNA gene of *Tropheryma whippelii*. Eur J Clin Microbiol Infect Dis 18:62, 1999.

49. Maiwald M, von Herbay A, Persing DH, et al: *Tropheryma whippelii* DNA is rare in the intestinal mucosa of patients without other evidence of Whipple disease. Ann Intern Med 134:115, 2001.

50. Puite RH, Tesluk H: Whipple's disease. Am J Med 19:383, 1955.

51. Gross JB, Wollaeger EE, Sauer WG, et al: Whipple's disease: A report of four cases, including two in brothers, with observations on pathologic physiology, diagnosis, and treatment. Gastroenterology 36:65, 1959.

52. Dykman DD, Cuccherini BA, Fuss IJ, et al: Whipple's disease in a father-daughter pair. Dig Dis Sci 44:2542, 1999.

53. Marth T, Roux M, von Herbay A, et al: Persistent reduction of complement receptor-3 alpha-chain expressing mononuclear blood cells and transient inhibitory serum factors in Whipple's disease. Clin Immunol Immunopathol 72:217, 1994.

54. Marth T, Neurath M, Cuccherini BA, Strober W: Defects of monocyte interleukin 12 production and humoral immunity in Whipple's disease. Gastroenterology 113:442, 1997.

55. Feurle GE, Dörken B, Schopf E, Lenhard V: HLA-B27 and defects in the T-cell system in Whipple's disease. Eur J Clin Invest 9:385, 1979.

56. Dobbins WO: HLA antigens in Whipple's disease. Arthritis Rheum 30:102, 1987.

57. Bai JC, Mota AH, Maurino E, et al: Class I and class II HLA antigens in a homogeneous Argentinean population with Whipple's disease: Lack of association with HLA-B27. Am J Gastroenterol 86:992, 1991.

58. Olivieri I, Brandi G, Padula A, et al: Lack of association with spondyloarthritis and HLA-B27 in Italian patients with Whipple's disease. J Rheumatol 28:1294, 2001.

59. Kirkpatrick PM, Kent SP, Mihas A, Pritchett P: Whipple's disease: Case report with immunological studies. Gastroenterology 75:297, 1978.

60. Martin FF, Vilseck J, Dobbins WO, et al: Immunological alterations in patients with treated Whipple's disease. Gastroenterology 63:6, 1972.

61. Bjerknes R, Odegaard S, Bjerkvig R, et al: Whipple's disease: Demonstration of a persisting monocyte and macrophage dysfunction. Scand J Gastroenterol 23:611, 1988.

62. von Herbay A, Maiwald M, Ditton HJ, Otto HF: Histology of intestinal Whipple's disease revisited: A study of 48 patients. Virchows Arch 429:335, 1996.

63. Marth T, Kleen N, Stallmach A, et al: Dysregulated peripheral and mucosal Th1/Th2 response in Whipple's disease. Gastroenterology 123:1468, 2002.

64. Bassotti G, Pelli MA, Ribacchi R, et al: *Giardia lamblia* infestation reveals underlying Whipple's disease in a patient with longstanding constipation. Am J Gastroenterol 86:371, 1991.

65. Meier-Willersen HJ, Maiwald M, von Herbay A: Morbus Whipple in Assoziation mit opportunistischen Infektionen. [Whipple's disease associated with opportunistic infections]. Dtsch Med Wochenschr 118:854, 1993.

66. Fenollar F, Lepidi H, Gerolami R, et al: Whipple's disease associated with giardiasis. J Infect Dis 188:828, 2003.

67. Maiwald M, Meier-Willersen HJ, Hartmann M, von Herbay A: Detection of *Tropheryma whippelii* DNA in a patient with AIDS. J Clin Microbiol 33:1354, 1995.

68. Schneider T, Stallmach A, von Herbay A, et al: Treatment of refractory Whipple's disease with interferon-gamma. Ann Intern Med 129:875, 1998.

69. Enzinger FM, Helwig EB: Whipple's disease: A review of the literature and report of fifteen patients. Virchows Arch 336:238, 1963.

70. Fleming JL, Wiesner RH, Shorter RG: Whipple's disease: Clinical, biochemical, and histopathologic features and assessment of treatment in 29 patients. Mayo Clin Proc 63:539, 1988.

71. von Herbay A, Otto HF: Whipple's disease: A report of 22 patients. Klin Wochenschr 66:533, 1988.

72. von Herbay A, Otto HF: Abdominale Lymphome beim Morbus Whipple [Abdominal lymphoma in Whipple's disease]. Dtsch Med Wochenschr 114:2028, 1989.

73. Gillen CD, Coddington R, Monteith PG, Taylor RH: Extraintestinal lymphoma in association with Whipple's disease. Gut 34:1627, 1993.

74. Gruner U, Goesch P, Donner A, Peters U: Whipple disease and non-Hodgkin lymphoma. Z Gastroenterol 39:305, 2001.

75. MacDermott RP, Shephard JAO: Whipple's disease: Case record 37-1997. N Engl J Med 337:1612, 1997.

76. Albrecht T: Computertomographie abdominaler Lymphome bei Morbus Whipple [Computed tomography of the abdominal lymphomas in Whipple's disease]. Rofo Fortschr Geb Röntgenstr Neuen Bildgeb Verfahr 160:487, 1994.

77. Keinath RD, Merrell DE, Vlietstra R, Dobbins WO III: Antibiotic treatment and relapse in Whipple's disease: Long-term follow-up of 88 patients. Gastroenterology 88:1867, 1985.

78. Schnider PJ, Reisinger EC, Gerschlager W, et al: Long-term follow-up in cerebral Whipple's disease. Eur J Gastroenterol Hepatol 8:899, 1996.

79. Johnson L, Diamond I: Cerebral Whipple's disease: Diagnosis by brain biopsy. Am J Clin Pathol 74:486, 1980.

80. Adams M, Rhyner PA, Day J, et al: Whipple's disease confined to the central nervous system. Ann Neurol 21:104, 1987.

81. Louis ED, Lynch T, Kaufmann P, et al: Diagnostic guidelines in central nervous system Whipple's disease. Ann Neurol 40:561, 1996.

82. Gerard A, Sarrot-Reynauld F, Liozon E, et al: Neurologic presentation of Whipple disease: Report of 12 cases and review of the literature. Medicine (Baltimore) 81:443, 2002.

83. Lieb K, Maiwald M, Berger M, Voderholzer U: Insomnia for 5 years. Lancet 354:1966, 1999.

84. Verhagen WIM, Huygen PLM, Dalman JE, Schuurmans MMJ: Whipple's disease and the central nervous system: A case report and a review of the literature. Clin Neurol Neurosurg 98:299, 1996.

85. von Herbay A, Ditton HJ, Schuhmacher F, Maiwald M: Whipple's disease: Staging and monitoring by cytology and polymerase chain reaction analysis of cerebrospinal fluid. Gastroenterology 113:434, 1997.

86. Jeserich M, Ihling C, Holubarsch C: Aortic valve endocarditis with Whipple disease. Ann Intern Med 126:920, 1997.

87. Ratliff NB, McMahon JT, Naab TJ, Cosgrove DM: Whipple's disease in the porcine leaflets of a Carpentier-Edwards prosthetic mitral valve. N Engl J Med 311:902, 1984.

88. Dreier J, Szabados F, von Herbay A, et al: *Tropheryma whippelii* infection of an acellular porcine heart valve bioprosthesis in a patient who did not have intestinal Whipple's disease. J Clin Microbiol 42:4487, 2004.

89. Silvestry FE, Kim B, Pollack BJ, et al: Cardiac Whipple disease: Identification of Whipple bacillus by electron microscopy in the myocardium of a patient before death. Ann Intern Med 126:214, 1997.

90. Célard M, de Gevigney G, Mosnier S, et al. Polymerase chain reaction analysis for diagnosis of *Tropheryma whippelii* infective endocarditis in two patients with no previous evidence of Whipple's disease. Clin Infect Dis 29:1348, 1999.

91. Elkins C, Shuman TA, Pirolo JS: Cardiac Whipple's disease without digestive symptoms. Ann Thorac Surg 67:250, 1999.

92. Gubler JGH, Kuster M, Dutly F, et al: Whipple endocarditis without overt gastrointestinal disease: Report of four cases. Ann Intern Med 131:112, 1999.

93. Fenollar F, Lepidi H, Raoult D: Whipple's endocarditis: Review of the literature and comparisons with Q fever, *Bartonella* infection, and blood culture-positive endocarditis. Clin Infect Dis 33:1309, 2001.

94. Rubinow A, Canoso JJ, Goldenberg DL, et al: Arthritis in Whipple's disease. Isr J Med Sci .17:445, 1981.

95. O'Duffy JD, Griffing WL, Li CY, et al: Whipple's arthritis: Direct detection of *Tropheryma whippelii* in synovial fluid and tissue. Arthritis Rheum 42:812, 1999.

96. Altwegg M, Fleisch-Marx A, Goldenberger D, et al: Spondylodiscitis caused by *Tropheryma whippelii*. Schweiz Med Wochenschr 126:1495, 1996.

97. Frésard A, Guglielminotti C, Berthelot P, et al: Prosthetic joint infection caused by *Tropheryma whippelii* (Whipple's bacillus). Clin Infect Dis 22:575, 1996.

98. Balestrieri GP, Villanacci V, Battocchio S, et al: Cutaneous involvement in Whipple's disease. Br J Dermatol 135:666, 1996.

99. Williams JG, Edward DP, Tessler HH, et al: Ocular manifestations of Whipple disease: An atypical presentation. Arch Ophthalmol 116:1232, 1998.

100. Rickman LS, Freeman WR, Green WR, et al: Uveitis caused by *Tropheryma whippelii* (Whipple bacillus). N Engl J Med 332:363, 1995.

101. Geboes K, Ectors N, Heidbuchel H, et al: Whipple's disease: Endoscopic aspects before and after therapy. Gastrointest Endosc 36:247, 1990.

102. Silva MT, Macedo PM, Moura Nunes JF: Ultrastructure of bacilli and the bacillary origin of the macrophagic inclusions in Whipple's disease. J Gen Microbiol 131:1001, 1985.

103. Keren DF, Weisburger WR, Yardley JH, et al: Whipple's disease: Demonstration by immunofluorescence of similar bacterial antigens in macrophages from three cases. Johns Hopkins Med J 139:51, 1976.

104. Evans DJ, Ali MH: Immunocytochemistry in the diagnosis of Whipple's disease. J Clin Pathol 38:372, 1985.

105. Baisden BL, Lepidi H, Raoult D, et al: Diagnosis of Whipple disease by immunohistochemical analysis: A sensitive and specific method for the detection of *Tropheryma whipplei* (the Whipple bacillus) in paraffin-embedded tissue. Am J Clin Pathol 118:742, 2002.

106. Lepidi H, Costedoat N, Piette JC, et al: Immunohistological detection of *Tropheryma whipplei* (Whipple bacillus) in lymph nodes. Am J Med 113:334, 2002.

107. Ectors N, Geboes K, Devos R, et al: Whipple's disease: A histological, immunocytochemical and electron-microscopic study of the immune response in the small intestinal mucosa. Histopathology 21:1, 1992.

108. Dvorak AM: Ultrastructural monitoring of progress of Whipple's disease therapy. Dig Dis Pathol 2:81, 1989.

109. Sieracki JC, Fine G: Whipple's disease: Observations on systemic involvement: II. Gross and histologic observations. Arch Pathol 67:81, 1959.

110. Gross M, Jung C, Zoller WG: Detection of *Tropheryma whippelii* DNA (Whipple's disease) in faeces. Ital J Gastroenterol Hepatol 31:70, 1999.

111. Fenollar F, Fournier PE, Robert C, Raoult D: Use of genome selected repeated sequences increases the sensitivity of PCR detection of *Tropheryma whipplei*. J Clin Microbiol 42:401, 2004.

112. Lowsky R, Archer GL, Fyles G, et al: Diagnosis of Whipple's disease by molecular analysis of peripheral blood. N Engl J Med 331:1343, 1994.

113. Müller C, Stain C, Burghuber O: *Tropheryma whippelii* in peripheral blood mononuclear cells and cells of pleural effusion. Lancet 341:701, 1993.

114. Marth T, Fredricks D, Strober W, Relman DA: Limited role for PCR-based diagnosis of Whipple's disease from peripheral blood mononuclear cells. Lancet 348:66, 1996.

115. Fritscher-Ravens A, Swain CP, von Herbay A: Refractory Whipple's disease with anaemia: First lessons from capsule endoscopy. Endoscopy 36:659, 2004.

116. Ectors N, Geboes K, Wynants P, Desmet V: Granulomatous gastritis and Whipple's disease. Am J Gastroenterol 87:509, 1992.

117. Babaryka I, Thorn L, Langer E: Epithelioid cell granulomata in the mucosa of the small intestine in Whipple's disease. Virchows Arch 382:227, 1979.

118. Saint-Marc Girardin MF, Zafrani ES, Chaumette MT, et al: Hepatic granulomas in Whipple's disease. Gastroenterology 86:753, 1984.

119. Donaldson RM: Whipple's disease: Rare malady with uncommon potential. N Engl J Med 327:346, 1992.

120. von Herbay A, Ditton HJ, Schuhmacher F, et al: Molecular screening of DNA of *Tropheryma whippelii* in sarcoidosis [Abstract]. Pathol Res Pract 193:87, 1997.

121. Abdelmalek MF, Procop GW, Mitchell PS, Persing DH: Lack of association of sarcoidosis and intestinal lymphoma with *T. whippelii* infection [Abstract]. Gastroenterology 114: G1410, 1998.

122. Feurle GE, Marth T: An evaluation of antimicrobial treatment for Whipple's disease: Tetracycline versus trimethoprim-sulfamethoxazole. Dig Dis Sci 39:1642, 1994.

123. Knox DL, Bayless TM, Pittman FE: Neurologic disease in patients with treated Whipple's disease. Medicine (Baltimore) 55:467, 1976.

124. Feurle GE, Volk B, Waldherr R: Cerebral Whipple's disease with negative jejunal histology. N Engl J Med 300:907, 1979.

125. Ryser RJ, Locksley RM, Eng SC, et al: Reversal of dementia associated with Whipple's disease by trimethoprim-sulfamethoxazole: Drugs that penetrate the blood-brain barrier. Gastroenterology 86:745, 1984.

126. Cooper GS, Blades EW, Remler BF, et al: Central nervous system Whipple's disease: Relapse during therapy with trimethoprim-sulfamethoxazole and remission with cefixime. Gastroenterology 106:782, 1994.

127. Singer R, von Herbay A, Willig F: Successful treatment of cerebral Whipple's disease with rifampicin. Med Klinik 90:117, 1995.

128. Garas G, Cheng WS, Abrugiato R, Forbes GM: Clinical relapse in Whipple's disease despite maintenance therapy. J Gastroenterol Hepatol 15:1223, 2000.

129. Boulos A, Rolain JM, Raoult D: Antibiotic susceptibility of *Tropheryma whipplei* in MRC5 cells. Antimicrob Agents Chemother 48:747, 2004.

130. Cannon WR: Whipple's disease, genomics, and drug therapy. Lancet 361:1916, 2003.

131. Adler CH, Galetta SL: Oculo-facial-skeletal myorhythmia in Whipple's disease: Treatment with ceftriaxone. Ann Intern Med 112:467, 1990.

132. Simpson DA, Wishnow R, Gargulinski RB, Pawlak AM: Oculofacial-skeletal myorhythmia in central nervous system Whipple's disease: Additional case and review of the literature. Mov Disord 10:195, 1995.

133. Amarenco P, Roullet E, Hannoun L, Marteau R: Progressive supranuclear palsy as the sole manifestation of systemic Whipple's disease treated with pefloxacine. J Neurol Neurosurg Psychiatry 54:1121, 1991.

CHAPTER
104 Infectious Enteritis and Proctocolitis and Bacterial Food Poisoning

Ralph A. Giannella

Infectious diarrhea is a major cause of illness throughout the world. Diarrhea is the first or second most common cause of death in most developing countries; its greatest impact is on infants and children. In developing countries, prevalence rates of diarrhea are two to three times higher than in the United States, where there is an average of two episodes of diarrhea per year in children younger than 5 years of age. In Western countries, diarrhea leads to high morbidity with loss of time from school and work. Overall, physicians in the United States are consulted annually for 8.2 million diarrheal episodes.[1,2] A long list of complications, some mild and others life-threatening, can accompany infectious diarrhea. Medical costs and loss of productivity resulting from infectious diarrhea amount to more than $23 billion a year in the United States.

Our knowledge of infectious diarrheal disease has expanded exponentially in the past 2 decades. Advances have come from various disciplines to produce new understanding of these diseases. References 3 to 6 are excellent discussions of various aspects of enteric infections.

SUSCEPTIBILITY TO INTESTINAL INFECTION

Acquisition of an enteric infection is the result of the interaction of host factors that protect against infection and microbial virulence factors that function to overcome host defenses.

HOST DEFENSE FACTORS

Gastric Acidity

Ingested pathogenic bacteria and other pathogens first must survive passage through the stomach to infect the small or large intestine. In this regard, gastric acidity is the first line of defense.[7] Most bacterial pathogens are highly susceptible to low pH, and thus exposure to gastric acid significantly reduces the number of ingested viable bacteria. Gastric juice with a pH of less than 4.0 is rapidly bactericidal, whereas bacteria survive prolonged exposure to gastric juice from patients who are achlorhydric.[8] In experimental studies of cholera in healthy adults, clinical infection did not develop when as many as 10^{10} cholera bacteria were ingested, whereas as few as 10^4 Vibrio cholerae were able to produce disease when organisms were administered with sodium bicarbonate[9]; even fewer bacteria were necessary to produce clinical illness when organisms were directly instilled into the duodenum. Naturally occurring cholera also occurs more frequently in achlorhydric individuals.[10] The gastric barrier also may be of importance in preventing other enteric infections such as salmonellosis[11] and shigellosis.[12]

Intestinal Motility

Organisms surviving the milieu of the stomach enter the small intestine where normal propulsive motor activity clears them. Some bacteria elaborate toxins that impair intestinal motility.[13] In experimental animals it is often necessary to restrict intestinal motility with pharmacologic agents or with ligatures to allow enteropathogens to establish infection.[14]

Intestinal Microflora

The normal intestinal microflora, primarily in the colon, resist colonization of the intestine by newly introduced bacteria. Products elaborated by the resident microflora, including lactic acid and short-chain fatty acids, are toxic to many bacterial pathogens, and when the intestinal microflora are altered in instances such as administration of an antibiotic, the host may be more susceptible to intestinal infection (e.g., Clostridium difficile).[15] Alteration of intestinal flora by antibiotics also increases susceptibility to salmonellosis.[16,17]

Mucus

Mucus, in concert with intestinal motility, provides a nonspecific physical barrier to bacterial proliferation and mucosal colonization. Gastric mucus may act in conjunction with gastric acidity as the first line of enteric defense. Differences in the carbohydrate composition of intestinal mucus between immature and mature rats suggest that this difference in intestinal mucus might play a role in the reduced host defense of the immature animal,[18] perhaps by enhancing mucosal adhesion of pathogenic bacteria.

Systemic and Local Immune Mechanisms

The mucosal antibacterial immune response is quite complex and important in combating enteric pathogens. Secretory antibody in the intestine appears prior to serum antibody in response to intestinal infection with Shigella.[19] In cholera, there is a better correlation between the level of coproantibody and immune protection than there is with serum antibody and resistance to enteric infection with this pathogen[20]; however, both mucosal and systemic immune systems provide important protection against pathogenic bacteria. These immune responses may be directed against multiple targets. For example, the immune response against cholera may be antitoxic or antibacterial and originate from either the mucosal immune system (secretory IgA) or from the serum (IgG). Regardless, both serum and secretory antibodies exert their protective effects at the intestinal level, even though the serum components are produced outside the gut.

Other Factors

Breast-feeding also serves as a defense mechanism against bacterial enteropathogens. Breast-fed infants are less susceptible to bacterial diarrhea than are formula-fed infants.[21,22] Multiple factors are responsible for this protection. Breast milk contains secretory IgA antibodies against specific enteropathogens that survive passage through the gastrointestinal tract of infants.[23] Other components of breast milk such as lactoferrin, lysozyme, and lactoperoxidase also have anti-infective properties in vitro, and breast milk glycolipids may interfere with toxin or microbial adherence.[24]

BACTERIAL FACTORS

Bacterial pathogens have evolved various virulence factors and mechanisms that enable them to overcome host defenses, including adherence factors, enterotoxin and cytotoxin elaboration, mucosal invasion, and a variety of other factors.

Adherence

The ability of bacteria to adhere to host mucosal cells is a critical virulence factor in enterotoxin-producing and invasive bacteria as well as in enteroadherent Escherichia coli (EAEC) and enteropathogenic E. coli (EPEC). Bacterial adherence to host mucosal cells may be the predominant virulence factor, as in the case of EPEC; one of two important factors, (adherence plus toxin elaboration) in the case of enterotoxigenic organisms; or only one of several factors required for expression of full pathogenicity as seen in invasive organisms. Bacteria that cause disease by adhesion alone do not elaborate any of the traditional enterotoxins but rather adhere tightly to the mucosa of both the small and large intestine.[25] The classic

EPEC as well as the EAEC[26] are typical of this group. Other organisms, including enterotoxigenic *E. coli* and the invasive organisms *salmonellae* and *shigellae*, also must adhere to the intestinal surface to be fully pathogenic.

Studies on the mechanism by which EPECs cause diarrhea show that EPECs attach to the intestinal mucosa in a characteristic manner, producing ultrastructural changes known as *attaching-effacing lesions*[27] that lead to elongation and destruction of microvilli.[25,28] This pattern of bacterial binding to enterocytes also has been referred to as *attaching and effacing adherence*[27] and the particular morphologic alteration as *pedestal formation* (Fig. 104–1).[25]

The laboratory counterpart of mucosal colonization is adherence in tissue culture to various cell lines such as Hep-2 and HeLa. A characteristic form of *localized adherence* is observed only with classic EPEC serotypes. These events occur in the following three phases[29]:

1. Nonintimate attachment of EPEC to intestinal epithelial cells—attachment is mediated by a bundle-forming pilus associated with a large plasmid common to EPEC isolates
2. A signal transduction event that leads to cytoskeletal changes in the enterocyte via activation of protein kinase and the release of intracellular calcium
3. Intimate attachment of the bacterium to the host cell membrane—attachment is mediated by an outer membrane protein called *intimin*, which is encoded by the *eaeA* gene cluster on the EPEC chromosome[30]

The presence of a plasmid in EPEC serves to increase intimin production; this process is needed for localized adherence to occur.[31] EPEC strains with localized adherence produce acute diarrhea when these strains are administered to normal volunteers.[32] The role of the *eaeA* gene as a virulence factor in human EPEC infection has been confirmed in volunteer challenge studies.[33]

Enterotoxigenic organisms also require expression of bacterial adherence for proliferation of the organisms and colonization as well as for full expression of toxicity.[34] Enterotoxigenic *E. coli* (ETECs) adhere to the surface of the small bowel epithelium without penetrating the epithelial layer and do so by mechanisms different from those used by EPEC. The most important mechanism by which enterotoxigenic bacteria adhere to the intestinal mucosa is related to specific protein antigens on the surface of the bacterial cell known as *pili* or *fimbriae*, also referred to as *adherence antigens* or *colonization factor antigens*.[35] These pili bind to specific receptor sites on the surface of the intestinal cell via specific ligand-receptor interactions and are capable of hemagglutination in the presence of mannose.

The antigenic structure of the adherence pili determines the host specificity of the ETEC strains. For example, those bearing a K88 antigen are pathogenic for piglets, whereas others bearing K99 antigen cause disease in calves and lambs. ETEC adhesion antigens for humans include type 1,3,P and BFP pili.

Evidence that these colonization factors (e.g., pili and lectins) are important to the pathogenesis of *E. coli* diarrheal disease in animals is derived from the observations by Moon[36] that loss or gain of fimbriae by genetic manipulation results in the loss or gain of the ability to adhere to and colonize the intestine. Adherence not only permits colonization but also may facilitate the delivery of enterotoxin to the epithelium and may even enhance the ability of the organism to elaborate enterotoxin.[34,36]

Enterotoxin Production

Enterotoxins are polypeptides secreted by bacteria that alter intestinal salt and water transport without affecting mucosal morphology.[37,38] Many organisms elaborate enterotoxins (e.g., *V. cholerae*, *Shigella*, enterotoxigenic *E. coli*, and *Staphylococcus aureus*) and several enterotoxins may be elaborated by a single organism. Although most enterotoxins affect the small intestine, the colon also may be a target organ.

Several enterotoxin-producing organisms that cause food poisoning induce disease without requiring intestinal colonization. These include *S. aureus* and *Clostridium perfringens*, toxins of which are ingested preformed in food. These organisms do not need to colonize the intestine to establish disease, and this accounts for the brief incubation period characteristic of these illnesses.

Whether the enterotoxin is ingested preformed or first expressed within the intestinal lumen, the toxin-enterocyte or toxin–colonocyte interaction begins with the binding of the enterotoxin to a specific mucosal receptor. The toxin–receptor interaction increases the concentration of an intracellular mediator, resulting in alteration of salt and water flux. Thus far, three intracellular mediator systems have been shown to be involved in the pathogenesis of enterotoxigenic diarrhea. These are adenylate cyclase–cyclic adenosine monophosphate (cAMP), the guanylate cyclase–cyclic guanosine monophosphate (cGMP) systems, and intracellular calcium.[39,40] Alterations in these mediator systems have similar effects on transport processes to decrease the coupled influx of sodium and chloride and stimulate the active secretion of chloride from the cell into the intestinal lumen. Other intracellular mediator systems involved in the pathogenesis of bacterial diarrhea include protein kinase C and arachidonic acid metabolites, among others.

Cholera toxin (molecular weight ≈ 84,000 d), which stimulates adenylate cyclase, is a prototypical enterotoxin

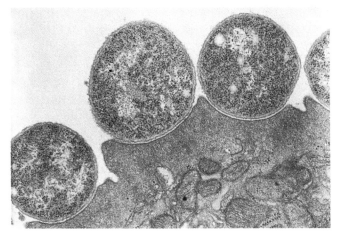

Figure 104–1 Electron micrograph of enteropathogenic *Escherichia coli* (EPEC) adherent to the jejunal mucosa and demonstrating the attaching and effacing lesion, also called *pedestal formation*. Tightly adherent *E. coli* are obliterating the brush border.

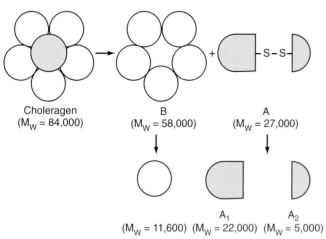

Choleragen
(M_W = 84,000)

B
(M_W = 58,000)

A
(M_W = 27,000)

A_1
(M_W = 11,600)

(M_W = 22,000)

A_2
(M_W = 5,000)

Figure 104–2 Subunit structure of cholera toxin (choleragen). M_W, molecular weight. (From Fishman PH: Action of cholera toxin: Events on the cell surface. In Field M, Fordtran JS, Schultz SG [eds]: Secretory Diarrhea. Bethesda, MD, American Physiological Society, 1980, p 86.)

(Fig. 104–2). We briefly discuss this toxin-enterocyte interaction because it is a well-understood model. Cholera toxin is composed of an A subunit surrounded by five B subunits that bind the toxin to a ganglioside (GM_1) receptor on the brush border membrane of the villus epithelial cell. The A subunit slowly penetrates the brush border membrane and is cleaved into two peptides, A_1 and A_2, linked by a disulfide bond. Reduction of this bond releases the active A_1 peptide that traverses the cell to the basolateral membrane, where it stimulates the ribosylation of G_s, the stimulatory subunit of a heterotrimeric G protein. This action results in the irreversible activation of G_s and an increase in cytosolic cAMP. This cAMP in turn activates cAMP-dependent kinases(s) that inhibit NaCl-coupled transport and stimulate chloride secretion.

In addition to cholera toxin, other important enterotoxins are those elaborated by E. coli.[41,42] Two classes of E. coli enterotoxins are known: heat-labile (LT) and heat-stable (ST) toxins. LT, which exists in two forms (LT-1 and LT-2, which differ by a few amino acid residues),[42] is a large-molecular-weight protein that causes diarrheal disease similar to, but less severe, than cholera. The subunit structure and mechanism of action of LT-1 and LT-2 also are similar to those of cholera toxin; although cholera toxin and LT bind to a glycolipid receptor, specifically GM_1, an additional glycoprotein receptor may exist for LT.[42]

Heat-stable enterotoxins also may be elaborated by E. coli. ST_as bind to brush border receptors on enterocytes and colonocytes, a receptor-guanylate cyclase, to increase intracellular levels of cGMP. ST_b is an unrelated enterotoxin elaborated by some E. coli pathogenic for pigs. Other organisms that elaborate highly homologous heat-stable enterotoxins include Yersinia enterocolitica, Citrobacter, and non-O1 vibrios.[42]

Cytotoxin Production

Cytotoxins are polypeptides that cause cell damage and death. Cytotoxins cause cell injury, inflammation, and intestinal secretion through inhibition of protein syn-

thesis or via a cascade involving one or more inflammatory mediator substances. Examples of organisms that produce cytotoxins include C. difficile (see Chapter 105),[15] some EPEC, enterohemorrhagic E. coli (EHEC), and Shigella.[43] The mechanisms by which cytotoxins cause cell injury, inflammation, and intestinal secretion are multiple and complex and include inhibition of protein synthesis, disruption of cellular actin and tight junction integrity, mitochondrial damage, and adenosine triphosphate depletion among others.

Mucosal Invasion

The mechanism of mucosal invasion involves invasion of enterocytes or colonocytes by the infecting organisms with subsequent intracellular multiplication, resulting in cell injury and possibly cell death. Shigellae are classic examples of invasive enteropathogens. Salmonella species, Campylobacter jejuni, Y. enterocolitica, and some (enteroinvasive) strains of E. coli invade intestinal cells and pass into the lamina propria where they elicit an inflammatory response and cause mucosal ulceration.[4,6]

Unlike enterotoxigenic organisms that favor colonization of the small intestine, invasive organisms primarily, but not exclusively, colonize the colon. In salmonellosis, the ileum is colonized in addition to the colon; in shigellosis, the small intestine is colonized transiently early in the course of the disease when watery diarrhea rather than dysentery is the predominant symptom.[44] Subsequently, colonization occurs in the colon and bloody diarrhea ensues. In the cases of shigellae and salmonellae, the ability to invade the gastrointestinal mucosa is of primary importance in the establishment of the enteric infection.[45,46]

Bacterial invasion alone is not sufficient to establish disease. Other properties of invading organisms are required. In the case of shigellae, the organisms also must multiply intracellularly. Thus, strains of Shigella flexneri that can invade but cannot multiply do not cause disease when fed to a susceptible host.[45] Intracellular multiplication of shigellae also involves lateral spread to adjacent intestinal cells and cell death. In the cases of salmonellae and Y. enterocolitica, however, the organisms penetrate into the lamina propria and may disseminate to extraintestinal sites. As a consequence of mucosal invasion and of the intramucosal multiplication of the organisms, an acute inflammatory reaction develops and mucosal ulceration can occur. Gross ulceration of the colonic mucosa commonly occurs in shigellosis, which accounts for dysenteric stools, but is much less common with Salmonella and Yersinia infections. Yersinia infection more commonly manifests with microscopic and minute ulcerations involving both the ileum and colon.

Some of the mechanisms by which invasive organisms induce intestinal secretion include increased intracellular calcium and products of inflammation such as prostaglandin and leukotriene metabolites, serotonin, substance P, interleukin (IL)-1, and reactive oxygen metabolites among others.

Other Factors

Other bacterial virulence factors, not as yet well defined, may modulate infectivity or the spectrum of illness, including the ability of bacteria to respond to chemotactic signals released by the mucosa, bacterial, elaboration of mucolytic enzymes to enable bacterial penetration of the intestinal cell, resistance to phagocytosis, and elaboration of substances that interfere with intestinal motility. The importance of these factors in modifying virulence is uncertain and they are not discussed further.

CLASSIFICATION OF BACTERIAL DIARRHEA

Acute bacterial diarrhea can be classified according to the mechanism by which the bacteria cause disease. These include the following:

1. Toxigenic—in which an enterotoxin is the major if not exclusive pathogenic mechanism
2. Cytotoxic—in which a cytotoxin induces acute inflammation and intestinal secretion
3. Invasive—in which the organism penetrates the mucosal surface as the primary event and induces acute inflammation, but enterotoxin may be produced as well
4. Enteroadherent—in which the cell cytoskeleton is altered

Many organisms elaborate enterotoxins that cause intestinal fluid and electrolyte secretion. As discussed earlier, the recognized diarrheal toxins can be grouped broadly into two categories: *enterotoxins*, which produce fluid secretion by activation of intracellular enzymes such as adenylate cyclase without any damage to the epithelial surface, and *cytotoxins*, which cause injury to the mucosal cell and induce fluid secretion. Diarrheal toxins produce two clinically recognizable acute diarrheal syndromes— noninflammatory (enterotoxin-induced) and inflammatory (cytotoxin-induced) diarrheas—which are discussed in the following section.

DIAGNOSIS OF INFECTIOUS DIARRHEAL DISEASE

EVALUATION OF THE PATIENT

The initial step in the diagnostic evaluation of a patient with acute diarrhea should be a thorough history and physical examination, the goals of which are to identify those patients who may be at risk of severe illness or susceptible to complications and those who will benefit from specific therapy. Most patients simply need rehydration therapy. Consideration of the patient's general health, severity and duration of illness, and the setting in which the illness was acquired should enable the clinician to determine who needs further evaluation (Fig. 104–3).

Patients who are debilitated, malnourished, immunocompromised, or have severe comorbid illnesses are at increased risk for complications of diarrhea and infection. They may require hospitalization and early diagnostic tests. Other patients who also require a more aggressive approach include those with systemic signs and evidence of an inflammatory diarrhea; illness lasting more than 3 to 4 days; a history or physical examination suggesting a disease process that will benefit from specific therapy; and infection with certain specific organisms (Table 104–1).[6]

Because the number of conditions that cause acute and chronic diarrhea is large, a useful method is to classify the diarrheal illness into one of two clinical syndromes: a watery, *noninflammatory* diarrheal syndrome and an *inflammatory* diarrheal syndrome (Table 104–2); a subgroup of the latter is the *proctitis* diarrheal syndrome. Categorization into one of these syndromes limits the number of potential causes and diagnostic tests that needs to be considered. This classification can usually be made on clinical grounds and with simple, inexpensive diagnostic tests.

In the United States, most of the cases of watery, noninflammatory diarrhea result in an illness that is self-

Table 104–1 Indications for Antimicrobial Therapy in Patients with Infectious Diarrhea

Bacterial infection
  Shigella
  Vibrio cholerae
  Clostridium difficile
  Traveler's diarrhea
  Salmonellosis (extraintestinal)
  Salmonellosis (with toxicity)
  Campylobacter diarrhea (prolonged)
Protozoal infection
  Giardia lamblia
  Entamoeba histolytica
Sexually transmitted diseases
  Gonorrhea
  Syphilis
  Chlamydia
Herpes simplex virus

From Park SI, Giannella RA: Approach to the adult patient with acute diarrhea. Gastroenterol Clin North Am 22:483, 1993.

Table 104–2 Characteristics That Help Distinguish Inflammatory from Noninflammatory Diarrhea

Characteristic	Inflammatory Diarrhea	Noninflammatory Diarrhea
Fecal leukocytes	Present	Absent
Clinical presentation	Bloody, small-volume diarrhea; left lower quadrant abdominal cramps; may be febrile and toxic	Large-volume, watery diarrhea; patients may have nausea, vomiting, cramps
Causes	*Shigella, Salmonella, Entamoeba histolytica, Campylobacter, Yersinia,* invasive *Escherichia coli, Clostridium difficile*	Viruses, *Vibrios, Giardia,* enterotoxigenic *E. coli,* enterotoxin-producing bacteria, food-borne gastroenteritis
Site of involvement	Colon	Small intestine
Diagnostic evaluation	Indicated	Indicated only if the patient is severely volume depleted or toxic appearing

From Park SI, Giannella RA: Approach to the adult patient with acute diarrhea. Gastroenterol Clin North Am 22:483, 1993.

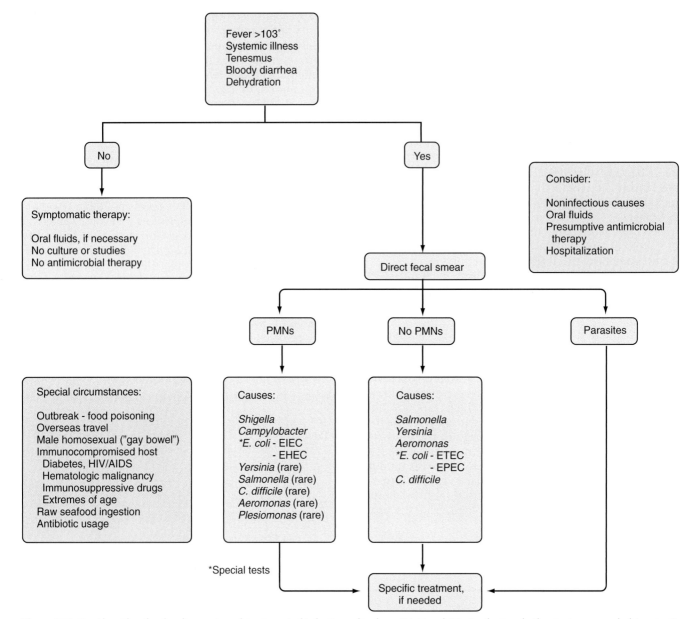

Figure 104–3 Algorithm for the diagnosis and treatment of infectious diarrhea. "No" and "Yes" refer to whether tests are needed (see text). AIDS, acquired immunodeficiency syndrome; EHEC, enterohemorrhagic *E. coli*; EIEC, enteroinvasive *E. coli*; EPEC, enteropathogenic *E. coli*; ETEC, enterotoxigenic *E. coli*; HIV, human immunodeficiency virus; PMN, polymorphonuclear neutrophil.

limited and does not require specific therapy. Evaluation of such patients is generally unrewarding and usually unnecessary. By contrast, many patients with acute inflammatory diarrhea are more ill, a specific pathogen frequently can be diagnosed, and antibiotic therapy may be beneficial.

Noninflammatory Diarrhea

Patients with noninflammatory diarrhea usually present with large-volume watery stools without blood or pus, or severe abdominal pain. These patients generally have few systemic signs or symptoms, and fever usually is absent. Abdominal cramping, nausea, and vomiting may occur. The most likely causes are viruses (rotavirus, Norwalk virus), enterotoxigenic *E. coli, V. cholerae*, staphylococcal and clostridial food poisoning, and *Giardia* and *Cryptosporidium* infections. Noninflammatory diarrheas gen-

erally do not require extensive evaluation. Pathogens causing noninflammatory diarrhea usually infect the small intestine and merely adhere to the mucosal surface without invading the epithelium or causing acute inflammation. Most of these organisms (e.g., cholera, rotavirus) elaborate enterotoxins that stimulate intestinal secretion, occasionally resulting in profound dehydration.

Inflammatory Diarrhea

Patients with inflammatory diarrhea usually present with multiple, small-volume stools that may be mucoid, grossly bloody, or both. Such patients may appear toxic and usually are febrile. Abdominal cramping may be severe. Because of the small stool volumes, these patients are less likely to be dehydrated than those with noninflammatory diarrhea. Physical findings may point to a specific diagnosis; some of these are listed in Table 104–3.

Table 104–3   Findings Suggesting the Causative Organisms for Some Inflammatory Diarrheas

Finding	Causative Organisms
Hemolytic-uremic syndrome	*Shigella*, enterohemorrhagic *Escherichia coli*
Reactive arthritis	*Salmonella*, *Shigella*, *Campylobacter*, *Yersinia*
Peritoneal signs	*Clostridium difficile*, enterohemorrhagic *E. coli*
Right lower quadrant tenderness	*Yersinia*
Thyroiditis, pericarditis, glomerulonephritis	*Yersinia*

From Park SI, Giannella RA: Approach to the adult patient with acute diarrhea. Gastroenterol Clin North Am 22:483, 1993.

Organisms causing inflammatory diarrheas usually affect the colon and either invade or elaborate cytotoxins resulting in an acute inflammatory reaction with disruption of the epithelial barrier, mucus, red blood cells, and white blood cells in the stool (see Table 104–2). Microbes causing this syndrome include *Shigella*, *Campylobacter*, EHEC, *C. difficile*, *Salmonella*, *Yersinia*, and *Entamoeba histolytica*. Fecal leukocytes (or positive stool lactoferrin test) indicate an acute inflammatory process, and sheets of polymorphonuclear leukocytes (PMNs) usually indicate colitis. The acute inflammatory diarrheal syndrome also can be of noninfectious etiology, such as ulcerative colitis, Crohn's disease, radiation or ischemic colitis, and diverticulitis. Table 104–4 lists the organisms that may be associated with the presence of fecal leukocytes.[47]

Proctitis Syndrome

Proctitis syndrome is characterized by frequent, painful bowel movements containing blood, pus, and mucus. The sensation of tenesmus usually is quite prominent, and rectal pain also may be prominent. Infectious causes include *Shigella*, herpes simplex virus type 2, and *Neisseria gonorrhoeae*. *Treponema pallidum* (syphilis), lymphogranuloma venereum, and *Chlamydia* venereum. The importance of this syndrome is that many of the causes have specific treatments. Noninfectious causes include idiopathic ulcerative proctitis, Crohn's proctitis, radiation proctitis, and solitary rectal ulcer syndrome.

LABORATORY DIAGNOSIS

Diagnostic Testing

After an adequate medical history and physical examination, the clinician should be able to classify the acute diarrheal illness as inflammatory or noninflammatory and determine its severity and whether complications are likely. The clinician also should be able to determine if diagnostic testing is needed and, if so, which tests should be used. In general, most episodes of acute diarrheal illness in the United States are self-limited; therefore, diagnostic testing should be kept to a minimum and treatment should be aimed at preventing dehydration. Investigations should be performed only if the result will influence management and outcome. Diagnostic testing

Table 104–4   Fecal Leukocytes in Intestinal Infections

Usually Present
Campylobacter
EHEC
EIEC
Shigella

Present or Absent
Aeromonas
Clostridium difficile (antibiotic-associated colitis)
EAggEC
Salmonella
Vibrio parahaemolyticus
Yersinia

Usually Absent
Bacillus cereus
Calicivirus, including Norovirus
Clostridium perfringens
DAEC
Entamoeba histolytica
EPEC
ETEC
Food poisoning
Giardia lamblia
Rotavirus and other viruses
Staphylococcus aureus
Vibrio cholerae
Other viruses

DAEC, diffusing adhering *Escherichia coli*; EAggEC, enteroaggregative *E. coli*; EHEC, enterohemorrhagic *E. coli*; EIEC, enteroinvasive *E. coli*; EPEC, enteropathogenic *E. coli*; ETEC, enterotoxigenic *E. coli*.

should be reserved for patients with severe illness, i.e., large-volume dehydrating diarrhea, severe abdominal pain, or a prolonged course (>3 days); patients with inflammatory diarrhea with bloody stools, systemic symptoms such as fever higher than 101°F or prostration; patients with history of recent travel to high-risk areas; and those at high risk for complications because of extremes of age, diabetes mellitus, and immunocompromise such as human immunodeficiency viral (HIV) infection or acquired immunodeficiency syndrome (AIDS), hematologic malignancy, or use of immunosuppressive medications (see Fig. 104–3).

Diagnostic testing for acute infectious diarrhea in the normal host includes stool cultures for bacterial pathogens including *E. coli* O157:H7, stool examination for ova and parasites, stool testing for *C. difficile* toxin, and stool examination for PMNs. More invasive investigations including flexible sigmoidoscopy with biopsies and upper gastrointestinal endoscopy with duodenal aspirate and biopsies are reserved for special situations, such as the immunocompromised host in whom stool examination has not yielded a diagnosis. Investigations should be focused to diagnose specific agents as suggested by the patient's history and physical examination.

Fecal Leukocytes

A particularly useful technique to focus the differential diagnosis is microscopic examination of the stool for PMNs (see Table 104–4). Invasive pathogens that primarily affect the colon, such as *Shigella* and *Campylobacter*, produce a "sea of polys," as well as red blood cells. The toxigenic organisms, viruses, and food-poisoning bacteria cause a watery stool that harbors few formed elements. A latex agglutination test for lactoferrin (a protein made by PMNs) in fecal specimens is available and provides a rapid and sensitive alternative to microscopy for the identification of inflammatory diarrhea.[48]

Salmonella, *Yersinia*, *Vibrio parahaemolyticus*, and *C. difficile* diarrhea have unpredictable findings with regard to fecal leukocytes depending on the degree of colonic involvement. Most cases show only occasional PMNs. An acute exacerbation of ulcerative or Crohn's colitis can produce a stool with many PMNs , thereby resembling bacillary dysentery. Although fecal microscopic examination is neither infallible nor even helpful in all cases, it is inexpensive and yields immediate information that can guide antibiotic therapy. Although the fecal lactoferrin test is slightly more expensive than microscopy for fecal leukocytes, it has several advantages, including ease, rapidity, and the absence of a requirement for a fresh stool specimen.

Stool Cultures

Stool cultures are ordered too frequently. In most microbiology laboratories, routine stool cultures are processed for *Shigella*, *Salmonella*, and *Campylobacter*. Other enteric pathogens such as *Yersinia*, *Vibrio*, and *E. coli* O157:H7 are not sought routinely. Therefore, if clinical suspicion is high, the microbiology department needs to be notified to search for these pathogens. Because of sporadic shedding of pathogens (nontyphoidal salmonellae, *Salmonella typhi*) and the fact that most episodes of acute diarrhea are caused by viruses, undetectable pathogens, or noninfectious causes, stool cultures infrequently are positive. At Massachusetts General Hospital, the isolation rate of bacterial pathogens from 2000 fecal cultures in 1980 was 2.4%.[49] In patients with severe diarrhea requiring hospitalization, the bacterial isolation rate from feces is somewhat higher, ranging from 27% to 43%,[50,51] and up to 58% in a study that used more advanced techniques.[52] Even in patients hospitalized for dysentery, the rate of positivity for microbiologic diagnosis is only 40% to 60%. In community patients with severe acute gastroenteritis (> four fluid stools per day lasting at least 3 days with at least one associated symptom), the yield of a stool culture and ova and parasite examination increased to 88%.[53] In outbreaks of gastroenteritis in the United States, only one half of the cases have a confirmed etiology, of which two thirds are bacterial in origin. These figures suggest that many cases of acute diarrhea are caused by unidentified pathogens.

When parasitic or protozoal infection is suspected, stool examination for cysts, trophozoites, larvae, or eggs should be performed. When either *Giardia* or cryptosporidia is suspected, a stool enzyme-linked immunosorbent assay (ELISA) should be requested. ELISA is done for rotaviruses or Norwalk viruses, but this test rarely is required in adults. Endoscopy may be useful to obtain aspirates and biopsies of the small bowel to detect *Giardia*, cryptosporidia, microsporidia, *Isospora belli*, or *Mycobacterium avium-intracellulare*. Flexible sigmoidoscopy can be useful in evaluating patients with proctitis, tenesmus, or sexually transmitted diseases or in identifying the pseudomembranes of *C. difficile*. In HIV-infected patients, colonoscopy with multiple biopsies is required to detect cytomegalovirus ulcers, which may be confirmed by the presence of "inclusion bodies" on biopsy.

It is not appropriate to request stool cultures and stool examination for ova and parasites for every patient with diarrhea. These tests should be performed only when the clinical suspicion is high that infection is the cause of diarrhea and the results of the stool tests will change management and influence outcome.

An algorithm for the diagnosis of acute diarrhea is presented to help determine which patients should be treated symptomatically and which require further diagnostic studies and treatment (see Fig. 104–3). Approximately 90% of cases of acute diarrhea fall into the "No" category.

TOXIGENIC PATHOGENS

The prototypical organisms in this group are *V. cholerae* and ETEC, both of which elaborate enterotoxins that cause dehydrating diarrhea. Diarrheal disease caused by *V. cholerae* and ETEC has the following characteristic: the entire disease results from intestinal fluid loss, which is related to the action of the enterotoxin on the small bowel epithelial cells. These organisms do not invade the mucosal surface; rather, they colonize the upper small bowel, "stick" to the epithelial cells, and elaborate an enterotoxin. Mucosal architecture remains intact, with no evidence of cellular destruction. The fecal effluent is watery and often voluminous, producing clinical features of dehydration. The origin of the fluid is the upper small bowel, where the enterotoxin has its greatest activity. Bacteremia is not a complication of toxigenic diarrhea.

CHOLERA

Cholera is a severe diarrheal disorder that can cause dehydration and death within 3 to 4 hours of onset. Stool output can exceed 1 L/hr, with daily fecal outputs of 15 to 20 L, if parenteral fluid replacement keeps up with losses. The acutely ill patient typically has marked signs of dehydration, poor skin turgor, "washerwoman's hands," absent pulses, reduced renal function, and hypovolemic shock.

Cholera is the prototypical toxigenic diarrhea. Its importance derives not necessarily from its clinical impact, because cholera is confined to certain areas of the world and tends to occur in epidemics, but from its role as a model of secretory diarrhea. More has been learned about pathophysiology—and normal intestinal function—from cholera than from any other intestinal disease. Treatment programs have been devised, including an oral rehydration regimen used to treat all major diarrheal illnesses; the cholera enterotoxin has been purified; the immunology and epidemiology of cholera have been clarified; and anticholera vaccines have been developed.

Microbiology

Vibrio cholerae is a Gram-negative, short, curved rod that looks like a comma. It is actively motile by means of a single polar flagellum. Vibrios are strongly aerobic and prefer alkaline and high-salt environments. The terminology and classification of *V. cholerae* are complex. Agglutination by antisera against the O1 antigen (cell wall polysaccharide) is used to characterize vibrios into O1 or non-O1 groups. They are then classified into serotypes based on the subspecificity of O1 antigen (A, B, C, i.e., Ogawa [A, B]; Inaba [A, C]; Hikojima [A, B, C]). *Biotype* refers to different phenotypic qualities (i.e., production of hemolysins, agglutination of various species of erythrocytes, resistance to polymyxin, and so forth). Toxigenic *V. cholerae* that agglutinate in O1 antiserum is the main cause of epidemic cholera. There are two major biotypes of *V. cholerae* O1: classic and El Tor. The latter strain is responsible for the current pandemic that began in 1961. El Tor vibrios are somewhat hardier than others in nature. Clinical disease is similar with both biotypes, although on average, El Tor infections are milder. The major serotypes associated with clinical disease are Inaba and Ogawa; a rare third type is Hikojima. The El Tor Inaba type is responsible for the current outbreak in South America. There also are unique O1 cholera strains (e.g., *V. parahaemolyticus* and *V. vulnificus*) that cause endemic disease along the Gulf Coast of the United States.[54]

A newly described toxigenic non-O1 strain, now designated *V. cholerae O139 Bengal*, was responsible for an epidemic that started in southern India and Bangladesh in late 1992 and spread rapidly to many other countries in Southeast Asia.[55,56] This strain was classified as a new serogroup because it did not react with antisera to the previously identified 138 serogroups.[56]

Cholera Toxin

All wild strains of *V. cholerae*, including O139, elaborate the same enterotoxin, a protein molecule with a molecular weight of 84,000d (see Fig. 104–2).[57] The structural genes for the cholera toxin are encoded by a filamentous bacteriophage.[58] Like the diphtheria toxin, the cholera toxin is composed of two types of subunits. Each toxin molecule contains five B subunits that encircle a single A subunit. The B subunit is responsible for binding to the receptor on the mucosa. The A subunit is responsible for activation of adenylate cyclase located on the basolateral cellular membrane. A second 10- to 30-kd LT has been described. This toxin alters intestinal permeability by acting on intestinal epithelial cell tight junctions; it has been called *zonula occludens toxin*.[59]

Epidemiology

For many centuries, the Bay of Bengal has been considered the "cradle of cholera." Western countries were relatively free of cholera epidemics until the 19th century, but since then, with the worldwide spread of the disease, six pandemics (across continents) have been reported. We are currently in the seventh pandemic, which started in 1961 in the Celebes Island in Indonesia and then made its way to the Philippines, Hong Kong, Japan, Korea, Thailand, India, Pakistan, and the Middle East, passing across the African continent to engulf the entire region, and, in 1991, spreading to South America. Although the overall number of cases of cholera in Latin America has subsided since 1991, outbreaks of *V. cholerae* have continued to occur sporadically throughout sub-Saharan Africa. During 1999, more than 200,000 cases of cholera were reported from Africa, accounting for 81% of the global total of cholera cases.[60]

The organism associated with the current pandemic is an El Tor biotype which, as mentioned earlier, generally causes a milder disease than that seen with the "classic" strains and with a higher frequency of inapparent infection.

The South American epidemic that began in Peru in January 1991 caused more than 1 million cases in its first 3 years. From 15,000 to 20,000 cases of cholera were reported each week during the peak of the epidemic, for a national incidence of 1:1000 persons. Unboiled drinking water, unwashed fruits or vegetables, and food or water from street vendors were implicated risk factors in this explosive outbreak.[63,64]

The epidemic of *V. cholerae* O139 Bengal that began in southern India and Bangladesh in late 1992 affected adults predominantly.[56] The clinical features of infection with the O139 Bengal strain were virtually indistinguishable from infection caused by *V. cholerae* O1.[65,66]

Cholera occurs sporadically along the Gulf Coast of the United States, primarily in Texas and Louisiana.[61] Among the millions of American travelers to endemic areas in foreign countries, only 41 imported cases of cholera were reported in the United States from 1961 to 1990, and none was associated with secondary spread. The current epidemic (more confined locale) in South America resulted in 151 cases of cholera in the United States: 26 cases in 1991, 103 in 1992, and 22 in 1993; only 1 death was reported.[62]

Contaminated water and food are the major vehicles for the spread of cholera. Infection by person-to-person contact is uncommon, and rarely do physicians, nurses, ward attendants, and laboratory workers who come in contact with the microorganism acquire clinical disease. The inoculum required to cause acute cholera is large, approximately 10^9 organisms. Even this number usually does not cause disease in a healthy person without bicarbonate or some other substance to buffer the acidity of the stomach. People with low gastric acidity, often associated with malnutrition, are more easily infected than those with normal acidity.

Humans are the only host for cholera vibrios. The carrier rate is approximately 5% after acute exposure, although long-term carriers are much less common. Cholera vibrios are harbored in the gallbladder, like *S. typhi*.

Pathogenesis

The clinical syndrome of cholera is caused by the action of the toxin on intestinal epithelial cells. Cholera toxin increases adenylate cyclase activity to result in elevated levels of cAMP in the intestinal mucosa, and this in turn causes intestinal secretion. Fluid loss in cholera originates in the small intestine. The most sensitive areas are the upper bowel, particularly the duodenum and upper jejunum; the ileum is less affected, and the colon usually is in a state of absorption and is relatively insensitive to the toxin. Diarrhea results because the large volume of fluid produced in the upper intestine overwhelms the absorptive capacity of the colon.

Attachment of *V. cholerae* to the intestinal mucosa is mediated by various surface components, including a fimbrial colonization factor known as *toxin-coregulated pilus*. The toxin-coregulated pilus attachment protein may play an important role in producing naturally occurring protective antibodies against *V. cholerae*.[67]

Despite the derivation of the term *cholera* (Greek: *chole*, bile), the appearance of choleric stools resembles "rice water"; that is, the stool has lost all pigment and becomes a clear fluid with small flecks of mucus. The electrolyte composition (Table 104–5) is isotonic with plasma, and the effluent has a low protein concentration. On microscopic examination there are no inflammatory cells, only small numbers of shed mucosal cells.

Cholera vibrios do not invade the mucosal surface, and bacteremia virtually is unknown in this disease. A biopsy specimen of the mucosa during acute cholera shows evidence of dehydration, with maintenance of normal architecture, in sharp contrast to the invasive and ulcerating lesions associated with *Salmonella* and *Shigella*.

Clinical Features

Like many other infectious diseases, there is a spectrum of clinical manifestations with *V. cholerae*—from an asymptomatic carrier state to a desperately ill patient with severe dehydration. The initial stage is characterized by vomiting and abdominal distention and is followed rapidly by diarrhea, which accelerates over the next few hours to frequent large volumes of rice water stools. All the clinical symptoms and signs can be ascribed to fluid and electrolyte losses. Patients present with profound dehydration and hypovolemic shock, usually leading to renal failure. The stool is isotonic with plasma, although there is an inordinate loss of potassium and bicarbonate, with resultant hypokalemic acidosis (see Table 104–5). Mild fever may be present, but there are no signs of sepsis.

Table 104–5	Electrolyte Concentrations of Choleric and Nonspecific Fecal Fluid and of Intravenous Fluids Used in Infectious Diarrheas

Type of Fluid	Electrolyte Concentrations, mmol/L			
	Sodium	**Potassium**	**Chloride**	**Bicarbonate**
Cholera stool				
Adult	124	16	90	48
Child	101	27	92	32
Nonspecific, child	56	25	55	14
Intravenous Therapy				
Lactated Ringer's solution	130	4	109	28*
5:4:1 solution†‡	129	11	97	44
2:1 solution§	141	—	94	47

*Equivalent concentration after lactate conversion.
†Add glucose, 110 mmol (20 g/L).
‡Intravenous solution that is 5 g of sodium chloride, 4 g of sodium bicarbonate, and 1 g of potassium chloride per liter.
§Solution that has a carbohydrate-to-sodium ratio of 2:1.

Immunologic Responses

After recovery from acute cholera, two serum antibodies can be demonstrated: a vibriocidal antibody directed against somatic antigen and an antitoxin antibody against the enterotoxin. Vibriocidal titers rise and fall rapidly during infection, and by 6 months only 1% of patients have high levels. In areas of high prevalence, such as the Indian subcontinent, the level of vibriocidal titer rises with age; by the 10th year of life, 50% of people have measurable titers. Protection is related to the presence and actual level of vibriocidal antibody. From these observations, it follows that acute cholera in endemic areas is a disease largely of young children, primarily those who lack vibriocidal antibody. Antitoxin titers rise somewhat slowly after acute infection and remain elevated for many months. The susceptibility of adults in areas endemic for the O139 Bengal strain of cholera indicates that the afflicted populations are immunologically naive and that prior exposure to *V. cholerae* O1 does not provide cross-protective immunity. Nevertheless, volunteer challenge studies indicate that an initial infection with O139 Bengal provides protection against recurrent disease.[65]

Elevation in titers of vibriocidal antibody may be caused by either actual infection with vibrios or asymptomatic carriage of vibrios. In field situations, the clinical case rate is approximately 0.26%; that is, for every clinical case of cholera there are approximately 400 asymptomatic people who have had contact with the organism, as demonstrated by a rise in vibriocidal antibody titers.

Treatment

Treatment of acute cholera is based on the physiologic principles of restoring fluid and electrolyte balance and maintaining intravascular volume. These objectives can be accomplished with intravenous solutions or oral fluids that contain electrolytes in isotonic concentrations (see Table 104–5). Particular attention is paid to administration of bicarbonate and potassium, which are lost excessively in cholera stool. An oral rehydration solution (ORS) has been developed for treating mild-to-moderate cases and is especially useful in developing countries (Table 104–6).[68]

The simple therapeutic principles of fluid replacement and antibiotics can save many lives. This knowledge has been available only in the past 30 years; before then the mortality rate for cholera was 50% to 75%. Application of these physiologic principles reduces the mortality rate in adults to less than 1%. Indeed, the mortality rate in the current epidemic in Peru is less than 1%. Children with cholera still have a mortality rate of 3% to 5% because of a lack of fluid reserve in the young child.

Antimicrobial agents are useful as ancillary measures to treat cholera because their use leads to reductions in stool output, duration of diarrhea, fluid requirements, and *Vibrio* excretion.[69] Tetracycline is recommended at a dose of 40 mg/kg/day orally up to a maximum of 4 g/day in four divided doses for 2 days. There is no proved value in lengthening the duration of treatment to 4 days. Single-dose therapy with ciprofloxacin results in a successful clinical response in 94% of patients infected with

Table 104–6 Compositions of Some Oral Hydration Beverages

	Sodium, mmol/L	Potassium, mmol/L	Chloride, mmol/L	Base, mmol/L	Carbohydrate, mmol/L	Osmolarity, mOsm/L
Rehydration						
WHO solution	90	20	80	10 (C)	111	310
Rehydralyte*	75	20	65	10 (C)	140	305
Maintenance						
Infalyte*	50	20	40	10 (B)	111	270
Lytren*	50	25	45	10 (C)	111	290
Pedialyte*	45	20	35	10 (C)	140	250
Resol*	50	20	50	11 (C)	111	270
Ricelyte*	50	25	45	11 (C)	30 (D)	200
Other liquids						
Apple juice	3	28	30	0	690[†]	730
Chicken broth	250	8	250	0	0	450
Cola	2	0.1	2	13 (B)	730[†]	750
Ginger ale	3	1	2	4 (B)	500[†]	540
Tea	0	0	0	0	0	5

*Ready to use.
[†]Combination of glucose and fructose.
B, bicarbonate; C, citrate; D, rice-syrup solids (g/L); WHO, World Health Organization.
Modified from Avery ME, Snyder JD: Oral therapy for acute diarrhea: The underused simple solution. N Engl J Med 323:891, 1990.

V. cholerae.[70,71] As a result of rising rates of resistance, tetracycline and doxycycline are often less effective than are the fluoroquinolones.[71,72] Alternative drugs include trimethoprim-sulfamethoxazole (TMP-SMX) and furazolidone.

Vaccines

Currently, no vaccines for the treatment of cholera are available in the United States. No cholera vaccination requirements exist for entry or exit in any country. Cholera vaccine is not recommended.

OTHER VIBRIOS

In addition to the cholera vibrios, at least nine other vibrios have important pathogenic significance.[61,73,74] These strains represent a diverse group of organisms that are morphologically and biochemically identical to *V. cholerae* but that do not agglutinate with the O group antiserum of the three cholera serotypes.[74,75] The non-O1 cholera vibrios produce several toxins and cause a wider range of infection than do cholera vibrios, including watery diarrhea, dysentery, wound infections, ear infections, and septicemia.[61,74]

The non-O1 cholera vibrios can be isolated from salty coastal waters of the United States, most commonly in the summer and fall when the temperature rises. Mollusks, particularly oysters, have a reported contamination rate of 10% to 15% and are the major source of non-O1 *Vibrio* disease; clams, mussels, and crabs also have been implicated.

Strains within the same species may produce different enterotoxins, cytotoxins, and hemolysins. The diversity of toxin production is matched by the diversity of clinical symptoms, which range from watery dehydrating diarrhea to frank dysentery. Some strains penetrate the intestinal mucosa and produce bacteremia, whereas others have been incriminated in wound infections after exposure to ocean water or handling raw seafood.[76]

In the Far East, non-O1 cholera vibrios have been associated mainly with severe dehydrating diarrhea. In Peru, serogroups O10 and O12 were isolated from patients with liquid diarrhea associated with mild-to-moderate dehydration.[77] In the United States, reported cases of disease caused by non-O1 cholera vibrios include wound and ear infections, septicemia, and infections of the lung and biliary tract.[74] The most common antecedent history is consumption of raw oysters within the previous 72 hours. In outbreaks, there is a high attack rate, with incubation periods that range from as short as 6 to 12 hours to as long as 3 days. A 1-week course of diarrheal illness is common. Because the gastrointestinal disease is self-limited and relatively benign in the United States, antibiotics are not recommended; however, septicemia, wound infections, and deep organ infections should be treated with appropriate antibiotics.

The incidence of *Vibrio* intestinal infections was studied among participants at an antimicrobial conference in New Orleans, many of whom had consumed raw oysters. Of 479 persons surveyed, 11% had a positive stool culture for vibrios, mainly *V. parahaemolyticus*, and approximately one third of those with a positive culture had diarrhea. Samples of local seafood, especially oysters, were found to harbor five different species of vibrios.[78] In the Chesapeake Bay area, the annual incidence of *Vibrio* infections related to consuming seafood is estimated to be 1.6 per 100,000 persons.[79]

Vibrio parahaemolyticus

V. parahaemolyticus causes an acute diarrheal disease after consumption of contaminated raw fish or shellfish. Recognized as an important pathogen in the Far East, *V. parahaemolyticus* also has been isolated in the United States, although the exact prevalence is unknown. Strains of *V. parahaemolyticus* produce a number of distinct hemolysins, the most significant of which appears to be responsible for the "Kanagawa phenomenon," which causes hemolysis of human red blood cells in Wagatsuma bacteriologic medium. Kanagawa-positive isolates are pathogenic for humans, whereas Kanagawa-negative strains are nonpathogenic and isolated from marine sources as part of their flora.

Pathogenic strains of *V. parahaemolyticus* produce a number of other toxins, including a lethal toxin that also is hemolytic. In some studies, these organisms produce an enterotoxin that causes fluid accumulation in the rabbit ileal loop model and a cytotoxic toxin that causes damage to HeLa cells. Some strains have the ability to invade the intestinal mucosa and cause bacteremia in experimental animals.[80]

Epidemiology

Many outbreaks of *V. parahaemolyticus* gastroenteritis have been reported in Japan; during the warm months, when the frequency of this infection is higher, this organism is responsible for most episodes of bacterial food poisoning in that country. Infections also have been documented in other countries in Asia as well as Australia and Great Britain. In the United States, there is a striking geographic association, with most cases occurring in coastal states such as Maryland, Massachusetts, Louisiana, New Jersey, and Washington. The organism is ubiquitous in marine waters and can be found along the coastlines of most countries in which cases have been reported.

The attack rate in epidemics varies from 24% to 86% of exposed persons. The mean incubation period for most outbreaks has been 13 to 23 hours, with a range of 4 to 48 hours. Most infections have been associated with seafish or sea water ingestion. Occasionally, boiled sardines, salted vegetables (contaminated from salt water), or crabs, shrimp, and oysters (both cooked and uncooked) have been incriminated. The common factor in most outbreaks appears to be a hiatus of several hours without proper refrigeration between catching the sea fish or mollusk and eating it.

Clinical Features

The diversity in toxins and virulence mechanisms is reflected in the variation in symptoms and signs observed in laboratory-confirmed outbreaks in the United States.[81,82] Explosive watery diarrhea is the cardinal manifestation in more than 90% of the cases. Abdominal cramps, nausea, vomiting, and headaches are common. Fever and chills occur in 25% to 50% of cases. Clinically, this illness resembles that produced by nontyphoidal *Salmonella*; however, in some cases a bloody dysenteric syndrome is observed, with fecal leukocytes and superficial mucosal ulcerations on sigmoidoscopic examination.

The duration of illness generally is short, with a median of 6 days (range, <1 to 30 days). Fatalities are rare and usually occur in persons with preexisting medical conditions. The diarrhea of *V. parahaemolyticus* usually is not as profuse as in *V. cholerae*, but hypotension and shock have been noted in some patients. Subclinical cases have been demonstrated in less than 1% of healthy persons. The infection is rare in the winter, suggesting that the carrier state is probably transient. The organism is no longer detectable in the stool once symptoms have resolved.

Treatment

Although explosive in onset, this disease generally is rather short-lived. Patients generally are treated symptomatically. The organism is sensitive to several antibiotics, including tetracycline, but there is no evidence that antimicrobial therapy has a role in management.

Additional Miscellaneous *Vibrio* Species

V. vulnificus is perhaps the most important noncholera *Vibrio* in the United States because of its severity of illness, especially in patients with underlying liver disease. The infection can be acquired as a wound infection in people swimming in salt waters or by direct consumption of seafood, usually raw oysters; the mortality rate of resulting septicemia is 50%. Because this infection can be lethal in patients with underlying liver disease, such persons should be warned to avoid eating raw seafood, especially oysters.[83]

Vibrio mimicus acquires its name from its similarity to cholera vibrios, even in producing an enterotoxin that resembles cholera toxin.[84] The organism has been isolated from patients in the United States with diarrhea, septicemia, or wound infections.[73] *Vibrio hollisae*, also known as enteric EF-13, is a rare isolate from stool and, occasionally, blood cultures. *Vibrio furnissii* is found in Asia. Its most celebrated outbreak was on an air flight from Tokyo to Seattle, during which 23 passengers developed severe diarrhea, resulting in one death and two hospitalizations.

Vibrio fluvialis, previously designated as enteric group EF-6, has been isolated from patients with severe watery diarrhea in Asia and the coastal United States.[73,74,79] The isolates produced a range of toxins, including an enterotoxin similar to classic cholera toxin. The organism is found only rarely in other parts of the world, including the United States. Bacteremia caused by *Vibrio metschnikovii* has been described in a limited number of cases and may be more common in patients with an underlying disease.[85] *Vibrio alginolyticus* is a rare cause of wound or ear infections and gastroenteritis.[73] *Vibrio damsela* is encountered rarely in wound infections.

AEROMONAS

Aeromonas species are ubiquitous environmental organisms found principally in fresh and brackish water, especially in the summer months. These organisms often are mistaken for coliforms in the laboratory and, as a result, reported incidence rates are falsely low. *Aeromonas* species are divided into two groups: psychrophilic (Greek: *psychros*, cold) aeromonads, which grow optimally at temperatures ranging from 22°C to 28°C, and mesophilic aeromonads, which grow best between 35°C and 37°C.[43] Psychrophilic strains usually are isolated from environmental water sources and fish; *Aeromonas salmonicida* is the most common strain in this group. Based on their phenotypic features, the mesophilic aeromonads are grouped into three complexes: *Aeromonas hydrophila*,

Aeromonas caviae, and *Aeromonas veronii*. All three of these *Aeromonas* species have been associated with human infections.[86,87] *Aeromonas* strains produce an array of toxins, including heat-labile enterotoxin, hemolysin, and cytotoxin.[88]

Epidemiology

Aeromonas infections are often associated with drinking untreated water, such as well water or spring water, just before the onset of symptoms.[89] Several studies have reported a high frequency of isolation of the organism from the stools of children with diarrhea; for example, the incidence of *Aeromonas* isolations in Western Australia was 10.2% in more than 1000 cases of childhood diarrhea, compared with 0.06% in control subjects.[90] Other studies have found a high carrier rate in healthy people, with a range of 0.7% to 3.2% and up to 27% in Thailand. The high carrier rate has raised some question about the pathogenicity of these organisms.[91]

Clinical Features

Aeromonas has long been recognized as a cause of wound infections after swimming in fresh or brackish water and of bacteremic or deep organ infections in immunocompromised hosts. In recent years, however, most isolates have come from intestinal infections. There is a range of illness, from mild diarrhea seen mostly in children to more severe cases that can require hospitalization. In a study from Western Australia, 22% of patients had blood and mucus in their stools, and one third required hospitalization for severe illness.[90] Most cases resolved within 1 week, but 37% of these children had symptoms for 2 or more weeks. In adults, chronic diarrhea is even more common, lasting an average of 42 days in the United States.[89]

Treatment

These organisms are consistently resistant to β-lactam antibiotics, such as penicillin, ampicillin, and first- or second-generation cephalosporins.[92] In fact, some cases of *Aeromonas* diarrhea have been activated apparently by prior treatment with ampicillin. *Aeromonas* species tend to be sensitive to TMP-SMX, third-generation cephalosporins, fluoroquinolones, tetracycline, and chloramphenicol. There is no convincing evidence that mild cases are improved by antibiotic treatment, but the duration of a chronic infection may be shortened by appropriate use of these drugs.

PLESIOMONAS SHIGELLOIDES

Plesiomonas shigelloides also is a member of the family Vibrionaceae but is isolated less frequently than *Aeromonas* in the United States.[86,91,93] Most cases have been associated with consumption of raw oysters or recent travel to Mexico or Asia.[94] Diarrhea ranges from mild and watery to severe colitis with visible blood. Abdominal pain often is prominent. Antibiotic sensitivity is similar to that of *Aeromonas*, but little information is available on the efficacy of treatment.

ESCHERICHIA COLI

E. coli are major components of the normal intestinal microflora in humans and animals. Although most strains are relatively harmless in the bowel, others possess virulence factors that are related to diarrheal disease. At least six types of *E. coli* intestinal pathogens have been recognized (Table 104–7). Their virulence factors include toxin production, adherence to epithelial cells, and invasiveness, each encoded by specific genetic elements (plasmids or chromosomal genes) that determine pathogenicity.

Enteropathogenic *Escherichia coli*

Severe epidemics of diarrhea raged in neonatal nurseries for decades, starting in the 1920s. Although uncommon in recent years, such outbreaks had a high mortality in infants. Approximately 14 serotypes were associated epidemiologically with neonatal diarrhea, including the well-known types O55, O111, and O119.[26] An analysis of published case-controlled studies and longitudinal surveys found that EPEC designated by serotype was recovered more frequently from sick children than from healthy control subjects.[26]

Table 104–7 Pathogenic Strains of *Escherichia coli* in the Intestine

Strains	Pathogenic Mechanisms	Persons Affected	Clinical Features
Enteropathogenic (EPEC)	Localized adherence O serogroups	Children Newborns in a nursery (outbreaks)	Watery diarrhea
Enterotoxigenic (ETEC)	Heat-labile and/or heat-stable toxin Adherence	Children in developing countries; travelers	Watery diarrhea
Enteroinvasive (EIEC)	Shiga-like toxin Epithelial cell invasion O serogroups (related to *Shigella*)	Children and adults Persons who ingest contaminated food and water (outbreaks)	Dysentery
Enterohemorrhagic (EHEC)	Shiga-like toxin (large quantities) O serogroups (usually O157:H7)	Children and adults Persons who ingest contaminated food, especially hamburger (outbreaks)	Bloody diarrhea Hemolytic-uremic syndrome
Enteroaggregative (EAggEC)	Aggregative adherence to Hep-2 cells	Children in developing countries	Watery diarrhea (acute) and persistent diarrhea
Diffusely adhering (DAEC)	Diffuse adherence to Hep-2 cells	Children in developing countries	Acute and persistent diarrhea

DAEC, diffusely adhering *E. coli*; EAggEC, enteroaggregative *E. coli*; EHEC, enterohemorrhagic *E. coli*; EIEC, enteroinvasive *E. coli*; EPEC, enteropathogenic *E. coli*; ETEC, enterotoxigenic *E. coli*; RBC, red blood cell; WBC, white blood cell.

These organisms adhere to the mucosal surface of the small and large intestine and cause dissolution of the glycocalyx and flattening and dissolution of the microvilli.[25,28] This results in a form of *localized adherence* resulting in a lesion called an *attaching and effacement lesion* (see Fig. 104–1) (this process is discussed earlier in "Bacterial Factors Involved in Intestinal Infection"). The mechanisms by which this attachment results in intestinal secretion is not understood clearly but includes alterations in enterocyte tyrosine kinase activity and intracellular calcium.

EPEC adherence factor is contained within a plasmid of the EPEC and has been used to construct a probe that, in turn, has been used to identify EPEC strains rapidly in stools of patients with diarrhea.[95] In a study from São Paulo, Brazil, *E. coli* adherence factor-positive classic EPEC was found in 26% of children with acute diarrhea; these organisms were the most common pathogens isolated from the children, exceeding rotavirus isolations in frequency.[96] EPEC strains are less frequent causes of diarrhea in industrialized countries but seem to be important pathogens in many developing countries, especially in children in the first 2 years of life.[97,98]

Resistance to antimicrobial drugs is common in *E. coli* adherence factor-positive classic EPEC strains.[96] Because most of these infections appear to be self-limited, there is no indication for antibiotic treatment, although non-absorbable antibiotics such as neomycin have been used in the past for neonates with severe EPEC diarrhea.

Enterotoxigenic *Escherichia coli*

Inspired by the discoveries in cholera, investigators directed their attention to *E. coli* as a cause of acute toxigenic diarrheal disease. Originally in India, and thereafter in many parts of the world, strains of *E. coli* were found to elaborate an enterotoxin similar to the toxin of *V. cholerae*.[99] ETEC is a group of *E. coli* distinct from EPEC serotypes. ETEC infections mostly are sporadic but may cause large outbreaks.

Pathologic Mechanism of Infection

ETEC is acquired by consuming contaminated food and liquids. The organisms first adhere to the surface of small intestinal enterocytes by mechanisms discussed earlier in the section "Bacterial Factors Involved in Intestinal Infection." They colonize the surface of the small bowel epithelium without penetrating the epithelial layer. As in cholera, there is neither mucosal damage nor bacteremia. Although a variety of specific pili are involved in adhesion of specific ETEC strains, all ETEC strains, whether pathogenic for humans or animals, elaborate similar enterotoxins.

Enterotoxins

Two types of enterotoxins are produced by ETEC.[29] The LT is a protein that is destroyed by heat and acid and has a molecular weight of approximately 80,000 d. It acts pathophysiologically like cholera toxin by activating adenylate cyclase, thereby causing secretion of fluid and electrolytes into the small intestinal lumen. LT also shares antigenic components with cholera toxin. The second toxin is heat stable (ST) and is able to withstand heating to 100°C. This toxin has a low molecular weight of approximately 2000 d, activates guanylate cyclase, and the resultant increase in cGMP induces intestinal secretion from both the small and large intestine. ST is really a family of toxins; the forms that cause disease most commonly in humans are $ST1_a$ and $ST1_b$ (which differ from each other by a few amino acid residues). ETEC strains may elaborate LT only, ST only, or both LT and ST. Not only do these toxins cause diarrhea in humans, but similar types of toxigenic *E. coli* also cause dehydrating diarrhea in domestic animals such as pigs, cows, and sheep.

Epidemiology

ETEC infections are acquired from other humans; animal strains of ETEC are rather host specific. The major vehicles of infection appear to be contaminated food and beverages. Infection occurs primarily in children, with the highest incidence in the tropics. There have been varying reports of ETEC infection in the United States, with high incidences in Chicago and Dallas and low figures in other American cities and Canada. Even in developing countries, the frequency of ETEC infection in children has varied from 15% to 50% of all diarrheal episodes. ETEC is the most common cause of diarrhea in travelers from North America and Northern Europe to areas of the developing world where diarrheal disease is prevalent. This pathogen also has become the leading bacterial etiology of outbreaks of gastroenteritis on cruise ships; water stored at overseas ports is the probable source of these ETEC infections.[100]

Clinical Features

ETEC infections are among the most common causes of diarrhea in children living in developing countries and travelers to these regions.[97] There is nothing distinctive about the clinical presentation of ETEC diarrhea. The incubation period is 24 to 48 hours, and the disease often begins with upper intestinal distress, followed shortly by watery diarrhea. The infection can be mild, with only a few loose bowel movements, or quite severe, mimicking cholera, with severe dehydration and even rice water stools. Indeed, the initial demonstration of such toxigenic diarrhea came from studies in Calcutta, India, of a serious form of diarrheal disease called *acute undifferentiated diarrhea*. Affected patients were admitted to the cholera ward until it was determined that vibrios were not present in their stools. ST-only strains cause a milder attack of diarrhea than do LT-producing strains, but affected patients have more vomiting and constitutional complaints.[101]

Immunity

Antibodies to the enterotoxins and colonization factors have been demonstrated in persons infected with ETEC. It appears that people residing in areas at high risk for ETEC infection acquire some mucosal immunity over time.[29] Thus, the risk that ETEC diarrhea would develop in students at a college in Mexico depended on their country of origin; those from South America had a relatively low risk of ETEC diarrhea, whereas those from North America had a high risk.[102]

Treatment

Most patients with ETEC diarrhea have only mild dehydration, but in children and older people even small amounts of intestinal purging can have serious consequences. The stool electrolyte losses in ETEC diarrhea are similar to those in cholera, and fluid replacement should follow the same principles. Although these organisms often are sensitive to many antimicrobial drugs, including TMP-SMX and quinolones, resistant isolates are being encountered increasingly.[100] Studies of patients with acute traveler's diarrhea have demonstrated shortening of the duration of diarrhea when effective antimicrobial therapy is initiated early in the course of illness.[103] Nevertheless, because most episodes of ETEC diarrhea are self-limited, treatment with antibiotics generally is not necessary.

Enteroinvasive E. coli

Originally described in Asia, enteroinvasive E. coli (EIEC) is recognized as a rare cause of dysentery. During 1971, there was an EIEC outbreak in the United States that was related to contaminated imported cheese.[104] Most episodes of EIEC infections are characterized by watery diarrhea; some patients experience a dysenteric syndrome, manifest as bloody mucoid diarrhea, tenesmus, fever, intestinal cramps, and multiple PMNs in the fecal effluent. EIECs have been recognized in at least eight E. coli serogroups, most of which are related biochemically and antigenically to Shigella. Other similarities to Shigella include the ability to invade epithelial cells and production of two toxins, a Shiga-like toxin (STX) and an enterotoxin. Diagnosis of EIEC in a routine bacteriologic laboratory is difficult and generally impractical. Surveys of EIEC in the United States have shown low isolation rates, except in a few celebrated outbreaks. Low rates of infection have been observed in some less developed countries,[97] although in Thailand the organism is common in children with diarrhea.[105]

Enterohemorrhagic E. coli

Acute hemorrhagic colitis, which first was recognized in two separate outbreaks in Michigan and Ohio in 1982,[106] has been associated mainly with a specific serotype of E. coli, O157:H7. This organism is estimated to be responsible for 0.6% to 2.4% of all cases of diarrhea and 15% to 36% of cases of hemorrhagic colitis in Canada, the United Kingdom, and the United States.[107] The spectrum of disease associated with E. coli O157:H7 includes bloody diarrhea, which is seen in as many as 95% of patients, nonbloody diarrhea, hemolytic-uremic syndrome (HUS), and thrombotic thrombocytopenic purpura. Currently, the class of EHEC includes more than 100 different serotypes.[108]

Epidemiology

EHEC has become the most commonly isolated pathogen from the stools of patients with bloody diarrhea in the United States.[109] The disease is most common in northern climates such as in Massachusetts, Minnesota, and the Pacific Northwest but occurs throughout the United States. It also is well known in Canada, Great Britain, and throughout Europe. Infections occur sporadically or in large outbreaks. The leading vehicle of infection is hamburger meat, although outbreaks have been associated with precooked meat patties, roast beef, salami, fresh-pressed apple cider, lettuce, alfalfa sprouts, and unpasteurized milk.[29,110-113] Water-borne outbreaks also have been associated with contaminated swimming pools and other recreational water bodies, well-water, and municipal water systems.[29] Person-to-person transmission probably has played a role in outbreaks in day-care centers and nursing homes.[107,114,115] Infection rates vary seasonally with a peak incidence from June to September.

EHEC strains are found in the fecal flora of a wide variety of animals, including cattle, sheep, pigs, goats, chickens, dogs, and cats. Many of these strains are of serotypes other than E. coli O157:H7. The most important reservoir of infection is cattle, hence, transmission via hamburger meat.

Virulence Factors

EHEC strains possess at least two virulence factors: an adherence mechanism causing attachment-effacement lesions similar to those seen with EPEC (see earlier) and two STX cytotoxins (I and II).[107,116] The toxins, which are identified either in stool samples or from culture of the organism itself, cause characteristic lesions in tissue culture lines such as Vero cells and HeLa cells. Some EHEC strains produce only STX I or II, whereas others produce both toxins. Most strains of E. coli O157:H7 possess the eaeA gene, which is associated with intimate attachment to the intestinal mucosa, as in EPEC (see earlier). They also produce enterohemolysin and are capable of using both heme and hemoglobin, a property that may enhance their virulence as well.[117] E. coli O157:H7 toxins may result in colitis that resembles ischemic colitis because they can cause endothelial damage, platelet aggregation, and microvascular fibrin thrombi.[118]

Clinical Features

After an incubation period of 1 to 14 days (mean, 3 to 4 days), there is the onset of watery nonbloody diarrhea associated with severe abdominal cramping and progression often to visibly bloody stools. Other symptoms include nausea, vomiting, low-grade fever, and chills. The development of frankly bloody diarrhea frequently results in admission to the hospital. Examination of the colon by endoscopy demonstrates a segmental colitis (i.e., friable inflamed mucosa with patchy erythema, edema, and superficial ulcerations). The process usually is most evident in the right colon (Fig. 104–4), but virtually any part of the colon may be affected, just as with idiopathic ischemic colitis. Plain radiographs of the abdomen may show subepithelial edema and hemorrhage ("thumbprinting"), usually in the ascending and transverse colon. Leukocytosis with a shift to the left usually is present, but anemia is uncommon unless infection is complicated by the development of HUS or thrombotic thrombocytopenic purpura.[107] Microscopic examination of the stool reveals red and white blood cells in low to moderate amounts. The median duration of diarrhea is 3 to 8 days, with longer durations in children and persons with bloody diarrhea.[107] A striking association has been noted between intestinal infection with

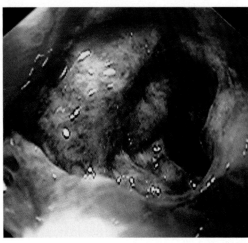

Figure 104–4 Colonoscopic appearance of the sigmoid colon in a patient with enterohemorrhagic *Escherichia coli* infection. The mucosa is edematous and violaceous, with diffuse subepithelial hemorrhage.

EHEC and HUS. In Minnesota, the incidence of HUS increased progressively during the 1980s to a current rate of 2.0 cases per 100,000 child-years. *E. coli* O157:H7 was isolated in 46% of children presenting with HUS. Risk factors for HUS include age younger than 5 years, attendance at a large day-care center, presence of bloody diarrhea, and a high white blood cell count.[110] Study from the British Isles showed that 95% of the cases of HUS had a prodromal diarrheal illness. The disease was seen most commonly in the summer. Most EHEC strains were O157:H7 or O157:H– (H not able to be typed) and approximately 30% of the isolates belonged to nine other serogroups of *E. coli*.[119,120] HUS is characterized by acute renal failure, microangiopathic hemolytic anemia, and thrombocytopenia.

Diagnosis

Several laboratory methods are used to diagnose EHEC infections. Because most isolates of *E. coli* O157:H7 do not ferment D-sorbitol, screening for this pathogen usually is done with sorbitol-MacConkey agar (SMAC). Sorbitol-negative colonies can then be serotyped with commercially available O157:H7 antisera. Such colonies should be sent to a reference laboratory for confirmation. The chances of obtaining a positive culture in stool depend on the time between the onset of symptoms and collection of the stool. Within 2 days of onset, virtually all stool specimens from EHEC-infected patients are positive for EHEC, whereas after 7 days only one third are positive.[121] In contrast, other studies have found that the median duration of excretion of EHEC is 17 to 29 days, with some patients shedding the bacterium for as long as 124 days.[29,122,123] *Shiga* toxin-producing *E. coli* (STEC) testing has been widely used but requires special facilities. Newer tests, including DNA probes, polymerase chain reaction (PCR), and enzyme immunoassays, can detect STEC I and II directly in stool specimens but are not in wide use. One report detailed use of peroxidase-labeled antibody directed against whole *E. coli* O157:H7 and subsequent immunohistochemical staining to identify the organisms on archival paraffin block tissue sec-

tions from patients with undiagnosed hemorrhagic colitis and ischemic colitis.[118]

Treatment

The desire to treat EHEC infections is understandable because of the presence of bloody diarrhea and concern that complications such as HUS will develop. Several reports, however, have raised concern that the risk of HUS is increased by antimicrobial therapy. In a murine model, certain antibiotics, notably ciprofloxacin, caused enhanced STX production by *E. coli* O157:H7 in vitro via the induction of bacteriophage encoded gene; this occurrence was associated with an increased death rate in treated mice.[124]

Antimicrobial therapy in humans does not appear to provide much benefit and may even be harmful. A randomized, controlled trial of TMP-SMX in children with *E. coli* O157:H7 enteritis found no effect of therapy on the duration of symptoms, pathogen excretion, or incidence of HUS.[125] One prospective cohort study identified 71 children with acute *E. coli* O157:H7 gastroenteritis of whom only 9 had been treated with antibiotics, however, 5 of the 10 children in whom HUS developed had received either TMP-SMX or a cephalosporin.[126] In this study, antibiotic therapy was associated with a significantly increased risk of HUS, but this conclusion has been challenged by others.[127,128] Because antibiotic use has not been shown to decrease morbidity resulting from EHEC and may increase the risk of HUS, it is not recommended that antibiotics be used routinely in the treatment of gastroenteritis if *E. coli* O157:H7 is the known or suspected cause. In cases of confirmed *E. coli* O157:H7 infection, patients should be followed closely for manifestations of HUS. Thorough cooking of ground beef is an important preventive measure.

Enteroaggregative *E. coli*

Unlike the localized adherence to Hep-2 cells seen with EPEC, some *E. coli* strains have been observed to adhere in an aggregative pattern with the bacteria clumping in a "stacked brick" pattern to the cell surface.[29] Although some investigations have implicated enteroaggregative E. coli (EAggEC) as a cause of acute and persistent diarrhea in children in developing countries,[29,129] other investigations have failed to find a significant association with diarrhea.[96,97,130] Up to one third of children infected with EAggEC have grossly bloody diarrhea. EAggEC has been associated with diarrhea in patients infected with HIV,[131] and EAggEC has been shown to be a cause of traveler's diarrhea.[132]

Volunteer challenge studies with different strains of EAggEC have yielded mixed results, suggesting that certain strains may be more virulent than others.[133] As yet, there have been no studies documenting the need for or efficacy of treatment of EAggEC infections. EAggEC include numerous serogroups that largely are distinct from those of EPEC. Certain serotypes such as O44:H18 appear to be more pathogenic than others.

Although there have been no controlled trials of therapy for EAggEC infections in children, a recent study of HIV-positive patients with diarrhea caused by EAggEC found a 50% reduction in stool output, fewer intestinal symptoms, and microbiologic eradication of the organism during treatment with ciprofloxacin.[134] Similarly, ciprofloxacin therapy of EAggEC resulted in a reduction of the duration of diarrhea in patients with traveler's diarrhea.[132]

INVASIVE PATHOGENS

Invasive organisms make their main impact on the host by invading the intestinal epithelium. Whereas the toxigenic organisms characteristically involve the upper intestine, the invasive pathogens target the lower bowel, particularly the distal ileum and colon. The main histologic finding with invasive pathogens is mucosal ulceration with an acute inflammatory reaction in the lamina propria. The principal pathogens in this group are *Salmonella*, *Shigella*, invasive *E. coli* (EIEC), *Campylobacter*, and *Yersinia*. There are important differences among these organisms, but they all share the property of mucosal invasion as the initiating event.

The precise mechanism of fluid production in invasive diarrhea is not known, but the following three theories have been invoked:

1. An enterotoxin may be responsible for fluid production, at least in the initial phase of the illness. Most *Shigella* strains elaborate an enterotoxin that differs significantly from cholera toxin but causes intestinal fluid and electrolyte secretion.[135] *Salmonella*, *Campylobacter*, and *Yersinia* strains elaborate enterotoxins.
2. Invasive organisms increase local synthesis of prostaglandins and cytokines at the site of the intense inflammatory reaction. In experimental animals, fluid secretion can be blocked by prostaglandin inhibitors such as indomethacin.[136] This theory suggests that prostaglandins are responsible for fluid secretion and subsequent diarrhea.
3. Damage to the epithelial surface may prevent reabsorption of fluids from the lumen. Transudation of fluid from a damaged intestine does not appear to be a significant factor[137,138]; however, colonic malabsorption of fluid, with a constant level of secretion, could contribute to the diarrhea.

SHIGELLA

Shigella organisms cause bacillary dysentery, a disease that has been described since early recorded history. The inhabitants of Athens in the second year of the Peloponnesian War were ravaged by dysentery. In the American Civil War, more than 1,700,000 soldiers suffered from dysentery, with 44,500 deaths. World War I also produced a high incidence of dysentery—3.7:1000 total casualties in France and up to 486:1000 casualties in East Africa. Although dysentery is a disease that becomes more prevalent in wartime, there is a constant endemic incidence in tropical countries as well as in temperate zones.

Microbiology

Shigellae comprise a group of Gram-negative enteric organisms that are included in the Enterobacteriaceae

and most closely resemble *E. coli*. They are differentiated from *E. coli* by being nonmotile, not producing gas from glucose, and generally being lactose negative. The following are four major subgroups:

- A: *Shigella dysenteriae*, 10 serotypes
- B: *Shigella flexneri*, 14 serotypes
- C: *Shigella boydii*, 18 serotypes
- D: *Shigella sonnei*, 1 serotype

Group A (*S. dysenteriae* 1), also known as the Shiga bacillus, produces the most severe form of dysentery. An outbreak in Central America in the late 1960s and early 1970s caused more than 10,000 deaths, mostly in young children. This organism has caused outbreaks in many developing countries in recent years. By contrast, *S. sonnei* produces the mildest disease.

There have been recent shifts in the incidence of dysentery and in the prevalence of specific serotypes. In the tropics, dysentery occurs mostly in late summer. In developed countries, such as the United States and those in Europe, the occurrence of dysentery has increased steadily, and the seasonal prevalence has shifted to winter. *S. flexneri* is the most common serotype in tropical countries, whereas in the United States and Europe, *S. sonnei* is the most common serotype. In the United States, for example, 60% to 80% of cases of bacillary dysentery are caused by *S. sonnei*.

Epidemiology

Shigellosis is a major diarrheal disease throughout the world, causing 10% to 20% of all cases of diarrhea from country to country. Dysentery occurs mostly in children between the ages of 6 months and 5 years, among whom the disease tends to be less severe than in adults; it is rare in infants younger than 6 months of age.

During infection, shigellae are present in large numbers in the feces. The route of infection is oral. The organisms survive best in alkaline conditions and are highly sensitive to heat and drying. Most transmission is person-to-person and is related to close human contact. There also have been dramatic epidemics related to ingestion of milk, ice cream, other foods, and occasionally water. A high incidence of infection occurs among laboratory workers who come in contact with this organism.

Measurements of inoculum size in volunteers reveal that 10^5 organisms produce an attack rate of 75%,[139] but increasing the inoculum size above this number does not increase the attack rate. There is not a good dose-response curve with *Shigella* (in contrast with *Salmonella*); indeed, dysentery can be produced with as few as 200 bacteria. The ability of *Shigella* species to survive in acidic conditions may account for the low inoculum that can produce disease.[140] Person-to-person transmission, facilitated by the low infective dose, accounts for rapid spread of *Shigella* in day-care centers and among people living in conditions of poor hygiene. These factors also explain the high frequency of dysentery among male homosexuals.

Pathogenicity

All strains of *Shigella* cause *dysentery*, a term that refers to a diarrheal stool that contains an inflammatory exudate composed of PMNs and blood. The exudative character of the stool is a point to be emphasized: This is not mere watery diarrhea but rather a loose bowel movement that contains pus. The inflammatory exudate is related to the main pathologic event: invasion of the colonic epithelium.

Humans are the only natural host for the dysentery organism, although monkeys and chimpanzees can become infected in captivity. Experimental infections can be produced in monkeys and guinea pigs. In experimental animal infections, the disease is made worse by starving the animals, feeding them antibiotics, or administering opium to reduce motility of the bowel.

The major site of attack of *Shigella* is the colon; scattered ulcerations can be seen in the terminal ileum as well. Invasion by *Shigella* is associated with a constellation of virulence factors that are related to various stages of invasion and lead eventually to death of the intestinal epithelial cell, focal ulcers, and inflammation of the lamina propria. These virulence factors are encoded by both chromosomal and plasmid genes, all of which are needed for the full expression of virulence. All virulent *Shigella*, as well as EIEC, contain large 120- to 140-megadalton plasmids, which are related to outer membrane proteins. Various loci encode for an invasion plasmid antigen (ipa), which seems to determine recognition of the epithelial cell; invasion factors (inv); and a series of vir proteins that are involved in regulation within the cell.[141] Having penetrated the mucosal surface, the organisms multiply within the epithelial cells and extend the infected area by "cell-to-cell transfer" of bacilli. Shigellae rarely penetrate beyond the intestinal mucosa and generally do not invade the bloodstream; however, bacteremia can occur in malnourished children and immunocompromised patients.

Although the initial lesions are confined to the epithelial layer, the local inflammatory response is severe, consisting of PMNs and macrophages. There is edema, microabscess formation, loss of goblet cells, degeneration

of normal cellular architecture, and mucosal ulceration. These events give rise to the characteristic clinical picture of bloody mucopurulent diarrhea. As the disease progresses, the lamina propria is involved extensively with the inflammatory response. Crypt abscess is a nonspecific but prominent feature (Fig. 104–5).

Cytotoxins

Initially, only *S. dysenteriae* 1 was known to elaborate an enterotoxin. This toxin, first identified by Shiga, has been shown to display a variety of biologic effects, depending on the experimental model used, including cytotoxicity, neurotoxicity in mice (seizures), and enterotoxicity (secretion of fluid and electrolytes). The neurotoxic properties may contribute to the seizures seen in some children with shigellosis. The toxin, which is a 75,000-dalton protein composed of two subunits, inhibits protein synthesis by irreversible inactivation of the 60S ribosomal subunit.[142] Inhibition of protein synthesis causes cytotoxicity and cell death. A toxin with similar antigenic and physiologic effects has been found in strains of *S. flexneri* and *S. sonnei*.[143]

Clinical Features

The classic presentation of bacillary dysentery is cramping abdominal pain, rectal burning, and fever, associated with multiple small-volume bloody mucoid bowel movements[142]; this full array, however, is not seen in all patients. The most constant findings are lower abdominal pain and diarrhea. Fever is present in approximately 40% of patients, and the typical dysenteric stool, consisting of blood and mucus, is present in only one third. Approximately one third of patients only have diarrhea without dysentery. Many patients demonstrate a biphasic illness. Initial symptoms are fever, abdominal pain, and watery diarrhea without gross blood; this stage may

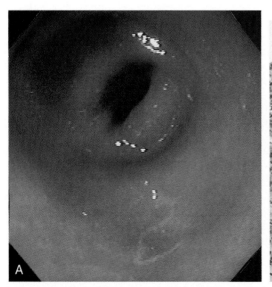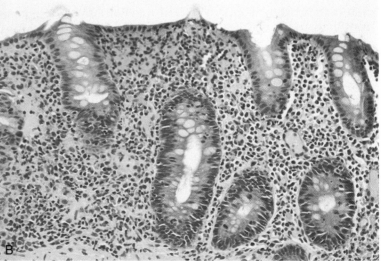

Figure 104–5 Shigellosis. *A*, Colonoscopic view of this rectum shows luminal narrowing and mucosal inflammation similar to that seen in ulcerative colitis. *B*, Histologic features include a severe inflammatory infiltrate of polymorphonuclear neutrophils and macrophages in the mucosa and submucosa. (*A* and *B*, From Wilcox CM: Atlas of Clinical Gastrointestinal Endoscopy. Philadelphia, WB Saunders, 1995.)

be related to the action of the enterotoxin on the small intestine. The second phase, which starts 3 to 5 days after onset, is characterized by tenesmus and small-volume bloody stools, corresponding to invasion of the colonic epithelium and acute colitis. A few patients have a toxic highly febrile illness associated with more severe colitis; even in this setting, bacteremia is distinctly uncommon. Malnutrition, especially in young children, and infection with *S. dysenteriae* 1 are associated with a more severe course. Among the intestinal complications of shigellosis are intestinal perforation and severe protein loss.

An extensive list of extraintestinal complications is associated with bacillary dysentery (Table 104–8).[144] Many patients complain of respiratory symptoms, such as cough and coryza, although pneumonia is rare. In young children, hypoglycemia may occur, and several neurologic findings can dominate the clinical picture, even before the diarrheal symptoms. Meningismus (the cerebrospinal fluid is normal) and seizures can occur with shigellosis, although there is no direct involvement of the central nervous system.[145,146] The meningismus and seizures have been related to the high fever, but they also can occur when the fever is not extraordinarily high. During the acute phase, HUS may occur.[147] Thrombocytopenia and a severe leukemoid reaction also have been reported.[148] A rash (rose spots) may occur during the acute phase of shigellosis.

After an acute attack of dysentery, usually 2 to 3 weeks after the onset, arthritis may appear. The presentation of joint pain or effusion usually is asymmetric and involves large joints. Joint complaints are present by themselves, not necessarily with other signs of Reiter's syndrome, and usually are associated with human leukocyte antigen (HLA)-B27; autoantibodies to this antigen cross-react with *Shigella* proteins, thereby resulting in circulating antibody-antigen complexes.[149]

The course of shigellosis varies. Children tend to have mild infections, lasting no more than 1 to 3 days. The average length of symptoms in adults is approximately 7 days. In more severe cases symptoms persist for 3 to 4 weeks and often are associated with relapses. Untreated bacillary dysentery, particularly when the course is prolonged, can be confused with ulcerative colitis.

Chronic carriers of *Shigella* have been identified; they may pass this organism in their feces for 1 year or more. Such carriers are distinctly uncommon, and usually they lose the organism spontaneously. Carriers of *Shigella* are prone to intermittent attacks of the disease, in contrast to *Salmonella* carriers, who rarely become reinfected with the strain they carry.

Diagnosis

The diagnosis of shigellosis should be suspected by the acute onset of the triad of lower abdominal pain, rectal burning, and diarrhea. Microscopic examination of stool is extremely useful and reveals multiple PMNs and red blood cells. This information should suggest bacillary dysentery, although the identification of the specific bacterial pathogen must await culture, because other microorganisms can cause the dysentery syndrome (e.g., *Campylobacter*, *V. parahaemolyticus*, *Salmonella*). Fecal specimens are the best source of a positive culture; blood and urine are only rarely positive in acute cases. Because *Shigella* species are fastidious, stool specimens or rectal swabs should be inoculated promptly into appropriate media. Sigmoidoscopy can confirm the diagnosis of colitis but is not necessary in most cases of shigellosis and is extremely uncomfortable in the setting of dysentery. Serologic and molecular tests are not useful for diagnosing acute cases of dysentery, although they are available for epidemiologic investigations.

A subacute presentation of dysentery can masquerade as ulcerative colitis (see later). The patient may have endured bloody diarrhea, cramps, and rectal pain for 2 to 4 weeks. Sigmoidoscopic findings are indistinguishable from those of patients with idiopathic ulcerative colitis (see Fig. 104–5), but a colonic biopsy may be helpful to differentiate the two.[150] With dysentery, the inflammatory process is acute (PMNs) and involves the entire lamina propria; also, colonic glands are straight without signs of regeneration. In ulcerative colitis, inflammation is chronic (lymphocytes) and involves mainly the lower one third of the lamina propria; colonic glands show signs of regeneration such as branching. Two major differences between dysentery and idiopathic ulcerative colitis are a positive stool culture for *Shigella* and dramatic improvement in symptoms after treatment of patients with dysentery with appropriate antimicrobial agents. When in doubt, treatment for shigellosis is recommended.

Deaths are rare in healthy persons, particularly adults, with bacillary dysentery; mortality is usually seen in young, often malnourished children or in debilitated patients, either the elderly or those with an immunodeficiency disease. A decreased level of consciousness and documented seizures are associated with a poor outcome in children.[145]

Treatment

The following general principles apply to the therapeutic approach to bacillary dysentery:
- Rehydration must be managed appropriately in any diarrheal disease, regardless of etiology; this maxim holds for dysentery.
- General supportive measures require attention; in the case of dysentery, children may have seizures related to high fever and electrolyte imbalance or meningismus.
- Antibiotic treatment is indicated for most patients with shigellosis.

Fluid and Electrolyte Therapy

Most patients with dysentery can be managed with oral rehydration. The indications for parenteral fluid replacement are marked diarrhea that leads to dehydration and severe vomiting that prevents oral replacement. High-volume diarrhea is seen occasionally with shigellosis and may result in severe dehydration and hypovolemia. Intravenous fluid replacement is indicated in this situation. Fluid losses can be replaced within a few hours by intravenous solutions and oral replacement should be encouraged as soon as possible (see Table 104–6). Antidiarrheal remedies generally are worthless and may even aggravate bacillary dysentery. Kaolin and pectate and other "water-binding" agents do not diminish stool volume or frequency.

Table 104–8 Complications and Unusual Manifestations of Bacterial Enterocolitis

Organism	Clinical Features
Shigella	Protein-losing enteropathy
	Meningitis and seizures (children)
	Pneumonitis
	Hemolytic-uremic syndrome (associated with *Shigella dysenteriae*)
	Thrombotic thrombocytopenic purpura
	Reactive arthritis*
	Erythema nodosum
	Post-dysenteric colitis
	Toxic megacolon
	Leukemoid reaction
	Appendicitis
	Myocarditis
	Postinfection irritable bowel syndrome
Nontyphi *Salmonella*	Bacteremia
	Extraintestinal infections
	Endocarditis
	Arthritis
	Osteomyelitis
	Pneumonia
	Arteritis
	Meningitis
	Chronic carrier state (1%)
	Cholecystitis, gallstones
	Postinfection colitis
	Toxic megacolon
	Postinfection irritable bowel syndrome
Salmonella typhi	Rose spot macules on the upper abdomen
	Myocarditis
	Intestinal and colonic ulceration, bleeding, and perforation
	Hepatosplenomegaly
	Bone marrow suppression
	Relapse of disease in 8-12%; may be more frequent in patients taking antibiotics, especially chloramphenicol
	Chronic carrier state (2-4%)
Campylobacter jejuni	Septic abortion
	Acute cholecystitis
	Pancreatitis
	Cystitis
	Guillain-Barré syndrome
	Reactive arthritis*
	Postinfection irritable bowel syndrome
	Toxic megacolon
Campylobacter fetus	Meningoencephalitis
	Septic arthritis
	Pneumonia
	Carditis
	Thrombophlebitis
	Mycotic aortic aneurysm
	Septic abortion
	Relapsing fever, chills, myalgias
Yersinia enterocolitica	Polyarthritis
	Reactive arthritis*
	Erythema nodosum (more common in women)
	Exudative pharyngitis
	Sepsis in patients with immunocompromise, cirrhosis, iron overload (especially patients treated with deferoxamine)
	Thyroiditis
	Pancarditis
	Glomerulonephritis
	Toxic megacolon
Clostridium difficile	Protein-losing colopathy
	Toxic megacolon
Enterohemorrhagic *Escherichia coli*	Thrombotic thrombocytopenic purpura
	Hemolytic-uremic syndrome
	Toxic megacolon
	Ischemic colitis
Vibrio vulnificus and *Vibrio alginolyticus*	Cellulitis
	Otitis media
	Sepsis and high mortality rate in patients with cirrhosis or who are immunocompromised

*Associated with HLA-B27. HLA, human leukocyte antigen.
Modified from Wolf D, Giannella RA: Antibiotic therapy for bacterial enterocolitis: A comprehensive review. Am J Gastroenterol 88:1667, 1993.

Antimicrobial Agents

The major determinant in the decision to use antibiotics is the severity of the illness. In practice, patients with moderate and severe cases of dysentery should receive antibiotic therapy. Mild cases often pass as self-limited events, without coming to a physician's attention. If such cases are seen in the clinic or in the physician's office, antibiotic therapy may not be required in light of the relatively benign course of infection. A reappraisal should be made when the culture report returns as positive for *Shigella*. In many cases, diarrhea has already ceased. Patients with persistent diarrhea should receive antibiotics. Ampicillin was previously the preferred antibiotic with TMP-SMX as an alternative choice; however, many strains, if not most, both in the United States and abroad now are resistant to these antibiotics. The quinolone antibiotics, such as ciprofloxacin, ofloxacin, and norfloxacin, are highly active in vitro against *Shigella* and are the drugs of choice. Single-dose therapy with 1 g of ciprofloxacin is as effective as two doses or a 5-day standard regimen in patients with *Shigella* infection; however, single-dose therapy proved less effective than multiple-dose regimens for patients with *S. dysenteriae* 1.[151] Problems with using quinolones in the treatment of *Shigella* include the high cost of the drugs and concern about cartilage damage in young children. Nalidixic acid is an alternative therapeutic agent that has produced good results, although resistance develops rapidly with widespread use of this drug.[152]

Because there is now increasing evidence of the skeletal safety of quinolones in children,[153] these drugs are being studied increasingly in pediatric populations. With single-dose pefloxacin therapy of infected children during an outbreak of multidrug-resistant *S. dysenteriae* 1 in Burundi, 91% of treated children became symptom free by day 5, and the remainder were substantially improved.[154] None of the children experienced any joint problems during the 4-week period of follow-up. Similarly, a double-blind trial of pivmecillinam compared with ciprofloxacin suspension for childhood shigellosis found that ciprofloxacin resulted in clinical responses in 80% of children, with no associated arthropathy.[155]

Although early animal and human volunteer studies indicated that the use of antimotility agents in the treatment of invasive diarrhea might lead to prolonged fever and pathogen carriage, a recent study has challenged this dictum. Treatment of dysenteric patients with a combination of the synthetic antidiarrheal agent loperamide and ciprofloxacin resulted in a significantly shortened duration of diarrhea and decreased number of stools when compared with ciprofloxacin alone.[156] The use of loperamide did not lead to prolonged fever or excretion of the pathogenic bacilli.

Antibiotics for shigellosis must be absorbed from the bowel to reach organisms within the intestinal wall and lamina propria, and the only effective delivery system is the bloodstream.[157] Nonabsorbable drugs, such as neomycin, kanamycin, paromomycin, colistin, and polymyxin, are clinically ineffective, despite in vitro sensitivity. Intravenous cefamandole also has proved disappointing. Curiously, amoxicillin, which is well absorbed and achieves higher serum levels than ampicillin, is not effective therapy for shigellosis.[158]

Chronic carriers of *Shigella* are rare. Postinfection carriage generally lasts less than 3 to 4 weeks and rarely exceeds 3 to 4 months. In circumstances in which eradication of the carrier state is deemed necessary, TMP-SMX or a fluoroquinolone should be used guided by antibiotic sensitivity results. Such treatment eliminates the carrier state in approximately 90% of patients.

Mild diarrhea and cramps may continue for days to weeks after treatment of bacillary dysentery, even when the organism is no longer present and the acute episode seems to have passed. These symptoms are not necessarily a cause for alarm, because the bowel may have sustained severe mucosal injury that requires time for repair. Approximately 10% of patients with shigellosis, however, may be left with these symptoms chronically, a condition called *postinfectious irritable bowel syndrome*.[159] Finally, shigellosis is highly contagious. Spread within a family is common. Secondary cases can occur in hospitals among other patients, nurses, and physicians. Careful hand washing and stool precautions are important to prevent dissemination of this disease.

NONTYPHOIDAL SALMONELLOSIS

Nontyphoidal salmonellosis refers to disease caused by any serotype of the genus *Salmonella*, with the exception of *S. typhi* and *S. paratyphi*. Approximately 2000 serotypes and variants are potentially pathogenic for animals and humans.

Microbiology

Salmonellae is a large group of Gram-negative bacilli that comprise one of the divisions in the family Enterobacteriaceae. Most strains are motile and produce acid and gas from glucose, mannitol, and sorbitol (except *S. typhi* and rare strains that produce only acid); they are active producers of hydrogen sulfide; and they are closely related to each other by somatic (O) and flagellar (H) antigens. These organisms are primarily intestinal pathogens, although some can be found in the bloodstream and internal organs of invertebrates; they are frequently isolated in sewage, river and sea water, and certain foods. Most salmonellae have a wide range of hosts.

The typing scheme for salmonellae is based on antigenic structure, but in recent years, the name of the strain has been derived from the city in which it was first isolated (e.g., Montevideo, Heidelberg, Dublin, Newport). Most salmonellae are flagellated; using the proper growth conditions, the H (flagellar) and O (somatic) antigens can be tested separately. In addition to H and O antigens, some strains, notably typhoid bacilli, have an additional somatic antigen associated with virulence (Vi). The Vi antigen prevents agglutination with O antigen. A positive correlation exists between virulence in mice and the amount of Vi antigen in a specific strain; however, this correlation does not carry over completely to humans, because even typhoid bacilli without measurable Vi antigen can be pathogenic for humans. A bacteriophage typing system against the Vi antigen is used for epidemiologic investigation of typhoid outbreaks. More than 70 anti-Vi phage types have been identified.

For convenience in the laboratory, a series of Kauff-mann-White serogroups that contain several serotypes was developed; these serotypes were based on shared antigens among the most common *Salmonella* types. Ninety percent of *Salmonella* pathogenic for humans falls into groups A to E, which contain 40 serotypes. The application of newer molecular methods to the taxonomy of salmonellae has revealed that all serotypes of *Salmonella* belong to one species that includes seven subspecies, which can be differentiated with biochemical tests. To avoid confusion with previous nomenclature, the new species *Salmonella enterica* was proposed.[160] Using this approach, the typhoid bacillus would be named *S. enterica* subspecies *enterica* serotype typhi. However, because this lengthy name is cumbersome, simpler acceptable versions are *S. typhi* or *S. enterica* serotype typhi.

Epidemiology

Salmonella is one of the great food-borne infections.[2] The major route of passage is by the 5 Fs: *f*lies, *f*ood, *f*ingers, *f*eces, and *f*omites. The disease can cause large outbreaks, which often are associated with common-source routes of spread. A frequent setting is an institutional supper or barbecue. Community outbreaks may persist for several months. For example, Riverside, California, experienced an epidemic involving 16,000 persons that raged for months and was related to a contaminated municipal water supply. The two most common serotypes in the United States are *Salmonella enteritidis* and *Salmonella typhimurium*. Although approximately 45,000 cases of salmonellosis are reported annually, these numbers reflect vast under-reporting, and it is estimated that 1.4 million cases of *Salmonella* food poisoning occur each year.[2] A recent pandemic of *S. enteritidis* infections has been noted, particularly in Great Britain and the United States. Eggs and poultry are the major sources of *Salmonella* infections.

Attack rates of *Salmonella* show a strong relationship to age. Children younger than 1 year of age have the highest attack rate, especially in the subset of infants 3 to 5 months old. The susceptibility of infants may be related to immunologic immaturity. There also are high attack rates and increased mortality in elderly persons. Nonhuman reservoirs play a crucial role in the transmission of the disease. In 500 outbreaks investigated over a 10-year period, almost 50% were related to animals or animal products. Poultry, meats, eggs, and dairy products were involved most frequently (Fig. 104–6).

Salmonellae have a tendency to colonize domestic animals. Poultry has the highest incidence of *Salmonella* carriage, particularly hens, chickens, and ducks. Vertical transmission via the transovarian route can occur in chickens, so even normal-appearing eggs can be contaminated with *Salmonella*. Pigs and cattle also may be heavily contaminated. Many of these animals can cohabit peacefully with salmonellae and usually are asymptomatic. Other creatures known to harbor *Salmonella* include buffalo, sheep, dogs, cats, rats, mice, guinea pigs, hamsters, seals, donkeys, turkeys, doves, pigeons, parrots, sparrows, lizards, whales, tortoises, house flies, ticks, lice, fleas, and cockroaches, to name but a few.

Commercially prepared foods may be contaminated with salmonellae: 40% of turkeys examined in California,

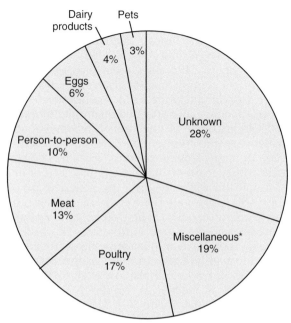

Figure 104–6 Source of infection in 500 human salmonellosis outbreaks between 1966 and 1975. *Includes over 50 sources that individually caused less than 3% of outbreaks. (Redrawn from the Centers for Disease Control, Salmonella Surveillance, Annual Summary, 1976. Washington, D.C., U.S. Department of Health, Education and Welfare, Public Health Service, 1977.)

50% of chickens in Massachusetts, and 20% of commercial egg whites have been shown in surveys to harbor these organisms. Large national and international outbreaks have been traced to commercially prepared chocolate balls, precooked roast beef, smoked whitefish, frozen eggs, ice cream, raw-milk cheese, alfalfa sprouts, cantaloupe, and powdered milk. Other commercial products not directly related to foods, such as carmine dye or brewer's yeast, also can be contaminated. Infected pets, especially turtles and lizards, have been implicated in the transmission of salmonellosis.

Pathogenic Mechanisms

Salmonellae attack the ileum and, to a lesser extent, the colon. They cause mild mucosal ulcerations and rapidly make their way through the epithelial surface to the lamina propria and then to the lymphatics and bloodstream and then rapidly spread to other organs by hematogenous dissemination. Histologic sections show edematous shortened crypts and invasion of the lamina propria by PMNs.

A series of pathogenic factors, each controlled by plasmids or chromosomal loci, are required for a fully pathogenic *Salmonella* strain. Specific plasmids encode for bacterial spread from Peyer's patches to other sites in the body.[161,162] Another virulence factor determines the ability of the strain to survive within macrophages after phagocytosis.[163] The outer membrane lipopolysaccharide and the Vi antigen are additional virulence factors. Another virulence factor imparts the ability of salmonellae to elicit transepithelial signaling to neutrophils,[164] which contribute to cell damage and secretion. Finally,

Salmonella strains produce enterotoxins that may play a role in diarrhea.[161,165,166]

The infectivity of a specific strain is related to its serotype and the inoculum size. For example, 10^5 *Salmonella newport* produces illness in some volunteers, whereas 10^9 *Salmonella pullorum* are unable to do so. The latter strain is poorly adapted to humans, as suggested by its rarity in clinical infections, but it is well adapted to chickens, from which it is frequently isolated. A dose-response curve has been determined for certain strains of *Salmonella*; an approximately 50% infection rate is seen with 10^7 organisms, whereas the infectivity rate rises to 90% with 10^9 organisms.

In experimental animals, the number of bacteria required to produce infections can be reduced by pre-treating the animals with antibiotics. Antibiotic exposure in humans also increases susceptibility to *Salmonella* infection.[167] In addition, reduced or absent gastric acid is known to increase susceptibility to infection, because acid in the stomach kills many of the challenge organisms.[140,141]

Predisposing Conditions

A number of associated conditions seems to increase the risk of salmonellosis (Table 104-9). The relationship between sickle cell anemia and *Salmonella* osteomyelitis is well known. Indeed, several forms of hemolytic anemia predispose to this infection, including malaria, bartonellosis, and louse-borne relapsing fever. The presumed mechanism of increased susceptibility is blockage of the reticuloendothelial system by macrophages that have ingested breakdown products of red blood cells, thereby reducing their ability to phagocytize salmonellae.[168] Patients with sickle cell anemia also have a decreased capacity to opsonize salmonellae because of defective activation of the alternative complement pathway.[169]

Neoplastic disease has been associated with an increased risk of salmonellosis. Leukemia, lymphoma, and disseminated malignancy appear to predispose

Table 104-9 Conditions That Predispose to *Salmonella* Infection

Achlorhydria
  Autoimmune gastritis
  Gastroduodenal surgery
Hemolytic anemia
  Bartonellosis
  Malaria
  Sickle cell disease
Immunosuppression
  AIDS
  Chemotherapy
  Glucocorticoid therapy
  Radiation
Malignancy
  Disseminated carcinoma
  Leukemia
  Lymphoma
Schistosomiasis
Ulcerative colitis

AIDS, acquired immunodeficiency syndrome.

patients to bloodstream invasion by this organism.[170] Use of glucocorticoids, chemotherapy, or radiation therapy also is associated with *Salmonella* sepsis. In AIDS patients, persistent *Salmonella* bacteremia, only temporarily yielding to antibiotic therapy, is related to the profound suppression of cell-mediated immunity.[171] Gastric surgery appears to be an important predisposing condition in the development of *Salmonella* infection. The obvious implication is that destruction of the gastric acid barrier enhances the host's susceptibility to infection.[7] All three species of schistosomiasis have been associated with invasive salmonellosis.[172] Salmonellae, as well as other Gram-negative bacteria, are capable of penetrating and multiplying within the parasites, which then serve as a source for recurrent bacteremia or bacilluria.

Ulcerative colitis may predispose to *Salmonella* infection and the carrier state, although this implication is based on only a few retrospective studies. One such analysis found that 5% of patients with idiopathic ulcerative colitis harbored *Salmonella* in their stools.[173]

Clinical Features

Although many serotypes of *Salmonella* are restricted to animals and have narrow host preferences, some strains are less fastidious and can cause serious human infection. *S. typhimurium* causes a spectrum of disease ranging from gastroenteritis to bacteremia; *S. newport* causes septicemia, and *S. typhi*, *S. paratyphi*, *S. schottmülleri*, and *S. hirschfeldii* (the last three known formerly as *S. paratyphi* A, B, and C, respectively) cause enteric (typhoid) fever.

Five clinical syndromes are seen with *Salmonella* (Table 104-10), including (1) *gastroenteritis*, noted in 75% of *Salmonella* infections; (2) *bacteremia*, with or without gastrointestinal involvement, seen in approximately 10% of cases; (3) *typhoidal* or *enteric fever*, seen with all typhoid and paratyphi strains and in approximately 8% of other *Salmonella* infections; (4) *localized infections* (e.g., bones, joints, meninges, and blood vessels), seen in approximately 5%; and (5) a *carrier state* in asymptomatic people (the organism usually is harbored in the gallbladder).[174]

The most common syndrome caused by *Salmonella* is *gastroenteritis*. The incubation period is usually 6 to 48 hours but can last as long as 7 to 12 days. Initial symptoms are nausea and vomiting, followed by abdominal cramps and diarrhea. The diarrhea usually lasts 3 or 4

Table 104-10 Relative Frequency of the Clinical Syndromes of *Salmonella* Infection

Syndrome	Frequency, %
Gastroenteritis—mild-to-severe and dehydrating ("dysenteric") colitis	75
Bacteremia—with or without gastroenteritis, endocarditis, arteritis, or AIDS	5-10
Typhoidal ("enteric fever")—with or without gastroenteritis	5-10
Localized—meninges, bones and joints, wounds, abscesses, gallbladder	5
Carrier state (>1 yr)	<1

AIDS, acquired immunodeficiency syndrome.

days and is accompanied by fever in approximately 50% of persons. In general, the pain of *Salmonella* gastroenteritis is located in the periumbilical area or the right lower quadrant. The diarrhea can vary from a few loose stools to dysentery with grossly blood and purulent feces to a cholera-like syndrome, which has been described in patients who are hypochlorhydric or achlorhydric.[11,175] Persistent fever or specific findings on physical examination suggest bacteremia or focal infection. *Salmonella* bacteremia is similar to sepsis caused by other Gram-negative bacteria, although there is an impression that it is less severe. Recurrent *Salmonella* bacteremia is seen in patients with AIDS.[171]

Once the organism invades the bloodstream, almost any organ can become involved. Meningitis, arteritis, endocarditis, osteomyelitis, wound infections, septic arthritis, and focal abscesses all have been reported.[174]

Patients become *chronic carriers* (defined as persistence for > 1 year) of nontyphoidal *Salmonella* as a consequence of either symptomatic or asymptomatic infections. The overall carrier rate is between 2:1000 and 6:1000 infected persons. Children, especially neonates, and patients older than 60 years tend to become carriers more frequently than do others. Also, structural abnormalities in the biliary tract, such as cholelithiasis, or the urinary tract, such as nephrolithiasis, predispose to and perpetuate the carrier state.[176]

Salmonella Colitis

Involvement of the colon in the course of *Salmonella* gastroenteritis probably is common, at least on the basis of animal studies and sigmoidoscopic examinations in select patients.[177] Although most patients with *Salmonella* present with mild diarrhea and watery bowel movements, colonic involvement may dominate the clinical picture; toxic megacolon and perforation due to *Salmonella* can occur.[178] Patients with *Salmonella* colitis typically have diarrhea for 10 to 15 days before the diagnosis is established. In contrast, patients with the usual form of gastroenteritis are symptomatic for 5 days or less. In the colonic form, diarrhea is more persistent, even though the organism may have disappeared from the feces on clinical presentation. Bowel movements are grossly bloody in approximately one half of the patients with *Salmonella* colitis. Sigmoidoscopic findings include hyperemia, granularity, friability, and ulcerations. Rectal biopsy specimens reveal mucosal ulcerations, hemorrhage, and crypt abscesses. Barium enema films confirm these findings and usually show pancolitis. In the acute period, there is no reliable method to distinguish idiopathic ulcerative colitis from *Salmonella* colitis, except by a positive stool culture. Any patient with an acute onset of colitis and no past history of colitis and with a duration of symptoms of 3 weeks or less should be considered to have infectious colitis; *Salmonella*, as well as EHEC, *Shigella*, *Campylobacter*, and *C. difficile,* are important diagnostic considerations.

The course of *Salmonella* colitis varies and can be as short as 1 week or as long as 2 to 3 months. The average duration of illness is 3 weeks. Complications include toxic megacolon, bleeding, and overwhelming sepsis.

It is important to recognize *Salmonella* colitis, so that inappropriate therapy is not administered. Glucocorticoids can exacerbate *Salmonella* colitis and result in silent perforation and septicemia. Finally, patients can be reassured of the self-limited course of *Salmonella* colitis as opposed to the chronic relapsing course of idiopathic ulcerative colitis.

Treatment

Although many antibiotics have been used to treat nontyphoidal *Salmonella* gastroenteritis, all have failed to alter the rate of clinical recovery. In fact, antibiotic therapy increases the frequency and duration of intestinal carriage of these organisms.[179] A review of 12 randomized trials found no differences in the duration of illness, diarrhea, or fever between patients treated with antibiotics and those treated with placebo.[180] Relapses were more common in those treated with antimicrobial agents, as were adverse drug reactions. It is thus apparent that antimicrobial therapy should not be used in most cases of *Salmonella* gastroenteritis.

Despite this general rule, antibiotics should be used when *Salmonella* gastroenteritis complicates certain conditions (Table 104–11), such as lymphoproliferative disorders; malignant disease; immunosuppressed states (AIDS and congenital or acquired forms); transplantation; known or suspected abnormalities of the cardiovascular system such as prosthetic heart valves, vascular grafts, aneurysms, and rheumatic or congenital valvular heart disease; foreign bodies implanted in the skeletal system; hemolytic anemias; the extreme ages of life; and pregnancy. In addition, patients with *Salmonella* gastroenteritis should be treated with antibiotics when they exhibit findings of severe sepsis (i.e., high fever, rigors, hypotension, decreased renal function, and systemic toxicity).

If a decision is made to initiate therapy in these select patients, the choice of drug may be problematic because of high levels of antibiotic resistance to ampicillin or TMP-SMX; currently, a fluoroquinolone is the drug of first choice. For patients with sensitive strains, ampicillin or

Table 104–11   Indications for Antibiotic Therapy in *Salmonella* Gastroenteritis

Abnormal cardiovascular system
   Aneurysms
   Prosthetic heart valves
   Valvular heart disease
   Vascular grafts
Extreme ages of life
Hemolytic anemia
Immunosuppression
   AIDS
   Congenital and acquired immunosuppressive disorders
   Glucorticoid treatment
   Organ transplants
Lymphoproliferative disorders
   Leukemia
   Lymphoma
Malignancies
Pregnancy
Prosthetic orthopedic devices
Sepsis

AIDS, acquired immunodeficiency syndrome.

TMP-SMX can be used (Table 104–12). The quinolones, particularly ciprofloxacin, are highly active in vitro and have shown good results in patients with enteric fever[181] and in chronic carriers.[182] Ciprofloxacin therapy in patients with uncomplicated *Salmonella* gastroenteritis, however, has led to a high relapse rate that is associated with more prolonged fecal excretion of salmonellae than seen in placebo-treated control subjects.[179] As might be expected, resistance to ciprofloxacin has been observed during therapy.[183]

Table 104–12 Antibiotic Therapy for Bacterial Enteropathogens in Adults

Organism/Syndrome	Recommended Antibiotics	Alternative Antibiotics
Shigella	Ciprofloxacin 500 mg twice daily × 3 days	Norfloxacin 400 mg twice daily × 3 days TMP-SMX 160 mg/800 mg twice daily × 3 days Nalidixic acid 1 g three times daily-four times daily × 5 days
Salmonella		
Gastroenteritis—uncomplicated	None	
Gastroenteritis—severe, immunocompromised patients, pregnant women, prostheses, cancer	Ciprofloxacin 500 mg twice daily × 7 days	TMP-SMX 160 mg/800 mg twice daily × 7 days Ceftriaxone 1 g IV twice daily × 7 days Tetracycline 500 mg four times daily × 7 days
Bacteremia and localized infection*		Cefotaxime, especially for meningitis or vascular infection, 2 g q 4-6 hr
	Chloramphenicol 50 mg/kg/day in four divided doses (not for use in vascular infections) Ampicillin 1 g q 4-6 hr Amoxicillin 1 g q 6-8 hr TMP 10/50 mg/kg/day + SMX 50 mg/kg/day in four divided doses	Ciprofloxacin 750 mg twice daily, especially long term for prevention of bacteremia relapse in patients with AIDS
Typhoid and enteric fevers	Chloramphenicol 500 mg PO or IV q 8 hr for at least 2 wk	Amoxicillin 1 g four times daily × 2 wk Ciprofloxacin 500 mg twice daily × 7-14 days TMP-SMX 160 mg/800 mg 1 or 2 tablets twice daily × 2 wk
Campylobacter jejuni		
Mild gastroenteritis	None	
Severe or prolonged gastroenteritis	Erythromycin 250 mg twice daily × 5 days	Ciprofloxacin 500 mg twice daily Norfloxacin 400 mg twice daily
Campylobacter fetus	Ampicillin and gentamicin IV	Erythromycin 0.25-1 g q 6 hr
Yersinia enterocolitica	Not usually required Tetracycline 500 mg four times daily TMP-SMX 160 mg/800 mg twice daily Ciprofloxacin 500 mg twice daily	Chloramphenicol 50 mg/kg/day in four divided doses An aminoglycoside
Escherichia coli		
Enteroinvasive	No controlled studies: consider empirical therapy Ciprofloxacin 500 mg twice daily Norfloxacin 500 mg twice daily	TMP-SMX 160 mg/800 mg twice daily
Enterotoxigenic	Ciprofloxacin 500 mg twice daily Norfloxacin 500 mg twice daily Rifaxamin 500 mg twice daily × 3 days	TMP-SMX 160 mg/800 mg twice daily
Enteropathogenic	No controlled studies: consider empirical therapy Ciprofloxacin 500 mg twice daily Norfloxacin 500 mg twice daily	TMP-SMX 160 mg/800 mg twice daily
Enterohemorrhagic	Unclear if antibiotics are effective; may be harmful	
Vibrio cholerae	Tetracycline 500 mg q 6 hr × 3 days	Ciprofloxacin 500 mg twice daily × 3 days Doxycycline 300 mg once or 100 mg once daily × 3 days
Vibrio parahaemolyticus	Supportive therapy	
Vibrio vulnificus and *Vibrio alginolyticus*	Tetracycline 500 mg four times daily or 0.5-1 g IV q 12 hr	Chloramphenicol 50 mg/kg/day four times daily Penicillin G > 20 million units/day IV

All antibiotics are administered orally unless otherwise indicated.
*Bacteremia is treated for 10-14 days; endocarditis and osteomyelitis are treated for ≥ 4-6 wk.
AIDS, acquired immunodeficiency syndrome; IV, intravenous; PO, orally; TMP-SMX, trimethoprim-sulfamethoxazole.
From Giannella RA: Treatment of acute infectious diarrhea. In Wolfe M (ed): Therapy of Digestive Disorders: A Companion to Sleisinger and Fordtran's Gastrointestinal and Liver Disease, 2nd ed. Elsevier, London. 2006.

During the past decade there has been an increase in the isolation of quinolone-resistant *Salmonella* isolates in Europe, especially from cattle.[184] The use of quinolones for veterinary use has been blamed for this rise in resistance. The strain of *S. typhimurium* known as definitive phage type 104 (DT104) often is multidrug resistant, but until recently, this strain has remained susceptible to the quinolones. Resistance to ceftriaxone of a *Salmonella* strain from livestock also has been observed recently in the United States.[185] As a consequence of the increasing levels of drug resistance, both domestically and internationally, antimicrobial therapy of *Salmonella* infections must be limited to high-risk patients and should be based on sensitivity testing.

TYPHOID FEVER

Typhoid (Greek: *typhos*, stupor or cloudy) fever is a febrile illness of prolonged duration, marked by hectic fever, delirium, persistent bloodstream infection, splenic enlargement, abdominal pain, and a variety of systemic manifestations. The illness caused by this pathogen differs from the nontyphoidal *Salmonella* infections in several respects. Typhoidal disease is not truly an intestinal disease and has more systemic than intestinal symptoms; it clearly differs from the usual form of gastroenteritis produced by nontyphoidal strains of *Salmonella*. *S. typhi* is remarkably adapted to humans, who represent the only natural reservoir; the other salmonellae are associated with animals.

Although *S. typhi* is the main cause of typhoid fever, other *Salmonella* serotypes occasionally produce a similar clinical picture, known variously as *typhoidal disease, enteric fever,* or *paratyphoid fever*. These serotypes are *S. paratyphi, S. schottmülleri* (formerly *S. paratyphi* B), and *S. hirschfeldii* (formerly *S. paratyphi* C), as well as others, such as *S. typhimurium*.

Microbiology

S. typhi is biochemically similar to other salmonellae and is distinguished primarily by its specific antigens. As a rule, this organism produces little or no gas from carbohydrates, elaborates only small amounts of hydrogen sulfide, and bears the Vi antigen on its surface. These markers should alert the laboratory to the possibility of this pathogen; confirmation of *S. typhi* is accomplished by serotyping.

Pathogenic Mechanisms

The pathologic events of typhoid fever are initiated in the intestinal tract after oral ingestion of typhoid bacilli.[16] The organism penetrates the small bowel mucosa and makes its way rapidly to the lymphatics, the mesenteric nodes, and, within minutes, the bloodstream. There is a paucity of local inflammatory findings, which explains the lack of intestinal symptoms at this early stage. This sequence of events is in marked contrast to that of other forms of salmonellosis and shigellosis, in which intestinal findings are prominent at the onset.

After the initial bacteremia, the organism is sequestered in macrophages and monocytic cells of the reticuloendothelial system. It undergoes multiplication and re-emerges several days later in recurrent waves of bacteremia, an event that initiates the symptomatic phase of infection. Now in great numbers, the organism is spread throughout the host and infects many organ sites. The intestinal tract may be seeded by direct bacteremic spread to Peyer's patches in the terminal ileum or via drainage of contaminated bile from the gallbladder, which often harbors large numbers of organisms.

Hyperplasia of the reticuloendothelial system, including lymph nodes, liver, and spleen, is characteristic of typhoid fever. The liver contains discrete micronodular areas of necrosis surrounded by macrophages and lymphocytes. Inflammation of the gallbladder is common and may lead to acute cholecystitis. Patients with preexisting gallbladder disease have a penchant for becoming carriers, because the bacillus becomes intimately associated with the existing chronic infection and may be incorporated within gallstones. Lymphoid follicles in the gut, such as Peyer's patches, become hyperplastic, with infiltration of macrophages, lymphocytes, and red blood cells. Subsequently, a follicle may ulcerate, penetrate through the submucosa to the intestinal lumen, and discharge large numbers of typhoid bacilli. As the bowel wall progressively is involved, it becomes paper-thin (most commonly in the terminal ileum), and is susceptible to perforation into the peritoneal cavity. Erosion into blood vessels produces severe intestinal hemorrhage.

Epidemiology

Improvements in environmental sanitation have reduced the incidence of typhoid fever in industrialized nations. Approximately 400 to 500 cases occur each year in the United States, chiefly in young people. Large-scale epidemics of typhoid occur on a regular basis in developing countries and are usually traced to contaminated food that is imported from an endemic area or to contaminated water supplies.[186]

Because *S. typhi* cohabits exclusively with humans, the appearance of a case could indicate the presence of a carrier. An investigation by public health authorities should be instituted to determine the source and the presence of other cases. As they are discovered, chronic carriers are registered with the health authorities, and the particular microorganism is phage-typed so that it can be traced in the event of an outbreak. Registered carriers represent only some of the potential reservoir, however, and do not take into account imported cases of typhoid, which represent more than 70% of the acute infections in the United States.[187]

Clinical Features

In its classic form without treatment, typhoid fever lasts about 4 weeks and evolves in a manner consistent with the pathologic events. The illness is described traditionally as a series of 1-week stages, although this pattern may be altered in mild cases and by antibiotic treatment.[188] The incubation period is generally 7 to 14 days, with wide variations at either extreme. During the *first week,* high fever, headache, and abdominal pain are common. The pulse is often slower than would be expected for the degree of fever, a finding referred to as *Faget's sign.*

Abdominal pain is localized to the right lower quadrant in most cases but can be diffuse. In approximately 50% of patients, there is no change in bowel habits; in fact, constipation is more common than diarrhea in children with typhoid fever. Near the end of the first week, enlargement of the spleen is noticeable, and an evanescent classic rash (rose spots) becomes manifest, most commonly on the chest.

During the *second week,* the fever becomes more continuous, and the patient looks sick and withdrawn. During the *third week,* the patient's illness evolves into the "typhoidal state," with disordered mentation and, in some cases, extreme toxemia. It is from this altered mental state that the term *typhoid* derives. In this period there is often intestinal involvement, manifested clinically by greenish "pea-soup" diarrhea and the dire complications of intestinal perforation and hemorrhage. The *fourth week* brings slackening of the fever and improvement in the clinical status, if the patient survives and recovers.

Typhoid fever is a less severe illness in previously healthy adults who seek medical attention for the earliest symptoms of fever, lassitude, and headache than it is in those who wait. Prompt diagnosis and appropriate therapy interrupt the classic 4-week scenario and produce an aborted illness consisting of little more than a few days of fever and malaise.

Because the typhoid bacillus is disseminated widely through recurrent waves of bacteremia, many organ sites can be involved. Patients with typhoid fever can have pneumonia, pyelonephritis, and metastatic infections of bone, large joints, and the brain. The gallbladder and liver are involved with inflammatory changes. Acute cholecystitis can occur during the initial 2 to 3 weeks, and jaundice, resulting from diffuse hepatic inflammation, has been observed in some patients.

The preeminent complications are intestinal hemorrhage and perforation.[189] These events are most likely to occur in the third week and during convalescence and are not related to the severity of the disease; they tend to occur in the same patient, however, with bleeding serving as a harbinger of possible perforation. Bleeding may be sudden and severe or a slow ooze. Before the availability of antibiotics, the frequency of hemorrhage was 20% in various series; it is less frequent since specific treatment has become available. Approximately 3% of patients with typhoid fever experience intestinal perforation, most commonly in the ileum.[190] Onset of perforation may be sudden, with signs of an acute abdomen, or there may be a leak of intraluminal contents to form an abscess in the lower quadrant or pelvis, producing a more insidious course.

After defervescence has occurred and the patient has apparently "ridden through the storm," a potential for recurrence remains. Relapse generally occurs 8 to 10 days after cessation of drug therapy and consists of a reenactment of the major manifestations. The organism is the same as the one that caused the original infection, with the identical antimicrobial susceptibility pattern.

Carriers

After 6 weeks, approximately 50% of typhoid victims still shed organisms in their feces. This figure declines progressively, and after 3 months only 5% to 10% are excreters; by 1 year the frequency is 1% to 3%.[191] The chronic carrier is identified by positive stool cultures for *S. typhi* at least 1 year after the acute episode or, in some cases, positive stool cultures without a documented history of disease. The probability of spontaneously aborting the carrier state is highly unlikely after this time. Chronic carriers are more common in older age groups, women (a 3:1 ratio of women to men), and persons with biliary disease. The organism usually is harbored in the gallbladder, although occasionally it is carried in the large intestine without involvement of the biliary tract.

Diagnosis

The diagnosis of typhoid fever is established by isolating the organism. Blood culture is the primary diagnostic test, is positive in 90% of patients during the first week, and remains positive for several weeks thereafter if the patient is untreated. Bone marrow culture also has a high yield, even in treated patients.[192] Stool cultures become positive in the second and third weeks. Sampling duodenal contents by a "string test" yields a positive culture in 70% of patients. By the third week, urine cultures reveal the organism in approximately 25% of patients. The titer of agglutinins against somatic (O) antigen (Widal test) rises during the second and third weeks of illness. An O titer of 1:80 or more in a nonimmunized person is suggestive of typhoid fever, and a titer of 1:320 usually is diagnostic in the appropriate clinical setting; a fourfold rise in titer provides stronger evidence. Although the H antigen is less specific than the O titer and is likely to be elevated from prior immunization or by infection with other enteric bacteria, an initial H antigen titer of 1:640 is strongly suggestive of typhoid fever. There are many false-positive and occasional false-negative Widal reactions, so that diagnosis based on a rise in titer alone is tenuous. Serologic tests have become available and permit rapid diagnosis of typhoid fever with a higher sensitivity and specificity relative to blood culture than the Widal test.[173] PCR assays for the diagnosis of *S. typhi* have been developed, but these are still research tools.

Treatment (see Table 104–12)

Drug resistance, mediated by plasmids, occurs among typhoid bacilli. Most strains are susceptible to chloramphenicol and ampicillin, although notable epidemics with strains resistant to either or both of these drugs have been reported in recent years. Hence, a great effort should be made in each case to isolate the organism and perform drug susceptibility tests. Chloramphenicol has high activity against most clinical isolates of typhoid bacilli. The response to therapy is remarkably constant, and defervescence regularly occurs 3 to 5 days after treatment is begun.[189] The clinical condition improves within 1 to 2 days, with decreased toxemia and slowly declining fever. In adults, chloramphenicol should be given in a total daily dose of 2g, administered in four equally divided doses by mouth. Occasionally, in very sick patients it may be necessary to give the drug by the intravenous route in the same total daily dose. Oral medication can be given after improvement in the clinical status. Chloramphenicol is well absorbed from the intestinal tract but is rather poorly absorbed from intramuscular sites; the intramuscular route is to be avoided. The duration of treatment is 2 weeks; prolongation of this treatment does not reduce the frequency of complications or carriers. Intestinal perforation and hemorrhage can occur during apparently successful treatment. Relapse may follow an otherwise uneventful course and should be treated with the same drug as was used initially.

Ampicillin has been recommended as alternative therapy but has been disappointing in comparison with chloramphenicol.[188,193] Amoxicillin, a closely related drug, provides better absorption and increased efficacy. Several studies have shown that amoxicillin, in doses of 4 g/day in four divided doses, has good activity. TMP-SMX also has been used in the therapy of typhoid fever with good results.

The advent of plasmid-mediated multidrug resistance and newer potentially more effective antimicrobial agents, such as the quinolones and third-generation cephalosporins, has led to a reevaluation of the treatment of typhoid fever. The fluoroquinolones, ciprofloxacin and ofloxacin, have been found to be highly effective therapy for infections caused by multidrug-resistant *S. typhi* and *S. paratyphi*. Long-term fecal carriage of *S. typhi* is a rare event in patients treated with quinolones. A 10- to 14-day course of a quinolone has proved highly effective for the treatment of enteric fever, with cure rates consistently close to 100%.[72] The only exception has been norfloxacin, which has provided slightly lower cure rates of 83% to 90%.[72] Defervescence generally occurs within 3 to 5 days of initiating therapy.

The optimal length of fluoroquinolone therapy for typhoid fever has not been fully elucidated. A number of studies have shown that courses of therapy ranging from 7 to 14 days provide a high degree of success. However, courses of therapy shorter than 5 to 6 days have been associated with unacceptable levels of failure.[72] The duration of fever before treatment, severity of infection at the time of presentation, and time to defervescence are factors that must be considered when determining the duration of fluoroquinolone therapy in a patient with enteric fever. Certain caveats should be made regarding the fluoroquinolones. The frequency of resistance of *S. typhi* to ciprofloxacin has been increasing gradually, especially in the Indian subcontinent, central Asia, and Vietnam.[186,194,195]

Third-generation cephalosporins such as cefotaxime, ceftriaxone, and cefoperazone also have been used successfully to treat typhoid fever; courses as short as 3 days have been shown to be as effective as the usual 10- to 14-day regimens.[196,197] By contrast, one trial that compared a 5-day course of ofloxacin with a 7-day course of cefixime found that the median fever clearance time was significantly longer and the rate of treatment failure was higher in children treated with cefixime.[198]

Glucocorticoids are administered for severe toxemia and fever and may produce a dramatic response in patients with profound sepsis.[199] Glucocorticoids should be given in high doses, 60 mg/day of prednisone divided into four doses, and tapered rapidly over the next 3 days. The wide experience with glucocorticoid treatment has failed to show any adverse effects, although the potential for masking intestinal perforation always is present.

Glucocorticoids should be reserved for patients with severe toxicity.

Studies have emphasized the importance of aggressive surgical intervention in typhoid fever.[190,200,201] Indications for surgery are progressive peritoneal signs or abscess formation. Closure of the perforation coupled with broad-spectrum antibiotics has resulted in reduced mortality from this dreaded complication.[201] However, the ileum may be riddled with multiple perforations, and resection may be required.

A chronic carrier who has been discharging *S. typhi* for longer than 1 year can be treated with antimicrobials in an attempt to eliminate the infection. The quinolone antibiotics, such as ciprofloxacin and norfloxacin, have become the treatment of choice in eradicating the carrier state.[202] Reappearance of the carrier state after such treatment generally is associated with gallbladder disease. Cholecystectomy eliminates the carrier state in 85% of carriers with gallstones or chronic cholecystitis but is recommended only for persons whose profession is incompatible with the typhoid carrier state, such as food handlers and health care providers.

Vaccines

Three types of typhoid vaccine are available currently. An acetone-inactivated vaccine affords 55% to 85% protection for 2 to 5 years, but this is not available in the United States. This relative immunity can be overcome by a large inoculum of bacilli. Local pain at the injection site and mild systemic reactions are common with this vaccine. A slightly less effective phenol-inactivated vaccine is available in the United States. A live attenuated *S. typhi* strain, Ty21a, which is given by mouth, produced 96% protection in an initial field trial in Alexandria,[203] but subsequent studies showed less impressive results.[204,205] Although the evidence is inconclusive, it appears that the live attenuated oral vaccine is protective. Because of its low toxicity and ease of administration, this vaccine should be used for travelers to high-risk areas particularly in the developing world. A fourth typhoid vaccine consists of purified Vi capsular polysaccharide and has demonstrated 75% efficacy in a large trial in Nepal.[206] This vaccine has fewer adverse effects than the killed whole cell parenteral vaccines.

CAMPYLOBACTER

The most important *Campylobacter* species found in human infections are *C. jejuni*, a major cause of diarrhea; *C. fetus*, which is generally found in immunocompromised patients; *C. coli*, a rare cause of gastroenteritis; and two new species, *C. cinaedi* and *C. fennelliae*, which are found in male homosexuals. Other species cause diarrhea on rare occasions: *C. hyointestinalis*, *C. upsaliensis*, and *C. laridis*.

The incidence and importance of human *Campylobacter* gastroenteritis have been recognized increasingly in recent years. It is estimated that 4% to 11% of all cases of diarrhea in the United States are caused by *C. jejuni*, and the isolation of *Campylobacter* often exceeds that of *Salmonella* and *Shigella*.[207]

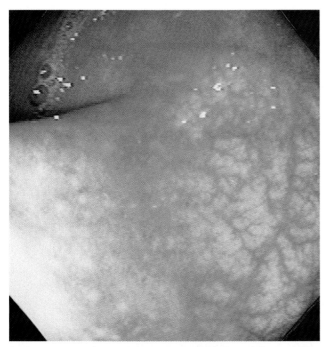

Figure 104-7 Colonoscopic appearance of *Campylobacter* colitis. The colitis is patchy, with areas of erythema and erosion (seen on the *left*). The rectal mucosa on the *right* is hyperemic, but without loss of the mucosal vascular pattern. (From Wilcox CM: Atlas of Clinical Gastrointestinal Endoscopy. Philadelphia, WB Saunders, 1995.)

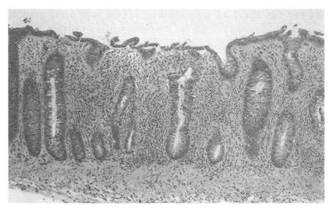

Figure 104-8 Photomicrograph of a patient with acute self limited colitis, the cause of which could have been *Campylobacter, Salmonella, Escherichia coli,* or any one of a number of other bacteria. The presence of inflammatory cells in the basal epithelium and straight glands without architectural distortion or branching helps differentiate acute colitis from chronic colitis. (Courtesy of Feldman's online Atlas, Current Medicine.)

The organism is isolated only rarely from fecal samples of asymptomatic persons, except in the tropics, where the incidence of *Campylobacter* infections is higher and there are many asymptomatic carriers.

Epidemiology

Transmission to humans appears to occur most commonly from infected animals and their food products. The reservoir for *Campylobacter* is enormous, because many animals can be infected, including cattle, sheep, swine, birds (poultry and others), and dogs. Furthermore, the organism has been isolated from fresh and salt water. Most human infections are related to consumption of improperly cooked or contaminated foods. Just as for *Salmonella,* chicken seems to be the major source, accounting for 50% to 70% of infections in some surveys.[208]

Clinical Features

The incubation period is 24 to 72 hours after organisms are ingested but can extend as long as 10 days. There is a wide spectrum of clinical illness, from frank dysentery to watery diarrhea to asymptomatic excretion.[209] Diarrhea and fever almost are invariable (90%). Abdominal pain is usually present (70%), and the patient may note bloody stools (50%). Constitutional symptoms such as headache, myalgia, backache, malaise, anorexia, and vomiting are frequent. Stool examination suggests colitis on the basis of fecal leukocytes and occult blood.[209] Endoscopy may reveal an inflammatory colitis (Figs. 104-7 and 104-8). The duration of illness usually is less than 1 week, although symptoms can persist for 2 weeks or more, and

relapses occur in as many as 25% of patients. Prolonged carriage of *Campylobacter* for 2 to 10 weeks after the onset of illness occurs in 16% of patients.[210]

Infections rarely may be complicated by gastrointestinal hemorrhage, toxic megacolon, pancreatitis, cholecystitis, HUS, bacteremia, meningitis, and purulent arthritis.[209] Postinfectious complications include reactive arthritis, usually in patients with the HLA-B27 phenotype, Guillain-Barré syndrome,[209,211] and immunoproliferative small intestinal disease.[212]

Diagnosis

Although certain clinical features suggest the diagnosis of *Campylobacter* rather than other pathogens, the diagnosis only can be established by culture. Features suggestive of *Campylobacter* infection are (1) a prodrome consisting of constitutional symptoms with coryza, headache, and generalized malaise; (2) a prolonged, often biphasic diarrheal illness presenting initially with diarrhea, followed by slight improvement and then by increasing severity; and (3) many white and red blood cells on microscopic examination of the stool.

The most reliable way to diagnose *Campylobacter* gastroenteritis is by stool culture. A selective isolation medium containing antibiotics must be used because *Campylobacter* organisms grow more slowly than do other enteric bacteria; the plates are grown at 42°C under CO_2 and reduced oxygen conditions. Dark-field or phase-contrast microscopy of fresh diarrheal stool shows the organism as a curved highly motile rod, with darting corkscrew movements.

Treatment (see Table 104-12)

Although *C. jejuni* is sensitive to erythromycin in vitro, three controlled therapeutic trials with this drug have shown no effect on the clinical course when compared with placebo.[213] One study showed some clinical benefit when the antibiotic was started within 3 days of the onset of symptoms. A delay in therapy beyond 4 days produces no clinical improvement; however, fecal excretion of the organism is reduced by erythromycin. The fluoroquinolone antibiotics, such as ciprofloxacin, also are active against these organisms.[214] Resistance to fluoroquinolones has been observed during the course of treatment for *Campylobacter* diarrhea.[215,216] Resistance to the fluoroquinolones is a major problem in some parts of the developing world. A study of U.S. military personnel in Thailand found that 50% of isolates were resistant to ciprofloxacin, whereas none was resistant to azithromycin.[217] A large study of human *Campylobacter* isolates in Minnesota found a rise in quinolone resistance from 1.3% to 10.2% between 1992 and 1998.[218] Factors associated with resistance of *Campylobacter* species to the quinolones include foreign travel and local patterns of fluoroquinolone use, especially if these agents are used in animal husbandry.[218,219] In locales where quinolone resistance is common, azithromycin has been shown to be superior to ciprofloxacin in decreasing the excretion of *Campylobacter* species and equivalent in terms of reducing the duration of symptoms.[217]

Mild cases of *Campylobacter* do not benefit from antibiotic therapy, but treatment should be given, early if possible, to patients with dysentery and those with high fever suggestive of bacteremia. Because of the difficulty in making an etiologic diagnosis on clinical grounds, a quinolone antibiotic should be used empirically because of its activity against *Campylobacter*, *Shigella*, and other enteric pathogens.

YERSINIA

Y. enterocolitica is an important intestinal pathogen that causes a spectrum of clinical illnesses from simple gastroenteritis to invasive ileitis and colitis.[220] It is a non-lactose-fermenting, urease-positive, Gram-negative rod. More than 50 serogroups and 5 biotypes have been identified.[220] Pathogenic mechanisms include the ability to invade epithelial cells and the production of a heat-stable enterotoxin, which is elaborated at 25°C but not at 37°C. Not all strains have these pathogenic properties.

The organism targets for invasion the epithelium overlying Peyer's patches, after which it proliferates within the follicles and spreads to the lamina propria. The abilities to attach to and penetrate epithelial cells are determined by the *inv* gene, which encodes a 103-kd protein known as *invasin*.[221]

Epidemiology

Yersinia gastroenteritis has been reported more frequently in Scandinavian and other European countries than in the United States. Several epidemics have been related to the consumption of contaminated milk and ice cream. The organism can be found in stream and lake water and has been isolated from many animals, including puppies, cats, cows, pigs, chickens, and horses. Animals, either as pets or food sources, are believed to be involved in the transmission of this disease.[222]

The serotypes most frequently involved in Scandinavia and Europe are 0:3 and 0:9, and Canada has many serotype 0:3 isolates.[223] Most of the isolates in the United States are serotype 0:8. Serogroups O:8 and O:5,27 have been responsible for most episodes of invasive disease in the United States.

Clinical Features

Several clinical syndromes have been described with *Yersinia* and tend to vary with the age of the patient and the underlying disease state.[220,224] Enterocolitis is the most common clinical condition, accounting for two thirds of all reported cases. This illness occurs most frequently in children younger than 5 years of age.[221,224] Presentation is nonspecific, with fever, abdominal cramps, and diarrhea, usually lasting 1 to 3 weeks. Microscopic examination of the fecal effluent reveals leukocytes and red blood cells in most instances. Profuse watery diarrhea, possibly related to the enterotoxin, also can occur. Diarrhea can persist for several weeks and may raise the possibility of inflammatory bowel disease. Radiographic findings, particularly in prolonged cases, are most intense in the terminal ileum and may resemble those of Crohn's disease[225]; most patients, however, have normal findings on endoscopy, intestinal biopsy, and barium studies.[223]

In children older than 5 years of age, mesenteric adenitis and associated ileitis have been described. Accompanying symptoms include nausea, vomiting, and aphthous ulcers in the mouth. Affected children often undergo a laparotomy, at which time enlarged mesenteric nodes and an ulcerated ileitis are observed. The condition may be confused clinically with acute appendicitis, although ultrasonography can be useful in separating these processes.[226] *Yersinia* is less likely to cause severe disease in adults, in whom acute diarrhea may be followed 2 to 3 weeks later by joint symptoms and rash (erythema nodosum or erythema multiforme), reminiscent of Reiter's syndrome. Reactive polyarthritis occurs in 2% of patients with yersiniosis, usually in persons positive for HLA-B27. *Yersinia* antigens can be detected in synovial fluid cells[227] and in intestinal mucosal biopsies, and specific IgA antibodies are found in the blood.[228]

Yersinia bacteremia is a relatively uncommon condition that is seen in patients with underlying diseases such as malignancy, diabetes mellitus, anemia, and liver disease. Metastatic foci can occur in bones, joints, and lungs.

The diagnosis of yersiniosis is established by culture of stool or body fluids. Because the organism resembles coliforms and therefore is easily missed on the culture plate, the laboratory should be advised of the suspicion of this infection. Serologic tests have proved useful in Europe and Canada[229] but have not provided much help for the cases reported in the United States.[230]

Treatment (see Table 104–12)

Y. enterocolitica strains are susceptible to several antimicrobial agents, including chloramphenicol, gentamicin, tetracycline, TMP-SMX, and fluoroquinolones, but they are resistant to penicillins and cephalosporins. There is no substantial evidence that antibiotics alter the course of the gastrointestinal infection[220,230]; indeed, the diagnosis often is established late in the course when the patient is improving spontaneously. Antibiotics should be used in more severe intestinal infections, particularly those masquerading as appendicitis. For the chronic relapsing form of diarrhea, antibiotic therapy has not proved useful. Septicemia in the immunocompromised patient is associated with a high mortality, with no apparent benefit from antibiotics, although treatment is mandatory in this setting.

VIRAL PATHOGENS

The major causes of acute gastroenteritis in the United States and in the rest of the world are viruses, which account for 30% to 40% of acute episodes of diarrhea. The leading human pathogens can be grouped into five categories: rotavirus, calicivirus including Norwalk virus, enteric adenovirus, astrovirus, and torovirus (Table 104–13).[231]

ROTAVIRUS

Rotavirus is a group of viruses that was discovered in 1973, in studies of Australian children with diarrhea in whom viral particles were identified in duodenal biopsy specimens by electron microscopy. Rotavirus infection is now recognized to be worldwide in distribution.

Microbiology

The virus measures 70 to 75 nanometers in diameter and contains a double-walled outer capsid (Fig. 104–9) and segmented double-stranded RNA. The virus has an icosahedral structure resembling the spokes of a wheel, hence the name "rota." Highly stable to heat, ether, and mild acids, the virus can be maintained in prolonged storage.

Three groups of rotavirus, A, B, and C, cause disease in humans. Group A rotavirus contains four common serotypes, which are the leading pathogens and cause severe gastroenteritis in young children worldwide.[231,232] Group B rotavirus is responsible for large outbreaks of

Table 104–13   Medical Importance and Epidemiologic and Clinical Features of Human Gastroenteritis Viruses

Virus	Medical Importance Demonstrated	Epidemiologic Features	Clinical Features	Laboratory Diagnostic Tests*
Rotavirus				
Group A	Yes	A major cause of endemic severe diarrhea in infants and young children worldwide (in winter in temperate zone)	Dehydrating diarrhea for 5-7 days; vomiting and fever are common	Immunoassay, electron microscopy, PAGE
Group B	Partially	Large outbreaks in adults and children in China	Severe watery diarrhea for 3-5 days	Electron microscopy, PAGE
Group C	Partially	Sporadic cases in young children worldwide	Similar to features of group A rotavirus	Electron microscopy, PAGE
Calicivirus	Yes	Causes diarrhea in children; associated with ingestion of contaminated shellfish and other foods in adults	Rotavirus-like illness in children; Norovirus-like in adults	Immunoassay, electron microscopy
Norovirus	Yes	Epidemics of vomiting and diarrhea in older children and adults; occurs in families, communities, and nursing homes; often associated with ingestion of shellfish, other food, or water	Acute vomiting, diarrhea, fever, myalgias, and headache lasting 1-2 days	Immunoassay, immune electron microscopy
Norwalk-like viruses (small, round structured viruses)	Partially	Similar to characteristics of Norovirus	Acute vomiting, diarrhea, fever, myalgias, and headache lasting 1-2 days	Immunoassay, immune electron microscopy
Enteric adenovirus	Yes	Endemic diarrhea of infants and young children	Prolonged diarrhea lasting 5-12 days; vomiting and fever	Immunoassay, electron microscopy with PAGE
Astrovirus	Yes	Causes diarrhea in children; reported in nursing homes	Watery diarrhea, often lasting 2-3 days, occasionally longer	Immunoassay, electron microscopy
Torovirus	Yes	Causes acute and persistent diarrhea in children; increased risk in immunocompromised children; occurs in community and hospital settings	Dehydrating, watery, occasionally bloody diarrhea with vomiting and abdominal pain; usually lasts 5-7 days	Immunoassay, electron microscopy

*Laboratory diagnostic tests, other than those for rotavirus group A, are usually available only in specialized research or diagnostic referral laboratories. Immunoassays are usually enzyme-linked immunosorbent assays or radioimmunoassays.
  PAGE, polyacrylamide-gel electrophoresis and silver staining of viral nucleic acid in stool.
  Modified from Blacklow NR, Greenberg HB: Viral gastroenteritis. N Engl J Med 325:252, 1991.

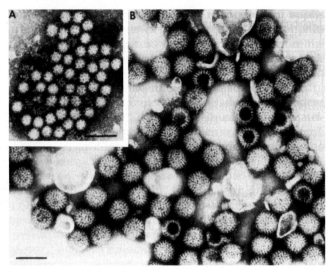

Figure 104–9 *A,* Electron micrograph of the Norovirus particle and aggregate from the stool of a volunteer to whom the Norwalk agent was administered. (Bar = 100 nm). *B,* Human rotavirus particles from the stool of an infant with gastroenteritis. The particles appear to have a double-shelled capsid. Occasional "empty" particles are seen. (Bar = 100 nm). (*A* and *B,* Courtesy of A. Kapikian, MD. Previously published in Lennete EH, Schmidt NJ: Diagnostic Procedures for Viral, Rickettsial, and Chlamydial Infections, 5th ed. New York, American Public Health Association, 1979, p 933.)

diarrhea in children and adults in China but is otherwise a rare isolate. Group C rotavirus causes disease in various parts of the world infrequently.

Pathology and Pathogenesis

Duodenal biopsy specimens of young children with rotavirus infection have demonstrated a patchy abnormality of the upper intestine.[233] In its severe form, the infection can produce denuded villi and flattening of the epithelial surface that can persist for 3 to 8 weeks. The morphologic changes are accompanied by physiologic abnormalities such as decreased xylose absorption and reduced brush border levels of disaccharidases. Rotavirus causes diarrhea by elaborating an enterotoxin and by activating the enteric nervous system, both of which stimulate intestinal secretion and diarrhea.[234,235]

Epidemiology

Rotavirus is responsible for childhood diarrhea in 35% of hospitalized and 10% to 30% of community-based cases.[232,236] The virus appears to be spread by the fecal-oral route. In temperate zones, the disease is more common in winter, but in the tropics it is endemic year-round. Within a family, the young child often is afflicted with clinical illness, whereas older siblings and adults can excrete the virus asymptomatically.

Clinical Features

Rotavirus causes a range of clinical illness from asymptomatic carriage to severe dehydration and even fatality.[237] The disease occurs principally in children 3 to 15 months of age; infections continue into the second year

of life but are less common thereafter. Mild infections with group A rotaviruses can develop in adults and usually are acquired from a sick child in the household. Vomiting often heralds the illness and is followed shortly by watery diarrhea. The incubation period is 1 to 3 days, and the average duration of illness is 5 to 7 days, although some instances of chronic diarrhea have been noted. Excretion of virus for as long as 3 to 8 weeks occurs in approximately one third of infected children.[238]

Diagnosis

Rapid diagnosis is achieved by detection of rotavirus antigen in the feces with several commercial immunoassays. PCR and nucleic acid probes also are available to detect the virus and identify its serogroups.[239,240]

Immunity

After infection with rotavirus, antibody develops in serum and intestinal secretions.[241] The antibody is active against the specific serotype and crosses over to other serotypes.[242,243] Natural rotavirus infection has a protective efficacy of 93% against recurrent rotavirus disease.[243] Levels of antibody in either serum or intestinal fluids do not correlate precisely with protection, a finding that has raised the possibility that cellular immunity plays a role as well.

Infants are protected for at least the first 3 months of life by maternal antibodies, although there is no convincing evidence that breast-feeding provides complete protection against this infection.[244] In addition to the possible protective role of maternal antibodies in breast milk, human milk mucin appears to have a potent antirotaviral activity in vitro and in a mouse model of infection.[245] The glycoprotein lactadherin binds specifically to all human rotavirus strains and inhibits their infectivity. Higher breast milk concentrations of lactadherin have been associated with protection against symptomatic rotavirus infection.[246]

Treatment

Because loss of fluids and electrolytes appears to be the main pathophysiologic event, rehydration is the mainstay of therapy for this infection. Field studies have established that the oral rehydration solutions (ORSs) consisting of glucose and electrolytes are effective in restoring fluid balance.[247] Rotavirus vaccines are derived from related animal rotaviruses or genetic reassortants of various human and animal strains.[248] A tetravalent rhesus-human reassortant rotavirus (RotaShield), which provided moderate protection against all severities of rotavirus gastroenteritis and excellent protection against severe dehydrating disease, was licensed for use among infants in the United States in 1998.[248] Post-licensing recognition of intussusception as an uncommon serious complication of the live attenuated rotavirus vaccine, however, led to the withdrawal of recommendations for its use.[249]

Antirotavirus immunoglobulin of bovine colostral origin has been found to be effective in reducing the duration of rotavirus infection and the amount of oral rehydration therapy required.[250]

CALICIVIRUS

Caliciviruses (Greek: *kalyx,* the cup of a flower) are single-stranded RNA viruses that are responsible for human and animal infections. Recent molecular studies have reclassified various enteric viruses (Norwalk, Snow Mountain, Montgomery, Sapporo, and so forth) and on the basis of genetic composition placed them in the taxonomic family of caliciviruses.[251]

The typical caliciviruses cause disease mainly in infants and young children.[252,253] Calicivirus disease is particularly common in day-care centers, where it accounts for more diarrhea than is attributed to bacterial infections.[252] The illness generally is mild and indistinguishable from that of rotavirus or even epidemic Norwalk disease.

Norovirus and Norwalk-Like Virus

Norwalk virus, newly named norovirus, was named for a 1968 outbreak of "winter vomiting disease" in Norwalk, Ohio. The group includes many small viruses, each named after the site of an outbreak of gastroenteritis: Norwalk, Hawaii, Snow Mountain, Montgomery, Taunton, Otofuke, and Sapporo. These small viral agents measure 27 to 35 nanometers,[254] and all contain a single structural protein with single-stranded RNA. This group of viruses is identified as the pathogen in approximately 40% of nonbacterial epidemics of diarrhea in the United States. The virus also has been encountered in Hawaii, England, Australia, and Japan.[231]

The Norwalk virus causes explosive epidemics of diarrhea that sweep through a community and have a high attack rate. The virus shows no respect for age and preys on virtually all age groups, except infants. Transmission occurs by person-to-person contact, primarily by the fecal-oral route. Raw shellfish also is a major source of infection; during an 8-month period in 1982, 103 outbreaks of Norwalk virus infection in New York State were related to ingestion of raw clams or oysters.[255] This virus is a major cause of outbreaks of gastroenteritis in camps, cruise ships, nursing homes, and hospitals.[256] It also can contaminate drinking water supplies.[257]

Pathology and Pathogenesis

The upper small intestine is the focus of attack. Intestinal biopsies reveal patchy mucosal lesions. Because the virus is so small, in contrast to rotavirus, Norwalk viral particles cannot be observed in electron microscopic sections, Among the physiologic abnormalities observed during illness are malabsorption of fat and xylose, diminished activity of intestinal disaccharidases, and delayed gastric emptying. Morphologic and physiologic abnormalities reverse within 1 to 2 weeks after infection.

Clinical Features

The disease has a spectrum of symptoms and signs, all mild. In one outbreak of the Norwalk agent, diarrhea was noted in 92% of proved cases, nausea in 88%, abdominal cramps in 67%, vomiting in 66%, and muscle aches in 56%.[258] Generally, the clinical illness lasts no longer than 24 to 48 hours.

Because the virus cannot be grown in the laboratory, the diagnosis can be established only by identifying viral antigen in the stool, and these tests currently are available only in research laboratories. The virus also can be seen in fecal effluent by using immune electron microscopy with the aid of serum from a convalescent subject (see Fig. 104–9). A monoclonal antibody-based ELISA and a PCR assay have been developed and can detect Norwalk virus in stool specimens.[259,260] Another option is an ELISA that can measure an IgM antibody response in serum, thereby suggesting a recent infection.

Immunity

Serum antibody titers are low in children, increase in adolescents, and are present in 60% of adults. Volunteer studies have revealed an unusual form of immunity that apparently is not related to antibody formation.[261] Volunteers who became sick during initial challenge were the same ones who became ill when rechallenged 24 to 42 months later. In contrast, those who resisted the initial challenge also resisted the subsequent challenge. Measurement of antibody in serum and intestinal juice showed higher levels of antibody in the volunteers who became ill on both the initial and subsequent challenges. This antibody had some protective value, albeit short-lived, because early rechallenge at 6 to 14 weeks after the initial dose produced protection in the subjects with antibody. Yet this protection did not persist, because the same group with antibody became ill when rechallenged several months later. Thus, it is postulated that nonimmune mechanisms in the intestine resist infection by this virus; repeated infections produce some protection, which is not permanent.

Treatment

No specific treatment for Norwalk virus infection is available. The disease is usually mild, but it can produce dehydration in elderly patients, who may require hospitalization.

ENTERIC ADENOVIRUS

Most adenoviruses cause upper respiratory infections, but a new group of fastidious strains, known as *serotypes 40* and *41*, which constitute subgenus F, are responsible for gastroenteritis in children younger than 2 years of age.[262] and in patients with AIDS. From 5% to 10% of childhood diarrhea is associated with enteric adenovirus. There is no seasonal occurrence.[232] Unlike rotavirus or Norwalk virus, infection with enteric adenovirus has a long incubation period of 8 to 10 days, and the illness can be prolonged for up to 2 weeks. Nosocomial and day-care center outbreaks are common and associated with high rates of asymptomatic infections.[263,264] Adults generally are protected from this infection, although it has been documented to cause diarrhea in immunocompromised individuals with AIDS. The virus cannot be cultured in available cell lines but can be visualized in stool by electron microscopy or with dot-blot hybridization or immunoassays. An enzyme immunoassay licensed by the U.S. Food and Drug Administration (Adenoclone) is available for detection of enteric adenoviruses in stool specimens.

ASTROVIRUS

Astrovirus is a small, nonenveloped, single-stranded RNA virus similar in structure to calicivirus.[265] In adults, the disease has relatively low infectivity, but in children it is a major cause of diarrheal illness. In a study from Thailand, astrovirus was second only to rotavirus as a cause of diarrhea in children.[266] There are at least seven viral serotypes. Antibody develops to many of these serotypes by 4 years of age, indicating that they probably cause infections frequently in childhood.

Astroviruses are responsible for outbreaks of diarrhea in day-care centers and communities with children younger than 12 months old.[264,267,268] The disease is characterized by watery or mucoid stools, nausea, vomiting, and occasionally fever, and tends to be milder than rotavirus diarrhea, with less than 6% of children becoming dehydrated.[266,268] Coinfections with other pathogens are common, and repeated infections may occur as a result of a lack of cross-protective immunity to the multiple serotypes of astrovirus. The virus can be recognized in stool specimens by means of electron microscopy, specific immunoassays, RNA probe hybridization, and PCR methodology, although all these tests remain research tools.[267,269] Treatment is supportive with an emphasis on oral rehydration.

TOROVIRUS

Toroviruses are enveloped single-stranded RNA viruses that cause enteric infections in animals,[270] and which in case-control studies have been demonstrated to cause diarrhea in children.[271,272] In a large prospective study of pediatric viral diarrhea, toroviruses accounted for 3% of episodes, a greater percentage than that for either the caliciviruses or astrovirus.[232] Although most diarrhea from toroviruses occurs in children younger than 2 years of age, older children, especially those who are immunocompromised, are at risk for symptomatic infections.[272]

Toroviruses have been associated with both acute and persistent (lasting > 14 days) diarrhea in children.[271,272] When torovirus has been encountered in children with persistent diarrhea, it is found often in association with other potential pathogens such as EAggEC. When compared with rotavirus infection, children infected with torovirus have less vomiting and more bloody diarrhea, although the latter symptom occurs in only 11% of patients. Toroviruses can be detected in stool specimens by electron microscopy or ELISA. As in other viral diarrheas, treatment is supportive. Fluid replacement is often required for as long as 1 week.[272]

SPECIAL SITUATIONS

HOSPITAL-ACQUIRED DIARRHEA

Acute diarrhea developing in the hospitalized patient may be due to infection with *C. difficile*, a side effect of various medications, ingestion of elixirs containing sorbitol or mannitol, or as a consequence of tube feedings. Antibiotic-associated diarrhea, from *C. difficile* infection, is the most common cause of acute diarrhea in hospitalized patients (see Chapter 105).[273,274] Diarrhea can range from mild illness to life-threatening disease associated with pseudomembranous colitis. This infection can follow treatment with almost any type of enteral or parenteral antibiotic. Because *C. difficile* infection is the single most common cause of diarrhea in hospitalized patients and *Salmonella*, *Shigella*, *Campylobacter*, and parasites are rarely the cause of diarrhea in hospitalized patients, the evaluation of patients in this setting with routine stool examinations for enteric pathogens and stool for ova and parasites is unrewarding and inappropriate.

ACUTE DIARRHEA IN PREGNANCY

Diarrhea in the pregnant patient is potentially a serious problem and infection must be excluded. Appropriate therapy is imperative for the health of both mother and fetus. Dehydration must be avoided because it can be deleterious to placental blood flow. The pregnant woman is at risk for infection with any enteric pathogen. In addition to the usual bacterial and viral pathogens, diarrhea and abdominal pain in the pregnant patient may be from malaria,[275] amoeba,[276] or *Giardia*.[277] In addition to dehydration, certain infectious agents have the ability to cause serious periparturitional complications.

Campylobacter infections in the pregnant patient may cause spontaneous abortion, prematurity, neonatal sepsis, neonatal enterocolitis, and death.[278] The incidence of complications associated with infectious diarrhea in the pregnant patient is unknown. One case series identified *Campylobacter* to be the most common bacterial enteric pathogen isolated from stool cultures of pregnant women with enteritis. Of nine patients infected with *Campylobacter*, two with nontyphoidal *Salmonella*, and one with *E. coli* O157:H7, one infection resulted in premature birth with neonatal sepsis and death and one neonate developed *C. jejuni* enterocolitis.[278]

Gastrointestinal infections can result in premature labor or spontaneous abortion probably as a result of bacteremia and placental infection. In other cases, infants may acquire the infection intrapartum by exposure at the introitus of asymptomatic carrier mothers. *S. sonnei* can occur in neonates born to mothers with asymptomatic shigellosis.[279] Diarrhea, failure to feed, and gastroenteritis, sometimes preceded by a respiratory illness, occurs 2 to 5 days after birth. Septicemia in neonates is more common than in the adult form of this disease. If diagnosed in the pregnant patient, treatment should probably be instituted (although there are no data on which to base this recommendation). Fluoroquinolones or TMP-SMX are not recommended in pregnancy, making ampicillin the choice with least risk to mother and fetus; ceftriaxone also may be used. Infections also may occur from an ascending, transcervical route, possibly resulting in a chorioamnionitis.[280] Salmonellosis in the pregnant patient also should be treated with antibiotics to protect against placental infection.

Treatment during pregnancy is problematic. Drug therapy poses a potential risk to the developing fetus, and such risk must be considered carefully prior to initiation. Sulfa drugs, fluoroquinolones, metronidazole, and tetracyclines should be avoided. Ampicillin and erythromycin are used widely and apparently safe. If mild, treatment of giardiasis can be delayed until after delivery; however, the infant should be closely observed for signs of failure to feed and diarrhea because infection of the fetus may occur during delivery.[277]

TRAVELER'S DIARRHEA

Diarrhea occurring among persons traveling from developed to developing countries is common and affects millions of people each year. Travelers from the United States to Mexico alone number more than 15 million annually, and attack rates in such travelers can be as high as 25% to 50%. Of those afflicted, nearly 30% are ill enough to stay in bed and another 40% must alter their scheduled activities.[281] Fortunately, 90% of cases are brief and self-limited, but 5% to 10% of patients acquire dysentery, and 1% to 2% of travelers will have persistent diarrhea lasting longer than 1 month; in some cases, diarrhea can last longer than 6 months and become a chronic illness (see later).

Microbiology

Traveler's diarrhea is a syndrome, not a specific illness, and is caused mainly by infectious microorganisms that are acquired from food and drink.[282-285] Infectious organisms can be identified in 60% to 80% of cases. Although an array of pathogens has been found, the leading culprits are various forms of *E. coli*, particularly ETEC (Table 104–14). As discussed earlier, this organism causes diarrhea by colonizing the small intestine and secreting heat-stable and/or heat-labile enterotoxins resulting in a secretory diarrhea. *Shigella* species have been encountered in approximately 10% of cases, although the rate of isolation varies from 0% to more than 20%. The disease caused by *Shigella* tends to be more severe than the usual form of traveler's diarrhea. Strains of *Campylobacter* are isolated in as many as 41% of cases, with higher rates during cooler seasons.[285-287] *Salmonella* organisms are

found in fewer than 5% of cases, although the frequency is higher among travelers to Asia than elsewhere. Rotavirus has been identified in approximately 10% of episodes of traveler's diarrhea when this pathogen is sought.[284,288] Among the parasites, *Giardia lamblia* and *Cryptosporidium* are the more common hazards to travelers. The protozoan parasite *Cyclospora cayetanensis* is responsible for traveler's diarrhea in visitors to a number of less developed countries, especially Nepal.[289]

More than one pathogen may be found in travelers with acute diarrhea (up to 15% in Mexico and 33% in Thailand). To confuse the issue further, no pathogens have been identified, despite careful laboratory study, in more than 40% of cases from all parts of the world, although a proportion of these respond to antibiotics, suggesting that unidentified bacteria may be responsible.

Epidemiology

The risk of developing traveler's diarrhea depends on the host's susceptibility, travel and eating habits, length of stay, and, most important, destination. Estimates of attack rates based on questionnaires filled out by returning travelers reveal substantial differences based on destination. Areas of the world having diarrhea attack rates of approximately 40% to 50% include Mexico, South and Central America, the Middle East, Southeast Asia, and Africa. Countries considered to be of moderate risk, with attack rates ranging from 10% to 20%, include most Caribbean islands, China, Japan, Mediterranean countries, Eastern Europe, and republics of the former Soviet Union. Areas with attack rates of less than 8% include Canada, Northern Europe, Australia, the United States, South Africa, the United Kingdom, Germany, and France.[290,291] In summarizing the experiences from 34 prospective studies, a somewhat greater risk emerges: median traveler's diarrhea rates of 53% (21% to 100%) in Latin America, 54% (21% to 100%) in Asia, and 54% (36% to 62%) in Africa.[292]

The national origin of the traveler is another important factor. At an international conference in Mexico held in 1968, participants from the United States and northern Europe had a 36% attack rate, compared with only 8% for colleagues from developing countries and 2% for local Mexicans.[293] Longer residence in a tropical country also leads to increased resistance to traveler's diarrhea, although a high risk of diarrhea persists during the first 2 years of residence.[289] Previous short-term travel to areas of high risk does not necessarily lead to protection.

The purpose of travel and the style of eating also are important factors that influence the risk of developing this illness. The greatest frequency of diarrhea occurs in people traveling as students or itinerant tourists, the lowest risk is in those visiting relatives, and an intermediate risk exists in business travelers.[288] Young travelers, particularly those ages 20 to 29 years, have the highest risk, whereas rates are lowest in persons older than 55 years of age.

Traveler's diarrhea is acquired through ingestion of fecally contaminated food or beverages. Younger travelers, missionaries, and tourists are at higher risk because of exposure to native foods, commercial eating establishments, and exposure to contaminated food and water.

Table 104–14 Relative Frequencies of Microbial Causes of Traveler's Diarrhea

Pathogen	Frequency, %	
	Average	*Range*
Enterotoxigenic *Escherichia coli*	40-60	0-72
Enteroadherent *E. coli*	15	NA
Campylobacter	10	0-41
Shigella	10	0-30
Rotavirus	5	0-36
Invasive *E. coli*	<5	0-5
Salmonella	<5	0-15
Vibrio	<5	0-30
Aeromonas	<5	0-30
Giardia lamblia	<5	0-6
Entamoeba histolytica	<5	0-6
Cryptosporidium	<5	NA
Cyclospora cayetanensis	<5	NA
Hafnia alvei	<5	0-16
No pathogen identified	40	22-83

NA, not available.

Travelers eating at private homes have the lowest risk. Dietary discretion is the first line of defense against acquiring traveler's diarrhea. Especially risky foods include uncooked vegetables, meat, and seafood; foods served steaming hot are the safest. Tap water, ice, unpasteurized milk and dairy products, and unpeeled fruits also are associated with an increased risk. Bottled carbonated beverages (especially flavored beverages), beer, wine, hot coffee, hot tea, and water boiled or appropriately treated with chlorine are relatively safe.

Clinical Features

In most cases, traveler's diarrhea is self-limited, and evaluation by a physician is not necessary. In cases that are prolonged or accompanied by fever, systemic manifestations, bloody stool, or occur in immunocompromised persons, evaluation should be done. The presence of dysentery, occult or gross blood, or fecal leukocytes on microscopic examination should prompt further diagnostic tests. It should be noted that many laboratories merely culture for *Salmonella*, *Shigella*, and *Campylobacter*, whereas enteric pathogens, such as *Yersinia* and enterotoxigenic and EHEC are not sought routinely. If there is concern for a specific pathogen, the laboratory should be alerted to look for it.

The disease does not begin immediately after the traveler's arrival but generally has its onset 2 to 3 days later.[282,288] Although most people have 3 to 5 loose stools per day, about 20% can have 6 to 15 watery bowel movements.[282,294] The average duration of illness in untreated subjects is 1 to 3 days, but a few unfortunate persons have persistent diarrhea throughout their stay. Watery loose stools are the most common complaint, with an array of associated symptoms (Table 104–15). From 2% to 10% of patients have fever, bloody stools, or both, and they are more likely to have shigellosis.[283] In general, persons with a milder clinical presentation, regardless of the pathogen, experience more rapid resolution of disease than those with more severe symptoms, but even mild disease can produce an illness that lasts 4 to 5 days. Despite the impressive list of symptoms, fewer than 1% of travelers are admitted to a local hospital, and no reports of death from diarrhea were recorded among several hundred

Table 104–15 Symptoms of Patients with Traveler's Diarrhea

Symptom	Percentage Affected
Gaseousness	79
Fatigue	74
Cramps	68
Nausea	61
Fever	56
Abdominal pain	55
Anorexia	53
Headache	39
Chills	38
Backache	35
Dizziness	34
Vomiting	29
Malaise	24
Arthralgias	23

thousand travelers from Switzerland.[288] Diarrhea persists in 1% to 3% of travelers for 30 days or longer.[294]

Treatment

In most cases of traveler's diarrhea, symptomatic therapy should be adequate. As for all forms of diarrhea, treatment entails fluid replacement and appropriate drugs. In most cases of traveler's diarrhea, severe dehydration seldom is encountered, and fluid losses generally can be replaced with soft drinks, fruit juices, bottled or carbonated beverages, hot broth, and soups. With severe diarrhea, ORSs should be used (see Table 104–6). Milk and dairy products should be avoided because of the common occurrence of lactose intolerance. Improvement in diarrhea should occur within 48 hours, and if bloody stools or systemic symptoms develop, travelers should seek medical attention.

Drug treatment is directed at either suppressing the pathogen with antibiotics or reducing fluid and electrolyte losses with antimotility/antisecretory agents. Antimotility drugs have enjoyed considerable popularity among tourists for providing relief from the intestinal indignities of travel, and their use is supported by good scientific studies.[295] Loperamide induces rapid improvement that is demonstrable even on the first day of therapy, with results that are significantly better than those of either placebo or bismuth subsalicylate.[295] Bismuth subsalicylate is an effective alternative treatment for mild-to-moderate traveler's diarrhea.[296] The most effective relief has been provided by a combination of an antimicrobial drug and an antimotility drug. In a study of travelers to Mexico, the combined use of loperamide and TMP-SMX curtailed diarrhea in 1 hour, compared with 30 hours when either drug was used alone or 59 hours with placebo.[297] Another study from Egypt, however, failed to show much benefit for the combination over the antibiotic alone.[298] Bismuth subsalicylate has antisecretory, antibacterial, and anti-inflammatory properties and also decreases the number of stools. It should not be used in combination with other antibiotic drugs because it reduces the bioavailability of tetracyclines and may do so with other antibiotics. Table 104–12 lists the antimicrobial therapy of specific enteric pathogens.

Several antibiotics have been used successfully to treat traveler's diarrhea. TMP-SMX or TMP alone reduced the duration of diarrhea from 93 hours to approximately 30 hours.[299] Ciprofloxacin was as effective as TMP-SMX[300]; results with a single dose of fluoroquinolones are encouraging.[301] The development of ciprofloxacin resistance in patients with *Campylobacter* enteritis has been associated with clinical relapse after treatment,[287] and in areas where fluoroquinolone resistant *C. jejuni* has become more common, azithromycin, rather than ciprofloxacin, should be used to treat traveler's diarrhea.[217] Several studies have shown that the nonabsorbable antibiotic, rifaximin, is as effective as a fluoroquinolone.[302,303] Because it is nonabsorbable, side effects should be rare.

Current recommendations for treatment are as follows: for mild-to-moderate diarrhea, generally fewer than four bowel movements per day without blood or fever, either loperamide or bismuth subsalicylate can be used effectively. For more severe diarrhea, the optimal therapy seems to be a combination of an antimotility drug and an effective antimicrobial drug.[304]

Prevention

Four approaches to preventing traveler's diarrhea are available: (1) avoidance of unsafe foods and beverages; (2) use of anti-infective drugs; (3) use of other medications such as antimotility/antisecretory agents; and (4) immunization. Precautions about eating habits should be observed, to prevent not only diarrhea but other food- and water-borne diseases. Bottled beverages generally are safe, although some epidemics have been associated with contaminated bottled drinks.[305,306] Carbonated beverages are safer than noncarbonated ones, due to the low pH (generally 4.0 to 5.0), which has antibacterial properties. Tea or coffee prepared with boiling water generally is safe if consumed while still hot. Because the venue of food consumption determines the risk of traveler's diarrhea, travelers are advised not to eat food from street vendors.

The high incidence of bacterial pathogens as a cause of traveler's diarrhea makes the use of prophylactic antibiotics tempting; however, safe eating and drinking habits are the traveler's best methods of prophylaxis. Even in high-risk areas, 50% to 60% of travelers will not get diarrhea. Prophylaxis should be recommended, however, for certain groups of people: persons with severe kidney, liver, or heart disease, insulin-dependant diabetes, inflammatory bowel disease, or those with gastrectomy, achlorhydria, or ileostomies, or those taking steroids or suffering with immunosuppressive illnesses. In addition, people for whom the trip will be ruined, important business plans disrupted, or the traveler who will not follow careful dietary practices benefit from prophylaxis.

Bismuth subsalicylate (Pepto-Bismol) significantly decreases the risk of developing traveler's diarrhea and prevents approximately 52% to 65% of the cases of diarrhea in high-risk areas. The most effective dosage is 2.1 g/day and should be given four times a day (at meals and at bedtime). Whereas prophylactic antibiotic therapy has a better success rate, bismuth subsalicylate has a more narrow and safer side effect profile. Side effects of this drug include transient blackening of the tongue and stool

and constipation. The salicylate portion of the molecule is absorbable and may result in toxicity, but this usually does not occur in the short courses given for prevention of traveler's diarrhea. Salicylate toxicity, however, should be considered in the elderly and in those already taking salicylates and avoided in patients with peptic ulcer disease or chronic renal failure.

Table 104–16 lists drugs used to prevent traveler's diarrhea. Various antibiotic regimens can prevent up to 70% to 80% of the episodes of traveler's diarrhea but do so at the expense of significant possible side effects. Various antibiotic regimens have been found to be effective. Use of antiparasitic agents or hydroxyquinone, however, has never been shown to be effective and should not be considered for prophylaxis. Side effects of antibiotic therapy vary and include skin rashes, photosensitivity, the rarer Stevens-Johnson syndrome, antibiotic-associated colitis, and vaginal candidiasis. In the individual patient, the broad use of antibiotics risks development of antimicrobial resistance, bacterial overgrowth, or persistent salmonellosis. Antidiarrheal agents and lactobacillus preparations are not useful prophylactically.

Chronic Diarrhea

In an unknown but small percentage of patients with traveler's diarrhea, the diarrhea becomes persistent and chronic. Such patients require evaluation. The differential diagnosis of chronic diarrhea in an individual whose diarrhea began with travel includes chronic infections as a result of bacteria, protozoa, or parasites, or postinfectious complications. Table 104–17 lists the potential causes of this syndrome.[19] Infectious etiologies should be evaluated first. *G. lamblia*, *C. cayetanensis*, and, rarely, *Shigella*, *Salmonella*, *I. belli*, or *C. jejuni* may be responsible for rare cases of persistent diarrhea in travelers.[294] In individuals with any exposure to antibiotics, a stool assay for *C. difficile* toxin should be included.

When infectious etiologies have been excluded, the possibility of malabsorption or tropical sprue should be considered. An abnormal complete blood count, prothrombin time, or Sudan stain for fecal fat or reduced serum levels of albumin, vitamin B_{12}, folate, or carotene may suggest this diagnosis. If upper gastrointestinal

---

Table 104–16 Drugs Used to Prevent Traveler's Diarrhea in Adults

Drug	Dose*	Comments
Bismuth subsalicylate	Two 262-mg tablets chewed well four times daily (with meals and at bedtime)	Not as effective as antimicrobial drugs; fewer side effects than other agents
Fluoroquinolone antibiotics		The most predictably effective antimicrobial drugs when susceptibilities are not known
Norfloxacin	400 mg daily	
Ciprofloxacin	500 mg daily	
Ofloxacin	300 mg daily	
Fleroxacin	400 mg daily	
Trimethoprim-sulfamethoxazole	160 mg of trimethoprim and 800 mg of sulfamethoxazole once daily	Resistance is common in tropical areas
Doxycycline	100 mg daily	Resistance is found in many areas of the world

*All drugs should be taken orally beginning on the day of arrival in the country one is visiting and continuing for 1-2 days after returning home, but none should be taken for >3 weeks.
From DuPont HL, Ericsson CD: Prevention and treatment of traveler's diarrhea. N Engl J Med 328:1821, 1993.

Table 104–17 Causes of Prolonged Diarrheal Illness after Travel

Persistent bacterial infection
  Salmonella
  Shigella
  Yersinia
  Campylobacter
  Aeromonas
  Escherichia coli (enteroinvasive)
Persistent protozoal infection
  Giardia
  Entamoeba histolytica
  Cryptosporidium
Antibiotic-associated colitis
Dietary intolerances
  Disaccharidase deficiency
  Altered diet with osmotic-induced diarrhea
Inflammatory bowel disease
Celiac sprue
Tropical sprue
Lymphocytic/collagenous colitis
Onset of chronic (presumably viral) enteritis/colitis
Post-infection irritable bowel syndrome

From Chak A, Banwell JG: Traveler's diarrhea. Gastroenterol Clin North Am 22:549, 1993.

endoscopy is done to search for small bowel pathogens, aspirates and biopsies can be obtained to exclude giardiasis, tropical sprue, or bacterial overgrowth.

In addition to tropical sprue, postinfectious syndromes developing after an acute diarrheal illness include the unmasking of previously subclinical illnesses such as celiac sprue, inflammatory bowel disease, or lymphocytic colitis. A syndrome called *postdysenteric colitis* may represent a postviral enteritis/colitis or a previously undiagnosed ulcerative colitis; endoscopically this entity appears similar to ulcerative colitis.

Despite extensive evaluation, some patients will have no identifiable cause for their chronic diarrhea. In such a case, postinfectious irritable bowel syndrome may be implicated.[159,307,308] Patients should be reassured, treated, and managed similarly to those patients with irritable bowel syndrome.

DIARRHEA IN THE ELDERLY

Diarrheal disease is a major cause of morbidity and mortality in adults older than 65 years of age.[309,310] The elderly are at increased risk for diarrhea and associated complications as a consequence of hypochlorhydria, intestinal motility disorders, underlying chronic medical diseases, immune senescence, and exposure to multiple medications, including antibiotics. A review of national mortality data found that most diarrheal deaths in the United States between 1979 and 1987 occurred in people older than 74 years of age (51%) and in adults ages 55 to 74 years (27%).[309] Elderly people living in long-term care facilities are at greater risk of death from diarrhea than are independent elderly.[309,311] Infectious diarrhea was the fourth most common infectious disease in residents of long-term care facilities.[312]

Microbiology

A number of infectious bacterial, viral, and parasitic agents can cause diarrhea in the elderly. In addition, noninfectious causes of diarrhea need to be considered, including medications such as laxatives or antacids, intestinal tumors that cause obstruction or produce secretory hormones, inflammatory bowel disease, malabsorption, and systemic illnesses including diabetes mellitus and thyrotoxicosis.[311]

A consistent association has been noted between advanced age and *C. difficile* infection.[313,314] Given the frequent need for hospitalization and the use of antimicrobial agents in the elderly, it is not surprising that *C. difficile* is the most commonly identified cause of diarrhea in the elderly. Mortality is no different in the elderly with *C. difficile* infection than it is in the young,[315] but older adults are more likely than younger people to have a severe event when exposed to EHEC[316] and *C. perfringens*.[317] In an outbreak of *E. coli* O157:H7 in a long-term care facility in Toronto in 1985, one third of the nursing home residents were infected, whereas only 13% of the employees developed diarrhea.[115] The elderly residents were also at substantially increased risk for mortality from EHEC in this study; 35% of the infected residents died, primarily from complications of HUS, whereas none of the infected staff members died. Elderly persons represented the only fatalities in a large outbreak of *E. coli* O157:H7 in Missouri.[316] As was demonstrated in Washington state,[126] the use of antibiotics for treatment of EHEC infections in the nursing home residents was associated with a threefold increased risk of death.[115]

Norwalk-like viruses are a common source of nursing home outbreaks and are responsible for substantial morbidity in the institutionalized elderly.[318] The elderly also are more likely than younger persons to have severe infections and to die from nontyphoidal salmonellosis and campylobacteriosis. Among the parasitic causes of diarrhea, *Cryptosporidium parvum* is a cause of morbidity in the elderly. In a Rhode Island hospital, a retrospective chart review of stool studies for *C. parvum* over a 5-year period showed that 36% of positive smears were in elderly patients, whereas 50% were in patients with HIV.[319] Most of the elderly with positive stool specimens acquired the infection in an institutional setting, and nearly one half were coinfected with *C. difficile*.

Clinical Features

Although the clinical manifestations of gastrointestinal infections in the elderly vary by pathogen, there are few major differences between the young and the old. Noteworthy is that the elderly are more likely to experience complications resulting from volume depletion. Dehydration may exacerbate other age-related complications such as delirium, electrolyte disturbances, renal insufficiency, malnutrition, and micronutrient deficiencies. If hemorrhagic colitis develops, the new blood loss superimposed on preexisting anemia can precipitate congestive heart failure, angina, or a myocardial infarction.

Diagnosis

Because many episodes of infectious diarrhea in the elderly are self-limited, supportive therapy is often all that is necessary. Signs of dehydration that are useful for evaluating young adults and children are often less reliable indicators of an elderly patient's hydration status. because older adults often have decreased skin elasticity, dry oral mucosa because of mouth breathing, and sunken eyes. Although it is important to take orthostatic vital signs, orthostatic changes generally do not occur until there has been substantial volume loss (>10%). Laboratory tests also are not especially helpful for diagnosing dehydration in the elderly. Although the ratio of blood urea nitrogen to creatinine, if elevated, suggests dehydration, this ratio is only a crude indicator of a patient's underlying volume status.

Noninfectious causes of diarrhea, such as use of magnesium-containing antacids, laxatives, stool softeners, and dietary supplements should be eliminated before embarking on a diagnostic evaluation; fecal impaction also should be excluded. Although stool cultures often are not helpful, except in outbreaks, stool studies for *C. difficile* toxin should be obtained, especially if the patient recently has received chemotherapy or antimicrobial treatment. Endoscopic procedures should be done if fecal occult blood tests are positive, invasive pathogens have been excluded, or symptoms are persistent or recurrent.

Treatment

If an elderly patient with diarrhea and dehydration is not severely dehydrated and is able to tolerate fluids by mouth, oral rehydration therapy is preferred over intravenous treatment. Patients who are severely dehydrated or unable to tolerate oral therapy should be rehydrated by the parenteral route. Antimicrobial therapy generally should be reserved for the treatment of specific infections such as shigellosis, invasive salmonellosis, or *C. difficile*.

DYSENTERY VERSUS ULCERATIVE COLITIS

The clinical distinction between bacillary or amebic dysentery and ulcerative colitis can be difficult. Two features distinguish dysentery, a condition also known as *acute self-limited colitis*, from an acute attack of idiopathic ulcerative colitis: a positive culture for a pathogen and a self-limited course without relapse. Positive bacteriologic culture is only encountered in 40% to 60% of reported cases.[52,150]

Histopathologic examination of colonic mucosa obtained by endoscopic biopsy can be helpful. Both the microbial form (dysentery) and the idiopathic form of acute colitis show edema, neutrophils in the lamina propria, and superficial cryptitis with preservation of the normal crypt pattern. Idiopathic ulcerative colitis, however, shows signs of chronicity such as crypt distortion and plasmacytosis in the lamina propria, which typically involves the base of the mucosa. Focal cryptitis and a mild increase in the cellularity of the lamina propria are found in both the microbial and idiopathic forms and can lead to confusion.[150]

In clinical practice, the main diagnostic problem is illustrated by a patient with severe acute colitis for several days, who has not responded to antibiotic therapy. Presumptive treatment should include a fluoroquinolone for

bacterial pathogens and metronidazole for protozoa. The decision to use other treatment, such as glucocorticoids, rests on the distinction between these diseases, and it may not be possible to make this distinction based on culture or histopathologic findings.

Certain pathogens involve principally the lower small bowel but may invade the colon as well; *Salmonella* and *Yersinia* make up this group. Although watery diarrhea is the usual manifestation, depending on the focus of infection, the spectrum extends from dehydrating diarrhea to frank colitis. Vibrios produce varying clinical manifestations, apparently related to the virulence factors in each infecting strain. *E. histolytica* attacks the large bowel and produces an invasive disease. Curiously, there is a paucity of PMNs in the stool, although occasional macrophages are present.

TREATMENT

FLUID THERAPY

Potentially devastating consequences of acute infectious diarrhea can result from fluid losses. Rehydration, prevention of ongoing gastrointestinal fluid loss, and replacement of electrolytes, therefore, are the initial goals of therapy. Toxigenic organisms, such as *V. cholerae*, certain strains of *E. coli* (ETEC), and rotavirus infection in children can result in extreme dehydration resulting from production of large amounts of isotonic fluid in the small bowel that overwhelms the ability of the colon to reabsorb it. "Nonspecific" diarrhea, usually caused by viruses, causes less fluid loss and a lower electrolyte concentration in the fecal effluent than does toxigenic diarrhea.

The traditional route of fluid administration has been intravenous, but ORSs, used widely in developing countries, can be used to rehydrate patients with moderate volume depletion.[68,69,320] Even in the United States, ORS is the treatment of choice for mild-to-moderate diarrhea in both children and adults and can be used in severe diarrhea after initial parenteral fluid replacement.[321] The effectiveness of ORS is a function of its electrolyte content which has been formulated specifically to replace stool losses. ORS also contains an actively transported substrate, commonly glucose. The use of ORS is based on the physiologic principle that glucose and other substrates enhance sodium absorption in the small intestine, even in the presence of secretory losses caused by bacterial toxins.

A variety of ORSs are available and are effective (see Table 104-6).[322] Even in patients who are vomiting, small increments of ORS can be given effectively. Patients with hypovolemic shock need intravenous hydration.

Although there is agreement on the value of ORS in treating dehydrating diarrhea, the specific formulation of electrolytes remains in dispute, particularly in treating well-nourished children in developed countries.[323,324] The two areas of dispute concern the appropriate sodium concentration and the osmolality of the solution. Some authorities have voiced concern that the concentration of sodium (90 mmol) in the standard ORS formulation may be too high and that it could cause hypernatremia and seizures.[249,320,325] This issue was examined in a study from Scotland in which children with acute diarrhea and mild dehydration were treated in a randomized fashion with solutions containing sodium concentrations of 35, 50, or 90 mmol and dextrose concentrations of 200, 111, and 110 mmol, respectively; all three formulations proved to be equally safe and effective.[326] Several authorities have recommended lower concentrations of sodium and a reduced osmolarity in ORS for children with diarrhea in developed countries.[249,320,325] A multicenter study of children with acute noncholera diarrhea found that treatment with a reduced-osmolarity, reduced-sodium ORS was associated with a lower total stool output, less total ORS intake, and a shortened duration of diarrhea than was treatment with the standard ORS.[327]

Additional criticisms of the traditional glucose-based ORS are that it fails to decrease the quantity and duration of diarrhea. An inexpensive alternative to glucose-based ORS is the substitution of starch derived from rice or cereals for glucose. Treatment with rice-based salt solutions produces lesser stool losses, a shorter duration of diarrhea, and greater fluid and electrolyte absorption than does glucose-based ORS in children and adults with diarrhea.[328] Recently, the addition of an amylase-resistant starch to ORS has been demonstrated to be even more effective in reducing the duration of diarrhea and fecal weight than was a rice flour-based ORS in patients with cholera.[329]

DIET

The traditional approach to any diarrheal illness is dietary abstinence, which restricts the intake of necessary calories, fluids, and electrolytes. Certainly, during an acute attack, the patient often finds it more comfortable to avoid high-fiber foods, fats, and spices because any oral consumption can provide a stimulus to defecation. Although giving the bowel a rest provides symptomatic relief, the patient must maintain intake with oral fluids containing calories and some electrolytes. On balance, it is better to eat judiciously during an attack of diarrhea than to restrict oral intake severely. In children, it is particularly important to restart feeding immediately after the child is able to accept oral intake.

It is wise to avoid milk and dairy products during the acute episode of diarrhea that may be complicated by secondary lactase deficiency. Ingestion of such items in this setting could potentiate fluid secretion and increase stool volume. Caffeine and methylxanthine-containing products should be avoided because the inhibition of phosphodiesterase can increase intracellular cAMP and result in increased intestinal secretion. Thus, coffee, strong tea, cocoa, and soft drinks such as the colas can potentiate abdominal cramps and diarrhea. Alcohol can irritate the intestine, and abstinence is recommended. In addition to the oral rehydration therapy outlined earlier, acceptable beverages for mildly dehydrated adults include fruit juices and various bottled soft drinks. It is advisable to "defizz" a carbonated drink by letting it stand in a glass before it is consumed. Soft, easily digestible foods are most acceptable to a patient with acute diarrhea. Secondary lactase deficiency and intolerance to lactose-containing foods can occur during and

after various small intestinal infections and can persist for up to one year.

ANTIMICROBIAL DRUGS

Less than 10% of cases of acute infectious diarrhea are benefited by treatment with antimicrobial drugs (see Table 104–12).[330] Infections in adults that benefit from specific therapy include *Shigella*, EIEC, *C. difficile*, traveler's diarrhea, *V. cholerae*, *E. histolytica*, *Giardia*, and some cases of *Salmonella*. There are conflicting reports concerning the efficacy of antimicrobial drugs in several important infections, such as those caused by *Campylobacter*; data are insufficient for infections caused by *Yersinia*, *Aeromonas*, vibrios, and several forms of *E. coli*. *Yersinia* infections probably do not benefit from treatment unless systemic illness is suspected. Antibiotic therapy is recommended for prolonged or severe cases of *Salmonella*, *Campylobacter*, *Aeromonas*, or *Plesiomonas* infections (see Tables 104–1 and 104–12).[71]

Empirical therapy may be recommended for persons with traveler's diarrhea and for patients with a febrile, dysenteric illness. If *Shigella* or *C. jejuni* is suspected, a fluoroquinolone is the drug of choice in adults. The issue of when antimicrobial therapy is appropriate for the management of acute diarrhea has been a vexing problem. Several studies have addressed this issue. Dryden and associates[53] studied empirical treatment in patients with severe, acute, community-acquired gastroenteritis (patients with > 4 stools per day for > 3 days and at least one associated symptom) and found that treatment with ciprofloxacin, 500 mg twice a day for 5 days, was associated with a reduction in the duration of diarrhea and other symptoms by more than 2 days, fewer failures, and significant clearing of pathogens when compared with placebo. Six weeks later, there was no difference in stool carriage of the pathogen (12%) nor any demonstrable antibiotic resistance. Goodman and colleagues[331] studied adults with acute diarrhea comparing ciprofloxacin, TMP-SMX, and placebo and found that ciprofloxacin, but not TMP-SMX, shortened the duration of diarrhea.[331] Similar findings have been noted in other studies of the empirical therapy of diarrhea.[332]

Based on these studies, a patient with severe community-acquired diarrhea, defined as a previously healthy person with diarrhea (>4 watery stools per day) lasting at least 3 days and at least one of the following symptoms—abdominal pain, fever, vomiting, myalgia, or headache—should receive an antimicrobial drug, preferably a fluoroquinolone. In such patients, there is a high likelihood that a bacterial pathogen will be isolated and treatment with an antibiotic will provide prompt relief of symptoms. In patients with bloody diarrhea, it is not possible to distinguish among *Shigella*, *Campylobacter*, and EHEC on clinical grounds. If symptoms of dysentery predominate, quinolone therapy is indicated. If dysentery is not present and if there is a reasonable possibility, based on epidemiologic evidence, that EHEC is the responsible pathogen, then antimicrobial therapy should be withheld until a microbiologic diagnosis can be established.[126]

The choice of antimicrobial drugs, when indicated, is based on in vitro sensitivity patterns, which are related to geographic prevalence. The fluoroquinolones, including norfloxacin, ciprofloxacin, and ofloxacin, possess broad-spectrum activity against virtually all important diarrheal pathogens (except *C. difficile*) and thus represent one of the best choices for treatment. Recommendations for antimicrobial therapy of specific infections are given in Table 104–12.[333] The optimal duration of antimicrobial therapy has not been defined with precision. Some authors recommend 3 days of treatment for diarrhea, others 5 days, and others 10 days; however, there are several studies of patients with severe diarrhea that suggest that a *single* dose is as effective as more prolonged therapy in cholera and shigellosis.[151,334-337]

NONSPECIFIC THERAPY

Literally hundreds of antidiarrheal nostrums can be found in pharmacies and assorted medical establishments throughout the world. Many products contain a combination of drugs, most of them therapeutically worthless and others potentially dangerous. Because most patients with infectious diarrhea, even with a recognized pathogen, have a mild self-limited course, specific treatment generally is not required. For more severe cases, as defined earlier, empirical antimicrobial therapy with a fluoroquinolone should be instituted, pending results of stool and blood cultures.

A variety of over-the-counter and prescription preparations are available for symptomatic relief of diarrhea and abdominal cramping (Table 104–18). Anticholinergics (dicyclomine [Bentyl], hyoscyamine [Levsin]) decrease intestinal motility and may provide relief of abdominal cramps but do not significantly alter diarrhea. Adsorbents such as attapulgite (Donnagel) kaolin, pectin, and activated charcoal decrease stool liquidity, but there

Table 104–18 Nonspecific Therapy for Infectious Diarrhea

Effective
Fluid
  Intravenous
  Oral rehydration therapy
Food
  Continue intake
  Avoid lactose, caffeine, and methylxanthines
Antimotility drugs
  Codeine, paregoric, tincture of opium
  Loperamide
  Diphenoxylate
Bismuth subsalicylate
Lactobacillus GG*
Zaldaride maleate†
Not Effective
Lactobacilli
Kaolin, pectin, charcoal
Anticholinergics
Cholestyramine
Hydroxyquinolones

*May be effective in children with rotaviral diarrhea.
†An antisecretory drug.

is no evidence that these preparations decrease intestinal fluid loss or number of bowel movements.

The opiate derivatives, loperamide and diphenoxylate-atropine, are particularly useful in controlling moderate to severe diarrhea. These agents decrease intestinal motor activity, decrease fluid secretion, enhance mucosal absorption, and increase anal sphincter tone. The overall effect is to enhance fluid transport, slow transit time, reduce fluid losses, and ameliorate abdominal cramping. They are effective and fairly safe.

Loperamide is arguably the best agent for acute diarrhea because it does not cross the blood–brain barrier, thereby reducing the risk for habituation or other central nervous system side effects. Treatment with loperamide produces rapid improvement, often within the first day of therapy.[297] The concern that an antimotility drug may exacerbate a case of dysentery[337] largely has been dispelled by clinical experience. Patients with shigellosis, even *S. dysenteriae* 1, have been treated inadvertently with loperamide as the only drug and have had a normal resolution of disease without evidence that the illness was prolonged or excretion of the pathogen was delayed.[295] These drugs however, generally should not be used in a patient with acute severe colitis, either infectious or noninfectious in origin.

Bismuth subsalicylate is an antisecretory agent with a low incidence of side effects, which is recommended to decrease stool liquidity and frequency.[296] The drug possesses both antimicrobial and antisecretory properties on the basis of the bismuth and salicylate moieties, respectively. In various trials of diarrhea among travelers in Mexico or West Africa, bismuth subsalicylate reduced the frequency of diarrhea significantly over placebo, but results generally were better when a high dose (4.2 g/day) was used.[338]

The combination of an antimicrobial drug and an antimotility drug provides the most rapid relief of diarrhea. In a study of travelers to Mexico, the combined use of loperamide and TMP-SMX curtailed diarrhea in 1 hour, compared with 30 hours with either drug alone or 59 hours with placebo.[297] Even with the severest diarrhea with fecal leukocytes or blood-tinged stool, the median duration of illness was 4.5 hours, a remarkable result in this setting. In a similar study involving U.S. military personnel in Egypt, loperamide added little to the efficacy of ciprofloxacin except in the initial 24 hours, when the combination was slightly better than the antibiotic alone.[298] Addition of loperamide to ciprofloxacin for the treatment of invasive diarrhea has led to a significantly shorter duration of diarrhea and a reduction in the median number of diarrheal stools.[156]

TUBERCULOSIS OF THE GASTROINTESTINAL TRACT

Any region of the gastrointestinal tract can be involved with tuberculosis. This occurrence still is prevalent in developing countries where tuberculosis is a common health problem. In recent years there has been an upsurge of gastrointestinal tuberculosis in the United States as a result of the influx of immigrants and the AIDS epidemic.

PATHOGENESIS

Mycobacterium tuberculosis is the pathogen responsible for most cases of intestinal tuberculosis. In some parts of the world, *Mycobacterium bovis*, an organism found in dairy products, still is responsible for some cases; however, *M. bovis* is an uncommon human pathogen in Western countries. The usual route of infection is direct penetration of the intestinal mucosa by swallowed organisms. In the past, intestinal tuberculosis was associated with active pulmonary infection and especially with active laryngeal involvement. Autopsies of patients with pulmonary tuberculosis, before the era of effective treatment, demonstrated intestinal involvement in 55% to 90% of fatal cases. There also was a higher risk of intestinal involvement with pulmonary cavitation and positive sputum smears, again reflecting the risk of a high inoculum of swallowed organisms. In modern series, however, pulmonary involvement is seen in less than 50% of patients with intestinal tuberculosis.[339,340] Indeed, the chest film is unremarkable in most patients now seen with intestinal tuberculosis.

CLASSIFICATION AND DISTRIBUTION OF DISEASE

The most frequent sites of intestinal involvement (75% of cases) are the ileum and cecum. Both sides of the ileocecal valve usually are involved, leading to incompetence of the valve, a finding that helps distinguish tuberculosis from Crohn's disease. Other locations of involvement, in order of frequency, are the ascending colon, jejunum, appendix, duodenum, stomach, esophagus, sigmoid colon, and rectum. Multiple areas of the bowel can be affected.

PATHOLOGY

The gross appearance of intestinal tuberculosis has been divided into the following three categories[339,340]:

1. *Ulcerative* lesions are seen in 60% of patients and consist of multiple superficial lesions confined largely to the epithelial surface. The process is highly virulent and in the past was associated with a high mortality rate.
2. *Hypertrophic* lesions occur in 10% of patients and manifests as scarring, fibrosis, and heaped-up mass lesions that mimic carcinoma.
3. *Ulcerohypertrophic* lesions are seen in 30% of patients, and in this type, mucosal ulcerations are combined with healing and scar formation.

At surgery, the bowel wall appears thickened, and there is an inflammatory mass surrounding the ileocecal region. Active inflammation is apparent, as are strictures and even fistula formation. The serosal surface is covered with multiple tubercles. The mesenteric lymph nodes frequently are enlarged and thickened. The mucosa itself is hyperemic, cobblestoned, edematous, and, in some cases, ulcerated. In contrast to Crohn's disease, the superficial ulcers tend to be circumferential, with the long axis perpendicular to the lumen. When these ulcers heal, the associated fibrosis causes stricture and stenosis of the lumen.

Histologically, the distinguishing lesion is a granuloma (Fig. 104–10). Caseation is not always seen, especially in the mucosa, although caseating granulomas are found with regularity in regional lymph nodes. The muscularis usually is spared. Sections of the involved region show acid-fast bacilli using the Ziehl-Neelsen stain in approximately one third of patients. The organism also can be recovered in a culture of the involved tissues.

CLINICAL FEATURES

Only some patients with intestinal tuberculosis have specific symptoms. The most common complaint is nonspecific chronic abdominal pain, reported in 80% to 90% of patients. Weight loss, fever, diarrhea or constipation, and blood in the stool may be present.[339-341] An abdominal mass, usually deep and posterior in the right lower quadrant of the abdomen, can be appreciated in approximately two thirds of patients. Laboratory findings include mild anemia with a normal white blood cell count. Complications include intestinal hemorrhage, perforation, obstruction, fistula formation, and malabsorption.[340,342] Perforation is uncommon but can occur, even during treatment. Intestinal obstruction is a more common finding and typically results from segmental and stenotic disease. Surgical intervention may be required to relieve obstruction despite appropriate drug therapy. Malabsorption can occur when obstruction leads to proximal bacterial overgrowth.

DIAGNOSIS

The definitive diagnosis of intestinal tuberculosis is made by identification of the organism in tissue, either by direct visualization with an acid-fast stain, by culture of the excised tissue, or by a PCR assay.[343] A presumptive diagnosis can be established in a patient with active pulmonary tuberculosis and radiologic and clinical findings that suggest intestinal involvement. Colonoscopic find-

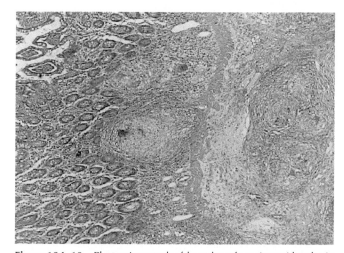

Figure 104–10 Photomicrograph of the colon of a patient with colonic tuberculosis, showing granulomas in the mucosa and submucosa.

ings, although nonspecific, consist of superficial areas of ulceration and a nodular friable mucosa.[341,343] The tuberculin skin test is less helpful, because a positive test does not necessarily mean active disease. In addition, many patients, especially older persons with weight loss and inanition and those with AIDS, have a negative skin test in the face of active intestinal tuberculosis.

Radiologic examination of the bowel reveals a thickened bowel wall with distortion of the mucosal folds, ulcerations, varying degrees of bowel stenosis, and pseudopolyp formation (Fig. 104–11).[344,345] Computed tomography may show preferential thickening of the ileocecal valve and medial wall of the cecum, extension to the terminal ileum, and massive lymphadenopathy with central necrosis.[344] The cecum is contracted with disease on both sides of the valve, and the valve itself often is distorted and incompetent; conification of the cecum, as seen on barium enema, is characteristic of tuberculosis and is referred to as *Stierlin's sign.* Tuberculosis tends to involve short segments of the intestine with stenosis and fistula formation. In the hypertrophic form a mass can be seen that resembles a cecal carcinoma. Calcified mesenteric lymph nodes and an abnormal chest film are other findings that aid in the diagnosis of intestinal tuberculosis.

Several diseases can resemble intestinal tuberculosis. Crohn's disease gives virtually all of the changes of intestinal tuberculosis, except for the presence of the organism, which makes the definitive diagnosis of mycobacterial infection. *Y. enterocolitica* can produce mesenteric adenopathy, ulcerations, and thickening of the bowel mucosa. Usually, this infection has a shorter history and resolves spontaneously. Involvement of the cecum with carcinoma or amebiasis can be confused with tuberculosis. Syphilis and lymphogranuloma venereum should be considered, but intestinal involvement with these infections is now uncommon.

TREATMENT

Standard antituberculosis treatment gives a high cure rate for intestinal tuberculosis. There are no controlled studies to determine the optimal therapy or duration, but extrapolation from other forms of extrapulmonary tuberculosis suggests that a three-drug regimen for a period of 12 months would be adequate treatment. The drugs are isoniazid (300 mg/day), pyrazinamide (15 to 30 mg/kg/day), and rifampin (600 mg/day). In AIDS patients, either ethambutol (15 mg/kg) or streptomycin (15 mg/kg) should be added. Moreover, the course of intestinal tuberculosis in AIDS is more prolonged and may require treatment with second-line drugs because of the high frequency of resistant organisms.

In the past, surgical intervention often was required for intestinal tuberculosis, especially in cases involving the ileocecal region.[346,347] Obstruction and fistula formation were the leading indications for surgery. In the current era, most fistulas and ulcerative complications respond to medical management, but mass lesions associated with the hypertrophic form still may necessitate an operative approach, because they can lead to luminal compromise with complete obstruction.[339,342] Surgery also may be necessary when free perforation, confined perforation with abscess formation, or massive hemorrhage occur. Because of its similarity to carcinoma of the cecum, undiagnosed ileocolonic tuberculous disease may prompt exploratory laparotomy and right hemicolectomy, although minimal resection is required for tuberculous disease because the condition often improves dramatically with appropriate drug therapy; colonoscopy has reduced the need for diagnostic laparotomy. Postoperative pulmonary complications are more common in patients with than without concomitant active pulmonary tuberculosis[347] and include obstruction, enterocutaneous fistula, perforation, wound infection, and bleeding.[339,347]

BACTERIAL FOOD POISONING

Food poisoning is defined as an illness caused by the consumption of food contaminated with bacteria, bacterial toxins, parasites (e.g., trichinosis), viruses (e.g., hepatitis), or chemicals (e.g., amanitine with ingestion of mushrooms). Food poisoning caused by bacteria constitutes 75% of the outbreaks and 86% of cases in the United States for which an etiology can be determined[348]; however, only 42% of such outbreaks fulfill the microbiological standards for a confirmed etiology. The Centers for Disease Control and Prevention (CDC) recorded 2751 food-borne outbreaks occurring from 1993 to 1997, affecting 86,000 persons[348]; however, unreported cases

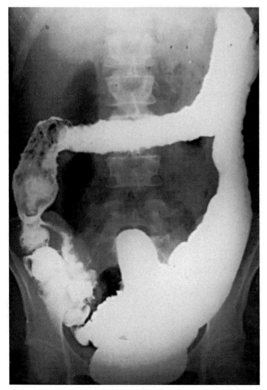

Figure 104–11 Film from a barium enema of a patient with colonic tuberculosis showing extensive involvement of the cecum and ascending and transverse colon. The ulcerated, narrowed, ahaustral appearance is typical of granulomatous infiltration of the bowel. (Courtesy of H. I. Goldberg, MD, San Francisco, CA.)

and unidentified microorganisms probably increase the incidence by 10 to 100 times.

A food-borne disease outbreak is defined by two criteria: (1) similar illness, usually gastrointestinal, in two or more persons, and (2) epidemiologic or laboratory investigation that implicates food as the source. An extensive list of agents has been associated with food-borne illness syndromes (Table 104–19).[348] The major recognized causes of bacterial food poisoning are C. perfringens; S. aureus; Vibrio, including V. cholerae and V. parahaemolyticus; Bacillus cereus; Salmonella; Clostridium botulinum; Shigella; E. coli O157:H7; and certain species of Campylobacter, Yersinia, Listeria, and Aeromonas. Other bacteria, such as group A streptococcus and Listeria monocytogenes, have been implicated in some outbreaks (see Table 104–19).

Salmonella outbreaks predominate and constitute more than one half of confirmed cases of food-borne illness, in part because of its ease of recognition and general awareness of physicians and the public about the organism. E. coli is the next most frequent cause of food-borne outbreaks, followed closely by C. perfringens, S. aureus, and Shigella. Several pathogens rarely are reported, namely B. cereus and V. parahaemolyticus, but have been well studied in certain parts of the world. Their contribution to food-borne diarrheal illness in the United States has been recognized only recently, and their recovery from stool or food requires special laboratory procedures.

Approach to the Patient

A thorough history should provide clues to the etiology of the food-borne illness (Table 104–20). Details to be elicited should include the food ingested (Table 104–21); the time period between ingestion and onset of symptoms; the number of people who ingested the food and how many became ill; and the preparation and storage of the suspected food (e.g., picnic, home canning, restaurant).

Some food-borne illnesses are more common during certain seasons.[349] For example, during the summer months illnesses due to bacteria such as Salmonella, Shigella, and S. aureus are prevalent. Illnesses due to C. jejuni are more common in the spring and fall. C. perfringens outbreaks occur least often in the summer. Infections due to B. cereus and Norwalk virus occur year round.

In addition to considering the organism and its vector, one must also take into account the susceptibility of the host. Persons with liver disease have an annual rate

Table 104–19 Estimates of Rates of Food-Borne Illnesses and Mortality in the United States

Pathogen	Estimated Total No. of Cases	Food-Borne Transmission, %	No. of Deaths	Case Fatality Rate
Bacterial				
Brucella	1,554	50	11	0.0071
Campylobacter	2,453,926	80	124	0.0000
Escherichia coli				
O157:H7 (EHEC)	73,480	85	61	0.0008
Non-O157:H7 (EHEC)	36,740	85	30	0.0008
Listeria monocytogenes	2,518	99	504	0.2001
Salmonella				
S. typhi	824	80	3	0.0036
Nontyphoidal	1,412,498	95	582	0.0004
Shigella	448,240	20	70	0.0002
Noncholera Vibrio	7,880	65	20	0.0025
Vibrio vulnificus	94	50	37	0.3936
Yersinia enterocolitica	96,368	90	3	0.0000
Toxin Mediated				
Bacillus cereus	27,360	100	0	0.0000
Clostridium botulinum (food botulism)	58	100	4	0.0690
Clostridium perfringens	248,520	100	7	0.0000
Food poisoning				
Staphylococcal	185,060	100	2	0.0000
Streptococcal	50,920	100	0	0.0000
Parasitic				
Cryptosporidium parvum	300,000	10	66	0.0002
Cyclospora cayetanensis	16,264	90	0	0.0000
Giardia lamblia	2,000,000	10	10	0.0000
Toxoplasma gondii	225,000	50	750	0.0033
Trichinella spiralis	52	100	0	0.0000
Viral				
Astrovirus	3,900,000	1	10	0.0000
Norovirus and Norwalk-like viruses	23,000,000	40	310	0.0000
Rotavirus	3,900,000	1	30	0.0000
Hepatitis A virus	83,391	5	83	0.0010
Total	38,629,641	—	1809	0.0000

EHEC, enterohemorrhagic Escherichia coli.
From Mead PS, Slutsker L, Dietz V, et al: Food-related illness and death in the United States. Emerg Infect Dis 5:607, 1999.

Table 104–20 Features of Bacterial Food Poisoning

Organism	Common Vehicles	Median Incubation, hrs (Range)	Primary Toxin	Clinical Features	Median Duration, days (Range)	Secondary Attack Rate, %	Sources of Diagnostic Material
Bacillus cereus	Fried rice, vanilla sauce, cream, meatballs, boiled beef, barbecued chicken	2 (1-16) 9 (6-14)	Heat stable Heat labile	V, C, D D, C, V	0.4 (0.2-0.5) 1 (1-2)	0 0	Vomitus, stool, implicated food
Campylobacter jejuni	Milk, chicken, beef	48 (24-240)	?	D, F, C, B, H, M, N, V	7 (2-30)	25	Stool, rectal swab
Clostridium perfringens	Beef, turkey, chicken	12 (8-22)	Heat labile	D, C (N, V F rare)	1 (0.3-3)	0	Stool, rectal swab; food, food-contact surfaces
Escherichia coli	Salads, beef	24 (8-44) 96 (24-120)	Heat labile Heat stable Verotoxin	D, C, N, H, F, M F, M, D, C B, C, F, hemolytic-uremic syndrome	3 (1-4)	0	Stool, rectal swab
Listeria monocytogenes	Milk, raw vegetables, cole slaw, dairy products, poultry, beef	?	?	D, F, C, N, V, B	?	10	Stool, rectal swab
Salmonella	Eggs, meat, poultry	24 (5-72)	—	D, C, N, V, F, H, B (rare), enteric fever	3 (0.5-14)	30-50	Stool, rectal swab from patients and food preparers; raw food
Shigella	Milk, salads (potato, tuna, turkey)	24 (7-168)	—	C, F, D, B, H, N, V	3 (0.5-14)	40-60	Stool, rectal swab from patients, food preparers; implicated food
Staphylococcus aureus	Ham, pork, canned beef, cream-filled pastry	3 (1-6)	Heat stable	V, N, C, D, F (rare)	1 (0.3-1.5)	0	Stool, vomitus; food or food-contact surfaces; nose, hands, purulent lesion on food preparer
Vibrio parahaemolyticus	Seafood, rarely salt water or salted vegetables	12 (2-48)	?	D, C, N, V, H, F, B (rare)	3 (2-10)	0	Stool, rectal swab; food, food-contact surfaces; seawater
Yersinia enterocolitica	Chocolate milk or raw milk, pork	72 (2-144)	Heat stable	F, C, D, V, pharyngitis, arthritis, mesenteric adenitis, rashes	7 (2-30)	20	Stool from food preparer

B, bloody diarrhea; C, cramping abdominal pain; D, diarrhea; F, fever; H, headache; M, myalgia; N, nausea; V, vomiting; TCBS, thiosulfate citrate bile salts sucrose.
From Snydman DR: Food poisoning. In Gorbach SL, Bartlett JG, Blacklow NR (eds): Infectious Diseases. Philadelphia, WB Saunders, 1992, p 771.

Table 104–21 Organisms and Food-Borne Diseases Associated with Specific Foods or Beverages

Food	Associated Organisms and Diseases
Beef and pork	*Salmonella*
	Staphylococcus aureus
	Clostridium perfringens
	EHEC
	Bacillus cereus
	Yersinia enterocolitica
	Listeria monocytogenes
	Brucella
	Trichinella spiralis
Carbonated drinks	Heavy metal poisoning
Chinese food	*Bacillus cereus* (in fried rice)
	Monosodium glutamate poisoning
Eggs	*Salmonella*
	Staphylococcus aureus
Fish	*C. botulinum*
	Ciguatera poisoning
	Scombroid poisoning
	Diphyllobothrium latum
	Anisakiasis
Honey	*Clostridium botulinum*
Milk and cheese	*Salmonella*
	Campylobacter
	EIEC and EHEC
	Yersinia enterocolitica
	Group A streptococci
	Brucella
	Listeria monocytogenes
Poultry	*Salmonella*
	Staphylococcus aureus
	Campylobacter
	Clostridium perfringens
	Listeria monocytogenes
Shellfish	*Vibrio parahaemolyticus*
	Vibrio cholerae (O1 and non-O1)
	Hepatitis A
	Norovirus and Norwalk-like viruses
	Paralytic shellfish poisoning
	Neurotoxic shellfish poisoning
Vegetables	*Clostridium botulinum*
	Salmonella
	Shigella
	B. cereus
	Norovirus

EHEC, enterohemorrhagic *Escherichia coli*; EIEC, enteroinvasive *E. coli*.
From Bishai WR, Sears CL: Food poisoning syndromes. Gastroenterol Clin North Am 22:579, 1993.

of illness from *V. vulnificus* 80 times greater, and a death rate 200 times greater, than those of adults without liver disease.[350] Patients with compromised immune symptoms, such as chronic renal insufficiency, malignancy, diabetes, or iron overload states or those on glucocorticoids are probably also at increased risks of infection and death.[351] Gastric acidity, as discussed earlier, is a natural defense mechanism against infection that may be compromised by prior gastric surgery, or use of proton pump inhibitors.

The presenting symptom complex may give a clue to the etiologic organism. Symptom complexes may be classified as (1) nausea and vomiting; (2) noninflammatory diarrhea; (3) inflammatory diarrhea; (4) neurologic symptoms; and (5) systemic or miscellaneous symptoms.

This section deals with *C. perfringens*, *S. aureus*, *Listeria*, *B. cereus*, and botulism; the other bacterial agents are discussed in previous sections. Table 104–20 lists the characteristics of the more common types of bacterial food poisoning.

STAPHYLOCOCCUS AUREUS

Coagulase-positive *S. aureus* is the third most common cause of food poisoning in the United States; before 1973, it was the leading cause.

Microbiology

Five immunologically distinct enterotoxins have been associated with food-poisoning strains of *S. aureus*. These enterotoxins, termed *A*, *B*, *C*, *D*, and *E*, are heat-resistant polypeptides. When they are tested in a rat intestinal loop model, net secretion of water and electrolytes is observed.[352] Enterotoxins induce vomiting when fed to monkeys or human volunteers.

Epidemiology

Staphylococcal food poisoning has a short incubation period ($\approx$3 hours), with a range of 1 to 6 hours. The disease usually is clustered within a family or group, with a high attack rate. Many foods have been implicated in this form of food poisoning; however, foods with a high-salt concentration (e.g., ham or canned meat) or a high-sugar content (e.g., custard and cream) selectively favor the growth of staphylococci. The major mode of transmission is from a food handler to the food product. Involved foods usually have been cut, sliced, grated, mixed, or ground by workers who are carriers of toxin-producing strains of *S. aureus*.

Pathogenic Mechanisms

Three requisites for staphylococcal food poisoning are (1) contamination of a food with enterotoxin-producing staphylococci; (2) suitable growth requirements of the food for the organism: and (3) suitable time and temperature for the organism to multiply. The emetic dose of enterotoxin A or B for humans has been estimated to be between 1 and 25 µg.

Clinical Features

Symptoms of staphylococcal food poisoning are primarily profuse vomiting, nausea, and abdominal cramps, often followed by diarrhea occurring 1 to 4 hours after ingestion of a suspect meal. Vomiting is the dominant initial symptom and can lead to a severe metabolic alkalosis. Fever is unusual. Rarely, hypotension and marked prostration occur. Fatalities are unusual, and recovery is complete within 24 to 48 hours. Diagnosis is made based on the typical presentation occurring a few hours following the ingestion of typical foods. Most people with staphylococcal food poisoning do not consult a physician. More severe cases may require supportive care, particularly rehydration and correction of alkalosis. No specific therapy is available.

CLOSTRIDIUM PERFRINGENS

C. perfringens is a major food-borne pathogen that produces vomiting and diarrhea. The disease is caused by an enterotoxin elaborated by strains of C. perfringens type A. A more severe and often lethal food-borne illness, known variously as enteritis necroticans (Darmbrand) and pigbel, is caused by C. perfringens type C (see later).

Microbiology

Clostridia are Gram-positive, spore-forming, obligate anaerobes that can be found in the normal intestinal flora of humans and animals and in the soil. Although an anaerobe, C. perfringens is remarkably aerotolerant and survives exposure to oxygen for as long as 72 hours. C. perfringens produces 12 toxins that are mostly active in tissues, as well as several enterotoxins. The food poisoning syndrome is caused by a heat-labile protein enterotoxin, better termed a secretory cytotoxin, which is a structural component of the spore coat and is formed during sporulation; as other enterotoxins, it causes fluid accumulation in the rabbit ileal loop model presumably by altering membrane ion permeability.[353] Unlike cholera and E. coli enterotoxins, clostridial enterotoxin has its maximum activity in the ileum, inhibits glucose transport, damages the intestinal epithelium, and causes protein loss into the intestinal lumen.[354]

Epidemiology and Pathogenic Mechanisms

Epidemics of C. perfringens are characterized by high attack rates, with a large number of affected persons, usually 40 to 50 per outbreak. The incubation period varies from 8 to 14 hours but can be as long as 22 hours. In almost every outbreak of clostridial food poisoning, roasted, boiled, stewed, or steamed meats or poultry is the vehicle of infection. Usually, the meat is cooked in bulk so that heat gain and internal pressure are insufficient to kill the spores. The implicated food invariably undergoes a period of inadequate cooling, which allows the spores to germinate. The organism proliferates rapidly at temperatures between 15°C and 50°C. Unless the food is reheated to a very high temperature, it will contain many viable organisms.

Clinical Features

C. perfringens food poisoning is characterized by watery diarrhea, severe cramping abdominal pain, and frequently, vomiting that begins 8 to 24 hours after the incriminating meal. Fever, chills, headache, or other signs of infection usually are absent. The illness is of short duration, usually less than 24 hours. Rare fatalities have been recorded in debilitated or hospitalized patients.[355] No specific treatment is required for this illness.

Enteritis Necroticans

Enteritis necroticans is a disease that was described originally in post–World War II Germany, in an outbreak affecting more than 400 people who consumed rancid meat. Similar outbreaks, associated with the consumption of poorly cooked pork, have been described in New Guinea and are labeled pigbel.[356] The disease is caused by strains of C. perfringens type C. A β toxin is produced that, in malnourished patients, cannot be inactivated by the usual intestinal proteases and causes transmural intestinal wall necrosis. Intestinal perforation, sepsis, and hemorrhage result in a 40% mortality rate. Fortunately, this disease is rare. In the uncomplicated case, treatment is symptomatic and supportive.

Outbreaks of pigbel have been related to consumption of pig in large native feasts. The pig is improperly cooked, and large quantities are consumed over 3 or 4 days. Other cases, most often in children younger than 10 years of age, occur in villages. Enteritis necroticans associated with the consumption of chitterlings is encountered rarely in the United States.[357]

LISTERIA

Listeria are Gram-positive highly motile bacilli that are relatively heat resistant. They have been isolated from the intestinal tracts of humans and animals and from sewage and well water. Cases can occur as part of an outbreak or on a sporadic basis. In reported epidemics, the vehicles of infection have been raw and pasteurized milk, soft cheeses, cole slaw, shrimp, rice salad, pork dishes, and raw vegetables.[358,359] Listeria can be cultured from raw poultry, beef, or pork; prepackaged meat products; cheeses; and raw vegetables.[360]

Listeriosis usually is a systemic disease associated with bacteremia that can seed the meninges, heart valves, or body organs. Intestinal symptoms such as diarrhea and cramping often precede fever and bacteremia. Immunocompetent hosts occasionally develop gastroenteritis characterized by fever, headache, abdominal pain, nausea, and diarrhea; this form of listeriosis usually is not complicated by bacteremia.[361]

Among the food-borne pathogens, Listeria have been associated with the highest mortality rates; 70 deaths were reported from 1983 to 1987, for a case-fatality rate of 27%. Neurologic sequelae may occur in a sizeable proportion of survivors of central nervous system listeriosis. The propensity of the organism to attack immunosuppressed persons and pregnant women may account for the severity of the infection.

BACILLUS CEREUS

B. cereus is an aerobic, spore-forming, Gram-positive rod that has been associated with two clinical types of food poisoning—a diarrhea syndrome and a vomiting syndrome.[362] The organisms responsible for the two syndromes produce different toxins and have different epidemiologies.

Diarrhea Syndrome

Diarrhea results from an enterotoxin that causes intestinal secretion by activation of adenylate cyclase in intestinal epithelial cells, similar to the action of cholera toxin.

The median incubation period appears to be 9 hours, with a range of 6 to 14 hours. The clinical illness is characterized by diarrhea (96%), generalized cramps (75%), and vomiting (23%).[362] Fever is uncommon. The duration of illness ranges from 20 to 36 hours, with a median of 24 hours. The original report of *B. cereus* as a cause of diarrheal disease was associated with consumption of contaminated meatballs, but strains of *B. cereus* associated with diarrhea have been found in approximately 25% of many foods sampled, including cream, pudding, meat, spices, dried potatoes, dried milk, vanilla sauces, and spaghetti sauces, all of which are contaminated before cooking.[363] If the food is prepared so that the temperature is maintained at 30°C to 50°C, vegetative growth is permitted. Spores can survive extreme temperatures, and when allowed to cool relatively slowly, they germinate, multiply, and elaborate toxin. There is no evidence that human carriage of the organism or other means of contamination plays a role in transmission.

Whether the diarrheogenic heat-labile enterotoxin actually is ingested or produced in vivo is not known; however, the incubation of diarrheal illness is too long for preformed toxin, and a large inoculum (10^6) is required to cause illness, observations that suggest that intestinal colonization is required. Usually, no therapy is required because of the short duration of symptoms.

Vomiting Syndrome

Although the organism associated with the vomiting disease appears to be the same as the one causing diarrhea, a different type of toxin has been implicated.[364] The emetic syndrome results from ingestion of a preformed enterotoxin that is stable to heat. The emetic syndrome is more common than the diarrheal syndrome. Cell-free culture filtrates from these strains do not produce intestinal secretion, but they produce vomiting when fed to rhesus monkeys.

The vomiting syndrome has a short incubation period of approximately 2 hours. Virtually all affected persons have vomiting and abdominal cramps. Diarrhea is present in only one third. The duration of illness ranges from 8 to 10 hours, with a median of 9 hours; the illness usually is mild and self-limited, so no specific therapy is required. Nearly all reported cases involving the vomiting toxin have implicated fried rice as the vehicle.[362]

In England, almost 90% of uncooked rice was found to be colonized by *B. cereus*, although the number of organisms was relatively low.[365] The disease has been ascribed to the common practice in Chinese restaurants of allowing large portions of boiled rice to drain unrefrigerated to avoid clumping. Flash-frying during the final preparation of the fried rice does not produce enough heat to destroy apparently preformed heat-stable toxin. It appears that the emetic illness is caused by preformed toxin, because the incubation period is short, and there is an extremely high attack rate approaching 100% in outbreaks.

BOTULISM

Botulism is a rare food-borne disease resulting from exposure to neurotoxins secreted by strains of *Clostridium botulinum*. Between 1993 and 1997, there were 13 outbreaks of botulism in the United States, accounting for 56 cases and 1 death.[348] Although food-borne botulism is relatively uncommon, it is the most lethal of all the bacterial toxin-mediated food-borne diseases and the only one for which specific effective therapy is available.

Epidemiology

During the past few decades, food-borne botulism has become the least common form of botulism, trailing after wound and infant botulism. Food-borne botulism develops after the ingestion of preformed toxin in improperly preserved canned vegetables, salsas, meats, and fish. A disproportionate number of recent cases have occurred in the Pacific Northwest and Alaska, and cases have been associated with native American foods such as whale or seal that have been fermented or preserved with traditional methods. Recent outbreaks in the United States have been associated with baked potatoes, cheese sauce, beef stew, and garlic cooking oil.[366]

Infant botulism develops in infants whose gastrointestinal tract becomes colonized with live *C. botulinum* bacteria, which secrete small amounts of botulinum toxin. Absorption of low concentrations of the toxin leads to lethargy, poor feeding, constipation, diminished muscle tone, and a weak cry. The source of the botulinum toxin is not clear; household dust, soil, and honey in feedings have been suggested as possible sources. It is recommended that honey not be given to infants.

Pathogenic Mechanisms

C. botulinum and closely related species of clostridia produce heat-resistant spores that are capable of surviving food preservation techniques that destroy nonsporulating organisms. The seven serologically distinct botulinum toxins are designated with the letters *A* to *G*. Neutralization by type-specific serologic reagents is used to differentiate the serotypes. Types A, B, and E are responsible for most human cases of botulism.[367] Neurotoxin-producing strains of *Clostridium butyricum* and *Clostridium baratii* are less commonly responsible for human botulism. Toxin production occurs in the presence of anaerobic, low-solute, and low-acid conditions.

C. botulinum usually is unable to replicate in the mature human gut, although the toxin is acid stable and easily traverses the gastric barrier intact. After absorption, the botulinum toxin binds irreversibly to presynaptic cholinergic nerve endings of the cranial and peripheral nerves, thereby resulting in inhibition of the release of acetylcholine and the characteristic clinical syndrome that results from the blockade of voluntary motor and autonomic cholinergic junctions.

Clinical Features

Ingestion of botulinum toxin initially results in gastrointestinal symptoms, including nausea, vomiting, abdominal pain, and diarrhea, usually within 18 to 36 hours after toxin ingestion.[366] Once neurologic symptoms develop, constipation is common. Dry mouth, diplopia, and blurred vision are followed by dysarthria, dysphonia, dysphagia, and peripheral muscle weakness. The typical symmetrical descending paralysis starts with the cranial nerves and then affects the upper extremities, respiratory muscles, and, finally, lower extremities. Respiratory muscle paralysis may result in respiratory failure and death if mechanical ventilation is not instituted; higher cortical functions are unaffected.

Diagnosis

Botulism should be suspected in any patient with the acute onset of gastrointestinal, autonomic nervous system, and cranial nerve dysfunction, especially if the patient recently has consumed foods that were home canned. Results of magnetic resonance imaging or computed tomography of the brain and lumbar puncture are normal in patients with botulism, whereas electromyography may show characteristic abnormalities. If foodborne botulism is suspected, stool, serum, and implicated foods should be tested for botulinum neurotoxin by the mouse inoculation test.

Treatment

Supportive therapy with mechanical ventilation has helped to reduce mortality rates from botulism greatly during the past several decades. The diagnosis of botulism must be considered early in any case of unexplained paralysis, and antitoxin should be administered if the diagnosis is credible. The trivalent equine botulinum antitoxin is available only through the CDC, which maintains supplies of antitoxin at sites around the country for immediate release in case of an emergency. To obtain the antitoxin, physicians need to contact their state health department's emergency hotline or the CDC directly (telephone no. 1-800-232-4636).

Speed is of the essence, because the antitoxin cannot displace the toxin once it has bound to the presynaptic nerve terminal; it serves only to bind free circulating toxin. Once symptoms have developed, the usefulness of the antitoxin is reduced greatly. In a large retrospective analysis of 134 cases of botulinum toxin A-mediated disease, patients who received antitoxin therapy early in the course had a mortality rate of 10%, as opposed to a mortality rate of 15% in those who received the antitoxin more than 24 hours after the onset of symptoms and 46% in those who did not receive antitoxin at all.[368] Moreover, patients who received antitoxin stayed in the hospital an average of 10 days, compared with 56 days for the untreated group.

The current recommendation is to administer a single 10-mL dose of intravenous antitoxin to each exposed person. This recommendation is based on the calculation that each vial has enough neutralizing antibody (for types A, B, and E) to bind a titer of toxin that is 100 times greater than the highest titer documented to date by the CDC.

BACILLUS ANTHRACIS

Although most anthrax infections are the result of cutaneous exposure to or inhalation of infected spores, the ingestion of infected animal tissue can lead to gastrointestinal disease.

Microbiology

Bacillus anthracis is an aerobic, Gram-positive, spore-forming, nonmotile bacillus that is found in soil. Endospores can remain dormant in soil for many years. Anthrax spores germinate in nutrient-rich environments. Vegetative anthrax bacilli elaborate an antiphagocytic polyglutamyl capsule and a toxin complex that is composed of protective antigen, lethal factor, and edema factor.[369] Protective antigen acts as the binding site for the lethal and edema factors. The lethal factor stimulates macrophages to release tumor necrosis factor-α and IL-1, which contribute to death from toxemia in anthrax infections characterized by high-grade bacteremia.

Epidemiology

The consumption of endospore-contaminated meat from infected animals is the primary mode of transmission of gastrointestinal anthrax. Point source outbreaks within households are common. This form of anthrax never has been conclusively documented in the United States, presumably because livestock are vaccinated for anthrax in regions endemic for the disease and because animals routinely are inspected by federal and state meat inspectors. In 2000, an outbreak of gastrointestinal illness characterized by diarrhea, abdominal pain, and fever was identified in two family members who had consumed meat from a carcass that was found to be contaminated with *B. anthracis*.[370] Fortunately, the infections were mild and self-limited.

Pathogenic Mechanisms

Entry of endospores through the gastrointestinal mucosa initiates infection. Macrophages phagocytose ingested endospores, which then germinate to form vegetative bacteria in mesenteric lymph nodes. The bacteria are then released from the macrophages, multiply in the local lymphatic systems, and enter the bloodstream. The release of the exotoxin complexes results in local tissue damage with massive edema, mucosal ulcerations, and the development of systemic toxemia.

Clinical Features

Approximately 1 to 7 days after the ingestion of raw or undercooked meat from infected animals, nausea, vomiting, abdominal pain, and fever develop. Patients often rapidly develop worsening symptoms characterized by bloody diarrhea, diffuse abdominal pain with rebound tenderness, and, occasionally, hematemesis. Ascites, which may be purulent, develops 2 to 4 days later. More than 50% of episodes are fatal, with death occurring as a consequence of toxemia, intestinal perforation, or shock from hemorrhage and fluid losses.

Oropharyngeal anthrax is a less common form of infection that develops when spores are deposited in the oropharynx. Symptoms include fever, a severely sore throat, and dysphagia, which may progress to respiratory distress. Examination often reveals swelling of the neck, lymphadenitis, and pharyngeal ulcers covered by a pseudomembrane. Despite the relatively severe symptoms, this form of infection tends to be milder than the gastrointestinal disease and rarely is fatal.

Treatment and Prevention

Because some strains of *B. anthracis* contain an inducible β-lactamase, initial therapy should consist of ciprofloxacin. Because there is a higher risk of mortality in severe cases, the addition of rifampin or clindamycin, or both, is recommended in these situations. Penicillin and doxycycline are both highly active against *B. anthracis* in the absence of resistance. An anthrax vaccine, consisting of a sterile filtrate of an attenuated strain of the organism, is available to the U.S. military but not to civilians.

FISH POISONING

Food poisoning due to marine toxins in fish is a common worldwide problem. The commonest of these are ciguatera and scombroid poisoning.[371,372]

CIGUATERA

Ciguatera (Spanish: *cigua*, sea snail) poisoning manifests with a combination of gastrointestinal and neurologic symptoms and findings. It accounts for approximately one half of fish-related outbreaks in the United States. Ciguatera poisoning occurs most commonly in the coastal regions of the United States; however, in this age of air transport of foods, cases can occur inland as well. It is especially common in the tropics and subtropics.

More than 400 different species of fish have been associated with ciguatera poisoning, including grouper, red snapper, amberjack, and dolphin. The illness is caused by the consumption of fish containing toxins produced by dinoflagellates. Fish consume the dinoflagellates that elaborate the toxin(s) that subsequently are stored in fish flesh and viscera. The toxin is concentrated up the food chain as small fish are consumed by larger fish. The fish are not affected by the toxins; they do not appear spoiled and taste normal. The commonest toxin involved is ciguatoxin, a marine saponin, but a number of toxins can be involved.[373] The toxins are both heat and acid resistant and survive preservation (freezing) and preparation (cooking) procedures.

As mentioned, the usual manifestation involves a combination of gastrointestinal and neurologic symptoms. Gastrointestinal symptoms occur 3 to 6 hours after eating contaminated fish and usually involve a combination of nausea, vomiting, abdominal cramps, and diarrhea. Sweating and headaches also may occur. A variety of neurologic symptoms occur 3 to 72 hours after ingestion and include paresthesias, blurred vision, nerve palsies, cold dysesthesia, and so forth. Cardiovascular symptoms also may occur and include bradycardia, heart block, and hypotension. Variations in the symptom complex and in the severity of individual symptoms may occur depending on the type of fish eaten and presumably on the type and quantity of toxin or toxins consumed.

Diarrhea is the result of toxin-stimulated intestinal secretion mediated by changes in intracellular calcium. Neurologic symptoms are a consequence of alterations in voltage-dependent neural sodium channels. The illness may persist up to one month and, rarely, may last up to one year. Approximately 3% to 20% of patients may have chronic effects, such as fatigue, myalgias, and headaches. Chronic symptoms may be aggravated or triggered by ingestion of caffeine or alcohol. Fatalities are rare and usually result from cardiovascular collapse.

The diagnosis is a clinical one based on clinical suspicion and the compatible signs and symptoms: There is no available confirmatory test, no specific treatment, and treatment is supportive. Intravenous mannitol may be helpful in severe cases.

SCOMBROID

Scombroid poisoning is a common but under-reported illness. It also is misdiagnosed frequently as a fish "allergy." It occurs after the consumption of fish that has been poorly refrigerated or improperly stored, allowing bacterial proliferation and the accumulation of histamine. Bacteria decarboxylate histidine in the muscle of fish, producing high levels of histamine. The fish do not appear spoiled but may taste "peppery." The histamine is not destroyed by cooking or freezing. The illness can occur after ingestion of either fresh or canned fish or consumption of foods such as tuna salad or tuna burgers. The most common fish involved are dark meat fish such as tuna, mackerel, and bonito, but scombroid poisoning also may occur with mahi-mahi, bluefish, swordfish, or salmon ingestion.

The usual clinical presentation begins as soon as 1 hour after ingestion of the contaminated fish. Symptoms and signs include flushing, warmth, erythematous skin rash, pruritus, palpitations, and tachycardia. Patients also may experience headache, blurred vision, and respiratory distress. Occasionally respiratory distress may occur from facial and lingual swelling. The illness usually resolves spontaneously within 12 hours without any sequelae. Diagnosis is a clinical one based on the signs and symptoms just described. Plasma histamine levels, if measured acutely, may be elevated. Treatment mainly is supportive, but H-1 antihistamines may be helpful.

ACKNOWLEDGMENT

This chapter succeeds the chapter in the previous edition by Davidson H. Hamer and Sherwood L. Gorbach, entitled "Infectious Diarrhea and Bacterial Food Poisoning." I wish to acknowledge that I have drawn heavily on the material from their chapter, and many portions of the original chapter remain.

REFERENCES

1. Garthright WE, Archer DL, Kvenberg JE: Estimates of incidence and costs of intestinal infectious diseases in the United States. Public Health Rep 103:107, 1988.
2. Mead PS, Slutsker L, Dietz V, et al: Food-related illness and death in the United States. Emerg Infect Dis 5:607, 1999.
3. Diagnosis and management of foodborne illnesses: A primer for physicians and other health care professionals. MMWR 53:RR-4:1, 2004.

4. Robinson PK, Giannella RA, Taylor MB: Infectious diarrheas. In Taylor MB (ed): Gastrointestinal Emergencies, 2nd ed. Baltimore, Williams & Wilkins, 1997, p 649.
5. Wolf D, Giannella RA: Antibiotic therapy for bacterial enterocolitis. Am J Gastroenterol 88:1667, 1993.
6. Park SI, Giannella RA: Approach to the adult patient with acute diarrhea. Gastroenterol Clin North Am 22:483, 1993.
7. Giannella RA, Broitman SA, Zamcheck N: The influence of gastric acidity on bacterial and parasitic enteric infections. Ann Intern Med 78:271, 1973.
8. Giannella RA, Broitman SA, Zamcheck N: Gastric acid barrier to ingested microorganisms in man: In vivo and in vitro studies. Gut 13:251, 1972.
9. Hornick RB, Music SI, Wenzel R, et al: The Broad Street pump revisited: Response of volunteers to ingested *Cholera vibrios*. Bull NY Acad Med 47:1181, 1971.
10. Gitelson S: Gastrectomry, achlorhydria, and cholera. Isr J Med Sci 7:663, 1977.
11. Giannella RA, Broitman SA, Zamcheck N: Salmonella enteritis: I. Role of reduced gastric secretion in pathogenesis. Am J Dig Dis 11:1000, 1971.
12. DuPont HL, Hornick RB, Snyder MJ, et al: Immunity in shigellosis: I. Response of man to attenuated strains of *Shigella*. J Infect Dis 125:5, 1972.
13. Justus PG, Martin JL, Goldberg DA, et al: Myoelectrical effects of *C. difficile*: Motility-altering factor distinct from its cytotoxin and enterotoxin in rabbits. Gastroenterology 83:836, 1982.
14. Formal SB, Dammin GJ, LaBrec EH, et al: Experimental shigellosis infection: Characteristics of a fatal infection in guinea pigs. J Bacteriol 75:604, 1958.
15. Lyerly DM, Krivan HC, Wilkins TD: *C. difficile*: Its disease and toxins. Clin Microbiol Rev 1:1, 1988.
16. Hornick RB, Greisman SE, Woodward TE, et al: Typhoid fever: Pathogenesis and immunologic control. N Engl J Med 283:686, 1970.
17. Bohnhoff M, Miller CP: Enhancing susceptibility to *Salmonella* infection in streptomycin-treated mice. J Infect Dis 111:117, 1962.
18. Shub MD, Pang KY, Swann DA, et al: Age-related changes in chemical composition and physical properties of mucous glycoproteins from rat intestine. Biochem J 215:405, 1983.
19. Davies A: An investigation into the serologic properties of dysentery stools. Lancet 2:1009, 1922.
20. Freter R: Intestinal immunity: Studies of the mechanism of action of intestinal immunity in experimental cholera. Tex Rep Biol Med 27:299, 1969.
21. Goldman AS, Garza C, Nicholas B, et al: Immunological factors in human milk during the first year of lactation. J Pediatr 100:563, 1982.
22. Mata LJ, Urrutia JJ, Fernandez R, et al: Shigellosis in breast-fed Guatemalan Indian neonates. Am J Dis Child 117:142, 1969.
23. Kenny JF, Boesman MI, Michaels RH, et al: Bacterial and viral coproantibodies in breast-fed infants. Pediatr 39:202, 1967.
24. Hanson LA, Anderson B, Carlson B, et al: Defense of mucosal membranes by antibodies, receptor analogues, and non-specific host factors. Infection 13:S166, 1985.
25. Rothbaum R, McAdams AJ, Giannella RA, Partin JL: A clinicopathologic study of enterocyte-adherent *E. coli*: A cause of protracted diarrhea in infants. Gastroenterology 83:441, 1982.
26. Levine MM, Edelman R: Enteropathogenic *Escherichia coli* of classic serotypes associated with infant diarrhea: Epidemiology and pathogenesis. Epidemiol Rev 6:31, 1984.
27. Moon HW, Whipp SC, Argenzio RA, et al: Attaching and effacing activities of rabbit and human *E. coli* in pig and rabbit intestine. Infect Immun 41:1340, 1983.
28. Ulshen MH, Rollo JL: Pathogenesis of *E. coli* gastroenteritis: Another mechanism. N Engl J Med 302:99, 1980.
29. Nataro JP, Kaper JB: Diarrheagenic *Escherichia coli*. Clin Microbiol Rev 11:142, 1998.
30. Donnenberg MS, Kaper JB: Enteropathogenic *Escherichia coli*. Infect Immun 60:3953, 1992.
31. Jerse AE, Kaper JB: The *eae* gene of enteropathogenic *Escherichia coli* encodes a 94-kilodalton membrane protein, the expression of which is influenced by the EAF plasmid. Infect Immun 59:4302, 1991.
32. Levine MM, Nataro JP, Karch H, et al: The diarrheal response of humans to some classic serotypes of enteropathogenic *Escherichia coli* is dependent on a plasmid encoding an enteroadhesiveness factor. J Infect Dis 152:550, 1985.
33. Donnenberg MS, Tacket CO, James SP, et al: Role of the *eaeA* gene in experimental enteropathogenic *Escherichia coli* infection. J Clin Invest 92:1412, 1993.
34. Smith HW, Linggood MA: Observations on the pathologic properties of the K88, Hly, and Ent plasmids of *E. coli* with particular reference to porcine diarrhea. J Med Microbiol 4:467, 1971.
35. Evans DG, Silver RP, Evans DJ Jr, et al: Plasmid-controlled colonization factor associated with virulence in *Escherichia coli* enterotoxigenic for humans. Infect Immun 12:656, 1975.
36. Moon HW: Luminal and mucosal factors of small intestine affecting pathogenic colonization. In Field M, Fordtran JS, Schultz S (eds): Secretory Diarrhea. Bethesda, MD, American Physiological Society, 1980, p 119.
37. Carpenter CC: Cholera and other enterotoxin-related diarrheal disorders. J Infect Dis 126:551, 1972.
38. Finkelstein RA: Cholera. Crit Rev Microbiol 2:553, 1973.
39. Giannella RA, Drake KW: Effect of purified *E. coli* heat-stable enterotoxin on intestinal cyclic nucleotide metabolism and fluid secretion. Infect Immun 24:19, 1979.
40. Field M: Mechanisms of action of cholera and *E. coli* enterotoxins. Am J Clin Nutr 32:189, 1979.
41. Levine MM: *E. coli* that cause diarrhea. J Infect Dis 155:377, 1987.
42. Cohen MB, Giannella RA: Enterotoxigenic *E. coli*. In Blaser M, Smith P, Ravdin J, et al (eds): Infections of the Gastrointestinal Tract, 2nd ed. Philadelphia, Lippincott Williams & Wilkins, 2002, p 579.
43. O'Brein AD, Holmes RK: *Shiga* and *Shiga*-like toxins. Microbiol Rev 51:775, 1987.
44. Rout WR, Formal SB, Giannella RA: Pathophysiology of *Shigella* diarrhea in the rhesus monkey: Intestinal transport, morphological and bacteriological studies. Gastroenterology 68:270, 1975.
45. LaBrec EH, Schneider H, Magnani IJ, et al: Epithelial cell penetration as an essential step in the pathogenesis of bacillary dysentery. J Bacteriol 88:1503, 1964.
46. Giannella RA, Formal SB, Dammin GJ, et al: Pathogenesis of salmonellosis: Studies of fluid secretion, mucosal invasion, and morphological reaction in rabbit intestine. J Clin Invest 52:441, 1973.
47. Calubrian O, Domenico P, Klein N, Cunha B: The significance of fecal leukocytes in infectious disease. Hosp Physician Feb:56, 1990.
48. Guerrant RL, Araujo V, Soares E, et al: Measurement of fecal lactoferrin as a marker of fecal leukocytes. J Clin Microbiol 30:1238, 1992.
49. Koplan JP, Fineberg HV, Ferraro MJB, et al: Value of stool cultures. Lancet 2:413, 1980.
50. Rowland MG, Davies H, Patterson S, et al: Viruses and diarrhea in West Africa and London: A collaborative study. Trans R Soc Trop Med Hyg 72:95, 1978.
51. Watson B, Ellis M, Mandal B, et al: A comparison of the clinic-pathological features with stool pathogens in patients

hospitalized with the symptom of diarrhoea. Scand J Infect Dis 18:553, 1986.

52. Jewkes J, Larson HE, Price AB, et al: Aetiology of acute diarrhea in adults. Gut 22:388, 1981.

53. Dryden MS, Gabb RJ, Wright SK: Empirical treatment of severe acute community-acquired gastroenteritis with ciprofloxacin. Clin Infect Dis 22:1019, 1996.

54. Blake PA, Allegra DT, Snyder JD, et al: Cholera: A possible endemic focus in the United States. N Engl J Med 310:305, 1980.

55. Ramamurthy T, Garg S, Sharma R, et al: Emergence of novel strain of Vibrio cholerae with epidemic potential in southern and eastern India. Lancet 341:703, 1993.

56. Cholera Working Group: Large epidemic of cholera-like disease in Bangladesh caused by Vibrio cholerae 0139 synonym Bengal. Lancet 342:387, 1993.

57. Johnson JA, Salles CA, Panigrahi P, et al: Vibrio cholerae 0139 synonym Bengal is closely related to Vibrio cholerae El Tor but has important differences. Infect Immun 62:2108, 1994.

58. Waldor MK, Mekalanos J: Lysogenic conversion by a filamentous phage encoding cholera toxin. Science 272:1910, 1996.

59. Fasano A, Baudry B, Pumplin DW, et al: Vibrio cholerae produces a second enterotoxin which affects intestinal tight junctions. Proc Natl Acad Sci U S A 88:5242, 1991.

60. World Health Organization. Cholera, 1999. Wkly Epidemiol Rec 75:249, 2000.

61. Morris JG, Black RE: Cholera and other vibrios in the United States. N Engl J Med 312:343, 1985.

62. Update: Vibrio cholerae 01-Western hemisphere, 1991-1994, and V. cholerae 0139-Asia, 1994. MMWR Morb Mortal Wkly Rep 44:215, 1995.

63. Ries AA, Vugia DJ, Beingolea L, et al: Cholera in Piura, Peru: A modern urban epidemic. J Infect Dis 166:1429, 1992.

64. Mujica OJ, Quick RE, Palacios AM, et al: Epidemic cholera in the Amazon: The role of produce in disease risk and prevention. J Infect Dis 169:1381, 1994.

65. Morris JG, Losonsky GE, Johnson JA, et al: Clinical and immunologic characteristics of Vibrio cholerae 0139 Bengal infection in North American volunteers. J Infect Dis 171:903, 1995.

66. Basu A, Garg P, Datta S, et al: Vibrio cholerae 0139 in Calcutta, 1992-1998: Incidence, antibiograms, and genotypes. Emerg Infect Dis 6:139, 2000.

67. Herrington DA, Hall RH, Losonsky G, et al: Toxin, toxin-coregulated pili and the toxR regulon are essential for Vibrio cholerae pathogenesis in humans. J Exp Med 168:1487, 1989.

68. World Health Organization: Guidelines for cholera control. Geneva, Switzerland, World Health Organization, Programme for Control of Diarrhoeal Disease. WHO/CCD/SER/80.4 Rev. 2, 1991.

69. Centers for Disease Control and Prevention: Update: Cholera—Western Hemisphere, and recommendations for treatment of cholera. MMWR Morb Mortal Wkly Rep 40:562, 1991.

70. Gotuzzo E, Seas C, Echevarria J, et al: Ciprofloxacin for the treatment of cholera: A randomized, double-blind, controlled clinical trial of a single daily dose in Peruvian adults. Clin Infect Dis 20:1485, 1995.

71. Khan WA, Bennish ML, Seas C, et al: Randomised controlled comparison of single-dose ciprofloxacin and doxycycline for cholera caused by Vibrio cholerae 01 or 0139. Lancet 348:296, 1996.

72. Hamer DH, Gorbach SL: Use of the quinolones for the treatment and prophylaxis of bacterial infections. In Andriole VT (ed): The Quinolones, 3rd ed. San Diego, Academic Press, 2000.

73. Hlady WG, Klontz KC: The epidemiology of Vibrio infections in Florida, 1981-1993. J Infect Dis 173:1176, 1996.

74. Blake PA, Weaver RE, Hollis DG: Diseases of humans (other than cholera) caused by vibrios. Annu Rev Microbiol 34:341, 1980.

75. Hughes JM, Hollis DG, Gangarosa EJ, et al: Non-cholera vibrio infections in the United States. Ann Intern Med 88:602, 1978.

76. Shapiro RL, Altekruse S, Hutwagner L, et al: and the Vibrio Working Group: The role of Gulf Coast oysters harvested in warmer months in Vibrio vulnificus infections in the United States, 1988-1996. J Infect Dis 178:752, 1998.

77. Dalsgaard A, Albert MJ, Taylor DN, et al: Characterization of Vibrio cholerae non-01 serogroups obtained from an outbreak of diarrhea in Lima, Peru. J Clin Microbiol 33:2715, 1995.

78. Lowry PW, McFarland LM, Peltier BH, et al: Vibrio gastroenteritis in Louisiana: A prospective study among attendees of a scientific congress in New Orleans. J Infect Dis 160:978, 1989.

79. Hoge CW, Watsky D, Peeler RN, et al: Epidemiology and spectrum of vibrio infections in a Chesapeake Bay community. J Infect Dis 160:985, 1989.

80. Calia FM, Johnson DE: Bacteremia in suckling rabbits after oral challenge with Vibrio parahaemolyticus. Infect Immun 11:1222, 1975.

81. Daniels NA, MacKinnon L, Bishop R, et al: Vibrio parahaemolyticus infections in the United States, 1973-1998. J Infect Dis 181:1661, 2000.

82. Daniels NA, Ray B, Easton A, et al: Emergence of a new Vibrio parahaemolyticus serotype in raw oysters: A prevention quandary. JAMA 284:1541, 2000.

83. Klontz KC, Lieb S, Schreiber M, et al: Syndromes of Vibrio vulnificus infections: Clinical and epidemiologic features in Florida cases, 1981-1987. Ann Intern Med 109:318, 1988.

84. Shandera WX, Johnston JM, Davis BR, et al: Disease from infection with Vibrio mimicus, a newly recognized Vibrio species. Ann Intern Med 99:169, 1983.

85. Hansen W, Freney J, Benyagoub H, et al: Severe human infections caused by Vibrio metschnikovii. J Clin Microbiol 31:2529, 1993.

86. Janda JM, Abbott SL: Unusual food-borne pathogens: Listeria monocytogenes, Aeromonas, Plesiomonas, and Edwardsiella species. Clin Lab Med 19:553, 1999.

87. Namdari H, Bonnone EJ: Microbiologic and clinical evidence supporting the role of Aeromonas caviae as a pediatric enteric pathogen. J Clin Microbiol 28:837, 1990.

88. Namdari H, Bottone EJ: Cytotoxin and enterotoxin production as factors delineating enteropathogenicity of Aeromonas caviae. J Clin Microbiol 28:1796, 1990.

89. Holmberg SD, Schell WL, Fanning GR, et al: Aeromonas infections in the United States. Ann Intern Med 105:683, 1986.

90. Gracey M, Burke V, Robinson J: Aeromonas-associated gastroenteritis. Lancet 2:1304, 1982.

91. Holmberg SD, Farmer JJ III: Aeromonas hydrophila and Plesiomonas shigelloides as causes of intestinal infections. Rev Infect Dis 6:633, 1984.

92. Jones BL, Wilcox MH: Aeromonas infections and their treatment. J Antimicrob Chemother 35:453, 1995.

93. Brenden RA, Miller A, Janda JM: Clinical disease spectrum and pathogenic factors associated with Plesiomonas shigelloides infections in humans. Rev Infect Dis 10:303, 1988.

94. Holmberg SD, Wachsmuth K, Hickman-Brenner FW, et al: Plesiomonas enteric infections in the United States. Ann Intern Med 105:690, 1986.

95. Jerse AE, Martin WC, Galen JE, et al: Oligonucleotide probe for detection of the enteropathogenic Escherichia coli (EPEC) adherence factor of localized adherent EPEC. J Clin Microbiol 28:2842, 1990.

96. Tardelli TA, Rassi V, MacDonald KL, et al: Enteropathogens associated with acute diarrheal disease in urban infants in Sao Paulo, Brazil. J Infect Dis 164:331, 1991.

97. Levine MM, Ferreccio C, Prado V, et al: Epidemiologic studies of *Escherichia coli* diarrheal infections in a low socioeconomic level peri-urban community in Santiago, Chile. Am J Epidemiol 138:849, 1993.

98. Germani Y, Bégaud E, Duval P, et al: Prevalence of enteropathogenic, enteroaggregative, and diffusely adherent *Escherichia coli* among isolates from children with diarrhea in New Caledonia. J Infect Dis 174:1124, 1996.

99. Clements JD, Finkelstein RA: Immunological cross-reactivity between a heat-labile enterotoxin of *Escherichia coli* and subunits of *Vibrio cholerae* enterotoxin. Infect Immun 21:1036, 1978.

100. Daniels NA, Neimann J, Karpati A, et al: Traveler's diarrhea at sea: Three outbreaks of waterborne enterotoxigenic *Escherichia coli* on cruise ships. J Infect Dis 181:1491, 2000.

101. Merson MH, Sack RB, Islam S, et al: Disease due to enterotoxigenic *Escherichia coli* in Bangladeshi adults: Clinical aspects and a controlled trial of tetracycline. J Infect Dis 141:702, 1980.

102. Evans DJ Jr, Ruiz-Palacios G, Evans DG, et al: Humoral immune response to the heat-labile enterotoxin of *Escherichia coli* in naturally acquired diarrhea and antitoxin determination by passive immune hemolysis. Infect Immun 16:781, 1977.

103. Mattila L, Peltola H, Siitonen A, et al: Short-term treatment of traveler's diarrhea with norfloxacin: A double-blind, placebo-controlled study during two seasons. Clin Infect Dis 17:779, 1993.

104. Tulloch EF, Ryan KJ, Formal SB: Invasive enteropathic *Escherichia coli* dysentery: An outbreak in 28 adults. Ann Intern Med 79:13, 1973.

105. Taylor DN, Echeverria P, Sethabutr O, et al: Clinical and microbiologic features of *Shigella* and enteroinvasive *Escherichia coli* infections detected by DNA hybridization. J Clin Microbiol 26:1362, 1988.

106. Riley LW, Remis RS, Helgerson SD, et al: Hemorrhagic colitis associated with a rare *Escherichia coli* serotype. N Engl J Med 308:681, 1983.

107. Su C, Brandt LJ: *Escherichia coli* O157:H7 infection in humans. Ann Intern Med 123:698, 1995.

108. Griffin PM, Mead PS, Sivapalaswingam S: E. *coli* O157:H7 and other enterohemorrhagic *E. coli*. In Blaser MJ, Smith PD, Ravdin JI, et al (eds): Infections of the Gastrointestinal Tract, 2nd ed. Philadelphia, Lippincott Williams & Wilkins, 2002, p 627.

109. Slutzker LA, Ries AA, Green JG, et al: *Escherichia coli* O157:H7 diarrhea in the United States: Clinical and epidemiological features. Ann Intern Med 126:505, 1997.

110. Martin DL, MacDonald KL, White KE, et al: The epidemiology and clinical aspects of the hemolytic-uremic syndrome in Minnesota. N Engl J Med 323:1161, 1990.

111. Bell BP, Goldoft M, Griffin PM, et al: A multistate outbreak of *Escherichia coli* O157:H7-associated bloody diarrhea and hemolytic-uremic syndrome from hamburgers: The Washington experience. JAMA 272:1349, 1994.

112. Keene WE, Hedberg K, Herriot DE, et al: A prolonged outbreak of *Escherichia coli* O157:H7 infections caused by commercially distributed raw milk. J Infect Dis 176:815, 1997.

113. Besser RE, Lett SM, Weber JT, et al: An outbreak of diarrhea and hemolytic-uremic syndrome from *Escherichia coli* O157:H7 in fresh-pressed apple cider. JAMA 269:2217, 1993.

114. Belongia EA, Osterholm MT, Soler JT, et al: Transmission of *Escherichia coli* O157:H7 infection in Minnesota child day-care facilities. JAMA 269:883, 1993.

115. Carter AO, Borczyk AA, Carlson JAK, et al: A severe outbreak of *Escherichia coli* O157:H7-associated hemorrhagic colitis in a nursing home. N Engl J Med 317:1496, 1987.

116. Karmali MA: Infection by verocytotoxin-producing *Escherichia coli*. Clin Microbiol Rev 2:15, 1989.

117. Law D, Kelly J: Use of heme and hemoglobin by *Escherichia coli* O157 and other *Shiga*-like toxin-producing *E. coli* serogroups. Infect Immun 63:700, 1995.

118. Su C, Brandt LJ, Alt E, et al: The immunohistological diagnosis of *E. coli* O157:H7: Possible association with colonic ischemia. Am J Gastroenterol 93:1055, 1998.

119. Milford DV, Taylor CM, Guttridge B, et al: Haemolytic-uraemic syndromes in the British Isles 1985-1988—association with verocytotoxin-producing *Escherichia coli*: I. Clinical and epidemiological aspects. Arch Dis Child 65:716, 1990.

120. Kleanthous H, Smith HR, Scotland SM, et al: Haemolytic-uraemic syndromes in the British Isles, 1985-1988—association with verocytotoxin-producing *Escherichia coli*: II. Microbiological aspects. Arch Dis Child 65:722, 1990.

121. Tarr PI, Neill MA, Clausen CR, et al: *Escherichia coli* O157:H7 and the hemolytic-uremic syndrome: Importance of early cultures in establishing the etiology. J Infect Dis 162:553, 1990.

122. Shah S, Hoffman R, Shillam P, et al: Prolonged fecal shedding of *Escherichia coli* O157:H7 during an outbreak at a day care center. Clin Infect Dis 23:835, 1996.

123. Karch H, Russman H, Schmidt H, et al: Long-term shedding and clonal turnover of enterohemorrhagic *Escherichia coli* O157 in diarrheal disease. J Clin Microbiol 33:1602, 1995.

124. Zhang X, McDaniel AD, Wolf LE, et al: Quinolone antibiotics induce *Shiga* toxin-encoding bacteriophages, toxin production, and death in mice. J Infect Dis 181:664, 2000.

125. Proulx F, Turgeon JP, Delage G, et al: Randomized, controlled trial of antibiotic therapy for *Escherichia coli* O157:H7 enteritis. J Pediatr 121:299, 1992.

126. Wong CS, Srdjan J, Habeeb RL, et al: The risk of hemolytic-uremic infections. N Engl J Med 342:1930, 2000.

127. Safdar N, Said A, Gangnon RE, Maki DG: Risk of hemolytic-uremic syndrome after antibiotic treatment of *E. coli* O157:H7 enteritis. JAMA 288: 996, 2002.

128. Molbak K, Mead PS, Griffin PM: Antimicrobial therapy in patients with *E. coli* O157:H7 infection. JAMA 288:1014, 2002.

129. Cravioto A, Tello A, Navarro A, et al: Association of *Escherichia coli* Hep-2 adherence patterns with type and duration of diarrhoea. Lancet 337:262, 1991.

130. Gunzberg ST, Chang BJ, Elliott SJ, et al: Diffuse and enteroaggregative patterns of enteric *Escherichia coli* isolated from aboriginal children from the Kimberley region of Western Australia. J Infect Dis 167:755, 1993.

131. Wanke CA, Mayer H, Weber R, et al: Enteroaggregative *Escherichia coli* as a potential cause of diarrheal disease in adults infected with human immunodeficiency virus. J Infect Dis 178:185, 1998.

132. Glandt M, Adachi JA, Mathewson JJ, et al: Enteroaggregative *Escherichia coli* as a cause of traveler's diarrhea: Clinical response to ciprofloxacin. Clin Infect Dis 29:335, 1999.

133. Nataro JP, Yikang D, Cookson S, et al: Heterogeneity of enteroaggregative *Escherichia coli* virulence demonstrated in volunteers. J Infect Dis 171:465, 1995.

134. Wanke CA, Gerrior J, Blais V, et al: Successful treatment of diarrheal disease with enteroaggregative *Escherichia coli* in adults infected with human immunodeficiency virus. J Infect Dis 178:1369, 1998.

135. Keusch GT, Grady GF, Mata LJ, et al: Pathogenesis of shigella diarrhea: I. Enterotoxin production by *Shigella dysenteriae*: I. J Clin Invest 51:1212, 1972.

136. Gots RE, Formal SB, Giannela RA: Indomethacin inhibition of *Salmonella typhimurium*, *Shigella flexneri*, and cholera-mediated rabbit ileal secretion. J Infect Dis 130:280, 1974.

137. Kinsey MD, Dammin GJ, Formal SB, Giannella RA: The role of altered intestinal permeability in the pathogenesis of *Salmonella* diarrhea in the Rhesus monkey. Gastroenterology 71:429, 1976.

138. Giannella RA, Rout WR, Formal SB, Collins H: The role of plasma filtration in the intestinal fluid secretion mediated with infection with *Salmonella typhimurium*. Infect Immun 13:470, 1976.

139. DuPont HL, Levine MM, Hornick RB, et al: Inoculum size in shigellosis and implications for expected mode of transmission. J Infect Dis 159:1126, 1989.

140. Gorden J, Small PLC: Acid resistance in enteric bacteria. Infect Immun 61:364, 1993.

141. Philipon A, Sansonetti PJ: Shigellosis: Innate mechanisms of inflammatory destruction of the intestinal epithelium, adaptive immune response, and vaccine development. Crit Rev Immunol 23:371, 2003.

142. Acheson DWK, Keusch GT: *Shigella* and enteroinvasive *Escherichia coli*. In Blaser MJ, Smith PD, Ravdin JI, et al (eds): Infections of the Gastrointestinal Tract. New York, Raven Press, 1995, p 763.

143. Keusch GT, Jacewicz M: The pathogenesis of shigella diarrhea: VI. Toxin and antitoxin in *Shigella flexneri* and *Shigella sonnei* infections in humans. J Infect Dis 135:552, 1977.

144. Barrett-Connor E, Conner JD: Extra-intestinal manifestations of shigellosis. Am J Gastroenterol 52:234, 1970.

145. Khan WA, Dhar U, Salam MA, et al: Central nervous system manifestations of childhood shigellosis: Prevalence, risk factors, and outcome. Pediatrics 103:E18, 1999.

146. Daoud AS, Zaki M, al-Mutari G, et al: Childhood shigellosis: Clinical and bacteriological study. J Trop Med Hyg 93:275, 1990.

147. Koster FT, Boonpucknavig V, Sujaho S, et al: Renal histopathology in the hemolytic-uremic syndrome following shigellosis. Clin Nephrol 21:126, 1984.

148. Butler T, Islam M, Bardhan PK: The leukemoid reaction in shigellosis. Am J Dis Child 138:162, 1984.

149. Tsuchiya N, Husby G, Williams RC, et al: Autoantibodies to the HLA-B27 sequence cross-react with the hypothetical peptide from the arthritis-associated *Shigella* plasmid. J Clin Invest 86:1193, 1990.

150. Nostrant TT, Kumar NB, Appleman HD: Histopathology differentiates acute self-limited colitis from ulcerative colitis. Gastroenterology 92:318, 1987.

151. Bennish ML, Salam MA, Khan WA, et al: Treatment of shigellosis: III. Comparison of one- or two-dose ciprofloxacin with standard 5-day therapy—a randomized, blinded trial. Ann Intern Med 117:727, 1992.

152. Khalil K, Khan SR, Mazhar K, et al: Occurrence and susceptibility to antibiotics of *Shigella* species in stools of hospitalized children with bloody diarrhea in Pakistan. Am J Trop Med Hyg 58:800, 1998.

153. Burkhardt JE, Walterspiel JN, Schaad UB: Quinolone arthropathy in animals versus children. Clin Infect Dis 25:1196, 1997.

154. Gendrel D, Moreno JL, Nduwimana M, et al: One-dose treatment of pefloxacin for infection due to multidrug-resistant *Shigella dysenteriae* type 1 in Burundi. Clin Infect Dis 24:83, 1997.

155. Salam MA, Dhar U, Khan AK, et al: Randomised comparison of ciprofloxacin suspension and pivmecillinam for childhood shigellosis. Lancet 352:522, 1998.

156. Murphy GS, Bodhidatta L, Echeverria P, et al: Ciprofloxacin and loperamide in the treatment of bacillary dysentery. Ann Intern Med 118:582, 1993.

157. Haltalin KC, Nelson JD, Hinton LV, et al: Comparison of orally absorbable and nonabsorbable antibiotics in shigellosis. J Pediatr 2:708, 1968.

158. Nelson JD, Haltalin KC: Amoxicillin less effective than ampicillin against *Shigella* in vitro and in vivo: Relationship of efficacy to activity in serum. J Infect Dis 129:S222, 1974.

159. Wang LH, Fang XC, Pan GZ: Bacillary dysentery as a causative factor of irritable bowel syndrome and its pathogenesis. Gut 53:1096, 2004.

160. Le Minor L, Popoff MY: Designation of *Salmonella enterica* sp. nov., non. Rev., as the type and only species of the genus *Salmonella*. Int J Sys Bacteriol 37:465, 1987.

161. Finley BB, Heffron F, Falkow S: Epithelial cell surfaces induce *Salmonella* proteins required for bacterial adherence and invasion. Science 243:940, 1989.

162. Zhang S, Kingsley RA, Santos RL, et al: Molecular pathogenesis of *Salmonella enterica* serotype *Tyhimurium*-induced diarrhea. Infec Immun 71:1, 2003.

163. Fields PI, Groisman EA, Heffron F: A *Salmonella* locus that controls resistance to microbial proteins from phagocytic cells. Science 243:1059, 1989.

164. McCormick BA, Miller SI, Carnes D, et al: Transepithelial signaling to neutrophils by salmonellae: A novel virulence mechanism for gastroenteritis. Infect Immun 63:2302, 1995.

165. Wallis TS, Starkey WG, Stephen J, et al: Enterotoxin production by *Salmonella typhimurium* strains of different virulence. J Med Microbiol 21:19, 1986.

166. Chopra AK, Huang JH, Xu XJ, et al: Role of *Salmonella* enterotoxin in overall virulence of the organism. Microb Pathogen 27:155, 1999.

167. Pavia AT, Shipman LD, Wells JG, et al: Epidemiologic evidence that prior antimicrobial exposure decreases resistance to infection by antimicrobial-sensitive *Salmonella*. J Infect Dis 161:255, 1990.

168. Kaye D, Gill FA, Hook EW: Factors influencing host resistance to *Salmonella* infections: The effects of hemolysis and erythrophagocytosis. Am J Med Sci 254:205, 1967.

169. Hand WL, King NL: Serum opsonization of salmonella in sickle cell anemia. Am J Med 64:388, 1977.

170. Han T, Sokal JE, Neter E: Salmonellosis in disseminated malignant diseases. N Engl J Med 276:1045, 1967.

171. Glaser JB, Morton-Kute L, Berger SR: Recurrent *Salmonella typhimurium* bacteremia associated with the acquired immune deficiency syndrome. Ann Intern Med 102:189, 1985.

172. Rocha H, Brazil S, Kirk JW, et al: Prolonged *Salmonella* bacteremia in patients with *Schistosoma mansoni* infection. Arch Intern Med 128:254, 1971.

173. Lindeman RJ, Weinstein L, Levitan R, et al: Ulcerative colitis and intestinal salmonellosis. Am J Med Sci 254:855, 1967.

174. Rubin HR, Weinstein L: Salmonellosis: Microbiologic, Pathologic, and Clinical Features. New York, Stratton Intercontinental, 1977.

175. Gray JI, Trueman AM: Severe *Salmonella* gastroenteritis associated with hypochlorhydria. Scot Med J 16:255, 1971.

176. Musher DN, Rubenstein AD: Permanent carriers of nontyphosa salmonellae. Arch Intern Med 132:869, 1973.

177. Mandal BK, Mani V: Colonic involvement in salmonellosis. Lancet 1:887, 1976.

178. Deppisch LM, Grans CA: Salmonellosis: A cause of toxic megacolon. J Clin Gastroenterol 12:605, 1990.

179. Neill MA, Opal SM, Heelan J, et al: Failure of ciprofloxacin in convalescent fecal excretion after acute salmonellosis: Experience during an outbreak in health care workers. Ann Intern Med 114:195, 1991.

180. Sirinavin S, Garner P: Antibiotics for treating *Salmonella* gut infections. Cochrane Library 2000.114:195, 1991.

181. Stanley PJ, Flegg PJ, Mandal BK, et al: Open study of ciprofloxacin in enteric fever. J Antimicrob Chemother 23:789, 1989.

182. Cherubin CE, Kowalski J: Nontyphoidal *Salmonella* carrier state treated with norfloxacin. Ann Intern Med 85:100, 1990.

183. Piddock LJV, Whale K, Wise R: Quinolone resistance in *Salmonella*: Clinical experience. Lancet 1:1459, 1990.

184. Malorny B, Schroeter A, Helmuth R: Incidence of quinolone resistance over the period 1986 to 1998 in veterinary *Salmonella* isolates from Germany. Antimicrob Agents Chemother 43:2278, 1999.

185. Fey PD, Safranek TJ, Rupp ME, et al: Ceftriaxone-resistant *Salmonella* infection acquired by a child from cattle. N Engl J Med 342:1242, 2000.

186. Tarr PE, Kuppens L, Jones TC, et al: Considerations regarding mass vaccination against typhoid fever as an adjunct to sanitation and public health measures: Potential use in an epidemic in Tajikistan. Am J Trop Med Hyg 61:163, 1999.

187. Mermin JH, Townes JM, Gerber M, et al: Typhoid fever in the United States, 1985-1994: Changing risks of international travel and antimicrobial resistance. Arch Intern Med 158:633, 1998.

188. Stuart BM, Pullen RL: Typhoid: Clinical analysis of 360 cases. Arch Intern Med 78:629, 1946.

189. Woodward TE, Smadel JE: Management of typhoid fever and its complications. Ann Intern Med 60:144, 1964.

190. Butler T, Knight J, Nath SK, et al: Typhoid fever complicated by intestinal perforation: A persisting fatal disease requiring surgical management. Rev Infect Dis 7:244, 1985.

191. Kaye D, Merselis JG, Connolly CS, et al: Treatment of chronic carriers of *Salmonella typhosa* with ampicillin. Ann N Y Acad Sci 145:429, 1967.

192. Gilman RH, Terminel M, Levine MM, et al: Relative efficacy of blood, urine, rectal swab, bone-marrow, and rose-spot cultures for recovery of *Salmonella typhi* in typhoid fever. Lancet 1:1211, 1975.

193. Robertson RP, Wahab MFA, Raasch FO: Evaluation of chloramphenicol and ampicillin in *Salmonella* enteric fever. N Engl J Med 278:171, 1968.

194. Chitnis V, Chitnis D, Verma S, et al: Multidrug-resistant *Salmonella typhi* in India. Lancet 354:514, 1999.

195. Wain J, Hoa NTT, Chinh NT, et al: Quinolone-resistant *Salmonella typhi* in Vietnam: Molecular basis of resistance and clinical response to treatment. Clin Infect Dis 25:1404, 1997.

196. Soe GB, Overturf GD: Treatment of typhoid fever and other systemic salmonelloses with cefotaxime, ceftriaxone, cefoperazone, and other new cephalosporins. Rev Infect Dis 9:719, 1987.

197. Acharya G, Butler T, Ho M, et al: Treatment of typhoid fever: Randomized trial of a three-day course of ceftriaxone versus a fourteen-day course of chloramphenicol. Am J Trop Med Hyg 52:162, 1995.

198. Phuong CXT, Kneen R, Anh NT, et al: A comparative study of ofloxacin and cefixime for treatment of typhoid fever in children. Pediatr Infect Dis J 18:245, 1999.

199. Hoffman SL, Punjabi NH, Kumala S, et al: Reduction of mortality in chloramphenicol-treated severe typhoid fever by high-dose dexamethasone. N Engl J Med 310:83, 1984.

200. Bitar R, Tarpley J: Intestinal perforation in typhoid fever: An historical and state-of-the-art review. Rev Infect Dis 7:257, 1985.

201. Mock CN, Amaral J, Visser LE: Improvement in survival from typhoid ileal perforation: Results of 221 operative cases. Ann Surg 215:244, 1992.

202. Rodriguez-Noriega E, Andrade-Villanueva J, Amaya-Tapia G: Quinolones in the treatment of *Salmonella* carriers. Rev Infect Dis 11:S1179, 1989.

203. Wahdan MH, Serie C, Cerisier Y, et al: A controlled field trial of live *Salmonella typhi* Ty 21a oral vaccine against typhoid: Three-year results. J Infect Dis 145:292, 1982.

204. Levine MM, Ferreccio C, Black RE, et al: Chilean Typhoid Committee: Large-scale field trial of Ty21a live oral typhoid vaccine in enteric-coated capsule formulation. Lancet 1:1049, 1987.

205. Hirschel B, Wurthrich R, Somaini B, et al: Inefficacy of the commercial live oral Ty 21a vaccine in the prevention of typhoid: Three-year results. J Infect Dis 145:292, 1982.

206. Acharya IL, Lowe CU, Thapa R, et al: Prevention of typhoid fever in Nepal with the Vi capsular polysaccharide of *Salmonella typhi*. N Engl J Med 317:1101, 1987.

207. Altekruse SF, Stern NJ, Fields PI, et al: *Campylobacter jejuni*: An emerging foodborne pathogen. Emerg Infect Dis 5:28, 1999.

208. Deming MS, Tauxe RV, Blake PA, et al: *Campylobacter* enteritis at a university: Transmission from eating chicken and from cats. Am J Epidemiol 126:526, 1987.

209. Mishu Allos B, Blaser MJ: *Campylobacter jejuni* and the expanding spectrum of related infections. Clin Infect Dis 20:1092, 1995.

210. Kapperud G, Lassen J, Ostroff SM, et al: Clinical features of sporadic *Campylobacter* infections in Norway. Scand J Infect Dis 24:741, 1992.

211. Rees JH, Soudain SE, Gregson NA, et al: *Campylobacter jejuni* infection and Guillain-Barré syndrome. N Engl J Med 333:1374, 1995.

212. Lecuit M, Abachin W, Martin A, et al: Immunoproliferative small intestinal disease associated with *Campylobacter jejuni*. N Engl J Med 350:239, 2004.

213. Levine MM: Antimicrobial therapy for infectious diarrhea. Rev Infect Dis 8:S207, 1986.

214. Pichler HET, Diridl G, Stickler K, et al: Clinical efficacy of ciprofloxacin compared with placebo in bacterial diarrhea. Am J Med 82(S4A):329, 1987.

215. Segreti J, Gootz TD, Goodman LJ, et al: High-level quinolone resistance in clinical isolates of *Campylobacter jejuni*. J Infect Dis 165:667, 1992.

216. Wretlind B, Stromberg A, Ostlund L, et al: Rapid emergence of quinolone resistance in *Campylobacter jejuni* in patients treated with norfloxacin. Scand J Infect Dis 24:685, 1992.

217. Kuschner RA, Trofa AF, Thomas RJ, et al: Use of azithromycin for the treatment of *Campylobacter* enteritis in travelers to Thailand, an area where ciprofloxacin resistance is prevalent. Clin Infect Dis 21:536, 1995.

218. Smith KE, Besser JM, Hedberg CW, et al: Quinolone-resistant *Campylobacter jejuni* infections in Minnesota, 1992-1998. N Engl J Med 340:1525, 1999.

219. Talsma E, Goettsch WG, Nieste HLJ, et al: Resistance in *Campylobacter* species: Increased resistance to fluoroquinolones and seasonal variation. Clin Infect Dis 29:845, 1999.

220. Naktin J, Beavis KG: *Yersinia enterocolitica* and *Yersinia pseudotuberculosis*. Clin Lab Med 19:523, 1999.

221. Isberg RR, Leong JM: Cultured mammalian cells attach to the invasion protein of *Yersinia* pseudotuberculosis. Proc Natl Acad Sci U S A 85:6682, 1988.

222. Ackers M-L, Schoenfeld S, Markman J, et al: An outbreak of *Yersinia enterocolitica* O:8 infections associated with pasteurized milk. J Infect Dis 181:1834, 2000.

223. Simmonds SD, Noble MA, Freeman HJ: Gastrointestinal features of culture-positive *Yersinia enterocolitica* infection. Gastroenterology 92:112, 1987.

224. Ostroff SM, Kapperud G, Lassen J, et al: Clinical features of sporadic *Yersinia enterocolitica* infections in Norway. J Infect Dis 166:812, 1992.

225. Vantrappen G, Pouette E, Geboes K: *Yersinia* enteritis and enterocolitis: Gastroenterological aspects. Gastroenterology 72:220, 1977.

226. Puylaert JBCM, Cermeijden RJ, Van Der Werf SDJ, et al: Incidence and sonographic diagnosis of bacterial ileocaecitis masquerading as appendicitis. Lancet 2:84, 1989.

227. Granforb K, Jalkanan S, Von Essen R, et al: *Yersinia* antigens in synovial fluid cells from patients with reactive arthritis. N Engl J Med 320:216, 1989.

228. DeKoning J, Heesemann J, Hoogkamp-Korstanje JAA, et al: *Yersinia* in intestinal biopsy specimens from patients with seronegative spondyloarthropathy: Correlation with specific serum IgA antibodies. J Infect Dis 159:109, 1989.

229. Bottone EJ, Sheehan DJ: *Yersinia enterocolitica*: Guidelines for serologic diagnosis of human infections. Rev Infect Dis 5:898, 1982.

230. Paim CH, Gillis F, Tuomanen E, et al: Placebo-controlled double-blind evaluation of trimethoprim-sulfamethoxazole treatment of *Yersinia enterocolitica* gastroenteritis. J Pediatr 104:308, 1984.

231. Blacklow NR, Greenberg HB: Viral gastroenteritis. N Engl J Med 325:252, 1991.

232. Waters V, Ford-Jones EL, Petric M, et al: Etiology of community-acquired pediatric viral diarrhea: A prospective longitudinal study in hospitals, emergency departments, pediatric practices, and child care centers during the winter rotavirus outbreak, 1997 to 1998. Pediatr Infect Dis J 19:843, 2000.

233. Davidson GP, Barnes GL: Structural and functional abnormalities of the small intestine in infants and young children with rotavirus enteritis. Acta Paediatr Scand 68:181, 1979.

234. Lundgren O, Peregrin AT, Persson K, et al: Role of the enteric nervous system in the fluid and electrolyte secretion of rotavirus diarrhea. Science 287:491, 2000.

235. Morris AP, Estes MK: Microbes and microbial toxins: Paradigm for microbial-mucosal interactions: VIII. Pathological consequences of rotavirus infection and its enterotoxin. Am J Physiol 281:G303, 2001.

236. Rodriguez WJ, Kim HW, Brandt CD, et al: Longitudinal study of rotavirus infection and gastroenteritis in families served by a pediatric medical practice: Clinical and epidemiologic observations. Pediatr Infect Dis J 6:170, 1987.

237. Zheng BJ, Lo SKF, Tam JSL, et al: Prospective study of community-acquired rotavirus infection. J Clin Microbiol 27:2083, 1989.

238. Richardson S, Grimwood K, Gorrell R, et al: Extended excretion of rotavirus after severe diarrhoea in young children. Lancet 351:1844, 1998.

239. Wilde J, Yolken R, Willoughby R, et al: Improved detection of rotavirus shedding by polymerase chain reaction. Lancet 337:323, 1991.

240. Gouvea V, Allen JR, Glass RI, et al: Detection of group B and C rotaviruses by polymerase chain reaction. J Clin Microbiol 29:519, 1991.

241. Matson DO, O'Ryan ML, Herrera I, et al: Fecal antibody responses to symptomatic and asymptomatic rotavirus infections. J Infect Dis 167:577, 1993.

242. Brussow H, Wechau H, Lerner L, et al: Seroconversion patterns to four human rotavirus serotypes in hospitalized infants with acute rotavirus gastroenteritis. J Infect Dis 161:1105, 1990.

243. Ward RL, Bernstein DI, for the U.S. Rotavirus Vaccine Efficacy Group: Protection against rotavirus disease after natural rotavirus infection. J Infect Dis 169:900, 1994.

244. Glass RI, Stoll BJ, Wyatt RG, et al: Observations questioning a protective role for breast-feeding in severe rotavirus diarrhea. Acta Paediatr Scand 75:713, 1986.

245. Yolken RH, Peterson JA, Vonderfecht SL, et al: Human milk mucin inhibits rotavirus replication and prevents experimental gastroenteritis. J Clin Invest 90:1984, 1992.

246. Newburg DS, Peterson JA, Ruiz-Palacios GM, et al: Role of human-milk lactadherin in protection against symptomatic rotavirus infection. Lancet 351:1160, 1998.

247. Santosham M, Burns B, Nadkarni V, et al: Oral rehydration therapy for acute diarrhea in ambulatory children in the United States: A double-blind comparison of four different solutions. Pediatrics 76:159, 1985.

248. Centers for Disease Control and Prevention: Rotavirus vaccine for the prevention of rotavirus gastroenteritis among children. MMWR Morb Mortal Wkly Rep 48(Suppl RR2):1, 1999.

249. Centers for Disease Control and Prevention. Intussusception among recipients of rotavirus vaccine: United States, 1998-1999. MMWR Morb Mortal Wkly Rep 48:577, 1999.

250. Sarker SA, Casswall TH, Mahalanabis D, et al: Successful treatment of rotavirus diarrhea in children with immunoglobulin from immunized bovine colostrum. Pediatr Infect Dis J 17:1149, 1998.

251. Green KY, Ando T, Balayan MS, et al: Taxonomy of the caliciviruses. J Infect Dis 181(Suppl. 2):S322, 2000.

252. Matson DO, Estes MK, Glass RI, et al: The occurrence of calicivirus-associated diarrhea in children attending day care centers. J Infect Dis 159:71, 1989.

253. O'Ryan ML, Mamani N, Gaggero A, et al: Human caliciviruses are a significant pathogen of acute sporadic diarrhea in children of Santiago, Chile. J Infect Dis 182:1519, 2000.

254. Jiang X, Graham DY, Wang K, et al: Norwalk virus genome cloning and characterization. Science 250:1580, 1990.

255. Morse DL, Guzewich JJ, Hanrahan JP, et al: Widespread outbreaks of clam- and oyster-associated gastroenteritis: Role of Norwalk virus. N Engl J Med 314:678, 1986.

256. Fankhauser RL, Noel JS, Monroe SS, et al: Molecular epidemiology of Norwalk-like viruses in outbreaks of gastroenteritis in the United States. J Infect Dis 178:1571, 1998.

257. Kukkula M, Maunula L, Silvennoinen E, et al: Outbreak of viral gastroenteritis due to drinking water contaminated by Norwalk-like viruses. J Infect Dis 180:1771, 1999.

258. Kuritsky JN, Osterhold MT, Greenberg HB, et al: Norwalk gastroenteritis: A community outbreak associated with bakery product consumption. Ann Intern Med 100:519, 1984.

259. Moe CL, Gentsch J, Grohmann G, et al: Application of PCR to detect Norwalk virus in fecal specimens from outbreaks of gastroenteritis. J Clin Microbiol 32:642, 1994.

260. Herrmann JE, Blacklow NR, Matsui SM, et al: Monoclonal antibodies for detection of Norwalk virus antigen in stools. J Clin Microbiol 33:2511, 1995.

261. Johnson PC, Mathewson JJ, DuPont HL, et al: Multiple-challenge study of host susceptibility to Norwalk gastroenteritis in U.S. adults. J Infect Dis 161:18, 1990.

262. Kotloff KL, Losonsky GA, Morris JG Jr, et al: Enteric adenovirus infection and childhood diarrhea: An epidemiologic study in three clinical settings. Pediatrics 84:219, 1989.

263. Van R, Wun CC, O'Ryan ML, et al: Outbreaks of human enteric adenovirus types 40 and 41 in Houston day care centers. J Pediatr 120:516, 1992.

264. Lew JF, Moe CL, Monroe SS, et al: Astrovirus and adenovirus associated with diarrhea in children in day care settings. J Infect Dis 164:673, 1991.

265. Kurtz JB, Lee TW: Astroviruses: Human and animal. In Novel Diarrhoea Viruses. CIBA Foundation Symposium 128. Chichester, England, John Wiley, 1987, p 92.

266. Herrmann JE, Taylor DN, Echeverria P, et al: Astroviruses as a cause of gastroenteritis in children. N Engl J Med 324:1757, 1991.

267. Mitchell DK, Monroe SS, Jiang X, et al: Virologic features of an astrovirus diarrhea outbreak in a day care center revealed by reverse transcriptase-polymerase chain reaction. J Infect Dis 172:1437, 1995.

268. Naficy AB, Rao MR, Holmes JL, et al: Astrovirus diarrhea in Egyptian children. J Infect Dis 182:685, 2000.

269. Moe CL, Allen JR, Monroe SS, et al: Detection of astrovirus in pediatric stool samples by immunoassay and RNA probe. J Clin Microbiol 29:2390, 1991.

270. Koopmans M, Horzinek MC: Toroviruses of animals and humans: A review. Adv Virus Res 43:233, 1994.

271. Koopmans MPG, Goosen ESM, Lima AM, et al: Association of torovirus with acute and persistent diarrhea in children. Pediatr Infect Dis J 16:504, 1997.

272. Jamieson FB, Wang EEL, Bain C, et al: Human torovirus: A new nosocomial gastrointestinal pathogen. J Infect Dis 178: 1263, 1998.

273. McFarland LV, Mulligan ME, Kwok RYY, et al: Nosocomial acquisition of C. difficile infection. N Engl J Med 320:204, 1989.

274. Siegel D, Edelstein P, Nachamkin I: Inappropriate testing for diarrheal disease in the hospital. JAMA 263:979, 1990.

275. Prien-Larsen J, Stjernquist M: Malaria in pregnancy. Acta Obstet Gynecol Scand 72:496, 1993.

276. Kerrigan K: Fulminant amoebic colitis in pregnancy. Trop Doctor 21:46, 1991.

277. Hill D: *Giardia lamblia*. In Mandel G, Bennett J, Dolin R (eds): Principles and Practice of Infectious Disease. New York, Churchill Livingstone, 1995, p 2487.

278. Simor A, Ferro S: *Campylobacter jejuni* infection occurring during pregnancy. Eur J Clin Microbiol Infect Dis 9:142, 1990.

279. Armor S: Periparturitional shigellosis. Neb Med J 75:239, 1990.

280. Rebarber A, Star Hampton B, Lewis V, Bender S: Shigellosis complicating preterm premature rupture of membranes resulting in congenital infection and preterm delivery. Obstet Gynecol 100:1063, 2002.

281. Gorbach SL, Edelman R (eds): Travelers' Diarrhea: National Institutes of Health Consensus Development Conference. Rev Infect Dis 8(Suppl 2):S109, 1986.

282. Gorbach SL, Kean BH, Evans DG, et al: Travelers' diarrhea and toxigenic *Escherichia coli*. N Engl J Med 292:933, 1975.

283. Black RE: Pathogens that cause travelers' diarrhea in Latin America and Africa. Rev Infect Dis 12(Suppl 1):S131, 1990.

284. Steffen R, Collard F, Tornieporth N, et al: Epidemiology, etiology, and impact of traveler's diarrhea in Jamaica. JAMA 281:811, 1999.

285. Dupont HL, Ericsson CD: Prevention and treatment of traveler's diarrhea. N Engl J Med 328:1821, 1993.

286. Mattila L, Siitonen A, Kyronseppa H, et al: Seasonal variation in etiology of travelers' diarrhea. J Infect Dis 165:385, 1992.

287. Petruccelli BP, Murphy GS, Sanchez JL, et al: Treatment of traveler's diarrhea with ciprofloxacin and loperamide. J Infect Dis 165:557, 1992.

288. Steffen R: Epidemiologic studies of travelers' diarrhea, severe gastrointestinal infections, and cholera. Rev Infect Dis 8(Suppl 2):S122, 1986.

289. Shlim DR, Hoge CW, Rajah R, et al: Persistent high risk of diarrhea among foreigners in Nepal during the first 2 years of residence. Clin Infect Dis 29:613, 1999.

290. Steffen R, van der Linde F, Gyr K, et al: Epidemiology of diarrhea in travelers. JAMA 249:1176, 1983.

291. MacDonald K, Cohen M: Epidemiology of traveler's diarrhea: Current perspectives. Rev Infect Dis 8(Suppl 2): S117, 1986.

292. Black RE: Epidemiology of travelers' diarrhea and relative importance of various pathogens. Rev Infect Dis 12(Suppl 1): S73, 1990.

293. Lowenstein MS, Balows A, Gangarosa EJ: Turista at an international congress in Mexico. Lancet 1:529, 1973.

294. DuPont HL, Capsuto EG: Persistent diarrhea in travelers. Clin Infect Dis 22:124, 1996.

295. Johnson PC, Ericsson CD, DuPont HL, et al: Comparison of loperamide with bismuth subsalicylate for the treatment of acute travelers diarrhea. JAMA 255:757, 1986.

296. Gorbach SL: Bismuth therapy in gastrointestinal diseases. Gastroenterology 99:863, 1990.

297. Ericsson CD, DuPont HL, Mathewson JJ, et al: Treatment of travelers' diarrhea with sulfamethoxazole and trimethoprim and loperamide. JAMA 263:257, 1990.

298. Taylor DN, Sanchez JL, Candler W, et al: Treatment of travelers' diarrhea: Ciprofloxacin plus loperamide compared with ciprofloxacin alone. Ann Intern Med 114:731, 1991.

299. DuPont HL, Evans DG, Rios N, et al: Prevention of travelers' diarrhea with trimethoprim-sulfamethoxazole. Rev Infect Dis 4:533, 1982.

300. Ericsson CD, Johnson PC, DuPont HL, et al: Ciprofloxacin or trimethoprim-sulfamethoxazole as initial therapy for travelers' diarrhea. Ann Intern Med 106:216, 1987.

301. Salam I, Katelaris P, Leigh-Smith S, et al: Randomised trial of single-dose ciprofloxacin for travellers' diarrhoea. Lancet 344:1537, 1994.

302. DuPont HL, Jiang Z-D, Ericsson CD, et al: Rifaximin versus ciprofloxacin for the treatment of traveler's diarrhea: A randomized, double-blind clinical trial. Clin Infect Dis 33:1807, 2001.

303. Steffen R, Sack DA, Riopel L, et al: Therapy of traveler's diarrhea with rifaximin on various continents. Am J Gastroenterol 98:1073, 2003.

304. Adachi JA, Ostrosky-Zeichner L, DuPont HL, et al: Empirical antimicrobial therapy for traveler's diarrhea. Clin Infect Dis 31:1079, 2000.

305. Harris JR: Are bottled beverages safe for travelers [editorial]? Am J Public Health 72:787, 1982.

306. Chak A, Banwell JG: Traveler's diarrhea. Gastroenterol Clin North Am 22:549, 1993.

307. Spiller RC: Postinfectious irritable bowel syndrome. Gastroenterology 124:1662, 2003.

308. Neal KR, Barker L, Spiller RC: Prognosis in post-infectious irritable bowel syndrome: A 6-year follow up study. Gut 51: 410, 2002.

309. Lew JF, Glass RI, Gangarosa RE, et al: Diarrheal deaths in the United States, 1979 through 1987: A special problem for the elderly. JAMA 265:3280, 1991.

310. Gangarosa RE, Glass RI, Lew JF, et al: Hospitalizations involving gastroenteritis in the U.S., 1985: The special burden of the disease among the elderly. Am J Epidemiol 135:281, 1992.

311. Bennett RG, Greenough WB: Approach to acute diarrhea in the elderly. Gastroenterol Clin North Am 22:517, 1993.

312. Garibaldi RA, Brodine S, Matsumiya S, et al: Infections among patients in nursing homes. N Engl J Med 305:731, 1981.

313. Aronsson B, Mollby R, Nord CE: Antimicrobial agents and *Clostridium difficile* in acute enteric disease: Epidemiological data from Sweden, 1980-1982. J Infect Dis 151:476, 1985.

314. Brown E, Talbot G, Axelrod P, et al: Risk factors for *Clostridium difficile* toxin-associated diarrhea. Infect Control Hosp Epidemiol 11:283, 1990.

315. Brandt LJ, Grenwald DA, Koches KA, et al: *Clostridium difficile* colitis in the elderly. Am J Gastroenterol 94:3263, 1999.

316. Swerdlow DL, Woodruff BA, Brady RC, et al: A waterborne outbreak in Missouri of *Escherichia coli* O157:H7 associated with bloody diarrhea and death. Ann Intern Med 117:812, 1992.

317. Borriello SP, Barclay FE, Welch AR, et al: Epidemiology of diarrhoea caused by enterotoxigenic *Clostridium perfringens*. J Med Microbiol 20:363, 1985.

318. Gordon SM, Oshiro LS, Jarvis WR, et al: Foodborne Snow Mountain agent gastroenteritis with secondary person-to-person spread in a retirement community. Am J Epidemiol 131:702, 1990.

319. Neill MA, Rice SK, Ahmad NV, et al: Cryptosporidiosis: An unrecognized cause of diarrhea in elderly hospitalized patients. Clin Infect Dis 22:168, 1996.

320. Avery ME, Snyder JD: Oral therapy for acute diarrhea: The underused simple solution. N Engl J Med 13:891, 1990.

321. Santosham M, Daum AS, Dillman L, et al: Oral rehydration therapy of infantile diarrhea: A controlled study of well-

nourished children hospitalized in the United States and Panama. N Engl J Med 306:1071, 1982.

322. Calligaro I: Treatment of acute diarrhea in children. Am Pharm NS32(11):29-34, 1992.

323. Guarino A, Albano F, Guandalini S, et al: Oral rehydration: Toward a real solution. J Pediatr Gastroenterol Nutr 33: S2, 2001.

324. Thillainayagam AV, Hunt JB, Farthing MJG: Efficacy of oral rehydration therapy: Is low osmolality the key? Gastroenterology 114:197, 1998.

325. Santosham M, Greenough WB: Oral rehydration therapy: A global perspective. J Pediatr 118:544, 1991.

326. Cutting WA, Belton NR, Gray JA, et al: Safety and efficacy of three oral rehydration solutions for children with diarrhoea (Edinburgh 1984-1985). Acta Paediatr Scand 78:253, 1989.

327. International Study Group on Reduced-Osmolarity ORS solutions: Multicentre evaluation of reduced-osmolarity oral rehydration salts solution. Lancet 345:282, 1995.

328. Gore SM, Fontaine O, Pierce NF: Impact of rice based oral rehydration solution on stool output and duration of diarrhoea: Meta-analysis of 13 clinical trials. BMJ 304:287, 1992.

329. Ramakrishna BS, Venkataraman S, Srinivasan P, et al: Amylase-resistant starch plus oral rehydration solutions for cholera. N Engl J Med 342:308, 2000.

330. Savarino SJ, Levine MM: Specific and nonspecific treatment of diarrhea. In Gorbach SL, Bartlett JG, Blacklow NR (eds): Infectious Diarrhea. Philadelphia, WB Saunders 1992, p 638.

331. Goodman LJ, Trenholme GM, Kaplan RL, et al: Empiric antimicrobial therapy of domestically acquired acute diarrhea in urban adults. Arch Intern Med 150:541, 1990.

332. Wistrom J, Norrby SR: Fluoroquinolones and bacterial enteritis: When and for whom? J Antimicrob Chemother 36:23, 1995.

333. Giannella RA: Treatment of intestinal infections. In Wolfe M (ed): Therapy of Digestive Disorders, 2nd ed. Philadelphia, Elsevier, 2006.

334. Islam MR: Single-dose tetracycline in cholera. Gut 28:1029, 1987.

335. Oldfield EC III, Bourgeois AL, Omar AK, et al: Empirical treatment of Shigella dysentery with trimethoprim: Five-day course versus single dose. Am J Trop Med Hyg 37:616, 1986.

336. Butler T, Lolekha S, Rasidi C, et al: Treatment of acute bacterial diarrhea: A multicenter international trial comparing placebo with fleroxacin given as a single dose or once daily for 3 days. Am J Med 94(Suppl. 3A):187S, 1993.

337. DuPont HL, Hornick RB: Adverse effect of Lomotil therapy in shigellosis. JAMA 226:1525, 1990.

338. DuPont HL, Sullivan P, Pickering LK, et al: Symptomatic treatment of diarrhea with bismuth subsalicylate among students attending a Mexican university. Gastroenterology 73:715, 1977.

339. Horvath KD, Whelan RL: Intestinal tuberculosis: Return of an old disease. Am J Gastroenterol 93:692, 1998.

340. Marshall JB: Tuberculosis of the gastrointestinal tract and peritoneum. Am J Gastroenterol 88:989, 1993.

341. Shah S, Thomas V, Mathan M, et al: Colonoscopic study of 50 patients with colonic tuberculosis. Gut 33:347, 1992.

342. McGee GS, Williams LF, Potts J, et al: Gastrointestinal tuberculosis: Resurgence of an old pathogen. Am Surg 55:16, 1989.

343. Kim KM, Lee A, Choi YK, et al: Intestinal tuberculosis: Clinicopathologic analysis and diagnosis by endoscopic biopsy. J Gastroenterol 93:606, 1998.

344. Balthazar EJ, Gordon R, Hulnick D: Ileocecal tuberculosis: CT and radiologic evaluation. Am J Roentgenol 154:499, 1990.

345. Park SJ, Han JK, Kim JS, et al: Tuberculous colitis: Radiologic-colonoscopic correlation. Am J Roentgenol 175:121, 2000.

346. Bentley G, Webster JHH: Gastrointestinal tuberculosis: A 10-year review. Br J Surg 54:90, 1967.

347. Chen W-S, Su W-J, Wang H-S, et al: Large bowel tuberculosis and possible influencing factors for surgical prognosis: 30 years' experience. World J Surg 21:500, 1997.

348. Olson SJ, MacKinnon LC, Goulding JS, et al: Surveillance for foodborne-disease outbreaks-United States, 1993-1997. MMWR Morb Mortal Wkly Rep 49(Suppl. SS-1):1, 2000.

349. Bishai W, Sears CL: Food poisoning syndromes. Gastroenterol Clin North Am 22:579, 1993.

350. Centers for Disease Control and Prevention: Vibrio vulnificus infections associated with raw oyster consumption, Florida 1891-1992. MMWR 42:405, 1993.

351. Johnston IM, Becker SI, McFarland LM: Vibrio vulnificus: Man and the sea. JAMA 253:2850, 1985.

352. Sullivan R, Asano T: Effects of staphylococcal enterotoxin B on intestinal transport in the rat. Am J Physiol 222:1793, 1971.

353. Duncan CL, Strong DH: Clostridium perfringens type A food poisoning: I. Response of the rabbit ileum as an indication of enteropathogenicity of strains of Clostridium perfringens in monkeys. Infect Immun 3:167, 1971.

354. McDonel JL, Duncan CL: Regional localization of activity of Clostridium perfringens type A enterotoxin in the rabbit ileum, jejunum, and duodenum. J Infect Dis 136:661, 1977.

355. Thomas M, Noah ND, Male GE, et al: Hospital outbreak of Clostridium perfringens food poisoning. Lancet 1:1046, 1977.

356. Murrell TGC, Egerton JR, Rampling A, et al: The ecology and epidemiology of the pigbel syndrome in man in New Guinea. J Hyg Camb 64:375, 1966.

357. Petrillo TM, Beck-Sagué CM, Songer JG, et al: Enteritis necroticans (pigbel) in a diabetic child. N Engl J Med 342:1250, 2000.

358. Schlech WF III: Foodborne listeriosis. Clin Infect Dis 31:770, 2000.

359. Schuhat A, Deaver KA, Wenger JD, et al: Role of foods in sporadic listeriosis: I. Case-control study of dietary risk factors. JAMA 267:2041, 1992.

360. Pinner RW, Schuchat A, Swaminathan B, et al: Role of foods in sporadic listeriosis: II. Microbiologic and epidemiologic investigation. JAMA 267:2046, 1992.

361. Aureli P, Fiorucci GC, Caroli D, et al: An outbreak of febrile gastroenteritis associated with corn contaminated by Listeria monocytogenes. N Engl J Med 342:1236, 2000.

362. Terranova W, Blake PA: Bacillus cereus food poisoning. N Engl J Med 298:143, 1978.

363. Gilbert RJ, Parry JM: Serotypes of Bacillus cereus from outbreaks of food poisoning and from routine foods. J Hyg Camb 78:69, 1977.

364. Melling J, Capel BJ, Turnbull PCB, et al: Identification of a novel enterotoxigenic activity associated with Bacillus cereus. J Clin Pathol 29:938, 1976.

365. Mortimer PR, McCann G: Food poisoning episodes associated with Bacillus cereus in fried rice. Lancet 1:1043, 1974.

366. Crane JK: Preformed bacterial toxins. Clin Lab Med 19:583, 1999.

367. Shapiro RL, Hatheway C, Swerdlow DL: Botulism in the United States: A clinical and epidemiologic review. Ann Intern Med 129:221, 1998.

368. Tacket CO, Shandera WX, Mann JM, et al: Equine antitoxin use and other factors that predict outcome in type A foodborne botulism. Am J Med 76:794, 1984.

369. Dixon TC, Meselson M, Guillemin J, Hanna PC: Anthrax. N Engl J Med 341:815, 1999.

370. Human ingestion of *Bacillus anthracis*-contaminated meat—Minnesota, August 2000. MMWR Mort Morb Wkly Rep 49:813, 2000.

371. Morris JG: Natural toxins associated with fish and shellfish. In Blaser M, Smith P, Ravdin J, et al. (eds): Infections of the Gastrointestinal Tract, 2nd ed. Philadelphia, Lippincott Williams & Wilkins, 2002, p 215.

372. Barbier HMJ, Diaz JH: Prevention and treatment of toxic seafood-borne diseases in travelers. J Travel Med 10:29, 2003.

373. Vernoux JP, Lewis RJ: Isolation and characterization of Caribbean ciguatoxins from the horse-eye Jack (*Caranx latus*). Toxicon 35:889, 1997.

CHAPTER

105 Antibiotic-Associated Diarrhea, Pseudomembranous Enterocolitis, and *Clostridium difficile-*Associated Diarrhea and Colitis

Ciarán P. Kelly and J. Thomas Lamont

ANTIBIOTIC-ASSOCIATED DIARRHEA

Diarrhea is a common side effect of antibiotic use and may result from a variety of mechanisms.[1] The most common type of diarrhea, often called *simple antibiotic-associated diarrhea* (AAD), is believed to result from a disturbance of the normal colonic microflora leading to alterations in bacterial degradation of nonabsorbed carbohydrates and bile salts. Colonic bacteria ferment the complex carbohydrates in dietary fiber and other carbohydrates that are not absorbed in the small intestine, and the fermentation products are then metabolized and absorbed in the colon. Disruption of this process by antibiotic therapy is believed to cause osmotic diarrhea. Bile salts are known to stimulate fluid secretion by the colonic mucosa, and another mechanism for AAD may be reduced bacterial degradation of bile salts within the colonic lumen. Other mechanisms that may account for AAD include stimulation of intestinal motility

through the motilin-like effect of erythromycin, an allergic reaction, or infection with other microorganisms including *Clostridium perfringens* type A, *Staphylococcus aureus,* and *Salmonella enterica.*[2-4] The genotype of *C. perfringens* that causes AAD appears to be distinct from those that induce food poisoning.[3,5] Type A strains isolated from patients with AAD carry the *C. perfringens* enterotoxin (*CPE*) gene on a plasmid, whereas those that cause food poisoning have a chromosomal *CPE* gene. *S. aureus* was identified as a cause of severe AAD and enterocolitis prior to the identification of *Clostridium difficile-*associated diarrhea.[2,6] However, since the advent of sensitive and specific testing for *C. difficile,* few cases of *S. aureus* AAD have been confirmed, and the true role played by this pathogen in AAD is unclear.

AAD complicates 2% to 5% of antibiotic treatment courses, but the incidence varies depending on the antibiotic used; it is more common, for example, during therapy with ampicillin (5% to 10%), amoxicillin-

Table 105–1   Differences Between Antibiotic-Associated Diarrhea Caused by *Clostridium difficile* and Antibiotic-Associated Diarrhea from Other Causes

Characteristic	Diarrhea from *C. difficile* Infection	Diarrhea from Other Causes
Most commonly implicated antibiotics	Clindamycin, cephalosporins, penicillins	Clindamycin, cephalosporins, or amoxicillin-clavulanate
History	Usually no relevant history of antibiotic intolerance	History of diarrhea with antibiotic therapy is common
Clinical features		
Diarrhea	May be florid; evidence of colitis with cramps, fever, and fecal leukocytes is common	Usually moderate in severity (i.e., "nuisance diarrhea") without evidence of colitis
Findings on CT or colonoscopy	Evidence of colitis is common	Usually normal
Complications	Hypoalbuminemia, anasarca, toxic megacolon; relapse may occur after treatment with metronidazole or vancomycin	Usually none except occasional cases of dehydration
Results of assay for *C. difficile* toxin	Positive	Negative
Epidemiologic pattern	May be epidemic or endemic in hospitals or long-term care facilities	Sporadic
Treatment		
Withdrawal of implicated antibiotic	May resolve but often persists or progresses	Usually resolves
Antiperistaltic agents	Contraindicated	Often useful
Oral metronidazole or vancomycin	Prompt response	Not indicated

From Bartlett JG: Clinical practice: Antibiotic-associated diarrhea. N Engl J Med 346:334, 2002.

clavulanate (10% to 25%), or cefixime (15% to 20%) and less common during therapy with fluoroquinolones (1% to 2%) or trimethoprim-sulfamethoxazole (<1%).[7-9]

Most cases of AAD are mild and self-limited. Pseudomembranous colitis is absent, and significant complications are rare. *C. difficile* infection accounts for less than 10% of AAD cases but is an important pathogen to identify because it often requires specific antimicrobial therapy and may lead to life-threatening complications, as discussed in the following section. A comparison between the clinical features of AAD due to *C. difficile* and cases from other causes is presented in Table 105–1.

The management of simple AAD consists of discontinuing the inciting antibiotic if symptoms are moderately severe, or poorly tolerated. If necessary, antiperistaltic agents (e.g., loperamide) may be used to provide symptom relief. In contrast, antiperistaltic agents are contraindicated for *C. difficile*-associated diarrhea because of concern for exacerbating toxin-mediated colonic mucosal injury or precipitating toxic megacolon. Because AAD is believed to result from an alteration of the normal colonic microflora, a variety of probiotic agents have been evaluated for its treatment and prevention. In a double-blind, controlled clinical trial, coadministration with antibiotics of oral capsules containing viable *Saccharomyces boulardii* reduced the incidence of AAD in hospitalized patients from 22% to 9.5% in the placebo and *S. boulardii* group, respectively (*P* = 0.04).[10] Another randomized, placebo-controlled trial, however, failed to demonstrate a beneficial effect for *S. boulardii* in an elderly population of antibiotic recipients.[11] *Lactobacillus* species, and in particular *Lactobacillus rhamnosus* GG, also have been studied in clinical trials of AAD. In one study, *Lactobacillus* GG was effective in reducing the incidence of AAD in children being treated for respiratory tract infections to 5% compared with a 16% incidence in the placebo group[12]; other clinical trials of *Lactobacillus* GG have yielded negative results.[13] A meta-analysis examined the results of randomized, double-blind, placebo-controlled trials of probiotic therapy for AAD published between 1966 and 2000.[14] In all, 9 such studies were identified, including 4 studies using *S. boulardii* and 4 using *Lactobacillus* GG. The combined odds ratio for AAD in the probiotic-treated groups was 0.37 compared with placebo (95% confidence interval, 0.26 to 0.53; *P* < 0.001). For *S. boulardii*, the odds ratio in favor of active treatment over placebo was 0.39 (0.25 to 0.62; *P* < 0.001) and for lactobacilli, 0.34 (0.19 to 0.61; *P* < 0.01). A second meta-analysis yielded similar results.[15] Thus, the weight of published evidence suggests that probiotic agents such as *S. boulardii* and lactobacilli, when used in combination with antibiotics, reduce the risk for AAD. The prophylactic use of a probiotic agent may be especially advantageous in individuals with a history of susceptibility to AAD.

PSEUDOMEMBRANOUS ENTEROCOLITIS

Pseudomembranous enterocolitis was a rare entity in the medical literature before the advent of antibiotic therapy. In recent decades, pseudomembranous colitis has emerged as a frequent complication of antibiotic use, and almost all cases are now caused by infection with toxin-producing strains of *C. difficile*.

A case report by Finney published in 1893 is considered to be the first description in the medical literature of pseudomembranous enterocolitis.[9,16] In that instance, fatal pseudomembranous inflammation of the small intestine followed surgery in a debilitated young woman with gastric outlet obstruction caused by peptic ulcer disease. The presence of an inflammatory pseudomembrane overlying the intestinal mucosa characterizes pseudomembranous colitis (when the colon alone is involved) or pseudomembranous enterocolitis (when the small intestine also is involved).[9] The pseudomembrane comprises inflammatory and cellular debris and forms visible patches of yellow or gray exudate that obscure the underlying mucosa. In early lesions, a 1- to 2-mm area of punctate ulceration may be visible. Classic lesions consist of ovoid plaques of 2 to 10 mm in diameter separated by areas of normal or hyperemic mucosa. Histologically, the pseudomembrane can be seen to emanate from a central area of epithelial ulceration to form the mucosal plaques. In more severe cases, the areas of ulceration and the overlying pseudomembranes may combine to cover large areas of mucosa.

Risk factors for the development of pseudomembranous enterocolitis in the absence of *C. difficile* infection include intestinal surgery, intestinal ischemia, and other enteric infections. During the 1940s to the 1970s, most reported cases of pseudomembranous enterocolitis occurred following abdominal or pelvic surgery.[17,18] Bartlett has identified numerous descriptions of pseudomembranous enterocolitis in the medical literature associated with a wide variety of other intestinal disorders including *Shigella* infection, Crohn's disease, neonatal necrotizing enterocolitis, intestinal obstruction, Hirschprung's disease, and colonic carcinoma.[7,9] Intestinal ischemia can result in histologic changes similar to those observed in severe *C. difficile* colitis, although well-defined characteristic patchy pseudomembranes usually are not seen. Severe systemic insults including shock, advanced renal failure, spinal fracture, extensive burns, heavy metal poisoning, and hemolytic-uremic syndrome have also been implicated in the development of pseudomembranous enterocolitis. A potential common etiologic factor shared by many of these disorders is hypoperfusion of the intestinal mucosa leading to tissue necrosis and epithelial ulceration.

A number of other infectious agents has been implicated to cause pseudomembranous colitis in the absence of *C. difficile* infection, most notably *S. aureus*.[2,3,6] Prior to the identification of *C. difficile* as the most common cause of pseudomembranous colitis, *S. aureus* frequently was identified in stool cultures of patients with postoperative pseudomembranous enterocolitis. This finding led to the use of oral vancomycin, which proved to be an effective therapy.[6] In retrospect, it is difficult to ascertain to what extent the efficacy of vancomycin reflected its activity against staphylococcal infection or against unrecognized infection with *C. difficile*. Currently, 2% to 3% of patients with antibiotic-associated pseudomembranous colitis have negative tests for *C. difficile* and its toxins in stool specimens despite use of the most sensitive available assays; it remains unclear what proportion of these patients have false-negative tests for *C. difficile* or instead have an alternative infectious etiology for their pseudomembranous colitis.

CLOSTRIDIUM DIFFICILE-ASSOCIATED DIARRHEA AND COLITIS

C. difficile, an anaerobic, gram-positive, spore-forming, toxigenic bacillus, was first isolated in 1935 from the fecal flora of healthy neonates.[19] The organism passed into obscurity until 1978, when the association between toxins released by this organism and antibiotic-induced pseudomembranous colitis first was reported.[20,21] Since that time, the incidence of *C. difficile* infection has increased dramatically, and the organism is now recognized as the primary cause of nosocomial infectious

diarrhea in developed countries.[22,23] The incidence of nosocomial *C. difficile*-associated diarrhea is approximately 0.7:1000 hospital discharges with reported infection rates of 0.1 to 30:1000 patients in nonepidemic settings.[24-29] The reported incidence of community-acquired *C. difficile* AAD is substantially lower, ranging from 8 to 12 cases per 100,000 person-years.[30,31] Knowledge of the epidemiology, pathogenesis, and treatment of disease caused by *C. difficile* has increased dramatically during the past 25 years but has not yet led to any substantial decline in the frequency of *C. difficile* diarrhea and colitis.

PATHOGENESIS AND EPIDEMIOLOGY

The requirements for *C. difficile* to infect at-risk individuals are as follows: (1) alteration of the normal colonic microflora by antibiotics or other antimicrobial agents; (2) oral ingestion of *C. difficile* or its spores with resultant intestinal colonization; and (3) toxin release into the colonic lumen with subsequent intestinal injury and inflammation. Several host factors, particularly the immune response to *C. difficile* toxins, determine whether a patient remains an asymptomatic carrier or develops a spectrum of disease ranging from mild diarrhea to life-threatening pseudomembranous colitis (Fig. 105–1).[32]

Alteration of the Colonic Microflora

Alteration of the resident colonic microflora, usually a result of antimicrobial therapy, is the common initial event that predisposes to *C. difficile* infection. The protective barrier provided by the normal stable intestinal microflora frequently is referred to as *colonization resistance*. Removal of this barrier by antibiotics and subsequent infection with *C. difficile* originally was demonstrated in animal models.[33-35] *C. difficile* also can colonize the intestine of "germ-free" mice but are eliminated after these animals are inoculated with fecal flora from normal mice; this experiment clearly confirmed the importance of the normal flora in preventing colonization.[34] "Colonization resistance" can be demonstrated in vitro where the growth of *C. difficile* is inhibited by fecal extracts from healthy adults but not by sterile extracts.[36]

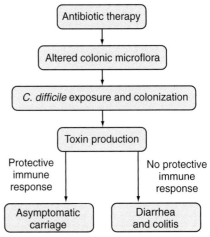

Figure 105–1 Pathogenesis of *Clostridium difficile*-associated diarrhea and colitis. (From Kyne L, Farrell R, Kelly CP: *Clostridium difficile*. Gastroenterol Clin North Am 30:753, 2001.)

Human neonates and infants have poor colonization resistance because they have not yet developed a stable complex colonic microflora.[37,38] Colonization rates with *C. difficile* of 25% to 80% have been reported in infants and children up to 24 months of age, but despite large concentrations of toxins in the feces, they rarely develop *C. difficile*-associated diarrhea.[39] Absence of toxin receptor expression on the immature colonic epithelium is a possible explanation of the carrier state in infants and children.[40] As discussed later, the carrier state in infancy produces an important host immune response that may influence the outcome of infection later in adult life.

Almost all antimicrobial agents can predispose to *C. difficile* diarrhea and colitis, including vancomycin and metronidazole.[41,42] However, the precise risks associated with individual agents are difficult to establish.[43-45] The frequency of association of specific antibiotics is related to their frequency of use, their route of administration, and their effect on the colonic microflora.[43,45] Antibiotics frequently associated with *C. difficile* infection and diarrhea include clindamycin, cephalosporins, ampicillin, and amoxicillin (Table 105–2).[44,46-48] Cancer chemotherapy agents that possess antibacterial properties and bowel preparation regimens (prior to colonoscopy or colonic surgery) also may result in sufficient disturbance of the intestinal microflora to allow colonization with *C. difficile*.[49]

Hospital Epidemiology of *Clostridium difficile* Infection

Chronic intestinal carriage rates in healthy adults are low (0% to 3% in American and European populations).[28,50,51] Furthermore, it is unclear whether carriage is a temporary or permanent state.[42] In contrast, hospital inpatients treated with antibiotics have reported colonization rates of 15% to 21%.[23,28,52-54] Thus, the hospital environment is a major source of *C. difficile* infection. Infected stool, environmental surfaces, inanimate objects, and the hands of health care workers all represent potential sources of infection with *C. difficile* and its spores in the hospital setting.[23,54] Thus, in one study, *C. difficile* was acquired in 3.2 days by patients who shared a room with a *C. difficile*-positive roommate compared with 18.9 days by patients in single rooms or with roommates who were culture negative.[52] In the same study, *C. difficile* was cultured from the hands of 59% of hospital workers caring for patients with positive *C. difficile* cultures and from bedrails, toilets, floors, call buttons, and other surfaces in the rooms of *C. difficile*-infected patients. Asymptomatic carriers rarely develop *C. difficile*-associated diarrhea, but they can serve as an important source of spread in the hospital environment.[55] In one study, 29% of environmental cultures taken from the rooms of symptom-free carriers were positive for *C. difficile*, compared with only 8% of cultures from rooms of culture-negative patients.[52] *C. difficile* strains causing infection in other hospital inpatients also have been linked to asymptomatic carriers.[56]

In antibiotic-treated animals, the infective dose of toxigenic *C. difficile* may be as low as two organisms.[21] If human susceptibility is similar, control of *C. difficile* infection in hospitals will continue to be a major challenge since up to 10^9 organisms per gram are excreted in liquid feces.[57,58] Furthermore, highly resistant spores of *C. difficile* may persist for many months in hospital units and can result in infection if ingested.[57]

Although it is not possible currently to eradicate *C. difficile* and its spores from the hospital environment, certain control measures have been recommended to reduce the prevalence of *C. difficile*-associated diarrhea (Table 105–3).[59] Hospital inpatients with *C. difficile*-associated diarrhea should be bedded in private rooms whenever possible to reduce patient-to-patient spread. Strict enteric precautions and regular handwashing after patient contact should be observed, because *C. difficile* can be cultured from the hands of health care workers after as many as 60% of contacts with infected patients.[52] A controlled trial of using vinyl disposable gloves during patient contact also led to a reduced incidence of *C. difficile* diarrhea.[61] Thorough environmental disinfection with agents effective against *C. difficile*, such as sodium hypochlorite, alkaline glutaraldehyde, or ethylene oxide, should be performed after discharge of infected patients.[60]

Table 105–3 Practice Guidelines for the Prevention of *Clostridium difficile* Diarrhea

1. Limit the use of antimicrobial drugs.
2. Wash hands between contact with all patients.
3. Use enteric (stool) isolation precautions for patients with *C. difficile* diarrhea.
4. Wear gloves when contacting patients with *C. difficile* diarrhea or their environment.
5. Disinfect objects contaminated with *C. difficile* with sodium hypochlorite, alkaline glutaraldehyde, or ethylene oxide.
6. Educate the medical, nursing, and other appropriate staff members about the disease and its epidemiology.

From Fekety R: Guidelines for the diagnosis and management of *Clostridium difficile*-associated diarrhea and colitis. American College of Gastroenterology, Practice Parameters Committee. Am J Gastroenterol 92:739, 1997.

Table 105–2 Antimicrobial Agents that Predispose to *Clostridium difficile*-Associated Diarrhea and Colitis

Frequently	Less Frequently	Rarely or Never
Ampicillin and amoxicillin	Tetracyclines	Parenteral aminoglycosides
Cephalosporins	Sulfonamides	Metronidazole
Clindamycin	Macrolides (including erythromycin)	Bacitracin
	Chloramphenicol	Vancomycin
	Trimethoprim	
	Fluoroquinolones	

Adapted from Kelly CP, LaMont JT: Treatment of *Clostridium difficile* diarrhea and colitis. In Wolfe MM (ed): Gastrointestinal Pharmacotherapy. Philadelphia, WB Saunders, 1993, p 199.

Hospital outbreaks of *C. difficile*-associated diarrhea occur frequently and likely result from the close approximation of susceptible individuals (i.e., elderly and infirm patients) taking antibiotics who are then exposed to the pathogen either in the hospital environment or through person-to-person spread. Antibiotic therapy with metronidazole or vancomycin is not recommended as a disease control measure.[62] The incidence of *C. difficile* diarrhea can be reduced by avoiding the unnecessary use of broad-spectrum antibiotics. In the future, increasing individual and herd immunity to *C. difficile* by vaccination or by passive immunotherapy may become a viable approach to reducing the prevalence of this common nosocomial disease.[59,63-65] Prophylactic measures such as the use of bacterial and yeast probiotic agents or toxin binders in high-risk hospital patients also warrant further investigation.[66-69]

Clostridium difficile Toxins A and B

C. difficile diarrhea and colitis are caused by toxins, not by bacterial invasion of the colonic mucosa. Pathogenic strains of *C. difficile* produce two structurally similar protein exotoxins, toxin A and toxin B, which are the major known virulence factors of this bacterium. The genes encoding toxin A and toxin B reside in a 19.6-kb chromosomal region called the *C.* difficile *pathogenicity locus* (Fig. 105–2).[70-74] This locus comprises the genes encoding toxin A (*tcdA*) and B (*tcdB*) as well as two putative regulatory genes (*tcdC* and *tcdD*).[73-77] The *tcdD* gene product appears to up-regulate toxin transcription by complexing with RNA polymerase that binds to the toxin promoter regions. The *tcdC* gene is transcribed in the opposite direction to *tcdA*, *tcdB*, and *tcdD*, and its gene product is more abundant during exponential bacterial growth, a situation in which toxin production is low.[75] These findings have led to speculation that *tcdC* may encode a toxin gene repressor. The fifth gene of the pathogenicity locus, *tcdE*, encodes a protein of undetermined function, although some data support the theory that it may act to lyse cell walls, thereby releasing toxins A and B into the colonic lumen.[78]

Toxins A and B both belong to the large clostridial cytotoxin family, share a number of structural features, and are 49% identical at the amino acid level.[74,79-81] The *tcdA* gene encodes a polypeptide of 2710 amino acids (deduced molecular mass, 308,128 d) and the *tcdB* gene encodes a protein of 2366 amino acids (269,711 d). Both toxins carry an *N*-terminal enzymatic domain that mediates their toxic effects on mammalian cells, a central hydrophobic region that may act as a transmembrane domain to facilitate toxin entry into the cytoplasm, and a C-terminal domain consisting of a series of repeated sequences that are believed to mediate toxin binding to receptors on intestinal cell membranes (Fig. 105–3). Both toxins possess similar enzymatic activities and are UDP-glucose hydrolases and glucosyltransferases. Following internalization into the host cell cytoplasm, the toxins catalyze the transfer and covalent attachment of a glucose residue from UDP-glucose to a conserved threonine amino acid on small (20 to 25 kd), guanosine triphosphate-binding, rho proteins. The rho family of proteins are part of the Ras protein superfamily, are expressed in all eukaryotic cells, and act as intracellular signaling molecules to regulate cytoskeletal organization and gene expression. The rho proteins, RhoA, Cdc42, and Rac, are substrates for both toxins A and B, whereas Rap is a substrate for toxin A only.[74,82-84] Glucosylation of rho proteins by the toxins leads to disordered cell signaling, disorganization of the cytoskeleton, disruption of protein synthesis, cell rounding, and cell death.[74,85] Both toxins also activate NF-κB and MAP kinases in target cells leading to the release of proinflammatory cytokines including interleukin (IL)-1β, tumor necrosis factor-α, and IL-8.[85,86] These cellular proinflammatory effects likely contribute to the marked intestinal inflammatory

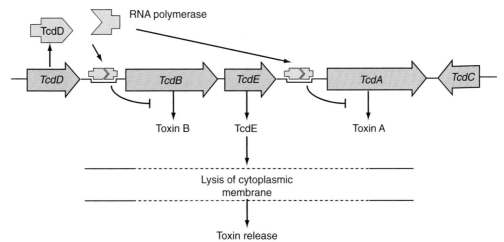

Figure 105–2 *Clostridium difficile* pathogenicity locus. The pathogenicity locus of *C. difficile* is a 19.6-kb segment carrying five genes (*TcdA-E*), including the genes encoding toxin A (*TcdA*) and toxin B *(TcdB)*. *TcdD* appears to activate toxin A and toxin B transcription by forming a complex with RNA polymerase that binds to *TcdA* and *TcdB* promoter regions. *TcdC* appears to act as a negative regulator of toxin production, and *TcdE* may mediate toxin release through its ability to disrupt the bacterial cytoplasmic membrane. (From Warny M, Kelly CP: Pathogenicity of *Clostridium difficile* toxins. In Hecht G [ed]: Microbial Pathogenesis and the Intestinal Epithelial Cell. Washington, DC, ASM Press, 2003, p 503.)

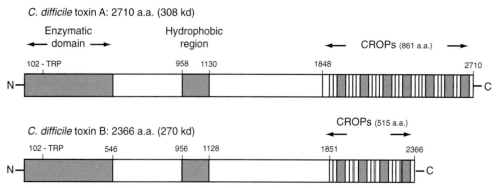

Figure 105–3 Structure of *Clostridium difficile* toxins. Toxin A and toxin B share three similar domains: (1) an *N*-terminal enzymatic domain responsible for cytotoxicity that carries a conserved tryptophan residue (Trp-102) probably involved in binding to uridine diphospho (UDP)-glucose; (2) a central, major hydrophobic region of 172 amino acids (a.a.) that is highly conserved and may act as a transmembrane domain to facilitate exit from endosomes into the cytoplasm; (3) a C-terminal binding domain composed of contiguous repeating units also known as clostridial repetitive oligopeptides (CROPs). Toxin A carries 30 CROPs whereas toxin B carries 19. They include sequences of 50 amino acids (represented in orange) and 21 amino acids (represented in white). (From Warny M, Kelly CP: Pathogenicity of *Clostridium difficile* toxins. In Hecht G [ed]: Microbial Pathogenesis and the Intestinal Epithelial Cell. Washington, DC, ASM Press, 2003, p 503.)

response that is evident in *C. difficile*-associated diarrhea and pseudomembranous colitis.

Toxin A is an inflammatory enterotoxin that induces intestinal fluid secretion, increased mucosal permeability, and marked enteritis and colitis when injected into the intestinal lumen of animals.[85] Toxin A also possesses cytotoxic activity against cultured cells.[87,88] Toxin B is an extremely potent cytotoxin but has minimal enterotoxic activity in animals, initially suggesting that toxin B did not contribute to diarrhea and colitis in humans.[87,89-91] It is now known, however, that toxins A and B cause injury and electrophysiologic changes in human colonic explants in vitro. In fact, toxin B is 10 times more potent than toxin A in inducing both of these changes.[92] In a chimeric animal model for *C. difficile* toxin-induced injury to the human intestinal mucosa in which human intestinal xenografts were transplanted subcutaneously into immunodeficient mice and then the mice were injected with toxin A or toxin B; toxin B was equivalent to toxin A in its ability to cause tissue injury and an acute intestinal inflammatory response.[93] Furthermore, toxin A⁻/toxin B⁺ strains of *C. difficile* have been isolated from patients with diarrhea and pseudomembranous colitis.[94-97] Thus, toxin B now is considered to be a major factor in the pathogenesis of *C. difficile*-associated diarrhea and colitis in humans.

The Immune Response to *Clostridium difficile*

Serum IgG and IgA antibodies against *C. difficile* toxins are found in more than 50% of healthy children and adults.[98-102] Mucosal IgA antitoxin antibodies also are detectable in more than 50% of human colonic secretions, and in one study, these antibodies inhibited binding of toxin A to its intestinal receptors.[100,102] Immunization against *C. difficile* toxins protects animals from *C. difficile* colitis.[103] Because immunized animals still are colonized by toxigenic *C. difficile*, it appears that this protection is the result of toxin neutralization, a situation that may be similar to the asymptomatic carrier state in humans.[53]

There is considerable evidence linking high serum IgG antitoxin A antibody concentrations and protection against *C. difficile*-associated diarrhea and colitis.[59,63-65] Recurrent *C. difficile* diarrhea has been associated with low serum antitoxin antibody concentrations both in children and in adults.[98,102,104,105] In one study, patients with *C. difficile* diarrhea and a low level of serum IgG against toxin A had a 48-fold greater risk of recurrence compared with patients who had high antitoxin concentrations (Fig. 105–4).[106] High serum IgG antitoxin A concentrations also have been identified in asymptomatic carriers of toxigenic *C. difficile*. In a prospective study of nosocomially acquired *C. difficile*, 51% of infected patients remained asymptomatic.[53] At the time of colonization, serum levels of IgG antibody against toxin A were three times higher in the asymptomatic group compared with patients who developed diarrhea (see Fig. 105–4). The immune response to toxin B has not yet been correlated strongly with specific clinical outcomes. Nonetheless, toxin B is immunogenic in humans, and antibody responses to toxin B may play a role in immune protection against *C. difficile*-associated diarrhea.[59,64,65]

Other Risk Factors for *Clostridium difficile* Infection

In addition to antimicrobial therapy, older age and increased comorbidity are important risk factors for *C. difficile* infection.[107] In England and Wales, 75% of reported *C. difficile* infections between 1992 and 1996 occurred in patients aged 65 years or older.[50] Data from the United States also demonstrate that age is an independent risk factor for this infection.[108,109] The elderly particularly are predisposed to infection with *C. difficile* because of increased nosocomial exposure and frequent courses of antibiotics and a reduced ability of their polymorphonuclear leukocytes to phagocytose these organisms.[110] In one study of antibiotic recipients, patients with severe underlying disease at the time of hospital admission were eight times more likely to develop *C. difficile* infection compared with patients who were less severely ill.[53] Other reported risk factors for *C. difficile*

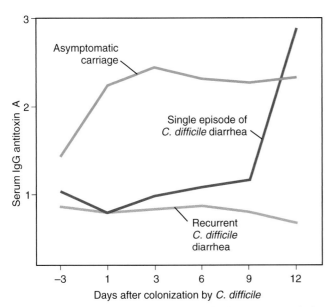

Figure 105–4 Serum IgG antitoxin A antibody response and clinical outcome of infection with *Clostridium difficile*. Patients with nosocomial *C. difficile* diarrhea were studied prospectively, and serum IgG antitoxin A antibody concentrations were measured by enzyme-linked immunosorbent assay (ELISA) at regular intervals. A correlation was observed between the IgG response to toxin A and the clinical outcome of infection. Asymptomatic carriers mounted an early memory immune response to toxin A. By contrast, no significant increase in serum IgG antitoxin A was found in patients who experienced recurrent *C. difficile* diarrhea. In those who had a single episode of diarrhea, IgG antitoxin A levels generally were increased on day 12 of their first episode. Thus, a serum antibody response to toxin A during *C. difficile* infection is associated with protection against symptoms or against recurrent diarrhea. (Adapted from Kyne L, Warny M, Qamar A, Kelly CP: Association between antibody response to toxin A and protection against recurrent *Clostridium difficile* diarrhoea. Lancet 357:189, 2001.)

infection include the use of a nasogastric tube, gastrointestinal procedures, acid antisecretory medications, intensive care unit stay, and length of hospital stay.[43] The strengths of the associations of these risk factors with *C. difficile* vary from study to study. These factors often are markers of disease severity, older age, or both, and the significance of their association with *C. difficile* may be lost after controlling for these confounding variables.[53,107,109]

Patients undergoing cytotoxic chemotherapy for malignancy are at risk for *C. difficile*-associated diarrhea and colitis for a number of reasons including frequent antibiotic use, nosocomial exposure to *C. difficile,* and the severity of their underlying disease.[111,112] Even in the absence of antibiotic use, antineoplastic chemotherapy predisposes to *C. difficile* infection; methotrexate is the most commonly implicated agent.[49] Presumably this predisposition reflects the ability of chemotherapeutic drugs to alter the colonic microflora and reduce *C. difficile* colonization resistance. *C. difficile*-associated diarrhea has also been reported in patients undergoing immunosup-

pressive therapy in the setting of solid organ or bone marrow transplantation.[113,114] Patients with human immunodeficiency virus (HIV) infection also are at risk for *C. difficile*-associated diarrhea due to multiple risk factors, including frequent prophylactic and therapeutic antibiotic use, hospitalization, and immunocompromise.[115-118] *C. difficile* colitis behaves the same in patients with acquired immunodeficiency syndrome as it does in control groups.[118] As a result, testing for *C. difficile* should be a part of the diagnostic evaluation in patients with HIV infection, diarrhea, and a history of current or recent antibiotic treatment.

Patients with inflammatory bowel disease (IBD) are at increased risk for *C. difficile* infection.[119,120] Infection with a broad range of enteric pathogens including *C. difficile*, *Campylobacter*, and *Salmonella* species can precipitate or mimic disease relapse in IBD. *C. difficile* is the most commonly identified specific pathogen in IBD patients in North America and Europe, however, and is present in as many as 5% to 19% of patients with relapse in some case series.[121,122] Some IBD patients with *C. difficile* infection do not have a history of recent antibiotic use, suggesting that IBD itself may cause sufficient alterations in the colonic microenvironment to negate the colonization resistance of the normal colonic microflora.[121,122] The possibility of enteric infection with *C. difficile* or other pathogens should be considered in patients with an increase in IBD disease activity. If *C. difficile* infection is identified, antimicrobial therapy with metronidazole or vancomycin is indicated in combination with other IBD therapies.

CLINICAL FEATURES

Clinical manifestations of *C. difficile* infection range from asymptomatic carriage to mild or moderate diarrhea to life-threatening pseudomembranous colitis. Asymptomatic carriage of *C. difficile* is common in hospitalized patients. Several large epidemiologic studies indicate that 10% to 16% of hospital inpatients receiving antibiotics in high-risk units are carriers.[28,52,53,55,123] Despite the fact that most of the *C. difficile* isolates from carriers are toxin producing, the carriers do not develop symptomatic disease.[28,55] As mentioned earlier, the host immune response to *C. difficile* toxins appears to be instrumental in protecting carriers from *C. difficile* diarrhea.[104]

In patients who develop diarrhea with *C. difficile*, symptoms usually begin soon after colonization. The incubation period is usually less than a week, with a median time of onset of approximately 2 days.[28,52,53,124] Colonization may occur during ongoing antibiotic treatment or after a course of antibiotics. Olson and associates[26] reported that 96% of patients with symptomatic *C. difficile* infection had received antibiotics within 14 days of the onset of diarrhea and that all had received an antibiotic within the previous 3 months.

C. difficile diarrhea typically is associated with the frequent passage of loose or watery bowel movements. Mucus or occult blood may be present, whereas melena and hematochezia are rare. Some patients may present with fever, leukocytosis, and cramping abdominal pain.[125] Because *C. difficile* is not an invasive pathogen, extraintestinal manifestations of *C. difficile* infection such as septic arthritis, bacteremia, or splenic abscess are extremely rare.[126-129] An oligoarticular, asymmetrical, nondeforming, large-joint arthropathy, similar to that seen in other infectious colitides, sometimes is seen.[130]

Patients with more severe disease may develop a colonic ileus or toxic dilatation and present with minimal or even no diarrhea.[125] In the absence of diarrhea, the only clues to the diagnosis may be high fever, moderate or marked (e.g., leukemoid) polymorphonuclear leukocytosis, lower or diffuse abdominal pain, tenderness, and distention.

Abdominal plain films may reveal a dilated colon (>7 cm in its greatest diameter) or toxic megacolon. Patients with colonic dilatation also may have small bowel ileus with air-fluid levels mimicking intestinal obstruction or ischemia. In such cases, a computed tomographic scan of the abdomen may be a useful diagnostic test, although in general, it reveals nonspecific features common to ischemic, infectious, and inflammatory colitides (Fig. 105–5).[131] Radiologic features of pseudomembranous colitis include mucosal edema, thumbprinting, thickened colonic wall, pancolitis, and pericolonic inflammation with or without ascites, and with little or no small bowel involvement other than ileus.[132] Flexible sigmoidoscopy or colonoscopy is sometimes indicated (see later) when the diagnosis remains unclear after initial evaluation. Complications of severe *C. difficile* colitis include dehydration, hypoalbuminemia, electrolyte disturbances, toxic megacolon, bowel perforation, and death.[60,125]

DIAGNOSIS

The diagnosis of *C. difficile* diarrhea or colitis is based on a history of recent or current antimicrobial therapy, development of diarrhea or other evidence of acute colitis, and demonstration of infection by toxigenic *C. difficile*, usually by detection of toxin A or B, or both, in a stool sample.[47,60]

Diagnostic Tests for *Clostridium difficile* Infection

The diagnosis of *C. difficile* diarrhea should be considered in any patient with acute diarrhea who has received antibiotics within the previous 3 months and especially in anyone whose diarrhea began 72 hours or more after hospitalization. Approximately 40% of patients with *C. difficile* diarrhea at tertiary referral centers are symptomatic on admission to the hospital.[52,53,133] In this setting, a history of recent discharge or transfer from another hospital or nursing home may suggest the diagnosis.

Testing of solid or formed stools for *C. difficile* toxin is not recommended because only patients with diarrhea require treatment.[47,52,53,60,123] Treatment of asymptomatic carriers with antimicrobial agents against *C. difficile* is not recommended because it may prolong the carrier state[62]; neither is follow-up stool testing for *C. difficile* indicated in an asymptomatic patient who has had a recent episode of *C. difficile* diarrhea. Stool carriage of this organism following an episode of *C. difficile* diarrhea may persist for 3 to 6 weeks even after cessation of all symptoms.[134] Because asymptomatic carriers may act as a hidden reservoir for *C. difficile* infection, especially in hospitals and nursing homes, universal precautions should be followed for all patients to reduce the likelihood of patient-to-patient spread of nosocomial infectious disease.

If *C. difficile* diarrhea is suspected, a freshly passed stool should be submitted immediately to the laboratory in a clean watertight container to be tested for the presence of fecal toxin A or B. Anaerobic storage or the use of transport media does not improve diagnostic accuracy and therefore is not necessary.[54] Storage at ambient temperatures can result in denaturation of fecal toxin; samples should therefore be tested immediately or refrigerated or frozen, pending later testing.[135]

A variety of laboratory tests are available to diagnose infection with toxigenic *C. difficile*, but enzyme immunoassays (EIAs) to detect toxin antigens in stool are currently used most frequently (Table 105–4). These tests have the advantages of being relatively inexpensive, quick (12 to 24 hours), and highly specific, although their relatively low sensitivity (≈90%) leads to some false-negative results. The tissue culture cytotoxicity assay is more sensitive and has greater diagnostic accuracy, but it is more costly and time consuming (48 to 72 hours).

Tissue Culture Cytotoxicity Assay

The gold standard diagnostic test to identify *C. difficile* toxins in stool is the tissue culture cytotoxicity assay.[136-138] By inactivating rho proteins (as discussed earlier) toxins A and B cause a disintegration of the actin cytoskeleton of the cells in tissue culture, leading to a characteristic cell rounding. A suspension of diarrheal stool diluted in phosphate-buffered saline is centrifuged, filtered, and then added to a monolayer of cultured cells, usually fibroblasts or Chinese hamster ovary cells. The monolayer is examined at 24 hours and again at 48 hours for cell rounding. The specificity of a positive result is established by preincubating an aliquot of the patient's stool

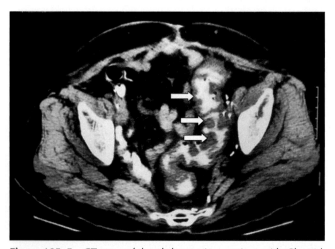

Figure 105–5 CT scan of the abdomen in a patient with *Clostridium difficile* colitis. Marked thickening of the colonic wall in the sigmoid colon and an accordion-like pattern, produced by a series of broad edematous colonic haustral folds, are evident (*arrows*). (From Linevsky JK, Kelly CP: *Clostridium difficile* colitis. In Lamont JT [ed]: Gastrointestinal Infections: Diagnosis and Management. New York, Taylor & Francis Group, LLC, 1997, p 293.)

Table 105–4 Stool Tests for the Diagnosis of *Clostridium difficile* Infection

Test	Detects	Advantages	Disadvantages
Cytotoxin assay	Toxin B	Gold standard; highly sensitive and specific	Requires tissue culture facility; takes 24-48 hr
Enzyme immunoassay	Toxin A and/or B	Fast (2-6 hr); easy to perform; highly specific	Neither as sensitive nor as specific as the cytotoxin assay
Latex agglutination assay	Bacterial enzyme (glutamate dehydrogenase)	Fast; inexpensive; easy to perform	Poor sensitivity and specificity
Culture	Toxigenic and nontoxigenic *C. difficile*	Sensitive; allows strain typing in epidemics	Requires anaerobic culture; not specific for toxin-producing strains; takes 2-5 days
Polymerase chain reaction	Toxin A or B genes in isolates or directly in feces	Highly sensitive and specific	Requires expertise in molecular diagnostic techniques

Adapted from Linevsky JK, Kelly CP: *Clostridium difficile* colitis. In Lamont JT (ed): Gastrointestinal Infections: Diagnosis and Management. New York, Taylor & Francis Group, LLC, 1997, p 293.

specimen with specific neutralizing antitoxin antibody; stool that gives a positive result when tested alone and becomes negative after incubation with antitoxin antibody is a true positive. False-positive results may result from pathogens other than *C. difficile* and from non-*C. difficile* enterotoxins.

The cytotoxicity assay is highly sensitive (67% to 100%) and specific (85% to 100%), if performed under optimal conditions; however, sensitivity may be reduced by inactivation of toxins during transport and storage, by the age and type of cell line used, and by diluting the stool.[54,135,139-141] Therefore, a negative cytotoxicity test does not completely exclude *C. difficile* as the cause of diarrhea. The main disadvantages of the cytotoxicity assay are that it is relatively expensive, requires a cell culture facility, and needs at least 24 hours for the test result to be available.

Enzyme-Linked Immunoassays

Commercially available EIAs are used widely for the detection of toxin A or toxins A and B of *C. difficile* in stool specimens.[136-138,142,143] These assays detect toxin A and/or toxin B by their interaction with either a monoclonal antibody or polyclonal antiserum that specifically recognizes toxin epitopes. EIAs are easier to perform than is the cytotoxicity test, are relatively inexpensive, and results may be available within 2 to 6 hours. Although they have high specificity (75% to 100%) for toxins, their main drawback is that they are less sensitive than the cytotoxicity test (63% to 99%). In addition, some EIA kits detect only toxin A in which case diarrhea due to a toxin A⁻/toxin B⁺ strain of *C. difficile* will be falsely negative.[96] For this reason, commercial kits that detect both toxins A and B have a slight advantage over those that detect toxin A alone.[143]

Clostridium difficile *Culture*

Stool culture for *C. difficile* is sensitive (89% to 100%) but is not specific for toxin-producing strains of the bacterium. In vitro testing for toxin production by isolates cultured from toxin-negative stools can improve specificity, but this is not a routine laboratory procedure and is costly and time consuming. One advantage of culturing *C. difficile* is that it permits strain typing of individ-

ual isolates; therefore, it is useful in tracking hospital outbreaks for epidemiologic studies.[55,91]

Polymerase Chain Reaction for Detection of Toxin Genes

Polymerase chain reaction (PCR), using specific primers based on the genes for toxins A and B, can detect toxigenic *C. difficile* in clinical isolates.[144-152] PCR is highly sensitive (100%) and specific (96.7% to 100%), but technically demanding. PCR may require initial culture of *C. difficile* (although PCR methods for the detection of toxin genes directly in feces have been described).[147-151] Using a nested PCR assay on stool samples, Alonso and colleagues[152] reported 99% concordance with the cytotoxicity assay and a sensitivity and specificity of 96.3% and 100%, respectively. Application of PCR methods in the clinical laboratory requires expertise in molecular diagnostic techniques and may not prove to be any more rapid or less expensive than stool cytotoxicity assay.

Sigmoidoscopy and Colonoscopy

Neither sigmoidoscopy nor colonoscopy is required for diagnosis in most patients with *C. difficile* diarrhea.[60] Endoscopy is helpful, however, when the diagnosis is in doubt or when disease severity demands rapid diagnosis. Sigmoidoscopy may be normal in patients with mild diarrhea or may demonstrate nonspecific colitis in moderate cases. The finding of colonic pseudomembranes in a patient with AAD is virtually pathognomonic for *C. difficile* colitis (Fig. 105–6).[47,153] These pseudomembranes appear as yellow, gray, or white plaques 2 to 5 mm in diameter, and in some areas they can coalesce to cover large areas of the mucosal surface. Sigmoidoscopy may not be sufficient to identify all patients with pseudomembranous colitis; approximately 15% to 20% will not have pseudomembranes in the rectosigmoid but will have pseudomembranes in the more proximal areas of the colon.[154] Other nonspecific endoscopic findings include erythema, edema, friability, small ulcerations, and erosions.

In mild disease, colonic mucosal biopsies may be normal or demonstrate only mild and nonspecific acute inflammatory changes with neutrophil infiltration. In

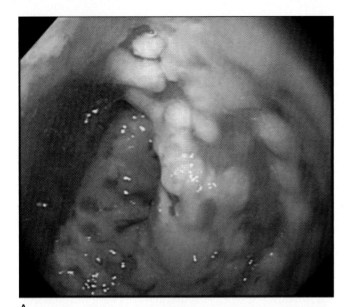

A

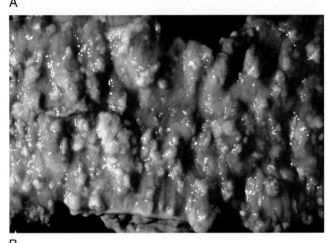

B

Figure 105–6 Colonoscopic image of pseudomembranous colitis (*A*) and a colon resection specimen from a patient with severe, refractory *Clostridium difficile* diarrhea and colitis (*B*). Characteristic raised adherent yellow plaques that vary in size from 2 to 5 mm are visible on the colonic mucosa. In some areas, coalescing pseudomembranes are evident. There is some erythema of the colonic mucosa between the pseudomembranes, but the epithelium is intact. (*A*, From Kwon JH, Kelly CP: *Clostridium difficile* and antibiotic-associated diarrhea. In Bayless RM, Diehl AM [eds]: Advanced Therapy in Gastroenterology and Liver Disease, 5th ed. Hamilton, Ontario, Canada, BC Decker, 2005, p 302; and *B*, From Kelly CP, Pothoulakis C, LaMont JT: *Clostridium difficile* colitis. N Engl J Med 330:257, 1994.)

more severe cases, colonic histology shows focal ulceration of the mucosa associated with the eruption of inflammatory cells and necrotic debris that covers the area of ulceration, the so-called summit or volcano lesion (Fig. 105–7).[47,155]

Miscellaneous Laboratory Tests

Many patients with acute *C. difficile* diarrhea develop a polymorphonuclear leukocytosis with a left shift. Occasionally a "leukemoid" reaction with an extremely high white blood cell count of 20,000 to 90,000 cells/mm^3 is

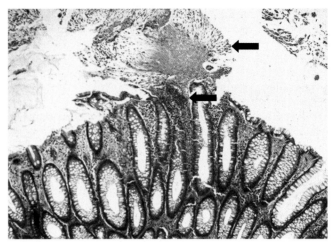

Figure 105–7 Histologic image of an endoscopic biopsy specimen from a patient with pseudomembranous colitis showing a "summit" or "volcano" lesion. Focal ulceration of the colonic mucosa is evident (*lower arrow*), with exudation of a pseudomembrane made up of inflammatory cells, fibrin, and necrotic debris (*upper arrow*). The adjoining mucosa is intact. (From Kelly CP, Pothoulakis C, LaMont JT: *Clostridium difficile* colitis. N Engl J Med 330:257, 1994.)

Table 105–5 Treatment of *Clostridium difficile* Diarrhea and Colitis

1. Discontinue inciting antibiotic if possible
2. Provide supportive therapy (see text)
3. Confirm the diagnosis
4. Prescribe specific therapy if symptoms are severe or persistent:
   Metronidazole orally for 10-14 days (drug of choice)
   Vancomycin orally for 10-14 days if
     Diarrhea does not improve during metronidazole treatment
     Patient cannot tolerate metronidazole
     Patient is pregnant or <10 yr of age
     Diarrhea and colitis are severe
5. If patient cannot tolerate oral medication: metronidazole 500 mg, every 6 hours intravenously

Adapted from Fekety R: Guidelines for the diagnosis and management of *Clostridium difficile*-associated diarrhea and colitis. American College of Gastroenterology, Practice Parameters Committee. Am J Gastroenterol 92:739, 1997.

seen, usually in patients with severe diarrhea accompanied by fever, dehydration, and pseudomembranous colitis. Serum albumin may be decreased, especially in severe colitis, probably secondary to an acute protein-losing colopathy. Rarely, patients with protein-losing colopathy and severe hypoalbuminemia may present with peripheral edema or ascites.

TREATMENT

Mild-to-Moderately Severe *Clostridium difficile* Diarrhea and Colitis

The first step in the management of *C. difficile* diarrhea and colitis is to discontinue the precipitating antibiotics if possible (Table 105–5).[60] Diarrhea resolves in approximately 15% to 25% of patients without specific anti-*C. difficile* therapy.[26,156] Conservative therapy alone, however, is not appropriate in patients who are severely ill or who have only mild-to-moderate illness but who also have multiple medical problems. It is difficult, if not impossible, to predict who will improve and who will have ongoing or worsening symptoms after just discontinuation of antibiotics and conservative management. In patients with active infections elsewhere (e.g., pneumonia and urinary tract infection) and in whom antibiotic therapy must be continued, the antibiotic regimen should be switched to agents with a relatively low likelihood of exacerbating *C. difficile* diarrhea, for example, parenteral aminoglycosides, trimethoprim, erythromycin or rifampicin (see Table 105–2).[46] Antimotility agents such as diphenoxylate plus atropine (Lomotil), loperamide (Imodium), or narcotics are best avoided because they may impair clearance of toxin from the colon and worsen toxin-induced colonic injury or precipitate ileus and toxic dilatation of the colon.[60,157-159] Treatment of asymptomatic carriers with antimicrobial agents against *C. difficile* is not recommended because it may prolong the carrier state.[62]

Many antimicrobial agents show activity against *C. difficile* in vitro[160-166]; however, clinical resistance to cefoxitin is commonplace among patients with this infection, even though cefoxitin is used in selective media to culture *C. difficile*.[167] Clindamycin resistance also is seen in clinical isolates and has been associated with some nosocomial outbreaks.[168] There is increasing evidence of fluoroquinolone resistance among nosocomial *C. difficile* isolates, with 7% of 198 clinical isolates in a series from France showing varying levels of resistance related to point mutations in gyrA or gyrB.[169] Fortunately, resistance to metronidazole is rare, and resistance to vancomycin is essentially nonexistent. In one study of 186 clinical isolates, all were sensitive to both metronidazole and vancomycin with minimum inhibiting concentrations (MICs) of 0.5 to 4 mg/mL.[167] In another series from Spain, 6% of 415 isolates showed intermediate sensitivity to metronidazole (i.e., MIC >16 mg/mL).[170] However, this partial resistance pattern was not clonal and was not sustained in serial culture. These findings suggest an acquired tolerance rather than genetically determined metronidazole resistance. Many antimicrobial agents, such as ampicillin or amoxicillin, which have in vitro activity against *C. difficile*, are common causes of *C. difficile*-associated diarrhea in clinical practice.[161,171] This observation illustrates the fact that in vitro sensitivity testing alone is a poor predictor of therapeutic efficacy in this disease. The preclinical efficacy of therapeutic agents for *C. difficile*-associated diarrhea has been assessed in clindamycin-exposed Syrian hamsters.[66,162,165,172,173] These animals develop a fulminant and fatal cecitis when exposed to toxigenic *C. difficile* after administration of clindamycin. Historically, this animal model has provided a reliable indication of the effectiveness of therapeutic agents for *C. difficile* infection and diarrhea.

Specific antibiotic therapy to eradicate *C. difficile* is required in patients with severe symptoms or in those whose symptoms persist despite discontinuation of antibiotic treatment. The most effective antimicrobials for the treatment of *C. difficile* diarrhea are metronidazole (250 to 500 mg three or four times a day for 10 to 14 days) and vancomycin (125 to 500 mg four times a day for 10 to 14 days) (Table 105–6).[174] Bacitracin, teicoplanin, and fusidic acid also have been used to treat acute infection but have few if any advantages over metronidazole or vancomycin. In a systematic review, none of these alternative antibiotics were superior in terms of response rates.[175] The advantages and disadvantages of specific therapeutic agents are discussed in the following sections.

Metronidazole

Metronidazole generally is recommended as the drug of first choice for acute *C. difficile* diarrhea and colitis.[60,176] It is inexpensive ($0.50 per 250-mg tablet) and is highly effective for the treatment of this condition. Several clinical studies have demonstrated that metronidazole therapy results in the resolution of diarrhea and colitis in more than 95% of patients treated.[26,160,175] In a prospective, randomized trial of acute *C. difficile* infection, metronidazole (250 mg four times a day for 10 days) was as effective as vancomycin (500 mg four times daily for 10 days) in terms of response and recurrence rates.[156]

Metronidazole, unlike vancomycin, is well absorbed in the upper intestine following oral administration. Fecal concentrations are low or absent in healthy individuals or asymptomatic carriers of *C. difficile*, but higher fecal concentrations are observed in patients with *C. difficile* colitis. In patients with acute colitis, metronidazole may be secreted through an inflamed intestinal mucosa or rapid transit in the upper intestine may result in its decreased absorption.[177-179] Intravenous metronidazole

Table 105–6   Comparison of Metronidazole and Vancomycin for the Treatment of *Clostridium difficile* Diarrhea

Variables	Metronidazole	Vancomycin
Dose	250-500 mg	125-500 mg
Frequency	tid or qid	qid
Duration	10-14 days	10-14 days
Route	Oral or intravenous	Oral
Response rate	>95%	>95%
Cost (10-day oral course)	$20	$800
Disadvantages	Systemic side effects; rare resistant strains of *C. difficile*	Encourages growth of nosocomial vancomycin-resistant bacteria

Adapted from Kelly CP, LaMont JT: Treatment of *Clostridium difficile* diarrhea and colitis. In Wolfe MM (ed): Therapy of Digestive Disorders. Philadelphia, WB Saunders, 2000, p 513.

(500 mg four times per day) may be used in patients who cannot tolerate oral medication, because it is excreted into bile and accumulates in bactericidal levels in the inflamed colon.[177]

Oral metronidazole therapy usually is well tolerated but can be associated with systemic side effects.[179] In one report of more than 600 patients receiving metronidazole for C. difficile diarrhea only 1% experienced significant side effects.[26] Adverse effects include nausea, a metallic taste, a disulfiram-like reaction with alcohol, and a peripheral sensory neuropathy with prolonged therapy. Metronidazole may potentiate the action of warfarin, resulting in prolongation of the prothrombin time. Metronidazole is usually not used in pregnant and nursing women because of chromosomal abnormalities, unknown effects on fetal organogenesis, and reports of tumorigenicity in rodents. Its safety in children has not been documented. Enigmatically, metronidazole has been identified as the antibiotic agent responsible for causing some cases of C. difficile diarrhea, demonstrating the importance of reduced colonization resistance in the pathophysiology of C. difficile-associated diarrhea.[180-182]

Vancomycin

Vancomycin was introduced for the treatment of C. difficile-associated diarrhea and colitis in 1978,[183] and its pharmacokinetic properties make it an ideal agent for the treatment of this infection. When given orally, vancomycin is neither absorbed nor metabolized significantly, and as a result high concentrations in the colonic lumen are achieved. The efficacy of vancomycin in the treatment of C. difficile colitis has been demonstrated in controlled trials.[51,156,183,184] Improvement in diarrhea usually is evident within 72 hours of initiating therapy, and complete resolution of symptoms occurs in most patients (96% overall) by the end of a 10-day treatment course.[175] In 122 patients treated with vancomycin at one institution, the response rate, drug intolerance rate, and relapse rate were 99%, 1%, and 10%, respectively.[26]

Fekety and coworkers[185] demonstrated that vancomycin at a dose of 125 mg four times a day is as effective as vancomycin 500 mg four times a day. The lower dose is recommended for patients with mild-to-moderate colitis, and the higher dose for critically ill patients (i.e., those with ileus, colonic dilatation, or fulminant pseudomembranous colitis). Vancomycin may be administered by mouth, nasogastric tube, or even by enema.[26,60] However, it should not be given intravenously for treatment of C. difficile infection because effective colonic luminal concentrations are not obtained following parenteral administration.[186,187]

Oral vancomycin is not absorbed appreciably, and as a result systemic side effects are rare. Despite its many advantages, vancomycin now is considered a second-line agent for the treatment of C. difficile because of its higher cost (a 10-day course may cost as much as $800) and concerns regarding the spread of vancomycin-resistant enterococci.[176] Vancomycin therapy is recommended, however, for infections that fail to respond to metronidazole, for patients who are intolerant of metronidazole, patients with fulminant pseudomembranous colitis, patients who are pregnant, or children younger than 10 years of age.[60,176]

Other Antimicrobial Agents

Bacitracin (25,000 units four times daily for 7 to 10 days) is less effective than metronidazole or vancomycin for the treatment of C. difficile diarrhea, with an overall response rate of only 80% and a relapse rate of 30%.[184,188-190] In randomized therapeutic trials, teicoplanin, 100 mg twice a day for 10 days, was as effective as vancomycin for the treatment of C. difficile diarrhea.[191,192] Teicoplanin, however, is relatively expensive and is not available for oral administration in the United States. Fusidic acid has been tested in a limited number of patients but appears to be less effective than metronidazole or vancomycin and is associated with a relapse rate of approximately 28%.[192,193] Treatment with colestipol, an ion exchange resin that binds toxins (10 g four times daily), is associated with a low response rate (36%) and is not recommended as primary therapy.[51]

Severe Pseudomembranous Colitis

Severe pseudomembranous colitis occurs in only 3% to 5% of patients with C. difficile infection but is associated with a mortality rate of up to 65%.[129,194,195] Many patients who develop fulminant C. difficile disease already have substantial comorbid disease and often are critically ill.[196,197] Diarrhea may be minimal or absent because of ileus, and patients may present with abdominal pain, peritoneal signs, colonic dilatation, leukocytosis, and a clinical picture of progressive sepsis.[88,157,198] Prompt diagnosis and aggressive therapy are necessary to avoid substantial morbidity and mortality.

The first step is to discontinue precipitating antibiotics if possible and start therapy with metronidazole or vancomycin. Although there are no published data indicating that vancomycin is superior to metronidazole for the treatment of severe C. difficile colitis, vancomycin often is used as a first-line agent in critically ill patients.[60] Intravenous metronidazole should be given if oral medication is not tolerated. Intravenous vancomycin is not recommended, for the reasons mentioned earlier. In the presence of ileus, vancomycin (500 mg every 6 hours) may be administered via nasogastric tube with intermittent clamping of the tube.[26] For critically ill patients, a combination of antibiotics administered by various routes may be indicated. Six of eight patients with severe ileus were treated successfully using a combination of vancomycin administered by nasogastric tube, intravenous metronidazole, and vancomycin-retention enemas (500 mg of vancomycin in 100 mL of normal saline administered every 6 hours via a Foley catheter inserted into the rectum). Patients treated with this regimen responded within 5 to 17 days.[26] Intracecal infusion of vancomycin has been reported but is not recommended because of the risks associated with placement of a narrow-bore tube over a guidewire at colonoscopy in patients with severe active colitis.[199]

Passive immunization with pooled human immunoglobulin has been used empirically in patients with severe colitis who were not responsive to metronidazole or vancomycin. As discussed earlier, patients with severe or prolonged C. difficile diarrhea have low serum and fecal concentrations of antibody against C. difficile toxins.[53,98,102,104-106] Intravenous infusion of normal pooled human immunoglobulin (400 mg/kg body weight) increases serum IgG antitoxin concentrations and has been used successfully to treat a small number of patients with severe *C. difficile* colitis.[105,200,201]

Emergency surgery sometimes is required in patients with severe colitis not responding to medical therapy and in whom bowel perforation is impending or has occurred.[132,195,197,198,202] The operation of choice is usually a subtotal colectomy with temporary ileostomy. Surgical intervention in this setting is associated with a high perioperative mortality rate, making the decision to operate difficult. Grundfest-Bronitowski and associates[197] reported an overall mortality rate of 42% in a series of patients undergoing surgery for fulminant, severe *C. difficile* infection. In another series of five patients with toxic megacolon, subtotal colectomy and ileostomy were successful in only one patient.[203]

Recurrent *Clostridium difficile* Diarrhea

One of the most difficult clinical problems in treating patients with *C. difficile* infection is the high incidence of recurrences.[60,204,205] The numerous treatment approaches described in this section indicate that no single measure is widely effective in preventing further recurrences. Multiple episodes of recurrent *C. difficile*-associated diarrhea are not uncommon, and more than 10 bouts of recurrence have occurred in some patients. Approximately 15% to 30% of patients successfully treated with vancomycin or metronidazole relapse after completion of their initial antibiotic therapy.[69,106,175,205,206] The clinical features of recurrence are similar to the initial attack with watery diarrhea, cramping abdominal pain, or fever occurring 2 to 10 days after discontinuing therapy. Late recurrences are less common but may occur for up to 2 months after stopping antibiotic treatment. The diagnosis of recurrent *C. difficile*-associated diarrhea is confirmed by stool toxin assay. In patients with typical symptoms of recurrence, therapy can be reinstituted while awaiting stool assay results. Prompt therapy is especially important in patients whose initial attack of *C. difficile* diarrhea was severe, because they are more likely to suffer from severe and recurrent disease, presumably because of their inadequate immune response to *C. difficile* toxins.[65,106]

Bacteriologic typing studies demonstrate that symptomatic recurrence may result from reinfection with either the same or a different strain of *C. difficile* that caused the initial episode.[207,208] Resistance to metronidazole or to vancomycin is seldom if ever an important factor in recurrence. For example, Bartlett and colleagues were unable to demonstrate in vitro vancomycin resistance in 23 isolates of *C. difficile* from relapsing patients.[209] In some patients, *C. difficile* can be cultured from the stools, during successful vancomycin therapy, and these patients may be more likely to relapse than those in whom eradication of the pathogen occurs during therapy.[207] However, *C. difficile* can also be cultured from the stools during and after successful antibiotic treatment in patients who do not relapse.[134] Culture positivity during symptomatic improvement may reflect the persistence of antibiotic-resistant spores. In one study, 18 of 22 patients with recurrence were noted to have colonic diverticula, leading to the speculation that spores may survive in diverticula where they escape the normal cleansing action of diarrhea and may not be exposed to the high luminal concentration of antibiotics.[204] However, reinfection by bacteria and spores through the usual fecal-oral route is a more likely mechanism of recurrence.[208]

Conservative Therapy

In a report of 20 patients with clindamycin-associated pseudomembranous colitis, published before the discovery of vancomycin as effective therapy, all patients eventually recovered when clindamycin was stopped.[210] An important advantage to this form of management is that recurrence of diarrhea or colitis does not occur, probably because stopping all antimicrobial agents allows for restoration of the colonic microflora and subsequent *C. difficile* colonization resistance. Some patients with mild symptoms of recurrence have been managed conservatively, without specific antibiotic treatment, but this approach is not appropriate for elderly or infirm patients with moderate or severe symptoms.

Repeat Treatment with Vancomycin or Metronidazole

Patients with recurrence typically are treated with a second course of the same antibiotic used to treat the initial attack, but treatment is usually for 14 days; this has a success rate of about 40%. Patients with one recurrence have a substantial risk of further recurrences, and in two independent studies, patients with one or more previous recurrences had a subsequent recurrence rate of greater than 50% following standard therapy with metronidazole or vancomycin.[69,106]

Prolonged or Tapering and Pulsed Antibiotic Therapy

The use of tapering- and pulsed-regimen antibiotic therapies is based on the theory that recurrence is caused by persistence of antibiotic-resistant spores, which then convert to vegetative toxin-producing forms when antibiotic therapy is discontinued. Administration of vancomycin or metronidazole every other day or every third day allows the spores to vegetate on the off days and then be susceptible to antibiotics. Tedesco and colleagues[204] treated 22 patients with multiple recurrences of *C. difficile* colitis using tapered doses of vancomycin for a 3-week period, followed by every-other-day therapy for 1 week and every third day for an additional week. All patients responded symptomatically and remained well during a mean follow-up period of 6 months. The rationale for this approach is suspect, however, because there is no known mechanism for spores to sense the presence or absence of antibiotics in their environment. An alternative explanation is that maintenance therapy over a prolonged period reduces the likelihood of reinfection when treatment eventually is terminated. It is interesting that toxin production by *C. difficile* does not occur during the early exponential growth phase of the bacterium but rather in the subsequent stationary phase.[75] Hence, after active *C. difficile* toxin-induced diarrhea and colitis have been controlled by treatment with metronidazole or vancomycin, 24 to 72 hours is needed for the bacteria to reinitiate toxin production.

Binding Resins

Anion-exchange binding resins, which bind to toxins in the bowel lumen, have been proposed as a possible alternative to antimicrobial therapy. Clinical studies have been performed using colestipol and cholestyramine. For colestipol the symptomatic response in patients with acute *C. difficile* colitis was a disappointing 36% compared to a placebo response rate of 22%.[51,175] Cholestyramine therapy yielded a somewhat better overall response rate of 68%,[51,175,211] but this still compares poorly with response rates of more than 95% with vancomycin or metronidazole. Therefore, binding resins are not used as primary therapy for *C. difficile* colitis but may be beneficial in treating recurrence. Tedesco treated 11 patients with relapsing *C. difficile* colitis with tapering doses of vancomycin plus colestipol 5 g every 12 hours.[212] Because anion-exchange resins bind vancomycin and other drugs, they must be taken at least 2 or 3 hours apart from the vancomycin, making combination therapy cumbersome.[213]

Tolevamer is a soluble anionic polymer designed to bind *C. difficile* toxins. In preclinical studies tolevamer strongly inhibited the cytotoxicity and enterotoxicity of *C. difficile* toxins and was superior to metronidazole in protecting hamsters from death caused by *C. difficile* cecitis.[66] In a phase II human clinical trial, results with tolevamer were similar to those of vancomycin when used as primary treatment for mild or moderately severe infection.[67] Although not yet approved for clinical use, tolevamer may provide a safe, effective, nonantibiotic agent for treatment and prevention of *C. difficile* infection. This agent does not have antibiotic properties and therefore should not delay reconstitution of the normal colonic microflora.

Probiotic Therapy

Probiotic agents are an attractive therapeutic option for recurrent *C. difficile* infection, because restoration of the colonization resistance of the normal colonic microflora can lead to permanent eradication of *C. difficile* from the colon. This is in contrast to treatment with antimicrobial agents that further delay recolonization by normal colonic bacteria. Bacteriotherapy has been reported in patients with recurrent infection using enemas of fresh feces from a healthy relative or rectal infusions of a mixture of 10 different aerobic and anaerobic bacteria.[214,215] The defined bacterial mixture led to bowel colonization with *Bacteroides* species, as well as prompt elimination of *C. difficile,* suggesting that *Bacteroides* may be one of the organisms that normally protects against pathogenic colonization with *C. difficile.* Another probiotic therapy for *C. difficile* diarrhea is the oral administration of a nontoxigenic strain of *C. difficile* that was reported to be effective in two patients with relapsing *C. difficile* diarrhea.[216] Preclinical studies are underway to characterize a nontoxigenic strain of *C. difficile* that may be suitable for administration as a prophylactic agent to prevent infection with toxigenic *C. difficile* in hospital patients who are receiving antibiotics.[68]

Lactobacillus species have been used widely as probiotics. In an open-label study, *Lactobacillus* strain GG was reported to be effective in preventing diarrhea in patients with recurrent *C. difficile* colitis.[217] A subsequent controlled clinical trial, however, did not demonstrate that *Lactobacillus* GG was effective in protecting against AAD in hospital patients.[218]

The yeast *S. boulardii* is used widely as a probiotic agent in continental Europe and is now available in the United States without prescription.[10,219] In a double-blind, controlled clinical trial, coadministration of oral capsules containing viable *S. boulardii* with antibiotics significantly reduced the incidence of AAD in hospitalized patients (from 22% on placebo to 9.5% in the *S. boulardii* group; $P = 0.04$).[10] In that study, however, few patients had *C. difficile*-associated diarrhea. A second randomized, placebo-controlled trial examined the efficacy of *S. boulardii* in combination with either vancomycin or metronidazole in patients with *C. difficile* diarrhea.[69] Diarrhea recurrence rates were similar in subjects treated during their first episode of *C. difficile* diarrhea (19% in the *S. boulardii* group vs. 24% in the placebo group; $P = 0.86$). In contrast, patients with a history of recurrent *C. difficile* diarrhea who received *S. boulardii* had fewer recurrences than the placebo group (35% and 65%, respectively; $P = 0.04$). In a subsequent study *S. boulardii* (500 mg twice daily for 28 days) only reduced relapse rates (from 50% to 17%; $P = 0.05$) in patients treated with high-dose vancomycin (500 mg four times a day for 10 days) but not in patients on other antibiotic regimens.[220] These controlled clinical trials indicate that *S. boulardii* is safe and effective in some patients with a history of recurrent *C. difficile*-associated diarrhea, but its protective effects are not uniform.

Immunization Against
Clostridium difficile *Toxins*

As described earlier, there is considerable evidence that some individuals have protective immunity against *C. difficile*-associated diarrhea and that protection is associated with higher antitoxin antibody concentrations in serum, intestinal secretions, or both.[53,59,64,65,102,104-106] Leung and coworkers reported on six children with multiple relapses of *C. difficile*-associated diarrhea who had low concentrations of serum IgG antibody to toxin A.[105] Five of these children were treated with intravenous immune globulin at a dose of 400 mg/kg, which contains high-titer IgG antitoxin A. Treatment was followed by resolution of symptoms. Similar results also have been reported by other investigators.[201] A *C. difficile* vaccine has been produced containing inactivated toxoid A and B. In early clinical trials, this vaccine was immunogenic,[221,222] and in a small case series, vaccination was associated with resolution of recurrent *C. difficile* diarrhea in three subjects.[223] Further studies are needed to determine whether passive or active immunization against *C. difficile* and its toxins can be effective in treating patients with refractory or recurrent disease. If effective, these therapeutic approaches also may be useful in preventing *C. difficile*-associated diarrhea in high-risk individuals such as elderly and infirm patients receiving antibiotic therapy in hospital.

Approach to Management of Recurrent
Clostridium difficile *Diarrhea*
and Colitis

The management of a first episode of recurrent *C. difficile*-associated diarrhea does not differ greatly from treat-

Table 105–7 Approach to Management of Recurrent *Clostridium difficile* Colitis

First Relapse

Confirm diagnosis

Symptomatic treatment if symptoms are mild

10- to 14-day course of metronidazole (or vancomycin) if symptoms are moderate or severe

Second Relapse

Confirm diagnosis

Vancomycin* taper

    125 mg q 6 hr for 7 days

    125 mg q 12 hr for 7 days

    125 mg qd for 7 days

    125 mg qod for 7 days

    125 mg q 3 days for 7 days

Further Relapse

Therapy with microorganisms, e.g., bacteriotherapy; *Saccharomyces boulardii,* in combination with metronidazole or vancomycin

or Vancomycin 125 mg q 6 hr plus cholestyramine 4 g twice daily[†]

or Vancomycin 125 mg q 6 hr and rifampicin 600 mg twice daily

or Intravenous immunoglobulin

---

*Metronidazole may be substituted for vancomycin, although there are no published data regarding its efficacy in this treatment regimen.

[†]Since cholestyramine binds vancomycin, oral doses of these two agents must be separated by 2-3 hours, making this regimen difficult to implement.

Adapted from Linevsky JK, Kelly CP: *Clostridium difficile* colitis. In Lamont JT (ed): Gastrointestinal Infections: Diagnosis and Management. New York, Taylor and Francis Group, LLC, 1997, p 293.

---

ment of an initial episode (Table 105–7).[131] Stool samples should be obtained to reconfirm infection with toxigenic *C. difficile*. Patients with mild symptoms of recurrence may be able to be managed conservatively without additional antibiotic treatment, just like patients with a primary episode. If symptoms persist or are severe, a 14-day course of metronidazole or vancomycin should be administered. If a second recurrence occurs, other treatment approaches should be considered. Tedesco and associates proposed a tapering and pulsed antibiotic regimen that is well tolerated and frequently successful.[204,224] If this fails, a wide range of other approaches have been described, some of which are summarized in Table 105–7. Unfortunately, with the exception of the probiotic agent *S. boulardii*, none of these treatment options has been evaluated in randomized, controlled trials. In some instances, multiple recurrences develop, and a variety of different regimens must be used before the organism is finally eradicated. In such cases, prolonged therapy with oral vancomycin (125 mg once or twice daily) is a pragmatic and effective means to prevent further recurrences. This approach is indicated in high-risk patients in whom symptomatic recurrence might be life threatening or in individuals who have consistently failed other measures, including multiple antibiotic regimens and probiotics.

REFERENCES

1. Hogenauer C, Hammer HF, Krejs GJ, Reisinger EC: Mechanisms and management of antibiotic-associated diarrhea. Clin Infect Dis 27:702, 1998.
2. Altemeier WA, Hummel RP, Hill EO: Staphylococcal enterocolitis following antibiotic therapy. Ann Surg 157:847, 1963.
3. Borriello SP, Larson HE, Welch AR, et al: Enterotoxigenic *Clostridium perfringens*: A possible cause of antibiotic-associated diarrhoea. Lancet 1:305, 1984.
4. Olsen SJ, DeBess EE, McGivern TE, et al: A nosocomial outbreak of fluoroquinolone-resistant salmonella infection. N Engl J Med 344:1572, 2001.
5. Sparks SG, Carman RJ, Sarker MR, McClane BA: Genotyping of enterotoxigenic *Clostridium perfringens* fecal isolates associated with antibiotic-associated diarrhea and food poisoning in North America. J Clin Microbiol 39:883, 2001.
6. Khan MY, Hall WH: Staphylococcal enterocolitis: Treatment with oral vancomycin. Ann Intern Med 65:1, 1966.
7. Bartlett JG: Clinical practice: Antibiotic-associated diarrhea. N Engl J Med 346:334, 2002.
8. Wistrom J, Norrby SR, Myhre EB, et al: Frequency of antibiotic-associated diarrhoea in 2462 antibiotic-treated hospitalized patients: A prospective study. J Antimicrob Chemother 47:43, 2001.
9. Bartlett JG: Pseudomembranous enterocolitis and antibiotic-associated diarrhea. In Feldman M, Friedman LS, Sleisenger MH (eds): Sleisenger and Fordtran's Gastrointestinal and Liver Disease, 7th ed. Philadelphia, WB Saunders, 2002, p 1914.
10. Surawicz CM, Elmer GW, Speelman P, et al: Prevention of antibiotic-associated diarrhea by *Saccharomyces boulardii*: A prospective study. Gastroenterology 96:981, 1989.
11. Lewis SJ, Potts LF, Barry RE: The lack of therapeutic effect of *Saccharomyces boulardii* in the prevention of antibiotic-related diarrhoea in elderly patients. J Infect 36:171, 1998.
12. Arvola T, Laiho K, Torkkeli S, et al: Prophylactic *Lactobacillus* GG reduces antibiotic-associated diarrhea in children with respiratory infections: A randomized study. Pediatrics 104:e64, 1999.
13. Thomas MR, Litin SC, Osmon DR, et al: Lack of effect of *Lactobacillus* GG on antibiotic-associated diarrhea: A randomized, placebo-controlled trial. Mayo Clin Proc 76:883, 2001.
14. D'Souza AL, Rajkumar C, Cooke J, Bulpitt CJ: Probiotics in prevention of antibiotic associated diarrhoea: Meta-analysis. BMJ 324:1361, 2002.
15. Cremonini F, Di Caro S, Nista EC, et al: Meta-analysis: The effect of probiotic administration on antibiotic-associated diarrhoea. Aliment Pharmacol Ther 16:1461, 2002.
16. Finney JMT: Gastroenterostomy for cicatrizing ulcer of the pylorus. Bull Johns Hopkins Hosp 4:53, 1893.
17. Wakefield RD, Sommers SD: Fatal membranous staphylococcal enteritis in surgical patients. Ann Surg 138:249, 1953.
18. Dixon CF, Weismann RE: Acute pseudomembranous enteritis or enterocolitis: A complication following intestinal surgery. Surg Clin North Am 28:99, 1948.
19. Hall IC, O'Toole E: Intestinal flora in newborn infants: With a description of a new pathogenic anaerobe, *Bacillus difficilis*. Am J Dis Child 49:390, 1935.
20. Bartlett JG, Chang TW, Gurwith M, et al: Antibiotic-associated pseudomembranous colitis due to toxin-producing clostridia. N Engl J Med 298:531, 1978.
21. Larson HE, Price AB, Honour P, Borriello SP: *Clostridium difficile* and the aetiology of pseudomembranous colitis. Lancet 1:1063, 1978.
22. Guerrant RL, Hughes JM, Lima NL, Crane J: Diarrhea in developed and developing countries: Magnitude, special settings, and etiologies. Rev Infect Dis 12(Suppl 1):S41, 1990.
23. McFarland LV: Epidemiology of infectious and iatrogenic nosocomial diarrhea in a cohort of general medicine patients. Am J Infect Control 23:295, 1995.
24. Alfa MJ, Du T, Beda G: Survey of incidence of *Clostridium difficile* infection in Canadian hospitals and diagnostic approaches. J Clin Microbiol 36:2076, 1998.

25. Lai KK, Melvin ZS, Menard MJ, et al: *Clostridium difficile*-associated diarrhea: Epidemiology, risk factors, and infection control. Infect Control Hosp Epidemiol 18:628, 1997.

26. Olson MM, Shanholtzer CJ, Lee JT Jr, Gerding DN: Ten years of prospective *Clostridium difficile*-associated disease surveillance and treatment at the Minneapolis VA Medical Center, 1982-1991. Infect Control Hosp Epidemiol 15:371, 1994.

27. Samore MH: Epidemiology of nosocomial *Clostridium difficile* diarrhoea. J Hosp Infect 43(Suppl):S183, 1999.

28. Samore MH, DeGirolami PC, Tlucko A, et al: *Clostridium difficile* colonization and diarrhea at a tertiary care hospital. Clin Infect Dis 18:181, 1994.

29. Struelens MJ, Maas A, Nonhoff C, et al: Control of nosocomial transmission of *Clostridium difficile* based on sporadic case surveillance. Am J Med 91(Suppl):138S, 1991.

30. Hirschhorn LR, Trnka Y, Onderdonk A, et al: Epidemiology of community-acquired *Clostridium difficile*-associated diarrhea. J Infect Dis 169:127, 1994.

31. Levy DG, Stergachis A, McFarland LV, et al: Antibiotics and *Clostridium difficile* diarrhea in the ambulatory care setting. Clin Ther 22:91, 2000.

32. Kyne L, Farrell R, Kelly CP: *Clostridium difficile*. Gastroenterol Clin North Am 30:753, 2001.

33. Onderdonk AB, Cisneros RL, Bartlett JG: *Clostridium difficile* in gnotobiotic mice. Infect Immun 28:277, 1980.

34. Wilson KH, Freter R: Interaction of *Clostridium difficile* and *Escherichia coli* with microfloras in continuous-flow cultures and gnotobiotic mice. Infect Immun 54:354, 1986.

35. Wilson KH, Silva J, Fekety FR: Suppression of *Clostridium difficile* by normal hamster cecal flora and prevention of antibiotic-associated cecitis. Infect Immun 34:626, 1981.

36. Borriello SP, Barclay FE: An in vitro model of colonisation resistance to *Clostridium difficile* infection. J Med Microbiol 21:299, 1986.

37. Borriello S P: 12th C. L. Oakley Lecture: Pathogenesis of *Clostridium difficile* infection of the gut. J Med Microbiol 33:207, 1990.

38. Larson HE, Barclay FE, Honour P, Hill ID: Epidemiology of *Clostridium difficile* in infants. J Infect Dis 146:727, 1982.

39. Kelly CP, LaMont JT: *Clostridium difficile* infection. Annu Rev Med 49:375, 1998.

40. Eglow R, Pothoulakis C, Itzkowitz S, et al: Diminished *Clostridium difficile* toxin A sensitivity in newborn rabbit ileum is associated with decreased toxin A receptor. J Clin Invest 90:822, 1992.

41. Hecht JR, Olinger EJ: *Clostridium difficile* colitis secondary to intravenous vancomycin. Dig Dis Sci 34:148, 1989.

42. Saginur R, Hawley CR, Bartlett JG: Colitis associated with metronidazole therapy. J Infect Dis 141:772, 1980.

43. Bignardi GE: Risk factors for *Clostridium difficile* infection. J Hosp Infect 40:1, 1998.

44. Gorbach SL: Antibiotics and *Clostridium difficile*. N Engl J Med 341:1690, 1999.

45. Ambrose N: The effects of single doses of antibiotics on faecal flora with a reference to their mode of excretion. J Drug Dev 1:233, 1989.

46. Spencer RC: The role of antimicrobial agents in the aetiology of *Clostridium difficile*-associated disease. J Antimicrob Chemother 41(Suppl C):21, 1998.

47. Kelly CP, Pothoulakis C, LaMont JT: *Clostridium difficile* colitis. N Engl J Med 330:257, 1994.

48. Kelly CP, LaMont JT: Treatment of *Clostridium difficile* diarrhea and colitis. In Wolfe MM (ed): Gastrointestinal Pharmacotherapy. Philadelphia, WB Saunders, 1993, p 199.

49. Anand A, Glatt AE: *Clostridium difficile* infection associated with antineoplastic chemotherapy: A review. Clin Infect Dis 17:109, 1993.

50. Djuretic T, Wall PG, Brazier JS: *Clostridium difficile*: An update on its epidemiology and role in hospital outbreaks in England and Wales. J Hosp Infect 41:213, 1999.

51. Mogg GA, Arabi Y, Youngs D, et al: Therapeutic trials of antibiotic-associated colitis. Scand J Infect Dis Suppl 22:41, 1980.

52. McFarland LV, Mulligan ME, Kwok RY, Stamm WE: Nosocomial acquisition of *Clostridium difficile* infection. N Engl J Med 320:204, 1989.

53. Kyne L, Warny M, Qamar A, Kelly CP: Asymptomatic carriage of *Clostridium difficile* and serum levels of IgG antibody against toxin A. N Engl J Med 342:390, 2000.

54. Gerding DN, Johnson S, Peterson LR, et al: *Clostridium difficile*-associated diarrhea and colitis. Infect Control Hosp Epidemiol 16:459, 1995.

55. Shim JK, Johnson S, Samore MH, et al: Primary symptomless colonisation by *Clostridium difficile* and decreased risk of subsequent diarrhoea. Lancet 351:633, 1998.

56. Clabots CR, Johnson S, Olson MM, et al: Acquisition of *Clostridium difficile* by hospitalized patients: Evidence for colonized new admissions as a source of infection. J Infect Dis 166:561, 1992.

57. Fekety R, Kim KH, Brown D, et al: Epidemiology of antibiotic-associated colitis: Isolation of *Clostridium difficile* from the hospital environment. Am J Med 70:906, 1981.

58. Hoffman P: *Clostridium difficile* in hospitals. Curr Opin Infect Dis 7:471, 1994.

59. Kyne L, Kelly C: Prospects for a vaccine for *Clostridium difficile*. BioDrugs 10:173, 1998.

60. Fekety R: Guidelines for the diagnosis and management of *Clostridium difficile*-associated diarrhea and colitis. American College of Gastroenterology, Practice Parameters Committee. Am J Gastroenterol 92:739, 1997.

61. Johnson S, Gerding DN, Olson MM, et al: Prospective, controlled study of vinyl glove use to interrupt *Clostridium difficile* nosocomial transmission. Am J Med 88:137, 1990.

62. Johnson S, Homann SR, Bettin KM, et al: Treatment of asymptomatic *Clostridium difficile* carriers (fecal excretors) with vancomycin or metronidazole: A randomized, placebo-controlled trial. Ann Intern Med 117: 297, 1992.

63. Kelly CP: Immune response to *Clostridium difficile* infection. Eur J Gastroenterol Hepatol 8:1048, 1996.

64. Giannasca PJ, Warny M: Active and passive immunization against *Clostridium difficile* diarrhea and colitis. Vaccine 22:848, 2004.

65. Wilcox M, Minton J: Role of antibody response in outcome of antibiotic-associated diarrhoea. Lancet 357:158, 2001.

66. Kurtz CB, Cannon EP, Brezzani A, et al: GT160-246, a toxin binding polymer for treatment of *Clostridium difficile* colitis. Antimicrob Agents Chemother 45:2340, 2001.

67. Louie T, Peppe J, Watt CK, et al: A phase 2 study of the toxin binding polymer Tolevamer in patients with *Clostridium difficile*-associated diarrhea [Abstract]. Gastroenterology 126:A511, 2004.

68. Sambol SP, Merrigan MM, Tang JK, et al: Colonization for the prevention of *Clostridium difficile* disease in hamsters. J Infect Dis 186:1781, 2002.

69. McFarland LV, Surawicz CM, Greenberg RN, et al: A randomized placebo-controlled trial of *Saccharomyces boulardii* in combination with standard antibiotics for *Clostridium difficile* disease. JAMA 271:1913, 1994.

70. Braun V, Hundsberger T, Leukel P, et al: Definition of the single integration site of the pathogenicity locus in *Clostridium difficile*. Gene 181:29, 1996.

71. Cohen SH, Tang YJ, Silva J Jr: Analysis of the pathogenicity locus in *Clostridium difficile* strains. J Infect Dis 181:659, 2000.

72. Hammond GA, Johnson JL: The toxigenic element of *Clostridium difficile* strain VPI 10463. Microb Pathol 19:203, 1995.

73. Hammond GA, Lyerly DM, Johnson JL: Transcriptional analysis of the toxigenic element of *Clostridium difficile*. Microb Pathog 22:143, 1997.

74. Warny M, Kelly CP: Pathogenicity of *Clostridium difficile* toxins. In Hecht G (ed): Microbial Pathogenesis and the Intestinal Epithelial Cell. Washington, DC, ASM Press, 2003, p 503.

75. Dupuy B, Sonenshein AL: Regulated transcription of *Clostridium difficile* toxin genes. Mol Microbiol 27:107, 1998.

76. Mani N, Dupuy B: Regulation of toxin synthesis in *Clostridium difficile* by an alternative RNA polymerase sigma factor. Proc Natl Acad Sci U S A 98:5844, 2001.

77. Moncrief JS, Barroso LA, Wilkins TD: Positive regulation of *Clostridium difficile* toxins. Infect Immun 65:1105, 1997.

78. Tan KS, Wee BY, Song KP: Evidence for holin function of *tcdE* gene in the pathogenicity of *Clostridium difficile*. J Med Microbiol 50:613, 2001.

79. Barroso LA, Wang SZ, Phelps CJ, et al: Nucleotide sequence of *Clostridium difficile* toxin B gene. Nucleic Acids Res 18:4004, 1990.

80. Dove CH, Wang SZ, Price SB, et al: Molecular characterization of the *Clostridium difficile* toxin A gene. Infect Immun 58:480, 1990.

81. von Eichel-Streiber C, Laufenberg-Feldmann R, Sartingen S, et al: Cloning of *Clostridium difficile* toxin B gene and demonstration of high *N*-terminal homology between toxin A and B. Med Microbiol Immunol 179:271, 1990.

82. Chaves-Olarte E, Weidmann M, von Eichel-Streiber C, Thelestam M: Toxin A and B from *Clostridium difficile* differ with respect to enzymatic potencies, cellular substrate specificities and surface binding to cultured cells. J Clin Invest 100:1734, 1997.

83. Just I, Selzer J, Wilm M, et al: Glucosylation of Rho proteins by *Clostridium difficile* toxin B. Nature 375:500, 1995.

84. Just I, Wilm M, Selzer J, et al: The enterotoxin from *Clostridium difficile* (ToxA) monoglucosylates the Rho proteins. J Biol Chem 270:13932, 1995.

85. Pothoulakis C: Pathogenesis of *Clostridium difficile*-associated diarrhoea. Eur J Gastroenterol Hepatol 8:1041, 1996.

86. Warny M, Keates AC, Keates S, et al: p38 MAP kinase activation by *Clostridium difficile* toxin A mediates monocyte necrosis, IL-8 production, and enteritis. J Clin Invest 105:1147, 2000.

87. Sullivan NM, Pellett S, Wilkins TD: Purification and characterization of toxins A and B of *Clostridium difficile*. Infect Immun 35:1032, 1982.

88. Triadafilopoulos G, Pothoulakis C, O'Brien MJ, LaMont JT: Differential effects of *Clostridium difficile* toxins A and B on rabbit ileum. Gastroenterology 93:273, 1987.

89. Lyerly DM, Saum KE, MacDonald DK, Wilkins TD: Effects of *Clostridium difficile* toxins given intragastrically to animals. Infect Immun 47:349, 1985.

90. Mitchell TJ, Ketley JM, Haslam SC, et al: Effect of toxin A and B of *Clostridium difficile* on rabbit ileum and colon. Gut 27:78, 1986.

91. Pothoulakis C, Barone LM, Ely R, et al: Purification and properties of *Clostridium difficile* cytotoxin B. J Biol Chem 261:1316, 1986.

92. Riegler M, Sedivy R, Pothoulakis C, et al: *Clostridium difficile* toxin B is more potent than toxin A in damaging human colonic epithelium in vitro. J Clin Invest 95:2004, 1995.

93. Savidge TC, Pan WH, Newman P, et al: *Clostridium difficile* toxin B is an inflammatory enterotoxin in human intestine. Gastroenterology 125:413, 2003.

94. Kato H, Kato N, Katow S, et al: Deletions in the repeating sequences of the toxin A gene of toxin A-negative, toxin B-positive *Clostridium difficile* strains. FEMS Microbiol Lett 175:197, 1999.

95. Kato H, Kato N, Watanabe K, et al: Identification of toxin A-negative, toxin B-positive *Clostridium difficile* by PCR. J Clin Microbiol 36:2178, 1998.

96. Limaye AP, Turgeon DK, Cookson BT, Fritsche TR: Pseudomembranous colitis caused by a toxin A−B+ strain of *Clostridium difficile*. J Clin Microbiol 38:1696, 2000.

97. Lyerly DM, Barroso LA, Wilkins TD, et al: Characterization of a toxin A-negative, toxin B-positive strain of *Clostridium difficile*. Infect Immun 60:4633, 1992.

98. Aronsson B, Granstrom M, Mollby R, Nord CE: Serum antibody response to *Clostridium difficile* toxins in patients with *Clostridium difficile* diarrhoea. Infection 13:97, 1985.

99. Johnson S, Gerding DN, Janoff EN: Systemic and mucosal antibody responses to toxin A in patients infected with *Clostridium difficile*. J Infect Dis 166:1287, 1992.

100. Kelly CP, Pothoulakis C, Orellana J, LaMont JT: Human colonic aspirates containing immunoglobulin A antibody to *Clostridium difficile* toxin A inhibit toxin A-receptor binding. Gastroenterology 102:35, 1992.

101. Viscidi R, Laughon BE, Yolken R, et al: Serum antibody response to toxins A and B of *Clostridium difficile*. J Infect Dis 148:93, 1983.

102. Warny M, Vaerman JP, Avesani V, Delmee M: Human antibody response to *Clostridium difficile* toxin A in relation to clinical course of infection. Infect Immun 62:384, 1994.

103. Kim PH, Iaconis JP, Rolfe RD: Immunization of adult hamsters against *Clostridium difficile*-associated ileocecitis and transfer of protection to infant hamsters. Infect Immun 55:2984, 1987.

104. Bacon AE III, Fekety R: Immunoglobulin G directed against toxins A and B of *Clostridium difficile* in the general population and patients with antibiotic-associated diarrhea. Diagn Microbiol Infect Dis 18:205, 1994.

105. Leung DY, Kelly CP, Boguniewicz M, et al: Treatment with intravenously administered gamma globulin of chronic relapsing colitis induced by *Clostridium difficile* toxin. J Pediatr 118:633, 1991.

106. Kyne L, Warny M, Qamar A, Kelly CP: Association between antibody response to toxin A and protection against recurrent *Clostridium difficile* diarrhoea. Lancet 357:189, 2001.

107. Brandt LJ, Kosche KA, Greenwald DA, et al: *Clostridium difficile*-associated diarrhea in the elderly. Am J Gastroenterol 94:3263, 1999.

108. Brown E, Talbot GH, Axelrod P, et al: Risk factors for *Clostridium difficile* toxin-associated diarrhea. Infect Control Hosp Epidemiol 11:283, 1990.

109. McFarland LV, Surawicz CM, Stamm WE: Risk factors for *Clostridium difficile* carriage and *C. difficile*-associated diarrhea in a cohort of hospitalized patients. J Infect Dis 162:678, 1990.

110. Bassaris HP, Lianou FE, Legakis NJ, et al: Interaction between *Clostridium difficile* and polymorphonuclear leukocytes from the elderly and postoperative cancer patients: Phagocytosis and bacterial function. Med Microbiol Immunol 173:49, 1984.

111. Blot E, Escande MC, Besson D, et al: Outbreak of *Clostridium difficile*-related diarrhoea in an adult oncology unit: risk factors and microbiological characteristics. J Hosp Infect 53:187, 2003.

112. Kyne L, Sougioultzis S, McFarland LV, Kelly CP: Underlying disease severity as a major risk factor for nosocomial *Clostridium difficile* diarrhea. Infect Control Hosp Epidemiol 23:653, 2002.

113. Keven K, Basu A, Re L, et al: *Clostridium difficile* colitis in patients after kidney and pancreas-kidney transplantation. Transpl Infect Dis 6:10, 2004.

114. Tomblyn M, Gordon L, Singhal S, et al: Rarity of toxigenic *Clostridium difficile* infections after hematopoietic stem cell transplantation: Implications for symptomatic management of diarrhea. Bone Marrow Transplant 30:517, 2002.

115. Pulvirenti JJ, Mehra T, Hafiz I, et al: Epidemiology and outcome of *Clostridium difficile* infection and diarrhea in HIV infected inpatients. Diagn Microbiol Infect Dis 44:325, 2002.

116. Barbut F, Meynard JL, Guiguet M, et al: *Clostridium difficile*-associated diarrhea in HIV-infected patients: Epidemiology and risk factors. J Acquir Immune Defic Syndr Hum Retrovirol 16:176, 1997.

117. Tumbarello M, Tacconelli E, Leone F, et al: *Clostridium difficile*-associated diarrhoea in patients with human immunodeficiency virus infection: A case-control study. Eur J Gastroenterol Hepatol 7:259, 1995.

118. Lu SS, Schwartz JM, Simon DM, Brandt LJ: *Clostridium difficile*-associated diarrhea in patients with HIV positivity and AIDS: A prospective controlled study. Am J Gastroenterol 89:1226, 1994.

119. LaMont JT, Trnka YM: Therapeutic implications of *Clostridium difficile* toxin during relapse of chronic inflammatory bowel disease. Lancet 1:381, 1980.

120. Bolton RP, Sherriff RJ, Read AE: *Clostridium difficile*-associated diarrhoea: A role in inflammatory bowel disease? Lancet 1:383, 1980.

121. Meyer AM, Ramzan NN, Loftus EV Jr, et al: The diagnostic yield of stool pathogen studies during relapses of inflammatory bowel disease. J Clin Gastroenterol 38:772, 2004.

122. Mylonaki M, Langmead L, Pantes A, et al: Enteric infection in relapse of inflammatory bowel disease: Importance of microbiological examination of stool. Eur J Gastroenterol Hepatol 16:775, 2004.

123. Gerding DN, Olson MM, Peterson LR, et al: *Clostridium difficile*-associated diarrhea and colitis in adults. A prospective case-controlled epidemiologic study. Arch Intern Med 146:95, 1986.

124. Johnson S, Clabots CR, Linn FV, et al: Nosocomial *Clostridium difficile* colonisation and disease. Lancet 336:97, 1990.

125. Triadafilopoulos G, Hallstone AE: Acute abdomen as the first presentation of pseudomembranous colitis. Gastroenterology 101:685, 1991.

126. Feldman RJ, Kallich M, Weinstein MP: Bacteremia due to *Clostridium difficile*: Case report and review of extraintestinal *C. difficile* infections. Clin Infect Dis 20:1560, 1995.

127. Pron B, Merckx J, Touzet P, et al: Chronic septic arthritis and osteomyelitis in a prosthetic knee joint due to *Clostridium difficile*. Eur J Clin Microbiol Infect Dis 14:599, 1995.

128. Studemeister AE, Beilke MA, Kirmani N: Splenic abscess due to *Clostridium difficile* and *Pseudomonas paucimobilis*. Am J Gastroenterol 82:389, 1987.

129. Kyne L, Merry C, O'Connell B, et al: Factors associated with prolonged symptoms and severe disease due to *Clostridium difficile*. Age Ageing 28:107, 1999.

130. Wolf LE, Gorbach SL, Granowitz EV: Extraintestinal *Clostridium difficile*: Ten years' experience at a tertiary-care hospital. Mayo Clin Proc 73:943, 1998.

131. Linevsky JK, Kelly CP: *Clostridium difficile* colitis. In LaMont JT (ed): Gastrointestinal Infections: Diagnosis and Management. New York, Marcel Dekker, 1997, p 293.

132. Cleary RK: *Clostridium difficile*-associated diarrhea and colitis: Clinical manifestations, diagnosis, and treatment. Dis Colon Rectum 41:1435, 1998.

133. Kyne L, Merry C, O'Connell B, et al: Community-acquired *Clostridium difficile* infection. J Infect 36:287, 1998.

134. Issack MI, Elliott TS: *Clostridium difficile* carriage after infection. Lancet 335:610, 1990.

135. Brazier JS: The diagnosis of *Clostridium difficile*-associated disease. J Antimicrob Chemother 41(Suppl C):29, 1998.

136. Barbut F, Kajzer C, Planas N, Petit JC: Comparison of three enzyme immunoassays, a cytotoxicity assay, and toxigenic culture for diagnosis of *Clostridium difficile*-associated diarrhea. J Clin Microbiol 31:963, 1993.

137. Merz CS, Kramer C, Forman M, et al: Comparison of four commercially available rapid enzyme immunoassays with cytotoxin assay for detection of *Clostridium difficile* toxin(s) from stool specimens. J Clin Microbiol 32:1142, 1994.

138. Whittier S, Shapiro DS, Kelly WF, et al: Evaluation of four commercially available enzyme immunoassays for laboratory diagnosis of *Clostridium difficile*-associated diseases. J Clin Microbiol 31:2861, 1993.

139. Peterson LR, Kelly PJ: The role of the clinical microbiology laboratory in the management of *Clostridium difficile*-associated diarrhea. Infect Dis Clin North Am 7:277, 1993.

140. Tichota-Lee J, Jaqua-Stewart MJ, Benfield D, et al: Effect of age on the sensitivity of cell cultures to *Clostridium difficile* toxin. Diagn Microbiol Infect Dis 8:203, 1987.

141. Walker RC, Ruane PJ, Rosenblatt JE: Comparison of culture, cytotoxicity assays, and enzyme-linked immunosorbent assay for toxin A and toxin B in the diagnosis of *Clostridium difficile*-related enteric disease. Diagn Microbiol Infect Dis 5:61, 1986.

142. Doern GV, Coughlin RT, Wu L: Laboratory diagnosis of *Clostridium difficile*-associated gastrointestinal disease: Comparison of a monoclonal antibody enzyme immunoassay for toxins A and B with a monoclonal antibody enzyme immunoassay for toxin A only and two cytotoxicity assays. J Clin Microbiol 30:2042, 1992.

143. Lyerly DM, Neville LM, Evans DT, et al: Multicenter evaluation of the *Clostridium difficile* TOX A/B TEST. J Clin Microbiol 36:184, 1998.

144. Alonso R, Munoz C, Pelaez T, et al: Rapid detection of toxigenic *Clostridium difficile* strains by a nested PCR of the toxin B gene. Clin Microbiol Infect 3:145, 1997.

145. Kato N, Ou CY, Kato H, et al: Identification of toxigenic *Clostridium difficile* by the polymerase chain reaction. J Clin Microbiol 29:33, 1991.

146. Wren B, Clayton C, Tabaqchali S: Rapid identification of toxigenic *Clostridium difficile* by polymerase chain reaction. Lancet 335:423, 1990.

147. Boondeekhun HS, Gurtler V, Odd ML, et al: Detection of *Clostridium difficile* enterotoxin gene in clinical specimens by the polymerase chain reaction. J Med Microbiol 38:384, 1993.

148. Green GA, Riot B, Monteil H: Evaluation of an oligonucleotide probe and an immunological test for direct detection of toxigenic *Clostridium difficile* in stool samples. Eur J Clin Microbiol Infect Dis 13:576, 1994.

149. Gumerlock PH, Tang YJ, Meyers FJ, Silva J Jr: Use of the polymerase chain reaction for the specific and direct detection of *Clostridium difficile* in human feces. Rev Infect Dis 13:1053, 1991.

150. Gumerlock PH, Tang YJ, Weiss JB, Silva J Jr: Specific detection of toxigenic strains of *Clostridium difficile* in stool specimens. J Clin Microbiol 31:507, 1993.

151. Kato N, Ou CY, Kato H, et al: Detection of toxigenic *Clostridium difficile* in stool specimens by the polymerase chain reaction. J Infect Dis 167:455, 1993.

152. Alonso R, Munoz C, Gros S, et al: Rapid detection of toxigenic *Clostridium difficile* from stool samples by a nested PCR of toxin B gene. J Hosp Infect 41:145, 1999.

153. Kwon JH, Kelly CP: *Clostridium difficile* and antibiotic-associated diarrhea. In Bayless RM, Diehl AM (eds): Advanced Therapy in Gastroenterology and Liver Disease, 5th ed. Hamilton, Ontario, Canada, BC Decker, 2005, p 302.

154. Tedesco FJ, Corless JK, Brownstein RE: Rectal sparing in antibiotic-associated pseudomembranous colitis: A prospective study. Gastroenterology 83:1259, 1982.

155. Price AB, Davies DR: Pseudomembranous colitis. J Clin Pathol 30:1, 1977.

156. Teasley DG, Gerding DN, Olson MM, et al: Prospective randomised trial of metronidazole versus vancomycin for

Clostridium difficile-associated diarrhoea and colitis. Lancet 2:1043, 1983.

157. Burke GW, Wilson ME, Mehrez IO: Absence of diarrhea in toxic megacolon complicating *Clostridium difficile* pseudo-membranous colitis. Am J Gastroenterol 83:304, 1988.

158. Novak E, Lee JG, Seckman CE, et al: Unfavorable effect of atropine-diphenoxylate (Lomotil) therapy in lincomycin-caused diarrhea. JAMA 235:1451, 1976.

159. Walley T, Milson D: Loperamide-related toxic megacolon in *Clostridium difficile* colitis. Postgrad Med J 66:582, 1990.

160. Peterson LR, Gerding DN: Antimicrobial agents. In Rambaud JC, Ducluzeau R (eds): *Clostridium difficile*-Associated Intestinal Diseases. Paris, Springer-Verlag, 1990, p 115.

161. Bartlett JG, Taylor NS, Chang T, Dzink J: Clinical and laboratory observations in *Clostridium difficile* colitis. Am J Clin Nutr 33:2521, 1980.

162. Bartlett JG, Chang TW, Onderdonk AB: Comparison of five regimens for treatment of experimental clindamycin-associated colitis. J Infect Dis 138:81, 1978.

163. Clabots CR, Shanholtzer CJ, Peterson LR, Gerding DN: In vitro activity of efrotomycin, ciprofloxacin, and six other antimicrobials against *Clostridium difficile*. Diagn Microbiol Infect Dis 6:49, 1987.

164. Dzink J, Bartlett JG: In vitro susceptibility of *Clostridium difficile* isolates from patients with antibiotic-associated diarrhea or colitis. Antimicrob Agents Chemother 17:695, 1980.

165. Fekety R, Silva J, Toshniwal R, et al: Antibiotic-associated colitis: Effects of antibiotics on *Clostridium difficile* and the disease in hamsters. Rev Infect Dis 1:386, 1979.

166. Young GP, Ward PB, Bayley N, et al: Antibiotic-associated colitis due to *Clostridium difficile*: Double-blind comparison of vancomycin with bacitracin. Gastroenterology 89:1038, 1985.

167. Drummond LJ, McCoubrey J, Smith DG, et al: Changes in sensitivity patterns to selected antibiotics in *Clostridium difficile* in geriatric inpatients over an 18-month period. J Med Microbiol 52:259, 2003.

168. Johnson S, Samore MH, Farrow KA, et al: Epidemics of diarrhea caused by a clindamycin-resistant strain of *Clostridium difficile* in four hospitals. N Engl J Med 341:1645, 1999.

169. Dridi L, Tankovic J, Burghoffer B, et al: gyrA and gyrB mutations are implicated in cross-resistance to ciprofloxacin and moxifloxacin in *Clostridium difficile*. Antimicrob Agents Chemother 46:3418, 2002.

170. Pelaez T, Alcala L, Alonso R, et al: Reassessment of *Clostridium difficile* susceptibility to metronidazole and vancomycin. Antimicrob Agents Chemother 46:1647, 2002.

171. Fekety R, Silva J, Armstrong J, et al: Treatment of antibiotic-associated enterocolitis with vancomycin. Rev Infect Dis 3(Suppl):S273, 1981.

172. Bartlett JG, Onderdonk AB, Cisneros RL, Kasper DL: Clindamycin-associated colitis due to a toxin-producing species of *Clostridium* in hamsters. J Infect Dis 136:701, 1977.

173. Browne RA, Fekety R Jr, Silva J Jr, et al: The protective effect of vancomycin on clindamycin-induced colitis in hamsters. Johns Hopkins Med J 141:183, 1977.

174. Kelly CP, LaMont JT: Treatment of *Clostridium difficile* diarrhea and colitis. In Wolfe MM (ed): Therapy of Digestive Disorders. Philadelphia, WB Saunders, 2000, p 513.

175. Zimmerman MJ, Bak A, Sutherland LR: Review article: Treatment of *Clostridium difficile* infection. Aliment Pharmacol Ther 11:1003, 1997.

176. Recommendations for preventing the spread of vancomycin resistance. In Recommendations of the Hospital Infection Control Practices Advisory Committee (HICPAC). Am J Infect Control 23:87, 1995.

177. Bolton RP, Culshaw MA: Faecal metronidazole concentrations during oral and intravenous therapy for antibiotic associated colitis due to *Clostridium difficile*. Gut 27:1169, 1986.

178. Ings RM, McFadzean JA, Ormerod WE: The fate of metronidazole and its implications in chemotherapy. Xenobiotica 5:223, 1975.

179. Bartlett JG: Metronidazole. Johns Hopkins Med J 149:89, 1981.

180. Bingley PJ, Harding GM: *Clostridium difficile* colitis following treatment with metronidazole and vancomycin. Postgrad Med J 63:993, 1987.

181. Saginur R, Hawley CR, Bartlett JG: Colitis associated with metronidazole therapy. J Infect Dis 141:772, 1980.

182. Thomson G, Clark AH, Hare K, Spilg WG: Pseudomembranous colitis after treatment with metronidazole. BMJ 282:864, 1981.

183. Keighley MR, Burdon DW, Arabi Y, et al: Randomised controlled trial of vancomycin for pseudomembranous colitis and postoperative diarrhoea. BMJ 2:1667, 1978.

184. Young GP, Ward PB, Bayley N, et al: Antibiotic-associated colitis due to *Clostridium difficile*: Double-blind comparison of vancomycin with bacitracin. Gastroenterology 89:1038, 1985.

185. Fekety R, Silva J, Kauffman C, et al: Treatment of antibiotic-associated *Clostridium difficile* colitis with oral vancomycin: Comparison of two dosage regimens. Am J Med 86:15, 1989.

186. Kleinfeld DI, Sharpe RJ, Donta ST: Parenteral therapy for antibiotic-associated pseudomembranous colitis. J Infect Dis 157:389, 1988.

187. Oliva SL, Guglielmo BJ, Jacobs R, Pons VG: Failure of intravenous vancomycin and intravenous metronidazole to prevent or treat antibiotic-associated pseudomembranous colitis. J Infect Dis 159:1154, 1989.

188. Chang TW, Gorbach SL, Bartlett JG, Saginur R: Bacitracin treatment of antibiotic-associated colitis and diarrhea caused by *Clostridium difficile* toxin. Gastroenterology 78:1584, 1980.

189. Dudley MN, McLaughlin JC, Carrington G, et al: Oral bacitracin versus vancomycin therapy for *Clostridium difficile*-induced diarrhea: A randomized double-blind trial. Arch Intern Med 146:1101, 1986.

190. Tedesco FJ: Bacitracin therapy in antibiotic-associated pseudomembranous colitis. Dig Dis Sci 25:783, 1980.

191. de Lalla F, Nicolin R, Rinaldi E, et al: Prospective study of oral teicoplanin versus oral vancomycin for therapy of pseudomembranous colitis and *Clostridium difficile*-associated diarrhea. Antimicrob Agents Chemother 36:2192, 1992.

192. Wenisch C, Parschalk B, Hasenhundl M, et al: Comparison of vancomycin, teicoplanin, metronidazole, and fusidic acid for the treatment of *Clostridium difficile*-associated diarrhea. Clin Infect Dis 22:813, 1996.

193. Cronberg S, Castor B, Thoren A: Fusidic acid for the treatment of antibiotic-associated colitis induced by *Clostridium difficile*. Infection 12:276, 1984.

194. Jobe BA, Grasley A, Deveney KE, et al: *Clostridium difficile* colitis: An increasing hospital-acquired illness. Am J Surg 169:480, 1995.

195. Rubin MS, Bodenstein LE, Kent KC: Severe *Clostridium difficile* colitis. Dis Colon Rectum 38:350, 1995.

196. Anand A, Bashey B, Mir T, Glatt AE: Epidemiology, clinical manifestations, and outcome of *Clostridium difficile*-associated diarrhea. Am J Gastroenterol 89:519, 1994.

197. Grundfest-Broniatowski S, Quader M, Alexander F, et al: *Clostridium difficile* colitis in the critically ill. Dis Colon Rectum 39:619, 1996.

198. Morris JB, Zollinger RM Jr, Stellato TA: Role of surgery in antibiotic-induced pseudomembranous enterocolitis. Am J Surg 160:535, 1990.

199. Pasic M, Jost R, Carrel T, et al: Intracolonic vancomycin for pseudomembranous colitis. N Engl J Med 329:583, 1993.

200. Salcedo J, Keates S, Pothoulakis C, et al: Intravenous immunoglobulin therapy for severe *Clostridium difficile* colitis. Gut 41:366, 1997.

201. Wilcox MH: Descriptive study of intravenous immunoglobulin for the treatment of recurrent *Clostridium difficile* diarrhoea. J Antimicrob Chemother 53:882, 2004.

202. Bradbury AW, Barrett S: Surgical aspects of *Clostridium difficile* colitis. Br J Surg 84:150, 1997.

203. Synnott K, Mealy K, Merry C, et al: Timing of surgery for fulminating pseudomembranous colitis. Br J Surg 85:229, 1998.

204. Tedesco FJ, Gordon D, Fortson WC: Approach to patients with multiple recurrences of antibiotic-associated pseudomembranous colitis. Am J Gastroenterol 80:867, 1985.

205. Kyne L, Kelly CP: Recurrent *Clostridium difficile* diarrhoea. Gut 49:152, 2001.

206. McFarland LV, Surawicz CM, Rubin M, et al: Recurrent *Clostridium difficile* disease: Epidemiology and clinical characteristics. Infect Control Hosp Epidemiol 20:43, 1999.

207. Walters BA, Roberts R, Stafford R, Seneviratne E: Relapse of antibiotic-associated colitis: Endogenous persistence of *Clostridium difficile* during vancomycin therapy. Gut 24:206, 1983.

208. Wilcox MH, Fawley WN, Settle CD, Davidson A: Recurrence of symptoms in *Clostridium difficile* infection: Relapse or reinfection? J Hosp Infect 38:93, 1998.

209. Bartlett JG, Tedesco FJ, Shull S, et al: Symptomatic relapse after oral vancomycin therapy of antibiotic-associated pseudomembranous colitis. Gastroenterology 78:431, 1980.

210. Tedesco FJ, Barton RW, Alpers DH: Clindamycin-associated colitis: A prospective study. Ann Intern Med 81:429, 1974.

211. Kreutzer EW, Milligan FD: Treatment of antibiotic-associated pseudomembranous colitis with cholestyramine resin. Johns Hopkins Med J 143:67, 1978.

212. Tedesco FJ: Treatment of recurrent antibiotic-associated pseudomembranous colitis. Am J Gastroenterol 77:220, 1982.

213. Taylor NS, Bartlett JG: Binding of *Clostridium difficile* cytotoxin and vancomycin by anion exchange resins. J Infect Dis 141:92, 1980.

214. Tvede M, Rask-Madsen J: Bacteriotherapy for chronic relapsing *Clostridium difficile* diarrhoea in six patients. Lancet 1:1156, 1989.

215. Persky SE, Brandt LJ: Treatment of recurrent *Clostridium difficile*-associated diarrhea by administration of donated stool directly through a colonoscope. Am J Gastroenterol 95:3283, 2000.

216. Seal D, Borriello SP, Barclay F, et al: Treatment of relapsing *Clostridium difficile* diarrhoea by administration of a nontoxigenic strain. Eur J Clin Microbiol 6:51, 1987.

217. Gorbach SL, Chang TW, Goldin B: Successful treatment of relapsing *Clostridium difficile* colitis with *Lactobacillus* GG. Lancet 2:1519, 1987.

218. Thomas MR, Litin SC, Osmon DR, et al: Lack of effect of *Lactobacillus* GG on antibiotic-associated diarrhea: A randomized, placebo-controlled trial. Mayo Clin Proc 76:883, 2001.

219. Elmer GW, Surawicz CM, McFarland LV: Biotherapeutic agents: A neglected modality for the treatment and prevention of selected intestinal and vaginal infections. JAMA 275:870, 1996.

220. Surawicz CM, McFarland LV, Greenberg RN, et al: The search for a better treatment for recurrent *Clostridium difficile* disease: Use of high-dose vancomycin combined with *Saccharomyces boulardii*. Clin Infect Dis 31:1012, 2000.

221. Kotloff KL, Wasserman SS, Losonsky GA, et al: Safety and immunogenicity of increasing doses of a *Clostridium difficile* toxoid vaccine administered to healthy adults. Infect Immun 69:988, 2001.

222. Aboudola S, Kotloff KL, Kyne L, et al: *Clostridium difficile* vaccine and serum immunoglobulin G antibody response to toxin A. Infect Immun 71:1608, 2003.

223. Sougioultzis S, Kyne L, Drudy D, et al: *Clostridium difficile* toxoid vaccine in recurrent *C. difficile*-associated diarrhea [Abstract]. Gastroenterology 126(Suppl 2):A512, 2004.

224. McFarland LV, Elmer GW, Surawicz CM: Breaking the cycle: Treatment strategies for 163 cases of recurrent *Clostridium difficile* disease. Am J Gastroenterol 97:1769, 2002.

CHAPTER
106 Intestinal Protozoa

Christopher D. Huston

Intestinal protozoa traditionally have been considered important pathogens in the developing world where food and water hygiene are poor. A basic knowledge of the intestinal protozoa that cause human disease, however, is of growing importance to physicians practicing medicine in the United States, Canada, and Europe as a result of increasing world travel, globalization of the world's economy, and the growing number of chronically immunosuppressed people. These epidemiologic changes are especially pertinent for patients with acquired immunodeficiency syndrome (AIDS) and organ transplant recipients, in whom microsporidia, *Cryptosporidium* species, *Isospora belli*, and *Cyclospora cayetanensis* are leading causes of chronic diarrhea worldwide. *Cryptosporidium parvum*, *I. belli*, and *C. cayetanensis* recently have been recognized as frequent pathogens in immunocompetent individuals as well, and recent food and water-borne outbreaks in the United States and Canada raise questions about the safety of our increasingly complex water and food supplies. Our understanding of the biology of these organisms is still rudimentary but is rapidly changing. For example, it has only been recognized recently that *Entamoeba histolytica*, the cause of amebic dysentery, and the nonpathogenic intestinal ameba *Entamoeba dispar* are distinct species, and the *Cryptosporidium* species of medical importance were reclassified in 2002. The emergence of these pathogens as major causes of disease in the developed world has stimulated a growing number of basic science investigations. This chapter summarizes major recent advances in our understanding of the intestinal protozoa, with an emphasis on clinical epidemiology and disease characteristics and optimal approaches to accurate diagnosis and treatment.

ENTAMOEBA HISTOLYTICA

EPIDEMIOLOGY

E. histolytica was first linked causally to amebic colitis and liver abscess by Lösch in 1875 and was named by Schaudinn in 1903 for its ability to destroy host tissues. In 1925, Emil Brumpt proposed the existence of a second, morphologically identical nonpathogenic *Entamoeba* species, *E. dispar*, to explain why only a few people infected with what was then termed *E. histolytica* develop invasive disease. Although Brumpt's hypothesis was not accepted during his lifetime, it is now clear that he was correct, and *E. histolytica* has been reclassified to include two morphologically indistinguishable species: *E. histolytica*, the cause of invasive amebiasis, and *E. dispar*, a nonpathogenic intestinal commensal parasite (see later section).[1]

E. histolytica is a parasite of global distribution, but most of the morbidity and mortality from amebiasis occur in Central and South America, Africa, and the Indian subcontinent.[2] Fortunately, most of the 500 million individuals worldwide previously believed to be asymptomatic *E. histolytica* cyst passers actually are infected with *E. dispar*. The best current estimate is that *E. histolytica* causes 34 to 50 million symptomatic infections annually worldwide, resulting in between 40,000

and 100,000 deaths each year.[3,4] In Dhaka, Bangladesh, where diarrheal diseases are the leading cause of childhood death, 55% of children studied prospectively were infected with *E. histolytica* during 2 years of follow-up.[5]

E. histolytica has a simple, two-stage life cycle consisting of an infectious cyst and a motile trophozoite (Fig. 106–1). The mature cyst form measures 5 to 20 μm in diameter and contains four nuclei. The ameboid trophozoite, which is responsible for tissue invasion, measures 10 to 60 μm (Fig. 106–2) and contains a single nucleus with a central karyosome (Fig. 106–3). The cysts are relatively resistant to chlorination and desiccation and survive in a moist environment for several weeks. Infection occurs following ingestion of cysts in fecally contaminated food or water. Within the lumen of the small intestine, a quadrinucleate cyst undergoes nuclear followed by cytoplasmic division, giving rise to eight trophozoites.[6] Only about 10% of infected individuals develop invasive disease that is characterized by invasion of the colonic epithelium by trophozoites.[1] Trophozoites that gain access to the bloodstream may spread hematogenously to establish infection at distant sites (most commonly liver abscess, as discussed in Chapter 79). Why some individuals develop invasive disease while others remain asymptomatic remains unexplained, but both parasite and host differences are likely to be important. For example, amebic liver abscess is primarily a

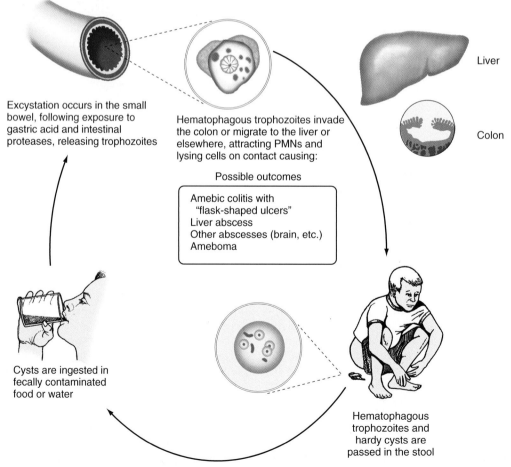

Excystation occurs in the small bowel, following exposure to gastric acid and intestinal proteases, releasing trophozoites

Hematophagous trophozoites invade the colon or migrate to the liver or elsewhere, attracting PMNs and lysing cells on contact causing:

Liver

Colon

Possible outcomes

Amebic colitis with "flask-shaped ulcers"
Liver abscess
Other abscesses (brain, etc.)
Ameboma

Cysts are ingested in fecally contaminated food or water

Hematophagous trophozoites and hardy cysts are passed in the stool

Figure 106–1 Life cycle of *Entamoeba histolytica*. PMNs, polymorphonuclear neutrophils. (From Petri WA, Sing U, Ravdin JI: Enteric amebiasis. In Guerrant RL, Walker DH, Weller PF [eds]: Tropical Infectious Diseases: Principles, Pathogens, and Practice. Philadelphia, WB Saunders, 1999.)

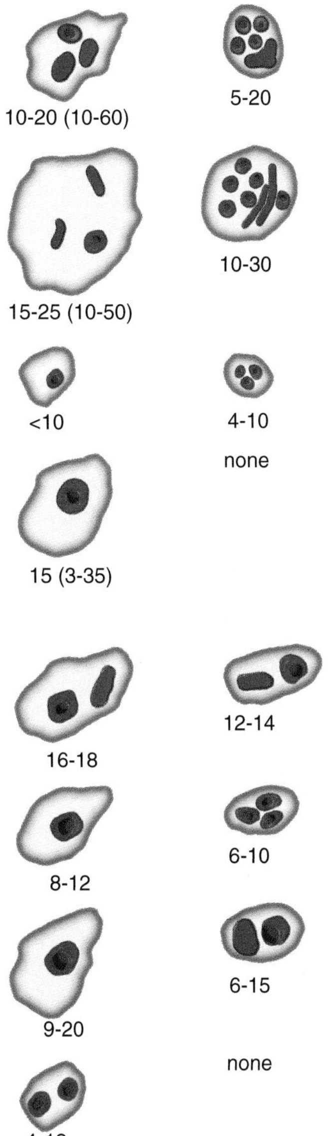

	Human pathogen	Estimated frequency	Trophozoite morphology and usual size range in μm	Cyst morphology and usual size range in μm	Characteristic features
Entamoeba histolytica	Yes	1-10%	10-20 (10-60)	5-20	Central punctate karyosome, erythrophagocytosis Indistinguishable from E. dispar and E. moshkovskii
E. coli	No	3-20%	15-25 (10-50)	10-30	Large size, 5 to 8 nuclei; splinter-like chromatoid bodies Eccentric karyosome distinguishes trophozoite from E. histolytica and E. dispar
E. hartmanni	No	?	<10	4-10	Small size
E. gingivalis	No	10-90% (mouth)	15 (3-35)	none	Oral trophozoite only
E. polecki	Uncertain	rare	16-18	12-14	Uninucleate cyst with large karyosome May represent multiple species
Endolimax nana	No	10-33%	8-12	6-10	Vesiculate nucleus
Iodamoeba butschlii	No	5-8%	9-20	6-15	"I" cyst (see text)
Dientamoeba fragilis*	Uncertain	4-10%	4-12	none	Binucleate trophozoites with a connecting thread

Figure 106–2 Amebae that infect the human gastrointestinal tract. E, Entamoeba (From Ravdin Jl, Guerrant RL: Current problems in the diagnosis and treatment of amebic infections. Curr Clin Trop Infect Dis 7:82, 1986.)

*Dientamoeba fragilis was initially classified as an ameba, but is more closely related to the flagellates (trichomonads) based on morphologic studies and phylogenetic analyses.

disease of adult men, and some studies suggest that susceptibility to both intestinal and hepatic amebiasis is linked to human leukocyte antigen (HLA) class II alleles.[7,8]

PATHOGENESIS, PATHOLOGY, AND IMMUNOLOGY

Both amebic factors and the host's inflammatory response contribute to tissue destruction during invasive amebiasis. Microscopy studies have defined a step-wise progression of disease.[9-11] After excystation within the lumen of the small intestine, trophozoites adhere to colonic mucins and epithelial cells, largely via an amebic galactose/N-acetyl-D-galactosamine inhibitable surface lectin.[12-14] Cysteine proteinases secreted by the trophozoites then facilitate tissue invasion by degrading human colonic mucus and extracellular matrix proteins.[15-18] Further disruption of the colonic epithelium results directly from contact-dependent cytolysis of epithelial and immune cells and from an acute epithelial cell inflammatory response with recruitment of neutrophils and immune-mediated tissue damage.[12,19-23]

The cecum and ascending colon are affected most commonly, although in severe disease the entire colon may be involved. On gross examination, pathology can range from mucosal thickening to multiple punctate ulcers with normal intervening tissue (Fig. 106–4), to frank necrosis. The depth of invasion of amebic trophozoites often halts at the level of the muscularis mucosa. Subsequent lateral spread of amebae and degradation of extracellular matrix proteins by proteases secreted by the trophozoites undermine the overlying epithelium, result-

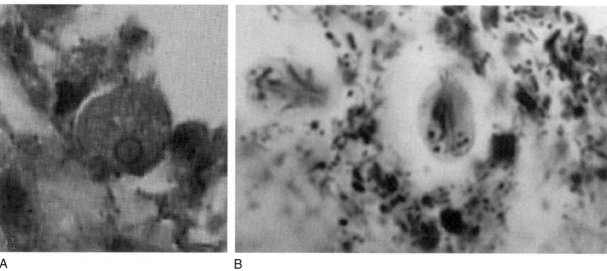

A   **B**

Figure 106–3 *A,* An *Entamoeba histolytica* trophozoite in a stool specimen. Note the nucleus with a prominent central karyosome. *B, Giardia lamblia* cyst in stool. (Original magnification ×400.)

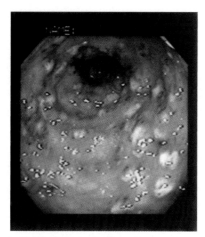

Figure 106–4 Colonoscopic findings in a patient with amebic colitis. Multiple punctate ulcers are visible.

ing in the clean-based, flask-shaped ulcers (see Fig.106–1) that characterize amebic colitis.[24,25] Early in infection, an influx of neutrophils is typical, but, in well-established ulcers, few inflammatory cells are seen.[11,24-26] Organisms may be seen ingesting red blood cells (erythrophagocytosis). At distant sites of infection (e.g., liver abscess), similar pathologic characteristics include central liquefaction of tissue surrounded by a minimal mononuclear cell infiltrate.[25-27]

Because more than 90% of individuals colonized with *E. histolytica* spontaneously clear the infection within 1 year, an effective immune response to amebiasis seems to develop.[28] Furthermore, children with fecal antiamebic lectin IgA have short-lived protection from subsequent intestinal infection.[5,29] The role of IgA in protection is not certain, however, and the contributions of humoral and cellular immunity to protection from amebiasis remain unknown. Nearly everyone with invasive amebiasis develops a systemic and a mucosal humoral immune response.[30-35] Antibodies alone are unable to clear estab-lished infection, since asymptomatic cyst passers remain infected for months after development of antiamebic antibodies.[28,30] Passive immunization experiments in a severe combined immunodeficient (SCID) mouse model of liver abscess, however, suggest an important role for preexisting humoral immunity in protection from infec-tion.[36] Reports that individuals receiving corticosteroids may be at increased risk of severe amebic colitis suggest that cellular immunity also plays an important role in control of *E. histolytica* infection.[37,38] Despite these obser-vations, no increase in the severity of disease in patients with AIDS has been observed. In fact, in a mouse model of amebic colitis, disease was exacerbated by CD4$^+$ T cells.[39]

CLINICAL FEATURES

Infection with *E. histolytica* results in one of three outcomes. Approximately 90% of infected cyst-passing individuals remain asymptomatic. The other 10% of infections result in invasive amebiasis usually character-ized by dysentery (amebic colitis) or, in a few cases, extraintestinal disease (most commonly amebic liver abscess) (see Chapter 79).[1,28]

When epidemiologic risk factors are present, amebic dysentery should be considered in the differential diag-nosis of occult or grossly bloody diarrhea. In the United States, immigrants from or travelers to endemic regions, male homosexuals, and institutionalized individuals are at greatest risk for amebiasis. In addition, malnourished patients, infants, the elderly, pregnant women, and patients receiving corticosteroids may be at increased risk for fulminant disease.[2,37,38] Of interest, patients with AIDS are not at increased risk for invasive amebiasis.

The major diagnostic challenge for the clinician seeing a patient with amebic colitis is to distinguish the illness from other causes of bloody diarrhea. The differential diagnosis includes causes of bacterial dysentery (e.g., *Shigella, Salmonella,* and *Campylobacter* species and

Table 106–1 Comparison of Amebic Colitis and Invasive Bacterial Dysentery

Feature	Amebic Colitis	Invasive Bacterial Dysentery
Immigration from or travel to an endemic area	Yes	Sometimes
Usual duration of symptoms	>7 days	2-7 days
Diarrhea	94-100%	100%
Fecal occult blood	100%	40%
Abdominal pain	12-80%	~50%
Weight loss	Common	Unusual
Fever >38°C	Minority	Majority

Adapted from Huston CD, Petri WA: Amebiasis. In Rakel R (ed): Conn's Current Therapy 2001. Philadelphia, WB Saunders, 2001.

enteroinvasive or enterohemorrhagic *Escherichia coli*), and noninfectious diseases, including inflammatory bowel disease, and ischemic colitis.[2,40] In contrast with bacterial dysentery, which typically begins abruptly, amebic colitis has a gradual onset over 1 to several weeks (Table 106–1). Although more than 90% of patients with amebic colitis present with diarrhea, abdominal pain without diarrhea may occur. The presence or absence of abdominal pain, tenesmus, and fever is highly variable. Weight loss is common with amebic colitis because of the chronicity of the illness, and only microscopic blood is present in the stool of most patients.[2,40,41]

The most feared complication of amebic dysentery, acute necrotizing colitis with toxic megacolon, occurs in 0.5% of cases. This complication manifests as an acute dilatation of the colon, and 40% of patients die from bacterial sepsis unless the megacolon is recognized promptly and treated surgically.[42,43] Unusual complications include the formation of enterocutaneous, rectovaginal, and enterovesicular fistulas and ameboma. Ameboma, due to intraluminal granulation tissue, can cause bowel obstruction and mimic carcinoma of the colon.[2,40]

Although a history of dysentery is often obtained in patients with amebic liver abscess (see Chapter 79), most of these patients do not have coexistent dysentery.[44-46] Other extraintestinal sites of infection rarely occur and typically result either from direct extension of liver abscesses (e.g., amebic pericarditis or lung abscess) or hematogenous spread (e.g., brain abscess).[2,47]

DIAGNOSIS

Since patients with amebiasis treated in error with glucocorticoids for inflammatory bowel disease may develop fulminant colitis, accurate initial diagnosis is critical, especially if patients have epidemiologic risk factors.[37,38] The gold standard for the diagnosis of amebic colitis remains colonoscopy with biopsy, and colonoscopy should be performed when noninfectious causes of bloody diarrhea are strong considerations in the differential diagnosis. Since the cecum and ascending colon are most frequently affected in amebiasis, colonoscopy is preferred to sigmoidoscopy. Classically, multiple punctate ulcers measuring 2 to 10 mm are seen with normal intervening tissue (see Fig. 106–4); the colonic epithelium, however, may simply appear indurated with no visible ulcerations, and, in severe cases, where the ulcers have coalesced, the epithelium may appear necrotic or resem-

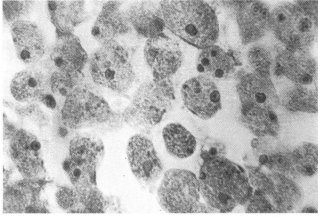

Figure 106–5 Amebic colitis. This high-power view of colon biopsy specimen shows multiple amebic trophozoites, many of which have ingested red blood cells (erythrophagocytosis). Nonpathogenic ameba do not exhibit erythrophagocytosis. (From the photo collection of the late Harrison Juniper, MD.)

ble that of ulcerative colitis. Histologic examination of a biopsy specimen taken from the edge of an ulcer reveals amebic trophozoites and a variable inflammatory infiltrate (Figs. 106–5 and 106–6).[25] Identification of amebae can be aided by periodic acid–Schiff staining of biopsy tissue, which stains trophozoites magenta.

Stool examination for ova and parasites, the traditional method for diagnosis of amebiasis, should no longer be relied on. Although the presence of amebic trophozoites with ingested erythrocytes strongly correlates with *E. histolytica* infection, these rarely are present.[48] In the absence of hematophagous trophozoites, microscopy cannot distinguish *E. histolytica* from *E. dispar*. Difficulty in distinguishing other nonpathogenic amebae (see later) and white blood cells from *E. histolytica* also limits the specificity of stool microscopy.[49] Furthermore, the sensitivity of microscopy for identification of amebae is at best 60% and may be reduced by delays in processing of stool samples.[49,50] The primary utility of stool microscopy for ova and parasites in a patient with diarrhea, therefore, is to evaluate for other parasitic causes of diarrhea.

Noninvasive methods to accurately differentiate *E. histolytica* from *E. dispar* include stool culture with isoenzyme analysis, serum antibody titers, polymerase chain reaction (PCR), and an enzyme-linked immunosorbent assay (ELISA) that detects the amebic lectin antigen in stool samples.[51-61] Of these, only serum antibody titers and the stool ELISA are widely available for clinical use.

Because serum antiamebic antibodies do not develop in patients infected with *E. dispar*, serologic tests for amebiasis accurately distinguish *E. histolytica* and *E. dispar* infection. Seventy-five percent to 85% of patients with

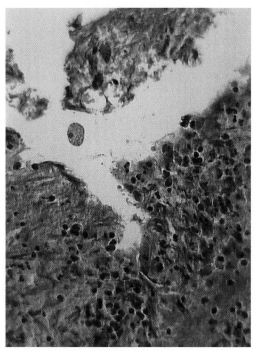

Figure 106–6 Colonic biopsy specimen from a patient with amebic colitis. Note the amebic trophozoite and ulcer with a surrounding inflammatory infiltrate. (Hematoxylin-eosin, ×100.)

acute amebic colitis have detectable antiamebic antibodies on presentation, and convalescent titers develop in more than 90% of patients.[31,32,62] For amebic liver abscess, 70% to 80% of patients have detectable antibody titers on presentation, and convalescent titers develop in greater than 90% of patients. Because antiamebic antibodies can persist for years, however, a positive result must be interpreted with care.[31] For individuals with known epidemiologic risks, a positive result simply may represent infection in the distant past. In the setting of recent travel to an endemic region and a positive antibody titer, diagnosis is confirmed by an appropriate response to antiamebic treatment.

The most specific test clinically available for the diagnosis of amebiasis is a stool ELISA to detect the *E. histolytica* adherence lectin. Only one of the many ELISA tests developed thus far (*E. histolytica* II test, TechLab, Blacksburg, VA) accurately distinguishes *E. histolytica* from *E. dispar*.[50,57,58] This test's specificity when compared with the gold standard of stool culture followed by isoenzyme analysis was greater than 90%, and it was greater than 85% sensitive under optimal conditions.[58] In other studies, the sensitivity of this method has been less impressive, emphasizing the need for rapid processing of stool samples.[63,64] Prior to initiation of treatment, amebic lectin antigen also can be detected in the serum of more than 90% of patients with amebic liver abscess.[65]

TREATMENT

Agents for treatment of amebiasis are categorized as luminal or tissue amebicides on the basis of the location of their antiamebic activity (Table 106–2). The luminal amebicides include iodoquinol, diloxanide furoate, and

Table 106–2 Amebicidal Agents Currently Available in the United States*

Amebicidal Agent	Advantages	Disadvantages
Luminal Amebicides		
Paromomycin (Humatin)	7-day treatment course; may be useful during pregnancy	Frequent gastrointestinal side effects; rare ototoxicity and nephrotoxicity
Iodoquinol (Yodoxin)	Inexpensive and effective	20-day treatment course; contains iodine; rare optic neuritis and atrophy with prolonged use
Diloxanide furoate (Furamide)		Available in the United States only from the CDC; frequent gastrointestinal side effects; rare diplopia
For Invasive Intestinal Disease Only		
Tetracyclines, erythromycin		Not effective for liver abscesses; frequent gastrointestinal side effects; tetracyclines should not be administered to children or pregnant women
For Both Invasive Intestinal and Extraintestinal Amebiasis		
Metronidazole (Flagyl)	Drug of choice for amebic colitis and liver abscess	Anorexia, nausea, vomiting, and metallic taste in nearly one third of patients; disulfiram-like reaction with alcohol; rare seizures
Tinidazole (Tindamax)	Alternative to metronidazole	Recently approved for distribution in the United States; side effects are similar to those with metronidazole
Nitazoxanide (Alinia)	Useful alternative if intolerant of metronidazole/tinidazole	Limited clinical data for amebiasis; rare and reversible conjunctival icterus
Chloroquine (Aralen)	Useful only for amebic liver abscess	Occasional headache, pruritus, nausea, alopecia, and myalgias; rare heart block and irreversible retinal injury

*Also see Chapter 79.
CDC, Centers for Disease Control and Prevention.
Adapted from Huston CD, Petri WA: Amebiasis. In Rakel R (ed): Conn's Current Therapy 2001. Philadelphia, WB Saunders, 2001.

paromomycin.[66,67] Of these, paromomycin, a nonabsorbable aminoglycoside, is preferred because of its safety, short duration of required treatment, and superior efficacy. Its major side effect is diarrhea. Approximately 85% of asymptomatic patients are cured with one course of paromomycin, and, because it is nonabsorbable and has moderate activity against trophozoites that have invaded the colonic mucosa, it also may be useful for single-drug treatment of mild invasive disease during pregnancy.[68,69] The tissue amebicides include metronidazole, tinidazole, nitazoxanide, erythromycin, and chloroquine.[67,70] Of these, metronidazole and tinidazole are the drugs of choice, with cure rates higher than 90%.[71] The new antiparasitic nitazoxanide appears to be efficacious, but data are limited to small trials.[70,72,73] Erythromycin has no activity against amebic liver disease, and chloroquine has no activity against intestinal disease.[74]

Because an estimated 10% of asymptomatic cyst passers develop invasive disease, *E. histolytica* carriers should be treated.[1,4] For noninvasive disease, treatment with a luminal agent alone is adequate (e.g., paromomycin, 25 to 35 mg/kg/day in three divided doses for 7 days).[67] Patients with amebic colitis should be treated with an oral nitroimidazole (either metronidazole, 500 to 750 mg three times daily for 10 days, or tinidazole, 800 mg three times daily for 5 days) followed by a luminal agent such as paromomycin to prevent recurrent disease.[67,71] At the doses required, gastrointestinal side effects develop in approximately 30% of patients.[71] Because of severe gastrointestinal side effects, simultaneous treatment with a nitroimidazole and a luminal agent generally is not recommended. Most patients with colitis respond promptly with resolution of diarrhea in 2 to 5 days.[2] Despite conflicting reports on the safety of the nitroimidazoles for the developing fetus during pregnancy, women with severe disease during pregnancy should probably be treated without delay. As discussed in Chapter 79, metronidazole, 750 mg three times a day for 10 days, followed by a luminal agent, also is the treatment of choice for amebic liver abscess.[67,74]

CONTROL AND PREVENTION

Prevention and control of *E. histolytica* infection depends on interruption of fecal-oral transmission. Water can be made safe for drinking and food preparation by boiling (for 1 minute), halogenation (with chlorine or iodine), or filtration.[6] In the United States and Europe, modern water treatment facilities effectively remove *E. histolytica*. The importance of safe drinking water is highlighted by an outbreak of amebiasis in Tbilisi, Republic of Georgia, where there is an ongoing water-borne epidemic due to decay of water treatment facilities following the demise of the Soviet Union.[75] More important, in most of the developing world, no modern water treatment facilities exist and none are likely to be constructed in the foreseeable future. Recent data suggest that naturally acquired immunity to intestinal amebiasis provides short-lived protection against reinfection, giving hope that a vaccine may be feasible.[5,29] Because humans and some higher nonhuman primates are the only known hosts for *E. histolytica*, a vaccine that successfully

prevents colonization might enable eradication of the disease.[76]

OTHER INTESTINAL AMEBAE

Eight species of commensal amebae commonly infect the human gastrointestinal tract (see Fig. 106–2). These include *E. dispar*, *Entamoeba moshkovskii*, *Entamoeba coli*, *Entamoeba hartmanni*, *Entamoeba gingivalis*, *Entamoeba polecki*, *Endolimax nana*, and *Iodamoeba butschlii*. *Dientamoeba fragilis* (discussed in following section), previously thought to be an ameba, is more closely related to the flagellated protozoan *Trichomonas vaginalis* than to the true amebae.[6] With the exception of *E. gingivalis*, which has no known cyst stage, all of these true amebae have simple two-stage life cycles, consisting of an infectious cyst form and a motile trophozoite form.[6] All but *E. dispar* can be differentiated from *E. histolytica* using light microscopy based on characteristic features of the cyst and trophozoite forms (see Fig. 106–2). *E. dispar* must be differentiated from *E. histolytica* based on antigenic or genetic differences.[1]

E. dispar is a nonpathogenic protozoan parasite that is morphologically indistinguishable from *E. histolytica* by light microscopy (see Fig. 106–2).[1] An estimated 450 million people worldwide are infected with *E. dispar*, and infection with *E. dispar* is approximately 10 times more prevalent than *E. histolytica* infection.[1,3,4] Although *E. dispar* has been demonstrated to cause mucosal ulcerations in animal models, it has not been demonstrated to cause human disease and does not require treatment.[1] *E. moshkovskii*, thought to be a free-living ameba, has cysts and trophozoites indistinguishable from those of *E. histolytica* and *E. dispar*. A recent study showing high prevalence (21.1%) of *E. moshkovskii* infection in Bangladeshi children suggests that humans may be a frequent host for this organism.[77] The primary clinical significance of *E. dispar* and *E. moshkovskii* is that they must be distinguished from *E. histolytica* to enable accurate diagnosis of invasive amebiasis. PCR to amplify small ribosomal RNA (not clinically available) and ELISAs using monoclonal antiamebic antibodies to detect specific *E. histolytica* antigens make accurate diagnosis possible (see the section on *E. histolytica* diagnosis).[52-61]

Besides *E. dispar*, *Entamoeba coli* is the intestinal commensal most frequently mistaken for *E. histolytica*. *E. coli* trophozoites contain a single nucleus with a prominent karyosome that usually is eccentric in location, distinguishing them from *E. histolytica*/*E. dispar* trophozoites, which have a centrally located karyosome. In addition, the cyst form of *E. coli* typically contains five to eight nuclei (see Fig. 106–2). *E. coli* is nonpathogenic and requires no specific treatment; however, it is a valuable marker of fecal-oral exposure and can be found concurrently with *E. histolytica* in 10% to 30% of patients in endemic regions.[6]

E. hartmanni was classified as "small race" *E. histolytica* for many years. It is now recognized as a nonpathogen and requires no treatment. The trophozoites resemble those of *E. histolytica* except for their small size (<10 μm).[6]

E. gingivalis is the only ameba found in the oral cavity, where it lives in the anaerobic environment of the gingival crease. The trophozoite is identical in size to that of *E. histolytica* and contains a single nucleus with a prominent central karyosome (see Fig. 106–2). No cyst form of *E. gingivalis* has been identified, and oral-oral contact is believed to be the mode of transmission.[6,78] *E. gingivalis* is associated with poor dental hygiene and periodontal disease, but a causal relationship to periodontitis has not been proven,[78] except perhaps in AIDS patients, in whom treatment with metronidazole has been reported to be effective.[79]

E. polecki, a parasite characterized by a uninucleated cyst, is primarily a parasite of pigs and monkeys that sometimes infects humans. Recent data suggest that several distinct uninucleated cyst-producing *Entamoeba* species can infect humans and it has been proposed that these organisms collectively be termed *E. polecki*–like.[80] Infection is rare except in Papua, New Guinea, where as many as 30% of children were found to be colonized in one study.[81] At present, specific treatment of *E. polecki*-like infections is not recommended routinely, but persons with heavy burdens of this parasite may develop nonspecific gastrointestinal symptoms and might benefit from treatment. Good clinical responses to metronidazole and diloxanide furoate have been reported.[82]

E. nana is another nonpathogenic intestinal ameba that frequently infects humans.[6] The distribution of *E. nana* is worldwide, but it is most common in the tropics where 5% to 33% of individuals are infected.[83,84] Infection requires no specific treatment but serves as a useful marker for fecal-oral exposure. *E. nana* trophozoites can be distinguished from those of *E. histolytica* by their vesiculate nucleus, large irregular karyosome, and relatively small size (8 to 12 μm).[6] *I. butschlii* is a nonpathogenic intestinal ameba passed by the fecal-oral route. Its trophozoites contain a single nucleus with a large karyosome (which is distinct from the punctate karyosome of *E. histolytica*). *I. butschlii* cysts contain a single nucleus and a large, eccentric glycogen mass that stains with iodine (hence the name *Iodamoeba*). *I. butschlii* infection requires no treatment.[6]

GIARDIA LAMBLIA

EPIDEMIOLOGY

Giardia lamblia is a ubiquitous flagellated intestinal protozoan. Van Leeuwenhoek accurately described its motile trophozoite form in 1681, but it was not until 1915 that Stiles named the species.[6] The life cycle of *Giardia* consists of an infectious cyst form and a motile trophozoite (Fig. 106–7). The cyst is oval (8 to 12 μm long by 7 to 10 μm wide); contains four nuclei; and has a rigid outer wall that protects it from dehydration, extremes of tem-

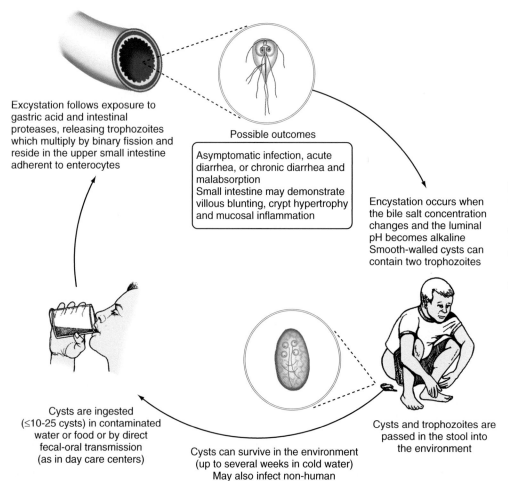

Excystation follows exposure to gastric acid and intestinal proteases, releasing trophozoites which multiply by binary fission and reside in the upper small intestine adherent to enterocytes

Possible outcomes

Asymptomatic infection, acute diarrhea, or chronic diarrhea and malabsorption
Small intestine may demonstrate villous blunting, crypt hypertrophy and mucosal inflammation

Encystation occurs when the bile salt concentration changes and the luminal pH becomes alkaline
Smooth-walled cysts can contain two trophozoites

Cysts are ingested (≤10-25 cysts) in contaminated water or food or by direct fecal-oral transmission (as in day care centers)

Cysts can survive in the environment (up to several weeks in cold water)
May also infect non-human mammalian species

Cysts and trophozoites are passed in the stool into the environment

Figure 106–7 Life cycle of *Giardia lamblia*. (From Hill DR, Nash TE: Intestinal flagellate and ciliate infections. In Guerrant RL, Walker DH, Weller PF [eds]: Tropical Infectious Diseases: Principles, Pathogens, and Practice. Philadelphia, WB Saunders, 1999.)

perature, and chlorination (Fig. 106–8). *Giardia* cysts can survive in cold water for several weeks.[6,85] Ingestion of as few as 10 to 25 cysts can result in infection.[85] Excystation occurs after ingestion, following exposure to stomach acid and intestinal proteases; each cyst gives rise to two trophozoites. *Giardia* trophozoites (see Fig. 106–3*B*) are pear-shaped (10 to 20 μm long by 7 to 10 μm wide), contain two nuclei, have eight flagella for locomotion, and replicate by binary fission. The trophozoites live in the duodenum where they adhere to enterocytes. Trophozoites eventually encyst following exposure to alkaline conditions or bile salts and are excreted in the stool to complete the life cycle.[85]

Analysis of DNA restriction fragment length polymorphisms has demonstrated tremendous variability of *Giardia* isolates from humans and other mammals, and different *G. lamblia* isolates have been shown to have different pathogenicity in experimental human infections.[86,87] Common patterns are observed among *Giardia* isolates from humans, beavers, and other mammals, however, suggesting that these animals do not have their own species of *Giardia* and can serve as a reservoir for human disease.[86]

G. lamblia is the most frequently identified intestinal parasite in the United States. (It was identified in 7.2% of stool samples examined by state health departments in 1987.[88]) Giardiasis occurs in both endemic and epidemic forms via water-borne, food-borne, and person-to-person transmission.[89-95] Worldwide, *Giardia* infects infants more commonly than adults and in highly endemic regions, essentially all children are infected by 2 to 3 years of age.[96,97] In the developing world, it is likely that recurrent infantile diarrhea caused by giardiasis contributes significantly to malnutrition.[96] In the United States, children in day care facilities and sexually active homosexual men have the greatest risk of infection.[88,98] During a yearlong longitudinal study at a U.S. day care center, *Giardia* cysts were identified at some time in the stool of more than 30% of children.[95] Additional risk factors for infection include drinking untreated surface water, a shallow well

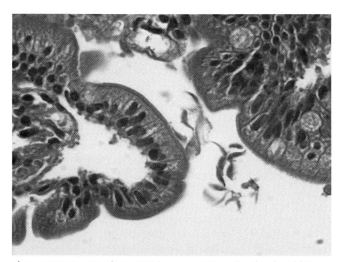

Figure 106–8 Giardiasis. High-power view of a duodenal biopsy specimen showing many trophozoites near the surface of the epithelium between villi. (Courtesy of the Carlo Denegri Foundation, Turin, Italy.)

as a residential water source, swimming in any natural body of fresh water, and contact with a person with giardiasis or a child in day care.[90]

PATHOGENESIS, PATHOLOGY, AND IMMUNOLOGY

Giardia causes malabsorptive diarrhea by an unknown mechanism. Trophozoites adhere (perhaps by suction) to the epithelium of the upper small intestine, using a disk structure located on their ventral surface.[6,85] There is no evidence that trophozoites invade the mucosa.[99] Studies using electron microscopy have shown damage to the mucosal brush border.[85,100] On biopsy, pathologic changes range from an entirely normal-appearing duodenal mucosa (except for adherent trophozoites), as was found in more than 96% of biopsy specimens in one large study, to severe villus atrophy with a mononuclear cell infiltrate that resembles celiac sprue.[99,101,102] The severity of diarrhea appears to correlate with the severity of the pathologic change.[85]

The host immune response plays a critical role in limiting the severity of giardiasis. When infected with *Giardia*, individuals with common variable immunodeficiency develop severe, protracted diarrhea and malabsorption with sprue-like pathologic changes that resolve with treatment.[102] Both a systemic and mucosal humoral immune response can be measured consistently following *Giardia* infection. High parasite-specific serum IgM, IgG, and IgA titers can be detected, and secretory IgA (s-IgA) can be detected in saliva and in breast milk of infected mothers.[103-105] Animal studies suggest that both early and late immune responses are important for control of *Giardia* infections. Interleukin (IL)-6 is important in the early immune response to *Giardia* in mice, as are mast cells, which may function as IL-6 producers or via another mechanism.[106-108] In a B-cell-deficient transgenic mouse model, infection does not resolve, confirming the importance of the humoral immune response for clearance of established infections.[109] *Giardia* vary in expression of a group of cysteine-rich surface proteins (termed *variant surface proteins*) in culture, and, in experimental human infections, *G. lamblia* isolates have been shown to undergo antigenic variation after approximately 2 weeks (roughly the time required to mount an initial antibody response).[110] Although the role of the variant surface proteins has not been established, antigenic variation may enable *Giardia* to evade the host immune response.[111]

The importance of a cellular immune response is also clear from animal studies. Athymic nude mice are unable to control *Giardia muris* infection, but reconstitution with immune spleen cells results in partial control. On immune reconstitution, however, severe inflammatory changes and villus atrophy develop in the intestine, suggesting that the immune response to infection may contribute to pathology.[112]

CLINICAL FEATURES

The clinical manifestations of *Giardia* vary greatly, ranging from asymptomatic infection to severe, chronic

Table 106–3   Frequency of Symptom(s) in Patients with Giardiasis[93,99,103]

Symptom(s)	Frequency (%)
Diarrhea	32-100
Fatigue	22-97
Abdominal pain/cramps	75-83
Flatulence/bloating	58-79
Weight loss	60
Anorexia	45
Vomiting	17-26
Fever	12-21

diarrhea with malabsorption. In one large study of biopsy-proven giardiasis, only 32% of patients had diarrhea, and most patients had nonspecific gastrointestinal complaints.[99] Reported symptoms, in order of decreasing frequency, include diarrhea, fatigue, abdominal cramps, bloating, malodorous stool, flatulence, weight loss, fever, and vomiting (Table 106–3).[93,103] During a food-borne outbreak, the mean duration of diarrhea was 16 days, but symptoms resolved spontaneously in nearly one half of infected individuals after 7 to 8 days.[93]

As mentioned earlier, the severity of illness depends on both host and parasite factors. Different *Giardia* isolates have different abilities to cause disease during experimental human infections.[87] Furthermore, certain populations, including children younger than 2 years of age and patients with hypogammaglobulinemia, are more likely to develop serious disease.[96,102] Despite the importance of cellular immunity for controlling infection in animal models and the increased risk of *Giardia* infection among sexually active homosexual men, severe infections that are resistant to treatment or an increased frequency of giardiasis have been noted only rarely in patients with AIDS.[113] Several recent reports, however, do suggest that *Giardia* infection may be more severe or refractory to treatment in patients with advanced AIDS.[114,115]

DIAGNOSIS

Examination of concentrated, iodine-stained wet stool preparations and modified-trichrome-stained permanent smears has been the conventional approach to identifying *Giardia* infections (see Fig. 106–3*B*). Because cysts and trophozoites are present only intermittently in the stool, however, the sensitivity is only approximately 50%, even with examination of multiple specimens.[101] With direct sampling of duodenal contents (e.g., duodenal aspiration or the "string test"), sensitivity can be improved to approximately 80% (see Fig. 106–8).[101] Identification of trophozoites with small intestinal biopsy specimens requires careful examination of multiple microscope fields to ensure accuracy.[99]

Numerous molecular tests based on ELISAs or direct immunofluorescent antibody (DFA) microscopy now are commercially available to diagnose giardiasis in stool samples.[116-118] These assay kits all work well, with sensitivities greater than 90% and specificities approaching 100%.[118] Given the inability to exclude giardiasis even

with repeated conventional stool examinations and the difficulties of duodenal sampling, the first diagnostic test performed to evaluate for *Giardia* infection should be a stool ELISA or DFA. The primary role of endoscopy is evaluation for other pathologic conditions.

TREATMENT

Metronidazole, 250 mg orally three times a day for 5 days, is the preferred treatment for giardiasis.[67] At this relatively low dosage, metronidazole is generally well tolerated and is 80% to 95% effective at eradicating *Giardia*.[119] The most common side effects are nausea, a metallic taste, and a disulfiram-like reaction with alcohol. Nitazoxanide appears to be at least as effective as metronidazole and has the advantage of being available in a liquid formulation for use in pediatric patients. The recommended dosage in children is 100 mg (ages 12 to 47 months) or 200 mg (age > 4 years) twice daily, and in adults is 500 mg twice daily for 3 days.[70,73,120] Alternative regimens include (1) tinidazole (2 g orally for one dose); (2) quinacrine (2 mg/kg three times a day for 5 days (maximum 300 mg per day); (3) furazolidone (100 mg orally four times a day for 7 to 10 days); or (4) paromomycin (25 to 35 mg/kg/day in three divided doses for 7 days). Simple and effective single-dose treatment with tinidazole has been used for years in Europe and the developing world and has recently been approved by the U.S. Food and Drug Administration.[67] Because paromomycin is not absorbed and there have been conflicting reports regarding the safety of metronidazole and tinidazole for the developing fetus, paromomycin may be useful for treatment of giardiasis during pregnancy.[67]

Many patients have prolonged lactose intolerance following *Giardia* infection, which can mimic ongoing infection. Therefore, the diagnosis should be reconfirmed prior to repeating therapy. For people in whom therapy fails, repeat treatment with the same drug (e.g., with higher doses of metronidazole) or combination therapy with metronidazole and quinacrine may work.[115,119] Nitazoxanide alone may also be effective.[121,122] When treatment repeatedly fails, patients should be evaluated for common variable immunodeficiency.[102,119]

CONTROL AND PREVENTION

Control of giardiasis relies on interruption of fecal-oral transmission. Water can be made safe for drinking and food preparation by boiling (for 1 minute), halogenation (with chlorine or iodine preparations), or filtration.[6,119] Because of the low infectious dose of *Giardia* cysts and the poor hygiene of infants and children, person-to-person spread in day care centers is much more difficult to control. Temporarily removing infected children who are ill from day care is ineffective, perhaps because many infected children remain asymptomatic and go unrecognized.[123] In the developing world, endemic giardiasis is unlikely to be controlled until facilities for adequate filtration of water and disposal of sewage become available. A *Giardia* vaccine comprised of killed *G. lamblia* trophozoites has been licensed for use in cats and dogs, but there have been few studies addressing human vaccination for giardiasis.[124] Reduced susceptibility of some people living in endemic areas suggests that vaccination may be possible.[125]

DIENTAMOEBA FRAGILIS

Dientamoeba fragilis is a binucleate organism with an ameboid trophozoite that measures 4 to 12 μm in diameter (see Fig. 106–2). No cyst form has been identified. The organism was initially classified as an ameba but is more closely related to the flagellates (trichomonads) based on morphologic studies and phylogenetic analyses of small-subunit ribosomal RNA gene sequences. The mode of transmission remains unknown. The absence of a cyst form makes direct fecal-oral transmission unlikely, because the trophozoite is killed by gastric acid. Because of an association with *Enterobius vermicularis* (pinworm), some have hypothesized that it is carried in pinworm eggs.[126] Infection with *D. fragilis* is common throughout the world. *D. fragilis* was identified in 0.5% of all stool samples examined in a large U.S. study, and the prevalence has been as high as 20% to 50% in selected populations.[88,127-130]

The role of *D. fragilis* as a pathogen has been controversial. *D. fragilis* trophozoites do not invade tissue, and many individuals infected with *D. fragilis* remain asymptomatic.[126] Furthermore, the organism is often identified in the presence of other intestinal parasites, making its role in disease unclear.[127,129,130] Several studies of patients infected only with *D. fragilis* have found an association with diarrhea, abdominal pain, nausea, weight loss, anorexia, flatus, and malaise that resolved only after eradication.[128,131,132] Treatment with iodoquinol, metronidazole, and tetracycline has been effective.[128,132,133]

BLASTOCYSTIS HOMINIS

Blastocystis hominis is an intestinal protozoan parasite that commonly infects the human colon. It is of uncertain taxonomic classification. Diameter ranges from 3 to 30 μm. In culture, *B. hominis* has ameboid, vacuolated, and granular forms.[6,134] Recently, a cyst form has also been identified.[135]

The distribution of *B. hominis* is worldwide, but infection is most common in the tropics.[84,88,136-138] In a large study of intestinal parasitism in the United States, *B. hominis* was identified in 2.6% of stool specimens submitted to state health departments. More than 70% of positive samples were from California.[88] Among American travelers and expatriates, the prevalence often exceeds 30%.[84,138]

The significance of *B. hominis* as a pathogen remains controversial. Although several studies have suggested an association with irritable bowel syndrome, cause or effect has not been established, and *B. hominis* infection is not more common among patients with gastrointestinal complaints than among asymptomatic control subjects in most series.[84,138-141] In addition, the parasite burden does not correlate with symptoms.[84,136] Nevertheless, multiple studies have used iodoquinol, 650 mg orally

three times a day for 20 days, or metronidazole, 750 mg orally three times a day for 10 days, for treatment of symptomatic patients, with an overall improvement rate of about 50%.[83,142] This clinical improvement may actually be due to treatment of unrecognized infections due to other organisms, since many people infected with *B. hominis* simultaneously harbor known pathogens.[127,143,144]

CRYPTOSPORIDIUM SPECIES

EPIDEMIOLOGY

First recognized by Tyzzer as a gastric infection in mice in 1907, *Cryptosporidium* species are tiny intracellular apicomplexan protozoan parasites (2 to 5 μm) that infect the gastrointestinal epithelium of a wide range of vertebrates. *C. parvum* is the species that most frequently infects mammals, including humans. It was first found in mice and was distinguished from *Cryptosporidium muris* (the gastric species) by its location in the small intestine and slightly smaller size. Based on genetic and biologic differences, *C. parvum* human genotype (genotype 1 or genotype H) was renamed *Cryptosporidium hominis* in 2002. The name *Cryptosporidium parvum* has been retained for the bovine genotype (genotype 2). Together, *C. hominis* and *C. parvum* cause most human infections, but occasionally other species may cause human disease (especially in immunocompromised patients).[145]

The cryptosporidia were brought to prominent medical attention only in the early 1980s because of the devastating disease they cause in patients with advanced human immunodeficiency virus (HIV) infection. However, *Cryptosporidium* species are increasingly recognized as a cause of self-limited diarrhea, usually lasting 1 to 4 weeks in immunocompetent patients.[146,147] In developing countries, children younger than 5 years of age are most frequently affected.[148] In industrialized countries, because *Cryptosporidium* oocysts are small and highly chlorine resistant, cryptosporidiosis has been associated with water-borne epidemics, including numerous chlorinated swimming pool outbreaks and the largest waterborne outbreak ever recorded that infected more than 400,000 Milwaukee residents in 1993.[149,150] A low infectious dose and ready person-to-person spread have also resulted in epidemics in hospitals and day care centers.[151,152] In rural areas, zoonotic infections from direct contact with farm animals have been reported.[153]

PATHOGENESIS, PATHOLOGY, AND IMMUNOLOGY

On ingestion of an infectious dose that may be as low as 1 to 10 hardy oocysts, excystation and release of sporozoites occur in the lumen of the small bowel. The sporozoites then attach to the intestinal microvillus border, triggering host cell cytoskeletal rearrangement and extension of the host cell membrane around the sporozoite. The result is an intracellular but extracytoplasmic "feeder" vacuole in which the sporozoite receives nutrients, matures into the merozoite form, and reproduces asexually. On release into the intestinal lumen, the merozoites either can infect nearby cells, perpetuating the cycle of asexual reproduction and clinical symptoms, or mature into gametocytes and begin sexual reproduction. The life cycle is completed when the microgamete penetrates the macrogamete to form a zygote, which develops into a sporozoite-containing oocyst. The infectious oocysts then are either excreted in the feces or can excyst and reinfect the intestinal epithelium. Rarely, parasites have been identified within the biliary, respiratory, and even the conjunctival epithelium in immunocompromised patients.[6] By far, the most common extraintestinal site is in the biliary tract where infection is believed to result from the intraluminal spread of parasites.

Animal and human studies suggest that both humoral and cellular immune responses aid in the control of *Cryptosporidium* infections. Cryptosporidial diarrhea is much more severe, if not intractable, in patients with immunoglobulin deficiency, lymphocytic malignancies, or low CD4 counts associated with HIV infection than it is in immunocompetent persons.[147,154,155]

CLINICAL FEATURES

After a 1-week incubation period (range, 2 to 14 days), a watery, noninflammatory diarrheal illness typically lasts for 10 to 14 days in immunocompetent hosts. Nausea, vomiting, abdominal pain, and mild fever also may be seen. Respiratory symptoms, pancreatitis, and biliary involvement are rare, the latter occurring in HIV-infected individuals (see Chapter 32). Brief recurrence of diarrhea may be seen after improvement.[150,156]

In immunocompromised patients, particularly those with very low CD4 lymphocyte counts, cryptosporidial diarrhea can be cholera-like, protracted (often for the duration of severe immunocompromise), and fatal.[147]

DIAGNOSIS

Because cryptosporidial infection usually will not be detected in the laboratory unless a test for it is specifically requested, the most important element in diagnosis is to consider it in all patients with diarrhea lasting longer than 5 to 7 days and to request special fecal studies for *Cryptosporidium*. Because *Cryptosporidium* is spread in water, it is reasonable to consider cryptosporidiosis in the same clinical settings that one considers the diagnosis of giardiasis. In addition, it should be considered as a potential cause of persistent diarrhea in immunocompromised patients.

Traditionally, cryptosporidial oocysts have been detected with a modified acid-fast stain of the stool (which can also detect *Cyclospora* and *Isospora*).[157] As with giardiasis, ELISA or DFA tests of the stool have replaced microscopy as the diagnostic test of choice. Numerous commercial kits employing either method have been developed that have sensitivity and specificity in excess of 90%. One should remember, however, that these immunodiagnostic tests may be of limited value in testing environmental samples since there is some cross-reactivity with nonhuman cryptosporidial oocysts.[118]

Occasionally, cryptosporidiosis is diagnosed with intestinal biopsy.

Serologic tests are helpful primarily in epidemiologic studies, especially since these tests may be negative at the time of initial clinical presentation and often persist after infection is resolved. Finally, abdominal ultrasound and computed tomographic scanning may be helpful in diagnosing acalculous cholecystitis and cholangiopathies, which may, in immunocompromised individuals, be caused by cryptosporidia. Specific diagnosis, however, requires histopathology, and so endoscopic retrograde cholangiopancreatography with brushing or biopsy of the duct and ampulla usually is necessary.

TREATMENT

Nitazoxanide, a new antiparasitic with broad-spectrum antiprotozoal and antihelminthic activity, is the only known drug with consistent efficacy for treatment of cryptosporidiosis in immunocompetent patients.[70,72,158,159] Unfortunately, failure is common in immunocompromised patients such as those with advanced HIV infection, although some studies have shown benefit.[160] The recommended dosage in children is 100 mg (ages 12 to 47 months) or 200 mg (age >4 years) twice daily, and in adults is 500 mg twice daily for 3 days. Nitazoxanide generally is well tolerated. Yellow sclerae caused by drug deposition is rare and resolves after nitazoxanide is discontinued. Additional treatment options in immunocompromised patients not responsive to nitazoxanide may include the nonabsorbable aminoglycoside paromomycin, or paromomycin in combination with azithromycin.[161]

Most important in treating HIV-infected patients with cryptosporidiosis is highly active antiretroviral therapy (HAART), because improvement of cryptosporidiosis is dependent on improvement in the CD4 lymphocyte counts in immunocompromise. Finally, papillotomy may be required for biliary obstruction and papillary stenosis caused by cryptosporidiosis in immunocompromised patients (see Chapter 32). This procedure improves the obstruction but does not reduce the parasite burden.

CONTROL AND PREVENTION

Most important in control and prevention of this difficult protozoan infection is education regarding boiling or careful filtration of water (i.e., filter pores must be <1 μm in diameter). In addition, scrupulous enteric precautions are required in institutions such as hospitals, day care centers, or extended care facilities for the elderly. These precautions are especially important since chlorine is ineffective in reducing oocyst viability. One study examined *C. parvum* oocyst viability following exposure to common hospital disinfectants. Of the disinfectants tested, only 2% glutaraldehyde was effective at reducing viability, and it only worked for the lowest concentration of oocysts and when treatment was for at least 10 hours. Because glutaraldehyde is corrosive, endoscopic equipment exposed to *Cryptosporidium* cannot be immersed for sufficient time, causing concern for hospital disinfection practices.[162]

Finally, because of the potential substantial long-term impact of cryptosporidial infection on growth and development, control of cryptosporidiosis is critical to child health in developing areas and must receive high priority worldwide in programs directed at improved water and sanitation.[163,164]

CYCLOSPORA CAYETANENSIS

EPIDEMIOLOGY

Although recognized by Schaudinn as a cause of enteritis in moles in 1901, *Cyclospora* was first described by Ashford in 1979 in three patients in Papua, New Guinea.[165] *Cyclospora* then was seen increasingly in AIDS patients who had protracted diarrhea and in immunocompetent patients with persistent diarrhea in New York City, the Caribbean, among expatriates in Nepal, and in an outbreak among house staff in a Chicago hospital.[166-168] Its definitive sporulation and naming as *Cyclospora cayetanensis* was reported by Ortega and associates in 1993.[169] Ribosomal DNA analysis of phylogenetic relationships suggest that *Cyclospora* is closely related to *Eimeria*.[170]

Cyclospora infection is usually highly seasonal (in summer or wet months) and is probably spread via fecal contamination of water and vegetables.[171,172] *Cyclospora* again was brought to prominent attention throughout the United States and Canada with repeated outbreaks of diarrheal illnesses occurring in more than 2000 patients every year from 1996 through 2000 in association with consumption of the late spring shipment of Guatemalan raspberries.[173,174]

PATHOGENESIS, PATHOLOGY, AND IMMUNOLOGY

The pathogenesis, pathology, and immunology of *Cyclospora* appear to be similar to those described for *Cryptosporidium*, although *Cyclospora* has not been as thoroughly studied as *Cryptosporidium*. One important distinction is that, unlike *Cryptosporidium*, which is promptly infectious when it is excreted in the stool, *Cyclospora* requires development outside the host before it becomes infectious. Consequently, the risk of secondary person-to-person spread, which is common with cryptosporidial infections, is not described with *Cyclospora* infections. An additional difference is that, unlike the numerous mammalian hosts for cryptosporidial infections that also may infect humans, the animal reservoir(s) for *Cyclospora* are poorly understood at present.

The histopathologic changes seen in *Cyclospora* infections are, again, similar to those seen with cryptosporidiosis, with villus blunting and mild inflammatory infiltrate in the lamina propria predominately in the small bowel.[175]

CLINICAL FEATURES

The clinical presentation of *Cyclospora* infection also is indistinguishable from that described earlier with *Cryptosporidium* infections, with the exception of more prominent severe generalized fatigue and malaise with *Cyclospora* infections even in immunocompetent individuals. *Cyclospora* diarrhea typically lasts for 1 to 3 weeks and may be associated with significant weight loss. Finally, also as seen with cryptosporidiosis, protracted diarrhea and acalculous cholecystitis also may occur with *Cyclospora* infection in HIV-infected individuals.

DIAGNOSIS

As with *Cryptosporidium*, one must consider the diagnosis of *Cyclospora* in individuals with protracted diarrhea. Diagnosis is best made at present with the acid-fast stain. *Cyclospora* oocysts are nearly twice the size of those of *Cryptosporidium* (4 to 10 μm).[176] In addition, *Cyclospora* exhibits striking blue-green autofluorescence when examined under fluorescence microscopy, a characteristic that may have contributed to its initial confusion with cyanobacteria.[177] Improved diagnostic methods using PCR have been developed but are currently not available for clinical use.[178]

TREATMENT

In contrast with *Cryptosporidium* infections, *Cyclospora* infections are readily treatable even in immunocompromised patients. The drug of choice is trimethoprim-sulfamethoxazole at a dosage of 160/800 mg twice daily for 1 week. Treatment promptly eradicates the organism and relieves symptoms.[179,180] This treatment is similarly effective in patients with AIDS, although maintenance therapy with a single dose of trimethoprim-sulfamethoxazole three times per week may be needed to prevent relapse.[181] Recent data show that ciprofloxacin provides a reasonable alternative in patients unable to tolerate trimethoprim-sulfamethoxazole.[182] Nitazoxanide also appears to be effective.[72]

CONTROL AND PREVENTION

Although readily treatable, *Cyclospora* infections are extremely difficult to control or prevent because of our limited ability to detect low infectious doses of oocysts, which may contaminate products such as raspberries and from which the organism is extremely difficult to eradicate. From limited studies, the organism also appears to be relatively chlorine resistant and thus poses challenges to effective water treatment, much like those seen with *Cryptosporidium*. Elucidation of the reservoir of *Cyclospora* will undoubtedly enhance our ability to prevent and control the spread of this highly infectious parasite. For example, it remains unclear why it is only the spring rather than the fall shipment of raspberries from Guatemala that consistently has posed problems with spread of *Cyclospora* infections. Whether this is related to migration of an avian reservoir has been postulated but not proven.[183] Consistent with this postulate is the reported isolation of *Cyclospora* oocysts from chickens in several studies.[171,172]

ISOSPORA BELLI

EPIDEMIOLOGY

A relative of *Cyclospora* and *Eimeria*, *I. belli* is much larger, with elliptical oocysts measuring 20 to 30 μm long and containing two visible sporocysts that are acid-fast. Like *Cyclospora*, *Isospora* oocysts appear to require sporulation outside of the human host before they become infectious. There are no known nonhuman hosts for *I. belli*, and its distribution appears to be throughout tropical areas around the world. *Isospora* is a less common cause of diarrhea in children in developing areas than is *Cryptosporidium* and is seen more often in older children, in immunocompromised patients, and in institutionalized children in North America.[184,185]

PATHOGENESIS, PATHOLOGY, AND IMMUNOLOGY

The pathogenesis, pathology, and immunology of *Isospora* infections, although less thoroughly studied, appear to be similar to those of *Cryptosporidium* and *Cyclospora* infections.

CLINICAL FEATURES

Similar to *Cryptosporidium* and *Cyclospora* infections, *Isospora* characteristically produces a self-limiting diarrheal illness in immunocompetent individuals and in travelers to tropical areas, with watery diarrhea and abdominal pain lasting 2 to 4 weeks. In immunocompromised patients, *Isospora* may produce a protracted sprue-like illnesses with malabsorption, weight loss, and prolonged diarrhea.[185] As with *Cryptosporidium* and *Cyclospora*, acalculous cholecystitis has also been reported in patients with AIDS and *Isospora* infections.

DIAGNOSIS

The diagnosis of *Isospora* should be suspected in immunocompetent patients with diarrhea lasting longer than 5 to 7 days, especially following travel to tropical or developing areas, and in immunocompromised patients with persistent diarrhea. Unlike other protozoan infections, *Isospora* infections may be associated with peripheral eosinophilia and with Charcot-Leyden crystals in the stool. The diagnosis of *Isospora* relies on identification of the large, oval oocysts (20 to 30 μm by 10 to 19 μm) on microscopic examination of concentrated fecal specimens by acid-fast staining. Oocysts also may be seen on small bowel biopsy. In contrast with *Cryptosporidium*

and *Cyclospora* infections, *Isospora* organisms have been observed invading beyond the epithelium into the lamina propria.[145,186]

TREATMENT

As with *Cyclospora*, *Isospora* infections are readily treated with trimethoprim/sulfamethoxazole. For immunocompromised patients, the dosage is 160/800 mg orally four times a day for 10 days, and then two times a day for 3 weeks, with both symptomatic and parasitologic responses, even in patients with AIDS.[67] For immunocompetent adults, trimethoprim/sulfamethoxazole, 160/800 mg two times a day for 10 days, is adequate. As previously described with *Cyclospora*, maintenance suppressive therapy may be required in patients with AIDS.[180] Alternatives to trimethoprim/sulfamethoxazole may include ciprofloxacin.[182]

CONTROL AND PREVENTION

Prevention and control of *Isospora* infections will likely require improved sanitation in tropical areas.

MICROSPORIDIA

EPIDEMIOLOGY

Microsporidia, the nontaxonomic term for *Enterocytozoon bieneusi*, *Encephalitozoon* (old *Septata*) *intestinalis*, and several other nonintestinal pathogens of the phylum Microspora, are important causes of diarrhea, mainly in patients with impaired cell-mediated immunity from AIDS or organ transplantation.[187,188] *E. bieneusi* causes approximately 90% of cases.[189] Microsporidia are identified in as many as 50% of AIDS patients with chronic diarrhea and are the most commonly identified diarrheal pathogen in most series.[188] The prevalence of infection is strongly correlated with decreasing CD4 T-lymphocyte counts, although cases in individuals with CD4 cell counts greater than 200 cells mm^3 are not uncommon.[147,189,190] The pathogenic role of microsporidia in immunocompetent persons is less clear, but it is distinctly less common. Likewise, the reservoir and modes of transmission are not certain.[191-193] Epidemiologic data suggest that water-borne, person-to-person, and possibly sexual transmission occur.

PATHOGENESIS, PATHOLOGY, AND IMMUNOLOGY

Although *E. bieneusi* enters only the cytoplasm of enterocytes, *E. intestinalis* forms a parasitophorous vacuole in enterocytes, endothelial cells, fibroblasts, and macrophages and may disseminate to the kidney, prostate gland, and upper respiratory tract. Typically intestinal pathology is marked by villus atrophy, crypt hyperplasia, and mild inflammation in the lamina propria.[187] The importance of cellular immunity in determining both infection and illness with intestinal microsporidia is indicated by its striking predominance in immunocompromised individuals after organ transplant or in those with AIDS.

CLINICAL FEATURES

Primarily limited to immunocompromised patients, microsporidia cause chronic watery, noninflammatory diarrhea and weight loss, occasionally with abdominal pain, nausea, vomiting, fever, and acalculous cholecystitis or even sclerosing cholangitis.[187] *E. intestinalis* also may cause colitis and dissemination, especially to the kidneys or less often to sinuses, bronchi, conjunctivae, or prostate.[194] Cases of self-limited diarrhea in travelers or health professionals rarely have been reported.[191-193]

DIAGNOSIS

Most laboratories use a modified trichrome stain to identify microsporidia in stool specimens.[195] This method requires considerable skill and has limited sensitivity because of the small size of the spores (1×1.5 μm) (*E. intestinalis* is slightly larger). Sensitivity can be improved by initially screening samples with fluorescent chitin stains such as Fungi-Fluor chitin stain or Uvitex 2B and confirming positive results by modified trichrome staining.[196,197] In addition, Gram stain and electron microscopy may identify the organisms in intestinal biopsy specimens. Sensitive PCR methods have been developed that enable species differentiation, but use of these methods is currently limited to research applications.[193,198]

TREATMENT

E. intestinalis infections (≈10% of cases) respond well to albendazole, 400 mg twice or three times daily for 3 weeks to 3 months.[67] The response of *E. bieneusi* to albendazole is poor, but data indicate that oral fumagillin, 20 mg three times daily for 2 weeks, may be effective for treatment of intestinal *E. bieneusi* infection in immunocompromised patients.[199] Side effects of treatment including neutropenia and thrombocytopenia are frequent and, given the limited clinical data available, this treatment should be undertaken with caution. As with all opportunistic infections in patients with AIDS, effective antiretroviral therapy (i.e., HAART) is essential for controlling microsporidial infections.

CONTROL AND PREVENTION

Because the reservoir and transmission of microsporidia remain unclear, control measures are primarily directed toward appropriate sanitary precautions and handwashing.

TRYPANOSOMA CRUZI (AMERICAN TRYPANOSOMIASIS OR CHAGAS' DISEASE)

EPIDEMIOLOGY

Although symptomatic, Chagas' disease has been confined to South and Central America, at least four autochthonous (indigenous) cases, as well as occasional laboratory-acquired and imported cases of acute Chagas' disease, have occurred in the United States. Increasing numbers of immigrants are presenting with chronic Chagas' disease, however, and pose distinct risks for transmission of Chagas' disease.[200] In patients surviving acute infection with *Trypanosoma cruzi* in whom the chronic form of illness develops, myocardial disease is the most common manifestation. Megaesophagus and megacolon are the most common intestinal manifestations of American trypanosomiasis. Small intestinal dilatation and aperistalsis also are seen. At postmortem examination, even in patients with asymptomatic *T. cruzi* involvement of the intestine, the small intestine has a significant reduction in submucosal and myenteric autonomic plexuses.

American trypanosomiasis could prove to be a significant health problem in the United States. There is a large reservoir of *T. cruzi* infection in animals in the southern United States. Infection has been detected in animals in Arizona, California, New Mexico, Texas, Louisiana, Georgia, Florida, and Maryland; the epidemiologically important insects, the reduviid bugs of the Triatominae group, have the same wide geographic distribution. Infection is transmitted when the reduviid bug infected with *T. cruzi* bites the victim. On biting, the arthropod discharges feces. The parasite is then introduced through the skin when the patient scratches the bite. The apparent difference between the South American reduviid bugs and those found in the United States is that the species in the United States do not defecate on biting, suggesting that infection follows exposure of the mucous membranes to insect feces independent of a bite.

PATHOGENESIS, PATHOLOGY, AND IMMUNOLOGY

Metacyclic trypanosomes are deposited with the feces of the bug during the time it is taking a blood meal. Characteristically, deposition occurs on or near mucous membranes, particularly on the outer canthus of the eye or around the nose or lips. The invading organisms are phagocytosed by histiocytes in the corium and enter the adipose and subcutaneous muscle cells, where they change into the intracellular or amastigote form. The amastigotes multiply intracellularly and, at variable intervals in response to unknown triggers; then they transform into the extracellular bloodstream form or trypomastigote, killing the infected cells and being discharged into the blood and lymphatic circulation to spread to diverse areas of the body. On entry into cells in target organs, the trypomastigotes change back into amastigotes and the cycle begins again.

The signs and symptoms of Chagas' disease are the result of both direct tissue injury and autoimmune damage. Intracellular multiplication of amastigotes results in lysis of both host cells and direct tissue damage as large numbers of parasites escape into the circulation. A brisk immune response occurs that is against the exposed trypomastigotes in the bloodstream. This response does not cure the infection but ultimately suppresses the recurrent parasitemia. Nerve and cardiac epitopes have been shown to cross-react with *T. cruzi* antigens, however, and are believed to trigger chronic autoimmune destruction of cardiac myocytes and the submucosal and myenteric plexuses.

The end result is cardiomyopathy and enteromegaly (Fig. 106–9), which at times may be massive. Immunosuppression as a consequence of chemotherapy or AIDS can reactivate chronic *T. cruzi* infection, causing brain abscesses or acute disease.

CLINICAL FEATURES

Acute Chagas' disease occurs most often in children. It is characterized by high fever and marked edema, particularly with a periorbital distribution, but often involving the entire body. In patients with acute Chagas' disease, the periorbital edema of one or both eyes is striking and is referred to as *Romaña's sign*. The victim may appear to be suffering from myxedema. There usually is enlargement of the thyroid gland, lymph nodes, and salivary glands, and hepatosplenomegaly is present. The acute stage lasts 20 to 30 days.

Chronic Chagas' disease depends on the major organ involvement within the body. Most commonly the symptoms are cardiac, manifested primarily as arrhythmias and congestive heart failure. With megaesophagus, the history is indistinguishable from that of achalasia. With megacolon (see Fig. 106–9), infrequent bowel movements or chronic constipation are the cardinal symptoms. With dilatation of the small intestine, diarrhea or constipation may occur; the markedly dilated bowel may cause abdominal distention and evidence of weight loss.

DIAGNOSIS

Routine laboratory data provide no clue to the diagnosis of Chagas' disease. Diagnosis of acute disease depends on demonstration of the trypanosome forms on blood smears during periods when the amastigotes rupture cells. During febrile periods, if the blood smear results are negative, inoculation of a patient's blood into a guinea pig leads to proliferation of trypanosomes that frequently can be recovered and identified. Amastigote forms may be detected in bone marrow, the spleen, or enlarged lymph nodes.

The most usual immunologic method for diagnosis of American trypanosomiasis is complement fixation. Other immunologic tests are under investigation but not widely applied. Xenodiagnosis has been used but is relatively insensitive, identifying fewer than 50% of patients infected with chronic Chagas' disease. In this technique, trypanosome-free laboratory reduviid bugs are allowed to bite suspected victims. The trypanosomes multiply

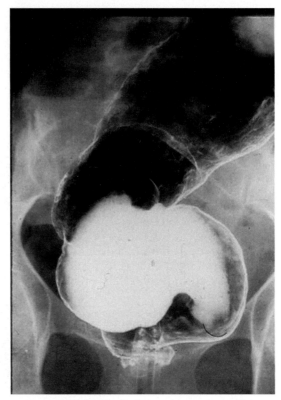

Figure 106–9   Film from a barium enema examination revealing megarectum and megasigmoid in a patient with Chagas' disease. This complication is caused by autoimmune destruction of the submucosal and myenteric nerve plexuses that is believed to be a consequence of a cross-reaction of nerve epitopes with an antigen from *Trypanosoma cruzi*.

rapidly in the intestinal tract of the insect, and examination of the intestine reveals flagellated trypanosomes in 10 to 30 days. Immunologic and PCR-based assays also have been developed.[200]

TREATMENT

Nifurtimox, 8 to 10 mg/kg daily in four divided doses for 90 to 120 days, or benznidazole, 5 to 7 mg/kg daily in two divided doses for 30 to 90 days, can be used for treatment of Chagas' disease.[67] Both are subject to availability problems, have limited efficacy, and are associated with significant side effects including gastrointestinal symptoms in 40% to 70% of patients (nausea, vomiting, abdominal pain, and anorexia) and frequent neurologic sequelae.[201] Patients with achalasia caused by Chagas' disease may be treated with either brusque pneumatic dilatation of the esophagus or esophagomyotomy. Occasionally, aperistaltic segments of intestine that are responsible for symptoms may need be resected.

CONTROL AND PREVENTION

Control and prevention require improved housing, use of insecticides and netting, and screening blood for antibody in endemic areas.

ACKNOWLEDGMENT

I acknowledge Dr. Owen's chapter in the sixth edition, from which the "*Trypanosoma cruzi* (American trypanosomiasis or Chagas' disease)" section was adapted, and Dr. Richard Guerrant, with whom I originally wrote this chapter for the seventh edition.

REFERENCES

1. Diamond LS, Clark CG: A redescription of *Entamoeba histolytica* Schaudinn, 1903 (Emended Walker, 1911) separating it from *Entamoeba dispar* Brumpt, 1925. J Euk Microbiol 40:340, 1993.
2. Haque R, Huston CD, Hughes M, et al: Amebiasis. N Engl J Med 348:1565, 2003.
3. Walsh JA: Problems in recognition and diagnosis of amebiasis: Estimation of the global magnitude of morbidity and mortality. Rev Infect Dis 8:228, 1986.
4. WHO/PAHO/UNESCO: Report: A consultation with experts on amoebiasis. Mexico City, Mexico, 28-29 January, 1997. WHO Epidemiol Bull 18:13, 1997.
5. Haque R, Duggal P, Ali IM, et al: Innate and acquired resistance to amebiasis in Bangladeshi children. J Infect Dis 186:547, 2002.
6. Katz M, Despommier DD, Gwadz R: Parasitic Diseases, 2nd ed. New York, Springer-Verlag, 1989, p 301.
7. Duggal P, Haque R, Roy S, et al: Influence of human leukocyte antigen class II alleles on susceptibility to *Entamoeba histolytica* infection in Bangladeshi children. J Infect Dis 189:520, 2004.
8. Arellano J, Perez-Rodriguez M, Lopez-Osuna M, et al: Increased frequency of HLA-DR3 and complotype SCO1 in Mexican mestizo children with amoebic abscess of the liver. Parasite Immunol 18:491, 1996.
9. Takeuchi A, Phillips BP: Electron microscope studies of experimental *Entamoeba histolytica* infection in the guinea pig: I. Penetration of the intestinal epithelium by trophozoites. Am J Trop Med Hyg 24:34, 1975.
10. Beaver PC, Blanchard JL, Seibold HR: Invasive amebiasis in naturally infected New World and Old World monkeys with and without clinical disease. Am J Trop Med Hyg 39:343, 1988.
11. Chadee K, Meerovitch E: *Entamoeba histolytica*: Early progressive pathology in the cecum of the gerbil (*Meriones unguiculatus*). Am J Trop Med Hyg 34:283, 1985.
12. Ravdin JI, Guerrant RL: Role of adherence in cytopathogenic mechanisms of *Entamoeba histolytica*: Study with mammalian tissue culture cells and human erythrocytes. J Clin Invest 68:1305, 1981.
13. Chadee K, Petri WA Jr, Innes DJ, Ravdin JI: Rat and human colonic mucins bind to and inhibit the adherence lectin of *Entamoeba histolytica*. J Clin Invest 80:1245, 1987.
14. Petri WA Jr, Smith RD, Schlesinger PH, et al: Isolation of the galactose binding lectin of *Entamoeba histolytica*. J Clin Invest 80:1238, 1987.
15. Moncada D, Keller K, Chadee K: *Entamoeba histolytica* cysteine proteinases disrupt the polymeric structure of colonic mucin and alter its protective function. Infect Immun 71:838, 2003.
16. Keene WE, Petitt MG, Allen S, McKerrow JH: The major neutral proteinase of *Entamoeba histolytica*. J Exp Med 163:536, 1986.
17. Li E, Yang WG, Zhang T, Stanley SL Jr: Interaction of laminin with *Entamoeba histolytica* cysteine proteinases and its effect on amebic pathogenesis. Infect Immun 63:4150, 1995.
18. Que X, Reed SL: Cysteine proteinases and the pathogenesis of amebiasis. Clin Microbiol Rev 13:196, 2000.
19. Leippe M, Ebel S, Schoenberger OL, et al: Pore-forming peptide of pathogenic *Entamoeba histolytica*. Proc Nat Acad Sci U S A 88:7659, 1991.
20. Huston CD, Houpt ER, Mann BJ, et al: Caspase 3-dependent killing of host cells by the parasite *Entamoeba histolytica*. Cell Microbiol 2:617, 2000.
21. Seydel KB, Li E, Zhang Z, Stanley SL: Epithelial cell-initiated inflammation plays a crucial role in early tissue damage in amebic infection of human intestine. Gastroenterology 115:1446, 1998.
22. Zhang Z, Wang L, Seydel KB, et al: *Entamoeba histolytica* cysteine proteinases with interleukin-1 beta converting enzyme (ICE) activity cause intestinal inflammation and tissue damage in amoebiasis. Mol Microbiol 37:542, 2000.
23. Eckmann L, Reed SL, Smith JR, Kagnoff MF: *Entamoeba histolytica* trophozoites induce an inflammatory cytokine response by cultured human cells through the paracrine action of cytolytically released interleukin-1 alpha. J Clin Invest 96:1269, 1995.
24. Brandt H, Perez-Tamayo R: The pathology of human amebiasis. Hum Pathol 1:351, 1970.
25. Amebiasis (*Entamoeba histolytica*). In Cotran RS, Kumar V, Robbins SL: Robbins Pathologic Basis of Disease, 4th ed. Philadelphia, WB Saunders, 1989, p 397.
26. Chadee K, Meerovitch E: The pathology of experimentally induced cecal amebiasis in gerbils (*Meriones unguiculatus*): Liver changes and amebic liver abscess formation. Am J Pathol 119:485, 1985.
27. Chadee K, Meerovitch E: The Mongolian gerbil (*Meriones unguiculatus*) as an experimental host for *Entamoeba histolytica*. Am J Trop Med Hyg 33:47, 1984.
28. Gathiram V, Jackson TFHG: A longitudinal study of asymptomatic carriers of pathogenic zymodemes of *Entamoeba histolytica*. South Afr Med J 72:669, 1987.
29. Haque R, Ali IM, Sack RB, et al: Amebiasis and mucosal IgA antibody against the *Entamoeba histolytica* adherence lectin in Bangladeshi children. J Infect Dis 183:1787, 2001.
30. Choudhuri G, Prakash V, Kumar A, et al: Protective immunity to *Entamoeba histolytica* infection in subjects with anti-amoebic antibodies residing in a hyperendemic zone. Scand J Infect Dis 23:771, 1991.
31. Krupp IM: Antibody response in intestinal and extraintestinal amebiasis. Am J Trop Med Hyg 19:57, 1970.
32. Ortiz-Ortiz L, Zamacona G, Sepulveda B, Capin NR: Cell-mediated immunity in patients with amebic abscess of the liver. Clin Immunol Immunopathol 4:127, 1975.
33. del Muro R, Acosta E, Merino E, et al: Diagnosis of intestinal amebiasis using salivary IgA antibody detection. J Infect Dis 162:1360, 1990.
34. Aceti A, Pennica A, Celestino D, et al: Salivary IgA antibody detection in invasive amebiasis and in asymptomatic infection. J Infect Dis 164:613, 1991.
35. Abou el-Magd I, Soong CJ, el-Hawey AM, Ravdin JI: Humoral and mucosal IgA antibody response to a recombinant 52-kDa cysteine-rich portion of the *Entamoeba histolytica* galactose-inhibitable lectin correlates with detection of native 170-kDa lectin antigen in serum of patients with amebic colitis. J Infect Dis 174:157, 1996.
36. Cieslak PR, Virgin HW IV, Stanley SL Jr: A severe combined immunodeficient (SCID) mouse model for infection with *Entamoeba histolytica*. J Exp Med 176:1605, 1992.
37. Kanani SR, Knight R: Relapsing amoebic colitis of 12 years' standing exacerbated by corticosteroids. BMJ 2:613, 1969.
38. Kanani SR, Knight R: Amoebic dysentery precipitated by corticosteroids. BMJ 3:114, 1969.
39. Houpt ER, Glembocki DJ, Obrig TG, et al: The mouse model of amebic colitis reveals mouse strain susceptibility to infec-

tion and exacerbation of disease by CD4[+] T cells. J Immunol 169:4496, 2002.

40. Huston CD, Petri WA: Amebiasis. In Rakel RE, Bope ET (eds): Conn's Current Therapy, 2001. Philadelphia, WB Saunders, 2001, p 50.

41. Speelman P, McGlaughlin R, Kabir I, Butler T: Differential clinical features and stool findings in shigellosis and amoebic dysentery. Trans R Soc Trop Med Hyg 81:549, 1987.

42. Ellyson JH, Bezmalinovic Z, Parks SN, Lewis FR Jr: Necrotizing amebic colitis: A frequently fatal complication. Am J Surg 152:21, 1986.

43. Aristizabal H, Acevedo J, Botero M: Fulminant amebic colitis. World J Surg 15:216, 1991.

44. Kapoor OP, Joshi VR: Multiple amoebic liver abscesses: A study of 56 cases. J Trop Med Hyg 75:4, 1972.

45. Katzenstein D, Rickerson V, Braude A: New concepts of amebic liver abscess derived from hepatic imaging, serodiagnosis, and hepatic enzymes in 67 consecutive cases in San Diego. Medicine 61:237, 1982.

46. Nordestgaard AG, Stapleford L, Worthen N, et al: Contemporary management of amebic liver abscess. Am Surg 58:315, 1992.

47. Kapoor OP, Shah NA: Pericardial amoebiasis following amoebic liver abscess of the left lobe. J Trop Med Hyg 75:7, 1972.

48. Gonzalez-Ruiz A, Haque R, Aguirre A, et al: Value of microscopy in the diagnosis of dysentery associated with invasive *Entamoeba histolytica*. J Clin Pathol 47:236, 1994.

49. Krogstad DJ, Spencer HC, Healy GR, et al: Amebiasis: Epidemiologic studies in the United States 1971-1974. Ann Intern Med 88:89, 1978.

50. Haque R, Neville LM, Hahn P, Petri WA Jr: Rapid diagnosis of *Entamoeba* infection by using *Entamoeba* and *Entamoeba histolytica* stool antigen detection kits. J Clin Microbiol 33:2558, 1995.

51. Sargeaunt PG, Williams JE, Greene JD: The differentiation of invasive and noninvasive *Entamoeba histolytica* by isoenzyme electrophoresis. Trans R Soc Trop Med Hyg 72:519, 1978.

52. Strachan WD, Chiodini PL, Spice WM, et al: Immunological differentiation of pathogenic and non-pathogenic isolates of *Entamoeba histolytica*. Lancet 1:561, 1988.

53. Troll H, Marti H, Weiss N: Simple differential detection of *Entamoeba histolytica* and *Entamoeba dispar* in fresh stool specimens by sodium acetate-acetic acid-formalin concentration and PCR. J Clin Microbiol 35:1701, 1997.

54. Blessman J, Buss H, Ton Nu PA, et al: Real-time PCR for detection and differentiation of *Entamoeba histolytica* and *Entamoeba dispar* in fecal samples. J Clin Microbiol 40:4413, 2002.

55. Britten D, Wilson SM, McNerney R, et al: An improved colorimetric PCR-based method for detection and differentiation of *Entamoeba histolytica* and *Entamoeba dispar* in feces. J Clin Microbiol 35:1108, 1997.

56. Petri WA Jr, Jackson TFHG, Gathiram V, et al: Pathogenic and nonpathogenic strains of *Entamoeba histolytica* can be differentiated by monoclonal antibodies to the galactose-specific adherence lectin. Infect Immun 58:1802, 1990.

57. Haque R, Kress K, Wood S, et al: Diagnosis of pathogenic *Entamoeba histolytica* infection using a stool ELISA based on monoclonal antibodies to the galactose-specific adhesin. J Infect Dis 167:247, 1993.

58. Haque R, Ali IK, Akther S, Petri WA Jr: Comparison of PCR, isoenzyme analysis, and antigen detection for diagnosis of *Entamoeba histolytica* infection. J Clin Microbiol 36:449, 1998.

59. Ong SJ, Cheng MY, Liu KH, Horng CB: Use of the ProSpecT microplate enzyme immunoassay for the detection of pathogenic and non-pathogenic *Entamoeba histolytica* in faecal specimens. Trans R Soc Trop Med Hyg 90:248, 1996.

60. Jelinek T, Peyerl G, Loscher T, Nothdurft HD: Evaluation of an antigen-capture enzyme immunoassay for detection of *Entamoeba histolytica* in stool samples. Eur J Clin Microbiol Infect Dis 15:752, 1996.

61. Mirelman D, Nuchamowitz Y, Stolarsky T: Comparison of use of enzyme-linked immunosorbent assay-based kits and PCR amplification of rRNA genes for simultaneous detection of *Entamoeba histolytica* and *E. dispar*. J Clin Microbiol 35:2405, 1997.

62. Ravdin JI, Jackson TFHG, Petri WA Jr, et al: Association of serum antibodies to adherence lectin with invasive ameabiasis and asymptomatic infection with pathogenic *Entamoeba histolytica*. J Infect Dis 162:768, 1990.

63. Gatti S, Swierczynski G, Robinson F, et al: Amebic infections due to the *Entamoeba histolytica-Entamoeba dispar* complex: A study of the incidence in a remote rural area of Ecuador. Am J Trop Med Hyg 67:123, 2002.

64. Gonin P, Trudel L: Detection and differentiation of *Entamoeba histolytica* and *Entamoeba dispar* isolates in clinical samples by PCR and enzyme-linked immunosorbent assay. J Clin Microbiol 41:237, 2003.

65. Haque R, Mollah NU, Ali IKM, et al: Diagnosis of amebic liver abscess and intestinal infection with the TechLab *Entamoeba histolytica* II antigen detection and antibody tests. J Clin Microbiol 38:3235, 2000.

66. McAuley JB, Herwaldt BL, Stokes SL, et al: Diloxanide furoate for treating asymptomatic *Entamoeba histolytica* cyst passers: Fourteen years' experience in the United States. Clin Infect Dis 15:464, 1992.

67. Drugs for parasitic infections. Med Lett Drugs Ther April 1:1, 2002.

68. Blessmann J, Tannich E: Treatment of asymptomatic intestinal *Entamoeba histolytica* infection. N Engl J Med 347:1384, 2002.

69. McAuley JB, Juranek DD: Paromomycin in the treatment of mild-to-moderate intestinal amebiasis. Clin Infect Dis 15:551, 1992.

70. Nitazoxanide (*Alinia*)—a new anti-protozoal agent. Med Lett Drugs Ther 45:29, 2003.

71. Bassily S, Farid Z, El-Masry NA, Mikhail EM: Treatment of intestinal *E. histolytica* and *G. lamblia* with metronidazole, tinidazole, and ornidazole: A comparative study. J Trop Med Hyg 90:9, 1987.

72. Diaz E, Mondragon J, Ramirez E, Bernal R: Epidemiology and control of intestinal parasites with nitazoxanide in children in Mexico. Am J Trop Med Hyg 68:384, 2003.

73. Rossignol JF, Ayoub A, Ayers MS: Treatment of diarrhea caused by *Giardia intestinalis* and *Entamoeba histolytica* or *Entamoeba dispar*: A randomized, double-blind placebo-controlled study of nitazoxanide. J Infect Dis 184:381, 2002.

74. Powell SJ, Wilmot AJ, Elsdon-Dew R: Further trials of metronidazole in amoebic dysentery and amoebic liver abscess. Ann Trop Med Parasitol 61:511, 1967.

75. Barwick RS, Uzicanin A, Lareau S, et al: Outbreak of ameabiasis in Tblisi, Republic of Georgia, 1998. Am J Trop Med Hyg 67:623, 2002.

76. Huston CD, Petri WA Jr: Host-pathogen interaction in ameabiasis and progress in vaccine development. Eur J Clin Microbiol Infect Dis 17:601, 1998.

77. Ali IKM, Hossain MB, Roy S, et al: *Entamoeba moshkovskii* infections in children in Bangledesh. Emerg Infect Dis 9:580, 2003.

78. Petri WA Jr, Singh U, Ravdin JI: Enteric amebiasis. In Guerrant RL, Walker DH, Weller PF (eds): Tropical Infectious Diseases: Principles, Pathogens, and Practice. Philadelphia, Churchill Livingstone, 2000, p 685.

79. Lucht E, Evengard B, Skott J, et al: *Entamoeba gingivalis* in human immunodeficiency virus type 1-infected patients with periodontal disease. Clin Infect Dis 27:471, 1998.

80. Verweij JJ, Polderman AM, Clark CG: Genetic variation among human isolates of uninucleated cyst-producing *Entamoeba* species. J Clin Microbiol 39:1644, 2001.

81. Desowitz RS, Barnish G: *Entamoeba polecki* and other intestinal protozoa in Papua, New Guinea, Highland children. Ann Trop Med Parasitol 80:399, 1986.

82. Salaki JS, Shirey JL, Strickland GT: Successful treatment of symptomatic *Entamoeba polecki* infection. Am J Trop Med Hyg 28:190, 1979.

83. Qadri SM, al-Okaili GA, al-Dayel F: Clinical significance of *Blastocystis hominis*. J Clin Microbiol 27:2407, 1989.

84. Herwaldt BL, de Arroyave KR, Wahlquist SP, et al: Infections with intestinal parasites in Peace Corps volunteers in Guatemala. J Clin Microbiol 32:1376, 1994.

85. Hill DR: *Giardia lamblia*. In Mandell GL, Bennett JE, Dolin R (eds): Principles and Practice of Infectious Diseases. Philadelphia, Churchill Livingstone, 2000, p 2888.

86. Nash TE, McCutchan T, Keister D, et al: Restriction-endonuclease analysis of DNA from 15 *Giardia lamblia* isolates obtained from humans and animals. J Infect Dis 152:64, 1985.

87. Nash TE, Herrington DA, Losonsky GA, Levine MM: Experimental human infections with *Giardia lamblia*. J Infect Dis 156:974, 1987.

88. Kappus KD, Lundgren RG Jr, Juranek DD, et al: Intestinal parasitism in the United States: Update on a continuing problem. Am J Trop Med Hyg 50:705, 1994.

89. Moore GT, Cross WM, McGuire D, et al: Epidemic giardiasis at a ski resort. N Engl J Med 281:402, 1969.

90. Dennis DT, Smith RP, Welch JJ, et al: Endemic giardiasis in New Hampshire: A case-control study of environmental risks. J Infect Dis 167:1391, 1993.

91. Isaac-Renton JL, Cordeiro C, Sarafis K, Shahriari H: Characterization of *Giardia duodenalis* isolates from a waterborne outbreak. J Infect Dis 167:431, 1993.

92. Isaac-Renton JL, Lewis LF, Ong CS, Nulsen MF: A second community outbreak of waterborne giardiasis in Canada and serological investigation of patients. Trans R Soc Trop Med Hyg 88:395, 1994.

93. Osterholm MT, Forfang JC, Ristinen TL, et al: An outbreak of foodborne giardiasis. N Engl J Med 304:24, 1981.

94. White KE, Hedberg CW, Edmonson LM, et al: An outbreak of giardiasis in a nursing home with evidence for multiple modes of transmission. J Infect Dis 160:298, 1989.

95. Pickering LK, Woodward WE, DuPont HL, Sullivan P: Occurrence of *Giardia lamblia* in children in day care centers. J Pediatr 104:522, 1984.

96. Farthing MJ, Mata L, Urrutia JJ, Kronmal RA: Natural history of *Giardia* infection of infants and children in rural Guatemala and its impact on physical growth. Am J Clin Nutr 43:395, 1986.

97. Fraser D, Dagan R, Naggan L, et al: Natural history of *Giardia lamblia* and *Cryptosporidium* infections in a cohort of Israeli Bedouin infants: A study of a population in transition. Am J Trop Med Hyg 57:544, 1997.

98. Peters CS, Sable R, Janda WM, et al: Prevalence of enteric parasites in homosexual patients attending an outpatient clinic. J Clin Microbiol 24:684, 1986.

99. Oberhuber G, Kastner N, Stolte M: Giardiasis: A histologic analysis of 567 cases. Scand J Gastroenterol 32:48, 1997.

100. Chavez B, Gonzalez-Mariscal L, Cedillo-Rivera R, Martinez-Palomo A: *Giardia lamblia*: In vitro cytopathic effect of human isolates. Exp Parasitol 80:133, 1995.

101. Kamath KR, Murugasu R: A comparative study of four methods for detecting *Giardia lamblia* in children with diarrheal disease and malabsorption. Gastroenterology 66:16, 1974.

102. Ament ME, Rubin CE: Relation in giardiasis to abnormal intestinal structure and function in gastrointestinal immunodeficiency syndromes. Gastroenterology 62:216, 1972.

103. Soliman MM, Taghi-Kilani R, Abou-Shady AF, et al: Comparison of serum antibody responses to *Giardia lamblia* of symptomatic and asymptomatic patients. Am J Trop Med Hyg 58:232, 1998.

104. Nayak N, Ganguly NK, Walia BN, et al: Specific secretory IgA in the milk of *Giardia lamblia*-infected and uninfected women. J Infect Dis 155:724, 1987.

105. Rosales-Borjas DM, Diaz-Rivadeneyra J, Dono-Leyva A, et al: Secretory immune response to membrane antigens during *Giardia lamblia* infection in humans. Infect Immun 66:756, 1998.

106. Zhou P, Li E, Zhu N, et al: Role of interleukin-6 in the control of acute and chronic *Giardia lamblia* infections in mice. Infect Immun 71:1566, 2003.

107. Bienz M, Dai WJ, Welle M et al: Interleukin-6-deficient mice are highly susceptible to *Giardia lamblia* infection but exhibit normal intestinal immunoglobulin A responses against the parasite. Infect Immun 71:1569, 2003.

108. Li E, Zhou P, Ziva P, Singer SM: Mast cell dependent control of *Giardia lamblia* infections in mice. Infect Immun 72:6642, 2004.

109. Stager S, Muller N: *Giardia lamblia* infections in B cell-deficient transgenic mice. Infect Immun 65:3944, 1997.

110. Nash TE, Herrington DA, Levine MM, et al: Antigenic variation of *Giardia lamblia* in experimental human infections. J Immunol 144:4362, 1990.

111. Nash TE: Antigenic variation in *Giardia lamblia* and the host's immune response. Philos Trans R Soc Lond B Biol Sci 352:1369, 1997.

112. Hill DR: Giardiasis: Issues in diagnosis and management. Infect Dis Clin North Am 7:503, 1993.

113. Smith PD, Lane HC, Gill VJ, et al: Intestinal infections in patients with AIDS. Ann Intern Med 108:328, 1988.

114. Aronson NE, Cheney C, Rholl V, et al: Biliary giardiasis in a patient with human immunodeficiency virus. J Clin Gastroenterol 33:167, 2001.

115. Nash TE, Ohl CA, Thomas E, et al: Treatment of patients with refractory giardiasis. Clin Infect Dis 33:22, 2001.

116. Alles AJ, Waldron MA, Sierra LS, Mattia AR: Prospective comparison of direct immunofluorescence and conventional staining methods for detection of *Giardia* and *Cryptosporidium* spp. in human fecal specimens. J Clin Microbiol 33:1632, 1995.

117. Zimmerman SK, Needham CA: Comparison of conventional stool concentration and preserved-smear methods with Merifluor *Cryptosporidium/Giardia* Direct Immunofluorescence Assay and ProSpecT *Giardia* EZ Microplate Assay for detection of *Giardia lamblia*. J Clin Microbiol 33:1942, 1995.

118. Garcia LS, Shimizu RY: Evaluation of nine immunoassay kits (enzyme immunoassay and direct fluorescence) for detection of *Giardia lamblia* and *Cryptosporidium parvum* in human fecal specimens. J Clin Microbiol 35:1526, 1997.

119. Hill DR, Nash TE: Intestinal flagellate and ciliate infections. In Guerrant RL, Walker DH, Weller PF (eds): Tropical Infectious Diseases: Principles, Pathogens, and Practice. Philadelphia, Churchill Livingstone, 2000, p 703.

120. Ortiz JJ, Ayoub A, Gargala G, et al: Randomized clinical study of nitazoxanide compared to metronidazole in the treatment of symptomatic giardiasis in children in Northern Peru. Alim Pharm Ther 15:1409, 2001.

121. Adagu IS, Nolder D, Warhurst DC, Rossignol JF: In vitro activity of nitazoxanide and related compounds against isolates of *Giardia intestinalis*, *Entamoeba histolytica*, and *Trichomonas vaginalis*. J Antimicrob Chemother 2002:103, 2002.

122. Abboud P, Lemee V, Gargala G, et al: Successful treatment of metronidazole- and albendazole-resistant giardiasis with nitazoxanide in a patient with acquired immunodeficiency syndrome. Clin Infect Dis 32:1792, 2001.

123. Bartlett AV, Englender SJ, Jarvis BA, et al: Controlled trial of *Giardia lamblia*: Control strategies in day care centers [published erratum appears in Am J Public Health 1991 Oct;81(10):1251]. Am J Public Health 81:1001, 1991.

124. Olson ME, Ceri H, Morck DW: *Giardia* vaccination. Parasitol Today 16:213, 2000.

125. Faubert GM: The immune response to *Giardia*. Parasitol Today 12:140, 1996.

126. Johnson EH, Windsor JJ, Clark CG: Emerging from obscurity: Biological, clinical, and diagnostic aspects of *Dientamoeba fragilis*. Clin Microbiol Rev 17:553, 2004.

127. Markell EK, Udkow MP: *Blastocystis hominis*: Pathogen or fellow traveler? Am J Trop Med Hyg 35:1023, 1986.

128. Millet V, Spencer MJ, Chapin M, et al: *Dientamoeba fragilis*, a protozoan parasite in adult members of a semicommunal group. Dig Dis Sci 28:335, 1983.

129. Millet VE, Spencer MJ, Chapin MR, et al: Intestinal protozoan infection in a semicommunal group. Am J Trop Med Hyg 32:54, 1983.

130. Spencer MJ, Millet VE, Garcia LS, et al: Parasitic infections in a pediatric population. Pediatr Infect Dis 2:110, 1983.

131. Shein R, Gelb A: Colitis due to *Dientamoeba fragilis*. Am J Gastroenterol 78:634, 1983.

132. Spencer MJ, Garcia LS, Chapin MR: *Dientamoeba fragilis*: An intestinal pathogen in children? Am J Dis Children 133:390, 1979.

133. Dardick KR: Tetracycline treatment of *Dientamoeba fragilis*. Conn Med 47:69, 1983.

134. Keystone JS, Kozarsky P: *Isospora bella, Sarcocystis* species, *Blastocystis hominis*, and *Cyclospora*. In Mandell GL, Bennett JE, Dolin R (eds): Principles and Practice of Infectious Diseases. Philadelphia, Churchill Livingstone, 2000, p 2915.

135. Stenzel DJ, Stein B, Lengy J: A cyst-like stage of *Blastocystis hominis*. Int J Parasitol 21:613, 1991.

136. Doyle PW, Helgason MM, Mathias RG, Proctor EM: Epidemiology and pathogenicity of *Blastocystis hominis*. J Clin Microbiol 28:116, 1990.

137. Nimri LF: Evidence of an epidemic of *Blastocystis hominis* infections in preschool children in northern Jordan. J Clin Microbiol 31:2706, 1993.

138. Shlim DR, Hoge CW, Rajah R, et al: Is *Blastocystis hominis* a cause of diarrhea in travelers? A prospective controlled study in Nepal. Clin Infect Dis 21:97, 1995.

139. Giacometti A, Cirioni O, Fiorentini A, et al: Irritable bowel syndrome in patients with *Blastocystis hominis* infection. Eur J Clin Microbiol Infect Dis 18:436, 1999.

140. Yakoob J, Jafri W, Jafri N, et al: Irritable bowel syndrome—in search of an etiology: Role of *Blastocystis hominis*. Am J Trop Med Hyg 70:383, 2004.

141. Udkow MP, Markell EK: *Blastocystis hominis*: Prevalence in asymptomatic versus symptomatic hosts. J Infect Dis 168:242, 1993.

142. Grossman I, Weiss LM, Simon D, et al: *Blastocystis hominis* in hospital employees. Am J Gastroenterol 87:729, 1992.

143. Markell EK, Udkow MP: Association of *Blastocystis hominis* with human disease? J Clin Microbiol 28:1085, 1990.

144. Markell EK: Is there any reason to continue treating *Blastocystis* infections? Clin Infect Dis 21:104, 1995.

145. Xiao L, Fayer R, Ryan U, Upton SJ: *Cryptosporidium* taxonomy: Recent advances and implications for public health. Clin Microbiol Rev 17:72, 2004.

146. Current WL, Reese NC, Ernst JV, et al: Human cryptosporidiosis in immunocompetent and immunodeficient persons: Studies of an outbreak and experimental transmission. N Engl J Med 308:1252, 1983.

147. Navin TR, Weber R, Vugia DJ, et al: Declining CD4$^+$ T-lymphocyte counts are associated with increased risk of enteric parasitosis and chronic diarrhea: Results of a 3-year longitudinal study. J Acquir Immune Defic Syndr Hum Retrovirol 20:154, 1999.

148. Newman RD, Sears CL, Moore SR, et al: Longitudinal study of *Cryptosporidium* infection in children in northeastern Brazil. J Infect Dis 180:167, 1999.

149. LeChevallier MW, Norton WD, Lee RG: Occurrence of *Giardia* and *Cryptosporidium* spp. in surface water supplies. Appl Environ Microbiol 57:2610, 1991.

150. Mackenzie WR, Hoxie NJ, Proctor ME, et al: A massive outbreak in Milwaukee of *Cryptosporidium* infection transmitted through the public water supply. N Engl J Med 331:161, 1994.

151. Koch KL, Phillips DJ, Aber RC, Current WL: Cryptosporidiosis in hospital personnel: Evidence for person-to-person transmission. Ann Intern Med 102:593, 1985.

152. Cordell RL, Addiss DG: Cryptosporidiosis in child care settings: A review of the literature and recommendations for prevention and control. Pediatr Infect Dis J 13:311, 1994.

153. Miron D, Kenes J, Dagan R: Calves as a source of an outbreak of cryptosporidiosis among young children in an agricultural closed community. Pediatr Infect Dis J 10:438, 1991.

154. Winkelstein JA, Marino MC, Ochs H, et al: The X-linked hyper-IgM syndrome: Clinical and immunologic features of 79 patients. Medicine (Baltimore) 82:373, 2003.

155. Gentile G, Venditti M, Micozzi A, et al: Cryptosporidiosis in patients with hematologic malignancies. Rev Infect Dis 13:842, 1991.

156. Chen XM, Keithly JS, Paya CV, La Russo NF: Cryptosporidiosis. N Engl J Med 346:1723, 2002.

157. Greenberg P, Koch J, Cello J: Diagnosis of *Cryptosporidium parvum* in patients with severe diarrhea and AIDS. Dig Dis Sci 41:2286, 1996.

158. Rossignol JF, Ayoub A, Ayers MS: Treatment of diarrhea caused by *Cryptosporidium parvum*: A prospective randomized, double-blind, placebo-controlled study of nitazoxanide. J Infect Dis 184:103, 2001.

159. Amadi B, Mwiya M, Musuku J, et al: Effect of nitazoxanide on morbidity and mortality in Zambian children with cryptosporidiosis: A randomised controlled trial. Lancet 360:1375, 2002.

160. Rossignol JF, Hidalgo H, Feregrino M, et al: A double-blind placebo-controlled study of nitazoxanide in the treatment of cryptosporidial diarrhoea in AIDS patients in Mexico. Trans R Soc Trop Med Hyg 92:663, 1998.

161. White AC, Chappell CL, Hayat CS, et al: Paromomycin for cryptosporidiosis in AIDS: A prospective, double-blind trial. J Infect Dis 170:419, 1994.

162. Cleaning and disinfection of equipment for gastrointestinal flexible endoscopy: Interim recommendations of a working party of the British Society of Gastroenterology. Gut 29:1134, 1988.

163. Guerrant DI, Moore SR, Lima AAM, et al: Association of early childhood diarrhea and cryptosporidiosis with impaired physical fitness and cognitive function four to seven years later in a poor urban community in Northeast Brazil. Am J Trop Med Hyg 61:707, 1999.

164. Checkley W, Epstein LD, Gilman RH, et al: Effects of *Cryptosporidium parvum* infection in Peruvian children: Growth faltering and subsequent catch-up growth. Am J Epidemiol 148:497, 1998.

165. Ashford RW: Occurrence of an undescribed coccidian in man in Papua, New Guinea. Ann Trop Med Parasitol 73:497, 1979.

166. Huang P, Weber JT, Sosin DM, et al: The first reported outbreak of diarrheal illness associated with *Cyclospora* in the United States. Ann Intern Med 123:409, 1995.

167. Long EG, Ebrahimzadeh A, White EH, et al: Alga associated with diarrhea in patients with acquired immunodeficiency syndrome and in travelers. J Clin Microbiol 28:1101, 1990.

168. Update: Outbreaks of *Cyclospora cayetanensis* infection—United States and Canada, 1996. MMWR Morb Mortal Wkly Rep 45:611, 1996.

169. Ortega YR, Sterling CR, Gilman RH, et al: *Cyclospora* sp: A new protozoan pathogen of humans. N Engl J Med 328:1308, 1993.

170. Relman DA, Schmidt TM, Gajadhar A, et al: Molecular phylogenetic analysis of *Cyclospora*, the human intestinal pathogen, suggests that it is closely related to *Eimeria* species. J Infect Dis 173:440, 1996.

171. Sherchand JB, Cross JH, Jimba M, et al: Study of *Cyclospora cayetanensis* in health care facilities, sewage water, and green leafy vegetables in Nepal. Southeast Asian J Trop Med Public Health 30:58, 1999.

172. Sherchand JB, Cross JH: Emerging pathogen *Cyclospora cayetanensis* infection in Nepal. Southeast Asian J Trop Med Public Health 32:143, 2001.

173. Herwaldt BL, Ackers ML: An outbreak in 1996 of cyclosporiasis associated with imported raspberries: The *Cyclospora* working group. N Engl J Med 336:1548, 1997.

174. Herwaldt BL, Beach MJ: The return of *Cyclospora* in 1997: Another outbreak of cyclosporiasis in North America associated with imported raspberries. Cyclospora Working Group. Ann Intern Med 130:210, 1999.

175. Connor BA, Shlim DR, Scholes JV, et al: Pathologic changes in the small bowel in nine patients with diarrhea associated with a coccidia-like body. Ann Intern Med 119:377, 1993.

176. Berlin OG, Novak SM, Porschen RK, et al: Recovery of *Cyclospora* organisms from patients with prolonged diarrhea. Clin Infect Dis 18:606, 1994.

177. Varea M, Clavel A, Doiz O, et al: Fuchsin fluorescence and autofluorescence in *Cryptosporidium*, *Isospora*, and *Cyclospora* oocysts. Int J Parasitol 28:1881, 1998.

178. Varma M, Hester JD, Schaeffer FW, et al: Detection of *Cyclospora cayetanensis* using a quantitative real-time PCR assay. J Microbiol Methods 53:27, 2003.

179. Hoge CW, Shlim DR, Ghimire M, et al: Placebo-controlled trial of co-trimoxazole for *Cyclospora* infections among travellers and foreign residents in Nepal. Lancet 345:691, 1995.

180. Pape JW, Verdier RI, Johnson WD: Treatment and prophylaxis of *Isospora bella* infection in patients with the acquired immunodeficiency syndrome. N Engl J Med 320:1044, 1989.

181. Pape JW, Verdier RI, Boncy M, et al: *Cyclospora* infection in adults infected with HIV: Clinical manifestations, treatment, and prophylaxis. Ann Intern Med 121:654, 1994.

182. Verdier RI, Fitzgerald DW, Johnson WD, Pape JW: Trimethoprim-sulfamethoxazole compared with ciprofloxacin for treatment and prophylaxis of *Isospora bella* and *Cyclospora cayetanensis* infection in HIV-infected patients: A randomized, controlled trial. Ann Intern Med 132:885, 2000.

183. Osterholm MT: Cyclosporiasis and raspberries—lessons for the future. N Engl J Med 336:1597, 1997.

184. Godiwala T, Yaeger R: *Isospora* and traveler's diarrhea. Ann Intern Med 106:908, 1987.

185. DeHovitz JA, Pape JW, Boncy M, Johnson WD: Clinical manifestations and therapy of *Isospora bella* infection in patients with the acquired immunodeficiency syndrome. N Engl J Med 315:87, 1986.

186. Brandborg LL, Goldberg SB, Briedenbach WC: Human coccidiosis—a possible cause of malabsorption: The life cycle in small-bowel mucosal biopsies as a diagnostic feature. N Engl J Med 283:1306, 1970.

187. Bryan RT, Weber R, Schwartz DA: Microsporidiosis. In Guerrant RL, Walker DH, Weller PF (eds): Tropical Infectious Diseases: Principles, Pathogens, and Practice. Philadelphia, Churchill Livingstone, 2000, p 840.

188. Didier ES: Microsporidiosis. Clin Infect Dis 27:1, 1998.

189. Sobottka I, Schwartz DA, Schottelius J, et al: Prevalence and clinical significance of intestinal microsporidiosis in human immunodeficiency virus-infected patients with and without diarrhea in Germany: A prospective coprodiagnostic study. Clin Infect Dis 26:475, 1998.

190. Hutin YJF, Sombardier MN, Liguory O, et al: Risk factors for intestinal microsporidiosis in patients with human immunodeficiency virus infection: A case-control study. J Infect Dis 178:904, 1998.

191. Sandfort J, Hannemann A, Gelderblom H, et al: *Enterocytozoon bieneusi* infection in an immunocompetent patient who had acute diarrhea and who was not infected with the human immunodeficiency virus. Clin Infect Dis 19:514, 1994.

192. Albrecht H, Sobottka I: *Enterocytozoon bieneusi* infection in patients who are not infected with human immunodeficiency virus. Clin Infect Dis 25:344, 1997.

193. Muller A, Bialek R, Kamper A, et al: Detection of microsporidia in travelers with diarrhea. J Clin Microbiol 39:1630, 2001.

194. Sobottka I, Albrecht H, Schafer H, et al: Disseminated *Encephalitozoon (Septata) intestinalis* infection in a patient with AIDS: Novel diagnostic approaches and autopsy-confirmed parasitological cure following treatment with albendazole. J Clin Microbiol 33:2948, 1995.

195. Weber R, Bryan RT, Owen RL, et al: Improved light-microscopical detection of microsporidia spores in stool and duodenal aspirates. The Enteric Opportunistic Infections Working Group. N Engl J Med 326:161, 1992.

196. Berlin OG, Conteas CN, Porschen RK: Rapid epifluorescent technique to detect microsporidia. AIDS 10:1175, 1996.

197. van Gool T, Snijders F, Reiss P, et al: Diagnosis of intestinal and disseminated microsporidial infections in patients with HIV by a new rapid fluorescence technique. J Clin Pathol 46:694, 1993.

198. Menotti J, Cassinat B, Porcher R, et al: Development of a real-time polymerase-chain-reaction assay for quantitative detection of *Enterocytozoon bieneusi* DNA in stool specimens from immunocompromised patients with intestinal microsporidiosis. J Infect Dis 187:1469, 2003.

199. Molina JM, Tourneur M, Sarfati C, et al: Fumagillin treatment of intestinal microsporidiosis. N Engl J Med 346:1963, 2002.

200. Kirchhoff LV: American trypanosomiasis. In Guerrant RL, Walker DH, Weller PF (eds): Tropical Infectious Diseases: Principles, Pathogens, and Practice. Philadelphia, Churchill Livingstone, 2000.

201. Kirchhoff LV: Changing epidemiology and approaches to therapy for Chagas' disease. Curr Infect Dis Rep 5:59, 2003.

CHAPTER
107 Intestinal Worms

David E. Elliott

Parasitic worms are found worldwide, and modern travel, emigration, and consumption of "exotic" cuisines allow intestinal helminths to appear in any locale. Travel history is a critical, but often overlooked, aspect of the patient interview. Many helminths survive for decades within a host, so even a remote history of visits to or emigration from countries where they are endemic is important. Fresh food is flown around the world and frequently consumed raw, as a result of which patients now can acquire tropical helminths without leaving their industrialized temperate cities. Physicians need to remain alert to the possibility of infection with these organisms because some cause severe disease that requires years to develop or occurs only under special circumstances. For example, patients may have occult *Strongyloides stercoralis* until treatment with glucocorticoids causes fulminant disease; occult *Clonorchis sinensis* until they develop cholangiocarcinoma; or occult *Schistosoma mansoni* until the occurrence of portal hypertension and bleeding from esophageal varices.

In developed countries, we usually stumble across the diagnosis of an intestinal helminth rather than because we actively pursue it. Helminths are complex organisms well adapted to their hosts; like quiet house guests, most cause no symptoms. Worms rarely cause diarrhea and, in most studies, patients with multiple worm infections do not have looser stools than do noninfected individuals. Many medical laboratories do not assay formed stool routinely for parasite eggs. Lack of diarrhea, however, does

not imply lack of helminths, and so physicians need to communicate their concerns of possible helminthic infection to laboratory personnel. A phone call to the local laboratory before the sample is sent can improve diagnostic results dramatically. Occasionally, alarmed patients may bring proglottids or whole worms that they passed with their stools. These specimens should be fixed in 5% aqueous formalin and sent for identification.[1] All specimens should be handled carefully with full precautions to avoid accidental exposure.

Some helminthic infections are difficult to diagnose, especially when the worm burden is light. Diagnosis may require serologic evaluation, analysis of multiple stools, or use of concentration techniques, in addition to a high level of physician awareness. For example, *S. stercoralis* eggs do not appear in the stool and diagnosis is best made serologically. *Ancylostoma caninum* causes eosinophilic enteritis, but doesn't lay eggs when infecting humans.

Although some helminths can cause severe disease, this is unusual. Most individuals colonized with these organisms have no symptoms or illness attributable to the parasites. Only with heavy infections does disease usually result. Well-adapted worms usually act more as commensals than as pathogens. It is even possible that exposure to helminths affords some protection against disease because of excessive immune reactions.[2,3] Helminths induce immune regulatory pathways.[4] Recent studies in mice and rats show that exposure to helminths can be used to prevent or treat colitis,[2,5-8] insulin-dependent diabetes,[9] and autoimmune encephalitis.[10,11] Studies in humans show that helminth exposure improves ulcerative colitis[12] and probably Crohn's disease[13,14] and that helminth eradication increases atopy.[15] Although it remains important to treat helminth infections when they are discovered, further research on these organisms may enable discovery of new approaches to treat immune-mediated disease.

This chapter is divided into three sections: nematodes (roundworms), cestodes (tapeworms), and trematodes (flukes or flatworms). For the most part, each worm is addressed separately, noting its epidemiology, life cycle, clinical manifestations, diagnosis, and treatment.

NEMATODES

ASCARIS LUMBRICOIDES (See also Chapter 79)

Ascaris lumbricoides is the largest of the nematode parasites that colonize humans. Females can grow to 49 cm (19 inches).[16] The name *lumbricoides* alludes to its resemblance to earth worms (*Lumbricus* sp.). The parasite is acquired by ingesting its eggs. *Ascaris* can cause intestinal obstruction and biliary symptoms. Treatment is albendazole.

Epidemiology

A. lumbricoides has a worldwide distribution, although these parasites are most numerous in underdeveloped countries and in areas with poor sanitation. About 25% of the world's population (1.5 billion people) harbor *A. lumbricoides*.[17] Children acquire the parasite by playing in dirt contaminated with eggs, whereas adults most often acquire the infection by farming or eating raw vegetables from plants fertilized with untreated sewage. Pigs harbor *Ascaris suum*, which is closely related to *A. lumbricoides*, but cross infection is rare.[18]

Life Cycle

Humans obtain the parasite by ingesting embryonated eggs that contain third-stage larvae. Freshly deposited fertilized eggs incubate in the soil for 10 to 15 days while the embryo develops and molts twice. The eggs become infective after this incubation period. The eggs are remarkably stable, can survive freezing, and can remain viable for 7 to 10 years. The eggs are resistant to most chemical treatments, including pickling, but they die rapidly in boiling water.

Once ingested, eggs hatch in the duodenum and release their larvae, which penetrate the intestinal wall and enter the mesenteric venules and lymphatics. Larvae migrating with portal blood pass to the liver, through the sinusoids to the hepatic veins, and then through the right heart to enter the lungs. Larvae migrating via the lymphatics pass through mesenteric lymph nodes to the thoracic duct and enter the superior vena cava to arrive in the lungs. The larvae then lodge in the pulmonary capillaries and break into the alveoli, where they molt twice while growing to 1.5 mm in length. Larvae then ascend the tracheobronchial tree, and, arriving in the hypopharynx, they are again swallowed and pass into the small intestine, where they molt again and finally mature.

Mature male *A. lumbricoides* worms are smaller (10 to 30 cm) than mature females (20 to 49 cm). Worms mate in the small intestine and females deposit about 200,000 eggs a day. Adult worms live for about 1 year (6 to 18 months). Because their eggs require incubation in the soil to become infective, *Ascaris* does not multiply in the host. Continued infection requires repeat ingestion of embryonated eggs.

Clinical Features and Pathophysiology

A. lumbricoides produces no symptoms in most infected persons. Often, worms are found unexpectedly on endoscopy or eggs are identified in stool specimens of patients with symptoms not directly attributable to the worms. Disease usually develops only in those with heavy worm burdens: pulmonary, intestinal, and hepatobiliary ascariasis are well described.

Pulmonary ascariasis (*Ascaris* pneumonia) develops 4 to 16 days after ingesting infective eggs as the larva migrate into the alveoli and elicit an inflammatory response that can cause consolidation. The pneumonia usually is self-limited but can be life threatening.

Large numbers of mature worms can cause severe intestinal symptoms, including abdominal pain, distention, nausea, and vomiting. The most common complication of intestinal ascariasis is partial or complete small bowel obstruction; such patients often have a history of passing mature worms in their stool or vomitus. Patients with intestinal obstruction generally have more than 60 worms,[19] and the fortunately rare fatal cases often have more than 600 worms. Fatality results from intestinal necrosis caused by obstruction, intussusception, or volvulus (Fig. 107–1).[20]

A. lumbricoides are highly motile. Mature worms may enter the ampulla of Vater and migrate into the bile or pancreatic ducts (Fig. 107–2),[21] causing biliary pain, obstructive jaundice, ascending cholangitis, acalculous cholecystitis, or acute pancreatitis.[16] The worms may move in and out of the papilla, producing intermittent symptoms and fluctuating laboratory tests. Recurrent ascending cholangitis or acute pancreatitis from ascaria-

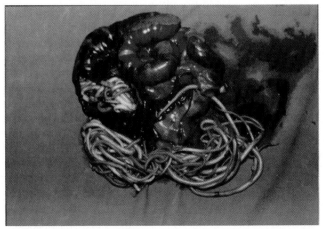

Figure 107–1   Small intestinal obstruction caused by *Ascaris lumbricoides*. (From Wasadikar PP, Kulkarni AB: Intestinal obstruction due to ascariasis. Br J Surg 84:410, 1997.)

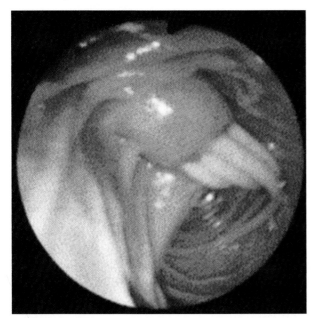

Figure 107–2 Endoscopic view of the duodenum showing four *Ascaris lumbricoides* in the ampulla. (From van den Bogaerde JB, Jordaan M: Intraductal administration of albendazole for biliary ascariasis. Am J Gastroenterol 92:1531, 1997.)

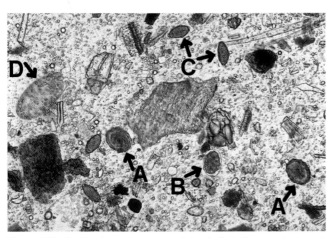

Figure 107–3 Stool specimen containing helminth eggs. *A, Ascaris lumbricoides. B,* Hookworm. *C, Trichuris trichiura. D, Fasciolopsis buski.* (A-D, Courtesy of Mae Melvin, MD, Atlanta, GA.)

sis is rare in highly developed western countries and can be fatal if the diagnosis is not entertained.[22]

Diagnosis

Often it is an alarmed patient that discovers *Ascaris* after passing a motile adult worm with a bowel movement. The worms, however, usually do not cause diarrhea. Most patients do not have specific symptoms or eosinophilia.

Ascaris eggs are visible in direct smears of stool (Fig. 107–3). The eggs begin to appear in the stool about 2 months after initial exposure. Fertilized eggs are 35 × 55 μm and have a thick shell and outer layer; females also lay unfertilized eggs that are larger (90 × 44 μm) and have a thin shell and outer layer. *Ascaris* eggs that lose their outer layer resemble the eggs of hookworms.

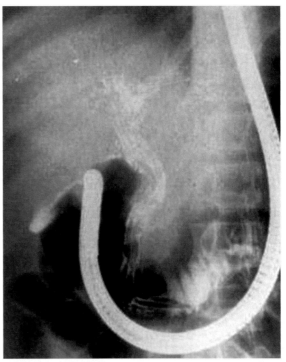

Figure 107–4 Endoscopic retrograde cholangiopancreatography showing several *Ascaris lumbricoides* in the common bile duct. (From van den Bogaerde JB, Jordaan M: Intraductal administration of albendazole for biliary ascariasis. Am J Gastroenterol 92:1531, 1997.)

Adult worms may be seen endoscopically or identified on upper gastrointestinal series as long linear filling defects within the small bowel. The worms retain barium after it has cleared from the patient's gastrointestinal tract, producing linear opacities. Similar findings are seen on endoscopic retrograde cholangiopancreatography (ERCP) if a worm is in the bile or pancreatic duct (Fig. 107–4). *Ascaris* also has a characteristic appearance on ultrasound examination of the biliary tree or pancreas: they appear as long linear echogenic strips that do not cast acoustic shadows, and in cross section they have a "bull's eye" appearance.[23,24]

Treatment

Asymptomatic colonization with *A. lumbricoides* is treated easily with a single 400-mg oral dose of albendazole. Albendazole inhibits glucose uptake and microtubule formation, effectively paralyzing the worms. Albendazole is poorly absorbed but is teratogenic; therefore, its use should be avoided in pregnant women. When possible, treatment should be delayed until after delivery. Patients with pulmonary ascariasis should be treated with glucocorticoids to reduce the pneumonitis and be given two 400-mg doses of albendazole 1 month apart to kill any worms migrating through tissues. Albendazole can cause nausea, vomiting, and abdominal pain.

Intestinal ascariasis with obstruction often can be treated conservatively with fluid resuscitation, nasogastric decompression, antibiotics, and one dose of albendazole. Surgery is not required unless the patient develops signs of volvulus, intussusception, or peritonitis. If the bowel is viable at surgery, an enterotomy allows intraoperative removal of worms. Albendazole can be held until after the obstruction resolves and then is used to eradicate any remaining organisms.

Hepatobiliary ascariasis also can be treated conservatively with fluid resuscitation, bowel rest, and antibiotics.[25] Worms in the bile duct are not effectively treated with albendazole because it is poorly absorbed and not concentrated in the bile. This feature of albendazole is beneficial because intraductal paralyzed worms, unable to pass through the sphincter of Oddi, could become trapped in the bile duct. Patients with hepatobiliary ascariasis should be treated with albendazole each day for several days since the worms become susceptible only when they migrate out of the duct. Ascending cholangitis, acute obstructive jaundice, or acute pancreatitis requires emergent ERCP with worm extraction from the ducts by balloon, basket, or forceps.

STRONGYLOIDES STERCORALIS
(See also Chapter 79)

Strongyloides stercoralis is a free-living tropical and semi-tropical soil helminth that has a larval form that penetrates intact skin. As a parasite, *Strongyloides* lives in the intestine and lays eggs that hatch while still in the gut. Filariform larvae develop within the intestine, migrate along defined paths, and mature to increase the number of adult parasites in the host. Immunosuppression and glucocorticoid treatment cause a fulminant reproduction of parasites that can prove fatal. Treatment is ivermectin.

Epidemiology

S. stercoralis is endemic in tropical and semitropical regions but also can be acquired in rural southeastern United States and northern Italy. *Strongyloides* exists as a free-living organism that does not require a host to replicate. Improved sanitation does not remove the risk of acquiring the parasite from soil. Patients from endemic areas, military veterans that served in Asia, and prisoners of war are at high risk of having subclinical strongyloidiasis.

Life Cycle

Adult male and female *S. stercoralis* live in the soil and lay eggs that hatch rhabditiform larvae. Rhabditiform larvae develop in the soil into mature adults, to complete the life cycle of this worm. Rhabditiform larvae also may develop into longer (500 μm) infective filariform larvae. Filariform larvae can penetrate any area of skin that contacts the soil, after which they migrate through the dermis to enter the vasculature. The larvae circulate in the venous blood until they reach the lungs, where they break into the alveoli and ascend the bronchial tree. The worms then are swallowed with saliva and pass with into the small bowel, where they embed in the jejunal mucosa and mature. Female *S. strongyloides* can lay fertile eggs by parthenogenesis and, therefore, do not require males to reproduce. The eggs hatch within the small bowel and rhabditiform larvae migrate into the lumen. Rhabditiform larvae, not eggs, are passed in the stool.

A critical feature of *S. stercoralis* infection is that rhabditiform larvae can develop into infective filariform larvae within the intestine. Filariform larvae are able to reinfect ("autoinfect") the patient, thereby increasing the parasite burden and permitting prolonged colonization. Subclinical strongyloidiasis may exist for many decades after the host has left an endemic area.

Clinical Features and Pathophysiology

Most patients with *S. stercoralis* have no abdominal symptoms. Patients may have a serpiginous urticarial rash (larva currens) caused by the rapid (5 to 10 cm/hr) dermal migration of filariform larvae. This rash often occurs on the buttocks from larvae entering the perianal skin after they exit the anus during autoinfection. A study of prisoners of war found this creeping eruption to be a far more common symptom of chronic strongyloidiasis than were gastrointestinal complaints.[26] Occasionally, patients have nausea, abdominal pain, or unexplained occult gastrointestinal blood loss due to *S. stercoralis*. The parasite also may cause colonic inflammation that resembles ulcerative colitis but is more right-sided and with a strong eosinophilic infiltrate.[27,28]

While the parasite burden remains balanced, symptoms are minimal or absent. Immunosuppression or glucocorticoid administration upsets this balance. Previously asymptomatic but chronically infected patients develop fulminant, potentially fatal strongyloidiasis from massive autoinfection.[29] The mechanisms that permit massive autoinfection are unknown, but one theory holds that chemotherapy or immunosuppression decreases local eosinophils that may help constrain the parasites. In addition, glucocorticoids may act directly on the parasites to increase the development of infective filariform larvae.[30] Cyclosporine may be partially toxic for *S. stercoralis* and appears to suppress autoinfection during the period of its use.[31]

Massive autoinfection produces disseminated fulminant strongyloidiasis. Migrating filariform larvae injure the intestinal mucosa and carry luminal bacteria into the bloodstream, resulting in polymicrobial sepsis with enteric organisms; *Streptococcus bovis* endocarditis or meningitis may result.[32] Numerous larvae migrating through the lungs cause pneumonitis, and worms may arrive in unusual locations such as the brain. Fulminant strongyloidiasis frequently is fatal.

Diagnosis

Patients with chronic strongyloidiasis often are asymptomatic. Peripheral blood eosinophils may be elevated, but a normal eosinophil count does not argue against infection with this parasite. Currently, the best method for detecting exposure is enzyme-linked immunosorbent assay (ELISA) for IgG antibodies against *S. stercoralis*. This assay is performed by the Centers for Disease Control and Prevention in the United States and is 95% sensitive[33]; sensitivity may be lower for travelers than for immigrants.[34] False-positive reactions can occur in patients exposed to other helminthic parasites.[35] Serologic positivity may indicate prior exposure to *S. stercoralis* and not necessarily active infection. Because chronic strongyloidiasis can remain subclinical and difficult to detect for decades, however, treatment of seropositive patients is warranted. Indeed, some argue that patients even suspected of having strongyloidiasis should be treated empirically before glucocorticoid therapy.[36]

Active infection can be diagnosed by finding rhabditiform larvae in direct smears of the stool, although this is an insensitive method. A 10-fold more sensitive technique is to spread stool on an agar plate and look for serpentine tracks left by migrating larvae.[37] Intestinal biopsy is very insensitive.

Treatment

Chronic strongyloidiasis is best treated with one dose of ivermectin, 200 μg/kg given orally; this dose is used in both adult and pediatric patients. Ivermectin is better tolerated than thiabendazole. Ivermectin paralyzes the intestinal adult worms by interfering with interneuron-motorneuron transmission but has no effect on migrating larvae. Patients can develop recurrent infection from migrating larvae; a repeat dose after 2 weeks reduces this concern. Patients with fulminant, disseminated strongyloidiasis complicating acquired immunodeficiency syndrome require repeat doses 2, 15, and 16 days after the first dose.

PARACAPILLARIA (CAPILLARIA) PHILIPPINENSIS

Capillariasis is acquired by eating raw fish that are infected with the parasite.[38] The nematode causing capillariasis has been renamed from *Capillaria philippinensis* to *Paracapillaria philippinensis*,[39] but by any name it is deadly. The parasite replicates in the host, creating an ever-increasing number of intestinal worms. Patients develop protein-losing, spruelike diarrhea with progressive emaciation and anasarca that ultimately leads to death. Treatment is albendazole.

Epidemiology

The first known human case of capillariasis was reported in 1964. It remains a rare but deadly parasitic infection. From 1965 through 1968, an epidemic in the rural Philippines involved 229 cases, with an overall mortality rate of 30%.[40] As the name implies, *P. philippinensis* is endemic in the Philippines, but it also is endemic in Thailand, and cases occur in Japan, Taiwan, Egypt, and Iran.

Life Cycle

Birds, not humans, are the natural hosts for *P. philippinensis*. In the avian small intestine, the larvae mature into adults. The adults are quite small, measuring up to 3.9 mm for males and 5.3 mm for females. Adult worms mate and produce eggs. Eggs are deposited in bird droppings into ponds and rivers and are swallowed by fish to complete the life cycle.

People become infected with the worm by eating raw or undercooked fresh or brackish water fish that contain the parasite larvae. Some female adult *P. philippinensis* are larviparous and produce infective larvae instead of eggs. These larvae then mature in the small intestine and increase the parasite burden. This pathway of autoinfection permits a massive increase in parasite numbers. A

rhesus monkey initially fed 27 larvae had more than 30,000 worms by 162 days of infection.[41]

Clinical Features and Pathophysiology

Capillariasis produces a progressive spruelike illness. Symptoms begin with vague abdominal pain and borborygmi. Two or three weeks after infection, patients begin to have diarrhea. Initially intermittent, diarrhea becomes persistent and increasingly voluminous. Patients rapidly waste from escalating steatorrhea and protein-losing enteropathy. Eventually they manifest emaciation, anasarca, and hypotension; diarrhea produces severe hypokalemia. If untreated, patients die from cardiac failure or secondary bacterial sepsis usually about 2 months after the onset of symptoms.

The progressive disease is believed to result from an ever-increasing number of poorly adapted intestinal parasites. In autopsy studies, the jejunal intestinal mucosa showed flattened, denuded villi with numerous plasma cells, lymphocytes, macrophages, and neutrophils infiltrating the lamina propria.[38]

Diagnosis

Diagnosis is made by finding eggs and larvae in stool specimens. No serologic tests for capillariasis are available. Symptomatic patients have detectable eggs in their stool. The eggs are easily confused with those of *Trichuris trichiura*, but *T. trichiura* eggs have prominent bipolar plugs that appear cut off in *P. phillipinensis*.[38]

Treatment

Capillariasis requires extended antihelminthic treatment with albendazole 200 mg orally twice a day for 10 days or mebendazole 200 mg orally twice a day for 20 days to prevent recurrence. Albendazole is better tolerated than mebendazole, which can cause headache, diarrhea, and abdominal pain. Extended treatment is necessary because the larvae are resistant to these agents. Both albendazole and mebendazole are teratogenic in rats, but no increase in birth defects was noted in women treated with mebendazole who were unaware they were pregnant.

HOOKWORMS (NECATOR AMERICANUS, ANCYLOSTOMA DUODENALE, AND ANCYLOSTOMA CANINUM)

Worldwide, an estimated 1 billion people are infected with hookworm, usually by *Necator americanus, Ancylostoma duodenale,* or a mixture of both. Hookworm is acquired by skin contact with contaminated soil. Moderate infection can cause iron deficiency. Hookworm should be suspected in patients with eosinophilia and iron deficiency anemia. The dog and cat parasite, *A. caninum,* is a cause of eosinophilic enteritis. Treatment is albendazole.

Necator americanus and *Ancylostoma duodenale*
Epidemiology

N. americanus and *A. duodenale* infect about 20% of the world population. The geographic distribution of the two

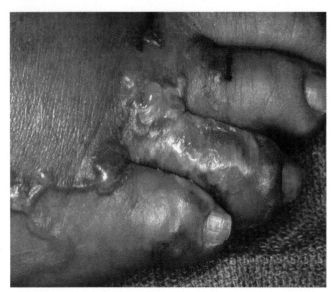

Figure 107–5 A patient's foot with a serpiginous rash caused by hookworm larvae migrating through dermis. (Courtesy of the University of Iowa Department of Dermatology, Iowa City, IA.)

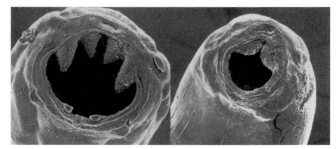

Figure 107–6 View of the buccal cavities of *Ancylostoma duodenale* and *Necator americanus*. (From Hotez PJ, Pritchard DI: Hookworm infection. Sci Am 272:70, 1995.)

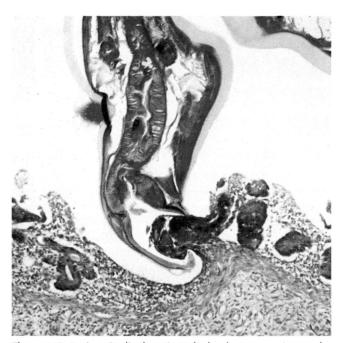

Figure 107–7 Longitudinal section of a hookworm grazing on the intestinal mucosa. (Courtesy of Wayne M. Meyers, Washington, DC.)

species overlaps extensively, but *N. americanus* predominates in the Americas, South Pacific, Indonesia, southern India, and central Africa, whereas *A. duodenale* is more common in north Africa, the Middle East, Europe, Pakistan, and northern India. *Ancylostoma ceylonicum* usually infects cats but also causes some human hookworm infections. Hookworm infection is acquired by contacting soil contaminated with human waste. Hookworm is endemic in tropical-to-warm temperate areas that lack sufficient sewage facilities. Indigenous hookworm infection has been largely eradicated in the United States, although small pockets of transmission still exist.[42]

Life Cycle

Infective third-stage hookworm larvae penetrate intact skin, for example, between the toes of bare feet while walking on contaminated ground. Larvae migrate through the dermis to reach blood vessels. This migration can cause a pruritic, serpiginous rash called *cutaneous larva migrans* (Fig. 107–5). *Ancylostoma braziliense* normally infects dogs and cats but produces a similar rash during its ineffective dermal wandering in humans and is the usual cause of cutaneous larva migrans; *N. americanus, A. duodenale, and A. braziliense* all may cause cutaneous larva migrans. Larvae of *N. americanus* and *A. duodenale* enter blood vessels in the skin and migrate with venous flow through the right heart to the lungs. *A. duodenale* larvae may arrest their migration and become dormant for many months before proceeding to the lungs.[43] In the lungs, larvae penetrate the alveoli and enter the air space, after which they migrate up the pulmonary tree, are swallowed with saliva, and pass into the small intestine, where they mature. Patients also can acquire *A. duodenale* by directly ingesting larvae crawling on contaminated fresh vegetables. Adult worms develop large buccal cavities and graze on the intestinal mucosa, ingesting epithelial cells and blood (Figs. 107–6 and 107–7). Adults are about 1 cm long and can live for up

to 14 years. Mature worms mate and lay eggs. Each female *N. americanus* and *A. duodenale* lays about 10,000 and 20,000 eggs a day, respectively. Eggs are deposited with feces in moist, shady soil, where they hatch to release larvae. The larvae molt twice, after which they move to the soil surface and seek a suitable host.

Clinical Features and Pathophysiology

Light infections with *N. americanus* and *A. duodenale* cause no symptoms.[44] The major consequence of moderate and heavy hookworm infection is iron deficiency. Adult worms feed on intestinal epithelial cells and blood. The closely related *A. caninum* (see later) secretes anticoagulant peptides that inhibit clotting factors[45] and platelet aggregation,[46] thereby preventing hemostasis and permitting the hematophagous parasites to feed on host blood. Intestinal blood loss is estimated to be 0.01 to 0.04 mL/day per adult *N. americanus* and 0.05 to 0.3 mL/day per adult *A. duodenale*.[47] With a moderate number of worms, this blood loss becomes appreciable

(Table 107–1). Iron deficiency results when iron loss outstrips iron absorption.[48] The average North American diet is high in iron, so anemia may not develop, and males with a diet high in iron (>20 mg/day) can tolerate up to 800 adult hookworms without developing anemia.

Diagnosis

Hookworms produce numerous eggs that can be identified on direct smears of formalin-fixed stool (see Fig. 107–3). Evaluation of three stool specimens obtained on separate days should permit the diagnosis of hookworm; however, light infections may require concentration techniques. Eggs mature rapidly at room temperature and may hatch to release larvae. It is difficult to distinguish *N. americanus* eggs from those of *A. duodenale* simply by morphology. The eggs of *Trichostrongylus orientalis* can be mistaken as hookworm eggs.

Treatment

Albendazole 400 mg given orally as a single dose is adequate treatment for hookworm. Mebendazole 100 mg orally twice daily for 3 days also is effective but not as well tolerated. *A. duodenale* larvae can remain in a dormant state for months before maturing and causing relapse, a situation that is treated with a repeat course of albendazole or mebendazole.

Ancylostoma caninum

Epidemiology and Life Cycle

Ancylostoma caninum is a common hookworm of dogs and cats. It has worldwide distribution and is prevalent in the northern hemisphere. The parasite exists in areas with adequate sanitation, because dogs and cats indiscriminately defecate in yards, parks, and sandboxes. The life cycle of *A. caninum* is similar to that of *A. duodenale* and the worm can be acquired orally; however, *A. caninum* does not fully mature in the human host, so no eggs are produced.

Clinical Features and Pathophysiology

A. caninum is a well-recognized cause of cutaneous larva migrans, a distinctive, serpiginous rash caused by an abortive migration of the parasite in an unsupportive host. *A. caninum* also can cause eosinophilic enteritis, although not all eosinophilic enteritis is caused by this parasite (see Chapter 26). Patients with eosinophilic enteritis from *A. caninum* are often dog owners and present with colicky mid-abdominal pain and peripheral eosinophilia[49] but do not recall having cutaneous larva migrans. Intestinal biopsies show high numbers (>45/high-power field) of mucosal eosinophils.[50] Eosinophilic inflammation is most prevalent in distal small bowel and, unlike eosinophilic gastroenteritis, is absent in the stomach. On endoscopy of the terminal ileum, patients may have scattered, small, superficial aphthous ulcers and mucosal hemorrhage.[51] Serologic evidence suggests that *A. caninum* also may be a cause of abdominal pain without eosinophilia or eosinophilic enteritis.[49]

Diagnosis

Diagnosis of *A. caninum* infection is difficult. The parasite never fully matures, does not lay eggs, and is hard to detect. Serologic tests for *A. caninum* are research tools not routinely available at the time of this writing.

Treatment

Albendazole 400 mg as a single oral dose or mebendazole 100 mg orally twice daily for 3 days is adequate to treat *A. caninum* infection. Given for brief periods, these drugs are quite safe. Patients with distal small bowel eosinophilic enteritis not attributable to another cause may benefit from empirical treatment for *A. caninum*.

WHIPWORM (*TRICHURIS TRICHIURA*)

Trichuris trichiura, commonly called "whipworm," has worldwide distribution. People acquire *Trichuris* by ingesting embryonated parasite eggs. Most individuals have no symptoms, although heavy infections are associated with a dysentery-like syndrome. Treatment is mebendazole.

Epidemiology

An estimated 800 million people harbor *T. trichiura*. It occurs in temperate as well as tropical countries and remains prevalent in areas with suboptimal sanitation. In one equatorial Cameroon province, 97% of the school-age children had *T. trichiura*.[52] Whipworm eggs are sensitive to desiccation, so prevalence is low in desert climates.

Life Cycle

T. trichiura has a simple life cycle. Colonization occurs by ingesting the parasite egg, each of which contains one developed larva. The eggs "hatch" in the intestine, and larvae migrate to the cecum, mature, mate, and lay eggs. This process takes about 8 to 12 weeks. Adults worms are approximately 3 cm in length and have a thin tapered anterior region so that the worm resembles a whip (Fig. 107–8). A mature female worm lays about 20,000 eggs per day and can live for 3 years. Eggs are deposited with feces into the soil. Over the next 2 to 6 weeks, one larva develops within each egg, but the egg is not infective until it has fully embryonated. Therefore, *T. trichiura* does not multiply in the host and is not directly transmitted to other persons.

Table 107–1	Iron Losses in Women: Comparison of Loss Due to Hookworm and Physiologic Losses*	
Condition	**Iron Loss, mg/day**
Menstruation	0.44
Pregnancy	2.14
Lactation	0.23
"Moderate" hookworm infection	
Necator americanus (60-200 worms)	1.10
Ancylostoma duodenale (20-100 worms)	2.30

*Losses shown are in addition to the basal iron loss of 0.72 mg/day. Adapted from Stoltzfus R., Dreyfus ML, Chwaya HM, Albonico M: Hookworm control as a strategy to prevent iron deficiency. Nutr Rev 55:223, 1997.

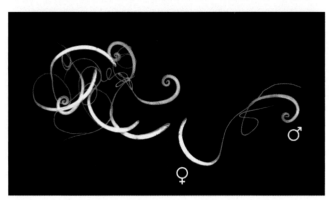

Figure 107–8 Adult male and female whipworms (*Trichuris* species).

Clinical Features and Pathophysiology

Most individuals with *T. trichiura* infection have no symptoms attributable to the parasite. Most people in an endemic area are colonized by small numbers (<15) of worms, and for them the parasite is a commensal organism rather than a pathogen. Some people harbor hundreds or even thousands of worms,[53] and they are the ones who develop symptoms[54]; this bimodal distribution of infection persists after patients are treated and then become reinfected naturally, suggesting that unique host factors (genetic or behavioral) help determine the worm burden in an individual.

Rectal prolapse can occur in children with extremely high numbers of *T. trichiura* worms.[55] Some individuals with numerous worms have mucoid diarrhea and occasional bleeding, a combination of symptoms called the *Trichuris dysentery syndrome* (TDS). Children with this condition appear to have growth retardation[56], however, studies attributing these symptoms to *T. trichiura* are difficult to interpret because individuals with TDS often are socioeconomically deprived and may be coinfected with other pathogens.

Colonic biopsies from children with TDS show little or no pathology compared with those of healthy local children,[57] other than an increase in mast cells[58] and in the number of cells that express tumor necrosis factor-α and calprotectin.[59]

A different but closely related species, *Trichuris muris*, infects mice. Mouse strains that react to the parasite with a strong Th2 response, characterized by production of interleukin (IL)-4, IL-5, and IL-13, are able to expel the worms, whereas strains that respond with a type 1 (Th1) response (interferon [IFN]-γ) have difficulty expelling the worms.[60] Blocking IL-4 makes resistant strains susceptible and blocking IFN-γ makes susceptible strains resistant to chronic infection with *T. muris*.[61] The type of immune response developed by inbred mice to *T. muris* is an important factor in determining length and intensity of infection. A similar response in humans may explain why some people repeatedly acquire heavy infections, whereas others carry only a few worms.

Diagnosis

Diagnosis is made by identifying *T. trichiura* eggs in stool specimens. *Trichuris* eggs are $23 \times 50\ \mu m$ in size and have characteristic "plugs" at each end (see Fig. 107–3).

Treatment

T. trichiura is treated with mebendazole 100 mg twice a day for 3 days; alternatively, patients can take albendazole 400 mg each day for 3 days. Heavily infected patients may require 7 days of treatment.[62] Single-dose treatment with a combination of albendazole (400 mg) and ivermectin (200 µg/kg) also appears quite effective, with cure rates of up to 80% and egg reduction rates of 94%.[63,64]

PINWORM (*ENTEROBIUS VERMICULARIS*)

Enterobius vermicularis, commonly called "pinworm," is the most common helminthic parasite encountered by primary care providers in developed nations. It is acquired by ingesting parasite eggs. Most people have no symptoms from the parasite. Diagnosis is made by the cellophane tape test. Treatment is mebendazole for the affected patient and for all family members.

Epidemiology

E. vermicularis is a quintessential intestinal parasite with no geographic constraints. It is transmissible by close contact with colonized individuals. People have had pinworm for thousands of years, and before modern sanitation, colonization by pinworm probably was universal. *E. vermicularis* eggs were identified in a 10,000-year-old human stool (coprolite) found in Utah.[65] The pinworm *Enterobius gregorii*, originally thought to be a separate species of pinworm,[66,67] actually may be just a young adult form of *E. vermicularis*.[68]

People of every socioeconomic group may acquire pinworm infection, and it remains quite prevalent. School-age children are colonized most commonly, thereby permitting other household members to acquire the parasite. Crowding and institutionalization promote acquisition. Eggs can survive in the environment for approximately 15 to 20 days and are resistant to chlorinated water (e.g., swimming pools).

Pinworm remains common in many areas but appears to be decreasing in prevalence. A survey of positive cellophane tape tests (see later) in New York City documented a sharp decline in positivity from 57 out of 248 tests in 1971 to 17 of 165 in 1978 to 0 of 38 in 1986.[69] Similar trends are reported from California.

Life Cycle

E. vermicularis has a simple life cycle with a "hand-to-mouth" existence. The worm is acquired by ingesting parasite eggs. Most often these eggs are on the hands of the host; however, the small eggs also may become airborne, inhaled, and then swallowed.

Eggs hatch in the duodenum, releasing larvae that molt twice as they mature and then migrate to the cecum and ascending colon (Fig. 107–9). Adult parasites are small: males measure 0.2×2 to 5 mm and females measure 0.5×8 to 13 mm. After mating, gravid females migrate to the rectum. During the night, egg-laden females migrate out of the anal canal and onto the perianal skin. Each female deposits up to 17,000 eggs, which mature rapidly, becoming infective within 6 hours. Pinworm infection fre-

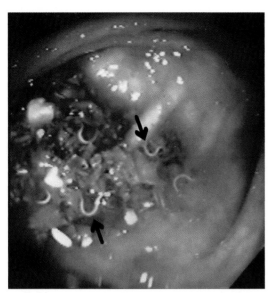

Figure 107–9 Pinworms (*Enterobius vermicularis*) (*arrows*) found on screening colonoscopy of an institutionalized man.

quently causes perianal itching, and scratching gathers eggs onto the hands, promoting reinfection and transmission to others.

Clinical Features and Pathophysiology

E. vermicularis is an extremely well-adapted parasite that produces no specific symptoms in most colonized persons. Most symptoms are minor such as pruritus ani and restless sleeping. Pinworm does not cause eosinophilia or appendicitis, although one case report implicated a heavy synchronous *E. vermicularis* exposure with development of eosinophilic colitis in a homosexual man.[70]

Vulvovaginitis is more frequent in girls with pinworm than girls without this infection. Vulvovaginitis may be caused by migration of the worms into the introitus and genital tract. Dead worms and eggs encased in granulomas have been found in the cervix, endometrium, fallopian tubes, and peritoneum, attesting to the migratory effort of female worms.[71] Ectopic enterobiasis is rare and causes no or little overt pathology.

Diagnosis

E. vermicularis eggs are not plentiful in stool. This may account for the low prevalence rates determined by studies that use only stool specimens. The National Institutes of Health cellophane tape test is the classic diagnostic test for pinworm. A 2- to 3-inch piece of clear tape is applied serially to several perianal areas in the morning before washing. The tape is then applied to a glass slide. Microscopic evaluation demonstrates parasite eggs that measure 30×60 µm, have a thin shell, and appear flattened on one side. Three to seven daily samples are needed to exclude pinworm infection.

Treatment

Pinworm actually requires no treatment unless the patient is symptomatic. It is highly transmittable, however, and for that reason should be expunged. *E. ver-*

micularis is treated readily with a single 100-mg dose of mebendazole or a 400-mg dose of albendazole. Reinfection is common, and patients should receive a second treatment after 15 days. All members of the family should be treated and clothes and bed linens washed. Albendazole and mebendazole are teratogenic and should not be given to pregnant women.

TRICHINELLA SPECIES (See also Chapter 79)

Trichinosis is a systemic illness caused by any of the five closely related *Trichinella* species. People acquire the parasite by ingesting larvae present in raw or undercooked meat such as pork. Trichinosis has both intestinal and systemic phases characterized sequentially by nausea and diarrhea, fever, myalgia, and periorbital edema. Intense exposure can cause death due to severe myositis, neuritis, and thrombosis. Treatment is albendazole and glucocorticoids.

Epidemiology

Trichinosis is acquired by eating raw or undercooked meat that contains parasite larvae. Domestic pigs are the most common carriers. Human disease is caused by five closely related *Trichinella* species: *Trichinella spiralis*, *Trichinella pseudospiralis*, *Trichinella britovi*, *Trichinella nelsoni*, and *Trichinella nativa*; these species can be distinguished using molecular approaches.[72] *Trichinella* has worldwide distribution with *T. spiralis* and *T. pseudospiralis* in the Americas, Europe, and Russia; *T. britovi* in Europe, North Africa, the Middle East, and Asia; *T. nelsoni* in equatorial Africa; and *T. nativa* in the Arctic and subarctic regions. *T. nativa* is resistant to freezing. Each of the *Trichinella* species can infect any mammal, and *T. pseudospiralis* also can infect birds.

Trichinosis was much more common in the United States than it is now. In the late 1940s, about 400 cases per year of symptomatic trichinosis were reported to various health agencies, and this number dropped to an average of 14.4 cases per year in the period of 1997-2001[73]; reports from Germany show a similar pattern.[74] This decrease is explained by two major factors: first is the strong admonition to thoroughly cook all pork products, and second is a change in farming practice to now feed pigs only grain. Trichinosis is a re-emerging illness in eastern Europe, however, related in part to relaxation of regulations.[75]

Currently, most reported cases involve a discrete exposure. For example, a 1991 outbreak in Wisconsin involved 40 people who ate pork sausage from one shop. A 1995 outbreak in Idaho involved 10 people who ate cougar jerky.[76] In France, several outbreaks have resulted from eating raw horse meat.[77] This emphasizes that all mammals including herbivores can transmit *Trichinella*.

Life Cycle

The same host harbors both the adult and larval forms of *Trichinella*.[78] People acquire the parasite by eating raw or undercooked meat that contains encapsulated parasite larvae. Each cyst dissolves in the digestive tract, releasing one larva that invades the small intestinal mucosa, and lives within the cytoplasm of about 45 villus cells (Fig. 107–10). Larvae mature rapidly and mate within 30 hours. Adults are minute, with males measuring 60 µm × 1.2 mm and females measuring 90 µm × 2.2 mm. Females are viviparous and begin releasing larvae about 1 week after initial ingestion. Adults are short-lived, producing larvae for only 4 weeks, by which time they are expelled by the host.

The larvae live longer. Larvae measure 6 × 100 µm and enter the blood and lymphatic vessels. They are distributed through the body but develop only within striated muscle. The larva enters a striated muscle fiber but does not kill the myocyte. Instead, it induces the cell to transform into a novel "nurse cell" that houses and feeds the parasite. The larva grows and develops into the infective stage in about 5 weeks. A capsule forms around the coiled larvae as it awaits ingestion by another carnivore. The encapsulated larva remain viable for many years.

Clinical Features and Pathophysiology

Although most infections with *Trichinella* are asymptomatic, significant exposure produces illness and even death.[79] Clinical trichinosis has two phases caused by the enteral (adult) and parenteral (larval) stages of the parasite. Intestinal symptoms result from enteritis caused by adult worms that have embedded themselves in the intestinal epithelium. Enteritis produces abdominal pain, nausea, vomiting, diarrhea, and low-grade fever. Intestinal symptoms begin about 2 days to 1 week and peak at 2 weeks after ingestion of contaminated meat. The timing and severity of symptoms vary with intensity of exposure. The intestinal phase of trichinosis often is misdiagnosed as viral gastroenteritis or "food poisoning."

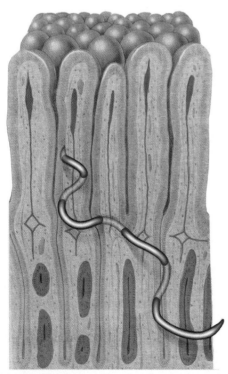

Figure 107–10 Illustration of *Trichinella spiralis* coiled through enterocytes in the small intestine.

T. spiralis also infects mice and rats, permitting detailed study of the intestinal phase of infection.[80] Mice begin to expel adult worms about 2 weeks after initial infection. Th2 cytokines (IL-4 and IL-5) promote worm expulsion. Expulsion of adult worms results from focal immune attack, increased secretions, and enhanced intestinal motility; T lymphocytes, eosinophils, and mast cells assist this primary response. Rats previously exposed to *T. spiralis* rapidly expel the parasite on rechallenge, a protection likely resulting from an immediate-type hypersensitivity response to the parasite triggered by IgE-armed mast cells.

The parenteral phase of trichinosis begins with the birth of migratory larvae about 1 week after ingestion of the contaminated meat. Larvae migrate into muscle and other organs such as the brain, spinal cord, and heart, evoking inflammatory responses; high fever, myalgia, periorbital edema, dysphagia, headache, and paresthesia result. Symptoms peak about 4 to 5 weeks after initial exposure and can take months to resolve. The severity and timing of symptoms vary with the intensity of exposure. Many patients develop systemic complaints without prior intestinal symptoms.

The inflammatory response to migrating larvae produces myositis. Patients have eosinophilia and an elevated creatine phosphokinase level. An intense exposure can cause fatal myocarditis, neuritis, and vasculitis/thrombosis. Patients are at highest risk of death between the 3rd and 6th week after exposure. Because trichinosis is rare, index cases often are misdiagnosed initially. Multiple individuals presenting in a narrow time frame and with similar and compatible symptoms should prompt consideration of trichinosis as the diagnosis.

Diagnosis

Trichinella cannot by diagnosed by stool examination or intestinal biopsy. *Trichinella* species do not lay eggs. No larvae are present in stool specimens. Even with heavy infections, adult worms are too infrequent to be found by random biopsy. Diagnosis is made by muscle biopsy demonstrating larvae within nurse cells. Diagnosis also can be made by serology. Acute and convalescent serum samples confirm a rise in anti-*Trichinella* antibody. ELISA usually detect IgG antibody against the muscle-stage larvae excretory-secretory antigens. Peak antibody production occurs after about 2 months and lasts for years.

Treatment

Although adults are short lived, treatment with albendazole 400 mg twice a day or mebendazole 5 mg/kg/day for 10 to 15 days is warranted.[81] Treatment abbreviates the production of larvae by adult worms. Addition of glucocorticoids reduces inflammation and systemic symptoms; however, glucocorticoids given in the absence of a benzimidazole can prolong the intestinal phase, increasing the number of larvae released.

ANISAKIS SIMPLEX

Anisakis simplex and another anisakid, *Pseudoterranova decipiens*, can infect people and transiently cause abdominal pain, hematemesis, or intestinal inflammation. Anisakis infection also is a cause of food allergy. It is acquired by eating raw or undercooked fish. Usually, no treatment is required.

Epidemiology and Life Cycle

A. simplex and *P. decipiens* infect fish and marine mammals. People become accidental hosts by eating raw or pickled fish. Instances of anisakiasis have become more common with the increased popularity of eating raw fish (e.g., sushi and sashimi). Many species of salt-water fish harbor *A. simplex* including herring, mackerel, salmon, plaice, and even squid. The parasite initially infects crustaceans that are consumed by fish. The fish are then eaten by marine mammals that serve as definitive hosts for the intestinal worm. Adult intestinal worms lay eggs that are passed with the fish feces. The eggs hatch to release larvae that infect crustaceans and renew the life cycle.

Clinical Features and Pathophysiology

A. simplex and *P. decipiens* cause transient infections in humans. Anisakids do not reach full maturity and therefore produce no eggs. The most common gastrointestinal symptom is acute severe stomach pain with nausea and hematemesis shortly after eating raw fish. Endoscopy may demonstrate a small larva partially penetrating the gastric or intestinal wall.[82,83] Rarely, *A. simplex* can enter the intestinal wall and cause a strong inflammatory reaction that may mimic acute appendicitis[84] or Crohn's disease.

A. simplex is a potent allergen. Many cases of seafood (fish) allergy actually may be reaction to *A. simplex*,[85] including anaphylaxis from well-cooked marine fish.[86]

Diagnosis and Treatment

A history of recent (within 3 days) ingestion of raw fish and compatible symptoms suggests anisakiasis. Diagnosis is made by finding larvae on endoscopy or in surgically excised specimens. Gastric anisakiasis is diagnosed by endoscopy, and endoscopic removal of the anisakid alleviates symptoms. Intestinal anisakiasis usually involves the terminal ileum. Surgery is performed on patients that present with symptoms of acute small bowel obstruction or peritonitis.[87]

A. simplex and P. decipiens infections are transient because the parasites do not survive in humans. Therefore, treatment with an antelminthic is not needed.

CESTODES

DIPHYLLOBOTHRIUM SPECIES

Fish tapeworm (*Diphyllobothrium* species) is the largest parasite of humans, reaching lengths of up to 40 feet (12 m). People acquire the parasite by eating raw or undercooked fresh water fish. *Diphyllobothrium latum* absorbs dietary cobalamin and can cause vitamin B$_{12}$ deficiency over time. Treatment is albendazole.

Epidemiology

D. latum is most common, but other *Diphyllobothrium* species (e.g., *Diphyllobothrium dendriticum*) can colonize humans.[88] *D. latum* is endemic in northern Europe, Russia, and Alaska. Fish tapeworm has been reported in Africa, Japan, Taiwan, Australia, South America, North America, and Canada.[89]

Life Cycle

Fish tapeworm has a complex life cycle with two intermediate hosts. Parasite eggs that reach fresh water embryonate and then release free-swimming larvae called *coracidia*. Coracidia are ingested by water fleas (*Cyclops* and *Diaptomus*) and develop into procercoid larvae. Fresh-water fish eat these small crustaceans, and the parasite changes into the infective plerocercoid form. If an infected fish is consumed by another fish, the plerocercoid larva simply migrates into the flesh of the second fish. Trout, salmon, pike, perch, and whitefish all can harbor *D. latum*. The plerocercoid larva embed in fish muscle and organs, growing to 2 cm in length. People acquire the parasite by eating raw or undercooked fish. *D. latum* also can colonize many other mammals such as dogs, cats, bears, and seals. In mammals, the ingested plerocercoid larva attaches to the wall of the small intestine and matures into an adult worm. A long chain of proglottids, called the *strobila*, develops off the scolex (Fig. 107–11). *D. latum* is the largest parasite of humans, reaching 40 feet (12 m) in length. The proglottids release eggs into the lumen that pass with the feces.

Clinical Features and Pathophysiology

Fish tapeworm is not invasive and causes no direct symptoms. The worm obtains nutrients by absorbing luminal contents through its surface. *D. latum* produces a sub-

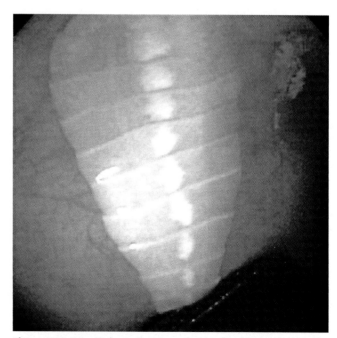

Figure 107–11 Endoscopic view of part of a fish tapeworm (the strobila with mature proglottids) in the cecum in a middle-aged woman with watery diarrhea after a fishing trip in Northern Canada. She also frequently ate sushi. The worm, which was several feet long, was residing in the small intestine and was retrieved by suction. She was treated successfully with praziquantel. (Courtesy of Roy Joseph, MD, Denton, TX.)

stance that splits vitamin B_{12} from intrinsic factor in the intestine,[90] interfering with host absorption of the vitamin. The tapeworm also avidly absorbs vitamin B_{12}, effectively competing with its host. *D. latum* is long-lived and, over time, can cause significant vitamin B_{12} deficiency in patients with limited dietary cobalamin. Rarely, severe vitamin B_{12} deficiency results in megaloblastic anemia and neurologic symptoms.

Diagnosis and Treatment

Fish tapeworm is diagnosed by identifying *D. latum* eggs in stool specimens. Occasionally, proglottids are passed that also are diagnostic. Praziquantel is effective in a single oral dose of 10 mg/kg. Patients should be warned that they may pass a rather long worm 2 to 5 hours after taking the medication. Albendazole 400 mg each day for 3 days also kills the tapeworms.

TAENIA SAGINATA AND *TAENIA SOLIUM*

An estimated 50 million people are colonized with beef (*Taenia saginata*) or pork (*Taenia solium*) tapeworm. Colonization occurs by eating raw or undercooked meat infested with cysticerci. Tapeworms usually cause no symptoms and may surprise an endoscopist who finds the unsuspected jejunal inhabitant. Ingestion of *T. solium* eggs causes cysticercosis, a potentially fatal disease. Treatment is praziquantel or albendazole.

Epidemiology

Beef and pork tapeworm occur where livestock are exposed to untreated human waste and people eat raw or undercooked meat. Both parasites have a worldwide distribution, although infections originating in the United States and Europe are rare. Beef tapeworm is endemic in Africa, the Middle East, Eastern Europe, Asia, and Latin America. Pork tapeworm is endemic in Africa, India, China, Asia, and Latin America. *T. solium* is rare in Muslim countries where pork consumption is prohibited. *T. solium* is considered an eradicable parasite,[91] although progress in such eradication is slow; livestock vaccination may assist this goal.[92]

Life Cycle

Adult tapeworms release gravid proglottids, each containing up to 100,000 eggs. Proglottids and eggs are passed with the stool. Proglottids of *T. saginata* remain motile and may crawl out of the feces, prompting patient alarm. Untreated human waste used to fertilize fields allows cattle to eat infective eggs on vegetation. Free-ranging pigs are coprophagous and directly consume poorly disposed human waste. Ingested eggs release an embryo (oncosphere) that penetrates the intestinal wall and enters the blood vessels or lymphatics. The parasites are carried to subcutaneous tissue, muscle, and organs where they develop into cysticerci. The cysticerci can live for several years, until human consumption of infected meat. Once in human intestine, the cysticercus evaginates to form a scolex that serves as the anterior attachment point of the tapeworm to the mucosa of the proximal jejunum. The worm develops over several

months as proglottids form and mature in a chain behind the scolex. This long tapelike chain is called the *strobila*. Beef tapeworms can reach 4 to 10 m, and pork tapeworms 2 to 4 m in length. Mature gravid proglottids break away from the distal end of the worm and pass with the stool to complete the life cycle. Adult worms can live in the small intestine for 25 years.

Clinical Features and Pathophysiology

Most people colonized with adult *T. saginata* or *T. solium* are asymptomatic. Colonization usually is limited to one worm that obtains nutrients by absorbing luminal contents through its surface. Motile proglottids may crawl out of the anus or "swim" in the toilet eliciting immediate concern. Rarely, acute biliary or pancreatic duct obstruction can occur if proglottids migrate into these sites.

The most feared complication of *T. solium* infection is cysticercosis,[93] which occurs when people inadvertently consume *T. solium* eggs. Just as in pigs, the eggs release oncospheres that penetrate the intestinal wall, disseminate through the body, and form cysticerci. Cysticerci produce localized inflammation in the brain, spinal cord, eye, and heart with dire consequences. Neurocysticercosis is a common cause of epilepsy in countries where *T. solium* is endemic. An estimated 50,000 people die of neurocysticercosis each year. Because the disease occurs after ingestion of parasite eggs, neurocysticercosis in a patient who has not visited or emigrated from an endemic country should prompt an effort to identify local carriers.

Diagnosis

Beef and pork tapeworm is diagnosed by identifying eggs or proglottids in stool specimens. The eggs of the two species are indistinguishable microscopically. The proglottids of *T. saginata* are 2 cm long and have more than 12 uterine branches, whereas those of *T. solium* measure 1.2 cm and have fewer than 10 uterine branches.[89] Egg and proglottid production can be sporadic, necessitating repeated stool tests. Cysticercosis usually is diagnosed by computed tomography (CT) or magnetic resonance imaging and confirmed by serology using a larval cyst antigen–specific immunoblot assay.

Treatment

Praziquantel is effective in a single oral dose of 10 mg/kg. Albendazole 400 mg each day for 3 days also kills the tapeworms. The worms usually break apart and are passed as sections of disintegrating strobilae. Patients with cysticercosis should be treated with albendazole 15 mg/kg each day for 8 days to kill the cysticerci. Local inflammation transiently increases as cysticerci die and thus seizures may occur or worsen as neurocysticercosis is treated. The addition of glucocorticoids prevents exacerbation of neurocysticercosis during therapy.

HYMENOLEPIS NANA AND *HYMENOLEPIS DIMINUTA*

Hymenolepis nana (dwarf tapeworm) is the smallest, but most common, tapeworm that colonizes humans. It can be transmitted directly from person to person. Self-inoculation or internal autoinfection permits accumulation of a large number of worms that can cause anorexia, abdominal pain, and diarrhea. *Hymenolepis diminuta* (rodent tapeworm) is larger and rarely colonizes humans. It is acquired by ingesting infected insects and usually causes no symptoms. Treatment is praziquantel.

Epidemiology

H. nana is the most common tapeworm of humans. Unlike other tapeworms, it can be transmitted from person to person without the need of an intermediate host. Dwarf tapeworm has a worldwide distribution. Prevalence is highest in warm and arid regions. A survey of Egyptian children found that 16% carried *H. nana*,[94] and it was found in 54% of individuals within a coastal Australian aboriginal community.[95] In the United States, a 1987 survey of state diagnostic laboratories found that 900 of 216,000 submitted stool specimens demonstrated *H. nana*, with 34 states reporting positive specimens.[42] *H. nana* also colonizes mice and rats; however, the strains that colonize people appear to differ from those of rodents.

Human colonization with *H. diminuta* is rare but also enjoys a worldwide distribution. Rats and mice are the parasite's usual hosts. Humans, usually young children, acquire rodent tapeworm by ingesting fleas, grain beetles, mealworms, or cockroaches infested with larval forms of the parasite. The incorporation of beetles in traditional oriental medications also permits transmission of *H. diminuta*.[96]

Life Cycle

H. nana does not require an intermediate insect host. Ingested eggs release oncospheres that invade the small intestinal mucosa, lodge within the lymphatics of the villi, and then develop into cysticercoid larvae. Each cysticercoid larva then ruptures into the lumen and evaginates to form a scolex that attaches to the mucosa of the ileum. The worms mature growing a strobila or chain of developing proglottids. Adult worms average 2 cm in length and have about 200 proglottids, each containing about 150 eggs; the most distal proglottids disintegrate to release eggs into the lumen. About 20 to 30 days after initial ingestion, the worm begins to shed eggs in the stool; eggs shed in the stool are infective immediately. *H. nana* adults live for only 4 to 6 weeks, but self-inoculation or internal autoinfection allows colonization to persist for years. Limited sanitation or poor hand-washing permits transmission to others.

Like other *Hymenolepis* species, *H. nana* can infect insects and form cysticercoid larvae. Ingestion of infected fleas, beetles, mealworms, or cockroaches allows transmission of *H. nana*; however, acquisition by this pathway is rare. Most transmission is by direct ingestion of eggs.

H. diminuta requires intermediate insect hosts. Insects ingest eggs as they consume rodent droppings. The eggs release oncospheres that penetrate into the insect's viscera and form cysticercoid larvae. Rats and mice that eat infected insects acquire the tapeworm. People acquire rodent tapeworm the same way, by eating infected insects. Once in the intestine, the cysticercoid larva evaginates to form a scolex that attaches to the ileal mucosa.

The worm matures, growing a strobila that reaches a length of up to 90 cm. The most distal proglottids disintegrate, releasing eggs into the intestinal lumen.

Clinical Features and Pathophysiology

Most people colonized with *H. nana* or *H. diminuta* have no symptoms; however, self-inoculation or internal autoinfection can cause heavy infections with *H. nana* resulting in anorexia, abdominal pain, and diarrhea.

Mice can harbor *H. nana*, permitting investigation of the mechanisms that limit worm density. It appears that a Th1 IFN-γ response provides protective immunity against cysticercoid larvae,[97,98] and a Th2 response involving IgE and mast cells assists in the expulsion of adult worms.[99,100]

Diagnosis and Treatment

Dwarf or rodent tapeworm is diagnosed by finding parasite eggs in the stool. *H. nana* eggs measure 30 to 47 μm in diameter. The eggs of the much less prevalent *H. diminuta* are larger and measure 56 to 86 μm in diameter. Examination of several stool specimens taken on different days are needed to identify low-level colonization. Adults of both parasites can be killed with a single oral dose of praziquantel at 25 mg/kg; however, eggs escape this treatment. Therefore, patients with *H. nana* infection should be retreated in 1 week. Family members also should be examined and considered for treatment.

DIPYLIDIUM CANINUM

Dipylidium caninum (dog tapeworm) is a common parasite of household pets that rarely colonizes children. It is acquired by eating fleas that contain parasite cysticercoid larvae. Dog tapeworm causes no symptoms, but parents who find proglottids crawling in their child's diaper understandably seek medical evaluation. Treatment is praziquantel.

Echinococcus species also are tapeworms of dogs. Ingestion of *Echinococcus granulosus*, *Echinococcus multilocularis*, or *Echinococcus vogeli* eggs causes severe disease due to formation of hydatid cysts (see Chapter 79).

Epidemiology

D. caninum is the most common tapeworm of domesticated dogs and cats. It has a worldwide distribution. People acquire dog tapeworm by inadvertently ingesting fleas infected with the parasite. Most cases involve infants and young children who have close contact with their pets.

Life Cycle

Parasite eggs are ingested by the larval form of fleas that inhabit dogs or cats. Each egg releases an oncosphere that penetrates the gut wall and develops into a cysticercoid larva within the insect's viscera. The insect larva then develops into an adult flea that can distribute the cysticercoid larva to other animals. Dogs, cats, and occasionally children ingest infected adult fleas. Once in the intestine, the cysticercoid larva evaginates to form a scolex that attaches to the mucosa of the small intestine. The worm matures, forming a strobila or chain of developing proglottids that trails behind the scolex. The adult worm measures 10 to 70 cm in length. Gravid proglottids detach from the distal end of the worm and pass with the stool. The proglottids look like cucumber seeds (12 × 3 mm), are motile, and occasionally crawl out of the anus. They can be mistaken for maggots. As they dry, they release small packets that contain 5 to 15 eggs.

Clinical Features and Pathophysiology

Because people do not often eat fleas, colonization is limited. Low numbers of dog tapeworms cause no symptoms. *D. caninum* is discovered when children or their parents find motile proglottids crawling in a diaper, underwear, or stool.

Diagnosis and Treatment

D. caninum is identified by its characteristic proglottid that looks like a moving cucumber seed. The proglottids often are mistaken for adult pinworms (*E. vermicularis*) because that parasite is much more common. Stool examination for egg packets usually is unrewarding.

D. caninum causes a self-limited colonization that spontaneously clears, and dog tapeworm requires no treatment. Most patients and their families, however, prefer that the parasite be expunged actively and so treatment is given with a single oral dose of praziquantel, 10 mg/kg, or niclosamide 500 mg (chewable tablet).

TREMATODES (See also Chapter 79)

INTESTINAL FLUKES (*FASCIOLOPSIS BUSKI,* *HETEROPHYES* SPECIES, AND *ECHINOSTOMA* SPECIES)

Most intestinal trematodes have a broad host range, and more than 50 different species are capable of colonizing humans.[101] Many of these are geographically restricted and are acquired because of specific indigenous dietary behaviors. The more common intestinal trematodes are *Fasciolopsis buski*, *Heterophyes* species, and *Echinostoma* species.

Fasciolopsis buski

F. buski is the largest intestinal trematode that colonizes humans; adults measure 7.5 cm long and 2 cm wide. *F. buski* is endemic in southeast Asia and Indonesia and is acquired by ingesting metacercariae encysted on fresh water plants. The metacercariae excyst in the duodenum and attach to the small intestinal mucosa. Within 3 months, they mature to adult flatworms and begin to lay eggs. The eggs pass with feces into fresh water and embryonate. Each egg releases a ciliated miracidium that seeks a suitable snail to infect. The miracidium enters the snail and develops into a sporocyst that asexually multiplies and releases numerous cercariae. The cercariae swim to fresh water plants, and each encysts to form a metacercaria on the plant surface, awaiting ingestion by a mammal.

Adult *F. buski* live for about 1 year and cause no symptoms in most colonized people.[102] Histology of jejunal biopsy specimens along with carbohydrate, fat, and protein absorption were normal in one study of patients harboring *F. buski*[103]; however, in 1952, a 15-year-old Thai girl, hospitalized for diarrhea and abdominal pain, died of anasarca with more than 470 adult worms in her small intestine.[104] Diagnosis is by finding parasite eggs in the stool (see Fig. 107–3). Treatment is one 15 mg/kg dose of praziquantel given orally.

Heterophyes Species

Heterophyes species and the closely related *Metagonimus yokogawai* are small flatworms measuring about 1.0 to 1.7 mm in length by 0.3 to 0.6 mm in width. *Heterophyes heterophyes* is endemic in west Africa, Egypt, Israel, Turkey, China, Japan, Taiwan, and the Philippines. *Heterophyes nocens* is endemic in Japan and Korea. *M. yokogawai* is endemic in Siberia, the Balkans, China, Korea, and Japan. People acquire these parasites by eating raw or undercooked fish that contain metacercariae. In the United States, a case of *H. heterophyes* involved a Pennsylvania woman who ate sushi flown in from Asia.[105] The metacercariae ingested with raw fish excyst in the intestine, attach to the small intestinal mucosa, and develop into adults. The adults lay eggs that are deposited with feces passed into fresh or brackish water. The eggs release miracidia that swim in search of a suitable snail. A miracidium enters a snail and develops into a sporocyst that asexually multiplies and releases numerous cercariae. The cercariae swim away from the snail in search of a fish to infect. Either fresh-water or salt-water fish feeding in brackish outlets can become infected.

These parasites produce no specific symptoms in most people. Occasional heavy infections cause mild abdominal pain and mucoid diarrhea. The worms attach at the villus crypts and produce a localized eosinophilic inflammation. Rarely, parasite eggs may enter blood vessels and lymphatics, producing distant granulomatous reactions. Diagnosis is by finding eggs in the stool, which may require concentration techniques. The eggs of *Heterophyes* species appear similar to those of *M. yokogawai*. Treatment of the trematodes is a single 20-mg/kg oral dose of praziquantel.

Echinostoma Species

There are at least 16 species of *Echinostoma* that can colonize humans.[106] Adults are 2 to 6 mm in length and 1 to 1.5 mm in width, depending on the species. *Echinostoma* species are endemic in Taiwan, Korea, Thailand, Japan, Indonesia, and the Philippines. One outbreak of probable echinostomiasis involved 18 of 20 American travelers returning from Kenya.[107] People acquire *Echinostoma* by eating raw or undercooked fresh water mollusks or fish infected with metacercariae. The ingested metacercariae excyst in the intestine, attach to the small intestinal mucosa, and develop into adults. The adults lay eggs that are deposited into fresh water with the feces. The eggs embryonate and then hatch, each releasing a miracidium that swims in search of a suitable snail. A miracidium enters a snail and develops into a sporocyst that asexually multiplies and releases numerous cercariae. Depending on the species, the *Echinostoma* cercariae swim away from the snail in search of another mollusk or fish to infect.

Although *Echinostoma* species produce no symptoms in most people, these parasites may cause epigastric pain, abdominal cramps, and diarrhea.[107] Diagnosis is by finding eggs in the stool. Echinostoma eggs resemble those of *F. buski* but are smaller. Treatment is one 25-mg/kg dose of praziquantel given orally.

LIVER FLUKES (*CLONORCHIS SINENSIS, OPISTHORCHIS* SPECIES, AND *FASCIOLA* SPECIES)

Clonorchis sinensis, Opisthorchis viverrini, and *Opisthorchis felineus*

C. sinensis and *Opisthorchis* species are closely related parasites that have similar life cycles and cause similar diseases. *C. sinensis* is endemic in China, Hong Kong, Taiwan, and North Vietnam. *Opisthorchis viverrini* is endemic in Thailand and Laos. *Opisthorchis felineus* is endemic in Russia and Ukraine. People acquire these parasites by eating metacercariae present in raw or under-cooked fish. The metacercariae excyst in the stomach and duodenum as the fish is digested. The worms migrate along the mucosa to the ampulla of Vater and into the biliary tree, where they grow into adults. Leaf-shaped adult *C. sinensis* measure 5 mm wide × 2.5 cm long × 1 mm thick. Opisthorchis is smaller. The adult parasites lay eggs that pass with the bile into the intestinal lumen to be excreted. The eggs are ingested by fresh-water snails where they hatch, releasing miracidia that develop into sporocysts. Each sporocyst asexually reproduces within the snail, eventually producing numerous cercariae. The cercariae exit the snail and swim in search of a suitable fish to invade. The parasites encyst as metacercariae in the muscles of the fish, awaiting ingestion by a mammalian host.

Most infections with *C. sinensis* or *Opisthorchis* are asymptomatic. With heavy exposures, patients develop fever, malaise, hepatic tenderness, and eosinophilia,[108] symptoms and signs that abate as the worms mature and begin laying eggs in the bile ducts. In a few patients, these parasites may cause relapsing cholangitis (see Chapter 79). The worms elicit a fibrotic and adenomatous reaction in the smaller branches of the biliary ducts and can produce localized obstruction and hepatic abscess. The flukes also may migrate into the pancreatic duct and cause pancreatitis.

The most important complication of chronic infection with *C. sinesis* or *O. viverrini* is cholangiocarcinoma.[109] Infection with these parasites dramatically increases the risk of developing this otherwise rare cancer (Table 107–2)[110-114]: Parasites damage the bile duct, causing desquamation followed by hyperplasia, adenomatous hyperplasia, periductal fibrosis, dysplasia, and finally cholangiocarcinoma.[115] Cancer may result from increased sensitivity to carcinogens. Hamsters infected with *O. viverrini* develop cholangiocarcinoma when treated with subcarcinogenic doses of dimethylnitrosamine. *C. sinensis* and *O. viverrini* may sensitize patients to dietary or endogenously produced *N*-nitroso compounds and thereby increase the risk for cholangiocarcinoma.[116] A 1977 study found that 26% of Chinese immigrants relocating to New York had *C. sinensis*.[117] Because of the increased cancer risk associated with these parasites, it is advisable to look for them in any patient from an endemic area.[118]

Diagnosis is by finding parasite eggs in the stool or duodenal aspirate. Symptomatic patients may have curvilinear lucencies in the bile and pancreatic ducts on ERCP.[119] Ultrasound findings include increased periductal echogenicity and floating echogenic foci in the gallbladder.[120] The recommended treatment is praziquantel 25 mg/kg every 8 hours for a total of three doses. Heavy infections may require 2 days of therapy.[121] An alternative treatment is albendazole 10 mg/kg twice a day for 7 days. Albendazole is teratogenic and should not be given to pregnant women.

Fasciola hepatica and *Fasciola gigantica*

F. hepatica has a worldwide distribution, whereas *F. gigantica* is endemic in Hawaii, Asia, India, the Middle East, and Africa. Both species infect sheep, goats, and cattle as their normal hosts. Humans acquire these parasites by ingesting metacercariae encysted on fresh-water plants such as watercress. The metacercariae excyst in the small intestine, penetrate through the bowel wall, and enter the peritoneal cavity, where they migrate to the liver, penetrate the capsule, and travel through the hepatic parenchyma in search of a bile duct. They reside within the bile ducts, reaching maturity within 3 or 4 months,

Table 107–2 Reported Relative Risks of Cholangiocarcinoma in Patients with *Clonorchis* or *Opisthorchis* Infection

Parasite	Reference	Relative Risk
Clonorchis sinensis	110	3.1
	111	6.5
	112	6.0
Opisthorchis viverrini	113	5.0
	114	
	Light*	1.7
	Medium†	3.2
	Heavy‡	14.0

*<1500 eggs per gram of stool.
†1501-6000 eggs per gram of stool.
‡>6000 eggs per gram of stool.

after which they lay eggs. Adult *F. hepatica* are 1.3 × 4 cm in size and *F. gigantica* grow up to 7 cm in length. Adults of both species are only 1 mm thick and resemble leaves. *Fasciola* are long-lived—one documented infection persisted for 16 years.[122] Adults lay eggs that pass with the bile into the intestinal lumen from which they are excreted. On reaching fresh water, *Fasciola* eggs embryonate, hatch, and release miracidia that swim in search of a suitable snail. A miracidium enters a snail and develops into a sporocyst that asexually multiplies, eventually releasing numerous cercariae. The cercariae swim to a fresh-water plant and encyst on the wall, awaiting ingestion by a mammal.

Fasciola infections usually are asymptomatic. In the acute phase, patients can have abdominal pain and hepatomegaly as the parasites penetrate the intestinal wall and hepatic capsule. Abdominal CT scan may show low-density areas in the periphery of the liver. Patients also develop symptoms from migration of the parasites to other sites such as subcutaneous fat.[123] Acute symptoms wane as the parasites enter the bile ducts. During the chronic phase of fascioliasis, patients may have symptoms of intermittent biliary obstruction and cholangitis. Rarely, patients develop pancreatitis. ERCP may show curvilinear lucencies in the bile duct (Fig. 107–12).[124]

Diagnosis is by finding eggs in the stool. However, *Fasciola* release low numbers of eggs, making this test insensitive. Duodenal or bile aspirates also can demonstrate

eggs. The most sensitive method to detect *Fasciola* infection is ELISA for antibodies against the worms[125]; antibody titer drops after successful drug treatment.

Unlike other trematodes, *Fasciola* are resistant to praziquantel. Triclabendazole is the drug of choice for fascioliasis. In one study, a single oral dose of triclabendazole (10 mg/kg) cured 79% of patients as measured by fecal egg counts and ELISA.[126]

BLOOD FLUKES (*SCHISTOSOMA MANSONI, SCHISTOSOMA JAPONICUM, SCHISTOSOMA MEKONGI, SCHISTOSOMA INTERCALATUM*)

Visceral (hepatosplenic and intestinal) schistosomiasis is caused by *Schistosoma mansoni*, *Schistosoma japonicum*, *Schistosoma mekongi*, and *Schistosoma intercalatum*. Schistosomes infect more than 200 million people worldwide. People acquire the parasite through contact with contaminated water. Visceral schistosomiasis can cause colitis and fibrosis of the portal vein, producing portal hypertension. Treatment is praziquantel.

Epidemiology

Schistosomes are tropical parasites with a worldwide distribution. *S. mansoni* is endemic in regions of Africa, the Middle East, Puerto Rico, the Dominican Republic, Central America, and South America. *S. japonicum* is endemic in China, Indonesia, the Philippines and Thailand. *S. mekongi* is endemic in Laos and Cambodia. *S. intercalatum* is endemic in Africa. In most countries in which schistosomes are endemic, some regions have a high prevalence of infection, whereas in other areas the parasite is absent. Schistosomes live in tropical snails for part of their life cyle. It is the distribution of these snails that helps define the geographic limits of schistosomes.

Construction of water reservoirs and irrigation canals has expanded the snail habitat in many countries, a practice that has increased the risk of acquiring schistosomiasis. Mice and other mammals can harbor schistosomes and may allow spread of the parasite even with improved sanitation,[127] making it difficult to eradicate; nonetheless, Japan successfully eradicated *S. japonicum*, and *S. mansoni* is vanishing from some areas of Puerto Rico.[128]

Life Cycle

Schistosome worms are acquired by contacting fresh water infested with parasite cercariae. Cercariae are fork-tailed, microscopic larvae that swim through the water in search of a suitable mammalian host. On finding this host, they penetrate through intact skin, shed their tails, and transform into schistosomula that are covered with a double lipid-bilayer tegument; this tegument thwarts most immunologic attacks. Schistosomula migrate into blood vessels where they are swept with the venous flow through the right heart into the lungs. They migrate through the pulmonary capillaries, flow through the left heart into the systemic circulation, and eventually reach the liver, where they mature, mate, and migrate distally against venous flow in the portal system. The 2-cm female is partly ensheathed by the shorter male and the

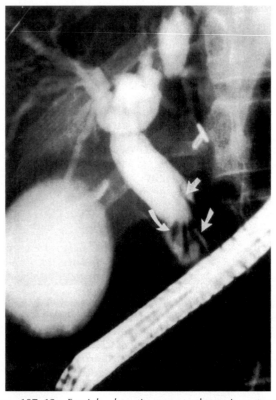

Figure 107–12 *Fasciola hepatica* on endoscopic retrograde cholangiopancreatography appearing as curvilinear lucencies (*arrows*) in the distal bile duct. A leaf-shaped fluke was extracted from the bile duct. (From Veerappan A, Siegel JH, Podany J, et al: Fasciola hepatica pancreatitis: Endoscopic extraction of live parasites. Gastrointest Endosc 37:473, 1991.)

"couple" reside together within the mesenteric veins. *S. mansoni* and *S. intercalatum* prefer to dwell in the vessels drained by the inferior mesenteric vein, whereas *S. japonicum* and *S. mekongi* prefer the vessels drained by the superior mesenteric vein.

The worms remain in the mesenteric vessels, consuming blood and nutrients and depositing eggs. *S. mansoni* lays 250 eggs and *S. japonicum* lays 3500 eggs per worm pair each day. Many of the eggs pass through the intestinal wall and enter the lumen of the bowel. The eggs pass with the stool, and if deposited in fresh water, hatch to release ciliated miracidia. Miracidia swim in search of a suitable tropical snail to infect. After penetrating into the snail's foot process, a miracidium transforms into a primary (mother) sporocyst. Secondary sporocysts bud off the primary sporocyst, migrate to the snail's liver, and mature. Cercariae bud off the secondary sporocysts, exit the snail, and swim in search of a permissive mammalian host.

Clinical Features and Pathophysiology

Dermal invasion and migration by infecting cercariae usually produce no symptoms. Patients with repeated contact may develop a mild papular rash, in contrast to the intensely pruritic papular rash that develops after exposure to avian schistosomes such as *Trichobilharzia ocellata*. These avian trematodes infect waterfowl but are unable to live in mammals, and so the cercariae/schistosomula die in a person's skin, eliciting an immunologic response that produces "swimmer's itch." Swimmer's itch is common in the Great Lakes region and has occurred as far north as Iceland.[129] Swimmer's itch is not dangerous, but repetitive scratching can cause a secondary cellulitis.

Schistosomula migrate through the body without producing symptoms. Juvenile and adult worms evade immune attack elegantly since their tegument is coated with histocompatibility and blood group antigens derived from the host. The tegument contains immunoglobulin receptors and proteases that may help cleave any bound antibody. Moreover, schistosomes produce several proteins that prevent complement, neutrophils, macrophages, or lymphocytes from injuring them.[130] Such immune evasion allows adult worms to survive in the blood vessels without causing much direct damage. The average life span of worms is thought to be about 5 years, but there are documented cases of adult worms surviving for more than 35 years after individuals had left an endemic area.[131]

Schistosome worms release eggs each day throughout their long life, and it is the parasite's eggs that cause disease. Whereas the adult worms evade immune responses, the schistosome eggs invite one, exuding antigens that trigger a strong cell-mediated Th2 immune response.

Katayama fever is the classic presentation of acute schistosomiasis. It results from a brisk early immune response to schistosome eggs that occurs within the first 2 weeks of egg deposition or from about 35 to 50 days after contacting water heavily infested with cercariae. Symptoms are caused by circulating immune complexes and resemble those of serum sickness. Patients have fever, malaise, arthralgia, myalgia, cough, and diarrhea with the additional finding of a marked eosinophilia. Serum aminotransferase levels are normal, and eggs usually are absent from the stool. *S. japonicum* releases the largest number of eggs and causes the most intense acute schistosomiasis reaction, with fatality rates approaching 25%. Most people do not develop acute schistosomiasis, but in those that do and survive, symptoms resolve as the infection enters the chronic phase.

Each schistosome egg secretes antigens that provoke a focal granulomatous inflammatory reaction that helps move the egg from the inside of a capillary, through the intestinal wall, and out into the lumen.[132] Thus, inflammation actually benefits the parasite. Passage of eggs through the bowel wall causes intestinal schistosomiasis with occult blood in the stools or even bloody diarrhea. Patients also may have tenesmus and tenderness over the sigmoid colon. Patients with *S. mansoni* can develop colitis with inflammatory pseudopolyps (Fig. 107–13) composed of numerous eosinophils and occasional eggs, a picture that may resemble Crohn's disease or ulcerative colitis.[133] *S. japonicum* prefers to dwell in veins drained by the superior mesenteric vein and lays thousands of eggs at a time. *S. japonicum* can produce upper abdominal pain unrelated to meals, gastric bleeding, and pyloric obstruction due to inflammation and fibrosis.

About half of the eggs pass out of the body; the other half lodge in the host's tissues and cause the pathology of chronic schistosomiasis. Eggs are carried by the portal flow and lodge in the liver. Other eggs lodge in the

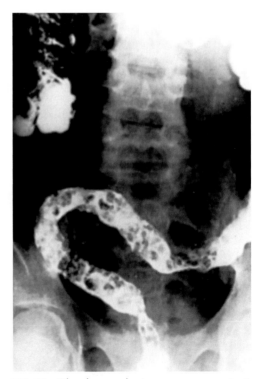

Figure 107–13 Film from a barium enema examination of a 20-year-old Egyptian man with bloody diarrhea and tenesmus. Multiple polypoid lesions due to *Schistosoma mansoni* are seen throughout the rectosigmoid, which is displaced out of the pelvis by a large pericolic abscess. (From Reeder MM, Hamilton LC: Radiologic diagnosis of tropical diseases of the gastrointestinal tract. Radiol Clin North Am 7:57, 1969.)

mesenteric and portal veins or remain in the intestinal wall. In these locations, the eggs elicit granulomatous inflammation with eosinophils, macrophages, lymphocytes, fibroblasts, and mast cells (Fig. 107–14). Eosinophils account for 50% of the schistosome egg granuloma cell population. Eosinophils degranulate, depositing major basic protein that produces an eosinophilic halo around the eggs termed the *Splendore-Hoeppli phenomenon.* Eosinophils likely assist in killing the miracidia that is protected by the tough egg shell. After 1 or 2 weeks the miracidium dies, antigen release wanes, and the granuloma involutes to leave a fibrotic scar.

Over the years, the daily production of eggs, granulomas, and scars accumulates enough damage to produce disease. Eggs that lodge in the hepatic and portal vessels produce a unique pattern of scarring called *Symmers' pipestem fibrosis,* in which the vessels become fibrotic, resembling clay pipe stems on cross section; this process causes the presinusoidal venous obstruction and portal hypertension characteristic of hepatosplenic schistosomiasis. Patients typically have an enlarged left hepatic lobe, splenomegaly, and thrombocytopenia due to platelet sequestration. Hepatocellular function remains normal because the blood supply to the liver is maintained by increased hepatic artery flow. Patients have normal serum aminotransferase levels and mildly elevated alkaline phosphatase and gamma-glutamyl transferase. Patients with hepatosplenic schistosomiasis do not develop cirrhosis unless coinfected with hepatitis B or C and so lack stigmata of hepatic insufficiency. The classic presentation of decompensated hepatosplenic schistosomiasis is variceal hemorrhage.

Hepatosplenic schistosomiasis results from accumulated injury and requires prolonged, moderately intense infection. Patients with hepatosplenic schistosomiasis typically are adolescent to late 20s in age and have had schistosomiasis for 5 to 15 years. Compensated disease improves, however, after schistosomes are killed by drug therapy, permitting the portal tributaries to heal and remodel.[134,135]

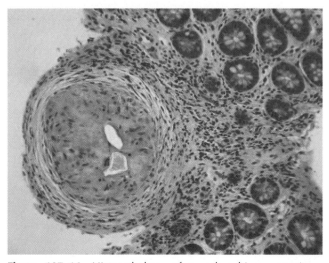

Figure 107–14 Histopathology of a colon biopsy specimen from a patient with schistosomiasis showing a schistosome egg granuloma.

Schistosome eggs also can lodge in other sites besides the intestine, liver, spleen, and splanchnic venous circulation. Eggs may percolate through portocaval collateral vessels, lodge in the pulmonary capillaries, and over time cause pulmonary hypertension and cor pulmonale. Eggs may enter the vertebral venous plexus and become emboli to the spinal cord or brain. Granulomatous inflammation in the central nervous system can result in conus equinus syndrome, transverse myelitis, or schistosomal cerebritis.

Patients with schistosomiasis may present with recurrent bacteremia. Adult schistosome worms may ingest enteric bacteria transiently present in the portal circulation, harbor these bacteria, and serve as reservoirs for infection. Recurrent *Salmonella* infection is particularly common in patients with schistosomiasis.[136]

Schistosomiasis may cause membranoproliferative glomerulonephritis or focal glomerulosclerosis with proteinuria, nephrotic syndrome, and end-stage renal disease. Schistosomal nephropathy results from deposition of immune complexes of parasite antigens and antibodies, and the renal disease can be progressive even if the parasites are killed with drug therapy.[137]

Diagnosis

Schistosome eggs are present in stool, but not in high numbers. The classic method for detecting the eggs is the Kato-Katz thick smear.[138] This technique is not performed as part of the standard ova and parasite test, and standard evaluation is not sensitive enough to find the relatively rare schistosome eggs. Even Kato-Katz thick smears are not highly sensitive and are unlikely to detect patients with very low levels of infection.

Most patients with intestinal schistosome infections are asymptomatic; patients come to medical attention during evaluation of mild anemia, occult blood in the stools, or unexpected variceal hemorrhage. On endoscopy, a patient may have inflammatory polyps that contain eggs,[133] but usually the intestinal mucosa appears normal. Subtle changes in the vascular pattern may result from egg emboli that produce a terminal curling of the small blood vessels.[139] Biopsy of the rectum can demonstrate eggs, especially when the biopsy is crushed between two glass slides and the whole biopsy specimen is surveyed microscopically (Fig. 107–15). Evaluation of six crush biopsies is more sensitive than of two Kato-Katz smears for *S. mansoni.*[140]

Although eggs lodge in the liver and cause portal hypertension, liver biopsy is an insensitive method for detecting schistosomiasis. Liver biopsy should not be used solely to test for schistosomiasis but rather to stage comorbid disease such as viral hepatitis B or C.

Present or past exposure to schistosomes is detectable by serology. Antischistosome antibodies are detected by ELISA using adult microsomal antigens. Sensitivity varies depending on whether the infecting schistosome is the same species as that used to prepare the antigens. The ELISA uses *S. mansoni* microsomal antigens, so immunoblot tests employing antigens from *S. japonicum* and *Schistosoma hematobium* (urinary schistosomiasis) also are performed.[141] The antibody assay also is useful to diagnose acute schistosomiasis (Katayama fever) because there are few or no eggs in the stool during the peak of

Table 107–3 World Health Organization Criteria for Staging Hepatosplenic Schistosomiasis*

Liver Parenchymal patterns on ultrasonography and Image Pattern (IP) scores

Pattern	Sonographic Appearance	IP Score
A	Normal structure	0
	*Patterns observed in schistosomiasis**	
B	'Starry sky' (diffuse echogenic foci)	1
C	Highly echogenic 'ring echoes', which correspond to the 'pipe stems' seen in a scan perpendicular to the one in which rings are seen	2
D	Highly echogenic 'ruff' around the portal bifurcation and main stem	4
E	Highly echogenic 'patches' extending* from the main portal vein and branches into the parenchyma	6
F	Highly echogenic 'bands' and 'streaks', extending from the main portal vein and its bifurcation to the liver surface, where they retract the organ surface.	8
	Patterns indicating pathology different from periportal fibrosis. If these are present, no score is given.	
X	Diffusely coarse liver texture, irregular liver surface, distorted hepatic veins, rounded caudal liver edge	–
Y	Diffusely increased liver echogenicity, loss of highly reflective edges of peripheral portal branches, possibly distal sound extinction, rounded caudal liver edge	–
Z	Other liver abnormalities	–

Periportal Thickening (PT) Score

If liver parenchyma shows indications of periportal fibrosis

Assign a preliminary PT score of 1

Continue the examination

Measure the thickness of the wall of the second order portal branches

Calculate the mean wall thickness (both walls) for the two (or three) vessels measured.

Adjust results for body height

normal range	2 SD or less above mean	score = 0
increased	> 2SD but ≤ 4 SD above mean	score = 3
much increased	> 4S above mean	score = 7

This gives the intermediate PT score

Calculate the final PT score

Add the preliminary PT score to the intermediate PT score

This gives a <u>final PT score in the range 1 (1 + 0) to 8 (1 + 7)</u>

Portal Hypertension (PH) Score

Portal vein diameter: Adjust the value for height

Normal	increase 0 to ≤ 2 SD	score = 0
Dilatation	increase 2 to ≤ 4SD	score = 4
Marked dilatation	increase > 4 SD	score = 6

Collateral veins

no collateral vessel detected	score = 0
collaterals detected	score = 4

Ascites

None detected	score = 0
Ascites present	score = 3

Calculate the final Portal Hypertension (PH) score

This is the sum of the above three scores:

Portal vein score	0 - 6
+ Collateral vein score	0 - 4
+ Ascites score	<u>0 - 3</u>
= **Portal Hypertension score**	0 - 13

Interpretation of the final score

IP score	PT score	PH score	Interpretation
0	0	0	No sign of periportal fibrosis
1	1	0	Incipient periportal fibroses not excluded
2	1	0	Periportal fibrosis possible
4	1	0	Periportal fibrosis probable
2	4,8	0	Periportal fibrosis
4	4,8	0	Periportal fibrosis
6	1,4,8	0	Advanced periportal fibrosis
8	1,4,8	0	Advanced periportal fibrosis
4-8	1,4,8	3-13	Advanced periportal fibrosis + portal hypertension

Also see Figure 79–4.

*Staging is determined by assessing degree of parenchymal changes, periportal thickening, and portal hypertension.

†Combined patterns can exist and are assigned an IP score corresponding to the highest IP score of the 2 or 3 patterns.

Adapted from Abdel-Wahab MF, Esmat G, Milad M, et al: Characteristic sonographic pattern of schistosomal hepatic fibrosis. Am J Trop Med Hyg 40:72, 1989.

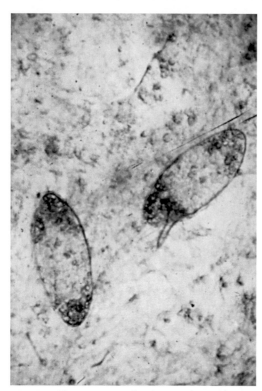

Figure 107–15 Photomicrograph of a crush preparation of the rectum demonstrating *Schistosoma mansoni* eggs in the colon mucosa. ×200. (Courtesy of C. M. Knauer, MD, San Jose, CA.)

the reaction. The ELISA does not distinguish active from prior infections; therefore, it is most useful for diagnosis in recent travelers rather than in expatriates. Because, schistosomes can be long-lived, one-time treatment of antibody-positive patients is reasonable.

Active infection can be demonstrated by detecting the circulating schistosome gut-associated protein antigens, circulating cathodic antigen (CCA) and circulating anodic antigen (CAA) in the patient's serum.[142] Serologic detection of CCA and CAA has an equivalent or higher sensitivity than does the Kato-Katz thick smear, but each test misses some low-level infections.[143] Measurement of circulating antigens also may prove useful to document response to treatment[144]; however, these tests are not yet commercially available in the United States.

Abdominal ultrasound is an important additional test in hepatosplenic schistosomiasis. Ultrasound evaluation documents periportal fibrosis, splenomegaly, portal blood flow, and collateral vessels. Periportal fibrosis has a characteristic appearance: multiple echogenic areas each with central echolucency.[145,146] A complex scoring system exists that uses a liver parenchyma image pattern (IP), a portal thickening (PT), and a portal hypertension (PH) score to stage the disease (Table 107–3).[147]

Treatment

Praziquantel is the drug of choice to treat schistosomiasis. It is the safest schistosomicide in current use. Praziquantel given orally in three doses of 20 mg/kg, each 4 hours apart (total dose, 60 mg/kg), gives the best cure rates (60% to 98%), depending on the series. Eggs continue to be shed in the stool for up to 2 weeks after drug treatment, because eggs that were deposited before treat-

ment can take this long to work through the intestinal wall. Patients who are not cured with a single course of praziquantel have a dramatic decrease in egg counts and will respond to a second course of treatment. Periportal fibrosis improves after the worms are killed, halting the daily deluge of eggs and permitting the portal tributaries to heal and remodel.[134,135]

REFERENCES

1. Little MD: Laboratory diagnosis of worms and miscellaneous specimens. Clin Lab Med 11:1041, 1991.
2. Elliott DE, Urban JF, Argo CK, Weinstock JV: Does the failure to acquire helminthic parasites predispose to Crohn's disease? FASEB J 14:1848, 2000.
3. Yazdanbakhsh M, Kremsner PG, van Ree R: Allergy, parasites, and the hygiene hypothesis. Science 296:490, 2002.
4. Elliott DE, Summers RW, Weinstock JV: Helminths and the modulation of mucosal inflammation. Curr Opin Gastroenterol 21:51, 2005.
5. Elliott D, Li J, Blum A, et al: Exposure to schistosome eggs protects mice from TNBS-induced colitis. Am J Physiol 284: G385, 2003.
6. Khan WI, Blennerhasset PA, Varghese AK, et al: Intestinal nematode infection ameliorates experimental colitis in mice. Infect Immun 70:5931, 2002.
7. Moreels TG, Nieuwendijk RJ, De Man JG, et al: Concurrent infection with *Schistosoma mansoni* attenuates inflammation-induced changes in colonic morphology, cytokine levels, and smooth muscle contractility of trinitrobenzene sulphonic acid induced colitis in rats. Gut 53:99, 2004.
8. Elliott DE, Setiawan T, Metwali A, et al: *H. polygyrus* inhibits established colitis in IL-10-deficient mice. Eur J Immunol 34:2690, 2004.
9. Cooke A, Tonks P, Jones FM, et al: Infection with *Schistosoma mansoni* prevents insulin-dependent diabetes mellitus in non-obese diabetic mice. Parasite Immunol 21:169, 1999.
10. Sewell D, Qing Z, Reinke E, et al: Immunomodulation of experimental autoimmune encephalomyelitis by helminth ova immunization. Int Immunol 15:59, 2003.
11. La Flamme AC, Ruddenklau K, Backstrom BT: Schistosomiasis decreases central nervous system inflammation and alters the progression of experimental autoimmune encephalomyelitis. Infect Immun 71:4996, 2003.
12. Summers RW, Elliott DE, Urban JF Jr, et al: Trichuris therapy for active ulcerative colitis: A randomized trial. Gastroenterology 128:825, 2005.
13. Summers RW, Elliott DE, Qadir K, et al: *Trichuris suis* seems to be safe and possibly effective in the treatment of inflammatory bowel disease. Am J Gastroenterol 98:2034, 2003.
14. Summers RW, Elliott DE, Thompson RA, et al: Trial of helminthic ova in active Crohn's disease. Gastroenterology 126:A75, 2004.
15. van den Biggelaar AH, Rodrigues LC, van Ree R, et al: Long-term treatment of intestinal helminths increases mite skin-test reactivity in Gabonese schoolchildren. J Infect Dis 189: 892, 2004.
16. Khuroo MS: Ascariasis. Gastroenterol Clin North Am 25:553, 1996.
17. Chan MS, Medley GF, Jamison D, Bundy DA: The evaluation of potential global morbidity attributable to intestinal nematode infections. Parasitology 109:373, 1994.
18. Anderson TJ, Jaenike J: Host specificity, evolutionary relationships, and macrogeographic differentiation among *Ascaris* populations from humans and pigs. Parasitology 115:325, 1997.

19. de Silva NR, Guyatt HL, Bundy DA: Worm burden in intestinal obstruction caused by *Ascaris lumbricoides*. Trop Med Int Health 2:189, 1997.

20. Wasadikar PP, Kulkarni AB: Intestinal obstruction due to ascariasis. Br J Surg 84:410, 1997.

21. van den Bogaerde JB, Jordaan M: Intraductal administration of albendazole for biliary ascariasis. Am J Gastroenterol 92:1531, 1997.

22. Maddern GJ, Dennison AR, Blumgart LH: Fatal *Ascaris* pancreatitis: An uncommon problem in the west. Gut 33:402, 1992.

23. Khuroo MS, Zargar SA, Mahajan R, et al: Sonographic appearances in biliary ascariasis. Gastroenterology 93:267, 1987.

24. Schulman A: Ultrasound appearances of intra- and extrahepatic biliary ascariasis. Abdom Imaging 23:60, 1998.

25. Gonzalez AH, Regalado VC, Van den Ende J: Noninvasive management of *Ascaris lumbricoides* biliary tact migration: A prospective study in 69 patients from Ecuador. Trop Med Int Health 6:146, 2001.

26. Gill GV, Bell DR: *Strongyloides stercoralis* infection in former Far East prisoners of war. BMJ 2:572, 1979.

27. Weight SC, Barrie WW: Colonic *Strongyloides stercoralis* infection masquerading as ulcerative colitis. J R Coll Surg Edinb 42:202, 1997.

28. Al Samman M, Haque S, Long JD: Strongyloidiasis colitis: A case report and review of the literature. J Clin Gastroenterol 28:77, 1999.

29. Keiser PB, Nutman TB: *Strongyloides stercoralis* in the immunocompromised population. Clin Microbiol Rev 17:208, 2004.

30. Genta RM: Dysregulation of strongyloidiasis: A new hypothesis. Clin Microbiol Rev 5:345, 1992.

31. Palau LA, Pankey GA: Strongyloides hyperinfection in a renal transplant recipient receiving cyclosporine: Possible *Strongyloides stercoralis* transmission by kidney transplant. Am J Trop Med Hyg 57:413, 1997.

32. Link K, Orenstein R: Bacterial complications of strongyloidiasis: *Streptococcus bovis* meningitis. South Med J 92:728, 1999.

33. Loutfy MR, Wilson M, Keystone JS, Kain KC: Serology and eosinophil count in the diagnosis and management of strongyloidiasis in a non-endemic area. Am J Trop Med Hyg 66:749, 2002.

34. Sudarshi S, Stumpfle R, Armstrong M, et al: Clinical presentation and diagnostic sensitivity of laboratory tests for *Strongyloides stercoralis* in travellers compared with immigrants in a non-endemic country. Trop Med Int Health 8:728, 2003.

35. Siddiqui AA, Berk SL: Diagnosis of *Strongyloides stercoralis* infection. Clin Infect Dis 33:1040, 2001.

36. Klein RA, Cleri DJ, Doshi V, Brasitus TA: Disseminated *Strongyloides stercoralis*: A fatal case eluding diagnosis. South Med J 76:1438, 1983.

37. Jongwutiwes S, Charoenkorn M, Sitthichareonchai P, et al: Increased sensitivity of routine laboratory detection of *Strongyloides stercoralis* and hookworm by agar-plate culture. Trans R Soc Trop Med Hyg 93:398, 1999.

38. Cross JH: Intestinal capillariasis. Clin Microbiol Rev 5:120, 1992.

39. Moravec F: Redescription and systematic status of *Capillaria philippinensis*, an intestinal parasite of human beings. J Parasitol 87:161, 2001.

40. Detels R, Gutman L, Jaramillo J, et al: An epidemic of intestinal capillariasis in man: A study in a Barrio in Northern Luzon. Am J Trop Med Hyg 18:676, 1969.

41. Cross JH, Banzon T, Clarke MD, et al: Studies on the experimental transmission of *Capillaria philippinensis* in monkeys. Trans R Soc Trop Med Hyg 66:819, 1972.

42. Kappus KD, Lundgren RGJ, Juranek DD, et al: Intestinal parasitism in the United States: Update on a continuing problem. Am J Trop Med Hyg 50:705, 1994.

43. Nawalinski TA, Schad GA: Arrested development in *Ancylostoma duodenale*: Course of a self-induced infection in man. Am J Trop Med Hyg 23:895, 1974.

44. Pritchard DI, Brown A: Is *Necator americanus* approaching a mutualistic symbiotic relationship with humans? Trends Parasitol 17:169, 2001.

45. Stassens P, Bergum PW, Gansemans Y, et al: Anticoagulant repertoire of the hookworm *Ancylostoma caninum*. Proc Natl Acad Sci U S A 93:2149, 1996.

46. Chadderdon RC, Cappello M: The hookworm platelet inhibitor: Functional blockade of integrins GPIIb/IIIa (α2bβ3) and GPIa/IIa (α2β1) inhibits platelet aggregation and adhesion in vitro. J Infect Dis 179:1235, 1999.

47. Roche M, Layrisse M: The nature and causes of "hookworm anemia." Am J Trop Med Hyg 15:1029, 1966.

48. Stoltzfus RJ, Dreyfuss ML, Chwaya HM, Albonico M: Hookworm control as a strategy to prevent iron deficiency. Nutr Rev 55:223, 1997.

49. Croese J, Loukas A, Opdebeeck J, Prociv P: Occult enteric infection by *Ancylostoma caninum*: A previously unrecognized zoonosis. Gastroenterology 106:3, 1994.

50. Walker NI, Croese J, Clouston AD, et al: Eosinophilic enteritis in northeastern Australia: Pathology, association with *Ancylostoma caninum*, and implications. Am J Surg Pathol 19:328, 1995.

51. Croese J, Fairley S, Loukas A, et al: A distinctive aphthous ileitis linked to *Ancylostoma caninum*. J Gastroenterol Hepatol 11:524, 1996.

52. Ratard RC, Kouemeni LE, Ekani BM, et al: Ascariasis and trichuriasis in Cameroon. Trans R Soc Trop Med Hyg 85:84, 1991.

53. Bundy DA, Cooper ES, Thompson DE, et al: Predisposition to *Trichuris trichiura* infection in humans. Epidemiol Infect 98:65, 1987.

54. Stephenson LS, Holland CV, Cooper ES: The public health significance of *Trichuris trichiura*. Parasitology 121(Suppl):S73, 2000.

55. Jung RC, Beaver PC: Clinical observations on *Trichocephalus trichiurus* (whipworm) infestation in children. Pediatrics 8:548, 1951.

56. Cooper ES, Bundy DA, MacDonald TT, Golden MH: Growth suppression in the *Trichuris* dysentery syndrome. Eur J Clin Nutr 44:285, 1990.

57. MacDonald TT, Choy MY, Spencer J, et al: Histopathology and immunohistochemistry of the caecum in children with the *Trichuris* dysentery syndrome. J Clin Pathol 44:194, 1991.

58. Cooper ES, Spencer J, Whyte-Alleng CA, et al: Immediate hypersensitivity in colon of children with chronic *Trichuris trichiura* dysentery. Lancet 338:1104, 1991.

59. MacDonald TT, Spencer J, Murch SH, et al: Immunoepidemiology of intestinal helminthic infections: II. Mucosal macrophages and cytokine production in the colon of children with *Trichuris trichiura* dysentery. Trans R Soc Trop Med Hyg 88:265, 1994.

60. Else KJ, Hultner L, Grencis RK: Cellular immune responses to the murine nematode parasite *Trichuris muris*. II. Differential induction of TH-cell subsets in resistant versus susceptible mice. Immunology 75:232, 1992.

61. Else KJ, Finkelman FD, Maliszewski CR, Grencis RK: Cytokine-mediated regulation of chronic intestinal helminth infection. J Exp Med 179:347, 1994.

62. Sirivichayakul C, Pojjaroen-Anant C, Wisetsing P, et al: The effectiveness of 3, 5, or 7 days of albendazole for the treatment of *Trichuris trichiura* infection. Ann Trop Med Parasitol 97:847, 2003.

63. Ismail MM, Jayakody RL: Efficacy of albendazole and its combinations with ivermectin or diethylcarbamazine (DEC) in the treatment of *Trichuris trichiura* infections in Sri Lanka. Ann Trop Med Parasitol 93:501, 1999.

64. Belizario VY, Amarillo ME, de Leon WU, et al: A comparison of the efficacy of single doses of albendazole, ivermectin, and diethylcarbamazine alone or in combinations against *Ascaris* and *Trichuris* species. Bull World Health Organ 81:35, 2003.

65. Fry GF, Moore JG: *Enterobius vermicularis*: Ten thousand-year-old human infection. Science 166:1620, 1969.

66. Hugot JP: *Enterobius gregorii* (Oxyuridae, Nematoda), a new human parasite. Ann Parasitol Humaine Comparee 58:403, 1983.

67. Chittenden AM, Ashford RW: *Enterobius gregorii* Hugot 1983: First report in the U.K. Ann Trop Med Parasitol 81:195, 1987.

68. Hasegawa H, Takao Y, Nakao M, et al: Is *Enterobius gregorii* Hugot, 1983 (Nematoda: Oxyuridae) a distinct species? J Parasitol 84:131, 1998.

69. Vermund SH, MacLeod S: Is pinworm a vanishing infection? Laboratory surveillance in a New York City medical center from 1971 to 1986. Am J Dis Child 142:566, 1988.

70. Liu LX, Chi J, Upton MP, Ash LR: Eosinophilic colitis associated with larvae of the pinworm *Enterobius vermicularis*. Lancet 346:410, 1995.

71. Sinniah B, Leopairut J, Neafie RC, et al: Enterobiasis: A histopathological study of 259 patients. Ann Trop Med Parasitol 85:625, 1991.

72. Appleyard GD, Zarlenga D, Pozio E, Gajadhar AA: Differentiation of *Trichinella* genotypes by polymerase chain reaction using sequence-specific primers. J Parasitol 85:556, 1999.

73. Roy SL, Lopez AS, Schantz PM: Trichinellosis surveillance—United States, 1997-2001. MMWR Surveill Summ 6:1, 2003.

74. Hinz E: Trichinellosis and trichinellosis control in Germany. Southeast Asian J Trop Med Public Health 22(Suppl):329, 1991.

75. Pozio E: New patterns of *Trichinella* infection. Vet Parasitol 98:133, 2001.

76. Moorhead A, Grunenwald PE, Dietz VJ, Schantz PM: Trichinellosis in the United States, 1991-1996: Declining but not gone. Am J Trop Med Hyg 60:66, 1999.

77. Ancelle T, Dupouy-Camet J, Desenclos JC, et al: A multifocal outbreak of trichinellosis linked to horse meat imported from North America to France in 1993. Am J Trop Med Hyg 59:615, 1998.

78. Despommier DD: *Trichinella spiralis* and the concept of niche. J Parasitol 79:472, 1993.

79. Capo V, Despommier DD: Clinical aspects of infection with *Trichinella* species. Clin Microbiol Rev 9:47, 1996.

80. Finkelman FD, Shea-Donohue T, Goldhill J, et al: Cytokine regulation of host defense against parasitic gastrointestinal nematodes: Lessons from studies with rodent models. Annu Rev Immunol 15:505, 1997.

81. Dupouy-Camet J, Kociecka W, Bruschi F, et al: Opinion on the diagnosis and treatment of human trichinellosis. Expert Opin Pharmacother 3:1117, 2002.

82. Ikeda K, Kumashiro R, Kifune T: Nine cases of acute gastric anisakiasis. Gastrointest Endosc 35:304, 1989.

83. Deardorff TL, Kayes SG, Fukumura T: Human anisakiasis transmitted by marine food products. Hawaii Med J 50:9, 1991.

84. Kark AE, McAlpine JC: Anisakiasis ("herring worm disease") as a cause of acute abdominal crisis. Br J Clin Pract 48:216, 1994.

85. del Pozo MD, Moneo I, de Corres LF, et al: Laboratory determinations in *Anisakis simplex* allergy. J Allergy Clin Immunol 97:977, 1996.

86. Audicana MT, Ansotegui IJ, de Corres LF, Kennedy MW: *Anisakis simplex*: Dangerous—dead and alive? Trends Parasitol 18:20, 2002.

87. Caramello P, Vitali A, Canta F, et al: Intestinal localization of anisakiasis manifested as acute abdomen. Clin Microbiol Infect 9:734, 2003.

88. Dick TA, Nelson PA, Choudhury A: Diphyllobothriasis: Update on human cases, foci, patterns and sources of human infections and future considerations. Southeast Asian J Trop Med Public Health 32(Suppl 2):59, 2001.

89. Schantz PM: Tapeworms (cestodiasis). Gastroenterol Clin North Am 25:637, 1996.

90. Nyberg W: The influence of *Diphyllobothrium latum* on the vitamin B_{12} intrinsic factor complex: II. In vitro studies. Acta Med Scand 167:189, 1960.

91. Centers for Disease Control and Prevention: Recommendations of the International Task Force for Disease Eradication. MMWR 42:1, 1993.

92. Lightowlers MW, Gauci CG, Chow C, et al: Molecular and genetic characterisation of the host-protective oncosphere antigens of taeniid cestode parasites. Int J Parasitol 33:1207, 2003.

93. Garcia HH, Gonzalez AE, Evans CA, Gilman RH: Cysticercosis Working Group in Peru: *Taenia solium* cysticercosis. Lancet 362:547, 2003.

94. Khalil HM, el Shimi S, Sarwat MA, et al: Recent study of *Hymenolepis nana* infection in Egyptian children. J Egypt Soc Parasitol 21:293, 1991.

95. Reynoldson JA, Behnke JM, Pallant LJ, et al: Failure of pyrantel in treatment of human hookworm infections (*Ancylostoma duodenale*) in the Kimberley region of northwest Australia. Acta Trop 68:301, 1997.

96. Chu GS, Palmieri JR, Sullivan JT: Beetle-eating: A Malaysia folk medical practice and its public health implications. Trop Geogr Med 29:422, 1977.

97. Asano K, Okamoto K: Murine T cell clones specific for *Hymenolepis nana*: Generation and functional analysis in vivo and in vitro. Int J Parasitol 21:891, 1991.

98. Asano K, Muramatsu K: Importance of interferon-gamma in protective immunity against *Hymenolepis nana* cysticercoids derived from challenge infection with eggs in BALB/c mice. Int J Parasitol 27:1437, 1997.

99. Watanabe N, Nawa Y, Okamoto K, Kobayashi A: Expulsion of *Hymenolepis nana* from mice with congenital deficiencies of IgE production or of mast cell development. Parasite Immunol 16:137, 1994.

100. Conchedda M, Bortoletti G, Gabriele F, et al: Immune response to the cestode *Hymenolepis nana*: Cytokine production during infection with eggs or cysts. Int J Parasitol 27:321, 1997.

101. Liu LX, Harinasuta KT: Liver and intestinal flukes. Gastroenterol Clin North Am 25:627, 1996.

102. Plaut AG, Kampanart-Sanyakorn C, Manning GS: A clinical study of *Fasciolopsis buski* infection in Thailand. Trans R Soc Trop Med Hyg 63:470, 1969.

103. Jaroonvesama N, Charoenlarp K, Areekul S: Intestinal absorption studies in *Fasciolopsis buski* infection. Southeast Asian J Trop Med Public Health 17:582, 1986.

104. Sadun EH, Maiphoom C: Studies on the epidemiology of the human intestinal fluke, *Fasciolopsis buski* (Lankester) in central Thailand. Am J Trop Med Hyg 2:1070, 1953.

105. Adams KO, Jungkind DL, Bergquist EJ, Wirts CW: Intestinal fluke infection as a result of eating sushi. Am J Clin Pathol 86:688, 1986.

106. Huffman JE, Fried B: Echinostoma and echinostomiasis. Adv Parasitol 29:215, 1990.

107. Poland GA, Navin TR, Sarosi GA: Outbreak of parasitic gastroenteritis among travelers returning from Africa. Arch Intern Med 145:2220, 1985.

108. Koenigstein RP: Observations on the epidemiology of infections with *Clonorchis sinensis*. Trans R Soc Trop Med Hyg 42:503, 1949.

109. Anonymous: Infection with liver flukes (*Opisthorchis viverrini*, *Opisthorchis felineus*, and *Clonorchis sinensis*). IARC Monogr Eval Carcinog Risks Hum 61:121, 1994.

110. Gibson JB: Parasites, liver disease, and liver cancer. IARC Sci Publ 1:142, 1971.

111. Kim YI, Yang DH, Chang KR: Relationship between *Clonorchis sinensis* infestation and cholangiocarcinoma of the liver in Korea. Seoul J Med 15:247, 1974.

112. Chung CS, Lee SK: An epidemiological study of primary liver carcinomas in Busan area with special reference to clonorchiasis. Korean J Pathol 10:33, 1976.

113. Parkin DM, Srivatanakul P, Khlat M, et al: Liver cancer in Thailand: I. A case-control study of cholangiocarcinoma. Int J Cancer 48:323, 1991.

114. Haswell-Elkins MR, Mairiang E, Mairiang P, et al: Cross-sectional study of *Opisthorchis viverrini* infection and cholangiocarcinoma in communities within a high-risk area in northeast Thailand. Int J Cancer 59:505, 1994.

115. Kim YI: Liver carcinoma and liver fluke infection. Arzneimittelforschung 34:1121, 1984.

116. Haswell-Elkins MR, Satarug S, Elkins DB: *Opisthorchis viverrini* infection in northeast Thailand and its relationship to cholangiocarcinoma. J Gastroenterol Hepatol 7:538, 1992.

117. Kammerer WS, Van Der Decker JD, Keith TB, Mott KE: Clonorchiasis in New York City Chinese. Trop Doct 7:105, 1977.

118. Schwartz DA: Cholangiocarcinoma associated with liver fluke infection: A preventable source of morbidity in Asian immigrants. Am J Gastroenterol 81:76, 1986.

119. Leung JW, Sung JY, Chung SC, Metreweli C: Hepatic clonorchiasis—a study by endoscopic retrograde cholangiopancreatography. Gastrointest Endosc 35:226, 1989.

120. Choi D, Hong ST, Lim JH, et al: Sonographic findings of active *Clonorchis sinensis* infection. J Clin Ultrasound 32:17, 2004.

121. Harinasuta T, Pungpak S, Keystone JS: Trematode infections: Opisthorchiasis, clonorchiasis, fascioliasis, and paragonimiasis. Infect Dis Clin North Am 7:699, 1993.

122. Reinhard GH, Graf V, Augustin HJ: Chronic fascioliasis with destructive cholangitis. Fortschr der Med 109:737, 1991.

123. Arjona R, Riancho JA, Aguado JM, et al: Fascioliasis in developed countries: A review of classic and aberrant forms of the disease. Medicine 74:13, 1995.

124. Veerappan A, Siegel JH, Podany J, et al: Fasciola hepatica pancreatitis: Endoscopic extraction of live parasites. Gastrointest Endosc 37:473, 1991.

125. Hillyer GV, Soler de Galanes M, Rodriguez-Perez J, et al: Use of the Falcon assay screening test–enzyme-linked immunosorbent assay (FAST-ELISA) and the enzyme-linked immunoelectrotransfer blot (EITB) to determine the prevalence of human fascioliasis in the Bolivian Altiplano. Am J Trop Med Hyg 46:603, 1992.

126. Apt W, Aguilera X, Vega F, et al: Treatment of human chronic fascioliasis with triclabendazole: Drug efficacy and serologic response. Am J Trop Med Hyg 52:532, 1995.

127. Sene M, Bremond P, Herve JP, et al: Comparison of human and murine isolates of *Schistosoma mansoni* from Richard-Toll, Senegal, by isoelectric focusing. J Helminthol 71:175, 1997.

128. Hillyer GV, Soler de Galanes M: Seroepidemiology of schistosomiasis in Puerto Rico: Evidence for vanishing endemicity. Am J Trop Med Hyg 60:827, 1999.

129. Kolarova L, Skirnisson K, Horak P: *Schistosome cercariae* as the causative agent of swimmer's itch in Iceland. J Helminthol 73:215, 1999.

130. Fishelson Z: Novel mechanisms of immune evasion by *Schistosoma mansoni*. Mem Inst Oswaldo Cruz 90:289, 1995.

131. Hornstein L, Lederer G, Schechter J, et al: Persistent *Schistosoma mansoni* infection in Yemeni immigrants to Israel. Isr J Med Sci 26:386, 1990.

132. Doenhoff MJ, Hassounah O, Murare H, et al: The schistosome egg granuloma: Immunopathology in the cause of host protection or parasite survival? Trans R Soc Trop Med Hyg 80:503, 1986.

133. el-Masry NA, Farid Z, Bassily S, et al: Schistosomal colonic polyposis: Clinical, radiological, and parasitological study. J Trop Med Hyg 89:13, 1986.

134. Doehring-Schwerdtfeger E, Abdel-Rahim IM, Kardorff R, et al: Ultrasonographical investigation of periportal fibrosis in children with *Schistosoma mansoni* infection: Reversibility of morbidity twenty-three months after treatment with praziquantel. Am J Trop Med Hyg 46:409, 1992.

135. Boisier P, Ramarokoto CE, Ravaoalimalala VE, et al: Reversibility of *Schistosoma mansoni*-associated morbidity after yearly mass praziquantel therapy: Ultrasonographic assessment. Trans R Soc Trop Med Hyg 92:451, 1998.

136. Rocha H, Kirk JW, Hearey CD Jr: Prolonged *Salmonella* bacteremia in patients with *Schistosoma mansoni* infection. Arch Intern Med 128:254, 1971.

137. Martinelli R, Pereira LJ, Brito E, Rocha H: Clinical course of focal segmental glomerulosclerosis associated with hepatosplenic *Schistosomiasis mansoni*. Nephron 69:131, 1995.

138. Elliott DE: Schistosomiasis. Pathophysiology, diagnosis, and treatment. Gastroenterol Clin North Am 25:599, 1996.

139. Sanguino J, Peixe R, Guerra J, et al: Schistosomiasis and vascular alterations of the colonic mucosa. Hepatogastroenterology 40:184, 1993.

140. Abdel-Hafez MA, Bolbol AH: Fibre-optic sigmoidoscopy compared with the Kato technique in diagnosis and evaluation of the intensity of *Schistosoma mansoni* infection. Trans R Soc Trop Med Hyg 86:641, 1992.

141. Tsang VC, Wilkins PP: Immunodiagnosis of schistosomiasis. Immunol Invest 26:175, 1997.

142. de Jonge N, Kremsner PG, Krijger FW, et al: Detection of the schistosome circulating cathodic antigen by enzyme immunoassay using biotinylated monoclonal antibodies. Trans R Soc Trop Med Hyg 84:815, 1990.

143. van Lieshout L, Panday UG, de Jonge N, et al: Immunodiagnosis of *Schistosomiasis mansoni* in a low endemic area in Surinam by determination of the circulating antigens CAA and CCA. Acta Trop 59:19, 1995.

144. De Clercq D, Sacko M, Vercruysse J, et al: Assessment of cure by detection of circulating antigens in serum and urine, following schistosomiasis mass treatment in two villages of the Office du Niger, Mali. Acta Trop 68:339, 1997.

145. Abdel-Wahab MF, Esmat G, Milad M, et al: Characteristic sonographic pattern of schistosomal hepatic fibrosis. Am J Trop Med Hyg 40:72, 1989.

146. De Jesus AR, Miranda DG, Miranda RG, et al: Morbidity associated with *Schistosoma mansoni* infection determined by ultrasound in an endemic area of Brazil, Caatinga do Moura. Am J Trop Med Hyg 63:1, 2000.

147. Ultrasound in Schistosomiasis: A Practical Guide to the Standardized Use of Ultrasonography for the Assessment of Schistosomiasis-related Morbidity. 2000; *http://www.who.int/tdr/publications/publications/ultrasound.htm*

CHAPTER
108 Crohn's Disease

Bruce E. Sands

Idiopathic inflammatory bowel disease (IBD) comprises those conditions characterized by a tendency for chronic or relapsing immune activation and inflammation within the gastrointestinal tract. Crohn's disease and ulcerative colitis are the two major forms of idiopathic IBD. Less common but increasingly recognized are the atypical microscopic colitides, primarily collagenous colitis and lymphocytic colitis. Other chronic inflammatory conditions of the intestine share some features of presentation and pathogenesis but have identifiable etiologies. These disorders include diversion colitis, bypass enteropathy, radiation colitis, and drug-induced colitides. The two major forms of IBD share many clinical and epidemiologic characteristics, suggesting that underlying causation may be similar. Indeed, more than occasionally Crohn's disease cannot be distinguished from ulcerative colitis on clinical grounds, yet the two diseases are distinct syndromes with divergent treatment and prognosis.

Crohn's disease is a condition of chronic inflammation potentially involving any location of the alimentary tract from mouth to anus, but with a propensity for the distal small bowel and proximal large bowel. Inflammation in Crohn's disease often is discontinuous along the longitudinal axis of the gut and may involve all layers from mucosa to serosa. Affected persons usually experience diarrhea and abdominal pain, often accompanied by weight loss. Frequent complications include stricture and fistula formation, which often necessitate surgery. Numerous extraintestinal manifestations also may be present. The etiology of Crohn's disease is incompletely understood, and therapy, although generally effective in alleviating the symptoms, is not curative.

HISTORY

Although the eponym "Crohn's disease" has gained general acceptance in recent decades, clear clinicopathologic reports of the same process date back at least 2 centuries. Morgagni provided a description of intestinal inflammation characteristic of Crohn's disease in 1761.[1] Only after the identification of the tubercle bacillus by Koch in 1882 was it possible to describe persons with ileocecal disease similar to intestinal tuberculosis but lacking the organism. Such reports were provided by Fenwick (1889),[1] Dalziel (1913),[2] Weiner (1914), Moschcowitz and Wilensky (1923 and 1927), and Goldfarb and Suissman (1931).[3] In 1932, the landmark publication of Crohn and his colleagues Ginzburg and Oppenheimer called attention to "terminal ileitis" as a distinct entity and chronic disease.[4] This term was soon deemed unsuitable, however, when it became apparent that the disease process might involve the colon. Patients, too, misunderstood and were frightened by the "terminal" nature of their illness. The term *regional enteritis* embraced the focal nature of the process but failed to incorporate knowledge of the possibility of disparate sites of involvement within the gastrointestinal tract, including the small and large bowel in combination[5] and large bowel in isolation.[6] The term *granulomatous enterocolitis* lost acceptance when it became clear that granulomas were not a sine qua non of the diagnosis. In the end, the name *Crohn's disease* has been adopted to encompass the many clinical presentations of this pathologic entity. But for the alphabetic priority these authors chose, Crohn's disease might well have been "Ginzburg's" or "Oppenheimer's" disease.

EPIDEMIOLOGY

Accurate comparisons of epidemiologic data on the incidence and prevalence of Crohn's disease are hampered by a lack of gold standard criteria for diagnosis and inconsistent case ascertainment. The invasiveness and expense of diagnostic modalities ensure that diagnosed cases represent only a fraction of the diseased population. Studies relying on the observations of large referral centers may be biased toward reporting more aggressive forms of the disease, thereby underestimating its true incidence.

Misclassification of disease also is problematic. Historically, unidentified infections, later recognized by improved culture and diagnostic techniques, may have accounted for some portion of cases, particularly among persons with a single episode of disease. At times, differentiating Crohn's disease from ulcerative colitis may be difficult, especially at the time of diagnosis and before the passage of time has allowed distinctive disease characteristics to become manifest. Reassignment of a diagnosis of Crohn's disease or ulcerative colitis may be as high as 10% in the first 2 years after diagnosis.[7]

Despite these methodologic limitations, distinct and reproducible geographic and temporal trends in incidence have been observed. In both Europe and North America, higher incidence rates have been noted in more northern latitudes. For example, age-adjusted annual incidence rates of 6 and 10 cases per 100,000 persons have been reported in Northern Alberta[8] and Southeastern Norway,[7] respectively, whereas estimates of incidence rates reached only 0.9 per 100,000 in Spain[9] and 3.4 per 100,000 in Italy.[10] A recent systematic review noted an incidence in North America ranging from 3.1 to 14.6 per 100,000 person-years.[11] A north-south gradient similar to that observed in Europe has been noted in the United States[12] and even within the state of California itself, with estimated incidence rates of 7.0 and 3.6 per 100,000 in northern and southern California, respectively.[13,14] Recent estimates of incidence across Europe have confirmed prior observations of a north-south gradient, but the differential is now less than previously observed, perhaps because of increasing rates in the south and stabilization of rates in the north.[15]

In Japan, the incidence rate has remained low, with estimates between 0.08 and 0.5 per 100,000,[16,17] whereas in Australia and New Zealand, incidence rates have ranged from 1.75 to 2.1 per 100,000.[18,19] Crohn's disease is thought to be extremely rare in much of South America and Africa,[20] with the exception of South Africa, where

the most recent estimate of the incidence rate for the white population is 2.6 per 100,000; it is considerably lower among the nonwhite population.[21] Estimates from less affluent nations, however, are likely to be influenced by decreased access to health care. Genetic and environmental factors in these regions are therefore difficult to disentangle.

In regions where incidence estimates have been studied over long periods, a sharp rise in incidence was observed from the mid-1950s to the early 1970s, followed by stabilization of the rate since the 1980s. This trend has been shown most clearly in population-based studies in the United States and Denmark. In Olmsted County, Minnesota, the incidence rate rose from approximately 3 per 100,000 in 1954-1963 to nearly 8 per 100,000 in 1964-1973.[22] In Copenhagen County, Denmark, the rise has been even more precipitous, with a sixfold increase in incidence between 1962 and 1987, from less than 1 to 4.1 per 100,000 per year.[23] The factors contributing to these trends have not been completely elucidated but probably do not reflect merely improved diagnostic capabilities with discovery of greater numbers of mild cases; this possibility is negated by the observation that death rates from Crohn's disease in six geographically diverse countries also increased from the 1950s to the 1970s.[24] These trends are explained best by one or more environmental factors, although which of these has been the driving force remains elusive (see later).

Studies throughout the world have shown a small excess risk of Crohn's disease among women. Most reports show a female-to-male ratio between unity and 1.2:1. Some studies have noted a trend from unity to increasing female risk over the past 5 decades.[22] This slight difference in risk may be explained by hormonal or lifestyle factors and stands in contrast with the nearly equal or even slight male predominance seen in ulcerative colitis.

Crohn's disease is diagnosed most frequently among persons aged 15 to 30 years, although the age of diagnosis may range from early childhood through the entire lifespan. Population-based studies from recent years have shown the median age of diagnosis to be approximately 30 years.[22,25] Conflicting information may be found regarding trends in the age of diagnosis. In Olmsted County, Minnesota, younger age groups, particularly between ages 20 and 29 years, account for the rise in incidence over the 1960s and 1970s.[22] In contrast, population-based studies in Uppsala, Sweden[26] and Copenhagen, Denmark[25] have observed a trend toward increasing median age at diagnosis. In Stockholm, the median age of diagnosis has increased from 25 years in 1960-1964 to 32 years in 1985-1989. These findings reflect a larger proportion of patients diagnosed when older than age 60 years. Indeed, many, though not all, studies have shown a smaller second peak in incidence later in life, generally in the 7th decade.[27] This second peak may be the result of ascertainment bias because of more frequent contact with medical care and more frequent evaluation of older patients. Differences in clinical presentation among younger and older patients suggest that distinct risk factors are operative at different ages at onset.[28] The pathologic findings in young and old patients are not different, although some studies have identified a greater proportion of colonic and distal disease among older patients,[27] whereas ileal disease predominates in younger patients.[29]

ETIOLOGY AND PATHOGENESIS

INITIATING EVENTS

In light of the nature of the pathologic findings in Crohn's disease (see later) and ulcerative colitis, it has long been clear that IBD represents a state of sustained immune response. The question arises as to whether this is an appropriate response to an unrecognized pathogen or an inappropriate response to an innocuous stimulus. Over the decades, many infectious agents have been proposed as the cause of Crohn's disease including *Chlamydia*, *Listeria monocytogenes*, cell wall–deficient *Pseudomonas* species, reovirus, and many others. Paramyxovirus (measles virus) has been implicated etiologically in Crohn's disease as a cause of granulomatous vasculitis and microinfarcts of the intestine[30]; a proposed association between early measles vaccination and Crohn's disease has been largely disproved.[31] Another suggestion has been that the commensal flora, although normal in speciation, possess more subtle virulence factors, such as enteroadherence, that cause or contribute to IBD.[32]

Among the most enduring hypotheses is that *Mycobacterium paratuberculosis* is the causative agent of Crohn's disease. This notion dates to Dalziel's observation in 1913 that idiopathic granulomatous enterocolitis in humans is similar to Johne's disease, a granulomatous bowel disease of ruminants caused by *M. paratuberculosis*.[33] *M. paratuberculosis* is extremely fastidious in its culture requirements, and some proponents of this hypothesis have speculated that the presence of *M. paratuberculosis* as a spheroplast may confound efforts to confirm the theory. Efforts to confirm this theory have included attempts to culture the organism; demonstrate it by immunohistochemistry, in situ hybridization, and polymerase chain reaction methodology; and empiric treatment with antimycobacterial antibiotics. Most investigation in this area has been inconclusive, providing insufficient evidence to either prove or reject the hypothesis.

Experiments in genetic animal models of IBD have suggested strongly that in a genetically susceptible host, one need not invoke a classic pathogen as the cause of IBD, but rather nonpathogenic commensal enteric flora are sufficient to induce a chronic inflammatory response. In diverse models, animals raised under germ-free conditions show diminished or delayed expression of the IBD phenotype.[34] On introduction of defined bacterial flora, however, the expected phenotype of bowel inflammation becomes manifest (Fig. 108–1).[34] Recent advances in our understanding of the genetic bases of Crohn's disease suggest that diverse bacterial agents are capable of fueling the inflammation of Crohn's disease (see later).

In light of the diversity of substances and bacteria within the intestinal lumen, it is remarkable that the gut is not perpetually inflamed. The presence of low-level physiologic inflammation within the healthy intestinal mucosa represents a state of preparedness to deal with potentially harmful agents; a more vigorous response would not be appropriate if directed toward the innocuous commensal flora of the gut. Inflammation is kept in check through an active process termed *immune tolerance*. Tolerance is mediated in part by subsets of CD4[+] helper T cells that are generated in the intestinal mucosa and secrete the down-regulatory cytokines, transforming growth factor (TGF)-β_1 and interleukin (IL)-10. Two specific T cell populations—T regulatory 1 (Tr1) and T helper 3 (Th3) cells—appear to have similar roles in maintaining mucosal tolerance in the intestine.[35] As in the animal models of IBD, evidence in humans who have IBD also points to an over-responsiveness of mucosal T cells to the enteric flora.[36]

When an antigenic challenge occurs, or when tolerance is broken, the immune response may be skewed toward cell-mediated immunity or toward humoral immunity with the production of characteristic cytokine profiles by CD4[+] T cell populations. Th1 cells are characterized by their production of a typical cytokine profile of IL-2 and interferon (IFN)-γ. Th1 responses support cell-mediated immunity and a delayed hypersensitivity-type response. Th2 cells, in contrast, evoke humoral immunity and antibody production and elaborate IL-4, IL-5, IL-10, and other cytokines.[37] In normal hosts, the nature of the response, Th1 or Th2, depends on the characteristics of the pathogen and of the antigen-presenting cell, as well as intrinsic characteristics of the host. In the dysregulated immune response of IBD, however, immune response is sustained. Most animal models of IBD are Th1 models. These models include the IL-2 -/- mouse, the IL-10 -/- mouse, and the CD45RB[hi] severe combined immune deficiency ("SCID") mouse transfer model. In Crohn's disease, CD4[+] T cells have a Th1 cytokine profile, whereas in ulcerative colitis, the cytokine profile is that of a Th2 response, although lacking in IL-4 expression.[38]

Animal models have demonstrated that a broad array of genetic alterations may result in the stereotypic responses of Th1- or Th2-like IBD. In these models, the sustained nature of the inflammation is the result of either abnormal barrier function (dominant negative N-cadherin mouse,[39] intestinal trefoil factor -/- mouse,[40] mdr1a -/- mouse[41]) or immune dysregulation (IL-2 -/- mouse,[42] IL-10 -/- mouse,[43] human leukocyte antigen [HLA]-B27 rat,[44] and others). With the description now of three distinct genes associated with Crohn's disease, which collectively do not account for all cases of the disease, it is clear that the same phenomenon will apply in human IBD, namely, that diverse genetic perturbations may result in two main disease phenotypes characterized as Crohn's disease or ulcerative colitis. In addition, the animal models point to the likelihood that interactions among many genes will be important in disease expression, because the expression of the IBD phenotype is specific to the strain of animal into which the genetic variant is bred. An intriguing observation in humans is that bone marrow transplantation may cure Crohn's disease,[45] whereas small bowel transplantation may not.[46] This observation suggests that immunologic defects, rather than defects intrinsic to the bowel, may be paramount.

The sustained nature of the immune response in IBD may have diverse causes. *Poor intestinal barrier function* may permit continued exposure of lamina propria lym-

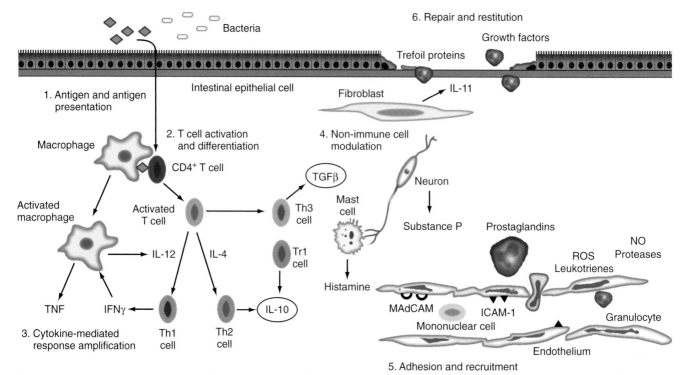

Figure 108–1 Pathogenesis of Crohn's disease. Mucosal inflammation is triggered by an antigen (1) believed to be bacterial in origin. Antigen-presenting cells, including macrophages, process the antigen and present it in the context of a major histocompatibility complex class II molecule to CD4+ T cells, leading to activation and differentiation (2). T cells may differentiate as T helper 1 (Th1), Th2, Th3, or T regulatory 1 (Tr1) cells. Interleukin (IL)-10 produced by Th2 and Tr1 cells and transforming growth factor (TGF)-β released locally by Th3 cells down-regulate inflammation. The T cell-derived cytokine IL-4 leads to Th2 differentiation, whereas the macrophage-derived cytokine IL-12 promotes Th1 differentiation of T cells. Macrophages are stimulated by interferon (IFN)-γ, produced by Th1 cells, leading to further release of IL-12, as well as release of tumor necrosis factor (TNF) and other proinflammatory cytokines (3). Nonimmune cells also modulate the immune response (4). Fibroblasts produce IL-11 and other regulatory cytokines, whereas neurons help regulate the immune response by stimulating release of histamine from mast cells and by secreting substance P, both of which may increase vascular permeability locally. Granulocytes and mononuclear cells are recruited into the mucosa in a highly coordinated fashion through the expression of integrins on leukocyte and adhesion molecules, such as mucosal addressin cellular adhesion molecule (MAdCAM) and intercellular adhesion molecule-1 (ICAM-1) on the endothelial cell (5). Once present in the mucosa, these cells release injurious and proinflammatory substances, including prostaglandins, leukotrienes, proteases, reactive oxygen species (ROS), and nitric oxide (NO). Finally, mucosal healing may occur through a process of restitution and repair (6). (Adapted from Sands BE: Novel therapies for inflammatory bowel disease. Gastroenterol Clin North Am 28:323, 1999.)

phocytes to antigenic stimuli from the lumen. Poor barrier function also may be a factor in the onset of Crohn's disease, because such patients have increased intestinal permeability preceding clinical relapse of disease.[47] Moreover, increased intestinal permeability is found in a subset of these patients' apparently healthy family members, which suggests a further genetic contribution to altered intestinal permeability.[48] Alternatively, a sustained exaggerated inflammatory reaction may result from an *ineffective immune response*—resulting from a variety of defects—to an ever-present stimulus, as occurs in a number of conditions in humans in which there is a known immunologic defect. For example, patients with chronic granulomatous disease have a defect in oxidative metabolism of granulocytes that results in a Crohn's-like inflammatory response in the bowel. Finally, the sustained nature of the inflammation may result from a *programmed over-responsiveness* to a persistent stimulus. Consistent with this theory is the finding that the mucosal T cells in patients with Crohn's disease have defective apoptosis.[49] This finding could account for the sustained nature of inflammation in IBD, because pro-

grammed cell death of lymphocytes is a normal mechanism for dampening immune response. In diverse animal models of colitis and in Crohn's disease, agents that restore apoptosis of T lymphocytes are therapeutic.[49]

The interaction between T cells and macrophages also is critical to the pathogenesis of Crohn's disease. Both cell types are found together in the earliest lesions of Crohn's disease. The antigens that perpetuate the inflammatory response are taken up by macrophages. Degradation of antigen within proteosomes in macrophages results in presentation of an epitope in the context of the class II major histocompatibility complex (MHC). Interaction between MHC class II and the T cell receptor (CD3) results in antigen-specific interaction between the macrophage and the CD4+ T cell. This event is necessary, but not sufficient, to activate the T cell. A second costimulatory signal is needed as well, because binding of CD3 to MHC class II without a costimulatory signal may result in anergy or apoptosis. Important costimulatory signals include binding of tumor necrosis factor (TNF) to TNF receptor, CD40 to CD40 ligand, and B7 to CD28. Activation of T cells leads to production of IL-2, an important growth factor for T cells. The nature of the costimulatory signal also influences the differentiation of T cells into Th1, Th2, or Th3 cells.

AMPLIFICATION AND TISSUE REACTION

On activation, macrophages further shape and amplify the immune response by producing IL-2 and the proinflammatory cytokines IL-1 and TNF. IL-12 is likely to be a master cytokine in shaping Th1 responses and may be a highly effective target for future therapies.[50] Within mononuclear cells, the key nuclear transcription factor is nuclear factor-kappa B (NFκB), which regulates the transcription of IL-1, IL-6, IL-8, TNF, and other peptides central to the inflammatory response.[51] NFκB is regulated tightly within the cell. In the inactive state, NFκB is held in the cytoplasm, bound to inhibitory κBα. During cell activation after receptor binding, various kinases phosphorylate inhibitory κBα, thereby leading to its degradation. NF-κB is then released, permitting translocation to the nucleus, where it binds to the promoter regions of numerous genes that support the inflammatory response. Such genes include those that encode proinflammatory cytokines such as TNF, adhesion molecules, and chemokines.[52] In addition to being essential to the formation of granulomas, TNF causes neutrophil activation and, along with IFN-γ, induces the expression of MHC class II on intestinal epithelial cells. Finally, TNF and other proinflammatory cytokines contribute to the expression of adhesion molecules on the endothelial cells of the intestinal vasculature.

Expression of adhesion molecules is critical to amplify the immune response, because the resident populations of granulocytes and mononuclear cells alone do not account for the vigorous inflammatory reaction characterizing IBD. Adhesion molecules on the leukocyte surface and their ligands on the endothelium of venules in the lamina propria interact in a coordinated multistep process that permits trafficking of inflammatory cells into the mucosa. First, a weak interaction between selectins on the leukocyte surface and the endothelium leads to rolling of the leukocytes along the endothelium. Second, in the presence of chemokines such as IL-8, activation occurs, and integrins are expressed on the leukocyte surface. Third, interactions between leukocyte integrins and immunoglobulin-like cellular adhesion molecules on the endothelial surface lead to spreading of the cell and diapedesis.[53] Specificity is conferred by the presence of tissue-specific cellular adhesion molecules. The integrins α4β7 and αEβ7 are of special importance in IBD, because the corresponding ligands—mucosal addressin cellular adhesion molecule and E-cadherin—are gut specific. Mucosal addressin cellular adhesion molecule is expressed constitutively on the endothelium of venules in the lamina propria,[54] whereas binding of αEβ7 on intestinal lymphocytes to E-cadherin on intestinal epithelium permits localization of intraepithelial lymphocytes. Antibodies to the α4 subunit of integrin have proven to be therapeutic in some patients with Crohn's disease.[55,56]

Once recruited to the lamina propria, mononuclear cells and granulocytes elaborate a variety of injurious and proinflammatory substances that ultimately cause tissue destruction. These substances include prostaglandins, reactive oxygen metabolites, nitric oxide, leukotrienes, and proteases. Collagenase and matrix metalloproteinases play a pivotal role in the tissue destruction seen in IBD.[57] Counterbalancing these destructive substances are other substances that promote epithelial restitution and repair, including IL-11, trefoil peptides, and growth factors such as epidermal growth factor and keratinocyte growth factor.

GENETICS

The argument for a genetic predisposition to IBD begins with the observation that family members of affected persons are at greatly increased risk of developing IBD. The relative risk among first-degree relatives is 14 to 15 times higher than that of the general population.[58] Roughly one of five patients with Crohn's disease will report having at least one affected relative. Many families have more than one affected member, and although there is a tendency within families for either ulcerative colitis or Crohn's disease to be present exclusively, mixed kindreds also occur, suggesting the presence of some shared genetic traits as a basis for both diseases; ethnicity plays a role as well. Eastern European (Ashkenazi) Jews are at a twofold to fourfold higher risk of developing IBD than non-Jews in the same geographic location and are at greater risk of having multiple affected family members. Studies of monozygotic and dizygotic twins suggest that genetic composition is a more powerful determinant for Crohn's disease than for ulcerative colitis: The concordance rate among monozygotic twins is as high as 67% for Crohn's disease, but only 13% to 20% for ulcerative colitis; most studies have suggested that concordance of disease location[48,59,60] and disease behavior[61] are higher than one would expect by chance. Finally, some subclinical markers of Crohn's disease, including anti-*Saccharomyces cerevisiae* antibodies,[62] are more frequent among apparently healthy family members of Crohn's disease probands than among the general population.

With the sequencing of the entire human genome, as well as remarkable progress in genome-wide scans for regions of IBD linkage, specific IBD genes have been identified. The presence of a locus on chromosome 16 (the IBD1 locus) had been confirmed repeatedly to be linked to Crohn's disease, indicating the presence of a Crohn's disease gene in this region.[63] Two independent groups have identified the IBD1 locus as the *NOD2* (*n*ucleotide-binding *o*ligomerization *d*omain 2) gene, also known as *CARD15* (*c*aspase-recruitment *d*omain 15).[64,65] Persons with disease-associated allelic variants on both chromosomes have a 40-fold relative risk of Crohn's disease compared with those lacking variant *NOD2/CARD15* genes, whereas heterozygous individuals have a sevenfold relative risk of Crohn's disease.[65] Studies have associated genetic polymorphisms of *NOD2/CARD15* with younger onset of disease, ileal location of disease, and increased likelihood of stricture formation.[66-69] It has been estimated that as many as 20% to 30% of cases of Crohn's disease may bear abnormal *NOD2/CARD15*. Nevertheless, the penetrance of *NOD2/CARD15* is estimated to be less than 1%[70]; that is, disease-related allelic variants of the gene may be found in a large number of individuals who do not have Crohn's disease. This strongly suggests that environmental factors, as yet incompletely elucidated, play a significant role in the expression of the Crohn's disease phenotype (see later).

The discovery of the association of *NOD2/CARD15* with Crohn's disease has opened a remarkable window into the pathogenesis of Crohn's disease. The gene product of *NOD2/CARD15* is a cytosolic protein that functions as an intracellular sensor of bacteria. Specifically, the cytosolic protein is now known to bind muramyl dipeptide (MurNAc-L-Ala-D-isoGln), a component of bacterial peptidoglycan.[71,72] The NOD2/CARD15 protein is found in both monocytes and enterocytes, specifically in Paneth cells,[73] which lie within the crypts and produce the endogenous antimicrobial peptides called *defensins*. The *NOD2/CARD15* gene consists of two CARD domains, a nucleotide binding domain (NBD), and 10 leucine-rich repeats (LRR). The allelic variants most commonly associated with Crohn's disease in European and American populations include two missense mutations (Arg702Trp, Gly908Arg) and one frameshift insertion leading to early truncation of the protein (Leu1007fsinsC). These and other more rare polymorphisms primarily affect the ability of the LRR to interact with RICK (Rip-like interacting CLARP kinase, also called *Rip-2* or *CARDIAK*). In normal function, the interaction of NOD2/CARD15 and

RICK mediates binding to IKK, an inhibitor of NFκB, and results in the activation of NFκB, thereby effecting inflammation. Paradoxically, then, genetic polymorphisms of NOD2/CARD15 might be expected to diminish inflammation because of decreased activation of NFκB, whereas NFκB is up-regulated in tissue inflamed by Crohn's disease.

This apparent paradox has yet to be unraveled completely, but diverse lines of investigation have suggested possible explanations. First, RICK, in addition to its interaction with NOD2/CARD15, lies downstream of the toll-like receptors (TLR) 2, 3, and 4, which bind lipopolysaccharide, peptidoglycan, and double-stranded RNA, respectively.[74] It has been hypothesized that the failure of NOD2 to activate RICK may contribute to a compensatory increase in activation of RICK through the TLR pathways. Second, *NOD2/CARD15* has been shown to mediate anti-inflammatory signals induced by TLR2 ligands such as peptidoglycan. Conversely, defective *NOD2/CARD15* results in defective release of the anti-inflammatory cytokine IL-10 from mononuclear cells[75] Therefore, it is conceivable that the proinflammatory effects of bacteria, mediated through other TLRs, combined with the down-regulation of IL-10 production because of defective signaling through TLR2, produces exaggerated inflammation to otherwise nonpathogenic bacteria. Similarly, NOD2 inhibits TLR2-mediated Th1 responses, whereas NOD2 deficiency leads to increased TLR2-mediated activation of NFκB (Fig. 108–2).[76] Third,

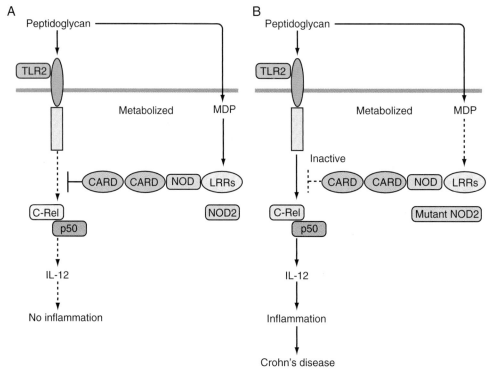

Figure 108–2 A proposed model of the role of mutant NOD2 in the pathogenesis of Crohn's disease, in which mutant NOD2 cannot block toll-like receptor 2 (TLR2). *A*, Data presented by Watanabe and colleagues[76] support a model whereby NOD2 normally senses muramyl dipeptide (MDP), a breakdown product of bacterial peptidoglycan produced in the cytosol, and limits TLR2 signaling activated by peptidoglycan at the cell surface. This affects activation of the NFκB subunit c-Rel, leading to modulation in the production of interleukin (IL)-12 and tempering of the inflammatory response to intestinal flora. *B*, Mutant NOD2 in Crohn's disease is unable to sense MDP. A key constraint on the TLR2 pathway is thereby removed, which leads to enhanced IL-12 production, provocation of inflammation, and propagation of disease. CARD, caspase recruitment domain; LRRs, leucine-rich repeats. (From O'Neill LA: How NOD-ing off leads to Crohn disease. Nat Immunol 5:776, 2004.)

NOD2 protein and TAK1 (TGF-β activated kinase 1) reciprocally activate each other. NOD2 inhibits TAK1 induced activation of NFκB, whereas the defective LRR domain of NOD2 associated with Crohn's disease is less effective in inhibiting the activation of NFκB by TAK1.[77] Fourth, NOD protein expression may enhance apoptosis by caspases, which regulate the proliferation of T cells, thereby limiting immune responses.[78] Finally, it has been noted that when NOD2/CARD15 is expressed, the production of β-defensins, which are antibacterial proteins produced by Paneth cells, is defective in Crohn's patients, suggesting a link with variant NOD2.[79]

Two additional genes have recently been associated with Crohn's disease. The first, the OCTN (organic cation transporter) gene, is located at the previously identified IBD5 locus on chromosome 5q31[80,81] The second, DLG5, located on chromosome 10q23,[82] may play a role in maintaining normal cellular structure. Other loci suggested to have linkage to IBD include regions on chromosomes 1p,[83] 1q, 3p, 3q, 6p, and 7. The 6p region, though not as strongly associated as IBD1, is of interest because it is the site of the HLA genes and the TNF gene. Crohn's disease has been associated with a variety of HLA class II genes, albeit inconsistently.

ENVIRONMENT

Although the greatest relative risk of Crohn's disease is found among first-degree relatives of affected persons, particularly siblings of the proband, environmental factors also are important. As noted earlier, the rising incidence of Crohn's disease over many decades highly suggests an environmental contribution to the expression of disease. Epidemiologic studies have examined numerous risk factors for Crohn's disease. Most studies have found breast-feeding to be protective for IBD, presumably by playing a role in early programming of immune responses in the developing gastrointestinal tract. Occupations associated with outdoor physical labor are relatively under-represented among Crohn's patients, and Crohn's disease has been associated with higher socioeconomic status,[84] presumably because of relative underexposure to diverse environmental antigens in the course of childhood. Many, but not all, studies have discerned an increased risk of Crohn's disease among women who use oral contraceptives. Nonsteroidal anti-inflammatory drugs (NSAIDs) have been implicated not only in exacerbations of IBD but also as a potential precipitant of new cases, perhaps by increasing intestinal permeability. Increased intake of refined sugars and a paucity of fresh fruits and vegetables in the diet have been associated with the development of Crohn's disease. It is conceivable that this observation may be confounded by exacerbation of symptoms in patients with mild disease because of increased dietary fiber intake and subsequent avoidance of these food items before diagnosis.

Smoking is one of the more notable environmental factors for IBD. Ulcerative colitis is largely a disease of ex-smokers and nonsmokers, whereas Crohn's disease is more prevalent among smokers, and smokers have more surgery for their disease and a greater risk of relapse after resection. The reasons for the divergent effect of smoking on Crohn's disease and ulcerative colitis are poorly understood but may include effects on intestinal permeability, cytokine production, and clotting in the microvasculature.

Many patients report a correlation between disease exacerbations and stress. Although depression and anxiety are a common reaction to illness, Crohn's disease has not been shown to be caused by stress or by an anxious personality.[85] The mind-body connection between emotional states or stress and intestinal inflammation in IBD is slowly being revealed, however, and in animal models of IBD, animals under stress are more prone to exacerbation of gut inflammation.[86]

A virtually unexplored area is the connection between environmental and genetic factors in the expression of disease. One initial venture into this area is the finding of a differential increase in intestinal permeability among first-degree relatives of Crohn's disease probands when given NSAIDs as compared with control subjects given NSAIDs.[87]

PATHOLOGY

Focal intestinal inflammation is the hallmark pathologic finding in Crohn's disease. This tendency for focal inflammation is evident in focal crypt inflammation, focal areas of marked chronic inflammation, the presence of aphthae and ulcers on a background of little or no chronic inflammation, and the interspersing of segments of involved bowel with segments of uninvolved bowel. Even within a single biopsy specimen one may see a pronounced variability in the degree of inflammation. The presence of focally enhanced gastritis, characterized by a focal perifoveolar or periglandular lymphomonocytic infiltrate, is a common finding that occurs in 43% of unselected patients with Crohn's disease.[88] This finding underscores the focal nature of the inflammation, despite the strong potential for inflammation to occur anywhere along the longitudinal axis of the gut. To a certain extent, the nature of the findings and the depth of inflammatory changes depend on the chronicity of the inflammation.

EARLY FEATURES

Because of the variable and often long delay between the onset of the disease process and its diagnosis, it rarely is possible to observe the evolution of pathology from the earliest events. Studies of recurrent Crohn's disease after ileal resection have offered a window into the sequence of pathologic changes in the disease.[89] The earliest characteristic lesion of Crohn's disease is the *aphthous ulcer*. These superficial ulcers are minute, ranging in size from barely visible to 3 mm, and are surrounded by a halo of erythema.[90] In the small intestine, aphthous ulcers arise most often over lymphoid aggregates with destruction of the overlying M cells. In the colon, aphthae may occur without an endoscopically visible central erosion and may be associated with lymphoepithelial complexes.[91] Crohn's disease typically occurs in normal mucosa, although villus blunting may be seen in the surrounding mucosa.[90] Aphthous ulcers represent focal areas of immune activation. The M cells and underlying lymphoid aggregates are primary locations for antigen sampling and antigen presentation, so it is not surprising that HLA-DR is strongly expressed on the follicle-associated epithelium of the aphthous ulcer.[92] Furthermore, contact with luminal contents is a key factor in the development of aphthous ulcers in Crohn's disease. Aphthous ulcers heal in bowel excluded from the fecal stream by ileostomy, whereas re-establishing intestinal continuity leads to their recurrence[93]; these observations provide strong evidence for the role of luminal factors in the early pathogenesis of Crohn's disease.

The presence of *granulomas* (Fig. 108–3), although highly characteristic of Crohn's disease, is neither unique to Crohn's disease nor universally found. Noncaseating granulomas, like aphthous lesions, are believed to be an early finding.[94] Estimates of the prevalence of granulomas in Crohn's disease have varied greatly, ranging from 15% in endoscopic series[91] to as high as 70% in surgical series.[95] Whether granulomas are found appears to be in part a matter of how hard one looks and how much tissue is available to examine; the more tissue sampled, the larger the specimen, and the more levels taken for histopathology, the more likely granulomas are to be found. Granulomas may be discovered in involved and uninvolved bowel, in any layer of the gut, and in mesenteric lymph nodes. Granulomas also may be found outside the intestinal tract, such as in the skin, eye, and liver, but extraintestinal granulomas are rare; occasionally, they may be recognized as millet seed–like nodules on the serosal surface at laparotomy. The granulomas of Crohn's disease are sarcoid-like, consisting of collections of epithelioid histiocytes and a mixture of other inflammatory cells such as lymphocytes and eosinophils; giant cells occasionally are seen. The granulomas usually are sparse, scattered, and not well formed. In contrast with the granulomas of tuberculosis, there is little or no central necrosis, and acid-fast stains and mycobacterial cultures are negative. It also is important to distinguish the granulomas of Crohn's disease from those that may occur in association with an injured crypt. The latter represent a response to mucin released from injured goblet cells and may be found in ulcerative colitis and other conditions.

Regardless of whether granulomas are found, the granulomatous inflammation of Crohn's disease represents a particular process involving characteristic cell types and regulation by specific cytokines and adhesion molecules. TNF is the key cytokine in the formation of granulomas. Appreciation of this fact led to the concept of anti-TNF therapies as a treatment for Crohn's disease (see later).

LATER FEATURES

Resected specimens of intestine may show localized foci of architectural distortion unaccompanied by chronic inflammation, an observation that suggests early superficial lesions such as aphthae may be transient and reversible.[96] When the disease becomes chronic, however, aphthae may coalesce into larger ulcers with a stellate appearance. Linear or serpiginous ulcers may form when multiple ulcers fuse in a longitudinal direction. With linear and transverse coalescence of ulcers, the classic cobblestoned appearance may result, as networks of ulcers surround areas of relatively normal mucosa and prominent submucosal edema. Ulcers also may extend down to the muscularis propria.

A prevailing generalization is that intestinal inflammation in Crohn's disease is a transmural process, in contrast to the more superficial inflammation of ulcerative colitis. The transmural nature of the inflammation, however, cannot be appreciated on superficial endoscopic biopsy, and in resected specimens it tends to be focal. Transmural involvement is observed less commonly than is disease of the mucosa and submucosa, but to the extent that transmural disease is noted, it is highly consistent with a diagnosis of Crohn's disease. Dense lymphoid aggregates may enlarge the submucosa. At times lymphoid aggregates also may be seen just outside the muscularis propria. The presence of lymphoid aggregates in both the submucosa and external to the muscularis propria are a reliable sign of Crohn's disease even when granulomas are not seen.[96] Lymphoid aggregates occasionally may be seen within the muscularis propria, most often adjacent to the myenteric plexus.

Large ulcers, sinus tracts, and strictures are late features of Crohn's disease. Sinuses and fistulas represent extensions of fissures; sinus tracts end blindly, and fistulas enter epithelial-lined organs such as bowel, skin, bladder, or vagina. Intramural sinus tracts are recognized easily on barium studies. With penetration of inflammation to the serosa, serositis may occur, resulting in adhesion of bowel to loops of small bowel, colon, or other adjacent organs. As a result of the chronicity of the inflammatory process, free perforation is much less common than walled-off

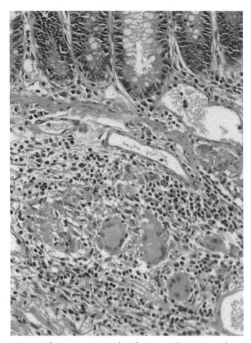

Figure 108–3 Photomicrograph of a granuloma in a biopsy specimen obtained from a patient with Crohn's disease. Note the loosely formed collection of cells, consisting of multinucleated giant cells and mononuclear cells, including T cells and epithelioid macrophages. Central caseation is not seen. (Courtesy of Gregory Lauwers, MD, Boston, MA.)

perforation or contained intra-abdominal abscesses or fistula formation. Fissures and fistulas are lined by neutrophils and surrounded by histiocytes and a mononuclear cell infiltrate; partial epithelialization also is frequently observed, perhaps reflecting partial healing.

Fibrosis is another transmural aspect of the disease. Fibrosis may be evident grossly as irregular thickening of the bowel wall and, along with hypertrophy of the muscularis mucosa, may contribute to the development of strictures. TGF-β is released locally in the presence of inflammation and is a cytokine critical for restitution and healing. In Crohn's disease, however, TGF-β may be a double-edged sword. Fibroblasts isolated from the lamina propria produce primarily type III collagen in response to TGF-$β_1$, and in the inflamed tissues of Crohn's disease, significantly greater amounts of type III collagen are produced in response to this cytokine.[97] Thus, a cytokine essential to the healing process also is implicated in fibrogenesis in Crohn's disease.

OTHER FEATURES

At the anatomic level, one of the most characteristic findings of Crohn's disease is the presence of *fat wrapping*. This finding is highly characteristic of Crohn's disease and refers to the "creeping" of mesenteric fat onto the serosal surface of the bowel. Surgeons have long taken fat wrapping as a reliable indicator of the presence of diseased tissue, an observation borne out by careful study. Mesenteric adipose tissue hypertrophy and creeping fat are recognized early in the course of disease at laparotomy or laparoscopy. Locally, fat wrapping correlates with the presence of underlying acute and chronic inflammation, as well as transmural inflammation in the form of lymphoid aggregates.[98] Of note, expression of peroxisome proliferator-activated receptor γ, a pivotal mediator in the regulation of adipose tissue homeostasis, is increased greatly in Crohn's tissues.[99] In turn, adipocytes may participate in the inflammatory process of Crohn's disease by producing TNF and other inflammatory mediators.

At the microscopic level, the finding of *pyloric metaplasia*, normally a response to peptic ulcer disease when found in the duodenum, strongly suggests a diagnosis of Crohn's disease when found in the terminal ileum. Careful descriptive immunopathology of areas of pyloric metaplasia reveals the presence of an ulcer-associated cell lineage. Budlike glandular structures arise adjacent to areas of ulceration and are distinguished by production of epidermal growth factor in acinar cells of the nascent gland and by trefoil proteins (see Chapter 1) in the more superficial cells lining the tract. Epidermal growth factor and trefoil proteins, in turn, may promote restitution of the epithelium in adjacent mucosal ulceration.[100]

CLINICAL FEATURES

DISEASE LOCATION

Crohn's disease has a predilection for the distal small bowel and proximal large bowel. Nearly one half of all patients have disease affecting both ileum and colon.

Another one third have disease confined to the small bowel, primarily the terminal ileum and in some cases including the jejunum as well.[25] Isolated jejunal involvement is rare. Gross involvement of the esophagus, stomach, or duodenum also is rare and almost always is seen in association with disease of the distal small bowel or colon. Focally enhanced acute and chronic inflammation may be seen in gastric biopsies in patients with Crohn's disease either with or without gross involvement of the stomach.[101] From 20% to 25% of patients have disease confined to the colon. The discontinuous nature of the disease makes possible many variations in disease location, leading to considerable differences in the clinical presentation. The disease usually stays confined to the segment in which it presents, but anatomic localization may vary over time, generally by involvement of additional segments of the alimentary tract, reflecting gross involvement with a disease that has the potential to affect any segment of the gastrointestinal tract.

CLINICAL PRESENTATION

The presentation of Crohn's disease may be subtle and varies considerably. Factors contributing to this variability include the location of disease within the gastrointestinal tract, the intensity of inflammation, and the presence of specific intestinal and extraintestinal complications. Compared with ulcerative colitis, abdominal pain is a more frequent and persistent complaint. Pain may be intermittent and colicky or sustained and severe and is attributable to inflammation, abscess and obstruction. Some patients may experience symptoms that are mild but long-standing or that are atypical. Such patients are more likely to experience a delay in diagnosis in excess of a year. In the past, a mean delay in diagnosis of 3.3 years from the onset of symptoms was reported,[102] but with improved diagnostic methods, and perhaps heightened awareness of the disease, more recent series have described delays of less than 1 year. Occasionally, radiologic and endoscopic findings are subtle, precluding definitive diagnosis even among patients with typical symptoms. Fecal occult blood may be found in approximately one half of patients, but in contrast with ulcerative colitis, gross rectal bleeding is uncommon, and acute hemorrhage is rare.[103] Constitutional symptoms, particularly weight loss and fever, or growth retardation in children, may be prominent and occasionally are the sole presenting features of Crohn's disease.

Typical Presentations

Disease of the ileum, often accompanied by involvement of the *cecum*, may present insidiously. Some patients present with a small bowel obstruction, perhaps precipitated by impaction of indigestible foods such as raw vegetables or fruit. Many years of subclinical inflammation may progress to fibrotic stenosis, with the subsequent onset of intermittent colicky pain, sometimes accompanied by nausea and vomiting. Physical examination may reveal fullness or a tender mass in the right hypogastrium during obstructive episodes. Patients with an active inflammatory component to their disease more often present with anorexia, loose or frequent stools, and weight loss; their examination may reveal fever or evidence of malnutrition. Occasionally, a patient may present with acute right lower quadrant pain, mimicking appendicitis.

Colonic disease may involve mainly the right colon or may extend distally to involve most or all of the colon (*extensive or total colitis*). In patients with Crohn's colitis, tenesmus is a less frequent complaint than in patients with ulcerative colitis, because the rectum often is not involved or may be less severely inflamed than other colonic segments. The typical presenting symptom of colonic disease is diarrhea, occasionally with passage of obvious blood. The severity of the diarrhea tends to correlate with both the extent of colitis and the severity of inflammation, and the presentation may range from minimally altered bowel habits to fulminant colitis. Abdominal pain may be present to a greater extent than is seen in ulcerative colitis. Systemic manifestations such as weight loss and malaise also may be prominent.

Although most patients with Crohn's colitis have relative or complete sparing of the rectum, *proctitis* may be the initial presentation in some cases. Among a series of 96 patients with idiopathic proctitis, 13.6% progressed to develop Crohn's disease, usually within 3 years of initial presentation.[104]

Perianal disease is another common presentation of Crohn's disease. In as many as 24% of patients with Crohn's disease, perianal disease precedes intestinal manifestations with a mean lead time of 4 years.[105] More often, however, perianal disease occurs concomitantly with or after the onset of the symptoms of luminal disease. Perianal findings may be categorized as skin lesions, anal canal lesions, and perianal fistulas.[106] Skin lesions include maceration, superficial ulcers, and abscesses. Anal canal lesions include fissures, ulcers, and stenosis. The anal fissures of Crohn's disease tend to be placed more eccentrically than the usual idiopathic fissures, which generally occur in the midline. In most cases, anal stricture is asymptomatic, but occasionally obstruction may occur, particularly if stool consistency improves in the course of treatment. Deeper abscesses may arise secondary to fistulas, especially when the internal os is located high in the rectum.

Unusual Presentations

Upper gastrointestinal tract Crohn's disease is uncommon in the absence of disease beyond the ligament of Treitz. Approximately one third of patients with proximal Crohn's disease do not have evidence of distal Crohn's disease at the time of diagnosis, but virtually all develop distal disease in time.[107] Patients with proximal Crohn's disease tend to be younger at the time of diagnosis and more often present with abdominal pain and malaise.[107] Patients with upper tract disease do not undergo surgery more often than do patients with lower tract disease alone, but the length of bowel that is resected tends to be greater.[107] *Gastroduodenal Crohn's disease* presents as *Helicobacter pylori*–negative peptic ulcer disease, with dyspepsia or epigastric pain as the primary symptoms. When outflow obstruction occurs because of stricture formation or edema, early satiety, nausea, vomiting, and weight loss may predominate.

Esophageal Crohn's disease is rare, occurring in less than 2% of patients. The presenting symptoms may include dysphagia, odynophagia, substernal chest pain, and heartburn. These symptoms may be progressive and lead to profound weight loss.[108] Aphthous ulcers may sometimes be found in the mouth and posterior pharynx. Esophageal stricture and even esophagobronchial fistula may complicate the course. An intriguing observation is that HLA-DR expression frequently is seen in the esophageal epithelium of patients with Crohn's disease even when the disease is located more distally in the gastrointestinal tract, perhaps indicating widespread immunologic activation of the gastrointestinal mucosa.[109]

Crohn's disease confined solely to the jejunum and ileum is unusual and may be impossible to differentiate from *ulcerative jejunoileitis*, a distinct condition that occasionally may respond to a gluten-free diet (see Chapter 101). Frank malabsorption and steatorrhea often occur. When the disease is confined to a short segment of intestine or has features consistent with Crohn's disease, initial management should be based on the presumed diagnosis of Crohn's disease.

Controversy continues to surround the diagnosis of *Crohn's disease of the appendix*. When idiopathic granulomatous inflammation is confined to the appendix, the presentation most often resembles that of acute appendicitis and occasionally periappendiceal abscess. The condition is rare, but the lack of disease in other locations of bowel portends a favorable prognosis, with a postoperative recurrence rate as low as 6%[110]; some authors suggest that granulomatous appendicitis should be considered an entity separate from Crohn's disease.[110]

DISEASE BEHAVIOR

Clinical observation suggests that disease behavior in Crohn's disease may be divided roughly into two categories: aggressive fistulizing disease and indolent cicatrizing disease denoted by fibrostenotic stricture[111]; a third subset of patients appear to develop neither behavior over long periods of observation. Moreover, these distinctions are not always neat. Both fistula and stricture may occur simultaneously in the same patient, as in the patient with a fistula arising behind a terminal ileal stricture, or at different times. Nevertheless, a distinctive cytokine profile of increased IL-1β and IL-1 receptor antagonist levels in intestinal tissues from patients with nonpenetrating, noncicatrizing disease suggests that distinct pathogenetic mechanisms operate among these groups.[112]

Fistula and Abscess

Fistulas are frequent manifestations of the transmural nature of Crohn's disease. Immune activation triggers the release of a variety of proteases and matrix metalloproteinases[113] that may contribute directly to tissue destruction, sinus tract formation, and, finally, penetration to adjacent tissues. *Perianal fistulas* are common and are estimated to occur in 15% to 35% of patients (Fig. 108–4A). When the fistula arises from an anal gland, a low-lying

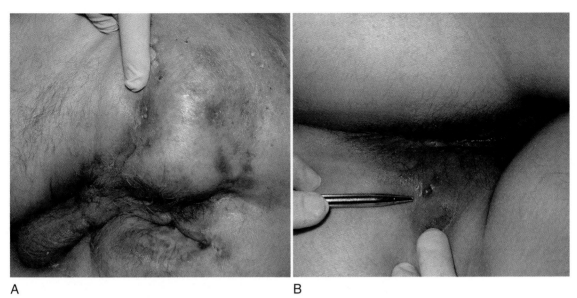

A   B

Figure 108–4 *A,* Perianal fistula in a woman with Crohn's disease. *B,* Multiple healed perineal fistulas that, when active, drained into the buttock and perineum; healing was associated with hyperpigmentation of the skin surrounding the fistulous opening. (*A* and *B,* Courtesy of Lawrence J. Brandt, MD, Bronx, NY.)

perianal fistula is the most common result. Such fistulas often are minimally symptomatic and may resolve with local care alone. Surprisingly, not all perianal fistulas occur in the setting of active rectal inflammation. In some cases, perianal fistulization may be extensive, forming a network of passages and extending to multiple openings that may include not only the perianal region but also the labia or scrotum, buttocks, or thighs (Fig. 108–4*B*).

Fistulas from one segment of the gastrointestinal tract to another also occur frequently. Enteroenteric, enterocolonic, and colocolonic fistulas often are asymptomatic. Much more rarely, colonic disease penetrates normal duodenum or stomach to form a coloduodenal or cologastric fistula. Affected patients may have feculent vomiting. If the fistula tracks posteriorly from the terminal ileum to the retroperitoneum, the ensuing phlegmon may ensnare the ureter (usually the right ureter), causing noncalculous hydronephrosis. Such patients often present with thigh pain or a limping gait. Deeper penetration yields the classic, but fortunately rare, circumstance of a psoas abscess. Affected patients typically present with right flank discomfort, fever, and a gait similar to those with ureteral entrapment.

Fistula to the vagina may occur with penetration from a severely inflamed rectal vault anteriorly (i.e., *rectovaginal fistula*) or from the small bowel. *Rectovaginal fistulas* tend to occur among women who have had a hysterectomy, permitting direct extension to the adjacent vaginal cuff without the interfering presence of the uterus. Patients present with foul, persistent vaginal discharge and occasionally with passage of flatus or frank stool per vagina. Patients also may complain of dyspareunia or perineal pain. The vaginal os of the fistula may be difficult to visualize, but palpation may elicit tenderness of the posterior vaginal wall. Fistulas arising from terminal ileal disease often occur in the setting of an ileal stricture, back pressure and stasis perhaps contributing to the process.

Enterovesicular or *colovesicular fistulas* may present as recurrent polymicrobial urinary tract infection or as frank pneumaturia and fecaluria. These fistulas are notoriously difficult to heal by nonsurgical means, but the resulting cystitis may be controlled with antibiotics. *Enterocutaneous fistulas* to the anterior abdomen, often occurring after surgery, may be especially troublesome. A classic presentation of Crohn's disease is the onset of an enterocutaneous fistula after appendectomy for what had been presumed to be appendicitis. Often the tract of the fistula will follow the planes of dissection to the abdominal surface.

It has been estimated that as many as one fourth of all patients with Crohn's disease will present with an intra-abdominal abscess at some time in their lives.[114] This figure is much less than one would imagine in light of the high frequency of fistulas. For the most part, inflamed serosal surfaces adhere to innocent serosa, thereby containing what would be an otherwise free perforation. The classic presentation of an intra-abdominal abscess is that of a patient with spiking fevers and focal abdominal tenderness or localized peritoneal signs. Unfortunately, many of the patients at highest risk for perforation or abscess also are on glucocorticoids, which are notorious for suppressing peritoneal signs and fever and masking the presentations of infection. Therefore, a high level of suspicion must be maintained. When free perforation and peritonitis do occur, the situation is life threatening.

Stricture

Stricture is another characteristic complication of Crohn's disease. Strictures represent long-standing inflammation and may occur in any segment of the gastrointestinal tract in which inflammation has been active. Strictures do not develop in all patients with inflammatory disease but are likely to recur, most often at the anastomosis, in patients who undergo bowel resection

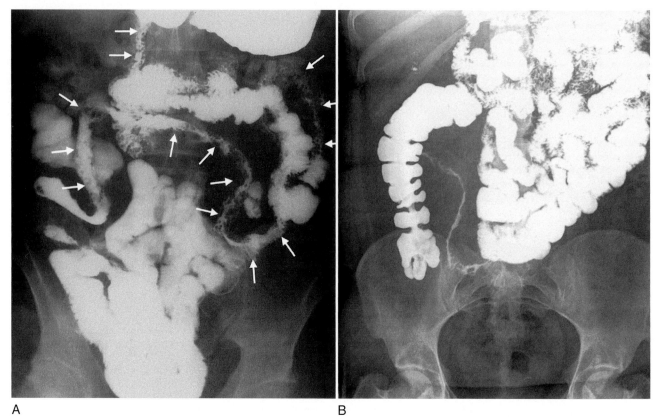

A   B

Figure 108–5   Barium examination of the small intestine in two patients with Crohn's disease. Barium studies continue to play an important role in the evaluation of patients with Crohn's disease. *A*, Multiple areas of narrowed small intestine are noted (*arrows*) with a classic cobblestone appearance of the mucosa. Note also the separation of bowel loops. *B*, A "string sign" is noted in the right lower quadrant. This classic radiologic sign of a markedly narrowed bowel segment amid widely spaced bowel loops results from spasm and edema associated with active inflammation rather than fibrostenosis; the typical string sign resolves transiently with administration of glucagon, which relieves smooth muscle spasm. (*A* and *B*, Courtesy of Jack Wittenberg, MD, Boston, MA.)

because of a stricture. These observations suggest that additional unidentified factors play a role in stricture formation. Strictures are usually silent until the luminal caliber is small enough to cause relative obstruction. Symptoms may include colicky postprandial abdominal pain and bloating, punctuated by more severe episodes, and often culminating in complete obstruction. However, not all obstructive presentations are caused by fibrotic strictures. The classic radiologic "string sign" of a markedly narrowed bowel segment amidst widely spaced bowel loops (Fig. 108–5) is a result of spasm and edema associated with active inflammation rather than fibrostenosis; the typical string sign transiently resolves with administration of glucagon, which relieves smooth muscle spasm. Short of demonstrating a clear response to anti-inflammatory therapy or reviewing a surgical specimen, the clinician may find it extremely difficult to differentiate a fibrostenotic from an inflammatory stricture. All strictures must be considered with suspicion, and biopsies of a stricture need to be pursued vigorously, because some strictures will harbor cancer.

CLASSIFICATION OF DISEASE

A major need in the clinical investigation of Crohn's disease is the ability to define subgroups of patients with distinctive, if not unique, characteristics. The ability to define such subgroups of patients with distinct prognoses could add tremendous power to the investigation of new therapies and to genetic studies. In light of the wide heterogeneity of demographic, anatomic, and disease behavior characteristics, however, distilling the numerous possible phenotypes into simple categories is a formidable task. The Vienna Classification of Crohn's Disease is one proposed scheme that incorporates the patient's age at onset, disease location, and disease behavior into a schema with 24 potential subgroups.[115] It is not surprising that in this scheme, significant associations are noted between age at diagnosis and location and between disease behavior and location, along with a trend toward an association between age at diagnosis and disease behavior.[116] Increasingly, subclinical characteristics such as serologic markers and genetic profiles will be utilized for their prognostic values in projecting outcomes in this heterogeneous disease.

PATHOPHYSIOLOGY OF COMMON SYMPTOMS AND SIGNS

Diarrhea is the most common complaint among patients with Crohn's disease. Increased stool frequency and decreased stool consistency arise through alterations in mucosal function and intestinal motility. In any given patient, multiple factors are likely to contribute to diarrhea. Altered fluid and electrolyte absorption and secretion may decrease stool consistency. Increased mucosal permeability from mucosal inflammation may result in exudation of protein and fluids. Increased production of prostaglandins, biogenic amines, cytokines, neuropeptides, and reactive oxygen metabolites all contribute to these alterations. An imbalance in the luminal concentration of bile salts relative to dietary fat may result in either bile salt–induced diarrhea or steatorrhea in the setting of ileal dysfunction or resection (see Chapter 98). Bacterial overgrowth may occur behind strictured bowel and contribute to malabsorption (see Chapter 99). Disordered colonic motility is seen in the setting of chronic inflammation and also contributes to diarrhea. Occasionally, medications used to treat Crohn's disease may exacerbate diarrhea. Diarrhea can occur with olsalazine, which may induce a secretory diarrhea, and any of the 5-aminosalicylates (5-ASAs), which rarely may induce a paradoxical flare of Crohn's disease.

The pathophysiology of *abdominal pain* in Crohn's disease is not well understood. Multiple lines of investigation have provided tantalizing clues about the connection between the nervous system and Crohn's disease, although the relationship among the enteric nervous system, inflammation, and immune activation in Crohn's disease is quite complex. Stretch receptors in the bowel wall may be stimulated as a food bolus passes through stenotic bowel, leading to abdominal pain and possibly vomiting. Visceral pain may result from inflammation of the serosa. The ganglia of the myenteric plexuses in the intestine in Crohn's disease have been noted to be increased in size and number, possibly indicating neural dysfunction.[117] Substance P binding may participate in the expression of pain. Substance P receptors have been found in increased numbers around the lymphoid follicles in the microvasculature and on enteric neurons in Crohn's disease, even in locations distant from active inflammation.[118] Enteroglia, support cells of the enteric nervous system, express MHC class II antigens in Crohn's disease, raising the possibility that they participate in the inflammatory process as antigen-presenting cells.[119]

Weight loss and *malnutrition* are often seen in patients with Crohn's disease and contribute to the complaints of weakness, irritability, malaise, and easy fatigability that are so common. In children, malnutrition may manifest as growth retardation. A host of specific nutritional deficiencies may be found even among patients in long-standing remission,[120,121] including iron, folic acid, vitamin B_{12}, calcium, magnesium, zinc, and, particularly in the setting of malabsorption from small bowel disease, fat-soluble vitamins. Potential contributing factors for these deficiencies are numerous and include inadequate intestinal absorption among patients with extensive small bowel disease or resection; increased protein losses through exudation from inflamed bowel; specific medications (e.g., decreased calcium absorption with glucocorticoids; malabsorption of fat, fat-soluble vitamins, and calcium with cholestyramine; folate malabsorption with sulfasalazine); and increased energy and protein requirements resulting from the catabolic state induced by

intense inflammation. Moreover, unrecognized infection can be a major contributing factor beyond the catabolism induced by the disease itself. Bypassing of small bowel by enteroenteric or enterocolonic fistulas also may contribute to undernutrition. The most important factor in weight loss, however, is poor oral intake. Most often, poor intake results from fear of eating induced by postprandial abdominal pain or diarrhea and restriction of activities associated with meals. Decreased intake occasionally may be a consequence of unnecessarily restrictive diets imposed by the physician or the patient in an effort to control symptoms. Weight loss disproportionate to the burden of disease should raise the suspicion of occult malignancy.

Anorexia, nausea, and *vomiting* also may contribute to weight loss and poor nutrition. As with other symptoms of Crohn's disease, diverse mechanisms may be contributory. TNF originally was discovered as a cytokine capable of inducing cachexia in patients with malignancy and sepsis. Indeed, serum levels of TNF in severely ill patients with Crohn's disease may be high enough to contribute to anorexia. Delayed gastric emptying may be a causative factor for these symptoms in as many as one third of children with Crohn's disease[122] and reflects an unexpectedly high rate of gastroduodenal Crohn's disease. Anorexia, nausea, or vomiting also may be caused by drugs used to treat the disease, including metronidazole, sulfasalazine, 6-mercaptopurine (6-MP), azathioprine, and methotrexate.

Fever associated with active Crohn's disease usually is low grade and may occasionally be the presenting complaint; increased production of proinflammatory cytokines, including IL-1, IL-6, and TNF, likely are contributory. When spiking, high, or persistent fevers occur, the clinician needs to consider an infectious etiology and undertake an evaluation appropriate to the clinical picture. Rarely, such fever patterns are manifestations of Crohn's disease activity alone without superimposed illness or even abscess formation.

Anemia is found in one third of patients with Crohn's disease, primarily as a consequence of iron deficiency from blood loss. Macrocytic anemia also may result from vitamin B_{12} deficiency because of ileal disease or resection or bacterial overgrowth or, less commonly, from folate deficiency because of proximal small bowel disease or sulfasalazine therapy. Overproduction of IFN-γ, TNF, or IL-1 may inhibit erythropoietin production, contributing to anemia resistant to iron supplementation.[123]

EXTRAINTESTINAL MANIFESTATIONS

In addition to penetrating and cicatrizing complications that may arise in patients with Crohn's disease, numerous complications may occur distant from the bowel. It is estimated that one fourth of all patients with Crohn's disease will have an extraintestinal manifestation of IBD.[124] Many of these complications are common to both Crohn's disease and ulcerative colitis and indeed to other nonidiopathic inflammatory conditions of the bowel. For example, patients with ileal Crohn's disease are at increased risk of cholelithiasis, but patients with extensive ulcerative colitis are at nearly the same risk.[125] In

Crohn's disease, however, the major risk factor for this complication appears to be the number of prior ileal resections.[126] In large series, extraintestinal manifestations are found to occur more frequently in Crohn's disease than in ulcerative colitis and are more common among patients with colonic involvement than in patients with no colonic inflammation. One fourth of those affected will have more than one manifestation.[127,128] Conceptually, these extraintestinal manifestations may be categorized as those associated with small bowel disease or large bowel disease and those that occur in association with active bowel disease or independent of the state of inflammation. Some complications occur as a direct result of the bowel disease, such as nephrolithiasis resulting from oxalate malabsorption. In the case of inflammatory mucocutaneous, joint, and ocular manifestations, the pathogenesis is an influx of mononuclear cells activated in the gut, but homing aberrantly to the involved extraintestinal organs.[129]

Musculoskeletal Manifestations

Among the most common extraintestinal manifestations are disorders of the bones and joints. Clubbing of the fingernails is a common and innocuous finding. More consequential are arthritic manifestations, which are observed more frequently in patients with Crohn's disease than in those with ulcerative colitis. In a study of 976 patients with ulcerative colitis and 483 patients with Crohn's disease, pauciarticular arthropathy (type I, affecting four or fewer joints) occurred in 3.6% of patients with ulcerative colitis and in 6.0% of those with Crohn's disease.[130] In most patients, joint symptoms occurred in the setting of a relapse of bowel symptoms. Polyarticular arthropathy (type II, with five or more joints affected) occurred in 2.5% of patients with ulcerative colitis and 4.0% of those with Crohn's disease.[130] Among patients with Crohn's disease, nearly one half had joint symptoms in association with a relapse in bowel disease. Intriguingly, distinct HLA genotypes are associated with these two types of peripheral arthropathy—type I: HLA-DRB1*0103, B*35 and B*27; and type II: HLA-B*44.[131]

Other reports indicate that peripheral arthralgias occur in 16% to 20% of patients with Crohn's disease,[132] most strongly in association with colonic disease.[128] Patients tend to have waxing and waning joint pain and stiffness in association with flares of bowel disease. Joints may be involved in an asymmetrical or migratory fashion. With rare exception, the disease is nondeforming and often is accompanied by skin complications (erythema nodosum) and eye complications (uveitis). Rheumatoid factor typically is negative in these patients. Knee and ankle joints often are affected first, but elbows, wrists, proximal interphalangeal, metacarpophalangeal, and metatarsophalangeal joints may be involved subsequently.[132] Patients who have undergone ileocecal resection for their disease tend to have fewer arthritic complications after their surgery.[133]

Axial arthropathies are less common than peripheral arthropathies and occur in 3% to 6% of patients with IBD. Spondylitis associated with IBD, like idiopathic ankylosing spondylitis, presents as insidious low back pain and morning stiffness that is improved by exercise.

As many as 75% of patients with Crohn's disease and spondylitis may be positive for HLA-B27. Iritis may occur in association with this manifestation. Bilateral symmetrical sacroiliitis without progression to spondylitis is more common than spondylitis and is reported to occur in 4% to 18% of patients.[132] In one study, radiologic findings of sacroiliitis were detected in 29% of patients with Crohn's disease, although only 3% had symptoms of sacroiliitis.[134]

More rare rheumatologic complications include granulomatous vasculitis,[135] periostitis, and amyloidosis. In addition, a septic joint, although a rare complication of Crohn's disease, should be kept in mind. A septic hip joint is a striking, devastating, and fortunately rare complication of a psoas abscess that extends directly to the acetabular capsule.

Glucocorticoids used to treat Crohn's disease may be a cause of joint pain. Withdrawal of glucocorticoids may lead to pseudoarthritis, with diffuse joint aches that gradually resolve. Adrenal insufficiency should be considered in such patients. Aseptic necrosis of the hip and other joints may occur with or without the use of glucocorticoids and may be disabling.[136] Osteomyelitis may occur as a result of direct extension by a fistula, usually to the pelvis, or may be a recurrent problem distant from the site of inflammation, presumably through hematogenous spread of bacteria.[137]

Metabolic bone disease is common in Crohn's disease; osteopenia (T score on dual energy x-ray absorptiometry between −2.49 and −1.0) or osteoporosis (T score lower than −2.5) occurs in 30% to 60% of patients. Morbidity as a consequence of increased susceptibility to bone fractures includes debilitating and painful vertebral crush fractures, which may occur even in children with Crohn's disease. Although glucocorticoid use is the main risk factor for this metabolic bone disease in ulcerative colitis, low bone mineral density is a feature of Crohn's disease even at diagnosis.[138] Contributing factors include malabsorption of calcium and vitamin D; smoking[139]; and perhaps the effects of proinflammatory cytokines such as TNF, IL-1, and IL-6 on osteoclasts, some of which may be genetically determined.[140]

Mucocutaneous Manifestations

The most common skin lesions associated with IBD are *pyoderma gangrenosum* and *erythema nodosum*. Neither condition is found solely in IBD, and the finding of one or the other lesion is not specific for either major form of IBD.[141] Pyoderma gangrenosum appears first as a papule, pustule, or nodule, most often on the leg or occasionally around a stoma, and progresses to an ulcer with undermined borders. Pyoderma may, however, occur virtually anywhere on the body. The ulcer typically has a violaceous rim and crater-like holes pitting the base. The phenomenon of pathergy, or the development of large ulcers in response to minor trauma, is characteristic of pyoderma gangrenosum and the skin lesions of Behçet's syndrome.[142] Healing is associated with a classically cribriform, or pocked, scar. In Crohn's disease pyoderma gangrenosum often occurs without an associated flare of bowel symptoms.

In contrast with pyoderma gangrenosum, erythema nodosum is much more frequently seen in women than in men. Like pyoderma gangrenosum, many other diseases are associated with erythema nodosum, including *Streptococcus* or *Yersinia* infection, tuberculosis, leprosy, fungal infections, Behçet's syndrome, and sarcoidosis. The classic appearance is of tender subcutaneous nodules with an erythematous or dusky appearance, most often seen on the pretibial region. There is a strong association with arthropathy. Erythema nodosum often presents during exacerbations of bowel disease and tends to improve with treatment of the underlying bowel disease. If possible, erythema nodosum lesions should not be biopsied because biopsied lesions tend to scar, whereas spontaneously resolving lesions heal without scar formation.

Aphthous ulcers of the mouth are common among patients with Crohn's disease and ulcerative colitis but are also frequently seen among otherwise healthy persons.[143] As the most cephalad point of the gastrointestinal tract, the mouth rarely may be involved directly by the granulomatous inflammation of Crohn's disease. Angular cheilitis is seen in nearly 8% of patients with Crohn's disease.[143]

A rare manifestation is *metastatic Crohn's disease*, granulomatous inflammation of the skin remote from the gastrointestinal tract but histologically identical to the primary bowel lesion.[144] Described cases have included lesions behind the ears, in the perineum, and on the legs, penis, and vulva. Other rare skin manifestations of Crohn's disease include leukocytoclastic vasculitis,[145] Sweet's syndrome (neutrophilic dermatosis),[146] cutaneous polyarteritis nodosa, and epidermolysis bullosa acquisita. Some reports have suggested an increased occurrence of psoriasis among patients with Crohn's disease.[147]

Ocular Manifestations

Ocular manifestations are estimated to occur in 6% of patients with Crohn's disease.[148] *Episcleritis* is more common in Crohn's disease than in ulcerative colitis, consists of injection of the sclera and conjunctiva, and does not affect visual acuity. Episodes tend to occur in association with active bowel disease. *Scleritis* involves deeper layers of the eye and also occurs most often in parallel with active bowel disease but may cause lasting damage if untreated. *Uveitis* usually presents with headache, deep eye pain, lacrimation, blurred vision, and photophobia, as a consequence of iridospasm. Physical examination findings include meiosis and ciliary flush. Visual acuity is preserved unless the posterior segment becomes involved. In contrast with the uveitis associated with ankylosing spondylitis, the presentation of uveitis in patients with IBD often is insidious, with bilateral involvement and extension to the posterior segment.[149] Slit-lamp examination demonstrates an inflammatory "flare" in the anterior chamber. At least one report suggests that children with Crohn's colitis frequently have asymptomatic anterior chamber inflammation.[150] Other ocular complications of Crohn's disease include a particular corneal injury referred to as *keratopathy* and night blindness resulting from malabsorption of vitamin A.

Hepatobiliary Manifestations

Gallstones are found in more than 25% of men and women with Crohn's disease, representing a relative risk of 1.8 compared with the general population.[126] Asymptomatic and mild elevations of liver biochemical tests often are seen in Crohn's disease, but few of these patients develop clinical evidence of cirrhosis. Primary sclerosing cholangitis more often is associated with ulcerative colitis but may occur in 4% of patients with Crohn's disease, usually those with colonic involvement.[151] In patients with Crohn's disease, the inflammatory changes most often are confined to the small biliary radicals and, therefore, the presentation is usually one of abnormal liver biochemical tests, *pericholangitis* on liver biopsy, and a normal cholangiogram.[151] Other hepatobiliary complications of Crohn's disease include fatty liver and autoimmune hepatitis.

Renal and Genitourinary Manifestations

In addition to the direct complications of perforating Crohn's disease with encroachment on the bladder and other genitourinary structures, and inflammatory entrapment of the ureter, *uric acid* and *oxalate stones* are common in patients with Crohn's disease. In the setting of fat malabsorption resulting from intestinal resection or extensive small bowel disease, luminal calcium binds free fatty acids, thereby decreasing the calcium that is available to bind and clear oxalate. Increased oxalate is absorbed as the sodium salt, resulting in hyperoxaluria and calcium oxalate stone formation. Uric acid stones are believed to result from volume depletion and a hypermetabolic state. More rare complications include membranous nephropathy, glomerulonephritis, and renal amyloidosis. Penile and vulvar edema also have been reported, but the mechanism for these occurrences is unknown.

Coagulation and Vascular Complications

A *prothrombotic tendency* has been noted in both major forms of IBD. Patients may present with venous thromboembolism or, much less commonly, arterial thrombosis. The hypercoagulable state may arise from many possible causes. Contributing factors may include thrombocytosis; increased levels of fibrinogen, fibrinopeptide A, factor V, and factor VIII; antithrombin III deficiency; and free protein S deficiency; all are related to active bowel inflammation. Circulating immune complexes, increased levels of plasminogen activator inhibitors, decreased levels of tissue plasminogen activator, and spontaneous platelet aggregation may be present independent of bowel inflammation. Increased prevalence of the factor V Leiden mutation has been observed by some[152] but not other investigators.[153] Defective methylenetetrahydrofolate reductase is more prevalent among patients with IBD than it is in the general population.[154] This finding, along with folate and vitamin B_{12} deficiency, is linked to hyperhomocysteinemia, which in turn predisposes to thrombosis. In more than one half of patients who experience thrombosis, however, no predisposing factor can be identified.[155]

Other Manifestations

Clinically significant disease of the lungs,[156] heart, pancreas, and nervous system[157] in association with Crohn's disease is unusual, but reported. Subclinical lung involvement may be much more common than is apparent, perhaps reflecting the commonality of bronchus-associated lymphoid tissue and gut-associated lymphoid tissue.[156] Cardiomyopathy may result from a variety of nutrient deficiencies in patients with marked malabsorption. Pleuropericarditis, myocarditis, and endocarditis may occur rarely.[158] Acute pancreatitis,[159] granulomatous pancreatitis,[160] and pancreatic insufficiency[161] also have been reported.

DIFFERENTIAL DIAGNOSIS

Establishing a diagnosis of Crohn's disease usually is straightforward once it is considered. Nevertheless, a large number of alternative diagnoses may be considered during various stages of the evaluation. Reports are legion of other diseases mistakenly diagnosed as Crohn's disease and of Crohn's disease mistaken for other diseases. Misdiagnoses may be attributed to the protean presentations of Crohn's disease, which include considerable variability among patients with distinct anatomic distributions of disease, different degrees of inflammation, and the variable presence of intestinal complications and extraintestinal manifestations. There are a number of clinical situations in which Crohn's disease should enter the differential diagnosis. These clinical presentations include diarrhea or abdominal pain, especially when localized to the right lower quadrant; evidence of intestinal inflammation on radiologic or endoscopic studies; the discovery of an intestinal stricture or fistula arising from the bowel; and evidence of inflammation or granulomas on intestinal histology. Categories of causation that overlap with Crohn's disease in clinical presentation include functional bowel disorders, primarily irritable bowel syndrome; immune-mediated diseases, particularly other colitides and most importantly ulcerative colitis; medications, especially NSAIDs; vascular disorders, notably ischemic bowel disease and collagen vascular diseases; neoplasia, including carcinoma and lymphoma; infectious diarrheas, gut inflammation, or granulomas; and miscellaneous other diseases and syndromes, including diverticular disease. Once the presence of bowel inflammation has been confirmed, the differential diagnosis may focus on presentation according to the anatomic location of the findings (Table 108–1).

ESTABLISHING THE DIAGNOSIS AND EVALUATION OF DISEASE

No single symptom, sign, or diagnostic test establishes the diagnosis of Crohn's disease. Rather the diagnosis is established through a total assessment of the clinical presentation with confirmatory evidence from radiologic, endoscopic, and, in most cases, pathologic findings. The initial evaluation includes a thorough history taking, physical examination, and simple laboratory tests. History taking focuses on the key symptoms and their severity and duration. Specific points to be covered should include recent travel history, use of antibiotics and other medications, diet, and sexual activity. Family history of IBD may raise the level of suspicion but, when found, does not guarantee the diagnosis. The review of systems should elicit extraintestinal manifestations and weight loss. Fever may be associated with the underlying disease or a suppurative complication. A careful examination of the abdomen for signs of obstruction, tenderness, or a mass should be undertaken. Thorough inspection of the perineum and a rectal examination may disclose findings highly suggestive of the underlying diagnosis or gross or occult blood.

Laboratory data may be normal, but anemia and hypoalbuminemia should be assessed. Anemic patients should undergo further evaluation to define the contributions of iron, folate, or vitamin B_{12} deficiencies. The white blood cell count may be normal or elevated; an increased number of band forms suggests the possibility of a pyogenic complication. In the patient with vague symptoms suggestive of irritable bowel syndrome, an elevated C-reactive protein or erythrocyte sedimentation rate, although not specific for IBD, may prompt further investigation. Stool studies should include culture, examination for ova and parasites, and testing for *Clostridium difficile* toxin and should be performed before endoscopy or barium studies. Serology for *Entamoeba histolytica* should be considered in selected patients.

Ultimately, the diagnosis of Crohn's disease is confirmed by findings on barium studies, endoscopy, and usually histopathology. Barium studies accurately define the anatomic location of disease and can discern evidence of active inflammation. A small bowel follow-through study is the primary modality when small bowel disease is suspected (see Fig. 108–5), although capsule endoscopy is increasingly being used for this indication (see later). For most situations, small bowel enema, or enteroclysis, adds little additional information and may in fact miss gastroduodenal findings at the expense of increased cost and morbidity from discomfort associated with the use of a nasogastric tube, increased radiation exposure, and possibly sedation.[162] Barium studies are especially useful to delineate the late transmural complications of Crohn's disease, but typical findings may be seen early in the disease as well. Early findings include aphthous ulcers, a coarse villus mucosal pattern, and thickened folds.[163] Submucosal edema may be evident as thickening or flattening of the valvulae conniventes, whereas transmural edema manifests as widening of the separation between bowel loops. Ulcers most often occur on the mesenteric border with consequent pseudosacculation of the antimesenteric border because of shortening of the mesenteric portion.[163] Later findings include a cobblestone appearance resulting from edema and inflammation of relatively spared islands of mucosa separated by intersecting longitudinal and transverse knifelike clefts of ulceration.[163] Still later, one may discern fistulas, sinus tracts, and fixed strictures.

Other radiologic studies also may provide useful information. Computed tomography (CT) studies do not demonstrate mucosal detail and often appear normal early in the course of the disease (Fig. 108–6). Nevertheless, CT is of great value in discerning extraluminal features.[164] As the disease progresses, mesenteric lymphadenopathy and transmural thickening of the bowel are usually seen. CT is highly sensitive for detecting

Table 108–1 Differential Diagnosis of Crohn's Disease

Differential Diagnosis of Ileitis	Henoch-Schönlein purpura
Backwash ileitis in ulcerative colitis	Intestinal ischemia (focal segmental ischemia: acute enteritis,
Drug-related	chronic enteritis, stricture; chronic mesenteric ischemia)
Ischemic (oral contraceptives, ergotamine, amphetamines,	Vasculitis (polyarteritis nodosa, Churg-Strauss syndrome,
phenylephrine, cocaine)	systemic lupus erythematosus, Takayasu's arteritis,
NSAID-related ulcer or stricture	Wegener's granulomatosis, lymphomatoid granulomatosis,
Gynecologic disorders	giant cell arteritis, rheumatoid vasculitis, thromboangiitis
Ectopic pregnancy	obliterans)
Endometriosis	**Differential Diagnosis of Colitis**
Ovarian cyst or tumor	Acute self-limited colitis
Ovarian torsion	Behçet's disease
Pelvic inflammatory disease	Chronic granulomatous disease
Tubo-ovarian abscess	Crohn's colitis
Ileitis associated with spondyloarthropathy	Diversion colitis
Infection	Diverticulitis
Actinomycosis israelii	Drug-related intestinal inflammation (NSAIDs, gold,
Anisakis simplex	penicillamine)
Cryptococcosis	Eosinophilic gastroenteritis
Cytomegalovirus	Graft-vs.-host disease
Histoplasma capsulatum	Indeterminate colitis
Mycobacterium avium complex	Infections
Mycobacterium tuberculosis	*Aeromonas pleisioides*
Neutropenic enterocolitis	Amebiasis
Salmonella	*Campylobacter*
Yersinia enterocolitica	*Clostridium difficile*
Yersinia pseudotuberculosis	Cytomegalovirus
Infiltrative disorders	*Escherichia coli* (enterohemorrhagic, enteroinvasive)
Amyloidosis	*Mycobacterium tuberculosis*
Eosinophilic gastroenteritis	*Salmonella*
Other Inflammatory disorders	Schistosomiasis
Appendiceal abscess	*Shigella*
Appendicitis	Strongyloidiasis
Cecal diverticulitis	*Yersinia enterocolitica*
Lymphoid nodular hyperplasia	Ischemic colitis (transient ischemic colitis, chronic ischemic
Neoplasms	colitis, ischemic stricture, ischemic colitis with toxic
Carcinoid tumor	megacolon)
Cecal or ileal adenocarcinoma	Microscopic colitis
Lymphoma	Collagenous colitis
Lymphosarcoma	Lymphocytic colitis
Metastatic cancer	Radiation colitis
Radiation enteritis	Sarcoidosis
Torsion of the appendiceal epiploica	Segmental colitis associated with diverticular disease
Vascular disorders	Solitary rectal ulcer syndrome
Behçet's syndrome	Ulcerative colitis

NSAID, nonsteroidal anti-inflammatory drug.
From Sands BE: From symptom to diagnosis: Clinical distinctions among various forms of intestinal inflammation. Gastroenterology 126:1518, 2004.

differences in tissue densities. Therefore, the detection on CT of even small amounts of air in the bowel wall or adjacent structures is highly suggestive of perforating disease. Fibrofatty proliferation of the mesentery, the radiologic correlate of creeping fat seen at laparotomy, may be noted.[165] CT is the essential study for identifying suppurative complications of Crohn's disease, such as intra-abdominal and retroperitoneal abscess.

Other potentially useful modalities include ultrasound, magnetic resonance imaging (MRI), and scintigraphy. Ultrasound is used primarily to exclude other causes of abdominal pain, including biliary and gynecologic causes. Continuing advances in transabdominal ultrasound,[166] endosonography,[167] and vascular flow studies[168] may in time provide improved diagnostic accuracy and

grading of activity in Crohn's disease. MRI may provide visualization of complex perianal fistulas superior to that of pelvic CT.[169] As technology improves, MRI may provide imaging of the abdomen equal or superior to CT without exposure to ionizing radiation[170] and also may prove useful in demonstrating response to treatment.[171] Ultrasound- and CT-guided percutaneous drainage of intra-abdominal abscesses is a safe and effective alternative to surgical drainage in well-selected patients.[172] A growing body of evidence suggests that leukocyte scintigraphy may be a useful diagnostic study in Crohn's disease. Among children with suspected IBD, ^{99m}Tc leukocyte scintigraphy is highly sensitive in identifying abnormalities in patients with just mild inflammation on biopsy and a normal small bowel follow-through.[173] Lower radi-

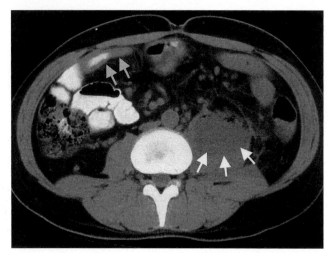

Figure 108–6 Abdominal computed tomography (CT) of a patient with Crohn's disease. This image was obtained from the same patient whose small bowel follow-through study is seen in Figure 108-5A. A left psoas muscle abscess (*white arrows*), arising from penetrating disease extending from adjacent bowel, was missed on small bowel follow-through. Thickened small bowel (*gray arrows*), minor retroperitoneal lymphadenopathy and fatty proliferation of the mesentery are also seen. (Courtesy of Jack Wittenberg, MD, Boston, MA.)

ation exposure is an advantage of this technique over barium studies.

Because of its ability to visualize the mucosa directly and permit biopsy for histopathology, endoscopy complements radiologic techniques. Many of the same mucosal features seen on barium studies are also recognized on endoscopy, including aphthous ulcers, mucosal edema, cobblestoning, and luminal narrowing (Fig. 108–7). The visual impression of demarcated lesions on a background of normal mucosa is easily recognized in early or mild disease. Rectal sparing is more specific before treatment has been initiated. The discontinuous segmental nature of the disease is an important clue to the diagnosis and has a high positive predictive value.[174] Intubation and biopsy of the terminal ileum should be attempted in all patients having colonoscopy and greatly increase the sensitivity and specificity of the examination.[175] There is growing interest in the potential role of wireless capsule endoscopy in detecting small bowel lesions of Crohn's disease.[176] The presence of significant bowel stricture should be excluded radiologically before attempting capsule endoscopy because the rate of retained capsule may be as high as 25% and obstruction is possible.[177] In general, the diagnostic accuracy of colonoscopy and histologic interpretation is increased substantially by obtaining multiple biopsies from both

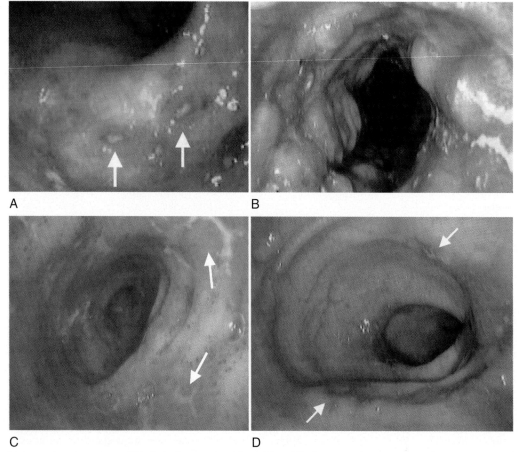

Figure 108–7 Endoscopic appearance of Crohn's disease. A wide variety of findings may be seen on endoscopy, in part depending on the duration and severity of the disease. *A,* Typical aphthous ulcers (*arrows*), consisting of a central white depression surrounded by a slightly elevated, erythematous rim only a few millimeters in diameter. *B,* Findings more typical of advanced disease, with erythema, edema, and a cobblestone appearance. *C,* Stellate ulcers (*arrows*) in the terminal ileum. *D,* Discrete ulcers (*arrows*) with normal intervening mucosa, typical of the patchy inflammation seen in Crohn's disease.

involved and uninvolved sites. The use of jumbo forceps should be considered to improve sampling of the submucosa. Balloon dilatation of strictures is another application of endoscopy in Crohn's disease that may delay or spare the need for surgery.

DIFFERENTIATING CROHN'S DISEASE FROM ULCERATIVE COLITIS

When IBD is confined to the colon, the main diagnostic distinction is between Crohn's colitis and ulcerative colitis. As noted earlier, ulcerative colitis and Crohn's disease share many similarities in epidemiology and clinical manifestations. The distinction between these diseases is becoming increasingly important with regard to choices of surgical and medical therapies. Patients with features of both diseases are said to have *indeterminate colitis*, a vague term applied in various ways among different centers. As many as 10% of patients presenting with IBD are considered to have indeterminate colitis. A diagnosis of indeterminate colitis has particular implications for surgical therapy, because patients undergoing ileoanal pouch construction for indeterminate colitis have a relatively high likelihood of developing Crohn's-like complications of the pouch.[178] Histology, when applied without attention to clinical features, has a high

likelihood of yielding a diagnosis of indeterminate colitis.[179,180] Therefore, the entire clinical picture must be considered for accurate diagnosis (Table 108–2). Discriminating features for Crohn's disease include the presence of small bowel disease, predominantly right colonic disease, rectal sparing, fistulization (with the exception of rare rectovaginal fistulas in ulcerative colitis), major perineal complications, and granulomas. In cases initially labeled as indeterminate, the true diagnosis usually becomes clear with the passage of time.

With an incomplete understanding of the environmental and genetic determinants that produce a clinical phenotype of Crohn's disease or ulcerative colitis, immunologic markers are being explored as a means of differentiating the two diseases. The presence in serum of perinuclear antineutrophil cytoplasmic antibody (pANCA) and antiglycan antibodies to mannan (a constituent of the cell wall of baker's yeast anti-*Saccharomyces cerevisiae* antibody [ASCA]) correlate with the diagnosis of ulcerative colitis and Crohn's disease, respectively.[181-183] The specificity of each of these serologic markers is approximately 85%, but sensitivity is considerably lower at 50% to 65%, with considerable variation among assays performed in different laboratories. In addition, pANCA may be found in approximately 15% of patients with Crohn's disease, particularly among patients with an ulcerative colitis-like phenotype.[184] Combining the two

Table 108–2 Differentiation of Crohn's Colitis from Ulcerative Colitis

Variable	Crohn's Colitis	Ulcerative Colitis
Mucosal lesions	Aphthous ulcers are common in early disease; late disease is notable for stellate, "rake," "bear claw," linear, or serpiginous ulcers; cobblestoning	Microulcers are more common than larger ulcers Pseudopolyps are more common
Distribution	Often discontinuous and asymmetric with skipped segments and normal intervening mucosa, especially in early disease	Continuous, symmetric, and diffuse, with granularity or ulceration found throughout the involved segments of colon; periappendiceal inflammation (cecal patch) is common even when the cecum is not involved
Rectum	Completely, or relatively, spared	Typically involves the rectum with proximal involvement to a variable extent
Ileum	Often involved ($\approx$75% of cases of Crohn's disease)	Not involved, except as "backwash" ileitis in ulcerative pancolitis
Depth of inflammation	Submucosal, mucosal, and transmural	Mucosal; not transmural except in fulminant disease
Serosal findings	Marked erythema and creeping fat (the latter is virtually pathognomonic)	Absent, except in severe colitis or toxic megacolon
Complications	Perianal findings are often prominent, including large anal skin tags and deep fissures; perianal fistulas are often complex	Perianal findings are not prominent (any fissures or fistulas are uncomplicated)
Strictures	Often present	Rarely present; suggestive of adenocarcinoma
Fistulas	Perianal, enterocutaneous, rectovaginal, enterovesicular, and other fistulas may be present	Not present, except rarely for rectovaginal fistula
Granulomas	Present in 15-60% of patients (higher frequency in surgical specimens than in mucosal pinch biopsies)	Generally not present (microgranulomas may be associated with ruptured crypt abscesses)
Other histologic features	Crypt abscesses may be present Hallmark is focally enhanced inflammation, often on a background of normal mucosa	Crypt abscesses and ulcers are the defining lesions Ulceration on a background of inflamed mucosa
Serology	pANCA positive in 20-25%; ASCA positive in 41-76%	pANCA positive in 60-65%; ASCA positive in 5%

ASCA, anti-*Saccharomyces cerevisiae* antibody; pANCA, perinuclear antineutrophil cytoplasmic antibody.
From Sands BE: From symptom to diagnosis: Clinical distinctions among various forms of intestinal inflammation. Gastroenterology 126:1518, 2004.

assays improves specificity but at the further expense of sensitivity.[181] Thus, serologic testing for pANCA and ASCA currently is an adjunct to diagnosis in selected cases—one additional piece of evidence to be considered but not definitive in establishing the diagnosis. Additional serologic markers such as anti-OmpC (outer membrane porin C) and anti-I2 may further increase sensitivity and diagnostic value.[185] Increasingly, serologic markers are recognized as providing prognostic information; for example, patients with Crohn's disease who are ASCA positive have a higher rate of surgery and require surgery earlier in the course of disease, independent of disease location and smoking.[186,187]

ASSESSING DISEASE ACTIVITY

In daily practice, usually it is sufficient to follow the patient's symptoms and signs with treatment. Rarely is it necessary to subject the patient to repeated radiologic studies or colonoscopies to ascertain disease activity, and disease location tends to be stable over time. Repeat studies are undertaken when symptoms have increased substantially or have changed and are suspected to arise not from persistent intestinal inflammation but from other causes such as infection, a complication, or from a functional disorder. In clinical research, however, more quantitative evaluations are needed. Composite scoring systems, most commonly the Crohn's Disease Activity Index (CDAI) (Table 108–3), are used in an attempt to integrate the many possible features of the disease. Other disease activity indices include the van Hees index,[188] the Cape Town index,[189] the Harvey-Bradshaw index,[190] the International Organization of IBD (or Oxford) index,[191] the St. Marks Crohn's index,[192] the De Dombal's index,[193] the Talstad index,[194] and a Crohn's disease activity index for survey research.[195] Specialized indices have been developed for use in children.[196,197] These indices vary in the features included in the scoring system, but most include a combination of subjective symptoms and objective findings on examination and laboratory testing. A great deal of interobserver variation has been noted,[198] and in fibrostenotic disease, indices that rely more heavily on subjective measurements may poorly reflect bowel inflammation as a cause of symptoms.[199] Other approaches have included use of disease activity indices that focus on a specific outcome, such as perianal disease,[200,201] endoscopic findings,[202] or achieving an individual goal of therapy.[203] Each of these approaches has advantages and disadvantages, but all have their application in research rather than in clinical practice.

Another approach with some merit is the measurement of biologic markers of disease inflammation. The erythrocyte sedimentation rate and serum acute phase response proteins such as C-reactive protein and orosomucoid may be useful in tracking disease activity but lack sensitivity and specificity. Another approach is to measure the serum levels of cytokines, cytokine receptors, and adhesion molecules that are proximate to the expression of acute-phase reactants. Examples include IL-6, IL-1, soluble IL-2 receptor, and soluble intercellular adhesion molecule-1.[204] As with the acute-phase reactants, these tests also lack sensitivity and specificity. Direct measurements of intestinal immune activation in a mucosal sample could enhance sensitivity and specificity but are inconvenient, invasive, and, if dependent on biopsy, subject to variability and poor standardization. Quantification of radiolabeled leukocytes in stool appears to be a sensitive and fairly specific indicator of mucosal inflammation but is cumbersome to perform and exposes the patient to radiation. More recently, fecal excretion of calprotectin, a protein found in neutrophils, has been shown to be a sensitive marker of bowel inflammation that also may correlate with relapse of quiescent disease.[205]

Ultimately, it is desirable to measure the patient's overall state of well-being, or subjective health status.

Table 108–3   Crohn's Disease Activity Index (CDAI)*

Variable	Scale	Weight
Liquid or very soft stools	Daily stool count is summed for 7 days	2
Abdominal pain	Sum of 7 days of daily ratings as 0 = none, 1 = mild, 2 = moderate, 3 = severe	5
General well-being	Sum of 7 days of daily ratings as 0 = generally well, 1 = slightly below par, 2 = poor, 3 = very poor, 4 = terrible	7

Features of extraintestinal disease	Presence of any of the following during the 7 days:
	    Arthritis or arthralgia
	    Skin or mouth lesions, including pyoderma gangrenosum, erythema
	        nodosum, aphthous stomatitis
	    Iritis or uveitis
	    Anal fissure, fistula, or perirectal abscess
	    Other external fistula
	    Fever >100°F
		20 each

Opiates for diarrhea	0 = no, 1 = yes	30
Abdominal mass	0 = none, 2 = questionable, 5 = definite	10
Hematocrit	Men: 47−hematocrit Women: 42−hematocrit	6
Body weight	100 × [1 − (body weight/standard weight)]	1

*To calculate the CDAI, the scale is multiplied by the weighting factor for each variable and then all eight weighted variables are added. For research purposes, remission is defined as a CDAI score of <150 and severe disease is defined as a CDAI score of >450.
From Best WR, Becktel JM, Singleton JW, et al: Development of a Crohn's disease activity index. National Cooperative Crohn's Disease Study. Gastroenterology 70:439, 1976.

Health-related quality of life may be measured with generic instruments, which focus on various domains of health common to many disease states, or with disease-specific instruments, which focus on specific domains relevant to the disease of interest. The Inflammatory Bowel Disease Questionnaire, the most widely accepted disease-specific instrument, measures separate domains for bowel, social, systemic, and emotional function.[206]

TREATMENT

GOALS

Because neither medical nor surgical therapy provides a cure, the primary goals of therapy are to induce and maintain remission. In achieving these goals, the intention is to ameliorate symptoms and improve the patient's quality of life. Therefore, it is essential to consider the adverse consequences of therapy, particularly with regard to any durable consequences of short-term treatment and adverse effects of maintenance therapy. Other goals may be specific to the individual patient, such as healing a fistula or achieving normal growth in a child. Maintaining adequate nutrition may at times be a challenge and is an important goal in all patients.

MEDICAL THERAPY

Aminosalicylates

In the United States, aminosalicylates are used in the treatment of ulcerative colitis and in mild-to-moderate Crohn's disease. Sulfasalazine, the parent compound of all aminosalicylates used in IBD, was developed as a treatment for rheumatoid arthritis but was serendipitously found to improve the bowel symptoms of patients with colitis who were treated for associated arthropathy. Later, a classic experiment by Azad Khan and colleagues determined that 5-ASA (mesalamine) rather than sulfapyridine was the therapeutic moiety of sulfasalazine.[207] Most of the adverse effects of sulfasalazine are due to its sulfapyridine moiety, which serves as a carrier for the 5-ASA portion of the molecule; release of 5-ASA from sulfapyridine depends on azoreductase activity of the colonic flora, thereby ensuring its delivery to the colon. Because almost the entire dose of the 5-ASA compound is absorbed in the upper gastrointestinal tract when given orally, and the beneficial effects of 5-ASAs depend on topical delivery to affected mucosa, diverse means of overcoming proximal intestinal absorption of 5-ASA were developed. These delivery systems include enemas or suppositories, which deposit the drug in the left colon or rectum; encoating with protective materials that release the drug in a pH-dependent manner to achieve controlled (Pentasa) or delayed (Asacol) delivery; and diazo-bonding the drug to a second 5-ASA molecule (olsalazine) or to an inert carrier (balsalazide). The site of delivery of coated preparations depends largely on the properties of the coating material used and its pH sensitivity. Some preparations (Pentasa) release half of the dose in the small bowel and the remainder in the colon, whereas other preparations release mesalamine in the distal terminal ileum and beyond. Diazo-bonded preparations have release profiles closely resembling that of sulfasalazine.

Numerous therapeutic mechanisms have been attributed to aminosalicylates, including inhibition of T cell proliferation, presentation of antigen to T cells, and antibody production by B cells; inhibition of macrophage and neutrophil adhesion; and decreased production of IL-1 and TNF. The aminosalicylates are excellent free radical scavengers and inhibit cyclooxygenase and production of prostaglandin E_2.[208] Many of these effects appear to be mediated through down-regulation of NFκB activity.[209]

Most studies have shown sulfasalazine to be superior to placebo in inducing remission in active Crohn's disease, when the colon is the primary site affected.[210] Efficacious doses, as used in the National Cooperative Crohn's Disease Study (NCCDS), are in the range of 4 to 6 g/day (1 g/15 kg body weight).[210] The European Cooperative Crohn's Disease Study (ECCDS) found sulfasalazine 3 g/day to provide no significant benefit in achieving remission.[211] Early studies with controlled-release mesalamine (Pentasa) at doses less than 2 g/day failed to show efficacy in the treatment of mild-to-moderate active Crohn's disease.[212,213] A much larger study of 466 patients with mild-to-moderate Crohn's disease compared daily doses of 1, 2, and 4 g with placebo for 16 weeks. The 43% remission rate on 4 g of mesalamine was statistically and clinically superior to the placebo response rate of 18%.[214] Notably, ileal disease responded best to the 4 g/day dose, thereby suggesting that mesalamine provides a potential benefit over sulfasalazine in treating this subgroup of patients. Subsequent trials of similar design, however, failed to show benefit over placebo; although the treatment effect was of similar magnitude, the placebo response was larger than the originally observed 18%. More recently, a meta-analysis failed to demonstrate a clinically significant benefit of Pentasa 4 g/day in patients with mild-to-moderate Crohn's disease.[215] Furthermore, numerous studies with a variety of preparations have failed to demonstrate prevention of relapses of Crohn's disease with 5-ASA compounds.[216] Therefore, although maintenance therapy with mesalamine often is prescribed in Crohn's disease, little data justify the expense and inconvenience of this practice.

In summary, sulfasalazine 4 to 6 g/day may be useful in the treatment of mild-to-moderate colonic Crohn's disease, whereas the role of mesalamine is uncertain. The small margin of benefit and relatively slow onset of effect (4 to 8 weeks) must be weighed against the excellent safety profile of these agents (Table 108–4).

Antibiotics

Antibiotics have a clear role in treating pyogenic complications of Crohn's disease. On the basis of relatively little evidence, antibiotics also are used to treat perineal disease, fistulas, and active Crohn's disease. The largest reported experience has been with metronidazole. The anaerobic flora affected by metronidazole may have particular importance in the pathogenesis of Crohn's disease.[36] Perhaps the clearest demonstration of this principle is a study of postsurgical prophylaxis after ileal resection. In this disease model, which in some ways may

Table 108–4 Safety Profiles of Agents Used to Treat Crohn's Disease

Agent	Adverse Effects	Use in Pregnancy*	Use While Nursing*
5-Aminosalicylates (5-ASAs)			
Sulfasalazine	Anorexia, dyspepsia, nausea/vomiting; hemolysis; neutropenia, agranulocytosis; folate deficiency; reversible male infertility; neuropathy; see also sulfa-free 5-ASAs	No evidence of teratogenicity; normal fetal growth; take with folic acid	Negligible amounts are excreted in breast milk; safe for term neonates
Sulfa-free (mesalamine, olsalazine, balsalazide)	Headache; drug fever; rash; paradoxical exacerbation of diarrhea; pancreatitis; hepatitis; pericarditis; pneumonitis; nephritis; secretory diarrhea (olsalazine)	No evidence of teratogenicity; normal fetal growth	Found in breast milk in low concentrations; rare watery diarrhea in breast-fed infants
Antibiotics			
Metronidazole	Anorexia, nausea/vomiting, dysgeusia; disulfiram-like effect; peripheral neuropathy; reversible neutropenia	Questionable teratogenicity, normal fetal growth	Found in breast milk; with rare exception, should not be used
Ciprofloxacin	Nausea/vomiting; headache; restlessness; rash; pseudomembranous colitis; elevated aminotransferases; spontaneous tendon rupture	Theoretical teratogenic potential; insufficient data in humans	Found in breast milk; should not be used
Glucocorticoids			
Classic	Sleep and mood disturbance, acne, striae, hirsutism, adrenal suppression, proximal myopathy, glucose intolerance, hypertension, narrow-angle glaucoma, cataracts, pseudotumor cerebri, infection, edema, impaired wound healing, growth retardation, bone loss, aseptic necrosis	No evidence of teratogenicity in humans; more frequent stillbirths and reduced fetal birthweight when used for other diseases; may be used for severe disease	Safe for breast-feeding
Novel (controlled ileal-release budesonide)	Adrenal suppression at doses of 9 mg/day and higher in two divided doses, but frequency of classic glucocorticoid adverse effects similar to placebo	No data available	No data available
Immune Modulators			
6-Mercaptopurine, azathioprine	Nausea; drug fever, rash, arthralgias; leukopenia; thrombocytopenia; bone marrow suppression; pancreatitis; hepatitis; infection; lymphoma (?)	Teratogenic in animals, but large series in renal transplantation and various diseases do not show an increase in frequency of birth defects; evidence for fetal growth retardation and prematurity; isolated cases of neonatal immune and bone marrow suppression; limited experience in IBD appear favorable; may be used for severe disease	Small amounts are excreted in breast milk; breast-feeding not recommended
Methotrexate	Anorexia, nausea/vomiting; leukopenia; megaloblastic anemia; alopecia; hepatic fibrosis; interstitial pneumonitis; neuropathy	Highly teratogenic, particularly in first trimester; abortifacient	Small amounts are excreted in breast milk; breast-feeding not recommended
Cyclosporine	Reversible or irreversible decrease in renal function; hypertension; tremor, headache, paresthesias, seizure; hypertrichosis; gingival hyperplasia; hepatotoxicity; infection; lymphoma	Significant levels in fetal circulation; does not appear to be teratogenic; frequencies of intrauterine growth retardation and premature delivery are increased, especially at higher doses; little reported experience in IBD	Excreted in breast milk; breast-feeding not recommended
Biologic Response Modifiers			
Infliximab	Upper respiratory tract and other infections; disseminated tuberculosis; increased risk of systemic fungal infection and infection with other intracellular pathogens; acute or delayed hypersensitivity reactions; antinuclear antibodies, anti-double-stranded DNA antibodies, lupus-like reaction; demyelinating disease; contraindicated in CHF because of increased mortality; lymphoma	Limited data in humans	No data available

CHF, congestive heart failure; IBD, inflammatory bowel disease.
*Adapted from Connell WR: Safety of drug therapy for inflammatory bowel disease in pregnant and nursing women. Inflammatory Bowel Dis 2:33, 1996; and Sands BE: Therapy of inflammatory bowel disease. Gastroenterology 118(Suppl 1):S72, 2000.

replicate the earliest events in the initiation of Crohn's disease, high-dose metronidazole (20 mg/kg/day for 3 months) demonstrated a prophylactic effect on endoscopic and clinical recurrence at 1 year, with numerical but not statistical advantages at 2 and 3 years of follow-up.[217] In this study, as in clinical usage, side effects (including gastrointestinal upset, nausea, dysgeusia, and peripheral neuropathy) were common.

Open-label experience suggests that metronidazole 20 mg/kg/day is beneficial in healing perineal fistulas.[218] Fistulas tend to recur with cessation of therapy, but long-term use is limited by side effects. Studies of metronidazole in active Crohn's disease generally have not demonstrated benefit but have suggested better outcomes in subgroups of patients with colonic involvement.[219,220]

Ciprofloxacin is used increasingly to treat Crohn's disease. One study found ciprofloxacin 1 g/day to be equivalent to mesalamine 4 g/day in achieving remission of mild-to-moderate active Crohn's disease at week 6, with more than one half of the patients in each group achieving remission.[221] Another study compared the combined use of ciprofloxacin and metronidazole, 1 g each, against methylprednisolone for active Crohn's disease. The antibiotic combination was comparable with glucocorticoids in achieving remission over 12 weeks.[222] A more recent study failed to detect additional efficacy of the same dual antibiotic regimen over placebo when added to controlled ileal-release budesonide; however, a trend toward benefit was noted in the subgroup of patients with colonic disease.[223]

Preliminary evidence suggests that clarithromycin monotherapy also may be useful in treating active disease.[224] Additional interest in clarithromycin is sparked by its role as part of a highly effective treatment for atypical mycobacterial infection. Studies of antimycobacterial therapy, however, have not shown consistent benefit. A study of quadruple therapy (rifampicin, ethambutol, dapsone, and clofazimine) showed significantly fewer relapses when compared with placebo among patients with inactive disease treated for 9 months.[225] Radiologic or endoscopic healing was not observed, however, suggesting that this therapy was not curative. Other antimycobacterial regimens have failed to produce either short-term or durable benefit, thus far failing to fulfill Koch's postulates for disease causation.

In summary, antibiotics may play an adjunctive role in the treatment of Crohn's disease and, in selected patients, may be useful in treating perineal disease, enterocutaneous fistulas, or active colonic disease. As the antigenic determinants of the intestinal flora are further elucidated, more directed antibiotic approaches may be feasible.

Glucocorticoids

Glucocorticoids play a central yet vexing role in the treatment of Crohn's disease. Early favorable series of glucocorticoid treatment led to the validation of their short-term efficacy in the NCCDS (prednisone 0.5 to 0.75 mg/kg/day for initial treatment of active disease with the dose adjusted according to CDAI)[210] and the ECCDS (6-methylprednisolone 48 mg/day in the first week, tapered to 12 mg by week 6, and held at 8 mg for remis-

sion up to 2 years).[211] In usual practice, patients with mild-to-moderate disease that does not respond to primary therapy and those with moderately severe symptoms are treated initially with 40 to 60 mg of prednisone and then tapered off the drug over a period of 6 to 12 weeks. Response rates are high, approximately 80% by 1 month.[226] When doses are pushed as high as 1 mg/kg/day for up to 7 weeks, 92% of patients may achieve clinical remission.[227] The onset of response is rapid, usually within the first 3 weeks of treatment. Patients with severely active disease usually respond to intravenous administration of glucocorticoids.[228]

Numerous anti-inflammatory and immunosuppressive effects have been attributed to glucocorticoids to account for their efficacy. These effects include inhibition of the expression of proinflammatory cytokines, adhesion molecules, MHC class II molecules, leukotrienes, elastase, collagenase, and nitric oxide synthase. Glucocorticoids bind to a cytoplasmic receptor found in all cells and then enter the nucleus to bind glucocorticoid-response elements on the chromosomal DNA, thereby producing a variety of downstream physiologic effects.[229] The anti-inflammatory effects of glucocorticoids may follow from down-regulation of NFκB and induction of inhibitory κB.[230] Direct cellular effects also may occur, with reduced phagocytic activity of neutrophils and, in some situations, apoptosis of lymphocytes.[229]

Unfortunately, the beneficial effects of glucocorticoids come at the expense of frequent and often severe adverse effects (see Table 108–4). The most common side effects are troubling neuropsychiatric symptoms (mood disturbance and insomnia) and cosmetic effects (acne, cushingoid appearance, hair loss, and hirsutism). Still more serious are metabolic consequences, such as adrenocortical suppression, glucose intolerance, myopathy, and bone loss. The risk of infectious complications is increased, particularly at doses of prednisone higher than 40 mg; doses lower than 10 mg confer no appreciable increased risk of infection.[231] This unfavorable risk profile makes prolonged use of glucocorticoids hazardous.

Furthermore, glucocorticoids are not effective as long-term therapy. A meta-analysis of maintenance glucocorticoid therapy in Crohn's disease failed to detect benefit at 6, 12, or 24 months in the prevention of relapse.[232] Conversely, once glucocorticoids are introduced, they are unable to be discontinued without recurrent symptoms in many patients, even with gradual tapering; this problem is referred to as *glucocorticoid dependence*. Among patients with Crohn's disease who received glucocorticoids for the first time, no response (*glucocorticoid resistance*) was seen in 20% in the first 30 days.[226] Among the 80% who were complete or partial responders, 55% had a prolonged response, whereas 45% relapsed or were unable to taper off treatment within 1 year.[226] Clinical factors associated with glucocorticoid dependence include smoking, younger age at onset, colonic location, and non-fibrostenotic disease.[233] Mechanisms that may contribute to glucocorticoid resistance include up-regulation of the multidrug resistance (*mdr*) gene[234] and increased serum levels of glucocorticoid-binding globulin.[235] Moreover, only 29% of patients who achieve clinical remission on glucocorticoids also achieve endoscopic remission.[227] This finding suggests that the effect of glucocorticoids in most patients is to suppress symptoms when given in doses above a threshold that may vary among patients and even in the same patient over time.

Principles of glucocorticoid use in Crohn's disease include the following:

1. *Use an effective dose*—Underdosing at the start of therapy typically leads to dose escalation and prolonged dosing to achieve a response.
2. *Do not overdose*—Patients who do not benefit from 40 to 60 mg are unlikely to benefit from increased or prolonged oral dosing. Such patients require intravenous dosing or treatment with another rapidly acting agent, such as infliximab (see later).
3. *Do not treat for excessively short periods*—Doses should not be tapered too quickly once symptoms have been controlled. Very brief courses of glucocorticoids (≤3 weeks) are likely to result in a rebound flare.
4. *Do not treat for excessively long periods*—Patients in whom a second glucocorticoid taper fails shortly after a first should be considered candidates for glucocorticoid-sparing immune modulators. Glucocorticoids should not be begun without a strategy in mind for terminating treatment.
5. *Anticipate side effects*—Bone loss in particular may be anticipated with even short-term use. Strategies to preserve bone density should be undertaken early (Fig. 108–8).

In an attempt to limit the unintended systemic effects of glucocorticoid therapy, novel glucocorticoids have been developed. *Budesonide* possesses glucocorticoid receptor affinity equal or superior to that of traditional glucocorticoids and also takes advantage of enhanced first-pass metabolism by the liver to limit systemic exposure. A controlled ileal-release formulation of budesonide targets the terminal ileum and right colon. Studies have demonstrated 9 mg/day of this preparation to be superior to placebo and mesalamine[236,237] and nearly as effective as prednisolone in achieving remission, but with fewer side effects. Pushing the dose higher results in better efficacy but at the expense of increasing adrenocortical suppression and side effects.[238] Budesonide treatment in asymptomatic patients delays the time to relapse slightly, but the rate of relapse at 1 year is not less than that for placebo.[238,239] Similarly, budesonide 3 or 6 mg/day after ileal or ileocecal resection does not improve the recurrence rate at 1 year.[240,241] Therefore, lack of a maintenance effect is consistent for both novel and traditional glucocorticoids. In light of its superior therapeutic response compared with mesalamine, and its relative safety, budesonide may be considered as first-line therapy for patients with active ileal, ileocecal, or right colonic disease. In addition, some patients who are dependent on conventional glucocorticoids may be switched successfully to budesonide, with the potential benefits of decreased systemic glucocorticoid exposure.[242]

In summary, glucocorticoids are effective for the short-term control of symptoms of Crohn's disease but are neither effective nor safe for long-term maintenance of response. In patients with disease that is refractory to or dependent on glucocorticoids, steroid-sparing strategies should be considered, including immune modulators or surgery.

Thiopurine Agents

The thiopurine antimetabolites *azathioprine* and *6-MP* have been considered treatments for Crohn's disease since the initial report of Brooke and colleagues describing healing of fistulas with azathioprine.[243] Another decade would pass before the efficacy of this class of drugs was demonstrated in a randomized, controlled trial by Present and colleagues.[203] Earlier studies were marred by either insufficient power or incomplete understanding of adequate dosing and the slow onset of action of these agents.

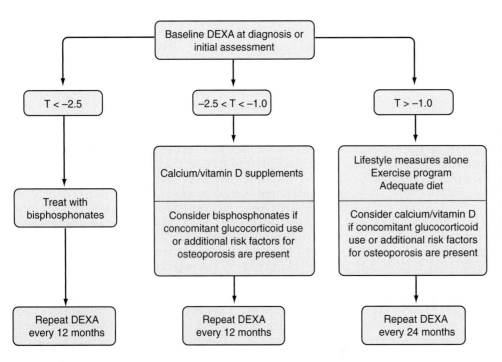

Figure 108–8 Management of metabolic bone disease in Crohn's disease. T, T score; DEXA, dual-energy x-ray absorptiometry. (From Silverberg MS, Steinhart AH: Bone density in inflammatory bowel disease. Clin Perspect Gastroenterol 3:117, 2000.)

A meta-analysis of studies of azathioprine and 6-MP in Crohn's disease has provided the best summary of the effects of these drugs. For active disease, treatment produced an odds ratio of response of 3.09 (95% confidence interval [CI], 2.45-3.91) compared with placebo, with improved response when treatment was continued for at least 17 weeks.[244] Convincing evidence of benefit also was seen in maintenance of remission (odds ratio over placebo, 2.27; 95% CI, 1.76-2.93),[244] glucocorticoid sparing[245,246] (odds ratios for active disease, 3.69; 95% CI, 2.12-6.42, and for quiescent disease, 4.64; 95% CI, 1.00-21.54),[244] and improvement in fistulas (odds ratio, 4.64; 95% CI, 1.50-13.20).[244] Overall, approximately one half to two thirds of patients may respond to thiopurine therapy. In contrast with glucocorticoids, mucosal healing frequently is seen with adequate dosing of these agents.[247]

In clinical practice, azathioprine and 6-MP are used virtually interchangeably with the exception of dosing. Azathioprine generally is used in doses of 2 to 2.5 mg/kg/day, whereas 6-MP is given in doses of 1 to 1.5 mg/kg/day. Much is known about the metabolism of 6-MP and azathioprine (Fig. 108–9). Azathioprine is a prodrug that is converted in part to 6-MP through nonenzymatic means and into a variety of other immunologically active and inert metabolites. Xanthine oxidase converts 6-MP to 6-thiouric acid, in competition with hypoxanthine phosphoribosyltransferase. The former pathway accounts for an important drug interaction with allopurinol, a xanthine oxidase inhibitor. Concurrent treatment with allopurinol and a thiopurine agent necessitates a dose reduction of at least one third if leukopenia is to be avoided.

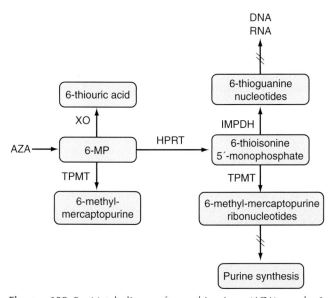

Figure 108–9 Metabolism of azathioprine (AZA) and 6-mercaptopurine (6-MP). AZA is converted to 6-MP nonenzymatically. HPRT, hypoxanthine phosphoribosyltransferase; IMPDH, inosine monophosphate dehydrogenase; TPMT, thiopurine methyltransferase; XO, xanthine oxidase. (From Dubinsky M, Lamothe S, Yang HY, et al: Pharmacogenomics and metabolite measurement for 6-mercaptopurine therapy in inflammatory bowel disease. Gastroenterology 118:705, 2000.)

Thiopurine methyltransferase (TPMT) plays a key role in the metabolic pathway. Variations in TPMT activity, which are largely determined genetically, account for preferential shunting of 6-MP to the production of 6-methylmercaptopurine when enzyme activity is normal or high. Persons who are homozygous for a recessive mutation that results in inactivation of TPMT (≈1:300 persons) produce exceedingly high levels of 6-thioguanine (6-TG) nucleotides. These persons are unlikely to tolerate thiopurine agents at all and tend to have profound leukopenia and other limiting adverse effects. In contrast, persons who are TPMT heterozygous (≈10% of the population) are likely to have moderately high levels of 6-TG nucleotides. They usually require lower doses of drug but are much more likely to respond. A steady state in the production of erythrocyte 6-TG nucleotides is reached 2 weeks after dosing.[248] The reported positive correlation between erythrocyte 6-TG nucleotides and therapeutic response offers the possibility of both monitoring adherence to the drug regimen and optimizing dosing of these agents.[249] Correlations between higher levels of 6-TG nucleotides and leukopenia and between metabolite levels and response to therapy may explain the clinical observation that patients who achieve mild leukopenia are more likely to respond to therapy.[250] However, leukopenia is not necessary to achieve a therapeutic response.

The relevant mechanisms of action of azathioprine and 6-MP are not clearly understood. Metabolites of both agents inhibit de novo synthesis of purine ribonucleotides and thereby inhibit cell proliferation. Azathioprine and its metabolites may have immunosuppressive properties beyond those of the metabolites produced in common with 6-MP. Both drugs inhibit cell-mediated immunity. The thiopurines cause a reduction in the number of circulating natural killer cells over many months, perhaps accounting for the slow onset of action of these agents.[251] More recently, azathioprine and 6-MP have been shown to activate Rac1 when costimulation of CD4+ T lymphocytes occurs via CD28, effecting apoptosis of the cell and diminishing the immune response.[252]

A study of intravenous loading of azathioprine found no acceleration of the time to response over oral dosing.[248] Unexpectedly, the oral dosing arm of the study with azathioprine 2 mg/kg/day achieved a maximum rate of remission of 24% (discontinuation of prednisone and CDAI < 150) by week 8. The remission rate did not increase over an additional 8 weeks of follow-up, thus contradicting the long-held notion of a prolonged time to response. The study did not, however, address improvement beyond the 16th week of treatment.

In clinical trials, adverse events severe enough to result in withdrawal have been seen in 8.9% of patients.[244] Nausea often is reported in the first weeks of treatment but gradually subsides. Allergic reactions consisting of fever, rash, or arthralgias, usually within a few weeks of introducing the drug, are seen in 2% of patients. Pancreatitis, observed in 3% to 7%, is another idiosyncratic reaction and usually occurs in the first month of therapy. The presentation may be subtle, with nausea and vague dyspepsia, or may be one of classic epigastric pain with radiation to the back. If serum amylase and lipase levels are followed closely, symptoms sometimes may be noted to precede the discovery of laboratory abnormalities. When recognized promptly, discontinuation of the drug leads to resolution of pancreatitis. Rechallenge with either drug should not be attempted because recurrent pancreatitis is certain to occur. Elevated serum aminotransferase levels develop in as many as 9% of patients and have been correlated with the presence of very high levels of 6-methylmercaptopurine.[249] More serious cholestatic hepatitis is rare, occurring in less than 1% of patients.[253]

Bone marrow suppression is another concern with thiopurine agents. A 27-year, retrospective, single-center study of 739 IBD patients treated with azathioprine found 28 patients (3.8%) to have developed leukopenia (white blood cell count $<3 \times 10^9/\text{mm}^3$), 9 of whom (1.2%) had severe leukopenia (white blood cell count $< 2 \times 10^9/\text{mm}^3$).[254] Three of these patients became pancytopenic, and two died of sepsis. In another retrospective report of 396 patients treated with 6-MP, 2% experienced leukocyte counts below $3.5 \times 10^9/\text{mm}^3$.[255] Although leukopenia occurs early among patients with low TPMT activity, it may not be related solely to TPMT genotype and may occur at any time during therapy.[255] For this reason, it is advisable to continue monthly monitoring of the complete blood count for the duration of therapy and more frequently in the weeks after introducing the drug or increasing dosage. Temporary cessation of therapy for a week or two and an adjustment in the dose usually suffice to bring the leukocyte count within the normal range. Careful monitoring of the leukocyte count also should be performed during a tapering regimen of glucocorticoids. Concurrent treatment with glucocorticoids may raise the leukocyte count, but as the glucocorticoid is discontinued, leukopenia may arise.

Infections may occur in the setting of thiopurine therapy. With long-term treatment as many as 1.8% of patients may experience a severe infection, not necessarily in the setting of leukopenia.[253] Patients treated concurrently with glucocorticoids may be at greater risk of serious infection, including cytomegalovirus. Treatment should be interrupted when serious infections occur, although the effect of the drug will endure for weeks.

The question of whether patients with IBD who are treated with 6-MP or azathioprine are at increased risk of malignancy is unresolved. Immunosuppressive regimens given to patients after organ transplantation and for other immune-mediated conditions are associated with an excess risk of malignancy, particularly non-Hodgkin's lymphoma. Such regimens have included azathioprine, often administered in high doses and in conjunction with other immunosuppressive agents. The combined long-term experience at two centers involving treatment of 1151 patients with IBD failed to reveal an excess risk of cancer but did include a single case of diffuse histiocytic lymphoma of the brain.[253,256] Most cancers in treated patients were colorectal cancers assumed to be a consequence of the underlying IBD itself. Such studies cannot confirm or exclude a possible association with non-Hodgkin's lymphoma, however, because of the rarity of lymphoma and the unsettled question of whether Crohn's disease itself confers an increased risk of lymphoma. Nevertheless, if there is an increased risk of lymphoma with immunosuppressive therapy, studies suggest that the absolute risk is small.[257] For the properly selected patient, the small risk of lymphoma does not outweigh the benefits of improved quality of life and possibly of increased life expectancy.[258]

Azathioprine and 6-MP should be considered for patients with active Crohn's disease in whom first-line therapies fail or in whom glucocorticoids cannot be tapered off successfully. Patients who are treated with antibiotics for a fistula and who cannot tolerate or do not respond to these agents also may be considered for treatment with a thiopurine agent. The introduction of thiopurine medications should be timed with their slow onset of action in mind. Many patients require an initial tapering regimen of glucocorticoids used as a fast-acting agent to complement azathioprine or 6-MP. Thiopurine therapy also may be considered for the postsurgical prophylaxis of Crohn's disease. Although conflicting data exist about the efficacy of this approach,[259,260] the benefits in preventing recurrence may outweigh the risks of these agents in patients who are deemed to have a high likelihood of future resections. Given the favorable efficacy of thiopurine agents and their relative safety, there is increasing interest in introducing these agents earlier in the course of the disease. Evidence suggests that the addition of 6-MP is advantageous for children who require even a first course of glucocorticoids shortly after diagnosis.[261] It is unclear whether thiopurine therapy prevents or delays the occurrence of fibrostenotic complications of Crohn's disease, and it is possible to see the slow progression of a stricture in patients who otherwise have been asymptomatic on such therapy for many years.

Once treatment has begun and proved to be effective, the question of how long to continue therapy inevitably arises. A recent report demonstrated a clinical relapse rate of 50% 3 years after withdrawal of azathioprine in patients who had been in remission for at least 5 years on the drug.[262] In large referral centers it is common for patients to be treated with azathioprine or 6-MP for many years. The decision to withdraw thiopurine therapy should be undertaken after discussion between physician and patient of possible risks and benefits.

Methotrexate

Methotrexate has long been used to treat psoriasis and rheumatoid arthritis. A randomized, controlled trial studied patients with chronically active Crohn's disease despite at least 3 months of prednisone (at least 12.5 mg/day) and with at least one failed attempt to taper off treatment.[263] All patients were brought to a 20 mg/day dose of prednisone to standardize therapy, with separate stratification for patients in whom the dose of prednisone was increased and for those in whom the dose had dropped to 20 mg before entry. Subjects then received either weekly injections of methotrexate 25 mg intramuscularly or placebo while executing a tapering prednisone regimen over 16 weeks. Overall, 39.4% of patients assigned to methotrexate achieved remission off prednisone compared with 19.1% of placebo-treated patients.[263] Most patients responded by the 8th week of treatment. Although the remission rates in the methotrexate-treated high- and low-prednisone group were nearly equal (39.0% and 40.0%, respectively), the remission rate for placebo-treated patients in the high-prednisone dose group was 10.0%, compared with 35.3% in the low-dose group.[263] This result often is misconstrued as showing that methotrexate works well for patients on high doses of prednisone but not for those on low doses of prednisone, but it merely shows an unexpectedly high placebo response rate among patients dependent on low doses of glucocorticoids.

Methotrexate also is beneficial in maintaining remission. A follow-up study randomized patients who achieved remission on methotrexate 25 mg intramuscularly once weekly to receive either placebo injections or weekly injections of methotrexate 15 mg. At week 40, 65% of patients treated with methotrexate were still in remission, compared with 39% of placebo-treated patients ($P = .04$).[264] Treatment was well tolerated. Among patients who relapsed on the lower maintenance dose, more than one half were able to achieve remission again with resumption of a 25-mg dose. If the 16 weeks of induction therapy are included, the combined duration of therapy was nearly 1 year, with some patients in selected practices treated successfully for more than 4 years. Although oral dosing would be more convenient for long-term administration, this route is unreliable because of variable intestinal absorption, particularly in the presence of small bowel disease.

Although methotrexate is a folate antagonist, the drug often is given with folic acid 1 to 2 mg/day to prevent nausea and stomatitis. Therefore, other modes of action are likely responsible for its efficacy. The drug possesses a variety of other immune-modulating and anti-inflammatory effects, including inhibition of IL-1, IL-2, IL-6, and IL-8 and induction of adenosine, which has direct immunosuppressive properties.[265]

In addition to stomatitis and nausea, diarrhea, hair loss, and mild leukopenia may occur with methotrexate. Serum aminotransferase elevations sometimes may be seen but correlate poorly with the more serious complication of hepatic fibrosis. Liver biopsy is performed routinely in patients with psoriasis after cumulative doses of 1.5, 3, and 5 g have been administered, but these guidelines have not been widely adopted in patients with rheumatoid arthritis, in whom the risk of hepatic fibrosis appears to be lower. Obesity and alcohol intake correlate with fibrosis. Methotrexate interacts with sulfa medications and with azathioprine and 6-MP to cause severe leukopenia. Rare but potentially life-threatening interstitial pneumonitis may present as cough and dyspnea of insidious onset. Early detection, cessation of methotrexate, and treatment with glucocorticoids are essential. Finally, methotrexate is a potent abortifacient and is strongly teratogenic. Women of childbearing capacity must use methotrexate only with highly effective contraception.

Methotrexate may be considered as an alternative to the thiopurine analogs, particularly among patients who do not tolerate these drugs. Some patients who do not respond to 6-MP may respond to methotrexate.[266] In addition to its proven role as a glucocorticoid-sparing agent, methotrexate may be considered as a treatment for active disease, although its value for this indication is less clear.[267]

Other Immune Modulators

There appears to be little role for *cyclosporine* in Crohn's disease. A series of uncontrolled and randomized, controlled trials has shown high doses of cyclosporine to be efficacious in treating inflammatory disease and fistulas but at an unacceptably high cost in adverse effects. Moreover, lower doses, although somewhat safer, are not effective in maintaining remission.[268] For virtually all indications, equally effective and less hazardous medications are available. *Tacrolimus* is absorbed more reliably from the intestine than is cyclosporine and has a similar mode of action via inhibition of calcineurin, thereby diminishing T cell activation.[269] Preliminary data suggest that tacrolimus may be useful in treating glucocorticoid-resistant disease, and a randomized, controlled trial has demonstrated efficacy in healing fistulas.[270,271] The drug may also be effective as a topical agent for oral or perineal disease.[272] *Mycophenolate mofetil*, like azathioprine and 6-MP, inhibits purine synthesis. Because of the similarity of these agents in mode of action, mycophenolate mofetil had been considered primarily as an alternative treatment for patients intolerant of or resistant to treatment with azathioprine. Studies have shown disappointing efficacy, however, and the role of mycophenolate mofetil in Crohn's disease remains unclear.

Infliximab

Infliximab is the first biologic response modifier shown to be effective in Crohn's disease. This chimeric monoclonal anti-TNF antibody had an unsuccessful history as an investigational antisepsis agent before its use in Crohn's disease was explored. Despite conflicting reports regarding the importance of TNF in IBD, the Dutch investigator van Deventer posited that in light of the critical role of TNF in granuloma formation, an anti-TNF agent might prove efficacious for granulomatous bowel disease. Open-label trials subsequently demonstrated rapid and prolonged improvement in disease activity, accompanied in many cases by mucosal healing.[273-275]

A randomized, controlled trial provided strong confirmation of the initial impression of efficacy. Patients with moderate-to-severe Crohn's disease were randomized to an initial infusion of placebo or 5, 10, or 20 mg/kg of infliximab (then called *cA2*).[276] Qualifying patients had moderate-to-severe Crohn's disease (CDAI, 220 to 400) despite treatment with aminosalicylates (59%), oral glucocorticoids (59%), or 6-MP or azathioprine (37%). Approximately one half of the studied patients had prior segmental intestinal resections, and the group had a mean duration of disease in excess of 10 years. The major end point was clinical response, defined as a decrease in the CDAI of 70 or more points at week 4.

All treatment groups had results significantly better than those with placebo (placebo response rate of 17%), with the highest rate of response seen in the 5-mg/kg group (81%).[276] A smaller but still significant proportion of patients had a clinical response by week 12 (48% for 5 mg/kg vs. 12% for placebo). The proportion of patients in clinical remission (CDAI < 150 and a decrease in CDAI of ≥ 70 points) at week 4 also was significantly higher among the 5-mg/kg group (33%) compared with the placebo group (4%). Time to response for nearly all patients was 2 weeks. Clinical improvement was accompanied by improvement in health-related quality of life and decreases in serum C-reactive protein levels.

Coincidental healing of enterocutaneous fistulas in some patients led to a separate randomized, controlled trial of infliximab for this indication.[276] Patients with draining enterocutaneous fistulas were enrolled and followed for closure of 50% or more of the fistulas at two successive visits 1 month apart. More than one half of the patients had more than one fistula, and 90% of the fistulas were perianal. Infliximab in a dose of 5 or 10 mg/kg or placebo was infused at weeks 0, 2, and 6. Among patients assigned to infliximab 5 mg/kg, 68% achieved the primary end-point, compared with 26% of those given placebo ($P = 0.0002$).[277] Complete closure of all fistulas was observed in 55% of patients given infliximab 5 mg/kg but in only 13% of placebo-treated patients. In patients who achieved the primary end-point, the median duration of response was 3 months.[277]

Limited information regarding the efficacy of repeated dosing was available before the commercial release of infliximab in the United States. Subsequently, maintenance dosing every 8 weeks was demonstrated to maintain response in patients with fistulizing and nonfistulizing disease.[278,279] Other important observations from these studies included the demonstration of the steroid-sparing effect of infliximab, and sustained improvement in quality of life out to the 54-week duration of these studies. In addition, patients who failed to respond to induction dosing were unlikely to respond to additional repeated dosing. Finally, the ability to restore response by escalating the dose in patients who lose response in the course of therapy was noted in both studies.

The mode of action of infliximab is likely to be more involved than its nominal binding of TNF. The antibody may bind and clear soluble TNF but also binds to cell-bound TNF. Through the latter mechanism, infliximab has been shown to induce apoptosis of cells expressing membrane TNF. Present hypotheses regarding the efficacy of infliximab favor the ability to control the mucosal immune response by causing apoptosis of these cells.[280-282]

Treatment with infliximab usually is well tolerated. In clinical trials, antibodies to infliximab (ATI) (also referred to as *human antichimeric antibodies*) developed in 13% of infliximab-treated patients with Crohn's disease. Patients in whom ATI develop are more likely—although not uniformly so—to experience acute infusion reactions, which may include chest tightness, dyspnea, rash, and hypotension. ATI are less likely to develop in patients treated concomitantly with glucocorticoids or immune modulators, providing a justification for continuing methotrexate, azathioprine, or 6-MP, even when the patient has failed these treatments. Delayed hypersensitivity reactions, consisting of severe polyarthralgia, myalgia, facial edema, urticaria, or rash, are unusual complications that may occur 3 to 12 days after an infusion.[283] High ATI concentrations appear in such patients after the occurrence of such reactions but are not necessarily found before reinfusion. The major risk factor for delayed hypersensitivity appears to be a long delay (probably ≥ 6 months) between infusions, thereby priming an anamnestic antibody response.[283] Delayed hypersensitivity appears to be less common when the induction regimen is a series of three infusions, and when an immune modulator is given concurrently.[283] Anti-double-stranded DNA antibodies develop in 9% of treated patients, but lupus-like reactions are rare. As with ATI, anti-double-stranded DNA antibodies are less likely to occur if an immune modulator is given with infliximab. Upper respiratory infections occur with greater frequency during treatment with infliximab. In the course of treatment of enterocutaneous fistulas, perianal abscesses may arise from superficial healing and closure of an infected pocket. Any patient suspected of having a pyogenic complication of Crohn's disease or any serious infection should undergo adequate drainage and treatment with antibiotics before starting or continuing infliximab. Reactivation of tuberculosis has been observed with anti-TNF therapies, including infliximab, and has resulted in disseminated disease and death. Therefore, all patients should be screened for pulmonary tuberculosis before starting therapy. In clinical trials totaling roughly 500 patients, lymphoma developed in 4 patients with rheumatoid arthritis and 1 with Crohn's disease. It remains difficult to disentangle the potential confounding effects of other drugs and baseline risk in assessing causality and magnitude of risk for non-Hodgkin's lymphoma with infliximab. Infliximab is rated as a class B agent for use in pregnancy, and although the rate of birth defects does not appear to be elevated in the small number of pregnancies that have been reported to have occurred while on therapy, use during pregnancy has not been routine.

Selection of patients is the key to using infliximab safely, effectively, and appropriately (Fig. 108–10). Patients without objective findings of inflammation or with fibrostenotic disease are unlikely to benefit, whereas treating patients with an undrained abscess is likely to be unsafe. Appropriate patients generally will not have responded to other therapies, including immune modulators. Patients selected in this way are likely to require repeated dosing with infliximab to control disease over long periods. For the occasional patient who has a prolonged response to induction therapy with infliximab, dosing at long intervals on flare should be undertaken only with full consideration of the possible formation of ATI, subsequent increased risk of dose-limiting infusion reactions, and possible loss of response.

Adjunctive Therapies

Many other therapies are used to control the symptoms and adverse consequences of Crohn's disease. Antidiarrheal and anticholinergic agents may help alleviate symptoms. Patients with ileal disease or resection may require parenteral vitamin B_{12} supplementation or cholestyramine 1 to 4 g/day to control bile salt diarrhea. Iron supplementation also may be needed. Smoking cessation should be vigorously pursued as a means of improving long-term outcomes.[284] Bone loss should be anticipated as a potentially serious complication in all patients. Bone density should be checked at diagnosis and at regular intervals thereafter, with appropriate medical management of bone loss (see Fig. 108–8).

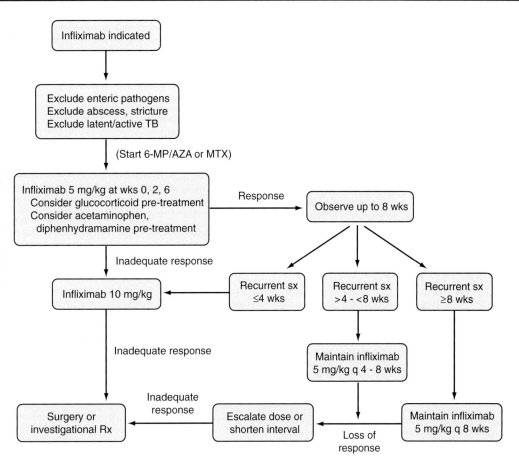

Figure 108–10 Proposed guidelines for the treatment of Crohn's disease with infliximab. AZA, azathioprine; 6-MP, 6-mercaptopurine; MTX, methotrexate; TB, tuberculosis; sx, symptoms; Rx, therapy. (Adapted from Sands BE: Therapy of inflammatory bowel disease. Gastroenterology 118[Suppl]:S68, 2000.)

Novel Therapies

Recent progress in understanding the pathogenesis of Crohn's disease has borne fruit in the development of a wide variety of novel therapeutic agents. In addition to holding real promise for safer and more effective therapy in the future, clinical trials of novel therapeutics offer access to these agents for patients whose disease has exhausted approved therapies. Promising agents under investigation include anti-IL-12 antibodies,[285] antiadhesion molecule antibodies such as natalizumab,[55] and growth factors.[286] Human growth hormone given with a high-protein diet has shown preliminary efficacy but cannot be recommended without further evaluation of safety and efficacy.[287] Alternative approaches to TNF inhibition are being explored, including adalimumab, a human anti-TNF antibody.[288] Such an agent should, in theory, be less antigenic than infliximab. Open-label studies with thalidomide, which has antiangiogenic properties in addition to destabilizing TNF messenger RNA, are promising, but the potent teratogenicity of this agent precludes widespread use.[289,290] Probiotic therapies are being examined as a safe means of modulating the intestinal immune response in IBD.[291]

Some novel agents defy conventional understanding of the pathogenesis of Crohn's disease. Porcine whipworm (*Trichuris suis*) has been administered as a possible treatment for both Crohn's disease and ulcerative colitis, with promising effect and excellent safety and tolerability.[292] Theoretically, this iatrogenic helminthic infestation might counter the prevailing Th1 dominant responses of Crohn's disease by invoking Th2 responses. Recombinant granulocyte-macrophage colony stimulating factor, or sargramostim, has been tried as a therapeutic agent for Crohn's disease on the hypothesis that defective innate immune responses, rather than defects in the adaptive immune response, are a contributing factor to Crohn's disease.[293] Administering sargramostim may, in theory, bolster the innate immune response by stimulating neutrophil function. Although the hypotheses underlying these unusual therapies have yet to be proven, *T. suis* and sargramostim have shown potential in early-phase clinical trials.

NUTRITIONAL THERAPY

Nutritional therapy in Crohn's disease conceivably has two purposes: repletion of nutrients and treatment of the primary disease (see Chapter 16). Specific deficits should be identified and corrected. Protein-calorie malnutrition should be addressed, preferably with enteral supplementation. Many, but not all, patients with Crohn's disease are lactose intolerant and may require increased calcium supplementation. Total parenteral nutrition may be considered for patients with severe malnutrition before surgery or for selected patients with severe Crohn's disease as a primary therapy in combination with bowel rest.[121] Patients with short bowel syndrome from multiple small bowel resections may require enteral nutrition with defined diets; rarely, patients with severe short bowel syndrome may require life-long total parenteral nutrition.

A meta-analysis has found defined enteral diets to be inferior to glucocorticoids in achieving clinical response,[294] but defined enteral diets still may be useful in children for whom glucocorticoids are undesirable.[121] Elemental diets do not appear to be superior to polymeric diets.[294] Children even may be taught to receive nocturnal feedings after self-intubation with a nasogastric tube. Long-term tolerance may be poor, however, and disease tends to recur when the patient's usual diet is reintroduced. Self-reported food intolerances are common among patients with Crohn's disease,[295] but exclusion diets have not been shown to be beneficial.[296] Elimination of multiple food items may lead to serious malnutrition. Patients with a stricture may tolerate roughage poorly or may experience complete intestinal obstruction. Increasingly, specific nutrients are being considered for their therapeutic properties. Examples include a delayed release formulation of fish oil,[297] in which the active component is eicosapentaenoic acid, and so-called prebiotic nutrients, which facilitate the growth of beneficial flora.

SURGICAL THERAPY

Surgery plays an integral role in the treatment of Crohn's disease, both to control symptoms and treat complications. By the 20th year from the onset of symptoms, roughly three fourths of patients will have had surgery.[298] Depending on the prevalent medical culture in the country of study, the rate of surgery within 3 years of diagnosis varies from 25% to 45%. From 25% to 38% of patients require a second surgery by 5 years after the first, and about one third of patients who need a second surgery eventually require a third.[299] Because of the high likelihood of recurrence after segmental resection, the guiding principle of surgery in Crohn's disease is preservation of intestinal length and function. Taking wide margins does not reduce the likelihood of recurrent disease and, with repeated resection, may contribute to intestinal failure. Procedures may be categorized as resections with or without anastomosis, external (i.e., stoma) or internal bypass surgery, and a variety of surgical approaches for repair or resection of a fistula.[300] Stricturoplasty rather than resection may be appropriate for patients with multiple fibrotic, nonphlegmonous strictures of the small bowel and for patients with short bowel syndrome or at risk for this complication because of prior resections.[300] Although 80% of patients who undergo ileocecal resection have evidence of endoscopic recurrence in the neo-terminal ileum within 1 year of surgery,[89] the time to symptomatic recurrence usually is several years. Recurrent disease almost always occurs proximal to the anastomosis. Recurrence after proctocolectomy and permanent ileostomy is relatively uncommon.

Indications for surgery include complications such as intra-abdominal abscess, medically intractable fistula, fibrotic stricture with obstructive symptoms, toxic megacolon, hemorrhage, and cancer.[301] Patients with symptoms refractory to medical therapy should also be considered for surgery, particularly when the patient remains glucocorticoid-dependent or refractory despite optimal medical therapy. Among children, a well-timed bowel resection may be indicated for growth failure. In patients with indeterminate colitis for whom colectomy and ileal pouch-anal anastomosis is being considered, there is a high rate of pouch failure. Therefore, thorough preoperative assessment should be completed to ascertain the correct diagnosis.[302] In selected cases with rectal sparing and lack of fistulizing behavior, ileal pouch–anal anastomosis or ileorectal anastomosis may be considered (see Chapter 110).[303,304] Increasing facility with laparoscopic approaches to Crohn's disease may reduce the operative morbidity and improve the safety of surgery.[305,306]

COSTS OF CARE

Substantial medical and societal costs are incurred in the course of Crohn's disease. A recent study from Sweden showed that although ulcerative colitis is twice as prevalent as Crohn's disease, the total combined medical and societal costs of Crohn's disease are twice that of ulcerative colitis.[307] An analysis of data from a population-based cohort in the United States found projected lifetime costs of medical care to exceed $40,000 when median charges were applied.[308] Surgery generated the largest proportion of costs (44%), but nearly two thirds of patient time was spent off medical therapies, largely reflecting surgically induced remission.[308] Short of a cure, safe, well-tolerated, effective, and inexpensive means of maintaining remission should provide the greatest economic impact in the care of patients with the disease.

CROHN'S DISEASE IN THE LIFE CYCLE

CHILDREN AND ADOLESCENTS

Approximately 25% of new Crohn's disease diagnoses are made in persons younger than 20 years of age. In most respects, Crohn's disease has the same pathophysiology and clinical features in children as it does in adults. The special consequences of Crohn's disease in children and adolescents relate to the vulnerability of this population to disturbances in physical growth, sexual maturation, and psychosocial development. Deceleration of growth velocity may precede gastrointestinal symptoms in as many as 20% of children.[309] Correction of nutritional deficits and vigorous treatment of inflammation will lead to normal growth and development in most children with Crohn's disease. The potential for glucocorticoids to cause mood disturbances and cosmetic side effects may have dire implications for the child's psychosocial development, but their role in decreasing height velocity has been questioned.[310] Increasingly, immune modulators are being incorporated into pediatric treatment regimens as a means of minimizing glucocorticoid use.[261,311]

In evaluating disease, medical personnel must be particularly sensitive to the trauma of intrusive and sometimes painful examinations and procedures that are done routinely in adults. Sadly, children with Crohn's disease also are subject to the vicissitudes of their social circumstances: underinsured children are more likely to present with more severe disease, undoubtedly because of poor access to medical care and prolonged delays in diagnosis.[312] As much as possible, children with Crohn's disease should be permitted to function normally in school and extracurricular activities, although special accommodations may sometimes need to be arranged.

SEXUALITY, FERTILITY, AND PREGNANCY

Crohn's disease affects many persons in the peak of their reproductive years. Studies have varied in the assessment of female fertility in Crohn's disease, showing either no difference from the general population or a slight decrease. Studies that have detected diminished fertility generally have correlated this finding with increased disease activity. Contributing factors may include true infertility or a conscious decision to avoid childbearing. In men and women, decreased libido from symptoms such as diarrhea, abdominal pain, and fatigue is not uncommon; in women, dyspareunia from rectovaginal fistula may play an additional role. Except for reversible sperm abnormalities caused by sulfasalazine, men with Crohn's disease have normal fertility.

The effect of pregnancy on the course of Crohn's disease depends on the status of the disease at conception. Women with quiescent disease at conception have the same rate of relapse as nonpregnant women. Among women with active disease at conception, the "one third rule" applies: one third improve, one third worsen, and one third have unchanged symptoms during their pregnancy.[313] HLA disparity at both DRB1 and DQ between mother and fetus is strongly associated with improvement in IBD symptoms during pregnancy.[314] Postpartum relapses are uncommon and tend to be mild.

Most pregnancies carried by women with Crohn's disease are normal. Among the small number of women who experience stillbirth, spontaneous abortion, or premature labor, two thirds had active disease during the pregnancy. The rate of cesarean section is not increased compared with that of the general population, and perineal complications occur infrequently among women who deliver vaginally with an episiotomy.[315,316] For a review of the safety of medical therapies in pregnancy and nursing, see Table 108–4.

THE AGING PATIENT

Compared with younger patients diagnosed with Crohn's disease, older patients are more likely to have colonic disease, and in particular, distal colonic disease.[317] As with children, the presentation may be subtle; extraintestinal symptoms may predominate, and diagnosis may be delayed. Medical management is essentially no different for the older patient, but the clinician more often must consider the variety of other conditions prevalent among older patients when choosing therapies. Thus, for example, older persons treated with glucocorticoids are at increased risk for hypertension, hypokalemia, and confusion.[318] Glucocorticoids also tend to complicate

the management of diabetes. Antibiotics may diminish vitamin K production by intestinal flora and cause an excessively prolonged prothrombin time with warfarin therapy. Anticholinergic drugs may induce urinary retention, altered mental status, or glaucoma.

PROGNOSIS

MORBIDITY

The natural history of Crohn's disease is a moving target, continuously changing as therapeutic strategies improve. The course is highly variable and difficult to predict for a given patient. Population-based studies from Scandinavia provide the best information regarding the course of disease. In the first year after diagnosis, the cumulative relapse rate is high, approaching 50%, with 10% of patients having a chronic relapsing course.[319] Thereafter, patients generally are true to their own history: The rate of relapse in the first 2 years of the disease correlates with the risk of relapse in the ensuing 5 years.[320] Symptomatically active disease in the preceding year yields a high likelihood of active disease in the next year. Conversely, a year in which symptoms are quiescent has an 80% probability of being followed by another year without exacerbation.[320] Over a 4-year period, the same analysis has shown that 22% of patients remain in remission, 25% experience chronically active symptoms, and 53% have a course that fluctuates between active and inactive disease.[320] Although most persons continue to lead productive lives, the course of the disease may be punctuated by periods of poor productivity. Over time, approximately 10% of patients may be disabled by their disease.

CANCER

The estimated risk of colorectal cancer in Crohn's disease has varied widely, ranging from no risk above that of the general population to an estimated standardized incidence ratio as high as 26.6.[321] When Crohn's disease involves the large bowel, the excess risk of colorectal cancer appears to be similar to that in ulcerative colitis of similar extent.[321] The characteristics and prognosis of colorectal cancer in Crohn's disease also are similar to those for colorectal cancer in ulcerative colitis.[322] For these reasons, surveillance colonoscopy has been recommended as a means of early detection.[323] A thinner caliber colonoscope may be required to traverse narrowed bowel. Segments of bowel excluded by diversion procedures are at greatly increased risk of developing cancer and present a great challenge to early detection.

Little controversy surrounds the increased risk of small bowel adenocarcinoma associated with long-standing disease or bypassed loops of the small intestine. Despite a roughly 12-fold relative risk, small bowel cancers remain rare, because of the extremely low incidence of this disease in the general population.[324]

The association between Hodgkin's and non-Hodgkin's lymphoma and Crohn's disease remains unclear. Studies relying on cases at referral centers have found an increased risk of lymphoma, whereas population-based studies have not. The most likely explanations are either a referral bias or an increased risk confined to patients with more severe disease.[321]

Squamous cell carcinomas may arise in association with a chronic fistula to the skin. Some studies also have found an association between Crohn's disease and respiratory cancers,[324] perhaps attributable to increased smoking behavior.

MORTALITY

Population-based studies generally have shown a modestly increased mortality rate in Crohn's disease.[325-329] Mortality appears to be highest in the first 4 or 5 years after diagnosis, with a 15-year survival rate that is 93.7% of that of the general population.[327,328] Patients with proximal small bowel disease may have a higher risk of mortality, whereas those with ileal or ileocecal disease have a lower risk, comparable to the general population.[327,329] The excess mortality may be ascribed to complications of Crohn's disease, including colorectal cancer.

COPING WITH CROHN'S DISEASE

Although the old myths surrounding psychopathology as an underlying cause of IBD have long been debunked, coping with diarrhea, pain, malaise, and decreased energy takes a toll on all persons who suffer from Crohn's disease as well as on their families. Depression and anxiety often diminish daily functioning that already may be impaired by the physical manifestations of the disease; psychosocial functioning, of course, has a large impact on the patient's quality of life.[330] Patients cite concerns about lack of energy, loss of control, body image, fear and isolation, feeling unclean, and not reaching their full potential.[331] The medical provider can help greatly in alleviating these concerns by providing accurate and plentiful information. Lay organizations such as the Crohn's and Colitis Foundation of America provide valuable resources in support of affected persons and their families (http://www.ccfa.org). An attitude of hopefulness is warranted, as an astounding number of therapeutic innovations—and someday perhaps a cure—unfold.

REFERENCES

1. Kirsner JB: Historical aspects of inflammatory bowel disease. J Clin Gastroenterol 10:286, 1988.
2. Dalziel TK: Thomas Kennedy Dalziel 1861-1924. Chronic interstitial enteritis. Dis Colon Rectum 32:1076, 1989.
3. Baron JH: Inflammatory bowel disease up to 1932. Mt Sinai J Med 67:174, 2000.
4. Crohn BB, Ginzburg L, Oppenheimer GD: Regional ileitis, a pathological and clinical entity. JAMA 99:1323, 1932.
5. Brooke BN: Granulomatous diseases of the intestine. Lancet 2:745, 1959.
6. Lockhart-Mummery HE, Morson BC: Crohn's disease (regional enteritis) of the large intestine and its distinction from ulcerative colitis. Gut 1:87, 1960.
7. Moum B, Ekbom A, Vatn MH, et al: Inflammatory bowel disease: Re-evaluation of the diagnosis in a prospective population-based study in southeastern Norway. Gut 40:328, 1997.
8. Pinchbeck BR, Kirdeikis J, Thomson AB: Inflammatory bowel disease in northern Alberta: An epidemiologic study. J Clin Gastroenterol 10:505, 1988.
9. Martinez-Salmeron JF, Rodrigo M, de Teresa J, et al: Epidemiology of inflammatory bowel disease in the Province of Granada, Spain: A retrospective study from 1979 to 1988. Gut 34:1207, 1993.
10. Ranzi T, Bodini P, Zambelli A, et al: Epidemiological aspects of inflammatory bowel disease in a north Italian population: A 4-year prospective study. Eur J Gastroenterol Hepatol 8:657, 1996.
11. Loftus EV Jr, Schoenfeld P, Sandborn WJ: The epidemiology and natural history of Crohn's disease in population-based patient cohorts from North America: A systematic review. Aliment Pharmacol Ther 16:51, 2002.
12. Sonnenberg A, McCarty DJ, Jacobsen SJ: Geographic variation of inflammatory bowel disease within the United States. Gastroenterology 100:143, 1991.
13. Kurata JH, Kantor-Fish S, Frankl H, et al: Crohn's disease among ethnic groups in a large health maintenance organization. Gastroenterology 102:1940, 1992.
14. Hiatt RA, Kaufman L: Epidemiology of inflammatory bowel disease in a defined northern California population. West J Med 149:541, 1988.
15. Shivananda S, Lennard-Jones J, Logan R, et al: Incidence of inflammatory bowel disease across Europe: Is there a difference between north and south? Results of the European Collaborative Study on Inflammatory Bowel Disease (EC-IBD). Gut 39:690, 1996.
16. Morita N, Toki S, Hirohashi T, et al: Incidence and prevalence of inflammatory bowel disease in Japan: Nationwide epidemiological survey during the year 1991. J Gastroenterol 30(Suppl 8):1, 1995.
17. Yoshida Y, Murata Y: Inflammatory bowel disease in Japan: Studies of epidemiology and etiopathogenesis. Med Clin North Am 74:67, 1990.
18. Eason RJ, Lee SP, Tasman-Jones C: Inflammatory bowel disease in Auckland, New Zealand. Aust N Z J Med 12:125, 1982.
19. Anseline PF: Crohn's disease in the Hunter Valley region of Australia. Aust N Z J Surg 65:564, 1995.
20. Mayberry J, Mann R: Inflammatory bowel disease in rural sub-Saharan Africa: Rarity of diagnosis in patients attending mission hospitals. Digestion 44:172, 1989.
21. Wright JP, Froggatt J, O'Keefe EA, et al: The epidemiology of inflammatory bowel disease in Cape Town 1980-1984. S Afr Med J 70:10, 1986.
22. Loftus EV Jr, Silverstein MD, Sandborn WJ, et al: Crohn's disease in Olmsted County, Minnesota, 1940-1993: Incidence, prevalence, and survival. Gastroenterology 114:1161, 1998.
23. Munkholm P, Langholz E, Nielsen OH, et al: Incidence and prevalence of Crohn's disease in the county of Copenhagen, 1962-87: A sixfold increase in incidence. Scand J Gastroenterol 27:609, 1992.
24. Delco F, Sonnenberg A: Commonalities in the time trends of Crohn's disease and ulcerative colitis. Am J Gastroenterol 94:2171, 1999.
25. Munkholm P: Crohn's disease--occurrence, course and prognosis: An epidemiologic cohort-study. Dan Med Bull 44:287, 1997.
26. Ekbom A, Helmick C, Zack M, Adami HO: The epidemiology of inflammatory bowel disease: A large, population-based study in Sweden. Gastroenterology 100:350, 1991.
27. Andres PG, Friedman LS: Epidemiology and the natural course of inflammatory bowel disease. Gastroenterol Clin North Am 28:255, 1999.

28. Sandler RS, Eisen GM: Epidemiology of inflammatory bowel disease. In Kirsner JB (ed): Inflammatory Bowel Disease. Philadelphia, WB Saunders, 2000, p 89.

29. Polito JM II, Childs B, Mellits ED, et al: Crohn's disease: Influence of age at diagnosis on site and clinical type of disease. Gastroenterology 111:580, 1996.

30. Wakefield AJ, Pittilo RM, Sim R, et al: Evidence of persistent measles virus infection in Crohn's disease. J Med Virol 39:345, 1993.

31. Davis RL, Kramarz P, Bohlke K, et al: Measles-mumps-rubella and other measles-containing vaccines do not increase the risk for inflammatory bowel disease: A case-control study from the Vaccine Safety Datalink Project. Arch Pediatr Adolesc Med 155:354, 2001.

32. Masseret E, Boudeau J, Colombel JF, et al: Genetically related *Escherichia coli* strains associated with Crohn's disease. Gut 48:320, 2001.

33. Van Kruiningen HJ: Lack of support for a common etiology in Johne's disease of animals and Crohn's disease in humans. Inflamm Bowel Dis 5:183, 1999.

34. Fiocchi C: Inflammatory bowel disease: Etiology and pathogenesis. Gastroenterology 115:182, 1998.

35. MacDonald TT: Effector and regulatory lymphoid cells and cytokines in mucosal sites. Curr Top Microbiol Immunol 236:113, 1999.

36. Duchmann R, May E, Heike M, et al: T cell specificity and cross reactivity towards enterobacteria, bacteroides, bifidobacterium, and antigens from resident intestinal flora in humans. Gut 44:812, 1999.

37. Romagnani S: T-cell subsets (Th1 versus Th2). Ann Allergy Asthma Immunol 85:9, 2000; quiz, 18, 21.

38. Fuss IJ, Heller F, Boirivant M, et al: Nonclassical CD1d-restricted NK T cells that produce IL-13 characterize an atypical Th2 response in ulcerative colitis. J Clin Invest 113:1490, 2004.

39. Hermiston ML, Gordon JI: Inflammatory bowel disease and adenomas in mice expressing a dominant negative *N*-cadherin. Science 270:1203, 1995.

40. Mashimo H, Wu DC, Podolsky DK, Fishman MC: Impaired defense of intestinal mucosa in mice lacking intestinal trefoil factor. Science 274:262, 1996.

41. Panwala CM, Jones JC, Viney JL: A novel model of inflammatory bowel disease: Mice deficient for the multiple drug resistance gene, *mdr1a*, spontaneously develop colitis. J Immunol 161:573, 1998.

42. Sadlack B, Merz H, Schorle H, et al: Ulcerative colitis-like disease in mice with a disrupted interleukin-2 gene. Cell 75:253, 1993.

43. Kuhn R, Lohler J, Rennick D, et al: Interleukin-10-deficient mice develop chronic enterocolitis. Cell 75:263, 1993.

44. Hammer RE, Maika SD, Richardson JA, et al: Spontaneous inflammatory disease in transgenic rats expressing HLA-B27 and human beta 2m: An animal model of HLA-B27-associated human disorders. Cell 63:1099, 1990.

45. Lopez-Cubero SO, Sullivan KM, McDonald GB: Course of Crohn's disease after allogeneic marrow transplantation. Gastroenterology 114:433, 1998.

46. Sustento-Reodica N, Ruiz P, Rogers A, et al: Recurrent Crohn's disease in transplanted bowel. Lancet 349:688, 1997.

47. D'Inca R, Di Leo V, Corrao G, et al: Intestinal permeability test as a predictor of clinical course in Crohn's disease. Am J Gastroenterol 94:2956, 1999.

48. Peeters M, Nevens H, Baert F, et al: Familial aggregation in Crohn's disease: Increased age-adjusted risk and concordance in clinical characteristics. Gastroenterology 111:597, 1996.

49. Sturm A, Fiocchi C: Life and death in the gut: More killing, less Crohn's. Gut 50:148, 2002.

50. Neurath MF, Fuss I, Kelsall BL, et al: Antibodies to interleukin 12 abrogate established experimental colitis in mice. J Exp Med 182:1281, 1995.

51. Neurath MF, Pettersson S: Predominant role of NF-kappa B p65 in the pathogenesis of chronic intestinal inflammation. Immunobiology 198:91, 1997.

52. Barnes PJ, Karin M: Nuclear factor-kappaB: A pivotal transcription factor in chronic inflammatory diseases. N Engl J Med 336:1066, 1997.

53. Walzog B, Gaehtgens P: Adhesion molecules: The path to a new understanding of acute inflammation. News Physiol Sci 15:107, 2000.

54. Briskin M, Winsor-Hines D, Shyjan A, et al: Human mucosal addressin cell adhesion molecule-1 is preferentially expressed in intestinal tract and associated lymphoid tissue. Am J Pathol 151:97, 1997.

55. Ghosh S, Goldin E, Gordon FH, et al: Natalizumab for active Crohn's disease. N Engl J Med 348:24, 2003.

56. Sandborn WJ, Colombel JF, Enns R, et al: Natalizumab induction and maintenance therapy for Crohn's disease. N Engl J Med 353:1912, 2005.

57. von Lampe B, Barthel B, Coupland SE, et al: Differential expression of matrix metalloproteinases and their tissue inhibitors in colon mucosa of patients with inflammatory bowel disease. Gut 47:63, 2000.

58. Binder V: Genetic epidemiology in inflammatory bowel disease. Dig Dis 16:351, 1998.

59. Satsangi J, Grootscholten C, Holt H, Jewell DP: Clinical patterns of familial inflammatory bowel disease. Gut 38:738, 1996.

60. Bayless TM, Tokayer AZ, Polito JM II, et al: Crohn's disease: Concordance for site and clinical type in affected family members—potential hereditary influences. Gastroenterology 111:573, 1996.

61. Colombel JF, Grandbastien B, Gower-Rousseau C, et al: Clinical characteristics of Crohn's disease in 72 families. Gastroenterology 111:604, 1996.

62. Sendid B, Quinton JF, Charrier G, et al: Anti-*Saccharomyces cerevisiae* mannan antibodies in familial Crohn's disease. Am J Gastroenterol 93:1306, 1998.

63. Hugot JP, Laurent-Puig P, Gower-Rousseau C, et al: Mapping of a susceptibility locus for Crohn's disease on chromosome 16. Nature 379:821, 1996.

64. Ogura Y, Bonen DK, Inohara N, et al: A frameshift mutation in NOD2 associated with susceptibility to Crohn's disease. Nature 411:603, 2001.

65. Hugot JP, Chamaillard M, Zouali H, et al: Association of NOD2 leucine-rich repeat variants with susceptibility to Crohn's disease. Nature 411:599, 2001.

66. Cuthbert AP, Fisher SA, Mirza MM, et al: The contribution of NOD2 gene mutations to the risk and site of disease in inflammatory bowel disease. Gastroenterology 122:867, 2002.

67. Hampe J, Grebe J, Nikolaus S, et al: Association of NOD2 (CARD 15) genotype with clinical course of Crohn's disease: A cohort study. Lancet 359:1661, 2002.

68. Lesage S, Zouali H, Cezard JP, et al: CARD15/NOD2 mutational analysis and genotype-phenotype correlation in 612 patients with inflammatory bowel disease. Am J Hum Genet 70:845, 2002.

69. Abreu MT, Taylor KD, Lin YC, et al: Mutations in NOD2 are associated with fibrostenosing disease in patients with Crohn's disease. Gastroenterology 123:679, 2002.

70. Zhou Z, Lin XY, Akolkar PN, et al: Variation at NOD2/CARD15 in familial and sporadic cases of Crohn's disease in the Ashkenazi Jewish population. Am J Gastroenterol 97:3095, 2002.

71. Inohara N, Ogura Y, Fontalba A, et al: Host recognition of bacterial muramyl dipeptide mediated through NOD2: Implications for Crohn's disease. J Biol Chem 278:5509, 2003.

72. Girardin SE, Boneca IG, Viala J, et al: Nod2 is a general sensor of peptidoglycan through muramyl dipeptide (MDP) detection. J Biol Chem 278:8869, 2003.

73. Lala S, Ogura Y, Osborne C, et al: Crohn's disease and the NOD2 gene: A role for Paneth cells. Gastroenterology 125:47, 2003.

74. Kobayashi K, Inohara N, Hernandez LD, et al: RICK/Rip2/CARDIAK mediates signalling for receptors of the innate and adaptive immune systems. Nature 416:194, 2002.

75. Netea MG, Kullberg BJ, de Jong DJ, et al: NOD2 mediates anti-inflammatory signals induced by TLR2 ligands: Implications for Crohn's disease. Eur J Immunol 34:2052, 2004.

76. Watanabe T, Kitani A, Murray PJ, Strober W: NOD2 is a negative regulator of toll-like receptor 2-mediated T helper type 1 responses. Nat Immunol 5:800, 2004.

77. Chen CM, Gong Y, Zhang M, Chen JJ: Reciprocal cross-talk between Nod2 and TAK1 signaling pathways. J Biol Chem 279:25876, 2004.

78. Inohara N, Nunez G: NODs: Intracellular proteins involved in inflammation and apoptosis. Nat Rev Immunol 3:371, 2003.

79. Fellermann K, Wehkamp J, Herrlinger KR, Stange EF: Crohn's disease: A defensin deficiency syndrome? Eur J Gastroenterol Hepatol 15:627, 2003.

80. Rioux JD, Daly MJ, Silverberg MS, et al: Genetic variation in the 5q31 cytokine gene cluster confers susceptibility to Crohn disease. Nat Genet 29:223, 2001.

81. Peltekova VD, Wintle RF, Rubin LA, et al: Functional variants of OCTN cation transporter genes are associated with Crohn disease. Nat Genet 36:471, 2004.

82. Stoll M, Corneliussen B, Costello CM, et al: Genetic variation in DLG5 is associated with inflammatory bowel disease. Nat Genet 36:476, 2004.

83. Cho JH, Nicolae DL, Ramos R, et al: Linkage and linkage disequilibrium in chromosome band 1p36 in American Chaldeans with inflammatory bowel disease. Hum Mol Genet 9:1425, 2000.

84. Sonnenberg A: Occupational distribution of inflammatory bowel disease among German employees. Gut 31:1037, 1990.

85. Addolorato G, Capristo E, Stefanini GF, Gasbarrini G: Inflammatory bowel disease: A study of the association between anxiety and depression, physical morbidity, and nutritional status. Scand J Gastroenterol 32:1013, 1997.

86. Qiu BS, Vallance BA, Blennerhassett PA, Collins SM: The role of CD4+ lymphocytes in the susceptibility of mice to stress-induced reactivation of experimental colitis. Nat Med 5:1178, 1999.

87. Zamora SA, Hilsden RJ, Meddings JB, et al: Intestinal permeability before and after ibuprofen in families of children with Crohn's disease. Can J Gastroenterol 13:31, 1999.

88. Parente F, Cucino C, Bollani S, et al: Focal gastric inflammatory infiltrates in inflammatory bowel diseases: Prevalence, immunohistochemical characteristics, and diagnostic role. Am J Gastroenterol 95:705, 2000.

89. Rutgeerts P, Geboes K, Vantrappen G, et al: Natural history of recurrent Crohn's disease at the ileocolonic anastomosis after curative surgery. Gut 25:665, 1984.

90. Rickert RR, Carter HW: The "early" ulcerative lesion of Crohn's disease: Correlative light and scanning electron-microscopic studies. J Clin Gastroenterol 2:11, 1980.

91. Okada M, Maeda K, Yao T, et al: Minute lesions of the rectum and sigmoid colon in patients with Crohn's disease. Gastrointest Endosc 37:319, 1991.

92. Fujimura Y, Kamoi R, Iida M: Pathogenesis of aphthoid ulcers in Crohn's disease: Correlative findings by magnifying colonoscopy, electron microscopy, and immunohistochemistry. Gut 38:724, 1996.

93. Rutgeerts P, Goboes K, Peeters M, et al: Effect of faecal stream diversion on recurrence of Crohn's disease in the neoterminal ileum. Lancet 338:771, 1991.

94. Kelly JK, Sutherland LR: The chronological sequence in the pathology of Crohn's disease. J Clin Gastroenterol 10:28, 1988.

95. Chambers TJ, Morson BC: The granuloma in Crohn's disease. Gut 20:269, 1979.

96. Riddell RH: Pathology of idiopathic inflammatory bowel disease. In Kirsner JB (ed): Inflammatory Bowel Disease. Philadelphia, WB Saunders, 2000, p 427.

97. Stallmach A, Schuppan D, Riese HH, et al: Increased collagen type III synthesis by fibroblasts isolated from strictures of patients with Crohn's disease. Gastroenterology 102:1920, 1992.

98. Borley NR, Mortensen NJ, Jewell DP, Warren BF: The relationship between inflammatory and serosal connective tissue changes in ileal Crohn's disease: Evidence for a possible causative link. J Pathol 190:196, 2000.

99. Desreumaux P, Ernst O, Geboes K, et al: Inflammatory alterations in mesenteric adipose tissue in Crohn's disease. Gastroenterology 117:73, 1999.

100. Wright NA, Poulsom R, Stamp G, et al: Trefoil peptide gene expression in gastrointestinal epithelial cells in inflammatory bowel disease. Gastroenterology 104:12, 1993.

101. Oberhuber G, Puspok A, Oesterreicher C, et al: Focally enhanced gastritis: A frequent type of gastritis in patients with Crohn's disease. Gastroenterology 112:698, 1997.

102. Higgens CS, Allan RN: Crohn's disease of the distal ileum. Gut 21:933, 1980.

103. Belaiche J, Louis E, D'Haens G, et al: Acute lower gastrointestinal bleeding in Crohn's disease: Characteristics of a unique series of 34 patients. Belgian IBD Research Group. Am J Gastroenterol 94:2177, 1999.

104. Langevin S, Menard DB, Haddad H, et al: Idiopathic ulcerative proctitis may be the initial manifestation of Crohn's disease. J Clin Gastroenterol 15:199, 1992.

105. Baker WN, Milton-Thompson GJ: The anal lesion as the sole presenting symptom of intestinal Crohn's disease. Gut 12:865, 1971.

106. Buchmann P, Alexander-Williams J: Classification of perianal Crohn's disease. Clin Gastroenterol 9:323, 1980.

107. Wagtmans MJ, Verspaget HW, Lamers CB, van Hogezand RA: Clinical aspects of Crohn's disease of the upper gastrointestinal tract: A comparison with distal Crohn's disease. Am J Gastroenterol 92:1467, 1997.

108. D'Haens G, Rutgeerts P, Geboes K, Vantrappen G: The natural history of esophageal Crohn's disease: Three patterns of evolution. Gastrointest Endosc 40:296, 1994.

109. Oberhuber G, Puspok A, Peck-Radosavlevic M, et al: Aberrant esophageal HLA-DR expression in a high percentage of patients with Crohn's disease. Am J Surg Pathol 23:970, 1999.

110. Richards ML, Aberger FJ, Landercasper J: Granulomatous appendicitis: Crohn's disease, atypical Crohn's, or not Crohn's at all? J Am Coll Surg 185:13, 1997.

111. Greenstein AJ, Lachman P, Sachar DB, et al: Perforating and non-perforating indications for repeated operations in Crohn's disease: Evidence for two clinical forms. Gut 29:588, 1988.

112. Gilberts EC, Greenstein AJ, Katsel P, et al: Molecular evidence for two forms of Crohn disease. Proc Natl Acad Sci U S A 91:12721, 1994.

113. Heuschkel RB, MacDonald TT, Monteleone G, et al: Imbalance of stromelysin-1 and TIMP-1 in the mucosal lesions of children with inflammatory bowel disease. Gut 47:57, 2000.

114. Ribeiro MB, Greenstein AJ, Yamazaki Y, Aufses AH Jr: Intra-abdominal abscess in regional enteritis. Ann Surg 213:32, 1991.

115. Gasche C, Scholmerich J, Brynskov J, et al: A simple classification of Crohn's disease: Report of the Working Party for the World Congresses of Gastroenterology, Vienna 1998. Inflamm Bowel Dis 6:8, 2000.

116. Urayama S, Chang EB: Mechanisms and treatment of diarrhea in inflammatory bowel diseases. Inflamm Bowel Dis 3:114, 1997.

117. Dvorak AM, Silen W: Differentiation between Crohn's disease and other inflammatory conditions by electron microscopy. Ann Surg 201:53, 1985.

118. Mantyh CR, Vigna SR, Bollinger RR, et al: Differential expression of substance P receptors in patients with Crohn's disease and ulcerative colitis. Gastroenterology 109:850, 1995.

119. Geboes K, Collins S: Structural abnormalities of the nervous system in Crohn's disease and ulcerative colitis. Neurogastroenterol Motil 10:189, 1998.

120. Geerling BJ, Badart-Smook A, Stockbrugger RW, Brummer RJ: Comprehensive nutritional status in patients with long-standing Crohn disease currently in remission. Am J Clin Nutr 67:919, 1998.

121. Han PD, Burke A, Baldassano RN, et al: Nutrition and inflammatory bowel disease. Gastroenterol Clin North Am 28:423, 1999.

122. Gryboski JD, Burger J, McCallum R, Lange R: Gastric emptying in childhood inflammatory bowel disease: Nutritional and pathologic correlates. Am J Gastroenterol 87:1148, 1992.

123. Schreiber S, Howaldt S, Schnoor M, et al: Recombinant erythropoietin for the treatment of anemia in inflammatory bowel disease. N Engl J Med 334:619, 1996.

124. Veloso FT, Carvalho J, Magro F: Immune-related systemic manifestations of inflammatory bowel disease: A prospective study of 792 patients. J Clin Gastroenterol 23:29, 1996.

125. Lorusso D, Leo S, Mossa A, et al: Cholelithiasis in inflammatory bowel disease: A case-control study. Dis Colon Rectum 33:791, 1990.

126. Lapidus A, Bangstad M, Astrom M, Muhrbeck O: The prevalence of gallstone disease in a defined cohort of patients with Crohn's disease. Am J Gastroenterol 94:1261, 1999.

127. Danzi JT: Extraintestinal manifestations of idiopathic inflammatory bowel disease. Arch Intern Med 148:297, 1988.

128. Farmer RG, Hawk WA, Turnbull RB Jr: Clinical patterns in Crohn's disease: A statistical study of 615 cases. Gastroenterology 68:627, 1975.

129. Salmi M, Jalkanen S: Endothelial ligands and homing of mucosal leukocytes in extraintestinal manifestations of IBD. Inflamm Bowel Dis 4:149, 1998.

130. Orchard TR, Wordsworth BP, Jewell DP: Peripheral arthropathies in inflammatory bowel disease: Their articular distribution and natural history. Gut 42:387, 1998.

131. Orchard TR, Thiyagaraja S, Welsh KI, et al: Clinical phenotype is related to HLA genotype in the peripheral arthropathies of inflammatory bowel disease. Gastroenterology 118:274, 2000.

132. Gravallese EM, Kantrowitz FG: Arthritic manifestations of inflammatory bowel disease. Am J Gastroenterol 83:703, 1988.

133. Orchard TR, Jewell DP: The importance of ileocaecal integrity in the arthritic complications of Crohn's disease. Inflamm Bowel Dis 5:92, 1999.

134. Scott WW Jr, Fishman EK, Kuhlman JE, et al: Computed tomography evaluation of the sacroiliac joints in Crohn disease: Radiologic/clinical correlation. Skeletal Radiol 19:207, 1990.

135. Wakefield AJ, Sankey EA, Dhillon AP, et al: Granulomatous vasculitis in Crohn's disease. Gastroenterology 100:1279, 1991.

136. Freeman HJ, Freeman KJ: Prevalence rates and an evaluation of reported risk factors for osteonecrosis (avascular necrosis) in Crohn's disease. Can J Gastroenterol 14:138, 2000.

137. Bousvaros A, Marcon M, Treem W, et al: Chronic recurrent multifocal osteomyelitis associated with chronic inflammatory bowel disease in children. Dig Dis Sci 44:2500, 1999.

138. Ghosh S, Cowen S, Hannan WJ, Ferguson A: Low bone mineral density in Crohn's disease, but not in ulcerative colitis, at diagnosis. Gastroenterology 107:1031, 1994.

139. Dresner-Pollak R, Karmeli F, Eliakim R, et al: Increased urinary N-telopeptide cross-linked type 1 collagen predicts bone loss in patients with inflammatory bowel disease. Am J Gastroenterol 95:699, 2000.

140. Schulte CM, Dignass AU, Goebell H, et al: Genetic factors determine extent of bone loss in inflammatory bowel disease. Gastroenterology 119:909, 2000.

141. Lebwohl M, Lebwohl O: Cutaneous manifestations of inflammatory bowel disease. Inflamm Bowel Dis 4:142, 1998.

142. Finkel SI, Janowitz HD: Trauma and the pyoderma gangrenosum of inflammatory bowel disease. Gut 22:410, 1981.

143. Lisciandrano D, Ranzi T, Carrassi A, et al: Prevalence of oral lesions in inflammatory bowel disease. Am J Gastroenterol 91:7, 1996.

144. Hackzell-Bradley M, Hedblad MA, Stephansson EA: Metastatic Crohn's disease: Report of three cases with special reference to histopathologic findings. Arch Dermatol 132:928, 1996.

145. Zlatanic J, Fleisher M, Sasson M, et al: Crohn's disease and acute leukocytoclastic vasculitis of skin. Am J Gastroenterol 91:2410, 1996.

146. Travis S, Innes N, Davies MG, et al: Sweet's syndrome: An unusual cutaneous feature of Crohn's disease or ulcerative colitis. The South West Gastroenterology Group. Eur J Gastroenterol Hepatol 9:715, 1997.

147. Lee FI, Bellary SV, Francis C: Increased occurrence of psoriasis in patients with Crohn's disease and their relatives. Am J Gastroenterol 85:962, 1990.

148. Hopkins DJ, Horan E, Burton IL, et al: Ocular disorders in a series of 332 patients with Crohn's disease. Br J Ophthalmol 58:732, 1974.

149. Lyons JL, Rosenbaum JT: Uveitis associated with inflammatory bowel disease compared with uveitis associated with spondyloarthropathy. Arch Ophthalmol 115:61, 1997.

150. Hofley P, Roarty J, McGinnity G, et al: Asymptomatic uveitis in children with chronic inflammatory bowel diseases. J Pediatr Gastroenterol Nutr 17:397, 1993.

151. Rasmussen HH, Fallingborg JF, Mortensen PB, et al: Hepatobiliary dysfunction and primary sclerosing cholangitis in patients with Crohn's disease. Scand J Gastroenterol 32:604, 1997.

152. Over HH, Ulgen S, Tuglular T, et al: Thrombophilia and inflammatory bowel disease: Does factor V mutation have a role? Eur J Gastroenterol Hepatol 10:827, 1998.

153. Zauber NP, Sabbath-Solitare M, Rajoria G, Mogan G: Factor V Leiden mutation is not increased in patients with inflammatory bowel disease. J Clin Gastroenterol 27:215, 1998.

154. Mahmud N, Molloy A, McPartlin J, et al: Increased prevalence of methylenetetrahydrofolate reductase C677T variant in patients with inflammatory bowel disease, and its clinical implications. Gut 45:389, 1999.

155. Solem CA, Loftus EV, Tremaine WJ, et al: Venous thromboembolism in inflammatory bowel disease. Am J Gastroenterol 99:97, 2004.

156. Fireman Z, Osipov A, Kivity S, et al: The use of induced sputum in the assessment of pulmonary involvement in Crohn's disease. Am J Gastroenterol 95:730, 2000.

157. Elsehety A, Bertorini TE: Neurologic and neuropsychiatric complications of Crohn's disease. South Med J 90:606, 1997.

158. Levine JB: Extraintestinal manifestations of inflammatory bowel disease. In Kirsner JB (ed): Inflammatory Bowel Disease. Philadelphia, WB Saunders, 2000, p 397.

159. Weber P, Seibold F, Jenss H: Acute pancreatitis in Crohn's disease. J Clin Gastroenterol 17:286, 1993.

160. Barthet M, Hastier P, Bernard JP, et al: Chronic pancreatitis and inflammatory bowel disease: True or coincidental association? Am J Gastroenterol 94:2141, 1999.

161. Hegnhoj J, Hansen CP, Rannem T, et al: Pancreatic function in Crohn's disease. Gut 31:1076, 1990.

162. Bernstein CN, Boult IF, Greenberg HM, et al: A prospective randomized comparison between small bowel enteroclysis and small bowel follow-through in Crohn's disease. Gastroenterology 113:390, 1997.

163. Scotiniotis I, Rubesin SE, Ginsberg GG: Imaging modalities in inflammatory bowel disease. Gastroenterol Clin North Am 28:391, 1999.

164. Gore RM, Balthazar EJ, Ghahremani GG, Miller FH: CT features of ulcerative colitis and Crohn's disease. AJR Am J Roentgenol 167:3, 1996.

165. Herlinger H, Furth EE, Rubesin SE: Fibrofatty proliferation of the mesentery in Crohn disease. Abdom Imaging 23:446, 1998.

166. Gasche C, Moser G, Turetschek K, et al: Transabdominal bowel sonography for the detection of intestinal complications in Crohn's disease. Gut 44:112, 1999.

167. Cho E, Mochizuki N, Ashihara T, et al: Endoscopic ultrasonography in the evaluation of inflammatory bowel disease [Abstract]. Endoscopy 30(Suppl 1):A94, 1998.

168. Ludwig D, Wiener S, Bruning A, et al: Mesenteric blood flow is related to disease activity and risk of relapse in Crohn's disease: A prospective follow-up study. Am J Gastroenterol 94:2942, 1999.

169. Hussain SM, Outwater EK, Joekes EC, et al: Clinical and MR imaging features of cryptoglandular and Crohn's fistulas and abscesses. Abdom Imaging 25:67, 2000.

170. Low RN, Francis IR, Politoske D, Bennett M: Crohn's disease evaluation: Comparison of contrast-enhanced MR imaging and single-phase helical CT scanning. J Magn Reson Imaging 11:127, 2000.

171. Madsen SM, Thomsen HS, Schlichting P, et al: Evaluation of treatment response in active Crohn's disease by low-field magnetic resonance imaging. Abdom Imaging 24:232, 1999.

172. Sahai A, Belair M, Gianfelice D, et al: Percutaneous drainage of intra-abdominal abscesses in Crohn's disease: Short and long-term outcome. Am J Gastroenterol 92:275, 1997.

173. Charron M, Di Lorenzo C, Kocoshis S: Are ^{99m}Tc leukocyte scintigraphy and SBFT studies useful in children suspected of having inflammatory bowel disease? Am J Gastroenterol 95:1208, 2000.

174. Pera A, Bellando P, Caldera D, et al: Colonoscopy in inflammatory bowel disease: Diagnostic accuracy and proposal of an endoscopic score. Gastroenterology 92:181, 1987.

175. Marshall JK, Hewak J, Farrow R, et al: Terminal ileal imaging with ileoscopy versus small-bowel meal with pneumocolon. J Clin Gastroenterol 27:217, 1998.

176. Lo SK: Capsule endoscopy in the diagnosis and management of inflammatory bowel disease. Gastrointest Endosc Clin North Am 14:179, 2004.

177. Kastin DA, Buchman AL, Barrett T, et al: Strictures from Crohn's disease diagnosed by video capsule endoscopy. J Clin Gastroenterol 38:346, 2004.

178. Koltun WA, Schoetz DJ Jr, Roberts PL, et al: Indeterminate colitis predisposes to perineal complications after ileal pouch-anal anastomosis. Dis Colon Rectum 34:857, 1991.

179. Shivananda S, Hordijk ML, Ten Kate FJ, et al: Differential diagnosis of inflammatory bowel disease: A comparison of various diagnostic classifications. Scand J Gastroenterol 26:167, 1991.

180. Riegler G, Arimoli A, Esposito P, et al: Clinical evolution in an outpatient series with indeterminate colitis. Dis Colon Rectum 40:437, 1997.

181. Quinton JF, Sendid B, Reumaux D, et al: Anti-*Saccharomyces cerevisiae* mannan antibodies combined with antineutrophil cytoplasmic autoantibodies in inflammatory bowel disease: prevalence and diagnostic role. Gut 42:788, 1998.

182. Ruemmele FM, Targan SR, Levy G, et al: Diagnostic accuracy of serological assays in pediatric inflammatory bowel disease. Gastroenterology 115:822, 1998.

183. Sutton CL, Yang H, Li Z, et al: Familial expression of anti-*Saccharomyces cerevisiae* mannan antibodies in affected and unaffected relatives of patients with Crohn's disease. Gut 46:58, 2000.

184. Vasiliauskas EA, Plevy SE, Landers CJ, et al: Perinuclear antineutrophil cytoplasmic antibodies in patients with Crohn's disease define a clinical subgroup. Gastroenterology 110:1810, 1996.

185. Landers CJ, Cohavy O, Misra R, et al: Selected loss of tolerance evidenced by Crohn's disease-associated immune responses to auto- and microbial antigens. Gastroenterology 123:689, 2002.

186. Vasiliauskas EA, Kam LY, Karp LC, et al: Marker antibody expression stratifies Crohn's disease into immunologically homogeneous subgroups with distinct clinical characteristics. Gut 47:487, 2000.

187. Forcione DG, Rosen MJ, Kisiel JB, Sands BE: Anti-*Saccharomyces cerevisiae* antibody (ASCA) positivity is associated with increased risk for early surgery in Crohn's disease. Gut 53:1117, 2004.

188. van Hees PA, van Elteren PH, van Lier HJ, van Tongeren JH: An index of inflammatory activity in patients with Crohn's disease. Gut 21:279, 1980.

189. Wright JP, Marks IN, Parfitt A: A simple clinical index of Crohn's disease activity--the Cape Town index. S Afr Med J 68:502, 1985.

190. Harvey RF, Bradshaw JM: A simple index of Crohn's disease activity. Lancet 1:514, 1980.

191. Myren J, Bouchier IA, Watkinson G, et al: The OMGE Multinational Inflammatory Bowel Disease Survey 1976-1982: A further report on 2,657 cases. Scand J Gastroenterol Suppl 95:1, 1984.

192. Willoughby JM, Kumar P, Beckett J, Dawson AM: A double-blind trial of azathioprine in Crohn's disease. Gut 12:864, 1971.

193. De Dombal FT, Burton IL, Clamp SE, Goligher JC: Short-term course and prognosis of Crohn's disease. Gut 15:435, 1974.

194. Talstad I, Gjone E: The disease activity of ulcerative colitis and Crohn's disease. Scand J Gastroenterol 11:403, 1976.

195. Sandler RS, Jordan MC, Kupper LL: Development of a Crohn's index for survey research. J Clin Epidemiol 41:451, 1988.

196. Hyams JS, Ferry GD, Mandel FS, et al: Development and validation of a pediatric Crohn's disease activity index. J Pediatr Gastroenterol Nutr 12:439, 1991.

197. Lloyd-Still JD, Green OC: A clinical scoring system for chronic inflammatory bowel disease in children. Dig Dis Sci 24:620, 1979.

198. de Dombal FT, Softley A: IOIBD report no 1: Observer variation in calculating indices of severity and activity in Crohn's disease. International Organisation for the Study of Inflammatory Bowel Disease. Gut 28:474, 1987.

199. Papi C, Ciaco A, Bianchi M, et al: Correlation of various Crohn's disease activity indexes in subgroups of patients with primarily inflammatory or fibrostenosing clinical characteristics. J Clin Gastroenterol 23:40, 1996.

200. Allan A, Linares L, Spooner HA, Alexander-Williams J: Clinical index to quantitate symptoms of perianal Crohn's disease. Dis Colon Rectum 35:656, 1992.

201. Irvine EJ: Usual therapy improves perianal Crohn's disease as measured by a new disease activity index. McMaster IBD Study Group. J Clin Gastroenterol 20:27, 1995.

202. Mary JY, Modigliani R: Development and validation of an endoscopic index of the severity for Crohn's disease: A prospective multicentre study. Groupe d'Etudes Therapeutiques des Affections Inflammatoires du Tube Digestif (GETAID). Gut 30:983, 1989.

203. Present DH, Korelitz BI, Wisch N, et al: Treatment of Crohn's disease with 6-mercaptopurine: A long-term, randomized, double-blind study. N Engl J Med 302:981, 1980.

204. Nielsen OH, Vainer B, Madsen SM, et al: Established and emerging biological activity markers of inflammatory bowel disease. Am J Gastroenterol 95:359, 2000.

205. Tibble JA, Sigthorsson G, Bridger S, et al: Surrogate markers of intestinal inflammation are predictive of relapse in patients with inflammatory bowel disease. Gastroenterology 119:15, 2000.

206. Guyatt G, Mitchell A, Irvine EJ, et al: A new measure of health status for clinical trials in inflammatory bowel disease. Gastroenterology 96:804, 1989.

207. Azad Khan AK, Piris J, Truelove SC: An experiment to determine the active therapeutic moiety of sulphasalazine. Lancet 2:892, 1977.

208. MacDermott RP: Progress in understanding the mechanisms of action of 5-aminosalicylic acid. Am J Gastroenterol 95:3343, 2000.

209. Bantel H, Berg C, Vieth M, et al: Mesalazine inhibits activation of transcription factor NF-kappaB in inflamed mucosa of patients with ulcerative colitis. Am J Gastroenterol 95:3452, 2000.

210. Summers RW, Switz DM, Sessions JT Jr, et al: National Cooperative Crohn's Disease Study: Results of drug treatment. Gastroenterology 77:847, 1979.

211. Malchow H, Ewe K, Brandes JW, et al: European Cooperative Crohn's Disease Study (ECCDS): Results of drug treatment. Gastroenterology 86:249, 1984.

212. Rasmussen SN, Lauritsen K, Tage-Jensen U, et al: 5-Aminosalicylic acid in the treatment of Crohn's disease: A 16-week double-blind, placebo-controlled, multicentre study with Pentasa. Scand J Gastroenterol 22:877, 1987.

213. Mahida YR, Jewell DP: Slow-release 5-amino-salicylic acid (Pentasa) for the treatment of active Crohn's disease. Digestion 45:88, 1990.

214. Singleton JW, Hanauer SB, Gitnick GL, et al: Mesalamine capsules for the treatment of active Crohn's disease: Results of a 16-week trial. Pentasa Crohn's Disease Study Group. Gastroenterology 104:1293, 1993.

215. Hanauer SB, Stromberg U: Oral Pentasa in the treatment of active Crohn's disease: A meta-analysis of double-blind, placebo-controlled trials. Clin Gastroenterol Hepatol 2:379, 2004.

216. Lang KA, Peppercorn MA: Medical therapy for Crohn's disease. In Kirsner JB (ed): Inflammatory Bowel Disease. Philadelphia, WB Saunders, 2000, p 557.

217. Rutgeerts P, Hiele M, Geboes K, et al: Controlled trial of metronidazole treatment for prevention of Crohn's recurrence after ileal resection. Gastroenterology 108:1617, 1995.

218. Brandt LJ, Bernstein LH, Boley SJ, Frank MS: Metronidazole therapy for perineal Crohn's disease: A follow-up study. Gastroenterology 83:383, 1982.

219. Sutherland L, Singleton J, Sessions J, et al: Double-blind, placebo-controlled trial of metronidazole in Crohn's disease. Gut 32:1071, 1991.

220. Ursing B, Alm T, Barany F, et al: A comparative study of metronidazole and sulfasalazine for active Crohn's disease: The Cooperative Crohn's Disease Study in Sweden: II. Result. Gastroenterology 83:550, 1982.

221. Colombel JF, Lemann M, Cassagnou M, et al: A controlled trial comparing ciprofloxacin with mesalazine for the treatment of active Crohn's disease. Groupe d'Etudes Therapeutiques des Affections Inflammatoires Digestives (GETAID). Am J Gastroenterol 94:674, 1999.

222. Prantera C, Zannoni F, Scribano ML, et al: An antibiotic regimen for the treatment of active Crohn's disease: A randomized, controlled clinical trial of metronidazole plus ciprofloxacin. Am J Gastroenterol 91:328, 1996.

223. Steinhart AH, Feagan BG, Wong CJ, et al: Combined budesonide and antibiotic therapy for active Crohn's disease: A randomized controlled trial. Gastroenterology 123:33, 2002.

224. Leiper K, Morris AI, Rhodes JM: Open-label trial of oral clarithromycin in active Crohn's disease. Aliment Pharmacol Ther 14:801, 2000.

225. Prantera C, Kohn A, Mangiarotti R, et al: Antimycobacterial therapy in Crohn's disease: Results of a controlled, double-blind trial with a multiple antibiotic regimen. Am J Gastroenterol 89:513, 1994.

226. Munkholm P, Langholz E, Davidsen M, Binder V: Frequency of glucocorticoid resistance and dependency in Crohn's disease. Gut 35:360, 1994.

227. Modigliani R, Mary JY, Simon JF, et al: Clinical, biological, and endoscopic picture of attacks of Crohn's disease: Evolution on prednisolone. Groupe d'Etude Therapeutique des Affections Inflammatoires Digestives. Gastroenterology 98:811, 1990.

228. Shepherd HA, Barr GD, Jewell DP: Use of an intravenous steroid regimen in the treatment of acute Crohn's disease. J Clin Gastroenterol 8:154, 1986.

229. Rubin RH, Ikonen T, Gummert JF, Morris RE: The therapeutic prescription for the organ transplant recipient: the linkage of immunosuppression and antimicrobial strategies. Transpl Infect Dis 1:29, 1999.

230. Thiele K, Bierhaus A, Autschbach F, et al: Cell specific effects of glucocorticoid treatment on the NF-kappaBp65/Ikappa-Balpha system in patients with Crohn's disease. Gut 45:693, 1999.

231. Stuck AE, Minder CE, Frey FJ: Risk of infectious complications in patients taking glucocorticosteroids. Rev Infect Dis 11:954, 1989.

232. Steinhart AH, Ewe K, Griffiths AM, et al: Corticosteroids for maintaining remission of Crohn's disease. Cochrane Database Syst Rev 2000(2):CD000301.

233. Franchimont DP, Louis E, Croes F, Belaiche J: Clinical pattern of corticosteroid-dependent Crohn's disease. Eur J Gastroenterol Hepatol 10:821, 1998.

234. Farrell RJ, Murphy A, Long A, et al: High multidrug resistance (P-glycoprotein 170) expression in inflammatory bowel disease patients who fail medical therapy. Gastroenterology 118:279, 2000.

235. Mingrone G, DeGaetano A, Pugeat M, et al: The steroid resistance of Crohn's disease. J Investig Med 47:319, 1999.

236. Thomsen OO, Cortot A, Jewell D, et al: A comparison of budesonide and mesalamine for active Crohn's disease. International Budesonide-Mesalamine Study Group. N Engl J Med 339:370, 1998.

237. Greenberg GR, Feagan BG, Martin F, et al: Oral budesonide as maintenance treatment for Crohn's disease: A placebo-controlled, dose-ranging study. Canadian Inflammatory Bowel Disease Study Group. Gastroenterology 110:45, 1996.

238. Greenberg GR, Feagan BG, Martin F, et al: Oral budesonide for active Crohn's disease. Canadian Inflammatory Bowel Disease Study Group. N Engl J Med 331:836, 1994.

239. Lofberg R, Rutgeerts P, Malchow H, et al: Budesonide prolongs time to relapse in ileal and ileocaecal Crohn's disease: A placebo-controlled one-year study. Gut 39:82, 1996.

240. Hellers G, Cortot A, Jewell D, et al: Oral budesonide for prevention of postsurgical recurrence in Crohn's disease. The IOIBD Budesonide Study Group. Gastroenterology 116:294, 1999.

241. Ewe K, Bottger T, Buhr HJ, et al: Low-dose budesonide treatment for prevention of postoperative recurrence of Crohn's disease: A multicentre randomized placebo-controlled trial. German Budesonide Study Group. Eur J Gastroenterol Hepatol 11:277, 1999.

242. Cortot A, Colombel JF, Rutgeerts P, et al: Switch from systemic steroids to budesonide in steroid-dependent patients with inactive Crohn's disease. Gut 48:186, 2001.

243. Brooke BN, Hoffmann DC, Swarbrick ET: Azathioprine for Crohn's disease. Lancet 2:612, 1969.

244. Pearson DC, May GR, Fick GH, Sutherland LR: Azathioprine and 6-mercaptopurine in Crohn disease: A meta-analysis. Ann Intern Med 123:132, 1995.

245. Candy S, Wright J, Gerber M, et al: A controlled double-blind study of azathioprine in the management of Crohn's disease. Gut 37:674, 1995.

246. Ewe K, Press AG, Singe CC, et al: Azathioprine combined with prednisolone or monotherapy with prednisolone in active Crohn's disease. Gastroenterology 105:367, 1993.

247. D'Haens G, Geboes K, Ponette E, et al: Healing of severe recurrent ileitis with azathioprine therapy in patients with Crohn's disease. Gastroenterology 112:1475, 1997.

248. Sandborn WJ, Tremaine WJ, Wolf DC, et al: Lack of effect of intravenous administration on time to respond to azathioprine for steroid-treated Crohn's disease. North American Azathioprine Study Group. Gastroenterology 117:527, 1999.

249. Dubinsky MC, Lamothe S, Yang HY, et al: Pharmacogenomics and metabolite measurement for 6-mercaptopurine therapy in inflammatory bowel disease. Gastroenterology 118:705, 2000.

250. Colonna T, Korelitz BI: The role of leukopenia in the 6-mercaptopurine-induced remission of refractory Crohn's disease. Am J Gastroenterol 89:362, 1994.

251. Pedersen BK, Beyer JM: A longitudinal study of the influence of azathioprine on natural killer cell activity. Allergy 41:286, 1986.

252. Tiede I, Fritz G, Strand S, et al: CD28-dependent Rac1 activation is the molecular target of azathioprine in primary human CD4+ T lymphocytes. J Clin Invest 111:1133, 2003.

253. Present DH, Meltzer SJ, Krumholz MP, et al: 6-Mercaptopurine in the management of inflammatory bowel disease: Short- and long-term toxicity. Ann Intern Med 111:641, 1989.

254. Connell WR, Kamm MA, Ritchie JK, Lennard-Jones JE: Bone marrow toxicity caused by azathioprine in inflammatory bowel disease: Twenty-seven years of experience. Gut 34:1081, 1993.

255. Colombel JF, Ferrari N, Debuysere H, et al: Genotypic analysis of thiopurine S-methyltransferase in patients with Crohn's disease and severe myelosuppression during azathioprine therapy. Gastroenterology 118:1025, 2000.

256. Connell WR, Kamm MA, Dickson M, et al: Long-term neoplasia risk after azathioprine treatment in inflammatory bowel disease. Lancet 343:1249, 1994.

257. Farrell RJ, Ang Y, Kileen P, et al: Increased incidence of non-Hodgkin's lymphoma in inflammatory bowel disease patients on immunosuppressive therapy but overall risk is low. Gut 47:514, 2000.

258. Lewis JD, Schwartz JS, Lichtenstein GR: Azathioprine for maintenance of remission in Crohn's disease: Benefits outweigh the risk of lymphoma. Gastroenterology 118:1018, 2000.

259. Hanauer SB, Korelitz BI, Rutgeerts P, et al: Postoperative maintenance of Crohn's disease remission with 6-mercaptopurine, mesalamine, or placebo: A two-year trial. Gastroenterology 127:723, 2004.

260. Ardizzone S, Maconi G, Sampietro GM, et al: Azathioprine and mesalamine for prevention of relapse after conservative surgery for Crohn's disease. Gastroenterology 127:730, 2004.

261. Markowitz J, Grancher K, Kohn N, et al: A multicenter trial of 6-mercaptopurine and prednisone in children with newly diagnosed Crohn's disease. Gastroenterology 119:895, 2000.

262. Treton X, Bouhnik Y, Mary JY, et al: Azathioprine withdrawal in patients with Crohn's disease maintained on prolonged remission under treatment is associated with a high risk of relapse [Abstract]. Gastroenterology 126(Suppl 2):A113, 2004.

263. Feagan BG, Rochon J, Fedorak RN, et al: Methotrexate for the treatment of Crohn's disease. The North American Crohn's Study Group Investigators. N Engl J Med 332:292, 1995.

264. Feagan BG, Fedorak RN, Irvine EJ, et al: A comparison of methotrexate with placebo for the maintenance of remission in Crohn's disease. North American Crohn's Study Group Investigators. N Engl J Med 342:1627, 2000.

265. Cronstein BN, Naime D, Ostad E: The antiinflammatory mechanism of methotrexate: Increased adenosine release at inflamed sites diminishes leukocyte accumulation in an in vivo model of inflammation. J Clin Invest 92:2675, 1993.

266. Mack DR, Young R, Kaufman SS, et al: Methotrexate in patients with Crohn's disease after 6-mercaptopurine. J Pediatr 132:830, 1998.

267. Lemann M, Chamiot-Prieur C, Mesnard B, et al: Methotrexate for the treatment of refractory Crohn's disease. Aliment Pharmacol Ther 10:309, 1996.

268. Feagan BG, McDonald JW, Rochon J, et al: Low-dose cyclosporine for the treatment of Crohn's disease. The Canadian Crohn's Relapse Prevention Trial Investigators. N Engl J Med 330:1846, 1994.

269. Gerber DA, Bonham CA, Thomson AW: Immunosuppressive agents: Recent developments in molecular action and clinical application. Transplant Proc 30:1573, 1998.

270. Sandborn WJ, Present DH, Isaacs KL, et al: Tacrolimus for the treatment of fistulas in patients with Crohn's disease: A randomized, placebo-controlled trial. Gastroenterology 125:380, 2003.

271. Fellermann K, Ludwig D, Stahl M, et al: Steroid-unresponsive acute attacks of inflammatory bowel disease: Immunomodulation by tacrolimus (FK506). Am J Gastroenterol 93:1860, 1998.

272. Casson DH, Eltumi M, Tomlin S, et al: Topical tacrolimus may be effective in the treatment of oral and perineal Crohn's disease. Gut 47:436, 2000.

273. Derkx B, Taminiau J, Radema S, et al: Tumour necrosis factor antibody treatment in Crohn's disease. Lancet 342:173, 1993.

274. van Dullemen HM, van Deventer SJ, Hommes DW, et al: Treatment of Crohn's disease with anti-tumor necrosis factor chimeric monoclonal antibody (cA2). Gastroenterology 109:129, 1995.

275. Baert FJ, D'Haens GR, Peeters M, et al: Tumor necrosis factor alpha antibody (infliximab) therapy profoundly downregulates the inflammation in Crohn's ileocolitis. Gastroenterology 116:22, 1999.

276. Targan SR, Hanauer SB, van Deventer SJ, et al: A short-term study of chimeric monoclonal antibody cA2 to tumor necrosis factor alpha for Crohn's disease. Crohn's Disease cA2 Study Group. N Engl J Med 337:1029, 1997.

277. Present DH, Rutgeerts P, Targan S, et al: Infliximab for the treatment of fistulas in patients with Crohn's disease. N Engl J Med 340:1398, 1999.

278. Hanauer SB, Feagan BG, Lichtenstein GR, et al: Maintenance infliximab for Crohn's disease: The ACCENT I randomised trial. Lancet 359:1541, 2002.

279. Sands BE, Anderson FH, Bernstein CN, et al: Infliximab maintenance therapy for fistulizing Crohn's disease. N Engl J Med 350:876, 2004.

280. Di Sabatino A, Ciccocioppo R, Cinque B, et al: Defective mucosal T cell death is sustainably reverted by infliximab in a caspase-dependent pathway in Crohn's disease. Gut 53:70, 2004.

281. Lugering A, Schmidt M, Lugering N, et al: Infliximab induces apoptosis in monocytes from patients with chronic active Crohn's disease by using a caspase-dependent pathway. Gastroenterology 121:1145, 2001.

282. Van den Brande JM, Braat H, van den Brink GR, et al: Infliximab but not etanercept induces apoptosis in lamina propria T-lymphocytes from patients with Crohn's disease. Gastroenterology 124:1774, 2003.

283. Hanauer SB, Rutgeerts PJ, D'Haens G, et al: Delayed hypersensitivity to infliximab (Remicade) reinfusion after 2- to 4-year interval without treatment [Abstract]. Gastroenterology 116:A731, 1999.

284. Cosnes J, Carbonnel F, Carrat F, et al: Effects of current and former cigarette smoking on the clinical course of Crohn's disease. Aliment Pharmacol Ther 13:1403, 1999.

285. Mannon PJ, Fuss IJ, Mayer L, et al: Anti-IL-12 Crohn's Disease Study Group. Anti-interleukin-12 antibody for active Crohn's disease. N Engl J Med 351:2069, 2004.

286. Sands BE: Novel therapies for inflammatory bowel disease. Gastroenterol Clin North Am 28:323, 1999.

287. Slonim AE, Bulone L, Damore MB, et al: A preliminary study of growth hormone therapy for Crohn's disease. N Engl J Med 342:1633, 2000.

288. Stack WA, Mann SD, Roy AJ, et al: Randomised controlled trial of CDP571 antibody to tumour necrosis factor-alpha in Crohn's disease. Lancet 349:521, 1997.

289. Ehrenpreis ED, Kane SV, Cohen LB, et al: Thalidomide therapy for patients with refractory Crohn's disease: An open-label trial. Gastroenterology 117:1271, 1999.

290. Vasiliauskas EA, Kam LY, Abreu-Martin MT, et al: An open-label pilot study of low-dose thalidomide in chronically active, steroid-dependent Crohn's disease. Gastroenterology 117:1278, 1999.

291. Malchow HA: Crohn's disease and *Escherichia coli*: A new approach in therapy to maintain remission of colonic Crohn's disease? J Clin Gastroenterol 25:653, 1997.

292. Summers RW, Elliott DE, Qadir K, et al: *Trichuris suis* seems to be safe and possibly effective in the treatment of inflammatory bowel disease. Am J Gastroenterol 98:2034, 2003.

293. Dieckgraefe BK. Korzenik JR: Treatment of active Crohn's disease with recombinant human granulocyte-macrophage colony-stimulating factor. Lancet 360:1478, 2002.

294. Griffiths AM, Ohlsson A, Sherman PM, Sutherland LR: Meta-analysis of enteral nutrition as a primary treatment of active Crohn's disease. Gastroenterology 108:1056, 1995.

295. Ballegaard M, Bjergstrom A, Brondum S, et al: Self-reported food intolerance in chronic inflammatory bowel disease. Scand J Gastroenterol 32:569, 1997.

296. Pearson M, Teahon K, Levi AJ, Bjarnason I: Food intolerance and Crohn's disease. Gut 34:783, 1993.

297. Belluzzi A, Brignola C, Campieri M, et al: Effect of an enteric-coated fish-oil preparation on relapses in Crohn's disease. N Engl J Med 334:1557, 1996.

298. Mekhjian HS, Switz DM, Watts HD, et al: National Cooperative Crohn's Disease Study: Factors determining recurrence of Crohn's disease after surgery. Gastroenterology 77:907, 1979.

299. Whelan G, Farmer RG, Fazio VW, Goormastic M: Recurrence after surgery in Crohn's disease: Relationship to location of disease (clinical pattern) and surgical indication. Gastroenterology 88:1826, 1985.

300. Strong S, Fazio VW: The surgical management of Crohn's disease. In Kirsner JB (ed): Inflammatory Bowel Disease. Philadelphia, WB Saunders, 2000, p 658.

301. Hurst RD, Molinari M, Chung TP, et al: Prospective study of the features, indications, and surgical treatment in 513 consecutive patients affected by Crohn's disease. Surgery 122:661, 1997.

302. Sagar PM, Dozois RR, Wolff BG: Long-term results of ileal pouch-anal anastomosis in patients with Crohn's disease. Dis Colon Rectum 39:893, 1996.

303. Panis Y, Poupard B, Nemeth J, et al: Ileal pouch/anal anastomosis for Crohn's disease. Lancet 347:854, 1996.

304. Pastore RL, Wolff BG, Hodge D: Total abdominal colectomy and ileorectal anastomosis for inflammatory bowel disease. Dis Colon Rectum 40:1455, 1997.

305. Alabaz O, Iroatulam AJ, Nessim A, et al: Comparison of laparoscopically assisted and conventional ileocolic resection for Crohn's disease. Eur J Surg 166:213, 2000.

306. Wu JS, Birnbaum EH, Kodner IJ, et al: Laparoscopic-assisted ileocolic resections in patients with Crohn's disease: Are abscesses, phlegmons, or recurrent disease contraindications? Surgery 122:682, 1997.

307. Blomqvist P, Ekbom A: Inflammatory bowel diseases: Health care and costs in Sweden in 1994. Scand J Gastroenterol 32:1134, 1997.

308. Silverstein MD, Loftus EV, Sandborn WJ, et al: Clinical course and costs of care for Crohn's disease: Markov model analysis of a population-based cohort. Gastroenterology 117:49, 1999.

309. Kanof ME, Lake AM, Bayless TM: Decreased height velocity in children and adolescents before the diagnosis of Crohn's disease. Gastroenterology 95:1523, 1988.

310. Motil KJ, Grand RJ, Davis-Kraft L, et al: Growth failure in children with inflammatory bowel disease: A prospective study. Gastroenterology 105:681, 1993.

311. Markowitz J, Grancher K, Mandel F, Daum F: Immunosuppressive therapy in pediatric inflammatory bowel disease: Results of a survey of the North American Society for Pediatric Gastroenterology and Nutrition. Subcommittee on Immunosuppressive Use of the Pediatric IBD Collaborative Research Forum. Am J Gastroenterol 88:44, 1993.

312. Spivak W, Sockolow R, Rigas A: The relationship between insurance class and severity of presentation of inflammatory bowel disease in children. Am J Gastroenterol 90:982, 1995.

313. Korelitz BI: Inflammatory bowel disease and pregnancy. Gastroenterol Clin North Am 27:213, 1998.

314. Kane S, Kisiel J, Shih L, et al: HLA disparity determines disease activity through pregnancy in women with inflammatory bowel disease. Am J Gastroenterol 99:1523, 2004.

315. Brandt LJ, Estabrook SG, Reinus JF: Results of a survey to evaluate whether vaginal delivery and episiotomy lead to perineal involvement in women with Crohn's disease. Am J Gastroenterol 90:1918, 1995.

316. Illnyckyji A, Blanchard JF, Rawsthorne P, et al: Perianal Crohn's disease and pregnancy: Role of the mode of delivery. Am J Gastroenterol 94:3274, 1999.

317. Tokayer AZ, Brandt LJ: Idiopathic inflammatory bowel disease in the elderly. In Kirsner JB (ed): Inflammatory Bowel Disease. Philadelphia, WB Saunders, 2000, p 335.

318. Akerkar GA, Peppercorn MA, Hamel MB, Parker RA: Corticosteroid-associated complications in elderly Crohn's disease patients. Am J Gastroenterol 92:461, 1997.

319. Moum B, Ekbom A, Vatn MH, et al: Clinical course during the first year after diagnosis in ulcerative colitis and Crohn's disease: Results of a large, prospective population-based study in southeastern Norway, 1990-1993. Scand J Gastroenterol 32:1005, 1997.

320. Munkholm P, Langholz E, Davidsen M, Binder V: Disease activity courses in a regional cohort of Crohn's disease patients. Scand J Gastroenterol 30:699, 1995.

321. Lewis JD, Deren JJ, Lichtenstein GR: Cancer risk in patients with inflammatory bowel disease. Gastroenterol Clin North Am 28:459, 1999.

322. Ribeiro MB, Greenstein AJ, Sachar DB, et al: Colorectal adenocarcinoma in Crohn's disease. Ann Surg 223:186, 1996.

323. Friedman S, Rubin PH, Bodian C, et al: Screening and surveillance colonoscopy in chronic Crohn's colitis. Gastroenterology 120:820, 2001.

324. Persson PG, Karlen P, Bernell O, et al: Crohn's disease and cancer: A population-based cohort study. Gastroenterology 107:1675, 1994.

325. Ekbom A, Helmick CG, Zack M, et al: Survival and causes of death in patients with inflammatory bowel disease: A population-based study. Gastroenterology 103:954, 1992.

326. Gollop JH, Phillips SF, Melton LJ III, Zinsmeister AR: Epidemiologic aspects of Crohn's disease: A population-based study in Olmsted County, Minnesota, 1943-1982. Gut 29:49, 1988.

327. Munkholm P, Langholz E, Davidsen M, Binder V: Intestinal cancer risk and mortality in patients with Crohn's disease. Gastroenterology 105:1716, 1993.

328. Persson PG, Bernell O, Leijonmarck CE, et al: Survival and cause-specific mortality in inflammatory bowel disease: A population-based cohort study. Gastroenterology 110:1339, 1996.

329. Probert CS, Jayanthi V, Wicks AC, Mayberry JF: Mortality from Crohn's disease in Leicestershire, 1972-1989: An epidemiological community-based study. Gut 33:1226, 1992.

330. Turnbull GK, Vallis TM: Quality of life in inflammatory bowel disease: The interaction of disease activity with psychosocial function. Am J Gastroenterol 90:1450, 1995.

331. Casati J, Toner BB, de Rooy EC, et al: Concerns of patients with inflammatory bowel disease: A review of emerging themes. Dig Dis Sci 45:26, 2000.

CHAPTER
109 Ulcerative Colitis

Chinyu Su and Gary R. Lichtenstein

Ulcerative colitis (UC) is a chronic inflammatory disorder of the gastrointestinal tract that affects the large bowel and is a major disorder under the broad group of inflammatory bowel diseases (IBDs). Dr. Samuel Wilks is credited with being the first to describe this disorder in 1859 when he described this entity as "idiopathic colitis" and recognized it as distinct from the then more common bacillary dysentery.[1] He also reported the pathologic finding of dilated and thinned colon with severe universal inflammation in a patient with this condition.[2] In 1909, Hawkins described the chronic and relapsing nature of the disease course, and the "stealthy hemorrhage" onset of distal disease in which bleeding often occurred in the presence of constipation.[3] In that same year, Sir Arthur Hurst gave a more complete description of UC, including its sigmoidoscopic appearances and differentiation from bacillary dysentery.[4] Its etiology remained controversial, however, and an infectious or psychosomatic origin was considered the primary cause. The discovery of the double-helix by Watson and Crick in the 1950s paved the era of genetic research, and in the last several decades, immunology has taken on the central stage of research in the pathogenesis of UC. At present, the precise etiology of UC is unknown but is thought to be multifactorial, involving genetic, immunologic, and environmental factors. It is also now evident that patients with UC may have a broad spectrum of clinical presentations and extraintestinal manifestations. Although UC is not associated with an increased mortality compared with the general population, the disease can lead to substantial morbidity and direct and indirect health care costs. Fortunately, significant advances have been made since the initial description of UC regarding management of the disease and its associated complications, including medical therapies and surgical techniques.

EPIDEMIOLOGY

The incidence and prevalence of UC vary with geographic location and ethnicity. Rigorous epidemiologic studies have been limited by several potential issues. The diagnosis of UC may be difficult due to its variation in clinical manifestations, and in some regions, the common occurrence of infectious colitis that can mimic UC. Differences in health care systems also contribute to the inaccurate estimation of cases, and reliable determination of the epidemiology of UC for a particular population may not be possible. With improved diagnostic techniques and increased awareness, UC is now recognized worldwide. Despite this increased recognition, however, most of the available epidemiologic data derive from population- or hospital-based studies conducted in North America and northern Europe.

In general, there has been a distinct north-south gradient in risk. The areas with the highest rates of reported incidence and prevalence of UC include North America, England, northern Europe, and Australia (Tables 109–1 and 109–2). In North America, the incidence rates range from 6.0 to 14.3 cases per 100,000 person-years, and the

Table 109–1 Incidence of Ulcerative Colitis in Various Geographic Regions

Region	Period of Study	Incidence (per 100,000 person-years)
North America		
Alberta	1981	6.0
Manitoba	1987-1996	14.3-15.6
California	1980-1981	10.9
Minnesota	1984-1993	8.3
Europe		
Scandinavia	1980-1999	9.2-20.3
Great Britain	1985-1994	13.9
Northern Europe	1988-1994	3.2-11.8
Southern Europe	1980-1994	1.5-9.6
Asia		
Israel	1987-1992	Not available
India	1999-2000	6.0
Japan	1991	1.9
Korea	1992-1994	1.2
Africa		
South Africa	1980-1984	0.6-5.0
Central and South America	1987-1993	1.2-2.2

Adapted from Loftus EV: Clinical epidemiology of inflammatory bowel disease: Incidence, prevalence, and environmental influences. Gastroenterology 126:1504, 2004.

Table 109–2 Prevalence of Ulcerative Colitis in Various Geographic Regions

Region	Period of Study	Prevalence (per 100,000 persons)
North America		
Alberta	1981	37.5
Manitoba	1994	169.5
Minnesota	2001	246
Europe		
Scandinavia	1987	161.2
Great Britain	1995-1996	122-243
Northern Europe	1984	24.8
Southern Europe	1988-1992	21.4-121
Asia		
Israel	1980-1985	55.2-70.6
India	1999	44.3
Japan	1991	18.1
Korea	1997	7.6
Singapore	1985-1996	6.0

Adapted from Loftus EV: Clinical epidemiology of inflammatory bowel disease: Incidence, prevalence, and environmental influences. Gastroenterology 126:1504, 2004.

prevalence ranges from 37 to 246 cases per 100,000 persons.[5] In Europe, the incidence rates range from 1.5 to 20.3 cases per 100,000 person-years, and the prevalence ranges from 21 to 243 cases per 100,000 persons.[5] The disease has been considered more common in northern Europe, although recent studies suggest that the incidence of UC in southern Europe is comparable to that in northern Europe.[6] In contrast, studies have reported significantly lower annual incidence rates of 0.6 to 6 per 100,000 persons in other parts of the world, including Asia, Africa, and Latin America.[5]

The overall incidence of UC has remained relatively stable over the past 3 decades; however, there appears to be geographic variation in this time frame. Although the incidence rates in North America, England, and Sweden have remained unchanged or declined, those in southern Europe have increased.[7] These time trends are in contrast with those of Crohn's disease, which has shown an increase in incidence across geographic regions.

There appears to be a marked ethnic variation in the incidence of UC. One ethnic group with high incidence of this disease is the Jewish population. Incidence rates of UC among Jews have been shown to be several-fold higher than in the non-Jewish population across various geographic regions. In the United States, for example, the annual incidence of UC among Jews is 13 cases per 100,000 person-years compared with 3.8 per 100,000 among non-Jewish whites.[7] Within Israel, Ashkenazi Jews have a higher incidence than do Sephardic Jews, but a lower incidence than in the United States and northern Europe, suggesting that environmental factors also play an etiologic role.

UC traditionally has been considered extremely uncommon in minorities, but recent studies have disputed this notion. Early studies reported that UC was rare in blacks. Most of these studies, however, were conducted in regions with limited black populations, and more recent studies suggest an increasing incidence of UC among African Americans. By the late 1970s, the incidence rates were comparable between whites and non-whites in the United States.[8,9] An increase in incidence of UC also has been observed among blacks in South Africa, although the incidence rate still remains lower than that for South African whites.[10]

UC in Asia generally is less common than in the Western countries. The prevalence and annual incidence rates for UC in Japan have remained relatively stable at about 5.5 cases per 100,000 persons and 0.36 to 0.5 cases per 100,000 persons, respectively[11]; this stability is in contrast with the rising incidence of Crohn's disease in the Japanese population. Limited data also suggest similar findings in the Chinese and Korean populations.[12,13] The prevalence of UC in India has been reported to be substantially lower than that among Europeans,[14] although an accurate assessment of its epidemiology is hampered by several of the aforementioned issues. In contrast to the limited data on the indigenous South Asians, several studies have demonstrated that South Asian immigrants in England are more likely to have UC than are European natives.[14-16] This changing epidemiology with immigrant population from low-risk to high-risk geographic regions supports the concept of environmental influence on disease development.

UC may present at all ages, although diagnosis before the age of 5 years or after 75 years is uncommon. The peak incidence of UC occurs in the 2nd and 3rd decades of life. Studies have reported a second, smaller peak in the elderly, between the ages of 60 and 70 years. This second peak is less pronounced than that for Crohn's disease. Most studies have not shown any gender difference in the occurrence of UC and a male-to-female ratio of nearly 1:1 applies to all age groups.

Certain lifestyle and socioeconomic factors have been associated with the development of UC. It is more common in industrialized than in underdeveloped countries and among urban than rural populations. Within a defined population, there may be a slightly higher incidence of disease among those of higher socioeconomic stratum. As mentioned before, studies of immigrants to high-risk geographic regions have shown increases in their incidence rates of UC compared with the incidence rate for the same ethnic groups living in their native countries. Together, these observations support the notion that environmental factors influence the development of UC.

ETIOLOGY AND PATHOGENESIS

The etiology of UC is presently unknown but is likely multifactorial. The currently held paradigm involves the complex interaction of three elements: genetic susceptibility, host immunity, and environmental factors. Dysregulation of the enteric immune response in genetically predisposed individuals leads to the development of acute and chronic inflammation and the pathologic feature of mucosal damage. The specific inciting antigens for the inflammatory process have yet to be identified, but several sources have been suggested, including pathogenic and commensal microorganisms, metabolic byproducts of these agents, and normal epithelial structures.

GENETICS

Genetic factors have been linked to the development of UC. Supporting this association is the observation that family history is one of the most important risk factors for developing the disease. The familial incidence of UC has been recognized for many years. The figures vary widely among different studies, but about 10% to 20% of patients have at least one other affected family member.[17] This familial association generally occurs in first-degree relatives. The relative risk of the same disease in a sibling of an individual with UC has been estimated as between 7 and 17 based on North American and European studies. Parents, offspring, and second-degree relatives appear to be at a lower risk for developing UC than are first-degree relatives. Data from the United States suggest a preponderance of parent-sibling combinations, but in the United Kingdom, the disease is shared more commonly by siblings.

Furthermore, this familial association is greater in Jews who are known to have a higher incidence of IBD. The lifetime risk of developing disease is threefold higher among first-degree relatives of Jewish patients compared with relatives of non-Jewish patients.[18] A similar increase in risk also has been observed in relatives of patients with early onset of disease. This familial association contrasts with the low incidence of UC among spouses of patients with IBD in most series. Although reports of IBD in both husband and wife are rare, a study of 30 conjugal instances of IBD found a higher frequency of husband-wife pairs, both of whom developed disease after cohabitation, thus suggesting a shared environmental exposure.[19]

Studies on the clinical characteristics of familial disease also have shown that the onset of disease in a child is noted at a much earlier age than in the affected parent, but there is a high degree of concordance between affected siblings for age of onset. This observation of the younger age of onset in the offspring of an affected patient may have genetic basis, such as inheritance from parents of a greater number of putative susceptibility genes, or may be due just to earlier recognition by parents and physicians. For all affected first-degree relatives within a family, there is a high concordance for type of disease (UC vs. Crohn's disease), extent of disease, and occurrence of extraintestinal manifestations.[20]

The strongest evidence of a genetic influence for UC is derived from twin studies. In three large European twin pair studies, approximately 6% to 16% of monozygotic twin pairs had concordant UC compared with 0% to 5% of dizygotic twin pairs.[21-23] These concordance rates are substantially lower than those for Crohn's disease, suggesting that genetic determinants, although important, play a less significant role than in Crohn's disease. No twin pair demonstrated both UC and Crohn's disease, further supporting the genetic basis of these disorders.

Numerous studies have examined the effect of family history on disease location. In UC, no consistent correlation has been observed in the studies that examined disease extent (e.g., left-sided vs. extensive colitis) and the presence or absence of a positive family history of UC.[24]

The inheritance of UC cannot be described by a simple mendelian model. It is likely that multiple genes are involved and that different genes may confer susceptibility, disease specificity, and phenotype. Linkage studies have suggested that there are susceptibility genes for UC on chromosomes 2, 3, 6, 7, and 12.[25,26] The IBD2 locus on chromosome 12 appears to have the strongest linkage demonstrated in studies involving large numbers of families with UC.[27] The recently identified *NOD2/CARD15* gene mutations located on chromosome 16 associated with Crohn's disease have not been associated with UC. Similar to Crohn's disease, a recent study has linked the C3435T polymorphism for the human multidrug resistance 1 (*MDR1*) gene to susceptibility for UC.[28] The *MDR1* gene product P-glycoprotein is highly expressed in intestinal epithelial cells and serves an important barrier function against xenobiotics. Animals deficient for the *MDR1a* gene develop a spontaneous colitis resembling UC,[29,30] which can be prevented by antibiotics. Individuals with the single nucleotide mutation C3435T, which is associated with a lower P-glycoprotein expression in the intestine,[31] are at an increased risk for developing UC.[32] In contrast to *NOD2/CARD15*, the frequency of this polymorphism in patients with Crohn's disease is similar to that in control subjects.

There also are genes that appear to influence disease behavior independently of susceptibility genes. The best studied of these are the human leukocyte antigen (HLA) alleles. One allele of HLA-DR2 (*DRB1*1502*) appears to be involved in disease susceptibility in Japanese and Jewish populations. Several centers have reported an association between severe disease and a rare allele of HLA-DR1 (*DRB1*0103*). In some studies, the HLA-DR3, DQ2 haplotype is associated with extensive colitis, especially among women. Among the Jewish population, the perinuclear antineutrophil antibody (pANCA) is a marker for the *DRB*1502* allele of HLA-DR2, but in non-Jewish whites, this antibody is associated with the HLA-DR3 DQ2-tumor necrosis factor (TNF)-α_2 haplotype.

ENVIRONMENTAL FACTORS

Several infectious organisms, including mycobacterial and viral agents, have been implicated in the pathogenesis of IBD, an association postulated mostly for Crohn's disease. No specific infective organism, however, has been isolated consistently from patients with UC, and therefore, it is unlikely that the disease is caused by a single common infectious agent.

Several clinical and experimental observations also have suggested the involvement of intestinal microflora in the pathogenesis of IBD. It has been suggested that components of the normal intestinal flora may initiate or contribute to the development of the chronic inflammatory state. It is possible that products of the commensal flora promote inflammation in the presence of an impaired mucosal barrier or injury to the mucosa.[33] Studies have shown reduced numbers of anaerobic bacteria and *Lactobacillus* spp. both in experimental colitis and in patients with active UC but not quiescent disease.[34] Colitis can be prevented or abrogated by administering *Lactobacillus* spp. in animal models.[35,36] Furthermore, studies have shown that both animal models of colitis and patients with IBD have reduced tolerance toward their own intestinal flora.[37,38] In germ-free conditions, the onset of inflammation in many experimental models of colitis is reduced or prevented.[39] These observations in aggregate support the notion that normal intestinal flora may modulate the chronic, low-grade inflammation in the normal physiologic state and that the host tolerance in health to these normal flora is lost during inflammation.

In addition to infective agents, several other environmental factors have been proposed as contributing etiologic factors of UC. The best characterized environmental factor associated with UC is cigarette smoking. Multiple studies consistently have shown that UC is more common among nonsmokers than among current smokers, with the relative risk of UC in nonsmokers ranging from 2 to 6[40]; this association is independent of genetic background and gender. Furthermore, there may be a dose-response relationship, with the disease more common in current light smokers than in heavy smokers. This relationship is consistent with observations that clinical improvement with nicotine therapy in patients with UC appear to be limited to those treated with high doses of nicotine but not those receiving lower doses. This risk of developing UC with smoking is particularly high for former smokers, especially within the first 2 years of smoking cessation. The rebound effect also is higher for former heavy smokers than for former light smokers.[41]

Smokers also appear to have reduced rates of hospitalization for UC and reduced rates of pouchitis following colectomy.[42] Studies on the role of passive smoking in UC have yielded conflicting results. In one case-controlled study, childhood exposure to tobacco significantly decreased the adult risk of UC by 50%,[43] whereas another study reported approximately a twofold increase in the incidence of UC among children of smokers compared with children of nonsmokers.[44]

Multiple mechanisms have been postulated to account for the apparent protective effect of active smoking on UC. These include modulation of cellular and humoral immunity, changes in cytokine levels, increased generation of free oxygen radicals, and modification of eicosanoid-mediated inflammation. Smoking also may have an effect on mucus production by the colonic mucosa, and alter colonic mucosal blood flow and gut motility. No single mechanism, however, can explain the clinical observation of the beneficial influence of smoking on UC and its adverse effect on Crohn's disease (see Chapter 108).

Other environmental risk factors that have been suggested as perhaps influencing the development of UC include diet (wheat, maize, cow's milk, refined sugar, fruit and vegetables, alcohol), oral contraceptives, food additives (silicon dioxide), toothpaste, and breast feeding[7]; none, however, has been shown conclusively to be associated with UC. Early reports implicated food allergy, especially milk allergy, as a potential etiology of UC.[45-47] A subsequent study also found a positive relationship between allergy to cow's milk in infants and later development of UC.[48] It is difficult, however, to define a causal relationship due to recall bias and the possibility that early symptoms of disease may have altered diet. Clinical observations further argue against dietary allergy as a potential cause of UC, including the lack of response to bowel rest during a severe attack of disease,[49] and anecdotal case reports that bowel diversion with an ileostomy was not effective in treating active UC. At present, there is little evidence that milk or any other food plays a primary role in the etiology of UC.

The influence of oral contraceptives on UC first was implicated in case reports of colitis developing after these agents were introduced.[50-52] In a British population-based study, there was a slight increase in UC among contraceptive users, but the association became insignificant after adjusting for social class and smoking habits.[53] A subsequent meta-analysis also failed to show a significant association, with a pooled relative risk of 1.29 (95% confidence interval [CI]; 0.94-1.77) for developing UC with oral contraceptive use.[54] Breast-feeding has been suggested to be protective against the development of UC[55]; however, this protective benefit is weak and not shown by other studies.[56,57]

Studies have consistently demonstrated a negative association between appendectomy and subsequent development of UC[58,59]; as for smoking, an opposite association appears to be the case for Crohn's disease. The mechanisms for this protective effect of appendectomy on UC are unknown. It is possible that removal of appendiceal-associated lymphoid tissues may abrogate certain pathologic alterations in mucosal immune responses and therefore prevent the onset of UC. Alternatively, the absence of those lymphoid tissues merely may characterize an immune response distinct from UC. The former hypothesis is suggested by a population-based study that found a lower incidence rate of UC after appendectomy compared with that before appendectomy.[60]

IMMUNOPATHOGENESIS

The prevailing theory of the pathogenesis of UC emphasizes the role of enteric immune response. The physiologic state of the intestine is one of constant low-grade inflammation in response to environmental stimuli such as bacterial products or endogenous factors. Breaches in this well-regulated mucosal immune system lead to the chronic uncontrolled mucosal inflammation observed in UC. In this regard, immunologic mechanisms in the pathogenesis of UC involve both humoral and cell-mediated responses.

Humoral Immunity

Histologic examination of the inflamed colon indicates a marked increase in the number of plasma cells. This increase is not uniform among cells producing different classes of immunoglobulins. The largest proportional increase occurs in IgG synthesis, which has the highest pathogenic potential among antibody classes. The increase in IgG synthesis in UC is most pronounced in the IgG_1 and IgG_3 subclasses, in contrast to Crohn's disease, in which the increase in IgG_2 synthesis is more prominent.[61,62] This disparity in the local IgG subclass response likely reflects differences in antigenic stimuli or host immunoregulatory responses between the two groups of IBD patients.

The increased IgG synthesis in IBD may represent polyclonal stimulation; however, patients with UC frequently have circulating antibodies to dietary, bacterial, and self-antigens that are mostly of the IgG isotype, usually the IgG_1 subclass. Many of these antibodies are thought to be epiphenomena because the serum antibody titers do not correlate with clinical parameters. Nevertheless, the known cross-reaction between enterobacterial antigens and colonic epithelial epitopes may be an important triggering event, even though, later in the course of the disease, the serum antibody titer to either the bacterial or the colonic antigen may be unimportant.

The concept that UC is an autoimmune disease is supported by its increased association with other autoimmune disorders, including thyroid disease, diabetes, and pernicious anemia.[63] Patients with UC have varying levels of autoantibodies to lymphocytes, ribonucleic acid, smooth muscle, gastric parietal cell, and thyroid antibodies; these are neither tissue nor disease specific. Antibodies to epithelial cell-associated components, which specifically recognize intestinal antigen, also have been described.[64] The best characterized intestinal autoantigen

is an epithelial antigen of 40-kd size found in normal colonic epithelium.[63] This autoantigen is recognized by IgG eluted from the inflamed colonic mucosa of patients with UC and is a component of the tropomyosin family of cytoskeletal proteins.[65] This autoantibody has the potential to activate complement in vivo, but direct evidence of antibody-induced cytotoxicity has not been observed. The antibody response to this 40-kd protein appears to be unique to UC and is not found in Crohn's disease or other inflammatory conditions. This autoantigen shares an epitope with antigens found in the skin, bile duct, eyes, and joints,[66,67] sites frequently involved in the extraintestinal manifestations of UC. The precise pathogenic significance of this autoantibody in UC remains unclear at present.

An autoantibody that has received significant attention is pANCA.[68] This autoantibody is present in 60% to 85% of patients with UC.[69,70] It is synthesized within the lamina propria and is of the IgG_1 subclass. The antigen to which the pANCA is directed has not yet been determined with certainty, and a variety of putative antigens have been proposed, including nuclear histone and nonhistone proteins. The most recent evidence suggests that the antigen is a 50-kd nuclear envelope protein that is specific to myeloid cells.[71] Just as with other autoantibodies found in patients with UC, the pathogenic relevance of pANCA in this disorder is unknown. In fact, the prevailing thought is that pANCA has no pathogenic role in UC but that it may serve as a potential marker of susceptibility and genetically distinct subsets of UC. The level of pANCA titer does not correlate with disease activity but may decline in patients with long-standing remission or in patients who have had colectomy for at least 10 years. Studies have suggested that pANCA may be associated with a more aggressive disease course[72] and the development of pouchitis following ileal pouch-anal anastomosis (IPAA) in patients with UC.[73]

Cellular Immunity

Immune dysregulation in UC also involves cell-mediated immunity. The mucosal T cells can be divided into two anatomically different groups: lamina propria lymphocytes and intraepithelial lymphocytes (IELs). Immune cells within the lamina propria consist of a mixture of cell types, including T cells, B cells, macrophages, and dendritic cells. The most common immune cells are IgA-secreting plasma cells. Lamina propria lymphocytes express surface adhesion molecules, $\alpha4\beta7$, that provide a homing signal for peripheral immune cells to the mucosal sites.[74] Most investigators have found a similar distribution of T cell subsets (CD4+, CD8+ within the lamina propria in patients with UC compared with that in controls).[75] Lamina propria lymphocytes have been reported to be cytotoxic to autologous colonic epithelial cells, but the exact mechanisms are unknown and the results have not been confirmed.[76] Helper function mainly has involved the effects of T cells on immunoglobulin production by B cells, but the results have been varied and do not provide firm evidence for an underlying immune abnormality in UC. Studies using nonspecific mitogens have found diminished suppressor activity during active disease only, but an antigen-induced suppressor assay has shown that patients with UC in remission exhibited suppressor defects to a range of mycobacterial and enterobacterial antigens.[77] This phenomenon of antigen-induced suppression was predominantly CD8[+] cell dependent and correlated with a poor response to skin testing with purified protein derivative; these defects were limited to the peripheral blood and not lamina propria lymphocytes.

In patients with UC, the absolute number of IELs is normal or reduced. Most of these cells are CD8[+] cells, and the function of IELs has not been well characterized. It has been suggested that they are cytotoxic and also may be active in suppressing local immune response. In patients with UC, the proportion of IELs using the γδ T cell receptor may increase.[78] However, the function and significance of γδ T cells are unknown.

Regardless of their functional status, mucosal T cells within the lamina propria and epithelium as well as peripheral blood T cells display a variety of activation markers, suggesting an activated memory phenotype.[79] Studies have suggested that T cell receptor repertoire is altered in active IBD.[80] Studies have also shown restricted Vβ usage, but there is no distinct pattern when compared with T cells from healthy lamina propria.

Although T cell mediated immunity has attracted the most attention in the pathogenesis of UC, nonspecific cellular immunity also is altered. In patients with active disease, there is an overproduction of circulating monocytes as well as mucosal macrophages.[81] The inflamed mucosa of patients with UC also exhibits infiltration of substantial numbers of granulocytes.

Epithelial Cells

Intestinal epithelial cells serve barrier functions and play a role in enteric immunity. Colonocytes express class II antigens and can function as antigen-presenting cells.[82] In addition, they also express cytokine receptors, secrete various cytokines and chemokines, and express leukocyte adhesion molecules.[83-86] Thus, abnormalities in colonic epithelial cells can contribute to the development of UC. Patients with UC have an increased turnover rate of colonic epithelium,[87] and other abnormalities of epithelial cells include a reduced metabolism of short-chain fatty acids, especially butyrate, abnormal membrane permeability,[88] and altered composition of glycoprotein mucus produced by the colonic epithelium.[89] The role of epithelial cells in the pathogenesis of IBD is supported further by animal modes of colitis using disruption of colonic epithelium.[90]

Consequences of Immune Activation

Activation of macrophages, lymphocytes, and colonic epithelial cells leads to the release of a variety of cytokines and mediators that further amplify the immune and inflammatory response of UC and result in tissue damage. Based on the cytokines they produce, CD4[+] T cells have been divided into two major immune phenotypes: T helper 1 (Th1) and T helper 2 (Th2). The Th1 response is characterized by cell-mediated immunity and is associated with the production of interleukin (IL)-2 and interferon (IFN)-γ. The differentiation of T cells along a Th1 pathway is stimulated by IL-12 generated in response to

exposure to infectious agents. The Th2 response is characterized by the production of cytokines IL-4, IL-5, and IL-10, which amplify the humoral immune response. Th1 and Th2 subsets reciprocally down-regulate each other through cytokine production.[91] Both Th1 and Th2 pathways can be regulated by unique regulatory T cells (Th3, T regulatory 1) subsets that produce IL-10 and transforming growth factor-β and down-regulate inflammation.[92] Macrophages in the inflamed colon in patients with active UC synthesize IL-1β, TNF, and IL-6, whereas lamina propria T cells probably produce IL-2 and IFN-γ. This immune response can be up-regulated further by presentation of antigen to CD4[+] lymphocytes by colonic epithelial cells that express HLA class II antigens.[82] Release of these cytokines also may lead to other abnormalities seen in UC, such as increased epithelial cell permeability and collagen synthesis. Alteration of endothelium by a variety of cytokines may result in local ischemia. Increased expression of endothelial adhesion molecules in response to inflammatory mediators recruits circulating granulocytes and monocytes to the inflamed tissues, thus further perpetuating the inflammatory response. Elevated cytokine levels within the mucosa also stimulate the release of metalloproteinase from fibroblasts with subsequent matrix degradation. Mucosal concentrations of many mediators have been shown to be elevated in patients with active UC, including leukotrienes, thromboxane, platelet-activating factor, nitric oxide, and reactive oxygen metabolites.[93] These mediators, which are mostly released from active macrophages and neutrophils, contribute to inflammation and mucosal injury, alter epithelial cell permeability, and interfere with iron transport, thereby further contributing to diarrhea. Diarrhea in UC also is caused by complement activation and the release of kinins and other inflammatory mediators from mast cells and eosinophils (see Chapter 2).

PSYCHOGENIC FACTORS

Psychosomatic factors first were implicated in the pathogenesis of UC in the 1930s,[94] but there is no good direct evidence to support this concept. Since introduction of glucocorticoids for treating patients with UC and the focus on immunologic aspects of the pathogenesis of the disease in the 1950s, this previously widely held notion has diminished in popularity.

Experimental studies have helped identify mechanisms of the proinflammatory potential of stress in animal models of colitis.[94] When applied prior to the introduction of proinflammatory stimuli, stress has been shown to increase the severity of colonic inflammation in rats. This particular response has been shown not to be mediated by either vasopressin or corticotropin-releasing factor. In addition, stress has been shown to increase intestinal permeability directly in rats via cholinergic nerves and to potentiate intestinal inflammation in this particular situation There are indeed studies reporting that psychosocial stress increases the risk of relapse in patients with quiescent UC.[95,96] Conversely, many of the psychologic features observed in patients with UC are likely secondary to this chronic disease process. It is important for physicians to be aware of this phenomenon when managing these patients.

PATHOLOGY

At the time of initial presentation, approximately 45% of patients with UC have disease limited to the rectosigmoid, 35% have disease extending beyond the sigmoid but not involving the entire colon, and 20% of patients have pancolitis.[97] The disease typically is most severe distally and progressively less severe more proximally. In contrast to Crohn's disease, continuous and symmetrical involvement is the hallmark of UC (Fig. 109–1), with sharp transition between diseased and uninvolved segments of bowel. There are a few exceptions to this general rule. First, medical therapy may result in areas of sparing. For example, topical enema therapy may lead to near complete healing of disease in the rectum and distal sigmoid colon in patients with newly diagnosed UC. Second, up to 75% of patients with left-sided UC may have appendiceal inflammation and patchy inflammation in the cecum,[98] resembling the skip pattern characteristic of Crohn's disease. These patterns of rectal sparing and skip lesions may lead to a misdiagnosis of Crohn's disease.

Macroscopically, the mucosa in UC appears hyperemic, edematous, and granular in mild disease. As disease progresses, the mucosa becomes hemorrhagic with visible punctate ulcers. These ulcers may enlarge and extend into the lamina propria. They often are irregular with overhanging edges or may be linear along the line of the teniae coli. Epithelial regeneration with recurrent attacks results in the formation of pseudopolyps, which is typical of long-standing UC but that also may be seen in acute

disease (Fig. 109–2). Another characteristic appearance of long-standing disease is atrophic and featureless colonic mucosa, associated with shortening and narrowing of the colon. Patients with severe disease may develop acute dilatation of the colon, and these cases are characterized by thin bowel wall and grossly ulcerated mucosa with only small fragments or islands of mucosa remaining. With perforation, a fibrinopurulent exudate may be seen on the serosal surface of the bowel.

Microscopically, the early stage of UC is marked by edema of the lamina propria and congestion of capillaries and venules, often with extravasation of red blood cells. This is followed by an acute inflammatory cell infiltrate of neutrophils, lymphocytes, plasma cells, and macrophages. There also may be increased numbers of eosinophils and mast cells. Neutrophilic infiltration of colonic crypts gives rise to cryptitis and ultimately to crypt abscess with neutrophilic accumulations in the crypt lumina. This migration of neutrophils from the circulation into the lamina propria occurs in response to a variety of chemoattractants, including chemotactic peptides of colonic bacteria, IL-8, activated complement, platelet-activating factor, and leukotriene B_4. The cryptitis is associated with discharge of mucus from goblet cells and increased epithelial cell turnover. Thus, the acute inflammatory infiltration results in the characteristic histopathology of goblet cell mucin depletion, formation of exudates, and epithelial cell necrosis. None of these histologic findings, however, is specific for UC.

Inflammation in UC characteristically is confined to the mucosa, in contrast to the transmural involvement of Crohn's disease. The inflammatory changes typically end at the luminal aspect of the muscularis mucosa. With increasing inflammation, however, the surface epithelial cells become flattened and eventually ulcerate. Deep ulceration may undermine the surrounding epithelium.

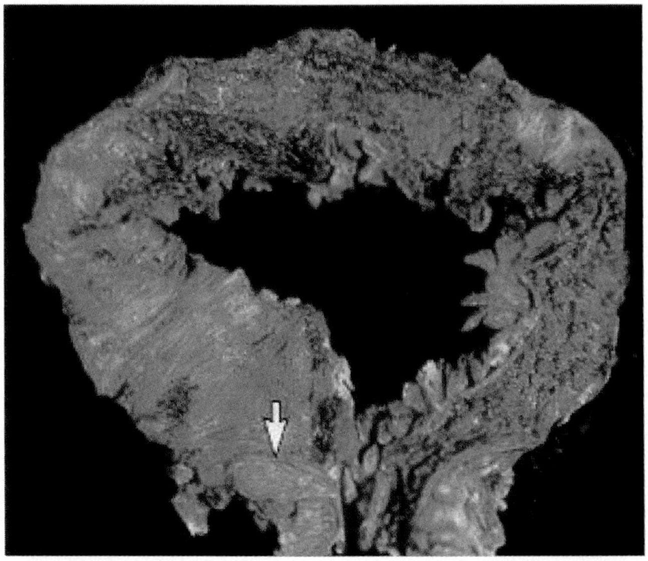

Figure 109–1 Total colectomy specimen from a patient with ulcerative colitis. The colon shows diffuse mucosal inflammation that extends proximally from the rectum without interruption to the transverse colon. The mucosal pattern in the terminal ileum and cecum (*arrow*) is normal. The distal mucosa is erythematous and friable with many ulcers and erosions. (Courtesy of Feldman, online Gastro Atlas, Current Medicine).

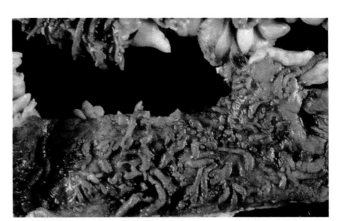

Figure 109–2 Surgical specimen of resected colon from a patient with severe ulcerative colitis showing numerous inflammatory polyps (pseudopolyposis). Pseudopolyps are most common in ulcerative colitis but also may be seen in Crohn's disease, ischemia, and other ulcerative conditions of the colon. These blunt or finger-like lesions develop as by-products of ulcers that penetrate into the submucosa, leaving islands of adjacent regenerative mucosa. Although the intervening areas of colonic mucosa are ulcerated, pseudopolyps can persist even when inflammation has abated and the mucosa has healed. (Courtesy of Feldman, online Gastro Atlas, Current Medicine).

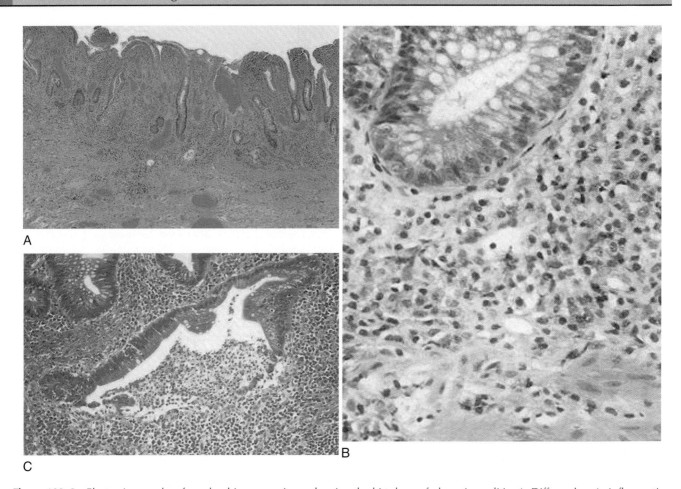

Figure 109–3 Photomicrographs of a colon biopsy specimen showing the histology of ulcerative colitis. *A,* Diffuse chronic inflammation of the lamina propria and crypt distortion are present. These features are important in differentiating ulcerative colitis from acute "self-limited" colitis. *B,* The base of a single distorted colonic crypt. There is a large number of "basal" plasma cells between the crypt and the muscularis mucosae, another important finding that helps differentiate acute from chronic colitis. *C,* A single crypt abscess. The bottom of this distorted crypt has been destroyed by an aggregate of polymorphonuclear neutrophils. This finding is not specific for ulcerative colitis and may be seen in Crohn's disease and other types of colitis. (Courtesy of Feldman, online Gastro Atlas, Current Medicine).

At this stage of the disease, some inflammation and vascular congestion may be present in the submucosa, and ulceration may extend into the muscularis mucosa. Whereas this deeper involvement may be confused with Crohn's disease, it usually presents diffusely rather than with the fissuring pattern of transmural inflammation that characterizes Crohn's disease.

During the healing phase of UC, the inflammatory infiltrate subsides and epithelial regeneration takes place. Epithelial cells undergoing regenerative changes become cuboidal with eccentric, large nuclei, and prominent nucleoli. These features may be confused with dysplasia. Thus, a diagnosis of dysplasia in UC should be made with caution in the presence of acute inflammation. Accordingly, surveillance colonoscopy (see "Dysplasia and Colorectal Cancer" section) should be performed during a period of remission.

A classic histologic feature of chronic quiescent UC is crypt architectural distortion or actual dropout of glands (Fig. 109–3). Architectural changes include branching or bifid glands, wide separation among glands, and shortened glands that do not extend down to the muscularis mucosa. Whereas architectural alteration is a prominent feature of chronic quiescent UC, the histologic abnor-

malities may revert to normal after mild flares in the early course of disease. Another characteristic feature of chronic quiescent UC is Paneth cell metaplasia, with the presence of Paneth cells beyond the hepatic flexure, where they typically are absent. Other nonspecific chronic changes seen in UC include neuronal hypertrophy and fibromuscular hyperplasia of the muscularis mucosa. Varying degrees of acute and/or chronic inflammation of the lamina propria may be present in chronic quiescent disease. A thin band of predominantly lymphocytic inflammation occasionally may be seen deep to the muscularis mucosa, presenting diagnostic challenges.

Most of these findings are not specific for UC. Features that reflect chronicity and thus argue against a diagnosis of infectious or acute self-limited colitis include distorted crypt architecture, crypt atrophy, increased intercrypt spacing to fewer than 6 crypts per millimeter, an irregular mucosal surface, basal lymphoid aggregates, and a chronic inflammatory infiltrate.[99,100] Histologic severity of inflammation does not necessarily correlate with clinical disease activity in patients with UC and patients may be relatively symptom free, while histology reveals significant inflammation.

CLINICAL FEATURES

Patients with UC may present with a variety of symptoms. Common symptoms include diarrhea, rectal bleeding, passage of mucus, tenesmus, urgency, and abdominal pain. In more severe cases, fever and weight loss may be prominent. The symptom complex tends to differ according to the extent of disease.[101] Patients with proctitis often have local symptoms of tenesmus, urgency, mucus, and bleeding, whereas patients with extensive colitis may have more diarrhea, weight loss, fever, clinically significant blood loss, and abdominal pain. In general, the severity of the symptoms correlates with the severity of the disease; however, active disease may be found at endoscopy in patients who are otherwise asymptomatic.

The onset of UC typically is slow and insidious. Symptoms have usually been present for weeks or months by the time the patient seeks medical attention. The median interval between the onset of symptoms and diagnosis of UC is approximately 9 months.[102] Some patients with UC may present much more acutely, with symptoms mimicking infectious colitis. Indeed, it is not uncommon to find a patient who had onset of UC after a documented gastrointestinal infection, such as *Salmonella* or *Clostridium difficile*. This observation raises the question as to whether the infection revealed preexisting but silent disease or was actually the initiating factor.

SYMPTOMS

Rectal Bleeding

Rectal bleeding is common in UC. The characteristic of the bleeding is determined by the location of the disease. Patients with proctitis usually complain of passing fresh blood, either separately from the stool or streaked on the surface of a normal or hard stool.[103] This symptom often is mistaken for bleeding from hemorrhoids. In contrast to hemorrhoidal bleeding, patients with ulcerative proctitis often pass a mixture of blood and mucus and may even be incontinent. Patients with proctitis also often complain of the frequent and urgent need to defecate, only to pass small quantities of blood and mucus without fecal matter.

When the disease extends proximal to the rectum, blood usually is mixed with stool or there may be grossly bloody diarrhea. When the disease activity is severe, patients pass liquid stool containing blood, pus, and fecal matter. This stool is often likened to anchovy sauce, and some patients with this symptom do not actually recognize that they are passing blood. Unless the patient has severe disease, the passage of blood clots is unusual and suggests other diagnoses such as a tumor. Active UC that is sufficient to cause diarrhea almost always is associated with macroscopic blood. The diagnosis needs to be questioned if visible blood is absent.

Diarrhea

Diarrhea is common but not always present in patients with UC. Up to 30% of patients with proctitis or proctosigmoiditis may complain of constipation and hard stools.[103] Most patients with active disease complain of frequent passage of loose or liquid stools and may have nocturnal diarrhea. Fecal urgency, sensation of incomplete evacuation, and fecal incontinence also are common, especially when the rectum is severely inflamed. Diarrhea in this setting often is accompanied by passage of large quantities of mucus, blood, and pus.

The pathophysiology of the diarrhea in UC involves several mechanisms, but failure to absorb salt and water is perhaps the predominant factor.[104] This failure results from reduced Na^+/K^+, ATPase pump activity, increased mucosal permeability, and altered membrane phospholipids. High mucosal concentrations of lipid inflammatory mediators, which are detected in UC, have been shown to stimulate chloride secretion in normal colon, and it is possible that these mediators also contribute to diarrhea by increasing mucosal permeability. Urgency and tenesmus, which are common symptoms when the rectum is inflamed, are caused by poor compliance and loss of the reservoir capacity of the inflamed rectum.[105] With severe inflammation, the urgency can be sufficiently acute as to cause incontinence.

Colonic motility is altered by inflammation, and there is rapid transit through the inflamed colon. With left-sided disease, distal transit is rapid, but there is actual slowing of proximal transit,[106] which may help explain the constipation that is commonly seen in patients with distal colitis. Prolonged transit times in the small intestine also occur in the presence of active colonic inflammation.[106]

Abdominal Pain

Many patients with UC complain of abdominal pain with active disease, but pain generally is not a prominent symptom. Patients may experience vague lower abdominal discomfort, an ache in the left iliac fossa, or intermittent abdominal cramping preceding bowel movements and often persisting transiently after defecation. Severe cramping and abdominal pain can occur in association with severe attacks of the disease. The cause of the pain is unclear but may relate to increased tension within the inflamed colonic wall during muscular contraction. Patients with active proctitis also frequently complain of tenesmus and urgency associated with painful straining and passage of mucus and blood with only scanty stools.

Other Symptoms

Disease of moderate or severe activity often may be associated with systemic symptoms. Patients may develop anorexia and nausea and, in severe attacks, actually may vomit. These symptoms, as well as protein loss through inflamed mucosa, hypercatabolism, and down-regulation of albumin synthesis caused by the inflammation, account for weight loss and hypoalbuminemia that may be profound. Fever, an additional catabolic factor, usually accompanies severe attacks but is typically of a moderate degree. Patients also may complain of symptoms from anemia and hypoalbuminemia, including fatigue, dyspnea, and peripheral edema. A few patients may present with extraintestinal manifestations, such as acute arthropathy, episcleritis, and erythema nodosum. These manifestations typically parallel the activity of colitis.

SIGNS

Patients with mild or even moderately severe disease exhibit few abnormal physical signs. They are usually well nourished and well appearing and show no signs of chronic disease. Indeed, these patients can appear deceptively well. Weight should always be recorded, and, for children and adolescents, both height and weight should be plotted on developmental growth charts. The affected portion of the colon may be tender on abdominal palpation, but this generally is mild and not associated with rebound or guarding. Bowel sounds are normal. Digital rectal examination also is frequently normal, but the rectal mucosa may feel "velvety" and edematous; the anal canal may be tender; and there may be blood on withdrawal of the examining finger.

Patients with severe attacks also may appear well, but most are ill with tachycardia, fever, orthostasis, and weight loss. The abdomen typically is soft with only mild tenderness over the diseased segment. Abdominal tenderness may become diffuse and moderate with more severe disease. Bowel sounds may be normal or hyperactive but diminish with progressive disease. In fulminant colitis, the abdomen often becomes distended and firm, with absent bowel sounds and signs of peritoneal inflammation.

There may be aphthoid ulceration of the oral mucosa. Clubbing of the fingernails is a frequent manifestation of chronic disease. Peripheral edema may occur secondary to hypoalbuminemia. Minor perianal disease may be present but is never as severe as is seen in patients with Crohn's disease. Signs of extraintestinal manifestations also may be present.

LABORATORY FINDINGS

Laboratory findings in UC are nonspecific and reflect the severity of the underlying disease. Patients with active proctitis and proctosigmoiditis often have normal laboratory test results. Patients with limited distal disease often pass visible blood in the stool, but the amount of blood loss typically is small and anemia, if present, is mild. Patients with active extensive disease or severe distal disease may demonstrate laboratory abnormalities. Hematologic changes, including anemia, leukocytosis and thrombocytosis, reflect active disease. In contrast, patients with quiescent UC typically manifest no laboratory abnormalities. Iron deficiency anemia may be present because of chronic blood loss. Anemia also may be present secondary to bone marrow suppression resulting from chronic inflammation or medications, such as azathioprine, 6-mercaptopurine (6-MP), and sulfasalazine.

Mild or moderate attacks rarely are associated with any biochemical disturbance. Hypokalemia, metabolic alkalosis, and elevated serum creatinine may be present in severe flares of UC, reflecting volume depletion. Hypoalbuminemia may be seen with both acute and chronic disease. Minor elevations in serum levels of aspartate aminotransferase or alkaline phosphatase also are frequently associated with severe disease, but these changes are transient and return to normal when the disease enters into remission. These abnormalities probably reflect a combination of fatty liver, sepsis, and poor nutrition. Persistently elevated liver biochemical tests, especially serum alkaline phosphatase, are seen in about 3% of patients with UC and should lead to further investigation, particularly to exclude the presence of primary sclerosing cholangitis (PSC) (see Chapter 65).

Serum inflammatory markers including erythrocyte sedimentation rate (ESR) and C-reactive protein (CRP) may be elevated in active disease. These abnormalities are typically absent or minimal in patients with mildly to moderately active disease. Elevation in these inflammatory parameters is neither sensitive nor specific for UC; however, measuring them may be useful in clinical practice to assess disease activity in individual patients, particularly if these values are normal during periods of inactive disease. For following clinical changes, CRP is more sensitive than ESR because of the shorter half-life of CRP.

NATURAL HISTORY AND PROGNOSIS

Most (80%) patients with UC have a disease course characterized by intermittent flares interposed between variable periods of remission. The duration of relapse-free periods varies greatly from patient to patient. More than 50% of patients present with mild disease at their first attack, and 6% to 19% of patients have severe disease at presentation.[107,108] Following the initial flare, 40% to 65% of patients have an intermittent course, and 5% to 10% of patients have a chronic continuous course.[109,110] Up to 10% of patients have a severe first attack ultimately requiring colectomy.[107] In population-based studies, the proportion of patients with active disease remains relatively constant over years, with approximately 50% of all patients being in remission at any time point during follow-up (Fig. 109–4).[97,109] Twenty-five years after the diagnosis of UC, 90% of patients still have a relapsing course (Fig. 109–5)[97]; however, disease activity in the preceding years predicts the subsequent chance of disease activity. The probability of remaining in remission for 1 year after a relapse has been estimated at 30%. After being in remission for 1 year, the risk of relapse decreases to 20% for the following year. Few patients (1%) diagnosed with UC have only one attack followed by a relapse-free course,[109] and they likely represent misdiagnosed infectious colitis.

Factors influencing disease relapse and remission include bacterial and viral infections, the use of nonsteroidal anti-inflammatory drugs (NSAIDs) and antibiotics, smoking, seasonality, and psychosocial stress. Both the severity and extent of disease are important prognostic factors for the first attack of UC. In general, patients with disease that is limited to the distal colon do better than those with extensive colitis. UC diagnosed in the elderly generally has been thought to present with more severe initial attacks, but this belief has not been observed consistently.

The rate of colectomy varies in studies, in part related to the different proportions of patients with extensive versus limited disease. The probability of colectomy is highest in the first year of diagnosis. In one Scandinavian study, the colectomy rate was 10% within the first year of diagnosis, 3% in the second year, and approximately 1% per year thereafter.[109] In general, the overall colectomy rate is 24% at 10 years and 30% at 25 years (see Fig.

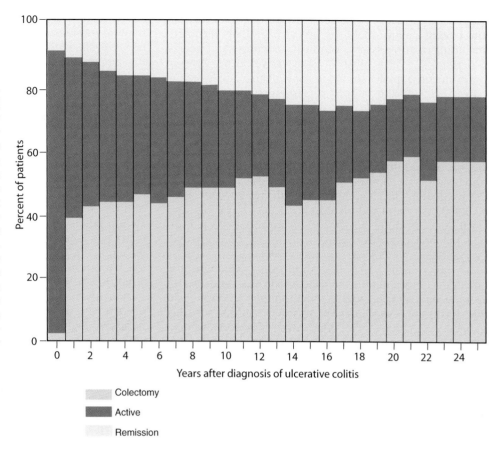

Figure 109–4 Percentage of patients with ulcerative colitis who had active disease, were in remission, or who have had colectomy each year after diagnosis. After a few years, the proportion of patients in remission remains relatively constant, with approximately 50% of all patients being in remission at any time point during follow-up. The proportion of patients with active disease gradually decreases to about 30%, and approximately 30% of patients undergo colectomy within 25 years after diagnosis. (Adapted from Langholz E, Munkholm P, Davidsen M, et al: Course of ulcerative colitis: Analysis of changes in disease activity over years. Gastroenterology 107:3, 1994.)

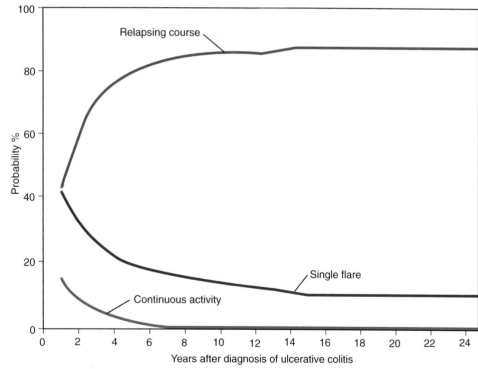

Figure 109–5 Cumulative probabilities for various disease courses after diagnosis of ulcerative colitis. At 25 years after the diagnosis, 90% of patients had an intermittent course with remission and relapses. The cumulative probability of a completely relapse-free course decreased rapidly with time to approximately 10% after 25 years. Similarly, the cumulative probability of a continuously active course was low—1% after 5 years and 0.1% after 25 years. (Adapted from Langholz E, Munkholm P, Davidsen M, et al: Course of ulcerative colitis: Analysis of changes in disease activity over years. Gastroenterology 107:3, 1994.)

109–4).[97] The probability of colectomy is related to the extent of disease at diagnosis. In one study, one third of patients with pancolitis underwent colectomy within the first year of diagnosis compared with less than 8% of patients with limited disease.[109] This difference disappears after the first year, however, and the subsequent disease course is similar for all patients.

Disease extent may progress over time. In patients initially presenting with proctitis or proctosigmoiditis, disease extension occurs in approximately 10% to 30% of patients at 10 years after diagnosis.[107,111,112] Less commonly, extensive colitis regresses over time with treatment.

Despite the burden of a chronic illness, more than 90% of patients with UC are able to maintain capacity for work after 10 years of disease.[97] Limited data suggest that the overall quality of life is not impaired significantly, including marital issues, physical activities, and social function.[97,108,113] For most patients, however, the disease may affect the quality of life to some degree during acute flares. Even during periods of remission, patients may remain anxious for fear of relapse and may alter their lifestyle to accommodate the unpredictable nature of the disease.

Despite the morbidity of UC, mortality associated with the disease has dropped dramatically since the late 1950s and 1960s. The mortality for a severe attack of UC was approximately 35% before the introduction of glucocorticoid therapy and now is less than 2%. Long-term survival does not differ significantly from that expected for age-matched controls, even with the risk of colorectal cancer that attends long-standing colitis.

Mortality from UC has diminished dramatically since the introduction of glucocorticoids, and death from severe attacks now is uncommon. Patients with UC have life expectancy comparable to that of the general population.[107,110,114] One large study from Sweden did show a trend toward excess mortality, especially from unrelated disease[115]; however, this observation has not been confirmed in other studies. Two studies from the United Kingdom and Denmark reported at most a small increase in mortality in patients with UC.[116,117] Mortality risk is greatest in the elderly and in patients with extensive colitis at diagnosis, mostly related to postoperative complications within the first 2 years of disease and to other comorbidities. Therefore, life insurance premiums for patients with UC should not be markedly higher than those for the general population.

DIAGNOSIS

Currently, there is no single test that allows the diagnosis of UC with acceptable sensitivity and specificity. Thus, the diagnosis relies on a combination of compatible clinical features, endoscopic appearances, and histologic findings. Stool cultures should be obtained to exclude infection with routine bacterial pathogenic organisms; assay for toxins A and B of *C. difficile*, and examinations for ova and parasites also should be performed. Infection with *Escherichia coli* O157:H7 should be considered and requires special stool cultures (or molecular probes). Similarly, special cultures for gonococcus or *Chlamydia* may be necessary in selected cases. In immunosuppressed patients, the possibility of opportunistic infection of the colon must be excluded (see "Differential Diagnosis" section). A diagnosis of UC should be questioned if there is only a single episode of acute illness or the histopathology findings are nonspecific and lack signs of chronicity.

ENDOSCOPY

The diagnosis of UC can be strongly suggested by sigmoidoscopy in most cases. In patients presenting with their first attack of UC, sigmoidoscopy with biopsies usually is sufficient to confirm the diagnosis, thereby allowing initiation of therapy. In patients with active flares, sigmoidoscopy is best performed in the unprepared bowel so the earliest signs of UC can be detected without the hyperemia that is frequently present because of preparative enemas.

Colonoscopy is not recommended in patients with active disease for fear of perforation. In general, endoscopic examination should be avoided in patients with severe disease. If endoscopy is necessary, care must be taken to avoid excessive distention.

After active disease has been controlled in a patient with newly diagnosed UC, colonoscopy should be performed to establish the extent of the disease and to exclude Crohn's disease. Multiple biopsy specimens should be taken from throughout the colon to map the histologic extent of disease and to confirm the diagnosis if there is concern about Crohn's disease.[118] Additionally, intubation and biopsy of the terminal ileum should be attempted to exclude the presence of Crohn's disease.

In patients with an established diagnosis of UC who present with a typical flare, sigmoidoscopy usually is not necessary. Sigmoidoscopy combined with histologic evaluation, however, may be useful for assessing disease severity, particularly when therapeutic response is in question. Colonoscopy may be similarly useful, especially in patients whose symptoms seem out of proportion to the known extent of disease. Additionally, colonoscopy is essential for colorectal cancer surveillance (see "Dysplasia and Colorectal Cancer" section).

The hallmark of UC is symmetrical and continuous inflammation that begins in the rectum and extends proximally without interruption for the entire extent of disease. The earliest endoscopic sign of UC is a decrease or loss of the normal vascular pattern, with erythema and edema of the mucosa (Fig. 109–6). In fact, distortion or loss of vascular markings may be the only endoscopic evidence of UC in patients with quiescent disease. As the disease progresses, the mucosa becomes granular and friable. With more severe inflammation, the mucosa may be covered by yellow-brown mucopurulent exudates associated with mucosal ulcerations. In UC, mucosal ulcerations occur in areas of inflammation; vary in size from a few millimeters to several centimeters; and may be punctate, annular, linear, or serpiginous. Finally, severe UC is associated with mucosa that bleeds spontaneously, and there may be extensive areas of denuded mucosa from severe mucosal ulcerations with diffuse colitis (see Fig. 109–6). Marked edema may at times lead to luminal narrowing.

In patients with long-standing UC, pseudopolyps may be present. Inflammatory pseudopolyps develop in active disease and result from inflamed, regenerating epithelium that is interposed among ulcerations. These inflammatory pseudopolyps give the colonic mucosa a cobblestone appearance. With repeated inflammation that is followed by healing, these pseudopolyps remain during quiescent disease and usually do not regress with treatment. Endoscopically, pseudopolyps typically are small, soft, pale, fleshy, and glistening; however, they may be large, sessile, or pedunculated and may have surface ulcerations. Differentiation of these benign pseudopolyps from neoplastic polyps may be difficult and requires histologic confirmation.

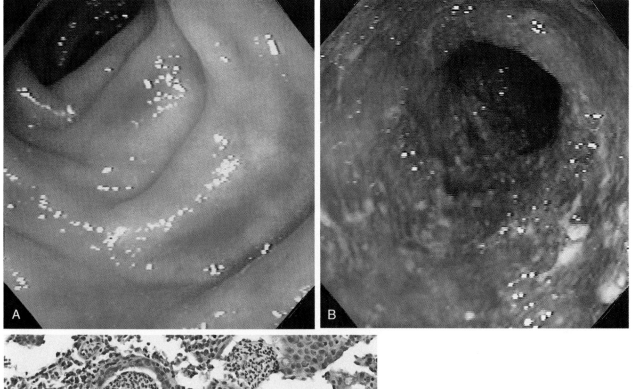

Figure 109–6 Spectrum of severity of ulcerative colitis. *A*, Colonoscopic findings in mild ulcerative colitis demonstrating edema, loss of vascularity, and patchy subepithelial hemorrhage. *B*, Colonoscopic findings in severe ulcerative colitis with loss of vascularity, hemorrhage, and mucopus. The mucosa is very friable, with spontaneous bleeding as well as bleeding after the mucosa is touched by the endoscope. *C*, Histology showing a severe acute and chronic inflammatory process, with multiple crypt abscesses.

(Continued)

There is a loss of the normal colonic architecture with long-standing inflammation that is characterized by muscular hypertrophy, loss of the normal haustral fold pattern, decreased luminal diameter, and shortening of the colon; a resultant featureless appearance of the colon in chronic UC gives rise to the so-called lead pipe seen on barium enema examination. Strictures occasionally may be present in patients with chronic UC and result from focal muscular hypertrophy associated with inflammation. However, malignancy must be excluded in patients with UC who have strictures, particularly those with long strictures without associated inflammation and those proximal to the splenic flexure.

RADIOLOGY

Patients with a severe attack of UC should have a supine plain film of the abdomen.[119] The presence of intraperi-

toneal air may be missed on plain abdominal films, however, and CT radiography has demonstrated a better diagnostic yield than plain abdominal radiography for detecting disease complications and extent. In the presence of severe disease, the luminal margin of the colon (i.e., the interface between the colonic mucosa and the luminal gas) becomes edematous and irregular. Thickening of the colonic wall often is apparent on a plain film, and prognostic signs such as mucosal islands (islands of residual mucosa surrounded by extensive deep ulcerations), small bowel distention, and colonic dilatation can be detected (Fig. 109–7). Plain films also are useful for detecting the presence of fecal material. Inflamed colon seldom contains feces, and no fecal material is present when the whole colon is involved. It is common, however, for a patient with left-sided disease to have proximal constipation (Fig. 109–8). Thus, a plain film can give considerable information with respect to the extent of disease. The presence of marked colonic dilata-

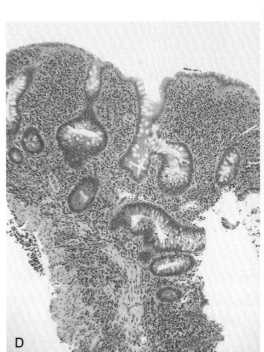

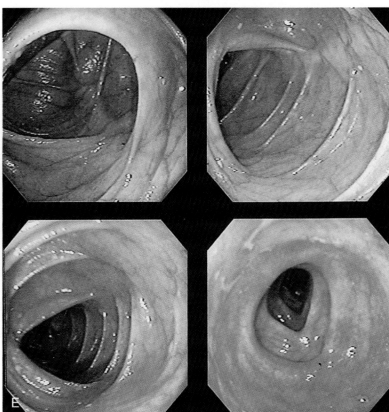

Figure 109–6, cont'd *D,* The colonic architecture is distorted, with a loss of crypts and abnormal branching of the crypts. Recognition of the disordered architecture is useful in differentiating acute from chronic colitis. *E,* Surveillance colonoscopy in a patient with chronic ulcerative colitis. The ascending colon (*top left*), transverse colon (*top right*), and descending colon (*bottom left*) are normal, but the sigmoid colon shows active inflammation (*bottom right*). *F,* A biopsy specimen of the normal-appearing colon demonstrates abnormal architecture with shortened crypts and no active colitis.

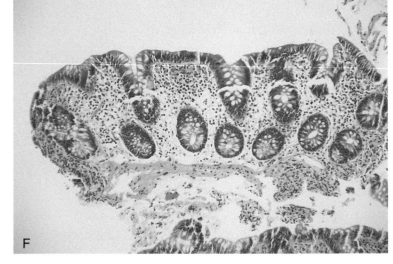

tion suggests fulminant colitis or toxic megacolon. A plain abdominal film also may detect unsuspected free air and is especially useful in following the daily progress of a patient on high-dose glucocorticoid therapy in whom such a complication may be masked.

With the advent of endoscopy, barium studies have become less frequently used in the care of patients with UC. Barium studies of the colon remain important, however, and may be superior to colonoscopy for certain indications, for example, the evaluation of colonic strictures; barium enema provides information on their location, length, and diameter and allows visualization of the entire colon when strictures preclude advancement of the colonoscope. Upper gastrointestinal barium study and small bowel follow-through with peroral pneumo-

colon (air-contrast visualization of the terminal ileum) should be performed to exclude Crohn's disease. Recently, magnetic resonance (MR) imaging enterography has been used to visualize the small bowel without the need for oral contrast agents; its role in IBD is evolving.

The earliest radiologic change of UC seen on barium studies is fine mucosal granularity (Fig. 109–9). The mucosal line becomes irregular and is not as sharp as that of a normal colon. With increasing severity, the mucosal line becomes thickened and irregular, and superficial ulcers are well shown en face. Deep ulceration can appear as "collar-stud" or "collar-button" ulcers in tangent, which indicates that the ulceration has extended through the mucosa to the muscularis propria (Fig. 109–10).

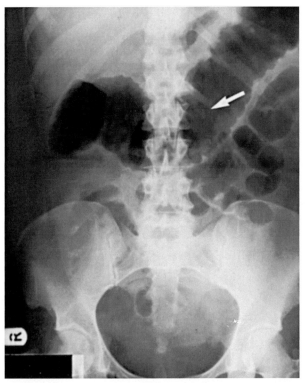

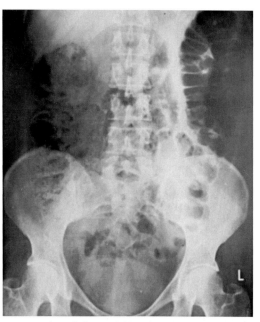

Figure 109–8 Plain abdominal film of a patient with mild left-sided ulcerative colitis showing a stool-filled proximal colon.

Figure 109–7 Plain abdominal film of a patient with severe ulcerative colitis. The transverse colon is dilated (*arrow*), the colon wall is thickened, and mucosal islands are visible. In addition, distended loops of small bowel are apparent.

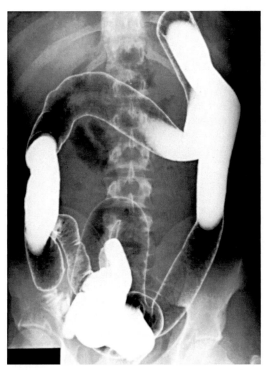

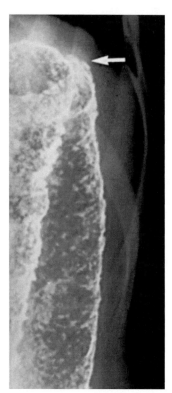

Figure 109–9 A double-contrast barium enema in a patient with long-standing ulcerative colitis indicated by a marked loss of haustration. The mucosa is finely granular throughout the colon, consistent with mildly active disease. The terminal ileum is normal.

Figure 109–10 A double-contrast barium enema in a patient with active ulcerative colitis. This localized view of the splenic flexure shows multiple ulcers. At the flexure itself there is deep ulceration appearing as a "collar-button" ulcer (*arrow*).

Haustral folds may be normal in mild disease but become edematous and thickened as disease progresses. Loss of haustrations also can occur, especially in patients with long-standing disease (see Fig. 109–11). Since lack of haustrations can be a normal appearance for the left colon, this sign is relevant for only the ascending and transverse colon. With long-standing disease, loss of haustration may lead to a featureless and tubular appearance of the colon. Other chronic changes are shortening of the colon and widening of the presacral space as seen on a lateral film of the rectum. Pseudopolyps may be present and often are filiform. In the presence of active changes, these pseudopolypoid changes can resemble a cobblestone pattern (Fig. 109–11).

DIFFERENTIAL DIAGNOSIS

A variety of inflammatory and noninflammatory diseases of the colon can mimic UC and need to be considered in making the diagnosis. This differential diagnosis can be grouped broadly into three categories: Crohn's disease,

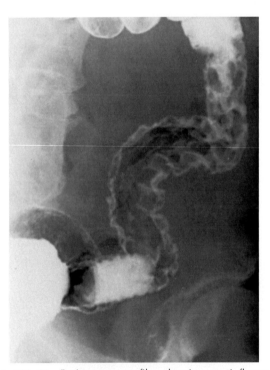

Figure 109–11 Barium enema film showing postinflammatory polyps in a shortened sigmoid and descending colon in a patient with active ulcerative colitis.

infectious causes, and noninfectious causes (Table 109–3). Crohn's disease should be excluded in all patients given a diagnosis of UC, and colonoscopy with multiple biopsies is important in this regard. The presence of skip lesions or granulomas supports a diagnosis of Crohn's disease. Other endoscopic features distinguishing UC from Crohn's disease are listed in Table 109–4. It is not uncommon for patients with ileal Crohn's disease also to have rectal involvement, and these patients may present with symptoms of proctitis rather than symptoms of small intestinal involvement. In patients with limited proctitis or diffuse pancolitis, it may be impossible to differentiate these two IBDs. Thus it is advisable to obtain radiologic assessment of the small intestine in all patients with colonic disease, particularly in those with pancoli-

Table 109–3 Differential Diagnosis of Ulcerative Colitis

Infectious Causes
Salmonella
Shigella
Escherichia coli O157:H7
Campylobacter jejuni
Yersinia enterocolitica
Entamoeba histolytica
Clostridium difficile
Aeromonas hydrophila
Listeria monocytogenes
Neisseria gonorrhoeae
Chlamydia
Cytomegalovirus
Herpes simplex virus
Schistosomiasis
Non-Infectious Causes
Crohn's disease
Diverticulitis
Ischemic colitis
Radiation colitis
Behçet's disease
Diversion colitis
Neutropenic colitis (typhlitis)
Microscopic colitis
    Collagenous colitis
    Lymphocytic colitis
Eosinophilic colitis
Graft-versus-host disease
Drugs or toxins
    Nonsteroidal anti-inflammatory drugs
    Chemotherapy
    Penicillamine
    Gold
Acute self-limited colitis
Solitary rectal ulcer syndrome

Table 109–4 Endoscopic Differentiation of Ulcerative Colitis and Crohn's Disease

Variable	Ulcerative Colitis	Crohn's Disease
Distribution	Diffuse inflammation that extends proximally from the anorectal junction	Rectal sparing, frequent "skip" lesions
Inflammation	Diffuse erythema, early loss of vascular markings with mucosal granularity or friability	Focal and asymmetric, "cobblestoning"; granularity and friability less common
Ulceration	Small ulcers in a diffusely inflamed mucosa; deep, ragged ulcers in severe disease	Aphthoid ulcers, linear/serpiginous ulceration; intervening mucosa is often normal
Colonic lumen	Often narrowed in long-standing chronic disease; "tubular colon"; strictures are rare	Strictures are common

tis or limited proctitis on colonoscopy and elevated inflammatory makers or hypoalbuminemia on laboratory tests. A definitive diagnosis of Crohn's disease may require the development of small bowel disease or perianal complications. Approximately 10% of patients are diagnosed with "indeterminate" colitis when the distinction between Crohn's disease and UC cannot be made. These patients should be managed as if they had UC, until more characteristic features of Crohn's disease appear. The key points in the differential diagnosis between UC and Crohn's disease are summarized in Tables 109–4 and 109–5.

Another major category of differential diagnosis for UC is infection (see Chapter 104). As mentioned previously, newly diagnosed UC may present as part of a well-documented episode of infectious colitis. It is unknown if the infection prompts the UC or simply unmasks underlying UC that previously had subclinical activity. Patients with documented UC in clinical remission also

may develop acute infectious colitis and present with symptoms of flare of UC. Thus, infections need to be excluded with each episode of disease exacerbation. The most common organisms causing infectious colitis are *Salmonella*, *Shigella*, and *Campylobacter*. Patients with infectious colitides usually have a more acute onset of symptoms than do patients with a flare of UC, and have a prominence of abdominal pain; they also may report diarrheal illness in contacts. The sigmoidoscopic appearance of infectious colitis may be indistinguishable from that of UC, but the histologic appearance usually is helpful in differentiating infectious acute colitis from a more chronic condition. The presence of a chronic inflammatory infiltrate, architectural disturbances, and basal lymphoid aggregates favors a diagnosis of UC, and these features distinguish infectious colitis from UC with a probability of 80%, albeit with considerable interobserver variation.[99,100] Other bacterial infectious colitides include infection with *E. coli* O157:H7, which can occur

Table 109–5 Features That Distinguish Ulcerative Colitis from Major Differential Diagnoses

Diagnosis	Clinical Features	Radiologic Aspects	Histologic Aspects
Ulcerative colitis	Bloody diarrhea	Extends proximally from rectum; fine mucosal ulceration	Distortion of crypts; acute and chronic diffuse inflammatory cell infiltrate; goblet cell depletion; crypt abscesses; lymphoid aggregates
Crohn's colitis	Perianal lesions common; may be associated with ileitis; frank bleeding is less frequent than in ulcerative colitis	Segmental disease; rectal sparing; strictures, fissures, ulcers, fistulas; small bowel involvement	Focal inflammation; submucosal involvement; granulomas; goblet cell preservation; transmural inflammation; fissuring
Ischemic colitis	Occurs in the elderly; sudden onset, often painful; usually resolves spontaneously in several days	Segmental splenic flexure and sigmoid involvement is most common with "thumbprinting" early and ulceration after 24-72 hr; rectal involvement is rare	Mucosal necrosis with "ghost cells"; congestion with red blood cells; hemosiderin and fibrosis (chronic disease)
Microscopic colitis	Watery diarrhea; normal appearing mucosa at colonoscopy	Usually normal	Chronic inflammatory infiltrate; increased intraepithelial lymphocytes (lymphocytic colitis) and subepithelial collagen band (collagenous colitis)
Infectious colitis	Sudden onset; identifiable source in some cases (e.g., *Salmonella*); pain may predominate (e.g., *Campylobacter*); pathogens are present in stool	Usually normal	Crypt architecture is usually normal; edema, superficial neutrophilic infiltrate, crypt abscesses
Pseudomembranous colitis	May be a history of antibiotic use; characteristic pseudomembranes may be seen on sigmoidoscopy; *Clostridium difficile* toxin is detectable in stools	Edematous; shaggy outline	May resemble acute ischemic colitis; shows "summit" lesions of fibrinopurulent exudate
Amebic colitis	Travel to endemic area; amebae may be detected in a fresh stool specimen	Discrete ulcers; ameboma or strictures	Similar to ulcerative colitis; amebae present in lamina propria or in flask-shaped ulcers, identified by periodic acid–Schiff stain
Gonococcal proctitis	Rectal pain; pus	Granular changes in rectum	Intense polymorphonuclear neutrophil infiltration; purulent exudate; gram-negative diplococci

in outbreaks or sporadically. Patients with this infection, particularly children and the elderly, may develop associated hemolytic-uremic syndrome or thrombotic thrombocytopenic purpura. Because the diagnosis requires a special culture medium and cannot be made on routine stool cultures, clinicians need to have a high index of suspicion and specifically request such a test. Recent development of molecular probes may facilitate the ability to establish this diagnosis. *Yersinia* infections may cause enteritis, enterocolitis, or colitis and may last for several months before resolving spontaneously. The diagnosis is made on the basis of stool culture or a rising titer of serum antibody. Other less common bacterial infections causing colitis include *Aeromonas hydrophila* and *Listeria monocytogenes*; the former is usually associated with drinking untreated water.

A history of antibiotic use suggests pseudomembranous colitis associated with *C. difficile* (see Chapter 105). This infectious colitis can present with diarrhea and may be superimposed on a relapse of UC. Thus, appropriate stool studies for toxin analysis are necessary even in patients with established UC who present with an exacerbation to exclude superimposed *C. difficile* infection. *C. difficile* toxins have been found in the stools of up to 28% of patients with IBD.[120,121] *C. difficile* infection can occur in the absence of antibiotics, especially in the elderly and in hospitalized patients. Thus, it is important to exclude *C. difficile* infection in hospitalized patients who do not respond to medical therapy as expected or who suddenly lose their initial response to treatment. Patients with *C. difficile* infections often present with watery diarrhea and have the characteristic pseudomembranes at colonoscopy. This infection may cause severe colitis that progresses to toxic megacolon and bowel perforation.

In patients from endemic areas, certain protozoal and parasitic infections need to be considered (see Chapters 106 and 107). Amebic colitis tends to have a more prolonged course than do most bacterial colitides, but amebiasis is not a cause of chronic colitis. Schistosomal colitis may be chronic, diffuse, exhibit pseudopolyps, and involve the rectum. The presence of ova in a biopsy specimen confirms the diagnosis. Other infectious causes of a bloody diarrhea include opportunistic infections of the colon in immunosuppressed patients (see Chapters 32 and 33). Cytomegalovirus (CMV) infection has been reported in patients with UC, typically those with long-standing disease who are being treated with glucocorticoids or immunosuppressants; the diagnosis of CMV infection should be considered whenever patients with UC on glucocorticoids either fail to respond as expected or lose their response to treatment. CMV colitis in steroid-naive patients also has been described.[122] Patients with CMV colitis often present with abdominal pain and bloody diarrhea and have discrete deep ulcerations on colonoscopy; however, CMV colitis may present with diffuse inflammation. Because the clinical presentation of CMV colitis may be indistinguishable from a flare of UC, a high index of suspicion is needed to make the diagnosis. Endoscopic biopsies should be obtained from both the mucosa and ulcer bed. Careful histologic examination for giant cells with intranuclear inclusion is important to confirm the diagnosis. *Mycobacterium avium* complex usually causes patchy rather than diffuse inflam-

mation. Sexually transmitted causes of proctitis, including gonorrhea, *Chlamydia*, and lymphogranuloma venereum, usually do not cause diarrhea and are associated with large volumes of watery pus, especially gonorrhea. These diagnoses are made clinically and confirmed by appropriate cultures as well as histologic appearance on rectal biopsy specimens.

Other noninfectious causes of colitis that should be considered in the differential diagnosis of UC include diverticulitis, ischemia, radiation, collagenous colitis, lymphocytic colitis, and drug-induced colitis. Diverticulitis and ischemic colitis often present acutely or subacutely, but most of the noninfectious colitides have prolonged presentations that may extend for several months. Acute diverticulitis most commonly occurs in the sigmoid colon and does not involve the rectum (see Chapter 114). When the inflammation does extend to the rectum, it tends to be patchy and involves only the upper rectum. This appearance is more likely to be confused with Crohn's disease than UC. Ischemic colitis usually occurs in the elderly (see Chapter 111). The classic distribution is segmental involvement in the "watershed" areas around the splenic flexure or sigmoid colon; ischemic proctitis also has been described. Radiation colitis usually occurs in patients who have been given radiation therapy for uterine, cervical, or prostate cancer. The location of disease depends on the sites of irradiation but typically involves the sigmoid or rectum. The onset of symptoms often corresponds to the radiation therapy but may develop years afterward (see Chapter 38). Microscopic colitis, including lymphocytic and collagenous colitis, can present with symptoms similar to those of UC but should be distinguished readily from UC by the normal endoscopic appearance and characteristic histopathology (see Chapter 121). A drug history must always be taken in a patient with colitis. NSAIDs, gold, and penicillamine all have been implicated in causing colitis.

Patients with UC may present with symptoms similar to those of irritable bowel syndrome, colonic neoplasm, solitary rectal ulcer syndrome, diverticular disease, and factitious diarrhea. These diagnoses do not give rise to diffuse inflammation in the colon and therefore should be distinguished easily from UC on endoscopy (see Chapters 114, 115, 119, 121, and 122).

ASSESSMENT OF DISEASE ACTIVITY

Assessment of disease activity is important for prognostication and therapeutic decision making. Several instruments have been developed to allow standardized evaluation of disease activity for UC. Although none is accepted universally as standard, one of the most commonly used for this purpose is that of Truelove and Witts.[123] This classification categorizes patients into having mild, moderate, or severe disease based on a combination of clinical findings and laboratory parameters, including frequency of bowel movements, rectal bleeding, fever, tachycardia, anemia, and elevated ESR (Table 109–6). The Truelove and Witts classification is reliable and simple to use in clinical practice, although it is most applicable for patients with extensive colitis and may not

Table 109–6 Truelove and Witts Classification of Ulcerative Colitis

Mild
<4 stools/day, without or with only small amounts of blood
No fever
No tachycardia
Mild anemia
ESR < 30 mm/hr

Moderate
Intermediate between mild and severe

Severe
>6 stools/day, with blood
Fever > 37.5°C
Heart rate > 90 beats/min
Anemia with hemoglobin < 75% of normal
ESR > 30 mm/hr

ESR, erythrocyte sedimentation rate.
Adapted from Truelove SC, Witts LJ: Cortisone in ulcerative colitis: Final report on a therapeutic trial. BMJ 2:1041, 1955.

Table 109–7 Ulcerative Colitis Disease Activity Index*

Variable/Score	Criteria
Stool Frequency	
0	Normal
1	1-2 stools/day > normal
2	3-4 stools/day > normal
3	>4 stools/day > normal
Rectal Bleeding	
0	None
1	Streaks of blood
2	Obvious blood
3	Mostly blood
Mucosal Appearance	
0	Normal
1	Mild friability
2	Moderate friability
3	Exudation, spontaneous bleeding
Physician Global Assessment	
0	Normal
1	Mild
2	Moderate
3	Severe

*Range: 0–12.

Table 109–8 Endoscopic and Histologic Assessment of Disease Activity

Score	Criteria
Endoscopic Assessment	
0	Normal mucosa
1	Loss of vascular pattern
2	Granular, nonfriable mucosa
3	Friability on rubbing
4	Spontaneous bleeding, ulceration
Histologic Assessment	
0	Normal
1	No significant inflammation—possibly architectural changes of chronic disease and small foci of lymphocytes but no acute inflammation, crypt abscesses, or epithelial destruction
2	Mild to moderate inflammation—edema, vascularity, increased acute and chronic inflammatory cells but intact epithelium
3	Severe inflammation—heavy infiltrate of acute and chronic inflammatory cells, crypt abscesses, ulceration of surface epithelium, purulent exudate

Other scales have also been developed, many of which are modifications of the Truelove and Witts classification and the Ulcerative Colitis Disease Activity Index.[127-129] None of these disease activity instruments has ever been formally validated. There also are many endoscopic and histologic scales of grading the severity of colitis (Table 109–8).[130,131] Endoscopic findings do not always correlate with clinical symptoms, but such correlations generally are more consistent within individuals. Thus, although therapeutic decisions are based primarily on clinical status, it may be useful to follow sigmoidoscopic mucosal appearance over time in an individual patient if the clinical response to treatment is uncertain.

In addition to the typical categorization of disease activity into mild, moderate, and severe, an important subgroup is fulminant colitis. Patients with severe colitis who appear toxic, with fever higher than 101°F, tachycardia, abdominal distention, signs of localized or generalized peritonitis, and leukocytosis, are considered to have fulminant colitis. Toxic megacolon is said to occur when there is radiologic evidence of colon dilatation to greater than 6 cm in an acutely ill patient. Fulminant colitis and toxic megacolon are clinical diagnoses, and endoscopic examination should be avoided in patients with severe or fulminant colitis because of the risk of inducing megacolon or perforation.

MEDICAL THERAPY

The goals of therapy of UC are (1) to induce remission; (2) to maintain remission; (3) to maintain adequate nutrition; (4) to decrease disease- and treatment-related complications; and (5) to improve the quality of life. The current management strategy focuses on using appropriate medical therapy and optimizing timing of surgery.

Several factors should be considered in determining the optimal therapy for patients with UC (Fig. 109–12). Current therapeutic strategies can be classified broadly based on disease activity into those that treat active

adequately reflect disease severity in patients with limited colitis. Additionally, the Truelove and Witts classification does not take into account endoscopic findings in assessing the disease severity.

A numerical disease activity instrument that is more useful for patients with limited disease and for conducting clinical trials is the Ulcerative Colitis Disease Activity Index.[124-126] This index is the sum of scores from four components: stool frequency, rectal bleeding, sigmoidoscopic findings, and physician's global assessment (Table 109–7). This disease activity index ranges from 0 to 12, with the higher total scores representing more severe disease. In general, a patient is considered to be in remission if the Ulcerative Colitis Disease Activity Index score is equal or less than 2 and to have severe disease if the score is greater than 10. Clinical response generally is accepted to be reflected by a decrease by 3 points from the patient's initial baseline score.

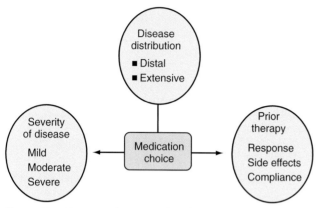

Figure 109–12 Considerations of medical therapies for ulcerative colitis.

Table 109–9 Induction Therapy for Ulcerative Colitis Depending on Disease Severity

Mild disease	Moderate disease	Severe disease
5-aminosalicylates	5-aminosalicylates	IV glucocorticoids
Topical (distal colitis)	Topical (distal colitis)	IV cyclosporine
Oral (distal/ extensive colitis)	Oral (distal/ extensive colitis)	IV infliximab
Combination	Combination	
	Glucocorticoids	
	Topical (distal)	
	Oral (distal/extensive)	
	Combination	
	Azathioprine or 6-mercaptopurine	

IV, intravenous.

Table 109–10 Maintenance Therapy for Ulcerative Colitis

Preparation	Type
5-Aminosalicylates	Topical (distal) Oral (distal/ extensive)
Azathioprine or 6-mercaptopurine	—

disease (induction therapy) (Table 109–9) and those that prevent recurrence of disease once remission is achieved (maintenance therapy) (Table 109–10). This concept of induction of remission and maintenance of remission forms the basis of our evaluation of the efficacy of a specific therapy. The extent of disease in any given patient is an important consideration to help determine the route of administration of medication. Enema preparations may be used alone or in combination with systemic therapy for patients with left-sided disease or disease distal to splenic flexure. Proctitis or disease limited to the rectum may be treated with suppositories or foam preparations. Other important factors to consider are prior response to or side effects from a specific medication and patient compliance. These factors might favor or preclude the use of a specific agent.

Given the chronic nature of UC, medications need to be both efficacious and well accepted by patients from the standpoints of safety and ease of administration. The mainstay of medical therapy focuses on regimens that alter host response to decrease mucosal inflammation. Therapies that target other aspects of the systemic inflammatory process or manipulate the enteric flora also have been developed to treat UC.

AMINOSALICYLATES

Oral Aminosalicylates

Sulfasalazine consists of an antibacterial component, sulfapyridine, bonded by an azo bond to a salicylate, 5-aminosalicylic acid (5-ASA, mesalamine) (Fig. 109–13).[132] The benefit of sulfasalazine for the treatment of IBD was discovered serendipitously in 1942 by Nana Svartz when patients with UC receiving this medication for "rheumatoid" arthritis noted improvement in colitic symptoms[133]; these individuals had peripheral arthropathy associated with their IBD. Research subsequently established that 5-ASA is the principal therapeutic moiety of sulfasalazine in IBD and that the sulfapyridine component of the parent drug serves as an inactive carrier largely preventing 5-ASA from absorption in the small intestine and allowing it to be released in the colon.[134,135] Approximately 90% of sulfasalazine reaches the colon, and only a small amount is absorbed in the small bowel. On reaching the colon, the enzyme azoreductase, which is elaborated by colonic bacteria, cleaves the azo bond to release the active constituent moiety, 5-ASA. After 5-ASA is absorbed from the colon, 20% of the compound undergoes hepatic acetylation, forming *N*-acetyl 5-ASA, and is excreted in the urine.

Sulfasalazine is the first line of therapy and is effective for inducing remission in patients with mild-to-moderate UC,[132,136] but it has not been evaluated in a randomized, controlled fashion in patients with severely active disease. At a dose of 3 to 6 g/day, sulfasalazine induces remission in 39% to 62% of patients with mild-to-moderate UC, about twice the remission rate of placebo-treated patients.[137,138]

Various formulations and controlled-release systems (Table 109–11; see also Fig. 109–13) have been developed to deliver 5-ASA to specific sites of the gastrointestinal tract without the sulfapyridine moiety, which is thought to be responsible for most of the side effects. Olsalazine (Dipentum) is a 5-ASA dimer linked by an azo bond and is formulated in gelatin capsules. Balsalazide (Colazal) consists of a 5-ASA monomer linked to a biologically inactive carrier molecule, 4-aminobenzoyl-β-alanine. Similar to sulfasalazine, 5-ASA is released from olsalazine and balsalazide in the colon on cleavage of the azo bond via the bacterial enzyme azoreductase. Approximately 99% of the drug is delivered intact to the colon, and its metabolites are cleared rapidly in the urine. Two commonly used mesalamine preparations allow delivery of 5-ASA before the drug reaches the colon: (1) Pentasa, which uses ethylcellulose-coated microgranules that release mesalamine from the duodenum throughout the small bowel and the colon (≈50% of 5-ASA is released in the

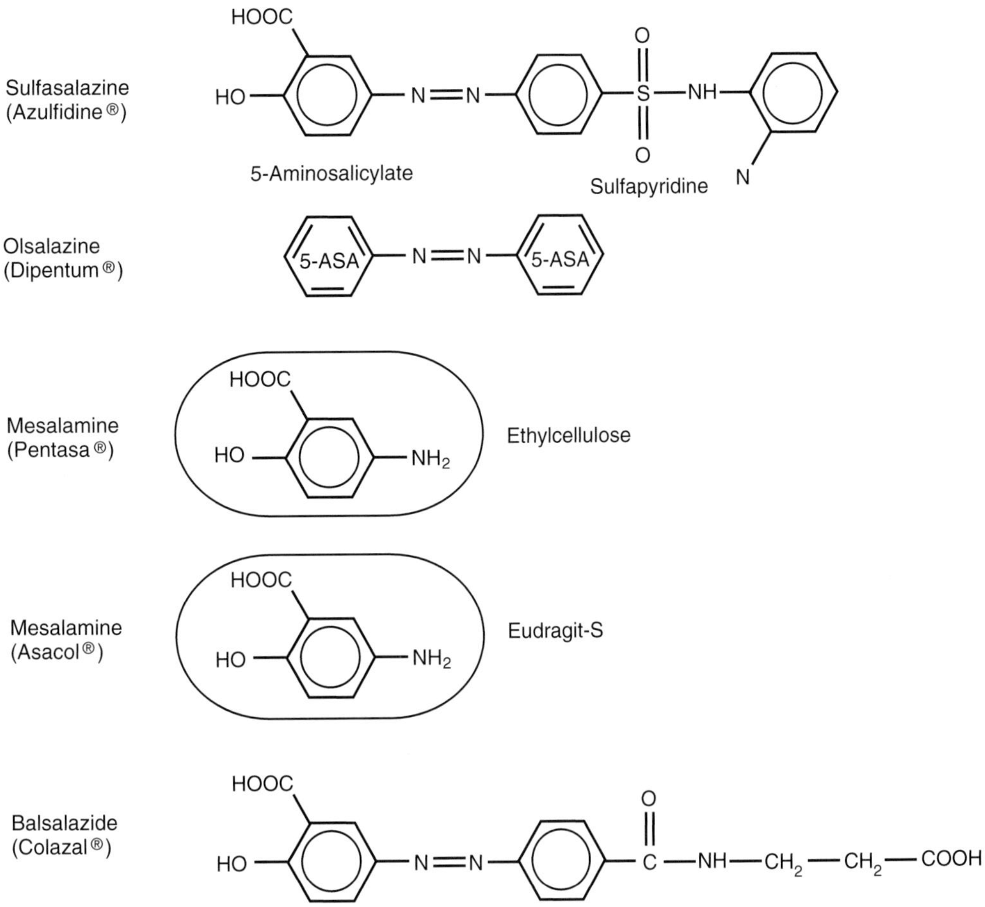

Figure 109–13 Molecular structures of 5-aminosalicylate (5-ASA) preparations.

Table 109–11 Oral 5-Aminosalicylic Acid (5-ASA) Preparations and Sites of Delivery in the Gastrointestinal Tract

Drug	Formulation	Site of Delivery
Prodrugs		
Sulfasalazine	Sulfapyridine + 5-ASA	Colon
Olsalazine (Dipentum)	5-ASA dimer	Colon
Balsalazide (Colazal)	4-aminobenzoyl β-alanine + 5-ASA	Colon
Mesalamine Preparations		
Asacol Claversal Salofalk	pH sensitive, resin coated, delayed release	Distal ileum, colon
Rowasa	Enema	Distal colon
Canasa	Suppository	Rectum
Pentasa	Ethylcellulose-coated microgranules, controlled release	Duodenum to colon

small intestine, while the remainder is released in the colon): and (2) Asacol, which is a Eudragit-S-coated mesalamine tablet that is released at a pH greater than 7, usually in the distal ileum and the colon (with Asacol, ≈15% to 30% of mesalamine is released into the small bowel).

These oral 5-ASA derivatives and mesalamines have been shown to be superior to placebo for mildly to mod-erately active UC.[138-141] There may be a trend toward ther-apeutic benefit of these newer 5-ASA compounds over sulfasalazine, but the various preparations appear to be comparable in efficacy.[138,141] Balsalazide has been shown to have superior efficacy and more rapid response com-pared with other mesalamine agents.[142,143] In a random-ized, controlled study, balsalazide 6.75 g daily, a dose equivalent to mesalamine 2.4 g daily, achieved higher rates of remission and better tolerance compared with pH-dependent mesalamine 2.4 g daily.[142] It has been sug-gested that the greatest benefit of balsalazide is in patients with newly diagnosed left-sided UC.[143]

More important than the specific 5-ASA preparation used is the dose-dependent response when 5-ASA is used as an induction therapy for active UC.[138,141] For this indi-cation, mesalamine is not effective at doses lower than 2 g daily, and there is an increased response at doses of 4 to 4.8 g daily. This dose of Asacol is comparable to 12 g/day of sulfasalazine, which is impractical in clinical practice because of the high probability of intolerance. No controlled trial has evaluated the use of aminosalicy-lates for severely active UC, but they are generally thought not to be effective in severely active disease.

Once remission is achieved, sulfasalazine and other 5-aminosalicylates are effective in maintaining it.[144-147] This benefit appears to be dose dependent for sulfasalazine with a dose of 2 g/day often employed to balance both efficacy and adverse side effects.[144] Such a dose-dependent response, however, has not been found with the other 5-ASA preparations, and at doses of 1.5 to

4.8 g/day, remission can be maintained in more than 50% of patients.[148] Sulfasalazine may have a slight but statistically significant therapeutic superiority relative to the newer 5-ASAs in maintaining remission that is not sustained over a 12-month duration.[148] A double-blind, randomized, controlled trial comparing two doses of balsalazide (1.5 g twice daily and 3 g twice daily) with mesalamine 0.5 g three times daily for 6 months reported a remission rate of 77.5% with the higher dose of balsalazide compared with remission rates of 56.8% and 43.8% with mesalamine and the lower dose of balsalazide, respectively.[149] In general, the same dose of mesalamine or 5-ASA derivative that achieves induction of remission is recommended for maintenance therapy, though this recommendation has not been formally tested in a randomized, placebo-controlled fashion.

Common side effects of sulfasalazine include fever, rash, nausea, vomiting, and headaches (Table 109-12). Other less common but important side effects of sulfasalazine include hypersensitivity reactions, reversible sperm abnormalities, and impairment of folate absorption. Approximately 15% of patients on sulfasalazine develop significant side effects that require discontinuation of the medication. Up to 90% of patients who are intolerant to sulfasalazine, however, can tolerate mesalamine.[150] In clinical trials, the newer 5-ASA preparations and balsalazide have been shown to be better tolerated than sulfasalazine,[141,151,152] although the adverse event profiles during maintenance therapy appear to be similar for 5-ASA preparations and sulfasalazine.[148] Sulfasalazine may impair folate absorption (by competitively inhibiting the jejunal enzyme, folate conjugase) thereby contributing to anemia. Folate supplementation should be prescribed to patients receiving sulfasalazine. Olsalazine is associated with drug-induced diarrhea in up to 10% of patients, which often limits its use. It has been noted that if olsalazine is ingested with meals and continued despite the side effect of diarrhea, its incidence can be lessened substantially to 3%. In fact, a systematic review of oral 5-ASA for maintenance of remission in UC found olsalazine to be significantly inferior to sulfasalazine, and this reduced efficacy was related mostly to a significantly higher rate of withdrawals because of adverse events.[148] Oral mesalamine preparations do not appear to have significant dose-dependent toxicity.

Topical Aminosalicylates

Topical aminosalicylates can be administered in the form of 5-ASA enemas, 5-ASA suppositories, and, in Europe, 5-ASA foam. The use of enemas allows the medication to be delivered up to the level of the splenic flexure in about 95% of individuals, and the suppositories are used to treat disease up to 15 to 20 cm from the anal verge.

Topical mesalamine derivatives may be used as an alternative monotherapy or as an adjunctive therapy to oral agents in patients with left-sided colitis. They are effective for inducing remission in patients with mild to moderately active distal UC, without a clear dose-response effect[153,154] in nonrefractory patients. The standard dosing regimens used to induce remission are 1 to 4 g of enema nightly or mesalamine suppositories 1 to 1.5 g either nightly or in divided doses throughout the day. Mesalamine enemas have been shown to be comparable to oral sulfasalazine in the treatment of active distal UC, with fewer side effects.[155] Similar efficacies have been demonstrated for mesalamine enemas regardless of whether the 1-, 2-, or 4-g formulation is used for the induction of remission in patients with mild-to-moderate left-sided UC not requiring concurrent corticosteroids. In fact, mesalamine enemas are perceived to be even more effective than topical steroid enemas in this setting.[154,156] A combination of topical and oral mesalamine also may be more effective than oral mesalamine alone,[157] suggesting a dose-response effect. In patients with limited proctitis, mesalamine suppositories, 500 mg administered twice daily, have been shown to be beneficial for treating active disease.[158] Mesalamine foam has a more uniform distribution and longer persistence in the distal colon compared with mesalamine enemas. The foam preparation has been shown to provide better patient acceptance than the enema preparation,[159] but mesalamine foams currently are not available in the United States.

Topical mesalamine preparations are effective for maintaining remission in patients with left-sided UC or proctitis.[153,154] The effective maintenance dosing interval ranges from nightly to every 3 days. Topical mesalamine is as effective as oral mesalamine,[160] and the combination of topical and oral mesalamine may be more effective than oral mesalamine alone as a maintenance regimen; in patients who received oral therapy alone and those who received combination therapy for 1 year, relapse rates of 69% and 39%, respectively, were seen.[161]

Table 109–12 Side Effects of Sulfasalazine and 5-Aminosalicylates

Dose-Related Side Effects	Non–Dose-Related Side Effects
Nausea, vomiting, dyspepsia	Hypersensitivity skin rashes (occasionally with photosensitivity)
Anorexia	Fever
Headache	Arthralgia
Alopecia	Hemolytic anemia (Heinz bodies)
Back pain	Agranulocytosis, aplastic anemia
Folate malabsorption (with sulfasalazine)	Pancreatitis
	Hepatitis
	Male infertility (with sulfasalazine)
	Colitis
	Fibrosing alveolitis, pulmonary eosinophilia
	Pericarditis, myocarditis

GLUCOCORTICOIDS

Systemic Glucocorticoids

At doses equivalent to 40 to 60 mg/day of prednisone, glucocorticoids are effective first-line therapy for moderate-to-severe flares of UC.[123,162-166] The use of doses higher than 60 mg/day is associated with increased side effects without appreciable clinical benefit and thus should be avoided. The addition of sulfasalazine to corticosteroids in moderately to severely active UC does not offer any incremental benefit. Although no study has directly compared the efficacy of oral and parenteral glucocorticoids, the latter commonly are used in severe disease. No adequately designed controlled study has been performed to confirm the clinical impression that continuous infusion of parenteral glucocorticoids is superior to pulse therapy.

The use of adrenocorticotropin (ACTH) has been suggested as an alternative to conventional glucocorticoid therapy in active UC in small studies.[167] One double-blind, randomized, controlled trial suggested that intravenous ACTH was more effective than intravenous hydrocortisone for the treatment of severely active UC only in steroid-naive patients[168]; this observation has not been confirmed. Because most patients with severely active flares have been treated previously with glucocorticoids, ACTH rarely is used in clinical practice. A noteworthy complication of ACTH therapy is bilateral adrenal hemorrhage.

Glucocorticoids have no maintenance benefits in patients with UC. Steroid-dependent patients, or individuals who are unable to taper off glucocorticoids without experiencing disease exacerbation, benefit from the addition of steroid-sparing agents. There has been no trial to date assessing mesalamine therapy and its efficacy to maintain remission induced with glucocorticoids. The long-term remission rate in patients who required parenteral glucocorticoids for severe UC is approximately 50%.[169] Immunomodulatory agents as discussed subsequently should be considered in patients who are steroid dependent, require two courses of glucocorticoids for induction of clinical response or remission within 1 year, or require parenteral glucocorticoids to induce remission.

Glucocorticoids are associated with many mild and serious side effects in patients with IBD (Table 109–13). These side effects occur commonly and involve nearly every organ system. Every effort should be made to minimize glucocorticoid use and exposure.

Budesonide is a new glucocorticoid preparation that is structurally different from prednisone. The presence of $16\alpha,17\alpha$-acetyl side chains allows enhanced topical anti-inflammatory activity and affinity for glucocorticoid receptors compared with prednisone.[170] In addition, it has an approximately 90% first-pass metabolism in the liver and erythrocytes and is converted to metabolites that have little or no biologic activity. The resultant low systemic bioavailability translates to significantly less toxicity compared with traditional glucocorticoids. Entocort is a controlled-ileal-release oral budesonide preparation. It consists of Eudragit-L-coated microgranules with an internal ethylcellulose component that releases budesonide at pH above 5.5. Approximately 50% to 80% of

Table 109–13 Side Effects of Glucocorticoids

System	Side Effects
Metabolic	Electrolyte imbalance, hypokalemia Fluid retention Hypertension Hyperglycemia, secondary diabetes Hyperlipidemia, altered fat distribution
Musculoskeletal	Osteoporosis Osteonecrosis Myopathy
Endocrine	Adrenal insufficiency Cushingoid appearance
Gastrointestinal	Dyspepsia Dysphagia (candidiasis)
Neuropsychiatric	Depression Insomnia Anxiety, mood swings Psychosis
Ocular	Cataracts Glaucoma
Skin	Striae Acne Purpura, ecchymoses, petechiae Impaired wound healing
Pediatric	Growth failure
Infectious complications	Various pathogens

budesonide is absorbed in the ileocecal region. There currently is no oral formulation of budesonide that provides optimal release characteristics for the entire length of the colon. A small uncontrolled study has suggested that Budenofalk, which is not available in the United States, may be effective for prednisone-dependent UC[171]; however, controlled studies have not shown the benefit of oral budesonide for the treatment of active UC.[172]

Topical Glucocorticoids

Topical glucocorticoids in liquid and foam formulations are effective short-term therapy for active UC distal to the splenic flexure.[173,174] Foam preparations often are tolerated better by patients and may be easier to retain than liquid preparations. As mentioned previously, topical glucocorticoids have been found to be less effective than topical mesalamine for inducing remission of distal UC[156]; however, the combination of topical corticosteroids and topical mesalamine often is more efficacious than either alone in the short-term treatment of distal UC.[175]

Whereas systemic absorption of glucocorticoids with topical therapy is significantly less than that with oral administration, prolonged treatment with topical steroids still may be associated with steroid-related side effects and should be avoided. As mentioned previously, budesonide is a new potent corticosteroid with a rapid first-pass metabolism. Budesonide enemas, which are currently not available in the United States, have been shown to be effective for the treatment of active distal UC in several controlled trials. In a double-blind, randomized, controlled trial of patients with active distal UC, budesonide, 2 mg/100 mL for 6 weeks, resulted in a remission rate of 19% compared with 4% in patients receiving placebo therapy ($P < 0.05$).[176] Subsequent trials have shown budesonide enema to be as efficacious as or even superior to prednisolone enema without resultant depression of endogenous cortisol levels.[177-179] Budesonide enema perhaps is inferior in efficacy to mesalamine enema[180] but clearly presents an alternative to treatment of distal UC. The optimal dose for budesonide enema consistently has been shown to be 2 mg/100 mL once daily.[176,177,181] Budesonide in foam preparation also has been shown to have comparable efficacy with traditional hydrocortisone foam for the treatment of active proctosigmoiditis.[182] Additional studies are needed to determine the effect of longer term topical budesonide use. As with other steroid preparations, budesonide enema is not effective for maintaining remission in UC.[181]

IMMUNOMODULATORS

Azathioprine and 6-Mercaptopurine (6-MP)

Of the various immunomodulatory agents, the most widely used are azathioprine and 6-MP. These two agents are purine analogs that interfere with nucleic acid metabolism and cell growth and exert cytotoxic effects on lymphoid cells. They are both inactive prodrugs with subtle structural differences. Azathioprine is nonenzymatically converted to 6-MP, which is then metabolized through a series of enzymatic pathways to both active and inactive metabolites (Fig. 109–14). The two primary metabolites of 6-MP are 6-thioguanine nucleotides (6-TGNs) and 6-methylmercaptopurine (6-MMP). The 6-TGN metabolites are thought be responsible for the immunomodulatory action of azathioprine and 6-MP and their bone marrow suppression property, whereas hepatotoxicity is thought to be related to 6-MMP. One key enzyme involved in the biotransformation of 6-MP is thiopurine methyltransferase (TPMT) which converts 6-MP to its inactive metabolites, 6-MMP and methylmercaptopurine ribonucleotides. There is a population polymorphism in the *TPMT* gene.[183] Whereas most of the population (89%) has a homozygous wild-type *TPMT*, 11% and 0.3% of the population have heterozygous and homozygous mutations in *TPMT* genotype, respectively. These individuals have decreased-to-absent enzyme activity. The clinical significance of this genetic polymorphism lies in that inherited differences in TPMT may be responsible for

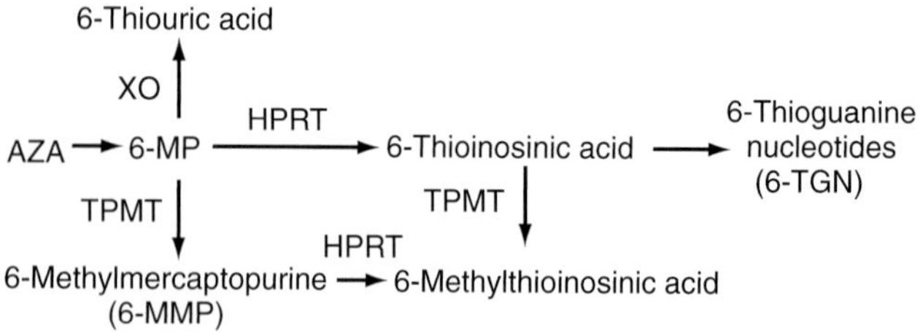

most of the variability in drug response observed among individuals.

Four controlled studies (Table 109–14) have demonstrated efficacy of azathioprine in the treatment of active UC.[184-187] Available data also suggest their benefit in steroid sparing and maintenance of remission in patients with UC.[188-192] An uncontrolled study found that 6-MP therapy allowed reduction or cessation of glucocorticoids in 61% of patients with steroid-dependent UC.[188] As a maintenance agent, continued azathioprine therapy resulted in a 1-year relapse rate of 36% in patients with remission achieved by azathioprine compared with a relapse rate of 59% in patients who discontinued azathioprine following azathioprine-induced remission.[190] The relapse rate has been reported to be as high as 87% in one retrospective review of 105 patients treated with 6-MP for chronic refractory UC, in which complete clinical remission was achieved in 65% of the patients.[193] A small, randomized, but open-label study, however, suggested that azathioprine monotherapy was at best comparable to high-dose sulfasalazine (6 g daily) as maintenance therapy following steroid-induced remission in patients with severely active UC.[194]

From the efficacy standpoint, patients with steroid-dependent UC who are able to achieve remission with azathioprine and mesalamine and discontinue glucocorticoids can be maintained in remission with azathioprine alone.[191] Another important indication for azathioprine or 6-MP is maintenance of remission induced by intravenous cyclosporine.[195-197] The addition of azathioprine or 6-MP to oral cyclosporine eliminates the need for colectomy in up to 80% of patients at 6 months following response to intravenous therapy.[195,196]

The optimal dose of azathioprine or 6-MP for treating UC is unclear, and there has been no formal dose-ranging study reported in the literature. The effective doses for 6-MP and azathioprine generally are 1-1.5 mg/kg/day and 2-2.5 mg/kg/day, respectively.[198] At these doses, however, there still may be nonresponders and higher doses may be necessary. Induction of leukopenia had been advocated for dose optimization,[199] but this practice was not supported in subsequent studies.[200-202] The use of monitoring metabolite levels may be beneficial in determining the optimal dose of azathioprine or 6-MP. Retrospective studies have suggested that erythrocyte 6-TGN levels greater than 235 to 250 pmol/8 × 10⁸ erythrocytes (red blood cells) correlate with a greater likelihood of clinical response in patients treated with azathioprine or 6-MP for IBD.[201,203] Most of the patients in those studies had Crohn's disease, and whether this positive correlation between clinical response and 6-TGN level applies to patients with UC as well is unknown.[203,204] Retrospective studies have suggested the benefit of monitoring 6-TGN metabolite levels to optimize azathioprine or 6-MP dosing.[203,205] The incorporation of 6-TGN metabolite measurement in patients receiving azathioprine or 6-MP therapy for IBD in general is controversial and represents an evolving area of clinical practice. It probably is most useful for identifying reasons for nonresponse to therapy and for suspected noncompliance. If used, metabolite levels should be determined at least 2 weeks following dose adjustment to allow sufficient time for the metabolites to reach steady-state.

Figure 109–14 Metabolism of azathioprine (AZA) and 6-mercaptopurine (6-MP). HPRT, hypoxanthine phosphoribosyltransferase; TPMT, thiopurine methyltransferase; XO, xanthine oxidase.

Table 109–14   Randomized, Controlled Trials of Azathioprine (AZA) for Ulcerative Colitis

Reference	Treatment Indication	No. of Patients	AZA Dose	Duration of Therapy (mo)	Response in Treatment Group, No. (%)	Response in Control Group, No. (%)	P Value
Induction of Remission							
185	Active disease	80	2.5 mg/kg/day	1	31/40 (78)	27/40 (68)[†]	0.45
186	Active disease	20	2.5 mg/ kg/day	3	6/10 (60)	8/10 (80)*	NS
Maintenance of Remission							
185	Quiescent disease	80	1.5-2.5 mg/kg/day	11	16/40 (40)	9/40 (23)[†]	0.18
190	Quiescent disease	67	100 mg/day (mean)	12	21/33 (64)	14/34 (41)[†]	0.04
Steroid Sparing							
190	Steroid-dependent or chronic, active disease	12	100 mg/day (mean)	12	2/7 (29)	3/5 (60)[†]	NS
187	Steroid-dependent disease	30	1.5 mg/kg/day	6	NR	NR[†]	<0.05
184	Steroid-dependent disease	44	2-2.5 mg/kg/day	6	NR	NR[†]	<0.001
189	Steroid-dependent disease	52	2 mg/kg/day	6	15/27 (58)	6/25 (26)[‡]	0.04
191	Steroid-dependent disease	70	2.2 mg/kg/day	24	25/34 (74)	27/36 (75%)[§]	NS

*Control group treated with sulfasalazine.
[†]Control group received placebo.
[‡]Control group received mesalamine 3.2 g/day.
[§]Control group received AZA 2.2 mg/kg/day and olsalazine 1.5 g/day.
NR, not reported; NS, not significant.
Adapted from Su C, Lichtenstein GR: Treatment of inflammatory bowel disease with azathioprine and 6-mercaptopurine. Gastroenterol Clin North Am 33:209, 2004.

Given the controversies regarding the optimal doses for azathioprine and 6-MP therapy, there is no standard guideline regarding initial dosing and its subsequent adjustment. There are two general alternate approaches. The first is to start the medication at 50 mg daily and increase by 25 mg every 1 to 2 weeks while monitoring for cytopenia, a potential toxicity of therapy. The second approach is to determine *TPMT* genotype or phenotype before initiating therapy. The active metabolites, 6-TGNs, also are responsible for myelosuppression with therapy, and patients with *TPMT* mutation or decreased *TPMT* enzyme activity are more likely to experience this toxicity because of preferential shunting of 6-MP metabolism toward the excessive production of 6-TGN.[206] Thus, identifying *TPMT* polymorphism before initiating azathioprine or 6-MP therapy may decrease the risk of myelotoxicity. Patients with homozygous wild-type *TPMT* or normal (to high) *TPMT* enzyme activity level can receive these agents starting at the weight-based optimal dose of 2.5 mg/kg/day for azathioprine or 1.5 mg/kg/day for 6-MP. It has been suggested by some investigators that in patients with heterozygous *TPMT* mutation or intermediate enzyme activity level, 6-MP or azathioprine should be started at 50% of the weight-based optimal dose. Alternative therapy should be considered in individuals with homozygous mutations for *TPMT*. Others[207] have suggested that there should be no differentiation between those who have the wild type (full enzyme activity) or who are heterozygotes (intermediate enzyme activity) because the positive predictive value as to whether those patients in the intermediate enzyme activity group will develop myelosuppression is low. Regardless of whether an individual has the knowledge of *TMPT* genotype or phenotype, continued frequent monitoring of complete blood counts remains necessary, because only 27% of all patients with leukopenia will have *TPMT* mutations present.[208]

Azathioprine and 6-MP therapy have a delayed onset of action. The mean time to clinical response with azathioprine or 6-MP therapy in patients with UC has been reported to be 3 to 4 months in uncontrolled studies,[192,209] a figure that is similar to the 17 weeks' response time to clinical benefit in placebo-controlled trials of azathioprine or 6-MP therapy for active Crohn's disease.[210] Intravenous loading of azathioprine at 40 mg/kg for 36 hours does not shorten the time required for a therapeutic response in patients with Crohn's disease.[202] Such practice presumably would have the same results if attempted in patients with UC.

Since azathioprine or 6-MP therapy is associated with a number of potentially significant toxicities, its duration of therapy should be determined weighing clinical benefit against these potential toxicities. The optimal duration of maintenance therapy with azathioprine or 6-MP currently is unknown in patients with UC. In patients with Crohn's disease, the maintenance benefit of azathioprine or 6-MP can be observed for at least 5 years.[211,212] Based on these data in Crohn's disease and the paucity of alternative maintenance therapies, in patients with UC in whom remission is maintained on azathioprine or 6-MP, treatment generally is continued indefinitely as long as there is no significant adverse side effect.

Common side effects of azathioprine and 6-MP therapy include nausea, vomiting, bone marrow suppression, pancreatitis, allergic reactions, and infections (Table 109–15).[213,214] Bone marrow suppression occurs in 2% to 5% of patients.[213,215] It is dose dependent and manifests primarily as leukopenia, although all three cell lines may be affected. This hematologic toxicity may increase with concurrent use of sulfasalazine or antibiotics.[201,216-218] It is known that mesalamine can interact with the enzyme TPMT, leading to increased levels of 6-TGN, and that this interaction has been associated with leukopenia. Bone marrow suppression is managed with dose reduction or medication withdrawal. Routine monitoring of complete blood count with differentials is necessary for patients receiving azathioprine or 6-MP and should be continued for the entire duration of therapy. Allergic reactions to azathioprine or 6-MP usually manifest as fever, rash, and arthralgia and resolve following discontinuation of medications.[215,219] Recurrence of similar reactions occurs with medication challenge, although individuals who develop allergic reactions to one agent may be able to tolerate subsequent challenge with the other.[220] Pancreatitis also is idiosyncratic and dose independent.[215,221,222] It usually occurs during the first month of therapy and is reversible on drug withdrawal.

Abnormal liver chemistry tests may develop on azathioprine or 6-MP therapy and usually resolve following drug withdrawal.[223] Because liver biopsy is not performed routinely, the pattern of hepatic injury, if any, in these patients is unknown. Cholestasis with inflammation, nodular regenerative hyperplasia, and peliosis hepatis have been reported with azathioprine and 6-MP therapy.[215,223] As is the case for complete blood counts, routine monitoring of liver chemistry tests is recommended. An increased risk of malignancy, primarily lymphoma, has been reported, but not consistently.[215,224,225] The lymphoma that develops in patients with IBD receiving these immunomodulatory agents appears to be associated with Epstein-Barr virus.[226]

Cyclosporine

Cyclosporine A is a potent inhibitor of cell-mediated immunity. Its use in UC is primarily in patients with severe, steroid-refractory disease. There has only been one randomized, placebo-controlled trial evaluating the efficacy of intravenous cyclosporine in severe UC. In this study of 20 patients who did not respond to at least 7

days of intravenous hydrocortisone, 9 (82%) of the 11 patients receiving continuous intravenous infusion of cyclosporine at 4 mg/kg/day responded compared with none of the 9 patients receiving placebo therapy.[127] The response was rapid, at a mean of 7 days. After the therapy was converted to oral cyclosporine, 44% of those patients who responded initially required colectomy during the 6-month follow-up period.[227] The addition of azathioprine or 6-MP in patients who have responded to intravenous cyclosporine reduces the rate of relapse or colectomy.[195,196] Thus, cyclosporine can be considered a bridge therapy to control active disease while waiting for elective surgery or the onset of action of azathioprine or 6-MP. Intravenous cyclosporine monotherapy may be equally as effective as intravenous glucocorticoids in patients with severely active UC, thus potentially minimizing toxicities of combination therapy.[228] With the addition of azathioprine, long-term remission at 1 year may be more likely in patients who initially respond to intravenous cyclosporine monotherapy than in those who respond to intravenous corticosteroids.

Because most of the serious adverse effects of cyclosporine, which are discussed subsequently, are dose dependent, intravenous doses lower than 4 mg/kg that still can achieve efficacy would be desirable. One randomized, controlled trial has shown that a dose of 2 mg/kg is as effective as 4 mg/kg given intravenously in patients with severely active UC, judged by clinical response rates, time to response, and short-term colectomy rates.[229] The mean plasma cyclosporine levels were 237 ng/mL in patients receiving the 2 mg/kg dose and 332 ng/mL in patients receiving the 4 mg/kg dose. As expected, the higher dose resulted in a higher incidence of hypertension, albeit not a statistically significant one. Thus, high-dose intravenous cyclosporine dose not appear to provide additional clinical benefit over low-dose therapy in the treatment of severe UC. Initiating therapy at 2 mg/kg may be reasonable, but regardless of the dose used, careful monitoring of plasma cyclosporine trough levels is necessary.

Cyclosporine has been associated with many adverse effects, including paresthesias, tremor, headache, hypertrichosis, and gingival hyperplasia (Table 109–16). Other potentially serious toxicities include hypertension, seizures, electrolyte and abnormal liver-associated

Table 109–15 Side Effects of Azathioprine and 6-Mercaptopurine

Bone marrow suppression
Pancreatitis
Nausea, abdominal pain, diarrhea
Hypersensitivity reactions (fever, rash, arthralgia)
Abnormal liver biochemical test results
Infections
Lymphoma

Table 109–16 Side Effects of Cyclosporine

Hypertension
Tremor
Renal insufficiency
Electrolyte abnormalities
Headache
Hirsutism
Gingival hyperplasia
Paresthesia
Nausea, vomiting, diarrhea
Hepatotoxicity
Infections
Seizure
Anaphylaxis
Opportunistic infections

chemistry abnormalities, nephrotoxicity, anaphylaxis, and opportunistic infections. These complications are mostly dose dependent. Severe complications have been reported in up to 12% of patients with UC.[230] Thus, careful monitoring for side effects is critical during cyclosporine therapy. Baseline serum electrolytes, creatinine, cholesterol, and liver chemistry values should be measured. Cyclosporine therapy should be avoided in patients with an impaired creatinine clearance to minimize severe nephrotoxicity. Patients with a serum cholesterol lower than 120 mg/dL should receive nutritional support to improve their cholesterol level before initiating cyclosporine therapy, because a low cholesterol level is associated with an increased risk of seizures. During intravenous therapy, cyclosporine levels should be monitored daily, and the dose should be adjusted to achieve a trough concentration (measured 1 hour prior to dosing) between 200 and 400 ng/mL as determined by high-pressure liquid chromatography. Serum electrolytes and serum creatinine levels should be monitored daily or every other day. The dose of cyclosporine also should be decreased when the serum creatinine increases by 20% to 30% over baseline. If patients respond to intravenous cyclosporine, the route of administration can be changed to oral therapy with 2 mg of oral agent for 1 mg of intravenous cyclosporine. The drug can be administered in two divided doses daily. Drug monitoring during oral cyclosporine therapy includes weekly trough cyclosporine levels and weekly to biweekly electrolytes and creatinine levels. Oral cyclosporine should be continued for 3 to 6 months, while waiting for surgery or for azathioprine or 6-MP to take effect. Patients on long-term cyclosporine therapy should receive *Pneumocystis carinii* pneumonia prophylaxis with trimethoprim-sulfamethoxazole.

Methotrexate

Methotrexate is a folic acid antagonist and has both antimetabolite and anti-inflammatory properties. Early reports suggested potential benefit of methotrexate administered intramuscularly or orally in UC.[231,232] The only randomized, placebo-controlled trial, however, failed to demonstrate efficacy of methotrexate for the treatment of active UC.[233] In this study of 67 patients with chronic active UC, oral methotrexate at 12.5 mg/wk for 9 months was comparable with placebo therapy in the rate of achieving first remission, relapse following remission, time to first remission, and the mean steroid dose. It is unknown if methotrexate at higher doses administered intramuscularly or subcutaneously may be beneficial in induction or maintenance of remission in UC. Given the absence of data supporting its efficacy, methotrexate cannot at this time be considered a standard therapy for UC.

Other Immunomodulators

Alternative immunomodulators have been explored for patients who do not tolerate or have not responded to the aforementioned immunosuppressants. Mycophenolate mofetil has similar pharmacodynamic properties as azathioprine and 6-MP but a more rapid onset of action. A pilot study of patients with chronic active UC receiving concomitant prednisolone found azathioprine to be superior to mycophenolate mofetil throughout the 1-year study period, with remission rates at 1 year of 100% versus 88%, respectively.[234] Uncontrolled studies reported less than 50% remission rates with mycophenolate mofetil therapy in patients with steroid-dependent UC[235,236] and the intolerance rate was high.[235] A substantial number of patients developed adverse effects necessitating drug withdrawal, including recurrent upper respiratory tract infection, bacterial meningitis, depression, and migraine headache.[234,236]

Tacrolimus is another immunosuppressant with actions similar to cyclosporine. In contrast to cyclosporine, it has a 100-fold greater potency and a more rapid onset of action. One small study suggested benefit of tacrolimus in patients with steroid-refractory IBD when administered intravenously, then orally, and with concomitant azathioprine and mesalamine.[237] An alternative is to administer oral tacrolimus alone without intravenous induction and to add azathioprine for maintenance therapy in the responders.[238] This approach has been reported to have a response within 1 to 2 weeks and a remission rate of 67% at 12 weeks.[239] The overall colectomy rate, however, was 34%, and 50% of the patients with a minimum follow-up of 2 years required a colectomy.[238] There have not been any studies directly comparing tacrolimus and cyclosporine. Furthermore, tacrolimus can result in a number of toxicities as in cyclosporine therapy, including nephrotoxicity, electrolyte abnormalities, nausea, diarrhea, headache, tremors, paresthesias, insomnia, alopecia, hirsutism, and gingival hyperplasia.[238,239] Thus, the use of these alternative immunomodulators is currently not incorporated into standard practice.

ANTIBIOTICS

Antibiotics have a limited role in the management of UC, and most controlled studies have not demonstrated their benefit either in active disease or maintenance of remission.[240-244] The most commonly used antibiotics in this setting are metronidazole and ciprofloxacin. One randomized, controlled trial found oral tobramycin to be superior to placebo as a short-term adjunctive therapy to glucocorticoids for active UC.[245] Another randomized, controlled trial reported a modest benefit for the addition of ciprofloxacin for 6 months in patients with UC refractory to mesalamine and corticosteroids.[246] Recent data have been published on a poorly absorbed (<0.4%) antibiotic, Rifaximin, for treatment of steroid refractory UC and have demonstrated efficacy over placebo. At present the data showing efficacy of antibiotics for treatment of patients with UC are not as convincing as are the data for treatment of Crohn's disease. Thus, at present the primary role of antibiotics in the treatment of UC is in the management of its suppurative complications.

PROBIOTICS

Probiotics are living organisms in foods and dietary supplements that beneficially affect the host by improving its intestinal microbial balance.[247] A probiotic can be a specific nonpathogenic strain of a bacterial species or a mixture of multiple species and strains. An example of the latter is VSL#3, which contains four strains of *Lactobacillus* (*Lactobacillus acidophilus, Lactobacillus delbrueckii* subspecies *bulgaricus, Lactobacillus plantarium,* and *Lactobacillus casei*), three strains of *Bifidobacterium* (*Bifidobacterium infantis, Bifidobacterium longum, Bifidobacterium breve*), and one strain of *Streptococcus* (*Bifidobacterium salivarius* subspecies *thermophilus*).

For patients with mildly to moderately active UC, open-label pilot studies reported remission rates of 63% to 71% with *Saccharomyces boulardii*[248] and VSL#3,[249] respectively. As a maintenance therapy, a specific strain of *E. coli,* Nissle 1917, was equally effective as low-dose mesalamine in preventing relapse in two randomized, controlled trials of 236 patients with UC in clinical remission.[250,251] A different probiotic preparation using fermented milk that contains two strains of bifidobacteria and *L. acidophilus* also has been found effective in maintaining remission in patients with UC in a small randomized, controlled trial.[252] Alteration of the composition of the fecal flora by probiotic therapy has been shown in an uncontrolled study in which VSL#3 was administered to patients with quiescent UC. This probiotic maintenance therapy resulted in clinical relapses in 25% of the patients over 12 months,[253] and the fecal concentrations of the nonpathogenic bacterial species contained in VSL#3 increased significantly throughout the entire duration of therapy, starting as early as 20 days after initiation of therapy. Controlled trials comparing probiotic regimens to higher doses of mesalamine are necessary before routine use of probiotics as a maintenance therapy in patients with UC.

NUTRITIONAL THERAPY

Short-chain fatty acids, especially butyrate, have been shown to be the main energy substrate for colonocytes. Butyrate metabolism accounts for approximately 70% of colonocyte oxygen utilization. The suggestion that there is an impairment of colonocyte oxidation of short-chain fatty acids in UC led to therapeutic investigations on this form of nutritional therapy. Indeed, placebo-controlled studies have found butyrate enemas to be beneficial in treating mildly active left-sided colitis.[254-256]

Fish oils containing eicosapentaenoic acid have been found to attenuate colitis in animal models of colitis, probably via protecting the integrity of colonic mucosa, suppressing the inflammatory response, or both.[257-259] In a small, placebo-controlled, cross-over study of patients with mild-to-moderate UC, treatment with fish oil resulted in a 56% reduction in disease activity compared with a 4% reduction in controls ($P < 0.05$).[260] This benefit has not been confirmed in other studies, and a benefit in maintaining remission has not been observed.[261-263] Furthermore, compliance is limited because of side effects and the odor of the fish oil preparation.

In contrast to Crohn's disease where bowel rest and total parenteral nutrition may improve disease, multiple studies have not found total parenteral nutrition with or without bowel rest to have any therapeutic advantage in patients with UC.[264,265] Parenteral nutrition, however, may offer nutritional benefit in these patients.

In general it is important to provide adequate nutrition to patients with UC who are about to undergo surgery. However, nutrition is no more effective than placebo for use as primary therapy for the treatment of active UC.

OTHER THERAPIES

Nicotine

Based on the observation that smoking is associated with a decreased risk of UC and that a former smoker with active colitis may gain clinical benefit on resuming smoking, nicotine has been used to treat patients with this disease. Randomized, controlled trials have shown some benefit of transdermal nicotine in the treatment of active UC.[266-269] When administered at the highest tolerated dosage of 22 mg/day or less for 4 weeks in patients with mildly to moderately active UC, transdermal nicotine resulted in clinical improvement in 39% of patients compared with 9% of patients who received placebo therapy ($P = 0.007$).[266] As a single therapy, however, transdermal nicotine was not as effective as low-dose prednisolone.[270] Common side effects included nausea, lightheadedness, itching, and tremor. Topical nicotine therapy has fewer side effects and may be an alternative. Pilot studies have shown topical nicotine to be beneficial in patients with distal UC, but no large, randomized, controlled trial has been performed[271,272] and transdermal nicotine has not been found to be effective as a maintenance therapy.[273] Thus, based on the available data on clinical efficacy and the overall poor patient tolerability, the use of nicotine cannot be considered part of standard armamentarium for treating UC.

Heparin

Heparin, a group of sulfated glycosaminoglycans, has both anti-inflammatory and immunomodulatory properties in addition to its well-known anticoagulant activity. The exact mechanism whereby heparin may ameliorate UC remains uncertain. An anticoagulant benefit, however, may not be responsible, because similar efficacy has not been observed in patients with IBD when treated with warfarin. Because of their negative charge, the glycosaminoglycans that constitute heparin have varied biologic effects, including significant anti-inflammatory actions and augmentation of the peptide growth factors involved in intestinal mucosal repair and regeneration. Based on reports of fortuitous improvement in patients with UC receiving heparin for treatment of deep venous thromboses, pilot studies have suggested that unfractionated heparin may be effective for inducing remission in patients with severe, refractory UC.[274,275] Compared with glucocorticoids as a first-line therapy, however, small randomized, controlled trials have reported conflicting results.[276,277] Intravenous heparin therapy was associated with substantial bleeding complications. Low-molecular-weight heparin offers advantages over unfractionated heparin in its route of administration, and preliminary studies suggested a benefit of low-molecular-weight heparin in the treatment of active UC.[278,279]

Unfortunately, this finding was not confirmed in a large, placebo-controlled trial of patients with mildly to moderately active UC receiving low-molecular-weight heparin for 6 weeks.[280]

Biologic Therapy

Recent advances in our understanding of the pathogenesis of IBD have resulted in the development of therapies targeted at specific molecules or mediators involved in the inflammatory processes of these diseases. Most studies evaluating the efficacy of these agents have been performed in patients with Crohn's disease, and only limited data are available for patients with UC.

Antitumor Necrosis Factor Antibody Therapy

TNF is a key proinflammatory cytokine that has been demonstrated to play a role in several disease states, including IBD. Elevated TNF concentrations have been found in inflamed intestine in patients with Crohn's disease and UC, and stool and mucosal concentrations of TNF in patients with IBD have been shown to correlate with clinical disease activity.

Infliximab (Remicade) is a chimeric monoclonal antibody of IgG$_1$ subclass directed against human TNF-α. It consists of 75% human and 25% murine components (Fig. 109–15). The efficacy of infliximab in Crohn's disease is well established,[281-284] and it is approved by the U.S. Food and Drug Administration for the treatment of Crohn's disease and ulcerative colitis. The efficacy of infliximab in Crohn's disease is thought to operate via a multitude of mechanisms, including antagonizing the activity of TNF-α,[285,286] initiating cytotoxicity on immune cells,[287] and inducing T-cell apoptosis.[288,289]

Controlled and uncontrolled data suggest that infliximab may be beneficial in the treatment of active UC, providing rapid response and perhaps having a steroid-sparing effect.[290-294] In one small randomized, controlled trial that was terminated early because of difficulties with enrollment, 4 of the 8 patients with severe steroid-refractory UC receiving one infusion of infliximab at 5, 10, or 20 mg/kg dose had clinical response at 2 weeks after infusion, compared with none of the 3 patients receiving placebo infusions.[295,296] In a subsequent study of 42 patients with moderately active steroid-refractory UC, remission rates at week 6 after the initial infusion were comparable between patients who received two infusions of 5 mg/kg of infliximab 2 weeks apart and did not result in higher clinical remission rates than patients who received placebo therapy 2 and 6 weeks after the initial infusion.[297]

Recently presented preliminary results from two large multicenter, multicountry randomized, double-blind trials (ACTI and ACTII) showed efficacy of infliximab therapy in UC.[298,299] In these two similarly designed trials, 728 patients with moderately to severely active UC who failed conventional therapy were randomized to placebo, infliximab 5 mg/kg, or infliximab 10 mg/kg at weeks 0, 2, and then every 8 weeks for one year. In the ACTI trial where all patients were either refractory to or intolerant of glucocorticoids and/or azathioprine and/or 6-mercaptopurine, clinical response was achieved at week 30 in 52% and 51% of patients receiving infliximab 5 mg/kg and 10 mg/kg, respectively. The rates of clinical remission at week 30 were 34% and 37% in the two respective groups. These results were significantly higher than the response and remission rates of 30% and 16%, respectively, in patients receiving placebo therapy. Treatment with infliximab was also shown to have steroid-sparing and mucosal healing properties. These data have led to the approval of infliximab by the Food and Drug Administration for patients with moderately to severely active UC who have had an inadequate response to conventional therapy. Infliximab is now accepted as part of the standard treatment options in patients with UC.

Antiadhesion Molecule Therapy

Several agents directed at blocking adhesion molecules have been evaluated for the treatment of UC. These molecules are glycoproteins expressed on the surfaces of endothelial cells and lymphocytes. Adhesion molecules are important in cellular trafficking in IBD and other diseases, in which immune and inflammatory cells from the periphery are recruited into sites of inflammation. Among these, natalizumab is a humanized IgG$_4$ monoclonal antibody against lymphocyte adhesion molecules, α4 integrins. A pilot study of 10 patients with active UC suggested clinical benefit with a single infusion of 3 mg/kg of natalizumab.[300] Another antiadhesion molecule agent is MLN-02 (formerly called *LDP-02*), a humanized IgG$_1$ monoclonal antibody to α4β7 integrin. In a phase 2 study, two infusions of 0.5 mg/kg of MNL-02 administered 29 days apart were found to be effective in achieving both clinical remission and response at 6 weeks after the initial infusion in patients with moderately active UC.[301]

Other Biologic Therapies

IL-2 is one of the major cytokines produced by Th1 cells. Given the predominance of Th2-driven immune phenomena, two agents designed to block the binding of IL-2 to its receptor have been examined for potential efficacy in UC. Daclizumab, a humanized monoclonal antibody against the IL-2 receptor (CD25), has been suggested to be beneficial in patients with refractory UC in a small open-label pilot study.[302] A potential clinical benefit also has been reported with basiliximab, a chimeric monoclonal antibody to the IL-2 receptor, in a small, uncontrolled study of patients with steroid-refractory

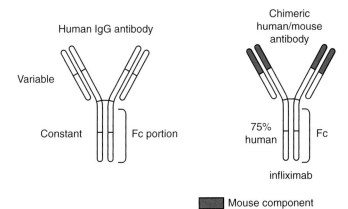

Figure 109–15 Structural diagram of antitumor necrosis factor antibody therapy using infliximab.

UC.[303] Along the emphasis on T cell-mediated immune response in the pathogenesis of UC, a humanized monoclonal antibody to CD3, visilizumab, has shown promise in a pilot study in hospitalized patients with UC whose disease failed to respond to intravenous glucocorticoids.[304]

Other biologic therapies include agents targeted at tissue repair and restitution following mucosal injury. In this regard, epidermal growth factor (EGF) is a potent mitogenic peptide that stimulates cell proliferation in the gastrointestinal tract. A preliminary study showed EGF enemas at a dose of 5 µg daily for 2 weeks to be effective in treating mild-to-moderate left-sided UC when administered along with oral mesalamine (remission rate 83% in active treatment vs. 8% in placebo group; $P < 0.001$).[305] In contrast, another potent stimulant of intestinal epithelial cells, repifermin (keratinocyte growth factor-2) was not found to be more effective than placebo when administered intravenously in patients with active UC in a phase 2 dose-ranging study.[306] Further studies are clearly necessary to confirm some of these early promising findings.

Cytapheresis

Active UC is characterized by activation and infiltration of leukocytes in the colonic mucosa. Since leukocyte-derived inflammatory cytokines play an important role in the initiation and perpetuation of the inflammatory process, reduction of peripheral blood levels of leukocytes has been proposed as a therapeutic option for treating the disease. Several methods of depleting peripheral blood leukocytes have been developed and have been shown to hold promise in the treatment of severely active UC in both controlled and uncontrolled studies.[307-314] The primary benefit of these leukocyte apheresis therapies appears to be as adjunctive therapy, allowing steroid taper and possibly maintaining remission; however, leukocytapheresis is an intensive therapy and the practicalities of its use still need to be addressed. Use of leukocytapheresis in the treatment of UC should be reserved to the clinical trial setting until data from large-scale, randomized, controlled trials are available.

Nuclear Hormone Receptor Agonist

Peroxisome proliferator-activated receptor-gamma is a nuclear hormone receptor that is best known for its role in regulating metabolism and adipocyte differentiation. It also has been shown to have immunomodulatory and anti-inflammatory properties in multiple sites, including the colon.[315-318] A pilot clinical trial has reported potential benefit of a ligand for this receptor, rosiglitazone, in the treatment of patients with mildly to moderately active UC, with a response rate of 54% and a remission rate 27% after 12 weeks of therapy.[319] A multicenter, randomized, controlled trial currently is ongoing to evaluate its efficacy in UC.

SURGICAL THERAPY

Removal of the colon and rectum cures UC. Common indications for surgical therapy of UC are medically refractory disease, intractable disease with an impaired quality of life, and unacceptable side effects from medical therapy (Table 109–17). Other indications for surgery include uncontrolled hemorrhage, toxic megacolon, perforation, dysplasia or carcinoma, systemic complications, and growth retardation. The goals of surgical treatment are to remove the diseased colon while preserving continence and sexual function. Elimination of the potential risk of colorectal cancer is also important. The role of prophylactic proctocolectomy in patients with long-standing extensive UC is controversial. Whereas most clinicians do not routinely recommend proctocolectomy solely for the purpose of prophylaxis against colorectal cancer, patients should be informed of the limitations of our current colonoscopic surveillance program (see Chapters 119 and 120).

There are multiple surgical options for UC (see Chapter 111), including subtotal colectomy with ileostomy, colectomy with ileorectal anastomosis, proctocolectomy with Brooke ileostomy, proctocolectomy with continent ileostomy, restorative proctocolectomy with ileal pouch anal anastomosis (IPAA), and proctocolectomy with ileal pouch-anal transition zone anastomosis (Fig. 109–16). The choice of operation is based on several factors, including the indication and urgency of surgery, the age and general health of the patient, the status of anal function, and the patient's preference of functional outcome and lifestyle.

Subtotal colectomy with ileostomy is the least extensive of these operations wherein most of the colon is removed, a Hartman pouch or a mucous fistula is created for the remaining colon, and an end-ileostomy is created. Subtotal colectomy with ileostomy typically is performed in patients requiring emergent surgery for severe, fulminant colitis. This operation has the advantage of allowing restorative surgery in the future. Colectomy with ileorectal anastomosis is similar to subtotal colectomy with ileostomy but maintains bowel continuity. Many patients continue to have attacks of colitis and the retained rectal stump is at risk of developing colorectal cancer. Thus, lifelong endoscopic surveillance of the rectum is necessary for patients who elect this type of operation.

Total proctocolectomy with a permanent Brooke end ileostomy is one of the earliest operations performed for UC. Removal of the entire colon and rectum eliminates any future disease and risk of colorectal cancer. The primary disadvantage of this operation is the presence of the permanent ileostomy, which may not be acceptable from the standpoint of quality of life for some patients. Proctocolectomy with Brooke ileostomy is the operation

Table 109–17	Indications for Surgery in Ulcerative Colitis

Uncontrollable colonic hemorrhage
Toxic megacolon
Colonic perforation
Medically-refractory disease
Intolerable or unacceptable side effects from medical therapy
Colonic dysplasia or carcinoma
Systemic complications
Growth retardation

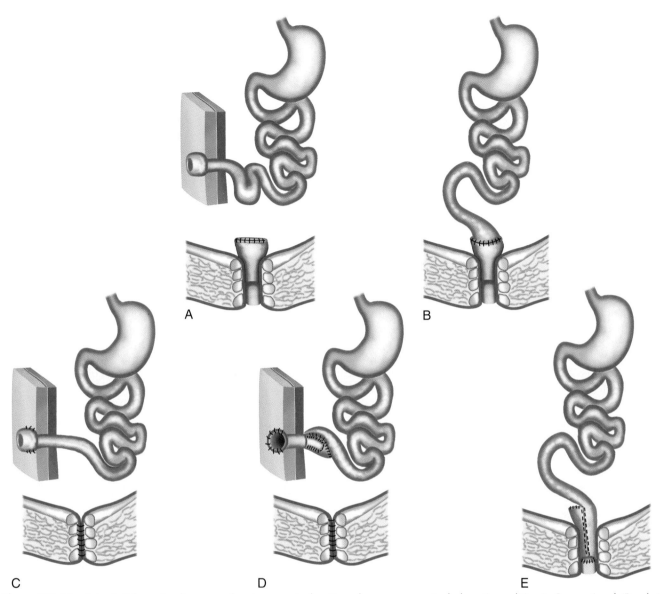

Figure 109–16 *A* to *E,* Schematic diagrams of various surgical options for management of ulcerative colitis. *A,* Conventional (Brooke) ileostomy with a subtotal colectomy and a Hartman pouch. *B,* Subtotal colectomy with ileorectal anastomosis. *C,* Conventional (Brooke) ileostomy with a total proctocolectomy. *D,* Continent ileostomy (Koch pouch) with total proctocolectomy. *E,* Restorative proctocolectomy with ileal pouch anal anastomosis. (*A-E,* Adapted from Blumberg D, Beck DE: Surgery for ulcerative colitis. Gastroenterol Clin North Am 31:219, 2002.)

of choice for elderly patients, those with anal dysfunction, and those who do not wish to have a restorative proctocolectomy.

Proctocolectomy with continent ileostomy (Koch pouch) was developed as an alternative to the conventional end ileostomy.[320] In this surgery, loops of small bowel are used to create an intra-abdominal pouch with an intussuscepted ("nipple") valve. This pouch allows storage of stool contents and is attached to the abdominal wall with a flush ostomy opening. The stool contents in the pouch are emptied by inserting a catheter through the stoma. Because of technical challenges associated with this operation (e.g., slippage of the nipple valve) and the development of restorative procedures, proctocolectomy with continent ileostomy rarely is performed.

Restorative proctocolectomy with IPAA is currently the operation of choice for most patients with UC who require elective colectomy. In this procedure, the entire

colon and rectum are removed with preservation of the anal sphincters, and a pouch is constructed from approximately 20 cm of the distal ileum (see Fig. 109–18). Bowel continuity is established by anastomosing this pouch with the anal canal. An IPAA usually is performed as a two-stage operation, during the first stage of which a temporary diverting ileostomy is created to allow the ileal pouch to heal. This operation can be performed as a single-stage operation; however, there have been reports suggesting a higher rate of obstruction and sepsis when this is done.[321] The ileostomy is then reversed after approximately 2 to 4 months. Proctocolectomy with IPAA presents technical challenges and may not be suitable or technically feasible for all patients. Most reports suggest satisfactory quality of life following IPAA surgery.[322] Mean stool frequency ranges from 4 to 9 bowel movements per day, including 1 or 2 nocturnal stools. Nocturnal seepage occurs in approximately 20%

of patients in the early postoperative period and is infrequent after the first year. Rates of complications following IPAA surgery vary widely.[323] In one large series from 1995 of more than 1000 patients undergoing restorative proctocolectomy and IPAA, most of whom had UC, the overall morbidity rate was 63% (early complications 28%, late complications 51%).[322] These numbers likely will be lower as experience grows with this type of surgery. These complications, covered in Chapter 110, include obstruction, sepsis, abscess, anastomotic leak, pouchitis resulting in pouch failure, fecal incontinence, and sexual and urinary dysfunction. Thus, this surgery is best performed in centers with considerable experience with the operation and in the management of pouch dysfunction.

A widely performed modification of proctocolectomy with IPAA is proctocolectomy with ileal pouch-anal transition zone anastomosis. This technically less complex surgery involves stapling the ileal pouch to the distal rectum in close proximity to the dentate line (1 to 4 cm), thereby eliminating the need to perform rectal mucosectomy. This type of surgery may carry a lower risk for fecal incontinence and may be performed as a single-stage operation without a temporary diverting ileostomy. Controversy exists as to whether the retained transitional epithelium is at risk for developing dysplasia and carcinoma.[324]

MANAGEMENT OF SPECIFIC COMPLICATIONS

An algorithm for the management of patients with active UC of mild to moderate severity is outlined in Figure 109–17. The management of severely active UC is shown in Figure 109–18.

TOXIC MEGACOLON

Toxic megacolon is defined as acute colonic dilatation with a colon diameter of greater than 6 cm (on radiologic examination) and loss of haustrations in a patient with a severe attack of colitis.[325,326] Maximal colonic dilatation most frequently is observed in the transverse colon. This complication of UC results from extension of colonic inflammation beyond the mucosa to the underlying tissues including the muscularis propria. Loss of contractility from the inflammatory reaction leads to the accumulation of gas and fluid within the lumen and subsequent colonic dilatation.

Toxic megacolon occurs in approximately 5% of severe flares of UC. It frequently is encountered early in the course of disease and may be the initial presentation. Nearly 50% of patients with toxic megacolon develop this complication within 3 months of their diagnosis.[327] Toxic

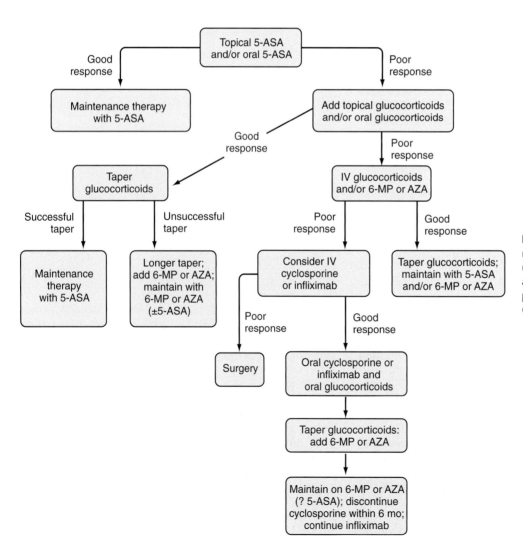

Figure 109–17 Management of mildly-to-moderately active ulcerative colitis. 5-ASA, 5-aminosalicylate; AZA, azathioprine; IV, intravenous; 6-MP, 6-mercaptopurine.

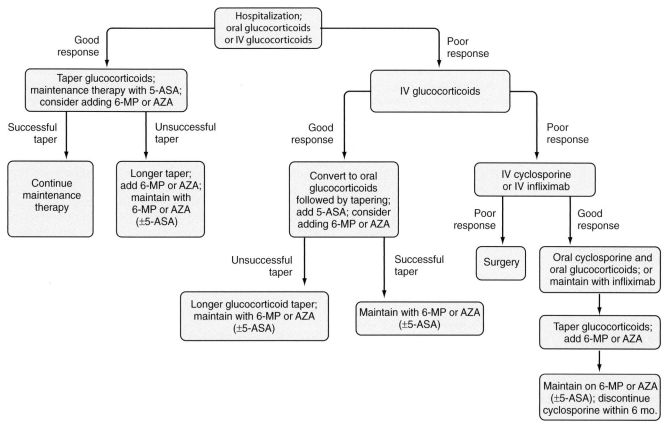

Figure 109–18 Management of severely active ulcerative colitis. 5-ASA, 5-aminosalicylate; AZA, azathioprine; IV, intravenous; 6-MP, 6-mercaptopurine.

megacolon usually occurs in patients with extensive colitis, but patients with disease limited to the left colon also can develop it. Precipitating factors for toxic megacolon include electrolyte imbalance (particularly hypokalemia), use of antimotility drugs including anticholinergic agents and narcotics, and procedures such as barium enema and colonoscopy performed during a severe attack.[328] These procedures should be avoided in the presence of a severe flare of UC. With clinical deterioration, patients may develop fever, tachycardia, hypotension, diffuse abdominal distention and tenderness, and decreased bowel sounds. Other laboratory parameters reflecting progressive severe systemic inflammation include marked leukocytosis, metabolic alkalosis, and electrolyte disturbances.

Medical management for toxic megacolon is directed at treating the underlying inflammation, restoring colonic motility, and preventing free colonic perforation. If colonic dilatation occurs during the initial presentation of UC, intravenous glucocorticoids and fluid replacement should be initiated and electrolyte abnormalities should be corrected. Reduction of fluid and air within the gastrointestinal tract may be achieved through bowel rest and nasogastric decompression. Other conservative management approaches include maneuvers to reduce abdominal distention by allowing the redistribution and/or passage of colon gas. Gas tends to rise and fill the most superiorly located bowel segment (i.e., the transverse colon) if the patient is in the supine position.

Encouraging patients to move about or rotating patients who are bed bound, the use of knee-elbow position when prone, and the insertion of a rectal tube all have been suggested to be helpful in reducing bowel distention.[329,330] Systemic antibiotics often are empirically administered, because mortality from toxic megacolon correlates with the development of sepsis.[331] Approximately 50% of acute dilatation resolves with medical therapy.[330,332] However, since the presence of colonic perforation is the most important predictor of mortality (44% in patients undergoing emergent colectomy after perforation compared with 2% in patients undergoing colectomy without perforation),[333] an important aspect of management is to determine optimal timing of surgical intervention. In general, patients who do not improve after 48 to 72 hours of medical therapy should undergo surgery.[330] Close clinical observation for signs of impending perforation is critical. Patients with progressive abdominal distention, development of rebound tenderness, or hemodynamic instability should undergo immediate colectomy. For patients who achieve remission on medical therapy, subsequent management is controversial. In one series, nearly 50% of patients treated successfully for toxic megacolon eventually required colectomy for intractable disease.[334] Thus, some clinicians recommend elective colectomy following resolution of toxic megacolon.

Free perforation also may develop in the absence of colonic dilatation. This complication is rare, occurring in 1% of patients with UC without toxic megacolon.[332,335]

Classic physical findings of peritonitis may be absent, largely because of the masking effect of glucocorticoids, but most patients have a marked deterioration in overall clinical condition after perforation. It is important to examine for the hepatic dullness every day in patients with severe colitis on high-dose glucocorticoids because they may have a free perforation and not have the classic signs of peritonitis. A daily plain film of the abdomen also is recommended for the same purpose. As with toxic megacolon, patients with extensive colitis appear to be at greatest risk for this complication. The segment most at risk for free perforation is the sigmoid colon. The mortality associated with free perforation in patients with UC has been reported to be more than 50%.[335] Thus, the possibility of free perforation must be considered in patients with fulminant UC, particularly if there is deterioration in general condition, even in the absence of colonic dilatation.

STRICTURES

Colonic strictures complicating UC develop in approximately 5% of patients.[336] This complication most commonly occurs in patients with extensive and long-standing colitis. Patients with colonic strictures usually present with alterations in bowel habits, both constipation and diarrhea. Clinically significant obstruction is rare. Colonic strictures complicating UC typically are short (2 to 3 cm in length), occur distal to the splenic flexure, and represent hypertrophy and thickening of muscularis mucosa rather than fibrosis.[336] There needs to be a high index of suspicion of malignancy in patients with colonic strictures associated with UC, especially when they are located proximal to the splenic flexure.[337] One series reported malignancy in 24% of colonic strictures in patients with UC.[336] Moreover, cancer associated with strictures tends to be more advanced than cancers not associated with strictures in patients with UC. Endoscopic appearance cannot reliably distinguish benign colonic strictures from malignant strictures and multiple biopsies are recommended at colonoscopy. Because carcinoma may not be detected on mucosal biopsies, however, surgical resection of the stricture is advised, particularly in patients with long-standing UC.

DYSPLASIA AND COLORECTAL CANCER

Patients with UC have an increased risk of colorectal cancer. This risk is dependent on several factors, the most important being the duration and extent of the disease. Other risk factors include PSC, family history of colon cancer, age at diagnosis of disease, severity of inflammation, and possibly backwash ileitis.[338-342] The incidence of colon cancer in UC varies depending primarily on the duration and extent of the disease but has been estimated at approximately 7% to 10% at 20 years of disease and as high as 30% after 35 years of disease.[343] Thus, in general, the risk of CRC may be estimated to increase within the range of 0.5% to 1.0% per year after 8 to 10 years of disease in patients with extensive UC.[343]

Although prophylactic colectomy can virtually eliminate the risk of colorectal cancer, patients often are unwilling to undergo surgery, particularly if there is no other indication for colectomy. Thus, colonoscopic surveillance programs have been developed in an effort to reduce the risk of colorectal cancer associated with UC. The primary goal of surveillance colonoscopy is to detect dysplasia, defined as unequivocal neoplastic epithelium, because currently it is the most important marker to detect concurrent or subsequent cancer. Dysplasia can be classified histologically and endoscopically into several groups, each with different prognostic implications. Histologic assessment is classified as negative, indefinite, and positive for dysplasia. Two grades of dysplasia are recognized: low (Fig. 109–19A) and high (Fig. 109–19B).[344] Endoscopically, dysplasia can be characterized as flat or raised based on the appearance of the surface of the dysplastic area. Flat dysplasia represents most of the dysplasia

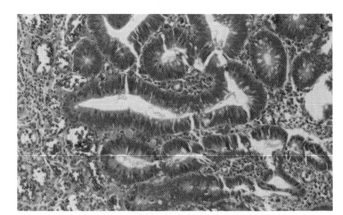

A

B

Figure 109–19 Photomicrograph of a colon biopsy specimen showing the histologic features of dysplasia. *A,* Low-grade dysplasia is characterized by nuclear enlargement, crowding, and hyperchromasia in the colonic epithelial cells. Nuclei are stratified but remain in the basal half of the cells. There is some depletion of mucin. *B,* In high-grade dysplasia, the changes are more pronounced. Nuclei are stratified to the surface, and there is a marked increase in nuclear pleomorphism. Branching of the glands in a cribriform pattern and scattered cell necrosis is shown. No mucin goblets are evident. (Courtesy of Feldman, online Gastro Atlas, Current Medicine).

detected in patients with UC. Raised dysplasia is also termed *dysplasia-associated lesion or mass* (DALM) and can be found as a polypoid lesion, mass, plaque, or stricture.

In a landmark study, Blackstone and associates[345] identified 12 patients with DALMs during surveillance colonoscopies, of whom 7 (58%) subsequently were found to have colon cancer. Subsequent studies have confirmed this high incidence of developing invasive carcinoma,[346-348] including the finding of carcinoma on immediate colectomy in up to 50% of patients with DALMs.[349] A systematic review of 10 surveillance studies of 1225 patients reported that 10 (42%) of 24 patients with high-grade dysplasia who underwent immediate colectomy had synchronous cancer, and 15 (32%) of 47 patients who were found to have high-grade dysplasia after an initially normal colonoscopy subsequently were found to have cancer.[349] Thus, the presence of a DALM lesion or high-grade dysplasia appears to be highly predictive of concurrent or subsequent colon cancer, and colectomy is recommended for these patients.

DALMs consist of a heterogeneous group of dysplastic lesions and can broadly be categorized into adenoma-like DALMs and nonadenoma-like DALMs based on their endoscopic and histologic appearances. Several small series reported that adenoma-like DALMs carry a low risk for developing cancer and that they may be managed conservatively without immediate colectomy.[350-352] A prospective follow-up study compared the outcomes of 24 patients in one of 3 groups: (1) UC and adenoma-like DALMs (located within an area of colitis but with no other areas of flat dysplasia or cancer); (2) patients with UC and coincidental sporadic adenomas (located proximal to the extent of colitis); and (3) patients without UC but with sporadic adenomas.[353] All polyps were managed conservatively with complete polypectomy followed by colonoscopic surveillance. During the follow-up period, the proportion of patients with adenoma-like DALMs developing further adenomas (58%) was similar to those in the other two groups of patients, and no cancer was found, suggesting that these polypoid, adenoma-like DALMs follow a relatively benign course comparable to that of sporadic adenomas unrelated to colitis. Another prospective study also supported the practice of polypectomy for dysplastic polypoid lesions without flat dysplasia adjacent to the polyps or throughout the colon in patients with UC.[354] Thus, conservative management with complete polypectomy and endoscopic surveillance has become an increasingly accepted alternative to the traditional recommendation of colectomy in patients with UC and adenoma-like DALMs.

The predictive value of low-grade dysplasia for the development of more advanced lesions varies among studies. In the aforementioned systematic review of 10 studies in the literature, the risk of synchronous cancer at immediate colectomy was 19% (3 of 16) in patients with low-grade dysplasia.[349] In patients with newly diagnosed low-grade dysplasia after a previously normal surveillance colonoscopy, 16% later progressed to high-grade dysplasia, DALM, or cancer (8%), whereas 29% of patients with untreated low-grade dysplasia found at the initial surveillance colonoscopy progressed to high-grade dysplasia, DALM, or cancer (13%). In a single center study of 46 UC patients with flat low-grade dysplasia on

surveillance colonoscopy, unexpected advanced neoplasia occurred in 4 (24%) of 17 patients who underwent immediate colectomy.[355] Five additional cases of cancer at stage II or higher occurred despite surveillance examinations. These findings suggest that patients with low-grade dysplasia are at relatively high risk of developing more advanced lesions or cancer. However, in two European studies with a total of 89 patients, only 3% to 10% of patients with low-grade dysplasia later developed high-grade dysplasia, DALM, or cancer after 10 years of follow-up.[356,357] Thus, some experts have advocated a more conservative approach for low-grade dysplasia.

Most authorities recommend annual to biannual colonoscopy with biopsies in patients with UC extending beyond proctitis who have disease for 8 to 10 years.[358,359] Examinations should be performed during periods of inactive disease so as not to allow inflammation and reactive change to obscure the picture. Four-quadrant biopsies should be obtained every 10 cm and from any potentially dysplastic lesion. Thus, performing proper surveillance requires extensive biopsies. In fact, it has been estimated that at least 18 jumbo biopsies are required to achieve 95% probability of identifying dysplasia or cancer if it is present.[360] Because the goal of surveillance colonoscopy is to detect dysplasia before cancer develops, a minimum of 64 biopsies are required to detect highest rate of dysplasia anywhere in the colon with 95% confidence.

A successful surveillance program also depends on appropriate management based on findings on colonoscopy and biopsies. Colectomy is recommended for flat dysplasia, either low-grade or high-grade, or invasive carcinoma (Fig. 109–20).[342,349,361] Focal low-grade dysplasia may be managed by continued surveillance colonoscopy, whereas colectomy is recommended for patients with multifocal low-grade dysplasia.

The management of polypoid lesions identified on surveillance colonoscopy is summarized in Figure 109–21. Polypoid lesions identified outside of underlying colitis are considered coincidental sporadic adenoma and can be treated with complete polypectomy if technically feasible. These patients should continue to receive surveillance colonoscopy annually or biannually.

For pedunculated or sessile polypoid lesions within regions of colitis, endoscopic polypectomy should be performed. In addition to multiple random biopsies at regular intervals throughout the entire colon as mentioned earlier, biopsies should be obtained from the area around the polyp site. If the polypectomy is not complete, surgical resection is necessary. If the polypectomy is complete and there is dysplasia in the surrounding mucosa or the rest of the colon, colectomy should be advised because of the high association with synchronous carcinoma and subsequent development of invasive cancer.[345,349]

Alternatively, if polypectomy is complete and there is no dysplasia in the surrounding mucosa or the rest of the colon, this polypoid dysplastic lesion can be considered an adenoma-like DALM. In this scenario, patients should be advised of the uncertainty regarding optimal management of adenoma-like DALMs.[362] Recent studies have suggested that conservative management with complete endoscopic polypectomy followed by careful colono-

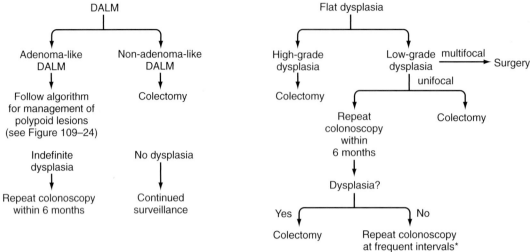

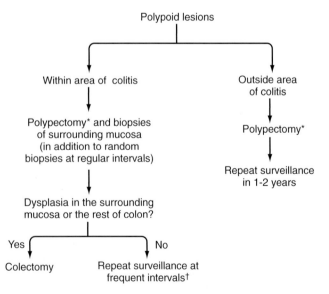

*Ideal frequency has not been determined.

Figure 109–20 Recommended algorithm for management of DALM, flat dysplasia, indefinite dysplasia or no dysplasia on surveillance colonoscopy. DALM, dysplasia-associated lesion or mass.

scopic surveillance may be an acceptable alternative to the traditional recommendation of colectomy.[353,354] If the polyp is pedunculated with a well-defined stalk, endoscopic resection with continued surveillance at an increasing interval (e.g., 6 months initially) generally is considered adequate. If the polyp is sessile, the same practice may be used provided that the patient understands it is controversial.[354] Decisions should be individualized. Other factors that should be taken into consideration include age (lesions in younger patients are more likely to be related to disease rather than sporadic adenomas), duration of disease, severity and course of disease, family history of CRC, and personal history of PSC.[353,362]

Colonoscopic surveillance is fraught with many potential pitfalls, including sampling error, interobserver vari-

*If polypectomy is incomplete, patients should undergo surgery.
†Ideal frequency has not been determined.

Figure 109–21 Recommended algorithm for management of polypoid lesions.

ability for determining dysplasia, and difficulty detecting and differentiating dysplastic lesions from other lesions. Thus, techniques have been developed to enhance the diagnostic accuracy of surveillance colonoscopy in patients with UC. These techniques include the use of magnifying and chromoendoscopy, in which tissue stains are applied to the gastrointestinal mucosal surface at endoscopy to better enhance or characterize specific findings.[363-365] Use of magnifying and chromoendoscopy as an adjunct to conventional colonoscopy has been shown, in comparison with conventional colonoscopy, to increase the rate of detecting dysplasia and has been shown to have both a sensitivity and specificity of 93% for differentiating neoplastic and non-neoplastic lesions.[363] In addition, research has investigated the use of molecular, genetic, and immunohistochemical markers to enhance diagnostic accuracy of colitis-associated dysplasia. Although both sporadic colon cancer and IBD-associated malignancy follow a similar pathway from dysplasia to carcinoma,[366] recent studies have shown differences in the prevalence and timing of certain molecular events between these two groups of neoplasias. Some of these differences in colitis-associated dysplasia include infrequent and late mutations in the APC and β-catenin genes, more frequent and early abnormalities in the 3p (von Hippel–Lindau gene locus), p53, and p16 loci, and higher prevalence of Sialyl-Tn antigen expression.[367-374]

POUCHITIS

Pouchitis is the most common long-term complication of colectomy with IPAA (see Chapter 110). Pouchitis is said to occur when there is nonspecific inflammation of the ileal reservoir, resulting in variable clinical symptoms resembling those of UC. Pouchitis occurs in up to 7% to 51% of patients undergoing restorative proctocolectomy for UC.[375,376] The incidence is highest during the first 6 months after closure of loop ileostomy. The pathophysiology of pouchitis is not well understood but is likely multifactorial. Several etiologic mechanisms have been postulated including fecal stasis, recurrent UC, Crohn's disease, mucosal ischemia, and viral infection; another postulated mechanism is an ongoing immune process that may be recurrent UC, misdiagnosed Crohn's disease, or an overlap or other form of IBD.[377,378]

Characteristic symptoms of pouchitis include increased bowel frequency, rectal bleeding, abdominal cramping, rectal urgency, tenesmus, and fecal incontinence.[379] Other associated symptoms are fever, malaise, arthralgias, and erythema nodosum. Endoscopic evaluation may reveal mucosal erythema, edema, granularity, friability, petechiae, loss of vascular pattern, erosions, and superficial ulcerations. Deep and irregularly shaped ulcers characteristic of Crohn's disease may be present. Histologically, pouchitis is marked by an acute inflammatory infiltrate with mucosal ulceration and crypt abscesses in addition to chronic inflammation with villus atrophy and crypt hyperplasia. Similar to UC, the diagnosis of pouchitis is based on a constellation of clinical symptoms, endoscopic appearances, and histologic features.[378,380] Acute pouchitis is defined when symptoms are present for fewer than 4 weeks, whereas symptoms lasting more than 4 weeks are considered to be from chronic pouchitis.[378] More than 20% of patients have chronic continuous symptoms, but less than 10% will have severe chronic pouchitis requiring long-term maintenance therapy.[376]

The presence of pANCA has been associated with the development of chronic pouchitis following IPAA surgery for UC.[381] A subsequent prospective study measuring pANCA titers at the time of colectomy for UC found a higher incidence of pouchitis during follow-up in patients with a positive pANCA compared with patients with a negative pANCA (42% vs. 20%; $P = 0.09$).[382] The cumulative risk of developing chronic pouchitis among patients with high-level pANCA (56%) before colectomy was significantly higher than in patients with negative, low, or medium levels of pANCA (16% to 22%; $P = 0.005$). Thus, pANCA may be useful for identifying patients at risk for developing chronic pouchitis after IPAA surgery and who may require more aggressive medical therapy for treating pouchitis. Another predictor of developing pouchitis after IPAA is PSC, which is present in approximately 5% of patients with UC. In a retrospective study of more than 1000 patients who had IPAA for UC, at least one episode of pouchitis developed in 32% of patients without PSC and 63% of patients with PSC.[383] In patients with PSC, the cumulative risk of pouchitis at 10 years after IPAA was 79% compared with 46% in patients without PSC.

The mainstay of therapy for pouchitis is antibiotics. In the only placebo-controlled trial of antibiotics for the treatment of chronic active pouchitis, metronidazole at 1200 mg/day for 7 days resulted in an overall response rate of 73% compared with 9% for placebo.[384] Ciprofloxacin at 1 g/day for 2 weeks also is effective for the treatment of acute pouchitis and has been shown to be superior to metronidazole in efficacy and tolerability in a randomized, controlled trial.[385] Alternative regimens include topical metronidazole, amoxicillin/clavulanic acid, combination of ciprofloxacin and metronidazole, and combination of ciprofloxacin and rifaximin.[386-388] For patients who are on chronic therapy, cycling of multiple antibiotics at weekly intervals may help overcome bacterial resistance.

The second-line option for treating pouchitis is topical and oral mesalamines.[380,389] However, the use of these agents is based on uncontrolled studies and anecdotal experiences. Topical and systemic corticosteroids can be used for patients with pouchitis that do not respond to antibiotics and mesalamines. In a randomized, controlled trial, budesonide enema (2 mg/100 mL) nightly had similar efficacy as, but fewer side effects than, metronidazole (1 g/day) in the treatment of acute pouchitis.[390] Immunosuppressive and biologic therapies, including cyclosporine enema, azathioprine, and infliximab, also have been reported to be beneficial and may be considered in patients whose pouchitis is refractory to the conventional therapies.[391,392]

Probiotic therapy is another option. In a placebo-controlled trial, 40 patients with quiescent chronic pouchitis were randomized to either an oral probiotic preparation (VSL#3) or placebo for 9 months. The relapse rate of probiotic-treated patients was 15% compared with 100% in the placebo group, and all patients who discontinued probiotics had a relapse within 3 months.[393] This benefit has been replicated in another study and extended to prophylaxis of pouchitis onset by initiating probiotic therapy immediately following ileostomy closure.[394,395]

Other nonconventional therapies include nutritional replacement using known energy substrates for the bowel and bismuth carbomer enema. Bismuth has been used to treat pouchitis with varying results. An open-label study reported benefit of bismuth carbomer enemas in 10 (83%) of 12 patients with chronic pouchitis.[396] However, a placebo-controlled study failed to show benefit.[397] Another uncontrolled study reported improvement in 11 of 13 patients with chronic pouchitis treated with chewable bismuth subsalicylate tablets,[398] but this finding has not been confirmed in controlled trials.

In the only randomized comparison of glutamine and butyrate suppositories in patients with chronic pouchitis after withdrawal of all conventional therapies, 60% of patients treated with glutamine 1 g twice daily for 3 weeks entered remission compared with 33% of patients receiving butyrate 40 mM twice daily.[399] The results for bismuth carbomer enemas have been conflicting but do not appear to be effective treatment for chronic active pouchitis.[396,397] Finally, surgical options such as ileal pouch excision or reconstruction should be considered in cases refractory to medical therapies or cases in which the frequency or chronicity of pouchitis compromises the patient's quality of life.[400]

EXTRAINTESTINAL MANIFESTATIONS

Patients with UC commonly present with a wide range of systemic and local problems that may add to the complexity of treatment. These extraintestinal manifestations may affect virtually every organ system, but the most commonly involved organs are the skin, eyes, mouth, joints, and liver (Table 109–18). These extraintestinal complications are often classified by their relations to the activity of the colitis, but they may occur before, during,

Table 109–18 Common Extraintestinal Manifestations of Ulcerative Colitis

System	Manifestations
Musculoskeletal	Peripheral arthropathy
	Ankylosing spondylitis
	Sacroiliitis
	Osteopenia
	Osteoporosis
	Osteomalacia
	Osteonecrosis
Dermatologic	Erythema nodosum
	Pyoderma gangrenosum
	Oral ulcerations
	Angular stomatitis
	Aphthous stomatitis
	Pyostomatitis vegetans
	Psoriasis
	Sweet's syndrome (acute febrile neutrophilic dermatosis)
Ophthalmologic	Uveitis/iritis
	Episcleritis
	Scleritis
	Conjunctivitis
	Retinal vascular disease
Hematologic	Iron deficiency anemia
	Autoimmune hemolytic anemia
	Anemia of chronic disease
	Leukocytosis or thrombocytosis
	Leukopenia or thrombocytopenia
	Hypercoagulable state
	Coagulation abnormalities
Hepatobiliary	Steatosis
	Primary sclerosing cholangitis
	Pericholangitis
	Cholangiocarcinoma
	Autoimmune hepatitis

or following exacerbations of bowel disease. Manifestations that parallel disease activity usually improve on treatment of the colitis.

DERMATOLOGIC

The most common skin manifestations of UC are complications of drug treatment. These include hypersensitivity, photosensitivity, and urticarial rashes related to sulfasalazine and less commonly to mesalamines. Patients receiving glucocorticoids often develop acne, which can be distressing cosmetically. Other common dermatologic manifestations associated with UC are erythema nodosum and pyoderma gangrenosum. Erythema nodosum occurs in 2% to 4% of patients with UC. Its activity typically parallels the activity of the underlying bowel disease. Erythema nodosum also may occur as a drug reaction to the sulfapyridine component of sulfasalazine. It classically presents as single or multiple tender, raised, erythematous nodules on the extensor surfaces of the lower extremities. If possible, the diagnosis should be made clinically without biopsy, because biopsy

is associated with increased tendency to scar formation. Erythema nodosum usually responds to treatment of the UC. Severe or refractory cases may require systemic glucocorticoids or immunosuppressive therapy. Pyoderma gangrenosum is less frequent than erythema nodosum and occurs in 1% to 2% of patients. It is usually related to the activity of colitis but may present or persist despite inactive bowel disease. Lesions may be single or multiple and usually occur on the trunk or extremities but may develop on the face, breast, or sites of trauma, including stoma and intravenous sites.[401] The classic lesion begins as erythematous pustules or nodules that break down, ulcerate, and coalesce into a larger, tender, burrowing ulcer with irregular, violaceous edges.[402] Although the appearance can be dramatic, the ulcers are sterile. Histopathologically, pyoderma has the features of a sterile abscess with a marked neutrophilic infiltration. Pyoderma gangrenosum may resolve with treatment of the underlying colitis. Most cases usually respond to intralesional glucocorticoid injections or topical therapy with cromolyn sodium, mesalamine, glucocorticoids, or tacrolimus.[402-404] More severe cases may require systemic glucocorticoids, immunosuppressants, such as cyclosporine, azathioprine, methotrexate, and tacrolimus, dapsone, or infliximab.[405,406] Other less common skin manifestations associated with UC include Sweet's syndrome or acute febrile neutrophilic dermatosis, and pyodermite végétante Hallopeau. The latter has a similar presentation to pyoderma gangrenosum but also involves the mouth.

OCULAR

The two most common ocular manifestations associated with UC are episcleritis and uveitis, occurring in 5% to 8% of patients. Episcleritis is characterized by painless hyperemia of the sclera and conjunctiva without loss of vision. It typically parallels the activity of bowel disease and usually responds to anti-inflammatory therapy. In contrast, uveitis presents as an acute or subacute painful eye with visual blurring and often photophobia and headache. There is no significant change in visual acuity unless the posterior uveal structures or the retina is involved. Temporal correlation of uveitis with the activity of the colitis is less predictable than with episcleritis. Uveitis should receive prompt treatment with local steroid ocular drops to prevent progression to blindness. The occurrence of uveitis increases with the dose and duration of glucocorticoid usage. Glucocorticoid therapy can also lead to posterior subcapsular cataracts. Thus, patients receiving steroid therapy should be advised to undergo annual ophthalmologic examination.

ORAL

At least 10% of patients with UC develop oral aphthous ulcers. These lesions usually occur with flares of colitis and resolve on control of the bowel disease. Angular stomatitis and a sore tongue may be seen in patients with deficiencies of iron or other micronutrients (see Chapter 15). A rare oral lesion that may be seen in patients with

UC is pyostomatitis (pyoderma) vegetans, which appears as a pustular eruption of the oral mucosa resulting in a cobblestone appearance.[407]

MUSCULOSKELETAL

Musculoskeletal abnormalities associated with UC can be broadly grouped into rheumatologic disorders and metabolic bone diseases. Peripheral arthropathy occurs in 5% to 20% of patients with UC. The risk of arthropathy increases with the extent of colonic disease. Peripheral arthropathy can be classified into two distinct types (Table 109–19).[408] Type 1 is asymmetrical and pauciarticular, affecting fewer than five joints and typically involving the large joints (knees, elbows, ankles). It usually manifests as acute, self-limited episodes that parallel the underlying bowel disease activity. Type 2 arthropathy is symmetrical and polyarticular, affecting five or more joints and typically involving the small joints. This type presents with persistent symptoms independent of the colitis activity. Both forms are nondeforming and seronegative. The involved joints are swollen, erythematous, and hot. Peripheral arthropathy usually responds to treatment of the colitis. Rest, physical therapy, intra-articular glucocorticoid injections, and therapeutic arthrocentesis also may help control symptoms.

Axial arthropathy occurs less frequently than does peripheral arthropathy in patients with UC, and includes sacroiliitis and spondylitis. Isolated sacroiliitis occurs in 10% to 15% of patients, but the incidence may be higher based on MR imaging. It does not usually parallel the activity of the bowel disease. The typical symptom is low back pain, but some patients may be asymptomatic. Most patients with sacroiliitis are HLA-B27 negative and do not progress to ankylosing spondylitis. Ankylosing spondylitis occurs in 1% to 2% of patients with UC, and most of these patients are HLA-B27 positive. Symptoms of ankylosing spondylitis may appear long before or after the onset of the intestinal symptoms and are independent of the activity of colitis. Patients often experience severe onset of back pain at a young age, usually associated with morning stiffness and exacerbated by periods of rest. The course of ankylosing spondylitis is progressive, resulting in permanent skeletal damage. Radiologic films in early stages may be normal or show only minimal sclerosis. Advanced stages are characterized by a "bamboo spine," with squaring of vertebral bodies, bony proliferation, and ankylosis. Treatment of axial arthropathy is similar to that for peripheral arthropathy, except that control of the underlying colitis does not alter the progressive nature of ankylosing spondylitis. Clinical success with anti-TNF therapy also has been reported.[409]

Patients with UC may develop low bone mineral density, owing to several factors, including glucocorticoid therapy, low physical activity, and possibly inflammatory cytokines. In general, individuals with UC who have not been treated with glucocorticoids are not considered to be at increased risk of osteopenia or osteoporosis. Bone densitometry (dual-energy x-ray absortiometry [DEXA] scan) at 1- to 2-year intervals is recommended for individuals who have received glucocorticoids at high dose or for long duration. Osteonecrosis, also known as *avascular* or *aseptic necrosis of bone* or *osteochondritis dissecans*, is a less common but serious complication in patients with UC. Patients typically present with joint swelling and pain exacerbated by motion. Most cases involve the hips and are bilateral, but the knees and shoulders may be affected. The most important risk factor for osteonecrosis is glucocorticoid therapy, with one series reporting a 4% incidence of osteonecrosis within 6 months of glucocorticoid therapy in patients with IBD.[410] The concurrent use of total parenteral nutrition is another risk factor. Early diagnosis by MR imaging or bone scan is essential for proper treatment, including medical management, cortical decompression, and arthroplasty.

HEPATOBILIARY

A wide range of hepatobiliary complications is associated with UC. Mild elevations in serum aminotransferase and alkaline phosphatase levels are common in severe attacks of UC. In most cases, the levels return to normal once remission is achieved. These abnormalities are thought to be related to a combination of factors, including malnutrition, sepsis, and fatty liver. An excess of fat in the hepatocytes is found in 60% of patients who undergo urgent colectomy for severe colitis.

The most important hepatobiliary complication associated with UC is PSC, which occurs in approximately 3% of patients (see Chapter 65). PSC is a chronic inflammatory disease of the biliary tree resulting in fibrosis and

Table 109–19 Types of Peripheral Arthropathy Associated with Ulcerative Colitis (UC)

Feature	Type 1 (Pauciarticular)	Type 2 (Polyarticular)
Frequency in UC	35%	24%
Number of joints affected	<5	≥5
Joints affected	Mainly large joints	Mainly small joints
Joints affected	Knee > ankle > wrist > elbow > MCP > hip > shoulder	MCP > knee > PIP > wrist > ankle > elbow > shoulder
Duration of attacks	<10 wk (median 5 wk)	Months to years (median 3 yr)
Association with bowel disease activity	Parallel	Independent

MCP, metacarpophalangeal joint; PIP, proximal interphalangeal joint.
Adapted from Su C, Judge TA, Lichtenstein GR: Extraintestinal manifestations of inflammatory bowel disease. Gastroenterol Clin North Am 31:307, 2002.

eventual cirrhosis and hepatic failure. Either or both intrahepatic and extrahepatic ducts may be involved. It is characterized radiologically by beading, irregularity, and stricturing of the bile ducts. The diagnosis of PSC is made on either endoscopic retrograde cholangiography or MR cholangiography. A liver biopsy may support the diagnosis but rarely is diagnostic. The classic histopathology of PSC on liver biopsy is the "onion skin" pattern with concentric fibrosis around the small bile ducts and ultimately obliteration of the ducts. The histologic appearance can be variable, however, ranging from chronic inflammatory infiltration in the portal tracts to cirrhosis. PSC should be excluded in patients with UC who have persistently abnormal liver tests or evidence of chronic liver disease. PSC is independent of the underlying colitis and it usually follows a progressive course after many years of stable disease. Unfortunately, no treatment has been shown definitively to be effective. Ursodeoxycholic acid may slow disease progression. Patients with a dominant extrahepatic biliary stricture may benefit from endoscopic dilatation or stent placement. Patients who develop end-stage liver disease require liver transplantation. Additionally, patients with PSC are at a significantly increased risk of cholangiocarcinoma.

HEMATOLOGIC

The occurrence of hypercoagulability is a well-recognized complication of UC. The incidence of thromboembolic events in patients with UC varies widely in different studies but most commonly manifest as deep venous thrombosis or pulmonary embolism; renal artery thrombosis, cerebrovascular accidents, coronary artery thrombosis, and venous thrombosis of mesenteric, portal, and hepatic vessels all have been reported.[411-413] The cause of the thromboembolism is multifactorial. Physiologically, microvascular activation of coagulation is present in the inflammatory states of colitis. A variety of coagulation and platelet abnormalities may be present in patients with UC, particularly those with severe disease, and include thrombocytosis; increased levels of fibrinogen, coagulation factors V and VIII and plasminogen activator inhibitor; and decreased levels of antithrombin III, proteins C and S, factor V Leiden, and tissue plasminogen activator. Although there is no increased frequency of specific coagulation abnormalities in patients with UC, there may be an increased incidence of factor V Leiden mutation in patients with thromboembolic complications associated with UC.[414-416] Patients with these complications should be treated with anticoagulants, just as in other patient populations. Although there may be concerns of an increased risk of gastrointestinal bleeding with anticoagulation, it generally is safe and rarely is complicated by colonic bleeding.

Another common hematologic complication is anemia. The anemia in patients with UC may be a result of chronic gastrointestinal blood loss, chronic disease, folate deficiency from sulfasalazine therapy, or autoimmune hemolysis. Autoimmune hemolytic anemia, usually Coombs positive, may be related to sepsis or glucose-6-phosphate dehydrogenase deficiency in patients on sulfasalazine.

OTHER MANIFESTATIONS

Secondary systemic amyloidosis is a rare but serious complication associated with UC.[417] Amyloidosis in these patients usually affects the kidney and presents with proteinuria followed by nephrotic syndrome and subsequent renal insufficiency. Diagnosis is made with a fat pad aspiration, or alternatively, biopsies from the liver, rectum, or kidney. Pericarditis, pleuropericarditis, and constrictive pericarditis have been reported in patients with UC,[418-421] although this complication also may be related to mesalamine therapy.[422,423] The pathogenesis of these complications is unknown, and their true association with UC is uncertain. Patients with UC may also develop abnormalities in pulmonary function, including an increase in functional reserve capacity and a decrease in diffusion capacity.[424] Other pulmonary diseases that have been described in patients with UC include bronchiectasis, bronchiolitis, fibrosing alveolitis, pulmonary fibrosis, and pulmonary vasculitis.[425-427]

REFERENCES

1. Wilks S: Lectures on Pathological Anatomy. London, Ongman, Brown, Green, Longman, & Roberts, 1859.
2. Wilks S: Morbid appearances in the intestines of Miss Bankes. Med Times Gazette 1859, p 264.
3. Hawkins HP: An address on the natural history of ulcerative colitis and its bearing on treatment. BMJ 765, 1909.
4. Hurst AF: Ulcerative colitis. Guy Hosp Rep 71:26, 1909.
5. Loftus EV Jr: Clinical epidemiology of inflammatory bowel disease: Incidence, prevalence, and environmental influences. Gastroenterology 126:1504, 2004.
6. Shivananda S, Lennard-Jones J, Logan R, et al: Incidence of inflammatory bowel disease across Europe: Is there a difference between north and south? Results of the European Collaborative Study on Inflammatory Bowel Disease (EC-IBD). Gut 39:690, 1996.
7. Sandler RS, Loftus EV: Epidemiology of inflammatory bowel diseases. In Sartor RB, Sandborn WJ (eds): Kirsner's Inflammatory Bowel Diseases, 6th ed. Philadelphia, WB Saunders, 2004, p 245.
8. Calkins BM, Lilienfeld AM, Garland CF, et al: Trends in incidence rates of ulcerative colitis and Crohn's disease. Dig Dis Sci 29:913, 1984.
9. Hiatt RA, Kaufman L: Epidemiology of inflammatory bowel disease in a defined northern California population. West J Med 149:541, 1988.
10. Wright JP, Froggatt J, O'Keefe EA, et al: The epidemiology of inflammatory bowel disease in Cape Town 1980-1984. S Afr Med J 70:10, 1986.
11. Yoshida Y, Murata Y: Inflammatory bowel disease in Japan: Studies of epidemiology and etiopathogenesis. Med Clin North Am 74:67, 1990.
12. Lee YM, Fock K, See SJ, et al: Racial differences in the prevalence of ulcerative colitis and Crohn's disease in Singapore. J Gastroenterol Hepatol 15:622, 2000.
13. Yang SK, Hong WS, Min YI, et al: Incidence and prevalence of ulcerative colitis in the Songpa-Kangdong District, Seoul, Korea, 1986-1997. J Gastroenterol Hepatol 15:1037, 2000.
14. Probert CS, Jayanthi V, Rampton DS, et al: Epidemiology of inflammatory bowel disease in different ethnic and religious groups: Limitations and aetiological clues. Int J Colorectal Dis 11:25, 1996.

15. Probert CS, Jayanthi V, Pinder D, et al: Epidemiological study of ulcerative proctocolitis in Indian migrants and the indigenous population of Leicestershire. Gut 33:687, 1992.

16. Carr I, Mayberry JF: The effects of migration on ulcerative colitis: A three-year prospective study among Europeans and first- and second- generation South Asians in Leicester (1991-1994). Am J Gastroenterol 94:2918, 1999.

17. Satsangi J, Jewell DP, Rosenberg WM, et al: Genetics of inflammatory bowel disease. Gut 35:696, 1994.

18. Yang H, McElree C, Roth MP, et al: Familial empirical risks for inflammatory bowel disease: Differences between Jews and non-Jews. Gut 34:517, 1993.

19. Laharie D, Debeugny S, Peeters M, et al: Inflammatory bowel disease in spouses and their offspring. Gastroenterology 120:816, 2001.

20. Satsangi J, Grootscholten C, Holt H, et al: Clinical patterns of familial inflammatory bowel disease. Gut 38:738, 1996.

21. Orholm M, Binder V, Sorensen TI, et al: Concordance of inflammatory bowel disease among Danish twins: Results of a nationwide study. Scand J Gastroenterol 35:1075, 2000.

22. Thompson NP, Driscoll R, Pounder RE, et al: Genetics versus environment in inflammatory bowel disease: Results of a British twin study. BMJ 312:95, 1996.

23. Tysk C, Lindberg E, Jarnerot G, et al: Ulcerative colitis and Crohn's disease in an unselected population of monozygotic and dizygotic twins: A study of heritability and the influence of smoking. Gut 29:990, 1988.

24. Lee JC, Lennard-Jones JE: Inflammatory bowel disease in 67 families each with three or more affected first-degree relatives. Gastroenterology 111:587, 1996.

25. Satsangi J, Parkes M, Louis E, et al: Two-stage genome-wide search in inflammatory bowel disease provides evidence for susceptibility loci on chromosomes 3, 7, and 12. Nat Genet 14:199, 1996.

26. van Heel DA, Satsangi J, Carey AH, et al: Inflammatory bowel disease: Progress toward a gene. Can J Gastroenterol 14:207, 2000.

27. Parkes M, Barmada MM, Satsangi J, et al: The IBD2 locus shows linkage heterogeneity between ulcerative colitis and Crohn disease. Am J Hum Genet 67:1605, 2000.

28. Schwab M, Schaeffeler E, Marx C, et al: Association between the C3435T MDR1 gene polymorphism and susceptibility for ulcerative colitis. Gastroenterology 124:26, 2003.

29. Panwala CM, Jones JC, Viney JL: A novel model of inflammatory bowel disease: Mice deficient for the multiple drug resistance gene, *mdr1a*, spontaneously develop colitis. J Immunol 161:5733, 1998.

30. Maggio-Price L, Shows D, Waggie K, et al: *Helicobacter bilis* infection accelerates and *H. hepaticus* infection delays the development of colitis in multiple drug resistance-deficient (mdr1a−/−) mice. Am J Pathol 160:739, 2002.

31. Hoffmeyer S, Burk O, von Richter O, et al: Functional polymorphisms of the human multidrug-resistance gene: Multiple-sequence variations and correlation of one allele with P-glycoprotein expression and activity in vivo. Proc Natl Acad Sci U S A 97:3473, 2000.

32. Schwab M, Schaeffeler E, Marx C, et al: Association between the C3435T *MDR1* gene polymorphism and susceptibility for ulcerative colitis. Gastroenterology 124:26, 2003.

33. Chadwick VS, Anderson RP: Inflammatory products of commensal bacteria and gastrointestinal disorders. Dig Dis 8:253, 1990.

34. Fabia R, Ar'Rajab A, Johansson ML, et al: Impairment of bacterial flora in human ulcerative colitis and experimental colitis in the rat. Digestion 54:248, 1993.

35. Schultz M, Veltkamp C, Dieleman LA, et al: *Lactobacillus plantarum* 299V in the treatment and prevention of spontaneous colitis in interleukin-10-deficient mice. Inflamm Bowel Dis 8:71, 2002.

36. Fabia R, Ar'Rajab A, Johansson ML, et al: The effect of exogenous administration of *Lactobacillus reuteri* R2LC and oat fiber on acetic acid-induced colitis in the rat. Scand J Gastroenterol 28:155, 1993.

37. Duchmann R, Kaiser I, Hermann E, et al: Tolerance exists towards resident intestinal flora but is broken in active inflammatory bowel disease (IBD). Clin Exp Immunol 102:448, 1995.

38. Duchmann R, Schmitt E, Knolle P, et al. Tolerance toward resident intestinal flora in mice is abrogated in experimental colitis and restored by treatment with interleukin-10 or antibodies to interleukin-12. Eur J Immunol 26:934, 1996.

39. Sartor RB: Microbial influences in inflammatory bowel diseases: Role in pathogenesis and clinical implications. In Sartor RB, Sandborn WJ (eds): Kirsner's Inflammatory Bowel Diseases, 6th ed. Philadelphia, WB Saunders, 2004, p 138.

40. Boyko EJ, Perera DR, Koepsell TD, et al: Effects of cigarette smoking on the clinical course of ulcerative colitis. Scand J Gastroenterol 23:1147, 1988.

41. Lindberg E, Tysk C, Andersson K, et al: Smoking and inflammatory bowel disease: A case control study. Gut 29:352, 1988.

42. Merrett MN, Mortensen N, Kettlewell M, et al: Smoking may prevent pouchitis in patients with restorative proctocolectomy for ulcerative colitis. Gut 38:362, 1996.

43. Sandler RS, Sandler DP, McDonnell CW, et al: Childhood exposure to smoke and risk of ulcerative colitis. Am J Epidemiol 135:603, 1992.

44. Lashner BA, Shaheen NJ, Hanauer SB, et al: Passive smoking is associated with an increased risk of developing inflammatory bowel disease in children. Am J Gastoenterol 88:356, 1993.

45. Truelove SC: Ulcerative colitis provoked by milk. BMJ 5220:154, 1961.

46. Wright R, Truelove SC: A controlled therapeutic trial of various diets in ulcerative colitis. BMJ 5454:138, 1965.

47. Andersen AFR: Ulcerative colitis—an allergic phenomenon. Am J Dig Dis 9:91, 1942.

48. Glassman MS, Newman LJ, Berezin S, et al: Cow's milk protein sensitivity during infancy in patients with inflammatory bowel disease. Am J Gastroenterol 85:838, 1990.

49. McIntyre PB, Powell-Tuck J, Wood SR, et al: Controlled trial of bowel rest in the treatment of severe acute colitis. Gut 27:481, 1986.

50. Bonfils S, Hervoir P, Girodet J, et al: Acute spontaneously recovering ulcerating colitis (ARUC): Report of six cases. Am J Dig Dis 22:429, 1977.

51. Heron HC, Khubchandani IT, Trimpi HD, et al: Evanescent colitis. Dis Colon Rectum 24:555, 1981.

52. Kilpatrick ZM, Silverman JF, Betancourt E, et al: Vascular occlusion of the colon and oral contraceptives: Possible relation. N Engl J Med 278:438, 1968.

53. Vessey M, Jewell D, Smith A, et al: Chronic inflammatory bowel disease, cigarette smoking, and use of oral contraceptives: Findings in a large cohort study of women of childbearing age. BMJ 292:1101, 1986.

54. Godet PG, May GR, Sutherland LR: Meta-analysis of the role of oral contraceptive agents in inflammatory bowel disease. Gut 37:668, 1995.

55. Corrao G, Tragnone A, Caprilli R, et al: Risk of inflammatory bowel disease attributable to smoking, oral contraception and breastfeeding in Italy: A nationwide case-control study. Cooperative Investigators of the Italian Group for the Study of the Colon and the Rectum (GISC). Int J Epidemiol 27:397, 1998.

56. Whorwell PJ, Holdstock G, Whorwell GM, et al: Bottle feeding, early gastroenteritis, and inflammatory bowel disease. BMJ 1:382, 1979.

57. Gilat T, Hacohen D, Lilos P, et al: Childhood factors in ulcerative colitis and Crohn's disease: An international cooperative study. Scand J Gastroenterol 22:1009, 1987.

58. Rutgeerts P, D'Haens G, Hiele M, et al: Appendectomy protects against ulcerative colitis. Gastroenterology 106:1251, 1994.

59. Smithson JE, Radford-Smith G, Jewell GP: Appendectomy and tonsillectomy in patients with inflammatory bowel disease. J Clin Gastroenterol 21:283, 1995.

60. Hallas J, Gaist D, Sorensen HT: Does appendectomy reduce the risk of ulcerative colitis? Epidemiology 15:173, 2004.

61. Kett K, Rognum TO, Brandtzaeg P: Mucosal subclass distribution of immunoglobulin G-producing cells is different in ulcerative colitis and Crohn's disease of the colon. Gastroenterology 93:919, 1987.

62. Scott MG, Nahm MH, Macke K, et al: Spontaneous secretion of IgG subclasses by intestinal mononuclear cells: Differences between ulcerative colitis, Crohn's disease, and controls. Clin Exp Immunol 66:209, 1986.

63. Snook JA, de Silva HJ, Jewell DP: The association of autoimmune disorders with inflammatory bowel disease. Q J Med 72:835, 1989.

64. Aronson RA, Cook SL, Roche JK: Sensitization to epithelial antigens in chronic mucosal inflammatory disease: I. Purification, characterization, and immune reactivity of murine epithelial cell-associated components (ECAC). J Immunol 131:2796, 1983.

65. Das KM, Dasgupta A, Mandal A, et al: Autoimmunity to cytoskeletal protein tropomyosin: A clue to the pathogenetic mechanism for ulcerative colitis. J Immunol 150:2487, 1993.

66. Bhagat S, Das KM: A shared and unique peptide in the human colon, eye, and joint detected by a monoclonal antibody. Gastroenterology 107:103, 1994.

67. Das KM, Vecchi M, Sakamaki S: A shared and unique epitope(s) on human colon, skin, and biliary epithelium detected by a monoclonal antibody. Gastroenterology 98:464, 1990.

68. Saxon A, Shanahan F, Landers C, et al: A distinct subset of antineutrophil cytoplasmic antibodies is associated with inflammatory bowel disease. J Allergy Clin Immunol 86:202, 1990.

69. Seibold F, Slametschka D, Gregor M, et al: Neutrophil autoantibodies: A genetic marker in primary sclerosing cholangitis and ulcerative colitis. Gastroenterology 107:532, 1994.

70. Shanahan F: Neutrophil autoantibodies in inflammatory bowel disease: Are they important? Gastroenterology 107:586, 1994.

71. Terjung B, Spengler U, Sauerbruch T, et al: "Atypical p-ANCA" in IBD and hepatobiliary disorders react with a 50-kilodalton nuclear envelope protein of neutrophils and myeloid cell lines. Gastroenterology 119:310, 2000.

72. Vecchi M, Bianchi MB, Sinico RA, et al: Antibodies to neutrophil cytoplasm in Italian patients with ulcerative colitis: Sensitivity, specificity, and recognition of putative antigens. Digestion 55:34, 1994.

73. Sandborn WJ, Landers CJ, Tremaine WJ, et al: Antineutrophil cytoplasmic antibody correlates with chronic pouchitis after ileal pouch-anal anastomosis. Am J Gastroenterol 90:740, 1995.

74. Hamann A, Andrew DP, Jablonski-Westrich D, et al: Role of alpha 4-integrins in lymphocyte homing to mucosal tissues in vivo. J Immunol 152:3282, 1994.

75. Senju M, Wu KC, Mahida YR, et al: Two-color immunofluorescence and flow cytometric analysis of lamina propria lymphocyte subsets in ulcerative colitis and Crohn's disease. Dig Dis Sci 36:1453, 1991.

76. Gibson PR, van de Pol E, Pullman W, Doe WF: Lysis of colonic epithelial cells by allogeneic mononuclear and lymphokine activated killer cells derived from peripheral blood

77. and intestinal mucosa: Evidence against a pathogenic role in inflammatory bowel disease. Gut 29:1076, 1988.

77. Dalton HR, Hoang P, Jewell DP: Antigen induced suppression in peripheral blood and lamina propria mononuclear cells in inflammatory bowel disease. Gut 33:324, 1992.

78. Trejdosiewicz LK, Smart CJ, Oakes DJ, et al: Expression of T-cell receptors TcR1 (gamma/delta) and TcR2 (alpha/beta) in the human intestinal mucosa. Immunology 68:7, 1989.

79. Raedler A, Fraenkel S, Klose G, et al: Elevated numbers of peripheral T cells in inflammatory bowel diseases displaying T9 antigen and Fc alpha receptors. Clin Exp Immunol 60:518, 1985.

80. Duchmann R, Strober W, Alling DW, et al: T-cell receptor Vβ gene expression in inflammatory bowel disease lamina propria lymphocytes: Evidence for altered Vβ gene usage. Inflamm Bowel Dis 1:184, 1995.

81. Meuret G, Bitzi A, Hammer B: Macrophage turnover in Crohn's disease and ulcerative colitis. Gastroenterology 74:501, 1978.

82. Mayer L, Shlien R: Evidence for function of Ia molecules on gut epithelial cells in man. J Exp Med 166:1471, 1987.

83. Reinecker HC, Podolsky DK: Human intestinal epithelial cells express functional cytokine receptors sharing the common gamma c chain of the interleukin-2 receptor. Proc Natl Acad Sci U S A 92:8353, 1995.

84. Watanabe M, Ueno Y, Yajima T, et al: Interleukin-7 is produced by human intestinal epithelial cells and regulates the proliferation of intestinal mucosal lymphocytes. J Clin Invest 95:2945, 1995.

85. Jung HC, Eckmann L, Yang SK, et al: A distinct array of proinflammatory cytokines is expressed in human colon epithelial cells in response to bacterial invasion. J Clin Invest 95:55, 1995.

86. Huang GT, Eckmann L, Savidge TC, et al: Infection of human intestinal epithelial cells with invasive bacteria upregulates apical intercellular adhesion molecule-1 (ICAM)-1) expression and neutrophil adhesion. J Clin Invest 98:572, 1996.

87. Allan A, Bristol JB, Williamson RC: Crypt cell production rate in ulcerative proctocolitis: Differential increments in remission and relapse. Gut 26:999, 1985.

88. Gibson PR, van de PE, Barratt PJ, et al: Ulcerative colitis—a disease characterised by the abnormal colonic epithelial cell? Gut 29:516, 1988.

89. Podolsky DK, Isselbacher KJ: Glycoprotein composition of colonic mucosa: Specific alterations in ulcerative colitis. Gastroenterology 87:991, 1984.

90. Hermiston ML, Gordon JI: Inflammatory bowel disease and adenomas in mice expressing a dominant negative N-cadherin. Science 270:1203, 1995.

91. Powrie F, Coffman RL: Cytokine regulation of T-cell function: Potential for therapeutic intervention. Immunol Today 14:270, 1993.

92. Smith KM, Eaton AD, Finlayson LM, et al: Oral tolerance. Am J Respir Crit Care Med 162:S175, 2000.

93. Boughton-Smith N, Pettipher R: Lipid mediators and cytokines in inflammatory bowel disease. Eur J Gastroenterol Hepatol 2:241, 1990.

94. Drossman DA, Ringel Y: Psychosocial factors in ulcerative colitis and Crohn's disease. In Sartor RB, Sandborn WJ (eds): Kirsner's Inflammatory Bowel Diseases, 6th ed. Philadelphia, WB Saunders, 2004, p 340.

95. Levenstein S, Prantera C, Varvo V, et al: Stress and exacerbation in ulcerative colitis: A prospective study of patients enrolled in remission. Am J Gastroenterol 95:1213, 2000.

96. Bitton A, Sewitch MJ, Peppercorn MA, et al: Psychosocial determinants of relapse in ulcerative colitis: A longitudinal study. Am J Gastroenterol 98:2203, 2003.

97. Langholz E, Munkholm P, Davidsen M, et al: Course of ulcerative colitis: Analysis of changes in disease activity over years. Gastroenterology 107:3, 1994.
98. D'Haens G, Geboes K, Peeters M, et al: Patchy cecal inflammation associated with distal ulcerative colitis: A prospective endoscopic study. Am J Gastroenterol 92:1275, 1997.
99. Surawicz CM, Belic L: Rectal biopsy helps to distinguish acute self-limited colitis from idiopathic inflammatory bowel disease. Gastroenterology 86:104, 1984.
100. Allison MC, Hamilton-Dutoit SJ, Dhillon AP, et al: The value of rectal biopsy in distinguishing self-limited colitis from early inflammatory bowel disease. Q J Med 65:985, 1987.
101. Both H, Torp-Pedersen K, Kreiner S, et al: Clinical appearance at diagnosis of ulcerative colitis and Crohn's disease in a regional patient group. Scand J Gastroenterol 18:987, 1983.
102. Pimentel M, Chang M, Chow EJ, et al: Identification of a prodromal period in Crohn's disease but not ulcerative colitis. Am J Gastroenterol 95:3458, 2000.
103. Rao SS, Holdsworth CD, Read NW: Symptoms and stool patterns in patients with ulcerative colitis. Gut 29:342, 1988.
104. Sandle GI, Higgs N, Crowe P, et al: Cellular basis for defective electrolyte transport in inflamed human colon. Gastroenterology 99:97, 1990.
105. Rao SS, Read NW, Davison PA, et al: Anorectal sensitivity and responses to rectal distention in patients with ulcerative colitis. Gastroenterology 93:1270, 1987.
106. Rao SS, Read NW, Brown C, et al: Studies on the mechanism of bowel disturbance in ulcerative colitis. Gastroenterology 93:934, 1987.
107. Sinclair TS, Brunt PW, Mowat NA: Nonspecific proctocolitis in northeastern Scotland: A community study. Gastroenterology 85:1, 1983.
108. Edwards FC, Truelove SC: The course and prognosis of ulcerative colitis. Gut 41:299, 1963.
109. Hendriksen C, Kreiner S, Binder V: Long-term prognosis in ulcerative colitis—based on results from a regional patient group from the county of Copenhagen. Gut 26:158, 1985.
110. Stonnington CM, Phillips SF, Zinsmeister AR, et al: Prognosis of chronic ulcerative colitis in a community. Gut 28:1261, 1987.
111. Ayres RC, Gillen CD, Walmsley RS, et al: Progression of ulcerative proctosigmoiditis: Incidence and factors influencing progression. Eur J Gastroenterol Hepatol 8:555, 1996.
112. Powell-Tuck J, Ritchie JK, Lennard-Jones JE: The prognosis of idiopathic proctitis. Scand J Gastroenterol 12:727, 1977.
113. Hendriksen C, Binder V: Social prognosis in patients with ulcerative colitis. BMJ 281:581, 1980.
114. Ritchie JK, Powell-Tuck J, Lennard-Jones JE: Clinical outcome of the first ten years of ulcerative colitis and proctitis. Lancet 1:1140, 1978.
115. Brostrom O, Monsen U, Nordenwall B, et al: Prognosis and mortality of ulcerative colitis in Stockholm County, 1955-1979. Scand J Gastroenterol 22:907, 1987.
116. Card T, Hubbard R, Logan RF: Mortality in inflammatory bowel disease: A population-based cohort study. Gastroenterology 125:1583, 2003.
117. Winther KV, Jess T, Langholz E, et al: Survival and cause-specific mortality in ulcerative colitis: Follow-up of a population-based cohort in Copenhagen County. Gastroenterology 125:1576, 2003.
118. Pera A, Bellando P, Caldera D, et al: Colonoscopy in inflammatory bowel disease: Diagnostic accuracy and proposal of an endoscopic score. Gastroenterology 92:181, 1987.
119. Buckell NA, Williams GT, Bartram CI, et al: Depth of ulceration in acute colitis: Correlation with outcome and clinical and radiologic features. Gastroenterology 79:19, 1980.
120. Greenfield C, Aguilar R Jr, Pounder RE, et al: *Clostridium difficile* and inflammatory bowel disease. Gut 24:713, 1983.
121. Mylonaki M, Langmead L, Pantes A, et al: Enteric infection in relapse of inflammatory bowel disease: Importance of microbiological examination of stool. Eur J Gastroenterol Hepatol 16:775, 2004.
122. Pfau P, Kochman ML, Furth EE, et al: Cytomegalovirus colitis complicating ulcerative colitis in the steroid-naive patient. Am J Gastroenterol 96:895, 2001.
123. Truelove SC, Witts LJ: Cortisone in ulcerative colitis: Final report on a therapeutic trial. BMJ 2:1041, 1955.
124. Schroeder KW, Tremaine WJ, Ilstrup DM: Coated oral 5-aminosalicylic acid therapy for mildly to moderately active ulcerative colitis: A randomized study. N Engl J Med 317:1625, 1987.
125. Sutherland LR, Martin F: 5-Aminosalicylic acid enemas in treatment of distal ulcerative colitis and proctitis in Canada. Dig Dis Sci 32:64S, 1987.
126. Sutherland LR, Martin F, Greer S, et al: 5-Aminosalicylic acid enema in the treatment of distal ulcerative colitis, proctosigmoiditis, and proctitis. Gastroenterology 92:1894, 1987.
127. Lichtiger S, Present DH, Kornbluth A, et al: Cyclosporine in severe ulcerative colitis refractory to steroid therapy. N Engl J Med 330:1841, 1994.
128. Rachmilewitz D: Coated mesalazine (5-aminosalicylic acid) versus sulphasalazine in the treatment of active ulcerative colitis: A randomised trial. BMJ 298:82, 1989.
129. Powell-Tuck J, Day DW, Buckell NA, et al: Correlations between defined sigmoidoscopic appearances and other measures of disease activity in ulcerative colitis. Dig Dis Sci 27:533, 1982.
130. Baron JH, Connell AM, Lennard-Jones JE: Variation between observers in describing mucosal appearances in proctocolitis. BMJ 5375:89, 1964.
131. Truelove SC, Richards WC: Biopsy studies in ulcerative colitis. BMJ 4979:1315, 1956.
132. Baron JH, Connell AM, Lennard-Jones JE: Sulphasalazine and salicylazosulphadimidine in ulcerative colitis. Lancet 1:1094, 1962.
133. Svartz N: Salazopyrin, a new sulfanilamide preparation. Acta Med Scand 110:577, 1942.
134. Azad Khan AK, Piris J, Truelove SC: An experiment to determine the active therapeutic moiety of sulphasalazine. Lancet 2:892, 1977.
135. Van Hees PA, Bakker JH, van Tongeren JH: Effect of sulphapyridine, 5-aminosalicylic acid, and placebo in patients with idiopathic proctitis: A study to determine the active therapeutic moiety of sulfasalazine. Gut 21:632, 1980.
136. Dick AP, Grayson MJ, Carpenter RG, et al: Controlled trial of sulphasalazine in the treatment of ulcerative colitis. Gut 5:437, 1964.
137. Sutherland L, Roth D, Beck P, et al: Oral 5-aminosalicylic acid for inducing remission in ulcerative colitis. Cochrane Database Syst Rev CD000543, 2000.
138. Sutherland LR, May GR, Shaffer EA: Sulfasalazine revisited: A meta-analysis of 5-aminosalicylic acid in the treatment of ulcerative colitis. Ann Intern Med 118:540, 1993.
139. Meyers S, Sachar DB, Present DH, et al: Olsalazine sodium in the treatment of ulcerative colitis among patients intolerant of sulfasalazine: A prospective, randomized, placebo-controlled, double-blind, dose-ranging clinical trial. Gastroenterology 93:1255, 1987.
140. Sninsky CA, Cort DH, Shanahan F, et al: Oral mesalamine (Asacol) for mildly to moderately active ulcerative colitis: A multicenter study. Ann Intern Med 115:350, 1991.
141. Sutherland L, MacDonald JK: Oral 5-aminosalicylic acid for induction of remission in ulcerative colitis. Cochrane Database Syst Rev CD000543, 2003.
142. Green JR, Lobo AJ, Holdsworth CD, et al: Balsalazide is more effective and better tolerated than mesalamine in the treat-

ment of acute ulcerative colitis. The Abacus Investigator Group. Gastroenterology 114:15, 1998.

143. Pruitt R, Hanson J, Safdi M, et al: Balsalazide is superior to mesalamine in the time to improvement of signs and symptoms of acute mild-to-moderate ulcerative colitis. Am J Gastroenterol 97:3078, 2002.

144. Azad Khan AK, Howes DT, Piris J, et al: Optimum dose of sulphasalazine for maintenance treatment in ulcerative colitis. Gut 21:232, 1980.

145. Misiewicz JJ, Lond MB: Controlled trial of sulphasalazine in maintenance treatment of ulcerative colitis. Lancet 2:185, 1965.

146. Kiilerich S, Ladefoged K, Rannem T, et al: Prophylactic effects of olsalazine versus sulphasalazine during 12 months' maintenance treatment of ulcerative colitis. The Danish Olsalazine Study Group. Gut 33:252, 1992.

147. Hanauer S, Schwartz J, Robinson M, et al: Mesalamine capsules for treatment of active ulcerative colitis: Results of a controlled trial. Pentasa Study Group. Am J Gastroenterol 88:1188, 1993.

148. Sutherland L, Roth D, Beck P, et al: Oral 5-aminosalicylic acid for maintenance of remission in ulcerative colitis. Cochrane Database Syst Rev CD000544, 2002.

149. Kruis W, Schreiber S, Theuer D, et al: Low-dose balsalazide (1.5 g twice daily) and mesalazine (0.5 g three times daily) maintained remission of ulcerative colitis but high-dose balsalazide (3.0 g twice daily) was superior in preventing relapses. Gut 49:783, 2001.

150. Giaffer MH, O'Brien CJ, Holdsworth CD: Clinical tolerance to three 5-aminosalicylic acid releasing preparations in patients with inflammatory bowel disease intolerant or allergic to sulphasalazine. Aliment Pharmacol Ther 6:51, 1992.

151. Mansfield JC, Giaffer MH, Cann PA, et al: A double-blind comparison of balsalazide, 6.75 g, and sulfasalazine, 3 g, as sole therapy in the management of ulcerative colitis. Aliment Pharmacol Ther 16:69, 2002.

152. Loftus EV Jr, Kane SV, Bjorkman D: Systematic review: Short-term adverse effects of 5-aminosalicylic acid agents in the treatment of ulcerative colitis. Aliment Pharmacol Ther 19:179, 2004.

153. Marshall JK, Irvine EJ: Rectal aminosalicylate therapy for distal ulcerative colitis: A meta-analysis. Aliment Pharmacol Ther 9:293, 1995.

154. Cohen RD, Woseth DM, Thisted RA, et al: A meta-analysis and overview of the literature on treatment options for left-sided ulcerative colitis and ulcerative proctitis. Am J Gastroenterol 95:1263, 2000.

155. Kam L, Cohen H, Dooley C, et al: A comparison of mesalamine suspension enema and oral sulfasalazine for treatment of active distal ulcerative colitis in adults. Am J Gastroenterol 91:1338, 1996.

156. Campieri M, Gionchetti P, Belluzzi A, et al: Efficacy of 5-aminosalicylic acid enemas versus hydrocortisone enemas in ulcerative colitis. Dig Dis Sci 32:67S, 1987.

157. Safdi M, DeMicco M, Sninsky C, et al: A double-blind comparison of oral versus rectal mesalamine versus combination therapy in the treatment of distal ulcerative colitis. Am J Gastroenterol 92:1867, 1997.

158. Danish 5-ASA Group: Topical 5-aminosalicylic acid versus prednisolone in ulcerative proctosigmoiditis: A randomized, double-blind multicenter trial. Dig Dis Sci 32:598, 1987.

159. Campieri M, Paoluzi P, d'Albasio G, et al: Better quality of therapy with 5-ASA colonic foam in active ulcerative colitis: A multicenter comparative trial with 5-ASA enema. Dig Dis Sci 38:1843, 1993.

160. Andreoli A, Spinella S, Levenstein S, et al: 5-ASA enema versus oral sulphasalazine in maintaining remission in ulcerative colitis. Ital J Gastroenterol 26:121, 1994.

161. d'Albasio G, Pacini F, Camarri E, et al: Combined therapy with 5-aminosalicylic acid tablets and enemas for maintaining remission in ulcerative colitis: A randomized double-blind study. Am J Gastroenterol 92:1143, 1997.

162. Lennard-Jones JE, Longmore AJ, Newell AC: An assessment of prednisone, salazopyrine, and topical hydrocortisone used as outpatient treatment for ulcerative colitis. Gut 1:217, 1960.

163. Baron JH, Connell AM, Kanaghinis TG, et al: Outpatient treatment of ulcerative colitis. Comparison between three doses of oral prednisone. BMJ 5302:441, 1962.

164. Truelove SC, Jewell DP: Intensive intravenous regimen for severe attacks of ulcerative colitis. Lancet 1:1067, 1974.

165. Truelove SC, Willoughby CP, Lee EG, Kettlewell MG: Further experience in the treatment of severe attacks of ulcerative colitis. Lancet 2:1086, 1978.

166. Jarnerot G, Rolny P, Sandberg-Gertzen H: Intensive intravenous treatment of ulcerative colitis. Gastroenterol 89:1005, 1985.

167. Kaplan HP, Portnoy B, Binder HJ, et al: A controlled evaluation of intravenous adrenocorticotropic hormone and hydrocortisone in the treatment of acute colitis. Gastroenterology 69:91, 1975.

168. Meyers S, Sachar DB, Goldberg JD, et al: Corticotropin versus hydrocortisone in the intravenous treatment of ulcerative colitis: A prospective, randomized, double-blind clinical trial. Gastroenterology 85:351, 1983.

169. Kornbluth A, Marion JF, Salomon P, et al: How effective is current medical therapy for severe ulcerative and Crohn's colitis? An analytic review of selected trials. J Clin Gastroenterol 20:280, 1995.

170. Thalen BA, Axelsson BI, Andersson PH, et al: 6 alpha-Fluoro- and 6 alpha,9 alpha-difluoro-11 beta,21-dihydroxy-16 alpha,17 alpha-propylmethylenedioxypregn-4-ene-3,20-dione: Synthesis and evaluation of activity and kinetics of their C-22 epimers. Steroids 63:37, 1998.

171. Keller R, Stoll R, Foerster EC, et al: Oral budesonide therapy for steroid-dependent ulcerative colitis: A pilot trial. Aliment Pharmacol Ther 11:1047, 1997.

172. Lofberg R, Danielsson A, Suhr O, et al: Oral budesonide versus prednisolone in patients with active extensive and left-sided ulcerative colitis. Gastroenterology 110:1713, 1996.

173. Truelove SC: Treatment of ulcerative colitis with local hydrocortisone hemisuccinate sodium: A report on a controlled therapeutic trial. BMJ 2:1072, 1958.

174. Watkinson G: Treatment of ulcerative colitis with topical hydrocortisone hemisuccinate sodium. BMJ 2:1077, 1958.

175. Mulder CJ, Fockens P, Meijer JW, et al: Beclomethasone dipropionate (3 mg) versus 5-aminosalicylic acid (2 g) versus the combination of both (3 mg/2 g) as retention enemas in active ulcerative proctitis. Eur J Gastroenterol Hepatol 8:549, 1996.

176. Hanauer SB, Robinson M, Pruitt R, et al: Budesonide enema for the treatment of active, distal ulcerative colitis and proctitis: A dose-ranging study. U.S. Budesonide Enema Study Group. Gastroenterology 115:525, 1998.

177. Danish Budesonide Study Group: Budesonide enema in distal ulcerative colitis: A randomized dose-response trial with prednisolone enema as positive control. Scand J Gastroenterol 26:1225, 1991.

178. Danielsson A, Hellers G, Lyrenas E, et al: A controlled randomized trial of budesonide versus prednisolone retention enemas in active distal ulcerative colitis. Scand J Gastroenterol 22:987, 1987.

179. Lofberg R, Ostergaard TO, Langholz E, et al: Budesonide versus prednisolone retention enemas in active distal ulcerative colitis. Aliment Pharmacol Ther 8:623, 1994.

180. Lemann M, Galian A, Rutgeerts P, et al: Comparison of budesonide and 5-aminosalicylic acid enemas in active distal ulcerative colitis. Aliment Pharmacol Ther 9:557, 1995.

181. Lindgren S, Lofberg R, Bergholm L, et al: Effect of budesonide enema on remission and relapse rate in distal ulcerative colitis and proctitis. Scand J Gastroenterol 37:705, 2002.

182. Bar-Meir S, Fidder HH, Faszczyk M, et al: Budesonide foam vs. hydrocortisone acetate foam in the treatment of active ulcerative proctosigmoiditis. Dis Colon Rectum 46:929, 2003.

183. Weinshilboum RM, Sladek SL: Mercaptopurine pharmacogenetics: Monogenic inheritance of erythrocyte thiopurine methyltransferase activity. Am J Hum Genet 32:651, 1980.

184. Kirk AP, Lennard-Jones JE: Controlled trial of azathioprine in chronic ulcerative colitis. BMJ 284:1291, 1982.

185. Jewell DP, Truelove SC: Azathioprine in ulcerative colitis: Final report on controlled therapeutic trial. BMJ 4:627, 1974.

186. Caprilli R, Carratu R, Babbini M: Double-blind comparison of the effectiveness of azathioprine and sulfasalazine in idiopathic proctocolitis: Preliminary report. Am J Dig Dis 20:115, 1975.

187. Rosenberg JL, Wall AJ, Levin B, et al: A controlled trial of azathioprine in the management of chronic ulcerative colitis. Gastroenterology 69:96, 1975.

188. Adler DJ, Korelitz BI: The therapeutic efficacy of 6-mercaptopurine in refractory ulcerative colitis. Am J Gastroenterol 85:717, 1990.

189. Ardizzone S, Samolvico F, Bollani S, et al: Azathioprine is more effective than oral 5-ASA in the treatment of steroid-dependent ulcerative colitis [Abstract]. Gastroenterology 120:A127, 2001.

190. Hawthorne AB, Logan RF, Hawkey CJ, et al: Randomised controlled trial of azathioprine withdrawal in ulcerative colitis. BMJ 305:20, 1992.

191. Mantzaris GJ, Sfakianakis M, Archavlis E, et al: A prospective, randomized observer-blind 2-year trial of azathioprine monotherapy versus azathioprine and olsalazine for the maintenance of remission of steroid-dependent ulcerative colitis. Am J Gastroenterol 99:1122, 2004.

192. Ardizzone S, Molteni P, Imbesi V, et al: Azathioprine in steroid-resistant and steroid-dependent ulcerative colitis. J Clin Gastroenterol 25:330, 1997.

193. George J, Present DH, Pou R, et al: The long-term outcome of ulcerative colitis treated with 6-mercaptopurine. Am J Gastroenterol 91:1711, 1996.

194. Sood A, Midha V, Sood N, et al: Azathioprine versus sulfasalazine in maintenance of remission in severe ulcerative colitis. Indian J Gastroenterol 22:79, 2003.

195. Cohen RD, Stein R, Hanauer SB: Intravenous cyclosporin in ulcerative colitis: A five-year experience. Am J Gastroenterol 94:1587, 1999.

196. Fernandez-Banares F, Bertran X, Esteve-Comas M, et al: Azathioprine is useful in maintaining long-term remission induced by intravenous cyclosporine in steroid-refractory severe ulcerative colitis. Am J Gastroenterol 91:2498, 1996.

197. Domenech E, Garcia-Planella E, Bernal I, et al: Azathioprine without oral ciclosporin in the long-term maintenance of remission induced by intravenous ciclosporin in severe, steroid-refractory ulcerative colitis. Aliment Pharmacol Ther 16:2061, 2002.

198. Sandborn WJ: A review of immune modifier therapy for inflammatory bowel disease: Azathioprine, 6-mercaptopurine, cyclosporine, and methotrexate. Am J Gastroenterol 91:423, 1996.

199. Colonna T, Korelitz BI: The role of leukopenia in the 6-mercaptopurine-induced remission of refractory Crohn's disease. Am J Gastroenterol 89:362, 1994.

200. Markowitz J, Grancher K, Mandel F, et al: Relationship of leukopenia to 6-MP induced remission of Crohn's disease [Abstract]. J Pediatr Gastroenterol Nutr 27:A8, 1998.

201. Dubinsky MC, Lamothe S, Yang HY, et al: Pharmacogenomics and metabolite measurement for 6-mercaptopurine therapy in inflammatory bowel disease. Gastroenterology 118:705, 2000.

202. Sandborn WJ, Tremaine WJ, Wolf DC, et al: Lack of effect of intravenous administration on time to respond to azathioprine for steroid-treated Crohn's disease. North American Azathioprine Study Group. Gastroenterology 117:527, 1999.

203. Cuffari C, Hunt S, Bayless T: Utilisation of erythrocyte 6-thioguanine metabolite levels to optimise azathioprine therapy in patients with inflammatory bowel disease. Gut 48:642, 2001.

204. Su C, Wang S, Deren J, et al: Measurement of 6-TG levels in patients with IBD: Are all groups identical? [Abstract]. Gastroenterology 122:A78, 2002.

205. Dubinsky MC, Yang H, Hassard PV, et al: 6-MP metabolite profiles provide a biochemical explanation for 6-MP resistance in patients with inflammatory bowel disease. Gastroenterology 122:904, 2002.

206. Lennard L, Van Loon JA, Weinshilboum RM: Pharmacogenetics of acute azathioprine toxicity: Relationship to thiopurine methyltransferase genetic polymorphism. Clin Pharmacol Ther 46:149, 1989.

207. Lichtenstein GR: Use of laboratory testing to guide 6-mercaptopurine/azathioprine therapy. Gastroenterology 127:1558, 2004.

208. Colombel JF, Ferrari N, Debuysere H, et al: Genotypic analysis of thiopurine S-methyltransferase in patients with Crohn's disease and severe myelosuppression during azathioprine therapy. Gastroenterology 118:1025, 2000.

209. Steinhart AH, Baker JP, Brzezinski A, et al: Azathioprine therapy in chronic ulcerative colitis. J Clin Gastroenterol 12:271, 1990.

210. Sandborn W, Sutherland L, Pearson D, et al: Azathioprine or 6-mercaptopurine for inducing remission of Crohn's disease. Cochrane Database Syst Rev CD000545, 2000.

211. Kim PS, Zlatanic J, Korelitz BI, et al: Optimum duration of treatment with 6-mercaptopurine for Crohn's disease. Am J Gastroenterol 94:3254, 1999.

212. Fraser AG, Orchard TR, Jewell DP: The efficacy of azathioprine for the treatment of inflammatory bowel disease: A 30-year review. Gut 50:485, 2002.

213. Connell WR, Kamm MA, Ritchie JK, et al: Bone marrow toxicity caused by azathioprine in inflammatory bowel disease: Twenty-seven years of experience. Gut 34:1081, 1993.

214. Su CG, Stein RB, Lewis JD, et al: Azathioprine or 6-mercaptopurine for inflammatory bowel disease: Do risks outweigh benefits? Dig Liver Dis 32:518, 2000.

215. Present DH, Meltzer SJ, Krumholz MP, et al: 6-Mercaptopurine in the management of inflammatory bowel disease: Short- and long-term toxicity. Ann Intern Med 111:641, 1989.

216. Lewis LD, Benin A, Szumlanski CL, et al: Olsalazine and 6-mercaptopurine-related bone marrow suppression: A possible drug-drug interaction. Clin Pharmacol Ther 62:464, 1997.

217. Lowry PW, Szumlanski CL, Weinshilboum RM, et al: Balsalazide and azathioprine or 6-mercaptopurine: Evidence for a potentially serious drug interaction. Gastroenterology 116:1505, 1999.

218. Szumlanski CL, Weinshilboum RM: Sulphasalazine inhibition of thiopurine methyltransferase: Possible mechanism for interaction with 6-mercaptopurine and azathioprine. Br J Clin Pharmacol 39:456, 1995.

219. Korelitz BI, Zlatanic J, Goel F, et al: Allergic reactions to 6-mercaptopurine during treatment of inflammatory bowel disease. J Clin Gastroenterol 28:341, 1999.

220. Cheng BK, Lichtenstein GR: Are individuals with Crohn's disease who are intolerant to 6-mercaptopurine able to tol-

erate azathioprine? [Abstract]. Gastroenterology 118:A1336, 2000.

221. Warman JI, Korelitz BI, Fleisher MR, et al: Cumulative experience with short- and long-term toxicity to 6-mercaptopurine in the treatment of Crohn's disease and ulcerative colitis. J Clin Gastroenterol 37:220, 2003.

222. Haber CJ, Meltzer SJ, Present DH, et al: Nature and course of pancreatitis caused by 6-mercaptopurine in the treatment of inflammatory bowel disease. Gastroenterology 91:982, 1986.

223. Bouhnik Y, Lemann M, Mary JY, et al: Long-term follow-up of patients with Crohn's disease treated with azathioprine or 6-mercaptopurine. Lancet 347:215, 1996.

224. Lewis JD, Bilker WB, Brensinger C, et al: Inflammatory bowel disease is not associated with an increased risk of lymphoma. Gastroenterology 121:1080, 2001.

225. Connell WR, Kamm MA, Dickson M, et al: Long-term neoplasia risk after azathioprine treatment in inflammatory bowel disease. Lancet 343:1249, 1994.

226. Dayharsh GA, Loftus EV Jr, Sandborn WJ, et al: Epstein-Barr virus–positive lymphoma in patients with inflammatory bowel disease treated with azathioprine or 6-mercaptopurine. Gastroenterology 122:72, 2002.

227. Kornbluth A, Lichtiger S, Present D, et al: Long-term results of oral cyclosporin in patients with severe ulcerative colitis: A double-blind randomized multicenter trial [Abstract]. Gastroenterology 106:A714, 1994.

228. D'Haens G, Lemmens L, Geboes K, et al: Intravenous cyclosporine versus intravenous corticosteroids as single therapy for severe attacks of ulcerative colitis. Gastroenterology 120:1323, 2001.

229. Van Assche G, D'Haens G, Noman M, et al: Randomized, double-blind comparison of 4 mg/kg versus 2 mg/kg intravenous cyclosporine in severe ulcerative colitis. Gastroenterology 125:1025, 2003.

230. Stein R, Cohen R, Hanauer S: Complications during cyclosporine therapy for inflammatory bowel disease [Abstract]. Gastroenterology 112:A1096, 1997.

231. Kozarek RA, Patterson DJ, Gelfand MD, et al: Methotrexate induces clinical and histologic remission in patients with refractory inflammatory bowel disease. Ann Intern Med 110:353, 1989.

232. Baron TH, Truss CD, Elson CO: Low-dose oral methotrexate in refractory inflammatory bowel disease. Dig Dis Sci 38:1851, 1993.

233. Oren R, Arber N, Odes S, et al: Methotrexate in chronic active ulcerative colitis: A double-blind, randomized, Israeli multicenter trial. Gastroenterology 110:1416, 1996.

234. Orth T, Peters M, Schlaak JF, et al: Mycophenolate mofetil versus azathioprine in patients with chronic active ulcerative colitis: A 12-month pilot study. Am J Gastroenterol 95:1201, 2000.

235. Ford AC, Towler RJ, Moayyedi P, et al: Mycophenolate mofetil in refractory inflammatory bowel disease. Aliment Pharmacol Ther 17:1365, 2003.

236. Fellermann K, Steffen M, Stein J, et al: Mycophenolate mofetil: Lack of efficacy in chronic active inflammatory bowel disease. Aliment Pharmacol Ther 14:171, 2000.

237. Fellermann K, Ludwig D, Stahl M, et al: Steroid-unresponsive acute attacks of inflammatory bowel disease: Immunomodulation by tacrolimus (FK506). Am J Gastroenterol 93:1860, 1998.

238. Fellermann K, Tanko Z, Herrlinger KR, et al: Response of refractory colitis to intravenous or oral tacrolimus (FK506). Inflamm Bowel Dis 8:317, 2002.

239. Hogenauer C, Wenzl HH, Hinterleitner TA, et al: Effect of oral tacrolimus (FK 506) on steroid-refractory moderate/severe ulcerative colitis. Aliment Pharmacol Ther 18:415, 2003.

240. Davies PS, Rhodes J, Heatley RV, et al: Metronidazole in the treatment of chronic proctitis: A controlled trial. Gut 18:680, 1977.

241. Gilat T, Suissa A, Leichtman G, et al: A comparative study of metronidazole and sulfasalazine in active, not severe, ulcerative colitis. An Israeli multicenter trial. J Clin Gastroenterol 9:415, 1987.

242. Mantzaris GJ, Archavlis E, Christoforidis P, et al: A prospective, randomized, controlled trial of oral ciprofloxacin in acute ulcerative colitis. Am J Gastroenterol 92:454, 1997.

243. Mantzaris GJ, Hatzis A, Kontogiannis P, et al: Intravenous tobramycin and metronidazole as an adjunct to corticosteroids in acute, severe ulcerative colitis. Am J Gastroenterol 89:43, 1994.

244. Chapman RW, Selby WS, Jewell DP: Controlled trial of intravenous metronidazole as an adjunct to corticosteroids in severe ulcerative colitis. Gut 27:1210, 1986.

245. Burke DA, Axon AT, Clayden SA, et al: The efficacy of tobramycin in the treatment of ulcerative colitis. Aliment Pharmacol Ther 4:123, 1990.

246. Turunen UM, Farkkila MA, Hakala K, et al: Long-term treatment of ulcerative colitis with ciprofloxacin: A prospective, double-blind, placebo-controlled study. Gastroenterology 115:1072, 1998.

247. Fuller R: Probiotics in man and animals. J Appl Bacteriol 66:365, 1989.

248. Guslandi M, Giollo P, Testoni PA: A pilot trial of *Saccharomyces boulardii* in ulcerative colitis. Eur J Gastroenterol Hepatol 15:697, 2003.

249. Fedorak RN, Gionchetti P, Campieri M, et al: VSL3 probiotic mixture induces remission in patients with active ulcerative colitis [Abstract]. Gastroenterology 124:A377, 2003.

250. Kruis W, Schutz E, Fric P, et al: Double-blind comparison of an oral *Escherichia coli* preparation and mesalazine in maintaining remission of ulcerative colitis. Aliment Pharmacol Ther 11:853, 1997.

251. Rembacken BJ, Snelling AM, Hawkey PM, et al: Nonpathogenic *Escherichia coli* versus mesalazine for the treatment of ulcerative colitis: A randomised trial. Lancet 354:635, 1999.

252. Ishikawa H, Akedo I, Umesaki Y, et al: Randomized controlled trial of the effect of bifidobacteria-fermented milk on ulcerative colitis. J Am Coll Nutr 22:56, 2003.

253. Venturi A, Gionchetti P, Rizzello F, et al: Impact on the composition of the faecal flora by a new probiotic preparation: Preliminary data on maintenance treatment of patients with ulcerative colitis. Aliment Pharmacol Ther 13:1103, 1999.

254. Scheppach W: Treatment of distal ulcerative colitis with short-chain fatty acid enemas: A placebo-controlled trial. German-Austrian SCFA Study Group. Dig Dis Sci 41:2254, 1996.

255. Vernia P, Marcheggiano A, Caprilli R, et al: Short-chain fatty acid topical treatment in distal ulcerative colitis. Aliment Pharmacol Ther 9:309, 1995.

256. Scheppach W, Sommer H, Kirchner T, et al: Effect of butyrate enemas on the colonic mucosa in distal ulcerative colitis. Gastroenterology 103:51, 1992.

257. Empey LR, Jewell LD, Garg ML, et al: Fish oil-enriched diet is mucosal protective against acetic acid-induced colitis in rats. Can J Physiol Pharmacol 69:480, 1991.

258. Marotta F, Chui DH, Safran P, et al: Shark fin enriched diet prevents mucosal lipid abnormalities in experimental acute colitis. Digestion 56:46, 1995.

259. Nieto N, Torres MI, Rios A, et al: Dietary polyunsaturated fatty acids improve histological and biochemical alterations in rats with experimental ulcerative colitis. J Nutr 132:11, 2002.

260. Aslan A, Triadafilopoulos G: Fish oil fatty acid supplementation in active ulcerative colitis: A double-blind, placebo-controlled, crossover study. Am J Gastroenterol 87:432, 1992.

261. Lorenz R, Weber PC, Szimnau P, et al: Supplementation with n-3 fatty acids from fish oil in chronic inflammatory bowel

disease: A randomized, placebo-controlled, double-blind cross-over trial. J Intern Med 225(Suppl):225, 1989.

262. Hawthorne AB, Daneshmend TK, Hawkey CJ, et al: Treatment of ulcerative colitis with fish oil supplementation: A prospective 12-month randomised controlled trial. Gut 33:922, 1992.

263. Greenfield SM, Green AT, Teare JP, et al: A randomized controlled study of evening primrose oil and fish oil in ulcerative colitis. Aliment Pharmacol Ther 7:159, 1993.

264. McIntyre PB, Powell-Tuck J, Wood SR, et al: Controlled trial of bowel rest in the treatment of severe acute colitis. Gut 27:481, 1986.

265. Dickinson RJ, Ashton MG, Axon AT, et al: Controlled trial of intravenous hyperalimentation and total bowel rest as an adjunct to the routine therapy of acute colitis. Gastroenterology 79:1199, 1980.

266. Sandborn WJ, Tremaine WJ, Offord KP, et al: Transdermal nicotine for mildly to moderately active ulcerative colitis: A randomized, double-blind, placebo-controlled trial. Ann Intern Med 126:364, 1997.

267. Pullan RD, Rhodes J, Ganesh S, et al: Transdermal nicotine for active ulcerative colitis. N Engl J Med 330:811, 1994.

268. Guslandi M, Frego R, Viale E, et al. Distal ulcerative colitis refractory to rectal mesalamine: Role of transdermal nicotine versus oral mesalamine. Can J Gastroenterol 16:293, 2002.

269. Sandborn WJ: Nicotine therapy for ulcerative colitis: A review of rationale, mechanisms, pharmacology, and clinical results. Am J Gastroenterol 94:1161, 1999.

270. Thomas GA, Rhodes J, Ragunath K, et al: Transdermal nicotine compared with oral prednisolone therapy for active ulcerative colitis. Eur J Gastroenterol Hepatol 8:769, 1996.

271. Green JT, Thomas GA, Rhodes J, et al: Nicotine enemas for active ulcerative colitis: A pilot study. Aliment Pharmacol Ther 11:859, 1997.

272. Sandborn WJ, Tremaine WJ, Leighton JA, et al: Nicotine tartrate liquid enemas for mildly to moderately active left-sided ulcerative colitis unresponsive to first-line therapy: A pilot study. Aliment Pharmacol Ther 11:663, 1997.

273. Thomas GA, Rhodes J, Mani V, et al: Transdermal nicotine as maintenance therapy for ulcerative colitis. N Engl J Med 332:988, 1995.

274. Evans RC, Wong VS, Morris AI, et al: Treatment of corticosteroid-resistant ulcerative colitis with heparin: A report of 16 cases. Aliment Pharmacol Ther 11:1037, 1997.

275. Folwaczny C, Wiebecke B, Loeschke K: Unfractioned heparin in the therapy of patients with highly active inflammatory bowel disease. Am J Gastroenterol 94:1551, 1999.

276. Ang YS, Mahmud N, White B, et al: Randomized comparison of unfractionated heparin with corticosteroids in severe active inflammatory bowel disease. Aliment Pharmacol Ther 14:1015, 2000.

277. Panes J, Esteve M, Cabre E, et al: Comparison of heparin and steroids in the treatment of moderate and severe ulcerative colitis. Gastroenterology 119:903, 2000.

278. Torkvist L, Thorlacius H, Sjoqvist U, et al: Low-molecular-weight heparin as adjuvant therapy in active ulcerative colitis. Aliment Pharmacol Ther 13:1323, 1999.

279. Vrij AA, Jansen JM, Schoon EJ, et al: Low-molecular-weight heparin treatment in steroid-refractory ulcerative colitis: Clinical outcome and influence on mucosal capillary thrombi. Scand J Gastroenterol Suppl 234:41, 2001.

280. Bloom S, Kiilerich S, Lassen MR, et al: Low molecular weight heparin (tinzaparin) vs. placebo in the treatment of mild to moderately active ulcerative colitis. Aliment Pharmacol Ther 19:871, 2004.

281. Targan SR, Hanauer SB, van Deventer SJ, et al: A short-term study of chimeric monoclonal antibody cA2 to tumor necrosis factor alpha for Crohn's disease. Crohn's Disease cA2 Study Group. N Engl J Med 337:1029, 1997.

282. Sands BE, Anderson FH, Bernstein CN, et al: Infliximab maintenance therapy for fistulizing Crohn's disease. N Engl J Med 350:876, 2004.

283. Hanauer SB, Feagan BG, Lichtenstein GR, et al: Maintenance infliximab for Crohn's disease: The ACCENT I randomised trial. Lancet 359:1541, 2002.

284. Present DH, Rutgeerts P, Targan S, et al: Infliximab for the treatment of fistulas in patients with Crohn's disease. N Engl J Med 340:1398, 1999.

285. Siegel SA, Shealy DJ, Nakada MT, et al: The mouse/human chimeric monoclonal antibody cA2 neutralizes TNF in vitro and protects transgenic mice from cachexia and TNF lethality in vivo. Cytokine 7:15, 1995.

286. Knight DM, Trinh H, Le J, et al: Construction and initial characterization of a mouse-human chimeric anti-TNF antibody. Mol Immunol 30:1443, 1993.

287. Scallon BJ, Moore MA, Trinh H, et al: Chimeric anti-TNF-alpha monoclonal antibody cA2 binds recombinant transmembrane TNF-alpha and activates immune effector functions. Cytokine 7:251, 1995.

288. van Deventer SJ: Review article: Targeting TNF alpha as a key cytokine in the inflammatory processes of Crohn's disease—the mechanisms of action of infliximab. Aliment Pharmacol Ther 13(Suppl 4):3-8; discussion 38:3, 1999.

289. Lugering A, Schmidt M, Lugering N, et al: Infliximab induces apoptosis in monocytes from patients with chronic active Crohn's disease by using a caspase-dependent pathway. Gastroenterology 121:1145, 2001.

290. Chey WY, Hussain A, Ryan C, et al: Infliximab for refractory ulcerative colitis. Am J Gastroenterol 96:2373, 2001.

291. Gornet JM, Couve S, Hassani Z, et al: Infliximab for refractory ulcerative colitis or indeterminate colitis: An open-label multicentre study. Aliment Pharmacol Ther 18:175, 2003.

292. Kohn A, Prantera C, Pera A, et al: Anti-tumour necrosis factor alpha (infliximab) in the treatment of severe ulcerative colitis: Result of an open study on 13 patients. Dig Liver Dis 34:626, 2002.

293. Mamula P, Markowitz JE, Brown KA, et al: Infliximab as a novel therapy for pediatric ulcerative colitis. J Pediatr Gastroenterol Nutr 34:307, 2002.

294. Su C, Salzberg BA, Lewis JD, et al: Efficacy of anti-tumor necrosis factor therapy in patients with ulcerative colitis. Am J Gastroenterol 97:2577, 2002.

295. Sands BE, Podolsky DK, Tremaine WJ, et al: Chimeric monoclonal anti-tumor necrosis factor antibody (cA2) in the treatment of severe, steroid-refractory ulcerative colitis (UC) [Abstract]. Gastroenterology 110: A1008, 1996.

296. Sands BE, Tremaine WJ, Sandborn WJ, et al: Infliximab in the treatment of severe, steroid-refractory ulcerative colitis: A pilot study. Inflamm Bowel Dis 7:83, 2001.

297. Probert CS, Hearing SD, Schreiber S, et al: Infliximab in moderately severe glucocorticoid resistant ulcerative colitis: A randomised controlled trial. Gut 52:998, 2003.

298. Sandborn WJ, Rachmilewitz D, Hanauer SB, et al: Infliximab induction and maintenance therapy for ulcerative colitis: the ACT II trial. Gastroenterology 128:A104, 2005 (In press, N Engl J Med).

299. Rutgeerts P, Feagan BG, Olson A, et al: A randomized placebo-controlled trial of infliximab therapy for active ulcerative colitis: ACT1 trial (N Engl J Med, in press).

300. Gordon FH, Hamilton MI, Donoghue S, et al: A pilot study of treatment of active ulcerative colitis with natalizumab, a humanized monoclonal antibody to alpha-4 integrin. Aliment Pharmacol Ther 16:699, 2002.

301. Feagan B, Greenberg G, Wild G, et al: Treatment of ulcerative colitis with a humanized antibody to the alpha-4-beta-7 integrin. N Engl J Med 352:2499, 2005.

302. Van Assche G, Dalle I, Noman M, et al: A pilot study on the use of the humanized anti-interleukin-2 receptor antibody

daclizumab in active ulcerative colitis. Am J Gastroenterol 98:369, 2003.

303. Creed TJ, Norman MR, Probert CS, et al: Basiliximab (anti-CD25) in combination with steroids may be an effective new treatment for steroid-resistant ulcerative colitis. Aliment Pharmacol Ther 18:65, 2003.

304. Plevy S, Salzberg B, Van Assche G, et al: A humanized anti-CD3 monoclonal antibody, visilizumab, for treatment of severe steroid-refractory ulcerative colitis: Results of a phase I study [Abstract]. Gastroenterology 126:A75, 2004.

305. Sinha A, Nightingale J, West KP, et al: Epidermal growth factor enemas with oral mesalamine for mild-to-moderate left-sided ulcerative colitis or proctitis. N Engl J Med 349:350, 2003.

306. Sandborn WJ, Sands BE, Wolf DC, et al: Repifermin (keratinocyte growth factor-2) for the treatment of active ulcerative colitis: A randomized, double-blind, placebo-controlled, dose-escalation trial. Aliment Pharmacol Ther 17:1355, 2003.

307. Sasaki M, Tsujikawa T, Fujiyama Y, et al: Leukocytapheresis therapy for severe ulcerative colitis. Ther Apheresis 2:101, 1998.

308. Sawada K, Ohnishi K, Fukui S, et al: Leukocytapheresis therapy, performed with leukocyte removal filter, for inflammatory bowel disease. J Gastroenterol 30:322, 1995.

309. Shimoyama T, Sawada K, Hiwatashi N, et al: Safety and efficacy of granulocyte and monocyte adsorption apheresis in patients with active ulcerative colitis: A multicenter study. J Clin Apher 16:1, 2001.

310. Kohgo Y, Hibi H, Chiba T, et al: Leukocyte apheresis using a centrifugal cell separator in refractory ulcerative colitis: A multicenter open label trial. Ther Apher 6:255, 2002.

311. Hanai H, Watanabe F, Takeuchi K, et al: Leukocyte adsorptive apheresis for the treatment of active ulcerative colitis: A prospective, uncontrolled, pilot study. Clin Gastroenterol Hepatol 1:28, 2003.

312. Naganuma M, Funakoshi S, Sakuraba A, et al: Granulocytapheresis is useful as an alternative therapy in patients with steroid-refractory or -dependent ulcerative colitis. Inflamm Bowel Dis 10:251, 2004.

313. Suzuki Y, Yoshimura N, Saniabadi AR, et al: Selective granulocyte and monocyte adsorptive apheresis as a first-line treatment for steroid naive patients with active ulcerative colitis: A prospective uncontrolled study. Dig Dis Sci 49:565, 2004.

314. Sawada K, Muto T, Shimoyama T, et al: Multicenter randomized controlled trial for the treatment of ulcerative colitis with a leukocytapheresis column. Curr Pharm Des 9:307, 2003.

315. Katayama K, Wada K, Nakajima A, et al: A novel PPAR gamma gene therapy to control inflammation associated with inflammatory bowel disease in a murine model. Gastroenterology 124:1315, 2003.

316. Tanaka T, Kohno H, Yoshitani S, et al: Ligands for peroxisome proliferator-activated receptors alpha and gamma inhibit chemically induced colitis and formation of aberrant crypt foci in rats. Cancer Res 61:2424, 2001.

317. Saubermann LJ, Nakajima A, Wada K, et al: Peroxisome proliferator-activated receptor gamma agonist ligands stimulate a Th2 cytokine response and prevent acute colitis. Inflamm Bowel Dis 8:330, 2002.

318. Desreumaux P, Dubuquoy L, Nutten S, et al: Attenuation of colon inflammation through activators of the retinoid X receptor (RXR)/peroxisome proliferator-activated receptor gamma (PPARgamma) heterodimer: A basis for new therapeutic strategies. J Exp Med 193:827, 2001.

319. Lewis JD, Lichtenstein GR, Stein RB, et al: An open-label trial of the PPAR-gamma ligand rosiglitazone for active ulcerative colitis. Am J Gastroenterol 96:3323, 2001.

320. Myrvold HE: The continent ileostomy. World J Surg 11:720, 1987.

321. Penna C, Daude F, Parc R, et al: Previous subtotal colectomy with ileostomy and sigmoidostomy improves the morbidity and early functional results after ileal pouch-anal anastomosis in ulcerative colitis. Dis Colon Rectum 36:343, 1993.

322. Fazio VW, Ziv Y, Church JM, et al: Ileal pouch-anal anastomoses complications and function in 1005 patients. Ann Surg 222:120, 1995.

323. Blumberg D, Beck DE: Surgery for ulcerative colitis. Gastroenterol Clin North Am 31:219, 2002.

324. Negi SS, Chaudhary A, Gondal R: Carcinoma of pelvic pouch following restorative proctocolectomy: Report of a case and review of the literature. Dig Surg 20:63, 2003.

325. Lennard-Jones JE, Ritchie JK, Hilder W, et al: Assessment of severity in colitis: A preliminary study. Gut 16:579, 1975.

326. Bartram CI: Radiology in the current assessment of ulcerative colitis. Gastrointest Radiol 1:383, 1977.

327. Roys G, Kaplan MS, Juler GL: Surgical management of toxic megacolon. Am J Gastroenterol 68:161, 1977.

328. Hartong WA, Arvanitakis C, Skibba RM, et al: Treatment of toxic megacolon: A comparative review of 29 patients. Am J Dig Dis 22:195, 1977.

329. Marion JF, Present DH: The modern medical management of acute, severe, ulcerative colitis. Eur J Gastroenterol Hepatol 9:831, 1997.

330. Panos MZ, Wood MJ, Asquith P: Toxic megacolon: The knee-elbow position relieves bowel distention. Gut 34:1726, 1993.

331. Strauss RJ, Flint GW, Platt N, et al: The surgical management of toxic dilatation of the colon: A report of 28 cases and review of the literature. Ann Surg 184:682, 1976.

332. Greenstein AJ, Aufses AH Jr: Differences in pathogenesis, incidence, and outcome of perforation in inflammatory bowel disease. Surg Gynecol Obstet 160:63, 1985.

333. Greenstein AJ, Sachar DB, Gibas A, et al: Outcome of toxic dilatation in ulcerative and Crohn's colitis. J Clin Gastroenterol 7:137, 1985.

334. Grant CS, Dozois RR: Toxic megacolon: Ultimate fate of patients after successful medical management. Am J Surg 147:106, 1984.

335. Greenstein AJ, Barth JA, Sachar DB, et al: Free colonic perforation without dilatation in ulcerative colitis. Am J Surg 152:272, 1986.

336. Gumaste V, Sachar DB, Greenstein AJ: Benign and malignant colorectal strictures in ulcerative colitis. Gut 33:938, 1992.

337. Reiser JR, Waye JD, Janowitz HD, et al: Adenocarcinoma in strictures of ulcerative colitis without antecedent dysplasia by colonoscopy. Am J Gastroenterol 89:119, 1994.

338. Rutter M, Saunders B, Wilkinson K, et al: Severity of inflammation is a risk factor for colorectal neoplasia in ulcerative colitis. Gastroenterology 126:451, 2004.

339. Brentnall TA, Haggitt RC, Rabinovitch PS, et al: Risk and natural history of colonic neoplasia in patients with primary sclerosing cholangitis and ulcerative colitis. Gastroenterology 110:331, 1996.

340. Askling J, Dickman PW, Karlen P, et al: Family history as a risk factor for colorectal cancer in inflammatory bowel disease. Gastroenterology 120:1356, 2001.

341. Heuschen UA, Hinz U, Allemeyer EH, et al: Backwash ileitis is strongly associated with colorectal carcinoma in ulcerative colitis. Gastroenterology 120:841, 2001.

342. Itzkowitz SH, Harpaz N: Diagnosis and management of dysplasia in patients with inflammatory bowel disease. Gastroenterology 126:1634, 2004.

343. Lewis JD, Deren JJ, Lichtenstein GR: Cancer risk in patients with inflammatory bowel disease. Gastroenterol Clin North Am 28:459, 1999.

344. Riddell RH, Goldman H, Ransohoff DF, et al: Dysplasia in inflammatory bowel disease: Standardized classification

with provisional clinical applications. Hum Pathol 14:931, 1983.

345. Blackstone MO, Riddell RH, Rogers BH, et al: Dysplasia-associated lesion or mass (DALM) detected by colonoscopy in long-standing ulcerative colitis: An indication for colectomy. Gastroenterology 80:366, 1981.

346. Butt JH, Konishi F, Morson BC, et al: Macroscopic lesions in dysplasia and carcinoma complicating ulcerative colitis. Dig Dis Sci 28:18, 1983.

347. Lennard-Jones JE, Melville DM, Morson BC, et al: Precancer and cancer in extensive ulcerative colitis: Findings among 401 patients over 22 years. Gut 31:800, 1990.

348. Rosenstock E, Farmer RG, Petras R, et al: Surveillance for colonic carcinoma in ulcerative colitis. Gastroenterology 89:1342, 1985.

349. Bernstein CN, Shanahan F, Weinstein WM: Are we telling patients the truth about surveillance colonoscopy in ulcerative colitis? Lancet 343:71, 1994.

350. Nugent FW, Haggitt RC, Gilpin PA: Cancer surveillance in ulcerative colitis. Gastroenterology 100:1241, 1991.

351. Medlicott SA, Jewell LD, Price L, et al: Conservative management of small adenomata in ulcerative colitis. Am J Gastroenterol 92:2094, 1997.

352. Connell WR, Lennard-Jones JE, Williams CB, et al: Factors affecting the outcome of endoscopic surveillance for cancer in ulcerative colitis. Gastroenterology 107:934, 1994.

353. Engelsgjerd M, Farraye FA, Odze RD: Polypectomy may be adequate treatment for adenoma-like dysplastic lesions in chronic ulcerative colitis. Gastroenterology 117:1288, 1999.

354. Rubin PH, Friedman S, Harpaz N, et al: Colonoscopic polypectomy in chronic colitis: Conservative management after endoscopic resection of dysplastic polyps. Gastroenterology 117:1295, 1999.

355. Ullman T, Croog V, Harpaz N, et al: Progression of flat low-grade dysplasia to advanced neoplasia in patients with ulcerative colitis. Gastroenterology 125:1311, 2003.

356. Befrits R, Ljung T, Jaramillo E, et al: Low-grade dysplasia in extensive, long-standing inflammatory bowel disease: A follow-up study. Dis Colon Rectum 45:615, 2002.

357. Lim CH, Dixon MF, Vail A, et al: Ten-year follow-up of ulcerative colitis patients with and without low-grade dysplasia. Gut 52:1127, 2003.

358. Kornbluth A, Sachar DB: Ulcerative colitis practice guidelines in adults. American College of Gastroenterology, Practice Parameters Committee. Am J Gastroenterol 92:204, 1997.

359. Winawer S, Fletcher R, Rex D, et al: Colorectal cancer screening and surveillance: Clinical guidelines and rationale—update based on new evidence. Gastroenterology 124:544, 2003.

360. Rubin CE, Haggitt RC, Burmer GC, et al: DNA aneuploidy in colonic biopsies predicts future development of dysplasia in ulcerative colitis. Gastroenterology 103:1611, 1992.

361. Judge TA, Lewis JD, Lichtenstein GR: Colonic dysplasia and cancer in inflammatory bowel disease. Gastrointest Endosc Clin North Am 12:495, 2002.

362. Bernstein CN: ALMs versus DALMs in ulcerative colitis: Polypectomy or colectomy? Gastroenterology 117:1488, 1999.

363. Kiesslich R, Fritsch J, Holtmann M, et al: Methylene blue-aided chromoendoscopy for the detection of intraepithelial neoplasia and colon cancer in ulcerative colitis. Gastroenterology 124:880, 2003.

364. Jaramillo E, Watanabe M, Befrits R, et al: Small, flat colorectal neoplasias in long-standing ulcerative colitis detected by high-resolution electronic video endoscopy. Gastrointest Endosc 44:15, 1996.

365. Rutter MD, Saunders BP, Schofield G, et al: Pancolonic indigo carmine dye spraying for the detection of dysplasia in ulcerative colitis. Gut 53:256, 2004.

366. Vogelstein B, Fearon ER, Hamilton SR, et al: Genetic alterations during colorectal-tumor development. N Engl J Med 319:525, 1988.

367. Itzkowitz SH, Young E, Dubois D, et al: Sialosyl-Tn antigen is prevalent and precedes dysplasia in ulcerative colitis: A retrospective case-control study. Gastroenterology 110:694, 1996.

368. Karlen P, Young E, Brostrom O, et al: Sialyl-Tn antigen as a marker of colon cancer risk in ulcerative colitis: Relation to dysplasia and DNA aneuploidy. Gastroenterology 115:1395, 1998.

369. Benhattar J, Saraga E: Molecular genetics of dysplasia in ulcerative colitis. Eur J Cancer 31A:1171, 1995.

370. Odze RD, Brown CA, Hartmann CJ, et al: Genetic alterations in chronic ulcerative colitis-associated adenoma-like DALMs are similar to non-colitic sporadic adenomas. Am J Surg Pathol 24:1209, 2000.

371. Fogt F, Vortmeyer AO, Stolte M, et al: Loss of heterozygosity of the von Hippel-Lindau gene locus in polypoid dysplasia but not flat dysplasia in ulcerative colitis or sporadic adenomas. Hum Pathol 29:961, 1998.

372. Fogt F, Vortmeyer AO, Goldman H, et al: Comparison of genetic alterations in colonic adenoma and ulcerative colitis-associated dysplasia and carcinoma. Hum Pathol 29:131, 1998.

373. Walsh SV, Loda M, Torres CM, et al: P53 and beta catenin expression in chronic ulcerative colitis–associated polypoid dysplasia and sporadic adenomas: An immunohistochemical study. Am J Surg Pathol 23:963, 1999.

374. Harpaz N, Peck AL, Yin J, et al: p53 protein expression in ulcerative colitis-associated colorectal dysplasia and carcinoma. Hum Pathol 25:1069, 1994.

375. Dozois RR, Goldberg SM, Rothenberger DA, et al: Restorative proctocolectomy with ileal reservoir. Int J Colorectal Dis 1:2, 1986.

376. Stahlberg D, Gullberg K, Liljeqvist L, et al: Pouchitis following pelvic pouch operation for ulcerative colitis. Incidence, cumulative risk, and risk factors. Dis Colon Rectum 39:1012, 1996.

377. Nicholls RJ, Banerjee AK: Pouchitis: Risk factors, etiology, and treatment. World J Surg 22:347, 1998.

378. Sandborn WJ: Pouchitis following ileal pouch-anal anastomosis: Definition, pathogenesis, and treatment. Gastroenterology 107:1856, 1994.

379. Hurst RD, Molinari M, Chung TP, et al: Prospective study of the incidence, timing, and treatment of pouchitis in 104 consecutive patients after restorative proctocolectomy. Arch Surg 131:497, 1996.

380. Mahadevan U, Sandborn WJ: Diagnosis and management of pouchitis. Gastroenterology 124:1636, 2003.

381. Sandborn WJ, Landers CJ, Tremaine WJ, et al: Antineutrophil cytoplasmic antibody correlates with chronic pouchitis after ileal pouch-anal anastomosis. Am J Gastroenterol 90:740, 1995.

382. Fleshner PR, Vasiliauskas EA, Kam LY, et al: High level perinuclear antineutrophil cytoplasmic antibody (pANCA) in ulcerative colitis patients before colectomy predicts development of chronic pouchitis after ileal pouch-anal anastomosis. Gut 49:671, 2001.

383. Penna C, Dozois R, Tremaine W, et al: Pouchitis after ileal pouch-anal anastomosis for ulcerative colitis occurs with increased frequency in patients with associated primary sclerosing cholangitis. Gut 38:234, 1996.

384. Madden MV, McIntyre AS, Nicholls RJ: Double-blind crossover trial of metronidazole versus placebo in chronic unremitting pouchitis. Dig Dis Sci 39:1193, 1994.

385. Shen B, Achkar JP, Lashner BA, et al: A randomized clinical trial of ciprofloxacin and metronidazole to treat acute pouchitis. Inflamm Bowel Dis 7:301, 2001.

386. Nygaard K, Bergan T, Bjorneklett A, et al: Topical metronidazole treatment in pouchitis. Scand J Gastroenterol 29:462, 1994.

387. Gionchetti P, Rizzello F, Venturi A, et al: Antibiotic combination therapy in patients with chronic, treatment-resistant pouchitis. Aliment Pharmacol Ther 13:713, 1999.

388. Mimura T, Rizzello F, Helwig U, et al: Four-week open-label trial of metronidazole and ciprofloxacin for the treatment of recurrent or refractory pouchitis. Aliment Pharmacol Ther 16:909, 2002.

389. Gionchetti P, Amadini C, Rizzello F, et al: Review article: Treatment of mild to moderate ulcerative colitis and pouchitis. Aliment Pharmacol Ther 16(Suppl 4):13, 2002.

390. Sambuelli A, Boerr L, Negreira S, et al: Budesonide enema in pouchitis: A double-blind, double-dummy, controlled trial. Aliment Pharmacol Ther 16:27, 2002.

391. Winter TA, Dalton HR, Merrett MN, et al: Cyclosporin A retention enemas in refractory distal ulcerative colitis and "pouchitis." Scand J Gastroenterol 28:701, 1993.

392. Viscido A, Habib FI, Kohn A, et al: Infliximab in refractory pouchitis complicated by fistulae following ileo-anal pouch for ulcerative colitis. Aliment Pharmacol Ther 17:1263, 2003.

393. Gionchetti P, Rizzello F, Venturi A, et al: Oral bacteriotherapy as maintenance treatment in patients with chronic pouchitis: A double-blind, placebo-controlled trial. Gastroenterology 119:305, 2000.

394. Gionchetti P, Rizzello F, Helwig U, et al: Prophylaxis of pouchitis onset with probiotic therapy: A double-blind, placebo-controlled trial. Gastroenterology 124:1202, 2003.

395. Mimura T, Rizzello F, Helwig U, et al: Once-daily high-dose probiotic therapy (VSL#3) for maintaining remission in recurrent or refractory pouchitis. Gut 53:108, 2004.

396. Gionchetti P, Rizzello F, Venturi A, et al: Long-term efficacy of bismuth carbomer enemas in patients with treatment-resistant chronic pouchitis. Aliment Pharmacol Ther 11:673, 1997.

397. Tremaine WJ, Sandborn WJ, Wolff BG, et al: Bismuth carbomer foam enemas for active chronic pouchitis: A randomized, double-blind, placebo-controlled trial. Aliment Pharmacol Ther 11:1041, 1997.

398. Tremaine W, Sandborn W, Kenan ML: Bismuth subsalicylate tablets for chronic antibiotic-resistant pouchitis [Abstract]. Gastroenterology 114:A1101, 1998.

399. Wischmeyer P, Pemberton JH, Phillips SF: Chronic pouchitis after ileal pouch-anal anastomosis: Responses to butyrate and glutamine suppositories in a pilot study. Mayo Clin Proc 68:978, 1993.

400. Kuhbacher T, Schreiber S, Runkel N: Pouchitis: Pathophysiology and treatment. Int J Colorectal Dis 13:196, 1998.

401. Finkel SI, Janowitz HD: Trauma and the pyoderma gangrenosum of inflammatory bowel disease. Gut 22:410, 1981.

402. Callen JP: Pyoderma gangrenosum. Lancet 351:581, 1998.

403. Powell RJ, Holbrook MR, Stevens A: Pyoderma gangrenosum and its treatment. Lancet 350:1720, 1997.

404. Lyon CC, Stapleton M, Smith AJ, et al: Topical tacrolimus in the management of peristomal pyoderma gangrenosum. J Dermatol Treat 12:13, 2001.

405. Friedman S, Marion JF, Scherl E, et al: Intravenous cyclosporine in refractory pyoderma gangrenosum complicating inflammatory bowel disease. Inflamm Bowel Dis 7:1, 2001.

406. Galun E, Flugelman MY, Rachmilewitz D: Pyoderma gangrenosum complicating ulcerative colitis: Successful treatment with methylprednisolone pulse therapy and dapsone. Am J Gastroenterol 81:988, 1986.

407. Van Hale HM, Rogers RS III, Zone JJ, et al: Pyostomatitis vegetans: A reactive mucosal marker for inflammatory disease of the gut. Arch Dermatol 121:94, 1985.

408. Orchard TR, Wordsworth BP, Jewell DP: Peripheral arthropathies in inflammatory bowel disease: Their articular distribution and natural history. Gut 42:387, 1998.

409. Keyser FD, Mielants H, Veys EM: Current use of biologicals for the treatment of spondyloarthropathies. Expert Opin Pharmacother 2:85, 2001.

410. Vakil N, Sparberg M: Steroid-related osteonecrosis in inflammatory bowel disease. Gastroenterology 96:62, 1989.

411. Miehsler W, Reinisch W, Valic E, et al: Is inflammatory bowel disease an independent and disease-specific risk factor for thromboembolism? Gut 53:542, 2004.

412. Talbot RW, Heppell J, Dozois RR, et al: Vascular complications of inflammatory bowel disease. Mayo Clin Proc 61:140, 1986.

413. Schapira M, Henrion J, Ravoet C, et al: Thromboembolism in inflammatory bowel disease. Acta Gastroenterol Belg 62:182, 1999.

414. Liebman HA, Kashani N, Sutherland D, et al: The factor V Leiden mutation increases the risk of venous thrombosis in patients with inflammatory bowel disease. Gastroenterology 115:830, 1998.

415. Papa A, Danese S, Grillo A, et al: Review article: Inherited thrombophilia in inflammatory bowel disease. Am J Gastroenterol 98:1247, 2003.

416. Guedon C, Cam-Duchez V, Lalaude O, et al: Prothrombotic inherited abnormalities other than factor V Leiden mutation do not play a role in venous thrombosis in inflammatory bowel disease. Am J Gastroenterol 96:1448, 2001.

417. Greenstein AJ, Sachar DB, Panday AK, et al: Amyloidosis and inflammatory bowel disease: A 50-year experience with 25 patients. Medicine (Baltimore) 71:261, 1992.

418. Patwardhan RV, Heilpern RJ, Brewster AC, et al: Pleuropericarditis—an extraintestinal complication of inflammatory bowel disease: Report of three cases and review of literature. Arch Intern Med 143:94, 1983.

419. Rheingold OJ: Inflammatory bowel disease and pericarditis [Letter]. Ann Intern Med 82:592, 1975.

420. Mukhopadhyay D, Nasr K, Grossman BJ, et al: Pericarditis associated with inflammatory bowel disease. JAMA 211:1540, 1970.

421. Oxentenko AS, Loftus EV, Oh JK, et al: Constrictive pericarditis in chronic ulcerative colitis. J Clin Gastroenterol 34:247, 2002.

422. Gujral N, Friedenberg F, Friedenberg J, et al: Pleuropericarditis related to the use of mesalamine. Dig Dis Sci 41:624, 1996.

423. Ishikawa N, Imamura T, Nakajima K, et al: Acute pericarditis associated with 5-aminosalicylic acid (5-ASA) treatment for severe active ulcerative colitis. Intern Med 40:901, 2001.

424. Godet PG, Cowie R, Woodman RC, et al: Pulmonary function abnormalities in patients with ulcerative colitis. Am J Gastroenterol 92:1154, 1997.

425. McKee AL, Rajapaksa A, Kalish PE, et al: Severe interstitial pulmonary fibrosis in a patient with chronic ulcerative colitis. Am J Gastroenterol 78:86, 1983.

426. Forrest JA, Shearman DJ: Pulmonary vasculitis and ulcerative colitis. Am J Dig Dis 20:482, 1975.

427. Mahadeva R, Walsh G, Flower CD, et al: Clinical and radiological characteristics of lung disease in inflammatory bowel disease. Eur Respir J 15:41, 2000.

CHAPTER
110 Ileostomy, Colostomy, and Pouches

Robert R. Cima and John H. Pemberton

Proctocolectomy and permanent ileostomy return most patients with chronic ulcerative colitis (UC) to excellent health and remove premalignant mucosa in patients with chronic UC or familial adenomatous polyposis (FAP). Many of the inconveniences and dangers formerly associated with an ileal stoma have been eliminated by improved surgical techniques, a wider range of better stomal appliances, and more effective education of patients.[1]

Between 1930 and 1950, the metabolic consequences of ileostomy became apparent, as did the frequent mechanical complications caused by "ileostomy dysfunction." Better understanding of fluid, electrolyte, and blood replacement resolved the first problem while newer techniques of ileostomy construction resolved the second.[2,3] Before these advances, ileostomies were made by withdrawal of the intestine through the abdominal wall, the serosal surface of ileum then being sutured to the skin. Ileostomy dysfunction resulted from the serositis following exposure of the serosal surface to stomal effluent. The mucosa of the ileum, however, is not susceptible to inflammation after a similar exposure, and a solution therefore was conceptually simple: evert the mucosal surface of the bud and suture the mucosa to the skin, as was described simultaneously early in the 1950s in the United Kingdom and United States. This modification is commonly referred to as a *Brooke ileostomy* (Fig. 110–1).[1] Development of new ileostomy appliances quickly led to better acceptance by patients and, ulti-

mately, to excellent long-term results.[4] Enterostomal therapy was introduced in the 1960s as an additional allied health support, and ileostomy societies have blossomed in most countries, providing a lay component of support to treatment of patients with stomas.

Brooke ileostomies are incontinent by definition, and during the 1960s, Nils Kock, a Swedish surgeon, developed the first effective alternative to this incontinent ileostomy.[5] The "Kock pouch" procedure featured an ileal pouch, a nipple valve, and an ileal conduit, which led to a cutaneous stoma that, because an appliance was not needed, could be made flush with the skin. The Kock pouch was used in selected patients with chronic UC and FAP.[6]

Stimulated by patients' acceptance, surgeons explored other alternatives to the incontinent ileal stoma with its ever-present external appliance. The ileoanal pull-through operation was resurrected, with an important technical modification: the addition of an ileal reservoir.[7,8] This procedure offered the advantages of a normal exit for stool and preservation of the anal sphincters. Indeed, the use of this procedure in thousands of patients has revealed ileal pouch-anal anastomosis (IPAA) to be the procedure of choice in most patients requiring proctocolectomy for chronic UC or FAP.

Although the Brooke ileostomy had become the usual operation after a colectomy in the United Kingdom and the United States, ileorectostomy was standard in continental Europe and South America. Indeed, these differ-

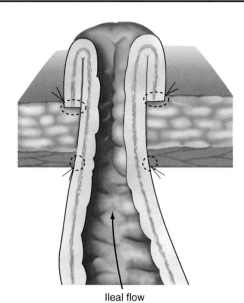

Ileal flow

Figure 110–1 Anatomy of the Brooke ileostomy. The mucosa is everted and sewn to the skin. No serosal surface is therefore exposed to intestinal content.

ent attitudes continue to influence approaches to the newer operations. This chapter details the pathophysiologic and clinical implications of colectomy per se and describes the options for control of enteric content. There are three surgical options after total colectomy in patients with chronic UC and FAP: (1) proctocolectomy with the terminal Brooke ileostomy, (2) IPAA, and (3) ileorectostomy. The Kock pouch and IPAA are contraindicated in patients with Crohn's colitis, but the option of segmental colectomy is available.

PATHOPHYSIOLOGIC CONSEQUENCES OF PROCTOCOLECTOMY

FECAL OUTPUTS AFTER PROCTOCOLECTOMY

After a colectomy with any type of ileostomy, the absence of the colon obviously prevents its reabsorption of electrolytes and water. Usually, this creates no major pathophysiologic disturbance, but some important principles should be remembered. A normal colon absorbs at least 1000 mL of water and 100 mEq of sodium chloride each day,[9] and the healthy colon can increase absorption more than 5 L/day[10] when presented with increased amounts of fluid. Also, the colon has a greater capacity than the small intestine to conserve sodium chloride when a person is salt depleted. For example, under conditions of extremely low salt intake, sodium losses in normal stool can be reduced to 1 or 2 mEq/day,[11] whereas patients with ileostomies have obligatory sodium losses of 30 to 40 mEq/day.[12,13]

Well-functioning conventional (Brooke) ileostomies discharge 300 to 800 g of material daily, 90% of which is water.[12,13] Continent ileostomies and IPAAs have similar volumes of effluent.[14] Foods containing substantial unabsorbable residue increase the total ileostomy output by increasing the amount of solids discharged. Although many anecdotes are reported on the effect of foods on the volume and consistency of stomal effluents, the response to specific foods varies from one patient to another, and changes usually are minimal.[15]

FUNCTIONAL SEQUELAE

When oral intakes of sodium, chloride, and fluid are adequate, patients with ileostomies do not become depleted in volume or electrolytes; negative sodium balance, however, may follow periods of diminished oral intake, vomiting, or excess perspiration.[16] In addition, chronic oliguria is to be anticipated, even with established ileostomies, because normal stools contain approximately 100 mL of water, whereas ileostomies lose 500 to 600 mL/day.[6,17] Patients with ileostomies also have lower urinary Na^+/K^+ ratios because of compensatory renal conservation of sodium and water. These changes in the composition of urine presumably contribute to the increased frequency of urolithiasis ($\approx$5%) in patients with ileostomies,[18] whose stones are predominantly composed of urate or calcium salts.

When an ileostomy is accompanied by resection of the terminal ileum, abnormalities of bile acid reabsorption, malabsorption of vitamin B_{12} (see Chapters 97 and 98), steatorrhea, and more than expected losses of fluid ($\geq$1 L/day) may result. These abnormalities usually do not follow a colectomy that is performed for chronic UC or FAP because the ileum, being free of disease, is preserved. Resection for Crohn's colitis may require removal of additional diseased ileum with the possible consequences of malabsorption and even short bowel syndrome, depending on the length of small bowel removed (see Chapters 98 and 100).

Colectomy also reduces the exposure of bile acids to the metabolic effects of the fecal flora, and after ileostomy, secondary bile acids largely disappear from bile; no metabolic consequences of significance have been recognized in this situation.[19,20] The flora of ileostomy effluents have quantitative (10^4 to 10^7 organisms per milliliter) and qualitative characteristics that are intermediate between those of feces and those of normal ileal contents[21-23]; the presence of a reservoir, Kock pouch, or IPAA predisposes to a more fecal-like flora.

The principal pathophysiologic sequelae of colectomy with ileostomy are mainly the potential consequences of a salt-losing state; patients should be advised to use salt liberally and to increase their fluid intake, especially at times of stress, in hot weather, and after vigorous exercise. A balanced salt solution (Gatorade or Powerade) is a good source of balanced electrolytes. The limited ability of the small intestine to absorb sodium and water, however, means that stomal volumes also increase when the oral intake is increased.[13]

CLINICAL CONSEQUENCES OF PROCTOCOLECTOMY

After successful proctocolectomy, life expectancy is slightly below normal for the first few years owing to complications of the stoma and to intestinal obstruction;

after ileorectostomy for FAP or chronic UC, particularly the former, cancer may develop in the retained rectum. In general, however, the long-term mortality rate in patients after proctocolectomy and conventional ileostomy is the same as for a matched normal population.[24] Ninety percent of patients with conventional ileostomies who responded to a survey rated the results of their operation as excellent and claimed little inconvenience.[4] Almost all were able to lead normal lives and enjoy normal sexual relationships; a few patients avoided certain strenuous physical activities.

The metabolic consequences of a proctocolectomy per se should be the same regardless of whether a conventional ileostomy or an alternative procedure is performed. Patients in whom an ileostomy alternative achieves an excellent result will have a better quality of life than will patients with a stoma because the former will not need to wear an ileostomy appliance. Indeed, when the Brooke ileostomy and IPAA were compared, patients with IPAA experienced significant advantages in performing daily activities and appeared to enjoy a better quality of life.[25] There are certain special complications of the newer operations, however, including incontinence (Kock pouch), pelvic infections and sepsis, and pouchitis (ileal pouch anal anastomosis), which are discussed later.

COMPLICATIONS AND MANAGEMENT OF THE CONVENTIONAL BROOKE ILEOSTOMY

Major long-term complications relate to malfunctioning ileostomies, prestomal ileitis, and irritation of the peristomal skin. If the ileostomy was improperly constructed (a less frequent problem with newer techniques), the stoma may become obstructed. *Obstruction* leads to cramping abdominal pain, increased ileal discharge (up to 4 L/day), and fluid and electrolyte depletion. Excessive ileal output arises, at least in part from increased intestinal secretion as the result of dilatation of the intestine proximal to the obstructed stoma. Stomal obstruction usually can be demonstrated by examining the stoma with the little finger or by endoscopy with a narrow endoscope. Radiologic studies reveal a dilated ileum proximal to the point of obstruction. Many obstructed ileostomies require reconstruction, and at operation, ulcerations often are found in the resected terminal ileum; their pathogenesis is unclear but probably relates in some way to the mechanical consequences of obstruction.

Prestomal ileitis is a much less common problem than is stomal obstruction. Patients with this complication exhibit the features of mechanical obstruction, but, in addition, have signs of systemic toxicity (e.g., fever, tachycardia, and anemia).[26,27] In prestomal ileitis, the ileum has numerous punched-out ulcers, sometimes extending to the serosa. It is not clear whether prestomal ileitis has a different pathogenesis from the changes that follow simple mechanical obstruction of the stoma; both complications involve ileum that was normal histologically at the time of colectomy. "Backwash ileitis," seen typically in chronic UC, does not predispose to either prestomal ileitis or obstruction. Conversely, patients who have had colectomy and ileostomy for Crohn's

disease experience problems with the ileal stoma more frequently perhaps because transmural inflammation involves the new terminal ileum. In some instances, it may be difficult to determine whether stomal dysfunction results from mechanical obstruction or recurrent Crohn's disease.

Most people with an ileostomy lead a normal life and eat a normal diet; poorly digestable foods (e.g., nuts, corn, some fruits, lightly cooked vegetables) may obstruct the stoma and should be eaten in moderation, after careful chewing.[4] Some patients experience continuing difficulties managing their ileostomy. These problems vary in severity, some being minor inconveniences and others being significant drawbacks to the success of the operation. Mechanical difficulties because of a poorly fitting stomal appliance may cause excoriation of the skin around the ileostomy or may even erode the stoma to produce a fistula. Occasionally, a peristomal abscess or peristomal hernias may develop, and a small number of pregnant women develop prolapse of the stoma. Some patients complain of unpleasant odors arising from the ileostomy bag, especially after eating certain foods, such as onions and beans. Because most odor arises from bacterial action on the contents of the appliance, however, the problem may be offset by frequent emptying of the appliance and by adding sodium benzoate or chlorine tablets to the bag. Oral bismuth subgallate also controls odor, but doubts exist as to whether its long-term use is justified, as questions of neurotoxicity and encephalopathy have been raised.[28,29]

Trained stomal therapists and lay societies of ileostomy patients can be helpful with numerous aspects of postoperative care. Education of the patient is best started before surgery; meetings with others who have undergone ileostomy and referral to specialized texts can allay many fears and uncertainties.[30,31] The United Ostomy Association (36 Executive Park, Suite 120, Irvine, CA 92714, www.uoa.org) publishes an excellent series of booklets dealing with all aspects of life for the ileostomy patient. These materials also are of great help to nursing staffs in the absence of registered enterostomal therapists. The location of therapists can be obtained from the Wound Ostomy and Continence Nurses Society (4700 W. Lake Ave, Glenview, IL 60025; www.wocn.org).

CONTINENT ILEOSTOMY (KOCK POUCH)

Clearly, one of the major (social) drawbacks to ileostomy could be eliminated if a continent stoma were possible. Nils Kock reasoned that a pouch and nipple valve constructed of terminal ileum could store ileal content internally until emptied voluntarily by passage of a large, soft catheter several times daily, thereby obviating the need for an external appliance (Fig. 110–2).[5] The first such operations were reported in 1969, and the results were promising[5]; however, the nipple valve sometimes failed, usually because it slipped out of the pouch, and led to incontinence. Techniques gradually improved, and the most recent approaches have been more successful, providing continence in most patients. In two series, more than 90% of patients were continent for gas and feces, (i.e., never requiring an appliance).[6,32] This high success

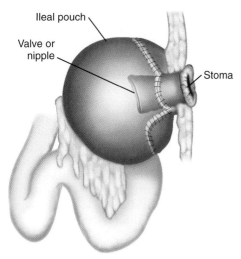

Figure 110–2 The continent ileostomy. The pouch is formed from a loop of ileum, folded on itself as a U, and sutured along the antimesenteric borders. The two limbs making up the pouch are then incised, exposing the mucosa, and the nipple valve is fashioned. The pouch is closed and positioned as shown underneath the abdominal wall. Note that the stoma is flush with the skin. (© Copyright 1991, Mayo Clinic, Rochester, Minnesota.)

Ileal pouch

Valve or nipple

Stoma

rate, however, is achieved at the price of additional operations in most patients for nipple or pouch dysfunction, fistula, or stricture.

Long-term follow-up has shown excellent acceptance by most patients with functioning pouches.[6,32,33] In as many as half of all patients with Kock pouches, however, incontinence develops, usually during the first year. Risk factors have been examined by the Mayo Clinic group: older (age >50 years), overweight men who had a conventional ileostomy converted to a pouch were most at risk, whereas young (<30 years), nonobese women having a pouch fashioned as a primary procedure had a risk of nipple valve failure estimated at less than 10%.[6] Nonspecific inflammation, "pouchitis," developed in as many as 30% of patients with the Kock pouch.[22,34] The signs and symptoms of Kock pouch pouchitis—abdominal cramps, difficult intubation, increased output, and bleeding from the pouch—are features comparable with pouchitis after IPAA; antibiotics usually relieve symptoms promptly.[22] In more than three decades since the Kock procedure was first performed, there is only one report of cancer occurring in the pouch.[35]

Although many patients were satisfied with the Kock pouch, the fundamental mechanical problem of the nipple valve design prevented widespread acceptance of the procedure. A continent ileostomy, the T pouch, has been developed to combat this problem. Its design[36] avoids slippage of the intussusceptive nipple valve constructed in the traditional Kock pouch. In the T pouch, the valve mechanism is made by securing an isolated distal ileal segment into a serosal lined trough formed by the base of two adjacent ileal segments. Around this isolated valve segment the high volume/low pressure reservoir is fashioned. Once constructed, the distal end of the valve mechanism is brought up through the skin as a stoma. Only a few patients have had T-pouches con-

structed and the results are promising, but long-term follow-up is required to assess the structural integrity and clinical success of the new valve design.

Given the wide acceptance of the IPAA, continent ileostomy operations are performed rarely and used mainly in patients who have had a proctocolectomy and ileostomy and who desire enteric continence. The contributions of Nils Kock to the current surgical approaches to proctocolectomy, however, provide the foundation for the current major alternatives to ileostomy.

ILEAL POUCH-ANAL ANASTOMOSIS

IPAA is now the procedure of choice for most patients who require proctocolectomy for chronic UC or FAP. IPAA is not considered suitable for patients with Crohn's disease, although this recommendation now is being questioned.[37,38] The operation has several major advantages: (1) nearly all mucosal disease is removed (in contrast to ileorectostomy); (2) the normal route for elimination is maintained (a permanent stoma is not required); (3) the anal sphincters are undisturbed; and (4) the pelvic dissection, being less extensive than in cancer operations, should not endanger innervation of the sexual organs. The general principle of ileoanal anastomosis was first described in 1947, and its revival was influenced by the success of pediatric surgeons in children with Hirschsprung's disease.[7] Early approaches used a straight pull-through and sutured the ileum directly to the anal verge.[39] Although results in children were encouraging, excessive stool frequency and anal seepage were unacceptable to many adult patients.[40] Subsequently, the operation was modified to include one of several forms of ileal pouch. The basics are as follows: An abdominal colectomy is performed; the distal rectal mucosa is excised from the underlying upper internal anal sphincter and lower rectal cuff, which is left in place; an ileal pouch is fashioned; and the ileal reservoir is sutured or stapled to the midanal canal, anastomosing the ileal mucosa to the anoderm. A diverting ileostomy is usually required for 2 to 3 months until the anastomosis heals completely. At a second operation 8 to 12 weeks later, the diverting ileostomy is closed.

The Mayo Clinic has acquired considerable experience with IPAA, having performed such operations at last report more than 2200 times.[41-43] Although pouches of different configurations have been advocated by various surgical groups in the past, the pouch routinely used today is the J-pouch because of its ease of construction and reliable function (Fig. 110–3).

LONG-TERM RESULTS

IPAA is a complex, sophisticated operation, and complications occur frequently. The overall morbidity rate still hovers between 25% and 30%. Failure, however, is rare, even in those who suffer a postoperative complication, and at the Mayo Clinic, 94% of patients with IPAA have a successful outcome. It is just as important to understand the complications of restorative proctocolectomy, how to avoid them, and what to do if they occur as it is to know

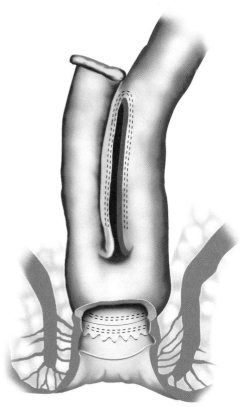

Figure 110–3 The anatomy of the most commonly used type of ileal pouch, the J-pouch. A pouch approximately 12 to 15 cm in length is constructed by opening the common wall between the two limbs of the "J" formed from the distal terminal ileum. The apex is then anastomosed to the upper anal canal.

how to select appropriate patients and how to perform the procedure rapidly and accurately. Although it is not discussed any further here, the key to successful outcome is a surgeon who performs the operation effortlessly; the operation struggled through is the one fraught with complications and sometimes with failure.

Complications

Pelvic infection is a serious complication that occurs in the early postoperative period in about 5% of patients with chronic UC.[41-43] Computed tomography (CT) is useful for demonstrating pelvic fluid collections or phlegmon. Patients with pelvic phlegmon usually respond to conservative treatment with broad-spectrum antibiotics and bowel rest, whereas patients with a pelvic abscess should undergo CT-guided drainage, if technically feasible, or laparotomy and drainage. The frequency of pelvic abscess is declining owing to increased experience with the procedure and to the construction of a shorter rectal cuff.

Abdominal sepsis, an ominous development, occurs in 6% of patients with IPAA.[41-43] Ultimately, 41% of patients who underwent laparotomy for control of abdominal sepsis required pouch excision. Moreover, normal pouch function was achieved in only 29% of patients requiring reoperation. However, among septic patients who did not require reoperation, but rather had aggressive nonsurgical management, 92% had satisfactory pouch function over the long term.

Closure of temporary ileostomies also may be associated with complications. Peritonitis occurred in 4% of patients and postoperative intestinal obstruction in 12% of patients. Proximal and distal serosal tears during stoma mobilization, in addition to anastomotic leaks, are important causes of peritonitis. If all extraperitoneal bowel (afferent and efferent limbs and the stoma itself) is resected, however, the chance of leaving an unrecognized perforation is nearly eliminated.

Almost all patients have a weblike stricture of the ileoanal anastomosis on returning for ileostomy closure. This stricture generally can be dilated digitally without difficulty. If the pouch retracts under anastomotic tension, heavy scarring and a long, fibrotic stricture result. This type of stricture is manifested by increased straining over stools, a sensation of incomplete pouch evacuation, or a high stool frequency (>10 to 12 stools per day). Repeated anal dilatation may prevent progression of the stricture.

Clinical Results

Following an IPAA, the average stool frequency is six stools during the day, with one stool at night. Daytime and nocturnal stool frequency and the ability to discriminate flatus from stool remain stable over time, whereas the need for stool bulking and hypomotility agents declines. The lower stool frequencies 6 months after surgery compared with the frequency in the early postoperative period are likely attributable to increased pouch capacity over time.

Major fecal incontinence (> twice per week) occurs in 5% of patients during the day and 12% during sleep. In contrast, minor episodes of nocturnal incontinence occur in up to 30% of patients at least 1 year after the operation. A pad must be worn by 28% of patients for protection against seepage. Minor perianal skin irritation is reported by 63% of patients.

Patients older than 50 years of age have a higher daytime stool frequency (eight per day) than do patients younger than age 50 years (six per day). Men and women have similar stool frequencies postoperatively, but women have more episodes of fecal soilage during the day and night.

Seventy-eight percent of patients with excellent continence 1 year after surgery remain unchanged at 10 years; 20% experience minor incontinence; and 2% have poor control. Of patients with minor incontinence at 1 year, 40% remain unchanged, 40% improve, and 20% worsen by 10 years. Nocturnal fecal spotting increases during the 10-year period, but not significantly.

Pouchitis

A wide range of quoted incidences suggests that the level of clinical suspicion and the diagnostic criteria for pouchitis vary greatly.[23,44,45] Of note, patients with preoperative extraintestinal manifestations of chronic UC had significantly higher rates of pouchitis than patients without such manifestations (39% with preoperative symptoms and 26% without).[45] Most patients with apparent pouchitis have intermittent symptoms or respond well to therapy. In a few, however, symptoms are severe and persistent enough to lead to surgical removal of the pouch. Patients present with increased volumes of output, bleeding, discomfort from the pouch, and general symptoms similar to those of the initial disease. Fever, anemia, and dehydration as a result of diarrhea may be variably present; fecal incontinence also is common. Extraintestinal dermatologic and rheumatologic manifestations are seen occasionally.[45]

In a patient with pouchitis, endoscopy shows the pouch mucosa to be reddened, swollen, and often ulcerated. The mucosa is friable and bleeds readily from minor trauma during endoscopy; inflammatory changes usually are confined to the pouch but also can be seen in the adjacent ileum. Biopsies show a range of acute and chronic inflammatory changes depending on severity. A disease activity index combining clinical, endoscopic, and histologic features has been developed (Table 110–1).[46] Although some early reports suggested that there was a relationship between pouchitis and perinuclear antineutrophil cytoplasmic antibodies, the serum marker most closely associated with chronic UC, on evaluation of 102 patients with ileal pouches revealed no such association.[47]

Exclusion of possible etiologies that may require specific treatment is essential. The following points must be remembered: Patients with ileal pouches are not immune

Table 110–1   Pouchitis Disease Activity Index*

Criteria	Score
Clinical	
Postoperative stool frequency	
Usual	0
1 or 2 stools/day more than usual	1
≥3 stools/day more than usual	2
Rectal bleeding	
None or rare	0
Present daily	1
Fecal urgency/abdominal cramps	
None	0
Occasional	1
Usual	2
Fever (>100°F)	
Absent	0
Present	1
Endoscopic	
Edema	1
Granularity	1
Friability	1
Loss of vascular pattern	1
Mucus exudate	1
Ulceration	1
Acute Histologic	
Polymorphonuclear leukocyte infiltration	
Mild	1
Moderate + crypt abscess	2
Severe + crypt abscess	3
Ulceration per low-power field (average)	
<25%	1
≥25%, ≤50%	2
>50%	3

*Pouchitis is defined as a total score of ≥7.
Adapted from Sandborn WJ, Tremaine WJ, Batts KP, et al: Pouchitis after ileal pouch-anal anastomosis: A pouchitis disease activity index. Mayo Clin Proc 69:409, 1994.

to superimposed specific enteric infections; stool culture and microscopy for parasites are appropriate. Recurrent Crohn's disease is always a major concern. The clinical features of the underlying inflammatory bowel disease (IBD) need to be reviewed carefully, including gross and histologic examination of the resected bowel. Because a small but definite proportion of colitis falls into an "unclassifiable" group, some patients with previously unrecognized Crohn's disease present with pouchitis as the presentation of (recurrent) Crohn's disease. Surgical complications, such as a strictured anastomosis with partial obstruction to outflow from the pouch, need to be looked for carefully and treated by dilatation if present.

Treatment

If diarrhea alone is the major complaint, treatment with simple antidiarrheal measures may be all that is required. For more severely symptomatic patients, a variety of empiric treatments have emerged. When the condition was first encountered in continent ileostomies, anecdotal evidence was that constant drainage would help, based on the assumption that stasis was an important predisposing factor.[22] Stasis should be a lesser factor after IPAA, although incomplete emptying (e.g., with the S pouch) or a persistent anastomotic stricture may need to be excluded. Metronidazole, 500 mg twice daily for 28 days, has been used often as a first line of treatment. The response to metronidazole or other broad-spectrum antibiotics usually is dramatic. Some patients relapse after initial therapy with antibiotics, and they require subsequent courses of treatment. In general, antibacterial agents against anaerobes have been most successful.

When antibiotics are ineffective, treatment should consist of regimens that are effective in IBD: glucocorticoid enemas, aminosalicylates, mesalamine enemas, and even systemic glucocorticoids. There is evidence that bismuth subsalicylate (Pepto-Bismol) 270 mg daily for 3 weeks is effective in patients with antibiotic-resistant pouchitis. Most patients unresponsive to antibiotics improve on one of these programs. Severe recurrent disease or major extraintestinal symptoms rarely require pouch removal.

Possible Etiologies

Acute, nonspecific inflammation of ileal pouches apparently reflects the propensity of the patient for IBD. Thus, pouchitis is much more common in patients with IBD than it is in patients with FAP. Still, patients operated on for FAP are not completely protected from pouchitis. The nonspecific pathologic features of pouchitis are important because pouchitis may result from different causes.[48]

Histopathology of healthy and diseased pouches[49,50] has shown that chronic inflammation is usual, even when the patient is asymptomatic. Villus architecture is distorted, and colonic metaplasia is present in biopsies from most pouches even in the absence of severe acute inflammation. Thus, these changes are considered natural sequelae of the altered anatomy, just as the histologic changes of experimental and clinical blind-loop syndrome have been attributed to bacterial overgrowth.

Other possible causes of pouchitis have little support, including damage by bile acids or their bacterial metabolites (because dihydroxy bile acids are intestinal secretagogues and cellular toxins)[51] and short-chain fatty acids (SCFAs). There is an increasing body of evidence that normal colonic mucosa uses SCFAs as a source of calories, and some authors have proposed that IBD can result when the colon is deprived of SCFAs.[52] The clearest clinical experiment that tests this hypothesis is "diversion colitis." Harig and coworkers proposed that diversion colitis is caused by deprivation of SCFAs.[53] Support for the proposal is provided by the observation that diversion colitis improves in response to SCFA enemas. Ileal pouches contain high concentrations of SCFAs (≤100 mM), however, and a state of deprivation seems unlikely. Indeed, pouchitis has worsened or shown no predictable response to SCFA enemas.[54] In a detailed evaluation of luminal factors, fecal concentrations of bacteria, bile acids, and SCFAs were similar in patients with or without pouchitis.[51] Pouchitis has no relationship to the presence or absence of backwash ileitis at the time of proctocolectomy.[55]

The overall experience with pouchitis is that 40% of patients with a pouch will never have pouchitis; 40% will have a single episode; 15% will have intermittently recurring episodes; and 5% or less will develop chronic pouchitis.[48]

Possible Sequelae

Although the prevalence of chronic pouchitis is low, the possible consequences of chronic inflammation of the neorectum, especially dysplasia and malignant change, arouse concern. Cancer has been reported in the pouch and in the pelvis after IPAA, most likely the result of malignant degeneration of a dysplastic rectal cuff.[56] Morphologic and biochemical changes occur in the ileal mucosa of pouches, including villus blunting, chronic inflammatory infiltrates, variable transition to production of a colonic type of mucus (sulfomucins), and increased cellular proliferation.[57] Observations based on long-term follow-up (mean of 6.3 years) proposes three patterns of mucosal adaptation[50]: approximately one half of the patients showed mild villus atrophy and minimal inflammation; slightly fewer had transient moderate or severe atrophy and inflammation with intervals of recovery; and approximately 10% had permanent subtotal or total villus atrophy with chronic inflammation. In this study, low-grade dysplasia developed in three of eight patients in the last group and as early as 2 years postoperatively in one patient. The patients at risk are those with chronic pouchitis.

Pouch Failure

Large series have reported failure rates between 2% and 12% and in the Mayo clinic series, 6% of patients ultimately require pouch excision or construction of a permanent ileostomy. The most frequent causes of pouch failure, either alone or in combination, include pelvic sepsis, high stool volumes, Crohn's disease, and uncontrollable fecal incontinence; pouchitis is the sole cause in 2% of all patients. Of the patients in whom the pouch fails, failure occurs within 1 year in 75%, by 2 years in 12%, and 3 years in 12%. Thus, failure after IPAA occurs within several years after the operation and is the result of a combination of early or late complications of the procedure.

Quality of Life

Often, quality of life is the deciding factor for patients choosing a particular operation for chronic UC. Several studies that analyzed the outcome of surgery for chronic UC have demonstrated that most patients are satisfied with the operation and lead a normal life-style regardless of the procedure.

In one study of quality of life after a Brooke ileostomy or IPAA for chronic UC and FAP, patients were highly satisfied with either operation (Brooke ileostomy, 93%; IPAA, 95%).[25] Daily activities (e.g., sexual life, participation in sports, social interaction, work, recreation, family relationships, travel), however, were more likely to be adversely affected with a Brooke ileostomy than by IPAA.

Sexual Dysfunction

Impotency and retrograde ejaculation developed in 1.5% and 4% of men, respectively. Dyspareunia developed in 7% of women postoperatively. Of note, 49% of women noted sexual dysfunction preoperatively, yet sexual activity increased dramatically after IPAA because of an improvement in general health.

CONTROVERSIES

Double-Stapled Versus Hand-Sewn Anastomosis

Much of the debate whether to staple the anastomosis or not has evolved because functional outcomes should be improved if the anal transition zone (or more recently, "columnar cuff" [CC]) is preserved. Does preserving the CC enhance continence after IPAA? In nonrandomized trials, a stapled anastomosis has been equated with better outcome, which in turn has been attributed to less injury of the anal sphincters; preservation of the CC and hence anal sensory discrimination; and preservation of the rectoanal inhibitory reflex. To determine if stapled IPAA conferred any advantage over hand-sewn IPAA, we conducted a randomized study at the Mayo Clinic in which 41 patients were randomized to double-stapled (17 patients) or hand-sewn (15 patients) technique.[58] In the stapled group, 1.5 to 2.0 cm of CC was preserved, whereas complete mucosectomy was performed in the hand-sewn group. Overall, complications were the same in the two groups. Stool frequency and rates of fecal incontinence during the day and night were similar between the groups; however, fewer patients treated with the double-stapled technique had nocturnal incontinence. Moreover, resting and squeezing anal sphincter pressures were preserved better after double-stapling.

Role of Defunctioning Ileostomy

The most feared complication of IPAA is pelvic sepsis; therefore, a defunctioning ileostomy after pouch construction usually is performed to minimize its occurrence.[59] Whereas pelvic sepsis complicates 6% of IPAA procedures at the Mayo Clinic, the rates reported in the literature vary between 0% and 25%. Although the incidence of pelvic sepsis is relatively low at the Mayo Clinic, when it occurs, it is responsible for a significant proportion of the failed pouches.[60]

Protagonists of defunctioning ileostomies argue that diverting stomas allow the anal sphincter and ileal mucosa to recover before restoration of intestinal continuity and that patients have a short-lived experience of a stoma to appreciate fully the ultimate benefit of IPAA. Use of a loop ileostomy does not appear to protect the patient fully from pelvic sepsis; however, its presence makes it easier to manage a patient with pelvic sepsis. Among the patients at the Mayo Clinic who required laparotomy to control sepsis, 41% lost the pouch ultimately, and only 29% ever recovered ileoanal function. However, if no reoperation was required, 92% of patients with sepsis eventually had a functioning pouch.[60]

Supporters of a one-stage procedure believe that an IPAA can be performed without increased risk of pelvic sepsis.[61-66] A one-stage procedure avoids an ileostomy and a second hospitalization and operation, lowers the total cost, and results in a shorter hospital stay and perhaps a decreased incidence of small bowel obstruction. In the large single-surgeon study reported by Sugerman and associates, there were no differences in the complication rates and functional outcomes of patients who had not had a diverting ileostomy compared with those who had a diverting ileostomy[61]; there also was no relationship to steroid use.[61,63,67] Whereas there might be no significant difference in the complication rate in patients without a diverting ileostomy, one study has suggested that the severity of complications was greater in those patients without a protecting ileostomy.[68] Although it is our practice to perform a diverting ileostomy in all patients undergoing an IPAA, in properly selected patients who have uncomplicated procedures performed by experienced surgeons, a one-stage IPAA might be appropriate. The surgeon and patient care team must be attentive to the early signs of pelvic sepsis and aggressively investigate the possibility of a pouch or an anastomotic leak and intervene as needed.

ADDITIONAL ISSUES

Risk of Cancer

Patients with chronic UC are at risk of developing adenocarcinoma of the colon.[69] This risk increases as the duration of disease and the extent of colonic involvement increase. Any surgery that leaves behind diseased colonic mucosa puts the patient at risk of developing dysplasia or neoplasia in the residual colonic mucosa. The risk of developing a carcinoma in the residual colonic mucosa may be related directly to the amount of residual mucosa remaining in situ.

Complete excision of the rectal mucosa during IPAA substantially decreases the risk of dysplasia. With the widespread acceptance of stapled IPAA, the residual cuff epithelium (CE) is reduced to less than 1 cm or nearly eliminated. Studies such as that by Tsunoda and colleagues, which demonstrated the presence of dysplasia in mucosectomy specimens, have been used as evidence to support the use of routine complete mucosal resection.[70] Opposite conclusions were drawn by Ziv and associates after stapled IPAA.[71] To make this topic even more complex, several studies report that viable mucosa is present in the rectal muscular cuff after mucosal resection. In one such study, islands (rests) of mucosa were present despite "complete" mucosal resection.[72] The incidence of dysplasia in the retained rectal mucosa, or distal rectal doughnut, after double-stapled ileoanal anastomosis is approximately 1%.

The question of follow-up of the CE has been addressed by several investigators. The Cleveland Clinic reported its experience with 254 patients who underwent double-stapled IPAA and had follow-up with annual postsurgical CE biopsy.[71] During a mean follow-up of 2 years, low-grade dysplasia was found in eight patients (3%). Repeat biopsies confirmed dysplasia in only two of these eight patients. Significant correlation was seen between CE dysplasia and presence of dysplasia or cancer of the large bowel before surgery; there was no association with age, sex, duration of the disease, anastomotic technique, or length of rectal cuff. The risk of dysplasia in the residual CE was 25% or 10%, respectively, in patients who had cancer or had dysplasia in the original proctocolectomy specimen.

Detection of neoplastic change in the pouch itself is another reason to perform follow-up in patients with IPAA. A subgroup of patients has been identified, in whom the mucosa of the pelvic pouch develops severe villus atrophy.[50] These patients seem to have a significantly higher incidence of dysplasia compared with patients without villus atrophy (71% vs. 0%). The former group may be at greater risk of developing carcinoma and may require more intensive follow-up with regular pouch endoscopy and biopsy.

To date, there have been a small number of case reports of carcinomas arising in ileal pouches or in the region of the anastomosis.[73-75] Surprisingly, many of these cancers have arisen in patients who have undergone a complete mucosectomy with hand-sewn anastomosis. Given the known occurrence of dysplasia in pouch mucosa and the rare reports of cancers arising in pouches, routine clinical and endoscopic surveillance should be performed in patients after their IPAA.

Fertility and Pregnancy

Most patients who present for surgery with chronic UC are in their child-bearing years. Although a number of centers have reported on women becoming pregnant after IPAA, functional results as well as obstetric implications, including the impact of IPAA surgery on fertility or fecundity (the ability to become pregnant), have not been analyzed easily.[42,76,77] In a large population-based study in Sweden, the rate of pregnancy in women who had undergone an IPAA was reduced significantly.[78] Moreover, of the post-IPAA patients who became pregnant, 29% of pregnancies occurred only after in vitro fertilization (IVF) compared to the 1% expected IVF rate for all births. The basis of this decreased fertility is unknown, but the authors believed that anatomic changes in the pelvis may be a contributing factor. In a follow-up study, the same authors looked at female fecundity before and after operations for FAP.[79] Some of the women had an IPAA, whereas others had an ileorectostomy. The women with an ileorectostomy had a fecundity rate similar to the general population; however, fecundity dropped to 54%

following IPAA. Until further studies are done to confirm and clarify these findings, young women considering undergoing IPAA should be informed of the possibility of decreased fertility.

IPAA and Indeterminate Colitis

Among 1519 consecutive patients with chronic UC undergoing IPAA between January of 1981 and December of 1995, 82 (5%) of patients had features of "indeterminate colitis" (IC), including unusual distribution of inflammation, deep linear ulcers, neural proliferation, transmural inflammation, fissures, and creeping fat.[80] We found that 12 (15%) of 82 IC patients eventually developed Crohn's disease during follow-up, whereas only 26 (2%) of 1437 chronic UC patients developed Crohn's disease.[80] The probability of remaining free of CD at 10 years was 98% of patients with chronic UC and only 81% in the IC patients. After IPAA, patients with IC who did not develop Crohn's disease experienced long-term outcomes nearly identical to those of patients with chronic UC; that is, nearly 85% had functioning pouches 10 years after the operation. Crohn's disease, however, regardless of whether it develops and is diagnosed after the IPAA operations for chronic UC or IC, is associated with poor long-term outcomes. Whether patients with IC need to be managed expectantly for the development of Crohn's disease needs further study.

ABDOMINAL COLECTOMY AND ILEORECTAL ANASTOMOSIS

The aim of a colectomy with an ileorectal anastomosis (IRA) is to extirpate most of the diseased colonic mucosa, thus reducing the risks of hemorrhage, dilatation, megacolon perforation, and malignant degeneration, while allowing the rectum to retain continence for stool and gas. The rationale for an IRA is that the operation avoids a permanent stoma, minimizes or eliminates injury to the pelvic nerves, and is easy to perform; other operations, if they become necessary, are not precluded.[81-83] The rationale against the operation, however, is nearly as convincing. Subsequent proctectomy is required in 6% to 37% of patients; poor results have been reported in up to 50%; and the risk of developing carcinoma in the retained rectum approaches 17% after 27 years.[84,85] In patients with Crohn's disease and minimal or no rectal involvement, IRA with excision of the diseased colon is an appropriate operation.

PATIENT SELECTION

Patients are candidates for IRA if the rectum is distensible, if the disease (chronic UC, Crohn's) involves the rectum only minimally, and if patients are willing to undergo follow-up screening for rectal cancer. Patients of any body habitus may undergo IRA. Although there is no maximum age that contraindicates an ileorectostomy, functional results related to poor sphincter function must be considered in older patients, especially in older female patients.

COMPLICATIONS

Operative mortality for elective IRA has been reported to vary between 2% and 8%.[86] Almost all deaths have been caused by anastomotic leakage, which affects 3% of patients; small bowel obstruction complicates the recovery of about 15%. Although sexual function in men usually is preserved postoperatively, up to 50% of women have experienced postoperative dyspareunia.

PHYSIOLOGY

The primary attraction of an IRA is that the major anatomic mechanisms responsible for maintaining continence are retained: The rectal reservoir, the pelvic floor, and the internal and external anal sphincters are preserved. The absorptive capacity of the proximal colon is lost, however, and ileal content is continuously presented to the rectal remnant.

The rectum should be compliant and large to allow passive accommodation. Compliance depends on rectal wall elasticity, and in active inflammatory disease, compliant accommodation is impaired.[87] Moreover, the smaller the rectum, the greater the elasticity coefficient; patients with active chronic UC have a smaller rectum than do controls.[88] Therefore, the lesser the mucosal inflammation and elasticity coefficient, the better the compliance and the fewer the stools per day. Sphincteric function in patients with IRA differs little from that in normal people.

After an IRA, patients with quiescent rectal disease should be able to absorb water and sodium in the rectal segment. Moreover, with quiescent disease, the rectum is capacious and distensible, resulting in low stool frequency and little or no incontinence. Conversely, if the rectal mucosa is inflamed, absorption is impaired and fecal volume is greater; moreover, the more inflamed the mucosa, the less capacious and distensible will be the rectum, and increased stool frequency, urgency, and incontinence will follow.

The best measure of successful clinical outcome after an IRA is the rate of subsequent proctocolectomy because of persistence or recurrence of disease or the occurrence of rectal cancer. The reported late proctectomy rate for persistence or recurrence of disease varies greatly, from 5% to 58%. The probability that a patient with chronic UC will have a good result after IRA—that is, will not require steroids, be in good general health, and have an acceptable stool frequency with no incontinence—is approximately 50%. The risk of cancer developing in the retained rectum is about 5% at 15 years after operation; this increases to 15% by 30 years.[82,85,86] Unfortunately, these cancers typically are of advanced grade and stage compared with the usual colorectal cancer. Those operated on for FAP must, of course, undergo close surveillance for cancer.

The quality of life after IRA has been reported to be good; patient satisfaction is high, and an active, productive life-style can be preserved.[89] Overall satisfaction is tempered, however, by the fact that patients often believe that they have not been cured because they must undergo frequent follow-up examinations.

COLOSTOMY IN THE MANAGEMENT OF INFLAMMATORY BOWEL DISEASE

For patients with chronic UC, colostomy has no role either electively or emergently. Resection of the rectosigmoid, coloanal anastomosis, and cecoanal anastomosis are operations for chronic UC mentioned here only to be condemned.[90-92] Urgent or emergent intervention for decompensating or fulminating chronic UC is best managed by abdominal colectomy, Brooke ileostomy, and either oversewing the rectum or establishing a rectal mucous fistula.

Colostomy is only a slightly better choice for patients with Crohn's colitis. Segmental resection, although associated with higher recurrence rates, is an acceptable alternative to abdominal colectomy and ileorectostomy, if there is a significant length of normal colon adjacent to the diseased segment. It was taught to remove the involved segment together with the colon proximal to this segment and to perform an ileocolostomy, but it makes more sense in a patient with Crohn's disease of the distal sigmoid colon alone to resect only the sigmoid colon and anastomose the descending colon to the rectum, rather than performing an abdominal colectomy and ileorectostomy.

LAPAROSCOPY

The most important change in surgical practice related to all of these procedures is the application of laparoscopic techniques. Minimal access colon surgery began in the early 1990s; however, improvements in image technology and instrumentation have only recently facilitated complex colorectal procedures. At the Mayo Clinic, this approach has now been used in more than 70 patients with chronic UC since an initial pilot study in seven patients reported in 2001.[93] Indications for operative intervention are not changed by the laparoscopic approach. In a case-matched series of 40 patients undergoing laparoscopic IPAA (LAP), IPAA being matched to two open controls, and controlling for disease, age, gender, body mass index (BMI), and date of operation,

the LAP group exhibited significant benefits, in time, to (1) ingesting clear liquids (1 vs. 3 days; $P < .001$); (2) eating a regular diet (3 vs. 4 days; $P < .001$); and (3) regaining bowel function (2 vs. 3 days; $P < .001$).[94] Moreover, duration of narcotic use was shorter in the LAP group ($P < .001$), and length of stay was reduced (4 vs. 7 days; $P < .001$). LAP patients had longer operative times (270 vs. 192 minutes; $P < 0.001$), but operative time decreased with experience and now averages 180 to 210 minutes. Other authors also are seeing these advantages.[95,96]

SUMMARY OF RISK-BENEFIT ANALYSIS

CONVENTIONAL ILEOSTOMY

The Brooke ileostomy is safe and reliable and has broad applicability to patients with IBD who require proctocolectomy. It is not, however, entirely free of complications (Table 110–2). Up to 30% of patients have a septic complication; 20% to 25% require stomal revision; 15% have recurrent small bowel obstruction; and stomal dysfunction can occur in up to 30% of cases. These data should be kept in mind when evaluating the alternative procedures.

ILEORECTAL ANASTOMOSIS

The primary benefit of an IRA is that the rectum is undisturbed by the operative dissection; the normal pathway of defecation is left in situ; and the incidence of bladder or sexual problems is low. Moreover, there is no perineal wound (see Table 110–2). In many patients, the overall functional results are reasonably good. The major problem with an IRA is that actual or potentially diseased mucosa is left in situ. In a few patients, inflammatory changes do resolve, but in most, the disease process continues unabated. The sequelae of leaving disease behind include (1) poor anastomotic healing, which is responsible for the relatively higher mortality after IRA than after continent ileostomy and IPAA; (2) continued need for

Table 110–2 Comparison of Surgical Options after Colectomy

	Stoma	Continence	Mortality, %	Overall Morbidity, %	Small Bowel Obstruction, %	Perineal Wound Complication, %	Stools Per 24 Hours	Failure, %	All Disease Removed?	Cancer Risk, %	Disease Indication
Brooke ileostomy	Yes	No	<1.0	19-70	15	33	NA	—	Yes	0	CD (?UC, FAP)
Ileorectal anastomosis	No	Yes	2.5-8.0	16-20	15	NA	1-3	24-60	No	15 (30 yr)	CD, UC
Continent ileostomy	Yes	Yes	<1.0	15-60	7	35	3-5	50	Yes	†	UC, FAP
Ileal pouch-anal anastomosis	No	Yes	<1.0	30-50	22	NA	5-7	8	Yes*	*	UC, FAP

Maximum follow-up time is 13 years. NA, not appropriate.
Disease indication: CD, Crohn's disease; FAP, familial adenomatous polyposis; UC, ulcerative colitis.
*Ten instances of neoplasia in the cuff or pouch after ileal pouch-anal anastomosis have been reported in more than 12,000 cases.
†Two cancers in Kock pouches (continent ileostomies) have been reported.

anti-inflammatory therapy; (3) continued bleeding and mucus discharge; (4) incontinence and high stool frequency when inflammation flares up; and (5) the possibility of malignant degeneration.

CONTINENT ILEOSTOMY

The major benefit of the Kock pouch is that, although a stoma is constructed, discharge is controlled without the need for an external appliance. Moreover, in patients with chronic UC, all disease is removed. The principal problem with continent ileostomy is the high rate of complications, usually involving the nipple valve, and leading to incontinence or to complete outflow obstruction; these complications, in turn, almost always require another operation. As with the Brooke ileostomy, a perineal wound accompanies this operation; the wound fails to heal promptly in about one third of patients. This operation is rarely performed today because the success of IPAA has made it obsolete.

ILEAL POUCH-ANAL ANASTOMOSIS

The major benefit of IPAA is that it successfully restores fecal continence in most patients; the major problem is the high complication rate of approximately 30%. Occasional incontinence appears early in almost all patients after operation, particularly at night. Major episodes of daytime incontinence affect approximately 10% of patients, but this frequency declines to almost zero after 4 years. Other complications are pelvic infection, stricture, fistula, sinus tracts, pouch leakage, and small bowel obstruction. As surgeons' experience with the operation has broadened, these surgical complications have decreased in frequency. Although nonspecific inflammation of the pouch, or pouchitis, is the most important current drawback, in most patients it is treated effectively and simply with antibiotics. When severe and recurrent, pouchitis can lead to failure of the operation; this is uncommon. Despite these problems, the benefits of IPAA are clear: all disease is removed, the patient does not have a stoma, and anal defecation is voluntary and controlled.

REFERENCES

1. Hill GL (ed): Historical introduction. In Ileostomy: Surgery, Physiology, and Management. New York, Grune & Stratton, 1976, p 1.
2. Brooke BN: Management of ileostomy including its complications. Lancet 2:102, 1952.
3. Turnbull RB: Symposium on chronic ulcerative colitis: Management of ileostomy. Am J Surg 86:617, 1953.
4. Roy PH, Sauer WG, Beahrs OH, Farrow GN: Experience with ileostomies: Evaluation of long-term rehabilitation in 497 patients. Am J Surg 119:77, 1970.
5. Kock NG: Intra-abdominal reservoir in patients with permanent ileostomy: Preliminary observations on a procedure resulting in fecal continence in five ileostomy patients. Arch Surg 99:223, 1969.
6. Dozois RR, Kelly KA, Beart RW Jr, Beahrs OH: Continent ileostomy: The Mayo Clinic experience. In Dozois RR (ed): Alternatives to Conventional Ileostomy. Chicago, Year Book, 1985, p 180.
7. Ravitch MM, Sabiston DC: Anal ileostomy with preservation of the sphincter. Surg Gynecol Obstet 84:1095, 1947.
8. Beart RW Jr, Metcalf AM, Dozois RR, Kelly KA: The J ileal pouch-anal anastomosis: The Mayo Clinic Experience. In Dozois RR (ed): Alternatives to Conventional Ileostomy. Chicago, Year Book, 1985, p 384.
9. Phillips SF, Giller J: Contribution of the colon to electrolyte and water conservation in man. J Lab Clin Med 81:733, 1973.
10. Debongnie JC, Phillips SF: Capacity of the human colon to absorb fluid. Gastroenterology 74:698, 1978.
11. Dole VP, Dahle LK, Cotzias G, et al: Dietary treatment of hypertension: Clinical and metabolic studies of patients on the rice-fruit diet. J Clin Invest 29:1189, 1950.
12. Kramer P: The effect of varying sodium loads on the ileal excreta of human ileostomized subjects. J Clin Invest 45:1710, 1966.
13. Kanaghinis T, Lubran M, Coghill NF: The composition of ileostomy fluid. Gut 4:322, 1963.
14. Metcalf AM, Phillips SF: Ileostomy diarrhea. Clin Gastroenterol 15:705, 1986.
15. Kramer P, Kearney MS, Ingelfinger FJ: The effect of specific foods and water loading on the ileal excreta of ileostomized human subjects. Gastroenterology 42:535, 1962.
16. Gallagher ND, Harrison DD, Skyring AP: Fluid and electrolyte disturbances in patients with long established ileostomies. Gut 3:219, 1962.
17. Clarke AM, Chirnside A, Hill GL, et al: Chronic dehydration and sodium depletion in patients with established ileostomies. Lancet 2:740, 1967.
18. Clarke AM, McKenzie RG: Ileostomy and the risk of urinary uric acid stones. Lancet 2:395, 1969.
19. Morris JS, Low-Beer TS, Heaton KW: Bile salt metabolism and the colon. Scand J Gastroenterol 8:425, 1973.
20. Gadacz TR, Kelly KA, Phillips SF: The Kock ileal pouch: Absorptive and motor characteristics. Gastroenterology 72:1287, 1977.
21. Gorbach SL, Nahas L, Weinstein L: Studies of intestinal microflora: IV. The microflora of ileostomy effluent: A unique microbial etiology. Gastroenterology 53:874, 1967.
22. Kelly DG, Phillips SF, Kelly KA, et al: Dysfunction of the continent ileostomy: Clinical features and bacteriology. Gut 24:193, 1983.
23. O'Connell PR, Rankin DR, Weiland LH, Kelly KA: Enteric bacteriology, absorption, morphology, and emptying after ileal pouch-anal anastomosis. Br J Surg 73:909, 1986.
24. Watts JM, de Dombal FT, Goligher JC: Long-term complications and prognosis following major surgery for chronic ulcerative colitis. Br J Surg 53:1014, 1966.
25. Pemberton JH, Phillips SF, Ready RR, et al: Quality of life after Brooke ileostomy and ileal pouch-anal anastomosis. Ann Surg 209:620, 1989.
26. Phillips SF: Metabolic consequences of a stagnant loop at the end of the small bowel. World J Surg 11:763, 1987.
27. Knill-Jones RP, Morson B, Williams R: Prestomal ileitis: Clinical and pathological findings in five cases. Q J Med 39:287, 1970.
28. Sparberg M: Bismuth subgallate as an effective means for control of ileostomy odor: A double-blind study. Gastroenterology 66:476, 1974.
29. Report from the Australian Drug Evaluation Committee. Adverse effects of bismuth subgallate. Med J Aust 2:664, 1974.
30. Lennenberg E, Rowbotham JL: The Ileostomy Patients: A Descriptive Study of 1425 Persons. Springfield, IL, Charles C Thomas, 1970.
31. Sparberg M: The Ileostomy Case. Springfield, IL, Charles C Thomas, 1971.
32. Kock NG, Mynvold HE, Nilsson LO, Phillipson BN: Continent ileostomy: The Swedish experience. In Dozois RR (ed): Alter-

natives to Conventional Ileostomy. Chicago, Year Book, 1985, p 163.

33. Mullen P, Behrens D, Chalmers T, et al: Barnett continent intestinal reservoir: Multicenter experiences with an alternative to the Brooke ileostomy. Dis Colon Rectum 38:573, 1995.

34. Kelly DG, Branon ME, Phillips SF, Kelly KA: Diarrhea after continent ileostomy. Gut 21:711, 1980.

35. Cox CL, Butts DR, Roberts MP, et al: Development of invasive adenocarcinoma in a long-standing Kock continent ileostomy: Report of a case. Dis Colon Rectum 40:500, 1997.

36. Kaiser AM, Stein JP, Beart RW: T-pouch: A new valve design for a continent ileostomy. Dis Colon Rectum 45:411, 2002.

37. Panis Y, Poupard B, Nemeth J, et al: Ileal pouch/anal anastomosis for Crohn's disease. Lancet 347:854, 1996.

38. Regimbeau JM, Panis Y, Pocard M, et al: Long-term results of ileal pouch-anal anastomosis for colorectal Crohn's disease. Dis Colon Rectum 44:769, 2001.

39. Stryker SJ, Dozois RR: The ileoanal anastomosis: Historical perspectives. In Dozois RR (ed): Alternatives to Conventional Ileostomy. Chicago, Year Book, 1985, p 225.

40. Coran AG: Straight endorectal pull-through of the ileum for the management of benign disease of the colon and rectum in children and adults. In Dozois RR (ed): Alternatives to Conventional Ileostomy. Chicago, Year Book, 1985, p 335.

41. Pemberton JH, Kelly KA, Beart RW Jr, et al: Ileal pouch-anal anastomosis for chronic ulcerative colitis: Long-term results. Ann Surg 206:504, 1987.

42. Farouk R, Pemberton JH, Wolff BG, et al: Functional outcomes after ileal pouch-anal anastomosis for chronic ulcerative colitis. Ann Surg 231:919, 2000.

43. Dozois RR, Kelly KA: J ileal pouch-anal anastomosis for chronic ulcerative colitis: Complications and long-term outcome in 1310 patients. Br J Surg 85:800, 1998.

44. Fleshman JW, Cohen A, McLeod RS, et al: The ileal reservoir and ileo-anal anastomosis procedure: Factors affecting technical and functional outcome. Dis Colon Rectum 31:10, 1988.

45. Lohmuller JL, Pemberton JH, Dozois RR, et al: Pouchitis and extraintestinal manifestations of inflammatory bowel disease after ileal pouch-anal anastomosis. Ann Surg 211:622, 1990.

46. Sandborn WJ, Tremaine WJ, Batts KP, et al: Pouchitis after ileal pouch-anal anastomosis: A pouchitis disease activity index. Mayo Clin Proc 69:409, 1994.

47. Aisenberg J, Legnani PE, NIlubol N, et al: Are pANCA, ASCA, or cytokine gene polymorphisms associated with pouchitis? Long-term follow-up in 102 ulcerative colitis patients. Am J Gastroenterol 99:432, 2004.

48. Sandborn WJ: Pouchitis following ileal pouch-anal anastomosis: Definition, pathogenesis, and treatment. Gastroenterology 107:1856, 1994.

49. Apel R, Cohen Z, Andrews CW, et al: Prospective evaluation of early morphological changes in pelvic ileal pouches. Gastroenterology 107:435, 1994.

50. Veress B, Reinholt FP, Lindquist K, et al: Long-term histomorphological surveillance of the pelvic ileal pouch: Dysplasia develops in a subgroup of patients. Gastroenterology 109:1090, 1995.

51. Sandborn WJ, Tremaine WJ, Batts KP, et al: Fecal bile acids, short-chain fatty acids, and bacteria after ileal pouch-anal anastomosis do not differ in patients with pouchitis. Dig Dis Sci 40:1474, 1995.

52. Roediger WEW: The colonic epithelium in chronic ulcerative colitis—an energy deficiency disease? Lancet 2:712, 1980.

53. Harig JM, Soergel KH, Komorowski RA, Wood CM: Treatment of diversion colitis with short chain fatty acid irrigation. N Engl J Med 320:23, 1989.

54. DeSilva HJ, Ireland A, Kettlewell M, et al: Short-chain fatty acids irrigation in severe pouchitis [Letter]. N Engl J Med 321:1416, 1989.

55. Gustavsson S, Weiland LH, Kelly KA: Relationship of backwash ileitis to ileal pouchitis after ileal pouch-anal anastomosis. Dis Colon Rectum 30:25, 1987.

56. Stern H, Walfisch S, Mullen B, et al: Cancer in an ileoanal reservoir: A new late complication. Gut 31:473, 1990.

57. DeSilva HJ, Millaro PR, Kettlewell M, et al: Mucosal characteristics of pelvic ileal pouches. Gut 32:61, 1991.

58. Reilly WT, Pemberton JH, Wolff BG, et al: Randomized prospective trial comparing ileal pouch-anal anastomosis (IPAA) performed by excising the anal mucosa to IPAA performed by preserving the anal mucosa. Ann Surg 225:666, 1997.

59. Galandiuk S, Wolff BG, Dozois RR, Beart RW Jr: Ileal pouch-anal anastomosis without ileostomy. Dis Colon Rectum 34:870, 1991.

60. Galandiuk S, Scott NA, Dozois RR, et al: Ileal pouch-anal anastomosis: Reoperation for pouch-related complications. Ann Surg 212:446, 1990.

61. Sugerman HJ, Sugerman EL, Meador JG, et al: Ileal pouch anal anastomosis without ileal diversion. Ann Surg 232:530, 2000.

62. Heuschen UA, Hinz U, Allemeyer EH, et al: One- or two-stage procedure for restorative proctocolectomy: Rationale for a surgical strategy in chronic ulcerative colitis. Ann Surg 234:788, 2001.

63. Hosie KB, Grobler SP, Keighley MR: Temporary loop ileostomy following restorative proctocolectomy. Br J Surg 79:33, 1992.

64. Tjandra JJ, Fazio VW, Milsom JW, et al: Omission of temporary diversion in restorative proctocolectomy: Is it safe? Dis Colon Rectum 36:1007, 1993.

65. Matikainen M, Santavirta J, Hiltunen K: Ileoanal anastomosis without a covering ileostomy. Dis Colon Rectum 33:384, 1990.

66. Sugerman HJ, Newsome HH, Decosta G, et al: Stapled ileoanal anastomosis for chronic ulcerative colitis and familial polyposis without a temporary diverting ileostomy. Ann Surg 213:606, 1991.

67. Cohen Z, McLeod RS, Stephen W, et al: Continuing evolution of the pelvic pouch procedure. Ann Surg 216:506, 1992.

68. Williamson MER, Lewis WG, Sagar PM, et al: One-stage restorative proctocolectomy without temporary ileostomy for chronic ulcerative colitis: A note of caution. Dis Colon Rectum 40:1019, 1997.

69. Langholz E, Munkholm P, Davidsen M, et al: Colorectal cancer risk and mortality in patients with chronic ulcerative colitis. Gastroenterology 103:1444, 1992.

70. Tsunoda A, Talbot IC, Nicholls RJ: Incidence of dysplasia in the anorectal mucosa in patients having restorative proctocolectomy. Br J Surg 77:506, 1990.

71. Ziv Y, Fazio VW, Sirimarco MT, et al: Incidence, risk factors, and treatment of dysplasia in the anal transition zone after ileal pouch-anal anastomosis. Dis Colon Rectum 37:1281, 1994.

72. Haray PN, Amamath B, Weiss EG, et al: Low malignant potential of the double-stapled ileal pouch-anal anastomosis. Br J Surg 83:1406, 1996.

73. Laureti S, Ugolini F, D'Errico A, et al: Adenocarcinoma below ileoanal anastomosis for chronic ulcerative colitis: Report of a case and review of the literature. Dis Colon Rectum 45:418, 2002.

74. Hassan C, Zullo A, Speziale G, et al: Adenocarcinoma of the ileoanal pouch anastomosis: An emerging complication? Int J Colorectal Dis 18:276, 2003.

75. Heuschen UA, Heuschen G, Autschbach F, e al: Adenocarcinoma in the ileal pouch: Late risk of cancer after restorative proctocolectomy. Int J Colorectal Dis 16:126, 2001.

76. Nelson H, Dozois RR, Kelly KA, et al: The effect of pregnancy and delivery on ileal pouch-anal anastomosis functions. Dis Colon Rectum 32:384, 1989.

77. Juhasz ES, Fozard, B, Dozois RR, et al: Ileal pouch-anal anastomosis function following childbirth: An extended evaluation. Dis Colon Rectum 38:59, 1995.

78. Olsen KO, Joelsson M, Laurberg S, et al: Fertility after ileal pouch-anal anastomosis in women with ulcerative colitis. Br J Surg 86:493, 1999.

79. Olsen KO, Juul S, Bulow S, et al: Female fecundity before and after operation for familial adenomatous polyposis. Br J Surg 90:227, 2003.

80. Yu CS, Pemberton JH, Larson D: Ileal pouch-anal anastomosis in patients with IC: Long-term results. Dis Colon Rectum 43:1487, 2000.

81. Aylett SO: Three hundred cases of diffuse chronic ulcerative colitis treated by total colectomy and ileo-rectal anastomosis. BMJ 1:1001, 1966.

82. Grundfest SF, Fazio V, Weiss RA, et al: The risk of cancer following colectomy and IRA for extensive mucosal chronic ulcerative colitis. Ann Surg 193:9, 1981.

83. Watts JM, Hughes SR: Chronic ulcerative colitis and Crohn's disease: Results after colectomy and IRA. Br J Surg 64:77, 1977.

84. Adson MA, Cooperman AM, Farrow GM: Ileorectostomy for ulcerative disease of the colon. Arch Surg 104:424, 1972.

85. Johnson WR, McDermott FT, Hughes ESR, et al: The risk of rectal carcinoma following colectomy in chronic ulcerative colitis. Dis Colon Rectum 26:44, 1983.

86. Baker WNW, Glass RE, Ritchie JK, Aylett SO: Cancer of the rectum following colectomy and IRA for chronic ulcerative colitis. Br J Surg 65:862, 1978.

87. Denis PH, Colin R, Galmiche JP, et al: Elastic properties of the rectal wall in normal adults and in patients with chronic ulcerative colitis. Gastroenterology 77:45, 1979.

88. Farthing MJG, Lennard-Jones JE: Sensibility of the rectum to distension and the anorectal distension reflex in chronic ulcerative colitis. Gut 19:64, 1978.

89. Mignon M, Bonfils S: Altered physiology in chronic ulcerative colitis patients with IRA. In Dozois RR (ed): Alternatives to Conventional Ileostomy. Chicago, Year Book, 1985, p 61.

90. Clark CG, Ward MWM: The place of isolated rectal excision in the treatment of chronic ulcerative colitis. Br J Surg 67:653, 1980.

91. Roediger WEW, Pihl E, Hughes E: Preserving the ascending colon as an alternative support option in chronic ulcerative colitis. Surg Gynecol Obstet 54:348, 1982.

92. Varma JS, Browning GGP, Smith AW, et al: Mucosal proctectomy and colo-anal anastomosis for distal ulcerative proctocolitis. Br J Surg 74:381, 1987.

93. Young-Fadok TM, Dozois ED, Sandborn WJ, Tremaine WJ: A case-matched study of laparoscopic proctocolectomy and ileal pouch-anal anastomosis (IPAA) versus open IPAA for chronic ulcerative colitis [Abstract]. Gastroenterology 120:A452, 2001.

94. Hahnloser D, Young-Fadok TM: Earlier postoperative spontaneous diuresis in laparoscopic versus open total proctocolectomy and ileal pouch-anal anastomosis. Surg Endosc 17(Suppl):S238, 2003.

95. Ky AJ, Sonoda T, Milsom JW: One-stage laparoscopic restorative proctocolectomy: An alternative to the conventional approach? Dis Colon Rectum 45:207, 2002.

96. Kienle P, Weitz J, Benner A, et al: Laparoscopically assisted colectomy and ileoanal pouch procedure with and without protective ileostomy. Surg Endosc 17:716, 2003.

CHAPTER
111 Intestinal Ischemia

Lawrence J. Brandt

Intestinal ischemia produces a broad spectrum of disorders, depending on the onset, duration, and cause of the injury; the area and length of bowel affected; the vessel involved; and the degree of collateral blood flow. Variability in these factors influences not only the presentation of the ischemic event but also its treatment and outcome. Ischemic injury may be acute or chronic, and it may be caused by a disturbance in the arterial supply or venous drainage of the bowel and involve the small intestine, the colon, or both. Since the development and widespread use of colonoscopy, angiography, computed tomography (CT), and other imaging modalities, various types of ischemic injury to the gastrointestinal tract have been recognized and increasingly appreciated (Table 111–1; see also Tables 111–2 and 111–4). Our concepts of their pathogenesis, diagnosis, and management have been so altered since the 1980s that much of what has been written in the past is no longer applicable. In this chapter I describe the spectrum of ischemic damage to the gastrointestinal tract and discuss the management of these conditions in light of recent advances.

ANATOMY OF THE SPLANCHNIC CIRCULATION

The celiac axis (CA), superior mesenteric artery (SMA), and inferior mesenteric artery (IMA) supply almost all of the blood flow to the digestive tract.[1] There is marked variability of vascular anatomy among individuals, but typical patterns have emerged from anatomic dissections and abdominal angiographic studies.

CELIAC AXIS

The CA (Fig. 111–1) arises from the anterior aorta and typically gives rise to three major branches: the left gastric artery, the common hepatic artery, and the splenic artery. The common hepatic artery gives rise to the gastroduodenal, right gastroepiploic, and superior pancreaticoduodenal arterial branches; the splenic artery gives off pancreatic and left gastroepiploic arterial branches.

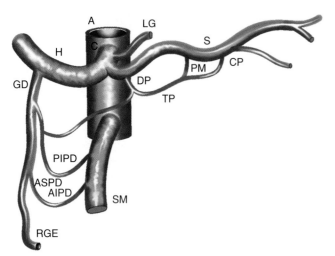

Figure 111–1 Diagram of typical celiac axis anatomy. A, aorta; AIPD, anterior inferior pancreaticoduodenal artery; ASPD, anterior superior pancreaticoduodenal artery; C, celiac axis; CP, caudal pancreatic artery; DP, dorsal pancreatic artery; GD, gastroduodenal artery; H, common hepatic artery; LG, left gastric artery; PIPD, posterior inferior pancreaticoduodenal artery; PM, pancreata magna; RGE, right gastroepiploic artery; S, splenic artery; SM, superior mesenteric artery; TP, transverse pancreatic artery. (From Nebesar RA, Kornblith PL, Pollard JJ, Michels NA: Celiac and Superior Mesenteric Arteries: A Correlation of Angiograms and Dissections. Boston, Little, Brown, 1969.)

Table 111–1	Types and Approximate Frequencies of Intestinal Ischemia

Type	**Frequency, %**
Colon ischemia	70-75
Acute mesenteric ischemia	20-25
Focal segmental ischemia	5
Chronic mesenteric ischemia	5
Mesenteric venous thrombosis	Included in above*

*Mesenteric venous thrombosis may manifest as colon ischemia, acute mesenteric ischemia, or as focal segmental ischemia. The frequency of mesenteric venous thrombosis is rising as computed tomography is performed more commonly.

The CA and its branches supply the stomach, duodenum, pancreas, and liver.

SUPERIOR MESENTERIC ARTERY

The SMA (Fig. 111–2) has its origin from the anterior aorta near the neck of the pancreas. It gives rise to four major vessels: the inferior pancreaticoduodenal, middle colic, right colic, and ileocolic arteries, as well as to a series of jejunal and ileal branches, all of which supply their named portions of intestine. These intestinal branches typically form a series of arcades, and from the terminal arcade, numerous straight vessels arise that enter the intestinal wall.

INFERIOR MESENTERIC ARTERY

The IMA (Fig. 111–3) arises 3 to 4 cm above the aortic bifurcation close to the inferior border of the duodenum.

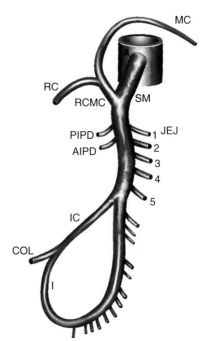

Figure 111–2 Diagram of typical superior mesenteric artery anatomy. A, aorta; AIPD, anterior inferior pancreaticoduodenal artery; COL, colic branches; I, ileal branches; IC, ileocolic artery; JEJ, jejunal branches; MC, middle colic artery; PIPD, posterior inferior pancreaticoduodenal artery; RC, right colic artery; SM, superior mesenteric artery. (From Nebesar RA, Kornblith PL, Pollard JJ, Michels NA: Celiac and Superior Mesenteric Arteries: A Correlation of Angiograms and Dissections. Boston, Little, Brown, 1969.)

It branches into the left colic artery, gives off multiple sigmoid branches, and terminates as the superior rectal artery. The IMA and its branches supply the large intestine from the distal transverse colon to the proximal rectum. The distal rectum is supplied by branches of the internal iliac (hypogastric) artery.

COLLATERAL AND ANASTOMOTIC CIRCULATION

Abundant collateral circulation to the stomach, duodenum, and rectum accounts for the paucity of ischemic events in these areas. The major anastomosis between the CA and the SMA is formed from the superior pancreaticoduodenal branch of the CA and the inferior pancreaticoduodenal branch of the SMA. These vessels constitute the pancreaticoduodenal arcade and provide blood to the duodenum and the pancreas. The splenic flexure and sigmoid colon have limited anastomoses, and ischemic damage is more common in these locations. There are three potential paths of communication between the SMA and IMA: (1) the marginal artery of Drummond, which is closest to and parallel with the wall of the intestine; (2) the central anastomotic artery, a larger and more centrally placed vessel; and (3) the arc of Riolan, an artery in the base of the mesentery. In the presence of SMA or IMA occlusion, a large collateral termed the *meandering artery* may be identified angiographically and represents a dilated central anastomotic artery or arc of Riolan (Fig.

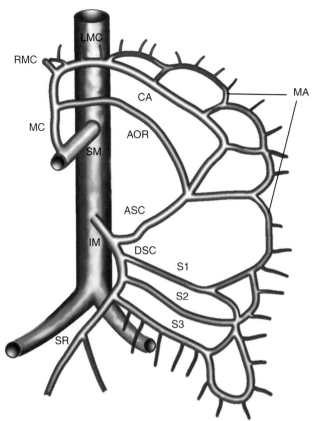

Figure 111–3 Diagram of typical inferior mesenteric artery anatomy. AOR, arc of Riolan; ASC, ascending branch of the left colic artery; CA, central artery; DSC, descending branch of the left colic artery; IM, inferior mesenteric artery; LMC, left branch of middle colic artery; MA, marginal artery; MC, middle colic artery; RMC, right branch of middle colic artery; S1, S2, S3, sigmoid branches; SM, superior mesenteric artery; SR, superior rectal artery. (From Nebesar RA, Kornblith PL, Pollard JJ, Michels NA: Celiac and Superior Mesenteric Arteries: A Correlation of Angiograms and Dissections. Boston, Little, Brown, 1969.)

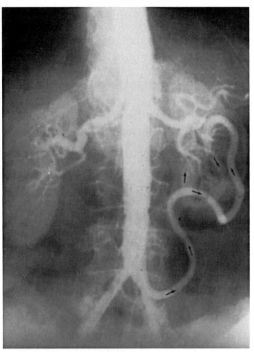

Figure 111–4 A flush aortogram of a patient with superior mesenteric artery (SMA) occlusion. The presence of a prominent meandering artery indicates that the collateral channels have been present for some time and that the occlusion is not acute. The *arrows* show the direction of flow from the inferior mesenteric artery to the SMA. (From Boley SJ, Brandt LJ, Veith FJ: Ischemic disorders of the intestines. Curr Probl Surg 15:29, 1978.)

111–4). It is critical to determine the direction of flow within a meandering artery before sacrificing the IMA, such as during aortic aneurysm surgery, lest the IMA be the main vessel supplying blood to the small bowel because of an occluded SMA.

PATHOPHYSIOLOGY AND PATHOLOGY

Ischemic injury of the intestine results from deprivation of oxygen and nutrients necessary for cellular integrity. Remarkably, the bowel can tolerate a 75% reduction of mesenteric blood flow and oxygen consumption for 12 hours with no changes on light microscopy, because only one fifth of the mesenteric capillaries is open at any time, and when oxygen delivery is decreased, the bowel adapts by increasing oxygen extraction.[2] Below a critical level of blood flow, however, these compensatory mechanisms are overwhelmed and no longer protective.

When a major vessel is occluded, collaterals open immediately in response to the drop in arterial pressure distal to the obstruction and remain open so long as pressure in the vascular bed distal to the obstruction remains below systemic pressure. After several hours of ischemia, however, vasoconstriction develops in the obstructed bed, elevating its pressure and reducing collateral flow. If sustained for a prolonged period, the vasoconstriction can become irreversible and persist even after correction of the cause of the ischemic event. Such persistent vasoconstriction explains the operative findings of progressive bowel ischemia after cardiac function has been optimized and in the absence of arterial or venous obstruction.

Blood flow is affected by a variety of systemic, humoral, local, and neural influences. The sympathetic nervous system, mainly via α-adrenergic receptors, is of primary importance in maintaining resting splanchnic arteriolar tone; other vasoactive substances, including angiotensin II, vasopressin, and prostaglandins, also have been implicated in the pathogenesis of ischemic injury.

Ischemic damage results both from hypoxia during the period of ischemia and reperfusion injury when blood flow is re-established. More reinjury from brief ischemia appears during reperfusion, but as the ischemic period lengthens, hypoxia becomes more detrimental than reperfusion[3]; the injury after 3 hours of ischemia and 1 hour of reperfusion is more severe than that after 4 hours of ischemia. Reperfusion injury has been attributed to many factors, including reactive oxygen radicals. When molecular oxygen is reduced in univalent steps, superoxide, hydrogen peroxide, and hydroxyl radicals are formed. These oxygen radicals damage an array of molecules found in tissues, including nucleic acids, membrane lipids, enzymes, and receptors; such widespread damage can result in cell lysis, impaired cell function, and necrosis on reperfusion of ischemic tissues.

A potent source of oxygen radicals in ischemic, reperfused tissue is the enzyme xanthine oxidase (XO), the rate-limiting enzyme in nucleic acid degradation. In nonischemic tissue, this enzyme exists as a dehydrogenase (XDH) that uses nicotinamide adenine dinucleotide rather than O_2 as the electron acceptor during purine oxidation; as a result, it does not produce oxygen radicals. During ischemia, XDH is converted to XO with production of reactive oxygen radicals. Inhibition of XO by allopurinol dramatically attenuates the epithelial cell necrosis and the increased microvascular permeability seen during reperfusion.

Neutrophils are another source of reactive oxygen metabolites. During reperfusion, XO-derived oxidants initiate the production and release of leukotriene B_4 and platelet-activating factor, which lead to neutrophil adherence and migration. The adherent leukocytes mediate microvascular injury by release of proteases and physical disruption of the endothelial barrier. Oxygen radical scavengers (superoxide dismutase, dimethyl sulfoxide), XO inhibitors, and agents that inhibit leukocyte adherence and migration have been shown experimentally to protect various organs against reperfusion injury but are not yet used clinically because, in large measure, they must be given before or coincident with the ischemic injury to have protective effects.[3]

ACUTE MESENTERIC ISCHEMIA

Intestinal ischemia can be classified as acute or chronic and of venous or arterial origin. In the acute forms, intestinal viability is threatened, whereas in the chronic forms, blood flow is inadequate to support the functional demands of the intestine. Acute mesenteric ischemia (AMI) is much more common than the chronic type, and arterial disease is more frequent than venous disease. Arterial forms of AMI include SMA embolus (SMAE), nonocclusive mesenteric ischemia (NOMI), SMA thrombosis (SMAT), and focal segmental ischemia (FSI) (Table 111–2). Acute mesenteric venous thrombosis (MVT) and FSI are the venous forms of AMI.

AMI results from inadequate blood flow to all or part of the small intestine and may involve the right half of the colon because its blood supply is from the SMA. Regardless of the cause of the ischemic insult, the end results are similar: a spectrum of bowel injury that ranges from transient alteration of bowel function to transmural gangrene. Clinical manifestations vary with the extent and severity of ischemic injury and, to a lesser degree, with its cause.

INCIDENCE

AMI accounts for about 0.1% of admissions to our tertiary care center. This figure has risen over the past 30 years, owing to increased recognition of the disorder, an aging population, and the widespread use of intensive care units with the salvage of patients who previously would have died from cardiovascular conditions but who now survive to develop AMI as a delayed consequence of their primary disease.

Most series of AMI reported in the late 1970s and early 1980s showed that SMAE was responsible for 40% to 50%, NOMI for 20% to 30%, and SMAT for 10% to 20% of cases. More recently, the incidence of NOMI has declined, likely because intensive care unit monitoring enables prompt correction of hypotension and blood volume deficits, and the widespread use of calcium channel blockers and other systemic vasodilators may protect the vascular bed from spasm. Today, SMAE is the most common cause of AMI.

CLINICAL FEATURES

Early identification of AMI requires a high index of suspicion, especially in patients older than 50 years of age who have long-standing congestive heart failure (particularly if poorly controlled), cardiac arrhythmias, recent myocardial infarction, or hypotension. The development of sudden abdominal pain in a patient with any of these risk factors should suggest the diagnosis of AMI. Younger individuals, however, are not without risk of AMI, especially if they are taking vasoactive medications (e.g., phenylephrine, amphetamines, triptans), using cocaine, or have underlying thrombophilia. Hence, unexplained, persistent, and severe abdominal pain should prompt consideration of AMI as an explanation for the pain. A history of postprandial abdominal pain in the weeks to months preceding the acute onset of severe abdominal pain is associated only with SMAT.

Almost all patients with AMI have acute abdominal pain. Early in the course of disease, the pain of AMI is far more impressive than the physical findings. Initially, the pain is severe, but the abdomen usually is flat, soft, and most often not tender or less tender than expected based on the magnitude of the pain. Sudden, severe abdominal pain accompanied by rapid and often forceful bowel evacuation, especially with minimal or no abdominal signs, strongly suggests SMAE. A more indolent and less striking onset is more typical of MVT, whereas with NOMI, appreciation of abdominal pain may be overshadowed by the precipitating disorders, such as hypotension, acute congestive heart failure, acute hypo-

Table 111–2	Causes and Approximate Frequencies of Acute Mesenteric Ischemia

Cause	Frequency, %
SMA embolus	50
Nonocclusive mesenteric ischemia	25
SMA thrombosis	10
Mesenteric venous thrombosis	10
Focal segmental ischemia	5

SMA, superior mesenteric artery.

volemia, or cardiac arrhythmias. Pain is absent in as many as 25% of patients with NOMI.

Unexplained abdominal distention or gastrointestinal bleeding may be the only indications of AMI when pain is absent, especially when due to NOMI. Distention, although absent early in the course of AMI, is often the first sign of intestinal infarction. The stool contains occult blood in 75% of patients. Right-sided abdominal pain associated with the passage of maroon or bright red blood in the stool, although characteristic of colon ischemia, also may be seen with AMI, because the blood supply to both the right colon and small bowel originates from the SMA. Elderly patients with AMI have been reported to develop mental confusion acutely in as many as 30% of cases.[4] Patients who survive cardiopulmonary resuscitation and who then develop recurrent bacteremia or sepsis should be suspected of having had NOMI, which resulted in a segment of bowel with subacute ischemic injury, acting as a portal for bacterial translocation.[5] Although episodes of sepsis may be treated successfully with antibiotics, the length of damaged bowel must be removed to prevent recurrent sepsis.

Although abdominal findings early in the course of intestinal ischemia are minimal or absent, increasing tenderness, rebound tenderness, and muscle guarding reflect progressive loss of intestinal viability. Such abdominal findings strongly indicate the presence of infarcted bowel. The rate of progression from the onset of abdominal pain to intestinal infarction varies, not with the specific cause of ischemia but with the severity of the ischemic insult; MVT generally has a more indolent, or so-called tumbleweed, course than do the arterial causes of AMI.

LABORATORY FEATURES AND DIAGNOSIS

On admission to the hospital, approximately 75% of patients with AMI have leukocytosis above 15,000 cells/mm[3] and about 50% have metabolic acidemia. A normal white blood cell (WBC) count cannot be used to exclude early AMI, just as a high WBC count does not make the diagnosis. Elevated levels of serum phosphate, D-lactate, amylase, and other enzymes have been noted, as have high peritoneal fluid amylase and intestinal alkaline phosphatase activity, but the sensitivity and specificity of these markers of intestinal ischemia have not been established.[6] More specific intestinal enzymes including diamine oxidase, hexosaminidase, glutathione S-transferase,[7] and intestinal fatty acid binding protein[8] also lack sufficient sensitivity and specificity to diagnose AMI. Moreover, serum markers, when elevated, usually indicate late-stage disease.

Although poorly sensitive (30%) and nonspecific, plain films of the abdomen still are obtained in evaluating patients with suspected AMI. Plain films of the abdomen usually are normal in AMI before infarction. Later on, formless loops of small intestine, ileus, "thumbprinting" of the small bowel or right colon (Fig. 111–5), or still later, pneumatosis and portal or mesenteric vascular gas may be seen. In one study, the mortality rate of patients with normal plain film studies was 29%, whereas it was 78% in those with abnormal findings.[9] The primary

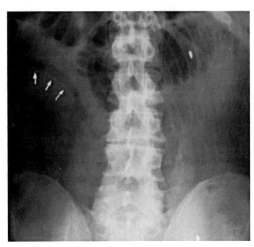

Figure 111–5 Plain film of the abdomen shows an ileus and a formless, fixed loop of small intestine (arrows) in a patient with acute mesenteric ischemia due to superior mesenteric artery embolus.

purpose of plain films (or CT scans) is to exclude causes of abdominal pain other than ischemia that might mandate a different therapeutic approach.

Duplex scanning and Doppler flowmetry can be used to evaluate patients suspected of having AMI, but these techniques are limited in their clinical use by the following factors:

1. Only the proximal portions of the major splanchnic vessels can be studied reliably, not the peripheral vasculature.
2. Vessel occlusions are not diagnostic of intestinal ischemia since complete occlusions can be seen in asymptomatic individuals.
3. Blood flow though the SMA is highly variable, which makes interpretation difficult.
4. NOMI, which accounts for approximately 25% of AMI, cannot be diagnosed reliably by ultrasound.

CT has largely replaced plain film study of the abdomen for diagnosis today and is used to identify arterial and venous thromboses as well as ischemic bowel.[10-13] Findings on CT include colon dilatation, bowel wall thickening, abnormal bowel wall enhancement, lack of enhancement of arterial vasculature with timed intravenous contrast injections, arterial occlusion, venous thrombosis, engorgement of mesenteric veins, intramural gas and mesenteric or portal venous gas (Fig. 111–6), infarction of other organs, ascites, and signs related to the cause of the infarcted bowel such as hernia.[10] There are three relatively specific findings of AMI that are better depicted on CT scans compared with plain films: (1) gas in the bowel wall or portal system; (2) acute embolic infarction of other intra-abdominal organs; and (3) thrombi in the mesenteric vessels.[11] Unfortunately, the early signs on CT are nonspecific and the late signs reflect necrotic bowel. In a study comparing CT findings in 39 patients who had AMI proven at surgery with 24 patients suspected of AMI that was disproved at surgery, the finding of arterial or venous thrombosis, intramural or portal venous gas, focal lack of bowel wall enhancement, or liver or splenic infarcts had a sensitivity and specificity of 64% and 92%, respectively.[12] However, the presence of

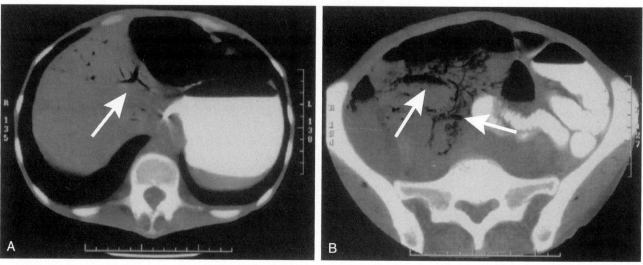

Figure 111–6   Computed tomography (CT) scans of a patient with acute mesenteric ischemia showing gas *(arrow)* in the portal veins *(A)* and gas *(arrows)* in the wall of the intestine, mesentery, and mesenteric vessels *(B)*. Pneumatosis intestinalis is a late sign of ischemic injury, connotes bowel necrosis, and mandates exploration.

just one imaging criterion was needed for a study to be "positive," and thus the predictive value of traditional scanning may not be as high as reported.

CT angiography has been shown to be promising in the diagnosis of AMI, and in one study, the added CT angiographic findings were believed to alter clinical management in 19% of 62 patients by making the diagnosis of AMI when CT alone did not.[14] Magnetic resonance (MR) angiography is another of the newer imaging techniques used to diagnose AMI that not only can image the vasculature but may perhaps be useful in determining metabolic consequences of inadequate blood flow.[15]

Laparoscopy may be useful, but it can be misleading because early in ischemic injury, blood may be shunted to the serosa, giving a normal appearance to the outside of the bowel while the mucosa may be necrotic. Moreover, laparoscopy is potentially dangerous because SMA blood flow decreases when intraperitoneal pressure exceeds 20 mm Hg.

Selective mesenteric angiography, frequently with papaverine infusion, currently is the mainstay of diagnosis and initial treatment of both occlusive and nonocclusive forms of AMI, and should be performed promptly if AMI is suspected or diagnosed on other imaging tests. Sensitivity and specificity of mesenteric angiography for diagnosing AMI in most studies are 90% to 100% and 100%, respectively.[16] Opponents of routine angiography for patients suspected of having AMI cite several problems with this approach: (1) difficulties in performing these studies in critically ill patients may make angiography impractical and contribute to inordinate delays in surgery; (2) the large number of negative examinations done to identify patients with AMI early in the course of disease is considered by some to offset the value of the study; and (3) the most serious potential drawback is the possible critical delay in surgical correction of vascular insufficiency because angiography is not available. Proponents of angiography accept that the large number of negative angiographic studies is necessary if diagnoses are to be made early enough to improve survival. Prompt

laparotomy, however, is indicated in patients with suspected AMI if angiography cannot be performed expeditiously. More controversial is the need for angiography in a patient with suspected AMI and signs of peritonitis. Since such signs usually connote infarcted bowel, the most compelling reason for angiography, namely, diagnosis of AMI while the effects of intestinal ischemia are still reversible, is no longer relevant. Angiography nonetheless still plays an important role in this situation because it can diagnose AMI and its cause and provide a "roadmap" for revascularization and access for serial postoperative angiographic studies.

MANAGEMENT

Our approach to the management of AMI is based on several observations. First, if the diagnosis is not made before intestinal infarction, the mortality rate is 70% to 90%. Second, diagnosis of both the occlusive and nonocclusive forms of AMI can be made in most patients by angiography. Third, vasoconstriction, which may persist even after the cause of the ischemia is corrected, is the basis of NOMI and a contributing factor in the other forms of AMI. Finally, vasoconstriction can be relieved by vasodilators infused into the SMA. The cornerstones of our approach, therefore, are the earlier and more liberal use of angiography and the incorporation of intra-arterial papaverine in the treatment of both occlusive AMI and NOMI.

Patients older than 50 years of age who have the risk factors previously described and younger patients, especially those with atrial fibrillation, vasculitis, a coagulation disorder, and those on vasoactive medications, who seek medical attention for sudden, severe abdominal pain that lasts longer than several hours, should be suspected of having AMI. These patients should be managed according to the algorithm shown in Figure 111–7. Less absolute indications for inclusion into this protocol consist of unexplained acute abdominal distention, colonoscopic

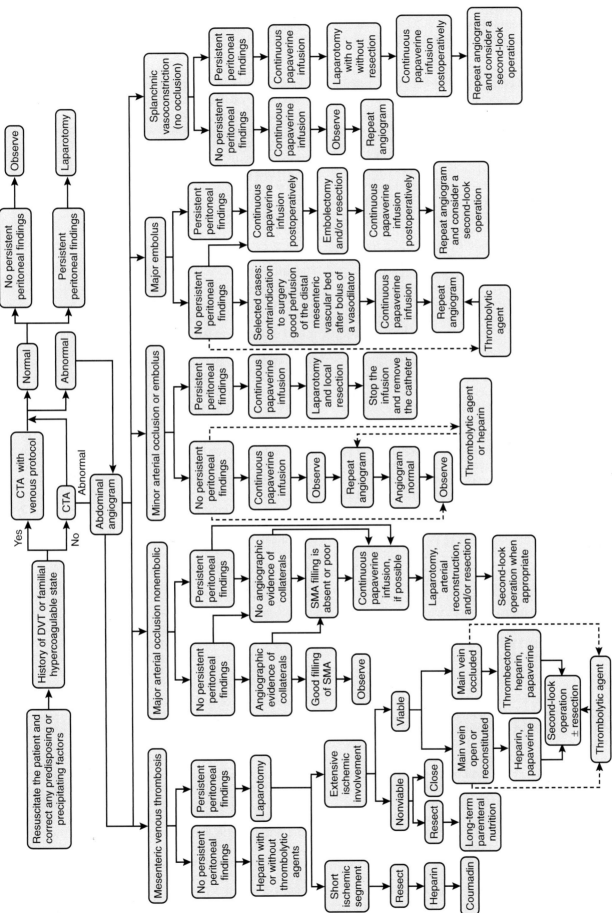

Figure 111–7   Algorithm for the diagnosis and treatment of intestinal ischemia. CTA, computed tomographic angiogram; DVT, deep venous thrombosis; SMA, superior mesenteric artery. Solid lines show accepted management plan; dotted lines show alternative management plan. (Modified from Brandt LJ, Boley SJ: AGA technical review on intestinal ischemia: American Gastrointestinal Association. Gastroenterology 118:954, 2000; corrected version in Gastroenterology 119:281, 2000.)

evidence of isolated right-sided colonic ischemia, and acidosis without an identifiable cause.

Initial management of patients suspected of having AMI includes resuscitation and diagnostic imaging studies. Resuscitation includes relief of acute congestive heart failure and correction of hypotension, hypovolemia, and cardiac arrhythmias. Broad-spectrum antibiotics are given immediately because of the high incidence of positive blood cultures in AMI and because they reduce the extent and severity of ischemic injury in experimental animals.[17] There are no randomized, controlled studies showing the benefit of antibiotics in AMI, and it is unlikely that such studies will ever be done. After resuscitation, plain films or CT scan of the abdomen are obtained, not to establish the diagnosis of AMI but rather to exclude other causes of abdominal pain. A normal plain film or CT scan does not exclude AMI; ideally, patients are studied before radiologic signs appear because these connote irreversibly damaged bowel. If no alternative diagnosis is made on these studies, selective SMA angiography is performed. Based on the angiographic findings and the presence or absence of peritoneal signs, the patient is treated according to the algorithm in Figure 111-7.

Even when the decision to operate has been based on clinical grounds, preoperative angiography should be performed to manage the patient properly at and after laparotomy. Relief of mesenteric vasoconstriction is essential to the treatment of emboli, thromboses, and the nonocclusive "low-flow" states. Infusion of papaverine through the angiography catheter in the SMA is used to relieve mesenteric vasoconstriction preoperatively and postoperatively. The papaverine is infused by pump at a constant rate of 30 to 60 mg/hr; papaverine concentrations may vary with the need for fluid restriction.

Although most of the papaverine infused into the mesenteric bed is cleared during one pass through the liver, blood pressure and cardiac rate and rhythm must be monitored constantly. Some patients with liver disease may exhibit a drop in blood pressure with this dose of papaverine, but the most common cause of hypotension during the papaverine infusion is catheter dislodgment. Patients who have a sudden drop in blood pressure should have the papaverine replaced with saline or glucose solution and promptly undergo plain film imaging of the abdomen to confirm the catheter's location. If the catheter has come out of the SMA, it should be replaced and the papaverine restarted. The clinical and angiographic responses of the patient to the vasodilator determine the duration of therapy.

Laparotomy is performed in AMI to restore arterial flow obstructed by embolus or thrombosis or to resect irreparably damaged bowel or both. Embolectomy, thrombectomy, or arterial bypass precedes evaluation of intestinal viability because bowel that initially appears infarcted may show surprising recovery after adequate blood flow is restored. In the operating room, intestinal viability can be assessed clinically, by qualitative or quantitative surface fluorescence or by Doppler ultrasonography.[18]

Short segments of bowel that are nonviable or questionably viable after revascularization are resected, and a primary anastomosis is performed. If extensive portions of the bowel are of questionable viability, however, only the clearly necrotic bowel is resected and re-exploration (second look) is planned for within 12 to 24 hours. The interval between the first and second operations is used both to allow better demarcation between viable and nonviable bowel and to attempt to improve intestinal blood flow by using intra-arterial papaverine and by maximizing cardiac output.

The use of anticoagulants in the management of AMI is controversial. Anticoagulation with heparin may cause intestinal or intraperitoneal hemorrhage and, except for MVT, should not be used routinely in the immediate postoperative period; 48 hours after embolectomy or arterial reconstruction, when thrombosis is frequent, anticoagulation is appropriate.

Specific Types of Acute Mesenteric Ischemia[16]

Superior Mesenteric Artery Emboli (SMAE)

SMAE are responsible for 40% to 50% of AMI episodes. Emboli usually originate from a left atrial or ventricular mural thrombus. Many patients with SMAE have had previous peripheral artery emboli, and approximately 20% have synchronous emboli. SMAE lodge at points of normal anatomic narrowing, usually immediately distal to the origin of a major branch. Angiography typically reveals a rounded filling defect with nearly complete obstruction to flow. Mesenteric atherosclerosis is usually not as severe as in SMAT. Emboli proximal to the origin of the ileocolic artery are considered "major" emboli. "Minor" emboli are those that lodge in the SMA distal to the takeoff of the ileocolic artery or in the distal branches of the SMA (Fig. 111-8).

Various therapeutic approaches have been proposed for SMAE, depending on the presence or absence of peritoneal signs, whether the embolus is partially or completely occluding, and whether the embolus is above the origin of the ileocolic artery or more distal. Therapy for SMAE has included surgical revascularization, intra-arterial perfusion with vasodilators or thrombolytic agents, and anticoagulation.[16] In the absence of peritoneal signs, minor SMA emboli have been treated successfully with all of these agents without the need for surgery. Patients with major emboli usually are explored after papaverine infusion is begun. Nonoperative therapy using only papaverine infusion is employed if there are significant contraindications to surgery, no peritoneal signs, and adequate perfusion of the vascular bed distal to the embolus after a bolus of vasodilator into the SMA.

Exploratory laparotomy is mandatory when peritonitis is present; embolectomy and bowel resection are performed as necessary. If possible, intra-arterial papaverine is begun before surgery and is continued during surgery. If no second look is planned, infusion is continued for 12 to 24 hours postoperatively; persistent vasospasm is excluded by angiography before removal of the catheter (see Fig. 111-8). If a second operation is planned, the infusion is continued through the second procedure until vasoconstriction has been shown by angiography to have ceased. Recognition of persistent vasoconstriction has prompted some authorities to recommend routine use of

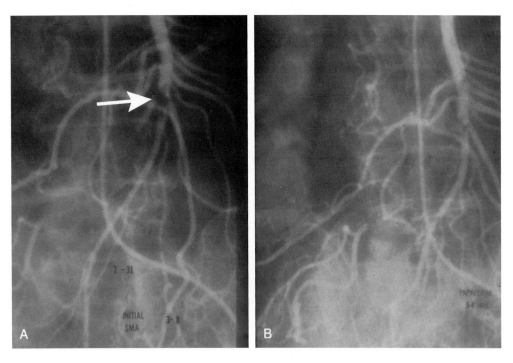

Figure 111–8 *A,* Superior mesenteric artery (SMA) angiogram in a 71-year-old man with abdominal pain showing an embolus occluding the SMA at the level of the origin of the right colic artery *(arrow).* Vasoconstriction is noted distal to the embolus. *B,* Repeat angiogram done 24 hours after SMA embolectomy and preoperative and postoperative papaverine infusions into the SMA. Vasodilatation is seen, and all vessels are patent except for a distal jejunal branch.

intra-arterial papaverine in all patients with SMAE; the best survival rates are seen in patients treated in this way.[16]

Thrombolytic therapy using streptokinase, urokinase, or recombinant tissue plasminogen activator has been used in small series of patients with some success. Thrombolytic therapy is most likely to be successful when the embolus is partially occluding or is minor and the study is performed within 12 hours of the onset of symptoms.[19]

Nonocclusive Mesenteric Ischemia (NOMI)

NOMI is responsible for 20% to 30% of AMI and usually is due to splanchnic vasoconstriction consequent to a preceding cardiovascular event. AMI may appear hours to days after the event, and vasoconstriction, which initially is reversible, may persist even after the precipitating event has been corrected. Precipitating causes for NOMI include acute myocardial infarction, congestive heart failure, arrhythmias, shock, cirrhosis, and chronic kidney disease (especially when dialysis is required).

NOMI is diagnosed by angiography using four criteria: (1) narrowing of the origins of SMA branches; (2) irregularities in the intestinal branches; (3) spasm of the arcades; and (4) impaired filling of intramural vessels. Patients with these signs who are neither in shock nor on vasopressors and who do not have pancreatitis can be considered to have NOMI (Fig. 111–9).

SMA infusion of papaverine is begun as soon as the diagnosis is made. Operation is performed if peritoneal signs are present, and the infusion is continued during and after exploration. Necrotic bowel is resected; it is better to leave bowel of questionable viability and perform a second-look operation than to perform massive enterectomy, because compromised but viable bowel often improves with supportive measures. The infusion is continued as for second-look operations following embolectomy.

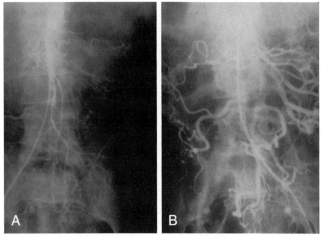

Figure 111–9 Superior mesenteric angiogram in a patient with nonocclusive mesenteric ischemia (NOMI) following a bout of gastrointestinal hemorrhage and shock. *A,* The pretreatment film shows the diffuse vasoconstriction of NOMI. *B,* Marked vasodilatation is evident on the repeat study after 48 hours of an intra-arterial papaverine infusion. (From Brandt LJ, Boley SJ: Ischemic intestinal syndromes. Adv Surg 15:1, 1981.)

When papaverine infusion is used as the only treatment for NOMI in patients without signs of peritonitis, it is continued for 24 hours, and repeat angiography is performed 30 minutes after changing the papaverine infusion to normal saline. Papaverine infusion is maintained and angiography repeated daily until there is no roentgenographic evidence of vasoconstriction and the patient's clinical findings resolve. Infusions, usually discontinued after 24 hours, have been given for as long as 5 days.

Acute Superior Mesenteric Artery Thrombosis (SMAT)

Acute SMAT occurs in areas of severe atherosclerotic narrowing, most often at the origin of the SMA. The acute ischemic episode may be superimposed on chronic mesenteric ischemia (CMI), and 20% to 50% of patients have a history of postprandial abdominal pain and weight loss during the weeks to months preceding the acute event. Evidence of coronary, cerebrovascular, or peripheral arterial insufficiency is common.

SMAT is demonstrated on flush aortography, which usually shows occlusion of the SMA 1 to 2 cm from its origin. Some distal filling of the SMA via collaterals is common. Branches both proximal and distal to the obstruction may show localized or diffuse vasoconstriction. In patients with abdominal pain, no abdominal tenderness, and complete occlusion of the SMA on aortography, it is important, though difficult, to distinguish between acute thrombosis and long-standing, coincidental chronic occlusion. Prominent collaterals between the SMA and other major splanchnic vessels indicate chronic SMA occlusion. If there is good filling of the SMA, the occlusion is considered to be chronic and the abdominal pain unrelated to mesenteric vascular disease (see Fig. 111–4). The absence of collateral vessels or the presence of collaterals with inadequate filling of the SMA indicates an acute occlusion and demands prompt intervention. If possible, an angiographic catheter is placed in the proximal SMA, and papaverine infusion is begun before surgery is undertaken.

At surgery, necrotic bowel is resected and remaining bowel is revascularized. Papaverine infusion is continued throughout the operative period, and management is the same as for SMAE. There are but few reports of use of thrombolytic agents or percutaneous angioplasty for SMAT.

Complications

Complications of angiography and prolonged infusion of vasodilator drugs include transient acute tubular necrosis following angiography, local hematomas at the arterial puncture sites, dislodgment of catheters, and fibrin clots on the arterial catheter. Infusion for more than 5 days has not had significant systemic effects.

Results

Although mortality rates of 70% to 90% are reported for AMI through the 1980s for patients diagnosed and treated conventionally, the suggested approach described here can reduce these catastrophic figures. The best survival is reported in series in which angiography has been used routinely in the management of AMI.[20-25]

In our tertiary medical center, more than 50% of the patients with AMI treated according to our approach survived, and more than 75% have lost less than 1 m of intestine. The importance of early diagnosis is emphasized by the survival of 90% of patients who had AMI but no signs of peritonitis and who had angiography early in their course. Ideally, all patients with AMI should be studied when plain films of the abdomen and CT scan-

ning are normal and before signs of an acute surgical abdomen and laboratory evidence of infarction appear. *Diagnosis before the occurrence of intestinal infarction is the most important factor in improving survival of patients with AMI.*

MESENTERIC VENOUS THROMBOSIS

MVT occurs as an acute, subacute, or chronic disorder. It is only since the development of recent imaging techniques that these various forms of MVT have been recognized; previously, only acute MVT was known, and diagnosis was made at laparotomy or autopsy.

INCIDENCE

In early studies, MVT was believed to be the major cause of AMI, but most of these cases probably represented NOMI. Today, only 5% to 10% of patients with AMI have MVT, and the reported mean age of these individuals is younger, 48 to 60 years, than of those with other forms of AMI.

PREDISPOSING CONDITIONS (Table 111–3)

Previously, a cause of MVT was identified in fewer than half of patients. The discoveries of the primary and secondary hypercoagulable states and with use of estro-

---

Table 111–3 Conditions Associated with Mesenteric Venous Thrombosis

Hypercoagulable states
    Activated protein C resistance
    Antithrombin deficiency
    Protein C deficiency
    Protein S deficiency
    Methyltetrahydrofolate deficiency
    Estrogen use (oral contraceptives, hormone replacement therapy)
    Polycythemia vera
    Thrombocytosis
    Neoplasms
Peripheral deep venous thrombosis
Pregnancy
Portal hypertension
    Cirrhosis
    Congestive splenomegaly
    After sclerotherapy of esophageal varices
Inflammation
    Diverticulitis
    Pancreatitis
    Peritonitis (e.g., appendicitis, perforated viscus)
    Inflammatory bowel disease
    Pelvic or intra-abdominal abscess
Postoperative state or trauma
    Blunt abdominal trauma
    Splenectomy and other postoperative states
Decompression sickness

gens for contraception and hormone replacement have enabled identification of the cause in almost 90% of patients.[26]

PATHOPHYSIOLOGY

The location of the initial thrombus within the mesenteric venous circulation varies with the cause. MVT secondary to cirrhosis, neoplasm, or operative injury begins at the site of obstruction and extends peripherally, whereas thrombosis of primary hypercoagulable states starts in smaller branches and propagates into the major trunks. Intestinal infarction is rare unless the branches of the peripheral arcades and the vasa recta are involved. When collateral circulation is inadequate and venous drainage from a segment of bowel is compromised, the affected intestine becomes congested, edematous, cyanotic, and thickened with intramural hemorrhage. Serosanguineous peritoneal fluid heralds early hemorrhagic infarction. Arterial vasoconstriction can be marked, but pulsations persist up to the bowel wall. The occurrence of transmural infarction may make it impossible to differentiate venous from arterial occlusion.

CLINICAL FEATURES

MVT can have an acute, subacute (weeks to months), or chronic onset; except for late complications, the latter is asymptomatic. As many as 60% of patients have a history of peripheral vein thromboses.[27]

Acute MVT presents with abdominal pain in more than 90% of patients and, as with acute arterial ischemia, the pain initially is out of proportion to the physical findings. The mean duration of pain before admission is 5 to 14 days but may be more than 1 month in as many as 25% of individuals.[28] Other symptoms, including nausea and vomiting, occur in more than 50%. Lower gastrointestinal bleeding, bloody diarrhea, or hematemesis occurs in 15% and indicates bowel infarction. Fecal occult blood is found in more than half of instances during the course of MVT. Initial physical findings vary at different stages and with different degrees of ischemic injury, but guarding and rebound tenderness develop as bowel infarction evolves. Most patients have a temperature higher than 38°C (100.4°F), and 25% exhibit signs of septic shock.

Subacute MVT describes the condition in patients who have abdominal pain for weeks to months but no intestinal infarction. Subacute MVT can be due either to extension of thrombosis at a rate rapid enough to cause pain but that permits collaterals to develop, thus preventing infarction, or to acute thrombosis of venous drainage sufficient to permit recovery from ischemic injury. The diagnosis usually is made on imaging studies ordered to diagnose other conditions. Nonspecific abdominal pain usually is the only symptom of subacute MVT, and physical examination and laboratory tests are normal. Some patients who present with subacute MVT ultimately develop intestinal infarction; this blurs the distinction between the acute and subacute forms of MVT. At autopsy, coexistent new and old thromboses have been found in nearly half of the patients.

Chronic MVT is seen in patients who are asymptomatic at the time of thrombosis but who may develop gastrointestinal bleeding from varices.[29] Most patients who bleed do so from gastroesophageal varices secondary to portal or splenic vein thrombosis, and they have physical findings of portal hypertension. Laboratory studies may show secondary hypersplenism with pancytopenia or thrombocytopenia.

DIAGNOSIS

Acute Mesenteric Venous Thrombosis

The absence of specific symptoms, signs, or laboratory results and the typical variability in the course of the disease make it difficult to diagnose acute MVT preoperatively. Abdominal plain film signs of MVT are similar to those of other forms of AMI and almost always reflect the presence of infarcted bowel. Barium enemas are of little diagnostic value, because MVT unusually involves the colon. Characteristic findings on small bowel series include marked thickening of the bowel wall due to congestion and edema with separation of loops and thumbprinting.

Selective mesenteric arteriography can establish a definitive diagnosis before bowel infarction, can differentiate venous thrombosis from arterial forms of ischemia, and can provide access for vasodilator therapy. Angiographic findings of acute MVT include thrombus in the SMV with partial or complete occlusion; failure to visualize the SMV or portal vein; slow or absent filling of the mesenteric veins; arterial spasm; failure of the arterial arcades to empty; reflux of contrast medium into the artery; and prolonged blush in the involved segment.[30]

Ultrasonography, CT, and MR imaging all have been used to demonstrate thrombi in the SMV and the portal vein.[31,32] CT can diagnose MVT in more than 90% of patients and is the diagnostic study of choice. Specific findings include thickening and enhancement of the bowel wall; enlargement of the SMV; a central lucency in the lumen of the vein (representing a thrombus); a sharply defined vein wall with a rim of increased density; and dilated collateral vessels in a thickened mesentery (Fig. 111–10). When MVT is diagnosed on CT scanning, angiography may not be necessary, but in selected symptomatic patients it better delineates thrombosed veins and provides access for intra-arterial vasodilators. Esophagogastroduodenoscopy and colonoscopy rarely are helpful, because the duodenum and colon are infrequently involved. As in other forms of AMI, laparoscopy may be useful either when other studies are contraindicated or in concert with imaging tests.[33]

The diagnosis of MVT usually has been made at laparotomy, where its hallmarks are serosanguinous peritoneal fluid, dark red to blue-black edematous bowel, thickening of the mesentery, good arterial pulsations in the involved segment, and thrombi in cut mesenteric veins. At this stage, some degree of intestinal infarction invariably has occurred. When persons suspected to have AMI exhibit clinical features suggesting MVT, contrast-enhanced CT is performed before SMA angiography, although this recommendation is becoming moot as CT

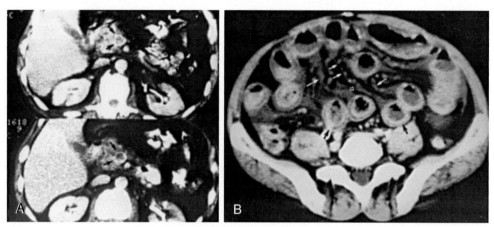

Figure 111–10 Superior mesenteric venous thrombosis. *A,* Abdominal computed tomography (CT) with intravenous contrast demonstrating an enlarged superior mesenteric vein with a central lucency in the lumen, representing the thrombus. The vein wall is sharply defined with a rim of increased density surrounding the thrombus *(arrows). B,* Abdominal CT with intravenous contrast agent showing thickening and persistent enhancement of the bowel wall *(black arrows)* and dilated collateral vessels within a thickened mesentery *(white arrows).* (From Boley SJ, Brandt LJ: Ischemic disorders of the intestines. Surg Clin North Am 72:194, 1992.)

angiography is increasingly used as the initial imaging test.

Chronic Mesenteric Venous Thrombosis

Because chronic MVT is asymptomatic or presents as gastrointestinal bleeding, the diagnostic evaluation is directed toward determining the cause of the bleeding. Endoscopy and appropriate imaging studies should identify the cause and site of bleeding and the extent of thrombosis.

TREATMENT

Acute Mesenteric Venous Thrombosis

Most patients with acute MVT initially are believed to have some form of AMI and are treated as discussed in the sections above and as outlined in the algorithm of Figure 111–7. In asymptomatic persons in whom the diagnosis is made on a CT scan done for other than abdominal pain, either 3 to 6 months of anticoagulation or no therapy in some cases is reasonable. In symptomatic individuals, treatment is determined by the presence or absence of peritoneal signs; signs of peritonitis mandate laparotomy and resection of infarcted bowel. If long segments of questionably viable bowel are found, papaverine is infused, and if arterial spasm is relieved and the SMV or portal vein is visualized, thrombectomy and/or a second look may be attempted to determine whether resection should be performed. Following surgery, heparin should be administered. Immediate heparinization for 7 to 10 days has been shown to diminish recurrence and progression of thrombosis and to improve survival.[34,35] In the absence of peritoneal signs, immediate heparinization followed by a 3- to 6-month course of warfarin may be all that is needed. A comparison of patients who were treated surgically with those managed medically suggested that nonoperative management is a reasonable option provided the diagnosis on CT scan is certain and there is no transmural necrosis or

perforation.[36] A few case reports have documented the use of thrombolytic agents in the treatment of acute MVT.

Current recommendations for the duration of anticoagulation are not supported by evidence-based data, but rather on conventional practice. If an underlying hypercoagulable state is found, lifelong treatment with warfarin is advised. If no underlying thrombophilic state is documented, a 3- to 6-month course of therapy is believed to be sufficient.

Chronic Mesenteric Venous Thrombosis

Treatment of chronic MVT is aimed at controlling bleeding, usually from esophageal varices. Sclerotherapy, variceal banding, portosystemic shunts, devascularization procedures, and bowel resection all have a place in treating selected patients. No treatment is indicated for patients with asymptomatic chronic MVT.

PROGNOSIS

Mortality associated with acute MVT is lower than that for other forms of AMI and varies from 20% to 50%. Recurrence rates of 20% to 25% fall to about 15% if heparin therapy is begun promptly. The natural history of chronic MVT is not known, but from postmortem studies it appears that almost 50% of patients with MVT have no bowel infarction and many have no symptoms.

FOCAL SEGMENTAL ISCHEMIA OF THE SMALL INTESTINE

Vascular insults to short segments of small intestine produce a broad spectrum of clinical features without the life-threatening complications associated with more extensive ischemia. The causes of FSI include atheromatous emboli, strangulated hernias, immune complex disorders and vasculitis, blunt abdominal trauma, segmental venous thrombosis, radiation therapy, and oral contraceptives, among others. With FSI there is usually adequate collateral circulation to prevent transmural infarction; the most common lesion is partial bowel wall necrosis with invasion by intestinal bacteria. FSI may present as acute enteritis, chronic enteritis, or a stricture. In the acute pattern, abdominal pain often simulates acute appendicitis. Physical findings are those of an "acute abdomen," and an inflammatory mass may be palpated. The chronic enteritis pattern may resemble Crohn's disease with cramping abdominal pain, diarrhea, fever, and weight loss. Roentgenographic findings also may resemble those of Crohn's disease except that FSI occurs anywhere in the small bowel, whereas Crohn's disease mainly affects the terminal ileum. The most common presentation is chronic small bowel obstruction from a stricture with intermittent abdominal pain, distention, and vomiting. Bacterial overgrowth in the dilated loop proximal to the obstruction may produce a "blind loop" syndrome. Radiologic studies typically reveal a smooth tapered stricture of variable length with an abrupt change to normal bowel distally and dilated bowel proximally. Treatment of FSI is resection of the involved bowel.

COLON ISCHEMIA

Colon ischemia (CI) is a frequent disorder of the large bowel in older persons and is the most common form of intestinal ischemic injury. It comprises a spectrum (Table 111–4) including (1) reversible colopathy (submucosal or intramural hemorrhage); (2) transient colitis; (3) chronic colitis; (4) stricture; (5) gangrene; and (6) fulminant, universal colitis. The initial presentation usually is the same among these types and does not necessarily predict the course of disease, with the exception of ischemia involving the ascending colon. This latter pattern may simultaneously involve the small intestine, usually is caused by SMAE or NOMI, may have associated shock, and carries a mortality rate of more than 50%.[37,38]

INCIDENCE

The incidence of CI is underestimated, because many patients suffer only mild or transient damage and do not seek medical attention. Also, CI is frequently misdiag-

Table 111–4 Types and Approximate Frequencies of Colon Ischemia in Patients Seen at a Tertiary Referral Hospital

Type	Frequency, %*
Reversible colopathy	30-40
Transient colitis	15-20
Chronic ulcerating colitis	20-25
Stricture	10-15
Gangrene	15-20
Fulminant universal colitis	<5

*Because of the approximate nature of the frequencies, the total of the frequencies of all types of colon ischemia adds up to more than 100%.

nosed and confused with other disorders, notably inflammatory bowel disease. In our tertiary care hospital, CI accounts for approximately 1:2000 hospital admissions and is seen in approximately 1:100 flexible sigmoidoscopies and colonoscopies. A recent study using medical claims data from a large health care organization calculated a crude incidence rate of 7.2 cases per 100,000 person-years of observation in the general population, in contrast to 42.8 cases per 100,000 person-years for patients with irritable bowel syndrome (IBS). After adjustment for age, sex, and calendar year, the incidence of CI in people with IBS was 3.4 times higher than it was in persons without IBS.[39] In the general population, CI has no sex predilection, and more than 90% of patients with CI of noniatrogenic causes are older than 60 years of age. CI affecting young persons has been documented in case reports or series of a few patients and usually has been due to vasculitis, coagulation disorders, illicit use of cocaine, and a variety of iatrogenic causes, including a wide variety of medications such as estrogens, serotonergic agonists and antagonists, sumatriptan, and methamphetamine.

PATHOPHYSIOLOGY AND CAUSES

CI can result from alterations in the systemic circulation or anatomic or functional changes in the local mesenteric vasculature (Table 111–5). In most cases, no specific cause for the ischemia is identified, and such episodes are viewed as localized nonocclusive ischemia, perhaps secondary to small-vessel disease. Abnormalities on angiography rarely correlate with clinical manifestations of disease, but age-related abnormalities in the splanchnic vessels, including narrowings of small vessels, tortuosity of the long colic arteries, and fibromuscular dysplasia (FMD) of the superior rectal artery, may contribute to CI. The colon is particularly susceptible to ischemia, perhaps owing to its relatively low blood flow, its unique decrease in blood flow during periods of functional activity, and its sensitivity to autonomic stimulation. What triggers the episode of CI, however, usually is not known.

PATHOLOGY

Morphologic changes after CI vary with the duration and severity of the injury. The mildest injury is mucosal and submucosal hemorrhage and edema, with or without partial necrosis and ulceration of the mucosa. With more severe injury, chronic ulcerations, crypt abscesses, and pseudopolyps develop, changes that may mimic inflammatory bowel disease (Fig. 111–11)[40]; pseudomembranes also may be seen. Iron-laden macrophages and submucosal fibrosis are characteristic of ischemic injury. With severe ischemia, the muscularis propria is replaced by fibrous tissue, forming a stricture. The most severe form of ischemic damage causes transmural infarction.

CLINICAL FEATURES AND DIAGNOSIS

CI usually presents with sudden, cramping, mild, left lower abdominal pain; an urgent desire to defecate; and

Table 111–5 Causes of Colon Ischemia

Allergy	Iatrogenic causes
Amyloidosis	Surgical
Cardiac failure or arrhythmias	Aneurysmectomy
Emboli	Aortoiliac reconstruction
Arterial	Barium enema
Cholesterol	Colectomy with inferior mesenteric artery ligation
Atrial myxoma	Colon bypass
Hematologic disorders and coagulopathies	Colonoscopy
Activated protein C resistance	Exchange transfusions
Antithrombin deficiency	Gynecologic operations
Paroxysmal nocturnal hemoglobinuria	Lumbar aortography
Polycythemia vera	Medications and drugs
Protein C and S deficiencies	Alosetron
Prothrombin 20210A mutation	Cocaine
Sickle cell disease	Danazol
Infection	Digitalis
Bacteria (*Escherichia coli* O157:H7)	Ergot
Parasites (*Angiostrongylus costaricensis*)	Estrogens
Viruses (hepatitis B virus, cytomegalovirus)	Flutamide
Inferior mesenteric artery thrombosis	Glycerin enema
Long-distance running	Gold salts
Pancreatitis	GoLYTELY
Pheochromocytoma	Immunosuppressive agents
Ruptured ectopic pregnancy	Interferon-α
Shock	Methamphetamine
Strangulated hernia	Nonsteroidal anti-inflammatory drugs
Trauma (blunt or penetrating)	Penicillin
Vasculitis and vasculopathy	Phenylephrine
Buerger's disease	Pit viper toxin
Fibromuscular dysplasia	Progestins
Kawasaki's disease	Pseudoephedrine
Polyarteritis nodosa	Psychotropic drugs
Rheumatoid vasculitis	Saline laxatives
Systemic lupus erythematosus	Sumatriptan
Takayasu's arteritis	Tegaserod
Volvulus	Vasopressin

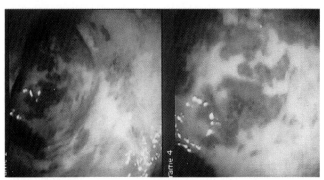

Figure 111–11 Colonoscopic view of deep ulcerations in the colon of a patient with colon ischemia who was misdiagnosed as having Crohn's disease.

passage within 24 hours of bright red or maroon blood or bloody diarrhea. Bleeding is not sufficient to require transfusion. Mild-to-moderate abdominal tenderness usually is present over the involved segment of bowel.

The splenic flexure, descending colon, and sigmoid are affected most commonly (Fig. 111–12). Certain causes tend to affect particular segments: systemic low-flow states, the right colon; local nonocclusive ischemic injuries, the "watershed" areas (the splenic flexure and

rectosigmoid); and ligation of the IMA, the sigmoid. The length of affected bowel also depends on the cause: atheromatous emboli involve short segments, and nonocclusive injuries involve longer portions of colon.

If CI is suspected and the patient has no signs of peritonitis and an unrevealing abdominal plain film or a CT scan showing only a thickened segment of colon, colonoscopy should be performed on the unprepared colon within 48 hours of the onset of symptoms. During colonoscopy and barium enema examination, care should be taken not to overdistend the colon because high intraluminal pressure diminishes intestinal blood flow and may aggravate ischemic damage, particularly in patients with vasculitis.[41] Colonoscopy is preferable to barium enema because it is more sensitive in diagnosing mucosal abnormalities and biopsy specimens may be obtained. Hemorrhagic nodules seen at colonoscopy represent bleeding into the submucosa and are equivalent to thumbprints on barium enema studies. (Fig. 111–13). Segmental distribution of these findings, with or without ulceration, is highly suggestive of CI, but the diagnosis of CI cannot be made conclusively in a single study unless mucosal gangrene is seen (Fig. 111–14). Recently, a colonoscopic finding called the *colon single-stripe sign* has been described in patients with CI, referring to a single

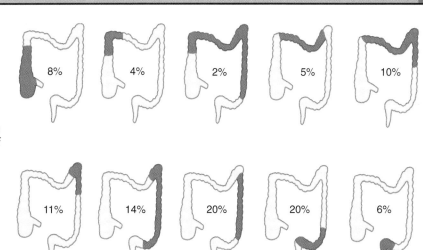

Figure 111–12 Schematic of patterns of colon ischemia showing the percentage of involvement of each pattern in a total of 250 cases.

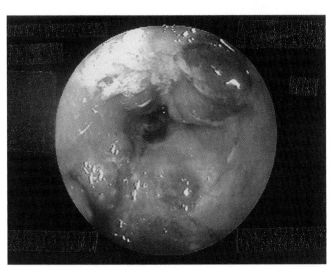

Figure 111–13 Colonoscopic equivalent of a thumbprint, caused by submucosal hemorrhage and edema, in a patient with colonic ischemia.

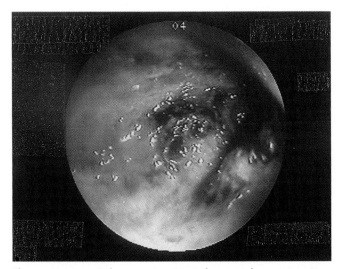

Figure 111–14 Colonoscopic view of mucosal gangrene in a patient with colonic ischemia. The necrotic epithelium appears black against the relatively healthy tissue.

line of erythema with erosion/ulceration oriented along the longitudinal axis of the colon; it had a 75% histopathologic yield in making the diagnosis of ischemic injury and signified a milder course than did a circumferential ulcer.[42] Segmental disease, rectal sparing, and rapid spontaneous evolution usually resulting in resolution of disease are characteristics of CI.

The initial diagnostic study should be performed within 48 hours, because thumbprinting disappears within days as the submucosal hemorrhages are resorbed or the overlying mucosa sloughs. Studies performed 1 week after the initial study should reflect evolution of the injury—either normalization of the colon or replacement of the thumbprints with a segmental ulcerative colitis-type pattern (Fig. 111–15). Universal colonic involvement, however, favors true ulcerative colitis, whereas fistula formation suggests Crohn's disease. Occasionally, an abundant inflammatory response can produce heaping-up of mucosa and submucosa that resembles a stricture or neoplasm (Fig. 111–16).

At the time of symptom onset, colon blood flow typically has returned to normal; therefore, mesenteric angiography usually is not indicated. An exception to this rule is when the clinical presentation does not allow a clear distinction to be made between CI and AMI or perhaps when only the ascending colon is involved. Administration of air during flexible sigmoidoscopy or a limited colonoscopy can be used to reveal thumbprinting not otherwise visible on abdominal plain films; thumbprints stand out as relatively radiodense nodules against the radiolucency of the administered air. Nodules in the left colon or throughout the colon imply CI, whereas nodules isolated to the ascending colon suggest the possibility of otherwise silent SMA disease and the need for evaluation of the mesenteric vasculature.

CLINICAL COURSE AND MANAGEMENT
(Fig. 111–17)

When CI is diagnosed and physical examination does not suggest gangrene or perforation, the patient is treated expectantly. Parenteral fluids are administered and the

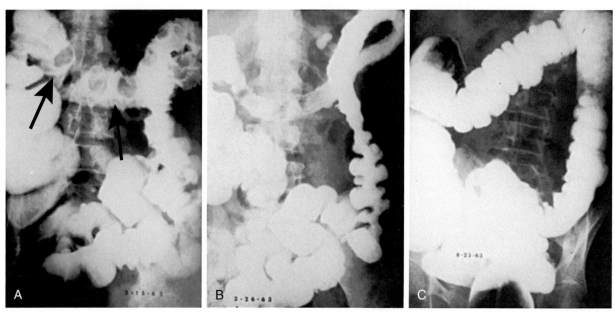

Figure 111–15 Films from serial barium enema examinations in a patient with reversible ischemic damage to the transverse colon and splenic flexure. *A,* Initial study shows dramatic thumbprints *(arrows)* throughout the area of involvement. *B,* Eleven days later, the thumbprints are gone, and the involved colon has the appearance of segmental colitis. *C,* Five months after the onset, the colon has returned to normal. The patient was asymptomatic by 3 weeks after the onset of her illness. (From Boley SJ, Schwartz SS: Colonic ischemia: Reversible ischemic lesions. In Boley SJ, Schwartz SS, Williams LF [eds]: Vascular Disorders of the Intestines. New York, Appleton-Century-Crofts, 1971, p 589.)

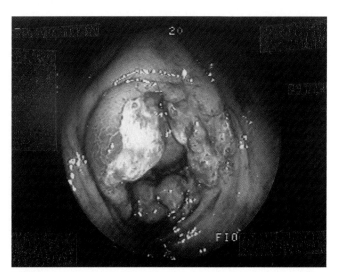

Figure 111–16 Colonoscopic view of colon ischemia resembling neoplasia of the cecum in a patient with metastatic cancer treated with interleukin-2 and interferon-α. The inflamed, edematous mass was thought to be due to neoplasia. The lesion resolved spontaneously after just 5 days. (From Sparano JA, Dutcher JP, Kaleya R, et al: Colonic ischemia complicating immunotherapy with interleukin-2 and interferon-α. Cancer 68:1538, 1991.)

bowel is placed at rest. Broad-spectrum antibiotics are given to "cover" the fecal flora because in experimental models, antibiotics reduce the extent and severity of bowel damage. No randomized, controlled, blinded trials have been done to prove the validity of this recommendation. Cardiac failure and arrhythmias are treated, and medications that may cause mesenteric vasoconstriction

are withdrawn. If the colon appears distended, it is decompressed with a rectal tube. Serial imaging tests or endoscopic evaluations of the colon and continued monitoring of the hemoglobin level, WBC count, and electrolyte levels are indicated until the patient's condition stabilizes.

Increasing abdominal tenderness, guarding, rebound tenderness, rising temperature, and paralytic ileus indicate colonic infarction and demand immediate laparotomy and colon resection if appropriate. At operation, mucosal injury may be extensive, despite normal-looking serosa, and the extent of resection should be guided by the distribution of disease as seen on preoperative studies rather than the appearance of the serosal surface of the colon at the time of operation.

In more than half of patients with CI, the disease is reversible. Generally, the symptoms of CI resolve within 48 to 72 hours and the colon heals in 1 to 2 weeks. With severe injury, it may take 1 to 6 months for the colon to heal; however, during this time the patient is usually asymptomatic. Symptoms that persist for more than 2 weeks are associated with a higher incidence of acute complications and irreversible disease: gangrene and perforation, segmental ulcerating colitis, or stricture.

Gangrene

Abdominal tenderness with fever and signs of peritonitis suggests infarction and the need for emergent laparotomy.

Segmental Ulcerating Colitis

Segmental ulcerating colitis may be seen with any of the following clinical patterns: recurrent fevers and sepsis; continuing or recurrent bloody diarrhea; and persistent

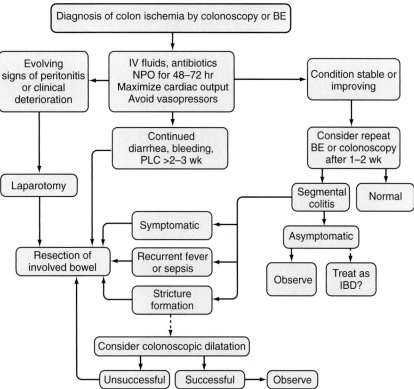

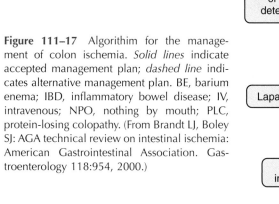

Figure 111–17 Algorithim for the management of colon ischemia. *Solid lines* indicate accepted management plan; *dashed line* indicates alternative management plan. BE, barium enema; IBD, inflammatory bowel disease; IV, intravenous; NPO, nothing by mouth; PLC, protein-losing colopathy. (From Brandt LJ, Boley SJ: AGA technical review on intestinal ischemia: American Gastrointestinal Association. Gastroenterology 118:954, 2000.)

or chronic diarrhea with protein-losing colopathy. Patients who are asymptomatic or minimally symptomatic but have endoscopic evidence of persistent disease should undergo follow-up colonoscopy to determine whether the colitis is healing, becoming chronic, or forming a stricture. Recurrent fever, leukocytosis, and septicemia suggest unhealed segmental colitis and, if found, mandates elective resection of the ischemic segment of bowel. Patients with persistent diarrhea, bleeding, or protein-losing colopathy of more than 2 weeks' duration are at high risk of perforation, and resection is indicated. Patients who present with segmental ulcerating colitis are frequently misdiagnosed as having inflammatory bowel disease. Response to oral steroid therapy usually is poor and may be associated with an increased incidence of perforation. Success has been achieved with fatty acid enemas and corticosteroids given per rectum (Dr. L. Brandt, personal observation). Patients whose symptoms cannot be controlled medically should have a segmental resection, which usually is curative.

Ischemic Stricture

Ischemic strictures that produce no symptoms can be observed. Some disappear over 12 to 24 months with no therapy. Of course, resection is required for those that cause obstruction. There is limited experience with endoscopic dilatation of ischemic strictures, although I have had success in a few cases using this technique.

Universal Fulminant Colitis

Sudden onset of a "toxic universal colitis picture" with signs of peritonitis and a rapidly progressive course are typical of universal fulminant colitis, a rare variant of CI. Total abdominal colectomy with ileostomy usually is required.

SPECIAL CLINICAL PROBLEMS

Colon Ischemia in Patients with Carcinoma of the Colon and Other Potentially Obstructive Lesions

Fewer than 10% of patients with CI have a distal and potentially obstructing lesion or disorder. In half the cases, carcinoma of the colon is present, whereas in the remaining half, diverticulitis, volvulus, fecal impaction, postoperative stricture, prior ischemic stenosis, or radiation stricture is seen. Typically, the associated lesion is distal, and there is a segment of normal colon between the distal lesion and the proximal colitis (Fig. 111–18).

Colon Ischemia Complicating Aortic Surgery

CI complicates elective aortic surgery in up to 7% and surgery for ruptured abdominal aortic aneurysms in up to 60% of cases.[43] CI is responsible for approximately 10% of the deaths after aortic replacement. Factors that contribute to postoperative CI include aneurysmal rupture, hypotension, operative trauma to the colon, hypoxemia, arrhythmias, prolonged cross-clamp time, and improper management of the IMA during aneurysmectomy. Tonometric determination of intramural pH of the sigmoid before and after cross-clamping the aorta has been used successfully to predict which patients will develop CI after aneurysmectomy.[44]

Because postoperative CI is serious and difficult to diagnose early, colonoscopy should be performed within 2 to 3 days after surgery for a ruptured abdominal aortic aneurysm or in patients with a prolonged cross-clamping time, a patent IMA on preoperative aortography, nonpulsatile flow in the hypogastric arteries during surgery, or postoperative diarrhea. If CI is identified, oral feeding and liquids are stopped and antibiotic therapy is begun; clinical deterioration requires reoperation. At surgery, all ischemic colon must be resected.

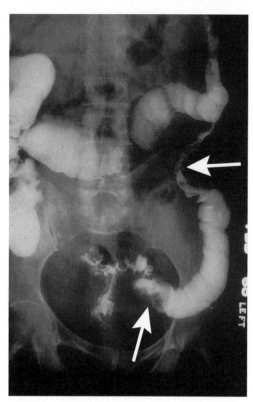

Figure 111–18 Film from a barium enema demonstrating a narrowed segment of colon ischemia *(upper arrow)* proximal to a carcinoma in the distal sigmoid *(lower arrow).* The area of colon between the lesion and the ischemic segment is normal. (From Boley SJ, Brandt LJ, Veith FJ: Ischemic disorders of the intestines. Curr Probl Surg 15:1, 1978.)

CHRONIC MESENTERIC ISCHEMIA (INTESTINAL ANGINA)

CMI is uncommon, accounting for less than 5% of intestinal ischemic diseases; it almost always is caused by mesenteric atherosclerosis, although rare causes such as collagen vascular disease and inflammatory vasculopathy are known. There is no specific association between CMI and smoking, although 75% of patients with CMI have a history of smoking.[45] Abdominal pain is likely caused by ischemia in the small intestine as blood is "stolen" from this organ to meet the increased demand for gastric blood flow as food enters the stomach.[46] This rationale for why the pain occurs so soon after eating, when food still remains in the stomach, is preferable to the historic explanation that a fixed and limited blood supply is incapable of meeting the increased metabolic demands of the small intestine during digestion.

The cardinal clinical feature of CMI is abdominal cramping discomfort that usually occurs within 30 minutes after eating, gradually increases in severity, and then slowly resolves over 1 to 3 hours. Although minimal at first, abdominal pain progressively increases in severity over weeks to months. The association of pain with meals leads to fear of eating with resultant weight loss. Nausea, bloating, episodic diarrhea, and malabsorption or constipation may occur, but it is the weight loss and relation of the abdominal pain to the meals that charac-

terize this syndrome. Early in the course of disease, if patients do not eat, they remain pain free; pain occurs only after eating or during a meal. Later, pain may become continuous, and this portends intestinal infarction. Uncommon presentations of CMI include antral ulcerations that are unassociated with *Helicobacter pylori* and that do not heal on therapy with proton pump inhibitors; gastroparesis (that resolves after revascularization); and acalculous cholecystitis. Approximately one third to one half of patients have evidence of cardiac, cerebral, or peripheral vascular disease. Physical findings are usually limited, but patients with advanced disease may appear cachectic. The abdomen typically remains soft and nontender even during painful episodes, although distention may be appreciated. An abdominal bruit is common but nonspecific.

Diagnosis of CMI is difficult because of the vague nature of the complaints and the lack of a specific diagnostic test. Abdominal plain films and CT scans are usually normal, although vascular calcification may be present. Endoscopic inspection of the gastrointestinal tract usually reveals it to be normal, and random biopsies of the upper tract may show only nonspecific abnormalities; a diagnostic clue may be antral ulcerations that are unassociated with *H. pylori* and that do not heal on acid-suppression therapy. Barium studies are normal or show nonspecific evidence of either malabsorption or a motility disturbance. Rarely, radionuclear emptying tests may show delayed gastric emptying. Duplex ultrasonography can be used to identify splanchnic artery stenoses but not to establish the diagnosis of CMI.[47] Elevated peak systolic velocity in the SMA and CA of 275 and 200 cm/sec, respectively, is a reliable sign of at least 70% stenosis of these vessels.[48] Duplex ultrasonography and phase-contrast cine MR imaging of the SMA and CA have been used to measure the effect of eating on mesenteric blood flow, all based on the principle that eating normally increases blood flow to the small intestine, whereas in CMI, this fails to occur; however, postprandial studies are no better than fasting examinations, especially at lesser degrees of vascular stenosis.[48] More experience with these provocative tests is needed before firm conclusions about their diagnostic usefulness can be made. Duplex ultrasonography, MR angiography, and even traditional mesenteric angiography all merely reveal anatomic limitations of splanchnic blood flow and do not establish the presence or absence of intestinal ischemia.

In the absence of any specific, reliable, diagnostic test, diagnosis of CMI is based on clinical symptoms, in combination with radiologic demonstration of an occlusive process of the splanchnic vessels, and, to a great measure, the exclusion of other gastrointestinal disorders. Angiography should show occlusion of two or more splanchnic arteries to allow the diagnosis of CMI; however, such occlusions, even of all three vessels, do not by themselves make the diagnosis of CMI, because they may be present with no corresponding clinical symptoms. In most patients with CMI, at least two of the three splanchnic vessels either are completely obstructed or severely stenosed. In a review of series of patients with CMI,[45] 91% had occlusion of at least two vessels and 55% had involvement of all three; 7% and 2% had isolated occlusion of the SMA and CA, respectively.

CMI is not considered to require urgent therapy, although acute complete occlusion of the gastrointestinal blood supply may occur if thrombosis is superimposed on already narrowed arteries. A patient with the typical pain of CMI and unexplained weight loss whose diagnostic evaluation has excluded other gastrointestinal disease (Fig. 111–19) and whose angiogram shows occlusive involvement of at least two of the three major arteries should undergo revascularization.

Surgical revascularization has been the traditional method of therapy for patients with CMI. Since the early 1980s, percutaneous transluminal mesenteric angioplasty (PTMA) alone or with stent insertion has been used as alternative therapy but is reported only in small numbers of patients. Whether surgery or PTMA is better will be determined by their relative success in relieving symptoms and the durability of such relief. The results of surgical revascularization for CMI vary in different reports, depending on the nature of the operations used, the number of vessels revascularized, and whether concurrent operations such as aortic reconstruction are performed.

The true efficacy of surgical revascularization and PTMA is difficult to determine because of the varied criteria used by different investigators to define a successful outcome. Thus, some authors use graft or vessel patency rates, whereas others define success by relief of symptoms, recurrence rates, or long-term survival. A tabulation of 17 series of surgical revascularization for CMI totaling 614 patients yielded perioperative mortality rates that ranged from 0%[49-54] to 16%,[55] success rates of 59%[56] to 100%[50-54] and recurrence rates of 0%[49,50,54,55,57,58] to 26.5%.[59] Most recent series have reported mortality rates below 10%, success rates of more than 90%, and recur-

rence rates generally lower than 10%.[16] Several long-term studies have shown that patients surviving surgical revascularization have cumulative 5-year survival rates of approximately 80% to 90%.[16]

The initial success rates of PTMA are similar to those of surgical revascularization. The experience with PTMA is more limited but has been achieved in patients often considered too high risk for a surgical procedure. In 10 representative series of PTMA for CMI, totaling 128 patients, clinical success rates (i.e., relief of symptoms) have varied from 63%[60] to 100%,[61] with little mortality.[16] Recurrence of symptoms, however, has been much higher than after surgical revascularization, varying from 10% to 67% in the larger series.[16] More recently, intraluminal stenting has been added to PTMA in an attempt to decrease the incidence of recurrent stenoses. Too few patients have been treated in this fashion to permit a conclusion as to its long-term value in managing patients with CMI.

Patients with CMI who are otherwise relatively healthy probably should be treated by surgical revascularization; poorer risk patients should have an initial attempt at PTMA with or without stenting to relieve symptoms. If, however, the use of stents proves to reduce the recurrence rates of PTMA close to those of surgical revascularization, PTMA may become the method of choice.

VASCULITIS AND ANGIOPATHY OF THE SPLANCHNIC CIRCULATION

Inflammation and necrosis can affect splanchnic blood vessels of all sizes: arteries, veins, the vasa recta, arterioles, and venules.[62] Symptoms depend on the size of the involved vessel. Polyarteritis nodosa and rheumatoid arthritis affect medium and large vessels and, clinically, may be indistinguishable from AMI caused by emboli or thromboses, except for associated systemic features such as renal failure, cutaneous nodules, or a positive rheumatoid factor.

The vasa recta and intramural arteries and arterioles may be affected in systemic vasculitides. With vasculitis, the ischemic injury typically involves small segments of the intestine. Abdominal pain, fever, gastrointestinal bleeding, diarrhea, and intestinal obstruction are common. Ulceration and stricture formation are common, but with small-vessel involvement perforation is less frequent.

Typically, vasculitis is caused by immune complex deposition in the walls of vessels, which leads to activation of the complement system and an inflammatory reaction; aneurysm formation, vessel rupture and bleeding, vascular occlusion, thrombosis, and/or fibrosis may ensue. A variety of vasculitides are discussed in the following sections.

ALLERGIC GRANULOMATOUS ANGIITIS (CHURG-STRAUSS SYNDROME)

Allergic granulomatous angiitis is a disorder that is typified by asthma, glomerulonephritis, eosinophilia, and granulomatous inflammation associated with antineutrophil cytoplasmic autoantibodies.[63] Necrotizing vasculitis affects small- and medium-sized vessels and

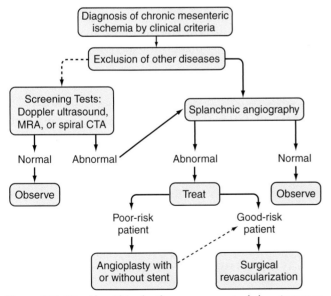

Figure 111–19 Algorithim for the management of chronic mesenteric ischemia. *Solid lines* indicate accepted management plan; *dashed line* indicates alternative management plan. CTA, computed tomographic angiogram; MRA, magnetic resonance angiography. (From Brandt LJ, Boley SJ: AGA technical review on intestinal ischemia: American Gastrointestinal Association. Gastroenterology 118:954, 2000.)

involves the gastrointestinal tract in almost half the patients. As in other vasculitides, abdominal pain and bleeding secondary to ischemia are the usual manifestations. Glucocorticoid therapy usually is effective.

BEHÇET'S DISEASE

Behçet's disease (see Chapter 34) is characterized by oral and genital ulcers, recurrent iritis or chorioretinitis, and skin lesions. It is most often seen in Eastern Mediterranean men and is strongly associated with the B51 allele. Small-vessel vasculitis accounts for much of the damage, but large-vessel involvement of both arteries and veins is not uncommon. Gastrointestinal disease, present in 50% of patients, typically affects the ileocecal area, although involvement of the esophagus and small intestine has been reported.[64] Attacks are recurrent and usually self-limited; they do not cause a chronic disorder, except for the uveitis. The most common gastrointestinal symptoms are abdominal pain, diarrhea, and bleeding; deep ulcers are responsible for the most common intestinal complications, i.e., severe bleeding and perforation. Mortality is low in Behçet's disease; however, intestinal perforation is one of the common causes of death. Therapy with glucocorticoids, immunosuppressive agents, and colchicine has been tried, with varying success.

BUERGER'S DISEASE

Also called *thromboangiitis obliterans,* Buerger's disease involves medium-sized and small peripheral arteries and veins, especially the infrapopliteal vessels; foot claudication and rubor are the most frequent symptoms. It is largely a disease of men, especially those who have smoked cigarettes from an early age, and typically has its onset before 50 years of age; there is a distinct absence of other atherosclerotic risk factors. Intestinal involvement is unusual, but most common is involvement of the vessels supplying the small intestine.[65] In the acute lesion, inflammation spreads outward from the thrombus-endothelium interface through the vessel wall. Later, microabscesses, necrotizing granulomas, and multinucleated giant cells occur in the thrombus, after which the thrombus organizes and becomes occlusive. Intestinal involvement usually requires resection.

COGAN'S SYNDROME

Cogan's syndrome is a rare disorder of young people characterized by vasculitis of the conjunctiva, cornea, and cochlea.[66] Although this vasculitis usually is localized, it is considered to be a hypersensitivity reaction to an unknown viral agent, and the disease can become disseminated. Three percent to 10% of patients develop gastrointestinal symptoms, with diarrhea and bloody stools. High-dose glucocorticoids, and occasionally cytotoxic agents, are required. Vascular surgery may be needed after inflammation is controlled.

FIBROMUSCULAR DYSPLASIA

FMD is a rare angiopathy that is neither related to atherosclerosis nor to inflammation.[67] Its cause is unknown, although genetic factors may play a role and there is an association with cigarette smoking and hypertension. There are several types of FMD depending on which arterial layer is involved—intima, media, or adventitia. The renal arteries are most commonly involved followed by the carotid and vertebral arteries and then other vascular beds including the mesenteric arteries. Splanchnic involvement may manifest with symptoms of AMI or CMI.[68] Diagnosis is based on the same techniques used to image other vascular disorders; the classic "string of beads" appearance is typical of only the medial type of FMD whereas aneurysms and dissection are known complications of all types. Therapy consists of percutaneous transluminal angioplasty, surgical revascularization, and resection of necrotic bowel as indicated.

HENOCH-SCHÖNLEIN PURPURA

Henoch-Schönlein (see Chapter 34) purpura typically affects children aged 4 to 7 years of age. It is characterized by IgA immune complexes deposited within the small vessels of the skin, gastrointestinal tract, joints, and kidneys and is often preceded by an upper respiratory infection. The classic clinical triad consists of palpable purpura (usually below the waist), arthritis (knees and ankles), and abdominal pain; the gastrointestinal tract is involved in up to 75% of patients.[69] Abdominal pain and gastrointestinal bleeding are the most common gastrointestinal symptoms and are caused by mucosal and submucosal hemorrhage; a submucosal hematoma may be the lead point of an intussusception. Gastrointestinal involvement may be documented by endoscopy[70] or by CT study.[71] The disease is usually self-limited, but the outlook may be less favorable in adults, in large measure because of the development of renal failure.

HYPERSENSITIVITY VASCULITIS

Hypersensitivity vasculitis uncommonly involves the splanchnic vasculature, and, in contrast with necrotizing vasculitis, which involves arteries, affects mainly the postcapillary venules. A large variety of causes are known to trigger this disorder, including infections (*Streptococcus, Staphylococcus,* hepatitis B virus, influenza virus, cytomegalovirus, mycobacteria, and rickettsiae), drugs, and chemicals.

KAWASAKI'S DISEASE

Kawasaki's disease, also called *infantile febrile mucocutaneous lymph node syndrome,* is a necrotizing vasculitis of medium-sized arteries.[72] It manifests as fever, rash on the palms and soles, desquamation, conjunctival congestion, "strawberry" tongue, and cervical lymphadenopathy in infants and children. Many have nausea, vomiting, abdominal pain, and diarrhea, and they may suffer ileus, small bowel obstruction, bleeding, and perforation. Death may be due to coronary artery aneurysms and myocardial infarction. Treatment is aspirin for the acute phase and large intravenous doses of gamma globulin for the prevention of coronary artery aneurysms.

KÖHLMEIER-DEGOS DISEASE (MALIGNANT ATROPHIC PAPULOSIS)

Köhlmeier-Degos disease is a rare form of progressive occlusive vascular disease of young men that affects the small- and medium-sized arteries, mainly those of the skin and intestine.[73] Typically, skin lesions of porcelain-white, punctate scars with erythematous borders are found on the trunk and upper extremities. The rash is followed, within months to years, by the development of abdominal pain and spontaneous intestinal perforation. Thrombosis of small- and medium-sized vessels is found, without inflammatory cell infiltration. There is no known therapy for this disease, and it is generally fatal.

POLYARTERITIS NODOSA

Polyarteritis nodosa (see Chapter 34) is a necrotizing vasculitis of medium- and small-sized arteries characterized by aneurysms at branch points. Abdominal symptoms are reported in up to half of patients with the disorder, most frequent of which is abdominal pain, usually from ischemia.[74] Involvement of the small bowel is most common, followed by lesions of colon, liver, and pancreas. Diagnosis is suggested by typical angiographic findings of aneurysms in the mesenteric, renal, and hepatic vasculature. Treatment with glucocorticoids and cyclophosphamide or azathioprine has improved survival greatly.

Vasculitis resembling polyarteritis also is associated with hepatitis B and C virus infections.[75,76] Fifty percent of patients with classic polyarteritis are hepatitis B surface antigen positive, but unlike classic polyarteritis, only small arteries are involved. Patients develop a polyarteritis picture following the viral infection, presumably from deposition of antigen-associated immune complexes on the vessel wall.

RHEUMATOID VASCULITIS

Rheumatoid vasculitis affects the gastrointestinal tract in approximately 10% of patients, usually those who have subcutaneous nodules and who are seropositive for rheumatoid factor.[77] As with all vasculitides, ischemia manifests with abdominal pain, bleeding, perforation, and gangrene. Other diseases have been noted in association with rheumatoid arthritis, including atrophic gastritis, gastric antral vascular ectasia (GAVE), inflammatory bowel disease, collagenous colitis, and amyloidosis.

SYSTEMIC LUPUS ERYTHEMATOSUS

Systemic lupus erythematosus (see Chapter 34) affects the gastrointestinal system in about half of cases and may involve any of the hollow and solid gastrointestinal organs.[62] The most common symptoms are nausea, vomiting, and abdominal pain, but diarrhea, malabsorption, pseudo-obstruction, peritonitis, pancreatitis, protein-losing enteropathy, and ascites are also well-known occurrences. The systemic nature of the disorder makes differential diagnosis complicated, but vasculitis-induced ischemia underlies many of the presentations. The vasculitis typically involves small vessels and causes FSI and gastrointestinal bleeding, both of which are associated with high mortality rates if not diagnosed promptly.

TAKAYASU'S DISEASE

Takayasu's disease ("pulseless disease") is an idiopathic chronic inflammatory disorder that most often affects the aorta and its branches in young women of Asian heritage; it is unusual that the splanchnic vessels are involved.[78] Fibrotic occlusion of the involved vessels is the end result of the inflammatory process. Takayasu's disease rarely has been associated with Crohn's disease and ulcerative colitis, and in the serum of some of these patients, antibodies to both colonic mucosa and aorta have been detected. Treatment is large doses of glucocorticoids prior to reconstructive surgery. The 5-year survival rate is higher than 90%.

ACKNOWLEDGMENT

The author is indebted to Dr. Scott J. Boley, who for decades has been laying the groundwork for this chapter and who played a critical role in preparing earlier editions.

REFERENCES

1. Kornblith PL, Boley SJ, Whitehouse BS: Anatomy of the splanchnic circulation. Surg Clin North Am 72:1, 1992.
2. Boley SJ, Freiber W, Winslow PR, et al: Circulatory responses to acute reduction of superior mesenteric arterial flow. Physiologist 12:180, 1969.
3. Zimmerman BJ, Granger DN: Reperfusion injury. Surg Clin North Am 72:65, 1992.
4. Finucane PM, Arunachalam T, O'Dowd J, et al: Acute mesenteric infarction in elderly patients. J Am Geriatr Soc 37:355, 1989.
5. Gaussorgues P, Guerugniand PY, Vedrinne JM, et al: Bacteremia following cardiac arrest and cardiopulmonary resuscitation. Intensive Care Med 14:575, 1988.
6. Kurland B, Brandt LJ, Delany HM: Diagnostic tests for intestinal angina. Surg Clin North Am 72:85, 1992.
7. Khurana S, Corbally MT, Manning F, et al: Glutathione S-transferase: A potential new marker of intestinal ischemia. J Pediatr Surg 37:1543, 2002.
8. Kanda T, Fujii H, Tani T, et al: Intestinal fatty acid-binding protein is a useful diagnostic marker for mesenteric infarction in humans. Gastroenterology 110:339, 1996.
9. Ritz JP, Runkel N, Berger G, et al: [Prognostic factors in mesenteric infarct]. Zentralblatt Chir 122:332, 1997.
10. Yamada K, Saeki M, Yamaguchi T, et al: Acute mesenteric ischemia: CT and plain radiographic analysis of 26 cases. Clin Imaging 22:34, 1998.

11. Lee R, Tung HKS, Cheung SCW, et al: CT in acute mesenteric ischemia. Clin Radiol 58:279, 2003.

12. Taourel PG, Deneuville M, Pradel JA, et al: Acute mesenteric ischemia: Diagnosis with contrast-enhanced CT. Radiology 199:632, 1996.

13. Smerud MJ, Johnson CD, Stephens DH: Diagnosis of bowel infarction: A comparison of plain films and CT scans in 23 cases. AJR Am J Roentgenol 154:99, 1990.

14. Kirkpatrick IDC, Kroeker MA, Greenberg HM: Biphasic CT with mesenteric CT angiography in the evaluation of acute mesenteric ischemia: Initial experience. Radiology 229:91, 2003.

15. Li KC, Pelc LR, Dalman RL, et al: In vivo magnetic resonance evaluation of blood oxygen saturation in the superior mesenteric vein as a measure of the degree of acute blood flow reduction in the superior mesenteric artery: findings in a canine model. Acad Radiol 4:21, 1997.

16. Brandt LJ, Boley SJ: AGA technical review on intestinal ischemia: American Gastrointestinal Association. Gastroenterology 118:954, 2000.

17. Jamieson WG, Pliagus G, Marchuk S, et al: Effect of antibiotic and fluid resuscitation upon survival time in experimental intestinal ischemia. Surg Gynecol Obstet 167:103, 1988.

18. Horgan PG, Gorey JF: Operative assessment of intestinal viability. Surg Clin North Am 72:143, 1992.

19. Schoenbaum SW, Pena C, Koenigsberg P, et al: Superior mesenteric artery embolism: Treatment with intraarterial urokinase. J Vasc Interv Radiol 3:485, 1992.

20. Boley SJ, Sprayregen S, Siegelman SS, et al: Initial results from an aggressive roentgenological and surgical approach to acute mesenteric ischemia. Surgery 82:848, 1977.

21. Boley SJ, Feinstein FR, Sammartano R, et al: New concepts in the management of emboli of the superior mesenteric artery. Surg Gynecol Obstet 153:561, 1981.

22. Clark RA, Gallant TE: Acute mesenteric ischemia: Angiographic spectrum. AJR Am J Roentgenol 142:555, 1984.

23. Boos S: [Angiography of the mesenteric artery 1976-1991: A change in the indications during mesenteric circulatory disorders?]. Radiologe 32:154, 1992.

24. Bottger T, Schafer W, Weber W, et al: [Value of preoperative diagnosis in mesenteric vascular occlusion: A prospective study]. Langenbecks Arch Chir 375:278, 1990.

25. Czerny M, Trubel W, Claeys L, et al: [Acute mesenteric ischemia]. Zentralbl Chir 122:538, 1997.

26. Harward RTS, Green D, Bergan JJ, et al: Mesenteric venous thrombosis. J Vasc Surg 9:328, 1989.

27. Clavien PA, Durig M, Harder F: Venous mesenteric infarction: A particular entity. Br J Surg 75:252, 1988.

28. Font VE, Hermann RE, Longworth DL: Chronic mesenteric venous thrombosis: Difficult diagnosis and therapy. Cleve Clin J Med 56:823, 1989.

29. Warshaw AL, Gongliang J, Ottinger LW: Recognition and clinical implications of mesenteric and portal vein obstruction in chronic pancreatitis. Arch Surg 123:410, 1987.

30. Clark AZ, Gallant TE: Acute mesenteric ischemia: Angiographic spectrum. AJR Am J Radiol 142:555, 1984.

31. Clavien PA, Huber O, Mirescu D, et al: Contrast-enhanced CT scan as a diagnostic procedure in mesenteric ischemia due to mesenteric venous thrombosis. Br J Surg 76:93, 1989.

32. Al Karawi MA, Quaiz M, Clark D, et al: Mesenteric vein thrombosis, non-invasive diagnosis and followup (US + MRI) and non-invasive therapy by streptokinase and anticoagulants. Hepatogastroenterology 37:507, 1990.

33. Cho YP, Jung SM, Han MS, et al: Role of diagnostic laparoscopy in managing acute mesenteric venous thrombosis. Surg Laparosc Endosc Percutan Tech 13:215, 2003.

34. Rhee RY, Gloviczki P, Mendonca CT, et al: Mesenteric venous thrombosis: Still a lethal disease in the 1990s. J Vasc Surg 20:688, 1994.

35. Grieshop RJ, Dalsing MC, Cikrit DF, et al: Acute mesenteric venous thrombosis: Revisited in a time of diagnostic clarity. Am Surg 57:573, 1991.

36. Brunaud L, Antunes L, Collinet-Adler S, et al: Acute mesenteric venous thrombosis: Case for nonoperative management. J Vasc Surg 34:673, 2001.

37. Sakai L, Keltner R, Kaminski D: Spontaneous and shock-associated ischemic colitis. Am J Surg 140:755, 1980.

38. Guttormson NL, Bubrick MP: Mortality from ischemic colitis. Dis Colon Rectum 26:462, 1983.

39. Cole JA, Cook SF, Sands BE, et al: Occurrence of colon ischemia in relation to irritable bowel syndrome. Am J Gastroenterol 99:486, 2004.

40. Brandt LJ, Boley SJ, Goldberg L, et al: Colitis in the elderly. Am J Gastroenterol 76:239, 1981.

41. Church JM: Ischemic colitis complicating flexible endoscopy in a patient with connective tissue disease. Gastrointest Endosc 41:181, 1995.

42. Zuckerman GR, Prakash C, Merriman RB, et al: The colon single-stripe sign and its relationship to ischemic colitis. Am J Gastroenterol 98:2018, 2003.

43. Zelenock GB, Strodel WE, Knol JA, et al: A prospective study of clinically and endoscopically documented colonic ischemia in 100 patients undergoing aortic reconstructive surgery with aggressive colonic and direct pelvic revascularization, compared with historic controls. Surgery 106:771, 1989.

44. Schiedler MG, Cutler BS, Fiddian-Green RG: Sigmoid intramural pH for prediction of ischemic colitis during aortic surgery: A comparison with risk factors and inferior mesenteric artery stump pressures. Arch Surg 122:881, 1987.

45. Moawad J, Gewertz BL: Chronic mesenteric ischemia: Clinical presentation and diagnosis. Surg Clin North Am 77:357, 1997.

46. Poole JW, Sammartano RJ, Boley SJ: Hemodynamic basis of the pain of chronic mesenteric ischemia. Am J Surg 153:171, 1987.

47. Moneta GL: Screening for mesenteric vascular insufficiency and follow-up of mesenteric artery bypass procedures. Semin Vasc Surg 14:186, 2001.

48. Gentile AT, Moneta GL, Lee RW, et al: Usefulness of fasting and postprandial duplex ultrasound examinations for predicting high-grade superior mesenteric artery stenosis. Am J Surg 169:476, 1995.

49. Beebe HG, MacFarlane S, Raker EJ: Supraceliac aortomesenteric bypass for intestinal ischemia. J Vasc Surg 5:749, 1987.

50. Calderon M, Reul GJ, Gregoric ID, et al: Long-term results of the surgical management of symptomatic chronic intestinal ischemia. J Cardiovasc Surg (Torino) 33:723, 1992.

51. Christiansen MG, Lorentzen JE, Schroeder TV: Revascularization of atherosclerotic mesenteric arteries: Experience in 90 consecutive patients. Eur J Vasc Surg 8:297, 1994.

52. Gentile AT, Moneta GL, Taylor LM Jr, et al: Isolated bypass to the superior mesenteric artery for intestinal ischemia. Arch Surg 129:926, 1994.

53. Johnston KW, Lindsay TF, Walker PM, et al: Mesenteric arterial bypass grafts: Early and late results and suggested surgical approach for chronic and acute mesenteric ischemia. Surgery 118:1, 1995.

54. Wolf YG, Verstandig A, Sasson T, et al: Mesenteric bypass for chronic mesenteric ischemia. Cardiovasc Surg 6:34, 1998.

55. Van Damme H, Creemers E, Limet E: [Surgical treatment of chronic mesenteric ischemia]. Acta Gastroenterol Belg 52:406, 1989.

56. Sandmann W, Bohner H, Kneiemeyer HW, et al: [Chronic mesenteric ischemia]. Dtsch Med Wochenschr 119:979, 1994.

57. Geelkerken RH, vanBockel H, deRoos WK, et al: Chronic mesenteric vascular syndrome: Results of reconstructive surgery. Arch Surg 126:1101, 1991.

58. Moawad J, McKinsey JF, Wyble CW, et al: Current results of surgical therapy for chronic mesenteric ischemia. Arch Surg 132:613, 1997.

59. Hollier LH, Bernatz PE, Pairolero PC, et al: Surgical management of chronic intestinal ischemia: A reappraisal. Surgery 90:940, 1981.

60. Matsumoto AH, Tegtmeyer CJ, Fitzcharles EK, et al: Percutaneous transluminal angioplasty of visceral arterial stenoses: Results and long-term clinical follow-up. J Vasc Interv Radiol 6:165, 1995.

61. Roberts L Jr, Wertman DA, Mills SR, et al: Transluminal angioplasty of the superior mesenteric artery: An alternative to surgical revascularization. AJR Am J Roentgenol 141:1039, 1983.

62. Bailey M, Chapin W, Licht H, et al: The effects of vasculitis on the gastrointestinal tract and liver. Gastroenterol Clin North Am 27:747, 1998.

63. Lhote F, Guillevin L: Polyarteritis nodosa, microscopic polyangiitis, and Churg-Strauss syndrome: Clinical aspects and treatment. Rheum Dis Clin North Am 21:911, 1995.

64. Lee RG: The colitis of Behçet's syndrome. Am J Surg Pathol 10:888, 1986.

65. Lie JT: Visceral intestinal Buerger's disease. Int J Cardiol 66S:249, 1998.

66. Haynes G, Kaiser-Kupfer M, Mason P, et al: Cogan's syndrome. Medicine 59:426, 1980.

67. Slovut DP, Olin JW. Fibromuscular dysplasia. N Engl J Med 350:1862, 2004.

68. Guill CK, Benavides DC, Rees C, at al: Fatal mesenteric fibromuscular dysplasia: A case report and review of the literature. Arch Intern Med 164:1148, 2004.

69. Robson WL, Leung AK: Henoch-Schönlein purpura. Adv Pediatr 41:163, 1994.

70. Nakasone H, Hokama A, Fukuchi J, et al: Colonoscopic findings in an adult patient with Henoch-Schönlein purpura. Gastrointest Endosc 52:392, 2000.

71. Jeong YK, Ha HK, Yoon CH, et al: Gastrointestinal involvement in Henoch-Schönlein syndrome: CT findings. AJR Am J Roentgenol 168:965, 1997.

72. Kawasaki T: Clinical features of Kawasaki's syndrome. Acta Paediatr Jpn 25:79, 1983.

73. Fruhwirth J, Mischinger HJ, Werkgartner G, et al: Köhlmeier-Degos disease with primary intestinal manifestation. Scand J Gastroenterol 10:1066, 1997.

74. Bassel K, Harford W: Gastrointestinal manifestations of collagen-vascular disease. Semin Gastrointest Dis 6:228, 1995.

75. Deny P, Guillevin L, Bonacorsi S, et al: Association between hepatitis C virus and polyarteritis nodosa. Clin Exp Rheumatol 10:319, 1992.

76. Guillevin L, Lhote F, Cohen P, et al: Polyarteritis nodosa related to hepatitis B virus: A prospective study with long-term observation of 41 patients. Medicine 74:238, 1995.

77. Scott DGI, Baco PA, Tribe CR: Systemic rheumatoid vasculitis: A clinical laboratory study of 50 cases. Medicine 60:288, 1981.

78. Sharma BK, Jain S, Sagar S: Systemic manifestations of Takayasu arteritis: The expanding spectrum. Int J Cardiol 54S:149, 1996.

CHAPTER
112 Ulcers of the Small and Large Intestine

Anil B. Nagar and Deborah D. Proctor

Ulcers of the small and large intestine are rare, yet are responsible for a broad spectrum of diseases. Ulcers may occur singly as in solitary rectal ulcer syndrome (SRUS) or diffusely as in enteropathy-type intestinal T cell lymphoma (ETL), and clinical presentations vary with location and degree of intestinal involvement, ranging from anemia and hypoproteinemia to abdominal pain, hemorrhage, obstruction, and perforation. This chapter is divided into two sections: (1) isolated intestinal ulcers, including nonspecific solitary ulcers of the small intestine, SRUS, stercoral ulcers, and nonsteroidal anti-inflammatory drug (NSAID)-induced ulcerations; and (2) syndromes of diffuse intestinal ulceration, including ulcerative enteritis, refractory celiac disease, and ETL. The syndromes of diffuse intestinal ulceration still have a poor prognosis, although our understanding of them has been increased by the demonstration in affected patients of abnormal, monoclonal intestinal T lymphocytes with chromosomal abnormalities. Because of the length and relative inaccessibility of the small intestine, diagnosis of these entities remains challenging; however, enteroscopy and capsule endoscopy have improved greatly our ability to evaluate the small intestine.

ISOLATED ULCERS

NONSPECIFIC OR IDIOPATHIC SMALL INTESTINAL ULCERATION

Solitary ulcers of the small intestine can result from a wide variety of causes (Table 112–1). Solitary ulcers beyond the duodenum that cannot be explained on the basis of any known etiology are referred to as nonspecific or idiopathic intestinal ulcers. Such solitary nonspecific ulcers are rare, with an incidence of 4:100,000.[1]

Clinical Features

Patients with nonspecific ulcers of the small intestine present most commonly with symptoms of intermittent small bowel obstruction but also may present with abdominal pain, perforation, or acute or chronic gastrointestinal blood loss. Symptoms may be present from a few days to many years before diagnosis. In a review of the Mayo Clinic experience with 59 cases of small intestinal ulcers over the 22 years ending in 1979, Boydstun and associates[1] identified only six cases in which enteric-coated potassium chloride supplements were probably the cause. Focal intestinal ulceration in these cases results from ischemia caused by high local concentrations of potassium. The ischemic injury caused by potassium manifests the entire spectrum of ischemic injury from merely submucosal edema to ulceration, perforation, and circumferential stenosis. These lesions are no longer observed because this formulation of potassium is no longer available. The remaining 53 patients (89.8%) had no identifiable cause of ulceration. Patients ranged in age from 17 to 77 years, with most presenting in the 5th and 6th decades of life; no gender predominance was found. The most common presenting symptom was intermittent small bowel obstruction (63%). Physical findings ranged from nonspecific abdominal tenderness and distention to an acute abdomen, resulting from intestinal perforation. Laboratory evaluation was notable only for anemia in one half the patients. Radiologic studies localized the ulcer in a minority of patients.

Pathology

In the Mayo Clinic series,[1] the ileum was the most common location of nonspecific ulceration (78%), whereas perforation (13 cases) occurred most commonly in the jejunum (78%). At surgery, 41 patients were found

Table 112–1 Causes of Small Intestinal Ulceration

Categories	Specific Causes
Infectious	Bacteria, viruses, fungi, parasites
Inflammatory	Crohn's disease, Behçet's syndrome, granulomatous enteritis, sarcoidosis
Collagen-vascular disease, vasculopathy and multisystem disease	Autoimmune enteropathy, vasculitis (e.g., polyarteritis nodosum, systemic lupus erythematosus, giant cell arteritis, Churg-Strauss syndrome, Henoch-Schönlein purpura) polymyositis-dermatomyositis, thrombotic thrombocytopenic purpura, mixed connective tissue disease, reactive arthritis, Sjögren's disease
Drugs	Aspirin, NSAIDs, antimetabolites, chemotherapeutic agents, BCG, antibiotics, slow-release potassium
Celiac sprue	Refractory celiac sprue, ulcerative enteritis
Hypersensitivity	Food allergies
Ischemia	Mesenteric ischemia, vascular abnormalities
Radiation	Therapeutic, accidental
Traumatic	Incarcerated hernia, stomal ulceration, intussusception, foreign body ingestion
Toxic	Heavy metal poisoning
Neoplastic	Primary, metastatic; angiocentric T cell lymphoma
Congenital	Duplications, stenoses
Metabolic	Uremia
Malnutrition	
Hyperacidity	Zollinger-Ellison syndrome, heterotopic gastric mucosa
Tropical sprue	
Mucosal lesions	Lymphocytic enterocolitis, eosinophilic gastroenteritis
Hypogammaglobulinemia	
Nongranulomatous chronic idiopathic enterocolitis	
Cryptogenic multifocal ulcerous stenosing enteritis	

BCG, bacille Calmette-Guérin; NSAID, nonsteroidal anti-inflammatory drug.

to have solitary ulcers, five patients had two ulcers, and six patients had more than three ulcers. Ulcer size varied between 0.3 and 5 cm. On pathologic examination, the ulcers were predominantly antimesenteric and, in some cases, associated with a fibrous scar that narrowed the lumen. Microscopy revealed nonspecific chronic inflammation that ended abruptly at the ulcer edge. The intervening bowel and vasculature were normal.[1]

Treatment

All patients were treated with segmental resection; only two had recurrent ulceration 2 and 10 years after initial diagnosis and resection. Vascular disease, central nervous system disease, infection, trauma, and hormonal influences all have been postulated as possible causes of primary nonspecific ulcerations; however, the cause or causes remain unknown. In the absence of more recent reviews, it is impossible to determine the current incidence rate of these ulcers.

SOLITARY RECTAL ULCER SYNDROME

SRUS is an uncommon disorder of evacuation that affects patients of all ages and is characterized by rectal ulceration, erythema or mass associated with straining at defecation, rectal prolapse, a feeling of incomplete evacuation, and typical histologic features. The diagnosis often is delayed due to lack of awareness of the disorder.

Pathogenesis

The pathogenesis of SRUS is uncertain, and there is a spectrum of disease with a variety of causes. A large sub-group of patients strain excessively during defecation, and some have a behavioral disorder. Occult or overt rectal prolapse with paradoxical contraction of the pelvic floor appears to be involved in most patients.[2] Evidence of inappropriate pelvic floor contraction is shown in electromyographic and video proctographic studies.[2] It has been suggested that mucosal trauma can arise from the pressure of prolapsed mucosa against a closed anal canal[3] and that straining during defecation results in prolapse and high fecal voiding pressures that reduce local blood flow causing ischemia and ulceration.[3] The mucosa of the anterior wall of the rectum, 7 to 10 cm above the anal verge, is the most common area of prolapse into the anal canal, and this corresponds to the usual location of ulceration in SRUS. SRUS has been associated with use of ergotamine suppositories and after radiation therapy, further supporting a pathogenic role for ischemia.[4,5] Moreover, the successful treatment of SRUS using biofeedback has been associated with an increase in local blood flow, additionally suggesting that SRUS may be associated with reduced rectal blood flow from impaired extrinsic autonomic cholinergic nerve activity.[6]

The association of SRUS and rectal prolapse is not entirely clear, with the incidence of associated rectal prolapse varying from 13% to 94%.[7] It is assumed that the ulcer develops as a result of local trauma to the apex of the prolapse, either because of manual attempts to reduce the prolapse digitally, or contractions of the external anal sphincter when the mucosa prolapses through the anal canal.[3] Du Boulay and colleagues[8] have shown that the histology of the rectal mucosa is similar to that seen at other sites of mucosal prolapse, suggesting that prolapse of the mucosa alone rather than the entire rectal wall is important in SRUS pathogenesis. Ischemia results in fibromuscular obliteration of the lamina propria and the formation of an ulcer. Once the ulcer is formed, it may further exacerbate the urge to defecate; this urge, along with straining and changes in local blood flow, combine to cause persistent symptoms and chronic ulceration.

Clinical Features

Patients with SRUS have a varied presentation, but most complain of constipation with a feeling of incomplete evacuation and straining at defecation with the passage of mucus and blood; there may be evidence of internal or external rectal prolapse. Men and women are equally affected, and although most patients present in young adulthood, 25% of patients are older than 60 years of age when they initially seek medical attention.[9] The mean duration of symptoms is long, ranging from 3.5 to 5 years, possibly reflecting a delay in diagnosis.

Diagnosis and Pathology

Diagnosis of SRUS is based on clinical symptoms along with endoscopic findings and typical histology. Sigmoidoscopy usually demonstrates a single 1-cm ulcer on the anterior rectal wall within 10 cm of the anal verge. The ulcer may have a polypoid appearance (Fig. 112–1), and multiple ulcers are seen in 30% of patients. In a few patients only mucosal erythema and hyperemia are seen. Differential diagnosis includes inflammatory bowel disease, malignancy, ischemic colitis, medications, and infections. Endorectal ultrasound demonstrates thickening of the wall of the rectum, particularly the muscularis propria. Defecation proctography may be used to demonstrate rectal prolapse.

Biopsies always should be taken from the ulcer margin or abnormal appearing mucosa. In 1969, Madigan and Morson[10] first described the histologic features of SRUS that include mucosal thickening with elongation and distortion of the glands, edema of the lamina propria, and fibrosis and extension of smooth muscle fibers upward between the crypts (Fig. 112–2). The misplaced and dysplastic-appearing glands in the submucosa may be misinterpreted as carcinoma and must be interpreted with caution and within the appropriate clinical context.

Treatment

Asymptomatic patients may not require any treatment and in some individuals, SRUS may resolve spontaneously. Treatment includes improving bowel habits, use of local agents, biofeedback, and surgery. The addition of fiber as a bulking agent along with habit training to reduce straining may result in symptomatic improvement in patients with mild disease. Local agents such as topical steroids and sulfasalazine are not effective. Sucralfate enemas and human fibrin sealant have been effective in small studies.[11] Argon plasma coagulation has been used to treat hemorrhage from SRUS; continued treatment with argon plasma coagulation has been associated with symptomatic and endoscopic improvements.[12]

Behavioral therapy or biofeedback is the first line of therapy for those with more severe disease and improves symptoms in more than 50% of patients; ulcer healing, however, is seen in but a few patients. This therapy aims at bowel habit training with normalization of pelvic floor coordination. Jarrett and associates demonstrated that biofeedback resulted in improved rectal blood flow, which was associated with a successful clinical outcome.[6]

Surgery is indicated in patients with severe disease who do not respond to medical or biofeedback therapy. Surgical procedures include operations for rectal prolapse, excision of the ulcer, or colostomy. Long-term results of surgery in 60 patients followed for more than 12 months were reviewed by Sitzler and colleagues.[13] Only 55% to 60% of patients had a satisfactory long-term outcome

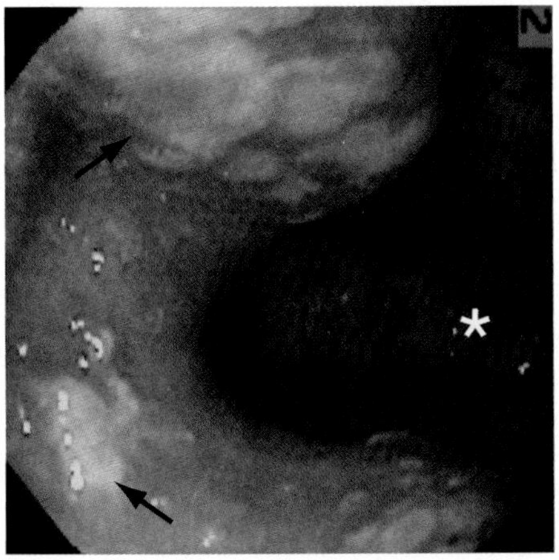

Figure 112–1 Endoscopic photograph obtained during colonoscopy in a 40-year-old patient with solitary rectal ulcer syndrome. The endoscopic findings show a large (4 × 3 cm) ulcer in the distal rectum located 3 cm above the anal verge. The ulcer margins have a polypoid appearance. The *black arrows* show exudative material within the nodularity of the ulcer; the *white star* is over the colonic lumen. Histologic findings were typical of solitary rectal ulcer syndrome.

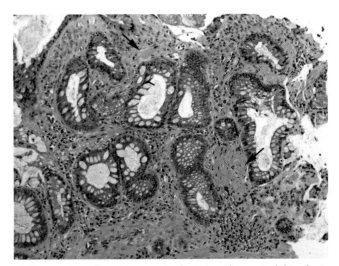

Figure 112–2 Photomicrograph depicting the typical histologic appearance of solitary rectal ulcer. This high-power view shows disorganized crypts with reactive epithelium, mild inflammation in the lamina propria, and smooth muscle fibers abnormally present in the mucosa (*arrows*). The last finding represents hyperplasia of the muscularis mucosa, a frequent histologic finding in this condition. (Courtesy of Marie E. Robert, MD, New Haven, CT.)

from antiprolapse operations; anterior resection failed in four of seven patients. Colostomy is frequently required in patients whose initial surgery fails.[13]

STERCORAL ULCERS OF THE COLON

Stercoral ulcers result from pressure necrosis of the mucosa caused by the direct effect of a hard fecal mass. The pressure of the hard fecal mass (scybalum) over time results in local ischemic necrosis and ulceration and may eventuate in perforation. These ulcers are rare and usually asymptomatic, until presentation with lower gastrointestinal bleeding or colonic perforation. Maurer and coworkers observed that 3.2% of colonic perforations in their series were caused by stercoral ulcers.[14]

Chronic constipation is the major risk factor for stercoral ulceration and, although described in patients of all ages, it is more common among elderly patients with factors that may be associated with constipation.[15] Constipation and fecal impaction are observed commonly, but complications of stercoral ulceration are relatively uncommon. Serpell and Nicholls[16] reviewed 64 cases of stercoral perforation of the colon. The median age of these patients was 60 years, and 23% of them were nursing home residents. Factors that increase constipation and formation of a scybalum, such as antacids containing aluminum hydroxide, use of narcotic analgesics, constipating sedatives, and chronic renal failure, were observed in patients who developed ulceration.[16] Why a stercoral develops is unclear, although several factors predispose the left colon to stercoral ulceration, including dehydrated and hard feces, a relatively narrow-diameter colon with high pressure, and relatively low blood supply.

Patients usually present with peritonitis and findings of an acute abdomen, due to ulcer perforation.[16] An abdominal mass is sometimes palpable. Plain films of the abdomen may demonstrate pneumoperitoneum, fecal loading, or calcified scybala. Nonperforating ulcers can present with lower gastrointestinal bleeding. Caution must be used in disimpacting patients with hard fecal masses in the rectum, because removal of the mass may result in severe hemorrhage if the underlying blood vessel in the ulcer base is torn from the tamponading stool.

The antimesenteric border of the colon is most commonly involved, usually in the sigmoid or proximal rectum. Ulcers usually are large, irregular, and sharply demarcated and may be single or multiple. The ulcers conform to the contour of the impacted scybala and result from ischemic pressure necrosis. A rounded or ovoid perforation may be seen in the center of the ulcer where colonic thinning is maximum. Necrotic colonic mucosa with acute and chronic inflammation is noted on histology.[15] Differential diagnosis includes spontaneous colonic perforation, malignancy, ischemia, and infections.

Perforated stercoral ulcers require emergency laparotomy with resection of the affected colonic segment. A Hartmann operation is the preferred procedure, and along with extensive peritoneal lavage, is associated with a lower mortality than other surgical procedures.[14,16] Nonperforating stercoral ulcers may respond to antibiotics

and aggressive treatment of constipation, although surgical resection remains the only definitive treatment.

NSAID-INDUCED ULCERATION OF THE SMALL INTESTINE

NSAIDs are among the most frequently prescribed drugs in the world, and their side effects largely involve the gastrointestinal tract. The gastric effects of NSAIDs are discussed in Chapter 49.

Clinical Features

It has been recognized that a variety of NSAIDs can cause jejunal and ileal inflammation and ulceration.[17] The spectrum of small intestinal disease caused by NSAIDs varies from occult blood and protein loss in the absence of symptoms to hypoalbuminemia, anemia, diarrhea, and weight loss. Symptoms of partial small bowel obstruction such as vomiting and colicky abdominal pain may be seen secondary to the development of diaphragm-like strictures.

In addition to these clinically apparent presentations, NSAIDs may cause more subtle changes in the small intestine known as *NSAID enteropathy*. Increased intestinal permeability, inflammation, and subtle bleeding can be demonstrated via nuclear medicine techniques in many patients on NSAIDs in whom anemia and hypoalbuminemia can develop subsequently.

Pathology

In an autopsy study, Allison and associates established that small intestinal ulcerations distal to the duodenum were prevalent in NSAID users. Of 713 patients studied, NSAIDs had been prescribed to 249 in the 6 months before death; 8.4% of the NSAID users had ulcerations of the small intestine compared with only 0.6% of the NSAID nonusers. Although no information is available regarding morbidity caused by NSAIDs during life, 3 of the NSAID users had died of small intestinal perforation.[18]

The pathologic appearance of NSAID-induced ulceration is nonspecific in that the lesions can be single or multiple and range from tiny punched-out ulcers to confluent areas of deep ulceration with stricture formation. The intervening mucosa is normal. NSAID ulcers cannot be distinguished from nonspecific or idiopathic intestinal ulcerations on the basis of gross or microscopic pathologic appearance. Ulcerations rarely are associated with diaphragm-like strictures in patients with long-standing NSAID use, and this has been referred to as *diaphragm disease*; diaphragms are thin, concentric strictures that comprise mucosa and submucosa with or without submucosal fibrosis.

Mechanism of Injury

The mechanisms of NSAID-induced injury to the small bowel are not completely understood and may involve both systemic and local effects (Fig. 112–3). Bjarnason and associates demonstrated that NSAIDs cause increased intestinal permeability in humans, as measured by loss of chromium[51]-labeled proteins into the intestine.[19] In

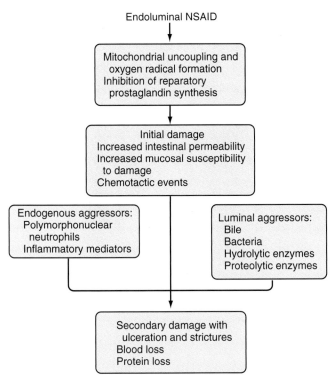

Figure 112–3 Hypothetical sequence of events involved in the pathogenesis of nonsteroidal anti-inflammatory drug (NSAID) enteropathy. (From Aabakken L: Small bowel side effects of nonsteroidal anti-inflammatory drugs. Eur J Gastroenterol Hepatol 11:383, 1999.)

another study, 33 (67%) of 49 patients taking oral NSAIDs were found to have intestinal inflammation, as measured by scintigraphic assessment of indium[111]-labeled white blood cell accumulation in the small bowel and fecal excretion of indium[111].[20] Nineteen of the 32 patients who also underwent simultaneous scanning with ^{99m}Tc-labeled red blood cells showed blood loss at sites identical to where intestinal inflammation was demonstrated. Quantitation of blood loss in eight patients was found to be comparable with that seen in colorectal cancer. Increased intestinal permeability and low-grade inflammation with blood and protein loss is referred to as *NSAID enteropathy.*

Bjarnason and coworkers[19] have suggested that the topical phase of injury to the small intestine is a cyclooxygenase (COX)-independent mechanism and is due to the ability of NSAIDs to uncouple mitochondrial oxidative phosphorylation. This uncoupling leads to a reduction of adenosine triphosphate production and leakage of calcium (Ca^{2+}) from mitochondria. Sequelae of this process include increased cytosolic Ca^{2+}, damage to mitochondria with increased production of reactive oxygen species, and disturbed sodium/potassium (Na^+/K^+) ratios with cellular osmotic imbalance, resulting in a loss of control of intercellular junctions and increased permeability. Inappropriate contact with enterocytes of luminal contents, such as bile acids, pancreatic secretions, bacteria, and food antigens, results in neutrophil chemotaxis causing nonspecific inflammation and ulceration as a systemic response to the initial injury. In addition, the concomitant COX inhibition that occurs with all COX-nonselective NSAIDs, regardless of the route of administration, may result in decreased prostaglandin synthesis and an alteration in mucosal blood flow that may potentiate ulceration (see Fig. 112–3).[21] Enterohepatic circulation of NSAIDs also may contribute to injury. Selective COX-2 inhibitors have a significantly reduced risk for gastrointestinal injury, although it is yet unclear if they are completely free of small bowel injury. Using capsule endoscopy, Goldstein and colleagues found significantly less small bowel injury in healthy subjects taking a selective COX-2 inhibitor compared with naproxen.[22]

Diagnosis

Despite the use of esophagogastroduodenoscopy, colonoscopy, and barium contrast studies, no source of blood loss is found in one half of patients with iron-deficiency anemia who are taking NSAIDs. In one reported case, intraoperative Sonde enteroscopy revealed an ulcerated and strictured area of the ileum in a transfusion-dependent patient in whom prior conventional investigations had been unrevealing.[23] Lengeling and coworkers demonstrated that routine ileocolonoscopy can identify ulcerative ileitis possibly caused by NSAID use.[24] Tibble and associates demonstrated that fecal excretion of calprotectin, a nondegraded neutrophil cytosolic protein, can be used to assess intestinal inflammation and may therefore be a practical method for diagnosing NSAID enteropathy. This method has been found to significantly correlate with fecal excretion of indium 111.[25] Capsule endoscopy[26] has increased our ability to diagnose small bowel ulceration and diaphragm disease (Fig. 112–4) but must be used cautiously in patients with suspected strictures.

Treatment

Although avoidance of NSAIDs is the most effective therapy for NSAID enteropathy, experimental studies show that metronidazole reduces inflammation and occult blood loss without changing intestinal permeability.[27] Sulfasalazine also has been shown to reduce intestinal inflammation, as measured by fecal indium-labeled neutrophil excretion,[28] suggesting that active mediators of inflammation as well as anaerobes normally found in the small intestine may play a role in the pathogenesis of NSAID injury to the small bowel. COX-2 selective inhibitors thus far have not been found to increase small bowel permeability and may be substituted in patients injured by nonselective NSAIDs. Although prostaglandin E analogs prevent NSAID-induced gastric and duodenal injury, their effect on the distal small bowel is unknown.

DIFFUSE ULCERATIONS

ULCERATIVE ENTERITIS, REFRACTORY CELIAC SPRUE, AND ENTEROPATHY-TYPE INTESTINAL T CELL LYMPHOMA

Definitions

Diffuse small intestinal ulcerations can complicate celiac sprue and can occur in patients without known celiac

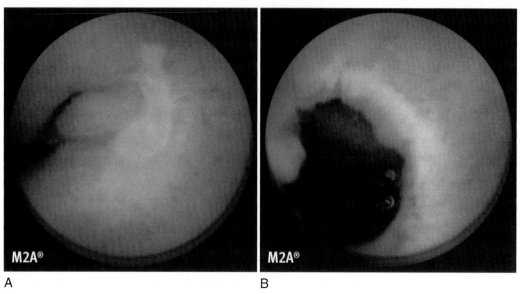

Figure 112–4   *A,* Nonsteroidal anti-inflammatory drug (NSAID) ulcer in the small intestine seen at capsule endoscopy. *B,* NSAID membranous stricture from the same patient shown in *A;* the patient was taking a nonselective cyclooxygenase inhibitor. (From Halpern M, Jacob H: Atlas of Capsule Endoscopy. Norcross, Given Imaging, 2002.)

sprue who present with sprue-like symptoms and have either flat or normal intervening intestinal mucosa but are refractory to gluten withdrawal. These syndromes have been variously termed *ulcerative jejunitis, chronic ulcerative nongranulomatous jejunoileitis,* or *idiopathic chronic ulcerative enteritis.*[29] The term *ulcerative enteritis* is used in this discussion. Refractory celiac sprue itself encompasses a heterogeneous group of patients and is discussed more fully in Chapter 101. For the purposes of this discussion, *refractory celiac sprue* refers to patients with (1) small intestinal histology or antibodies consistent with celiac sprue; (2) severe, persistent malabsorption, often with diffuse small intestinal ulcerations despite strict adherence to a gluten-free diet; and (3) no histologic evidence of lymphoma.[30-32] T cell lymphoma can complicate established celiac sprue or can manifest de novo with multiple intestinal ulcerations and malabsorption in patients without known underlying celiac sprue but with small intestinal biopsies that demonstrate villus atrophy. This syndrome, ETL, has only been recognized by the World Health Organization International Classification Project recently as a specific disorder,[33] and also is discussed in Chapter 28.

These subjects are confusing because even though the patients share clinical and histologic similarities, and ulcerative enteritis and refractory celiac sprue have a heightened risk of progressing to T cell lymphoma, these clinical syndromes are rare and, until recently, diagnoses have been based on varying criteria. Molecular and genetic evidence now support these clinical syndromes being linked by intestinal intraepithelial T cell lymphocyte abnormalities.[30,31,34,35] In addition, it appears that many of these patients have previously undiagnosed celiac sprue .[30,36,37]

Background

The association of malabsorption and lymphoma was reported first in 1937. In 1949, two patients with small

intestinal ulcerations and sprue-like symptoms were described, and the term *ulcerous jejunoileitis* was coined. Over the next 4 decades, several case reports prompted a registry to be established noting clinical and histologic similarities among patients with ulcerative enteritis, refractory celiac sprue, and intestinal T cell lymphoma. Unable to identify any connection between these clinical syndromes, the nomenclature and case reports were simply descriptive.[29,35] Beginning in the 1980s, evidence in favor of underlying celiac sprue as the predisposing factor for ulcerative enteritis, refractory celiac sprue, and ETL in many patients began emerging from registries,[29,37] genotyping studies,[36] and literature reviews.[32,38]

In addition to clinical reports, several molecular biology studies have linked celiac sprue, refractory celiac sprue, ulcerative enteritis, and ETL via intra-epithelial T cell lymphocyte abnormalities.[30,31,34,35,39] In 1985, DNA analysis was used to show that, in four patients with celiac sprue, multiple small intestinal ulcers, and lymphoma, the intraepithelial T cells were monoclonal.[40] Subsequently, polymerase chain reaction (PCR) and immunophenotypic analysis have been used to demonstrate that the intestinal intraepithelial T cells consist of a monoclonal, phenotypically aberrant population of cells in ETL, ulcerative enteritis, and refractory celiac sprue.[30,31,34,35,41] In 1995, Murray and colleagues[35] used PCR amplification in patients with ETL to show that the neoplastic T cells shared the same monoclonal T cell receptor gene rearrangements as did the T cell population in the adjacent nonlymphomatous intestinal mucosa. In 1997, Ashton-Key and coworkers[34] confirmed these findings and further demonstrated that the intraepithelial T cell population was monoclonal in the ulcers and in the nonulcerated intervening intestinal mucosa in patients with ulcerative enteritis, as well as in tumor cells from subsequent lymphoma cases. They concluded that refractory celiac sprue and ulcerative enteritis were in fact cryptic T cell lymphomas. Cellier and colleagues[31] further demonstrated that in patients with refractory celiac sprue, ulcerative enteritis, and ETL, the intraepithelial T cells were phenotypically abnormal. The abnormal T cells were medium to large sized and expressed intracytoplasmic CD3 but lacked cell surface expression of CD3-TCR complexes, CD4, and CD8; T cells in uncomplicated celiac disease tend to be CD3[+], CD4[−], and CD8[+]. Bagdi and colleagues[30] additionally demonstrated a second, less common type of tumor cell that was small, monomorphic, and expressed CD3[+], CD4[−], CD8[+], and CD56[+]. All tumor cells contained TIA-1 cytotoxic granules that along with granzyme B are believed to be at least partially responsible for the epithelial damage in these diseases. In 2002, Farstad and coinvestigators[41] identified another marker, CD30, previously identified on Epstein Barr virus-infected cells and B and T cell lymphomas, but of unknown function, on intraepithelial lymphocytes in seven patients with refractory celiac sprue, three with ETL. They suggested that the presence of CD30[+] T cells might allow the early detection of overt lymphoma even in lymphocytes remote from tumor, although an accompanying editorial cautioned on use of this marker alone as a prognostic indicator.

Zettl and coworkers, also in 2002,[42] used comparative genomic hybridization to demonstrate that ETL tumor cells had chromosomal imbalances in 87% of cases, 58% showing gains on chromosome 9q, and 16% on chromosome 1q; recurrent genetic losses occurred on chromosomes 8p, 13q, and 9p. Chromosome 8p is of particular importance because it has a gene implicated in apoptosis or cell death, and with loss of this genetic material, decreased apoptosis of intraepithelial T cell lymphocytes might contribute to the accumulation of T cells in celiac sprue and the subsequent development of ETL.[42] Taking chromosomal analysis a step further, Verkarre and associates[43] in 2003 performed the first cytogenetic study in refractory celiac sprue and demonstrated that the intraepithelial T lymphocytes in refractory celiac sprue have a partial trisomy of 1q22q44. These authors suggested that this gain on chromosome 1q, previously demonstrated to be present in 16% of cases of ETL, may be an early event on the way to malignant transformation of T cells in refractory celiac sprue.

Although the origin of the abnormal intestinal intraepithelial T cells remains controversial, elegant work by Blumberg and colleagues[44] in 1993 showed that most normal human small intestinal intraepithelial T lymphocytes were derived from an oligoclonal expansion of a limited number of α/β T-cell clones. In 2001,[45] it was demonstrated that the stimulation of intestinal epithelial cells by interferon-γ, either alone or in combination with tumor necrosis factor, markedly increased the secretion of several chemoattractants for T lymphocytes, thus indicating that epithelial cells play a role in mediating normal and inflammatory T cell responses to mucosal antigens. In another study,[46] the expansion and hyperplasia of T cells in refractory celiac sprue were shown to be regulated by interleukin (IL)-15. In 10 patients with refractory celiac sprue, IL-15 was markedly overexpressed in intestinal epithelial cells as well as in the lamina propria, inducing clonal expansion of intra-epithelial lymphocytes and initiating T cell cytotoxicity against intestinal epithelial cells. This study suggested that inhibiting this enterocyte-derived IL could be a potential treatment option for refractory celiac sprue.[46]

Clinical Features

The age of patients with ulcerative enteritis, refractory celiac sprue, and ETL ranges from 18 to 80 years, most patients presenting in their 40s or later. Women are affected slightly more commonly than are men in a ratio of 1.6:1.0. Patients with either the new onset of, or long-standing, proved celiac sprue, may present with worsening malabsorption and abdominal pain that are increasingly unresponsive to a gluten-free diet. Another group of patients presents with unexplained malabsorption and abdominal pain and have either a flat or otherwise normal-appearing small intestinal biopsy but never respond to a gluten-free diet. Malabsorption, diarrhea, and weight loss are conspicuous, often severe, and may be present for years. Alternatively, patients may present more acutely with complications, including gastrointestinal hemorrhage, perforation, or intestinal obstruction secondary to stricture formation.[29-31,34,35,46-48]

Physical examination reveals profound weight loss, cachexia and signs of severe malabsorption, steatorrhea, and protein-losing enteropathy. Abdominal tenderness may be mild, diffuse, or severe. Hepatomegaly and splenic atrophy may be present. Peripheral lymphadenopathy is unusual, but an abdominal mass may occur in patients who have developed lymphoma.[33] Dermatitis herpetiformis, a condition usually associated with celiac disease, may be observed. Signs and symptoms of anemia may occur as a result of chronic nutritional deficiency or acute gastrointestinal hemorrhage. Intestinal perforation typically leads to signs of peritonitis. When intestinal obstruction has occurred, there may be acute vomiting and abdominal distention.[29-31,34,35,46-48]

Laboratory Diagnosis

The laboratory abnormalities reflect the diarrhea, severe malabsorption, and complications of the disease. Findings include iron-deficiency or macrocytic anemia, prolongation of the prothrombin time, electrolyte abnormalities consistent with the degree of dehydration, hypoalbuminemia, hypocalcemia, hypomagnesemia, hypocholesterolemia, and low serum carotene levels. Stool abnormalities include increased volume, mild to severe steatorrhea, increased fecal α_1-antitrypsin excretion, and a positive fecal occult blood test. The D-xylose test usually is abnormal.[29-31,34,35]

Serum antigliadin, antiendomysial, and tissue transglutaminase antibodies, typically present in celiac sprue, may be present or absent in ulcerative enteritis, refractory celiac sprue, or ETL. In a literature review[49] of refractory celiac sprue, only 6 of 11 patients tested were IgA antigliadin antibody positive, and 8 of 14 patients were antiendomysial antibody positive. These results are quite different from the typical serologic pattern in uncomplicated celiac sprue, where antiendomysial antibodies are reported to have close to 100% specificity and become negative with prolonged gluten withdrawal. Although not necessary for diagnosis, HLA-DQ2 or DQ8 genes will be found in most patients with one of these clinical syndromes.[32,36]

Pathology

In ulcerative enteritis and refractory celiac sprue, ulcers are diffuse, more commonly located in the jejunum and ileum than in the duodenum, and are histologically benign. The ulcers range from 1 mm to 3.5 cm, are rarely solitary, and are well circumscribed. Some of the ulcers are superficial, extending to the muscularis mucosa, but usually they extend to the muscularis propria and occasionally through it, thus causing perforation. In most cases, the intraepithelial T lymphocytes express intracytoplasmic CD3[+] and are surface CD3[−], CD4[−], and CD8[−]; CD8[+] or coexpression of both CD8 and CD56 occur in a minority of cases. PCR analysis of the T cell receptor γ-chain gene demonstrates monoclonality of the T lymphocytes consistent with cryptic T cell lymphomas.[30,31,39]

Overt T cell lymphoma can present either as multiple ulcers or as an ulcerated mass. Tumor cells can be demonstrated in both ulcerated and nonulcerated areas of the intestine.[29-31,33-35,40]

The grossly normal intestinal mucosa adjacent to or distant from either a benign- or malignant-appearing ulcer can show either normal villus architecture or partial or total villus atrophy with crypt hyperplasia and an increased number of intraepithelial lymphocytes (Fig. 112–5). Features of inflammatory bowel disease are absent, and there is no evidence of an infectious process.[29-31,34,40]

Reports describing the histology of endoscopically normal gastric and colonic mucosa in patients with refractory celiac sprue have demonstrated widespread distribution of abnormal lymphocytes throughout the gastrointestinal tract; lymphocytic gastritis and lymphocytic and collagenous colitis have been reported.[50,51] In patients with refractory celiac sprue and concurrent lymphocytic gastritis or lymphocytic colitis, gastric and colonic T cells were monoclonal, immunophenotypically abnormal, and identical to duodenal and jejunal T cells. T cells in gastric and colonic biopsies in patients with refractory celiac sprue without lymphocytic gastritis or colitis tend to have a polyclonal gene rearrangement.[50]

Endoscopy

Because the ulcers most commonly are located distal to the duodenum, direct visualization of the jejunum and ileum is necessary and can be accomplished via capsule endoscopy or push enteroscopy or operative enteroscopy. The major advantages of capsule endoscopy are ease of use and visualization of the entire small intestine in 80% to 90% of patients during the 8-hour acquisition time.[26] High-quality capsule endoscopy images demonstrate villus atrophy and small intestinal erosions and ulcerations (Fig. 112–6). The capsule needs to be used cautiously in patients with known or suspected strictures.

The major advantage of push enteroscopy over operative enteroscopy is that procedure time is usually less than 1 hour; the chief limitation is that the depth of insertion generally is only to the mid- or distal jejunum. During push enteroscopy, biopsies should be taken both of the ulcerated areas and the grossly normal intervening small intestinal mucosa.[31,34] The major advantage of operative enteroscopy is that the endoscopist and surgeon can function in a coordinated fashion in the operating theater by identifying and immediately resecting any involved areas.

Occasional patients with ulcerative enteritis, refractory celiac sprue, and ETL also have gastric or colonic ulcers[29] that can be identified on routine endoscopy. Biopsies of normal gastric and colonic mucosa also should be obtained, because reports have demonstrated abnormal lymphocytic involvement throughout the gastrointestinal tract.[50,51]

Radiology

Radiologic abnormalities are common in these clinical syndromes. Barium contrast study of the small bowel or enteroclysis may show flat intestinal mucosa or other

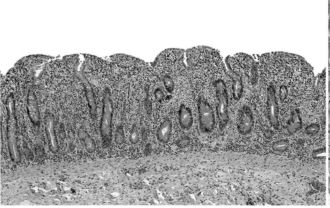

A

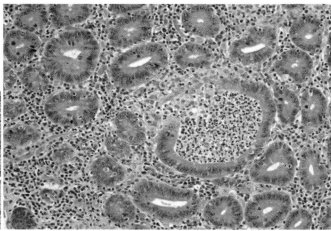

B

Figure 112–5 Full-thickness biopsy specimen of the jejunum in a patient with long-standing, severe refractory celiac sprue. *A*, Low-power view. The mucosal architecture shows complete villus flattening with crypt hyperplasia (severe mucosal lesion). There is an increase in the number of intraepithelial lymphocytes. The lamina propria is expanded by inflammatory cells that extend beneath the base of the crypts. *B*, High-power view. Polymorphonuclear neutrophils are destroying an epithelial crypt. In other areas, small ulcers were present. (*A* and *B*, Courtesy of Marie E. Robert, MD, New Haven, CT.)

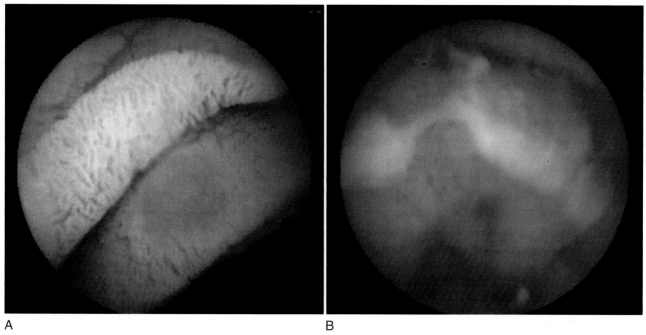

A   B

Figure 112–6   *A,* Capsule endoscopy photograph of a patient with refractory celiac sprue and multiple erosions (ulcerative enteritis) in the duodenum and jejunum. The capsule image shows villus atrophy and an erosion in the mid-jejunum. *B,* Capsule endoscopy photograph of another patient with refractory celiac sprue and ulcerative enteritis. The capsule image shows an ileal ulceration with exudate, located in the ileum. Duodenal biopsies revealed a clonal T cell population. (*A,* Courtesy of Jeffrey P. Baker, MD, Toronto; *B,* Courtesy of Moshe Rubin, MD, and Peter Green, MD, NY.)

evidence of malabsorption, such as hypersecretion or mucosal effacement. Separation and thickening of small intestinal loops, ulcerations, or a mass may be seen (Fig. 112–7). Strictures may be single or multiple and appear as areas of luminal narrowing alternating with more dilated portions of small bowel. The abnormal changes tend to be more noticeable in the proximal small intestine. Computed tomography may show nonspecific thickening and separation of small bowel loops, a small spleen, enlarged or cavitated mesenteric lymph nodes, or metastatic disease.[29,31]

Treatment and Prognosis

Although the magnitude is difficult to assess, patients with ulcerative enteritis and refractory celiac sprue have a significantly increased risk of progressing to frank lymphoma, at least 33% for patients with ulcerative enteritis as noted in one literature review.[38] In another study of 39 patients with refractory celiac sprue, 31% developed lymphoma and 44% died within a median follow-up period of 42 months.[52]

All patients initially should be treated with fluid and electrolyte replacement. Total parenteral nutrition can improve nutritional status in severely malnourished patients. If small intestinal biopsies show villus atrophy and there is no evidence of ETL, patients should be placed on a strict gluten-free diet, although it is impossible to predict which patients will respond to gluten withdrawal alone.[49] In patients with villus atrophy and ETL, adherence to a strict gluten-free diet is a logical, although unproved, recommendation, because patients with celiac

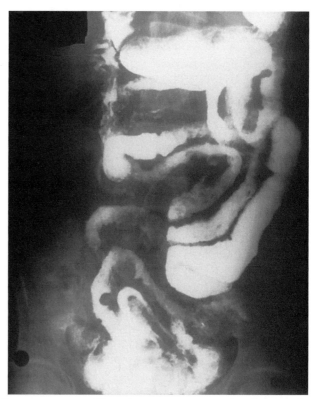

Figure 112–7   Small bowel series in a patient with refractory celiac sprue and ulcerative enteritis. There is diffuse involvement of the small intestine with multiple ulcerations and separation and thickening of the loops of jejunum and ileum. (Courtesy of Christophe Cellier, MD, PhD, Paris.)

sprue who adhere to a strict gluten-free diet may have a reduced risk of developing ETL.[53]

In patients with refractory celiac sprue or ulcerative enteritis, after gluten withdrawal fails, glucocorticoids often are tried, with varying success. Patients who do respond to glucocorticoids often remain steroid dependent.[31,34] With the knowledge that these syndromes are cryptic T cell lymphomas, open-label studies have been undertaken using immunosuppressant therapy. In patients with refractory celiac sprue, prednisone and azathioprine are more promising than cyclosporine as demonstrated in several trials (Fig. 112–8).[47,48] Exploratory laparotomy should be considered in select cases of refractory celiac sprue or ulcerative enteritis, especially if a complication such as perforation, obstruction, or hemorrhage occurs. In view of reports of widespread gastrointestinal involvement with abnormal T lymphocytes,[50,51] elective surgical resection usually is neither indicated nor possible, especially in a severely malnourished patient. However, in the rare patient with localized involvement, surgical resection of the involved bowel offers a good chance for survival.[29,34]

Patients with overt lymphoma usually are treated with a combination of surgical resection and chemotherapy. Although there have been a few reported cases of long-term survivors, most patients with ETL die within a short time of diagnosis, often from intestinal complications, sepsis, or poor nutritional status (see Chapter 28).[33]

With the recognition that refractory celiac sprue, ulcerative enteritis, and ETL all are characterized by proliferation of an aberrant monoclonal population of T cells, therapy targeted to the abnormal T cell population at an early stage no doubt will be possible in the near future.

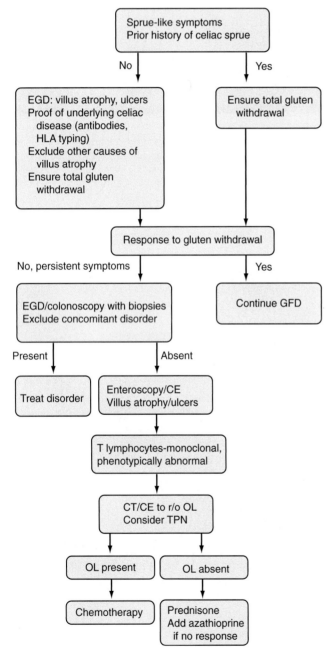

Figure 112–8 Algorithm for the diagnosis and management of ulcerative enteritis and refractory celiac sprue. CE, capsule endoscopy; CT, computed tomography; EGD, esophagogastroduodenoscopy; GFD, gluten-free diet; HLA, human leukocyte antigen; OL, overt lymphoma; r/o, rule out; TPN, total parenteral nutrition.

REFERENCES

1. Boydstun JS, Gaffey TA, Bartholomew LG: Clinicopathologic study of nonspecific ulcers of the small intestine. Dig Dis Sci 26:911, 1981.
2. Halligan S, Nicholls RJ, Bartram CI: Proctographic changes after rectopexy for solitary rectal ulcer syndrome and preoperative predictive factors for a successful outcome. Br J Surg 82:314, 1995.
3. Womack NR, Williams NS, Holmfield JH, Morrison JF: Pressure and prolapse: The cause of solitary rectal ulceration. Gut 28:1228, 1987.
4. Eckardt VF, Kanzler G, Remmele W: Anorectal ergotism: Another cause of solitary rectal ulcers. Gastroenterology 91:1123, 1986.
5. Crowe J, Stellato TA: Radiation-induced solitary rectal ulcer. Dis Colon Rectum 28:610, 1985.
6. Jarrett ME, Emmanuel AV, Vaizey CJ, Kamm MA: Behavioural therapy (biofeedback) for solitary rectal ulcer syndrome improves symptoms and mucosal blood flow. Gut 53:368, 2004.
7. Tjandra JJ, Fazio VW, Church JM, et al: Clinical conundrum of solitary rectal ulcer. Dig Colon Rectum 35:227, 1992.
8. Du Boulay CE, Fairbrother J, Isaacson PG: Mucosal prolapse syndrome: A unifying concept for solitary rectal ulcer syndrome and related disorders. J Clin Pathol 36:1264, 1983.
9. Vaizey CJ, van den Bogaerde JB, Emmanuel AV, et al: Solitary rectal ulcer syndrome. Br J Surg 85:1617, 1998.
10. Madigan MR, Morson BC: Solitary ulcer of the rectum. Gut 10:871, 1969.
11. Zargar SA, Khuroo MS, Mahajan R: Sucralfate retention enemas in solitary rectal ulcer. Dis Colon Rectum 34:455, 1991.
12. Stoppino V, Cuomo R, Tonti P, et al: Argon plasma coagulation of hemorrhagic solitary rectal ulcer syndrome. J Clin Gastroenterol 37:392, 2003.
13. Sitzler PJ, Kamm MA, Nicholls RJ, McKee RF: Long-term outcome of surgery for solitary rectal ulcer syndrome. Br J Surg 85:1246, 1998.

14. Maurer CA, Renzulli P, Mazzucchelli L, et al: Use of accurate diagnostic criteria may increase incidence of stercoral perforation of the colon. Dis Colon Rectum 43:991, 2000.

15. Gekas P, Schuster MM: Stercoral perforation of the colon: Case report and review of the literature. Gastroenterology 80:1054, 1981.

16. Serpell JW, Nicholls RJ: Stercoral perforation of the colon. Br J Surg 77:1325, 1990.

17. Bjarnason I, Hayllar J, Macherson AJ, et al: Side effects of non-steroidal anti-inflammatory drugs on the small and large intestine in humans. Gastroenterology 104:1832, 1993.

18. Allison MC, Howatson AG, Torrance CJ, et al: Gastrointestinal damage associated with the use of nonsteroidal anti-inflammatory drugs. N Engl J Med 327:749, 1992.

19. Bjarnason I, Williams P, So A, et al: Intestinal permeability and inflammation in rheumatoid arthritis: Effects of non-steroidal anti-inflammatory drugs. Lancet 2:1171, 1984.

20. Bjarnason I, Zanelli G, Prouse P, et al: Blood and protein loss via small intestinal inflammation induced by non-steroidal anti-inflammatory drugs. Lancet 2:711, 1987.

21. Somasundaram S, Hayllar H, Rafi S, et al: The biochemical basis of non-steroidal anti-inflammatory drug-induced damage to the gastrointestinal tract: A review and a hypothesis. Scand J Gastroenterol 30:289, 1995.

22. Goldstein JI, Eisen G, Lewis B, et al: Celecoxib is associated with fewer small bowel lesions than naprosyn + omeprazole in healthy subjects as determined by capsule endoscopy. Am J Gastroenterol 98(Suppl):S297, 2003.

23. Achanta KK, Petros JG, Cave DR, et al: Use of intraoperative enteroscopy to diagnose nonsteroidal anti-inflammatory drug injury to the small intestine. Gastrointest Endosc 49:544, 1999.

24. Lengeling RW, Mitros FA, Brennan JA, Schulze KS: Ulcerative ileitis encountered at ileo-colonoscopy: Likely role of nonsteroidal agents. Clin Gastroenterol Hepatol 1:160, 2003.

25. Tibble JA, Sigthorsson G, Foster R, et al: High prevalence of NSAID enteropathy as shown by a simple faecal test. Gut 45:362, 1999.

26. Pennazio M, Santucci R, Rondonotti E, et al: Outcome of patients with obscure gastrointestinal bleeding after capsule endoscopy: report of 100 consecutive cases. Gastroenterology 126:643, 2004.

27. Bjarnason I, Hayllar J, Smethurst P, et al: Metronidazole reduces intestinal inflammation and blood loss in non-steroidal anti-inflammatory drug induced enteropathy. Gut 33:1204, 1992.

28. Bjarnason I, Hopkinson N, Zanelli G, et al: Treatment of non-steroidal anti-inflammatory drug-induced enteropathy. Gut 31:777, 1990.

29. Baer AN, Bayless TM, Yardley JH: Intestinal ulceration and malabsorption syndromes. Gastroenterology 79:754, 1980.

30. Bagdi E, Diss TC, Munson P, et al: Mucosal intra-epithelial lymphocytes in enteropathy-associated T-cell lymphoma, ulcerative jejunitis, and refractory celiac disease constitute a neoplastic population. Blood 94:260, 1999.

31. Cellier C, Delabesse E, Helmer C, et al: Refractory sprue, coeliac disease, and enteropathy-associated T-cell lymphoma. Lancet 356:203, 2000.

32. Biagi F, Corazza GR: Defining gluten refractory enteropathy. Eur J Gastroenterol Hepatol 13:561, 2001.

33. Gale J, Simmonds PD, Mead GM, et al: Enteropathy-type intestinal T-cell lymphoma: Clinical features and treatment of 31 patients in a single center. J Clin Oncol 18:795, 2000.

34. Ashton-Key M, Diss TC, Pan L, et al: Molecular analysis of T-cell clonality in ulcerative jejunitis and enteropathy-associated T-cell lymphoma. Am J Pathol 151:493, 1997.

35. Murray A, Cuevas EC, Jones DB, et al: Study of the immuno-histochemistry and T-cell clonality of enteropathy-associated T cell lymphoma. Am J Pathol 146:509, 1995.

36. Howell WM, Leung ST, Jones DB, et al: HLA-DRB, -DQA, and -DQB polymorphism in celiac disease and enteropathy-associated T-cell lymphoma: Common features and additional risk factors for malignancy. Hum Immunol 43:29, 1995.

37. Swinson CM, Slavin G, Coles EC, et al: Coeliac disease and malignancy. Lancet 1:111, 1983.

38. Biagi F, Lorenzini P, Corazza GR: Literature review on the clinical relationship between ulcerative jejunoileitis, coeliac disease, and enteropathy-associated T-cell lymphoma. Scand J Gastroenterol 35:785, 2000.

39. Daum S, Weiss D, Hummel M, et al: Frequency of clonal intraepithelial T lymphocyte proliferations in enteropathy-type intestinal T cell lymphoma, coeliac disease, and refractory sprue. Gut 49:804, 2001.

40. Isaacson PG, O'Connor NTJ, Spencer J, et al: Malignant histiocytosis of the intestine: A T-cell lymphoma. Lancet 2:688, 1985.

41. Farstad IN, Johansen FE, Vlatkovic L, et al: Heterogeneity of intraepithelial lymphocytes in refractory sprue: Potential implications of CD30 expression. Gut 51:372, 2002.

42. Zettl A, Ott G, Makulik A, et al: Chromosomal gains at 9q characterize enteropathy-type T-cell lymphoma. Am J Pathol 161:1635, 2002.

43. Verkarre V, Romana SP, Cellier C, et al: Recurrent partial trisomy 1q22-q44 in clonal intraepithelial lymphocytes in refractory celiac sprue. Gastroenterology 125:40, 2003.

44. Blumberg RS, Yockey CE, Gross GC, et al: Human intestinal intraepithelial lymphocytes are derived from a limited number of T cell clones that utilize multiple Vβ T cell receptor genes. J Immunol 150:5144, 1993.

45. Shibahara T, Wilcox JN, Couse T, et al: Characterization of epithelial chemoattractants for human intraepithelial lymphocytes. Gastroenterology 120:60, 2001.

46. Mention JJ, Ahmed MB, Begue B, et al: Interleukin 15: A key to disrupted intraepithelial lymphocyte homeostasis and lymphomagenesis in celiac disease. Gastroenterology 125:730, 2003.

47. Maurino E, Niveloni S, Chernavsky A, et al: Azathioprine in refractory sprue: Results from a prospective, open-label study. Am J Gastroenterol 97:2595, 2002.

48. Goerres MS, Meijer JW, Wahab PJ, et al: Azathioprine and prednisone combination therapy in refractory coeliac disease. Aliment Pharmacol Ther 18:487, 2003.

49. Ryan BM, Kelleher D: Refractory celiac disease. Gastroenterology 119:243, 2000.

50. Verkarre V, Asnafi V, Lecomte T, et al: Refractory celiac sprue is a diffuse gastrointestinal disease. Gut 52:205, 2003.

51. Robert ME, Ament ME, Weinstein WM: The histologic spectrum and clinical outcome of refractory and unclassified sprue. Am J Surg Pathol 24:676, 2000.

52. Cellier C, Lecomte T, Afchain P, et al: Refractory celiac disease: Factors associated with overt lymphomatous transformation and survival [Abstract]. Gastroenterology 126:A246, 2004.

53. Collin P, Reunala T, Pukkala E, et al: Coeliac disease-associated disorders and survival. Gut 35:1215, 1994.

CHAPTER
113 Appendicitis

George A. Sarosi, Jr., and Richard H. Turnage

HISTORICAL NOTES

Recognition of the appendix in acute abdominal syndromes is a recent event in the history of medicine. The first anatomic mention of the appendix was made by Leonardo da Vinci in the early 15th century, but it was not until 1711 that the first clearly recognizable case report of appendicitis was recorded by the German surgeon Lorenz Heister.[1] Throughout the 18th and 19th centuries, the prevailing medical opinion was that acute abdominal pain and right lower quadrant inflammation was a consequence of inflammation of the cecum or its surrounding tissues. The modern description of the pathophysiology of appendicitis and the role of the appendix in acute abdominal syndromes dates to 1886, the year Reginald Fitz presented a paper to the Massachusetts Medical Society in which he coined the term *appendicitis* and espoused early surgical intervention as its appropriate treatment.[2] The first appendectomy for acute appendicitis actually had been performed by Lawson Tait in 1880 but was not reported until 1890.[3]

EPIDEMIOLOGY

Appendicitis is the most common acute abdominal emergency seen in developed countries. The crude incidence rate of appendicitis in the United States for all age groups is 11:10,000 individuals per year[4]; similar rates are noted in other developed countries. Inexplicably, the rates of appendicitis are as much as 10 times lower in many less developed African countries.[5] The incidence rate of the disease peaks between 15 and 19 years of life at 48.1:10,000 population per year and falls to about 5:10,000 population per year by age 45 years, after which it remains constant.[4] Men are at greater risk than women with a case ratio in most series of 1.4:1. The lifetime risk of appendicitis has been estimated at 8.6% in men and 6.7% in women.[4] Approximately 250,000 appendectomies are performed each year in the United States for a diagnosis of acute appendicitis, despite the fact that incidence rates of appendicitis have been declining over the last 50 years.[6] Between 1989 and 2000, a 15% decrease in the overall incidence of appendicitis was noted in an English study[7]; similar trends have been noted in the United States and in Canada.[4,8] The explanation for this decrease has not yet been elucidated.

ANATOMY AND EMBRYOLOGY

The vermiform appendix and the cecum are best thought of as a single anatomic unit. Developmentally part of the midgut, the appendix and cecum form between the 8th and 12th weeks of gestation as a bud arising from the midgut loop, before the ascending colon has become delineated. Congenital malformations of the appendix such as agenesis and duplication are rare. With an average length of 9 cm,[9] the origin of the appendix varies and the appendix may assume any of the positions of a clock hand with the center considered the appendiceal origin. Unlike the rest of the colon, the appendix has a complete longitudinal muscle layer. The blood supply of the appendix is found in a separate mesentery, the mesoappendix, and consists of an appendicular branch of the ileocolic branch of the superior mesenteric artery. The lymphatic drainage of the appendix occurs via the ileocolic lymph nodes and is shared with the terminal ileum and right colon.

Although the right colon is fixed in the retroperitoneum, the appendix and cecum have a more varied position within the abdomen. The position of the appendix depends on a number of factors, including the degree of cecal descent and peritoneal fixation, the configuration of the cecum, the appendiceal length, the degree of development of the pericecal fossae, associated adhesions, and the habitus of the individual.[10] Typically the location of the appendix is described as retrocecal, pelvic, subcecal, or paraileal (Fig. 113–1). The position of the appendix has important clinical implications. The classic progression of symptoms requires irritation of the parietal peritoneum by a mobile appendix; as many as 60% may have a retrocecal or pelvic position, resulting in an atypical clinical presentation of acute appendicitis.

The classic surface anatomy of the appendix was described by McBurney in the late 19th century.[11] McBurney's point is located at the junction of the lateral and middle thirds of a line drawn from the right anterior superior iliac spine to the umbilicus. Classically, this surface marking has been important in both the diagnosis and treatment of acute appendicitis; however, two studies have shown that the appendix is located within 5 cm of McBurney's point in less than 50% of the cases.[12,13] This anatomic finding helps explain why pain or tenderness located at McBurney's point is not found in all cases of appendicitis.

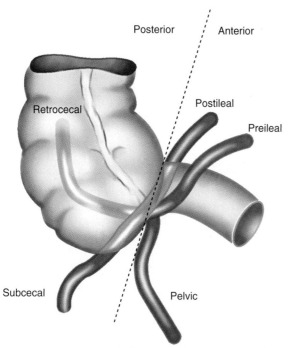

Figure 113–1 Positions of the appendix. (From Buschard K, Kjaeldgaard A: Investigation and analysis of the position, fixation, length, and embryology of the vermiform appendix. Acta Chir Scand 139:293, 1973.)

PATHOLOGY

Acute appendicitis is classified as acute, gangrenous, or perforated. The earliest gross findings of acute appendicitis are injection of the serosal blood vessels and edema of the appendiceal wall. In more advanced cases, the serosal surface appears dull and is covered by fibrinopurulent exudates. Over time, focal areas of gangrene develop marked by greenish and black discoloration of the wall; with perforation, focal necrosis of the appendiceal wall develops and adjacent abscesses form.[14]

Microscopically each of these forms of appendicitis has distinctive characteristics. In acute or suppurative appendicitis, a neutrophilic infiltrate involves the muscularis propria layer circumferentially and is accompanied by acute inflammation and ulceration of the mucosa, edema and microabscesses in the appendicular wall, and vascular thrombosis. The hallmarks of gangrenous appendicitis are transmural inflammation of the appendix with focal areas of wall necrosis. Vascular thrombosis is more prominent in gangrenous than in suppurative appendicitis. The presence of mucosal inflammation alone ("catarrhal" inflammation) is more characteristic of infectious enteritis or colitis and is not considered evidence of acute appendicitis; for the microscopic diagnosis of appendicitis to be made, inflammation must extend to the muscularis propria.[15]

PATHOGENESIS

Despite more than 100 years of study, there still is no single explanation for all cases of appendicitis. The classic hypothesis is that obstruction of the appendiceal lumen by either a fecalith or lymphoid hyperplasia produces an increase in intraluminal pressure, which in turn results in venous hypertension, ischemia of the appendiceal wall, and subsequent bacterial invasion of the appendix with necrosis and perforation. Experimental evidence in animal models exists to support this hypothesis of the etiology of acute appendicitis.[16] This hypothesis, however, does not explain all cases of appendicitis. Review of pathologic series shows that luminal obstruction is found in the minority of cases. Fecaliths are present in only 8% to 44% of cases of acute appendicitis, with most series at the lower end of the range,[14,15,17] and lymphoid hyperplasia is more common in noninflamed appendices than in acute appendicitis.[18] Other causes of luminal obstruction such as foreign bodies, tumors, and fibrous bands are uncommon. Finally, direct measurement of intraluminal pressure at appendectomy for appendicitis reveals an elevated pressure only in a few cases.[19]

An alternative hypothesis for the etiology of appendicitis is based on the concept that either bacterial or viral enteric infection leads to mucosal ulceration of the appendix and subsequent bacterial invasion from the normal colonic flora. This theory is supported by the finding that up to 75% of cases of appendicitis demonstrate well-defined superficial mucosal ulceration. Furthermore, mucosal ulceration is a more consistent finding than dilation of the appendix or fecaliths and is found earlier in the course of appendicitis.[20] Additional support for the role of infection in the etiology of appendicitis is found in two lines of epidemiologic evidence. The first is based on the hygiene theory of appendicitis advocated by Barker in the mid 1980s.[21] According to this hypothesis, changes in sanitation tied to the Industrial Revolution resulted in decreased enteric infections in infancy with subsequent decreased immunity to the same infections later in childhood and young adulthood. Acquisition of these infections later in life was believed to predispose people to appendicitis, thus explaining the rise in the incidence rates of appendicitis in the first half of the century. The decrease in the overall rate of enteric infections over the last half of the century explains the overall decline in appendicitis. The second line of epidemiologic evidence supporting the role of infection in the etiology of appendicitis is the seasonal variance in incidence rate of appendicitis and the occurrence of temporal and spatial clusters of appendicitis, both hallmarks of infectious diseases.[22] It is important to recognize, however, that no specific infectious agent has been linked with appendicitis, suggesting that infection is not the complete story.

A decrease in dietary fiber intake (the fiber hypothesis) also has been proposed as the cause of appendicitis. According to this hypothesis, decreased dietary fiber causes firm stool and an increased enteric transit time, resulting in more fecaliths and more appendicitis. This hypothesis was believed to explain both the rise in appendicitis rates in the early 20th century and the marked differences in appendicitis rates between developed Western countries and undeveloped African countries. Doubt has been cast on this hypothesis, however, for several reasons. First, despite falling dietary fiber in urban Africans, appendicitis rates have not risen markedly.[23] Second, the rates of appendicitis in the Western world have fallen without changes in dietary fiber intake. Finally, a prospective series from Africa demonstrated continued high-fiber intake even in patients with appendicitis.[24]

It is likely that any one of several different inciting events such as luminal obstruction, infection, or trauma may initiate breakdown of the appendiceal mucosa, resulting in bacterial invasion. The end result is appendicitis.

DIAGNOSIS

Diagnosis of appendicitis remains a significant clinical challenge because of the many different entities that manifest with acute abdominal pain and the relatively nonspecific initial presentation of the disease. Because the natural history of appendicitis is a time-dependent progression to perforation, there is some urgency in making a prompt and accurate diagnosis. Not all causes of acute abdominal pain, however, require surgical intervention, and a negative appendectomy carries some risks for the patient including adhesion formation, infection, and postoperative disability. Table 113–1 illustrates many

Table 113–1 Diagnoses that Mimic Appendicitis*

Diagnosis	Findings that Help Differentiate from Appendicitis
Bacterial or viral enteritis	Nausea, vomiting, and diarrhea are severe; pain usually develops after vomiting
Mesenteric adenitis	Fever is uncommon; WBC count is usually normal; duration of symptoms is longer; RLQ physical findings are less marked
Pyelonephritis	High fever and rigors are common; marked pyuria or bacteriuria; urinary symptoms; abdominal rigidity is less marked
Renal colic	Pain radiates to the right groin; significant hematuria; character of the pain is clearly colic
Acute pancreatitis	Pain and vomiting are more severe; tenderness is less well localized; serum amylase and lipase levels are elevated
Crohn's disease	History of similar attacks; diarrhea is more common; palpable mass is more common
Cholecystitis	Pain and tenderness are greater; radiation of pain is to right shoulder; nausea is more marked; liver biochemical tests are more likely to be abnormal; history of prior attacks is common
Meckel's diverticulitis	Very difficult to distinguish preoperatively from appendicitis
Cecal diverticulitis	Difficult to distinguish preoperatively; symptoms are milder and of longer duration; CT scan is helpful
Sigmoid diverticulitis	Older patient; radiation of pain is to suprapubic area, not RLQ; fever and WBC count are higher; change in bowel habits is more common
Small bowel obstruction	Prior abdominal surgery; colicky pain; vomiting and distention are more marked; RLQ localization is uncommon
Ectopic pregnancy	Positive pregnancy test; menstrual irregularity; characteristic progression of symptoms is absent; syncope
Ruptured ovarian cyst	Occurs mid-menstrual cycle; WBC count is normal; nausea and vomiting are less common; sudden onset of pain
Ovarian torsion	Vomiting is more marked; occurs at same time as pain; progression of symptoms is absent; mass often is palpable
Acute salpingitis or tubo-ovarian abscess	Longer duration of symptoms; pain begins in lower abdomen; history of STD, vaginal discharge, and marked cervical tenderness often are present

*Major clinical entities in the differential diagnosis of right lower quadrant abdominal pain and clinical features that help differentiate them from acute appendicitis.

CT, computed tomography; RLQ, right lower quadrant; STD, sexually transmitted disease; WBC, white blood cell.

of the common diagnoses that may mimic acute appendicitis. Compounding this diagnostic challenge is that there is no single symptom, finding, or laboratory test that is completely sensitive or specific for appendicitis.[25]

CLINICAL FEATURES

A detailed history and careful physical examination remain cornerstones of the diagnosis of acute appendicitis. Although no single item of the history, in isolation, will reliably enable the diagnosis, the combination of the classic symptoms and a typical progression of symptoms coupled with right lower quadrant tenderness allows good diagnostic accuracy. In the classic presentation of acute appendicitis, patients first note vague poorly localized epigastric or periumbilical discomfort, typically not severe and often attributed to "gastric upset." Patients commonly report feeling that a bowel movement should make the pain better, a sensation known as the *downward urge*.[26]

Diarrhea sometimes is seen with appendicitis, but this is not common. Within 4 to 12 hours of the onset of pain, most patients also note nausea, anorexia, vomiting, or some combination of these three symptoms. The nausea usually is mild to moderate, and most patients have only a few episodes of emesis. If vomiting is the major symptom, the diagnosis of appendicitis should be questioned. Likewise, emesis preceding the onset of pain should suggest other diagnoses.[25] Many patients report a mild fever or chills; high fevers or significant rigors are uncommon. The patient's abdominal pain typically increases in intensity, and a characteristic shift in the pain to the right lower quadrant occurs over 12 to 24 hours. The character of the pain becomes achy and more localized. Localization of the pain to the right lower quadrant is a valuable finding when present and occurs in more than 80% of patients with appendicitis.[25]

On physical examination, most patients appear slightly ill. Tachycardia is uncommon with simple appendicitis but may be seen with complicated appendicitis. Most patients with simple appendicitis have a temperature lower than 100.5°F; temperature higher than 100.5°F is most often associated with perforated or gangrenous appendicitis.[17] Patients with appendicitis, like other patients with peritonitis, tend to lie still rather than move about. Right lower quadrant tenderness and rigidity, both voluntary and involuntary, are common findings on abdominal palpation. Localized right lower quadrant tenderness is an important finding when present, but its absence does not exclude appendicitis. A variety of methods exist to elicit localized right lower quadrant peritonitis, including the "cough sign" (the presence of point tenderness with a cough), percussion tenderness, and formal elicitation of rebound tenderness. Although all of these techniques are reasonably sensitive, a small study showed rebound tenderness to be the most accurate predictor of the localized peritonitis associated with appendicitis.[27]

Additional findings that may be helpful in accurately diagnosing appendicitis include the psoas sign, the obturator sign, Rovsing's sign, and rectal tenderness. The psoas sign is sought by having a supine patient flex the right hip against resistance or by passively flexing and extending the right hip with the patient in the left lateral decubitus position. Pain with either of these maneuvers is believed to result from irritation of the underlying psoas muscle by an inflamed retroperitoneal appendix. The obturator sign is elicited by internally and externally rotating the flexed right hip. Pain is believed to arise from an inflamed pelvic appendix irritating the obturator internus muscle. Rovsing's sign is the finding of right lower quadrant pain during palpation or when left-sided rebound tenderness is elicited. All of these findings are valuable when present, but their absence does not exclude appendicitis.[25]

The typical presentation of appendicitis can be easy to diagnose but is encountered in only 50% to 60% of cases. An atypical presentation of appendicitis occurs for a variety of reasons. The classic migration of periumbilical pain to the right lower quadrant is believed to result from irritation of the parietal peritoneum in the right lower quadrant by the inflamed appendix. In cases of retrocecal or pelvic appendicitis, this irritation may not occur. Atypical presentations of appendicitis are particularly common in patients who are at the extremes of age, pregnant, or immunosuppressed, including those with acquired immunodeficiency syndrome (AIDS) and a low CD4 cell count.

Appendicitis in infants and young children remains a difficult diagnostic challenge because of difficulties in obtaining an accurate history. In young patients, the characteristic history of pain is difficult to elicit, and nonspecific findings of vomiting, lethargy, and irritability tend to predominate. Physical examination is difficult to perform because of poor patient cooperation, and localized right lower quadrant tenderness is found in less than 50% of cases.[28] In addition, the characteristic laboratory findings often are not present; for example, leukopenia is as common as leukocytosis in young infants[29]; as a result, errors in diagnosis are common, and the frequency of complicated appendicitis is as high as 40% to 70%.[30]

The diagnosis of appendicitis in elderly patients also is a challenge. The classic pattern of pain migration, right lower quadrant tenderness, fever, and leukocytosis is observed less frequently in older patients with appendicitis.[29] Older patients also tend to present to medical attention in a delayed time frame compared with younger patients. For all of these reasons, the complication and perforation rates can be as high as 63% in patients older than 50 years of age.[31]

The presentation of appendicitis during pregnancy also is associated with an atypical clinical presentation, particularly as the pregnancy progresses. In one series, only 57% of pregnant women with appendicitis had the classic progression of pain.[32] Nausea and vomiting tend to be more common in pregnant women with appendicitis but are also common findings during normal pregnancy. Fever and leukocytosis are less commonly seen in pregnant women than in other patient groups, and the value of leukocytosis is obscured by the physiologic leukocytosis of pregnancy. Although right-sided abdominal pain and tenderness are found in more than 90% of pregnant women with appendicitis, pain is located in the right lower quadrant only 75% of the time.[32]

Immunocompromised patients in general, and patients with AIDS in particular, represent a challenging group in which to diagnose appendicitis. Abdominal pain in patients with AIDS is common, with reported rates of 12% to 50%. The range of diagnoses responsible for this pain is greater than in the non-AIDS patient and includes opportunistic infections and malignancies. Although patients with AIDS and appendicitis usually present with classic symptoms, there often is a history of chronic abdominal pain. Diarrhea is a more common presenting symptom of appendicitis in human immunodeficiency virus-positive patients, and leukocytosis is relatively uncommon. Declining CD4 counts are associated with delays in presentation to medical attention and increased perforation rates.[33] Despite the challenges of diagnosing appendicitis in patients with AIDS, the surgical outcomes with appropriate treatment are quite good, with no mortalities and a 13% complication rate in the largest series, comparable with outcomes in patients without AIDS.[33]

LABORATORY STUDIES

Laboratory findings in acute appendicitis include a variety of markers of acute inflammation. An elevated total white blood cell count (WBC) in the range of 11,000 to 17,000/mm^3 is seen in approximately 80% of patients, but the specificity for acute appendicitis versus other causes of acute abdominal pain is poor.[17,34] An elevated proportion of granulocytes in the total WBC or an elevated total neutrophil count ("left shift") also is seen in the vast majority of patients with appendicitis but also is not specific for appendicitis.[34] C-reactive protein, an acute-phase reactant synthesized by the liver, is believed to rise within 12 hours of the development of an acute inflammatory process. Although elevated in 50% to 90% of cases of appendicitis, C-reactive protein levels are nonspecific when cut-off values of 5 to 25 mg/L are used.[35] A urinalysis often is obtained in patients with acute appendicitis to exclude urinary tract infections, but mild abnormalities, either pyuria or hematuria, are present in about 50% of cases of appendicitis.[36]

The value of laboratory investigations in diagnosing acute appendicitis has been a matter of some debate. In patients with a classic presentation by history and physical examination, many authors believe that there is little additional information obtained from laboratory studies. When all cases of appendicitis are considered, however, adding laboratory studies such as WBC, left shift, and C-reactive protein have been shown to improve diagnostic accuracy.[34,37] When clinical findings are compared with inflammatory markers, the markers are stronger predictors of appendicitis than are individual historical or physical findings. Direct comparison of WBC and C-reactive protein suggests that total WBC or total granulocyte count is more sensitive and accurate than C-reactive protein for detecting acute appendicitis.[35,37] The diagnostic performance of inflammatory markers is even better in identifying patients with perforated appendicitis.

All patients suspected of having acute appendicitis should have a complete blood count and in women of childbearing age, a pregnancy test should be obtained. The value of other laboratory tests such as amylase, liver tests, or urinalysis lies in helping exclude other diagnoses that may mimic acute appendicitis.

IMAGING STUDIES

Traditionally, there has been little role for routine imaging studies in patients suspected of having acute appendicitis. As is stated in the classic text *Cope's Early Diagnosis of the Acute Abdomen,* over reliance on laboratory tests and radiologic evaluations often misleads the clinician, especially if the history and physical examination are less than diligent and complete.[26] In 50% to 60% of cases, the diagnosis of appendicitis requires no imaging studies and can be made on clinical grounds alone.[38,39] When diagnosis is less certain, a variety of imaging tests has been used to help confirm or exclude the diagnosis of acute appendicitis: plain abdominal films, abdominal ultrasound, radionuclide scans, and abdominal and pelvic computed tomography (CT).

Plain abdominal radiography often is the initial imaging test for patients with acute abdominal pain. Findings on plain films of the abdomen consistent with appendicitis include a radiopaque right lower quadrant coprolith; gas in the appendix (which may be a normal finding); focal right lower quadrant ileus or a sentinel loop; loss of the right psoas shadow, a right lower quadrant soft tissue mass, and gas bubbles; the latter two findings suggest perforation and abscess formation.[10] All of these findings are suggestive but not definitive for appendicitis. In a prospective study in which plain abdominal films were ordered on all patients suspected of having appendicitis, the films changed clinical management in only 6% of cases.[40] Plain abdominal films should be used in the evaluation of acute appendicitis only when bowel obstruction or gastrointestinal perforation are thought to be likely. Their role in the routine evaluation of appendicitis should be discouraged.

Abdominal ultrasound has been used to image the acute abdomen for nearly 2 decades. Although ultrasound is considered the imaging test of choice for biliary and gynecologic diseases, its importance in the diagnosis of acute appendicitis remains controversial. The ultrasound characteristics of appendicitis are well defined. With a 5- or 7.5-MHz transducer, the technique of graded compression is used to displace the mobile loops of bowel in the right lower quadrant. The diagnosis of appendicitis can be made confidently if a 7-mm or thicker noncompressible blind-ended loop of bowel is identified (Fig. 113–2). A shadowing appendicolith, pericecal inflammation, or a localized pericecal fluid collection all are suggestive of appendicitis.[41] Appendicitis is excluded during ultrasound by visualization of a normal appendix. A normal appendix, however, is demonstrated less than 50% of the time even by experienced sonographers, thus reducing the value of a negative ultrasound study.[42] The reported sensitivity of ultrasound in the diagnosis of appendicitis in adults is 85% and its specificity is 92% in a collected review.[43] Ultrasound appears to be more sensitive and specific in children than in adults, with sensitivity and specificity greater than 90% in most series.[42]

There are some important limitations to the usefulness of ultrasound in the diagnosis of appendicitis. All ultra-

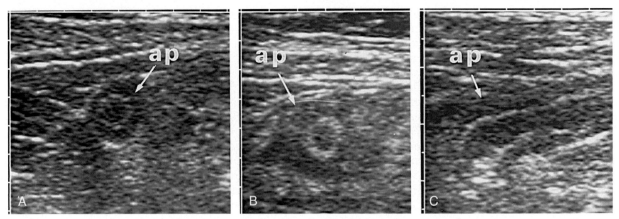

Figure 113–2   Transverse (*A* and *B*) and longitudinal (*C*) ultrasonograms of the right lower quadrant demonstrating a swollen, noncompressible appendix (ap) proved at operation to be acute appendicitis. (*A-C*, Courtesy of Roy A. Filly, MD.)

sound-based techniques are operator dependent. These excellent results cited above were achieved in dedicated trials performed by interested and experienced ultrasonographers. In one multicenter trial focused on the diagnosis of the acute abdomen, the "real world" sensitivity of ultrasound fell to 55%.[44] Ultrasound also is less sensitive in patients with a body mass index greater than 25 and those with perforated appendicitis.[41,45] Finally, ultrasound is more useful in confirming than in excluding the diagnosis of appendicitis, reducing its clinical usefulness in patients with a low pretest probability of appendicitis.

Radionuclide scanning has been advocated to help in the diagnosis of uncertain cases of appendicitis. Two major techniques are used, either HMPAO (^{99m}Tc-hexamethylpropyleneamine oxime)-labeling of the patient's leukocytes, or technetium 99-labeled antigranulocyte antibodies. In both of these techniques, an accumulation of the radionuclide in the right lower quadrant is considered positive for appendicitis. The reported sensitivity of radionuclide scanning is 91% to 94%, with specificities in the 82% to 94% range.[46,47] Limitations of these techniques remain their lack of availability in all hospitals, the relatively long time required to perform them, and operator dependence in the interpretation of the scans.

Abdominal CT scans are considered the imaging study of choice in nonclassic cases of appendicitis and with the development of rapid helical and multidetector CT scanners, CT imaging increasingly is used as the first test to evaluate patients with acute abdominal pain. CT has long been considered valuable in making the diagnosis of appendiceal abscess, and CT-based therapy of these abscesses has become common. Over the last decade, a number of authors have advocated broadening the use of CT scans to assist in the diagnosis of atypical appendicitis. A wide variety of techniques have been used for appendiceal protocol CT scans that differ in terms of the amount of the abdomen scanned, the thickness of the individual cuts, and the types of contrast used. Several conclusions have emerged from these studies: thin (5-mm) cuts are better than thick (10-mm) cuts,[48] and enteric contrast improves accuracy.

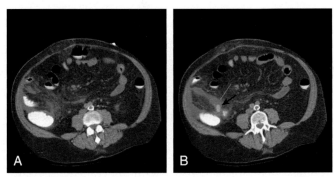

Figure 113–3   *A*, Diffuse inflammatory changes in the mesentery surrounding the distal ileum and cecum. *B*, A fecolith is shown in the appendiceal lumen (*arrow*). (*A* and *B*, Courtesy of William R. Brugge, MD, Boston, MA.)

CT findings consistent with appendicitis include an inflamed, distended (>6 mm) appendix that fails to fill with contrast or air (Fig. 113–3), often accompanied by an appendicolith or appendiceal wall thickening. Periappendiceal inflammation, cecal apical thickening, and peri-cecal fluid collections are associated findings in appendicitis.[49] Visualization of a normal appendix or the finding of alternative intra-abdominal pathology constitutes a negative study. The performance of appendiceal CT has been impressive (Table 113–2), with sensitivity rates of 92% to 100% and specificity rates of 87% to 98%. The best results occur when enteric contrast is administered both by mouth and per rectum and contrast opacification of the cecum occurs. Limitations of CT scanning for appendicitis include the time required for enteric contrast to fill the bowel, decreased sensitivity in patients with low body fat content, allergic reactions to intravenous contrast agents, exposure to ionizing radiation, and cost.

In patients in whom a diagnosis of appendicitis cannot be confidently made based on clinical history, physical examination, and laboratory findings, the best imaging study has not been clearly determined. Based on current evidence, however, it would appear that CT scanning is more sensitive and specific and less operator dependent

Table 113–2   Contrast Techniques and Reported Outcomes in Appendiceal CT Scans

Contrast Technique	Accuracy, %	Sensitivity, %	Specificity, %
No contrast[104,105]	85-97	87-99	85-99
PO and IV[48,61,106]	90-99	92-98	83-98
PO and rectal[107,108]	94-98	100	85-95
Rectal[109,110]	98	98	98

IV, intravenous; PO, oral.

in adults. In pregnant women and in very thin patients, especially in institutions with experienced ultrasonographers, abdominal ultrasound is probably an alternative first imaging study in atypical cases of appendicitis. In pediatric patients, when the diagnosis of appendicitis cannot be confidently made after evaluation by a pediatric surgeon, ultrasound should be the first imaging test selected. This recommendation is based on the increased sensitivity of ultrasound in children and the theoretical 10-fold increase in lifetime cancer risk engendered by exposure of children to ionizing radiation.[50] In patients of any age, the initial step in evaluating patients with suspected acute appendicitis should be evaluation of the patient by an experienced surgeon because this diagnostic evaluation is at least as accurate as any imaging study.[51]

CLINICAL SCORING SYSTEMS AND COMPUTER-AIDED DIAGNOSIS

Based on data that suggest that examiner experience improves diagnostic accuracy in acute appendicitis, a variety of scoring systems have been devised over the last 15 years to aid in the diagnosis of appendicitis. Most of these scoring systems assign numeric weights to findings from history, physical examination, and laboratory values in an attempt to predict the probability of appendicitis. More than 10 different scoring systems have been published, all of which purport to reduce errors in diagnosis and negative appendectomy rates. In an examination of the performance of multiple published scoring systems on a single well-defined patient data set, the ability of the scoring systems to predict appendicitis was disappointing.[52] The ability of scoring systems to perform well when applied to patient populations other than the population for which they had been developed remains a problem with these systems. Other studies have reported similar results looking at individual scores.[53,54] At this point there is no universally applicable scoring system for the diagnosis of acute appendicitis.

DIAGNOSTIC LAPAROSCOPY

An additional investigation proposed to assist in making the diagnosis in equivocal cases of acute appendicitis is diagnostic laparoscopy. Inserting a laparoscope into the abdomen allows direct visualization of the appendix without appendectomy, if the appendix is normal. The appeal of this approach is greatest in women of childbearing age in whom gynecologic causes of acute abdom-

inal pain may cloud the diagnosis and often are amenable to laparoscopic treatment. In two prospective studies of diagnostic laparoscopy for cases of possible appendicitis, gynecologic causes of pain were found in 48% to 73% of women with a normal appendix.[55,56] Because there is weak evidence to suggest appendectomy may predispose women to tubal infertility,[57] avoidance of unnecessary appendectomies is desirable in women of childbearing age. Diagnostic laparoscopy has been used in two prospective series to nearly eliminate negative appendectomies in women of childbearing age.[55,58]

Despite these promising results, some cautionary notes must be sounded. Most studies of diagnostic laparoscopy report examinations performed under general anesthesia, making this a resource intensive test when compared with imaging studies. Although diagnostic laparoscopy can be performed under local anesthesia, technical constraints reduce its success rate. For example, in gynecologic pelvic laparoscopy performed under local anesthesia, failure to obtain complete visualization of the pelvis occurred in up to 15 % of the cases.[59] This incomplete examination rate compares poorly with CT scanning. Currently, diagnostic laparoscopy cannot be recommended over appendiceal protocol CT scanning as an initial test but probably should be used as a supplement to CT or ultrasound evaluations when the results of these tests are equivocal.

DIAGNOSTIC ACCURACY

The concept of diagnostic accuracy refers to the fact that not all patients with a preoperative diagnosis of appendicitis are found to have acute appendicitis at operation. Because of the time-dependent risk of appendiceal perforation with its resultant increase in complications, there is some urgency in making the diagnosis of appendicitis. As a result, treatment decisions are often made in the presence of incomplete clinical information. An appendectomy is termed *negative* when a normal appendix is found at exploration for acute appendicitis. Traditionally an inverse relationship has been found between the frequency of negative appendectomies and the frequency of perforation at operation. Studies have shown that an increased diagnostic accuracy at operation results in an increased perforation rate.[60] This tradeoff was believed to be a consequence of the increased time required to confirm the etiology of acute abdominal pain in the absence of any specific test for appendicitis. In the interests of avoiding complications, the standard teaching has been to accept a certain negative appendectomy rate to improve patient outcomes. In most series without the use of diagnostic imaging, a negative appendectomy rate of 10% to 30% with a perforation rate of 10% to 25% was believed to represent a "good" balance[4,17,39]; in these series, the negative appendectomy rate was higher in women than in men.

In recent years, there appears to be a trend toward improved diagnostic accuracy without concomitant increases in perforation risk, through the use of imaging studies to aid in the diagnosis of appendicitis. In several series in which CT scanning has been used selectively or universally in cases of presumed appendicitis, negative appendectomy rates have been reduced to 4% to 8% without an increase in the perforation rate.[39,61-66] The improvement in diagnostic accuracy has been observed in all patient groups, but most notably in women and children. These results suggest that with diagnostic imaging, it may be possible to increase our diagnostic certainty without exposing patients to an increased risk of perforation. Whether a policy of increased use of imaging studies in the diagnosis of appendicitis will prove to be cost-effective is not yet clear, but early data suggest it may be if enough negative explorations can be avoided.[67] As a result of all of these recent diagnostic modalities, a new approach to the patient with acute abdominal pain and suspected appendicitis is emerging. A suggested management approach is outlined in Figure 113–4. The goal of this new approach using imaging techniques and laparoscopy is to eliminate in-hospital observation as a tool for improving diagnostic accuracy, because the time required to increase diagnostic certainty may increase the likelihood of complications.

A strong incentive exists for avoiding negative appendectomies beyond diagnostic pride. Complication rates between 5% and 15% have been reported with the removal of a normal appendix, most of which are infectious, including wound, pulmonary, and urinary tract infections. A 1.3% risk of small bowel obstruction is reported in the series with the longest follow-up.[68] Of patients found to have a normal appendix at operation, about 12% are found to have another surgical disease. An additional 18% to 20% have intra-abdominal findings that can explain their symptoms but are nonsurgical, the most common causes being ileitis or ileocolitis, mesenteric adenitis, or right ovarian cystic disease.[69] An additional advantage of using CT scanning in atypical appendicitis is that many of these diagnoses can be made by this technique.[39] In as many as 60% of patients with negative appendectomies, no diagnosis can be made even with a subsequent evaluation.

COMPLICATIONS

The major complication of untreated appendicitis is perforation, with resultant peritonitis, abscess, and portal pylephlebitis. Overall, the perforation rate is between 10% and 30% in most series; however, the rate of perforation varies widely with age and is most common at the

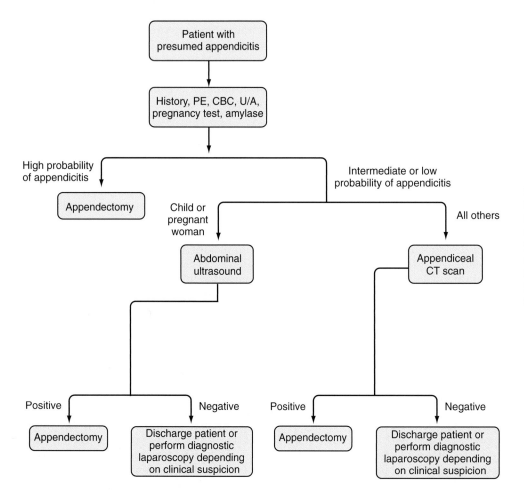

Figure 113–4   A proposed diagnostic and therapeutic algorithm for the patient with presumed appendicitis in which diagnostic imaging is used to avoid hospital admissions for observation. CBC, complete blood count; PE, physical examination; U/A, urinalysis.

extremes of age. Perforation rates as high as 90% have been reported in children younger than 2 years of age,[28] and adults older than age 70 have perforation rates of between 50% and 70%.[31,60] Persons between the ages of 10 and 30 years have the lowest perforation rates, generally between 10% and 20%. The risk of perforation appears to increase as the duration of illness increases, particularly after 24 hours. Perforation of the appendix is a consequence of delay in diagnosis, and several studies have shown that patients with perforation have symptoms that average 30 hours longer do than patients with simple appendicitis.[70] Much of this delay appears to be a result of delay in presentation to medical attention rather than delay in medical decision making, but patients with perforation often have atypical presentations of their appendicitis.[70]

Patients with perforation are more likely to have significant fever, leukocytosis, and physical findings of peritonitis than are patients with uncomplicated appendicitis. Although perforation often can be predicted preoperatively based on the presence of these findings, not all patients with these findings have perforation.[71] Free perforation into the peritoneal cavity results in findings of diffuse peritonitis and can be associated with free intraperitoneal air on abdominal plain films. Patients with generalized peritonitis from appendicitis are difficult to distinguish preoperatively from patients with other causes of diffuse peritonitis.

An abscess develops after perforation if the perforated appendix is walled off from the remainder of the peritoneal cavity because of its retroperitoneal location, or by loops of small bowel, or omentum. A localized collection of inflammatory tissue or phlegmon initially forms, and subsequently a true abscess develops. On physical examination, patients with an abscess often have a palpable right lower quadrant mass.

The most severe complication of appendiceal perforation is septic thrombophlebitis of the portal vein, also known as *portal pylephlebitis*. Although more common early in the 20th century, there are still cases of this disease today; diverticulitis is now the most common cause.[72] This rare complication should be considered in a patient with appendicitis who presents with high fever and mild jaundice. Treatment of pylephlebitis is control of the inciting infection and long-term (4- to 6-week) antibiotic therapy. The major organisms are gram-negative enteric aerobes and anaerobes. Even with aggressive therapy, the incidence of hepatic abscesses following pylephlebitis is 50%, with mortality rates of 30% to 50%.[73]

TREATMENT

Treatment of acute appendicitis is and remains appendectomy. Little has changed since Fitz and McBurney advocated early operative treatment of appendicitis in the late 19th century. Appendectomy is recommended, even though some cases of appendicitis may resolve spontaneously. At this time we have no prospective ability to identify self-limited cases, and to wait for resolution places patients at risk for perforation and the resultant life-threatening complications. Although small studies have demonstrated that most cases improve with intravenous antibiotics alone, more than 35% of the patients relapse in 1 year.[74] Appendectomy is a surgical urgency, not a true emergency. Patients with appendicitis should be given intravenous fluids to correct intravascular volume depletion and electrolyte imbalances; intravenous antibiotics to decrease wound infection rates; and taken to the operating room when they are stable. Brief periods may be taken to optimize the patient's concomitant medical conditions for operation, but long delays increase the rate of perforation and compromise patient outcomes.

Two standard operative approaches exist for performing an appendectomy, either open appendectomy or laparoscopic appendectomy. The gold standard is the open appendectomy, performed though a muscle-splitting right lower quadrant incision; either an oblique or a transverse skin incision may be used. The appendix is identified and removed even if it is found to be normal. If normal, it is removed primarily to prevent future diagnostic confusion and an exploration is carried out to identify other intra-abdominal causes of the patient's symptoms. If other surgical pathology is found at exploration, this incision may be extended or a separate incision performed to address the process at hand. In advanced cases with severe inflammation, cecectomy may be required.[75] Any abscesses present are drained and the abdomen is irrigated and closed.

The other approach to appendectomy is the laparoscopic appendectomy. First described by Semm in 1983,[76] this procedure has been the subject of considerable study since then. The technique of laparoscopic appendectomy has become standardized and typically is performed via a three-trocar technique. After gaining access to the abdomen, the appendix and then the entire abdomen are inspected. If the appendix is inflamed, an appendectomy is performed. If other intra-abdominal surgical pathology is found, it can be treated laparoscopically, or an appropriate open surgical procedure can be performed.

It remains controversial whether laparoscopic appendectomy is superior to open appendectomy. There now have been more than 20 randomized, controlled trials and 5 recent meta-analyses, including an analysis by the Cochrane collaboration, comparing the two procedures[77-81]; all of these studies have remarkably similar conclusions. Both procedures are safe and effective in the treatment of nonperforated appendicitis. After laparoscopic appendectomy, patients require less pain medication, and they return to normal activity about 1 week sooner than after open appendectomy. The wound infection rate is 50% lower than after open appendectomy, but there may be an increased rate of intra-abdominal abscesses. The hospital course after laparoscopic appendectomy is 0.7 days shorter, and patients resume a normal diet at about the same time as after open appendectomy. Laparoscopic appendectomy takes more time to perform and is associated with higher equipment costs. At this point it is not possible to say that one procedure is superior to another for all patients; however, for some patient groups, particularly those who need a rapid return to work, and those with an uncertain diagnosis, laparoscopic appendectomy is preferable.

An exception to the statement that all patients with appendicitis require urgent appendectomy is the patient with perforation and a palpable right lower quadrant mass. These patients usually have extensive periappendiceal inflammation or abscess formation. In patients with a palpable mass who do not have diffuse peritonitis or toxicity, initial management can be operative or nonoperative. Although data are limited, there is a suggestion that early operative intervention may be associated with a higher complication rate.[82,83] With initial nonoperative management, patients are placed on bowel rest, given intravenous fluids and antibiotics, and a CT scan of the abdomen is obtained. If a single abscess 3 cm or larger is discovered, percutaneous drainage of the abscess under CT guidance is performed. If multiple abscesses are found or the patient does not improve within 24 to 48 hours of conservative therapy, operative drainage of the abscess is performed. Success rates of 88% to 95% have been reported with initial nonoperative management.[82,83] Following resolution of the acute illness in older patients in whom a perforated cecal cancer is a possibility, colonoscopy or barium enema should be performed. Data from our own institution suggest that the incidence of appendiceal or cecal cancer in patients older than 60 years of age who present with acute appendicitis may exceed 20% (unpublished data). Most authors recommend interval appendectomy when the acute inflammation has resolved (6 to 12 weeks later); however, the role of interval appendectomy remains controversial because the rate of recurrent appendicitis is less than 20% at 1 year.

TREATMENT OUTCOMES

The modern treatment of simple acute appendicitis is associated with excellent outcomes. The mortality rate from acute appendicitis in one large series is 0.08% with a complication rate of 5%.[17] Older series have reported mortality rates of 0.2% with a complication rate of 6%.[4] Patients typically are hospitalized for 24 to 48 hours after open appendectomy and 24 to 36 hours after laparoscopic appendectomy. Patients usually return to full activity 2 weeks after laparoscopic appendectomy and 3 weeks after open appendectomy.[78]

Morbidity and mortality attributable to appendicitis increase markedly with complicated appendicitis and, in particular, with perforation. Mortality rates of 1% to 4% and complication rates of 12% to 25% have been reported for perforated appendicitis.[84] In patients older than 70 years of age in whom both perforation and significant medical comorbidity are common, mortality has been reported to be as high as 32%.[31] Patients with perforated appendicitis often have a stormy postoperative course, with intra-abdominal abscesses and need for reoperation.

MISCELLANEOUS TOPICS

THE APPENDIX AND ULCERATIVE COLITIS

There are now more than 20 epidemiologic studies suggesting that appendectomy may protect against the development of ulcerative colitis; a similar relationship is not seen with Crohn's disease. A recent meta-analysis of 17 case control studies suggests that the relative risk of developing ulcerative colitis after appendectomy is about 0.3 that of controls.[85] Although these data come from case control studies and questions can be raised about the appropriateness of the controls, this conclusion has been confirmed in one of the two large cohort studies performed.[86] Some researchers have suggested that appendectomy may attenuate the course of active ulcerative colitis.[87,88] In a mouse model of autoimmune colitis similar to ulcerative colitis, removal of the appendix early in life resulted in significant attenuation of colonic inflammation.[89] Although these findings are far from conclusive, they provide important insights into both ulcerative colitis and possibly the immune function of the appendix.

CROHN'S DISEASE OF THE APPENDIX

Although the appendix frequently is involved in patients with Crohn's disease of the ileum or colon, isolated Crohn's disease of the appendix is quite rare.[90] Crohn's appendicitis is difficult to distinguish from the more usual acute appendicitis preoperatively, although commonly patients with Crohn's disease of the appendix have a longer history of pain. Treatment of appendiceal Crohn's disease is appendectomy, which can be accomplished with a low rate of postoperative fistula formation.[91] The clinical course of Crohn's disease isolated to the appendix appears to be much more benign than typical Crohn's disease. Because isolated Crohn's disease of the appendix is quite rare, any patient found to have Crohn's appendicitis should undergo evaluation of the remainder of the gastrointestinal tract for evidence of Crohn's disease.

RECURRENT AND CHRONIC APPENDICITIS

Recurrent appendicitis is the clinical scenario in which a patient with pathologically confirmed acute appendicitis relates one or more prior episodes with identical symptoms that resolved without surgical intervention. This diagnosis remains somewhat controversial but has been documented in clinical series.[92] This diagnosis presupposes that some cases of appendicitis can resolve without medical intervention. Series of such cases exist in the radiologic literature where patients with imaging findings consistent with appendicitis have rapid resolution of their symptoms without treatment. The percentage of cases of appendicitis that resolve spontaneously is unknown, but estimates have been made in the range of 6% to 8%. In small series of patients with spontaneous resolution of appendicitis, the recurrence rate is approximately 40%.[93] No prospective means of identifying spontaneously resolving appendicitis have been identified; therefore, all cases of appendicitis should be treated surgically. The existence of recurrent appendicitis serves as a reminder not to discount the diagnosis of appendicitis in patients just because of prior similar abdominal pain.

Chronic appendicitis is the pathologic findings of fibrosis and chronic inflammation in the presence of a clinical syndrome consistent with appendicitis. Many of these patients report previous episodes of pain and the relief of their symptoms after appendectomy.[94] This is not a common problem, and caution should used in applying this diagnosis to patients with poorly characterized chronic abdominal pain because most of these patients are unlikely to improve with appendectomy.

DIVERTICULITIS OF THE APPENDIX

Diverticula of the appendix are uncommon, with a reported incidence in appendectomy specimens of 0.004% to 2.1%.[95,96] Two forms of diverticula exist: congenital and acquired. True congenital diverticula are quite rare, but acquired diverticula are found in 1% to 2% of appendectomy specimens.[97] Although the etiology of acquired diverticula is unclear, they are believed to be pulsion diverticula, like colonic diverticula. Appendiceal diverticula typically come to clinical attention as an incidental finding on barium enema, CT scan, or at surgical exploration.[98] Acute inflammation (diverticulitis) of appendiceal diverticula produces a clinical picture that mimics acute appendicitis, making diverticulitis of the appendix a difficult preoperative diagnosis. A few characteristics of appendiceal diverticulitis are different from those of appendicitis. Diverticulitis typically occurs in patients in the 4th decade of life rather than in the 1st or 2nd decades and tends to manifest more insidiously with many days of pain prior to presentation.[99] CT scanning can make the diagnosis readily. Appendiceal diverticulitis is more likely to perforate than is the usual case of appendicitis, making surgery rather than nonoperative management the treatment of choice to avoid the complications associated with appendiceal perforation.

EPITHELIAL MALIGNANCIES OF THE APPENDIX

Tumors of the appendix are rare and are found in approximately 1% of appendix specimens submitted for pathologic examination.[96] Most appendiceal tumors are carcinoid tumors and are discussed elsewhere (see Chapter 30). The incidence rate of epithelial malignancies of the appendix has been estimated to be 0.12:1,000,000 per annum.[100] The two types of epithelial malignancies of the appendix are mucinous adenocarcinoma or cystadenocarcinoma and colonic-type (nonmucinous) adenocarcinoma. Mucin-producing tumors are approximately twice as common as non-mucin-producing tumors.[101] Non–mucin-producing tumors of the appendix typically manifest a clinical picture indistinguishable from that of acute appendicitis, with acute right lower quadrant pain and tenderness. On CT scan, findings of a soft tissue mass or an appendix greater than 15 mm in diameter should raise the suspicion of an appendiceal cancer.[102] In contrast, fewer than one third of mucinous appendiceal adenocarcinomas present as acute appendicitis.[103] More commonly, these lesions are found incidentally on imaging studies as a cystic right lower quadrant mass or in a patient with increasing abdominal girth secondary to pseudomyxoma peritonei. The optimal treatment of all adenocarcinomas of the appendix is right hemicolectomy, either as a primary operation or as a secondary operation when adenocarcinoma of the appendix is noted on pathologic examination of an appendectomy specimen. Overall survival of adenocarcinoma of the appendix is approximately 60% at 5 years and appears to be a function of tumor stage at presentation.[101]

INCIDENTAL OR PROPHYLACTIC APPENDECTOMY

The lifetime risk of appendicitis at birth is about 1 in 12, and declines to 1 in 35 by 35 years of age. The greatest risk of appendicitis in a given year occurs over the 2nd decade of life when the risk is about 0.25% per year.[4] Although appendicitis is the most common cause of emergent abdominal surgery, given the low lifetime risk of appendicitis, elective prophylactic appendectomy cannot be recommended. Incidental appendectomy, the removal of a normal appendix at the time of other abdominal surgery was, at one time, the leading cause of appendectomy in women. In light of the falling incidence of appendicitis, the enthusiasm for incidental appendectomy has declined. In operations where it will not add morbidity, however, a case may exist for incidental appendectomy in patients younger than 30 years of age. In older patients, the low residual lifetime risk of appendicitis makes incidental appendectomy difficult to defend.

REFERENCES

1. Williams GR: Presidential address: A history of appendicitis, with anecdotes illustrating its importance. Ann Surg 197:495, 1983.
2. Golden RL, Fitz RH: Appendicitis, and the Osler connection: A discursive review. Surgery 118:504, 1995.
3. Seal A: Appendicitis: A historical review. Can J Surg 24:427, 1981.
4. Addiss DG, Shaffer N, Fowler BS, et al: The epidemiology of appendicitis and appendectomy in the United States. Am J Epidemiol 132:910, 1990.
5. Walker AR, Segal I: Appendicitis: An African perspective. J R Soc Med 88:616, 1995.
6. Series 13: Ambulatory and Inpatient Procedures in the United States, 1996. Hyattsville, Md, National Center for Health Statistics, 2004.
7. Kang JY, Hoare J, Majeed A, et al: Decline in admission rates for acute appendicitis in England. Br J Surg 90:1586, 2003.
8. Al Omran M, Mamdani M, McLeod RS: Epidemiologic features of acute appendicitis in Ontario, Canada. Can J Surg 46:263, 2003.
9. Schumpelick V, Dreuw B, Ophoff K et al: Appendix and cecum: Embryology, anatomy, and surgical applications. Surg Clin North Am 80:295, 2000.
10. Beneventano TC, Schein CJ, Jacobson HG: The roentgen aspects of some appendiceal abnormalities. AJR Am J Roentgenol 96:344, 1966.
11. McBurney C: Experience with early operative interference in cases of diseases of the vermiform appendix. N Y Med J 21:676, 1889.
12. Ramsden WH, Mannion RA, Simpkins KC, et al: Is the appendix where you think it is—and if not does it matter? Clin Radiol 47:100, 1993.

13. Karim OM, Boothroyd AE, Wyllie JH: McBurney's point—fact or fiction? Ann R Coll Surg Engl 72:304, 1990.

14. Gray GF Jr, Wackym PA: Surgical pathology of the vermiform appendix. Pathol Annu 21:111, 1986.

15. Carr NJ: The pathology of acute appendicitis. Ann Diagn Pathol 4:46, 2000.

16. Pieper R, Kager L, Tidefeldt U: Obstruction of appendix vermiformis causing acute appendicitis: An experimental study in the rabbit. Acta Chir Scand 148:63, 1982.

17. Hale DA, Molloy M, Pearl RH, et al: Appendectomy: A contemporary appraisal. Ann Surg 225:252, 1997.

18. Chang AR: An analysis of the pathology of 3003 appendices. Aust N Z J Surg 51:169, 1981.

19. Arnbjornsson E, Bengmark S: Obstruction of the appendix lumen in relation to pathogenesis of acute appendicitis. Acta Chir Scand 149:789, 1983.

20. Sisson RG, Ahlvin RC, Harlow MC: Superficial mucosal ulceration and the pathogenesis of acute appendicitis. Am J Surg 122:378, 1971.

21. Barker DJ: Rise and fall of Western diseases. Nature 338:371, 1989.

22. Andersson R, Hugander A, Thulin A, et al: Clusters of acute appendicitis: Further evidence for an infectious aetiology. Int J Epidemiol 24:829, 1995.

23. Walker AR, Segal I: Effects of transition on bowel diseases in sub-Saharan Africans. Eur J Gastroenterol Hepatol 9:207, 1997.

24. Naaeder SB, Archampong EQ: Acute appendicitis and dietary fibre intake. West Afr J Med 17:264, 1998.

25. Wagner JM, McKinney WP, Carpenter JL: Does this patient have appendicitis? JAMA 276:1589, 1996.

26. Silen W: Cope's Early Diagnosis of the Acute Abdomen. New York, Oxford University Press, 1991.

27. Golledge J, Toms AP, Franklin IJ, et al: Assessment of peritonism in appendicitis. Ann R Coll Surg Engl 78:11-14, 1996.

28. Rothrock SG, Pagane J: Acute appendicitis in children: Emergency department diagnosis and management. Ann Emerg Med 36:39, 2000.

29. Paajanen H, Mansikka A, Laato M et al: Are serum inflammatory markers age dependent in acute appendicitis? J Am Coll Surg 184:303, 1997.

30. Nance ML, Adamson WT, Hedrick HL: Appendicitis in the young child: A continuing diagnostic challenge. Pediatr Emerg Care 16:160, 2000.

31. Franz MG, Norman J, Fabri PJ: Increased morbidity of appendicitis with advancing age. Am Surg 61:40, 1995.

32. Andersen B, Nielsen TF: Appendicitis in pregnancy: Diagnosis, management, and complications. Acta Obstet Gynecol Scand 78:758, 1999.

33. Flum DR, Steinberg SD, Sarkis AY, et al: Appendicitis in patients with acquired immunodeficiency syndrome. J Am Coll Surg 184:481, 1997.

34. Andersson RE, Hugander AP, Ghazi SH, et al: Diagnostic value of disease history, clinical presentation, and inflammatory parameters of appendicitis. World J Surg 23:133, 1999.

35. Hallan S, Asberg A: The accuracy of C-reactive protein in diagnosing acute appendicitis—a meta-analysis. Scand J Clin Lab Invest 57:373, 1997.

36. Puskar D, Bedalov G, Fridrih S, et al: Urinalysis, ultrasound analysis, and renal dynamic scintigraphy in acute appendicitis. Urology 45:108, 1995.

37. Andersson RE: Meta-analysis of the clinical and laboratory diagnosis of appendicitis. Br J Surg 91:28, 2004.

38. Horton MD, Counter SF, Florence MG, et al: A prospective trial of computed tomography and ultrasonography for diagnosing appendicitis in the atypical patient. Am J Surg 179:379, 2000.

39. Rao PM, Rhea JT, Rattner DW, et al: Introduction of appendiceal CT: Impact on negative appendectomy and appendiceal perforation rates. Ann Surg 229:344, 1999.

40. Boleslawski E, Panis Y, Benoist S, et al: Plain abdominal radiography as a routine procedure for acute abdominal pain of the right lower quadrant: Prospective evaluation. World J Surg 23:262, 1999.

41. Birnbaum BA, Jeffrey RB Jr: CT and sonographic evaluation of acute right lower quadrant abdominal pain. AJR Am J Roentgenol 170:361, 1998.

42. Guillerman RP, Brody AS, Kraus SJ: Evidence-based guidelines for pediatric imaging: The example of the child with possible appendicitis. Pediatr Ann 31:629, 2002.

43. Orr RK, Porter D, Hartman D: Ultrasonography to evaluate adults for appendicitis: Decision making based on meta-analysis and probabilistic reasoning. Acad Emerg Med 2:644, 1995.

44. Franke C, Bohner H, Yang Q, et al: Ultrasonography for diagnosis of acute appendicitis: Results of a prospective multicenter trial. Acute Abdominal Pain Study Group. World J Surg 23:141, 1999.

45. Josephson T, Styrud J, Eriksson S: Ultrasonography in acute appendicitis: Body mass index as selection factor for US examination. Acta Radiol 41:486, 2000.

46. Barron B, Hanna C, Passalaqua AM, et al: Rapid diagnostic imaging of acute, nonclassic appendicitis by leukoscintigraphy with sulesomab, a technetium 99m-labeled antigranulocyte antibody Fab' fragment. LeukoScan Appendicitis Clinical Trial Group. Surgery 125:288, 1999.

47. Rypins EB, Kipper SL: ^{99m}Tc-hexamethylpropyleneamine oxime (Tc-WBC) scan for diagnosing acute appendicitis in children. Am Surg 63:878, 1997.

48. Weltman DI, Yu J, Krumenacker J Jr, et al: Diagnosis of acute appendicitis: Comparison of 5- and 10-mm CT sections in the same patient. Radiology 216:172, 2000.

49. Rao PM, Rhea JT, Novelline RA: Helical CT of appendicitis and diverticulitis. Radiol Clin North Am 37:895, 1999.

50. Hall EJ: Lessons we have learned from our children: Cancer risks from diagnostic radiology. Pediatr Radiol 32:700, 2002.

51. Kosloske AM, Love CL, Rohrer JE, et al: The diagnosis of appendicitis in children: Outcomes of a strategy based on pediatric surgical evaluation. Pediatrics 113:29, 2004.

52. Ohmann C, Yang Q, Franke C: Diagnostic scores for acute appendicitis. Abdominal Pain Study Group. Eur J Surg 161:273, 1995.

53. Macklin CP, Radcliffe GS, Merei JM, et al: A prospective evaluation of the modified Alvarado score for acute appendicitis in children. Ann R Coll Surg Engl 79:203, 1997.

54. Jahn H, Mathiesen FK, Neckelmann K, et al: Comparison of clinical judgment and diagnostic ultrasonography in the diagnosis of acute appendicitis: Experience with a score-aided diagnosis. Eur J Surg 163:433, 1997.

55. Larsson PG, Henriksson G, Olsson M, et al: Laparoscopy reduces unnecessary appendicectomies and improves diagnosis in fertile women: A randomized study. Surg Endosc 15:200, 2001.

56. Van Den Broek WT, Bijnen AB, van Eerten PV, et al: Selective use of diagnostic laparoscopy in patients with suspected appendicitis. Surg Endosc 14:938, 2000.

57. Coste J, Job-Spira N, Fernandez H, et al: Risk factors for ectopic pregnancy: A case-control study in France, with special focus on infectious factors. Am J Epidemiol 133:839, 1991.

58. Van Den Broek WT, Bijnen AB, van Eerten PV, et al: Selective use of diagnostic laparoscopy in patients with suspected appendicitis. Surg Endosc 14:938, 2000.

59. Zupi E, Marconi D, Sbracia M, et al: Is local anesthesia an affordable alternative to general anesthesia for minilaparoscopy? J Am Assoc Gynecol Laparosc 7:111, 2000.

60. Wen SW, Naylor CD: Diagnostic accuracy and short-term surgical outcomes in cases of suspected acute appendicitis. Can Med Assoc J 152:1617, 1995.
61. Schuler JG, Shortsleeve MJ, Goldenson RS, et al: Is there a role for abdominal computed tomographic scans in appendicitis? Arch Surg 133:373, 1998.
62. Applegate KE, Sivit CJ, Salvator AE, et al: Effect of cross-sectional imaging on negative appendectomy and perforation rates in children. Radiology 220:103, 2001.
63. Bendeck SE, Nino-Murcia M, Berry GJ, et al: Imaging for suspected appendicitis: Negative appendectomy and perforation rates. Radiology 225:131, 2002.
64. Brandt MM, Wahl WL: Liberal use of CT scanning helps to diagnose appendicitis in adults. Am Surg 69:727, 2003.
65. DeArmond GM, Dent DL, Myers JG, et al: Appendicitis: Selective use of abdominal CT reduces negative appendectomy rate. Surg Infect 4:213, 2003.
66. Pena BM, Taylor GA, Fishman SJ, et al: Effect of an imaging protocol on clinical outcomes among pediatric patients with appendicitis. Pediatrics 110:1088, 2002.
67. Rao PM, Rhea JT, Novelline RA, et al: Effect of computed tomography of the appendix on treatment of patients and use of hospital resources. N Engl J Med 338:141, 1998.
68. Andersson RE: Small bowel obstruction after appendicectomy. Br J Surg 88:1387, 2001.
69. Lau WY, Fan ST, Yiu TF, et al: Negative findings at appendectomy. Am J Surg 148:375, 1984.
70. Temple CL, Huchcroft SA, Temple WJ: The natural history of appendicitis in adults: A prospective study. Ann Surg 221: 278, 1995.
71. Oliak D, Yamini D, Udani VM, et al: Can perforated appendicitis be diagnosed preoperatively based on admission factors? J Gastrointest Surg 4:470, 2000.
72. Drabick JJ, Landry FJ: Suppurative pylephlebitis. South Med J 84:1396, 1991.
73. Plemmons RM, Dooley DP, Longfield RN: Septic thrombophlebitis of the portal vein (pylephlebitis): Diagnosis and management in the modern era. Clin Infect Dis 21:1114, 1995.
74. Eriksson S, Granstrom L: Randomized controlled trial of appendicectomy versus antibiotic therapy for acute appendicitis. Br J Surg 82:166, 1995.
75. Sarkar R, Bennion RS, Schmit PJ, et al: Emergent ileocecectomy for infection and inflammation. Am Surg 63:874, 1997.
76. Semm K: Endoscopic appendectomy. Endoscopy 15:59, 1983.
77. Garbutt JM, Soper NJ, Shannon WD, et al: Meta-analysis of randomized controlled trials comparing laparoscopic and open appendectomy. Surg Laparosc Endosc 9:17, 1999.
78. Hellberg A, Rudberg C, Kullman E, et al: Prospective randomized multicentre study of laparoscopic versus open appendicectomy. Br J Surg 86:48, 1999.
79. Temple LK, Litwin DE, McLeod RS: A meta-analysis of laparoscopic versus open appendectomy in patients suspected of having acute appendicitis. Can J Surg 42:377, 1999.
80. Golub R, Siddiqui F, Pohl D: Laparoscopic versus open appendectomy: A meta-analysis. J Am Coll Surg 186:545, 1998.
81. Sauerland S, Lefering R, Neugebauer EA: Laparoscopic versus open surgery for suspected appendicitis. Cochrane Database Syst Rev CD001546, 2002.
82. Brown CV, Abrishami M, Muller M, et al: Appendiceal abscess: Immediate operation or percutaneous drainage? Am Surg 69:829, 2003.
83. Oliak D, Yamini D, Udani VM, et al: Initial nonoperative management for periappendiceal abscess. Dis Colon Rectum 44:936, 2001.
84. Margenthaler JA, Longo WE, Virgo KS, et al: Risk factors for adverse outcomes after the surgical treatment of appendicitis in adults. Ann Surg 238:59, 2003.
85. Koutroubakis IE, Vlachonikolis IG, Kouroumalis EA: Role of appendicitis and appendectomy in the pathogenesis of ulcerative colitis: A critical review. Inflamm Bowel Dis 8:277, 2002.
86. Andersson RE, Olaison G, Tysk C, et al: Appendectomy and protection against ulcerative colitis. N Engl J Med 344:808, 2001.
87. Radford-Smith GL, Edwards JE, Purdie DM, et al: Protective role of appendicectomy on onset and severity of ulcerative colitis and Crohn's disease. Gut 51:808, 2002.
88. Cosnes J, Carbonnel F, Beaugerie L, et al: Effects of appendicectomy on the course of ulcerative colitis. Gut 51:803, 2002.
89. Mizoguchi A, Mizoguchi E, Chiba C, et al: Role of appendix in the development of inflammatory bowel disease in TCR-α mutant mice. J Exp Med 184:707, 1996.
90. Richards ML, Aberger FJ, Landercasper J: Granulomatous appendicitis: Crohn's disease, atypical Crohn's, or not Crohn's at all? J Am Coll Surg 185:13, 1997.
91. Prieto-Nieto I, Perez-Robledo JP, Hardisson D et al: Crohn's disease limited to the appendix. Am J Surg 182:531, 2001.
92. Barber MD, McLaren J, Rainey JB: Recurrent appendicitis. Br J Surg 84:110, 1997.
93. Cobben LP, de Van Otterloo AM, Puylaert JB: Spontaneously resolving appendicitis: Frequency and natural history in 60 patients. Radiology 215:349, 2000.
94. Mattei P, Sola JE, Yeo CJ: Chronic and recurrent appendicitis are uncommon entities often misdiagnosed. J Am Coll Surg 178:385, 1994.
95. Friedlich M, Malik N, Lecompte M, et al: Diverticulitis of the appendix. Can J Surg 47:146, 2004.
96. Collins DC: Seventy-one thousand human appendix specimens: A final report, summarizing forty years' study. Am J Proctol 14:265, 1963.
97. Phillips BJ, Perry CW: Appendiceal diverticulitis. Mayo Clin Proc 74:890, 1999.
98. Chiou YY, Pitman MB, Hahn PF, et al: Rare benign and malignant appendiceal lesions: Spectrum of computed tomography findings with pathologic correlation. J Comput Assist Tomogr 27:297, 2003.
99. Place RJ, Simmang CL, Huber PJ Jr: Appendiceal diverticulitis. South Med J 93:76, 2000.
100. McCusker ME, Cote TR, Clegg LX, et al: Primary malignant neoplasms of the appendix: A population-based study from the surveillance, epidemiology, and end-results program, 1973-1998. Cancer 94:3307, 2002.
101. Ito H, Osteen RT, Bleday R, et al: Appendiceal adenocarcinoma: Long-term outcomes after surgical therapy. Dis Colon Rectum 47:474, 2004.
102. Pickhardt PJ, Levy AD, Rohrmann CA Jr, et al: Primary neoplasms of the appendix manifesting as acute appendicitis: CT findings with pathologic comparison. Radiology 224:775, 2002.
103. Deans GT, Spence RA: Neoplastic lesions of the appendix. Br J Surg 82:299, 1995.
104. Kaiser S, Frenckner B, Jorulf HK: Suspected appendicitis in children: US and CT—a prospective randomized study. Radiology 223:633, 2002.
105. Lane MJ, Liu DM, Huynh MD, et al: Suspected acute appendicitis: Nonenhanced helical CT in 300 consecutive patients. Radiology 213:341, 1999.
106. Jacobs JE, Birnbaum BA, Macari M, et al: Acute appendicitis: Comparison of helical CT diagnosis focused technique with oral contrast material versus nonfocused technique with oral and intravenous contrast material. Radiology 220:683, 2001.
107. Funaki B, Grosskreutz SR, Funaki CN: Using unenhanced helical CT with enteric contrast material for suspected appendicitis in patients treated at a community hospital. AJR Am J Roentgenol 171:997, 1998.

108. Rao PM, Rhea JT, Novelline RA, et al: Helical CT technique for the diagnosis of appendicitis: Prospective evaluation of a focused appendix CT examination. Radiology 202:139, 1997.

109. Garcia Pena BM, Mandl KD, Kraus SJ, et al: Ultrasonography and limited computed tomography in the diagnosis and management of appendicitis in children. JAMA 282:1041, 1999.

110. Rao PM, Rhea JT, Novelline RA, et al: Helical CT combined with contrast material administered only through the colon for imaging of suspected appendicitis. AJR Am J Roentgenol 169:1275, 1997.

CHAPTER
114 Diverticular Disease of the Colon

Jeffrey M. Fox and Neil H. Stollman

The earliest description of the pathology of chronic diverticulosis traditionally has been attributed to Cruveilhier in 1849, although an earlier description by Sir Erasmus Wilson was noted in an editorial comment in *Lancet* in 1840.[1] Occasional reports of the condition appear in the literature of the 19th century. The role of surgery in the treatment of acute diverticulitis was defined by Mayo and associates in 1907. The presence of uncomplicated pseudodiverticula, herniations of the mucosa and submucosa through the muscularis of the colon, was defined as diverticulosis on radiologic studies by Case in 1914. The role of diet in the pathogenesis of diverticulosis was advanced in the landmark paper by Painter and Burkitt in 1971.[2] Our knowledge of the epidemiology and clinical behavior of diverticular disease has grown rapidly over the past few decades, in large measure due to advances in imaging technology. The incidence of this disorder is increasing in the Western world.[3-5] In 1998, diverticular disease resulted in total medical costs of $2.499 billion (direct costs: $2.358 billion; indirect costs: $141 million) and accounted for 230,058 hospital stays (with diverticular disease as the primary diagnosis only); 147,785 outpatient hospital visits; 165,343 emergency department visits; and 2,216,519 physician office visits.[6] Despite the morbidity observed in symptomatic patients, most patients (80%) with diverticulosis remain asymptomatic throughout their lifetime. This observation raises the question as to whether a largely asymptomatic disorder, present in a majority of the elderly population, is in fact a "disease." Moreover, because more elderly people have diverticulosis than do not, one can speculate if it is even

an abnormality and not just a normal phenomenon of aging. This chapter reviews the epidemiology, pathophysiology, clinical presentation, and treatment of diverticular disease of the colon.

EPIDEMIOLOGY

Because most patients are asymptomatic, the true incidence and prevalence of diverticulosis are difficult to ascertain. Autopsy series may underestimate prevalence if small diverticula are missed, whereas series using barium enema (BE) for diagnosis may overestimate the condition and lead to selection bias because the study usually is done to investigate symptoms.[7] Recent studies report overall prevalence rates for diverticulosis of 12% to 49%.[8] The incidence of diverticular disease clearly increases with age, ranging from less than 10% in those younger than 40 years of age to an estimated 50% to 66% of patients 80 years of age and older.[9] Diverticulosis appears to be just as common in men and women,[10] although men may have a higher incidence of diverticular bleeding and women may have more episodes of obstruction or stricture.[11]

Diverticulosis, with its striking geographic variation, has been termed a *disease of Western civilization*. The disorder is extraordinarily rare in rural Africa and Asia; conversely, the highest prevalence rates are seen in the United States, Europe, and Australia.[2] Within a given country, the prevalence of colonic diverticula also may vary among ethnic groups. In Singapore, the annual

Table 114–1 Factors that Influence the Risk for Diverticulosis

Risk	Risk Factor
Increased	Increasing age
	Dietary meat intake
	Living in Western countries (e.g., United States, Western Europe, Australia)
	Connective tissue diseases
Decreased	Dietary fiber intake
	Living in predominantly rural Asian or African countries (e.g., Kenya, Jordan, Thailand)
Equivocal or none	Gender
	Alcohol
	Smoking
	Colorectal cancer
	Polycystic kidney disease

incidence of diverticulitis in Chinese inhabitants was 0.14 cases per million; in European inhabitants the rate was 5.41 per million.[12] Japanese-born individuals who migrated to and lived in Hawaii have diverticulosis at autopsy 52% of the time, much more frequently than those remaining in Japan.[13] As an individual country becomes more urbanized over time, an increase in diverticulosis seems to follow, as has been shown in Singapore and Israel.[14,15] This observation may be attributable in part to a "Westernization" of diet with an increase in meat ingestion and a diminution of fiber intake as a country becomes more industrialized.[10] Aside from age, geography, and ethnicity, other inherited and acquired risk factors have been associated with the presence of diverticulosis (Table 114–1). The role of dietary fiber is detailed later in this chapter. There is no conclusive evidence that diverticular disease is associated with colorectal cancer.

Much of the sentinel data on the natural history of diverticulosis was reported by Parks in Belfast in the 1960s and 1970s,[9,16] although these data suffer from the selection bias of studying only symptomatic patients. Parks observed that patients with many diverticula were, on average, older than those with few diverticula, suggesting that the number of diverticula in an individual increases with age. In contrast, patients with total colonic involvement were, on average, younger than those with segmental disease, suggesting that the pattern of colon involvement may be determined early on and remain more or less fixed. A study of barium enemas (BEs) performed an average of 4.4 years apart in patients with diverticulosis demonstrated no apparent progression of disease in most patients.[17]

PATHOLOGIC ANATOMY

Diverticula tend to form in loosely parallel rows along the colonic lumen, mainly adjacent to the taenia coli. This tendency likely results from a relative weakness of the muscle wall at sites where the vasa recta penetrate the circular muscle to provide blood supply to the submucosa and mucosa. Weakness at these sites is believed to allow the mucosa and submucosa to herniate outward from the lumen, leading to diverticula formation. Because they do not involve the muscle layer itself but rather are hernia-

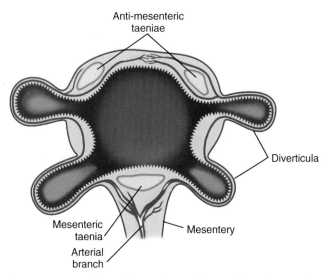

Figure 114–1 Colonic diverticula and their relationship to the taenia coli.

tions of the mucosa and submucosa through a defect in the muscularis, colonic diverticula are, strictly speaking, *pseudo*diverticula (Fig. 114–1). In this chapter, the incorrect, but traditional, terms *diverticulum* (singular) and *diverticula* (plural) are used rather than pseudodiverticulum and pseudodiverticula.

Diverticula can vary in number from one to literally hundreds. The typical size of a diverticulum is 3 to 10 mm in diameter, but they can exceed 2 cm. Giant colonic diverticula have been described, with sizes up to 25 cm. Most giant diverticula are discovered incidentally, are single, located in the sigmoid colon, and are asymptomatic, rarely manifesting with infection, obstruction, or perforation.[18]

Diverticula can occur anywhere in the colon, and the segment typically involved depends highly on geography. In Western countries, diverticula occur mainly in the left colon, with up to 90% of patients having involvement of the sigmoid colon and only 15% having right-sided involvement with or without the left colon involved.[1,9,19] In contrast, right-sided involvement is predominant in Asian countries. The ascending colon is involved in about 75% of patients in Singapore[14,20] compared with only 25% who have sigmoid disease. In Japan, the prevalence of right-sided diverticulosis found on BE doubled (from 10% to 20%) in the last 2 decades, a period over which left colon involvement remained the same (≈4%).[21] The structural morphology of the diverticula found on both sides of the colon appears to be identical worldwide. Although the precise factors causing the segmental predominance of left colon involvement in the West and right colon in the East are not known, both environmental (e.g., dietary) and genetic factors are believed to play roles. Additionally, a blending of genetic and cultural lineages could explain why many people in the United States develop pancolonic diverticulosis.

ETIOLOGY AND PATHOGENESIS

Investigations directed at elucidating the etiology of colonic diverticulosis have focused mainly in three areas: (1) altered colonic wall structure; (2) abnormal motility producing increased intraluminal pressures; and (3) the role of dietary fiber. All three mechanisms likely contribute to diverticular formation.

COLONIC WALL STRUCTURE

Early gross descriptions of colons bearing diverticula reported thickening of the muscle wall and shortening of the taenia, with a resulting accordion-like pleating of the folds. This appearance, called *myochosis*, is corroborated by the colonoscopic appearance in which markedly thickened folds are seen. Routine histology, however, does not reveal muscle hypertrophy. Electron microscopic studies confirm that the colonic walls in patients with diverticulosis have structurally normal muscle cells but contain a greater than 200% increase in elastin deposition between the muscle cells in the taenia relative to controls.[22] The elastin is laid down in a contracted form, resulting in shortening of the taenia and bunching of the circular muscle. An increase in type III collagen synthesis in patients with diverticulosis also has been described, raising the possibility that age-related changes in collagen composition play an etiologic role.[23] In addition to an overall increase in the collagen content, an overexpression of a tissue inhibitor of metalloproteinases has been identified in colons with diverticula.[24] Because matrix metalloproteinases are believed to regulate deposition of extracellular matrix proteins, an increase in their regulatory molecule (tissue inhibitor) might explain the increase in elastin and collagen deposition found in diverticular colons. The importance of gut wall connective tissue also is underscored by the higher rate of diverticulosis reported in patients with connective tissue disorders, such as Ehlers-Danlos syndrome, Marfan syndrome, and scleroderma.[5]

MOTILITY

Early investigations using manometry demonstrated higher resting, postprandial and neostigmine-stimulated luminal pressures in patients with diverticulosis compared with controls.[25,26] Based on simultaneous manometry and cineradiography, Painter proposed a theory of segmentation, postulating that contraction of the colon at haustral folds caused the colon to act not as a continuous tube, but as a series of discrete "little bladders" which led to excessively high pressures within each segment.[26,27] He further suggested that the Western diet may alter colonic motility to augment hypersegmentation, thereby increasing the tendency to form diverticula. More recently, using flexible endoscopy to accurately place manometric catheters within the sigmoid colon, the motility abnormalities previously described have been confirmed.[28] Further, patients with symptomatic diverticular disease have been reported to have higher motility indices than either asymptomatic patients or normals.[29] In addition to increased contraction amplitude, another study found retropropagation of contractile waves in diverticular segments of colon, indicating that motility in these patients may be abnormal in both magnitude and direction.[30] With respect to right colon diverticula, an Asian study has confirmed elevated resting and stimulated luminal pressures in the presence of proximal colon diverticulosis.[31] Although the demonstration of abnormal motility and elevated intraluminal pressures in the diverticular colon has been consistent, the physiologic basis for these abnormalities is less clear. An increased activity of excitatory cholinergic nerves and a decreased activity of nonadrenergic, noncholinergic inhibitory nerves, the latter in part mediated by nitric oxide, have been demonstrated in diverticular colons compared with control colons.[32] In contrast, a study of the tachykinin neurotransmitter system showed a *decreased* contractility of circular muscle induced by substance P in diverticular colons compared with normal ones.[33] An imbalance in the normal excitatory and inhibitory influences favoring excitation may result in the observed increased tonicity observed in colons with diverticulosis.

DIETARY FIBER

The wide geographic variation of diverticular disease, with higher prevalence in countries with a Westernized diet, has long suggested a dietary factor in its pathogenesis. Low intake of dietary fiber has been strongly suspected to be the main dietary factor behind these geographic differences. Burkitt and Painter were early proponents of this theory, labeling diverticulosis a "deficiency disease" that, like scurvy, should be avoidable with dietary changes.[2] In one important study, they demonstrated that United Kingdom residents who consumed a refined, low-fiber Western diet, had stool transit times more than twice as slow and stool weights significantly less than those of rural Ugandans eating a very high-fiber diet.[34] The long intestinal transit time and smaller volume stools were believed to allow an increase in intraluminal pressure, thus predisposing to diverticular herniation, whereas bulkier stools were associated with less colonic contraction and lower wall pressures. Although more recent studies in Western cohorts have failed to confirm this finding in humans consistently, corroborative animal data do exist. Wistar rats who were fed low-fiber diets developed diverticula 45% of the time, compared with only 9% of those on high-fiber diets.[35] In humans, other observational evidence exists with respect to the etiologic role of fiber in diverticulosis. In the United States, fiber intake decreased by 28% during from 1909 to 1975,[5] a period of dramatic increase in the prevalence of diverticular disease. In a British study, a group of vegetarians on a high-fiber diet had a lower prevalence of diverticulosis than did nonvegetarians (12% vs. 33%).[36] Dietary influences for diverticulosis may have different effects on the right and left sides of the colon. Right-sided diverticular disease was shown in an Asian study to have no association with fruit and vegetable intake or supplemental fiber intake but to be strongly associated with meat consumption.[37] Whether these associations apply to Westerners with right-sided diverticulosis is not known. The potential role of fiber in the treatment of diverticular disease is addressed later in this chapter.

UNCOMPLICATED DIVERTICULOSIS

Most patients with diverticulosis will remain asymptomatic throughout their lifetimes and many cases go undetected. Others have symptoms attributed to their disease but lack serious or life-threatening features; these patients with symptomatic uncomplicated diverticular disease (SUDD) are discussed later. Patients with bleeding, diverticulitis, and other associated complications such as obstruction, stricture, or fistulization are described in the section on symptomatic complicated diverticular disease.

ASYMPTOMATIC DIVERTICULOSIS

Asymptomatic diverticulosis usually is an incidental finding in patients undergoing evaluation for other indications, such as occult blood loss or colon cancer screening. With an increasing number of people undergoing endoscopic screening for colon cancer, more such asymptomatic patients are likely to be found. There is no clear indication for any therapy or follow-up in these patients. A possible *prophylactic* benefit of a high-fiber diet has been suggested in two publications of 47,888 male health professionals followed over 4 years, and in whom 385 (0.75%) new cases of symptomatic diverticular disease were identified.[38,39] A dietary review found an inverse association between dietary fiber intake and the risk of subsequently developing clinically evident diverticular disease. The study also noted that fruit and vegetable fiber, or insoluble fiber, had a greater protective effect than did cereal fiber. Conversely, diets high in fat and red meat were associated with an increased risk of diverticular disease. Although prospective randomized trials are lacking, these findings suggest that patients with asymptomatic diverticulosis may benefit from increasing their fruit and vegetable fiber intake while decreasing their fat and red meat consumption, a sensible life-style change that likely provides other salutatory health benefits as well.

SYMPTOMATIC UNCOMPLICATED DIVERTICULAR DISEASE

Clinical Features

Some patients come to clinical attention because of nonspecific abdominal complaints and are found to have diverticulosis coli. A causal relationship between the diverticulosis and the abdominal symptoms often is difficult to establish. If there are features that are consistent with a diverticular source, however, and there is no evidence of a serious inflammatory condition, patients may be defined as having SUDD. Most such patients present with left lower quadrant pain; the British refer to this condition as *painful diverticular disease*. The pain often is exacerbated by eating and diminished by defecation or the passage of flatus. Patients also may report other symptoms of colonic dysfunction, including bloating, constipation, diarrhea, or the passage of mucus per rectum. Physical examination may be normal, or reveal fullness or mild tenderness in the left lower quadrant, but frank rebound or guarding is absent. Because rates of occult bleeding in diverticulosis are similar to those in healthy controls, a positive fecal occult blood test *never* should be attributed to diverticulosis.[40] Other laboratory studies should be normal.

Because a BE can characterize the number, size, and location of diverticula, it previously had been a commonly used initial study in such patients. BE, however, may be insufficient to rule out competing diagnoses such as malignancy in patients with diverticulosis. In symptomatic patients in whom a double-contrast BE showed sigmoid diverticulosis, a subsequent colonoscopy confirmed only 55% of neoplastic lesions that were suspected on the BE, whereas eight polyps and three malignancies were identified on colonoscopy that were missed on the BE (24% false-negative rate for BE).[41] Although the BE may remain useful in certain cases, particularly if a colonoscopy cannot be performed safely or completely, endoscopic evaluation (Fig. 114–2) has assumed a

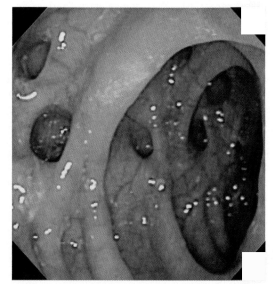

Figure 114–2 Colonoscopic view of the sigmoid colon in a patient with symptomatic uncomplicated diverticulosis.

primary role in the evaluation of most patients, particularly to exclude neoplasia. It once was believed to be unsafe to perform colonoscopy in patients with diverticulosis because of an increased risk of perforation; however, it was demonstrated that manometrically measured "burst pressures" for diverticula far exceed the usual pressures encountered during routine sigmoidoscopy or colonoscopy, even with the endoscope pressing against the wall or with heavy air insufflation.[42] These data and many years of clinical experience have demonstrated the relative safety of evaluating patients with abdominal symptoms by endoscopy. Caution should be exercised in patients with suspected or proved diverticulitis, however, because of a theoretical risk of perforating the wall of a diverticulum that has lost its integrity due to inflammation. In all patients, air insufflation should be minimized and excessive force in advancing the endoscope should be avoided.

The diverticula-laden colon can be challenging for the endoscopist to navigate because of spasm, luminal narrowing, fixation from prior inflammation and fibrosis, or confusion between luminal and diverticular openings. A number of solutions have been proposed to alleviate this problem. The use of a smaller diameter "pediatric" colonoscope can be useful for difficult colons. One group has reported a success rate of more than 90% with a pediatric colonoscope in cases in which an adult colonoscope could not be passed through the sigmoid, 44% of which had diverticulosis.[43] When colonoscopy with standard and pediatric colonoscopes were compared head-to-head, the reason for failure to complete the examination was thought to be stenosing diverticular disease in 12 of 14 patients with the standard colonoscope, compared with 2 of 8 with the pediatric colonoscope.[44] A technique involving distention of the lumen with 100 to 300 mL of water, coined the "sigmoid floatation maneuver," was said to have facilitated colonoscopy in six technically difficult cases of severe diverticular disease.[45]

Occasionally, an endoscopist encounters an inverted diverticulum, where a diverticular dome protrudes into the lumen instead of out of it. These inversions often resemble polyps endoscopically, although they may be distinguished by their normal overlying mucosa, broad base, and location within a bed or row of diverticula. They are soft appearing when manipulated with the endoscope tip or a biopsy forceps ("pillow sign") and may be reducible. On BE, inverted diverticula appear as broad-based sessile polyps with a characteristic central umbilication.[46] Although it is not always possible to distinguish such a diverticulum from a polyp, when inverted diverticula are encountered, removal should be avoided. Inadvertent colonoscopic diverticulectomy has been reported;[47] interestingly, these patients had uneventful recoveries with conservative therapy.

The presenting symptoms of SUDD overlap considerably with those of irritable bowel syndrome (IBS). Some authorities have postulated that diverticula are, in fact, a late consequence of IBS. In a Danish cohort of IBS patients, one third of whom had diverticula, no difference in symptoms or prognosis was detected between those with diverticula and those without diverticula over more than 5 years of follow-up.[48] This finding led the investigators to conclude that there is no basis to consider SUDD as a separate entity from IBS. Ritchie reported that there was a similarity of pain sensation from rectal balloon distention in patients with IBS and those with diverticulosis.[49] Whether these two disorders are distinct entities is unknown and probably not clinically important, because both are treated in a similar fashion with equally good prognoses.

Treatment

Aside from the reported preventive effect of dietary fiber described earlier, fiber also is a mainstay of treatment for SUDD. Many uncontrolled trials of fiber in SUDD have been reported, all limited by a high placebo response rate. A randomized, double-blind trial from Oxford University showed a statistically significant decrease in bowel symptoms relative to controls in patients with SUDD who were placed on a high-fiber diet[50]; the separation between treatment and control groups, however, was not noted until the 3 month follow-up evaluation. It is important to instruct patients to start fiber supplementation at a low dose and slowly increase the dose, because patients initially can worsen from diarrhea, gas, or bloating if the fiber dose is started too high or quickly. Because it often can take months to improve, as demonstrated in the above study, the initial adverse symptoms can discourage patients from adhering to the fiber supplements if they are not counseled properly. In contrast, another study of fiber supplementation in patients with diverticular disease showed no significant improvement in overall symptoms, although decreased transit time and increased stool frequency were documented.[51] Despite these conflicting data and the certainty that diverticula do not regress with an increased fiber intake, some amelioration of symptoms in patients with SUDD often can be seen with a high-fiber diet.

The hypermotility of the colon in diverticulosis suggests that anticholinergic or antispasmodic medications such as dicyclomine or hyoscyamine might improve symptoms by diminishing muscular contraction. Nonetheless, there are no adequately controlled therapeutic trials documenting such a benefit. Intravenous glucagon has been reported to offer short-term relief of pain, presumably as a result of smooth muscle relaxation.[51] There is no rationale for the use of antibiotics or narcotic analgesics in uncomplicated diverticular disease.

Surgical intervention generally is not considered for patients with truly uncomplicated diverticulosis, because the risks of surgery outweigh the benefits in most cases. Some patients with subclinical or "smoldering" diverticulitis may present with pain in a characteristic pattern for diverticulitis, however, but show no signs of systemic inflammation, such as fever or leukocytosis. In a cohort of such patients from the Mayo Clinic who underwent sigmoid resection with primary anastomosis for their symptoms without signs or laboratory markers of systemic inflammation, 76% of the resected specimens had evidence of acute or chronic diverticular inflammation.[52] This finding underscores the importance of clinical follow-up and an open mind regarding those patients with apparently uncomplicated disease whose symptoms do not improve with conservative treatment.

COMPLICATED DIVERTICULOSIS

Diverticulitis, defined as inflammation, infection, or both associated with diverticula, is probably the most common clinical manifestation of this disorder, affecting an estimated 10% to 25% of patients with diverticula.[9] It generally is believed to be the result of perforation of a single diverticulum.[53] When this results in a localized phlegmon, the term *uncomplicated diverticulitis* is used. *Complicated diverticulitis* refers to cases associated with abscess, free perforation with peritonitis, fistula, or obstruction.[54] Besides diverticulitis, the other major form of complicated diverticular disease is bleeding, which is discussed later in this chapter.

UNCOMPLICATED DIVERTICULITIS

Pathophysiology

The process by which a diverticulum becomes inflamed has been likened to that causing appendicitis, in which the sac becomes obstructed by inspissated stool in its neck. The fecolith abrades the mucosa of the sac, causing low-grade inflammation and further blocking drainage. Histologically, one of the earliest signs of inflammation is hyperplasia of the mucosal lymphoid tissue and lymphoid tissue aggregation at the apex of the involved sac.[55] The obstructed diverticulum predisposes to expansion of the normal bacterial flora, diminished venous outflow with localized ischemia, and altered mucosal defense mechanisms. One such alteration is a defective CD2 pathway-induced apoptosis, which has been found in lamina propria lymphocytes in patients with diverticulitis, possibly leading to an up-regulation of the local immune response in these patients similar to that seen in patients with Crohn's disease and ulcerative colitis.[56] The cascade of events initiated by obstruction allows bacteria to breach the mucosa and extend the process through the full wall thickness, ultimately leading to perforation.[57] The extent and localization of the perforation determine its clinical behavior. Microperforations may remain very well localized, contained by the pericolic fat and mesentery, and cause small pericolic abscesses. A larger perforation can allow a more extensive abscess to form, which may track longitudinally around the bowel wall. This process can lead to a large inflammatory mass, fibrosis, extension to other organs, or fistulas. Free perforation into the peritoneum causing frank bacterial or fecal peritonitis can be life-threatening but fortunately is uncommon, with a population incidence of 4 cases per 100,000 population per year.[3,58] Hinchey and associates have described a staged grading system reflecting the severity of perforation (Table 114–2).[59]

Clinical Features

Patients with acute diverticulitis typically present with left lower quadrant abdominal pain, reflecting the propensity for this disorder to occur in the sigmoid colon in Western countries; a redundant sigmoid colon, however, may manifest with suprapubic or right-sided pain. In contrast, Asian patients with diverticulitis have predominantly right-sided symptoms, corresponding to the location of their diverticula.[60] The pain may be intermittent or constant and frequently is associated with a change in bowel habits, either diarrhea or constipation.[61] Anorexia, nausea, and vomiting also may occur. Dysuria and urinary frequency can result from bladder irritation by the adjacent inflamed sigmoid colon.

Physical examination usually discloses localized tenderness, generally in the left lower quadrant; however, as noted, right-sided signs do not preclude the possibility of diverticulitis. Guarding and rebound tenderness may be present, as may a tender, cylindrical, palpable mass. Bowel sounds typically are depressed but may be normal in mild cases or increased in the presence of obstruction. Rectal examination may disclose tenderness or a mass, particularly with a low-lying pelvic abscess. Fever is present in most patients, whereas hypotension and shock are unusual. The white blood cell (WBC) count frequently is elevated, although one study reported a normal WBC count with no left shift in 46% of patients.[61] No other laboratory abnormalities are routinely helpful, although other laboratory tests can help to rule out other diagnostic possibilities in select patients.

The differential diagnosis for diverticulitis is extensive. Acute appendicitis is the misdiagnosis most frequently made in patients with diverticulitis, particularly with right-sided disease. In Hong Kong, where awareness of right-predominant diverticulosis presumably is high, 34 of 35 patients with right-sided diverticulitis initially were believed to have acute appendicitis.[60] Although appendicitis is, on average, a disease of younger patients than is acute diverticulitis, there is a wide range of ages for both. Clinical suspicion for one must remain high when diagnosing the other on clinical grounds. Other common diagnoses that need to be excluded include inflammatory bowel disease; other forms of colitis (infectious or ischemic); colorectal cancer; peptic ulcer disease; and gynecologic conditions such as pelvic inflammatory disease, ovarian cyst rupture, and ovarian torsion. Occasionally, diverticulitis can occur concomitantly with other diseases; in one study of patients admitted to the

Table 114–2 Hinchey Classification of Colonic Diverticular Perforation

Stage	Definition
I	Confined pericolic abscess
II	Distant abscess (retroperitoneal or pelvic)
III	Generalized peritonitis due to rupture of a pericolic or pelvic abscess (noncommunicating with the colonic lumen because of obliteration of the diverticular neck by inflammation)
IV	Fecal peritonitis due to free perforation of a diverticulum (communicating with the colonic lumen)

hospital with diverticulitis, 7% were later found also to have a colon malignancy.[62]

Diagnosis

Most patients with acute diverticulitis present with signs and symptoms sufficient to justify the clinical diagnosis and institution of empiric therapy. Clinical diagnosis can, however, occasionally be inaccurate, and emergency surgery for presumed diverticulitis, without the benefit of radiologic confirmation, carries a misdiagnosis rate as high as 34% to 67%.[63] Therefore, radiologic studies to confirm the diagnosis of diverticulitis should be employed, particularly if invasive intervention may be required.

Plain Films

An erect chest film, together with erect and supine abdominal films, should be performed on patients with significant abdominal pain. The erect chest film has the dual purpose of detecting pneumoperitoneum, which has been reported to be present in up to 11% of patients with acute diverticulitis[64] and to assess cardiopulmonary status in a generally elderly population with frequent comorbid illness. Abdominal films are abnormal in 30% to 50% of patients with acute diverticulitis,[64,65] with findings that include bowel dilation from obstruction or ileus, or a soft tissue density suggesting an abscess.

Contrast Enema Examinations

As mentioned, contrast BE (Fig. 114–3) had been the diagnostic standard for diverticulitis and its complications for many years. Because the use of barium in the setting of an intestinal perforation carries a risk of barium peritonitis, only water-soluble contrast enemas (e.g., Gastrografin) should be used in the setting of acute diverticulitis. A gentle, single-contrast study should be performed and terminated once significant findings of diverticulitis have been discovered, with visualization of the entire colon deferred to a later date; air (double)-contrast studies are not indicated. Findings considered *diagnostic* of diverticulitis include demonstration of extravasated contrast material outlining an abscess cavity, an intramural sinus tract, or a fistula.[1,66] Extensive diverticulosis, spasm, mucosal thickening or spiking, or deformed sacs, although suggestive of diverticulitis, are not conclusive. An extraluminal mass compressing bowel is said to be the most common finding in severe diverticulitis,[67] although this finding is not specific for this diagnosis. Obviously, in the *absence* of diverticula or associated findings, the diagnosis must be reconsidered. Contrast enema has been shown to have a sensitivity of 62% to 94% for detecting acute diverticulitis, with false-negative results in 2% to 15%.[54,68]

Computed Tomography

Because diverticulitis is mainly an extraluminal disease, luminal contrast studies may be inaccurate. Computed tomography (CT) (Fig. 114–4) has now replaced contrast enema as the diagnostic procedure of choice for acute diverticulitis. CT has the ability both to image mural and extraluminal disease and to enable therapy with percutaneous drainage of abscesses. Abdominal and pelvic scanning ideally is performed with water-soluble contrast, given both orally and rectally, and with intravenous contrast, when not contraindicated. CT criteria for diverticulitis include the presence of diverticula with pericolic infiltration of fatty tissue (often appearing as fat "stranding"), colonic wall thickening, and abscess formation. The earliest large series of CT findings in diverticulitis reported the finding of pericolic fat inflammation in 98%, diverticula in 84%, a colonic wall thickness greater than 4 mm in 70%, and an abscess in 35%.[69] Contrast enemas in the same patients underestimated the extent of disease in 15 (41%) of 37 cases. Numerous subsequent trials comparing these two modalities in patients with suspected

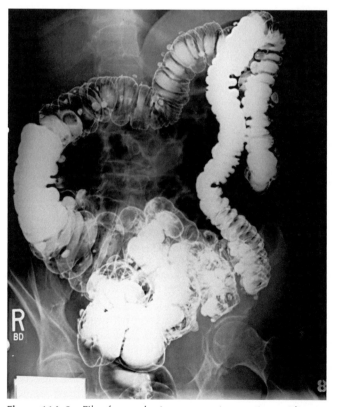

Figure 114–3 Film from a barium enema in a patient with pancolonic diverticulosis. There is marked redundancy and overlapping of the sigmoid colon, which obscures the definition of intraluminal lesion.

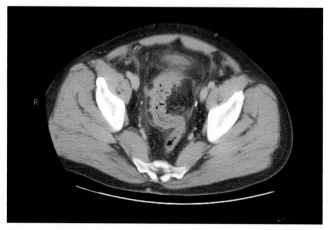

Figure 114–4 Computed tomography scan of a patient with acute diverticulitis showing colon wall thickening, a mass adjacent to the sigmoid, and "stranding" of the fat.

diverticulitis consistently have reported CT sensitivities of 93% to 98% and specificities of 75% to 100%, significantly more accurate than contrast enemas.[66,70,71] CT also has been found to be highly sensitive and specific for right-sided diverticulitis and in helping to differentiate diverticulitis from colorectal cancer of the ascending colon and cecum.[72,73] Although some reports show a lower sensitivity of CT for diverticulitis,[74,75] it is increasingly becoming clear that, when diagnosis is in doubt or clinical deterioration occurs, CT is the best primary radiologic diagnostic modality. Conversely, in patients with mild disease and in whom the diagnosis is straightforward, CT scanning may not be necessary.

Ultrasonography

Based on its relatively low cost, convenience, and non-invasive nature, ultrasonography (US) has been advocated as a potentially useful diagnostic modality in diverticulitis. Characteristic findings implying active inflammation include bowel wall thickening, presence of diverticula or abscesses, and hyperechogenicity of the bowel wall. US has a reported sensitivity of 84% to 98% and specificity of 80% to 93%.[76,77] One study of 71 patients with suspected diverticulitis who underwent US reported a negative predictive value of 100%.[78] A trial comparing US with CT revealed equally good accuracy.[79] US also is useful in female patients to exclude gynecologic pathology. Despite these encouraging data, US remains highly operator dependent, especially for detecting interloop abscesses, air-filled abscesses, or disease complications posterior in the abdomen that are hard to visualize. US therefore remains a second-line diagnostic tool to be used in select circumstances or for research purposes.

Magnetic Resonance Imaging

With limited resolution secondary to motion artifact introduced by peristalsis and respiration, the potential role of magnetic resonance imaging remains to be demonstrated. Whether decreased scan times and intraluminal contrast agents will overcome these limitations remains to be seen.

Endoscopy

Because of the risk of perforation, either from the instrument itself or air insufflation, endoscopy generally is avoided in the initial evaluation of patients with suspected acute diverticulitis. A limited rigid or flexible sigmoidoscopy with minimal air insufflation may be helpful to exclude alternative diagnoses, such as inflammatory bowel disease, carcinoma, or ischemic colitis. As noted earlier, once the acute setting has passed, a colonoscopy should be electively performed to confirm the presence of diverticula and to exclude competing diagnoses, particularly neoplasia.

Treatment

One of the initial decisions regarding patients with diverticulitis involves a determination of the need for hospitalization. Factors to be considered include severity of illness, ability to tolerate oral intake, comorbid diseases, and available outpatient support systems (e.g., a reliable

family). An appropriate patient for outpatient management would be one with mild symptoms, no peritoneal signs, the ability to take oral fluids, and a supportive home network. These patients should be treated with a clear liquid diet and antibiotics. When cultured, most diverticular abscesses grow mixed aerobic and anaerobic infections, the most common single organisms being *Escherichia coli*, *Streptococcus* spp., and *Bacteroides fragilis*.[80] Therefore, oral antibiotics with broad-spectrum coverage, such as amoxicillin/clavulanate, sulfamethoxazole/trimethoprim with metronidazole, or a fluoroquinolone with metronidazole, are reasonable choices.[81] Other medical treatments, such as rifaximin, mesalazine, and probiotics, show promise as alternative therapies and may play a role in preventing recurrent diverticulitis, but need further study.[82] Patients treated as outpatients should have close follow-up. They should be instructed to call the physician for increasing pain, fever, or inability to tolerate oral fluids, each of which could indicate the development of complications and the need for hospitalization. Symptomatic improvement generally should be evident within 2 to 3 days, at which time the diet may be slowly advanced. Antibiotic treatment should be continued for 7 to 10 days.

Patients with uncomplicated diverticulitis who are elderly or immunosuppressed, have severe comorbidities, or demonstrate high fever or significant leukocytosis should be hospitalized. Although data imply that early consultation with a subspecialist improves quality of care in the inpatient management of diverticulitis,[83] this is probably not necessary for many straightforward cases. Bowel rest with either clear liquids or nothing by mouth should be instituted. Intravenous fluid therapy to restore intravascular volume, balance electrolytes, and ensure adequate urinary output should be initiated. Broad-spectrum intravenous antibiotics should be started. Recommended combination regimens include anaerobic coverage with metronidazole or clindamycin and gram-negative coverage with an aminoglycoside, monobactam, or a third-generation cephalosporin.[81] Single-agent coverage with intravenous second-generation cephalosporins or beta-lactamase inhibitor combinations, such as ampicillin/sulbactam or ticarcillin/clavulanate, are reasonable alternatives. Symptomatic improvement with decreasing fever and leukocytosis should be observed within 2 to 4 days, at which point diet may be advanced. If improvement continues, patients may be discharged but should complete a 7- to 10-day oral antibiotic course. Failure to improve with conservative medical therapy warrants a diligent search for complications, consideration of alternative diagnoses, and surgical consultation. Most patients hospitalized with acute diverticulitis respond to conservative medical therapy, but it has been estimated that 15% to 30% require surgery during the hospital admission.[1,5,16,54] Surgery may be necessary when pain, fever, and leukocytosis do not respond to days of antibiotics and supportive care. If surgery is planned and complicated disease (e.g., abscess) is ruled out, resection of the diseased segment of bowel with primary anastomosis is the most commonly performed operation, usually in a single-stage procedure. The main requirements in performing a single-stage procedure are the ability to perform bowel preparation and technical feasibility, usually determined by the extent of extramural inflammation. The entire sigmoid colon should be removed (in left-sided disease) because this is the most common location for initial disease and recurrence. The distal resection margin should be the proximal rectum and the anastomosis should be free of tension to decrease risk of anastomotic leak.[84] For uncomplicated diverticulitis, laparoscopic sigmoid colectomy has gained increasing enthusiasm[85] and has significant advantages over open techniques with respect to length of stay and postoperative in-hospital morbidity.[86] Medical and surgical management of complications such as perforation, abscess, fistula, or obstruction are discussed later in this chapter.

Special Topics

Recurrent Diverticulitis

For patients who respond well to conservative therapy, the issues of likelihood of recurrence and elective prophylactic surgical resection arise. The risk of recurrent symptoms following an attack of acute diverticulitis has been reported to range from 7% to 45%,[1,5,16,54] with one half of second attacks occurring within 1 year. Recurrent attacks have been said to be less likely to respond to medical therapy and have a higher mortality rate.[16,54] Elective resection generally is recommended after two attacks of uncomplicated diverticulitis,[84,85,87] although this recommendation is now being challenged, many experts preferring to wait for two or more attacks before advising surgery. Recent studies have begun to show a decrease in recurrence rates of diverticulitis and symptomatic diverticular disease in patients treated with mesalamine,[88] rifaximin, and combinations of these agents.[89,90] Most patients report having a good functional outcome and low rates of recurrent disease after elective resection for recurrent diverticulitis.[88] In considering an elective sigmoid resection, relevant variables include the severity and responsiveness of the attack(s), the general health of the patient, the risk to the patient of a subsequent attack, and the risk of the resection itself. The latter factor may be lessened by the increasing use of the laparoscopic approach in many patients. Additionally, up to 10% of patients will have symptomatic recurrent diverticulitis after surgical resection, and reoperation may be required in 2% to 3%.[54,84,91,92] In patients undergoing resection for diverticulitis, higher recurrence rates occur when the sigmoid colon is used for the distal resection margin, rather than the rectum.[93] Therefore, it is recommended to resect the entire distal colon whenever possible, forming the distal anastomosis with the proximal rectum and the proximal anastomosis with a noninflamed, non-diverticula-bearing portion of colon.[54,84]

The Young Patient

Diverticulitis is relatively uncommon in patients younger than 40 years of age, representing 2% to 5% of all patients with diverticulitis.[1,16] As such, it is often missed or mistaken for other diagnoses, such as appendicitis or inflammatory bowel disease. Like diverticulitis in older patients, the disease is mainly sigmoid in location, although one report has described a right-sided predominance in young Israelis.[94] There seems to be a significant male predominance in young patients.[1,95] Attacks often are more severe, with 88% of younger patients requiring urgent surgery during their initial attack, and recurrence and complication rates that are higher than in older patients.[1,95] When patients with acute diverticulitis are managed nonoperatively, youth is an independent risk factor for poor outcome in subsequent course,[96] possibly due to delay in diagnosis. For these reasons, some authors advocate elective segmental colectomy in a healthy young person after one well-documented episode of diverticulitis[54,87,96]; others have questioned this approach.[84,94,97]

The Immunocompromised Patient

Diverticulitis may manifest more subtly in immunocompromised patients and represents a more difficult diagnostic challenge than in those with a normal immune system. Although diverticulitis in such patients does not appear to be more common, it appears to have graver consequences. One study reported that 24% of non-immunosuppressed patients needed surgery for diverticulitis, whereas 100% of immunosuppressed ones required surgery.[98] Immunocompromised patients have a higher rate of free perforation (43% vs. 14%), need for surgery (58% vs. 33%), and postoperative mortality (39% vs. 2%) than do noncompromised patients.[99] In solid organ (e.g., heart, lung, and kidney) transplant populations, mortality from diverticulitis has been found to be extremely high, ranging from 25% to 100%.[100-102] Because of this high risk, many authorities advocate elective resection after an initial episode of diverticulitis in an immunosuppressed patient.[7,87]

Right-Sided Diverticulitis

In Western countries, diverticulitis of the ascending colon or cecum is uncommon, because of the relatively low prevalence of diverticula in these portions of the colon. Nonetheless, right-sided diverticulitis should be part of the differential diagnosis for any patient with right lower quadrant symptoms. In Asia, right-sided diverticulitis is the predominant form of diverticulitis. Especially in younger patients, the diagnosis of right-sided diverticulitis is more difficult to make than is left-sided disease and is virtually indistinguishable clinically from acute appendicitis. Clinical factors that might be helpful to distinguish diverticulitis from appendicitis in a person of Asian ethnicity who might therefore have right-sided diverticulitis are that patients with diverticulitis tend to be older and have a lower frequency of nausea and vomiting than patients with appendicitis.[103] Radiologically, right-sided diverticulitis and appendicitis also are easily confused, especially when a local abscess is present (Fig. 114–5). There is an estimated preoperative misdiagnosis rate in right-sided colon inflammatory conditions of 40% to 92%.[103,104] Even with excellent imaging, the diagnosis of right-sided diverticulitis frequently is made at laparotomy. When the proper diagnosis is made preoperatively, treatment of right-sided disease is the same as for left-sided diverticulitis. One study suggested better overall responsiveness of right-sided diverticulitis to medical therapy alone, even after multiple attacks.[105] The much more common complication associated with right colonic diverticula is hemorrhage, discussed later in this chapter.

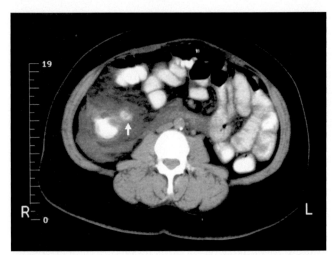

Figure 114–5   Computed tomography scan of a patient with a right lower quadrant abscess (*arrow*). The differential diagnosis of this finding includes right-sided diverticulitis and appendicitis.

COMPLICATED DIVERTICULITIS

Abscess

When perforation of a colonic diverticulum occurs, the ability of the pericolic tissues to control the spread of the inflammatory process determines subsequent clinical behavior and treatment. A localized phlegmon initially develops with a limited spread. Further spread can lead to the formation of larger local or distant abscesses (Hinchey stages I and II, respectively). When abscess contents spread diffusely in the peritoneum causing purulent or fecal peritonitis (Hinchey stages III and IV, respectively), it can lead to sepsis and death if the patient does not undergo urgent surgical intervention. Clinical signs suggesting abscess formation include a tender mass on physical examination, persistent fever, or leukocytosis despite an adequate trial of appropriate intravenous antibiotics. Once an abscess is suspected, radiologic evaluation with a CT scan is the best modality for confirming the diagnosis and following its course over time.

Small pericolic abscesses (stage I) often can be treated conservatively with broad-spectrum antibiotics and bowel rest.[84] In one series of patients with diverticulitis, 7 of 10 patients with pericolic abscesses responded successfully to conservative treatment.[106] This favorable prognosis may result from maintenance of a fistula between the abscess and the colon lumen, thus permitting spontaneous internal drainage. Noninterventional management of abscesses should be considered only in stable patients who demonstrate unequivocal improvements in pain, fever, tenderness, and leukocytosis over the first few days of therapy.

CT-guided percutaneous drainage of abdominal abscesses has assumed a prominent complementary role with surgery (Fig. 114–6). The immediate advantage of percutaneous catheter drainage is rapid control of sepsis and patient stabilization without the need for general anesthesia. It often eliminates the need for a multiple-stage procedure with colostomy,[107] instead allowing for temporary palliative drainage and subsequent single-stage resection in 3 to 4 weeks. Success rates of CT-guided drainage for stabilizing patients and safely allowing for subsequent single-stage procedures range from 74% to 80%.[108,109] An urgent surgical procedure is required in the 20% to 25% of patients in whom the abscess is multiloculated, anatomically inaccessible, or not resolving with percutaneous drainage.

In cases where surgical intervention is necessary, the approach has evolved over the last half century. Historically, three-stage management was preferred for complicated diverticulitis of any severity. Stage I involved a proximal colostomy and drainage of abscesses; stage II was for resecting the diseased bowel (colostomy maintained to protect anastomosis); and stage III was to restore bowel continuity. Although the multiple-stage surgical approach to diverticular disease was effective for management of abscesses, generally it is desirable to limit the number of laparotomies to minimize morbidity and duration of hospitalization. Additionally, only about one half of patients undergoing proximal-end colostomy have the colostomy reversed because of the technical difficulties and the risks of anastomotic leakage and mortality.[110] In the last few decades, two-stage management (e.g., primary resection of diseased bowel with proximal end colostomy and oversewing of the distal stump [also referred to as the *Hartmann procedure*]) and, increasingly, management with a single operation (i.e., resection with primary anastomosis) have become the preferred surgical approaches. The switch to fewer operations has been made without a discernable compromise in overall outcomes relative to three-stage approaches.[111] Single-stage management, which is fast becoming the standard for elective management of uncomplicated diverticulitis, also is being used increasingly in appropriate patients with complicated diverticulitis. To do so, bowel preparation is believed to be necessary. When free perforation is ruled out, bowel preparation is performed prior to the operation with either a 1-day polyethylene glycol-electrolyte lavage or a traditional 2- or 3-day mechanical preparation; both types of preparation have been shown to have similar outcomes in a randomized trial.[112] In the setting of urgent or emergent surgery when free perforation is a concern, bowel lavage may be performed "on table," thereby allowing a primary anastomosis to be performed in a single stage.[113,114] Regardless of approach, surgery for complicated diverticulitis has evolved into a relatively safe procedure with one of the highest success rates of any of the common gastrointestinal procedures.[115]

Free Perforation

Peritonitis (Hinchey stages III or IV) is a surgical emergency and requires urgent operative intervention. Although uncommon in the antibiotic era, mortality from generalized peritonitis associated with diverticulitis has been reported in the 12% to 26% range.[116] Early identification of free perforation is critical. CT scan can confirm the diagnosis in ambiguous cases, but an abdominal series showing free intraperitoneal air combined with high clinical suspicion are sufficient to justify exploration. Broad-spectrum intravenous antibiotics, such as a second- or third-generation cephalosporin and metronidazole, should be instituted immediately.

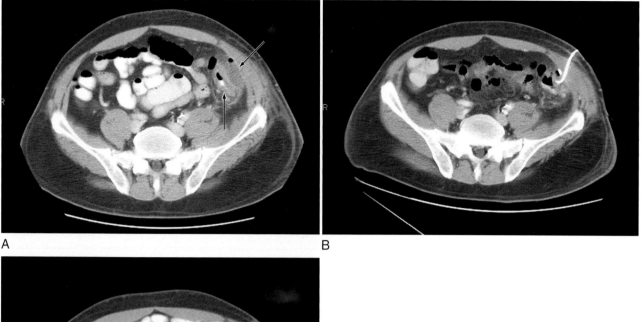

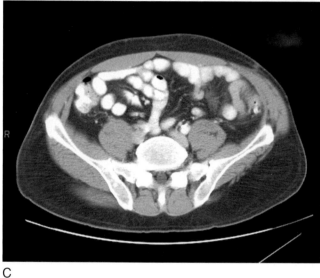

Figure 114–6 Computed tomography (CT) scans with CT-guided percutaneous drainage of an abdominal abscess complicating acute diverticulitis. *A,* Arrows point to the abscess arising from the sigmoid colon. *B,* A drainage catheter has been inserted into the abscess. The patient also was treated with intravenous antibiotics. *C,* The catheter has been removed and the abscess has resolved.

For more confined abscesses, the surgical options are the following:

1. *Primary resection* of the diseased sigmoid colon with either the Hartmann procedure (two-stage) or primary colorectal anastomosis (single-stage).
2. *Secondary resection* with the initial operation to create a diverting colostomy and suture the perforation, if possible, and subsequent procedure(s) to resect the diseased colon and restore bowel continuity.

There is no clear consensus whether primary or secondary resection is more beneficial for peritonitis from diverticulitis. Retrospective studies suggest an advantage for primary over secondary resection with respect to morbidity and mortality.[116,117] Two randomized trials comparing primary with secondary resection yielded conflicting results, with neither appearing to be clearly superior.[118,119] Practically, the decision of primary or secondary resection is made intraoperatively based on the extent of disease, the difficulty of bowel mobilization, the degree of peritoneal contamination, and the surgeon's expertise. In most cases of free perforation, at least two separate operations are necessary regardless of whether primary or secondary resection is performed. As noted

previously, in many cases, restoration of the anastomosis is not possible and the colostomy is left indefinitely. Cases of peritonitis also require pelvic drainage, clearance of the rectum of fecal material when possible, and mobilization of the splenic flexure to perform a tension-free anastomosis. Placement of ureteral stents prophylactically can help prevent accidental ureteral injury during the operation.[115]

Fistula

When a diverticular phlegmon or abscess extends or ruptures into an adjacent organ, a fistula can occur. Fistulas are believed to develop in fewer than 5% of patients with diverticulitis but are present in about 20% of those who require surgery for diverticulitis.[120] In a Cleveland Clinic review of 84 patients seen over 26 years with internal fistulas caused by diverticular disease, 65% were colovesical.[121] There was a 2:1 male predominance, attributed to the protection given the bladder by the uterus. In one series, pneumaturia was present in 57% and fecaluria in 42%[122]; the latter is pathognomonic for colovesical fistula. Cystoscopy, cystography, and BE can be useful, though demonstration of the actual fistula often is difficult. In both of the above series, single-stage operative resection with fistula closure and primary anastomosis could be performed in 75% of patients. Presumably, single-stage management is possible so frequently in the presence of fistulas to extracolonic organs because the fistula has effectively "decompressed" the inflammatory process. Colovaginal fistulas are the next most common internal fistula after colovesical fistula, representing approximately 25% of all cases.[121] The passage of stool or flatus per the vagina is pathognomonic. Frequent vaginal infections or copious discharge should prompt consideration of the diagnosis. Many patients with colovaginal fistula have undergone a previous hysterectomy. Treatment is surgical resection of the diseased segment of colon with repair of the contiguous organ, which generally can be performed as a single-stage procedure.[84] Coloenteric, colouterine, and coloureteral fistulas occur much less commonly than colovesical and colovaginal fistulas. Spontaneous colocutaneous fistulas are rare and more frequently follow surgical repair. Other rare fistula types that have been reported as a presumed or documented complication of diverticulitis include colocholecystal, coloappendiceal, and colosalpingal. Although diverticular disease is a common cause of fistula from the colon to adjacent organs, other conditions such as inflammatory bowel disease, pancreatitis, radiation enteritis and colitis, and malignancy also can cause fistulas and these diagnoses must be considered when a fistula involving the colon is discovered.

Obstruction

Obstruction may accompany diverticular disease either acutely or chronically. During an attack of acute diverticulitis, partial colonic obstruction can occur because of luminal narrowing from the pericolic inflammation, compression from abscess formation, or both. Obstruction can be confirmed with a gentle water-soluble contrast enema in a patient not suspected to have free perforation,[120] while simultaneously excluding an obstructing sigmoid neoplasm. Complete obstruction is unusual. Colonic ileus or pseudo-obstruction also can occur, as can small bowel obstruction if a loop of small intestine becomes incorporated into the inflammatory mass. These conditions usually improve with effective medical therapy including antibiotics, bowel rest, and nasogastric suction. Surgical intervention may be required for persistent obstruction from acute diverticulitis not responding to medical therapy. Ideally, a modified bowel preparation with gentle irrigation enemas and/or low-dose oral laxatives given over a period of a few days can be given preoperatively,[120] thereby allowing the possibility of primary anastomosis in some cases. In cases when bowel preparation is not possible, a Hartmann procedure usually is performed.

Recurrent attacks of diverticulitis, which may be subclinical, can initiate chronic stricturing of the colonic wall without ongoing inflammation. In such cases, high-grade or complete obstruction can occur. A contrast enema can help distinguish benign stricture from neoplasm. Colonoscopy also plays an important diagnostic role, and one group investigating strictures with colonoscopy was able to distinguish benign from malignant etiology in 67% of patients.[123] Strictures in which malignancy cannot be excluded despite colonoscopic and radiologic examinations should undergo surgical resection. A trial of endoscopic dilation therapy can reasonably be attempted in patients in whom neoplasm is believed to be sufficiently excluded and in whom *acute* diverticulitis is not a concern. Balloon dilation success rates for benign colonic strictures have been reported in the 67% to 79% range.[124,125] Colonic metal stents may have a role in treating obstruction complicating diverticular disease, particularly in providing temporary decompression to allow for bowel preparation and subsequent single-stage resection without diversion.[126]

DIVERTICULAR HEMORRHAGE

Diverticulosis, angioectasias (vascular ectasias), colitis, neoplasms, and hemorrhoids are responsible for most cases of lower gastrointestinal bleeding.[19,127-130] Diverticular hemorrhage is the most common identifiable cause of significant lower gastrointestinal bleeding, accounting for 30% to 40% of cases with confirmed sources.[131,132] It often is difficult, however, to make a precise determination of the source of bleeding and conclusive evidence of the cause of bleeding is available only in a minority of cases,[127,128] either by visualizing an actively bleeding lesion endoscopically or by identifying extravasation from a specific site angiographically. More frequently, circumstantial evidence is used to suggest diverticulosis as the source of hemorrhage. Clinical features suggestive of diverticular hemorrhage include copious bright red or maroon blood per rectum, the presence of diverticulosis on colonoscopy or radiologic studies, exclusion of an upper gastrointestinal source, and exclusion of alternative colonic sources. These clinical criteria, suggested by Quinn in 1960, are nonspecific and will be met by various lesions other than diverticula, most notably angioectasias.

EPIDEMIOLOGY

Severe hemorrhage has been reported to occur in 3% to 5% of patients with diverticulosis.[19,133,134] Despite the fact that most diverticula are in the left colon in Western individuals, the site of bleeding diverticula has been believed to be in the proximal colon in more than one half of patients.[135-137] A large series of 180 Asian patients with diverticular hemorrhage reported a higher bleeding rate and greater need for surgery with right-sided compared with left-sided disease.[137]

PATHOPHYSIOLOGY

To study the pathogenesis of diverticular bleeding, Meyers and colleagues used sophisticated microangiographic techniques on resected colon specimens from patients with arteriographically documented bleeding diverticula.[138] Three-dimensional histologic reconstructions demonstrated consistent findings of intimal thickening and medial thinning of the vasa recta as it coursed over the dome of the diverticulum. They proposed that these changes led to a segmental weakening of the artery, thus predisposing to its rupture. This arterial lesion was absent in diverticula that did not bleed. What predisposes to this arterial change and what precipitates its rupture are unknown. Inflammation does not appear to be a contributing factor, because it is not found histologically in bleeding diverticula that were resected. This absence might explain why bleeding rarely complicates diverticulitis.

Nonsteroidal anti-inflammatory drugs (NSAIDs) have been implicated in lower intestinal, and specifically diverticular, bleeding. A large prospective series of patients with lower intestinal bleeding reported a risk of bleeding with NSAIDs equal to that of duodenal ulcer.[139] An overall increased risk of diverticular bleeding also was found at the 4-year follow-up of a large study of health professionals who had been free of diverticulosis at baseline.[140] In addition to having a higher rate of complications from diverticulosis, such as bleeding and perforation, patients taking NSAIDs also appear to have more severe complications.[141-143] Hence, patients who have an episode of diverticular bleeding and are concurrently taking NSAIDs should be urged to discontinue them. Whether patients with diverticulosis without a prior bleeding episode should be counseled as well to avoid NSAIDs is less clear. In a multicenter trial of patients randomized to naproxen (conventional NSAID) or rofecoxib (cyclooxygenase [COX]-2 selective agent), the relative risk of lower intestinal bleeding from all causes was 0.46 in patients taking rofecoxib relative to the naproxen group.[144] Whether hemorrhage specifically from diverticula is reduced by replacing NSAIDs with COX-2 selective agents is unknown, and the cost-effectiveness of this approach has not been established.

CLINICAL FEATURES

Diverticular hemorrhage typically manifests as abrupt, painless hematochezia. Because the bleeding is arterial, the volume of blood usually is moderate or large, an observation that can help distinguish diverticular hemorrhage from other common causes of rectal bleeding. Patients often pass red or maroon clots; melena is unusual. Because the bleeding is overt, neither a positive fecal occult blood test nor iron-deficiency anemia should be attributed to diverticular hemorrhage. Natural history studies report that bleeding ceases spontaneously in 70% to 80% of patients, and rebleeding rates range from 22% to 38%.[133,134,137] The chance of a third bleeding episode can be as high as 50%,[133] leading many to recommend surgical resection after a second bleeding episode, similar to the management of recurrent diverticulitis.[87]

DIAGNOSIS AND MANAGEMENT

The diagnosis and treatment of patients with lower intestinal bleeding in general have been reviewed comprehensively elsewhere (see Chapter 13).[130,145] The algorithm in Figure 114–7 summarizes the management of patients

with bleeding diverticula. In unstable patients, volume and blood product resuscitation require immediate attention. Excluding an upper gastrointestinal source by nasogastric lavage or upper endoscopy is warranted because 10% to 15% of patients with hematochezia have an upper tract cause. If bleeding is massive or the patient remains unstable after attempted resuscitation, early angiography to attempt bleeding localization and surgical consultation should be obtained.

A stable patient with suspected active or recent diverticular bleeding should undergo bowel preparation for a colonoscopy. The ability to identify a diverticular source, to exclude alternative diagnoses, and to provide therapy of actively bleeding lesions support colonoscopy as a primary investigation in this setting. Rapid (over 3 to 4 hours) oral or nasogastric purge with a balanced electrolyte solution provides a safe and effective bowel preparation; a dose of metoclopramide before initiation may improve tolerance to the lavage.[146] If diverticulosis is not found on colonoscopy, alternative diagnoses should be entertained. If diverticula are found but bleeding has stopped and no other colonic causes are found, diverticular hemorrhage is often diagnosed presumptively and the patient should be instructed to avoid NSAIDs and anticoagulants, if possible. As noted, most patients with diverticular hemorrhage do not rebleed.

The endoscopic identification of active bleeding or stigmata of recent hemorrhage from a specific site (Fig. 114-8) is evident in about 10% to 20% of colonoscopic examinations for diverticular bleeding and is very useful. The appearance of nonbleeding stigmata (i.e., visible vessel or adherent clot within a diverticulum) may permit one to estimate the future risk of hemorrhage from that site,[147] although this concept has not been validated as well in the colon as it has for peptic ulcer bleeding. However, identification of a bleeding site allows endoscopic therapy to be applied. The use of epinephrine injection alone[148] or in combination with other therapies such as heater probe coagulation,[149] bipolar coagulation,[150-152] endoclips,[153] fibrin sealant,[154] and band ligation[155] all have been shown in small case series to achieve hemostasis safely in patients with diverticular bleeding.[144] If endoscopic therapy is not effective or durable, localizing the site facilitates directed therapy with angiography or segmental surgical resection.

In the absence of randomized trials, the true effectiveness of endoscopic treatment for diverticular hemorrhage is not known. In a retrospective study, Jensen and colleagues were able to identify definite bleeding sources in 10 of 48 patients with suspected diverticular bleeding.[152] These lesions were treated with epinephrine and cauterized with bipolar coagulation. None of the endoscopically treated patients had recurrent bleeding or required surgery. These results were compared with 17 historic controls who had bleeding stigmata but no endoscopic therapy, 9 of whom rebled and 6 of whom required surgery. Although this study has limitations, it is the most compelling support of urgent endoscopic therapy for diverticular hemorrhage to date. Stigmata of active or recent hemorrhage are not common findings at endoscopy, however, and endoscopic therapy only is relevant to a minority of patients. Another group at the Mayo Clinic with an approach to lower intestinal bleed-

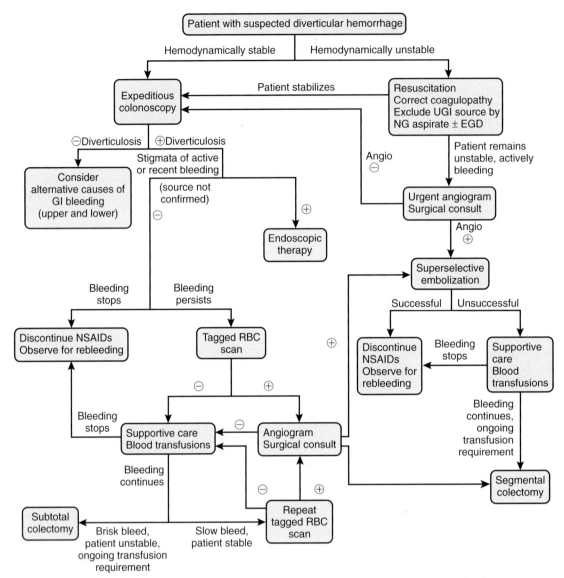

Figure 114–7 Algorithim for the management of patients with bleeding diverticula. EGD, esophagogastroduodenoscopy; GI, gastrointestinal; NSAIDs, nonsteroidal anti-inflammatory drugs; NG, nasogastric; UGI, upper gastrointestinal.

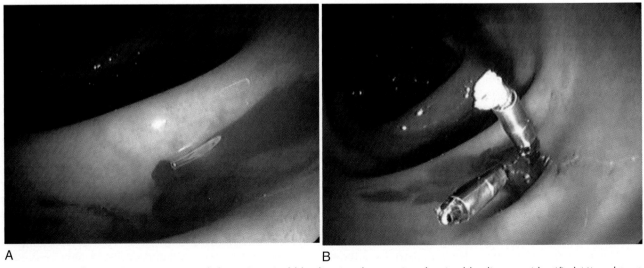

Figure 114–8 Colonoscopy in a patient with lower intestinal bleeding in whom a site of active bleeding was identified (*A*) and treated successfully with placement of two clips (*B*). (*A* and *B*, Courtesy of Janak Shah.)

ing similar to Jensen's group reported that urgent colonoscopy (i.e., performed <12 hours after admission) was no more effective at identifying bleeding stigmata than colonoscopy performed later in the hospitalization.[156] It seems reasonable to perform colonoscopy within the first 12 to 48 hours of admission in most cases.

When active bleeding is present but colonoscopy fails to allow localization or treatment of a bleeding source, further evaluation with nuclear scintigraphy ("tagged red blood cell scan") or angiography can be undertaken, taking into account local availability and expertise. A third radiographic option, enhanced CT, also has shown promise for identifying active lower intestinal bleeding sources, though its role has yet to be defined.[157] Nuclear scintigraphy (Fig. 114–9) has many theoretical advantages in the evaluation of lower intestinal bleeding.[158] It is noninvasive, technically simple, relatively inexpensive, and sensitive to bleeding rates as low as 0.1 mL/min. Scintigraphy can identify only the site, not the etiology of the bleeding, and it has no therapeutic potential. Furthermore, some studies have questioned its accuracy.[159] Given its sensitivity and relative simplicity, however, many centers use scintigraphy prior to angiography to minimize the chance of a negative angiogram and to help select a specific artery for injection.[160] Angiography has a theoretical sensitivity for lower intestinal bleeding rates

of 0.5 mL/min. Advantages of angiography are identification of the site of bleeding accurately enough to direct segmental surgical resection and therapeutic capability. Although angiographic embolization had previously been felt to carry a risk of bowel infarction, superselective embolization (Fig. 114–10), or embolization of distal arterial branches, has been demonstrated to be both effective (67% to 100% with lasting hemostasis) and relatively safe (ischemia rates < 20%).[161-163] Where available, arterial embolization increasingly is becoming the nonsurgical therapy of choice when endoscopic methods are not possible.

Surgery in lower intestinal bleeding usually is avoided until endoscopic or angiographic therapies fail or are unavailable. Because diverticular bleeding stops spontaneously in most patients, surgical management infrequently is required. The primary indications for operative management are large transfusion requirements, recurrent hemorrhage either refractory or not amenable to therapy, or hemodynamic instability unresponsive to resuscitation. When surgery is necessary, a partial colectomy is preferred to a subtotal colectomy whenever possible. Segmental resection can be performed if the bleeding site is identified clearly from a therapeutically unsuccessful angiographic or endoscopic procedure *or* when the extent of diverticulosis is proved to be confined

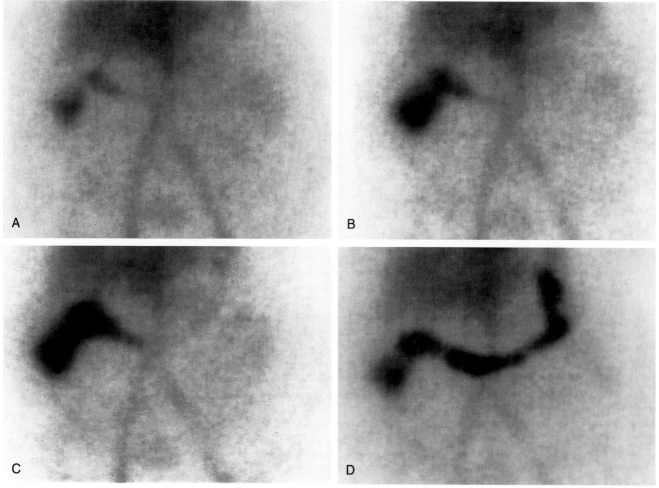

Figure 114–9   Nuclear scintigraphy scan in a patient with lower intestinal bleeding. A site of bleeding is identified in the patient's right lower quadrant.

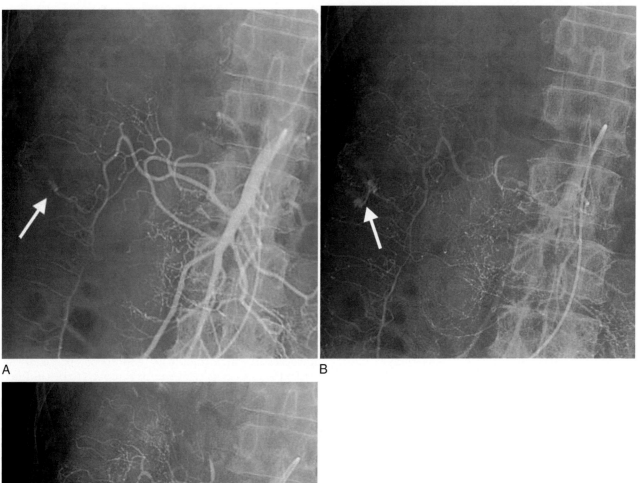

A

B

C

Figure 114–10 Selective angiography of the superior mesenteric artery in a patient with lower intestinal bleeding due to diverticulosis. The bleeding site is identified *(A, arrow)* and embolized with microcoils *(B, arrow). C,* The coils are seen *(arrow)* in the bleeding vessel and the extravasation of contrast material has stopped.

to a specific segment of the colon. The rebleeding rate was 6% in seven series of patients who underwent segmental resections for angiographically documented bleeding sites.[164] As noted, however, it is often difficult to identify an extravasation site angiographically. One series found that angiography resulted in a successful directed resection in only 12% of patients.[165] In patients with persistent, life-threatening bleeding and no identification of a likely bleeding site, a subtotal or "blind" colectomy may be required as a last resort. These patients have had an extremely high morbidity and mortality,[166] possi-

bly because of the multiple invasive tests leading to that end and the resultant delay in definitive management. Additionally, a blind colectomy runs the risk of not resecting the bleeding lesion when the source is more proximal and has a high risk of anastomotic failure.[135] Nonetheless, more recent literature has shown morbitity and mortality rates of a subtotal colectomy not to differ from those of a "blind" hemicolectomy, where the site of the bleeding is not identified.[167,168] Clearly, a close collaborative relationship between the gastroenterologist and the surgeon is paramount in managing such patients.

ACKNOWLEDGMENT

Dr. Stollman gratefully acknowledges the contributions of Jeffrey B. Raskin, MD, who inspired his interest in this field and has provided guidance, mentoring, and insight throughout.

REFERENCES

1. Nathan BN: Who first described colonic diverticula? Can J Surg 34:203, 1991.
2. Painter NS, Burkitt DP: Diverticular disease of the colon: A deficiency disease of Western civilization. BMJ 2:450, 1971.
3. Kang JY, Hoare J, Tinto A, et al: Diverticular disease of the colon--on the rise: A study of hospital admissions in England between 1989/1990 and 1999/2000. Aliment Pharmacol Ther 17:1189, 2003.
4. Makela J, Kiviniemi H, Laitinen S: Prevalence of perforated sigmoid diverticulitis is increasing. Dis Colon Rectum 45:955, 2002.
5. Schwesinger WH, Page CP, Gaskill HV III, et al: Operative management of diverticular emergencies: Strategies and outcomes. Arch Surg 135:558, 2000; discussion 562.
6. Sandler RS, Everhart JE, Donowits M, et al: The burden of selected digestive diseases in the United States. Gastroenterology 122:1500, 2002.
7. Schoetz DJ Jr: Uncomplicated diverticulitis: Indications for surgery and surgical management. Surg Clin North Am 73:965, 1993.
8. Delvaux M: Diverticular disease of the colon in Europe: Epidemiology, impact on citizen health and prevention. Aliment Pharmacol Ther 18(Suppl 3):71, 2003.
9. Parks TG: Natural history of diverticular disease of the colon. Clin Gastroenterol 4:53, 1975.
10. Jun S, Stollman N: Epidemiology of diverticular disease. Best Pract Res Clin Gastroenterol 16:529, 2002.
11. McConnell EJ, Tessier DJ, Wolff BG: Population-based incidence of complicated diverticular disease of the sigmoid colon based on gender and age. Dis Colon Rectum 46:1110, 2003.
12. Kyle J, Adesola, AD, Tinckler, LF, deBeaux, J: Incidence of diverticulitis. Scand J Gastroenterol 2:77, 1967.
13. Stemmermann GN, Yatani R: Diverticulosis and polyps of the large intestine: A necropsy study of Hawaii Japanese. Cancer 31:1260, 1973.
14. Lee YS: Diverticular disease of the large bowel in Singapore: An autopsy survey. Dis Colon Rectum 29:330, 1986.
15. Levy N, Stermer E, Simon J: The changing epidemiology of diverticular disease in Israel. Dis Colon Rectum 28:416-8, 1985.
16. Parks TG: Natural history of diverticular disease of the colon: A review of 521 cases. BMJ 4:639, 1969.
17. Horner JL: Natural history of diverticulosis of the colon. Am J Dig Dis 3:343, 1958.
18. Levi DM, Levi JU, Rogers AI, et al: Giant colonic diverticulum: An unusual manifestation of a common disease. Am J Gastroenterol 88:139, 1993.
19. Reinus JF, Brandt LJ: Vascular ectasias and diverticulosis: Common causes of lower intestinal bleeding. Gastroenterol Clin North Am 23:1, 1994.
20. Chia JG, Wilde CC, Ngoi SS, et al: Trends of diverticular disease of the large bowel in a newly developed country. Dis Colon Rectum 34:498, 1991.
21. Miura S, Kodaira S, Shatari T, et al: Recent trends in diverticulosis of the right colon in Japan: Retrospective review in a regional hospital. Dis Colon Rectum 43:1383, 2000.
22. Whiteway J, Morson BC: Elastosis in diverticular disease of the sigmoid colon. Gut 26:258, 1985.
23. Bode MK, Karttunen TJ, Makela J, et al: Type I and III collagens in human colon cancer and diverticulosis. Scand J Gastroenterol 35:747, 2000.
24. Mimura T, Bateman AC, Lee RL, et al: Up-regulation of collagen and tissue inhibitors of matrix metalloproteinase in colonic diverticular disease. Dis Colon Rectum 47:371, 2004.
25. Arfwidsson S, Knock NG, Lehmann L, Winberg T: Pathogenesis of multiple diverticula of the sigmoid colon in diverticular disease. Acta Chir Scand 63:1, 1964.
26. Painter NS: The aetiology of diverticulosis of the colon with special reference to the action of certain drugs on the behaviour of the colon. Ann R Coll Surg Engl 34:98, 1964.
27. Painter NS, Truelove SC, Ardran GM, Tuckey M: Segmentation and the localization of intraluminal pressures in the human colon, with special reference to the pathogenesis of colonic diverticula. Gastroenterology 49:169, 1965.
28. Trotman IF, Misiewicz JJ: Sigmoid motility in diverticular disease and the irritable bowel syndrome. Gut 29:218, 1988.
29. Cortesini C, Pantalone D: Usefulness of colonic motility study in identifying patients at risk for complicated diverticular disease. Dis Colon Rectum 34:339, 1991.
30. Bassotti G, Battaglia E, Spinozzi F, et al: Twenty-four hour recordings of colonic motility in patients with diverticular disease: Evidence for abnormal motility and propulsive activity. Dis Colon Rectum 44:1814, 2001.
31. Sugihara K, Muto T, Morioka Y: Motility study in right-sided diverticular disease of the colon. Gut 24:1130, 1983.
32. Tomita R, Fujisaki S, Tanjoh K, Fukuzawa M: Role of nitric oxide in the left-sided colon of patients with diverticular disease. Hepatogastroenterology 47:692, 2000.
33. Liu L, Shang F, Markus I, Burcher E: Roles of substance P receptors in human colon circular muscle: Alterations in diverticular disease. J Pharmacol Exp Ther 302:627, 2002.
34. Burkitt DP, Walker AR, Painter NS: Effect of dietary fibre on stools and the transit-times, and its role in the causation of disease. Lancet 2:1408, 1972.
35. Fisher N, Berry CS, Fearn T, et al: Cereal dietary fiber consumption and diverticular disease: A lifespan study in rats. Am J Clin Nutr 42:788, 1985.
36. Gear JS, Ware A, Fursdon P, et al: Symptomless diverticular disease and intake of dietary fibre. Lancet 1:511, 1979.
37. Lin OS, Soon MS, Wu SS, et al: Dietary habits and right-sided colonic diverticulosis. Dis Colon Rectum 43:1412, 2000.
38. Aldoori WH, Giovannucci EL, Rimm EB, et al: A prospective study of diet and the risk of symptomatic diverticular disease in men. Am J Clin Nutr 60:757, 1994.
39. Aldoori WH, Giovannucci EL, Rockett HR, et al: A prospective study of dietary fiber types and symptomatic diverticular disease in men. J Nutr 128:714, 1998.
40. Nakama H, Fattah AS, Zhang B, et al: Association of diverticulosis coli and vascular ectasias and the results of fecal occult blood test. Hepatogastroenterology 47:1277, 2000.
41. Boulos PB, Karamanolis DG, Salmon PR, Clark CG: Is colonoscopy necessary in diverticular disease? Lancet 1:95, 1984.
42. Brayko CM, Kozarek RA, Sanowski RA, Howells T: Diverticular rupture during colonoscopy: Fact or fancy? Dig Dis Sci 29:427, 1984.
43. Bat L, Williams CB: Usefulness of pediatric colonoscopes in adult colonoscopy. Gastrointest Endosc 35:329, 1989.
44. Kaffes AJ, Mishra A, Ding SL, et al: A prospective trial of variable stiffness pediatric vs. standard instrument colonoscopy. Gastrointest Endosc 58:685, 2003.
45. Falchuk ZM, Griffin PH: A technique to facilitate colonoscopy in areas of severe diverticular disease. N Engl J Med 310:598, 1984.

46. Glick SN: Inverted colonic diverticulum: Air contrast barium enema findings in six cases. AJR Am J Roentgenol 156:961, 1991.

47. Ladas SD, Prigouris SP, Pantelidaki C, Raptis A: Endoscopic removal of inverted sigmoid diverticulum: Is it a dangerous procedure? Endoscopy 21:243, 1989.

48. Otte JJ, Larsen L, Andersen JR: Irritable bowel syndrome and symptomatic diverticular disease: Different diseases? Am J Gastroenterol 81:529, 1986.

49. Ritchie J: Similarity of bowel distension characteristics in the irritable colon syndrome and diverticulosis. Gut 18:A990, 1977.

50. Brodribb AJ: Treatment of symptomatic diverticular disease with a high-fibre diet. Lancet 1:664, 1977.

51. Ornstein MH, Littlewood ER, Baird IM, et al: Are fibre supplements really necessary in diverticular disease of the colon? A controlled clinical trial. BMJ 282:1353, 1981.

52. Horgan AF, McConnell EJ, Wolff BG, et al: Atypical diverticular disease: Surgical results. Dis Colon Rectum 44:1315, 2001.

53. Berman LG, Burdick D, Heitzman ER, Prior JT: A critical reappraisal of sigmoid peridiverticulitis. Surg Gynecol Obstet 127:481, 1968.

54. Roberts P, Abel M, Rosen L, et al: Practice parameters for sigmoid diverticulitis: The Standards Task Force American Society of Colon and Rectal Surgeons. Dis Colon Rectum 38:126, 1995.

55. Morson BC: Pathology of diverticular disease of the colon. Clin Gastroenterol 4:37, 1975.

56. Boirivant M, Marini M, Di Felice G, et al: Lamina propria T cells in Crohn's disease and other gastrointestinal inflammation show defective CD2 pathway-induced apoptosis. Gastroenterology 116:557, 1999.

57. Williams RA, Davis I.P: Diverticular disease of the colon. In Haubrick WS, Schaffner F (eds): Bockus Gastroenterology. Philadelphia, WB Saunders, 1995, p 1637.

58. Hart AR, Kennedy HJ, Stebbings WS, Day NE: How frequently do large bowel diverticula perforate? An incidence and cross-sectional study. Eur J Gastroenterol Hepatol 12:661, 2000.

59. Hinchey EJ, Schaal PG, Richards GK: Treatment of perforated diverticular disease of the colon. Adv Surg 12:85, 1978.

60. Markham NI, Li AK: Diverticulitis of the right colon—experience from Hong Kong. Gut 33:547, 1992.

61. Ambrosetti P, Robert JH, Witzig JA, et al: Acute left colonic diverticulitis: A prospective analysis of 226 consecutive cases. Surgery 115:546, 1994.

62. Bahadursingh AM, Virgo KS, Kaminski DL, Longo WE: Spectrum of disease and outcome of complicated diverticular disease. Am J Surg 186:696, 2003.

63. Wexner SD, Dailey TH: The initial management of left lower quadrant peritonitis. Dis Colon Rectum 29:635, 1986.

64. Kourtesis GJ, Williams RA, Wilson SE: Surgical options in acute diverticulitis: Value of sigmoid resection in dealing with the septic focus. Aust N Z J Surg 58:955, 1988.

65. Morris J, Stellato TA, Lieberman J, Haaga JR: The utility of computed tomography in colonic diverticulitis. Ann Surg 204:128, 1986.

66. Doringer E: Computerized tomography of colonic diverticulitis. Crit Rev Diagn Imaging 33:421, 1992.

67. McKee RF, Deignan RW, Krukowski ZH: Radiological investigation in acute diverticulitis. Br J Surg 80:560, 1993.

68. Shrier D, Skucas J, Weiss S: Diverticulitis: An evaluation by computed tomography and contrast enema. Am J Gastroenterol 86:1466, 1991.

69. Hulnick DH, Megibow AJ, Balthazar EJ, et al: Computed tomography in the evaluation of diverticulitis. Radiology 152:491, 1984.

70. Ambrosetti P, Jenny A, Becker C, et al: Acute left colonic diverticulitis—compared performance of computed tomography and water-soluble contrast enema: Prospective evaluation of 420 patients. Dis Colon Rectum 43:1363, 2000.

71. Werner A, Diehl SJ, Farag-Soliman M, Duber C: Multi-slice spiral CT in routine diagnosis of suspected acute left-sided colonic diverticulitis: A prospective study of 120 patients. Eur Radiol 13:2596, 2003.

72. Jang HJ, Lim HK, Lee SJ, et al: Acute diverticulitis of the cecum and ascending colon: The value of thin-section helical CT findings in excluding colonic carcinoma. AJR Am J Roentgenol 174:1397, 2000.

73. Jang HJ, Lim HK, Lee SJ, et al: Acute diverticulitis of the cecum and ascending colon: Thin-section helical CT findings. AJR Am J Roentgenol 172:601, 1999.

74. Johnson CD, Baker ME, Rice RP, et al: Diagnosis of acute colonic diverticulitis: Comparison of barium enema and CT. AJR Am J Roentgenol 148:541, 1987.

75. Stefansson T, Nyman R, Nilsson S, et al: Diverticulitis of the sigmoid colon: A comparison of CT, colonic enema, and laparoscopy. Acta Radiol 38:313, 1997.

76. Verbanck J, Lambrecht S, Rutgeerts L, et al: Can sonography diagnose acute colonic diverticulitis in patients with acute intestinal inflammation? A prospective study. J Clin Ultrasound 17:661, 1989.

77. Zielke A, Hasse C, Nies C, et al: Prospective evaluation of ultrasonography in acute colonic diverticulitis. Br J Surg 84:385, 1997.

78. Wilson SR, Toi A: The value of sonography in the diagnosis of acute diverticulitis of the colon. AJR Am J Roentgenol 154:1199, 1990.

79. Pradel JA, Adell JF, Taourel P, et al: Acute colonic diverticulitis: Prospective comparative evaluation with US and CT. Radiology 205:503, 1997.

80. Brook I, Frazier EH: Aerobic and anaerobic microbiology in intra-abdominal infections associated with diverticulitis. J Med Microbiol 49:827, 2000.

81. Chow AW: Appendicitis and diverticulitis. In Hoeprich PD, Jordan MC, Ronald AR (eds): Infectious Diseases: A Treatise of Infectious Processes. Philadelphia, JB Lippincott, 1994, p 878.

82. Tursi A: Acute diverticulitis of the colon: Current medical therapeutic management. Expert Opin Pharmacother 5:55, 2004.

83. Zarling EJ, Piontek F, Klemka-Walden L, Inczauskis D: The effect of gastroenterology training on the efficiency and cost of care provided to patients with diverticulitis. Gastroenterology 112:1859, 1997.

84. Wong WD, Wexner SD, Lowry A, et al: Practice parameters for the treatment of sigmoid diverticulitis: The Standards Task Force American Society of Colon and Rectal Surgeons. Dis Colon Rectum 43:290, 2000.

85. Kohler L, Sauerland S, Neugebauer E: Diagnosis and treatment of diverticular disease: Results of a consensus development conference. The Scientific Committee of the European Association for Endoscopic Surgery. Surg Endosc 13:430, 1999.

86. Guller U, Jain N, Hervey S, et al: Laparoscopic vs open colectomy: Outcomes comparison based on large nationwide databases. Arch Surg 138:1179, 2003.

87. Stollman NH, Raskin JB: Diagnosis and management of diverticular disease of the colon in adults. Ad Hoc Practice Parameters Committee of the American College of Gastroenterology. Am J Gastroenterol 94:3110, 1999.

88. DiMario F, Aragona G, Leandro G, et al: Efficacy of mesalamine in the treatment of symptomatic diverticular disease. Dig Dis Sci 50:581, 2005.

89. Tursi A, Brandimarte G, Daffina R: Long-term treatment with mesalamine and rifaximin versus rifaximin alone for patients with recurrent attacks of acute diverticulitis of colon. Dig Liver Dis 34:510, 2002.

90. Tursi A: Acute diverticulitis of the colon—current medical therapeutic management. Expert Opin Pharmacother 5:55, 2004.

91. Thorn M, Graf W, Stefansson T, Pahlman L: Clinical and functional results after elective colonic resection in 75 consecutive patients with diverticular disease. Am J Surg 183:7, 2002.

92. Frizelle FA, Dominguez JM, Santoro GA: Management of post-operative recurrent diverticulitis: A review of the literature. J R Coll Surg Edinb 42:186, 1997.

93. Thaler K, Dinnewitzer A, Mascha E, et al: Long-term outcome and health-related quality of life after laparoscopic and open colectomy for benign disease: Determinants of recurrence after sigmoid resection for uncomplicated diverticulitis. Surg Endosc 17:1404, 2003.

94. Reisman Y, Ziv Y, Kravrovitc D, et al: Diverticulitis: The effect of age and location on the course of disease. Int J Colorectal Dis 14:250, 1999.

95. Konvolinka CW: Acute diverticulitis under age forty. Am J Surg 167:562, 1994.

96. Chautems RC, Ambrosetti P, Ludwig A, et al: Long-term follow-up after first acute episode of sigmoid diverticulitis: Is surgery mandatory?—a prospective study of 118 patients. Dis Colon Rectum 45:962, 2002.

97. Spivak H, Weinrauch S, Harvey JC, et al: Acute colonic diverticulitis in the young. Dis Colon Rectum 40:570, 1997.

98. Perkins JD, Shield CF III, Chang FC, Farha GJ: Acute diverticulitis: Comparison of treatment in immunocompromised and nonimmunocompromised patients. Am J Surg 148:745, 1984.

99. Tyau ES, Prystowsky JB, Joehl RJ, Nahrwold DL: Acute diverticulitis: A complicated problem in the immunocompromised patient. Arch Surg 126:855, 1991.

100. Lederman ED, Conti DJ, Lempert N, et al: Complicated diverticulitis following renal transplantation. Dis Colon Rectum 41:613, 1998.

101. Maurer JR: The spectrum of colonic complications in a lung transplant population. Ann Transplant 5:54, 2000.

102. Khan S, Eppstein AC, Anderson GK, et al: Acute diverticulitis in heart and lung transplant patients. Transpl Int 14:12, 2001.

103. Nirula R, Greaney G: Right-sided diverticulitis: A difficult diagnosis. Am Surg 63:871, 1997.

104. Violi V, Roncoroni L, Boselli AS, et al: Diverticulitis of the caecum and ascending colon: An unavoidable diagnostic pitfall? Int Surg 85:39, 2000.

105. Komuta K, Yamanaka S, Okada K, et al: Toward therapeutic guidelines for patients with acute right colonic diverticulitis. Am J Surg 187:233, 2004.

106. Ambrosetti P, Robert J, Witzig JA, et al. Incidence, outcome, and proposed management of isolated abscesses complicating acute left-sided colonic diverticulitis: A prospective study of 140 patients. Dis Colon Rectum 35:1072, 1992.

107. Saini S, Mueller PR, Wittenberg J, et al: Percutaneous drainage of diverticular abscess: An adjunct to surgical therapy. Arch Surg 121:475, 1986.

108. Stabile BE, Puccio E, van Sonnenberg E, Neff CC: Preoperative percutaneous drainage of diverticular abscesses. Am J Surg 159:99, 1990.

109. Schechter S, Eisenstat TE, Oliver GC, et al: Computerized tomographic scan-guided drainage of intra-abdominal abscesses: Preoperative and postoperative modalities in colon and rectal surgery. Dis Colon Rectum 37:984, 1994.

110. Desai DC, Brennan EJ Jr, Reilly JF, Smink RD Jr: The utility of the Hartmann procedure. Am J Surg 175:152, 1998.

111. Hackford AW, Schoetz DJ Jr, Coller JA, Veidenheimer MC: Surgical management of complicated diverticulitis: The Lahey Clinic experience, 1967 to 1982. Dis Colon Rectum 28:317, 1985.

112. Fleites RA, Marshall JB, Eckhauser ML, et al: The efficacy of polyethylene glycol-electrolyte lavage solution versus traditional mechanical bowel preparation for elective colonic surgery: A randomized, prospective, blinded clinical trial. Surgery 98:708, 1985.

113. Lee EC, Murray JJ, Coller JA, et al: Intraoperative colonic lavage in nonelective surgery for diverticular disease. Dis Colon Rectum 40:669, 1997.

114. Wedell J, Banzhaf G, Chaoui R, et al: Surgical management of complicated colonic diverticulitis. Br J Surg 84:380, 1997.

115. Wolff BG, Devine RM: Surgical management of diverticulitis. Am Surg 66:153, 2000.

116. Krukowski ZH, Matheson NA: Emergency surgery for diverticular disease complicated by generalized and faecal peritonitis: A review. Br J Surg 71:921, 1984.

117. Nagorney DM, Adson MA, Pemberton JH: Sigmoid diverticulitis with perforation and generalized peritonitis. Dis Colon Rectum 28:71, 1985.

118. Kronborg O: Treatment of perforated sigmoid diverticulitis: A prospective randomized trial. Br J Surg 80:505, 1993.

119. Zeitoun G, Laurent A, Rouffet F, et al: Multicentre, randomized clinical trial of primary versus secondary sigmoid resection in generalized peritonitis complicating sigmoid diverticulitis. Br J Surg 87:1366, 2000.

120. Rothenberger DA, Wiltz O: Surgery for complicated diverticulitis. Surg Clin North Am 73:975, 1993.

121. Woods RJ, Lavery IC, Fazio VW, et al: Internal fistulas in diverticular disease. Dis Colon Rectum 31:591, 1988.

122. McBeath RB, Schiff M Jr, Allen V, et al: A 12-year experience with enterovesical fistulas. Urology 44:661, 1994.

123. Forde KA, Treat MR: Colonoscopy in the evaluation of strictures. Dis Colon Rectum 28:699, 1985.

124. Kozarek RA: Hydrostatic balloon dilation of gastrointestinal stenoses: A national survey. Gastrointest Endosc 32:15, 1986.

125. Blomberg B, Rolny P, Jarnerot G: Endoscopic treatment of anastomotic strictures in Crohn's disease. Endoscopy 23:195, 1991.

126. Tamim WZ, Ghellai A, Counihan TC, et al: Experience with endoluminal colonic wall stents for the management of large bowel obstruction for benign and malignant disease. Arch Surg 135:434, 2000.

127. Boley SJ, DiBiase A, Brandt LJ, Sammartano RJ: Lower intestinal bleeding in the elderly. Am J Surg 137:57, 1979.

128. Potter GD, Sellin JH: Lower gastrointestinal bleeding. Gastroenterol Clin North Am 17:341, 1988.

129. Gostout CJ, Wang KK, Ahlquist DA, et al: Acute gastrointestinal bleeding: Experience of a specialized management team. J Clin Gastroenterol 14:260, 1992.

130. Elta GH: Urgent colonoscopy for acute lower GI bleeding. Gastrointest Endosc 59:402, 2004.

131. Longstreth GF: Epidemiology and outcome of patients hospitalized with acute lower gastrointestinal hemorrhage: A population-based study. Am J Gastroenterol 92:419, 1997.

132. Peura DA, Lanza FL, Gostout CJ, Foutch PG: The American College of Gastroenterology Bleeding Registry: Preliminary findings. Am J Gastroenterol 92:924, 1997.

133. McGuire HH Jr, Haynes BW Jr: Massive hemorrhage for diverticulosis of the colon: Guidelines for therapy based on bleeding patterns observed in fifty cases. Ann Surg 175:847, 1972.

134. Zuckerman GR, Prakash C: Acute lower intestinal bleeding: II. Etiology, therapy, and outcomes. Gastrointest Endosc 49:228, 1999.

135. Casarella WJ, Kanter IE, Seaman WB: Right-sided colonic diverticula as a cause of acute rectal hemorrhage. N Engl J Med 286:450, 1972.

136. McGuire HH Jr: Bleeding colonic diverticula: A reappraisal of natural history and management. Ann Surg 220:653, 1994.

137. Wong SK, Ho YH, Leong AP, Seow-Choen F: Clinical behavior of complicated right-sided and left-sided diverticulosis. Dis Colon Rectum 40:344, 1997.

138. Meyers MA, Alonso DR, Gray GF, Baer JW: Pathogenesis of bleeding colonic diverticulosis. Gastroenterology 71:577, 1976.

139. Wilcox CM, Alexander LN, Cotsonis GA, Clark WS: Nonsteroidal anti-inflammatory drugs are associated with both upper and lower gastrointestinal bleeding. Dig Dis Sci 42:990, 1997.

140. Aldoori WH, Giovannucci EL, Rimm EB, et al: Use of acetaminophen and nonsteroidal anti-inflammatory drugs: A prospective study and the risk of symptomatic diverticular disease in men. Arch Fam Med 7:255, 1998.

141. Goh H, Bourne R: Non-steroidal anti-inflammatory drugs and perforated diverticular disease: A case-control study. Ann R Coll Surg Engl 84:93, 2002.

142. Wilson RG, Smith AN, Macintyre IM: Complications of diverticular disease and non-steroidal anti-inflammatory drugs: A prospective study. Br J Surg 77:1103, 1990.

143. Campbell K, Steele RJ: Non-steroidal anti-inflammatory drugs and complicated diverticular disease: A case-control study. Br J Surg 78:190, 1991.

144. Laine L, Connors LG, Reicin A, et al: Serious lower gastrointestinal clinical events with nonselective NSAID or coxib use. Gastroenterology 124:288, 2003.

145. Zuccaro G Jr: Management of the adult patient with acute lower gastrointestinal bleeding: American College of Gastroenterology Practice Parameters Committee. Am J Gastroenterol 93:1202, 1998.

146. Jensen DM, Machicado GA: Diagnosis and treatment of severe hematochezia: The role of urgent colonoscopy after purge. Gastroenterology 95:1569, 1988.

147. Foutch PG, Rex DK, Lieberman DA: Diverticular bleeding: Are nonsteroidal anti-inflammatory drugs risk factors for hemorrhage and can colonoscopy predict outcome for patients? Am J Gastroenterol 90:1779, 1995.

148. Bertoni G, Conigliaro R, Ricci E, et al: Endoscopic injection hemostasis of colonic diverticular bleeding: A case report. Endoscopy 22:154, 1990.

149. Johnston J, Sones J: Endoscopic heater probe coagulation of the bleeding colonic diverticulum. Gastrointest Endosc 32:160, 1986.

150. Savides TJ, Jensen DM: Colonoscopic hemostasis for recurrent diverticular hemorrhage associated with a visible vessel: A report of three cases. Gastrointest Endosc 40:70, 1994.

151. Foutch PG, Zimmerman K: Diverticular bleeding and the pigmented protuberance (sentinel clot): Clinical implications, histopathological correlation, and results of endoscopic intervention. Am J Gastroenterol 91:2589, 1996.

152. Jensen DM, Machicado GA, Jutabha R, Kovacs TO: Urgent colonoscopy for the diagnosis and treatment of severe diverticular hemorrhage. N Engl J Med 342:78, 2000.

153. Hokama A, Uehara T, Nakayoshi T, et al: Utility of endoscopic hemoclipping for colonic diverticular bleeding. Am J Gastroenterol 92:543, 1997.

154. Andress HJ, Mewes A, Lange V: Endoscopic hemostasis of a bleeding diverticulum of the sigma with fibrin sealant. Endoscopy 25:193, 1993.

155. Farrell JJ, Graeme-Cook F, Kelsey PB: Treatment of bleeding colonic diverticula by endoscopic band ligation: An in-vivo and ex-vivo pilot study. Endoscopy 35:823, 2003.

156. Smoot RL, Gostout CJ, Rajan E, et al: Is early colonoscopy after admission for acute diverticular bleeding needed? Am J Gastroenterol 98:1996, 2003.

157. Yamaguchi T, Yoshikawa K: Enhanced CT for initial localization of active lower gastrointestinal bleeding. Abdom Imaging 28:634, 2003.

158. O'Neill BB, Gosnell JE, Lull RJ, et al: Cinematic nuclear scintigraphy reliably directs surgical intervention for patients with gastrointestinal bleeding. Arch Surg 135:1076, 2000.

159. Hunter JM, Pezim ME: Limited value of technetium 99m-labeled red cell scintigraphy in localization of lower gastrointestinal bleeding. Am J Surg 159:504,. 1990.

160. Alavi A, Ring EJ: Localization of gastrointestinal bleeding: superiority of ^{99m}Tc sulfur colloid compared with angiography. AJR Am J Roentgenol 137:741, 1981.

161. DeBarros J, Rosas L, Cohen J, et al: The changing paradigm for the treatment of colonic hemorrhage: Superselective angiographic embolization. Dis Colon Rectum 45:802, 2002.

162. Gordon RL, Ahl KL, Kerlan RK, et al: Selective arterial embolization for the control of lower gastrointestinal bleeding. Am J Surg 174:24, 1997.

163. Gady JS, Reynolds H, Blum A: Selective arterial embolization for control of lower gastrointestinal bleeding: Recommendations for a clinical management pathway. Curr Surg 60:344, 2003.

164. Browder W, Cerise EJ, Litwin MS: Impact of emergency angiography in massive lower gastrointestinal bleeding. Ann Surg 204:530, 1986.

165. Cohn SM, Moller BA, Zieg PM, et al: Angiography for preoperative evaluation in patients with lower gastrointestinal bleeding: Are the benefits worth the risks? Arch Surg 133:50, 1998.

166. Setya V, Singer JA, Minken SL: Subtotal colectomy as a last resort for unrelenting, unlocalized, lower gastrointestinal hemorrhage: Experience with 12 cases. Am Surg 58:295, 1992.

167. Farner R, Lichliter W, Kuhn J, et al: Total colectomy versus limited colonic resection for acute lower intestinal bleeding. Am J Surg 178:587, 1999.

168. Renzulli P, Maurer CA, Netzer P, et al: Subtotal colectomy with primary ileorectoscopy is effective for unlocalized, diverticular hemorrhage. Lagenbeck's Arch Surg 387:67, 2002.

CHAPTER
115 Irritable Bowel Syndrome

Nicholas J. Talley

Irritable bowel syndrome (IBS) is important because of its high prevalence, substantial morbidity, and enormous costs.[1-3] In the United States, approximately 12% of patients seen by primary care physicians have IBS, but it is likely that this frequency is an underestimate.[4-6] In gastrointestinal practices, more than one third of patients have functional gastrointestinal disorders, IBS being the most frequent diagnosis.[7] Because a substantial proportion of gastroenterology practice comprises patients with IBS or other functional gastrointestinal disorders, it is essential that clinicians develop expertise in diagnosing and treating IBS. The diagnosis of IBS rests on making a positive clinical diagnosis from the history; that tests often are not needed represents an important conceptual advance.[8] There is increasing evidence that at least a subset of IBS has an organic gastrointestinal tract basis.[9] Nonetheless, only symptom-directed therapy rather than disease-modifying treatments are available; the evidence base for current therapy has strengthened considerably with the publication of well-performed meta-analyses (see later). In this chapter, current knowledge of the epidemiology and pathophysiology of IBS is reviewed to provide a rational basis for its diagnosis and therapy.

DEFINITIONS

IBS is characterized by the presence of abdominal discomfort or pain associated with disturbed defecation.[3] Bloating or visible abdominal distention often are present in patients with IBS but are not considered essential symptoms for diagnosis.[3]

In a classic study from the United Kingdom, Manning and associates first reported that six symptoms were more frequent in those subsequently documented to have IBS, although only four were statistically significant in the initial report (Table 115-1).[10] Later studies showed that these symptoms were specific, but not sensitive, for identifying IBS and were of greater diagnostic value in women.[11,12] In an effort to build on the diagnostic utility of the Manning criteria, the Rome (I and II) criteria were created following a formal consensus process to provide a standard for clinical research (see Table 115-1).[3] Despite limited data on validity, it was proposed subsequently that the Rome criteria be used in clinical practice.[1] Comparisons of the criteria have shown that both the Rome I and Rome II criteria identify similar patient populations, although the Rome II criteria appear to be more restrictive in some studies.[13-15] The Manning criteria identify additional patients with IBS-like symptoms who arguably also should be classified as true IBS.[13-15]

Table 115–1   Comparison of the Major Diagnostic Criteria for the Irritable Bowel Syndrome (IBS)

Manning Criteria	Rome I Criteria	Rome II Criteria
Abdominal pain that is relieved after a bowel movement* Looser stool at pain onset* More frequent stools at pain onset* Abdominal distention (visible)* Sensation of incomplete rectal evacuation Passage of mucus	≥3 mo of continuous or recurrent symptoms of abdominal pain or discomfort relieved with defecation or associated with change in frequency or consistency of stool *and* Disturbed defecation (≥ 2 of the following): Altered stool frequency Altered stool form (hard or loose/watery) Altered stool passage (straining or urgency, feeling of incomplete evacuation) Passage of mucus Bloating or feeling of abdominal distention	≥ 12 wk, which need not be consecutive, in the preceding 12 mo of abdominal discomfort or pain that has at least 2 of the 3 following features: Relieved with defecation Onset associated with a change in frequency of stool Onset associated with a change in stool form

*Significant discriminators in original report.
Adapted from Drossman DA, Corrazziari E, Talley NJ, et al: Rome II: The Functional Gastrointestinal Disorders, 2nd ed. McLean, VA, Degnon, 2000; and Manning AP, Thompson WG, Heaton KW, Morris AF: Towards positive diagnosis of the irritable bowel. BMJ 2:653, 1978.

CLINICAL FEATURES

HISTORY

Abdominal Discomfort or Pain

IBS should not be diagnosed in the absence of abdominal discomfort or pain.[3] Distinguishing discomfort from pain can be problematic for both the patient and physician, however, because of the strong influence of cultural issues. In the United States, what a physician may label as mild pain often is considered discomfort by the patient. The pain or discomfort in IBS typically is relieved by defecation, or its onset is associated with an increase or decrease in stool frequency or looser or harder stools. The pain often is poorly localized, waxes and wanes, may be aggravated by eating, and can occur in any part of the abdomen, although it more typically is located in the lower abdomen; it may be referred to different areas in the abdomen or to the chest or back. Exacerbation of pain by life events or difficult life situations is common. Abdominal discomfort or pain that is continuous or unrelated to defecation or induced by menstruation, urination, or physical activity is unlikely to be caused by IBS.

Constipation and Diarrhea

Patients with IBS experience constipation, diarrhea or alternating constipation or diarrhea; typically bowel symptoms are variable and intermittent.[3] The terms *constipation* and *diarrhea* may reflect a wide variety of different symptom experiences to different patients, and so whenever a patient uses them, an exploration of their meaning is required.[16] Any combination of infrequent defecation, passage of hard stools, excessive straining, feelings of incomplete rectal evacuation, or rectal discomfort may be referred to as constipation, whereas increased stool frequency, urgency, or the passage of liquid or watery stools, or even more frequent small hard stools, may be referred to as diarrhea by the patient. Stool form can be measured objectively and graded by patient or physician; the Bristol stool form scale now is routinely used in clinical trials, and changes in stool form (at the

extreme ends of the scale) roughly correlate with colonic transit time.[17,18]

Bloating and Visible Distention

A feeling of bloating is common in IBS, and its site can be difficult for the patient to localize. Visible abdominal distention is characteristic but less common; it can be objectively measured and usually is not imagined.[19] Gas can mean excess bloating, belching, flatus, or even reflux symptoms to the patient. Again, it is important that patients are asked to explain the meaning of the terms they are using to describe their symptoms.

Noncolonic Symptoms

Other clinical features can help support the diagnosis of IBS but in themselves are not diagnostic. Nausea is common and at least one third of patients with IBS have epigastric discomfort or pain (dyspepsia).[1,8] Extracolonic symptoms including headache, backache, impaired sleep, fatigue, increased urinary frequency or urgency, and dyspareunia are more common in patients with IBS but have no accepted diagnostic value.[1,20] Comorbid anxiety or depression, and fibromyalgia also are associated with IBS.[1]

Chronicity

For a confident diagnosis of IBS, symptoms should have been present for at least 6 months; IBS may accompany other chronic disorders. For example, IBS is present in one third or more of patients with inflammatory bowel disease in remission.[21] A number of different conditions may cause transient bowel symptoms including pregnancy, dietary indiscretion, food poisoning, traveler's diarrhea, bed rest, weight loss, and acute stress (nervous diarrhea); these should be distinguished from the chronic, recurrent symptoms of IBS.

PHYSICAL EXAMINATION

The physical examination in IBS usually is normal, although deep tenderness over the colon may be appreciated. Abdominal wall pain should be excluded clinically; if tensing the abdominal wall muscles increases abdominal tenderness, this suggests a point of localized abdominal wall abnormality (Carnett's test).[22,23] Ovarian cancer also needs to be considered in any middle-aged or older woman presenting with new-onset IBS-like symptoms.[24] A pelvic examination may, therefore, be relevant to determine if there is any irregular, fixed pelvic mass.

EPIDEMIOLOGY

IBS is a common disorder all over the world.[15,25] Epidemiologic studies have defined the prevalence and identified potential risk factors for IBS, but there remains a lack of adequate data on the incidence of IBS (the rate of development of IBS in those previously unaffected).

PREVALENCE

Prevalence estimates for IBS have varied anywhere from 3% to 20% in the United States, with similar results reported elsewhere; however, prevalence estimates are influenced substantially by the definition applied. For example, Saito and associates noted in Olmsted County, Minnesota, that the prevalence of IBS varied from 8% to 22% depending on the criteria used.[26]

Younger people have a higher prevalence of IBS in the community. Generally, it is believed that IBS is uncommon in the elderly, but population-based studies indicate IBS increases with advancing age. Thus, for example, using three or more of the Manning criteria to define IBS, the prevalence of IBS in Olmsted County ranged from 8% in those 65 to 74 years of age to more than 12% in those older than 85 years.[27] Obviously, organic disease is more prevalent in elderly persons and could account for some of the reported IBS-like symptoms, but it seems likely that IBS in the elderly is often underdiagnosed or misclassified as diverticular disease, by example.[28]

GENDER AND RACE

The gender specific prevalence rates are approximately two female to one male in most studies, and all population-based studies have reported a female predominance.[15,29] Healthy women have greater rectal sensitivity, slower colonic transit, and smaller stool outputs than do men, which may explain why certain symptoms, such as straining and passage of hard stools, seem to be more common in women.[30,31] In clinical practice in the United States, women outnumber men, which partly is explained by increased health care-seeking behavior among women; this appears to be culturally derived, because data from India indicate more men than women present for care of IBS in that part of the world; this does not mean that more men than women have IBS in the general population in India.[27]

The prevalence of IBS generally is similar in whites and blacks, although some data have suggested it may be lower in Hispanics than in non-Hispanic whites in the United States.[32,33] IBS is common in China, Japan, South America, and the Indian subcontinent. Indeed, IBS is common and its prevalence comparable in all countries where it has been studied.[34-37]

SUBGROUPS

Subdividing IBS based on the predominant symptom pattern is attempted commonly, but little data are available on IBS prevalence by symptom subgroup. Moreover, it is unclear if those with one predominant symptom (i.e., diarrhea or constipation), if followed long enough, eventually develop the other (i.e., constipation or diarrhea), but some data from primary care support this contention.[38] Also, definitions of IBS subgroups remain arbitrary and have not been based on pathophysiologic data, and different definitions have been used in different studies. Nonetheless, in a study from Olmsted County, Minnesota, 5.5% of the population had diarrhea-predominant IBS and 5% constipation-predominant IBS; both diarrhea and constipation-type symptoms occurred in 5%, whereas 4% did not meet strict criteria for either constipation or diarrhea.[39] Another population-based study found higher rates of constipation in community subjects with IBS.[40]

INCIDENCE AND DISAPPEARANCE OF SYMPTOMS

The onset rate of IBS was 67 per 1000 person-years by applying the Manning criteria to a cohort in Olmsted County that was surveyed at a 12- to 20-month interval.[41] This study did not exclude people with a past history of IBS, however, and hence this is not the true incidence rate. Another study reported that the incidence of a clinical diagnosis of IBS in Olmsted County was 0.2% per year, which reflects the lower end of the incidence rate because people with IBS symptoms who did not seek consultation were not able to be included in this calculation.[42]

In a follow-up study in Olmsted County, 38% of subjects meeting the definition of IBS at entry did not meet these criteria 12 to 20 months later.[41] The actual prevalence of IBS did not change from year to year, however, because the disappearance of symptoms in some patients with IBS was balanced by others who developed IBS. Among those losing IBS in the community, there also may be a subset in whom symptoms evolve to reflect another functional gastrointestinal disorder, especially dyspepsia.[43] Data on the flux of symptom groups in clinic patients, however, are sparse. Hence, IBS usually is a chronic disorder, although symptoms frequently are variable.

RISK FACTORS

The best accepted risk factor for IBS is bacterial gastroenteritis.[44-46] Depression,[47] adverse life events and hypochondriasis,[48] female gender, younger age, and prolonged duration of diarrhea following the initial attack[49] have been reported to increase the risk of postinfectious IBS. Bacterial factors also may be important, and there is evidence to suggest postinfectious IBS more commonly follows infection with *Campylobacter* than with other pathogens. Other possible risk factors for IBS include an affluent childhood environment,[50] estrogen use postmenopausally,[51] recent antibiotic use,[52] food intolerance,[53,54] and extraintestinal somatic symptoms.[54] In contrast, oral glucocorticoid users may be at a lower risk of IBS.[55] IBS is associated with an approximately threefold increased risk of ischemic colitis[56]; however, a cause-and-effect relationship has not been established and the absolute risk remains very small (43 per 100,000 person years).

HEALTH CARE SEEKING

Understanding why a patient is presenting for care is important in terms of planning appropriate management strategies. The rate of health care seeking for IBS may in part be affected by health care access; consulting rates in the United States have varied between 25% and 46%, but up to 40% of patients do not have easy access to health care in this country.[57] In Australia, consulting rates have been 73% where health care access essentially is universal.[57]

Drivers of health care seeking remain poorly documented.[57] The severity and chronicity of symptoms, in particular abdominal pain, partly promote health care seeking.[58,59] IBS patients are more concerned about their health and more fearful of illness, suggesting that anxiety about their illness may be another factor.[57] Children of a parent with IBS may see physicians more frequently than those who do not have a parent with IBS.[60] They also are more likely to report poorer health in childhood as well as greater parental attention and receipt of gifts or rewards for being ill, suggesting there may have been early childhood programming of abnormal illness behavior.[61] Those who seek medical attention tend to be more disturbed psychologically than nonconsultors,[62-65] and those who consult for IBS also are more likely to consult about relatively minor complaints as well as other nongastrointestinal somatic symptoms.[57] There remain other unknown factors that must be important, however, because these psychological factors still seem to poorly explain observed health care-seeking rates.[57]

EXCESS ABDOMINAL SURGERY

There is evidence that patients with IBS are at risk of undergoing excess surgery.[66-68] In a large health maintenance organization study, patients with IBS, compared with controls, reported more cholecystectomies (12% vs. 4%), appendectomies (21% vs. 12%), and hysterectomies (33% vs. 17%); IBS was associated independently with these operations.[66] A full explanation for these findings is uncertain, but presumably, some of this excess surgery reflects misdiagnosis and inappropriate intervention.[69] It is also possible that IBS could predispose to an excess of certain diseases that lead to surgery. For example, constipation is associated with an increased risk of gallstones,[70] but whether this association applies to constipation-predominant IBS is uncertain. Some surgeons continue to

believe that patients with IBS-type symptoms respond favorably to intra-abdominal surgery, although the evidence is anecdotal and probably reflects a placebo response.[69]

IMPACT ON QUALITY OF LIFE AND COSTS

A systematic review concluded that there was good evidence for a decrease in health-related quality of life (QOL) in patients with moderate-to-severe IBS[71] and that the QOL in IBS is impaired to a degree comparable with other chronic disorders such as depression or gastroesophageal reflux disease. The impact of IBS on QOL indicates that IBS deserves serious attention and therapeutic intervention; the data are more conflicting in terms of the impact of IBS on QOL in nonconsultors.[71]

IBS is associated with substantial costs because of days lost from work, excess physician visits, diagnostic testing, and use of medications.[72-74] Patients with IBS miss three times as many days from work as do those without bowel symptoms.[75] There are at least 2.4 to 3.5 million physician visits annually in the United States for IBS, with a minimum of 2.2 million prescriptions written.[76] A comprehensive burden of illness study in the United States estimated that IBS cost $1.6 billion in direct costs and a staggering $19.2 billion in indirect costs.[77]

PATHOPHYSIOLOGY

A number of different mechanisms have been implicated in the pathogenesis of IBS including abnormal motility, visceral hypersensitivity, low-grade inflammation, and stress.[1,8,78] Genetic factors could modulate the processing of gut signals centrally and the inflammatory and immune responses locally, possibly predisposing to IBS. It seems reasonable to postulate that for IBS to manifest, several abnormalities (multiple "hits") may need to occur. Some authors, therefore, conceptualize IBS as "a discrete collection of organic bowel diseases,"[8] whereas other experts are concerned about "organification" of IBS because it may reduce the emphasis on the biopsychosocial model[1,79] and imply that biologic factors are not sufficient to cause the disease. It seems likely in IBS that an understanding of the individual, including his or her psychosocial nature and response to environmental factors influences the expression of any biologic determinants (Fig. 115-1). Regardless, further major therapeutic advances in the field seem unlikely to occur until the specific biologic basis for symptoms is identified better.

ALTERED COLONIC AND SMALL BOWEL MOTILITY

In IBS, diarrhea may occur from multiple colonic mechanisms including increased high-amplitude propagated contractions (HAPCs), an enhanced gastrocolic response (prolonged rectosigmoid motor activity in response to a meal), or rectal hypersensitivity.[80-82] Constipation may be secondary to increased segmental (nonpropulsive) contractions or decreased HAPCs.[83,84] Colonic and small

Figure 115–1 A conceptual model depicting the relationship between early life, psychosocial factors, physiology, symptom experience, and behavior and outcome. IBS, irritable bowel syndrome. (Adapted from Drossman D, Camilleri M, Mayer E, Whitehead W: AGA technical review on irritable bowel syndrome. Gastroenterology 123: 2108, 2002.)

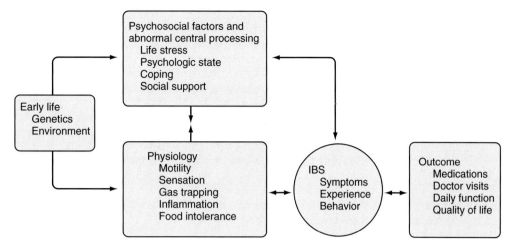

bowel transit has been documented to be delayed in IBS with constipation and accelerated in IBS with diarrhea, but not all studies concur.[1,85]

Abdominal pain in IBS also may be associated with HAPCs.[86] A greater increase in phasic contractions in the terminal ileum and colon has been observed following distention, fatty meals, and cholecystokinin in patients with IBS (Fig. 115–2A).[87] Discrete clusters of jejunal contractions also have been noted with increased frequency and duration in IBS (Fig. 115–2B), and have been associated with pain in limited numbers of IBS patients.[87]

Colonic motility in IBS can be increased by stress, anger, or instillation of deoxycholic acid, but this increase, alhtough greater than in controls, is not specific[1]; a greater increase in colonic phasic contractions has been observed following corticotropin-releasing hormone (CRH),[88] and this is improved by a CRH antagonist.[89] Patients with IBS also have greater small bowel motor stimulation than do controls after cholecystokinin infusion, a fatty meal, or ileal distention.[90] Autonomic dysfunction also has been reported in IBS patients with sympathetic adrenergic dysfunction associated with diarrhea and vagal dysfunction with constipation.[91]

Unfortunately, none of these motility parameters can be used as a diagnostic marker for IBS, and there remains no consensus on the exact patterns of motor derangement that actually induce constipation or diarrhea. It is possible that the motor abnormalities observed are secondary rather than primary in this disorder.

VISCERAL HYPERSENSITIVITY

More than 30 years ago, balloon distention in the rectum was shown to induce pain at lower volumes in patients with IBS[92]; this has been confirmed in multiple studies using the barostat balloon that controls for changes in compliance, leading to the suggestion that colonic hypersensitivity is a useful biologic marker of IBS.[93,94] Visceral hypersensitivity may explain the fact that IBS patients seem more likely than controls to be aware of the presence of gas or intestinal contractions after meals or stress. Visceral hypersensitivity probably is confined to the gut because somatic pain thresholds are normal, although not all studies agree.[95-97]

Visceral hypersensitivity is not a universal finding in patients with IBS but affects about 60% of patients (Fig. 115–3).[98] In contrast to control subjects, patients with IBS and normal baseline visceral hypersensitivity may have rectal hypersensitivity induced by repeated distention of the sigmoid colon.[99] This suggests that in IBS there is abnormal sensitization within the dorsal horn of the spinal cord or higher up in the central nervous system. Putative neurotransmitters that are of relevance include serotonin, neurokinins, and calcitonin gene-related peptide.[100] The N-methyl-D-aspartate (NMDA) receptor also may be important because it modulates central (spinal cord) neuronal excitability.[101] Visceral sensitivity, at least in the esophagus, can be reduced by a NMDA receptor antagonist. It is possible that inflammation is responsible for the sensitization in a subset with IBS, as discussed later; however, some of this decreased threshold to balloon distention may be attributed to hypervigilance or excessive attention to, or fear of, a painful stimulus.[102]

ABNORMAL GAS PROPULSION AND EXPULSION

Ambulatory monitoring of abdominal girth has revealed that the abdomen swells during the day, peaking in the late evening but decreasing on lying down; this phenomenon often is exaggerated in IBS.[103] Retention of gas following gas infusion into the small intestine is greater in patients with IBS than it is in healthy controls.[104] Furthermore, in those with IBS, intestinal gas infusion induces more discomfort than it does in controls when subjects are asked to voluntarily suppress passing the gas.[104] During gas infusion, IBS patients, in contrast to healthy controls, involuntarily suppress their abdominal wall muscle contraction, which may explain their tendency to become distended; this could reflect an abnormal intestinal-somatic reflex response.[105] Bacterial overgrowth has been speculated to contribute to bloating in IBS, but this is not established with certainty.[106] Intravenous neostigmine has been demonstrated to clear retained intestinal gas and to reduce abdominal symptoms in patients with IBS and functional bloating.[107] Physical activity may also enhance gas transit[108] and thus is to be encouraged.

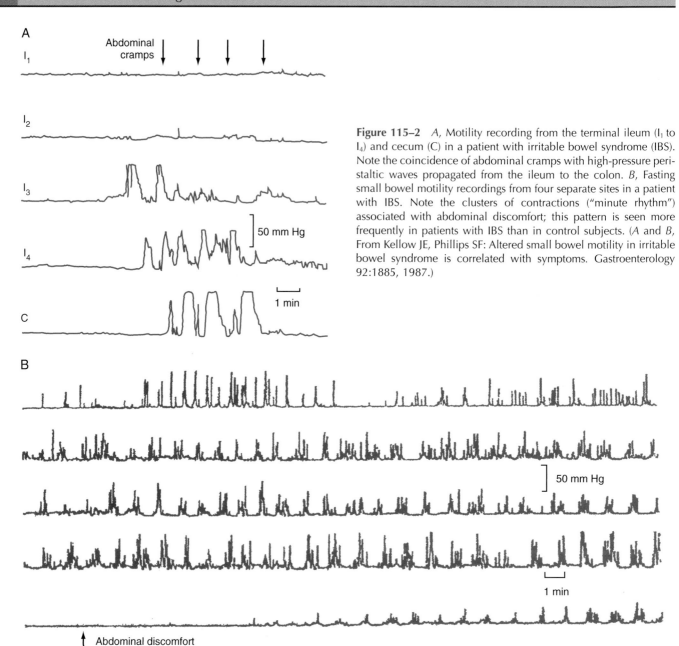

Figure 115–2   *A,* Motility recording from the terminal ileum (I_1 to I_4) and cecum (C) in a patient with irritable bowel syndrome (IBS). Note the coincidence of abdominal cramps with high-pressure peristaltic waves propagated from the ileum to the colon. *B,* Fasting small bowel motility recordings from four separate sites in a patient with IBS. Note the clusters of contractions ("minute rhythm") associated with abdominal discomfort; this pattern is seen more frequently in patients with IBS than in control subjects. (*A* and *B,* From Kellow JE, Phillips SF: Altered small bowel motility in irritable bowel syndrome is correlated with symptoms. Gastroenterology 92:1885, 1987.)

LOCAL INFLAMMATION

The normal intestine is chronically in a state of inflammation, which occurs because of the balance between commensal enteric organisms and the host immune system. Inflammatory cells, including mast cells,[109-111] and activated T lymphocytes[112,113] are increased above normal in the mucosa in a subset of patients with IBS, suggesting a low-grade inflammatory bowel disease may be present. Furthermore, lymphocytic infiltration of the myenteric plexus associated with neuron degeneration has been observed in severe IBS,[114] as have increased mast cells in the muscularis externa.[115] The cause of these abnormalities is unknown, but infections, abnormal bacterial flora, bile, or food antigens all could be contributors.

From 7% to 30% of patients who have recovered from a proved episode of bacterial enteritis may develop IBS.[44-49,116] One study, however, has suggested that those with preexisting IBS who develop gastroenteritis may be more likely to seek medical consultation, thereby inflating the apparent risk estimates of this group.[117] If the illness lasts more than 3 weeks or there are organisms involved that are toxigenic, then the risk of postinfectious IBS is increased.[116] Furthermore, those with psychological distress may have a further increased risk of postinfective IBS.[45,47,48] In those who develop postinfectious IBS, there are increases in CD3, CD4, and CD8 T lymphocytes, macrophages, and enteroendocrine (enterochromaffin) cells (Fig. 115–4).[47,112] Increased small intestinal permeability as demonstrated by the lactulose/mannitol test also has been reported to occur in

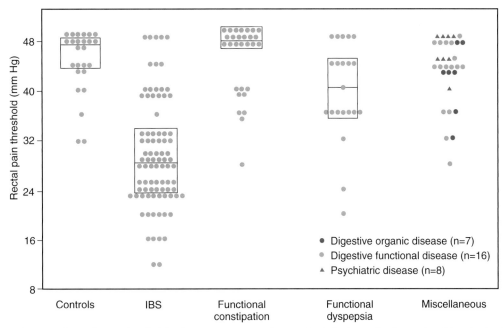

Figure 115–3   Distribution of rectal pain thresholds (distention pressure in mm Hg inducing pain) for each subject in the following groups: asymptomatic controls, irritable bowel syndrome (IBS), functional constipation, functional dyspepsia, and a miscellaneous group. *Black bars* and *boxes* represent median ±25% of patients. At the level of 40 mm Hg, the sensitivity of the rectal barostat to separate IBS patients from normal subjects and non-IBS patients was 95% and its specificity was 71.8%. (From Bouin M, Plourde V, Boivin M, et al: Rectal distention testing in patients with irritable bowel syndrome: Sensitivity, specificity, and predictive values of pain sensory thresholds. Gastroenterology 122:1771, 2002.)

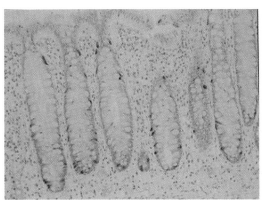

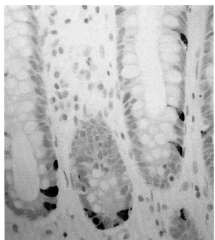

Figure 115–4   Enteroendocrine (enterochromaffin) cell hyperplasia in a rectal biopsy obtained from a patient with postinfective irritable bowel syndrome 3 months after *Campylobacter* enteritis. Synaptophysin-positive cells are brown, with blue hematoxylin counterstain. (Courtesy of S. Dunlop, MD, and R. Spiller, MD, Nottingham, UK.)

postinfectious IBS[112,116]; however, this test is confounded by intestinal transit and bacterial overgrowth, and whether abnormal intestinal permeability occurs remains speculative.

Colonic inflammation is associated with the production of a number of important mediators including 5-hydroxytryptamine (5-HT), prostaglandins, bradykinins, adenosine and nerve growth factors, to name a few.[8] The abnormal release of 5-HT may have a central role in the manifestations of IBS.[118] More than 95% of 5-HT is located in the enteroendocrine cells of the intestine. 5-HT is released from these cells following stroking or increased pressure, for example after a meal; 5-HT then acts on primary intrinsic afferent neurons to initiate the peristaltic reflex by activation of ascending excitation and descending inhibition.[8] The 5-HT then is primarily retaken up by a specific serotonin transporter (SERT) expressed in the enterocytes. There is some evidence that an exaggerated release of 5-HT in IBS can occur after a meal.[119] Furthermore, it has been observed in rectal biopsies that 5-HT molecular signaling may be abnormal in IBS; in one study, 5-HT reuptake was reduced in IBS and also in ulcerative colitis compared with controls, although 5-HT release was unaffected and the numbers of enteroendocrine cells were unchanged.[120] The findings were similar in IBS patients with constipation or diarrhea leading to the hypothesis that in IBS there is increased availability of mucosal 5-HT that can induce diarrhea, but if there is desensitization of 5-HT receptors, this leads to constipation or an alternating bowel pattern.[120]

FOOD INTOLERANCE AND ALLERGY

Many patients with IBS attribute their symptoms to certain foods, with wheat, dairy products, citrus fruits, potatoes, onions, and chocolate most frequently implicated.[121,122] In an uncontrolled trial, one half of the patients with IBS reported improvement with elimination diets.[53]

Wheat Intolerance or Allergy

Substantial amounts of wheat are eaten in the Western countries, 10% to 15% of which is not digested by human enzymes.[8] Furthermore, subtle forms of gluten intolerance may be present in some people with IBS who do not have any overt evidence of celiac sprue (see Chapter 101).[123] In the absence of a definitive diagnosis of celiac sprue, however, a gluten-free diet cannot be recommended in IBS, at present.[8]

Sugar Malabsorption

Symptoms of IBS can be confused with those of lactose intolerance.[124] Lactose intolerance occurs with varying prevalence depending on one's ethnic group and is seen in 10% of populations of northern European descent, 40% to 60% of those of Asian decent, 90% of Chinese, and 60% to 80% of Africans. In acquired hypolactasia, there is some residual ability to digest small amounts of lactose and because most people do not ingest more than 12.5 g of lactose a day, they do not suffer from this ingestion.[125] Unless a lactose-intolerant patient regularly ingests substantial amounts of lactose, lactose intolerance cannot be the explanation for the symptoms.[126]

Fructose and sorbitol malabsorption may contribute to IBS symptoms in some patients; however, fructose-sorbitol malabsorption, with a prevalence of 30% in those with IBS, may be no more common in IBS than in the background population.[127,128,129]

ABNORMAL COLONIC FLORA AND BACTERIAL OVERGROWTH

It has been suggested that the colonic flora could be abnormal in a subset of patients with IBS, resulting in increased colonic fermentation, production of excess gas, and development of symptoms in those who are otherwise predisposed.[130] This has led to an interest in probiotic therapy for IBS.

Others have reported that there is a high prevalence of small bowel bacterial overgrowth in IBS, based on hydrogen breath testing and the clinical response to nonabsorbable antibiotics.[131,132] Abnormal hydrogen breath test results may occur because of transit abnormalities,

however, and it is unclear how often bacterial overgrowth is documented by quantitative culture in patients with IBS who have abnormal breath tests.[133,134]

CENTRAL DYSREGULATION

Visceral afferent signals from the gut reach the brainstem and thalamus and are only consciously perceived occasionally, although there may be some subliminal registration of low-intensity signals.[1] Abnormal modulation of visceral afferent signals may occur at multiple levels in visceral, spinal, and central regions. Based on cerebral blood flow changes, functional brain imaging studies (functional magnetic resonance imaging or positron-emission tomography [PET]) have suggested that there are alterations in the brain response to visceral stimuli in IBS. In IBS patients, greater activation of the mid-cingular cortex, an area that processes visceral signals, has been reported following delivered or anticipated rectal distention.[135,136] This could explain why anxiety or stress may enhance perception of visceral pain, whereas relaxation or distraction decreases pain in IBS. Using hypnosis to selectively alter noxious stimuli, PET scanning revealed significant changes in anterior cingulate cortex activity.[137] Sex differences in brain networks concerned with anti-nociceptive and autonomic responses following rectal distention in IBS also have been observed.[138]

PSYCHOLOGICAL FACTORS

Psychological and psychiatric comorbidity is increased in those with IBS, but this association is not just explained by consultation bias.[1,63-65,139-141] In patients with IBS, a history of sexual, physical, or emotional abuse also is reported more often than in those without IBS.[142-145] Abuse has not been shown to alter rectal sensation[146] but may modulate central brain responses to pain.[147] Patients with IBS are more likely to report greater lifetime and daily stressful events than are those with organic disease or healthy controls and may be more susceptible to stress-altering gastrointestinal function.[1] Childhood stress may be particularly important.[78] In rats, maternal separation in the perinatal period induces an anxiety state and is associated with visceral hypersensitivity.[78] Furthermore, in rats, moderately severe stress leads to the release of corticotropin-releasing factor and acceleration of colonic transit.[148] Sustained stress could, therefore, be important in both the onset and persistence of IBS.

GENETICS

Limited, but increasing, evidence points to at least a small hereditary component of IBS. There is clustering of IBS in families.[149,150] Twin studies generally have shown that there is a greater concordance of IBS in monozygotic compared with dizygotic twins, suggesting a moderate genetic component, although the environmental component probably is greater.[151,152] Potential candidate genes have been reported to be associated with IBS, but further confirmatory evidence is required and their functional

Table 115–2   Alarm Features Considered Potentially Relevant in the Diagnosis of Organic Disease as Opposed to Irritable Bowel Syndrome

History	Physical Examination
New onset after age 50 years	Occult or overt blood on rectal examination
Weight loss	Signs of anemia
Blood in the stool	Abdominal mass
Fever	Signs of bowel obstruction
Nighttime symptoms (waking the patient from sleep)	Signs of malabsorption
Persistent diarrhea	Signs of thyroid dysfunction
Severe chronic constipation	Arthritis (active)
Recurrent vomiting	Dermatitis herpetiformis or pyoderma
Progressive dysphagia	gangrenosum
Travel history to locations with endemic parasitic diseases	
Family history of colon cancer, inflammatory bowel disease, or celiac sprue	

Adapted from Olden KW: Diagnosis of irritable bowel syndrome. Gastroenterology 122:1701, 2002.

significance unraveled. For example, patients with IBS have been reported to have significantly lower frequencies of the high producer genotypes of interleukin (IL)-10. A lower amount of this anti-inflammatory cytokine might predispose to greater inflammation in response to an infectious insult in IBS[153]; others have failed to confirm these observations.[154] In IBS with constipation, polymorphisms of the α_2-adrenoreceptors ($\alpha_2$ac del 322-325 and α_2a C-1291G) have been observed.[155] In the 5HT$_{2A}$ receptor, the C allele of the 102 T/G polymorphism and the A allele of the −1438 G/A polymorphism were reported to be associated with IBS, but the data are unconvincing.[156] Associations with polymorphisms of the promoter region of the serotonin transporter gene in IBS have not been consistent.[155,157]

Table 115–3   Prevalence of Organic Disease in Patients Meeting Symptom-Based Criteria for Irritable Bowel Syndrome

Organic GI Disease	IBS Patients, %	General Population, %
Inflammatory bowel disease	0.51-0.98	0.3-1.2
Colorectal cancer	0-0.51	0-6 (varies with age)
Celiac sprue	4.7	0.25-0.5
Gastrointestinal infection	0-1.5	NA
Thyroid dysfunction	6	5-9
Lactose malabsorption	22-26	25

GI, gastrointestinal; NA, not applicable.
Data from Cash B, Schoenfeld P, Chey W: The utility of diagnostic tests in irritable bowel syndrome patients: A systematic review. Am J Gastroenterol 97:2812, 2002.

DIAGNOSIS

In patients who present with IBS-like symptoms, there are a number of "alarm" features (or "red flags") that clearly warrant prompt investigation, including any history of bleeding or evidence of anemia clinically, a history of unexplained weight loss, unexplained vomiting, progressive dysphagia, a family history of malignancy, and new-onset symptoms in older age (Table 115–2).[124,158,159] Not all traditional alarm features, however, have been documented to have adequate diagnostic utility. For example, nighttime symptoms are common in IBS and appear not to discriminate IBS from organic disease,[158] although most physicians would still investigate patients who were being awakened in the middle of the night by pain or those with nocturnal diarrhea. Any patient 50 years of age or older requires a structural colonic evaluation, if not previously completed. The preference remains colonoscopy to exclude other disease and, in particular, colon cancer. Although older persons may develop IBS, the risk of organic disease increases with age. Furthermore, colon cancer screening in those 50 years of age and older, even with no symptoms, currently is recommended in the United States.

Patients who meet the Rome criteria for IBS and who have no alarm features are unlikely to have another cause for their presentation other than IBS. For example, Vanner and associates evaluated 98 patients who met the Rome I criteria with no alarm features, of whom 50% had been referred because of diagnostic uncertainty.[160] The Rome I criteria had a positive predictive value of up to 100% in this setting, although their sensitivity was only 65%. Another study reported that three or more Manning criteria in the absence of alarm features correctly diagnosed 96% of cases of IBS.[158]

A systematic review found six studies that had evaluated the value of diagnostic tests in IBS.[9] The results, based on limited numbers of referred patients, suggested that IBS patients do not have an increased risk of most organic diseases compared with non-IBS controls (Table 115–3). Extensive investigations to exclude most possibilities are not only expensive but have the danger of reinforcing abnormal illness behavior. There also is the real risk of uncovering findings that are irrelevant to the diagnosis but which precipitate yet more expensive and even dangerous investigations.

Traditional screening tests that have low yields in IBS patients include a full blood count, renal and liver function testing, thyroid function testing, and evaluation of three fresh stool samples for parasites; even though these are inexpensive tests they can be reassuring for both patient and physician if negative or normal.[8] Low-grade Crohn's disease can be missed. An elevated C-reactive protein may indicate the presence of undiagnosed Crohn's disease but often is negative in this setting. Fecal calprotectin has been shown to discriminate IBS from Crohn's disease with excellent sensitivity and specificity.[161,162] In contrast, evaluation of the small bowel either radiologically or via capsule endoscopy has a very low yield in the setting of typical IBS symptoms without alarm features; only if there is concern should such investigations be considered. Hydrogen breath testing to identify lactose intolerance or small bowel bacterial overgrowth cannot be endorsed routinely.[8] Bile salt malabsorption causing diarrhea in the setting of IBS occurs uncommonly, and a therapeutic trial of cholestyramine is probably more useful than a 75-seleno-homocholic acid-taurine (Se-CAT) test.[8,163,164] If diarrhea is persistent, colonoscopy with biopsy may be considered, although the yield of colonic biopsy remains low, and this test is probably not cost-effective.[9] In a setting of severe constipation, exclusion of pelvic outlet obstruction with anorectal manometry including balloon expulsion testing should be considered because this may alter management.[1,2,8]

Routine testing for celiac sprue is a consideration. Data from the United Kingdom have reported there was a seven-fold increased risk of celiac sprue in patients with IBS; up to 5% of patients with symptoms consistent with IBS had celiac sprue compared with 0.5% of controls[165]; however, much lower rates have been observed in the United States.[166] Decision analysis suggests that testing is cost-effective unless the prevalence of celiac sprue falls to less that 1% in those with IBS-like symptoms.[167] A screening test in those on a normal diet (antiendomysial or tissue transglutaminase antibody) followed by duodenal biopsies in those with a positive test should be considered, unless the background prevalence of celiac sprue is very low in the patient population being seen. Latent celiac sprue (antibody positive, biopsy normal) may respond to a gluten-free diet, but its prevalence in IBS is unclear.[123]

In summary, the diagnosis of IBS can be made based on the history (with particular attention to presence or absence of the Rome criteria) and in the absence of any red flags (alarm features). A normal physical examination can be reassuring for patient and physician. In this setting, the patient who responds to an empiric trial of therapy for IBS does not require any further diagnostic evaluation (Fig. 115–5).[159] Those who fail to respond should undergo more extensive evaluation, depending on the predominant symptoms.

MANAGEMENT

EDUCATION AND SUPPORT

IBS tends to be a life-long disorder, and establishment of a strong physician–patient relationship is key to providing the best clinical care (Table 115–4).[8] Indeed, patients with IBS often perceive their physician as having a highly negative medical belief about the disorder and this perception per se impedes best care.[168,169] Other common patient perceptions of the care they receive include that they have been mislabeled as psychologically disturbed and that they have not been provided with adequate medical information or support.[168,169] A good physician–patient relationship has been associated with reduced use of medical services.[170]

It is important to discover why the patient has decided to visit at this time. The reasons can vary: new life stressors; exacerbating factors in the diet or changes in medications; increased fear of serious disease; and the development of treatable psychiatric comorbidity. A hidden agenda such as seeking disability or new narcotic abuse sometimes may explain the consulting behavior. In terms of providing optimal reassurance, it is important first to educate the patients and then to actively reassure them. Patients typically want to understand why their symptoms have occurred; they also want to obtain validation that their symptoms are "real." Specific education classes designed for those with IBS appear to be useful therapeutic interventions,[171,172] although randomized,

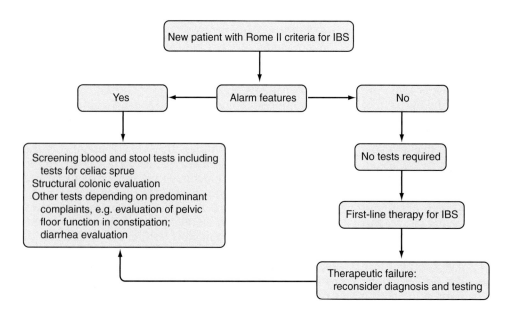

Figure 115–5 Algorithm for diagnostic testing for irritable bowel syndrome (IBS). (Adapted from Cash BD, Chey WD: Irritable bowel syndrome: An evidence-based approach to diagnosis. Aliment Pharmacol Ther 19:1235, 2004.)

Table 115–4   Management Recommendations for Irritable Bowel Syndrome

Make a positive diagnosis based on symptoms and the absence of alarm features
Establish the effect of illness on the patient and on the patient's psychosocial resources (e.g., family support)
Establish if there is a comorbid psychiatric disease or an unresolved major loss or trauma
Assess the patient's expectations and hidden fears (e.g., find out why he or she has presented now despite long-standing symptoms) and try to address all concerns
Provide education, including an understandable explanation of why symptoms might arise, emphasizing that the patient is not alone in his or her suffering and the prognosis is benign
Provide firm reassurance, emphasizing that the symptoms are known to be real (not just "in the patient's head") and that irritable bowel syndrome is a recognized bowel disease
Avoid giving mixed messages (e.g., by reassuring the patient and then ordering extensive tests without an adequate explanation)
Avoid repeated tests unless a new development of structural disease is suspected (e.g., presentation with new alarm features)
Base treatment on the principle of patient-based responsibility for care
Set realistic treatment goals; consider referral to a patient support group
Organize a continuing care strategy if symptoms have been chronic or disabling
Consider psychological treatments for patients with moderate-to-severe symptoms

Adapted from Talley N, Spiller RC: Irritable bowel syndrome: A little understood organic bowel disease? Lancet 360:555, 2002.

Table 115–5   Treatment of Irritable Bowel Syndrome: A Stepped-Care Approach

Step	Severity of Symptoms	Level of Care	Clinical and Psychological Issues	Management
1	Mild	Primary	Fear of serious disease, anxiety, worry, stress	Positive diagnosis; explanation; reassurance; dietary management; regular follow-up
2	Moderate	Secondary	Uncertainty regarding diagnosis; disturbed lifestyle	Reinforce above measures Stress management; target drugs to specific complaints, e.g., anticholinergic agent (pain), tegaserod (constipation, pain), loperamide (diarrhea)
3	Severe	Tertiary	Coexistent psychiatric disease; possible secondary gain; disability, chronic pain	Avoid overtesting; low-dose tricyclic antidepressant, or SSRI; alosetron (severe diarrhea); treat depression, anxiety; referral to pain clinic

SSRI, selective serotonin reuptake inhibitor.
Adapted from Drossman DA, Thompson WG: The irritable bowel syndrome: Review and a graduated multicomponent treatment approach. Ann Intern Med 116:1009, 1992.

controlled trials have not been done to prove the effectiveness of these interventions.

A stepped-care approach depending on the severity of the presenting symptoms provides a useful guide for considering therapies (Table 115–5).[173]

DIET

The standard of care for IBS typically has been a high-fiber diet.[174-178] Data from the available randomized, controlled trials, however, indicate that fiber is not helpful for pain or diarrhea, although it may benefit constipation and provide some global symptom benefit.[179,180] The best evidence for fiber supplements comes from those studies of soluble fiber, mainly psyllium[180]; wheat bran has been no better than placebo in IBS. Fiber supplements often are better tolerated than diet change alone. The key to taking fiber and fiber supplements is to begin at a low dose and increase very slowly. This reduces the problems of excessive bloating, gas, and pain that typically are aggravated by increased fiber. For example, most of the powder fiber supplements contain about 3 to 6 g of fiber. If the goal is to supplement approximately 10 to 15 g

of fiber in total, the amount should be increased by 3 to 6 g every 1 to 2 weeks.

Many patients with IBS suspect that food intolerance may be relevant to their symptoms. It is useful to determine the amounts of milk and milk products being consumed to decide whether lactose intolerance testing should be considered. Clinical experience suggests that even in the setting of a diagnosis of lactose intolerance and typical IBS symptoms, more often than not, the IBS symptoms persist despite withdrawal of all lactose in the diet, indicating that this is the chance overlap of common conditions. Fructose consumption has increased dramatically in the United States and in other developed countries; excess fructose could lead to some IBS-like symptoms that might be relieved by exclusion of this sugar (Table 115–6).[127–129] Reducing fatty foods, gas-producing foods, or caffeine or alcohol also may be helpful for some patients, but controlled trials to support this recommendation are lacking.

Exclusion diets can be useful in some cases. One randomized trial measured IgG antibodies to foods and then excluded those IgG positive foods from the diet in the active arm of the trial; in the sham arm, other foods from the diet were excluded in a blinded fashion.[181]

Table 115–6 Carbohydrate Composition of Common Foods

Food Items	Fructose, g*	Sorbitol, g*
Apples	≤ 6.0	≤ 1.0
Pears	≤ 8.9	≤ 4.5
Bananas	≤ 3.8	0
Sweet cherries	≤ 7.2	≤ 12.6
Strawberries	≤ 2.5	0
Grapes	≤ 10.5	0
Plums	≤ 4.0	≤ 2.8
Prunes	≤ 23	≤ 15
Dates	≤ 31	0
Peaches	≤ 1.5	≤ 1.3
Apple juice	6-8	0.3-1.0
Pear juice	5-9	1.1-2.6
Orange juice	≤ 5.3	0
Honey (100 g or 3 tbsp)	35	0
Sugar-free gum and mints	0	1.3-2.2 per piece

*Per 100-g edible portion.
Adapted from Dunlop SP, Jenkins D, Spiller RC: Distinctive clinical, psychological, and histological features of postinfective irritable bowel syndrome. Am J Gastroenterol 98:1578, 2003.

The exclusion of foods with a positive IgG antibody response provided therapeutic benefit in both diarrhea- and constipation-predominant IBS. Other studies of food exclusion diets have suggested that in diarrhea-predominant IBS, a proportion of patients will respond. Cromoglycate did show some benefit in one trial of patients with positive skin prick tests to foods, but these results remain to be confirmed.[182]

It has been suggested that abnormal colonic flora could be relevant in the pathogenesis of IBS, which has led to the interest in using probiotics to try and naturally alter the flora. Some initial small trials produced promising results with *Bifidobacterium infantis*, *Lactobacillus plantarum*, and VSL #3,[183,184] but the findings have been variable.[185] This variation may reflect the dose used, whether live or dead organisms were given, and other unknown factors.

ANTISPASMODICS AND ANTICHOLINERGICS

In the United States, anticholinergics (dicyclomine, propantheline, belladonna, and hyoscyamine) continue to be used commonly for IBS.[177] A meta-analysis of 23 randomized, controlled trials concluded that antispasmodics were superior to placebo in the treatment of IBS.[186] Overall, there was an improvement of abdominal pain and IBS global symptoms in the pooled analyses[186]; however, the quality of most of these trials was low, the results were mixed and publication bias cannot be excluded. Moreover, only the anticholinergic antispasmodics are available in the United States, and these do not have any well-established efficacy.[177] Non-anticholinergic antispasmodics, unavailable in the United States, include mebeverine (a smooth muscle relaxant), selective calcium channel blockers (e.g., pinaverium), and opiate agonists (e.g., trimebutine). Anticholinergics clinically seem most useful for those with postprandial pain when taken 30 minutes prior to eating. No advantage of sublingual or suppository over oral anticholinergic preparations has been documented in IBS.

LAXATIVES

The efficacy of this class of drugs for constipation-predominant IBS is uncertain. No randomized, controlled trials of laxatives in IBS are available. Osmotic laxatives often are prescribed but can aggravate bloating and pain. Polyethylene glycol, although not approved for this indication, does seem useful in practice, particularly if constipation is troublesome despite other therapy.[187,188] Stimulant laxatives are probably safer than has been appreciated, but they often induce abdominal cramping or pain and generally seem unsatisfactory for patients with IBS.[189]

ANTIDIARRHEALS

Loperamide is established to be efficacious based on randomized, controlled trials in IBS with diarrhea; however, this agent does not improve abdominal pain or bloating. The number of patients needed to treat to prevent one occurrence [NNT], a statistical technique to enable comparisons of efficacy, is 1 for loperamide[179,190-192]: Loperamide is most effective when taken prophylactically, rather than being taken after diarrhea has occurred; doses of loperamide range from 2 to 16 mg/day, and high doses seem safe. Diphenoxylate has not been tested in IBS but probably is similarly efficacious. Codeine phosphate because of its side effects (dizziness, nausea, sedation), and high-risk of inducing dependence should be avoided in IBS.

Anecdotally, bile salt-sequestering agents (e.g., cholestyramine) seem to help diarrhea in IBS in some cases, possibly because of underlying bile salt malabsorption. It is best begun at a low dose and built up slowly to four times daily if needed. Bismuth subsalicylate anecdotally is also useful for diarrhea control in IBS but must be used intermittently because of concerns about bismuth toxicity.

SEROTONIN RECEPTOR DRUGS

The serotonin type 4 receptor agonist tegaserod is a prokinetic drug that has efficacy in constipation-predominant IBS. The drug accelerates small bowel and colonic transit, stimulates intestinal secretion, and may have some visceral analgesic actions.[193,194] It is approved for use only in women with IBS because of the lack of adequate efficacy data in men.[195-199] The NNT with tegaserod has been calculated to be between 8 and 14.[177,199] The standard dose is 6 mg twice daily. It improves global symptoms and especially constipation in IBS; it is not efficacious if diarrhea is predominant. The drug seems to be well tolerated, with diarrhea and headache being the main side effects.[200] Although rare cases of ischemic colitis have been reported in association with the use of tegaserod, this probably reflects the general increased risk of ischemic colitis in those with IBS rather than an adverse drug effect.[201]

Alosetron is a 5-HT$_3$ antagonist that is efficacious in women with severe diarrhea-predominant IBS.[202] The NNT has been calculated to be 7,[202] and it has been shown to improve QOL.[203] The starting dose is 1 mg daily. In the United States, it is available only via a restricted prescribing program because of concern for ischemic colitis and severe constipation.[204] The dose can be increased to 1 mg twice daily after 4 weeks if symptoms are not controlled and there have been no side effects. Ischemic colitis occurs in 0.1% and is drug-related but usually transient and without irreversible consequence; up to 50% of patients with alosetron-associated ischemic colitis required hospitalization.[205] Constipation occurs in one third of alosetron-treated patients. The prescription of the drug is absolutely contraindicated in IBS patients with any history of constipation or a thrombotic tendency. Pharmacogenomic data suggest that alosetron may be more efficacious in those with the long homozygous polymorphism of the *SERT* transporter gene, but this needs confirmation.[206] Cilansetron is another 5-HT$_3$ antagonist that appears to be efficacious in women and men with diarrhea-predominant IBS, and it too has been linked with a small risk of ischemic colitis.[194]

ANTIDEPRESSANTS AND ANXIOLYTICS

The tricyclic antidepressants appear to be efficacious in IBS but may improve global well-being more than symptoms.[207] Meta-analyses have reported the NNT was between 3 and 4, although these studies included a number of low-quality and potentially flawed trials.[177,208] A large randomized, controlled trial of desipramine (from 50 to 150 mg) versus placebo in female patients showed that 60% were responders to the tricyclic versus 47% to placebo; this difference failed to reach significance in the intention-to-treat analysis but was significant in the per protocol analysis.[209] When using an antidepressant in IBS, it is recommended to start it at a low dose (e.g., 10 to 25 mg of desipramine or nortriptyline) and increase the dose by 10 to 25 mg weekly, aiming for a dose of 50 mg initially; many patients do not require full antidepressant dosing (unless comorbid depression is present). Tricyclic antidepressants tend to be constipating and, therefore, may be of most benefit in diarrhea-predominant IBS, although the data supporting this are unclear. Adverse events with tricyclic antidepressants are a problem. Approximately 1 in 3 to 1 in 4 treated patients develops side effects, with 1 in 22 having potentially serious reactions; up to 40% discontinue use or change therapy because of intolerance.[210]

The selective serotonin reuptake inhibitors (SSRIs) cause fewer side effects than the tricyclic antidepressants, but the randomized, controlled trials in IBS have reported conflicting results. In one trial that lacked a placebo arm, paroxetine was compared with usual care in IBS patients and shown to improve QOL but not abdominal pain.[211] Other studies showed some benefit for pain or no effect on pain[212,213]; the findings remain inconsistent. It is possible that SSRIs may be more beneficial in constipation-

predominant IBS because they accelerate small bowel transit.[214]

Benzodiazepines may have a small benefit over placebo in IBS, but the evidence for this is very weak.[176] Because of habituation, this class of drugs generally should be avoided.

MISCELLANEOUS DRUGS

Three weeks of oral prednisone (30 mg/day) failed to improve postinfectious IBS symptoms in one placebo-controlled trial.[215] Anticonvulsants have analgesic properties; gabapentin may have some therapeutic value for pain of IBS anecdotally, but phenytoin was not shown to be beneficial in a randomized trial.[216] Beta blockers may inhibit colonic motor function, but neither atenolol nor timolol were better than placebo in small trials.[217,218] Leuprolide is a gonadotrophin-releasing hormone analog that was superior to placebo in terms of reducing abdominal pain and nausea[219,220]; however, the entry criteria for these studies were vague and side effects of chemical castration were significant; this drug cannot be routinely recommended. Colchicine increases spontaneous bowel movements and decreases colonic transit time,[221] but its role in IBS with constipation is unknown. Misoprostol may be helpful for refractory constipation,[222] but no controlled trials in IBS are available. Domperidone and erythromycin are prokinetic agents used predominantly in the upper gastrointestinal tract and probably are not efficacious in IBS.[176]

Octreotide reduces intestinal transit time, secretion, and sensation in IBS[223] but is impractical to use for diarrhea in IBS. Clonidine, an α_2-receptor agonist, may be useful in diarrhea-predominant IBS because it enhances rectal compliance and reduces fasting colonic motor activity[224]; however, significant side effects, particularly postural hypotension, sedation, fluid retention, and depression, limit its use. Nonabsorbable antibiotics such as neomycin and rifaximin appear to be superior to placebo in IBS in very short-term treatment studies, but long-term results are unavailable and any benefit of the drug for IBS remains in dispute.[131,132]

There is no convincing evidence that either simethicone[225] or charcoal works for excessive gas in IBS.[226,227] Beano (α-galactosidase) may reduce flatus but not other IBS symptoms.[228] Malodorous flatus may respond to zinc acetate, bismuth subsalicylate, or a bulky charcoal cushion device.[229-231]

PSYCHOLOGICAL TREATMENTS

Psychotherapy, hypnotherapy, and cognitive behavioral therapy (CBT) have been proposed to be useful treatments for IBS.[1] A systematic review concluded that only hypnotherapy was of established benefit because of methodologic limitations.[232] Hypnotherapy may improve cognition in IBS.[233] Better efficacy data have since appeared for CBT,[79,209] albeit not in all controlled trials.[234] There are no head-to-head studies comparing the different psychological interventions. Based on the available literature, IBS patients with abdominal pain, diarrhea, and psychological distress appear most likely to have a beneficial response to such intervention, particularly if the symptoms have been of short duration and have waxed and waned.[1] Patients with constant abdominal pain do poorly with psychological treatment.[1] Indeed, symptoms tend not to improve; rather, the ability to cope with IBS seems to drive any global benefit. The major advantage of psychological treatment is that despite the initial expense, long-term benefits may be cost offsetting.[211]

ALTERNATIVE TREATMENTS

Many different alternative remedies are used by patients with IBS.[235] In one high-quality randomized, controlled study, Chinese herbal medicine (comprising a combination of 20 herbs) was superior to placebo, although this requires confirmation[236] and the risks of using multiple herbal concoctions continues to be of concern.[237] An ayurvedic preparation also was superior to placebo,[238] but the data here remain limited. Ginger and aloe are used often, but there are no controlled trials in IBS.[235] Whether pancreatic enzymes help remains unknown, although a small double-blind cross-over study suggests some benefit for postprandial bloating.[239] Acupuncture may reduce rectal hypersensitivity,[240,241] but efficacy is not established in controlled trials.

PROGNOSIS

In clinical practice, once a diagnosis of IBS has been made, it usually requires no revision despite prolonged follow-up. In 112 consecutive IBS patients followed through their medical records for a median of 29 years, survival in IBS was not different from expected, although 9% developed organic disease a median of 15 years after diagnosis.[170] Among 75 patients with a clinical diagnosis of IBS followed up for 10 to 13 years, none had another explanation uncovered for their symptoms, yet 92% had not had symptom resolution; 47% had undergone a repeat structural colonic evaluation to no avail.[242] Some IBS patients have spontaneous improvement over time, but usually IBS is a relapsing disorder. The presence of excessive psychological distress or anxiety, as well as a long duration of complaints, tends to indicate a poorer prognosis.[1]

REFERENCES

1. Drossman D, Camilleri M, Mayer E, Whitehead W: AGA technical review on irritable bowel syndrome. Gastroenterology 123:2108, 2002.
2. Camilleri M, Heading RC, Thompson WG: Consensus report: Clinical perspectives, mechanisms, diagnosis, and management of irritable bowel syndrome. Aliment Pharmcol Ther 16:1407, 2002.
3. Drossman DA, Corrazziari E, Talley NJ, et al: Rome II: The Functional Gastrointestinal Disorders, 2nd ed. McLean, VA, Degnon, 2000.
4. Longstreth GF, Burchette RJ: Family practitioners' attitudes and knowledge about irritable bowel syndrome: Effect of a trial of physician education. Fam Pract 20:670, 2003.
5. Thompson WG, Heaton KW, Smyth GT, Smyth C: Irritable bowel syndrome: The view from general practice. Eur J Gastroenterol Hepatol 97:689, 1997.
6. Wilson S, Roberts L, Roalfe A, et al: Prevalence of irritable bowel syndrome: A community survey. Br J Clin Pract 54:495, 2004.
7. Russo MW, Gaynes BN, Drossman DA: A national survey of practice patterns of gastroenterologists with comparison to the past two decades. J Clin Gastroenterol 29:339, 1999.
8. Talley N, Spiller RC: Irritable bowel syndrome: A little understood organic bowel disease? Lancet 360:555, 2002.
9. Cash B, Schoenfeld P, Chey W: The utility of diagnostic tests in irritable bowel syndrome patients: A systematic review. Am J Gastroenterol 97:2812, 2002.
10. Manning AP, Thompson WG, Heaton KW, Morris AF: Towards positive diagnosis of the irritable bowel. BMJ 2:653, 1978.
11. Hammer J, Talley NJ: Diagnostic criteria for the irritable bowel syndrome. Am J Med 107(Suppl):5S, 1999.
12. Talley NJ, Phillips SF, Melton LJ III, et al: Diagnostic value of the Manning criteria in irritable bowel syndrome. Gut 31:77, 1990.
13. Boyce PM, Koloski NA, Talley NJ: Irritable bowel syndrome according to varying diagnostic criteria: Are the new Rome II criteria unnecessarily restrictive for research and practice? Am J Gastroenterol 95:3176, 2000.
14. Hillila MT, Farkkila MA: Prevalence of irritable bowel syndrome according to different diagnostic criteria in a nonselected adult population. Aliment Pharmacol Ther 20:339, 2004.
15. Saito Y, Schoenfeld P, Locke GR: The epidemiology of irritable bowel syndrome in North America: A systematic review. Am J Gastroenterol 97:1910, 2002.
16. Talley NJ, Weaver AL, Zinsmeister AR, Melton L Jr: Self-reported diarrhea: What does it mean? Am J Gastroenterol 89:1160, 1994.
17. Lewis SJ, Heaton KW: Stool form scale as a useful guide to intestinal transit time. Scand J Gastroenterol 32:920, 1997.
18. Degen LP, Phillips SF: How well does stool form reflect colonic transit? Gut 39:109, 1996.
19. Reilly BP, Bolton MP, Lewis MJ, et al: A device for 24-hour ambulatory monitoring of abdominal girth using inductive plethysmography. Physiol Meas 23:661, 2002.
20. Whitehead WE, Palsson O, Jones KR: Systematic review of the comorbidity of irritable bowel syndrome with other disorders: What are the causes and implications? Gastroenterology 122:1140, 2002.
21. Minderhoud IM, Itta M, Oldenburg B, et al: IBS-like symptoms in patients with inflammatory bowel disease in remission: Relationships with quality of life and coping behavior. Dig Dis Sci 49:469, 2004.
22. Costanza CD, Longstreth GF, Liu AL: Chronic abdominal wall pain: Clinical features, health care costs, and long-term outcome. Clin Gastroenterol Hepatol 2:395, 2004.
23. Srinivasan R, Greenbaum DS: Chronic abdominal wall pain—a frequently overlooked problem: Practical approach to diagnosis and management. Am J Gastroenterol 97:824, 2002.
24. Webb PM, Purdie DM, Grover S, et al: Symptoms and diagnosis of borderline, early, and advanced epithelial ovarian cancer. Gynecol Oncol 92:232, 2004.
25. Talley NJ: Irritable bowel syndrome: Definition, diagnosis, and epidemiology. Baillieres Best Pract Res Clin Gastroenterol 13:371, 1999.
26. Saito YA, Talley NJ, Melton LJ III, et al: The effect of new diagnostic criteria for irritable bowel syndrome on community

prevalence estimates. Neurogastroenterol Motil 15:687, 2003.

27. Talley NJ, O'Keefe EA, Zinsmeister AR, Melton LJ III: Prevalence of gastrointestinal symptoms in the elderly: A population-based study. Gastroenterology 102:895, 1992.

28. Bennett G, Talley NJ: Irritable bowel syndrome in the elderly. Best Pract Res Clin Gastroenterol 16:63, 2002.

29. Thompson WG: Gender differences in irritable bowel symptoms. Eur J Gastroenterol Hepatol 9:299, 1997.

30. Lee OY, Mayer EA, Schmulson M, et al: Gender-related differences in IBS symptoms. Am J Gastroenterol 96:2184, 2001.

31. Houghton LA, Lea R, Jackson N, Whorwell PJ: The menstrual cycle affects rectal sensitivity in patients with irritable bowel syndrome but not healthy volunteers. Gut 50:471, 2002.

32. Taub E, Cuevas JL, Cook EW III, et al: Irritable bowel syndrome defined by factor analysis: Gender and race comparisons. Dig Dis Sci 40:2647, 1995.

33. Zuckerman M, Guerra L, Drossman D, et al: Comparison of bowel patterns in Hispanics and non-Hispanic whites. Dig Dis Sci 40:1763, 1995.

34. Gwee KA, Wee S, Wong ML, Png DJ: The prevalence, symptom characteristics, and impact of irritable bowel syndrome in an Asian urban community. Am J Gastroenterol 99:924, 2004.

35. Lau EM, Chan FK, Ziea ET, et al: Epidemiology of irritable bowel syndrome in Chinese. Dig Dis Sci 47:2621, 2002.

36. Lule GN, Amayo EO: Irritable bowel syndrome in Kenyans. East Afr Med J 79:360, 2002.

37. Olubuyide IO, Olawuyi F, Fasanmade AA: A study of irritable bowel syndrome diagnosed by Manning criteria in an African population. Dig Dis Sci 40:983, 1995.

38. Mearin F, Balboa A, Badia X, et al: Irritable bowel syndrome subtypes according to bowel habit: Revisiting the alternating subtype. Eur J Gastroenterol Hepatol 15:165, 2003.

39. Mearin F, Baro E, Roset M, et al: Clinical patterns over time in irritable bowel syndrome: Symptom instability and severity variability. Am J Gastroenterol 99:113, 2004.

40. Talley NJ, Zinsmeister AR, Melton LJ III: Irritable bowel syndrome in a community: Symptom subgroups, risk factors, and health care utilization. Am J Epidemiol 142:76, 1995.

41. Talley N, Weaver A, Zinsmeister A, Melton LJ III: Onset and disappearance of gastrointestinal symptoms and functional gastrointestinal disorders. Am J Epidemiol 136:165, 1992.

42. Locke GR III, Yawn BP, Wollan PC, et al: Incidence of a clinical diagnosis of the irritable bowel syndrome in a United States population. Aliment Pharmacol Ther 19:1025, 2004.

43. Agreus L, Svardsudd K, Talley NJ, et al: Natural history of gastroesophageal reflux disease and functional abdominal disorders: A population-based study. Am J Gastroenterol 96:2905, 2001.

44. Ilnyckyj A, Balachandra B, Elliott L, et al: Post-traveler's diarrhea irritable bowel syndrome: A prospective study. Am J Gastroenterol 98:596, 2003.

45. Gwee KA, Graham JC, McKendrick MW, et al: Psychometric scores and persistence of irritable bowel after infectious diarrhoea. Lancet 347:150, 1996.

46. Dunlop SP, Jenkins D, Neal KR, Spiller RC: Relative importance of enterochromaffin cell hyperplasia, anxiety, and depression in postinfectious IBS. Gastroenterology 125:1651, 2003.

47. Dunlop SP, Jenkins D, Spiller RC: Distinctive clinical, psychological, and histological features of postinfective irritable bowel syndrome. Am J Gastroenterol 98:1578, 2003.

48. Gwee KA, Leong YL, Graham C, et al: The role of psychological and biological factors in postinfective gut dysfunction. Gut 44:400, 1999.

49. Neal KR, Hebden JM, Spiller RC: Prevalence of gastrointestinal symptoms six months after bacterial gastroenteritis and risk factors for development of the irritable bowel syndrome: Postal survey of patients. BMJ 314:779, 1997.

50. Howell S, Talley NJ, Quine S, Poulton R: The irritable bowel syndrome has origins in the childhood socioeconomic environment. Am J Gastroenterol 99:1572, 2004.

51. Ruigomez A, Garcia Rodriguez LA, Johansson S, Wallander MA: Is hormone replacement therapy associated with an increased irritable bowel syndrome? Maturitas 44:133, 2003.

52. Mendall MA, Kumar D: Antibiotic use, childhood affluence and irritable bowel syndrome (IBS). Eur J Gastroenterol Hepatol 10:59, 1998.

53. Nanda R, James R, Smith H, et al: Food intolerance and the irritable bowel syndrome. Gut 30:1099, 1989.

54. Locke GR III, Zinsmeister AR, Talley NJ, et al: Risk factors for irritable bowel syndrome: Role of analgesics and food sensitivities. Am J Gastroenterol 95:157, 2000.

55. Huerta C, Garcia Rodriguez LA, Wallander MA, Johansson S: Users of oral steroids are at a reduced risk of developing irritable bowel syndrome. Pharmacoepidemiol Drug Saf 12:583, 2003.

56. Cole JA, Cook SF, Sands BE, et al: Occurrence of colon ischemia in relation to irritable bowel syndrome. Am J Gastroenterol 99:486, 2004.

57. Koloski N, Talley N, Boyce P: Predictors of health care seeking for irritable bowel syndrome and nonulcer dyspepsia: A critical review of the literature on symptom and psychosocial factors. Am J Gastroenterol 96:1340, 2001.

58. Koloski NA, Talley NJ, Huskic SS, Boyce PM: Predictors of conventional and alternative health care seeking for irritable bowel syndrome and functional dyspepsia. Aliment Pharmacol Ther 17:841, 2003.

59. Talley N, Boyce P, Jones M: Predictors of health care seeking for irritable bowel syndrome: A population-based study. Gut 41:394, 1997.

60. Levy RL, Whitehead WE, Von Korff MR, Feld AD: Intergenerational transmission of gastrointestinal illness behavior. Am J Gastroenterol 95:451, 2000.

61. Whitehead WE, Winget C, Fedoravicius AS, et al: Learned illness behavior in patients with irritable bowel syndrome and peptic ulcer. Dig Dis Sci 27:202, 1982.

62. Hu WHC, Wong W-M, Lam CLK, et al: Anxiety but not depression determines health care-seeking behaviour in Chinese patients with dyspepsia and irritable bowel syndrome: A population-based study. Aliment Pharmacol Ther 16:2081, 2002.

63. Smith RC, Greenbaum DS, Vancouver JB, et al: Psychosocial factors are associated with health care seeking rather than diagnosis in irritable bowel syndrome. Gastroenterology 98:293, 1990.

64. Drossman DA, McKee DC, Sandler RS, et al: Psychosocial factors in the irritable bowel syndrome: A multivariate study of patients and nonpatients with irritable bowel syndrome. Gastroenterology 95:701, 1988.

65. Whitehead WE, Bosmajian L, Zonderman AB, et al: Symptoms of psychologic distress associated with irritable bowel syndrome. Gastroenterology 95:709, 1988.

66. Longstreth GF, Yao JF: Irritable bowel syndrome and surgery: A multivariate analysis. Gastroenterology 126:1665, 2004.

67. Kennedy TM, Jones RH: Epidemiology of cholecystectomy and irritable bowel syndrome in a UK population. Br J Surg 87:1658, 2000.

68. Hasler WL, Schoenfeld P: Systematic review: Abdominal and pelvic surgery in patients with irritable bowel syndrome. Aliment Pharmacol Ther 17:997, 2003.

69. Talley NJ: Unnecessary abdominal and back surgery in irritable bowel syndrome: Time to stem the flood now? Gastroenterology 126:1899, 2004.

70. Veysey MJ, Thomas LA, Mallet AI, et al: Colonic transit influences deoxycholic acid kinetics. Gastroenterology 121:812, 2001.

71. El-Serag HB, Olden KW, Bjorkman D: Health-related quality of life among persons with irritable bowel syndrome: A systematic review. Aliment Pharmacol Ther 16:1171, 2002.

72. Inadomi JM, Fennerty MB, Bjorkman D: Systematic review: The economic impact of irritable bowel syndrome. Aliment Pharmacol Ther 18:671, 2003.

73. Longstreth GF, Wilson A, Knight K, et al: Irritable bowel syndrome, health care use, and costs: A U.S.-managed care perspective. Am J Gastroenterol 98:600, 2003.

74. Leong SA, Barghout V, Birnbaum HG, et al: The economic consequences of irritable bowel syndrome: A U.S. employer perspective. Arch Intern Med 163:929, 2003.

75. Drossman D, Li Z, Andruzzi E, et al: U.S. householder survey of functional gastrointestinal disorders: Prevalence, sociodemography, and health impact. Dig Dis Sci 38:1569, 1993.

76. Sandler RS: Epidemiology of irritable bowel syndrome in the United States. Gastroenterology 99:409, 1990.

77. Sandler R, Everhart J, Donowitz M, et al: The burden of selected digestive diseases in the United States. Gastroenterology 122:1500, 2002.

78. Mayer EA, Collins SM: Evolving pathophysiologic models of functional gastrointestinal disorders. Gastroenterology 122:2032, 2002.

79. Drossman DA: The "organification" of functional GI disorders: Implications for research. Gastroenterology 124:6, 2003.

80. Clemens CH, Samsom M, Van Berge Henegouwen GP, Smout AJ: Abnormalities of left colonic motility in ambulant nonconstipated patients with irritable bowel syndrome. Dig Dis Sci 48:74, 2003.

81. Chey WY, Jin HO, Lee MH, et al: Colonic motility abnormality in patients with irritable bowel syndrome exhibiting abdominal pain and diarrhea. Am J Gastroenterol 96:1499, 2001.

82. Steens J, Van Der Schaar PJ, Penning C, et al: Compliance, tone, and sensitivity of the rectum in different subtypes of irritable bowel syndrome. Neurogastroenterol Motil 14:241, 2002.

83. Vassallo MJ, Camilleri M, Phillips SF, et al: Colonic tone and motility in patients with irritable bowel syndrome. Mayo Clin Proc 67:725, 1992.

84. Cole SJ, Duncan HD, Claydon AH, et al: Distal colonic motor activity in four subgroups of patients with irritable bowel syndrome. Dig Dis Sci 47:345, 2002.

85. Hutchinson R, Notghi A, Smith NB, et al: Scintigraphic measurement of ileocaecal transit in irritable bowel syndrome and chronic idiopathic constipation. Gut 36:585, 1995.

86. Clemens CH, Samsom M, Roelofs JM, et al: Association between pain episodes and high-amplitude propagated pressure waves in patients with irritable bowel syndrome. Am J Gastroenterol 98:1838, 2003.

87. Kellow JE, Phillips SF: Altered small bowel motility in irritable bowel syndrome is correlated with symptoms. Gastroenterology 92:1885, 1987.

88. Fukudo S, Nomura T, Hongo M: Impact of corticotropin-releasing hormone on gastrointestinal motility and adrenocorticotropic hormone in normal controls and patients with irritable bowel syndrome. Gut 42:845, 1998.

89. Sagami Y, Shimada Y, Tayama J, et al: Effect of a corticotropin-releasing hormone receptor antagonist on colonic sensory and motor function in patients with irritable bowel syndrome. Gut 53:958, 2004.

90. Kellow JE, Phillips SF, Miller LJ, Zinsmeister AR: Dysmotility of the small intestine in irritable bowel syndrome. Gut 29:1236, 1988.

91. Aggarwal A, Cutts TF, Abell TL, et al: Predominant symptoms in irritable bowel syndrome correlate with specific autonomic nervous system abnormalities. Gastroenterology 106:945, 1994.

92. Ritchie J: Pain from distension of the pelvic colon by inflating a balloon in the irritable colon syndrome. Gut 14:125, 1973.

93. Bouin M, Plourde V, Boivin M, et al: Rectal distention testing in patients with irritable bowel syndrome: Sensitivity, specificity, and predictive values of pain sensory thresholds. Gastroenterology 122:1771, 2002.

94. Mertz H, Naliboff B, Munakata J, et al: Altered rectal perception is a biological marker of patients with irritable bowel syndrome. Gastroenterology 109:40, 1995.

95. Verne GN, Robinson ME, Price DD: Hypersensitivity to visceral and cutaneous pain in the irritable bowel syndrome. Pain 93:7, 2001.

96. Chang L, Mayer EA, Johnson T, et al: Differences in somatic perception in female patients with irritable bowel syndrome with and without fibromyalgia. Pain 84:297, 2000.

97. Cook IJ, van Eeden A, Collins SM: Patients with irritable bowel syndrome have greater pain tolerance than normal subjects. Gastroenterology 93:727, 1987.

98. Delvaux M: Role of visceral sensitivity in the pathophysiology of irritable bowel syndrome. Gut 51(Suppl 1):67, 2002.

99. Munakata J, Naliboff B, Harraf F, et al: Repetitive sigmoid stimulation induces rectal hyperalgesia in patients with irritable bowel syndrome. Gastroenterology 112:55, 1997.

100. Buéno L, Fioramonti J, Garcia-Villar R: Pathobiology of visceral pain: Molecular mechanisms and therapeutic implications: III. Visceral afferent pathways: A source of new therapeutic targets for abdominal pain. Am J Physiol Gastrointest Liver Physiol 278:G670, 2000.

101. Willert RP, Woolf CJ, Hobson AR, et al: The development and maintenance of human visceral pain hypersensitivity is dependent on the N-methyl-D-aspartate receptor. Gastroenterology 126:683, 2004.

102. Whitehead WE, Palsson OS: Is rectal pain sensitivity a biological marker for irritable bowel syndrome: Psychological influences on pain perception. Gastroenterology 115:1263, 1998.

103. Quigley EMM: From comic relief to real understanding: How intestinal gas causes symptoms. Gut 52:1659, 2003.

104. Serra J, Azpiroz F, Malagelada JR: Mechanisms of intestinal gas retention in humans: Impaired propulsion versus obstructed evacuation. Am J Physiol Gastrointest Liver Physiol 281:G138, 2001.

105. Tremolaterra F, Serra J, Azpiroz F, et al: Bloating and abdominal wall dystony [Abstract]. Gastroenterology 126:A53, 2004.

106. Lin HC: Small intestinal bacterial overgrowth: A framework for understanding irritable bowel syndrome. JAMA 292:852, 2004.

107. Caldarella MP, Serra J, Azpiroz F, Malagelada J: Prokinetic effects in patients with intestinal gas retention. Gastroenterology 122:1748, 2002.

108. Dainese R, Serra J, Azpiroz F, Malagelada J: Effects of physical activity on intestinal gas transit and evacuation in healthy subjects. Am J Med 116:536, 2004.

109. Weston AP, Biddle WL, Bhatia PS, Miner PB Jr: Terminal ileal mucosal mast cells in irritable bowel syndrome. Dig Dis Sci 38:1590, 1993.

110. O'Sullivan M, Clayton N, Breslin NP, et al: Increased mast cells in the irritable bowel syndrome. Neurogastroenterol Motil 12:449, 2000.

111. Talley NJ, Butterfield JH: Mast cell infiltration and degranulation in colonic mucosa in the irritable bowel syndrome. Am J Gastroenterol 91:1675, 1996.

112. Spiller RC, Jenkins D, Thornley JP, et al: Increased rectal mucosal enteroendocrine cells, T lymphocytes, and increased gut permeability following acute *Campylobacter enteritis* and in post-dysenteric irritable bowel syndrome. Gut 47:804, 2000.

113. Chadwick VS, Chen W, Shu D, et al: Activation of the mucosal immune system in irritable bowel syndrome. Gastroenterology 122:1778, 2002.

114. Tornblom H, Lindberg G, Nyberg B, Veress G: Full-thickness biopsy of the jejunum reveals inflammation and enteric neuropathy in irritable bowel syndrome. Gastroenterology 123:1972, 2002.

115. Hiatt RB, Katz L: Mast cells in inflammatory conditions of the gastrointestinal tract. Am J Gastroenterol 37:541, 1962.

116. Spiller RC: Postinfectious irritable bowel syndrome. Gastroenterology 124:1662, 2003.

117. Parry SD, Stansfield R, Jelley D, et al: Is irritable bowel syndrome more common in patients presenting with bacterial gastroenteritis? A community-based, case-control study. Am J Gastroenterol 98:327, 2003.

118. Crowell MD, Shetzline MA, Moses PL, et al: Enterochromaffin cells and 5-HT signaling in the pathophysiology of disorders of gastrointestinal function. Curr Opin Investig Drugs 5:55, 2004.

119. Houghton LA, Atkinson W, Whitaker RP, et al: Increased platelet depleted plasma 5-hydroxytryptamine concentration following meal ingestion in symptomatic female subjects with diarrhoea predominant irritable bowel syndrome. Gut 52:663, 2003.

120. Coates MD, Mahoney CR, Linden DR, et al: Molecular defects in mucosal serotonin content and decreased serotonin reuptake transporter in ulcerative colitis and irritable bowel syndrome. Gastroenterology 126:1657, 2004.

121. Whorwell P, Lea R: Dietary treatment of the irritable bowel syndrome. Curr Treat Options Gastroenterol 7:307, 2004.

122. Niec AM, Frankum B, Talley NJ: Are adverse food reactions linked to irritable bowel syndrome? Am J Gastroenterol 93:2184, 1998.

123. Wahnschaffe U, Ullrich R, Riecken EO, Schulzke JD: Celiac disease-like abnormalities in a subgroup of patients with irritable bowel syndrome. Gastroenterology 121:1329, 2001.

124. Olden KW: Diagnosis of irritable bowel syndrome. Gastroenterology 122:1701, 2002.

125. Suarez FL, Savaiano DA, Levitt MD: A comparison of symptoms after the consumption of milk or lactose-hydrolyzed milk by people with self-reported severe lactose intolerance. N Engl J Med 333:1, 1995.

126. Parker TJ, Woolner JT, Prevost AT, et al: Irritable bowel syndrome: Is the search for lactose intolerance justified? Eur J Gastroenterol Hepatol 13:219, 2001.

127. Nelis GF, Vermeeren MA, Jansen W: Role of fructose-sorbitol malabsorption in the irritable bowel syndrome. Gastroenterology 90:1016, 1990.

128. Ledochowski M, Widner B, Bair H, et al: Fructose- and sorbitol-reduced diet improves mood and gastrointestinal disturbances in fructose malabsorbers. Scand J Gastroenterol 35:1048, 2000.

129. Skoog SM, Bharucha AE: Dietary fructose and gastrointestinal symptoms. Am J Gastroenterol 99:2046, 2004.

130. Madden JA, Hunter JO: A review of the role of the gut microflora in irritable bowel syndrome and the effects of probiotics. Br J Nutr 88(Suppl 1):S67, 2002.

131. Pimentel M, Chow EJ, Lin HC: Normalization of lactulose breath testing correlates with symptom improvement in irritable bowel syndrome: A double-blind, randomized, placebo-controlled study. Am J Gastroenterol 98:412, 2003.

132. Pimentel M, Chow EJ, Lin HC: Eradication of small intestinal bacterial overgrowth reduces symptoms of irritable bowel syndrome. Am J Gastroenterol 95:3503, 2000.

133. Hasler WL: Lactulose breath testing, bacterial overgrowth, and IBS: Just a lot of hot air? Gastroenterology 125:1898, 2003.

134. O'Leary C, Quigley EMM: Small bowel bacterial overgrowth, celiac disease, and IBS: What are the real associations? Am J Gastroenterol 98:720, 2003.

135. Mertz H, Morgan V, Tanner G, et al: Regional cerebral activation in irritable bowel syndrome and control subjects with painful and nonpainful rectal distention. Gastroenterology 118:842, 2000.

136. Naliboff BD, Derbyshire SW, Munakata J, et al: Cerebral activation in patients with irritable bowel syndrome and control subjects during rectosigmoid stimulation. Psychosom Med 63:365, 2001.

137. Rainville P, Duncan GH, Price DD, et al: Pain affect encoded in human anterior cingulate but not somatosensory cortex. Science 1997:968, 1997.

138. Naliboff BD, Berman S, Chang L, et al: Sex-related differences in IBS patients: Central processing of visceral stimuli. Gastroenterology 124:1738, 2003.

139. Locke GR III, Weaver AL, Melton LJ III, Talley NJ: Psychosocial factors are linked to functional gastrointestinal disorders: A population-based nested case-control study. Am J Gastroenterol 99:350, 2004.

140. Koloski NA, Talley NJ, Boyce PM: Does psychological distress modulate functional gastrointestinal symptoms and health care seeking? A prospective, community cohort study. Am J Gastroenterol 98:789, 2003.

141. Talley NJ, Boyce PM, Jones M: Is the association between irritable bowel syndrome and abuse explained by neuroticism? A population-based study. Gut. 42:47, 1998.

142. Drossman DA, Leserman J, Nachman G, et al: Sexual and physical abuse in women with functional or organic gastrointestinal disorders. Ann Intern Med 113:828, 1990.

143. Talley NJ, Fett SL, Zinsmeister AR, Melton LJ: Gastrointestinal tract symptoms and self-reported abuse: A population-based study. Gastroenterology 107:1040, 1994.

144. Drossman DA, Talley NJ, Leserman J, et al: Sexual and physical abuse and gastrointestinal illness: Review and recommendations. Ann Intern Med 123:782, 1995.

145. Talley NJ, Fett SL, Zinsmeister AR: Self-reported abuse and gastrointestinal disease in outpatients: Association with irritable bowel-type symptoms. Am J Gastroenterol 90:366, 1995.

146. Ringel Y, Whitehead WE, Toner BB, et al: Sexual and physical abuse are not associated with rectal hypersensitivity in patients with irritable bowel syndrome. Gut 53:838, 2004.

147. Ringel Y, Drossman DA, Turkington TG, et al: Regional brain activation in response to rectal distension in patients with irritable bowel syndrome and the effect of a history of abuse. Dig Dis Sci 48:1774, 2003.

148. Tache Y: Corticotropin-releasing factor receptor antagonists: Potential future therapy in gastroenterology? Gut 53:919, 2004.

149. Locke GR III., Zinsmeister AR, Talley NJ, et al: Familial association in adults with functional gastrointestinal disorders. Mayo Clin Proc 75:907, 2000.

150. Kalantar JS, Locke GR III, Zinsmeister AR, et al: Familial aggregation of irritable bowel syndrome: A prospective study. Gut 52:1703, 2003.

151. Levy RL, Jones KR, Whitehead WE, et al: Irritable bowel syndrome in twins: Heredity and social learning both contribute to etiology. Gastroenterology 121:799, 2001.

152. Morris-Yates A, Talley NJ, Boyce PM, et al: Evidence of a genetic contribution to functional bowel disorder. Am J Gastroenterol 93:1311, 1998.

153. Gonsalkorale WM, Perrey C, Pravica V, et al: Interleukin 10 genotypes in irritable bowel syndrome: Evidence for an inflammatory component? Gut 52:91, 2003.

154. van der Veek P, Kroon Y, van der Berg M, et al: Role of tumor necrosis factor-alpha and interleukin-10 gene polymorphisms in irritable bowel syndrome. Am J Gastroenterol 100:2510, 2005.

155. Kim HJ, Camilleri M, Carlson PJ, et al: Association of distinct α_2-adrenoceptor and serotonin transporter polymorphisms

with constipation and somatic symptoms in functional gastrointestinal disorders. Gut 53:829, 2004.

156. Pata C, Erdal E, Yazc K, et al: Association of the −1438 G/A and 102 T/C polymorphism of the 5-Ht2A receptor gene with irritable bowel syndrome 5-Ht$_{2A}$ gene polymorphism in irritable bowel syndrome. J Clin Gastroenterol 38:561, 2004.

157. Pata C, Erdal ME, Derici E, et al: Serotonin transporter gene polymorphism in irritable bowel syndrome. Am J Gastroenterol 97:1780, 2002.

158. Hammer J, Eslick G, Howell S, et al: Diagnostic yield of alarm features in irritable bowel syndrome and functional dyspepsia. Gut 53:666, 2004.

159. Cash BD, Chey WD: Irritable bowel syndrome: An evidence-based approach to diagnosis. Aliment Pharmacol Ther 19:1235, 2004.

160. Vanner SJ, Depew WT, Paterson WG, et al: Predictive value of the Rome criteria for diagnosing the irritable bowel syndrome. Am J Gastroenterol 94:2912, 1999.

161. Tibble J, Teahon K, Thjodleifsson B, et al: A simple method for assessing intestinal inflammation in Crohn's disease. Gut 47:506, 2000.

162. Tibble JA, Sigthorsson G, Foster R, et al: Use of surrogate markers of inflammation and Rome criteria to distinguish organic from nonorganic intestinal disease. Gastroenterology 123:450, 2002.

163. Sinha L, Liston R, Testa HJ, Moriarty KJ: Idiopathic bile acid malabsorption: Qualitative and quantitative clinical features and response to cholestyramine. Aliment Pharmacol Ther 12:839, 1998.

164. Wildt S, Norby Rasmussen S, et al: Bile acid malabsorption in patients with chronic diarrhoea: Clinical value of SeHCAT test. Scand J Gastroenterol 38:826, 2003.

165. Sanders DS, Carter MJ, Hurlstone DP, et al: Association of adult coeliac disease with irritable bowel syndrome: A case-control study in patients fulfilling ROME II criteria referred to secondary care. Lancet 358:1504, 2001.

166. Locke GRI, Murray JA, Zinsmeister AR, et al: Celiac disease serology in irritable bowel syndrome and dyspepsia: A population-based case-control study. Mayo Clin Proc 79:476, 2004.

167. Spiegel BM, DeRosa VP, Gralnek IM, et al: Testing for celiac sprue in irritable bowel syndrome with predominant diarrhea: A cost-effectiveness analysis. Gastroenterology 126: 1721, 2004.

168. Dixon-Woods M, Critchley S: Medical and lay views of irritable bowel syndrome. Fam Pract 17:108, 2000.

169. Bertram S, Kurland M, Lydick E, et al: The patient's perspective of irritable bowel syndrome. J Fam Pract 50:521, 2001.

170. Owens DM, Nelson DK, Talley NJ: The irritable bowel syndrome: Long-term prognosis and the physician-patient interaction. Ann Intern Med 122:107, 1995.

171. Saito YA, Prather CM, Van Dyke CT, et al: Effects of multidisciplinary education on outcomes in patients with irritable bowel syndrome. Clin Gastroenterol Hepatol 2:576, 2004.

172. Colwell LJ, Prather CM, Phillips SF, Zinsmeister AR: Effects of an irritable bowel syndrome educational class on health-promotion behaviors and symptoms. Am J Gastroenterol 93:901, 1998.

173. Drossman DA, Thompson WG: The irritable bowel syndrome: Review and a graduated multicomponent treatment approach. Ann Intern Med 116:1009, 1992.

174. Mertz HR: Irritable bowel syndrome. N Engl J Med 349:2136, 2003.

175. Thompson WG: Review article: The treatment of irritable bowel syndrome. Aliment Pharmacol Ther 16:1395, 2002.

176. Talley NJ: Evaluation of drug treatment in irritable bowel syndrome. Br J Clin Pharmacol 56:362, 2003.

177. Brandt L, Bjorkman D, Fennerty M, et al: An evidence-based approach to the management of irritable bowel syndrome in North America. Am J Gastroenterol 97(Suppl):S7, 2002.

178. Fass R, Longstreth GF, Pimentel M, et al: Evidence- and consensus-based practice guidelines for the diagnosis of irritable bowel syndrome. Arch Intern Med 161:2081, 2001.

179. Jailwala J, Imperiale TF, Kroenke K: Pharmacologic treatment of the irritable bowel syndrome: A systematic review of randomized, controlled trials. Ann Intern Med 133:136, 2000.

180. Bijkerk CJ, Muris JWM, Knotterus JA, et al: Systematic review: The role of different types of fibre in the treatment of irritable bowel syndrome. Aliment Pharmacol Ther 19:245, 2004.

181. Atkinson W, Gurney R, Sheldon TA, Whorwell PJ: Do food elimination diets improve irritable bowel syndrome? A double-blind trial based on IgG antibodies to food [Abstract]. Gastroenterology 124:A29, 2003.

182. Stefanini GF, Bazzocchi G, Prati E, et al: Efficacy of oral disodium cromoglycate in patients with irritable bowel syndrome and positive skin prick tests to foods. Lancet 1:207, 1986.

183. Nobaek S, Johansson ML, Molin G, et al: Alteration of intestinal microflora is associated with reduction in abdominal bloating and pain in patients with irritable bowel syndrome. Am J Gastroenterol 95:1231, 2000.

184. Kim HJ, Camilleri M, McKinzie S, et al: A randomized controlled trial of a probiotic, VSL#3, on gut transit and symptoms in diarrhoea-predominant irritable bowel syndrome. Aliment Pharmacol Ther 17:895, 2003.

185. Sen S, Mullan MM, Parker TJ, et al: Effect of *Lactobacillus plantarum* 299v on colonic fermentation and symptoms of irritable bowel syndrome. Dig Dis Sci 47:2615, 2002.

186. Poynard T, Regimbeau C, Benhamou Y: Meta-analysis of smooth muscle relaxants in the treatment of irritable bowel syndrome. Aliment Pharmacol Ther 15:355, 2001.

187. DiPalma JA, DeRidder PH, Orlando RC, et al: A randomized, placebo-controlled, multicenter study of the safety and efficacy of a new polyethylene glycol laxative. Am J Gastroenterol 95:446, 2000.

188. Corazziari E, Badiali D, Bazzocchi G, et al: Long-term efficacy, safety, and tolerability of low daily doses of isosmotic polyethylene glycol electrolyte balanced solution (PMF-100) in the treatment of functional chronic constipation. Gut 46:522, 2000.

189. Wald A: Is chronic use of stimulant laxatives harmful to the colon? J Clin Gastroenterol 36:386, 2003.

190. Efskind PS, Bernklev T, Vatn MH: A double-blind placebo-controlled trial with loperamide in irritable bowel syndrome. Scand J Gastroenterol 31:463, 1996.

191. Lavo B, Stenstam M, Nielsen AL: Loperamide in treatment of irritable bowel syndrome: A double-blind placebo-controlled study. Scan J Gastroenterol Suppl 130:77, 1987.

192. Cann PA, Read NW, Holdsworth CD, Barends D: Role of loperamide and placebo in management of irritable bowel syndrome (IBS). Dig Dis Sci 29:239, 1984.

193. Prather CM, Camilleri M, Zinsmeister AR, et al: Tegaserod accelerates orocecal transit in patients with constipation-predominant irritable bowel syndrome. Gastroenterology 118:463, 2000.

194. Talley NJ: Pharmacologic therapy for the irritable bowel syndrome. Am J Gastroenterol 98:750, 2003.

195. Muller-Lissner SA, Fumagalli I, Bardhan KD, et al: Tegaserod, a 5-HT$_4$ receptor partial agonist, relieves symptoms in irritable bowel syndrome patients with abdominal pain, bloating and constipation. Aliment Pharmacol Ther 15:1655, 2001.

196. Nyhlin H, Bang C, Elsborg L, et al: A double-blind, placebo-controlled randomized study to evaluate the efficacy, safety, and tolerability of tegaserod in patients with irritable bowel syndrome. Scand J Gastroenterol 39:119, 2004.

197. Kellow JE, Lee OY, Chang FY, et al: An Asia-Pacific, double blind, placebo-controlled, randomized study to evaluate the efficacy, safety, and tolerability of tegaserod in patients with irritable bowel syndrome. Gut 52:671, 2003.

198. Novick J, Miner P, Krause R, et al: A randomized, double-blind, placebo-controlled trial of tegaserod in female patients suffering from irritable bowel syndrome with constipation. Aliment Pharmacol Ther 16:1877, 2002.

199. Evans BW, Clark WK, Moore DJ, Whorwell PJ: Tegaserod for the treatment of irritable bowel syndrome. Cochrane Database Syst Rev CD003960, 2004.

200. Tougas G, Snape WJ Jr, Otten MH, et al: Long-term safety of tegaserod in patients with constipation-predominant irritable bowel syndrome. Aliment Pharmacol Ther 16:1701, 2002.

201. Wooltorton E: Tegaserod (Zelnorm) for irritable bowel syndrome: Reports of serious diarrhea and intestinal ischemia. Can Med Assoc J 170:1908, 2004.

202. Cremonini F, Delgado-Aros S, Camilleri M: Efficacy of alosetron in irritable bowel syndrome: A meta-analysis of randomized controlled trials. Neurogastroenterol Motil 15:79, 2003.

203. Watson ME, Lacey L, Kong S, et al: Alosetron improves quality of life in women with diarrhea-predominant irritable bowel syndrome. Am J Gastroenterol 96:455, 2001.

204. Lembo A, Weber HC, Farraye FA: Alosetron in irritable bowel syndrome: Strategies for its use in a common gastrointestinal disorder. Drugs 63:1895, 2003.

205. Miller DP, Alfredson T, Cook SF, et al: Incidence of colonic ischemia, hospitalized complications of constipation, and bowel surgery in relation to use of alosetron hydrochloride. Am J Gastroenterol 98:1117, 2003.

206. Camilleri M, Atanasova E, Carlson PJ, et al: Serotonin-transporter polymorphism pharmacogenetics in diarrhea-predominant irritable bowel syndrome. Gastroenterology 123:425, 2002.

207. Talley NJ: Antidepressants in IBS: Are we deluding ourselves? Am J Gastroenterol 99:921, 2004.

208. Jackson JL, O'Malley PG, Tomkins G, et al: Treatment of functional gastrointestinal disorders with antidepressant medications: A meta-analysis. Am J Med 108:65, 2000.

209. Drossman D, Toner BB, Whitehead WE, et al: Cognitive-behavioral therapy versus education and desipramine versus placebo for moderate to severe functional bowel disorders. Gastroenterology 125:19, 2003.

210. Clouse RE, Lustman PJ, Geisman RA, Alpers DH: Antidepressant therapy in 138 patients with irritable bowel syndrome: A five-year clinical experience. Aliment Pharmacol Ther 8:409, 1994.

211. Creed F, Fernandes L, Guthrie E, et al: The cost-effectiveness of psychotherapy and paroxetine for severe irritable bowel syndrome. Gastroenterology 124:303, 2003.

212. Tabas G, Beaves M, Wang J, et al: Paroxetine to treat irritable bowel syndrome not responding to high-fiber diet: A double-blind, placebo-controlled trial. Am J Gastroenterol 99:914, 2004.

213. Kuiken SD, Tytgat GN, Boeckxstaens GE: The selective serotonin reuptake inhibitor fluoxetine does not change rectal sensitivity and symptoms in patients with irritable bowel syndrome: A double-blind, randomized, placebo-controlled study. Clin Gastoenterol Hepatol 1:219, 2003.

214. Gorard DA, Libby GW, Farthing MJG: Influence of antidepressants on whole gut orocaecal transit times in health and irritable bowel syndrome. Aliment Pharmacol Ther 8:159, 1994.

215. Dunlop SP, Jenkins D, Neal KR, et al: Randomized, double-blind, placebo-controlled trial of prednisolone in post-infectious irritable bowel syndrome. Aliment Pharmacol Ther 18:77, 2003.

216. Greenbaum DS, Ferguson RK, Kater LA, et al: A controlled therapeutic study of the irritable bowel syndrome: Effect of diphenylhydantoin. N Engl J Med 288:13, 1973.

217. Fielding JF: Timolol treatment in the irritable bowel syndrome. Digestion 22:155, 1981.

218. McIntyre AS, Burnham WR, Thompson DG: Atenolol in irritable bowel syndrome. Lancet 1:8575, 1988.

219. Mathias JR, Clench MH, Abell TL, et al: Effect of leuprolide acetate in treatment of abdominal pain and nausea in premenopausal women with functional bowel disease: A double-blind, placebo-controlled, randomized study. Dig Dis Sci 43:1347, 1998.

220. Mathias JR, Clench MH, Reeves-Darby VG, et al: Effect of leuprolide acetate in patients with moderate to severe functional bowel disease: Double-blind, placebo-controlled study. Dig Dis Sci 39:1155, 1994.

221. Verne GN, Davis RH, Robinson ME, et al: Treatment of chronic constipation with colchicine: Randomized, double-blind, placebo-controlled, crossover trial. Am J Gastroenterol 98:1112, 2003.

222. Roarty TP, Weber F, Soykan I, McCallum RW: Misoprostol in the treatment of chronic refractory constipation: Results of a long-term open label trial. Aliment Pharmacol Ther 11:1059, 1997.

223. Schewetz I, Naliboff B, Munakata J, et al: Anti-hyperalgesic effect of octreotide in patients with irritable bowel syndrome. Aliment Pharmacol Ther 19:123, 2004.

224. Camilleri M, Kim DY, McKinzie S, et al: A randomized, controlled exploratory study of clonidine in diarrhea-predominant irritable bowel syndrome. Clin Gastroenterol Hepatol 1:111, 2003.

225. Friis H, Bode S, Rumessen JJ, Gudmand-Hoyer E: Effect of simethicone on lactulose-induced H_2 production and gastrointestinal symptoms. Digestion 49:227, 1991.

226. Suarez FL, Furne J, Springfield J, Levitt MD: Failure of activated charcoal to reduce the release of gases produced by the colonic flora. Am J Gastroenterol 94:208, 1999.

227. Potter T, Ellis C, Levitt M: Activated charcoal: In vivo and in vitro studies of effect on gas formation. Gastroenterology 88:620, 1985.

228. Ganiats TG, Norcross WA, Halverson AL, et al: Does Beano prevent gas? A double-blind crossover study of oral alpha-galactosidase to treat dietary oligosaccharide intolerance. J Fam Pract 39:441, 1994.

229. Suarez FL, Furne JK, Springfield J, Levitt MD: Bismuth subsalicylate markedly decreases hydrogen sulfide release in the human colon. Gastroenterology 114:923, 1998.

230. Suarez FL, Springfield J, Levitt MD: Identification of gases responsible for the odour of human flatus and evaluation of a device purported to reduce this odour. Gut 43:100, 1998.

231. Fink RN, Lembo AJ: Intestinal gas. Curr Treat Options Gastroenterol 4:333, 2001.

232. Talley NJ, Owens BK, Boyce P, Paterson K: Psychological treatment for irritable bowel syndrome: A critique of controlled treatment trials. Am J Gastroenterol 91:277, 1996.

233. Gonsalkorale WM, Toner BB, Whorwell PJ: Cognitive change in patients undergoing hypnotherapy for irritable bowel syndrome. J Psychosom Res 56:271, 2004.

234. Boyce PM, Talley NJ, Balaam B, et al: A randomized controlled trial of cognitive behavior therapy, relaxation training, and routine clinical care for the irritable bowel syndrome. Am J Gastroenterol 98:2209, 2003.

235. Spanier JA, Howden CW, Jones MP: A systematic review of alternative therapies in the irritable bowel syndrome. Arch Intern Med 163:265, 2003.

236. Bensoussan A, Talley NJ, Hing M, et al: Treatment of irritable bowel syndrome with Chinese herbal medicine: A randomized controlled trial. JAMA 280:1585, 1998.

237. Langmead L, Rampton DS: Review article: Herbal treatment in gastrointestinal and liver disease—benefits and dangers. Aliment Pharmacol Ther 15:1239, 2001.

238. Yadav SK, Jain AK, Tripathi SN, Gupta JP: Irritable bowel syndrome: Therapeutic evaluation of indigenous drugs. Indian J Med Res 90:496, 1989.

239. Suarez F, Levitt MD, Adshead J, Barkin JS: Pancreatic supplements reduce symptomatic response of healthy subjects to a high fat meal. Dig Dis Sci 44:1317, 1999.

240. Xing J, Larive B, Mekhail N, Soffer E: Transcutaneous electrical acustimulation can reduce visceral perception in patients with the irritable bowel syndrome: A pilot study. Altern Ther Health Med 10:38, 2004.

241. Xiao WB, Liu YL: Rectal hypersensitivity reduced by acupoint TENS in patients with diarrhea-predominant irritable bowel syndrome: A pilot study. Dig Dis Sci 49:312, 2004.

242. Adeniji OA, Barnett CB, DiPalma JA: Durability of the diagnosis of irritable bowel syndrome based on clinical criteria. Dig Dis Sci 49:572, 2004.

CHAPTER
116 Intestinal Obstruction and Ileus

Richard H. Turnage, Maureen Heldmann, and Philip Cole

Impairment to the aboral passage of intestinal contents may result from either mechanical obstruction or failure of normal intestinal motility in the absence of an obstructing lesion (*ileus*). Intestinal obstruction may be categorized according to the degree of obstruction to the flow of intestinal contents (*partial* or *complete*), the absence or presence of intestinal ischemia (*simple* or *strangulated*), and the site of obstruction (*small intestinal* or *colonic*). These distinctions have prognostic and therapeutic relevance. For example, complete or strangulated obstruction requires urgent operative management, whereas partial small intestinal obstruction may, in selected cases, be managed successfully without laparotomy. A *closed-loop obstruction* refers to a mechanical obstruction in which both the proximal and distal parts of the involved intestinal segment are occluded. This condition has a particularly high risk of strangulation, necrosis, and perforation.

SMALL INTESTINAL OBSTRUCTION

ETIOLOGY

The three most common causes of small bowel obstruction (SBO) are postoperative intra-abdominal adhesions, hernias, and neoplasms. A more comprehensive list of causes of intestinal obstruction is shown in Table 116–1.

Intra-abdominal Adhesions

The most common cause of SBO is intra-abdominal adhesions following laparotomy; such adhesions account for one half to three fourths of all cases.[1] Peritoneal adhesions are common after laparotomy and are exacerbated by intra-abdominal infection, ischemia, and the presence of foreign bodies, including suture material.

Adhesive SBO is a relatively frequent complication of laparotomy, as illustrated by several population-based and large case studies. For example, the risk of adhesive SBO after appendectomy is about 1% with 30 years of follow-up,[2] whereas the risk after partial or subtotal colectomy is as high as 18%.[3,4] Beck and associates, in a population-based study, found that the risk of intestinal obstruction was 14.3% following operations in which there was resection and reanastomosis of the intestine.[5] The frequency of adhesive SBO after gynecologic operations is similar to that of appendectomy except for cesarean delivery, in which the risk of subsequent SBO is approximately 1 per 2000 procedures.[6] Lower abdominal or pelvic procedures have a higher risk of postoperative adhesive obstruction than do upper abdominal procedures, such as cholecystectomy and gastrectomy.[7] Furthermore, the risk of SBO is greatest in the first several years following the index procedure, although patients may develop intestinal obstruction up to 30 years postoperatively.[2-4,8]

Table 116–1 Causes of Intestinal Obstruction

Type of Obstruction	Causes
Intrinsic	Congenital: atresia, stenosis
	Inflammatory: diverticulitis, inflammatory bowel disease, ischemic injury, radiation injury, drugs and chemicals, postanastomotic
	Intussusception
	Obstruction: polypoid neoplasm, gallstone, foreign body, bezoars, feces
	Neoplasm
Extrinsic	Congenital bands
	Adhesions
	Hernias
	Volvulus
	Carcinomatosis
	Endometriosis
	Abscess

Hernias

Hernias are the second most common cause of SBO, and account for about one fourth of all cases.[1,9] Fevang and colleagues reported that 30% of 877 patients undergoing operation for SBO had an incarcerated hernia as the cause of their obstruction.[1] The studies quoted[1,9] may overestimate the frequency in which hernias cause SBO because they consider only patients who had an operation for intestinal obstruction and not patients treated nonsurgically, as in most instances of partial adhesive obstruction and obstruction from Crohn's disease. This hypothesis is consistent with the experience of Miller and coworkers, who reported that hernias accounted for only 2% of all admissions for SBO, whereas adhesions and Crohn's disease caused 74% and 7%, respectively, of SBO admissions.[10]

SBO may be caused both by internal (paraduodenal, obturator, intermesenteric) and external (inguinal, femoral, umbilical, and incisional) hernias; the latter is a much more common cause than the former. In either case, SBO from hernias has a particularly high risk of strangulation, failure to resolve spontaneously, and recurrence when not corrected surgically.[9,11] In one retrospective series of 47 patients, the incidence of strangulated obstruction was 33% for patients whose obstructions were caused by hernias and only 8% for patients with adhesive obstruction.[9] This increased risk of obstruction and strangulation is due at least in part to the rigid fascial defect through which the herniated intestine passes. Femoral hernias, in particular, pose a high risk of intestinal obstruction and strangulation.[11,12] In these cases, the herniated intestine passes through the femoral canal, which is bound anteriorly and medially by the ileopubic tract as it inserts into the pectineus fascia, posteriorly by the pectineus fascia and the superior ramus of the pubis, and laterally by the femoral vessels.

Although SBO from a "groin" hernia may occur at any age, it is particularly prevalent in the elderly. The median age of adults presenting with incarcerated groin hernias in a study of 147 patients was 70 years.[12] In another series, 43% of adults presenting with incarcerated groin hernias were older than 60 years of age.[13] Advanced age, con-comitant chronic illnesses, and treatment delay are associated with unfavorable outcomes in patients with SBO from hernias, just as with SBO from other causes.[11-14]

Internal hernias may be congenital (e.g., paraduodenal) or acquired (e.g., hernias through mesenteric defects created in the performance of intestinal anastomoses). Although unusual, the occurrence of SBO in a patient without a prior laparotomy or external evidence of an incarcerated hernia should suggest this as one of the potential causes of the obstruction. The 3% incidence of internal herniation of the Roux limb after gastric bypass for weight loss is a particularly important example of an internal hernia, given the frequency in which this procedure is performed today.[15,16] Congenital and acquired internal hernias are discussed in greater detail in Chapter 93.

Various authors have reported the herniation of a portion of the intestinal wall (Richter's hernia) or a whole segment of the intestine through a laparoscopic trocar site with resultant bowel obstruction.[17,18] The incidence of trocar site hernias after laparoscopic fundoplication or cholecystectomy is 1% to 3%, whereas SBO is significantly less common; trocar site hernias occur at 10-mL port sites positioned at or close to the midline.[18,19] SBO after laparoscopic herniorrhaphy usually is due to herniation of the bowel through a defect in the peritoneal closure during a transabdominal preperitoneal herniorrhaphy (TAPP). In these instances, the bowel is tethered by adhesions between the partially peritoneal-covered prosthesis and the intestine, with formation of a kink or a point of torsion. In one series of 3229 laparoscopic herniorrhaphies, only 4 patients developed obstruction, all of whom had a TAPP approach.[20]

Neoplasms

In contrast to colonic tumors with resultant obstruction, neoplasms are a relatively unusual cause of SBO and account for about 5% to 10% of cases.[9,10,21] In patients who present with SBO without prior laparotomy or physical evidence of a hernia, half have malignant neoplasms as the cause.[22] Most commonly, the small bowel becomes obstructed by extrinsic compression or local invasion or both from advanced gastrointestinal or gynecologic malignancies, a mechanism accounting for 92% of neoplastic SBOs in a Mayo Clinic series.[9] The two most common primary malignancies causing SBO in a series of 32 patients were colorectal and ovarian adenocarcinoma, accounting for 41% and 28% of cases, respectively.[21] A significant percentage of patients with a history of intra-abdominal malignancies who present with SBO, however, have peritoneal adhesions as the cause of their obstruction. In one series, Edna and Bjerkeset found that more than half of 41 patients who developed SBO after operations for colorectal cancer had peritoneal adhesions as the cause.[3] Hematogenous metastases from breast adenocarcinoma, melanoma, or Kaposi's sarcoma also may involve the intestine with subsequent obstruction. Primary neoplasms of the small bowel are the cause of SBO in less than 3% of cases. Both carcinoid tumors (see Chapter 30) and adenocarcinoma (see Chapter 118) have been reported as the most common malignancy of the small intestine to cause symptoms of obstruction.

PATHOPHYSIOLOGY

The duration and degree of obstruction and the presence and severity of ischemia determine the local and systemic consequences of intestinal obstruction. The intestinal mucosa is an important and early site of injury in both simple and strangulated intestinal obstruction. Microscopic evidence of epithelial injury occurs within the first 4 to 6 hours of simple intestinal obstruction and progresses to focal epithelial necrosis as the duration increases to 8 to 12 hours.[23] Strangulated obstruction markedly exacerbates the mucosal injury with extensive mucosal necrosis and sloughing within 180 minutes of strangulation.[24]

Intestinal obstruction causes the profound accumulation of fluid and swallowed air within the lumen proximal to the obstruction. Impaired water and electrolyte absorption and enhanced secretion cause the net movement of isotonic fluid from the intravascular space into the intestinal lumen.[25] The accumulation of swallowed air, and to a lesser extent hydrogen, carbon dioxide, and methane generated by bacterial overgrowth within the obstructed bowel, contributes to intestinal dilatation.[26]

The failure of normal intestinal motility with SBO allows the overgrowth of bacteria within the small intestine and loss of the normally increasing concentration gradient of bacteria from the jejunum to the ileum. In one study using a porcine model of ileal obstruction, there was a 10,000-fold increase in the concentration of *Escherichia coli* in the ileum and a 40 million-fold increase in the jejunum when compared with counts in normal controls.[27] Data in humans and in animals suggest that the overgrowth of enteric bacterial flora occurs within a few hours of obstruction and is maximal by 24 hours.[28]

Experimental and clinical evidence suggests that bacterial overgrowth is an important part of the pathophysiology of intestinal obstruction. Disruption of the ecologic balance of the normal enteric microflora is associated with the translocation of bacteria to mesenteric lymph nodes and systemic organs in laboratory and clinical situations.[29-31] In one study by Deitch, enteric bacteria, particularly *E. coli*, were cultured from mesenteric lymph nodes in nearly 60% of patients with simple intestinal obstruction compared with only 4% of mesenteric lymph nodes from controls.[31] These observations are consistent with the experimental observations of Samel and associates, who described the translocation of bacteria into the submucosa within 36 minutes of simple intestinal obstruction; in the setting of ischemia, bacteria were noted within the submucosa within 11 minutes.[32] These data are consistent with the hypothesis that translocating enteric bacteria contribute to the systemic infections and septic consequences of SBO.[31,32] Furthermore, bacterial overgrowth within the obstructed intestine also may contribute to the hypersecretion of fluid by the intestinal mucosa. Heneghan and colleagues found that ileal obstruction in germ-free animals caused intestinal distention without hypersecretion, suggesting that a bacterial-derived enterotoxin may be the mediator of intestinal hypersecretion.[33]

The systemic manifestations of SBO are related, at least in part, to hypovolemia and the inflammatory response incited by ischemic or gangrenous intestine. Hypovolemia primarily is due to the loss of fluids into the intestinal lumen, bowel wall, and peritoneal cavity. When combined with anorexia and vomiting, a marked reduction in intravascular volume results. Intestinal ischemia or infarction markedly exacerbates the loss of intravascular fluid both locally into the bowel as well as systemically through a generalized microvascular "leak." The generation and activation of pro-inflammatory mediators, such as neutrophils, complement, cytokines, eicosanoids, and oxygen-derived free radicals, have been linked to remote organ failure and mortality associated with intestinal ischemia and reperfusion injury.

CLINICAL FEATURES

History

Patients with SBO classically present with the acute onset of cramping mid-abdominal pain, vomiting, obstipation, and abdominal distention. The magnitude of symptoms depends on the degree of obstruction (i.e., complete or partial) and the site and duration of the obstruction. Typically, patients describe paroxysms of periumbilical pain occurring at 4- to 5-min intervals for proximal obstructions and less frequently for more distal obstructions. With prolonged obstruction, the cramping pain subsides as the motility in the distended intestine is inhibited. The development of continuous severe pain, particularly when localized, strongly suggests the presence of strangulated obstruction with intestinal ischemia. Closed-loop obstructions are associated with the sudden onset of severe, unremitting abdominal pain. Patients with proximal intestinal obstructions have profuse vomiting, more frequent pain, and minimal abdominal distention; distal obstructions typically are associated with less frequent vomiting and much more abdominal distention. The emesis of patients with SBO often is feculent because of the increased bacterial count in the obstructed gut.

Although obstipation is considered the sine qua non of SBO, patients with partial obstruction may continue to pass flatus and stool. Even patients with complete SBO evacuate the bowel distal to the obstruction.

Physical Examination

Auscultation of the abdomen reveals periods of increasing bowel sounds separated by intervals of relative quiet. The quality of the bowel sounds usually is described as high pitched or musical. *Borborygmi*, or rumbling bowel sounds that are audible at a distance, may be heard and correspond with paroxysms of abdominal cramping pain. In the setting of prolonged obstruction, bowel sounds disappear as intestinal motility decreases.

Abdominal tenderness with guarding or other evidence of peritonitis suggests strangulated obstruction and necessitates urgent laparotomy. Closed-loop obstruction may present with pain out of proportion to the physical findings much like that of acute mesenteric ischemia. Early in the course of a closed-loop obstruction, acute mesenteric ischemia likely results from venous obstruction and increased intraluminal pressure in the involved bowel; arterial compromise develops later on as the process progresses. Occult rectal bleeding suggests mucosal ulceration that may be the result of intestinal ischemia or a mucosal lesion such as adenocarcinoma. The presence of a tender mass at the site of an inguinal, femoral, or umbilical hernia strongly suggests that this is the etiology of the obstruction. Erythema of the overlying skin suggests the presence of strangulation as is shown in Figure 116–1.

The patient's heart rate, blood pressure, and temperature may provide insight into the systemic response to the obstruction. The most common systemic manifestations of intestinal obstruction are related to hypovolemia and include tachycardia, tachypnea, altered mental status, oliguria, and ultimately hypotension. These findings, particularly when unresponsive to volume repletion, suggest strangulated obstruction. With the exception of clinical evidence of a complete obstruction, none of these physical findings is sufficiently reliable to predict the presence of *early* intestinal strangulation.

RADIOLOGY

Abdominal Films

After history and physical examination, plain abdominal films should be obtained on patients suspected of having SBO. Films taken with the patient in the supine position and in the upright (or lateral decubitus) position may (1) confirm the diagnosis of intestinal obstruction; (2) localize the obstruction to the small intestine or colon; and (3) provide evidence of the degree of obstruction (i.e., partial or complete). Abdominal films taken with the patient recumbent often demonstrate distended small intestine with an abnormal gas pattern, whereas abdominal films taken with the patient in an upright position often reveal multiple air-fluid levels within distended loops of bowel resembling an inverted "U" (Fig. 116–2). The presence of air-fluid levels in dilated small bowel loops alone is insufficient to distinguish early complete or partial SBO from ileus. In this setting, attention should be paid to the pattern of gas within the colon. The absence of gas within the colon is consistent with a complete SBO, whereas gas present in a normal or slightly distended colon may be seen in early complete SBO, partial SBO, or ileus. Lappas and coworkers[34] reviewed 12 abdominal radiologic findings associated with SBO and found that the combination of air-fluid levels of different heights in the *same* bowel loop and a mean air-fluid level diameter of 2.5 cm or greater was most predictive of a high-grade partial or complete SBO. As the duration and severity of intestinal obstruction increase, plain films also may demonstrate a thickened intestinal wall or pneumatosis intestinalis (a finding diagnostic of gangrenous bowel).

The limitations of abdominal plain films in determining the presence of intestinal obstruction are well recognized; 20% to 30% of patients have equivocal or normal studies.[35,36] Furthermore, radiology alone does not localize the site or establish etiology of the obstruction. False-negative films are most likely to occur with low-grade, proximal, or closed-loop obstructions, in which cases fluoroscopic contrast studies or computed tomography (CT) may be diagnostic.

Contrast Studies

Fluoroscopic studies of the gastrointestinal tract with enteral contrast agents (barium sulfate or diatrizoate [Gastrografin]) have been used to evaluate patients suspected of having SBO, particularly when the clinical presentation is atypical and the abdominal plain films are nondiagnostic. Contrast examinations with barium sulfate have been shown to provide "useful" information (i.e., definite diagnosis, no obstruction, high grade or complete obstruction) in 50% to 80% of patients studied.[37] Other studies have suggested that the movement of orally administered diatrizoate into the colon within 6 to 24 hours may predict patients most likely to respond to nonoperative management.[38,39]

In our practice, fluoroscopic contrast studies are limited to those patients suspected of having partial SBO complicating Crohn's disease, radiation enteritis, or malignancy. In these instances, barium sulfate provides excellent definition of the site of obstruction and thus is preferred. In patients with chronic partial SBO, fluoroscopic imaging of the obstruction may be facilitated by the performance of barium enteroclysis, which has 86% to 100% accuracy for characterizing the site of chronic SBO (Fig. 116–3).[36] This study is, of course, contraindicated in patients with complete or high-grade SBO and in those with clinical evidence of strangulation or perforation.

Computed Tomography

Many studies now support the use of abdominal CT to evaluate patients suspected of having SBO. In addition to being more accurate than abdominal plain films and flu-

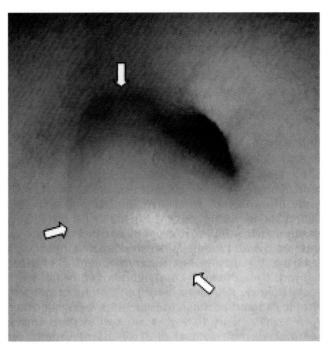

Figure 116–1   The periumbilical region of a patient with an incarcerated umbilical hernia. Erythema of the skin overlying the hernia mass (*arrows*) strongly suggests strangulation of the contents of the hernia, which in this case was omentum.

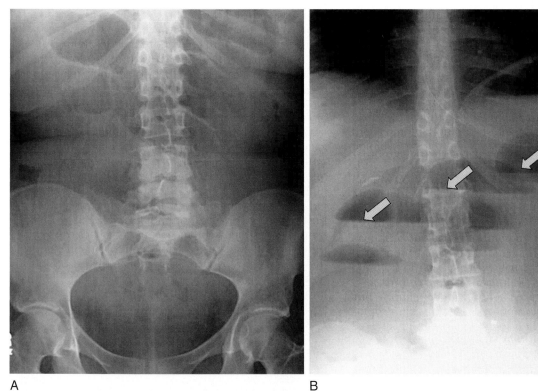

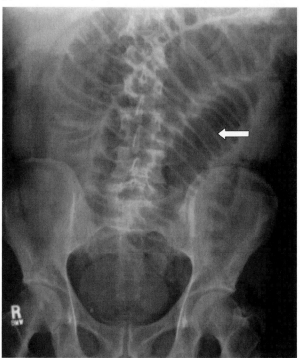

Figure 116–2 Abdominal plain film of a patient with a complete small bowel obstruction (SBO) in the supine (*A*) and upright (*B*) positions. The supine abdominal film demonstrates centrally located dilated loops of small intestine without gas in the colon or rectum. The upright abdominal film demonstrates multiple air-fluid levels (*arrows*). *C*, An abdominal film of a patient with another high-grade SBO demonstrating markedly dilated small intestine with prominent plica circulares (*arrow*).

oroscopic contrast studies of the bowel, CT allows assessment of the entire abdomen for alternative diagnoses or complications of intestinal obstruction.[35,40-42] The authors of these studies recommend CT to evaluate patients suspected of having SBO when the clinical presentation or abdominal films are nondiagnostic or confusing.

CT usually is performed with intravenous and enteral contrast; however, in patients with a high-grade SBO, fluid-filled, distended loops of small bowel are readily apparent in the absence of enteral contrast. Moderate grades of obstruction can be studied with antegrade enteral CT contrast administered 30 minutes to 2 hours prior to scanning; intravenous contrast aids in assessment of the bowel wall for signs of edema or ischemia. The findings suggestive of mechanical SBO are shown in Table 116–2. Demonstration of a transition zone with dilated loops of bowel filled with gas, fluid or both, proximal to an obstruction, and collapsed loops of bowel distal to an obstruction strongly supports the diagnosis of intestinal obstruction (Fig. 116–4). The "small bowel feces" sign, which refers the presence of particulate matter admixed with gas within the dilated bowel lumen proximal and collapsed bowel distal to a mechanical transition, has a high specificity for subacute or low-grade SBO. CT is 90% to 95% sensitive, 96% specific, and 95% accurate in determining the presence of complete or high-grade SBO and provides information regarding the site and cause of obstruction in up to 95% of instances (Fig. 116–5). Low-grade or intermittent bowel obstruction remains a diagnostic challenge, however, with some studies reporting a diagnostic accuracy of about 50% in these instances.[35,40-43] CT enteroclysis and magnetic resonance (MR) imaging enteroclysis combine the advantages of active luminal small bowel distention with mural and extraenteric evaluation and have been shown to raise the accuracy for detection of small intestinal diseases to nearly 100%.[44-46]

CT also is accurate in determining the presence of a strangulated obstruction or closed-loop obstruction. A U-shaped or C-shaped dilated bowel loop with a radial distribution of stretched mesenteric vessels converging toward a torsion point ("whirl sign") is characteristic of a closed-loop obstruction (Fig. 116–6A).[47,48] Intestinal ischemia is suggested by high-density or striated bowel wall thickening, altered mural enhancement, inflammatory changes and hemorrhage in the mesentery, ascites, or pneumatosis intestinalis (see Fig. 116–6B). The sensitivity, specificity, and accuracy of these criteria to predict strangulated obstruction range from 83% to 94%.[49,50]

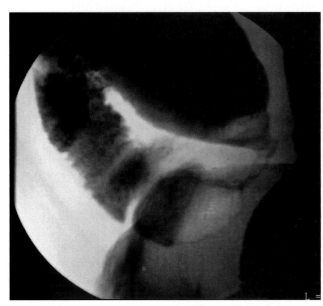

Figure 116–3 Barium contrast study of the small intestine (enteroclysis) in a patient with an ischemic stricture of the ileum. Note the focal stenosis with proximal dilatation of the intestine.

LABORATORY FEATURES

The complete blood count in patients with SBO often reveals a slight leukocytosis. Although significant neutrophilia and left shift are more common in patients with strangulated obstruction than in patients with simple

Table 116–2 Computed Tomography (CT) Findings in Patients with Simple Complete, Closed-Loop, and Strangulated Small Intestinal Obstruction

Type of Obstruction	Findings
Simple obstruction, complete (Fig. 116–4) or partial (Fig. 116–5)	Proximal bowel dilatation, discrete transition zone with collapsed distal small bowel and no passage of oral contrast beyond the transition zone
	Little gas or fluid in colon
Closed-loop obstruction (see Fig. 116–6A)	
Bowel wall changes	U-shaped, distended, fluid-filled bowel loop
	Whirl sign—tightly twisted mesentery around a collapsed bowel segment
	Beak sign—fusiform tapering at the site of obstruction
	Two adjacent collapsed round, oval, or triangular loops of bowel at the site of obstruction
Mesenteric changes	Fixed radial distribution of several dilated bowel loops with stretched and thickened mesenteric vessels converging toward the point of obstruction
Strangulated obstruction (see Fig. 116–6B)	
Bowel wall changes	Bowel wall thickening with increased attenuation on unenhanced images
	Target or halo sign—concentric rings of slightly different densities
	Pneumatosis intestinalis
	Poor enhancement or lack of enhancement of the bowel wall with intravenous contrast
	Serrated beak configuration of the obstructed bowel loop
Mesenteric changes	Changes range from haziness and blurring of the mesenteric vessels to obliteration of the mesentery and its vessels caused by mesenteric congestion and hemorrhage
	Diffuse engorgement of mesenteric vasculature
	Unusual course of the mesenteric vasculature
Other changes	Large amount of ascites

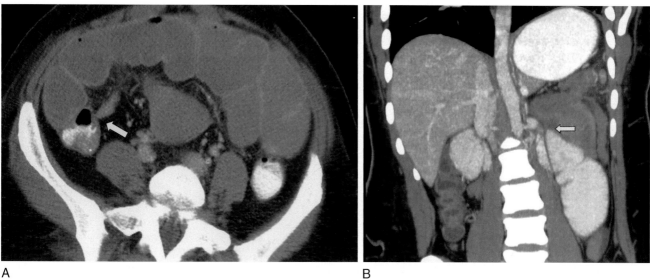

Figure 116–4   Abdominal computed tomography (CT) images of two patients with adhesive small bowel obstruction (SBO). The image on the left (A) shows fluid-filled loops of ileum proximal to a transition point at the site of obstruction (*arrow*); decompressed bowel is seen distal to the obstruction. The image on the right (B) is from a patient with a complete SBO of the proximal jejunum; the markedly dilated, contrast-filled jejunum tapers to the point of complete obstruction (*arrow*). This patient's abdominal plain film had demonstrated no gas in the abdomen.

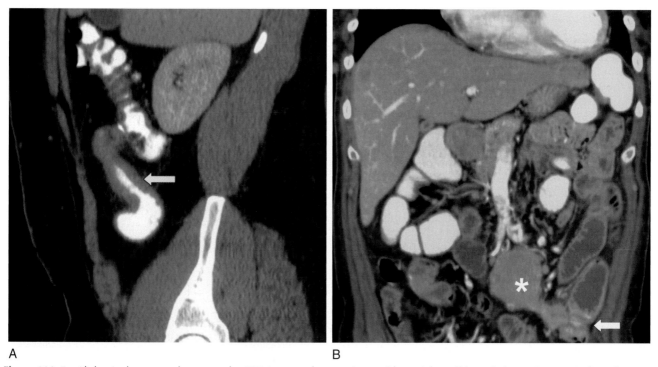

Figure 116–5   Abdominal computed tomography (CT) images of two patients with partial small bowel obstruction. *A,* Crohn's disease is suggested by the markedly thickened ileal wall with a long stenotic region (*arrow*). *B,* A focal stenosis of the ileum (*arrow*) is noted with a large mass of metastatic carcinoid and mesenteric lymphadenopathy (*). This CT image corresponds to the operative image in Figure 116–8.

obstruction, the predictive value of this parameter is too low to be useful as a sole determinant of strangulation. Vomiting and the profound loss of intravascular fluid that accompanies SBO may alter serum electrolyte composition and impair renal function. Serum levels of amylase, lactate dehydrogenase, phosphate, and potassium may be elevated in patients with strangulated bowel; however, these parameters also lack sufficient predictive value to allow differentiation between simple intestinal obstruction and strangulated obstruction at a stage prior to frank intestinal necrosis and peritonitis.[51]

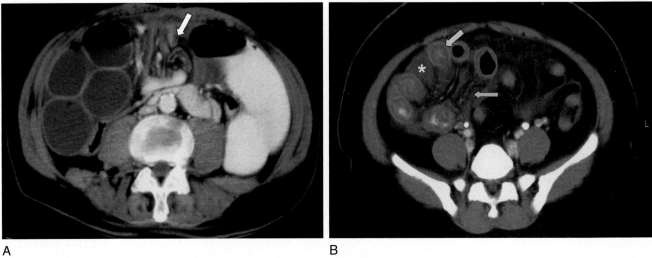

A   B

Figure 116–6   Abdominal computed tomography (CT) images of patients with intestinal obstruction. *A,* A patient with a closed-loop obstruction in which the small intestine twisted around omentum that was adherent to the anterior abdominal wall *(arrow).* Note the massively dilated loops of contrast-filled proximal intestine on the right side of the abdomen and the fluid-filled loops of bowel containing no contrast on the left. In the center of the abdomen is a tightly twisted segment of bowel ("whirl sign") consisting of the site of torsion with obstruction of the afferent and efferent limbs of the intestine. *B,* A patient with strangulated obstruction, evidence of which includes bowel wall thickening *(blue arrow),* mesenteric stranding *(green arrow),* and ascites *(asterisk).*

TREATMENT AND OUTCOME

Resuscitation and Initial Management

The first step in the management of patients with SBO is restoration of intravascular volume by the infusion of isotonic fluids. A Foley catheter is placed to allow rapid and ongoing assessment of the adequacy of fluid resuscitation. Central venous catheterization or even pulmonary arterial catheterization may be required to guide fluid management, especially in patients with cardiac or renal disease. Serum electrolytes should be measured and abnormalities corrected. Metabolic acidosis suggests profound intravascular volume depletion with or without gangrenous bowel, and when refractory to fluid resuscitation, strongly suggests strangulated obstruction. A nasogastric tube should be placed to decompress the stomach and minimize further intestinal distention from swallowed air. Decompression of the stomach also may serve to reduce the discomfort associated with gastric distention and the risk of aspiration. Following these initial measures, subsequent therapeutic decisions depend primarily on whether obstruction is complete, partial, or accompanied by evidence of strangulation. This axiom is reflected in the algorithm presented in Figure 116–7.

Complete Small Intestinal Obstruction

Complete SBO necessitates early laparotomy. Preoperative preparation includes the intravenous administration of broad-spectrum antibiotics directed toward gram-negative aerobes and anaerobes. Second-generation cephalosporins such as cefoxitin or cefotetan are commonly used agents. The rationale for early laparotomy in patients with complete obstruction is based on three observations: (1) the low likelihood of resolution of complete SBO with nonoperative management; (2) the high risk of strangulation for complete SBO; and (3) the diffi-

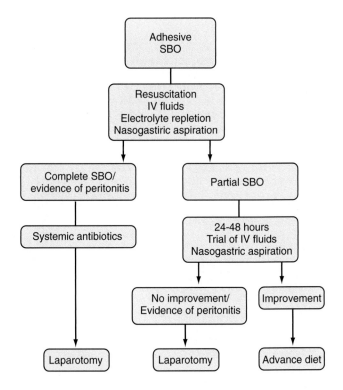

Figure 116–7   Algorithm for the management of a patient with adhesive small bowel obstruction (SBO). Patients with SBO secondary to a hernia should undergo urgent exploration, reduction, and repair of the hernia, and are not candidates for nonoperative management.

culty in detecting strangulated obstruction by clinical parameters until very late in the course of the disease.[51,52]

In a series of 149 patients with complete SBO, 84% required laparotomy because of either failure to resolve the obstruction or the appearance of obvious clinical evidence of strangulation.[51] In another series in which 24 patients with complete SBO and no signs of strangulation were managed nonoperatively, 18 came to operation within 48 hours—13 for failure to improve and 5 for suspected strangulation.[53]

The overall incidence of intestinal strangulation in patients with SBO (complete or partial) ranges from 8% to 22%[54]; however, nearly half of patients with complete SBO have strangulated bowel.[51] Patients with SBO due to hernias are at particularly high risk of strangulation. This high risk, combined with the very low likelihood of spontaneous resolution, mandates an operative approach to all patients with SBO related to hernias.

Differentiating patients with early strangulated SBO from those with simple complete SBO is not possible with currently available clinical parameters. The classic features of strangulated obstruction are leukocytosis, tachycardia, localized abdominal tenderness, and fever. The more of these classic findings present, the greater the probability of gangrenous bowel; however, 5% to 15% of patients with gangrenous bowel have none of these findings.[53] In a study by Sarr and colleagues[51] of 51 patients with complete SBO, no preoperative clinical parameter was predictive of strangulation. Even the clinical judgment of experienced senior surgeons predicted the presence of strangulation in less than half of the patients in whom strangulation was present. Furthermore, only 1 of 10 patients in whom strangulation was predicted correctly had an early, reversible ischemic lesion. In the study by Sarr and colleagues, the preoperative assessment of simple complete SBO was correct in only 69% of cases, and nonoperative treatment of complete SBO was associated with a 31% risk of delayed definitive treatment of strangulated obstruction.[51]

The operative management of complete SBO entails relief of the obstruction and resection of any gangrenous bowel. The point of obstruction often can be identified by a transition zone of dilated intestine proximal, and decompressed bowel distal, to the point of obstruction (Fig. 116–8). In the absence of frankly necrotic intestine, viability should be assessed several minutes following the release of the obstruction by inspection (return of normal color, peristalsis, and arterial pulsation in the vasa recta), fluorescein fluorimetry, and/or Doppler flowmetry. A number of laboratory and clinical studies have shown clinical assessment alone to be inaccurate in predicting long-term viability of reperfused bowel, and hence various adjunctive techniques have been investigated, of which laser Doppler flowmetry has the highest accuracy and is the most readily available.

Partial Small Intestinal Obstruction

Selected patients with partial SBO from intra-abdominal adhesions may be treated nonoperatively, provided there is significant clinical improvement within 24 to 48 hours of presentation and no clinical evidence of gangrenous bowel. Patients managed nonoperatively should receive intravenous fluid and electrolyte restoration and gastric decompression as described earlier. It is imperative that these patients be examined frequently and evidence of clinical deterioration, or even the failure to promptly improve, should mandate urgent operative management (see algorithm in Fig. 116–7).

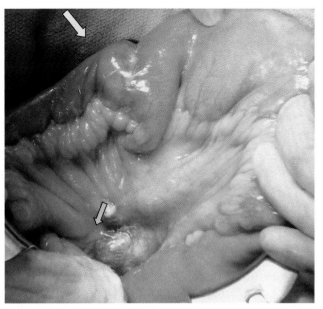

Figure 116–8 Transition point (*white arrow*) in a patient undergoing surgery for small bowel obstruction from a carcinoid tumor of the small intestine with metastases to lymph nodes within the underlying mesentery (*blue arrow*). The dilated bowel proximal and decompressed bowel distal to the transition point are readily apparent. This intraoperative photograph is from the same patient as the CT image in Figure 116–5B.

Although the likelihood of gangrenous bowel in patients with partial SBO is very low (0/91 patients in one series[54]) when compared with instances of complete SBO (21/51 in one series[51]), patients with partial SBO who present with severe abdominal pain or physical findings suggestive of peritonitis should be resuscitated and undergo urgent laparotomy. A similar approach should be taken for patients who develop these symptoms during a period of nonoperative management.

The success of nonoperative treatment of patients with partial SBO has been well documented. In two series, 65% and 81% of patients with partial SBO were managed successfully without an operation.[52,53] Eighty-five to 95% of patients whose partial SBOs ultimately resolve show substantial improvement within the first 48 hours of treatment.[52,53] Hence patients managed nonoperatively should demonstrate substantial improvement within the first 24 to 48 hours of treatment. If after 48 hours of nonoperative management, resolution has not occurred, operative management is indicated.

Whether the placement of a long intestinal tube into the small bowel improves the likelihood of successful nonoperative management is controversial. A prospective, randomized trial of short versus long intestinal tubes published in 1995 by Fleshner and coworkers[55] found no significant difference in outcome of patients managed with a standard nasogastric tube compared with those treated with a long intestinal tube. Hospitalization for patients successfully treated with long intestinal tubes was longer than that of patients treated with a nasogastric tube (4.6 vs. 2.8 days; $P < 0.001$).[55] If long intestinal tubes have a place in the management of patients with SBO, it is in those with multiple prior episodes of intestinal obstruction from adhesions, radiation enteritis, or complex Crohn's disease and not in those presenting with their first episode of adhesive intestinal obstruction.

Other studies have examined the ability of orally administered diatrizoate to enhance the likelihood of successful nonoperative management of SBO. In one of the earliest prospective, randomized trials Assalia and associates[56] found that the average time to the passage of stool (6.2 vs. 23.3 hours) and the average hospital stay (2.2 vs. 4.4 days) was less for patients receiving 100 mL of diatrizoate orally (*n* = 59) when compared with those treated with nasogastric aspiration and intravenous fluid alone (*n* = 48). A subsequent prospective, randomized study of 104 patients with adhesive SBO found that oral diatrizoate reduced the need for operative management of patients who had failed 48 hours of nonoperative management by 74%.[57] Not all studies, however, have found diatrizoate to be beneficial in the treatment of patients with SBO. A prospective, randomized trial by Fevang and colleagues found that the oral administration of a barium and diatrizoate mixture had no effect on the likelihood of resolution or length of hospital stay when compared with a control group receiving standard nonoperative treatment.[58] Similar results were reported in a prospective, randomized trial of 50 patients with adhesive partial SBO.[59] It is postulated that the high osmolarity of diatrizoate (1900 mOsm/L, about six times that of extracellular fluid) promotes the movement of fluid from the intestinal wall and vasculature into the bowel lumen, thereby increasing the pressure gradient across the obstruction. It also has been suggested that diatrizoate dilutes the intestinal contents at the site of obstruction and improves intestinal motility by reducing bowel wall edema.[57]

Although there is increasing experience with the laparoscopic management of adhesive SBO, less than half of these cases can be managed exclusively by laparoscopy because the dense adhesions obscure the point of obstruction.[60-62] For those patients managed successfully by laparoscopy, the advantages include an earlier time to discharge, a faster return to full activity, and perhaps decreased perioperative morbidity.[60-62] The retrospective data comparing open and laparoscopic techniques are impaired by the selection bias created when patients with extensive adhesions or other complications require laparotomy—an event that occurs in at least 50% of instances in which laparoscopy is attempted.

Results of Treatment

The outcome of patients with SBO may be considered in terms of immediate risk of morbidity and mortality and long-term risk of recurrent obstruction. Fevang and colleagues documented the early risks of SBO in a retrospective study of 877 patients. Over the entire period of the study, 1960 to 1995, the risk of death associated with intestinal obstruction was 5.2%; this risk was significantly reduced in the last 5 years of the study period. Advanced age, premorbid illnesses, and nonviable strangulated bowel all markedly increased the risk of mortality (odds ratio = 4 for each of these conditions). Causes of death included massive bowel infarction (29%), pulmonary failure (21%), and cardiac disease (15%). Overall, 23% of patients developed one or more postoperative complica-

tions, with pulmonary, cardiac, and urinary complications predominating. In the study by Fevang and colleagues, the median hospital stay for patients with SBO was about 7 days; advanced age, nonviable strangulated bowel, and treatment delays all were associated with greater lengths of hospitalization.[1]

Once a patient develops adhesive SBO, the likelihood of recurrent obstruction is 30% to 50% over a 10-year follow-up period.[63-65] It is unclear if nonoperative management adversely affects the incidence of recurrent obstruction.[63-65] Miller and coworkers related the likelihood of recurrent obstruction to the pattern of peritoneal adhesions: patients developing obstruction from a single adhesive band had a 25% risk of recurrence compared with a 49% incidence of recurrence for patients with dense, matted adhesions.[63]

SPECIAL CONSIDERATIONS

Early Postoperative Obstruction

SBO in the early postoperative period may be difficult to distinguish from normal postoperative ileus. The incidence of early postoperative SBO was shown by Stewart and associates to be 0.7% in 8098 patients undergoing laparotomy.[66] The operations associated with the highest incidence of postoperative obstruction were those on the small intestine (3%), left colectomy or proctectomy (2.9%), and appendectomy for perforated appendicitis (1.7%). Upper abdominal operations, such as hepatobiliary procedures, had the lowest risk of early postoperative SBO (0.06%).[66] A study by Ellozy and colleagues reported that nearly 10% of 225 patients developed early postoperative SBO after operations on the small intestine and colon.[67]

Patients with early postoperative SBO present with nausea and vomiting, abdominal distention, and abdominal pain as early as the fourth to eighth postoperative day. These patients usually have a partial SBO, and plain abdominal films demonstrate dilated loops of small intestine with air-fluid levels. The study will be interpreted as normal or nonspecific in as many as 10% to 27% of cases. Barium contrast and abdominal CT studies define the site of obstruction in 65% to 70% of cases.[68,69] Furthermore, abdominal CT demonstrates the presence of an intra-abdominal abscess that may be either the cause of a mechanical obstruction or a contributor to the development of paralytic ileus. *The most important clinical feature differentiating early postoperative SBO from postoperative ileus is the occurrence of obstructive symptoms after an initial return of bowel function and resumption of oral intake.*

Management of patients with early postoperative SBO begins with intravascular volume resuscitation and nasogastric aspiration. In one series, nearly 80% of 101 patients had spontaneous resolution of their symptoms after an average of 6 days; only 4% of patients required more than 2 weeks of treatment.[69] In another series, 20 of 23 cases resolved with nonoperative management alone, all within 6 days of treatment.[67] Strangulated obstruction is rare.[68,69] Patients who develop SBO early after laparoscopy must be suspected of having had a portion of their intestine herniate through a trocar site and, as such, they require urgent operative relief of their obstruction.

Small Bowel Obstruction in Patients with Malignancy

Peritoneal spread of gastrointestinal and gynecologic malignancies are important causes of SBO. Several retrospective studies have shown that 25% to 50% of patients with ovarian cancer develop malignant bowel obstruction from progressive encasement of the bowel and its mesentery by ovarian carcinomatosis.[70,71] In both colorectal[72] and ovarian[71] cancer, the risk of developing malignant SBO is linked strongly to the stage of the disease. For example, Ellis and coworkers found that only 18% of patients who developed SBO after undergoing colectomy for early-stage colon cancer had recurrent cancer as the cause of their SBO, whereas carcinomatosis was the cause of obstruction in 82% of patients with more advanced disease.[72] Similarly, Tunca and associates found that only 15% of patients with stage I ovarian cancer eventually developed malignant SBO compared with 35% of patients with more advanced disease.[71] In the absence of recurrent malignancy, SBO may result from postoperative, intraperitoneal adhesions or fibrosis from radiation therapy.

The time from the initial diagnosis of malignancy to the development of SBO also is of prognostic significance. Patients who develop SBO within the first year of their initial diagnosis should be suspected of having a malignant etiology, whereas those who develop SBO after being disease free for an extended period are more likely to have adhesive obstruction. Low and colleagues[73] reported that gadolinium-enhanced MR imaging may accurately differentiate malignant from benign causes of SBO in patients with a history of malignant disease. In this study, the sensitivity, specificity, and accuracy of MR imaging for detecting malignant obstruction was 90% to 93%, 89% to 95%, and 92%, respectively.[73]

Because most instances of SBO from recurrent malignancies are incurable, the goal of treatment is to improve the quality of life for a patient with a limited life expectancy. In these instances, the purpose of surgery is to relieve the symptoms of obstruction. Factors to consider in planning operative therapy include the chance of successful palliation, the risk of repeat obstruction, the quality of life for the patient after surgery, the ability to administer future chemotherapy, and the risk of operative morbidity and mortality. Surgical options include resection with reanastomosis, surgical bypass with an enteroenterostomy, or diverting ileostomy. In most instances, the patient's symptoms can be palliated. For example, in one retrospective study of 64 patients with recurrent ovarian cancer, the obstruction was relieved surgically in 84% of cases and 71% were able to tolerate a diet for at least 60 days postoperatively. The median survival of patients in whom the obstruction was relieved was about 12 months.[74] Others have reported similar results, with 40% to 60% of patients surviving more than 1 year.[75,76]

Intussusception

Intussusception is the invagination of a proximal segment of bowel (intussusceptum) into an adjacent distal segment (intussuscipiens), as shown in Figure 116–9. Although more often recognized as a cause of SBO in children, about 5% of cases of intussusception occur in adults.[77] In contrast to children, in whom there rarely is an anatomic abnormality of the intestine, intussusception in adults is associated with an underlying pathologic process in more than 90% of cases.[77,78] The most common lesions associated with intussusception in adults are neoplasms, inflammatory lesions, and Meckel's diverticula. In one review of 48 adults with intussusception, 36 were caused by neoplasms.[78] Malignant neoplasms were found in at least half of adults with colocolic intussusceptions and enteroenteric intussusceptions.[77,78]

Patients with intussusception present with intermittent cramping abdominal pain, vomiting, and, to a lesser extent, diarrhea. They may have occult or overt rectal bleeding. Often, symptoms are present for several weeks prior to presentation. In one series, an abdominal mass was palpable in 42% of patients.[78] The right lower quadrant of the abdomen may feel "empty" on palpation because the distal ileum and cecum have invaginated into the ascending colon and hence into the right upper quadrant; this empty right lower quadrant of the abdomen is referred to as *Dance's sign*.

Ultrasonography is the primary initial diagnostic tool in children; air contrast enemas are reserved for those children in whom intussusception is found by ultrasound or when the clinical suspicion of intussusception is exceptionally high.[79-81] In adults, the procedure of choice is CT scanning (Fig. 116–10). Diagnostic patterns on CT include (1) a *target lesion*, characterized by an intraluminal soft-tissue density mass with an eccentrically placed fatty area of CT attenuation that represents the intussusception and the intussuscepted mesentery, respectively; (2) a *reniform mass*, with a high attenuation peripherally and lower attenuation centrally, and explained by the invaginated intussusception surrounded by thickened small bowel; and (3) a *sausage-shaped mass*, with alternating areas of low and high attenuation representing closely spaced bowel wall, mesenteric fat, and/or intestinal fluid and gas.[82]

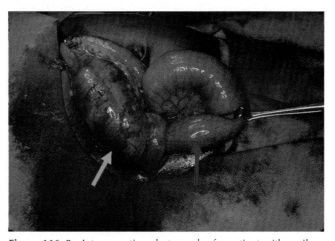

Figure 116–9 Intraoperative photograph of a patient with an ileocolic intussusception. The ileum (intussusceptum, *blue arrow*) is seen entering the ascending colon (intussuscipiens, *green arrow*). (Courtesy of Feldman's online Atlas, Current Medicine.)

Sixty to 80% of children with ileocolic intussusception can be managed successfully at the time of diagnosis by hydrostatic reduction with contrast enema. The success of this technique diminishes substantially as the duration of symptoms exceeds 24 hours. When hydrostatic reduction is unsuccessful or unavailable, manual reduction of the intussusception with careful inspection of the involved intestine is necessary. Intestinal resection is reserved for those instances in which the bowel is nonviable.

The association of neoplasms and other intestinal pathology with intussusception in adults mandates resection of the involved bowel and makes hydrostatic or pneumatic reduction unreasonable. Primary resection without attempting reduction is the preferred treatment for colonic intussusception, including ileocecal intussusception. For lesions involving the right colon, a right hemicolectomy is performed. When the intussusception involves only the small intestine, resection is the preferred operative approach, although manual reduction of the intussusception with careful palpation of the intestinal wall may allow the surgeon to limit the amount of bowel resected.

Gallstone Ileus

Gallstone ileus is an unusual cause of intestinal obstruction, accounting for about 1% to 4% of all cases.[83,84] This complication of cholelithiasis is more common in the elderly and in two studies occurred in patients with an average age of 73 and 77 years.[85,86] The term *gallstone ileus* is a misnomer, because this condition represents a true mechanical obstruction of the intestine by a gallstone or gallstones within the lumen of the bowel. Most commonly, gallstones large enough to cause obstruction enter the bowel via a cholecystoduodenal fistula. As the stone migrates through the gastrointestinal tract it produces intermittent obstruction, with resultant

waxing and waning of symptoms that confound early diagnosis. The most common site of obstruction is the ileum (60%), followed by the jejunum (15%), stomach (15%), colon (5%), and duodenum (5%). In the absence of an intestinal stricture, a gallstone of at least 2 cm is required to cause intestinal obstruction, and stones as large as $7 \times 4 \times 3$ cm have been reported (Fig. 116–11).

Diagnosis of gallstone ileus is delayed in up to half of the patients because of nonspecific and inconsistent symptoms. Only 50% to 70% of patients have clinical features of SBO; some patients may present with diarrhea.[87] The classic radiologic features of gallstone ileus include pneumobilia, intestinal obstruction, aberrant gallstone location, and a change in the location of a previously observed stone.[88] Only about 10% of gallstones are sufficiently calcified to be visualized radiologically.

Treatment of gallstone ileus is focused on removing the obstructing stone, which may be accomplished by operative enterolithotomy.[88,89] Endoscopic removal of stones with or without lithotripsy also has been reported.[90] In general, enterolithotomy alone is the appropriate initial treatment given the emergent nature of this procedure, the advanced age of many of these patients, and the frequent occurrence of a complex right upper quadrant mass containing the cholecystoenteric fistula. Together, these factors argue against identification and repair of the fistula at the time of emergent laparotomy for SBO. Doko and coworkers[85] found that attempts to relieve the obstruction and repair the biliary-enteric fistula in a single operation were associated with a 61% incidence of complications. It has been estimated that as many as 17% of patients develop recurrent gallstone ileus or other biliary complications after enterolithotomy alone and, therefore, elective cholecystectomy with repair of the fistula usually is performed when the patient has recovered from the initial operative procedure.[87] Of note, however, Lobo and associates reported 11 elderly patients

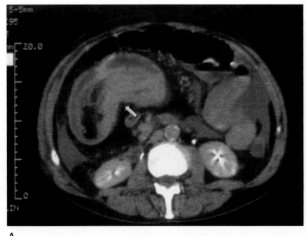
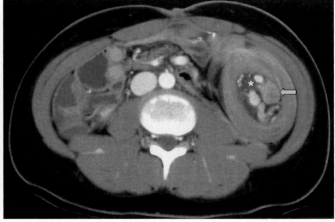

A   B

Figure 116–10 Abdominal computed tomography (CT) scans of two patients with ileocolic intussusceptions. *A,* CT scan from a patient with an ileocolic intussusception due to adenocarcinoma of the cecum demonstrating the reniform-shaped mass (*arrow*) with alternating areas of low and high attenuation representing closely spaced bowel wall, mesenteric fat, and/or intestinal fluid and gas. *B,* In this CT scan from another patient, the target lesion pattern is shown, consisting of the intussuscepted ileum (*arrow*) with associated mesentery (*asterisk*).

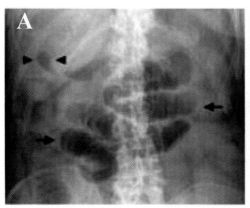
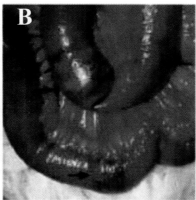
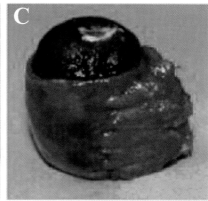

Figure 116–11 Gallstone ileus in a 78-year-old woman with a 2-week history of nausea and vomiting. *A,* Plain film of the abdomen revealing characteristic features of gallstone ileus, including air in the biliary tree (*arrowheads*) and dilated loops of small intestine (*arrows*); an obstructing stone was not seen on this plain film examination. At exploratory laparotomy, 2 obstructing gallstones were identified in the jejunum (*B*) with adjacent perforations and fecal contamination of the peritoneal cavity. The stones were removed by enterolithotomy and segmental resection of the jejunum (*C*). In addition, the cholecystoduodenal fistula was repaired and cholecystectomy was performed. (From Besselink MG and Kroeze J, Mayo Clin Proc 80:699, 2005).

presenting with gallstone ileus who were treated with enterolithotomy alone, none of whom developed subsequent biliary symptoms when followed for a median period of 46 months.[83]

Midgut Volvulus

Midgut volvulus from intestinal rotational anomalies is an important cause of SBO, particularly in neonates. The anatomy and embryology that underlie the development of duodenal obstruction from Ladd's bands and midgut volvulus is discussed in greater detail in Chapter 93. It is worth reiterating, however, that the most common anomaly is nonrotation in which there is inadequate counterclockwise rotation of the midgut loop around the superior mesenteric artery (SMA). This results in the duodenojejunal junction and the entire small intestine being located to the right of the midline. The colon resides in the left abdomen with the cecum near the midline. The narrow mesenteric pedicle predisposes the patient to midgut volvulus and the peritoneal attachments (Ladd's bands), which extend anterior and lateral to the duodenum to fix the cecum to the posterior body wall, may obstruct the duodenum.

Fifty to 75% of malrotations are detected during the first month of life, and more than 90% are discovered within the first year because of clinical evidence of duodenal obstruction (from Ladd's bands) or midgut volvulus. Infants with duodenal obstruction from Ladd's bands present with signs of gastric and proximal duodenal obstruction, including bilious vomiting with minimal abdominal distention. Midgut volvulus also presents with obstructive signs often complicated by signs of intestinal ischemia. Occult gastrointestinal bleeding is a common early finding, and if transmural necrosis develops, acidosis, thrombocytopenia, and frank sepsis may ensue.

The high risk of intestinal ischemia and necrosis from midgut volvulus and the associated high mortality rate mandate aggressive diagnosis and management of neonatal SBO. A plain abdominal film demonstrates a distended stomach and proximal duodenal bulb with a paucity of small bowel gas. An upper gastrointestinal contrast study is diagnostic by demonstrating malpositioning of the duodenojejunal junction to the right of the midline with the small intestine on the right and the cecum and ascending colon to the left. The contrast study also may demonstrate a characteristic corkscrew or coiled appearance in the third or fourth portions of the duodenum (Fig. 116–12*A*). A contrast enema demonstrates the colon on the left side of the abdomen and the small intestine positioned to the right (see Fig. 116–12*B*).

Treatment of intestinal malrotation, whether manifested by duodenal obstruction from Ladd's bands or midgut volvulus, is surgical. In the latter case, the diagnosis should be followed immediately by laparotomy, because a delay of even hours may mean the difference between viable or infarcted intestine. Operative repair of malrotation is achieved by the performance of the Ladd procedure, which consists of the following parts:

1. Relief of the midgut volvulus and division of the peritoneal bands that tether the cecum, small bowel mesentery, mesocolon, and duodenum around the base of the SMA. This allows the mesenteric leaves to open widely and is associated with a very low incidence of recurrent volvulus.
2. Division of the Ladd's peritoneal bands to relieve the extrinsic compression and obstruction of the distal duodenum. This is accomplished by meticulous and complete mobilization of the entire duodenum with division of all anterior, lateral and posterior attachments.

An appendectomy is often performed to eliminate future confusion from acute appendicitis developing in an abnormally positioned appendix.

COLONIC OBSTRUCTION

ETIOLOGY

The most common causes of colonic obstruction are malignancy, volvulus, and stricture secondary to diver-

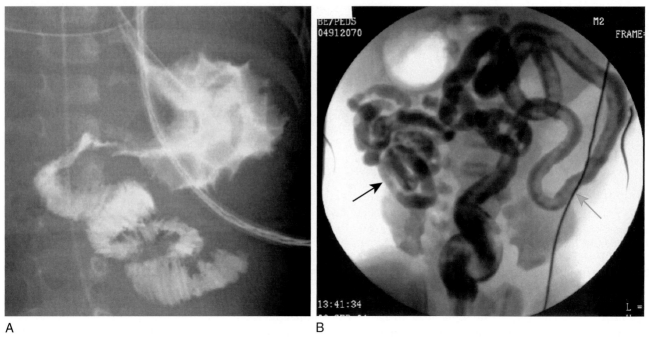

A   B

Figure 116–12 *A,* Representative film from upper gastrointestinal fluoroscopy with barium contrast in a patient with intestinal malrotation. The image demonstrates failure of the third part of the duodenum to cross the midline and the corkscrew appearance of the proximal jejunum. *B,* Barium contrast study in a patient with intestinal malrotation demonstrating the small bowel to the right (*black arrow*) and the colon to the left of the midline (*blue arrow*).

ticulitis. These three pathologic conditions account for about 90% of instances of colorectal obstructions. Less frequent causes include Crohn's disease, endometriosis, intussusception, extrinsic tumors, and fecal impaction.

Adenocarcinoma

Malignant neoplasms, nearly all of which are adenocarcinoma, cause more than 50% of all cases of colonic obstruction. About 20% of patients with colorectal cancer present with obstructive symptoms, and half of these require emergency operative decompression. Three fourths of obstructing adenocarcinomas occur distal to the splenic flexure, many within reach of a flexible sigmoidoscope.[91] Carcinomas of the left colon most commonly manifest as a scirrhous tumor causing progressive stenosis of the lumen, whereas cancers located in the right colon grow as a polypoid or fungating mass that obstructs the colon on reaching a size that occludes the lumen or by acting as a lead point of a colonic intussusception.

Volvulus

Colonic volvulus (Latin, *volvere,* to roll or turn) is the axial twisting of the colon on its vascular pedicle. A closed-loop obstruction typically is produced with ischemia resulting from twisting of the vascular pedicle and the increased wall tension from distention. In the United States and other Western countries, colonic volvulus causes 1% to 4% of all cases of intestinal obstruction and 10% to 15% of colonic obstructions. In Eastern Europe

and parts of Africa and Asia, volvulus is responsible for 20% to 50% of all cases of intestinal obstruction.

The sigmoid colon and cecum are the most frequent sites of colonic volvulus, accounting for about 75% and 22% of all cases, respectively. Rare sites of colonic volvulus involve the transverse colon (2%) and the splenic flexure (<1%). The anatomic factors necessary for the development of volvulus include a redundant segment of bowel that is freely movable within the peritoneal cavity and close approximation of two points of fixation of the colon. In sigmoid volvulus, the redundant sigmoid colon is fixed across a narrow base by the lateral peritoneal attachments proximally and the rectum distally. Failure of fusion of the parietal peritoneum to the cecum and ascending colon allows the formation of a cecal volvulus in which the distal ileum, cecum, and ascending colon rotate and twist or fold upward (the latter is termed a *cecal bascule*). In either case, vascular compromise leads to gangrene and perforation. Volvulus of the transverse colon is uncommon and is related to the congenital or surgical absence of supporting ligaments and tissues, including the gastrocolic, splenocolic, and phrenicocolic ligaments.

Diverticulitis and Other Causes of Benign Colonic Strictures

Benign colonic strictures occur most commonly as a consequence of diverticulitis and less commonly at the site of a surgical anastomosis. These benign colonic strictures account for less than 10% of instances of colonic obstruction. Furthermore, obstruction accounts for only about 10% of the complications related to diverticular disease (see Chapter 114).

PATHOPHYSIOLOGY

The competency of the ileocecal valve is of great importance in the pathophysiology of colonic obstruction. When the ileocecal valve is competent, the cecum cannot decompress fluid and gas into the small bowel, resulting in a closed-loop obstruction and ultimately ischemia of the colonic wall. In the setting of colonic obstruction, the cecum is the part of the colon that is most susceptible to ischemia because of the direct relationship between wall tension and the radius of a sphere as defined by LaPlace's law

$$T = P \times R$$

where T is tension on the wall, P is pressure, and R is the radius. Thus, as fluid and gas accumulate within the obstructed colon, intraluminal pressure increases. Wall tension is greatest at the site of greatest radius, which, in the colon, is the cecum. Generally, acute dilatation of the cecum to 10 cm suggests colonic wall ischemia is likely, and a diameter greater than 13 cm suggests perforation is imminent.

CLINICAL FEATURES

Many of the clinical manifestations of colonic obstruction are similar regardless of the etiology. Periumbilical or hypogastric pain and abdominal distention are the two most common presenting features. The pain varies from a vague discomfort to the excruciating pain of peritonitis. Severe unremitting pain suggests gangrenous bowel and mandates urgent laparotomy. Patients may experience either diarrhea (reflecting the passage of liquid stool around an obstructing lesion) or obstipation, depending on the degree and location of the obstruction.

Benign and Malignant Colonic Strictures

Patients with left-sided colonic tumors or benign fibrotic strictures often will have noted a change in stool caliber over the preceding months. Blood in the stool, or an iron deficiency anemia, is highly suggestive of carcinoma, as is the occurrence of weakness, weight loss, and anorexia. Vomiting, when present, usually is a late finding. The symptoms of malignant- and diverticular-associated colonic obstruction often are insidious in onset, with a median duration of 3 months. One fourth of patients have symptoms from 6 to 24 months before diagnosis.[91]

Colonic Volvulus

Acute abdominal distention is the most common presentation for patients with colonic volvulus and is present in two thirds of patients. About 20% of patients have abdominal pain, nausea, vomiting, and constipation. In one series of 228 patients with colonic volvulus, 10% presented in shock.[92] The duration of symptoms for patients with colonic volvulus is significantly less than that of patients with a malignant or diverticular stricture. In a series by Grossman and colleagues, the average duration of symptoms prior to evaluation was 73 hours.[92] In another report, patients with sigmoid volvulus had symptoms for an average of 5 days prior to presentation.[93]

Patients with sigmoid volvulus are often in the 6th to 8th decades of life and frequently have concomitant chronic illnesses, such as cardiac, pulmonary, and renal disease, that significantly influence their outcome.[92,94-96] Males develop sigmoid volvulus more commonly than do females. Chronic constipation and laxative abuse as well as mental illnesses also are common. In a large series of patients with sigmoid volvulus, 30% had a history of psychiatric disease and 13% were institutionalized at the time of diagnosis.[96] Abdominal tenderness is present in less than one third of patients with volvulus, and severe pain or signs of peritonitis suggest impending or actual colonic necrosis and perforation.

Patients with cecal volvulus tend to be younger than patients with sigmoid volvulus and often have a history of prior abdominal operations. There is a slight female predominance of cecal volvulus. Case reports document the occurrence of cecal volvulus in pregnant and puerperal women and in children. Nearly one third of patients with cecal volvulus have a concomitant partially obstructing lesion located more distally in the colon. A history of chronic constipation and laxative use also is a frequent finding in patients with cecal volvulus.

DIAGNOSIS

Benign and Malignant Colonic Strictures

The initial diagnostic approach to patients suspected of having colonic obstruction is similar to that of patients with SBO. Plain abdominal films taken in the supine and upright or decubitus positions should be obtained to localize the site of the obstruction, to determine whether the obstruction is partial or complete, and to allow differentiation of Ogilvie's syndrome, ileus, and mechanical small or large bowel obstruction. Small bowel distention may be evident on abdominal films of colonic obstruction depending on the competency of the ileocecal valve (Fig. 116–13).

Further diagnostic studies are predicated on the presence or absence of peritonitis and the degree of obstruction (i.e., partial or complete). Patients with peritonitis should undergo resuscitation and urgent laparotomy without additional diagnostic procedures, whereas patients without evidence of strangulated bowel and an abdominal film suggestive of distal obstruction should undergo a water-soluble contrast enema to confirm and localize the obstruction (Fig. 116–14). The use of water-soluble contrast media obviates the risk of barium peritonitis in the case of unrecognized perforation. The fine mucosal detail provided by air contrast barium studies is not required for patients with an acute obstruction because the main purposes of this study are to document the presence of obstruction and to localize it.

Although colonoscopy may be useful in patients with partial colonic obstructions, it has little role in the initial evaluation of patients suspected of having complete obstruction. The insufflation of air or carbon

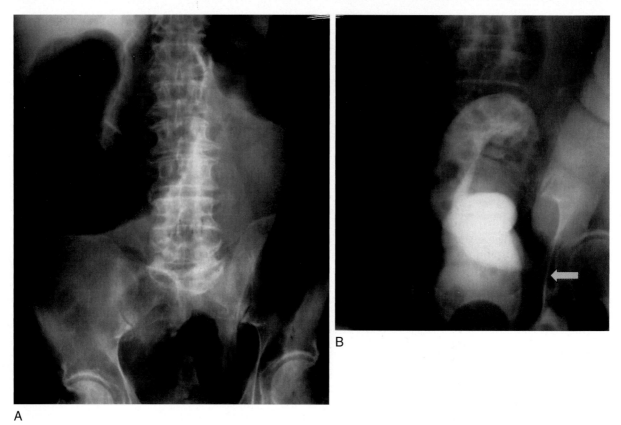

Figure 116–13 Abdominal film of a patient with high-grade colonic obstruction and a competent ileocecal valve (*A*). Note the markedly distended, gas-filled colon without dilatation or gas in the small intestine. The etiology of this patient's colonic obstruction was a left inguinal hernia which is demonstrated on the water-soluble contrast enema (*B*). Although a common cause of small intestinal obstruction, inguinal hernias rarely obstruct the colon. The *arrow* demonstrates the point of obstruction of the sigmoid colon as it traverses the inguinal canal.

dioxide through the endoscope into the obstructed bowel may worsen colonic distention and precipitate perforation.[97]

Colonic Volvulus

The plain abdominal film of a sigmoid volvulus demonstrates a markedly dilated sigmoid colon and proximal colon with minimal gas in the rectum. The classic radiologic feature of sigmoid volvulus is a distended ahaustral sigmoid loop (i.e., "bent inner-tube" appearance), the apex of which often is directed toward the patient's right shoulder (Fig. 116–15).[98] The classic radiologic features of cecal volvulus include (1) a massively dilated cecum located in the epigastrium or left upper quadrant; (2) a coffee-bean appearance of the distended cecum; (3) distended loops of small bowel suggesting SBO; and (4) a single, long air-fluid level present on upright or decubitus films (Fig. 116–16).[99] In these instances, the massively distended cecum extends across the abdominal midline and is "directed" toward the patient's left upper quadrant or left mid-abdomen. Although these classic radiologic findings of colonic volvulus are seen in only 40% to 60% of cases,[94,96,98,99] the diagnosis of colonic volvulus can be made with abdominal radiographs alone in as many as 85% of instances.[95] The radiologic appearance of trans-

verse colon volvulus is not specific and shows only colonic dilatation.

In patients with suspected sigmoid or cecal volvulus and an equivocal plain abdominal film, a water-soluble contrast enema may be helpful by demonstrating a point of torsion (i.e., a mucosal spiral pattern, or "bird's beak sign") (Fig. 116–17). In patients with abdominal films most consistent with a sigmoid volvulus, initial rigid or flexible proctosigmoidoscopy may allow prompt decompression of the volvulus.

TREATMENT AND OUTCOME

Benign and Malignant Colonic Strictures

Resuscitation of patients with colonic obstruction includes the restoration of intravascular volume, correction of electrolyte abnormalities, and nasogastric aspiration. The urgency with which the obstruction must be decompressed depends on the degree of obstruction (partial or complete) and the presence (or absence) of clinical evidence of strangulation.

The goals of operative management are threefold: (1) to decompress the obstructed colon promptly; (2) to treat the obstructing lesion definitively; and (3) to re-establish

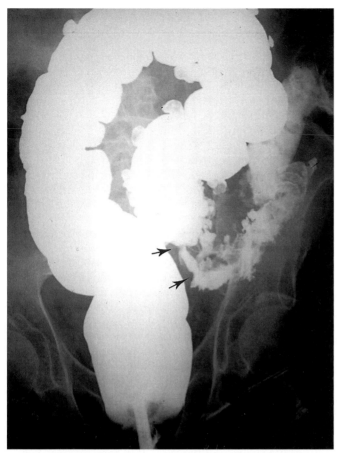

Figure 116–14 Representative film from a contrast enema of a patient with high-grade sigmoid obstruction from a stricture (*arrows* identify the proximal and distal extent of the stricture). Although this patient has multiple diverticula within the sigmoid colon, differentiation of this benign diverticular stricture from a malignant stricture is not possible based on this study alone.

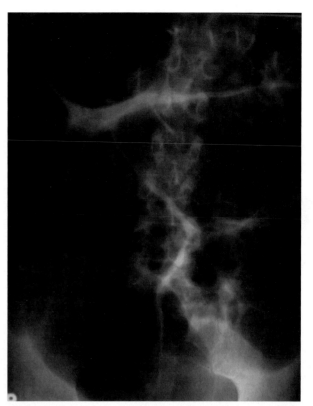

Figure 116–15 Abdominal film from a patient with a sigmoid volvulus. Note the massively dilated colon with a classic "bent-inner tube" appearance emanating from the pelvis toward the right upper quadrant of the abdomen.

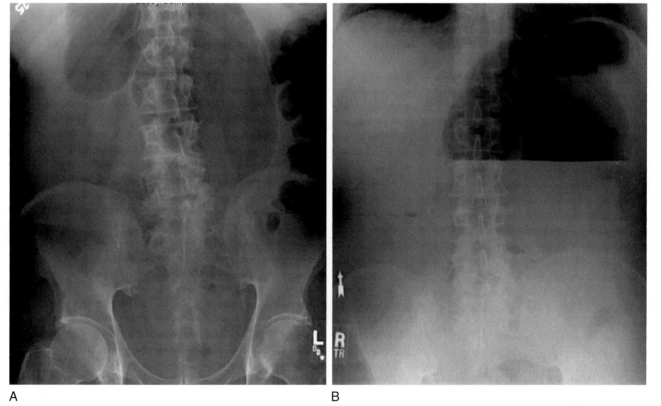

A   B

Figure 116–16 Supine (*A*) and upright (*B*) abdominal films of a patient with a cecal volvulus. The film taken in the supine position (*A*) shows a massively dilated cecum located in the epigastrium and left upper quadrant, whereas the upright film (*B*) shows a long air-fluid level extending across much of the upper abdomen.

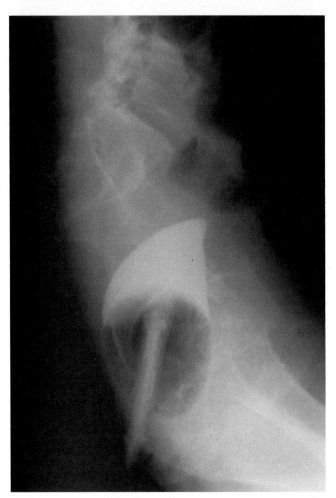

Figure 116–17   Representative film from a contrast enema of a patient with a sigmoid volvulus demonstrating a characteristic "bird's beak" obstruction at the junction between the sigmoid colon and the rectum.

intestinal continuity. All three of these goals may or may not be obtainable at the initial operation. Patients with partially obstructing benign or malignant strictures and no evidence of peritonitis may undergo semielective resection of the stricture after resuscitation and nasogastric aspiration. The conversion of an emergent operation to a semielective procedure allows subsequent preparation of the colon for primary anastomosis and therefore lowers operative risk. As with patients with SBO, the absence of substantial clinical improvement within 24 hours mandates urgent decompression of the obstructed colon, either operatively or, if possible, through the endoscopic placement of a colonic stent. Complete colonic obstruction necessitates emergent operative decompression.

Obstructions located proximal to the splenic flexure are most frequently adenocarcinomas and can be treated with right hemicolectomy and primary ileocolic anastomosis in all but the most unfit patients.[91] This operation accomplishes all three goals of treatment and can be performed on unprepared bowel with minimal increase in postoperative complications. Surgical options in

obstructed patients who are medically unable to withstand resection include tube cecostomy, colostomy, or loop ileostomy; we prefer the last one. The presence of nonviable colon necessitates resection in even the most severely compromised patient. In this instance, resection with end ileostomy and distal mucous fistula obviates the risk of performing an anastomosis in a grossly contaminated field or in a critically ill patient in whom the risk of anastomotic dehiscence may be particularly high.

Obstruction at or distal to the splenic flexure may be either adenocarcinoma or a diverticular stricture, differentiation of which may be difficult at the time of laparotomy. Patients who are medically fit with relatively small tumors or inflammatory masses of the left colon or sigmoid may undergo left or sigmoid colectomy with an end colostomy and closure of the distal bowel or the creation of a distal mucous fistula. The advantages of this approach are twofold: (1) immediate resection of the tumor or the inflammatory mass, which may promote a more rapid convalescence than if the lesion had been left in situ; and (2) avoidance of an anastomosis in an unprepared left colon, which diminishes postoperative complications such as wound infection, anastomotic dehiscence, and sepsis. The disadvantage of this approach is that it requires a subsequent laparotomy to restore intestinal continuity. In a review of seven series comprising more than 300 patients, Deans and colleagues found that the mortality rate of this approach was 8.7%, similar to the 9.2% mortality rate for patients undergoing initial diverting colostomy with subsequent colonic resection.[91] A major disadvantage of the staged approach is that 25% to 64% of these patients never have intestinal continuity restored.[91,100]

Two less commonly employed operative approaches to patients with inflammatory or neoplastic obstructions of the left colon are (1) primary resection with on-table colonic lavage and immediate anastomosis; and (2) subtotal colectomy with ileoproctostomy.[101,102] These approaches allow resection of the tumor and immediate restoration of intestinal continuity, with mortality rates and anastomotic leak rates similar to that of primary resection with colostomy.

Recently, studies have reported the successful use of endoscopically placed self-expanding metal stents to relieve malignant colonic obstruction prior to definitive resection or to palliate obstructive symptoms in patients with advanced disease. This approach allows for mechanical bowel preparation with subsequent primary anastomosis, treatment of significant concomitant medical illnesses, or both.[103] Several reviews have documented relief of colonic obstruction using endoscopically placed stents in up to 80% to 90% of patients in whom this technique is attempted.[103,104] The complications associated with colonic stent placement include perforation (4%), stent migration (10%), and recurrent obstruction (10%). Less frequent and less serious complications include fecal impaction, stent fracture, fistula formation, stent dislodgment, tenesmus, and bleeding.[105-107]

Regardless of the approach, emergent operations to relieve distal colonic obstruction are associated with greater morbidity and mortality risks than those performed electively. Smothers and coworkers also found that patients requiring emergent operations for obstructing colon cancer had greater rates of perioperative morbidity and mortality than would have been predicted based on the stage of disease alone.[108] Other authors have related the higher rates of morbidity and mortality in patients requiring emergent operations for malignant colon obstructions to the advanced age of these patients, the presence of concomitant medical conditions, relative ischemia in the obstructed bowel, fecal loading, intraoperative contamination, and technical difficulties in managing the distended colon.[100]

Colonic Volvulus

The initial management of patients with sigmoid volvulus without evidence of peritonitis is proctoscopic decompression and placement of a rectal tube into the obstructed bowel. Ballantyne compiled the results of 19 American series totaling 595 patients treated nonoperatively and found that proctoscopy, either alone or combined with a rectal tube, successfully reduced the volvulus in 70% to 80% of attempts.[94] Two other large series reported successful proctoscopic decompression of sigmoid volvulus in 83% to 93% of patients.[92,93] Placement of a rectal tube for 48 hours may minimize the possibility of early recurrence. Successful reduction of sigmoid volvulus also has been reported with colonoscopy; however, the procedure must be performed carefully with minimal insufflation of air (or preferably carbon dioxide) to minimize the risk of perforation of the distended, inflamed bowel. Brothers and associates warned of the difficulty in adequately examining the colonic mucosa in the emergent setting, thus possibly delaying appropriate management.[97]

Endoscopic reduction of sigmoid volvulus alone is associated with a recurrence rate of 25% to 50%.[92-94,97] Hence, elective sigmoid resection and coloproctostomy, or in medically compromised patients, end colostomy, should follow proctoscopic decompression and mechanical preparation of the bowel. Recurrence rates with this approach are 3% to 6%.[92,94,97] Patients requiring emergent laparotomy for strangulated sigmoid volvulus require sigmoid resection with end colostomy and a Hartmann pouch.

The role of initial nonoperative management of patients with cecal volvulus is less well defined than that of sigmoid volvulus. Although colonoscopy has been employed successfully to reduce cecal volvulus, the risk of perforation of the thinned, often ischemic cecum is substantial, as is the danger of missing a segment of necrotic bowel with delay in definitive resection.[97] Options for the operative management of cecal volvulus include cecopexy, cecostomy, and resection. Detorsion alone, or when combined with appendectomy, is associated with a high recurrence rate.[109] Others have favored the performance of a cecopexy in which the right colon is anchored to the peritoneum of the right paracolic gutter with or without a cecostomy.[110] Right colectomy with primary ileo-transverse colostomy effectively prevents recurrent volvulus and is the procedure of choice for most surgeons, including us. Ballantyne and colleagues reported 27 patients with cecal volvulus who were treated with resection and primary anastomosis with no operative mortality and no recurrence in 5 years of follow-up.[95]

Overall the mortality rate for patients with colonic volvulus is about 8% to 14%, the presence of gangrenous bowel being a major predictor of death[92]; the colonic wall is gangrenous in 15% to 20% of patients with cecal or sigmoid volvulus.[92,95,96] In a review of 18 American studies involving 229 patients with sigmoid volvulus, the mortality rate for patients with gangrenous bowel was 80%, whereas only 10% of patients without colonic necrosis died.[95] In a more recent study, the mortality rate for patients with gangrenous colonic volvulus was 25%.[92]

ILEUS

ETIOLOGY

Ileus refers to the failure of aboral passage of intestinal contents in the absence of mechanical obstruction. Livingston and Passaro defined it as "the functional inhibition of propulsive bowel activity, irrespective of pathogenetic mechanism."[111] The most common cause of ileus is abdominal or retroperitoneal surgery; other causes of ileus include inflammatory, metabolic, neurogenic, and medications (Table 116–3) (see Chapter 117).

Postoperative ileus is an inevitable response to laparotomy and a principal reason for delayed resumption of oral intake, prolonged hospitalization, and increased costs after abdominal operations.[112] The annual economic impact of postoperative ileus in the United States has been estimated to be about $1 billion. Normally, gastrointestinal function returns after laparotomy in an

Table 116–3 Causes of Ileus

Category	Specific Causes
Drugs	Narcotics, phenothiazines, diltiazem, anticholinergic agents, clozapine
Electrolyte abnormalities	Hypokalemia, hyponatremia, hypomagnesemia, hypermagnesemia, hypocalcemia, hypercalcemia
Intestinal ischemia	Mesenteric arterial embolus or thrombosis, mesenteric venous thrombosis, chronic mesenteric ischemia
Intra-abdominal inflammation	Appendicitis, diverticulitis, perforated duodenal ulcer
Iatrogenic	Laparotomy, laparoscopy
Retroperitoneal inflammation or hemorrhage	Lumbar compression fracture, acute pancreatitis, pyelonephritis
Infection	Intra-abdominal or systemic sepsis
Thoracic diseases	Lower rib fractures, lower lobe pneumonia, myocardial infarction

orderly and predictable manner: Small bowel motility returns first, within the first 24 hours of the procedure; and gastric and colonic motility return in 24 to 48 hours and 48 to 72 hours, respectively. A delay in the return of normal gastrointestinal function should initiate a search for a complication such as intra-abdominal infection, systemic disorders (e.g., sepsis or electrolyte disturbances), or drug-related effects, especially from narcotics or psychotropic agents.

PATHOPHYSIOLOGY OF POSTOPERATIVE ILEUS

The pathophysiology of postoperative ileus involves a complex interaction of inhibitory neuroenteric reflexes, including increased efferent inhibitory sympathetic activity; inflammation within the bowel wall; the local and systemic release of inhibitory gastrointestinal peptides and endogenous opioids; and the use of exogenous opioids for anesthesia and postoperative analgesia.[111,113]

Inhibitory Neural Reflexes

Incision through the abdominal wall and manipulation of the intestine alter normal basal electrical activity of the gut by activating inhibitory sympathetic reflexes via afferent somatic and splanchnic nerves.[113,114] The release of norepinephrine by efferent sympathetic splanchnic nerves inhibits acetylcholine release from excitatory neurons in the myenteric plexus, thereby causing relaxation of the intestinal wall.[115] The efficacy of thoracic epidural-administered local anesthetics in attenuating postoperative ileus is thought to be related to the disruption of afferent and efferent inhibitory neural reflexes.[116,117] Tache and coworkers[118] and others[119,120] have proposed a central neural hypothesis, in which laparotomy causes the central release of corticotrophin-releasing factor in the paraventricular nucleus of the hypothalamus and the dorsal vagal complex, which then triggers efferent inhibitory motor pathways to inhibit gastrointestinal motility.

Local Inflammation Within the Bowel Wall

Evidence in animal models of postoperative ileus suggests that local inflammation within the bowel wall is an important cause of postoperative ileus. These studies indicate that abdominal surgery activates a population of macrophages residing in the muscularis propria of the bowel with subsequent release of pro-inflammatory cytokines and chemokines. These cytokines, in turn, recruit and activate leukocytes to release pro-inflammatory mediators that subsequently inhibit enteric smooth muscle function for sustained periods of time postoperatively.[121-123] A study by Kalff and associates[124] extended these laboratory findings to humans by showing that laparotomy (1) activated a population of resident macrophages within the muscularis propria of the jejunum; (2) caused the expression of messenger RNA for interleukin (IL)-6, IL-1β, tumor necrosis factor-α, cyclooxygenase-2, and inducible nitric oxide synthase in the muscularis, but not mucosa; (3) recruited leukocytes into the muscularis propria of the jejunum; and (4) impaired jejunal muscle contractility.

Endogenous and Exogenous Opioids

Endogenous opioids are released into the bloodstream during major operations[125,126] and opioids are exogenously administered for pain relief in the perioperative and postoperative periods.[127,128] Both inhibit gastrointestinal motility and are thought to be of major importance in the development of postoperative ileus.[125-128]

Endogenous opioids (e.g, met- and leu-enkephalins, μ-endorphin, and dynorphin) are present in neurons of the myenteric and submucosal plexus, where they activate membrane-bound receptors on enteric myocytes and the terminals of sympathetic and sensory peripheral neurons.[129] Activation of the μ_2-opioid receptors in the gastrointestinal tract impairs motility, whereas activation of μ_1-receptors in the central nervous system mediates the analgesic effects of opioids.[130,131] At least in part, μ-receptor activation alters gastrointestinal motility by inhibiting the release of acetylcholine from cholinergic neurons.[128,132] At therapeutic doses, morphine and other opioid analgesics are selective for μ-receptor subtypes when compared with δ- and κ-receptors, although they do not differentiate for the specific classes of μ-receptors (i.e., μ_1 vs. μ_2).[133]

Morphine inhibits the organized, spike potentials associated with propulsion and normal gastrointestinal motility. In primates, low doses of morphine increase the frequency of random, nonpropagating spike potentials and contractions within the colon, whereas higher doses inhibit all electrical and contractile activity of the colon.[134] In humans recovering from laparotomy, morphine disrupts the normal pattern of recovery of colonic motility electrical activity by inducing the development of phasic stationary, nonmigrating colonic spike potentials.[135]

CLINICAL FEATURES AND DIAGNOSIS

The principal clinical findings of patients with ileus include poorly localized abdominal pain, abdominal distention, nausea, vomiting, and obstipation. These clinical manifestations, including the abdominal pain, may be difficult to distinguish from those associated with mechanical bowel obstruction. The absence of bowel sounds is not a consistent feature of nonobstructive ileus, although "rushes and tinkles" and borborygmi usually are not heard.

Differentiation of ileus from mechanical SBO usually is possible based on consideration of the entire clinical picture and the presence of gas in the stomach, small intestine, and colon on abdominal plain films. In those cases in which the abdominal plain film is nondiagnostic, fluoroscopic contrast studies of the gastrointestinal tract and CT may confirm the diagnosis. CT offers the additional benefit of delineating other intra-abdominal inflammatory processes, such as abscesses, acute pancreatitis, or retroperitoneal hemorrhage, that may contribute to nonmechanical bowel dysfunction. The passage of CT contrast into the colon within 4 hours excludes SBO and favors ileus as the etiology of a patient's intestinal dysmotility.

TREATMENT AND OUTCOME

The treatment of ileus following uncomplicated laparotomy involves limiting oral intake, the maintenance of intravascular volume, and the correction of electrolyte abnormalities, particularly hypokalemia. If accompanied by abdominal distention, nausea, or vomiting, a nasogastric tube should be placed. If ileus is prolonged (>3 to 5 days), a thorough search for an underlying cause must be undertaken. Review of the patient's medications may reveal drugs known to be associated with impaired intestinal motility, especially opiates. Measurement of serum electrolytes may demonstrate hypokalemia, hypocalcemia, hypomagnesemia or hypermagnesemia, or other electrolyte disturbances commonly associated with ileus. CT may reveal the presence of an intra-abdominal abscess or other evidence of peritoneal sepsis, as well as the presence of postoperative obstruction.

Nasogastric Intubation

Several randomized clinical studies have shown that nasogastric decompression does not shorten the time to the first bowel movement or decrease the time to oral intake in patients who have undergone laparotomy. Moreover, it has been suggested that inappropriate use of nasogastric decompression may contribute to postoperative respiratory complications such as atelectasis and pneumonia.[136,137] These studies are consistent with recent clinical experience that has nearly abolished the routine use of nasogastric aspiration after uncomplicated abdominal operations.

Pharmacologic Agents

Nonsteroidal Anti-inflammatory Drug Therapy

The administration of nonsteroidal anti-inflammatory drugs (NSAIDs) has been shown to decrease the frequency of postoperative nausea and vomiting and improve gastrointestinal transit in several experimental and clinical studies.[138,139] This beneficial effect is due, at least in part, to a 20% to 30% reduction in the amount of opioids required by patients given perioperative NSAIDs.[140] An additional benefit may be gained by the anti-inflammatory effects of some of these agents.

Modulation of Sympathetic and Parasympathetic Input

In humans, attempts to reduce inhibitory adrenergic signals while promoting cholinergic signals have been either unsuccessful in promoting the resolution of postoperative ileus,[141] or have been limited by the occurrence of uncomfortable and even potentially dangerous adverse effects.[142,143] The epidural administration of local anesthetics block afferent and efferent inhibitory reflexes, including inhibitory sympathetic efferent signals. They have the added benefit of blocking the afferent stimuli that triggers the catabolism that characterizes the response to surgery. Thoracic epidural injections with bupivacaine hydrochloride have been shown to significantly reduce the duration of postoperative ileus when compared with systemic opioid therapy alone in patients undergoing laparotomy.[144-147] The location of the epidural

catheter is important, low-thoracic or lumbar epidurals lacking the beneficial effects of thoracic epidurals.[144,146,148,149] Furthermore, shorter periods of epidural anesthesia (24 hours) are not as effective as longer periods (48 to 72 hours).[148] Several studies, including prospective trials, have found that epidural anesthetics alone (e.g., bupivacaine) are more effective in reducing the duration of postoperative ileus than are epidural opioids or the combination of local anesthetics and epidural opioids.[144,147,149]

Prokinetic Agents

Metoclopramide hydrochloride is a cholinergic agonist and dopamine antagonist that initiates phase 3 of the interdigestive migrating motor complex. Although it has been the subject of numerous randomized, controlled trials, none has demonstrated a significant benefit on the duration of postoperative ileus.[150-152]

Erythromycin is a macrolide antibiotic that binds to and stimulates the motilin receptor on small intestinal smooth muscle cells. Two prospective, randomized trials have examined the effect of erythromycin on the duration of postoperative ileus, with neither demonstrating a beneficial effect.[153,154]

Cisapride is a serotonin receptor agonist that promotes the release of acetylcholine from the myenteric plexus. Although several randomized clinical trials demonstrated a reduction in duration of ileus, others failed to demonstrate a benefit. This agent was removed from the market because of potentially fatal cardiac effects.[155]

Octreotide is a somatostatin analog that inhibits the secretion of several gastrointestinal hormones. In one canine study, octreotide was shown to shorten the duration of postoperative ileus.[156] However, clinical studies are lacking.

Multimodal Treatment of Postoperative Ileus

Multimodal approaches to postoperative ileus have been developed to take advantage of the additive effects of various single-modality interventions such as thoracic epidural analgesia with local anesthetics, opioid-sparing analgesia, minimally invasive operative techniques, and early nutrition. Thus, use of continuous thoracic epidural analgesia with local anesthetics, early oral feeding, and mobilization may reduce the duration of postoperative ileus to only 1 to 2 days after colonic surgery.[157]

REFERENCES

1. Fevang BT, Fevang J, Stangeland L, et al: Complications and death after surgical treatment of small bowel obstruction: A 35-year institutional experience. Ann Surg 231:529, 2000.
2. Andersson RE: Small bowel obstruction after appendectomy. Br J Surg 88:1387, 2001.
3. Edna TH, Bjerkeset T: Small bowel obstruction in patients previously operated on for colorectal cancer. Eur J Surg 164:587, 1998.
4. Nieuwemhuijzen M, Reijnen MM, Kuijpers JH, et al: Small bowel obstruction after total or subtotal colectomy: A 10-year retrospective review. Br J Surg 85:1242, 1998.

5. Beck DE, Opelka FG, Bailey HR, et al: Incidence of small-bowel obstruction and adhesiolysis after open colorectal and general surgery. Dis Colon Rectum 42:241, 1999.

6. Al-Took S, Platt R, Tulandi T: Adhesion-related small-bowel obstruction after gynecologic operations. Am J Obstet Gynecol 180:313, 1999.

7. Matter I, Khalemsky L, Abrahamson J, et al: Does the index operation influence the course and outcome of adhesive intestinal obstruction? Eur J Surg 163:767, 1997.

8. Ellis H, Moran BJ, Thompson JN, et al: Adhesion-related hospital readmissions after abdominal and pelvic surgery: A retrospective cohort study. Lancet 353:1476, 1999.

9. Mucha P Jr: Small intestinal obstruction. Surg Clin North Am 67:597, 1987.

10. Miller G, Boman J, Shrier I, et al: Etiology of small bowel obstruction. Am J Surg 180:33, 2000.

11. Rai S, Chandra SS, Smile SR: A study of the risk of strangulation and obstruction in groin hernias. Aust N Z J Surg 68:650, 1998.

12. Alvarez JA, Baldonedo RF, Bear IG, et al: Incarcerated groin hernias in adults: Presentation and outcome. Hernia 8:121, 2004.

13. Kulah B, Kulacoglu I, Oruc T, et al: Presentation and outcome of incarcerated external hernias in adults. Am J Surg 181:101, 2001.

14. Fevang B, Fevang J, Soreide O, et al: Delay in operative treatment among patients with small bowel obstruction. Scand J Surg 92:131, 2003.

15. Podnos YD, Jimenez JC, Wilson SE, et al: Complications after laparoscopic gastric bypass: A review of 3464 cases. Arch Surg 138:957, 2003.

16. Higa KD, Ho T, Boone KB: Internal hernias after laparoscopic Roux-en-Y gastric bypass: Incidence, treatment, and prevention. Obes Surg 13:350, 2003.

17. Hass BE, Schrager RE: Small bowel obstruction due to Richter's hernia after laparoscopic procedures. J Laparoendosc Surg 3:421, 1993.

18. Bowrey D, Blom D, Crookes P, et al: Risk factors and prevalence of trocar site herniation after laparoscopic fundoplication. Surg Endosc 15:663, 2001.

19. Azurin D, Go L: Trocar site herniation following laparoscopic cholecystectomy and the significance of an incidental pre-existing umbilical hernia. Am Surg 61:1343, 1995.

20. Phillips E, Arregui M, Carroll B, et al. Incidence of complications following laparoscopic hernioplasty. Surg Endosc 9:16, 1995.

21. Miller G, Boman J, Shrier I, et al: Small-bowel obstruction secondary to malignant disease: An 11-year audit. Can J Surg 43:353, 2000.

22. McCloy C, Brown T, Bolton J, et al: The etiology of intestinal obstruction in patients without prior laparotomy or hernia. Am Surg 64:1343, 1998.

23. Kabaroudis A, Papaziogas B, Koutelidakis I, et al: Disruption of the small intestine mucosal barrier after intestinal occlusion: A study with light and electron microscopy. J Invest Surg 16:23, 2003.

24. Fevang J, Ovrebo K, Svanes K, Rokke O: Endotoxin and cytokine release in strangulation obstruction and in partial occlusion of the mesenteric artery in pigs. Eur. Surg Res 21:26, 1999.

25. Shields R: The absorption and secretion of fluid and electrolytes by the obstructed bowel. Br J Surg 52:774, 1965.

26. Levitt MD: Volume and composition of intestinal gas determined by means of an intestinal wash out technique. N Engl J Med 284:1394, 1971.

27. Roscher R, Oettinger W, Beger HG: Bacterial microflora, endogenous endotoxin, and prostaglandins in SBO. Am J Surg 155:348, 1988.

28. Bishop RF, Allcock EA: Bacterial flora of the small intestine in acute intestinal obstruction. BMJ 1:766, 1960.

29. Berg RD, Garlington AW: Translocation of certain indigenous bacteria from the gastrointestinal tract to the mesenteric lymph nodes and other organs in a gnotobiotic mouse model. Infect Immunol 23:403, 1979.

30. Deitch EA, Maejima K, Berg RD: Effect of oral antibiotics and bacterial overgrowth on the translocation of the gastrointestinal tract microflora in burned rats. J Trauma 25:385, 1985.

31. Deitch EA: Simple intestinal obstruction causes bacterial translocation in man. Arch Surg 124:699, 1989.

32. Samel S, Keese M, Kleczka M, et al: Microscopy of bacterial translocation during small bowel obstruction and ischemia in vivo: A new animal model. BMC Surg 2:6, 2002.

33. Heneghan JB, Robinson JWL, Menge H, et al: Intestinal obstruction in germ-free dogs. Eur J Clin Invest 11:285, 1981.

34. Lappas JC, Reyes BL, Maglinte DDT: Abdominal radiography findings in small bowel obstruction: Relevance to triage for additional diagnostic imaging. AJR Am J Roentgenol 176:167, 2001.

35. Maglinte DD, Reyes BL, Harmon BH, et al: Reliability and role of plain film radiography and CT in the diagnosis of small-bowel obstruction. AJR Am J Roentgenol 167:1451, 1996.

36. Shrake PD, Rex DK, Lappas JC, et al: Radiographic evaluation of suspected small bowel obstruction. Am J Gastroenterol 86:175, 1991.

37. Riveron FA, Obeid FN, Horst HM, et al: The role of contrast radiography in presumed bowel obstruction. Surgery 106:496, 1989.

38. Biondo S, Pares D, Mora L, et al: Randomized clinical study of Gastrografin administration in patients with adhesive small bowel obstruction. Br J Surg 90:542, 2003.

39. Blackmon S, Lucius C, Wilson JP, et al: The use of water-soluble contrast in evaluating clinically equivocal small bowel obstructions. Am Surg 66:238, 2000.

40. Megibow AJ, Balthazar EJ, Cho KC, et al: Bowel obstruction: Evaluation with computed tomography. Radiology 180:313, 1991.

41. Balthazar EJ: Computed tomography of small bowel obstruction. AJR Am J Roentgenol 162:255, 1994.

42. Suri S, Gupta S, Sudhakar PJ, et al: Comparative evaluation of plain films, ultrasound and CT in the diagnosis of intestinal obstruction. Acta Radiol 40:422, 1999.

43. Peck JJ, Milleson T, Phelan J: The role of computed tomography with contrast and small bowel follow-through in management of small bowel obstruction. Am J Surg 177:375, 1999.

44. Boudiaf M, Jaff A, Soyer P et al: Small bowel diseases: Prospective evaluation of multidetector row helical CT enteroclysis in 107 consecutive patients. Radiology 233:338, 2004.

45. Umschaden HW, Szolar D, Gasser J, et al: Small bowel disease: Comparison of MR enteroclysis image with conventional enteroclysis and surgical findings. Radiology 215:717, 2000.

46. Schmidt S, Leopori D, Meuwly JY, et al: Prospective comparison of MR enteroclysis with multi-planar spiral CT enteroclysis: Interobserver agreement and sensitivity by means of "sign-by-sign" correlation. Eur Radiol 13:1303, 2003.

47. Khurana B: The whirl sign. Radiology 226:69, 2003.

48. Makita O, Ikushima I, Matsumoto N, et al: CT differentiation between necrotic and non-necrotic small bowel in closed loop and strangulating obstruction. Abdom Imag 24:120, 1999.

49. Ha HK, Kim JS, Lee MS, et al: Differentiation of simple and strangulated small bowel obstruction: Usefulness of known CT criteria. Radiology 204:507, 1997.

50. Balthazar EJ, Liebeskind ME, Macari M: Intestinal ischemia in patients in whom small bowel obstruction is suspected: Evaluation of accuracy, limitations and clinical implications of CT in diagnosis. Radiology 205:519, 1997.

51. Sarr MG, Bulkley GB, Zuidema GD: Preoperative recognition of intestinal strangulation obstruction: Prospective evaluation of diagnostic capability. Am J Surg 145:176, 1983.

52. Brolin RE, Krasna MJ, Mast BA: Use of tubes and radiographs in the management of small bowel obstruction. Ann Surg 206:126, 1987.

53. Peetz DJ, Gamelli RL, Pilcher DB: Intestinal intubation in acute, mechanical small-bowel obstruction. Arch Surg 117:334, 1982.

54. Brolin RE: Partial small bowel obstruction. Surgery 95:145, 1984.

55. Fleshner PR, Siegman MG, Slater GI, et al: A prospective, randomized trial of short versus long tubes in adhesive small-bowel obstruction. Am J Surg 170:366, 1995.

56. Assalia A, Schein M, Kopelman D, et al: Therapeutic effect of oral Gastrografin in adhesive, partial small-bowel obstruction: A prospective randomized trial. Surgery 115:433, 1994.

57. Choi HK, Chu KW, Law WL: Therapeutic value of Gastrografin in adhesive small bowel obstruction after unsuccessful conservative treatment: a prospective randomized trial. Ann Surg 236:1, 2002.

58. Fevang BT, Jensen D, Fevang J, et al: Upper gastrointestinal contrast study in the management of small bowel obstruction: A prospective randomized study. Eur J Surg 166:39, 2000.

59. Feigin E, Seror D, Szold A, et al: Water-soluble contrast material has no therapeutic effect on postoperative small-bowel obstruction: Results of a prospective, randomized clinical trial. Am J Surg 171:227, 1996.

60. Luque-deLeon E, Metzger A, Tsiotos GG, et al: Laparoscopic management of small bowel obstruction: indications and outcome. J Gastroenterol Surg 2:132, 1998.

61. Wullstein C, Gross E: Laparoscopic compared with conventional treatment of acute adhesive small bowel obstruction. Br J Surg 90:1147, 2003.

62. Nagle A, Ujiki M, Denham W, et al: Laparoscopic adhesiolysis for small bowel obstruction. Am J Surg 187:464, 2004.

63. Miller G, Boman J, Shrier I, et al: Natural history of patients with adhesive small bowel obstruction. Br J Surg 87:1240, 2000.

64. Barkan H, Webster S, Ozeran S: Factors predicting the recurrence of adhesive small-bowel obstruction. Am J Surg 170:361, 1995.

65. Landercasper J, Cogbill TH, Merry WH, et al: Long-term outcome after hospitalization for small-bowel obstruction. Arch Surg 128:76, 1993.

66. Stewart RM, Page CP, Brender J, et al: The incidence and risk of early postoperative small bowel obstruction: A cohort study. Am J Surg 154:643, 1987.

67. Ellozy SH, Harris MT, Bauer JJ, et al: Early postoperative small-bowel obstruction: A prospective evaluation in 242 consecutive abdominal operations. Dis Colon Rectum 45:1214, 2002.

68. Quatromoni JC, Rosoff L, Halls JM, et al: Early postoperative small bowel obstruction. Ann Surg 191:72, 1980.

69. Pickleman J, Lee RM: The management of patients with suspected early postoperative small bowel obstruction. Ann Surg 210:216, 1989.

70. Dvoretsky PM, Richards KA, Angel A, et al: Survival time, causes of death, and tumor: Treatment related morbidity in 100 women with ovarian cancer. Hum Pathol 19:1273, 1988.

71. Tunca JC, Buchler DA, Mack EA: The management of ovarian cancer-caused bowel obstruction. Gynecol Oncol 12:186, 1981.

72. Ellis CN, Boggs HW Jr, Slagle GW, et al: Small bowel obstruction after colon resection for benign and malignant diseases. Dis Colon Rectum 34:367, 1991.

73. Low RN, Chen SC, Barone R: Distinguishing benign from malignant bowel obstruction in patients with malignancy: Findings at MR imaging. Radiology 228:157, 2003.

74. Pothuri B, Vaidya A, Aghajanian C, et al: Palliative surgery for bowel obstruction in recurrent ovarian cancer: An updated series. Gynecol Oncol 89:306, 2003.

75. Walsh HPJ, Schofield PF: Is laparotomy for small bowel obstruction justified in patients with previously treated malignancy? Br J Surg 71:933, 1984.

76. Ketcham AS, Hoye RC, Pilch YH, et al: Delayed intestinal obstruction following treatment for cancer. Cancer 25:406, 1970.

77. Azar T, Berger DL: Adult intussusception. Ann Surg 226:134, 1997.

78. Nagorney DM, Sarr MG, McIlrath DC: Surgical management of intussusception in the adult. Ann Surg 193:230, 1981.

79. Shields WE, Maves CK, Hedlung GL, et al: Air enema for diagnosis and reduction of intussusception: Clinical experience and pressure correlates. Radiology 181:169, 1991.

80. DiFiore JW: Intussusception. Semin Pediatr Surg 8:214, 1999.

81. Verschelden P, Filiatrault D, Garel L, et al: Intussusception in children: Reliability of US in diagnosis—a prospective study. Radiology 184:741, 1992.

82. Merine D, Fishman EK, Jones B: Enteroenteric intussusception: CT findings in nine patients. AJR Am J Roentgenol 148:1129, 1987.

83. Lobo DL, Jobling JC, Balfour TW: Gallstone ileus: Diagnostic pitfalls and therapeutic successes. J Clin Gastroenterol 30:72, 2000.

84. Clavien PA, Richon J, Burgan S, et al: Gallstone ileus. Br J Surg 77:737, 1990.

85. Doko M, Zovak M, Kopljar M, et al: Comparison of surgical treatments of gallstone ileus: Preliminary report. World J Surg 27:400, 2003.

86. Pavlidis TE, Atmatzidis KSW, Papziogas BT, et al: Management of gallstone ileus. J Hepatobiliary Pancreat Surg 10:299, 2003.

87. Reisner RM, Cohen JR: Gallstone ileus: A review of 1001 reported cases. Am Surg 60:441, 1994.

88. van Hillo M, van der Vliet JA, Wiggers T, et al: Gallstone obstruction of the intestine: An analysis of ten patients and a review of the literature. Surgery 101:273, 1987.

89. Franklin ME Jr, Dorman JP, Schuessler WW: Laparoscopic treatment of gallstone ileus: A case report and review of the literature. J Laparoendosc Surg 4:265, 1994.

90. Lubbers H, Mahlke R, Lankisch PG: Gallstone ileus: Endoscopic removal of a gallstone obstructing the upper jejunum. J Intern Med 246:593, 1999.

91. Deans G, Krukowski Z, Irwin S: Malignant obstruction of the left colon. Br J Surg 81:1270, 1994.

92. Grossmann EM, Longo WE, Stratton MD, et al: Sigmoid volvulus in Department of Veterans Affairs Medical Centers. Dis Colon Rectum 43:414, 2000.

93. Arnold GJ, Nance FC: Volvulus of the sigmoid colon. Ann Surg 177:527, 1973.

94. Ballantyne GH: Review of sigmoid volvulus: history and results of treatment. Dis Colon Rectum 25:494, 1982.

95. Ballantyne GH, Brandner MD, Beart RW Jr, et al: Volvulus of the colon: incidence and mortality. Ann Surg 202:83, 1985.

96. Ballantyne GH: Review of sigmoid volvulus: Clinical patterns and pathogenesis. Dis Colon Rectum 25:823, 1982.

97. Brothers TE, Strodel WE, Eckhauser F: Endoscopy in colonic volvulus. Ann Surg 206:1, 1987.

98. Agrez M, Cameron D: Radiology of sigmoid volvulus. Dis Colon Rectum 24:510, 1981.

99. Haskin PH, Teplick SK, Teplick JG, et al: Volvulus of the cecum and right colon. JAMA 245:2433, 1981.

100. Deen K, Madoff R, Goldberg S, et al: Surgical management of left colon obstruction. J Am Coll Surg 187:573, 1998.

101. Murray JJ, Schoetz DJ Jr, Coller JA, et al: Intraoperative colonic lavage and primary anastomosis in nonelective colon resection. Dis Colon Rectum 34:527, 1991.

102. Brief DK, Brener BJ, Goldenkranz R, et al: Defining the role of subtotal colectomy in the treatment of carcinoma of the colon. Ann Surg 213:248, 1991.

103. Dauphine C, Tan P, Bert R, et al: Placement of self-expanding metal stents for acute malignant large-bowel obstruction. Ann Surg Oncol 9:575, 2002.

104. Meisner S, Hensler M, Knop F, et al: Self-expanding metal stents for colonic obstruction: Experience from 104 procedures in a single center. Dis Colon Rectum 47:444, 2004.

105. Khot UP, Wenk L, Murali K, et al: Systematic review of the efficacy and safety of colorectal stents. Br J Surg 89:1096, 2002.

106. McDoff R, Dykes S: What's new with colon and rectal surgery. J Am Coll Surg 198:91, 2004.

107. Law W, Choi H, Lee Y, et al: Palliation for advanced malignant colorectal obstruction by self-expanding metallic stents: Prospective evaluation of outcomes. Dis Colon Rectum 47:39, 2004.

108. Smothers L, Hynan L, Fleming J, et al: Emergency surgery for colon cancer. Dis Colon Rectum 46:24, 2003.

109. Burke JB, Ballantyne GH: Cecal volvulus: Low mortality at a city hospital. Dis Colon Rectum 27:737, 1984.

110. Anderson JR, Welch GH: Acute volvulus of the right colon: An analysis of 69 patients. World J Surg 10:336, 1986.

111. Livingston EH, Passaro EP: Postoperative ileus. Dig Dis Sci 35:121, 1990.

112. Prasad M, Matthews JB: Deflating postoperative ileus. Gastroenterology 117:489, 1999.

113. Holte K, Kehlet H: Postoperative ileus: Progress towards effective management. Drugs 62:2603, 2002.

114. Condon RE, Cowles VE, Schulte WJ, et al: Resolution of postoperative ileus in humans. Ann Surg 203:574, 1986.

115. Dubois A, Weise VK, Kopin IJ: Postoperative ileus in the rat: Physiology, etiology and treatment. Ann Surg 178:781, 1973.

116. Liu S, Carpenter RL, Neal JM: Epidural anesthesia and analgesia: Their role in postoperative outcome. Anesthesiology 82:1474, 1995.

117. Steinbrook RA: Epidural anesthesia and gastrointestinal motility. Anesth Analg 86:837, 1998.

118. Tache Y, Monnikes H, Bonaz B, et al: Role of CRF in stress-related alterations of gastric and colonic motor function. Ann N Y Acad Sci 697:233, 1993.

119. De Winter BY, Boeckxstaens GE, De Man JG, et al: Effect of adrenergic and nitrergic blockade on experimental ileus in rats. Br J Pharmacol 120:464, 1997.

120. Zittel TT, Lloyd KC, Rothenhofer I, et al: Calcitonin gene-related peptide and spinal afferents partly mediate postoperative colonic ileus in the rat. Surgery 123:518, 1998.

121. Kalff JC, Schraut WH, Simmons RL, et al: Surgical manipulation of the gut elicits an intestinal muscularis inflammatory response resulting in paralytic ileus. Ann Surg 228:652, 1998.

122. Kehlet H. Postoperative ileus. Gut 47(Suppl 4):85, 2000.

123. de Jonge WJ, van den Wijngaard RM, The FO, et al: Postoperative ileus is maintained by intestinal immune infiltrates that activate inhibitory neural pathways in mice. Gastroenterology 125:1137, 2003.

124. Kalff JC, Turler A, Schwarz NT, et al: Intra-abdominal activation of a local inflammatory response within the human muscularis externa during laparotomy. Ann Surg 237:301, 2003.

125. Brix-Christensen V, Goumon Y, Tonnesen E, et al: Endogenous morphine is produced in response to cardiopulmonary bypass in neonatal pigs. Acta Anaesthesiol Scand 44:1204, 2000.

126. Yoshida S, Ohta J, Yamasaki K, et al: Effect of surgical stress on endogenous morphine and cytokine levels in the plasma after laparoscopic or open cholecystectomy. Surg Endosc 14:137, 2000.

127. Pappagallo M: Incidence, prevalence, and management of opioid bowel dysfunction. Am J Surg 182(Suppl):S11, 2001.

128. Kurz A, Sessler DI: Opioid-induced bowel dysfunction: Pathophysiology and potential new therapies. Drugs 63:649, 2003.

129. Kromer W: Endogenous opioids, the enteric nervous system, and gut motility. Dig Dis 8:361, 1990.

130. Manara L, Bianchetti A: The central and peripheral influences of opioids on gastrointestinal propulsion. Annu Rev Pharmacol Toxicol 25:249, 1985.

131. Manara L, Bianchi G, Ferretti P, et al: Inhibition of gastrointestinal transit by morphine in rats results primarily from direct drug action on gut opioid sites. J Pharmacol Exp Ther 237:945, 1986.

132. DeLuca A, Coupar IM: Insights into opioid actions in the intestinal tract. Pharmacol Ther 69:103, 1996.

133. Friedman JD, Dello Bueno FA: Opioid antagonists in the treatment of opioid-induced constipation and pruritus. Ann Pharmacother 35:85, 2001.

134. Ferraz AAB, Cowles VE, Condon RE, et al: Opioid and non-opioid analgesic drug effects on colon contractions in monkeys. Dig Dis Sci 40:1417, 1995.

135. Frantzides CT, Cowles V, Salaymeh B, et al: Morphine effects on human colonic myoelectric activity in the postoperative period. Am J Surg 163:144, 1995.

136. Cheatham ML, Chapman WC, Key SP, et al: A meta-analysis of selective versus routine nasogastric decompression after elective laparotomy. Ann Surg 221:469, 1995.

137. Saga PM, Kruegener G, MacFie J: Nasogastric intubation and elective abdominal surgery. Br J Surg 79:1380, 1992.

138. Cheng G, Cassissi C, Drexler PF, et al: Salsalate, morphine and postoperative ileus. Am J Surg 171:85, 1996.

139. Ferraz AA, Cowles VE, Condon RE, et al: Nonopioid analgesics shorten the duration of postoperative ileus. Am Surg 61:1079, 1995.

140. Merry B, Power W: Perioperative NSAIDs: Towards greater safety. Pain Rev 2:268, 1995.

141. Heimbach DM, Crout JR: Treatment of paralytic ileus with adrenergic neuronal blocking drugs. Surgery 69:582, 1971.

142. Kleinfeld D: Edrophonium used for vagotonic action. JAMA 223:922, 1973.

143. Kreis ME, Kasparek M, Zittell TT, et al: Neostigmine increases postoperative colonic motlity in patients undergoing colorectal surgery. Surgery 130:449, 2001.

144. Liu SS, Carpenter RL, Mackey DC, et al: Effects of perioperative analgesic technique on rate of recovery after colon surgery. Anesthesiology 83:757, 1995.

145. Bredtmann RD, Herden HN, Teichmann W, et al: Epidural analgesia in colonic surgery: Results of a randomized prospective study. Br J Surg 77:638, 1990.

146. Neudecker J, Schwenk W, Junghans T, et al: Randomized controlled trial to examine the influence of thoracic epidural analgesia on postoperative ileus after laparoscopic sigmoid resection. Br. J Surg 98:1292, 1999.

147. Jorgensen H, Fomsgaard JS, Dirks J, et al: Effect of epidural bupivacaine versus combined epidural bupivacaine and morphine on gastrointestinal function and pain after major gynaecological surgery. Br J Anaesth 87:727, 2001.

148. Steinbrook RA: Epidural anesthesia and gastrointestinal motility. Anesth Analg 86:837, 1998.

149. Asantila R, Eklund P, Rosenberg PH: Continuous epidural infusion of bupivacaine and morphine for postoperative analgesia after hysterectomy. Acta Anaesthesiol Scand 35:513, 1991.

150. Jepsen S, Klaerke A, Nielsen PH, et al: Negative effect of metoclopramide in postoperative adynamic ileus: A prospective, randomized, double-blind study. Br J Surg 73:290, 1986.

151. Davidson ED, Hersh T, Brinner RA, et al: The effects of metoclopramide on postoperative ileus: A randomized double-blind study. Ann Surg 190:27, 1979.

152. Seta ML, Kale-Pradham PB: Efficacy of metoclopramide in postoperative ileus after exploratory laparotomy. Pharmacotherapy 10:1181, 2001.

153. Smith AJ, Nissan A, Lanouette NM, et al: Prokinetic effect of erythromycin after colorectal surgery: Randomized, placebo-controlled, double-blind study. Dis Colon Rectum 43:333, 2000.

154. Bonacini M, Quiason S, Reynolds M, et al: Effect of intravenous erythromycin on postoperative ileus. Am J Gastroenterol 88:208, 1993.

155. Tonini M, De Ponti F, Di Nucci A, et al: Review article: Cardiac adverse effects of gastrointestinal prokinetics. Aliment Pharmacol Ther 13:1585, 1999.

156. Cullen JJ, Eagon JC, Kelly KA: Gastrointestinal peptide hormones during postoperative ileus: Effect of octreotide. Dig Dis Sci 39:1179, 1994.

157. Holte K, Kehlet H: Postoperative ileus: Progress towards effective management. Drugs 62:2603, 2002.

CHAPTER
117 Acute and Chronic Pseudo-obstruction

Michael Camilleri

Acute and chronic pseudo-obstruction represent a vast array of conditions that are encountered commonly in clinical practice. Acute presentations require coordinated management with the help of interventionalists, internists, and surgeons. Chronic conditions require coordinated management with experts in dietetics and nutrition; further studies are needed to develop improved pharmacotherapies. Significant advances in management of parenteral nutrition and its complications, use of enteral support, and advances in isolated small intestinal transplantation provide life support for these patients, and the gastroenterologist is key in orchestrating the best modality and timing of treatment.

The functions of small intestinal and colonic smooth muscle are controlled mainly by the intrinsic and extrinsic nerves of the gastrointestinal tract (Fig. 117–1), the interstitial cells of Cajal (ICC), and, to a lesser degree, by gastrointestinal hormones (see Chapters 94 and 95).

The human small bowel and colon display widely divergent patterns of absorption, motility, and transit. Propulsive, peristaltic activity can move luminal contents over long distances of the small intestine almost as rapidly as contents are moved through the esophagus. The small intestine facilitates emptying from the stomach, mixes chyme with digestive enzymes and bile, and delivers residue to the colon. The last action is accomplished by the ileum via a specialized type of contraction (giant migrating, or "power," contraction) wave analogous to the high-amplitude colonic contractions that propagate at rates reaching approximately 2 cm/sec and are responsible for mass movements in the colon.

Intermittent, or "bolus," emptying from the small intestine ensures there is sufficient time for salvage of remaining nutrients in the small intestine. The small intestine and colon also set up feedback inhibitory reflexes (e.g., ileal brake) that retard proximal motor functions such as gastric emptying. These feedback mechanisms involve hormones such as enteroglucagon, glucagon-like peptides, and peptide YY.

Patients with small intestine dysmotility also usually have abnormal motor function of other parts of the gastrointestinal tract. Dysmotility of the small intestine and colon has a wide range of clinical manifestations, regardless of the underlying cause of the disorder. At one end of the spectrum patients may be asymptomatic, and at the other end of the spectrum they may have chronic intestinal pseudo-obstruction (CIP). Intestinal pseudo-obstruction is defined as a clinical syndrome characterized by impaired intestinal propulsion, which may resemble intestinal obstruction, but for which no mechanical cause is found. It may involve the small or large bowel and presents in acute, subacute, or chronic forms. This clinical definition is used because its precise underlying pathophysiologic processes are unclear. The definition also fits a broad range of clinical conditions, from constipation to the more complex and severe clinical syndrome CIP.

This chapter focuses on the acute form of (predominantly) colonic pseudo-obstruction that is associated with bowel dilatation and on the chronic form that typically affects the small bowel. Chronic colonic pseudo-obstruction manifests as slow transit constipation and

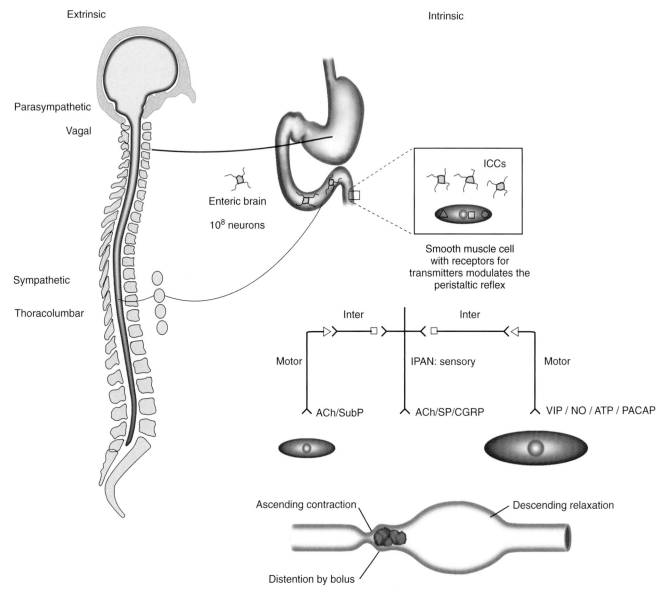

Figure 117–1 Extrinsic and intrinsic control of intestinal motility. The enteric nervous system controls stereotypical motor functions such as the migrating motor complex and the peristaltic reflex; enteric control is modulated by the extrinsic parasympathetic and sympathetic nerves, which respectively stimulate and inhibit nonsphincteric muscle. ACh, acetylcholine; IPAN, intrinsic primary afferent neuron; SP, substance P; CGRP, calcitonin gene-related peptide; VIP, vasoactive intestinal peptide; NO, nitric oxide; ATP, adenosine triphosphate; PACAP, pituitary adenylate cyclase-activating polypeptide. (From Camilleri M, Delgado-Aros S: Dysmotility of the small and large intestine. In Yamada T, Alpers DH, Kaplowitz N, et al [eds]: The Atlas of Gastroenterology, 3rd ed. Philadelphia, Lippincott Williams & Wilkins, 2003, p 298.)

colonic inertia and are addressed elsewhere in this book (see Chapters 12 and 95).

EPIDEMIOLOGY

The prevalence of small intestine dysmotility is unknown but varies according to the underlying disease and seems to be less frequent in comparison with esophageal, gastric, or colonic dysmotility. The literature documents several hereditary diseases associated with (1) smooth muscle degeneration, including familial visceral myopathies (FVMs) and childhood visceral myopathies (CVMs); and (2) diseases with myenteric plexus degener-

ation, including familial visceral neuropathies (FVNs). All of these disorders are encountered rarely, even in tertiary care centers. A small number of such families, mostly whites and, less often, African Americans[1] and Latinos,[2] has been reported. The epidemiology of small bowel pseudo-obstruction is unknown. These rare familial disorders are discussed in the first part of this chapter.

Conversely, congenital and acquired colonic diseases are understood more clearly. Hirschsprung's disease, the prototypic congenital colonic dysmotility disorder, affects 1 in 5000 births (see Chapter 93). Constipation affects about 12% to 15% of the population, with an equal split between functional constipation and organic evacuation disorders.

NEURAL CONTROL OF SMALL INTESTINAL AND COLONIC MOTILITY

The enteric nervous system (ENS) consists of vast ganglionated plexuses located in the wall of the gastrointestinal tract[3]; the most important functionally are the myenteric and submucosal plexuses. In association with the muscle layers, the networks of ICC are recognized as the likely pacemakers activating neuromuscular function. The ENS consists of approximately 100 million neurons in higher mammals, a number roughly equal to the number of neurons in the spinal cord. Histologic and electrophysiologic studies[4,5] of the intestinal tract have characterized the properties of the neurons and the transmitters mediating its functions, including the peristaltic reflex, and the neuroimmune interactions between neurons and inflammatory cells.

In terms of small bowel and colonic motility, ontogenically, the ENS develops in utero by migration of neural crest cells to the developing alimentary canal. Migration, colonization, differentiation, and maintenance or survival of neural crest cells are regulated by specific signaling molecules that include transcription factors (e.g., Mash1), neurotrophic factors (e.g., the glial-derived neurotrophic factor [GDNF] and its receptor subunits), and the neuregulin signaling system.

Precursor cells arise from three axial levels of the neural crest: vagal, rostrotruncal, and lumbosacral[6] levels. The enteric neurons mainly arise from the vagal neural crest of the developing hindbrain and colonize the gut by migration in a rostrocaudal direction. Vagal crest cells, however, are not restricted to a particular intestinal region. Some enteric neurons arrive in the hindgut from the lumbosacral level via a caudorostral wave of colonization. Rarely, the migrating cells do not reach the entire gut; usually this affects the terminal portion of the bowel, as in classic forms of Hirschsprung's disease (see Chapter 93).[7] The neural crest cells that migrate and colonize the gut become neuroblasts or neuronal support cells, glioblasts. However, *differentiation* into neurons and glial cells seems not to take place until the cells have reached their final destinations in the gut. Movement through the gut mesenchyme, survival in the gut, and differentiation into mature cells are influenced by contacts of precursor cells with the *microenvironment*, other cells in the mesenchyme, neural crest-derived cells, and the extracellular matrix. The latter provides directional and differentiation signals such as GDNF, which ensures survival of committed neuroblasts.

Enteric serotonergic neurons appear so early in development that they coexist in primordial enteric ganglia with still-dividing neural precursors. Serotonin (5-HT), acting via the 5-HT_{2B} receptor strongly promotes development of neurons at specific times and affects the development of late-arising enteric neurons.

CHRONIC INTESTINAL PSEUDO-OBSTRUCTION

CIP is a syndrome that suggests mechanical obstruction of the small or large bowel in the absence of an anatomic lesion that obstructs the flow of intestinal contents. Segments of affected bowel appear dilated on radiologic studies. In contrast, a similar motor disorder of small bowel or colon unassociated with dilatation is referred to as *chronic intestinal dysmotility*.

ETIOLOGY

There are a number of variations in the etiology and course of CIP. CIP is usually secondary to an underlying disorder affecting neuromuscular function, although rare familial cases have been described. Neuropathic causes include amyloidosis, diabetes mellitus, and paraneoplastic syndromes; scleroderma is an example of a myopathic process. Combinations of neuropathic and myopathic etiologies also occur in scleroderma and in amyloidosis. In general, small intestine dysmotility may be secondary to neuropathy or myopathy, and evidence now suggests that some cases may be characterized by abnormalities of the ICC, the pacemakers of the intestine.

Neuropathology in Enteric Neuropathies

The following section summarizes the reported morphologic and molecular features in enteric neuropathies that result in gut dysmotility in the absence of systemic or easily identified neuromuscular disorders such as autonomic neuropathies, parkinsonism, and multiple sclerosis. Many of the features may be present in the same tissue specimen, such as inflammation, apoptosis and degeneration. It is unlikely that a different mechanism is responsible for each feature, and there is a limited morphologic phenotype of the histopathology of these disorders. A combination of molecular derangements may contribute to the degenerative process that leads to enteric neuronal loss, including disorders of intracellular Ca^{2+} signaling, mitochondrial dysfunction, oxidative stress, and alterations in signal transduction pathways.

Table 117–1 lists the pathologic features that have been described in enteric neuropathies. For detailed descriptions of the morphologic and molecular pathology and the clinical observations and implications of these observations, the reader is referred to a recent review.[8]

Role of the Interstitial Cells of Cajal

The ICC function as the intestinal pacemaker cells. The proto-oncogene *c-kit* encodes for a tyrosine kinase recep-

Table 117–1   *Pathologic Features in Enteric Neuropathies*

Aganglionosis
Interstitial cell pathology
Intestinal neuronal dysplasia
Mitochondrial dysfunction
Neural degeneration
Neural inflammation
Neuronal hyperplasia and ganglioneuromas
Neuronal intranuclear inclusions and apoptosis

tor that facilitates the development of the ICC. ICC typically are surrounded by collagen fibers and have close contact with smooth muscle cells via gap junctions. Gap junctions allow for transmission of pacemaking activity, a consequence of spontaneous oscillation in resting membrane potentials that is unaffected by the effects of 10^{-6} M verapamil, an L-type calcium channel blocker. This characteristic proves that they are not simply smooth muscle cells, but they have self-generating ability to initiate the electrical potential that spreads through the muscle layer. All cell types express muscarinic receptor types M_2 and M_3, neurokinin receptors NK_1 and NK_3, and inhibitory receptor VIP_1.[9]

In clinical studies, a relative deficiency of c-kit–positive cells has been reported in Hirschsprung's disease, CIP,[10,11] gastrointestinal stromal tumors, and multiple gastrointestinal autonomic tumors.[12] There also is a well-documented observation of delayed maturation of ICC.[13]

Megacolon in adults also has been associated with abnormal morphology and ultrastructure of ICC. Faussone-Pellegrini and associates demonstrated the presence of normal ICC with several branches in the dilated transverse colon but abnormal ICC (e.g., paucity of mitochondria) in the nondilated descending colon.[14]

In patients with acquired slow transit constipation, unassociated with colonic dilatation, the number of ICC in the muscle layers of the sigmoid colon is lower (Fig. 117–2) compared with control colons resected for a variety of other indications. Moreover, confocal images of the colons from patients with acquired slow transit constipation show that the ICCs have irregular surface markings, a paucity of branches,[15] and reduced c-kit staining of myenteric plexus cells, consistent with a reduction in the number of ICC or their tyrosine kinase content.

Primary Causes

Primary causes of CIP are rare compared with secondary dysmotilities and may be familial or sporadic.

Familial Visceral Myopathies

FVM is a group of genetic diseases characterized by degeneration and fibrosis of gastrointestinal smooth muscle and, in one type, also of urinary smooth muscle. There are at least three reported types of FVM based on gross lesions of the gastrointestinal tract and the pattern of inheritance (Table 117–2). There are mitochondrial DNA disorders in FVM type II, and this condition also is called *mitochondrial neurogastrointestinal encephalopathy* (MNGIE), or *oculogastrointestinal neuropathy*. On routine pathology, there is no difference in histologic findings among the three types of FVM.[16] Degenerating muscle cells appear pale, poorly defined, and fragmented; become surrounded by collagen; and take on a vacuolated appearance. Special histochemical stains may identify giant mitochondria as ragged red fibers in skeletal muscle or in affected bowel; cytochemistry can identify mitochondrial enzyme deficiencies in MNGIE or FVM-II.

FVM-II or MNGIE. The enzymes in the mitochondrial respiratory chain are encoded by nuclear and mitochondrial DNA. Mitochondria are involved in the production of energy (adenosine triphosphate), the generation of reactive oxygen species, and the initiation of

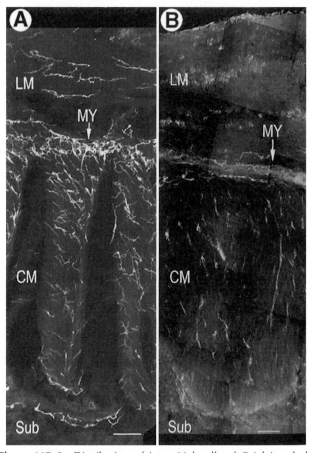

Figure 117–2 Distribution of interstitial cells of Cajal in whole transverse mounts of the sigmoid colon in a normal control section (*A*) and in a patient with slow transit constipation (*B*). CM, circular muscle; LM, longitudinal muscle; MY, myenteric; Sub, submucosal. (*A* and *B*, From He CL, Burgart L, Wang L, et al: Decreased interstitial cell of Cajal volume in patients with slow-transit constipation. Gastroenterology 118:14, 2000.)

apoptosis. The disorders are inherited as sporadic, autosomal dominant, autosomal recessive, or X-linked. These are diverse diseases characterized by mitochondrial abnormalities in skeletal muscle, which manifest as the classic "ragged red fibers" on a Gomorra trichrome stain. The metabolic abnormality involves cells in other tissues: central and peripheral nervous system, gut and enteric neurons, heart, kidney, liver, thyroid, pancreas, bone marrow, and others.[17] Selected mutations in the mitochondrial 16,569 base pair genome result in several pathologic disorders and syndromes that may affect two or more of these organs. Description of all of the syndromes is beyond the scope of this chapter.

Patients present with skeletal muscle pain and cramps, systemic lactic acidosis with elevated circulating muscle enzyme levels (e.g., creatine phosphokinase [CPK], alanine aminotransferase [ALT], and aldolase), and, as mentioned earlier, ragged red fibers on modified Gomorra stain. Special stains for the respiratory muscle enzymes can identify the precise functional defect. Thus, for example, succinate dehydrogenase–positive fibers appear "ragged blue" (because of the cytochemical stain of the enzyme), and staining of the adjacent tissue section with cytochrome c oxidase demonstrates a deficiency in the

Table 117–2   Classification of Familial Visceral Myopathies

Features	Type I	Type II (MNGIE)	Type III
Mode of transmission	Autosomal dominant	Autosomal recessive; sporadic cases	Autosomal recessive
Gross abnormalities	Esophageal dilatation, megaduodenum, redundant colon, and megacystis	Gastric dilatation, slight dilatation of the entire small intestine with numerous diverticula	Marked dilatation of the entire digestive tract from esophagus to rectum
Histology	Degeneration and fibrosis of both muscle layers	Same as type I	Same as type I
Clinical manifestations			
Age at onset	After the 1st decade	Adolescence	Middle age
Percent with symptoms	<50	>75	>75
Symptoms of CIP	Variable severity	Severe plus pain	Classic CIP
Extragastrointestinal features	Megacystis, uterine inertia, and mydriasis	Ptosis and external ophthalmoplegia, muscle pain, peripheral neuropathy, and deafness	None observed
Treatment, prognosis	Surgery in some cases; prognosis good	No effective medical or surgical treatment; prognosis poor	Same as type II

CIP, chronic intestinal pseudo-obstruction; MNGIE, mitochondrial neurogastrointestinal encephalopathy.

Table 117–3   Classification of Familial Visceral Neuropathies

Features	Type I	Type II
Mode of transmission	Autosomal dominant	Autosomal recessive
Gross abnormalities	Dilatation of various lengths of small intestine, often distal small bowel; megacolon; gastroparesis	Hypertrophic pyloric stenosis, dilated and short small intestine, malrotation of small intestine
Histology	Degeneration of argyrophilic neurons and decreased numbers of nerve fibers	Deficiency of argyrophilic neurons and increased number of neuroblasts
Clinical manifestations		
Age at onset	Any age	Infancy
Percent with symptoms	>75	100
Symptoms of CIP	67% CIP	All symptoms
Extragastrointestinal features	None	Malformation of CNS, patent ductus arteriosus in some cases
Treatment, prognosis	No effective medical or surgical treatment; prognosis fair	No effective medical or surgical treatment; prognosis poor

CIP, chronic intestinal pseudo-obstruction; CNS, central nervous system.

latter enzyme, implying a gene defect in the control of the complex IV respiratory chain proteins.[17] In the intestine, there is hypertrophy of the circular muscle layer, atrophy of the longitudinal muscle, and megamitochondria in myenteric neurons and muscle cells demonstrating the ubiquity of mitochondrial defects in these tissues.[18]

Screening tests for MNGIE are measurement of serum lactic acid, muscle enzymes, and thymidine phosphorylase in circulating leukocytes.[19] The last test is based on mutations identified in the gene for thymidine phosphorylase in 21 probands with MNGIE.[19]

Familial Visceral Neuropathies

FVN is a group of genetic diseases characterized by degeneration of the myenteric plexus (Table 117–3). There are at least two distinct phenotypes of FVN, types I and II,[20] and there are a number of syndromic congenital neuropathies that may be classified broadly[21] as follows:

1. *Disorders of colonization* by migrating neural crest–derived neurons, as in Hirschsprung's disease, that are related to abnormalities in the *RET* gene (the gene for tyrosine kinase) and GDNF, or the disorder of endothelin (ET)-3 and its receptor, ET-B.

2. *Disorders of differentiation* of enteric nerves, as in intestinal ganglioneuromatosis related to a specific germline point mutation in *RET* at codon 918 of exon 16 (M918T) or codon 883 (A883F) in multiple endocrine neoplasia (MEN) 2b syndrome.

3. Disorders of the survival or maintenance of enteric nerves, as in hypoganglionosis and possibly congenital achalasia, which can result from one of several mechanistic derangements of ligands (e.g., 5-HT or neurotrophin-3) and their receptors (e.g., 5-HT_{2B} and tyrosine kinase C) or transcription factors (e.g., SOX_{10}).

Disturbances in these genetic mechanisms result in syndromic dysmotilities such as Hirschsprung's disease,

Waardenburg-Shah syndrome (piebaldism, neural deafness, megacolon), MEN 2A or 2B, and idiopathic hypertrophic pyloric stenosis. Visceral neuropathy may result in bowel dilatation, although this dilatation generally is less frequent or less severe than in visceral myopathy.

Hirschsprung's disease, a relatively common condition affecting 1 in 5000 live births and causing intestinal obstruction in neonates and megacolon in infants and adults, is often associated with mutations in genes encoding ligands/receptors, such as GDNF-Ret or ET-3-ETB. Hirschsprung's disease is discussed in detail in Chapter 93.

MEN 2B is a serious congenital neuropathic condition associated with tumors of the neuroendocrine system. It presents with severe constipation or megacolon, diarrhea (when associated with enterocolitis), or obstruction, often in infancy.[22] Other external stigmata of MEN 2B are a characteristic facies with "blubbery lips" from mucosal neuromas, marfanoid habitus, medullated corneal nerve fibers, and medullary thyroid carcinoma; the last develops eventually in almost all patients. In MEN 2B, intestinal pathology shows transmural intestinal ganglioneuromatosis (i.e., massive proliferations of neural tissue such as neurons, supporting cells, and nerve fibers) that appears as thickened nerve trunks among mature nerve cells.

Other FVNs. There are a few reported families that do not fit into the two types of FVN discussed previously and that may be associated either with generalized neurologic disease or with mental retardation, calcification of basal ganglia or hypertrophy of nerve fibers, and an absence of ganglion cells.

Childhood Visceral Myopathies

CVMs have been recognized as two distinctive forms of disease (Table 117–4). These two diseases differ from FVM in their clinical manifestations and modes of inheritance. Degeneration and fibrosis of gastrointestinal and urinary smooth muscle can be detected in both types of CVM[23] and result in bowel dilatation, ureteropelvicaliectasis or megacystis.

Non-familial Visceral Myopathy (Sporadic Hollow Visceral Myopathy). The nonfamilial type of visceral myopathy is uncommon, and a careful family history must be obtained in these patients to exclude a diagnosis of FVM.

Idiopathic Non-familial Visceral Neuropathy (Sporadic Hollow Visceral Neuropathy or Chronic Idiopathic Intestinal Pseudo-obstruction)

Non-FVN, or chronic idiopathic intestinal pseudo-obstruction, typically results from myenteric plexus damage by chemicals, drugs, or viral infections. Infants, young children, and adults are affected. Delayed gastric emptying has been observed after viral gastroenteritis, which may cause permanent damage to the myenteric plexus in some patients. Debinski and associates have documented such a syndrome in association with herpes viral elements in the myenteric plexus of patients with pseudo-obstruction.[24]

Patients with non-FVN usually have disturbed motility of the entire gastrointestinal tract; the urinary tract usually is unaffected. The intestine may be dilated and shows active, nonperistaltic or incoordinated contractions on barium examination. In contrast, patients with visceral myopathies tend to have inactive dilated intestine. Histologic examination of the myenteric plexus reveals a reduction in the number or abnormal morphology of neurons that are enlarged, with thick, irregular, clubbed processes. Hypertrophy of one or both muscle layers of the muscularis propria also may be observed.

In a study of 40 patients with chronic idiopathic intestinal pseudo-obstruction, intestinal phasic pressure studies were abnormal but routine histology of the gastrointestinal tract was normal in patients whose tissue was available for analysis.[25] Slow transit of chyme through the stomach or small bowel[26] provides an objective means to noninvasively suspect dysmotility.

Secondary Causes of Small Intestinal Dysmotility

Secondary causes of small intestine dysmotility are summarized in Table 117–5 and are discussed in the following sections.

Scleroderma (Progressive Systemic Sclerosis). Intestinal pseudo-obstruction is a well-described gastrointestinal complication of scleroderma.[27,28] The small bowel is the second most frequently involved gastrointestinal organ in scleroderma, after the esophagus. Radiologic

---

Table 117–4 Classification of Childhood Visceral Myopathies

Features	Type I	Type II*
Mode of transmission	Possibly autosomal recessive	Possibly autosomal recessive
Gross abnormalities	Dilatation of entire gastrointestinal tract	Short, malrotated small intestine and malfixation of microcolon
Histology	Degeneration and fibrosis of gastrointestinal and urinary smooth muscle cells	Vacuolar degeneration of gastrointestinal and urinary smooth muscle cells
Clinical manifestations		
Age of onset	Infancy and young childhood	Infancy
Gender	Both male and female	Predominantly female
Symptoms of CIP	Constipation, distention with or without CIP	Obstipation, intestinal pseudo-obstruction
Extragastrointestinal features	Megacystis and megaureter	Megacystis and megaureter
Treatment, prognosis	No effective treatment; prognosis poor	No effective treatment; prognosis poor

*Megacystis-microcolon-intestinal hypoperistalsis.
CIP, chronic intestinal pseudo-obstruction.

Table 117–5   Manifestations of Gastrointestinal Dysmotility in Systemic Diseases

Disease	Gastrointestinal Manifestations					
	Pharynx	**Esophagus**	**Stomach**	**Small Intestine**	**Colon**	**Anorectum**
Collagen vascular						
Scleroderma	—	Dilatation, aperistalsis of lower 2/3, incompetent LES	Gastroparesis	Dilatation with narrowed valvulae conniventes, PCI	Dilatation; loss of haustra, PCI, wide-mouthed diverticula	Reduced IAS tone
Dermatomyositis/ polymyositis	Decreased UES tone, aspiration	Dilatation, dysmotility of proximal portion	Gastroparesis rarely	Megaduodenum, distal dilatation rarer	Dilatation	—
SLE	—	Aperistalsis	—	—	Dilatation, ischemia	—
Mixed CTD	—	Dilatation, lower 2/3, aperistalsis	Not involved	Megaduodenum	Diverticula	—
Neuromuscular						
Diabetic neuropathy	Decreased peristalsis	Decreased peristalsis, normal LES	Dilatation, gastroparesis	Delayed, normal, or rapid transit	Dilatation	Decreased sensation, low IAS pressure, low EAS pressure
Parkinsonism	Impaired peristalsis	Diffuse spasm, dilatation, aperistalsis	Gastroparesis	Dilatation	Dilatation, sigmoid volvulus	—
Spinal cord injury	—	—	Gastroparesis infrequently	Increased gas	Delayed transit, left-sided colon dysfunction	Pelvic floor dysfunction; decreased sensation, IAS, EAS
Neurofibromatosis	—	—	Gastroparesis infrequently	Dilatation	Dilatation	—
Paraneoplastic neuropathy	—	Aperistalsis, achalasia	Gastroparesis	Dilatation, dysmotility	Dilatation, constipation	—
Myotonic dystrophy	Decreased peristalsis, low UES tone	Decreased peristalsis, dilatation	Gastroparesis, dilatation	Dilatation	Dilatation	EAS dysfunction
Duchenne dystrophy	Decreased peristalsis	Dilatation	Dilatation, rare gastroparesis	Dilatation	Dilatation	—
Amyloidosis	—	Aperistalsis, incomplete LES relaxation	Gastroparesis	Dilatation	Dilatation	—
Infections						
Chagas' disease	—	Dilatation, aperistalsis, incomplete LES relaxation	Dilatation	Proximal dilatation	Dilatation	Low IAS
Endocrine						
Hypothyroidism	—	—	Gastroparesis	—	Constipation	—
Hypoparathyroidism	—	—	Gastroparesis	—	Constipation	—

CTD, connective tissue disease; EAS, external anal sphincter; IAS, internal anal sphincter; LES, lower esophageal sphincter; PCI, pneumatosis cystoides intestinalis; SLE, systemic lupus erythematosus; UES, upper esophageal sphincter.

evidence of gastric sclerosis, intestinal sclerosis, or both occurs in 40% of scleroderma patients. Barium examination reveals dilatation of the duodenum and jejunum, delayed barium transit, and narrow, tightly packed valvulae conniventes, despite bowel dilatation, producing an accordion-like appearance.[27] Wide-necked diverticula may be seen but are more frequent in the colon. An uncommon and potentially serious finding is pneumatosis cystoides intestinalis, which usually signifies a poor prognosis.

Degeneration of smooth muscle and its replacement by collagen is responsible for the small bowel dysmotility in scleroderma. The circular muscle is involved more often than is the longitudinal muscle layer.[27,29] The submucosal and myenteric plexuses appear normal by hematoxylin and eosin staining and on silver stains, but studies with more specialized stains have not been reported. Small bowel dysmotility leads to bacterial overgrowth, resulting in steatorrhea, malabsorption, and weight loss.

Disturbances of small bowel motility[30,31] and transit[32] result in delayed gastric emptying, small bowel transit, or both. There is absence of the interdigestive migrating motor complex (MMC), low-amplitude clusters of propagated and nonpropagated contractions (<10 mm Hg fasting and postprandially),[33] abnormally prolonged MMC cycle, diminished activity of phase III, hypomotility of the fed pattern,[31] and antral hypomotility (characterized by low-amplitude contractions, typically <40 mm Hg). Gastric emptying may be delayed by resistance to flow in the dilated, hypomotile small intestine, even if the stomach itself is unaffected. Patients with scleroderma but without gastrointestinal involvement demonstrate normal small bowel manometry[33] and normal small bowel transit time.

Oral erythromycin was effective in short-term studies that evaluated gastric emptying and symptoms in an open-label study of scleroderma patients.[34] Octreotide, a long-acting somatostatin analog, induces phase III activity and may reduce bacterial overgrowth and symptoms.[30] Octreotide should be used at least 2 hours after the last meal of the day to induce an MMC and potentially clear residue and bacterial overgrowth into the colon.

Dermatomyositis and Polymyositis. The gastrointestinal tract is involved in one half of patients with these diseases. Esophageal involvement causes dysphagia, which often is a presenting symptom, but weakness and atrophy of skeletal muscles and an associated skin rash typically are present. Megaduodenum and delayed intestinal transit of barium are prominent features. Autopsy findings have shown atrophy and fibrosis of intestinal smooth muscle, suggesting a visceral myopathy.

Systemic Lupus Erythematosus. Abdominal pain is the most common gastrointestinal symptom in systemic lupus erythematosus (SLE), occurring in 10% to 20% of patients. Autopsy studies disclose a 60% to 70% prevalence of previous peritoneal inflammation, but documented cases of serositis as the sole cause of abdominal pain are rare. *Lupus enteritis* is the term used to describe bowel changes from SLE-induced vasculitis of small blood vessels, which in turn causes ischemia and leads to intestinal mucosal ulceration, edema, and hemorrhage. Smooth muscle dysfunction secondary to ischemia results in dysfunction and results in dilatation of the small bowel and ileus. In severe cases, there is necrosis of the bowel wall with perforation or infarction.

Diagnosis of SLE enteritis is made radiologically. Small bowel changes include dilatation, coarsened folds, and thumbprinting secondary to submucosal edema and hemorrhage. Diarrhea occurs in 5% to 10% of SLE patients. Unusual intestinal manifestations can cause diagnostic difficulties, for example, SLE may simulate Crohn's ileitis or cause a severe protein-losing enteropathy in association with vasculitis and basement membrane thickening seen on full-thickness jejunal biopsy. In a series of five patients with SLE, intestinal hypomotility associated with reduced bladder capacity and bilateral ureteral distention was found in four patients, and aperistalsis of the esophagus in three patients. Treatment, which consisted of high-dose glucocorticoids, parenteral nutrition, promotility agents, and antibiotics, led to remission of both CIP and urinary abnormalities in all cases. Antroduodenal manometry performed in two patients after remission showed increased intestinal motility. One patient died, and postmortem examination showed intestinal vasculitis.[35]

Mixed Connective Tissue Disease. Mixed connective tissue disease is a clinical entity characterized by overlapping features of scleroderma, polymyositis, and rheumatoid arthritis with antinuclear antibody against ribonucleoprotein. The extent of gastrointestinal involvement is unknown but esophageal involvement is most common. Duodenal and jejunal dilatation are seen radiologically, and pneumatosis cystoides intestinalis may complicate severe disease.[36]

Diabetes Mellitus. Many diabetics experience diarrhea, which has a variety of causes (e.g., bacterial overgrowth, pancreatic exocrine insufficiency, bile salt malabsorption, impaired absorption or secretion). Early radiologic studies of the small bowel demonstrated variable findings, including normal, delayed, or rapid transit. Similarly discrepant results are found using the hydrogen breath test, and there is a poor correlation of rapid transit (based on hydrogen breath testing) with diarrhea. The small bowel may be affected in patients presenting with the gastroparesis syndrome, and this involvement can be detected by manometry,[37] prolonged transit,[32] or, rarely, by dilated intestine.

Demyelination of the proximal vagus nerve and sympathetic nerves supplying the bowel occurs in diabetes. The intrinsic nervous system of the gut appears to be unaffected, because no morphologic abnormalities of the myenteric or submucosal plexuses have been observed; however, studies in animal models and a single case report of a patient requiring pancreas-renal transplant showed degeneration of the ICC.[38] Although thickening of the small bowel muscle layers and eosinophilic hyaline bodies in smooth muscle cells have been observed,[39] most authorities believe that myopathy is not a cause of gastrointestinal dysmotility in patients with diabetes.

Motility studies of the small bowel in patients with diabetes have shown mixed results. Normal MMCs are found in many patients with documented gastroparesis. Abnormalities that have been demonstrated include absence of intestinal phase III, MMCs originating in the distal duodenum or jejunum, and incoordinated bursts of nonpropagated contractions (Fig. 117-3).[37] The clinical relevance of these abnormal findings is uncertain. In one study, there was no correlation between abnormal transit time and manometric abnormalities. Hyperglycemia, which can delay gastric emptying, induces intestinal phase III-like activity and alters orocecal transit time even in healthy subjects; however, the relevance of these findings to diabetic bowel dysmotility is not clear. Among community diabetics, constipation and use of laxatives are significantly more common than in age- and gender-matched controls.[40,41] Constipation is probably multifactorial in diabetes, as it is in nondiabetic patients[42]; acute

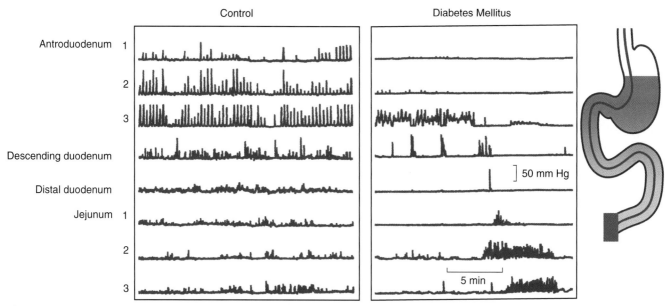

Figure 117–3   Gastroduodenal motility in health and in diabetes mellitus. These postprandial tracings show normal-amplitude, irregular contractility in a healthy control and a paucity of antral contractions, tonic contractions at the pylorus (3rd tracing), and development of a fasting-like migrating motor complex pattern in the small intestine in a patient with diabetes mellitus. These features are suggestive of a neuropathic disorder. (Adapted from Camilleri M: Medical treatment of chronic intestinal pseudo-obstruction. Pract Gastroenterol 15:10, 1991.)

hyperglycemia does not significantly affect colonic motor function or tone.

Parkinson's Disease. Symptoms of gastrointestinal dysmotility are common in patients with Parkinson's disease. High dysphagia, nausea, bloating, constipation, and difficulty with evacuation of stool occur frequently.[43] Dilatation of the small bowel may be seen radiologically.[44] Small bowel dysmotility does occur; however, its frequency is not known. Manometric studies in patients with Parkinson's disease reveal infrequent or even absent MMCs, hypomotility in the fed state, and an increased incidence of retrograde and tonic contractions compared with controls.[45] The contribution of these abnormalities to symptoms is not clear.

The pathogenesis of small bowel dysmotility is unknown in Parkinson's disease. Lewy bodies, which are neurons containing cytoplasmic hyaline inclusions, originally were identified in the brain and are highly characteristic of Parkinson's disease; they have not been reported in the small bowel, although they have been found in the myenteric plexus of the esophagus and colon in patients with dysphagia and megacolon.[46] Dopaminergic neurons are reported to be deficient in colons of patients with parkinsonism and constipation.[47]

Therapy for patients with Parkinson's disease includes drugs that adversely affect gut motility such as dopamine agonists and anticholinergics. Symptoms are as common in untreated as in treated patients, however, suggesting that the disease itself is the primary factor producing dysmotility and resultant symptoms.[43]

Spinal Cord Injury. Extrinsic denervation of the small bowel by spinal cord injury usually produces only mild and probably insignificant small intestinal dysmotility.

The only changes revealed in manometric studies performed in a group of patients with spinal cord injury were a greater number of phase III contractions beginning in the duodenum rather than in the antrum in patients with high spinal cord lesions.[48] Patients with injury to the lower spinal cord demonstrated no abnormal findings consistent with preservation of bowel innervation from the vagus and third thoracic sympathetic levels. One report described a woman with cervical spinal stenosis and paraplegia who displayed normal MMCs but a twofold to threefold prolonged interval between MMCs.

Immediately after spinal cord injury, a state of spinal shock develops, characterized by complete loss of all sensory, motor, and reflex function below the level of injury. Paralytic ileus with abdominal distention follows and usually resolves in a few days. In the long term, postprandial abdominal distention and discomfort occur in more than 40% of patients with spinal cord injury, symptoms that likely are due to constipation. Many stable spinal cord injury patients exhibit increased amounts of gas in the small and large intestine on routine abdominal plain films. Colonic dysmotility is well recognized and is responsible for the common problems of constipation and difficulty with evacuation in these patients.[49] Spinal cord injury decreases colonic motility; although the postprandial colonic response is present, it is suboptimal and confined to the descending colon.[50] In patients with spinal cord injury, rectal compliance and resting anal sphincter pressures are lower than normal values, and ramp rectal inflation demonstrates patterns of sphincter activity similar to that recorded in the patients' cystometrograms. There was no definite relationship of bowel function to the findings on anorectal manometry in these patients. Rehabilitation goals include continence of stool, simple willful independent defecation, and prevention of gastrointestinal complications. Individualized, person-centered bowel care includes diet, laxatives, enemas, suppositories, and scheduling of bowel care to initiate defecation and accomplish fecal evacuation. Digital-rectal stimulation is a technique used during bowel care to open the anal sphincter and facilitate reflex peristalsis.[51]

Neurofibromatosis (von Recklinghausen Disease). Gastrointestinal neurofibromas are most commonly found in the small intestine. They are reported to occur in up to 10% of patients with neurofibromatosis, but their true incidence is probably underestimated because they generally are asymptomatic. Small bowel neurofibromas may be single or multiple and are found most frequently in the ileum. These tumors are submucosal and may become quite large and extend to the serosa. Their presence usually is established by a small bowel series. Mucosal ulceration can cause acute or chronic bleeding. Mechanical small bowel obstruction or intussusception requires exploratory surgery.

CIP has been described in one patient with neurofibromatosis. Small bowel manometry was abnormal, and small bowel transit was markedly delayed.[26] Pathologic studies of the nerves and muscles in the small bowel are lacking in this disease. In the colon, neurogenic changes consisting of nerve fiber proliferation in the myenteric and submucosal plexuses were found in a patient with megacolon.[52]

Paraneoplastic Visceral Neuropathy. CIP has been reported in association with small cell carcinoma of the lung,[53-56] and carcinoid tumors.[57,58] This phenomenon represents a paraneoplastic syndrome caused by visceral neuropathy. The small bowel, like the colon, shows widespread neuronal and axonal degeneration of the myenteric and submucosal plexuses. There also is mononuclear cell infiltration and Schwann cell proliferation.[55] There are no metastases to the bowel in this syndrome. These patients often have antineuronal nuclear (anti-Hu) antibodies that can now be detected by an immunofluorescence-based assay. The antibody is postulated to be directed toward an epitope that is shared between the neuronal elements within the ENS and the underlying malignancy.[55] Among patients with neurologic manifestations associated with small cell lung cancer and antineuronal nuclear antibodies, 12% had gastrointestinal disturbances, such as achalasia, gastroparesis, and CIP.

Pseudo-obstruction symptoms are the presenting features in patients with visceral neuropathy and small cell carcinoma. The lung cancer usually is occult, is missed on chest film, and often is found at autopsy or by chest computed tomography (CT) and mediastinoscopy. The small bowel usually is not dilated on radiologic studies, but there is some delay of barium passage through the small bowel. Small bowel manometry shows features suggestive of neuropathy, such as bursts of intestinal contractions that are poorly coordinated or propagated.[54,55] In older patients with intestinal pseudo-obstruction or feeding intolerance of unknown cause and recent onset, a malignancy, especially small cell carcinoma of lung,

must be suspected. A screening blood test using antineuronal enteric antibody or anti-Hu, has high specificity.[55] If positive, a CT scan of the chest and mediastinoscopy may be necessary to confirm the diagnosis. Histopathology of the bowel demonstrates an inflammatory infiltrate of the myenteric plexus, typically composed of CD4+ and CD8+ T lymphocytes.[59]

Myotonic Muscular Dystrophy. Myotonic muscular dystrophy is a slowly progressive disease characterized by myotonia or difficulty in muscle relaxation. In addition to muscle wasting, affected patients often have a nasal voice as a result of pharyngeal and palatal weakness, early onset of cataracts, and cardiac conduction defects. Dysphagia is the most common gastrointestinal symptom and results from esophageal involvement. Diarrhea and abdominal cramping occur in up to one third of those affected. Malabsorption and steatorrhea have been reported in a few cases. Constipation also is frequent and can alternate with diarrhea. Intestinal pseudo-obstruction is rare. The small bowel may demonstrate abnormal but nonspecific radiologic changes including dilatation, diminished motility, and delayed transit of barium.[60]

Dysmotility of the small intestine may play a significant role in the production of intestinal symptoms. In a group of 10 patients with myotonic muscular dystrophy who had symptoms of intestinal dysmotility but normal small bowel contrast examinations, abnormal small bowel motility was found in all. Manometric findings included low-amplitude contractions in fasting and fed states, retrograde propagation of MMC phase III, interruption of phase III, and increased incidence of tonic contractions.[61] Spontaneous pneumoperitoneum, megacolon, and low-amplitude small bowel contractions also have been documented. In one patient with chronic pseudo-obstruction and a dilated small bowel, manometry revealed an increased maximal rate of low-amplitude duodenal contractions.

Histologically, small intestine smooth muscle discloses changes similar to those found in dystrophic skeletal muscle, including cells that are swollen, partially destroyed, decreased in size, and replaced by fat. Using a silver stain, degenerative changes of the myenteric plexus of the colon were found in a patient with megacolon,[62] indicating that intestinal dysmotility may be caused by smooth muscle as well as enteric nerve dysfunction. In most patients with myotonic muscular dystrophy, the predominant cause of dysmotility appears to be smooth muscle damage.

Duchenne Muscular Dystrophy. Duchenne muscular dystrophy is a severe, pseudohypertrophic muscular dystrophy that has an X-linked recessive pattern and affects boys early in childhood. Skeletal and cardiac fibers are infiltrated and eventually replaced by connective tissue and fat; smooth muscle of the gastrointestinal tract is involved similarly. Histologic changes consist of degeneration and atrophy of smooth muscle fibers and separation of fibers by connective tissue.[63] The myenteric plexus is not involved.

Despite typical dystrophic changes in the small bowel in most postmortem specimens, gastrointestinal symptoms usually are related to dysmotility of the esophagus and stomach, which are more severely affected than is the small bowel. Dysphagia is the predominant symptom (36% in one series), followed less often by vomiting, diarrhea, and constipation.[63] Orocecal transit time is normal in asymptomatic subjects; however, severe bowel dysmotility can occur. Episodes of acute intestinal pseudo-obstruction, manifested by abdominal distention, persistent vomiting, and gastric or small bowel dilatation, can be life threatening.[64] CIP also has been reported in Duchenne dystrophy.[65] Nitrergic innervation (nitric oxide–containing nerves) of the gut is deficient in an animal model of Duchenne dystrophy, suggesting that there is deficiency in the ability to relax muscle; in fact, the tone of the stomach is increased under basal conditions.

Amyloidosis. Amyloid protein is deposited in the small bowel in all forms of amyloidosis: primary, secondary, myeloma-associated, and familial or hereditary forms. The severity of dysmotility is related to the amount and distribution of amyloid deposited. In all forms, amyloid is deposited in blood vessel walls, leading to ischemic ulcers, infarction, and occasionally perforation.

Gastrointestinal disease is present in as many as 60% of patients with reactive or secondary (AA) amyloidosis.[66] The most common disease causes of reactive amyloidosis are chronic degenerative arthropathies, particularly rheumatoid arthritis (which accounts for ≈50% of cases) and less often ankylosing spondylitis and psoriatic arthritis. Gastrointestinal involvement appears to be less common in AL amyloidosis, with biopsy-diagnosed and clinically apparent disease occurring in only 8% and 1%, respectively, of 769 patients in a retrospective review from the Mayo Clinic.[67] Hepatic involvement is much more common, being seen in as many as 70% of patients.

Neuromuscular infiltration initially affects the intrinsic nervous system and results in a neuropathic process[68] that is characterized by uncoordinated contractions of normal amplitude.[69] At a later stage, tissue wall infiltration results in a myopathic process with low-amplitude contractions that typically are associated with significantly prolonged transit as in other systemic disorders such as scleroderma.

Neuropathic and myopathic variants of amyloid have been demonstrated pathologically and may be related in part to the type of amyloid fibrils.[70] One report, for example, evaluated 16 patients with amyloidosis and intestinal pseudo-obstruction (13 with AA, 2 with AL, and 1 with dialysis-related amyloidosis).[70] Inexplicably, the patients with AA amyloidosis tended to have amyloid deposits in the myenteric plexus without appreciable muscle infiltration, whereas the other patients had diffuse and extensive infiltration and replacement of the muscularis propria throughout the gastrointestinal tract. In primary and myeloma-associated forms of amyloidosis, the muscle layers of the small bowel are affected more severely than is the mucosa, resulting in dysmotility. In the secondary and hereditary forms, the mucosa is involved predominantly, resulting in malabsorption. Amyloid deposits are found infrequently in the myenteric plexus, although in hereditary forms, familial amyloidosis neuropathy may result from deposition in the major nerve trunks supplying the bowel.[71]

Gastrointestinal symptoms in amyloidosis include diarrhea, constipation (which often is present for years and then is followed by diarrhea), malabsorption, and pseudo-obstruction. Diarrhea can occur without malabsorption and may improve with antibiotic therapy.[72] Radiologically, there is coarsening of the small bowel mucosal pattern, dilatation, and diminished motility with prolonged transit of barium.[73] These changes are nonspecific and can resemble those of scleroderma.

In a group of patients with amyloidosis of various types, orocecal transit time was prolonged to more than twice that of controls. With heavy infiltration of the small bowel muscle layers, acute intestinal pseudo-obstruction may occur and is a serious and often fatal complication.[74]

Chagas' Disease. Chronic infection with *Trypanosoma cruzi* leads to destruction of the submucosal and myenteric plexuses along the entire length of the gastrointestinal tract. Megacolon and megaesophagus are the most common presentations, although the small bowel may be similarly affected with megaduodenum and megajejunum. Small intestine manometric studies in these patients demonstrate normal frequency of the MMC, but the velocity of propagation of the activity front is slowed significantly, to about one half that of normal.[75] Patients with small bowel involvement may be asymptomatic despite significant neuronal destruction. Diarrhea, constipation, or intestinal pseudo-obstruction can occur. The early phase of gastric emptying of liquids is abnormally rapid in Chagas' disease patients with megaduodenum, which suggests that increased duodenal receptivity may have a significant effect on the gastroduodenal transfer of liquids.[76]

Thyroid Disease. Thyroid dysfunction may present primarily as gastrointestinal disease with a variety of disparate symptoms depending on whether the patient is hyperthyroid or hypothyroid.[77,78] Intestinal dysmotility (associated with change in the frequency of the slow wave oscillations of smooth muscle electrical potential) results from the altered thyroid state and has been considered to be the cause of symptoms. Thus, in the duodenum, slow wave frequencies are increased in hyperthyroid patients and decreased in hypothyroid patients. These abnormalities return to normal after correction of the thyroid dysfunction.

Hyperthyroidism. Early radiologic studies using the crude barium meal test reported both rapid gastric emptying and rapid small bowel transit in hyperthyroidism. Later studies using the hydrogen breath test confirmed a rapid orocecal transit time; this is, however, a consequence of accelerated small bowel transit, because the rate of gastric emptying actually is normal.[77,79,80] Hyperthyroid patients may present with diarrhea and mild malabsorption[77,78]; more than 25% of hyperthyroid patients excrete more than 7 g of fat in their stool daily. Malabsorption apparently is caused by decreased contact time of luminal contents with small bowel mucosa as a result of rapid transit; this abnormality improves after correction of the hyperthyroid state.

Hypothyroidism. Gastric emptying time is delayed significantly in hypothyroidism[81] In contrast to hyperthyroidism, small bowel transit is slowed significantly in patients with hypothyroidism.[77] With adequate hormone replacement, transit may be normalized. Many hypothyroid patients develop constipation, which probably results from colonic dysmotility. A manometric study in one patient revealed decreased amplitude of small bowel contractions and an overall decreased motility index.[82] With severe hypothyroidism (i.e., myxedema), paralytic ileus and intestinal pseudo-obstruction can occur.

Hypoparathyroidism. The mechanism by which parathyroid hormone affects gastrointestinal motility is not known; however, calcium is essential for smooth muscle contraction, and hypocalcemia may impair gut contractile activity. Intestinal pseudo-obstruction and malabsorption have been reported with small bowel dysmotility in hypoparathyroid subjects. Barium studies reveal dilated loops of small bowel and prolonged transit time such patients. Symptoms improve with calcium administration.

Drug-Induced Changes in Motility of the Small Intestine. Many drugs profoundly affect gastrointestinal motility. Although the colon usually is recognized as the main target organ for drug-induced dysmotility, the small bowel is also affected frequently. Phenothiazines and some antiparkinsonian drugs decrease colonic and small bowel motility and can cause constipation, colonic pseudo-obstruction, and adynamic ileus. Tricyclic antidepressants in particular are noted for causing ileus. The anticholinergic agents atropine and scopolamine and related belladonna alkaloids decrease intestinal tone as well as the amplitude and frequency of peristaltic contractions.

Opiate analgesics are well known to suppress motility throughout the gastrointestinal tract, particularly the colon. Morphine enhances the amplitude of nonpropulsive small bowel contractions and markedly decreases propulsive contractions by its effects on μ-opiate receptors on intestinal muscle cells. The duodenum and the jejunum are more prone to these effects than is the ileum. The net effect is delayed small bowel transit. Morphine and nalbuphine significantly delay small bowel transit compared with placebo.

Calcium channel antagonists, especially verapamil, cause constipation in up to 20% of patients. Small bowel transit time in subjects taking verapamil was unchanged from pretreatment values; however, transit through the colon was slowed, an effect that likely accounts for the constipation seen with this drug.

Clonidine, an α$_2$-adrenergic agent used as an antihypertensive, prolongs orocecal transit of liquids. A comprehensive dose-response study of the transit of solids, however, did not show any significant effects on gastric small bowel or colonic transit in healthy individuals or in patients with diarrhea-predominant irritable bowel syndrome when treated with this drug.

Octreotide is a long-acting synthetic analog of somatostatin. In normal individuals, it increases the frequency of MMCs by shortening the duration of phase II. It was shown to be useful in the short term in a small group of scleroderma patients with pseudo-obstruction by inducing phase III contractions and possibly reducing small bowel bacterial overgrowth.[30] When given after a meal, intravenous somatostatin interrupts the fed pattern of motility and induces bursts of propagated activity similar to phase III in health and disease. Octreotide retards small bowel transit in health when given prior to meals.

Celiac Sprue. Intestinal pseudo-obstruction occurs in association with celiac sprue, but the mechanism is unclear.[83] Dilated small bowel loops with delayed passage of barium are observed radiologically. In one patient who underwent exploratory laparotomy with full-thickness jejunal biopsy, the nerves and muscle coats appeared normal on both light and electron microscopy.[83] Parenteral nutrition may be required during prolonged pseudo-obstruction.

Jejunal Diverticulosis. Diverticula can occur anywhere in the small intestine, but they are most common in the jejunum. Like their counterparts in the colon, they represent herniations through the mesenteric side of the bowel and usually are acquired. Jejunal diverticulosis is associated with many diseases, including scleroderma, celiac sprue, Fabry's disease, FVM-II (mitochondrial cytopathy), and Cronkhite-Canada syndrome. Patients present with diarrhea, steatorrhea, weight loss, and megaloblastic anemia, most commonly from bacterial overgrowth. CIP occurs in jejunal diverticulosis and can mimic mechanical obstruction.[28] Abnormal myenteric plexuses have been described with silver staining, but it is unclear whether they are a cause or effect of the diverticulosis.

Radiation Injury. Ionizing radiation damages all structures of the small intestine, including the mucosa, blood vessels, connective tissue, enteric nerves, and smooth muscle. Radiation damage to the bowel can be separated into acute and chronic injury. The threshold radiation dose to induce inflammation or pseudo-obstruction is unclear.

Acute Injury. Above a certain threshold dose of radiation to the abdomen, nausea, vomiting, abdominal pain, and diarrhea are common. These symptoms abate soon after exposure is discontinued. Reversible changes in small bowel absorptive function have been considered as the main cause of diarrhea in these patients. Small bowel dysmotility may play a significant role in acute radiation enteropathy. Decreased intestinal motility, particularly in the distal small bowel, with both fasting and feeding, may persist up to 1 month after the last exposure to radiation.[84,85]

Motility studies in humans in the acute phase of radiation sickness have not been performed, but one study demonstrated accelerated small bowel transit in a group of patients undergoing abdominopelvic irradiation compared with their pretreatment values[86]; more than 75% of the patients exhibited diarrhea during treatment.

Chronic Injury. Delayed gastrointestinal complications may occur months, years, or even decades after radiation exposure. Both neuronal and muscular structures of the small bowel are affected in these patients, and the resulting dysmotility leads to bacterial overgrowth, diarrhea, and malabsorption. Edema, atrophy, and fibrosis of smooth muscle fibers are characteristic histologic findings.[87] The myenteric plexus can appear normal on routine staining; however, proliferation of submucosal neurons with extension into the circular muscle coat has been observed.[87]

Gastrointestinal symptoms from previous radiation damage have been attributed to altered gut motility. Recurrent episodes of intestinal pseudo-obstruction have been observed many years after received abdominal radiation and is associated with malnutrition.[87] On gastrointestinal manometry, failure of a liquid-solid meal to induce postprandial motility, and delayed initiation and reduced intensity of MMCs during nocturnal fasting were observed.[88] Small bowel contrast studies show dilated loops of bowel with air-fluid levels and thickened bowel wall. Manometric evaluation in one patient revealed normal MMCs in the proximal duodenum, decreased amplitude and frequency of contractions in the distal duodenum, and absence of peristaltic contractions in the jejunum. Subsequent histologic examination of the bowel suggested smooth muscle damage as the cause of dysmotility.[87]

Diffuse Lymphoid Infiltration. Four cases of CIP in association with diffuse lymphoid infiltration of the small bowel have been described.[89] All four patients were women who presented with diarrhea at an early age. Histology revealed lymphocytic infiltration of the lamina propria, muscularis propria, and myenteric plexus. The infiltrates were demonstrated to be polyclonal by immunochemical stains, reflecting a pseudolymphoma rather than a true neoplasm. The myenteric plexus appeared normal with routine and silver stains. An absence of smooth muscle cells was found in areas of lymphoid infiltration.

Idiopathic Myenteric Ganglionitis. Ganglionitis refers to a marked lymphoplasmacellular infiltrate in the myenteric plexus,[90] which may be associated with paraneoplastic (lung cancer, ganglioneuroblastoma),[91] infectious (e.g., herpes), or neurologic disorders; some cases appear to be idiopathic. Histologic examination of colonic and ileum specimens reveal prominent lymphoplasmacellular (CD4$^+$ and CD8$^+$ T lymphocytes) infiltration within the myenteric plexus, a marked decrease in a wide array of neuronal peptides/transmitters, and marked myenteric neuron damage. Other cases have shown that the infiltrate was eosinophil-predominant. Neurons in the myenteric ganglia expressed the potent eosinophil chemoattractant interleukin 5. Some patients responded symptomatically to systemic glucocorticoid therapy.[92]

Jejunoileal Bypass. Recurrent episodes of intestinal pseudo-obstruction can occur in patients after jejunoileal bypass for morbid obesity. Plain films reveal massively dilated small bowel loops and occasional pneumatosis cystoides intestinalis. Bacterial overgrowth of the bypassed small intestine causes this enteropathy; small bowel cultures typically grow fecal flora and anaerobes similar to those described in blind-loop syndrome.

Anorexia Nervosa and Bulimia. Delayed gastric emptying of solids and orocecal transit time are well-established abnormalities in patients with anorexia or bulimia.[93] Whole-gut transit time, measured by radiopaque markers, is also significantly delayed, especially in anorexia, compared with controls.[93] Electrolyte abnormalities (e.g., hypokalemia) may occur secondary to nutritional deficiencies or concomitant diuretic abuse. Typically, the motility disorder is less significant than the underlying psychological and nutritional manifestations of the disease.

CLINICAL FEATURES

With a few exceptions, most patients with small intestine dysmotility have similar clinical manifestations regardless of the underlying causes for the dysmotility. The spectrum of clinical manifestations varies widely, but there are features that typify neuropathic and myopathic intestinal dysmotility (Table 117-6).

Patients may have recurrent symptoms of postprandial cramping, periumbilical, and epigastric abdominal pains; abdominal bloating; easy satiety; anorexia; weight loss; nausea; and vomiting. Symptoms usually are aggravated by eating. Diarrhea can occur in patients with bacterial overgrowth and malabsorption. In severe cases, patients have recurrent episodes of abdominal pain, vomiting, and distention, a "pseudo-obstruction syndrome" that mimics mechanical obstruction.

Plain abdominal films of patients with intestinal pseudo-obstruction during exacerbation show multiple air-fluid levels and dilatation of the small intestine. The prevalence and severity of recurrent obstructive episodes vary from patient to patient and from episode to episode in the same patient. Some patients have episodes that are not associated with bowel dilatation or air-fluid levels; such presentations are more likely in neuropathic

Table 117-6 Typical Features of Neuropathic and Myopathic Small Intestinal Dysmotility

Feature	Neuropathic Dysmotility	Myopathic Dysmotility
Symptoms	Early satiety, bloating, constipation	Early satiety, bloating, constipation, diarrhea
Bowel sounds	Hyperactive, high-pitched	Inactive, infrequent
Intestinal dilatation	±	+++
Diverticulosis and bacterial overgrowth	±	++
Autonomic features	++	Absent
Contraction amplitude	Normal	Low (<10 mm Hg)
Response to prokinetic agents	++	±
Need for enteral or parenteral nutrition	±	+++
Consider isolated small bowel transplant	±	++

Key: +, often; ++, more often; +++, most often; ±, maybe.

pseudo-obstruction. Dilatation and bacterial overgrowth are more common in myopathic diseases.

Findings on physical examination vary according to the severity of symptoms. The patients may be cachectic and malnourished because they are unable to take in adequate nutrients or because they have malabsorption from bacterial overgrowth in the small intestine. The abdomen may be distended and mildly tender. Bowel sounds are inactive and infrequent in patients with smooth muscle dysfunction but are hyperactive and high-pitched in patients with neuropathic dysfunction. Borborygmi may be detected in some patients. In less symptomatic patients, abdominal examination may be normal. In patients with CIP, during an obstructive episode, abdominal examination may be indistinguishable from that with a true mechanical obstruction.

Symptoms of dysmotility of other parts of the gastrointestinal tract or other organs may occur as well, depending on their underlying diseases. Megacystis and megaureters are commonly seen in FVM-I and CVM; these patients may have urinary retention and infection. Mydriasis, ptosis, and external ophthalmoplegia may be seen in patients with certain forms of FVM (e.g. mitochondrial cytopathy). Ataxia, dysautonomia, and neurologic symptoms may be seen in patients with certain forms of visceral neuropathies.

In the secondary forms of small intestine dysmotility, patients may also have systemic manifestations of the underlying disease (e.g., scleroderma, muscular dystrophies, autonomic neuropathy). These are important clinical clues in patients in whom the underlying disease has not yet been diagnosed. A careful systems review is essential to diagnose or exclude problems in the skin, eyes, joints, and autonomic nervous system (questions regarding vision in response to bright lights, postural dizziness, sweating, bladder and sexual function).

COMPLICATIONS

Malnutrition

Malnutrition occurs in patients with severe dysmotility of the small intestine as a result of inadequate intake of food (often secondary to pain) and vomiting. The patients may be anemic due to iron, folate, and vitamin B_{12} deficiency. Serum cholesterol, calcium, and albumin levels may be low typically in patients with malabsorption secondary to bacterial overgrowth. In severe cases, particularly in patients with familial or sporadic forms of hollow visceral myopathy, long-term parenteral nutrition may be the only method to provide adequate nutrients.

Small Intestinal Bacterial Overgrowth

Bacterial overgrowth in the small intestine (see Chapter 99) may complicate severe intestinal (typically myopathic) dysmotility.[94] These patients have malabsorption and steatorrhea, which causes additional weight loss, and the small intestine usually is dilated and atonic. The diagnosis can be made by culturing an intestinal aspirate for both aerobic and anaerobic bacteria. Many different

species can be found, and the total concentration of bacteria generally exceeds 10^5 colony-forming units (cfu) aerobic organisms/mL or 10^3 cfu anaerobic organisms per milliliter. Another approach to diagnosing bacterial overgrowth is the timed analysis of excretion in the breath of volatile metabolites produced by intraluminal bacteria. Measurement of expired labeled $^{14}CO_2$ after oral administration of ^{14}C-labeled substrates (e.g., D-xylose) and of breath hydrogen after administration of nonlabeled substrates both have been used for this purpose. In the presence of myopathic dysmotility, the ^{14}C-D-xylose breath test may be less accurate than culture of duodenal aspirates.[95] The patients may have macrocytic anemia caused by vitamin B_{12} deficiency, and typically they have elevated serum levels of folate. Tetracycline, metronidazole, ciprofloxacin, or rifaximin can be used for 7 to 10 days intermittently to treat patients with intestinal bacterial overgrowth, depending on the frequency of recurrence of diarrhea. In some cases, an antibiotic may need to be given for 1 week of every 3 to 4 weeks. Abdominal bloating may improve with antibiotics in some patients.

Pneumatosis Cystoides Intestinalis

Pneumatosis cystoides intestinalis (see Chapter 121) is a rare condition characterized by multiple, gas-filled cysts in the wall of the small and large intestine. Pneumoperitoneum may occur. Pneumatosis cystoides intestinalis can occur in some patients with small intestine dysmotility and dilatation. In most cases, this condition is an incidental finding on plain films. The pathogenesis is not known, and there is no specific treatment for this condition, although supplemental oxygen by nares or mask may help resolve the cysts. Surgery should be avoided unless there is a complication such as intestinal obstruction, because it usually causes deterioration of the patient's condition.

DIAGNOSIS

Diagnostic approaches for patients with small intestine dysmotility are outlined in Table 117–7.

Laboratory Tests

A complete blood count may reveal anemia and macrocytosis as a result of malnutrition and bacterial overgrowth. Blood chemistries also reflect malnutrition and malabsorption. Diabetic patients have hyperglycemia, and hypoparathyroid patients may have hypocalcemia. Patients with connective tissue disease have a positive antinuclear antibody or SCL-70. Patients with thyroid disease have changes in serum triiodothyronine, thyroxine, and thyroid-stimulating hormone levels. Muscular dystrophy or mitochondrial cytopathy patients may have elevated CPK and isoenzymes. Hemagglutination and complement fixation for Chagas' disease may be positive in patients who have lived in Central or South America.

Antineuronal nuclear antibody (ANNA) should be sought in patients with a smoking history to exclude

Table 117–7 Diagnostic Studies for Patients with Small Intestinal or Colonic Dysmotility

Types of Studies	Specific Tests
Blood	Complete blood count
	Blood chemistries, including blood sugar
	Antinuclear antibodies
	Thyroid tests: triiodothyronine, thyroxin, thyroid-stimulating hormone
	Serum creatine phosphokinase and isoenzymes
	Hemagglutination and complement fixation for Chagas' disease
	ANNA or antibodies for paraneoplastic process
Radiologic	Plain abdominal films (in patients with abdominal distention)
	Radiopaque marker intestinal transit study
	Upper gastrointestinal series and small bowel follow through
	Enteroclysis with fluoroscopy
	Barium enema
	Scintigraphic gastric, small intestinal and colonic transit studies
	Intravenous pyelogram
	CT scan of chest and abdomen
	CT enterography
Other	Skeletal muscle biopsy
	Cultures and bacterial counts of small intestine aspirates
	Small intestinal or colonic manometric study
	Anorectal manometry and balloon expulsion test
	Histologic studies of full-thickness biopsy specimens to examine smooth muscle and myenteric plexus by special silver stain, immunohistochemistry, and confocal microscopy of enteric plexuses

ANNA, antineuronal nuclear antibody; CT, computed tomography.

paraneoplastic pseudo-obstruction. Blood lactate, pyruvate (signs of acidosis), CPK, ALT (muscle damage), and leucocyte thymidine phosphorylase are screening tests for mitochondrial cytopathy.

Radiology

Plain abdominal films are useful in patients who complain of abdominal distention and bloating, because they may show gaseous distention of the areas affected by severe dysmotility, which usually are dilated. Dilatation is more commonly seen in myopathic than in neuropathic dysmotility.

Enteroclysis, or small bowel enema, is useful to detect lesions in the small intestine and rule out mechanical obstruction. Experienced radiologists can identify structural lesions in the small intestine in up to 98% of patients with mechanical obstruction. Rarely, obstruction may be missed on barium studies but revealed by small bowel manometry.[96]

Measurement of Intestinal Transit with Radiopaque Markers

Radiopaque markers that move with the colonic contents are robust measures of transit. Hinton and colleagues[97] measured gastrointestinal transit times using 2- to 5-mm polythene pellets containing barium sulfate (these have been replaced by the commercially available Sitzmarks). In normal subjects, all but one had passed 80% of the markers by the 5th day after ingestion, but none had passed 80% by the end of the first day.

Segmental colonic transit can also be measured with daily abdominal plain films after a single dose of radiopaque markers. Metcalf and coworkers[98] simplified the method so that only one study with a fast film, high-kV technique would be necessary, and radiation exposure therefore was minimal. By this method, radiopaque markers are taken in fixed numbers (24 per day), at the same time (arbitrarily, 9:00 AM) each day for 3 days. On the 4th day, again at the same time, a film is taken. The method works on the assumption that a 24-hour sampling interval approximates continuous observation. Rapid transit can cause all the markers to be lost in the feces before radiologic studies on the 4th day; conversely, in slow transit, all 72 markers may be present on the single film. A film on day 7 can then give more information.

Measurement of Intestinal Transit with Scintigraphy

The transit of gamma-emitting radioisotopes through the colon can be quantified using a gamma camera linked to a computerized recording and processing system.[99] In contrast to radiologic methods, the isotope can be monitored for long periods without increasing radiation exposure. Using this noninvasive approach,[100] a good correlation was found between stool consistency and colonic transit; the correlation is clearly influenced, however, by the extremes of transit and form, with little predictive value from stool that is not watery or extremely hard. Radioisotopic transit is useful particularly for gastric emptying and colonic transit but is less accurate for small bowel transit.

Other Studies

Skeletal (striated) muscle biopsy may be needed in patients suspected of having muscular dystrophy or mitochondrial cytopathy. Cultures of small bowel aspirates should be obtained for culture and sensitivity in patients with clinically suspected bacterial overgrowth (e.g., a compatible history with steatorrhea, bloating, and elevated serum folate levels) in whom there is a poor response to antibiotics. Small intestine manometry is indicated if there is no known underlying disease and the nature of the dysmotility (myopathy vs. neuropathy) is unclear.

If a full-thickness biopsy of the dysfunctional part of the intestine is available, careful pathologic examination for abnormalities in the smooth muscle or myenteric plexus with special trichrome and silver stains must be performed. The most informative evaluation now includes assessment of the neurotransmitters by immunohistochemistry and morphologic assessment of the ICC using confocal microscopy—that is, microscopy that allows several "depths" of view of the three-dimensional myenteric plexus to be reconstructed for better assessment of neural structures and their content.

Small Intestinal Manometric Studies

A low-compliance water infusion technique, miniature transducers, and radiotelemetry have been combined to measure phasic pressure activity in the stomach and small bowel. Impedance measurements provide pressure profiles from closely spaced sensors, although it is unclear whether these will enhance the diagnostic capability of manometry.

The small intestine has a unique pattern of motility. During fasting, there is a cyclical pattern of motility, the MMC.[101] The MMC is divided into three phases. Phase I is a quiescent period that lasts for about 15 to 30 minutes. Phase II, which lasts for about 60 minutes, is a period of intermittent contractions that increase in frequency with time until phase III is initiated. During phase III, which lasts for 4 to 10 minutes, there are intense contractions that propagate aborally from the duodenum to the ileum. After phase III, the small intestine become quiescent again (i.e., enters phase I) to start a new cycle of the MMC. This cyclical pattern continues until the subject eats. After eating, the MMC is replaced by frequent, intermittent, irregular contractions, or the fed pattern. The fed pattern usually lasts for 2 to 6 hours, depending on the size of the meal eaten; after it is complete, the fasting pattern, or MMC, returns.

Myopathic Pattern. In patients with smooth muscle dysfunction or degeneration, manometry demonstrates a decrease in amplitude of contractions in the affected segment. This pattern generally is found during both the fasting and fed periods. The fed pattern also is associated with reduced frequency of contractions, in part a result of reduced gastric emptying. Weston and associates showed that in myopathic disorders, antral amplitudes usually are less than 40 mm Hg and duodenal amplitudes are less than 10 mm Hg.[32]

Neuropathic Pattern. Neurologic disorders tend to produce disorganization and incoordination of motor activity that typically is of normal amplitude. The MMC is often absent or abnormal in these patients. An abnormal rate of migration, as well as retrograde propagation of the activity front (phase III), also may be noted. Activity fronts may appear to be normal proximally and then to arrest or disappear in the more distal segments of the small intestine. In neurologic intestinal disorders, the normal fed pattern may not replace the fasted pattern, and MMC-like activity persists postprandially (normally, the MMC activity should be abolished for 1 hour per 200 kcal ingested) and the frequency of antral contractions in the first hour is typically less than 1/min in neuropathic disorders, in contrast to the average 2/min (range 1 to 3/min) in healthy controls.[33] These abnormalities in frequency reflect dysregulation by the enteric or extrinsic nervous system.

Mechanical Obstruction Pattern. Recurring intense contractions followed by periods of motor quiescence have been observed radiologically in the intestine proximal to an obstruction. This phenomenon can be detected manometrically as clustered contractions[102] or simultaneous prolonged contractions in conjunction with periods of intervening quiescence lasting longer than 1 minute. Manometry is not the usual way to establish the diagnosis of mechanical obstruction, but these patterns should alert the physician to the possibility of mechanical obstruction and mandate a careful small bowel barium study (e.g., enteroclysis).

Overall, small intestine manometry lacks the specificity to diagnose the underlying disease, other than suggesting the nature of the pathophysiologic process.

DIFFERENTIATION FROM MECHANICAL OBSTRUCTION

Patients with severe dysmotility of the small intestine may develop CIP. Partial small bowel obstruction from adhesions, tumors, intussusception, or stricture can mimic CIP. Features listed in Table 117–8 help differentiate these two entities. Enteroclysis, a careful small bowel series with fluoroscopy, or CT enterography are probably most helpful to differentiate CIP from mechanical obstruction. Manometry has proven useful in one series[96]; however, in many cases, exploratory laparoscopy may be necessary to exclude an obstructing lesion. CT enterography[103] and capsule endoscopy[104] rapidly are becoming essential preoperative procedures, given their ability to detect obstruction. Patients undergoing capsule endoscopy must be cautioned that failure to pass the capsule may require operation, but that such failure usually is caused by an obstruction that would require surgery anyway.

TREATMENT

Medical Treatments

Drug Therapy to Improve Small Intestinal Motility

In terms of drug therapy (Table 117–9), from an evidence-based perspective, the most effective orally active med-

Table 117–8   Differentiation of Chronic Intestinal Pseudo-obstruction from Mechanical Intestinal Obstruction

Variable	Chronic Pseudo-obstruction	Mechanical Obstruction
Bowel symptoms	Diarrhea or constipation	Constipation and obstipation
Other gastrointestinal symptoms	Possibly dysphagia or symptoms of gastroparesis	No esophageal or gastric problems
Symptoms between attacks	Abdominal pain, nausea, vomiting, or dysphagia	Usually none
Patient's appearance	Cachectic	Seldom cachectic
Urinary tract	May have retention and infection	No urinary symptoms
Systemic disease	Symptoms and signs of systemic disease	None
Family history	May be positive	None
Plain abdominal film	Air throughout small intestine and colon	No air beyond point of obstruction
Esophagogram	May show esophageal aperistalsis and dilatation	Normal
UGI and SBFT	Gastroparesis and megaduodenum	Intestine dilated above obstruction
Enteroclysis	No obstructing lesion	Obstructing lesion
Barium enema	May show redundant colon or wide-mouthed diverticula	Obstructing lesion
IVU	Megacystis or megaureter	Normal
Esophageal manometry	Diminished LES tone and low-amplitude contractions in distal 2/3 (myopathy); incoordination (neuropathy)	Normal
Jejunal manometry	Fasting—absence of MMC, and presence of low-amplitude contractions (myopathy), fed (<1/min), inactive fed pattern with MMCs (neuropathy)	Clusters, or simultaneous prolonged contractions, during fasting and fed periods, but MMCs during fasting
Exploratory laparotomy	No obstructing lesion found	Obstructing lesion

IVP, intravenous pyelography; LES, lower esophageal sphincter; MMC, migrating motor complex; SBFT, small bowel follow through; UGI, upper gastrointestinal.

Table 117–9   Mechanisms of Action of Prokinetic Agents

Medication Class	Examples	Mechanism
5-HT$_4$ agonist	Metoclopramide, tegaserod, cisapride	Activates intrinsic cholinergic neuron
Dopamine-2 antagonist	Metoclopramide, domperidone	Inhibits dopaminergic neurons which are inhibitory; antiemetic by central nervous system action
Macrolide	Erythromycin	Activates intrinsic motilin receptor or cholinergic neurons
Somatostatin	Octreotide	Activates somatostatinergic neurons

5-HT, 5-hydroxytryptamine (serotonin).

ication for small intestine dysmotility is cisapride, which decreased the transit time of a meal through the small bowel both in normal subjects and in patients with neuropathic forms of chronic intestinal dysmotility.[105-107]

In a small, short-term study, octreotide, a somatostatin analog, stimulated intestinal motility, possibly reduced bacterial overgrowth, and improved abdominal symptoms in patients with scleroderma.[30] Other open-labeled studies confirmed the long-term effectiveness of octreotide with erythromycin in the treatment of CIP. Some data, however, show that octreotide retards gastric[108] and small bowel transit in health, and many authorities use the drug to induce MMC-like contractions at least 2 hours after the last meal of the day to "sweep" residue out of the intestine toward the colon and thereby avoid bacterial overgrowth.

Symptomatic and Supportive Treatments

Abdominal pain, bloating, nausea, and vomiting in patients with small intestine dysmotility are often related to eating. Most of these symptoms can be minimized by manipulating the amount, nature, and frequency of meals. Patients need to ingest sufficient calories without overloading the inefficient bowel: a useful rule of thumb is 25 cal/kg of the patient's ideal body weight per day. Adult patients should consume 1500 to 1800 cal/day divided into three or four equal feedings. Depending on the patient's level of symptoms, one half or more of the calories may come from supplemental formulas because a liquid meal empties faster from the stomach and probably progresses more easily through the small bowel than does a solid meal. These formulas are lactose-free and contain the daily requirements of vitamins and minerals. When patients still feel full several hours after the first meal of the day, it is important that they restrict oral intake to fluids for the remainder of the day and not force themselves to eat subsequent meals that will only aggravate their symptoms. There is no documented advantage to using elemental formulas and, in general, 1 kcal/mL solutions are better tolerated than those with higher calorie content.

Cisapride was the mainstay of long-term treatment. Patients with vagal dysfunction (e.g., diabetic, postvagotomy) appeared to respond less well to this drug than those with no autonomic dysfunction (idiopathic pseudo-obstruction).[106] In the long term, 60% of patients appeared to benefit from cisapride, an improvement that persisted for up to 1 year[107]; efficacy was not tested beyond 1 year.

Since cisapride is not easily available, other prokinetic agents are now used, including erythromycin, 250 mg three times a day before meals; metoclopramide, 10 mg three times a day before meals; or tegaserod, 2 to 6 mg before meals, and octreotide, 50 µg at least 2 hours after the final meal of the day. The evidence for these approaches is limited, however, and the drug trial should be stopped if there are adverse effects or lack of efficacy. Recurrent symptoms and signs of intestinal pseudo-obstruction may occur, in which case nasogastric suction and intravenous fluids are needed. When obstructive symptoms and pain persist or occur several times per week despite dietary manipulation, the alternatives are either enteral feeding via a laparoscopically or endoscopically placed jejunal feeding tube or long-term parenteral nutrition to improve the patient's symptoms and nutritional state. Regrettably, in our experience, the former approach is more effective in patients with gastroparesis than in those with pseudo-obstruction.

Abdominal pain unrelated to eating is uncommon in patients with small intestine dysmotility, and the presence of significant pain that is *unrelated* to meals should raise questions about the diagnosis. During episodes of obstruction, patients may require parenteral administration of narcotics such as morphine or meperidine. Long-term narcotic use should be discouraged, however, because patients may become addicted and narcotics may further disturb gastrointestinal motility. Tramadol and gabapentin sometimes are prescribed for such pain, but these medications also may retard intestinal transit; there are conflicting data on their transit effects in otherwise healthy people and virtually no data in patients with intestinal pseudo-obstruction.[109-111]

Constipation is common in patients who also have colon involvement. It is important to make certain that these patients have a good bowel movement at least once every few days, because constipation tends to increase symptoms of intestinal dysmotility. We prescribe 30 to 60 mL (or two tablets three times a day) of milk of magnesia per day. Enemas may be used if the patients have had no bowel movement for 3 days. Bulk-forming laxatives should be avoided in patients with severe small intestine dysmotility because they tend to worsen symptoms.

Treatment of Secondary Causes

A few types of secondary small intestine dysmotility, such as hypothyroidism, celiac sprue, and drug-induced dysmotility, can be treated specifically with thyroid replacement, a gluten-free diet, and discontinuation of the offending drugs, respectively. There are no specific treatments for most of the secondary causes of small intestine dysmotility.

Surgical Treatment

Patients who have dysmotility limited to short segments of the small intestine, such as those with megaduodenum, have a better prognosis than those with dysmotility throughout the length of the bowel, because the dysfunctional segment can be resected or bypassed.[112]

Megaduodenum, which is commonly seen in FVM-I and scleroderma, has been surgically treated using a side-to-side duodenojejunostomy, which usually gives symptomatic relief to most patients. In some patients with a massively dilated duodenum, this procedure may be inadequate to drain the duodenum. In these cases, resection of as much of the duodenum as possible with preservation of the papilla of Vater and anastomosis of the opened jejunum to the cut edge of duodenum may be required.

For patients with long segments of small intestine dysmotility, there is no effective surgical treatment. Unnecessary surgery may create adhesions and additional difficulties. Venting decompression by percutaneous jejunostomy, minilaparotomy, or laparoscopy provides symptom relief and reduces hospitalization rates for recurrent exacerbations of pseudo-obstruction.[113,114] In the past, enterectomy was performed rarely for pseudo-obstruction[115]; this is considered now only in the context of intestinal transplantation.

Small Bowel Transplantation

Small bowel transplantation has become a reality with the introduction of effective immunosuppression (chiefly sirolimus, tacrolimus, and mycophenolate). In a review of the world experience for the period 1985-1997, survival of all patients and grafts was approximately 60%, approximately three fourths of whom did not require parenteral nutrition support.[116] Adults seemed to fare less well than children, however, with an actuarial survival for patients and grafts of 48% and 36%, respectively, at 3 years in adults. In reaching a decision about transplantation, it is important to recall that the 3-year survival of patients on home total parenteral nutrition (TPN) is 85%.[117] More recent data using isolated small bowel transplantation show that the 3-year patient and graft survival, particularly in those treated with sirolimus, is close to 75%.[118]

Several factors limit the success of small bowel transplantation and may result in death: infections (including cytomegalovirus and Epstein-Barr virus, which account for ≈50% of deaths), rejection (≈8% of deaths), technical problems, and lymphoproliferative disease (20% to 40% deaths in different programs). The latter is particularly linked to Epstein-Barr virus infection, use of OKT3 immunosuppression, and glucocorticoids.[119] The high patient survival and parenteral nutrition–free survival achieved after isolated intestinal transplantation have reduced complications from infection related to immunosuppression and have resulted in a renewed enthusiasm for intestinal transplantation. Concurrently, sirolimus treatment has reduced graft loss drastically. Parenteral nutrition–associated liver disease has been shown to be reversible with intestinal transplantation. Optimizing parenteral nutrition regimens is key to patient management; if liver dysfunction in patients receiving parenteral nutrition becomes refractory to treatment, there should be prompt consideration for isolated intestinal transplantation.[118] In general, small bowel transplantation still is restricted to life-saving situations, such as necrotizing enterocolitis, intestinal failure (short bowel syndrome), inability to be maintained on TPN, and rarely

CIP in young patients who have TPN-related or other liver failure and who lack intravenous access for TPN.

In the future, gastroenterologists may be involved in the management of patients after small bowel transplantation. First, specialized zoom-video endoscopy needs to be evaluated further to determine if enlarged crypt areas, and villus blunting or flattening correlate with histologic evidence of rejection. Second, severe rejection (mucosal necrosis with loss of villi) has a grave prognostic significance (11% graft survival, 18% patient survival) and may be an indication for removal of the graft. Third, living-related small bowel transplantation technically is feasible and has been reported to be followed by complete functional adaptation of the graft. Fourth, lymphoproliferative disease may present during follow-up.[120,121]

ACUTE COLONIC PSEUDO-OBSTRUCTION

Acute colonic pseudo-obstruction, also referred to as *Ogilvie's syndrome*, presents as intestinal ileus with massive bowel dilatation and occurs typically in critically ill medical and surgical patients. Toxic megacolon, a complication of inflammatory bowel disease, is discussed in Chapter 109 and megacolon due to Chagas' disease (infection by *T. cruzi*) is discussed briefly below and in Chapter 106.

PATHOPHYSIOLOGY AND MECHANISMS

Table 117–10 summarizes the mechanisms of acute intestinal pseudo-obstruction proposed to date.

Local stimuli result in an inhibitory reflex that result in ileus, for which the splanchnic nerves provide both the afferent and efferent pathways. Local stimuli, including handling of intestine during experimental surgery, results in massive monocyte infiltration of the bowel wall, and inflammatory mediators such as ICAM-1, MCP-1, iNOS, and COX-2 messenger RNA are up-

Table 117–10 Proposed Pathophysiologic Mechanisms for Acute Intestinal Pseudo-obstruction

Reflex motor inhibition through splanchnic afferents in response to noxious stimuli
Excess sympathetic (inhibitory) motor input to the intestine (does not contract)
Excess parasympathetic (excitatory) motor input to the intestine (does not relax)
Decreased parasympathetic (excitatory) motor input to the intestine (does not contract)
Excess stimulation of peripheral μ opioid receptors by endogenous or exogenous opioids (initially intestinal activation, followed by prolonged inhibition preventing contraction)
Inhibition of nitric oxide release from inhibitory motoneurons (intestine does not relax to allow peristalsis)

From Delgado-Aros S, Camilleri M: Pseudo-obstruction in the critically ill. In Scholmerich J (ed): Bailliere's Best Practice and Research in Clinical Gastroenterology: Gastrointestinal Disorders and the Critically Ill, Vol 17. London, Elsevier, 2003, p 427.

regulated during the first 18 hours postmanipulation. The degree of postoperative ileus correlates with the intestinal inflammatory response.

Several studies have identified the release of endogenous opioids after surgery and related them to the inflammatory response to surgery. The frequent use of narcotics to treat postsurgical pain may aggravate the "normal" postoperative ileus and may induce acute intestinal pseudo-obstruction.[122] Opioids inhibit nitric oxide (NO) release from inhibitory motoneurons in vitro and delay transit in vivo. Mechanisms and management of acute postoperative ileus are the subject of intense investigation[123] and search for novel therapies (e.g., alvimopan, a μ antagonist).[124]

CLINICAL FEATURES

Acute intestinal pseudo-obstruction usually presents in patients with an underlying severe clinical disorder, such as stroke, myocardial infarction, peritonitis, and sepsis, or after a variety of surgical procedures including orthopedic surgery, cesarean section, and cardiovascular or lung surgery. Systemic diseases that affect the neuromuscular component of the gastrointestinal tract, such as amyloidosis, may first present with an acute episode of intestinal pseudo-obstruction .

The characteristic clinical feature of intestinal pseudo-obstruction is severe abdominal distention, with absence of passage of stool or gas. Up to 41% of patients with intestinal pseudo-obstruction, however, still pass some gas or even present with diarrhea during the episode. Because many patients present after abdominal surgery and bowel cleansing, the absence of bowel movements is not a diagnostically useful symptom. Nausea and vomiting may be present, and nasogastric aspiration usually is ineffective and does not result in major air or fluid withdrawal because the functional obstruction affects the colon. Abdominal discomfort is usually present, but frequently the distention is painless and there is no associated abdominal tenderness. In fact, the presence of abdominal pain and tenderness may be a sign of perforation or ischemia. Frequent clinical evaluation in combination with white blood cell count and abdominal radiography are key to identify bowel perforation.

Bowel sounds vary from absent to hyperactive, and, in many cases, are high pitched and suggestive of mechanical obstruction.[125]

RADIOLOGY

The hallmark of this disease is dilatation of the colon on a plain abdominal film. When plain abdominal films demonstrate air in all colonic segments, including the rectosigmoid, the condition can be differentiated from mechanical obstruction. The dilatation preferentially affects the cecum and ascending and transverse colon, although the left colon including the rectum also may be dilated. The small bowel also is involved in some cases. Absence or effacement of haustration and air-fluid levels frequently is observed in colonic obstruction or pseudo-obstruction.[125] Free air usually is a radiologic sign of intestinal perforation. Free air in association with pneumatosis intestinalis, however, may not be associated with perforation and does not necessarily mandate surgical exploration.

The maximal diameter of the cecum on abdominal films varies in the literature from 7 to 25 cm. Cecal diameter may be of important prognostic value and has implications in management (see later).

Alternatives to contrast enemas are judicious proctosigmoidoscopy, which may provide diagnosis and decompression, although not without complications, and CT of the abdomen, which has a sensitivity of 96% and specificity of 93%.

PROGNOSIS

Mortality Rate

The mortality rate of patients with acute colonic pseudo-obstruction varies from 0 to 32% and is partly determined by comorbidity.[125,126] Older patients, poor clinical condition, and surgical treatment for acute pseudo-obstruction are associated with an increased mortality risk. There are no randomized clinical trials comparing surgical with medical treatment to clarify whether surgery itself or selection bias influences the mortality associated with surgical treatment. Intestinal ischemia or perforation, which occurs in approximately 1 in 6 to 7 cases, is associated with a 50% increase in the risk of death.[125]

The diameter of the colon may be another risk factor for mortality. When surgical decompression is used in mechanically obstructed patients with a cecal diameter greater than 9 cm, there is a dramatic reduction in mortality.[127] This is the basis for the use of the 9-cm cut-off as a sign of "impending perforation" in patients with acute colonic pseudo-obstruction. In Vanek and Al-Salti's review, perforation rates for cecal diameters less than 12 cm, 12 to 14 cm, or above 14 cm were 0, 7%, and 23%, respectively.[125] Mortality also was associated with the duration of delay to decompression: 15% in those decompressed less than 4 days after onset of dilatation, 27% when the decompression occurred after 4 to 7 days, and 73% after the 7th day.

PREVENTION

Laparoscopy and regional anesthesia may help reduce postsurgical ileus.[128] Bowel dysfunction is more pronounced with codeine compared with other opioids, and use of transdermal opioids may prevent major postsurgical ileus in these patients. Selective peripheral opioid antagonists, which antagonize the gastrointestinal effects of systemic opioids without diminishing their analgesic effect, may have a potential role in preventing postsurgical or opioid-related ileus (see section on treatment).

TREATMENT

With correction of reversible potential causes or associated imbalances, such as infection, hypovolemia, hypox-

emia, abnormal electrolytes (especially potassium and calcium levels), and use of medications that may induce ileus, the ileus usually disappears in 2 to 6 days in 83% to 96% of patients (Table 117–11).[125] Intravenous saline and glucose solutions for hydration should be sufficient because of the short-lived and reversible nature of the dysfunction in most cases. In patients with prolonged acute colonic pseudo-obstruction, parenteral or enteral[129] nutrition may be necessary. Rectal tubes are not useful except when the sigmoid is involved. Enemas may facilitate "cleaning" of the colon but have not shown any efficacy except for diatrizoate (Gastrografin) enemas in anecdotal reports. Moreover, enemas may precipitate colonic perforation.[125] When the diameter of the cecum is greater than 9 cm and is not reduced after treatment of known potential causes, decompression should be performed within the first 72 hours after diagnosis[125] to reduce the risk of ischemia, perforation, and death.

Medical Decompression

Adrenergic blockers and the acetylcholinesterase inhibitor neostigmine have been tested over several years, typically in open-label studies. A variety of adverse events have been described after intravenous administration of 2 to 2.5 mg of neostigmine, the most frequent being abdominal cramps in 17% of patients, excessive salivation in 13%, sweating in 4%, nausea or vomiting in 4%, and transient bradycardia in 6%. We recommend a starting dose of 1 mg rather than 2 mg to decrease the likelihood of bradycardia.

Table 117–11 Clinical Management of Acute Colonic Pseudo-obstruction
Diagnose acute intestinal pseudo-obstruction when there is acute massive intestinal (usually colonic) dilatation (cecal diameter ≥7 cm on abdominal plain films) and mechanical obstruction is excluded
Treat reversible underlying conditions (e.g., infection, hypotension) and correct any imbalance of electrolytes
Nothing by mouth; intravenous fluids, and nasogastric tube if nausea or vomiting are present
Rectal tube if the sigmoid colon is involved
Daily abdominal plain film, white blood cell count, and serum electrolytes
Presence of abdominal pain and tenderness associated with an elevated white blood cell count suggests intestinal perforation
Prompt surgery if perforation is suspected
If after 72 hr of conservative measures, the cecal diameter is >9 cm and there are no contraindications to neostigmine: infuse neostigmine (1-2 mg) intravenously over 3 to 5 min (with electrocardiographic and vital sign monitoring and patient in supine position during and for at least 60 min after the infusion); use atropine to reverse bradycardia; repeat infusion after 4 hr if no response or if recurrence of dilatation
Endoscopic decompression if there is no response to neostigmine
Percutaneous cecostomy/surgery if other measures fail to decrease cecal distention

From Delgado-Aros S, Camilleri M: Pseudo-obstruction in the critically ill. In Scholmerich J (ed): Bailliere's Best Practice and Research in Clinical Gastroenterology: Gastrointestinal Disorders and the Critically Ill, Vol 17. London, Elsevier, 2003, p 427.

Although prompt decompression of the colon after administration of neostigmine often is clinically obvious, as the patient passes gas or develops abdominal cramping, it has not been shown that such volume decompression by passage of gas reduces the risk of perforation and mortality in these patients. Nonetheless, if conservative measures fail, it is a safe choice in selected patients whose cecal diameter is greater than 9 cm for 72 hours. Contraindications for its use are heart rate less than 60 beats/min and/or systolic blood pressure less than 90 mm Hg; active bronchospasm; serum creatinine concentration greater than 3 mg/dL; and signs of bowel perforation. A second administration of neostigmine should be considered if there is partial or no response to the first trial or if there is recurrence of the ileus after the initial response.

Acute colonic pseudo-obstruction may be associated with the use of narcotics to treat pain; recently developed peripherally restricted μ-opioid antagonists such as methyl-naltrexone and alvimopan (referred to in some papers as ADL 8-2698) may improve postoperative or opioid-related ileus without reversing analgesia or inducing withdrawal symptoms.[124,130,131] Although these results may not apply to patients with acute colonic pseudo-obstruction, peripheral μ-opioid antagonists should be tested in the future.

Erythromycin, metoclopramide, and cisapride have been subjects of anecdotal reports, but none of these drugs has been tested formally in the setting of acute colonic pseudo-obstruction.

Endoscopic Decompression

Colonoscopic decompression can be achieved technically in patients presenting with acute colonic pseudo-obstruction at high risk of cecal perforation. Colonoscopic decompression has not been shown to improve the outcome of these patients, however, and colonoscopy of an unprepared bowel may distend the colon further and lead to perforation.[125]

Randomized, controlled trials of the efficacy of colonoscopic decompression are lacking and resolution of ileus, perforation, and mortality rates are similar with colonoscopic decompression and conservative treatment alone.

Endoscopic decompression should be considered as a third-line treatment option in patients with acute colonic pseudo-obstruction with high risk of cecal perforation when conservative and pharmacologic maneuvers have failed. Rectal decompression may be helpful if the sigmoid colon is dilared.

Nonsurgical Cecostomy

In view of the high rate of recurrence of colonic dilatation after endoscopic decompression, alternative techniques to decompress the colon have been proposed to avoid surgery in these patients. Percutaneous cecostomy has been reported to be successful in several case reports, but is associated with significant morbidity. Percutaneous cecostomy has been performed with endoscopic assistance.[132]

Surgical Decompression

Surgical decompression, which includes cecostomy, colostomy, or resection, is associated with poorer outcome,[125] possibly because it is usually resorted to in patients with more severe disease in whom conservative or other measures have failed. Surgery is essential when perforation or peritonitis are suspected.

COLONIC PSEUDO-OBSTRUCTION AND MEGACOLON

Megacolon and megarectum are descriptive terms, without etiologic or pathophysiologic implications. Megacolon has been defined on radiologic study as a diameter of >6.5 cm for the rectosigmoid or descending colon; >8 cm for the ascending colon; and >12 cm for the cecum. Megacolon can be caused by aganglionosis (Hirschsprung's disease), can be idiopathic (complicating chronic constipation of any cause) or may be a manifestation of a diffuse gastrointestinal dysmotility (intestinal pseudo-obstruction). Note that megacolon does not include simple elongation (dolichocolon) of the colon.

In *congenital megacolon* (Hirschsprung's disease), colonic dilatation results from functional obstruction (usually of the rectum) caused by a congenital absence of the intramural neural plexuses that mediate relaxation (aganglionosis). This results in a narrow segment of the large intestine, that is, one that fails to relax. Hirschsprung's disease is discussed in detail in Chapter 93.

Acquired megacolon can complicate any of the many causes of constipation, and megacolon may be assumed to be acquired when it can be ascertained that colonic dilatation was not present on some earlier examination. A common background for acquired megacolon is colonic inertia, which is common at both extremes of life. In children, this form can be confused with the congenital condition.

Worldwide, infection with T. cruzi (Chagas' disease) is the most common form of acquired megacolon. In this condition, the dilated segment of colon is abnormal, because of destruction of the ENS by the organism's neurotoxin. Although originally confined to the South American continent, it is now estimated that there are 350,000 T. cruzi-seropositive persons in the United States, one third of whom are thought to have chronic Chagas' disease. Some patients acquire megacolon as part of a generalized intestinal pseudo-obstruction.

CHRONIC COLONIC PSEUDO-OBSTRUCTION

Chronic colonic pseudo-obstruction manifests as either slow-transit constipation (see Chapters 12 and 95) or as part of the spectrum of CIP or megacolon (see earlier).

REFERENCES

1. Newton WT: Radical enterectomy for hereditary megaduodenum. Arch Surg 96:549, 1968.
2. Byrne WJ, Cipel L, Euler AR, et al: Chronic idiopathic intestinal pseudo-obstruction syndrome in children: Clinical characteristics and prognosis. J Pediatr 90:585, 1977.
3. Wood JD, Grundy D: Little brain–big brain: V. Neurogastroenterol Motil 10:377, 1998.

4. Thuneberg L: Interstitial cells of Cajal: intestinal pacemaker cells? Adv Anat Embryol Cell Biol 71:1, 1982.

5. Furness JB, Kunze WA, Clerc N: Nutrient tasting and signaling mechanisms in the gut: II. The intestine as a sensory organ—neural, endocrine, and immune responses. Am J Physiol 277:G922, 1999.

6. Pomeranz HD, Rothman TP, Gershon MD: Colonization of the post-umbilical bowel by cells derived from the sacral neural crest: Direct tracing of cell migration using an intercalating probe and a replication-deficient retrovirus. Development 111:647, 1991.

7. Fu CG, Muto T, Masaki T, Nagawa H: Zonal adult Hirschsprung disease. Gut 39:765, 1996.

8. De Giorgio R, Camilleri M: Human enteric neuropathies: Morphology and molecular pathology. Neurogastroenterol Motil 16:515, 2004.

9. Ward SM, Harney SC, Bayguinov JR, et al: Development of electrical rhythmicity in the murine gastrointestinal tract is specifically encoded in the tunica muscularis. J Physiol 505:241, 1997.

10. Vanderwinden JM, Rumessen JJ, Liu H, et al: Interstitial cells of Cajal in human colon and in Hirschsprung disease. Gastroenterology 111:901, 1996.

11. Isozaki K, Hirota S, Miyagawa J, et al: Deficiency of *c-kit*⁺ cells in patients with a myopathic form of chronic idiopathic intestinal pseudo-obstruction. Am J Gastroenterol 92:332, 1997.

12. Hirota S, Isozaki K, Moriyama Y, et al: Gain-of-function mutations of *c-kit* in human gastrointestinal stromal tumors. Science 279:577, 1998.

13. Kenny SE, Vanderwinden JM, Rintala RJ, et al: Delayed maturation of the interstitial cells of Cajal—a new diagnosis for transient neonatal pseudoobstruction: Report of two cases. J Pediatr Surg 33:94, 1998.

14. Faussone-Pellegrini MS, Fociani P, Buffa R, Basilisco G: Loss of interstitial cells and a fibromuscular layer on the luminal side of the colonic circular muscle presenting as megacolon in an adult patient. Gut 45:775, 1999.

15. He CL, Burgart L, Wang L, et al: Decreased interstitial cell of Cajal volume in patients with slow-transit constipation. Gastroenterology 118:14, 2000.

16. Mitros FA, Schuffler MD, Teja K, et al: Pathologic feature of familial visceral myopathy. Hum Pathol 13:825, 1982.

17. Mueller LA, Camilleri M, Emslie-Smith AM: Mitochondrial neuro-gastrointestinal encephalomyopathy: manometric and diagnostic features. Gastroenterology 116:959, 1999.

18. Perez-Atayde AR, Fox V, Teitelbaum JE, et al: Mitochondrial neurogastrointestinal encephalo-myopathy: Diagnosis by rectal biopsy. Am J Surg Pathol 22:1141, 1998.

19. Nishino I, Spinazzola A, Hirano M: Thymidine phosphorylase gene mutations in MNGIE, a human mitochondrial disorder. Science 283:689, 1999.

20. Chokhavatia S, Anuras S: Neuromuscular disease of the gastrointestinal tract. Am J Med Sci 301:201, 1991.

21. Milla PJ: Endothelins, pseudo-obstruction and Hirschsprung disease. Gut 44:148, 1999.

22. Carney JA, Go VL, Sizemore GW, et al: Alimentary tract ganglioneuromatosis: A major component of the syndrome of multiple endocrine neoplasia type 2b. N Engl J Med 295:1287, 1976.

23. Bonsib SM, Fallon B, Mitros FA, et al: Urologic manifestations of patients with visceral myopathy. J Urol 132:1112, 1984.

24. Debinski HS, Kamm MA, Talbot IC, et al: DNA viruses in the pathogenesis of sporadic chronic idiopathic intestinal pseudo-obstruction. Gut 41:100, 1997.

25. Stanghellini V, Camilleri M, Malagelada J-R: Chronic idiopathic intestinal pseudo-obstruction: Clinical and intestinal manometric findings. Gut 28:5, 1987.

26. Camilleri M, Brown ML, Malagelada J-R: Impaired transit of chyme in chronic intestinal pseudoobstruction: Correction by cisapride. Gastroenterology 91:619, 1986.

27. Schuffler MD, Rohrmann CA, Chaffer RG, et al: Chronic intestinal pseudoobstruction: A report of 27 cases and review of the literature. Medicine 60:173, 1981.

28. Hirsh EH, Brandenburg D, Hersh T, Brooks WS Jr: Chronic intestinal pseudo-obstruction. J Clin Gastroenterol 3:247, 1981.

29. Schuffler MD, Beagle RG: Progressive systemic sclerosis of the gastrointestinal tract and hereditary hollow visceral myopathy: Two distinguishable disorders of intestinal smooth muscle. Gastroenterology 77:664, 1979.

30. Soudah HC, Hasler WL, Owyang C: Effect of octreotide on intestinal motility and bacterial overgrowth in scleroderma. N Engl J Med 325:1461, 1991.

31. Greydanus MP, Camilleri M: Abnormal postcibal antral and small bowel motility due to neuropathy or myopathy in systemic sclerosis. Gastroenterology 96:110, 1989.

32. Greydanus MP, Camilleri M, Colemont LJ, et al: Ileocolonic transfer of solid chyme in small intestinal neuropathies and myopathies. Gastroenterology 99:158, 1990.

33. Weston S, Thumshirn M, Wiste J, Camilleri M: Clinical and upper gastrointestinal motility features in systemic sclerosis and related disorders. Am J Gastroenterol 93:1085, 1998.

34. Fiorucci S, Distrutti E, Bassotti G, et al: Effect of erythromycin administration on upper gastrointestinal motility in scleroderma patients. Scand J Gastroenterol 29:807, 1994.

35. Perlemuter G. Chaussade S. Wechsler B, et al: Chronic intestinal pseudo-obstruction in systemic lupus erythematosus. Gut 43:117, 1998.

36. Norman DA, Fleischmann RM: Gastrointestinal systemic sclerosis in serologic mixed connective tissue disease. Arthritis Rheum 21:811, 1978.

37. Camilleri M, Malagelada J-R: Abnormal intestinal motility in diabetics with gastroparesis syndrome. Eur J Clin Invest 14:420, 1984.

38. He CL, Soffer EE, Ferris CD, et al: Loss of interstitial cells of Cajal and inhibitory innervation in insulin-dependent diabetes. Gastroenterology 121:427, 2001.

39. Whalen GE, Soergel KH, Geenen JE: Diabetic diarrhea: A clinical and pathophysiological study. Gastroenterology 56:1021, 1969.

40. Maleki D, Locke GR III, Camilleri M, et al: Gastrointestinal symptoms among persons with diabetes in the community. Arch Intern Med 160:2808, 2000.

41. Janatuinen E, Pikkarainen P, Laakso M, Pyorala K: Gastrointestinal symptoms in middle-aged diabetic patients. Scand J Gastroenterol 28:427, 1993.

42. Maleki D, Camilleri M, Burton DD, et al: Pilot study of pathophysiology of constipation among community diabetics. Dig Dis Sci 43:2373, 1998.

43. Edwards LL, Pfeiffer RF, Quigley EMM, et al: Gastrointestinal symptoms in Parkinson's disease. Mov Disord 6:151, 1991.

44. Lewitan A, Nathanson L, Slade WR: Megacolon and dilatation of the small bowel in parkinsonism. Gastroenterology 17:367, 1952.

45. Bozeman T, Anuras S, Hutton T, et al: Small intestinal manometry in Parkinson's disease. Gastroenterology 99:1202, 1990.

46. Kupsky WJ, Grimes MM, Sweeting J, et al: Parkinson's disease and megacolon: Concentric hyaline inclusions (Lewy bodies) in enteric ganglion cells. Neurology 37:1253, 1987.

47. Singaram C, Ashraf W, Gaumnitz EA, et al: Dopaminergic defect of enteric nervous system in Parkinson's disease patients with chronic constipation. Lancet 346:861, 1995.

48. Fealey RD, Szurszewski JH, Meritt JL, et al: Effect of spinal cord transection on human upper gastrointestinal motility and gastric emptying. Gastroenterology 87:69, 1984.

49. Bruninga K, Camilleri M: Colonic motility and tone after spinal cord and cauda equina injury. Am J Gastroenterol 92:891, 1997.

50. Fajardo NR, Pasiliao RV, Modeste-Duncan R, et al: Decreased colonic motility in persons with chronic spinal cord injury. Am J Gastroenterol. 98:128, 2003.

51. Stiens SA, Bergman SB, Goetz LL: Neurogenic bowel dysfunction after spinal cord injury: Clinical evaluation and rehabilitative management. Arch Phys Med Rehabil 78:S86, 1997.

52. Feinstat T, Tesluk H, Schuffler MD, et al: Megacolon and neurofibromatosis: A neuronal intestinal dysplasia. Gastroenterology 86:1573, 1984.

53. Schuffler MD, Baird HW, Fleming CR, et al: Intestinal pseudoobstruction as the presenting manifestation of small-cell carcinoma of the lung. Ann Intern Med 98:129, 1983.

54. Sodhi N, Camilleri M, Camoriano JK, et al: Autonomic function and motility in intestinal pseudoobstruction caused by paraneoplastic syndrome. Dig Dis Sci 34:1937, 1989.

55. Lennon VA, Sas DF, Busk MF, et al: Enteric neuronal autoantibodies in pseudoobstruction with small-cell lung carcinoma. Gastroenterology 100:137, 1991.

56. Lee H-R, Lennon VA, Camilleri M, Prather CM: Paraneoplastic gastrointestinal motor dysfunction: Clinical and laboratory characteristics. Am J Gastroenterol 96:373, 2001.

57. Chinn JS, Schuffler MD: Paraneoplastic visceral neuropathy as a cause of severe gastrointestinal motor dysfunction. Gastroenterology 95:1279, 1988.

58. Gerl A, Storck M, Schalhorn A, et al: Paraneoplastic chronic intestinal pseudoobstruction as a rare complication of bronchial carcinoid. Gut 33:1000, 1992.

59. De Giorgio R, Barbara G, Stanghellini V, et al: Clinical and morphofunctional features of idiopathic myenteric ganglionitis underlying severe intestinal motor dysfunction: A study of three cases. Am J Gastroenterol 97:2454, 2002.

60. Simpson AF, Khilnani MT: Gastrointestinal manifestations of the muscular dystrophies. AJR Am J Roentgenol 125:948, 1975.

61. Nowak TV, Anuras S, Brown BP: Small intestinal motility in myotonic dystrophy patients. Gastroenterology 86:808, 1984.

62. Yoshida MM, Krishnamurthy S, Wattchow DA: Megacolon in myotonic dystrophy caused by a degenerative neuropathy of the myenteric plexus. Gastroenterology 95:820, 1988.

63. Jaffe KM, McDonald CM, Ingman E, et al: Symptoms of upper gastrointestinal dysfunction in Duchenne muscular dystrophy: Case-control study. Arch Phys Med Rehabil 71:742, 1990.

64. Barohn RJ, Levine EJ, Olson JO, et al: Gastric hypomotility in Duchenne's muscular dystrophy. N Engl J Med 319:15, 1988.

65. Leon SH, Schuffler MD, Kettler M, et al: Chronic intestinal pseudoobstruction as a complication of Duchenne's muscular dystrophy. Gastroenterology 90:455, 1986.

66. Okuda Y, Takasugi K, Oyama T, et al: Amyloidosis in rheumatoid arthritis: Clinical study of 124 histologically proven cases. Ryumachi 34:939, 1994.

67. Menke DM, Kyle RA, Fleming CR, et al: Symptomatic gastric amyloidosis in patients with primary systemic amyloidosis. Mayo Clin Proc 68:763, 1993.

68. Battle WM, Rubin MR, Cohen S, Snape WJ: Gastrointestinal motility dysfunction in amyloidosis. N Engl J Med 301:24, 1979.

69. Camilleri M, Malagelada J-R, Stanghellini V, et al: Gastrointestinal motility disturbances in patients with orthostatic hypotension. Gastroenterology 88:1852, 1985.

70. Tada S, Iida M, Yao T, et al: Intestinal pseudo-obstruction in patients with amyloidosis: Clinicopathologic differences between chemical types of amyloid protein. Gut 34:1412, 1993.

71. Gilat T, Revach M, Sohar E: Deposition of amyloid in the gastrointestinal tract. Gut 10:98, 1969.

72. Feurle GE: Pathophysiology of diarrhea in patients with familial amyloid neuropathy. Digestion 36:13, 1987.

73. Legge DA, Carlson HC, Wollaeger EE: Roentgenologic appearance of systemic amyloidosis involving gastrointestinal tract. AJR Am J Roentgenol 110:406, 1970.

74. Wald A, Kichler J, Mendelow H: Amyloidosis and chronic intestinal pseudoobstruction. Dig Dis Sci 26:462, 1981.

75. Oliveira RB, Meneghelli UG, de Godoy RA, et al: Abnormalities of interdigestive motility of the small intestine in patients with Chagas' disease. Dig Dis Sci 28:294, 1983.

76. Troncon LE, Aprile LR, Oliveira RB, Iazigi N: Abnormally rapid gastric emptying of an isosmotic liquid meal in patients with megaduodenum. Dig Dis Sci. 45:2145, 2000.

77. Shafer RB, Prentiss RA, Bond JH: Gastrointestinal transit in thyroid disease. Gastroenterology 86:852, 1984.

78. Miller LJ, Gorman C, Go V: Gut-thyroid interrelationships. Gastroenterology 75:901, 1978.

79. Wegener M, Wedmann B, Langhoff T, et al: Effect of hyperthyroidism on the transit of a caloric solid-liquid meal through the stomach, the small intestine, and the colon in man. J Clin Endocrinol Metab 75:745, 1992.

80. Wiley ZD, Larigne ME, Liu KM, et al: The effect of hyperthyroidism on gastric emptying rates and pancreatic exocrine and biliary secretion in man. Dig Dis Sci 23:1008, 1978.

81. Kahraman H, Kaya N, Demircali A, et al: Gastric emptying time in patients with primary hypothyroidism. Eur J Gastroenterol Hepatol 9:901, 1997.

82. Duret RL, Bastenie MD: Intestinal disorders in hypothyroidism: Clinical and manometric study. Am J Dig Dis 16:723, 1971.

83. Dawson DJ, Sciberras CM, Whitwell H: Coeliac disease presenting with intestinal pseudoobstruction. Gut 25:1003, 1984.

84. Otterson MF, Sarna SK, Lee MB: Fractionated doses of ionizing radiation after postprandial small intestinal motor activity. Dig Dis Sci 37:709, 1992.

85. Summers RW, Glenn CE, Flatt AJ, et al: Does irradiation produce irreversible changes in canine jejunal myoelectric activity? Dig Dis Sci 37:716, 1992.

86. Fernandez-Banares F, Villa S, Esteve M, et al: Acute effects of abdominopelvic irradiation on the orocecal transit time: Its relation to clinical symptoms and bile salt and lactose malabsorption. Am J Gastroenterol 86:1771, 1991.

87. Perino LE, Schuffler MD, Mehta SJ, et al: Radiation-induced recurrent intestinal pseudoobstruction. Gastroenterology 91:994, 1986.

88. Husebye E, Hauer-Jensen M, Kjorstad K, Skar V: Severe late radiation enteropathy is characterized by impaired motility of proximal small intestine. Dig Dis Sci 39:2341, 1994.

89. McDonald GB, Schuffler MD, Kadin ME, et al: Intestinal pseudoobstruction caused by diffuse lymphoid infiltration of the small intestine. Gastroenterology 89:882, 1985.

90. De Giorgio R, Barbara G, Stanghellini V, et al: Clinical and morphofunctional features of idiopathic myenteric ganglionitis underlying severe intestinal motor dysfunction: A study of three cases. Am J Gastroenterol 97:2454, 2002.

91. Schobinger-Clement S, Gerber HA, Stallmach T: Autoaggressive inflammation of the myenteric plexus resulting in intestinal pseudoobstruction. Am J Surg Pathol 23:602, 1999.

92. Schappi MG, Smith VV, Milla PJ, Lindley KJ: Eosinophilic myenteric ganglionitis is associated with functional intestinal obstruction. Gut 52:752, 2003.

93. Kamal N, Chami T, Andersen A, et al: Delayed gastrointestinal transit times in anorexia nervosa and bulimia nervosa. Gastroenterology 101:1320, 1991.

94. Vantrappen G, Janssens J, Hellemans J, et al: The interdigestive motor complex of normal subjects and patients with

bacteria overgrowth of the small intestine. J Clin Invest 59:1158, 1977.

95. Valdovinos MA, Camilleri M, Thomforde GM, Frie C: Reduced accuracy of ^{14}C-D-xylose breath test for detecting bacterial overgrowth in gastrointestinal motility disorders. Scand J Gastroenterol 28:963, 1993.

96. Frank JW, Sarr MG, Camilleri M: Use of gastroduodenal manometry to differentiate mechanical and functional intestinal obstruction: an analysis of clinical outcome. Am J Gastroenterol 89:339, 1994.

97. Hinton JM, Lennard-Jones JE, Young AC: A new method for studying gut transit times using radiopaque markers. Gut 10:842, 1969.

98. Metcalf AM, Phillips SF, Zinsmeister AR, et al: Simplified assessment of segmental colonic transit. Gastroenterology 92:40, 1987.

99. Proano M, Camilleri M, Phillips SF, et al: Transit of solids through the human colon: Regional quantification in the unprepared bowel. Am J Physiol 258:G856, 1990.

100. Degen L, Phillips SF: How well does stool form reflect colonic transit? Gut 39:109, 1996.

101. Szurszewski JH: A migrating electric complex of the canine small intestine. Am J Physiol 217:1757, 1969.

102. Summers RW, Anuras S, Green J: Jejunal manometry patterns in health, partial intestinal obstruction, and pseudo-obstruction. Gastroenterology 85:1290, 1983.

103. Reittner P, Goritschnig T, Petritsch W, et al: Multiplanar spiral CT enterography in patients with Crohn's disease using a negative oral contrast material: Initial results of a noninvasive imaging approach. Eur Radiol 12:2253, 2002.

104. Mow WS, Lo SK, Targan SR, et al: Initial experience with wireless capsule enteroscopy in the diagnosis and management of inflammatory bowel disease. Clin Gastroenterol Hepatol 2:31, 2004.

105. Abell TL, Camilleri M, DiMagno EP, et al: Long-term efficacy of oral cisapride in symptomatic upper gut dysmotility. Dig Dis Sci 36:616, 1991.

106. Camilleri M, Balm RK, Zinsmeister AR: Determinants of response to a prokinetic agent in neuropathic chronic intestinal motility disorder. Gastroenterology 106:916, 1994.

107. Camilleri M, Balm RK, Zinsmeister AR: Symptomatic improvement with one-year cisapride treatment in neuropathic chronic intestinal dysmotility. Aliment Pharmacol Ther 10:403, 1996.

108. Foxx-Orenstein A, Camilleri M, Stephens D, Burton D: Effect of a somatostatin analogue on gastric motor and sensory functions in healthy humans. Gut 52:1555, 2003.

109. Freye E, Latasch L: Effects of tramadol and tilidine/naloxone on oral-caecal transit and pupillary light reflex. Arzneimittelforschung 50:24, 2000.

110. Wilder-Smith CH, Hill L, Spargo K, Kalla A: Treatment of severe pain from osteoarthritis with slow-release tramadol or dihydrocodeine in combination with NSAIDs: A randomised study comparing analgesia, antinociception and gastrointestinal effects. Pain 91:23, 2000.

111. Field MJ, Oles RJ, Lewis AS, et al: Gabapentin (Neurontin) and S-(+)-3-isobutylgaba represent a novel class of selective antihyperalgesic agents. Br J Pharmacol 121:1513, 1997.

112. Anuras S, Shirazi S, Faulk DL, et al: Surgical treatment of familial visceral myopathy. Ann Surg 189:306, 1979.

113. Pitt HA, Mann LL, Berquist WE, et al: Chronic intestinal pseudo-obstruction: Management with total parenteral nutrition and a venting enterostomy. Arch Surg 120:614, 1985.

114. Murr MM, Sarr MG, Camilleri M: The surgeon's role in the treatment of chronic intestinal pseudo-obstruction. Am J Gastroenterol 90:2147, 1995.

115. Mughal MM, Irving MH: Treatment of end-stage chronic intestinal pseudo-obstruction by subtotal enterectomy and home parenteral nutrition. Gut 29:1613, 1988.

116. Grant D: Intestinal transplantation: 1997 report of the international registry. Intestinal Transplant Registry. Transplantation 67:1061, 1999.

117. Howard L, Malone M: Current status of home parenteral nutrition in the United States. Transplant Proc 28:2691, 1996.

118. Fishbein TM, Kaufman SS, Florman SS, et al: Isolated intestinal transplantation: Proof of clinical efficacy. Transplantation 76:636, 2003.

119. Madariaga JR, Reyes J, Mazariegos G, et al: The long-term efficacy of multivisceral transplantation. Transplant Proc 32:1219, 2000.

120. Farmer DG, McDiarmid SV, Yersiz H, et al: Improved outcome after intestinal transplantation: An 8-year, single-center experience. Transplant Proc 32:1233, 2000.

121. Younes BS, McDiarmid SV, Martin MG, et al: The effect of immunosuppression on post-transplant lymphoproliferative disease in pediatric liver transplant patients. Transplantation 70:94, 2000.

122. Pappagallo M: Incidence, prevalence, and management of opioid bowel dysfunction. Am J Surg 182:11S, 2001.

123. Behm B, Stollman N: Postoperative ileus: Etiologies and interventions. Clin Gastroenterol Hepatol 1:71, 2003.

124. Taguchi A, Sharma N, Saleem RM, et al: Selective postoperative inhibition of gastrointestinal opioid receptors. N Engl J Med 345:935, 2001.

125. Vanek VW, Al-Salti M: Acute pseudo-obstruction of the colon (Ogilvie's syndrome): An analysis of 400 cases. Dis Colon Rectum 29:203, 1986.

126. Geller A, Petersen BT, Gostout CG: Endoscopic decompression for acute colonic pseudo-obstruction. Gastrointest Endosc 44:144, 1996.

127. Lowman RM, Davis L: An evaluation of cecal size in impending perforation of the cecum. Surg Gynecol Obstet 16:711, 1956.

128. Rodgers A, Walker N, Schug S, et al: Reduction of postoperative mortality and morbidity with epidural or spinal anaesthesia: Results from overview of randomised trials. BMJ 321:1493, 2000.

129. Fukatsu K, Zarzaur BL, Johnson CD, et al: Enteral nutrition prevents remote organ injury and death after a gut ischemic insult. Ann Surg 233:660, 2001.

130. Yuan CS, Foss JF, O'Connor M, et al: Methylnaltrexone for reversal of constipation due to chronic methadone use: A randomized controlled trial. JAMA 283:367, 2000.

131. Liu SS, Hodgson PS, Carpenter RL, et al: ADL 8-2698, a trans-3,4-dimethyl-4-(3-hydroxyphenyl) piperidine, prevents gastrointestinal effects of intravenous morphine without affecting analgesia. Clin Pharmacol Ther 69:66, 2001.

132. Ramage JI, Bharucha AE, Baron TH: Percutaneous endoscopic cecostomy for recurrent Ogilvie's syndrome. Am J Gastroenterol 97:S175, 2002.

CHAPTER

118 Small Intestinal Neoplasms

Anil K. Rustgi

EPIDEMIOLOGY

Benign and malignant neoplasms of the small bowel account for only a small fraction of all gastrointestinal neoplasms. Approximately two thirds of small bowel neoplasms are malignant, but account for only 1.1% to 2.4% of gastrointestinal malignancies. In comparison, approximately 70% of gastrointestinal malignancies originate in the colon and rectum, nearly 11% arise in the esophagus, and about 16% are gastric.[1-5] Fewer than 2500 cases of small bowel cancer are diagnosed annually in the United States, and fewer than 1000 patients succumb to their disease each year.[1-5]

Worldwide, a particularly high-incidence region of small bowel cancer is New Zealand, involving the Maori; low-incidence regions are found in Asia and Africa. Small bowel cancers are more common in males than females; the incidence in males is 0.5 to 1.5/100,000 and in females is 0.2 to 1.0/100,000.[1-6] Small bowel cancers are more common in the elderly population, with most cases occurring after 60 years of age.[1-6] Socioeconomic factors do not appear to play a role in the incidence of small bowel cancer. Small bowel malignancies comprise a wide variety of tumors, 95% of which are adenocarcinomas, carcinoids, lymphomas, and sarcomas.[6,7] Small bowel adenocarcinomas and carcinoids are more common in African Americans than among whites.[4,8] Based on the National Cancer Data Base[9] and the National Cancer Institute's Surveillance, Epidemiology, and End Results Program,[3] adenocarcinoma is the most common small bowel malignancy, with an annual incidence in the United States of 3.9 cases per million persons. Most patients affected with small bowel adenocarcinoma are in their 50s or 60s at the time of diagnosis. Small bowel adenocarcinomas occur throughout the intestine, with

55% found in the duodenum, about 18% in the jejunum, 13% ileum, and the remaining 14% not specified in terms of location.[10,11]

Carcinoids (see Chapter 30) are the second most frequently diagnosed small intestinal malignancy, with an annual incidence of 2.9 cases per million persons in the United States and an average age at diagnosis of 55 to 60 years. The most common sites of extranodal lymphomas are the stomach and small intestine (see Chapter 28). Benign small bowel neoplasms include adenomas, lipomas, and leiomyomas, among others. Table 118–1 provides a listing of benign and malignant small bowel neoplasms.

PATHOLOGY

Neoplasms of the small intestine can arise from any of the cells that make up this organ. Thus, small bowel tumors may be of epithelial or nonepithelial origin. Adenomas and adenocarcinomas are derived from mucosal glands; leiomyomas and leiomyosarcomas arise from smooth muscle; carcinoids arise from argentaffin cells; nerve sheath cells give rise to neurilemmomas and malignant schwannomas; neurons are the cell of origin of neurofibromas and neurofibrosarcomas; hemangiomas and angiosarcomas are derived from the vasculature; fibromas and fibrosarcomas arise from fibroblasts; lymphomas originate from lymphocytes in the mucosa and Peyer's patches; and gastrointestinal stromal tumors (GISTs) are believed to arise from mesenchymal cells in the submucosa.

Adenocarcinomas comprise nearly 35% to 50% of all primary malignant small intestinal neoplasms, followed by carcinoid tumors (20% to 40%), lymphomas (14%), and sarcomas (11% to 13%).[8,9] Small intestinal lymphomas (discussed in Chapter 28) are most common in the terminal ileum; adenocarcinomas more often arise proximally; carcinoid tumors (see Chapter 30) almost always are in the ileum; and sarcomas are distributed evenly throughout the small intestine, with a slight predilection for the jejunum. Approximately 75% of primary small bowel carcinoids are less than 1.5 cm in diameter at the time of diagnosis, and approximately 30% of patients with carcinoid tumors have multifocal disease.

Table 118–1 Some Benign and Malignant Small Intestinal Neoplasms

Benign	Malignant
Adenoma	Adenocarcinoma
Leiomyoma	Carcinoid
Lipoma	Lymphoma
Lymphangioma	Low-grade B cell lymphoma
Fibroma	Immunoproliferative small intestinal neoplasms
Hemangioma	Enteropathy-associated T cell lymphoma
Neurofibroma	Metastatic tumors
Neurilemmoma	Sarcoma
	Leiomyosarcoma
	Liposarcoma
	Fibrosarcoma
	Neurofibrosarcoma
	Angiosarcoma

Table 118–2 Staging of Small Bowel Adenocarcinoma

Stage	Tumor (T)	Node (N)	Metastasis (M)	Percentage of Cases at Presentation
0	Tis	N0	M0	2.7
1	T1/T2	N0	M0	12
2	T3/T4	N0	M0	27
3	Any T	N1	M0	26
4	Any T	Any N	M1	32.3

Tis, tumor in-situ.

Small intestinal cancer is classified further according to the World Health Organization scheme as adenocarcinoma in situ, mucinous (colloid) adenocarcinoma, signet cell carcinoma, squamous cell carcinoma, adenosquamous carcinoma, small cell carcinoma, and undifferentiated carcinoma. Staging of small intestinal cancer is according to the TNM (tumor, lymph node, metastasis) staging system from the American Joint Commission on Cancer and International Union Against Cancer (Table 118–2).

Benign neoplasms may be found throughout the small intestine, but some patterns are apparent. For example, adenomas are distributed evenly throughout the small intestine, although there is a slightly higher frequency of these lesions in the duodenum and ileum. Fibromas and lipomas are more common in the ileum, and 80% to 90% of hemangiomas and neurofibromas are distributed evenly between the jejunum and ileum. Adenomas arise from mucosal glands, and although they begin as sessile growths, they become polypoid in most instances. Adenomas account for approximately one third of all benign small intestinal neoplasms. Adenomas may be divided into tubular, villous, and tubulovillous types on the basis of histologic examination. Villous adenomas are not as common as tubular neoplasms and usually are larger, more often sessile, located in the second portion of the duodenum, and have undergone malignant degeneration at the time of diagnosis in 40% to 45% of cases.

Leiomyomas are benign smooth muscle neoplasms that originate from the smooth muscle wall of the muscularis mucosa or muscularis propria. They account for up to 40% of benign small intestinal neoplasms. Leiomyomas may grow intraluminally, extraluminally, or both. As they grow, leiomyomas may undergo necrosis and hemorrhage, which can be severe at times. Histologically, they comprise bundles of spindle-shaped smooth muscle cells with rare or absent mitoses; more than two mitoses per high-powered field or any nuclear pleomorphism is indicative of a leiomyosarcoma. Lipomas occur most often in the ileum, arise from the submucosa, and tend to grow intraluminally. Lipomas rarely bleed, but if large enough, they may cause intestinal obstruction and intussusception (Fig. 118–1).

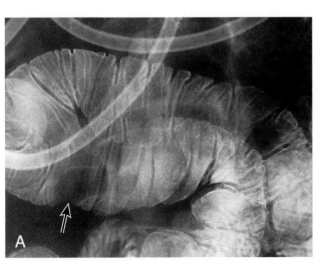
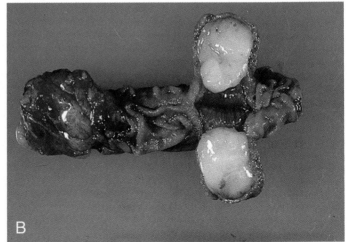

Figure 118–1 *A*, Film from an enteroclysis demonstrating a smooth, submucosal lesion that was found to be lipoma *(arrow)*. *B*, Surgical resection specimen of a lipoma from another patient who presented with intussusception and bleeding. (*A* and *B*, Courtesy of Igor Laufer, MD, Philadelphia, PA.)

ETIOLOGY AND RISK FACTORS

Although the small intestine constitutes nearly 75% of the gastrointestinal tract and approximately 90% of its mucosal surface, only 1% of gastrointestinal adenocarcinomas arise from the small bowel. There is no single hypothesis or set of experimental data to explain the paucity of small bowel adenocarcinomas compared with colonic, gastric, pancreatic, and esophageal adenocarcinomas, which is rather remarkable given the overlapping geographic- and age-related distribution of small bowel and colon cancers. Although speculative, the following notions have been advanced to help explain the low rates of small bowel malignancy[12]:

1. Fewer bacteria, especially anaerobic species, to convert bile acids to carcinogens[13,14]
2. Increased intraluminal pH, which may prevent the formation of nitrosamines that are so evident in the acidic environment of the stomach[15,16]
3. Mucosal hydrolases, such as benzpyrene hydroxylase, which convert potential carcinogens into less carcinogenic moieties[17]
4. Rapid transit through the small bowel, which may limit contact between potential carcinogens and the mucosa[13]
5. Dilution of carcinogens in the liquid chyme of the small intestine
6. Different rates of mucosal cell turnover between the small and large intestines—small intestinal mucosal cells are lost and renewed extremely rapidly, and therefore, cells harboring gene mutations are continually being shed[18,19]
7. Higher concentrations of secretory IgA and mucosal T lymphocytes to provide immune surveillance against abnormal epithelial cells[18]

Experimental evidence supports the notion that the small intestine affords a protective milieu against malignant transformation. For example, in *BDF1* mice, exposure to various carcinogens (e.g., *N*-nitroso-*N*-methylurea [NMU], *N*-nitroso-*N*-ethylurea [NEU], 1-2-dimethylhydrazine [DMH], and *N*-nitrosodimethylamine [NDMA]) incites apoptosis (programmed cell death) in the stem cell compartment of small intestinal crypts, whereas damaged stem cells of colonic crypts survive and proliferate on exposure to the same carcinogens, with only limited apoptosis.[20] Moreover, comparison of specific DNA adducts (a chemical bond between a carcinogen and DNA; adducts reflect DNA damage) from the mucosa of human small intestine and colon obtained at surgery has led to the observation that total DNA adducts are nearly 30 times greater in the colon than in the small intestine.[21,22] DNA adducts are crucial in malignant neoplastic development and progression. It has been noted that in the inbred mouse strain B10.O20, small intestinal adenocarcinomas develop after exposure in utero to NEU, whereas such neoplasms do not develop in other mouse strains. A putative gene that may account for this phenomenon, called *ssicl* (for susceptibility to small intestinal cancer), maps to the distal arm of mouse chromosome 4.[23] The most commonly studied mouse model for small intestinal polyposis is the murine intestinal neoplasia (Min) mouse, a breed that was subjected to chemical mutagens and then crossbred, resulting in a phenotype in which adenomatous polyps in the small intestine developed to a greater extent than did adenomatous polyps in the colon.[24] Min represents the murine ortholog of the APC gene and the phenotype resembles, but does not precisely recapitulate, all aspects of familial adenomatous polyposis (FAP)[25]; in humans with FAP, colonic polyposis predominates and small intestinal neoplasms are less common. Subsequent germline inactivation of the APC gene in embryonic stem cells resulted in mice with more colonic adenomatous polyps, including aberrant crypt foci, although the small intestinal phenotype still predominated.[26,27] Min mice ultimately succumb to anemia from gastrointestinal bleeding. Min mice have been used for the study of chemopreventive strategies with aspirin, nonsteroidal anti-inflammatory drugs, and selective cyclooxygenase-2 inhibitors, although none of these approaches appears to be relevant for small intestinal neoplasms as of yet.[28] Whether chemoprevention may be applicable to ameliorating the number and size of duodenal adenomatous polyps in patients with FAP remains under investigation.

Insights into the pathogenesis of malignant small intestinal neoplasms have been gained through molecular genetic approaches. Detailed analysis of small bowel adenocarcinomas reveals a profile reminiscent of colonic adenocarcinomas. There is activation of oncogenes, inactivation of tumor suppressor genes, and dysregulation of cell cycle proteins. Mutation in the *Ki-ras* oncogene has been described in nearly 40% of small bowel adenocarcinomas. Tumor suppressor gene inactivation, by virtue of mutation or loss of heterozygosity, has been noted in p53 (65%), APC (5%), and p16 (90%).[29-34] Abnormalities also have been noted in the p21 and p27 cyclin-dependent kinase inhibitors. Other genetic abnormalities include increased expression of the erbB2[neu] protein and microsatellite instability (MSI),[35,36] the latter of which is the signature of tumors in hereditary nonpolyposis colorectal cancer (HNPCC). As such, it is likely that the accumulation of genetic alterations promotes transformation of a small bowel adenoma into an adenocarcinoma, as well as growth of the adenocarcinoma itself. GISTs (see Chapter 29) harbor mutations in the *c-kit* oncogene, the functional consequence of which is aberrant cell growth.[37,38] *C-kit*, also designated as *CD117*, is a tyrosine kinase receptor that is overexpressed in GISTs.[38] Rarely, GISTs involve mutations in the platelet-derived growth factor receptor (PDGFR).[39]

SMALL BOWEL ADENOCARCINOMA

Despite the low incidence of malignant small intestinal neoplasms, several factors have been identified that contribute to the development of these tumors (Table 118-3). Small intestinal adenocarcinomas are more common in populations that consume diets high in animal fat and protein.[40,41] There is a twofold increase in the relative risk of small bowel adenocarcinomas in patients who eat red meat at least once a week, although the risk does not increase with further increases in meat intake. There is a correlation between the occurrence of small bowel adenocarcinomas and ingestion of smoked or cured foods, with an odds ratio of 1.7 : 1 if such foods

Table 118–3 Risk Factors for Small Intestinal Tumors

Major	Minor
African American ethnicity	Anal cancer
Male gender	Cholecystectomy
Celiac sprue	High-fat diet
Crohn's disease	Hodgkin's disease
Increasing age	Squamous cell
Inherited adenomatous and	cancer of the
hamartomatous polyposis	skin
syndromes	Wilms' tumor
Familial adenomatous polyposis	
Hereditary nonpolyposis colorectal	
cancer	
Peutz-Jeghers syndrome	

are eaten one to three times per month and an odds ratio of 2.1:1 if they are consumed daily. No association has been observed between the incidence of small intestinal adenocarcinoma and consumption of fruits and vegetables or use of tobacco or alcohol. Several carcinogens, including bracken fern and *N*-methyl-*N*-nitro-*N'*-nitrosoguanidine (MNNG), have been associated with the development of small bowel adenomas and adenocarcinomas in rodent models.[42] Bile acids may play a role in the development of small bowel adenocarcinoma, especially in the duodenum.[43] In patients with FAP, adenomatous polyps develop within the duodenum and around the ampulla of Vater, and adenocarcinoma of the proximal small bowel is the leading cause of cancer death in patients who have undergone colectomy for FAP.[44,45] There may be additive or synergistic effects between bile acids and germline APC mutations to foster the high predilection of duodenal polyps and adenocarcinoma in FAP.

Small bowel adenocarcinomas appear to progress through an adenoma-adenocarcinoma sequence just as colorectal adenocarcinomas, and all small bowel adenomas should be regarded as precancerous.[46] Approximately one third of all spontaneous small bowel adenomas contain a malignant component, although the percentage varies greatly among published studies.[9] Neoplasms located at the ampulla of Vater tend to be larger, are more likely to be villous rather than tubular, and are more likely to undergo malignant transformation than are other small intestinal neoplasms.[47-49] Other etiologic factors (see Table 118–3) for the development of small bowel adenocarcinomas are Crohn's disease (see Chapter 108),[50-52] celiac sprue (see Chapter 101),[53] and HNPCC (see Chapter 119), the latter of which is associated with MSI.[54]

Patients with Peutz-Jeghers (PJ) syndrome develop hamartomatous polyps in the small intestine and colon in addition to the hallmark orocutaneous melanin spots (see Chapter 119).[55] These polyps are especially common in the jejunum, and adenocarcinoma can arise within adenomatous foci in the hamartoma. Mutations in the *LKB1* gene, which encodes a serine threonine kinase, fosters the development of such polyps, a concept that has been investigated in cell culture and mouse models.[56-59] Other hamartomatous polyposis syndromes (see Chapter 119) include juvenile polyposis, Cowden's

syndrome, Bannayan-Ruvalcaba-Riley syndrome, Devon family syndrome, and Cronkhite-Canada syndrome; all of these may be associated with a variety of polyps in the small bowel, although without increased risk of small bowel malignancy.

CLINICAL FEATURES

Most neoplasms of the small intestine are not associated with symptoms and are diagnosed either late in their course or incidentally at laparotomy or autopsy. The general absence of symptoms can be ascribed to the distensibility of the small bowel wall and the liquid nature of its luminal contents. If a lesion (or lesions) lead(s) to symptoms, the presentation depends upon the pathology of the neoplasm and its location. At least 50% of benign lesions remain asymptomatic, whereas 70% to 90% of malignant lesions are associated with symptoms. No symptoms or signs are specific for either benign or malignant tumors, however, and even though the duration of symptoms tends to be shorter for patients with a malignancy than for those with benign lesions, months may elapse before the diagnosis is made.

If a lesion becomes large enough, a patient may present with cramping periumbilical pain, bloating, and nausea with emesis resulting from mechanical small bowel obstruction. Small bowel obstruction is the most common presentation for benign lesions and occurs in as many as 70% of such cases. Obstruction may result from either luminal constriction or intussusception. In fact, a benign small bowel neoplasm is the most common cause of intussusception in adults. Whereas adenomas, adenocarcinomas, and lymphomas tend to grow into the lumen, they may grow through the submucosa and muscle, often becoming large before a diagnosis is made; these lesions also may cause volvulus. As many as 80% of malignant tumors are associated with abdominal pain, although the pain is not caused by obstruction. Back pain in a patient with a primary malignant small bowel lesion suggests spread to the retroperitoneum. Mechanisms of back pain include hemorrhage into the tumor, invasion of enteric ganglia, ischemia, and serosal involvement.

Gastrointestinal bleeding, usually chronic, is the second most common symptom of neoplasms of the small intestine. Bleeding occurs in 20% to 50% of patients with benign lesions (e.g., leiomyomas) and, less commonly, in patients with malignant lesions. Massive hemorrhage is more common with sarcomas (e.g., GISTs) than it is with carcinomas, carcinoid tumors, or lymphomas. Weight loss is rare in patients with benign lesions, but, along with anorexia, is noted in 50% of patients with malignancies. Intestinal perforation also is rare in patients with benign lesions but occurs in 10% of patients with sarcomas and lymphomas. Periampullary lesions may result in jaundice or pancreatitis. In patients with carcinoid tumors, symptoms of the carcinoid syndrome typically do not develop in the absence of hepatic metastases, and, even with hepatic lesions, 28% to 50% of patients with such tumors remain free of the carcinoid syndrome (see Chapter 30).

The physical examination may not reveal small intestinal malignancies, although up to 25% of such patients may have a palpable abdominal mass. Twenty-five percent of patients with malignancy also may present with the findings of obstruction-distention, borborygmi, a palpable mass, and diffuse mild-to-moderate abdominal tenderness. Some patients may have a positive fecal occult blood test, although the incidence of this positivity is highly variable and ranges from 10% to 70%; other patients may present with jaundice secondary to either biliary obstruction or hepatic replacement by metastases. Cachexia, hepatomegaly, and ascites may be present in patients with advanced metastatic disease.

DIAGNOSIS

Laboratory studies are of limited utility in the diagnosis of neoplasms of the small intestine, especially in patients with localized disease. In patients with gastrointestinal blood loss, microcytic anemia eventually develops. Patients with biliary tract compromise have elevated serum alkaline phosphatase and bilirubin levels, and those with extensive hepatic disease have elevated lactate dehydrogenase and aminotransferase levels and decreased serum albumin levels. The only tumor marker that has been evaluated routinely in patients with neoplasms of the small intestine, especially in those with adenocarcinoma, is serum carcinoembryonic antigen; the level of carcinoembryonic antigen usually is not elevated in the absence of hepatic metastases. Similarly, for patients with carcinoid tumors, 5-hydroxyindole acetic acid is a useful marker, but it is cleared by the liver after the first pass from the primary tumor and levels in urine are not elevated until hepatic metastases are extensive. There are specific immunoperoxidase (staining) and cell surface (flow cytometry) markers for lymphomas. Abdominal plain films usually are nondiagnostic, although in patients with an acute presentation they may reveal bowel obstruction or free air. Barium contrast studies, including an upper gastrointestinal series with a small bowel follow-through (SBFT) remain the primary radiologic means of diagnosing small bowel neoplasms,[60] although increasing interest is being directed to capsule endoscopy (see later). The upper gastrointestinal series with SBFT is abnormal in approximately 50% to 80% of patients with small bowel neoplasms and can define the neoplasm in 30% to 44% of cases; this figure increases to 90% if an enteroclysis study (small bowel enema) is performed.[61] Barium enema may demonstrate lesions in the distal and terminal ileum if there is sufficient reflux of contrast through the ileocecal valve.

Small bowel adenocarcinomas produce intraluminal lesions, often with an "apple-core" appearance similar to that seen with colorectal carcinomas, and with ulceration; an apple-core lesion also may be seen with metastatic carcinoma (Fig. 118-2). Sarcomas tend to produce an intraluminal "bulge," with intact overlying mucosa and a large extraluminal component that displaces loops of bowel. A carcinoid tumor can have the appearance of focal mural nodularity, typically in the distal ileum, however, progressive disease is associated with fixation of bowel loops and loss of the normal mucosal pattern, which may be from fibrosis or ischemic injury and which may mimic Crohn's disease. Lymphomas may demon-

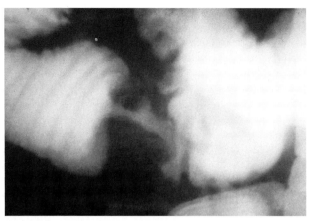

Figure 118-2 Film from a small bowel follow through demonstrating an "apple-core" appearance caused by a metastatic lesion to the small intestine from a scirrhous gastric cancer. (Courtesy of Igor Laufer, MD, Philadelphia, PA.)

strate a variety of appearances, including multiple nodules or polyps, a spruelike pattern, or intraluminal or extraluminal masses possibly with fistula formation. Benign lesions typically appear as submucosal filling defects.

Abdominal computed tomography (CT) facilitates localization of small bowel abnormalities and is especially useful for detecting extraluminal disease; it is suboptimal, however, for detecting small intraluminal or mucosal lesions. Ultrasound and magnetic resonance imaging do not have major roles in the diagnosis of small bowel lesions. Angiography is of limited value except for delineating lesions with a vascular component and for localizing a site of severe hemorrhage. A technetium-labeled red blood cell scan also may be helpful in locating the source of active gastrointestinal bleeding but alone cannot diagnose the presence of a neoplasm.

Endoscopic evaluation usually is limited to the duodenum, which may be visualized through either a forward- or side-viewing endoscope; the terminal ileum may be visualized via colonoscopy. Small bowel enteroscopy is helpful as an adjunct to barium studies and particularly is useful in the evaluation of patients with gastrointestinal bleeding caused by a benign or malignant small bowel tumor. Intraoperative enteroscopy may be useful in selected cases. Although gaining popularity in the diagnosis of small bowel Crohn's disease and mucosal vascular lesions as a cause of gastrointestinal bleeding,[62] swallowed radiotelemetry videocapsules also may be useful to transmit images of benign or malignant bowel wall lesions (Fig. 118-3); Benign lesions now are the second most common cause of diagnosed gastrointestinal bleeding on capsule endoscopy.

TREATMENT

BENIGN NEOPLASMS

Therapy of benign neoplasms of the small intestine usually consists of resection, either via an endoscope or at laparotomy, as determined by the size, growth pattern, and location of the lesion. Most adenomas may be adequately removed at surgery by segmental resection, although if there is any evidence of malignant degeneration, the margins of resection should be extended and draining lymph nodes should be excised. Pedunculated duodenal adenomas may be snared through the endoscope and removed. Endoscopic mucosal resection has

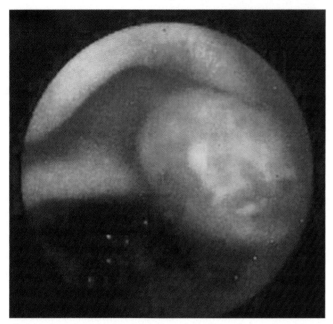

Figure 118–3 Capsule endoscopy view of an ulcerated mass in a patient who presented with gastrointestinal bleeding. Four ulcerated, bleeding masses were found throughout the small bowel; these were confirmed at surgery and found to be sarcomas. (Courtesy of Ann Marie Joyce, MD, Philadelphia, PA.)

been used to remove sessile duodenal adenomas. If an adenoma involves the ampulla, it may be necessary to perform a sphincterotomy or sphincteroplasty before surgery for diagnosis and for biliary/pancreatic decompression or after local resection to reduce the risk of postoperative stricture formation. Larger periampullary or ampullary lesions, which are more likely to harbor malignancy, may require pancreaticoduodenectomy (Whipple's procedure), the decision for which is facilitated by histopathology of frozen sections. Patients must undergo periodic surveillance following removal of an adenoma, especially if it is a villous adenoma, because there is a significant chance of recurrence; however, survival is excellent for these patients. Endoscopic ultrasound (EUS) is a useful technique to diagnose ampullary adenomas and for surveillance as well. EUS can detect small ampullary tumors and can reveal invasion into contiguous structures, adjacent lymph nodes, and vascular invasion.[63]

EUS also is helpful in discerning whether submucosal lesions are benign or malignant and to define the size, growth pattern, and blood supply of a mucosal or submucosal lesion; leiomyomas and GISTs can be differentiated by fine-needle aspiration and staining for *c-kit*, for example (Fig. 118–4). The polyps of PJ syndrome may be managed by either endoscopic or surgical resection. Hemangiomas and leiomyomas are best approached by segmental resection, if possible.

MALIGNANT NEOPLASMS

Adenocarcinomas

In many patients, a preoperative diagnosis is made endoscopically, and most patients undergo surgical explo-

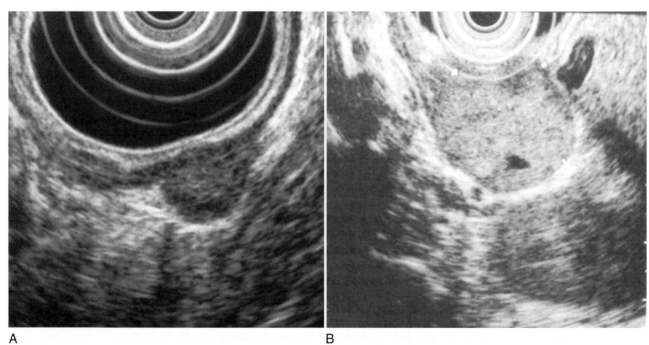

A   B

Figure 118–4 *A*, Endoscopic ultrasonography in two patients with a gastrointestinal stromal tumor (GIST). *A*, A benign GIST appears as small (<3 cm), homogeneous, hypoechoic lesion arising, most commonly, within and contained within the muscularis propria layer. *B*, A malignant GIST appears as large (>3 cm), inhomogeneous lesions arising within the muscularis propria and with possible extension into other wall layers and surrounding structures. (*A* and *B*, Courtesy of Gregory Ginsberg, MD, Philadelphia, PA.)

ration and resection. Patients whose primary lesions arise in the first or second portion of the duodenum usually are treated by pancreaticoduodenectomy, although there is no evidence that the outcome with this procedure, when it is technically feasible, is superior to that with segmental resection. Segmental resection usually is sufficient for patients with tumors arising from the third and fourth portions of the duodenum. Even when faced with large tumors and positive lymph nodes, surgeons typically resect the lesion to provide symptomatic relief. Segmental resection is associated with low postoperative morbidity and good long-term outcome. Operative mortality rates have improved over the last decade and are under 5%. Patients with jejunal or ileal tumors tend to undergo cancer-directed surgery.

Prognosis of intestinal adenocarcinoma is determined by resectability, pathologic status of the resection margins, histologic grade, and presence or absence of lymph node involvement. The overall 5-year survival rate ranges from 20% to 35%.[64] In one series of 67 patients, the 5-year survival rate for patients who underwent resection was 54%. Further analysis demonstrated that patients with tumor limited to the mucosa and submucosa had a 5-year survival rate of 100%, whereas 5-year survival rates for patients with disease extending to the serosa, regional lymph nodes, or distant sites were 52%, 45%, and 0%, respectively.[63] In a separate study, patients with favorable prognostic features of negative lymph nodes and negative surgical margins, well-differentiated or moderately differentiated histologic grade, and a primary lesion limited to the duodenum or ampulla had an actuarial 5-year survival rate of 80%, whereas patients who lacked these features had a 5-year survival rate of 38%.[64] Furthermore, although postoperative radiation therapy to the tumor bed increased local control of tumor, such therapy did not enhance survival, because patients still succumbed to distant metastatic disease.

The jejunum and ileum are the sites involved in more than 50% of cases of adenocarcinoma of the small intestine. Most of these tumors are technically resectable, although lymph node metastases are common and therefore resection for cure may not be possible. As for more proximal lesions, the overall 5-year survival rate is 20% to 30%. Prognostic factors are similar to those for duodenal lesions; 5-year survival rates are 45% to 70% in patients with negative lymph nodes but only 12% to 14% in those with lymph node involvement.[65]

Although some patients may benefit from adjuvant therapy, the benefit of routine adjuvant chemotherapy or radiation therapy, or both, has yet to be confirmed[66]; 5-fluorouracil, doxorubicin, and mitomycin C are employed in the adjuvant setting and also for unresectable tumors.[67] Radiation therapy is fraught with the side effects caused by radiation-induced enteritis (see Chapter 38). Future directions may involve the correlation of genetic and biochemical abnormalities in tumors, with stratification of patients to different therapeutic modalities.[68]

It is conceivable that functional genomics and proteomics may lead to the identification of new biomarkers for small bowel malignancies, thereby permitting earlier detection, monitoring of recurrent disease, and the development of new therapeutics. Such strategies are investigational currently, and it is likely lessons will be acquired from similar approaches in other gastrointestinal cancers and applied to neoplasms of the small intestine.

Sarcomas

Both genetic and environmental factors predispose to gastrointestinal sarcomas. Patients with neurofibromatosis (heritable neurofibromas accompanied by germline *NF1* mutations), and Li-Fraumeni syndrome (heritable breast cancers and sarcomas accompanied by germline *p53* tumor suppressor gene mutations) are at increased risk for sarcomas. Patients with FAP are predisposed to desmoid tumors that can invade the small bowel. Environmental risk factors include exposure to radiation, thoratrast, estrogens, anabolic steroids, and insecticides. Of all gastrointestinal sarcomas, nearly 30% occur in the small bowel (60% to 70% occur in the stomach). Nonspecific symptoms may occur, and advanced stages are associated with abdominal pain or obstruction and gastrointestinal bleeding. Diagnosis is facilitated by barium studies, abdominal CT scan, capsule enteroscopy, and EUS (for proximal duodenal sarcomas).

Sarcomas in the small bowel (as throughout the gastrointestinal tract) include GISTs, gastrointestinal autonomic nerve tumors, leiomyosarcomas (most common small bowel sarcoma), liposarcomas, malignant fibrous histiocytoma, angiosarcomas, and Kaposi's sarcomas. The subset of sarcomas that lack S-100, express CD34 (a hematopoietic stem cell marker), and *CD117* (*c-kit*) are called *GISTs*. *C-kit* mutations in the protein's juxtamembrane domain are found in 60% of GISTs and are associated with higher-grade tumors with more frequent recurrences and higher mortality than when *c-kit* is absent. *C-kit* mutations confer a growth advantage to the cell harboring such mutations. Age, mitotic index, and size are independent prognostic factors; gastric location, size (<5 cm), low mitotic count, and proliferative index are favorable prognostic variables. Leiomyosarcomas display smooth muscle differentiation, for example, expression of muscle-specific antigen (HHF-35), desmin, or actin; lack of CD117 also is characteristic. Due to differences in immunocytochemical markers, it may be better to classify small bowel sarcomas as leiomyosarcomas with smooth muscle markers, GISTs, sarcomas with neurologic markers, and other less common lesions. Gross inspection cannot distinguish a benign from a malignant smooth muscle neoplasm, so if any such neoplasm is to be operated on, wide excision is required. Lymph node resection, however, usually is not necessary for leiomyosarcomas because they metastasize only rarely to lymph nodes. Hence, most of these tumors can be resected. The 5-year survival rate is approximately 50%, and the major prognostic variables include tumor grade and surgical resectability.[69-72] Even with extensive disease, resection or bypass may offer considerable palliation. Rarely, isolated hepatic metastases are found and may be resected or embolized. Resection of isolated pulmonary disease may result in a 5-year survival rate of 20%. Five- and 10-year survival data for patients who underwent palliative resection are 25% and 6%, respectively. In comparison, 5- and 10-year survival data for patients who had resections with curative intent are 50% and 35%, respectively. No benefit has been demonstrated yet for either adjuvant chemotherapy or radiation therapy. For patients with unresectable disease, doxorubicin-based regimens offer the best tumor response, although the median duration of the benefit is short, and the prognosis remains poor.

Imatinib (Gleevec), a protein tyrosine kinase inhibitor targeted originally to the PDGFR, inhibits *c-kit* and the tyrosine kinase fusion protein product of *Bcr-Abl*, which is involved in the pathogenesis of chronic myeloid leukemia (CML). Originally approved for CML, where imatinib was found to normalize leukocyte and platelet counts in more than 80% of patients in a trial of 700 patients,[73] imatinib was approved in 2002 for unresectable and metastatic GISTs.[74] Administered orally, imatinib is well tolerated with minimal nausea, vomiting, edema, and diarrhea. A phase 2 trial evaluated nearly 150 patients with unresectable or metastatic GISTs[74] and found that tumors were reduced dramatically in 54% of patients and remained stable in 28% of patients.

Lymphomas and Carcinoids

For a discussion of the management of lymphomas and carcinoids, see Chapters 28 and 30.

Metastatic Cancer

Despite the rarity of primary small intestinal malignancies, the small bowel frequently is involved by metastatic disease. Metastatic lesions may produce symptoms of intestinal obstruction as well as bleeding and abdominal

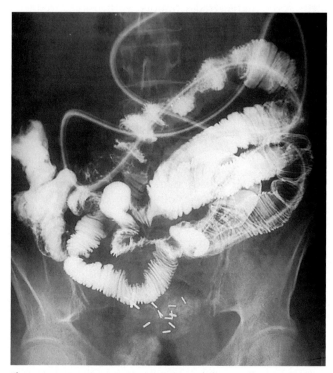

Figure 118–5 Contrast examination of the small intestine in a patient with partial small bowel obstruction and extensive extramucosal disease caused by metastatic lung cancer. Contrast has been delivered through a Miller-Abbot tube (Courtesy of Igor Laufer, MD, Philadelphia, PA.)

pain. The primary tumor that most often metastasizes to the small intestine is melanoma; 60% of patients with melanoma have metastases in the gastrointestinal tract. Virtually any other extra-abdominal or intra-abdominal malignancy (e.g., lung, breast, colon, stomach) may metastasize or extend directly to the small bowel (Fig. 118–5), and palliative resection may be considered in any but the most advanced cases. Systemic therapy may be offered if effective chemotherapy exists for the primary lesion; however, survival rates for these patients are poor because of the extensive tumor burden.

REFERENCES

1. Neugut AI, Marvin MR, Rella VA, et al: An overview of adenocarcinoma of the small intestine. Oncology 11:529, 1997.
2. Neugut AI, Jacobson JS, Suh S, et al: The epidemiology of cancer of the small intestine. Cancer Epidemiol Biomarkers Prev 7:243, 1998.
3. Chow JS, Chen CC, Ahsan H, et al: A population-based study of the incidence of malignant small bowel tumors: SEER, 1973-1990. Int J Epidemiol 25:722, 1996.
4. DiSario JA, Burt RW, Vargas H, et al: Small bowel cancer: Epidemiological and clinical characteristics from a population-based registry. Am J Gastroenterol 89:699, 1994.
5. Bhutani MS, Gopalswamy N: A multicenter experience in the United States with primary malignant tumors of the small intestine. Am J Gastroenterol 89:460, 1994.
6. Parkin DM, Whelan SL, Ferlay J, et al (eds): Cancer Incidence in Five Continents, Vol VII. Lyon, France, IARC Scientific Publications, 1997, p 143.
7. Severson RK, Schenk M, Gurney JG: Increasing incidence of adenocarcinomas and carcinoid tumors of the small intestine in adults. Cancer Epidemiol Biomarkers Prev 5:81, 1996.
8. Weiss NS, Yang C: Incidence of histologic types of cancer of the small intestine. J Natl Cancer Inst 78:653, 1987.
9. Howe JR, Karnell LH, Scott-Conner C: Adenocarcinoma of the small bowel. Cancer 86:2693, 1999.
10. North JH, Pack MS: Malignant tumors of the small intestine: A review of 144 cases. Am Surg 66:46, 2000.
11. Lowenfels AB, Sonni A: Distribution of small bowel tumors. Cancer Lett 3:83, 1997.
12. Chow WH, Linet MS, McLaughlin JK, et al: Risk factors for small intestine cancer. Cancer Causes Control 4:163, 1993.
13. Hill MJ, Drasar BS, Hawksworth G, et al: Bacteria and aetiology of cancer of the large bowel. Lancet 1:95, 1971.
14. Laquer GL: Carcinogenetic effects of cyad meal and cycasin in germ-free rats. Fed Proc 23:1386, 1964.
15. Potten CS: Clonogenic, stem and carcinogen-target cells in small intestine. Scand J Gastroenterol 104(Suppl):3, 1984.
16. Potten CS: The significance of spontaneous and induced apoptosis in the gastrointestinal tract of mice. Cancer Metastasis Rev 11:179, 1992.
17. Wartenberg LW: Carcinogen detoxifying mechanisms in the gastrointestinal tract. Gastroenterology 51:932, 1996.
18. Boyle WJ, Brenner DA: Molecular and cellular biology of the small intestine. Curr Opin Gastroentrol 11:121, 1995.
19. Bieganski T: Biochemical, physiological and pathophysiological aspects of intestinal diamine oxidase. Acta Physiol Pol 34:139, 1983.
20. Kim SH, Roth KA, Moser AR, et al: Transgenic mouse models that explore the multistep hypothesis of intestinal neoplasia. J Cell Biol 123:877, 1993.
21. Potten CS, Li YQ, O'Connor PJ, Winton DJ: A possible explanation for the differential cancer incidence in the intestine,

based on distribution of the cytotoxic effects of carcinogens in the murine large bowel. Carcinogenesis 12:2305, 1992.

22. Hamada K, Umemoto A, Kajikawa A, et al: Mucosa specific DNA adducts in human small intestine: A comparison with the colon. Carcinogenesis 15:2677, 1994.

23. Fineman RJA, Demant P: A gene for susceptibility to small intestinal cancer, *ssic1*, maps to the distal part of mouse chromosome 4. Cancer Res 55:3179, 1995.

24. Moser AR, Pitot HC, Dove WF: A dominant mutation that predisposes to multiple intestinal neoplasia in the mouse. Science 247:322, 1990.

25. Su LK, Kinzler KW, Vogelstein B, et al: Multiple intestinal neoplasia caused by a mutation in the murine homolog of the *APC* gene. Science 256:668, 1992.

26. Fodde R, Edelmann W, Yang K, et al: A targeted chain-termination mutation in the mouse *Apc* gene results in multiple intestinal tumors. Proc Natl Acad Sci U S A 91:8969, 1994.

27. Smits R, Kielman MF, Breukel C, et al: Apc1638T—a mouse model delineating critical domains of the adenomatous polyposis coli protein involved in tumorigenesis and development. Genes Dev 13:1309, 1999.

28. Oshima M, Dinchuk JE, Kargman SL, et al: Suppression of intestinal polyposis in *Apc* delta716 knockout mice by inhibition of cyclooxygenase 2 (COX-2). Cell 87:803, 1996.

29. Arber N, Shapira I, Ratan J, et al: Activation of c-K-*ras* mutations in human gastrointestinal tumors. Gastroenterology 118:1045, 2000.

30. Rashid A, Hamilton SR: Genetic alterations in sporadic and Crohn's-associated adenocarcinomas of the small intestine. Gastroenterology 113:123, 1997.

31. Arber N, Hibshoosh H, Yasui W, et al: Abnormalities in the expression of cell cycle related proteins in tumors on the small bowel. Cancer Epidemiol Biomarkers Prev 12:1101, 1999.

32. Sellner F: Investigation on the significance of the adenoma-carcinoma sequence in the small bowel. Cancer. 66:702, 1990.

33. Trejo LE, Shaked M, Hibshoosh H, et al: Cell cycle abnormalities in small bowel tumors in Israel. Gastroenterology 118:1546, 2000.

34. Zhu L, Kim K, Domenico R, et al: Adenocarcinoma of duodenum and ampulla of Vater: Clinicopathology study and expression of p53, c-neu, TGF-alpha, CEA, and EMA. J Surg Oncol 61:100, 1996.

35. Hibi K, Kondo K, Akiyama S, et al: Frequent genetic instability in small intestine carcinomas. Jpn J Cancer Res 61:698, 1995.

36. Keller G, Rotter M, Vogelstein H, et al: Microsatellite instability in adenocarcinomas of the upper gastrointestinal tract. Am J Pathol 14:593, 1995.

37. Hirota S, Isozaki K, Moriyama Y, et al: Gain-of-function mutations of *c-kit* in human gastrointestinal stromal tumors. Science 279:577, 1998.

38. Nakahara M, Isozaki K, Hirota S, et al: A novel gain-of-function mutation of *c-kit* gene in gastrointestinal stromal tumors. Gastroenterology 115:1090, 1998.

39. Chompret A, Kannengiesser C, Barrois M, et al: PDGFRA germline mutation in a family with multiple cases of gastrointestinal stromal tumor. Gastroenterology 126:318, 2004.

40. Negri E, Bosetti C, La Vecchia C, et al: Risk factors for adenocarcinoma of the small intestine. Int J Cancer 82:171, 1999.

41. Chow WH, Linet MS, McLaughlin JK, et al: Risk factors for small intestine cancer. Cancer Causes Control 4:164, 1993.

42. Martin MS, Martin F, Justabo E, et al: Susceptibility of inbred rats to gastric and duodenal carcinomas induced by *N*-methyl-*N*-nitro-*N'*-nitrosoguanidine. J Natl Cancer Inst 53:837, 1974.

43. Ross RK, Hartnett NM, Bernstein L, et al: Epidemiology of adenocarcinomas of the small intestine: Is bile a small bowel carcinogen? Br J Cancer 63:143, 1991.

44. Spigelman AD, Talbot IC, Penna C, et al: Evidence for adenoma-carcinoma sequence in the duodenum of patients with familial adenomatous polyposis. J Clin Pathol 47:709, 1994.

45. Offerhaus GJA, Giardiello FM, Krush AJ, et al: The risk of upper gastrointestinal cancer in familial adenomatous polyposis. Gastroenterology 102:1980, 1993.

46. Rose DM, Hochwald SN, Klimstra DS, et al: Primary duodenal adenocarcinoma: A ten-year experience with 79 patients. J Am Coll Surg 182:89, 1996.

47. Wilson JM, Melvin DB, Gray GF: Primary malignancies of the small bowel: A report of 96 cases and a review of the literature. Ann Surg 180:175, 1974.

48. Shulten MF, Dyesu R, Beal JM: Villous adenoma of the duodenum: A case report and review of the literature. Am J Surg 130:90, 1976.

49. Bremer EH, Battaile WG, Bulle PH: Villous adenoma of the upper gastrointestinal tract: Clinical review and report of a case. Am J Gastroenterol 50:135, 1968.

50. Sigel JE, Petras RE, Lashner BA, et al: Intestinal adenocarcinoma in Crohn's disease. Am J Surg Pathol 23:651, 1999.

51. Munkholm P, Langholz E, Davidsen M, et al: Intestinal cancer risk and mortality in patients with Crohn's disease. Gastroenterology 105:1716, 1993.

52. Lewis JD, Deren JJ, Lichtenstein GR: Cancer risks in patients with inflammatory bowel disease. Gastroenterol Clin North Am 28:459, 1999.

53. Pricolo VE, Mangi AA, Aswad B, et al: Gastrointestinal malignancies in patients with celiac sprue. Am J Surg 176:344, 1998.

54. Rodriguez-Bigas MA, Vasen HFA, Lynch HT, et al: Characteristics of small bowel carcinoma in hereditary nonpolyposis colorectal cancer. Cancer 83:240, 1998.

55. Hizawa K, Iida M, Matsumoto T, et al: Neoplastic transformation arising in Peutz-Jeghers polyposis. Dis Colon Rectum 36:953, 1993.

56. Ylikorkala A, Rossi DJ, Korsisaari N, et al: Vascular abnormalities and deregulation of VEGF in Lkb1-deficient mice. Science 293:1323, 2001.

57. Miyoshi H, Nakau M, Ishikawa TO, et al: Gastrointestinal hamartomatous polyposis in Lkb1 heterozygous knockout mice. Cancer Res 62:2261, 2002.

58. Bardeesy N, Sinha M, Hezel AF, et al: Loss of the Lkb1 tumour suppressor provokes intestinal polyposis but resistance to transformation. Nature 419:162, 2002.

59. Nakau M, Miyoshi H, Seldin MF, et al: Hepatocellular carcinoma caused by loss of heterozygosity in *Lkb1* gene knockout mice. Cancer Res 62:4549, 2002.

60. Ekberg O, Ekholm S: Radiography in primary tumors of the small bowel. Acta Radiol 21:79, 1980.

61. Maglinte DDT, Hall R, Miller RE, et al: Detection of surgical lesions of the small bowel by enteroclysis. Am J Surg 147:225, 1984.

62. Costamagna G, Shah SK, Riccioni ME, et al: A prospective trial comparing small bowel radiographs and video capsule endoscopy for suspected small bowel disease. Gastroenterology 123:999, 2002.

63. Tio TL, Mulder CJ, Eggink WF: Endosonography in staging early carcinoma of the ampulla of Vater. Gastroenterology 102:1392, 1992.

64. Veyrieres M, Paillet P, Hay JM: Factors influencing long-term survival in 100 cases of small intestine primary adenocarcinoma. Am J Surg 173:237, 1997.

65. Lai ECS, Doty JE, Irving C, Tompkins RK: Primary adenocarcinoma of the duodenum: Analysis of survival. World J Surg 12:695, 1988.

66. Barnes G Jr, Romero L, Hess KR, Curley SA: Primary adenocarcinoma of the duodenum: Management and survival in 67 patients. Ann Surg Oncol 1:73, 1994.

67. Crawey C, Ross P, Norman A, et al: The royal Marsden experience of small bowel adenocarcinoma treated with protracted venous infusion 5-fluorouracil. Br J Cancer 78:508, 1998.

68. Arber N, Hibshoosh H, Yasui W, et al: Abnormalities in the expression of cell cycle-related proteins in tumors of the small bowel. Cancer Epidemiol Biomarkers Prev 12:1101, 1999.

69. Conlon KC, Casper ES, Brennan MF: Primary gastrointestinal sarcomas: Analysis of prognostic variables. Ann Surg Oncol 2:26, 1995.

70. DeMatteo RP, Lewis JJ, Leung D, et al: Two hundred gastrointestinal stromal tumors: Recurrence patterns and prognostic factors for survival. Ann Surg 231:51, 2000.

71. Mudan SS, Conlon KC, Woodruff JM, et al: Salvage surgery for patients with recurrent gastrointestinal sarcoma: Prognostic factors to guide patient selection. Cancer 88:66, 2000.

72. Dougherty MJ, Compton C, Talbert M, Wood WC: Sarcomas of the gastrointestinal tract: Separation into favorable and unfavorable prognostic groups by mitotic count. Ann Surg 214:569, 1991.

73. Kantarijan H, Sawyers C, Hochhaus A, et al: Hematologic and cytogenetic responses to imatinib mesylate in chronic myelogenous leukemia. N Engl J Med 346:645, 2002.

74. Demetri GD, Mehren M, Blanke CD, et al: Efficacy and safety of imatinib mesylate in advanced gastrointestinal stromal tumors. N Engl J Med 347:472, 2002.

CHAPTER
119 Colonic Polyps and Polyposis Syndromes

Steven H. Itzkowitz and Jeremy Rochester

A gastrointestinal polyp is a discrete mass of tissue that protrudes into the lumen of the bowel. A polyp may be characterized by its gross appearance according to the presence or absence of a stalk, its overall size, and whether it is one of multiple similar masses occurring elsewhere in the gastrointestinal tract. Regardless of these features, however, specific definition rests on the histologic characteristics.

Because of their protrusion into the bowel lumen and the stresses of the fecal stream to which they are exposed, polyps may cause symptoms: they may ulcerate and bleed; abdominal pain may result when a peristaltic wave propels a polyp downstream, thereby stretching its blood supply and nerve fibers; and large polyps rarely may even obstruct the intestine. Symptomatic polyps are uncommon, and the greatest concern with polyps is their potential to become malignant. The bulk of evidence supports the hypothesis that most colonic cancers arise within previously benign adenomatous polyps. Only a small percentage of all colonic adenomas progress to carcinoma, however, and because colonic polyps are so common in the industrialized world, universal detection and removal pose practical and economic problems. To manage colonic polyps appropriately, therefore, the physician must understand the differences in pathogenesis and natural history of the distinct pathologic categories of these lesions.

COLONIC POLYPS

Colonic polyps may be divided into two major groups: neoplastic (the adenomas and carcinomas) and nonneoplastic (Table 119–1). The adenomas and carcinomas share a common characteristic—cellular dysplasia—but they may be subdivided according to the relative contribution of certain microscopic features. The nonneoplastic polyps may be grouped into several distinct categories, including hyperplastic polyps, "mucosal polyps," juvenile polyps, inflammatory polyps, and others. Submucosal lesions also may impart a polypoid appearance to the overlying mucosa and therefore are briefly mentioned even though they are not true polyps.

NEOPLASTIC (ADENOMATOUS AND MALIGNANT POLYPS)

Pathology

Histologic Features

Adenomatous polyps are tumors of benign neoplastic epithelium that may either be pedunculated (i.e., attached by a stalk) or sessile (i.e., attached by a broad base with little or no stalk). The neoplastic nature of adenomas is apparent by histologic examination of their glandular architecture. *Tubular adenomas* are the most common subgroup and are characterized by a complex network of branching adenomatous glands (Fig. 119–1*A*). In *villous adenomas*, the adenomatous glands extend straight down from the surface to the center of the polyp, thereby creating long, finger-like projections (see Fig. 119–1*B*). *Tubulovillous* (villoglandular) *adenomas* manifest a combination of these two histologic types. A polyp is assigned a histologic type on the basis of its predominant glandular pattern, and in practice, pure villous adenomas are quite rare. According to the World Health Organization, adenomas are classified as *tubular* if at least 80% of the glands are of the branching, tubule type and as *villous* if at least 80% of the glands are villiform.[1] Tubular ade-

Table 119–1 Classification of Colorectal Polyps

Neoplastic Mucosal Polyps
Benign (adenoma)
  Serrated
  Tubular
  Tubulovillous
  Villous
Malignant (carcinoma)
  Noninvasive
    Carcinoma in situ
    Intramucosal
  Invasive
Non-neoplastic Mucosal Polyps
Hyperplastic
Mucosal polyp (normal mucosa in a polypoid configuration)
Juvenile (retention)
Peutz-Jeghers
Inflammatory
Submucosal Lesions
Colitis cystica profunda
Pneumatosis cystoides intestinalis
Lymphoid polyp (benign and malignant)
Lipoma
Carcinoid
Metastatic neoplasms
Other lesions

nomas account for 80% to 86% of adenomatous polyps, tubulovillous for 8% to 16%, and villous adenomas for 3% to 16%.[2,3] Tubular adenomas usually are small and exhibit mild dysplasia, whereas villous architecture is more often encountered in large adenomas and tends to be associated with more severe degrees of dysplasia (Table 119–2).

By definition, all colorectal adenomas are dysplastic. Adenomatous epithelium is characterized by abnormal cellular differentiation and renewal, resulting in hypercellularity of colonic crypts with cells that possess variable amounts of mucin and that are hyperchromatic, with elongated nuclei arranged in a "picket fence" pattern. These cytologic alterations confer an increased basophilic appearance to the adenomatous epithelium on conventional hematoxylin-eosin staining. Although the predominant cell type is an immature goblet cell or columnar cell, adenomas may contain other cell types, such as neuroendocrine cells, Paneth cells, squamous morules, and, rarely, melanocytes. On cross section, the inner contour of an adenomatous gland lumen usually is smooth, in contrast to the serrated appearance of a hyperplastic gland lumen (see later).

The dysplasia exhibited by all adenomas can be graded subjectively on the basis of certain cytologic and archi-

Table 119–2 Relative Frequency of Adenomas: Relation of Histologic Type to Size of Adenoma and Degree of Dysplasia

Type of Adenoma	Size of Adenoma* %			Degree of Dysplasia† %		
	<1 cm	*1-2 cm*	*>2 cm*	*Mild*	*Moderate*	*Severe*
Tubular	77	20	4	88	8	4
Tubulovillous	25	47	29	58	26	16
Villous	14	26	60	41	38	21

*Adapted from Muto T, Bussey HJR, Morson BC: The evolution of cancer of the colon and rectum. Cancer 36:2251, 1975.
†Adapted from Konishi F, Morson BC: Pathology of colorectal adenomas: A colonoscopic survey. J Clin Pathol 35:830, 1989.

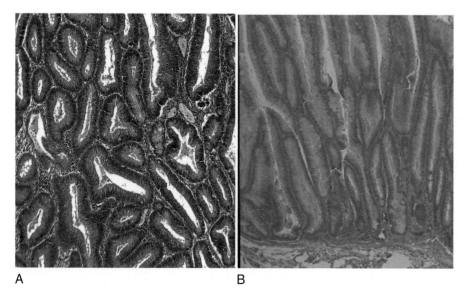

A   B

Figure 119–1 Comparison of tubular and villous histology. *A*, Tubular adenomas consist of branched, crowded glands arranged in a complex cerebriform pattern. (Used with permission by Jae H. Lim and Kevin M. Ishioka, Brown Medical School. Digital Photography: http://www.brown.edu/Courses/Digital_Path/.) *B*, Villous histology is marked by glands that are long, finger-like fronds typically projecting from the polyp stroma to the surface without much branching. In the center two crypts, the adenomatous epithelium at the top has not yet fully replaced the normal epithelium at the bottom. (From The Internet Pathology Laboratory for Medical Education, Florida State University College of Medicine. http://www-medlib.med.utah.edu/WebPath/webpath.html. © 1994-2006 Edward C. Klatt, MD.)

tectural features into three categories: mild, moderate, and severe. Some polyps may contain the entire spectrum from mild to severe dysplasia, but in all cases, the adenoma is classified according to its most dysplastic focus. In cells that exhibit *mild dysplasia,* the nuclei in the cell maintain their basal polarity but are hyperchromatic, slightly enlarged, and elongated, yet uniform in size, without prominent nucleoli (Fig. 119–2). There often is loss of goblet cell mucin. Architecturally, the glands manifest branching and budding and become more crowded. With *moderate dysplasia,* nuclei become stratified and pleomorphic with prominent nucleoli, along with further loss of goblet cell mucin and increased glandular crowding. *Severe dysplasia* (see Fig. 119–2) is characterized by further stratification and pleomorphism of nuclei, more numerous and prominent nucleoli, increased nuclear-cytoplasmic ratios, and extreme glandular crowding. With further cell proliferation within the crypt, cells pile up, lose polarity, and create glands within glands, giving a disorderly cribriform appearance termed *carcinoma in situ* (Fig. 119–3). Most pathologists group severe dysplasia and carcinoma in situ, considering them both as high-grade dysplasia[2]; one reason for this grouping is to avoid using the term *carcinoma* for these lesions because they often can be managed endoscopically rather than surgically (see later). Indeed, it is now common practice to categorize dysplasia in colorectal adenomas into only two grades: *low-grade* dysplasia, which includes mild and moderate dysplasia, and *high-grade* dysplasia, which comprises severe dysplasia and carcinoma in situ.

Carcinoma in situ is characterized by intracryptal cell proliferation that leaves intact the basement membrane surrounding the gland. If a focus of neoplastic cells grows beyond the basement membrane and into the lamina propria of the mucosa, the lesion is termed *intramucosal carcinoma* (see Fig. 119–3). Both carcinoma in situ and intramucosal carcinoma are noninvasive lesions without metastatic potential, because lymphatics are not present in the colonic mucosa above the level of the muscularis mucosae.[4] Because clinical confusion often arises on encountering these two entities, it has been suggested that both carcinoma in situ and intramucosal carcinoma be reported as "noninvasive carcinoma" to avoid unnecessarily aggressive management. Only when a focus of neoplastic cells has spread through the muscularis mucosae is the lesion considered *invasive carcinoma* (see Fig. 119–3). An adenoma that contains a focus of invasive carcinoma commonly is referred to as a *malignant polyp* (see later).

Mild dysplasia is found in 70% to 86% of adenomatous polyps, moderate dysplasia in 18% to 20%, severe dysplasia (carcinoma in situ) in 5% to 10%, and invasive carcinoma in 5% to 7%.[3,5,6] Higher grades of dysplasia are more common in adenomas of larger size and greater villous content,[2] and adenomas with severe dysplasia are more likely to contain foci of invasive cancer.

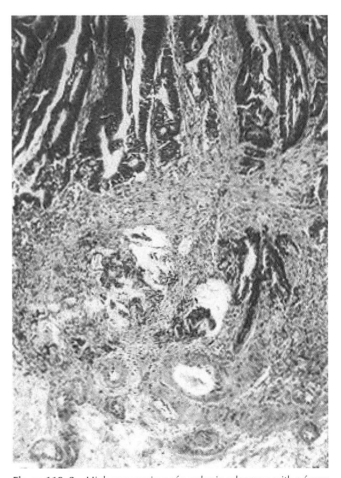

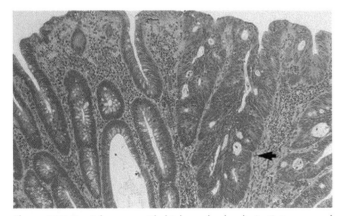

Figure 119–2 Adenoma with high-grade dysplasia (intramucosal carcinoma). This photomicrograph shows a section of adenoma with a focus of high-grade dysplasia (*arrow*). The focus has a complicated glandular architecture but does not show the desmoplastic stroma seen in invasive carcinomas. (From Boland CR: The Colon, Rectum, and Anus. *In* Feldman M (ed): Gastroenterology and Hepatology: The Comprehensive Visual Reference. Philadelphia, Churchill Livingstone, 1996.)

Figure 119–3 High-power view of a colonic adenoma with a focus of invasive carcinoma showing a desmoplastic stroma that is separating the carcinomatous tubules. There is also cautery artifact present, and the invasive tumor is present at the endoscopic resection margin. (From Boland CR: The Colon, Rectum, and Anus. *In* Feldman M (ed): Gastroenterology and Hepatology: The Comprehensive Visual Reference. Philadelphia, Churchill Livingstone, 1996.)

Adenoma Size

Adenomas are categorized into three size groups: <1 cm, 1 to 2 cm, and >2 cm.[5] Overall, most adenomas are smaller than 1 cm, but the size distribution of adenomas may vary greatly among studies, depending on study design, age of the study population, and location of the adenomas within the colon. Thus, in autopsy series, which describe a presumably asymptomatic population dying of other causes, only 13% to 16% of adenomas are larger than 1 cm,[7-9] whereas surgical and colonoscopic series that include symptomatic or higher-risk patients report a higher prevalence (26% to 40%) of adenomas larger than 1 cm.[2,3,5] In countries where the prevalence of colon cancer is high, adenomas tend to be larger than in low-prevalence countries.[10,11] Adenoma size increases as a function of age,[8,12,13] even in low-prevalence countries,[10] and larger adenomas are more common in distal colonic segments.[2,5,8]

Diminutive Polyps

Diminutive polyps measure 5 mm or less in diameter and are commonly encountered during endoscopy. An earlier concept that these lesions were almost always nonneoplastic has been revised based on several flexible sigmoidoscopic and colonoscopic studies in which 30% to 50% of diminutive polyps were found to be adenomatous[14-18]; despite the frequency of adenomatous change, however, they represent little if any threat of cancer. Earlier studies found that less than 1% of diminutive polyps were villous or contained a focus of severe dysplasia and that they almost never harbored invasive carcinoma.[14-16,18] In a more recent analysis of 4381 diminutive polyps, 4.4% contained severe dysplasia or villous components, although still only 0.1% had invasive carcinoma.[19] Moreover, in a retrospective study of predominantly asymptomatic people with diminutive adenomas found on flexible sigmoidoscopy, full colonoscopy identified a synchronous proximal adenoma in only 33% of subjects, and most of the proximal lesions were smaller than 5 mm.[20] Likewise, prospective colonoscopic studies confirm only a 24% to 34% prevalence of proximal adenomas in asymptomatic patients with distal diminutive polyps (of all histologic types)[21,22]; the likelihood of finding proximal adenomas is greater when the distal polyp is larger than 5 mm.[21] Diminutive adenomas manifest little, if any, appreciable growth over time.[23,24] A population-based study that involved fulgurating small polyps (even those up to 1 cm in size) without obtaining initial histologic identification reported that the subsequent risk for colorectal cancer and overall survival was no worse than in the general population.[25] Thus, taken together, these observations indicate that diminutive polyps, even when they prove to be adenomas, have little biologic or clinical significance. Nonetheless, the fact that these tiny polyps often are missed by computed tomographic (CT) colonography (or virtual colonoscopy; see later), has provided some fuel to the debate of how safe it is if these lesions go undetected. An important exception to the rule of the innocuous nature of diminutive adenomas is in the setting of hereditary nonpolyposis colorectal cancer (HNPCC), where even small adenomas already can display advanced pathologic features such as villous histology or high-grade dysplasia (see later).

Malignant Potential of Adenomatous Polyps

The three principal features that correlate with malignant potential for an adenomatous polyp are size, histologic type, and degree of dysplasia (Table 119–3). Although higher rates of malignant transformation are found when

Table 119–3 Malignant Potential of Adenomatous Polyps

	Surgical Polypectomies*		Colonoscopic Polypectomies[†]	
Variable	*Total No.*	*No. with Carcinoma (%)*	*Total No.*	*No. with Carcinoma (%)*
Adenoma size				
<1 cm	1479	19 (1.3)	1661	8 (0.5)
1-2 cm	580	55 (9.5)	2738	125 (4.6)
>2 cm	430	198 (46.0)	1387	150 (10.8)
Histologic type				
Tubular	1880	90 (4.8)	3725	104 (2.8)
Tubulovillous	383	86 (22.5)	1542	130 (8.4)
Villous	243	99 (40.7)	519	49 (9.5)
Degree of dysplasia[‡]				
Mild	1734	99 (5.7)	NA	NA
Moderate	549	99 (18.0)	NA	NA
Severe	223	77 (34.5)	NA	NA

*Adapted from Muto T, Bussey HJR, Morson BC: The evolution of cancer of the colon and rectum. Cancer 36:2251, 1975.
[†]Adapted from Shinya H, Wolff VI: Morphology, anatomic distribution and cancer potential of colonic polyps. Ann Surg 190:679, 1979.
[‡]This category refers to the most extensive degree of dysplasia *outside* the area of carcinoma but within the polyp. However, by convention, because an adenoma is classified according to the most severe grade of dysplasia, if carcinoma is present, it is considered a malignant polyp regardless of the degree of surrounding dysplasia.
NA, not available.

Table 119–4 Relation of Adenoma Size, Histologic Type, and Degree of Dysplasia to Invasive Carcinoma

	Percent with Carcinoma					
	Histologic Type			Degree of Dysplasia		
Adenoma Size, cm	Tubular	Tubulovillous	Villous	Mild	Moderate	Severe
<1	1	4	10	0.3	2	27
1-2	10	7	10	3	14	24
>2	35	46	53	42	50	48

Adapted from Muto T, Bussey HJR, Morson BC: The evolution of cancer of the colon and rectum. Cancer 36:2251, 1975.

the source of the pathologic material is mainly from surgical polypectomies[5] rather than colonoscopic polypectomies,[6] the malignant potential is correlated directly with larger adenoma size, more villous histology, and higher degrees of dysplasia. These three histopathologic criteria usually are interdependent, so it is difficult to assign a primary premalignant role to any one of them. For example, although only 1.3% of all adenomas smaller than 1 cm may harbor a cancer (see Table 119–3), if these small lesions have a predominant villous component or contain a focus of severe dysplasia, the cancer rate rises to 10% or 27%, respectively (Table 119–4). A small (<1 cm), tubular, mildly dysplastic adenoma is highly unlikely to harbor a focus of invasive cancer. Nonetheless, although this type of lesion is innocuous in itself, once removed, it often is considered a marker of an individual who is at (low) risk for developing a recurrent adenoma (discussed later). Since adenomas that are larger than 1 cm, have villous architecture, or manifest high-grade dysplasia or carcinoma represent a more biologically hazardous group, the term *adenoma with advanced pathology* (AAP) often is applied to adenomas that display any of these features.

Other Adenoma Variants

Flat Adenomas. A subset of adenomas termed *flat adenomas* by Muto and coworkers[26] is receiving increasing attention as a potentially important lesion. Macroscopically, a flat adenoma is either completely flat or slightly raised and may contain a central depression. Typically less than 1 cm in diameter, these lesions can be missed easily at endoscopy. This potential risk has prompted investigators, particularly in Japan, to adapt better methods of detection that involve the use of dye-spraying (chromoendoscopy) to generate a contrast relief-map image of the mucosa, or magnification colonoscopy, for enhanced visualization.[27] In studies without the use of such specialized endoscopic techniques, flat adenomas accounted for 8.5% to 12% of all adenomas and could be multiple.[28-30] Prospective studies of Western populations aided by the use of chromoendoscopy found that 6.8% to 36% of all detected adenomas were flat. Compared with lesions that were polypoid, these flat polyps tended to be smaller and to have increased rates of high-grade dysplasia and early cancer.[31-33] Indeed, it has been suggested that flat adenomas may have distinct biologic and chromosomal profiles.[32,34] In contrast, re-evaluation

of adenomas removed during the National Polyp Study found no increased risk of high-grade dysplasia in polyps classified as flat based on histologic features.[35] Future studies may help define whether broader acceptance of chromoendoscopy by endoscopists in Western countries will result in higher detection rates of flat adenomas, lower colorectal cancer incidence, or both following colonoscopy. A hereditary flat adenoma syndrome in four families described by Lynch and colleagues[36] subsequently was confirmed to be a variant of familial adenomatous polyposis (FAP) (see later).

The natural history of flat adenomas is not known. It is possible that they give rise to typical polypoid adenomas. Alternatively, the facts that residual flat adenoma tissue can be found adjacent to flat carcinomas, that some studies have observed a substantial incidence of high-grade dysplasia in these small lesions, and that flat adenomas have a lower incidence of *k-ras* mutations compared with polypoid adenomas, suggest that malignant progression from flat adenomas may not necessarily involve a polypoid phase.[37] It is possible that flat adenomas are the precursors of the long-recognized but uncommon small de novo colon carcinomas.[38]

Serrated Adenomas. Serrated adenomas are polyps that share features of both adenomatous and hyperplastic polyps. Originally called *mixed hyperplastic-adenomatous polyps*, these lesions are characterized by colonic crypts with a saw-tooth, serrated configuration resembling that of hyperplastic polyps; because of nuclear atypia, they are considered adenomas. This is discussed further in the section on hyperplastic polyps.

Aberrant Crypts. Investigations of human and carcinogen-treated rat colonic mucosa have disclosed a putative preneoplastic lesion called the *aberrant crypt*.[39] Found within macroscopically normal mucosa, aberrant crypts may occur individually or as small, slightly raised foci. They can be identified in methylene blue–stained whole mounts of colonic mucosa using a low-power lens (Fig. 119–4) or with a magnifying endoscope.[40] When viewed from above, the lumina of aberrant crypts are elliptical and irregular rather than circular. Aberrant crypt foci have become useful biomarkers in animal studies of colon carcinogenesis and chemoprevention. It is not clear, however, whether these lesions are valid surrogate intermediate end-point markers for adenomas or whether the results of these experimental manipulations can be extrapolated to humans. Human aberrant crypts often are hyperplastic; however, when dysplastic, they may represent the earliest detectable preneoplastic lesions. This notion is supported by molecular studies indicating that dysplastic, but not hyperplastic, aberrant crypts manifest mutations in the adenomatous polyposis coli (*APC*) gene (see later).[41]

Pathogenesis

Histogenesis

Adenomatous polyps are thought to arise from a failure in a step, or steps, of the normal process of cell proliferation and cell death (apoptosis). The initial aberration appears to arise in a single colonic crypt in which the proliferative compartment, instead of being confined to the crypt base, is expanded throughout the entire crypt. This disturbance results in a so-called *unicryptal adenoma.* The DNA-synthesizing cells at the surface are not sloughed into the lumen, as normally occurs, and they accumulate in a downward infolding manner, interposing themselves between normal preexisting crypts. New adenomatous glands then are created either by further infolding or by branching. Thus, the unicryptal adenoma is believed to arise from a monoclonal expansion of an abnormal cell, and as the adenoma enlarges, the adenomatous cell population becomes polyclonal. Evidence for this concept comes from studying intestinal tissues from an extremely rare patient with *FAP* who was an XO/XY mosaic.[42] Analysis of Y chromosome expression in the intestinal mucosa

of this individual revealed that normal crypts of the small and large intestine and even unicryptal adenomas were monoclonal (either XO or XY), whereas at least 76% of very small microadenomas were polyclonal. Whether the same situation also applies to sporadic adenoma development is not clear at present and is the subject of some debate.[43]

Adenoma-Carcinoma Hypothesis

It is generally accepted that most, if not all, colon cancers originate within previously benign adenomas. Rarely, colon cancers may develop de novo in apparently flat, nonadenomatous epithelium although, as noted earlier, even these lesions might conceivably arise from preexisting flat adenomas. Evidence in support of the adenoma-carcinoma sequence comes from epidemiologic, clinical, pathologic, and molecular studies.

Epidemiologic Evidence. The prevalence of adenomas within a population, and the prevalence of people with multiple adenomas, geographically parallels the prevalence of colon cancer.[10] Indeed, adenoma prevalence increases in migrants from low-risk to high-risk colon cancer regions (see Chapter 120). The prevalence rates for both adenomatous polyps and cancer increase with age, and age distribution curves indicate that the development of adenomas precedes that of carcinomas by 5 to 10 years.[5,44]

Clinicopathologic Evidence. The most compelling evidence for the adenoma-carcinoma sequence is the fact

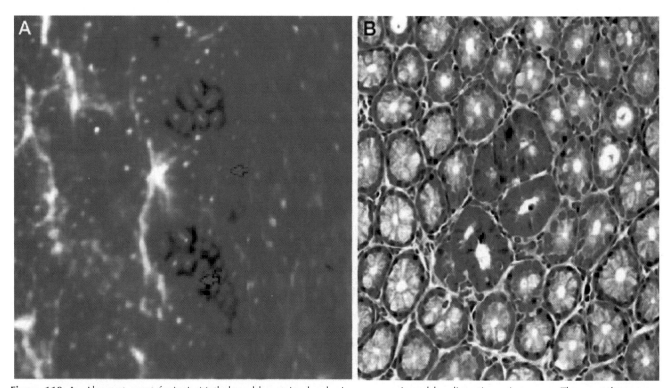

Figure 119–4 Aberrant crypt foci. *A,* Methylene blue-stained colonic mucosa viewed by dissecting microscopy. The crypt lumens are viewed on end and appear as white spots. The aberrant crypt foci (*arrows*) have widened diameters, increased staining, and slit-like lumens. *B,* Histologic examination of these aberrant crypt foci reveals dysplasia. These tiny microscopic adenomas are associated with bi-allelic inactivation of the APC gene. (Reprinted by permission from Macmillan Publishers Ltd: Modern Pathology. From Redston M: Carcinogenesis in the GI tract: From morphology to genetics and back again. Mod Pathol 14:236, copyright 2001).

that in patients with FAP who have hundreds to thousands of adenomas, the development of colorectal cancer is inevitable. For individuals in the general population without an inherited predisposition to colon cancer, perhaps the best evidence that adenomas give rise to carcinomas comes from endoscopic intervention studies. The National Polyp Study (see later) demonstrated that colonoscopic removal of adenomas results in a much lower than expected incidence of subsequent colorectal cancer.[45] In addition, screening proctosigmoidoscopy can lower the expected incidence of[46,47] and mortality from[48,49] rectal cancer. Pathology-based studies frequently describe the presence of remnant adenoma tissue within colon cancers. Conversely, small foci of cancer are extremely rare in normal mucosa but commonly are found in adenomas, particularly in those that are larger, more dysplastic, and more highly composed of villous elements (see Tables 119–3 and 119–4). Furthermore, the site distribution within the colon is similar for large adenomas and colon cancers. In addition, adenomatous polyps are found in one third of surgical specimens that contain a single colon cancer and in more than two thirds of specimens that contain more than one synchronous cancer.

Molecular Genetic Evidence. Molecular genetic studies provide some of the strongest experimental support for the adenoma-carcinoma hypothesis. The progression from adenoma to carcinoma results from an accumulation of molecular genetic alterations involving, among other changes, activation of oncogenes, inactivation of tumor suppressor genes, and participation of so-called stability genes[50] (see Chapter 120). The K-*ras* oncogene commonly undergoes point mutations at particular sites within the gene, thereby endowing it with the ability to transform cells. Only 9% of small adenomas exhibit K-*ras* gene mutations, compared with 58% of adenomas larger than 1 cm and 47% of colon cancers[51]; therefore, K-*ras* activation may act at an intermediate stage in tumorigenesis, perhaps contributing to a polypoid growth pattern. The fact that a large number of adenomas and cancers do not have K-*ras* gene mutations indicates that other genetic events also must play a role.

Tumor suppressor genes that normally function to suppress tumor development frequently are inactivated in colorectal neoplasms by mutation or allelic deletion, thereby promoting tumorigenesis. The loss of function of tumor suppressor genes on chromosomes 5q, 18q, and 17p are critical for colorectal tumorigenesis. The *APC* gene, which resides on the long arm of chromosome 5, is considered the "gatekeeper" for the process of colon carcinogenesis.[52] Mutation or loss of this gene is believed to be the crucial first step that confers susceptibility to colonic adenomas in patients with FAP as well as in people with sporadic adenomas. The APC protein plays an important role in colonic epithelial cell homeostasis (see later). Other tumor suppressor genes are located on chromosome 18q, in a region where the *DCC* (deleted in colon cancer) gene resides. Loss of function of *DCC*, or other nearby tumor suppressor genes, seems to contribute to later stages of adenoma progression, because allelic deletion at this locus occurs in only 11% to 13% of small tubular or tubulovillous adenomas but increases to 47% of adenomas with foci of cancer and 73% of frank colon

cancers.[51] Allelic deletion of chromosome 17p, at the locus that contains the *p53* gene, is the most common region of allelic loss in colorectal cancers. Because adenomas seldom manifest 17p deletion,[51] this alteration probably occurs as a late step in the adenoma-carcinoma progression. Perhaps the most compelling molecular evidence that colon carcinomas arise from previous adenomas is that when cancer cells arise in a malignant adenoma, they share the identical pattern of molecular alterations as the neighboring adenoma cells, but in addition, they acquire further mutations that are presumably critical for malignant behavior.[53]

Although oncogenes and tumor suppressor genes enhance the adenoma-carcinoma process by directly stimulating cell proliferation and inhibiting cell death, stability genes, or caretakers, normally keep genetic alterations to a minimum, and thus, when they are inactivated by mutation or loss, they permit mutations in other target genes to occur at a higher rate.[50] Examples of stability genes include the DNA mismatch repair (MMR) and base-excision repair (BER) genes responsible for repairing subtle mistakes that are made during DNA replication. Germline mutations of DNA MMR genes (such as *hMLH1*, *hMSH2*, *hMSH6*) occur in individuals with HNPCC, whereas inheritance of a mutated BER gene (e.g., *MUTYH*, also known as *MYH*), is responsible for a type of attenuated adenomatous polyposis (see later).

Pathways of Colon Carcinogenesis

It is useful to consider the process of colon carcinogenesis in two general stages: the formation of the adenoma, termed *tumor initiation*, and the progression of the adenoma to carcinoma, termed *tumor progression* (Fig. 119–5). It is believed that most, if not all, adenomas arise from an initial loss of *APC* gene function, and for that to happen, epithelial cells have to lose the function of both *APC* alleles (so-called two hits). In patients with FAP, one *APC* allele is inherited in a mutated form (*germline mutation*) from the affected parent. Adenomas arise when the

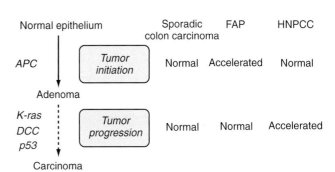

Figure 119–5 Pathways of colon carcinogenesis. Adenomas develop as a consequence of factors involved in tumor initiation, and progress to carcinomas because of factors that act as tumor promoters. A simplified theory comparing the two hereditary colon cancer syndromes suggests that the tumor initiation phase is accelerated in familial adenomatous polyposis (FAP) patients, accounting for numerous polyps. In contrast, the tumor progression phase is accelerated in hereditary nonpolyposis colorectal cancer (HNPCC) patients, accounting for the often rapid progression of adenomas to carcinoma.

second, normal copy of the *APC* gene from the unaffected parent either is lost or mutated (*somatic mutation*). Because individuals affected with FAP are born with the first hit, they develop polyps at a much younger age and in much greater number than does the general population. As such, FAP can be considered a condition of accelerated tumor initiation. Despite this abnormal initiation rate, once adenomas form in patients with FAP, it is believed that each adenoma tends to display a normal progression to carcinoma. Thus, the inevitable progression to cancer in FAP is more a consequence of the numerous polyps than of any increased premalignant potential of the individual adenoma. In the general population, sporadic adenomas arise as a consequence of two acquired somatic mutations of the *APC* gene. Because two acquired hits are statistically less likely than one acquired hit, sporadic adenomas tend to occur later in life and to be fewer in number than the polyps in patients with FAP.

Another major molecular pathway for colon carcinogenesis involves mutations in DNA MMR genes (see Chapter 120). This is the predominant pathway in patients with HNPCC. Mutations in these enzymes result in a characteristic molecular phenotype termed *microsatellite instability* (MSI), a phenomenon that is observable in colon cancer cells from approximately 85% of HNPCC colon cancers but in only 15% of sporadic colon cancers. Although its name implies a lack of polyps, HNPCC colon cancers do arise from preexisting adenomas. It is believed that the number of adenomas that occurs in patients with HNPCC is similar to that in the general population but that HNPCC is marked by an accelerated tumor progression stage, so the few adenomas that do arise often manifest advanced pathology (villous features, high-grade dysplasia) even at small sizes.[54] Indeed, adenomas in patients with HNPCC often manifest MSI[55] even in their earliest stages of formation. Because these adenomas tend to progress more rapidly to carcinoma,[56,57] surveillance intervals for colonoscopy following removal of adenomas in HNPCC patients should be shortened (see later; see also Chapter 120).

Epidemiology and Etiology

Prevalence of Adenomas

The prevalence of adenomatous polyps is affected by four major factors: (1) the inherent risk for colon cancer in the population, (2) age, (3) gender, and (4) family history of colorectal cancer. The frequency of colon adenomas varies widely among populations, but it tends to be higher in populations at greater risk for colon cancer (Table 119–5).[10] One illustrative example is to compare the very high adenoma prevalence in Japanese living in Hawaii (a very high risk area for colon cancer) with the much lower adenoma prevalence in Japanese who still reside in Japan, an area of much lower risk. Even within Japan itself, adenoma prevalence correlates quite well with colon cancer prevalence in different prefectures of the country. Data from autopsy series provide an approximation of adenoma prevalence. In populations at low risk for colon cancer, adenoma prevalence rates are lower than 12% (see Table 119–5), whereas in most intermediate- and high-risk populations, adenomas are found in 30% to 40% of the population, and rates as high as 50% to 60% have been observed.[7,58,59] One half to two thirds of people older than 65 years of age in high-risk areas may harbor colonic adenomas.[7,58,60]

The true prevalence rate of adenomatous polyps within an asymptomatic living population is only now being elucidated because, until recently, colonoscopy was not performed on healthy individuals in the absence of gastrointestinal symptoms. Approximately 27% to 32% of asymptomatic average-risk individuals older than 50 years of age undergoing screening colonoscopy will have an adenoma, and 6% to 10% will have an AAP[61-64] (Table 119–6). By comparison, colonoscopic screening of asymptomatic individuals between 40 and 49 years of age revealed prevalence rates of only 8.7% for tubular adenomas and 3.5% for AAP or cancer.[65] Colonoscopic series indicate that men have a 1.5 relative risk of adenomas compared with age-matched women,[65,66] thus confirming earlier observations in autopsy series.[8,11]

The prevalence of adenomas is higher in older people, particularly those older than 60 years of age. In fact, age is the single most important independent determinant of

Table 119–5 Prevalence of Adenomatous Polyps in Various Populations

Population	Prevalence of Colon Cancer	Men, Age in Years			Women, Age in Years		
		20-39	40-59	60+	20-39	40-59	60+
Hawaiian-Japanese	Very high	50	69	64	0	71	58
U.S. (New Orleans)							
Whites	High	0	39	47	0	10	35
Blacks	High	19	26	52	0	27	41
Brazil (São Paulo)	Intermediate	5	14	30	8	14	23
Japan							
Akita	Intermediate	21	31	46	0	8	37
Miyagi	Low	1	9	23	4	9	17
Costa Rica (San José)	Low	0	6	13	2	4	9
Colombia (Cali)	Low	2	7	18	2	10	15

From Correa P: Epidemiology of polyps and cancer. In Morson BC (ed): The Pathogenesis of Colorectal Cancer. Philadelphia, WB Saunders, 1978, p 126.

Table 119–6 Prevalence of Adenomas and Cancer in Asymptomatic Individuals Older Than 50 Years of Age: Results of Screening Studies

Study Design	Screening Colonoscopy		CT Colonography or Colonoscopy	Fecal DNA or FOBT*
	Ref 61	*Ref 62*	*Ref 63*	*Ref 64*
No. of patients	3121	1994	1233	4404
Mean age, yr	62.9	59.8	57.8	68.8
Male gender, %	96.8	58.9	59	44.6
% with family history of CRC	13.9	—	2.6	14
% with adenomas				
Any	31.9	—	13.6[†]	27
Advanced	9.6	6.1	—	9.7
High-grade dysplasia	1.6	—	—	0.9
≥10 mm	4.9	2.5	3.9	5.2
Villous	2.9	—	—	3.2
Cancer	1	0.6	0.2	0.7

*Patients with positive results were evaluated by colonoscopy.
[†]Includes adenomas ≥6 mm only.
CRC, colorectal cancer; FOBT, fecal occult blood test.

Table 119–7 Anatomic Distribution of Colorectal Adenomatous Polyps

Type of Series	Anatomic Site of Colorectal Polyps (%)				
	Cecum and Ascending	*Transverse*	*Descending*	*Sigmoid*	*Rectum*
Autopsy					
All adenomas[7,9,59]	34	26	10	19	10
Adenomas >1 cm[7]	34	11	14	16	21
Colonoscopy					
Asymptomatic[68]	23	24	24	24	5
Symptomatic[3]	8	14	19	47	12

adenoma prevalence[7,11,12,58-60,65-71] both in high-risk and low-risk regions of the world (see Table 119–5). Not only is advancing age associated with a higher prevalence rate of adenomas but it also correlates with a greater likelihood for multiple polyps, adenomas with more severe degrees of dysplasia, and, in some studies, larger adenoma size.

Adenoma prevalence also is higher in individuals with a positive family history of colorectal cancer and adenomas,[72-74] particularly if more than one relative is affected with colorectal neoplasia, and if the affected relative is young.

Race, per se, does not appear to be an independent determinant of adenoma prevalence. Adenomas seldom develop in blacks who reside in South Africa, whereas for African Americans living in New Orleans, the adenoma prevalence rate is comparable to the prevalence rate for that city's high-risk white population.[10]

Incidence of Adenomas

Estimating the incidence rate of new adenomas requires examining the colon of individuals at more than one point in time. Two types of endoscopic studies lend themselves to this analysis: postpolypectomy (or post-cancer resection) surveillance studies, and interval examinations in persons who initially had a negative examination. Of course, for both types of studies, the small but measurable miss rate of adenomas may contribute to the rate of apparent incident adenomas (see "Detection of Adenomas"). For the purposes of this discussion, adenomas found in individuals after polypectomy are considered recurrences (see "Postpolypectomy Management"), whereas those that are found in individuals after an initial negative colonoscopy are considered incident adenomas. In this latter group of subjects, the incidence of new adenomas varies from 24% to 41%.[66] In one study, patients underwent colonoscopy twice on the same day to clear the colon of all potentially missed adenomas, and 38% were found to have new adenomas when recolonoscoped 2 years later.[75] Three-year follow-up sigmoidoscopy after an initial negative examination in the Prostate, Lung, Colorectal, and Ovarian (PLCO) Cancer Screening Trial found a 3.1% incidence of all adenomas and 0.8% incidence of advanced adenomas or cancer.[76] Only one study has performed follow-up colonoscopy in average-risk, asymptomatic individuals who originally did not have adenomas at colonoscopy.[77] At a mean interval of 5.5 years, the incidence rate of adenomas was 27%, and the rate for AAPs was less than 1%.

Anatomic Distribution

The distribution of adenomatous polyps within the colon differs, depending on the method of investigation (Table 119–7). In autopsy series that approximate the normal distribution in presumably asymptomatic subjects, adenomas are distributed uniformly throughout the colorectum; this even distribution has been confirmed in colonoscopic investigations of asymptomatic subjects.[23,58] Large adenomas in autopsy series have a distal predominance, in the region where most colon cancers arise, thereby supporting the adenoma-carcinoma hypothesis. Likewise, adenomas detected in surgical and colonoscopic studies of symptomatic people also display a left-sided predominance, indicating that distal adenomas are more likely to come to clinical attention. In older individuals, particularly those older than 60 years of age, adenoma distribution demonstrates a shift toward more proximal colonic locations. This phenomenon, which is based on both autopsy[11,12,59,71] and colonoscopic studies of symptomatic[78] as well as asymptomatic subjects,[22,61,62,67,69,79] has importance for choosing appropriate colon cancer screening approaches (see Chapter 120).

Risk Factors for Adenoma Susceptibility

Evidence is mounting to suggest that both heredity and environment contribute to colonic adenoma susceptibility. Indeed, the interplay between genetic predisposition and environmental factors supports a hypothesis proposed by Hill many years ago concerning adenoma causation, which was based mainly on epidemiologic and histopathologic observations.[80] He postulated that genetic susceptibility to colonic adenomas is extremely common throughout the world. For adenomas to form and then progress to cancer, several environmental factors, presumably dietary, must act in concert. One factor would be responsible for the initial development of adenomas, another would enhance the growth of adenomas, and one or more carcinogens or tumor promoters would finally give rise to cancer.

Inherited Susceptibility to Adenomatous Polyps

There is a strong genetic component to the well-defined hereditary polyposis (FAP) and nonpolyposis (HNPCC) colon cancer syndromes that exhibit a mendelian pattern of inheritance (see later); however, 95% of common (sporadic) adenomas and carcinomas arise in people who do not have these syndromes. In the past, this observation was interpreted to mean that genetic predisposition played only a minor role in most colonic neoplasms. Epidemiologic studies, however, have revealed a twofold to threefold greater risk for colon cancer in probands who have a first-degree relative affected by colonic cancer or adenoma.[72,81] Several studies have found a similar increase in risk for adenomas in first-degree relatives of people with adenomas.[72,81] Moreover, data from the National Polyp Study indicate that siblings and parents of patients with adenomatous polyps are at an increased risk for colon cancer, particularly when the adenoma proband is younger than 60 years of age.[82] There is even a suggestion that adenomas in patients with a family history of colorectal cancer have faster growth rates.[83]

It is now estimated that as much as 10% to 30% of colon cancers are familial, implying the possibility of susceptibility genes that give rise to common colon cancers.[72] Indeed, several genes have been identified that may contribute to so-called common familial risk. These include a germline mutation in the *APC* gene at codon 1307 (I1307K) that appears to predispose Ashkenazi Jewish populations to colon cancer; mutations of the DNA MMR gene *hMSH6*, a type I transforming growth factor (TGF)-β receptor allele—TβR-I(6A); and polymorphisms of certain genes involved in metabolism of nutrients and environmental agents, such as methylenetetrahydrofolate reductase and *N*-acetyltransferases 1 and 2.[72,84] In addition, germline mutations of *APC* at codon E1317Q, and other genes involved in the APC pathway, such as β-*catenin* and *AXIN1*, as well as the DNA mismatch repair genes *hMLH1* and *hMSH2*, also have been implicated in the predisposition to multiple adenomas.[85] The identification of genes responsible for common susceptibility to colonic adenomas is an area for considerable research.

Dietary and Lifestyle Risk Factors

Although genetic predisposition clearly plays a role in colorectal carcinogenesis, diet and life-style factors also contribute. It is estimated that as much as a third to a half of colon cancer risk and a fourth to a third of distal colon adenoma risk might be avoidable by modification of dietary and life-style habits.[86] For the most part, dietary factors that correlate with a predisposition to colon cancer (see Chapter 120) also are associated with a risk for colonic adenomas.[86-87] Factors that have each been correlated with an increased adenoma risk include excess dietary fat, excess alcohol intake, obesity, and cigarette smoking. Curiously, low calcium intake, despite being associated with increased risk for colon cancer, does not appear to confer risk for adenomas (although as discussed later, calcium supplementation does seem to lower adenoma recurrences). Factors that have shown the most consistent protective effect against adenomas in epidemiologic studies include dietary fiber, plant foods, and carbohydrate. Indeed, analysis of dietary questionnaires from patients in the prospective PLCO Trial found that those with the highest fiber intake had a 27% lower risk of adenomas compared with those who had the lowest fiber intake.[88] Other protective measures include increased physical activity, increased intake of calcium, and high-folate intake. An analysis of an asymptomatic, predominantly male veteran population that underwent screening colonoscopy found that smoking and moderate-to-heavy alcohol use increased risk, whereas cereal fiber intake, vitamin D intake, and use of nonsteroidal anti-inflammatory drugs (NSAIDs) decreased risk factors for advanced colonic neoplasia (AAPs and colon cancer).[89]

Unfortunately, the rather attractive hypothesis that proper diets would reduce colon cancer risk has not been substantiated when tested in prospective, interventional studies.[90] Indeed, dietary changes administered over 2 to 4 years have failed to significantly reduce recurrent or incident adenomas in several studies that tested (1) reductions in fat with increases in fiber, fruits, and vegetables; (2) combinations of low-fat with wheat bran and/or β-carotene supplements; (3) supplements of wheat bran fiber with vitamins C and E; and (4) a complex supplement of calcium, vitamin C, vitamin E, and selenium.

Unlike these null studies, there are four classes of chemopreventive compounds that have shown protective effects against colon adenomas and/or cancers: NSAIDs, calcium, hormone replacement therapy (HRT), and selenium. Of these, aspirin and NSAIDs are the most well-established agents. Greater than 90% of the more than 110 studies of various animal models and more than 35 epidemiologic studies confirm a significant reduction in colorectal adenomas, cancers, and cancer-associated mortality among aspirin or NSAID users.[90] For example, the Nurses' Health Study, a prospective cohort study of 27,077 nurses, found that regular use of aspirin was associated with a lower risk of developing colorectal adenomas.[91] Three randomized, prospective trials investigating the use of aspirin to prevent colorectal adenomas have shown decreased rates of adenoma recurrence in the study groups compared with placebo. In one trial, that was terminated early because of significant results, 635 patients with a history of curative resection of colorectal cancer and randomized to 325 mg/day of aspirin (or placebo) were found to have a significant reduction in incident adenomas after a mean of 12.8 months.[92] Another trial in patients with prior colorectal adenomas compared 81 mg/day or 325 mg/day of aspirin with placebo and found that the 81-mg dose reduced the relative risk of developing adenomas and advanced adenomas by 19% and 41%, respectively, with a similar, but not significant, trend found with the higher dose.[93] The 1-year results of a trial comparing two doses of lysine acetylsalicylate with placebo found a significant reduction in recurrence of adenomas larger than 5 mm in both treatment groups but a greater effect with the higher dose.[94] In the Physicians' Health Study, administration of aspirin 325 mg every other day over 5 years showed no reduction compared with placebo in advanced adenomas or colon cancers.[95] NSAIDs act by inhibiting cyclooxygenase (COX)-1 and COX-2 enzymes, which thereby reduces cellular proliferation, enhances apoptosis, and reduces angiogenesis; other COX-independent effects also are operative. Based on these observations as well as studies showing that selective COX-2 inhibition reduces the number of adenomas in patients with FAP (see later), large-scale prospective studies of COX-2 inhibitors (celecoxib and rofecoxib) have been undertaken.[96] Unfortunately, adverse cardiovascular side effects have limited the use of these agents, but any reduction in sporadic adenomas will be an important proof of principle regarding COX inhibition in colon carcinogenesis.

Calcium supplements have been shown in two randomized placebo-controlled phase III studies to reduce adenoma recurrence by approximately 19% to 34%, with effects noticed even after 1 year of supplementation.[97,98] It has even been suggested that calcium supplements may have a more pronounced effect on advanced adenomas.[99] The mechanism for this protective effect likely is multifactorial because calcium has been shown to decrease proliferation of colonic epithelial cells and to inhibit mucosal injury induced by bile acids and carcinogens in the fecal stream. Calcium may act by neutralizing the mutagenic effects of bile acids on the colonic mucosa or by directly inhibiting epithelial cell proliferation.

In a study investigating chemoprevention of skin cancer, selenium supplements were associated with a 58% reduction in colon cancer incidence as a secondary endpoint.[90] This result has prompted additional trials to evaluate the effects of selenium on recurrent adenoma formation. Finally, HRT has been associated in many studies with an approximate 20% reduction in colon cancer risk and a protective effect against colonic adenomas.[90] As with NSAIDs, the adverse side effects of HRT often outweigh the chemopreventive effects of these agents. The results of other ongoing studies of ursodeoxycholic acid, folate with or without aspirin, and celecoxib with or without selenium for polyp prevention are awaited anxiously.[96]

Conditions Associated with Adenomatous Polyps

A variety of clinical circumstances have been associated with adenomatous polyps. Of the conditions listed in the following discussions, the predisposition to have or to develop adenomas is strongest for patients with ureterosigmoidostomies, acromegaly, and *Streptococcus bovis* bacteremia. Patients with any of these three conditions should undergo a thorough colorectal examination and, in the former two conditions, periodic surveillance should be considered (although the frequency of such examinations is not well defined). As for the other conditions, the data are either conflicting or the risk is not strong enough to recommend a policy of surveillance.

Ureterosigmoidostomy Sites. Patients who have undergone a urinary diversion procedure with implantation of the ureters into the sigmoid colon are at particularly high risk for development of neoplastic lesions at the ureterosigmoidostomy sites.[100] At least 29% of such patients develop colonic neoplasms, usually close to the stoma, after this procedure. Adenomatous polyps and carcinomas have been found after mean latent periods of 20 and 26 years, respectively. Lesions that resemble juvenile polyps and inflammatory polyps also have been reported at ureterosigmoidostomy sites. It has been suggested that these lesions are produced by the generation of *N*-nitrosamines from urinary amines in the presence of fecal flora. In view of the extremely high frequency of neoplasia in this setting, these patients should undergo life-long colonoscopic surveillance in keeping with the long latent period between the implantation of the ureters and the subsequent development of colonic neoplasia.

Acromegaly. Patients with acromegaly have an increased tendency to develop colon cancers and adenomas.[101-103] Although these studies involve few subjects, consistently high prevalence rates of 5% to 25% for colon cancer and 14% to 35% for adenomatous polyps have been observed in patients with acromegaly. The risk for colonic neoplasia may be higher in younger acromegalics,[101] those with a family history of colon cancer,[102] those with multiple skin tags (acrochordons),[103] and those with previous colorectal adenomas.[104] The mechanism for enhanced colonic neoplasia in this disease is not clear but probably relates to increased growth hormone and/or insulin-like growth factor (IGF)-1 levels. In nonacromegalics, high serum levels of IGF-1 have been correlated with an increased risk of colorectal cancer.[105] In acromegalics, high serum IGF-1 levels have been correlated with increased epithelial cell proliferation,[106] and increased recurrence rates of colorectal adenomas.[104] Other studies in acromegalics, however, have not found that blood levels of growth hormone or IGF-1 correlated with the presence of neoplasms,[103] and the risk of neoplasia was actually greater in cured acromegalics than in those with active disease.[102]

Streptococcus bovis *Bacteremia.* Bacteremia and endocarditis caused by *S. bovis* have been associated with colorectal carcinoma, adenomatous polyps, and even FAP.[107-109] The fecal carrier rate of this organism is higher in people with adenomas or carcinomas than in those with benign colonic diseases or in normal controls.[109] In animal models, *S. bovis,* or even an extract of its bacterial cell wall antigens, increased the expression of markers associated with early colon carcinogenesis.[110] It has been suggested that patients with *S. bovis* bacteremia have thorough colonic examination to exclude a neoplasm. Endocarditis caused by *Streptococcus agalactiae* (an organism that seldom is pathogenic in adults) has been reported in two patients, each of whom had a rectal villous adenoma with foci of carcinoma.[111]

Skin Tags. The correlation between colonic neoplasia and the presence and multiplicity of acrochordons in acromegalic patients led to the question of whether skin tags (usually located on the upper trunk or axillae) could serve as a cutaneous marker of colonic polyps in the general population. Although a significant correlation was found between the presence of skin tags and adenomatous polyps in prospective studies of symptomatic patients presenting for colonoscopy, no such correlation was found in asymptomatic patients and in members of familial polyposis kindreds.[112] Thus, acrochordons do not appear to be useful markers for polyps in average-risk asymptomatic persons.

Atherosclerosis and Cholesterol. An association between adenomatous polyps and atherosclerosis has been documented by necropsy studies, one of which noted a correlation between the degree of atherosclerosis and the multiplicity, size, and degree of dysplasia of adenomas.[113] This observation suggests that these two common conditions of westernized populations share certain risk factors, possibly elevated serum cholesterol levels. A cause-effect relation between serum cholesterol concentration and adenomatous polyps, however, has not been established. Curiously, patients with colon cancer often have low serum cholesterol levels that apparently precede the development of cancer[114] and are, therefore, not simply a metabolic consequence of the cancer.

Breast Cancer. Epidemiologic investigations have found an association between cancers of the breast and colon in terms of prevalence and mortality rates.[115] Case-control studies, however, have found little or no increased risk for adenomatous polyps in women who have had breast cancer. Moreover, asymptomatic women whose only risk factor for colonic neoplasia was a personal history of breast cancer had an identical prevalence of adenomas compared with a control group.[116] Loss of the *BRCA1* tumor suppressor gene, which is important for predisposition to some hereditary breast and ovarian cancers, does not appear to play a role in colon carcinogenesis.[117] Therefore, unless future studies determine otherwise, a personal history of breast cancer should not be considered a risk factor for colonic adenomas.

Cholecystectomy. In some studies, cholecystectomy has been associated with an increased risk for colon cancer, although this increase is only modest and applies mainly to women and to proximal colonic lesions.[118] It is postulated that in the absence of the gallbladder, there is enhanced delivery of bile acids to the colon and possibly a shift from primary to secondary bile acids that enhances the proliferative activity of the colonic mucosa. In general, however,, case-control studies have not found an increased risk for adenomatous polyps among patients who have had cholecystectomy,[119] nor was this a risk factor for advanced adenomas or colon cancer among asymptomatic male veterans.[89]

Diagnosis of Adenomatous Polyps

Symptoms and Signs

Most patients with colonic polyps either have no symptoms referable to the gastrointestinal tract or have nonspecific intestinal symptoms. In individuals with symptoms that can be attributed to colonic polyps, the most common presenting symptom is occult or overt rectal bleeding. Histopathologic observations suggest that in contrast to colonic carcinomas, which exhibit considerable surface erosion, the generally less rigid adenomas maintain the integrity of their surface epithelium but may bleed into the polyp stroma.[120] These findings help explain the clinical impression that bleeding from polyps is intermittent and usually does not cause fecal occult blood loss or anemia.

Other symptoms that have been attributed to colonic polyps are constipation, diarrhea, and flatulence. Constipation or decreased stool caliber is more likely to be caused by bulky lesions in the distal colon. Large colonic polyps may be associated with cramping lower abdominal pain from intermittent intussusception. Unless these widely prevalent symptoms disappear with the removal of the polyp, they must be attributed to other causes.

A syndrome of *secretory diarrhea* with considerable and sometimes life-threatening water and electrolyte depletion occasionally has been observed in patients with villous adenomas.[121] Tumors that produce this syndrome are typically larger than 3 to 4 cm in diameter and are almost always located in the rectum or rectosigmoid, providing little surface area distal to the tumor for reabsorption of fluid and electrolytes. In contrast to the absorption of water and sodium and secretion of potassium by normal colonic mucosa, secretory villous adenomas exhibit a net secretion of water and sodium and an exaggerated secretion of potassium.[122] A tumor-derived secretagogue has been postulated to account for the secretory diarrhea in this syndrome that mimics cholera.

Detection

Colorectal polyps usually are clinically silent. They typically are detected either in asymptomatic people being screened for colorectal neoplasia or incidentally during investigation for symptoms ostensibly referable to the colon or evaluation of unexplained iron deficiency anemia. A more complete discussion of colorectal cancer screening can be found in Chapter 120. This section addresses the issue of adenoma detection using the available screening modalities.

Fecal Occult Blood Testing

The actual frequency of bleeding from adenomas is difficult to determine. Less than 10% of people who report frank rectal bleeding will be found to have a significant adenoma (i.e., >1 cm or carcinoma in situ) as the cause.[123,124] In general, polyps smaller than 1 cm do not bleed. This dictum is supported by quantitative measurements of fecal blood loss in people with known adenomas that indicate only those with adenomas larger than 1.5 to 2.0 cm lose more than the usual amounts of blood, regardless of the location of the polyp within the colon.[125] Thus, less than 40% of patients with known adenomas show positive fecal occult blood testing (FOBT) results,[125-127] the higher rates occurring primarily in patients with larger and distal polyps. Newer immunochemical tests for fecal occult blood, and a more sensitive guaiac-based test, can enhance the sensitivity for detecting adenomas larger than 1 cm,[128] but their place in screening has not been established yet. Newer tests that use immunochemical rather than guaiac-based technology to detect occult blood are beginning to show promise for detecting clinically important colorectal neoplasms.[129]

When asymptomatic individuals undergo colon cancer screening with guaiac-based FOBTs, about 1% to 3% of asymptomatic adults older than 40 years of age have a positive result.[130] Less than one half of these people have a colorectal neoplasm, and among the lesions found, adenomas outnumber carcinomas by 3:1. Thus the proportions of all positive guaiac tests attributable to colonic neoplasms (i.e., positive predictive values) are 30% to 35% for adenomas and 8% to 12% for cancer.[131] Despite the predominance of adenomas among lesions detected, 75% of adenomas may still be missed by guaiac testing (i.e., false-negative values) unless they are large or located in the distal portion of the colon. Positive test results for occult blood 1 to 2 years after a negative search will detect some of these missed polyps.[132] Because small polyps seldom bleed and their rate of detection by occult blood testing is low, sigmoidoscopy has been recommended to complement FOBTs.

Sigmoidoscopy

For several decades, sigmoidoscopy was the mainstay of endoscopic colon cancer screening. Rigid sigmoidoscopy would detect polyps (of all histologic types) in about 7% of asymptomatic individuals older than 40 years of age,[133] whereas the flexible sigmoidoscope would find polyps in 10% to 15%, principally because a greater length of bowel could be examined.[134,135] Screening sigmoidoscopy has been demonstrated to reduce mortality from distal rectosigmoid cancers by as much as 60% to 75% based on several retrospective case-control studies.[74] Conclusions of three large-scale prospective studies of screening sigmoidoscopy—the PLCO Study in the United States,[76] the United Kingdom Flexible Sigmoidoscopy Screening Trial,[136] and a "once-only" sigmoidoscopy trial in Italy[137]—are awaited. Baseline findings of the U.K. study were that 12% and 0.3% of subjects between ages 55 and 64 years were found to have distal adenomas and distal

cancers, respectively.[136] The Italian study found an 11% prevalence of distal adenomas in the same age group. In the meantime, the increasing use of colonoscopy in the United States has resulted in a marked reduction in screening sigmoidoscopy examinations.

Barium Enema

Although large polyps are detected readily by either the single-contrast or double-contrast barium enema, the latter technique maximizes the detection of small polyps.[138] The detection of adenomas by barium enema is dependent on size. In the National Polyp Study, the detection rate of adenomas smaller than 5 mm, 6 to 10 mm, and larger than 10 mm was 32%, 53%, and 48%, respectively.[139] Common sources of error include inadequate cleansing of the colon, which contributes to the 5% to 10% false-positive rate, and diagnostic difficulty caused by the presence of diverticulosis, redundant bowel, or poor mucosal coating, which results in a 10% false-negative rate. Because of these issues, as well as the fact that barium enema never has been formally tested as a colon cancer screening tool, the use of barium enema for colon cancer screening has all but been abandoned in favor of colonoscopy or CT colonography (see later).

Colonoscopy

Colonoscopy is preferred to double-contrast barium enema examination for adenoma detection because it has enhanced diagnostic accuracy as well as therapeutic capability. This diagnostic superiority has been demonstrated in studies of patients with known polyps[139,140] as well as in symptomatic patients found to have negative findings on proctosigmoidoscopic and barium enema examinations.[141] Despite its reputation as the gold standard for adenoma detection, colonoscopy has some limitations. Colonoscopy fails to reach the cecum in up to 10% of cases; it usually requires patient sedation; and it carries a higher cost than barium enema or sigmoidoscopy. Colonoscopy also can miss neoplasms, especially those located at flexures or behind folds. In general, adenomas that are missed tend to be small. One study of tandem colonoscopies performed by two experienced endoscopists estimated that the first examination could miss up to 15% of small polyps (<8 mm) but none of the larger polyps.[142] A similar study reported an overall miss rate for adenomas of 24%, with a miss rate for adenomas smaller than 5 mm, 6 to 9 mm, and larger than 10 mm of 27%, 13%, and 6%, respectively.[143] A more recent study using CT colonography as the reference standard demonstrated that colonoscopy can miss 12% of adenomas larger than 10 mm.[144] In the National Polyp Study, the miss rate for adenomas was 20%, all of which were smaller than 1 cm.[139] These limitations notwithstanding, the use of colonoscopy as a primary screening method has gained acceptance to the point where it has been incorporated into colorectal cancer screening guidelines[145] and currently is endorsed by governmental agencies.

The likelihood of finding an adenoma by colonoscopy for various clinical indications has been reviewed.[146] The baseline frequency of adenomas in asymptomatic individuals older than 50 years of age is 29%. As mentioned earlier, older age and male gender were strong predictors of adenoma prevalence; 38% of males older than age 60 were found to have an adenoma, and 10% of them had a large (>1 cm) adenoma. The yield of finding adenomas is independent of the indication for the colonoscopy, such as a positive FOBT, a positive family history of colorectal cancer, nonemergent rectal bleeding, or other intestinal symptoms. Thus, adenomas often are serendipitous findings in a population in which these lesions are frequent baseline findings.

CT Colonography

Also known as *virtual colonoscopy*, CT colonography involves scanning the colon with a helical or spiral CT scanner to produce both two-dimensional and three-dimensional images of the colon and rectum. Patients undergo a standard bowel preparation and the colon is distended with air while images are taken with the patient in both the supine and prone positions without sedation. In this rapidly emerging field, a number of studies have compared the performance characteristics of CT colonography with standard optical colonoscopy for the detection of polyps.[147] Factors affecting detection rates include the polyp prevalence rate in the population being studied; the

experience of the radiologist; and technical aspects including bowel preparation techniques, software, and the use of single-row or multirow scanners. In high-prevalence populations that included symptomatic patients, the sensitivity for detecting polyps ranged from 29% to 59% for small polyps, 47% to 82% for medium polyps, and 63% to 92% for large polyps (Fig. 119–6). Studies of cohorts with low polyp prevalences fared less well, with sensitivities ranging from 32% to 58% and specificities of 90% for polyps larger than 6 mm in diameter.[148,149] In the only large study to date involving a pure asymptomatic screening population, CT colonography had a sensitivity of 86% for polyps 5 to 9 mm and 92% for polyps larger than 10 mm in the hands of highly skilled radiologists and with patients ingesting oral contrast prior to the study (so-called fecal tagging) to facilitate distinguishing stool from mucosal abnormalities.[150] Indeed, the use of fecal tagging without a cathartic prep for CT colonography is feasible and might conceivably enhance patient compliance.[151] In all studies, the detection of polyps smaller than 5 mm by CT colonography has been consistently low. Nonetheless, there are instances where CT

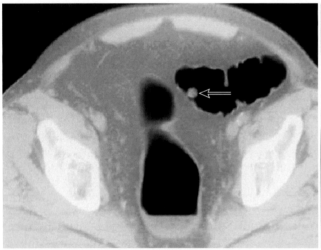

A

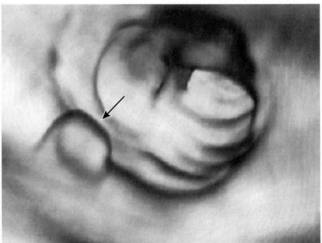

B

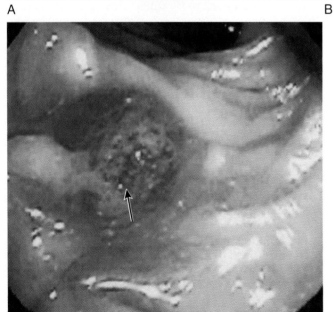

C

Figure 119–6 Sigmoid polyp detected by CT colonography (virtual colonoscopy). Images of the polyp (*arrows*) by standard two-dimensional CT scan (*A*), CT colonography with three-dimensional reconstruction (*B*), and regular colonoscopy (*C*). (*A-C*, From Fenlon HM, Nunes DP, Schroy PC, et al: A comparison of virtual and conventional colonoscopy for the detection of colorectal polyps. N Engl J Med 341:1496, 1999.)

colonography detected polyps and even cancers that were missed by colonoscopy.[144,150] It remains unclear how frequently CT colonoscopy (with its attendant radiation exposure) should be performed in a healthy screening population. Further studies will help determine the role for this rapidly emerging technology in colorectal cancer screening.

Newer Methods for Adenoma Detection

Based on our knowledge of molecular genetic alterations in colon carcinogenesis, a noninvasive method for detecting altered human DNA in stool has been developed.[152,153] In initial studies of patients with colon cancer, the sensitivity of the test was approximately 65%. In a large, multicenter study of average-risk, asymptomatic individuals older than 50 years of age, the sensitivity for colon cancer was 52% with specificity of 95%.[64] This study demonstrated that stool DNA analysis was three to four times more sensitive than FOBT for detecting invasive cancers and adenomas with high-grade dysplasia. Further enhancements of this promising technology are being developed in an effort to offer an alternative approach for noninvasive colon cancer screening. The use of chromoendoscopy to aid in the diagnosis of flat adenomas may be a useful adjunct to colonoscopy (see earlier). Further population and intervention studies are required before the full impact of these tests on colorectal cancer screening can be determined.

Management

Proper management of the patient with adenomatous polyps requires an understanding of the natural history of untreated adenomas, the relationship between multiple adenomas and carcinomas, and the course of patients after treatment (polypectomy).

Natural History

Little is known about adenoma growth rate, primarily because with the advent of endoscopy, polyps now are removed readily, thereby interrupting the natural history of their growth. Thus, our limited knowledge about polyp growth rate has been pieced together from two main types of studies: longitudinal follow-up studies on patients with unresected polyps and studies that compare the age distribution of people with adenomas with that of people with carcinomas.

The Untreated Adenoma. Longitudinal studies of people with untreated adenomas afford the most direct picture of the natural history of adenomas. In general, however, studies of this kind have been retrospective and either involved few patients or suffered from a lack of histologic confirmation of the index polyp. Despite these drawbacks, it appears that the adenoma-to-carcinoma progression is rather slow, requiring several years to unfold. Muto and associates reported that in 14 individuals with unresected polyps, it took at least 5 years and often more than 10 years for histologically proven adenomas to progress to cancer.[5] The size of the index polyp affects the interval to carcinoma, because larger adenomas are more likely than smaller ones to develop or already contain a focus of cancer. But even starting with a 1-cm polypoid tumor of unknown histology, serial

barium enema measurements have suggested that it may take 2 to 5 years for cancer to develop[154] and that the cumulative risk of cancer at the polyp site is 2.5% at 5 years, 8% at 10 years, and 24% at 20 years after diagnosis.[155] Other radiologic studies indicate that in adenomas with growth rates that are as rapid as those of cancer, doubling times are still longer than 4 to 6 months.[156,157]

Smaller polyps are likely to require even more time to progress to cancer, and even after several years, many adenomas do not enlarge. For example, in a study involving 213 asymptomatic people with rectal polyps of unknown histology ranging in size from 0.2 to 1.5 cm, serial rigid sigmoidoscopies over 3 to 5 years detected only two cancers, and only 4% of the polyps grew larger; the other 96% of polyps remained unchanged, got smaller, or disappeared.[158] Also, over a 3-year period, adenomas smaller than 1 cm did not significantly change size, and those that were 5 to 9 mm actually showed slight regression.[159] In another endoscopic study, histologically proven diminutive adenomas were left in place for 2 years, after which time only one half of them enlarged, but none grew to more than 0.5 cm or developed severe dysplasia or cancer.[23] By contrast, other investigators reported that of 30 rectosigmoid polyps 3 to 9 mm left in place, but measured every 6 months for 2 years, none regressed in size, although only 3 showed a fast growth rate (2 to 4 mm per year).[160] A mathematical model, using assumptions based on doubling-time calculations from serial barium enemas, predicts that a diminutive polyp (<0.5 cm) requires 2 to 3 years to reach 1-cm size.[161] A recent computational analysis of data from the National Polyp Study, where initial adenoma rates were high but incidence rates were low, also supports the notion that adenomas can regress.[162] Despite evidence of polyp regression or slow growth rates, from a clinical management standpoint, any polyp that is detected should be removed.

Age Distribution Studies. Additional, albeit indirect, support of the rather slow growth of adenomas comes from studies that have compared the mean age of people with adenomas with that of people with carcinomas. For instance, studies from St. Mark's Hospital in London and from the National Polyp Study in the United States indicate that the mean age of people with a single adenoma is about 4 to 5 years younger than those with a colon cancer.[5,163] A similar analysis in FAP patients has shown that patients with adenomas are about 12 years younger than those with colon cancer.[5] The mean age of male veterans with AAP or colon cancer found by screening colonoscopy was 65.1 years, compared with 62.7 years for those without any polyps.[89] Kozuka and colleagues estimated that the transition period for adenomas with mild dysplasia to cancer is 8 years, whereas the interval for adenomas with severe dysplasia to become malignant is 3.6 years.[44] Finally, Eide calculated that over a 10-year period, there is only a 2.5% risk that an adenoma-bearing person will develop colon cancer, but this risk would be greater if the adenoma were large or villous.[164]

Multiple Adenomas and Carcinomas

For proper patient management and design of cancer screening and surveillance programs, it is important to know the frequency with which adenomas coexist with other adenomas or carcinomas. The term "multiple adenomas" (or carcinoma) simply means 2 or more neoplasms and should not be confused with the "multiple adenomatous polyposis syndrome" that is characterized by hundreds of polyps (see below). An adenoma or carcinoma that is diagnosed at the same time as an index colorectal neoplasm is called a *synchronous* lesion, whereas one that is diagnosed at least 6 months later (a somewhat arbitrary limit) is considered *metachronous.*

The adenomatous polyp itself commonly is regarded as a marker of a neoplasm-prone colon. Indeed, 30% to 50% of colons with one adenoma will contain at least one other synchronous adenoma, especially in the older age groups.[5,12,16] The risks of colon cancer and of high-grade dysplasia both rise with the number of adenomas present (Table 119–8) and approach 100% in people with FAP.

A synchronous adenoma can be found in 30% of colons that harbor a carcinoma[5,165-167] and in 50% to 85% of those that harbor two or more synchronous cancers.[5,165,168,169] If the synchronous adenoma is diagnosed preoperatively and is distant from the carcinoma, the surgical approach may have to be adapted to the particular circumstances.[165] For this reason, preoperative colonoscopy is strongly recommended before the resection of any colorectal carcinoma. Also, the presence of a synchronous adenoma in a patient with colon cancer increases the risk for developing subsequent colon cancer.[5,166] Similarly, a synchronous adenoma in a patient

with a colonic polyp places that person at greater risk for developing metachronous polyps[170] and cancer.[170,171]

Initial Management

If a polyp is detected by barium enema or CT colonography, a colonoscopy is recommended to afford the simultaneous opportunities to remove the polyp and search for synchronous neoplasms. When a polyp is encountered during sigmoidoscopy, it should be removed to establish its histologic type. If the polyp is hyperplastic, most authorities do not recommend a full colonoscopy,[172] although this is controversial (see "Hyperplastic Polyps").

There is some debate as to whether rectosigmoid adenomas found at sigmoidoscopy are markers for proximal colonic neoplasia and thereby prompt the need for a full colonoscopy. This controversy applies particularly to patients who have only a single, small, tubular adenoma with low-grade dysplasia. Some studies indicate that in this subset of patients, colonoscopy does not discover a substantial number of proximal AAPs or cancers,[173-175] nor is there a subsequent risk of developing proximal cancer among those who do not undergo colonoscopy.[176,177] In contrast, two screening colonoscopy studies suggest that the odds of finding advanced proximal neoplasia even with a small, single, tubular adenoma, is 2.6-fold to 4-fold that of finding no distal pathology[61,79] (Table 119–9). Some authors have estimated that by not doing

Table 119–8 Correlation Between the Number of Adenomas and Associated Carcinomas or High-Grade Dysplasia

No. of Adenomas per Patient	St. Mark's Hospital[5]		National Polyp Study[2]	
	No. of Patients	% of Patients with Carcinoma	No. of Patients	% of Patients with High-Grade Dysplasia
1	1331	30	1093	7
2	296	52	430	10
3	83	57	166	19
4	40	50	83	17
5	13	77	40	20
≥6	25	80	55	20

Table 119–9 Frequency of Advanced Proximal Neoplasia Related to Findings in the Distal Colon

	Frequency of Advanced Proximal Neoplasia					
	Ref 61*		Ref 62*		Ref 79†	
Findings in Distal Colon	Percent	Odds Ratio (95% CI)	Percent	Relative Risk (95% CI)	Percent	Odds Ratio (95% CI)
No distal polyps	2.7	1.0	1.5	1.0	5.3	1.0
Distal hyperplastic polyp	2.8	1.1 (0.6-2.1)	4.0	2.6 (1.1-5.9)	—	—
Distal adenoma	6.8	2.6 (1.7-4.1)	7.1	4.0 (1.9-8.3)	5.0	1.26 (0.81-1.98)
Distal advanced neoplasm			11.5	6.7 (3.2-16.6)		
Tubular adenoma >1 cm	8.6	3.2 (1.5-6.8)	—	—	4.5	1.66 (1.10-2.52)
Villous features	12.5	4.7 (2.1-10.4)	—	—	12.1	2.46 (1.60-3.77)
High-grade dysplasia	11.4	4.5 (1.5-13.4)	—	—	—	—
Invasive cancer	25.0	9.8 (3.6-26.4)	—	—	—	—

*Screening colonoscopy study.
†Screening sigmoidoscopy followed by colonoscopy.
CI, confidence interval.

colonoscopy for a distal, nonadvanced adenoma, 36% of advanced proximal neoplasms would be missed.[178] Furthermore, 52% of patients with advanced proximal neoplasia have no distal adenoma,[61] and 70% of proximal colon cancers lack a distal marker lesion.[179] These observations have provided the incentive to consider colonoscopy as a primary screening modality. For the time being, recommended guidelines are to individualize the approach to these patients.[172] Since risk factors for finding advanced proximal neoplasia are increasing age,[61,62,79] a positive family history of colorectal cancer,[61,79] and male gender,[62] performing colonoscopy in these individuals on the basis of finding a distal, small, tubular adenoma would seem prudent. A risk index that stratified patients into low, intermediate, or high risk based on the type and size of distal colonic polyps as well as patient age and male sex was able to predict the risk of proximal advanced colonic neoplasia.[180]

There is little debate that if sigmoidoscopy reveals more than one adenoma, or a distal AAP, then a full colonoscopy is warranted because of the higher likelihood of finding synchronous proximal advanced neoplasms (see Table 119–9). Because negative biopsy results from a fractional sample of a polyp cannot possibly rule out cancer, total excision of a polyp is the only method of providing a thorough and accurate histologic diagnosis. For larger polyps, this may require piecemeal excision, and for sessile growths, injection of saline into the polyp base can assist with complete endoscopic resection. After apparent complete removal of a large adenoma, it is advisable to repeat the colonoscopy in 3 to 6 months to document the completeness of the excision.[172] If a polyp cannot be completely excised after two or three endoscopic sessions, surgical therapy is recommended.

Based on the previous discussion, screening colonoscopy is gaining acceptance in the United States as a primary screening tool, although many other countries with more limited resources do not yet subscribe to this philosophy. Two large-scale European trials are underway to evaluate the use of selective colonoscopy in patients based on the findings of a single sigmoidoscopy performed about the age of 60 years.[136,137] After screening sigmoidoscopy, 5% to 8% of patients were referred for colonoscopy based on the finding of high-risk lesions or multiple polyps. Of these patients 15% to 18% were found to have proximal adenomas, 5% advanced proximal adenomas, and fewer than 1% to have cancer. Follow-up data regarding the incidence and mortality of colorectal cancer in these patients, as well as the results of the PLCO Cancer Screening Trial,[76] will provide additional data from prospective trials on the utility of screening sigmoidoscopy.

Management of the Malignant Polyp

The term *malignant polyp* refers to an adenoma in which a focus of carcinoma has invaded beyond the muscularis mucosae into the submucosa (see earlier). This term is not applied to adenomas containing either carcinoma in situ or intramucosal carcinoma because these lesions are not invasive and carry no metastatic potential. Rarely, polyps may consist entirely of carcinoma. These so-called polypoid carcinomas usually are considered a subset of malignant polyps, and they most likely represent a previous adenoma that is completely replaced by carcinoma.

Sometimes islands of benign adenomatous epithelium are found beneath the muscularis mucosae, and care must be taken not to mistake such "pseudocarcinomatous invasion" for true invasive carcinoma; this important distinction may be difficult particularly in the rare instance when the ectopic benign epithelium exhibits features of high-grade dysplasia. Ectopic benign epithelium is seen more often in larger pedunculated polyps, particularly in the sigmoid colon. Because the distinction between carcinoma in situ and invasive carcinoma will influence both management and prognosis, it is crucial that tissue be properly oriented for pathologic examination and that close communication takes place among endoscopist, surgeon, and pathologist.

The endoscopic removal of the vast majority of colorectal polyps raises two central and related questions: Is endoscopic polypectomy alone adequate therapy for the malignant polyp? If not, what features of the polyp can predict the presence of residual disease or subsequent recurrence? The answers are vital because they determine the decision for subsequent surgical resection of bowel.

Complete endoscopic removal of an adenoma with noninvasive carcinoma is curative. The decision regarding therapy becomes much more difficult when polyps contain invasive carcinoma. Although most of these lesions are treated adequately by endoscopic polypectomy, approximately 10% of patients will experience an adverse outcome[181] defined as residual cancer in the bowel wall or in lymph nodes either at the time of polypectomy or on follow-up examination. This rate of failure is comparable to that of the precolonoscopic era when adenomas were larger and underwent more complete surgical resection.[181] Because malignant polyps account for only 5% of all adenomas, and because not all patients who have had colonoscopic removal of malignant polyps have had surgical resection or are available for follow-up, conclusions often are based on small numbers.

Notwithstanding these limitations, combined experience has identified certain favorable and unfavorable histopathologic features of a colonoscopically resected malignant polyp that can be used to classify a patient as being at low or high risk for an adverse outcome (Table 119–10). If none of these unfavorable risk factors is found, the patient is considered to have been cured by the endoscopic polypectomy. This principle applies even to endoscopically removed polypoid carcinomas, which have been associated with a surprisingly good outcome when not complicated by any unfavorable histopathologic features. If one or more unfavorable features is found in a malignant polyp (see Fig. 120–21), the chance of an adverse outcome rises to about 10% to 25%.[182] In such cases, surgical resection usually should be performed, taking into account the risk of operative mortality in elderly patients with comorbid illnesses.[172]

Several aspects of defining these risk factors demand close collaboration between endoscopists and pathologists. First, some malignant polyps contain only a small focus of poorly differentiated carcinoma, and therefore meticulous pathologic analysis is essential. Second, identification of vessel invasion by cancer cells in malignant polyps may be difficult, in which case special stains of vascular endothelium can be used for clarification. Third,

Table 119–10   Risk Factors for Adverse Outcomes in Patients with Malignant Polyps

Risk Factor	Favorable Feature	Unfavorable Feature
Degree of differentiation	Well or moderate	Poor
Invasion of veins or lymphatics	Absent	Present
Polypectomy margin	Clear or >2-mm margin	Involved
Invasion of submucosa of bowel wall	Absent	Present

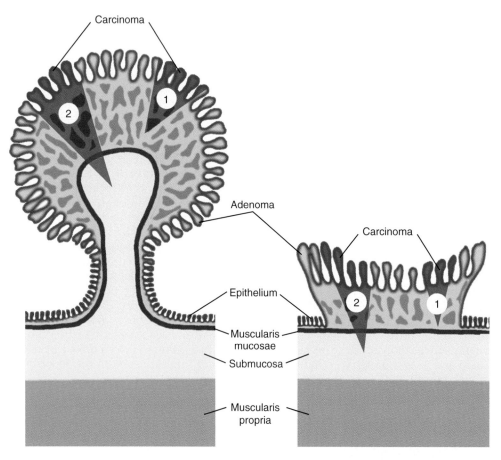

Figure 119–7 Carcinoma in situ versus invasive cancer. Carcinoma is considered intramucosal or carcinoma in situ, as indicated by the area labeled "1" either in a pedunculated adenoma (*left*) or in a sessile adenoma (*right*). This lesion, as a rule, does not metastasize. Carcinoma in an adenomatous polyp is considered invasive when it breaches the muscularis mucosae, as indicated by the area labeled "2." Invasive cancer in a pedunculated polyp is unlikely to metastasize, and it is managed differently from invasive cancer in a sessile polyp, which often requires surgical resection.

although the polypectomy margin may be found on microscopy to contain cancer cells, some studies suggest that if the endoscopist believes that a complete excision was achieved, surgical resection may not be necessary because the electrocautery may have effectively destroyed residual tumor in the bowel wall.[183] Finally, when judging the adequacy of endoscopic polypectomy, the issue of submucosal invasion is important. A pedunculated polyp differs anatomically from a sessile polyp in that the submucosa of the former projects up into the stalk, whereas the submucosa of the latter is in direct continuity with the bowel wall proper (Fig. 119–7). If cancer in a pedunculated polyp is confined to the submucosa of the stalk and all other histologic features are favorable, surgery is not indicated because the chance of an adverse outcome from endoscopic polypectomy is less than the operative mortality. Once the submucosa of the bowel wall is involved with cancer (a situation that

occurs more readily in sessile polyps), the chance of an adverse outcome often outweighs the operative mortality, thereby justifying surgical resection. Furthermore, because endoscopic technique purposely avoids cutting deep into the bowel wall submucosa, there are few published examples of sessile lesions that have been completely excised endoscopically with clear margins and no other unfavorable features.

Deciding on the optimal plan of management after polypectomy involves weighing the risks of morbidity and mortality from potential residual or recurrent cancer against the risks of morbidity and mortality from a surgical attempt to cure any such residual disease or lymph node metastasis. A few general recommendations, however, are offered. If excision of an adenoma is complete, endoscopic polypectomy alone is adequate therapy for adenomas that contain carcinoma in situ, pedunculated adenomas that harbor well-differentiated or moderately differentiated invasive carcinoma, and polypoid carcinomas. Resectional surgery is indicated for malignant polyps in which the invasive carcinoma (1) is poorly differentiated, (2) involves endothelium-lined channels (lymphatics, blood vessels), (3) extends to or within 2 mm of the polypectomy margin, or (4) involves the submucosa of the colonic wall (including all sessile adenomas). Clearly the ultimate plan of therapy must be individualized according to each patient's medical condition. For most patients with malignant polyps, polypectomy without surgical resection seems adequate, with the caveat that postpolypectomy endoscopic surveillance be incorporated into the patient's health care.

Postpolypectomy Management

Polyp Recurrence Rates. Although patients in whom a colorectal adenoma has been excised completely are likely to develop subsequent (metachronous) neoplasms, the frequency and time course of this future transformation are not well understood. In long-term retrospective studies, the cumulative risk of adenoma recurrence is nearly linear, being 20% at 5 years after polypectomy and rising to 50% after 15 years (Fig. 119–8).[184] Information on this subject is inexact because earlier studies were primarily retrospective, involved short follow-up periods, and differed in endoscopic indications. Moreover, recurrence rates tend to be somewhat inflated because lesions missed during the index colonoscopy may be considered recurrences. With these caveats in mind, it is estimated that one third of people who have undergone polypectomy develop recurrent adenomas.[185-187] The recurrence rate at 1 year is as low as 5% to 15%[184,187] but more realistically ranges from 30% to 45% based on prospective colonoscopy studies.[185,188-191] In the National Polyp Study, the overall adenoma recurrence rate was 42% for patients who underwent surveillance colonoscopy at 1 and 3 years after index polypectomy compared with 32% in the group that was examined only at 3 years.[45] There is general consensus that recurrent adenomas typically are smaller and less likely to harbor advanced pathology than are index adenomas.

Can histopathologic features of adenomas at the time of the index polypectomy be used to help predict recurrence of adenomas? Virtually all studies agree that the presence of multiple index adenomas is an important predictor of subsequent adenoma (and carcinoma) recurrence[184,185,187,192,193] (see Fig. 119–8). This dictum applies despite negative findings on colonoscopy 1 year after polypectomy.[188] Some studies suggest that polyp size greater than 1 cm,[186,187,193] severe dysplasia,[194] villous histology,[187,192] and older age[185,187] also are risk factors for adenoma recurrence, but the relative importance of each of these factors independently is uncertain.

It can be argued that the most clinically important recurrence is an AAP. Some studies have reported a 6.3% to 7.0% recurrence rate for AAP over a 4-year follow-up period.[190] In the National Polyp Study, the recurrence rate of advanced adenomas was 3.3%, regardless of whether patients underwent colonoscopy at 1 and 3 years, or only 3 years, after polypectomy. The cumulative incidence of AAP was 4% at 3 years and 8% at 6 years of follow-up. Independent predictors for AAP at follow-up included: more than three adenomas at index colonoscopy, and age older than 60 years at the time of adenoma diagnosis with a parent who had colorectal cancer.[195] In the presence of these two risk factors, cumulative AAP recurrence rates rose to 10% at 3 years and 20% at 6 years of follow-up. The individuals at lowest risk for developing AAP were those with a single adenoma diagnosed when younger than 60 years of age. Another colonoscopic follow-up study reported that multiple adenomas at the index colonoscopy increased the risk of AAP, but also found that adenoma size greater than 1 cm and proximal location were additional risk factors.[193]

Effect of Polypectomy on Colorectal Cancer Incidence. If adenomas are the precursor to colon cancer, then removing them should decrease the subsequent incidence of colon cancer. Indeed, several uncontrolled and case-control series strongly suggest that distal colorectal cancers can be prevented and mortality reduced by screening proctosigmoidoscopy.[46-49] Other studies found that removal of adenomas by polypectomy was associated with an increased incidence of colon cancer.[196-198] Because these retrospective studies did not establish a polyp-free colon (or always consider adenoma size and histology), however, the higher colon cancer rate might reflect malignant progression of other adenomas that had not been removed. Two studies from the Mayo Clinic also did not establish a polyp-free colon at the time of polypectomy.[25,171] Despite these observations, if the removed polyps were small (<1 cm), there was no greater risk for subsequently developing colon cancer,

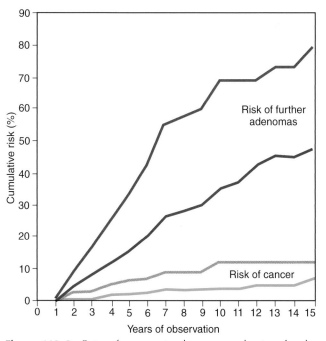

Figure 119–8 Rate of recurrent adenomas and rate of colon cancers after adenoma removal. The risk of developing further adenomas (*orange, purple*) or cancer (*blue, green*) is higher in patients who initially underwent removal of multiple adenomas (*orange, blue*) rather than a single adenoma (*purple, green*). (Modified from Morson BC, Bussey HJR: Magnitude of risk for cancer in patients with colorectal adenomas. Br J Surg 72[Suppl]: S23, 1985.)

whereas the removal of large adenomas was associated with a greater risk of subsequent colorectal cancer, again supporting the concept that advanced neoplasms at index polypectomy are predictors of subsequent neoplasia. Important observations also come from the St. Marks Hospital study in which rectal adenomas were removed without any subsequent examinations.[176] If the index polyp was a small, tubular adenoma, there was no greater risk of subsequent cancer anywhere in the colon, whereas the risk was significantly increased if the index adenoma was large or contained villous elements. Others have shown a marked reduction in colon cancer incidence related to polypectomy.[199]

The most valid study design to address this issue is a prospective colonoscopic study in which an adenoma-free colon is established and patients are followed for subsequent development of colonic neoplasms. The National Polyp Study is a landmark study in this regard. This was a prospective, multicenter, randomized trial in which a cohort of 1418 patients underwent a "clearing" colonoscopy to remove one or more adenomas and was then followed at specific intervals for a mean of 5.9 years. During the follow-up period, five early asymptomatic cancers were detected, representing only 10% to 24% of the expected incidence compared with three historical reference groups.[45] Two other studies (from Norway and Italy) confirm that colonoscopic polypectomy was associated with a 75% to 80% reduction in subsequent colorectal cancer incidence.[200,201] In a smaller study, the Funen Adenoma Follow-up Study, it was found that although the incidence of subsequent colon cancers was not reduced by polypectomy, the mortality was reduced.[202] In summary, these studies indicate that the adenoma is a marker of a neoplasm-prone colon and that colonoscopic clearing of all adenomas is of considerable benefit.

Frequency of Surveillance Colonoscopy. The National Polyp Study has taught us that performing follow-up colonoscopy at 1 year is a low-yield proposition, as others have observed using sigmoidoscopy.[199] It also is worth realizing that an endoscopic examination of the colorectum may afford protection against colon cancer for 6 to 10 years.[47,48] Moreover, it has been proposed that a single lifetime sigmoidoscopy at about age 55 to 60 years could be standard policy for colon cancer screening, with referral of patients for colonoscopy and subsequent surveillance only if the sigmoidoscopy discloses a distal adenoma with advanced features.[136]

A consensus statement for postpolypectomy surveillance guidelines has been generated by the major gastroenterology medical societies.[145] A complete colonoscopy should be performed at the time of polypectomy, clearing the colon of all existing adenomas; this may take more than one session for large or multiple polyps. The interval before the next surveillance colonoscopy is based on the patient's category of recurrent adenoma risk (Table 119–11). If the patient is in the high-risk group for adenoma recurrence, repeat colonoscopy is performed in 3 years to check for metachronous adenomas. For low-risk patients, repeat colonoscopy should be performed in 5 years. After one negative follow-up surveillance colonoscopy, the subsequent surveillance interval can be

Table 119–11 Risk Factors for Developing an Adenoma with Advanced Pathology or a Colorectal Cancer after Colonoscopic Polypectomy

Low risk
  1 or 2 small (<1 cm) tubular adenomas
  No family history of colorectal neoplasia
High risk
  Multiple (≥3) adenomas
  Large adenoma (>1 cm)
  Adenoma with a villous component
  Adenoma with high-grade dysplasia
  First-degree relative with colorectal cancer

increased to 5 years. Adherence to this plan is predicted to be cost-effective.[172]

NON-NEOPLASTIC

Pathologically, whereas neoplastic polyps are part of an identifiable spectrum, non-neoplastic polyps fall into several distinct and unrelated groups, including *hyperplastic polyps, mucosal polyps, juvenile polyps, Peutz-Jeghers polyps, inflammatory polyps,* and many other submucosal lesions (see Table 119–1).

Hyperplastic Polyps

The most common non-neoplastic polyp in the colon is the hyperplastic polyp, referred to by some pathologists as metaplastic polyps. Hyperplastic polyps usually are small; their average size is less than 5 mm and they seldom are greater than 10 mm, although larger hyperplastic polyps have been reported.

Histologic Features
Hyperplastic polyps typically are small sessile lesions that are grossly indistinguishable from small adenomatous polyps. Microscopically, the colonic crypts are elongated and the epithelial cells assume a characteristic papillary configuration (Fig. 119–9). The epithelium is made up of well-differentiated goblet and absorptive cells. The cytologic atypia that is characteristic of adenomatous polyps is not seen. Mitoses and DNA synthesis are limited to the base of the crypts, and orderly cell maturation is preserved. The epithelial cell and attendant pericryptal sheath fibroblast make up an epithelial-mesenchymal unit that migrates up the colonic crypt. In contrast to adenomatous polyps, in which the epithelium and fibroblast appear to be immature, this tissue is better differentiated, and abundant collagen is synthesized in the basement membrane.[203] It is thought that the migration of epithelial cells up the colonic crypt is slow and that hyperplastic polyps develop from the failure of mature cells to detach normally.[204]

Polyps that display features of both hyperplastic and adenomatous transformation have been described. These mixed hyperplastic-adenomatous polyps account for about 13% of hyperplastic polyps.[205] When this type of polyp exhibits larger size, prominent architectural

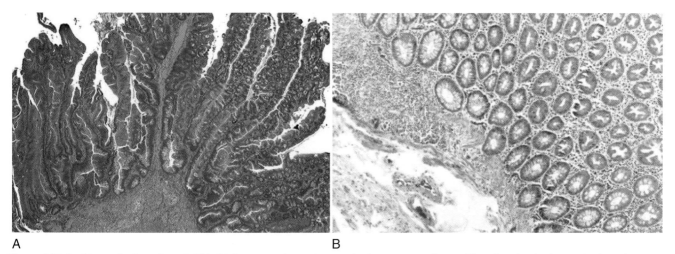

Figure 119–9 Hyperplastic polyp. *A*, This high-power photomicrograph demonstrates the papillary fronds of a hyperplastic polyp, consisting of elongated epithelial cells with large amounts of mucus. The nuclei retain their basal orientation and demonstrate no atypia. (From Fontelo P et al: Online Courses: Virtual Gastrointestinal Endoscopic Biopsy Course: www.afip.org.) *B*, This photomicrograph demonstrates the characteristic "starfish" appearance of hyperplastic glands cut in cross section. Again, the orderly appearance of the nuclei, the generous cytoplasmic-to-nuclear ratio, and the abundance of secreted mucus at the surface of the polyp (*top*) can be readily appreciated. (From Pathology Education Resources Laboratory, Indiana University School of Medicine, http://erl.pathology.iupui.edu/, © 1997-1998 Indiana University.)

distortion, nuclear atypia, and upper crypt zone mitoses, it usually is considered more adenomatous than hyperplastic, and is termed a *serrated adenoma*. Evidence is mounting to support the concept of a distinct *serrated polyp neoplasia pathway*.[206,207] Hyperplastic polyps may give rise to serrated adenomas by a subtle form of genomic instability related to a specific type of DNA replication error. These lesions can then give rise to the approximate 10% of colon cancers that manifest low levels of microsatellite instability,[208] and there is evidence that sporadic cancers with high levels of MSI also arise from a serrated neoplasia pathway involving the activation of the *Braf* oncogene with subsequent methylation silencing of *hMLH1*.[207]

For the most part, true sporadic hyperplastic polyps are considered to have little if any intrinsic malignant potential; however, it is important to consider that hyperplastic polyps and neoplastic lesions can appear in the same colon, suggesting that the two may be pathogenetically related. Indeed, a germline mutation of the *APC* gene (E1317Q) has been associated with an unusually large number of colorectal hyperplastic polyps in association with adenomas.[209] Coexisting hyperplastic and adenomatous polyps are common also in the setting of a strong family history of colorectal cancer, including HNPCC.[210] Hyperplastic polyps of concern are those that are large (>1 cm), numerous (>20), located in the proximal colon, and associated with a family history of colon cancer.[207]

Prevalence

The prevalence of hyperplastic polyps is not known with precision, but these growths are common. In colonoscopic examinations of asymptomatic patients older than 50 years of age, hyperplastic polyps were found in 9% to 10%,[67,68] although this frequency may be higher (30% to 31%) among male veterans.[69,211] Sigmoidoscopic screening of asymptomatic relatives of adenoma-prone kindreds revealed 26% with hyperplastic polyps, a prevalence that

was essentially identical (28%) to that of asymptomatic spouse controls.[212] Autopsy data report a prevalence rate of 20% to 35%.[8,12,60]

The frequency of hyperplastic polyps depends largely on the site of the colon being examined and on the age of the patient. Autopsy studies repeatedly observe a distal predominance of hyperplastic polyps.[8,11,12,70] Of course, sigmoidoscopic studies, which focus on the distal colon and rectum, find more hyperplastic polyps, but even screening colonoscopy studies detect more hyperplastic polyps in the distal than in the proximal colon.[62] Among all diminutive polyps (<5 mm) removed during colonoscopy, hyperplastic polyps outnumber adenomatous polyps in the rectum and sigmoid, whereas adenomas predominate in the remainder of the colon.[15,213] The prevalence of hyperplastic polyps increases with age.[10,54,70] There also is an association between hyperplastic polyp prevalence and colon cancer prevalence (Table 119–12), although this correlation is not as firm as the association between adenomas and colon cancers, nor does it necessarily imply any premalignant potential to the hyperplastic polyp itself. Data suggest that current smoking is a risk factor for hyperplastic polyps.[89]

Management

Hyperplastic polyps remain small, usually are sessile, and seldom if ever cause symptoms. Inasmuch as they are not likely to give rise to cancer, little is gained by removing them, but because they cannot be distinguished from neoplastic or serrated polyps simply by gross examination, they usually are removed. Given their usual predominance in the distal colorectum, finding hyperplastic polyps in this location is not an alarming finding, particularly in the elderly. Therefore, the bulk of evidence does not support a policy of proximal polyp hunting by colonoscopy in patients with hyperplastic polyps in the rectosigmoid.[74,77,172,214-216] A systematic review of the subject found that in asymptomatic individuals, a

Table 119–12 Prevalence of Hyperplastic Polyps

| | | Prevalence Rate of Polyps, % | | | | | |
| | | Men, Age in Years | | | Women, Age in Years | | |
Population	Prevalence of Colon Cancer	20-39	40-59	60+	20-39	40-59	60+
Hawaiian-Japanese U.S. (New Orleans)	Very high	50	69	84	0	57	73
Whites	High	11	19	13	—	25	30
Blacks	High	10	18	14	6	7	9
Brazil (São Paulo)	Intermediate	14	26	40	12	23	31
Japan							
Akita	Intermediate	0	2	2	0	2	8
Miyagi	Low	1	2	2	0	0	3
Costa Rica (San José)	Low	0	7	7	5	1	9
Colombia (Cali)	Low	6	17	11	2	9	16

From Correa P: Epidemiology of polyps and cancer. In Morson BC (ed): The Pathogenesis of Colorectal Cancer. Philadelphia, WB Saunders, 1978, p 126.

distal hyperplastic polyp is associated with a 21% to 25% risk for any proximal neoplasia and a 4% to 5% risk of advanced proximal neoplasia, thus justifying colonoscopy.[217] While we await additional data on this subject, current guidelines do not recommend performing colonoscopy for a distal hyperplastic polyp, nor do such patients need to be entered into a regular surveillance program for detecting subsequent neoplasms.[172] Serrated adenomas are much less common than hyperplastic polyps, accounting for less than 1% of all polyps and between 1% and 11% of adenomas.[207] The prevalence of high-grade dysplasia and cancer in these lesions, however, may be as high as 5% to 16%.[207] Thus, surveillance intervals for serrated adenomas, although not yet defined, should follow that of other adenomas, bearing in mind their possibly more rapid progression.

MUCOSAL

The colon frequently harbors excrescences or mammillations of tissue that histologically are normal mucosa. In these instances, the submucosa has elevated the normal tissue overlying it. These lesions may be termed *mucosal polyps*, and their presence has no clinical significance. Mucosal polyps always are small and may constitute 8% to 20% of the material recovered in a collection of colonoscopic biopsies.

JUVENILE

Juvenile polyps (Fig. 119–10) are mucosal tumors that consist primarily of an excess of lamina propria and dilated cystic glands, rather than an overabundance of epithelial cells as seen in adenomatous and hyperplastic polyps, and therefore they are classified as hamartomas. The appearance of distended, mucus-filled glands, inflammatory cells, and edematous lamina propria has prompted some observers to call these lesions *retention polyps*. Juvenile polyps appear to be acquired lesions because they seldom are seen in the first year of life and are most common from ages 1 to 7 years; occasion-

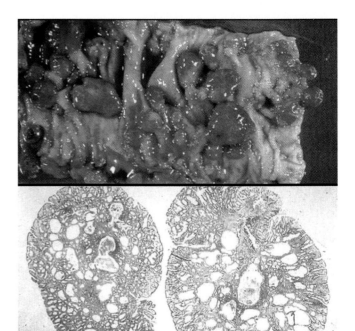

Figure 119–10 Juvenile polyps. (*Top*) Resection specimen of a colon harboring multiple juvenile polyps. (*Bottom*) Histologic photomicrograph revealing the characteristic large cystic spaces of this lesion. (From Demetris AJ, Finkelstein SD, Nalensnik MA, et al: Slide Carousel of GI Pathology Course for Medical Students. http://www.pathology.pitt.edu/lectures/gi/. © Department of Pathology, University of Pittsburgh School of Medicine.)

ally they are found in adults. Juvenile polyps more often are single than multiple, usually are pedunculated, and tend to range in size from 3 mm to 2 cm. Because these polyps tend to be in the rectum and to develop a stalk, they may prolapse during defecation and even slough. In addition, the stroma contains a generous vascular supply, which explains the considerable blood loss suffered by some patients. Because of the high likelihood of bleeding and prolapse, removal of juvenile polyps is suggested.

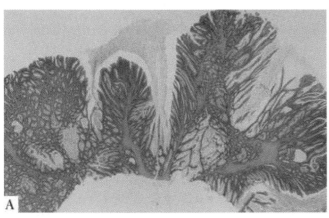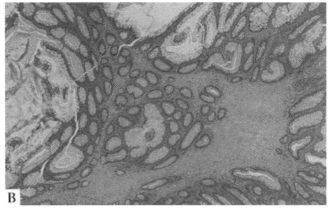

Figure 119–11 Low-power (*A*) and high-power (*B*) photomicrographs of a Peutz-Jeghers polyp. In this type of polyp, the glandular epithelium is supported by an arborizing framework of well-developed smooth muscle that is contiguous with the muscularis mucosae. (From Boland CR: The Colon, Rectum, and Anus. *In* Feldman M (ed): Gastroenterology and Hepatology: The Comprehensive Visual Reference. Philadelphia, Churchill Livingstone, 1996.)

Juvenile polyps have essentially no malignant potential when single,[218] and they tend not to recur. Although approximately 20% of individual juvenile polyps in the rectum may be associated with proximal polyps, proximal adenomas are rare, and the subsequent rate of dying of or developing colorectal cancer is no greater than these rates for the general population, even without specific surveillance.[218] When juvenile polyps are multiple (see "Juvenile Polyposis Syndrome"), however, the risk of developing cancer is present, because adenomatous epithelium may be present in some juvenile polyps or because of a coexistent adenoma.

PEUTZ-JEGHERS

The Peutz-Jeghers polyp is a unique hamartomatous lesion characterized by glandular epithelium supported by an arborizing framework of well-developed smooth muscle that is contiguous with the muscularis mucosae (Fig. 119–11). The smooth muscle bands fan out into the head of the polyp and become progressively thinner as they project toward its surface. A Peutz-Jeghers polyp differs from a juvenile polyp in that the lamina propria is normal, and the characteristic architecture of the lesion derives chiefly from its abnormal smooth muscle tissue. These polyps almost always are multiple, and their distinctive appearance, in association with the extraintestinal manifestations, makes Peutz-Jeghers syndrome easily identifiable. This type of polyp seldom is found in the colon in the absence of generalized polyposis (see later).

INFLAMMATORY (PSEUDOPOLYPS)

Inflammatory polyps are found in the regenerative and healing phases of inflammation. They usually are formed by full-thickness ulceration of epithelium followed by a regenerative process that leaves the mucosa in bizarre polypoid configurations. Less commonly, inflammatory polyps may represent relatively normal mucosa sitting amidst re-epithelialized ulcerations. Inflammatory polyps may be large and solitary, mimicking a neoplastic mass, or they may form mucosal bridges that span the lumen. Multiple lesions may mimic a polyposis syndrome. The term *pseudopolyp* is used to distinguish them from neoplastic lesions, but in reality these are true polypoid protuberances. Histologically, inflammation and exuberant granulation tissue may be seen in the early postinflammatory period, but later the polyp may resemble normal mucosa.

Any form of severe colitis, including chronic inflammatory bowel disease (ulcerative colitis, Crohn's disease),[219] amebic colitis,[220] ischemic colitis, or bacterial dysentery, may give rise to inflammatory polyps. In chronic schistosomiasis, multiple inflammatory polyps that contain granulation tissue, eggs, or adult worms commonly are seen.[221] The significance of these polyps, which have no intrinsic neoplastic potential, is that they often appear in diseased colons that are at high risk for developing colon cancer (ulcerative colitis, schistosomiasis); therefore, they must be distinguished from neoplastic lesions that do carry premalignant potential. Giant or grouped pseudopolyps may cause colonic obstruction.

Rare cases of multiple and recurrent inflammatory gastrointestinal polyps that produce pain and obstruction have been reported on a sporadic and even a familial basis.[222] These lesions are found primarily in the ileum, may be very large, and may even cause intussusception. Cap polyposis is another rare condition, characterized by inflammatory polyps with elongated crypts, a mixed inflammatory infiltrate in the lamina propria, and a surface cap of fibrinopurulent exudate.[223] Although cap polyposis may be confused endoscopically with inflammatory bowel disease, mucosal prolapse has been suggested as a possible underlying etiology.

SUBMUCOSAL LESIONS

Colitis Cystica Profunda

Colitis cystica profunda (see Chapter 121) is a rare lesion consisting of dilated, mucus-filled glands in the submucosa that may form solitary or multiple polyps. The typical lesion is a solitary polyp smaller than 3 cm that most commonly is found in the rectum in the setting of chronic inflammation. Prior surgical procedures and ulcerative proctitis have been linked to the pathogenesis of this abnormality. The involved epithelium shows no evidence of dysplasia. The primary significance of this lesion is that it must be recognized and distinguished from colloid carcinoma, which may look similar histologically, because a mistaken diagnosis of colloid carcinoma could lead to inappropriate radical surgery.[224] The lesion is presumably caused by displacement of normal colonic glands to beneath the epithelium during the healing of a surgical wound or inflammation. Rarely, the polyps may become large or be recurrent and can even produce colon obstruction. It has been suggested that the pathologic picture and clinical presentation of colitis cystica profunda are similar to those of the so-called solitary rectal ulcer and that both may be produced by rectal prolapse.[224]

Pneumatosis Cystoides Intestinalis

Multiple gas-filled cysts are occasionally encountered within the submucosa of the colon (and small intestine) and may produce a polypoid appearance. The diagnosis of pneumatosis cystoides intestinalis (see Chapter 121) may be made on full-thickness pathologic sections or by the characteristic radiologic or endoscopic appearance of the intramural gas-filled cysts. The diagnosis is substantiated at endoscopy if the cysts collapse after aspiration with a sclerotherapy needle or by unroofing them with a biopsy forceps. This condition may produce a variety of symptoms, some of which are suggestive of colitis, but it also may be associated with vague symptoms or remain asymptomatic.[225]

Two forms of pneumatosis intestinalis have been recognized. One type (pneumatosis linearis) may be associated with a fulminant mucosal process, such as inflammatory or ischemic bowel disease in adults or necrotizing enterocolitis in children. In these fulminant settings, in which the condition often is fatal, it is thought that the cysts result from invasion of the submucosa by gas-forming bacteria. The more common type is seen in adults and is more typically a chronic or incidental finding, and it even may be associated with an asymptomatic pneumoperitoneum. Pneumatosis cystoides intestinalis is associated with chronic obstructive pulmonary disease and may be seen in patients with scleroderma. The genesis of the gas-filled cysts in these benign settings is incompletely understood, but it has been demonstrated that gas within the bowel lumen diffuses into the cysts, which may contribute to their maintenance. Oxygen therapy results in the resolution of these cysts,[226] but the pathophysiologic basis of this response is by no means clear. The natural history can be deduced only from a small number of cases, but the disease may persist for months.[225-227] A single course of oxygen therapy (often as little as 5 to 6 L/min of oxygen) can result in resolution of symptoms for a long time. Antibiotics are of no benefit.

Other Submucosal Lesions

Any lesion beneath the colon mucosa may elevate the overlying epithelium to produce a polypoid appearance. Lymphoid tissue is present throughout the colon, and hypertrophied follicles may be mistaken for a pathologic mucosal process. Benign lymphoid polyps even may grow large enough to produce symptoms (pain, bleeding) or may become pedunculated. Multiple benign lymphoid polyps may be found as normal variants, particularly in children (Fig. 119–12). The principal importance of benign lymphoid polyps is in their distinction from malignant lymphoid lesions. Malignant lymphoma[228] and chronic lymphocytic leukemia[229] can manifest as multiple colonic polyposis.

The colon is the most common gastrointestinal site for lipomas, which tend to be solitary, but may be multiple, submucosal lesions. Lipomas usually are asymptomatic and detected incidentally. The low density of fat may give the lesions a characteristic radiologic appearance, and their soft, deformable nature is helpful to the colonoscopist in making the diagnosis grossly. Colonic lipomas are most frequent in the right colon and tend to occur on or near the ileocecal valve.[230] Removal of these lesions usually is unnecessary.

Important tumors such as carcinoids (see Chapter 30), metastatic neoplasms (especially melanoma), and other rare cancers may produce submucosal lesions without distinctive identifying characteristics. Other submucosal lesions may be detected incidentally, including fibromas,

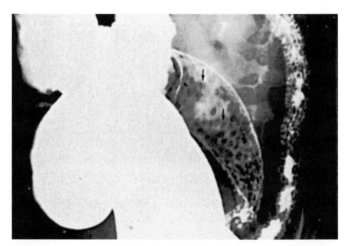

Figure 119–12 Lymphoid polyps of the colon in a child. This spot film of the sigmoid colon from a barium enema examination demonstrates diffuse lymphoid hyperplasia. Many of these polyps display characteristic umbilication (*arrows*). Lymphoid hyperplasia may be a normal variant in some children; a malignant lymphoma also may rarely present a similar radiologic appearance.

neurofibromas, leiomyomas, granular cell tumors, hemangiomas, and endometriosis.

GASTROINTESTINAL POLYPOSIS SYNDROMES

Gastrointestinal polyposis refers to the presence of numerous polypoid lesions throughout the gastrointestinal tract. The polyposis syndromes are distinct entities clinically and pathologically that have been sorted into recognizable categories over the past century (Table 119–13). Most of these syndromes are inherited, and most are associated with an increased colon cancer risk, but all are classified on the basis of the histologic type of polyp and the clinical presentation. Recent advances in genetics have not only permitted a more accurate understanding of the relationships among these syndromes, but the genes responsible for these conditions, particularly the adenomatous polyposis syndromes, have provided insight into the genetic basis of sporadically occurring colon cancer.

POLYPOSIS SYNDROMES

The inherited adenomatous polyposis syndromes include several entities that are characterized by the development of large numbers of adenomatous polyps in the colon. The identification of the *APC* gene set the stage for understanding how colon cancers arise, and also permitted proper classification of Gardner's syndrome, attenuated adenomatous polyposis coli (AAPC), and many cases of Turcot's syndrome as variants of classic familial adenomatous polyposis (FAP) (Table 119–14). More recently,

Table 119–13 Classification of Gastrointestinal Polyposis Syndromes

Inherited Polyposis Syndromes
Adenomatous polyposis syndromes
  Familial adenomatous polyposis
  Variants of familial adenomatous polyposis
    Gardner's syndrome
    Turcot's syndrome
    Attenuated adenomatous polyposis coli
  Familial tooth agenesis syndrome
  Bloom's syndrome
  MYH polyposis
Hamartomatous polyposis syndromes
  Peutz-Jeghers syndrome
  Juvenile polyposis
  Syndromes related to juvenile polyposis
    Cowden's disease
    Bannayan-Ruvalcaba-Riley syndrome
  Rare hamartomatous polyposis syndromes
    Hereditary mixed polyposis syndrome
    Intestinal ganglioneuromatosis and neurofibromatosis
    Devon family syndrome
    Basal cell nevus syndrome
Noninherited Polyposis Syndromes
Cronkhite-Canada syndrome
Hyperplastic polyposis syndrome
Lymphomatous polyposis
Nodular lymphoid hyperplasia

Table 119–14 Familial Adenomatous Polyposis Syndromes: Clinical Variants

Variant	Polyps	Extraintestinal Abnormalities	Gene Mutation
Classic FAP	Colonic adenomas (thousands) Duodenal and ampullary adenomas Gastric fundic gland polyps Jejunal and ileal adenomas Ileal lymphoid polyps	Mandibular osteomas Dental abnormalities	*APC* gene (usually truncated protein)
Gardner's variant	Same as FAP	Osteomas of mandible, skull, long bones CHRPE Dental impactions, supernumerary teeth Desmoid tumors Epidermoid cysts Fibromas, lipomas Thyroid, adrenal tumors	*APC* gene
Turcot's variant	Colonic adenomas (may be fewer than in classic FAP)	Medulloblastoma Glioblastoma multiforme* CHRPE	*APC* gene DNA mismatch repair genes*
Attenuated APC	Colonic adenomas (>100; proximal colon) Duodenal and ampullary adenomas Gastric fundic gland polyps	Mandibular osteomas (rare)	*APC* gene 5′ and 3′ regions; E1317Q mutation

*May be more appropriately classified under hereditary nonpolyposis colon cancer (HNPCC) (see Chapter 120).
APC, adenomatous polyposis coli; CHRPE, congenital hypertrophy of the retinal pigment epithelium; FAP, familial adenomatous polyposis.

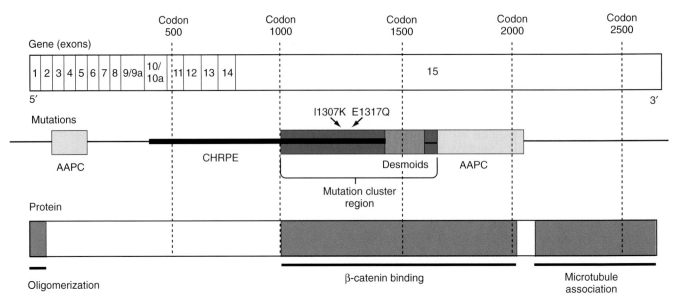

Figure 119–13   Schematic diagram of the APC gene, its mutations, and functional domains of the protein. The gene consists of 15 exons. Mutations associated with attenuated adenomatous polyposis coli (AAPC) occur in the 5′ and 3′ regions of the gene. Congenital hypertrophy of the retinal pigment epithelium (CHRPE) lesions are only seen with mutations downstream of exon 9. The mutation cluster region is in the center of the gene, where most mutations give rise to florid polyposis. Desmoid tumors are associated with the region shown. The I1307K and E1317Q mutations give rise to a milder phenotype. Domains of the APC protein responsible for oligomerization, β-catenin binding, and microtubule association are shown along the bottom. (Modified from Goss KH, Groden J: Biology of the adenomatous polyposis coli tumor suppressor. J Clin Oncol 18:1967, 2000.)

the *MYH* base-excision repair gene has been identified as an important cause of multiple colonic adenomas.

Familial Adenomatous Polyposis

Genetics

FAP is the most common adenomatous polyposis syndrome. It is inherited as an autosomal dominant disease with 80% to 100% penetrance, and an estimated prevalence of 1 in 5000 to 7500.[231] In this condition, one mutated *APC* allele is inherited as a germline mutation from the affected parent, and adenomas develop when the second allele (from the unaffected parent) becomes mutated or lost. The identification of the gene responsible for FAP began in 1986 with the investigation of a patient who had multiple congenital malformations and a deleted portion of the long arm of chromosome 5 that was identified cytogenetically.[232] Genetic mapping studies and restriction fragment length polymorphism (RFLP) analysis in 1987 led to the localization of the FAP gene in the 5q21-q22 region.[233,234] At the same time, RFLP analysis suggested that one of the two alleles for the FAP gene frequently was lost in sporadically occurring colorectal cancers. The fact that a lost gene might contribute to tumor progression suggested that the FAP locus might encode for a tumor suppressor gene.[235]

In 1991, the *APC* gene responsible for FAP was cloned by two collaborating groups and reported simultaneously.[236-238] The large size of this gene (encoding 2844 amino acids) may account for the relatively high frequency of new mutations. Germline mutations are found in patients with FAP and Gardner's syndrome, and in most instances, the mutations create a stop codon resulting in a truncated protein. The germline mutations are dispersed throughout the 5′ half of the gene, whereas somatic mutations of *APC* tend to accumulate in the mutation cluster region (Fig. 119–13).[239]

The APC protein is a multifaceted regulator of colonic epithelial cell homeostasis and participates in processes of cell proliferation, migration, differentiation, apoptosis, and chromosomal segregation.[240] The proximal portion of the APC protein contains regions that enable oligomerization as well as binding to proteins that regulate the actin cytoskeleton, thereby affecting cell morphology, polarity, and migration. In its central portion, the APC protein binds to β-catenin, a protein that normally maintains cell-cell junctions by anchoring a cell surface adhesion molecule, E-cadherin. In normal cells, APC forms a complex with other proteins (axin, conductin, and the GSK3B serine-threonine kinase) to bind β-catenin. This binding results in phosphorylation of β-catenin, which subsequently undergoes down-regulation in the cytoplasm. If mutations occur in the β-catenin-binding region, however, β-catenin no longer is down-regulated, allowing it to enter the nucleus where it acts in conjunction with other transcription factors to up-regulate target genes that then promote adenoma formation. Similarly, germline mutations of axin recently were discovered to cause a multiple colonic adenoma phenotype (see later). The carboxy-terminal portion of

APC contains a domain that contributes to proper chromosomal segregation and cytoskeleton regulation. Because the vast majority of *APC* mutations truncate the protein, this has the dual effect of disrupting the constitutive breakdown of β-catenin, leading to activation of cancer-associated genes, and creating abnormal chromosomal segregation, leading to chromosomal instability.

Clinical Features

Colonic. Classic FAP is characterized by the progressive development of hundreds to thousands of adenomatous polyps in the large intestine. A patient who inherits an *APC* mutation usually does not develop adenomas until approximately 10 to 12 years of age; rarely, however, polyps appear in the first decade of life. In one early series of FAP cases, the average age at onset of polyps was 25 years, but symptoms did not appear until the age of 33 years. The average age for the diagnosis of adenomas was 36 years, for cancer 39 years, and for death from cancer, 42 years; 90% of FAP cases have been identified by 50 years of age.[241] A more recent study that focused on early screening reported that 50% of FAP gene carriers will have polyps at sigmoidoscopy by approximately 15 years of age.[242]

FAP begins with a small number of polyps, and the number increases progressively until the colon becomes studded with adenomas. All varieties of adenomatous polyps may be seen, including tubular, tubulovillous, and villous adenomas. The number of macroscopic polyps in a colectomy specimen averages 1000 but may be tens of thousands. Germline mutations of *APC* gene between codons 1250 and 1464 have been associated with more profuse carpeting of the colon (Fig. 119–14), whereas mutations elsewhere in the gene result in fewer colorectal polyps (Fig. 119–15).[243] Histologic examination of the colon reveals numerous microscopic adenomas as well, the smallest of which may involve a single colonic crypt. The size and number of polyps correspond to the latent period between the onset of clinical disease and the time of detection; tumors tend to be more numerous in symptomatic probands than in asymptomatic younger relatives discovered by screening. Most polyps are small (<1 cm), and, individually, these polyps are identical to adenomatous polyps found in the general population.

Colorectal cancer should be considered an inevitable consequence in the natural history of FAP, appearing approximately 10 to 15 years after the onset of polyposis. Colon cancer is unusual in adolescence, but it has been diagnosed as early as 9 years of age.[244] The cancers have the same pathologic grades of malignancy and the same distribution within the colon as are seen in the general population, except that multiple simultaneous cancers are much more frequent (48% of cases).[241] Despite attention to screening and surveillance, approximately 25% of patients with FAP will have colon cancer at the time of colectomy.[245]

Upper Gastrointestinal. Because FAP patients are born with a germline *APC* mutation in all cells of the body, tumors frequently develop in other organs besides the colon. For example, polyps in the stomach and small intestine are present in almost all FAP patients (Fig.

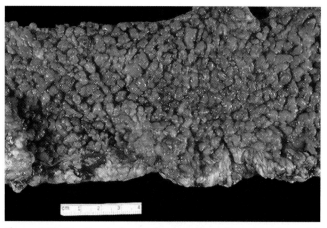

Figure 119–14   Surgical resection specimen from a patient with familial adenomatous polyposis (FAP). Patients with FAP have multiple adenomatous polyps often carpeting the colon, as demonstrated in this specimen. This close-up view demonstrates the presence of innumerable polyps, all of which are adenomas and may contain villous elements or carcinoma. A total colectomy is the only reasonable management in this situation. (Courtesy of Arnold Markowitz, MD, New York, NY.)

119–16).[246] Gastric polyps occur in 30% to 100% of patients, and curiously, most polyps in the stomach are non-neoplastic fundic gland polyps. These polyps are typically 1- to 5-mm sessile growths characterized microscopically by hyperplasia of fundic glands and microcysts. They may appear in the first decade of life, even before other gastrointestinal adenomas develop. Epithelial dysplasia can be seen in approximately 25% of fundic gland polyps in patients with FAP and results from mutations of the *APC* gene.[247] Gastric adenomas are uncommon and occur in approximately 5% of FAP patients, usually in the gastric antrum. The development of gastric adenocarcinoma in FAP patients is quite rare in the United States[247,248] but is higher in Japan, where the gastric cancer rate in the general population is higher.[249] Microcarcinoids also may be found in the stomach.[250]

Duodenal adenomas occur in 60% to 90% of FAP patients and the incidence increases with age.[251] There is a propensity for adenomas to involve the periampullary region and even to obstruct the pancreatic or biliary ductal system, resulting in pancreatitis. As many as 50% to 85% of FAP patients manifest adenomatous change of the papilla of Vater (see Fig. 119–16).[246,251] As a consequence, a 4% to 12% lifetime incidence of duodenal cancer (usually periampullary) has been reported[246] with relative risks of 124 to 331.[248,251] Collectively, these adenocarcinomas are the major cause of cancer death after prophylactic colectomy in FAP patients. The risk estimates for duodenal adenocarcinoma may be somewhat inflated by older prevalence studies, because under endoscopic surveillance a rather low rate of duodenal and ampullary adenoma progression to carcinoma has been observed.[252] Regardless, it is advisable to perform screening and surveillance of the stomach and duodenum.

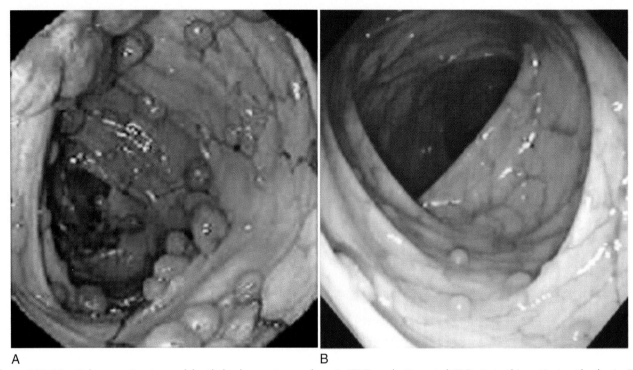

A   B

Figure 119–15   Colonoscopic views of familial adenomatous polyposis (FAP) and attenuated FAP. *A,* In this patient with classic FAP, polyposis is not florid; there were hundreds of polyps in the colon. *B,* In this patient with attenuated FAP, there are fewer polyps than in classic FAP and they are smaller. (*A* and *B,* courtesy of Arnold Markowitz, MD, New York, NY.)

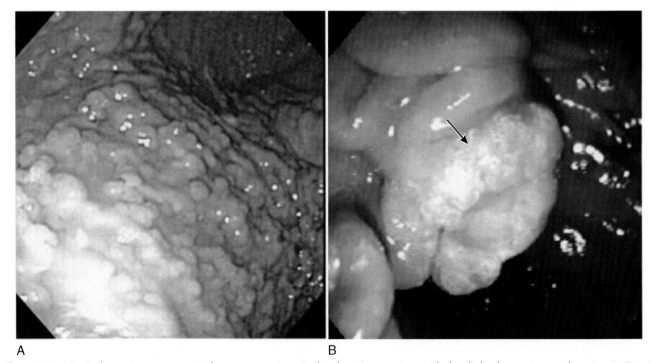

A   B

Figure 119–16   Endoscopic appearance of upper gastrointestinal polyps in a patient with familial adenomatous polyposis. *A,* Gastric fundic gland polyposis with numerous, small polyps distributed diffusely throughout the stomach. *B,* Adenomatous change on the papilla of Vater (*arrow*). These lesions may be subtle and require biopsy confirmation. (*A* and *B,* courtesy of Arnold Markowitz, MD, New York, NY.)

Although firm guidelines are not established, a suggested approach is outlined in Table 119–15. Jejunal adenomas have been detected in 40% and ileal adenomas in 20% of FAP patients. Fortunately, malignant transformation at these sites is rare,[246] but clinical vigilance is warranted and imaging with small bowel series or capsule endoscopy should be considered to examine the entire small intestine.[253] Likewise, attention should be given to surveillance of the distal ileum for neoplasia developing after subtotal colectomy or total proctocolectomy with ileal pouch anal anastomosis. Lymphoid hyperplasia may be present in the ileum in FAP patients and can be distinguished from adenomatous polyps only by biopsy.

Extraintestinal Features. Gardner's syndrome is a familial disease consisting of gastrointestinal polyposis and *osteomas* associated with a variety of benign soft tissue tumors and other extraintestinal manifestations (see Table 119–14). We now know that FAP and Gardner's syndrome are variable manifestations of a disease caused by mutations of the *APC* gene. Bone abnormalities include osteomas of the mandible, skull, and long bones, exostoses, and various dental abnormalities (including mandibular cysts, impacted teeth, and supernumerary teeth). When carefully sought, mandibular osteomas can be seen in up to 90% of patients with FAP even without other stigmata of Gardner's syndrome.[254] Radiologic examination of the mandible is a simple and noninvasive means to screen for young carriers of the FAP gene, but it is crucial to distinguish nonspecific sclerotic lesions in the mandible from true osteomas. Mandibular osteomas in FAP tend to be multiple, whereas nonspecific sclerotic bony lesions usually are single and located close to a diseased tooth. Osteomas can occur in children prior to the development of colonic polyposis. Because osteomas have no malignant potential, they are removed only for symptomatic or cosmetic reasons.

Table 119–15 Cancer Risks and Screening Recommendations in the Hereditary Polyposis Syndromes

Syndrome	Organ	Lifetime Risk of Cancer	Screening Recommendations
FAP, gene carriers	Colon cancer	Near 100%	Sigmoidoscopy annually; start at age 10-12 yr*
	Duodenal/periampullary cancer	5-12%	Upper GI endoscopy with forward- and side-viewing endoscopes q 1-3 yr; start at time of colectomy or age 20 yr
	Gastric cancer	≈0.5%	Same recommendation as for duodenal cancer
	Pancreatic cancer	≈2%	Possibly periodic abdominal ultrasound after age 20 yr
	Thyroid cancer	≈2%	Annual thyroid examination; start at age 10-12 yr
	CNS cancer	<1%	Annual physical examination; periodic head CT in members of affected families
	Hepatoblastoma	1.6%	Annual physical examination and hepatic ultrasound and α-fetoprotein for 1st decade of life
Peutz-Jeghers syndrome	All GI cancers	2-13%	Colonoscopy at symptom onset, or in late teenage years if the individual is asymptomatic; interval is determined by the number of polyps but at least q 3 yr; upper GI endoscopy q 2 yr; start at age 10 yr
	Small intestinal cancer	RR, 13	Annual Hgb; small bowel series or capsule endoscopy q 2 yr; start at age 10 yr
	Pancreatic cancer	RR, 100	Endoscopic or abdominal ultrasound q 1-2 yr; start at age 30 yr
	Breast cancer	RR, 8.8	Annual breast examination; mammogram q 1-3 yr; start at age 25 yr
	Uterine; ovarian cancer	RR, 8.0; 13	Annual pelvic examination; Pap smear and pelvic ultrasound; start at age 20 yr
	Sertoli cell tumor (testis)	Uncommon	Annual testicular examination beginning at age 10 yr; testis ultrasound if the patient has feminizing features
Juvenile polyposis	Colon cancer	<50%	Colonoscopy; start at symptoms or in early teens if the patient has no symptoms; interval is determined by the number of polyps, but at least q 3 yr
	Gastric, duodenal cancer	Rare	Upper GI endoscopy q 3 yr; start in early teens
Cowden's syndrome	Colon cancer	Little-none	No recommendations given
	Thyroid cancer	3-10%	Annual thyroid examination; start in teens
	Breast cancer	25-50%	Annual breast examination at age 25 yr; annual mammogram beginning at age 30 yr
	Uterine/ovarian cancer	Increase?	No recommendations given

*Sigmoidoscopy is used to identify a child with the FAP phenotype (i.e., polyps). If polyps are detected, colonoscopy usually is then performed to exclude proximal neoplasia.
CNS, central nervous system; CT, computed tomography; FAP, familial adenomatous polyposis; GI, gastrointestinal; Hgb, hemoglobin; RR, relative risk.
Adapted from Burt RW: Colon cancer screening. Gastroenterology 119:837, 2000.

Congenital hypertrophy of the retinal pigmented epithelium (CHRPE) has been reported in some families with FAP or Gardner's syndrome.[255,256] More than 90% of patients with Gardner's syndrome have pigmented ocular fundus lesions (vs. 5% of controls), which are likely to be multiple (63% have four or more lesions) and are bilateral in 87% of those affected.[255] Pigmented ocular fundus lesions are found in approximately half of the unaffected but at-risk first-degree relatives and have been identified in infants as young as 3 months old, suggesting that they are probably congenital. The presence of multiple, bilateral lesions appears to be a reliable marker for gene carriage in FAP, and their absence predicts lack of carriage if carrier relatives show CHRPE.[256] These marker lesions are asymptomatic curiosities that need not be sought in patients with an established diagnosis of FAP. CHRPE perhaps reflects the most accurate genotype-phenotype correlation in FAP patients; these lesions occur in patients with *APC* gene mutations distal to exon 9 up through the proximal portion of exon 15.[257]

A particularly serious complication of the adenomatous polyposis syndromes is the development of diffuse mesenteric fibromatosis, also called *desmoid tumors.* Desmoid tumors are reported in 4% to 32% of patients and rank second, after metastatic carcinoma, among lethal complications of the disease.[258] The absolute risk of desmoids in FAP patients has been estimated at 2.56/1000 person years, which is 825 times the risk in the general population.[258] Desmoid tumors often display familial aggregation; FAP patients who are first-degree relatives of a patient with FAP and a desmoid have a 2.5-fold greater risk for developing desmoid tumors than patients with FAP in general.[258] Predictors of increased desmoid risk include a germline mutation distal to codon 1399 and a strong family history of desmoids.[259] In this subset of patients, therefore, it would be prudent to incorporate abdominal imaging studies into their overall surveillance regimen, even though firm guidelines for desmoid tumor surveillance are not yet established. Desmoids occur when the disease-causing mutation is distal to codon 1444 of the *APC* gene (see Fig. 119–13). Curiously, recurrent desmoid tumors may manifest a somatic mutation of *APC* gene that is different from that of the initial tumor.[239] Commonly, desmoid tumors result from progressive growth of mesenteric fibroblasts that occurs after laparotomy (e.g., after prophylactic proctocolectomy), but they occasionally appear spontaneously. Desmoids cause gastrointestinal obstruction; constrict arteries, veins, or ureters; and are associated with a 10% to 50% mortality rate. Additional operative procedures usually are of no avail in this condition. Desmoid tumors may respond to radiation when localized and accessible.[260] Unfortunately, most tumors are in the mesentery in these patients, making radiation therapy impractical. Systemic chemotherapy occasionally may be successful.[261] Attempts at medical therapy have resulted in some modestly encouraging results. The NSAID sulindac, which can often cause colonic adenoma regression in FAP (see later), has resulted in partial tumor shrinkage in some patients but no response in others.[262,263] The antiestrogen drug tamoxifen has been effective in a few patients, as has progesterone.[264,265] None of these approaches is reliably effective in most patients, and the mechanism for their actions awaits explanation. For desmoids that significantly compromise the small bowel mesentery, small intestinal transplantation should be considered.

In addition to desmoid tumors, other soft tissue tumors are well described in FAP and Gardner's syndrome, including epidermoid cysts, fibromas, and lipomas. The epidermoid cysts, also called *inclusion cysts,* have erroneously been referred to as sebaceous cysts in the past. Epidermoid cysts are lined with normal epithelium and contain no sebaceous glands. When multiple epidermoid cysts appear before puberty in these kindreds, it is a harbinger of polyposis. Neoplasms of the biliary tree liver and adrenal glands also occur in these syndromes, and papillary carcinoma of the thyroid occurs in 1% of patients with FAP, predominantly in females.[266-269] Hepatoblastoma may affect young children in FAP families.

Genotype-Phenotype Correlations

Drawing precise genotype-phenotype correlations in FAP often is difficult because the identical *APC* gene mutation may give rise either to isolated colonic polyposis or to the extracolonic manifestations.[237] Moreover, an identical *APC* gene mutation can manifest quite different colonic and extracolonic phenotypic features among unrelated families.[270] Even within a single family, the disease may express itself variably in different individuals, including skipped generations and discordance in identical twins.[271] There are even some families that appear phenotypically to have FAP, but do not have mutations of the *APC* gene.[272] Additional genetic or environmental disease-modifying factors appear to be responsible for generating phenotypic variation. For example, in an animal model of human FAP in which the mouse *APC* gene has a germline mutation, a second gene, phospholipase A_2, was found to modify the number of polyps.[272] So far, studies do not substantiate phospholipase A_2 as a genetic modifier of human FAP. In other animal experiments, crossing mice with FAP with those who lack the COX-2 gene resulted in a substantial decrease in intestinal polyposis.[273] Indeed, COX-2 inhibitors cause adenoma regression in patients with FAP (see later). Thus, the FAP phenotype can be modified genetically and environmentally.

Despite the discrepancies in genotype-phenotype correlations, some general patterns have emerged (see Fig. 119–13). Profuse polyposis is found in the midportion of the gene (between codons 1250 and 1464, but especially around codon 1300), whereas a mild colonic phenotype is observed for mutations that affect the extreme proximal (5′) and distal (3′) ends of the *APC* gene responsible for attenuated FAP (see later), and for I1307K and E1317Q mutations. Desmoid tumors often, but not always, are seen with mutations just distal to the profuse polyposis region (between codons 1403 and 1578). CHRPE lesions are present with mutations distal to exon 9 (codons 463 to 1387). Papillary carcinoma of the thyroid is associated with mutations proximal to the mutation cluster region.[266]

Genetic Testing and Counseling

Genetic testing is an important component of the overall care of patients with FAP and their families, not so much for the management of the affected individual but to detect mutant gene carriers.[274] Approximately 20% of patients with FAP have a negative family history and represent new mutations at the *APC* locus.[241] Genetic testing is performed by extracting DNA from peripheral blood leukocytes. Sequencing offers the best sensitivity for mutations of the *APC* gene, but it is expensive and might detect variants of unknown clinical significance. Because most mutations of the *APC* gene result in a truncated protein product, the in vitro protein truncation test offers a useful method for detecting gene carriers. This assay is successful in about 80% of families tested and has the advantage of only requiring one affected individual. If successful in one family member, this test is nearly 100% accurate for identifying other gene carriers in that family.

An affected individual is tested first. Absence of a mutation in the affected individual suggests that genetic testing of at-risk relatives is not likely to yield clinically useful information and that the family should be screened by clinical tests. A positive protein truncation test allows at-risk relatives to be tested in a more focused manner and at lesser cost than with genetic testing. It is recommended that testing at-risk children be delayed until age 10 to 12 years, when clinical screening usually begins. Genetic testing of other family members is performed best within the context of a comprehensive genetic counseling program because it raises many issues such as psychological denial, survivor guilt, premature worrying if testing is performed at too young an age, intrafamily strife, employment discrimination, and medical insurability.[275]

Diagnosis and Screening

Patients with FAP may present with nonspecific symptoms, such as hematochezia, diarrhea, and abdominal pain. The key to the diagnosis and management of this disease, however, is to identify the presymptomatic individual, and this objective is achieved by the assiduous pursuit of the diagnosis in the relatives of affected patients. The diagnosis is made easily by sigmoidoscopy, given the often diffuse distribution of polyps, but colonoscopy may be preferred so that the full phenotype can be appreciated while excluding the presence of carcinoma elsewhere in the colon. The presence of more than 100 polyps and the confirmation that these are adenomas establish the diagnosis of FAP. Studies from St. Mark's Hospital in London on the natural history of FAP suggest that approximately 10 years elapses between the appearance of polyps and the development of cancer[241]; however, it is not advisable to delay surgery once the diagnosis is made, even in presymptomatic patients, except in individuals who have not completed puberty. Performing genetic testing at approximately age 10 to 12 years for at-risk individuals helps to streamline the clinical evaluation. In a family with a known mutation, children who test positive can then undergo a screening sigmoidoscopy to determine the status of their disease. If the gene test is negative, the child can be spared sigmoidoscopy, although it still might be prudent to perform sigmoidoscopy after adolescence just to offset the rare possibility of laboratory error.

Management

Surgery. Surgery is the only reasonable management option for colonic polyposis in FAP. The timing and extent of surgery are the major clinical considerations. Because any rectal mucosa that is left behind is at risk for developing carcinoma, the optimal treatment is to perform total proctocolectomy either with a conventional ileostomy or ileal pouch-anal anastomosis. For the most part, the latter operation in skilled hands is associated with little morbidity and is preferred by patients who must nonetheless be advised about the risk of decreased fertility among women undergoing this procedure.[276] For some patients, total proctocolectomy with conventional ileostomy is unacceptable, and they also do not want to chance the complications of an ileal pouch. In such cases, the decision to perform a subtotal colectomy with ileorectal anastomosis can be considered, bearing in mind that the rectal segment will remain at risk for carcinoma and the patient will have to comply with periodic surveillance examinations. In contrast to older patients who undergo ileorectal anastomosis, about one fifth of younger patients (median age of 35 years) with many rectal polyps will develop cancer in 5 to 23 years. According to the Mayo Clinic experience, among patients who are followed for more than 20 years, about three fifths develop carcinoma in the rectal stump despite semiannual sigmoidoscopic surveillance and fulguration of all polyps.[277] The prognosis in patients who develop rectal cancers in this setting is dismal; the 5-year disease-free survival rate has been reported to be 25%. In patients with ileorectal anastomosis, the risk of subsequent rectal cancer was higher in patients who had an *APC* mutation between codons 1250 and 1464, a finding that awaits confirmation in other studies.[278] These data provide a strong case for total proctocolectomy for FAP patients.

In spite of this ominous warning, others have advocated rectum-sparing operations and have achieved a reasonable degree of success. The Memorial Sloan-Kettering group in New York has advocated that a subtotal colectomy is safe for patients whose rectums are free of polyps. They also spare the rectum in patients with rectal polyps, carefully follow the patients and perform additional surgery as soon as malignant change is found.[279] The St. Mark's group in London reports satisfaction with rectum-sparing procedures for all patients with FAP and, furthermore, fulgurates only adenomas 5 mm or more in diameter at 3- to 6-month intervals. This group reported that 11 of 173 of their patients developed carcinoma in the rectum but that only 3 of the 11 have died of rectal cancer.[280] The Cleveland Clinic has advocated the use of colectomy with ileorectal anastomosis and reported an actuarial survivorship rate of 80% in 133 patients after 20 years, despite the presence of rectal polyps.[281] Other groups in the United States and Europe also prefer subtotal colectomy and ileoproctostomy, but approximately one quarter of patients treated this way have required a total proctectomy at a later date for cancer or intractable benign polyps.[282] It appears, therefore, that patients may elect the more limited procedure if they are willing to comply with rigorous follow-up (sigmoidoscopy every 3 to 6 months) and accept a risk of malignancy in the rectum of approximately 10%. The advent of effective medical therapy has provided new options for the surgical management of FAP, but as discussed in the next paragraph, rectal cancer can still occur despite adenoma regression.

Medical. Small adenomatous polyps in the rectum can be reversible lesions. Spontaneous regression of rectal polyps has been reported after subtotal colectomy and ileorectal anastomosis for FAP,[283] and this must be taken into account when one is evaluating the response of a rectal-sparing surgical procedure or medical treatment for this disease. Because of its antioxidant characteristics and its effects in experimental colon cancer, ascorbic acid (vitamin C, 3 g/day) was tried in patients with FAP who had undergone subtotal colectomy with ileorectal anastomosis at least 1 year earlier. A modest effect was observed, but it was neither consistent nor strong enough to advocate for general use.[284] Supplemental dietary calcium also was ineffective in polyposis patients.[285] A more ambitious trial has been reported in which 58 patients with FAP were treated with ascorbic acid (4 g/day), α-tocopherol (vitamin E, 400 mg/day), and supplemental fiber (22.5 g/day); a modest effect was seen after 2 years of therapy.[286]

A higher degree of enthusiasm has been generated for the use of NSAIDs in the treatment of colorectal polyps in FAP. Sulindac has been shown in both uncontrolled and controlled trials to decrease the number and size of colorectal adenomas in patients with FAP[79] who had intact colons as well as those with subtotal colectomy and ileorectal anastomosis. Unfortunately, maintaining these patients on sulindac does not protect them from developing rectal cancer, and the drug's effect on reducing adenomas is reversible on its discontinuation. Sulindac is less successful for controlling upper gastrointestinal neoplasia, and it does not appear to prevent the initial onset of adenomas in children who are genotypically affected with FAP.[287]

The mechanism by which sulindac causes colorectal adenoma regression in patients with FAP may relate in part to its ability to inhibit COX (prostaglandin synthase) activity and thereby to interfere with arachidonic acid metabolism. Since colorectal tumors (but not normal colonocytes) have high levels of COX-2 expression, it is possible that COX-2 inhibition by sulindac is responsible for adenoma regression.[288] Indeed, when mice carrying an *APC* mutation were bred with mice carrying a disrupted COX-2 gene, fewer polyps developed.[273] Sulindac also is capable of restoring the deficient cell death program (apoptosis) seen in colonocytes of patients with FAP, even without affecting colonocyte proliferation.[289] Since COX-2 overexpression can prevent apoptosis, it is possible that the benefit from sulindac relates to its ability to inhibit COX-2. Indeed, FAP patients with rectal adenomas treated with a selective COX-2 inhibitor also demonstrated a significant reduction in the number and size of adenomas.[290] Curiously, the sulfone derivative of sulindac has no inhibitory effect on either COX-1 or COX-2 enzymes, yet it too has been shown to cause rectal adenoma regression in FAP patients.[291]

Screening of Extracolonic Organs

Upper gastrointestinal screening should be performed at the time colonic adenomas are diagnosed or at least by age 20 (see Table 119–15).[72] A full evaluation of the entire small intestine should be performed at baseline. This can be done by small bowel series, capsule endoscopy, or perhaps by performing intraoperative small bowel enteroscopy at the time of initial proctocolectomy. Upper gastrointestinal polyps are rare prior to the onset of colonic disease, but side-viewing upper endoscopy should be performed in addition to conventional forward-viewing endoscopy because of its better visualization of the duodenal ampulla. The overall approach to upper gastrointestinal polyps is one of conservatism. Gastric polyps should be sampled to see if they are adenomas or fundic gland polyps with dysplasia. In the duodenum, villous adenomas, adenomas with high-grade dysplasia, large adenomas, and symptomatic adenomas, regardless of histology, should be removed. Endoscopic ablation of periampullary adenomas can be performed relatively safely by endoscopists skilled in this procedure, but regrowth of adenomatous tissue is common.[284] If duodenal polyps are small or few in number, surveillance can be performed every 1 to 3 years. The presence of worrisome duodenal adenomas or adenomatous change of the duodenal papilla warrants endoscopic inspection at more frequent intervals. Surgical resection of the duodenum, whether by local excision or pancreaticoduodenectomy, may be required in selected patients. Screening of other organs at risk for cancer is summarized in Table 119–15.

Variant Familial Adenomatous Polyposis Syndromes

Turcot's Syndrome (Glioma-Polyposis)

The term *Turcot's syndrome* applies to a syndrome of familial colonic polyposis with primary tumors of the central nervous system (see Table 119–14).[292,293] The phenotypic spectrum is broad, with colonic manifestations ranging from a single adenoma to profuse adenomatosis coli, and brain tumors representing different histopathologic types. Controversy exists as to whether this syndrome is inherited in an autosomal dominant or autosomal recessive manner. A comprehensive molecular diagnostic study of 14 Turcot's syndrome families has clarified that Turcot's syndrome kindreds fall into two groups based on their types of brain tumor and particular genetic alteration.[294] The more common group has germline mutations of the *APC* gene, and these patients tend to have medulloblastomas. In several cases, the brain tumor preceded the diagnosis of polyposis. The *APC* mutations were heterogeneous, with no association between specific mutations and the development of brain tumors. The inactivation of both *APC* alleles in brain tumor tissue implicates the *APC* gene in the pathogenesis of these neoplasms. The risk of cerebellar medulloblastoma in FAP was calculated to be 92 times that of the general population. In contrast, the second group of patients, including the family originally described by Turcot, had glioblastoma multiforme tumors. These individuals were found to have germline mutations in DNA MMR genes typical of HNPCC (see Chapter 120). Thus, Turcot's syndrome can be considered a true variant of FAP, although as with Gardner's syndrome, maintaining a separate designation may be superfluous. Because of familial clustering, once an individual with Turcot's syndrome has been identified, screening for affected family members should include colonoscopy as well as imaging studies of the brain (see Table 119–15).

Attenuated Adenomatous Polyposis Coli (AAPC)

Patients with classic FAP syndromes typically have tens to thousands of colonic adenomas. However, an attenuated form of FAP has been identified in which individuals manifest fewer adenomas that often have a flat rather than polypoid growth pattern and tend to cluster in the proximal colon.[295,296] As such, this condition may easily be confused with HNPCC (see Chapter 120). Although previously termed *hereditary flat adenoma syndrome*, this syndrome is more aptly named *attenuated FAP* by virtue of the existence of germline mutations of the very proximal and distal portions of the *APC* gene.[297] Like classic FAP, patients with AAPC are prone to develop multiple fundic gland polyps, duodenal and gastric adenomas, and even periampullary carcinoma[298]; however, colorectal cancers arise at a later age ($\approx$ 55 years) in AAPC patients than in those with classic FAP.

It is becoming increasingly clear that germline mutations not only in the *APC* gene but in other genes of the *APC* pathway, such as β-*catenin* and *axin*, can give rise to a multiple adenomatous polyposis phenotype.[299] Multiple colonic adenomas, colorectal cancer, and even hyperplastic polyps have been described in a Finnish family with familial tooth agenesis as a result of a germline mutation of *Axin2*.[300] Even more intriguing is the recent observation that germline defects in genes involved in DNA repair also can result in a phenotype that mimics AAPC. For example, numerous colonic adenomas have been described in a patient with Bloom's syndrome, a condition characterized by growth retardation, male sterility, facial erythema, and multiple cancers resulting from increased chromosomal breakage.[301] It appears that the genomic instability induced by mutations in the causative *BLM* gene affects the *APC* gene, thereby resulting in the polyposis phenotype.

Perhaps the most significant recent development in this field is the discovery that mutations of the *MYH* gene are a frequent cause of the multiple colorectal adenoma phenotype.[302] In fact, among patients with 15 to 100 adenomas, at least 30% have germline (usually biallelic) *MYH* mutations, whereas only 15% have germline *APC* mutations. When DNA is damaged, MYH acts in concert with other DNA base-excision repair enzymes to prevent mutations from occurring (Fig. 119–17). When MYH is defective, G:C → T:A transversions occur, and if this affects the *APC* gene, the resulting loss of APC function gives rise to multiple adenomas. Clinical features of MYH polyposis include multiple adenomas (usually between 5 and 100, rarely a florid polyposis), frequent development of colorectal cancer, and even some hyperplastic polyps. The phenotype occurs at a somewhat later age than does FAP. Gastric cancer, duodenal adenoma, osteoma, and CHRPE lesions have been described in patients with MYH mutations, but unlike FAP, MYH polyposis is an autosomal recessive disorder. Thus, genetic testing and counseling is directed more toward siblings and spouses than to parents or children. Surveillance guidelines for patients with MYH polyposis have not been established.

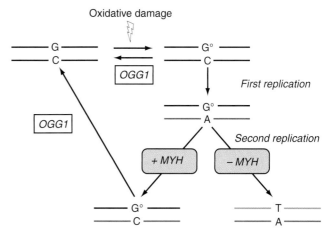

Figure 119–17 Function of the *MYH* gene in DNA base excision repair. Oxidative stress gives rise to 8-oxoguanine triphosphate, which is incorporated into DNA (G°). With the next DNA replication, DNA polymerase will preferentially insert adenine opposite G°, giving rise to G°:A mispairs, with G° in the template strand. In the presence of normal *MYH* gene function (+MYH), with the subsequent replication, adenine is removed and subsequent base-excision repair will convert G°:A to G°:C, which can then be repaired by OGG1 to GC. In the absence of *MYH* function (–MYH), G°:A mispairs remain uncorrected, giving rise to G:C → T:A transversion mutations.

Other Syndromes

Other familial syndromes in which a high incidence of colonic cancer is associated with a small number of colonic adenomas, such as Torre-Muir syndrome, are probably part of the spectrum of HNPCC and should not be confused with FAP or Gardner's syndrome.[303] A single family with gastric hyperplastic polyposis and a high incidence of gastric cancer has been described.[304] This rare condition is of interest because the gastric fundus may develop hyperplastic polyposis in FAP, but it is not known if this syndrome is linked in any way to FAP. Other patients have been described with multiple hyperplastic polyposis of the colon, some of whom had coexisting adenomas or a vague family history of polyposis, but again any pathologic relationship to FAP is speculative.[305] Six patients with multiple serrated adenomas have been described, four of whom had associated adenocarcinoma.[306] Further studies are needed to establish any genetic connection between serrated adenomatous polyposis and FAP.

Hamartomatous Polyposis Syndromes

Several discrete familial syndromes that are characterized by multiple hamartomatous polyps of the gastrointestinal tract have been described. These include Peutz-Jeghers syndrome, juvenile polyposis and related syndromes, and other rare syndromes (Table 119–16). Germline mutations of the *STK11/LKB1* gene account for Peutz-Jeghers syndrome, whereas the juvenile polyposis syndromes (JPSs) are associated with germline mutations of *BMPR1A* and *MADH4*. Each of these syndromes is associated with an increased risk of colorectal cancer, presumably because each of the genes responsible for the

Table 119–16   Familial Hamartomatous Polyposis Syndromes

Syndrome	Polyps	Location of Other GI Polyps	Features	Mutated Gene
Peutz-Jeghers syndrome	Hamartomas with bands of smooth muscle in the lamina propria	Small intestine Stomach Colon	Pigmented lesions (mouth, hands, feet) Ovarian sex cord tumors Sertoli tumors of the testes Airway polyps Pancreatic cancer Breast cancer Colon and esophageal cancer	STK11/LKB1
Juvenile polyposis	Juvenile polyps; also adenomas and hyperplastic polyps	Colon Small intestine Stomach	Colon cancer in some families Congenital abnormalities	MADH4, BMPR1A
Cowden's disease	Hamartomas with disorganized muscularis mucosae	Stomach Colon	Trichilemmomas and papillomas Other hamartomas Benign and malignant breast disease Benign and malignant thyroid disease	PTEN
Bannayan-Ruvalcaba Riley syndrome	Juvenile polyps	Colon Small intestine	Macroencephaly; developmental delay Penile pigmentation	PTEN
Neurofibromatosis	Neurofibromas	Small intestine Stomach Colon	von Recklinghausen's disease MEN 2B	NF1 RET

GI, gastrointestinal; MEN, multiple endocrine neoplasia.

hamartomatous polyposis syndromes behaves as tumor suppressor genes.

Peutz-Jeghers Syndrome

Peutz in 1921 and Jeghers in 1949 described the familial syndrome consisting of mucocutaneous pigmentation and gastrointestinal polyposis that now bears their names. Peutz-Jeghers syndrome (PJS) appears to be inherited as a single pleiotropic autosomal dominant gene with variable and incomplete penetrance.[307,308] Germline mutations of the STK11/LKB1, a serine threonine kinase gene on chromosome 19p, cause this syndrome,[309,310] but not all families with PJS are linked to this gene locus, suggesting genetic heterogeneity.

Early in infancy the characteristic mucocutaneous pigmentation of PJS may be noted. These deposits of melanin are found most commonly around the mouth, nose, lips, buccal mucosa, hands, and feet, and they also may be present in the perianal and genital regions (Fig. 119–18). The macular lesions are brown to greenish-black, are smooth and hairless, and, except for the buccal pigmentation, tend to fade at puberty. The clinician must distinguish these melanin deposits from ordinary freckles. Freckles are sparse near the nostrils and mouth, are absent at birth (but may occur in infancy), and never appear on the buccal mucosa. The presence of this pigmentation should alert the clinician to this syndrome, but the skin lesions and intestinal lesions occasionally are inherited separately.

Peutz-Jeghers polyps may increase in size progressively and cause small intestinal obstruction or intussusception that may occur as early as infancy. The polyps may be found in the stomach, small intestine, or colon, but they

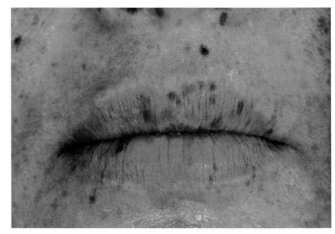

Figure 119–18 Mucocutaneous pigmentation of Peutz-Jeghers syndrome (From www.orl.cz/chorroby/ustni/vestibulum/vrozena.)

tend to be most prominent in the small intestine. Acute upper gastrointestinal bleeding and chronic fecal blood loss may complicate the disease. The average age of diagnosis in PJS is 23 to 26 years old. Carcinomas of the colon, duodenum, jejunum, and ileum have been reported in patients with PJS. Although it has been assumed that these cancers arise from rare foci of adenomatous epithelium that may develop within the Peutz-Jeghers polyps, recent evidence for loss of STK11/LKB1 expression in Peutz-Jeghers polyps even without dysplastic epithelium raises the possibility that the *STK11/LKB1* gene itself might be the gatekeeper to carcinogenesis in this syndrome, much like *APC* gene is the gatekeeper in FAP.[311,312] Colon polyps should be removed for histologic examination, but the relative inaccessibility of small intestinal polyps and the unpredictability of neoplastic complications make it difficult to have a routine surveillance program for small intestinal cancer.

Cancers throughout the gastrointestinal tract and other organs are quite common in familial PJS (see Table 119–16).[313] The mean age of diagnosis of cancer is approximately 40 to 50 years, with a 93% overall cumulative risk of developing cancer between 15 and 64 years of age. The cumulative risk of colon cancer is 36%, with similar rates for esophageal and pancreatic cancer. Ovarian cysts and distinctive ovarian sex cord tumors are seen in 5% to 12% of female patients with this syndrome.[314] The ovarian tumors are histologically unique and may occur in young patients. Hormonally active Sertoli cell testicular tumors with feminizing features may occur in young boys with PJS.[315] Breast cancers may be found in young women and may be bilateral,[316] and the magnitude of breast cancer risk in this syndrome is similar to other hereditary forms of breast cancer caused by germline mutations of *BRCA1* and *BRCA2*. Other tumors that may occur in this syndrome include pancreatic cancers in young patients and polyps or cancers of the biliary tree and gallbladder.[317] Thus, PJS confers an increased risk for cancer in a number of gastrointestinal and nonintestinal organs. Guidelines for screening are difficult to make but should be directed toward organs at risk for which early detection and treatment are reasonable, such as the entire gastrointestinal tract, gonads (in both sexes), and breasts (in women) (see Table 119–15). Videocapsule or intraoperative endoscopy of the entire gastrointestinal tract should be considered.

Tuberous sclerosis is characterized by the presence of hamartomatous lesions, with the classic triad of mental retardation, epilepsy, and adenoma sebaceum.[318] Hamartomatous polyps resembling Peutz-Jeghers polyps, as well as adenomatous polyps, may occur in this disease and often are located in the distal colon.

Juvenile Polyposis Syndrome

Juvenile polyps are distinctive hamartomas that usually are solitary and located principally in the rectums of children and occasionally in adults. They have a smooth surface and are covered by normal colonic epithelium. Juvenile polyposis (i.e., the presence of multiple juvenile polyps) is a diagnosis of exclusion. Other syndromes associated with juvenile polyps such as Cowden's disease and Bannayan-Riley-Ruvalcaba syndrome should be excluded (see later). Once that is done, JPS can be defined by any one of the following criteria: more than five juvenile polyps of the colon and rectum; juvenile polyps throughout the gastrointestinal tract; or any number of juvenile polyps in the gastrointestinal tract with a family history of juvenile polyps.[319] Often, JPS is considered when there is gastrointestinal polyposis in the absence of extraintestinal manifestations.

Juvenile polyposis typically causes gastrointestinal bleeding, intussusception, and obstruction. The clinical presentations of JPS and the FAP syndromes differ. Juvenile polyps produce symptoms in childhood, whereas the adenomatosis syndromes rarely present in childhood and usually become evident in early adult life. The average age of a patient with JPS is 4.5 years and 9.5 years in the nonfamilial and familial forms, respectively.[320]

The risk of colon and upper gastrointestinal cancer is increased in familial juvenile polyposis.[319] In a large Iowa kindred, 38% of affected individuals developed colon cancer and 21% developed upper gastrointestinal cancer.[321] Others report a somewhat lower risk estimate of 17% incidence of gastrointestinal malignancy.[322] Although juvenile polyps per se are not considered neoplastic, the synchronous adenomatous polyps and mixed juvenile-adenomatous polyps of these patients are what give rise to concern.[323,324] Thus, these polyps must be scrutinized by the pathologist for evidence of a mixed adenomatous appearance in the polyps or coexisting adenomas must be excluded, and kindreds with colorectal cancer should be subjected to careful colonoscopic surveillance.

JPS manifests autosomal dominant inheritance. Approximately 18% of cases will have a germline mutation of *MADH4 (SMAD4)*, a tumor suppressor gene involved in TGF-β signaling.[325] Knockout mouse models confirm that *MADH4* germline mutations predispose to gastrointestinal polyps and cancer.[319] Another 21% of JPS cases are caused by germline mutations of bone morphogenetic protein receptor 1A (*BMPR1A*), another member of the TGF-β superfamily that depends on MADH4 for signal transduction.

The diagnosis of JPS is made by endoscopy (see Table 119–15). Screening colonoscopy and upper endoscopy usually begins after 15 years of age if symptoms have not occurred already. Asymptomatic relatives also should be screened. Identification of a *MADH4* or *BMPR1A* mutation in a family helps guide screening, analogous to *APC* mutation testing. In general, juvenile polyps should be removed because of their tendency to bleed and obstruct. With a small number of polyps, periodic endoscopic polypectomy may be adequate. It has been suggested that surveillance endoscopy with polypectomy of the upper and lower gastrointestinal tracts be performed yearly until the patient is polyp free and then every 3 years.[319] For individuals with numerous juvenile polyps, colectomy should be considered. If subtotal colectomy with ileorectal anastomosis is chosen, the rectal segment must remain under surveillance. Family history must be defined in patients with multiple juvenile polyps to determine the sites of involvement and the history of neoplastic lesions. Gastric polyposis can be quite diffuse and cause anemia, posing a difficult management problem.

Syndromes Related to Juvenile Polyposis

Other conditions in which juvenile polyps are commonly encountered include Cowden's disease and Bannayan-Ruvalcaba-Riley syndrome, and it may be difficult to distinguish between the two. Germline mutations of *PTEN*, a tyrosine phosphatase protein that functions as a tumor suppressor, account for 81% and 57% of Cowden's disease and Bannayan-Ruvalcaba-Riley syndrome cases, respectively.[319]

Cowden's Disease. Although reported in only a very small number of families, Cowden's disease, or the multiple hamartoma syndrome, consists of hamartomatous polyps of the stomach, small intestine, and colon along with extraintestinal manifestations that include orocutaneous hamartomas, fibrocystic disease and cancer of the breast, nontoxic goiter, and thyroid cancer.[319] The hallmark of this autosomal dominant condition is the presence of multiple facial trichilemmomas, which arise from follicular epithelium and typically occur around the eyes, nose, and mouth. Gastrointestinal symptoms and colorectal cancer appear to be uncommon in this syndrome. The colorectal polyps in Cowden's disease are distinctive lesions characterized by disorganization and proliferation of the muscularis mucosae with nearly normal overlying colonic epithelium.[326] Ganglioneuromatosis of the colon and glycogenic acanthosis of the esophagus have been reported in association with Cowden's disease.[327] There does not appear to be an increased risk of gastrointestinal cancer; the major complication is cancer of the breast, uterus, and thyroid.

Bannayan-Ruvalcaba-Riley Syndrome. This rare autosomal dominant syndrome consists of hamartomatous gastrointestinal polyposis with macrocephaly, developmental delay and other developmental abnormalities, and pigmented spots on the penis.[328,329] Thyroiditis also has been described.

Rare Inherited Hamartomatous Polyposis Syndromes

Hereditary Mixed Polyposis Syndrome. A large kindred with a tendency to develop colonic polyps of mixed histologic types has been identified.[330] The disease appears to be confined to the colon. The earliest age of onset of polyps was 23 years, the median age of symptoms was 40 years, and the median age of colon cancer diagnosis was 47 years. The characteristic polyp was an atypical juvenile polyp, although some individuals had polyps of mixed histology and others had more than one histologic type of polyp including serrated adenomas. Linkage to chromosome 15q14-q22 has been described, in a region that overlaps with a possible colonic cancer gene, *CRAC1*.[331,332]

Intestinal Ganglioneuromatosis and Neurofibromatosis. Approximately 25% of patients with von Recklinghausen's syndrome (caused by *NF1* gene mutations) have neurofibromatosis involving the upper digestive tract with multiple submucosal neurofibromas or, less commonly, ganglioneuromas, that may cause dyspepsia, abdominal pain, or hemorrhage.[333] Gastrointestinal involvement usually is incidental and asymptomatic. Severe, uncontrolled symptoms have required surgical treatment in a few cases. Multiple intestinal ganglioneuromas also have been observed in families and individual cases unrelated to von Recklinghausen's disease.[334] Ganglioneuromas throughout the gastrointestinal tract can occur in patients with multiple endocrine neoplasia type 2B, related to mutations of the *RET* gene.[335]

Devon Family Syndrome. Multiple and recurrent inflammatory "fibroid polyps" of the stomach and intestine have been reported in a family.[336] These lesions, histologically distinct from juvenile polyps, may cause gastrointestinal obstruction, with symptoms beginning in adult life.

Basal Cell Nevus Syndrome. Basal cell nevus syndrome also is another syndrome that has been associated with multiple gastric hamartomatous polyps[337]; however, several kindreds have been reported without mention of gastrointestinal lesions.

NONINHERITED GASTROINTESTINAL POLYPOSIS SYNDROMES

Cronkhite-Canada Syndrome

In 1955, Cronkhite and Canada reported the first examples of an acquired, nonfamilial syndrome that now bears their names.[338] It is characterized by the presence of diffuse gastrointestinal polyposis, dystrophic changes in the fingernails, alopecia, cutaneous hyperpigmentation, diarrhea, weight loss, abdominal pain, and complications of malnutrition[339] (Fig. 119–19). Patients typically are middle aged or older (average 62 years) and present fairly acutely with a rapidly progressive illness consisting of chronic diarrhea and protein-losing enteropathy with the associated integumentary abnormalities. The diarrhea is attributable primarily to diffuse small intestinal mucosal injury, but bacterial overgrowth may be contributory. Gastrointestinal polyps are found in 52% to 96% of patients and range in location from the stomach to the rectum.[339] These polyps are hamartomas similar to the juvenile (retention) type, but unlike juvenile polyposis, the mucosa between polyps is histologically abnormal with edema, congestion, and inflammation. As is the case with juvenile polyps, there may be foci of adenomatous epithelium, which may confer a risk of carcinoma. Although adenomatous epithelium has been reported in these polyps and carcinoma has been reported to complicate this syndrome, malignant degeneration is the exception rather than the rule in this disease.[340]

The malabsorption syndrome is progressive in most patients, and the prognosis is poor because there is no specific therapy. It has been suggested that complete symptomatic remission occasionally may be achieved with the appropriate supportive management. In some cases, a variety of medical and surgical measures have been employed, making it difficult to identify the essential therapeutic modality(s). Glucocorticoids, anabolic steroids, antibiotics, and surgical resections have been tried in many of the patients in whom remissions have been reported. Despite this dilemma, aggressive nutritional support appears to be the most important factor influencing a favorable outcome. Enteral feeding (if possible) or parenteral feeding (if necessary) with sources of calories, nitrogen, and lipids, in addition to appropriate fluids, electrolytes, vitamins, and minerals, has resulted in complete symptomatic remissions with resolution of all of the ectodermal aberrations. Antibiotics may be beneficial when bacterial overgrowth contributes to the malabsorption. Although glucocorticoids have been used in some of the cases of symptomatic remission, the evidence to support their use is weak. Surgical therapy offers less

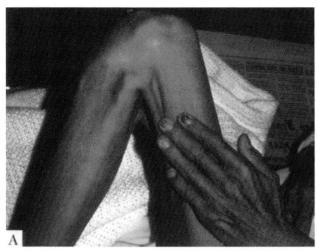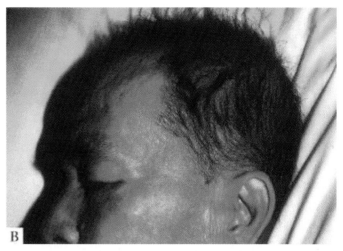

Figure 119–19   A patient with Cronkhite-Canada syndrome. This spontaneously arising noninherited polyposis syndrome is characterized by diffuse gastrointestinal hamartomatous polyposis, cutaneous hyperpigmentation, dystrophic changes in the fingernails (*A*), alopecia (*B*), and intestinal malabsorption. Similar to juvenile polyposis, adenomatous epithelium may occur in conjunction with hamartomas, conferring a risk of carcinoma. (From Boland CR: The Colon, Rectum, and Anus. *In* Feldman M (ed): Gastroenterology and Hepatology: The Comprehensive Visual Reference. Philadelphia, Churchill Livingstone, 1996.)

and is risky in these malnourished patients. One case of complete remission has been reported in a patient managed only with enteral administration of a nutritionally balanced complete liquid diet.[341] Attention should be paid to the possibility of secondary lactose or other disaccharide intolerance or protein-losing enteropathy in patients with diffuse small intestinal disease. Specific management awaits a better understanding of this perplexing syndrome.

Hyperplastic Polyposis Syndrome

Hyperplastic polyposis syndrome (HPS) is characterized by multiple, hyperplastic polyps in the colon. The World Health Organization definition of HPS is (1) at least 5 histologically diagnosed hyperplastic polyps proximal to the sigmoid colon, of which 2 are larger than 10 mm; or (2) any number of hyperplastic polyps occurring proximal to the sigmoid colon in an individual who has a first-degree relative with HPS; or (3) more than 30 polyps, but distributed throughout the colon.[342] The hyperplastic polyps in this syndrome tend to predominate in the distal colon, but the larger ones more frequently are located in the proximal colon. Adenomas frequently coexist, but colorectal cancer apparently is uncommon.[342] Colonoscopic surveillance every 1 to 3 years has been suggested. Shorter intervals might be considered in patients with AAPs. The genetic basis for this heterogeneous condition is not yet known.

Lymphomatous Polyposis

Lymphoma may present as multiple lymphomatous polyps of the gastrointestinal tract.[343] A variety of pathologic variants of Hodgkin's and non-Hodgkin's lymphomas may present this way, including immunoproliferative small intestinal disease. One variant worthy of mention is the mantle zone lymphoma (MZL),

which may produce nodular collections of proliferating lymphocytes in wide mantles that surround benign-appearing germinal centers.[344] The MZL has a characteristic histologic appearance and may have an indolent clinical course. These lesions are of importance because they require an adequate biopsy to distinguish them from true epithelial polyps and because of the possibility that MZL may have a prolonged clinical course of some prognostic significance.

Nodular Lymphoid Hyperplasia

Nodular lymphoid hyperplasia is a rare lymphoproliferative condition that is not related to a specific disease. It can be seen in healthy children (see Fig. 119–14) and also has been described in the terminal ileum of some patients with Gardner's syndrome and in some immunodeficiency syndromes, particularly IgA deficiency. These polyps, which are more common in the small intestine and measure approximately 3 to 6 mm, typically do not cause symptoms.

REFERENCES

1. Jass JR, Sobin LH (eds): World Health Organization: Histological Typing of Intestinal Tumours, 2nd ed. New York, Springer-Verlag, 1989.
2. O'Brien MJ, Winawer SJ, Zauber AG, et al: The National Polyp Study: Patient and polyp characteristics associated with high-grade dysplasia in colorectal adenomas. Gastroenterology 98:371. 1990.
3. Konishi F, Morson BCJ: Pathology of colorectal adenomas: A colonoscopic survey. J Clin Pathol 35:830, 1982.
4. Fenoglio CM, Kaye GI, Lane N: Distribution of human colonic lymphatics in normal, hyperplastic and adenomatous tissue. Gastroenterology 64:51, 1973.
5. Muto T, Bussey HJR, Morson BC: The evolution of cancer of the colon and rectum. Cancer 36:2251, 1975.

6. Shinya H, Wolff WI: Morphology, anatomic distribution, and cancer potential of colonic polyps. Ann Surg 190:679, 1979.

7. Rickert RR, Auerbach O, Garfinkel L, et al: Adenomatous lesions of the large bowel: An autopsy survey. Cancer 43:1847, 1979.

8. Williams AR, Balasooriya BAW, Day DW: Polyps and cancer of the large bowel: A necropsy study in Liverpool. Gut 23:835, 1982.

9. Arminski TC, McLean DW: Incidence and distribution of adenomatous polyps of the colon and rectum based on 1,000 autopsy examinations. Dis Colon Rectum 7:249, 1964.

10. Correa P: Epidemiology of polyps and cancer. In Morson BC (ed): The Pathogenesis of Colorectal Cancer. Philadelphia, WB Saunders, 1978, p 126.

11. Clark JC, Collan Y, Eide TJ, et al: Prevalence of polyps in an autopsy series from areas with varying incidence of large-bowel cancer. Int J Cancer 36:179, 1985.

12. Eide TJ, Stalsberg H: Polyps of the large intestine in northern Norway. Cancer 42:2839, 1978.

13. Johannsen LGK, Momsen O, Jacobsen NO: Polyps of the large intestine in Aarhus, Denmark: An autopsy study. Scand J Gastroenterol 24:799, 1989.

14. Granqvist S, Gabrielsson N, Sundelin P: Diminutive colonic polyps: Clinical significance and management. Endoscopy 1:36, 1979.

15. Tedesco FJ, Hendrix JC, Pickens CA, et al: Diminutive polyps: Histopathology, spatial distribution, and clinical significance. Gastrointest Endosc 28:1, 1982.

16. Gottlieb LS, Winawer SJ, Sternberg S, et al: National Polyp Study (NPS): The diminutive colonic polyp. Gastrointest Endosc 30:143, 1984.

17. Ryan ME, Parent K, Wyman JB, et al: Significance of diminutive colorectal polyps in 3282 flexible sigmoidoscopic examinations. Gastrointest Endosc 31:149, 1985.

18. Weston AP, Campbell DR: Diminutive colonic polyps: Histopathology, spatial distribution, concomitant significant lesions, and treatment complications. Am J Gastroenterol 90:24, 1995.

19. Church JM: Clinical significance of small colorectal polyps. Dis Colon Rectum 47:481, 2004.

20. Tripp MR, Morgan TR, Sampliner RE: Synchronous neoplasms in patients with diminutive colorectal adenomas. Cancer 60:1599, 1987.

21. Blue MG, Sivak MV Jr, Achkar E, et al: Hyperplastic polyps seen at sigmoidoscopy are markers for additional adenomas seen at colonoscopy. Gastroenterology 100:564, 1991.

22. Lieberman DA, Smith FW: Screening for colon malignancy with colonoscopy. Am J Gastroenterol 86:946, 1991.

23. Hoff G, Foerster A, Vatn MH, et al: Epidemiology of polyps in the rectum and colon: Recovery and evaluation of unresected polyps two years after detection. Scand J Gastroenterol 21:853, 1986.

24. Ueyama T, Kawamoto K, Iwashita I, et al: Natural history of minute sessile colonic adenomas based on radiographic findings. Dis Colon Rectum 38:268, 1995.

25. Spencer RJ, Melton LJ III, Ready RL, et al: Treatment of small colorectal polyps: A population-based study of the risk of subsequent carcinoma. Mayo Clin Proc 59:305, 1984.

26. Muto T, Kamiya J, Sawada T, et al: Small "flat adenoma" of the large bowel with special reference to its clinicopathologic features. Dis Colon Rectum 28:847, 1985.

27. Mitooka H: Flat neoplasms in the adenoma-carcinoma sequence in Japan. Semin Gastrointest Dis 11:238, 2000.

28. Lanspa SJ, Rouse J, Smyrk T, et al: Epidemiologic characteristics of the flat adenoma of Muto: A prospective study. Dis Colon Rectum 35:543, 1992.

29. Wolber RA, Owen DA: Flat adenomas of the colon. Hum Pathol 22:70, 1991.

30. Kubota O, Kino I, Kimura T, et al: Nonpolypoid adenomas and adenocarcinomas found in background mucosa of surgically resected colons. Cancer 77:621, 1996.

31. Rembacken BJ, Fujii T, Cairns A, et al: Flat and depressed colonic neoplasms: A prospective study of 1000 colonoscopies in the UK. Lancet 355:1211, 2000.

32. Saitoh Y, Waxman I, West AB, et al: Prevalence and distinctive biologic features of flat colorectal adenomas in a North American population. Gastroenterology. 120:1657, 2001.

33. Tsuda S, Veress B, Toth E, Fork FT: Flat and depressed colorectal tumours in a southern Swedish population: A prospective chromoendoscopic and histopathological study. Gut 51:550, 2002.

34. Richter H, Slezak P, Walch A, et al: Distinct chromosomal imbalances in nonpolypoid and polypoid colorectal adenomas indicate different genetic pathways in the development of colorectal neoplasms. Am J Pathol 163:287, 2003.

35. O'Brien MJ, Winawer SJ, Zauber AG, et al, and National Polyp Study Workgroup: Flat adenomas in the National Polyp Study: Is there increased risk for high-grade dysplasia initially or during surveillance? Clin Gastroenterol Hepatol 2:905, 2004.

36. Lynch HT, Smyrk TC, Watson P, et al: Hereditary flat adenoma syndrome: A variant of familial adenomatous polyposis? Dis Colon Rectum 35:411, 1992.

37. Owen DA: Flat adenoma, flat carcinoma, and de novo carcinoma of the colon. Cancer 77:3, 1996.

38. Shamsuddin AM: Microscopic intraepithelial neoplasia in large bowel mucosa. Hum Pathol 13:510, 1982.

39. Bird RP: Role of aberrant crypt foci in understanding the pathogenesis of colon cancer. Cancer Lett 93:55, 1995.

40. Takayama T, Katsuki S, Takahashi Y, et al: Aberrant crypt foci of the colon as precursors of adenoma and cancer. N Engl J Med 339:1277, 1998.

41. Jen J, Powell SM, Papadopoulos N, et al: Molecular determinants of dysplasia in colorectal lesions. Cancer Res 54:5523, 1994.

42. Novelli MR, Williamson JA, Tomlinson IPM, et al: Polyclonal origin of colonic adenomas in an XO/XY patient with FAP. Science 272:1187, 1996.

43. Shih IM, Wang TL, Traverso G, et al: Top-down morphogenesis of colorectal tumors. Proc Natl Acad Sci U S A 98:2640, 2001.

44. Kozuka S, Nogaki M, Ozeki T, et al: Premalignancy of the mucosal polyp in the large intestine: II. Estimation of the periods required for malignant transformation of mucosal polyps. Dis Colon Rectum 18:494, 1975.

45. Winawer SJ, Zauber AG, Gerdes H, et al: Prevention of colorectal cancer by colonoscopic polypectomy. N Engl J Med 329:1977, 1993.

46. Gilbertsen VA, Nelms JM: The prevention of invasive cancer of the rectum. Cancer 41:1137, 1978.

47. Müller AD, Sonnenberg A: Prevention of colorectal cancer by flexible endoscopy and polypectomy: A case-control study of 32,702 veterans. Ann Intern Med 123:904, 1995.

48. Selby JV, Friedman GD, Quesenberry CP Jr, et al: A case-control study of screening sigmoidoscopy and mortality from colorectal cancer. N Engl J Med 326:653, 1992.

49. Newcomb PA, Norfleet RG, Storer BE, et al: Screening sigmoidoscopy and colorectal cancer mortality. J Natl Cancer Inst 84:1572, 1992.

50. Vogelstein B, Kinzler KW: Cancer genes and the pathways they control. Nat Med 10:789, 2004.

51. Vogelstein B, Fearon ER, Hamilton S, et al: Genetic alterations during colorectal-tumor development. N Engl J Med 319:525, 1988.

52. Kinzler KW, Vogelstein B: Lessons from hereditary colorectal cancer. Cell 87:159, 1996.

53. Baker SJ, Preisinger AC, Jessup JM, et al: *p53* gene mutations occur in combination with 17p allelic deletions as late events in colorectal tumorigenesis. Cancer Res 50:7717, 1990.

54. Ahlquist DA: Aggressive polyps in hereditary nonpolyposis colorectal cancer: Targets for screening. Gastroenterology 108:1590, 1995.

55. Jacoby RF, Marshall DJ, Kailas S, et al: Genetic instability associated with adenoma to carcinoma progression in hereditary nonpolyposis colon cancer. Gastroenterology 109:73, 1995.

56. Vasen HFA, Nagengast FM, Meera Khan P: Interval cancers in hereditary non-polyposis colorectal cancer (Lynch syndrome). Lancet 345:1183, 1995.

57. Lindgren C, Liljegren A, Jaramillo E, et al: Adenoma prevalence and cancer risk in familial non-polyposis colorectal cancer. Gut 50:228, 2002.

58. Stemmermann GN, Yatani R: Diverticulosis and polyps of the large intestine: A necropsy study of Hawaii Japanese. Cancer 31:1260, 1973.

59. Chapman I: Adenomatous polypi of large intestine: Incidence and distribution. Ann Surg 157:223, 1963.

60. Sato E, Ouchi A, Sasano N, et al: Polyps and diverticulosis of large bowel in autopsy population of Akita prefecture, compared with Miyagi. Cancer 37:1316, 1976.

61. Lieberman DA, Weiss DG, Bond JH, et al: Use of colonoscopy to screen asymptomatic adults for colorectal cancer. N Engl J Med 343:162, 2000.

62. Imperiale TF, Wagner DR, Lin CY, et al: Risk of advanced proximal neoplasms in asymptomatic adults according to the distal colorectal findings. N Engl J Med 343:169, 2000.

63. Pickhardt PJ, Choi JR, Hwang I, et al: Computed tomographic virtual colonoscopy to screen for colorectal neoplasia in asymptomatic adults. N Engl J Med 349:2191, 2003.

64. Imperiale TF, Ransohoff DF, Itzkowitz SH, et al: Fecal DNA versus fecal occult blood for colorectal-cancer screening in an average-risk population. N Engl J Med 351:2704, 2004.

65. Imperiale TF, Wagner DR, Lin CY, et al: Results of screening colonoscopy among persons 40 to 49 years of age. N Engl J Med 346:1781, 2002.

66. Villavicencio RT, Rex DK: Colonic adenomas: Prevalence and incidence rates, growth rates, and miss rates at colonoscopy. Semin Gastrointest Dis 11:185, 2000.

67. Rex DK, Lehman GA, Hawes RH, et al: Screening colonoscopy in asymptomatic average-risk persons with negative fecal occult blood tests. Gastroenterology 100:64, 1991.

68. Johnson DA, Gurney MS, Volpe RJ, et al: A prospective study of the prevalence of colonic neoplasms in asymptomatic patients with an age-related risk. Am J Gastroenterol 85:969, 1990.

69. DiSario JA, Foutch PG, Mai HD: Prevalence and malignant potential of colorectal polyps in asymptomatic average-risk men. Am J Gastroenterol 86:941, 1991.

70. Coode PE, Chan KW, Chan YT: Polyps and diverticula of the large intestine: A necropsy survey in Hong Kong. Gut 26:1045, 1985.

71. Vatn MH, Stalsberg H: The prevalence of polyps of the large intestine in Oslo: An autopsy study. Cancer 49:819, 1982.

72. Burt RW: Colon cancer screening. Gastroenterology 119:837, 2000.

73. Gaglia P, Atkin WS, Whitelaw S, et al: Variables associated with the risk of colorectal adenomas in asymptomatic patients with a family history of colorectal cancer. Gut 36:385, 1995.

74. Winawer SJ, Fletcher RH, Miller L, et al: Colorectal cancer screening: Clinical guidelines and rationale. Gastroenterology 112:594, 1997.

75. Hixson LJ, Fennerty MB, Sampliner RE, et al: Two-year incidence of colon adenomas developing after tandem colonoscopy. Am J Gastroenterol 89:687, 1994.

76. Schoen RE, Pinsky PF, Weissfeld JL, et al: Prostate, Lung, Colorectal, and Ovarian Cancer Screening Trial Group: Results of repeat sigmoidoscopy 3 years after a negative exam. JAMA 290:41, 2003.

77. Rex DK, Cummings OW, Helper DJ, et al: Five-year incidence of adenomas after negative colonoscopy in asymptomatic average-risk persons. Gastroenterology 111:1178, 1996.

78. Granqvist S: Distribution of polyps in the large bowel in relation to age: A colonoscopic study. Scand J Gastroenterol 16:1025, 1981.

79. Levin TR, Palitz A, Grossman S, et al: Predicting advanced proximal colonic neoplasia with screening sigmoidoscopy. JAMA 281:1611, 1999.

80. Hill M: Etiology of the adenoma-carcinoma sequence. In Morson BC (ed): The Pathogenesis of Colorectal Cancer. Philadelphia, WB Saunders, 1978, p 153.

81. Burt RW: Hereditary aspects of colorectal adenomas. Cancer 70:1296, 1992.

82. Winawer SJ, Zauber AG, Gerdes H, et al: Risk of colorectal cancer in the families of patients with adenomatous polyps. N Engl J Med 334:82, 1996.

83. Almendingen K, Hofstad B, Vatn MH: Does a family history of cancer increase the risk of occurrence, growth, and recurrence of colorectal adenomas? Gut 52:747, 2003.

84. Potter JD: Colorectal cancer: Molecules and populations. J Natl Cancer Inst 91:916, 1999.

85. Fearnhead NS, Wilding JL, Winney B, et al: Multiple rare variants in different genes account for multifactorial inherited susceptibility to colorectal adenomas. Proc Natl Acad Sci U S A 101:15992, 2004.

86. Tomeo CA, Colditz GA, Willett WC, et al:. Harvard Report on Cancer Prevention, Vol 3: Prevention of colon cancer in the United States. Cancer Causes Control 10:167, 1999.

87. Peipins LA, Sandler RS: Epidemiology of colorectal adenomas. Epidemiol Rev 16:273, 1994.

88. Peters U, Sinha R, Chatterjee N, et al: Prostate, Lung, Colorectal, and Ovarian Cancer Screening Trial Project Team: Dietary fibre and colorectal adenoma in a colorectal cancer early detection programme. Lancet 361:1487, 2003.

89. Lieberman DA, Prindiville S, Weiss DG, et al: Risk factors for advanced colonic neoplasia and hyperplastic polyps in asymptomatic individuals. JAMA 290:2959, 2003.

90. Hawk ET, Levin B: Colorectal cancer prevention. J Clin Oncol 23:378, 2005.

91. Chan AT, Giovannucci EL, Schernhammer ES, et al: A prospective study of aspirin use and the risk for colorectal adenoma. Ann Intern Med 140:157, 2004.

92. Sandler RS, Halabi S, Baron JA, et al: A randomized trial of aspirin to prevent colorectal adenomas in patients with previous colorectal cancer. N Engl J Med 348:883, 2003.

93. Baron JA, Cole BF, Sandler RS, et al: A randomized trial of aspirin to prevent colorectal adenomas. N Engl J Med 348:891, 2003.

94. Benamouzig R, Deyra J, Martin A, et al: Daily soluble aspirin and prevention of colorectal adenoma recurrence: One-year results of the APACC trial. Gastroenterology 125:612, 2003.

95. Gann PH, Manson JE, Glynn RJ, et al: Low-dose aspirin and incidence of colorectal tumors in a randomized trial. J Natl Cancer Inst 85:1220, 1993.

96. Kelloff GJ, Schilsky RL, Alberts DS, et al: Colorectal adenomas: A prototype for the use of surrogate end points in the development of cancer prevention drugs. Clin Cancer Res 10:3908, 2004.

97. Baron JA, Beach M, Mandel JS, et al: Calcium supplements for the prevention of colorectal adenomas. N Engl J Med 340:101, 1999.

98. Bonithon-Kopp C, Kronborg O, Giacosa A, et al: Calcium and fibre supplementation in prevention of colorectal adenoma recurrence: A randomized intervention trial. European Cancer Prevention Organization Study Group. Lancet 356: 1300, 2000.

99. Wallace K, Baron JA, Cole BF, et al: Effect of calcium supplementation on the risk of large bowel polyps. J Natl Cancer Inst 96:893, 2004.

100. Stewart M, Macrae FA, Williams CB: Neoplasia and ureterosigmoidostomy: A colonoscopic survey. Br J Surg 69:414, 1982.

101. Delhougne B, Deneux C, Abs R, et al: The prevalence of colonic polyps in acromegaly: A colonoscopic and pathological study in 103 patients. J Clin Endocrinol Metab 80: 3223, 1995.

102. Brunner JE, Johnson CC, Zafar S, et al: Colon cancer and polyps in acromegaly: Increased risk associated with family history of colon cancer. Clin Endocrinol 32:65, 1990.

103. Ezzat S, Strom C, Melmed S: Colon polyps in acromegaly. Ann Intern Med 114:754, 1991.

104. Jenkins PJ, Frajese V, Jones AM, et al: Insulin-like growth factor I and the development of colorectal neoplasia in acromegaly. J Clin Endocrinol Metab 85:3218, 2000.

105. Ma J, Pollak M, Giovannucci E, et al: Prospective study of colorectal cancer risk in men and plasma levels of insulin-like growth factor (IGF)-1 and IGF-binding protein-3. J Natl Cancer Inst 91:620, 1999.

106. Cats A, Dullaart RP, Kleibeuker JH, et al: Increased epithelial cell proliferation in the colon of patients with acromegaly. Cancer Res 56:523, 1996.

107. Klein RS, Catalano MT, Edberg SC: *Streptococcus bovis* septicemia and carcinoma of the colon. Ann Intern Med 91:560, 1979.

108. Marshall JB, Gerhardt DC: Polyposis coli presenting with *Streptococcus bovis* endocarditis. Am J Gastroenterol 75:314, 1981.

109. Burns CA, McCaughey R, Lauter CB: The association of *Streptococcus bovis* fecal carriage and colon neoplasia: Possible relationship with polyps and their premalignant potential. Am J Gastroenterol 80:42, 1985.

110. Ellmerich S, Schöller M, Duranton B, et al: Promotion of intestinal carcinogenesis by *Streptococcus bovis*. Carcinogenesis 21:753, 2000.

111. Wiseman A, Rene P, Crelinsten GL: *Streptococcus agalactiae* endocarditis: An association with villous adenomas of the large intestine. Ann Intern Med 103:893, 1985.

112. Piette AM, Meduri B, Fritsch J, et al: Do skin tags constitute a marker for colonic polyps? A prospective study of 100 asymptomatic patients and meta-analysis of the literature. Gastroenterology 95:1127, 1988.

113. Stemmermann GN, Heilbrun LK, Nomura A, et al: Adenomatous polyps and atherosclerosis: An autopsy study of Japanese men in Hawaii. Int J Cancer 38:789, 1986.

114. Winawer SJ, Flehinger BJ, Buchalter J, et al: Declining serum cholesterol levels prior to diagnosis of colon cancer. JAMA 263:2083, 1990.

115. Porter JB, Walker AM, Jick H: Cancer of the breast, colon, ovary, and testis in the United States: Rates 1970-1978 from a hospital reporting system. Am J Public Health 74:585, 1984.

116. Rex DK, Sledge GW, Harper PA, et al: Colonic adenomas in asymptomatic women with a history of breast cancer. Am J Gastroenterol 88:2009, 1993.

117. Peelen T, de Leeuw W, van Lent K, et al: Genetic analysis of a breast-ovarian cancer family, with 7 cases of colorectal cancer linked to *BRCA1*, fails to support a role for *BRCA1* in colorectal tumorigenesis. Int J Cancer 88:778, 2000.

118. McFarlane MJ, Welch KE: Gallstones, cholecystectomy, and colorectal cancer. Am J Gastroenterol 88:1994, 1993.

119. Neugut AI, Murray TI, Garbowski GC, et al: Cholecystectomy as a risk factor for colorectal adenomatous polyps and carcinoma. Cancer 68:1644, 1991.

120. Sobin LH: The histopathology of bleeding from polyps and carcinomas of the large intestine. Cancer 55:577, 1985.

121. Shnitka TK, Friedman MHW, Kidd EG, et al: Villous tumors of the rectum and colon characterized by severe fluid and electrolyte loss. Surg Gynecol Obstet 112:609, 1961.

122. Duthie HL, Atwell JD: The absorption of water, sodium, and potassium in the large intestine with particular reference to the effects of villous papillomas. Gut 4:373, 1963.

123. Guillem JG, Forde KA, Treat MR, et al: The impact of colonoscopy on the early detection of colonic neoplasms in patients with rectal bleeding. Ann Surg 206:606, 1987.

124. Cheung PSY, Wong SKC, Boey J, et al: Frank rectal bleeding: A prospective study of causes in patients over the age of 40. Postgrad Med J 64:364, 1988.

125. Macrae F, St. John DJB: Relationship between patterns of bleeding and Hemoccult sensitivity in patients with colorectal cancers or adenomas. Gastroenterology 82:891, 1982.

126. Crowley ML, Freeman LD, Mottet MD, et al: Sensitivity of guaiac-impregnated cards for the detection of colorectal neoplasia. J Clin Gastroenterol 5:127, 1983.

127. Gabrielsson N, Granqvist S, Nilsson B: Guaiac tests detection of occult faecal blood loss in patients with endoscopically verified colonic polyps. Scand J Gastroenterol 20:978, 1985.

128. Allison JE, Tekawa IS, Ransom LJ, et al: A comparison of fecal occult blood tests for colorectal-cancer screening. N Engl J Med 334:155, 1996.

129. Nakajima M, Saito H, Soma Y, et al: Prevention of advanced colorectal cancer by screening using the immunochemical faecal occult blood test: A case-control study. Br J Cancer 89:23, 2003.

130. Simon JB: Occult blood screening for colorectal carcinoma: A critical review. Gastroenterology 88:820, 1985.

131. Winawer SJ, Schottenfeld D, Flehinger BJ: Colorectal cancer screening. J Natl Cancer Inst 83:243, 1991.

132. Hardcastle JD, Armitage NC, Chamberlain J, et al: Fecal occult blood screening for colorectal cancer in the general population: Results of a controlled trial. Cancer 58:397, 1986.

133. Moertel CG, Hill JR, Dockerty MB: The routine proctoscopic examination: A second look. Mayo Clin Proc 41:368, 1966.

134. Marks G, Boggs HW, Castro AF, et al: Sigmoidoscopic examinations with rigid and flexible fiberoptic sigmoidoscopes in the surgeon's office: A comparative prospective study of effectiveness in 1,012 cases. Dis Colon Rectum 22:162, 1979.

135. Winnan G, Berci G, Panish J, et al: Superiority of the flexible to the rigid sigmoidoscope in routine proctosigmoidoscopy. N Engl J Med 302:1011, 1980.

136. UK Flex. Sig. Screening Trial Investigators: Single flexible sigmoidoscopy screening to prevent colorectal cancer: Baseline findings of a UK multicenter randomized trial. Lancet 359: 1291, 2002.

137. Segnan N, Senore C, Andreoni B, et al: Baseline findings of the Italian multicenter randomized controlled trial of "once-only sigmoidoscopy"—SCORE. J Natl Cancer Inst 94:1763, 2002.

138. Ott DJ, Chen YM, Gelfand DW, et al: Single-contrast vs double-contrast barium enema in the detection of colonic polyps. AJR Am J Roentgenol 146:993, 1986.

139. Winawer SJ, Stewart ET, Zauber AG, et al: A comparison of colonoscopy and double-contrast barium enema for surveillance after polypectomy. N Engl J Med 342:1766, 2000.

140. Williams CB, Macrae FA, Bartrum CI: A prospective study of diagnostic methods in adenoma follow-up. Endoscopy 14:74, 1982.

141. Aldridge MC, Sim AJW: Colonoscopy findings in symptomatic patients without x-ray evidence of colonic neoplasms. Lancet 2:833, 1986.

142. Hixson LJ, Fennerty MB, Sampliner RE, et al: Prospective blinded trial of the colonoscopic miss rate of large colorectal polyps. Gastrointest Endosc 37:125, 1991.

143. Rex DK, Cutler CS, Lemmel GT, et al: Colonoscopic miss rates of adenomas determined by back-to-back colonoscopies. Gastroenterology 112:24, 1997.

144. Pickhardt PJ, Nugent PA, Mysliwiec PA, et al: Location of adenomas missed by optical colonoscopy. Ann Intern Med 141:352, 2004.

145. Winawer S, Fletcher R, Rex D, et al: Colorectal Cancer Screening and Surveillance: Clinical guidelines and rationale—update based on new evidence. Gastroenterology 124:544, 2003.

146. Rex DK: Colonoscopy: a review of its yield for cancers and adenomas by indication. Am J Gastroenterol 90:353, 1995.

147. van Dam J, Cotton P, Johnson CD, et al: AGA Future Trends Report: CT colonography. Gastroenterology 127:970, 2004.

148. Johnson CD, Toledano AY, Herman BA, et al: Computerized tomographic colonography: Performance evaluation in a retrospective multicenter setting. Gastroenterology. 125:688, 2003.

149. Cotton PB, Durkalski VL, Pineau BC, et al: Computed tomographic colonography (virtual colonoscopy): A multicenter comparison with standard colonoscopy for detection of colorectal neoplasia. JAMA 291:1713, 2004.

150. Pickhardt PJ, Choi JR, Hwang I, et al: Computed tomographic virtual colonoscopy to screen for colorectal neoplasia in asymptomatic adults. N Engl J Med. 349:2191, 2003.

151. Iannaccone R, Laghi A, Catalano C, et al: Computed tomographic colonography without cathartic preparation for the detection of colorectal polyps. Gastroenterology 127:1300, 2004.

152. Ahlquist DA, Skoletsky JE, Boynton KA, et al: Colorectal cancer screening by detection of altered human DNA in stool: Feasibility of a multitarget assay panel. Gastroenterology 119:1219, 2000.

153. Osborn NK, Ahlquist DA: Stool screening for colorectal cancer: Molecular approaches. Gastroenterology 128:192, 2005.

154. Figiel LS, Figiel SJ, Wieterson FK: Roentgenologic observation of growth rates of colonic polyps and carcinoma. Acta Radiol Diagn 3:417, 1965.

155. Stryker SJ, Wolff BG, Culp CE, et al: Natural history of untreated colonic polyps. Gastroenterology 93:1009, 1987.

156. Welin S, Youker J, Spratt JS Jr: The rates and patterns of growth of 375 tumors of the large intestine and rectum observed serially by double contrast enema study (Malmo technique). AJR Am J Roentgenol 90:673, 1963.

157. Tada M, Misaki F, Kawai K: Growth rates of colorectal carcinoma and adenoma by roentgenologic follow-up observations. Gastroenterol Jpn 19:550, 1984.

158. Knoernschild HE: Growth rate and malignant potential of colonic polyps: Early results. Surg Forum 14:137, 1963.

159. Hofstad B, Almendingen K, Vatn M, et al: Growth and recurrence of colorectal polyps: A double-blind three-year intervention with calcium and antioxidants. Digestion 59:148, 1998.

160. Bersentes K, Fennerty B, Sampliner RE, et al: Lack of spontaneous regression of tubular adenomas in two years of follow-up. Am J Gastroenterol 92:1117, 1997.

161. Carroll RLA, Klein M: How often should patients be sigmoidoscoped? A mathematical perspective. Prev Med 9:741, 1980.

162. Loeve F, Boer R, Zauber AG, et al: National Polyp Study Data: Evidence for regression of adenomas. Int J Cancer 111:633, 2004.

163. Winawer SJ, Zauber A, Diaz B: The National Polyp Study: Temporal sequence of evolving colorectal cancer from the normal colon. Gastrointest Endosc 33:167, 1987.

164. Eide TJ: Risk of colorectal cancer in adenoma-bearing individuals within a defined population. Int J Cancer 38:173, 1986.

165. Pagana TJ, Ledesman EJ, Mittelman A, et al: The use of colonoscopy in the study of synchronous colorectal neoplasms. Cancer 53:356, 1984.

166. Chu DZJ, Giacco G, Martin RG, et al: The significance of synchronous carcinoma and polyps in the colon and rectum. Cancer 57:445, 1986.

167. Langevin JM, Nivatvongs S: The true incidence of synchronous cancer of the bowel: A prospective study. Am J Surg 147:330, 1984.

168. Reilly JC, Rusin LC, Theuerkauf FJ Jr: Colonoscopy: Its role in cancer of the colon and rectum. Dis Colon Rectum 25:532, 1982.

169. Greenstein AJ, Heimann T, Sachar DB, et al: A comparison of multiple synchronous colorectal cancer in ulcerative colitis, familial polyposis coli, and de novo cancer. Ann Surg 203:123, 1986.

170. Morson BC, Bussey HJR: Magnitude of risk for cancer in patients with colorectal adenomas. Br J Surg 72(Suppl):S23, 1985.

171. Lotfi AM, Spencer RJ, Ilstrup DM, et al: Colorectal polyps and the risk of subsequent carcinoma. Mayo Clin Proc 61:337, 1986.

172. Bond JH: Polyp guideline: Diagnosis, treatment, and surveillance for patients with colorectal polyps. Am J Gastroenterol 95:3053, 2000.

173. Grossman S, Milos ML, Tekawa IS, et al: Colonoscopic screening of persons with suspected risk factors for colon cancer: II. Past history of colorectal neoplasms. Gastroenterology 96:299, 1989.

174. Zarchy TM, Ershoff D: Do characteristics of adenomas on flexible sigmoidoscopy predict advanced lesions on baseline colonoscopy? Gastroenterology 106:1501, 1994.

175. Wallace MB, Kemp JA, Trnka YM, et al: Is colonoscopy indicated for small adenomas found by screening flexible sigmoidoscopy? Ann Intern Med 129:273, 1998.

176. Atkin WS, Morson BC, Cuzick J: Long-term risk of colorectal cancer after excision of rectosigmoid adenomas. N Engl J Med 326:658, 1992.

177. Atkin WS, Saunders BP: Surveillance guidelines after removal of colorectal adenomatous polyps. Gut 51(Suppl V):v6-v9, 2002.

178. Schoen RE, Corle D, Cranston L, et al: Is colonoscopy needed for the nonadvanced adenoma found on sigmoidoscopy? Gastroenterology 115:533, 1998.

179. Dinning JP, Hixson LJ, Clark LC: Prevalence of distal colonic neoplasia associated with proximal colon cancers. Arch Intern Med 154:853, 1994.

180. Imperiale TF, Wagner DR, Lin CY, et al: Using risk for advanced proximal colonic neoplasia to tailor endoscopic screening for colorectal cancer. Ann Intern Med 139:959, 2003.

181. Wilcox GM, Anderson PB, Colacchio TA: Early invasive carcinoma in colonic polyps: A review of the literature with emphasis on the assessment of the risk of metastasis. Cancer 57:160, 1986.

182. Coverlizza S, Risio M, Ferrari A, et al: Colorectal adenomas containing invasive carcinoma: Pathologic assessment of lymph node metastatic potential. Cancer 64:1937, 1989.

183. Morson BC, Whiteway JE, Jones EA, et al: Histopathology and prognosis of malignant colorectal polyps treated by endoscopic polypectomy. Gut 25:437, 1984.

184. Morson BC: The evolution of colorectal carcinoma. Clin Radiol 35:425, 1984.

185. Neugut AI, Jacobson JS, Ahsan H, et al: Incidence and recurrence rates of colorectal adenomas: A prospective study. Gastroenterology 108:402, 1995.

186. Williams CB, Macrae FA: The St. Mark's neoplastic polyp follow-up study. Front Gastrointest Res 10:226, 1986.

187. Kronborg O, Hage E, Adamsen S, et al: Follow-up after colorectal polypectomy: II. Repeated examinations of the colon every 6 months after removal of sessile adenomas and adenomas with the highest degree of dysplasia. Scand J Gastroenterol 18:1095, 1983.

188. Waye JD, Braunfeld S: Surveillance intervals after colonoscopic polypectomy. Endoscopy 14:79, 1981.

189. Woolfson IK, Eckholdt GJ, Wetzel CR, et al: Usefulness of performing colonoscopy one year after endoscopic polypectomy. Dis Colon Rectum 33:389, 1990.

190. Schatzkin A, Lanza E, Corle D, et al: Lack of effect of a low-fat, high-fiber diet on the recurrence of colorectal adenomas. N Engl J Med 342:1149, 2000.

191. Alberts D, Martinez E, Roe DJ, et al: Lack of effect of a high-fiber cereal supplement on the recurrence of colorectal adenomas. N Engl J Med 342:1156, 2000.

192. Van Stolk RU, Beck GJ, Baron JA, et al: Adenoma characteristics at first colonoscopy as predictors of adenoma recurrence and characteristics at follow-up. Gastroenterology 115:13, 1998.

193. Martinez ME, Sampliner R, Marshall JR, et al: Adenoma characteristics as risk factors for recurrence of advanced adenomas. Gastroenterology 120:1077, 2001.

194. O'Brien M, Winawer SJ, Gottlieb LS, et al: Analysis of multiple determinants of significant dysplasia in colorectal adenomas. Gastrointest Endosc 31:148, 1985.

195. Winawer SJ: Colon surveillance for neoplasia. Gastrointest Endosc 49(Suppl):S63, 1999.

196. Kune GA, Kune S, Watson LF: History of colorectal polypectomy and risk of subsequent colorectal cancer. Br J Surg 74:1064, 1987.

197. Levi F, Randimbison L, LaVecchia C: Incidence of colorectal cancer following adenomatous polyps of the large intestine. Int J Cancer 55:415, 1993.

198. Simons BD, Morrison AS, Lev R, et al: Relationship of polyps to cancer of the large intestine. J Natl Cancer Inst 84:962, 1992.

199. Murakami, R, Tsukuma H, Kanamori S, et al: Natural history of colorectal polyps and the effect of polypectomy on occurrence of subsequent cancer. Int J Cancer 46:159, 1990.

200. This-Evensen E, Hoff GS, Sauar F, et al: Population-based surveillance by colonoscopy: Effect on the incidence of colorectal cancer. Telemark Polyp Study I. Scand J Gastroenterol 34:414, 1999.

201. Citarda F, Tomaselli G, Capocaccia R, et al: Efficacy in standard clinical practice of colonoscopic polypectomy in reducing colorectal cancer incidence. Gut 48:812, 2001.

202. Jørgensen OD, Kronborg O, Fenger C: The Funen Adenoma Follow-up Study: Incidence and death from colorectal carcinoma in an adenoma surveillance program. Scand J Gastroenterol 28:869, 1993.

203. Kaye GI, Pascal RP, Lane N: The colonic pericryptal fibroblast sheath: Replication, migration, and cytodifferentiation of a mesenchymal cell system in adult tissue. Gastroenterology 60:515, 1971.

204. Hayashi T, Yatani R, Apostol J, et al: Pathogenesis of hyperplastic polyps of the colon: A hypothesis based upon ultrastructural and in vitro cell kinetics. Gastroenterology 66:347, 1974.

205. Longacre TA, Fenoglio-Preiser CM: Mixed hyperplastic adenomatous polyps/serrated adenomas: A distinct form of colorectal neoplasia. Am J Surg Pathol 14:524, 1990.

206. Jass JR: Serrated adenoma and colorectal cancer. J Pathol 187:499, 1999.

207. Huang CS, O'Brien MJ, Yang S, et al: Hyperplastic polyps, serrated adenomas, and the serrated polyp neoplasia pathway. Am J Gastroenterol 99:2242, 2004.

208. Iino H, Jass JR, Simms LA, et al: DNA microsatellite instability in hyperplastic polyps, serrated adenomas, and mixed polyps: A mild mutator pathway for colorectal cancer? J Clin Pathol 52:5, 1999.

209. Frayling IM, Beck NE, Ilyas M, et al: The APC variants I1307K and E1317Q are associated with colorectal tumors, but not always with a family history. Proc Natl Acad Sci U S A 95:10722, 1998.

210. Liljegren A, Lindblom A, Rotstein S, et al: Prevalence and incidence of hyperplastic polyps and adenomas in familial colorectal cancer: Correlation between the two types of colon polyps. Gut 52:1140, 2003.

211. Foutch PG, DiSario JA, Pardy K, et al: The sentinel hyperplastic polyp: A marker for synchronous neoplasia in the proximal colon. Am J Gastroenterol 86:1482, 1991.

212. Cannon-Albright LA, Skolnick MH, Bishop DT, et al: Common inheritance of susceptibility to colonic adenomatous polyps and associated colorectal cancers. N Engl J Med 319:533, 1988.

213. Waye JD, Lewis BS, Frankel A, et al: Small colon polyps. Am J Gastroenterol 83:120, 1988.

214. Rex DK, Smith JJ, Ulbright TM, et al: Distal colonic hyperplastic polyps do not predict proximal adenomas in asymptomatic average-risk subjects. Gastroenterology 102:317, 1992.

215. Provenzale D, Garrett JW, Condon SE, et al: Risk for colon adenomas in patients with rectosigmoid hyperplastic polyps. Ann Intern Med 113:760, 1990.

216. Zauber AG, Winawer SJ, Diaz B, et al: The National Polyp Study: The association of colonic hyperplastic polyps and adenomas. Am J Gastroenterol 83:1060, 1988.

217. Dave S, Hui S, Kroenke K, et al: Is the distal hyperplastic polyp a marker for proximal neoplasia? J Gen Intern Med 18:128, 2003.

218. Nugent KP, Talbot IC, Hodgson SV, et al: Solitary juvenile polyps: Not a marker for subsequent malignancy. Gastroenterology 105:698, 1993.

219. Teague RH, Read AE: Polyposis in ulcerative colitis. Gut 16:792, 1975.

220. Berkowitz D, Bernstein LH: Colonic pseudopolyps in association with amebic colitis. Gastroenterology 68:786, 1975.

221. Nebel OT, El Masry NA, Castell DO, et al: Schistosomal disease of the colon: A reversible form of polyposis. Gastroenterology 67:939, 1974.

222. Anthony PP, Morris DS, Vowles KDJ: Multiple and recurrent inflammatory fibroid polyps in three generations of a Devon family: A new syndrome. Gut 25:854, 1984.

223. Géhénot M, Colombel JF, Wolschies E, et al: Cap polyposis occurring in the postoperative course of pelvic surgery. Gut 35:1670, 1994.

224. Levine DS: "Solitary" rectal ulcer syndrome: Are "solitary" rectal ulcer syndrome and "localized" colitis cystica profunda analogous syndromes caused by rectal prolapse? Gastroenterology 92:243, 1987.

225. Shallal JA, van Heerden JA, Bartholomew LG, et al: Pneumatosis cystoides intestinalis. Mayo Clin Proc 49:180, 1974.

226. Mirables M, Hinojosa J, Alonso J, et al: Oxygen therapy of pneumatosis coli: What is minimum oxygen requirement? Dis Colon Rectum 26:458, 1983.

227. Born A, Inouye T, Diamant N: Pneumatosis coli: Case report documenting time from x-ray appearance to onset of symptoms. Dig Dis Sci 26:855, 1981.

228. Mynster T, Hultberg B, Bülow S: Multiple lymphomatous polyposis of the colon and rectum. Scand J Gastroenterol 29:545, 1994.

229. Pescatore P, Benhamou Y, Raphael M, et al: Colonic polyposis as sole manifestation of chronic lymphocytic leukemia. J Clin Gastroenterol 18:248, 1994.

230. DeBeer RA, Shinya H: Colonic lipoma. Gastrointest Endosc 22:90, 1975.

231. Bussey HJR, Veale AMO, Morson BC: Genetics of gastrointestinal polyposis. Gastroenterology 74:1325, 1978.

232. Herrera L, Kakati S, Gibas L, et al: Brief clinical report: Gardner syndrome in a man with an interstitial deletion of 5q. Am J Med Genet 25:473, 1986.

233. Bodmer WF, Bailey CJ, Bodmer J, et al: Localization of the gene for familial adenomatous polyposis on chromosome 5. Nature 328:614, 1987.

234. Leppert M, Dobbs M, Scambler P, et al: The gene for familial polyposis coli maps to the long arm of chromosome 5. Science 238:1411, 1987.

235. Solomon E, Voss R, Hall V, et al: Chromosome 5 allele loss in human colorectal carcinomas. Nature 328:616, 1987.

236. Kinzler KW, Nilbert MC, Su LK, et al: Identification of FAP locus genes from chromosome 5q21. Science 253:661, 1991.

237. Nishisho I, Nakamura Y, Miyoshi Y, et al: Mutations of chromosome 5q21 genes in FAP and colorectal cancer patients. Science 253:665, 1991.

238. Groden J, Thliveris A, Samowitz W, et al: Identification and characterization of the familial adenomatous polyposis coli gene. Cell 66:589, 1991.

239. Miyaki M, Tanaka K, Kikuchi-Yanoshita R, et al: Familial polyposis: Recent advances. Crit Rev Oncol/Hematol 19:1, 1995.

240. Oving IM, Clevers HC: Molecular causes of colon cancer. Eur J Clin Invest 32:448, 2002.

241. Bussey HJR: Familial Polyposis Coli. Baltimore, Johns Hopkins Press, 1975.

242. Petersen GM, Slack J, Nakamura Y: Screening guidelines and premorbid diagnosis of familial adenomatous polyposis using linkage. Gastroenterology 100:1658, 1991.

243. Nagase H, Miyoshi Y, Horii A, et al: Correlation between the location of germ-line mutations in the *APC* gene and the number of colorectal polyps in familial adenomatous polyposis patients. Cancer Res 52:4055, 1992.

244. Naylor EW, Lebenthal E: Gardner's syndrome: Recent developments in research and management. Dig Dis Sci 25:945, 1980.

245. Jang YS, Steinhagen RM, Heimann TM: Colorectal cancer in familial adenomatous polyposis. Dis Colon Rectum 40:312, 1997.

246. Burt RW: Hereditary polyposis syndromes and inheritance of adenomatous polyps. Semin Gastrointest Dis 3:13, 1992.

247. Burt RW: Gastric fundic gland polyps. Gastroenterology 125:1462, 2003.

248. Offerhaus GJA, Giardiello FM, Krush AJ, et al: The risk of upper gastrointestinal cancer in familial adenomatous polyposis. Gastroenterology 102:1980, 1992.

249. Iwama T, Mishima Y, Utsunomiya J: The impact of familial adenomatous polyposis on the tumorigenesis and mortality at the several organs: its rational treatment. Ann Surg 217:101, 1993.

250. Watanabe H, Enjoji M, Yao T, et al: Gastric lesions in familial adenomatosis coli. Hum Pathol 9:269, 1978.

251. Debinski HS, Spigelman AD, Hatfield A, et al: Upper intestinal surveillance in familial adenomatous polyposis. Eur J Cancer 31A:1149, 1995.

252. Burke CA, Beck GJ, Church JM, van Stolk RU: The natural history of untreated duodenal and ampullary adenomas in patients with familial adenomatous polyposis followed in an endoscopic surveillance program. Gastrointest Endosc 49:358, 1999.

253. Caspari R, von Falkenhausen M, Krautmacher C, et al: Comparison of capsule endoscopy and magnetic resonance imaging for the detection of polyps of the small intestine in patients with familial adenomatous polyposis or with Peutz-Jeghers syndrome. Endoscopy 36:1054, 2004.

254. Bulow S, Sondergaard JO, Witt I, et al: Mandibular osteomas in familial polyposis coli. Dis Colon Rectum 27:105, 1984.

255. Blair NP, Trempe CL: Hypertrophy of the retinal pigment epithelium associated with Gardner's syndrome. Am J Ophthalmol 90:661, 1980.

256. Burn J, Chapman P, Delhanty J, et al: The UK northern region genetic register for familial adenomatous polyposis coli: Use of age of onset, congenital hypertrophy of the retinal pigment epithelium, and DNA markers in risk calculations. J Med Genet 28:289, 1991.

257. Olschwang S, Tiret A, Laurent-Puig P, et al: Restriction of ocular fundus lesions to a specific subgroup of *APC* mutations in adenomatous polyposis coli patients. Cell 75:959, 1993.

258. Gurbuz AK, Giardiello FM, Petersen GM, et al: Desmoid tumors in familial adenomatous polyposis. Gut 35:377, 1994.

259. Sturt NJH, Gallagher MC, Bassett P, et al: Evidence for genetic predisposition to desmoid tumors in familial adenomatous polyposis independent of the germline APC mutation. Gut 53:1832, 2004.

260. Kiel KD, Suit HD: Radiation therapy in the treatment of aggressive fibromatoses (desmoid tumors). Cancer 54:2051, 1984.

261. Tsukada K, Church JM, Jagelman DG, et al: Systemic cytotoxic chemotherapy and radiation therapy for desmoid in familial adenomatous polyposis. Dis Colon Rectum 34:1090, 1991.

262. Klein WA, Miller HH, Anderson M, et al: The use of indomethacin, sulindac, and tamoxifen for the treatment of desmoid tumors associated with familial polyposis. Cancer 12:2863, 1987.

263. Belliveau P, Graham AM: Mesenteric desmoid tumor in Gardner's syndrome treated by sulindac. Dis Colon Rectum 27:53, 1984.

264. Kingbrunner B, Ritter S, Domingo J, et al: Remission of rapidly growing desmoid tumors after tamoxifen therapy. Cancer 52:2201, 1983.

265. Lanari A: Effect of progesterone on desmoid tumors (aggressive fibromatosis). N Engl J Med 309:1523, 1983.

266. Truta B, Allen BA, Conrad PG, et al: Genotype and phenotype of patients with both familial adenomatous polyposis and thyroid carcinoma. Fam Cancer 2:95, 2003.

267. Painter TA, Jagelman DG: Adrenal adenomas and adrenal carcinomas in association with hereditary adenomatosis of the colon and rectum. Cancer 55:2001, 1985.

268. LeSher AR, Castronuovo JJ Jr, Filippone AL Jr: Familial polyposis coli and hepatocellular neoplasms. Surgery 105:668, 1989.

269. Garber JE, Li FP, Kingston JE, et al: Hepatoblastoma and familial adenomatous polyposis. J Natl Cancer Inst 80:1616, 1988.

270. Giardiello FM, Krush AJ, Petersen GM, et al: Phenotypic variability of familial adenomatous polyposis in 11 unrelated families with identical *APC* gene mutation. Gastroenterology 106:1542, 1994.

271. Stevenson JK, Reid BJ: Unfamiliar aspects of familial polyposis coli. Am J Surg 152:81, 1986.

272. Houlston R, Crabtree M, Phillips R, et al: Explaining differences in the severity of familial adenomatous polyposis and the search for modifier genes. Gut 48:1, 2001.

273. Oshima M, Dinchuk JE, Kargman SL, et al: Suppression of intestinal polyposis in $APC^{\Delta716}$ knockout mice by inhibition of cyclooxygenase 2 (COX-2). Cell 87:803, 1996.

274. Trimbath JD, Giardiello FM: Review article: Genetic testing and counselling for hereditary colorectal cancer. Aliment Pharmacol Ther 16:1843, 2002.

275. Lynch HT, Smyrk T, Lynch J, et al: Genetic counseling in an extended attenuated familial adenomatous polyposis kindred. Am J Gastroenterol 91:455, 1996.

276. Olsen KO, Juul S, Bulow S, et al: Female fecundity before and after operation for familial adenomatous polyposis. Br J Surg 90:227, 2003.

277. Moertel CG, Hill JR, Adson MA: Management of multiple polyposis of the large intestine. Cancer 28:160, 1971.

278. Bertario L, Russo A, Radice P, et al: Genotype and phenotype factors as determinants for rectal stump cancer in patients with familial adenomatous polyposis. Ann Surg 231:538, 2000.

279. Harvey JC, Quan SHQ, Stearns WW: Management of familial polyposis with preservation of the rectum. Surgery 84:476, 1978.

280. Bussey HJR, Eyers AA, Ritchie SM, et al: The rectum in adenomatous polyposis: The St. Mark's policy. Br J Surg 72:529, 1985.

281. Jagelman DG: Clinical management of familial adenomatous polyposis. Cancer Surv 8:159, 1989.

282. Skinner MA, Tyler D, Branum GE, et al: Subtotal colectomy for familial polyposis. Arch Surg 125:621, 1990.

283. Feinberg SM, Jagelman DG, Sarre RG, et al: Spontaneous resolution of rectal polyps in patients with familial polyposis following abdominal colectomy and ileorectal anastomosis. Dis Colon Rectum 31:169, 1988.

284. Bussey HJR, DeCosse JJ, Deschner EE, et al: A randomized trial of ascorbic acid in polyposis coli. Cancer 50:1434, 1982.

285. Stern HS, Gregoire RC, Kashtan H, et al: Long-term effects of dietary calcium on risk markers for colon cancer in patients with familial polyposis. Surgery 108:528, 1990.

286. DeCosse JJ, Miller HH, Lesser ML: Effect of wheat fiber and vitamins C and E on rectal polyps in patients with familial adenomatous polyposis. J Natl Cancer Inst 81:1290, 1989.

287. Giardiello FM, Yang VW, Hylind LM, et al: Primary chemoprevention of familial adenomatous polyposis with sulindac. N Engl J Med 346:1054, 2002.

288. Prescott SM, White RL: Self-promotion? Intimate connections between APC and prostaglandin H synthase-2. Cell 87:783, 1996.

289. Piazza GA, Kulchak Rahm AL, Krutzsch M, et al: Antineoplastic drugs sulindac sulfide and sulfone inhibit cell growth by inducing apoptosis. Cancer Res 55:3110, 1995.

290. Steinbach G, Lynch PM, Phillips RKS, et al: The effect of celecoxib, a cyclooxygenase-2 inhibitor, in familial adenomatous polyposis. N Engl J Med 342:1946, 2000.

291. Stoner GD, Budd GT, Ganapathi R, et al: Sulindac sulfone induced regression of rectal polyps in patients with familial adenomatous polyposis. Adv Exp Med Biol 407:45, 1999.

292. Turcot J, Despres JP, St. Pierre T: Malignant tumors of the central nervous system associated with familial polyposis of the colon: Report of two cases. Dis Colon Rectum 2:465, 1959.

293. Baughman FA, List CF, Williams JR, et al: The glioma-polyposis syndrome. N Engl J Med 281:1345, 1969.

294. Hamilton SR, Liu B, Parsons RE, et al: The molecular basis of Turcot's syndrome. N Engl J Med 332:839, 1995.

295. Leppert M, Burt R, Hughes JP, et al: Genetic analysis of an inherited predisposition to colon cancer in a family with a variable number of adenomatous polyps. N Engl J Med 322:904, 1990.

296. Lynch HT, Smyrk T, Lynch J, et al: Update on the differential diagnosis, surveillance and management of hereditary non-polyposis colorectal cancer. Eur J Cancer 31A:1039, 1995.

297. Spirio L, Olschwang S, Groden J, et al: Alleles of the *APC* gene: An attenuated form of familial polyposis. Cell 75:951, 1993.

298. Lynch HT, Smyrk TC, Lanspa SJ, et al: Upper gastrointestinal manifestations in families with hereditary flat adenoma syndrome. Cancer 71:2709, 1993.

299. Fearnhead NS, Wilding JL, Winney B, et al: Multiple rare variants in different genes account for multifactorial inherited susceptibility to colorectal adenomas. Proc Natl Acad Sci U S A 101:15992, 2004.

300. Lammi L, Arte S, Somer M, et al: Mutations in *AXIN2* cause familial tooth agenesis and predispose to colorectal cancer. Am J Hum Genet 74:1043, 2004.

301. Lowy AM, Kordich JJ, Gismondi V, et al: Numerous colonic adenomas in an individual with Bloom's syndrome. Gastroenterology 121:435, 2001.

302. Lipton L, Tomlinson I: The multiple colorectal adenoma phenotype and *MYH*, a base excision repair gene. Clin Gastroenterol Hepatol 2:633, 2004.

303. Graham R, McKee P, McGibbon D, et al: Torre-Muir syndrome: An association with isolated sebaceous carcinoma. Cancer 55:2868, 1985.

304. Seruca R, Carneiro F, Castedo S, et al: Familial gastric polyposis revisited. Cancer Genet Cytogenet 53:97, 1991.

305. Williams GT, Arthur JF, Bussey HJR, et al: Metaplastic polyps and polyposis of the colorectum. Histopathology 4:155, 1980.

306. Torlakovic E, Snover DC: Serrated adenomatous polyposis in humans. Gastroenterology 110:748, 1996.

307. Burdick D, Prior JT: Peutz-Jeghers syndrome: A clinicopathologic study of a large family with a 27-year follow-up. Cancer 50:2139, 1982.

308. Foley TR, McGarrity TJ, Abt AB: Peutz-Jeghers syndrome: A clinicopathologic survey of the "Harrisburg family" with a 49-year follow-up. Gastroenterology 95:1535, 1988.

309. Hemminki A, Markie D, Tomlinson I, et al: A serine/threonine kinase gene defect in Peutz-Jeghers syndrome. Nature 391:184, 1998.

310. Jenne DE, Reimann H, Nezu J, et al: Peutz-Jeghers syndrome is caused by mutations in a novel serine threonine kinase. Nat Genet 18:38, 1998.

311. Gruber SB, Entius MM, Petersen GM, et al: Pathogenesis of adenocarcinoma in Peutz-Jehgers syndrome. Cancer Res 58:5267, 1998.

312. Entius MM, Keller JJ, Westerman AM, et al: Molecular genetic alterations in hamartomatous polyps and carcinomas of patients with Peutz-Jeghers syndrome. J Clin Pathol 54:126, 2001.

313. Giardiello FM, Brensinger JD, Tersmette AC, et al: Very high risk of cancer in familial Peutz-Jeghers syndrome. Gastroenterology 119:1447, 2000.

314. Clement S, Efrusy ME, Dobbins WO III, et al: Pelvic neoplasia in Peutz-Jeghers syndrome. J Clin Gastroenterol 1979; 1:341.

315. Wilson DM, Pitts WC, Hintz RI, et al: Testicular tumors with Peutz-Jeghers syndrome. Cancer 57:2238, 1986.

316. Trau H, Schewach-Millet M, Fisher BK, et al: Peutz-Jeghers syndrome and bilateral breast carcinoma. Cancer 50:788, 1982.

317. Pedersen IR, Hartvigsen A, Hansen B, et al: Management of Peutz-Jeghers syndrome: Experience with patients from the Danish Polyposis Registry. Int J Colorect Dis 9:177, 1994.

318. Devroede G, Lemieux B, Masse S, et al: Colonic hamartomas in tuberous sclerosis. Gastroenterology 94:182, 1988.

319. Merg A, Howe JR: Genetic conditions associated with intestinal juvenile polyps. Am J Med Genet 129C:44, 2004.

320. Grotsky HW, Rickert RR, Smith WD, et al: Familial juvenile polyposis coli: A clinical and pathologic study of a large kindred. Gastroenterology 82:494, 1982.

321. Howe JR, Mitros FA, Summers RW: The risk of gastrointestinal carcinoma in familial juvenile polyposis. Ann Surg Oncol 5:751, 1998.

322. Coburn MC, Pricolo VE, DeLuca FG, et al: Malignant potential in intestinal juvenile polyposis syndromes. Ann Surg Oncol 2:386, 1995.

323. Goodman ZD, Yardley JH, Milligan FD: Pathogenesis of colonic polyps in multiple juvenile polyposis. Cancer 43:1906, 1979.

324. O'Riordain DS, O'Dwyer PJ, Cullen AF, et al: Familial juvenile polyposis coli and colorectal cancer. Cancer 68:889, 1991.

325. Howe JR, Roth S, Ringold JC, et al: Mutations in the smad4/dpc4 gene in juvenile polyposis. Science 280:1086, 1998.

326. Carlson GJ, Nivatvongs S, Snover DC: Colorectal polyps in Cowden's disease (multiple hamartoma syndrome). Am J Surg Pathol 8:763, 1984.

327. Lashner BA, Riddell RH, Winans CS: Ganglioneuromatosis of the colon and extensive glycogenic acanthosis in Cowden's disease. Dig Dis Sci 31:213, 1986.

328. Ruvalcaba RHA, Myhre S, Smith DW: Sotos syndrome with intestinal polyposis and pigmentary changes of the genitalia. Clin Genet 18:413, 1980.

329. DiLiberti JH, Weleber RG, Budden S: Ruvalcaba-Myhre-Smith syndrome: A case with probably autosomal dominant inheritance and additional manifestations. Am J Med Genet 15:491, 1983.

330. Whitelaw SC, Murday VA, Tomlinson IPM, et al: Clinical and molecular features of the hereditary mixed polyposis syndrome. Gastroenterology 112:327, 1997.

331. Jaeger EE, Woodford-Richens KL, Lockert M, et al: An ancestral Ashkenazi haplotype at the HMPS/CRAC1 locus on 15q13-q14 is associated with hereditary mixed polyposis syndrome. Am J Hum Genet 72:1261, 2003.

332. Tomlinson I, Rahman N, Frayling I, et al: Inherited susceptibility to colorectal adenomas and carcinoma: Evidence for a new predisposition gene on 15q14-q22. Gastroenterology 116:789, 1999.

333. Rutgeerts P, Hendricks H, Geboes K, et al: Involvement of the upper digestive tract by systemic neurofibromatosis. Gastrointest Endosc 27:22, 1981.

334. Hirata K, Kitahara K, Momosaka Y, et al: Diffuse ganglioneuromatosis with plexiform neurofibromas limited to the gastrointestinal tract involving a large segment of small intestine. J Gastroenterol 32:263, 1996.

335. Marsh DJ, Mulligan LM, Eng C: RET proto-oncogene mutations in multiple endocrine neoplasia type 2 and medullary thyroid carcinoma. Horm Res 47:168, 1997.

336. Allibone RO, Nanson JK, Anthony PP: Multiple and recurrent inflammatory fibroid polyps in a Devon family ("Devon polyposis syndrome"): An update. Gut 33:1004, 1992.

337. Schwartz RA: Basal cell nevus syndrome and gastrointestinal polyposis. N Engl J Med 299:49, 1978.

338. Cronkhite LW, Canada WJ: Generalized gastrointestinal polyposis: An unusual syndrome of polyposis, pigmentation, alopecia, and onychotrophia. N Engl J Med 252:1011, 1955.

339. Daniel ES, Ludwig SL, Lewin KJ, et al: The Cronkhite-Canada syndrome: An analysis of the pathologic features and therapy in 55 patients. Medicine 61:293, 1982.

340. Katayama Y, Kimura M, Konn M. Cronkhite-Canada syndrome associated with a rectal cancer and adenomatous changes in colonic polyps. Am J Surg Pathol 9:65, 1985.

341. Russell DM, Bhathal PS, St. John DJB: Complete remission in Cronkhite-Canada syndrome. Gastroenterology 85:180, 1983.

342. Ferrandez A, Samowitz W, DiSario JA, et al: Phenotypic characteristics and risk of cancer development in hyperplastic polyposis: Case series and literature review. Am J Gastroenterol 99:2012, 2004.

343. O'Briani DS, Kennedy MJ, Daly PA, et al: Multiple lymphomatous polyposis of the gastrointestinal tract. Am J Surg Pathol 13:691, 1989.

344. Triozzi PL, Borowitz MJ, Gockerman JP: Gastrointestinal involvement and multiple lymphomatous polyposis mantle-zone lymphoma. J Clin Oncol 4:866, 1986.

CHAPTER

120 Malignant Neoplasms of the Large Intestine

Robert S. Bresalier

Cancer of the colon and rectum (colorectal cancer [CRC]) is a major cause of cancer-associated morbidity and mortality in North America, Europe, and other regions with similar life-styles and dietary habits. CRC is the fourth most common newly diagnosed internal cancer overall in the United States, after cancers of the prostate, breast, and lung, and currently constitutes 10% of new cancers in men and 11% of new cancers in women. In 2006, there were an estimated 148,600 new CRC cases in the United States and 58,000 related deaths (a rate second only to that of lung cancer).[1] In the United States, CRC incidence rates in men and women are similar, although there appears to be a slight male predominance worldwide. Approximately 6% of the American population eventually will develop invasive colon or rectal cancer, and more than 6 million Americans who are alive today will die of the disease; an individual's lifetime risk of dying from CRC in the United States has been estimated to be 2.5%. Globally, CRC is the fourth most common cancer in men

and the third most common in women, with mortality paralleling incidence[2]; countries where CRC mortality was low before 1950 have reported substantial increases. Despite evidence that 5-year survival is 90% when CRC is diagnosed at an early stage, less than 40% of cases are diagnosed when the cancer is still localized.[3]

Rapid growth of knowledge about the molecular and biologic characteristics of CRC has provided useful insights into the pathogenesis of colonic neoplasms and cancer in general. New insights also have been gained in regard to primary prevention. Because CRC arises over long periods as the result of interactions between genetic predisposition and environmental insults, it has become possible to identify preneoplastic and early neoplastic lesions better and to improve survival rates. Rapidly evolving knowledge of CRC pathogenesis, especially in high-risk groups, is allowing the development of new tools to identify those who will benefit most from cancer surveillance and from adjuvant therapy following potentially curative surgery. After decades with limited options for treating advanced disease, new options for chemotherapy are now available.

Chapter 119 deals in detail with the principal premalignant colon lesion, the adenomatous polyp. In this chapter we examine what is known about factors that contribute further to the development of CRC, its predisposing conditions, biology, natural history, clinical presentation, diagnosis, and management. Current concepts and recent advances are stressed.

EPIDEMIOLOGY OF COLORECTAL CANCER

The frequency of CRC varies remarkably among different populations (Fig. 120–1).[4] Incidence rates are highest in the developed countries of North America, Australia, and New Zealand; intermediate in Europe; and low in Asia, South America, and especially sub-Saharan Africa.

Internationally, the incidence of colon cancer in men differs by a factor of almost 90 between areas with the extreme lowest and highest rates; the incidence of rectal cancer (cancer within 11 cm of the anus), differs by a factor of 13. CRC incidence also differs within countries, depending on region and population (Fig. 120–2). These differences are most likely due to differences in environmental factors, including dietary patterns (discussed later).

Although the incidences of colon and rectal cancer overall are parallel, geographic variation is more pronounced for colon cancer than for rectal cancer. High ratios of colon to rectal cancer (≥2 : 1) prevail in high-risk areas such as North America, whereas ratios below unity are often found in low-risk Asian and African populations. There is a steeper rise in the incidence of colon cancer for each unit increase in the incidence of rectal cancer in women compared with men. Although part of the regional variation in the ratios of colon to rectal cancer may arise from local conventions for classifying rectosigmoid tumors, these differences nonetheless

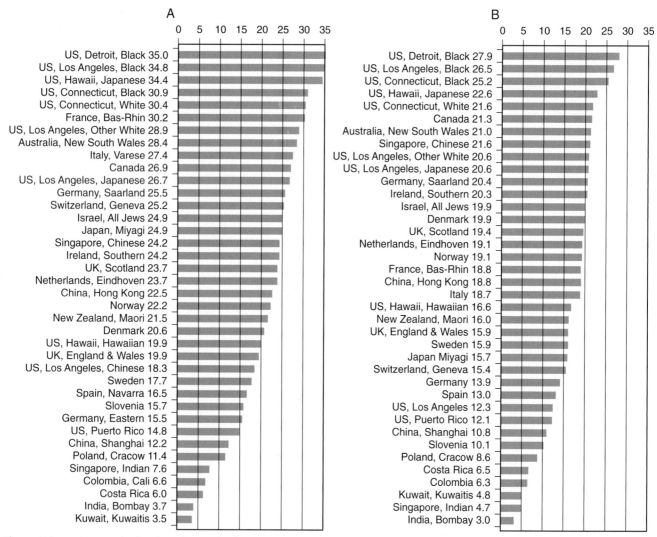

Figure 120–1 Age-standardized incidence of colon cancer per 100,000 population worldwide for men (A) and women (B). (A and B, Data from Parkin DM, Whelen SL, Ferlay J, et al: Cancer Incidence in Five Continents. [IARC Sci. Publ. No. 143]. Series. Lyon, International Agency for Research on Cancer, 1997.)

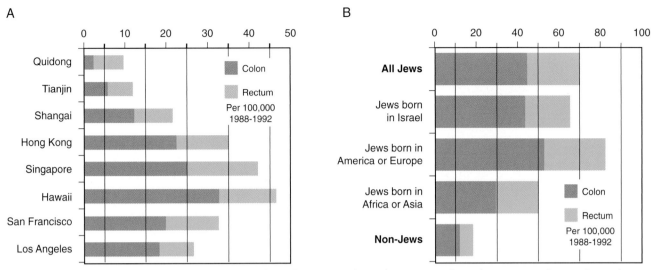

Figure 120–2 Age-standardized incidence of colon and rectal cancer in ethnic Chinese (*A*) and populations in Israel (*B*). Colorectal cancer incidence differs considerably within countries, depending on region and population, and in ethnic groups that migrate to areas with different diets and lifestyles. (*A* and *B*, Data from Parkin DM, Whelen SL, Ferlay J, et al: Cancer Incidence in Five Continents [IARC Sci. Publ. No. 143.] Series. Lyon, International Agency for Research on Cancer, 1997.)

suggest that colon and rectal cancer have related, but not identical, causes.

In the United States, the incidence of CRC also varies regionally. In general, rates in Southern and Western United States (except the San Francisco Bay area and Hawaii) are lower than the United States' average, whereas rates are highest in the Northeast and the North Central states. CRC incidence rates also are moderately higher for urban residents, although socioeconomic status is not a consistent risk factor for CRC in studies of the United States population. Although these regional differences in the United States have persisted over the long term, they gradually are fading, perhaps because of the increasing homogeneity of dietary patterns across the country.

Between 1950 and the mid-1980s, the incidence of colon cancer in the United States rose in the white population, whereas that of rectal cancer remained fairly stable. Mortality rates from CRC were stable among white men but decreased in white women. Both incidence and mortality rates for CRC increased substantially among the nonwhite population during this period.[5] CRC incidence and mortality have declined since 1985 in American adults at an average annual rate of 1.6% and 1.8%, respectively[3]; these trends are more evident in whites than blacks. Currently, both incidence and mortality rates for CRC are higher in the black population compared with the white population.[1]

The risk of CRC rises rapidly in populations that migrate from areas of low risk to areas of high risk. This pattern was demonstrated clearly in Japanese immigrants to Hawaii and to the continental United States during the 1950s and 1960s. Cancer rates for Issei (the migrating generation) rose over a short period to exceed those of native Japanese living in Japan, and the incidence rates for Nissei (their United States–born offspring) rose progressively to approximate those of the native white population. A similar upward displacement of CRC risk was

noted in Europeans who migrated to Australia after World War II and in Jews who migrated to Israel from low-risk areas in Yemen and North Africa. Longitudinal studies reveal that in many countries where CRC mortality rates were low before 1950, rates have increased sharply, whereas in countries where rates were high or moderate, they have decreased, stabilized, or increased slightly. Japan is a good example of this change: once a low-risk region for colon cancer, incidence rates have risen to equal or exceed those in North America and Europe.[4]

Studies of temporal trends by subsite location of large bowel cancer demonstrate that, for both sexes, incidence rates have increased for cancers of the right colon (cecum, ascending colon) and sigmoid colon and have decreased for cancers of the rectum; this change may reflect differing susceptibilities to neoplastic transformation in the proximal and distal colon. Currently in the United States, the prevalence of CRCs in whites is higher in the cecum and ascending colon (22% in men, 27% in women) and in the sigmoid colon (25% in men, 23% in women) than elsewhere in the large bowel (Fig. 120–3).

Descriptive epidemiology, including the study of temporal trends in CRC incidence, has played an important role in formulating hypotheses about the causes and pathogenesis of these lesions. Alterations in the subsite location of these tumors also have implications for clinical cancer detection; for example, the proportion of tumors beyond the reach of the sigmoidoscope increases with age.[5] Subsite distribution also may differ according to race.[6] These issues are discussed in subsequent sections.

ETIOLOGY AND CLUES ABOUT CAUSATION

Inter-regional differences in the incidence of CRC, including differences among population groups living in geographic proximity but with different life-styles, strongly suggest that environment plays a role in the

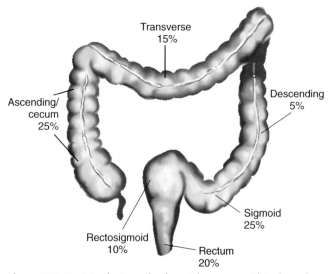

Figure 120–3 Distribution of colorectal cancers within the colon. Only approximately one half of cancers are within reach of the flexible sigmoidoscope.

Table 120–1	Factors That Potentially Influence Carcinogenesis in the Colon and Rectum*

Probably Related
High-fat and low-fiber consumption (adjusted for energy intake)[†]
Red meat consumption
Possibly Related
Beer and ale consumption (especially for rectal cancer)
Low dietary selenium
Environmental carcinogens and mutagens
Heterocyclic amines (from charbroiled and fried meat and fish)
Probably Protective
High-fiber consumption
Physical activity
Low body mass
Aspirin and NSAIDs
Calcium
Hormone replacement therapy (estrogen)
Possibly Protective[‡]
Yellow-green cruciferous vegetables
Carotene-rich foods
Vitamins C and E
Vitamin D
Cyclooxygenase-2 inhibitors

*Based on epidemiologic observations.
[†]Dietary fats and fiber are heterogeneous in composition, and not all fats or fiber components may play a role in causation or protection.
[‡]Based on limited data.
NSAIDs, nonsteroidal anti-inflammatory drugs.

development of this disease.[7] Migrant studies and rapid changes in incidence in countries assimilating Western practices support this concept. Strong circumstantial evidence exists for a link between diet and CRC. Population studies and animal studies have attempted to delineate the effects of various fats and proteins, carbohydrates, vegetable and fiber components, and micronutrients on the genesis of cancer of the large bowel (Table 120–1).

FAT, BILE ACIDS, AND BACTERIA

Several lines of evidence suggest that diets containing large proportions of fat predispose to CRC, especially in the descending and sigmoid colon. Colon cancer rates are high in populations whose total fat intake is high and are lower in those who consume less fat. On average, fat (saturated plus unsaturated) constitutes 40% to 45% of total calorie intake in Western countries with high rates of CRC, whereas in low-risk populations fat accounts for only 10% to 15% of dietary calories. Case-control and cohort studies also have suggested that the incidence and mortality rates from colon cancer, and in some cases rectal cancer, are positively correlated with dietary fat, but these findings are less convincing than data from descriptive epidemiologic studies. Differences may arise from methodologic limitations related to dietary history taking and a lack of sufficient variability in diet in communities from which subjects were drawn.

Early trials also often failed to take into account total energy intake. A prospective study assessed the relationship of meat, fat, and fiber intake among 88,751 women aged 34 to 59 years.[8] After adjustment for total energy intake, the intake of animal fat was significantly correlated with the risk of colon cancer. The intake ratio of red meat to chicken and fish was strongly associated with increased incidence of colon cancer, perhaps owing to differences in their fat composition. Similar findings have been reported that correlate the intake of saturated fat and the ratios of red meat to chicken and fish intake with both the incidence and recurrence of colorectal adenomas in women.[9] Cohort studies and a combined analysis of 13 case-control studies[10] that adjusted for total energy intake fail to provide clear-cut evidence for the association between dietary fat and CRC observed in earlier studies. Studies that specifically examine the association between intake of saturated/animal fat and CRC suggest a stronger association than with total fat.

Animal studies lend additional support for the role of dietary fat in the development of colon cancer. These studies usually involve the injection of carcinogens such as 1,2-dimethylhydrazine (DMH) or azoxymethane into rodents fed various diets. Animals fed a variety of polyunsaturated and saturated fats develop greater numbers of carcinogen-induced colonic adenocarcinomas than do those on low-fat diets. The amount and source of dietary fat may affect tumor development in such studies[11]; fatty acids derived from polyunsaturated fish oils (ω-3 fatty acids) and monosaturated olive oil may not promote tumors to the extent that other polyunsaturated fats do.

It has been proposed that dietary fat enhances cholesterol and bile acid synthesis by the liver, thereby increasing the amounts of these sterols in the colon. Colonic bacteria convert these compounds to secondary bile acids, cholesterol metabolites, and other potentially toxic metabolic compounds. Population studies demonstrate increased excretion of sterol metabolites and fecal bile acids in groups that consume a high-fat, low-fiber "Western" diet compared with other groups, and high fecal bile acid levels are found in some patients with CRC. Dietary fat also has been shown to increase the excretion of secondary bile acids in carcinogen-treated rats.

Secondary bile acids do not act as primary carcinogens, but as potent promoters of colon carcinogenesis in such animal models. Little is known about how lipid and sterol metabolites promote tumors, but both bile acids and free fatty acids have been shown to damage the colonic mucosa and increase the proliferative activity of its epithelium. Dietary consumption of high amounts of corn oil and beef fat increase colonic ornithine decarboxylase levels, which are associated with rapidly proliferating mucosa.

Activation of protein kinase C by bile acids in colonic mucosa also may represent an important intracellular event by which bile acids provoke a proliferative response. Bile acids may, in addition, induce release of arachidonate and conversion of arachidonic acid to prostaglandins in the mucosa, which may enhance cell proliferation.[12] Preclinical and clinical evidence indicate that nonsteroidal anti-inflammatory drugs (NSAIDs), which reduce prostaglandin synthesis, reduce the incidence of large bowel cancer (discussed later).[13,14] Inhibition of the inducible enzyme cyclooxygenase (COX)-2 may be particularly important in this regard.[15,16] Certain fatty acids could promote carcinogenesis by altering membrane fluidity after being incorporated into cell membranes. Bacterial enzymes such as 7-α-dehydroxylase (which converts cholic to deoxycholic acid), β-glucuronidase, nitroreductase, and azoreductase may be induced by a high-fat diet and also could convert compounds ingested in the diet to active carcinogens (see later).

An inverse relationship has been reported between physical activity and risk for CRC in men, whereas obesity is associated with elevated risk.[17] Serum cholesterol and β-lipoprotein levels have been positively correlated with the development of colorectal adenomas and carcinomas, but this association has not been demonstrated consistently, and serum cholesterol levels may decline before the development of colon cancer.

FIBER

Epidemiologic, case-control, and animal studies suggest that dietary fiber protects against the development of colon cancer. Dietary fiber is plant material that resists digestion and that is composed of a heterogeneous mix of carbohydrates (cellulose, hemicellulose, pectin) and noncarbohydrates (e.g., lignin). Although the protective role of fiber is not completely clear (owing to the lack of definition of fiber components in some studies), epidemiologic studies correlate high-fiber intake with a lower incidence of colorectal neoplasia.[18,19] The majority of both observational-epidemiologic and case-control studies support the protective effect of fiber-rich diets; however, these data do not define the relationship between fiber-rich food and the importance of nonfiber vegetable components, nutrients, and micronutrients in fruits and vegetables. The effect of fiber components on different portions of the large bowel also may vary. This may explain, in part, the inability to demonstrate a protective effect of fiber in several randomized, controlled trials that have examined the ability of fiber supplementation to prevent adenoma recurrence.[20,21]

Investigators postulate that fibers such as cereal bran exert their protective role by increasing stool bulk, thereby diluting carcinogens and promoters of carcinogenesis, enhancing their elimination, and minimizing their duration of mucosal contact by decreasing intestinal transit time. Increased fiber intake, in the form of whole wheat and rye bread, also reduces the concentration of fecal secondary bile acids and fecal mutagens in healthy subjects. Animal studies also have demonstrated a decreased incidence of colonic tumors in DMH-treated rats fed diets high in fiber and fiber components (wheat bran, cellulose, hemicellulose). Cellulose and hemicellulose decrease the levels of bacterial metabolic enzymes such as β-glucuronidase in experimental animals and may diminish the activation of carcinogens or cocarcinogens. Furthermore, some fiber components may bind to toxic or carcinogenic substances, perhaps decreasing their contact with the colonic mucosa. Fiber components also are fermented by fecal flora to short-chain fatty acids, thereby decreasing colonic pH and potentially inhibiting carcinogenesis.

CARCINOGENS AND FECAL MUTAGENS, VITAMINS, AND MICRONUTRIENTS

The possibility that specific genotoxic carcinogens may play a role in the genesis of CRC was raised when it was noted that the stools of certain persons exhibited mutagenic activity for bacteria in vitro. Mutagenic activity frequently is present in the feces of populations at high risk for large bowel cancer and is low or absent in low-risk populations. A specific group of highly unsaturated reactive compounds synthesized by colonic bacteria, fecapentaenes, may play a role in large bowel carcinogenesis. It also has been recognized that "charbroiled" meat and fish, and to a lesser extent fried foods, contain powerful mutagenic compounds. The structures of these compounds resemble a heterocyclic amine known to cause colon cancer in rodents. Metabolites similar to those of fried meat and fish are being sought as mutagens in human stools. A possible association between rectal cancer and beer and ale drinking also has been noted.[22] A twofold to threefold increase in CRC also has been observed in pattern and model makers in the automobile industry, but the specific carcinogenic agent has not yet been identified.

The exact nature of genotoxic carcinogens that may act in the human colon remains speculative, but the identification of such compounds could provide a basis for intervention and primary prevention of CRC. Limited data suggest that foods rich in carotene (vitamin A) and vitamin C could act as antioxidants in the chemoprevention of colon cancer, but prospective trials have failed to demonstrate such an effect. Other areas that merit further exploration in the prevention of CRC include the role of yellow-green cruciferous vegetables and micronutrients, including selenium salts, vitamin E, and folic acid. Recently, a good deal of attention has been given to a possible role for dietary calcium in colon cancer prevention (discussed later).

CALCIUM AND VITAMIN D

Epidemiologic, clinical, and laboratory evidence suggest that calcium intake may protect against carcinogenesis in the colon. The potential chemopreventive activity of calcium was suggested originally by epidemiologic studies reporting an inverse relationship between intake of vitamin D and calcium and CRC.[23] One study demonstrated that dietary calcium supplementation in the form of low-fat dairy foods may affect a variety of "intermediate biomarkers" thought to be associated with tumor progression in the colon.[24] The relationship between calcium intake and a lower incidence of colonic adenomas and carcinomas has not, however, uniformly been demonstrated. These conflicting findings may have arisen because of the difficulties inherent in dietary assessment and differences in intake of potentially confounding factors, including dietary components and putative chemopreventive agents.

Further credence to the beneficial effect of calcium in preventing large bowel cancer comes from numerous animal studies. Abnormal proliferation occurs in both neoplastic and preneoplastic lesions in the colon. The increase in colonocyte proliferation stimulated by intrarectal instillation of deoxycholate and free fatty acids or by dietary supplementation with cholic acid may be ameliorated by oral calcium supplementation in laboratory animals. Studies in rodents fed high-fat diets also demonstrate a reduction in the number of carcinogen-induced tumors in animals receiving supplemental calcium in their diet. This reduction may be true especially for tumors containing *K-ras* mutations, a finding also suggested by a recent study in humans. Ornithine decarboxylase, an enzyme involved in polyamine biosynthesis and elevated in preneoplastic states, is reduced in rat colonic mucosa incubated with calcium in vitro, and supplemental calcium suppresses elevated levels of this enzyme in the mucosa of elderly patients with adenomatous polyps.

It has been suggested that dietary calcium binds to ionized fatty acids and bile acids in the intestine, converting them to insoluble calcium compounds incapable of stimulating epithelial proliferation. Calcium increases fecal excretion of both phosphate and bile acids and modifies relative amounts of bile acids in bile.[25] In addition, calcium in milk products is capable of precipitating luminal cytotoxic surfactants, thereby inhibiting their effects on colonic mucosa. These potential beneficial effects of calcium have not been observed uniformly, however, and studies of the effects of calcium on the rectal mucosa have not always demonstrated a reduction in the proliferation rates. In other studies, calcium supplementation normalized the distribution of proliferating cells in the colonic crypt without affecting the rate of proliferation in the colorectal mucosa.

Vitamin D_3 metabolites and analogs have been shown to play an important role in the regulation of a number of important cellular processes, including proliferation, differentiation, and apoptosis, in addition to their established role in mineral homeostasis. These steroid compounds have rapid effects that do not involve gene transcription or protein synthesis, as well as genomic effects involving the vitamin D receptor and other transcription factors.[26] Effects of vitamin D and its metabolites have been demonstrated in normal and malignant colonocytes, and several potential mechanisms have been suggested by which these compounds might prevent carcinogenesis in the colon.

ARACHIDONIC ACID, EICOSANOIDS, AND CYCLOOXYGENASE-2

Clinical case-control and cohort studies have shown a 40% to 50% reduction in CRC-related mortality in individuals taking aspirin and other NSAIDs on a regular basis compared with those not taking these agents. The exact mechanism for cancer protection with these agents is unknown but may relate to altered synthesis of arachidonic acid metabolites (eicosanoids) that include prostaglandins, thromboxanes, leukotrienes, and hydroxy-eicosatetraenoic acids. These compounds modulate a number of signal transduction pathways that may affect cellular adhesion, growth, and differentiation.[16] COX (or prostaglandin-endoperoxide synthase) oxidizes arachidonic acid to prostaglandin G_2, reduces prostaglandin G_2 to prostaglandin H_2, and is the key enzyme responsible for production of prostaglandins and other eicosanoids.

This enzyme exists in two isoforms: COX-1 and COX-2. COX-1, the constitutive form of the enzyme, is present in most tissues and is involved in the physiologic production of prostaglandins to maintain normal homeostasis. COX-2 is induced by cytokines, mitogens, and growth factors, and its level has been shown to be elevated in both murine and human CRCs.[17,27-30] Expression of COX-2 is increased markedly in 85% to 95% of CRCs[27] and in experimental models of CRC. COX-2 inhibition prevents cancer development during both the initiation and promotion/progression stages of carcinogenesis.[31] Knockout of COX-2 results in suppression of intestinal polyposis in animal models of familial adenomatous polyposis (FAP).[17,29] It has been speculated that NSAIDs may reduce colon tumor formation through inhibition of prostaglandin-mediated proliferation, however, other evidence suggests that part of their effect may result from induction of programmed cell death or apoptosis. Overexpression of COX-2 has been demonstrated to decrease apoptosis, whereas COX-2 inhibition leads to an increase in apoptosis.[32]

One potential mechanism by which NSAIDs may induce apoptosis is through elevation of the prostaglandin precursor arachidonic acid. Increases in arachidonic acid after NSAID inhibition of COX stimulate conversion of sphingomyelin to ceramide, a mediator of apoptosis. NSAIDs also may inhibit the activation of genes by the nuclear hormone receptor peroxisome-proliferator-activated receptor δ (PPARδ) by disrupting the ability of this receptor to bind DNA.[33] PPARδ expression is elevated in CRCs and repressed by the APC gene product which is altered in CRC cells. The inhibition of PPARδ function enhances the ability of NSAIDs to induce apoptosis in colon cancer cells. PPARδ activates a variety of genes, including those involved in cellular growth and differentiation after exposure to a variety of ligands, such as eicosanoids. COX-2 inhibition could prevent production of these ligands and therefore prevent activation of PPARδ.

Other potential mechanisms by which COX-2 inhibition may affect tumor formation include alterations of cell adhesion to extracellular matrix proteins,[32] inhibition of tumor neovascularization (angiogenesis),[30] and reduction in carcinogen activation. A study[30] using the ApcΔ716 mouse, an animal model of FAP, demonstrated that treatment with the COX-2 specific inhibitor rofecoxib (Vioxx) was associated with a significant dose-dependent reduction in polyp number and size, as well as alterations in polyp morphology. COX-2 inhibition was associated with decreased levels of vascular endothelial growth factor (VEGF), and with lower rates of DNA replication.

In summary, environment and diet may affect the genesis of CRC, but their exact roles remain unclear. Their complex nature renders definition of the influence of individual environmental and dietary components difficult.

CHEMOPREVENTION

Chemoprevention (see Chapter 119) refers to the use of natural or synthetic agents to reverse, suppress, or prevent progression or recurrence of cancer.[34,35] This is a cornerstone of "primary prevention." Data on chemoprevention of CRC come from studies in laboratory animals (see earlier), observational epidemiologic studies, case-control studies, and randomized trials. Because the

natural history of CRC is protracted, clinical randomized trials often have concentrated on prevention of colorectal adenomas, which represent a form of intraepithelial neoplasia and are the precursors to carcinoma. The duration of the studies required, sample sizes necessary, cost, and ethical considerations make the use of cancer as an end point impractical.

This difficulty has led to an increasing use of surrogate "biomarkers" to study chemoprevention of CRCs. The hope is that use of such markers will lead to shorter, smaller, and less expensive trials.[35] To be valid, however, such biomarkers need to represent accurately the events involved in the process of carcinogenesis. When an intervention such as a chemopreventive agent is tested, there should be a clear relationship among the agent, modulation of the biomarker, and the development of cancer. Surrogate end points for cancer ideally should be validated in the context of clinical studies that use cancer as the ultimate end point. This is a difficult task because these are the very trials that such markers are designed to complement or replace.

There has been recent interest in the use of magnifying endoscopy to study aberrant crypt foci of the colon as possible markers in chemoprevention trials.[35] These foci consist of large, thick crypts that can be detected by chromoendoscopy using agents such as methylene blue (Fig. 120–4). Aberrant crypt foci, particularly those that are large and have dysplastic features, are thought to be precursors of adenomas in the colon. Standardization of techniques to identify and quantify these lesions is crucial to the successful interpretation of data from these trials.

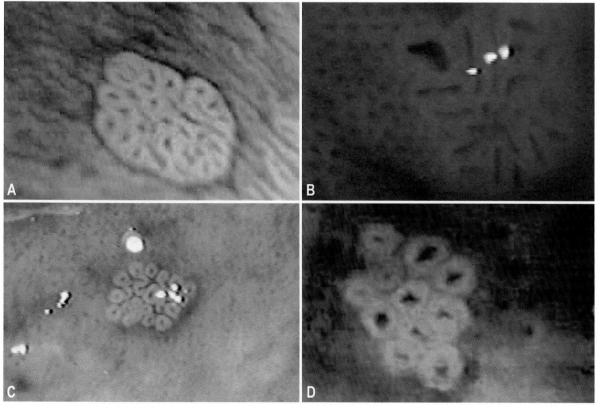

Figure 120–4   Four magnification colonoscopic views (*A-D*) of aberrant crypt foci. Aberrant crypt foci consist of large thick crypts, and are thought to be precursors of adenomas in the colon.

The potential benefit of low-fat, high-fiber diets based on descriptive epidemiology and case-control studies already has been discussed, but current data from prospective human trials are thus far equivocal or negative. Two large randomized trials examined the effects of fiber supplementation on adenoma recurrence. The Polyp Prevention Trial[21] randomized 2079 subjects with a history of colorectal adenomas to receive counseling together with a low-fat, high-fiber diet rich in fruits and vegetables or to receive their usual diet alone. The incidence of recurrent adenomas at 1 and 4 years, as determined by colonoscopy, was similar in both groups. In a study conducted by the Phoenix Colon Cancer Prevention Physician's Network,[20] 1429 patients with a history of colorectal adenoma were randomized to receive 2.0 g or 13.5 g of supplemental wheat bran per day. Colonoscopy failed to show a difference in the incidence of recurrent adenomas at a median follow-up of 34 to 36 months.

A large body of observational and laboratory studies suggests a role for dietary calcium supplementation in chemoprevention (mentioned earlier). A prospective double-blind placebo-controlled trial showed that supplemental calcium (3000 mg of calcium carbonate per day, equivalent to 1200 mg of elemental calcium) reduced the incidence and number of recurrent adenomas in subjects chosen for a recent history of such lesions.[36] The effect of calcium was modest: 19% reduction in adenoma recurrence and 24% reduction in the number of adenomas over 3 years, independent of age, sex, or dietary intake of calcium fat or fiber. Human trials using antioxidant vitamins A, C, and E have provided equivocal results, and current data do not support their routine use for colon cancer prevention in average-risk individuals.[37]

Folic acid and its metabolites play an important role in DNA synthesis, strand integrity, and methylation. Epidemiologic studies have found a lower incidence of CRC among those with high compared with low dietary folate intakes.[22,38,39] This protective effect also was suggested by the Nurse's Health Study,[38] in which high doses of folate (as part of multivitamin supplementation) given over several years were protective against CRC. A prospective randomized trial[40] failed, however, to demonstrate a protective effect of 1 mg/day of folate supplementation on adenoma recurrence when compared with placebo.

Epidemiologic, case-control, and prospective cohort trials suggest a protective effect against the development of CRC in women taking hormone (estrogen) replacement therapy.[41] It has been postulated that estrogen may protect against colon cancer development by decreasing production of secondary bile acids, by decreasing levels of insulin-like growth factor-1, or through as yet undetermined direct effects on colonic mucosal epithelial cells.

The most promising results come from trials using aspirin and NSAIDs for CRC prevention. Case-control and cohort studies have suggested that the risk for development of adenoma and carcinoma may be reduced substantially (40% to 50%) among aspirin and NSAID users, compared with controls.[14,15,35] A prospective cohort study among male health professionals[14] demonstrated that persons who take aspirin more than twice per week were at lower risk for CRC (relative risk, 0.68) than were controls, after accounting for a variety of potentially confounding factors. A randomized trial that assessed the effect of low-dose aspirin in an average-risk population demonstrated no significant reduction in the number of CRC cases during the first 6 years of follow- up[42]; longer follow-up may be necessary to demonstrate a significant aspirin effect on cancer development, because the Nurses' Health Study demonstrated that the benefits of aspirin may not be evident until after at least a decade of regular aspirin consumption.[15] Three prospective adenoma prevention trials (see later) now provide compelling evidence that aspirin use reduces the risk of colorectal adenoma development in individuals with a personal history of adenoma or carcinoma.[43-45]

Given the long natural history of CRC, prevention of adenoma recurrence after endoscopic removal often is used as an intermediate or surrogate end-point in chemoprevention trials.[35] In FAP, in which hundreds of adenomas occur in the colon and rectum, chemoprevention trials often use reductions of the number and size of adenomas as end points in short-term studies. Such trials have suggested a potential role for NSAIDs as chemopreventive agents in this setting. There is a significant decrease in the mean number and size of polyps in patients treated with the NSAID sulindac. In a small, randomized, double-blind, placebo-controlled trial of 22 patients with FAP, treatment with sulindac significantly reduced the number of colorectal polyps and their mean diameter during 9 months of treatment.[46] After 9 months of treatment, the number and diameter of polyps had decreased to 44% and 35% of respective baseline values. Three months after treatment was stopped, however, both the number and size of polyps had increased. A subsequent prospective cohort study[47] confirmed that long-term use of sulindac is effective in reducing the number of adenomas in patients with FAP. A 76% reduction in polyp number was seen at 1 year and was sustained (74% reduction) through 63 months of follow-up. Sulindac may not be effective, however, for primary prevention of adenoma development in genetically disposed individuals with FAP who have not yet developed macroscopic adenomas.[48]

A double-blind, placebo-controlled trial studied the effects of celecoxib (Celebrex), a selective COX-2 inhibitor, on colorectal polyps in patients with FAP.[49] Treatment with high doses of celecoxib for 6 months was associated with a significant reduction (28%) in the number of colorectal polyps compared with placebo (4.5%). This drug is now approved in the United States as an adjunct to standard therapy in patients with FAP.

It is unclear what the role of nonselective NSAIDs and COX-2 inhibitors will be in patients with sporadic adenomas and carcinomas. Trials are ongoing to determine their usefulness in preventing adenoma recurrence in this population. A randomized trial of aspirin versus placebo[44] demonstrated that daily use of 81 mg of aspirin was associated with a 19% reduction in adenoma occurrence and a 41% reduction in occurrence of advanced neoplasms (adenomas measuring at least 1 cm or with tubulovillous or villous features, severe dysplasia, or invasive cancer) compared with results of placebo treatment 3 years after removal of an index sporadic adenoma. A prospective, randomized trial in a higher risk group for adenoma recurrence, those with a previous history of sporadic CRC, demonstrated a 45% risk reduction in those taking 325 mg of aspirin daily compared with those taking placebo with a mean follow-up of almost 3 years.[43] Preliminary data from a randomized trial of the COX-2 inhibitor rofecoxib to prevent sporadic colorectal adenomas (the Adenomatous Polyp Prevention on Vioxx [APPROVe] trial)[50] suggest a significant reduction in adenoma recurrence at 1 and 3 years compared with placebo in subjects taking 25 mg of rofecoxib daily. This trial also demonstrated an increase in rofecoxib-associated cardiovascular adverse events beginning at 18 months. It is not clear whether the cardiovascular effects associated with rofecoxib in this trial are specific to this agent or represent an effect associated with use of COX-2 inhibitors in general. At least one study suggests that an increased cardiovascular risk is associated with celecoxib.

Other agents currently undergoing study for chemoprevention of colorectal neoplasia include the ornithine decarboxylase inhibitor difluoromethylornithine, the bile acid ursodiol, the 3-hydroxy-3-methylglutaryl-coenzyme A (HMG-CoA) reductase inhibitors such as pravastatin and lovastatin, epidermal growth factor receptor (EGFR) inhibitors, and matrix metalloproteinase (MMP) inhibitors.[35] Table 120–2 summarizes the status of current studies that examine the effect of chemopreventive agents on colorectal neoplasia.

Observational studies from around the world that compare different populations continue to find the risk of CRC to be lower among populations with high intakes of fruits and vegetables, as well as some vitamins and micronutrients. Migration studies strongly suggest an influence of diet and environmental influences on the incidence of CRC. It has been difficult to demonstrate similar effects in randomized, controlled chemoprevention trials. These trials ask narrowly defined questions and cannot easily assess complex interactions between dietary components or measure the effects of long-term alterations in dietary patterns on cancer per se. Nonetheless, these trials have provided exciting new data that may lead to primary prevention of CRC in the future.

BIOLOGY OF COLORECTAL CANCER

Current concepts concerning environmental causes for CRC have been discussed in the preceding sections. It has been suggested that carcinogens introduced into the bowel act in concert with other luminal factors (e.g., bile acid and other tumor promoters) to affect epithelial cells in the colonic mucosa; however, carcinogenesis is a multistage process. Cells must be genetically primed (through either hereditary disposition or genotoxic events) and induced to proliferate, after which they must pass through a series of stages en route to immortalization and uncontrolled growth. Our knowledge of this sequence of events in the colon, although fragmentary, is growing rapidly (see Chapter 3).

ABNORMAL CELLULAR PROLIFERATION

Abnormal cellular proliferation is a hallmark of neoplasia (see Chapter 3). Actively proliferating cells are more susceptible to initiators of carcinogenesis (primary carcinogens) and genetic alterations than are resting cells. In the normal colon, DNA synthesis occurs and cells divide and proliferate only in the lower and middle regions of the crypts. As cells normally migrate "upward" from deeper in the crypt, the number of cells that continue to proliferate decreases, and, on reaching the upper crypt region, they become terminally differentiated and can no longer divide. A substantial body of literature indicates that this sequence of events is disordered during the evolution of neoplastic lesions in the colon. Increased proliferative activity and characteristic differences in the distribution of triitiated thymidine–labeled cells (i.e., those that actively synthesize DNA) within the colonic crypts have been demonstrated and distinguish both "at risk" and affected members of kindreds with familial polyposis, as well as "nonpolyposis"-inherited colon cancer from lower risk groups. Correlations between rectal mucosal proliferation and the clinical and pathologic features of nonfamilial colorectal neoplasia also have been demonstrated. Conversely, populations at low risk of developing colon cancer, such as Seventh Day

Table 120–2 Efficacy of Chemoprotective Agents for Colorectal Neoplasia*

| | Observational Studies of Colon Cancer Incidence | | | Randomized Human Trials | | |
| | | | | Reduction in Mucosal Proliferation | Reduction in the Number of Polyps in Patients with FAP | Reduction in Number of Sporadic Adenomas |
Agent	Animal Studies	Case Control	Cohort Studies			
Aspirin/NSAID	+	+	+	NA	+	+
COX-2 inhibitors	+	NA	NA	+	+	⧖
Vitamins A, C, E	+	+	+	+	~	~
Calcium	+	+	+	~	NA	+
Fiber	+	+	+	+	~	–
Selenium	+	+	~	NA	–	NA
Fish oil	NA	+	NA	NA	+	NA
Organosulfur	+	NA	NA	NA	NA	NA

*The strength of evidence in the studies ranges from weak to strong as displayed from left to right in the table headings.
+, Most studies are positive for efficacy; –, most studies are negative for efficacy; ~, studies are equivocal for efficacy; ⧖, studies are ongoing.
COX, cyclooxygenase; FAP, familial adenomatous polyposis; NA, not available; NSAID, nonsteroidal anti-inflammatory drug.

Adventist vegetarians, have relatively quiescent proliferative activity in their colonic mucosa.

Disordered proliferative activity can be found in the colonic mucosa of rodents treated with a variety of chemical carcinogens, and increased proliferative activity is seen in animals whose colonic or rectal mucosa is exposed to tumor promoters such as secondary bile acids. Colonic epithelial cells also fail to repress DNA synthesis during epithelial renewal in ulcerative colitis (UC), a condition associated with an increased risk of CRC. Ornithine decarboxylase, an enzyme marker of rapid cellular proliferation, is present at high levels in the mucosa of members of familial polyposis kindreds, and levels increase in the colonic mucosa during chemically induced colonic carcinogenesis in rats. Ornithine decarboxylase increases in the colonic mucosa with age and is elevated in elderly patients with colonic adenomas. Experimental evidence also suggests that protein kinase C may be involved in the stimulation of colonic epithelial cell proliferation by tumor promoters. These findings have led to speculation that inhibitors of cellular proliferation may prove useful as anticancer drugs. NSAIDs and COX-2 inhibitors, for example, decrease proliferation and increase programmed cell death or apoptosis.[16,32]

A recent explosion of knowledge in the field of molecular genetics has demonstrated how alterations in proto-oncogenes and tumor suppressor genes may lead to disruption of mechanisms that regulate the normal cell cycle and cell proliferation. In some cases the cell is predisposed to abnormal proliferation by virtue of germline mutations (e.g., FAP). In other cases, somatic mutations occur as the result of complex interactions with environmental factors,[51] as detailed earlier.

MOLECULAR BIOLOGY AND BIOCHEMICAL CHANGES

Molecular Genetics

Tumor cells in the colon, as elsewhere, are characterized by heritable phenotypic changes that are the result of quantitative or qualitative alterations in gene expression (see Chapters 3 and 119). A large body of evidence demonstrates that CRCs are associated with an accumulation of such genetic alterations (Table 120–3; Fig. 120–5). Genetic changes that may lead to the development of CRC can be categorized into three major classes: alterations in proto-oncogenes, loss of tumor suppressor gene activity, and abnormalities in genes involved in DNA mismatch repair (MMR).[52,53] Adenomas and carcinomas arise in the context of genomic instability, by which epithelial cells acquire the number of mutations needed to attain a neoplastic state. Destabilization of the genome is a prerequisite to tumor formation and most

Table 120–3   Genes Altered in Sporadic Colorectal Cancer

Gene	Chromosome	Percentage of Tumors with Gene Alterations	Gene Class	Gene Function
K-ras	12	50	Proto-oncogene	Encodes guanine nucleotide-binding protein that regulates intracellular signaling
APC	5	70	Tumor suppressor	Regulation of β-catenin that is involved in activation of WnT/TcF signaling (activates c-myc, cyclin D$_1$)*; regulation of proliferation and apoptosis; interaction with E-cadherin (cell adhesion?)
DCC	18	70	Tumor suppressor?	Netrin-1 receptor; caspase substrate in apoptosis; cell adhesion
SMAD4 (DPC4, MADH4)	18	?	Tumor suppressor	Nuclear transcriptase factor in transforming growth factor (TGF-β1) signaling; regulation of angiogenesis; regulator of WAF1 promoter; downstream mediator of SMAD2
p53	17	75	Tumor suppressor	Transcription factor; regulator of cell cycle progression after cellular stress, of apoptosis, of gene expression, and of DNA repair
hMSH2	2	†	DNA mismatch repair	Maintains fidelity of DNA replication
hMLH1	3	†	DNA mismatch repair	Maintains fidelity of DNA replication
hMSH6	2	†	DNA mismatch repair	Maintains fidelity of DNA replication
TGF-β1 RII	3	‡	Tumor suppressor	Receptor for signaling in the TGF-β1 pathway; inhibitor of colonic epithelial proliferation, often mutated in tumors with MSI

*β-Catenin mutations (downstream of APC) are found in 16-25% of MSI colon cancers but not in microsatellite stable (MSS) cancers.
†Approximately 15% of sporadic colorectal cancers demonstrate MSI associated with alterations in mismatch repair genes (principally hMSH2 and hMLH1 but also hMSH3, hMSH6, hPMS1, and hPMS2).
‡Mutated in 73-90% of MSI colon cancers. Up to 55% of MSS colon cancer cell lines may demonstrate a TGF-β signaling blockage distal to TGF-β1 RII.
MSI, microsatellite instability; TGF-β, transforming growth factor-β.

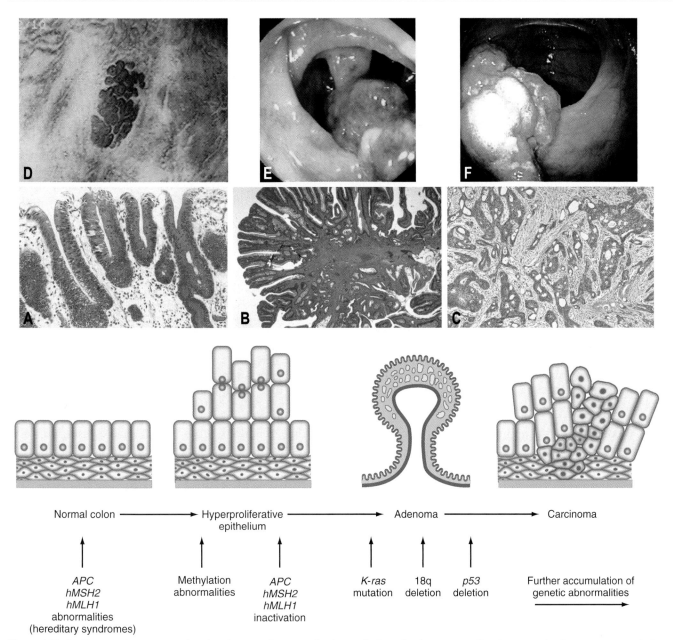

Figure 120–5 Proposed sequence of molecular genetic events in the evolution of colon cancer. Carcinomas arise from an accumulation of events the sequence of which has been defined. Alterations in *APC* or DNA mismatch repair genes may be inherited in the germline (FAP, HNPCC) or may be acquired after birth (somatic mutations). *Upper,* The *bottom row (A-C),* shows the histology and the *top row (D-F)* shows colonoscopic photographs. From left to right: Dysplastic aberrant crypt focus (*A* and *D,* with methylene blue staining); adenomatous polyp (*B* and *E*); and invasive carcinoma (*C* and *F*). HPNCC, hereditary monpolyposis colorectal cancer; FAP, familial adenomatous polyposis. (Aberrant crypt focus [*A* and *D*] reproduced from Takayama T. Katsucki S, Takahashi Y, et al: Aberrant crypt foci of the colon as precursors of adenoma and cancer. N Engl J Med 339:1277, 1998.)

commonly involves chromosomal instability with subsequent allelic loss, chromosomal amplifications and translocations, or increased rates of intragenic mutation in tandemly repeated DNA sequences known as microsatellites (microsatellite instability [MSI]).

Cellular proto-oncogenes are evolutionarily conserved human genes that contain DNA sequences homologous to those of acute transforming retroviruses. Many of these genes play a role in signal transduction and the normal regulation of cell growth. Inappropriate activation of these genes leads to abnormal transmission of regulatory messages from the cell surface to the nucleus that results in abnormal proliferation and, eventually, tumor formation. Three human *ras* genes—*K-ras, N-ras,* and *H-ras*—

encode guanine nucleotide-binding proteins that regulate intracellular signaling pathways. Approximately 65% of sporadic colorectal carcinomas have activating point mutations in a *ras* gene, most in *K-ras*. Most *ras* mutations appear to occur during intermediate stages of adenoma growth (see Chapter 119). *Ras* gene mutations occur in 47% of carcinomas, in 58% of adenomas larger than 1 cm, but in only 10% of adenomas smaller than 1 cm, suggesting that earlier events must contribute to neoplasia formation. Alterations in signal transduction may lead to abnormal cell growth and thus participate in neoplastic transformation, but activation of *ras* alone is not sufficient for progression to carcinoma. The exact functional relationship between *ras* mutations and carcinogenesis remains to be established, but understanding its role in stimulating proliferation may lead to the development of antitumor therapies aimed at interrupting signals that alter tumor cell growth.

Chromosomal abnormalities have been reported in CRCs for more than a decade, and abundant evidence has shown that allelic losses, particularly at chromosome locations 5q, 17p, and 18q, play major roles in the genesis of large bowel tumors.[52-57] A deletion within chromosome 5 in patients with FAP led to the identification of the *APC* gene on the long arm of this chromosome (5q21). Positional cloning identified a single tumor suppressor gene, which is mutated in both the germline of FAP patients and in sporadic colorectal tumors. The protein encoded by *APC* consists of 2843 amino acids. It is located at the basolateral membrane in colorectal epithelial cells, with expression that is increasingly pronounced as cells migrate up through the colonic crypt.

Somatic mutations of the *APC* gene occur in 60% to 80% of sporadic CRCs and adenomas, including the smallest dysplastic lesions. These mutations result in truncation of the APC protein in more than 98% of cases, a finding that has led to the development of clinically useful tests for genetic screening of FAP families.[58] Inactivation of both copies of the *APC* gene appears to be the "gatekeeping" event for the initiation of colorectal neoplasia. The *APC* gene product interacts with at least six other proteins, including glycogen synthetase 3-β (GSK-3β) and axin in the cytoplasm. Inactivation of this gene is required for net cellular proliferation and initiation of neoplasia in the colon.

APC functions to modulate extracellular signals that are transmitted to the nucleus through the cytoskeletal protein β-catenin as part of the Wnt signaling pathway (Fig. 120–6). Nuclear β-catenin binds to transcription factors in the nucleus that are members of the lymphoid enhancer factor-T cell factor (LEF/TCF) family including Tcf-4, which in turn activate various target genes (e.g., *c-myc*, cyclin D$_1$)[59] that affect cell cycling and growth. *APC* is a tumor suppressor gene that binds to β-catenin and causes its degradation through phosphorylation. Loss of *APC* function, therefore, leads to accumulation of β-catenin and unopposed stimulation through the Wnt-Tcf signaling pathway. This in turn leads to increased and unregulated proliferation and decreased programmed cell death (apoptosis). *APC* gene abnormalities also may lead to disruption of normal cell-cell adhesion through altered association with the cellular adhesion molecule E-cadherin. Disruption of *APC*-mediated regulation of transcriptional activation is critical for colorectal tumorigenesis and is achieved most commonly through inactivating mutations of both *APC* alleles; disruption also can occur through dominant mutations of the β-catenin gene that render β-catenin-Tcf-regulated transcription insensitive to the regulatory effects of normal wild-type *APC*.

Other genetic changes occur later in the adenoma-to-carcinoma sequence. Stepwise tumor progression is associated in more than 75% of cases with loss of the tumor suppressor gene activity located on chromosome 18q.

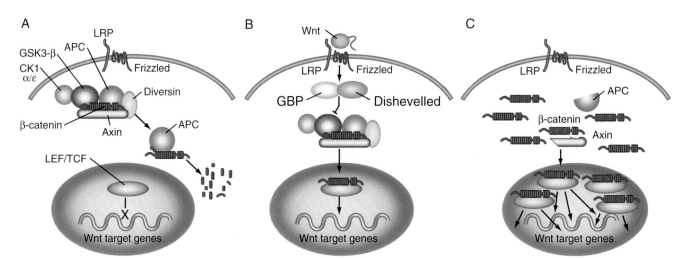

Figure 120–6 A model of Wnt signaling in normal and cancer cells. *A*, In the absence of Wnt signaling, APC, axin, and GSK3-β form a complex that results in β-catenin phosphorylation and degradation by a ubiquitin-dependent mechanism. *B*, Binding of Wnt to its cell surface receptor results in stabilization of β-catenin. Unphosphorylated β-catenin is able to translocate to the nucleus to form a complex with members of the LEF/TCF family and activates Wnt target genes. Frizzled and Dishevelled refer to gene products which participate in this pathway. *C*, Loss of or mutation of *APC* results in lack of β-catenin degradation and high levels of this protein in the cytoplasm and nucleus. Strong evidence exists that misregulation of Wnt target gene expression is crucial to transformation in colon cells. (From Waterman ML: Lymphoid enhancer factor/T cell factor expression in colorectal cancer. Cancer Metast Rev 23:41, 2004.)

Several candidate genes are present on this chromosome, and loss of chromosome 18 is associated with a poor prognosis.[60] One gene, designated *DCC* (deleted in CRC), originally was thought to be important because its loss from a stage II (Dukes B) cancer was associated in some studies with a worse prognosis; its role as an important tumor suppressor gene has been questioned.[55] *DPC4* (*SMAD4*) is another candidate tumor suppressor gene whose inactivation may play a role in development of CRC. *DPC4* belongs to the *SMAD* gene family involved in signal transduction pathways activated through the transforming growth factor (TGF)-β family receptors. Experimental inactivation of the mouse homologue *Dpc4* in a mouse model of adenomatous polyposis coli results in malignant progression of intestinal and colonic polyps initiated by loss of the *Apc* gene (the mouse homologue of *APC*).[61] Mutations in *SMAD4* and a related gene, *SMAD2*, have been reported in some sporadic CRCs.[62] Deletions of chromosome 17p involve the *p53* tumor suppressor gene, whose product normally prevents cells with damaged DNA from progressing from the G1 to the S phase in the cell cycle. Deletions within chromosome 17p are present in approximately 75% of CRCs. Loss of *p53* also may be associated with reduced apoptosis of damaged cells. Inactivation of the *p53* gene mediates the conversion from adenoma to carcinoma, a late and important event in colon carcinogenesis. Distant metastases from CRCs are associated with high fractional allelic loss and deletions of 17p and 18q. A distinct set of "metastasis suppressor genes" also has been postulated.[63]

Genomic instability creates a permissive state in which a cell acquires enough mutations to be transformed to a cancer cell. This is a common mechanism central to the development of most, if not all, colon cancers.[53] Several forms of genomic instability are common in colon cancer, including chromosome instability (CIN) and chromosome translocations; and MSI in which subtle sequence changes, including base substitutions, deletions, or insertions, lead to a hypermutable state (Fig. 120-7). Candidates responsible for CIN include genes responsible for the human mitotic checkpoint *hBUB1* and *hBUBR1*, genes involved in the DNA damage checkpoint *ATM*, *BRCA1* and *BRCA2*, *p53*, and *hRad17*, and genes that control centrosome number.

The significance of genomic instability in the pathogenesis of a subset of colon cancers became evident with the discovery of MSI in colon cancers associated with hereditary nonpolyposis colorectal cancer (HNPCC). Alterations in genes that help maintain DNA fidelity during replication are characteristic of patients with HNPCC.[53,64] Alterations in MMR genes designated *hMLH1*, *hPMS1*, *hPMS2*, *hMSH2*, *hMSH3*, and *hMSH6* may lead to the inability to repair base pair mismatches and result in DNA replication errors or MSI. Inactivation of the MMR system causes genomic instability by increasing the rate of polymerase-generated replication errors and degrading the fidelity of DNA replication, particularly at microsatellite repeat sequences.[53] MSI involves mutations or instability in short, tandemly repeated DNA sequences such as $(A)^n$, $(CA)^n$, and $(GATA)^n$. Such DNA sequences are found in several key genes that are important for maintaining normal cellular function (Table 120-4). The receptor for TGF-βRII, for example, often is mutated as the result of MSI.

Figure 120-7 Model of colon cancer formation in tumors that progress through the adenoma-to-carcinoma sequence along pathways marked by chromosomal instability (CIN) or microsatellite instability. ACF, aberrant crypt focus; MMR, mismatch repair; TGF, transforming growth factor. (From Grady WM: Genomic instability and colon cancer. Cancer Metast Rev 23:11, 2004.)

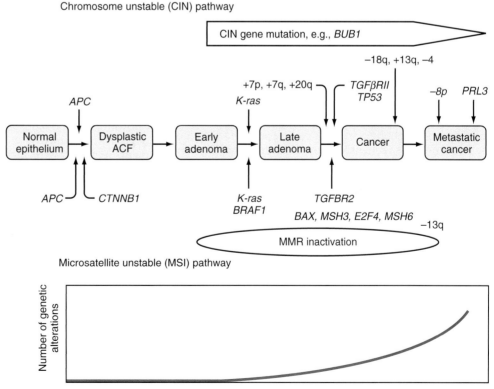

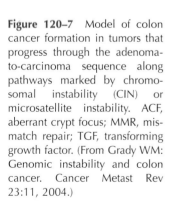

Table 120–4 Target Gene Mutations and Microsatellite Instability (MSI)

Target Gene	Frequency in Colon Cancers with MSI, %
TGF-β RII	73-90
BAX	41-52
Caspase 5	62
MSH 3	46-71
MSH 6	28-33
β-Catenin	16-25
IGFIIR	6-8
APC	70
E2F4	65

Most mutations cause frame shifts that prematurely truncate the protein, leading to inactivation of the affected allele.
Modified from Grady WM, Markowitz S: Genomic instability and colorectal cancer. Curr Opin Gastroenterol 16:62, 2000.

Multiple lines of evidence suggest that the TGF-β pathway is an important tumor-suppressing pathway in the colon and that alterations in this pathway lead to tumor development. Less frequently targeted genes include the insulin growth factor 2 receptor; Bax and caspase 5, proteins that regulate apoptosis; E2F4, a transcription factor; and MSH3 and MSH6, DNA MMR proteins. β-Catenin mutations are present in up to 25% of MSI colon cancers. MSI therefore leads to accumulation of mutations in vulnerable genes, eventually resulting in the acquisition of the malignant phenotype. Although a high frequency of MSI (instability at ≥40% of microsatellite loci) is characteristic of HNPCC, similar alterations can be found in about 15% of sporadic CRCs and also in premalignant lesions. MSI tumors remain diploid. Patients whose tumors demonstrate MSI may have a better prognosis[65] and respond differently to chemotherapy[66,67] than those whose tumors are characterized by chromosomal instability. Most patients with MSI colon cancers do not possess mutations in the known MMR genes; evidence indicates that MSI in these tumors may arise through epigenetic mechanisms.[68] Epigenetics is the study of clonal changes in gene expression without accompanying changes in DNA coding sequences. Epigenetic silencing is recognized now as an important mechanism in the evolution of a subgroup of CRCs. DNA methylation within promoters and alterations in histone modifications appear to be primary mediators of epigenetic inheritance in cancer cells. Hypermethylation of the hMLH1 promoter has been reported in up to 70% of sporadic MSI tumors.[68,69] In the large intestine, aberrant methylation may be an important early event in the age-related field defect observed in sporadic colorectal neoplasia. Aberrant methylation also contributes to tumor progression through a hypermethylator phenotype (CPG island methylator phenotype [CIMP]) responsible for most cases of MSI related to hMLH1 inactivation (associated with about 15% of sporadic CRCs).[68] DNA methylation and histone H3 lysine 9 hypoacetylation and methylation appear to form a mutually reinforcing loop that contributes to tumor supressor gene activation in CRCs.

Biochemical and Other Changes

Chapter 3 deals in depth with the biologic and biochemical changes that occur during the development of colorectal neoplasia. Alterations in cell surface and secreted proteins and glycoproteins, including a number of important cell adhesion molecules, are characteristic of CRCs.[70,71] Interactions between tumor cells themselves or between tumor cells and their environment may be homotypic (involving like molecules) or heterotypic (involving different adhesion molecules). Homotypic interactions often maintain the integrity of primary tumors by fostering adhesion between neighboring cells, whereas heterotypic interactions may occur between tumor cells and platelets, lymphocytes, vascular endothelial cells, and components of the basement membrane matrix. Most tumor-associated molecules represent quantitatively or qualitatively altered molecules found either on normal tissues or during development (e.g., oncofetal antigens such as carcinoembryonic antigen [CEA]). Many of these molecules appear to play a role in maintaining normal tissue homeostasis or targeting blood-borne cells to specific sites. Altered expression, therefore, may contribute to tumor invasion and metastasis.

MMPs (matrix metalloproteinase) are a family of extracellular matrix-degrading enzymes. Overexpression of MMP-1, -2, -3, -7, -9, -13, and MT1-MMP has been demonstrated in human CRCs. The degree of overexpression of some MMPs correlates with stage of disease, prognosis, or both.[72]

Metastasis is a multistage process by which tumor cells escape the primary tumor and establish secondary foci at distant sites (Fig. 120–8). Cells in the primary tumor must become vascularized (angiogenesis via vascular endothelial growth factors), escape the primary tumor by overcoming adhesive interactions (e.g., loss of E-cadherin) and disrupting basement membranes (metalloproteinases such as type IV collagenase, matrilysin, loss of tissue inhibitors of collagenase), and enter lymphatics and/or the circulation. In the bloodstream they must survive interactions with blood components and the immune system and be transported to distant organ sites (principally the liver). At distant sites, tumor cells adhere to target endothelia via specific interactions (e.g., tumor-associated sialoglycoproteins and endothelial selectins) (Fig. 120–9), extravasate, interact with the microenvironment (e.g., growth factors), and establish secondary tumor foci.

Tumor cell subpopulations with different metastatic potentials exist within the same primary tumor, and metastases result from the selective dissemination of those tumor cells that possess the ability to participate in all stages of this complex process. Several carbohydrate antigens have been studied in relation to their potential usefulness as diagnostic markers or in determining prognosis.[70,71,73-75]

FAMILIAL COLON CANCER

It has become increasingly clear that genetic predisposition plays a role in a substantial number of CRCs. Although it is convenient to categorize CRCs into

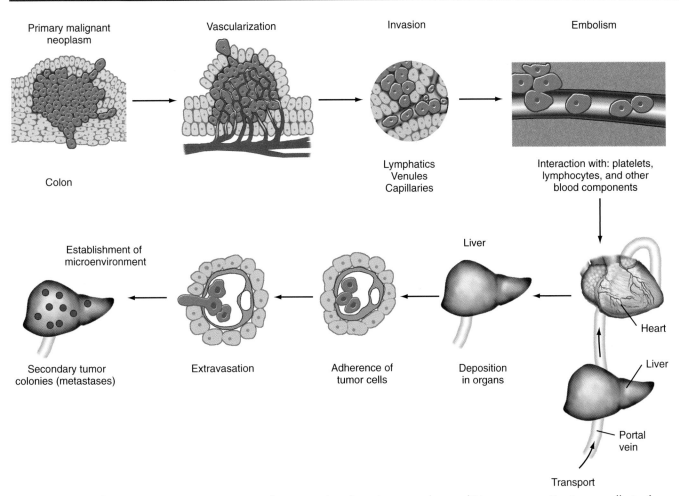

Figure 120–8 Colon cancer metastasis. Cancer cells metastasize through a complex, multistage process. For tumor cells to form metastatic foci at distant sites, they must complete all stages of this process.

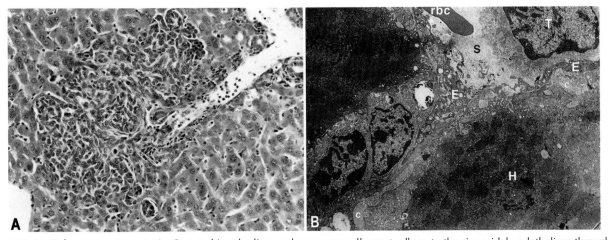

Figure 120–9 Colon cancer metastasis. On reaching the liver, colon cancer cells must adhere to the sinusoidal endothelium through specific interactions and then invade the parenchyma. *A,* Photomicrograph shows tumor cells invading the liver after extravasation from a blood vessel. *B,* Electron micrograph shows collagen bundles (c), rbc, red blood cell; S, sinusoid; tumor cells (T) adherent to sinusoidal endothelium (E) and invading between hepatocytes (H).

hereditary (or familial) and nonhereditary (or sporadic) types, it is more appropriate to assume that all cancers have genetic components, which may be inherited or acquired, to varying degrees. Accordingly, persons with familial colon cancer are born with an altered genome, and the environment may contribute additional geno-toxic events, leading to the malignant phenotype. In the case of "sporadic" cancers, multiple somatic mutations are contributed by the environment (see Chapter 3).

The role of heredity in the genesis of colon cancer is manifested most obviously in those with the heritable polyposis syndromes (FAP, Gardner's syndrome) dis-

Table 120–5   Amsterdam Criteria for Hereditary Nonpolyposis Colorectal Cancer

At least three relatives with colorectal cancer (one must be a first-degree relative of other two)
Colorectal cancer involving at least two generations
One or more colorectal cancer cases before age 50 yr

Criteria defined by the International Collaborative Group on Hereditary Nonpolyposis Colorectal Cancer.

Table 120–6   Bethesda Guidelines for Testing of Colorectal Tumors for Microsatellite Instability[76]

1. Individuals with cancer in families that meet the Amsterdam criteria (see Table 120–5)
2. Individuals with two HNPCC-related cancers, including synchronous and metachronous colorectal cancers or associated extracolonic cancers*
3. Individuals with colorectal cancer and a first-degree relative with colorectal cancer and/or HNPCC-related extracolonic cancer and/or a colorectal adenoma; one of the cancers diagnosed at age <45 yr and the adenoma diagnosed at age <40 yr
4. Individuals with colorectal cancer or endometrial cancer diagnosed at age <45 yr
5. Individuals with right-sided colorectal cancer with an undifferentiated pattern (solid/cribriform)† on histopathology diagnosed at age <45 yr
6. Individuals with signet ring cell-type colorectal cancer diagnosed at age <45 yr‡
7. Individuals with adenomas diagnosed at age <40 yr

*Endometrial, ovarian, gastric, hepatobiliary, or small intestinal cancer or transitional cell carcinoma of the renal pelvis or ureter.
†Poorly differentiated or undifferentiated carcinoma composed of irregular solid sheets of large eosinophilic cells and containing small glandlike spaces.
‡Composed of >50% signet ring cells.
HNPCC, hereditary nonpolyposis colorectal cancer.

cussed in Chapter 119. These syndromes are inherited in an autosomal dominant manner and are characterized by the presence of hundreds to thousands of colonic adenomas, with or without extracolonic tumors. Adenomas develop approximately a decade before the appearance of cancer, and virtually all affected persons eventually develop large bowel cancer if the colon is left in place. Nevertheless, these dramatic syndromes account for less than 1% of all cases of CRC.

HNPCC is an inherited disease in which colon cancers arise in discrete adenomas, but polyposis (i.e., hundreds of polyps) does not occur.[64,76,77] HNPCC accounts for approximately 6% of colonic adenocarcinoma. It is an autosomal dominant disorder with high penetration; approximately 80% are caused by germline mutations in genes responsible for repair of DNA errors called mismatches that occur during DNA replication (discussed earlier). During DNA synthesis, DNA polymerase may create single base-pair mismatches resulting in structural abnormalities (so-called loop-outs) involving unpaired bases. These alterations tend to occur at repetitive DNA sequences termed microsatellites. These errors are repaired by enzymes coded for by "MMR genes." The majority of reported germline mutations in DNA MMR genes have been associated with the *hMSH2* gene on chromosome 2 (40% to 50%) and the *hMLH1* gene on chromosome 3 (20% to 30%).

Mutations in *hMSH6*, *hPMS1*, and *hPMS2* also have been reported in a small number of patients. No locus has been identified, however, for many HNPCC families. The definition of HNPCC was standardized and most strictly defined by the International Collaborative Group on Hereditary Nonpolyposis CRC. These "Amsterdam criteria" (Table 120–5) include (1) at least three relatives with histologically verified CRC, one of them a first-degree relative of the other two (FAP excluded); (2) at least two successive generations affected; and (3) in one of the individuals, diagnosis of CRC before age 50 years. Because these criteria do not account for the frequent occurrence of extracolonic cancers in such families, or for small kindreds, broader clinical criteria have been developed, including the "Bethesda guidelines" published by a recent National Cancer Institute-sponsored workshop on HNPCC (Table 120–6).[77]

HNPCC families include members whose heritable cancer is limited to the colon and rectum (site-specific HNPCC, HNPCC type a, Lynch's syndrome I) and families whose members also are prone to cancer of the female genital tract and other sites (cancer family syndrome, HNPCC type b, Lynch's syndrome II) (Fig. 120–10). In HNPCC syndromes, discrete polyps, but not polyposis,

may antedate the cancers. Adenomas in the proximal colon sometimes may be flat or slightly raised lesions with foci of adenomatous change confined to the upper half of a crypt ("flat" adenomas). HNPCC is characterized by an autosomal dominant mode of genetic transmission, a tendency toward proximal sites of colon tumors, multiple primary malignancies (synchronous and metachronous), and a higher incidence of mucinous carcinomas (Table 120–7). These CRCs usually appear at age 40 to 50 years, 2 decades earlier than CRC in the general population. In a study of a small, defined population in central Finland, HNPCC accounted for 4% to 6% of CRCs identified. This figure is similar to estimates of Lynch and others for the U.S. population.

Patients with HNPCC and some unaffected family members have biologic markers that resemble those in patients with FAP syndromes. These markers include abnormal proliferative activity of colonic crypt cells, increased tetraploidy (twice the normal DNA content) in skin fibroblasts cultured in vitro, decreased degradation of fecal cholesterol, and cell-mediated immune defects in vitro that might interfere with the recognition of killing of incipient tumor cells in vivo. The genetic defect in HNPCC, however, results from loss of the *hMSH2* and *hMLH1* genes. Additional genes, such as *hPMS1*, *hPMS2*, and *hMSH6*, also may be involved, leading to increased susceptibility to mutation from failure to repair base pair mismatches.[64]

Although CRC syndromes with readily apparent patterns of inheritance currently account for only a small portion of total colon cancer cases, hereditary factors may be present in a larger proportion of cases.[78] Genetic susceptibility to CRC in the general population is suggested

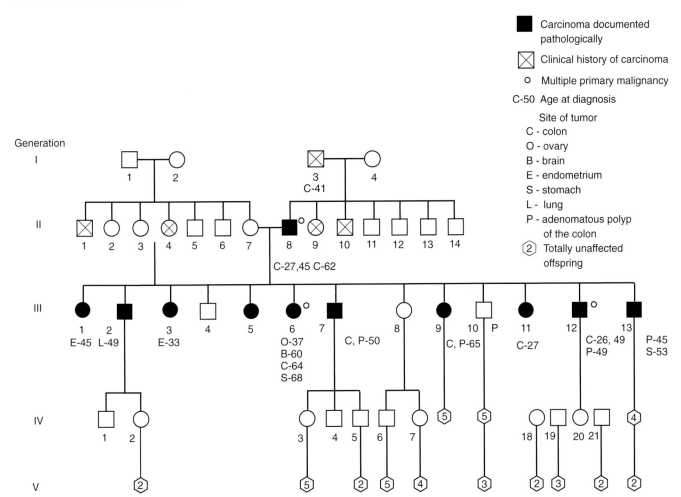

Figure 120–10   Pattern of inheritance of cancer in a familial aggregate with Lynch's syndrome II (HNPCC type b). Affected members were found in generations I, II, and III; members of generations IV and V were still young and at risk for developing carcinomas when the pedigree was obtained. (From Boland CR: Familial colonic cancer syndromes. West J Med 139:351, 1983.)

Table 120–7   Comparison of HNPCC and Sporadic Colorectal Cancer

Clinical Feature	HNPCC	Sporadic Colorectal Cancer
Mean age at diagnosis	45 yr	67 yr*
Multiple colon cancers	35%	4-11%
Synchronous	18%	3-6%
Metachronous	24%	1-5%
Proximal location†	72%	35%
Excess malignant tumors at other sites	Yes	No
Mucinous and poorly differentiated cancers	Common	Infrequent
Prognosis	Favorable‡	Variable

*Ninety percent of cancers in the general population are diagnosed in persons ≥50 yr of age (see Figure 120–11).
†Proximal to the splenic flexure; location of the initial cancer.
‡Patients whose tumors demonstrate microsatellite instability have a more favorable prognosis than those with microsatellite-stable tumors.
HNPCC, hereditary nonpolyposis colorectal cancer.

by the twofold to threefold increase in CRC in first-degree relatives of patients with "sporadic" adenomas and CRCs. The relative risk is even stronger when cancer occurs in family members younger than age 50 years. The precise role of genetic factors in this group and their interaction with the environment in the evolution of CRC remains to be defined.

PREDISPOSING FACTORS FOR COLORECTAL CANCER

The risk of developing CRC depends on a number of demographic factors (Table 120–8). The probable influence of diet and other environmental factors has been discussed (see Tables 120–1 and 2). Other factors include age, personal history of adenoma or of carcinoma, existence of predisposing diseases (particularly inflammatory bowel disease [IBD]), and family history (discussed earlier).

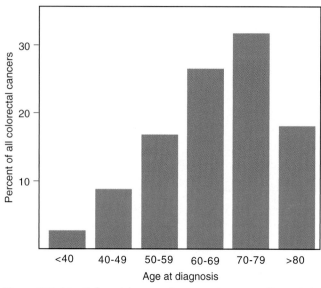

Figure 120–11 Colorectal cancer frequency by age at diagnosis in the United States. Ninety percent of cancers occur after age 50 years.

Table 120–8 Risk Factors for Colorectal Cancer

Age > 50 yr
High-fat, low-bulk diet*
Personal history of
    Colorectal adenomas (synchronous or metachronous)
    Colorectal carcinoma
Family history of
    Polyposis syndromes: FAP, Gardner's syndrome, Turcot's
      syndrome, Muir-Torre syndrome, Peutz-Jeghers syndrome,
      familial juvenile polyposis
    HNPCC
    First-degree relatives with colorectal cancer
Inflammatory bowel disease
    Ulcerative colitis[†]
    Crohn's disease[†]

*Based on descriptive epidemiology; data from case-control, cohort, and randomized trials are less convincing.
[†]Especially with high-grade dysplasia or dysplasia-associated mass lesions.
FAP, familial adenomatous polyposis; HNPCC, hereditary nonpolyposis colorectal cancer.

AGE

The risk of developing CRC rises sharply after age 40 years in the general population, with 90% of cancers occurring in persons aged 50 years and older (Fig. 120–11); a 50-year-old person has approximately a 5% chance of developing CRC if he or she survives to age 80 and a 2.5% risk of dying from the disease. This has important implications for screening, as discussed later in the chapter. Sporadic CRCs do arise in other age groups (3rd and 4th decades), however, and this diagnosis must be considered in younger persons with signs and symptoms characteristic of this disease, especially if they have a family history of colorectal neoplasia.

PRIOR ADENOMA AND CARCINOMA

Adenoma

Present evidence strongly indicates that most CRCs arise from preexisting adenomas (see Chapter 119). The risk of CRC increases with the number of adenomas, the most extreme example being the familial polyposis syndromes. Clinical and morphologic evidence suggest that, as adenomas grow larger, they progressively dedifferentiate, become dysplastic, and then become malignant. With increasing size or increasing villous architecture, the frequencies of nuclear atypia, dysplasia, and in situ or invasive carcinoma increase. Despite the potential for adenomas to evolve to carcinomas, however, the actual risk is unknown.

Adenomatous polyps are common, especially after age 50 years, in populations that consume a Western diet, but the prevalence of adenomas is high, compared with the incidence of cancer. It has been estimated that 29% of the living population older than 35 years in Norway have single or multiple colorectal adenomas. The annual conversion rate in those with adenomas (based on cancer incidence from multiple tumor registries in Norway) is 0.25%, indicating a moderate risk for developing CRC. The malignancy rate is higher in large adenomas, adenomas with villous architecture, and adenomas with cytologic nuclear atypia or dysplasia. The estimated annual rate of conversion to invasive cancer for persons bearing adenomas greater than 1 cm, villous components, or severe dysplasia is 3%, 17%, and 37%, respectively.

Carcinoma

People with CRC have an increased risk of harboring a second carcinoma (synchronous carcinomas) or of developing another one subsequently (metachronous carcinomas). The frequency of more than one carcinoma in the same person ranges between 2% and 6% (0.7% to 7.6% for synchronous cancers and 1.1% to 4.7% for metachronous ones). Most patients with simultaneous cancers have one in the proximal and the other in the distal colon. In the minority of patients with synchronous cancers, the two lesions are located in the same colonic segment. The degree of invasiveness of synchronous cancers often differs, and prognosis depends on the "worst-stage" lesion. Five-year survival rates for patients with synchronous cancers who have had the cancers resected are similar to those with single lesions. The interval between an initial cancer and a metachronous one may be considerable (lesions separated by as much as 23 years have been reported), but several studies note that 50% of metachronous cancers arise within 5 to 7 years of the index lesion. Second cancers often occur at a site remote from the initial lesion.

FAMILY HISTORY

The risk of CRC in first-degree relatives of those with sporadic CRC is increased twofold to threefold (see earlier). The risk is higher when adenoma or carcinoma has occurred in a relative at an early age or when more than one relative has had carcinoma. These factors have been taken into account in recent screening guidelines that stratify patients according to potential cancer risk.[78-83] FAP and its variants are inherited in an autosomal dominant manner, and without colectomy virtually all affected members with polyps eventually develop carcinoma. HNPCC also has an autosomal dominant pattern of inheritance.

Turcot's syndrome is a rare combination of inherited adenomatous polyposis and malignant brain tumors. Patients with Turcot's syndrome have been described who have germline mutations in the *APC* gene or mutations of *hMLH1* and *hPMS2* characteristic of HNPCC.[84] Inheritance is autosomal dominant.

Muir-Torre syndrome is a rare variant of HNPCC that manifests with multiple skin lesions, including sebaceous adenomas and carcinomas, basal cell and squamous cell carcinomas, and keratoacanthomas in addition to colonic adenomas and adenocarcinomas. MSI and loss of *hMLH1* and *hMSH2* expression has been noted in a high percentage of tumors occurring in the syndrome.

Peutz-Jeghers syndrome and the familial form of juvenile polyposis both have an increased risk of small and large bowel cancer (see Chapter 119). Peutz-Jeghers syndrome is an autosomal dominant disease, which in most families has been mapped to chromosome 19 p13.3 and the *STK11* gene (serine threonine kinase 11). Adenomatous changes have been reported in 3% to 6% of hamartomas from these patients. Extracolonic cancers are common and have been reported to occur in 50% to 90% of patients with Peutz-Jeghers syndrome (relative risk for all cancers was 15.2).[85] A significant increase has been reported for a variety of cancers in the esophagus, stomach, small intestine, pancreas, lung, breast, uterus, and ovary.

Familial juvenile polyposis is a rare autosomal dominant disease associated with polyps that may be limited to the colon or the stomach or that occur throughout the gastrointestinal tract.[86] The genetic basis of this syndrome is not understood, but germline mutations in a gene (*SMAD4*) located on chromosome 18q21.1 that encodes an intracellular mediator in the TGF-β signaling pathway have been identified in some affected patients. The *PTEN* gene located on chromosome 10 also has been linked to some cases. The presence of mixed juvenile and adenomatous polyps indicates which lesions have malignant potential.

INFLAMMATORY BOWEL DISEASE

Patients with idiopathic IBD (UC, Crohn's disease) are at increased risk for developing adenocarcinoma of the colon (see Chapters 108 and 109).[87-90] Actuarially derived (life table) cumulative cancer incidences from tertiary referral centers (Fig. 120–12) agree that the risk of cancer in patients with UC begins with a disease duration of 7 years and rises about 10% per decade, reaching approximately 30% at 25 years. Nonetheless, difficulties related to sources of referral, sampling, recognition and characterization of disease, differences in follow-up procedures, and methods used to detect neoplastic disease cloud many such studies. The assessed cancer risk for patients with UC followed in one private practice

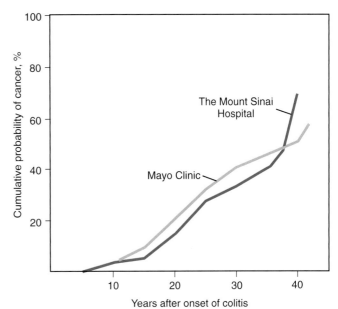

Figure 120–12 Cumulative probability of developing colorectal carcinoma in patients with ulcerative colitis seen at two tertiary referral centers. Data from primary care settings indicate a similar pattern but lower incidence rates (see text).

has been reported to be only 6.6% 26 years after onset of disease and 11.4% at 32 years. The true risk of developing colorectal carcinoma in UC must lie between predictions from tertiary centers and the primary care setting.

The risk of CRC for patients with UC correlates most closely with duration of disease. In a large group of patients with extensive disease who were followed prospectively, the risk of carcinoma per patient-year was zero before 10 years and 1 in 86 after 20 years. The risk is greatest in those with universal colitis.[87] Although it has been reported that the risk of cancer in left-sided disease (i.e., distal to the splenic flexure) begins approximately a decade later than with universal colitis, at least one surveillance study found no difference between these groups in the temporal development of preneoplastic dysplasia. The risk for patients with ulcerative proctitis is only slightly increased compared with that in the general population.

The risk of cancer is not related to severity of the initial attack of colitis, disease activity, or age at onset of colitis (independent of duration of disease). CRC in persons with UC appears to be a risk factor for CRC in their relatives without colitis.[88] Similarly, cancer in relatives without UC is a risk factor for those with colitis. There is an association of backwash ileitis with CRC in patients with UC who undergo proctocolectomy.[91] Cancer arising in the setting of UC traditionally has been thought to be a highly malignant lesion with a poor prognosis, but studies using matched controls from colon cancer populations without colitis have failed to show a significant difference in survival between the two groups.

The increased risk for CRC in patients with Crohn's disease or ileocolitis has been reported to be as much as 4 to 20 times that in the general population, although one cohort study failed to confirm an increased incidence of colon cancer in these patients.[92] Cancer may arise at an earlier age in these patients than in the general population. Many of these cancers are mucinous carcinomas; they may be present in surgically bypassed or strictured segments of colon.

Carcinomas do not develop de novo from normal mucosa but from mucosa that has undergone a sequence of morphologic changes that culminate in invasive carcinoma. As in precancerous adenomas, dysplasia is a precursor to carcinoma in IBD. Dysplasia includes abnormalities in crypt architecture and cytologic detail (Figs. 120–13 and 120–14). Epithelial crypts are reduced in number, irregularly branched, and crowded together ("back-to-back" glands). Cell nuclei may be enlarged and hyperchromatic, may have increased numbers of mitoses, and may be located at different levels in the cell, producing a "picket fence" appearance (pseudostratification). Dysplasia is classified by grade as mild (or low grade) to severe (or high grade) dysplasia.

Retrospective analyses report that 90% of resected colons from patients with UC and cancer contain dys-

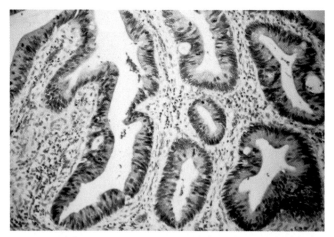

Figure 120–13 Photomicrograph of dysplasia in the setting of ulcerative colitis. The number of goblet cells is decreased. Glands are branched, irregular, and crowded together. Cell nuclei are hyperchromatic and occur at different levels, producing a pseudopalisading or "picket fence" appearance.

plastic mucosa somewhere in the colon, and 30% of patients with severe rectal or colonic dysplasia on resection or biopsy have coexistent carcinoma. Colonoscopic studies suggest that 25% of colons that demonstrate severe (high-grade) dysplasia on biopsy harbor a carcinoma. The incidence of dysplasia often is patchy, and it may be present in the colon but absent from the rectum.

Because the lack of uniformity of the definition of dysplasia may make interpretation of such data difficult, a multidisciplinary Inflammatory Bowel Disease-Dysplasia-Morphology Study Group developed a standardized classification for dysplasia arising in the setting of IBD. Several large prospective studies have attempted to determine the true risk of cancer in patients with colonic dysplasia and UC and the impact of screening programs for dysplasia.

Results suggest that biopsy surveillance programs can be effective in helping control the risk of carcinoma in patients with long-standing UC. The risk of cancer appears highest in those with high-grade dysplasia that arises in visible plaques or masses (dysplasia-associated lesion or mass [DALMs], as illustrated in Fig. 120–14). A computer cohort decision analysis suggested that surveillance should increase life expectancy for patients with UC.[93] Most investigators believe that patients who have UC for more than 7 to 8 years should undergo colonoscopy with multiple mucosal biopsies annually, to identify areas of dysplasia; they advocate colectomy for severe dysplasia or DALM. Because the significance of low-grade or moderate dysplasia is less clear, immediate resection for patients with these levels of dysplasia is controversial. Prophylactic colectomy also has been recommended as an option for those with disease of at least 10 years' duration. Studies employing flow cytometry have detected aneuploid cell populations in colons resected for UC with dysplasia or early cancer. Chromosomal alterations may occur early in UC-related neoplastic progression[94] and appear to precede the histologic development of dysplasia; relative loss of chromosome 18q also may be important in neoplastic progression.

Both dysplasia and increased risk of colon carcinoma have been reported in patients with Crohn's disease. As in UC, dysplasia appears in diseased colon segments, and

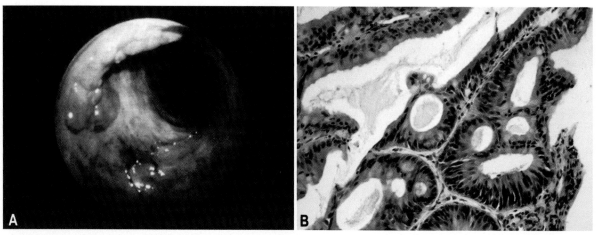

Figure 120–14 Plaque-like dysplasia-associated lesion or mass (DALM) in a patient with long-standing ulcerative colitis. *A,* Lesion as seen through the colonoscope. *B,* Biopsy specimen revealing high-grade dysplasia. DALM, dysplasia-associated lesion or mass.

its presence correlates with duration of disease. In one screening trial,[95] the finding of definite dysplasia was associated with age older than 45 years and increased symptoms. By life table analysis, the probability of detecting dysplasia or cancer after a negative screening colonoscopy was 22% by the fourth surveillance examination.

OTHER ASSOCIATIONS

Diverting bile to the lower small intestine, either surgically or by feeding cholestyramine, increases the yield of proximal colon tumors in carcinogen-treated animals. By analogy, cholecystectomy in humans could lead to increased delivery of secondary bile acids to the proximal bowel, and the possibility of an increase in colon cancer following cholecystectomy has been raised; although the clinical evidence for such an association is contradictory. Increased proliferative activity in the distal colonic mucosa has been demonstrated in patients who have undergone cholecystectomy, and an increased frequency of tubular adenomas has been observed in patients older than 60 years of age with a postcholecystectomy interval of more than 10 years, but an increased risk of colonic cancer for these patients has been both supported and refuted. There is no evidence that chronic use of cholestyramine is associated with an increased risk of colon cancer in humans.

A retrospective population-based cohort study that used the Swedish Inpatient Register evaluated almost 23,000 persons who had had cholecystectomy for up to 31 years after surgery.[96] Patients having had cholecystectomy had an increased risk of proximal intestinal adenocarcinoma, which declined with increasing distance from the common bile duct. The risk was significantly increased for adenocarcinoma of the small bowel and right colon but not the remaining colon or rectum.

PATHOLOGY, NATURAL HISTORY, AND STAGING

GROSS PATHOLOGY

The gross morphologic features of adenocarcinoma in the large bowel depend on the tumor's site. Carcinomas of the proximal colon, particularly those of the cecum and ascending colon, tend to be large and bulky, often outgrowing their blood supply and undergoing necrosis (Fig. 120–15). This polypoid configuration also may be found elsewhere in the colon and rectum. In the more distal colon and rectum, tumors more frequently involve a greater circumference of the bowel, producing an annular constriction or "napkin-ring" appearance (Fig. 120–16). The fibrous stroma of these tumors accounts for constriction and narrowing of the bowel lumen, whereas the circular arrangement of colonic lymphatics is responsible

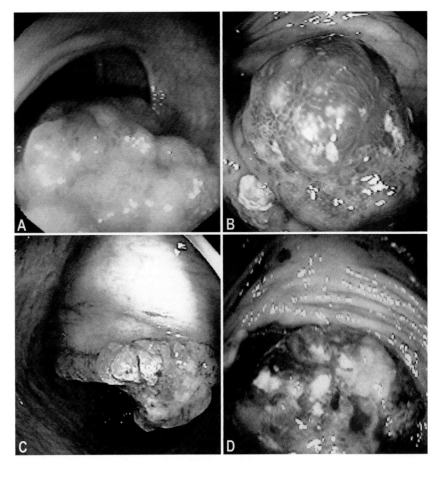

Figure 120–15 Carcinomas of the cecum seen at colonoscopy. Carcinomas of the proximal colon are often large and bulky polypoid lesions (*A* and *B*), involve the ileocecal valve (*C*), and may outgrow their blood supply and become necrotic (*D*).

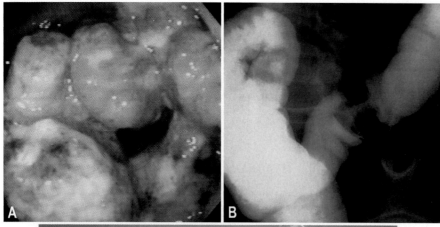

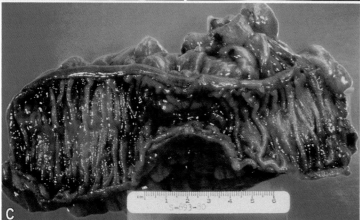

Figure 120–16 Obstructing carcinoma of the sigmoid colon. *A*, Colonoscopic view. *B*, Apple-core lesion seen on barium enema examination. *C*, Surgical specimen demonstrating an annular constriction or "napkin-ring" appearance.

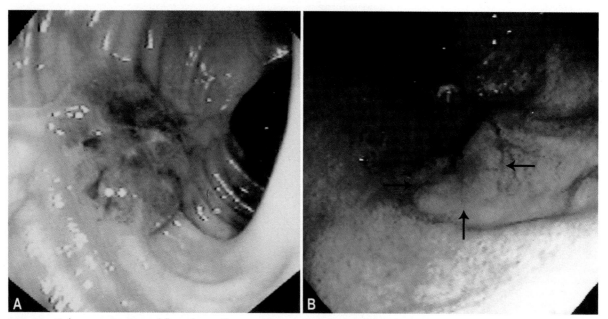

Figure 120–17 Colonoscopic view of flat, plaque-like carcinomas of the colon (*A*) and rectum (*B*) in patients with inflammatory bowel disease.

for their annular growth. These tumors also may become ulcerated. Occasionally, tumors have a flatter appearance with predominantly intramural spread (Fig. 120–17); the latter are seen most frequently in the setting of IBD. Morphologic features of CRCs have clinical, diagnostic, and prognostic implications.

HISTOLOGY

Carcinomas of the large bowel characteristically are adenocarcinomas that form moderately to well-differentiated glands and secrete variable amounts of mucin (Fig. 120–18). Mucin, a high-molecular-weight

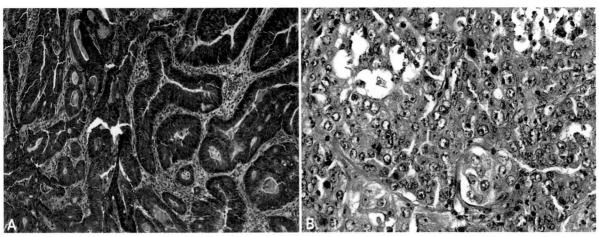

Figure 120–18   Histology of adenocarcinoma of the colon. *A,* Well-differentiated adenocarcinoma of the colon. Histologic sections stained with hematoxylin and eosin demonstrate crowded neoplastic glands containing variable amounts of mucin. *B,* Poorly differentiated adenocarcinoma of the colon.

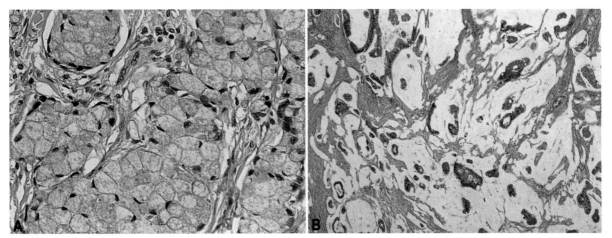

Figure 120–19   (*A*) Mucinous carcinomas of the colon as seen histologically include signet ring cell carcinoma in which a large vacuole of mucin displaces the nucleus and (*B*) colloid carcinoma with scattered nests of tumor cells floating in lakes of mucin.

glycoprotein, is the major product secreted by both normal and neoplastic glands of the colon and may be seen best with histochemical stains such as periodic acid–Schiff (PAS). In poorly differentiated tumors (see Fig. 120–18), gland formation and mucin production are present but less prominent. "Signet ring" cells, in which a large vacuole of mucin displaces the nucleus to one side, are a feature of some tumors (Fig. 120–19*A*). In approximately 15% of tumors, large lakes of mucin contain scattered collections of tumor cells (Fig. 120–19*B*). These mucinous or colloid carcinomas are most frequent in patients with HNPCC, with UC, and in patients whose carcinomas occur at an early age. Scirrhous carcinomas are uncommon and are characterized by sparse gland formation, with marked desmoplasia and fibrous tissue surrounding glandular structures. Sometimes tumors demonstrate a mixed histologic picture, with glands of varying degrees of differentiation.

Cancers other than adenocarcinomas account for less than 5% of malignant tumors of the large bowel. Tumors arising at the anorectal junction include squamous cell carcinomas, cloacogenic or transitional cell carcinomas, and melanomas (see Chapter 122). Primary lymphomas

and carcinoid tumors of the large bowel account for less than 0.1% of all large bowel neoplasms (see Chapters 28 and 30).

NATURAL HISTORY AND STAGING

CRCs begin as intramucosal epithelial lesions, usually arising in adenomatous polyps or glands. As cancers grow, they become invasive, penetrating the muscularis mucosae of the bowel and invading lymphatic and vascular channels to involve regional lymph nodes, adjacent structures, and distant sites. Although adenocarcinomas of the colon and rectum grow at varying rates, they most often have long periods of silent growth before producing bowel symptoms. The mean doubling time of colon cancers determined radiographically in one study was 620 days. Patterns of spread depend on the anatomy of the individual bowel segment as well as its lymph and blood supplies.

Cancers of the rectum advance locally by progressive penetration of the bowel wall. Extension of the primary tumor intramurally and parallel to the long axis of the bowel most often is limited, and lymphatic and hematogenous spread is unusual before penetration of the muscularis mucosae. Exceptions appear to be poorly differentiated tumors, which may metastasize lymphatically or hematogenously before penetrating the bowel. Because the rectum is relatively immobile and lacks a serosal covering, rectal cancers tend to spread contiguously to progressively involve local structures. Transrectal ultrasonography is useful in staging depth of rectal cancers. Because of the dual blood supply of the lower one third of the rectum, tumors arising here may metastasize hematogenously via the superior hemorrhoidal vein and portal system to the liver or by way of the middle hemorrhoidal vein and inferior vena cava to the lungs. The veins of the upper and middle thirds of the rectum drain into the portal system, and tumors in these segments first spread hematogenously to the liver. Occasionally, lumbar and thoracic vertebral metastases may result from hematogenous spread via portal-vertebral communications (i.e., Batson's vertebral venous plexuses).

Colon cancers may invade transmurally to penetrate the bowel wall and involve regional lymphatics and then distant nodes; lymphatic drainage generally parallels the arterial supply to a given bowel segment. The liver is the most common site of hematogenous spread from colon tumors via the portal venous system. Pulmonary metastases from colon cancer result, in general, from hepatic metastases.

On the basis of observations of what he believed to be an orderly progression of locoregional invasion by rectal cancers, Cuthbert Dukes proposed a classification in 1929, which has since been modified many times in attempts to increase its prognostic value for cancers of both the rectum and the colon. The most commonly employed modification of the Dukes system is that of Astler and Coller (Table 120–9). This classification uses the following designations:

A, tumors limited to the mucosa

B1, tumors extending into, but not through, the muscularis propria

B2, tumors penetrating the muscularis propria but without lymph node involvement

C, tumors with regional lymph node involvement

Stage C tumors are divided further into primary tumors limited to the bowel wall (C1) and those that penetrate the bowel wall (C2). By contrast, in the system proposed by the Gastrointestinal Tumor Study Group (GITSG), C1 lesions are those in which one to four regional lymph nodes contain tumor, and C2 lesions are those in which more than four lymph nodes contain tumor (see Table 120–9). Another modification, by Turnbull and associates, added a D category referring to distant metastases.

In an attempt to provide a uniform and orderly classification for CRCs, the American Joint Committee on Cancer (AJCC) has introduced the tumor-node-metastases (TNM) classification for CRC.[97] This system classifies the extent of the primary tumor (T), the status of regional lymph nodes (N), and the presence or absence of distant metastases (M). Cases are assigned the highest value of TNM that describes the full extent of disease and are grouped into five stages (0 through IV). The five stages have become important in uniformly ran-

domizing patients for therapeutic trials (Table 120–10) and have, in most cases, replaced the Dukes classification for CRC.

PROGNOSIS

Clinical and pathologic variables that may affect the prognosis of patients with CRC are outlined in Table 120–11. These variables are important in predicting clinical outcome and in designing optimal strategies for treatment and follow-up. Their identification has led to a progressive modification of the staging classifications for CRC. The roles of histologic differentiation, tumor size, location, configuration, degree of invasion, and lymph node status must be evaluated on the basis of prospective analyses of patients who undergo curative resections for CRC.

SURGICAL-PATHOLOGIC STAGING

The depth of transmural tumor penetration and the extent of regional lymph node spread are the most important determinants of prognosis (Fig. 120–20). Furthermore, the degree of bowel wall penetration affects prognosis, independently of lymph node status, and correlates with the number of involved nodes as well as with the incidence of local recurrence after surgical resection. The number of involved regional lymph nodes also correlates independently with outcome (Fig. 120–20B).

TUMOR MORPHOLOGY AND HISTOLOGY

The TNM classification (see Table 120–10) is based in part on the observation that, for most cancers, tumor size correlates with local and distant spread and, thus, indirectly with prognosis. Numerous studies suggest that CRC is an exception and that the size of the primary tumor per se does not correlate with prognosis. In fact, patients with exophytic or polypoid tumors appear to have a better prognosis than those with ulcerating or infiltrating tumors.

Tumor prognosis correlates with histologic grade: poor differentiation confers a worse prognosis than does a high degree of differentiation. Mucinous[71] and scirrhous carcinomas appear to be biologically more aggressive, and patients with these tumors do not survive as long as those who have other types of adenocarcinomas. Mucin-associated antigens may play a role in tumor progression and metastasis of colon cancer cells. Signet ring carcinomas have been reported to present at an advanced stage and to be highly invasive tumors.

Venous invasion by CRC (Fig. 120–21A) usually correlates with local recurrence after resection, visceral metastases, and decreased survival, but it may not be of independent prognostic value for tumors confined to the bowel wall. Although lymphatic invasion is associated with decreased survival, it is not clear whether this variable is independent of depth of tumor invasion and regional nodal metastasis. Perineural invasion (Fig. 120–21B) also is linked to increased local recurrence and

Table 120–9 Dukes Classification for Carcinoma of the Rectum and Its Modifications for Colorectal Carcinoma

Stage	Dukes, 1932 (Rectum)	Gabriel, Dukes, Bussey, 1935 (Rectum)	Kirklin et al, 1949 (Rectum + Sigmoid)	Astler-Coller, 1954 (Rectum + Colon)	Turnbull et al, 1967 (Colon)	Modified Astler-Coller (Gunderson, Sosin), 1974 (Rectum + Colon)	GITSG, 1975 (Rectum + Colon)
A	Limited to bowel wall	Limited to bowel wall	Limited to mucosa	Limited to mucosa	Limited to mucosa	Limited to mucosa	Limited to mucosa
B	Through bowel wall	Through bowel wall	—	—	Tumor extension into pericolic fat	—	—
B1	—	—	Into muscularis propria	Into muscularis propria	—	Into muscularis propria	Into muscularis propria
B2	—	—	Through muscularis propria	Through muscularis propria (and serosa)	—	Through serosa (m = microscopic; m + g = gross)	Through serosa
B3	—	—	—	—	—	Adherent to or invading adjacent structures	—
C	Regional nodal metastases	—	Regional nodal metastases	—	Regional nodal metastases	—	—
C1	—	Regional nodal metastases near primary lesion	—	Same as B1 + regional nodal metastases	—	Same as B1 + regional nodal metastases	1-4 regional nodes positive
C2	—	Proximal node involved at point of ligation	—	Same as B2 + regional nodal metastases	—	Same as B2 + regional nodal metastases	>4 regional nodes positive
C3	—	—	—	—	—	Same as B3 + regional nodal metastases	—
D	—	—	—	—	Distant metastases (liver, lung, bone) or parietal or adjacent organ invasion	—	—

GITSG, Gastrointestinal Tumor Study Group.

decreased survival, but such data are limited. The degree of inflammatory response and lymphocytic infiltration in and around a cancer may be related to outcome; increased inflammation, and immune reaction appear to confer a better prognosis, but, once again, the data are limited.

The prognosis of patients with CRC may be related to the DNA content of the primary tumor, since survival is shorter for patients with non-diploid or aneuploid tumors than for those whose tumor cells have a normal or diploid DNA content. Although the DNA content of the primary tumor may correlate with the potential for local or distant recurrence after primary resection, the value of routine flow cytometric measurements or image analysis of the DNA content of tumor cells for assessing clinical prognosis and planning treatment remains to be determined. Deletions in chromosomes 18q and 17p

(p53) may be important indicators of prognosis, independent of stage.[56,60] As indicated in Table 120–11, a growing number of other molecular markers also may predict prognosis or response to therapy.[60]

CLINICAL FEATURES

Whereas screening programs for CRC suggest that tumors diagnosed in asymptomatic patients are less advanced, assessment of the impact of early diagnosis on survival of asymptomatic persons awaits the results of prospective, randomized, controlled studies such as the Prostate, Lung, Colorectal and Ovarian (PLCO) Cancer Screening Trial.[98] Duration of symptoms may not correlate directly with prognosis, and some presenting symptoms (e.g., rectal bleeding) may be associated with better rates of survival.

Table 120–10 AJCC TNM Staging of Colorectal Cancer

Stage*	Criteria†
0	Carcinoma in situ: intraepithelial or invasion of lamina propria‡ (Tis N0 M0)
I	Tumor invades submucosa (T1 N0 M0)—Dukes A
	Tumor invades muscularis propria (T2 N0 M0)
II	Tumor invades through the muscularis propria into subserosa or into nonperitonealized pericolic or perirectal tissues (T3 N0 M0)—Dukes B
	Tumor perforates the visceral peritoneum or directly invades other organs or structures and/or perforates visceral peritoneum§ (T4 N0 M0)
III	Any degree of bowel wall perforation with regional lymph node metastasis
	N1: metastasis in 1-3 regional lymph nodes
	N2: metastasis in ≥4 regional lymph nodes
	Any T N1 M0—Dukes C
	Any T N2 M0
IV	Any invasion of bowel wall with or without lymph node metastasis, but with evidence of distant metastasis
	Any T
	Any N M1

*Stage II is subdivided into IIA (for T3 tumors) and IIB (for T4 tumors). Stage III is subdivided into IIIA (T1-T2 N1 M0), IIB (T3-T4 N1 M0), and IIIC (any T N2 M0). N1 lesions have 1-3 positive nodes; N2 tumors have ≥ 4 positive nodes. Smooth metastatic nodules in the pericolic or perirectal fat are considered lymph node metastases. Irregularly contoured metastatic nodules in the peritumoral fat are considered vascular invasion.
†Dukes B, which corresponds to stage II, is a composite of better (T3 N0 M0) and worse (T4 N0 M0) prognostic groups, as is Dukes C, which corresponds to stage III (Any T N1 M0 and Any T N2 M0).
‡Tis includes cancer cells confined within the glandular basement membrane (intraepithelial) or lamina propria (intramucosal) with no extension through the muscularis mucosae into the submucosa.
§Direct invasion in T4 includes invasion of other segments of the colorectum by way of serosa; e.g., invasion of the sigmoid colon by a carcinoma of the cecum.
AJCC, American Joint Committee on Cancer; NX, regional lymph nodes cannot be assessed; N0, no regional lymph node metastasis; MX, distant metastasis cannot be assessed; M0, no distant metastasis; M1, distant metastasis.
From the AJCC Cancer Staging Manual, 6th ed. New York, Springer-Verlag, 2002.

Table 120–11 Pathologic, Molecular, and Clinical Features that May Affect Prognosis in Patients with Colorectal Cancer

Feature or Marker	Effect on Prognosis
Pathologic	
Surgical-pathologic stage	
Depth of bowel wall penetration	Increased penetration diminishes prognosis
Number of regional nodes involved by tumor	1-4 nodes is better than > 4 nodes
Tumor morphology/histology	
Degree of differentiation	Well-differentiated is better than poorly differentiated
Mucinous (colloid) or signet ring cell histology	Diminished prognosis
Scirrhous histology	Diminished prognosis
Venous invasion	Diminished prognosis
Lymphatic invasion	Diminished prognosis
Perineural invasion	Diminished prognosis
Local inflammation and immunologic reaction	Improved prognosis
Tumor morphology	Polypoid/exophytic is better than ulcerating/infiltrating
Tumor DNA content	Increased DNA content (aneuploidy) diminishes prognosis
Tumor size	No effect in most studies
Molecular	
Loss of heterozygosity at chromosome 18q (*DCC, DPC4*)	Diminished prognosis
Loss of heterozygosity at chromosome 17p (*p53*)	Diminished prognosis
Loss of heterozygosity at chromosome 8p	Diminished prognosis
Increased labeling index for p21$^{WAF/CIP1}$ protein	Improved prognosis
Microsatellite instability	Improved prognosis
Mutation in *BAX* gene	Diminished prognosis
Clinical	
Diagnosis in asymptomatic patients	Possibly improved prognosis
Duration of symptoms	No demonstrated effect
Rectal bleeding as a presenting symptom	Improved prognosis
Bowel obstruction	Diminished prognosis
Bowel perforation	Diminished prognosis
Tumor location	May be better for colon than for rectum
	May be better for left colon than right colon tumors
Age < 30 yr	Diminished prognosis
Preoperative CEA	Diminished prognosis with a high CEA level
Distant metastases	Markedly diminished prognosis

CEA, carcinoembryonic antigen.

Figure 120–20 *A*, Survival probabilities according to the Dukes stage as modified by Astler-Coller (see Table 120–9) in patients undergoing potentially curative surgery for colorectal cancer. Expected survival among age- and sex-matched general populations is indicated by the straight line. *B*, Survival probabilities according to the number of nodes involved in patients with stage C colorectal carcinoma. Data using TNM staging confirm a substantial difference in 5-year survival between individuals with lesions 1 to 3 positive nodes (N1) and 4 or more positive nodes (N2).[151] (*A* and *B*, From Moertel CG, O'Fallon JR, Go VL, et al: The preoperative carcinoembryonic antigen test in the diagnosis, staging, and prognosis of colorectal cancer. Cancer 58:603, 1986.)

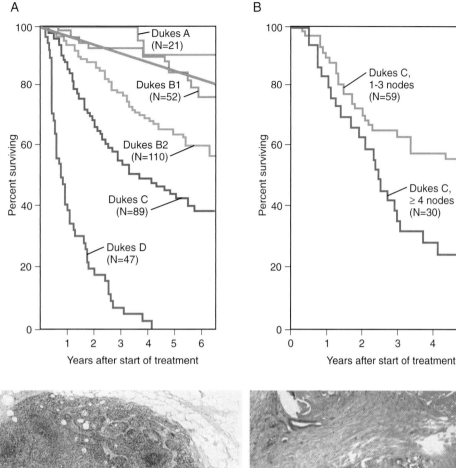

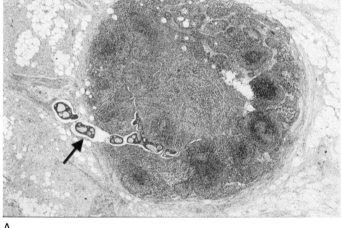

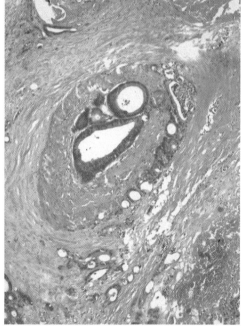

Figure 120–21 Pathologic features that may influence prognosis adversely include vascular invasion (*A*) and lymph node invasion (*B*). In *B*, high magnification microscopy demonstrates a lymph node containing adenocarcinoma cells. The arrow points to a lymphatic vessel containing tumor cells.

Bowel obstruction or perforation has been linked with poor prognosis. Patients who present with obstructing lesions may not be candidates for curative surgery and have higher rates of operative morbidity and mortality. Recurrence following "curative" surgery also is higher in patients who present with obstruction or perforation.

The location of the primary tumor may influence outcome. Disease-free survival at 3 years appears to be 2% to 14% higher after surgery for tumors of the left than of the right colon. Some studies suggest a survival advantage for patients with colon versus rectal cancers.

As many as 3% of CRCs arise before 30 years of age, and only 11% of such persons have a predisposing condition such as FAP or UC. The prognosis is worse than for older patients and is particularly poor in the pediatric age group. Poor prognosis may be related to a higher percentage of more advanced cancers and mucinous adenocarcinomas in these younger patients. Alternatively, patients with tumors demonstrating MSI appear to have a better prognosis irrespective of patient age.[65] Thus, whereas CRCs occur at a younger age in those with HNPCC, these individuals have a better prognosis than those with microsatellite-stable cancers.

Outcome has been shown to be related to the preoperative serum CEA level. Tumor recurrence is higher, and the estimated mean time to recurrence is shorter, in patients with Dukes B and C cancers who have high preoperative CEA levels. The preoperative CEA level may be of prognostic value only in patients with Dukes C CRCs who also have four or more involved lymph nodes (stage C2), but CEA level may not be indicative of survival probability in patients with Dukes A and B lesions or Dukes C lesions with fewer than four nodes involved. Expression of mucin-associated carbohydrate antigens other than CEA, such as sialyl Lewis[x], also may correlate with prognosis.[71,75] Expression of the carbohydrate-binding protein galectin-3 correlates with tumor progression in the colon and may confer a poor prognosis.[71,73]

Approximately one fourth of patients with CRC exhibit clinical evidence of hematogenous spread when seen initially, and one half of patients with CRC eventually develop metastases to a distant site, usually the liver; such metastases carry a poor prognosis at all times in the clinical course. The most important determinant of survival time for patients who present with liver metastases is the extent of hepatic involvement by tumor.

CLINICAL MANIFESTATIONS

Adenocarcinomas of the colon and rectum grow slowly and may be present as long as 5 years before symptoms appear. Persons with asymptomatic cancers often have occult blood loss from their tumors, and the bleeding rate increases with tumor size and degree of ulceration (Fig. 120–22).

Symptoms depend to some extent on the site of the primary tumor. Cancers of the proximal colon usually grow larger before they produce symptoms than do those of the left colon and rectum. Constitutional symptoms (fatigue, shortness of breath, angina) secondary to microcytic hypochromic anemia may be the principal presentation of right colon tumors. Less often, blood from right colon cancers is admixed with stool and appears as "mahogany feces." As a tumor grows, it produces vague abdominal discomfort or presents as a palpable mass. Obstruction is uncommon with these tumors because of the large diameters of the cecum and ascending colon, although cecal cancers may block the ileocecal valve and cause distal small bowel obstruction.

The left colon has a narrower lumen than the proximal colon, and cancers of the descending and sigmoid colon often involve the bowel circumferentially and cause obstructive symptoms. Patients may present with colicky abdominal pain, particularly after meals, and a change in bowel habits. Constipation may alternate with increased frequency of defecation, as small amounts of retained stool move beyond the obstructing lesion. Hematochezia is present more often with distal lesions than with proximal ones, and bright red blood passed per rectum or coating the surface of the stool is common with cancers of the left colon and rectum. Rectal cancers also cause obstruction and changes in bowel habits, including constipation, diarrhea, and tenesmus. Rectal cancers may invade the bladder, vaginal wall, or surrounding nerves, resulting in perineal or sacral pain, but this is a late occurrence.

Symptomatic patients with CRC often are misdiagnosed. Symptoms are ascribed to benign conditions such as diverticular disease (abdominal pain, bleeding, change in stool caliber), irritable bowel syndrome (abdominal

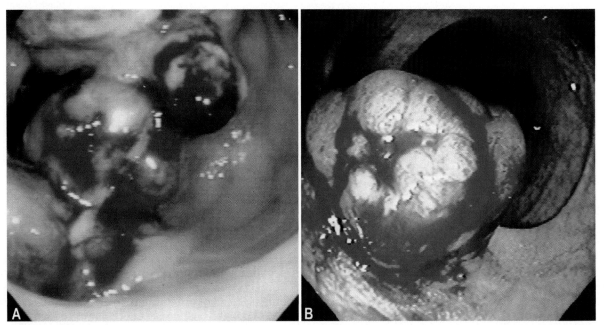

Figure 120–22   Colonoscopic view of bleeding carcinomas of the sigmoid colon (*A*) and cecum (*B*). Carcinomas of the colon often bleed intermittently. Patients may present with evidence of microcytic anemia or with hematochezia, depending on tumor site and the pattern of bleeding.

pain, change in bowel habits), or hemorrhoids (rectal bleeding) (Table 120–12). CRC should be considered when a patient, especially one older than 40 years of age, presents with hypochromic microcytic anemia or frank hematochezia and rectal bleeding. Too often, anemia in elderly people is ascribed to "chronic disease," only to be diagnosed later as a sign of advanced CRC. Abdominal pain—in any form—and bleeding also merit evaluation for cancer in this age group. Large bowel cancer may affect younger patients, particularly those with IBD or a strong family history for CRC and other cancers. Judicious evaluation of younger patients for CRC is therefore warranted when suggested by history and clinical presentation.

DIAGNOSIS AND SCREENING

TESTS WHEN COLORECTAL CANCER IS SUSPECTED

When CRC is suspected because of clinical signs and symptoms or when screening suggests the possibility of a large bowel tumor (discussed later), prompt endoscopic or radiologic diagnostic evaluation should be undertaken (Fig. 120–23). Colonoscopy is more accurate than air-contrast barium enema (ACBE), especially for detecting small lesions such as adenomas smaller than 1 cm; up to one half of adenomas larger than 1 cm may be missed by barium enema.[99,100] If colonoscopy is unavailable, technically difficult, or refused by the patient, an ACBE should be performed following sigmoidoscopy. ACBEs are more accurate than full-column barium enemas, not only for diagnosing cancers but also for detecting small

Table 120–12 Differential Diagnosis of Colorectal Cancer

Mass Lesions
Benign tumors (mucosal and submucosal)
Inflammatory masses
  Diverticulitis
  Infections (tuberculosis, amebiasis, fungal infections)
  Inflammatory bowel disease
  Ischemic colitis
  Solitary rectal ulcer
Strictures
Crohn's colitis
Ischemia
Radiation (late sequelae)
Rectal Bleeding
Diverticulosis
Hemorrhoids
Infectious colitis
Ischemic colitis
Solitary rectal ulcer
Inflammatory bowel disease
Abdominal Pain
Diverticulitis
Inflammatory bowel disease
Irritable bowel syndrome
Ischemic colitis
Changes in Bowel Habits
Infectious diarrhea
Inflammatory bowel disease
Irritable bowel syndrome
Medications

This list includes common clinical situations that initially may be confused with symptoms or signs of colorectal cancer, but it is not meant to be inclusive.

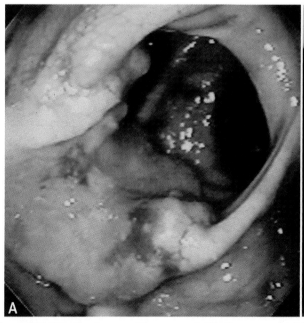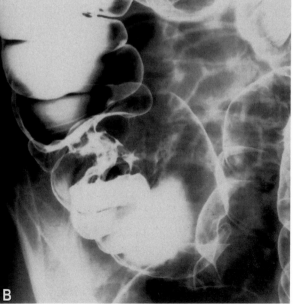

Figure 120–23 Carcinoma of the cecum infiltrating a cecal fold as seen by colonoscopy (*A*) and air-contrast barium enema (*B*).

adenomas, which often are present intercurrently. Neoplasms in the rectum and sigmoid colon are sometimes difficult to diagnose radiologically, and proctosigmoidoscopy should be used as a complement to double-contrast enema imaging. Flexible sigmoidoscopy (FS) is superior to rigid sigmoidoscopy.

If a carcinoma is detected radiologically or by sigmoidoscopy, a full colonoscopic examination should be done because of the high incidence of synchronous lesions and possible implications of the colonoscopic findings for the surgical treatment plan. As many as one half of the patients with proven cancers of the colon and rectum may harbor additional lesions, and for almost 10%, the operative plan will have to be modified as a result of preoperative colonoscopy.

PRINCIPLES OF SCREENING

Cancer prevention may be categorized as primary or secondary. *Primary prevention* refers to the identification of genetic, biologic, and environmental factors that are etiologic or pathogenetic and subsequent alteration of their effects on tumor development. Although several areas of study have been identified that may lead to primary prevention of large bowel cancer, available data do not yet provide a firm basis for the practical application of primary preventive measures. The goal of *secondary prevention* is to identify existing preneoplastic and early neoplastic lesions and to treat them thoroughly and expeditiously. The assumption is that early detection improves prognosis. In symptomatic patients it is important to minimize diagnostic delay. When the clinical setting suggests colorectal malignant disease (e.g., iron deficiency anemia in an elderly patient), prompt diagnostic evaluation should be undertaken. This approach pertains to individuals and small groups of patients seen in daily practice and is known as *case finding*. Screening

pertains to large populations. Screening an asymptomatic population for any disease is worthwhile if (1) the disease represents a major health problem; (2) effective therapy is available if the disease is found; (3) a sensitive and specific screening test is available that is readily acceptable to patients and physicians; and (4) the screening test is cost effective.

CRC fulfills at least the first two of these conditions, because it represents a major health problem, and localized lesions are curable by surgical resection. Furthermore, the prolonged natural history of colonic neoplasia affords time to detect and eliminate early neoplastic lesions before they reach an advanced, incurable stage. The challenge that remains is to develop effective, easily administered, and cost-effective screening tests for the disease. Current evidence indicates that screening for CRC reduces related mortality. This finding has resulted in a recommendation by the United States Preventive Services Task Force (USPSTF) that screening for CRC should be performed in all persons aged 50 years and older.[82] Almost all major health-related agencies have endorsed screening for CRC (Table 120–13), but the key questions of "who, how, and how often" remain a source of debate. In 1997, the Agency for Health Care Policy Research (AHCPR) authored a 48-page document, in which they set forth clinical practice guidelines for CRC screening, offering a variety of options for CRC screening (fecal occult blood test [FOBT], sigmoidoscopy, colonoscopy, ACBE) and providing a lengthy rationale for each.[101] These guidelines were updated in 2003.[102] The American Cancer Society (ACS) followed shortly thereafter with its own set of guidelines for CRC screening and surveillance. These guidelines provided recommendations in three major categories based on risk (average, moderate, and high). Moderate- and high-risk categories were subdivided further according to personal and family history of adenoma, carcinoma, or predisposing disease. *Average risk* is defined as all people 50 years or older who do not fall

Table 120–13 Guidelines for Screening Average Risk Individuals for Colorectal Cancer

Screening Tool	U.S. Preventive Services Task Force*	Multidisciplinary Expert Panel†	American Cancer Society‡
FOBT	Recommended annually	Recommended annually	Recommended annually as an option
Flexible sigmoidoscopy	Recommended at an unspecified interval	Recommended q 5 yr as an option	Recommended q 5 yr as an option
FOBT + flexible sigmoidoscopy	Annual FOBT + flexible sigmoidoscopy (interval not specified) recommended as an option	Annual FOBT + flexible sigmoidoscopy q 5 yr recommended as an option	Annual FOBT + flexible sigmoidoscopy q 5 yr recommended as an option
Colonoscopy	Recommended as an option at an unspecified interval	Recommended as an option q 10 yr	Recommended as an option q 10 yr
Double-contrast barium enema	Recommended as an option at an unspecified interval	Recommended as an option q 5 yr	Recommended as an option q 5 yr

*U.S. Preventive Services Task Force: Screening for colorectal cancer: Recommendations and rationale. Ann Intern Med 137:129, 2002.
†Winawer S, Fletcher R, Rex D, et al: Colorectal cancer screening and surveillance: Clinical guidelines and rationale—update based on new evidence. Gastroenterology 124:544, 2003. This approach is endorsed by numerous medical and surgical societies.
‡Smith RA, Cokkinides V, Eyre HJ: American Cancer Society guidelines for early detection of cancer, 2004. CA Cancer J Clin 54:41, 2004. This approach provides a menu of options, rather than recommending any specific option, to increase compliance with screening. FOBT should be done by the "take home sample" method. All positive tests should be followed up by colonoscopy.
FOBT, fecal occult blood test.

into moderate- or high-risk categories. This category encompasses 70% to 80% of individuals in the American population.

In 2001, the ACS updated its recommendations to offer a broader set of screening choices for different levels of CRC risk,[79] thereby allowing greater flexibility in achieving screening goals. This change was deemed necessary because evidence showed little progress in improving CRC screening rates.[103] Screening options included FOBT annually, FS every 5 years, annual FOBT plus FS every 5 years, double-contrast barium enema every 5 years, or colonoscopy every 10 years (see Table 120–13). These recommendations were modified slightly in 2002 with the addition of immunochemical FOBTs. The ACS recommendations are similar to updated guidelines issued by the USPSTF.[82] The USPSTF concluded that there is fair-to-good evidence that screening methods including FOBT, FS, combined FOBT and FS, colonoscopy, and barium enema were effective methods of reducing CRC mortality. Although each of the choices has inherent characteristics related to accuracy, prevention, potential costs, and risks, the concept is that any one of the tests is better than no test at all. Multiple options can be confusing, however, to both patients and physicians. Furthermore, the test options are not of equal efficacy, and such guidelines may lead to coverage of suboptimal testing by third-party payers.

The willingness of both patients and physicians to comply with recommendations for screening programs has a major impact on the effectiveness of CRC screening. Compliance by both potential screenees and physicians historically has been poor, and interventions to increase screening adherence have been disappointing.[104] The year 2000 goals set forth by the National Cancer Institute in 1996 called for 50% of the population older than 40 years of age to have had FOBT tests within the prior 2 years, a goal that was not met. Compliance rates generally are higher for FOBT than for sigmoidoscopy. Clinical trials report compliance rates of 50% to 80% for FOBT among volunteers,[105-110] but much lower rates (15% to 30%) are reported from community screening programs.[105] Data from the 1992 National Health Interview Survey indicated that only 17% and 26% of the population older than 49 years reported having a FOBT within the past 1 and 3 years, respectively, whereas the median adherence rate to programmatic offers of the FOBT was 40% to 50%, depending on the type of population. Adherence to recommended follow-up testing after an initial positive FOBT result also may be lower in the community setting than in larger screening trials. Up to one third of people who test positive may not respond to requests for follow-up. An analysis of diagnostic testing following a positive FOBT result in elderly medicine recipients[111] indicated that not only was compliance poor but follow-up diagnostic testing often was inadequate or improper. Unfortunately, compliance is often poorer among elderly persons, who are at greatest risk for colon cancer, and among minorities in whom mortality is high. Despite the availability of FS, most elderly patients are reluctant to have this test because of cost, discomfort, and fear.

While most physicians agree in principle with guidelines for sigmoidoscopic screening, many do not follow them with all patients. Reluctance to perform what is perceived as an uncomfortable and invasive procedure in asymptomatic persons, requirements for training, and limitations of time and resources contribute to reluctance on the part of primary care physicians. Compliance also is extremely important in any determination of cost effectiveness.[105,112]

Compliance with CRC screening has a major impact on the cost effectiveness of such programs. In one model, the cost per death prevented as the result of performing FOBTs increased from $225,000 to $331,000 as compliance decreased from 100% to 50%.[105] The FOBT is especially sensitive to the impact of compliance compared with other tests.[105,112]

In the absence of firm clinical data indicating which screening strategy provides the best balance of sensitivity, specificity, logistic feasibility, and cost, various mathematical models have been employed to examine this issue.[105,112-114] The cost-effectiveness of three screening strategies (annual FOBT, sigmoidoscopy every 5 years, or colonoscopy every 10 years) was compared using a computer model of 100,000 persons 50 years of age.[112] This model takes into account the costs of follow-up events. Positive FOBT results or adenomatous polyps found at sigmoidoscopy are worked up using colonoscopy. After polypectomy, colonoscopy is repeated every 3 years until no polyps are found. This study indicated that colonoscopy represented a cost-effective means of screening for CRC because it reduces mortality at relatively low incremental costs. Compliance rates render colonoscopy every 10 years the most cost-effective primary screening strategy for CRC, according to this study. Studies reviewed by the USPSTF indicate that CRC screening is likely to be cost effective (<$30,000 per additional year of life gained) regardless of the strategy chosen.[82,114,115]

The use of screening modalities for detection of adenomatous polyps is discussed in Chapter 119. Table 120–14 presents some of the characteristics of tests used to diagnose and screen for colorectal neoplasms.

SCREENING TECHNIQUES

Fecal Occult Blood Testing

Qualitative chromogen tests, which rely on the oxidative conversion of a colorless compound to a colored one in the presence of the pseudoperoxidase activity of hemoglobin, have been standardized employing guaiac-impregnated paper and developing solutions (hydrogen peroxide in denatured alcohol) and have been widely studied and utilized clinically (e.g., Hemoccult, Hemoccult II). These tests are available commercially, convenient, and inexpensive, however, their effectiveness in detecting occult blood in the stool depends on the degree of fecal hydration (increases sensitivity), amount of hemoglobin degradation during storage or by focal flora (decreases sensitivity), and the absence of interfering substances (e.g., ascorbic acid) that can either enhance or inhibit oxidation of the indicator dye.

Any foodstuff that contains compounds with pseudoperoxidase or peroxidase activity can produce a positive FOBT reaction. Red meat and peroxidase-

Table 120–14 Diagnostic and Screening Procedures for Colorectal Polyps and Cancers

Variables	Findings (%)
Proportion of adenomatous polyps and cancers that can be detected by various instruments (%)	
Rigid sigmoidoscope	30
Flexible sigmoidoscope (60 cm)	55
Colonoscope	95
Air-contrast barium enema	92
Single-column barium enema	85
False-negative rates (%)	
FOBT	40
Sigmoidoscopy*	15
Colonoscopy	5
Air-contrast barium enema	15
Single-column barium enema	30
False-positive rates (%)	
FOBT†	2
Air-contrast barium enema	3.5
Single-column barium enema	3
Complications (%)‡	
Bleeding rate with diagnostic colonoscopy	0.15
Bleeding rate with polypectomy	2
Perforation rate with diagnostic colonoscopy	0.2
Perforation rate with polypectomy	0.38
Perforation rate with sigmoidoscopy	0.011
Cost of each procedure (U.S. $)§	
FOBT	3.50
Flexible sigmoidoscopy	400.56
Colonoscopy	695.95
Colonoscopy with polypectomy	1003.76
Air-contrast barium enema	118.86
Single-column barium enema	159.77

*Rigid sigmoidoscopy may miss two or three times as many lesions as flexible sigmoidoscopy in examining the same bowel segment.
†A false-positive FOBT result will lead to additional work-up and charges. This needs to be considered in assessing the cost of a false-positive FOBT.
‡See Chapter 39.
§Costs are based on average Medicare payments in 2000. These do not reflect actual charges at a given institution or the costs of additional evaluation after a positive test.
FOBT, fecal occult blood test.
Data from Eddy DM, Nugent FW, Eddy JW, et al: Screening for colorectal cancer in a high-risk population: Results of a mathematical model. Gastroenterology 92:682, 1987; and Sonnenberg A, Delco F, Inadomi JM: Cost effectiveness of colonoscopy in screening for colorectal cancer. Ann Intern Med 133:573, 2000.

Table 120–15 Proper Performance of the Slide Guaiac Test for Fecal Occult Blood

1. For 3 days before and during testing, patients should avoid the following:
   Rare red meat
   Peroxidase-containing vegetables and fruit (e.g., broccoli, turnip, cantaloupe, cauliflower, radish)
   Certain medications (e.g., iron supplements, vitamin C, aspirin and other NSAIDs)
2. Two samples of each of three consecutive stools should be tested. (It is proper to sample areas of obvious blood.)
3. Slides should be developed within 4-6 days. Slides should not be rehydrated prior to developing (for average-risk screening). If slides are rehydrated, red meat must have been avoided (otherwise, too many false-positive results will occur).

NSAID, nonsteroidal anti-inflammatory drug.

Table 120–16 Features of the Slide Guaiac Test for Fecal Occult Blood

Advantages
Readily available
Convenient
Inexpensive
Good compliance in motivated patients
Disadvantages
Depends on the degree of fecal hydration
Affected by storage (hemoglobin degradation may occur)
Affected by tumor location
Causes of False-Positive Tests
Exogenous peroxidase activity
Red meat (nonhuman hemoglobin)
Uncooked fruits and vegetables (vegetable peroxidase; see Table 120–15)
Any source of GI blood loss (e.g., epistaxis, gingival bleeding, upper GI tract pathology, hemorrhoids)
Certain medications (see Table 120–15)
Causes of False-Negative Tests
Storage of slides
Degradation of hemoglobin by colonic bacteria
Ascorbic acid (vitamin C) ingestion
Improper sampling/developing
Lesion not bleeding at time of stool collection

GI, gastrointestinal; NSAIDs, nonsteroidal anti-inflammatory drugs.

containing foods (broccoli, turnips, cauliflower, radishes, cantaloupes), therefore, should be avoided for 3 days before and during testing. Although a drop of water added to the slide before development (rehydration) increases sensitivity, this is not recommended for screening average-risk populations, because it gives too many false-positive results. If rehydration is considered, dietary restriction to exclude peroxidase- and heme-rich foods is especially important. Some studies report false-positive FOBT results in patients who took a supplemental iron preparation, but recent studies have reported few or no false-positive FOBT results in those patients. Recommen-

dations for proper performance of these tests are listed in Table 120–15, and the advantages and limitations of the FOBT with the Hemoccult-type slide guaiac tests are outlined in Table 120–16.

CRCs and adenomas bleed intermittently, and detection of fecal occult blood by Hemoccult testing depends on the degree of blood loss. In general, 2 mL of blood in the stool is necessary to produce a positive result. Sampling multiple stool specimens is therefore likely to result in fewer false-negative evaluations. Sampling one specimen yields a 40% to 50% false-negative rate, which improves (i.e., false-negatives decrease) progressively as more stools are sampled. Two samples of each of three consecutive (daily) stools should therefore be tested. Location of the lesion also affects the ability to detect a cancer by Hemoccult testing. Right-sided cancers produce fewer false-negative tests than cancers elsewhere in the colon, because large bulky tumors bleed frequently. Potential "blind spots" of the Hemoccult test with high false-negative rates include the transverse and descending colon. The value of a positive FOBT result performed in conjunction with a digital rectal examination has been disputed, and this FOBT method is not recommended, largely because a single examination done in this way is not nearly as sensitive as the recommended method whereby three consecutive spontaneously passed stools are tested.[116] There also will be some false-positive results because digital rectal examination usually is not done in conjunction with dietary restrictions. Rehydration of Hemoccult cards increases

sensitivity but reduces specificity, and this method is not recommended for screening.[102]

In studies that have examined the potential benefit of FOBTs for detecting colorectal neoplasms in large populations, compliance has been in the range of 50% to 70%, although elderly patients—those at substantial risk for colon cancer—tend to be less compliant. The overall positivity rate ranges from 2% to 6% of those tested, and the positive predictive value is about 20% for adenomas and 5% to 10% for cancers. Most studies report that a large percentage of detected cancers are Dukes A and B lesions.

Large controlled studies of Hemoccult testing of asymptomatic patients in the general population have been reported from the United States,[107,117] Great Britain,[106] Scandinavia,[108-110] and France (Table 120–17).[118] These studies cite a rate of test positivity of 1% to 2.6% on first

Table 120–17   Controlled Trials of FOBTs in Screening Asymptomatic People for Colorectal Cancer (CRC)[106-110,116]

Variables	Trials				
	Minnesota	*Nottingham*	*Goteborg*	*Funen*	*New York*
Study population	46,000	152,850	28,000	61,933	22,000
Age	50-80 yr	50-74 yr	60-64 yr	45-74 yr	≥40 yr
Study design	Randomized: annual vs. biennial control	Randomized	Randomized	Randomized: biennial vs. control	Allocation by month assigned
Rehydration of test cards*	Yes—most	No	Yes—most	No	No
Compliance	Annual 75%; biennial 78%	50%	—	56%	—
Positivity rate	2.4% (nonhydrated) 9.8% (rehydrated)	1st screen: 2.1% 2nd screen: 1.2%	1st screen: 1.9% (nonhydrated); 5.8% (rehydrated) 2nd screen: 4.8% (prev. rehydrated); 8.0% (prev. nonhydrated)	1st screen: 1.0% 2nd screen: 0.8% 3rd screen: 0.9% 4th screen: 1.3% 5th screen: 1.8%	Regular attendees: 1.4% 1st screen: 2.6%
Positive predictive value for CRC	2.2% (rehydrated) 5.6% (nonhydrated)	1st screen: 9.9% 2nd screen: 11.9%	1st screen: 5.0% (nonhydrated) 2nd screen: 4.2% (rehydrated)	1st screen: 17.7% 2nd screen: 8.4%	10.7%
CRC mortality†	*18-yr follow-up:* 33% reduction for the annual group, 21% reduction for biennial group *CRC mortality/ 1000:* Annual—9.46 Biennial—11.19 Control—14.09 *Mortality ratio:* Annual—0.67 Biennial—0.79	*7- to 8-yr follow-up:* 15% reduction in cumulative CRC mortality Mortality ratio: 0.85	Not yet available	*10-yr follow-up:* 18% reduction in CRC mortality in the screened group Mortality ratio: 0.82	*10-yr follow-up:* 43% reduction in CRC mortality in the screened group

*Hemoccult test cards were used—rehydrated or nonhydrated.
†Reductions in mortality are relative risk reductions. A French trial using biennial FOBTs yielded a 16% reduction in CRC-related mortality in the screened group. The mortality ratio was 0.84 (confidence interval, 0.71-0.99) with 11 years of follow-up.[117]
FOBT, fetal occult blood test; prev., previously.

screen for nonhydrated slides and a predictive value for colonic neoplasms (adenomas plus carcinomas) of 22% to 58%. The positive predictive value for carcinomas alone is substantially less (5.6% to 18% for nonhydrated slides). Rehydration of slides with a drop of water before processing results in an increase in positivity and sensitivity but in a decrease in specificity and positive predictive value. Eighteen-year follow-up in the Minnesota trial[117] demonstrated a marked reduction in Dukes stage D cancers in the screened groups compared with the control group. Long-term follow-up of patients tested with Hemoccult in a large group practice setting (Kaiser-Permanente) yielded similar results. The predictive value of a positive test for colorectal carcinoma was 8% at 1 year, 10% at 2 years, and 11% at 4 years. Predictive value depends on what group is screened, and it may be increased in older age groups.

Mortality data are available from the Minnesota Study, a randomized, controlled trial that has provided the best evidence for the effectiveness of screening with FOBT.[107,117] After 13 years of follow-up, data indicate a 33% reduction in CRC-associated mortality with annual screening but an insignificant reduction of approximately 5% with biannual screening.[107] Approximately 80% of samples were rehydrated, yielding a high positivity rate of 9.8% (compared with 2.4% for nonhydrated slides). This resulted in a 38% rate of colonoscopy, leading some to suggest that a substantial portion of the mortality reduction resulted from chance detection through colonoscopy of nonbleeding cancers. This challenge has been refuted by the investigators, who find that only 6% to 11% of the mortality reduction was explained by chance detection.

Results of 18 years of follow-up now have been reported.[117] Cumulative 18-year CRC mortality remains 33% lower in the annual group than in the control group. The group tested with biennial screening now demonstrates a 21% lower CRC mortality than did the control group. Other randomized studies reported similar results. Data from Funen, Denmark, suggest an 18% decrease in CRC mortality during a 10-year study period,[108] and data from Nottingham, UK, also indicate a 15% reduction in mortality at 7.8 years' follow-up.[106] Data from New York suggest a 43% reduction in mortality in the screened group at 10 years.[119] A randomized French trial[117] also demonstrated a reduction in CRC mortality with biennial FOBT screening compared with a control population (mortality ratio, 0.84; 95% confidence interval, 0.71-0.99) in 11 years of follow-up; reduction is mortality was more pronounced in compliant individuals (mortality ratio, 0.67; 95% confidence interval, 0.56-0.81).

Methods that may decrease the false-positive FOBT rates while maintaining or increasing sensitivity currently are being refined and compared for efficiency with Hemoccult-type slide tests. Fecal immunochemical tests (FITs) are designed to detect human globin and are not affected by diet or drugs. One FIT, HemeSelect, showed good performance characteristics compared with standard heme-based FOBT tests in early studies and was used in a combination test to confirm positive Hemoccult Sensa (a sensitive guaiac-based test similar to Hemoccult) in a large managed care setting.[120] More recently, a FIT using a brush-based sampling technique and an immuno-gold membrane, which uses a dual antibody system specific for human hemoblobin, has undergone initial evaluation. Strategies that use an immunochemical-based FOBT have been shown to be cost-effective when used for colorectal cancer screening in Japan.

Proctosigmoidoscopy

The benefit of proctosigmoidoscopy in screening programs for CRC was suggested by several uncontrolled studies that used rigid proctosigmoidoscopy. Those studies suggested that proctosigmoidoscopy in asymptomatic average-risk persons might detect early-stage cancers and that detection and removal of adenomas could result in a lower than expected frequency of rectosigmoid cancers in the screened population.

Two case-control studies provided strong evidence that sigmoidoscopy can reduce CRC mortality. A study from the Kaiser-Permanente Medical Care Program[121] compared 261 members who died of cancer of the rectum or distal colon with 868 age- and sex-matched control subjects. Only 8.8% of case subjects had undergone screening by rigid sigmoidoscopy, compared with 24.2% of controls. Rigid sigmoidoscopy had no effect on mortality in another group whose lesions were beyond the reach of the sigmoidoscope. Furthermore, the beneficial effect of sigmoidoscopy extended 10 years. This and a second case-control study[122] indicate that sigmoidoscopy can result in a 70% to 80% reduction in mortality from cancers within reach of the sigmoidoscope. Because approximately 50% of all CRCs can be detected using the 60-cm flexible sigmoidoscope (see Fig. 120–3), these data suggest that periodic sigmoidoscopic screening could reduce overall CRC-related mortality by about one third. Because the flexible sigmoidoscope is superior to rigid instruments in detecting lesions, the flexible sigmoidoscope has replaced the rigid sigmoidoscope for CRC screening. A case-control study using FS and polypectomy[123] demonstrated a 60% reduction in colon cancer incidence associated with this procedure. Randomized, controlled trials are now underway to measure the effect of screening with FS on CRC mortality.[98,124] FS can be learned by nonphysicians and has been used successfully in screening programs that employ nurse practitioners[125]; wide variations in adenoma detection rates were observed, however, in the UK Flexible Sigmoidoscopy Screening Trial.[124] The PLCO study has enrolled 155,000 individuals in a recent prospective, randomized trial that compares FS to a usual-care control group.[98,126] Follow-up is planned through 2015 with cancer-related mortality as the major end point.

Colonoscopy, Barium Enema, and CT Colonography

Colonoscopy may well be the most effective tool for CRC screening, but data from prospective, randomized trials are lacking. The National Polyp Study of polypectomy and surveillance strongly suggested a reduction in CRC mortality as the result of removing adenomatous polyps.[127] It has been argued that colonoscopy is preferable to sigmoidoscopy, because there may be a substantial incidence of proximal colonic cancers and advanced adenomas beyond the reach of the sigmoidoscope.[128-131] Some of these individuals may not have distal findings on sigmoidoscopy that would trigger a subsequent colonoscopy. Two trials[130,131] suggested that approximately 50% of individuals with advanced proximal neoplasms (adenoma >1 cm; adenoma with villous features or dysplasia; cancer) have no distal neoplasms. Less than 2% of those who did not have distal neoplasms, however, had an advanced proximal lesion.[130] Given the need for colonoscopic follow-up, should FOBT or sigmoidoscopy be positive, colonoscopy may also prove to be cost-effective.[112]

ACBE has been included as an option in a variety of screening guidelines. No studies, however, have directly addressed the effectiveness of barium enema for colon cancer screening. Several studies have indicated that the sensitivity of ACBE is less than that of colonoscopy,[99,100] especially for detecting lesions less than 1 cm.

Computed tomography (CT) colonography, or "virtual" colonoscopy, involves the use of helical CT to generate high-resolution, two-dimensional images of the abdomen and pelvis. Three-dimensional images of the colon can be reconstructed by computer generation off-line (Figs. 120–24 and 120–25).[132,133] CT colonography has the potential advantage of being a rapid and safe method of providing full structural evaluation of the entire colon. Low sensitivity and specificity and the need for rapid high-resolution helical CT scanners have precluded its wide application for routine CRC screening, but software and techniques designed to improve the speed, accuracy, and reproducibility of results are emerging. Recognition of the importance of CRC screening has raised concerns over the ability of existing resources to handle

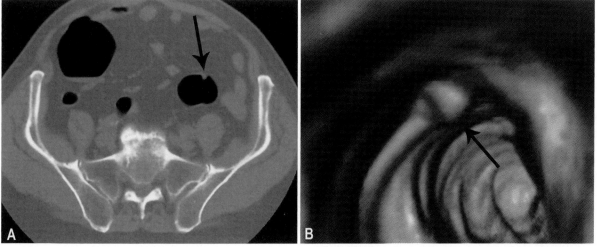

Figure 120–24 CT colonography (virtual colonoscopy). An 8-mm sigmoid polyp identified on an axial two-dimensional computed tomography (CT) image of the colon (*A, arrow*), and on an endoluminal three-dimensional reconstruction (*B*).

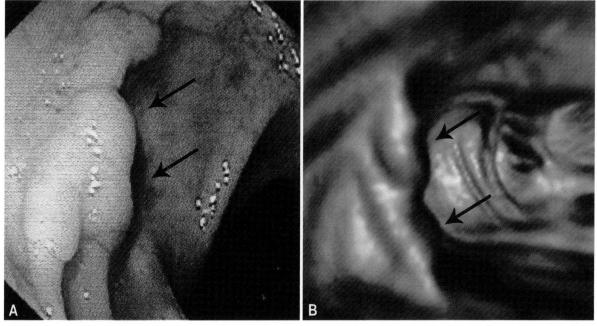

Figure 120–25 Representative views of a 2 cm sessile colon lesion seen on a fold. Lesion seen at colonoscopy (*A*) and on three-dimensional reconstruction (*B*).

the ensuing volume of expected procedures such as colonoscopy. CT colonography using CT or magnetic resonance imaging (MRI) could represent an alternate method with promise for the future.

The accuracy and potential of CT colonography as a screening tool for colorectal neoplasia has been hotly debated because initial studies yielded a wide range of sensitivity.[132-137] Two large recently published multicenter trials continued to fuel this controversy. One trial included 1233 asymptomatic individuals who underwent same-day virtual and optical colononoscopy.[136] This study employed multidetector CT scanners, three-dimensional endoluminal displays, and solid stool tagging and opacification of luminal fluid ("optical cleansing"). It demonstrated sufficiently high sensitivity (89% to 94%) and specificity (80% to 96%) for detecting polyps across a broad range of size categories (>6 to >10 mm) to warrant serious consideration as an option for screening. A second study of 600 individuals[137] reported a sensitivity for detecting even large polyps (55%) far below that of optical colonoscopy but used different technology and methods of analysis compared with the first study. Several key issues need to be addressed as the use of CT colonography becomes more widespread, principal among which is determination of the acceptable size cut-off of a lesion detected by CT colonography that will necessitate a follow-up colonoscopy. Other issues include the need for bowel preparation, the logistics of same-day colonoscopy, the ability to detect flat lesions, the impact on compliance, and cost-effectiveness. Methodologies that employ CT colonography without cathartic preparation and with "fecal tagging"[132] may make this a more attractive option for screening. CT colonography may also aid in detecting lesions located behind folds or near the anal verge.[138]

CARCINOEMBRYONIC ANTIGEN AND OTHER TUMOR MARKERS

A great deal of effort has been spent in search of serologic markers that would permit early detection and diagnosis of CRC. A variety of proteins, glycoproteins, and cellular and humoral substances have been studied as potential tumor markers, but none has been found specific for CRC. The most widely studied marker, CEA, may be useful in the preoperative staging and postoperative follow-up of patients with large bowel cancer, but it has a low predictive value for diagnosis in asymptomatic patients. The test's relatively low sensitivity and specificity combine to make it unsuitable for screening large asymptomatic populations. Several new protein and carbohydrate antigens are being examined and hold some promise in terms of specificity for preneoplastic and early neoplastic lesions in the colon[71,74]; their effectiveness for screening, however, remains to be determined. Promising approaches using genomic or proteomic techniques applied to biomarker discovery are being pursued that may result in practical clinical tests. One such approach involves the study of candidate genes or proteins assembled into panels of markers. Another "discovery-based approach" uses high through-put techniques that allow simultaneous assessment of tens of thousands of genes or proteins.[139]

GENETIC TESTING

A great deal of knowledge has been accumulated recently about genetic alterations that occur during colon carcinogenesis (discussed earlier), but specific tests are not currently available for most patients at risk for developing sporadic CRC. A molecular approach to CRC screening is attractive since it targets biologic changes that are fundamental to the neoplastic process. The feasibility of detecting altered DNA in stool has been demonstrated using a multitarget assay panel of molecular markers.[140] A recent multicenter study compared fecal DNA testing using such a panel with the FOBT and colonoscopy.[141] The fecal DNA panel consisted of 21 mutations: 3 in the K-ras gene, 10 in the APC gene, 8 in the p53 gene; the MSI marker BAT-26; and a marker of long DNA thought to reflect disordered apoptosis of cancer cells sloughed into the colonic lumen. Although most of the lesions identified by colonoscopy were not detected by either noninvasive test, multitargeted fecal DNA testing detected a higher proportion of important lesions compared with Hemoccult.

Genetic testing is now a reality for families with FAP (see Chapter 119).[78] Testing for altered products of the APC gene allows for early and accurate identification of family members at risk who require intensive surveillance. Proper genetic counseling, however, must be incorporated into the screening process.[58] Genetic testing for mutations in the hMSH2 and hMLH1 genes is appropriate when HNPCC is suspected but presents more difficulty than screening for FAP, because not all the genes involved have been identified, and the preferred method by which families should be screened has yet to be determined.[76,142] A generally accepted approach in individuals suspected of having HNPCC based on clinical criteria is first to perform MSI testing on the affected individual's tumor using a panel of microsatellite markers. Germline mutation testing for hMLH1 and hMSH2 is performed if the tumor is MSI-high (suggesting a mutation in an MMR gene). In cases in which HNPCC is strongly suspected based on clinical criteria, or when a mutation is established in a family member, germline testing is performed as a first step. If testing for hMLH1 and hMSH2 is negative, but HNPCC is strongly suspected, germline testing for hMSH6 can be performed. An allele of APC designated I1307K[143] is relatively infrequent in the general population but common in the Jewish population of Ashkenazi descent. There is a modest increase in the relative risk for CRC in those with this allele, but the penetrance for CRC is low compared with carrier frequencies, and genetic testing for I1307K is not recommended.

APPROACH TO SCREENING

Screening and case-finding approaches are different for patients in average-risk (>age 50 years) and high-risk groups. The latter group includes patients with long-standing UC, previous CRC, previous adenomas, female genital cancer, familial polyposis, HNPCC, and familial colon cancer. Data on the risk of CRC in women with a history of breast cancer are too limited at present to draw firm conclusions regarding appropriate screening intervals.

Average-Risk Group

Patients registered in a health care system should be categorized according to risk, so that appropriate screening can be added to other variables of medical evaluation. Relative risk should be assessed by family history and by personal history using questionnaires. A variety of options are available for screening average-risk individuals (≥50 years of age with no personal or family history of colorectal adenoma or carcinoma, and no personal history of IBD). These have been discussed previously, including guidelines from various health care agencies (see Table 120–13). Although yearly FOBTs or FS every 5 years is an individual option, it has been suggested that combining the two tests can increase the benefits of either test alone. The tests are complementary because the FOBT has the potential for detecting occult blood from a lesion anywhere in the colon, whereas FS can detect bleeding and nonbleeding lesions distal to the splenic flexure.

Colonoscopy every 10 years has the advantages of examining the entire colon and rectum and providing the opportunity to biopsy or remove lesions should they be found. Growing evidence indicates that colonoscopy is a cost-effective option with an acceptable risk profile. Several trials are now underway to examine colonoscopy for average-risk screening. A diagnostic evaluation is indicated for individuals with a positive FOBT result or distal neoplasm (adenoma, carcinoma) found at sigmoidoscopy. Colonoscopy is the diagnostic modality of choice. If colonoscopy is unavailable, not feasible, or not desired by the patient, double-contrast barium enema alone or in combination with FS is an acceptable alternative for evaluation of a positive FOBT result.

Screening should be accompanied by programs that educate patients and heighten physicians' awareness of the concepts and technologies involved in screening, diagnosis, treatment, and follow-up. The popular misconceptions that CRC is an incurable disease and that surgical intervention invariably leads to an impaired lifestyle, owing to a colostomy, must be discredited.

High-Risk Groups

Familial Adenomatous Polyposis and Familial Cancer

Screening of family members in kindreds with familial polyposis is discussed in Chapter 119. Screening should include genetic testing to detect abnormal (truncated) *APC* gene products if a diagnosis can be made by this method in one family member. Those who test positive should have annual or biannual FS, beginning at puberty, to assess for emergence of adenomas and to plan appropriate timing for colectomy. If genetic testing is unavailable, annual FS should begin at puberty. Genetic testing should always be combined with education and counseling of the individual as well as family members.

Patients with a family history of HNPCC must be examined colonoscopically, beginning at age 25 years, or at an age 5 years younger than that of the index case, because one cannot rely only on the FOBT in these very-high-risk patients. A reasonable approach is to perform colonoscopy every 2 years.[144] The search is primarily for the scattered adenomas that antedate carcinomas in these syndromes, and, for detection, colonoscopy is more sensitive than radiologic contrast studies. Genetic testing for HNPCC is now being introduced into clinical practice.[64,76,142] Genetic testing should be accompanied by counseling of the individual and the family members. The benefits of colonoscopic surveillance in patients with HNPCC mutations are suggested by screening trials.[145]

The approach to patients with a suggestive family history (e.g., one first-degree relative with colon cancer) is not firmly established. Whether these patients should be monitored in the same way as average-risk patients or be screened more rigorously remains to be determined. Some studies suggest that evidence supporting the use of colonoscopy as the first step in screening persons with one first-degree relative with CRC is insufficient, but other recent studies indicate that the risk may be sufficient to recommend colonoscopy, especially if adenoma or cancer in the index case occurred before age 60 years or if two first-degree relatives had an adenoma or cancer at any age. The ACS recommends that if CRC or adenomatous polyps occurred in any first-degree relative before age 60 years, or in two or more first-degree relatives at any age, then colonoscopy should be performed every 5 to 10 years, beginning at age 40 years, or 10 years before the youngest case in the immediate family.[80] In those with more than two affected first-degree relatives, special care should be taken to exclude the diagnosis of HNPCC, and periodic colonoscopy is advised.

Prior Adenomas or Colon Cancer

Table 120–18 lists the updated (2001) ACS guidelines for screening, surveillance, and early detection of colorectal adenomas and cancer for individuals at increased risk or at high risk of disease.[80] Although most of the ACS guidelines are in keeping with those of other agencies, surveillance of individuals with a personal history of adenomatous polyps deserves mention. The ACS suggests that those whose index lesion is a single adenoma less than 1 cm should have a follow-up colonoscopy 3 to 6 years after the initial polypectomy. If the examination is normal, the patient can be screened as per average-risk guidelines. In those with a large (>1 cm) adenoma, multiple adenomas, or adenomas with high-grade dysplasia or villous change, colonoscopy should be repeated within 3 years after the initial polypectomy. If normal, the examination should be repeated once again in 3 years. If it remains normal, then the patient can thereafter be screened as per average-risk guidelines. The guidelines for the latter group differ somewhat from previous ACS guidelines[79] and what is often practiced (colonoscopy 3 years after removal of an adenoma; if negative, colonoscopy every 5 years). Whether these guidelines will become standard practice remains to be determined. A discussion of surveillance of patients with a personal history of adenomas is provided in Chapter 119, and the

Table 120–18   Guidelines for the Surveillance of Cancer in People at Increased or High Risk

Risk Category	Age to Begin Surveillance	Recommendation	Comment
Increased Risk			
People with single, small (<1 cm) adenoma	3-6 yr after initial polypectomy	Colonoscopy*	If normal, patient can thereafter be screened as per guidelines for an average-risk person
People with a large (≥1 cm) adenoma, multiple adenomas, or adenomas with high-grade dysplasia or villous change	Within 3 yr after initial polypectomy	Colonoscopy*	If normal, repeat examination in 3 yr; if normal, the patient can thereafter be screened as per average risk guidelines
Personal history of curative-intent resection of colorectal cancer	Within 1 yr after cancer resection	Colonoscopy*	If normal, repeat examination in 3 yr; if normal, repeat examination q 5 yr
Either colorectal cancer or adenomatous polyps in any first-degree relative before age 60 yr, or in ≥2 first-degree relatives at any age (if not a hereditary syndrome)	Age 40 yr, or 10 yr before the age of the youngest case in the immediate family (whichever is sooner)	Colonoscopy*	Every 5-10 yr; colorectal cancer in relatives more distant than first-degree does not increase risk substantially above the average-risk group
High Risk			
Family history of FAP	Puberty	Early surveillance with flexible sigmoidoscopy, and counseling to consider genetic testing	If the genetic test is positive, colectomy is indicated; these patients are best referred to a center with experience in FAP management
Family history of HNPCC	Age 21 yr	Colonoscopy and counseling to consider genetic testing	If the genetic test is positive or if the patient has not had genetic testing, q 1-2 yr until age 40 yr, then annually; these patients are best referred to a center with experience in HNPCC management
Inflammatory bowel disease (ulcerative colitis; Crohn's colitis)	Cancer risk becomes significant 8 yr after the onset of pancolitis, or 12-15 yr after the onset of left-sided colitis	Colonoscopy with biopsies for dysplasia	Every 1-2 yr; these patients are best referred to a center with experience in inflammatory bowel disease surveillance and management

*If colonoscopy is unavailable, not feasible, or not desired by the patient, double-contrast barium enema (DCBE) alone, or the combination of flexible sigmoidoscopy and DCBE, is an acceptable alternative. The role of CT colonography as an alternative is being studied. Adding flexible sigmoidoscopy to DCBE may provide a more comprehensive diagnostic evaluation than DCBE alone in finding significant lesions. A supplementary DCBE may be needed if a colonoscopic examination fails to reach the cecum, and a supplementary colonoscopy may be needed if a DCBE identifies a possible lesion or does not adequately visualize the entire colorectum.
FAP, familial adenomatous polyposis; HNPCC, hereditary nonpolyposis colorectal cancer.
From Smith RA, von Eschenbach AC, Wender R, et al: American Cancer Society Guidelines for early detection guidelines for prostate, colorectal, and endometrial cancers. CA Cancer J Clin 1:51, 2001.

reader is referred there for a more detailed discussion of surveillance in this group.

Patients who have had a colon cancer resected should have colonoscopy performed 6 months to 1 year after surgery, followed by colonoscopy in 3 years. If the results are negative, colonoscopy should then be performed every 5 years (see Table 120–18). Serum CEA levels should be measured at regular intervals because postoperative CEA determinations may be cost-effective for detecting recurrent cancers. How long an asymptomatic patient who has had multiple negative examinations should be tested by various modalities is at present unclear. It should be noted that these recommendations are to some extent "educated guesses," and not all are based on prospective, randomized trials.

Inflammatory Bowel Disease

The appropriate surveillance schedule for patients with IBD has not been determined in long-term prospective trials. Colonoscopy combined with mucosal biopsy may be effective in detecting preneoplastic and early neoplastic lesions in patients with UC. The current recommendation is for colonoscopy every 1 or 2 years for patients who have had universal colitis for 8 years or left-sided UC for 12 to 15 years (see Table 120–18) (Fig. 120–26). Biopsies should be taken throughout the colon at 10-cm intervals, with special attention to areas that suggest a DALM. Although this biopsy procedure enables histology of only a small area of the colon, the short-term risk of carcinoma for patients with a negative biopsy is low. If dysplasia is high-grade or associated with a macroscopic lesion or

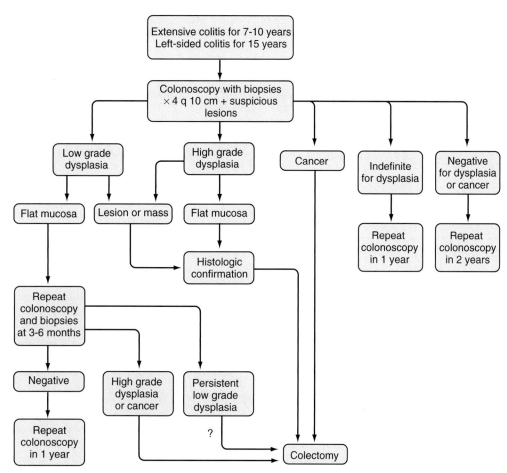

Figure 120–26 Algorithm for colonoscopic surveillance of patients with ulcerative colitis. "Histologic confirmation" refers to agreement by a second experienced pathologist that the biopsy specimen meets the criteria for dysplasia as defined by the Inflammatory Bowel Disease Dysplasia Morphology Study Group. (Modified from Ahnen DJ: Dysplasia and chronic ulcerative colitis. In Rustgi A [ed]: Gastrointestinal Cancers: Biology, Diagnosis, and Therapy. Philadelphia, JB Lippincott, 1995, p 399.)

mass, colectomy is recommended. A histologic diagnosis of low-grade dysplasia merits endoscopic follow-up at short intervals (e.g., at 3 to 6 months) as does an "indeterminate" reading resulting from active inflammation. Colectomy has been advocated by some for confirmed low-grade dysplasia. Patients with Crohn's disease of the colon should be evaluated endoscopically as dictated by symptoms, and special attention should be paid to strictured areas. Studies suggest a role for surveillance colonoscopy.[95]

INSURANCE COVERAGE FOR SCREENING

Based on evidence from several randomized trials, the Health Care Financing Administration (HCFA) decided to provide coverage for colon cancer screening procedures to medical beneficiaries beginning January 1, 1998. Coverage for average-risk individuals includes an annual FOBT and FS every 4 years. Barium enema is included as an option every 4 years in place of FS, after written justification. Colonoscopy is covered every 2 years for "high-risk" individuals (family history of CRC, personal history of adenoma or carcinoma, history of IBD, positivity for a recognized genetic marker of inherited CRC). After intense lobbying by several groups, Medicare now provides coverage for screening colonoscopy in average-risk individuals every 10 years or at an interval 4 years from

a previous sigmoidoscopy. This bill was signed December 21, 2000, and coverage was initiated July 1, 2001. Legislation requiring private insurers to cover CRC screening for any participant or beneficiary older than 50 years of age or those younger than 50 years who are at high risk for developing CRC has been adopted by 18 states. The American Gastroenterological Association and the Entertainment Industry Foundation's National CRC Research Alliance have issued the 2004 CRC Screening Legislation Report Card that analyzes the varied and complex state laws governing insurance for preventive CRC screening. The frequency of screenings complies with current Medicare CRC screening regulations.

SCREENING CAPACITY

It has been estimated that only half of the eligible U.S. population has been screened for CRC according to recommended guidelines. Efforts to increase compliance and screening recommendations should take into account the capacity to utilize various tests for screening and surveillance. A recent survey by the Centers for Disease Control and Prevention estimated that approximately 2.8 million FSs and 14.2 million colonoscopies were performed in the United States in 2002.[146] Physicians reported the capacity to perform an additional 6.7 million FS procedures and 8.2 million colonoscopies in 1 year. A forecasting model[147] using data from the U.S.

Census Bureau and Centers for Disease Control and Prevention survey indicated that capacity currently exists for widespread screening with the FOBT. The capacity for screening FS or colonoscopy depends on the proportion of available capacity used for CRC screening. Surveillance colonoscopy needs to be used appropriately as the availability of endoscopic resources decreases. A national survey of colorectal surveillance after polypectomy suggests that resources are being taxed by inappropriate surveillance practices that do not conform to current guidelines.[148] Risk stratification will become increasingly necessary as resources become limited.[149] Alternate screening modalities such as CT colonography may reduce demand for endoscopic procedures when used to screen low-risk groups but will result in increased demand for individuals trained in these techniques. The ability of CT colonography to reduce the demand for colonoscopy will also depend on the polyp size which generates a follow-up colonoscopy. Fecal DNA testing could increase compliance and reduce the need for screening colonoscopy if tests were sensitive and specific.[150] Currently available tests, however, do not perform well compared to colonoscopy.[141]

TREATMENT

SURGERY

Surgical resection is the treatment of choice for most CRCs. Preoperative colonoscopy should be performed, if possible, to rule out synchronous lesions, and serum CEA should be measured for staging and informed postoperative follow-up. Preoperative CT can be valuable for the evaluation of focal hepatic metastases if partial hepatectomy or regional hepatic artery infusion of chemotherapeutic agents is contemplated. CT also is useful for postoperative detection of pelvic recurrence in patients with rectosigmoid tumors. Transrectal ultrasonography is of value in the preoperative assessment of patients with rectal cancer.

The goal of surgery is wide resection of the involved segment of bowel, together with removal of its lymphatic drainage (Fig. 120–27). The extent of colonic resection is determined by the blood supply and distribution of regional lymph nodes. The resection should include a segment of colon at least 5 cm on either side of the tumor, although wider margins often are included because of obligatory ligation of the arterial blood supply. Extensive "super-radical" colonic and lymph node resection does not increase survival over that associated with segmental resection, and it increases morbidity. Minimally invasive laparoscopically assisted surgery may be an acceptable alternative to open surgery for colon cancer in selected patients.[150]

The approach toward rectal cancers depends on the location of the lesion. For lesions of the rectosigmoid and upper rectum, low anterior resection can be performed through an abdominal incision and primary anastomosis accomplished (Fig. 120–27F). Surgical treatment of rectal cancer should employ total mesorectal excision. This technique involves sharp dissection to create an avascular plane between the rectum, mesorectum (tissue surrounding the rectum which contains lymphatics and vascular structures), and the pelvic side wall. Using sharp dissection, the rectum and mesorectum can be delivered as a single unit. Mesorectal excision is associated with a lower local recurrence rate compared with blunt dissection of the rectum away from surrounding structures. Even for low rectal lesions, a sphincter-saving resection can be performed safely if a distal margin of at least 2 cm of normal bowel can be resected below the lesion, a goal now facilitated by end-to-end stapling devices. Tumor recurrence and survival are similar after sphincter-saving resections for rectal cancer and abdominoperineal resection (APR), if a 2-cm distal margin can be preserved in the former. The inability to obtain an adequate distal margin; the presence of a large, bulky tumor deep within the pelvis; and extensive local spread of rectal cancer all dictate the need for APR in which the distal sigmoid, rectosigmoid, rectum, and anus are removed through a combined abdominal and perineal approach and a permanent sigmoid colostomy is established.

In a patient with CRC, the primary tumor generally should be resected, even in the presence of distant metastases, to prevent obstruction or bleeding. In patients with advanced disease and multiple medical problems, repeated palliative fulguration of rectal tumors may be preferable to surgery. Modalities such as laser photoablation and argon plasma coagulation represent alternative means of palliation in these patients. Polypoid carcinomas may be removed endoscopically by snare polypectomy techniques (endoluminal resection).

Several studies indicate that although the age and physiologic status of a patient may affect operative mortality, advanced age per se does not affect tumor-associated mortality after surgery. Therefore, resection of cancer should not be limited or denied on the basis of age alone.

Postsurgical Follow-up

The incidence of recurrent colon cancer after surgical resection is high in persons who have serosal penetration or lymph node involvement by tumor. In addition, the incidence of metachronous CRC is 1.1% to 4.7%. Optimal strategies for surveillance after curative-intent surgery remain uncertain. It is not clear how often, or by what means, a patient should be evaluated following an apparently successful resection for cure. Colonoscopy is beneficial in the detection and removal of synchronous and metachronous adenomatous polyps in high-risk groups. History and physical examination, combined with CEA determinations at regular intervals, may provide a cost-effective benefit for detecting recurrent cancers. The sensitivity for detecting early recurrences is about 61% using either CT or CEA, but CT can be especially useful in examining the pelvis for recurrence after resection of rectosigmoid tumors. CT portography is an accurate method for detecting liver metastases if liver resection is considered. Immunoscintigraphy after administration of radiolabeled monoclonal antibodies raised against various tumor antigens, including CEA, may provide clinically significant information in staging patients prior to surgery or in detection of recurrent disease, but use of this modality has not been standard-

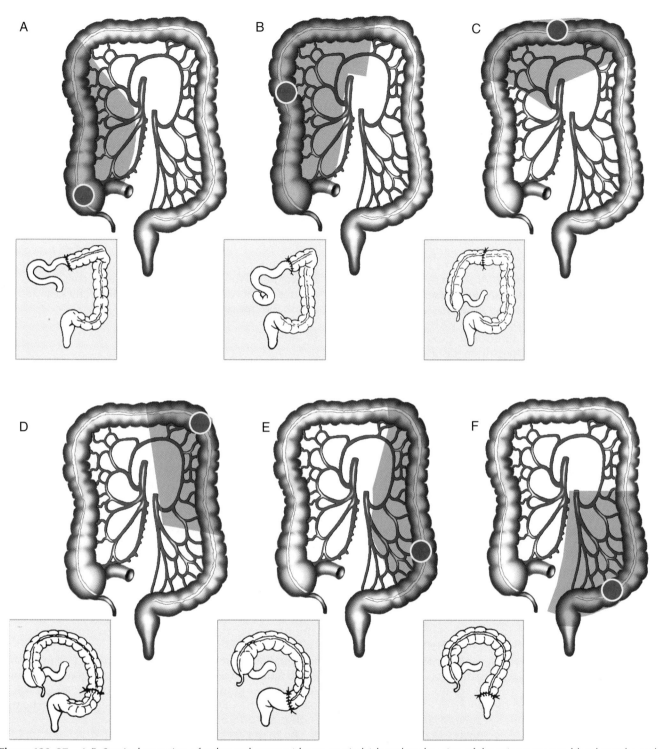

Figure 120–27   *A-F,* Surgical resection of colorectal cancer (shown as circle) based on location of the primary tumor, blood supply, and lymphatic drainage. Inset shows anatomy after resection of the tumor and anastomosis. (From Schrock T: Large intestine. In Way LW [ed]: Current Surgical Diagnosis and Treatment, 10th ed. New York, Lange, 1994.)

ized. The role of positron emission tomographic (PET) scanning currently is being evaluated. Magnetic resonance imaging (MRI) ultimately may produce the clearest delineation of hepatic metastases. Intraoperative ultrasonography (IOUS) now is being used to increase the ability to detect small and deep hepatic lesions that are not palpable during surgery.

Serial CEA determinations have been used to direct "second-look" surgical procedures. Measuring CEA levels at least every 2 months for the first 2 years after resection, and then every 4 months for the next 3 years, yields a small percentage of patients (≈5%) for whom CEA-directed second-look operations for recurrent carcinoma may be indicated. Survival following second-look procedures is high when surgeons have specialized training in oncologic surgery, but other surgeons have had more limited success, and long-term survival data are lacking. The concept of CEA-directed second-look laparotomy has been applied to resection of localized hepatic metastases.

Guidelines for colorectal surveillance after primary surgery with curative intent have been produced by a number of agencies.[151] All emphasize the importance of bowel surveillance with colonoscopy preoperatively, perioperatively, and at subsequent intervals. Other testing is not uniformly recommended or is recommended as dictated by symptoms or other findings.

Resection of Hepatic Metastases

The most common site of distant metastases from CRC is the liver. Synchronous metastases to the liver are evident at initial presentation in 10% to 25% of patients with colon cancer, and 40% to 70% of those whose cancers disseminate have hepatic involvement. Some 70% to 80% of hepatic metastases appear within 2 years after primary resection. The uniformly poor prognosis for patients with untreated hepatic metastases underlies an aggressive approach.[152,153] Hepatic resection is therefore recommended for certain candidates with hepatic metastasis from CRC. Candidates for resection of hepatic lesions are those whose primary tumor has been resected with curative intent and in whom where is no evidence of extrahepatic disease. The extent of liver involvement that is deemed resectable varies from tumor involving one lobe of the liver to focal disease in multiple lobes. The percentage of "resectable" liver metastases therefore varies in different series from 4.5% to 11% (5% to 6% in most series).

Modern techniques of anatomic dissection and hemostasis have resulted in operative mortality of about 2% in highly trained hands. Dissections along nonanatomic lines have permitted the resection of multiple lesions that previously might have been considered unresectable. Improved preoperative imaging, routine use of IOUS, application of new surgical techniques, and improved perioperative care have increased the number of patients undergoing successful hepatic resections for isolated hepatic metastases. Overall 5-year survival rates range from 20% to 45% in selected patients. The literature is difficult to interpret, however, because staging often is not uniform, and prospective controls are lacking. Furthermore, reported 2- and 3-year survival rates may not be valid, because recent data suggest that patients with unresected solitary liver lesions live at least 3 years. Long-term survival for those who undergo surgical resection of hepatic metastases depends on the absence of extrahepatic disease and adequate surgical margins. In some series, the stage of the primary lesion also is a significant prognostic variable. It is not evident whether patients with a solitary focus of metastasis live longer after resection than those who undergo resection of multiple metastases in the same lobe. It is clear, however, that patients with bilobar metastases are at increased risk for recurrence of metastasis in the liver after resection and that resection should not be attempted when more than four hepatic lesions are present. In patients whose tumor recurs after

hepatic resection, the liver is the initial site of recurrence in about 35%. Repeat hepatic resection for isolated metastases can result in long-term survival in selected persons. Improved survival after pulmonary resection of metastases from CRC has also been reported. Patients with up to three nodules in the lung who are surgical candidates should be considered for resection. Combined pulmonary and hepatic resection of metastatic disease has been used in selected cases.

Cryotherapy is a technique by which rapid freezing results in crystal formation with significant cellular damage and cell death. Tumors are frozen rapidly by means of a probe with IOUS guidance, so that malignant lesions can be ablated while the remaining liver tissue is preserved.[154] Radiofrequency ablation involves the use of radiofrequency energy to produce tissue destruction.[151] This is often done during an open surgical procedure employing ultrasound-guided needle electrodes that are inserted into the tumor. These are alternative approaches to treatment in patients whose liver metastases are unsuitable for surgical resection.

CHEMOTHERAPY

Adjuvant Chemotherapy

The prognosis for patients with CRC who undergo potentially curative surgery is correlated strongly with the stage of the primary tumor at surgery. Despite resection of all macroscopic tumor, patients whose primary tumor has penetrated the serosa or is associated with regional lymph node metastases at the time of surgery have high recurrence rates (Fig. 120–28; see also Table 120–9). The risk of relapse following surgery ranges from 20% to 30% for stage II disease to 50% to 80% for stage III disease. Patients who undergo aggressive surgical resection of isolated hepatic or pulmonary metastases also have high tumor recurrence rates in the liver, lung, and elsewhere. An effective adjuvant program to eradicate microscopic tumor foci is needed for such high-risk patients, who number 35,000 to 40,000 each year in the United States. The principle behind such adjuvant therapy is that treatment is most effective when tumor burden is minimal and cell kinetics are optimal. Data from numerous studies have now demonstrated delays in tumor recurrence and increases in survival for specific groups of patients with CRC who have received adjuvant therapy within 8 weeks of surgery.

The major advance in the adjuvant treatment of CRC came with the results of trials that explored the combination of 5-fluorouracil (5-FU) and levamisole. A large study assessed the benefit of this regimen in 1296 patients with resected colon cancer that either was locally invasive (Dukes B2; stage II) or had regional lymph node involvement (Dukes C; stage III). Therapy with 5-FU plus levamisole reduced the relative risk of cancer recurrence by 42%, and the overall death rate by 33% compared with surgery alone in patients with stage III disease. The results in patients with stage II disease were equivocal and too preliminary to allow firm conclusions to be drawn. Levamisole alone, the mechanism of action of which is not clearly understood, had no detectable effect. Data on all

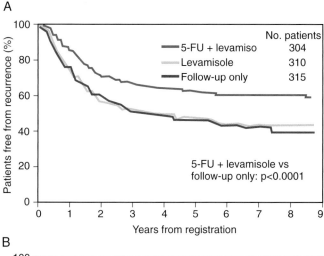

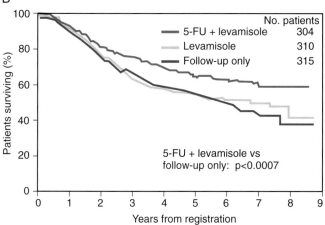

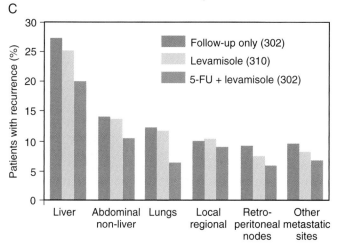

Figure 120–28   Adjuvant therapy of colon cancer in patients with Dukes C (stage III) disease. Effects of therapy with levamisole and 5-fluorouracil (5-FU) on tumor recurrence (*A*) and survival (*B*). *C*, Patterns of recurrence according to treatment arm. (From Moertel CG, Fleming TR, MacDonald JS, et al: Fluorouracil plus levamisole as effective adjuvant therapy after resection of stage III colon carcinoma: A final report. Ann Intern Med 122:321, 1995.)

929 eligible patients followed for 5 years or more confirm that 5-FU plus levamisole reduced the recurrence rate by 40% and the death rate by 33%.[155] The major effect was on reduction in recurrence at distant sites, such as the liver and the lungs. Based on these data, adjuvant therapy with 5-FU and levamisole is offered to patients with Dukes C (stage III) colon cancer.

The success of combinations of 5-FU and leucovorin for the treatment of advanced CRC led to a trial of this regimen in the adjuvant setting. Several trials suggested that this combination was successful in prolonging disease-free and overall survival.[156] Comparison of 5-FU/ levamisole and 5-FU/leucovorin for the adjuvant treatment of CRC in randomized clinical trials indicated an advantage in disease-free and overall survival in favor of 5-FU/ leucovorin.[157,158] Review of the combined data suggests that 5-FU/levamisole given for 1 year is an effective regimen, but 5-FU/leucovorin given for 6 months after "curative" surgery is superior with regard to convenience and efficacy. 5-FU/ leucovorin should therefore be considered the standard for adjuvant treatment of CRC. It is not clear whether patients with stage II, node-negative colon cancer should receive adjuvant chemotherapy, because the risk-benefit ratio in this case has not been established. Currently, the standard of care is to treat all patients with stage III disease and high-risk patients with stage II disease, with adjuvant therapy, although such treatment of the latter group is controversial.[159]

Recent trials have included patients with stage II and stage III (modified Dukes stages B2 and C) disease. Anatomic or biologic features may, in the future, define subsets of patients with stage II colon cancer who will benefit from adjuvant therapy. Such features may include colloid, signet ring, or poorly differentiated cancers, high preoperative CEA cell levels, aneuploid DNA content or high S phase, alterations in molecular markers, and the expression of certain tumor-associated antigens (e.g., sialyl-Tn, sialyl Lewis^x) or other genetic determinants (see section on prognostic factors). One analysis[60] indicated that retention of 18q alleles in microsatellite-stable cancers and mutation of the gene for TGF-β1 in cancers with high levels of MSI indicate a favorable outcome after adjuvant therapy with 5-FU–based regimens in patients with stage III colon cancer (Fig. 120–29). Tumor MSI status has also been shown to be a predictor of benefit from 5-FU–based adjuvant therapy for colon cancer.[67]

Other combined adjuvant chemotherapies for colon cancer currently are being studied, including regimens containing oxaliplatin and irinotecan. The use of combination therapies with either (1) irinotecan, 5-FU/ leucovorin (IFL), or (2) oxaliplatin, 5-FU/leucovorin (ROX) has demonstrated improved response and survival in advanced CRC (see later). A recent European trial (MOSAIC)[160] has documented significant improvement in three-year survival when oxaliplatin was added to 5-FU/ leucovorin in the FOLFOX regimen for patients with stage II and III colon cancer. Two U.S. cooperative trials will evaluate the addition of antiangiogenesis therapy with bevacizumab (Avastin) to chemotherapy.

Patients who have completed resection of isolated liver or lung metastases also should be offered adjuvant chemotherapy.[153] Portal infusion of chemotherapeutic

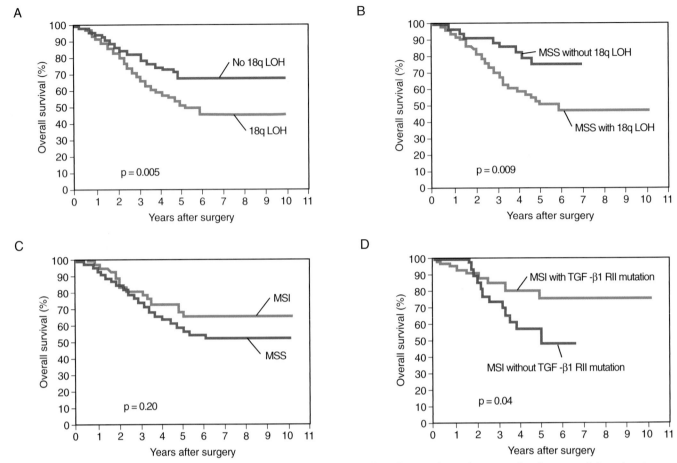

Figure 120–29 *A-D,* Molecular markers that predict a favorable outcome after adjuvant chemotherapy with 5-fluorouracil–based regimens. LOH, loss of heterozygosity; MSI, microsatellite instability; MSS, microsatellite stability; TGF-β1 RII, transforming growth factor-β1 receptor II. (From Watanabe T, Wu T-T, Catalano PJ, et al: Molecular predictors of survival after adjuvant chemotherapy for colon cancer. N Engl J Med 344:1196, 2001.)

agents as adjuvant therapy reduces liver metastasis,[161] but this approach has been limited to investigational use. Additional options include systemic regimens with activity in disseminated metastatic disease.

Adjuvant therapy for rectal cancer should be considered separate from that for colon cancer, because patterns of failure are different. Complete pelvic extirpation is common for patients with rectal cancer, because wide margins of resection may be difficult to obtain. Thus, local recurrence for stage II rectal cancer after primary resection approaches 25% to 30%, with a 50% or greater local recurrence rate in those with stage III tumors. Local recurrence is associated with significant morbidity, and patients with locally invasive rectal cancer are at high risk for systemic relapse. Studies during the past 2 decades have shown a significant decrease in local recurrence of rectal cancer in patients who receive moderate to high doses of preoperative and/or postoperative radiation (40 to 50 Gy) but little impact on systemic recurrence and survival.

Combined adjuvant radiation and chemotherapy has been used to address this potential for local and systemic recurrence. Encouraging results were seen in early prospective, randomized trials to evaluate the efficacy of combined-modality adjuvant therapy in patients with modified Dukes B2 and C (stages II and III) rectal cancer following curative surgery. A trial by the North Central Cancer Treatment Group evolved from this earlier work and strongly suggested that postsurgical combined-modality therapy decreases tumor relapse and improves survival over those with surgery alone or full-dose postoperative radiation therapy.[162] This trial randomized patients with stage II or stage III rectal cancer to receive postoperative radiation alone or radiation plus 5-FU and methyl-CCNU. After a median follow-up of more than 7 years, combined therapy significantly reduced local and overall recurrence and distant metastasis and improved patient survival over that compared with radiation alone (Fig. 120–30). Cancer-related deaths were reduced by 36% and the overall death rate by 29%. Combining protracted-infusion 5-FU with radiation therapy improved the effect of combined-treatment postoperative adjuvant therapy in patients with high-risk rectal cancer.[163] Based on these data, patients with resected

A

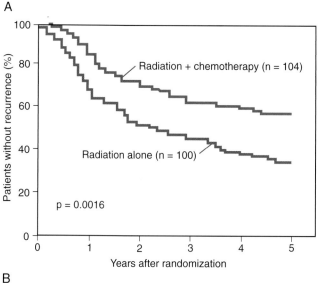

B

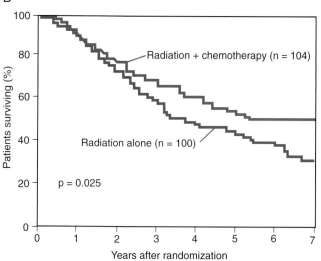

Figure 120–30 Combined-modality adjuvant therapy of stages II and III rectal cancer. Effects of radiation and chemotherapy on tumor recurrence (*A*) and survival (*B*). (From Krook JE, Moertel CG, Gunderson LL, et al: Effective adjuvant therapy for high-risk rectal carcinoma. N Engl J Med 324:709, 1991.)

the use of chemotherapeutic agents or radiation therapy prior to surgery in patients with advanced but locally confined malignancy. Neoadjuvant therapy allows radiation to be delivered in a nonoperated abdomen, reducing the chance of postoperative complications such as adhesions and bowel damage. Higher doses of preoperative (vs. postoperative) radiation can be delivered. Several trials are ongoing to evaluate the efficacy of preoperative versus postoperative multimodality adjuvant therapy (radiation and chemotherapy) for rectal cancer. Studies from Europe and the United States have suggested less toxicity from preoperative radiation therapy. A recent prospective, randomized European trial[165] comparing preoperative and postoperative combined-modality therapy demonstrated a significant reduction in local tumor relapse and less toxicity from preoperative combined-modality therapy compared with similar treatment given postoperatively. Oral capecitabine (Xeloda) is being studied as an enhancer of radiation therapy in the preoperative setting. Accurate endorectal ultrasound and MRI staging has allowed the appropriate use of preoperative therapy, enabling the exclusion of patients with early-stage disease.

Chemotherapy for Advanced Disease

Individuals presenting with operable CRCs have benefited from improvements in surgical techniques and advances in adjuvant chemotherapy. Approximately 30% to 40% of patients with CRC, however, have locoregionally advanced or metastatic disease on presentation. Furthermore, the 5-year survival rates for individuals with stages II and III CRC (82% and 57%, respectively) indicate that a significant portion of these individuals will have postsurgical recurrences and die from this disease. Systemic chemotherapy therefore is required for a large number of patients with advanced CRC.

5-FU is a fluoropyrimidine that, for four decades, has remained the mainstay of systemic chemotherapy for advanced CRC. 5-FU interacts with thymidylate synthetase and inhibits the methylation of deoxyuridylic to thymidylic acid, thereby inhibiting DNA synthesis. It has been administered as an oral agent, intravenously in bolus doses, or by continuous intravenous infusion, and is associated with response rates of approximately 15% to 20% in most studies when used as a single agent. Responses are often short-lived (4 to 5 months) and have not been associated with long-term survival. Toxicity of 5-FU includes myelosuppression, vomiting, diarrhea, and stomatitis and varies according to dose and mode of administration. Despite the recent approval of a number of new drugs for treatment of metastatic CRC, 5-FU remains a component of most regimens. Various regimens most often combine 5-FU with high-dose leucovorin (tetrahydrofolate), because leucovorin potentiates the binding of 5-FU to thymidylate synthetase and the combination is more effective than 5-FU alone.[166] Combined data from numerous trials indicate a twofold increase in tumor response rates with 5-FU/leucovorin compared with 5-FU alone (23% vs. 12%), and a small increase in survival.[167] The optimal doses of 5-FU and leucovorin and the optimal mode of administration (bolus

rectal cancer and transmural extension (stage II; Dukes B2) or with positive lymph nodes (stage III; Dukes C) should be considered for such combined-modality therapy.

Subsequent intergroup trials have attempted to identify the optimal chemotherapeutic agents and their best method of delivery.[164] These trials have compared a variety of chemotherapeutic agents in combination with postoperative radiation as adjuvant treatment of rectal cancer. Regimens include 5-FU alone, 5-FU/leucovorin, 5-FU/levamisole, 5-FU/leucovorin/levamisole, and more recently oxaliplatin/irinotecan. Comparisons also have included the relative benefits of continuous infusion 5-FU during preradiation and postradiation therapy phases versus bolus 5-FU during the nonradiation therapy portion. The term *neoadjuvant therapy* refers to vs. infusion) remain controversial, but continuous-infusion 5-FU appears to be superior to bolus regimens in terms of response rates, toxicity, and survival when compared with bolus regimens.[168] Capecitabine (Xeloda) is an oral fluoropyrimidine that is converted to 5-FU in tumor tissues. Two large phase III trials that compared capecitabine with bolus 5-FU suggest similar efficacy but fewer side effects associated with the oral agent.[169] Several phase III trials currently are comparing continuous-infusion 5-FU and capecitabine-based regimens. UFT, an oral 5-FU prodrug composed of a 1:4 fixed molar ratio of tegafur and uracil, is not approved currently for use in the United States.

After decades without significant change, the advent of a variety of new agents such as irinotecan (Camptosar), oxaliplatin (Eloxatin), and capecitabine, and molecular targeted agents such as cetuximab (Erbitux) and bevacizumab has led to a rapid evolution in the systemic treatment of CRC (Fig. 120–31). Second-line chemotherapy also has become standard for appropriate patients in whom first-line therapies have failed. The choice of therapy is individualized based on performance status, the type and timing of prior therapy, and the differing toxicity profiles of the drugs to be used in various regimens.

Irinotecan (CPT-11) is a potent inhibitor of topoisomerase 1, a nuclear enzyme involved in the unwinding of DNA during replication. Weekly treatment with irinotecan plus 5-FU/leucovorin was shown to be superior to the widely used regimen of 5-FU/leucovorin for stage IV metastatic colon cancer in terms response rate (39% vs. 21%), progression-free survival (7 vs. 4.3 months), and overall survival (14.4 vs. 12 months).[170] A second phase III trial confirmed these results,[171] and the combination of irinotecan, 5-FU and leucovorin (IFL) was approved as first-line treatment for advanced CRC. This regimen is associated with significant side effects because the side effects of irinotecan (diarrhea) and 5-FU (nausea, diarrhea, hematologic toxicity) overlap and may be especially severe with bolus 5-FU. A bimonthly regimen that combines leucovorin and 5-FU bolus and a 46-hour infusion at a high dose plus irinotecan (FOLFIRI) is another first-line therapy option for advanced or metastatic disease.

Oxaliplatin is a diaminocyclohexane platinum that, unlike other platinum compounds, does not cause nephrotoxicity and has activity against CRC. Several different combinations of biweekly bolus and infusional 5-FU, leucovorin, and oxaliplatin, collectively called FOLFOX, have been studied for treatment of advanced CRC. FOLFOX4 is a common regimen used worldwide that has been compared with IFL and IROX (irinotecan and oxaliplatin) in phase III trials.[168] The response rate with FOLFOX4 (45%) was significantly higher than that observed with IFL (31%) or IROX (35%). The median

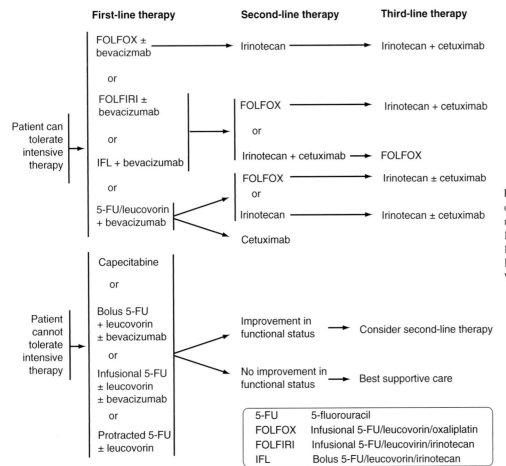

Figure 120–31 Options for chemotherapy for advanced or metastatic colon cancer. (From National Comprehensive Cancer Network: Clinical Practice Guidelines in Oncology. Colon Cancer, Version 1, 2005.)

overall survival durations for patients treated with IFL, FOLFOX4, and IROX were 15.0, 19.5, and 17.4 months, respectively, suggesting that regimens containing oxaliplatin may be options for first-line treatment of patients with advanced CRC. Recent guidelines from the National Comprehensive Cancer Network[153] recommend that primary therapy for metastatic disease in a patient with good tolerance consist of fluoropyrimidines (either 5-FU/leucovorin or capecitabine) and either irinotecan or oxaliplatin.

Bevacizumab is a recombinant humanized monoclonal IgG1 antibody that acts by binding all isoforms of circulating VEGF-A, and decreasing VEGF-A–mediated angiogenesis and vascular permeability. A recent phase III trial[168] compared IFL with IFL plus bevacizumab. When compared with IFL, the regimen containing bevacizumab resulted in an increase in overall response rate from 35% to 45% and extended median survival from 15.6 to 20.3 months. Bevacizumab recently was approved to be used in combination with intravenous 5-FU–based chemotherapy as first-line treatment of patients with metastatic CRC.

Cetuximab is a chimeric antibody directed against the EGFR, an important molecule involved with cell cycling, survival, invasion, and metastasis. It has been used, primarily in combination with irinotecan, in irinotecan-refractory patients.[170]

Selective infusion of chemotherapeutic agents into the hepatic arterial system may be employed to treat hepatic metastases. This method delivers more concentrated drug into the tumor capillary bed than do conventional means. The infusion catheter usually is implanted in the common hepatic artery (via the gastroduodenal artery) at the time of laparotomy. The development of implantable infusion pumps has led to increasing use of such therapy in major centers. Fluorinated pyrimidines, such as 5-FU and floxuridine (FUDR), have high hepatic extraction (80% to 95%), and it is thought that high concentrations of these drugs can be delivered with low systemic toxicity by direct hepatic arterial infusion. FUDR has received the most attention, and its continuous hepatic arterial infusion to treat hepatic metastases from CRC in patients not previously treated may achieve response rates of 54% to 83%. Criteria for response vary, however, and it is still unclear whether an impact on survival will be observed.

Randomized trials of systemic versus intrahepatic infusion of FUDR in patients with liver metastasis have shown significantly higher response rates for intrahepatic therapy, but again, the impact on survival remains unclear. Complications of the procedure, including arterial occlusion, local infection, and catheter leak, occur in a small number of patients. Morbidity of treatment consists of gastrointestinal tract inflammation and ulceration, hepatic injury with elevation in serum bilirubin and aminotransferases, and biliary ductal sclerosis, all of which may be substantial. It has been suggested that alternating hepatic intra-arterial FUDR and 5-FU may produce less toxicity than FUDR alone. Some investigators have combined hepatic artery occlusion or embolization with chemotherapeutic agents (chemoembolization) in an attempt to achieve better response rates in patients with extensive hepatic tumor.

IMMUNOTARGETED THERAPY AND IMMUNOTHERAPY

Use of monoclonal antibodies designed to modulate biologic processes key to tumor growth and behavior such as bevacizumab (directed against circulating VEGF), and cetuximab (directed against EGFR) already have been discussed. Both agents have been approved for treatment of advanced CRC.

Recent advances in immunology, molecular biology, and imaging have led to the development of radiolabeled monoclonal antibodies that can be used to detect CRC metastases (radioimmunodetection). These same antibodies can be linked to cytotoxic agents such as the A subunit of the plant toxin ricin, the toxin A chain of diphtheria, lymphokine-activated killer cells, and chemotherapeutic agents for immunotargeted therapy. Liposomes containing chemotherapeutic agents can be linked to monoclonal antibodies and delivered in a similar fashion. Most patients treated thus far with such therapy have had advanced disease, and further studies utilizing these agents in adjuvant therapy are needed.

Attempts to modulate the immune system of patients with metastatic disease also have been reported.[172] A large body of preclinical and clinical evidence has suggested that the immune system can be stimulated against malignant cells by means of active specific immunotherapy strategies. These approaches, including experimental cancer vaccine strategies, currently are limited to clinical trials but may hold promise for the future.

RADIOTHERAPY

Patients with rectal cancers whose tumors have penetrated the bowel wall or who have regional lymph node involvement are at 40% to 50% risk for local recurrence following resection of the primary tumor. Radiation therapy is used preoperatively or postoperatively to decrease local recurrence in those with high-risk rectal and rectosigmoid cancers (stages II and III lesions) or in a combined preoperative and postoperative "sandwich approach." This approach also is used to convert unresectable large tumors and those fixed to pelvic organs to resectable lesions. Radiation therapy occasionally may be useful for palliation of bleeding and pain resulting from advanced rectal disease. The possible advantages of radiation therapy must be balanced against its potential complications of radiation proctitis and small bowel damage (see Chapter 38).

Preoperative radiation alone reduces local recurrence in patients with rectal and rectosigmoid cancers, but there is no convincing evidence that it improves survival. Postoperative radiation therapy is generally restricted to patients at high risk for local recurrence of rectal cancer (penetration of the bowel wall, positive lymph nodes). Prospective but nonrandomized series show a substantial reduction in local recurrence for those receiving postoperative radiation therapy (6% to 8% for those receiving radiation vs. 40% to 50% for those receiving surgery alone). A randomized study also demonstrated results favoring radiation (an overall reduction in locoregional recurrence from 25% to 16%).[163] Distant metastases

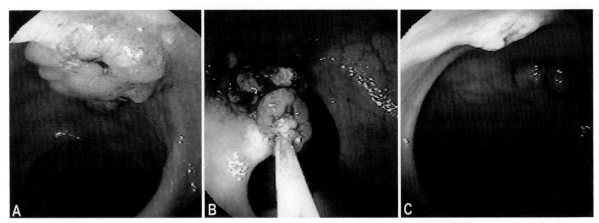

Figure 120–32 Colonoscopic views demonstrating removal of a polypoid carcinoma by snare cautery in a patient at high operative risk because of intercurrent illness. *A,* Polypoid carcinoma. *B,* Piecemeal removal by snare cautery. *C,* Site of lesion after removal.

remain a problem, however, and it is not clear whether survival is altered substantially. Given the recent demonstration of decreased recurrence and increased survival in patients with rectal cancer receiving combined preoperative or postoperative radiation and combination chemotherapy, this should be considered the treatment of choice for high-risk patients with transmural tumor extension or lymph node metastases.

ENDOSCOPIC THERAPY

Endoscopic therapy using the neodymium-yttrium-aluminum-garnet (Nd:YAG) laser or argon plasma coagulation has been used to recanalize the rectum as palliative therapy in patients with obstructing rectal cancers who are poor surgical risks or who have advanced stages of malignant disease; such palliation generally has been satisfactory. Reported complications are bleeding and perforation, but they are fewer than would be anticipated after surgery in these high-risk patients. Electrofulguration using a heater probe device has been reported under similar circumstances. Endoscopy with the use of snare cautery also may be used to remove polypoid lesions (Fig. 120–32), often in a piecemeal fashion.

Photodynamic therapy (PDT) also has been used to treat patients who are poor surgical risks. PDT involves the use of a photosensitizer that is taken up by the tumor and administered prior to photoradiation using a tuneable dye laser delivered through a flexible optical fiber. The photosensitizer porfimer sodium (Photofrin) has been approved by the U.S. Food and Drug Administration for palliation of esophageal cancers, but its use for rectal cancers has been more limited, given other available options. Limitations of PDT include cost and skin photosensitization.

Palliation of obstruction from colorectal lesions also may be accomplished by the use of expandable metal stents. Intraluminal stents are being used with increasing frequency for palliation and for relieving colorectal obstruction preoperatively, because repetitive treatments

as required for ablative therapies such as argon plasma coagulation and PDT are obviated.

OTHER MALIGNANT COLONIC TUMORS

Malignant tumors other than adenocarcinomas rarely originate in the large bowel. These include lymphomas, malignant carcinoid tumors, and leiomyosarcomas. In addition, lymphomas, leiomyosarcomas, malignant melanomas, and cancers of the breast, ovary, prostate, lung, stomach, and other organs can metastasize to the colon. Malignant carcinoid tumors are discussed in Chapter 30 and lymphomas in Chapter 28. Carcinomas of the anal canal are discussed in Chapter 122.

REFERENCES

1. Jemal A, Siegel R, Ward E, et al: Cancer statistics, 2006. CA Cancer J Clin 56:107, 2006.
2. Parkin DM, Pisani P, Ferlay J: Global cancer statistics. CA Cancer J Clin 49:33, 1999.
3. Ries LA, Wingo PA, Miller DS, et al: The annual report to the nation on the status of cancer, 1973–1977, with a special section on colorectal cancer. Cancer 88:2398, 2000.
4. Parkin DM, Whelen SL, Ferlay J, et al: Cancer Incidence in Five Continents (IARC Sci. Publ. No. 143). Series. Lyon, International Agency for Research on Cancer, 1997.
5. Cooper GS, Yuan Z, Landefeld CS, et al: A national population-based study of incidence of colorectal cancer and age: Implications for screening in older Americans. Cancer 75:775, 1995.
6. Demers RY, Severson RK, Schottenfeld D, Lazar L: Incidence of colorectal adenocarcinoma by anatomic subsite: An epidemiologic study of time trends and racial differences in the Detroit, Michigan area. Cancer 79:441, 1997.
7. Potter JD: Colorectal cancer: Molecules and populations. J Natl Cancer Inst 91:916, 1999.
8. Willett WC, Stampfer MJ, Colditz GA, et al: Relation of meat, fat, and fiber intake to the risk of colon cancer in a prospective study among women. N Engl J Med 323:1664, 1990.

9. Neugut AI, Garbowski GC, Lee WC, et al: Dietary risk factors for the incidence and recurrence of colorectal adenomatous polyps: A case-control study. Ann Intern Med 118:91, 1993.

10. Howe GR, Aronson KJ, Benito E, et al: The relationship between dietary fat intake and risk of colorectal cancer: Evidence from the combined analysis of 13 case-control studies. Cancer Causes Control 8:215, 1997.

11. Rao CV, Simi B, Wynn TT, et al: Modulating effect of amount and types of dietary fat on colonic mucosal phospholipase A_2, phosphatidylinositol-specific phospholipase C activities, and cyclooxygenase metabolite formation during different stages of colon tumor promotion in male F344 rats. Cancer Res 56:532, 1996.

12. Glinghammar B, Rafter J: Colonic luminal contents induce cyclooxygenase 2 transcription in human colon carcinoma cells. Gastroenterology 120:401, 2001.

13. Giovannucci E, Rimm EB, Stampfer MJ, et al: Aspirin use and the risk for colorectal cancer and adenoma in male health professionals. Ann Intern Med 121:241, 1994.

14. Giovannucci E, Egan KM, Hunter DJ: Aspirin and the risk of colorectal cancer in women. N Engl J Med 333:609, 1995.

15. Dannenberg AJ, Subbaramaiah K: Targeting cyclooxygenase-2 in human neoplasia: Rationale and promise. Cancer Cell 4:431, 2003.

16. Oshima M, Dinchuk JE, Kargman SL, et al: Suppression of intestinal polyposis in *APC* delta716 knockout mice by inhibition of cyclooxygenase 2 (COX-2). Cell 87:803, 1996.

17. Giovannucci E, Ascherio A, Rimm, AA, et al.: Physical activity, obesity, and risk for colon cancer and adenoma in men. Ann Intern Med 122:327, 1995.

18. Peters U, Sinha R, Chatterjee N, et al: Dietary fibre and colorectal adenoma in a colorectal cancer early detection programme. Lancet 361:1491, 2003.

19. Bingham SA, Day NE, Luben R, et al: Dietary fibre in food and protection against colorectal cancer in the European Prospective Investigation into Cancer and Nutrition (EPIC): An observational study. Lancet 361:1496, 2003.

20. Alberts DS, Martinez ME, Roe DJ, et al: Lack of effect of a high-fiber cereal supplement on the recurrence of colorectal adenomas. Phoenix Colon Cancer Prevention Physicians' Network. N Engl J Med 342:1156, 2000.

21. Schatzkin A, Lanza E, Corle D, et al: Lack of effect of a low-fat, high-fiber diet on the recurrence of colorectal adenomas. Polyp Prevention Trial Study Group. N Engl J Med 342:1149, 2000.

22. Baron JA, Sandler RS, Haile RW, et al: Folate intake, alcohol consumption, cigarette smoking, and risk of colorectal adenomas. J Natl Cancer Inst 90:57, 1998.

23. Bostick RM, Potter JD, Sellers TA, et al: Relation of calcium, vitamin D, and dairy food intake to incidence of colon cancer among older women. The Iowa Women's Health Study. Am J Epidemiol 137:1302, 1993.

24. Holt PR, Atillasoy EO, Gilman J, et al: Modulation of abnormal colonic epithelial cell proliferation and differentiation by low-fat dairy foods: A randomized controlled trial. JAMA 280:1074, 1998.

25. Alberts DS, Ritenbaugh C, Story JA, et al: Randomized, double-blinded, placebo-controlled study of effect of wheat bran fiber and calcium on fecal bile acids in patients with resected adenomatous colon polyps. J Natl Cancer Inst 88:81, 1996.

26. Kim KE, Brasitus TA: The role of vitamin D in normal and pathologic processes in the colon. Curr Opin Gastroenterol 17:184, 2001.

27. Kargman SL, O'Neill GP, Vickers PJ, et al: Expression of prostaglandin G/H synthase-1 and -2 protein in human colon cancer. Cancer Res 55:2556, 1995.

28. Hull MA, Fenwick SW, Chapple KS, et al: Cyclooxygenase-2 expression in colorectal cancer liver metastases. Clin Exp Metastasis 18:21, 2000.

29. Jacoby RF, Seibert K, Cole CE, et al: The cyclooxygenase-2 inhibitor celecoxib is a potent preventive and therapeutic agent in the min mouse model of adenomatous polyposis. Cancer Res 60:5040, 2000.

30. Oshima M, Murai N, Kargman S, et al: Chemoprevention of intestinal polyposis in the Apcdelta716 mouse by rofecoxib, a specific cyclooxygenase-2 inhibitor. Cancer Res 61:1733, 2001.

31. Reddy BS, Hirose Y, Lubet R, et al: Chemoprevention of colon cancer by specific cyclooxygenase-2 inhibitor, celecoxib, administered during different stages of carcinogenesis. Cancer Res 60:293, 2000.

32. Tsujii M, DuBois R: Alterations in cellular adhesion and apoptosis in epithelial cells overexpressing prostaglandin endoperoxide synthase 2. Cell 83:493, 1995.

33. He TC, Chan TA, Vogelstein B, Kinzler KW: PPARδ is an APC-regulated target of nonsteroidal anti-inflammatory drugs. Cell 99:335, 1999.

34. Janne PA, Mayer RJ: Chemoprevention of colorectal cancer. N Engl J Med 342:1960, 2000.

35. Hawk ET, Umar A, Viner JL: Colorectal cancer chemoprevention: An overview of the science. Gastroenterology 126:1423, 2004.

36. Baron JA, Beach M, Mandel JS, et al: Calcium supplements for the prevention of colorectal adenomas. Calcium Polyp Prevention Study Group. N Engl J Med 340:101, 1999.

37. Greenberg ER, Baron JA, Tosteson TD, et al: A clinical trial of antioxidant vitamins to prevent colorectal adenoma. Polyp Prevention Study Group. N Engl J Med 331:141, 1994.

38. Giovannucci E, Stampfer MJ, Colditz GA, et al: Multivitamin use, folate, and colon cancer in women in the Nurses' Health Study. Ann Intern Med 129:517, 1998.

39. Kim YI, Shirwadkar S, Choi SW, et al: Effects of dietary folate on DNA strand breaks within mutation-prone exons of the p53 gene in rat colon. Gastroenterology 119:151, 2000.

40. Cole BF, Baron JA, Sandler RS, et al: A randomized trial of folic acid to prevent colorectal adenomas. Proc Am Assoc Cancer Res (in press).

41. Grodstein F, Newcomb PA, Stampfer MJ: Postmenopausal hormone therapy and the risk of colorectal cancer: A review and meta-analysis. Am J Med 106:574, 1999.

42. Gann PH, Manson JE, Glynn RJ, et al: Low-dose aspirin and incidence of colorectal tumors in a randomized trial. J Natl Cancer Inst 85:1220, 1993.

43. Sandler RS, Halabi S, Baron JA, et al: A randomized trial of aspirin to prevent colorectal adenomas in patients with previous colorectal cancer. N Engl J Med 348:883, 2003.

44. Baron JA, Cole BF, Sandler RS, et al: A randomized trial of aspirin to prevent colorectal adenomas. N Engl J Med 348:891, 2003.

45. Benamouzig R, Deyra J, Martin A, et al: Daily soluble aspirin and prevention of colorectal adenoma recurrence: One-year results of the APACC trial. Gastroenterology 125:328, 2003.

46. Giardiello FM, Hamilton SR, Krush AJ, et al: Treatment of colonic and rectal adenomas with sulindac in familial adenomatous polyposis. N Engl J Med 328:1313, 1993.

47. Cruz-Correa M, Hylind LM, Romans KE, et al: Long-term treatment with sulindac in familial adenomatous polyposis: A prospective cohort study. Gastroenterology 122:641, 2002.

48. Giardiello FM, Yang VW, Hylind LM, et al: Primary chemoprevention of familial adenomatous polyposis with sulindac. N Engl J Med 346:1054, 2002.

49. Steinbach G, Lynch PM, Phillips RK, et al: The effect of celecoxib, a cyclooxygenase-2 inhibitor, in familial adenomatous polyposis. N Engl J Med 342:1946, 2000.

50. Bresalier R, Sandler RS, Bolognese J, et al: A randomized trial of rofecoxib to prevent colorectal adenomas: The APPROVe Trial. Gastroenterology (in press).

51. Lichtenstein P, Holm NV, Verkasalo PK, et al: Environmental and heritable factors in the causation of cancer: Analyses of cohorts of twins from Sweden, Denmark, and Finland. N Engl J Med 343:78, 2000.

52. Chung DC: The genetic basis of colorectal cancer: Insights into critical pathways of tumorigenesis. Gastroenterology 119:854, 2000.

53. Grady WM: Genomic instability and colon cancer. Cancer Metastasis Rev 23:11, 2004.

54. Jen J, Kim H, Piantadosi S, et al.: Allelic loss of chromosome 18q and prognosis in colorectal cancer. N Engl J Med 331:213, 1994.

55. Carethers JM, Hawn MT, Greenson JK, et al.: Prognostic significance of allelic loss at chromosome 18q21 for stage II colorectal cancer. Gastroenterology 114:1188, 1998.

56. Kahlenberg MS, Stoler DL, Rodriguez-Bigas MA, et al: *p53* tumor suppressor gene mutations predict decreased survival of patients with sporadic colorectal carcinoma. Cancer 88:1814, 2000.

57. Shibata D, Reale MA, Lavin P, et al: The DCC protein and prognosis in colorectal cancer. N Engl J Med 335:1727, 1996.

58. Giardiello FM, Brensinger JD, Petersen GM, et al: The use and interpretation of commercial *APC* gene testing for familial adenomatous polyposis. N Engl J Med 336:823, 1997.

59. Waterman ML: Lymphoid enhancer factor/T cell factor expression in colorectal cancer. Cancer Metastasis Rev 23:41, 2004.

60. Watanabe T, Wu TT, Catalano PJ, et al: Molecular predictors of survival after adjuvant chemotherapy for colon cancer. N Engl J Med 344:1196, 2001.

61. Takaku K, Oshima M, Miyoshi H, et al: Intestinal tumorigenesis in compound mutant mice of both Dpc4 (Smad4) and Apc genes. Cell 92:645, 1998.

62. Bresalier RS: Tumor progression in the intestine: Smad about you. Gastroenterology 115:1598, 1998.

63. Yoshida BA, Sokoloff MM, Welch DR, Rinker-Schaeffer CW: Metastasis-suppressor genes: A review and perspective on an emerging field. J Natl Cancer Inst 92:1717, 2000.

64. Chung DC, Rustgi AK: The hereditary nonpolyposis colorectal cancer NCER syndrome: Genetics and clinical implications. Ann Intern Med 138:560, 2003.

65. Gryfe R, Kim H, Hsieh ET, et al: Tumor microsatellite instability and clinical outcome in young patients with colorectal cancer. N Engl J Med 342:69, 2000.

66. Tajima A, Hess MT, Cabrera BL, et al: The mismatch repair complex hMutS alpha recognizes 5-fluorouracil-modified DNA: Implications for chemosensitivity and resistance. Gastroenterology 127:1678, 2004.

67. Ribic CM, Sargent DJ, Moore MJ, et al: Tumor microsatellite-instability status as a predictor of benefit from fluorouracil-based adjuvant chemotherapy for colon cancer. N Engl J Med 349:247, 2003.

68. Rashid A, Issa JP: CpG island methylation in gastroenterologic neoplasia: A maturing field. Gastroenterology 127:1578, 2004.

69. Deng G, Chen A, Hong J, et al: Methylation of CpG in a small region of the hMLH1 promoter invariably correlates with the absence of gene expression. Cancer Res 59:2029, 1999.

70. Bresalier RS: The biology of colorectal cancer metastasis. Gastroenterol Clin North Am 25:805, 1996.

71. Byrd JC, Bresalier RS: Mucins and mucin binding proteins in colorectal cancer. Cancer Metastasis Rev 23:77, 2004.

72. Zucker S, Vacirca J: Role of matrix metalloproteinases (MMPs) in colorectal cancer. Cancer Metastasis Rev 23:101, 2004.

73. Takenaka Y, Fukumori T, Raz A: Galectin-3 and metastasis. Glycoconj J 19:543, 2004.

74. Bresalier RS, Byrd JC, Tessler D, et al: A circulating ligand for galectin-3 is a haptoglobin-related glycoprotein elevated in individuals with colon cancer. Gastroenterology 127:741, 2004.

75. Sternberg LR, Byrd JC, Yunker CK, et al: Liver colonization by human colon cancer cells is reduced by antisense inhibition of MUC2 mucin synthesis. Gastroenterology 116:363, 1999.

76. Half EE, Bresalier R: Clinical management of hereditary colorectal cancer syndromes. Curr Opin Gastroenterol 20:32, 2004.

77. Rodriguez-Bigas MA, Boland CR, Hamilton SR, et al: A National Cancer Institute Workshop on Hereditary Nonpolyposis Colorectal Cancer Syndrome: Meeting highlights and Bethesda guidelines. J Natl Cancer Inst 89:1758, 1997.

78. Burt RW: Colon cancer screening. Gastroenterology 119:837, 2000.

79. Byers T, Nestle M, McTiernan A, et al: American Cancer Society guidelines on nutrition and physical activity for cancer prevention: Reducing the risk of cancer with healthy food choices and physical activity. CA Cancer J Clin 52:92, 2002.

80. Smith RA, von Eschenbach AC, Wender R, et al: American Cancer Society guidelines for the early detection of cancer: Update of early detection guidelines for prostate, colorectal, and endometrial cancers. Also: Update 2001—testing for early lung cancer detection. CA Cancer J Clin 51:38, 2001.

81. Smith RA, Cokkinides V, Eyre HJ: American Cancer Society guidelines for the early detection of cancer, 2004. CA Cancer J Clin 54:41, 2004.

82. Pignone M, Rich M, Teutsch SM, et al: Screening for colorectal cancer in adults at average risk: A summary of the evidence for the U.S. Preventive Services Task Force. Ann Intern Med 137:132, 2002.

83. Bond JH: Polyp guideline: Diagnosis, treatment, and surveillance for patients with colorectal polyps. Practice Parameters Committee of the American College of Gastroenterology. Am J Gastroenterol 95:3053, 2000.

84. Hamilton SR, Liu B, Parsons RE, et al: The molecular basis of Turcot's syndrome. N Engl J Med 332:839, 1995.

85. Giardiello FM, Brensinger JD, Tersmette AC, et al: Very high risk of cancer in familial Peutz-Jeghers syndrome. Gastroenterology 119:1447, 2000.

86. Carethers JM: Hamartomatous polyposis syndromes: Genetic pathways. Curr Opin Gastroenterol 18:1, 2002.

87. Ekbom A, Helmick C, Zack M, Adami HO: Ulcerative colitis and colorectal cancer: A population-based study. N Engl J Med 323:1228, 1990.

88. Nuako KW, Ahlquist DA, Mahoney DW, et al: Familial predisposition for colorectal cancer in chronic ulcerative colitis: A case-control study. Gastroenterology 115:1079, 1998.

89. Eaden JA, Abrams KR, Mayberry JF: The risk of colorectal cancer in ulcerative colitis: A meta-analysis. Gut 48:526, 2001.

90. Itzkowitz SH: Inflammatory bowel disease and cancer. Gastroenterol Clin North Am 26:129, 1997.

91. Heuschen UA, Henz U, Allemeyer EH, et al: Backwash ileitis is strongly associated with colorectal carcinoma in ulcerative colitis. Gastroenterology 120:841, 2001.

92. Persson PG, Karlen P, Bernell O, et al: Crohn's disease and cancer: A population-based cohort study. Gastroenterology 107:1675, 1994.

93. Provenzale D, Kowdley KV, Arora S, Wong JB: Prophylactic colectomy or surveillance for chronic ulcerative colitis? A decision analysis. Gastroenterology 109:1188, 1995.

94. Willenbucher RF, Zelman SJ, Ferrell LD, et al: Chromosomal alterations in ulcerative colitis-related neoplastic progression. Gastroenterology 113:791, 1997.

95. Friedman S, Rubin PH, Bodian C, et al: Screening and surveillance colonoscopy in chronic Crohn's colitis. Gastroenterology 120:820, 2001.

96. Lagergren J, Ye W, Ekbom A: Intestinal cancer after cholecystectomy: Is bile involved in carcinogenesis? Gastroenterology 121:542, 2001.

97. American Joint Committee on Cancer: Manual for Staging of Cancer, Colon, and Rectum, 6th ed. New York, Springer-Verlag 2002, p 113.

98. Prorok PC, Andriole GL, Bresalier RS, et al: Design of the Prostate, Lung, Colorectal and Ovarian (PLCO) Cancer Screening Trial. Control Clin Trials 21:273S, 2000.

99. Rex DK, Rahmani EY, Haseman JH, et al: Relative sensitivity of colonoscopy and barium enema for detection of colorectal cancer in clinical practice. Gastroenterology 112:17, 1997.

100. Winawer SJ, Stewart ET, Zauber AG, et al: A comparison of colonoscopy and double-contrast barium enema for surveillance after polypectomy. National Polyp Study Work Group. N Engl J Med 342:1766, 2000.

101. Winawer SJ, Fletcher RH, Miller L, et al: Colorectal cancer screening: Clinical guidelines and rationale. Gastroenterology 112:594, 1997.

102. Winawer S, Fletcher R, Rex D, et al: Colorectal cancer screening and surveillance: Clinical guidelines and rationale—update based on new evidence. Gastroenterology 124:544, 2003.

103. Centers for Disease Control and Prevention: Screening for colorectal cancer—United States. MMWR Morb Mortal Wkly Rep 48:116, 1999.

104. Vernon SW: Participation in colorectal cancer screening: A review. J Natl Cancer Inst 89:1406, 1997.

105. Lieberman DA: Cost-effectiveness model for colon cancer screening. Gastroenterology 109:1781, 1995.

106. Hardcastle JD, Chamberlain JO, Robinson MH, et al: Randomised controlled trial of faecal-occult-blood screening for colorectal cancer. Lancet 348:1472, 1996.

107. Mandel JS, Bond JH, Church TR, et al: Reducing mortality from colorectal cancer by screening for fecal occult blood. Minnesota Colon Cancer Control Study. N Engl J Med 328:1365, 1993.

108. Kronborg O, Fenger C, Worm J, et al: Causes of death during the first 5 years of a randomized trial of mass screening for colorectal cancer with fecal occult blood test. Scand J Gastroenterol 27:47, 1992.

109. Kewenter J, Asztely M, Ergaras B, et al: A randomized trial of fecal occult blood testing for early detection of colorectal cancer: Results of screening and rescreening 51325 subjects. In Miller AB, et al (eds): Cancer Screening. Cambridge, UK, Cambridge University Press, 1991, p 116.

110. Kronborg O, Fenger C, Olsen J, et al: Randomised study of screening for colorectal cancer with faecal-occult-blood test. Lancet 348:1467, 1996.

111. Lurie JD, Welch HG: Diagnostic testing following fecal occult blood screening in the elderly. J Natl Cancer Inst 91:1641, 1999.

112. Sonnenberg A, Delco F, Inadomi JM: Cost-effectiveness of colonoscopy in screening for colorectal cancer. Ann Intern Med 133:573, 2000.

113. Inadomi JM: Update on cost-effectiveness of screening for colorectal neoplasia. Curr Opin Gastroenterol 19:44, 2003.

114. Pignone M, Saha S, Hoerger T, Mandelblatt J: Cost-effectiveness analyses of colorectal cancer screening: A systematic review for the U.S. Preventive Services Task Force. Ann Intern Med 137:96, 2002.

115. U.S. Preventive Services Task Force: Screening for colorectal cancer: Recommendation and rationale. Ann Intern Med 137:129, 2002.

116. Collins JF, Lieberman DA, Durbin TE, et al. Accuracy of screening for fecal occult blood on a single stool sample obtained by digital rectal examination. Ann Intern Med 142:81, 2005.

117. Mandel JS, Church TR, Ederer F, Bond JH: Colorectal cancer mortality: Effectiveness of biennial screening for fecal occult blood. J Natl Cancer Inst 91:434, 1999.

118. Faivre J, Dancourt V, Lejeune C, et al: Reduction in colorectal cancer mortality by fecal occult blood screening in a French-controlled study. Gastroenterology 126:1674, 2004.

119. Winawer SJ, St John DJ, Bond JH, et al: Prevention of colorectal cancer: Guidelines based on new data. WHO Collaborating Center for the Prevention of Colorectal Cancer. Bull World Health Organ 73:7, 1995.

120. Allison JE, Tekawa IS, Ransom LJ, Adrain AL: A comparison of fecal occult-blood tests for colorectal-cancer screening. N Engl J Med 334:155, 1996.

121. Selby JV, Friedman GD, Quesenberry CP Jr, Weiss NS: A case-control study of screening sigmoidoscopy and mortality from colorectal cancer. N Engl J Med 326:653, 1992.

122. Newcomb PA, Norfleet RG, Storer BE, et al: Screening sigmoidoscopy and colorectal cancer mortality. J Natl Cancer Inst 84:1572, 1992.

123. Muller AD, Sonnenberg A: Prevention of colorectal cancer by flexible endoscopy and polypectomy: A case-control study of 32,702 veterans. Ann Intern Med 123:904, 1995.

124. Atkin W, Rogers P, Cardwell C, et al: Wide variation in adenoma detection rates at screening flexible sigmoidoscopy. Gastroenterology 126:1247, 2004.

125. Schoenfeld PS, Cash B, Kita J, et al: Effectiveness and patient satisfaction with screening flexible sigmoidoscopy performed by registered nurses. Gastrointest Endosc 49:158, 1999.

126. Schoen RE, Pinsky PF, Weissfeld JL, et al: Results of repeat sigmoidoscopy 3 years after a negative examination. JAMA 290:41, 2003.

127. Winawer SJ, Zauber AG, Ho MN, et al: Prevention of colorectal cancer by colonoscopic polypectomy. The National Polyp Study Workgroup. N Engl J Med 329:1977, 1993.

128. Rex DK, Chak A, Vasudeva R, et al: Prospective determination of distal colon findings in average-risk patients with proximal colon cancer. Gastrointest Endosc 49:727, 1999.

129. Schoen RE, Corle D, Cranston L, et al: Is colonoscopy needed for the nonadvanced adenoma found on sigmoidoscopy? The Polyp Prevention Trial. Gastroenterology 115:533, 1998.

130. Imperiale TF, Wagner DR, Lin CY, et al: Risk of advanced proximal neoplasms in asymptomatic adults according to the distal colorectal findings. N Engl J Med 343:169, 2000.

131. Lieberman DA, Weiss DG, Bond JH, et al: Use of colonoscopy to screen asymptomatic adults for colorectal cancer. Veterans Affairs Cooperative Study Group 380. N Engl J Med 343:162, 2000.

132. Iannaccone R, Laghi A, Catalano C, et al: Computed tomographic colonography without cathartic preparation for the detection of colorectal polyps. Gastroenterology 127:1300, 2004.

133. Chaoui A, Barish MA: Virtual colonoscopy: A new tool for colorectal cancer screening. Curr Opin Gastroenterol 17:78, 2001.

134. Johnson CD, Harmsen WS, Wilson LA, et al: Prospective blinded evaluation of computed tomographic colonography for screen detection of colorectal polyps. Gastroenterology 125:311, 2003.

135. Pineau BC, Paskett ED, Chen GJ, et al: Virtual colonoscopy using oral contrast compared with colonoscopy for the detection of patients with colorectal polyps. Gastroenterology 125:304, 2003.

136. Pickhardt PJ, Choi JR, Hwang I, et al: Computed tomographic virtual colonoscopy to screen for colorectal neoplasia in asymptomatic adults. N Engl J Med 349:2191, 2003.

137. Cotton PB, Durkalski VL, Pineau BC, et al: Computed tomographic colonography (virtual colonoscopy): A multicenter comparison with standard colonoscopy for detection of colorectal neoplasia. JAMA 291:1713, 2004.

138. Pickhardt PJ, Nugent PA, Mysliwiec PA, et al: Location of adenomas missed by optical colonoscopy. Ann Intern Med 141:352, 2004.

139. Ransohoff DF: Cancer: Developing molecular biomarkers for cancer. Science 299:1679, 2003.

140. Ahlquist DA, Skoletsky JE, Boynton KA, et al: colorectal cancer screening by detection of altered human DNA in stool: Feasibility of a multitarget assay panel. Gastroenterology 119:1219, 2000.

141. Imperiale TF, Ransohoff DF, Itzkowitz SH, et al: Fecal DNA versus fecal occult blood for colorectal-cancer screening in an average-risk population. N Engl J Med 351:2704, 2004.

142. Syngal S, Fox EA, Li C, et al: Interpretation of genetic test results for hereditary nonpolyposis colorectal cancer: Implications for clinical predisposition testing. JAMA 282:247, 1999.

143. Stern HS, Viertelhausen S, Hunter AG, et al: APC I1307K increases risk of transition from polyp to colorectal carcinoma in Ashkenazi Jews. Gastroenterology 120:392, 2001.

144. Jarvinen HJ, Mecklin JP, Sistonen P: Screening reduces colorectal cancer rate in families with hereditary nonpolyposis colorectal cancer. Gastroenterology 108:1405, 1995.

145. Jarvinen HJ, Aarnio M, Mustonen H, et al: Controlled 15-year trial on screening for colorectal cancer in families with hereditary nonpolyposis colorectal cancer. Gastroenterology 118:829, 2000.

146. Seeff LC, Richards TB, Shapiro JA, et al: How many endoscopies are performed for colorectal cancer screening? Results from CDC's survey of endoscopic capacity. Gastroenterology 127:1670, 2004.

147. Seeff LC, Manninen DL, Dong FB, et al: Is there endoscopic capacity to provide colorectal cancer screening to the unscreened population in the United States? Gastroenterology 127:1661, 2004.

148. Mysliwiec PA, Brown ML, Klabunde CN, Ransohoff DF: Are physicians doing too much colonoscopy? A national survey of colorectal surveillance after polypectomy. Ann Intern Med 141:264, 2004.

149. Imperiale TF, Wagner DR, Lin CY, et al: Using risk for advanced proximal colonic neoplasia to tailor endoscopic screening for colorectal cancer. Ann Intern Med 139:959, 2003.

150. Song K, Fendrick AM, Ladabaum U: Fecal DNA testing compared with conventional colorectal cancer screening methods: A decision analysis. Gastroenterology 126:1270, 2004.

151. Pfister DG, Benson AB III, Somerfield MR: Clinical practice: Surveillance strategies after curative treatment of colorectal cancer. N Engl J Med 350:2375, 2004.

152. Curley SA, Izzo F, Abdalla E, Vauthey JN: Surgical treatment of colorectal cancer metastasis. Cancer Metastasis Rev 23:165, 2004.

153. National Comprehensive Cancer Network: Clinical Practice Guidelines in Oncology. Colon Cancer, Version 1, 2005.

154. McCarty TM, Kuhn JA: Cryotherapy for liver tumors. Oncology (Williston Park) 12:979, 1998.

155. Moertel CG, Fleming TR, Macdonald JS, et al: Fluorouracil plus levamisole as effective adjuvant therapy after resection of stage III colon carcinoma: A final report. Ann Intern Med 122:321, 1995.

156. International Multicenter Pooled Analysis of Colon Cancer Trials (IMPACT) Investigators: Efficacy of adjuvant fluorouracil, leucovorin, and levamisole in Dukes B and C carcinoma of the colon: Results from the National Adjuvant Breast and Bowel Project C-4. Lancet 345:939, 2000.

157. Wolmark N, Rockette H, Mamounas E, et al: Clinical trial to assess the relative efficacy of fluorouracil and leucovorin, fluorouracil and levamisole, and fluorouracil, leucovorin, and levamisole in patients with Dukes B and C carcinoma of the colon: Results from National Surgical Adjuvant Breast and Bowel Project C-04. J Clin Oncol 17:3553, 1999.

158. O'Connell MJ, Laurie JA, Kahn M, et al: Prospectively randomized trial of postoperative adjuvant chemotherapy in patients with high-risk colon cancer. J Clin Oncol 16:295, 1998.

159. Gill S, Loprinzi CL, Sargent DJ, et al: Pooled analysis of fluorouracil-based adjuvant therapy for stage II and III colon cancer: who benefits and by how much? J Clin Oncol 22:1797, 2004.

160. Andre T, Boni C, Mounedji-Boudiaf L, et al: Oxaliplatin, fluorouracil, and leucovorin as adjuvant treatment for colon cancer. N Engl J Med 350:2343, 2004.

161. Liver Infusion Meta-analysis Group: Portal vein chemotherapy for colorectal cancer: A meta-analysis of 4000 patients in 10 studies. Liver Infusion Meta-analysis Group. J Natl Cancer Inst 89:497, 1997.

162. Krook JE, Moertel CG, Gunderson LL, et al: Effective surgical adjuvant therapy for high-risk rectal carcinoma. N Engl J Med 324:709, 1991.

163. O'Connell MJ, Martenson JA, Wieand HS, et al: Improving adjuvant therapy for rectal cancer by combining protracted-infusion fluorouracil with radiation therapy after curative surgery. N Engl J Med 331:502, 1994.

164. Ajlouni M: The role of radiation in adjuvant treatment of rectal cancer. Curr Opin Gastroenterol 17:86, 2001.

165. Sauer R, Becker H, Hohenberger W, et al: Preoperative versus postoperative chemoradiotherapy for rectal cancer. N Engl J Med 351:1731, 2004.

166. Sobrero AF, Aschele C, Bertino JR: Fluorouracil in colorectal cancer—a tale of two drugs: Implications for biochemical modulation. J Clin Oncol 15:368, 1997.

167. Piedbois P, Michaels S: For the Meta-analysis Group in Cancer: Survival benefit of 5FU/LV over 5FU bolus in patients with advanced colorectal cancer: An updated meta-analysis based on 2,751 patients. Proc Am Assoc Cancer Res 22:29, 2003.

168. Goldberg RM, Sargent DJ, Morton RF, et al: A randomized controlled trial of fluorouracil plus leucovorin, irinotecan, and oxaliplatin combinations in patients with previously untreated metastatic colorectal cancer. J Clin Oncol 22:23, 2004.

169. Hoff PM, Ansari R, Batist G, et al: Comparison of oral capecitabine versus intravenous fluorouracil plus leucovorin as first-line treatment in 605 patients with metastatic colorectal cancer: results of a randomized phase III study. J Clin Oncol 19:2282, 2001.

170. Saltz LB, Cox JV, Blanke C, et al: Irinotecan plus fluorouracil and leucovorin for metastatic colorectal cancer. Irinotecan Study Group. N Engl J Med 343:905, 2000.

171. Douillard JY, Cunningham D, Roth AD, et al: Irinotecan combined with fluorouracil compared with fluorouracil alone as first-line treatment for metastatic colorectal cancer: A multicentre randomised trial. Lancet 355:1041, 2000.

172. Mocellin S, Rossi CR, Lise M, Nitti D: Colorectal cancer vaccines: Principles, results, and perspectives. Gastroenterology 127:1821, 2004.

CHAPTER
121 Other Diseases of the Colon and Rectum

Arnold Wald

LYMPHOCYTIC AND COLLAGENOUS COLITIS

BACKGROUND

Lymphocytic and collagenous colitis are uncommon disorders characterized by chronic, watery diarrhea and histologic evidence of chronic mucosal inflammation in the absence of endoscopic or radiologic abnormalities of the colon. The two disorders are distinct histologically but have been grouped under the term *microscopic colitis*. They differ principally by the presence or absence of a thickened collagenous band, which is located in the colonic subepithelium in collagenous colitis.

The term *collagenous colitis* was used first in 1976 by Lindstrom in describing a middle-aged woman in whom evaluation for chronic diarrhea was normal except for colonic biopsies that showed a thickened band of subepi-

thelial collagen and increased lymphocytes in the lamina propria.[1] Histologically, the subepithelial collagen deposits resembled those in small intestinal mucosa of patients with collagenous sprue. The term *microscopic colitis* was used first in 1980 by Read and associates, who described a group of patients with chronic diarrhea of unknown origin, a subset of whom had a normal colonoscopy but abnormal histopathology on biopsy.[2] Later review showed that most of these patients had collagenous colitis, but some had increased lymphocytes in the lamina propria in the absence of a thickened collagen band. The term *lymphocytic colitis* was proposed in 1989 by Lazenby and associates[3] as a more specific histopathologic diagnosis to distinguish this entity from patterns of microscopic colitis in which other cellular elements such as eosinophils, mast cells, or neutrophils predominate.

Whether collagenous and lymphocytic colitis represent two ends of the spectrum of a single disorder or different entities remains uncertain, but their clinical presentations, evaluations, and treatments are similar.

EPIDEMIOLOGY

Both lymphocytic and collagenous colitis occur most commonly between ages 50 and 70 years, with a strong female predominance and frequent association with arthritis, celiac disease, and autoimmune disorders. In a large population-based study in Spain, the demographic features of both collagenous and lymphocytic colitis were similar: the disorders were found in 9.5 of every 100 patients with chronic watery diarrhea and normal-appearing mucosa on colonoscopy; the incidence rate of lymphocytic colitis was three times higher than that of collagenous colitis.[4] This last observation contrasts strikingly with published reports of more than 400 cases of collagenous colitis compared with more than 60 cases of lymphocytic colitis, a finding that suggests that there may be a publication bias. The overall mean annual incidence of both colitides was 4.2 per 100,000 inhabitants in Spain, similar to the rates from an epidemiologic study conducted in Sweden.[5] Although the incidence is clearly higher in older age groups, both entities have been reported in children and teenagers, in whom the clinical presentation is similar to that of adults.

PATHOLOGY

In both lymphocytic and collagenous colitis, there is a modest increase of mononuclear cells within the lamina propria and between crypt epithelial cells, consisting mainly of CD8+ T lymphocytes, plasma cells, and macrophages.[3] There may be flattening of the surface epithelial cells, a mild decrease in the number of goblet cells, Paneth cell hyperplasia, and an increased number of intraepithelial lymphocytes (Fig. 121–1). Neutrophils are not prominent, and cryptitis and crypt distortion are unusual.

In collagenous colitis, there is a thickened subepithelial collagen layer, which may be continuous or patchy (Fig. 121–2). In normal colon, the width of this collagen band is less than 4 to 5 µm, whereas in collagenous colitis, it is greater than 10 µm and averages 20 to 60 µm.[6] In normal colon, the subepithelial collagen band consists predominantly of type IV collagen, whereas in collagenous colitis, the band is composed of type VI collagen and tenascin as well as lesser amounts of types I and III collagen. Tenascin is a glycoprotein that is a marker of matrix remodeling and is a product of intestinal subepithelial myofibroblasts.[7] These changes are absent in lymphocytic colitis and suggest that the two main forms of microscopic colitis should be considered as separate disease entities. Although inflammatory changes occur diffusely throughout the colon, the characteristic collagen band thickening is highly variable, occurring in the cecum and transverse colon in more than 80% of cases and in the rectum in less than 30% of cases. Involvement of the left colon appears to be less intense than involvement of the right colon; nevertheless, multiple biopsies of the left colon above the rectosigmoid during flexible sigmoidoscopy are sufficient to make the diagnosis in approximately 90% of cases.[6] It is essential to emphasize that the diagnosis of collagenous colitis requires both mucosal inflammation and a thickened collagen band and that artifact resulting from poor orientation may give the mistaken appearance of a thickened basement membrane. It has been suggested that tenascin immunohistochemistry be used as a routine test in the diagnosis of microscopic colitis.[7]

ETIOLOGY AND PATHOGENESIS

The cause of lymphocytic and collagenous colitis is unknown. The most widely held hypothesis is that

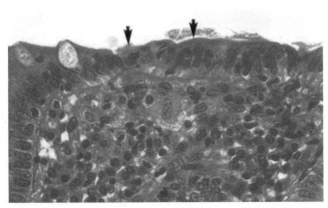

Figure 121–1 Histology of lymphocytic colitis. The arrows point to surface epithelial damage with increased numbers of intraepithelial lymphocytes. In addition, there is a superficial plasmacytosis without crypt distortion. Although a few intraepithelial neutrophils may be seen, widespread cryptitis is not a feature of lymphocytic colitis. (Courtesy of Feldman's online Atlas, Current Medicine.)

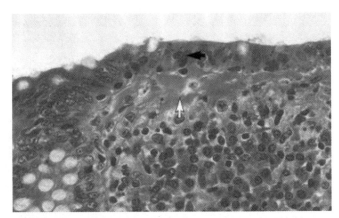

Figure 121–2 Histology of collagenous colitis. A thickened irregular subepithelial collagen table (*open arrow*) with patchy surface epithelial damage is shown. The surface epithelium also contains increased numbers of intraepithelial lymphocytes (*closed arrow*). In addition, there is a superficial plasmacytosis with prominent numbers of eosinophils. Crypt distortion and crypt abscesses are not usually seen in collagenous colitis. (Courtesy of Feldman's online Atlas, Current Medicine.)

they are inflammatory disorders arising from epithelial immune responses to intraluminal dietary or bacterial contents. This hypothesis is supported by the regression of inflammation following diversion of the fecal stream and recurrence of inflammation following restoration of intestinal continuity in three patients.[8] The identity of the inciting antigenic factors is uncertain, although medications,[9-11] bile salts, toxins, and infectious agents[12] have been postulated.

The strong association of rheumatologic diseases with microscopic colitis has raised the possibility that nonsteroidal anti-inflammatory drugs (NSAIDs) may play an etiologic role. One well-controlled study[13] found that chronic NSAID use occurred more frequently in patients with collagenous colitis than in age- and gender-matched controls (61% vs. 13%; $P < 0.02$), but this was not confirmed in another study.[14] One postulated mechanism by which NSAIDs may damage the colon is by increasing colonic permeability to allow luminal antigens to enter the lamina propria and promote inflammation. Because many patients with collagenous or lymphocytic colitis have not used NSAIDs and because NSAID use in older adults is common but these disorders are uncommon, other causes have been invoked including genetic susceptibility. Genetic susceptibility is supported by the finding that 12% of patients with microscopic colitis had a family history of inflammatory bowel disease (IBD).[11]

Approximately 20% to 30% of patients with celiac disease have been reported to have lymphocytic colitis, raising the possibility of similar pathogenetic mechanisms.[15] In 40% of patients with collagenous colitis, in one study, small intestinal biopsies were compatible with celiac disease,[16] although the frequency of celiac disease was only 2% of 45 patients with collagenous colitis[17] and 9% of 199 patients with lymphocytic colitis in another study.[11] Furthermore, patients with microscopic colitis do not respond to a gluten-free diet, and neither collagenous nor lymphocytic colitis is associated with human leukocyte antigens (HLAs) B8 and DR3, as is celiac disease. Finally, CD8+ T intraepithelial cells are predominant, in contrast to celiac disease in which CD3 and CD8 are prominent.

Because autoimmune disorders such as arthritis and thyroid abnormalities[11] have been described in patients with collagenous and lymphocytic colitis, there have been continued efforts to associate microscopic colitis with various autoimmune HLA haplotypes and serum markers. One small study showed that HLA-A1 antigens were expressed with increased frequency in lymphocytic but not collagenous colitis,[18] whereas another study showed similar abnormal expressions of HLA-DR antigens by mucosal epithelial cells in both conditions.[19] Whether such abnormalities are the cause or the result of these disorders is unknown. Another study found similarities in HLA-DQ loci between patients with celiac disease and patients with either lymphocytic or collagenous colitis.[20] Although gluten is not the inciting antigen in microscopic colitis, similar immune mechanisms may be involved in celiac disease and microscopic colitis.

The pathogenesis of the increased collagen band in collagenous colitis is unclear. It initially had been assumed that collagen synthesis is increased,[1] but colonic biopsies from patients with the disease showed decreased levels of interstitial collagenase, suggesting that reduced matrix degradation may contribute to the accumulation of matrix proteins.[21]

The mechanism of diarrhea in microscopic colitis is related to the severity of inflammation and not the extent or thickness of the collagen band. Perfusion studies have demonstrated defective active and passive absorption of sodium and chloride and reduced chloride-bicarbonate exchange in the colon[22]; two of six subjects had coexisting abnormalities of small intestinal fluid and electrolyte absorption. Other investigators have correlated colonic fluid absorption with the severity of inflammation.[23] A potential role for soluble mediators is suggested by a report that diarrhea was resolved by a histamine H_1 antagonist in a patient with microscopic colitis characterized by increased numbers of mast cells.[24] It has been suggested that bile acid malabsorption may contribute to diarrhea in patients with collagenous colitis and that treatment with a bile acid-binding resin such as cholestyramine may lead to a reduction in diarrhea. Bile acids are unlikely to cause the histologic changes observed in collagenous colitis, however, and a reduction in diarrhea was not associated with a decrease in colitis. Hormonal studies, including serum gastrin, vasoactive intestinal polypeptide, and urine 5-hydroxyindoleacetic acid levels, have been normal in microscopic colitis.

CLINICAL AND LABORATORY FEATURES

Patients with collagenous and lymphocytic colitis usually present with chronic watery diarrhea, with an average of eight stools each day, ranging in volume from 300 to 1700 g per 24 hours,[22] and associated with occasional fecal incontinence and abdominal cramps. Symptoms decrease with fasting.[5] Nausea, weight loss, and fecal urgency are variably present. Diarrhea generally is long-standing, lasting from months to years, with a fluctuating course of remissions and exacerbations. In one series of 172 patients, the median time from the onset of symptoms to diagnosis was 11 months,[17] whereas in another smaller series, the median time to diagnosis was 5.4 years.[14] Physical examination is usually unremarkable, and blood is not detected in the stool. Routine laboratory studies also are normal.

Examination of fresh stools showed fecal leukocytes in 55% of 116 patients with collagenous colitis.[17] Mild steatorrhea, mild anemia, low serum vitamin B_{12} levels, and hypoalbuminemia have been reported in varying numbers of patients but are not characteristic. Autoimmune markers that have been identified in patients with collagenous colitis include antinuclear antibodies (in up to 50%), perinuclear antineutrophil cytoplasmic antibodies (pANCA) (in 14%), rheumatoid factor, and increased C_3 and C_4 complement levels,[23] but none of these markers is of diagnostic value.

Colonoscopic examination is usually normal. Nonspecific abnormalities including patchy edema, erythema, friability, and an abnormal vascular pattern were reported in one study,[25] but the specificity or reproducibility of such findings is uncertain.

DIFFERENTIAL DIAGNOSIS

Infectious agents should be excluded by testing the stool for enteric pathogens, ova and parasites, and *Clostridium difficile* toxin. Many patients are incorrectly diagnosed with irritable bowel syndrome, a disorder that can be excluded by abnormal colonic biopsies and the finding of increased stool volume, both of which are uncharacteristic of irritable bowel syndrome.

Other diseases can produce colitis but should be distinguishable on histologic grounds. Acute infectious colitis is characterized by neutrophilic inflammation and decreased intraepithelial lymphocytes. Eosinophilic enterocolitis of the mucosal type is characterized by eosinophilic infiltration, shortened crypts, inflammation of the deeper parts of the lamina propria, and absence of increased intraepithelial lymphocytes. Amyloidosis has been mistaken for collagenous colitis, but its distribution includes the basement membranes of the crypts and blood vessels as well as the epithelium; confirmation can be made by histochemical staining. Mild cases of ulcerative colitis and Crohn's disease should present no diagnostic confusion in view of the characteristic endoscopic and histologic findings and absence of increased intraepithelial lymphocytes. Hormone-producing tumors, surreptitious laxative abuse, and hyperthyroidism can be excluded on clinical and biochemical grounds.

TREATMENT

There have been few controlled trials for either collagenous or lymphocytic colitis, and therapy is largely empirical. Evaluation of therapy is difficult, because both disorders usually exhibit a relapsing and remitting course over many years. No single agent works in all cases.[26]

About one third of patients respond to antidiarrheal agents, such as loperamide or diphenoxylate with atropine, as well as bulking agents such as psyllium or methylcellulose; clinical response is not associated with improvement of inflammation or collagen thickness. In an open-label trial of bismuth subsalicylate (8 chewable tablets per day for 8 weeks) in 12 patients, diarrhea resolved and stool weight was reduced within 2 weeks; in 9 patients colitis resolved with disappearance of the collagen band thickening.[27] Over a 7- to 28-month follow-up, 9 patients remained well, 2 were well but required retreatment, and 1 had persistent diarrhea. Both collagenous and lymphocytic colitis responded similarly, and there were no side effects of treatment; a controlled trial by the same investigators published only in abstract form confirmed these findings. Although the basis for its efficacy is unknown, bismuth subsalicylate possesses antidiarrheal, antibacterial, and anti-inflammatory properties; bismuth enemas have been reported to be effective in ulcerative colitis and chronic pouchitis.[28]

Other treatment trials for collagenous colitis and lymphocytic colitis have studied 5-aminosalicylate (mesalamine) compounds, glucocorticoids, and bile acid resins, alone or in combination; these agents appear to improve diarrhea and inflammation in some, but certainly not all, patients.[26] Although glucocorticoids given by either the oral or rectal route provide symptomatic improvement and decrease inflammation in more than 80% of cases, relapse usually occurs quickly after the drug is stopped.[5,29] Moreover, long-term use of glucocorticoids has undesirable effects, especially in older patients. The effectiveness of other immunosuppressants, such as azathioprine and 6-mercaptopurine, has been reported, but there are no sizable studies using these agents.[27,30]

Budesonide has been reported to be highly effective over a 6- to 8-week period in three placebo-controlled trials in patients with collagenous colitis.[31-33] Budesonide is a topically acting synthetic corticosteroid with both a high receptor-binding affinity in the mucosa and a high first-pass effect in the liver. In view of its proven efficacy, budesonide should be considered over 5-aminosalicylates or bile acid resins in patients who do not respond to antidiarrheal agents and bismuth subsalicylate.

The only report of surgery for collagenous colitis involved nine patients who underwent ileostomy for disabling refractory collagenous colitis, after which all had symptomatic and histologic remission.[26] In patients in whom intestinal continuity was restored, the disease recurred and of three patients who underwent proctocolectomy with ileal pouch-anal anastomosis, problematic diarrhea occurred. Ileostomy should be considered only as a last resort but appears to be effective in patients with disabling and refractory symptoms.

Based on available data, the treatment algorithm shown in Figure 121–3 is proposed.

DIVERSION COLITIS

BACKGROUND AND EPIDEMIOLOGY

Diversion colitis is an inflammatory process that occurs in diverted segments of the colon and rectum after surgical diversion of the fecal stream. The entity was first reported in 1981 by Glotzer and associates in 10 patients who had undergone ileostomy or colostomy for various indications other than IBD.[34] Since then, diversion colitis has been found in patients who have undergone surgical diversion for many indications, although diversion colitis has been reported to occur more commonly in patients with IBD (87%) than in those with noninflammatory conditions (28%).[35,36] The prevalence of diversion colitis has been underestimated because many patients are asymptomatic; however, histologic changes are likely to occur in diverted segments of the colon within months of surgical diversion.

PATHOLOGY

A spectrum of histologic changes has been described in diversion colitis, ranging from lymphoid follicular hyperplasia and mixed mononuclear and neutrophilic infiltration to severe inflammation with crypt abscesses, mucin granulomas, and Paneth cell metaplasia[37,38]; however, large ulcers and transmural changes are absent and crypt architecture generally is preserved. Endoscopic findings include erythema, friability, nodularity, edema, aphthous ulcerations, exudates, and frank bleeding, as in idiopathic

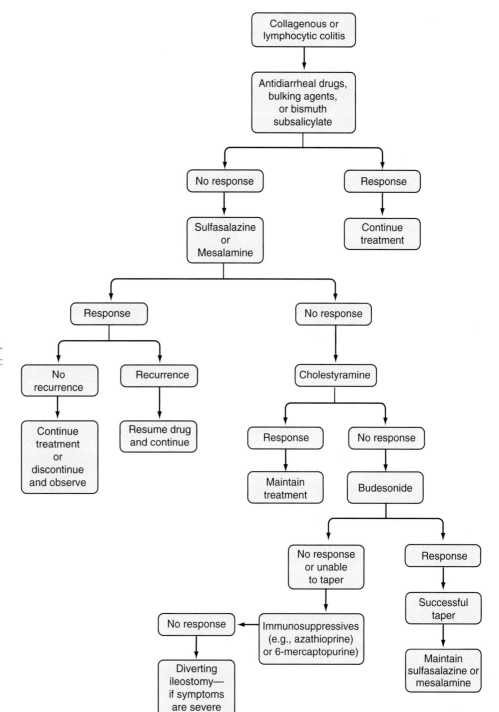

Figure 121–3 Approach to the treatment of collagenous or lymphocytic colitis.

PATHOGENESIS

Diversion colitis appears to be caused largely by the colonic epithelium suffering luminal nutrient deficiency. The principal nutrient substrates of colonic epithelium are luminal short-chain fatty acids (SCFAs), which are metabolic products of carbohydrate and peptide fermentation by anaerobic bacteria.[39,40] Roediger demonstrated

IBD. After extended periods following diversion, inflammatory pseudopolyps and strictures may develop.

that SCFAs are the major and preferred energy source for colonic epithelium and that the distal colon is more dependent on SCFAs for its metabolic needs than is the proximal colon.[41] Butyrate supplies the bulk of oxidative energy to the distal colon, whereas acetate, glutamine, and ketones provide alternative sources of energy. Harig and associates demonstrated that the excluded segments of colon contain negligible amounts of SCFAs and that infusion of glucose results in no appreciable anaerobic fermentation.[42] The number of obligate anaerobes is reduced in the excluded colon, consistent with reduced SCFA production.[43] Instillation of enemas containing

SCFAs resulted in disappearance of endoscopic changes within 4 to 6 weeks in four patients, although resolution of histologic abnormalities was slower and incomplete.[42]

Although SCFA deficiency has been widely accepted as the cause of diversion colitis, other observations suggest that SCFA deficiency may not be the entire etiologic explanation. First, studies in children indicate that SCFA enemas are not universally successful in treating diversion colitis.[44] Second, in germ-free rodents with surgical diversion and in patients receiving long-term parenteral nutrition or elimination diets (circumstances in which luminal SCFA concentrations are low), mucosal atrophy occurs rather than inflammation.[45] Third, inflammation does not occur in urinary colon conduits, where the fecal stream is diverted, and urine does not contain measurable SCFAs.[46] Finally, in a prospective, randomized, double-blind study of 13 patients with diversion colitis, butyrate enemas given for 14 days provided no improvement in either endoscopic or histologic parameters.[47] In a subsequent study by the same group, administration of SCFAs did not affect the bacterial population in the excluded colon.[48] Other luminal elements besides SCFA deficiency must play a role, but the nature of such factors is unknown.

DIAGNOSIS

The diagnosis of diversion colitis is based on the clinical picture, endoscopic findings, and histology. Diagnosis is relatively straightforward in a patient without preexisting IBD, but radiation colitis and ischemia should be considered in the appropriate clinical setting. Stool specimens for *C. difficile* toxin, ova and parasites, and cultures usually are adequate to exclude other etiologies.

In patients with a preoperative diagnosis of Crohn's disease, diversion colitis must be distinguished from recurrent IBD. Colonoscopic findings such as linear ulcers and possibly strictures are said to favor Crohn's disease, as do transmural inflammation, marked crypt architectural abnormalities, and epithelioid granulomas[35] Lymphoid hyperplasia occurs in both disorders but tends to be more prominent in diversion colitis.[49] If rectal involvement with Crohn's disease is absent prior to diversion, rectal inflammation is more likely to be caused by diversion than Crohn's disease.[2,35,50]

TREATMENT

The preferred treatment of diversion colitis is surgical restoration of colonic continuity, which rapidly reverses symptoms and histologic changes. If symptoms are moderate-to-severe and reanastomosis is not feasible, SCFA enemas containing a mixture of 60 mmol of acetate, 30 mmol of propionate, and 40 mmol of butyrate with 22 mmol of sodium chloride per liter are administered through the anus or mucous fistula twice daily for 4 weeks and then decreased to once or twice weekly.[42] Such preparations are not commercially available and must be formulated by compounding pharmacies, making it the most expensive of the nonsurgical options.[51] There are anecdotal reports that 5-aminosalicylate and hydrocorti-

sone retention enemas are effective as well.[52] Because they are available commercially, these agents are considered to be first-line therapies for most patients. One report suggested that intraluminal irrigation with soluble and insoluble fiber solutions improved endoscopic and histologic abnormalities and might be useful to reduce inflammation prior to surgical restoration of bowel continuity.[53]

NONSPECIFIC COLONIC ULCERS

Benign nonspecific ulcers of the colon are uncommon and the causes remain unknown. The most recent large review of the literature encompassed 127 patients and indicated that colonic ulcers occur at any age, with a peak incidence in the 4th and 5th decades and a slight female predominance.[54] Most of these ulcers occur in the proximal colon, virtually all are solitary and located on the antimesenteric side of the colon, and most are round and sharply demarcated from relatively normal surrounding mucosa (Fig. 121–4).[54,55] Histologically, there is nonspecific acute and chronic inflammation.[54]

PATHOGENESIS

The causes of nonspecific colonic ulcers are unknown. Hypotheses that have been advanced, but with little or no supporting evidence, include ischemia, cecal diverticulosis, and acid-peptic disease. Correlations with the use of drugs such as glucocorticoids, NSAIDs,[56,57] oral contraceptives, and oxyphenbutazone have been suggested, but causation has not been established and these drugs have not been implicated in most of the ulcers reported. It is likely that no single causative agent explains all cases. There have been reports of associations of non-

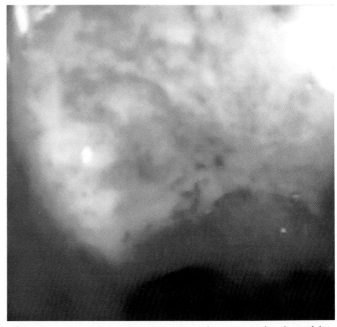

Figure 121–4 Endoscopic appearance of a nonspecific ulcer of the colon.

specific colon ulcers with chronic renal failure and renal transplantation,[58] Churg-Strauss syndrome,[59] Wegener's granulomatosis,[60] Behçet's disease, essential mixed cryoglobulinemia,[61] and systemic lupus erythematosus. Perhaps a mechanism common to all exists, but none has been identified.

CLINICAL FEATURES

The most frequent presenting symptoms are abdominal pain and bleeding. More than one half of patients with nonspecific colon ulcers present with acute or chronic abdominal pain, often in the right lower abdomen and mimicking appendicitis.[54] One third have lower gastrointestinal bleeding with hematochezia, and 16% present with an abdominal mass, most often when the ulcer is located in the left or sigmoid colon. A cecal ulcer should be suspected in a patient with gastrointestinal bleeding associated with a clinical picture consistent with appendicitis or in a patient with symptoms suggestive of pelvic inflammatory disease, ovarian disease, or Crohn's disease in the absence of these diseases.

DIAGNOSIS

Historically, nonspecific colonic ulcers usually were diagnosed at laparotomy after complications occurred. With the advent of endoscopy, many colonic ulcers are now diagnosed preoperatively and, in some cases, managed conservatively.

Colonoscopy is currently the diagnostic test of choice.[54] Flexible sigmoidoscopy is inadequate because most colonic ulcers are beyond the reach of the instrument. Abnormalities have been described in up to 75% of air-contrast barium enemas[54] and include mucosal irregularities, intraluminal filling defects or narrowing, a mass effect, or localized colonic spasm (Fig. 121–5). Roentgen findings are nonspecific, however, and diagnostically inferior to direct inspection by colonoscopy. Computed tomographic (CT) scans are most helpful in the presence of perforation or associated abscess formation.

The key to the diagnosis of these ulcers is the exclusion of diseases that are associated with ulceration; these include Crohn's disease, infections such as tuberculosis, *Entamoeba histolytica*, cytomegalovirus, and *Salmonella typhi*, stercoral ulcers, and solitary rectal ulcer syndrome. Amyloidosis[62] and neoplastic causes such as carcinoma and lymphoma are distinguished on histologic grounds but may not be distinguishable from nonspecific colonic ulcers on the basis of endoscopic appearance alone.

TREATMENT

Surgery is recommended for patients with ulcers complicated by perforation, significant gastrointestinal or intra-abdominal bleeding, and for those with persistent symptoms and failure of the ulcer to heal. In uncomplicated cases, however, an expectant approach has been advocated, with colonoscopy every 6 weeks to monitor healing. The most common surgical procedures are local

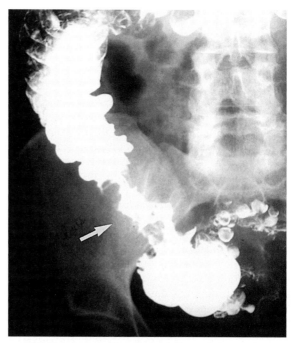

Figure 121–5 Nonspecific ulcer of the colon. Barium enema examination showing the lesion in Figure 121–4 (*arrow*). The initial interpretation was carcinoma of the ascending colon.

excision of the ulcer, oversewing of the ulcer if there is significant bleeding, and occasionally, more extensive resections of the affected colon.[54,63]

DIEULAFOY-TYPE COLONIC ULCERATION

In 1897, Georges Dieulafoy first described massive gastrointestinal bleeding emanating from a relatively enlarged ("persistent calibre") submucosal artery by way of a minute mucosal ulcer at the most superficial point of the vessel.[64] Although originally described in the stomach and most commonly occurring in the gastric fundus, identical lesions have been described in other gastrointestinal organs, including the colon and rectum.[65-67] In the colon, Dieulafoy-type lesions appear to have a strong male predominance and have been reported in all age groups.

Histologically, colonic Dieulafoy-type lesions are identical to those found elsewhere in the gastrointestinal tract. The submucosal artery is tortuous and hypertrophic, curving toward the mucosa. Inflammation is absent, and the solitary mucosal ulceration extends no deeper than the upper submucosal layer.

The clinical picture is one of acute and massive bleeding. Colonoscopy can identify the lesion in some cases[67] but is often difficult or impossible, especially when bleeding continues or thorough cleansing of the colon cannot be accomplished. Selective mesenteric angiography is the diagnostic study of choice, and surgical resection has been the principal form of therapy. Even after angiographic detection of the bleeding site, precise localization of the lesion is frequently difficult, and more extended resection often is required. In some cases, colonic lesions appear as pseudopolyps,[65] and successful treatment with sclerotherapy or electrocautery may obviate the need for surgery.[68]

CATHARTIC COLON

Cathartic colon is an infrequent and severe manifestation of chronic irritant laxative abuse. In 1943, Heilbrun first described radiologic abnormalities of the colon and terminal ileum associated with prolonged abuse of irritant cathartics.[69] Fewer than 50 cases have been reported in the literature, all in women with a duration of laxative abuse ranging from 10 to 70 years. It is important to emphasize that the term *cathartic colon* is based on barium enema characteristics and is not synonymous with prolonged use of laxatives or with laxative abuse. Indeed, misapplication of the term *cathartic colon* has led to inappropriate concerns over the chronic use of laxatives that, when used appropriately, is not associated with structural or functional damage to the colon. Cathartic colon is not the inevitable consequence of chronic laxative abuse, which may be associated with a variety of reversible symptoms as well as fluid and electrolyte abnormalities. In a review of 240 cases of chronic laxative abuse published in more than 70 reports, no case of cathartic colon was demonstrated.[70,71]

RADIOLOGIC AND PATHOLOGIC FEATURES

Heilbrun originally described the following characteristics in his original case report: loss of haustrations, pseudostrictures, dilated colon and terminal ileum, and gaping of the ileocecal valve[69]; similarities to the radiologic appearance of chronic ulcerative colitis were noted in this and subsequent studies. Characteristic changes are not always found throughout the colon, and there is a predilection for involvement of the ascending colon. Pathologic changes in resected specimens of cathartic colon have included mucosal atrophy, chronic inflammation with thickening of the muscularis mucosae, submucosal fatty infiltration, and mild fibrosis. Irreversible strictures and degenerative changes in intestinal neurons are absent. Neuronal changes have been found in patients with chronic laxative abuse, but these patients did not exhibit cathartic colon as defined here.[72]

DO LAXATIVES DAMAGE THE COLON?

The original suggestion that irritant laxatives, predominantly anthraquinones, damage the colon was based on studies in laboratory animals and in colons resected from laxative abusers.[73] Although mucosal atrophy and abnormalities of the enteric nervous system were described, the identities of the laxatives were not documented, nor was there information concerning preexisting conditions that might have prompted chronic use of laxatives.

Subsequent studies have reported changes in colonic epithelial cells and the submucosa in patients with long-term laxative abuse, and both anthraquinones and bisacodyl have been implicated[72]; however, the unclear nature and duration of laxative use and the inability to

exclude preexisting conditions make the significance of these observations uncertain. Studies in rodents and in chronically constipated women do not support the deleterious effect of anthraquinones on the ultrastructure of colonic nerves,[74,75] nor is there evidence to suggest that sennosides, bisacodyl, or related substances cause significant morphologic damage to the colonic enteric nervous system in either experimental animals or humans. Perhaps one or more laxatives that are no longer in use, such as podophyllin, may account for cases of cathartic colon, because no case of cathartic colon has been reported in persons who began to use or abuse irritant laxatives after 1960.[71]

CLINICAL FEATURES

Habitual laxative users and abusers often complain of abdominal discomfort, bloating, fullness, or inability to defecate completely without using laxatives. In the more severe cases, electrolyte and fluid abnormalities such as hypokalemia and hypovolemia are associated with excessive thirst and weakness. Uncommonly, protein-losing enteropathy has been reported. All symptoms are reversible on withdrawal of laxatives or conversion to a more appropriate regimen of laxative use, if there is no underlying diagnosis such as irritable bowel syndrome.

TREATMENT

Treatment of cathartic colon and symptoms of chronic laxative use is focused on reducing or eliminating irritant laxatives, substituting bulking or osmotic agents, and retraining the bowel. Although often thought to be irreversible, there is evidence that cathartic colon can partially or completely reverse after withdrawal of laxatives. In severe or refractory cases, subtotal colectomy or proctocolectomy has been effective.

The cathartic colon is of historic interest and is unlikely to be identified in current clinical practice. There is no evidence that currently used laxatives can produce this entity. The term *cathartic colon* should not be confused with "chronic laxative abuse syndrome," nor should the term imply that current laxatives are dangerous if used chronically but appropriately.

PSEUDOMELANOSIS COLI

Melanosis coli is a brownish discoloration of the colonic mucosa caused by the accumulation of pigment in macrophages of the lamina propria (Fig. 121–6). First described in the early 19th century, the term *melanosis coli* was coined by Virchow in 1857, because the pigment was considered to be melanin or a melanin-like substance. Subsequently, the pigment proved to be lipofuscin, both histochemically and ultrastructurally.[76,77] The term *pseudomelanosis coli*, though more accurate, has not been adopted widely.

The association between pseudomelanosis coli and chronic use of anthraquinone laxatives is established firmly and is supported further by the development of

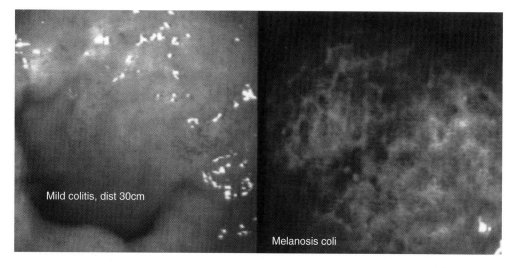

Figure 121–6 A colonoscopic view of pseudomelanosis coli associated with the chronic use of senna laxatives in a patient with ulcerative proctitis. There is little or no pseudomelanin pigment in the distal 30 cm of colon in the presence of active mild colitis (*left*), in contrast to the heavy pigmentation in the remaining colon (*right*). (Courtesy of Miguel Regueiro, MD, Pittsburgh, PA.)

characteristic pigmentation in laboratory animals after administration of anthraquinones.[78] Pseudomelanosis develops in more than 70% of persons who use anthraquinone laxatives (cascara sagrada, aloe, senna, rhubarb, and frangula), often within 4 months of use, with an average of 9 months. The condition is widely regarded as benign and reversible, and disappearance of the pigment generally occurs within 1 year of stopping laxatives.[79] Pseudomelanosis probably can result from other factors or exposure to other laxatives, however, and is not pathognomonic for anthraquinone use.

The pigment in pseudomelanosis coli is thought to originate from either macrophages or organelles within epithelial cells after damage by anthraquinone laxatives, which cause cells to die by apoptosis. Such a sequence of damage has been demonstrated in guinea pigs exposed to anthraquinones.[80] Histologically, the number and size of macrophages within the lamina propria are increased, and the greatest amount of pigment is found in macrophages furthest from the lumen. Abnormalities of colonic epithelial cells are noted on electron microscopy but not on light microscopy.[81]

Concern about a possible relationship between pseudomelanosis coli and the development of colonic neoplasms[82] has not been substantiated in a recent prospective case-control study.[83] Other confounding factors such as chronic constipation or dietary intake may account for an increased risk of colon cancer suggested by earlier studies.[84,85] Colonic neoplasms lack pigment-containing macrophages and are identified easily in patients with pseudomelanosis coli (Fig. 121–7).[86] Therefore, biopsies should be taken of any nonpigmented area of the colon in a patient with pseudomelanosis coli who undergoes colonoscopy.

CHEMICAL COLITIS

Damage to the colon has been reported after exposure to a number of rectally administered agents (Table 121–1), the better known of which are soaps and detergents used as "cleansing" enemas.[87,88] Other offending substances include hydrogen peroxide,[89] water-soluble contrast

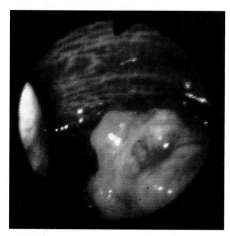

Figure 121–7 Pale colon cancer easily seen in contrast against the dark background of a colon with pseudomelanosis. The neoplasm is pale because it lacks pigment-containing macrophages. (Courtesy of Juergen Nord, MD, Tampa, FL.)

Table 121–1 Chemical Agents Associated with Colitis

Acetic acid
Alcohol
Ammonia
Caustic soda (sodium hydroxide)
Chloro-m-xylenol (Dettol)
Ergotamine
Formalin
Glutaraldehyde
Herbal medicines
Hydrofluoric acid
Hydrogen peroxide
Lye
Potassium permanganate
Radiocontrast agents (Hypaque, Renografin-76)
Soap
Sulfuric acid
Vinegar

agents such as sodium diatrizoate (Hypaque, Gastrografin),[90] vinegar, potassium permanganate, herbal medications,[91] glutaraldehyde,[92,93] formalin,[94] and alcohol.[95] Milder damage to the mucosa occurs after use of monobasic or dibasic sodium phosphate enemas[96] and bisacodyl suppositories. Colonic damage presumably occurs from a detergent, hypertonic, or direct toxic effect on the mucosa. The severity of the reaction depends on the type and concentration of the substance, the duration and extent of its contact with the mucosa, and perhaps the presence of underlying colonic disease.[97]

Soaps consist of a number of substances, including strong alkali, potash, phenol, and sodium and potassium salts of long-chain fatty acids. These agents produce liquefaction necrosis with mild to severe inflammation and saponification of the layers of the colon wall. Acute histologic changes include necrosis, leading, in more severe cases, to ulceration and formation of granulation tissue. Acute colitis may heal without residua or with fibrosis and scarring or progress to transmural necrosis and perforation. The severity of damage probably is related to the concentration of soap and duration of mucosal contact. Endoscopic findings have ranged from loss of the normal mucosal vascular pattern to aphthae to mucosal sloughing and ulceration.

Hydrogen peroxide enemas are no longer frequently used, but at one time they were employed to relieve meconium ileus and to remove fecal impactions. There are reports of severe damage associated with use of hydrogen peroxide, including severe colitis, pneumatosis coli, perforation, sepsis, and death.[89] Within minutes of contact, diffuse mucosal emphysema occurs, and after about 1 hour, the colon may become ischemic and eventually ulcerate (Fig. 121–8). Acute colitis has been reported after glutaraldehyde (Fig. 121–9).[92,93]

Colitis has been reported following the use of several hyperosmolar water-soluble contrast materials that often are employed to opacify the colon in cases of partial obstruction and to treat fecal impactions in adults.[90] Damage is believed to occur because of the hypertonicity of these agents, but the addition of Tween 80 to hyperosmolar agents to improve mucosal contrast may contribute to mucosal damage because of its detergent properties. Most reports of injury have occurred in the colon proximal to an obstruction and mainly in the right colon, suggesting that prolonged contact with these agents predisposes to mucosal injury.

PREVENTION AND TREATMENT

Proper cleaning and rinsing of endoscopes are required to minimize exposure of the patient to injurious disinfecting chemicals. Protocols require strict adherence to proper maintenance and adjustments in the rinse cycle of disinfecting machines.[93] Forced-air drying and rinsing of endoscope channels and the exterior of the instrument should ensure a chemical-free procedure.

Patients and health care professionals should be cautioned that soapsuds enemas should not be used. Rectal instillation of substances other than commercially available enemas for medicinal or ritualistic activities should be discouraged.

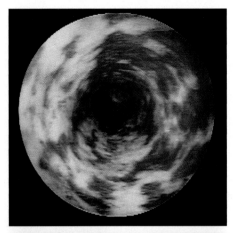

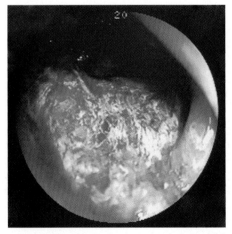

Figure 121–8 Colonoscopic photograph of hydrogen peroxide colitis in a patient to whom hydrogen peroxide was given to help remove a fecal impaction. Both panels show the so-called snow-white sign, referring to the appearance of the stark white necrotic mucosa. (Courtesy of Lawrence J. Brandt, MD, Bronx, NY.)

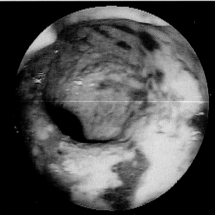

Figure 121–9 Colonoscopic photograph of glutaraldehyde colitis in a young man who had had a normal colonoscopy 3 hours before this photograph was taken. Colitis was caused by glutaraldehyde that had been used to disinfect the flexible sigmoidoscope after its previous use, but had not been sufficiently cleansed from the instrument. He complained of "agonizing" pain during the sigmoidoscopic examination and began to pass bright red blood 2 hours later. (Courtesy of Lawrence J. Brandt, MD, Bronx, NY.)

Treatment of chemical colitis is largely supportive, with intravenous fluids and broad-spectrum antibiotics. Surgery may be indicated in severe cases of bowel necrosis leading to gangrene or perforation. Most patients will recover completely after 4 to 6 weeks.

PNEUMATOSIS COLI (PNEUMATOSIS CYSTOIDES INTESTINALIS)

The term *pneumatosis coli* is synonymous with pneumatosis cystoides intestinalis when the disorder is limited to the colon. This uncommon disorder is characterized by multiple gas-filled cysts located in the submucosa and subserosa of the intestine. Pneumatosis cystoides intestinalis must be distinguished from pneumatosis linearis, or gas within the wall of the bowel, which usually is associated with bowel necrosis, signifies loss of bowel viability, and mandates surgery. Most cases of pneumatosis cystoides intestinalis occur in the jejunum and ileum, with only 6% of cases involving the colon. There is a propensity for involvement of the left side of the colon. Numerous conditions have been associated with pneumatosis coli, including appendicitis, Crohn's disease,[98] ulcerative colitis, diverticular disease, necrotizing enterocolitis, pseudomembranous colitis,[99] ileus,[100] and sigmoid volvulus. Pneumatosis also has been associated with nongastrointestinal conditions, including emphysema, collagen vascular diseases,[100,101] transplantation,[101] acquired immunodeficiency syndrome (AIDS),[102] glucocorticoid use, chemotherapy,[100] and certain medications. In AIDS, pneumatosis linearis may be associated with opportunistic infections of the colon and may resolve without surgery if the infection is treated successfully.[102] In approximately 20% of cases, there are no associated medical conditions and pneumatosis is considered primary.[103]

ETIOLOGY

Several theories have been suggested to explain the large and varied number of conditions associated with pneumatosis cystoides intestinalis. The most plausible theories are (1) the mechanical theory and (2) the bacterial theory.

According to the mechanical theory, intraluminal gas enters the bowel wall under pressure through a defect or potential defect in the intestinal mucosa. The mucosal defect may result from direct trauma or increased intraluminal pressure. This hypothesis could account for reports of pneumatosis after sigmoidoscopy without biopsy, cases of colitis, perforated duodenal ulcers, and jejunal diverticula and after intestinal anastomoses. The plausibility of this theory is diminished by the absence of a connection between the mucosa and the cysts and the presence of elevated levels of hydrogen gas in the cysts.[104]

The bacterial theory suggests that the cystic gas collections are the by-products of bacteria, specifically those that produce hydrogen. This theory has been supported by clinical observations and laboratory experiments. In laboratory animals, pneumatosis coli can be induced by injecting gas-forming bacteria into the bowel wall. In addition to local invasion of the intestinal wall, bacteria may produce gas cysts by manufacturing large amounts of hydrogen gas as a result of the fermentation of carbohydrates. Levitt and Olsson theorized that the high hydrogen tension in the colonic lumen leads to rapid diffusion into an intramural gas bubble and may cause N_2, O_2, and CO_2 to diffuse from the circulation into the gas bubble.[105] According to their theory, the gas bubble enlarges if there is continued diffusion of hydrogen into it. Indeed, high hydrogen content in the cysts has been documented,[106] and cysts regress in patients fed an elemental diet to decrease carbohydrate substrate for colonic bacteria. Two major observations argue against the bacterial theory of pneumatosis: (1) that bacteria are not cultured from cysts; and (2) with cyst rupture and pneumoperitoneum, peritonitis is not seen.

It is hypothesized that gas cysts can form by counterperfusion supersaturation of H_2 gas by which super H_2 production by colonic bacteria provides the condition for H_2 tension in the colonic lumen to approach the level of N_2 tension in the blood.[107] One such mechanism is exposure to drugs such as chloral hydrate that inhibit growth of H_2-consuming methanogenic bacteria in the colon to increase net H_2 production.[107] Another possible etiologic setting is the administration of a nonabsorbable carbohydrate such as lactulose, thereby increasing colonic hydrogen production in a setting where bacteria metabolizing H_2 are deficient.[108] Successful treatment with antibiotics[106,108] and colonic washouts also supports a bacterial etiology for pneumatosis coli.[109] In one study, stools from patients with pneumatosis coli were demonstrated to lack two major species of hydrogen-consuming bacteria.[104] Because hydrogen normally is produced only in the colon and not in the small intestine, pneumatosis coli may differ from pneumatosis intestinalis with respect to pathogenic mechanisms.

CLINICAL FEATURES AND DIAGNOSIS

The frequency of pneumatosis coli is highest in the 6th decade, with equal frequency in men and women.[103] In most cases, pneumatosis is an unexpected finding on abdominal plain films. The most common symptoms are diarrhea (68%), mucus discharge (68%), rectal bleeding (60%), and constipation (48%).[103] Approximately 3% of patients present with a complication of pneumatosis coli, including pneumoperitoneum, volvulus, intestinal obstruction, intussusception, tension pneumoperitoneum, and intestinal perforation. Physical examination may detect an abdominal mass, and rectal examination may reveal the cystic lesions. A plain abdominal film may identify radiolucent clusters or streaks along the bowel wall with pneumoperitoneum, if a cyst has ruptured. A markedly redundant sigmoid colon as well as the outline of the cysts or linear streaks may be seen on barium enema (Fig. 121–10).[103] Endoscopic examination with biopsy is necessary for definitive diagnosis, to exclude carcinoma, and to differentiate pneumatosis from familial adenomatosis polyposis[110] and from the thumbprinting of colon ischemia. The endoscopic appearance is of multiple cysts, which vary in size from a few millimeters to several centimeters (Fig. 121–11) and which on punc-

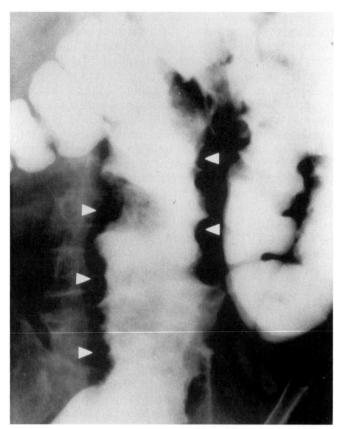

Figure 121–10   Single-contrast barium enema demonstrating the presence of gas-filled cysts in the wall of the colon characteristic of pneumatosis coli. (From Feldman M, Boland CR [eds]: Slide Atlas of Gastroenterology and Hepatology. Philadelphia, Current Medicine, 1996.).

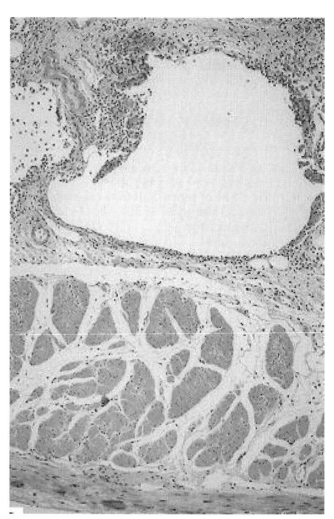

Figure 121–12   Histologic view of a large gas-filled cyst in the submucosa. These cysts are usually lined by histiocytes and multinucleated giant cells. Cysts also may be present in the subserosa. (Courtesy of Feldman's online Atlas, Current Medicine.)

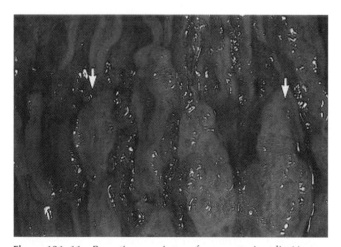

Figure 121–11   Resection specimen of pneumatosis coli. Numerous gas-filled cysts are seen in this surface view of the mucosa (*arrows*). (Courtesy of Feldman's online Atlas, Current Medicine.)

ture with a needle rapidly deflate. Endoscopic ultrasonography also has been used to establish the diagnosis in pneumatosis.[111]

PATHOLOGY

The cysts of pneumatosis cystoids resemble soap bubbles. They usually are thin-walled and unilocular and can occur separately or in clusters. They do not communicate with the intestinal lumen or with each other and have a spongy consistency that pops like a balloon when compressed. On cross section they appear shiny, honeycombed, and range in size from a few millimeters to several centimeters. Microscopically, the cysts have an endothelial lining that tends to gather and coalesce, forming multinucleate giant cells that increase in number as the cysts collapse, undergo fibrosis (Fig. 121–12) and are eventually sloughed, leaving the cysts without a lining. Progressive fibrosis leads to a decrease in the size of the cysts and ultimately to their obliteration. The connective tissue surrounding the cysts may show a granulomatous inflammatory reaction made up of eosinophils, lymphocytes, macrophages, and plasma cells. Subserosal cysts are surrounded by fibrous connective tissue and can produce adhesion of adjacent bowel loops. The mucosa in pneumatosis may be normal, or thinned and with or without ulcerations and inflammation where it is stretched over a cyst. Mucosal changes vary from mild focal abnormalities to extensive changes including granulomas, abnormal crypts with branching, shortening, cryptitis and abscesses, dilatation, and rupture.

TREATMENT

Because the natural history of pneumatosis is one of spontaneous regression in up to 50% of cases and because cysts may reappear after surgery, specific treatment is not recommended in asymptomatic individuals. Symptomatic patients may be treated successfully by breathing high-flow oxygen for several days[112] or by use of hyperbaric oxygen, especially in resistant cases[111]; high oxygen levels lead to replacement of hydrogen within the cysts and a corresponding reduction in the size of the cysts. Because cysts may recur after oxygen therapy,[112] a minimum of 48 hours of oxygen therapy is recommended to maximize the success rate. Metronidazole also has been used to treat pneumatosis coli, an observation that suggests that anaerobic bacteria play a role in the genesis of the disorder. Because cysts have been reported to recur after short courses of metronidazole,[109] treatment should continue until complete endoscopic resolution of the cysts is seen. In general, colonic resection is reserved for patients with complications such as intestinal obstruction and massive bleeding.

MALAKOPLAKIA

Malakoplakia is a rare chronic granulomatous disease first described by von Hansemann in 1901 and reported by Michaelis and Gutmann in 1902.[114] The term *malakoplakia* is derived from the Greek *"malakos"* (soft) and *"plakos"* (plaque) and reflects its usual appearance as a friable, yellow mucosal lesion. Microscopically, coliform bacteria are located in the cytoplasm of macrophages (von Hansemann bodies), and laminated intracytoplasmic inclusion bodies (Michaelis-Gutmann bodies) are considered the diagnostic features of this disorder.[114]

Malakoplakia may affect many organs, including lung, brain, adrenal glands, pancreas, bone, and the genitourinary tract. The most common sites of colonic involvement are the rectum, sigmoid, and right colon, in descending order of frequency.[116]

ETIOLOGY

The pathogenesis of malakoplakia is unknown. Proposed etiologies are infection, immunosuppression, systemic illness, neoplasia, and a genetic disorder. Evidence for an infectious etiology is based on the finding that some patients with malakoplakia have associated chronic infections. This was first described in the urologic form of malakoplakia in which more than 75% of patients were infected with *Escherichia coli*. This finding led to the belief that *E. coli* might be a primary cause of malakoplakia; however, other organisms also have been isolated, including *Klebsiella, Proteus, Mycobacterium, Staphylococcus*, and fungi,[117] suggesting that one infection is not the primary cause of the disease.

Other evidence points to a defect in macrophage killing as the cause of malakoplakia. Nondigested microorganisms are found within the lysosomes of macrophages in affected persons. Macrophages from these patients show a decrease in cyclic guanosine monophosphate, resulting in impaired bactericidal activity.[118] Peripheral blood monocytes also are found to have decreased bactericidal activity in malakoplakia. The defect in macrophage dysfunction may be reversed with the addition of a cholinergic agonist, both in vitro and in vivo.[119]

Malakoplakia has been reported in patients receiving chemotherapy and immunosuppressive therapy for organ transplantation.[120] Reversal of both macrophage abnormalities and clinical symptoms occurred after discontinuation of glucocorticoids and azathioprine.[121] Malakoplakia has been reported in various immune deficiency states such as primary hypogammaglobulinemia and AIDS.[122,123] Malakoplakia also has been associated with chronic systemic diseases such as systemic lupus erythematosus, ulcerative colitis, and sarcoidosis.[116]

There have been a substantial number of cases to support a neoplastic etiology for one form of malakoplakia.[124,125] In 1996, Bates and colleagues identified 19 cases of colorectal adenocarcinoma associated with malakoplakia,[125] which was present only in a focal area adjacent to the tumor, in contrast to cases not associated with a neoplasm, in which multiple organs may be affected. A possible genetic etiology was suggested by one report of colonic malakoplakia that clustered in a family.[126]

CLINICAL FEATURES AND DIAGNOSIS

Patients with malakoplakia usually present with abdominal pain, diarrhea, hematochezia, and fever.[116] Physical findings include a palpable rectal mass, abdominal mass, and weight loss. Diagnosis is by colonoscopy (and biopsy), which generally reveal the following three patterns of the disease:

1. Isolated rectosigmoid involvement, in which lesions appear as yellowish plaques that may be sessile, polypoid, and ulcerated; the colonic lumen may be strictured, and intestinal fistulas may occur, suggesting a diagnosis of cancer or Crohn's disease
2. Diffuse colonic involvement, which is characteristic of immunosuppressed patients
3. Focal lesions, which may be associated with an adenomatous polyp or cancer

Biopsy is essential to confirm the diagnosis and to exclude an underlying colonic malignancy (Fig. 121-13). Histology reveals the characteristic macrophages with voluminous cytoplasm containing the classic von Hansemann bodies (intracellular organisms) and Michaelis-Gutmann bodies (intracytoplasmic concentric laminated inclusion bodies). The histiocytes (also termed *von Hansemann cells*) must be distinguished from those found in fungal disease, leprosy, Whipple's disease, reticulum cell sarcoma, and macrophages harboring *Mycobacterium avium* complex.[123]

TREATMENT

Patients with newly diagnosed malakoplakia should undergo a thorough medical evaluation to determine if they are taking immunosuppressive medications or have coexisting medical illnesses or malnutrition. Tests of immune function and screening for associated bladder

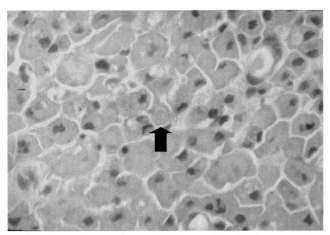

Figure 121-13 Histology of malakoplakia. Sheets of large pale cells characterize the histologic changes in malakoplakia. One of the histiocytes shows the characteristic ring-like Michaelis-Gutmann body (*arrow*) consisting of a central core of partially digested bacteria coated with iron and calcium phosphate. (Courtesy of Lawrence J. Brandt, MD, Bronx, NY.)

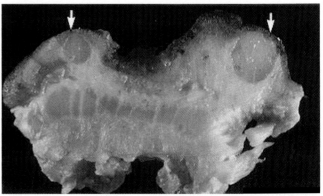

Figure 121-14 Resection specimen of colitis cystica profunda. Several submucosal cysts are filled with mucinous material (*arrows*). This entity occurs in the setting of chronic inflammatory bowel disease as well as the solitary rectal ulcer syndrome. These lesions have been confused with mucinous carcinomas, which also may be seen in chronic inflammatory bowel disease. (Courtesy of Feldman's online Atlas, Current Medicine.)

malakoplakia and colorectal cancer are prudent. Patients receiving immunosuppressive medications may improve after these medications are discontinued. Antibiotics such as trimethoprim-sulfamethoxazole and ciprofloxacin have been successful in treating malakoplakia.[127,128] Both antibiotics appear to kill the bacteria associated with malakoplakia and can penetrate the defective host macrophages. Cholinergic agents also may be useful in treating children with malakoplakia.[119] Surgical resection of the involved colon is recommended for cases associated with carcinoma or severe bleeding.

COLITIS CYSTICA PROFUNDA

Colitis cystica profunda is a rare disease characterized by mucin-filled cysts located in the submucosa of the large intestine (Fig. 121-14). The disease was first described in 1766 by Stark, who reported two cases associated with dysentery.[129] There are three patterns of disease: (1) localized with a polypoid lesion; (2) diffuse with multiple polypoid lesions; and (3) diffuse with a confluent sheet of cysts.

ETIOLOGY

The etiology of colitis cystica profunda is unknown, but several theories have been proposed. A possible congenital etiology is supported by several findings. In embryologic examinations, submucosal cysts have been found in multiple gastrointestinal locations. The occurrence of colitis cystica profunda in children and its association with other congenital conditions such as Peutz-Jeghers syndrome[130] also support a congenital origin for this disease. However, the absence of submucosal cysts in large autopsy series of infants and children reduces the plausibility of this etiology.

Colitis cystica profunda has been associated with acquired diseases that predispose to mucosal ulceration and inflammation, including ulcerative colitis,[131] Crohn's disease,[132] and infectious colitis.[133] Submucosal cysts also have been reported in areas exposed to local trauma, such as an intestinal anastomosis or colostomy.[134] Proctitis cystica profunda developed in rats treated with irradiation.[135] and at small bowel stomas also created in rats.[136]

Colitis cystica profunda has been found in association with adenocarcinoma of the colon, suggesting a neoplastic etiology. Several cases of adenocarcinoma of the stomach associated with gastritis cystica profunda have been reported.[137] In some reports, there is strong evidence of a causal link between cancer and colitis cystica profunda, because the submucosal cysts are often found adjacent to the adenocarcinoma, whereas adjacent benign mucosa is devoid of submucosal cysts.

The localized form of colitis cystica profunda is associated with rectal prolapse and solitary rectal ulcer syndrome.[129] Mucosal prolapse has been found in more than 50% of patients with the localized form of the disease. Trauma or ischemia caused by chronic traction on the mucosa and intramural vessels may play a role in the development of the submucosal cysts. Microscopic features of the localized form of the disease often include fibrosis of the lamina propria and hypertrophic muscle fibers, changes that are characteristic of solitary rectal ulcer syndrome (see Chapter 112).[138]

CLINICAL FEATURES AND DIAGNOSIS

Colitis cystica profunda affects men and women equally. The most common symptoms are rectal bleeding, mucus discharge, and diarrhea[129]; less common are tenesmus, abdominal pain, and rectal pain. Rarely, the patient may present with intestinal obstruction caused by the cysts.[139] At endoscopy, most lesions are located on the anterior rectal wall 6 to 7 cm from the anal verge. The lesions appear as polyps with overlying mucosa that may be

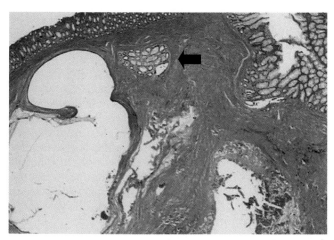

Figure 121–15   Histology of colitis cystica profunda showing the mucus-filled cysts and misplaced epithelium (*arrow*). (×5) (From Atlas of Gastrointestinal Pathology ED: Mitros FA. Gower Med Publ, New York, NY 1988.)

normal, inflamed, or ulcerated. Endoscopy may disclose an associated rectal prolapse in some cases. The endoscopic appearance of the lesions may be indistinguishable from a variety of lesions, including adenocarcinoma, adenomatous polyps, submucosal lipoma, neurofibroma, inflammatory pseudopolyps, pneumatosis coli, and endometriosis.[129] Barium enema may reveal radiolucent filling defects. Transrectal ultrasound may be useful in differentiating this disease from cancer and reveals hypoechoic cysts that may be surrounded by intact submucosa, unlike invasive cancer.[140] Biopsy is necessary to differentiate this lesion from a variety of inflammatory, neoplastic, and infectious conditions. On biopsy, the submucosa is seen to be thickened by the presence of the mucus-filled cysts (Fig. 121–15). The cysts usually communicate with the lumen through small openings in the mucosa. Although usually confined to the submucosa, cysts involving the muscularis propria and serosa have been reported. The surrounding connective tissue often shows chronic inflammation, and there may be extensive replacement of the lamina propria by fibroblasts.[138]

TREATMENT

A high-fiber diet and bowel retraining to avoid straining have led to regression of this disease in a few cases.[140] If fiber is not effective, polyethylene glycol solutions may be tried.[141] Glucocorticoid enemas also have been used with some success.[129] Most patients have been treated with surgery. In patients with associated rectal prolapse, repair of the prolapse alone may treat the colitis cystica profunda successfully, whereas for disease localized to the rectum, and in the absence of procidentia, local excision through a transanal approach is efficacious.[141] When the disease is localized to the rectum but is circumferential, total excision may be accomplished by mucosal sleeve resection and coloanal pull-through.[141] More diffuse lesions have been removed by segmental resection. Seg-

mental resection also may be necessary for large obstructing lesions and for lesions that cause hypokalemia, hypoalbuminemia, and severe anemia from chronic blood loss. A diverting colostomy may lead to regression of this disease and may be the best option for a patient with significant comorbidities.

NEUTROPENIC ENTEROCOLITIS (TYPHLITIS)

Neutropenic enterocolitis (typhlitis) is a potentially life-threatening condition associated with neutropenia related to chemotherapy. The entity was described initially by Wagner in 1970 in children undergoing chemotherapy for leukemia.[142] The disease commonly affects the ileum and cecum and may result in intestinal perforation. The frequency in persons at risk varies from 1% to 46%.[143] Neutropenic enterocolitis has been described after organ transplantation, with AIDS, and, in patients with leukemias treated with cytosine arabinoside, and with solid tumors treated with combination chemotherapy.[144-148]

ETIOLOGY

The cause of neutropenic enterocolitis may be multifactorial. The initial injury is an ulceration of the bowel mucosa with no associated inflammatory response. Mucosal injury may occur from leukemic infiltration, stasis of bowel contents, or mucosal ischemia from splanchnic vasoconstriction resulting from sepsis.[145,147,148] Certain drugs also may contribute to mucosal damage. Cytosine arabinoside can cause necrosis and delayed regeneration of intestinal glandular epithelium.[149] Vinca alkaloids used to treat leukemia also may contribute to cecal distention by damaging the myenteric plexus of the intestine. With mucosal injury in the setting of impaired host defenses, infectious colitis subsequently occurs. The infection is often polymicrobial; causative bacteria include *Escherichia coli*, *Staphylococcus aureus*, *Clostridia septicum*, and *Klebsiella* species[150]; fungal organisms such as *Aspergillus* and *Candida* also have been isolated.[150] In addition to transmural infection of the intestine, the cecum may become gangrenous and perforate as a result of increased distention and ischemia. The process may involve the ileum alone or both the ileum and cecum.[150]

CLINICAL FEATURES AND DIAGNOSIS

The most common presentation is with fever, diarrhea, nausea, vomiting, and abdominal pain in a patient receiving antineoplastic drugs.[151] Abdominal tenderness characteristically is localized to the right lower quadrant of the abdomen but may be absent or masked by drugs such as prednisone; localized tenderness may progress rapidly to diffuse signs of peritonitis as a result of intestinal perforation. Shock may occur as a result of bacteremia or intestinal perforation. On occasion, the sigmoid colon may be affected, further complicating the diagnosis.[152] Neutropenia is universal, and blood cultures

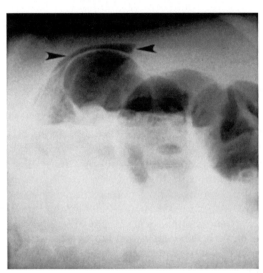

Figure 121–16 Left lateral decubitus plain film in a patient with neutropenic enterocolitis. The colon is dilated with a prominent intraluminal gas-fluid interface and free peritoneal air (*arrows*) resulting from cecal perforation. (From Hunger TB, Bjelland UJC: Gastrointestinal complications of leukemia and its treatment. AJR Am J Roentgenol 142:513, 1984.)

are positive in up to 50% of cases.[145,150] The differential diagnosis includes appendicitis, pseudomembranous colitis, ischemic colitis, volvulus, diverticulitis, and drug-induced diarrhea.

The diagnostic work-up should include a radiologic evaluation to exclude other diseases, confirm the diagnosis, and determine the severity of illness. Abdominal films may demonstrate dilated loops of small bowel with decreased air in the right lower quadrant and free intraperitoneal air if intestinal perforation has occurred (Fig. 121–16).[145] CT scans are most sensitive for establishing the diagnosis and help to exclude other conditions such as appendicitis and diverticulitis. The CT scan may reveal a thickened bowel wall, pneumatosis intestinalis, ascites, and free air.[153] Barium enema should be avoided because of the potential risk of perforation. Stool assay for *C. difficile* toxin should be performed routinely to exclude pseudomembranous *C. difficile* colitis.

TREATMENT

Management of neutropenic enterocolitis has varied. Approaches have included supportive measures alone, aggressive initial surgical resection, and combined medical and surgical treatment; successes and failures have been documented with all these approaches. In two studies, all patients treated medically recovered, whereas in another similar series, all patients managed medically died.[154] Clearly, successful management of patients with neutropenic enterocolitis needs to be individualized to optimize outcome.

In general, medical management includes broad-spectrum antibiotics, nasogastric suction, and bowel rest. Fluid resuscitation with isotonic solutions is critical for maintaining renal perfusion in the face of decreased

systemic vascular resistance from sepsis and intra-abdominal fluid sequestration. Close observation and serial abdominal and radiologic examinations are necessary to monitor the response to medical treatment. Antibiotics should have activity against enteric gram-negative organisms, gram-positive organisms, and anaerobes. Causative microorganisms include *Pseudomonas*, *S. aureus*, *E. coli*, and group A *Streptococcus*.[150] For patients who do not respond to antibacterial agents, amphotericin should be considered, because fungemia is common.[150] Blood transfusions may be necessary because the diarrhea is often bloody. Granulocyte-macrophage colony-stimulating factor to correct the neutropenia is a useful adjunct to medical therapy.[155] Early surgical intervention has been recommended in persons with a rapidly deteriorating course despite maximal medical therapy. Two series have shown a decreased mortality rate in patients with severe disease who are treated surgically compared with those treated medically.[154] For patients with complications such as frank gangrene, intestinal perforation, and shock despite vasopressor support, surgical intervention is mandatory.

Controversy surrounds the choice of operation. Gangrenous or perforated bowel should be resected. When the bowel is edematous with no vascular compromise and no signs of perforation, successful management has included no resection,[156] intestinal diversion with no resection,[154] and resection of the involved bowel. If resection is performed, construction of an ileostomy and mucous fistula may be the safest option, because intestinal anastomoses may be prone to breakdown in patients with neutropenia.[157] Because recurrences of neutropenic enterocolitis are common when chemotherapy is restarted, right hemicolectomy is recommended before chemotherapy is resumed.[147]

ENDOMETRIOSIS

Endometriosis, defined as the presence of endometrial tissue outside the uterine cavity and musculature, was first described by von Rokitansky in 1860. Most often, these ectopic tissues lie in the vicinity of the uterus. Endometriosis occurs in up to 15% of menstruating women and up to 30% of infertile women.[158] The initial description of nonpigmented endometriosis in 1986 resulted in increased recognition and a much higher prevalence of this disorder than appreciated previously.[159] In contrast to endometrial involvement of the female reproductive organs, gastrointestinal involvement is less common, usually asymptomatic, and clinically less important.[160] The most frequent intestinal organs involved are the rectosigmoid colon (96%), appendix (10%), and ileum (5%), with other organs involved uncommonly.[161] Intestinal endometriosis can mimic a wide variety of inflammatory, infectious, and neoplastic digestive disorders.[162]

ETIOLOGY AND PATHOGENESIS

Several hypotheses have been advanced to explain the ectopic location of endometrial tissue.[163-165] The most commonly accepted explanation is that of retrograde passage of endometrial tissue, which then implants and grows on pelvic organs and the peritoneum. From these sites, more distant implants arise via hematogenous or lymphatic dissemination; further dissemination may occur during surgical interventions. A less accepted hypothesis, which has fewer supporting data, is that of endometrial metaplasia, in which multipotential peritoneal mesothelial cells are induced by unknown factors to undergo metaplastic transformation to endometrial tissue.

Once implanted, endometrial tissue appears to be regulated by hormonal influences, so that estrogen promotes and progesterone inhibits growth. These repetitive cycles of growth and sloughing of tissue can lead to serosal irritation and progressive invasion of intestinal muscle with fibrosis and muscle hypertrophy. Thus, pain may arise from nerve impingement or serosal inflammation, whereas obstruction may result from luminal narrowing or intestinal kinking.

CLINICAL FEATURES

Endometriosis is found almost exclusively in women of childbearing age, with clinical onset usually between the ages of 20 and 45 years.[161] Women who experience symptoms or who undergo surgery for endometriosis beyond menopause presumably have chronic fibrosis or exacerbations induced by exogenous estrogens.

Although most women with endometrial implants on intestinal structures have no symptoms, those with serosal implants may complain of localized tenderness, low backache, or abdominal pain. Penetration of endometrial tissue into the bowel wall may produce constipation, diarrhea, and partial obstruction resulting in intermittent abdominal pain. Contrary to popular thinking, symptoms are not always cyclical and may not fluctuate with hormonal levels; nor are gastrointestinal symptoms necessarily associated with gynecologic symptoms. Rarely, hematochezia occurs when endometrial implants penetrate to the mucosa or when severe colonic fibrosis results in ischemia.[160] Less common presentations occur with more proximal colonic or small intestinal involvement and include acute appendicitis caused by an obstructing endometrioma, small bowel intussusception, and volvulus.[162,166]

DIAGNOSIS

The clinical diagnosis of intestinal endometriosis may be difficult because symptoms often are nonspecific and there may not be a close relationship between the symptoms and the menstrual cycle. Endometriosis should always be considered in women with recurrent abdominal pain and bowel symptoms, especially if they are in their reproductive years and have gynecologic complaints. Diagnosis is especially difficult because irritable bowel syndrome is so common in women.

An important component of the evaluation is a careful pelvic examination that includes combined rectovaginal palpation. Finding tender nodules or irregularities in the

cul-de-sac is highly suggestive of endometriosis. Because findings may vary considerably during the menstrual cycle, the pelvic examination should be performed immediately before and again after menstruation if no abnormalities were found initially.

It is rare to see endometrial implants on the colonic mucosa except when there is hematochezia. Thus, colonoscopy is often normal except for areas of extrinsic compression or strictures with intact mucosa.[167] More helpful is an air-contrast barium enema, which demonstrates submucosal polypoid masses or areas of noncircumferential narrowing of the lumen (Fig. 121–17). Diagnostic yield and accuracy may be enhanced by performance of these tests just before the onset of menses. CT scans (Fig. 121–18), ultrasonography, and magnetic resonance imaging all have been reported to assist with the diagnosis or assessment of the extent of endometrial involvement. High-resolution transvaginal and transrectal ultrasonography also may be useful in detecting small endometrial implants, particularly in the retroperitoneal pelvis.[168]

Definitive diagnosis of endometriosis often is made by laparoscopy or laparotomy with biopsy and is especially useful in patients with intestinal implants without pelvic involvement. The appreciation that endometrial tissue may be nonpigmented has increased the yield of these procedures considerably.[159]

The differential diagnosis of intestinal endometriosis includes inflammatory disorders such as Crohn's disease and ulcerative colitis with stricture; diverticulitis; infectious diseases such as ileocolonic tuberculosis and schis-

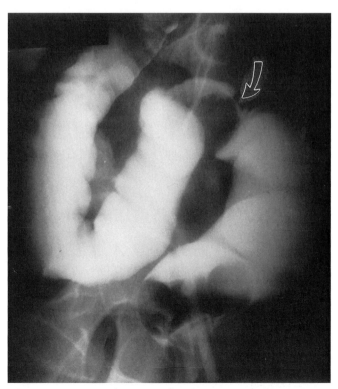

Figure 121–17 Single-contrast barium enema demonstrating a large, nodular, partially-obstructing endometrioma in the rectosigmoid colon (*arrow*). (Courtesy of Mark Peterson, MD, Pittsburgh, PA.)

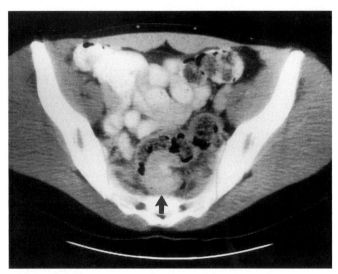

Figure 121–18 CT scan in the same patient as in Figure 121–17 showing the endometrial mass in the cul-de-sac (*arrow*) extending into the colon. (Courtesy of Mark Peterson, MD, University of Pittsburgh Medical Center, Pittsburgh, PA.)

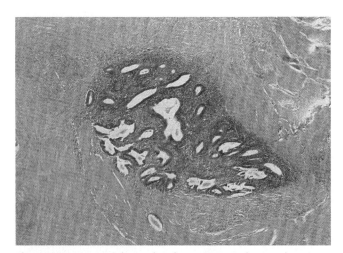

Figure 121–19 Histology of endometriosis. Endometrial stoma is seen around the glandular structures in the muscularis propria of the colon in a woman presenting with obstructive symptoms. The diagnosis of endometriosis was proved at surgery. (×10) (From Atlas of Gastrointestinal Pathology ED: Mitros FA. Gower Med Publ, New York, NY 1988.)

tosomiasis; benign and malignant neoplastic disorders; and colon ischemia.[162] It is important to emphasize that no radiologic or imaging finding is pathognomonic of endometriosis, that mucosal abnormalities that permit positive biopsies are rare, and that tissue for a definitive diagnosis is usually obtained only at laparotomy (Fig. 121–19).

TREATMENT

In general, when a diagnosis of serosal intestinal endometriosis is made, hormonal therapy is often the first therapeutic option, similar to the standard approach to pelvic endometriosis.[169,170] Low-dose estrogen-progestin compounds cause a pseudopregnancy state that results in decidualization of endometrial tissue and often relieves dysmenorrhea. Their use in more severe disease is questionable, however, and they generally are not recommended for symptomatic intestinal disease.

The most effective agents currently available are the synthetic androgen danazol and the gonadotropin-releasing hormone agonists.[171,172] Both act to decrease ovarian steroid synthesis by inhibiting pituitary release of follicle-stimulating hormone and luteinizing hormone. Although both are effective in decreasing pelvic pain associated with endometriosis and appear to decrease the size of endometrial implants, there are no studies of these agents in endometriosis-associated intestinal disease, and there is some concern that treatment may result in increased fibrosis and inadequate symptom resolution.[173,174] Ablation of endometrial implants on surfaces that can be visualized laparoscopically can be accomplished using carbon dioxide laser.[175]

For endometriosis that causes partial obstruction of the colon or small intestine, segmental resection of the involved area provides the best results and also serves to exclude an underlying carcinoma.[176-179] Resection can be performed by laparoscopic techniques or by open surgery, according to available expertise. If the patient is postmenopausal or if future pregnancies are not wanted, hysterectomy and bilateral salpingo-oophorectomy can be done at the time of resective surgery to minimize the risk of symptomatic disease in the future. Similar surgery also can be performed in premenopausal women who, despite medical therapy, have intractable symptoms.

REFERENCES

1. Lindstrom CG: "Collagenous colitis" with watery diarrhea: A new entity. Pathol Eur 11:87, 1976.
2. Read NW, Krejs GJ, Read MG, et al: Chronic diarrhea of unknown origin. Gastroenterology 68:264, 1980.
3. Lazenby AJ, Yardley JH, Giardiello FM, et al: Lymphocytic ("microscopic") colitis: A comparative histopathologic study with particular reference to collagenous colitis. Hum Pathol 20:18, 1989.
4. Fernandez-Banares F, Salas A, Forne M, et al: Incidence of collagenous and lymphocytic colitis: A 5-year population-based study. Am J Gastroenterol 94:418, 1999.
5. Olesen M, Eriksson S, Bohr J, et al: Microscopic colitis: a common diarrheal disease: An epidemiologic study in Orebro, Sweden, 1993-1998. Gut 53:346, 2004.
6. Tanaka M, Mazzoleni G, Riddell RH: Distribution of collagenous colitis: Utility of flexible sigmoidoscopy. Gut 33:65, 1992.
7. Salas A, Fernandez-Banares F, Casalots J, et al: Subepithelial myofibroblasts and tenascin expression in microscopic colitis. Histopathology 43:48, 2003.
8. Jarnerot G, Tysk C, Bohr J, Ericksson S: Collagenous colitis and fecal stream diversion. Gastroenterology 109:449, 1995.
9. Thomson RD, Lestina LS, Bensen SP, et al: Lansoprazole-associated microscopic colitis: A case series. Am J Gastroenterol 97:2908, 2002.
10. Berrebi D, Sautet A, Flejou JF, et al: Ticlopidine-induced colitis: A histological study including apoptosis. J Clin Pathol 51:280, 1998.

11. Olesen M, Eriksson S, Bohr J, et al: Lymphocytic colitis: A retrospective clinical study of 199 Swedish patients. Gut 53:536, 2004.

12. Anderson T, Anderson JR, Tvede M, Franzmann MB: Collagenous colitis: Are bacterial cytotoxins responsible? Am J Gastroenterol 88:375, 1993.

13. Riddell RH, Tanaka M, Mazzoleni G: Non-steroidal anti-inflammatory drugs as a possible cause of collagenous colitis: A case control study. Gut 33:683, 1992.

14. Goff JS, Barnett JL, Pelke T, Appelman HD: Collagenous colitis: Histopathology and clinical course. Am J Gastroenterol 92:57, 1997.

15. Wolber R, Owen D, Freeman H: Colonic lymphocytosis in patients with celiac sprue. Hum Pathol 21:1092, 1990.

16. Armes J, Gee DC, MaCrae FA, et al: Collagenous colitis: Jejunal and colorectal pathology. J Clin Pathol 45:784, 1992.

17. Zins BJ, Tremaine WJ, Carpenter HA: Collagenous colitis: Mucosal biopsies and association with fecal leukocytes. Mayo Clin Proc 70:430, 1995.

18. Giardiello FM, Lazenby AJ, Yardley JH, et al: Increased HLA A1 and diminished HLA A3 in lymphocytic colitis compared to controls and patients with collagenous colitis. Dig Dis Sci 37:496, 1992.

19. Sylwestrowicz T, Kelly JK, Hwang WS, et al: Collagenous colitis and microscopic colitis: The watery diarrhea-colitis syndrome. Am J Gastroenterol 84:763, 1989.

20. Fine KD, Do K, Schulte K, et al: High prevalence of celiac sprue-like HLA-DQ genes and enteropathy in patients with the microscopic colitis syndrome. Am J Gastroenterol 95:1974, 2000.

21. Aigner T, Neureiter D, Muller S, et al: Extracellular matrix composition and gene expression in collagenous colitis. Gastroenterology 113:136, 1997.

22. Bo-Linn GW, Vendrell DD, Lee E, Fordtran JS: An evaluation of the significance of microscopic colitis in patients with chronic diarrhea. J Clin Invest 75:1559, 1985.

23. Burgel N, Bojarski C, Mankertz J, et al: Mechanisms of diarrhea in collagenous colitis. Gastroenterology 123:433, 2002.

24. Baum CA, Bhatia P, Miner PB: Increased colonic mucosal mast cells associated with severe watery diarrhea and microscopic colitis. Dig Dis Sci 34:1462, 1998.

25. Richieri JP, Bonneau HP, Cano N, et al: Collagenous colitis: An unusual endoscopic appearance. Gastrointest Endosc 39:192, 1993.

26. Schiller LR: Diagnosis and management of microscopic colitis syndrome. J Clin Gastroenterol 38(Suppl 1):S27, 2004.

27. Fine KD, Lee EL: Efficacy of open-label bismuth subsalicylate for the treatment of microscopic colitis. Gastroenterology 114:2, 1998.

28. Ryder SD, Walker RJ, Jones H, Rhodes JM: Rectal bismuth subsalicylate as therapy for ulcerative colitis. Aliment Pharmacol Ther 4:333, 1990.

29. Munck LK, Kjeldsen J, Philipsen E, et al: Incomplete remission with short-term prednisolone treatment in collagenous colitis: A randomized study. Scand J Gastroenterol 38:606, 2003.

30. Pardi DS, Loftus EV Jr, Tremaine WJ, Sandborn WJ: Treatment of refractory microscopic colitis with azathioprine and 6-mercaptopurine. Gastroenterology 120:1483, 2001.

31. Baert F, Schmit A, D'Haens G, et al: Budesonide in collagenous colitis: A prospective double-blind, placebo-controlled trial with histological follow-up. Gastroenterology 122:20, 2002.

32. Miehlke S, Heymer P, Bethke B, et al: Budesonide treatment for collagenous colitis: A randomized double-blind, placebo-controlled multicenter study. Gastroenterology 123:978, 2002.

33. Bonderup OK, Hansen JB, Birket-Smith L, et al: Budesonide treatment of collagenous colitis: A randomized, double-blind, placebo-controlled trial with morphometric analysis. Gut 52:248, 2003.

34. Glotzer DJ, Glick ME, Goldman H: Proctitis and colitis following diversion of the fecal stream. Gastroenterology 24:211, 1981.

35. Korelitz BI, Cheskin LJ, Sohn N, Sommers SC: The fate of the rectal segment after diversion of the fecal stream in Crohn's disease: Its implications for surgical management. J Clin Gastroenterol 7:37, 1985.

36. Edwards CM, George B, Warren B: Diversion colitis: New light through old windows. Histopathology 34:1, 1999.

37. Yeong ML, Bethwaite PB, Prasad J, Isbister WH: Lymphoid follicular hyperplasia: A distinctive feature of diversion colitis. Histopathology 19:55, 1991.

38. Haque S, Eisen RN, West AB: The morphologic features of diversion colitis: Studies of a pediatric population with no other disease of the intestinal mucosa. Hum Pathol 24:211, 1993.

39. Cook SI, Sellin JH: Review article: Short-chain fatty acids in health and disease. Aliment Pharmacol Ther 12:507, 1998.

40. Mortensen PB, Clausen MR: Short-chain fatty acids in the human colon: Relation to gastrointestinal health and disease. Scand J Gastroenterol 216:132, 1996.

41. Roediger WEW: Utilization of nutrients by isolated epithelial cells of the rat colon. Gastroenterology 83:424, 1982.

42. Harig JM, Soergel KH, Komorowski RA, Wood CM: Treatment of diversion colitis with short-chain fatty acid irrigation. N Engl J Med 320:23, 1989.

43. Neut C, Colombel JF, Guillemot F, et al: Impaired bacterial flora in human excluded colon. Gut 30:1094, 1989.

44. Ordein JJ, DiLorenzo CD, Flores A, Hyman PE: Diversion colitis in children with severe gastrointestinal motility disorders. Am J Gastroenterol 87:88, 1992.

45. Morin CL, Ling V, Bourassa D: Small intestinal and colonic changes induced by a chemically defined diet. Dig Dis Sci 25:123, 1980.

46. Tomasino RM, Morello V, Latteri MA, et al: Histological and histochemical changes in the colon mucosa after ureterosigmoidostomy or colon conduit. Eur Urol 15:248, 1988.

47. Guillemot F, Colombel JF, Neut C, et al: Treatment of diversion colitis by short-chain fatty acids: Prospective and double-blind study. Dis Colon Rectum 34:861, 1991.

48. Neut C, Guillemot F, Gowerrousseau C, et al: Treatment of diversion colitis by short-chain fatty acids: Prospective and double-blind study. Gastroenterol Clin Biol 19:871, 1995.

49. Geraghty JM, Talbot IC: Diversion colitis: Histological features in the colon and rectum after defunctioning colostomy. Gut 32:1020, 1991.

50. Haas PA, Fox TA, Szilag EJ: Endoscopic examination of the colon and rectum distal to a colostomy. Am J Gastroenterol 85:850, 1990.

51. Eggenberger JC, Farid A: Diversion colitis. Curr Treat Options Gastroenterol 4:255, 2001.

52. Sartor RB, Murphy ME, Rydzak E: Miscellaneous inflammatory and structural disorders of the colon. In Yamada T (ed): Textbook of Gastroenterology, 3rd ed. Philadelphia, Lippincott Williams & Wilkins, 1999, p 1857.

53. deOliviera-Neto JP, de Aguilar-Nascomento JE: Intraluminal irrigation with fibers improves mucosal inflammation and atrophy in diversion colitis. Nutrition 20:197, 2004.

54. Ona FV, Allende HD, Vivenio R, et al: Diagnosis and management of nonspecific colon ulcer. Arch Surg 117:888, 1982.

55. Khawaja FI, Vakil N: Colonoscopy as an aid in the diagnosis of nonspecific ulcers of the colon. Gastrointest Endosc 33:43, 1987.

56. Kaufman HL, Fischer AH, Carroll M, Becker JM: Colonic ulceration associated with nonsteroidal anti-inflammatory drugs: Review of three cases. Dis Colon Rectum 39:705, 1999.

57. Buchman AL, Schwartz MR: Colonic ulceration associated with the systemic use of nonsteroidal anti-inflammatory medication. J Clin Gastroenterol 22:224, 1996.

58. Mills B, Zuckerman G, Sicard G: Discrete colon ulcers as a cause of lower gastrointestinal bleeding and perforation in endstage renal disease. Surgery 89:548, 1981.

59. Shimamoto C, Hirata I, Ohshiba S, et al: Churg-Strauss syndrome (allergic granulomatous angiitis) with peculiar multiple colonic ulcers. Am J Gastroenterol 85:316, 1990.

60. Wilson RT, Dean PJ, Upshaw JD, Wruble LD: Endoscopic appearance of Wegener's granulomatosis involving the colon. Gastrointest Endosc 33:388, 1987.

61. Baxter R, Nino-Murcia M, Bloom RJ, Kosek J: Gastrointestinal manifestations of essential mixed cryoglobulinemia. Gastrointest Radiol 13:160, 1988.

62. Hirata K, Sasaguri T, Kunoh M, et al: Solitary "amyloid ulcer" localized in the sigmoid colon without evidence of systemic amyloidosis. Am J Gastroenterol 92:356, 1997.

63. Shallman RW, Kuehner M, Williams GH, et al: Benign cecal ulcers. Dis Colon Rectum 28:732, 1985.

64. Dieulafoy G: Leçons clinique de l'Hotel-Dieu de Paris. Paris: Masson 2:1, 1897.

65. Gadenstatter M, Wetscher G, Crookes PF, et al: Dieulafoy's disease of the large and small bowel. J Clin Gastroenterol 27:169, 1998.

66. Nozae T, Kitamura M, Matsumata T, Sugimachi K: Dieulafoy-like lesions of colon and rectum in patients with chronic renal failure on long-term hemodialysis. Hepatogastroenterology 46:3121, 1999.

67. Dy NM, Gostout CJ, Balm RK: Bleeding from the endoscopically identified Dieulafoy lesion of the proximal small intestine and colon. Am J Gastroenterol 90:108, 1995.

68. Abdulian JD, Santoro MJ, Chen YK, Collen MJ: Dieulafoy-like lesion of the rectum presenting with exsanguinating hemorrhage: Successful endoscopic therapy. Am J Gastroenterol 88:1939, 1993.

69. Heilbrun N: Roentgen evidence suggesting enterocolitis associated with prolonged cathartic abuse. Radiology 41:486, 1943.

70. Leng-Peschlow E: Senna and its rational use. Pharmacology 44(Suppl 1):1, 1992.

71. Muller-Lissner S: What has happened to the cathartic colon? Gut 39:486, 1996.

72. Rieman JF, Zimmerman W: Ultrastructural studies of colonic nerve plexuses in chronic laxative abuse. Gastroenterology 74:1085, 1978.

73. Smith B: Effect of irritant purgatives on the myenteric plexus in man and the mouse. Gut 139:43, 1969.

74. Riecken EO, Zertz M, Ende C, et al: The effect of an anthraquinone laxative on colonic nerve tissue: A controlled trial in constipated women. Z Gastroenterol 28:660, 1990.

75. Wald A. Is chronic use of stimulant laxatives harmful to the colon? J Clin Gastroenterol 36:380, 2003.

76. Ghadially FN, Walley VM: Pigments of the gastrointestinal tract: A comparison of light microscopic and electron microscopic findings. Ultrastruct Pathol 19:213, 1995.

77. Benavides SR, Morgante PE, Monserrat AJ, et al: The pigment of melanosis coli: A lectin histochemical study. Gastrointest Endosc 46:131, 1997.

78. Walker NI, Bennett RE, Axelson RA: Melanosis coli: A consequence of anthraquinone-induced apoptosis of colonic epithelial cells. Am J Pathol 131:465, 1988.

79. Speare GS: Melanosis coli: Experimental observations of its production and elimination in twenty-three cases. Am J Surg 82:631, 1951.

80. Mengs U, Rudolph RL: Light and electron-microscopic changes in the colon of the guinea pig after treatment with anthranoid and non-anthranoid laxatives. Pharmacology 47(Suppl 1):172, 1993.

81. Balazs M: Melanosis coli: Ultrastructural study in 45 patients. Dis Colon Rectum 29:839, 1986.

82. Van Gorkom BAP, DeVries EGE, Karrenbeld A, Kleibeulier JH: Review article: Anthranoid laxatives and their potential carcinogenic effects. Aliment Pharmacol Ther 13:443, 1999.

83. Nusko G, Schneider B, Wittekind C, Hahn EG: Anthranoid laxative use is not a risk factor for colorectal neoplasia: Results of a prospective case control study. Gut 46:651, 2000.

84. Jacobs EJ, White E. Constipation, laxative use, and colon cancer among middle-aged adults. Epidemiology 9:385, 1998.

85. Roberts MC, Millikan RC, Galanko JA, et al: Constipation, laxative use, and colon cancer in a North Carolina population. Am J Gastroenterol 98:857, 2003.

86. Morganstern L, Shemen L, Allen W, et al: Melanosis coli: Changes in appearance when associated with colonic neoplasia. Arch Surg 118:62, 1983.

87. Hardin RD, Tedesco FJ: Colitis after Hibiclens enema. J Clin Gastroenterol 8:572, 1986.

88. Pike BF, Phillippi PJ, Lawson EH Jr: Soap colitis. N Engl J Med 285:217, 1971.

89. Bollen P, Goossens A, Hauser B, Vandenplas Y: Colonic ulcerations caused by an enema containing hydrogen peroxide. J Pediatr Gastroenterol Nutr 26:232, 1998.

90. Creteur V, Douglas D, Galante M, et al: Inflammatory colonic changes produced by contrast material. Radiology 147:77, 1983.

91. Segal I, Tim LO, Hamilton DG, et al: Ritual-enema-induced colitis. Dis Colon Rectum 22:195, 1979.

92. Stein BL, Lamoreux E, Miller M, et al. Glutaraldehyde-induced colitis. Can J Surg 44:113, 2001.

93. Fukunaga K, Khatibi A: Glutaraldehyde colitis: A complication of screening flexible sigmoidoscopy in the primary care center. Ann Intern Med 133:315, 2000.

94. Munoz-Navas M, Garcia-Villareal L: Caustic colitis due to formalin enema. Gastrointest Endosc 38:521, 1992.

95. Michopoulos S, Bouzakis H, Sotiropoulou M, et al: Colitis due to accidental alcohol enema: Clinicopathological presentation and outcome. Dig Dis Sci 45:1188, 2000.

96. Chan A, Depew W, Vanner S: Use of oral sodium phosphate colonic lavage solution by Canadian colonoscopists: Pitfalls and complications. Can J Gastroenterol 11:334, 1997.

97. Cappell MS: Colonic toxicity of administered drugs and chemicals. Am J Gastroenterol 99:1175, 2004.

98. John A, Dickey K, Fenwick J, et al: Pneumatosis intestinalis in Crohn's disease. Dig Dis Sci 37:813, 1992.

99. Tak P, Van Duinen C, Bun P, et al: Pneumatosis cystoides intestinalis with intestinal pseudo-obstruction: Resolution after metronidazole. Dig Dis Sci 37:949, 1992.

100. Knetchle S, Davidoff A, Rice R: Pneumatosis intestinalis: Clinical management and surgical outcome. Ann Surg 212:160, 1990.

101. Sequeira W: Pneumatosis cystoides intestinalis in systemic sclerosis and other diseases. Semin Arthritis Rheum 19:269, 1990.

102. Gelman SF, Brandt LJ: Pneumatosis intestinalis and AIDS: A case report and review of the literature. Am J Gastroenterol 93:646, 1998.

103. Gagliardi G, Thompson I, Hershman M, et al: Pneumatosis coli: A proposed pathogenesis based on study of 25 cases and review of the literature. Int J Colorectal Dis 11:11, 1996.

104. Christl S, Gibson G, Murgatroyd P, et al: Impaired hydrogen metabolism in pneumatosis cystoides intestinalis. Gastroenterology 104:392, 1993.

105. Levitt M, Olsson S: Pneumatosis cystoides intestinalis and high breath H_2 excretion: Insights into the role of H_2 in this condition. Gastroenterology 108:1560, 1995.

106. Read N, Al-Janabi N, Cann P: Is raised breath hydrogen related to the pathogenesis of pneumatosis coli? Gut 25:839, 1984.

107. Florin THJ: Alkyl halides, super hydrogen production, and the pathogenesis of pneumatosis cystoides coli. Gut 41:778, 1997.

108. Goodman RA, Riley TR: Lactulose-induced pneumatosis intestinalis and pneumoperitoneum. Dig Dis Sci 46:2549, 2001.

109. Ellis B: Symptomatic treatment of primary pneumatosis coli with metronidazole. BMJ 280:763, 1980.

110. Spigelman A, Williams C, Ansell J, et al: Pneumatosis coli: A source of diagnostic confusion. Br J Surg 77:155, 1990.

111. Shimada M, Ina K, Takahashi H, et al: Pneumatosis cystoides intestinalis treated with hyperbaric oxygen therapy: Usefulness of an endoscopic ultrasonic catheter probe for diagnosis. Intern Med 40:896, 2001.

112. Miralbes M, Hinojosa J, Aconso J, Berenguer J: Oxygen therapy in pneumatosis coli: What is the minimum oxygen requirement? Dis Colon Rectum 26:458, 1983.

113. von Hansemann D: Ulser Malakoplakia der Harnblase. Virch Arch Pathol Anat 173:302, 1903.

114. Michaelis L, Gutmann C: Ueber Einschlusse in Blasentumoren. Z Clin Med 47:208, 1902.

115. Lewin K, Harell G, Lee A, Crowley L: Malacoplakia—an electron-microscopic study: Demonstration of bacilliform organisms in malacoplakic macrophages. Gastroenterology 66:28, 1974.

116. Cipolletta L, Bianco M, Fumo F, et al: Malacoplakia of the colon. Gastrointest Endosc 41:225, 1995.

117. Stevens S, McClure J: The histochemical features of the Michaelis-Gutmann body and a consideration of the pathophysiological mechanisms of its formation. J Pathol 137:119, 1982.

118. Thorning D, Vaco R: Malacoplakia: Defect in digestion of phagocytosed material due to impaired vacuolar acidification? Arch Pathol 99:456, 1975.

119. Abdou N, NaPombejara C, Sagawa A, et al: Malacoplakia: Evidence for monocyte lysosomal abnormality correctable by cholinergic agonist in vitro and in vivo. N Engl J Med 297:1413, 1977.

120. Streem S: Genitourinary malacoplakia in renal transplant recipients: Pathogenic, prognostic, and therapeutic considerations. J Urol 132:10, 1984.

121. Biggar W, Crawford L, Cardella C, et al: Malacoplakia and immunosuppressive therapy: Reversal of clinical and leukocyte abnormalities after withdrawal of prednisone and azathioprine. Am J Pathol 119:5, 1985.

122. Mir-Madjlessi S, Tavassolie H, Kamalian N: Malakoplakia of the colon and recurrent colonic strictures in a patient with primary hypogammaglobulinemia: An association not previously described. Dis Colon Rectum 25:723, 1982.

123. Schwartz D, Ogden P, Blumberg H, et al: Pulmonary malakoplakia in a patient with the acquired immunodeficiency syndrome. Arch Pathol Lab Med 114:1267, 1990.

124. Pillay K, Chetty R: Malakoplakia in association with colorectal carcinoma: A series of four cases. Pathology 34:332, 2002.

125. Bates A, Dev S, Baithun S: Malakoplakia and Colorectal Adenocarcinoma. London, Department of Morbid Anatomy, London Hospital Medical College and Department of Histopathology, St Andrew's Hospital, 1996, p 171.

126. El-Mouzan M, Satti M, Al-Quorain A, El-Ageb A: Colonic malacoplakia—occurrence in a family: Report of cases. Dis Colon Rectum 31:390, 1988.

127. Van Furth R, Van't Wout J, Wertheimer P, Zwartendijk J: Ciprofloxacin for treatment of malacoplakia. Lancet 339:148, 1992.

128. Maderazo E, Berlin B, Marhardt C: Treatment of malacoplakia with trimethoprim-sulfamethoxazole. Urology 13:70, 1979.

129. Guest CB, Reznick RK: Colitis cystica profunda: Review of the literature. Dis Colon Rectum 32:983, 1989.

130. Anderson N, Rivera E, Flores D: Peutz-Jeghers syndrome with cervical adenocarcinoma and enteritis cystica profunda. West J Med 141:242, 1984.

131. Castleman B, McNeely BU: Case records of the Massachusetts General Hospital. Weekly clinicopathological exercises. N Engl J Med 286:147, 1972.

132. Aftalion B, Lipper S: Enteritis cystica profunda associated with Crohn's disease. Arch Pathol Lab Med 108:532, 1984.

133. Wayte D, Helwig E: Colitis cystica profunda. Am J Clin Pathol 48:159, 1967.

134. Rosen Y, Vallant J, Yermakov V: Submucosal cysts at a colostomy site: Relationship to colitis cystica profunda and reopening of a case. Dis Colon Rectum 19:453, 1976.

135. Hubmann F: Proctitis cystica profunda and radiation fibrosis in the rectum of the female Wistar rat after x-irradiation: A histopathological study. J Pathol 138:193, 1982.

136. Brynjolfsson G, Haley H: Experimental enteritis cystica in rats. Am J Clin Pathol 47:69, 1967.

137. Franzin G, Novelli P: Gastritis cystica profunda. Histopathology 5:535, 1981.

138. Levin D: "Solitary" rectal ulcer syndrome: Are "solitary" rectal ulcer syndrome and "localized" colitis cystica profunda analogous syndromes caused by rectal prolapse? Gastroenterology 92:243, 1987.

139. Bentley E, Chandrasoma P, Cohen H, et al: Colitis cystica profunda presenting with complete intestinal obstruction and recurrence. Gastroenterology 89:1157, 1985.

140. Petritsch W, Hinterleitner T, Aichbichler B, et al: Endosonography in colitis cystica profunda and solitary rectal ulcer syndrome. Gastrointest Endosc 41:382, 1995.

141. Beck DE: Surgical treatment for colitis cystica profunda and solitary rectal syndrome. Curr Treat Options Gastroenterol 5:231, 2002.

142. Wagner M, Rosenberg H, Ferbach D, Singleton E: Typhlitis: A complication of leukemia in childhood. AJR Am J Roentgenol 109:341, 1970.

143. Moir D, Bale P: Necropsy findings on childhood leukemia emphasizing neutropenic enterocolitis and cerebral calcification. Pathology 8:247, 1976.

144. Petruzzelli G, Johnson J, de Vries E: Neutropenic enterocolitis: A new complication of the head and neck cancer chemotherapy. Arch Otolaryngol Head Neck Surg 116:209, 1990.

145. Ettinghausen SE: Inflammatory disorders of the colon: Collagenous colitis, eosinophilic colitis, and neutropenic colitis. Surg Clin North Am 73:993, 1993.

146. Till M, Lee N, Soper W, Murphy R: Typhlitis in patients with HIV-1 infection. Ann Intern Med 116:998, 1992.

147. Keidan R, Fanning J, Gatenby R, Weese JL: Recurrent typhlitis: A disease resulting from aggressive chemotherapy. Dis Colon Rectum 32:206, 1989.

148. Paulino A, Kenney R, Forman E, Medeiros L: Typhlitis in a patient with acute lymphoblastic leukemia prior to the administration of chemotherapy. Am J Pediatr Hematol Oncol 16:348, 1994.

149. Slavin R, Dias M, Saral R: Cytosine arabinoside-induced gastrointestinal toxic alterations in sequential chemotherapeutic protocols. Cancer 42:1747, 1978.

150. Katz J, Wagner M, Gresik M, et al: Typhlitis: An 18-year experience and postmortem review. Cancer 65:1041, 1990.

151. Sloas M, Flynn P, Kaste S, Patrick C: Typhlitis in children with cancer: A thirty-year experience. Clin Infect Dis 17:484, 1993.

152. Abbasoglu O, Cakmakci M: Neutropenic enterocolitis in patients without leukemia. Surgery 113:113, 1993.

153. Vas W, Seeling R, Manhanta B, et al: Neutropenic colitis: Evaluation with computed tomography. CT J Comput Tomogr 12:211, 1988.

154. Moir C, Scudamore C, Benny W: Typhlitis: Selective surgical management. Am J Surg 151:563, 1986.

155. Kouroussis C, Samonis G, Androulakis N, et al: Successful conservative treatment of neutropenic enterocolitis complicating taxane-based chemotherapy. Am J Clin Oncol 23:309, 2000.

156. Mower W, Hawkins J, Nelson E: Neutropenic enterocolitis in adults with acute leukemia. Arch Surg 121:571, 1986.

157. Villar H, Warneke J, Peck M, et al: Role of surgical treatment in the management of complications of the gastrointestinal tract in patients with leukemia. Surg Gynecol Obstet 165:217, 1987.

158. Olive DL, Schwartz LB: Endometriosis: Medical progress. N Engl J Med 328:1759, 1993.

159. Jansen RP. Russel P: Nonpigmented endometriosis: Clinical, laparoscopic, and pathological definition. Am J Obstet Gynecol 155:1154, 1986.

160. Zwas FR, Lyon DT: Endometriosis: An important condition in clinical gastroenterology. Dig Dis Sci 36:353, 1991.

161. Weed JC, Ray JE: Endometriosis of the bowel. Obstet Gynecol 69:727, 1987.

162. Shah M, Tager D, Feller E: Intestinal endometriosis masquerading as common digestive disorders. Arch Intern Med 155:977, 1995.

163. Rock JA, Markham SM: Pathogenesis of endometriosis. Lancet 240:1264, 1992.

164. Bontis JN, Vavilis DT: Etiopathology of endometriosis. Ann N Y Acad Sci 816:305, 1997.

165. Oral E, Arici A: Pathogenesis of endometriosis. Obstet Gynecol Clin North Am 24:219, 1997.

166. Ferguson CM: Case records of the Massachusetts General Hospital. Weekly clinicopathological exercises. Case 28-1996. A 45-year-old woman with abdominal pain and a polypoid mass in the colon. N Engl J Med 335:807, 1996.

167. Bozdech JM: Endoscopic diagnosis of colonic endometriosis. Gastrointest Endosc 38:568, 1992.

168. Brosens I, Puttemans P, Campo R, et al: Noninvasive methods of diagnosis of endometriosis. Curr Opinion Obstet Gynecol 15:519, 2003.

169. Olive DL, Pritts EA: Treatment of endometriosis. N Engl J Med 345:266, 2001.

170. Kettel LM, Hummel WP: Modern medical management of endometriosis. Obstet Gynecol Clin North Am 24:361, 1997.

171. Berquist IA: Hormonal regulation of endometriosis and the rationales and effects of gonadotropin-releasing hormone agonist treatment: A review. Hum Reprod 10:446, 1995.

172. Hornstein MD, Yuzpe AA, Burry KA, et al: Prospective randomized double-blind trial of three versus six months of nafarelin therapy for endometriosis-associated pelvic pain. Fertil Steril 63:955, 1995.

173. Hall LLH, Malone JM, Ginsburg KA: Flare-up of endometriosis induced by gonadotropin-releasing hormone agonist leading to bowel obstruction. Fertil Steril 64:1204, 1995.

174. Hajiar LR, Kim W, Nolan GH, et al: Intestinal and pelvic endometriosis presenting as a tumor and associated with tamoxifen therapy: Report of a case. Obstet Gynecol 82:642, 1993.

175. Sutton C, Hill D: Laser laparoscopy in the treatment of endometriosis: A 5-year study. Br J Obstet Gynaecol 97:181, 1990.

176. Cameron IC, Rogers S, Collins MC, Reed MW: Intestinal endometriosis: Presentation, investigation, and surgical management. Int J Colorectal Dis 10:83, 1995.

177. Tran KT, Kuijpers HC, Willemsen WN, Bulten H: Surgical treatment of symptomatic rectosigmoid endometriosis. Eur J Surg 162:139, 1996.

178. Nozhat C, Nezhat F, Pennington E: Laparoscopic treatment of infiltrative rectosigmoid colon and rectovaginal septum endometriosis by the technique of videolaparoscopy and the CO_2 laser. Br J Obstet Gynaecol 99:664, 1992.

179. Redwine DB, Koning M, Sharpe DR: Laparoscopically assisted transvaginal segmental resection of the rectosigmoid colon for endometriosis. Fertil Steril 65:198, 1996.

CHAPTER
122 Diseases of the Anorectum

Tracy L. Hull

ANATOMY

The functional anal canal is 3 to 4 cm long beginning at the top of the anorectal ring (at the puborectalis sling) and extending down to the anal verge (anal orifice).[1] The top or upper anal canal is lined mostly with columnar epithelium, a continuation of the same type of tissue that lines the rectum. Some squamous epithelium starts to be intermixed with the columnar epithelium in the rectum at about 1 cm above the dentate line. This change to squamous epithelium is gradual, and the area 1 to 1.5 cm proximal to the dentate line is termed the *transitional zone*.[2] The dentate line is located in the mid-anal canal and is seen as a wavy line. Distal to the dentate line, the tissue is squamous epithelium, but is not like true skin since it has no hair, sebaceous glands, or sweat glands: it is commonly referred to as *anoderm*. The anoderm is thin, pale, and delicate, with the appearance of shiny, stretched skin. At the anal verge, the epithelium becomes thicker, and hair follicles begin to be seen (Fig. 122–1).[3]

Embryologically, the dentate line represents the junction between endoderm and ectoderm. Proximal to the dentate line, there is sympathetic and parasympathetic innervation; distally, the nerve supply is somatic.[3] Therefore, above the dentate line, pain sensation is negligible—a biopsy can be done painlessly above the dentate line.

However, below the dentate line anesthesia is needed to perform a biopsy.

The arterial supply of the anal area is from the superior, middle, and inferior hemorrhoidal arteries, which are continuations or branches of the inferior mesenteric, hypogastric, and internal pudendal arteries, respectively. Blood flow is not uniform to the entire circumference of the anus and is relatively less posteriorly. This differential flow is an important factor in the role postulated for ischemia in determining the chronicity of anal fissure.[4] The venous drainage from the anal canal is by both the systemic and portal systems. The internal hemorrhoidal plexus drains into the superior rectal veins, which drain into the inferior mesenteric vein and then into the portal vein. The distal part of the anal canal drains via the external hemorrhoidal plexus through the middle rectal and pudendal veins into the internal iliac vein (the systemic circulation).[2]

The lymphatic drainage of the anus changes at the dentate line. Proximally, the lymphatic drainage accompanies the blood vessels to the inferior mesenteric and periaortic nodes.[1-3] Distal to the dentate line, the lymph nodes drain to the inguinal nodes. Therefore, inguinal adenopathy can be seen with inflammatory and malignant disease of the lower anal canal.

Immediately proximal to the dentate line, the mucosa appears to have 6 to 14 pleats called the *columns of Mor-*

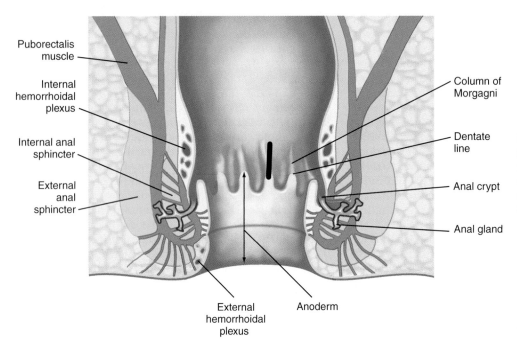

Puborectalis muscle

Internal hemorrhoidal plexus

Internal anal sphincter

External anal sphincter

Column of Morgagni

Dentate line

Anal crypt

Anal gland

External hemorrhoidal plexus

Anoderm

Figure 122–1 Schematic depiction of the anatomy of the anal region. The heavy vertical line denotes the transition zone that extends 1 to 1.5 cm proximal to the dentate line.

gagni. This configuration represents the funneling of the rectum as it narrows into the anal canal. Located at the base of the columns of Morgagni are anal crypts that lead to small rudimentary anal glands.[3] These glands may extend through the internal anal sphincter and, if their ducts are blocked, an anal abscess or fistula may develop (see Fig. 122–1).

The muscles surrounding the anal canal are important to maintain fecal continence. The internal anal sphincter is the thickened continuation of the circular smooth muscle of the rectum. This muscle is involuntary and composed of smooth muscle, which gives it a black hypoechoic appearance on anal ultrasound. The internal sphincter ends above the external sphincter.[3] The internal sphincter is important for continence, but partial division of the internal sphincter is possible without causing fecal incontinence. Division in the anterior or posterior position, however, could lead to stool leakage by creating an oval-shaped configuration in the distal anal canal. The oval shape allows gas and perhaps liquid stool to escape owing to its eccentricity. This is termed a *keyhole deformity* because the shape was thought to be reminiscent of the opening for the key in old-fashioned door locks.

The external anal sphincter is composed of a voluntary sheet of skeletal muscle, which is arranged as a tube surrounding the internal sphincter. It appears as a broad cylinder with mixed echogenicity on anal ultrasound. Proximally, the external sphincter is fused with the puborectalis muscle and, distally, it ends slightly past the internal sphincter.[1,3] Therefore, a groove can be palpated between the internal sphincter and external sphincter on digital examination that is referred to as the intersphincteric groove. The puborectalis is U-shaped and forms a sling that passes behind the lower rectum and attaches to the pubis. Therefore, it is prominent laterally and posteriorly but absent anteriorly. The anorectal ring is pal-

pable at the top of the anal canal, where the canal meets the rectum. It is composed of the puborectalis and the upper external and internal sphincters. The nerve supply to the external sphincter and puborectalis muscle is from the inferior rectal branch of the internal pudendal nerve (S2, S3, S4) and also from fibers of the fourth sacral nerve.[1,3]

EXAMINATION OF THE ANUS AND RECTUM

All routine comprehensive adult physical examinations should include a digital anal examination. When patients present with problems focused on the anorectal region or colon, a more comprehensive examination is indicated. Any examination of the anorectal region begins with a thorough history. This allows the patient to describe the symptoms and concerns, and the physician can develop rapport with the patient at this time. In turn, this will help alleviate the patient's potential apprehension and embarrassment during the examination. It is important to remember that many patients delay coming to the physician, even when they have significant problems, solely out of fear and embarrassment. Therefore, when doing the examination, *explaaation of each step* before it is done, along with a gentle touch, helps alleviate discomfort. It is equally important to avoid causing pain during the examination, particularly when looking for a fissure or anal abscess. Sometimes when an examination is too painful, doing it with some sedation or performing it in the operating room under anesthesia is appropriate.

Patients can be examined in the office in any of several positions, the most popular of which probably is the left lateral position. The patient is positioned on the examination table on his or her left side with the thighs and knees flexed. The buttocks should project slightly beyond the edge of the examination table. In some cases, an assistant is needed to retract the left buttock for optimal viewing.

In the knee-chest (or prone jackknife) position, the patient is on his or her knees with the arms folded and the shoulders and head on the examining table; some patients may be more comfortable resting on the left shoulder. Sometimes the examiner uses a special hydraulic table that has a shelf. The patient kneels on the shelf and drapes his or her chest over the main table. The table then is raised and its head is tipped down, propelling the buttocks forward and elevating them. This position allows the buttocks to be splayed apart for a clear view of the anus.

The dorsolithotomy position is the typical position used for the female gynecologic examination. It is also sometimes used to examine the anorectal region, particularly when looking for an anovaginal fistula.

During the examination, it is important to have all instruments available and have an assistant who additionally can help reassure the patient. Good lighting is essential to critically view the skin and to perform endoscopy of the anus and rectum.

INSPECTION

The examination begins with inspection of the skin. In some cases, looking at the patient's underwear will give a clue to the character of anal drainage or the presence of stool incontinence. As the buttocks are gently retracted, scars, skin abnormalities, stool, discharge of blood or pus, anal tags, warts, hemorrhoids, or lesions adjacent to or prolapsing from the anal canal are noted. The anus is inspected for gaping or scars, and the patient is asked to squeeze the anus to evaluate movement of the anal muscles. Next, the patient may be asked to strain so that the anal area can be examined for abnormal descent below its resting level (perineal descent syndrome). There is no exact measurement that correlates with disease on assessment of perineal descent during the physical examination. If, however, the anus elongates and descends instead of relaxing when the patient is asked to strain, this must be kept in mind if the patient is seeking treatment for symptoms that may correspond to defecatory dysfunction. Prolapse of the vagina or rectum, bulging hemorrhoids, or leakage of urine also should be noted during straining. In some instances, prolapse of the rectum may be seen only if the patient is placed on the toilet and asked to strain. Traction applied laterally to each side of the anal orifice with a gauze sponge will allow eversion of the distal anus for further inspection. This technique is particularly helpful in viewing a fissure without causing undo pain. Some examiners stroke the perianal skin with a cotton-tipped applicator to look for reflex contraction of the anal muscles (anocutaneous reflex) or check perianal sensation with a pinprick. These maneuvers give a crude determination of sphincter innervation. The surrounding skin of the buttocks, perivaginal region, base of the scrotum, and up to the tip of the coccyx should be viewed. Adenopathy in the inguinal region may be seen when certain infectious or neoplastic lesions are found distal to the dentate line.

PALPATION

Next, using a gloved and lubricated index finger, the examiner palpates the anal canal and perianal skin. Slow insertion and gentle pressure are appropriate. The index finger is swept all around the anal canal. Anal tone is noted, as are any scars, masses, or tenderness. Internal hemorrhoids are not palpable unless they are thrombosed. If insertion of the index finger is too painful, an attempt to apply pressure with the insertion finger on the wall opposite the area of tenderness may allow insertion of the finger. If the examination is still too painful, use of sedation or anesthesia may be warranted. Approximately 80% of the resting anal canal pressure is contributed by the internal anal sphincter. The external sphincter is evaluated by having the patient "squeeze" the anus around the examining finger.

Abnormalities sometimes appreciated in the anal canal include fistulous tracts, which feel like a cord or induration; the internal opening of a fistula, which may be appreciated as a knob of tissue in an otherwise smooth area of mucosa; cancers, which may be firm and hard; and ulcers, which feel uneven and craterous. Palpation anteriorly in a woman may reveal a rectocele or anterior defect in the sphincter complex.

Palpation of the distal rectum allows the detection of mass lesions, including polyps and cancers. Attention should be directed to the exact location of the lesion (i.e., anterior, posterior, right, left, or "in between"), and its size, mobility, and character (i.e., soft, ulcerated, hard, or pedunculated). Lesions outside the rectal wall also may be appreciated. The cervix can be felt through the anterior rectal wall in women, and the prostate should be examined in men. The character of the prostate should be noted, along with any hard nodularity that could represent cancer. Further studies are then ordered if needed. The mucosal wall should be assessed for its smoothness; in patients with proctitis, for example, the mucosa may feel rough and gritty.

In some patients with unexplained anal pain, the levator muscles should be palpated to determine if there is spasm or tenderness (*levator ani syndrome*). Similarly, the coccyx should be palpated between the examining internal index finger and the index finger of the opposite hand pressed over the external skin at the level of the coccyx. This maneuver is done to look for pain with motion (e.g., *coccygodynia*), as might be present with a coccygeal fracture.

The contents of the rectum should be assessed regarding the character and amount of stool. When the index finger is removed, any stool, blood, pus, or mucus on the glove should be noted.

ENDOSCOPY

The decision to perform endoscopy depends on the findings on history and physical examination. Endoscopy usually is necessary for the evaluation and exclusion of organic disease in patients with fecal incontinence, constipation, unexplained anal pain,[5] anemia, diarrhea, and rectal bleeding.

Anoscopy

Anoscopy allows visualization of the anal canal, dentate line, internal hemorrhoids, and distal rectum. This is the best method of viewing the anal canal. The anoscope is a short metal or plastic tubular device, usually with a beveled end. *An anoscope should NEVER be inserted or turned without the obturator in place.* Most adult anoscopes have a 2-cm diameter, but smaller ones are available. A fiberoptic light attachment provides optimal illumination; however, external lighting is used with some models.

The lubricated anoscope is inserted slowly as the examiner applies gentle pressure on the end of the obturator once the instrument has been fully advanced. The obturator is then removed, and the anal canal region is examined. To rotate the anoscope while it is in the canal, the obturator is replaced and the scope is turned. The obturator is then removed again and the scope is pulled back slowly to view the entire area. This includes the distal rectum, followed by the upper anal canal, down to the anoderm. To reinsert the scope and view another area, the obturator again must be replaced. Internal hemorrhoids can be seen bulging above the dentate line or prolapsing downward. Internal fistulous openings may be viewed, particularly along the dentate line. When the external skin is compressed, pus may be seen to bubble from the internal opening of a fistula. Rarely, the anoscope is needed to remove a low rectal polyp that cannot be removed through a flexible endoscope because of the low position of the polyp in the rectum or a difficult angulation on retroflexion of the endoscope.

Rigid Proctoscopy

Rigid proctosigmoidoscopy is performed mainly by colorectal surgeons today. The rigid proctoscope is 25 cm long and 11 to 20 mm in diameter and requires fiberoptic light for visualization. The instrument usually cannot be passed to its full extent into the rectosigmoid because of patient discomfort. Before insertion, the obturator is placed in the cylinder, and the instrument is lubricated. With the thumb of the examiner on the obturator, the instrument is advanced gently through the anal canal. The obturator is then removed, and the instrument is advanced under direct vision (to avoid perforation). The depth of insertion (usually from the anal verge) is noted. Examination is done during withdrawal of the instrument, usually while small puffs of air are supplied (by an external hand pump) to keep the rectum from collapsing. The appearance of the mucosa is noted.

Usually a patient has an enema before rigid proctoscopy so that the mucosa can be seen clearly. Exceptions to this rule are patients with proctitis or with suspected infections, in which case the virgin mucosa is inspected and stool is collected for cultures or other tests.

In the modern era of fiberoptic and video sigmoidoscopes, there are still some instances when a rigid proctoscope is superior. The proctoscope can measure the exact distance of a rectal tumor from the anal verge. It also can give the precise location of a lesion on the wall of the rectum. Such measurements are highly inaccurate with flexible instruments and are important for planning operative strategies. The rigid proctoscope is sometimes quicker and easier to use than a flexible scope when evaluating the rectum and doing a biopsy or aspirating fecal contents. Rigid biopsy forceps can be placed through the proctoscope. Caution must be used when doing biopsies with the rigid forceps anteriorly above 7 to 10 cm. This area corresponds to the intra-abdominal colon above the peritoneal reflection, and care must be taken to avoid perforation into the abdominal cavity. The biopsy forceps used with flexible endoscopes also can be used through the rigid proctoscope.

Flexible Sigmoidoscopy

The flexible sigmoidoscope is simply a shorter version of a colonoscope. It measures 60 cm in length. A formal bowel preparation used for colonoscopy usually is not done for flexible sigmoidoscopy; rather, two enemas are given before the examination. Sedation usually is not used, which is the reason why patients who have undergone both colonoscopy and flexible sigmoidoscopy report that the latter was more difficult.[6] As with colonoscopy, the lubricated tip of the sigmoidoscope is inserted and advanced under direct vision. The goal is to examine the left colon, which is reached 80% of the time.[7] Lesions can be biopsied, but the presence of polyps usually mandates full colonoscopy following a bowel preparation to exclude other polyps or cancer. The use of electrocautery and argon plasma coagulation usually is avoided during sigmoidoscopy if enemas have just been given, even if the preparation appears optimal, because intracolonic bowel explosions have occurred from ignition of bowel gas that has passed from the stool-containing proximal colon distally to the operative site.[8]

The exact role of flexible sigmoidoscopy is evolving. With the gradual shift of colorectal cancers to the more proximal colon over recent decades, flexible sigmoidoscopy is not adequate for colorectal cancer screening, and a complete colonic examination is needed. Flexible sigmoidoscopy, however, can be used to enhance the diagnostic capability of barium enema, which at times fails to visualize the distal rectum optimally because of the obscuring effect of the balloon needed to distend the colon and the catheter used to infuse the barium. Lesions of the rectum and sigmoid seen on radiologic studies also can be evaluated by flexible sigmoidoscopy. Flexible sigmoidoscopy permits serial examinations of the activity of proctosigmoiditis in patients with inflammatory bowel disease and allows rectosigmoid biopsies to be done. It is also the preferred endoscopic tool for surveying family members at risk for familial adenomatous polyposis (see Chapter 119).

HEMORRHOIDS

Hemorrhoids are perhaps the most misunderstood anorectal problem for patients and physicians alike. In clinical practice, patients use the term *hemorrhoid* to describe almost any anorectal problem, from pruritus ani to cancer.[9] In fact, hemorrhoids are a normal part of human anatomy,[10,11] in contrast to hemorrhoidal disease, which is manifested by prolapse, bleeding, and itching.[10] Hemorrhoids are dilated vascular channels located in three fairly constant locations: (1) left lateral, (2) right posterior, and (3) right anterior. Internal hemorrhoids originate above the dentate line and are covered with columnar or transitional mucosa. External hemorrhoids are located closer to the anal verge and are covered with squamous epithelium. Traditionally, internal hemorrhoids are classified into four grades: (1) first-degree hemorrhoids, which bleed with defecation; (2) second-degree hemorrhoids, which prolapse with defecation but return spontaneously to their normal position; (3) third-degree hemorrhoids, which prolapse through the anal canal at any time but especially with defecation, and can be replaced manually; and (4) fourth-degree hemorrhoids, which are prolapsed permanently.[11]

Although the exact incidence of hemorrhoidal disease is unknown, 10% to 25% of the adult population is thought to be affected.[12] Symptoms seem to be more common in older individuals, with a peak in prevalence at 45 to 65 years.

INTERNAL HEMORRHOIDS

It is speculated that internal hemorrhoids become symptomatic when their supporting structures become disrupted and the vascular anal cushions prolapse[13]; however, the exact pathogenesis is not clear. Hemorrhoids occur more frequently in people with constipation who have hard, infrequent stools.[14] Painless bleeding occurs, and red blood usually is seen on the toilet tissue or dripping into the toilet at the end of defecation. Sometimes the bleeding can be more substantial, and the blood can accumulate in the rectum, to be passed later as dark blood or clots.[11] When hemorrhoids prolapse, blood or mucus may stain a patient's underwear, and the mucus against the anal skin may lead to itching.[10]

The diagnosis of internal hemorrhoids is made with the beveled anoscope or by flexible sigmoidoscopy and retrograde view of the anorectal junction. The cushions can be seen to bulge into the anal lumen, or the tissue may prolapse out through the anal canal. Hemorrhoids may be symptomatic only intermittently and may look entirely normal if the patient is over a "flare."

Treatment

Treatment is based on the grade. Grade 1 and some early grade 2 internal hemorrhoids usually respond to dietary manipulation, along with avoidance of medications that promote bleeding, such as nonsteroidal anti-inflammatory drugs (NSAIDs). A high-fiber diet with 25 to 30 g of fiber daily should be introduced gradually into the diet and accompanied by six to eight glasses of fluid daily. Patients are encouraged to read the package regarding the amount of fiber per serving; for instance, a bowl of bran cereal can have 5 to 7 g of dietary fiber per serving.[15] Fiber supplementation with psyllium or hydrophilic colloid may be added to achieve the optimal amount of daily fiber if the amount of daily fiber is not sufficient.

Patients often are concerned that fiber supplementation will be "addictive" or that the package label calls the supplement a "laxative"; counseling about the goal of increasing the amount of dietary fiber helps them understand the importance of these agents. Fiber supplements can be started in a dose of 1 tsp daily for a week and then increased to 1 tbsp or more daily so as to allow the digestive tract to adjust to the increase in fiber. Patients are urged to avoid straining during defecation, reading while on the toilet, and deferring the urge to defecate for long periods of time. They should be encouraged to wipe the anal area gently after defecation with a moist facial tissue or baby wipes. Excessive scrubbing of the anus when showering or bathing is discouraged. Most over-the-counter agents are not efficacious, even though many patients report some relief of their symptoms with use of these products.[14] Sometimes docusate sodium or mineral oil can be prescribed if the stool is hard and does not respond to increased intake of fiber and fluid; laxatives and enemas rarely are needed.[15] Even patients who require more aggressive treatment of their hemorrhoids should be advised to increase their dietary fiber and fluids and to avoid straining during defecation to prevent recurrence after treatment.

When dietary manipulation does not work, more aggressive treatment may be needed. These measures can apply to grades 1, 2, and 3 internal hemorrhoids. Unless the patient has fourth-degree internal hemorrhoids, aggressive nonsurgical treatment usually is tried; most patients with fourth-degree hemorrhoids require surgical intervention. Most treatments are designed to affix the vascular cushion to the underlying sphincter. Options to achieve such fixation include injection with a sclerosing agent, rubber band ligation, cryotherapy, infrared photocoagulation, electrocoagulation, and application of a heater probe. These procedures can be performed in the office, usually after the patient has received an enema to evacuate the rectum of stool.

Sclerosing Agents

Injection therapy for hemorrhoids has been practiced for more than 100 years. The goal is to inject an irritant into the submucosa above the internal hemorrhoid at the anorectal ring (the area that does not have somatic innervation) to create fibrosis and prevent hemorrhoidal prolapse.[16] Usually less than 1 mL is needed to create a raised area. Many substances have been used, but sterilized arachis oils containing 5% phenol are the most popular.[16] This approach usually is advocated for first- and second-degree hemorrhoids.

Sclerotherapy can produce a dull pain for up to 2 days after injection. A rare but severe complication is life-threatening pelvic sepsis, which can occur 3 to 5 days after injection and usually is manifested by any combination of perianal pain or swelling, watery anal discharge, fever, leukocytosis, and other signs of sepsis. Prompt surgical intervention and intravenous antibiotics are mandatory.[16,17] Approximately 75% of patients with second-degree hemorrhoids improve after injection therapy.[18]

In patients with acquired immunodeficiency syndrome (AIDS), injection therapy may be favored over surgical treatments because of concerns about the patient's poor overall general condition. There also may be problems with wound healing for these patients. Successful treatment of second-, third-, and fourth-degree hemorrhoids without complications has been reported in patients with AIDS,[19] some of whom did require repeat treatment to manage persistent symptoms.

Rubber Band Ligation

Rubber band ligation (RBL) has become the most common office procedure for the treatment of second- and third-degree hemorrhoids.[20] Generally, this approach cannot be used with first-degree hemorrhoids, because there is insufficient tissue to pull into the bander. Treatment of fourth-degree hemorrhoids is almost never appropriate with this method.[18] Patients usually are asked to refrain from taking aspirin or NSAIDs for approximately 5 days before and after the treatment, to reduce the risk of bleeding. Rubber bands are applied to the rectal mucosa just proximal to the internal anal cushion. To avoid severe pain, bands are never placed on the external component, which is innervated by somatic fibers. There is disagreement as to how many bands should be placed at one time. Studies have shown that triple RBL is safe and effective at one sitting,[20,21] but many authorities believe that the severity of pain and risk of complications are less if one band is applied per visit.

Patients may experience discomfort after RBL; soaking in a sitz bath and taking acetaminophen usually constitute sufficient treatment. Immediate severe pain usually signals that the band has been placed too close to the dentate line and that it must be removed. After RBL, patients are instructed to increase the fiber in their diet and employ the other noninvasive bowel habit modifications discussed previously. Success is reported in 75% of patients with first-degree (when RBL can be performed) and second-degree hemorrhoids and in 65% of those with third-degree hemorrhoids. Repeat RBL is an option for patients who continue to have prolapsing tissue.

There can be important complications from RBL. Bleeding when the band with necrotic hemorrhoidal tissue comes off in 4 to 7 days may be severe and even life-threatening; severe bleeding occurs in about 1% of patients[21] and usually can be tamponaded by placing a large-caliber Foley catheter in the rectum, filling the balloon with 25 to 30 mL or more of fluid, and pulling the balloon tight against the top of the anal ring. If this approach fails, epinephrine can be injected at the bleeding site, but sometimes a suture is required to stop the bleeding. A more serious complication is sepsis. There have been five recorded deaths, two additional patients with life-threatening sepsis, and three cases of severe pelvic cellulitis following RBL of hemorrhoids.[17] The onset of sepsis usually is 2 to 8 days after RBL in otherwise healthy people. New or increasing anal pain, sometimes radiating down the leg, or difficulty voiding may be the first indications of a life-threatening infection. Immediate intravenous antibiotics and surgical débridement are required.

A few centers combine RBL with sclerotherapy to treat symptomatic second- and third-degree hemorrhoids.[20] Although this combination would seem to be advantageous intuitively, results are similar to those obtained with RBL only.

Cryotherapy

Cryotherapy freezes tissue, thereby destroying the hemorrhoidal plexus. Once a popular treatment, its use has declined because of the profuse, foul-smelling discharge resulting from necrosis of tissue. The procedure also can be painful, and healing can be prolonged.[22]

Infrared Photocoagulation

Infrared photocoagulation utilizes infrared radiation to coagulate the tissue, thereby leading to fibrosis. The device is applied for 1.5 seconds in two or three sites proximal to the hemorrhoidal plexus. Reported results for first- and second-degree hemorrhoids are as good as those reported for RBL or sclerotherapy.[18] One study reported a 10% relapse rate at 3 years in patients who had third-degree hemorrhoids and were treated with RBL at recurrence.[23] Pain and other complications are rare with infrared photocoagulation.

Electrocoagulation and Heater Probe

Use of thermal injury to fix the internal hemorrhoidal plexus is the basis for electrocoagulation and heater probe therapy. Both types of therapy compare favorably with rubber band ligation for the treatment of first- and second-degree hemorrhoids but have not gained popularity.

Surgery

Methods to reduce internal anal sphincter pressure in patients with internal hemorrhoids have been advocated in the past. These methods include internal sphincterotomy and manual dilatation of the anus (Lord's procedure) and are based on the general finding of an increase in resting anal canal pressure in patients with hemorrhoids[24]; these procedures, however, have not had widespread acceptance. One study of the Lord procedure to treat second- and third-degree internal hemorrhoids with a median follow-up of 17 years found a nearly 40% recurrence rate and a 52% rate of incontinence.[25] Lateral internal sphincterotomy occasionally is performed if patients have both a fissure and extensive hemorrhoids at the time of surgery for hemorrhoids.

Hemorrhoidectomy is the surgical procedure of choice for fourth-degree and some third-degree hemorrhoids and rarely is needed for first- or second-degree hemorrhoids. Hemorrhoidectomy can be done with local, regional, or general anesthesia. Whether the edges of the mucosa are closed or left open after excision of the hemorrhoidal tissue is a matter of preference, as results and postoperative pain are similar with either approach.[26] In one of the few long-term studies of hemorrhoidectomy, recurrent hemorrhoids were found in 26% at a median follow-up of 17 years,[25] but only 11% of patients needed an additional procedure.

Postoperative pain is the major drawback of hemorrhoidectomy. In an effort to reduce postoperative pain, topical and oral metronidazole have been used with success, although the mechanism of this action is not known.[27] Additionally, a new procedure was introduced in 1998 by Longo,[28] in which a circular stapler is used to fix the anal cushions in their correct positions. The mucosa is excised circumferentially just above the anorectal ring, thereby also interrupting the vascular supply to the cushion. This procedure is called the *procedure for prolapse of hemorrhoids* (PPH). It is usually used for third- and fourth-degree hemorrhoids. Results of the randomized multicenter U.S. experience, which compared PPH with the traditional excisional hemorrhoidectomy, showed that PPH-treated patients experienced significantly less pain and perhaps had better overall long-term results.[29] Another study comparing PPH with RBL found patients reported more pain and an increased risk of postoperative bleeding with PPH; however, more patients in the RBL group required excisional hemorrhoidectomy for persistent symptoms.[30]

PPH can have significant postoperative complications, of which bleeding and urinary retention are the most common.[29] Severe persistent postoperative pain can occur in one third of patients and may be related to placing the staple line too close to the dentate line.[31] Additionally, defecation urgency can be persistent in up to 28%. Perhaps the most feared complication is pelvic sepsis leading to death.[32] In summary, more data may be needed, but it appears that in some individuals PPH is superior to traditional hemorrhoidectomy in limiting postoperative pain.

Table 122–1 summarizes the treatment options for internal hemorrhoids.

EXTERNAL HEMORRHOIDS AND ANAL TAGS

External hemorrhoids are visible at the anal verge and actually represent residual redundant skin from previous episodes of external hemorrhoidal inflammation and edema. These skin tags typically occur in young and middle-aged adults and are easily seen when the buttocks are parted. They usually cause no symptoms and do not bleed, because they are covered with squamous epithelium; some people are uncomfortable during anal wiping due to irritation or the uncomfortable sensation of redundant tissue. Occasionally, external hemorrhoids interfere with perianal hygiene and cause itching and irritation. External hemorrhoids can be associated with acute pain from thrombosis.[13] The level of pain is variable, but patients may notice a rapidly increasing throbbing or

Table 122–1 Treatment Options for Internal Hemorrhoids

Type of Treatment	Hemorrhoid Grade	Success Rate, %	Comments
General			
Diet (increase in fiber and fluids) and habit modification	1-4	Unknown	Patients with all grades of hemorrhoids should follow these guidelines. Patients with high grades of hemorrhoids will need additional therapy.
Endoscopic			
Sclerosing agent	1-4	75	Life-threatening sepsis rarely may complicate therapy
			May be the favored treatment of patients with an acquired immunodeficiency (successful results even with grade 3 and 4 hemorrhoids)
Rubber band ligation	2 and 3	65-75	Grade 1 hemorrhoids are too small and grade 4 hemorrhoids are usually too large for this procedure
			Most commonly performed office procedure for hemorrhoids
			Life-threatening sepsis rarely may complicate therapy; 1% risk of severe hemorrhage when band sloughs
Cryotherapy	NA	NA	Currently not used because of the terrible odor that is produced as tissue necrosis occurs
Infrared coagulation	1 and 2	Same as for rubber band ligation	Equipment for the procedure is expensive
			Rare complications
Electrocoagulation or heater probe	1 and 2	Same as for rubber band ligation	Has not gained popularity as a treatment option
Surgical			
Anal dilation	NA	NA	No longer performed because of the high risk of fecal incontinence
Lateral internal sphincterotomy	All	NA	Only performed if an anal fissure is present and internal anal pressure is increased
			May be combined with an excisional hemorrhoidectomy if a fissure is present
Excisional hemorrhoidectomy	3 and 4	>75 on 10-year follow-up	Postoperative pain is pronounced
			External tags may be removed in the same surgical procedure
Procedure for prolapsing hemorrhoids*	3 and 4	Unknown; may be better than traditional excisional hemorrhoidectomy	New procedure
			Overall, significantly less postoperative pain than with excisional hemorrhoidectomy
			Bleeding can be a serious postoperative complication
			Some patients experience severe, persistent postoperative pain or defecation urgency
			Pelvic sepsis and death have been reported after this procedure

*Also called circular stapled hemorrhoidectomy.
NA, not applicable.

Table 122–2 Therapeutic Approach to Skin Tags and External Hemorrhoids

Condition	Approach
Skin tags	Delicate hygiene must be stressed—many patients wash the anal area too vigorously because of a feeling of inadequate cleanliness
	Reassurance
	Excise surgically if skin tags lead to problems with cleanliness or itching
	Unusual findings should be biopsied to rule out cancer
Thrombosed external hemorrhoids	Thrombosed hemorrhoid that is painful (usually in the first 48 hr from occurrence) can be excised or the thrombus enucleated
	A thrombosed hemorrhoid that recurs in the same location can be excised to prevent further recurrence
	0.3% nifedipine cream has been used to reduce the acute pain and to avoid surgery

burning pain accompanied by a new "lump" in the anal region. Sometimes the lump has a bluish discoloration caused by the clot. With time, a small area of necrosis may form over the lump followed by extrusion of the clot, with relief of the pain.

Treatment of external hemorrhoids usually is reassurance and proper anal hygiene, including delicate washing of the anal area and avoidance of aggressive wiping with harsh toilet tissue. Rarely is resection done; it is painful, and because of the swelling that accompanies any surgical excision, redundant tissue may persist after healing. The patient may feel the redundant tissue again and become upset about the "recurrence." When surgical excision is undertaken for internal hemorrhoids, as discussed earlier, any external component usually is excised at the same time.

The treatment of thrombosed hemorrhoids depends on the associated symptoms. With time, the pain associated with the acute thrombosis subsides. If the patient has minimal or moderate pain, sitz baths and analgesics are prescribed. For severe pain, the clot is removed under local anesthesia. Because of the high rate of recurrence with simple enucleation alone, some authorities recommend excising the entire thrombosis and overlying skin. This procedure also can be done in the office with scissors and local anesthesia.[33] The skin edges may be left open to heal by secondary intention.

Another successful therapy has been topical application of 0.3% nifedipine cream.[34] It is speculated that the success of this cream in reducing pain from thrombosed hemorrhoids results from anti-inflammatory and smooth muscle relaxing properties. It is used to relieve the initial pain and preclude the need for surgery.

Table 122–2 summarizes the treatment options for external hemorrhoids.

Special Considerations

Large, edematous, shiny perianal skin tags should alert the physician to the possibility of Crohn's disease. The tags may have a bluish discoloration. Careful history taking is indicated and further testing needed if there is any suspicion that the tags are not ordinary. Surgical excision of these Crohn's disease tags is to be avoided in almost every situation, because after surgery the patient usually is left with unhealed anal ulcers.

Patients who are infected with the human immunodeficiency virus (HIV) usually are treated as if they do not carry HIV, unless their immune status is significantly compromised. Previously mentioned was the use of scle-

rotherapy in this population.[19] In another study of 11 HIV-positive men with a mean CD4$^+$ count of 420/mm^3 and a mean follow-up of 6 months, no complications occurred after RBL of hemorrhoids, and symptoms improved in all.[35]

Pregnant women with problematic hemorrhoids usually are managed medically. Simply increasing the fiber and fluid intake and at times adding a stool softener is all that is needed. If a complication develops, such as acute prolapse with strangulation, surgical intervention in the operating room may be necessary.

Patients on anticoagulation including warfarin as well as other medications such as aspirin, enoxaparin, and clopidogrel also present a special challenge. There is no standard approach to treatment of this group of patients. Certainly it would be optimal to stop the medication for 5 to 7 days before any procedure and plan the treatment choice based on the grade of the hemorrhoid. For patients on warfarin with symptomatic hemorrhoids who cannot be off the medication for an extended period, transition to enoxaparin and cessation 12 hours before the procedure is an option. In my practice, I favor excisional therapy for this group because of the more controlled setting in the operating room; this is especially true if the most definitive treatment is desired.

ANAL FISSURE

An anal fissure is a longitudinal "cut" in the anoderm; it starts at the anal verge and can extend to the dentate line. More than 90% of anal fissures are located in the midposterior position of the anus; 10% are anterior. Any fissure not located in the anterior or posterior position or one that does not heal should alert the physician to the possibility of other diagnoses, such as Crohn's disease, tuberculosis, syphilis, cancer, a leukemic ulcer, or an HIV-related ulcer, which may be of viral or neoplastic origin.

The etiology of anal fissures is unknown. Using laser Doppler flowmetry, it has been shown that the posterior area of the anoderm is less well perfused than other areas of anoderm. There is speculation that increased tone in the internal sphincter muscle further reduces the blood flow to this area, especially at the posterior midline.[4] Based on these findings, fissures are thought to represent ischemic ulceration.[36] Trauma during defecation, especially with passage of a hard stool or explosive diarrhea, is believed to initiate the formation of a fissure.

Fissures usually are exquisitely tender, and the act of defecation is reported by patients to feel like passing razor blades. The history is classically one of *severe* pain during defecation. After defecation, patients may experience continued pain or burning for up to several hours. Bright red blood may be seen on the toilet tissue. On examination, a tender, edematous skin tag may be seen just distal to the fissure. Simply spreading the buttocks usually increases the pain and leads to anal sphincter muscle spasm. *A digital examination causes inhumane pain, increases the spasm, and should be avoided.* Once the fissure is healed or the pain has lessened, an examination can be done to exclude associated problems. If an examination is done and the anal canal is visualized, a hypertrophied anal papilla may be seen in patients with a chronic fissure. If the diagnosis is in doubt or the patient does not respond to treatment, an examination under anesthesia is indicated.

Fissures can be acute or chronic. Acute fissures are simply a split or crack in the anoderm, whereas chronic fissures show signs of chronicity, with rolled edges, fibrosis of the edges, deep ulceration with exposure of the underlying internal sphincter muscle, enlargement of the tissue at the dentate line (hypertrophied anal papilla), and edematous skin tags at the distal anal verge (Fig. 122–2).

Treatment of both acute and chronic anal fissures starts with dietary modification similar to the described conservative treatment of hemorrhoids. Patients are placed on a high-fiber diet with fiber supplements, and fluid intake is increased. Soaking in a sitz bath relaxes the sphincter and can provide some relief.[13] If needed, stool softeners are added. Acute fissures respond better to these measures than do chronic fissures.

The traditional surgical treatment of chronic anal fissure has come under intense scrutiny over the last 10 to 15 years. Because of concerns about alterations about fecal incontinence, pharmacologic therapy has gained popularity. One of the initial treatments was topical nitroglycerin to the anal region. A pea-sized amount of 0.2% to 0.4% nitroglycerin ointent with gradual escalation of the dose to three times daily is the most common way to use the medication. Headache is a significant adverse complaint,[37] and a gradual increase in dose may reduce this drawback. Patients should be cautioned to wear a finger cot or surgical glove when applying the ointment, to avoid absorption through the digital skin. Despite early successful clinical trials, long-term success rates have been questioned. A large systematic review found that healing of fissures with nitroglycerin was only marginally better than with placebo.[37] Another randomized trial found overall healing in about only one third of patients at 6 months.[38]

Calcium channel blockers (nifedipine and diltiazem) have been advocated because of their ability to relax the internal anal sphincter. Topical and oral agents have been studied, although far fewer studies are published for these agents than for nitroglycerin. In one pilot study, oral nifedipine, 20 mg twice daily, was reported to heal chronic anal fissures in 9 of 15 (60%) patients at 10 weeks; 10 patients experienced flushing, and 4 had mild headaches.[39] Topical 2% diltiazem gel has been used to treat nitroglycerin-resistant anal fissures in one study; of 39 fissures unhealed by nitroglycerin, 49% were healed at 8 weeks after diltiazem gel use.[38] This treatment modality requires further study to assess its place in the treatment algorithm.

The injection of botulinum toxin A, which inhibits acetylcholine release, into the internal sphincter close to a fissure was described first by Jost and Schimrigk in 1993.[41] Since then, this modality has gained popularity as a treatment for chronic anal fissure: In a study from Italy, 73% of anal fissures were healed at 8 weeks,[42] with no recurrences at a mean of 16 months later. Botulinum toxin injection also has been compared with topical nitroglycerin ointment; at 8 weeks, fissures were healed in 96% of patients injected with botulinum toxin and in 60% of those treated with nitroglycerin. In neither group was there a recurrence at a mean follow-up of 15 months.[43] Comparison of botulinum toxin with lateral internal sphincterotomy showed that at 1 year, more fissures were healed after surgery (94%) than with the injection (75%).[44] Long-term results may not be as optimal as hoped with botulinum injection. In one study of 57 patients, 22 (41%) had healed at a median of 42 months after botulinum injection.[45]

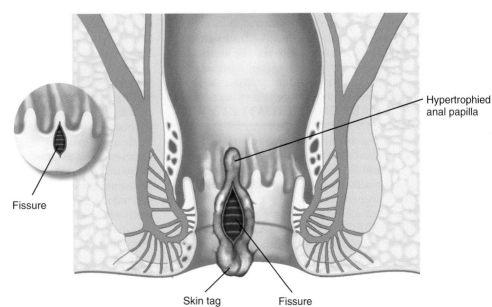

Figure 122–2 Schematic depiction of acute and chronic anal fissure. An acute fissure is depicted in the *inset* on the left as simply a split in the anoderm. A chronic fissure can show signs of chronicity with rolled edges, fibrosis, a hypertrophied anal papilla proximally, a tender distal skin tag, and exposed internal anal muscle.

Fissure

Hypertrophied anal papilla

Skin tag   Fissure

The standard treatment for chronic anal fissures has been lateral internal sphincterotomy. It remains the standard by which all other treatments must be measured. One long-term study found that among 2108 patients with anal fissures who underwent outpatient surgery with local anesthesia and intravenous sedation, the results were very good to excellent in 96% at a follow-up of 4 to 20 years. The rate of recurrent fissures was 1%. Permanent incontinence did not occur.[46] When performed correctly, lateral internal sphincterotomy still appears to be superior (and probably cheaper in the long-term) to any currently available medical treatment.[36,45]

An exception to the expected results with this approach was reported in a study comparing 0.2% isosorbide dinitrate ointment with lateral sphincterotomy.[48] An unusually high rate of healing of 89% (24 of 27 patients) at 2 years was found in the isosorbide dinitrate treatment group. The surgical treatment group demonstrated 100% healing at 2 years, but 15% of the patients (4 of 27) continued to have new alterations in continence at 2 years; 96% of the patients in both groups were female, which may have influenced these findings. Nonetheless, the authors made a reasonable point that perhaps the initial treatment should always be use of topical creams (as described previously) because of the potential for permanent alteration in continence with surgery; sphincterotomy would be reserved for patients whose fissures fail to heal with pharmacologic treatment.

Patients requiring special consideration are postpartum women. In one study, painful fissures developed in 29 (9%) of 313 postpartum primigravid women. Anal sphincter hypertonia was not seen in these patients,[49] and vaginal delivery is associated with anal trauma; hence, division of the anal sphincter in this setting may be detrimental. Of the 29 fissures, 27 healed with intensive medical treatment (which was not specified). The researchers suggested that if surgical intervention is needed in a postpartum woman with an anal fissure, an advancement flap (which raises a flap of healthy tissue to cover the open area) may be preferable to a lateral sphincterotomy.[50] Of historical interest is anal dilatation, or the Lord procedure. This procedure involves stretching the anal sphincter complex to rupture some of the fibers of the internal anal sphincter, thereby reducing the spasm and pressure that the internal sphincter muscle can generate at rest. The long-term problems involving soilage and incontinence of flatus and even stool have led to few indications for this procedure.

Table 122–3 lists the treatment options for anal fissures.

ABSCESSES AND FISTULAS

ABSCESSES

Almost all anorectal suppurative disease results from infection of the anal glands that extend from the anal crypts, located along the dentate line at the base of the columns of Morgagni. Acute infection can cause an abscess and lead to a chronic fistula-in-ano. Other causes include Crohn's disease, fissures that bore into the anal muscle, hematologic malignancies, tuberculosis, actinomycosis, trauma, foreign bodies, and anal surgery. The differential diagnosis also includes a pilonidal sinus, hidradenitis suppurativa, Bartholin's gland abscess, carcinoma, and lymphoma.

Because nearly all of the anal glands terminate in the intersphincteric plane, abscesses tend to originate in the intersphincteric space, from where they then can travel up, down, or circumferentially around the anus. Abscesses are classified according to where they extend to and may be perianal, ischiorectal, intersphincteric, or supralevator (Fig. 122–3). The most common type is the perianal abscess (40% to 50%), and the least common type is the supralevator abscess (2% to 9%).[51]

The diagnosis of anorectal abscess is based on typical symptoms and signs. Swelling, throbbing, and continuous pain are the most common symptoms. On examina-

Table 122–3 Treatment of Acute and Chronic Anal Fissure

Treatment	Comments
Acute	
Increase oral fluids, high-fiber diet, fiber supplements, sitz baths, and stool softeners if needed	Avoid digital rectal examination until the fissure is healed unless the diagnosis is in doubt (then examine in the operating room if needed)
	Usually responds to these measures
Chronic	
As above, usually with one of the following treatments added:	Also avoid digital examination unless the diagnosis is in doubt
0.2-0.4% Nitroglycerin cream applied to the anal area	Headache is major side effect
	Long-term success has been questioned
Calcium channel blockers (oral nifedipine or topical 2% diltiazem cream)	Seems promising but long-term success has been questioned
	Side effects (especially headache) may be less frequent than with nitroglycerin cream
Botulinum toxin A injected into anal muscle	Dose and exact injection site are not clear
	Expensive
	Long-term success is unknown
Lateral internal sphincterotomy	Traditional treatment
	Best results, with >90% long-term healing rate
	Durable
	May lead to fecal incontinence
Anal dilation (or Lord procedure)	Infrequently used because of the risk of fecal incontinence

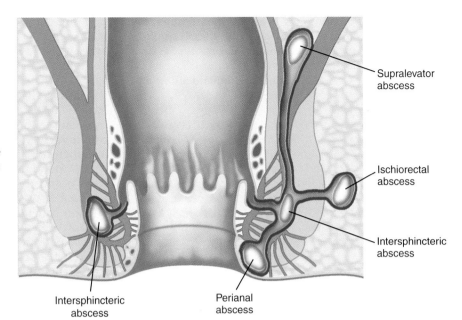

Figure 122–3 Schematic depiction of the classification of abscesses of the anal region based on the location.

Supralevator abscess

Ischiorectal abscess

Intersphincteric abscess

Intersphincteric abscess

Perianal abscess

tion, erythema or swelling may be seen. If the abscess is in the intersphincteric space, however, there may be no abnormal findings on the external skin. Nevertheless, a digital examination may be impossible because of pain, or a boggy area may be felt over the internal anal sphincter adjacent to the abscess. An ischiorectal abscess may produce pain in the buttock, but no abnormality may be appreciated on examination. The ischiorectal space is a potential space that can be large and therefore, pus may move upward rather than toward the skin.[51] Symptoms of a supralevator abscess may be intra-abdominal or urinary, and patients may have lower abdominal discomfort and urgency without any anorectal complaints or clinical findings. If the patient cannot be evaluated because the pain is severe or if no abnormality can be found on examination, the patient should undergo an examination under anesthesia. In elusive cases, an intra-anal ultrasound examination under anesthesia may be needed.

Treatment of an abscess in the perineal region requires incision and drainage. *Antibiotics alone are not adequate.* Failure to drain an abscess promptly can result in spread to adjacent spaces, and some necrotizing infections can be mutilating and life-threatening. Small abscesses can be drained in the office. The external opening should be made as close to the anal sphincter complex as possible without injuring it. Therefore, if a fistula develops, the fistulous tract will be short. The incision should be large enough or made in a cruciate fashion so that it will not close over before the inflammatory process has resolved. Packing should not be used, although some surgeons prefer to place a small "mushroom" catheter into the cavity to facilitate drainage. Large or high abscesses require drainage in the operating room.

It usually is not necessary to culture the pus. Hospitalization and intravenous antibiotics are reserved for patients who are immunocompromised or diabetic or who have signs of systemic infection, such as high fever. Patients should be followed closely to ensure that the process resolves.

FISTULA-IN-ANO

A fistula-in-ano is a tunnel that connects an internal opening, usually at an anal crypt at the base of the columns of Morgagni, with an external opening, usually on the perianal skin. A fistula-in-ano develops in 50% of patients who undergo incision and drainage of an abscess. Goodsall's rule can be used as a guide to find the internal opening of the fistula (Fig. 122–4). The rule states that when an imaginary line is drawn transversely through the center of the anus, external openings anterior to this line follow a radial (straight) path toward the anal canal and the diseased crypt; if the external opening is posterior to this line, the fistulous tract will curve and enter the anal canal in the posterior midline. Exceptions to the rule occur when an anterior opening curves around and is located in the posterior midline. In these cases, the external opening usually is several centimeters from the anal verge. This type of fistula is termed a *horseshoe fistula* because of its long, curved course. Because of the nature of the spaces around the anus, the fistulous tract can curve around and have an additional external opening anywhere along the tract on the opposite side.

The diagnosis of a fistula is made by seeing the drainage of blood, pus, and sometimes stool from its external opening. Some patients complain of perianal itching. If the tract seals over, pus may accumulate, and pain may develop. Long tracts can have secondary openings along their course. If the tract is chronic, it may be palpated as a cord under the skin. Pus sometimes may be expressed from the opening when the cord is palpated. Occasionally, anoscopy may reveal the internal opening of the fistula. Remembering Goodsall's rule can help the physician anticipate the probable location of the internal opening.

The differential diagnosis of fistula-in-ano is the same as for anal abscesses.

Treatment of fistula-in-ano is surgical intervention. The course of the fistulous tract influences the type of surgical treatment (Fig. 122–5). The most common treatment is a fistulotomy, or unroofing of the tunnel. Fistulotomy must be approached with caution if the tract traverses a substantial portion of the sphincter, in which case division would threaten continence. Most fistulas can be unroofed, however, and the base curetted and allowed to

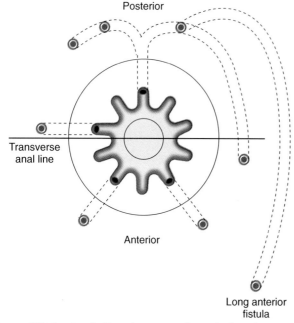

Figure 122–4   Goodsall's rule is a guide to finding the internal opening of a fistula-in-ano based on the location of the external opening and is important for surgical treatment. The rule states that when an imaginary line is drawn transversely through the center of the anus, external openings anterior to this line follow a radial (straight) path toward the anal canal and the diseased crypt. If the external opening is posterior to this line, the fistulous tract will curve and enter the anal canal in the posterior midline. Exceptions to the rule occur when an anterior opening curves around and then tracks to the posterior midline. In these cases, the external opening is usually several centimeters from the anal verge.

heal from the bottom up. The cure rate for uncomplicated fistulas not associated with Crohn's disease approaches 100%. Controversy exists as to whether fistulotomy should be done if a tract is found at the time a primary abscess is drained.[52]

A fistula that involves a substantial portion of the anal sphincter requires special treatment to avoid incontinence. Transanal advancement flaps are the most common surgical repair for these complex fistulas. Although initial success rates were higher, more recent studies found success rates varying from 67% to 77%.[53,54] Rates of incontinence after a flap repair range from 9% to 35%.[51,53] Alterations in continence tend to occur more often in patients older than 50 years.[55]

Fibrin adhesive made from autologous blood or commercial fibrin sealant has been used to close anal fistulas. The durable healing rate for cryptoglandular fistula was 23% in one study.[56] However, other studies have reported rates of 59% to 92%.[57,58] The fistulous tract is curetted aggressively, and the fibrin product is injected via the external opening until it is seen to emerge in the anal canal. Some surgeons prefer to place a suture over the internal opening to seal it off so that the fibrin is not dislodged by stool as the fibrin solidifies. No complications have been reported with this method, and continence is not affected. Retreatment for failures can be successful. The tract must be at least 1 cm long to allow sufficient length for the fibrin plug to adhere to the tract.

Direct closure of the internal opening for transsphincteric fistula has also been reported.[59] Of 106 patients reported by Athanasiadis and colleagues,[57] only 7 had persistent fistula, for an overall closure rate of 93.4%. The authors point out, however, that 24 of the 106 patients did require more than one operative procedure to obtain definitive fistula closure.

A seton is a rubber band–like material that is threaded through a fistula so that each end is tied loosely on the outside skin. Setons may be used to drain a fistulous tract before surgical repair to prevent the accumulation of pus;

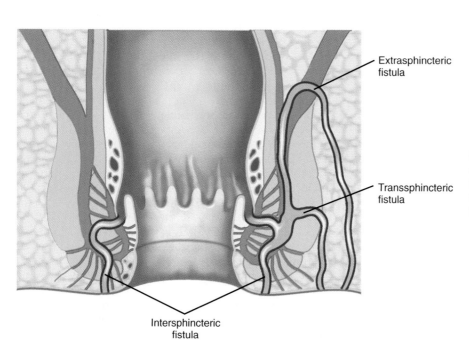

Figure 122–5   Schematic depiction of the classification of fistula-in-ano. Fistulotomy is not appropriate for extrasphincteric fistulas because it would leave the patient incontinent.

however, they also can be therapeutic if used as a cutting seton. In this latter approach, after the seton is placed, the skin alone (not the sphincter) is incised over the fistulous tract, and the seton is tightened gradually over several weeks so that it gradually cuts through the muscle. With gradual division of the muscle, the muscle will remain scarred in place and the ends will not spring back as they would when cut during a fistulotomy. This technique allows the fistulous tract to be unroofed gradually as the cut ends of the muscle scar close to their usual location, thereby minimizing the chance of incontinence.

It has been suggested that placing a loose seton until infection is controlled and removing it later can achieve significant healing. However, at a minimum of 10 years' follow-up with this treatment approach, 78% had recurrent sepsis.[60] Diligent follow-up and counseling need to be carried out if this treatment approach is chosen.

SPECIAL FISTULAS

Several types of fistula deserve special mention. Fistulas due to Crohn's disease are not cryptoglandular in origin but may be related to increased lymphoid tissue in the intersphincteric plane. They do not follow Goodsall's rule and usually are complex, with curved, multiple tracts. Any unusual fistula or nonhealing fistulotomy site should raise the possibility of Crohn's disease. Anal disease may be the first manifestation of Crohn's disease. Anorectal abscesses and suppuration may be less tender in patients with Crohn's disease than in some patients with cryptoglandular fistulas.[61] Treatment is tailored to the overall activity of the Crohn's disease (see Chapter 108). The goal is to improve the patient's quality of life; curing the Crohn's disease is not realistic, and healing the fistula may not be possible. Therefore, before treatment is started, the patient's gastrointestinal tract should be evaluated. In patients with severe colonic or rectal disease, the placement of a loose seton or mushroom catheter in an anal fistula may decrease symptoms; the seton or catheter may be left in indefinitely.[61] Some patients improve simply with the addition of oral metronidazole with or without ciprofloxacin.[62] The immunomodulator 6-mercaptopurine also has been used with some success. In one study one third of patients demonstrated clear improvement[63]; patients older than 40 years of age with new-onset perianal disease without true fistula were the best responders. Whether therapy with infliximab, a chimeric antibody to tumor necrosis factor, improves the healing of these difficult fistulas remains to be determined. In a study of 12 patients with anal fistula disease, 5 (42%) had a complete response rate[64]; of the remaining patients, 4 required surgical intervention and 3 had persistent fistula.

Fibrin glue products also have been used to treat fistulas associated with Crohn's disease, but the rate of success is low, with 31% healing in one study.[56]

Fistulotomy may be done for low fistulas with minimal anorectal involvement[61]; however, persistent nonhealing may be a problem. Advancement flaps have been used successfully to close Crohn's fistulas; there should be minimal anorectal involvement with Crohn's disease

when this type of repair is attempted. Despite the array of approaches, some patients have severe perianal sepsis and require fecal diversion with an ileostomy. In many, proctectomy is required later because of persistent discomfort or other problems. In general, surgical repair must be used with caution in anal fistulas in patients with Crohn's disease, and chronic, indwelling, loose setons are preferred to control symptoms of sepsis while preserving anal function.

In women with Crohn's disease, anovaginal fistulas present additional challenges. Traditionally, proctectomy or long-term seton drainage have been the accepted methods of treatment. Most such fistulas are too short to be amenable to fibrin glue. Surgical treatment with various flap repairs has been successful: In one study of 35 women, the initial success rate in selected women was 54%, with 68% healing after multiple flap procedures.[65,66]

Anovaginal fistulas not associated with Crohn's are also difficult to treat. Almost all are related to obstetric injury, with a few being cryptoglandular in origin. The local tissue usually is scarred and too rigid for successful treatment with advancement flaps. The anovaginal septum is usually very thin. Success is more likely if the sphincter is repaired in conjunction with repair of the fistula to give more tissue bulk to the anovaginal septum.[67]

Fistulas associated with radiation treatment, usually for cervical cancer, also are challenging. The first issue is to exclude recurrent cancer as the cause of the fistula. If the output of stool and gas per vagina is great, a stoma may be needed. A stoma also allows the tissue to soften, so additional treatment options can be evaluated. It may take up to 1 year for the area to become pliable enough for a reasonable attempt at surgical intervention to be undertaken. Repair with a flap can be attempted if the tissue looks normal and is pliable, but this rarely is the case. Resection of the rectum with anastomosis of healthy colon to the anus at the dentate line can be successful (coloanal anastomosis). Interposition of the gracilis muscle between the wall of the anorectum and vagina brings healthy tissue to the area and can lead to healing.

ANAL CANCER

Anal cancers are infrequent. They account for 1.5% of gastrointestinal cancers in the United States with 3500 new cases each year.[68] The incidence has increased 2% to 3% every year in the United States since the early 1980s.[69] Almost 80% are squamous cell cancers, 16% are adenocarcinomas, and 4% are other types.[70] Adenocarcinomas of the anal canal behave like adenocarcinomas of the rectum and are treated as such. Patients undergo abdominal-perineal resection with preoperative or postoperative chemoradiation therapy when the tumor is large or invasive or lymph nodes are positive for tumor.

Tumors arising in the distal anal canal usually are keratinizing squamous cell carcinomas. Those arising in the transitional mucosa frequently are nonkeratinizing squamous cell carcinomas. In the past, the two nonkeratinizing subtypes were referred to as *transitional cell* and *cloacogenic*. All anal carcinomas today are considered to be variants of squamous cell carcinoma, with various degrees of glandular/adnexal differentiation. The type previously called transitional cell carcinoma is composed of large cells, and the type previously referred to as cloacogenic carcinoma is composed of small cells,[71] but microscopically, these tumors may be heterogeneous, and it is not useful to subclassify them. Keratinizing and nonkeratinizing squamous cell cancers exhibit similar behavior. Anal bleeding is the most common symptom (45%), followed by the sensation of a mass (30%) or no symptoms (20%).[71] The development of anal cancer has been associated with infection with human papillomavirus, history of receptive anal intercourse, HIV infection, history of sexually transmitted diseases, history of cervical cancer, and use of immunosuppressive medication after solid organ transplantation.[72]

ANAL MARGIN CANCERS

Cancers arising distal to the anal verge (anal margin) are considered skin cancers and treated as such. Small lesions (<4 cm^2) with no fixation to deeper tissues are excised widely. Treated patients are then followed closely for 5 years. If the disease recurs, chemoradiation therapy is started. Invasive squamous cell cancer of the anal margin is treated with chemoradiation therapy.

ANAL CANAL CANCERS

In the past, standard treatment of anal canal cancers was abdominal-perineal resection with a permanent colostomy. In 1974, Nigro and colleagues presented the results of combined radiation and chemotherapy and showed that cure was possible without abdominal-perineal resection.[73] This led to a regimen of external-beam radiation with fluorouracil and mitomycin as the treatment of choice; surgery was reserved for residual cancer seen in the scar after treatment. Recently, cisplatin has been substituted for mitomycin in treatment trials, and complete response rates to combination treatment have been seen in 94% of patients. In one study, at a follow-up of 37 months, only 14% of patients required a colostomy for residual or recurrent disease.[71] With a follow-up mean of 5.6 years, another study found 30% of patients needed a stoma for recurrent or persistent disease.[74]

Patients with persistent or recurrent squamous cell carcinoma of the anal canal are treated with an abdominal-perineal resection. About 50% of such patients who undergo surgery can be cured.[71] Success has also been reported with an additional boost of radiation therapy combined with cisplatin-based chemotherapy.[71]

MELANOMA

Melanoma is as deadly in the anal region as elsewhere. Surgical excision offers the only chance for cure, and even this treatment has dismal results. Because of the poor success with any treatment, many investigators have questioned the use of abdominal-perineal resection for anal melanoma instead of wide local excision. In one

study 2/19 (10%) patients survived and the two patients who survived each had wide local excision.[75] The authors commented that anal ultrasound was valuable to guide treatment. They recommended that if ultrasound shows that the lesion can be excised, then wide excision should strongly be considered to avoid a permanent stoma, because most patients have regional or distant metastasis at presentation.[76]

BOWEN'S DISEASE

Bowen's disease is a confusing term in the literature. This entity generally is described as a dysplastic condition of the epithelium of the anal canal and perineal skin. It also is called squamous cell carcinoma in situ and thus is considered to be premalignant. Experts also refer to these lesions as anal squamous intraepithelial lesions (SILs) or anal intraepithelial neoplasia (AIN). There seems to be a progression from low-grade (AIN I) to high-grade (AIN III) lesions, similar to that observed in the cervix. In the literature, the relationship between Bowen's disease and AIN is not distinguished clearly, but it appears that Bowen's disease is AIN III. The lesion frequently is discovered at the time of pathologic examination of anal tissue obtained for an unrelated surgery.[77]

Disagreement continues regarding the treatment of Bowen's disease or high-grade AIN.[77] One approach involves directed therapy in the operating room: 3% acetic acid is painted on the distal rectal mucosa, anal mucosa, and perianal skin. Examination is then done with an operating microscope looking for patterns suggestive of high-grade dysplasia such as punctation and mosaicism. Then the tissue is painted with 10% iodine (Lugol's solution). Normal tissue will appear dark, whereas tissue that has high-grade intraepithelial changes appears yellow to tan. Directed destruction of tissue that has the characteristics of high-grade dysplasia is performed with electrocautery.[78] With use of this approach, no HIV-seronegative patient developed recurrent high-grade SIL; however, 79% of HIV-positive people had recurrent or persistent lesions.

Another approach reasons that because the condition stems from human papillomavirus (anal warts [see later]) as a predisposing factor,[79] the virus will remain in the "normal" tissue that is not excised. Accordingly, the best treatment option for patients with Bowen's disease (including HIV-positive patients) may be close observation, with regular biopsy of any suspicious areas to exclude invasive malignancy.[80,81]

PAGET'S DISEASE

This is a rare intraepithelial mucinous adenocarcinoma appearing as an erythematous, eczematoid plaque. It probably arises from the dermal apocrine sweat glands. The disease is more common in women than men and manifests with intractable itching. Diagnosis is by biopsy, and wide local excision is the treatment if invasion is not found. For invasive cancer, abdominal-perineal resection is the treatment of choice.

ANAL WARTS

Anal warts, or condylomata acuminata, are caused by the human papillomavirus (HPV). It is speculated that most squamous cell cancers of the anal area are caused by this virus. Condylomata affect 5.5 million Americans yearly and the prevalence is about 20 million.[82] Condylomata are caused by sexual transmission of HPV, although nonsexual transmission may be possible.[83] These lesions occur more frequently in men who have sex with men, immunosuppressed patients, following renal transplantation, and in individuals who have large numbers of sexual partners.[77] Multiple treatment modalities exist (see Table 122–4), but even when bulky lesions have resolved, the virus remains.

Podophyllin is a topical agent that is antimitotic. It requires repeated applications.[84] As a single agent, it results in cure rates of 50%.[84,85] Podophyllin cannot be used in the anal canal, however, and is poorly absorbed by keratinized lesions, which are characteristic of long-standing warts. The drug can cause skin irritation (severe necrosis and scarring have been reported) and is teratogenic in animals.

Trichloroacetic and dichloroacetic acid cause sloughing of tissue. These acids must be used with care to control the depth and size of the wound. They can be used in the anal canal. Cure rates of 75% have been reported with their use.[84,86]

Cryotherapy can be used in the anal canal. The depth and width of the wound must be monitored carefully. Success rates are similar to those associated with trichloroacetic acid.[84,87]

Topical 5-fluorouracil (5-FU) penetrates the skin and is used in a 5% cream. Success rates for 5-FU have ranged from 50% to 75%. Perhaps the best use of topical 5-FU is its biweekly application after surgical removal of warts to decrease rates of recurrence.[84,87]

Imiquimod cream is an immune response modifier that stimulates monocytes and macrophages to produce cytokines that affect cell growth and have an antiviral effect.[89] The cream is applied to the warts at bedtime three times a week for a total of 16 weeks. Imiquimod cannot be used for anal canal warts. The drug seems to work better for women than for men, with one study reporting clearance of warts in 72% of women compared with 33% of men.[90] Few side effects have been reported, although local skin irritation is seen.

Surgical excision and cautery yields the highest success rate, with cure rates of 63% to 91%; laser seems to offer no advantage over cautery. Disadvantages of cautery include the need for local or other forms of anesthesia and the presence of bioactive HPV in cautery-induced fumes.[84,91] Immune status seems to influence recurrence rates of recurrent condyloma. One study found significantly more recurrences in a shorter period for those with an immunocompromised status (defined as HIV-positive, those with leukemia, idiopathic lymphopenic syndrome, or organ transplant and those on chemotherapy).[92]

Interferon-α is approved by the U.S. Food and Drug Administration for injectional therapy of refractory condylomata acuminata. The dose is 1×10^6 units injected beneath a maximum of five lesions up to three times weekly for 3 to 8 weeks. Recurrence rates are 20% to 40%.[93] Topical interferon cream seems to be no better than placebo.[94] Surgery to eradicate the largest lesion, combined with topical or intralesional therapy, may decrease recurrence rates.

One promising therapy appears to be HspE7.[95] This is a novel fusion protein that combines immune stimulatory properties with an appropriate target antigen from

Table 122–4 Treatment Options for Anal Warts

Treatment	Success Rate, %	Comments
Podophyllin	20-50	May repeat applications if needed Skin irritation can occur Not used in the anal canal Poorly absorbed by keratinized lesions (most chronic warts are keratinized)
Trichloroacetic or dichloroacetic acid	75	Can be used in the anal canal Care is required to control the size of the slough
Cryotherapy	75	Can be used in the anal canal Care is required to limit the size of the wound Fumes from the therapy may contain active virus
Topical 5-fluorouracil	50-75	Probably best if used after surgical excision to decrease the incidence of recurrence
Imiquimod	75 in women 33 in men	Cannot be used in the anal canal; works better in women
Surgical excision (usually combined with cautery)	60-90	Fumes from the cautery may contain virus May need to be done in more than one session if a thick carpeting of lesions is present to avoid excising or burning excessive anoderm
Intralesional interferon-α injections	≈70	Injected into base of up to five warts three times a wk for 3-8 wk Approved by U.S. FDA for refractory condyloma
HspE7	Experimental	Promising treatment involving subcutaneous injections Fusion protein that combines immune-stimulating properties and a target antigen from human papillomavirus
External-beam radiation therapy	Variable	Reserved for giant cavitating condyloma called *Buschke-Lowenstein lesions* Used as the last resort, usually when bleeding or tissue invasion cannot be controlled

FDA, Food and Drug Administration.

HPV. In one study, HspE7 was broadly active for multiple HPV types. The warts were found to improve substantially, but usually did not disappear totally at 6 months' follow-up. Patients were HIV-negative and received three subcutaneous injections of HspE7. More studies are under way to further evaluate these findings.

Anogenital warts may affect immunocompromised patients, including those who are HIV-positive and transplant recipients. In such persons, the warts are more aggressive, recur earlier, and are more often dysplastic than in immunocompetent individuals. In HIV-positive patients, dysplasia and histologic evidence of HPV can occur in the absence of gross warts.[96] Gross warts should be treated as just discussed. Topical 5-FU cream and serial examinations, rather than extensive excision, have been advocated for HIV-positive patients with dysplasia.[96] Excision is reserved for patients with obvious lesions of the skin. Anal cytology (the "anal Pap test") has been considered in this group of patients, but as yet there are no firm recommendations for its use.

Buschke-Löwenstein tumors are a rare variant of anal warts. These lesions appear as giant condylomas that grow rapidly, invade locally, and cause extensive destruction of surrounding tissue. Treatment is surgical excision, if possible. These lesions also have responded to radiation therapy.[95]

Table 122–4 outlines the treatment options for anal warts.

PRURITUS ANI

Pruritus ani is an itch localized to the anus and perianal skin. Pruritus ani is categorized as either idiopathic or secondary. Idiopathic pruritus ani is diagnosed when no underlying etiology is found. Secondary pruritus ani results from an underlying disorder, and specific treatment leads to resolution of symptoms. Because pruritus ani is poorly understood, and an underlying premalignant lesion such as Bowen's disease or Paget's disease may be the cause of symptoms, all patients with pruritus ani deserve a thorough investigation.

In a prospective study, 109 patients were referred over a period of 2 years to a colorectal clinic for the primary symptoms of itching. On evaluation, 26 patients were found to have some form of colorectal or anal dysplasia, 56 had anorectal disease (most commonly fissures or hemorrhoids), and 27 had no identifiable etiologic disorder.[98] After surgical treatment of all patients with colorectal neoplasia, the itching resolved. Of the 56 patients with anorectal disease, 6 continued to have itching after medical or surgical treatment. All 27 of the patients with no obvious cause for their itching underwent conservative medical treatment, and 6 continued to have persistent symptoms.[98]

Thorough history taking and a physical examination are the starting points for evaluating patients with anal itching. Examination of the rectum and sigmoid colon should be included. The pattern of irritation should be noted, and consideration should be given to a biopsy of any abnormal skin. Usually, diet-induced pruritus is symmetrical, whereas infectious causes lead to an asymmetrical pattern of anal irritation. Leakage of stool or mucus because of fecal incontinence and leakage of mucus because of prolapse of the rectum or hemorrhoids can cause irritation and itching. Other causes include contact dermatitis, infections (such as candidiasis), parasites, systemic diseases (e.g., diabetes mellitus), diet (coffee, cola, chocolate, milk, beer, and others), and some medications. It has been said that dietary factors, especially any form of coffee, may be the most common culprit.[99] The exact mechanism whereby coffee may act as an irritant to the perianal skin is unclear, but perhaps for some persons, one of its metabolites can be irritating.

Any underlying disorder should be treated; however, in many patients the cause of pruritus ani may not be identified. These patients should be advised to modify their cleansing habits and to eliminate potential dietary culprits such as coffee, tea, and chocolate during a trial period. Most important is to convince the patient to stop "polishing" his or her anus. Frequently, the patient feels that the anal area is unclean, and he or she rubs the area vigorously, both for comfort and to try to clean the area more completely. Wiping gently with wet facial tissue or baby wipes is recommended. Avoiding soap and a washcloth in the shower may help. The patient should be instructed to use plain water and his or her hand to wash the perineum in the tub or shower. Creams or emulsifying ointments may be used instead of soap.[100] Perfumed soaps and astringents (such as witch hazel) should be avoided. A cotton ball placed by the anus and changed several times a day will absorb moisture and create a drier environment. A diet high in fiber with plenty of fluids (similar to the diet described for hemorrhoids) is recommended. A limited amount of 1% hydrocortisone cream can be used. Patients should be warned that chronic use of hydrocortisone will thin the anal skin and may lead to more problems.

Most patients respond to this regimen. Relapse is common and may require re-education of the patient. The physician should be aware that a previously overlooked underlying problem may be the cause of the pruritus and should take a fresh look at a patient who has a relapse. Assistance from a dermatologist also may be helpful and should be considered initially.[100]

Intradermal injection of methylene blue has been used successfully for the treatment of intractable idiopathic pruritus ani that has not responded to any other measures.[101]

ANAL STENOSIS

Anal stenosis is a narrowing of the anal canal. The condition may develop gradually after anorectal surgery, usually radical hemorrhoidectomy. Surgeons in the modern era have modified their surgical technique in an attempt to prevent this problem. Other causes include chronic anal fissure, inflammatory bowel disease (especially Crohn's disease), chronic diarrheal disease, habitual use of laxatives (mineral oil frequently is cited in lectures, but its mechanism is not clear), infections (tuberculosis, lymphogranuloma venereum, syphilis, and others), cancer, and irradiation.[102]

Treatment of anal stenosis depends on the degree of stenosis and associated symptoms. In mild stenosis, the examiner's finger can be placed just through the narrowing. Patients are placed on a high-fiber diet and bulking agents to produce stools that pass more easily, but patients must be cautioned to drink sufficient fluids so that they do not become constipated. Additionally, the bulky stools provide natural dilation. Gradual dilation by the patient (usually daily in the shower) with a commercial medical dilator or a smooth white candle also can produce improvement.[103] The candle should be devoid of fragrance and coloring, both of which could potentially be irritating to the anal skin.

In moderate stenosis, more force is required to insert the index finger. Patients may respond to dietary changes and graded dilations. The initial dilation may need to be done under anesthesia. If improvement is insufficient, surgery is indicated. Release of a stricture or a sphincterotomy may suffice. However, some patients may require an advancement flap.[103]

In severe stenosis, even the tip of the examiner's fifth finger cannot be inserted into the anal canal. There is loss of the anoderm, and surgical intervention is needed to deliver healthy tissue into the anal canal to compensate for this loss. Various advancement flaps are successful, and the type used depends on the patient's anatomy and the surgeon's preference.[103]

UNEXPLAINED ANAL PAIN

Unexplained anal pain refers to pain in the anorectal region in the absence of an underlying anatomic abnormality. Diagnosis is based almost entirely on the patient's symptoms. Confusing nomenclature has clouded the issue further.

Coccygodynia is a pain or ache in the tailbone and typically results from trauma to the coccyx or arthritis. Movement of the coccyx on digital rectal examination can reproduce the pain. Treatment in the acute setting includes sitz baths, NSAIDs, and stool softeners.[104] Glucocorticoid injections have been used in an attempt to reduce the pain. Rarely, removal of the coccyx is necessary.[105]

Levator ani syndrome and *proctalgia fugax* are probably not the same entity. In the literature, however, the terms often are used interchangeably, but incorrectly.

Levator ani syndrome affects women younger than 45 years of age. Episodes of pain are chronic or recurring and, by definition, occur during 12 weeks in the preceding year, with each episode lasting 20 minutes or more.[106] The discomfort is described as a vague tenderness or aching sensation high in the rectum. Discomfort usually does not awaken the patient from sleep and usually is worse after defecation and with sitting; walking or lying down seems to relieve the pain.[107] Symptoms have been attributed to spasm of the levator muscles. Physical examination may be normal, or the levator muscle may feel like a tight, tender band on rectal examination.[104]

Proctalgia fugax occurs in young men and "perfectionists." It is seen in early adulthood and subsides by middle age. The pain lasts seconds or minutes and then disappears. Pain is described as a sharp cramp or stabbing pain and may awaken the patient from sleep.[106,107] The pathogenesis is thought to involve anal smooth muscle

dysfunction, perhaps triggered by stressful events.[107] The frequency of proctalgia fugax may be increased in patients with other functional gastrointestinal complaints, such as unexplained abdominal pain, bloating, irritable bowel syndrome, and a sensation of incomplete evacuation. Physical examination is normal.[104,106,107]

Treatment of the levator ani syndrome and proctalgia fugax is controversial, and no single treatment works for all patients. Treatments for these disorders are grouped together, in part because of our incomplete understanding of the two conditions. Initial treatment is reassurance, sitz baths, perineal strengthening exercises, and regulation of bowel habits. These measures are usually effective.[104] Many other treatments have been proposed, including electrogalvanic stimulation,[108] levator massage, biofeedback,[109] drug therapies, acupuncture, and psychiatric evaluation.

In the past, the drug treatment of choice was benzodiazepines; however, because of their addictive potential and the chronic nature of these problems, the popularity of these drugs has declined. In the only randomized, controlled trial for proctalgia fugax, a salbutamol inhaler was used successfully.[110] Two puffs at the onset of pain were reported to lead to rapid relief.

Clonidine, an α_2 agonist, relaxes smooth muscle and has been used successfully.[111] The dose is 150 mg twice daily for 3 days, tapered to 75 mg twice daily for 2 days, and then 75 mg daily for 2 days. Diltiazem, a calcium antagonist, relaxes smooth muscle and also has been effective in a dose of 80 mg twice daily.[112] Topical nitroglycerin, 0.2% or 0.3%, applied at the onset of proctalgia fugax also has been used successfully.[113] A newer treatment involves linearly polarized near-infrared irradiation therapy and provides light, chemical, and thermal effects on the neuromuscular system and can alleviate pain.[112] One study used this treatment for patients with strongly tender points in each side of the rectum rather than the anal canal. Of 35 patients, 33 had good or excellent improvement after an average of 2.5 20-minute treatments.[112]

HIDRADENITIS SUPPURATIVA

Hidradenitis suppurativa is an inflammatory disease of the apocrine sweat glands and adjacent connective tissue. The initiating event is occlusion of the apocrine duct by a keratinous plug, leading to ductal dilation and stasis and then to secondary bacterial infection. The infection often ruptures into the surrounding soft tissue (Fig. 122–6). The chronic, cyclic nature of the disease ultimately leads to fibrosis and hypertrophic scarring of the skin. Commonly involved bacteria include *Streptococcus milleri*, *Staphylococcus aureus*, anaerobic streptococci, *Bacteroides* species,[115] *Escherichia coli*, *Klebsiella*, and *Proteus*.[116] The axilla is the most common site of disease, followed by the anogenital region. Clinical features include recurrent abscesses, chronic draining sinuses, and indurated, scarred skin and subcutaneous tissues. The spectrum of severity ranges from mild disease with spontaneous regression to severe involvement at multiple sites. Coexistent Crohn's disease occurs more frequently than expected, with a frequency of nearly 40% in one study.[117]

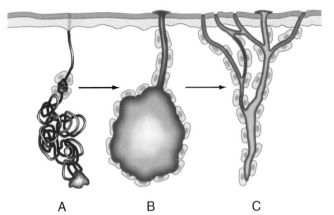

Figure 122–6 Hidradenitis suppurativa, an inflammatory disease of the apocrine sweat glands and adjacent connective tissue. *A,* The initiating event is occlusion of the apocrine duct by a keratinous plug. *B,* Bacteria are trapped beneath the keratinous plug and multiply to form an abscess, which can rupture into adjacent tissue. *C,* The end result is recurrent abscesses, chronic draining sinuses, and indurated scarred skin and subcutaneous tissues. Frequently, multiple tracts are interconnected and lead to the skin.

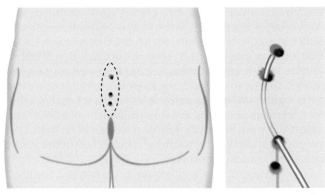

Figure 122–7 Pilonidal disease. On examination, there may be multiple pits or external openings in the intergluteal cleft proximal to the anus, as seen on the left. The openings frequently communicate with each other, as shown on the right. A probe can be passed between this network of tracts that communicate. Trapped loose hair is usually found in these tracts. One successful treatment option is to unroof all the tracts.

Diagnosis of hidradenitis suppurativa is based on the clinical presentation. Early symptoms include itching and erythema. Later, a firm, pea-sized nodule may be detected and may rupture spontaneously. The lesion heals with fibrosis but may recur adjacent to the original area. Over time, multiple abscesses and sinus tracts develop in the subcutaneous region to form a honeycomb-like pattern.[116] Discharge from the open areas may be serous or purulent.

Treatment consists initially of antibiotics active against *Staphylococcus.* Oral isotretinoin has been used successfully in mild cases.[118] Intralesional glucocorticoids, anti-androgen therapy,[116] and topical clindamycin[119] also have been used. Surgery is required for chronic disease. Apparent "cure" can be achieved by extensive excision of the involved area down to the soft tissue and with wide margins. The area is then closed with a skin graft or left to granulate.[120,121] New lesions can develop in untreated skin and close follow-up is needed.

PILONIDAL DISEASE

Pilonidal disease is an acquired problem that affects young adults after puberty. It occurs in the intergluteal cleft and may be confused with fistula-in-ano. The prevailing theory of pathogenesis is that hair in the cleft, along with desquamated epithelium, is propelled into the base of the cleft, where the barbs of hair shafts prevent them from being expelled, thereby setting up a granulomatous reaction, which creates a sinus.[122] With movement, the buttocks exert a drilling effect on the hair, driving them further into the sinus. Suppuration and abscess formation occur, with occlusion of the sinus by the accumulation of hair and debris. The unique hair distribution in affected persons is thought to play a role in the pathogenesis.[122] Free hair is found in the cyst or abscess cavity and also may be seen protruding from pits

in the intergluteal cleft. Symptoms may result from an acute abscess, chronic cyst, or draining sinuses. The diagnosis is made by identifying the abscess, which is characteristically several centimeters cephalad to the anus, or tiny openings in the intergluteal cleft over the sacrum (Fig. 122–7).

In mild cases, successful treatment has been achieved simply by shaving the hair on a regular basis (usually monthly) to prevent the hair from embedding in the intergluteal cleft. Any abscess requires immediate drainage. In patients with chronic disease, more extensive surgical treatment is needed. This usually consists of unroofing all sinus tracts with marsupialization; excision of the area with or without closure of the skin edges; or creation of advancement flaps, musculocutaneous flaps, or some variant of these.[122-126] When extensive surgical débridement is needed, vacuum-assisted closure devices have been shown to decrease length of time until the wound is healed.[127] Afterward, it is still necessary to shave the surrounding hair periodically to prevent recurrence. As with any other chronic draining fistula or sinus, squamous cell carcinoma may arise with long-standing disease.[128]

RECTAL FOREIGN BODY

Most foreign bodies in the rectum are not the result of oral ingestion. Accidental ingestion of a toothpick or a fishbone, however, may present as an abscess in the wall of the rectum or anus. More commonly, foreign bodies are placed into the rectum via the anus. Treatment (removal) often requires skill, trial and error, and luck to avoid a laparotomy. Most rectal foreign bodies result from sexual (erotic) stimulation or criminal assault. The history obtained from the patient is notoriously unreliable[129] as to what exactly the object is and how it was placed. If the patient indicates that the object was placed as a result of sexual assault, a full sexual assault examination is needed, including perianal brushings and sampling for sperm.[130] An abdominal film is useful to determine the size and location of the foreign body. If free air is seen, a laparotomy is almost unavoidable.

To remove the object, relaxation and sedation are needed. If removal cannot be accomplished in the office or emergency department with local anesthesia, the patient should be taken to the operating room for regional or general anesthesia. An important principle in removing the object via the anus is that the rectum exerts a traction vacuum effect on the foreign body. Therefore, passage of a well-lubricated Foley catheter will break the vacuum air seal and aid in removal of the object. Imagination is needed at times to remove the object via the anus. Obstetric forceps and an obstetric vacuum extractor have been used with success.[131] When a vacuum extractor is used, it is important to make sure that no rectal mucosa becomes trapped in the extractor. Another innovative approach is to put plaster of Paris into the foreign body (if it is a hollow object) and place a string into the plaster of Paris. The entire concoction is allowed to harden, and the string is pulled out with the foreign body.[130] Having the patient in the lithotomy position allows pressure to be applied simultaneously over the lower abdomen to facilitate expulsion of the foreign body. After any foreign body has been removed from the anus, sigmoidoscopic examination is needed to rule out a perforation. If the sigmoidoscopic examination is negative, a water-soluble contrast enema study should be done as well to exclude a perforation, even if the foreign body does not look capable of causing injury.[132] It is important to remember that the object that was used to place the foreign body in the rectum may have perforated the bowel.[132]

Laparotomy is reserved for cases of colonic perforation and objects that cannot be removed otherwise. After opening the abdomen, attempts still should be made to milk the object distally and expel it via the anus, by means of intra-abdominal manipulation. If this approach fails, a colotomy is done to retrieve the object. In many instances, simple closure of the colotomy is risky because of trauma from the attempts at removal and the additional trauma caused by the grinding of the object against the rectal wall. In these situations, a temporary colostomy may be needed. Following removal of the object via laparotomy, other perforations that may have occurred when the object was inserted still must be excluded.

REFERENCES

1. Keighley MRB, Williams NS: Surgical anatomy. In Surgery of the Anus, Rectum and Colon, 2nd ed. Philadelphia, WB Saunders, 1997, p 7.
2. Godlewski G, Prudhomme M: Embryology and anatomy of the anorectum. Surg Clin North Am 80:319, 2000.
3. Jorge JMN, Wexner SD: Anatomy and physiology of the rectum and anus. Eur J Surg 163:723, 1997.
4. Schouten WR, Briel JW, Auwerda JJA, Boerma MO: Anal fissure: New concepts in pathogenesis and treatment. Scand J Gastroenterol 31(Suppl 218):78, 1996.
5. American Gastroenterological Association Medical Position Statement on Anorectal Testing Techniques. Gastroenterology 116:732, 1999.
6. Ringel Y, Dalton CB, Brandt LJ, et al: Flexible sigmoidoscopy: The patient's perception. Gastrointest Endosc 55:315, 2002.
7. DiSario JA, Sanowski RA: Sigmoidoscopy training for nurses and resident physicians. Gastrointest Endosc 39:29, 1993.
8. Soussan EB, Mathieu N, Roque I, et al: Bowel explosion with colonic perforation during argon plasma coagulation for hemorrhagic radiation-induced proctitis. Gastrointest Endosc 57:412, 2003.
9. Orkin B, Young H: When are "hemorrhoids" really hemorrhoids? A prospective study. Dis Colon Rectum 43:A35, 2000.
10. Cirocco WC: A matter of semantics: Hemorrhoids are a normal part of human anatomy and differ from hemorrhoidal disease. Gastrointest Endosc 51:772, 2000.
11. Mazier WP: Hemorrhoids, fissures, and pruritus ani. Surg Clin North Am 74:1277, 1994.
12. Nelson RL, Abcarian H, Davis FG, et al: Prevalence of benign anorectal disease in a randomly selected population. Dis Colon Rectum 38:341, 1995.
13. Metcalf A: Anorectal disorders. Postgrad Med 98:81, 1995.
14. Pfenninger JL, Surrell J: Nonsurgical treatment options for internal hemorrhoids. Am Family Phys 52:821, 1995.
15. Orkin BA, Schwartz AM, Orkin M: Hemorrhoids: What the dermatologist should know. J Am Acad Dermatol 41:449, 1999.
16. Kaman L, Aggarwal S, Kumar R, et al: Necrotizing fasciitis after injection sclerotherapy for hemorrhoids. Dis Colon Rectum 42:419, 1999.
17. Barwell J, Watkins RM, Lloyd-Davies E, Wilkins DC: Life-threatening retroperitoneal sepsis after hemorrhoid injection sclerotherapy. Dis Colon Rectum 42:421, 1999.
18. MacRae HM, McLeod RS: Comparison of hemorrhoidal treatment modalities: A meta-analysis. Dis Colon Rectum 38:687, 1995.
19. Scaglia M, Delaini GG, Destefano I, Hulten L: Injection treatment of hemorrhoids in patients with acquired immunodeficiency syndrome. Dis Colon Rectum 44:401, 2001.
20. Chew SSB, Marshall L, Kalish L, et al: Short-term and long-term results of combined sclerotherapy and rubber band ligation of hemorrhoids and mucosal prolapse. Dis Colon Rectum 46:1232, 2003.
21. Armstrong DN: Multiple hemorrhoidal ligation: A prospective, randomized trial evaluating a new technique. Dis Colon Rectum 46:179, 2003.
22. Smith LE, Goodreau JJ, Fouty WJ: Operative hemorrhoidectomy versus cryodestruction. Dis Colon Rectum 22:10, 1979.
23. Linares Santiago E, Gomex Parra M, Mendoza Olivares FJ, et al: Effectiveness of hemorrhoidal treatment by rubber band ligation and infrared photocoagulation. Rev Esp Enferm Dig 93:238, 2001.
24. Loder PB, Kamm MA, Nicholls RJ, Phillips RKS: Haemorrhoids: Pathology, pathophysiology and aetiology. Br J Surg 81:946, 1994.
25. Konsten J, Baeten CGMI: Hemorrhoidectomy vs. Lord's method: 17-year follow-up of a prospective, randomized trial. Dis Colon Rectum 43:503, 2000.
26. Arbman G, Krook H, Haapaniemi S: Closed vs. open hemorrhoidectomy: Is there any difference? Dis Colon Rectum 43:31, 2000.
27. Nicholson TJ, Armstrong D: Topical metronidazole (10 percent) decreases posthemorrhoidectomy pain and improves healing. Dis Colon Rectum 47:711, 2004.
28. Longo A: Treatment of Hemorrhoid Disease by Reduction of Mucosa and Hemorrhoid Prolapse with Circular-Suturing Device: A New Procedure. Proceeding of the 6th World Congress of Endoscopic Surgery. Rome, June 3-6, 1998, p 777.
29. Senagore A, Singer M, Abcarian H: A Prospective, Randomized, Controlled, Multicenter Trial Comparing Stapled Hemorrhoidopexy and Ferguson Hemorrhoidectomy: One-Year

Results. Podium presentation at the American Society of Colon and Rectal Surgeons meeting. Chicago, June 3-8, 2002.

30. Peng BC, Jayne DG, Ho Y-H: Randomized trial of rubber band ligation vs. stapled hemorrhoidectomy for prolapsed piles. Dis Colon Rectum 46:291, 2003.

31. Carriero A, Longo A: Intraoperative, perioperative and postoperative complications of stapled hemorrhoidopexy. Osp Ital Chir 9:333, 2003.

32. Maw A, Eu K-W, Seow-Choen F: Retroperitoneal sepsis complicating stapled hemorrhoidectomy: Report of a case and review of the literature. Dis Colon Rectum 45:826, 2002,

33. Jongen J, Bach S, Stubinger SH, Bock J-U: Excision of thrombosed external hemorrhoid under local anesthesia: A retrospective evaluation of 340 patients. Dis Colon Rectum 46: 1226, 2003.

34. Perrotti P, Antropoli C, Molino D, et al:: Conservative treatment of acute thrombosed external hemorrhoids with topical nifedipine. Dis Colon Rectum 44:405, 2001.

35. Moore B, Fleshner P: Rubber band ligation for hemorrhoidal disease can be safely performed in select HIV-positive patients. Dis Colon Rectum 43:A32, 2000.

36. Schouten WR, Briel JW, Auwerda JJA, De Graaf EJR: Ischaemic nature of anal fissure. Br J Surg 83:63, 1996.

37. Nelson R: A systematic review of medical therapy for anal fissure. Dis Colon Rectum 47:422, 2004.

38. Richard CS, Gregoire R, Plewes EA, et al: Internal sphincterotomy is superior to topical nitroglycerin in the treatment of chronic anal fissure: Results of a randomized, controlled trial by the Canadian Colorectal Surgical Trials Group. Dis Colon Rectum 43:1048, 2000.

39. Cook TA, Humphreys MMS, Mortensen NJM: Oral nifedipine reduces resting anal pressure and heals chronic anal fissure. Br J Surg 86:1269, 1999.

40. Jonas M, Speake W, Scholefield JH: Diltiazem heals glyceryl trinitrate–resistant chronic anal fissures: A prospective study. Dis Colon Rectum 45:1091, 2002.

41. Jost W, Schimrig K: Use of botulinum toxin in anal fissure. Dis Colon Rectum 36:974, 1993.

42. Maria G, Cassetta E, Gui D, et al: A comparison of botulinum toxin and saline for the treatment of chronic anal fissure. N Engl J Med 338:217, 1998.

43. Brisinda G, Maria G, Bentivoglio AR, et al: A comparison of injections of botulinum toxin and topical nitroglycerin ointment for the treatment of chronic anal fissure. N Engl J Med 341:65, 1999.

44. Mentes BB, Irkorucu O, Akin M, et al: Comparison of botulinum toxin injection and lateral internal sphincterotomy for the treatment of chronic anal fissure. Dis Colon Rectum 46:232, 2003.

45. Minguez M, Herreros B, Espi A, et al: Long-term follow-up (42 months) of chronic anal fissure after healing with botulinum toxin. Gastroenterology 123:112, 2002.

46. Argov S, Levandovsky O: Open lateral sphincterotomy is still the best treatment for chronic anal fissure. Am J Surg 179:201, 2000.

47. Evans J, Luck A, Hewett P: Glyceryl trinitrate vs. lateral sphincterotomy for chronic anal fissure: Prospective, randomized trial. Dis Colon Rectum 44:93, 2001.

48. Parellada C: Randomized, prospective trial comparing 0.2 percent isosorbide dinitrate ointment with sphincterotomy in treatment of chronic anal fissure: A two-year follow-up. Dis Colon Rectum 47:437, 2004.

49. Corby H, Donnelly VS, O'Herlihy C, O'Connell PR: Anal canal pressures are low in women with postpartum anal fissure. Br J Surg 84:86, 1997.

50. Nyam DCNK, Wilson RG, Stewart AJ, et al: Island advancement flaps in the management of anal fissures. Br J Surg 82:326, 1995.

51. Janicke DM, Pundt MR: Anorectal disorders. Emerg Med Clin North Am 14:757, 1996.

52. Cox SW, Senagore AJ, Luchtefeld MA, et al: Outcome after incision and drainage with fistulotomy for ischiorectal abscess. Am Surg 63:686, 1997.

53. Mizrahi N, Wexner SD, Zmora O, et al: Endorectal advancement flap: Are there predictors of failure? Dis Colon Rectum 45:1616, 2002.

54. Sonoda T, Hull T, Piedmonte MR, Fazio VW: Outcomes of primary repair of anorectal and rectovaginal fistulas using the endorectal advancement flap. Dis Colon Rectum 45: 1622, 2002.

55. Schouten WR, Zimmerman DDE, Briel JW: Transanal advancement flap repair of transsphincteric fistulas. Dis Colon Rectum 42:1419, 1999.

56. Loungnarath R, Dietz DW, Mutch MG, et al: Fibrin glue treatment of complex anal fistulas has low success rate. Dis Colon Rectum 47:432, 2004.

57. Sentovich SM: Fibrin glue for all anal fistulas. J Gastrointest Surg 5:158, 2001.

58. Lindsey I, Smilgin-Humphreys MM, Cunningham C, et al: A randomized, controlled trial of fibrin glue vs. conventional treatment for anal fistula. Dis Colon Rectum 45:1608, 2002.

59. Athanasiadis S, Helmes C, Yazigi R, Kohler A: The direct closure of the internal fistula opening without advancement flap for transsphincteric fistulas-in-ano. Dis Colon Rectum 47:1174, 2004.

60. Buchanan GN, Owen HA, Torkington J, et al: Long-term outcome following loose-seton technique for external sphincter preservation in complex anal fistula. Br J Surg 91:476, 2004.

61. Sangwan YP, Schoetz DJ Jr, Murray JJ, et al: Perianal Crohn's disease. Dis Colon Rectum 39:529, 1996.

62. Solomon MJ, McLeod RS, O'Connor BI, et al: Combination ciprofloxacin and metronidazole in severe perianal Crohn's disease. Can J Gastroenterol 7:571, 1993.

63. Lecomte T, Contou J-F, Beaugerie L, et al: Predictive factors of response of perianal Crohn's disease to azathioprine or 6-mercaptopurine. Dis Colon Rectum 46:1469, 2003.

64. Poritz LS, Rowe WA, Koltun WA: Remicaide does not abolish the need for surgery in fistulizing Crohn's disease. Dis Colon Rectum 45:771, 2002.

65. Hull TL, Fazio VW: Surgical approaches to low anovaginal fistula in Crohn's disease. Am J Surg 173:95, 1997.

66. Hull TL, Fazio VW: Rectovaginal fistula in Crohn's disease. In Phillips RKS, Lunniss PJ (eds): Anal Fistula: Surgical Evaluation and Management. London, Chapman & Hall, 1996, p 143.

67. Tsang CBS, Madoff RD, Wong WD, et al: Anal sphincter integrity and function influences outcome in rectovaginal fistula repair. Dis Colon Rectum 41:1141, 1998.

68. Greenlee RT, Hill-Harmon MD, Murray T, Thun M: Cancer statistics, 2001. CA Cancer J Clin 51:15, 2001.

69. Franco EL: Epidemiology of anogenital warts and cancer. Obstet Gynecol Clin North Am 23:597, 1996.

70. Spratt JS: Cancer of the anus. J Surg Oncol 74:173, 2000.

71. Ryan DP, Compton CC, Mayer RJ: Carcinoma of the anal canal. N Engl J Med 342:792, 2000.

72. Maggard MA, Beanes SR, Ko CY: Anal canal cancer: A population-based reappraisal. Dis Colon Rectum 46:1517, 2003.

73. Nigro ND, Vaitkevicius VK, Considine B Jr: Combined therapy for cancer of the anal canal: A preliminary report. Dis Colon Rectum 17:354, 1974.

74. Nguyen WD, Mitchell KM, Beck DE: Risk factors associated with requiring a stoma for the management of anal cancer. Dis Colon Rectum 47:843, 2004.

75. Malik A, Hull TL, Floruta C: What is the best surgical treatment for anorectal melanoma? Int J Colorectal Dis 19:121, 2004.

76. Klas JV, Rothenberger DA, Wong WD, Madoff RD: Malignant tumors of the anal canal: The spectrum of disease, treatment, and outcomes. Cancer 85:1686, 1999.

77. Chang GJ, Welton ML: Anal neoplasia. Semin Colon Rectal Surg 14:111, 2003.

78. Chang GJ, Berry JM, Jay N, et al: Surgical treatment of high-grade anal squamous intraepithelial lesions: A prospective study. Dis Colon Rectum 45:453, 2002.

79. Sarmiento JM, Wolff BG, Burgart LJ, et al: Perianal Bowen's disease: Associated tumors, human papillomavirus, surgery, and other controversies. Dis Colon Rectum 40:912, 1997.

80. Brown SR, Skinner P, Tidy J, et al: Outcome after surgical resection for high-grade anal intraepithelial neoplasia (Bowen's disease). Br J Surg 86:1063, 1999.

81. Cleary RK, Schaldenbrand JD, Fowler JJ, et al: Perianal Bowen's disease and anal intraepithelial neoplasia. Dis Colon Rectum 42:945, 1999.

82. Cates W: Estimates of the incidence and prevalence of sexually transmitted diseases in the United States. American Social Health Association Panel. Sex Transm Dis 26:S2, 1999.

83. Wikstrom A: Clinical and serological manifestations of genital human papillomavirus infection. Acta Derm Venereol Suppl (Stockh) 193:1, 1995.

84. Congilosi SM, Madoff RD: Current therapy for current and extensive anal warts. Dis Colon Rectum 38:1101, 1995.

85. Greene I: Therapy for genital warts. Dermatol Clin 10:253, 1992.

86. Swerdlow DB, Salvati EP: Condyloma acuminatum. Dis Colon Rectum 14:226, 1971.

87. Godley MJ, Bradbeer CS, Gellan M, Thin RN: Cryotherapy compared with trichloroacetic acid in treating genital warts. Genitourin Med 63:390, 1987.

88. Krebs HB: Treatment of genital condylomata with topical 5-fluorouracil. Dermatol Clin 9:333, 1991.

89. Miller R, Birmachu E, Gerster J, et al: Imiquimod: Cytokine induction and antiviral activity. Int Antiviral News 3:111, 1995.

90. Schneider A, Sawada E, Gissmann L, Shah K: Human papillomaviruses in women with a history of abnormal Papanicolaou smears and their male partners. Obstet Gynecol 69:554, 1987.

91. King AR: Genital warts: Therapy. Semin Dermatol 11:247, 1992.

92. de la Fuente SG, Ludwig KA, Mantyh CR: Preoperative immune status determines anal condyloma recurrence after surgical excision. Dis Colon Rectum 46:367, 2003.

93. Browder JF, Araujo OE, Myer NA, Flowers FP: The interferons and their use in condyloma acuminata. Ann Pharmacother 26:42, 1992.

94. Kraus SJ, Stone KM: Management of genital infection caused by human papillomavirus. Rev Infect Dis 12:S620, 1990.

95. Goldstone SE, Palefsky JM, Winnett MT, Neefe JR: Activity of HspE7, a novel immunotherapy, in patients with anogenital warts. Dis Colon Rectum 45:502, 2001.

96. Karamanoukian R, De La Rosa J, Cosman B, et al: Conservative management of anal squamous dysplasia in patients with human immunodeficiency virus. Dis Colon Rectum 43:A5, 2000.

97. Sobrado CW, Mester M, Nadalin W, et al: Radiation-induced total regression of a highly recurrent giant perianal condyloma: Report of a case. Dis Colon Rectum 43:257, 2000.

98. Daniel GL, Longo WE, Vernava AM III: Pruritus ani: Causes and concerns. Dis Colon Rectum 37:670, 1994.

99. Friend WG: Pruritus ani. In Fazio VW (ed): Current Therapy in Colon and Rectal Surgery. Toronto, BC Decker, 1990, p 42.

100. Dasan S, Neill SM, Donaldson DR, Scott HJ: Treatment of persistent pruritus ani in a combined colorectal and dermatological clinic. Br J Surg 86:1337, 1999.

101. Farouk R, Lee PWR: Intradermal methylene blue injection for the treatment of intractable idiopathic pruritus ani. Br J Surg 84:670, 1997.

102. Aitola PT, Hiltunen K-M, Matikainen MJ: Y-V anoplasty combined with internal sphincterotomy for stenosis of the anal canal. Eur J Surg 163:839, 1997.

103. Liberman H, Thorson AG: Anal stenosis. Am J Surg 179:325, 2000.

104. Hull TL, Milsom JW: Pelvic floor disorders. Surg Clin North Am 74:1399, 1994.

105. Wesselmann U, Burnett AL, Heinberg LJ: The urogenital and rectal pain syndromes. Pain 73:269, 1997.

106. Whitehead WE, Diamant E, Enck P, et al: Functional disorders of the anus and rectum. Gut 45(Suppl II):II-55, 1999.

107. Vincent C: Anorectal pain and irritation: Anal fissure, levator syndrome, proctalgia fugax, and pruritis ani. Prim Care 26:53, 1999.

108. Hull TL, Milsom JW, Church J, et al: Electrogalvanic stimulation for levator syndrome: How effective is it in the long term? Dis Colon Rectum 36:731, 1993.

109. Gilliland R, Heymen JS, Altomare DF, et al: Biofeedback for intractable rectal pain: Outcome and predictors of success. Dis Colon Rectum 40:190, 1997.

110. Eckardt VF, Dodt O, Kanzler G, Bernhard G: Treatment of proctalgia fugax with salbutamol inhalation. Am J Gastroenterol 91:686, 1996.

111. Swain R: Oral clonidine for proctalgia fugax. Gut 28:1039, 1987.

112. Boquet J: Diltiazem for proctalgia fugax. Lancet 8496:1493, 1986.

113. Lowenstein B, Cataldo PA: Treatment of proctalgia fugax with topical nitroglycerin: Report of a case. Dis Colon Rectum 41:667, 1998.

114. Mibu R, Hotokezaka M, Mihara S, Tanaka M: Results of linearly polarized near-infrared irradiation therapy in patients with intractable anorectal pain. Dis Colon Rectum 46(Suppl):S50, 2003.

115. Parks RW, Parks TG: Pathogenesis, clinical features and management of hidradenitis suppurativa. Ann R Coll Surg Engl 79:83, 1997.

116. Brown TJ, Rosen T, Orengo IF: Hidradenitis suppurativa. South Med J 91:1107, 1998.

117. Church JM, Fazio VW, Lavery IC, et al: The differential diagnosis and comorbidity of hidradenitis suppurativa and perianal Crohn's disease. Int J Colorectal Dis 8:117, 1993.

118. Boer J, van Gemert MJP: Long-term results of isotretinoin in the treatment of 68 patients with hidradenitis suppurativa. J Am Acad Dermatol 40:73, 1999.

119. Jemec GBE, Wendelboe P: Topical clindamycin versus systemic tetracycline in the treatment of hidradenitis suppurativa. J Am Acad Dermatol 39:971, 1998.

120. Endo Y, Tamura A, Ishikawa O, Miyachi Y: Perianal hidradenitis suppurativa: Early surgical treatment gives good results in chronic or recurrent cases. Br J Dermatol 139:906, 1998.

121. Bocchini SF, Habr-Gama A, Kiss DR, et al: Gluteal and perianal hidradenitis suppurative: Surgical treatment by wide local excision. Dis Colon Rectum 46:944, 2003.

122. Schoeller T, Wechselberger G, Otto A, Papp C: Definite surgical treatment of complicated recurrent pilonidal disease with a modified fasciocutaneous V-Y advancement flap. Surgery 121:258, 1997.

123. Spivak H, Brooks VL, Nussbaum M, Friedman I: Treatment of chronic pilonidal disease. Dis Colon Rectum 39:1136, 1996.

124. Rosen W, Davidson JSD: Gluteus maximus musculocutaneous flap for the treatment of recalcitrant pilonidal disease. Ann Plast Surg 37:293, 1996.

125. Petersen S, Koch R, Stelzner S, et al: Primary closure techniques in chronic pilonidal sinus: A survey of the results of

different surgical approaches. Dis Colon Rectum 45:1458, 2002.

126. Urhan MK, Kucukel F, Topgul K, et al: Rhomboid excision and Limberg flap for managing pilonidal sinus: Results of 102 cases. Dis Colon Rectum 45:656, 2002.

127. McGuinness JG, Winter DC, O'Connell PR: Vacuum-assisted closure of a complex pilonidal sinus. Dis Colon Rectum 46:274, 2003.

128. Abboud B, Ingea H: Recurrent squamous cell carcinoma arising in sacrococcygeal pilonidal sinus tract: Report of a case and review of the literature. Dis Colon Rectum 42:525, 1999.

129. Mackinnon RPG: Removing rectal foreign bodies: Is the ventouse gender-specific [Letter]? Med J Aust 169:670, 1998.

130. Fry RD: Anorectal trauma and foreign bodies. Surg Clin North Am 74:1491, 1994.

131. Johnson SO, Hartranft TH: Nonsurgical removal of a rectal foreign body using a vacuum extractor: Report of a case. Dis Colon Rectum 39:935, 1996.

132. Losanoff JE, Kjossev KT: Rectal "oven mitt": The importance of considering a serious underlying injury. J Emerg Med 17:31, 1999.

SECTION
XI

Psychosocial Factors

CHAPTER

123 A Biopsychosocial Understanding of Gastrointestinal Illness and Disease

G. Richard Locke III

Perhaps the greatest achievement of the past decade has been the sequencing of the human genome. Some have argued that this sequence holds the key to understanding all of human disease. However, genetics is not destiny. Not all identical twins live life exactly the same way. Environmental factors come into play. Infections, toxins, early life experiences, success, failure, family, friends, religion, and politics all affect the way a person feels and their quality of life. In the long run the interaction of these factors, some biologic, some psychological, and others sociologic, all come together to give rise to human disease and illness.

This integration of factors, the biopsychosocial model, provides the opportunity to consider the patient as a whole person. All these factors affect the development and expression of disease as well as outcome. All these factors need to be considered in caring for the patient.

Much has been written about this model and its application to the functional gastrointestinal disorders (FGIDs). In these disorders, there is not a clear pathophysiology and the diagnosis is based on symptom-based definitions. Debate still exists as to the degree to which these are biologic versus psychological conditions. The biopsychosocial model is becoming the accepted way to view these disorders because it allows for all the potential issues to be considered.

In other areas of gastroenterology and hepatology, the biopsychosocial model has not been given much consideration. The emphasis remains on pathophysiology of disease. Disease can be diagnosed, treated, and either cured or ameliorated based on biologic principles. Yet very few diseases in gastroenterology are purely biological. Other areas of gastroenterology in addition to the FGID field would benefit from further consideration of psychosocial factors in the pathogenesis and natural history of disease.

The biopsychosocial model is not purely psychological either. Physicians have had an unfortunate history of classifying what they cannot explain as psychological. Many articles were written about the role of stress and personality in the development of peptic ulcer disease before *Helicobacter pylori* (HP) was discovered. When biologic findings are identified, they must be incorporated into the model.

This chapter provides an overview of the biopsychosocial model and its role in understanding gastrointestinal illness and disease. The goal is to highlight how this broad view can help clinicians as well as researchers on how best to help their patients and advance the treatment of illness.

CASE STUDY: A TYPICAL PATIENT IN A GASTROENTEROLOGY PRACTICE

Mrs. Jones is referred to a gastroenterologist by her internist because of abdominal pain. She says the pain has been present for about 3 months. It comes and goes without rhyme or reason. However, when it does come it is quite severe. She cannot function, and she basically has to go to bed. Some foods seem to bring it on but not consistently. Her bowels are irregular and she is losing weight. She had blood tests and a computed tomographic scan and these were normal. She worries that her primary physician thinks the problem is in her head. She knows the problem is real and wants to know what to do.

A common approach for gastroenterologists to take is to perform a careful history and physical examination and then create a differential diagnosis based on the pathophysiology of abdominal pain. Tests are ordered based on what is most likely to be present. Upper endoscopies with biopsies, colonoscopies with biopsies, small bowel radiography, urine porphyrins, and urine heavy metals all might be done to try to identify the cause of the disease. When all the tests are negative, the patients are told they do not have a gastrointestinal problem and are referred back to the primary provider.

Another approach is for the gastroenterologist to tell such patients that the yield of any test would be quite low and that they do not have anything to offer. They are referred back to the primary provider.

In a third approach, the gastroenterologist does the same as either of the first two approaches but then refers the patient to a psychiatrist or a psychologist with hope that he or she might be able to help.

In a fourth approach, the gastroenterologist explores the history a bit further. The patient has had pain off and on in the past, although mostly in the chest and joints but not in the belly. She has had urinary problems before but not bowel problems. She might give a history of abuse as a child or young adult; she may highlight the problems that she is having with her husband or her parent or her child or at work. She might later recognize that her pain seems to come on whenever she has to go to a family reunion. The gastroenterologist highlights these cognitive issues and leads the patient to a referral to a mental health professional.

In a fifth approach, the gastroenterologist may explore the psychosocial issues as noted earlier as well as past histories of infections or food reactions or symptoms in family members. The roles of visceral hypersensitivity, abnormal motility, subtle inflammation, and the brain-gut axis are discussed. The patient is offered therapy and a return appointment to assess response over time. A referral to a mental health professional is suggested in conjunction with the care provided in gastroenterology.

Patients such as Mrs. Jones are quite common in gastroenterology practices.[1] Each of these approaches is used. Which one is best? Best for the patient? Best for the gastroenterologist? Best for the primary care provider? Practice would be easy if there were randomized trials of management strategies for this situation, but there are not. Thus the clinician is faced with examining the existing models and deciding which one is best for an individual patient.

The first approach places emphasis on the biomedical model. The answer lies in tests and if the current tests are not useful, research will provide new insights into pathophysiology that will give rise to new tests and therapies. The second approach is rather nihilistic. The physician may be correct that he or she cannot help, but this may be due to a lack of interest on the part of the physician rather than an absence of insight by the medical profession. In the third and fourth models, the physician has recognized the role of psychological factors in the patient's condition; however, these are thought to be the only factors present. This schism of organic versus functional, or mind versus body, is prevalent in our thinking today. If the tests are negative, then the issue must be mental and help is needed. Many gastroenterologists feel inadequately trained to explore this psychological realm and referral to a mental health specialist is sought. Other gastroenterologists are more likely to explore these issues to open the door for further inquiry by the psychiatrist or psychologist. In the fifth approach the roles of physiology, psychology, and sociology are considered. A biopsychosocial model is developed to understand the patient's condition and a partnership among the patient, gastroenterologist, and mental health professional is developed.

THE BIOMEDICAL MODEL

In the classic biomedical model, disease is thought to arise from a series of molecular steps. Understanding these molecular steps leads to a better understanding of disease. It is hard to argue that this model has not been successful in our goal of understanding the pathogenesis of disease. This textbook provides an example of this approach. The basic underpinnings of gastrointestinal physiology and pathophysiology are discussed first, followed by the application of these principles to understanding diseases presented by each organ system. When confronted with a challenge, this model takes a reductionist approach[2-5]; that is, the goal is to reduce the problem to the specific abnormality that can be modified in an effort solve the problem.

The biomedical model has also appropriately emphasized early detection and intervention. Diseases are sought in their preclinical phase, and patients are encouraged to undergo tests and treatment to help prevent adverse outcomes down the road. Currently, gastroenterology is emphasizing colon cancer screening. Asymptomatic people are sought to have testing for early detection of precancerous lesions. If positive, these people, who are not sick or ill, are told they have a disease. Preventive therapies are suggested again, based on the pathophysiology of neoplasia. Although the goal is to eliminate human death and suffering, the focus is on the disease and its eradication. Certainly many patients with cancer have been helped using this approach. Cancer is not the only condition for which the biomedical model has been extremely helpful. This model has been successful in developing therapies of inflammatory bowel disease, viral hepatitis, peptic ulcer disease, and gastroesophageal reflux. No one yearns for the days of steroids, antibiotics and antacids.

However, patients do not present to health care providers with diseases. They may be worried about diseases, but they present with symptoms. Physicians try to understand these symptoms on the basis of the pathophysiology of disease. The clinician tries to translate the symptoms into a disease by using tests. By providing a disease label, the clinician can provide a more accurate prognosis and prescribe therapy. The symptoms provide an early warning system like a fire alarm. Once the disease is identified, the symptoms become less important. The therapy is directed toward curing the disease and the assumption is that this will in turn improve the symptoms.

Yet, symptoms are much more common than diseases, and there are a large number of symptoms that might be related to digestive disease. Between 1:5 and 1:10 adults report heartburn, chest pain, abdominal pain, constipation, bloating, or diarrhea.[6] In fact, two thirds of the population has at least one gastrointestinal symptom.[7] Only half of these people seek care for their symptom, and when they do, the usual testing will be negative.[8] How do we help these patients? At present the biomedical model does not provide a clear answer. The tendency had been to adopt a mind-body dualism. That is, when the biomedical approach cannot provide an answer, then the answer must be in the mind. The typical biomedical model keeps the mind and the body separate.

Certainly symptoms may be the result of a psychiatric disorder. Yet even these mental illnesses often have a biomedical basis and thus are not purely psychological. People with these conditions often do have some physiologic abnormalities. A purely psychiatric explanation is not appropriate either. A biopsychosocial model may be more helpful.

THE BIOPSYCHOSOCIAL MODEL

The biopsychosocial model was proposed by Engel in 1977 as a response to the divide he perceived between psychiatry and the other medical professions at that time.[9] Engel argued that the biopsychosocial model was needed to "provide a basis of understanding the determinants of disease and arriving at rational treatments and patterns of health care" and to "take into account the patient, the social context in which he lives, and the complementary system devised by society to deal with the disruptive effects of the illness, that is, the physician role and the health care system." The model sought to overcome the separation of mind and body. Conditions were the result of a multitude of interrelated factors. In addition, these factors had effects on each other: The psychological factors influence physiology and the physiology influences psychology.

An important concept is the difference between disease and illness (although the two are significantly intertwined).[4] As noted, the biomedical model focuses on disease, which traditionally has been something that physicians identify and measure whether on a laboratory test or a pathologic specimen. The biopsychosocial model places a greater emphasis on illness, which is what the patient experiences. Typically, the severity of the disease and the illness match; however, discordance can occur. Patients may have melena but stay home until they are dizzy or short of breath. Other people present with severe pain but have just a focal area of colonic inflammation. Figure 123–1 helps to illustrate this discordance.[4] A biopsychosocial model helps to explain why some people with symptoms develop illness and take on a "sick" role

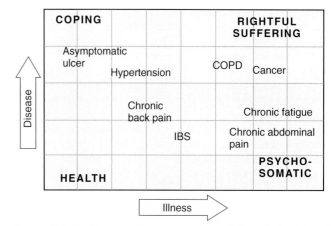

Figure 123–1 Conceptual representation of the relationship of illness with disease. Disease is a pathophysiologic process, whereas illness is what the patient with a disease actually experiences (see text for details). COPD, chronic obstructive pulmonary disease; IBS, irritable bowel syndrome. (From Drossman DA: Presidential Address: Gastrointestinal Illness and the Biopsychosocial Model. Psychosom Med 60:258, 1998.)

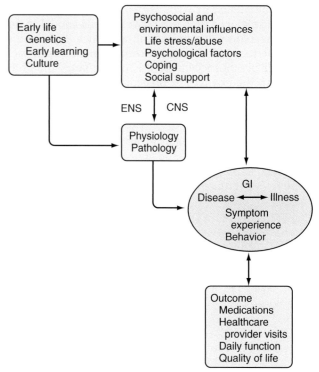

Figure 123–2 A biopsychosocial understanding of functional gastrointestinal disorders. Physiologic and psychosocial factors interact and affect each other in the development of the patient's illness. CNS, central nervous system; ENS, enteric nervous system; GI, gastrointestinal.

when others would consider the symptoms merely an aggravation of daily life.[9]

FUNCTIONAL GASTROINTESTINAL DISORDERS

A biopsychosocial model for FGIDs has been well articulated (Fig 123–2).[2] Certainly a genetic code places people at risk for specific diseases. Early in life they are exposed to infections and toxins, but they also learn from their parents and schoolmates. They may suffer from abuse, whether this be physical, sexual, or emotional. They will have life event stress both positive and negative. They will develop personality traits as a result of these gene-environment interactions. They will have different coping skills and have varying degrees of social support.

These factors all affect the function of the enteric nervous system and the brain-gut axis. Thus, people have varying thresholds for visceral sensation. Stimuli from the gastrointestinal tract may or may not give rise to signals that reach the cortex, and these signals may be sent to different parts of the brain. The sensory signal will then elicit a motor response both systemic and gastrointestinal specific. This change in physiology will give rise to symptoms of varying intensity.

Once the symptoms occur, the severity of illness that the patient experiences will again depend on psychosocial factors. Did they learn to stay home? Did they learn to express their emotions, or do they have alexithymia? Did they learn to fear disease and seek care? Do they think about the worst possibilities? Once they seek care, are they satisfied with their care or do they seek referral to other providers?

The key element of the biopsychosocial model is not just that biologic, psychological, and sociologic factors contribute to the illness but also they interact with each other. The psychosocial factors actually change the physiology and the changes in physiology affect psychological and social functioning.[2] You cannot experience an emotion or think a thought without biologic correlates (Fig 123–3).[5] When exposed to something threatening, we have an inner dialogue of automatic thoughts followed by anxiety that leads to autonomic nervous system activation. This process occurs with all perceived threats, whether real or imagined. These stresses go on to produce numerous changes in the neurobiology of the enteric nervous system.[10] The sympathetic and parasympathetic nervous systems, the hypothalamic-pituitary-adrenal axis, immune gut function, and viscerosomatic sensitivity all are modulated by exposure to stress. These can be reversible in the short term with an acute stress or more permanent with a chronic stress. For example, gastrointestinal symptoms are quite common in military veterans, and visceral hypersensitivity has been found in veterans recently returning from war.[11]

Certainly there is an abundant literature to support this model. The prototype condition is irritable bowel syndrome. Current evidence has shown a genetic component, an early life environment component, a post-infectious component, and a dietary component.[12-16] Associations have been identified with abuse, anxiety, depression, neuroticism, somatization, and sleep disturbance.[17-20] Health care seeking is strongly associated with psychosocial factors and quality of life.

This model also holds true for the other FGIDs such as chest pain and functional dyspepsia.[21-23] A similar biopsychosocial model has been proposed for children with recurrent abdominal pain.[24] There are comorbidities such as fibromyalgia, pelvic floor problems, and headaches. Early childhood issues related to feeding and elimination play a role, especially in constipation.[2,25]

These conditions have been labeled the FGIDs. Note the use of the term *disorder* rather than *disease*. "Disorders" as a phrase often connotes a psychological condition (e.g., attention deficit disorder, seasonal affective disorder, post-traumatic stress disorder). Why not use the phrase "disease?" Is it because the biomedical model does not have an answer as to a cause? Does the biomedical model hold a lock on what can be termed a disease? This is more than a semantic issue. Patients appreciate the validation that comes with the identification of a disease. Gastroesophageal reflux serves as an example. This condition has evolved from the symptom of heartburn to a disease with risk and need for intervention. Often the unspoken issue is that symptoms and disorders do not require treatment; the patient is expected to "live with it," whereas a disease means that patients have developed a problem no longer under their control. They need (rather than want) the assistance of a health care professional.

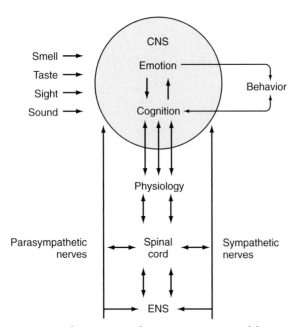

Figure 123–3 The interaction between environmental factors and the enteric nervous system. CNS, central nervous system; ENS, enteric nervous system. (From Wilhemson I: Brain-gut axis as an example of the bio-psycho-social model. Gut 47[Suppl 4]:iv5, 2000.)

GENERAL GASTROENTEROLOGY

Is the biopsychosocial model applicable to gastroenterology outside the field of FGID? Certainly, the enteric nervous system and the stress response affect hormonal secretion, immune function, and gut physiology, and these effects should occur in all conditions, not just the FGIDs. Substance abuse, alcohol addiction, mental illness, ineffective coping skills, and lack of social support each play a role in various digestive diseases. The biopsychosocial model enhances the provision of care in these situations. Although the literature regarding application of a biopsychosocial model to digestive disease in general is relatively sparse, many issues are worth highlighting.

Inflammatory bowel disease is clearly thought to be an organic condition, although the etiology is still not clear. Nonetheless, stress can affect the expression of the condition. Specifically, recent stressful life events have been associated with earlier time to relapse in ulcerative colitis.[26] Patients with Crohn's disease who report higher psychological distress and perceived stress are more likely to disagree with their physicians about the severity of their disease.[27] A person's social status may affect their access to therapy, and certainly a biopsychosocial model is needed to understand a patient's preference for ileal anal pouch anastomoses over ileostomies.

In acid peptic disorders, acute stress has an effect to increase gastric acid production and esophageal acid exposure.[21] This concept goes back to the original gastric fistula observations of Beaumont.[28] Years ago, peptic ulcer disease was thought to be associated with stress and personality type. Even though *H. pylori* has been shown to be a primary cause of peptic ulcer disease, stress continues to be an issue in idiopathic and even *H. pylori*-related ulcers[29,30]

In liver disease, most of the consideration for a biopsychosocial model comes with alcohol-related disease, especially in the area of liver transplantation for alcoholic cirrhosis. Certainly the psychosocial factors in the development of alcoholism are well known. However, other hepatic conditions can be affected by psychosocial factors. In a study of iatrogenic chronic viral hepatitis C infection, adjustment to illness was dependent on social factors, cognitive appraisals, adaptive tasks, and coping skills, thus emphasizing the need to develop a biopsychosocial model.[31] In another study, chronic psychosocial stress relevant to the type 1 personality was found to be associated with hepatitis severity.[32]

A biopsychosocial model helps understand the patient's need for coping skills and social support, even in patients with cancer. If the cancer is not curable, palliative care definitely follows a biopsychosocial model. Cancer pain is a prime example. Pain is not simply a reflection of biologic processes; it also is influenced by psychological and social factors.[33] The patient's mood and level of optimism may have an impact on outcome. Terminally ill patients place a significant burden on caregivers, and the caregiver in turn can have an effect on the patient. For example, caregivers often overestimate the severity of pain that a patient is experiencing, and when there is discordance between caregiver and patient, the patient is likely to report more anger, fatigue, poorer well-being, and lower quality of life.[34] When providing care to cancer patients at the end of life, biologic, psychologic, and social issues all are important.

For many areas of gastroenterology, the biopsychosocial model is not considered, yet such a model certainly can help. For example, patients with chronic pancreatitis often have significant pain and poor quality of life.[35] When the pain is difficult to treat, concerns about addiction often arise.[36] Because these patients may have a history of substance abuse, interpretation of the condition requires a full understanding of biopsychosocial factors.

Patients living on home parenteral nutrition also report poorer quality of life.[37,38] This, too, is associated with significant psychological distress, especially in children and adolescents. Eating is a highly social activity and the impact of not eating on the patient as a whole person needs to be considered.

IMPACT ON OUTCOME

Certainly a biopsychosocial model can help with the understanding of illness and suffering. Does this model improve outcome? Unfortunately the data needed to answer this question are scant. Certainly no randomized trial exists, nor are there extensive longitudinal studies. In a study of children with recurrent abdominal pain, the parent's willingness to accept a biopsychosocial model was positively associated with resolution of the abdominal pain during follow-up.[39]

Despite the appeal of the biopsychosocial model, incorporating it into practice and educating residents has been difficult.[40,41] In a survey of U.S. medical schools, 41% of schools used the term *biopsychosocial medicine* in the curriculum.[42] Much more needs to be done before this model is accepted into our approach to gastrointestinal illness and disease.

One strategy is to focus on the physician patient interaction.[43] Communication and a relationship-centered interview style have been shown to improve outcome in medicine in general. In FGIDs the strategy has included establishing a therapeutic relationship, eliciting and communicating the role of psychosocial factors, recognizing the patient's adaptations to chronic illness, and reinforcing healthy behaviors. Still, the application of this model in the management of disease is only in the early stages.

This chapter has introduced the concept of the biopsychosocial model and contrasted this model of illness to the traditional biomedical disease-based model. The usefulness of this model in understanding FGIDs has been highlighted. However, this model has not been used in other areas of gastroenterology. This has led to a continued dichotomy between the "organic" and "functional" gastrointestinal disorders. The goal for the future is to eliminate this schism. Research in the FGIDs is steadily increasing the pathophysiology of these disorders. Research in the organic conditions needs to increase our understanding of the psychosocial pathology of these conditions. Physicians cannot treat disease alone. Our patients are people. They come to us for help. Our goal is to help them in every way we can.

REFERENCES

1. Mitchell CM, Drossman DA: Survey of the AGA membership relating to patients with functional gastrointestinal disorders. Gastroenterology 92:1282, 1987.
2. Drossman DA: A biopsychosocial understanding of gastrointestinal illness and disease. In Feldman M, Friedman LS, Sleisenger MH (eds): Sleisenger and Fordtran's Gastrointestinal and Liver Disease: Pathophysiology, Diagnosis, Management, 7th ed. Philadelphia, WB Saunders, 2002, p 2373.
3. Drossman DA: Gastrointestinal illness and the biopsychosocial model. J Clin Gastroenterol 22:252, 1996.
4. Drossman DA: Presidential Address: Gastrointestinal Illness and the Biopsychosocial Model. Psychosom Med 60:258, 1998.

5. Wilhelmsen I: Brain-gut axis as an example of the bio-psycho-social model. Gut 47(Suppl 4):iv5; 2000; discussion, iv-10.

6. Locke GR: The epidemiology of functional gastrointestinal disorders in North America. Gastroenterol Clin North Am 25:1, 1996.

7. Drossman DA, Li Z, Andruzzi E, et al: U.S. householder survey of functional gastrointestinal disorders: Prevalence, sociodemography, and health impact. Dig Dis Sci 38:1569, 1993.

8. Kroenke K, Mangelsdorff AD: Common symptoms in ambulatory care: Incidence, evaluation, therapy, and outcome. Am J Med 86:262, 1989.

9. Engel GL: The need for a new medical model: A challenge for biomedicine. Science 196:129, 1977.

10. Mayer EA: The neurobiology of stress and gastrointestinal disease. Gut 47:861, 2000.

11. Dunphy RC, Bridgewater L, Price DD, et al: Visceral and cutaneous hypersensitivity in Persian Gulf war veterans with chronic gastrointestinal symptoms. Pain 102:79, 2003.

12. Levy RL, Whitehead WE, Von Korff MR, Feld AD: Intergenerational transmission of gastrointestinal illness behavior. Am J Gastroenterol 95:451, 2000.

13. Whitehead WE, Winget C, Fedoravicius AS, et al: Learned illness behavior in patients with irritable bowel syndrome and peptic ulcer. Dig Dis Sci 27:202, 1982.

14. Gwee KA, Graham JC, McKendrick MW, et al: Psychometric scores and persistence of irritable bowel after infectious diarrhoea. Lancet 347:150, 1996.

15. Atkinson W, Sheldon TA, Shaath N, Whorwell PJ: Food elimination based on IgG antibodies in irritable bowel syndrome: A randomised controlled trial. Gut 53:1459, 2004.

16. Morris-Yates A, Talley NJ, Boyce P, et al: Evidence of a genetic contribution to functional bowel disorder. Am J Gastroenterol 93:1311, 1998.

17. Drossman DA, McKee DC, Sandler RS, et al: Psychosocial factors in the irritable bowel syndrome: A multivariate study of patients and nonpatients with irritable bowel syndrome. Gastroenterology 95:701, 1988.

18. Drossman DA, Sandler RS, McKee DC, Lovitz AJ: Bowel patterns among subjects not seeking health care: Use of a questionnaire to identify a population with bowel dysfunction. Gastroenterology 83:529, 1982.

19. Drossman DA, Talley NJ, Leserman J, et al: Sexual and physical abuse and gastrointestinal illness: Review and recommendations. Ann Intern Med 123:782, 1995.

20. Whitehead WE, Bosmajian L, Zonderman AB, et al: Symptoms of psychologic distress associated with irritable bowel syndrome: Comparison of community and medical clinic samples. Gastroenterology 95:709, 1988.

21. Bradley LA, Richter JE, Pulliam TJ, et al: The relationship between stress and symptoms of gastroesophageal reflux: The influence of psychological factors. Am J Gastroenterol 88:11, 1993.

22. Locke GR III, Weaver AL, Melton LJ III, Talley NJ: Psychosocial factors are linked to functional gastrointestinal disorders: A population-based nested case-control study. Am J Gastroenterol 99:350, 2004.

23. Cheng C, Hui WM, Lam SK: Psychosocial factors and perceived severity of functional dyspeptic symptoms: A psychosocial interactionist model. Psychosom Med 66:85, 2004.

24. Hyams JS, Hyman PE: Recurrent abdominal pain and the biopsychosocial model of medical practice. J Pediatr 133:473, 1998.

25. Buxbaum E, Sodergren SS: A disturbance of elimination and motor development. Psychoanal Study Child 32:195, 1977.

26. Bitton A, Sewitch MJ, Peppercorn MA, et al: Psychosocial determinants of relapse in ulcerative colitis: A longitudinal study. Am J Gastroenterol 98:2203, 2003.

27. Sewitch MJ, Abrahamowicz M, Bitton A, et al: Psychosocial correlates of patient-physician discordance in inflammatory bowel disease. Am J Gastroenterol 97:2174, 2002.

28. Nutrition Classics: Beaumont W: Experiments and Observations on the Gastric Juice and the Physiology of Digestion, Plattsburgh, NY, FP Allen, 1833. Nutr Rev 35:144, 1977.

29. Levenstein S: Peptic ulcer at the end of the 20th century: Biological and psychological risk factors. Can J Gastroenterol 13:753, 1999.

30. Rosenstock SJ, Jorgensen T, Bonnevie O, Andersen LP: Does *Helicobacter pylori* infection explain all socio-economic differences in peptic ulcer incidence? Genetic and psychosocial markers for incident peptic ulcer disease in a large cohort of Danish adults. Scand J Gastroenterol 39:823, 2004.

31. Coughlan B, Sheehan J, Bunting B, et al: Evaluation of a model of adjustment to an iatrogenic hepatitis C virus infection. Br J Health Psychol 9:347, 2004.

32. Nagano J, Nagase S, Sudo N, Kubo C: Psychosocial stress, personality, and the severity of chronic hepatitis C. Psychosomatics 45:100, 2004.

33. Sutton LA, Porter LS, Keefe FJ: Cancer pain at the end of life: A biopsychosocial perspective. Pain 99:5, 2002.

34. Miaskowski C, Zimmer EF, Barrett KM, et al: Differences in patient's and family caregiver's perceptions of the pain experience influence patient and caregiver outcomes. Pain 72:217, 1997.

35. Wehler M, Nichterlein R, Fischer B, et al: Factors associated with health-related quality of life in chronic pancreatitis. Am J Gastroenterol 99:138, 2004.

36. Hung CI, Liu CY, Chen CY, et al: Meperidine addiction or treatment frustration. Gen Hosp Psych 23:31, 2001.

37. Pironi L, Paganelli F, Mosconi P, et al: The SF-36 instrument for the follow-up of health-related quality-of-life assessment of patients undergoing home parenteral nutrition for benign disease. Transplant Proc 36:255, 2004.

38. Engstrom I, Bjornestam B, Finkel Y: Psychological distress associated with home parenteral nutrition in Swedish children, adolescents, and their parents: Preliminary results. J Pediatr Gastroenterol Nutr 37:246, 2003.

39. Crushell E, Rowland M, Doherty M, et al: Importance of parental conceptual model of illness in severe recurrent abdominal pain. Pediatrics 112:1368, 2003.

40. Sadler JZ, Hulgus YF: Clinical problem solving and the biopsychosocial model. Am J Psychiatry 149:1315, 1992.

41. McClain T, O'Sullivan PS, Clardy JA: Biopsychosocial formulation: recognizing educational shortcomings. Acad Psychiatry 28:88, 2004.

42. Waldstein SR, Neumann SA, Drossman DA, Novack DH: Teaching psychosomatic (biopsychosocial) medicine in United States medical schools: Survey findings. Psychosom Med 63:335, 2001.

43. Larivaara P, Kiuttu J, Taanila A: The patient-centred interview: The key to biopsychosocial diagnosis and treatment. Scand J Prim Health Care 19:8, 2001.

CHAPTER

124 Palliative Medicine in Patients with Advanced Gastrointestinal and Hepatic Disease

Lisa Marr and David E. Weissman

DEFINITIONS

The purpose of this chapter is to review the physical and emotional care of patients with advanced and chronic, often life-limiting disease. Common gastrointestinal symptoms, important aspects of setting appropriate end-of-life goals, and communication skills are reviewed.

WHAT IS PALLIATIVE MEDICINE?

Palliative medicine is interdisciplinary care that aims to relieve suffering and improve quality of life not only for patients with advanced illness but also for their families.[1] Although often provided to patients with life-threatening illness not responsive to curative treatment,[2] it can be offered simultaneously with all other appropriate medical therapies up to and including aggressive, cure-oriented treatments.[1] In addition to the control of pain and other distressing symptoms, psychological, social, and spiritual needs are addressed as part of total patient care.[1] Because care near the end of life for complex physical and psychological problems cannot be provided by a single clinician, care is provided by a team that includes physicians, nurses, social workers, chaplains, and bereavement counselors. The interdisciplinary palliative care team works in concert with, and does not replace, the primary medical team. The ultimate goal of palliative medicine is to allow patients and their families to live as fully and symptom free as possible, in whatever time remains.

Palliative medicine recognizes that dying is a normal life cycle event and seeks neither to unnecessarily hasten nor postpone death but rather to focus care on patient-defined goals as death nears.[2] Most patients are able to articulate some or all of the following goals prior to death[3]:
- Freedom from pain and other distressing symptoms
- Having a sense of personal control over end-of-life decisions
- Avoiding inappropriate prolongation of dying
- Finding meaning and purpose in life
- Saying goodbye to friends and families

Palliative medicine and hospice care share the same philosophy of care. Unlike palliative medicine, however, hospice care in the United States is also a financial reimbursement system for the dying, largely defined by the Medicare Hospice Benefit (MHB). As such, hospice care has defined regulations and admission criteria. Under the MHB, patients are eligible for a specific set of services if (1) the physician certifies that the patient has less than 6 months to live, if the disease follows its usual course; and

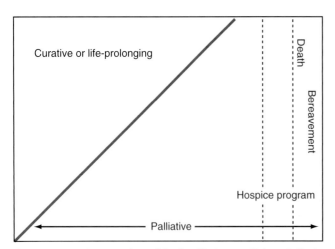

Figure 124–1 Integrated model of palliative medicine. Palliative care is not limited to hospice care, but may extend from the time a life-threatening illness is diagnosed through the patient's death and care of the bereaved family. (Adapted from Palliative Care Services: Report of the Subcommittee Branch on Institutional Program Guidelines. Canada, Health Services and Promotion Branch, Health and Welfare, 1989.)

(2) the goal of treatment is palliative rather than curative.[4] Although hospice care can be provided in special residential facilities or in long-term care facilities, more than 90% of hospice care in the United States is provided in the patient's home. There are no specific eligibility criteria for palliative care because there is no special defined reimbursement mechanism. The palliative care movement in the United States has developed largely in acute care hospitals and, more recently, in long-term care facilities. Therefore, all hospice care is palliative care, but not all palliative care is hospice care (Fig. 124–1). To truly provide seamless care of patients who are dying, communities need both palliative care and hospice services. More than 30 fellowships are now available for advanced physician training in palliative care, and board certification is available through the American Board of Hospice and Palliative Medicine.[5]

EXPLORING THE GOALS OF CARE

Exploring patient-defined goals of care is the first step in determining the most appropriate therapeutic interventions for a specific disease or symptom. An organized approach to goal setting can help both the clinician and patient achieve clearly articulated goals; this is best accomplished through a meeting with the patient and family or surrogate decision maker (Table 124–1). Prior to a goal-setting meeting, the clinician should review the disease course, response to prior treatments, and potential for further disease-modifying treatments and develop a realistic short- and long-term vision for the future clinical course, including a general sense of prognosis. With this in mind, the clinician can begin to review treatment options and help the patient decide which treatments are most likely to help meet his or her specific goals. All therapeutic options should be examined in light of the following question: *Does the intervention match or assist with the patient's treatment goals?*[6] As the burden of decision-making increases near the end of life,

it is important for physicians to understand their central role in helping patients make decisions. A model of shared decision making, in which the physician provides guidance and recommendations, generally is preferred to a paternalistic approach, or, at the opposite extreme, to one in which options are presented with no guidance.[7]

PROGNOSTICATION

Prognosis is a key piece of information that patients and families need as they are making decisions about proposed treatment plans near the end of life. Physicians often avoid providing prognostic information, however, and when pressed by patients, typically overestimate survival.[8] Overestimating prognosis or avoiding the discussion entirely (e.g., "only God can tell") typically is provided in a misguided attempt to protect the patient and family from bad news, but this approach results in false hope and delayed progression of the normal psychological coping mechanisms before and following death. Furthermore, if the imminence of death is not discussed honestly, patients will be more likely to accept costly, burdensome, and futile treatments.[9]

Prognostication guidelines are well-established for cancer.[10,11] The single best prognostic variable in cancer is performance status.[10,11] For example, patients with a Karnofsky Performance Status (KPS) of 40 (disabled; require special care and assistance) live on average less than 50 days, and patients with a KPS of 20 live an average of only 10 to 20 days[10] (Table 124–2). Put another way, patients who are spending more than 50% of the day resting or in bed generally have a prognosis of 3 months or less. Specific symptoms provide further information; symptoms with an independent predictive value for a poor prognosis are shortness of breath, anorexia, difficulty swallowing, and weight loss.[10]

Prognostic criteria for noncancer diagnoses have been published and are especially useful to help physicians know when to refer patients for hospice services.[12] Specific to gastroenterology, for example, general criteria have been established for chronic liver disease (Table 124–3). Beyond guidelines, some clinicians have advocated a simple test to determine when hospice services are appropriate by asking, "Would I be surprised if this patient died in the next 6 months?"[13]

No matter what type of cancer or noncancer fatal illness a person has, a "common final clinical pathway" occurs in most patients.[10] Signs and symptoms that predict a prognosis of "hours to days" are decreased and/or fluctuating levels of consciousness, a precipitous clinical decline, decreased oral intake, and inability to turn over in bed.[11] Patients close to death typically exhibit periods of apnea, retained oropharyngeal secretions (the "death rattle"), fever, and cool or mottled extremities.[11]

Discussing prognosis with patients and families is a key skill in palliative care. Physicians are advised to start by asking the patient if they previously have been given prognostic information; if they have a *sense of how much time is left;* and whether they would like to discuss prognosis. If a patient indicates that they do wish to discuss

Table 124–1 Process Steps for a Goal-Setting Family Meeting

1. Determine the reasons for convening a family conference.
   a. Clarify the goals of care and review the patient's medical condition.
   b. Decide on future levels of care and treatments, and resolve family conflicts.
2. Determine who should and who will be present for the conference.
   a. Include appropriate health care providers, e.g., nurse, chaplain, social worker, physician consultants, primary care physician, and so forth.
   b. Ask the patient, or health care power of attorney, who he or she would like to participate (e.g., the designated health care power of attorney, appropriate family members, clergy, lawyer, friend, and so forth).
3. Determine whether the patient has decision-making capacity.
   a. Able to understand information about diagnosis and treatment?
   b. Able to evaluate alternatives and compare risks and benefits?
   c. Able to communicate a choice, either verbally, in writing, or with a nod or gesture?
4. Choose the proper physical setting.
5. Introduce yourself, explain your relationship to the patient, and invite all participants to do the same.
6. Identify the legal decision maker, if available.*
7. Review the goals and purpose of the meeting.
8. Establish ground rules.
   a. Everyone will have the opportunity to talk.
   b. No interruptions are permitted.
9. Review the patient's current medical condition.
   a. "What is your understanding of ____'s present condition?" or "What have you been told about ____'s condition?"
   b. Review with the patient/family the current medical condition, e.g., expected prognosis and potential treatment plans. Avoid medical jargon.
   c. Invite questions.
   d. Defer treatment decision making until all questions about the patient's medical status have been asked to the extent possible.
10. Family discussion guidelines include the following:
    a. When the patient can speak for himself or herself,
       (1) Ask the patient what he or she is considering.
       (2) Ask the patient what type of support he or she would like from family members and from the health care team.
       (3) Invite discussion from other family members.
    b. When the patient cannot speak for himself or herself,
       (1) Describe the goal of substituted decision making, i.e., to speak on behalf of the patient by making those choices we believe the patient would make if he or she could speak.
       (2) Ask each family member what he or she believes the patient would choose if he or she were able to speak on his or her own behalf.
       (3) Ask each family member what his or her own wishes are for the patient.
       (4) Allow patients and families time alone, if they wish to talk before making a decision.
       (5) If there is a clear consensus of opinion, the meeting can be concluded. If there is no consensus, see No. 11.
11. Follow these guidelines when there is no consensus.
    a. Ask the family to discuss the issue on their own and schedule a follow-up meeting (use time as an ally).
    b. Ask each family member on what values his or her decision is based and how the decision will affect the patient and the other family members.
    c. Review again the goals you are trying to reach: What would the patient say if he or she were able to speak?
    d. Discuss other resources to support decision making.
12. Bring the conference to conclusion.
    a. Summarize the meeting for the family, including areas of agreement and disagreement.
    b. Decide if the decisions made lead to related issues that should be addressed while the family is present (e.g., "do not resuscitate" order, continuation or withdrawal of treatments, discharge planning).
    c. Provide a plan for follow-up, and offer to schedule further meetings with the family.
    d. Document a summary of the meeting in the medical record.
    e. Discuss relevant issues with all health team members.

*Note that laws governing surrogate decision making vary from state to state.
Adapted from Weissman DE, Ambuel B: Establishing treatment goals, withdrawing treatments. In Weissman DE, Ambuel B, Hallenback J (eds): Improving End-of-Life Care, 3rd ed. Milwaukee, Medical College of Wisconsin, 2000, p 101.

prognostic information, provide a broad estimate, *a few days to a few weeks* or *a few weeks to a few months,* rather than, *Mr. Jones, you have only 3 weeks to live.*[4] Once the time frame is presented, important future goals can be determined by asking, *What do you want/need to do in the time that is left?* (e.g., important events, saying goodbye to loved ones). This allows the clinician to "aim" the information at the level of the patient and family.[11]

COMMON THEMES IN PALLIATIVE MEDICINE

A complete review of symptoms commonly experienced by patients being cared for by palliative medicine physicians is beyond the scope of this chapter. Some of the most common symptoms experienced by patients with advanced gastrointestinal and hepatic disease, and

Table 124–2 Karnofsky Performance Status Scale

Status	Percentage Score	Criteria
Able to carry on normal activity and work; no special care is needed	100	Normal; no complaints; no evidence of disease
	90	Able to carry on normal activity; minor symptoms or signs of disease
	80	Normal activity with effort; some symptoms or signs of disease
Unable to work; able to live at home and care for most personal needs; varying amount of assistance is needed	70	Able to care for self; unable to carry on normal activity or do active work
	50	Requires considerable assistance and frequent medical care
Unable to care for self; requires equivalent of institutional or hospital care; disease may be progressing rapidly	40	Disabled; requires special care and assistance
	30	Severely disabled; hospitalization indicated, although death is not imminent
	20	Very sick; hospital admission is necessary; active supportive treatment is necessary
	10	Moribund; fatal processes progressing rapidly
	0	Dead

From Karnofsky DA, Abelman WH, Craver LP, Burchenal JH: The use of nitrogen mustards in the palliative treatment of carcinoma. Cancer 1:634, 1948.

Table 124–3 Suggested Criteria for Hospice Admission*

General Guidelines (apply to all diseases)—the patient should have all of the following:

The patient's condition is life-limiting, and the patient and/or family has been informed of this determination.

The patient and/or family has elected treatment goals directed toward relief of symptoms rather than cure of the underlying disease.

The patient has *either* of the following:
Documented progression of disease *or*
Diminished functional status

Guidelines for Liver Disease

The patient should not be a candidate for liver transplantation *and*

Prothrombin time >5 sec over control, *or* INR >1.5, *and* serum albumin <2.5 mg/dL *and*

One or more of the following:
Ascites refractory to diuretics and low-sodium diet *or* patient is noncompliant
Spontaneous bacterial peritonitis
Hepatorenal syndrome
Hepatic encephalopathy despite treatment
Recurrent variceal bleeding

Contributory factors that worsen prognosis:
Progressive malnutrition
Muscle wasting
Continued alcoholism
Primary liver cancer
Positive hepatitis B surface antigen

*Prognosis <6 months.
Adapted from Standards and Accreditation Committee: Medical Guidelines for Determining Prognosis in Selected Noncancer Diseases, 2nd ed. Arlington, Va, National Hospice Organization, 1996.

common gastrointestinal symptoms experienced by all patients at end of life, are discussed briefly in the following sections. As with all interventions, the benefit and burden of each treatment need to be evaluated in light of each patient's goals of care. If an intervention does not help advance an individual's goals of care, it should be withheld or withdrawn.[14]

ABDOMINAL PAIN

Freedom from pain is a central goal of palliative medicine. Abdominal pain may occur as one of three types: somatic, visceral, or neuropathic. Somatic pain typically is described as dull and achy; abdominal wall stretching from ascites is a common example. Patients describe visceral abdominal pain as either diffuse, as in peritonitis; referred, as in pain referred to the shoulder from hepatic disease; or colicky, as with bowel or bile duct obstruction.[15] Neuropathic abdominal pain arises from direct damage to peripheral or autonomic nerves near the spinal cord, the celiac or lumbar plexus, or more peripheral nerves. Neuropathic pain usually is described as burning, throbbing, sharp, or lancinating; abdominal pain from pancreatic cancer invading the celiac plexus is a common example.[15] It is important to make the distinction between pain types since treatments for each type of pain may be different. A thorough pain assessment is the first step. Questions to be asked include location, duration, temporal pattern, and pain modifiers.[16] Patients should be asked to rate the pain on a numeric or visual analog scale, or from "mild" to "severe" (Fig. 124–2). Other important questions are drug and nondrug treatments

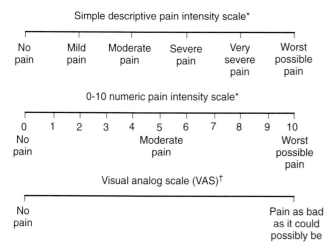

Simple descriptive pain intensity scale*

| No pain | Mild pain | Moderate pain | Severe pain | Very severe pain | Worst possible pain |

0-10 numeric pain intensity scale*

| 0 No pain | 1 | 2 | 3 | 4 | 5 Moderate pain | 6 | 7 | 8 | 9 | 10 Worst possible pain |

Visual analog scale (VAS)†

No pain   Pain as bad as it could possibly be

* If used as a graphic rating scale, a line 10 cm long is recommended.
† A line 10 cm long is recommended for VAS scales.

Figure 124–2 Pain intensity scales. (From Management of Cancer Pain: Adults. Rockville, MD, U.S. Department of Health and Human Services, Public Health Services, Agency for Health Care Policy and Research, 1994.)

Table 124–4 Short-Acting Opioid Equivalency Chart*

Short-Acting Drugs	Dose, mg Parenteral	Oral	Duration of Action, hr
Morphine	10	30	2-4
Hydromorphone	1.5	7.5	2-4
Oxycodone	—	30	2-4
Hydrocodone	—	30	2-4
Fentanyl	0.1	—	0.5-2

*Equianalgesic doses are approximate. Individual patient response must be observed.
Adapted from Max MB, Payne R (eds): Principles of Analgesic Use in the Treatment of Acute Pain and Cancer Pain, 4th ed. Glenview, Ill, American Pain Society, 1999.

that have been used, including their efficacy and toxicity. Finally, clinicians should assess the impact of the pain on the patients' activities of daily living; the patients' understanding of the cause of pain; and their specific goals for pain relief (e.g., improved sleep).[16]

Nonpharmacologic therapies (e.g., relaxation exercises, imagery, and judicious use of heat and cold) and over-the-counter medications (e.g., nonsteroidal anti-inflammatory drugs [NSAIDs] and acetaminophen) often are adequate for mild pain. Opioids are the drugs of choice for moderate to severe pain.[15] Short-acting opioids taken orally (morphine sulfate immediate release, hydrocodone, hydromorphone and oxycodone) reach their peak effect in 60 and 90 minutes and provide analgesic benefit for 2 to 4 hours (Table 124–4).[15] There is no ceiling dose of opioids, but combination products containing acetaminophen, aspirin or NSAIDs have a ceiling based on the toxicity profile of the nonopioid.[15]

Long-acting oral opioid preparations (morphine or oxycodone continuous release), provide 12 hours of analgesia.[15] Transdermal fentanyl offers 72 hours of pain relief and is a good option for patients with stable opioid requirements who cannot take oral medications.[17] Transdermal fentanyl takes 12 to 24 hours to reach full effect, and, similarly, analgesia and toxicities last for up to 24 hours after removal of a patch.[17] A small percentage of patients need patch replacement before 72 hours; cases of withdrawal occurring between 48 to 72 hours have been reported.[18] All patients receiving a long-acting preparation also need a short-acting opioid for breakthrough pain. One method for calculating the size of the dose for breakthrough pain is to take 10% to 20% of the 24-hour daily opioid dose, given every 1 to 4 hours as needed.[15] For example, if a patient is using 120 mg a day of long-acting morphine, an appropriate breakthrough dose would be morphine sulfate immediate release, 15 mg orally every 1 to 4 hours as needed.

The oral route is preferred for opioid administration based on availability, cost, and ease of use.[15] For those with difficulty swallowing, many of the short-acting oral opioids come in concentrated solutions.[15] Fentanyl also comes in a candy matrix on an applicator stick that can be twirled against the buccal mucosa for absorption; it has a quick onset and is an option for breakthrough pain.[15,19] Morphine and hydromorphone can be administered rectally, in the same dosages as used orally, with analgesic benefit similar to that in the oral route.[15] Of note, most long-acting oral morphine and oxycodone preparations are too large to put into nasogastric or gastric tubes and crushing them destroys the long-acting properties. There is no analgesic benefit of one long-acting oral preparation versus another.

Patients unable to take medications by oral, sublingual, transdermal, or rectal routes or patients in need of rapid pain control benefit from an intravenous or subcutaneous infusion.[15] Dosage by the subcutaneous route is equivalent to that by the intravenous route.[15] Morphine or hydromorphone can be given by the subcutaneous route, either as periodic injections or by a continuous infusion.[15] Intramuscular injections are never indicated; they are unnecessarily painful and absorption can be erratic.[15]

Opioid toxicities are predictable and often resolve without treatment. Opioids may cause nausea with initiation or dosage increase, but this almost always resolves within a few days. Nausea that occurs when patients have been on a stable dosage of opioid for a prolonged period (>1 week) rarely is related to the opioid but may occur in patients on very high doses.[20] There is no proven best treatment for opioid-induced nausea; starting with a low-cost available dopamine antagonist is a reasonable first step (e.g., prochlorperazine).

Pain is the antidote to the sedative effects of opioids, and respiratory depression represents the most serious end-result of opioid-induced sedation. Tolerance develops rapidly to opioid-induced sedation and thus, patients with severe pain easily may tolerate many grams per day of morphine or other opioids with no sedation or respiratory depression. Risk factors for respiratory depression include rapid intravenous bolus dosing, high doses in opioid-naïve patients, simultaneous use of other sedating medications, or poor hepatic or renal function. Patients with hepatic or renal insufficiency may need lower opioid doses given at longer intervals; short-acting opioids are preferred over long-acting agents in these patients. A physician's fear of causing respiratory depression in patients who are dying is not sufficient justification for withholding opioids; pain or palliative care experts should be consulted to assist in patient care.

Tolerance never develops to pruritus and constipation. Prophylaxis for opioid-induced constipation should begin at the onset of opioid therapy; preferred first treatment is a senna preparation. Pruritus is largely an idiosyncratic reaction, best treated by rotating opioids in hopes of finding a less itch-producing product. True allergic reactions are rare and are heralded by bronchospasm.

Tolerance to the analgesic effects of opioids is uncommon; in most patients, increasing pain indicates increasing pathology.[21] Physical dependence is universal—all patients on chronic opioids for more than several weeks can be expected to develop some signs of opioid withdrawal if the opioid is discontinued or an antagonist is administered.[22] A difficult diagnostic dilemma can arise in patients with underlying abdominal pain, because cramping abdominal pain is a symptom of opioid withdrawal. Psychological dependence (i.e., addiction) is rare in patients with chronic pain who have no history of addiction; the hallmark of addiction is the use of drugs despite harmful effects and loss of control of drug use.[22] A physician's fear of causing addiction in a dying patient is not a rational reason to withhold opioids.[22]

Many patients benefit from *adjuvant analgesics*, defined as nonopioid drugs used to enhance the effectiveness of opioids or drugs specifically used for neuropathic pain.[15] Examples include NSAIDs or corticosteroids for somatic pain[23] and tricyclic antidepressants and antiseizure drugs for neuropathic pain.[24] Anticholinergic drugs such as scopolamine or hyoscyamine may be used to help control abdominal visceral pain associated with intestinal obstruction (see "Intestinal Obstruction (Small and Large Bowel)").[11]

When oral and intravenous medications fail to provide adequate analgesia, anesthetic procedures should be explored, including autonomic blockade (e.g., celiac plexus block[25]) or epidural or intrathecal anesthesia.[26] All patients can benefit from nonpharmacologic treatments, including relaxation exercises, imagery, and judicious use of heat or cold.[27]

An abbreviated list of adjuvant analgesics for neuropathic pain is provided in Table 124–5; for a more comprehensive review, see reference 16.[15]

NAUSEA AND VOMITING

Nausea and vomiting are reviewed elsewhere (see Chapter 8). Nausea is reported in 50% to 60% of advanced cancer patients[28] and in 98% of patients admitted to an inpatient palliative care unit.[20] Whenever possible, finding the cause of nausea can assist in rational drug selection (Table 124–6). Because isolating a single cause is often difficult, a trial-and-error approach to drug and nondrug therapy, including use of combination drug therapies, is warranted.[29,30]

ANOREXIA AND CACHEXIA

Anorexia is defined as the loss of appetite, especially from disease; *cachexia* is defined as weight loss and wasting, particularly of muscle mass, and the general debility that can occur with chronic illness.[31] These entities often

Table 124–5 Adjuvant Therapies for Neuropathic Pain

Class	Example	Dose
Glucocorticoids	Dexamethasone	2-8 mg/day PO/IV in divided doses
Anticonvulsants	Gabapentin	300-3600 mg/day PO in divided doses
Tricyclic antidepressants	Amitriptyline	10-100 mg PO at bedtime
α₂-Adrenergic agonist	Clonidine	0.1-0.3 mg patch topically q24 hr
NMDA receptor antagonist	Methadone	See reference 15
Local anesthetics	Mexiletine	150-900 mg/day PO two to three times daily
GABA antagonist	Baclofen	5-10 mg PO three times daily

GABA, gamma-aminobutyric acid; IV, intravenous; NMDA, *N*-methyl-D-aspartate; PO, oral.
Adapted from Thomas JR, von Gunten CF: Pain in terminally ill patients: Guidelines for pharmacological management. CNS Drugs 17:621, 2003; and Weissman DE: Pain management. In Weissman DE, Ambuel B, Hallenback J (eds): Improving End-of-Life Care, 3rd ed. Milwaukee, Medical College of Wisconsin, 2000, p 23; and Abrahm JL: Pharmacologic Management of Cancer Pain. In Abrahm JL (ed): A Physician's Guide to Pain and Symptom Management in Cancer Patients. Baltimore, Johns Hopkins University Press, 2000, p 122.

Table 124–6 Targeted Treatment of Nausea

Etiology of Nausea	Drug Class and Examples
Stimulation of chemoreceptor trigger zone	Dopamine or serotonin antagonist (e.g., haloperidol 0.5-5 mg PO/SC/IV q 8 hr)
Anxiety	Benzodiazepine (lorazepam 0.5-1.5 mg PO/IV q 4-8 hours)
Gastroparesis	Metoclopramide (5-15 mg PO three times daily and at bedtime or 1 mg/kg/hr IV/SC)
Constipation	Laxatives (senna 1-4 PO twice daily)
Tumor-related elevated intracranial pressure	Glucocorticoid (dexamethasone 4-10 mg PO/IV two to four times daily)

IM, intramuscular; IV, intravenous; PO, oral; SC, subcutaneous.
Adapted from Bruera E, Sweeney C: Chronic nausea and vomiting. In Berger AM, Porentoy RK, Weissman DE (eds): Principles and Practice of Supportive Oncology, 2nd ed. Philadelphia, Lippincott-Raven, 2002, p 222; Hallenbeck J: Fast Fact and Concept #5 Treatment of Nausea and Vomiting. End-of-Life Palliative Education Resource Center: *www.eperc.mcw.edu.* 2000; and Storey P, Knight CF, Schonwetter RS (eds): Pocket Guide to Hospice/Palliative Medicine. Glenview, Ill, American Academy of Hospice and Palliative Medicine, 2003.

are combined into the *anorexia-cachexia syndrome*, a term usually referring to cancer-related anorexia and cachexia,[32] although this symptom complex can occur in patients with serious illness from any cause. Anorexia-cachexia syndrome is reported in up to 80% of cancer patients and represents a poorly understood neuroendocrine and metabolic disorder.[32,33]

Although the anorexia-cachexia syndrome itself is not painful, patients and families experience emotional suffering given the cultural significance of food intake; the loss of weight and inability to eat are a daily reminder of the illness experience and impending death.[33,34] The syndrome contributes to fatigue,[34] increased complications of antineoplastic treatments,[35] and decreased survival, with weight loss itself an independent risk factor for mortality.[33]

Aggressive nutritional supplementation in patients with advanced malignancy provides no survival benefit, no improvement in tumor shrinkage, and only minimal decrease in toxicity from antineoplastic treatments.[33] Patients and families often want to continue enteral or parenteral nutrition and hydration to provide the sense of "offering comfort" and to prevent their loved one from "starving to death."[35] Such attempts to provide artificial hydration and nutrition, however, may make the goal of comfort harder to achieve in the dying patient. Nasogastric and gastric tubes are uncomfortable and undignified; intravenous delivery of nutrition necessitates intravenous access; restraints are commonly needed; and such nutrition and hydration increase the patient's fluid volume, which in patients close to death may worsen ascites, pleural effusions, and peripheral edema.[36]

Appetite stimulants have a limited role in advanced cancer. Indications for starting an appetite stimulant include a prognosis of longer than 4 weeks combined with patient interest in regaining appetite. No drug has shown efficacy in prolonging survival or improving quality of life in population-based research, although individual patients may gain weight and have a greater sense of well-being.[34] The progestational agent megestrol acetate has been well studied.[11] At doses of 160 to 800 mg/day, megestrol results in a greater than 5% weight gain in 20% to 30% of advanced cancer patients, the weight gain being adipose tissue, not muscle[37]; if improvement is not seen in 2 to 4 weeks discontinuation of the drug is appropriate.[11] Glucocorticoids may lead to weight gain, but the well-known toxicities of these agents often preclude anything but their short-term use.[34] Other agents currently under investigation include eicosapentaenoic acid, dronabinol, testosterone, thalidomide, adenosine triphosphate, and NSAIDs.[11,38]

CONSTIPATION AND DIARRHEA

Constipation

Constipation is reported in more than 50% of patients on a palliative care or hospice unit,[39,40] a percentage that probably underestimates its true prevalence.[41] In seriously ill and dying patients, the most common precipitants of constipation are poor fluid intake, immobility, and use of opioid and anticholinergic medications; other possible causes need to be considered and are reviewed elsewhere (see Chapter 12).[11,39] More than 90% of patients on opioid medications experience constipation.[42] Opioids bind to receptors on the smooth muscle of the bowel, suppressing peristalsis and raising anal sphincter tone.[39] In one study, patients using transdermal fentanyl used less laxatives compared with those using oral morphine, indicating that transdermal fentanyl may be less constipating than other opioids.[43]

Although a stool softener may help lubricate hard stool, a bowel stimulant such as senna usually is necessary as both a prophylactic drug for opioid constipation and for initial therapy of established constipation. A commonly recommended regimen in the hospice literature is to start with senna, escalating as necessary; if no bowel movement is obtained in 3 days, bisacodyl or an enema (phospho-soda) is recommended.[44] More refractory constipation can be relieved with magnesium citrate, a sorbitol-based product, or small doses of polyethylene glycol.[39] Fiber supplements may lead to obstipation or obstruction and are not recommended for palliative care unless patients are also able to ingest large quantities of water.[39] Orally administered opioid antagonists may be effective in the reversal of opioid-related constipation in patients for whom these therapies are not effective.[45] When patients are actively dying, that is, death is expected within 1 to 2 weeks, and they have no abdominal symptoms, aggressive drug therapy to cause laxation on a regular basis is not indicated. In fact, use of laxatives that cause cramping or any use of suppositories or enemas usually increases patient discomfort and can be withheld (Table 124–7).

Table 124–7 Laxative Regimen for Constipation

Prophylaxis (e.g., patient starting opioids) or for recent mild constipation, start with
  Senna (±docusate sodium) 1-4 tablets PO twice daily
  Magnesium phosphate 15-80 mL PO daily in divided doses
For refractory constipation, check for fecal impaction, and start with
  Bisacodyl 5-15 mg/day PO
  If no response, use a bisacodyl suppository
For persisting refractory constipation, check for fecal impaction (see No. 4), and start with
  Magnesium citrate 8 oz *or*
  Lactulose, sorbitol, PEG solution, or enema
  Opioid antagonist (if patient is using exogenous opioids)— naloxone 0.8 mg PO twice daily, up to a maximum of 5 mg/day
For patients with a fecal impaction
  Use sedatives/analgesics to relieve the stress/pain of disimpaction
  Lubricate the rectum with a glycerin suppository or an oil-retention enema
  Manually disimpact the rectum
  Use enemas to clear the rectum
  Increase the daily oral laxative program

PEG, polyethylene glycol; PO, oral.
Adapted from Levy MH: Constipation and diarrhea in cancer patients: I. Prim Care Cancer 12:11, 1992; and Choi YS, Billings JA: Opioid antagonists: A review of their role in palliative care, focusing on use in opioid-related constipation. J Pain Symptom Manage 24:71, 2002.

Diarrhea

Diarrhea is less common than constipation and is reported in up to 10% of hospice patients.[39] Although the differential for diarrhea is broad, two common causes in the palliative care patient are overuse of laxative therapy or diarrhea secondary to leakage of stool around a fecal impaction.[39,41] Treatment is directed at the cause of diarrhea (Table 124–8). Octreotide is useful for refractory diarrhea (particularly with endocrine tumors such as VIPomas and gastrinomas), although it is quite costly.[46] Pancreatic enzyme replacement is helpful in cases of malabsorption following pancreatic cancer surgery. Cholestyramine and aspirin may be beneficial in radiation colitis-induced secretory diarrhea.[47] Opioids or opioid-like medications (e.g., loperamide) may offer the best symptomatic relief.

INTESTINAL OBSTRUCTION

Malignant bowel obstruction is seen most commonly as a complication of cancers of the colon, ovary, pancreas, and stomach.[48] Obstruction results from either intraluminal or extraluminal tumor. Benign causes, such as adhesions, post-radiation bowel damage, inflammatory bowel disease, opioid-induced impaction, or hernia also may cause obstruction (see Chapter 116).[48-50] Intestinal obstruction may occur in the small or large bowel or in both sites; multifocal obstructions are common.[49,50]

The symptoms of intestinal obstruction are nausea, vomiting, abdominal distention, constipation, and colicky abdominal pain.[51] Nasogastric suction is used to provide temporary relief; in many cases, just a few days of nasogastric suction may convert a complete obstruction to one that is partial or even resolve an obstruction. Surgery with a primary anastomosis, or stoma (e.g., colostomy, ileostomy), or endoluminal stenting is the preferred option for managing obstruction; the morbidity from major abdominal surgery in obstructed cancer patients is high.[52]

Nasogastric tubes are uncomfortable and therefore not desirable for long-term use. A venting gastrostomy tube is a less desirable option than directly bypassing the obstruction but can provide symptomatic relief and avoid the need for prolonged nasogastric intubation. Although partly digested food passes out of the tube, patients can still enjoy tastes and experience the psychological and communal benefit of eating.

Despite the advances in surgery and the growing use of endoluminal stents, such procedures will not be possible for many patients.[48] Medical management using drugs is effective at reducing the symptom burden of inoperable obstructions. The goals of pharmacologic therapy are a reduction in distressing symptoms; the avoidance of the need for parenteral hydration; and the removal of nasogastric suction. Pharmacologic treatments consist of a cocktail of drugs including opioids for abdominal pain, dopamine antagonist antiemetics such as phenothiazines or butyrophenones for nausea, and antisecretory drugs (anticholinergics, octreotide, or both) to reduce colicky pain and reduce intestinal secretions.[52-58] A prokinetic agent such as metoclopramide may provide relief for an incomplete or functional obstruction but should be avoided in complete obstruction.[52]

JAUNDICE, ASCITES, AND HEPATIC ENCEPHALOPATHY

Jaundice

Although jaundice is usually an ominous sign in patients with cancer, it may have a correctable cause.[59] The goal of pursuing a work-up of jaundice is to determine if there are conditions amenable to treatment in which the burden-to-benefit ratio is favorable, given the underlying extent of cancer. Interventional procedures for biliary obstruction, such as surgical bypass of the biliary tract or endoscopic placement of biliary stents, may be useful early in the disease course when patients have a good performance status, but their utility becomes less as performance status declines and the burden of stent placement with its potential for various complications increases.[59]

Pruritus commonly is associated with jaundice. Cool temperatures, lower humidity, and topical agents like astringents, moisturizers, and steroid creams may provide relief.[59] Both H_1 and H_2 antihistamines, phenothiazines, and bile acid resins have been used with some effectiveness (Table 124–9).[59] Opioid antagonists also have been used to treat pruritus, but their systemic use reverses analgesia in many patients receiving opioids.[60-64] Other drugs for pruritus and for which there is anecdotal experience include rifampicin, but its use may be limited by its risk for causing hepatitis.

Ascites

Between 15% and 50% of patients with cancer develop ascites, most commonly from ovarian, endometrial, breast, large bowel, stomach and pancreatic cancers.[59,65,66] Malignant ascites portends a poor prognosis, with a

---

Table 124–8 Etiology of Diarrhea and Helpful Therapeutic Agents

Etiology	Drug Class
Laxative overdose	Discontinue laxatives
Endocrine tumor	Octreotide 100-600 µg/24 hr SC/IV
Maldigestion	Pancreatic enzymes, 1-3 tablets before meals, 1 before snacks
Radiation enterocolitis	Cholestyramine 4 g PO three times daily Aspirin 325 mg PO q 4-6 hr
Ileal resection	Cholestyramine 4 g PO three times daily
Clostridium difficile colitis	Metronidazole 500 mg PO three times daily Vancomycin 125 mg PO four times daily
Any cause (symptomatic relief) except *C. difficile* colitis	Loperamide 4 mg PO stat, then 2 mg PO after each loose bowel movement, up to 16 mg/day

PO, oral; SC, subcutaneous.
Adapted from Mercadante S: Diarrhea, malabsorption, and constipation. In Berger AM, Porentoy RK, Weissman DE (eds): Principles and Practice of Supportive Oncology. Philadelphia, Lippincott-Raven, 2002, p 233; and Storey P, Knight CF, Schonwetter RS (eds): Pocket Guide to Hospice/Palliative Medicine. Glenview, Ill, American Academy of Hospice and Palliative Medicine, 2003.

Table 124–9   Therapy for Pruritus

Class	Drug(s)	Dose
Topical preparations	Calamine lotion, menthol-containing creams, colloidal oatmeal creams, hydrocortisone cream	Apply topically prn
Histamine H_1 receptor antagonist	Hydroxyzine	10-25 mg PO/IV q4-12 hours
Histamine H_2 receptor antagonist	Cimetidine	400 mg PO twice daily prn
Phenothiazines	Prochlorperazine	10 mg PO three times daily
Bile acid resins	Cholestyramine	4 g PO 1-4 times daily
Opioid antagonists	Naloxone	0.2 µg/kg/min IV
Rifamycin	Rifampin	300-450 mg/day PO (see text)

IV, intravenous; PO, oral; prn, as needed.
Adapted from Kichian K, Bain VG: Jaundice, ascites, and hepatic encephalopathy. In Doyle D, Hanks G, Cherny N, Calman K (eds): Oxford Textbook of Palliative Medicine, 4th ed. Oxford, Oxford University Press, 2004, p 507; and Storey P, Knight CF, Schonwetter RS (eds): Pocket Guide to Hospice/Palliative Medicine. Glenview, Ill, American Academy of Hospice and Palliative Medicine, 2003.

1-year survival of 40% and 3-year survival of less than 10%.[59] The well-known list of nonmalignant causes of ascites, including portal vein thrombosis, congestive heart failure, nephrotic syndrome, and pancreatitis, should be considered before assuming malignancy is the reason for the patient's ascites. Symptoms of ascites include an increase in abdominal girth, bloating, abdominal wall pain, nausea, anorexia, and dyspnea.

Evaluation of new ascites by paracentesis should be performed if the intervention will lead to a change in therapy or if the paracentesis will provide symptomatic benefit.

Repeated therapeutic paracentesis, with or without an indwelling peritoneal catheter, is the most commonly utilized invasive treatment for malignant ascites.[59] Peritoneovenous shunts have a better success rate in patients with nonmalignant ascites than in patients with malignant ascites but are infrequently used today.[67] Octreotide has been reported to provide symptomatic benefit in malignant ascites, but its cost may be prohibitive.[68]

Hepatic Encephalopathy

Hepatic encephalopathy due to hepatic metastases is uncommon unless there is an overwhelming liver tumor burden. Hepatic encephalopathy from direct cancer involvement of the liver is usually a terminal event; aggressive attempts at reversal are usually futile except for a very short-term benefit, which for some patients may be needed to help bring family closure. When death is near, clinicians should use opioid analgesics and other sedating medication liberally for control of distressing symptoms, even if such treatments worsen the encephalopathy. Family and staff counseling at this time

are important to ensure that all parties share the same goals of care.

GASTROINTESTINAL BLEEDING

Few events are as traumatic for families caring for their loved one as observing a massive gastrointestinal hemorrhage. If gastrointestinal bleeding is considered a likely future event, it is prudent to discuss care options and to develop a plan to provide patients and families a sense of control for what can seem to be an out-of-control situation. If the patient has advanced disease and is dying, the focus should be toward comfort rather than toward diagnostic and therapeutic interventions. Having dark-colored towels and sheets available to mask the bleeding is helpful, along with a sedating medication for emergency use (e.g., lorazepam or morphine).[11]

In conclusion, the interdisciplinary services offered by a palliative care team assist primary services in caring for patients with serious or life-threatening illness and their families. Unlike hospice, palliative care patients do not need a prognosis of 6 months or less to receive services. Common reasons for palliative medicine consultations include assistance with symptom management and exploration of the goals of care with patients and families. Many medical centers have or are developing palliative care services. The American Academy of Hospice and Palliative Medicine provides a list of palliative medicine and hospice physicians on their website (*www.aahpm.org*).

REFERENCES

1. The Center to Advance Palliative Care, *www.capc.org*
2. World Health Organization: Cancer pain relief and palliative care. Technical Report Series 804. Geneva: World Health Organization, 1990.
3. Putnam AT, Billings JA: Palliative medicine. In Ballantyne J, Fishman SM, Abdi S (eds): The Massachusetts General Hospital Handbook of Pain Management, 2nd ed. Philadelphia, Lippincott Williams & Wilkins, 2002, p 479.
4. Storey P, Knight C: UNIPAC One: The Hospice/Palliative Medicine Approach to End-of-Life Care, 2nd ed. New Rochelle, NY, Mary Ann Liebert, 2003, p 54.
5. American Board of Hospice and Palliative Medicine, *www.ABHPM.org*
6. Weissman DE, Ambuel B: Establishing treatment goals, withdrawing treatments. In Weissman DE, Ambuel B, Hallenback J (eds): Improving End-of-Life Care, 3rd ed. Milwaukee, Medical College of Wisconsin, 2000, p 101.
7. Quill TE, Brody H: Physician recommendations and patient autonomy: Finding a balance between physician power and patient choice. Ann Intern Med 125:763, 1996.
8. Christakis NA, Lamont EB: Extent and determinants of error in doctors' prognoses in terminally ill patients: prospective cohort study. BMJ 320:469, 2000.
9. Weeks JC, Cook EF, O'Day SJ, et al: Relationship between cancer patients' predictions of prognosis and their treatment preferences. JAMA 279:1709, 1998 [erratum 283:203, 2000].
10. Reuben DB, Mor V, Hiris J: Clinical symptoms and length of survival in patients with terminal cancer. Arch Intern Med 148:1586, 1988.
11. Storey P, Knight CF, Schonwetter RS (eds): Pocket Guide to Hospice/Palliative Medicine. Glenview, IL, American Academy of Hospice and Palliative Medicine, 2003.

12. Standards and Accreditation Committee Medical Guidelines Task Force: Medical Guidelines for Determining Prognosis in Selected Noncancer Diseases, 2nd ed. Arlington, VA, National Hospice Organization, 1996.

13. Lynn J, Schuster JL, Kabcenell A: Improving Care for the End of Life: A Sourcebook for Health Care Managers and Clinicans. New York, Oxford University Press, 2000.

14. Lo B: Futile interventions. In Lo B (ed): Resolving Ethical Dilemmas: A Guide for Clinicians, 2nd ed. Philadelphia, Lippincott Williams & Wilkins, 2000, p 72.

15. Thomas JR, von Gunten CF: Pain in terminally ill patients: Guidelines for pharmacological management. CNS Drugs 17:621, 2003.

16. Weissman DE: Pain management. In Weissman DE, Ambuel B, Hallenback J (eds): Improving End-of-Life Care, 3rd ed. Milwaukee, Medical College of Wisconsin, 2000, p 23.

17. Lehmann KA, Zech D: Transdernal fentanyl: clinical pharmacology. J Pain Symptom Manage 7(Suppl):S8, 1992.

18. Ripamonti C, Campa T, DeConno F: Withdrawal symptoms during chronic transdermal fentanyl administration managed with oral methadone. J Pain Symptom Manage 27:191, 2004.

19. Coluzzi PH, Schwartzberg L, Conroy JD, et al: Breakthrough cancer pain: A randomized trial comparing oral transmucosal fentanyl citrate (OTFC) and morphine sulfate immediate release (MSIR). Pain 91:123, 2001.

20. Bruera E, Seifert L, Watanabe S, et al: Chronic nausea in advanced cancer patients: A retrospective assessment of a metoclopramide-based antiemetic regimen. J Pain Symptom Manage 11:147, 1996.

21. Collin E, Poulain P, Gauvain-Piquard A, et al: Is disease progression the major factor in morphine "tolerance" in cancer pain treatment? Pain 55:319, 1993.

22. Sees KL, Clark HW: Opioid use in the treatment of chronic pain: Assessment of addiction. J Pain Symptom Manage 8:257, 1993.

23. Mercadante S, Casuccio A, Agnello A, et al: Analgesic effects of nonsteroidal anti-inflammatory drugs in cancer pain due to somatic or visceral mechanisms. J Pain Symptom Manage 17:351, 1999.

24. Farrar JT, Portenoy RK: Neuropathic cancer pain: The role of adjuvant analgesics. Oncology 15:1435, 2001.

25. Wong GY, Schroeder DR, Carns PE, et al: Effect of neurolytic celiac plexus block on pain relief, quality of life, and survival in patients with unresectable pancreatic cancer: A randomized, controlled trial. JAMA 291:1092, 2004.

26. Swarm RA, Karanikolos M, Cousins RJ: Anaesthetic techniques for pain control. In Doyle D, Hank SG, Cherny N, Calman K (eds): Oxford Textbook of Palliative Medicine, 4th ed. Oxford, Oxford University Press, 2004, p 378.

27. Abrahm JL: Nonpharmacologic strategies for pain and symptom management. In Abrahm JL (ed): A Physicians' Guide to Pain and Symptom Management in Cancer Patients. Baltimore, Johns Hopkins University Press, 2000, p 247.

28. Baines MJ: ABC of palliative care: Nausea, vomiting, and intestinal obstruction. BMJ 315:1148, 1997.

29. Bruera E, Sweeney C: Chronic nausea and vomiting. In Berger AM, Porentoy RK, Weissman DE (eds): Principles and Practice of Supportive Oncology, 2nd ed. Philadelphia, Lippincott-Raven, 2002, p 222.

30. Weissman DE: Nausea and vomiting. In Weissman DE, Ambuel B, Hallenback J (eds): Improving End-of-Life Care, 3rd ed. Milwaukee, Medical College of Wisconsin, 2000, p 62.

31. Hensyl WR (ed): Stedman's Medical Dictionary, 25th ed. Baltimore, Williams & Wilkins, 1990, pp 90, 226.

32. Strasser F: Pathophysiology of the anorexia/cachexia syndrome. In Doyle D, Hanks G, Cherny N, Calman K (eds): Oxford Textbook of Palliative Medicine, 4th ed. Oxford, Oxford University Press, 2004, p 520.

33. Bruera E: ABC of palliative care: Anorexia, cachexia, and nutrition. BMJ 315:1219, 1997.

34. Fainsinger RL, Pereira J: Clinical assessment and decision making in cachexia and anorexia. In Doyle D, Hanks G, Cherny N, Calman K (eds): Oxford Textbook of Palliative Medicine, 4th ed. Oxford, Oxford University Press, 2004, p 533.

35. Ambuel B, Weissman DE: Establishing treatment goals, withdrawing treatments. In Weissman DE, Ambuel B, Hallenback J (eds): Improving End-of-Life Care, 3rd ed. Milwaukee, Medical College of Wisconsin, 2000, p 103.

36. Lanuke K, Fainsinger RL, deMoissac D: Hydration management at the end of life. J Palliative Med 7:257, 2004.

37. Salacz M: Fast Fact and Concept #100: Megestrol Acetate and Cancer Anorexia Cachexia. www.eperc.mcw.edu, 2003.

38. Jatoi A, Loprinzi CL: Current management of cancer-associated anorexia and weight loss. Oncology 15:497, 2001.

39. Sykes N: Constipation and diarrhea. In Doyle D, Hanks G, Cherny N, Calman K (eds): Oxford Textbook of Palliative Medicine, 4th ed. Oxford, Oxford University Press, 2004, p 483.

40. Curtis EB, Krech R, Walsh TD: Common symptoms in patients with advanced cancer. J Palliat Care 7:25, 1991.

41. Mazuryk M: The clinical assessment of the patient with gastrointestinal symptoms. In Ripamonti C, Bruera E (eds): Gastrointestinal Symptoms in Advanced Cancer Patients. New York, Oxford University Press, 2002, p 17.

42. Mancini I, Bruera E: Constipation in advanced cancer patients. Support Care Cancer 6:356, 1998.

43. Radbruch L, Sabatowski R, Loick G, et al: Constipation and the use of laxatives: A comparison between transdermal fentanyl and oral morphine. Palliat Med 13:159, 2000.

44. Levy MH: Constipation and diarrhea in cancer patients: I. Prim Care Cancer 12:11, 1992.

45. Choi YS, Billings JA: Opioid antagonists: A review of their role in palliative care, focusing on use in opioid-related constipation. J Pain Symptom Manage 24:71, 2002.

46. Mercadante S: Diarrhea in terminally ill patients: Pathophysiology and treatment. J Pain Symptom Manage 10:298, 1995.

47. Mercadante S: Diarrhea, malabsorption, and constipation. In Berger AM, Porentoy RK, Weissman DE (eds): Principles and Practice of Supportive Oncology. Philadelphia, Lippincott-Raven, 2002, p 233.

48. Sainsbury R, Vaizey C, Pastorino U, et al: Surgical palliation. In Doyle D, Hanks G, Cherny N, Calman K (eds): Oxford Textbook of Palliative Medicine, 4th ed. Oxford, Oxford University Press, 2004, p 255.

49. Feuer DJ, Broadley KE, Shepherd JH, Barton DPJ: Systematic review of surgery in malignant bowel obstruction in advanced gynecologic and gastrointestinal cancer. Gynecol Oncol 75:313, 1999.

50. Ripamonti C, Bruera E: Palliative management of malignant bowel obstruction. Int J Gynecol Cancer 12:135, 2002.

51. Mercadante S: Pain in inoperable bowel obstruction. Pain Digest 5:9, 1995.

52. Ripamonti C, Mercadante S: Pathophysiology and management of malignant bowel obstruction. In Doyle D, Hanks G, Cherny N, Calman K (eds): Oxford Textbook of Palliative Medicine, 4th ed. Oxford, Oxford University Press, 2004, p 496.

53. Ripamonti C, Mercadante S, Groff L, et al: Role of octreotide, scopolamine butylbromide, and hydration in symptom control of patients with inoperable bowel obstruction and nasogastric tubes: A prospective randomized trial. J Pain Symptom Manage 19:23, 2000.

54. Mercadante S, Ripamonti C, Casuccio A, et al: Comparison of octreotide and hyoscine butylbromide in controlling gastrointestinal symptoms due to malignant inoperable bowel obstruction. Support Care Cancer 8:188, 2000.

55. Mercadante S, Maddaloni S: Octreotide in the management of inoperable bowel obstruction in terminal cancer patients. J Pain Symptom Manage 7:496, 1992.

56. Khoo D, Riley J, Waxman J: Control of emesis in bowel obstruction in terminally ill patients. Lancet 339:375, 1992.

57. Riley J, Fallon MT: Octreotide in terminal malignant obstruction of the gastrointestinal tract. Eur J Palliat Care 1:23, 1994.

58. Mangili G, Franchi M, Mariani A, et al: Octreotide in the management of bowel obstruction in terminal ovarian cancer. Gynecol Oncol 61:345, 1996.

59. Kichian K, Bain VG: Jaundice, ascites, and hepatic encephalopathy. In Doyle D, Hanks G, Cherny N, Calman K (eds): Oxford Textbook of Palliative Medicine, 4th ed. Oxford, Oxford University Press, 2004, p 507.

60. Khandelwal M, Malet PF: Pruritus associated with cholestasis: A review of pathogenesis and management. Dig Dis Sci 39:1, 1994.

61. Bergasa NV, Talbot T, Alling DW, et al: A controlled trial of naloxone infusions for the pruritus of chronic cholestasis. Gastroenterology 102:544, 1992.

62. Jones EA, Bergasa NV: The pruritus of cholestasis and the opioid system. JAMA 268:3359, 1992.

63. Wolfhagen FH, Sternieri E, Hop WC, et al: Oral naltrexone treatment for cholestatic pruritus: A double-blind, placebo-controlled study. Gastroenterology 113:1264, 1997.

64. Bergasa NV, Schmitt JM, Talbot TL, et al: Open-label trial of oral nalmefene therapy for the pruritus of cholestasis. Hepatology 27:679, 1998.

65. Runyon BA, Hoefs JC, Morgan TR: Ascitic fluid analysis in malignancy-related ascites. Hepatology 8:1104, 1988.

66. Lifshitz S: Ascites: Pathophysiology and control measures. Int J Radiat Oncol Biol Physiol 8:1423, 1982.

67. Holm A, Halpern NB, Aldrete JS: Peritovenous shunt for intractable ascites of hepatic, nephrogenic, and malignant causes. Am J Surg 158:162, 1989.

68. Cairns W, Malone R: Octreotide as an agent for the relief of malignant ascites in palliative care patients. Palliat Med 13:429, 1999.

CHAPTER

125 Complementary and Alternative Medicine Therapies in Gastrointestinal and Hepatic Disease

David J. Hass and Lawrence J. Brandt

DEFINITION AND EPIDEMIOLOGY

Complementary and alternative medicine (CAM) is defined broadly as medical practices neither taught widely in medical schools nor generally available in U.S. hospitals.[1] In recent years, the prevalence of CAM therapies has increased at an exponential rate both in national and international medical communities. A study by Eisenberg and associates[1] demonstrated that among the U.S. population, CAM use increased from 33.8% to 42.1% from 1990 to 1997. Estimated annual expenditures for CAM therapies are in excess of $27 billion, a sum that is equivalent to patients' out-of-pocket expenditures for all U.S. physician-based services.[1]

Ganguli and colleagues have reported that at least 50% of gastroenterology outpatients in a community setting implemented CAM therapies to help ameliorate their symptoms.[2] Given the widespread use of these modalities and the trend toward their increased utilization, an understanding of CAM therapies, including their potential risks and benefits, is necessary for the practicing gastroenterologist. A thorough knowledge of these practices allows physicians to provide comprehensive medical care and may help further a therapeutic rapport between physicians and their patients.

TYPES OF THERAPIES

There are a wide variety of CAM therapies, and those most commonly employed for gastrointestinal and hepatic disease are defined in Table 125–1. Regardless of the therapy employed, the overall philosophy of CAM takes a uniform holistic approach that all disease results from disturbances at a combination of physical, psychological, social, and spiritual levels. Thus, a CAM modality is used to restore balance and to facilitate the body's own healing responses, thereby ameliorating troublesome symptoms.[3]

DEMOGRAPHY

Certain patients are more likely to use CAM therapies than are others. Women and whites tend to utilize CAM more often than do men and African Americans, respec-

Table 125–1 Common Complementary and Alternative Medicine (CAM) Therapies for Gastrointestinal and Hepatic Diseases

CAM Therapy	Definition and Rationale
Acupuncture[130]	Based on the principles of Chinese medicine, "qi" is energy that circulates between organs along channels called *meridians*; through placement of needles at specifically defined locations (points), the flow of qi is restored to appropriate levels and the health of specific organs is improved
Ayurvedic medicine[131]	Holistic system of medicine from India that provides dietary and lifestyle recommendations to improve overall health
Colonic irrigation therapy	Cleansing of the colon through various oral and enema preparations to improve "digestive health"
Herbal medicine	Ingestion of various herbal therapies, supplements, or probiotics to improve physiologic function
Homeopathy[132]	Based on the principle "like should be cured with like"; administration of a diluted solution to the patient that, when given to a healthy person in an undiluted form, causes symptoms identical to those experienced by the ill person
Hypnosis	Induction of a deeply relaxed state, during which therapeutic suggestions are made to alter behavior and enhance relief of symptoms
Meditation/relaxation	A process of reflection and contemplation allowing one to focus thoughts to help alleviate symptoms
Reflexology	Areas on the feet correspond to organs of the body; massage and pressure applied to these regions can improve symptoms throughout the body

tively. Patients with higher levels of education, higher annual incomes, and comorbid medical conditions also are more likely to utilize CAM therapies.[1,2] Knowledge of these demographics assists the gastroenterologist in determining which patients are likely to be using these therapies, but it is also important to understand each patient's rationale and motivation for choosing a particular therapeutic modality.

RATIONALE FOR USE

Digestive disorders rank among the most common disease states for which people seek the advice of complementary practitioners. The attraction of CAM therapies is multifaceted. First, they provide patients who may not have a medical background with a sense of control over their own bodies and health. Second, CAM therapies provide patients with therapeutic alternatives when conventional medical therapies have failed to alleviate their symptoms or cure diseases, such as terminal cancer. Lastly, complementary therapies are attractive to patients who feel dissatisfied with the ways in which their physicians demonstrate understanding of their illnesses or handle their complaints.

GASTROINTESTINAL DISORDERS ADDRESSED BY CAM THERAPIES

This chapter focuses on the seven areas in gastroenterology and hepatology that are addressed most often by CAM therapies: (1) nausea and vomiting; (2) functional dyspepsia (FD); (3) irritable bowel syndrome (IBS); (4) inflammatory bowel disease (IBD); (5) diarrhea and constipation; (6) liver disease, specifically hepatitis B and C and alcoholic-induced liver injury; and (7) gastrointestinal malignancies. For each area, the data supporting the most frequently used CAM modalities are reviewed, along with their potential benefits and adverse effects.

NAUSEA AND VOMITING

Nausea and vomiting have a wide array of causes ranging from viral gastroenteritis to pregnancy (see Chapter 8). These symptoms can be quite distressing, and patients frequently resort to CAM therapies to seek symptomatic relief. In one study of pregnant women with these symptoms, 61% reported using CAM therapies for relief.[4] Several complementary modalities have been used to help ameliorate nausea and vomiting, ranging from herbal medicines to relaxation techniques. These therapies are summarized in Table 125–2.

Ginger (*Zingiber officinale*) is the herbal supplement most commonly employed to help relieve nausea and vomiting and derives its name from the Sanskrit word for horn, which describes the shape of the plant. Several mechanisms have been postulated to explain the antiemetic effect of ginger. Animal studies have demonstrated that 6-gingerol, a component of the herb, improves gastrointestinal motility.[5] Another component, galanolactone, is a 5-hydroxytryptamine-3 antagonist,[6] similar to ondansetron, an antiemetic agent used to treat chemotherapy-induced nausea and vomiting.

The antiemetic effect of ginger has been studied in various clinical conditions, including morning sickness, sea sickness, postchemotherapy nausea, and postoperative nausea. Although no more effective than placebo in the prevention of experimentally induced motion sickness, ginger has been documented to reduce vertigo induced by caloric stimulation of the vestibular apparatus within the inner ear.[7-9] In a systematic review of randomized clinical trials (RCTs) evaluating the efficacy of ginger for nausea and vomiting, Ernst and Pittler demonstrated that ginger is superior to placebo and equal in efficacy to metoclopramide for postoperative nausea and emesis. Furthermore, ginger relieved symptoms better than did placebo agents for the treatment of sea sickness, morning sickness of pregnancy, and chemotherapy-induced nausea and vomiting.[10] The dose of ginger prescribed in most of these studies ranged from 0.5 to 1 g/day.

Table 125–2 Complementary and Alternative Medicine (CAM) Therapies for Nausea and Vomiting

CAM Therapy	Proposed Mechanism of Action	Evidence	Adverse Effects
Ginger (*Zingiber officinale*)	Enhances GI motility; 5-HT$_3$ receptor antagonist[5,6]	Efficacy compared with placebo in RCTs for postoperative and chemotherapy-induced nausea, morning sickness, and sea sickness[10]	Inhibits thromboxane synthase, thereby causing an increased risk of bleeding with concurrent antithrombotic/antiplatelet agents[11]; safety in pregnancy unknown
Pyridoxine (vitamin B$_6$)	Unclear	RCTs demonstrate mixed results in the treatment of morning sickness[15]	Decreases serum levels of levodopa, phenobarbital, and phenytoin[16] Allergic reactions May cause peripheral neuropathy, dermatoses, photosensitivity, and dizziness if taken in excess (>250 mg/day)[17]
Acupuncture	Placement of needles at specifically defined locations (points) to restore the flow of "qi" and improve the health of specific organs	RCTs demonstrate efficacy for relief of symptoms following chemotherapy, surgery, and morning sickness[20-23]	Infections, perforations of internal organs, and spinal cord injury[24-32]
Relaxation therapy	Process of reflection and contemplation allows one to focus thoughts to help alleviate symptoms	Effective as an adjunctive therapy to standard antiemetic agents for chemotherapy-induced symptoms[33]	None reported

GI, gastrointestinal; 5-HT, 5-hydroxytryptamine; RCT, randomized controlled trial.

Although ginger appears to be a natural supplement worth considering, one must understand its potential adverse reactions before advocating it for relief of symptoms. First, ginger has been shown to inhibit platelet aggregation by inhibiting thromboxane synthase. Therefore, if patients are taking warfarin, aspirin, nonsteroidal anti-inflammatory drugs (NSAIDs), or clopidogrel concurrently, the risk of bleeding is increased.[11] Second, although not proven in animal studies, ginger has been documented to be potentially mutagenic in laboratory assays, thereby raising questions about the safety of the herbal supplement in pregnancy.[12,13]

Pyridoxine also has been prescribed to relieve the nausea and vomiting associated with pregnancy.[14] Utilization of this water-soluble vitamin was one of the most commonly employed CAM therapies in a survey of pregnant Canadian women with nausea and emesis, 29% of whom reported using pyridoxine.[4] Vutyavanich and colleagues reported a significant reduction in nausea, but no statistically significant reduction in vomiting, with pyridoxine, 30 mg daily, in an RCT.[15] Although the mechanism of action of pyridoxine is not established, certain drug interactions and adverse effects have been noted. Pyridoxine has been documented to decrease serum levels of levodopa, phenobarbital, and phenytoin when co-administered with these agents.[16] Allergic reactions to pyridoxine also have been documented, and when taken in excess (>250 mg/day), pyridoxine has been reported to cause peripheral neuropathy, dermatoses, photosensitivity, and dizziness.[17,18]

Acupuncture is another CAM modality commonly used to treat nausea and vomiting. In Chinese subjects, the P6 acupuncture point stimulated for relief of these symptoms is named *neiguan*, meaning medial pass. This acupuncture point is anatomically located three finger-breadths above the proximal palmar crease on the volar aspect of the wrist in the midline. To date, more than 30 published trials have evaluated the role of stimulating the P6 acupuncture point for relief of nausea and vomiting.[19] In a systematic review, acupuncture was demonstrated to be superior to placebo in ameliorating nausea and vomiting; the results were consistent despite numerous different investigators, patient populations, and various forms of acupuncture point stimulation.[18] These trials demonstrated that acupuncture effectively relieved nausea and emesis associated with chemotherapy,[20] surgery,[21,22] and pregnancy.[23]

The data supporting implementation of acupuncture/acupressure are impressive. In analyzing these data, however, gastroenterologists must recognize the difficulties of applying the methodology of RCTs with placebo controls to testing the efficacy of acupuncture. The nature of this complementary modality is such that each patient's regimen is individualized for relief of his or her specific symptoms, thereby precluding standardization of the treatment and calling into question the validity of the studies.

Several adverse events have been noted with acupuncture. Infection secondary to improper handling of needles or their re-use without sterilization has been suggested in the literature.[24] Transmission of hepatitis B virus (HBV), hepatitis C virus (HCV), and human immunodeficiency virus (HIV) has been reported.[25-27] Bacterial endocarditis secondary to *Propionibacterium acnes*[28] and bacteremia from *Staphylococcus aureus* and *Pseudomonas aeruginosa* with a consequent psoas abscess have been noted following acupuncture.[29] Two fatalities have been documented in which acupuncture was thought to have led to sepsis with staphylococcal organisms.[30] Although improperly sterilized needles seem to be the only risk factor for the aforementioned infections, it is difficult to prove that these infections were a direct result of acupuncture, as patients may not have divulged other potential risk factors that may be personally intimate (e.g., sexual preference, intravenous drug use).[32] Other risks associated with acupuncture therapy include perforation of an organ during placement of the needles; for example, pneumothorax, hemopericardium with tamponade, and spinal cord injury have been linked directly to acupuncture therapy.[24,31,32]

Lastly, relaxation therapies have been suggested as a CAM therapy for chemotherapy-induced nausea and vomiting. It has been reported that side effects related to chemotherapy are somewhat conditioned and are developed as a form of associative learning[33]; the anxiety experienced during chemotherapy sessions can serve as conditioning cues that lead to physiologic reactions. Through progressive muscle relaxation therapy, a patient's anxiety can be alleviated and physical symptoms averted. Relaxation therapies often are used as an adjunct to standard antiemetic medications.[32]

FUNCTIONAL DYSPEPSIA

Functional dyspepsia (FD) is defined as pain or discomfort in the epigastric area in the absence of demonstrable structural or physiologic abnormalities. Because symptoms tend to be short in duration and relatively mild, dyspepsia frequently is self-managed[34]; therefore, CAM therapies clearly are appealing. Herbal therapy has been a mainstay of complementary treatments for FD. The most common supplement therapies for FD, including

their active ingredients, proposed mechanisms of action, and adverse effects, are listed in Table 125–3.

Banana (Musa sapientum) has been evaluated for the treatment of FD in prospective open trials. This supplement is thought to promote gastric mucus secretion and has been documented to have antiulcerogenic properties in animals.[35] In a study by Arora and Sharma,[36] treatment with banana powder resulted in a reduction in symptoms in 75% of patients in the treatment group compared with 25% of those in the placebo group ($P < 0.05$). Causes of organic dyspepsia were excluded through various endoscopic and laboratory methods prior to study inclusion. The only adverse effect reported was pruritus in the treatment group.[36]

Capsaicin derived from the dried fruit of *Capsicum annuum* (red pepper), is an herbal supplement. Its mechanism of action is selective impairment of pain (C-type) fibers, which carry pain sensation to the central nervous system from the abdominal viscera.[37] In one study, 2.5 mg of red pepper powder given daily improved epigastric pain, nausea, and bloating, but placebo did not.[37] Although abdominal pain and diarrhea occurred initially in patients treated with capsaicin, these adverse effects were self-limited and of no serious clinical consequence.

Greater celandine (Chelidonium majus) was investigated in FD by Ritter and colleagues, in a randomized, double-blind, placebo-controlled trial.[38] Celandine accounted for a 34% reduction in symptoms compared with placebo ($P = 0.003$).[38] This agent is thought to contain a variety of alkaloids that also have a spasmolytic effect on smooth muscle.[39] Despite its apparent efficacy, celandine has many adverse effects, including xerostomia, insomnia, diarrhea, and fatigue. Idiosyncratic hepatotoxicity also

Table 125–3 Complementary and Alternative Medical Therapies for Functional Dyspepsia*

Herbal Supplement	Proposed Mechanism of Action	Evidence	Adverse Effects
Banana (Musa sapientum)	Antiulcerogenic; promotes gastric mucus secretion[35,36]	Open-label trial demonstrates efficacy[36]	Pruritus
Capsaicin (Capsicum annuum)	Selectively impairs the activity of nociceptive C-type pain fibers in the CNS[37]	RCT demonstrates efficacy compared with placebo[37]	Abdominal pain, diarrhea
Celandine (Chelidonium majus)	Contains alkaloids, which have a spasmolytic effect on smooth muscle[39]	RCT demonstrates efficacy compared with placebo[38]	Xerostomia, insomnia, diarrhea, fatigue, hepatotoxicity[40]
Liu-Jun-Zi-Tang	Increases gastric emptying; increases plasma somatostatin and gastrin levels; promotes gastric relaxation[34,41]	RCT demonstrates efficacy compared with placebo[41]	Interstitial pneumonitis[42]
Peppermint/caraway	Inhibits gastric smooth muscle contraction[43,44]	RCTs demonstrate efficacy compared with placebo[34,45]	Diarrhea, nausea, vomiting, allergic contact dermatitis, contact urticaria, asthma exacerbations, and atrial fibrillation[46-48]
Shenxiahewining	Unknown	RCT demonstrates efficacy compared with control medication (unclear if control was placebo)[34]	None reported
Tumeric (Curcuma longa)	Increases biliary secretion, promotes contraction of gallbladder; antispasmodic agent[49]	RCT demonstrates efficacy compared with placebo[34]	Nausea, vomiting, fatigue, headache

CNS, central nervous system; RCT, randomized controlled trial.
*Data adapted from Coon JT, Ernst E: Systematic review: Herbal medicinal products for non-ulcer dyspepsia. Aliment Pharmacol Ther 16:1689, 2002.

has been described with celandine but resolved without complication in most cases when the supplement was discontinued.[40]

Liu-Jun-Zi-Tang, also known as *TJ-43*, is a Chinese herbal medicine (CHM) that has been used frequently for relief of FD. The agent is a combination of several extracts including *Actractylodis laneae rhizoma, Ginseng radix, Pinelliae tuber, Hoelen, Zizyphi fructus, Aurantii nobilis pericarpium, Glycyrrhizae radix*, and *Zingiberis rhizoma*.[34] Multiple mechanisms of action have been proposed, including increased gastric emptying, increased serum levels of gastrin and somatostatin,[41] and relaxation of gastric smooth muscle.[42] A RCT of patients with FD compared TJ-43, 2.5 g three times per day, with placebo for 7 days. The treatment group displayed greater reductions in epigastric fullness, reflux, and nausea compared with the group treated with placebo ($P < 0.05$).[41] The only adverse event noted with use of TJ-43 was a case of drug-induced interstitial pneumonitis, which resolved after therapy was discontinued.[34]

Peppermint (Mentha piperita) and *caraway (Carum carvi)* are the supplements that have been investigated most thoroughly for the treatment of FD. Their proposed mechanism of action is thought to be inhibition of smooth muscle contractions by direct blockade of smooth muscle calcium channels.[43,44] Several placebo-controlled RCTs have compared variable fixed doses of these agents. The doses of these agents ranged from 180 to 270 mg and 100 to 150 mg daily for peppermint and caraway, respectively. In several trials a statistically significant improvement in symptoms such as bloating and epigastric pain was demonstrated when treatment groups were compared with placebo groups.[34,45] Adverse effects seen with these supplements include diarrhea, nausea, vomiting, allergic contact dermatitis, contact urticaria,[46] asthma exacerbations, and atrial fibrillation.[47,48]

Shenxiahewining is a mixture of Chinese herbs, specifically *Ginseng radix, Pinelliae tuber, Coptidis rhizoma, Zingiberis rhizoma exsiccatum*, and *Glycyrrhizae radix*, in a 3:9:3:3:3 ratio.[34] In a RCT performed in China, 92% of patients treated with shenxiahewining reported improvement in symptoms compared with 20% of a control group. No important adverse events were noted.[34]

Tumeric (Curcuma longa) is an agent that also has been documented to have therapeutic efficacy in alleviating FD. This agent is thought to increase biliary secretion, promote contraction of the gallbladder, and act as an antispasmodic.[49] In a placebo-controlled RCT performed in Thailand, tumeric (2 g/day) was found to significantly improve dyspeptic symptoms ($P = 0.003$).[34]

The data on the aforementioned supplement therapies suggest that some of those studied could be useful for patients with FD. Peppermint and caraway are the most extensively evaluated to date and, given their encouraging safety profiles, warrant further study.[34]

IRRITABLE BOWEL SYNDROME

IBS is defined as abdominal discomfort and altered bowel function in the absence of structural and biochemical abnormalities (see Chapter 115).[50] Symptoms include pain, bloating, cramping, constipation, and diarrhea. Gastroenterologists encounter this disease entity quite commonly, with frequencies in the population of 14% to 24% of women and 5% to 19% of men.[51] Patients with IBS often are frustrated that laboratory, radiologic, and endoscopic examinations fail to reveal an "organic" source of their discomfort, and they therefore often employ CAM therapies to help ameliorate their symptoms.

Many CAM therapies have been investigated for the treatment of IBS (Table 125–4). Herbal supplement therapy and the use of probiotics have been evaluated most extensively. Psyllium (*Plantago isphagula*) is the most commonly prescribed dietary supplement for patients with IBS. This fiber product acts as an osmotic bulking agent and decreases bowel transit time. There have been three placebo-controlled trials of psyllium use in IBS,[52-54] but only one fulfilled the five Rome criteria for appropriate study methodology (randomization, concealed allocation, placebo controlled, double blinding, and appropriate follow-up of study patients). Two additional trials compared psyllium with "active" agents, but neither trial was of high quality.[55,56] In general, the evidence that stool frequency, consistency, and ease of passage were better with psyllium than with placebo was modest, and there were no statistically significant differences in side effects among psyllium, lactulose, and placebo.

Although psyllium appears to be fairly harmless, allergic hypersensitivity reactions have been documented.[57] Impaired absorption of certain medications taken concomitantly, such as lithium and carbamazepine, has been reported.[58,59] Cases of acute esophageal obstruction also have occurred with psyllium-based agents, suggesting that dysphagia might preclude use of psyllium.[60]

Other supplemental therapies have been used for IBS. Peppermint oil, as previously discussed, is prescribed for its smooth muscle relaxant capabilities. In a meta-analysis by Pittler and Ernst,[61] peppermint oil improved symptoms of IBS compared with placebo treatment. Although statistical significance was demonstrated in this study, flaws in the methodology of the trials studied preclude evidence-based acceptance of the efficacy of peppermint oil in the treatment of IBS.

STW 5, an herbal preparation that contains bitter candytuft (*Iberis umbellate*), chamomile (*Matricaria chamomilla*), peppermint, caraway fruit, licorice root (*Glycyrrhiza glabra*), lemon balm leaves (*Melissa officinalis*), celandine (*Chelidonium majus*), angelica root (*Angelica archangelica*), and milk thistle (*Silybum marianum*), has been used to treat patients with IBS. Placebo-controlled RCTs have demonstrated STW 5 to improve symptoms of IBS and reduce the severity of abdominal pain.[62] Multiple mechanisms of action of STW 5 are postulated, with certain components thought to alter gastrointestinal motility, and others thought to act as smooth muscle relaxants.[58]

Although no adverse events have been reported for STW 5, individual components of the preparation are known to have potential toxicities. Specifically, celandine is known to be hepatotoxic at certain doses (>10 mg/day).[40] Chamomile is known to contain a coumarin derivative,

Table 125–4   Complementary and Alternative Medicine (CAM) Therapies for Irritable Bowel Syndrome

CAM Therapy	Proposed Mechanism of Action	Evidence	Adverse Effects
Psyllium	Osmotic bulking agent; decreases bowel transit time	RCT demonstrates efficacy for relief of constipation[50]	Allergic reactions, impaired absorption of some medications (lithium, carbamazepine), acute esophageal obstruction[53-60]
Peppermint oil	Inhibits smooth muscle contraction[43,44]	RCTs demonstrate possible efficacy compared with placebo, but methodologic flaws noted in studies[61]	Diarrhea, nausea, vomiting, allergic contact dermatitis, contact urticaria, asthma exacerbations, and atrial fibrillation[46-48]
STW 5 (see text)	Alters gastrointestinal motility; smooth muscle relaxant[43]	RCT demonstrates efficacy compared with placebo[62]	Hepatotoxicity, increased bleeding risk, potentiation of sedatives and anxiolytics, altered metabolism of drugs metabolized by CYP3A4 and uridine diphosphoglucuronosyl transferase[40,63-65]
Chinese herbal medicine	Unknown	RCT demonstrates efficacy compared with placebo[66]	None reported
Probiotic therapy	Alters intestinal microflora	RCT demonstrates efficacy compared with placebo[67,68]	None reported
Hypnotherapy	"Gut-related imagery"; patients' thoughts are focused toward changing gastrointestinal function[69]	RCT demonstrates efficacy compared with placebo[69]	None reported
Acupuncture	Placement of needles at specifically defined locations (points) to restore the flow of "qi" and to improve the health of specific organs	RCT demonstrates efficacy compared with sham[70] Data (only in abstract form) demonstrate greater efficacy than psyllium for relief of constipation[71]	Infections, perforations of internal organs, and spinal cord injury[24-32]
Homeopathy	Principle of "like should be cured with like"	Trend toward efficacy but statistical significance not reached[71]	None reported
Ayurvedic medicine	Holistic system of medicine from India that provides dietary and life-style recommendations to improve overall health	RCT demonstrates efficacy compared with placebo but with significant dropout rates in the trials[72]	None reported

CYP3A4, cytochrome P450 IIIA4; RCT, randomized, controlled trial.

which increases the risk of bleeding if prescribed concurrently with warfarin, aspirin, or NSAIDs. Chamomile also has been noted to potentiate the central nervous system depressant effects of benzodiazepines and barbiturates,[63,64] which often are prescribed to patients with IBS. Milk thistle is known to inhibit cytochrome P450 IIIA4 (CYP3A4) and uridine diphosphoglucuronosyl transferase and thus could alter the metabolism of many pharmacologic agents.[65]

CHM has been used for IBS symptoms, and RCTs have demonstrated a statistically significant benefit of its use over placebo. Patients treated with CHM reported improvement in their symptoms and less interference in their daily lives from IBS, with an overall improvement in their quality of life.[66]

Probiotics are microorganisms that promote health effects through adjustments of intestinal microflora (see Chapter 99).[67] Patients with infectious and inflammatory disease states such as pseudomembranous colitis and IBD use probiotics most commonly to ameliorate symptoms. Patients with IBS also have had benefit from these agents. Evidence from RCTs has demonstrated that ingestion of *Lactobacillus plantarum* resulted in significant reductions in abdominal pain and flatulence in patients with IBS.[68]

Hypnosis has been documented to have a significant therapeutic effect on symptoms of IBS. Through the use of "gut-directed imagery," whereby patients imagine they are inhibiting gastric secretion, an overall symptom improvement rate of 80% has been reported.[69] Clinical remission up to 3 months has been documented in patients with IBS treated with hypnotherapy. Acupuncture has been shown to be superior to sham therapy and fiber supplementation in patients with IBS.[70,71] Homeopathy has demonstrated a trend toward efficacy in IBS.[7] Lastly, Ayurvedic medicine (see Table 125–1) also has demonstrated efficacy in relief of symptoms from IBS. The trial of Ayurvedic medicine, however, had a large dropout rate and therefore should be interpreted with caution.[72]

INFLAMMATORY BOWEL DISEASE

The pathophysiology of Crohn's disease (CD) is not completely understood despite decades of research (see Chapter 108). An overactive intestinal mucosal immune system driven at least in part by a reaction to normal luminal flora is thought to be involved in the pathogenesis,[73] facilitated by failure of the mucosal epithelium to serve as an effective barrier to potential dietary and environmental toxins. Given the chronic and persistent nature of CD, many patients turn to CAM therapies when conventional therapies fail.

As mentioned earlier, probiotics frequently are employed by certain subgroups of patients with CD. Specifically, patients who have had a total proctocolectomy and creation of an ileal pouch-anal anastomosis (IPAA) have experienced the greatest benefit from these agents. Pouchitis in these patients occurs with a frequency of approximately 50% after 10 years (see Chapter 110).[74] Although the cause of pouchitis remains unknown, an alteration in enteric bacterial flora appears to play an important role.[74]

VSL #3 is a probiotic agent consisting of four strains of *Lactobacillus*, three strains of *Bifidobacterium*, and one strain of *Streptococcus*. In recent RCTs, administration of VSL #3 has been shown to reduce the frequency of pouchitis in IBD patients following IPAA, as well as to decrease the number of flares of pouchitis in patients known to have chronic pouchitis.[71,75] VSL #3 is thought to act by increasing tissue levels of interleukin-10, and decreasing levels of pro-inflammatory cytokines, such as interleukin-1 and tumor necrosis factor (TNF)-α.[76] No adverse events have been noted with administration of this compound.

Another probiotic worth mentioning is *Saccharomyces boulardii*. This organism, a nonpathogenic yeast originally isolated from the litchi fruit, has been documented to decrease the relapse rate of CD.[77] The mechanism by which *S. boulardii* exerts its beneficial effect on the intestine is by acting as a trophic agent on intestinal mucosa and triggering the release of immunoglobulin (Ig) A.[73] In one study, clinical relapses over a 6-month period were observed in 37% of patients who received mesalamine alone and in 6% of patients treated with mesalamine plus *S. boulardii*.[73]

Another supplemental therapy employed for the treatment of IBD is fish oil. Fish oil contains high amounts of ω-3 fatty acids, which serve as precursors of less pro-inflammatory cytokines than other fatty acids commonly found in many foods. In patients with ulcerative colitis and frequent disease exacerbations, disease activity scores were improved to a greater extent in patients who received fish oil than in those who consumed other forms of fat[78]; however, trials have failed to demonstrate that fish oil is effective in maintaining remission of ulcerative colitis.[79] Clinical trials evaluating the efficacy of fish oil in the treatment of CD have been disappointing, because no trial has documented fish oil to be effective in maintaining disease remission or lowering an individual patient's CD activity index.[78]

DIARRHEA AND CONSTIPATION

Altered bowel habits frequently lead to the use of CAM therapies. Within the discipline of complementary medicine, practitioners often group the symptoms of diarrhea and constipation together under the term *colonic health*. Although several CAM modalities have been reported to promote and improve colonic health, herbal supplements are considered the mainstay of treatment. These supplements range from anthraquinone-based stimulant laxatives, such as aloe (*Aloe barbadensis*,) to osmotic laxatives, such as magnesium citrate, to extracts of papaya (*Carica papaya*) and raspberry (*Rubus udaeus*). Those most commonly employed, including their proposed mechanisms of action, possible medication interactions, and reported adverse events, are listed in Table 125–5. As discussed later in this chapter, the lack of regulation of the supplement industry has permitted nonstandardization of the content and potency of many of these agents and thus should give practitioners pause before prescribing them.

Probiotics are also often employed to prevent diarrhea. A meta-analysis performed by D'Souza and colleagues described the clinical efficacy of various strains of *Lactobacillus* (*Lactobacillus bulgaricus, Lactobacillus acidophilus, Lactobacillus casei*, and *Lactobacillus GG*) and *S. boulardii* in the prevention of antibiotic associated diarrhea.[80] Castagliuolo and colleagues described the protective effects of *S. boulardii* on *Clostridium difficile*–induced diarrhea in humans; the mechanism of this action is the proteolytic digestion of toxin A and B molecules by a protease secreted by *S. boulardii*.[81] Another study reported that *S. boulardii* stimulates intestinal IgA in response to infection with *C. difficile*.[82] *S. boulardii* also has been shown to prevent relapses of pseudomembranous colitis and to maintain intestinal mucosal barrier function against enteropathogenic *Escherichia coli*.[83,84] VSL #3 has been demonstrated in a RCT to be effective in preventing radiation-induced diarrhea.[85]

Ernst and colleagues have reviewed the various CAM therapies that have been used for the treatment of constipation. Biofeedback, a treatment technique in which people are trained to use signals from their own bodies to help recognize a relaxed state (see Chapter 12), has demonstrated clear efficacy for the treatment of constipation.[86] Pelvic floor dyssynergia, which causes chronic constipation, is a result of the inappropriate contraction or failed relaxation of the puborectalis and external anal sphincter muscles during defecation. Pelvic floor dyssynergia is considered a form of "maladaptive learning,"[87] and biofeedback is thought to help retrain the body to alleviate symptoms.

Sensory training involves simulated defecation through the use of a water-filled balloon that is inserted into the rectum and then slowly withdrawn as the patient is asked to concentrate on relaxing the muscles that are behaving maladaptively.[87] Electromyography, which records muscle activity either from intraluminal probes or perianal surface electrodes, and anal manometry are alternative means by which sensory feedback can be provided to the patient with pelvic floor dyssynergia. More than 70% of adult patients with this disorder improve following biofeedback training.[87] Further studies are needed, however, to assess the long-term efficacy of biofeedback.

Table 125–5   Complementary and Alternative Therapies Promoting "Colonic Health"*[63]

Supplement	Proposed Mechanism of Action	Possible Drug Interactions	Adverse Effects
Aloe (Aloe barbadensis)	Anthracene stimulant laxative; increases bowel motility	Potentiation of cardiac glycosides; reduced action of glucocorticoids	Gastrointestinal spasm; bloating; hypokalemia; arrhythmia; pseudomelanosis coli
Apple pectin	Dietary fiber; binds bile acids	None reported	None reported
Cascara sagrada (Rhamnus purshiana)	Anthracene stimulant laxative; increases bowel motility	Potentiation of cardiac glycosides; reduced action of glucocorticoids	Gastrointestinal spasm; bloating; hypokalemia; arrhythmia; pseudomelanosis coli
Chamomile (Matricaria chamomilla)	Unknown mechanism	Increased risk of bleeding with concurrent warfarin, aspirin, or NSAIDs; potentiation of CNS depressant medications	Increased risk of bleeding; lethargy with potentiation of CNS depressants
Clove (Syzygium aromaticum)	Spasmolytic and local anesthetic	None reported	None reported
Echinacea	Promotes immune function through increases in T helper cell populations by increasing cytokine activity	Acetaminophen (secondary to glutathione depletion)	Allergic reactions; hepatotoxicity with concurrent acetaminophen
Fennel (Foeniculum vulgare)	Stimulates gastrointestinal motility; antispasmodic	None reported	Allergic reactions
Fenugreek (Trigonella foenum-graecum)	Unknown mechanism	Increased risk of bleeding with concurrent warfarin, aspirin, or NSAIDs	Increased risk of bleeding; galactorrhea (secondary to interaction at dopamine receptors)
Ginger (Zingiber officinale)	Enhances GI motility; 5-HT$_3$ receptor antagonist; inhibits platelet aggregation by inhibiting thromboxane synthase	Increased risk of bleeding with concurrent warfarin, aspirin, or NSAIDs, clopidogrel	Increased risk of bleeding
Hibiscus (Hibiscus sabdariffa)	Laxative (unknown mechanism)	None reported	None reported
Magnesium citrate	Osmotic laxative	None reported	Hypermagnesemia: prolonged QT interval on ECG, hypotension, hyporeflexia
Marshmallow (Althaea officinalis)	Immune stimulant, anti-inflammatory	May delay absorption of other medications	None reported
Oat bran (Avena sativa)	Decreases cholesterol and prostaglandin synthesis	None reported	None reported
Oregon grape (Berberis vulgaris)	Source of vitamin C; stimulates immune system; stimulates intestinal peristalsis	None reported	None reported
Papaya (Carica papaya)	Promotes healing of gastrointestinal ulceration and pancreatic function	Increased risk of bleeding with concurrent warfarin, aspirin, NSAIDs	Increased risk of bleeding; decreased testicular weight and interrupted estrus cycle in mice
Psyllium (Plantago isphagula)	Osmotic bulking agent; decreases bowel transit time; generates short-chain fatty acids	Impaired absorption of medications	Allergic reactions; impaired vitamin B$_{12}$, lithium, and carbamazepine absorption; esophageal obstruction
Raspberry (Rubus idaeus)	Unknown	None reported	None reported
Rhubarb (Rheum palmatum)	Anthracene stimulant laxative; increases bowel motility	Potentiation of cardiac glycosides; reduced action of glucocorticoids	Gastrointestinal spasm; bloating; hypokalemia; arrhythmia; pseudomelanosis coli
Senna (Cassia senna)	Anthracene stimulant laxative; increases bowel motility	Potentiation of cardiac glycosides; reduced action of glucocorticoids	Gastrointestinal spasm; bloating; hypokalemia; arrhythmia; pseudomelanosis coli
Spirulina	Green algae; contains magnesium	None reported	None reported
Valerian (Valeriana officinalis)	Spasmolytic agent	Interacts at GABA receptor; potentiation of CNS depressant medications	Lethargy; benzodiazepine-like withdrawal symptoms
Yellow dock (Rumex crispis)	Laxative (unknown mechanism)	None reported	None reported

*Derived from Hass DJ, Lewis JD: Quality of Manufacturer Provided Information on Safety and Efficacy Claims for Dietary Supplements. Submitted for publication 2004.
CNS, central nervous system; ECG, electrocardiogram; GABA, γ-aminobutyric acid; GI, gastrointestinal; 5-HT, 5-hydroxytryptamine; NSAIDs, nonsteroidal anti-inflammatory drugs.

Abdominal massage therapy has shown mixed results in the treatment of constipation. Ernst[88] reviewed the randomized trial data for abdominal massage as a treatment for constipation and found that, although some data suggested a significant increase in the number of days with bowel movements, and decrease in the number of episodes of fecal incontinence and number of enemas given, the trials were of poor quality and were methodologically flawed. The trials were not blinded and were subject to observer bias; only one study was randomized. Therefore, further RCTs are needed to determine whether massage is effective in patients with chronic constipation.

Homeopathy has been suggested to have clinical efficacy in the treatment of postoperative ileus. A meta-analysis of studies of patients with ileus after abdominal and gynecologic surgery revealed that homeopathic treatment with agents such as opium poppy (*Papaver somniferum L.*) and chaparral (*Raphanus sativus*) reduced the time to normal intestinal peristalsis significantly compared with placebo treatment.[89] The underlying principle of homeopathy is "like cures like," and these supplements, in diluted doses, are thought to ameliorate slowed intestinal transit because they themselves are known to cause constipation. This meta-analysis however, did not yield definitive conclusions, because several of the trials included were reported in publications that are not peer-reviewed, thereby raising suspicion as to the quality of the data.

LIVER DISEASE

CAM therapies are commonly used to treat conditions such as hepatitis B, hepatitis C, and alcoholic liver disease. One study of U.S. outpatients with chronic liver disease reported that 41% had used some form of CAM therapy in the preceding 4 weeks.[90] As with the other gastrointestinal conditions already discussed, most therapies used for chronic liver disease have been herbal supplements. Table 125–6 details the commonly employed supplements, their mechanisms of action, adverse events, and level of evidence to support their use.

Milk thistle (Silybum marianum), the CAM compound most frequently used for hepatic disease, has been employed for many disorders, including alcoholic liver disease, chronic viral hepatitis, and drug-induced hepatitis. Silymarin, the active ingredient, is derived from various parts of the milk thistle plant. Its mechanism of action is not defined fully but appears to be multifaceted. First, silymarin is thought to act as an antioxidant that prevents glutathione depletion.[91] Second, silymarin has anti-inflammatory activity and decreases leukotriene, prostaglandin, and TNF-α formation.[92] Lastly, in several animal studies, silymarin has been shown to block the proliferation of hepatic stellate cells and production of procollagen III, suggesting a role to slow fibrosis in chronic liver disease.[93]

Table 125–6   Complementary and Alternative Medicine (CAM) Therapies for Chronic Liver Disease

CAM Therapy	Proposed Mechanism of Action	Evidence	Adverse Effects
Milk thistle (*Silybum marianum*)	Antioxidant, anti-inflammatory, possibly antifibrotic effects[91-93]	Trials demonstrate improved serum aminotransferase levels compared with placebo; no data to support morbidity or mortality benefit[96,97]	Nausea, diarrhea, dyspepsia, headache, arthralgias, skin reactions, impotence, anaphylaxis; inhibits cytochrome P450 IIIA4 and uridine diphosphoglucuronosyl transferase[96,97]
S-Adenosyl-L-methionine	Participates in the synthesis of glutathione; acts as an antioxidant[97]	Trials of its use are methodologically flawed; no definitive data to support its use in alcoholic hepatitis	Dry mouth; nausea; akathisia; may block platelet aggregation in vitro
Chinese herbal medicine (CHM)	Antioxidant; inhibition of stellate cell activation in animal studies; increased interferon production[102,103]; inhibition of HBV DNA polymerase[105]	Trials suggesting that combination therapy with interferon and CHM increases clearance of HBsAg, HBeAg, and HBV DNA are methodologically flawed	Interstitial pneumonitis, autoimmune hepatitis, thrombocytopenic purpura[97]
Thymic extracts	Unknown	Trials suggest that combination therapy with interferon yields higher HCV virologic response rate than interferon alone or placebo[110]	Nausea, vomiting, rare thrombocytopenia[111]
Licorice (*Glycyrrhiza glabra*)	Activates cytochrome P450 phase I detoxification reactions; stimulates endogenous interferon; inhibits TNF-α[97,112]	RCTs demonstrate improvement in liver biochemical tests; no demonstrable morbidity or mortality benefit[113,114]	Pseudohyperaldosteronism effects: hypokalemia, sodium retention, hypertension; potential digitalis toxicity if taken concurrently[115]
Picrorrhiza kurroa	Antioxidant; anti-inflammatory; antiviral effects[97]	Only one trial details efficacy in acute HBV infection; paucity of data precludes recommendations[119]	None reported

HBeAg, hepatitis B e antigen; HBsAg, hepatitis B surface antigen; HBV, hepatitis B virus; HCV, hepatitis C virus; RCT, randomized controlled trial; TNF, tumor necrosis factor.

Silymarin has been evaluated in several trials of alcoholic liver disease (see Chapter 81). Ferenci and colleagues,[94] in a RCT of cirrhotic patients treated with 420 mg of silymarin versus placebo, demonstrated an improved 4-year survival in the treatment group compared with the placebo-treated group. Patients with alcoholic liver disease and early cirrhosis (Child-Turcotte-Pugh [CTP] class A) were more likely to benefit than were those with CTP class B or C. This trial, however, did not confirm a clear benefit of silymarin, because patients were not randomized properly; the placebo group contained patients with more advanced cirrhosis (CPT class C) than did the treatment group. In addition, the degree of abstinence from alcohol among the study participants was not followed, and the dropout rate was high. A larger, more rigorously defined study by Pares and colleagues[95] failed to demonstrate a survival benefit in alcoholic cirrhotic patients treated with 450 mg of daily silymarin compared with a group treated with placebo.

A systematic review of RCTs of silymarin in various hepatic disease states (hepatitis B, hepatitis C, alcoholic liver disease) also drew no firm conclusions about its therapeutic efficacy. Approximately one half of the trials demonstrated a significant biochemical response to silymarin, specifically a decrease in serum aminotransferase levels; however, this response did not translate into a statistically significant mortality or morbidity benefit. Favorable trends toward a decrease in the frequency of hepatic encephalopathy and gastrointestinal bleeding were suggested by these trials, but a statistically significant difference between those treated with silymarin and those treated with placebo was not reached.[96,97]

The reported adverse effects of silymarin include nausea, diarrhea, dyspepsia, headache, arthralgias, skin reactions, impotence, and anaphylaxis. Most important, milk thistle has been shown to inhibit CYP3A4 and uridine diphosphoglucuronosyl transferase, thereby leading to interactions with traditional prescription medications such as quinine, lidocaine, certain calcium channel blocking agents, and cyclosporine, all of which are metabolized in part by CYP3A4.[96,97]

S-Adenosyl-L-methionine (SAMe) acts as a methyl donor for many biochemical reactions and participates in the synthesis of glutathione, the predominant biochemical antioxidant.[98] This compound has been studied best in the treatment of alcoholic liver disease (see Chapter 81). A systematic review of eight placebo-controlled RCTs of patients treated for alcoholic liver disease revealed that SAMe had no statistically significant effect on mortality, liver-related mortality, or rate of liver transplantation.[97] The methodologic quality of these trials was poor. Further evaluation of SAMe in more properly designed trials is needed.[97] SAMe also has been evaluated in the treatment of cholestasis of pregnancy (see Chapter 37). In several controlled trials, SAMe reduced pruritus and serum bilirubin levels during pregnancy, thereby suggesting possible efficacy.[99] The safety of this agent in pregnancy has been demonstrated in RCTs.[100]

CHM is the most common CAM therapy employed for the treatment of HBV and the therapy that has been evaluated most rigorously. HBV is a significant global health problem (see Chapter 75).[101] Given the large number of people affected and high rate of endemic HBV infection in some parts of the world such as Asia, it is not surprising that CAM therapies are used frequently to treat illness associated with HBV.

Many different herbal combinations have been employed for the treatment of HBV infection. For example, TJ-9, known as *xiao-chai-hu-tang* in China, is a combination of seven herbs: bupleurum root, pinellia tuber, scutellaria root, jujube fruit, ginger rhizome, ginseng root, and glycyrrhiza root. This agent is thought to act as an antioxidant as well as an inhibitor of stellate cell fibrosis.[102,103] Another example of CHM is *Phyllanthus amarus*, the mechanism of action of which appears to be inhibition of HBV DNA polymerase.[104]

A systematic review of 9 randomized trials that evaluated CHM revealed that, compared with placebo treatment, the CHM compound *fuzheng jiedu tang* significantly increased the rate of clearance of hepatitis B surface antigen (HBsAg), hepatitis B e antigen (HBeAg), and HBV DNA. *P. amarus* and kurorinone were comparable to interferon treatment in clearing these serologic markers.[105] The quality of the aforementioned trials was poor, however, and thus no definitive conclusion can be reached at present regarding the efficacy of these agents for chronic HBV infection.

A review of the effects of CHM on asymptomatic HBsAg-positive carriers with normal aminotransferase levels evaluated three RCTs, all of which were of poor methodologic quality. The compound *Jianpi Wenshen* recipe was found to have beneficial effects on clearance of HBsAg, HBeAg, and seroconversion of HBeAg to antibody to HBeAg.[106] Given the flaws in the methodology of the trials evaluated, however, a recommendation for use of this agent cannot be endorsed without further investigation.

A meta-analysis of 27 RCTs compared CHM alone, CHM combined with interferon, and interferon alone for chronic HBV infection.[107] The absence of a strict placebo group in these trials is of concern. In China, where most CHM is used for HBV infection, CHM frequently is used as an adjunct or alternative to interferon therapy. Therefore, these trials were designed to assess the efficacy of CHM in conditions that replicate common clinical practice.[103] Patients who received CHM alone were more likely to clear HBsAg than were those treated with interferon alone. CHM was equivalent in efficacy to interferon in achieving clearance of HBeAg and HBV DNA. Patients who received combined therapy were more likely than those treated with interferon alone to achieve seroreversion for HBsAg and HBeAg, and to clear HBV DNA.[103]

Although these trials appear to favor the use of CHM as a potential adjunct therapy to interferon, most of the trials were of poor methodologic quality. In addition, most of the studies had a follow-up of only 3 months for assessing treatment outcomes. Furthermore, the studies that were reviewed were published in Chinese journals, and many details regarding blinding and randomization of the subjects in the trials were omitted from the publications, raising additional concerns regarding methodologic quality.[103]

CHM also has been studied for the treatment of HCV infection. A systematic review of 10 randomized trials evaluated the efficacy of CHM in patients with chronic

HCV infection. The results of the trials were disappointing in that none of the herbal agents employed was found to increase the rate of HCV RNA clearance. In addition, 9 of the 10 trials showed no improvement in serum aminotransferase levels.[108]

Adverse effects of CHM include hepatotoxicity; however, given the lack of manufacturing uniformity in content and potency of these agents, definitive causality has not been established.[109] Cases of interstitial pneumonitis, autoimmune hepatitis, and acute thrombocytopenic purpura also have been reported.[97]

Thymic extract efficacy and safety in the treatment of HCV infection has been evaluated in five RCTs. Patients who received thymosin-α1 (Tα1), a synthetic polypeptide, in combination with interferon therapy were more likely to have complete virologic response than were those patients treated with interferon alone or with placebo.[110] Reported adverse events included nausea and vomiting and one case of thrombocytopenia.[111]

Licorice (Glycyrrhiza glabra) has been evaluated as a possible CAM therapy for chronic HCV infection. The active component of licorice, glycyrrhizin, is thought to activate cytochrome P450 phase I detoxification reactions, stimulate endogenous interferon, and inhibit TNF-α.[97,112] Several RCTs have evaluated this compound for the treatment of HCV. Suzuki and colleagues[113] demonstrated that daily injections of Stronger Neo-Minophagen C, a compound of glycyrrhizin, glycine, and cysteine, decreased serum aminotransferase levels compared with placebo. A morbidity or mortality benefit was not demonstrated. Furthermore, the follow-up period in this trial was 1 month, making it extremely difficult to assess any long-term adverse effects of *G. glabra*. Given that this study was performed more than 20 years ago, the presence of HCV was not determined in the study population; inclusion criteria merely necessitated histologic evidence of chronic hepatitis. It is not clear, in fact, that the study population had HCV infection.

Another RCT evaluated the effects of *G. glabra* in patients with chronic HCV infection.[114] The efficacy of ursodeoxycholic acid combined with glycyrrhizin was compared with glycyrrhizin alone. There was a statistically significant biochemical improvement in the treatment group, but the trial lacked a placebo arm, and the outcome studied may not have been the most clinically meaningful to assess.

Adverse events with *G. glabra* are thought to be secondary to the active metabolite of licorice root, glycyrrhizin, which inhibits 11-β-hydroxysteroid dehydrogenase. This inhibition leads to a pseudoaldosterone effect, resulting in hypokalemia, sodium retention, and hypertension[115]; hypokalemia may increase the risk of toxicity from some drugs, such as digitalis.

Picrorrhiza kurroa is an Indian herb frequently used in traditional Ayurvedic medicine. It has been utilized for many gastrointestinal conditions and is used frequently for hepatic disease. The active ingredients, picroside and kutkoside,[116] are thought to act as antioxidants, anti-inflammatory agents, and inhibitors of proinflammatory cytokines.[97] Various studies have described possible cancer chemopreventive and antiviral qualities of these agents.[117,118] One trial demonstrated a beneficial biochemical effect of *P. kurroa* in reducing serum amino-

transferase levels in patients with acute HBV infection.[119] Clearly, more data are needed before any recommendation can be made regarding this agent.

GASTROINTESTINAL MALIGNANCIES

Estimates are that up to 64% of adult oncology patients have employed CAM therapies at some point during their treatment.[120] The motivation for use of these therapies in oncology patients is similar to the rationale cited by other patient populations. CAM therapies are appealing as a result of a failure of conventional medicine to control or cure disease, and they provide patients with a mechanism for feeling in more control of their therapeutic plan. Textbooks have been dedicated to this subject, and the discussion that follows highlights the most commonly employed CAM therapies.

A systematic review of studies of the beneficial effect of *green tea* consumption in reducing the incidence of gastrointestinal malignancy[121] demonstrated that green tea did help prevent colonic adenomatous polyp formation and chronic atrophic gastritis. No definitive supporting evidence, however, was found to conclude that green tea had a similar beneficial effect on the incidence of gastrointestinal malignancy.

Garlic is thought to inhibit the development of gastric cancer through several proposed mechanisms. An antibacterial effect against *Helicobacter pylori* has been demonstrated and is attributable to the thiosulfinate component of this agent.[122] Kaempferol, a flavonol present in high concentration in garlic, also contributes to the detoxification of carcinogenic compounds.[123] Published studies suggest that garlic may protect against the development of stomach and colon carcinomas. Most of the literature, however, consists of observational studies that cannot be used to confirm a therapeutic effect of garlic. Additional therapeutic intervention trials are needed to substantiate the claim that garlic is chemopreventive.[124]

Vitamins C and E are antioxidants that may reduce the incidence of colorectal cancer. In an epidemiologic study of colorectal cancer patients, long-term use of vitamins C and E did not provide a mortality benefit. In a subgroup analysis, however, use of vitamin C for more than 10 years was associated with a decreased risk of death from colorectal cancer before 65 years of age and a decreased risk of rectal cancer mortality at any age.[125]

Other dietary factors also could play a role in preventing malignancy. In Mediterranean countries there has been a lower incidence of breast, endometrial, colorectal, and prostate cancer compared with Western countries. These cancers have been postulated to have a relationship to diet, in that a low consumption of fruits and vegetables and a high consumption of red meat correlate with cancer incidence. A traditional Mediterranean diet contains low amounts of red meat and high amounts of fruits, vegetables, and olive oil. Some epidemiologists estimate by statistical modeling that up to 25% of colorectal cancer could be prevented in Western countries if diets were changed to reflect Mediterranean practices.[126]

Several CAM therapies have been implemented to help ameliorate pain in patients with metastatic disease. *Acupuncture* has shown promise for the treatment of pain associated with gastric cancer.[127] *Lycopodium clavatum*, a type of fern moss, has been reported to be effective as a homeopathic treatment for rectal cancer pain.[128] *Meditation and relaxation therapies* are practiced commonly by many cancer patients, not only to ameliorate physical pain but also to help cope with the depression that frequently accompanies malignant disease.

SAFETY AND REGULATION OF CAM THERAPIES

Because of the increasing popularity of CAM therapies, it is critically important that physicians understand their mechanisms of action as well as the data supporting their efficacy. It is equally important, however, that physicians understand the regulatory mechanisms, or lack thereof, that are in place for these modalities, so that effective safety measures can be employed to protect the welfare of patients.

Total yearly sales of herbal supplements are approximately $13.9 billion and steadily increasing in the United States. An estimated 15 million adults take prescription medications concurrently with herbal supplements.[1] Therefore, the safety of concurrent administration of herbal supplements and traditional allopathic medications is a concern to many physicians. In 1994, the U.S. Congress implemented the Dietary Supplement Health and Education Act (DSHEA). This legislation was developed to prevent the U.S. Food and Drug Administration (FDA) from regulating dietary supplements excessively and to ensure that safe and appropriately labeled supplements remain available to those persons who wish to use them.

DSHEA officially defines a "dietary supplement" as

A product (other than tobacco) that is intended to supplement the diet that bears or contains one or more of the following dietary ingredients: a vitamin, a mineral, an herb or other botanical, an amino acid, a dietary substance for use by man to supplement the diet by increasing total daily intake, or a concentrate, metabolite, constituent, extract or combination of these ingredients.[129]

Additional FDA guidelines specify that supplement manufacturers themselves are responsible for determining the safety of their products and for providing the evidence, if asked, to substantiate the claims made by their individual products. Approval from the FDA is not required prior to marketing of most of these agents, unless the supplement is deemed "new." A *new supplement* is defined as an agent not marketed prior to October 15th, 1994; however, no definitive list of products marketed before this date exists. Therefore, the responsibility rests with the manufacturer to determine if its product is in fact a new supplement. This rule creates an obvious conflict of interest in that new supplements require clinical research and capital expenditures to substantiate their efficacy, and manufacturers would prefer that supplement therapies be considered previously marketed.

Additionally, supplement manufacturers are not required to report adverse events that occur with use of their products. It is the responsibility of the FDA to prove that products are unsafe before their use can be restricted.[129] The FDA relies on physicians and other health care professionals to report suspected adverse events for an inquiry to be established for a particular agent. Therefore, it is of utmost importance that physicians be aware of their patients' use of supplements both to provide safe care and to know when to suspect adverse effects or medication interactions. Suspected adverse events or medication interactions can be reported online at http://www.fda.gov/medwatch.

REFERENCES

1. Eisenberg DM, Davis RB, Ettner SL, et al: Trends in alternative medicine use in the United States, 1990-1997. JAMA 280:1569, 1998.
2. Ganguli SC, Cawdron R, Irvine EJ: Alternative medicine use by Canadian ambulatory gastroenterology patients: Secular trend or epidemic? Am J Gastroenterol 99:319, 2004.
3. Zollman C, Vickers AJ: What is complementary medicine? In ABC of Complementary Medicine. New York, BMJ Books, 2000, p 1.
4. Hollyer T, Boon H, Georgousis A, et al: The use of CAM by women suffering from nausea and vomiting during pregnancy. BMC Complement Altern Med 2:5, 2002.
5. Yamahara J, Huang QR, Li Y, et al: Gastrointestinal motility enhancing effect of ginger and its active constituents. Chem Pharm Bull (Tokyo) 38:430, 1990.
6. Huang Q, Iwamoto M, Aoki S, et al: Anti-5-hydroxytryptamine-3 effect of galanolactone, diterpenoid isolated from ginger. Chem Pharm Bull (Tokyo) 39:397, 1991.
7. Koretz RL, Rotblatt M: Complementary and alternative medicine in gastroenterology: The good, the bad, and the ugly. Clin Gastroenterol Hepatol 2:957, 2004.
8. Stewart JJ, Wood MJ, Wood CD, Mims ME: Effects of ginger on motion sickness susceptibility and gastric function. Pharmacology 42:111, 1991.
9. Grøntved A, Hentzer E: Vertigo-reducing effect of ginger root: A controlled clinical study. Otorhinolaryngol Relat Spec 48:282, 1986.
10. Ernst E, Pittler MH: Efficacy of ginger for nausea and vomiting: A systematic review of randomized clinical trials. Br J Anaesth 84:367, 2000.
11. Srivastava KC: Aqueous extract of onion, garlic, and ginger inhibit platelet aggregation and alter arachidonic acid metabolism. Biomed Biochim Acta 43:335, 1984.
12. Abraham S, Abraham SK, Radhamony G: Mutagenic potential of the condiments, ginger and tumeric. Cytologia 41:591, 1976.
13. Soudamini KK, Unnikrishnan MC, Sukumaran K, Kuttan R: Mutagenicity and anti-mutagenicity of selected spices. Indian J Physiol Pharmacol 39:347, 1995.
14. Sahakian V, Rouse D, Sipes S, et al: Vitamin B$_6$ is effective therapy for nausea and vomiting of pregnancy. Obstet Gynecol 78:33, 1991.
15. Vutyavanich T, Wongtrangan S, Ruangsri R: Pyridoxine for nausea and vomiting of pregnancy: A randomized double-blind placebo-controlled trial. Am J Obstet Gynecol 173:881, 1995.
16. Vitamin B$_6$: Pyridoxine. In Lexi-comp.com—online, 1978-present.
17. Leklem JE: Vitamin B$_6$. In Machlin LJ (ed): Handbook of Vitamins, 2nd ed. New York, Marcel Dekker, 1991.
18. Schaumburg H, Kaplan J, Windebank A, et al: Sensory neuropathy from pyridoxine abuse: A new megavitamin syndrome. N Engl J Med 309:445, 1983.

19. Vickers AJ: Can acupuncture have specific effects on health? A systematic review of acupuncture antiemesis trials. J R Soc Med 89:303, 1996.

20. Dundee JW, Ghaly RG, Fitzpatrick KT, et al: Acupuncture to prevent cisplatin-associated vomiting. Lancet 1:1083, 1987.

21. Fry ENS: Acupressure and postoperative vomiting. Anaesthesia 41:661, 1986.

22. Ho RT, Jawan B, Fung ST, et al: Electro-acupuncture and postoperative emesis. Anaesthesia 45:327, 1990.

23. de Aloysio D, Penacchioni O: Morning sickness control in early pregnancy by Neiguan point acupressure. Obstet Gynecol 80:852, 1992.

24. Ernst E, White A: Life-threatening adverse reactions after acupuncture? A systematic review. Pain 71:123, 1997.

25. Rampes H, James R: Complications of acupuncture. Acupunct Med 13:26, 1995.

26. Kiyosawa K, Tanaka E, Sodeyama T: Transmission of hepatitis C in an isolated area in Japan. Gastroenterology 106:1596, 1994.

27. Vittecoq D, Mettetal JF, Rouzioux C, et al: Acute HIV infection after acupuncture treatments. N Engl J Med 320:250, 1989.

28. Scheel O, Sundsfjord A, Lunde P, Andersen BM: Endocarditis after acupuncture and injection treatment by a natural healer. JAMA 267:56, 1992.

29. Izatt E, Fairman M: Staphylococcal septicaemia with DIC associated with acupuncture. Postgrad Med J 53:285, 1977.

30. Pierik MG: Fatal staphylococcal septicemia following acupuncture: Report of two cases. RI Med J 82:251, 1982.

31. Hasegawa J, Noguchi N, Yamasaki J, et al: Delayed cardiac tamponade and hemothorax induced by an acupuncture needle. Cardiology 78:58, 1991.

32. Ernst E, Resch KL, White AR: The risks of acupuncture. Int J Risk Saf Med 6:179, 1195.

33. Freeman LW, Lawlis GF (eds): Mind-body interventions. In Mosby's Complementary and Alternative Medicine, a Research-Based Approach. St Louis, Mosby, 2001, p 146.

34. Coon JT, Ernst E: Systematic review: Herbal medicinal products for non-ulcer dyspepsia. Aliment Pharmacol Ther 16:1689, 2002.

35. Best R, Lewis DA, Nasser N: The antiulcerogenic activity of unripe plantain banana (*Musa* species). Br J Pharmacol 82:107, 1984.

36. Arora A, Sharma MP: Use of banana in non-ulcer dyspepsia. Lancet 335:612, 1990.

37. Bortolotti M, Coccia G, Grossi G, Miglioli M: The treatment of functional dyspepsia with red pepper. Aliment Pharmacol Ther 16:1075, 2002.

38. Ritter R, Schatton WFH, Gessner B et al: Clinical trial on standardized celandine extract in patients with functional epigastric complaints: Results of a placebo-controlled double-blind trial. Complement Ther Med 1:189, 1993.

39. Brinker F: Botanical review: *Chelidonium majus*. J Naturopath Med 3:93, 1992.

40. Benninger J, Schneider HT, Schuppan D, et al: Acute hepatitis induced by greater *Celandine* (*Chelidonium majus*). Gastroenterology 117:1234, 1999.

41. Tatsuta M, Iishi H: Effect of treatment with Liu-Jun-Zi-Tang (TJ-43) on gastric emptying and gastrointestinal symptoms in dyspeptic patients. Aliment Pharmacol Ther 7:459, 1993.

42. Hayakawa T, Arakawa K, Kase Y, et al: Liu-Jun-Zi-Tang, a kampo medicine, promotes adaptive relaxation in isolated guinea pig stomachs. Drugs Exp Clin Res 25:211, 1999.

43. Hillis JM, Aaronson PI: The mechanism of action of peppermint oil on gastrointestinal smooth muscle: An analysis using patch clamp electrophysiology and isolated tissue pharmacology in rabbit and guinea pig. Gastroenterology 101:55, 1991.

44. Forster HB, Niklas H, Lutz S: Antispasmodic effects of some medicinal plants. Planta Med 40:309, 1980.

45. May B, Kohler S, Schneider B: Efficacy and tolerability of a fixed combination of peppermint oil and caraway oil in patients suffering from functional dyspepsia. Aliment Pharmacol Ther 14:1671, 2000.

46. Wilkinson SM, Beck MH: Allergic contact dermatitis from menthol in peppermint. Contact Dermatitis 30:42, 1994.

47. Spurlock BW, Dailey TM: Shortness of (fresh) breath—toothpaste-induced bronchospasm. N Engl J Med 323:1845, 1990.

48. Thomas JG: Peppermint fibrillation. Lancet 1:222, 1962.

49. Chang HM, But PPH: Pharmacology and Applications of Chinese Materia Medica. Singapore, World Scientific, 1987.

50. Brandt LJ, Bjorkman D, Fennerty MB, et al: Systematic review on the management of irritable bowel syndrome in North America. Am J Gastroenterol 97(Suppl 11):S7, 2002.

51. Drossman DA, Whitehead WE, Camilleri M: The irritable bowel syndrome: A technical review for practice guideline development. Gastroenterology 112:2120, 1997.

52. Cheskin LJ, Kamal N, Crowell MD, et al: Mechanisms of constipation in older persons and effects of fiber compared with placebo. J Am Geriatr Soc 43:666, 1995.

53. Fenn GC, Wilkinson PD, Lee CE, et al: A general practice study of the efficacy of Regulan in functional constipation. Br J Clin Pract 40:192, 1986.

54. Ashraf W, Park F, Lof J, et al: Effects of psyllium therapy on stool characteristics, colon transit and anorectal function in chronic idiopathic constipation. Aliment Pharmacol Ther 9:639, 1995.

55. Dettmar PW, Sykes J: A multi-center, general practice comparison of ispaghula husk with lactulose and other laxatives in the treatment of simple constipation. Curr Med Res Opin 14:227, 1998.

56. Rouse M, Chapman N, Mahapatra M, et al: An open, randomized, parallel group study of lactulose versus ispaghula in the treatment of chronic constipation in adults. Br J Clin Pract 45:28, 1991.

57. Vaswani SK, Hamilton RG, Valentine MD, Adkinson NF Jr: Psyllium laxative–induced anaphylaxis. Allergy 51:266, 1996.

58. Perlman BB: Interaction between lithium salts and ispaghula husk. Lancet 335:416, 1990.

59. Skidmore-Rose L: Mosby's Handbook of Herbs and Natural Supplements. St. Louis, Mosby, 2001.

60. Noble JA, Grannis FW: Acute esophageal obstruction by a psyllium based laxative [Letter]. Chest 86:800, 1984.

61. Pittler MH, Ernst E: Peppermint oil for irritable bowel syndrome: A critical review and meta-analysis. Am J Gastroenterol 93:1131, 1998.

62. Madisch A, Holtmann G, Plein K, Hotz J: Treatment of irritable bowel syndrome with herbal preparations: Results of a double-blind, randomized, placebo-controlled, multi-center trial. Aliment Pharmacol Ther 19:271, 2004.

63. Gruenwald J (ed): PDR for Herbal Medicines. Montvale, NJ, Medical Economics, 2000.

64. O'Hara MA, Kiefer D, Farrell K, Kemper K: A review of 12 commonly used medicinal herbs. Arch Fam Med 7:532, 1997.

65. Venkataramanan R, Ramachandran V, Komoroski BJ, et al: Milk thistle, an herbal supplement, decreases the activity of CYP3A4 and uridine diphosphoglucuronosyltransferase in human hepatocyte cultures. Drug Metab Dispos 28:1270, 2000.

66. Bensoussan A, Talley NJ, Hing M, et al: Treatment of irritable bowel syndrome with Chinese herbal medicine: A randomized controlled trial. JAMA 280:1585, 1998.

67. Schaafsma G: State of the art concerning probiotic strains in milk products. IDF Nutr Newslett 5:23, 1996.

68. Nobaek S, Johansson M-L, Molin G, et al: Alteration of intestinal microflora is associated with reduction in abdominal

bloating and pain in patients with irritable bowel syndrome. Am J Gastroenterol 95:1231, 2000.

69. Whorwell PJ, Prior A, Colgan SM: Hypnotherapy in severe irritable bowel syndrome: Further experience. Gut 28:423, 1987.

70. Fireman Z, Segal A, Kopelman Y, et al: Acupuncture treatment for irritable bowel syndrome. Digestion 64:100, 2001.

71. Bolin T, Yiu T: Resistant constipation: A role for acupuncture? Aust N Z J Med 13:102, 1983.

72. Yadav SK, Jain AK, Tripathi SN, Gupta JP: Irritable bowel syndrome: Therapeutic evaluation of indigenous drugs. Indian J Med Res 90:496, 1989.

73. Podolsky DL: Inflammatory bowel disease. N Engl J Med 347:417, 2002.

74. Gionchetti P, Rizzelo F, Venturi A, et al: Oral bacteriotherapy as maintenance treatment in patients with chronic pouchitis: A double-blind, placebo-controlled trial. Gastroenterology 119:305, 2000.

75. Gionchetti P, Rizzelo F, Helwig U, et al: Prophylaxis of pouchitis onset with probiotic therapy: A double-blind, placebo-controlled trial. Gastroenterology 124:1202, 2003.

76. Ulisse, S, Gionchetti P, D'Alo D, et al: Expression of cytokines, inducible nitric oxide synthetase and matrix metalloproteinases in pouchitis: Effects of probiotic treatment. Am J Gastroenterol 96:2691, 2001.

77. Guslandi M, Mezzi G, Sorghi M, Testoni PA: *Saccharomyces boulardii* in maintenance treatment of Crohn's disease. Dig Dis Sci 45:1462, 2000.

78. Koretz RL: Immunonutrition: Can you be what you eat? Curr Opin Gastroentol 19:134, 2003.

79. Hawthorne AB, Daneshmend TK, Hawkey CJ, et al: Treatment of ulcerative colitis with fish oil supplementation: A prospective 12-month randomized, controlled trial. Gut 33:922, 1992.

80. D'Souza AL, Rajkumar C, Cooke J, Bulpitt CJ: Probiotics in prevention of antibiotic associated diarrhoea: Meta-analysis. BMJ 324:1361, 2002.

81. Castagliuolo I, Riegler MF, Valenick L, et al: *Saccharomyces boulardii* protease inhibits the effects of *Clostridium difficile* toxins A and B in human colonic mucosa. Infect Immunol 67:302, 1999.

82. Qamar A, Aboudola S, Warny M, et al: *Saccharomyces boulardii* stimulates intestinal immunoglobulin A immune response to *Clostridium difficile* toxin A in mice. Infect Immunol 69:2762-5, 2001.

83. McFarland LV, Surawicz CM, Greenberg RN, et al: A randomized placebo-controlled trial of *Saccharomyces boulardii* in combination with standard antibiotics for *Clostridium difficile* disease. JAMA 271:1913, 1994.

84. Czerucka D, Dahan S, Mograbi B, et al: *Saccharomyces boulardii* preserves the barrier function and modulates the signal transduction pathway induced in enteropathogenic *Escherichia coli*–infected T84 cells. Infection Immunol 68:5998, 2000.

85. Delia P, Sansotta G, Donato V, et al: Prevention of radiation-induced diarrhea with the use of VSL #3, a new high-potency probiotic preparation [Letter]. Am J Gastroenterol 97:2150, 2002.

86. Ernst E, Pittler MH, Stevinson C, White AR: The Desktop Guide to Complementary and Alternative Medicine. Edinburgh, Mosby, 2001.

87. Bassotti G, Chistolini F, Sietchiping-Nzepa F, et al: Biofeedback for pelvic floor dysfunction in constipation. BMJ 328:393, 2004.

88. Ernst E: Abdominal massage for chronic constipation: A systematic review of controlled clinical trials. Forsch Komplementärmed 6:149, 1999.

89. Barnes J, Resch KL, Ernst E: Homeopathy for postoperative ileus: A meta-analysis. J Clin Gastroenterol 25:628, 1997.

90. Seeff LB, Lindsay KL, Bacon BR, et al: Complementary and alternative medicine in chronic liver disease. Hepatology 34:596, 2001.

91. Mira L, Silva M, Manso CF: Scavenging of reactive oxygen species by silibinin dihemisuccinate. Biochem Pharmacol 48:753, 1994.

92. Carini R, Comoglio A, Albano E, Poli G: Lipid peroxidation and irreversible damage in the rat hepatocyte model: Protection by the silybin-phospholipid complex IdB 1016. Biochem Pharmacol 43:2111, 1992.

93. Boigk G, Stroedter L, Herbst H, et al: Silymarin retards collagen accumulation in early and advanced biliary fibrosis secondary to complete bile duct obliteration in rats. Hepatology 26:643, 1997.

94. Ferenci P, Dragosics B, Dittrich H, e al: Randomized controlled trial of silymarin treatment in patients with cirrhosis of the liver. J Hepatol 9:105, 1989.

95. Pares A, Planas R, Torres M, et al: Effects of silymarin in alcoholic patients with cirrhosis of the liver: Results of a controlled, double-blind, randomized and multicenter trial. J Hepatol 28:615, 1998.

96. Mulrow C, Lawrence V, Jacobs B, et al: Milk thistle: Effects on liver disease and cirrhosis and clinical adverse effects. Evidence Report/Technology Assessment No. 21. AHRQ publication No. 01-E025. Rockville, MD, Agency for Healthcare Research and Quality, 2000.

97. Levy C, Seeff LD, Lindor KD: Use of herbal supplements for chronic liver disease. Clin Gastroenterol Hepatol 2:947, 2004.

98. Rambaldi A, Gluud C: *S*-adenosyl-L-methionine for alcoholic liver diseases (Cochrane Review). In The Cochrane Library, issue 3. Chichester, UK, Wiley, 2004.

99. Hardy M, Coulter I, Morton SC, et al: *S*-Adenosyl-L-methionine for treatment of depression, osteoarthritis, and liver disease: Evidence Report/Technology Assessment No. 64, AHRQ Publication No. 02-E034. Rockville, MD, Agency for Healthcare Research and Quality, 2002.

100. Ribalta J: *S*-adenosyl-L-methionine in the treatment of patients with intrahepatic cholestasis of pregnancy: A randomized, double-blind, placebo-controlled study with negative results. Hepatology 13:1084, 1991.

101. Merican I, Guan R, Amarapuka D, et al: Chronic hepatitis B virus infection in Asian countries. J Gastroenterol Hepatol 15:1356, 2000.

102. Sakaida I, Matsumura Y, Akiyama S, et al: Herbal medicine Sho-saiko-to (TJ-9) prevents liver fibrosis and enzyme-altered lesions in rat liver cirrhosis induced by a choline deficient L-amino acid–defined diet. J Hepatol 28:298, 1998.

103. Kakumu S, Yoshioka K, Wakita T, et al: Effects of TJ-9 Sho-saiko-to (kampo medicine) on interferon gamma and antibody production specific for hepatitis B virus antigen in patients with type B chronic hepatitis. Int J Immunopharmacol 13:141, 1991.

104. Blumberg BS, Millman I, Venkateswaran PS, Thyagarajan SP: Hepatitis B virus and primary hepatocellular carcinoma: Treatment of HBV carriers with *Phyllanthus amarus*. Vaccine 8(Suppl):S86, 1990.

105. Liu JP, McIntosh H, Lin H: Chinese medicinal herbs for chronic hepatitis B (Cochrane Review). In The Cochrane Library, issue 3. Chichester, UK, Wiley, 2004.

106. Liu JP, McIntosh H, Lin H: Chinese medicinal herbs for asymptomatic carriers of hepatitis B virus infection (Cochrane Review). In The Cochrane Library, issue 3. Chichester, UK, Wiley, 2004.

107. McCulloch M, Broffman M, Gao J, Colford JM Jr: Chinese herbal medicine and interferon in the treatment of chronic hepatitis B: A meta-analysis of randomized, controlled trials. Am J Public Health 92:1619, 2002.

108. Liu JP, Manheimer E, Tsutani K, Gluud C: Medicinal herbs for hepatitis C virus infection (Cochrane Review). In The Cochrane Library, issue 3. Chichester, UK, Wiley, 2004.

109. Stedman C: Herbal hepatotoxicity. Semin Liver Dis 22:195, 2002.

110. Thompson Coon J, Ernst E: Complementary and alternative therapies in the treatment of chronic hepatitis C: A systematic review. J Hepatol 40:491, 2004.

111. Raymond RS, Fallon MB, Abrams GA: Oral thymic extract for chronic hepatitis C in patients previously treated with interferon: A randomized, double-blind, placebo-controlled trial. Ann Intern Med 129:797, 1998.

112. Abe N, Ebina T, Ishida N: Interferon induction by glycyrrhizin and glycyrrhetinic acid in mice. Microbiol Immunol 26:535, 1982.

113. Suzuki H, Ohta Y, Takino T, et al: Effects of glycyrrhizin on biochemical tests in patients with chronic hepatitis. Asian Med J 26:423, 1983.

114. Tsubota A, Kumada H, Arase Y, et al: Combined ursodeoxycholic acid and glycyrrhizin therapy for chronic hepatitis C virus infection: A randomized controlled trial in 170 patients. Eur J Gastroenterol Hepatol 11:1077, 1999.

115. Conn JW, Rovner DR, Cohen EL: Licorice-induced pseudoaldosteronism. JAMA 205:492, 1968.

116. Luper S: A review of plants used in the treatment of liver disease: I. Altern Med Rev 3:410, 1998.

117. Rajeshkumar NV, Kuttan R: Protective effect of Picroliv, the active constituent of *Picrorrhiza kurroa*, against chemical carcinogenesis in mice. Teratog Carcinog Mutagen 21:303, 2001.

118. Mehrotra R, Rawat S, Kulshreshtha DK, et al: In vitro studies on the effect of certain natural products against hepatitis B virus. Indian J Med Res 92:133, 1990.

119. Vaidya AB, Antarkar DS, Doshi JC, et al: *Picrorrhiza kurroa* (Kutaki) Royle ex Benth as a hepatoprotective agent: Experimental and clinical studies. J Postgrad Med 42:105, 1996.

120. Barraclough J (ed): Integrated Cancer Care: Holistic, Complementary, and Creative Approaches. New York, Oxford University Press, 2001.

121. Borrelli F, Capasso R, Russo A, Ernst E: Systematic review: Green tea and gastrointestinal cancer risk. Aliment Pharmacol Ther 19:467, 2004.

122. Jonkers D, van den Broek E, van Dooren I, et al: Antibacterial effect of garlic and omeprazole on *Helicobacter pylori*. J Antimicrob Chemther 43:837-839, 1999.

123. Hertog MGL, Hollman CH, Katan MB: Content of potentially anticarcinogenic flavanoids of 28 vegetables and 9 fruits commonly consumed in the Netherlands. J Agric Food Chem 40:2379, 1992.

124. Fleischauer AT, Arab L: Garlic and cancer: A critical review of the epidemiologic literature. J Nutr 131(3 Suppl):1032S, 2001.

125. Jacobs EJ, Connell CJ, Patel AV, et al: Vitamin C and vitamin E supplement use and colorectal cancer mortality in a large American Cancer Society cohort. Cancer Epidemiol Biomarkers Prev 10:17-23, 2001.

126. Trichopoulou A, Lagiou P, Kuper H, Trichopoulos D. Cancer and Mediterranean dietary traditions. Cancer Epidemiol Biomarkers Prev 9:869, 2000.

127. Dang W, Yang J: Clinical study on acupuncture treatment of stomach carcinoma pain. J Trad Chin Med 18:31, 1998.

128. Rajendran ES: Homeopathy as a supportive therapy in cancer. Homeopathy 93:99, 2004.

129. Lewis JD, Strom BL: Balancing safety of dietary supplements with the free market. Ann Intern Med 136:616, 2002.

130. Zollman C, Vickers AJ: Acupuncture. In: ABC of Complementary Medicine. New York, BMJ Books 12:15, 2000.

131. Ayurvedic Foundations—Dedicated to teaching authentic Ayurveda. Available at www.ayur.com/about.html.

132. Barnes JB, Resch KL, Ernst E: Homeopathy for postoperative ileus: A meta-analysis. J Clin Gastroenterol 25:628, 1997.

Index

Note: Page numbers followed by f indicate figures; those followed by n indicate notes; those followed by t indicate tables.